肿瘤组织病理学诊断

Diagnostic Histopathology of Tumors

（第3版）

上卷

注 意

医学在不断进步。虽然标准安全措施必须遵守,但由于新的研究和临床实践在不断拓展我们的知识,在治疗和用药方面做出某种改变也许是必需或适宜的。建议读者核对本书所提供的每种药品的生产厂商的最新产品信息,确认推荐剂量、服用方法与时间及相关的禁忌证。确定诊断、决定患者的最佳服药剂量和最佳治疗方式以及采取适当的安全预防措施是经治医师的责任,这有赖于他(她)们的个人经验和对每一位患者的了解。在法律允许的范围内,对于因与本书所包含的资料相关而引起的任何人身损伤或财产损失,出版商和编著者均不承担任何责任。

出版者

肿瘤组织病理学诊断

Diagnostic Histopathology of Tumors

（第3版）

上卷

主编 Christopher D.M. Fletcher
主译 回允中

北京大学医学出版社
Peking University Medical Press

图书在版编目（CIP）数据

肿瘤组织病理学诊断：第3版/（美）弗莱彻（Fletcher, C.D.M.）著；回允中译.
—北京：北京大学医学出版社，2009
书名原文：Diagnostic Histopathology of Tumors, Third Edition
ISBN 978-7-81116-794-8

Ⅰ.肿… Ⅱ.①弗… ②回… Ⅲ.肿瘤—诊断学：组织学（生物）：病理学 Ⅳ.R730.4

中国版本图书馆CIP数据核字（2009）第062721号

北京市版权局著作权合同登记号：图字：01-2007-4609

Diagnostic Histopathology of Tumors, 3rd edition
Christopher D.M. Fletcher
ISBN-13: 978-0-443-07434-9
ISBN-10: 0-443-07434-8

Copyright © 2007, Elsevier Limited. All rights reserved.

Authorized Simplified Chinese translation from English language edition published by the Proprietor.
978-981-272-068-9
981-272-068-5

Elsevier (Singapore) Pte Ltd.
3 Killiney Road, #08-01 Winsland House I, Singapore 239519
Tel: (65) 6349-0200, Fax: (65) 6733-1817
First Published 2009
2009年初版

Simplified Chinese translation Copyright © 2009 by Elsevier (Singapore) Pte Ltd and Peking University Medical Press. All rights reserved.

Published in China by Peking University Medical Press under special agreement with Elsevier (Singapore) Pte Ltd. This edition is authorized for sale in China only, excluding Hong Kong SAR and Taiwan. Unauthorized export of this edition is a violation of the Copyright Act. Violation of this Law is subject to Civil and Criminal Penalties.

本书简体中文版由北京大学医学出版社与Elsevier (Singapore) Pte Ltd.在中国境内（不包括香港特别行政区及台湾）协议出版。本版仅限在中国境内（不包括香港特别行政区及台湾）出版及标价销售。未经许可之出口，是为违反著作权法，将受法律之制裁。

肿瘤组织病理学诊断（第3版）

- 主　　译：回允中
- 出版发行：北京大学医学出版社（电话：010-82802230）
- 地　　址：(100191)北京市海淀区学院路38号 北京大学医学部院内
- 网　　址：http://www.pumpress.com.cn
- E-mail：booksale@bjmu.edu.cn
- 印　　刷：北京画中画印刷有限公司
- 经　　销：新华书店
- 责任编辑：马联华 畅晓燕 陈奋 李海燕　责任校对：杜悦　责任印制：郭桂兰
- 开　　本：889mm×1194mm 1/16　印张：62　字数：2109千字
- 版　　次：2009年8月第1版　2009年8月第1次印刷
- 书　　号：ISBN 978-7-81116-794-8
- 定　　价：1550.00元（上下卷）

版权所有，违者必究
（凡属质量问题请与本社发行部联系退换）

目录

著者名单	xi	
译校者名单	xv	
主译的话	xvii	
著者前言	xix	

上卷

1 **绪言** 1
Christopher D.M. Fletcher

2 **心脏和心包肿瘤** 7
Anton E. Becker

3 **脉管肿瘤** 41
Eduardo Calonje 和 Christopher D.M. Fletcher

4 **上呼吸道肿瘤** 83
 第一部分 鼻腔、副鼻窦和鼻咽 83
 Bruce M. Wenig
 第二部分 喉和气管 150
 Ben Z. Pilch

5 **肺和胸膜肿瘤** 181
Cesar A. Moran 和 Saul Suster

6 **口腔肿瘤** 215
The late D. Gordon MacDonald 和
Paul M. Speight

7 **涎腺肿瘤** 239
Wah Cheuk 和 John K.C. Chan

8 **食管和胃肿瘤** 327
Fiona Campbell、Gregory Y. Lauwers 和
Geraint T. Williams

9 **小肠和大肠（包括肛门部）肿瘤** 379
Jeremy R. Jass

10 **肝、胆囊和胆管肿瘤** 417
Sanjay Kakar 和 Linda D. Ferrell

11 **胰腺外分泌肿瘤** 463
Günter Klöppel 和 David S. Klimstra

12 **泌尿道肿瘤** 485
John N. Eble 和 Robert H. Young

13 **女性生殖道肿瘤** 567
 第一部分 卵巢、输卵管 567
     以及阔韧带和圆韧带
 Charles F. Zaloudek
 第二部分 子宫内膜 652
 George L. Mutter 和 Tan A. Ince
 第三部分 胎盘肿瘤和妊娠 672
     滋养细胞疾病
 Christopher P. Crum、Yonghee Lee 和
 David R. Genest
 第四部分 子宫肌层 683
 Marisa R. Nucci
 第五部分 宫颈 697
 Marisa R. Nucci、Kenneth R. Lee 和
 Christopher P. Crum
 第六部分 阴道 719
 Marisa R. Nucci
 第七部分 外阴 730
 Marisa R. Nucci

14 **男性生殖道肿瘤** 749
Jae Y. Ro、Mahul B. Amin、Kyu-Rae Kim 和
Alberto G. Ayala
 第一部分 前列腺和精囊 749
 第二部分 睾丸和睾丸周围组织 812
 第三部分 阴茎和阴囊 861

15 **腹膜肿瘤** 881
Philip B. Clement

16 **乳腺肿瘤** 903
Ian O. Ellis、Sarah E. Pinder 和 Andrew H.S. Lee

下卷

17	垂体肿瘤 M. Beatriz S. Lopes	971
18	甲状腺与甲状旁腺肿瘤 John K.C. Chan	997
	第一部分 甲状腺	997
	第二部分 甲状旁腺	1080
19	肾上腺肿瘤 Ernest E. Lack	1099
20	胰腺内分泌肿瘤 Günter Klöppel 和 Philipp U. Heitz	1123
21	淋巴网状系统肿瘤	1139
	第一部分 淋巴结 John K.C. Chan	1139
	第二部分 脾 Wah Cheuk 和 John K.C. Chan	1289
	第三部分 胸腺 Wah Cheuk 和 John K.C. Chan	1315
22	造血系统肿瘤 Jeffery L. Kutok	1363
23	皮肤肿瘤 Daniel J. Santa Cruz	1423
24	软组织肿瘤 Christopher D.M. Fletcher	1527
25	骨关节系统肿瘤 K. Krishnan Unni 和 Carrie Y. Inwards	1593
26	中枢神经系统肿瘤 M. Beatriz S. Lopes 和 Scott R. VandenBerg	1653
27	周围神经外胚层肿瘤 Christopher D.M. Fletcher	1733
28	自主神经系统（包括副神经节）肿瘤 Ernest E. Lack	1763
29	眼和眼附属器肿瘤 Robert Folberg	1781
30	耳肿瘤 Leslie Michaels	1813
31	肿瘤诊断中的电子显微镜检查 Bruce Mackay	1831
32	分子遗传学技术在诊断和预后中的应用 Janina A. Longtine 和 Jonathan A. Fletcher	1861
	索引	

著者名单

Mahul B. Amin MD
Chairman, Department of Pathology & Laboratory Medicine
Professor of Pathology at UCLA School of Medicine
Cedars-Sinai Medical Center
Los Angeles, CA, USA

Alberto G. Ayala MD
Deputy Chief of Service
Professor of Pathology, Weill Medical College of Cornell University
The Methodist Hospital;
Ashbel-Smith Professor Emeritus of Pathology
The University of Texas M.D. Anderson Cancer Center
Houston, TX, USA

Anton E. Becker MD PhD
Emeritus Professor of Cardiovascular Pathology
Academic Medical Center
University of Amsterdam
Netherlands

Eduardo Calonje MD DipRCPath
Director of Diagnostic Dermatopathology
Department of Dermato-Histopathology
St John's Institute of Dermatology
St. Thomas's Hospital
London, UK

Fiona Campbell BSc(Hons) MD FRCPath
Consultant Gastrointestinal Pathologist
Department of Pathology
Royal Liverpool University Hospital
Liverpool, UK

John K. C. Chan MBBS FRCPath FRCPA
Consultant Pathologist
Department of Pathology
Queen Elizabeth Hospital
Kowloon, Hong Kong

Wah Cheuk MD
Associate Consultant
Department of Pathology
Queen Elizabeth Hospital
Kowloon, Hong Kong

Philip B. Clement MD
Professor of Pathology
Department of Pathology
Vancouver General Hospital
Vancouver, BC, Canada

Christopher P. Crum MD
Professor of Pathology
Harvard Medical School;
Director, Women's and Perinatal Pathology
Brigham and Women's Hospital
Boston, MA, USA

John N. Eble MD FRCPA
Nordschow Professor of Laboratory Medicine
Professor & Chairman,
Department of Pathology & Laboratory Medicine
Indiana School of Medicine
Indianapolis, IN, USA

Ian O. Ellis BMedSci BM BS FRCPath
Professor of Cancer Pathology and Honorary Consultant Pathologist
Department of Histopathology
Nottingham University Hospitals NHS Trust
Nottingham, UK

Linda D. Ferrell MD
Professor and Vice Chair of Pathology
Director of Surgical Pathology
Department of Pathology
University of California,
San Francisco, CA, USA

Christopher D.M. Fletcher MD FRCPath
Director of Surgical Pathology
Brigham and Women's Hospital;
Chief of Onco-Pathology
Dana-Farber Cancer Institute;
Professor of Pathology
Harvard Medical School
Boston, MA, USA

Jonathan A. Fletcher MD
Director, Solid Tumor Cytogenetics
Department of Pathology
Brigham and Women's Hospital;
Associate Professor of Pathology and Pediatrics
Harvard Medical School
Boston MA, USA

Robert Folberg MD
Frances B. Geever Professor and Head
Department of Pathology
University of Illinois College of Medicine
Chicago, IL, USA

David R. Genest MD
Associate Professor of Pathology
Harvard Medical School;
Division of Women's and Perinatal Pathology
Brigham and Women's Hospital
Boston, MA, USA

Philipp U. Heitz MD
Emeritus Professor of Pathology
Department of Pathology
University of Zürich
Zürich, Switzerland

Tan A. Ince MD PhD
Instructor in Pathology
Harvard Medical School;
Associate Pathologist
Division of Women's and Perinatal Pathology
Department of Pathology
Brigham and Women's Hospital
Boston, MA, USA

Carrie Y. Inwards MD
Assistant Professor of Pathology and
Consultant, Division of Anatomic Pathology
Mayo Clinic College of Medicine
Rochester MN, USA

Jeremy R. Jass MD DSc FRCPath FRCPA
Canada Research Chair in Gastrointestinal Pathology
Department of Pathology
McGill University
Montreal, QC, Canada

Sanjay Kakar MD
Assistant Professor
Department of Pathology
UCSF and Veterans Administration Medical Center,
San Francisco, CA, USA

Kyu-Rae Kim MD PhD
Associate Professor
Department of Pathology
Asan Medical Center,
The University of Ulsan College of Medicine
Seoul, Korea

David S. Klimstra MD
Attending Pathologist and Chief of Surgical Pathology
Memorial Sloan-Kettering Cancer Center
Professor of Pathology and Laboratory Medicine
Weill Medical College of Cornell University
New York, NY, USA

Günter Klöppel MD PhD
Professor of Pathology and
Director of Department of Pathology
University of Kiel
Kiel, Germany

Jeffery L. Kutok MD PhD
Associate Professor of Pathology
Harvard Medical School;
Hematopathologist
Brigham and Women's Hospital
Boston, MA, USA

Ernest E. Lack MD
Director of Anatomic Pathology
Department of Pathology
Washington Hospital Center
Washington, DC, USA

Gregory Y. Lauwers MD
Director, Gastrointestinal Pathology Service
Department of Pathology
Massachusetts General Hospital;
Associate Professor of Pathology
Harvard Medical School
Boston, MA, USA

Andrew H. S. Lee MB BChir MRCP MRCPath
Consultant Histopathologist
Department of Histopathology
Nottingham University Hospitals
Nottingham, UK

Kenneth R. Lee MD
Associate Professor of Pathology
Harvard Medical School;
Boston, MA, USA

Yonghee Lee MD
Associate Professor of Pathology
Pochon CHA University College of Medicine
Bundang CHA General Hospital
Kyonggi-do, Korea

Janina A. Longtine MD
Chief, Molecular Diagnostics
Department of Pathology
Brigham & Women's Hospital;
Associate Professor of Pathology
Harvard Medical School
Boston, MA, USA

M. Beatriz S. Lopes MD
Professor of Pathology and Neurological Surgery
Department of Pathology - Neuropathology
University of Virginia School of Medicine
Charlottesville, VA, USA

The late D. Gordon MacDonald BDS PhD FRCPath FDSRCPS(G)
Formerly Professor in Oral Pathology and Honorary Consultant
Department of Oral Medicine & Pathology
Glasgow Dental Hospital
Glasgow, UK

Bruce Mackay MD PhD
Emeritus Professor of Pathology
University of Texas MD Anderson Cancer Center
Missouri City, TX, USA

Leslie Michaels MD FRCPath FRCP(C) FCAP
Professor Emeritus
Department of Histopathology
Royal Free and UCL Medical School
London, UK

Cesar A. Moran MD
Professor of Pathology, Director of Thoracic Pathology and Deputy Chairman
Department of Pathology
The University of Texas
MD Anderson Cancer Center
Houston TX, USA

George L. Mutter MD
Associate Professor of Medicine
Harvard Medical School;
Pathologist, Division of Women's and Perinatal Pathology
Department of Pathology
Brigham and Women's Hospital
Boston, MA, USA

Marisa R. Nucci MD
Associate Pathologist
Divisions of Women's and Perinatal Pathology and Surgical Pathology
Department of Pathology
Brigham and Women's Hospital;
Assistant Professor of Pathology
Harvard Medical School
Boston, MA, USA

Ben Z. Pilch MD
Associate Pathologist
Massachusetts General Hospital;
Associate Professor of Pathology
Harvard Medical School
Boston, MA, USA

Sarah E. Pinder MBChB FRCPath
Consultant Breast Pathologist
Histopathology Department
Addenbrooke's NHS Trust
Cambridge, UK

Jae Y. Ro MD PhD
Professor of Pathology
Department of Pathology
The Methodist Hospital
Weill Medical College of Cornell University
Houston, TX, USA

Daniel J. Santa Cruz MD
Cutaneous Pathology
WCP Laboratories Inc.
St Louis, MO, USA

Paul M. Speight BDS FDSRCPS(Glas) PhD FRCPath FDS RCS(Edin)
Professor of Oral and Maxillofacial Pathology
Department of Oral and Maxillofacial Pathology
School of Clinical Dentistry
University of Sheffield
Sheffield, UK

Saul Suster MD
Professor and Vice Chair
Director of Anatomic Pathology
The Ohio State University Hospital
Columbus, OH, USA

K. Krishnan Unni MB BS
Professor of Pathology and Orthopedics and Consultant, Division of Anatomic Pathology and Division of Orthopedic Oncology
Mayo Clinic College of Medicine
Rochester, MN, USA

Scott R. VandenBerg MD PhD
Professor of Pathology and Neurological Surgery
University of California School of Medicine,
San Francisco
San Francisco, CA, USA

Bruce M. Wenig MD
Chairman
Department of Pathology and Laboratory Medicine
Beth Israel Medical Center;
Professor of Pathology
Albert Einstein College of Medicine
New York, NY, USA

Geraint T. Williams BSc MD MRCR FRCP(Lond) FRCPath FMedSci
Professor of Pathology
Department of Pathology
Wales College of Medicine
Cardiff University
Cardiff, UK

Robert H. Young MD FRCPath
Director of Surgical Pathology
Department of Anatomic Pathology
Massachusetts General Hospital
Boston, MA, USA

Charles F. Zaloudek MD
Professor of Pathology
Department of Pathology
University of California, San Francisco
San Francisco, CA, USA

译校者名单

北京大学人民医院病理科

回允中　阚　秀　戴　林　沈丹华　谢大鹤　钱利华　鲍冬梅　陈定宝
孙昆昆　郑红芳　刘芳芳　王功伟　张晓波　高松源

北京大学临床肿瘤医院暨北京市肿瘤防治研究所病理科

薛卫成　刘毅强　时云飞　李香菊　董　彬　孙　宇　李忠武

哈尔滨医科大学第二附属医院病理科

杜金荣　韩丽姝　陈英准　李莹杰　韩桂萍　张艳梅　姜　影

大连医科大学

病理学教研室　　唐建武　李连宏　孙　雷
附属第一医院　　关宏伟
附属第二医院　　王莉芬

昆明医学院病理学教研室

王　芳　季语祝　沈　勤　庄利萍　郭　君　唐　莹　卜亚军

吉林大学第二医院病理科

高洪文

主译的话

Dr. Fletcher 主编的《肿瘤组织病理学诊断》(Diagnostic Histopathology of Tumors)一书自1995年首次出版以来，已两度再版，其第3版的中文译本即将与广大病理医生及相关临床医生见面。这是我主译的第七部诊断病理学巨著。十多年来，我为主译这些病理学巨著付出了许多，当然也从中学到了很多，获益匪浅。病理学涉及面很广，很多人感到知识匮乏，解决这个问题的必由之路就是"天天读"，除此以外没有捷径，这是病理学界许多同仁的共识。

《肿瘤组织病理学诊断》是一部好书——是一部按器官系统论述肿瘤组织病理学诊断的教科书。同其他病理学巨著一样，其每一章节均是从成百上千篇参考文献中提取精华撰写而成，是千千万万科学工作者常年辛勤劳动的结晶，这样的教科书自然具有权威性。我20年前的一篇个案报告竟然也被收入其中，作为参考文献引用（见本书377页参考文献416），就是一个很好的例证。

不断更新的教科书是你我永远的老师。值此《肿瘤组织病理学诊断》第3版中文版即将面世之际，我想在这里再次强调"请书会诊"(Textbook Consultation)的重要性。"请人会诊"(Human Consultation)固然重要，但在某种程度上，"请书会诊"似乎更为重要，尤其是在诊断有分歧的病例，无疑是可以选择的正确方法。对此，我想以高度富于细胞的子宫平滑肌瘤(highly cellular leiomyoma)为例说明这个问题。高度富于细胞的子宫平滑肌瘤是一种必须与子宫内膜间质肿瘤鉴别的、比较少见的子宫间叶性肿瘤。由于不太熟悉或根本不知道有这样一种疾病存在，"请人会诊"时诊断意见往往出入很大，不但不能解决问题，有时反而会令人无所适从。争论的焦点无非是：其是来源于平滑肌还是来源于子宫内膜间质，是良性肿瘤还是恶性肿瘤。高度富于细胞的子宫平滑肌瘤的组织学表现由于与子宫内膜间质肿瘤的组织学表现非常相似，容易被误诊为子宫内膜间质肿瘤。但是仔细观察会发现，其具有几个与子宫内膜间质肿瘤明显不同的特征（本书第684页仅寥寥数语就将此描述得清清楚楚），了解这些诊断和鉴别诊断要点，就不难做出正确诊断。此时，"请书会诊"不仅可以解决诊断问题，还能免除一些无谓的纷争。此外，千万不要忘记，在免疫组织化学染色不支持组织形态学诊断时，不能根据一个看似异常的免疫染色结果（尤其是阴性结果）来否定一个明确的形态学诊断，这是组织病理学诊断的重要原则之一。

毋庸置疑，病理医生在肿瘤诊断方面起着无与伦比的作用。由于所有肿瘤诊断均应采用严格的组织学标准，可以想见，在病理学诊断领域说"我说是就是"（金口玉言）的时代将一去不复返了！(The days of saying "It is what it is because I say it is" are gone! 见本书绪言部分)。诊断标准多数来源于经典的教科书，读书是为了实践，事实证明，读书可以明显提高病理学诊断水平。因此，我深切希望本书能为提高肿瘤组织病理学诊断水平做出应有的贡献。

本书的译者们为本书的出版付出了艰辛的劳动，在此表示深切的谢意。主译水平有限，错误在所难免，敬请读者批评指正。

北京大学人民医院 病理科
北京五洲女子医院 病理科
回允中
2009-03-26

著者前言

在本书第 2 版出版与第 3 版出版的 7 年间隔中，传统的形态学和免疫组织化学检查仍是卓越的、最可靠的和成本-效果最好的方法，诊断和预后评估仍然依靠它们做出，在多数情况下，肿瘤如何适当切除的决定也主要经由它们做出。在诸如分子遗传学诊断、基因表达谱和蛋白组学（proteomics）等更昂贵的现代技术可以应用的今天，当各种检查所得结果差异更大时——不仅在发达地区和发展中（或不发达的）地区之间（达到骇人听闻的程度），甚至在不同的发达国家或地区之间——在某种程度上，这些"传统"技术和解读方法的作用再一次得到认证。而上面提到的许多新技术也已经实现它们应用于临床的承诺。

的确，现在分子诊断的作用已经稳固确立。近些年来，分子诊断技术不断扩展，包括：敏感性试验，如在乳腺癌和结肠癌；神经胶质肿瘤的预测；追踪残留的微小疾病的更敏感方法，特别是在恶性淋巴造血系统肿瘤。分子诊断的这种广泛而又重要的作用在新的第 3 版全书中均有所反映，并且在 Janina Longtine 和 Jonathan Fletcher 撰写的第 32 章进行了特别讨论。也许最高层面的分子学进展是基于可重复的相关靶分子的确认的合理的靶向治疗不断增加。值得注意的是，这些靶分子多数是通过免疫组织化学检查（如 HER2/neu、c-kit 和 EGFR）确认的，至少开始时是这样的。然而，由于常常发生治疗对抗且不清楚对抗机制，为了选择最佳治疗方法，可能需要更多地依靠突变分析。近几年来，由于注意力已经集中到酪氨酸激酶上，一些持乐观态度的人希望：通过广泛筛选某种特定肿瘤的"着丝粒"（kinome），可以确认适当的激活靶点或易于干预的信号通路。在可预知的将来，这种技术还不太可能广泛应用，因此，在更好地了解治疗改变的相关性和激酶过表达或激活的真正机制之前，最好还是加以小心。

值得注意的是，从表面上看，肿瘤形态学分类和预测方法的进展步伐并没有明显减慢，而是继续发展并更加精确，这有助于不断提高解剖病理学的价值。这些进展多数已被收录在新版 WHO 分类中，后者在过去 5 年左右的时间中已经陆续发布。另外，与临床或治疗有关的"新的"肿瘤类型（或亚型）不断得到认可，形式上是各种各样的。本书第 3 版已根据这些新的信息进行了修订，有些章节是重新撰写的，特别是有关肝胆系统肿瘤、女性生殖道、造血系统和眼（及其附属器）章节的许多内容。

一如既往，所有的错误或遗漏都是我这个编者的责任。在这里，我首先要深深地感谢各位著者，他们对本书倾注了极大的热情，并为本书提供了大量高质量的素材。其次还要深深地感谢我的杰出的秘书 Kathleen Radzikowski，我还要感谢 Elsevier 的"主要负责人员"Michael Houston、Sheila Black 和 Bryan Potter，感谢他们的辛勤工作和大力支持。

Christopher D.M. Fletcher
Boston，2006
回允中译

绪言
Introduction

Christopher D. M. Fletcher 著
时云飞 薛卫成 译 回允中 校

在外科病理学甚至整个诊断组织病理学领域内，病理医师在肿瘤诊断方面所能起到的作用是无与伦比的。可惜，病人或非专业人员对此却一无所知，常常想当然地认为他们的诊断医师是外科医师、其他临床医师或肿瘤医师，这种误解也总是难免不同程度地反映在我们的某些同事身上！事实上，对于患有肿胀或肿块的任何病人来说，病理组织学报告才是诊断、预测临床经过和决定治疗的首要因素；当然，患有脓肿或血肿的病人可能是个例外。

对于做出及时、准确而又详尽的病理学报告的要求越来越高，特别是处于现今病理亚专业化日益发展和诉讼不断的社会中。肿瘤病理学和普通外科病理学正处于高速发展的阶段，这种需求反映在要增强对于从前未被认识的肿瘤类型或变型特征的认识，掌握并且应用不仅能够用于诊断，而且能为判断预后和了解发病机制提供客观帮助的新技术。外科病理医师的"信息库"在不断地扩充，这就要求我们查阅数量愈来愈多的亚专业化的杂志和教科书。我们编撰这部单独探讨有关各个系统肿瘤组织病理学诊断的教科书的目的就在于此，受邀参加本书编写的作者都是各个领域内公认的专家。我之所以采用"我们"一词，是想强调主编、作者和出版者之间在编写这本书中的密切合作，而所有的错误和疏漏，如同前两版一样，则完全由主编负责。我们必须承认，由于外科病理学发展神速，所以本书的一小部分内容难免过时，甚至到出版时就已被废弃！

本书应用的"tumor"一词原则上取其传统的描述性语义：也就是说，它既包括了肿瘤性病变，有时也包括了某些非肿瘤性肿块。有时我们无法确定某一病变是错构瘤性、增生性，还是肿瘤性病变，或者常常遇到至少是一个悬而未决而有争议的问题，此时本书常常采取一种实用而中性的原则。值得注意的是，有关肿瘤（neoplasm）目前尚无普遍认可的定义，因为单独强调克隆性并不充分，某些传统上被认为是反应性的病变也显示出具有单克隆性或寡克隆性改变，例如淋巴组织和滑膜病变。移植（异种移植物）模型具有生长能力可能是最令人信服的判断标准，但在常规情况下却无法应用！本书的重点依然是组织形态学，但是对于多数病变来说，还会提供基本的临床资料和相关的分子遗传学资料，因为这些资料对于准确分类非常有用。鉴别诊断的原则是（必要时进行适当的相互参照）着重描述那些具有特殊性或普遍性问题的肿瘤。

毋庸讳言，本书绪言一章确实为宣讲本人有关某些肿瘤病理学诊断常规实践的经验和观点提供了机会。下面提出的一些基本原理纯属本人观点，并非所有作者的共识。当然，其中某些建议也并非独创，只不过是外科病理学"约定俗成"的一些观点。我确信其中某些（尽管我不能确定是哪些观点！）属于 John Azzopardi 教授的观点，至少在欧洲是这样，John Azzopardi 教授是外科病理学领域中的一位伟大导师。如今在某些领域内认为这种宝贵的信息传承几乎没有什么价值，而作为执业的组织病理学医师，也被驱使常常专注于对诊断或预后做出比较客观或"科学"的评估。这一趋势充分反映在某些大型国际性学术会议中，表现为其内容被时髦的，但常常是昙花一现的各种技术、抗体、基因或突变分析所主导。就形态学和生物学行为而言，由于人类肿瘤较宿主更加易变、不可预测，而且更加特殊，所以注定需要有可靠的外科病理学诊断。外科病理学诊断主要依靠富有经验的病理医师进行仔细的光学显微镜检查，在适当或必要时应用现代技术辅助诊断。这种娴熟的形态学检查仍然是解剖病理学的金标准，至少在目前是这样。就其可靠性和成本效益而言，在近期内不大可能被超越。在诊断病理学的某些方面，我们的确会遇到不同程度的困扰，因此我们应该通过各种最有效的手段，朝着不断提高诊断的可重复性和客观性的方向进行不懈的努力。一个显而易见的事实是（至少在肿瘤医学中），外科病理学从未像现在这样起到至关重要的作用。临床医师希望得到（而且常常需要讨论）详细的病理学报告，这主要是由于组织病理学指标对于决定治疗具有非常重要的作用。在某些学术中心，常常认为外科病理学的专业知识是想当然的，尤以欧美为甚。这种看法应该受到谴责，否则长此以往必将削弱学术部门富有成效的培训工作，而且侧重点可能发生转移，进而导致重要的诊断技能日渐丢失。这种趋势部分地表现在资质认证前训练时间的缩短，以及从事基础研究的MD/PhDs和PhDs将重点放在了获取科研基金上，其结果之一是加大了在学术性医学中心中进行的大量研究与医院基本临床职责二者之间的距离。显然，要想增加真正的临床医学家的数量，就需要加大对于临床与衔接性研究的资助，并促进临床医师与实验室人员之间的相互尊重和合作。在这一点上，没人能比病理医师更适于这种合作。

下面我将尽量按照外科病理学实验室的流程，即从接收标本到签发报告，陈述一些指导性的原则。

在缺乏清楚而完整的临床资料的情况下，诊断肿瘤是鲁莽而又危险的，而且有时是不可能的。常常需要提醒我们的许多临床同事注意这样一个事实，有人在申请单中连有关年龄、性别、部位等这样简单的信息可能都不填写。这样做除了对于病人治疗可能产生负面影响以外，可能还存在是否遵守医院制度的问题。如果发现送到实验室的标本没有这些资料，那么作为合格的医务人员就应该毫不迟疑地与出现疏漏的医师或其同事联系。在得到所需要的充分信息之前，病理医师拒绝签发报告有时可能是恰当的。如果从前有任何肿瘤的病史，尤其是在同一解剖部位，则要求填写有关活检日期、诊断和（可获得的）相关的实验室检查结果。对于诊断所必需的辅助资料，即使没有要求也必须提供，例如骨肿瘤的放射学所见或血清生化检查。

准确而详细地描述一个大体肿瘤标本对于诊断、预后以及回顾性病理或临床研究至关重要，特别是对于根治性切除标本。在病理实验室首次检查切除标本时，通常是唯一能够准确测量肿瘤大小、重量、大致坏死范围以及与切缘距离的时机；一旦标本被剖开、切碎、固定或者扭曲变形，这些有用的信息将不复存在。同样，诸如肿瘤边缘类型（有包膜、局限性或浸润性）、出现卫星结节、波及（或累及）淋巴结以及播散或浸润邻近结构的范围等特征，都常常是在剖开标本时才能得到最好的确认。最后，病理报告中有关肿瘤的大体描述应当详细到使任何其他病理医师都能够构建出肿瘤清晰的大体图像。如果大体描述得好，即使没有看到组织切片，结合临床资料就有可能得到最后诊断，特别是对于那些比较常见的肿瘤。好的大体检查的其他重要作用是能够确保肿瘤取材充分。取材的方式和范围各异，取决于肿瘤的大小和解剖部位。但是，一般的做法是所有较大（或许>2 cm）的病变均应做连续切面，而所有显示不同表现的区域均应进行组织学检查。对于某些器官系统，根据大体检查所见要在最有可能发生浸润的肌层、浆膜或包膜部位仔细取材。由于现今盛行应用墨汁标记肿瘤切缘，有关这个问题我恳请大家要三思而行！几乎完全不考虑标本类型而一律选择墨汁来标记标本的做法，在某种程度上可能会导致浪费时间，因为所标记的往往是不相干的病变切缘，这种切缘或者没有复发的可能，或者就是有非常明显的恶性肿瘤或没有完全被切除，在大体检查时即可记录为切缘阳性（或至少从肿瘤学角度上看切除的不够充分）。有时候病变（或活检标本）太小，以致一个蜡块就足以完全包埋进行切片，这样的病例（即使不用墨汁染色）评估切缘根本不存在问题，然而却仍然有人应用墨汁进行标记。这种处理标本的趋势是很不理智的，常常失去了全面检查标本应有的益处，并且对于墨汁标记的有效性可能产生不良影响。但是，墨汁标记如果应用得当，其作用可能是无法估价的。

现在回到组织学诊断上，显然这是一个复杂的、常常具有器官特异性的过程，其细节将在本书各个章节中分别叙述。然而，仍可列出几项相关的准则。已经公认准则具有危险性，一味坚持应用这些准则会犯错误，因为每一项准则可能都有例外。不过，我仍认为这些准则能够提供有价值的指导原则。任何从前患有原发性（复发性）肿瘤的病人，均应复习以前的切片。这基于如下4个主要目的：（1）它是简单而实用的复查肿瘤类型的方法；（2）它便于评判肿瘤的组织学分级是否提高（或降低），由此可能影响临床预后；（3）这是唯一能够确定一个病人是否发生了两个独立的原发性肿瘤的方法，无论是同一类型的肿瘤还是不同类型的肿瘤。（4）有时这种复查能够提供重要的诊断线索，因为复发性或转移性肿瘤可能具有明显的表型改变或特异性分化能力的丧失，尤其是间叶性肿瘤。通过复习从前的组织学切片，有时会把一个怪异或似乎不能诊断的肿瘤变成一个简单病例！因此，应当牢记奥卡姆剃刀原理（principle of Occam's razor）：一个病人患有一种原发性肿瘤伴有奇特复发形态的可能性总是大于患有两种独立的原发性肿瘤的可能性。

第二项准则可能也是一项基本道理，我个人认为至关重要的是对于所有肿瘤的诊断都应该采用严格的组织学标准。除了专家根据经验做出诊断这种个别情况以外，任何依据个人想像主观诊断的做法都是不能接受的。如果同事或学员询问是如何做出这种诊断的，应该能够列举出诊断依据或标准，无论是阴性还是阳性所见；可以想见，"我说是就是"（金口玉言）的时代将一去不复返了！(The days of saying "It is what it is because I say it is" are gone!) 这样做的优点是：（1）增加诊断的一致性，从而便于决定治疗；（2）当分析已发表的资料或开始进行新的研究时（不论是临床研究还是病理学研究），我们才有可能进行比较，这是朝向了解肿瘤形态学和生物学行为迈出的至关重要的一步，尤其当需要进行大规模多中心研究时；（3）规定明确的诊断标准是培训病理医师唯一可靠的方式。为此，我们必须尽可能地推崇形态学的客观性，纵然外科病理学在某些方面仍然是一门保持一定主观性的科学。

第三项准则应该是众所周知的。应用苏木素－伊红（H&E）染色的肿瘤切片普遍适用于光学显微镜检查，在多数（但并非所有）情况下，首先应该在低倍镜下观察，因为低倍镜下表现对于区分良性和恶性病变常常能够提供最好的线索。诸如正常结构（常常是分叶状）是否保留、病变是否对称以及对于细胞构成和细胞核非典型性的总体印象等特征，对于鉴别良恶性很有帮助。相反，如果急于直接应用高倍镜观察，显然容易发现（然而也可能被引入歧途）各种肿瘤或假肿瘤性病变中的具有非典型性的细胞或令人忧虑的特征。这种现象的很好例证是，在任何位于黏膜或皮肤的反应性且常呈息肉状改变的病变中，其黏膜下或固有膜中几乎均可见到奇异性、常为多核的间质细胞，而且在各种软组织肿瘤中均可出现致密深染而不规则的变性（"老化"）细胞核。同样，出现单个或非常罕见的异常核分裂象也不一定就是恶性肿瘤：我会永远记得，在我做病理工作的第一年中，就在其他方面正常的增生期子宫内膜中见到过这样的核分裂象。

考虑到某些比较现代的技术已经应用到病理诊断实践中，本书将在每一章中提及与之相关的内容，而且将在第 32 章进行比较详细的讨论。免疫组化的应用到现在已有 25 年以上的历史，目前看来虽然不能再称之为现代，但是的确非常有用，然而必须根据实际情况进行解释。一个明确的形态学诊断从不允许一个看似异常的免疫染色结果将其否定，尤其是阴性结果。质量控制对于免疫组化发挥应有的作用至关重要，而且常要求每一个实验室都应该有一个"最低工作量"，尽管这个工作量究竟多大合适尚未完全确定。日常进行大量免疫组化染色而且工作人员也相对固定的实验室，要比那些规模较小、间断应用这项技术的实验室能够获得更加一致和高质量的染色结果。有关应用大量成组抗体或复杂免疫诊断流程的价值尚有争议，不过，在这个讲求成本－效益的年代，我的观点是根据 HE 染色形态学进行仔细地鉴别诊断分析，提出需要回答的特殊问题，再来决定是否应用免疫染色并选用抗体。过分扩大而盲目地应用成组抗体可能会造成误导或得出偏离的结果。应用的抗体越多，误导的可能性也就越大。同样，如果依赖免疫诊断流程（尤其是照搬某一个实验室的流程而不是你自己的流程），那么一个错误或假阳性（或阴性）的结果就可能会导致荒谬的诊断，而且这种免疫染色既耗时，又昂贵。目前，免疫组化的另一个重要作用就是越来越多地用于识别潜在的靶向治疗目标（例如 *c-kit* 或各种生长因子受体）。病理医师绝不要强迫自己进行这种检测，除非已经证明这种蛋白在某种特定的肿瘤类型中具有生物学相关性（通常是激活或突变），而且还必须有经过验证的可靠而且具有可重复性的用于这种目的的抗体。

在诸多较新的分子遗传学技术中，某些技术无疑已被证实（并将继续被证实）在肿瘤病理学中所具有的价值。但是应该记住以下两点：首先对于文献中发表的关于某种类型肿瘤的基因表达方式或核型异常，只有和形态学诊断对应时才有意义（或有效）。如果根据这些结果做出的诊断与形态学不一致，甚至相反，那么得出的结论就变得毫无价值。因此，组织病理学医师与基础研究人员之间的相互合作和彼此尊重是继续发展这些技术的先决条件。芯片技术（chip technology）允许对大宗肿瘤标本进行快速而详细的分子谱系研究，这种专业上的互动对于验证这些资料并从中提取最有应用价值的临床信息非常关键。不过，近年来许多基因组学表达谱的研究旨在鼓吹其新发现在诊断或预后方面的准确性，而对应用常规光学显微镜病理诊断却无帮助（仅有少数显著例外的情况），对于这一问题应该给予高度关注。这可能部分地反映了在这些研究工作中多数缺少有经验的病理医师的参与。其次，尽管最初认为分子和遗传学指标是有前景的，但是近些年来发现，除了某些情况（例如神经母细胞瘤中的 *N-myc* 扩增、许多白血病和肉瘤的细胞遗传学和分子学特征以及淋巴造血系统肿瘤中微小残留病灶的检测）之外，对于诊断和预后来说，它并不比仔细（或富有经验）的光学显微镜检查优越。因此，与所有需要进行评估的新技术相比，光学显微镜检查仍然是金标准。有关新技术更具客观性的说法值得商榷，这不只是因为存在费用和非专业性实验室试验可重复性差的问题，而且也是因为已经证实这些说法常常是错误的，例如以前曾经描述的所谓肿瘤特异性抗原或突变，或一度曾误以为 *p53* 表达是一种可靠的恶性表型标记物。

一旦做出诊断，病理学报告就必须规范，其指导作用远远超出一本书所能提供的信息。不过，重要的是要确保任何报告都能向临床医师提供尽可能多的有用的信息，在这种情形下，有越来越多的理由表明病理医师需要采用概要性（或模板性）报告格式，尤其是对于常见类型的肿瘤。按照这种格式报告，就不会遗漏关键的信息要点，而且使得临床医师能够最大限度地理解病理学报告。这不仅仅意味着报告中应该明确陈述肿瘤的类型、分级或分期（当可行时）以及切缘状况，而且也是提供有关临床特征综合信息的唯一机会，诸如生物学行为和理想的治疗方式，在适当的情况下还可以引用相关文献。对于少见的或者特殊的肿瘤，可能需要传递这种信息。至于外科病理医师是否提供治疗意见主要取决于医院环境和临床医师的胸襟和见识。然而，我的观点是外科病理医师绝对不要忘记，他们提供给临床的建议常常比较主观，可能明显不同于某些其他病理学专门研究的论述，在这种情况下，不应避讳提供任何其他专业知识或可用的背景资料。毋庸置疑，描述许多类型肿瘤临床特征和治疗结果的主要文章，至少最初都是发表在病理学杂志而不是临床杂志上。因此，外科病理医师常常会比临床医师更早获知最新发表的有关某种特定肿瘤诸多方面的信息。不过，也要防止病理医师"一言堂"的趋势，除非病理医师能够确保他们也浏览了相关的临床文献。

总结这篇绪言，我想提供一些适用于肿瘤诊断病理学的简单原则。其中多数是不言而喻而且可能是广为人知的。然而，令人惋惜的是这些原则却常常人被遗忘，值得引起注意。

1. 简单的统计学概率告诉我们，常见者就是常见；所以不要总是痴迷于少见而深奥（或令人兴奋！）的诊断，除非你确实已经排除了一个非常可能的诊断。这种陷阱的一个典型例证，就是评定发生在诸如上消化道或膀胱等内衬上皮的中空脏器的梭形细胞恶性肿瘤时，诊断肉瘤样（或梭形细胞）癌的可能性远远大于某些少见的肉瘤或癌肉瘤。

2. 如果在决定治疗之前难以确定病理诊断，病理医师从来不要惧怕要求得到较大的（或重复）活检标本。某些肿瘤活检标本实际上并不充分或不具有代表性。事实是我们的临床和放射学同道提供的活检标本有越来越小的倾向（冠以成本效应和方便病人的名义），这不仅限制了我们做出正确诊断的能力，而且也减少了提供有价值的预后信息的机会。这种趋势应当加以遏制，或至少应当受到质疑，或首先进行证实，尤其是因为术前肿瘤新辅助治疗的应用在不断增加，常常使得最终切除的标本缺乏诊断和预后意义。耗费数小时乃至数天，仍然犹豫不决，随后做出一个不确定的报告，或更糟糕的是做出一个不恰当的过于自信的报告，这就不如明确要求临床提供更多组织。有时，这无疑可以避免制定不恰当的治疗方案。在诊断报告中尽可能不要存在任何侥幸心理。

3. 病理医师应该从不惧怕承认他们不能诊断或不能对一个特定肿瘤进行分类这一事实。全球所有的病理医师有时都会从他人的诊断意见中受益。认为从不需要参考别人或专家诊断意见的病理医师是很危险的。外科病理学在不断的亚专业化，需要真正多面手的年代即将结束，这就更加需要参考他人的诊断意见。然而，总有一小部分人类肿瘤任何人都不能进行合理的归类。在这种情况下，即使分化方向不明确，也可能会（但不总是）有一些线索提示这种肿瘤的临床行为，不过这种线索只能被作为暂时的解释。实际上，一个肿瘤如果不能根据形态学可靠地归类，那么任何评估预后的尝试均不可信，充其量也不过是猜测而已！

4. 显然，上述观点的必然结果就是病理医师只能根据以往的所见、所学或所闻来做诊断。这给病理医师的诊断能力划定了清晰的界限，而且强调需要通过定期参加学术会议或日常阅览主要的专业杂志，跟上现今的不断进展。有人（日益在减少）一直把认识或重新分类诊断实体看成是毫无价值的"分解"，这是在铤而走险；有人试图强行将所有肿瘤诊断均纳入他们已经熟悉的范畴，这同样也是危险的。

5. 另外一点，表面上看来至少是与"不懂"这种状况有关，那就是病理医师（或就此而言对于任何其他执业医师）从来都不要惧怕承认错误。每一个病理医师至少偶尔都犯过错误，可能是微不足道或没有临床意义的错误，而且提出不同意见的任何人或许也有错误。我们的外科病理学专业是一种解释性的技巧或艺术，而不是简单的判断黑或白，因此不可避免地会出现凡人皆有的错误。就此而言，隐瞒或欺骗只会比承认诊断不当带来更大的麻烦。

6. 临床肿瘤医师常常认为癌症治疗的预后评估主要取决于肿瘤的分级和分期，而病理医师在肿瘤分级和分期评估方面可能具有重要作用。有些临床医师认为这些参数（尤其是分级）在没有具体诊断的情况下就能确定。从上述讨论来看，这显然是不明智的，外科病理医师应当抵制这种趋势。在许多器官系统，预后很可能是主要决定于准确的组织学分型，从来不要低估准确诊断的重要性。同样，对于某些类型的恶性肿瘤，进一步分级毫无意义，因为这些肿瘤类型本身不管组织学表现如何，总是能够表明生物学的低级别（例如婴儿纤维肉瘤）或高级别（例如胸膜恶性间皮瘤）。因此，重要的是要认识到在许多情况下分级（而且还常常包括分期）系统需要根据具体肿瘤类型进行裁定，泛化的分级方法无疑是危险的。同样，需要我们慎重对待的是，将突变分析作为临床治疗的预后因素时（例如胃肠道间质瘤和非小细胞性肺癌）必须经过认真验证，目前仍然局限于得到验证而又具有临床意义的肿瘤类型。在某些类型的肿瘤，由于相对缺乏重要的治疗进展，进而限制了比较尖端（而且昂贵）的诊断或预后技术的应用，这并不是我们所期望的结果。这种讨论还亟待解决什么是高级别肿瘤；这个问题并没有简单或明确的答案，但是下述例证可以为病理医师开拓思路并且促使我们对恶性肿瘤进行认真的评估和分析。仔细思考下面3个病人：第1例是一名60岁的男性，患有不能手术的支气管小细胞癌；我们知道这种肿瘤很可能迅速播散，而且他存活超过12个月的希望微乎其微。第2例是一名25岁的女性，患有大腿部局限性腺泡状软组织肉瘤；我们知道她的5年生存率可能为60%～70%，由于这种信息，她可以有稳定的恋爱关系并建立家庭，但是我们还知道她能活过45岁的几率小于15%，因为多数患有这种类型肿瘤的病人最终会发生远处转移。第3例是一名患有2级额叶星形细胞瘤的45岁病人；我们知道发生颅外扩散（转移）的危险非常小，但是术后复发的几率却非常高；我们还知道这种复发可能在5～10年内不断进展而致死。我认为完全有理由告知所有这3个病人他们患有生物学上高级别的肿瘤，然而临床医师、病理医师或研究人员对每一个病例的理解肯定是各不相同的，尤其是有关这些肿瘤固有的生物学行为。这些差别提示我们，至少在选择治疗方案时，需要根据生物学行为，而不是根据组织学分级来治疗肿瘤。

7. 最后，不言而喻，也许是最明确的一点，那就是在可行和安全的情况下，应该及时发出组织学报告，无论是对来自本院的标本还是来自千里之外病人的标本而言都是如此。外科病理学报告不仅是简单记录或刻板印证临床猜想的一种手段；对于肿瘤病理学而言，它几乎总是诊断的主宰因素和确定治疗方案的一个重要决策因素。病理学报告对于病人具有重大影响，虽然他们常常并不知道这个事实。奉劝任何一名没有认识到或没有准备承担这种职责的病理医师，最好还是考虑更换职业吧！

心脏和心包肿瘤
Tumors of the heart and pericardium

2

Anton E. Becker 著

谢大鹤 译 戴 林 校

引言	7	其他良性心脏肿瘤	30
临床表现	8	心脏和心包的恶性肿瘤	32
病理学	9	其他少见的心脏原发性肉瘤	35
心脏和心包的良性肿瘤	9	心脏和心包其他原发性恶性肿瘤	36

引言

心脏和心包的原发性肿瘤确属罕见,为此论点提供最佳注释者为美国陆海空三军病理学研究所(Armed Forces Institute of Pathology,AFIP)。1977年,除囊肿外,该研究所只收集到444例心脏和心包原发性肿瘤[1];然后,他们又根据1976—1993年间收录的386例原发性心脏肿瘤资料对原结果做出修订[2]。因此,即便是在一些大型专业的心血管病研究中心,这也都是相当冷僻的研究课题。

为使本章之论述更为客观、准确,可能须求助于三家具有不同背景的研究所,并对其所持论点进行比较研究。表2.1所示为AFIP的心脏肿瘤相对发病率,该表系根据Burke和Virmani 1996年的绘图所制[2]。表2.2之数据则取自《心脏肿瘤外科治疗:25年(1964—

表2.1 1976—1993年AFIP原发性心脏肿瘤的发病情况一览(囊肿和心包肿瘤除外)(adapted from Burke & Virmani[2])

婴幼儿和儿童[a] (n=55)				成人 (n=319)			
良性	(n=44)	恶性	(n=11)	良性	(n=193)	恶性	(n=126)
横纹肌瘤	20 (19)	横纹肌肉瘤	3 (1)	黏液瘤	110	血管肉瘤	32
纤维瘤	13 (8)	血管肉瘤	1 (0)	乳头状弹力纤维瘤	31	恶性纤维组织细胞瘤	15
黏液瘤	4 (0)	恶性纤维组织细胞瘤	1 (0)	血管瘤	15	骨肉瘤	13
血管瘤	2 (1)	平滑肌肉瘤	1 (1)	脂肪瘤样肥厚(房间隔)	12	平滑肌肉瘤	11
房室结间皮瘤	2 (1)	纤维肉瘤	1 (0)	房室结间皮瘤	8	纤维肉瘤	8
浦肯野细胞瘤	2 (1)	黏液肉瘤	1 (0)	纤维瘤	7	黏液肉瘤	7
畸胎瘤	1 (1)	不能分类者	3 (1)	脂肪瘤	2	横纹肌肉瘤	3
				副神经节瘤	2	滑膜肉瘤	4
				其他	6	脂肪肉瘤	2
						恶性神经鞘瘤	1
						不能分类者	30

[a] 指就医时年龄小于16岁的患者。
括弧内的数字表示初治年龄小于1岁的患者数量。

1989）经验之谈》一文[3]，作者分别来自美国 Texas 休斯敦的得克萨斯心脏病研究院（Texas Heart Institute）和 MD 安德森癌症研究中心（MD Anderson Cancer Institute, Houston）。表 2.3 所列之数据资料包括所有原发性心脏和心包肿瘤的病理材料和存档会诊标本，全部来自阿姆斯特丹学术医学中心（Academic Medical Center, Amsterdam）的心血管病理档案室。

调查结果表明：①原发性心脏肿瘤实属少见；②参与调查的研究所在此问题上的思维偏倚不仅关系到各种数据的绝对值，而且影响到各类肿瘤的（发生率）排序。但有两点是没有争议的：①迄今为止，最常见的心脏原发性肿瘤是心脏黏液瘤（表 2.4），但在婴幼和儿童，最常见的心脏原发性肿瘤则为横纹肌瘤。②从浸润性、破坏性生长伴潜在转移性的角度考虑，心脏原发性恶性肿瘤极为罕见，尤其是在婴幼儿和儿童。

表 2.2　原发性心脏肿瘤外科治疗 25 年之经验数据一览 (Adapted from Murphy et al. With permission from The Society of thoracic Surgeons[3]).

良性	(n=102)	恶性	(n=12)
黏液瘤	63	血管肉瘤	4
浦肯野细胞瘤	14	恶性纤维组织细胞瘤	2
横纹肌瘤	9	纤维肌肉瘤	1
纤维瘤	7	黏液肉瘤	1
脂肪瘤	4	平滑肌肉瘤	1
其他[a]	5	纤维肉瘤	1
		不能分类的肉瘤	2

[a] 包括血管瘤、血管瘤型错构瘤、静脉畸形、二尖瓣囊肿和肉芽肿。

表 2.3　阿姆斯特丹学术医学中心心血管病理档案室之原发性心脏和心包肿瘤一览

良性	(n=118)	恶性	(n=18)
黏液瘤	73	血管肉瘤	7
脂肪瘤	11	平滑肌肉瘤	3
横纹肌瘤	8	横纹肌肉瘤	3
乳头状弹力纤维瘤	8	黏液纤维肉瘤	2
血管瘤	6	间皮瘤	1
纤维瘤	5	淋巴瘤	1
浦肯野细胞瘤	2	恶性神经鞘瘤	1
副神经节瘤	2		
其他[a]	3		

[a] 包括纤维弹力型错构瘤型二尖瓣、血管脂肪纤维瘤样二尖瓣和房室结间皮瘤。

临床表现

对病理学家来说，重要的是要知道：心脏肿瘤的临床表现大都是非特异性的，其他很多疾病很可能有类似表现。这些表现大致可分为三大类：①全身性；②栓塞性；③心源性[4]。虽然这些临床表现主要是来自对心脏黏液瘤的临床经验总结，但对原发性心脏肿瘤临床表现的概念入门来说，还是具有普遍价值的。

全身性症状

心脏肿瘤的全身性症状表现多样，包括发热、极度虚弱和浑身不适。实验室检查异常项目有红细胞沉降率升高、高 γ 球蛋白血症、血小板增多或减少、红细胞数量增多、白细胞计数增多和贫血。这些全身性症状的形成机制尚未完全明了，但作为炎性反应的一部分，很可能与细胞活素（cytokine）的释放有关。

栓塞的表现

栓塞的形成可能源于肿瘤本身的碎片脱落，也可能是在肿瘤表面凝集形成的血栓脱落所致。如果是肿瘤碎片栓塞，则该肿瘤本身就有一个凸入心腔内的部分；而另一方面如果是血栓栓塞，则该肿瘤有可能长在心壁间，因其破坏了心内膜的完整性，继而就有可能导致心腔内附壁血栓形成。

要知道体动脉栓塞很可能是心脏肿瘤的首发症状，故在此情况下，病理医师就可大有用武之地。外周动脉的突然阻塞都应该提示这种可能性。因此，每一个栓子切除术标本都应给予认真检查，以确定肿瘤组织是否存在其中。但是，即便是只见有新鲜的血栓结构，病理报告上也不应除外源于心脏肿瘤的（心脏附壁）血栓栓子之可能性。且多发性体动脉栓塞（的临床表现）酷似全身性脉管炎或感染性心内膜炎，尤其是那些伴有明显全身症状的患者。

原发于右心腔的肿瘤可导致肺动脉栓塞，其临床表现与继发于静脉血栓形成的患者无异。

心源性表现

心源性事件的表现主要取决于该肿瘤的位置和大小。那些位于心肌间的肿瘤常以实质性占位取代心肌或以挤占心腔（容量）的形式损害心肌功能。而且，位于心壁间的肿瘤本身就可引起多种类型的心律失常，包括心房纤维性颤动和室颤。如是，猝死就很可能成为心脏肿瘤的首发症状。瘤体凸入心腔的心脏原发性肿瘤可能会导致栓塞，也可能会影响瓣膜功能。其症状和体征则

表2.4　不同研究系列报告之心脏黏液瘤的分布情况一览

研究机构及其统计概况	左心房	右心房	左心室	右心室	心瓣膜[a]
AFIP系列[2]：114例黏液瘤，占良性肿瘤的29%，两心房受累者2例（2%），多心腔受累者3例（3%）	83（73%） (MV：2) (LA+RA：2) (LA+LV：1) (LA+RA+MV：1)	22（19%）	2（2%） (LV+RV：1)	2（2%） (TV：1)	4（3.5%）
Mayo医学中心系列[5]（1954—1979）：68例黏液瘤，其中多发性黏液瘤3例	48（70.6%）	12（17.6%）	-	1（1.5%）	7（10.3%）
得克萨斯系列[3]（1964—1989）：63例黏液瘤，占良性肿瘤的61.8%	57（90.5%）	6（9.5%）	-	-	-
明尼苏达州立大学系列[6]（1959—1989）：51例黏液瘤，占良性肿瘤的50%	45（88.3%）	4（7.8%）	-	2（3.9%）	-
法国联合研究[7]（1961—1988）：444例黏液瘤，占良性肿瘤的92%，多发性黏液瘤5例	368（82.9%） (LA+RA：3) (LA+LV：1)	47（10.6%）	2（0.4%）	11（2.7%） (RV+RA：1)	11（2.7%）
日本调查材料[8]（1984—1989）：74例黏液瘤，占良性肿瘤总数的89.1%，无多发性黏液瘤	66（89.2%）	7（9.3%）	1（1.3%）	-	-
中国调查材料[9]（1962—1988）：633例黏液瘤，占良性肿瘤之97.8%，多发性黏液瘤26例	566（93.2%）	31（5.6%）	4（0.6%）	9（1.5%）	-
阿姆斯特丹学术医学中心心血管病理档案室：56例黏液瘤，占良性肿瘤的56.5%，多发性黏液瘤3例	61（83.5%）	8（11%）	1（1.4%）	3（4.1%）	-

[a]详见p16～17

MV：二尖瓣；LA：左心房；RA：右心房；LV：左心室；RV：右心室；TV：三尖瓣。

在很大程度上取决于受累心腔和肿瘤的大小。

最终可导致心脏压塞症状或体征的心包渗出大都与（心脏肿瘤）累及心外膜，亦或与原发性心包肿瘤有关。

病理学

本节将对原发性心脏肿瘤的良恶性鉴别做出说明。不过，这里所谓的"良性"之涵义与大脑原发性良性肿瘤有相似之处。生物学行为和明确的病理组织学形态可能是非浸润、非转移性肿瘤诊断的主要构件，但肿瘤的位置和大小可能会对患者的临床预后产生严重影响。而且，"良性"范畴内还应该包括一些在严格意义上未必是真性肿瘤的病变。实际上，其中有些就是现被认为是错构瘤而非真性肿瘤的病变。这远非是一个语义学的问题，因为如果患者的临床条件许可，在保守治疗下，此类病变中有些是会自行消退的。

心脏和心包的良性肿瘤
Benign tumors of the heart and pericardium

心脏黏液瘤　Cardiac myxoma

这是最常见的原发性心脏肿瘤（表2.1～2.3）。其中绝大部分病例（90%以上）的原发部位都是心房，尤其常见于左心房（表2.4）。

心脏黏液瘤大都起源于房间隔，靠近卵圆窝的位置，但发生在心房内其他位置者也有报道[5-11]。原发于心室者较为罕见。AFIP[1]和我们自己心血管病理档案室报告的发生率不寻常地增高（7.4%和5.5%），无疑与材料收集的偏倚有关。黏液瘤还可能起源于心瓣膜（参阅p16～17）；Mayo Clinic[5]报告的发生率（10.3%）与其他报告[6-9]相比，高得有点离谱。这纯属巧合，还是他们把别的病变（如乳头状弹力纤维瘤）也纳入其中尚不

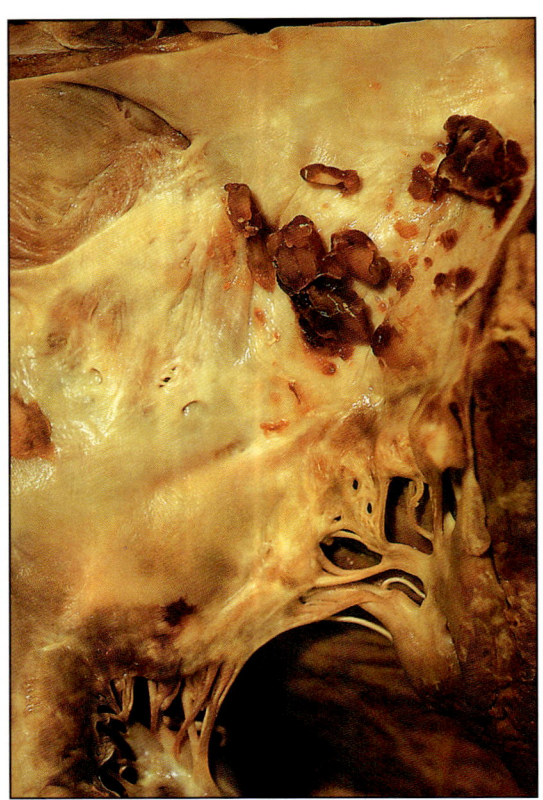

图2.1 一位70岁女性患者因一条腿突发剧痛入院，入院后很快就出现右侧半身不遂，并死于昏迷[10]。尸检示左心房多发性黏液瘤，体积相对较小（其右心房内有一大的带蒂黏液瘤，图中未显示）。

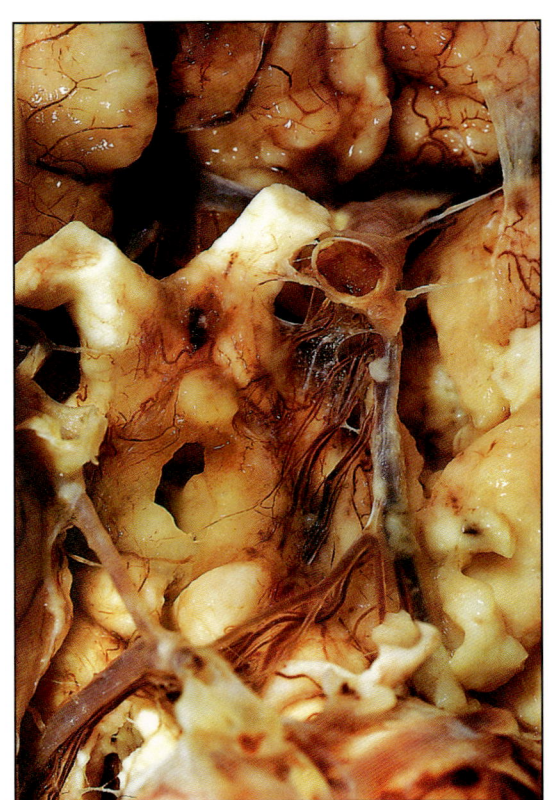

图2.2 与图2.1为同一患者。脑底面图示：颈内动脉被黏液瘤栓子堵塞。

得而知（另见p24）。多发性黏液瘤虽不多见，但其发生率之高，足以使这种多发性病变（multiplicity）不能被忽视（AFIP初版130名患者中有6例[1]，修订版为5/114例[2]；Mayo Clinic的这个数字为3/68[5]；Amsterdam Series 为3/73）。同样重要的是要认识到：多发性肿瘤未必局限在某一个心腔，很可能是黏液瘤综合征的一部分（参阅p16）。图2.1和2.2所示为一经典病例，该患者同时表现有肿瘤栓塞之戏剧性结局[10]。

大体病理形态

心脏黏液瘤可有梗，亦可无梗，但不管它是否具有发育完整的颈部，肿瘤大都有良好的活动性。黏液瘤大都表现为有多个分叶的息肉状肿物（图2.3），部分呈球状，为表面光滑的类球形肿物（图2.4）。色泽从灰白到暗红不等，不同侧面的色泽常有变换。偶可见表面血栓形成。肿瘤质软、脆，伴有特殊的凝胶状外观。虽然瘤体大部质地柔软、易碎，片状出血可致其色泽改变、体积增大、包膜紧张，但肿瘤基底部大都为均质实性、表面光滑、色泽灰白。有些黏液瘤质地坚实，偶有肉眼可见的钙化灶，甚至大部瘤体都由钙化灶构成，此即所谓石化（petrified）心脏黏液瘤（图2.5～2.7），但在临床

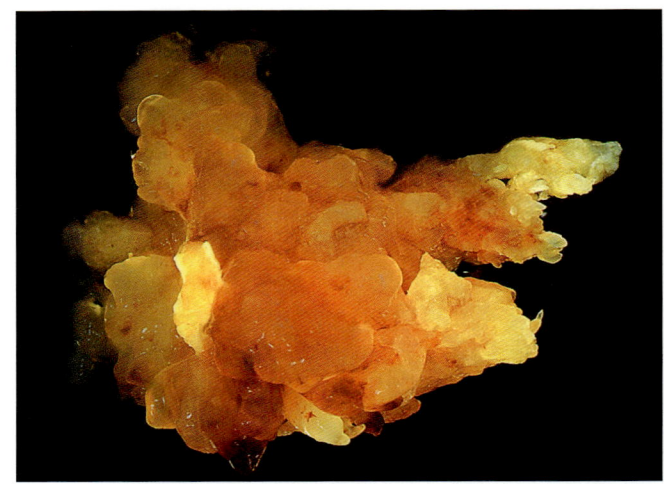

图2.3 起源于房间隔的左心房黏液瘤的手术标本，表现为有多个分叶的息肉状肿物。

上可能被误认为是心房血栓[12]。

因心脏黏液瘤切除后可能复发，故外科医生应将肿瘤连同其基底部一并切除。因此，心房黏液瘤的手术标本几乎肯定会带上一块结构完整的心房壁或房间隔。（标本上）找不到无肿瘤成分手术边缘的情况虽然极少发生，但在组织学诊断上，还是应该对此结构做出说明。此外，手术切除如果不完全，也无再次手术的迫切需求，因为黏液瘤的复发可以在用超声心动图做术后随诊时得到准确诊断。

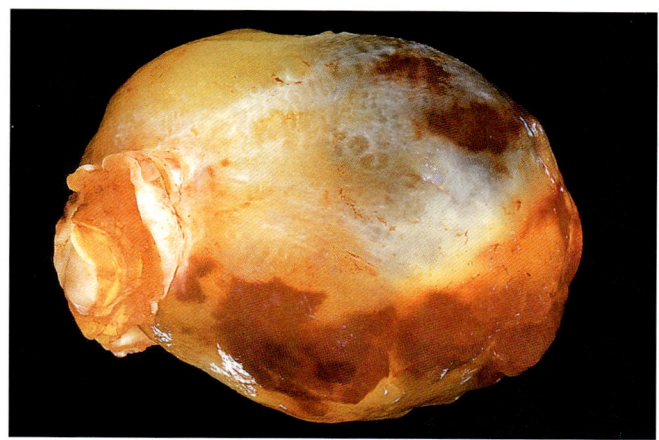

图2.4 发生在房间隔的左心房黏液瘤，瘤体呈球状，肿瘤表面光滑。

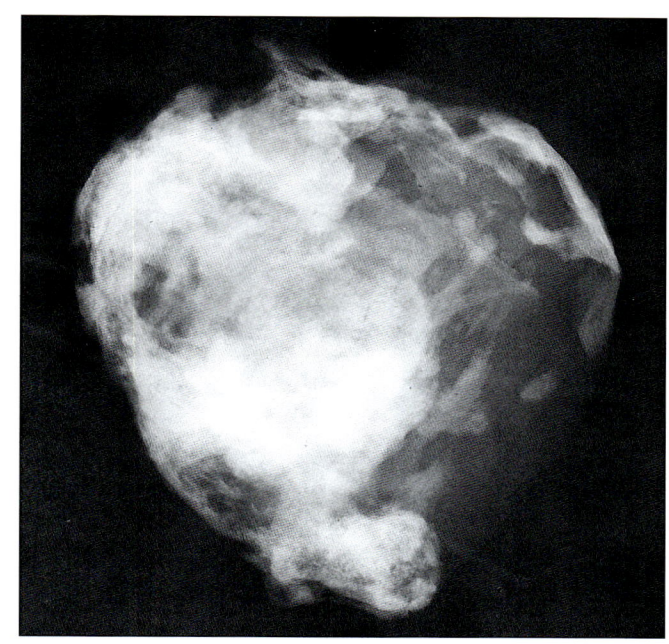

图2.6 与图2.5为同一患者标本，X线片显示（肿瘤）严重钙化。

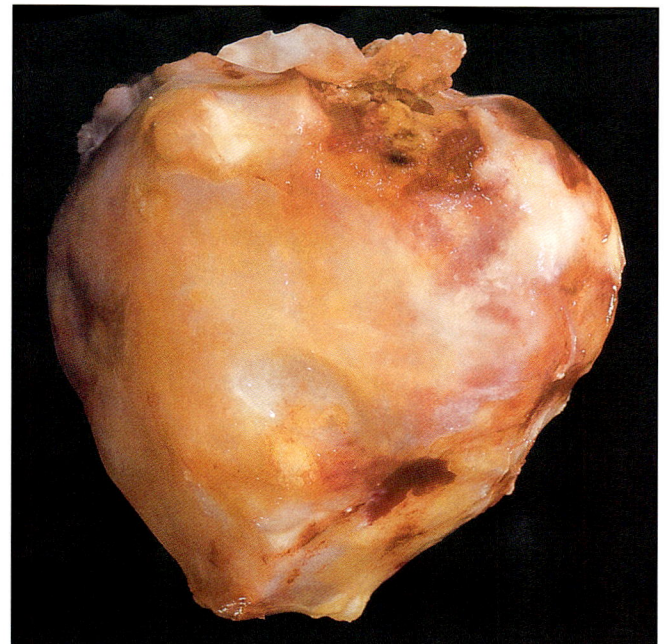

图2.5 石化心脏黏液瘤的大体形态，此手术切除标本原位于左心房。患者为48岁男性。

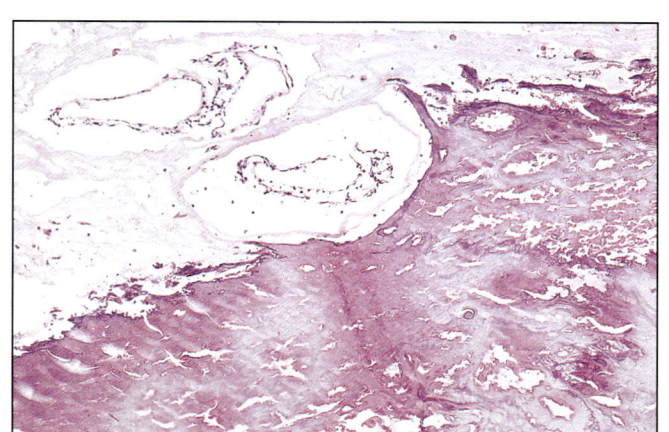

图2.7 图2.5所示标本之组织学形态，显示：黏液瘤细胞巢与一钙化灶相毗连，如是，可证明本病变之黏液瘤性质。

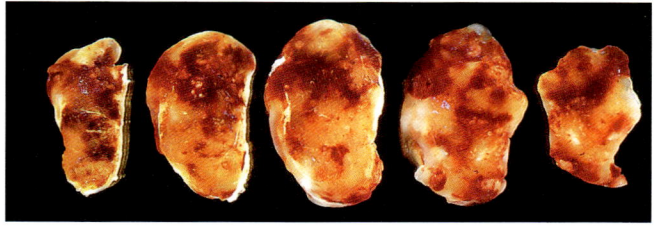

图2.8 球形黏液瘤手术标本之平行纵切面，显示：切面呈凝胶状，局部几乎为黏液状，并有反光，伴广泛片状出血。

心脏黏液瘤的切面呈凝胶状，局部近乎黏液状、有光泽，切面色泽可呈与表面相似的花斑状（图2.8）。肿瘤的靠周边部分大都因出血而呈暗红色。为了得到可靠、全面的病理组织学形态、继而取得准确的病理诊断，切片用组织块理应取自肿瘤的多个不同部位。这一点非常重要，因为它的唯一真正需要鉴别诊断的选项是一种伴有黏液样变的原发性恶性肿瘤（详见下文）。

病理组织学形态

显微镜下，心脏黏液瘤以大量黏液样基质和散在分布的细胞成分为其优势结构。后者由多种不同类型的细胞构成[13]，其中主要的细胞类型——即所谓"黏液瘤细胞"——现被认为是真肿瘤细胞[13-15]。这些细胞呈长梭形、多边形或星芒状（图2.9）。胞浆大多均质，偶有微小空泡，嗜伊红淡染。细胞核可为长形、圆形或卵圆形，特异性着色深浅不等。无核分裂象。那些大的多边形黏液瘤细胞偶被称为"蝶翅鳞状（lepidic）细胞"（lipis来

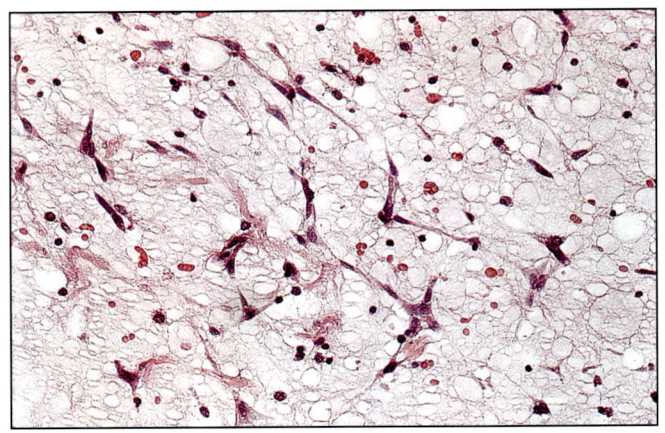

图2.9　显微镜切片展示出黏液瘤细胞形态的多形性。

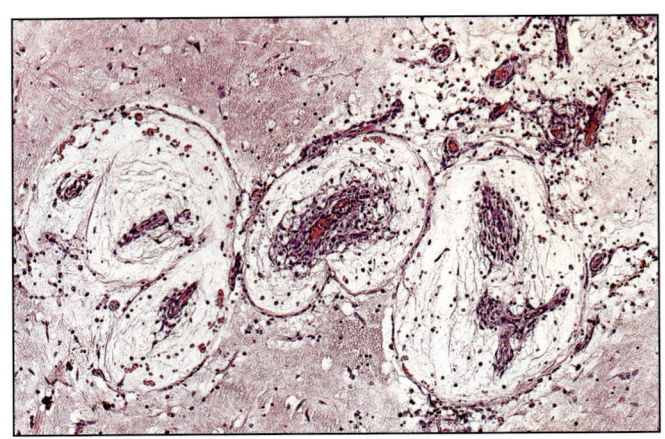

图2.11　镜下可见黏液瘤细胞典型的排列方式。瘤细胞相互交织成网状，并明显是围绕内皮细胞型毛细血管分布，但内皮细胞未必都很清楚。

自希腊语，意为"鳞屑"，此处特指覆于蝶翅上的鳞状物，这种类比相当富有想象力）。此术语是由Orr[16]于1942年引入，当时，他认为这些细胞起源于心内膜。在超微结构上，典型的黏液瘤细胞以胞浆中细胞器稀少为特征（图2.10），有数量不等的线粒体、光面和粗面内质网和胞浆微丝。后者包括两种类型：其中大部分是粗的（10 nm），无分支微丝，呈平行束状排列，无固定走向；第二类是细微丝(6～8 nm)，排列方式不规则。

黏液瘤细胞的排列方式多样。一种常见的方式是它们围绕仅被有内皮细胞的血管排列，或单层，或多层（图2.11）。瘤细胞可能相互交织成网状或以单链的形式出现。这些黏液瘤细胞群常常被包裹在一个大的、镜下几乎是空不着色的细胞外黏液样基质湖晕之中，而其周围基质则要浓密得多，嗜酸粉染，二者之间反差明显（图2.12）。黏液瘤细胞可能的排列方式还有小巢状（图2.13）和散在分布于黏液样基质中的单个瘤细胞（图2.14）。黏液瘤细胞可为多核，但在电镜下，可见其由几

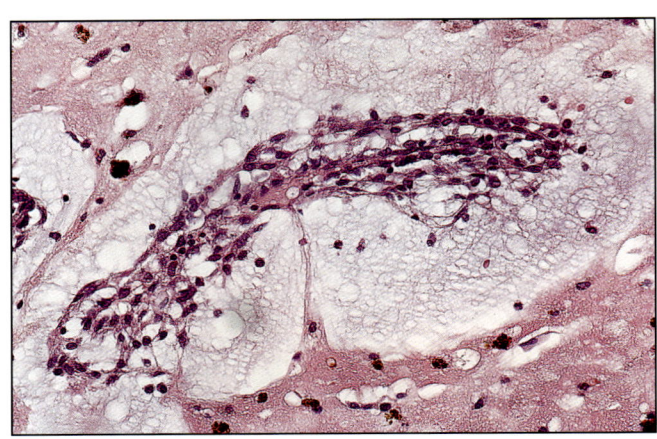

图2.12　如图2.11所示，这种排列方式常常伴随着一个大范围的黏液样组织晕环，该晕环与其周围嗜伊红染色更深的基质形成反差。

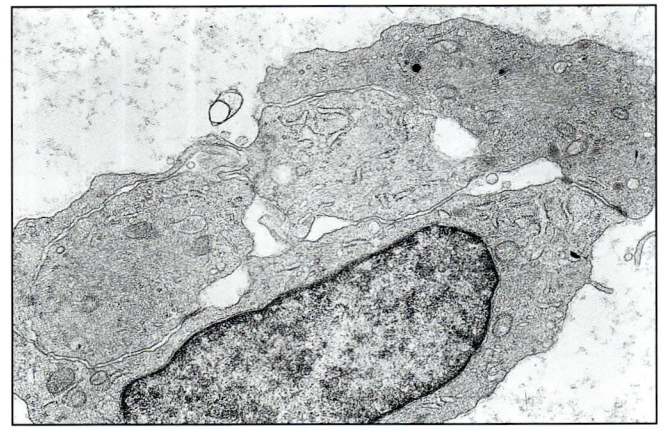

图2.10　几个紧密连接的典型黏液瘤细胞的超微结构：可见瘤细胞内细胞器稀少。胞浆基质中含有大量中间丝；细胞间可见细胞连接。

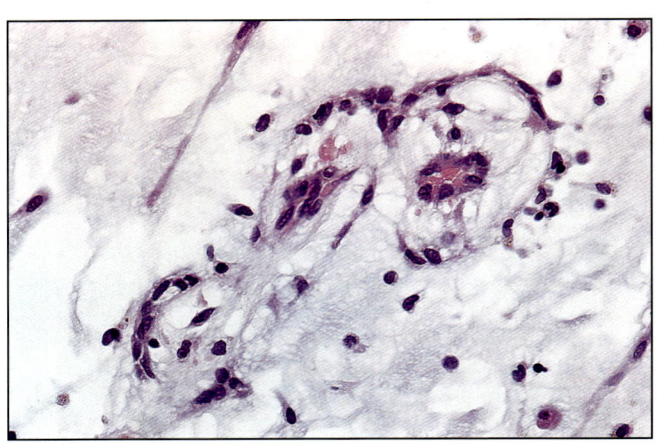

图2.13　镜下可见黏液瘤细胞排列方式的变化：从毛细血管周套袖状排列到小巢状分布。

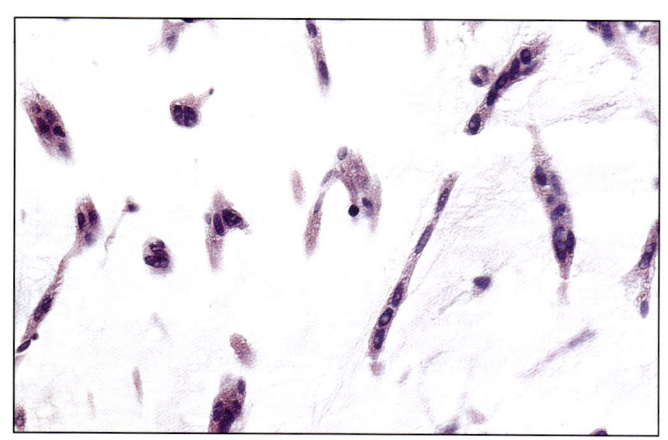

图2.14 显微照片图示：黏液瘤细胞以单个、零散的排列方式，弥漫性地分布于黏液样基质之中。

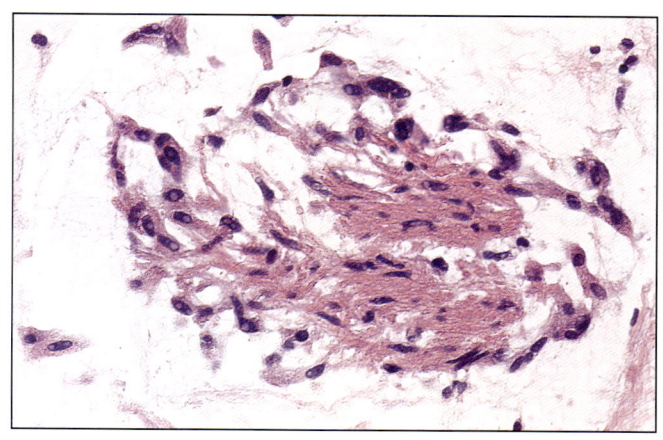

图2.15 显微照片图示：与形似平滑肌细胞的长梭形细胞密切连接在一起的"典型的"黏液瘤细胞。

个单核瘤细胞紧密挤在一起而形成[13]。偶可见由不同性质细胞围成的腺样腔隙（见下文）。肿瘤表面可能被覆着一层内皮细胞，亦可没有，但这几乎可以肯定是手术造成的人工假象。

因此，即便是在同一个黏液瘤之中，其瘤细胞的组织学和细胞学表现也是形态各异的。这一观点需要强调，因为病理医师受训用不同程度的、常暗含恶变之意的非典型性来评判肿瘤细胞。在心脏黏液瘤，为得到准确诊断，低倍镜下的组织形态之重要性远非高倍镜下仅能看到几个细胞的细胞学特征可比。同样需要反复强调的是：（黏液瘤中）核分裂象极为罕见（在56例黏液瘤中，没见到一个明确无误的核分裂象），故为临床实用计，可以说是不存在。实际上，如果发现有核分裂象，那就应该极端审慎地看待（良性）心脏黏液瘤的诊断（见下文）。

除了黏液瘤细胞，心脏黏液瘤中还可见很多其他类型的细胞。可能的情况是：这些间叶性细胞是一种分化上的表达，并无组织发生学意义[13]。最明显的例证就是那些类似纤维母细胞、肌纤维母细胞或平滑肌细胞的长梭形细胞的出现（图2.15）。这些细胞常与典型黏液瘤细胞和有明确内皮细胞被覆的血管腔有密切关系。

免疫组化染色[11,14]亦可突显上述各类细胞在免疫显型表达上的差异。用抗vWF（anti-van Willebrand factor，抗血管性血友病因子）和抗UEA-1（Ulex europaeus agglutinin Ⅰ，Ⅰ型荆豆凝集素）抗体做免疫组化染色，血管内皮细胞呈阳性反应[14,15,17,18]。黏液瘤细胞对波形蛋白呈强阳性，而抗vWF则为阴性，但这些细胞之间的黏液样基质中纤细的原纤维也可能为阳性。此外，那些直接紧紧围绕在血管内皮细胞周围分布的细胞对SMA（smooth muscle actin，平滑肌肌动蛋白）特异性单克隆抗体染色呈阳性反应者并不在少数。管壁呈结蛋白阳性的大血管大多分布在肿瘤基底部，某些梭形间质细胞亦可偶呈结蛋白阳性。我们用不同类型、标记肌动蛋白丝的单克隆抗体染色，发现这类细胞中有部分呈阳性；电镜下，这些细胞的部分胞浆中可见有纤细的胞浆微丝[13]；我们自己的观察为超微结构提供了有力的支持。同样，波形蛋白（一种57 kDa的中间丝）强阳性者则可能与电镜下看到的那些粗微丝有关。

心脏黏液瘤中出现腺样结构约占总数的5%，其被覆上皮从扁平到立方或柱状变化不等（图2.16～2.18）。这些细胞对阿新蓝、黏蛋白卡红和PAS（耐淀粉酶性）都呈阳性反应；细胞角蛋白（CK）免疫反应阳性[14,15]。这些细胞的超微结构特征是黏液分泌型上皮[14]（详见下文组织发生章节）。

在黏液瘤，出现巨噬细胞几乎是一种最为普遍的组织学现象，它们大都弥漫性地散在分布于黏液样间质之中，但以其基底部和出血部位最为集中（图2.19）。

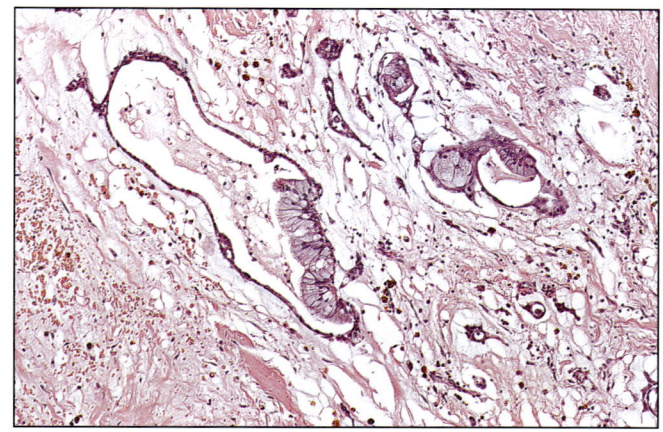

图2.16 心脏黏液瘤腺样结构的显微照片。可见由交替排列的扁平和柱状上皮被覆的管腔结构。（Courtesy of Dr R.J.van Suylen, Department of Pathology, Academic Hospital, Maastricht, The Netherlands.）

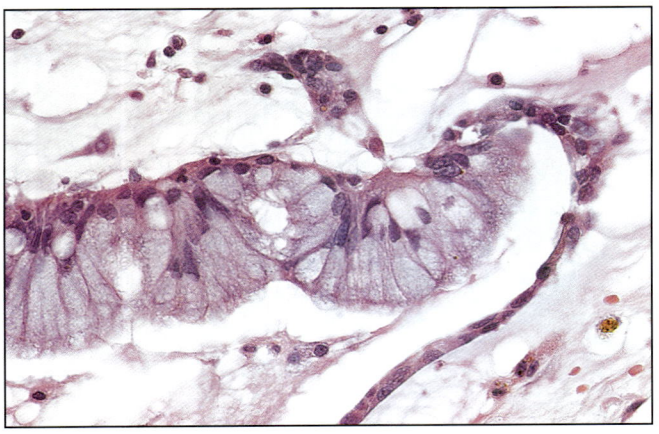

图2.17　图2.16之高倍镜图，显示：该柱状上皮的黏液分泌性质与肠上皮相似。

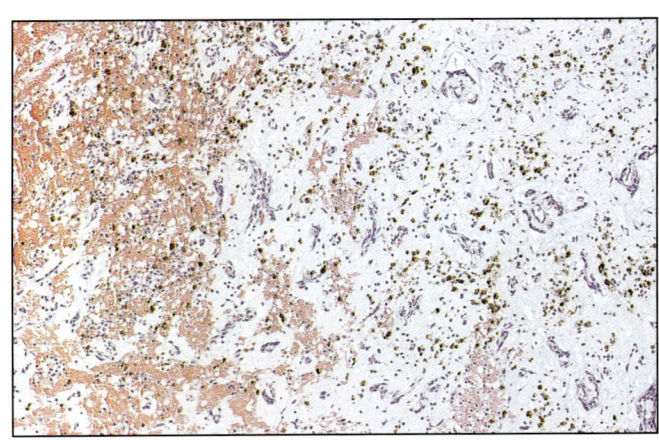

图2.19　显微镜图示：在新鲜出血灶周围，黏液瘤间质中散在分布有大量含铁血黄素吞噬细胞。

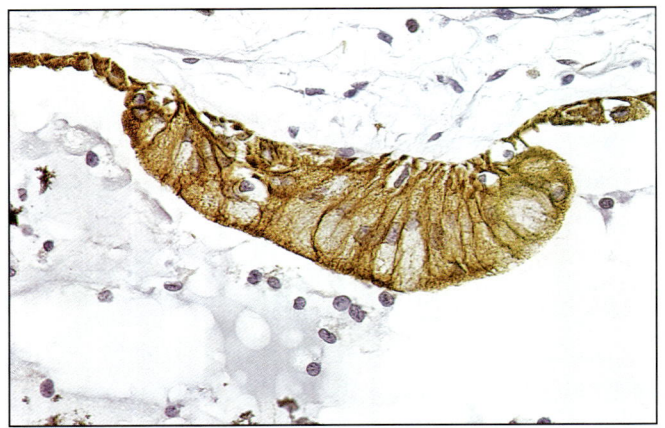

图2.18　免疫组化染色显示：黏液瘤细胞呈CK阳性。

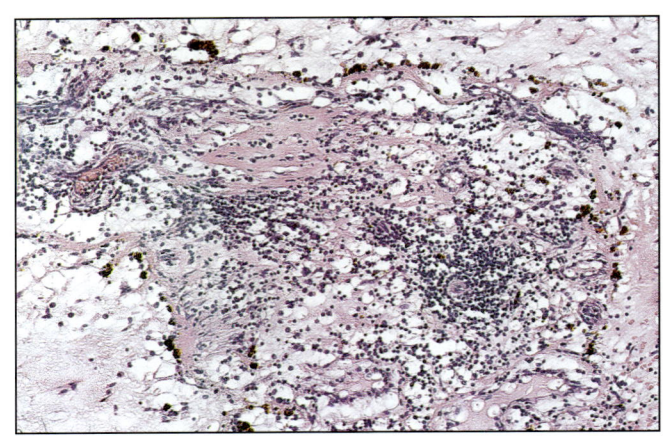

图2.20　显微镜图示：有大量淋巴细胞浸润之区域。

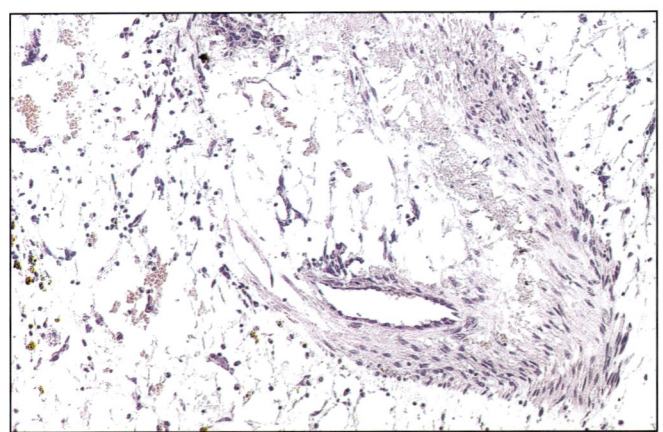

图2.21　黏液瘤基底部的大口径肌性动脉，该动脉中层像是被黏液瘤细胞所"虫蚀"。

淋巴细胞和浆细胞也是黏液瘤中常见的细胞类型（图2.20）。这些细胞主要聚集在肿瘤基底部，亦可见于肿瘤周围的心肌组织间。此外，偶可见有肥大细胞和灶状髓外造血细胞[10]。

黏液样基质本身呈阿新蓝强染，而且不受透明质酸酶预消化的影响；黏蛋白卡红和耐淀粉酶PAS染色可呈片状阳性。其中还含有数量不等、具有网状蛋白、胶原蛋白和弹性蛋白特征的结缔组织纤维。纤维组织是肿瘤蒂部最突出的成分，且多有大口径厚壁动脉进入蒂部。冠状动脉造影时偶可见到的所谓"肿瘤泛红现象（tumor blush）"，自有其在血管构架上的解剖学基础。这些动脉的中层大都被黏液瘤细胞侵蚀而呈虫蚀状（图2.21）。

在黏液瘤，间质出血几乎是最普遍的病变形式。手术标本的出血虽然比尸检标本略显突出[5]，但这些出血灶很可能是继发于腔内肿瘤活动性的损伤所致。陈旧性和新鲜出血的组织学证据就可定论；含铁血黄素吞噬细胞的聚集（图2.19）和被铁和钙包被的结缔组织纤维结节（所谓Gamma-Gandy小体，图2.22）就提供了这方面的证据。据称，心脏黏液瘤中的这些纤维硬化性结节可能与抗凝和/或抗血小板治疗有因果关系[19]。我不认同这种说法（Lie也持此观点[20]）。因为不管此前是否接受过治疗，只要你认真寻找，完全找不到这类结节的情况是非常少的。

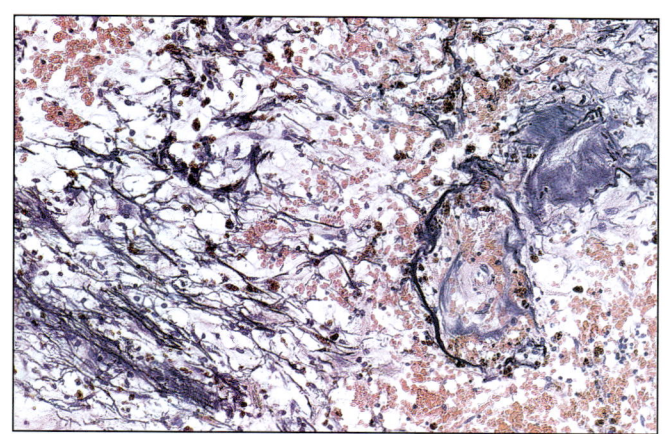

图2.22 黏液瘤间质中的Gamma-Gandy小体。由铁、钙包被的结缔组织纤维小体提供了此前为灶状出血的证据。

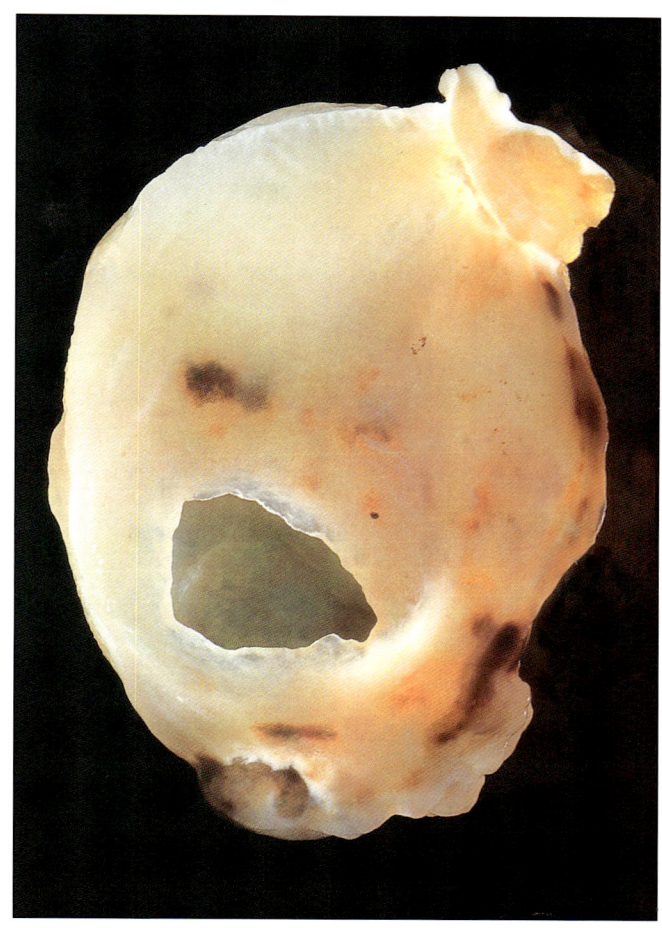

图2.23 手术切除的黏液瘤中充满清亮液体的囊腔显然是成于细胞外基质液化所致黏液瘤间质囊性变。

除了这些特殊的包被结节之外，镜下灶状钙化亦不少见。黏液瘤中的营养不良性（dystrophic）钙化偶可非常之广泛，以致整个瘤体变成钙石团块（图2.5～2.7）。

必须要强调指出：和细胞成分一样，黏液瘤间质也表现出广泛的部位间差异。明显为纤维性病变的区域和表现为黏液样间质液化——导致囊性变——的部位可能出现于同一肿瘤（图2.23）。这些囊肿中有些可能源于出血后发生纤维蛋白样（fibrinoid）间质改变，继而发展为纤维蛋白样变性（图2.24）。千万不要把纤维蛋白样变性与坏死混淆（另见复发性和"恶性"心脏黏液瘤一节）。

特别关注之处

心脏黏液瘤的某些特殊表现是为病理医师特别关注之处，值得在此简要讨论。

复发性和"恶性"心脏黏液瘤：心脏黏液瘤术后复发者虽不多见，但毫无疑问确是偶有发生（见Loire & Thermet 综述[21]）。正因如此，才推荐手术将黏液瘤连同其附着部位完整切除的做法[22,23]。但复发所涉及的机制问题基本还处在研究阶段。当然，据称，原发性黏液瘤手术切除不净、黏液瘤碎片在心脏组织中的种植均可导致术后复发。心脏黏液瘤的复发还被某些人视为"黏液瘤未必是良性"说法的证据[24]。不过，可能还有其他一些机制也在发挥作用。Loire和Thermet[21]根据他们自己的经验、文献综述，并详细分析后得出结论：发生在年轻人的复发性黏液瘤好像都有家族性倾向，其发生是因为它有所谓"黏液瘤综合征"（又称Carney综合征[25]或Swiss综合征[26]、遗传性心脏黏液瘤-皮肤色素沉

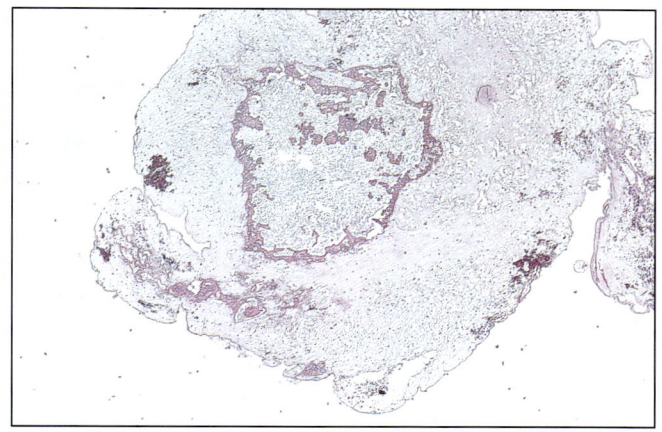

图2.24 镜下，有多处浅表和新鲜出血的黏液瘤之周边部位可见一囊样结构，囊内壁衬覆一层纤维蛋白样（fibrinoid）物质。

着-内分泌功能亢进）之多中心性病灶的基础（见下文）。这种情况下的复发率要远高于"散发"的心脏黏液瘤（21%对1%）[25]。而且，复发性肿瘤大都生长得更为迅速[27]，局部浸润也更加明显[28]。多中心性病变亦可通过以下事实说明：在这些患者，复发（性黏液瘤）可在

不只一个心腔同时发生（图 2.1）。

对黏液瘤综合征的认识亦可加深对某些"转移性"心脏黏液瘤的理解（见 Kotani 等[29]的个案报告及文献综述）。例如心脏黏液瘤术后出现皮肤黏液瘤，很可能是黏液瘤综合征的一部分，而不必视其为"皮肤转移"[30]。

当然，对心脏黏液瘤的潜在恶性问题确有严重争议。Loire[31]对所谓恶性病变的文献个案所做批评性综述就赞同早前的说法：即此类病变极可能代表了"被误读的身份"[1,5]。几乎所有恶性心脏黏液瘤的文献个案都能被归类为病理组织学诊断上的某种错误：或是误将尚未被认识的心脏肉瘤看作黏液瘤，或是将假性转移包块当真，其实这是黏液瘤碎片脱落所致栓塞、然后致缺血性梗死、继而累及动脉壁本身。几例未能被 Loire 归类者也都有符合逻辑的解释，恶性病变均被排除。不过，心脏黏液瘤恶变的可能性仍是一个值得关注的问题[32]。Kasugai[32]等人报道过一例具有典型良性形态、起源于左心房壁的心脏黏液瘤，而后来发生的几处转移性病变和左心房的一个复发性病灶，都表现为酷似所谓恶性纤维组织细胞瘤之黏液亚型（黏液纤维肉瘤）的形态特征。大家知道，在很多心脏黏液瘤病变，后者是潜在的鉴别诊断对象[33]。根据 Laya 等人的意见[33]，良性心脏黏液瘤和所谓恶性纤维组织细胞瘤黏液亚型二者之间鉴别的主要病理组织学形态特征是：（后者可见）多形性细胞呈灶状聚集、核分裂象、坏死和可见于黏液纤维肉瘤的广泛的血管增生，这些特征在心脏黏液瘤中是绝对看不到的。Kasugai 等人[31]也明确指出：我们从原发心脏肿瘤上切取的多个切片完全没有表现出任何恶性病变的证据，与随访标本的组织形态形成强烈反差。Scarpelli 等也报道一例具有腺样结构的心房黏液瘤，其被覆上皮呈 CK 阳性。原发肿瘤手术切除后 12 年发生脑转移[34]。该脑部肿瘤组织结构的优势成分是形状不规则、被覆黏液分泌型细胞的腺腔结构。这是首例具有腺样成分的心脏黏液瘤发生脑转移的文献个案，但是当然，你也可以怀疑此二者之间是否真的相关。

心脏黏液瘤的"恶性"与"被误读的身份"之争在可以预见的将来肯定是不会停止的。我们应清醒地看到：这样的文献个案是少之又少，但却被不同作者不只一次地加以引用，而每次引用都能很容易地对其少见的生物学行为做出选择性的解释。从实际应用来说，应该提醒病理医师的是：成人的心腔内肿瘤未必一定就是心脏黏液瘤。心脏原发性恶性肿瘤也可以类似的形式表现；黏液瘤的诊断被组织学形态大致确定之后，还应进一步做工作排除那些可能"被误读的特征"。至此，最重要的鉴别诊断就是软组织肉瘤的黏液型病变，如黏液样恶性纤维组织细胞瘤（黏液纤维肉瘤）和脂肪肉瘤（另见第 24 章）。

黏液瘤综合征：Schweizer-Cagianut 等人 1980 年报道了 Cushing 综合征合并少见的双侧肾上腺微小腺瘤样增生的一组家族性病例[35]。此后两年，他们追踪报告了其中一例已获诊眼睑"纤维瘤"的患者，原因是他 4 岁就出现半身轻瘫并死亡[36]。尸检诊断：一心脏黏液瘤（其同胞之一此前已获同样尸检诊断）、一眼睑黏液瘤而非纤维瘤、双侧乳腺多发性良性纤维腺瘤伴黏液瘤样变以及"口周及唇缘小雀斑样色素沉着"。Carney 等[37]认真地研究了这种少见的症状组合，并提出：这是一个由黏液瘤、斑点状色素沉着和内分泌功能亢进构成的综合征。根据家族性研究，他认为：其遗传模式很可能是常染色体显性遗传[38]。

现在，这种罕见综合征的冠名颇多，包括"Swiss 综合征"（因 Schweizer-Cagianut 报告的首例个案来自 Zurich, Swiitzerland）[26]、Carney 综合征[25]，以及首字母缩略词 NAMB 综合征（Nevi, Atrial myxoma, Mucocutaneous myxoma, Blue nevi）和 LAMB 综合征（Lentigines，余同上）。但正如 Carney[38]所指，后两个首字母缩略词的"巧妙构思要比临床病理的描述更为直白"。该综合征又名"家族性内分泌性黏液瘤着色斑病（myxolentiginosis）"，这是一个描述性名词，概括了该综合征的主要病症构成[39]。确实，该综合征包括来自皮肤黏膜、内脏和内分泌系统的多种病变及其不同组合形式。但它们未必会全都出现在同一患者身上。凡遇此类患者所应考虑到的病变有：心脏黏液瘤（强烈的多发倾向，见上文）、皮肤黏液瘤（单发或多发）、乳腺黏液样纤维腺瘤（单发或多发）、斑点状皮肤黏膜色素沉着（含雀斑痣、蓝痣或二者兼有）、沙粒体样黑色素性神经鞘瘤、原发性色素结节性肾上腺皮质疾病（含合并 Cushing 综合征者）、睾丸肿瘤（特别是 Sertoli 细胞瘤，大都为双侧和多中心性）和分泌生长激素的垂体瘤（可致巨人症或肢端肥大症）[38,40]。病理医师应该熟悉这种奇特的综合征，因为他们可能是有能力最早做出诊断的人。尤其是在复发性心脏黏液瘤患者，他们更应该和临床医师沟通，讨论黏液瘤综合征存在的可能性问题，临床医师未必意识到此综合征。正如 Carney 等[38]所指：如一家三代连续发生黏液瘤、斑点状色素沉着和内分泌功能亢进，则应推荐罹患此症者之直系血亲都应接受彻底检查以排除隐患。

起源于心脏瓣膜的黏液瘤：如上所述，人们对黏液瘤的心瓣膜起源问题一直存在争议，主要是因为 McAllister 和 Fenoglio 在其心脏肿瘤权威专著[1]中说"真性黏液瘤不会发生在心瓣膜上"。他们把发生在心瓣膜上的乳头状肿瘤归类为乳头状弹力纤维瘤，并把它描述为像是海葵，有多个乳头状叶片，经由一短梗附着在心内膜上（另见 p.24）。但此描述与文献报道的心瓣膜黏液瘤并不完全一致。而且，AFIP 最新资料中就包括 2 例起源于二尖瓣前叶和 1 例三尖瓣隔叶的黏液瘤（另见 Becker[10]）。

最近，经食管超声心动图已作为实用工具，被推广用来鉴别乳头状弹力纤维瘤和真性心瓣膜黏液瘤[41]。同时，病理医师必须要十分小心，千万不要把酷似黏液瘤样改变的心瓣膜（或心内膜）结节状结构异常说成是黏液瘤。一 4 岁儿童的主动脉瓣"黏液瘤"个案报道即可说明此观点[42]。

尽管如此，Wold and Lie[5] 还是报道了 7 例起源于心瓣膜的黏液瘤，都是出自 29 例尸检样本。其中 4 例起源于肺动脉瓣，其余 3 例分别起源于主动脉瓣、二尖瓣和三尖瓣。据他们说，其形态学特征与心房黏液瘤无异，但瓣膜黏液瘤常常很少形成细胞丛，合体瘤巨细胞也不多，瘤细胞很少在血管周围呈套袖状分布。据载[43]：一名 10 岁男童的三尖瓣黏液瘤未经瓣膜置换而被成功摘除。Cole[44] 和 Sharma 等人[45] 则提供了诊断明确的三尖瓣黏液瘤患者的完整的临床资料和文献综述，但未能出示肿瘤的病理组织学。他们报道的这两例个案均为男性，分别为 74 岁和 45 岁；病变均为一实性肿物，大小分别为 4cm×6cm 和 6cm×7cm，均借一短茎或一小蒂附着于三尖瓣隔叶之心房面。另据称[41]：一二尖瓣黏液瘤，3.3cm×3.2cm，借一短宽颈附着于二尖瓣后叶心房面。与此类似[46]，一 50 岁女性患者的黏液瘤发生在二尖瓣主动脉侧叶。以上各例都被病理组织学诊断为黏液瘤。

因此，有力的证据显示：黏液瘤可以，至少是偶可起源于心瓣膜。特别关注点之一：在这些黏液瘤文献个案中，位于右心者似比左心更常见；之二：瓣膜黏液瘤附着在房室瓣叶，或心房面，或心室面。

组织发生：过去曾有人认为黏液瘤是来自机化血栓——一个古老的概念[47,48]，时而喜获重生[49]，时而行将就木[50]。但现在的主流观点认为心脏黏液瘤是真性肿瘤。

长期以来，人们一直认为心脏黏液瘤起源于以胚胎残迹形式存在于心壁的原始多潜能间叶细胞[15,51-58]。大量研究也明确地展示出一个分化模式序列，强烈提示从原始间叶细胞到特化功能细胞之间的细胞适应（adaptation）或成熟（maturation）过程。心脏黏液瘤的免疫组化和细胞化学研究也支持这一概念[16,17,19,54]。用免疫染色技术可在内皮细胞和黏液瘤细胞之间做出鉴别。研究结果表明，与此前报告不同[55]，黏液瘤并非起源于内皮细胞，而是起源于原始的、可能具有 CD31 阳性内皮细胞分化潜能的心内膜下细胞[56]。间质细胞免疫显型表达上的差异强烈提示的分化过程，我们在创伤修复中已经非常熟悉[57]；此概念也得到下述现象的支持：大量第Ⅷa 因子阳性树突状细胞的发现提示有异常的机化血栓样分化[56]。因部分黏液瘤中含有很多星状细胞，它们对 Schwann 细胞、神经内分泌分化标记物 [S-100 蛋白、蛋白基因产物 9.5（PGP-9.5）、神经特异性烯醇化酶（NSE）和突触素（synaptophysin）] 呈阳性表达，故有人认为黏液瘤起源于心内膜感觉神经组织[58]。

迄今为止，心脏黏液瘤的细胞发生学研究已经发现了多种克隆和非克隆性异常。虽然这些研究最终可能会有助于加深对心脏黏液瘤组织发生的分子遗传学机制的理解，但就眼下情况来说，细胞遗传学研究在心脏黏液瘤的鉴别诊断上几乎没有什么实用价值可言[59,60]。

带有腺样腔隙的黏液瘤需要被特殊关注。这些细胞可能表现为黏液分泌型细胞，免疫组化示其 CK 阳性[16,61,62]。这些现象提示：黏液瘤的起源细胞应具有向上皮和向间叶分化的双向分化潜能。据此，有人就将心脏黏液瘤分类为错构瘤[61-64]。此概念得到一项研究的支持，该研究旨在评估其增生活性、转移潜能和癌基因的表达/肿瘤抑制基因产物；并得出结论说：结果符合一种反应性/错构瘤样过程[65]。

心脏横纹肌瘤　Cardiac rhabdomyoma

这是较为常见的心脏原发性肿瘤之一，最常见于婴幼儿和儿童（图 2.1～2.3）。心脏横纹肌瘤与结节性硬化（tuberous sclerosis，见下文）密切相关。临床表现变异极大。在部分患者，肿瘤可致死胎或围生期死亡[66,67]。另有一例报道巨大横纹肌瘤压迫比邻的冠状动脉并致宫内心肌梗死之个案[67]。

其余患者之临床病史则大都以心源性症状和体征为主，如心脏肥大、充血性心力衰竭或心律失常等。猝死和意外死亡者亦有报道[68,69]。心脏横纹肌瘤的临床重要性主要取决于瘤体的大小、单发还是多发，以及它是否凸入心腔。绝大多数横纹肌瘤都是多发性的，但未必一眼就能看到。本瘤的好发部位显然是心室：以左心室为最（几乎为 100%），其次是右心室，约占 80%[66]。心房受累则少得多（11/36 患者，约占 30%[66]），甚至更少 [33 名患者（3%）的 77 个横纹肌瘤中仅 1 个（1.3%）[70]]。据称：有起源于二尖瓣心室面的多发性小横纹肌瘤已被证实[71]。Schmincke[72] 于 1922 年首次描述的弥漫性横纹肌瘤病确有发生，但极为罕见。在此情况下，心肌弥漫性地被表现有横纹肌瘤细胞特征（见下文）的细胞所取代，虽然仍有形态大致正常的心肌细胞呈条索状或岛状存在[73]。在多发性横纹肌瘤的整个病变谱系中，这种现象极有可能代表了一种极端情况。

一般认为，任何示有心腔内肿物体征的婴幼儿很有可能患有横纹肌瘤（在此年龄段，黏液瘤极为罕见，见表2.1）。认识到这一点对临床非常重要，因为心脏横纹肌瘤的诊断一经成立，患者就不再具备手术指征，除非有心源性症状（见下文）。

大体病理形态

横纹肌瘤边界清楚，但无包膜，易与周围心肌相区别。其质地呈蜡样，色白至灰黄；瘤体从数毫米至几厘米不等。偶可见体积惊人者，其瘤体几乎将其所在心腔填满（图2.25）。

病理组织学形态

心脏横纹肌瘤的组织学形态很独特，瘤组织由形态怪异的肿胀肌细胞构成。瘤细胞质几乎是"空"的，细胞核连同细胞质团块被悬挂在细胞中央（图2.26），多条细胞质桥丝从此（呈放射状）延伸并与细胞膜连接，"蜘蛛样细胞（spider cell，图2.27）"也就因此而得名。高倍镜下，这些微细的细胞质桥丝上常可见心肌横纹。瘤细胞内含有糖原，酒精固定或冰冻切片上的PAS染色可突显之。本瘤所涉多糖之类型并不稳定，明显不同于糖原贮积病[74]。免疫组化结果和正常心肌相似，显示肌红蛋白、肌动蛋白、结蛋白和波形蛋白阳性，S-100蛋白阴性[75]。超微结构研究进一步证实了横纹肌瘤瘤细胞的肌源性质[66]。

间质成分大都稀少，但偶可出现明确的胶原性病灶。部分病变中可见与细胞坏死相关的钙化（图2.28）。患者的年龄越大，就越可能发生广泛钙化[76]。

特别关注之处

结节性硬化：人们对结节性硬化与心脏横纹肌瘤之间的密切相关已有共识。结节性硬化患者的超声心动图研究表明，合并心脏横纹肌瘤的发生率很高[77]。但在统计学上，儿童和婴幼儿之间却存在明显差异（58%对18%）。此现象可支持心脏横纹肌瘤自发性退化的概念（见下文）。据Fenoglio等[66]报道，在心脏横纹肌瘤系列尸检中，合并结节性硬化的发生率为37%。不过，此样本中的死胎和新生儿所占比例相当大，在此年龄组，很难做出组织学诊断。一项对来自三家儿童心脏病研究中心的33例婴幼及儿童所做的回顾性研究显示：其中30例都合并结节性硬化，占90.9%[70]。看来，在心脏横纹肌瘤患者，结节性硬化的准确发生率尚无法确定，究

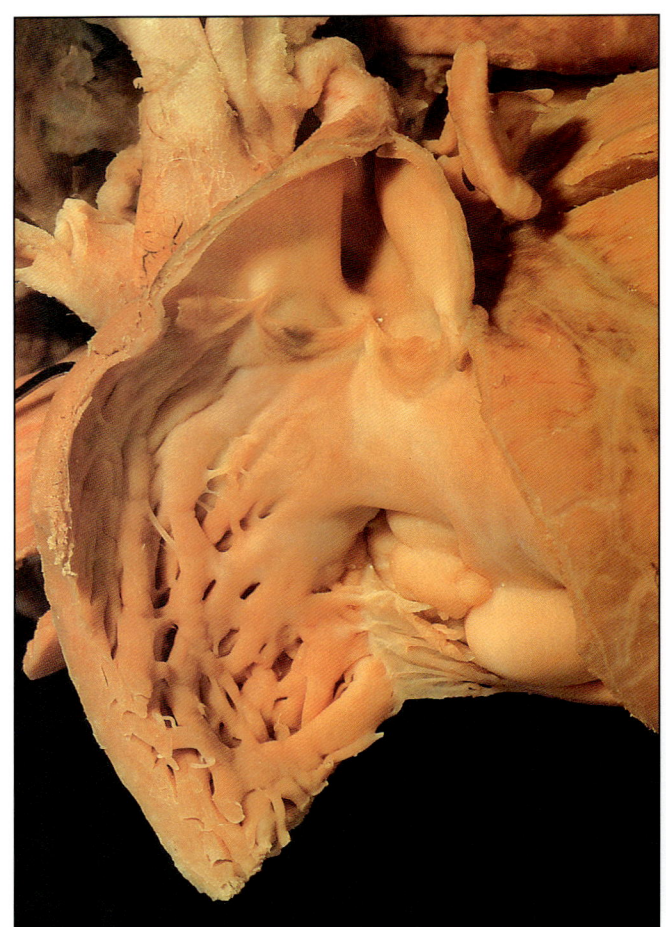

图2.25 肉眼可见右心房一巨大横纹肌瘤，自右房腔、经三尖瓣口突入右心室流入道口部。

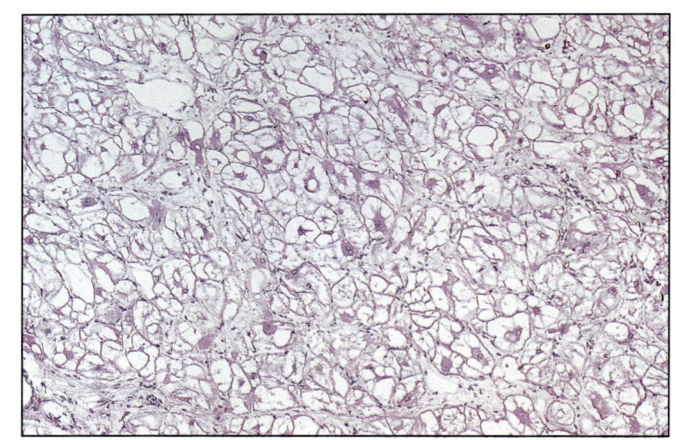

图2.26 镜下可见心脏横纹肌瘤特征性地由形态怪异的肿胀肌细胞构成。

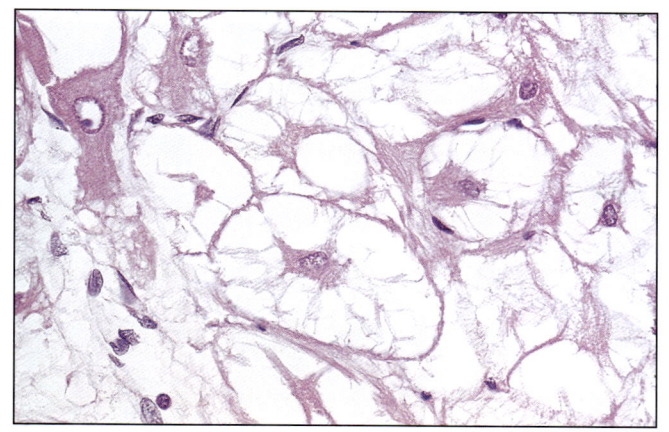

图2.27 心脏横纹肌瘤。标本同图2.26，高倍镜下可见典型的"蜘蛛样细胞"，细胞核和细胞质团块被悬挂在细胞中央，并借多条细胞质桥丝与细胞周边连接。

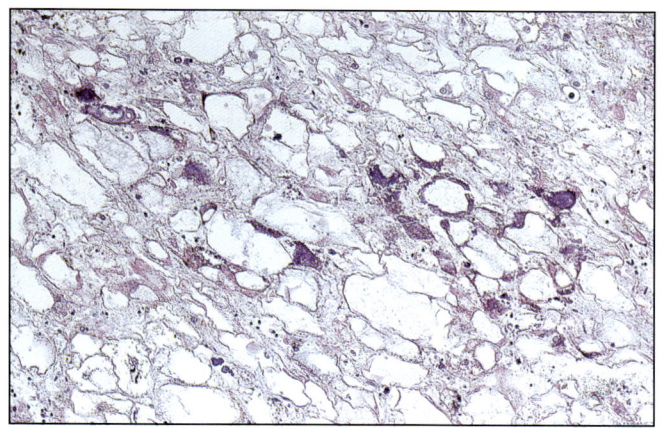

图2.28 与钙化相关的横纹肌瘤细胞渐进性坏死。

其原因，部分患者结节性硬化之症状和体征尚未显现而身先死之事可能部分地与之相关；否则，其发生率将会更高。Davies[78]明确指出：心脏横纹肌瘤总是合并有大脑结节性硬化，无论在临床上是否表现有相应的症状、体征。另据报道[79]，对5例婴幼儿出生前、后所做超声心动图显示患有心脏肿瘤，其后又做出结节性硬化的诊断[79]，此现象进一步强化了Davies的说法。

自发性退化：早在1923年Steinbiss就曾指出：合并结节性硬化的患者之心脏横纹肌瘤可以消退，并最终完全消失[74]。此论点现已被证实，并成为最高的临床准则[80-82]。一项十年（1984—1994）的结节性硬化患者回顾性评估显示：16例患者中有10例（62.5%）在初诊时即被确诊患有心脏横纹肌瘤。但在日后四次随访时发现心脏横纹肌瘤的数量在平稳减少：初诊时10名患者共有23个横纹肌瘤，第二、三、四次随访时的该数字组合分别是8与16、5与12、2与4[83]。实际上，根据超声心动图的评估结果，6岁以前就能看到心脏横纹肌瘤的完全自发性消退。因此，当某婴儿被发现有一心腔内肿物，但并无任何心源性症状或体征的话，就不必着急做手术，而应随诊观察，看该肿瘤能否自行消退。

这样的生物学行为支持以下概念：心脏横纹肌瘤，不管它是否合并结节性硬化，基本上都是错构瘤而非真性肿瘤。支持此概念的说法还有：相比单发性病变，多发性心脏横纹肌瘤的发生率明显占优，而且它们大都发生在婴幼儿。此外，Fenoglio等[84]还证实存在广泛的细胞连接，以桥粒和缝隙连接为特征，随机地遍布于细胞表面。但在正常心肌，这些细胞连接的排列方式却规整得多。提示：这些细胞出现了发育停滞，并失去了充分分化的能力。此观点得到Bruni等人[85]的支持，他们证实了两类细胞：一是典型的"蜘蛛样细胞"，二是可见大量肌原纤维、少量糖原和胞质空泡（内含有膜绑定糖原颗粒）的细胞。他们对此现象的解释：这是正常心肌细胞早期分化成熟的两个连续的阶段。有趣的是，正是沿着这条思路，遗传学研究现已将结节性硬化与定位在染色体9q34和最近的16q13.3上的杂合性丢失联系了起来；有人根据"相关错构瘤中相似等位基因丢失"的理论提出：这些基因现象可能起到了生长抑制剂的作用[86,87]。

鉴别诊断

由于肿胀肌细胞的形态怪异，所以在一般情况下，(心脏横纹肌瘤的)病理组织学诊断应该没有什么问题。不过，与糖原贮积病的鉴别偶可成为问题。但在后者，心肌组织学相当单调。尽管在肌原纤维周围会出现一圈空晕，但心肌的组织学结构大都没有改变，心肌细胞的形态也大都保持完好。横纹肌瘤的总的形态感觉就是无序：肌细胞形态怪异，瘤巨细胞的直径有时竟达80nm（图2.29）。

此外，不应将心脏横纹肌瘤和一种少见的"Purkinje细胞瘤"或"心肌细胞泡沫样变（foamy myocardial transformation，见下文）"的病变相混淆；不应混淆者还有一种少见的成熟心肌细胞错构瘤（hamartoma of mature cardiac myocyte）[88]，这种最近才被描述的病变缺少横纹肌瘤瘤细胞胞浆中的空泡。

心脏纤维瘤 Cardiac fibroma

心脏纤维瘤少见，但在婴幼和儿童却仍属最常见的肿瘤类型（表2.1）。位于华盛顿DC的AFIP对其23例住院病人所做临床病理相关性研究显示：患者的年龄跨度从日龄1天至56岁，平均13岁[89]。据我所知，年龄最大的患者为一77岁男性[90]。临床体征和症状主要取决于肿瘤的位置和大小。最突出的体征是心脏扩大，但

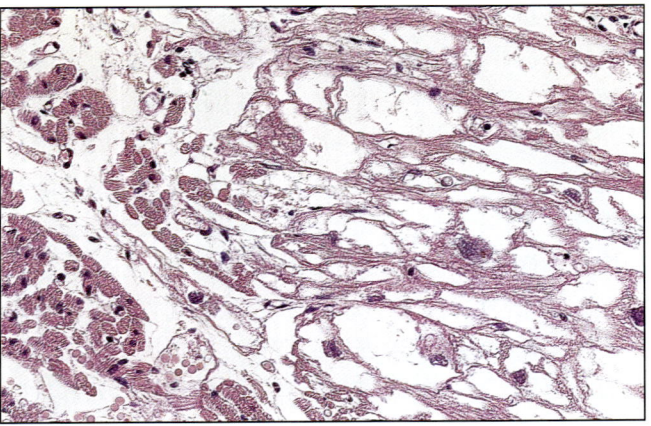

图2.29 照片突显了横纹肌瘤细胞异乎寻常地大，与其旁边的正常心肌细胞形成强烈反差。

其症状可能包括心力衰竭、心律失常、猝死、发绀和胸痛[89]。AFIP首期样本的10/17例患者的纤维瘤位于室间隔，这类患者或是症状明显（案载有室颤2例，充血性心力衰竭2例），或是猝死和意外死亡。而纤维瘤位于心室游离壁或心房者却可长期无症状。最终可出现瓣膜症状或心腔内阻塞症状。不过，有些游离壁纤维瘤的体积可大到与整个心脏相差无几，而患者却可仍无症状[91]。

大体病理形态

心脏纤维瘤之病变界清、实性、质硬、色白，与周围心肌分界清楚。不过，偶可见在心肌间广泛延伸、致使手术无法切净者[92]。此外，还有因肿瘤的位置、大小之故，完全切除手术是为不可行的情况，如室间隔几乎完全被纤维瘤所取代。

切面可见其纤维瘤样特征（图2.30），偶见肉眼可辨的钙化。

组织病理学

纤维瘤由结缔组织构成，还常混有多种不同的成分（图2.31-2.33）。其周边部即混有周围的心肌，故其镜下边界远不如其肉眼边界那么清楚。中心部位大都由玻璃样变的无细胞性胶原纤维构成（图2.32），而越靠近周边，细胞成分就越多（图2.33）。可出现弹力纤维，有时甚至还很丰富。"纤维弹力错构瘤"一词即源于此种特殊现象[93]。在纤维组织间偶可见心肌细胞，并见灶状聚集的未成熟细胞，很可能是髓外造血性质。镜下常可见灶状钙化（图2.34）。常见有囊性变，尤其是在肿瘤中心部位；这可能与毛细血管的数量大减有关。核分裂象极为罕见，即便是在细胞丰富处。而且，细胞丰富本身也不能被视为是恶性指征。

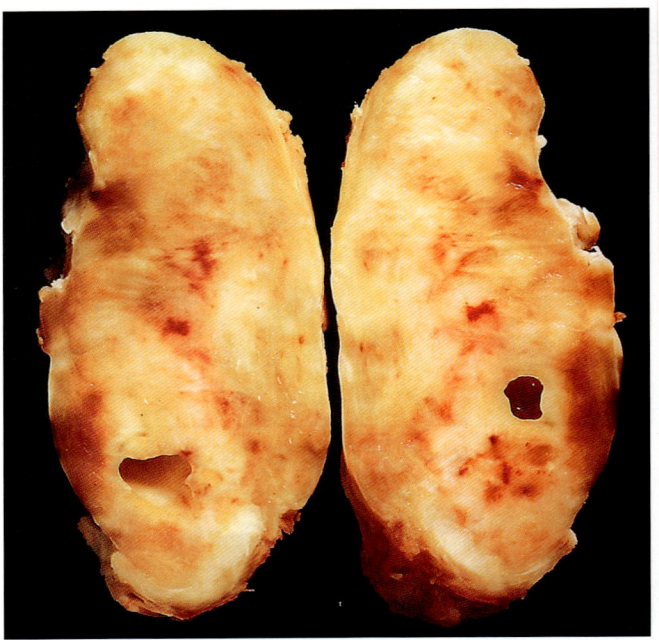

图2.30 心脏纤维瘤的切面显示其纤维瘤样性质，伴局部出血（可能是手术所致人工假象）和囊性变。

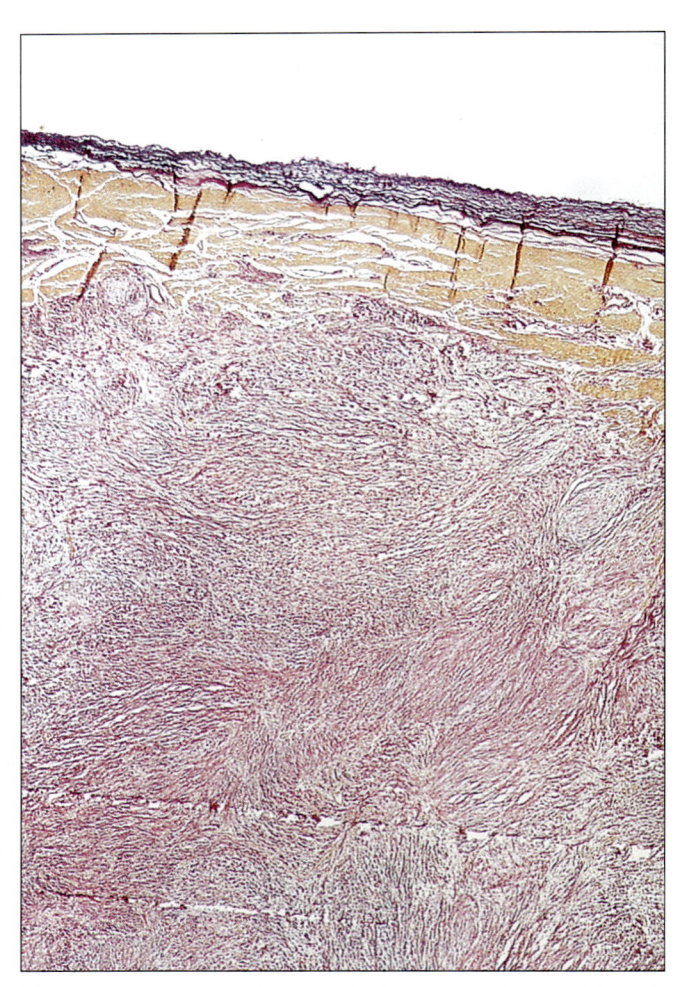

图2.31 镜下可见心脏纤维瘤的典型特征：在纤维瘤的周边部位，纤维瘤（成分）与存于此的心肌混合；覆在其表面的心内膜呈轻度纤维弹力型增厚（弹力组织染色）。

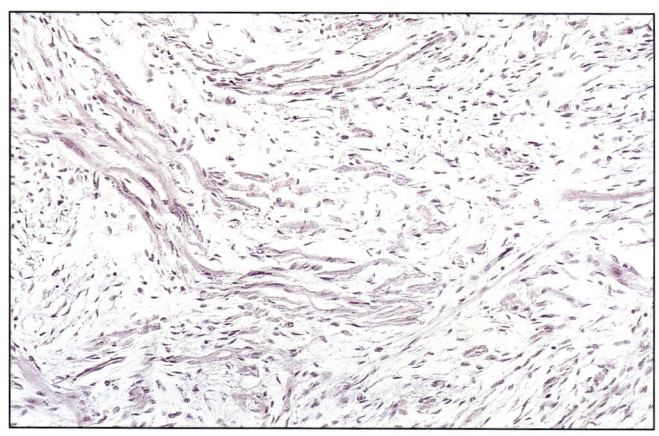

图2.32 在心脏纤维瘤的周边部分常可见走行方向不同、但聚集成束的梭形细胞（HE染色）。

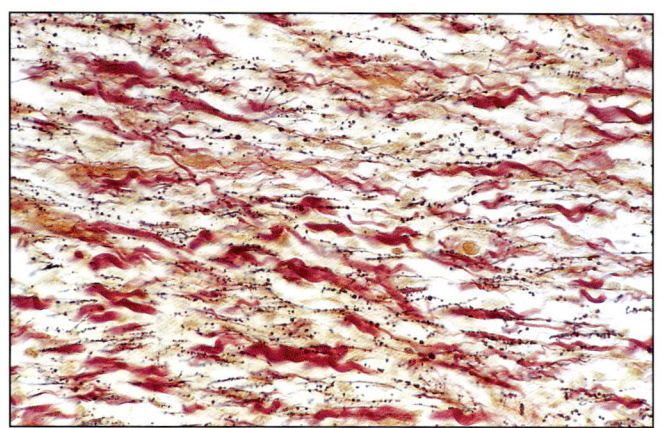

图2.33 心脏纤维瘤中心部位的优势成分常为粗大的胶原纤维和丛块状的弹力纤维片段（弹力组织染色）。

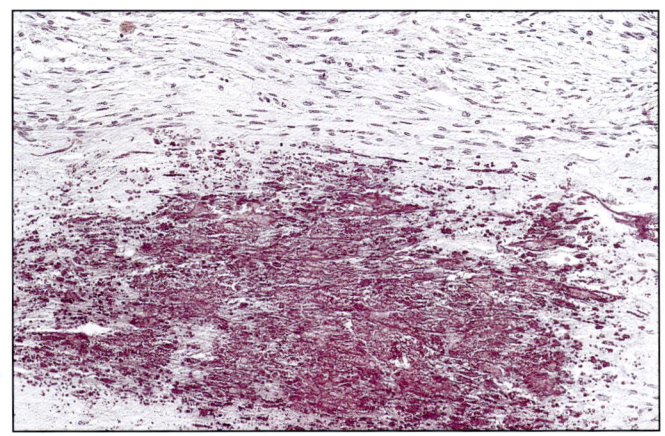

图2.34 镜下示有大片钙化变性的心脏纤维瘤。

上述病理组织学形态对心脏纤维瘤的诊断具有高度特征性。

特别关注之处

组织发生：电镜研究明确显示：心脏纤维瘤的主要细胞成分是纤维母细胞，分布于由黏多糖和胶原构成的基质之中[93,94]。Turi 等[94]还证实有中间型分化细胞的存在，胞浆中含有肌原纤维和丰富的粗面内质网。这些细胞以前曾被命名为肌纤维母细胞[95]，属于增生性纤维组织家族成员。鉴于纤维瘤病（fibromatosis）和心脏纤维瘤二者在自然病史以及光镜、电镜形态上表现出相似性，Turi 等[94]据此认为：二者系同一疾病过程，故"心脏纤维瘤病"显然是一个比心脏纤维瘤更为准确的名称。

上述考虑都与临床有关联。因为对一无症状患者而言，首要问题就是是否应该手术介入。据报道，一约6月龄婴儿的室间隔肿物经组织学诊断证实为心脏纤维瘤，临床部分切除术后14个月未见发展[96]。另有报道称，某婴儿之左心室后壁纤维瘤在其22月龄时接受次全切除术，术后7年无症状，且行动自如[97]。因此，你可以这样认为：患者有症状，手术介入才被认为有必要；如手术危及患者术后心功能，则就完全不具备心脏纤维瘤切除术的手术指征。

相关综合征：文献上可见少数合并有痣样基底细胞癌综合征（Gorlin 综合征）的心脏纤维瘤个案[97-101]；这在 Burke 等报道的 23 例个案中只见 1 例[89]。该综合征包括一系列发育异常：如肋骨和椎骨畸形、大头伴奇特面容、大脑镰钙化、下腭骨牙源性角化囊肿和多发性基底细胞癌[102]。但因临床表现多样，故确诊较困难。

心脏脂肪瘤　Cardiac lipoma

心脏脂肪瘤少见，McAllister 和 Fenoglio[1] 报道：在成人原发性心脏良性肿瘤中，其发病率为 18.6%，而 AFIP 新版系列中则为 6.2%[2]（表 2.1）。我们自己的样本中有 11 例脂肪瘤（9.3%，表 2.3）。此发生率的高低也可能与研究机构（如 AFIP）的偏倚有关。不过，在此问题上，应该引入几个疾病分类学概念：

1. 大家知道，心外膜的脂肪储备随年龄的增长而增加[103]；它们特征性地分布于右室前面、左右两侧房室沟和心外膜，并沿冠状动脉走行一线。而且，心外膜脂肪组织的大量增生常伴右室心肌和房间沟脂肪浸润。因此，人们就会问：脂肪组织究竟要聚集到何种程度，"脂肪瘤"的诊断才能成立？

2. 良性脂肪瘤样瘤的分类包括多种病变形式[104]，如孤立的边界清楚的脂肪瘤及其亚型、肌内和肌间脂肪瘤（又名浸润性脂肪瘤）以及一组弥漫性脂肪瘤病（另见第 24 章）。病变形式上的变化多端亦可见于"心脏脂肪瘤"。心脏孤立性脂肪瘤非常少见，已被定义为边界清楚、具有薄层完整包膜、由成熟脂肪细胞构成的肿瘤。据称，符合此定义的肿瘤或发生在心肌内，或在心外膜。后者大都在手术或尸检时才被发现[105]，但位于此处的巨大脂肪瘤偶可导致左心室功能障碍[106,107]，或因冠状动脉受累而引发需要手术的问题[108]。有人报道一极少见的猝死个案：患者女性，15 岁，多发性巨大脂肪瘤累及整个心脏，并危及所有心腔的功能[109]。AFIP 系列材料中包含 14 例脂肪瘤，多数患者的脂肪瘤并未引发心源性症状。但在某些情况下，患者可出现症状，其决定性因素是肿瘤的大小和位置。凸入心腔的心内膜下脂肪瘤可致瓣膜狭窄或关闭不全，而位于心壁间者则可导致心律失常和传导阻滞[110-117]。已有证据显示脂肪瘤与结节性硬化相关[1,118,119]。

3. 另一种类型的脂肪瘤即所谓"房间隔脂肪瘤样肥厚"，病变酷似横纹肌内"浸润型脂肪瘤"（见第 24 章）[120-122]。此病变最先由 Prior[120] 报道；其后，Page[121] 随机选择了 50 例尸检心脏材料，并做系统性研究后认定：这种病变极可能与心房间脂肪沉积的增加有关，是脂肪沉积随年龄增长而整体性增多的一部分；有人证明了它与体重增加之间的联系[122]。这种现象的极端例证可能被认定为"脂肪瘤样肥大"，但却未必会被视为疾病分类学上的一个实体。有人则质疑上述观点，理由是：该病变与其周围的心外膜脂肪沉积之间有明显分界；（病变中）含有不规则分布的肥大心肌细胞；而且在数量上，也不同于房间隔的通常的结构成分[123]。故而，Inoue 等人推荐使用"心脏脂肪瘤样错构瘤"一词[123]。尽管如此，房间沟内的脂肪过量聚集确有并发心律失常的倾向[1,119]。而这种心肌应激功能障碍可能缘于心肌萎缩和纤维化，伴局部大量脂肪沉积。这是在尸检和手术术时偶可遇到的现象[124]。

4. 房室瓣脂肪瘤性错构瘤是病理医师可能要面对的另一种极为罕见的病变。据我所知，文献有记载者尚不足 10 例[125]；二尖瓣、三尖瓣均可受累；年龄跨度在 2～76 岁。Behman 等[126] 报道的脂肪瘤样病变个案还累及乳头肌，并致瓣膜关闭不全。最后，文献上心脏和心包冬眠瘤的个案报道至少有 2 例[127,128]。

大体病理形态

综上所述，其大体形态基本上完全取决于"脂肪瘤"的类型。如果是有完整包膜的脂肪细胞聚集，则其大体形态与位于其他部位的脂肪瘤无异（图 2.35 和 2.36）。

如果是所谓的房间隔脂肪瘤样肥厚，病变大都首先见于右心房一侧。病变位于卵圆窝正上，呈明显的上缘突起状（图 2.37）。而卵圆窝本身则偶可因被突起的心房壁所遮掩而很难看到。切面上房间沟高度增厚，由灰黄色、常略显棕色的脂肪组织构成，并向其周围的心房心肌组织中浸润。仔细观察，常可在脂肪组织间见到原固有的心肌肌束。如瓣膜受累，则因其不均匀增厚而变形，在增厚处切面即可看出是脂肪组织（图 2.38）。

组织病理学

包膜完整的心脏脂肪瘤的病理组织学形态与身体其他部位者无异。在以成熟脂肪组织为优势成分的肿瘤结构中，偶可见心肌细胞、数量不等的结缔组织和血管。有些名称，如肌脂肪瘤、纤维脂肪瘤和血管脂肪瘤等大都与这些结构特征有直接关系。

在所谓房间隔脂肪瘤样肥大的病例，其组织学形态特征是：有大量分化成熟的脂肪细胞浸润，原固有心肌细胞或被取代，或已萎缩（图 2.39）。心肌结构保存最好的部分大都位于心内膜下，但在脂肪瘤深处亦可见有陷入其中的心肌细胞，看上去像是完全被脂肪组织所包围的孤岛。部分患者的病变好像是医源性的，更多发生于非瓣膜性心内膜上[129]。偶可见有分化成熟的脂肪细胞与空泡状、多球状脂肪细胞混合在一起的区域（图 2.40）。此外，亦可见颗粒状细胞，其光镜和电镜形态都酷似胚胎性脂肪细胞。

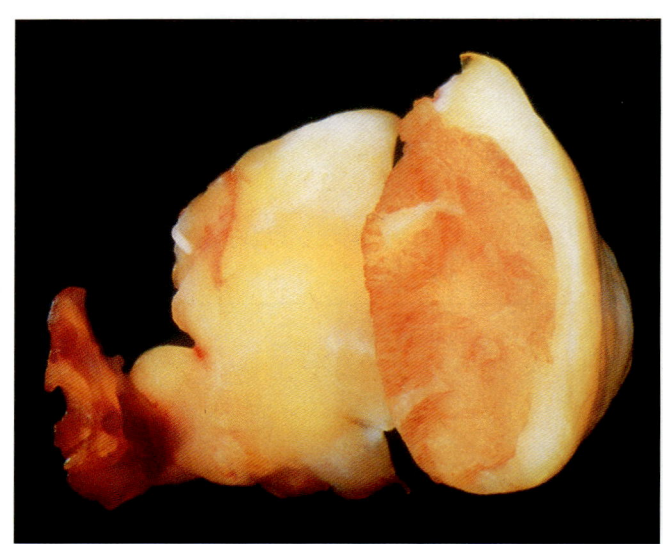

图2.35　图为一起源于右心室游离壁、延伸至室间隔腹面并凸入右室腔的脂肪瘤的手术切除标本[117]，其周边部分为实性脂肪组织团块，边缘为重度脂肪浸润的心肌组织。（Courtesy of Dr J. R. J. Elbers, Department of Pathology, St. Antonius Ziekenhuis, Nieuwegein, Utrecht, The Netherlands.）

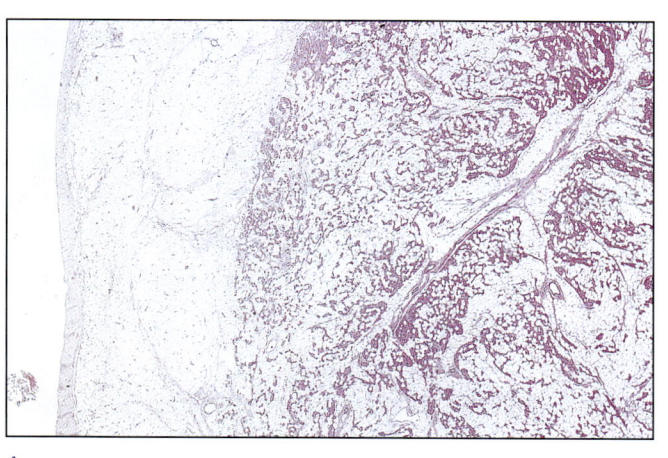 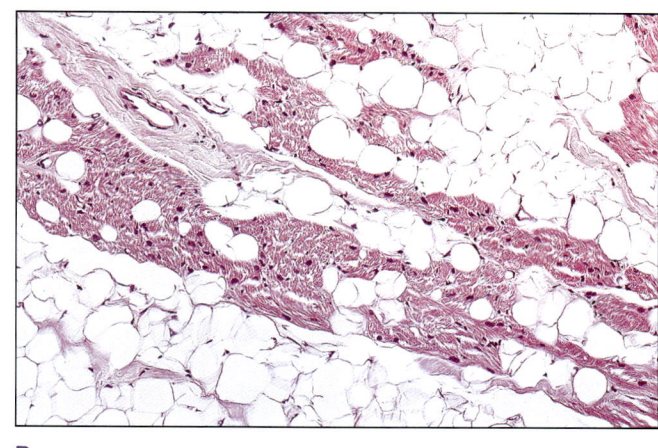

图2.36 脂肪瘤。镜下可见其表层区域由分化成熟的脂肪细胞构成,其下方是心肌浸润性脂肪瘤区域。

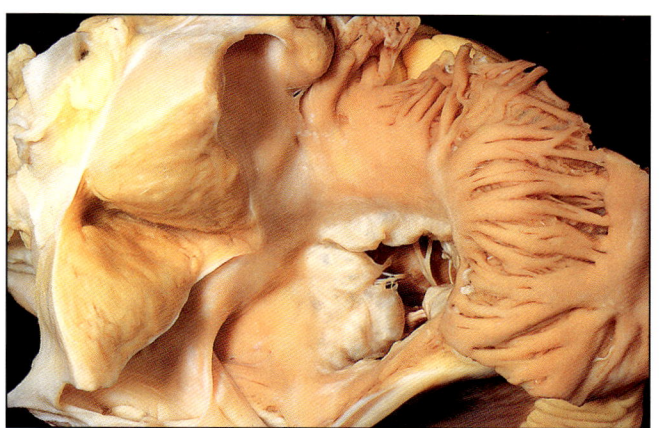 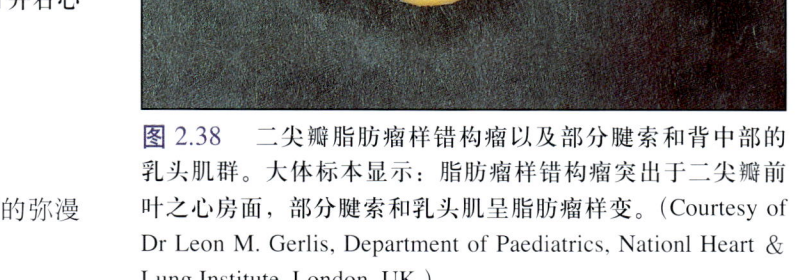

图2.37 房间隔脂肪瘤样肥厚。经由房间隔嵴切口打开右心房的心脏标本,切面可见脂肪组织。

图2.38 二尖瓣脂肪瘤样错构瘤以及部分腱索和背中部的乳头肌群。大体标本显示:脂肪瘤样错构瘤突出于二尖瓣前叶之心房面,部分腱索和乳头肌呈脂肪瘤样变。(Courtesy of Dr Leon M. Gerlis, Department of Paediatrics, Nationl Heart & Lung Institute, London, UK.)

心瓣膜脂肪瘤样错构瘤表现为成熟脂肪细胞的弥漫性浸润,几乎完全取代了原有的瓣膜组织结构。

特别关注之处

临床联系:如上所述,"真性"脂肪瘤大都没有什么症状,多是在常规体检时被发现。在婴幼儿和儿童,脂肪瘤极为罕见,如果出现,则可导致心壁增厚,继而使心腔变窄,甚至达到符合手术指征的程度。在此情况下,次全切除术可能要受制于解剖部位,但后期的随访结果仍可令人满意[130]。此外,它与结节性硬化之间可能存在的相关性应该时刻了然于胸。

现已明确,所谓房间隔脂肪瘤样肥大患者多可并发心律失常和心源性猝死[1,121,131]。如逢意外猝死,对此特殊病症组合的认识就很重要;但同时,病理医师应该加倍小心,勿对此症做出"过度诊断"。因为随着年龄的增长,脂肪组织在房间沟的聚集和在心房肌间的浸润都会逐渐增多[121],而且与脂肪组织在整个心外膜沉积数量的增加有关。具体到某一患者,要想确定此年龄性脂肪沉积能否导致其致命性心律失常,即便是不无可能,亦是非常之难。同时,病理医师可能会遇到房间隔的手术标本,或来自已知患有心律失常合并房间隔脂肪瘤样肥大的患者,或是令术者颇感困惑的术中偶见[124,132]。

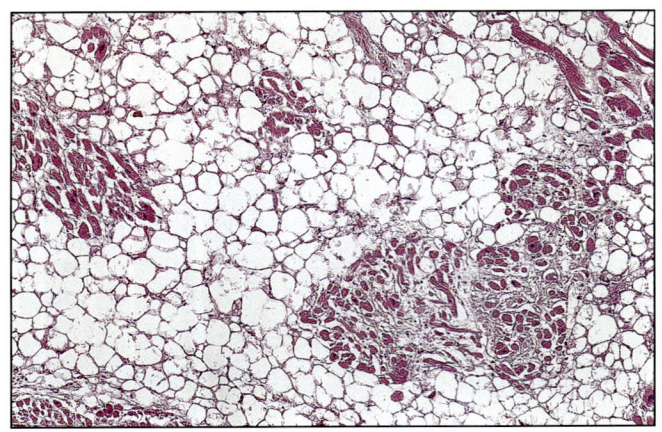

图2.39 房间隔脂肪瘤样增生的组织形态（其肉眼形态示于图2.37）显示：大量分化成熟的脂肪细胞浸润，伴局部残存心肌细胞。

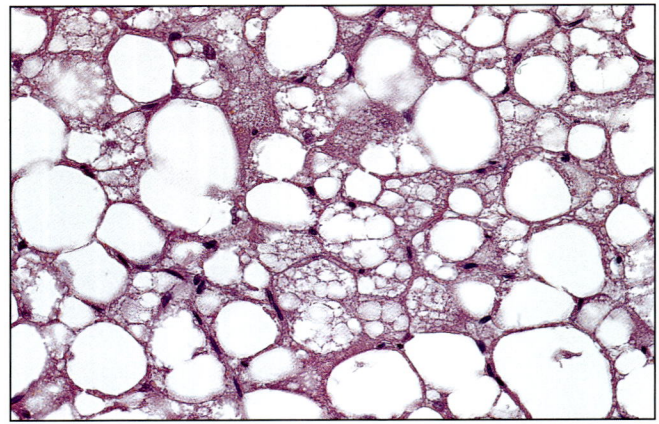

图2.40 与上图为同一标本。脂肪瘤样增生的组织形态显示：分化成熟的脂肪细胞与空泡状、多球状脂肪细胞混在一起的区域。

乳头状弹力纤维瘤　Papillary fibroelastoma

又名弹力纤维性乳头状瘤、心瓣膜乳头状瘤和巨大Lambl赘生物（见下文）。

自二维超声心动图技术推广以来，外科和临床经验表明：乳头状弹力纤维瘤是一种相对少见的病变。但据AFIP[1]指出：在所有成人原发性心脏良性肿瘤中，其发生率位列第三（17.4%，表2.1）。我们自己的记录是6.8%（表2.3）。"得克萨斯经验"系列[3]最近被扩大，囊括了1957年以来所有的病例[133]，但它并未提及本瘤。同样，来自法国[7]、日本[8]和中国[9]的文献也未见其踪影。另一方面，来自明尼苏达大学关于原发性心脏肿瘤的研究报告[6]却将"乳头状瘤"视为一种常见的原发性心脏肿瘤[以发生率高低为序排列位列第三（9.7%，12/124），在组织学良性的心脏肿瘤中占11.6%（12/103）]。看来，那些把"外生性"肿瘤都包括在内的研究中心就得出高发生率的结论，这反映了他们的固有偏倚，并非真实

情况。

尽管如此，这些乳头状瘤可发生在所有心瓣膜上，也可能是作为偶遇现象见于超声心动图检查（参见超声心动图特征的综述[134,135]）、手术或尸检。部分患者的肿瘤好像是医源性病变，更多发生于非瓣膜性心内膜上[129]；并偶可引发临床症状和体征，包括脑栓塞[136,137]或相关的心源性症状（参阅综述：乳头状弹力纤维瘤——一种"并不那么良性"的心脏肿瘤[138]）。据称，左心病变可能更具症状性，故更容易被超声心动图检出[139]。主动脉瓣部位具有潜在的危险性，此处的肿瘤有可能导致冠状动脉口阻塞或冠状动脉栓塞，实际上可引起急性心肌梗死[140-144]。

据文献记载，两例个案的弹力纤维瘤附着于各自的右室流出道[135,145]。乳头状弹力纤维瘤好发于成人，无明显峰值年龄段。发生于婴幼和儿童者仅偶有报告[144-146]。本文对其大体形态和组织学形态的精确描述将尽全力保证：乳头状弹力纤维瘤不会与黏液瘤样病变以及可能发生在儿童的其他瓣膜病变相混淆。

大体病理形态

弹力纤维瘤形似海葵[147]（图2.41），由一附着在心内膜上的线状花束构成，或无柄，或有一明显短蒂。瘤体大小不等，小者直径仅数毫米，大者直径则以厘米计（图2.42）。该肿瘤绝大多数都起源于心瓣膜，明显好发于主动脉瓣，但亦可见于两侧心房、心室壁的心内膜。在二尖瓣和三尖瓣，病变大都见于其心房面，且多在瓣叶的中间位置附近。但在主动脉瓣和肺动脉瓣，这些乳头状瘤在瓣叶心房面和心室面的发生几率大致相等；发生部位在瓣叶基部、还是游离缘也无明显差异。偶可见有多发性弹力纤维瘤患者。

组织病理学

其镜下形态具有高度特征性：其线状乳头轴心由一几乎没有细胞成分的胶原致密芯构成，偶被黏液瘤样基质包绕。有个案报告称：纤维性致密芯可出现软骨化生[148]；再外一圈是由粗的碎片状弹力纤维构成（图2.43）；最外表面被覆一层内皮细胞，可呈增生性改变[148]。其胶原性致密芯与心瓣膜的胶原成分相互连续。在同一肿瘤的不同线状乳头中，弹力纤维的数量和分布差异极大。

因其组织学形态颇具特色，故无真正的鉴别诊断问题。与心脏黏液瘤的相似性也仅限于包绕胶原致密芯周围的一圈疏松结缔组织及其明显的内皮细胞层（图2.44）。但如将整个病变都纳入视野，对鉴别诊断来说，就不应再构成问题。

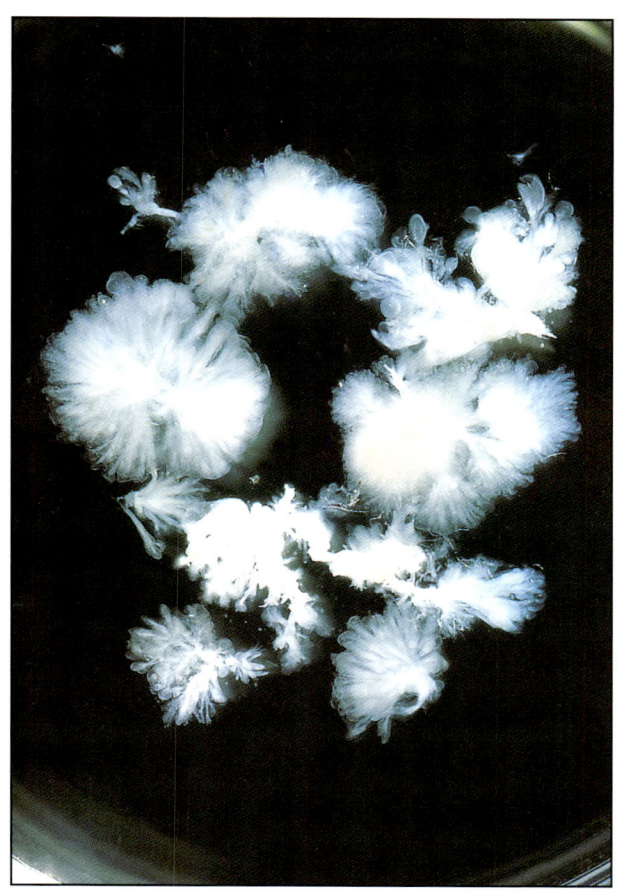

图2.41 乳头状弹力纤维瘤手术标本，患者49岁男性。首发症状为严重非典型性心绞痛型胸痛。超声心动图显示一与二尖瓣群相连的肿瘤。术中见该肿瘤附着于二尖瓣腱索。置于水中的大体标本（部分切除）可尽显其酷似海葵的乳头状形态。

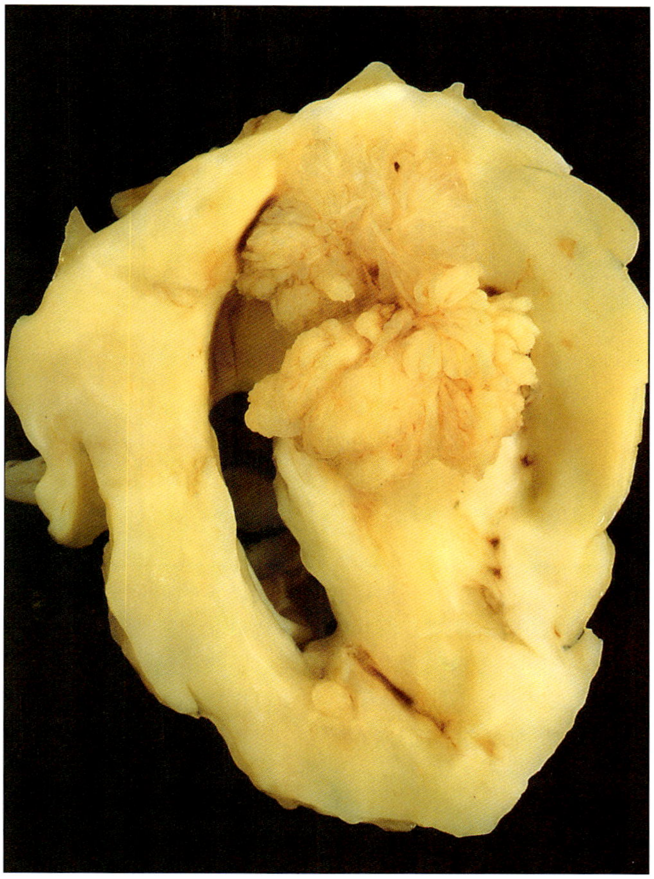

图2.42 一位于二尖瓣前叶心房面的巨大乳头状弹力纤维瘤之手术标本。(Reproduced with permission from Becher A E, Anderson RH 1983 Cardiac pathology. An integrated text and colour atlas. Gower, London, Fig.7.4.)

特别关注之处

本瘤之所以重要，是因为目前，其诊断基本上完全依靠二维超声心动图技术，患者本人可能并无症状。一旦临床诊断成立，接下来的问题就是应该怎么办，而且直接关系到这种乳头状增生性病变的性质问题。

McAllister和Fenoglio[1]认为乳头状弹力纤维瘤或是一种真性肿瘤，或是一种错构瘤。他们强调：因其组织学形态与正常乳头肌的腱索非常之相似，基本上复制了正常心内膜的所有成分，故应被视为一种错构瘤。但同时，他们也强调：乳头状弹力纤维瘤仅见于高龄个体，而不见于儿童（严格来讲，这里不是"不见"，而是"少见"），这一现象则不利于错构瘤的性质判断。上述观点以及乳头状弹力纤维瘤和所谓Lambl赘生物（成人尸体心瓣膜上的细小乳头状突起——译者注）在组织结构上的相似性，使得部分作者认为二者的组织发生机制相似：即心内膜对机械性损伤的一种反应性增生，并与年龄增长相关。故可用"巨大Lambl赘生物"一词取代

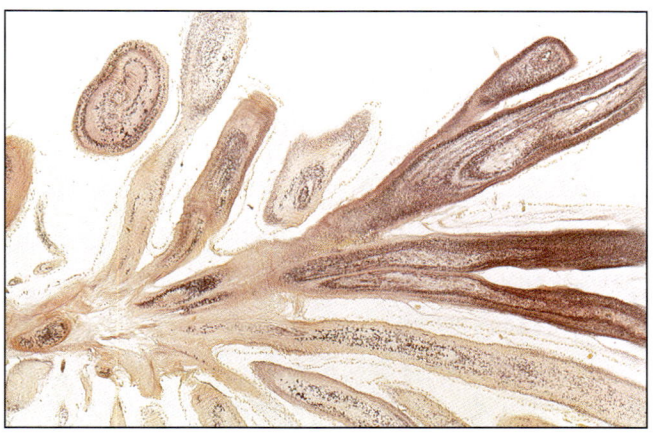

图2.43 乳头状弹力纤维瘤的组织学形态：呈多叶状，每叶都是由一几乎没有细胞成分的胶原致密芯和不规则形、丛状弹力纤维碎片构成；表面被覆一层内皮细胞（弹力纤维染色）。

乳头状弹力纤维瘤[149]。免疫组化研究也明确提示有表层内皮细胞的积极参与，伴基底膜物质的广泛形成[150]。Lambl赘生物虽然有很多鉴别性特征，但事实上还是有很多过渡形态存在，其中，两种病变之间的相似性还是很明显，而其间的差异则显得微不足道。

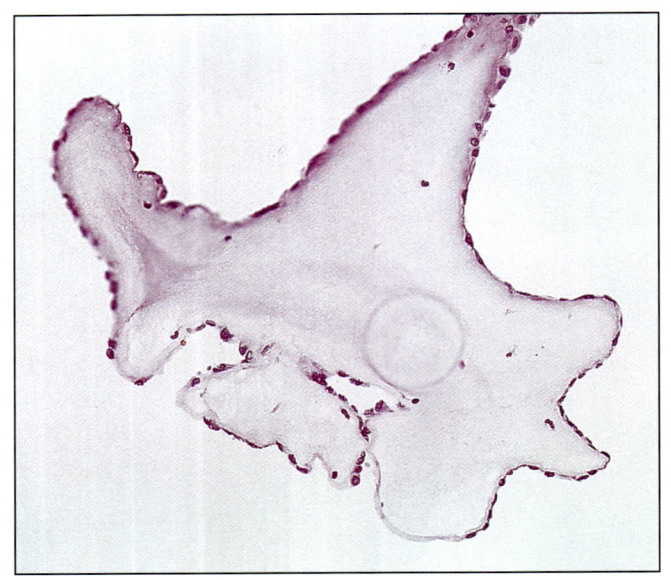

图2.44 乳头状弹力纤维瘤之一叶状乳头的周边部位，可见其黏液样基质，其表面形状由多个缺口状裂隙构成，并被覆有明显的内皮细胞层。本图所示与心脏黏液瘤之周边部位有某些相似之处，但其整体组织结构可以轻易地证明：这是乳头状弹力纤维瘤的一部分。

这并非没有临床意义，因有充分证据表明：乳头状弹力纤维瘤，尤其是位于左心的病变，可引起因体动脉栓塞所致的严重临床后果[138,151-153]。故，如发生猝死或意外心源性死亡，乳头状弹力纤维瘤就应被列入鉴别诊断对象的名单。迄今为止，我还没见过乳头状弹力纤维瘤术后复发的报道，虽然该病变大都只做局部切除，而不做瓣膜置换。

浦肯野细胞瘤　Purkinje cell tumor

这是一种独特而少见的病变，迄今为止仅有低龄婴儿患者的报道，明显好发于女性，并伴心动过速型心律失常。本瘤的性质尚无定论。实际上，有人坚持认为：它并非真性肿瘤，也不是来自浦肯野细胞，而是一种病因和发病机制都不明确的心肌病。这种不确定性的直接反映就是其名称的混乱：最常用的是婴儿心肌泡沫样变[157]、婴儿黄瘤样心肌病[155]、伴有组织细胞样变的婴儿心肌病[156]和婴儿组织细胞样心肌病[157]（参见Becker & Anderson的综述[158]）。Ferrans等[156]根据超微结构研究认为：这种病变代表心肌细胞发育早期阶段的一种存留现象。Silver等[159]认为：肌细胞没有完成原始阶段以后的成熟分化，而是变成了嗜酸瘤细胞（oncocytes）。他们认为，妊娠早期的病毒感染，如风疹病毒感染，或许是一种可能的原因。

Amini等[157]首先建议：本病变不应被视为一种心肌病，而是一种涉及外周浦肯野网的特殊病变。这是一个有趣的概念，因为稍早时，James等[160]曾经报道过一例与"心脏多灶性浦肯野细胞瘤"有关的婴儿猝死个案。随着电生理定位技术的发展和对儿童心律失常关注的增多，临床上，这种特殊病变在导致婴儿持续性室性心动过速方面的作用已获证明。Garson等[161]用外科方法追踪了14例这种特殊性质的病变，其中9例的病变为散在分布，4例为弥漫性地分布于左右两个心室。这14例"浦肯野细胞瘤"即是得克萨斯心脏病研究院和MD安德森癌症研究中心样本中的那些病例[3]（表2.2）。如此之高的发病率显然与以下两个因素相关：一是研究机构的集体偏倚，这些研究所的关注热点就是婴儿心律失常；二是有些研究所"原发性心脏肿瘤"研究课题的名下并不包括这些病变。我曾两次见到这种病变，两次都是尸检。第一例为7个月大女婴，时间是1980年（见Becker & Anderson专著[158]之图30.12和图30.13）；第二例见于1991年，也是一女婴，4周大（图2.45和图2.46）。

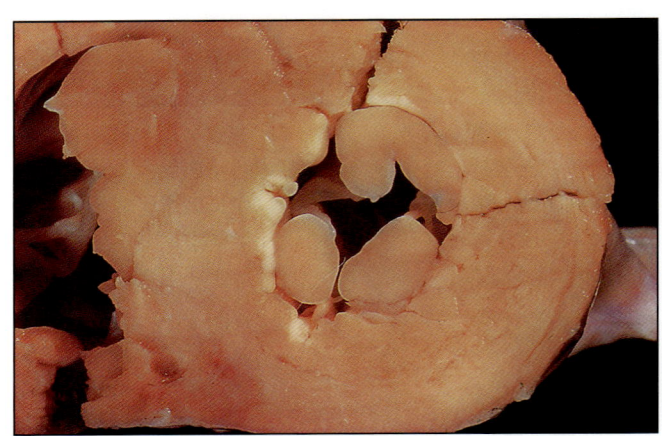

图2.45 浦肯野细胞瘤。患者为一意外猝死之4周龄女婴。心脏横断面示：心内膜下可见色泽棕灰的色斑。

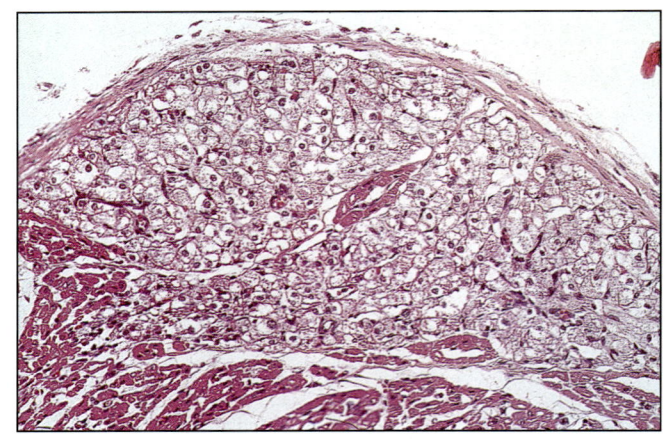

图2.46 浦肯野细胞瘤。图2.45之色斑处的组织形态，示：病变由轻度肿大、胞浆呈空泡状的细胞构成。

大体病理形态

浦肯野细胞瘤的病变或是边界清楚，或呈弥漫性改变，色泽或淡棕或发黄，或位于心内膜下（图2.45），或心外膜下[162]。病变部位无定，两心室均有分布，心房肌亦可受累。

组织病理学

其组织病理学形态亦颇具特色，故多可过目不忘[163]。病变所累区域内的心肌细胞肿胀（大小可为相邻正常心肌细胞的两倍）、圆形或多边形，胞浆略呈颗粒状，嗜伊红染色，并多呈明显空泡化（图2.46）。无核分裂象。因病变细胞呈泡沫状，故有人用"脂肪样"和"组织细胞样"冠之。

电镜下可见：胞浆颗粒是缘于线粒体数量增多和线粒体内空泡——线粒体肿胀和嵴变形。所有病变细胞内都包含有少量、多位于周边并有Z带的肌原纤维、桥粒和微丝（leptofibril）。这些病变细胞的肌源性概念即基于上述现象，同时也证明了它与周围型Purkinje细胞同源。而它类同于嗜酸瘤细胞转化之说，则是源于其胞浆内的大量线粒体聚集。

特别关注之处

在可以预见的未来，关于浦肯野细胞瘤组织发生问题的争论肯定不会有结果，但在临床方面，对持续性室性心动过速相关性Purkinje细胞瘤患婴的外科经验却强烈提示：该病变并非是一种进行性心肌病。根据对该病变的现有认识，将其视为一种心脏错构瘤并不牵强[162]。

在低龄婴儿，本病与心律失常的密切相关对病理医师来说也是一个重要命题。患婴所求助的研究中心如果不是对婴儿的这种心脏病学有专攻，他们大都不会要求对其做病理活检。每个病理医师或早或晚都可能会遇到低龄婴儿猝死的病例，但只要对本病保持警觉，便可做出正确诊断。

心脏畸胎瘤　Cardiac teratoma

迄今为止，最大的心脏畸胎瘤病例系列来自McAllister和Fenoglio[1]（78例良性肿瘤中11例，其中9例患者的年龄在1岁或以下）。与此相反，AFIP最新修订的报告[2]中仅有1例婴幼及儿童心脏畸胎瘤（表2.1），在47例良性心包肿瘤中也只有3例。心脏畸胎瘤明显好发于婴幼及儿童，且绝大多数患者为女性。

畸胎瘤大多为心包内肿瘤，附着于主动脉干和肺动脉干的根部，但心壁亦可受累（如明尼苏达大学描述的病例）[6]，并偶可以心肌间肿物的形式出现[163]。其临床症状、体征与其部位有关[163]。心脏增大是其突出特征，并常伴有心脏压迫症状和体征。心脏畸胎瘤确可迅速增大，并累及到前纵隔。通过超声心动图和扫描技术大都可获确诊，手术切除多可行。迄今为止，手术切除效果甚佳，即便是次全切除亦如是[6]。

大体病理形态

畸胎瘤大都位于心包内，有完整的蒂或无蒂，附着于心脏大动脉干根部。瘤体的大小变异颇大，但那些可引起临床注意者均已具相当尺寸，甚至数倍于心脏本身。瘤体呈分叶状，表面光滑。畸胎瘤切面呈多囊性，囊腔大小不等，内容液体，囊壁间可见实性病变区域；大体所见多与卵巢畸胎瘤无异。

组织病理学

理论上，畸胎瘤应包含所有三个胚层所衍生的组织成分。心脏畸胎瘤酷似发生于身体其他部位者，如卵巢（参见第13A章）。对病理医师来说，畸胎瘤的诊断虽非难事，但首先须除外恶性病变（见下文）。

特别关注之处

心脏畸胎瘤很少发生于心肌内。其在心包内的病变部位使得手术入路很清楚，多可被完整切除。术后随访效果亦多良好。至于本瘤何以好发于女性，依然不清楚。

就病理医师之关注而言，还有两项内容：其一是畸胎瘤与囊肿或囊性结构之间的鉴别。心包囊肿大多无症状，它们虽可呈多囊性，但其组织学形态却与畸胎瘤完全不同：囊肿壁由结缔组织构成，内面被覆单层扁平间皮细胞。另一潜在误诊是支气管源性囊肿——大都位于心肌间，镜下可见囊壁被覆典型的纤毛柱状或立方上皮，偶见鳞状上皮化生；囊壁本身则由数量不等的胶原纤维、平滑肌和软骨构成；其间可出现浆液或黏液性腺体，并偶见灶状淋巴细胞聚集。它与畸胎瘤的鉴别点是：病变中无其他组织成分。

其二，畸胎瘤的诊断一经确定，就应认真阅片，以除外那些（哪怕是最细微的）恶性证据。为此，须从肿瘤的多个不同部位取材，多做切片，这与身体其他部位畸胎瘤的处置原则类同。

心脏血管瘤　Cardiac angioma

在软组织肿瘤中，良性血管瘤是最常见者之一（见第3章），但在心脏，血管瘤却颇为少见（表2.1~2.3）。淋巴管瘤确属零星个案，不做详细讨论（AFIP样本中有2例心脏淋巴管瘤，一例在心包壁层；另一例在左心

室肌间 [1]）。

心脏血管瘤的临床表现取决于其病变的部位和瘤体大小。心脏的任何部位都可发生血管瘤，但明显以心包脏层为多发，并可导致心包积血 [164]。心肌血管瘤明显好发于室间隔和心室前壁；而心内膜下血管瘤则在所有四个心腔都有发生 [165]。这两个部位的血管瘤都可能导致心肌功能障碍 [166]，或最终导致充血性心力衰竭，或酷似心脏瓣膜病 [165]。有零星个案报告称：一名15岁女孩，表现有肺动脉流出道狭窄的症状体征，合并红细胞增多症，后被查出患有不宜手术的右心室血管瘤 [167]。此外，位于心壁内的血管瘤还可导致房室传导阻滞 [51]。在心内膜下部位，血管瘤一旦向内凸入心腔，则可酷似黏液瘤，尤以起源于房间隔者为甚 [51]。

心脏血管瘤大都根据其发生部位进行分类，但病变偶可表现为血管瘤病，呈弥漫性生长，广泛累及心脏之大部（图2.47）。

心脏血管瘤在任何年龄均可发生（McAllister & Fenoglio样本中15个患者的年龄跨度从7个月到80岁），但在婴儿，心脏血管瘤却极少出现症状 [168]。无性别差异。

大体病理形态

心脏血管瘤的大体形态与发生在身体其他部位的血管瘤无异。位于心腔内的血管瘤乍看上去，可能会给人以黏液瘤的感觉。

组织病理学

心脏血管瘤的组织形态与一般概念上的血管瘤无异（参见第3章）。最常见的组织学类型是毛细血管型（图2.48）和海绵状血管瘤。在心肌内膜活检，见到血管密度增加，再伴有间质纤维化，就是在提醒病理医生做出诊断（图2.49）。血管瘤的上皮样亚型似乎极为罕见，我只见过2例诊断明确的原发性心脏血管瘤个案：一例为上皮样血管瘤，患者为一62岁男性，患有慢性原发性高血压症，在心血管病常规体检做B超时发现一肿物附于房间隔，并凸入右心房 [169]。术前诊断为心脏黏液瘤。但病理组织学形态显示为典型的上皮样血管瘤（参见第3章，p51）。本瘤曾有多个名称（以"组织细胞样血管瘤"最为常见），但现在却被归类为以上皮样内皮细胞为共同特征的血管瘤家族成员之一 [170]。据信，上皮样血管瘤代表了（以上皮样内皮细胞为特征的血管瘤家族）谱系的良性端，而上皮样血管肉瘤（见第33页）则代表其恶性端 [171]。而此家族中介于两端之间者，即所谓上皮样血管内皮瘤（epithelioid hemangioendothelioma），此前曾被认为是一种低度恶性的血管肿瘤 [172]。但鉴于其全身转移率高达21%，而且在20名患者中有4人

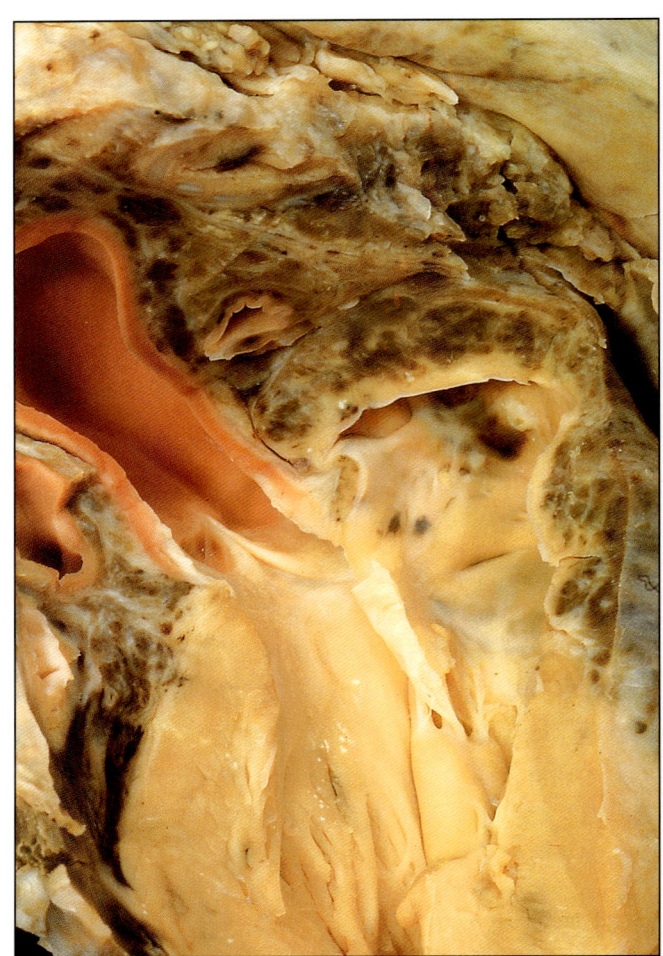

图2.47　弥漫性血管瘤病，病变广泛累及心脏和心包。患者为一4个月的男婴。图示：已被打开的左心房、左心室和主动脉被血管瘤完全覆盖。

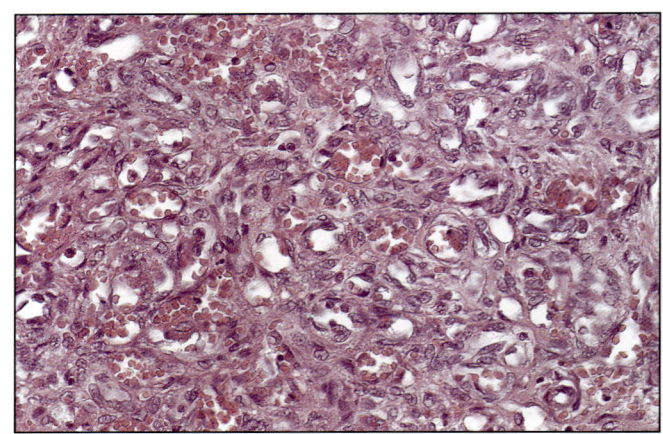

图2.48　典型的、基本上是良性的毛细血管瘤的组织形态（切片取自图2.47所示标本）。

（20%）直接死于本瘤，故最好将其视为完全恶性，而非交界型血管肿瘤 [173]。要想预言上皮样血管内皮瘤的恶性程度恐怕很难 [174]，而且有些病例的组织形态可能会与上皮样血管瘤多有交叠。有个案报道称，一名65

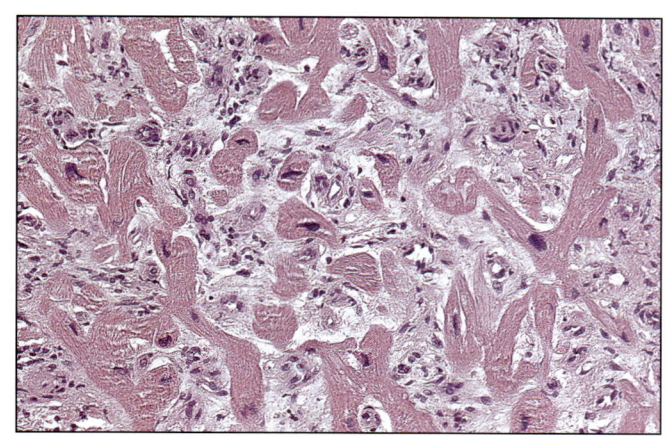

图2.49 心肌内膜活检,患者22岁男性,入院前1周感觉进行性呼吸困难,此前并无不适。临床诊断:心包炎(浆液性血性心包积液超过1升);超声心动图示:下壁心肌之大部见有罕见的毛玻璃样改变;冠状动脉造影示有血管盘旋。右心室(室间隔面)心肌内膜活检诊断为毛细血管型血管瘤,肥大的心肌细胞被弥漫性毛细血管瘤区间分隔。

最后,就是Luthringer等[176]提到的具有与"组织细胞样"(或上皮样)血管瘤有某些相似之处的病变,它们或附着于心壁内膜、心瓣膜,或自由浮动于心包腔内(升主动脉夹层动脉瘤之内容物就是其中之一)。这些病变由实性细胞团构成,并被纤维蛋白网包围(图2.50)。这些细胞呈圆形或多边形,胞浆嗜伊红染色,略呈泡沫状或呈空泡化;细胞边界清楚。故显示出一种组织细胞样或上皮样细胞的形态特征(图2.51)。免疫组化染色显示,与上皮样血管瘤细胞不同,这些细胞对内皮细胞标记物并不着色,而是对角蛋白呈阳性反应(图2.52)。我曾在一次心肌内膜活检中见到过这种病变,当时,我将其诊断为间皮细胞聚集,但其来源却一直在困扰着我(图2.50~2.52)。Luthringer等[176]也认同结节状间皮细胞增生的说法,但在组织来源的问题上一直含糊其辞。后继的研究认为,这些病变明显呈组织细胞样

岁男性左心房肿瘤患者,术前多次被诊断为黏液瘤。术后病理诊断为"组织细胞样血管瘤",但其组织形态呈交界型特征,与上述情况类似[175]。现在回过头来看,此例肿瘤极有可能是上皮样血管内皮瘤的实证。

Luthringer等[176]在其一篇题为"一种类似组织细胞样(上皮样)血管瘤的独特的心血管病变——提示有间皮参与的证据"的文章中提到的"组织细胞样"概念相当混杂。澄清它与本文的这些上皮样血管病变之间的差异具有重要临床意义(详见下文鉴别诊断章节)。

特别关注之处

生物学行为:心脏血管瘤的生物学行为与一般血管瘤相似。其生长潜能可能有限;虽已有自发性退化的报道[177],但如果不做手术切除,血管瘤将会持续存在下去。据称,心脏血管瘤完全切除术的预后甚佳[178]。

鉴别诊断:在心脏血管瘤,几乎没有什么重大的鉴别诊断问题。不过,还是应该在这些良性病变和扩张的血管之间做出鉴别。后者可见于心脏任何部位,但以心内膜下最为常见。组织学检查显示:扩张的血管丛中常有血栓形成,与痔疮所见类似。

另一种可能的错误是将血囊误诊为血管瘤。血囊几乎仅见于新生儿和婴儿,尤以三尖瓣和二尖瓣最为多见。实际上,所谓血囊并非是字面意义上真正的囊,而是瓣膜上兜住血液的憩室样结构,酷似一曲张的血管病变。

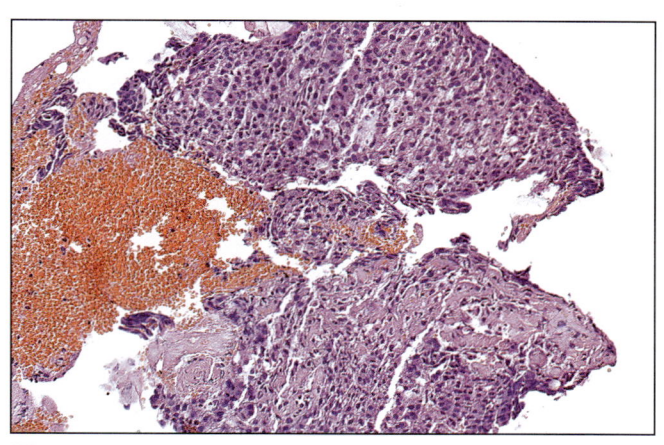

图2.50 心肌内膜活检,患者男性,23岁,非特异性胸疼,超声心动图显示:左心室收缩力减弱、冠状动脉造影正常,疑患心肌炎。组织学切片显示:在血液和纤维蛋白网中,可见心肌细胞和丛状分布的实性大细胞团。

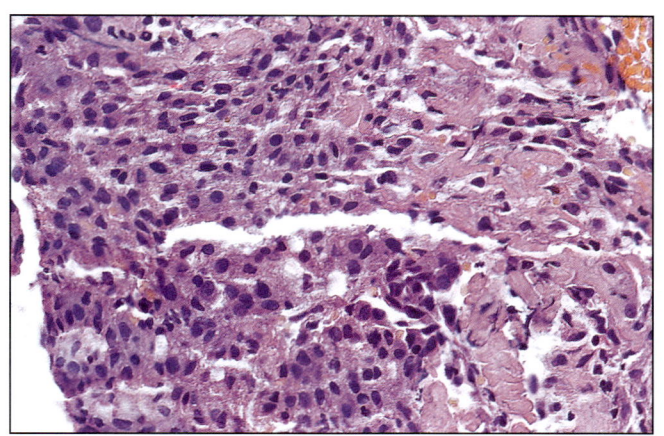

图2.51 图2.50之高倍镜观,示:这些丛状分布的大细胞呈多边形;胞浆细颗粒状,嗜酸淡红染色,偶有空泡化;细胞边界清楚。

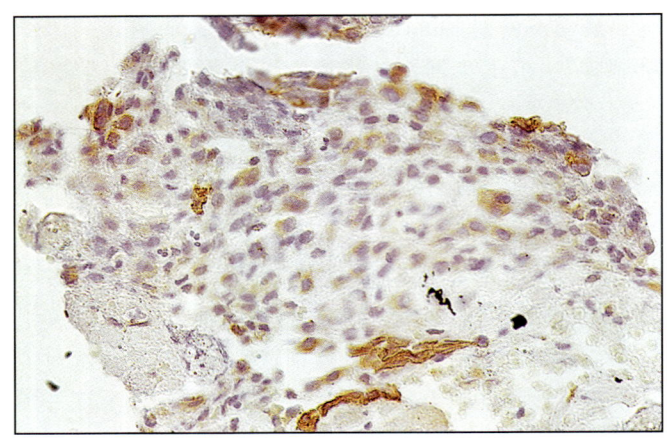

图2.52 图2.50切片之免疫组化染色,显示这些细胞呈CK阳性。这种病变酷似结节状间皮细胞增生,虽然它在心肌内膜活检中的出现尚存诸多悬疑,但不应将其视为原发性或转移性的恶性(肿瘤)。

特征,故建议冠以"间皮/单核细胞性偶发性心脏赘生物(mesothelial/monocytic incidental cardiac excrescence,MICE)"之名[179]。有报道称,所有这类个案好像都出现在心血管外科手术之后。既然如此,这些病变就不应该被误认为是原发性或转移性的恶性病变。

其他良性心脏肿瘤
Other benign cardiac tumors

房室结的(所谓)间皮瘤
Mesothelioma (so-called) of the atrioventricular node

本病变少见。据我所知,首例个案是由Armstrong和Mönckeberg[180]于1911年报道。1942年,Mahaim[181]认为,这种特殊肿瘤起源于在心脏胚胎发育过程中内陷入房室管的心外膜间皮细胞,此概念曾获普遍认同。在Mahaim之前,Rezek[182]曾指出:这种病变是内胚层起源,并非如Armstrong和Mönckeberg[180]所言是来自淋巴组织。免疫组化研究现已证实:其主要细胞成分对癌胚抗原(CEA)和CK的免疫染色呈阳性,提示为内胚层起源[183,184]。据此,该病变可能代表了移位的内胚层前肠组织,其发病机制可能与支气管源性囊肿相似[183]。这些现象印证了此前由Sopher、Spitz[184]和Travers[186]提出的概念。最近,有作者还发现了其中的神经内分泌成分,故认为这些病变代表了后鳃体易位[187]。在可以预见的未来,关于其组织发生学的争论无疑还将继续下去。

从临床角度看,必须要强调的是:迄今为止,文献个案的年龄跨度是从11个月至89岁,部分性或完全性房室传导阻滞为其最主要的临床特征,但猝死确可成为本瘤的首发现象[188-189]。一66岁患者之间皮瘤几乎完全取代了房室结,伴房内性传导阻滞、阵发性房性心律失常和自发性间歇性预激综合征,后者是被多条左侧传导旁路所易化[190]。

肉眼可见房间隔增厚,在房室结部位有或无轻度结节状隆起。用肉眼仔细观察,可见病变区域常呈多囊性改变。

镜下可见房室结区被一多囊性病变所取代,其中有囊腔、有导管,也有实性细胞巢(图2.53和2.54)。囊腔大小相差很多,其内衬细胞可单层、可多层、可呈扁平形、可呈立方状,常沿最内层囊壁呈栅栏状排列。瘤细胞呈抗淀粉酶PAS和阿新蓝染色阳性,这一结果并不会因用透明质酸酶做预消化而有所改变。此外,这些细胞对抗CEA免疫染色亦呈阳性反应。部分细胞巢的黏液染色为阴性,胞浆呈嗜伊红强染,类似于鳞状或移行上皮。这些细胞巢周围是由胶原和弹力纤维构成的致密结缔组织间质;鲜有可识别的房室结残迹。

电镜下可见两种主要的细胞类型[183]:第一类细胞以卵圆形胞体、大量桥粒和胞浆中含有大量张力原纤维束为特征,这些张力原纤维主要分布在细胞核周围;第二类细胞中含有中间丝和单层膜性致密颗粒,颗粒膜的部分区段与细胞表面膜融合,提示它具有分泌活性。

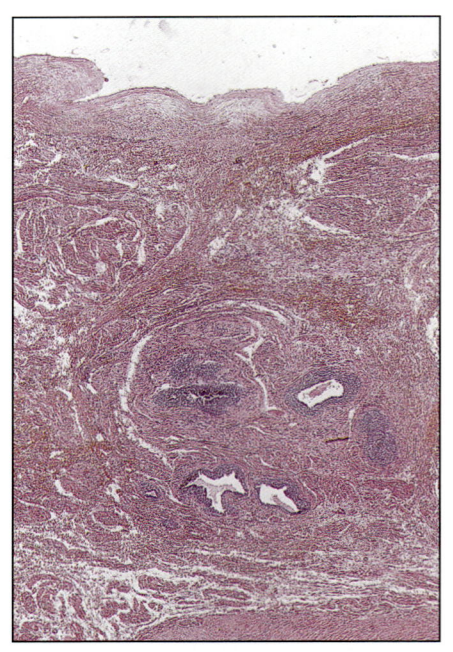

图2.53 房室结间皮瘤。该病变由很多小囊构成。(Courtesy of Dr J. E. Edwards, Cardiovascular Registry, United Hospital, St. Paul, MN, USA.)

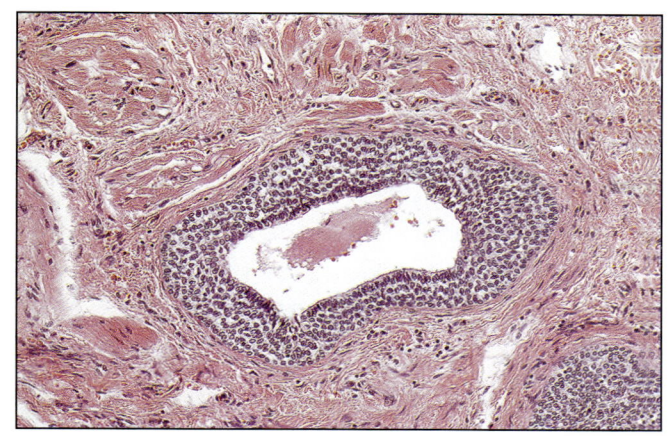

图 2.54 图 2.53 所示标本之高倍镜形态,显示内衬多层立方状上皮细胞,胞浆透明,沿囊壁内层呈栅栏状排列。

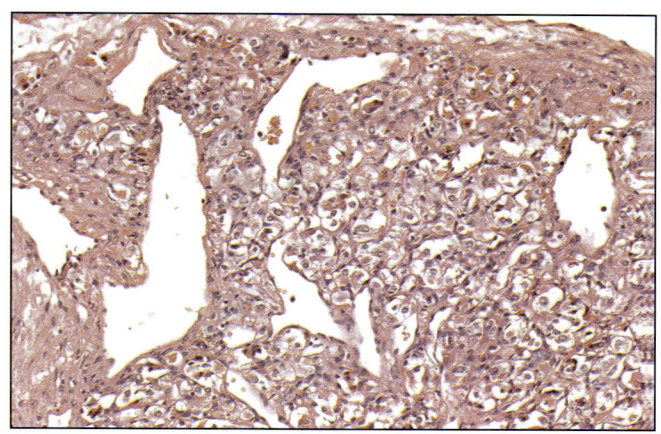

图 2.55 心脏副神经节瘤。患者 71 岁女性,有心房纤颤、高血压和心肌梗死病史。冠状动脉造影显示有三支性冠状动脉病,并在房间隔见一高度血管化区域。经食管超声心动图可见房间隔部位有一直径 5cm 的肿瘤。行体外循环下肿瘤切除术,但患者死于房间隔部位大出血。常规 HE 切片显示有宽大的血管空隙,嗜酸淡染的细胞聚集成 Zellballen 小体,周围是毛细血管网。(Courtesy of Dr R. J. van Suylen, Department of Pathology, Academic Hospital, Maastricht, The Netherlands.)

心脏副神经节瘤 Cardiac paraganglioma

心脏副神经节瘤起源于嗜铬性副神经节,该神经节位于心底、紧靠主动脉干和肺动脉干部位,由冠状动脉主干分支供血;"冠状动脉球"即因此而得名[191]。在 AFIP 图谱中,此类肿瘤被纳入肾上腺外副神经节相关系列[192]。首例心包内副神经节瘤(又名嗜铬细胞瘤或化学感受器瘤)个案由 Besterman 等[193] 于 1974 年报告。患者好发于年轻人。其临床表现虽然可能相当多样,但大都以去甲肾上腺素分泌过量所导致的症状和体征为主,如高血压[194-198]。

心脏副神经节瘤大都位于心外膜内,尤以左心房后下壁、房间沟和大动脉根部的心外膜表面位置居多,但亦可见于其他部位,如右或左冠状动脉邻中线处;亦有从房间沟内原发部位凸入心房腔的心脏副神经节瘤[199]——它们在二维超声心动图上酷似心房黏液瘤。此外,冠状动脉造影可能表现有"肿瘤泛红"现象,这是因局部血管密度增高所致。这种"泛红现象"虽非特异(心腔内血管瘤亦可出现类似现象),但因一般认为这种现象为黏液瘤所专属,故血管造影之所见很容易出现误导。不过,组织学研究很容易对其做出正确诊断。

肉眼上,心脏副神经节瘤质地均匀,色泽棕褐。镜下可见副神经节瘤的典型特征。病变主要由所谓主细胞构成,主细胞聚集成巢或称 Zellballen 小体,周围是毛细血管网和数量不等的结缔组织(图 2.55,并参阅第 28 章)。用 HE 常规染色如不能清楚展示这些特征,可用网硬蛋白染色突显之(图 2.56)。必要时,还可用神经内分泌分化的特异性标记物,如嗜铬粒蛋白(chromogranin, CgA)做免疫组化染色(图 2.57)。

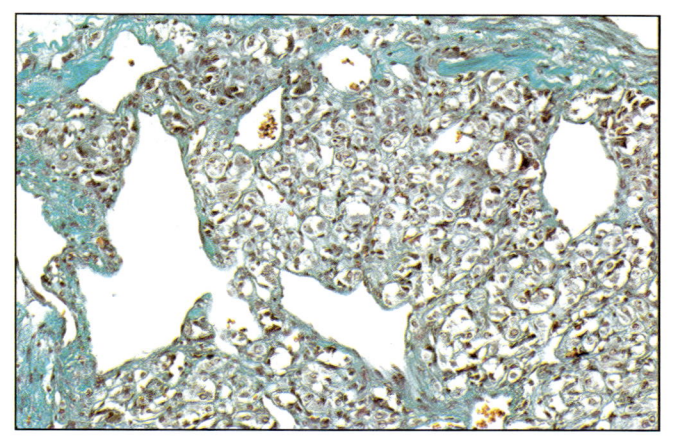

图 2.56 心脏副神经节瘤。Gomori 网硬蛋白染色很好地突显出典型的丛状结构。

心脏副神经节瘤的生物学行为或许可与颈动脉体副神经节瘤类比(参阅第 28 章),但因其太过罕见,不足以支持这方面的肯定结论。文献上 15 例个案中有 2 例发生转移[190],因此,其转移发生率就与颈动脉体瘤不相上下了[200]。同时,必须要指出:对病变性质尚无充分预案的手术风险极大。在这种情况下,术中大出血、术中死亡都是有可能的[199](另见图 2.55 所示病例档案)。

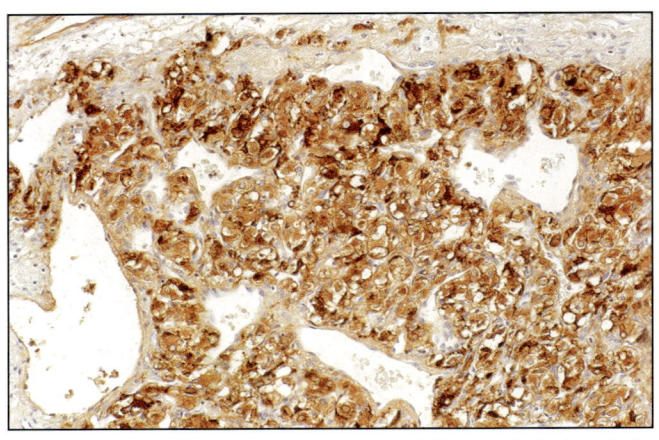

图2.57　心脏副神经节瘤。瘤细胞对嗜铬粒蛋白免疫组化染色呈强阳性。

心脏和心包的恶性肿瘤
Malignant tumors of the heart and pericardium

关于心脏原发性恶性肿瘤的调查向人们展示出一幅多彩的画面（表2.1～2.3）。1976—1993年AFIP系列[2]中恶性肿瘤在心脏、心包原发性肿瘤总数中约占37%；"得克萨斯经验"合计达11.7%[3]；而我们自己的心血管病理档案中包含18例心脏和心包原发性恶性肿瘤，在所有原发性肿瘤中占13.2%。毫无疑问，心脏恶性肿瘤发生率的宽幅差异显然是因三家研究机构的背景偏倚所致。Burke等[205]在修订1978年版AFIP系列[1]时又补充收集了75例原发性心脏肉瘤（40个外科病例），给人的总印象是血管肉瘤是最常见的原发性心脏肉瘤，但有调查报道[206,207]称：所谓恶性纤维组织细胞瘤的发病率与之相同。该研究系列包含1964—1989年间共21例原发性心脏肉瘤，其中7例确诊血管肉瘤，7例为恶性纤维组织细胞瘤[据有人判断，此结果基本上代表了此前的Murphy系列[3]（表2.2），之后在诊断上做出某些调整，并用得克萨斯大学胸外科的经验加以补充]，另外7例分别被诊断为横纹肌肉瘤（2）、平滑肌肉瘤（2）、未分化型肉瘤（1）、纤维黏液肉瘤（1）和黏液肉瘤（1）[206]。照此看来，在心脏原发性肉瘤中，恶性纤维组织细胞瘤的诊断只是在软组织肉瘤范围内做再检查和再分类的时候才得到认可[208]（参见第24章）。

恶性原发性心脏肿瘤章节还应包括原发性心包间皮瘤和原发性心脏淋巴瘤。但在以下章节仅就与心脏受累相关部分做重点详述。至于这两类肿瘤组织学特征的详细描述，读者可参阅本书有关章节。

颗粒细胞瘤　Granular cell tumor

心脏颗粒细胞瘤与发生在身体其他部位者（参阅第27章）属于同类，McAllister和Fenoglio[1]曾报道过3个成人病例；此后，另有4例已进入AFIP系列[2]。McAllister和Fenoglio[1]描述的病例最初都被诊断为横纹肌瘤。他们所提供的图像（图66）可明确澄清这确属误诊。同时，这些图像还使人模糊地联想到一种曾被冠以"浦肯野细胞瘤"之名加以描述的病变（见第26页）。组织化学和超微结构研究可以很好地解决这类鉴别诊断问题：所谓浦肯野细胞瘤的主细胞示有丰富的线粒体，而颗粒细胞瘤的瘤细胞胞浆中含有大的、PAS阳性的自噬体颗粒。

McAllister和Fenoglio[1]明确指出：他们收集这些肿瘤是因为它们会被误诊为横纹肌瘤，除此之外，它们"只是形态怪异，并无临床意义"。

神经纤维瘤　Neurofibroma

心脏神经纤维瘤极为罕见，如出现则常为von Recklinghausen病（多发性神经纤维瘤病）的一部分（参见第27章）。其可导致右室流出道阻塞[201]。

异位组织　Heterotopic tissues

在个别患者的心脏和心包中偶尔可见有岛状的胸腺或甲状腺组织[202,203]。无论是外科手术还是尸检，这些现象常为偶遇事件。我把一心脏外科手术中意外发现的罕见腺瘤样瘤病变也列在此标题下，该病变可弥漫性地分布在右心房心肌[204]。

血管肉瘤　Angiosarcoma

血管肉瘤可能是最常见的心脏原发性恶性肿瘤[209-212]。临床表现多样，但以充血性心力衰竭和呼吸困难最为突出[1,210]。原发性心脏血管肉瘤大都起源于右心，原发于心房者尤为多见[1,206]。一项在这些情况下临床病理形态谱系的研究显示：有两种主要形式：一是巨大阻塞性肿块，伴有明显的临床症状和体征；二是无明显症状的局部浸润型肿瘤，不常见[213]。发生于心包的病变在临床表现上酷似心包炎。

初诊时的平均年龄在40岁左右，但文献年龄跨度却在10～76岁。本病自然病史主要表现为临床病程短，患者大都会在出现症状后十个月内死于血管肉瘤。死亡原因几乎都与肿瘤对心脏的影响直接相关，如心脏压塞或心腔内阻塞。偶有存活较长者，现有两例个案报告[214,215]，他们的肿瘤都很大，都未能在心肺分流术下被完全切除，手术时也未见远端转移的证据。两位患者都接受了放疗，一名患者还接受了不足一疗程的化疗。他们二人在肿瘤切除术后未见复发的时间分别是 36 和 34 个月。其中一例在没有体外循环的情况下接受左心房血管肉瘤完全切除术，该患者术后 3 年，临床状态良好[216]。

临床上出现症状时，肿瘤大都已经扩散到无法实施根治术的程度了。其诊断可通过外科活检或心包液细胞学检查确定[211]。心脏血管肉瘤的诊断亦可经由心肌内膜活检做出[217]。

组织学形态变异颇大，从有肿瘤性血管结构的高分化病变，到异型性明显的梭形瘤细胞呈实性肿瘤性生长、完全看不到血管构型的低分化病灶都有。在低分化或未分化病变，第八因子相关抗原染色大都呈阴性，但其他内皮细胞标记物（如 CD31 和 CD34）多为阳性。如为阴性，则可求助于电镜，其结果常比免疫组化和细胞化学更有帮助。图 2.58 和 2.59 所示为一罕见的原发性上皮样血管肉瘤病变（参阅第 3 章，p. 66）。

一般情况下，如果肿瘤之大部都已纳入组织学观察范围，那诊断该肿瘤为血管肉瘤应该没有什么问题。主要的鉴别诊断问题，尤其是低分化血管肉瘤，是与其他类型的低分化肉瘤、纤维性（肉瘤样）间皮瘤和发生在心脏的转移性肿瘤之间的鉴别。

恶性纤维组织细胞瘤（无法分类的多形性肉瘤） Malignant fibrous histiocytoma (unclassified pleomorphic sarcoma)

据我所知，所谓心脏原发性恶性纤维组织细胞瘤的首例个案报道见于 1978 年[218]。这类肿瘤一直被视为最

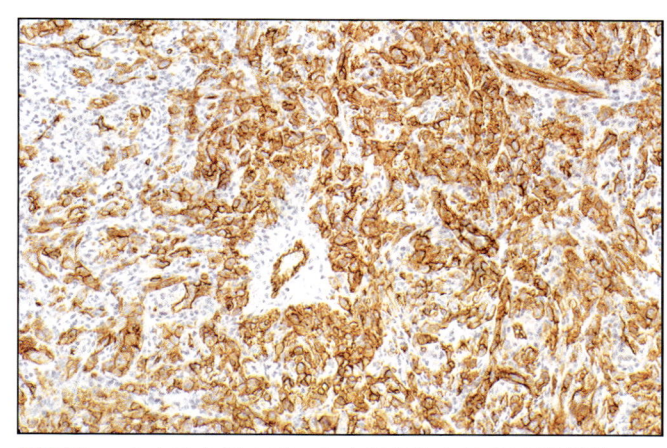

图2.59　上皮样血管肉瘤。免疫组化染色示CD34强阳性。

常见的软组织肉瘤之一；但在心脏，作为原发性肿瘤，它一般极为罕见。其名称尚有争议，所谓恶性纤维组织细胞瘤黏液样亚型，被命名为"黏液纤维肉瘤"或许更好些（见第 24 章关于恶性纤维组织细胞瘤的讨论）。

绝大多数心脏原发性多形性肉瘤都位于左心房，但位于左心室[206]、右心房[205] 和右心室[205] 的零星个案也都有报告。因其多发于左心房，故在临床上可能很容易被误诊为心房黏液瘤[35,219-221]。这对病理医师来说也一样，因为该肿瘤作为手术标本送达病理医师取材台时，标注明确为"黏液瘤"。对于稍欠经验者来说，它与黏液纤维肉瘤（即所谓恶性纤维组织细胞瘤的黏液样亚型）之间的鉴别诊断可能会遇到麻烦。因为肿瘤的优势成分为黏液样基质，散在其间的瘤细胞大都为梭形，呈链条状或丛状分布（参阅第 24 章）。不过，迄今为止，我还没有见过一例在组织形态上与心脏黏液瘤确有相似之处的黏液纤维肉瘤。恶性纤维组织细胞瘤黏液样亚型的病变中可见细胞密集区域，瘤细胞呈明显多形性，可见核分裂象、坏死和广泛的血管增生；除了黏液样基质以外，没有任何心脏黏液瘤的形态特征[35,221]。我曾见过两例最初被病理诊断为心脏黏液瘤的病例，二者都发生在非常见部位（一例起源于肺动脉瓣，一例起源于二尖瓣），二者都表现有黏液纤维肉瘤的典型形态特征：细胞核多形性、核分裂象和组织坏死。只是因为这 2 例肿瘤的"心源性和黏液瘤样"特征，才使得一位颇有经验的病理医师也会被引入歧途。不过，如有疑问，就从肿瘤的多个不同部位取材切片，可能对诊断大有助益。

位于左心房的肿瘤大都起源于后壁或房间隔，但其他部位亦可受累。多发性肿瘤也有报道[220]。整体预后不佳，另据根治术术后随访结果显示，至今有案可查的术后存活时间约在 10 ~ 60 个月之间[222]。肿瘤对放疗和化疗的反应性并无肯定结论，多数作者一致认为预后与治疗无关，系属天命[35,219]。局部复发常见，而且该肿

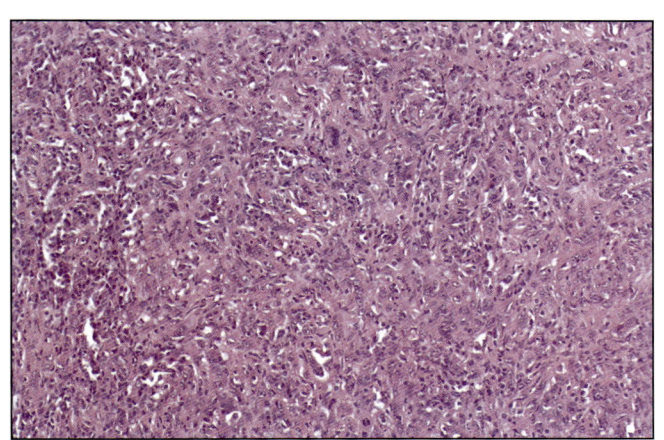

图2.58　上皮样血管肉瘤。肿瘤位于右心房并凸入心腔。肿瘤近乎实性，呈结节状生长，由索条状排列的上皮样瘤细胞构成，胞浆嗜酸性粉染，细胞核多形性明显。(Courtesy of Dr P.Pauwels, Laboratory of Pathology (Stishting PAMM), Catharina Ziekenhuis, Eindhoven, The Netherlands.)

瘤具有明显的局部浸润倾向[33,223]。Laya 等[33] 的综述报告指出：患者初诊时的平均年龄为 36 岁，比软组织肿瘤中的所谓恶性纤维组织细胞瘤患者的初诊年龄要小。

横纹肌肉瘤　Rhabdomyosarcoma

据 AFIP[1] 早期报告称，在最常见的成人心脏原发性恶性肿瘤中，心脏横纹肌肉瘤居于次席；但在其 1976—1993 年系列中仅含 3 例横纹肌肉瘤，这可能代表了诊断标准上的一种改变[2]。据载，该肿瘤可见于任何年龄，且无明显性别差异，但在儿童年龄组相对少见。一项对原发性心脏横纹肌肉瘤文献个案的调查显示，17 例 16 岁以下患者中，6 例在 1 岁或以下[224]。Burke 和 Virman[2] 收集了 3 例此年龄组的原发性横纹肌肉瘤，其中 1 例的初诊年龄小于 1 岁。据载[225]，一 8 岁男童患有罕见的葡萄状胚胎型横纹肌肉瘤，病变起源于二尖瓣之主动脉侧叶的心室面。我只见过一例心脏恶性横纹肌样瘤的个案报告，患者为一 6 个月大的女婴[226]。该肿瘤占据并扩展到整个左心室下侧壁，并将心包腔填充；镜下可见该肿瘤由多角形大细胞构成，胞浆嗜酸性红染，细胞核呈多形性，并常见有单个的嗜酸性胞浆包涵体。电镜观察显示，这些包涵体系由大量中间丝构成，正如 Hass（"恶性横纹肌样瘤"一词的命名者）等[227] 所言，这些病变与横纹肌肉瘤无关，学界对此已有共识。

患者的临床症状、体征与肿瘤的部位有关。常见有周身不适，且多合并心脏杂音和心律失常。横纹肌肉瘤可凸入心腔内，如是，则多呈息肉状；肿瘤亦可累及心包脏层和壁层。这两种情况几乎都是由于位于心肌内的肿瘤发展所致。在儿童年龄组，肿瘤大都起源于房间隔或室间隔（总计 35%）；但在成人，则多起源于左心房或右心室[224]。心脏横纹肌肉瘤的组织形态与身体其他部位软组织中的同类病变相似（参阅第 24 章）。图 2.60 所示为一例心脏原发性多形性横纹肌肉瘤。

心脏横纹肌肉瘤的自然过程甚危。据我所知，诊断一经确认，鲜有长期存活者，患者大都在确诊后一年内死亡。16 岁以下儿童的平均存活时间为 1.5 个月，成人为 6 个月[224]。

纤维肉瘤　Fibrosarcoma

与其他软组织肉瘤一样，"纤维肉瘤"的诊断备受挑战已有数十年之久。这种挑战与学界用现代技术、根据细胞类型对软组织肿瘤做更准确分类的持续追求有关；作为特殊病变实体，纤维肉瘤与恶性纤维组织细胞瘤之间的鉴别尤具代表性（参阅上文）。这种趋势在心脏原发性恶性肿瘤的系列报告中就有所反映。AFIP[1] 在

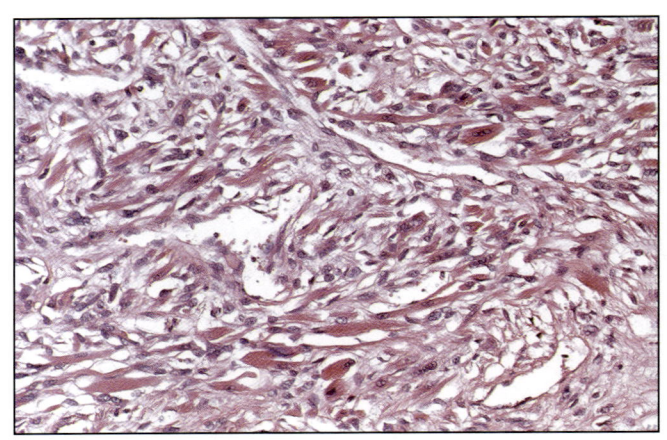

图 2.60　多形性横纹肌肉瘤。40 岁女性患者左心房壁一巨大肿瘤凸入左心房腔，并触及二尖瓣之主动脉侧瓣叶。多形性横纹肌肉瘤的组织学特征明显。注意：巨大的奇异型横纹肌母细胞。(Courtesy of Dr C.H.Heijmans, Laboratory of Pathology, Enschede, The Netherlands.)

其 1978 年系列中确诊了 14 例心脏原发性纤维肉瘤，没有恶性纤维组织细胞瘤的记载；但他们根据新收集个案所做修订新版中却记载了 6 例纤维肉瘤和 6 例恶性纤维组织细胞瘤[205]（见表 2.1）。不过，McAllister 和 Fenoglio[1] 确曾提到：上述 14 例被诊断为纤维肉瘤的病变中，5 例呈现所谓恶性纤维组织细胞瘤的形态指征："梭形瘤细胞呈席纹状或漩涡状排列，并可见瘤巨细胞"。此外，最近的一项外科研究系列确诊了 7 例恶性纤维组织细胞瘤，而无 1 例纤维肉瘤[206]。我们自己的材料中有 2 例黏液纤维肉瘤（另见表 2.3），讨论见"恶性纤维组织细胞瘤"标题下（见 p33）。

特殊部位纤维肉瘤的诊断与源于身体其他部位软组织肿瘤的适用标准相同（参阅第 24 章）。

未分化型肉瘤　Undifferentiated sarcoma

迄今为止，最大的研究系列系由 Burke 等[205] 报道。75 例心脏原发性肉瘤中，18 例被他们分类为"未分化型肉瘤"。这些肿瘤分别位于右 (n=4)、左 (n=5) 心房，右 (n=2)、左 (n=3) 心室和心包 (n=4)，其中一例已呈弥漫性生长。免疫组化染色显示：SMA、波形蛋白阳性，偶有瘤细胞呈 CK 阳性；但更有助于诊断的标记物却均为阴性。

总体上，这些患者的存活状态不佳。统计学上，分化型（即可被分类者）肉瘤与未分化型肉瘤［含未分化型病变 (n=18) 和恶性纤维组织细胞瘤 (n=6)］[205] 二者的存活率并无显著的统计学差异。最近，法国的一项以未分化型肉瘤为主的大型系列研究[228] 也发现：心脏肉瘤的组织学类型对其预后的影响甚微。

其他少见的心脏原发性肉瘤
Other rare primary sarcomas of the heart

平滑肌肉瘤　Leiomyosarcoma

1978年版AFIP[1]系列中仅一例平滑肌肉瘤，而1976—1993年系列中包括12例新病例，其中1例的确诊年龄还不满1岁[2]。得克萨斯心脏病研究院Murphy等[3]报道的143例外科患者中仅有1例平滑肌肉瘤；而此系列患者的随访[206]结果显示：在全部21例心脏原发性肉瘤中有2例平滑肌肉瘤。我们自己的18例心脏原发性恶性肿瘤的系列材料中有3例平滑肌肉瘤。此现象反映了本章在引言中提到的固有思维偏倚问题；它同样适用于法国最近的系列材料，其包含6例平滑肌肉瘤[228]，其中一名7个月大的男婴患有二尖瓣原发性多形性肉瘤[229]。与原文作者不同，我们能够证明其瘤细胞具有与抗SMA抗体1A4和CD34的免疫反应性[230]。鉴于此平滑肌细胞分化证据，我们认为，该肿瘤应分类为平滑肌肉瘤。偶有心脏平滑肌肉瘤细胞具有上皮样形态特征[231]。

平滑肌肉瘤高度恶性，可局部扩散，结局几乎总是难免一死[232,233]。其组织学诊断标准与其他部位同类病变相同（参阅第24章）。

脂肪肉瘤　Liposarcoma

心脏原发性脂肪肉瘤极为少见，AFIP[1]系列中仅有1例，有案可查的个案也只有11例[234]。迄今为止的文献个案表明其好发部位为一侧心房，其临床表现则与肿瘤所在部位直接相关。预后不佳，平均存活时间为8.3个月。转移常见，大多转移至肺和骨。

组织学诊断的适用标准与其他部位脂肪肉瘤相同（参阅第24章）。

骨肉瘤　Osteosarcoma

AFIP的一篇综述[235]曾指出：81例有切片存档的原发性心脏肉瘤中，9例具有骨肉瘤样分化；AFIP最近文献[2]则清点出13例骨肉瘤，在全部心脏原发性肉瘤中占9%。值得注意的是，这9例肿瘤都位于左心房，其中一例可能起源于二尖瓣。尽管其超声心动图表现并不典型，但因其部位的关系，临床上常被误诊为黏液瘤。此现象很重要，因其尤可突显以下观点的潜在危险：所有左心房肿物都被视为心脏黏液瘤。这些肿瘤预后全都不好，尽管外科姑息手术后有可能延长存活时间。迄今为止，所有被诊断为心脏原发性骨肉瘤的个案均已死亡。

心脏骨肉瘤的组织学诊断标准与身体其他部位骨肉瘤并无不同（参阅第25章）。

软骨肉瘤　Chondrosarcoma

我只查到3例心脏原发性软骨肉瘤的个案报道[236-238]。Muir和Seah报道的那例[236]材料最全。据载，患者为50岁女性，二尖瓣心脏原发性软骨肉瘤样间叶瘤（chondrosarcomatous mesenchymoma）。肿瘤的准确起源未明，但尸检报告倾向于其原发部位在左心室。镜下，肿瘤的主体部分由软骨肉瘤构成，但部分区域却表现为纤维肉瘤的特征，还有些部位可被解释为血管肉瘤样改变。

临床过程从开始出现症状（呼吸困难）到死亡历时约6个月。

滑膜肉瘤　Synovial sarcoma

在心脏，具有典型双相分化形态特征的原发性滑膜肉瘤非常少见[1]。有案可查[239]：一13岁男孩，其右心房一巨大肿物，有蒂，附着于房室环。术后镜检诊断为具有双相分化的恶性肿瘤，由上皮性腺体结构和梭形细胞性间质构成。免疫组化标记物染色，通过除外间皮瘤后，确认了滑膜肉瘤的诊断。至此，关于2例个案就有了质疑的空间：有关AFIP早期系列[1]中记载的那个完全适合双相间皮瘤诊断的个案，还有那例起源于所谓房室结间皮瘤的心脏滑膜肉瘤个案[240]。不管怎样，心脏原发性滑膜肉瘤是一种极为罕见的肿瘤。Nicholson等[239]对6例文献个案所做简要调查（包括他们自己的和上述两个有争议的病例）结果显示：发病年龄介于13～53岁，预后明显为差，此前已报个案的存活时间均不足一年。

恶性周围神经鞘瘤
Malignant peripheral nerve sheath tumor（MPNST）

在本书，此术语与下列名词同义："神经源性肉瘤"、"神经纤维肉瘤"、"恶性神经鞘瘤"。

在心脏，MPNST的组织病理学诊断与身体其他部位神经性软组织肉瘤的适用标准相同（参阅第27章）。AFIP[1]早期系列记载了4例此类恶性肿瘤患者，但无超微结构或免疫组化的证据；其中3例肿瘤的主体位于并覆盖右室流出道上，1例位于右心房。AFIP后期系列[2]又收集了2例，其中1例混有异源性横纹肌肉瘤成分。另有个案报道称[241]：一多发性心脏MPNST并腔内占位的51岁女性患者。我们见过一例确诊的MPNST (Courtesy of Dr P. Pauwels, Pathology Laboratory,

Catharina Hospital, Eindhoven, The Netherlands）肿瘤位于右心室，患者为一75岁女性。

心脏和心包其他原发性恶性肿瘤
Other primary malignant tumors of the heart and pericardium

间皮瘤　　Mesothelioma

心脏原发性恶性间皮瘤在已确诊的间皮瘤中占比不足5%。Chun等[242]从文献上收集到了大约120例；AFIP的1970年系列中有240例胸腔间皮瘤，其中局限于心脏、心包者仅8例[2]。因心脏间皮瘤很少有临床体征和症状，即便有也是非特异性的，故生前诊断的阳性率并不高[1,242-244]。虽然呼吸困难和心包积液常导致临床考虑本瘤，但转移性疾病的可能性显然要比心包原发性间皮瘤大得多。在这种情况下，鉴别诊断就要依靠脱落细胞学检查和组织活检。用这些方法，多可做出正确诊断；但细胞形态和组织结构的多样性偶可对恶性间皮瘤与转移性病变之间的鉴别构成干扰。不过，心包原发性间皮瘤的诊断与身体其他部位同类病变的标准基本相同（参阅第5章）。

据McAllister和Fenoglio说[1]，在疾病晚期，心包原发性间皮瘤侵犯表面心肌是一种常见现象；但肿瘤大片扩散到心内膜则被视为心脏原发性间皮瘤与其他各型肉瘤之间尸检鉴别的重要指征。我们自己的经验却反对此说（图2.61），图示肿瘤已广泛侵及左、右心室心肌，并累及心内膜，但并未在心腔内形成占位。

恶性畸胎瘤　　Malignant teratoma

AFIP早期系列[1]中有4例恶性畸胎瘤，患者都是1～4岁的儿童。确诊时，肿瘤业已广泛侵袭心脏，进行根治术已无可能。上述4名患儿均于出现症状后3个月内死亡。最近文献[2]又添一例内胚窦瘤，患者为一14个月大的女婴。

诊断须基于在背景良性的畸胎瘤中确认有某一类组织已经恶变。

心脏原发性淋巴瘤
Primary cardiac lymphoma

作为播散型恶性淋巴瘤的一部分，尤其是在疾病晚期，心脏受累似乎相当常见，尸检检出率几乎接近20%[245]。另一方面，心脏原发性淋巴瘤，即指首先起源于心脏的淋巴瘤，似乎极为罕见，当然是指在免疫功能正常的患者[246,248]。文献综述表明：心脏原发性淋巴瘤，包括低度、中度和高度病变，大都是B细胞性质。淋巴

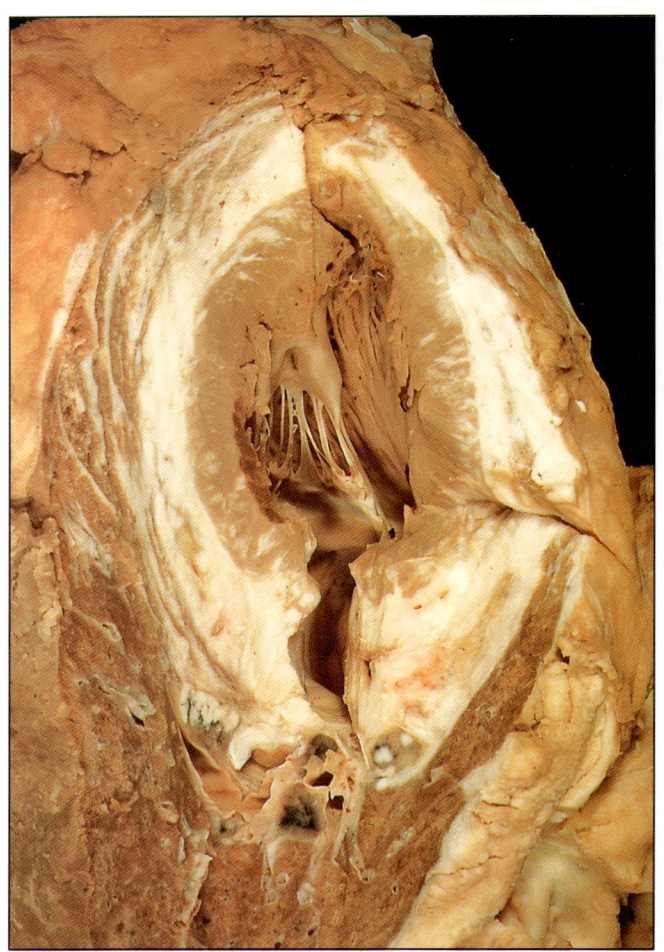

图2.61　一30岁女性患者的心脏标本。患者的首发体征为心包积液，经细胞学检查和病理活检诊断为间皮瘤。整个心脏都被间皮瘤所包围，累及左肺，并广泛侵袭心肌。图中所示为被打开的左心室。

瘤样病变大都以肿块形式起源于右心腔，多合并心包积液[248,249]。心包积液细胞学检查对绝大多数患者都有诊断意义。整体预后不佳，这在一定程度上，与对迟反应性心功能衰竭患者的诊断延误有关。治疗应与其他侵袭型恶性淋巴瘤相同。

其病理组织学诊断与一般淋巴瘤的适用标准相同（参阅第21章）。至此，应对心脏移植术后的"淋巴瘤"诊断做一警示。迄今的经验表明：心脏移植术后可能出现多种形态怪异的淋巴细胞增生，这很可能是病毒感染所致，未必具有异型性含义，切勿将其误诊为淋巴瘤。在这种情况下，病理医师对移植术后病理形态的复杂性的认识可能发挥关键作用。

参考文献

1. McAllister H A, Fenoglio J J Jr 1978 Tumors of the cardiovascular system. Atlas of tumor pathology, series 2, fascicle 15. Armed Forces Institute of Pathology, Washington, DC
2. Burke A, Virmani R 1996 Tumors of the heart and great vessels. Atlas of tumor pathology, series 3, fascicle 16. Armed Forces Institute of Pathology, Washington, DC
3. Murphy M C, Sweeney M S, Putnam J B Jr et al. 1990 Surgical treatment of cardiac tumours: a 25-year experience. Ann Thorac Surg 49: 612–618
4. Colucci W S, Braunwald E 1980 Primary tumors of the heart. In: Braunwald E (ed) Heart disease. A textbook of cardiovascular medicine. Saunders, Philadelphia, p 1502–1504
5. Wold L E, Lie J T 1980 Cardiac myxomas: a clinicopathologic profile. Am J Pathol 101: 219–234
6. Molina J E, Edwards J E, Ward H B 1990 Primary cardiac tumours: experience at the University of Minnesota. Thorac Cardiovasc Surg 38 (suppl. 2): 183–191
7. Blondeau Ph 1990 Primary cardiac tumours – French study of 533 cases. Thorac Cardiovasc Surg 38 (suppl. 2): 192–195
8. Sezai Y 1990 Tumours of the heart. Incidence and clinical importance of cardiac tumours in Japan and operative technique for left atrial tumours. Thorac Cardiovasc Surg 38 (suppl. 2): 201–204
9. Li G Y 1990 Incidence of clinical importance of cardiac tumours in China. Review of the literature. Thorac Cardiovasc Surg 38 (suppl. 2): 205–207
10. Becker A E 1973 Cardiac myxoma. Eur J Cardiol 1: 119–122
11. Burke A P, Virmani R 1993 Cardiac myxoma. A clinicopathologic study. Am J Clin Pathol 100: 671–680
12. Lie J T 1989 Petrified cardiac myxoma masquerading as organized atrial mural thrombus. Arch Pathol Lab Med 113: 742–745
13. Ferrans V J, Roberts W C 1973 Structural features of cardiac myxomas. Histology, histochemistry, and electron microscopy. Hum Pathol 4: 111–146
14. Goldman B I, Frydman C, Harpaz N et al. 1987 Glandular cardiac myxomas. Histologic, immunohistochemical, and ultrastructural evidence of epithelial differentiation. Cancer 59: 1767–1775
15. Johansson L 1989 Histogenesis of cardiac myxomas. An immunohistochemical study of 19 cases, including one with glandular structures, and review of the literature. Arch Pathol Lab Med 113: 735–741
16. Orr J W 1942 Endothelioma (pseudomyxoma) of heart. J Pathol Bacteriol 54: 125–128
17. Abenoza P, Sibley R K 1986 Cardiac myxoma with glandlike structures. An immunohistochemical study. Arch Pathol Lab Med 110: 736–739
18. Landon G, Ordoñez N G, Guarda L A 1986 Cardiac myxomas. An immunohistochemical study using endothelial, histiocytic, and smooth muscle cell markers. Arch Pathol Lab Med 110: 116–120
19. Kawano H, Sueyoshi N, Kawai S et al. 1993 The Gamna–Gandy body in cardiac myxoma. Cardiovasc Pathol 2: 93–96
20. Lie J T 1993 Gamna–Gandy body of the heart: petrified cardiac myxoma mimicking atrial thrombus. Cardiovasc Pathol 2: 97–98
21. Loire R, Thermet H 1991 Les récidives des myxomes intracardiaques. A propos de 6 patients sur 85 opérés. Ann Cardiol Angéiol 40: 1–7
22. Gerbode F, Keith W J, Hill J D 1967 Surgical management of tumours of the heart. Surgery 61: 94–101
23. Kabbani S S, Cooley D A 1973 Atrial myxoma. Surgical considerations. J Thorac Cardiovasc Surg 65: 731–737
24. Read R C, White H J, Murphy M L et al. 1974 The malignant potentiality of left atrial myxoma. J Thorac Cardiovasc Surg 67: 857–868
25. McCarthy P M, Piehler J M, Schaff H V et al. 1986 The significance of multiple, recurrent, and "complex" cardiac myxomas. J Thorac Cardiovasc Surg 91: 389–396
26. Hedinger C 1987 Kombination von Herzmyxomen mit primärer nodulärer Dysplasie der Nebennierenrinde, fleckenförmigen hauptpigmentierungen und myxoartigen Tumoren anderer Lokalisation – ein eigenartiger familiärer Symptomenkomplex ("Swiss syndrome"). Schweiz Med Wochenschr 117: 591–594
27. Meyer B J, Weber R, Jenzer H R et al. 1990 Rapid growth and recurrence of atrial myxomas in two patients with Swiss syndrome. Am Heart J 120: 220–222
28. Martin L W, Wasserman A G, Goldstein H et al. 1987 Multiple cardiac myxomas with multiple recurrences: unusual presentation of a "benign" tumour. Ann Thorac Surg 44: 77–78
29. Kotani K, Matsuzawa Y, Funahashi T et al. 1991 Left atrial myxoma metastasizing to the aorta, with intraluminal growth causing renovascular hypertension. Cardiology 78: 72–77
30. Oemus K, Rath F W 1990 Subkutane Metastasen eines Vorhofmyxoms? Fallbericht und Literaturübersicht. Zentralbl Allg Pathol 136: 189–197
31. Loire R 1991 Existe-t-il une malignité carcinologique des myxomes cardiaques? Arch Mal Coeur 84: 395–399
32. Kasugai T, Sakurai M, Yutani C et al. 1990 Sequential malignant transformation of cardiac myxoma. Acta Pathol Jpn 40: 687–692
33. Laya M B, Mailliard J A, Bewtra C et al. 1987 Malignant fibrous histiocytoma of the heart. A case report and review of the literature. Cancer 59: 1026–1031
34. Scarpelli M, Montironi R, Ricciuti R et al. 1997 Cardiac myxoma with glandular elements metastatic to the brain 12 years after the removal of the original tumor. Clin Neuropathol 16: 190–194
35. Schweizer-Cagianut M, Froesh E R, Hedinger C 1980 Familial Cushing's syndrome with primary adrenocortical microadenomatosis (primary adrenocortical nodular dysplasia). Acta Endocrinol 94: 529–535
36. Schweizer-Cagianut M, Salomon F, Hedinger C E 1982 Primary adrenocortical nodular dysplasia with Cushing's syndrome and cardiac myxomas. A peculiar familial disease. Virchows Arch [A] 397: 183–192
37. Carney J A, Gordon H, Carpenter P C et al. 1985 The complex of myxomas, spotty pigmentation, and endocrine overactivity. Medicine 64: 270–283
38. Carney J A, Hruska L S, Beauchamp G D et al. 1986 Dominant inheritance of the complex of myxomas, spotty pigmentation, and endocrine overactivity. Mayo Clin Proc 61: 165–172
39. Panossian D H, Marais G E, Marais H J 1995 Familial endocrine myxolentiginosis. Clin Cardiol 18: 675–678
40. Carney J A 1995 Carney complex: the complex of myxomas, spotty pigmentation, endocrine overactivity, and schwannomas. Semin Dermatol 14: 900–908
41. Zamorano J, Vilacosta I, Almeria C et al. 1993 Diagnosis of mitral valve myxoma by transesophageal echocardiography. Eur Heart J 14: 862–863
42. Görlach G, Hagel K J, Mulch J et al. 1986 Myxoma of the aortic valve in a child. J Cardiovasc Surg 27: 679–680
43. Pessotto R, Santini F, Piccin C et al. 1994 Cardiac myxoma of the tricuspid valve: description of a case and review of the literature. J Heart Valve Dis 3: 344–346
44. Cole D J, Hendren W G, Sink J D et al. 1989 Myxoma attached solely to the tricuspid valve. Am J Cardiol 64: 546–547
45. Sharma S C, Kulkarni A, Bhargava V et al. 1991 Myxoma of tricuspid valve. J Thorac Cardiovasc Surg 101: 938–939
46. Kulshrestha P, Rousou J A, Tighe D A 1995 Mitral valve myxoma: a case report and brief review of the literature. J Heart Valve Dis 4: 196–198
47. Thorel C 1915 Geschwülste des Herzens. Ergeb Allg Pathol Anat 17: 667–687
48. Husten K 1922 Über Tumoren und Pseudotumoren des Endocards. Beitr Pathol Anat 71: 132–169
49. Salyer W R, Page D L, Hutchins G M 1975 The development of cardiac myxomas and papillary endocardial lesions from mural thrombus. Am Heart J 89: 4–17
50. Lie J T 1989 The identity and histogenesis of cardiac myxomas. A controversy put to rest. Arch Pathol Lab Med 113: 724–726
51. Prichard R W 1951 Tumours of the heart: review of the subject and report of one hundred and fifty cases. Arch Pathol 51: 98–128
52. Stein A A, Mauro J, Thibodeau L et al. 1969 The histogenesis of cardiac myxoma: relation to other proliferative diseases of subendothelial vasoformative reserve cells. In: Sommers SC (ed) Pathology annual. Appleton-Century-Crofts, New York, vol 4, p 293–312
53. Feldman P S, Horvath E, Kovacs K 1977 An ultrastructural study of seven cardiac myxomas. Cancer 40: 2216–2232
54. Deshpande A, Venugopal P, Kumar A S et al. 1996 Phenotypic characterization of cellular components of cardiac myxoma: a light microscopy and immunohistochemistry study. Hum Pathol 27: 1056–1059
55. Morales A R, Fine G, Castro A et al. 1981 Cardiac myxoma (endocardioma). An immunocytochemical assessment of histogenesis. Hum Pathol 12: 896–899
56. Berrutti L, Silverman J S 1996 Cardiac myxoma is rich in factor XIIIa positive dendrophages: immunohistochemical study of four cases. Histopathology 28: 529–535
57. Gabbiani G, Ryan G B, Majno G 1971 Presence of modified fibroblasts in granulation tissue and their possible role in wound contraction. Experientia 27: 549–550
58. Krikler D M, Rode J, Davies M J et al. 1992 Atrial myxoma: a tumour in search of its origins. Br Heart J 67: 89–91
59. Richkind K E, Wason D, Vidaillet H J 1994 Cardiac myxoma characterized by clonal telomeric association. Genes Chromos Cancer 9: 68–71
60. Dijkhuizen T, van den Berg E, Molenaar W M et al. 1995 Rearrangements involving 12p12 in two cases of cardiac myxoma. Cancer Genet Cytogenet 82: 161–162
61. Schultrich S 1990 Zur Histogenese der kardialen Myxome an hand eines Myxoms mit drüsenartigen Strukturen. Pathologe 11: 220–223
62. Pucci A, Bartoloni G, Tessitore E et al. 2003 Cytokeratin profile and neuroendocrine cells in the glandular component of cardiac myxoma. Virchows Arch 443: 618–624
63. Mohr H J, Kolmerer K H 1959 Fibro-adenomatöses, schleimbildendes Hamartom in der rechten Herzkammer. Zentralbl Allg Pathol 100: 142–149
64. Vacek R 1963 Das intrakardiale Hamartoblastom. Zentralbl Allg Pathol 104: 383–391
65. Suvarna S K, Royd J A 1996 The nature of the cardiac myxoma. Int J Cardiol 57: 211–216
66. Fenoglio J J Jr, McAllister H A Jr, Ferrans V J 1976 Cardiac rhabdomyoma: a clinicopathologic and electron microscopic study. Am J Cardiol 38: 241–251
67. Geva T, Santini F, Pear W et al. 1991 Cardiac rhabdomyoma. Rare cause of fetal death. Chest 99: 139–143
68. Bohm N, Krebs G 1980 Solitary rhabdomyoma of the heart: clinically silent case with sudden, unexpected death in an 11-month-old boy. Eur J Pediatr 144: 167–173

69. Grellner W, Henssge C 1996 Multiple cardiac rhabdomyoma with exclusively histological manifestation. Forensic Sci Int 78: 1–5
70. Bosi G, Lintermans J P, Pellegrino P A et al. 1996 The natural history of cardiac rhabdomyoma with and without tuberous sclerosis. Acta Pediatr 85: 928–931
71. Pillai R, Kharma N, Brom A G et al. 1991 Mitral valve origin of pedunculated rhabdomyomas causing subaortic stenosis. Am J Cardiol 67: 663–664
72. Schmincke A 1922 Kongenitale Herzhypertrophie, bedingt durch diffuse Rhabdomyobildung. Beitr Pathol Anat 70: 513–515
73. Shrivastava S, Jacks J J, White R S et al. 1977 Diffuse rhabdomyomatosis of the heart. Arch Pathol Lab Med 101: 78–80
74. Fine G 1974 Primary tumors of the pericardium and heart. In: Edwards J E, Lev M, Abell M R (eds) The heart. Williams & Wilkins, Baltimore, p 189–210
75. Burke A P, Virmani R 1991 Cardiac rhabdomyomas: a clinicopathologic study. Mod Pathol 4: 70–74
76. Steinbiss W 1923 Zur Kenntnis der Rhabdomyome des Herzens und ihrer Beziehungen zur tuberösen Gehirnsklerose. Virchows Archiv [A] 243: 22–38
77. Smith H C, Waston G H, Patel R G et al. 1989 Cardiac rhabdomyomata in tuberous sclerosis: their course and diagnostic value. Arch Dis Child 64: 196–200
78. Davies M J 1975 Tumours of the heart and pericardium. In: Pomerance A, Davies M J (eds) The pathology of the heart. Blackwell, Oxford, p 423–440
79. Wallace G, Smith H C, Watson G H et al. 1990 Tuberous sclerosis presenting with fetal and neonatal cardiac tumours. Arch Dis Child 65: 377–379
80. Matsuoka Y, Nakati T, Kawaguchi K et al. 1990 Disappearance of a cardiac rhabdomyoma complicating congenital mitral regurgitation as observed by serial two-dimensional echocardiography. Pediatr Cardiol 11: 98–101
81. Farooki Z Q, Ross R D, Paridon S M 1991 Spontaneous regression of cardiac rhabdomyoma. Am J Cardiol 67: 897–899
82. Nir A, Tajik A J, Freeman W K et al. 1995 Tuberous sclerosis and cardiac rhabdomyoma. Am J Cardiol 76: 419–421
83. DiMario F J Jr, Diana D, Leopold H et al. 1996 Evolution of cardiac rhabdomyoma in tuberous sclerosis complex. Clin Pediatr 35: 615–619
84. Fenoglio J J Jr, Diana D J, Bowen T E et al. 1977 Ultrastructure of cardiac rhabdomyoma. Hum Pathol 8: 700–706
85. Bruni C, Prioleau P G, Ivey H H et al. 1980 New fine structural features of cardiac rhabdomyoma. Report of a case. Cancer 46: 2068–2073
86. Green A J, Johnson P H, Yates J R 1994 The tuberous sclerosis gene on chromosome 9q34 acts as a growth suppressor. Hum Mol Genet 3: 1833–1834
87. Green A J, Smith M, Yates J R 1994 Loss of heterozygosity on chromosome 16p13.3 in hamartomas from tuberous sclerosis patients. Nat Genet 6: 193–196
88. Burke A P, Ribe J K, Bajaj A K et al. 1998 Hamartoma of mature cardiac myocytes. Hum Pathol 29: 904–909
89. Burke A P, Rosado-de-Christenson M, Templeton P A et al. 1994 Cardiac fibroma: clinicopathologic correlates and surgical treatment. J Thorac Cardiovasc Surg 108: 862–870
90. Sakata K, Ohtaki A, Aiba M et al. 1997 Left ventricular fibroma in an aged patient: report of a case. Surg Today 27: 88–89
91. Tahernia A C, Bricker J T, Ott D A 1990 Intracardiac fibroma in an asymptomatic infant. Clin Cardiol 13: 506–512
92. Van der Hauwaert L G, Corbeel L, Maldague P 1965 Fibroma of the right ventricle producing severe tricuspid stenosis. Circulation 32: 451–456
93. Feldman P S, Meyer M W 1976 Fibroelastic hamartoma (fibroma) of the heart. Cancer 38: 314–323
94. Turi G K, Albala A, Fenoglio J J Jr 1980 Cardiac fibromatosis: an ultrastructural study. Hum Pathol 11: 577–579
95. Churg A M, Kahn L B 1977 Myofibroblasts and related cells in malignant fibrous and fibrohistiocytic tumours. Hum Pathol 8: 205–218
96. Bertolini P, Meisner J, Paek S U et al. 1990 Special considerations on primary cardiac tumours in infancy and childhood. Thorac Cardiovasc Surg 38: 164–167
97. Cotton J L, Kavey R E W, Palmier C E et al. 1991 Cardiac tumours and the nevoid basal cell carcinoma syndrome. Pediatrics 87: 725–727
98. Littler B O 1979 Gorlin's syndrome and the heart. Br J Oral Surg 17: 135–146
99. Harris S A, Large D M 1984 Gorlin's syndrome with a cardiac lesion and jaw cysts with some unusual histologic features: a case report and review of the literature. Int J Oral Surg 13: 59–64
100. Jones K L, Wolf P L, Jensen P et al. 1986 The Gorlin syndrome: a genetically determined disorder associated with cardiac tumour. Am Heart J 111: 1013–1015
101. Coffin C M 1992 Case I congenital cardiac fibroma associated with Gorlin syndrome. Pediatr Pathol 12: 255–262
102. Gorlin R J 1987 Nevoid basal-cell carcinoma syndrome. Medicine 66: 98–113
103. Reiner L, Mazzoleni A, Rodriguez F L 1955 Statistical analysis of epicardial fat weight in human hearts. Arch Pathol 60: 369–373
104. Enzinger F M, Weiss S W 1988 Soft tissue tumours, 2nd edn. Mosby, St Louis, p 301–345
105. Harjola P T, Ala-Kulju K, Ketonen P 1985 Epicardial lipoma. Scand J Thorac Cardiovasc 19: 181–183
106. Rokey R, Mulvagh S L, Cheirif J et al. 1989 Lipomatous encasement and compression of the heart: antemortem diagnosis by cardiac nuclear magnetic resonance imaging and catheterization. Am Heart J 117: 952–953
107. Verkkala K, Kupari M, Maamies T et al. 1989 Primary cardiac tumors – operative treatment of 20 patients. Thorac Cardiovasc Surg 37: 361–364
108. Reece I J, Cooley D A, Frazier O H et al. 1984 Cardiac tumors. J Thorac Cardiovasc Surg 66: 439–446
109. Li J, Ho S Y, Becker A E, Jones H 1998 Multiple cardiac lipomas and sudden death: a case report and literature review. Cardiovasc Pathol 7: 51–55
110. Estevez J M, Thompson D S, Levinson J P 1964 Lipoma of the heart. Arch Pathol 77: 638–642
111. Harada K, Seki I, Kobayashi H et al. 1980 Lipoma of the heart in a child. Clinical, echocardiographic, angiographic, and pathological features. Jpn Heart J 21: 903–910
112. Pansard Y, Hvass U, de Brux J L et al. 1985 Lipome du ventricule droit. Ann Chir 39: 403–407
113. Pilichowski P, Wolf J E, Delgove L et al. 1987 Lipome du ventricule gauche. Ann Chir 41: 85–88
114. Bellin M, Lermuziaux J N, Fabiani J N et al. 1987 Lipome du coeur. Ann Chir 41: 405–410
115. Anderson D R, Gray M R 1988 Mitral incompetence associated with lipoma infiltrating the mitral valve. Br Heart J 60: 169–171
116. Reynen K, Rein J, Wittekind C et al. 1993 Surgical removal of a lipoma of the heart. Int J Cardiol 40: 67–68
117. Wajon E M C J, Jaarsma W, Knaepen P J et al. 1992 Lipoma of the heart. Neth J Cardiol 2: 63–67
118. Murphy E S, Fujii Y, Yasuda A et al. 1958 The tuberous sclerosis complex: a study of a new case. Arch Pathol 65: 166–173
119. Lie J T 1991 Cardiac, pulmonary, and vascular involvements in tuberous sclerosis. Ann NY Acad Sci 615: 58–70
120. Prior J T 1964 Lipomatous hypertrophy of the cardiac interatrial septum. A lesion resembling hibernoma, lipoblastomatosis and infiltrating lipoma. Arch Pathol 78: 11–15
121. Page D L 1970 Lipomatous hypertrophy of the cardiac interatrial septum. Its development and probable clinical significance. Hum Pathol 1: 151–163
122. Burke A P, Litovsky S, Virmani R 1996 Lipomatous hypertrophy of the atrial septum presenting as a right atrial mass. Am J Surg Pathol 20: 678–685
123. Inoue T, Mohri N, Nagahara T et al. 1988 A case report of "lipomatous hypertrophy of the cardiac interatrial septum," with a proposal for a new term "lipomatous hamartoma of the cardiac atrial septum." Acta Pathol Jpn 38: 1588–1589
124. Bhattacharjee M, Neligan M C, Dervan P 1991 Lipomatous hypertrophy of the interatrial septum: an unusual intraoperative finding. Br Heart J 65: 49–50
125. Crotty T B, Edwards W D, Oh J K et al. 1991 Lipomatous hamartoma of the tricuspid valve: echocardiographic–pathologic correlations. Clin Cardiol 14: 262–266
126. Behman R, Williams G, Gerlis L et al. 1983 Lipoma of the mitral valve and papillary muscle. Am J Cardiol 51: 1459–1460
127. Kindblom L G, Svensson L 1977 Multiple hibernomas of the heart. A case report. Acta Pathol Microbiol Scand 85: 122–126
128. Heifetz S A, Parikh S R, Brown J W 1990 Hibernoma of the pericardium presenting as pericardial effusion in a child. Pediatr Pathol 10: 575–580
129. Kurup A N, Tazalaar H D, Edwards W D et al. 2002 Iatrogenic cardiac papillary fibroelastoma: a study of 12 cases (1990–2000). Hum Pathol 33: 1165–1169
130. Arciniegas E, Hakimi M, Farooki Z Q et al. 1980 Primary cardiac tumours in children. J Thorac Cardiovasc Surg 79: 582–591
131. Heggtveit H A, Fenoglio J J, McAllister H A 1976 Lipomatous hypertrophy of the interatrial septum. An assessment of 41 cases. Lab Invest 34: 318 (abstract)
132. Corbi P, Jebara V, Fabiani J N et al. 1990 Les tumeurs bénignes du coeur (à l'exception des myxomes). Expérience de neuf cas opérés. Ann Cardiol Angéiol 39: 433–436
133. Cooley D A 1990 Surgical treatment of cardiac neoplasms: 32 year experience. Thorac Cardiovasc Surg 38: 176–182
134. Klarich K W, Enriquez-Sarano M, Gura G M et al. 1997 Papillary fibroelastoma: echocardiographic characteristics for diagnosis and pathologic correlation. J Am Coll Cardiol 30: 784–790
135. Sun J P, Asher C R, Yang X S et al. 2001 Clinical and echocardiographic characteristics of papillary fibroelastomas: a retrospective and prospective study in 162 patients. Circulation 203: 2687–2693
136. McFadden P M, Lacy J R 1987 Intracardiac papillary fibroelastoma: an occult cause of embolic neurologic deficit. Ann Thorac Surg 43: 667–669
137. Gowda R M, Khan J A, Nair C K et al. 2003 Cardiac papillary fibroelastoma: a comprehensive analysis of 725 cases. Am Heart J 146: 404–410
138. Valente M, Basso C, Thiene G et al. 1992 Fibroelastic papilloma: a not-so-benign cardiac tumour. Cardiovasc Pathol 1: 161–166
139. Wolfe J T III, Finck S J, Safford R E et al. 1991 Tricuspid valve papillary fibroelastoma: echocardiographic characterization. Ann Thorac Surg 51: 116–118
140. Etienne Y, Jobic Y, Houel J F et al. 1994 Papillary fibroelastoma of the aortic valve with myocardial infarction: echocardiographic diagnosis and surgical excision. Am Heart J 127: 443–445
141. Grote J, Mugge A, Schafers H J et al. 1995 Multiplane transoesophageal detection of a papillary fibroelastoma of the aortic valve causing myocardial infarction. Eur Heart J 16: 426–429
142. Eckstein F S, Schafers H J, Grote J et al. 1995 Papillary fibroelastoma of the aortic valve presenting with myocardial infarction. Ann Thorac Surg 60: 206–208

143. Pasteuning W H, Zijnen P, van der Aa M A et al. 1996 Papillary fibroelastoma of the aortic valve in a patient with an acute myocardial infarction. J Am Soc Echocardiogr 9: 897–900
144. Deodhar A P, Tometzki A J, Hudson I N et al. Aortic valve tumor causing acute myocardial infarction in a child. Ann Thorac Surg 64: 1482–1484
145. Chang Y-S, Chu P-H, Jung S-M et al. 2005 Unusual cardiac papillary fibroelastoma in the right ventricular outflow tract. Cardiovasc Pathol 14: 104–106
146. de Menezes I C, Fragata J, Martins F M 1996 Papillary fibroelastoma of the mitral valve in a 3-year-old child: case report. Pediatr Cardiol 17: 194–195
147. Heath D, Thompson I M 1965 Papillary "tumours" of the left ventricle. Br Heart J 29: 950–954
148. Fishbein M C, Ferrans V J, Roberts W C 1975 Endocardial papillary elastofibromas. Histologic, histochemical, and electron microscopical findings. Arch Pathol Lab Med 99: 335–341
149. Pomerance A 1961 Papillary "tumours" of the heart valves. J Pathol Bacteriol 81: 135–140
150. Rubin M A, Snell J A, Tazelaar H D et al. 1995 Cardiac papillary fibroelastoma: an immunohistochemical investigation and unusual clinical manifestations. Mod Pathol 8: 402–407
151. Butterworth J S, Poindexter C A 1973 Papilloma of cusp of the aortic valve: report of a patient with sudden death. Circulation 48: 213–215
152. Topol E J, Biern R O, Reitz B A 1986 Cardiac papillary fibroelastoma and stroke. Echocardiographic diagnosis and guide to excision. Am J Med 80: 129–132
153. Kasarskis E J, O'Connor W, Earle G 1988 Embolic stroke from cardiac papillary fibroelastomas. Stroke 19: 1171–1173
154. Witzleben C L, Pinto M 1978 Foamy myocardial transformation in infancy. Arch Pathol Lab Med 102: 306–311
155. MacMahon E H 1971 Infantile xanthomatous cardiomyopathy. Pediatrics 48: 312–315
156. Ferrans V J, McAllister H A Jr, Haese W H 1976 Infantile cardiomyopathy with histiocytoid change in cardiac muscle cells: report of six patients. Circulation 53: 708–719
157. Amini M, Bosman C, Marino B 1980 Histiocytoid cardiomyopathy in infancy: a new hypothesis. Chest 77: 556–558
158. Becker A E, Anderson R H 1981 Pathology of congenital heart disease. Butterworths, London, p 407–412
159. Silver M M, Burns J E, Sethi R K et al. 1980 Oncocytic cardiomyopathy in an infant with oncocytosis in exocrine and endocrine glands. Hum Pathol 11: 598–605
160. James T N, Beeson C W II, Sherman E B et al. 1975 De subitaneis mortibus. XIII. Multifocal Purkinje cell tumors of the heart. Circulation 52: 333–344
161. Garson A Jr, Smith R T Jr, Moak J P et al. 1987 Incessant ventricular tachycardia in infants: myocardial hamartomas and surgical cure. J Am Coll Cardiol 10: 619–626
162. Kearney D L, Titus J L, Hawkins E P et al. 1987 Pathologic features of myocardial hamartomas causing childhood tachyarrhythmias. Circulation 75: 705–710
163. Farooki Z Q, Chang C H, Jackson W L et al. 1988 Intracardiac teratoma in a newborn. Clin Cardiol 11: 642–644
164. Stoupel E, Primo G, Kahn R J 1979 Cardiac tamponade with renal failure due to haemangioma of the heart. Acta Cardiol 34: 345–351
165. Chao J C, Reyes C V, Hwang M H 1990 Cardiac hemangioma. South Med J 83: 44–47
166. Weir I, Mills P, Lewis T 1987 A case of left atrial haemangioma: echocardiographic, surgical, and morphological features. Br Heart J 58: 665–668
167. Case records of the Massachusetts General Hospital. Weekly clinicopathological exercises 1983. Case 4 – 1983. A 15-year-old girl with a right ventricular mass. N Engl J Med 308: 206–214
168. Chang J S, Young M L, Chuu W M et al. 1992 Infantile cardiac hemangioendothelioma. Pediatr Cardiol 13: 52–55
169. de Nictolis M, Brancorsini D, Goteri G et al. 1996 Epithelioid haemangioma of the heart. Virchows Arch 428: 119–123
170. Rosai J, Gold J, Landy D 1979 The histiocytoid hemangiomas: a unifying concept embracing several previously described entities of skin, soft tissue, large vessels, bone and heart. Hum Pathol 10: 707–730
171. Fletcher C D M, Beham A, Bekir S et al. 1991 Epithelioid angiosarcoma of deep soft tissue: a distinctive tumor readily mistaken for an epithelial neoplasm. Am J Surg Pathol 15: 915–924
172. Weiss S W, Ishak K G, Dail D H 1986 Epithelioid hemangioendothelioma and related lesions. Semin Diagn Pathol 3: 259–287
173. Mentzel T, Beham A, Calonje E et al. 1997 Epithelioid hemangioendothelioma of skin and soft tissues: clinicopathologic and immunohistochemical study of 30 cases. Am J Surg Pathol 21: 363–374
174. Weiss S W, Enzinger F M 1982 Epithelioid hemangioendothelioma: a vascular tumor often mistaken for a carcinoma. Cancer 50: 970–981
175. Kuo T, Hsueh S, Su I et al. 1985 Histiocytoid hemangioma of the heart with peripheral eosinophilia. Cancer 55: 2854–2861
176. Luthringer D J, Virmani R, Weiss S W et al. 1990 A distinctive cardiovascular lesion resembling histiocytoid (epithelioid) hemangioma. Evidence suggesting mesothelial participation. Am J Surg Pathol 14: 993–1000
177. Palmer T E, Tresch D D, Bonchek L I 1986 Spontaneous resolution of a large, cavernous hemangioma of the heart. Am J Cardiol 58: 184–185
178. Tabry I F, Nassar V H, Rizk G et al. 1975 Cavernous haemangioma of the heart: case report and review of the literature. J Thorac Cardiovasc Surg 69: 415–420
179. Veinot J P, Tazelaar H D, Edwards W D, Colby T V 1994 Mesothelial/monocytic incidental cardiac excrescences: cardiac MICE. Mod Pathol 7: 9–16
180. Armstrong H, Mönckeberg J G 1911 Herzblock, bedingt durch primären Herztumor bei einem 5-jährigen Kinde. Dtsch Arch Klin Med 102: 144–166
181. Mahaim I 1942 Le coelethéliome tawarien bénin. Une tumeur sui generis du noeud de Tawara, avec bloc du coeur. Cardiologia 6: 57–82
182. Rezek P 1938 Über eine primäre epitheliale Geschwulst in der Gegend des Reizleitungssystems beim Menschen (Zugleich ein Beitrag zur Histiogenese seltener Herzgeschwülste). Virchows Arch [A] 301: 305–320
183. Linder J, Shelburne J D, Sorge J P et al. 1984 Congenital endodermal heterotopia of the atrioventricular node: evidence for the endodermal origin of so-called mesotheliomas of the atrioventricular node. Hum Pathol 15: 1093–1098
184. Burke A P, Anderson P G, Virmani R et al. 1990 Tumors of the atrioventricular nodal region. A clinical and immunohistochemical study. Arch Pathol Lab Med 114: 1057–1062
185. Sopher I M, Spitz W E 1971 Endodermal inclusion of the heart. So-called mesotheliomas of the atrioventricular node. Arch Pathol 92: 180–186
186. Travers H 1982 Congenital polycystic tumour of the atrioventricular node: possible familial occurrence and critical review of reported cases with special emphasis on histogenesis. Hum Pathol 13: 25–35
187. Cameselle-Teijeiro J, Abdulkader I, Soares P et al. 2005 Cystic tumor of the atrioventricular node of the heart appears to be the heart equivalent of the solid cell nests (ultimobranchial rests) of the thyroid. Am J Clin Pathol 123: 369–375
188. Wolf P L, Bing R 1965 The smallest tumor which causes sudden death. JAMA 194: 674–675
189. James T N, Galakhov I 1977 De subitaneis mortibus XXVI. Fatal electrical instability of the heart associated with benign congenital polycystic tumour of the atrioventricular node. Circulation 56: 667–678
190. Bharati S, Bauernfeind R, Josephson M 1995 Intermittent preexcitation and mesothelioma of the atrioventricular node: a hitherto undescribed entity. J Cardiovasc Electrophysiol 6: 823–831
191. Becker A E 1966 The glomera in the region of the heart and great vessels. A microscopic-anatomical and histochemical study. Pathol Eur 1: 410–424
192. Lack E E 1997 Tumors of the adrenal gland and extra-adrenal paraganglia. Atlas of tumor pathology, series 3, fascicle 19. Armed Forces Institute of Pathology, Washington DC
193. Besterman E, Bromley L L, Peart W S 1974 An intrapericardial phaeochromocytoma. Br Heart J 36: 318–320
194. Johnson T L, Shapiro B, Beierwaltes W H et al. 1985 Cardiac paragangliomas. A clinicopathologic and immunohistochemical study of four cases. Am J Surg Pathol 9: 827–834
195. Hui G, McAllister H A, Angelini P 1987 Left atrial paraganglioma: report of a case and review of the literature. Am Heart J 114: 1230–1234
196. Stowers S A, Gilmore P, Stirling M et al. 1987 Cardiac pheochromocytoma involving the left main coronary artery presenting with exertional angina. Am Heart J 114: 423–427
197. Shimoyama Y, Kawada K, Imamura H 1987 A functioning intrapericardial paraganglioma (pheochromocytoma). Br Heart J 57: 380–383
198. Chang C H, Lin P J, Chang J P et al. 1991 Intrapericardial pheochromocytoma. Ann Thorac Surg 51: 661–663
199. Aravot D J, Banner N R, Cantor A M et al. 1992 Location, localization and surgical treatment of cardiac pheochromocytoma. Am J Cardiol 69: 283–285
200. Gaylis H, Mieny C J 1977 The incidence of malignancy in carotid body tumours. Br J Surg 64: 885–889
201. Rosenquist G C, Krovetz L J, Haller J A Jr et al. 1970 Acquired right ventricular outflow obstruction in a child with neurofibromatosis. Am Heart J 79: 103–108
202. Lanks K W, Lautsch E V 1966 Pathogenesis of intramyocardial epithelial inclusion cysts. Arch Pathol 81: 365–367
203. Rose A G, Novitzky D, Price S K 1988 Heterotopic thyroid tissue in the heart. J Cardiovasc Pathol 1: 401–404
204. Natarajan S, Luthringer DJ, Fishbein MC 1997 Adenomatoid tumor of the heart: report of a case. Am J Surg Pathol 21: 1378–1380
205. Burke A P, Cowan D, Virmani R 1992 Primary sarcomas of the heart. Cancer 69: 387–395
206. Putnam J B Jr, Sweeney M S, Colon R et al. 1991 Primary cardiac sarcomas. Ann Thorac Surg 51: 906–910
207. Tazelaar H A, Locke T J, McGregor CGA 1992 Pathology of surgically excised primary cardiac tumors. Mayo Clin Proc 67: 957–965
208. Fletcher C D M 1992 Pleomorphic malignant fibrous histiocytoma: fact or fiction? A critical reappraisal based upon 159 tumors diagnosed as pleomorphic sarcoma. Am J Surg Pathol 16: 213–228
209. McAllister H A 1979 Primary tumours of the heart and pericardium. Pathol Ann 14: 325–355
210. Chitwood W R Jr 1988 Cardiac neoplasms: current diagnosis, pathology, and therapy. J Cardiac Surg 3: 119–154
211. Randall M B, Geisinger K R 1990 Angiosarcoma of the heart: pericardial fluid cytology. Diagn Cytopathol 6: 58–62
212. Löffler H, Grille W 1990 Classification of malignant cardiac tumours with respect to oncological treatment. Thorac Cardiovasc Surg 38 (suppl. 2): 196–199

213. Makhoul N, Bode F R 1995 Angiosarcoma of the heart: review of the literature and report of two cases that illustrate the broad spectrum of the disease. Can J Cardiol 11: 423–428
214. Sorlie D, Myhre E S, Stalsberg H 1984 Angiosarcoma of the heart. Unusual presentation and survival after treatment. Br Heart J 51: 94–97
215. Percy R F, Perryman R A, Amornmarn R et al. 1987 Prolonged survival in a patient with primary angiosarcoma of the heart. Am Heart J 113: 1228–1230
216. Hager W, Kremer K, Müller W 1970 Angiosarkom des Herzens. Dtsch Med Wochenschr 95: 680
217. Poletti A, Cocco P, Valente M et al. 1993 In vivo diagnosis of cardiac angiosarcoma by endomyocardial biopsy. Cardiovasc Pathol 2: 89–91
218. Shah A A, Churg A, Sbarbaro J A et al. 1978 Malignant fibrous histiocytoma of the heart presenting as an atrial myxoma. Cancer 42: 2466–2471
219. Weiss S W, Enzinger F M 1977 Myxoid variant of malignant fibrous histiocytoma. Cancer 39: 1672–1685
220. Ouzan J, Joundi A, Chapoutot L et al. 1990 Histiocytofibrome malin du coeur simulant un myxome de l'oreillette gauche. Arch Mal Coeur 83: 1011–1014
221. Pasquale M, Katz N M, Caruso A C et al. 1991 Myxoid variant of malignant fibrous histiocytoma of the heart. Am Heart J 122: 248–250
222. Korbmacher B, Doering C, Schulte H D et al. 1992 Malignant fibrous histiocytoma of the heart – case report of a rare left-atrial tumour. Thorac Cardiovasc Surg 40: 303–307
223. Wahba A, Liebold A, Birnbaum D E 1993 Recurrent malignant fibrous histiocytoma of the left atrium in a 27-year-old male. Eur J Cardiothorac Surg 7: 387–389
224. Hui K S, Green L K, Schmidt W A 1988 Primary cardiac rhabdomyosarcoma: definition of a rare entity. Am J Cardiovasc Pathol 2: 19–29
225. Hajar R, Roberts W C, Folger G M Jr 1986 Embryonal botryoid rhabdomyosarcoma of the mitral valve. Am J Cardiol 57: 376
226. Small E, Gordon G J, Barrett Dahms B 1985 Malignant rhaboid tumor of the heart in an infant. Cancer 55: 2850–2853
227. Haas J E, Palmer N F, Weinberg A G et al. 1981 Ultrastructure of malignant rhabdoid tumor of the kidney: a distinctive renal tumor in children. Hum Pathol 12: 646–657
228. Donsbeck A-V, Ranchere D, Coindre J M et al. 1999 Primary cardiac sarcomas: an immunohistochemical and grading study with long-term follow-up of 24 cases. Histopathology 34: 295–304
229. Itoh K, Matsumura T, Egawa Y et al. 1998 Primary mitral valve sarcoma in infancy. Pediatr Cardiol 19: 174–177
230. Becker A E, van der Wal A C 1998 Leiomyosarcoma on an infant's mitral valve. Pediatr Cardiol 19: 193
231. Pins M R, Ferrell M A, Madsen J C et al. 1999 Epithelioid and spindle cell leiomyosarcoma of the heart. Report of two cases and review of the literature. Arch Pathol Lab Med 123: 782–788
232. Antunes M J, Vanderdonck K M, Andrade C M et al. 1991 Primary cardiac leiomyosarcomas. Ann Thorac Surg 51: 999–1001
233. Fyfe A I, Huckell V F, Burr L H et al. 1991 Leiomyosarcoma of the left atrium: case report and review of the literature. Can J Cardiol 7: 193–196
234. Paraf F, Bruneval P, Balaton A et al. 1990 Primary liposarcoma of the heart. Am J Cardiovasc Pathol 3: 175–180
235. Burke A P, Virmani R 1991 Osteosarcomas of the heart. Am J Surg Pathol 51: 289–295
236. Muir C S, Seah C S 1966 Primary chondrosarcomatous mesenchymoma of the mitral valve. Thorax 21: 254–262
237. Tsai F C, Lin P J, Wu W J 1996 Primary chondrosarcoma of the heart: a case report. Chang Keng I Hsueh 19: 348–351
238. Miwa S, Konishi Y, Matsumoto M et al. 1997 Primary cardiac chondrosarcoma – a case report. Jpn Circ J 61: 795–797
239. Nicholson A G, Rigby M, Lincoln C et al. 1997 Synovial sarcoma of the heart. Histopathology 30: 349–352
240. Sheffield E A, Corrin B, Addis B J et al. 1988 Synovial sarcoma of the heart arising from a so-called mesothelioma of the atrioventricular node. Histopathology 12: 191–202
241. Guschmann M, Weng Y 1996 Primare multiple maligne Schwannome im Herzen – eine Raritat. Pathologe 17: 222–226
242. Chun P K C, Leeburg W T, Coggin J T et al. 1980 Primary pericardial epithelial mesothelioma causing acute myocardial infarction. Chest 77: 559–561
243. Sytman A L, MacAlpin R B 1971 Primary pericardial mesothelioma: report of 2 cases and review of the literature. Am Heart J 81: 760–769
244. Klima M, Spjut H J, Seybold W D 1976 Diffuse malignant mesothelioma. Am J Clin Pathol 65: 583–600
245. McDonnell P J, Mann R B, Bulkley B H 1982 Involvement of the heart by malignant lymphoma. A clinicopathologic study. Cancer 49: 944–951
246. Curtsinger C R, Wilson M J, Yoneda K 1989 Primary cardiac lymphoma. Cancer 64: 521–525
247. Zaharia L, Gill S 1991 Primary cardiac lymphoma. Am J Clin Oncol 14: 142–145
248. Chalabreysse L, Berger F, Leire R et al. 2002 Primary cardiac lymphoma in immunocompetent patients: a report of three cases and review of the literature. Virchows Arch 441: 456–461
249. Ceresoli G L, Ferreri A J, Bucci E et al. 1997 Primary cardiac lymphoma in immunocompetent patients: diagnostic and therapeutic management. Cancer 80: 1497–1506

脉管肿瘤
Vascular tumors

Eduardo Calonje 和 Christopher D. M. Fletcher 著

谢大鹤 译　戴 林 校

引言	41
良性血管肿瘤	41
反应性血管增生	41
血管扩张性病变	43
毛细血管瘤	45
海绵状血管瘤	48
上皮样血管瘤	51
深部血管瘤	54
中间恶性血管肿瘤	55
Kaposi样血管内皮瘤	56
网状血管内皮瘤	57
淋巴管内乳头状血管内皮瘤	57
复合性血管内皮瘤	58
Kaposi肉瘤（KS）	58
恶性血管肿瘤	62
上皮样血管内皮瘤	62
血管肉瘤	63
淋巴管肿瘤	67
血管周细胞肿瘤	70
血管球肿瘤	70
血管外皮瘤	72

引言

几乎没有哪一类肿瘤能像血管肿瘤那样，在组织形态和临床行为上表现出如此宽泛的谱系特征。其分类（之所以）能成为问题，不仅是因为在肿瘤和畸形（或所谓错构瘤）之间的划界尚属不明，而且更重要的是因为（血管）病变的良恶性鉴别实属不易。值得注意的是，同其他软组织肿瘤相比，在血管病变，细胞发生学和分子遗传学研究几乎未能提供任何有用的信息，这主要是因为血管肿瘤很难在（组织）培养中生长、发育；再有就是因为可用材料大都是混合性（生物）标本，人们无法将其非肿瘤性组织成分完全剔除。本章采用的是血管肿瘤的最新分类，其中包括最近被描述的病变实体，并根据生物学研究最新进展，对某些已知病变做重新分类（表3-1）。重点放在软组织和皮肤病变，因为这些部位血管肿瘤较为常见。其他器官的特殊血管肿瘤请参阅相关章节。

良性血管肿瘤 Benign tumors

反应性血管增生 Reactive vascular proliferations

血管内乳头状内皮细胞增生（Masson瘤） Intravascular papillary endothelial hyperplasia (Masson's tumor)

临床特征

血管内乳头状内皮细胞增生[1-5]是一种比较常见的反应性病变，是机化血栓的一种少见形式。它可见于三种不同情况：(1)仅累及某孤立扩张血管的单纯型病变（原发性）；(2)在多种原有病变（如血管瘤、痔疮和静脉曲张）基础上发生的局灶性病变（继发性）；(3)一种少见的与血肿并发的血管外病变[5]。外伤与上述任何形式的病变似均无稳定相关。典型的原发性病变表现为一无症状的蓝色结节，好发于年轻成人的指趾或头颈部，无性别差异。有报道称，此类病变亦可发生于乳腺，而

表3.1	脉管肿瘤的分类
血管 *良性肿瘤和瘤样病变* 反应性血管增生 　　乳头状内皮细胞增生（Masson瘤） 　　反应性血管内皮细胞瘤病 　　肾小球样血管瘤 　　杆菌性血管瘤病 血管扩张性病变 　　焰色痣（鲑鱼色斑、葡萄酒色痣） 　　蛛状痣 　　静脉湖 　　匐行性血管瘤 　　遗传性出血性毛细血管扩张（Osler-Weber- 　　　Rendu） 　　血管角质瘤 毛细血管瘤 　　亚型：　丛状血管瘤 　　　　　疣状血管瘤 　　　　　樱桃状血管瘤 　　　　　小叶性毛细血管瘤(化脓性肉芽肿) 海绵状血管瘤 　　亚型：　窦状血管瘤 动静脉血管瘤 　　亚型：　浅表（曲张动脉瘤） 　　　　　深部 微静脉型血管瘤 钉突样（靶样含铁血黄素沉着性）血管瘤 获得性弹力纤维性血管瘤 皮肤上皮样血管（瘤样）结节 上皮样血管瘤（嗜酸细胞增多性血管淋巴样增生） 静脉性血管瘤 梭形细胞血管瘤（血管内皮细胞瘤） 深部血管瘤 　　亚型：　肌内 　　　　　滑膜 　　　　　神经 　　　　　房室结 血管瘤病	*交界型血管肿瘤* 局部浸润型： 　　Kaposi样血管内皮瘤 　　巨细胞血管母细胞瘤 很少转移型： 　　网状血管内皮瘤 　　恶性血管内乳头状血管内皮瘤（Dabska瘤） 　　复合性血管内皮瘤 　　多形性血管内皮瘤 　　Kaposi肉瘤 *恶性血管肿瘤* 上皮样血管内皮瘤 血管肉瘤 　　亚型：　特发性（头颈部） 　　　　　合并淋巴水肿（"淋巴管肉瘤"） 　　　　　放射后 　　　　　软组织 　　　　　上皮样 "血管内膜"肉瘤 **淋巴管** 淋巴管瘤 　　亚型：　局限性淋巴管瘤 　　　　　海绵状淋巴管瘤/囊性水瘤 　　　　　良性淋巴管内皮瘤（获得性进行性 　　　　　　淋巴管瘤） 淋巴管瘤病 淋巴管肌瘤 淋巴管肌瘤病 **血管周细胞肿瘤** 血管球瘤 血管球血管瘤病 　　亚型：　浸润型血管球瘤 血管球血管肉瘤 所谓"血管外皮细胞瘤" 肌周细胞瘤

且，在这种情况下，它与血管肉瘤之间可能难以鉴别[6]。病变直径一般小于2cm，切除后很少复发。多发性病变并不常见，少数多发性个案与随后的β-干扰素治疗有关[7,8]。如果乳头状内皮细胞增生发生于原有血管病变基础之上，其临床表现则与原发性血管异常有关，而且该病变的范围趋向增大。这些继发性病变在理论上可发生于任何血管瘤基础之上，出现在任何解剖部位，但它与深部血管瘤，尤其是海绵状血管瘤的相关性尤为密切。

组织学形态

原发性病变多为边界清楚的出血性病变，仔细观察可见原固有的扩张血管腔，而且大都是薄壁静脉。继发性病变的形态取决于此前原位原发性病变的性质。在血管外病变，即便是在连续切片，也无明显血管结构可寻。所有（病变）形式的诊断性特征都是多发性小乳头状结构，被覆单层、扁平、无明显异型性的内皮细胞（图3.1），多无核分裂象；乳头芯由无细胞的玻璃样变性的胶原构成，其间偶有细小的毛细血管。在病变最早期，这些乳头似由纤维蛋白构成。虽然很多乳头都好像是游离于血管腔内，但其中部分乳头却附着于血管壁。乳头周围聚有大量红细胞，大都伴有血栓形成，并可表现有不同程度的机化。在血栓边缘地带，可见纤维蛋白样乳头形成的早期形态。

鉴别诊断

高分化血管肉瘤所在临床背景不同，而且一般都是血管外病变，并以浸润性或裂隙状生长方式、中重度

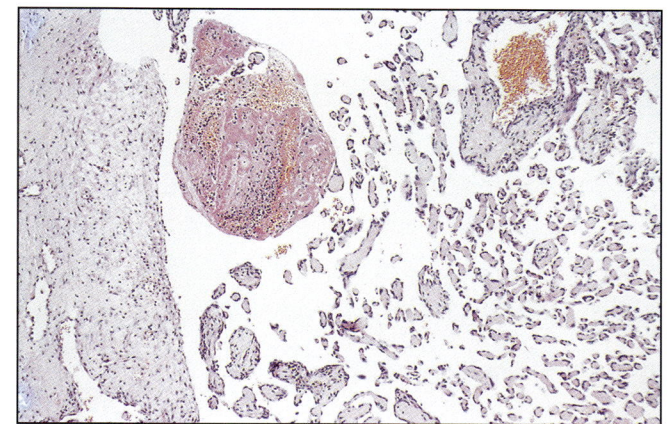

图3.1 Masson瘤（血管内乳头状内皮细胞增生）。注意：典型的半透明状乳头及其邻近的血栓。

细胞异型性、内皮细胞多层化和核分裂活跃为其特征。

反应性血管内皮细胞瘤病 Reactive angioendotheliomatosis

临床特征

直到20世纪80年代初，血管内皮细胞瘤病一直按惯例被分为恶性和良性两类。据信，认为有时仅根据临床表现和组织学形态，很难在二者之间做出鉴别。但现已明确：其恶性病变实际上是系统性亲血管性淋巴瘤（预后差，参阅第21章），与反应性病变完全无关；而后者确属起源于内皮细胞的自限性病变，一般仅局限于皮肤[9,10]。临床上，反应性血管内皮细胞瘤病非常少见，病变表现为红色斑疹、丘疹或斑块，而且可能合并有各种瘀斑、瘀点，但很少呈网状青斑（livedo，属小血管内膜炎，如冷凝球蛋白血症的大理石彩斑状皮肤病变，寒冷时发病，气温升高后消退—译者注）样改变。无年龄差异，但患者大都为成人，儿童很少受累[11]。本病可为特发性，亦可与多种系统性疾病有关，如副蛋白血症、肾病、淀粉样变性病、抗磷脂综合征、风湿性关节炎、肝硬化、风湿性多肌痛和结节病[10,12-16]。不过，与系统性疾病，尤其是与细菌性心内膜炎的相关性并不像此前所认为的那样密切。反应性血管内皮细胞瘤病的一个亚型被描述为：冷凝球蛋白血症患者的血管瘤病，伴管腔内冷凝蛋白沉积[17]。本病的临床病理谱系现已被扩展到涵盖其少见的局灶性病变，包括一个合并有周围血管动脉粥样硬化性疾病和医源性动静脉瘘的亚型，冠名为弥漫性皮肤血管瘤病[18-21]。

组织学形态

在真皮和皮下组织浅层，可见有多个排列密集的毛细血管丛（图3.2），毛细血管内皮细胞较正常者为大，无细胞异型性，管腔外被周细胞。很多病变具有明显的

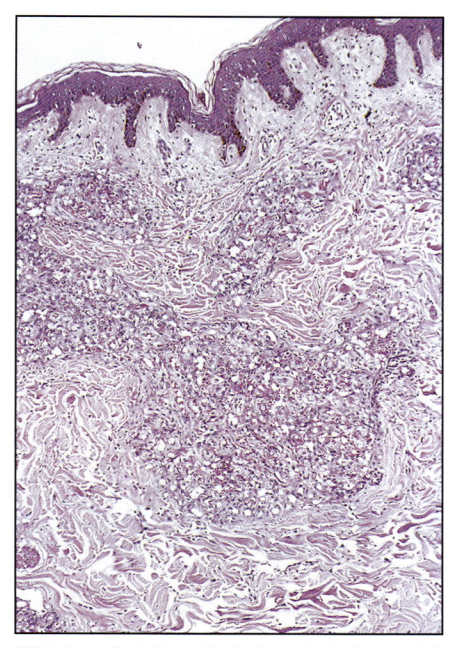

图3.2 反应性血管内皮细胞瘤病。可见多个形状不规则的毛细血管丛，丛中毛细血管排列紧密，贯通成形的程度不等。

小叶状结构。（肥大的）内皮细胞可能会将管腔闭塞，但无多层化现象。局部可见红细胞溢出，偶可见纤维素性血栓。真皮附近呈轻度慢性炎症，有时可伴有筋膜炎样改变。在伴有管腔内冷凝蛋白沉积的血管瘤病，很多毛细血管都被有折光性的嗜酸性血栓栓塞。在弥漫性真皮血管瘤病，可见大量尚未贯通成形的毛细血管增生。

肾小球样血管瘤 Glomeruloid hemangioma

肾小球样血管瘤是一种独特的反应性血管增生，可见于多中心性Castleman病和POEMS综合征（多发性神经病、器官肿大、内分泌病、M-球蛋白病和皮肤病变）患者[22-25]。临床上，患者表现为多发性皮肤血管瘤，组织学检查呈现樱桃状血管瘤或肾小球样血管瘤的形态特征，后者不太常见。镜下可见多个扩张的血管腔，尤其是在真皮浅层，腔内含有毛细血管丛，其形态酷似肾小球（图3.3）。毛细血管周围分布有周细胞和大圆形细胞，后者胞浆透明，偶可见PAS阳性的毛玻璃样小体，可能就是免疫球蛋白沉积物。这些大圆形细胞呈内皮细胞标记物阳性。肾小球样血管瘤病变中尚无人类疱疹病毒-8（HHV-8）的检出记录[26]。

血管扩张性病变 Vascular ectasias

与真性血管瘤不同，血管扩张性病变[27-29]并不表现为血管数量的增加，病变主要是由扩张的、固有的正常血管构成。但有些血管扩张性病变可能合并一个基础性的海绵状血管瘤或动静脉畸形[30]。血管扩张性病变包括焰色痣（鲑鱼色斑，葡萄酒色斑痣）、蛛状痣、静脉湖、匐

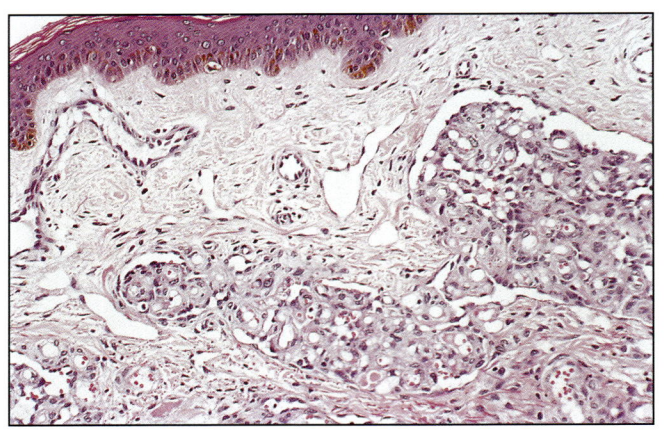

图3.3 肾小球样血管瘤。毛细血管丛呈小叶状凸入原有的血管管腔中。注意：（毛细血管之间大圆形细胞胞浆中的毛玻璃样）嗜酸性小球。

行性血管瘤和血管角质瘤。

焰色痣　Nevus flammeus

焰色痣包括鲑鱼色斑和葡萄酒色斑痣，这两种病变也被称为胎记（或胎痣），可见于约半数的新生儿[31]。鲑鱼色斑以粉红色、无凸起、位于头颈部、并随时间的推进而逐渐消退为其特征。与之相反，葡萄酒色斑痣则呈进行性生长，并无消退倾向，且可逐渐凸出体表。绝大多数焰色痣都是先天性病变，但文献上也有少数获得性病变的记载，包括一例发生在创伤后的个案[32]。家族性患者亦有发生，其（主控）基因已被定位于染色体5q[33,34]。在Sturge-Weber综合征（颅-眼-颜面血管瘤病综合征），葡萄酒色斑痣可能合并脑膜、大脑或视网膜的血管畸形；在Klippel-Trenaunay综合征（静脉曲张性骨肥大血管痣综合征），葡萄酒色斑痣可能合并肢体肥大、静脉曲张和部分静脉发育不全。后者如果合并动静脉瘘，则被称为Parke-Weber综合征。还有几种血管病变，尤其是化脓性肉芽肿和个别丛状血管瘤，可能会出现在葡萄酒色斑痣之中[35-37]。组织学上，这两种病变都表现为口径不等的真皮血管扩张（图3.4），

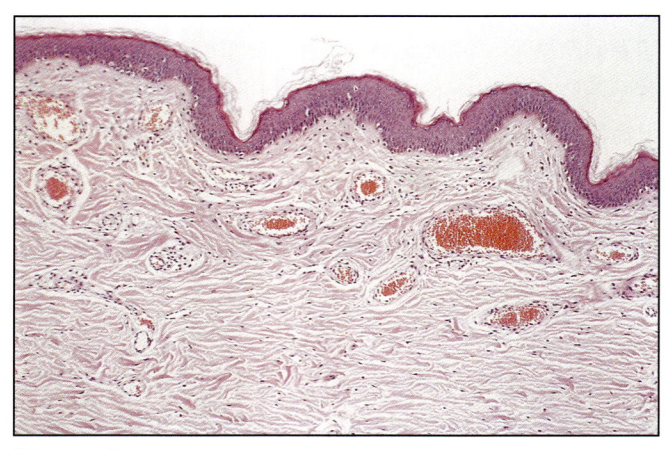

图3.4 葡萄酒色斑痣。扩张的薄壁血管均匀分布于真皮浅层。

在葡萄酒色斑痣，病变还常累及到皮下深层。

蛛状痣　Nevus araneus（spider nevus）

蛛状痣是非常常见的获得性病变，发病年龄跨度很宽，病变形态表现为红色针头样小丘疹，由此，有曲折血管向其四周发散。蛛状痣常并发于妊娠、慢性肝病和甲亢。典型的组织学形态是：在真皮浅层可见一扩张的、并与许多互相吻合的毛细血管沟通的厚壁动脉。

静脉湖　Venous lake

在老年人，静脉湖[38]是常见的静脉扩张性病变，阳光直射部位受累，尤其是面部，其中以唇、耳最为常见。组织学上，在真皮浅层可见一高度扩张的充血静脉，其周围环绕层数（厚薄）不等的平滑肌组织。

匐行性血管瘤　Angioma serpiginosum

匐行性血管瘤[39,42]是一种进展缓慢的少见病变，主要累及儿童，尤其是女孩下肢。皮损为微小的紫红色（斑点或）丘疹，呈螺旋状或匐行状排列；偶见线状排列者[43]。眼及中枢神经系统受累者多属个案[44,45]。家族性病例非常罕见[46]。单个病损的组织形态表现为真皮乳头中的小血管扩张。

遗传性出血性毛细血管扩张
Hereditary hemorrhagic telangiectasia（Osler-Weber-Rendu）

遗传性出血性毛细血管扩张[47]是一种常染色体显性遗传性疾病，以皮肤、黏膜和体内器官，尤其是胃肠道和肺出现多发性毛细血管扩张为特征。此病变可能合并有动静脉血管畸形。组织学上，受累脏器中可见有高度扩张的毛细血管和小静脉。

血管角质瘤　Angiokeratoma

血管角质瘤[48]并非真性血管肿瘤，而是代表一种合并有疣状表皮改变的浅表血管扩张性病变。临床可分为四型：

1. 与Fabry病（酰基鞘氨醇己三糖苷脂沉积症，伴性隐性遗传，临床表现为弥漫性皮肤血管角质瘤和发作性肢体疼痛；后期常有肾、心、脑血管的进行性损害—译者注）有关的弥漫性躯体血管角质瘤。其中，多发性血管角质瘤出现在儿童期晚期。Fabry病是因先天性溶酶体酶α-半乳糖苷酶A缺乏所致，但并非所有弥漫性躯体血管角质瘤患者都是Fabry病患者。同样的病变还可见于其他一些酶缺乏疾病，如α-L-岩藻糖苷酶[49]、β-甘露糖苷酶[50]、α-N-乙酰氨基半乳糖苷酶[51,52]、β-半乳糖苷酶[53]，亦可见于某些酶活性正常的患者[54]。

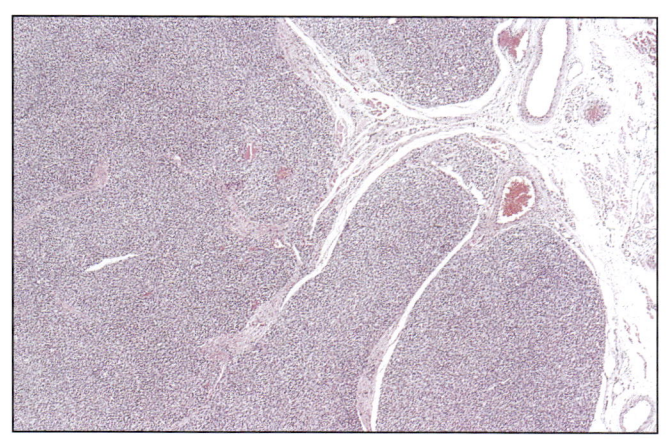

A

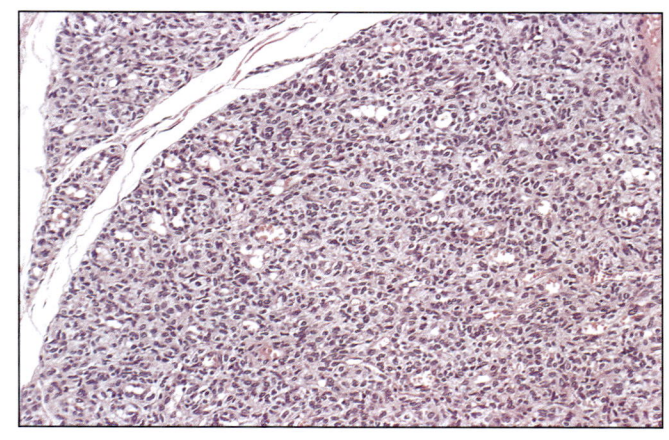

B

图3.5 毛细血管瘤（婴幼儿血管内皮细胞瘤）。注意其小叶状生长方式（A）和排列紧密的、基本尚未开通的毛细血管（B）。

2. Mibelli血管角质瘤，以双侧指、趾背面的丘疹为其特征[55]。
3. Fordyce血管角质瘤，专指发生在阴囊或是外阴的病变，后者较少见[56,57]。
4. 孤立性血管角质瘤[58]。

以上四型的组织学改变都一样。在Fabry病，表皮病变大都很轻，脂质沉积以胞浆空泡的形式出现在皮肤病变处的血管内皮细胞、周细胞和纤维母细胞[59]。它与疣状血管瘤之间的鉴别将在下文讨论。

毛细血管瘤 Capillary hemangioma

临床特征

毛细血管瘤[27-29,60]是婴幼儿期最为常见的良性血管肿瘤，每100个成活婴儿中就有1人罹病[29]，占所有血管瘤的32%～42%[27,60]。几乎所有脏器均可受累，但最常见于皮肤和软组织，尤以头颈部为最。

在婴幼儿，毛细血管瘤亦被称为婴幼儿细胞性血管瘤、婴幼儿血管内皮细胞瘤、草莓状痣或婴幼儿血管瘤。女性患者略多于男性。皮损表现为围生期的紫红色皮肤色斑，渐有隆起，此后数月至数年间，70%以上的病变都会逐渐消退[61]。大的病变多有损形象，但血管瘤若靠近机体关键结构，则可导致（相关疾病的）高发率。

组织学形态

毛细血管瘤的组织学特征随病变的进展而有所变化。低倍镜下，所有毛细血管瘤的总体结构，无论何种器官受累，都呈多叶状肿瘤形态（图3.5）。病变早期，小叶呈高度细胞性，由核分裂活跃的球形内皮细胞构成，这些内皮细胞围成微小、圆形、尚未开通的血管腔（图3.5）。因此，在病变最早期，肿瘤的内皮细胞性质很可能不会直接显现。随着病变的成熟，血管逐渐被开通，识别也就愈加容易；此后大都会出现管腔充血、内皮细胞变扁。在靠近肿瘤处，常可找到一支小的（通入肿瘤的）营养血管。比较陈旧性的病变则逐步被纤维化，其血管成分甚至会部分或全部消失。在婴幼儿病例，神经束膜的侵入并不少见，但这并不意味着它的恶性行为[62,63]。

网状蛋白染色有助于突显小管状的血管结构，尤其是在未成熟的实性病变（图3.6）。虽然在组织学上，未成熟的毛细血管瘤好像只是由内皮细胞构成，但电镜和免疫组化研究证实，其中还有大量其他种类的细胞，包括纤维母细胞、周细胞和肥大细胞[64-66]。如果能够证明每支血管周围有一层几乎完整的肌动蛋白阳性的周细胞，则有助于除外恶性病变。

肿瘤独具一种与胎盘微血管共有的免疫显型特征，特征性地表达GLUT-1（glucose transporter-1）和LeY（Lewis Y寡糖抗原，长I型多聚乳氨酸，胚泡表面表达，在胚胎发育和着床过程中起重要作用—译者注）阳性。GLUT-1，红细胞型葡萄糖转运蛋白，在这些病变中的表达贯彻其发展过程的始终[67,68]。因GLUT-1在其他类型儿童常见的血管肿瘤中并无表达，故此标记物的表达是一个有价值

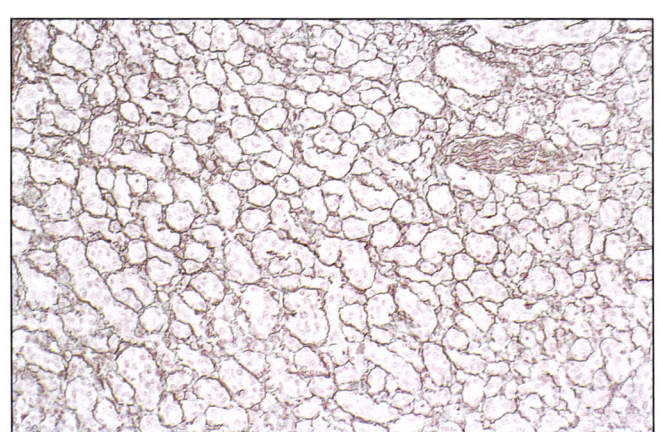

图3.6 毛细血管瘤。即便是在（毛细血管）开通程度最低的部位，网状蛋白染色亦能突显小管状（的血管）结构。

的鉴别诊断指标，尤其是在血管畸形的情况下，后者无 GLUT-1 表达。最近有研究显示：这些病变是由 CD133 阳性的内皮前体细胞构成的，至少部分如此[69]。此外，已有证据表明，幼年性毛细血管瘤具有克隆性[70,71]。

毛细血管瘤的各种亚型

丛状血管瘤
Tufted angioma (angiobla stoma of Nakagawa)

丛状血管瘤[72-77]是一种非常独特的与毛细血管瘤密切相关的良性血管肿瘤。作为一个病变实体，它首次被认可虽然是在 1976 年的英国文献，但同样的病变早在 1949 年就已被冠名"血管母细胞瘤"，见于日文文献[78]。

临床上，丛状血管瘤表现为一种获得性病变，绝大多数出现在低龄儿童的颈背部，少数见于黏膜部位[79]；无性别差异；个别病变可发生在成人。先天性病例非常之罕见[80]。有证据表明它偶有家族倾向[81]。病变进展缓慢，可经数年，呈边界不清的红色或棕红色斑疹、丘疹或呈结节状，病变大都柔软。偶有自发消退的个案报道[82,83]。其临床经过虽属良性，但因其病变过程的广泛性，要想完整切除几乎是不可能的；而且，肉眼皮损边缘之外的局部复发很常见。偶可发生 Kasabach-Merritt 综合征（婴儿血管瘤合并血小板减少性紫癜）[84,85]或许能表明（丛状血管瘤）与 Kaposi 样血管内皮细胞瘤之间的相关性或相似性（见 p56）。亦有合并血管畸形的报道[86]。

组织学形态：丛状血管瘤的最主要特征：在真皮和皮下组织浅层可见很多由毛细血管构成的圆形或卵圆形小叶，典型（小叶）以散在、互不连接的"炮弹头"形式分布（图 3.7）。单个小叶酷似草莓状痣的早期形态，由数量不等、尚未开通、但有周细胞环绕的无血毛细血管构成。血管内皮细胞形态大致正常，核分裂象少见。在局部，内皮细胞内可见结晶状、但性质未明的胞浆包涵体[87]。其独特的形态特征是：在某些肿瘤，小叶周围可见扩张的新月形淋巴样血管腔隙，故有人视其为血管内病变[88]；在个别病例的组织切片上，还可见 Kaposi 样血管内皮细胞瘤和丛状血管瘤之间重叠的现象[89,90]。

鉴别诊断：经常被混淆的病变是结节状 Kaposi 肉瘤；二者的鉴别要点是：丛状血管瘤可见"炮弹头"样结构模式，无（Kaposi 特征性的）梭形细胞群，网状蛋白染色下可见血管构型。Kaposi 样血管内皮细胞瘤（的病变范围）通常较大，也较为广泛，其中的小叶结构更具融合性。

疣状血管瘤 Verrucous hemangioma

疣状血管瘤[91-93]大都表现为儿童下肢的蓝黑色疣状病变。因其疣状形态，临床误诊者并不少见。组织学上，病变大都由真皮浅层大量扩张的毛细血管和偶尔可见的海绵状血管腔隙构成，并可向真皮深层和皮下组织扩展（图 3.8）。表皮则呈明显的棘皮症和角化过度改变。本瘤常有局部复发，须扩大切除以预防之。疣状血管瘤和血管角质瘤虽在外观上多有相似之处，但后者是一种血管扩张性病变，仅累及真皮乳头，单纯切除即可治愈。

樱桃状血管瘤
Cherry angioma (senile angioma, Campbell de Morgan spot)

樱桃状血管瘤[27]很常见，皮损为红色丘疹，位于中年以上成人的躯干和上肢；其数量随着年龄增长而增多。组织学上，以毛细血管扩张充血、小叶状结构和（病变）位于真皮乳头为特征。

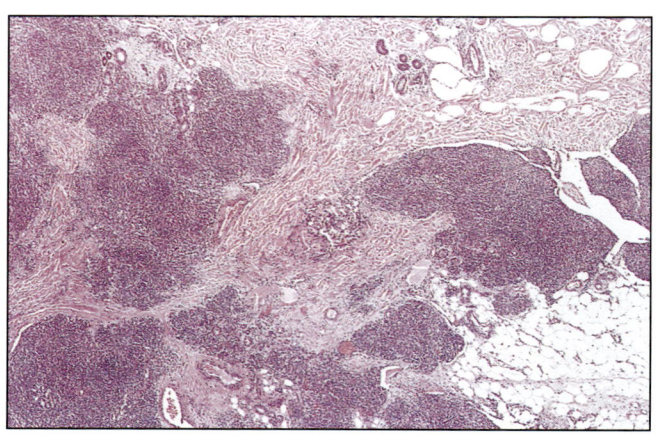

图3.7 丛状血管瘤。注意：分布不规则的毛细血管小叶及其周围的新月形血管腔隙（右上方）。

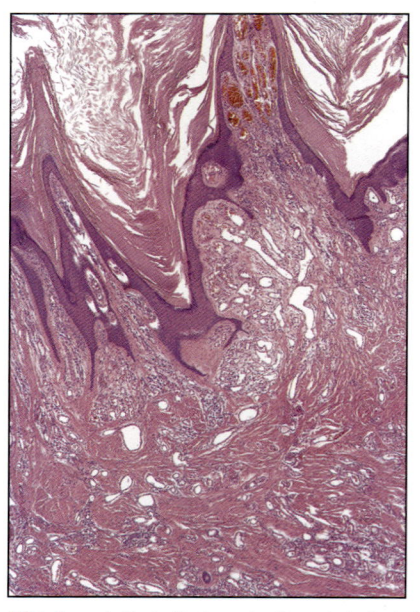

图3.8 疣状血管瘤。在明显过度角化的表皮下层，可见薄壁血管遍布真皮乳头和真皮深层。

小叶性毛细血管瘤（化脓性肉芽肿）
Lobular capillary hemangioma (pyogenic granuloma)

临床特征：化脓性肉芽肿[94,95]是一种很常见的皮肤和黏膜的血管病变，多年来被视为反应性或感染性病变。这种看法源自其广泛的浅表继发性感染（因多有溃疡形成），而且与创伤明显相关者占比1/3[96,97]。不过，其基本病变过程是小叶状血管增生，这种可能是肿瘤的病变可发生在深层和血管内（见下文），现已被恰当地重新命名为小叶性毛细血管瘤[98]。病变无明显年龄、性别差异；好发于手指和头颈部，尤以鼻、口腔黏膜为最。偶有先天性个案的报道[99,100]。典型病变形态呈一孤立、生长迅速、伴溃疡形成、出血性的息肉状蓝色结节，直径多小于2cm。偶有播散型（发疹型）化脓性肉芽肿的报道[101-103]。完全自发性消退者实无发生，而局部复发者可占10%，尤以不完全切除术后者多见，特别是发生在鼻间隔的病变。一种不常见现象是以多发性无蒂结节（卫星状）为特征的复发，主要发生于儿童和年轻人躯干[104,105]。化脓性肉芽肿偶可发生于葡萄酒色斑痣中[106,107]。有证据表明，化脓性肉芽肿样病变和使用卡培他滨（capecitabine，一种细胞周期特异性药物，本身无毒性，通过肿瘤相关性血管因子胸腺磷酸化酶在肿瘤所在部位转化为具有细胞毒性的氟尿嘧啶，从而降低氟尿嘧啶对正常细胞的损害—译者注）[108]、局部用全反维甲酸霜[109]和异维甲酸霜[110,111]治疗有关。

组织学形态：病变大都为外生性，有溃疡形成，周围是以棘皮症为特征的环形皮损。如果有溃疡形成，在皮损浅表部位则有大量急性炎性细胞浸润、肉芽组织增生，且多伴明显水肿；但在肿瘤中心却可见许多小叶状结构，它们都是由内皮细胞围成的细小毛细血管聚集而成，其中有些具有可辨认的管腔，有些则无（图3.9）。

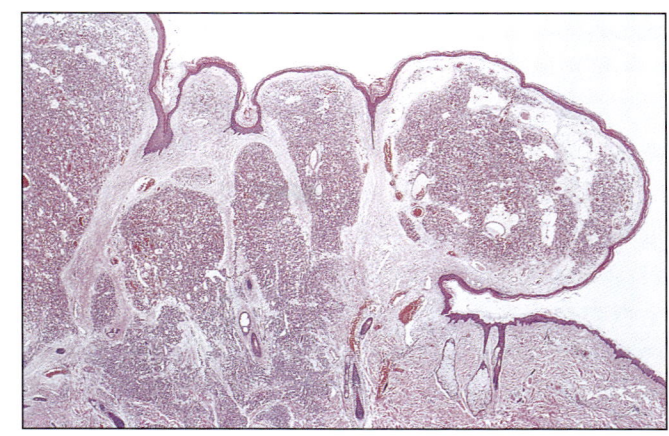

图3.9　化脓性肉芽肿。早期尚无溃疡性病变，低倍镜下可见典型的小叶状结构。

间质疏松、水肿。正常核分裂象可能很多，尤以黏膜病变为著（图3.10）。（瘤）细胞可呈轻中度异型性，尤其是发生在口腔[112]和结膜的病变；细胞异型性常在靠近溃疡表面处最为明显，究其性质则很可能是反应性的。偶可在局部区域见到围衬血管腔隙的内皮细胞呈上皮样改变。陈旧性病变可呈明显纤维化。（发生在）深部和血管内的化脓性肉芽肿大都没有类似于肉芽组织的病变成分。卫星状结节的组织形态与网状真皮、甚至与皮下组织的形态特征相似。用肌动蛋白做免疫组化染色可突显每支血管周围的一层周细胞。

各种亚型

妊娠性肉芽肿（granuloma gravidarum）指发生于妊娠女性牙龈上的同类病变，常在分娩后消退。皮下化脓性肉芽肿（subcutaneous pyogenic granuloma）表现为一无症状结节，主要累及上肢；除了与经典化脓性肉芽肿相关的继发性改变外，与经典型之组织学特征相同[113]。静脉内化脓性肉芽肿（intravenous pyogenic granuloma）是一种少见的类型，主要累及成人，尤其颈部和双手[114]，

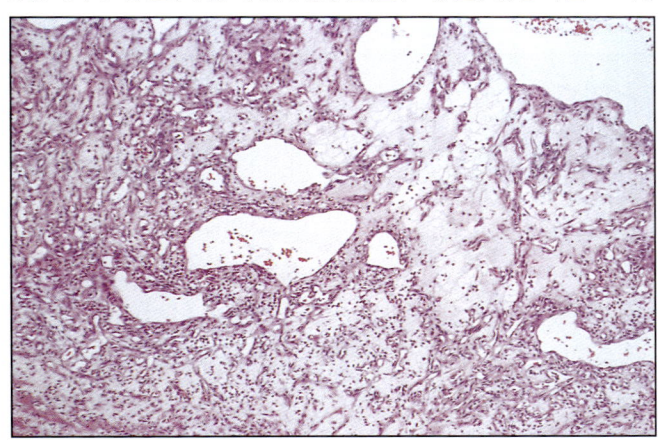

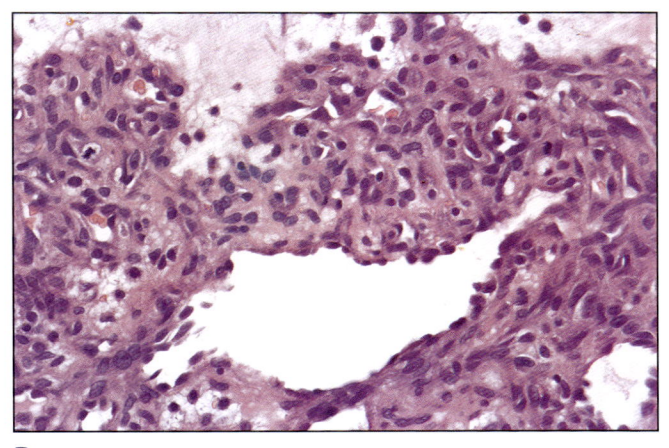

图3.10　化脓性肉芽肿。（A）溃疡性病变可见间质水肿和急性炎性细胞（浸润）。（B）尽管细胞高度密集，而且常见有（正常的）核分裂象，但内皮细胞核并无异型性或多层化现象。

未见继发性炎症性改变；临床行为良性。

鉴别诊断：传统上的鉴别诊断对象是高分化血管肉瘤和结节状Kaposi肉瘤。前者常边界不清，细胞异型性明显，并有胶原纤维束分隔其间。而后者则大都具有优势的梭形细胞成分，并伴裂隙状腔隙形成。但近年来，其主要鉴别诊断对象已变成杆菌性血管瘤病（bacillary angiomatosis），这是一种感染性血管增生性病变，其致病菌主要是一种革兰阴性细菌汉赛巴尔通体（Bartonella henselae），旧称汉赛罗克利巴体（Rochalimaea henselae）；其次是五日热巴尔通体（Bartonella quintana）[115,116]。这种病几乎无一例外地发生在获得性免疫功能缺陷综合征（AIDS）或其他免疫功能抑制性病患，极少见于正常个体。其准确诊断很重要，因其对抗生素治疗反应奇佳，尤其是红霉素。最近几年，由于针对致病菌的敏感性，HIV阳性患者常规接受预防性抗结核治疗，使得这种感染的发病率已明显减少。化脓性肉芽肿和杆菌性血管瘤病二者的病变结构很相似，但后者内皮细胞呈上皮样改变、肥胖且淡染；局灶性胞浆空泡；病变中随处可见丛状聚集的多形核白细胞及其核碎片、炎性细胞相关性颗粒状、嗜碱性或双染性物质（图3.11）；在Warthin-Starry或Giemsa染色下可见其中聚集有大量短杆菌。

海绵状血管瘤　Cavernous hemangioma

临床特征：与毛细血管瘤相比，海绵状血管瘤[27-29,60]虽然并不常见，但二者在发病年龄、好发性别和解剖分布相同；与前者不同的是，后者一般都比较大，（位置）比较深在，边界都不是很清楚，而且极少表现消退倾向。实际上，人体任何器官均可受累于海绵状血管瘤。相关的临床症状包括Mafucci综合征（多发性内生性软骨瘤、偶合并淋巴管瘤、多合并梭形细胞性血管瘤）、Kasabach-Merritt综合征（海绵状血管瘤伴血小板减少，可引发消耗性凝血）[117]和蓝色橡皮疱疹痣综合征（blue rubber bleb nevus syndrome），伴皮肤和消化道多发性血管瘤[118,119]。

组织学形态：海绵状血管瘤边界不清，由扩张程度不等、管壁厚薄不均、有扁平状内皮细胞衬覆的血管构成（图3.12）。局部常可见酷似毛细血管瘤的病变，尤其是在体表部位，很多病变其实就是毛细血管瘤和海绵状血管瘤的混合体。常见血栓形成、继发性营养障碍性钙化和轻度炎症。

海绵状血管瘤的各种亚型

窦状血管瘤　Sinusoidal hemangioma

临床特征：窦状血管瘤最近被视为海绵状血管瘤家族的一个独特类型[120]。其解剖分布颇广，尤以乳腺皮下组织为多见。但在此解剖部位，（它）可能被混淆为血管肉瘤。窦状血管瘤大多发生在中年，女性多见，皮损表现为位置浅表的蓝色结节。单纯切除即可治愈。

组织学形态：典型病变呈分叶状，边界相对清晰；病变由不规则形、窦样扩张的、充血的薄壁血管构成，低倍镜下呈典型筛窦状结构（图3.13）。背靠背的血管

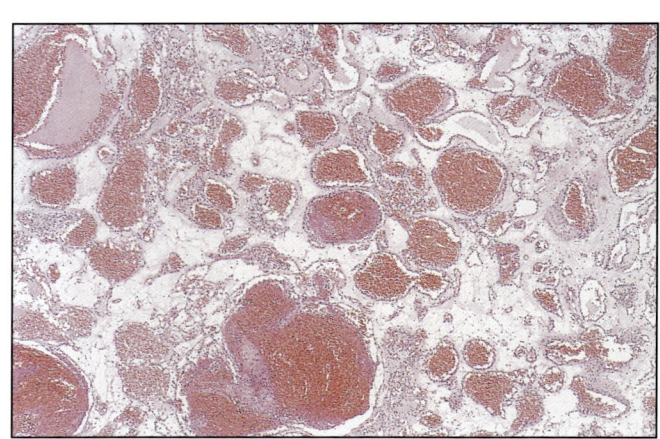

图3.12　海绵状血管瘤。（其中的）血管扩张、充血，局部可见血栓形成。

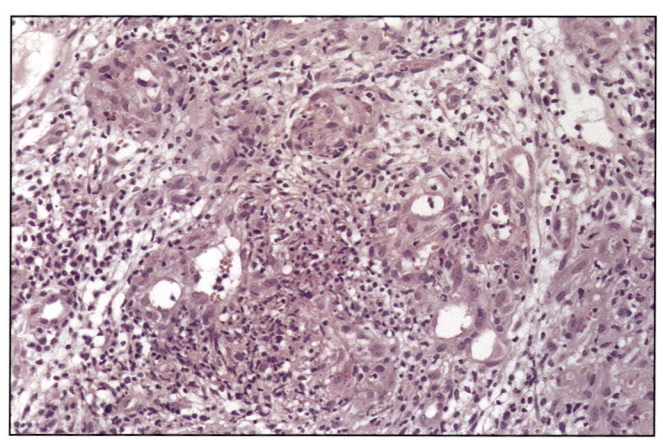

图3.11　杆菌性血管瘤病（bacillary angiomatosis）。注意：上皮样内皮细胞、伴随炎症和（细胞）核破裂碎片（图中央）。

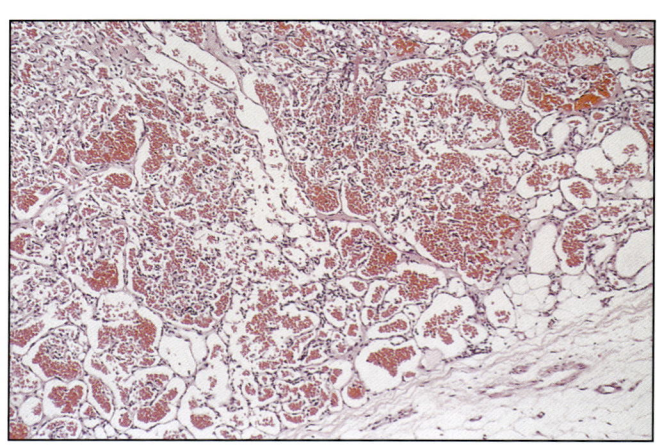

图3.13　窦状血管瘤。注意：成就筛窦状结构模式之血管壁的排列精巧。

之间会嵌入少量间质，其横断面就会形成假乳头状结构，这很容易使人想起Masson瘤（血管内乳头状内皮细胞增生）。血管内面大部被覆一层扁平的内皮细胞，并可见明显的局灶性细胞核轻度深染。血管周围常可见一层肌动蛋白阳性的血管周细胞。与普通型海绵状血管瘤一样，血栓形成伴营养不良性钙化甚是常见，可能是乳房影像学异常的主要原因。偶见中心性梗死。陈旧性病变可表现有血管纤维化和玻璃样变性。

鉴别诊断：鉴别诊断的主要对象是高分化血管肉瘤，尤其是发生在乳房的病变。乳房血管肉瘤是发生在实质内，而非是在真皮或皮下组织的病变，并具有明显的浸润性生长方式，而且，至少在局部可见明显的细胞核多形性和内皮细胞多层化。

动静脉血管瘤 Arteriovenous hemangioma

临床特征：动静脉血管瘤（动静脉畸形）[121-124]是一种不常见的病变，视病变深度可分为两种类型：深在型大都发生在青春期和年轻成人的头颈部或四肢，并伴有严重的动静脉分流和软组织肥厚。这种深在型病变所代表的可能是一种先天性畸形。其症状可能很严重，患者可能表现为心衰或Kasabach-Merritt综合征（海绵状血管瘤伴血小板减少性紫癜）。临床病理相关性研究，包括动脉造影，对明确诊断非常重要。不完全切除术后肿瘤仍持续生长、症状亦不见缓解者很是常见。

浅表型病变又名曲张型动脉瘤或肢端动静脉瘤[123]，其典型病变见于中老年人（多为男性）的头颈部（尤其是唇部）皮肤。皮损表现为一蓝紫色丘疹。一种以指、趾病变为表现形式的亚型已获证实[125]。部分病变与慢性肝病有关[126]。本瘤症状不多，主要有疼痛和间断性出血；（动静脉瘘）分流并非其常见的重要（临床）特征。浅表型动静脉血管瘤可与深在型病变伴生，此类病变无论在临床上还是在组织学上，都可能酷似Kaposi肉瘤（KS），故有假性KS或肢端皮肤血管炎（acroangiodermatitis，可并发动静脉瘘的皮肤血管炎）之称[127]。不过，同样的病变亦可见于由其他任何原因所导致的静脉瓣功能不全。

组织学形态：动静脉血管瘤的组织形态变异极大，深在型病变表现尤著；与其相比，浅表型病变的边界则大都很清楚。二型病变都表现为一种与不同口径动、静脉相应的厚壁和薄壁血管的混合体，并以薄壁静脉为优势成分（图3.14），用弹力纤维染色可突显之（图3.15）。某些肿瘤之局部可有与毛细血管瘤或海绵状血管瘤类似

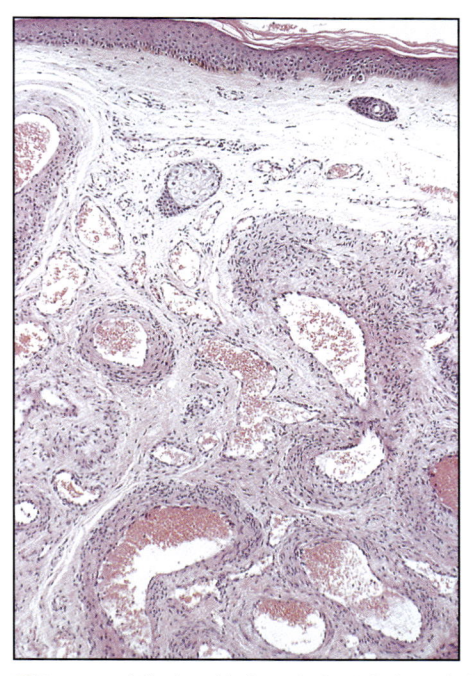

图3.14 动静脉血管瘤，浅表型病变，常有曲张型动脉瘤（蜿蜒状动脉瘤）之称。

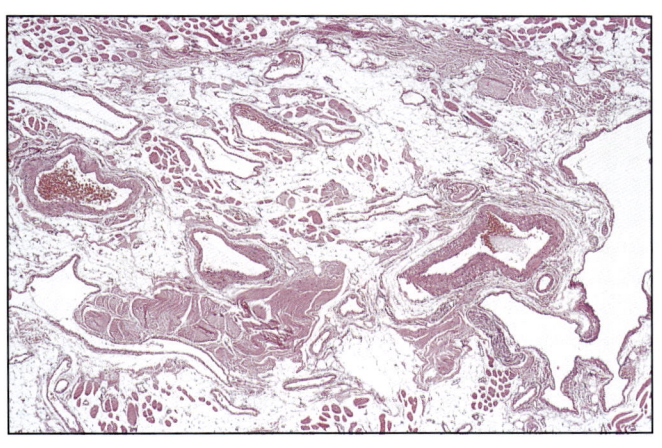

A

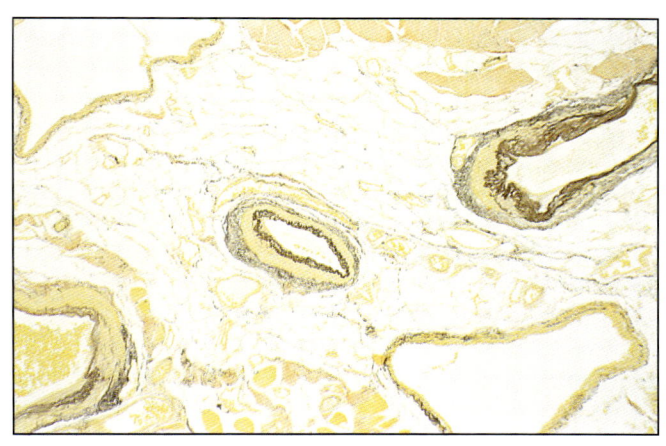

B

图3.15 动静脉血管瘤，深在型病变，系由很多大血管（A）构成，弹力VG染色可突显分布其壁间的弹力板（B）。

的病变结构。连续切片有助于显示动静脉吻合。局部血栓形成和间质钙化时有所见。要想在浅表型病变中确切证明有动脉存在大都非常困难。一般认为，这些血管可能是一种动脉化了的静脉，很多浅表型动静脉血管瘤很可能是真性静脉血管瘤[128]。

微静脉型血管瘤　Microvenular hemangioma

微静脉型血管瘤是一种独特的、据称是获得性静脉血管瘤病变形式之一的皮肤血管瘤[129,130]。皮损表现为红色或蓝紫色丘疹，主要见于年轻成人，尤其好发于四肢；儿童患者非常少见[131]。本病变无明显复发倾向。据称[132]：某（微静脉型血管瘤）个案原系POEMS综合征 [骨硬化性骨髓瘤，一种与浆细胞瘤有关的多系统病变，以多发性神经病 (P) 为主，另伴脏器肿大 (O)、内分泌病 (E)、M蛋白病 (M) 和皮肤病变 (S) 等] 患者[132]。组织学上（图3.16），肿瘤由不规则分支状薄壁小静脉构成，（小静脉）内覆单层内皮细胞，细胞核肥大；病变占据浅层和深层真皮，周围是硬化的胶原纤维束。这些血管呈有角分支状贯穿真皮层，而且其周围大都具有一层清晰可见的周细胞。病变底层可能更具分叶状结构。

钉突样血管瘤（靶样含铁血黄素沉着性血管瘤） Hobnail hemangioma（targetoid hemosiderotic hemangioma）

钉突样血管瘤[133-135]首次曾被描述为红色靶样含铁色素型血管瘤[133]，这是一种独特的皮肤血管瘤，好发于年轻或中年人的躯干和四肢，男性多见。其最初的描述冠名是鉴于其独特的临床表现——一种圆形小皮损，中央呈紫色，周围则环以从苍白渐变到瘀斑色的晕轮。但人们渐次发现：具有上述皮损形态的病例为数不多，而具有同样形态皮损者却可源于其他病因，如创伤[136]。据称，部分患者的皮肤病变呈周期性改变[137]。单纯切除即可治愈。

组织学上，在真皮浅层，可见不规则形扩张的薄壁血道，其内面被覆颇具特色、形态温和、状如钉突且呈局灶乳头状突起的内皮细胞（图3.17）。随着病变向真皮深层扩展，这些内皮细胞逐渐变扁平，渐行渐窄的血道将胶原纤维束分隔成片。周围间质中常可见溢出血管的红细胞和含铁血黄素沉积。我们认为：在所有以钉突样内皮细胞为特征之血管肿瘤家族谱系中，钉突样血管瘤位于其良性一端；此血管肿瘤家族成员还包括淋巴管内乳头状血管内皮瘤（papillary intralymphatic angioendothelioma, PILA，又名Dabska瘤）和网状血管内皮瘤（retiform hemangioendothelioma）[138]。其鉴别诊断问题将在淋巴管内乳头状血管内皮瘤一节中讨论（详见下文），但应强调指出的是：其组织学改变与放疗后可能出现的钉突样血管瘤几乎一样（p99）。免疫组化染色显示，在钉突样血管瘤，HHV-8呈稳定阴性[139]。

获得性弹力纤维性血管瘤　Acquired elastotic hemangioma

获得性弹力纤维性血管瘤是一种少见病变，好发于前臂和颈部皮肤的阳光暴露处，中老年女人多见[140]。皮损表现为一孤立性、无明显症状的小红斑。组织学上可见在真皮日光性弹性组织变性的大背景上，毛细血管

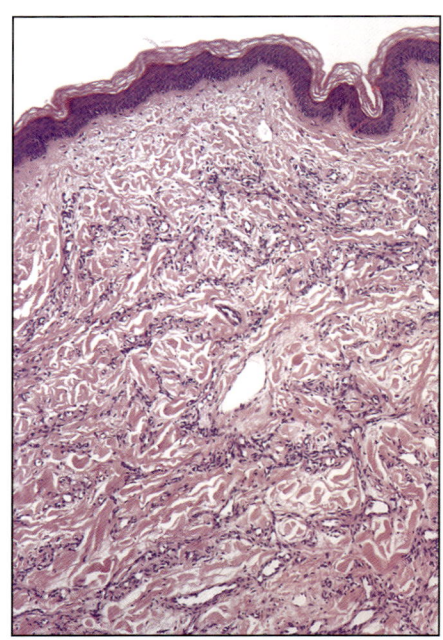

图3.16 微静脉型血管瘤。真皮胶原束之间可见血管成角分支。

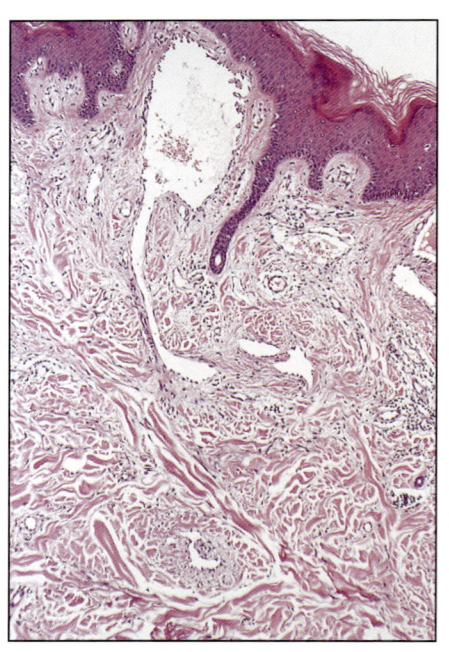

图3.17 钉突样血管瘤。血管腔面被覆的内皮细胞的细胞核凸向管腔，局部呈乳头状突起（图上方）。

在真皮浅层呈带状增生。

皮肤上皮样血管（瘤性）结节
Cutaneous epithelioid angiomatous nodule

临床表现：在上皮样血管瘤家族中，皮肤上皮样血管（瘤性）结节是一种最近才被描述的病变[141]。皮损表现为一丘疹或是一结节，好发于成年人，常常始于躯干，但时间不长旋即延扩至四肢和面部[141]。多发性病变罕见。无复发倾向。

组织学形态：镜下可见病灶呈孤立性、边界清、分叶状；病变由上皮样内皮细胞构成，这些内皮细胞肥大、淡粉染色，可具胞浆内腔（intracytoplasmic lumina），但血管腔的形成却非常之局限（图3.18）。尽管（瘤细胞的）实性生长方式令人不安，但其细胞核并无深染，亦无多形性。病变中可见轻度纤维化、含铁色素沉积和散在分布的炎性细胞，其中包括嗜酸性粒细胞。

鉴别诊断：皮肤上皮样血管结节与上皮样血管瘤的鉴别要点是：二者的临床表现不同；前者孤立的分叶状病变中，上皮样内皮细胞鲜有管腔形成，但可见少量炎细胞浸润。在杆菌性血管瘤病（bacillary angiomatosis）的分叶状结构中，内皮细胞的着色明显偏淡，并形成小的血管腔。而且病变中随处可见多形核中性粒细胞及其核尘的聚集，以及丛状聚集的无定形嗜碱性物质，其中聚集有大量短杆菌。

上皮样血管瘤（血管淋巴样增生伴嗜酸性粒细胞增多）
Epithelioid hemangioma (angiolymphoid hyperplasia with eosinophilia)

上皮样血管瘤有时又被称为血管淋巴样增生伴嗜酸性粒细胞增多[142]、假性或非典型性化脓性肉芽肿[143]、炎症性血管瘤样结节[143]、丘疹样血管形成（papular angioplasia）[144]、静脉内非典型血管增生[145]和组织细胞样血管瘤（histiocytoid hemangioma）[146]。对"组织细胞样血管瘤"的描述虽精准，但此名却颇具争议[147-150]，又因其最初定义不专，致其所含病变种类甚是宽泛，故现已渐被弃用[146]。上皮样血管瘤代表了以上皮样内皮细胞为特征的血管肿瘤家族病变谱系的良性端，此病变家族包括最近才被认识的皮肤上皮样血管（瘤样）结节（见上文）以及位于其恶性端的上皮样血管内皮瘤和上皮样血管肉瘤。虽然在多数情况下，上述各类肿瘤之间都能各归各类，但还是有少数个案表现出一定程度的病变重叠，尤其是在后两类恶性病变。上皮样血管瘤究竟是一种真性血管肿瘤，还是一种反应性病变，目前尚存争议；据称[151]，多种不同刺激，尤其是创伤，可致类似反应，但前一种观点已被广泛认同。

临床特征：上皮样血管瘤皮损的典型表现为单发或多发性皮肤红色小结节，好发于头颈部（耳周尤为多见）；好发年龄为中年成人，男性稍多[152,153]。皮损亦可发生于躯干、四肢，并可累及深部软组织。有个案报道称：病变亦可见于口腔黏膜[154-156]、舌[157,158]、乳腺[159]、淋巴结[160]、骨[161]、睾丸[162]，甚至可以发生于卵巢畸胎瘤之内[163]。发生在心脏的一组形态上相似、过去一直被视为上皮样血管瘤的病变，现称其组织来源可能是间皮或是组织细胞（见第2章）[164,165]。循环性嗜酸性粒细胞增多并不多见，但有报道称，其实际发生率可高达15%[150,152]。与Kimura病（嗜酸性粒细胞增生性淋巴肉芽肿）不同，上皮样血管瘤病变一般不累及淋巴结。多达1/3的患者可有局部复发，但从无远端转移发生[149,150,152,153]。有报道称，在HIV（艾滋病毒）感染者，原发性HHV-8（人疱疹病毒-8）感染可致一过性血管淋巴样增生（angiolymphoid hyperplasia）和Kaposi肉瘤[166]；但在上皮样血管瘤中从未检出有HHV-8[167]。凡具有与上皮样血管瘤中可见的组织学特征相似之病变，都极罕有与血管畸形相关[168]。

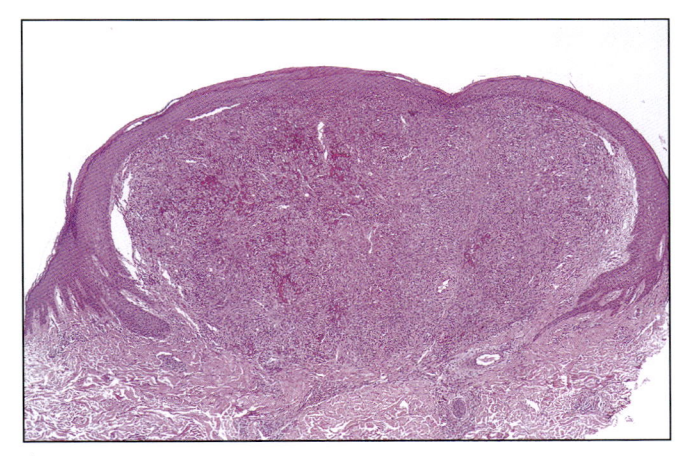

图3.18 上皮样血管（瘤样）结节。图为一以外生性结节为特征的病变（A），病变由排列紧密的上皮样血管内皮细胞构成（B）。

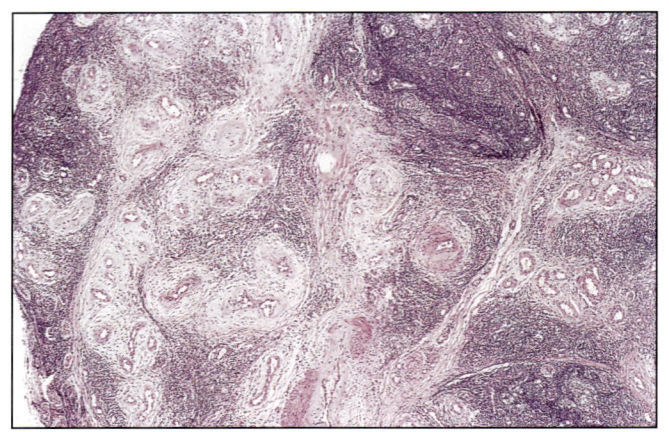

图3.19　上皮样血管瘤。可见或明或暗的分叶状结构和大量淋巴样细胞浸润。

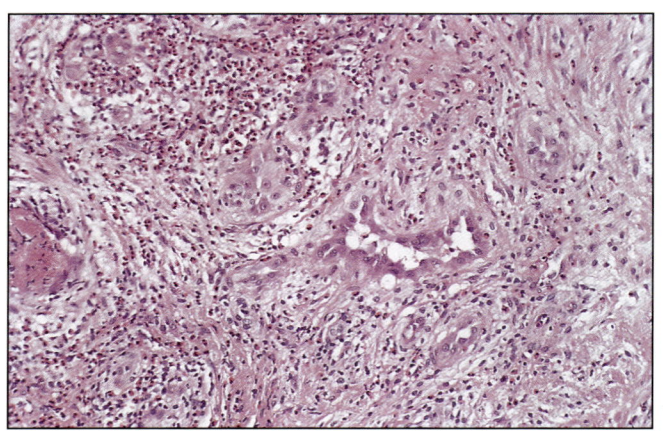

图3.20　上皮样血管瘤。可见上皮样内皮细胞极度肥大、局部胞浆空泡化；间质有大量嗜酸性粒细胞浸润。

组织学形态：皮损的边界大都清楚；病变由大量中小口径的薄壁血管构成，其内面被覆的内皮细胞肥大、胞浆丰富、嗜酸红染；细胞核呈卵圆形、空泡状、核仁不明显。至少在局部，病变中常可见小叶状结构（图3.19）。上皮样内皮细胞常凸入血管腔，形似钉突或墓碑（图3.20）。这些细胞可能有很多小的胞浆空泡，如有融合，即可形成所谓胞浆内脉管腔。核分裂象少见，细胞多形性也非其特征。偶有肌型厚壁血管发生黏液变性，并可见上皮样细胞呈实性巢状聚集。病变常可溯源到一支小动脉或静脉，整个病变常完全位于血管腔之内。偶有报道称：病变可溯源到大口径外周动脉[169,170]。这些（病变）血管周围多是由大量组织细胞、淋巴细胞、浆细胞、肥大细胞和嗜酸性粒细胞构成的重度炎性细胞浸润。偶有生发中心形成，但其发生率明显低于Kimura病。瘤细胞对内皮细胞标记物（免疫组化）呈着色反应，虽然发生在皮肤的病变之CK大都为阴性；但据称[161]：原发于骨的病变之CK却为阳性。

（上皮样血管瘤的）管腔内病变曾被描述为"静

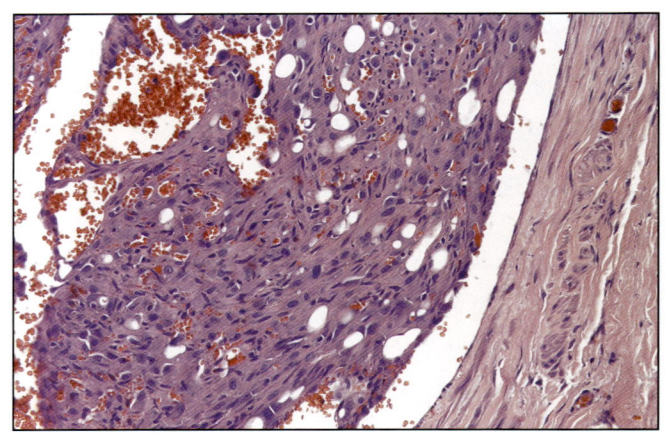

图3.21　静脉内非典型血管增生。这个发生在静脉腔内的病变由上皮样细胞和梭形细胞构成。

脉内非典型血管增生（intravenous atypical vascular proliferation）"[145]，现被认为是代表了多种不同形式的上皮样血管瘤；它好发于中青年成人，皮损呈一孤立性结节，好发部位在头颈部和上肢。与经典型上皮样血管瘤的不同之处在于：前者，在上皮样内皮细胞管道之间或周围，常混有大量梭形细胞（周细胞）成分——它进一步强化了这些病变的假恶性特征（图3.21）。至少我们的经验（及其原始文献[145]都）表明：本病变无明显复发倾向。

鉴别诊断：Kimura病不再被视为是上皮样血管瘤的同义词[171,175]，因为在临床上，前者主要累及年轻的东方男性，而且大都合并淋巴结病、嗜酸性粒细胞增多以及其他免疫介导性疾病的全身症状。组织学上，Kimura病的病变位置较深，有比较明显的纤维化，但最重要的是：其血管内皮细胞完全没有上皮样特征。嗜酸性粒细胞微脓肿随处可见。注射部位肉芽肿中没有上皮样细胞[176,177]。杆菌性血管瘤病中可见有胞浆淡染的上皮样细胞和大量中性粒细胞，而且同时可见嗜碱性染色的菌丛。上皮样血管内皮瘤的间质呈明显黏液样或玻璃样变性，瘤细胞呈条索状或巢状分布，而且难得一见有分化成形的血管腔。

静脉性血管瘤　Venous hemangioma

静脉性血管瘤现已被描述为一种发生在成人肠系膜、后腹膜和四肢骨骼肌的特殊的病变实体[178]。虽然在定义上（其发生部位）仅限于深部软组织，但根据我们的观察，（与之）类似病变可以同样的几率见于身体浅表部位，并偶可发生在内脏。"静脉性"血管瘤有时是放射学诊断用语，但此诊断的病理组织学相关性尚不明确。很多发生在骨骼肌内的病变可能更适于归类为肌内血管瘤（详见下文）。静脉性血管瘤由大量形状不规则、扩张或充血的肌型静脉构成（图3.22），其中偶有

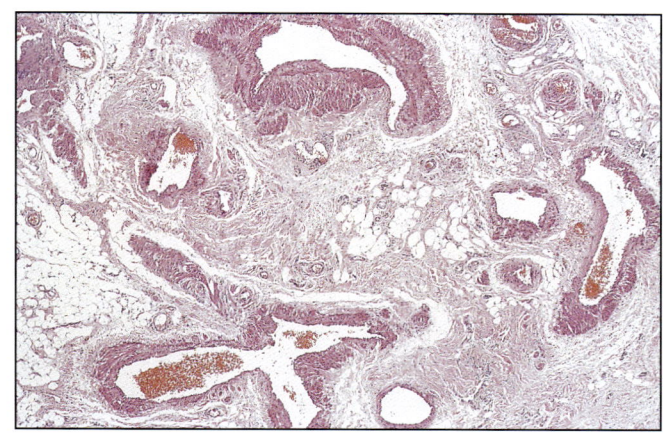

图3.22 静脉性血管瘤。此皮下病变系由大口径的薄壁静脉构成。

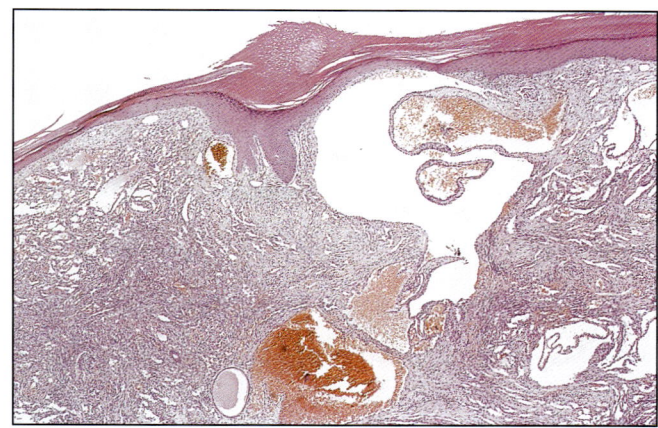

图3.23 梭形细胞血管瘤。可见实体性分布的梭形细胞区域和海绵状（血管瘤）病灶（伴有假乳头状结构）的混合形态之典型。

血栓形成。血栓中偶尔可见营养障碍性钙化。肿瘤之局部可有类似海绵状血管瘤之病变。

梭形细胞血管瘤（学称：梭形细胞血管内皮瘤）Spindle cell hemangoma（formerly spindle cell hemangioendothelioma）

临床特征：梭形细胞血管瘤是一种独特的血管肿瘤，1986年首报的冠名是红核梭形细胞血管内皮瘤（rubric spindle cell hemangioendothelioma），当时被认为是一种低度恶性血管肉瘤[179]。典型病变可呈单发，常为多发性蓝紫色结节，好发于四肢远端，尤其是双手的真皮或皮下组织；结节可有疼痛。病变可发生在骨骼肌，但非常罕见。梭形细胞血管瘤无明显性别差异，患者的年龄跨度很宽，但峰值在10～30岁左右。其临床经过缓慢；多发性病变患者的新、旧病灶之发生大都间隔多年[179-181]。这些曾被视为复发的新病变，似乎是在（旧病变）周围正常皮肤上重新发生的。自发性消退者只是偶发个案。多达10%的患者可合并其他异常，如淋巴水肿、早发性静脉曲张、Klippel-Trenaunay综合征（先天性毛细血管-静脉畸形伴骨肥大综合征）或Maffucci综合征（内生软骨瘤病合并多发性海绵状血管瘤）[179-183]。看来，这些病变与Maffuci综合征之间的相关性很可能比原先想像的要强得多[183]。将梭形细胞血管内皮瘤视为血管肉瘤之一型的根据是：某患者出现从原发灶向淋巴结的转移[179]。不过，此患者似乎患有另一种放射诱导型高度（低分化）肉瘤。最近有越来越多的证据显示：梭形细胞血管瘤是一种非肿瘤性病变，或是与局部血流异常相关，或是与血管畸形相伴[180,181,184,185]，故修订其名更为恰当。

组织学形态：组织学上，病变界线不清。主要由两种成分构成，其一是形状不规则、海绵状分布的薄壁血管腔，其二是主要由梭形细胞构成的实性病变（图3.23）。以血管腔内病变居优，且主要累及中等口径静脉者约占

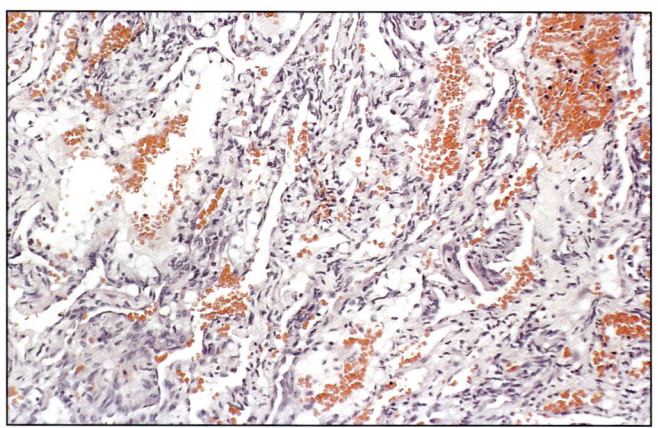

图3.24 梭形细胞血管瘤。可见明显空泡化的内皮细胞。

40%～50%。在肿瘤周边，常可见内膜纤维性增厚的、类似动静脉畸形的厚壁肌型血管。海绵状血管腔薄薄地被覆一单层内皮细胞，腔内可见机化血栓，并多有静脉石形成。（内皮细胞）常呈乳头状突起，乍看形似Masson瘤，但明显更具细胞性。实性病灶（主要）由分化良好的梭形细胞构成，胞浆少，嗜酸性红染；细胞核呈椭圆形或圆形；此外，还有少量上皮样细胞，其中，具有胞浆内大空泡的细胞数量因人而异（图3.24）。在这些实性病灶中，还常见有裂隙状血管腔。平滑肌细胞束不仅常出现在某些扩张血管腔的周围，而且也会见于实性病灶。偶可在局部见有退变性内皮细胞异型性。免疫组化染色：仅有血管腔内衬细胞和实性病灶中的上皮样细胞对内皮细胞标记物呈阳性着色；而梭形细胞大都仅呈波形蛋白阳性，少量呈肌动蛋白和/或结蛋白阳性。有报道称[180,187]，偶有病变呈现与上皮样血管内皮瘤混合之特征；不过，此类个案很可能是最近才被认识的所谓复合型血管内皮瘤（composite hemangioendothelioma）之实例（参阅p58）。

鉴别诊断：结节性Kaposi肉瘤一般都没有海绵状血管腔，也没有胞浆空泡化的上皮样细胞，其梭形细

胞的胞浆内可见透明小体；另外，HHV-8 免疫组化染色下，Kaposi 肉瘤的梭形细胞均呈阳性，而梭形细胞血管瘤之梭形细胞则均为阴性。

深部血管瘤　Deep hemangioma

肌内血管瘤　Intramuscular angioma

临床特征：肌内血管瘤，相对来说虽不多见，但在深在型软组织肿瘤中，却是发生几率最高者之一（图3.25）。任何年龄均可发病，峰值出现在青春期和年轻成人；无性别差异[188-190]。以发生率高低为序，其好发部位首推下肢，以下依次为头颈部、上肢和躯干。典型病变表现为一生长缓慢的肿块，常感疼痛，运动后尤甚。创伤对其发病似无影响，绝大多数患者的病变可能都是源于先天。X 线片上常可见有软组织钙化，其相应的病变或是静脉石，或是代谢性钙化。本病复发率高，约在 30%～50% 之间[188,190]，大都因首次手术切除不净所致。

组织学形态：传统上，肌内血管瘤的组织学分类都是根据（病变）管腔的口径和优势血管类型，将其分为小（毛细血管）型、大（海绵状）型和混合型三类[188]。但实际上，绝大多数病变都是混合型，均由毛细血管、静脉、小动脉、甚至淋巴样管腔构成[190]，以致对其进行可靠的亚型分类虽说不无可能，但也十分困难（图 3.26）。不过，单纯性毛细血管型肌内血管瘤主要见于头颈部，而肌内型淋巴管瘤则大都发生在躯干。所有肌内血管瘤中都可见数量不等、分化成熟的脂肪组织，此即该病变过去何以被称为浸润型血管脂肪瘤的原因[191]（图 3.27）。间质内常可见退化性或反应性肌膜核（sarcolemmal nuclei，又名核袋，原指去神经性萎缩的肌细胞）。早期报道所指其组织学分型与复发之间存在相关性之说并无实证，复发可能仅与手术切除是否彻底有关，反映了所有肌内型血管瘤（都具有）的浸润性特征，与其组织学类型无关[190]。

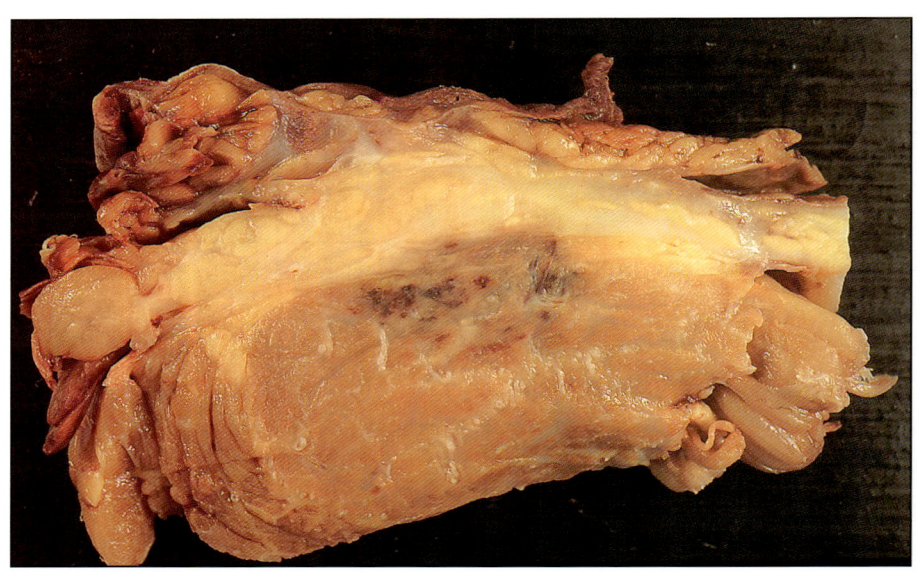

图3.25　肌内血管瘤。标本中心是被血栓栓塞的血管，其周围的肌肉因脂肪弥漫性浸润而显得苍白，所有这些病变在肿瘤中的分布均无定规。

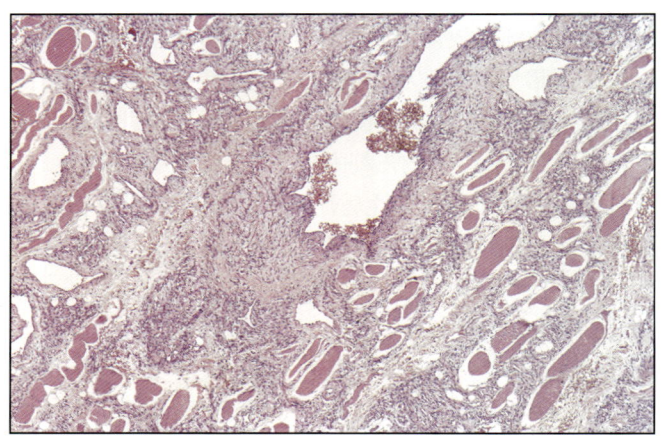

图3.26　肌内血管瘤。可见（病变是）由不同口径的血管构成的复杂混合体。

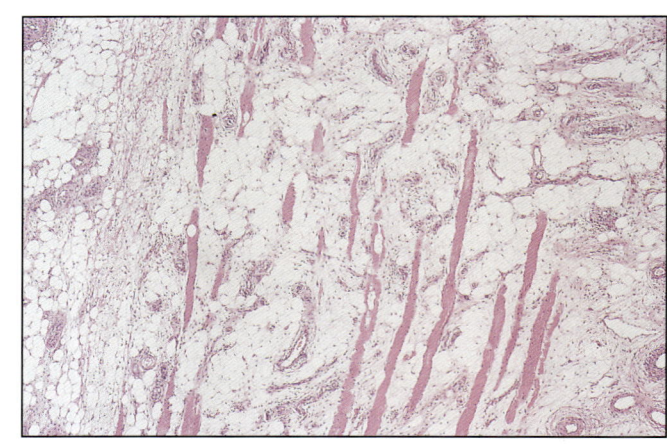

图3.27　肌内血管瘤。病变中大都可见大量脂肪细胞成分。

鉴别诊断：肌内血管瘤的组织学诊断虽说不难，但也必须与肌内脂肪瘤鉴别。后者的病程更长，复发可能性更小；而且其中的血管绝不会成为优势成分。单纯的毛细血管型肌内血管瘤偶可与血管肉瘤混淆，但前者常具有的分叶状结构、内皮细胞无异型性或复层化（之特征）可使鉴别不难。

滑膜血管瘤　Synovial hemangioma

滑膜血管瘤不常见，传统概念上，它包括起源于关节腔、滑囊、甚至腱鞘的肿瘤。不过，有建议说：此名称应保留给发生在前两个部位的病变[192]。滑膜血管瘤好发于年轻成人和儿童，尤其是男性。肿瘤生长缓慢，或无症状、或感疼痛；尤其好发于膝、肘，少见于手指[192]。那些累及周围软组织和骨骼的病变被视为血管瘤病的最佳例证。单纯性滑膜血管瘤的行为良性，术后无复发倾向。滑膜血管瘤中约半数表现为海绵状病变，余者可为毛细血管瘤、动静脉血管瘤或是纯静脉性血管瘤。

神经内血管瘤　Intraneural hemangioma

神经血管瘤极罕见，确诊无误之个案寥寥无几[193-195]。症状与受累神经有关，主要有疼痛、异样感觉和麻木。神经外衣、束膜和内膜可同时受累，且发生几率颇高[195]；有已累及四肢神经干的个案报道[195]，其中一例为三叉神经受累。组织学上，其病变形式多为海绵状血管瘤。

血管瘤病　Angiomatosis

血管瘤病并不常见，好发于儿童和青春期人群；以身体大片相互毗邻的组织受累和血管呈弥漫性增生为其特征[196]。偶可发现家族性病例[197]。该病变主要侵犯四肢，典型病变可（同时）累及多个组织层面，包括皮肤、皮下组织、肌肉、甚至（包括）骨。临床上，常见有受累肢体肥大，部分患者呈现血管角质瘤的临床特征[198]。合并内脏和中枢神经系统血管瘤者罕见。由于病变广泛，外科治疗很是困难，多有复发。来自不同机构的材料显示：其复发率在 60% ~ 90% 之间[197,198]。

据称，其组织学类型有二[197]，二者均可见增生的血管周围有大量分化成熟的脂肪组织，此特征或许可以证明血管瘤病可能的错构瘤性质。血管瘤病中最常见的结构模式是由静脉、海绵状血管腔和毛细血管混合而成，其中的静脉壁肌层不完整，程度不等，故显厚薄无序，形状无规。在大血管管壁内还常见丛状分布的小血管[197]。其次常见者则由细小毛细血管构成；而大口径的供血血管却难得一见（图 3.28）。上述两种结构模式中，均可见（病变在）神经周围的浸润（perineural invasion）。

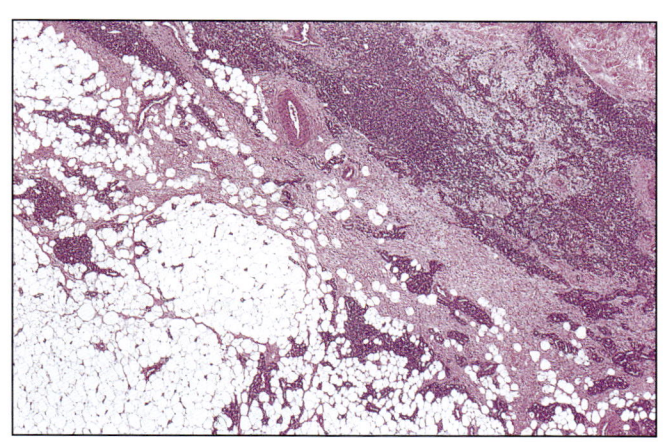

图 3.28　毛细血管型血管瘤病，可见脂肪组织弥漫性浸润筋膜。

肌内血管瘤和血管瘤病二者虽然在组织形态上非常相似，但前者常仅局限于某一组肌群，因此，密切联系临床是为病理鉴别诊断信心之源。深部动静脉畸形常具有血液分流的临床证据，组织学上则表现为静、动脉的混合；但这种表现仅可偶见于血管瘤病。

中间恶性血管肿瘤
Vascular tumors of intermediate malignancy

在其他病理学领域，低度或交界恶性的概念虽已明确，但在软组织肿瘤，尤其是血管肿瘤分类学中，这一概念的引入还只是最近的事（Fletcher 综述[199]）。血管内皮瘤一词最初是用来泛指一组良性（即婴儿型毛细血管瘤）和恶性（即血管肉瘤）血管肿瘤，现被用来特指此（血管肿瘤）新类别中的多种病变。严格来讲，所谓交界型肿瘤是指那些转移潜能虽然很低、但很确定的肿瘤（如网状血管内皮瘤）；那些无法根据组织形态准确判断其生物学行为的肿瘤偶被纳入其中。在软组织肿瘤 WHO 最新分类中，交界型肿瘤的概念再被扩展，将那些虽无远端转移潜能，但可局部浸润者也涵括在内[200]。在 WHO 分类中，低度或交界恶性肿瘤被分类为中间潜能型（intermediate potential）。被分类为局部浸润型的肿瘤包括 Kaposi 样血管内皮瘤和巨细胞性血管母细胞瘤。但巨细胞性血管母细胞瘤和多形性血管内皮瘤并未被 WHO 血管肿瘤分类工作组所采信，原因是这两种病变的个案报道数量太少，现有资料不足以对这些病变做准确分类。在本章，我们将其归入中间型肿瘤一类加以描述。而上皮样血管内皮瘤则因其高发病率和高死亡率，而被转列于恶性血管肿瘤项下（详见下文）。Kaposi 肉瘤是一种反应性病变还是真性肿瘤虽尚存争议，但我们仍将其视为中间恶性肿瘤。随着我们对神秘的交界型血管肿瘤认识

Kaposi 样血管内皮瘤
Kaposiform hemangioendothelioma

临床特征

Kaposi 样血管内皮瘤是一种独特而又少见的肿瘤，始见于婴儿腹膜后，但后来似乎更多地发生在四肢、胸壁、头颈部的皮下或深部软组织[201-204]；仅累及皮下者亦有发生[205,206]。患者大都在10岁以下，2岁以下者尤多，但成人病例亦有报道[207]。无性别差异。在部分患者，其发病率、死亡率与因肿瘤破坏性、浸润性生长所导致的合并症有关。在腹膜后，肿瘤常合并肠梗阻和黄疸；在其他部位，常与此肿瘤相伴者则为Kasabach-Merritt综合征（海绵状血管瘤伴血小板减少）。个别患者可合并骨和软组织的淋巴管瘤病。这些病变可能很难切除干净（因其解剖部位），但真性复发也很少发生。偶有报道称有淋巴结及其周围的转移[204]，但迄今为止尚未有远端转移的报道。

组织学形态

组织学上，Kaposi 样血管内皮瘤由大小不等的小叶构成，这些小叶以不规则形式向周围组织浸润，小叶间有纤维性间隔。腹膜后Kaposi样血管内皮瘤常累及胰腺、小肠和淋巴结等周围器官。肿瘤小叶由占比不同的短束状排列的高分化梭形细胞、裂隙状血管腔、充血毛细血管和散在其中的纤维素性血栓构成（图3.29）。偶可见小的上皮样细胞巢，尤其是发生在皮肤和软组织病变中。这些细胞内可含有含铁色素颗粒、玻璃样小体，甚至胞浆空泡。玻璃样小体亦可偶见于梭形细胞之内。炎性细胞大都稀少，核分裂象少见。肿瘤小叶周围可见扩张的血管。那些伴发淋巴管瘤病的病变中可见两种病变之间的过渡形态。免疫组化：肿瘤内皮细胞呈CD31、CD34和FLI-1（DNA结合翻译因子ETS家族成员，作为血管肿瘤标志物，Fli-1可能比CD31、CD34和VIIIRA因子更为敏感和特异，可用于鉴别上皮样血管肉瘤、癌及上皮样肉瘤 – 译者注）阳性；而GLUT-1（葡萄糖转运蛋白-1）和LeY（幼年型血管瘤相关抗原）阴性[204]。Von Willebrand因子（血管假性血友病因子，可协助血小板止血、运载第八因子）仅呈局灶阳性。梭形细胞对内皮细胞标记物（染色）呈不稳定阳性，肌动蛋白亦可呈局灶阳性。HHV-8至今未获证实。

鉴别诊断

其组织学形态与结节状Kaposi肉瘤颇为相似；但在临床上，除淋巴结型好发于淋巴结外，Kaposi肉瘤极少发生在儿童，且有多中心倾向。形态学上，结节状Kaposi肉瘤有较为明显慢性炎性细胞浸润，但无明显的小叶状结构；每个小叶周围亦无致密的纤维性间隔。婴儿型毛细血管瘤（"幼年型血管内皮瘤"参见第45页）是由管腔化不全的毛细血管（内皮细胞）实性结节所构成，其中并无梭形细胞成分。Kaposi样血管内皮瘤和血管肉瘤之间的鉴别点：前者没有细胞异型性，也没有（后者）独特的浸润性和相互吻合的管腔结构。

巨细胞性血管母细胞瘤
Giant cell angioblastoma

在"巨细胞性血管母细胞瘤"名下描述的病变是一种极为少见、具有局部浸润行为的、（组织结构）像是

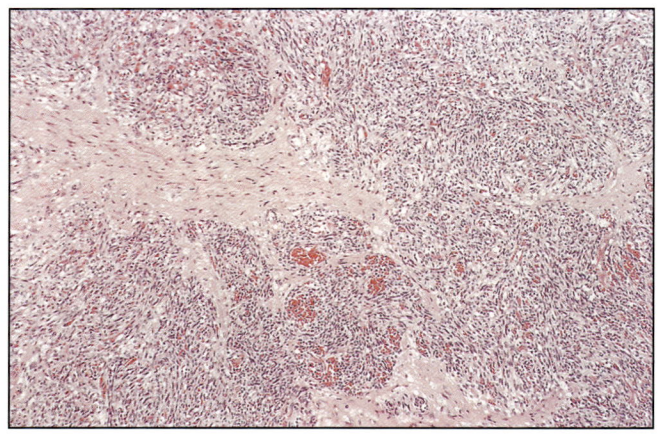

A

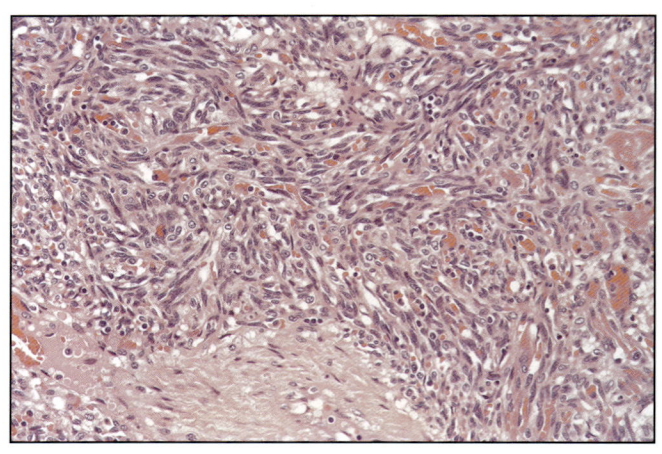

B

图3.29 Kaposi样血管内皮瘤。此梭形细胞血管瘤具有明显的小叶结构（A）；高倍镜下，可见与Kaposi肉瘤组织结构的相似之处以及纤维素性微血栓（B）。

很独特的血管肿瘤[208,209]。这些具有浸润性、先天性、或曰新生儿病变可见于身体多个不同部位。组织学上，肿瘤由束状、结节状分布的梭形细胞和肥大的组织样细胞构成，其间加杂有多核巨细胞，形态酷似肉芽肿。病变大都沿分支状血管腔分布，被覆的内皮细胞肥大。

网状血管内皮瘤
Retiform hemangioendothelioma

临床特征

网状血管内皮瘤是一种归入中间型的、罕有转移的少见病变[138,210,211]，但它却比PILA（Dabska瘤，乳头状淋巴管内血管内皮瘤）常见得多。这是一种生长缓慢的皮肤肿瘤，大都发生在年轻成人，无性别差异；好发于四肢，尤其是下肢远端。在极个别情况下，可发生在放疗之后或慢性淋巴水肿基础之上。多发性网状血管内皮瘤个案已有报道[212]。持续性局部复发常见，但转移至局部淋巴结者仅一例个案，还有一例转移到原发灶附近的软组织[213]。迄今为止，尚无远端扩散或肿瘤相关性死亡的病例报道。

组织学表现

网状血管内皮瘤是一种皮肤和/或皮下组织肿瘤，边界不清，组织形态酷似正常睾丸网；这种结构特征系因病变血管细长、并呈分支状而使然（图3.30），其内皮细胞呈单形性、钉突样突入管腔（图3.31）。约半数病变中可见明显的间质和管腔内淋巴细胞浸润。血管内皮细胞的胞浆量少，大都位于基底部，鲜有空泡形成。血管腔内偶可见有乳头，其轴心为透明变性胶原。大多数肿瘤中均可见由内皮细胞标记物着色阳性的单形性梭形细胞或上皮样细胞构成的实性细胞巢。

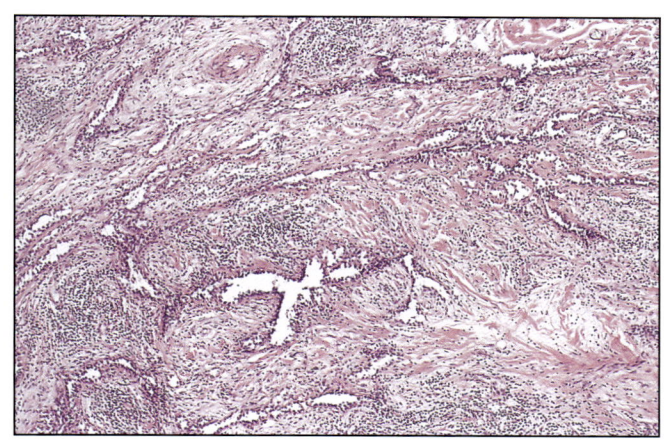

图3.30　网状血管内皮瘤。典型的分支状血管腔，伴大量淋巴细胞浸润。

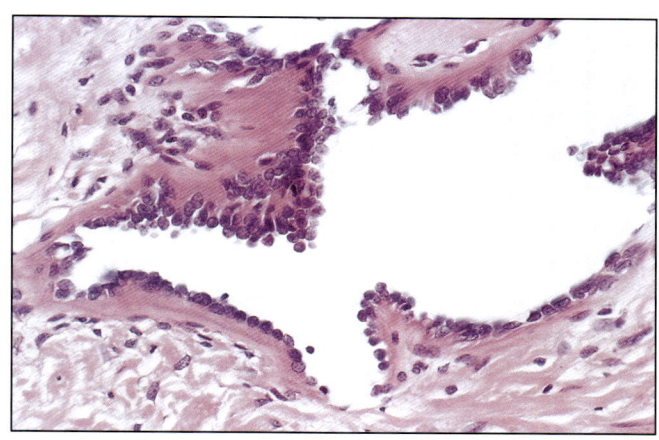

图3.31　网状血管内皮瘤。可见"钉突"样内皮细胞凸入管腔。

鉴别诊断

网状血管内皮瘤的鉴别诊断将在PILA一节叙述。

淋巴管内乳头状血管内皮瘤（血管内乳头状血管内皮瘤，Dabska瘤）
Papillary intralymphatic angioendo-thelioma（endovascular papillary angioendothelioma, Dabska tumor）

临床特征

淋巴管内乳头状血管内皮瘤（PILA）是一种少见的血管肿瘤。1969年，Dabska将其作为一种局部浸润、伴低度恶性潜能、主要累及婴幼及儿童的肿瘤加以描述[214]。但最新研究显示：患者中25%是成人[215]。无性别差异；身体各部位均可发病，但以四肢和躯干略多见[214,215]。在最初的系列报告中，至少有一例发生局部复发、局部淋巴结转移和死亡病例。但最近对12例文献个案中的8例随访显示：其中既没有局部复发，也没有远端转移[215]。现在看来，Dabska瘤是以钉突样细胞为特征的血管肿瘤家族成员之一，而钉突样形态本身可能是内皮细胞的高分化标志[216]。除网状血管内皮瘤外[138]，此肿瘤家族还包括一组现名为钉突样血管瘤[136]的良性病变，其首次描述被冠名为靶样含铁色素型血管瘤。现在看来，Dabska的原始病变系列中，至少有一部分今天很可能会分类到网状血管内皮瘤。故在有进一步系列材料问世之前，PILA的真正恶性潜能问题将不会有结论。在此存疑期间，应建议将肿瘤完全切除。

组织学表现

在采用严格诊断标准的前提下，部分研究者[215]和

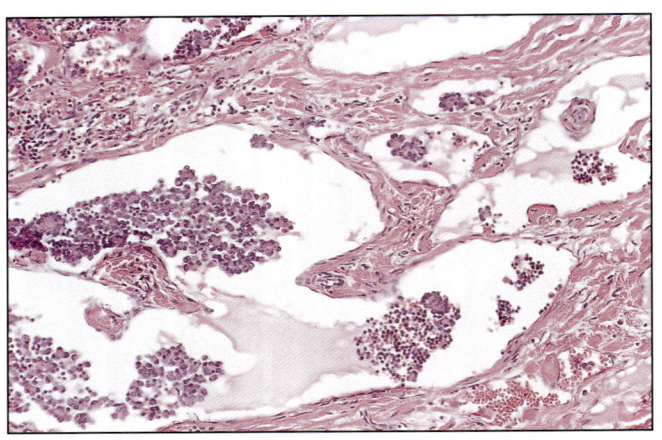

图 3.32 Dabska 瘤。海绵状淋巴管样腔隙中含有大量内皮细胞乳头和丛状聚集的淋巴细胞。

我们都认为：PILA 大都是由形状不规则的扩张血管构成，类似海绵状淋巴管瘤，但部分病变含有不规则分支状的小血管。PILA 常累及皮下组织。大量的淋巴细胞不仅见于周围间质，而且出现在血管腔内。部分病变血管内皮细胞的细胞核有明显异型性，但胞浆量很少，故形似典型钉突或是（向腔面突出的）火柴头。最具特征性者应属管腔内丛状内皮细胞乳头，乳头的透明轴心周围有淋巴细胞浸润（图 3.32）。其透明轴心似由肿瘤细胞合成的基底膜物质构成。最近有人根据免疫组化研究证据提出所谓"淋巴内皮分化"[215]一说，但此文章中 VEGFR-3（血管内皮细胞生长因子受体 3）的特异性并不可靠。

鉴别诊断

PILA 与网状血管内皮瘤二者在临床和组织学表现上有诸多相似之处，以致于有人称：后者可能是 PILA 的成人类型。不过，尽管二者在细胞学上非常相似，但 PILA 却没有后者的分支状结构，而且具有明显的丛状乳头结构；但在网状血管内皮瘤，丛状乳头结构最多也就是偶发而已。钉突样血管瘤主要发生在儿童和年轻成人，发病部位颇广，包括口腔。组织学上，其病变大都表浅、边界清楚、伴少量炎性细胞浸润和仅为灶状的钉突样内皮细胞。看不到大片的乳头状结构。血管肉瘤大都具有与此完全不同的临床背景，组织学上以不规则浸润性生长、内皮细胞异型性明显且多伴复层化血管为其特征。

复合性血管内皮瘤
Composite hemangioendothelioma

复合性血管内皮瘤[217]一词是最近专为一组好发于成人手、足的特殊血管病变而打造。有时可见其合并有淋巴水肿。文献报道有个案为先天性病变[218]。这些病变的生物学行为与网状血管内皮瘤类似，以多有局部复发而罕见转移为其特征。不过，我们曾见有经多年之后转化为高度血管肉瘤的偶发病例。组织学上，复合性血管内皮瘤一般是由良性、中间型和形态恶性的血管成分混合而成，其中以上皮样和网状血管内皮瘤的组合最为常见。很多病变中还含有（组织形态）无异于低度血管肉瘤的病灶（若换个环境，该处病变很可能是高度浸润性行为的形态指征）；有些病变中还可见梭形细胞血管瘤的形态特征。在一些仅具有良性成分的病变中，或可见具有淋巴管瘤结构特征的区域。

多形性血管内皮瘤
Polymorphous hemangioendothelioma

多形性血管内皮瘤[219,220]极为罕见，它在淋巴结中的发生几率远高于软组织。长期随访表明它具有转移能力，并可经历一险恶的临床过程。故有建议称：多形性血管内皮瘤实际上是血管肉瘤的一种少见亚型。组织学上，该肿瘤由实性细胞巢、血管瘤样结构和原始血管结构混合而成。多形性血管内皮瘤是否为一种独立的病变实体尚无定论。

Kaposi 肉瘤（KS） Kaposi sarcoma（KS）

KS[221-227]这一令人着迷的病变实体从首次被描述至今已逾百年；最近 20 年，因其多与艾滋病结伴而生，而成为重新点燃人们兴趣的话题。其细胞起源虽尚存争议，但多数证据都指为内皮细胞，尤其是淋巴管内皮为其主要的细胞成分[228-232]。不过，渐成主流的观点认为，KS 似由混合性细胞群构成。流行病学和临床病理多年的研究结果显示：其病因极有可能与某种感染性生物体有关，最早被视为肇事者的是几种病毒，包括巨细胞病毒[227,233,234]。1994 年，人们用 PCR 技术对 AIDS 相关性 KS 患者体内的疱疹病毒样 DNA 序列进行身份鉴定，最终获得突破[235]。自此，这一结果在所有类型的 KS，包括经典型和各种地方病型的患者的身上都被成功复制[236,237]。这种病毒现已被成功分离，可在电镜下成像，并被命名为 HHV-8[236,238-244]。其他一些肿瘤亦可从中检测出这种病毒，如 AIDS 相关性体腔淋巴瘤[236]、多中心性 Castleman 病[236]、免疫功能缺失的器官移植患者的非黑色素瘤性皮肤癌[241]和包括血管肉瘤在内的几种血管肿瘤[242]。但后几类肿瘤病毒检测的结果并不一致[243,244]，故未必具有病因学意义。所有类型KS病变中都能分离出这种新奇病毒一事本身，似乎就能对以下观点提供支持：流行病学和临床上有证据显示，KS是一种反应性的多灶性血管病变[245]。但另一方面，在KS多灶性病变中发现其单克隆性的研究报道[246]则坚持认为KS是一种肿瘤性病变，该病毒可能具有致瘤基因（oncogenic）的功能；但其他一些研究结果则不认同此种说法[247,248]，他们提出一种可能性：此病变过程很可能贯彻于前肿瘤形成（preneoplastic）期的始终。很显然，该问题的最终解决还需要更深入的研究。

临床特征

KS可分为以下几个临床类型[223,225-227]：

经典型地方性KS

病变为无痛性肿物，好发于四肢远端；患者大都是老年人，尤其是地中海周围地区或德裔犹太人中的男性，女性则很少受累。在此背景下，偶有家族性病例报道[223]。发展为全身性疾病者虽不多见，但有相当数量的患者合并有造血系统肿瘤，特别是non-Hodgkin淋巴瘤，这表明：此类患者还有合并免疫功能失调的可能性。

AIDS相关性KS

最初是以主要见于年轻男性艾滋病患者的播散型、浸润型疾病为其特征，但这并不绝对[223,225,226]。在西方（相对于非洲），艾滋病患者大都发生在同性恋高危人群。最常受累的脏器主要包括皮肤（图3.33）、消化道、淋巴结、肺和脾；其次，像肝、肾、眼、前列腺、心脏、膀胱、胆囊、甲状腺、胰腺和骨髓都可受到不同程度的侵犯[249,250]。但肌肉、骨骼和中枢神经系统的受累则非常少见，即便有，也难以察觉。皮肤病变的累及范围大都很广，并不仅局限于下肢。皮损以蓝紫色斑丘疹或结节为特征。黏膜，尤其是口腔黏膜受累很常见。HIV感染治疗技术的进步已明显降低了某些人群的KS发病率。

免疫抑制相关性KS[225,226,251,252]

少见，疾病表现为一种无痛性、偶为浸润性的病变；主要发生在曾接受免疫抑制治疗，尤其是肾移植相关治疗的患者。有时，免疫抑制剂停药或减量后，可见病变消退。

非洲KS

远在艾滋病成为流行时疫之前很多年，非洲KS在撒哈拉以南之非洲中部地区就已有流行；在某些国家，如乌干达，其发病率在该国"恶性肿瘤"中的占比就已经高达9%[225,226]。地方性非洲KS有两种主要类型：其一，发生在低龄儿童，伴全身淋巴结病，病情大都险恶[245,253,254]；其二，发生在中年人，尤其是男性，病情一般发展缓慢，好发于下肢。过去报道的浸润型病例中，至少有部分可能与HIV感染有关；现在，见于撒哈拉以南非洲KS中最常见的类型就是AIDS相关性KS（见上文）。

组织学形态：无论临床类型为何，所有KS的组织学表现都大致相似。根据KS某具体病变的发展，可将其分为三个各具特色、但可相互重叠的阶段：斑片期、斑块期和结节期。前两个阶段多见于艾滋病患者，并很可能作为早期病变被取活检。斑片期（patch）早期改变可能不太明显，很容易与炎症性皮肤病变混淆。在网状真皮层，尤其是在真皮浅层和固有血管、皮肤附属器周围，可见有参差不齐的小血管增生，其内皮细胞为单层，但有轻度异型性

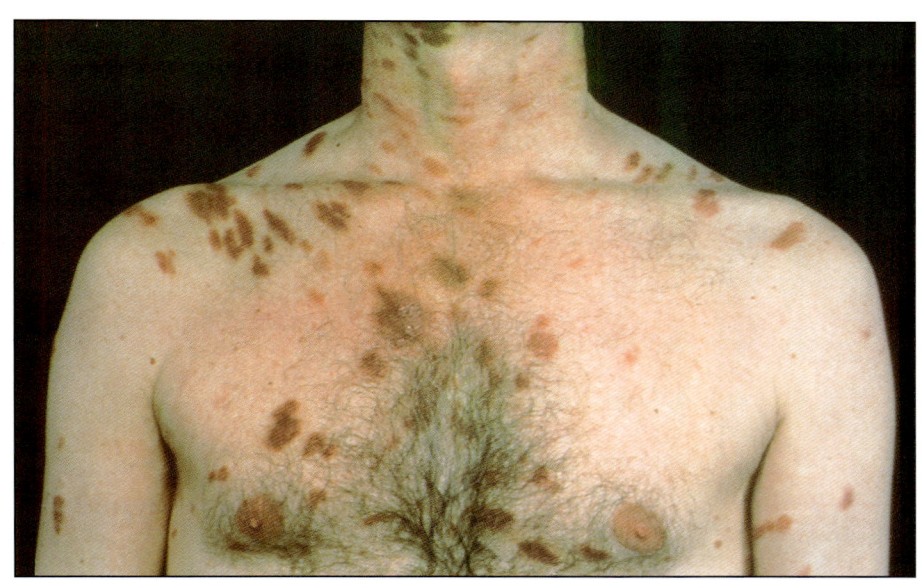

图3.33 Kaposi肉瘤。广泛的斑片期和斑块期病变。患者为年轻的同性恋男性艾滋病者。（Courtesy of St Johh's Institute of Dermatology, London, UK.）

（图 3.34）。这些血管具有与表皮平行排列的趋势。其周围可见渗出的红细胞伴含铁血黄素沉积和少量淋巴细胞、浆细胞等炎性细胞浸润（图 3.35）。后一种现象的出现虽不稳定，但却是有助于诊断的线索。正常血管和皮肤附属器可能突入这些新生的血管腔，有人把这种结构称为"海角征(promontory sign)"，但它并非为 KS 所特有。海角征还可见于其他许多良、恶性病变，包括良性淋巴管内皮瘤和血管肉瘤。某些局部，常酷似在血管肉瘤之所见，有大量胶原成分。梭形细胞仅可偶见于血管周围。斑块期（plaque）代表的是斑片期病变的扩大和发展，可累及整个网状真皮层，甚至波及皮下组织。梭形细胞成分明显增多，含铁血黄素沉积也更为突出（图 3.36）；嗜酸性透明小体随处可见。

结节型（nodular）KS 的病变边界清楚，主要累及真皮；肿瘤由交织状排列、形态单一的梭形细胞束构成，瘤细胞仅呈轻度异型性，但核分裂象却较为常见。在梭形细胞之间可见大量含有红细胞的裂隙状血管腔（图 3.37）。结节的周边部可见有扩张的血管。梭形细胞内、外常常可见有直径在 0.4~10 mm 的嗜酸性透明小体（图 3.38），它可能代表一种变性的红细胞[223,226,255]。嗜酸性透明小体虽可见于所有类型之 KS 病变，但在 AIDS 相关性 KS 中却更为常见。

KS 中的血管虽然可对各种内皮细胞标记物表现出

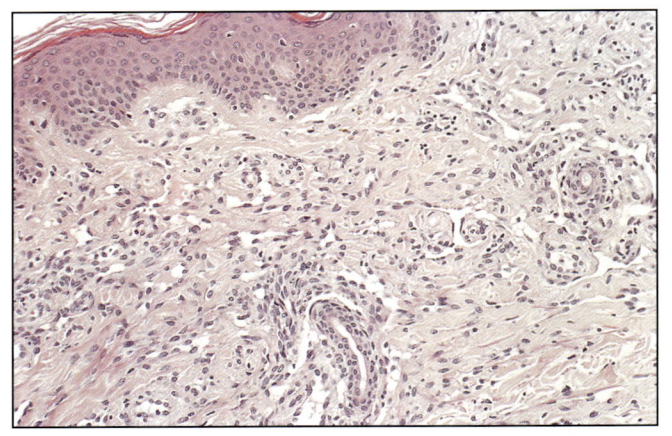

图 3.34 Kaposi 肉瘤的斑片期病变。可见大量排列紊乱的血管腔遍布整个真皮层和皮肤附属器周围。

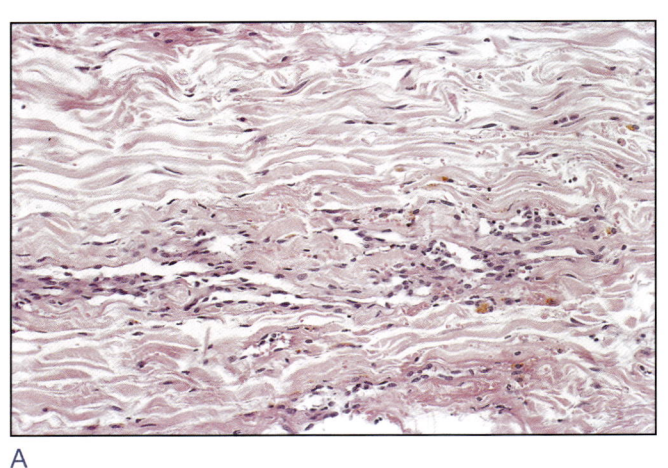
A

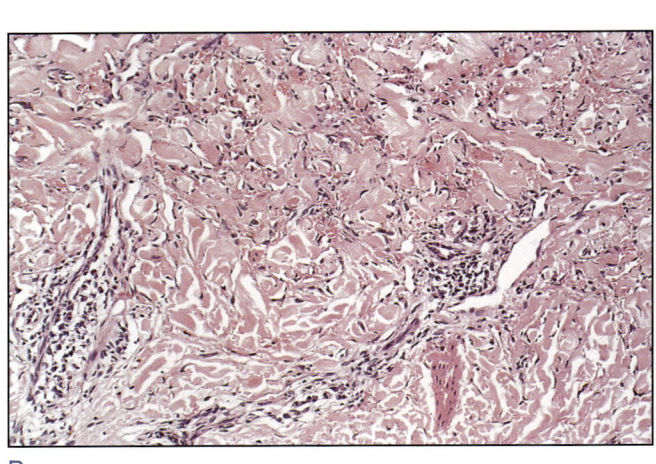
B

图 3.35 Kaposi 肉瘤的斑片期病变。这些血管腔有具有与表皮平行排列的趋势（A），并且大都伴有红细胞、浆细胞的渗出和含铁色素沉积（B）。

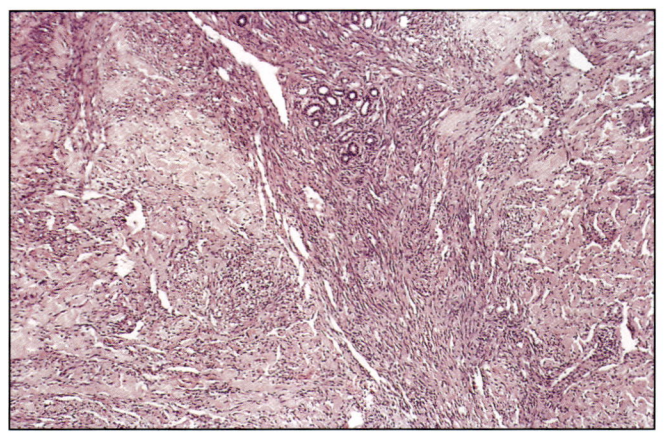

图 3.36 Kaposi 肉瘤的斑块期病变。可见其中的梭形细胞成分明显增多。

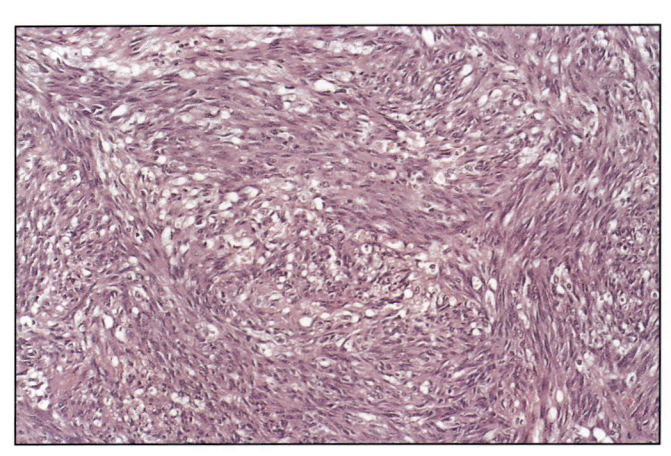

图 3.37 Kaposi 肉瘤的结节期病变。可见形态单一的梭形细胞沿裂隙状或筛网状血管腔排列。

不同程度的反应，但其中的梭形细胞成分对第八因子相关抗原却多为阴性，对 CD34（图 3.39）和 CD31 呈稳定而广泛的阳性。细胞多形性和坏死一般不是结节型 KS 的特征；血管和神经周围侵犯即便偶有发生，也极为罕见。所谓"淋巴管瘤样"型 KS[256,257] 代表的是经典的斑片期/斑块期病变。其中，分布于胶原束间的增生血管呈中度扩张，局部可类似良性淋巴管内皮瘤之形态（图 3.40）。所谓间变型 KS 主要见于前几年的非洲 KS 报道之中[221,258]，它是否存在尚存争议，其中大多数病变所代表的很可能是有明确恶性证据的其他肿瘤类型。不过，我们在非洲患者中见到过偶发、但证据确凿的多形性 KS 个案；有人还以经典型 KS 的间变化（anaplastic transformation of classic KS）为名报告了 5 例系列个案[259]。

最近，抗 HHV-8 潜伏核抗原 -1 的单克隆抗体（latent nuclear antigen-1 of HHV-8）已用于石蜡包埋活检[260,261]。这种标记物在 KS 诊断上的应用价值无可限量，因为它在 KS 所有临床类型中都呈稳定阳性（图 3.41）；而其他血管肿瘤则仅对 HHV-8 呈阳性表达。

鉴别诊断：病理组织学上，其鉴别诊断对象包括良性淋巴管内皮瘤、钉突样血管瘤、梭形细胞血管瘤、Kaposi 样血管内皮瘤、皮肤血管肉瘤、肢端皮血管炎、动脉瘤样良性纤维组织细胞瘤和所谓多核细胞血管组织细胞瘤（multinucleate cell angiohistiocytoma）。杆菌性血管瘤病和化脓性肉芽肿可能会在临床上与 KS 混淆，但它们之间在组织学上的鉴别大都没什么问题。

KS 和血管肉瘤二者都在胶原束间可见有裂隙状的新生血管腔分布，但后者表现有内皮细胞的多层化和明显细胞异型性。动脉瘤样良性纤维组织细胞瘤中可见泡沫细胞、多核巨细胞等，细胞多形性明显，但无裂隙状血管。肢端皮肤血管炎（acroangiodermatitis）[262] 由表浅血管丛中增生的小血管构成，多呈结节状分布，并伴有纤维化、含铁色素沉着和少量炎性细胞浸润。与 KS 斑片期病变不同，其新生血管比较小，排列似无不规则表现；病变不累及皮肤附属器，而且浆细胞也不多见。多核细胞血管组织细胞瘤的病变边界较清楚，并可见巨细胞和散在的、不无规则性且不在原有正常血管周围分布的血管。

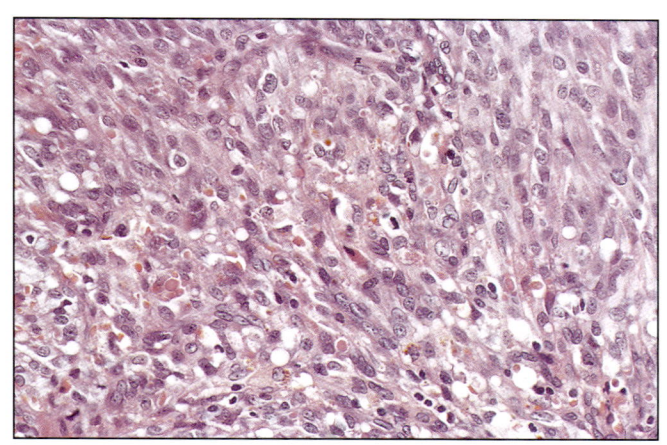

图 3.38　结节期 Kaposi 肉瘤，可见大量嗜酸性透明小体。

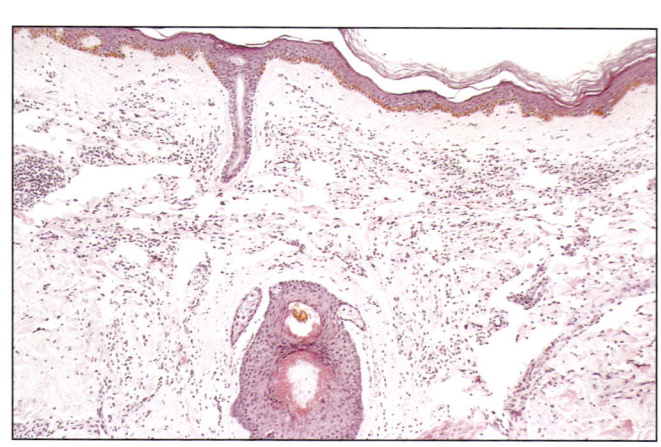

图 3.40　所谓"淋巴管瘤样"Kaposi 肉瘤，可见它与良性淋巴管内皮瘤有相似之处，但间质中可见有梭形细胞和炎性细胞。

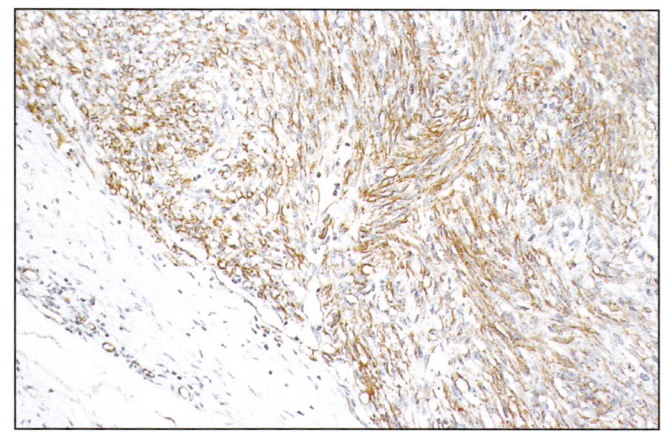

图 3.39　结节期 Kaposi 肉瘤，梭形细胞成分呈 CD34 稳定阳性。

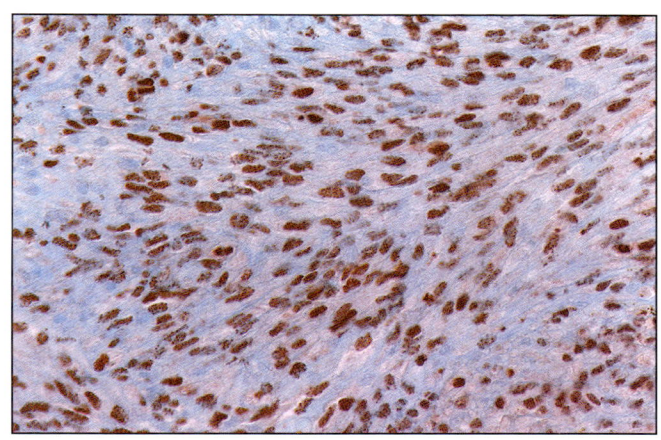

图 3.41　Kaposi 肉瘤，其梭形细胞的细胞核对 HHV-8 免疫组化染色呈强阳性。

恶性血管肿瘤

上皮样血管内皮瘤
Epithelioid hemangioendothelioma

临床特征

上皮样血管内皮瘤，1982年被视为软组织肿瘤中一种独立的病变实体[263]，是上皮样内皮细胞肿瘤家族中的一种低度恶性血管肿瘤[150,264]。但因其病情严重、死亡率高，我们视其为完全恶性[265]（详见下文）。此前，类似的病变和其他上皮样病变一起被归类在组织细胞样血管瘤项下[146,266]。同样的肿瘤亦可发生在其他器官，如肺（其曾用名为血管内细支气管肺泡瘤）[267]、肝[268]、骨[269]、胸、腹膜[270]、皮肤[271-274]、淋巴结[219]，甚至可发生在胃[275]、脑和脑膜[264]。在肺、肝和骨，多中心性病变常见（参阅第5、10、25章）。在软组织，30%～50%的病变起源于大中型血管，尤其是静脉[264-266,276]，故这类肿瘤可能发生在任何器官。上皮样血管内皮瘤的发病年龄范围很宽，但其峰值是中年人，很少发生在儿童[277]。发生在软组织的上皮样血管内皮瘤并无性别差异，但发生在肺、肝者却明显多见于女性；前者大都为单发，而发生在其他部位的肿瘤却大都是多中心性病变，可能会被误诊为转移。该肿瘤的临床表现取决于受累器官的性质；在软组织，其症状，如难治性疼痛，很可能与肿瘤对血管的压迫作用有关。30%的软组织上皮样血管内皮瘤患者可见转移。据文献载，其死亡率在17%（软组织）[265]、43%（肝）[268]和65%（肺）[264]不等。

组织学形态

低倍镜下，典型的上皮样血管内皮瘤着色浅淡、实性，有时可见间质呈深度玻璃样变性，起源于深部软组织者尤著。该肿瘤呈浸润性生长，边界大都不清；由圆形、多角形、间或短梭形内皮细胞构成；瘤细胞的胞浆量或多或少，呈玻璃样、嗜酸、粉染；细胞核呈空泡状，核仁不明显。瘤细胞呈条索状、小巢状或短梁状排列，周围是程度不等的透明变性或黏液样间质，其中常可见软骨样结构（图3.42）。胞浆中常可见明显的胞浆空泡，其中偶可含有红细胞，酷似原始的血管结构（图3.43），但构型完整的血管最多仅可见于局部。上皮样血管内皮瘤如起源于血管，瘤细胞向内可充斥管腔，向外则可浸透血管壁，并向周围组织浸润。原固有血管被（肿瘤）完全阻塞或阻断的情况常有发生。网状纤维染色可突显其中血管结构的管状构型（图3.44）。此外，营养障碍性钙化和骨化或可成为部分病变的突出特点[265,278]。

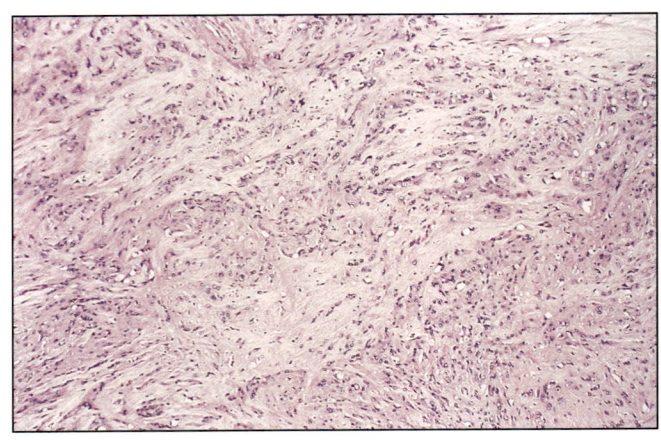

图3.42　上皮样血管内皮瘤。在透明变性的间质中可见瘤细胞呈典型的条索状生长方式。

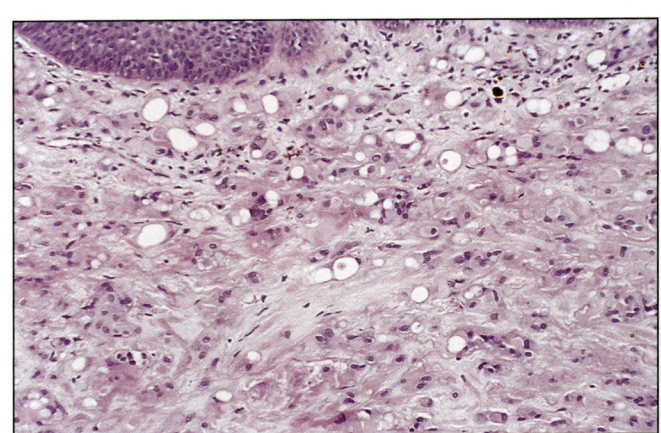

图3.43　上皮样血管内皮瘤，在此真皮病变中，可见明显的胞浆内腔以及腔内的红细胞。

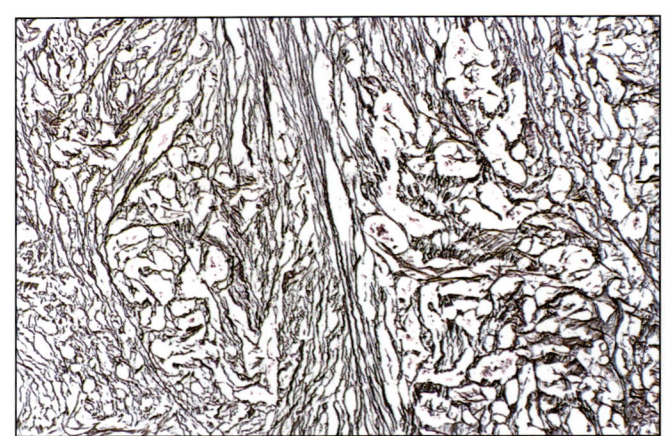

图3.44　上皮样血管内皮瘤，网状纤维染色可突显血管形成的结构构型。

间质的炎症反应一般并不明显，但在部分病变或可见明显的破骨细胞样巨细胞反应[278-280]。可成为上皮样血管内皮瘤之亚型者现已被描述为梭形细胞和组织（上皮样）细胞样血管内皮瘤。据称，迄今为止，仅在淋巴结和脾脏有此类个案的报道[150,219,281,282]。

虽然瘤细胞的异型性一般仅为轻度，核分裂象也不多见。但有时在同一病变中可见一形态谱：部分区域的瘤细胞不仅巢聚的数量多，而且异型性明显，核分裂象计数也高（图 3.45）[264,265]，甚至可在局部见到无异于上皮样血管肉瘤的病变。凡具此病变特征者之预后大都恶劣，该肿瘤即被标定为恶性[264,265]。在组织学特征和临床预后之间虽无明确相关，但核异型性明显、核分裂象计数高和血管肉瘤样病灶三者与临床预后差之间有正相关趋势。

免疫组化：上皮样血管内皮瘤大都表现有典型的血管免疫显型特征，并有内皮细胞标记物的表达，尤其是 CD31（图 3.46）和 von Willebrand 因子（血管性血友病因子）。多达 45% 的病变呈 α-SMA 阳性，26% 呈 CK 阳性（图 3.47）[265,283,284]。而与上皮性肿瘤不同，EMA 大都为阴性。CK 阳性最常见于发生在骨的病变，此处很可能反映了瘤细胞胞浆的中间丝含量高。对 2 例上皮样血管内皮瘤所做的细胞遗传学研究显示有 t(1;3)(p36.3;q25) 易位。

鉴别诊断

主要须与转移性或原发癌鉴别，尤其是在实质性脏器和骨骼。有助于鉴别的形态特征是：上皮样血管内皮瘤瘤细胞的胞浆空泡中可见红细胞，而不是黏液；再佐以对血管标记物的免疫染色呈阳性。此外，肉瘤瘤细胞核的多形性大都更为明显。在软组织，还要与上皮样肉瘤鉴别[286]；后者（的瘤细胞）一般都呈大片状生长（至少是在局部），胞浆空泡仅可偶见，CK、EMA 均为阳性，CD34 常为阳性；但对更具特异性的内皮细胞标记物染色，如 CD31 和 vWF 则都为阴性。病变间质有明显黏液变性的上皮样血管内皮瘤可能会与黏液样脂肪肉瘤和黏液样软骨肉瘤混淆。但后者具有明显的小叶状结构，无胞浆空泡，且 S-100 蛋白染色阳性。至于黏液样脂肪肉瘤，最佳鉴别点是识别典型的分支状血管构型和小的多泡状脂肪母细胞。

血管肉瘤　Angiosarcoma

血管肉瘤一词涵盖了此前被冠名为淋巴管肉瘤和恶性血管内皮瘤两种病变，原因是现在尚无可靠方法在血管和淋巴管内皮分化（或起源）之间做出鉴别。如具体到血管肉瘤个案，其分化可为单向或双向。本章主要讨论皮肤和软组织血管肉瘤，至于内脏的血管肉瘤将在有关章节中介绍。值得注意的是，深部软组织血管肉瘤曾被认为极为罕见，但近来却日渐增多，究其原因，可能是其特征性的上皮样细胞形态，过去很容易被误认为上皮或间皮分化。

皮肤血管肉瘤[287-292]的发生不外乎以下三个不同的

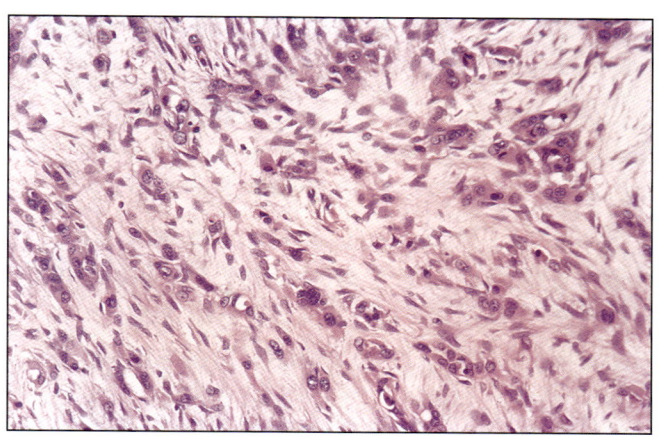

图 3.45　"恶性"上皮样血管内皮瘤，可见瘤细胞异型性明显，呈小灶状、实性丛状分布。

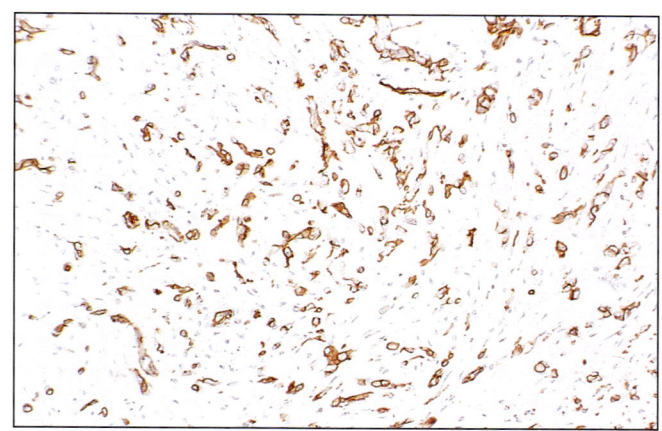

图 3.46　上皮样血管内皮瘤，CD31（JC70）是内皮细胞分化最敏感的免疫组化标记物之一。

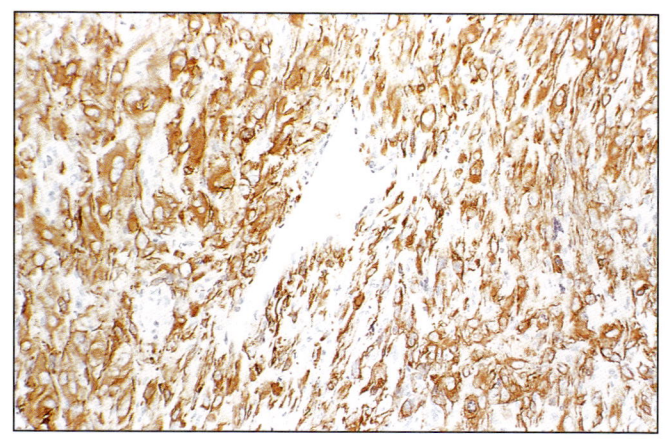

图 3.47　上皮样血管内皮瘤。CK 阳性很常见，虽然它不如上皮样血管肉瘤那样稳定。请注意，正常的内皮细胞呈阴性着色。

临床类型：(1) 头颈部特发性血管肉瘤；(2) 淋巴水肿相关性血管肉瘤；(3) 放疗后血管肉瘤。氯乙烯接触史常被视为肝血管肉瘤的相关因素之一，但在皮肤血管肉瘤，有此相关接触者仅为偶发个案[293]。血管肉瘤偶可发生在下述解剖部位和病变之中：发生在大血管[294]的血管瘤或血管畸形[295]、发生在神经[296]的神经纤维瘤病之丛状神经纤维瘤[297]、神经鞘瘤[296,298]，或见于恶性外周神经鞘瘤病变之局部[296,299]。在恶性生殖细胞瘤，血管肉瘤偶可作为其中之肉瘤样结构成分存在。血管肉瘤很少发生于儿童[300,301]。据称：偶有合并着色性干皮病的个案[302,303]。个别血管肉瘤患者还被确认合并有大疱性表皮松解症[304]、慢性静脉性溃疡[305]、病态肥胖[307]和痛风石[306]。还有报道称：在器官移植患者，（血管肉瘤的发生）与其免疫功能抑制有关，但在其发生机制中，HHV-8并无明显影响[308,309,309a]。

面部、颈部和头皮特发性血管肉瘤
Idiopathic angiosarcoma of the face, neck, and scalp

典型的特发性血管肉瘤好发于老年人，尤以男性居多；表现为多灶性、瘀伤样、红色略带紫色的皮损、斑块和结节，尤其好发于头皮和面部中心（图3.48）[287-292,310]。病变典型，但伴有面部弥漫性水肿者可能会被临床漏诊。预后极差，5年存活率仅在12%～33%[310,311]。一项针对面部、头皮和体内脏器的血管肉瘤的综合性研究显示：其总的5年存活率为24%[312]。死亡原因大都是局部病变的广泛浸润或广泛的远端（尤其是肺）转移。年轻患者的预后似乎要好些，放疗或可提高存活率[313,314]。

淋巴水肿相关型血管肉瘤[315-322]
Lymphedema-associated angiosarcoma

此型肿瘤常有淋巴管肉瘤之称，典型病变发生在乳房根治术并腋窝淋巴结清扫术后1～30年、已经或尚未接受放疗之女性的手臂（Stewart-Treves综合征）。此病与放疗诱导性血管肉瘤虽有重叠，但前者的病变大都发生在放疗野之外。临床上，未必都呈现有明显的淋巴水肿。淋巴水肿相关型血管肉瘤偶可见于其他类型的慢性淋巴水肿，如先天性淋巴水肿、医源性淋巴水肿、淋巴管畸形和丝虫性淋巴水肿。临床表现包括瘀斑样斑块、结节和受累肢体的大范围水（血）泡。预后与特发性血管肉瘤相似。

放疗后血管肉瘤[323-326]
Postradiation angiosarcoma

放疗后血管肉瘤原本少见，但现在却日渐增多，而且常常是在因良性或恶性病变而接受放疗之后多年才发生。迄今为止，最常见的是发生在皮肤的病变，其次发生在乳腺癌保乳手术后的乳腺实质。发生在乳腺皮肤的放疗后血管肉瘤一般都不伴有淋巴水肿，而且其潜伏期也比Stewart-Treves综合征要短[327]。部分乳腺血管肉瘤患者可能合并慢性淋巴水肿，其原因可能是疾病发展所致[328]。放疗后血管肉瘤的病因虽稍显平缓，但其预后却似与其他类型一般无二。

软组织血管肉瘤[291,329,330]
Soft tissue angiosarcoma

如上所述，深部软组织血管肉瘤虽曾被视为少见病，但现今的诊断却日渐增多。究其原因，可能是因绝大多数病变都表现有上皮样细胞形态，故而对其诊断标准和敏感性做出调整所致（详见下文）。软组织血管肉瘤最常见于老年人，尤以男性为多见；好发于下肢或腹腔（含腹膜后）。部分患者有放疗史。其5年存活率与皮肤病变差不多，最多也就是20%～30%。

组织学形态：各种临床类型血管肉瘤的组织形态特征非常相似，并表现出很宽的形态谱系：从有明确血管

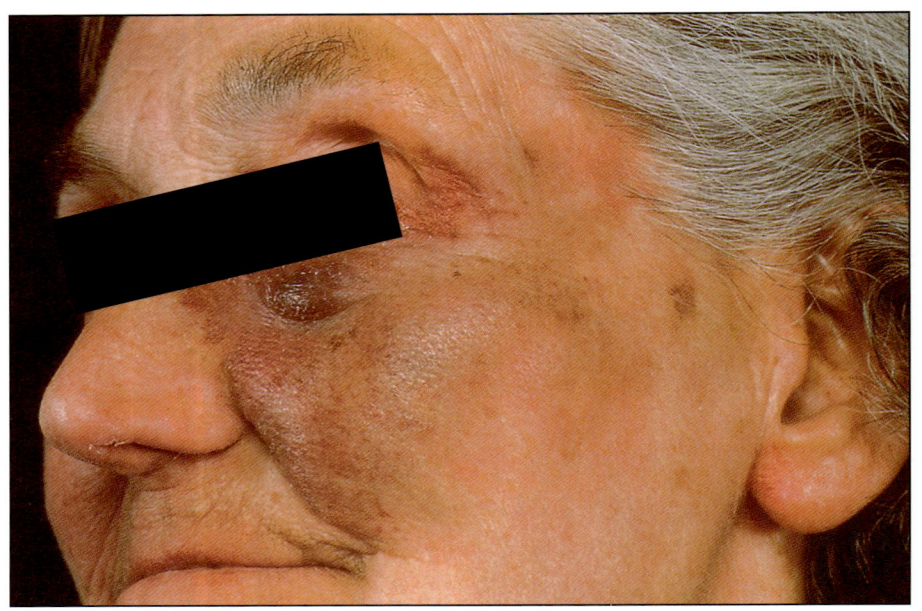

图3.48 皮肤血管肉瘤。发生于一老年患者头面部的典型瘀伤样病变。（Courtesy of St Johh's Institute of Dermatology, London, UK.）

形成的病灶，到分化很差、血管分化尚未成形的实性病变都有。典型病变是一种浸润型真皮肿瘤，由大量形状不整、互相吻合、散在分布于胶原束间的裂隙状血管腔构成（图3.49）；并可见皮下组织、骨骼肌甚至骨膜浸润。上述血管腔被覆的内皮细胞呈不同程度的多形性、核深染，并呈多层化、乳头状生长（图3.50）。正常和病理性核分裂象易见。实性病灶不少见，低分化病变多以实性瘤细胞巢结构居优，血管结构分化很少（图3.51）。在此情况下，网状纤维染色就十分有用，它可很好地突显血管分化的早期构型，因为新生血管都被一网硬蛋白鞘环绕。上皮样细胞成分居优的血管肉瘤约占5%（图3.52）[331]。有报道称：血管肉瘤偶可主要由颗粒细胞构成[332,333]。炎性细胞浸润常见，并可能很明显。据称：大量单核细胞浸润和预后良好呈正相关[310]，而核分裂计数高则与预后差呈正相关[334,335]；但我们认为，组织学特征（含分级）与预后之间并无可靠相关，而肿瘤的大小（或曰可切除性）似更为重要。

在低分化血管肉瘤，免疫组化染色或可有助于鉴别诊断，因其对各种内皮细胞标记物呈不同程度的阳性反应。虽有很多病变对第八因子相关抗原呈阴性反应，但对CD31、von Willebrand因子（单克隆抗体）（图3.53）或CD34（特异性稍差）染色的阳性率却很高。最近有报道称：在血管肿瘤诊断上，Ewing肉瘤标记物Fli-1的敏感性、特异性与CD31相当[336]；但我们感觉其特异性稍差。如能在电镜下找到内皮细胞的特征性细胞器，尤其是Weibel-Palade小体也行，但在皮肤血管肉瘤，W-P小体却难得一见。对4例深部和表浅血管肉瘤所做的细胞遗传学研究显示有复杂的染色体异常，主要累及第5、7、8、13、15、20、22号和Y染色体。

鉴别诊断：本章对血管肉瘤和良性血管肿瘤之间的鉴别已另有描述。非典型血管病变（p69）可发生在乳腺癌放疗后的乳房皮肤，并可被误诊为血管肉瘤[324]。

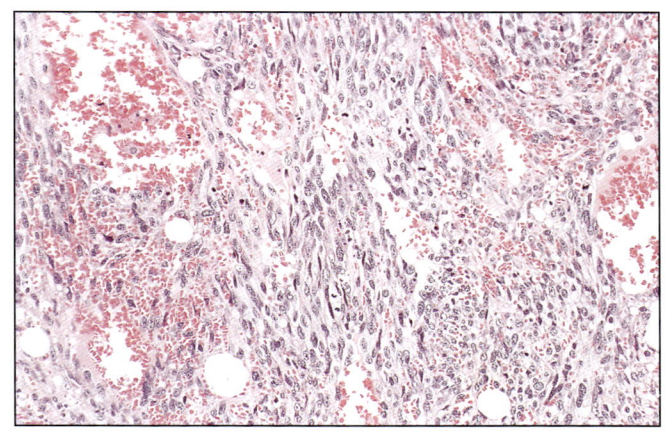

图3.51　低分化血管肉瘤。由梭形瘤细胞构成的实性癌巢，仅据此，诊断很难成立。

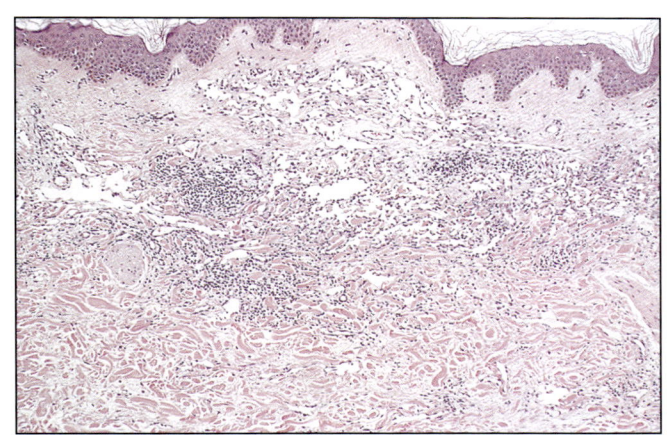

图3.49　皮肤血管肉瘤。可见大量裂隙状血管腔，分布于胶原纤维束间。

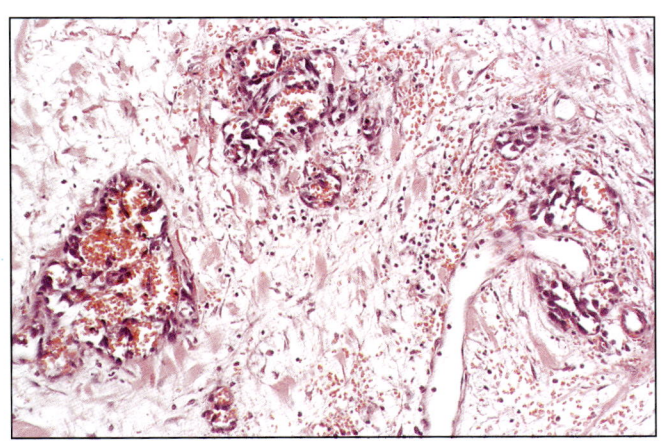

图3.50　皮肤血管肉瘤，病变中可见内皮细胞呈多层化和明显的细胞核异型性。

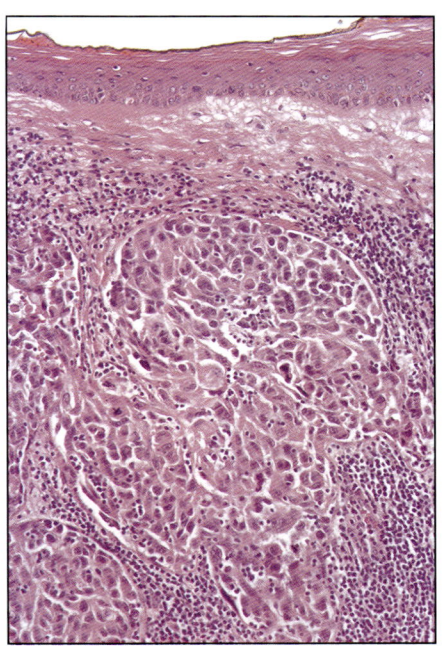

图3.52　皮肤上皮样血管肉瘤。如图所示之皮肤病变很容易被误诊为恶性黑色素瘤或癌。

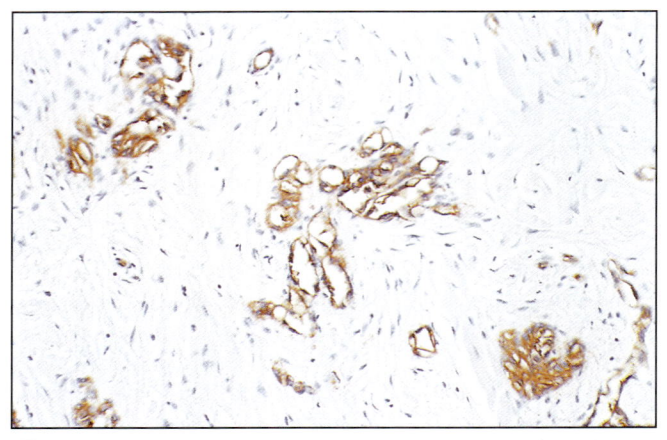

图3.53 淋巴水肿相关性血管肉瘤，病变位于足部，瘤细胞呈von Willebrand因子免疫组化染色阳性。

但前者系由局灶性增生的血管构成，病变血管的内皮细胞为单层，核深染，无核分裂象。低分化血管肉瘤（的组织像）与其他梭形细胞肉瘤、黑色素瘤和癌多有相似之处；在此情况下，网状纤维染色、免疫组化染色和（较少采用的）电镜就非常有助于正确诊断。一定要记住，在内皮细胞标记物中，荆豆凝集素Ⅰ（Ulex europaeus lectin type Ⅰ）在很多类型的癌中也呈阳性表达。

上皮样血管肉瘤 Epithelioid angiosarcoma

临床特征：上皮样血管肉瘤是一种独特而少见的肿瘤，代表上皮样血管肿瘤形态谱的恶性端[150,329]。上皮样血管肉瘤的构成几乎均为上皮样细胞，可以区别普通血管肉瘤之上皮样病灶。此组织学亚型最初见于甲状腺，尤其是地方性甲状腺肿的甲状腺[338,339]。对它在皮肤和软组织中的发生虽早已获认可，但被视为独立的病变实体还只是最近的事情[329]。上皮样血管肉瘤虽然大都发生在深部软组织（见上文），但也有偶发个案见于肾上腺[340]；据称，个别病变起源于诸如胸膜[270]、肺动脉[341]、乳腺[342]、骨[343]和阴道[344]等部位。皮肤[331,345]和软组织上皮样血管肉瘤好发于中老年人，男性尤为多见。肿瘤生长迅速，除可在部分患者见有皮肤出血性卫星病灶之外，很少有特异性临床表现。部分血管肉瘤表现为神经鞘瘤的恶变形态之一[298]；个别病变的发生还与异物[346]、动静脉瘘[330,347,348]或前期放疗[329,330,349]有关。起源于内脏的上皮样血管肉瘤偶可转移至皮肤[350]。绝大多数上皮样血管肉瘤的临床经过极具侵袭性，伴全身转移，且大都在确诊后2～3年内死亡。关于皮肤上皮样血管肉瘤的预后可获改善之说尚有待独立性认证。

组织学形态：上皮样血管肉瘤常见有坏死、出血、由大片状、实性分布的瘤细胞构成（图3.54）；瘤细胞呈上皮样；胞体大，呈圆形或卵圆形；胞浆丰富，嗜酸或双染；细胞核大、着色淡、空泡状，并有一明显的嗜酸性核仁。瘤细胞多形性虽不明显，但核分裂象很多见。部分瘤细胞内可见胞浆内空泡，其中偶含红细胞。血管形成可见于绝大多数病变，至少是在局部，并很少乳头状结构。部分病变显然是起源于大血管。网状纤维染色可突显管状的血管构型（图3.55）。免疫组化染色：几乎所有病变中的瘤细胞都对F-Ⅷ相关抗原和CD31呈阳性表达；CK阳性者约为50%，而EMA则仅在少数病变中呈局灶阳性。

鉴别诊断：上皮样血管肉瘤的鉴别对象必须包括几乎所有类型的上皮样恶性肿瘤，如转移癌、间皮瘤、恶性黑色素瘤、上皮样肉瘤和恶性上皮样神经鞘瘤，位于皮肤和软组织者尤然。鉴别要点：上皮样血管肉瘤的病变中大都可以找到胞浆内腔和血管形成的证据，最重要的是瘤细胞对内皮细胞特异性标记物（尤其是F-Ⅷ相关抗原和CD31）呈阳性表达。

"内膜"肉瘤 "Intimal" sarcomas

大血管的原发性肉瘤少见，文献个案的总数尚不足200[351-360]。血管壁肉瘤，尤其是见于诸如下腔静脉

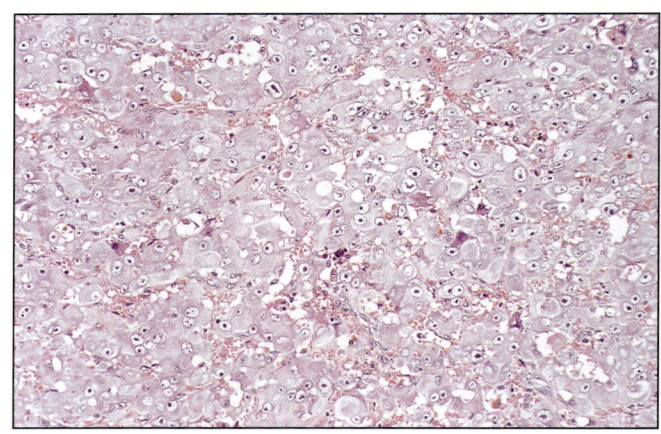

图3.54 上皮样血管肉瘤，注意瘤细胞的大片状生长方式及其非常明显的核仁。

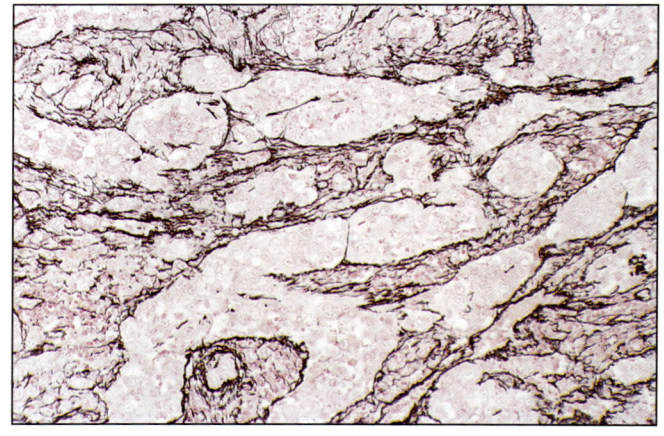

图3.55 上皮样血管肉瘤，网状纤维染色可突显血管形成的管状构型。

之类大静脉者，虽然多为平滑肌肉瘤[355]，但管腔肉瘤中的一部分可能是起源于内膜，内膜肉瘤即因此而得名。这类肿瘤主要见于主、肺动脉，是一种低分化的梭形细胞肉瘤；它们很少表现有内皮细胞分化的免疫组化证据，更多的是呈 SMA 阳性[360]；最近有研究称其骨桥蛋白（osteopontin）呈阳性[358]。不过，仅对波形蛋白呈阳性者占其大部。据此，有人认为：内膜肉瘤系起源于内膜的内皮细胞、纤维母细胞和肌纤维母细胞。实际上，内膜肉瘤仅好发于成人，预后极差。针对少数病变所做的比较基因组杂交技术（comparative genomic hybridization）研究显示：最稳定的细胞遗传学异常包括 12q13～14 的获得与扩增过表达[360]。

淋巴管肿瘤
Tumors of lymph vessels

淋巴管肿瘤比血管瘤少见得多，在所有脉管肿瘤中所占比例约为 4%[18]，其中绝大多数都是良性病变；而且，据信，其多为畸形，而并非真性肿瘤。淋巴管和血管肿瘤之间的鉴别并非都有可能，即便用免疫组化和电镜技术也无法鉴别二者；而且某些病变，如肌内血管瘤（上文）本身就是两种脉管成分的混合体。淋巴管瘤可分为五种主要类型：（1）海绵状淋巴管瘤；（2）囊性水瘤；（3）局限性淋巴管瘤；（4）获得性进行性淋巴管瘤（良性淋巴管内皮瘤）；（5）淋巴管瘤病。是否有毛细淋巴管瘤存在尚有存疑。

海绵状淋巴管瘤和囊性水瘤
Cavernous lymphangioma and cystic hydroma

临床特征

两种病变放在一起讨论是因为囊性水瘤可能仅为海绵状淋巴管瘤的一种亚型，其中有淋巴管的高度扩张。囊性水瘤好发部位的周边环境对其扩张大都阻力很少[361]。大多数病变发生在新生儿或 1 岁以内的婴儿，男女发病率相同[362-364]；偶可发现于成人[365]。囊性水瘤大都发生在颈部、腋窝和腹股沟，而海绵状淋巴管瘤亦可发生在口腔（尤其是舌）、四肢和腹腔（主要是肠系膜，其次是后腹膜）。虽然两种病变都可能局部复发，但尤以海绵状淋巴管瘤为常见。

组织学形态

真皮、皮下组织或深层组织中可见扩张的薄壁淋巴管，被覆的内皮细胞为扁平、单层，无异型性（图3.56），罕见有肥大或立方状上皮。管腔内可空无一物，亦可内容蛋白性淋巴液、淋巴细胞，偶有红细胞。周围间质中可见数量不等的淋巴细胞，偶可见淋巴滤泡。口径较大的管腔周围常可见不完整的平滑肌层（图3.57）。陈旧性病变则可出现明显纤维化。由于某些不明的原因，腹腔内淋巴管瘤的临床表现可能很急；组织学上，这类病变伴有明显的炎性反应、周围脂肪坏死和反应性病变[366]。

鉴别诊断

有时，可能无法与海绵状血管瘤鉴别，在伴有出血或管腔内红细胞时尤然。淋巴细胞聚集或可有助于淋巴管瘤的诊断。位于腹膜的病变须与囊性间皮瘤鉴别，后者囊腔大小相差更多，被覆上皮呈 CK 阳性，而对内皮细胞标记物则呈阴性表达。

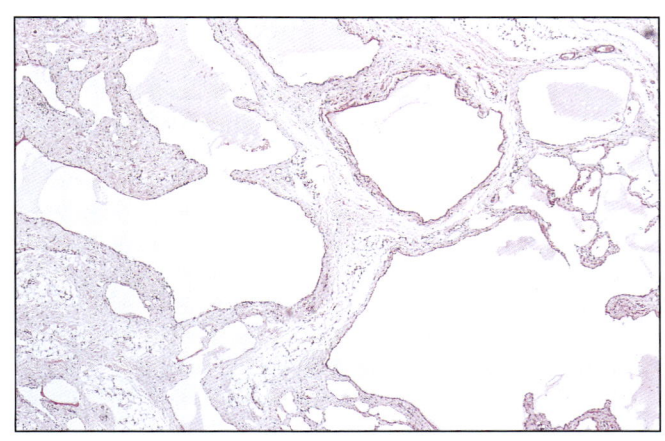

图3.56　海绵状淋巴管瘤。可见扩张的淋巴管，其管壁厚薄不等。

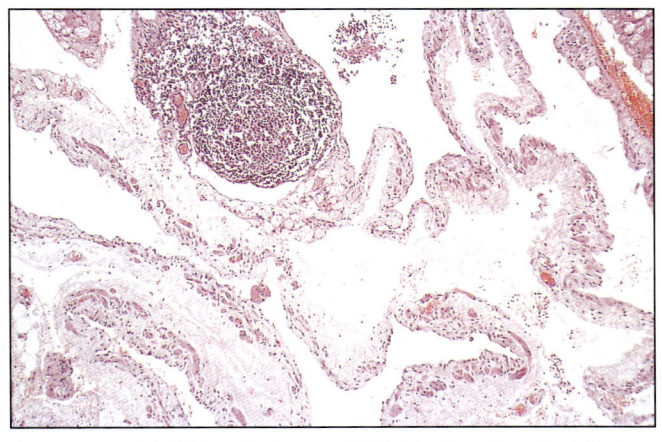

图3.57　海绵状淋巴管瘤，可见淋巴细胞聚集，部分管壁内可见明显的平滑肌（层）。

局限性淋巴管瘤
Lymphangioma circumscriptum

临床表现

局限性淋巴管瘤作为婴儿的一种发育畸形,常合并海绵状淋巴管瘤、囊性水瘤或淋巴管瘤病;或作为成人的一种获得性病变,常与放疗或慢性淋巴水肿有关[367-369]。后一种情况最好是被视为淋巴管扩张。无性别差异,可发生于身体任何部位,但以四肢多见。临床上,以出现大量无症状、局限性、内容清亮或血性液体的囊泡为特征。术后复发仅常见于发生在儿童的病变。

组织学形态

病变由皮肤浅层或真皮乳头中大量扩张的淋巴管构成,并伴覆盖其上方的表皮增生(图3.58)和周围间质淋巴细胞浸润。因系横断面之故,这些淋巴管几乎全都位于表层皮肤之内。有些病变,尤其是发生在儿童的局限性淋巴管瘤会与深部肌肉淋巴管相通;术中如不将其交通支结扎,则术后局部复发几率颇高[370]。

良性淋巴管内皮瘤(获得性进行性淋巴管瘤)
Benign lymphangioendothelioma (acquired progressive lymphangioma)

临床特征

良性淋巴管内皮瘤(获得性进行性淋巴管瘤)是一种少见的良性淋巴管畸形,虽然早在1970年它就被冠名血管内皮瘤(淋巴管型)[371]加以描述,但其后多年来,文献报道的个案并不是很多[372-375]。任何年龄均可罹患本病,但以中老年人最为多见;发病率男女相同。病变大都位于四肢,尤其是下肢,但亦可发生在面、背和腹部。临床上,病变呈单发性、边界清楚的红斑或斑块,虽可疑似瘀伤,但经年不退,并缓慢扩大。文献报道的多灶性进行性淋巴管瘤很可能是淋巴管瘤病个案[376]。有报道称:单纯切除术后复发者极为罕见,局部或次全切除术后,(病变)可自发性消退[377]。据称,偶有病变发生在放疗[378]和动脉造影[379]之后。

组织学形态

典型病变由横向排列的不规则薄壁管腔构成,它们在胶原纤维束间呈裂隙状生长,并相互吻合。这些管腔被覆单层扁平内皮细胞,其细胞异型性程度最高者仅至极轻度(图3.59)。管腔多为空腔,或仅含少量红细胞和/或蛋白性物质。这些管腔虽然大都位于真皮浅层,但病变扩散至真皮深层和皮下组织者时有所见。本病变不累及真皮乳头,也不像在局限性淋巴管瘤所见的那样与深部肌内淋巴管相通。

鉴别诊断

鉴于其管腔在胶原束间呈裂隙状生长方式,故首先就要与高分化血管肉瘤鉴别,尽管它们的临床表现各异。与后者鉴别的重要根据是:进行性淋巴管瘤的内皮细胞无异型性、无多层化、无核分裂象。Kaposi肉瘤斑片期临床表现为多灶性病变;在组织学上则表现为不规则形状的管腔围绕真皮固有血管和皮肤附属器周围生长,并伴浆细胞浸润、血管外漏出红细胞和含铁血黄素沉积。良性淋巴管内皮瘤和钉突样血管瘤的临床表现虽然不同,但二者的组织结构却可十分相似。但前者一般均无

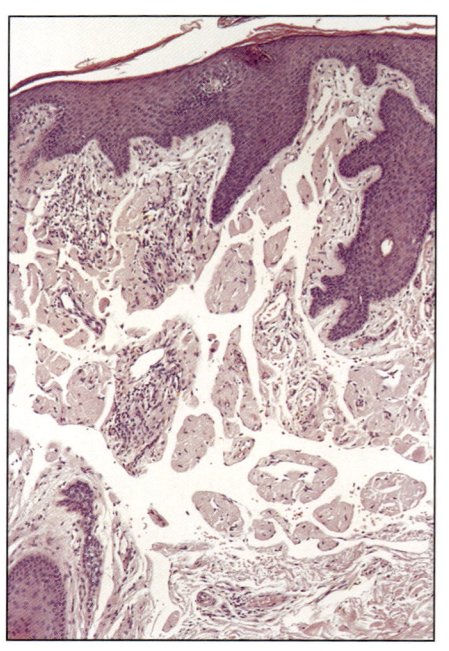

图3.59 良性淋巴管内皮瘤("进行性淋巴管瘤"),注意其在胶原束间裂隙状的生长方式及其完全没有异型性的内皮细胞。

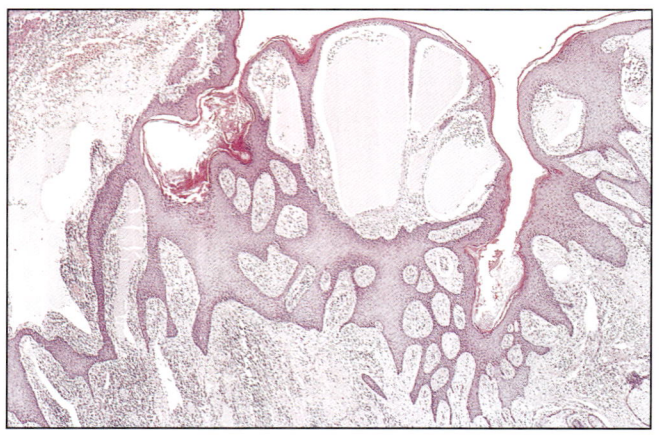

图3.58 局限性淋巴管瘤,真皮乳头内可见扩张的淋巴管及其所引发的炎性反应。

明显的钉突样内皮细胞,管腔内红细胞稀少,含铁色素沉积也大都不甚明显。

淋巴管瘤病　Lymphangiomatosis

淋巴管瘤病是一种非常少见的、以弥漫性累及实质性脏器、骨和/或软组织为特征的发育异常[380,381]。相当一部分患者的病变仅局限于某一肢体,伴或不伴骨骼受累[382]。典型病变发生在儿童,有时出生就已出现,无性别差异[381,382]。临床上,它可能与经典型血管瘤病或其他血管畸形重叠;在部分患者,不经血管造影便不能确诊。发生在软组织的淋巴管瘤病呈弥漫性、潮湿状且有波动感的肿胀性病变;它可与一皮肤瘘管相通,或偶呈与局限性淋巴管瘤病变无异之形态。与累及软组织和骨的淋巴管瘤病不同,内脏受累患者的预后大都不好[381]。

软组织型淋巴管瘤病的组织形态可能与海绵状淋巴管瘤或更多地是与良性淋巴管内皮瘤相似,典型病变伴有广泛的胶原裂隙状生长方式,与血管肉瘤有几分相似;但淋巴管要广泛得多,累及到真皮和皮下组织(图3.60)。还有一种现象,尤其是软组织型淋巴管瘤病,虽然管腔内几乎没有红细胞,但在间质中却可见大量含铁血黄素。陈旧性病变表现出明显的间质纤维化。

放疗后非典型脉管病变
Atypical vascular lesions after radiotherapy

血管瘤样病变很少出现在曾经的放疗野之内,而是大都发生在乳腺皮肤[324,383,385]。其中部分病变的组织形态可能表现出非典型特征,很可能被误诊为放疗后血管肉瘤,故为本文详述之要点。

这类病变大都发生在乳腺癌放疗后数年。就诱导时间而言,放疗之于非典型脉管病变的发生,大都短之于血管肉瘤[385]。临床表现并无特殊,从正常肤色到发红之间变化不等,大都呈多发性斑疹和丘疹。

组织学形态表现各异,病变偶可类似局限性淋巴管瘤[368]或良性淋巴管内皮瘤[378]。活检大多显示在浅层和/或深部真皮有形状不规则、扩张程度不等、被覆有单层内皮细胞的淋巴管样管腔。这些病变大都边界清楚,但可能具有裂隙状生长方式。这些管腔被覆的内皮细胞呈扁平状或稍有深染的钉突样改变,偶呈乳头状突起(图3.61)。无细胞核多形性,无细胞多层化,核分裂象也难得一见。

鉴别诊断对象包括高分化血管肉瘤、钉突样血管瘤和Kaposi肉瘤。与钉突样血管瘤的不同在于:放疗后脉管病变并不均匀,而且其病变管腔的主体部分未必都位于真皮浅层。但在某些情况下,单靠形态学是不可能做出鉴别的,最好还是根据放疗史定夺。与Kaposi肉

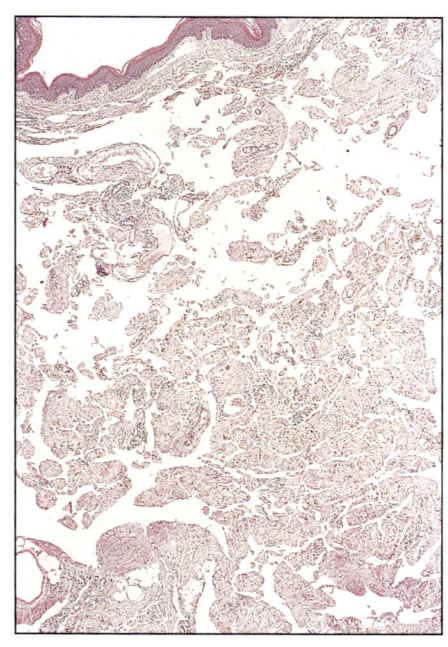

图3.60　淋巴管瘤病,在正常结构之间可见淋巴管呈非常广泛的弥漫性裂隙状生长。

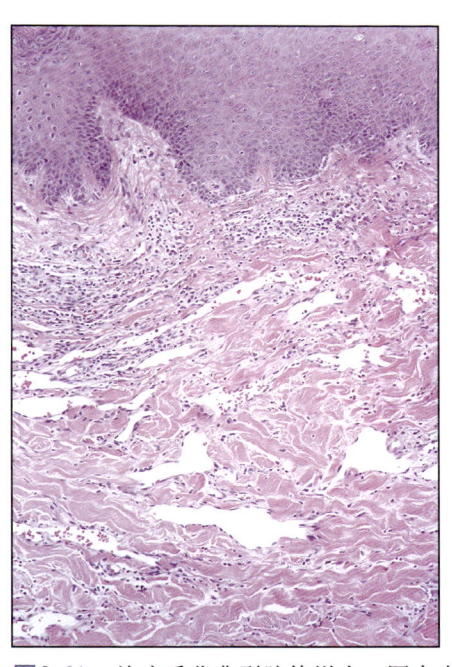

图3.61　放疗后非典型脉管增生。图中皮肤病变取自乳腺,病变由在结构上呈非典型性的淋巴样腔隙构成,但其内皮细胞既无多层化,也无多型性。

瘤的鉴别要点有:特殊的临床背景、无炎性反应、可见钉突样内皮细胞和局部乳头状突起。为与高分化血管肉瘤做鉴别,我们建议多做切片,仔细检查,以确认没有核分裂象和细胞异型性。

淋巴管肌瘤病　Lymphangiomyomatosis

淋巴管肌瘤病是一种非常少见的错构瘤性质的病变,以后腹膜、纵隔和肺实质(可见于70%的病例)

的淋巴管、淋巴结中的平滑肌弥漫性增生为特征[386-388]。病变如果很局限，则被视为淋巴管肌瘤。本病变几乎仅见于女性，而且是在育龄期间。该现象提示：激素在病变发生过程中的重要作用。但这种相关性尚存争议[388,390]。患者表现为呼吸困难、气胸和乳糜胸，受累范围广泛时，如果不做肺移植手术，本疾病常可致命[386-388]。现有共识认为：本病变可合并肾血管肌脂瘤，另有部分结节性硬化患者可罹患本病[388,391]。现有证据显示，部分淋巴管肌瘤病与16号染色体上结节性硬化基因复合体之一（TSC-2）的基因突变密切相关[392,393]。

镜下，病变由淋巴管以及环绕其周的丛状平滑肌细胞构成，平滑肌细胞分化程度高，胞浆略呈颗粒状，呈肌束状排列（图3.62）。免疫组化：这些细胞呈典型平滑肌细胞的免疫显型特征，另外，对HMB-45呈稳定阳性表达，这是一种黑色素瘤相关性标记物，可与黑色素前体糖蛋白反应[394]；类似的着色反应亦可见于MART-1（Melan-A，一种黑色素细胞分化抗原）染色[395]。能与其共享此免疫反应性者还有血管平滑肌脂肪瘤中的平滑肌成分（任何其他类型平滑肌都无此特性）和肺等部位的透明细胞（糖原）瘤。虽然这可能反映了它与不同蛋白的交叉反应，但它确可识别血管周平滑肌细胞的特殊亚型（即血管周上皮样细胞[396]，见第24章）；而且，这种免疫显型特征可能有助于鉴别诊断。

血管周细胞肿瘤
Tumors of perivascular cells

血管球肿瘤　Glomus tumors
临床特征

血管球肿瘤[397-399]起源于特化型、有温度调节功能、分布于动静脉吻合支（Sucquet-Hoyer吻合支）壁间的变异型平滑肌细胞。血管球肿瘤比较常见，好发于年轻成人；指（趾）甲下血管球瘤多见于女性，而发生在其他部位者则无明显性别差异。血管球肿瘤虽可发生在身体任何部位，包括黏膜和内脏，但以四肢，尤其是双手的真皮或皮下组织最为多见；瘤体直径多不足1cm。皮损呈紫蓝色结节状，并可伴有与触觉刺激有关的阵发性疼痛。组织学上实体性病变（下文）患者的最常见症状是疼痛。

偶可见多灶性病变，主要见于儿童，大都被认为是经常染色体显性方式遗传[400,401]。与多灶性、遗传性血管球瘤相关的基因组异常已被定位于第一号染色体p21-22[402,403]，并已被命名为glomulin（球管蛋白基因）[404]。多灶性病变形态常与海绵状血管瘤类似；但在临床上则可能与蓝色橡皮疱痣综合征中所见之皮损形态混淆。血管球肿瘤的发生部位所及范围颇广，包括气管、肺、纵隔、胃、小肠、结肠、直肠、肠系膜、骨骼、阴道、宫颈、翼突窝、肝、胰腺、卵巢，甚至还包括卵巢畸胎瘤，但上述部位所涉及患者的数量却很少[405,416]。偶有报道称，血管球瘤可起源于血管[417,418]或神经内[419]。文献对指（趾）甲下血管球瘤与von Recklinghausen病（神经纤维瘤病Ⅰ型）二者之间的相关性已有描述[420-422]。有散个案报道称：胃多发性血管球瘤伴血管内扩散，但其行为属良性[423]。特别要指出的是：尾骨球是一种正常的血管球体，直径可达数厘米，位于尾骨尖附近；如不经意间发现之，可能会与血管球瘤混淆[424]。

血管球肿瘤大多完全属良性病变，局部复发者非常罕见[399,425]。个别病变（见下文）的组织形态虽可令人担心，但恶性血管球瘤（或血管球肉瘤）是少之又少[426,430]。

组织学形态

血管球肿瘤大都边界清楚；组织学上由不同比例的血管球细胞、血管和平滑肌构成。迄今为止，血管球瘤（glomangioma）是血管球肿瘤中最为常见的一种类型，约占血管球肿瘤总数的60%（图3.63），其次是实体型血管球瘤（solid glomus tumor，图3.64，占比25%）和血管球肌瘤（glomangiomyomas，图3.65，15%）。典型的实体性血管球瘤由大量形态单一的圆形血管球细胞构成，胞浆嗜酸性，着色浅淡；细胞核大、圆形或卵圆形、有缺口，位于细胞中央，且形态一致；瘤细胞边界清楚，PAS强阳性。周围间质呈水肿样，亦可表现为广泛黏液变性。小血管散在分布于瘤细胞之间，但如无特殊染色，大都很难识别。据文献载，血管球肿瘤的个别类型可表现为嗜酸性变[431]或主要由上皮样细胞构成[432]。在血管球瘤和血管球肌瘤，血管球细胞所占比例各异，有些病变中仅可在血管周围见有薄薄的一层。在血管球肌瘤，

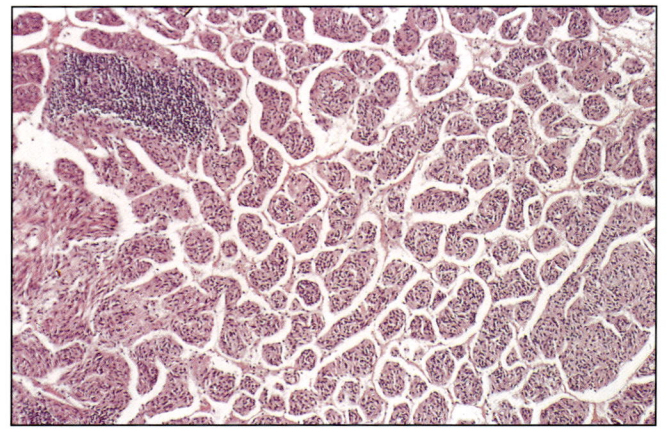

图3.62　淋巴管肌瘤病。可见沿大量淋巴样腔隙分布的平滑肌细胞结节，这些平滑肌细胞分化还好。

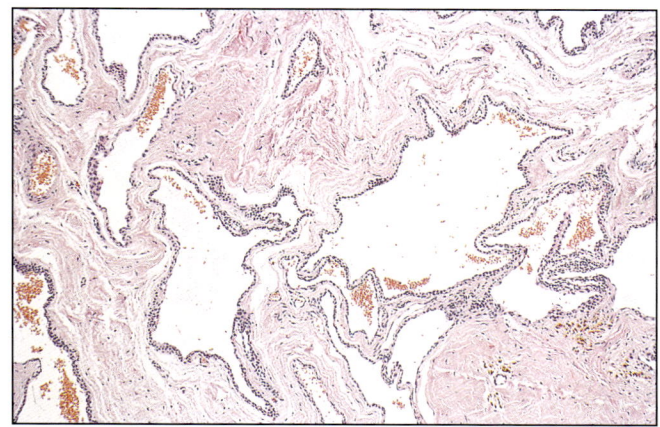

图3.63 血管球瘤，血管球肿瘤中最为常见的一种组织学类型，其间散在分布的血管球细胞有时并不醒目。

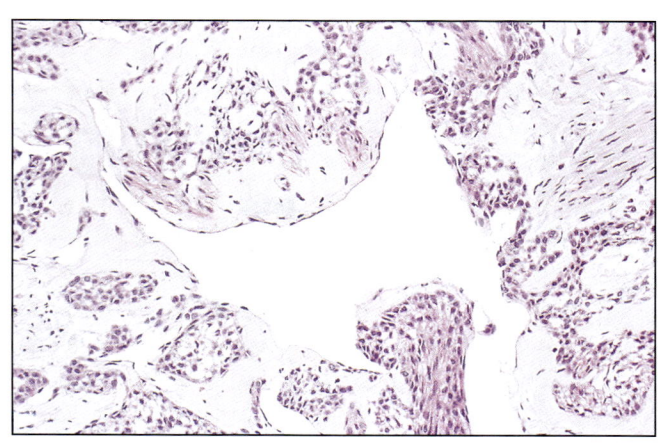

图3.65 血管球肌瘤，很多瘤细胞呈梭形，胞浆嗜酸染色。

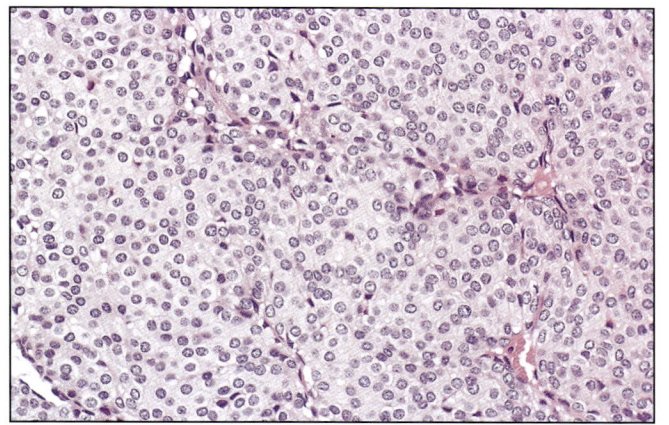

图3.64 实体型血管球瘤，表现有典型的血管球细胞形态，细胞边界清楚。

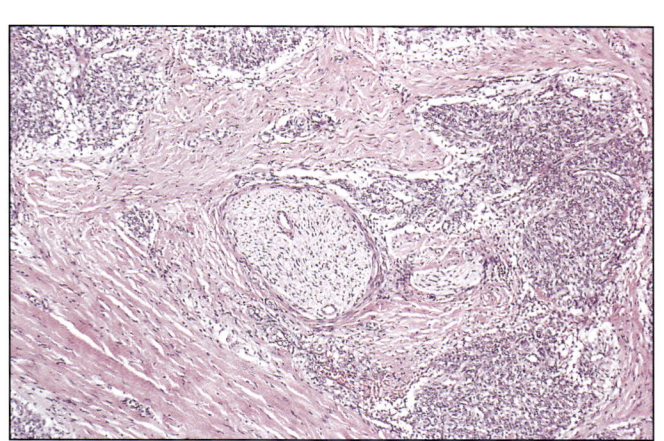

图3.66 浸润型血管球瘤，该病变取自大腿，肿瘤组织环绕并浸润股神经。

由高分化平滑肌构成的肿瘤成分所占比例也不稳定。在血管球瘤附近区域的正常血管周围，常可见成群的血管球细胞。

血管球血管瘤病（glomangiomatosis）被定义为一种兼具血管瘤特征和大量血管球细胞的肿瘤[430,433]。

所谓"浸润型血管球瘤"（图3.66）是一种少见类型，组织学上倒不失为典型的血管球瘤，但其病变位置大都深在，而且弥漫性地向周围软组织浸润[434,435]。因其术后局部复发率颇高，故准确识别非常重要。

免疫组化染色：典型的血管球瘤细胞呈 SMA（图3.67）和 MSA（肌肉特异性肌动蛋白）阳性，结蛋白染色偶呈局灶阳性[436-438]。CD34 亦可呈阳性[439]。

血管球肉瘤的诊断大都根据：镜下可见与明确为肉瘤样成分——圆形细胞肉瘤或平滑肌肉瘤样形态——并存的良性血管球瘤组织形态[426,430,440,441]。组织学诊断很困难，只是最近才有人提出定义恶性血管球瘤的确切标准[430]，标准如下：病变位置深在、肿瘤直径＞2cm、或非典型核分裂象、或中高度核级和≥5个核分裂象/50HPF。细胞核异型性明显、但无其他恶性指征者命名为共质体型（symplastic）血管球瘤。恶性潜能未定型血管球瘤被定义为：既不符合恶性血管球瘤的诊断标准，也不符合共质体型血管球瘤的诊断标准，但具有高度核分裂活性，而且病变位置表浅；或仅肿瘤直径一项超标，或仅具备病变位置深在一项恶性指标[430]。最大型系列研究报道指出：满足上述恶性转移标准者占比为38%[430]。

鉴别诊断

实体性血管球瘤与皮肤附属器肿瘤，尤其是与小汗腺腺瘤的鉴别，主要根据：后者可见有腺管分化、两类细胞群和上皮标记物免疫染色阳性。伴有假脉管形成的皮内痣至少在局部呈巢状结构，作为成熟证据，S-100蛋白染色呈阳性。

血管外皮瘤　Hemangiopericytoma

1942年，Stout 将所谓血管外皮瘤视为一种血管肿

血管周细胞肿瘤

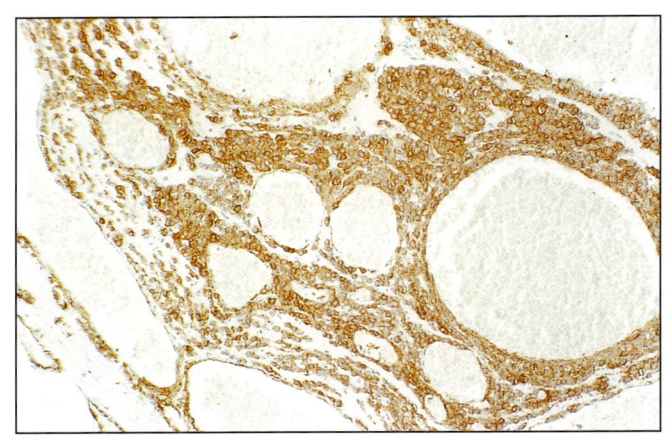

图3.67　血管球瘤，瘤细胞呈SMA普遍强阳性。

瘤，其组织来源是血管外皮细胞——血管周围的一种变异型平滑肌细胞[442]。这种说法的主要根据是：瘤细胞围绕分支状血管排列的结构模式，并在某种程度上（起码过去是）得到超微结构研究的支持[443-445]。但免疫组化研究却不支持此说，因为多数肿瘤（至少在成人）仅（和非特异性地）对波形蛋白和CD34呈阳性表达[446]，而对肌动蛋白或其他肌标记物则否[437,445,447]。

传统上，血管外皮瘤被分为成人和儿童两种类型，两型之间除了"外皮细胞瘤样"分支状血管模式之外，无论是在临床还是在病理上都很少共性；而上述结构模式特征却被多种其他类型的肿瘤所共享[448-450]。其中最为常见并能稳定共享此结构模式的肿瘤有：孤立性纤维瘤、滑膜肉瘤、婴儿型肌纤维瘤病、低度子宫内膜间质肉瘤、间叶性软骨肉瘤、深部良性纤维组织细胞瘤、和婴儿型纤维肉瘤。近年来，问题逐渐明朗：所谓婴儿型和成人型血管外皮瘤实际上是两种完全独立的病变实体，前者与婴儿型肌纤维瘤病密切相关，而后者的性质尚有争议，极有可能与孤立性纤维瘤同义（见第24章）。

按传统被诊断为成人型血管外皮瘤的病变似有相当的杂色性，这或许反映了其可重复性诊断标准的严重缺失。事实上，本人有机会查阅Stout的原始病案后发现：此实体可能从一开始就是个结构相当松散的异类混合体，这在缺少现代诊断技术的当时很容易理解。但作为结果，该术语就变成了一个诊断废纸篓之类的东西（与所谓"恶性纤维组织细胞瘤"相似），至今仍存有互不连续且尚无更好名称的亚型命名（详见下文）。与此同时，另一种理论也在持续升温，那就是真性血管外皮细胞病变存在的可能性（含Stout早期文献中的病案[441,452]）。这些病变，其中包括发生在成人的所谓"肌纤维瘤病"[452]，最好被分类在肌周细胞瘤项下，详细描述请见下文。

临床表现

据称，成人型血管外皮瘤好发于中老年人，男女发生率相等[453,454]。今天看来，按照过去的分类标准被纳入此类的病变中，多数或许可被视为占据其形态谱系之富细胞性一端的孤立性纤维瘤个案（参阅第24章）。其中还应包括那些位于盆腔和腹膜后、好像常见于成人女性并可能伴有因胰岛素样生长因子分泌所引发之低血糖症的细胞型病变[455]。据信，此独特的病变群中还包括那些起源于脑脊膜的病变（此前被称为血管母细胞性脑膜瘤，参阅第26章）[456,457]。但很多人坚持认为它们也是孤立性纤维瘤的细胞型病变；当然，就这些肿瘤类型的鉴别而言，现在好像还没有令人信服的鉴别标准。这些所谓的脑膜型血管外皮瘤的组织学分级虽然并不可靠，但其中很多最终都会发生浸润。对一般病理医生来说，一个相当实用的鉴别性特征就是：脑膜病变具有导致骨、腹腔内或肺（较少发生）转移的倾向，其潜伏期大都很长。

鼻窦血管外皮瘤（详细讨论参阅第4章）是一种显然是由肌样（肌动蛋白阳性）细胞构成的、组织学形态独特的亚型病变。主要发生在成人，特征是有局部复发倾向，但无转移[458,459]。

婴儿型血管外皮瘤可为先天性病变，亦可表现为一周岁之内发生的孤立性、多为深在性的真皮或皮下组织肿物[453,460,461]。部分患者可为多发性病变[461]，这进一步突显了它与婴儿型肌纤维瘤病之间的交叠。复发很常见，但其生物学行为一般仍属良性。偶有发生转移的个案报告[462]；但其所代表者可能是一种少见的多中心性病变形式，而非真性转移。其临床病理特征与婴儿型肌纤维瘤病其实无异；故目前的主流观点是：它们代表了同一病变实体的不同生长阶段或不同生长方式[460,461,463]。

肌周细胞瘤（myopericytoma），当前，我们倾向于用该名词涵盖那些被描述为成人型肌纤维瘤病的病变含血管球周细胞瘤（glomangiopericytoma）和肌周细胞瘤[452,463a]。我们还相信，该名词通常更适用于婴儿型肌纤维瘤病（见第24章）和见于成人的孤立性肌纤维瘤[464]。但术语上的这种变化被普遍接受尚需时日。作为一个病变群，这些病变最常发生于成人四肢的浅层软组织（尤其是下肢远端），虽然它们常常在出生时或儿童早期就已被发现。该病变可为单发或多发，时有疼痛感；局部复发者占10%～20%，但其中部分病变可能本来就是多灶性（或曰"场变型"）病变。有个案报道了一例导致肿瘤源性骨软化症（oncogenic osteomalacia）的血管球周细胞瘤[465]。恶性肌周细胞瘤非常罕见[463a,466]。

组织学形态

所谓成人型血管外皮瘤的组织形态与孤立性纤维瘤的细胞型病变无异（参阅第24章）。肿瘤边界大都清楚，多呈分叶状；由形态一致的瘤细胞构成，瘤细胞小、嗜碱性着色、卵圆形或梭形、细胞核呈卵圆形、细胞质边界不清。瘤细胞虽无特殊排列方式，但在很多薄壁、分支状血管周围的分布，形似典型的鹿角状分支结构（图3.68）。局灶性或弥漫性黏液样变和间质纤维化可为之特征。银染显示：肿瘤细胞位于血管腔之外，而且每个瘤细胞都外被一网状蛋白鞘。已被视为恶性指征的形态学特征包括细胞丰富密集、坏死出血以及核分裂象＞4个/10HPF[453]，后者是最重要的指征-上述标准与孤立性纤维瘤目前所采用的标准基本相同[467]。

婴儿型血管外皮瘤是一种多结节性肿瘤，其瘤细胞更具多形性，局部呈梭形或肌细胞样形态（图3.69）。核分裂象和灶状坏死是常见现象，如内皮下增生之所见，并可形似血管浸润。实际上，几乎所有病变中都可见由肥大梭形细胞构成的第二类肿瘤细胞群，这些瘤细胞具有肌样细胞特征，并呈α-SMA免疫染色阳性，呈微小结节状或束状分布。这就产生了一种或明或暗、难以与肌纤维瘤病的组织形态区别（但大都不太明显）的局部现象。

肌周细胞瘤包含一组具有连续性的病变形态谱：从具有肌纤维瘤病样形态的病变（图3.70）到酷似血管球瘤（图3.71）（但大都具有周细胞瘤样管腔）或血管平滑肌瘤的病变。所有病变都是由肌动蛋白阳性、有收缩性并表现出不同程度肌样细胞特征（梭形细胞或血管球样）的血管周细胞构成。很多病变都呈混合性形态，病变中除了血管周围梭形细胞呈嗜酸性着色，明显呈肌源性特征之外，余者均酷似肌纤维瘤病和所谓"血管外皮瘤"（图3.72）。血管周围常可见有（肿瘤主结节之外）类似的梭形细胞增生，尤其是在病变的周边区域，这些细胞的增生或是出现在外膜，或是内皮下层。如果不是

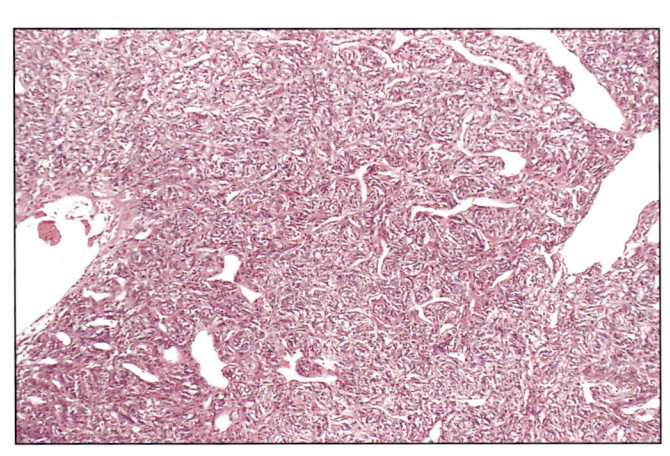

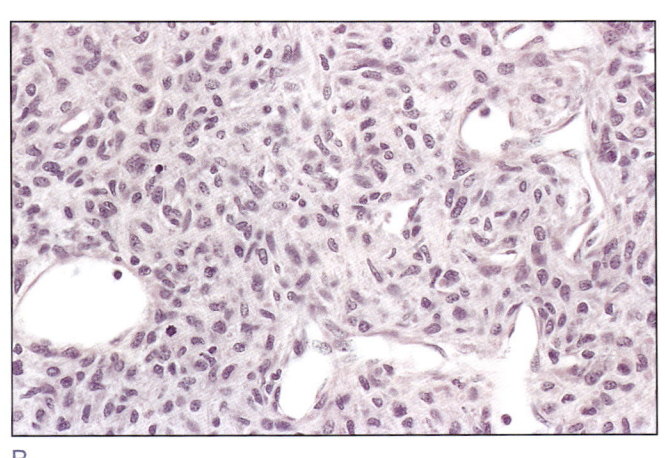

图3.68 所谓的血管外皮瘤。（A）典型的鹿角状分支血管、无序排列的瘤细胞、和无明显特征的纤维母细胞的细胞学形态。（B）细胞多形性大都不明显，即便是恶性病变：图示病变中的核分裂象记数多达15个/10HPF。其形态学表现与孤立性纤维瘤的细胞型病变无异。

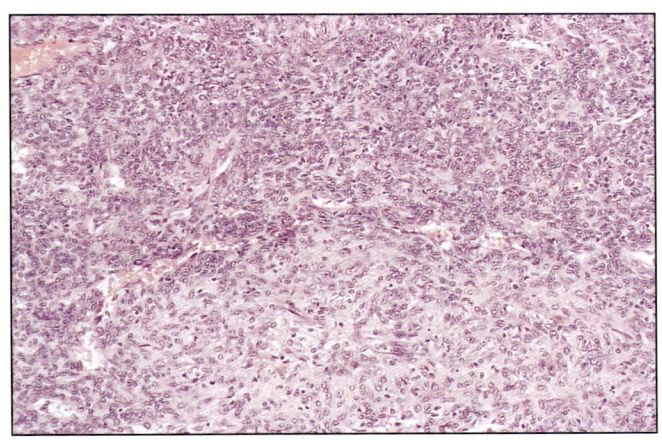

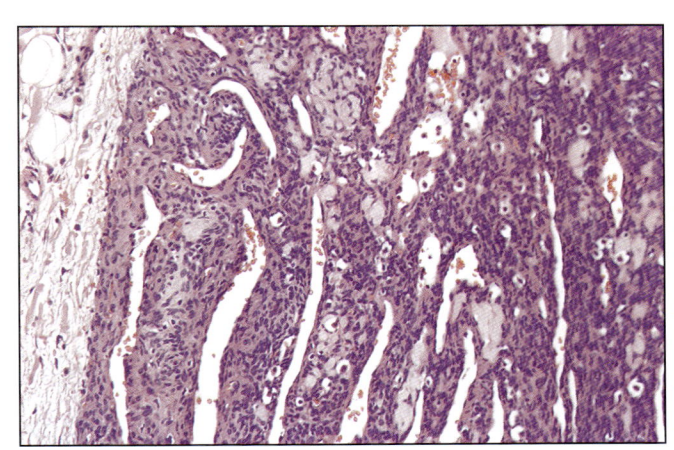

图3.69 婴儿型血管外皮瘤，局部可见瘤细胞转化为梭形、肌细胞样形态。

图3.70 肌周细胞瘤，该病变酷似肌纤维瘤病。注意：梭形瘤细胞的环血管排列方向。

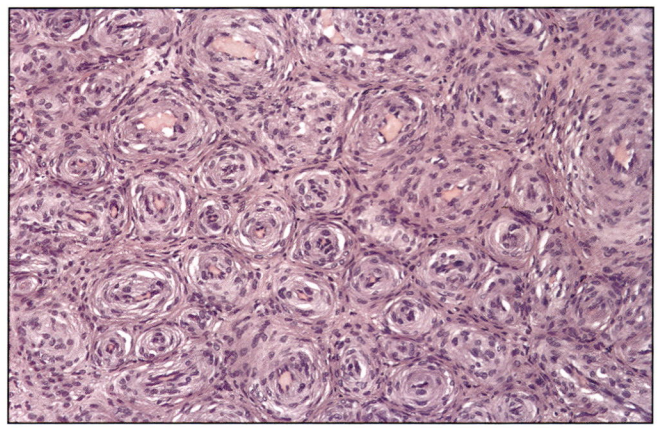

图3.71 肌周细胞瘤。在此形态谱系的最血管球化的一端，肌样梭瘤细胞围绕小血管呈同心圆状排列——这种形态是真性周细胞性病变。

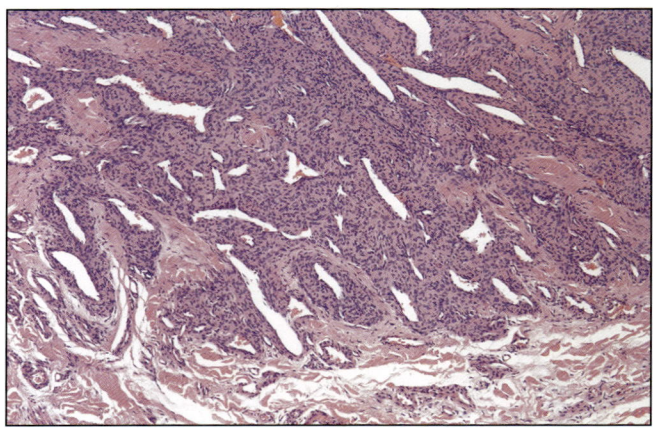

图3.72 肌周细胞瘤，该中间型病变由嗜酸性的、明显是围绕分支状血管排列的梭形瘤细胞构成。

在其上方见有完整的内皮细胞层，后一种形态酷似真性血管浸润；这也就是此前在婴儿型肌纤维瘤病和婴儿型血管外皮瘤中重点描述的形态特征（实际上，它们是同一形态谱系中的几个不同位点）。真性血管内肌周细胞瘤个案非常罕见[463a,468]。

鉴别诊断

随着免疫组化技术的发展，所谓血管外皮瘤的诊断已经逐渐成为被排斥的对象，因为很多肿瘤都表现有外皮细胞瘤样结构特征，至少是在局部[448,449]。其中主要包括：

- 滑膜肉瘤，呈双向分化特征，且EMA和CK阳性

- 间叶性软骨肉瘤，其中可见分化成熟的灶状软骨
- 深部良性纤维组织细胞瘤，它更具细胞多形性（表现有席纹状结构和炎性细胞浸润）
- 尿磷性间叶性肿瘤（phosphaturic mesenchymal tumor），有多种组织结构模式，而且大都伴有钙化和破骨细胞样巨细胞。

常常呈现出这种血管结构模式的其他肿瘤还有孤立性纤维瘤和婴儿型纤维肉瘤（参阅第24章），实际上，几乎任何类型的肉瘤都可能在局部间或表现有酷似所谓"血管外皮瘤"的结构特征。因此，这一诊断用词正在走进历史，即便想用，也须加倍小心！

参考文献

1. Salyer W R, Salyer D C 1975 Intravascular angiomatosis: development and distinction from angiosarcoma. Cancer 36: 995–1001
2. Clearkin K P, Enzinger F M 1976 Intravascular papillary endothelial hyperplasia. Arch Pathol Lab Med 100: 441–444
3. Kuo T T, Sayers C P, Rosai J 1976 Masson's "vegetant intravascular hemangioendothelioma": a lesion often mistaken for angiosarcoma. Study of seventeen cases located in the skin and soft tissues. Cancer 38: 1227–1236
4. Hashimoto H, Daimaru Y, Enjoji M 1983 Intravascular papillary endothelial hyperplasia. A clinicopathologic study of 91 cases. Am J Dermatopathol 5: 539–545
5. Pins M R, Rosenthal D I, Springfield D S et al. 1993 Florid extravascular papillary endothelial hyperplasia (Masson's pseudoangiosarcoma) presenting as a soft tissue sarcoma. Arch Pathol Lab Med 117: 259–263
6. Branton P A, Lininger R, Tavassoli F A 2003 Papillary endothelial hyperplasia of the breast: the great impostor for angiosarcoma: a clinicopathologic review of 17 cases. Int J Surg Pathol 11: 83–87
7. Reed C N, Cooper P H, Swerlick P A 1984 Intravascular papillary endothelial hyperplasia. Multiple lesions simulating Kaposi's sarcoma. J Am Acad Dermatol 10: 110–113.
8. Durieu C, Bayle-Lebey P, Gadroy A et al. 2001 Intravascular papillary endothelial hyperplasia: multiple lesions appearing in the course of treatment with interferon beta. Ann Dermatol Venereol 128: 1336–1338
9. Wick M R, Rocamora A 1988 Reactive and malignant "angioendotheliomatosis": a discriminant clinicopathological study. J Cutan Pathol 15: 260–271
10. McMenamin M E, Fletcher C D M 2002 Reactive angioendotheliomatosis: a study of 15 cases demonstrating a wide clinicopathologic spectrum. Am J Surg Pathol 26: 685–697
11. Brazzelli V, Baldini F, Vassallo C et al. 1999 Reactive angioendotheliomatosis in an infant. Am J Dermatopathol 21: 42–45
12. Ortonne N, Vignon-Pennamen M D, Majdalani G et al. 2001 Reactive angioendotheliomatosis secondary to dermal amyloid angiopathy. Am J Dermatopathol 23: 315–319
13. Creamer D, Black M M, Calonje E 2000 Reactive angioendotheliomatosis in association with the antiphospholipid syndrome. J Am Acad Dermatol 45: 903–906
14. Thai K E, Barrett W, Kossard S 2003 Reactive angioendotheliomatosis in the setting of antiphospholipid syndrome. Australas J Dermatol 44: 151–155
15. Tomasini C, Soro E, Pippione M 2000 Angioendotheliomatosis in a woman with rheumatoid arthritis. Am J Dermatopathol 22: 334–338
16. Shyong E Q, Gorevic P, Lebwohl M et al. 2002 Reactive angioendotheliomatosis and sarcoidosis. Int J Dermatol 41: 894–897
17. Le Boit P E, Solomon A R, Santa Cruz D J et al. 1992 Angiomatosis with luminal cryoprotein deposition. J Am Acad Dermatol 27: 969–973
18. Krell J M, Sánchez R L, Solomon A R 1994 Diffuse dermal angiomatosis: a variant of reactive cutaneous angioendotheliomatosis. J Cutan Pathol 21: 363–370
19. Kim S, Elenitsas R, James W D 2002 Diffuse dermal angiomatosis: a variant of reactive angioendotheliomatosis associated with peripheral vascular atherosclerosis. Arch Dermatol 138: 456–458

20. Kimyai-Asadi A, Nousari H C, Ketabchi N et al. 1999 Diffuse dermal angiomatosis: a variant of reactive angioendotheliomatosis associated with atherosclerosis. J Am Acad Dermatol 40: 257–259
21. Requena L, Farina M C, Renedo G et al. 1999 Intravascular and diffuse dermal reactive angioendotheliomatosis secondary to iatrogenic arteriovenous fistulas. J Cutan Pathol 26: 159–164
22. Chan J K C, Fletcher C D M, Hicklin G A et al. 1990 Glomeruloid hemangioma. A distinctive cutaneous lesion of multicentric Castleman's disease associated with POEMS syndrome. Am J Surg Pathol 14: 1036–1046
23. Yang S G, Cho K H, Bang Y-J et al. 1998 A case of glomeruloid hemangioma associated with multicentric Castleman's disease. Am J Dermatopathol 20: 266–270
24. Tsai C Y, Lai C H, Chan H L et al. 2001 Glomeruloid hemangioma – a specific marker of POEMS syndrome. Int J Dermatol 40: 403–406
25. Scheers C, Kolivras A, Corbisier A et al. 2002 POEMS syndrome revealed by multiple glomeruloid angiomas. Dermatology 204: 311–314
26. Obermoser G, Larcher C, Sheldon J A et al. 2003 Absence of human herpesvirus-8 in glomeruloid haemangioma associated with POEMS syndrome and Castleman's disease. Br J Dermatol 148: 1276–1278
27. MacCollum D W, Martin L W 1956 Hemangiomas in infancy and childhood. A report based on 6479 cases. Surg Clin North Am 36: 1647–1663
28. Watson W L, McCarthy W B 1940 Blood and lymph vessel tumors. A report of 1056 cases. Surg Gynecol Obstet 71: 569–588
29. Edgerton M T, Hiebert J M 1978 Vascular and lymphatic tumors in infancy, childhood and adulthood: challenge of diagnosis and treatment. Curr Probl Cancer 2: 4–44
30. Finley J L, Noe J M, Arndt K A et al. 1984 Port-wine stains. Morphologic variations and developmental lesions. Arch Dermatol 120: 1453–1455
31. Johnson S C, Hanke C W 2001 Unilateral acquired nevus flammeus in women. Cutis 67: 225–228
32. Adams D C, Lucky A W 2000 Acquired port-wine stains and antecedent trauma: case report and review of the literature. Arch Dermatol 136: 897–899
33. Berg J N, Quaba A A, Georgantopoulou A et al. 2000 A family with hereditary port wine stain. J Med Genet 37: E12
34. Breugem C C, Alders M, Salieb-Beugelaar G B et al. 2002 A locus for hereditary capillary malformations mapped on chromosome 5q. Hum Genet 110: 343–347
35. Askar I, Kilinc N, Yucetas A 2003 Pyogenic granuloma appearing on port-wine stain: a case report. Acta Chir Plast 45: 51–54
36. Valeyrie L, Lebrun-Vignes B, Descamps V et al. 2002 Pyogenic granuloma within port-wine stains: an alarming clinical presentation. Eur J Dermatol 12: 373–375
37. Kim H T, Choi E H, Ahn S K et al. 1999 Vascular tumors arising in port-wine stains: two cases of pyogenic granuloma and a case of acquired tufted angioma. J Dermatol 26: 813–816
38. Bean W B, Walsh J R 1956 Venous lakes. Arch Dermatol 74: 459–463
39. Stevenson J R, Lincoln C S 1967 Angioma serpiginosum. Arch Dermatol 95: 16–22
40. Frain-Bell W 1957 Angioma serpiginosum. Br J Dermatol 69: 251–268
41. Stevenson J R, Lincoln C S 1967 Angioma serpiginosum. Arch Dermatol 95: 16–22
42. Kumakiri M, Katoh N, Miura Y 1980 Angioma serpiginosum. J Cutan Pathol 7: 410–421
43. Al Hawsawi K, Al Aboud K, Al Aboud D et al. 2003 Linear angioma serpiginosum. Pediatr Dermatol 20: 167–168
44. Erbagci Z, Erbagci I, Erkilic S et al. 2004 Angioma serpiginosum with retinal involvement in a male: a possible role of continuous cold exposure. J Eur Acad Dermatol Venereol 18: 238–239
45. Gautier-Smith P C, Sanders M D, Sanderson K V 1971 Ocular and nervous system involvement in angioma serpiginosum. Br J Ophthalmol 55: 433–443
46. Marriot P J, Munro D D, Ryan T (1975) Angioma serpiginosum – familial incidence. Br J Dermatol 93: 701–706
47. Johnson W C 1976 Pathology of cutaneous vascular tumors. Int J Dermatol 15: 239–270
48. Imperial R, Helwig E B 1967 Angiokeratoma. A clinicopathological study. Arch Dermatol 95: 166–175
49. Epinette W W, Norins A L, Drew A L et al. 1973 Angiokeratoma corporis diffusum with α-L fucosidase deficiency. Arch Dermatol 107: 754–757
50. Rodríguez-Serna M, Botella-Estrada R, Chabás A et al. 1996 Angiokeratoma corporis diffusum associated with B-mannosidase deficiency. Arch Dermatol 132: 1219–1222
51. Kanzaki T, Yokota M, Irie F et al. 1993 Angiokeratoma corporis diffusum with glycopeptiduria due to deficient lysosomal α-N-acetylgalactosaminidase activity. Arch Dermatol 129: 460–465
52. Kodama K, Kobayashi H, Abe R et al. 2001 A new case of α-N-acetylgalactosaminidase deficiency with angiokeratoma corporis diffusum, with Meniere's syndrome amd without mental retardation. Br J Dermatol 144: 363–368
53. Ishibashi A, Tsuboi R, Shinmei M 1984 β-galactosidase and neuraminidase deficiency associated with angiokeratoma corporis diffusum. Arch Dermatol 120: 1344–1346
54. Holmes R C, Fensom A H, McKee P H et al. 1984 Angiokeratoma corporis diffusum in a patient with normal enzyme activities. J Am Acad Dermatol 10: 384–387
55. Haye K R, Rebello D J A 1961 Angiokeratoma of Mibelli. Acta Dermat Venereol 41: 56–60
56. Imperial R, Helwig E B 1967 Angiokeratoma of the scrotum (Fordyce type). J Urol 98: 379–387
57. Imperial R, Helwig E B 1967 Angiokeratoma of the vulva. Obstet Gynecol 29: 307–312
58. Lynch P J, Kosanovich N 1967 Angiokeratoma circumscriptum. Arch Dermatol 96: 665–668
59. Tarnowski W M, Hashimoto K 1969 New light microscopic findings in Fabry's disease. Acta Derm Venereol 49: 386–389
60. Coffin C M, Dehner L P 1993 Vascular tumors in children and adolescents: a clinicopathologic study of 228 tumors in 222 patients. Pathol Annu 28: 97–120
61. Lister W A 1938 The natural history of strawberry naevi. Lancet 1: 1429–1434
62. Perrone T 1985 Vessel-nerve intermingling in benign infantile hemangioendothelioma. Hum Pathol 16: 198–200
63. Calonje E, Mentzel T, Fletcher C D M 1995 Pseudomalignant perineural invasion in cellular ("infantile") capillary hemangiomas. Histopathology 26: 159–164
64. Taxy J B, Gray S R 1979 Cellular angiomas of infancy. An ultrastructural study of two cases. Cancer 43: 2322–2331
65. Gonzalez-Crussi F, Reyes-Mugica M 1991 Cellular hemangiomas ("hemangioendotheliomas") in infants. Light microscopic immunohistochemical and ultrastructural observations. Am J Surg Pathol 15: 769–778
66. Smoller B R, Apfelberg D B 1993 Infantile (juvenile) capillary hemangioma: a tumor of heterogeneous cellular elements. J Cutan Pathol 20: 330–336
67. North P E, Waner M, Mizeracki A et al. 2001 A unique microvascular phenotype shared by juvenile hemangiomas and human placenta. Arch Dermatol 137: 559–570
68. North P E, Waner M, Mizeracki A et al. 2000 GLUT1: a newly discovered immunohistochemical marker for juvenile hemangiomas. Hum Pathol 31: 11–22
69. Yu Y, Flint A F, Mulliken J B et al. 2004 Endothelial progenitor cells in infantile hemangioma. Blood 103: 1373–1375
70. Boye E, Yu Y, Paranya G et al. 2001 Clonality and altered behavior of endothelial cells from hemangiomas. J Clin Invest 107: 745–752
71. Walter J W, North P E, Waner M et al. 2002 Somatic mutation of vascular endothelial growth factor receptors in juvenile hemangioma. Genes Chromos Cancer 33: 295–303
72. Wilson-Jones E 1976 Malignant vascular tumours. Clin Exp Dermatol 1: 287–312
73. Wilson-Jones E, Orkin M 1989 Tufted angioma (angioblastoma). A benign progressive angioma, not to be confused with Kaposi's sarcoma or low-grade angiosarcoma. J Am Acad Dermatol 20: 214–225
74. Padilla R S, Orkin M, Rosai J 1987 Acquired "tufted" angioma (progressive capillary hemangioma). Am J Dermatopathol 9: 292–300
75. Herron M D, Coffin C M, Vanderhooft S L 2002 Tufted angiomas: variability of clinical morphology. Pediatr Dermatol 19: 394–401
76. Wong S N, Tay Y K 2002 Tufted angioma: a report of five cases. Pediatr Dermatol 19: 388–393
77. Okada E, Tamura A, Ishikawa O et al. 2000 Tufted angioma (angioblastoma): case report and review of 41 cases in the Japanese literature. Clin Exp Dermatol 25: 627–630
78. Cho K H, Kim S H, Park K C et al. 1991 Angioblastoma (Nakagawa) – is it the same as tufted angioma? Clin Exp Dermatol 16: 110–113
79. Kleinegger C L, Hammond H L, Vincent S D et al. 2000 Acquired tufted angioma: a unique vascular lesion not previously reported in the oral mucosa. Br J Dermatol 142: 794–799
80. Satter E K, Graham B S, Gibbs N F 2002 Congenital tufted angioma. Pediatr Dermatol 19: 445–447
81. Tille J C, Morris M A, Brundler M A et al. 2003 Familial predisposition to tufted angioma: identification of blood and lymphatic vascular components. Clin Genet 63: 393–399
82. Miyamoto T, Mihara M, Mishima E et al. 1992 Acquired tufted angioma showing spontaneous regression. Br J Dermatol 127: 645–648
83. Lam W Y, Mac-Moune Lai F, Look C N et al. 1994 Tufted angioma with complete regression. J Cutan Pathol 21: 461–466
84. Maguiness S, Guenther L 2002 Kasabach–Merritt syndrome. J Cutan Med Surg 6: 335–339
85. Enjolras O, Mulliken J B, Wassef M et al. 2000 Residual lesions after Kasabach–Merritt phenomenon in 41 patients. J Am Acad Dermatol 42: 225–235
86. Michel S, Hohenleutner U, Stolz W et al. 1999 Acquired tufted angioma in association with a complex cutaneous vascular malformation. Br J Dermatol 141: 1142–1144
87. Kumakiri M, Muramoto F, Tsukinaga I et al. 1983 Crystalline lamellae in the endothelial cells of a type of hemangioma characterised by the proliferation of immature endothelial cells and pericytes – angioblastoma (Nakagawa). J Am Acad Dermatol 8: 68–75
88. Fukunaga M 2000 Intravenous tufted angioma. APMIS 108: 287–292
89. Brasanac D, Janic D, Boricic I et al. 2003 Retroperitoneal kaposiform hemangioendothelioma with tufted angioma-like features in an infant with Kasabach–Merritt syndrome. Pathol Int 53: 627–631
90. Chu C Y, Hsiao C H, Chiu H C 2003 Transformation between Kaposiform hemangioendothelioma and tufted angioma. Dermatology 206: 334–337

91. Imperial R, Helwig E 1967 Verrucous hemangioma. A clinicopathologic study of 21 cases. Arch Dermatol 96: 247–253
92. Chan J K C, Tsang W Y W, Calonje E et al. 1995 Verrucous hemangioma. A distinctive but neglected variant of cutaneous hemangioma. Int J Surg Pathol 2: 171–176
93. Calduch L, Ortega C, Navarro V et al. 2000 Verrucous hemangioma: report of two cases and review of the literature. Pediatr Dermatol 17: 213–217
94. McGeoch A H 1961 Pyogenic granuloma. Aust J Dermatol 6: 33–40
95. Bhaskar S M, Jacoway J R 1961 Pyogenic granuloma. Clinical features, incidence, histology and result of treatment: report of 242 cases. J Oral Surg 24: 391–398
96. Patrice S J, Wiss K, Mulliken J B 1991 Pyogenic granuloma (lobular capillary hemangioma): a clinicopathologic study of 178 cases. Pediatr Dermatol 8: 267–276
97. Harris M N, Desai R, Chuang T Y et al. 2000 Lobular capillary hemangiomas: an epidemiologic report, with emphasis on cutaneous lesions. J Am Acad Dermatol 42: 1012–1016
98. Mills S E, Cooper P H, Fechner R E 1980 Lobular capillary hemangioma. The underlying lesion of pyogenic granuloma. A study of 73 cases from the oral and nasal mucous membranes. Am J Surg Pathol 4: 471–479
99. Ogunleye A O, Nwaorgu O G 2000 Pyogenic granuloma, a cause of congenital nasal mass: case report. Ann Trop Paediatr 20: 137–139
100. Willies-Jacobo L J, Isaacs H Jr, Stein M T 2000 Pyogenic granuloma presenting as a congenital epulis. Arch Pediatr Adolesc Med 154: 603–605
101. Nappi O, Wick M R 1986 Disseminated lobular capillary hemangioma (pyogenic granuloma). A clinicopathologic study of two cases. Am J Dermatopathol 8: 379–385
102. Wilson B B, Greer K E, Cooper P H 1989 Eruptive disseminated lobular capillary hemangioma (pyogenic granuloma). J Am Acad Dermatol 21: 391–394
103. Behne K, Robertson I, Weedon D 2002 Disseminated lobular capillary hemangioma. Australas J Dermatol 43: 297–300
104. Warner J, Wilson-Jones E 1968 Pyogenic granuloma recurring with multiple satellites. A report of 11 cases. Br J Dermatol 80: 218–227
105. Tursen U, Demirkan F, Ikizoglu G 2004 Giant recurrent pyogenic granuloma on the face with satellitosis responsive to systemic steroids. Clin Exp Dermatol 29: 40–41
106. Kim T H, Choi E H, Ahn S K et al. 1999 Vascular tumors arising in port-wine stains: two cases of pyogenic granuloma and a case of acquired tufted angioma. J Dermatol 26: 813–816
107. Askar I, Kilinc N, Yucetas A 2003 Pyogenic granuloma appearing on port-wine stain: a case report. Acta Chir Plast 45: 52–54
108. Piguet V, Borradori L 2002 Pyogenic granuloma-like lesions during capecitabine therapy. Br J Dermatol 147: 1270–1272
109. MacKenzie-Wood A R, Wood G 1998 Pyogenic granuloma-like lesions in a patient using topical tretinoin. Australas J Dermatol 39: 248–250
110. Exner J H, Dahod S, Pochi P E 1983 Pyogenic granuloma-like acne lesions during isotretinoin therapy. Arch Dermatol 119: 808–811
111. Hagler J, Hodak E, David M et al. 1992 Facial pyogenic granuloma-like lesions under isotretinoin therapy. Int J Dermatol 31: 199–200
112. Renshaw A A, Rosai J 1993 Benign atypical vascular lesions of the lip. A study of 12 cases. Am J Surg Pathol 17: 557–565
113. Cooper P H, Mills S E 1982 Subcutaneous granuloma pyogenicum. Lobular capillary hemangioma. Arch Dermatol 118: 30–33
114. Cooper P H, McAllister H A, Helwig E B 1979 Intravenous pyogenic granuloma. A study of 18 cases. Am J Surg Pathol 3: 221–228
115. LeBoit P E, Berger T G, Egbert B M et al. 1989 Bacillary angiomatosis. The histopathology and differential diagnosis of a pseudoneoplastic infection in patients with human immunodeficiency virus disease. Am J Surg Pathol 13: 909–920
116. Slater L N, Welch D F, Min K W 1992 *Rochalimaea henselae* causes bacillary angiomatosis and peliosis hepatis. Arch Intern Med 152: 602–606
117. Kasabach H H, Merritt K K 1961 Capillary hemangioma with extensive purpura. Report of a case. Am J Dis Child 59: 1063–1070
118. Fine R M, Derbes V J, Clark W H Jr 1961 Blue rubber bleb nevus. Arch Dermatol 84: 802–805
119. Rice S J, Fischer D S 1962 Blue rubber bleb nevus syndrome. Arch Dermatol 86: 502–511
120. Calonje E, Fletcher C D M 1991 Sinusoidal hemangioma: a distinctive benign vascular neoplasm within the group of cavernous hemangiomas. Am J Surg Pathol 15: 1130–1135
121. Girard C, Graham J H, Johnson W C 1974 Arteriovenous hemangioma (arteriovenous shunt): a clinicopathologic and histochemical study. J Clin Pathol 1: 73–87
122. Rusin L J, Harrel E 1976 Arteriovenous fistula. Cutaneous manifestations. Arch Dermatol 112: 1135–1138
123. Connelly M G, Winkelmann R K 1985 Acral arteriovenous tumor. Am J Surg Pathol 9: 15–21
124. Angervall L, Nielsen J M, Stener B et al. 1979 Concomitant arteriovenous vascular malformation in skeletal muscle. A clinical, angiographic and histologic study. Cancer 44: 232–238
125. Kadono T, Kishi A, Onishi Y et al. 2000 Acquired digital arteriovenous malformation: a report of six cases. Br J Dermatol 142: 362–365
126. Akiyama M, Inamoto N 2001 Arteriovenous haemangioma in chronic liver disease: clinical and histopathological features in four cases. Br J Dermatol 144: 604–609
127. Strutton G, Weedon D 1987 Acro-angiodermatitis: a simulant of Kaposi's sarcoma. Am J Dermatopathol 9: 85–89
128. Koutlas I G, Jessurun J 1994 Arteriovenous hemangioma: clinicopathological and immunohistochemical study. J Cutan Pathol 21: 343–349
129. Hunt S J, Santa Cruz D J, Barr R J 1991 Microvenular hemangioma. J Cutan Pathol 18: 235–240
130. Aloi F, Tomasini C, Pippione M 1993 Microvenular hemangioma. Am J Dermatopathol 15: 534–538
131. Sánz-Trelles A, Ojeda-Martos A, Jiménez-Fernández A et al. 1998 Microvenular hemangioma: a new case in a child. Histopathology 32: 89–90
132. Hudnall S D, Chen T, Brown K et al. 2003 Human herpesvirus-8-positive microvenular hemangioma in POEMS syndrome. Arch Pathol Lab Med 127: 1034–1036
133. Santa Cruz D J, Aronberg J 1988 Targetoid hemosiderotic hemangioma. J Am Acad Dermatol 19: 550–558
134. Guillou L, Calonje E, Speight P et al. 1999 Hobnail hemangioma: a pseudomalignant vascular lesion with a reappraisal of targetoid hemosiderotic hemangioma. Am J Surg Pathol 23: 97–105
135. Mentzel T, Partanen T A, Kutzner H 1999 Hobnail hemangioma ("targetoid hemosiderotic hemangioma"): clinicopathologic and immunohistochemical analysis of 62 cases. J Cutan Pathol 26: 279–286
136. Christenson L J, Stone M S 2001 Trauma-induced simulator of targetoid hemosiderotic hemangioma. Am J Dermatopathol 23: 221–223
137. Carlson J A, Daulad S, Godheart H P 1999 Targetoid hemosiderotic hemangioma – a dynamic vascular tumor: report of 3 cases with episodic and cyclic changes and comparison with solitary angiokeratomas. J Am Acad Dermatol 41: 215–224
138. Calonje E, Fletcher C D M, Wilson-Jones E et al. 1994 Retiform hemangioendothelioma: a distinctive form of low-grade angiosarcoma delineated in a series of 15 cases. Am J Surg Pathol 18: 115–125
139. Gutzmer R, Kaspari M, Herbst R A et al. 2002 Absence of HHV-8 DNA in hobnail hemangioma. J Cutan Pathol 29: 154–158
140. Requena L, Kutzner H, Mentzel T 2002 Acquired elastotic hemangioma: a clinicopathologic variant of hemangioma. J Am Acad Dermatol 47: 371–376
141. Brenn T, Fletcher C D M 2004 Cutaneous epithelioid angiomatous nodule: a distinct lesion in the morphologic spectrum of epithelioid vascular tumors. Am J Dermatopathol 26: 14–21
142. Wells G C, Whimster I W 1969 Subcutaneous angiolymphoid hyperplasia with eosinophilia. Br J Dermatol 81: 1–15
143. Wilson-Jones E, Bleehen S S 1969 Inflammatory angiomatous nodules with abnormal blood vessels occurring about the ears and scalp (pseudo or atypical pyogenic granulomas). Br J Dermatol 81: 804–816
144. Wilson-Jones E, Marks R 1970 Papular angioplasia. Vascular papules of the face and scalp simulating malignant vascular tumors. Arch Dermatol 102: 422–427
145. Rosai J, Akerman L R 1974 Intravenous atypical vascular proliferation. A cutaneous lesion simulating a malignant blood vessel tumor. Arch Dermatol 109: 714–717
146. Rosai J, Gold J, Landy R 1979 The histiocytoid hemangiomas. A unifying concept embracing several previously described entities of skin, soft tissue, large vessels, bone and heart. Hum Pathol 10: 707–730
147. Cooper P H 1988 Is histiocytoid hemangioma a specific pathologic entity? (editorial) Am J Surg Pathol 12: 815–817
148. Rosai J 1982 Angiolymphoid hyperplasia with eosinophilia of the skin. Its nosological position in the spectrum of histiocytoid hemangioma. Am J Dermatopathol 4: 175–184
149. Allen P W, Ramakrishna B, MacCormac L B 1992 The histiocytoid hemangiomas and other controversies. Pathol Annu 27 (part 1): 51–87
150. Tsang W Y W, Chan J K C 1993 The family of epithelioid vascular tumors. Histol Histopathol 8: 187–212
151. Fetsch J F, Weiss S W 1991 Observations concerning the pathogenesis of epithelioid hemangioma (angiolymphoid hyperplasia). Mod Pathol 4: 449–455
152. Olsen T G, Helwig E B 1985 Angiolymphoid hyperplasia with eosinophilia. A clinicopathologic study of 116 patients. J Am Acad Dermatol 12: 781–796
153. Castro C, Winkelmann R K 1974 Angiolymphoid hyperplasia with eosinophilia in the skin. Cancer 34: 1696–1705
154. Razquin S, Mayayo E, Citores M A et al. 1991 Angiolymphoid hyperplasia with eosinophilia of the tongue: report of a case and review of the literature. Hum Pathol 22: 837–839
155. Park Y, Chung J, Cho C G 2002 Angiolymphoid hyerplasia with eosinophilia of the tongue: report of a case and review of the literature. Oral Oncol 38: 103–106
156. Bartralot R, García-Patos V, Hueto J et al. 1996 Angiolymphoid hyperplasia with eosinophilia affecting the oral mucosa: report of a case and a review of the literature. Br J Dermatol 134: 744–748
157. Mariatos G, Gorgoulis V G, Laskaris G et al. 1999 Epithelioid hemangiomas (angiolymphoid hyperplasia with eosinophilia) in the oral mucosa. A case report and review of the literature. Oral Oncol 35: 435–438
158. Tsuboi H, Fujimura T, Katsuoka K 2001 Angiolymphoid hyperplasia with eosinophilia in the oral mucosa. Br J Dermatol 145: 365–366
159. Nair M, Aron M, Sharma M C 2000 Angiolymphoid hyperplasia with eosinophilia (epithelioid hemangioma) of the breast: report of a case. Surg Today 30: 747–749
160. Suster S 1987 Nodal angiolymphoid hyperplasia with eosinophilia. Am J Clin Pathol 88: 236–239

161. O'Connell J X, Kattapuram S V, Mankin H J et al. 1993 Epithelioid hemangioma of bone. A tumor often mistaken for low-grade angiosarcoma or malignant hemangioendothelioma. Am J Surg Pathol 17: 610–617
162. Banks E R, Mills S E 1990 Histiocytoid (epithelioid) hemangioma of the testis. The so-called vascular variant of "adenomatoid tumor." Am J Surg Pathol 14: 584–589
163. Madison J F, Cooper P H 1989 A histiocytoid (epithelioid) vascular tumor of the ovary: occurrence within a benign cystic teratoma. Mod Pathol 2: 55–58
164. Luthringer D J, Virmani R, Weiss S W et al. 1990 A distinctive cardiovascular lesion resembling histiocytoid/epithelioid hemangioma, evidence suggesting mesothelial participation. Am J Surg Pathol 14: 993–1000
165. Chan J K, Loo K T, Yau B K et al. 1997 Nodular histiocytic/mesothelial hyperplasia: a lesion potentially mistaken for a neoplasm in transbronchial biopsy. Am J Surg Pathol 21: 658–663
166. Oksenhendler E, Cazals-Hatem D, Schulz T F et al. 1998 Transient angiolymphoid hyperplasia and Kaposi's sarcoma after primary infection with human herpesvirus 8 in a patient with human immunodeficiency virus infection. N Engl J Med 338: 1585–1590
167. Jang K A, Ahn S J, Choi J H et al. 2001 Polymerase chain reaction (PCR) for human herpesvirus 8 and heteroduplex PCR for clonality assessment in angiolymphoid hyperplasia with eosinophilia and Kimura's disease. J Cutan Pathol 28: 363–367
168. Onishi Y, Ohara K 1999 Angiolymphoid hyperplasia with eosinophilia associated with arteriovenous malformation: a clinicopathological correlation with angiography and serial estimation of serum levels of renin, eosinophilic cationic protein and interleukin 5. Br J Dermatol 140: 1153–1156
169. Reed R J, Terazakis N 1972 Subcutaneous angiolymphoid hyperplasia with eosinophilia (Kimura's disease). Cancer 29: 489–497
170. Morton K, Robertson A J, Hadden W 1987 Angiolymphoid hyperplasia with eosinophilia: report of a case arising from the radial artery. Histopathology 11: 963–969
171. Kung I T, Gibson J B, Bannatyne P M 1984 Kimura's disease: a clinicopathological study of 21 cases and its distinction from angiolymphoid hyperplasia with eosinophilia. Pathology 16: 39–44
172. Urabe A, Tsuneyoshi M, Enjoji M 1987 Epithelioid hemangioma versus Kimura's disease. A comparative clinicopathologic study. Am J Surg Pathol 10: 758–766
173. Googe P B, Harris N L, Mihm M C J 1987 Kimura's disease and angiolymphoid hyperplasia with eosinophilia: two distinct clinicopathological entities. J Cutan Pathol 15: 263–271
174. Kuo T T, Shih L Y, Chan H L 1988 Kimura's disease, involvement of regional lymph nodes and distinction from angiolymphoid hyperplasia with eosinophilia. Am J Surg Pathol 12: 843–854
175. Chan J K C, Hui P K, Ng C S et al. 1989 Epithelioid haemangioma (angiolymphoid hyperplasia with eosinophilia) and Kimura's disease in Chinese. Histopathology 15: 557–574
176. Fawcett H A, Smith N P 1984 Injection site granuloma due to aluminium. Arch Dermatol 120: 1318–1322
177. Miliauskas J R, Mukherjee T, Dixon B 1993 Postimmunization (vaccination) injection-site reactions. A report of four cases and review of the literature. Am J Surg Pathol 17: 516–524
178. Weiss S W, Goldblum J R 2001 Soft tissue tumors, 4th edn. CV Mosby-Harcourt, Philadelphia, p 593
179. Weiss S W, Enzinger F M 1986 Spindle cell hemangioendothelioma, a low grade angiosarcoma resembling a cavernous hemangioma and Kaposi's sarcoma. Am J Surg Pathol 10: 521–530
180. Fletcher C D M, Beham A, Schmid C 1991 Spindle cell hemangioendothelioma: a clinicopathological and immunohistochemical study indicative of a non-neoplastic lesion. Histopathology 18: 291–301
181. Perkins P, Weiss S W 1996 Spindle cell hemangioendothelioma: an analysis of 78 cases with reassessment of its pathogenesis and biologic behavior. Am J Surg Pathol 20: 1196–1204
182. Scott G A, Rosai J 1988 Spindle cell hemangioendothelioma. Report of seven additional cases of a recently described vascular neoplasm. Am J Dermatopathol 10: 281–288
183. Fanburg J C, Meis-Kindblom J M, Rosenberg A C 1995 Multiple enchondromas associated with spindle-cell hemangioendotheliomas. An overlooked variant of Mafucci's syndrome. Am J Surg Pathol 19: 1029–1038
184. Imayama S, Murakamai Y, Hashimoto H et al. 1992 Spindle cell hemangioendothelioma exhibits the ultrastructural features of reactive vascular proliferation rather than of angiosarcoma. Am J Clin Pathol 97: 279–287
185. Ding J, Hashimoto H, Imayama S et al. 1992 Spindle cell hemangioendothelioma: probably a benign vascular lesion not a low-grade angiosarcoma. A clinicopathological, ultrastructural and immunohistochemical study. Virchow's Arch [A] 420: 77–85
186. Fletcher C D M 1996 Vascular tumors: an update with emphasis on the diagnosis of angiosarcoma and borderline vascular neoplasms. In: Weiss SW, Brooks JSJ (eds) Soft tissue tumors. Monographs in pathology. Williams & Wilkins, Baltimore, p 181–206
187. Zoltie N, Roberts P F 1989 Spindle cell haemangioendothelioma in association with epithelioid haemangioendothelioma. Histopathology 15: 544–546
188. Allen P W, Enzinger F M 1972 Hemangioma of skeletal muscle. An analysis of 89 cases. Cancer 29: 8–22
189. Fergusson I L 1972 Haemangiomata of skeletal muscle. Br J Surg 59: 634–637
190. Beham A, Fletcher C D M 1991 Intramuscular angioma: a clinicopathological analysis of 74 cases. Histopathology 18: 53–59
191. Lin J J, Lin F 1974 Two entities in angiolipoma. A study of 459 cases of lipoma with review of the literature on infiltrating angiolipoma. Cancer 34: 720–727
192. Devaney K, Vinh T Z, Sweet D E 1993 Synovial hemangioma: a report of 20 cases with differential diagnostic considerations. Hum Pathol 24: 737–745
193. Losli E J 1952 Intrinsic hemangioma of the peripheral nerves: a report of two cases and a review of the literature. Arch Pathol 53: 226–232
194. Wood M B 1980 Intraneural hemangioma: report of a case. Plast Reconstr Surg 65: 74–76
195. Vigna P A, Kusior M F, Collins M B et al. 1994 Peripheral nerve hemangioma. Potential for clinical aggressiveness. Arch Pathol Lab Med 118: 1038–1041
196. Rao V K, Weiss S W 1992 Angiomatosis of soft tissue. An analysis of the histologic features and clinical outcome in 51 cases. Am J Surg Pathol 16: 764–771
197. Howat A J, Campbell P E 1987 Angiomatosis: a vascular malformation of infancy and childhood. Report of 17 cases. Pathology 19: 377–382
198. Kraus M D, Lind A C, Alder S L et al. 1999 Angiomatosis with angiokeratoma-like features in children: a light microscopic and immunophenotypic examination of four cases. Am J Dermatopathol 21: 350–355
199. Fletcher C D M 1998 Borderline malignancy in soft tissue neoplasia – a meaningful concept? Pathol Case Rev 3: 100–104
200. Fletcher C D M, Unni K K, Mertens F 2002 World Health Organization classification of tumours. Pathology and genetics. Tumours of soft tissue and bone. IARC Press, Lyon
201. Tsang W Y W, Chan J K C 1991 Kaposi-like infantile hemangioendothelioma. A distinctive vascular neoplasm of the retroperitoneum. Am J Surg Pathol 15: 982–989
202. Tsang W Y W, Chan J K C, Fletcher C D M 1991 Recently characterized vascular tumours of skin and soft tissues. Histopathology 19: 489–501
203. Zukerberg L R, Nickoloff B J, Weiss S W 1993 Kaposiform hemangioendothelioma of infancy and childhood. An aggressive neoplasm associated with Kasabach–Merritt syndrome and lymphangiomatosis. Am J Surg Pathol 17: 321–328
204. Lyons L L, North P E, Lai F M M et al. 2004 Kaposiform hemangioendothelioma. A study of 33 cases emphasizing its pathologic, immunophenotypic, and biologic uniqueness from juvenile hemangioma. Am J Surg Pathol 28: 559–568
205. Vin-Christian K, McCalmont T H, Frieden I J 1997 Kaposiform hemangioendothelioma. An aggressive, locally invasive vascular tumor that can mimic hemangioma of infancy. Arch Dermatol 133: 1573–1578
206. Lai F M M, Choi P C L, Leung P C et al. 2001 Kaposiform hemangioendothelioma: five patients with cutaneous lesions and long follow-up. Mod Pathol 14: 1087–1092
207. Mentzel T, Mazzoleni G, Dei Tos A P et al. 1997 Kaposiform hemangioendothelioma in adults. Clinicopathologic and immunohistochemical analysis of three cases. Am J Clin Pathol 108: 450–455
208. Gonzalez-Crussi F, Choud P, Crawford S E 1991 Congenital infiltrating giant cell angioblastoma, a new entity? Am J Surg Pathol 15: 175–183
209. Vargas S O, Pérez-Atayde A R, Gonzalez-Crussi F et al. 2001 Giant cell angioblastoma: three additional occurrences of a distinct pathologic entity. Am J Surg Pathol 25: 185–196
210. Dufau J P, Pierre C, De SaintMaur P P et al. 1997 Hemangioendothelioma retiforme. Ann Pathol 17: 47–51
211. Fukunaga M, Endo Y, Masui F et al. 1996 Retiform haemangioendothelioma. Virchows Arch 428: 301–304
212. Duke D, Dvorak A, Harris T J et al. 1996 Multiple retiform hemangioendotheliomas. A low-grade angiosarcoma. Am J Dermatopathol 18: 606–610
213. Mentzel T, Stengel B, Katenkamp D 1997 Retiform hemangioendothelioma. Clinico-pathologic case report and discussion of the group of low-grade malignancy vascular tumors. Pathologe 18: 390–394
214. Dabska M 1969 Malignant endovascular papillary angioendothelioma of the skin in childhood. Clinicopathologic study of 6 cases. Cancer 24: 503–510
215. Fanburg-Smith J C, Michal M, Partanen T et al. 1999 Papillary intralymphatic angioendothelioma (PILA). A report of twelve cases of a distinctive vascular tumor with phenotypic features of lymphatic vessels. Am J Surg Pathol 23: 1004–1010
216. Manivel J C, Wick M R, Swanson P E et al. 1986 Endovascular papillary angioendothelioma of childhood: a vascular lesion possibly characterized by "high" endothelial cell differentiation. Hum Pathol 17: 1240–1244
217. Nayler S J, Rubin B P, Calonje E et al. 2000 Composite hemangioendothelioma: a complex low-grade vascular lesion mimicking angiosarcoma. Am J Surg Pathol 24: 352–361
218. Reis-Filho J S, Paiva M E, Lopes J M 2002 Congenital composite hemangioendothelioma: case report and reappraisal of the hemangioendothelioma spectrum. J Cutan Pathol 29: 226–231

219. Chan J K C, Frizzera G, Fletcher C D M et al. 1992 Primary vascular tumors of lymph nodes other than Kaposi's sarcoma. Analysis of 39 cases and delineation of two new entities. Am J Surg Pathol 16: 335–350
220. Nascimento A G, Keeney G L, Sciot R et al. 1997 Polymorphous hemangioendothelioma: a report of two cases, one affecting extranodal soft tissues, and review of the literature. Am J Surg Pathol 21: 1083–1089
221. Templeton A C 1981 Kaposi's sarcoma. Pathol Annu 16: 315–336
222. Gottlieb G J, Ackerman A B 1982 Kaposi's sarcoma: an extensively disseminated form in young homosexual men. Hum Pathol 13: 882–892
223. Gottlieb G J, Ackerman A B 1988 Kaposi's sarcoma: a text and an atlas. Lea & Febiger, Philadelphia
224. Dorfman R F 1984 Kaposi's sarcoma revisited. Hum Pathol 15: 1013–1017
225. Krigel R L, Friedman-Kien A E 1990 Epidemic Kaposi's sarcoma. Semin Oncol 17: 350–360
226. Chor P J, Santa Cruz D J 1992 Kaposi's sarcoma. A clinicopathologic review and differential diagnosis. J Cutan Pathol 19: 6–20
227. Tappero J W, Conant M A, Wolfe S F et al. 1993 Kaposi's sarcoma. Epidemiology, pathogenesis, histology, clinical spectrum, staging criteria and therapy. J Am Acad Dermatol 28: 371–395
228. Beckstead J H, Wood G S, Fletcher V 1985 Evidence for the origin of Kaposi's sarcoma from lymphatic endothelium. Am J Pathol 119: 294–300
229. Russell Jones R, Spaull J, Spry C et al. 1986 Histogenesis of Kaposi's sarcoma in patients with and without acquired immune deficiency syndrome (AIDS). J Clin Pathol 39: 742–744
230. Rutgers J L, Wieczorek R, Bonetti F et al. 1986 The expression of endothelial cell surface antigens by AIDS-associated Kaposi's sarcoma. Evidence for a vascular endothelial cell origin. Am J Pathol 122: 493–499
231. Regezi J A, MacPhail L A, Daniels T E et al. 1993 Human immunodeficiency virus-associated oral Kaposi's sarcoma. A heterogeneous cell population dominated by spindle-shaped endothelial cells. Am J Pathol 143: 240–249
232. Weninger W, Partanen T A, Breiteneder-Geleff S et al. 1999 Expression of vascular endothelial growth factor receptor-3 and podoplanin suggests a lymphatic endothelial cell origin of Kaposi's sarcoma tumor cells. Lab Invest 79: 243–251
233. Grody W W, Lewin K J, Naeim F 1988 Detection of cytomegalovirus DNA in classic and epidemic Kaposi's sarcoma by in situ hybridization. Hum Pathol 19: 524–528
234. Ioachim H L, Dorsett B, Melamed J et al. 1992 Cytomegalovirus, angiomatosis, and Kaposi's sarcoma: new observations of a debated relationship. Mod Pathol 5: 169–178
235. Chang Y, Cesarman E, Pessin M S et al. 1994 Identification of herpesvirus-like DNA sequences in AIDS-associated Kaposi's sarcoma. Science 266: 1865–1869
236. Cesarman E, Knowles D M 1997 Kaposi's sarcoma-associated herpesvirus: a lymphotropic human herpesvirus associated with Kaposi's sarcoma, primary effusion lymphoma and multicentric Castleman's disease. Semin Diagn Pathol 14: 54–66
237. Kennedy M M, Lucas S B, Jones R R et al. 1997 HHV-8 and Kaposi's sarcoma: a time cohort study. J Clin Pathol Mol Pathol 50: 96–100
238. Renne R, Zhong W, Herndier B et al. 1996 Lytic growth of Kaposi's sarcoma-associated herpesvirus (human herpesvirus 8) in culture. Nature Med 2: 342–346
239. O'Leary J J, Kennedy M M, McGee J O 1997 Kaposi's sarcoma associated herpes virus (KSHV/HHV8): epidemiology, molecular biology and tissue distribution. Molec Pathol 5: 4–8
240. Cesarman E, Knowles D M 1997 Kaposi's sarcoma-associated herpesvirus: a lymphotropic human herpesvirus associated with Kaposi's sarcoma, primary effusion lymphoma and multicentric Castleman's disease. Semin Diagn Pathol 14: 54–66
241. Boshoff C, Talbot S, Kennedy M et al. 1996 HHV-8 and skin cancers in immunosuppressed patients. Lancet 347: 338–339
242. McDonagh D P, Liu J, Gaffey M J et al. 1996 Detection of Kaposi's sarcoma-associated herpes virus-type DNA sequences in angiosarcoma. Am J Pathol 149: 1363–1368
243. Lebbe C, Pellet C, Avril M F et al. 1997 Sequences of human herpesvirus 8 are not detected in various non-Kaposi sarcoma vascular lesions. Arch Dermatol 133: 919–920
244. Lasota J, Miettinen M 1999 Absence of Kaposi's sarcoma-associated virus (human herpes virus-8) sequences in angiosarcoma. Virchow's Arch 434: 51–56
245. Bayley A C, Lucas S B 1990 Kaposi's sarcoma or Kaposi's disease? A personal reappraisal. In: Fletcher CDM, McKee PH (eds) The pathobiology of soft tissue tumours. Churchill Livingstone, Edinburgh, Ch. 7
246. Rabkin C S, Janz S, Lash A et al. 1997 Monoclonal origin of multicentric Kaposi's sarcoma lesions. N Engl J Med 336: 988–993
247. Delabesse E, Oksenhendler E, Lebbe C et al. 1997 Molecular analysis of clonality in Kaposi's sarcoma. J Clin Pathol 50: 664–668
248. Gill P S, Tsai Y C, Rao A P et al. 1998 Evidence for multiclonality in multicentric Kaposi's sarcoma. Proc Natl Acad Sci USA 95: 8257–8261
249. Moskowitz L B, Hensley G T, Gould E W et al. 1985 Frequency and anatomic distribution of lymphadenopathic Kaposi's sarcoma in the acquired immunodeficiency syndrome: an autopsy series. Hum Pathol 16: 447–456
250. Lemlich G, Schwam L, Lebwohl M 1987 Kaposi's sarcoma and acquired immunodeficiency syndrome: postmortem findings in twenty-four cases. J Am Acad Dermatol 16: 319–325
251. Gange R W, Wilson Jones E 1978 Kaposi's sarcoma and immunosuppressive therapy: an appraisal. Clin Exp Dermatol 3: 135–146
252. Stribling J, Weitzner S, Smith G V 1978 Kaposi's sarcoma in renal allograft recipients. Cancer 42: 442–446
253. Dutz W, Stout A P 1960 Kaposi's sarcoma in infants and children. Cancer 13: 684–693
254. Dorfman R F 1986 Kaposi's sarcoma. With special reference to its manifestations in infants and children and to the concepts of Arthur Purdy Stout. Am J Surg Pathol 10 (suppl. 1): 68–77
255. Kao G F, Johnson F B, Sulica V I 1990 The nature of hyaline (eosinophilic) globules and vascular slits of Kaposi's sarcoma. Am J Dermatopathol 12: 256–267
256. Gange R W, Wilson Jones E 1979 Lymphangioma-like Kaposi's sarcoma. A report of three cases. Br J Dermatol 100: 327–334
257. Cossu S, Satta R, Cottoni F et al. 1997 Lymphangioma-like variant of Kaposi's sarcoma. Clinicopathologic study of seven cases with review of the literature. Am J Dermatopathol 19: 16–22
258. O'Connell K M 1977 Kaposi's sarcoma: histopathological study of 159 cases from Malawi. J Clin Pathol 30: 687–695
259. Satta R, Cossu S, Massarelli G et al. 2001 Anaplastic transformation of classic Kaposi's sarcoma: clinicopathological study of five cases. Br J Dermatol 145: 847–849
260. Cheuk W, Wong K O, Wong C S et al. 2004 Immunostaining for human herpesvirus 8 latent nuclear antigen-1 helps distinguish Kaposi sarcoma from its mimickers. Am J Clin Pathol 121: 335–342
261. Robin Y M, Guillou L, Michels J J et al. 2004 Human herpesvirus 8 immunostaining: a sensitive and specific method for diagnosing Kaposi sarcoma in paraffin-embedded sections. Am J Clin Pathol 121: 330–334
262. Wilson Jones E, Cerio R, Smith N P 1990 Multinucleate cell angiohistiocytoma: an acquired vascular anomaly to be distinguished from Kaposi's sarcoma. Br J Dermatol 122: 651–653
263. Weiss S W, Enzinger F M 1982 Epithelioid hemangioendothelioma. A vascular tumor often mistaken for a carcinoma. Cancer 50: 970–981
264. Weiss S W, Ishak K G, Dail D H et al. 1986 Epithelioid hemangioendothelioma and related lesions. Semin Diagn Pathol 3: 259–287
265. Mentzel T, Beham A, Calonje E et al. 1997 Epithelioid hemangioendothelioma of skin and soft tissues: clinicopathologic and immunohistochemical study of 30 cases. Am J Surg Pathol 21: 363–374
266. Angervall L, Kindblom L-G, Karlsson K et al. 1985 Atypical hemangioendothelioma of venous origin. A clinicopathologic, angiographic, immunohistochemical and ultrastructural study of two endothelial tumors within the concept of histiocytoid hemangioma. Am J Surg Pathol 9: 504–516
267. Dail D H, Liebow A A, Gmelich J T et al. 1983 Intravascular, bronchiolar and alveolar tumor of the lung (IVBAT). Cancer 51: 452–464
268. Makhlouf H R, Ishak K G, Goodman Z D 1999 Epithelioid hemangioendothelioma of the liver: a clinicopathologic study of 137 cases. Cancer 85: 562–582
269. Tsuneyoshi M, Dorfman H D, Bauer T W 1986 Epithelioid hemangioendothelioma of bone. A clinicopathologic, ultrastructural and immunohistochemical study. Am J Surg Pathol 10: 754–764
270. Lin B T, Colby T, Gown A M et al. 1996 Malignant vascular tumors of the serous membranes mimicking mesothelioma. A report of 14 cases. Am J Surg Pathol 20: 1431–1439
271. Quante M, Patel N K, Hill S et al. 1998 Epithelioid hemangioendothelioma presenting in the skin. a clinicopathologic study of eight cases. Am J Dermatopathol 20: 541–546
272. Tyring S, Guest P, Lee P et al. 1989 Epithelioid hemangioendothelioma of the skin and femur. J Am Acad Dermatol 20: 362–366
273. Resnik K S, Kantor G R, Spielvogel R L et al. 1993 Cutaneous epithelioid hemangioendothelioma without systemic involvement. Am J Dermatopathol 15: 272–276
274. Polk P, Webb J M 1997 Isolated cutaneous epithelioid hemangioendothelioma. J Am Acad Dermatol 36: 1026–1028
275. Lee K C, Chan J K C 1988 Epithelioid haemangioendothelioma presenting as a gastric polyp. Histopathology 16: 335–337
276. Suster S, Moran C A, Koss M N 1994 Epithelioid hemangioendothelioma of the anterior mediastinum. Clinicopathologic, immunohistochemical and ultrastructural analysis of 12 cases. Am J Surg Pathol 18: 871–881
277. Roh H S, Kim Y S, Suhr K B et al. 2000 A case of childhood epithelioid hemangioendothelioma. J Am Acad Dermatol 42: 897–899
278. Kiryu H, Hashimoto H, Hori Y 1996 Ossifying epithelioid hemangioendothelioma. J Cutan Pathol 23: 558–561
279. Lamovec J, Sobel H, Zidon A et al. 1990 Epithelioid hemangioendothelioma of the anterior mediastinum with osteoclast-like giant cells. Am J Clin Pathol 93: 813–817
280. Williams S B, Bulter C B, Gilkey G W et al. 1993 Epithelioid hemangioendothelioma with osteoclast like giant cells. Arch Pathol Lab Med 117: 315–318
281. Silva E G, Philips M J, Langer B et al. 1986 Spindle and histiocytoid (epithelioid) haemangioendothelioma, primary in lymph node. Am J Clin Pathol 85: 731–735
282. Suster S 1992 Epithelioid and spindle-cell hemangioendothelioma of the spleen, report of a distinctive splenic vascular neoplasm of childhood. Am J Surg Pathol 16: 785–792
283. Van Haelst U J G M, Pruszczynski M, Ten Cate L N et al. 1990 Ultrastructural and immunohistochemical study of epithelioid

283. hemangioendothelioma of bone: coexpression of epithelial and endothelial markers. Ultrastruct Pathol 14: 141–149
284. Gray M F, Rosenberg A E, Dickersin G R et al. 1990 Cytokeratin expression in epithelioid vascular neoplasms. Hum Pathol 21: 212–217
285. Mendick M R, Nelson M, Pickering D et al. 2001 Translocation t(1;3)(p36.3;q25) is a nonrandom aberration in epithelioid hemangioendothelioma. Am J Surg Pathol 25: 684–687
286. Billings S D, Folpe A L, Weiss S W 2003 Epithelioid sarcoma-like hemangioendothelioma. Am J Surg Pathol 27: 48–57
287. Wilson Jones E 1964 Malignant angioendothelioma of skin. Br J Dermatol 76: 21–39
288. Girard C, Johnson W C, Graham J H 1970 Cutaneous angiosarcoma. Cancer 26: 868–883
289. Rosai J, Summer H W, Kostianovsky M et al. 1976 Angiosarcoma of the skin. A clinicopathologic and fine structural study. Hum Pathol 7: 83–109
290. Wilson Jones E 1976 Malignant vascular tumours. Clin Exp Dermatol 1: 287–312
291. Maddox J C, Evans H L 1981 Angiosarcoma of skin and soft tissues: a study of forty-four cases. Cancer 48: 1907–1921
292. Cooper P H 1987 Angiosarcomas of the skin. Semin Diagn Pathol 4: 2–17
293. Ghandur-Mnaymneh L, Gonzales M S 1981 Angiosarcoma of the penis with hepatic angiomas in a patient with low vinyl chloride exposure. Cancer 47: 1318–1324
294. Abratt R P, Williams M, Raff M et al. 1983 Angiosarcoma of the superior vena cava. Cancer 52: 740–743
295. Rossi S, Fletcher C D M 2002 Angiosarcoma arising in hemangioma/vascular malformation: report of four cases and review of the literature. Am J Surg Pathol 26: 1319–1329
296. Mentzel T, Katenkamp D 1999 Intraneural angiosarcoma and angiosarcoma arising in benign and malignant peripheral nerve sheath tumours: clinicopathological and immunohistochemical analysis of four cases. Histopathology 35: 114–120
297. Chaudhuri B, Ronan S G, Manaligod J R 1980 Angiosarcoma arising in a plexiform neurofibroma. Cancer 46: 605–610
298. McMenamin M E, Fletcher C D M 2001 Expanding the spectrum of malignant change in schwannomas: epithelioid malignant change, epithelioid malignant peripheral nerve sheath tumor and epithelioid angiosarcoma: a study of 17 cases. Am J Surg Pathol 25: 13–25
299. Morphopoulos G D, Banerjee S S, Ali H H et al. 1996 Malignant peripheral nerve sheath tumour with vascular differentiation: a report of four cases. Histopathology 28: 401–410
300. Kauffman S L, Stout A P 1961 Malignant hemangioendothelioma in infants and children. Cancer 14: 1186–1196
301. Lezana-del Valle P, Gerald W L, Tsai J et al. 1998 Malignant vascular tumors in young patients. Cancer 83: 1634–1639
302. Leake J, Sheehan M P, Rampling D et al. 1992 Angiosarcoma complicating xeroderma pigmentosum. Histopathology 21: 179–181
303. Marcon I, Collini P, Casanova M et al. 2004 Cutaneous angiosarcoma in a patient with xeroderma pigmentosum. Pediatr Hematol Oncol 21: 23–26
304. Schmutz J L, Kue E, Baylac F et al. 1998 Angiosarcoma complicating Hallopeau–Siemens-type epidermolysis bullosa. Br J Dermatol 138: 910–912
305. Al-Najjar A-W, Harrington C I, Slater D N 1986 Angiosarcoma: a complication of varicose leg ulceration. Acta Derm Venereol 66:167–170
306. Folpe A L, Johnston C A, Weiss S W 2000 Cutaneous angiosarcoma arising in a gouty tophus: report of a unique case and a review of foreign material-associated angiosarcomas. Am J Dermatopathol 22: 418–421
307. Azam M, Saboorian H, Bieligk S et al. 2001 Cutaneous angiosarcoma complicating morbid obesity. Arch Pathol Lab Med 125: 531–533
308. Kibe Y, Kishimoto S, Katoh N et al. 1997 Angiosarcoma of the scalp associated with renal transplantation. Br J Dermatol 136: 752–756
309. Ahmed I, Hamacher K L 2002 Angiosarcoma in a chronically immunosuppressed renal transplant recipient: report of a case and review of the literature. Am J Dermatopathol 24: 330–335
309a. Schmid H, Zeitz C 2005 Human herpesvirus 8 and angiosarcoma: analysis of 40 cases and review of the literature. Pathology 37: 284–287
310. Holden C A, Spittle M F, Wilson Jones E 1987 Angiosarcoma of the face and scalp, prognosis and treatment. Cancer 59: 1046–1057
311. Lydiatt W M, Shaha A R, Shah J P 1994 Angiosarcoma of the head and neck. Am J Surg 168: 451–454
312. Mark R J, Poen J C, Tran L M et al. 1996 Angiosarcoma. A report of 67 patients and a review of the literature. Cancer 77: 2400–2406
313. Pawlik T M, Paulino A F, McGinn C J et al. 2003 Cutaneous angiosarcoma of the scalp: a multidisciplinary approach. Cancer 98: 1716–1726
314. Morrison W H, Byers R M, Garden A S et al. 1995 Cutaneous angiosarcoma of the head and neck. A therapeutic dilemma. Cancer 76: 319–327
315. Stewart F W, Treves N 1948 Lymphangiosarcoma in postmastectomy lymphedema. A report of six cases in elephantiasis chirurgica. Cancer 1: 64–81
316. Woodward A H, Ivins J C, Soule E H 1972 Lymphangiosarcoma arising in chronic lymphedematous extremities. Cancer 30: 562–572
317. Alessi E, Sala F, Berti E 1986 Angiosarcomas in lymphedematous limbs. Am J Dermatopathol 8: 371–378
318. Capo V, Ozzello L, Fenoglio C M et al. 1985 Angiosarcomas arising in edematous extremities: immunostaining for factor VIII related antigen and ultrastructural features. Hum Pathol 16: 144–150
319. Danese C A, Grishman E, Oh C et al. 1967 Malignant vascular tumors of the lymphedematous extremity. Ann Surg 166: 245–253
320. Mackenzie D H 1971 Lymphangiosarcoma arising in chronic congenital and idiopathic lymphoedema. J Clin Pathol 24: 524–529
321. Woodward A H, Ivins J C, Soule E H 1972 Lymphangiosarcoma arising in chronic lymphedematous extremities. Cancer 30: 562–572
322. Krasagakis K, Hettmannsperger U, Tebbe B et al. 1995 Cutaneous metastatic angiosarcoma with a lethal outcome, following radiotherapy for a cervical carcinoma. Br J Dermatol 133: 610–614
323. Goette D K, Detlefs R L 1985 Postirradiation angiosarcoma. J Am Acad Dermatol 12: 922–926
324. Fineberg S, Rosen P P 1994 Cutaneous angiosarcoma and atypical vascular lesions of the skin and breast after radiation therapy for breast carcinoma. Am J Clin Pathol 102: 757–763
325. Karlsson P, Holmberg E, Johansson K A et al. 1996 Soft tissue sarcoma after treatment for breast cancer. Radiother Oncol 38: 25–31
326. Cafiero F, Gipponi M, Peressini A et al. 1996 Radiation-associated angiosarcoma. Diagnostic and therapeutic implications – two case reports and a review of the literature. Cancer 77: 2496–2502
327. Billings S D, McKenney J K, Folpe A L et al. 2004 Cutaneous angiosarcoma following breast-conserving surgery and radiation. Am J Surg Pathol 28: 781–788
328. Majeski J, Austin R M, Fitzgerald R H 2000 Cutaneous angiosarcoma in an irradiated breast after breast conservation therapy for cancer: association with chronic breast lymphedema. J Surg Oncol 74: 208–212
329. Fletcher C D M, Beham A, Bekir S et al. 1991 Epithelioid angiosarcoma of deep soft tissue: a distinctive tumor readily mistaken for an epithelial neoplasm. Am J Surg Pathol 15: 915–924
330. Meis-Kindblom J M, Kindblom L-G 1998 Angiosarcoma of soft tissue. A study of 80 cases. Am J Surg Pathol 22: 683–697
331. Marrogi A J, Hunt S J, Santa Cruz D J 1990 Cutaneous epithelioid angiosarcoma. Am J Dermatopathol 12: 350–356
332. McWilliam L J, Harris M 1985 Granular cell angiosarcoma of the skin: histology, electron microscopy and immunohistochemistry of a newly recognised tumor. Histopathology 9: 1205–1216
333. Hitchcock M G, Hurt M A, Santa Cruz D J 1994 Cutaneous granular cell angiosarcoma. J Cutan Pathol 21: 256–262
334. Naka N, Ohsawa M, Tomita Y et al. 1996 Prognostic factors in angiosarcoma: a multivariate analysis of 55 cases. J Surg Oncol 61: 170–176
335. Morgan M B, Swann M, Somach S et al. 2004 Cutaneous angiosarcoma: a case series with prognostic correlation. J Am Acad Dermatol 50: 867–874
336. Folpe A L, Chand E M, Goldblum J R et al. 2001 Expression of Fli-1, nuclear transcription factor, distinguishes vascular neoplasms from potential mimics. Am J Surg Pathol 25: 1061–1066
337. Schuborg C, Mertens F, Rydholm A et al. 1998 Cytogenetic analysis of four angiosarcomas from deep and superficial soft tissue. Cancer Genet Cytogenet 100: 52–56
338. Eckert F, Schmid U, Gloor F et al. 1986 Evidence of vascular differentiation in anaplastic tumours of the thyroid: an immunohistochemical study. Virchow's Arch [A] 410: 203–215
339. Eusebi V, Carcangiu M L, Dina R et al. 1990 Keratin positive epithelioid angiosarcoma of thyroid. A report of four cases. Am J Surg Pathol 14: 737–747
340. Wenig B M, Abbondanzo S L, Heffer C S 1994 Epithelioid angiosarcoma of the adrenal glands. Am J Surg Pathol 18: 62–73
341. Goldblum J R, Rice T W 1995 Epithelioid angiosarcoma of the pulmonary artery. Hum Pathol 26: 1275–1277
342. Macias-Martínez V, Murrieta-Tiburcio L, Molina-Cárdenas H et al. 1997 Epithelioid angiosarcoma of the breast. Clinicopathological, immunohistochemical and ultrastructural study of a case. Am J Surg Pathol 21: 599–604
343. Hasegawa T, Fujii Y, Seki K et al. 1997 Epithelioid angiosarcoma of bone. Hum Pathol 28: 985–989
344. McAdam J A, Stewart F, Reid R 1998 Vaginal epithelioid angiosarcoma. J Clin Pathol 51: 928–930
345. Prescott R J, Banerjee S S, Eyden B P et al. 1994 Cutaneous epithelioid angiosarcoma: a clinicopathological study of four cases. Histopathology 25: 421–429
346. Jennings T A, Peterson L, Axiotis C A et al. 1988 Angiosarcoma associated with foreign body material. Cancer 62: 2436–2444
347. Byers R J, McMahon R F T, Freemont A J et al. 1992 Epithelioid angiosarcoma arising in an arteriovenous fistula. Histopathology 21: 87–89
348. Wehrli B M, Janzen D L, Shokeir O et al. 1998 Epithelioid angiosarcoma arising in a surgically constructed fistula: a rare complication of chronic immunosuppression in the setting of renal transplantation. Am J Surg Pathol 22: 1154–1159
349. Seo I S, Min K W 2003 Postirradiation epithelioid angiosarcoma of the breast: a case report with immunohistochemical and electron microscopic study. Ultrastruct Pathol 27: 197–203
350. Val-Bernal J F, Figols J, Arce F P et al. 2001 Cardiac epithelioid angiosarcoma presenting as cutaneous metastases. J Cutan Pathol 28: 265–270
351. Sebenik M, Ricci A Jr, DiPasquale B et al. 2005 Undifferentiated intimal sarcoma of large systemic blood vessels: report of 14 cases with immunohistochemical profile and review of the literature. Am J Surg Pathol 29: 1184–1193
352. Herzberg A J, Pizzo S V 1988 Primary undifferentiated sarcoma of the thoracic aorta. Histopathology 13: 571–574
353. Haber L M, Truong L 1988 Immunohistochemical demonstration of the endothelial nature of aortic intimal sarcoma. Am J Surg Pathol 12: 798–802

354. Seelig M H, Klinger P J, Oldenburg W A et al. 1998 Angiosarcoma of the aorta: report of a case and review of the literature. J Vasc Surg 28: 732–737
355. Burke A P, Virmani R 1993 Sarcomas of the great vessels. A clinicopathologic study. Cancer 71: 1761–1773
356. Johansson L, Carlen B 1994 Sarcoma of the pulmonary artery: report of four cases with electron microscopic and immunohistochemical examinations, and review of the literature. Virchows Arch 424: 217–224
357. Nonomura A, Kurumaya H, Kono N et al. 1988 Primary pulmonary artery sarcoma. Report of two autopsy cases studied by immunohistochemistry and electron microscopy, and review of 110 cases reported in the literature. Acta Pathol Jpn 38: 883–896
358. Gaumann A, Petrow P, Mentzel T et al. 2001 Osteopontin expression in primary sarcomas of the pulmonary artery. Virchows Arch 439: 668–674
359. Santonja C, Martin-Hita A M, Dotor A et al. 2001 Intimal angiosarcoma of the aorta with tumour embolisation causing mesenteric ischaemia. Report of a case diagnosed using CD31 immunohistochemistry in an intestinal resection specimen. Virchows Arch 438: 404–407
360. Bode-Lesniewska B, Zhao J, Speel E J et al. 2001 Gains of 12q13-14 and overexpression of mdm2 are frequent findings in intimal sarcomas of the pulmonary artery. Virchows Arch 438: 57–65
361. Bill A H, Sumner D S 1965 A unified concept of lymphangioma and cystic hygroma. Surg Gynecol Obstet 120: 79–86
362. Gross R E, Goeringer C F 1939 Cystic hygroma of the neck. Report of twenty-seven cases. Surg Gynecol Obstet 69: 48–60
363. Harkin G A, Sabiston D C 1960 Lymphangioma in infancy and childhood. Surgery 47: 811–822
364. Chervenak F A, Issacson G, Blakemore K J et al. 1983 Fetal cystic hygroma. Cause and natural history. N Engl J Med 309: 822–825
365. De Perrot M, Rostan O, Morel P et al. 1998 Abdominal lymphangioma in adults and children. Br J Surg 85: 395–397
366. Hornick J L, Fletcher C D M 2005 Intra-abdominal cystic lymphangiomas obscured by marked superimposed reactive changes: clinicopathologic analysis of a series. Hum Pathol 36: 426–432
367. Peachey R D G, Lim C-C, Whimster I W 1970 Lymphangioma of the skin. A review of 65 cases. Br J Dermatol 83: 519–527
368. Flanagan B P, Helwig E B 1977 Cutaneous lymphangioma. Arch Dermatol 113: 24–30
369. Prioleau P G, Santa Cruz D J 1978 Lymphangioma circumscriptum following radical mastectomy and radiation therapy. Cancer 42: 1989–1991
370. Whimster I W 1976 The pathology of lymphangioma circumscriptum. Br J Dermatol 94: 473–486
371. Gold S C 1970 Angioendothelioma (lymphatic type). Br J Dermatol 82: 92–93
372. Wilson Jones E, Winkelmann R K, Zachary C B et al. 1990 Benign lymphangio-endothelioma. J Am Acad Dermatol 23: 229–235
373. Guillou L, Fletcher C D M 2000 Benign lymphangioendothelioma (acquired progressive lymphangioma): a lesion not to be confused with well-differentiated angiosarcoma and patch stage Kaposi's sarcoma. Am J Surg Pathol 24: 1047–1057
374. Grunwald M H, Amichai B, Avinoach I 1997 Acquired progressive lymphangioma. J Am Acad Dermatol 37: 656–657
375. Sevila A, Botella-Estrada R, Sanmartín O et al. 2000 Benign lymphangioendothelioma of the thigh simulating a low grade angiosarcoma. Am J Dermatopathol 22: 151–154
376. Watanabe M, Kishiyama K, Ohkawara A 1983 Acquired progressive lymphangioma. J Am Acad Dermatol 8: 663–667
377. Mehregan D R, Mehregan A H, Mehregan D A 1992 Benign lymphangioendothelioma: report of two cases. J Cutan Pathol 19: 502–505
378. Rosso R, Gianelli U, Carnevali L 1995 Acquired progressive lymphangioma of the skin following radiotherapy for breast carcinoma. J Cutan Pathol 22: 164–167
379. Kato H, Kadoya A 1996 Acquired progressive lymphangioma following femoral arteriography. Clin Exp Dermatol 21: 159–162
380. Asch M J, Cohen A H, Moore T C 1974 Hepatic and splenic lymphangiomatosis with skeletal involvement: report of a case and review of the literature. Surgery 76: 334–339
381. Ramani P, Shah A 1992 Lymphangiomatosis. Histological and immunohistochemical analysis of four cases. Am J Surg Pathol 16: 764–771
382. Singh Gomez C, Calonje E, Ferrar D W et al. 1995 Lymphangiomatosis of the limbs: clinicopathologic analysis of a series with a good prognosis. Am J Surg Pathol 19: 125–133
383. Díaz-Cascajo C, Borghi S, Weyers W et al. 1999 Benign lymphangiomatous papules of the skin after radiotherapy: a report of five new cases and review of the literature. Histopathology 35: 319–327
384. Requena L, Kutzner H, Mentzel T et al. 2002 Benign vascular proliferations in irradiated skin. Am J Surg Pathol 26: 328–337
385. Brenn T, Fletcher C D M 2005 Radiation-induced cutaneous atypical vascular lesions and angiosarcoma: Clinicopathologic analysis of 42 cases. Am J Surg Pathol 29: 983–996
386. Frack M D, Simon S, Dawson B H 1968 The lymphangiomyomatosis syndrome. Cancer 22: 428–437
387. Wolff M 1973 Lymphangiomyoma: clinicopathologic study and ultrastructural confirmation of its histogenesis. Cancer 31: 988–1007
388. Johnson S 1999 Rare diseases. I. Lymphangioleiomyomatosis: clinical features, management and basic mechanisms. Thorax 54: 254–264
389. Berger U, Khaghani A, Pomerance A et al. 1990 Pulmonary lymphangioleiomyomatosis and steroid receptors. An immunocytochemical study. Am J Clin Pathol 93: 609–614
390. Ohori N P, Yousem S A, Sonmez-Alpan E et al. 1991 Estrogen and progesterone receptors in lymphangioleiomyomatosis, epithelioid hemangioendothelioma, and sclerosing hemangioma of the lung. Am J Clin Pathol 96: 529–535
391. Torres V E, Bjornsson J, King B F et al. 1995 Extrapulmonary lymphangioleiomyomatosis and lymphangiomatous cysts in tuberous sclerosis complex. Mayo Clin Proc 70: 641–648
392. Smolarek T A, Wessner L L, McCormack F X et al. 1998 Evidence that lymphangiomyomatosis is caused by TSC2 mutations: chromosome 16p13 loss of heterozygosity in angiomyolipomas and lymph nodes from women with lymphangiomyomatosis. Am J Hum Genet 62: 810–815
393. Pacheco-Rodriguez G, Kristof A S, Stevens L A et al. 2002 Giles F. Filley lecture. Genetics and gene expression in lymphangioleiomyomatosis. Chest 121: 56S–60S
394. Chan J K C, Tsang W Y W, Pau M Y et al. 1993 Lymphangiomyomatosis and angiomyolipoma: closely related entities characterized by hamartomatous proliferation of HMB-45 positive smooth muscle. Histopathology 22: 445–455
395. Fetsch P A, Fetsch J F, Marincola F M et al. 1998 Comparison of melanoma antigen recognized by T cells (MART-1) to HMB-45: additional evidence to support a common lineage for angiomyolipoma, lymphangiomyomatosis and clear cell sugar tumor. Mod Pathol 11: 699–703
396. Pea M, Martignoni G, Zamboni G et al. 1996 Perivascular epithelioid cell. Am J Surg Pathol 20: 1149–1153
397. Bailey O T 1935 The cutaneous glomus and its tumors – glomangiomas. Am J Pathol 11: 915–935
398. Kohout E, Stout A P 1961 The glomus tumor in children. Cancer 14: 555–565
399. Tsuneyoshi M, Enjoji M 1982 Glomus tumor: a clinicopathologic and electron microscopic study. Cancer 50: 1601–1607
400. Pepper M C, Laubenheimer R, Cripps D J 1977 Multiple glomus tumours. J Cutan Pathol 4: 244–257
401. Happle R, Konig A 1999 Type 2 segmental manifestation of multiple glomus tumors: a review and reclassification of 5 case reports. Dermatology 198: 270–272
402. Boon L M, Brouillard P, Irrthum A et al. 1999 A gene for inherited cutaneous venous anomalies ("glomangiomas") localizes to chromosome 1p21-22. Am J Hum Genet 65: 125–133
403. Calvert J T, Burns S, Riney TJ et al. 2001 Additional glomangioma family link to chromosome 1p: no evidence for genetic heterogeneity. Hum Hered 51: 180–182
404. Brouillard P, Boom L M, Mulliken J B et al. 2002 Mutations in a novel factor, glomulin, are responsible for glomuvenous malformations ("glomangiomas"). Am J Hum Genet 70: 866–874
405. Kanwar Y S, Manaligod J R 1975 Glomus tumor of the stomach. An ultrastructural study. Arch Pathol 99: 392–397
406. Kim Y I, Kim J H, Suh R et al. 1989 Glomus tumor of the trachea. Report of a case with ultrastructural observations. Cancer 64: 881–886
407. Sunderraj S, Al-Kahalifa A A, Pal A K et al. 1989 Primary intra-osseous glomus tumor. Histopathology 14: 532–536
408. Geraghty J M, Everitt N J, Blundell J W 1991 Glomus tumour of the small bowel. Histopathology 19: 287–289
409. Harvey J A, Walker F 1987 Solid glomus tumor of the pterygoid fossa: a lesion mimicking an epithelial neoplasm of low-grade malignancy. Hum Pathol 18: 965–966
410. Koss M N, Hochholzer L, Moran C A 1998 Primary pulmonary glomus tumor: a clinicopathologic and immunohistochemical study of two cases. Mod Pathol 11: 253–258
411. Gaertner E M, Steinberg D M, Huber M et al. 2000 Pulmonary and mediastinal glomus tumors – report of five cases including a pulmonary glomangiosarcoma: a clinicopathologic study with literature review. Am J Surg Pathol 24: 1105–1114
412. Hirose T, Hasegawa T, Seki K et al. 1996 Atypical glomus tumor in the mediastinum: a case report with immunohistochemical and ultrastructural studies. Ultrastruct Pathol 20: 451–456
413. Jaiswal V R, Champine J G, Sharma S et al. 2004 Primary glomangioma of the liver: a case report and review of the literature. Arch Pathol Lab Med 128: 46–49
414. Miliauskas J R, Worthley C, Allen P W 2002 Glomangiomyoma (glomus tumor) of the pancreas: a case report. Pathology 34: 193–195
415. Gokten N, Peterdy G, Philpott T et al. 2001 Glomus tumor of the ovary: report of a case with immunohistiochemical and ultrastructural observations. Int J Gynecol Pathol 20: 390–394
416. Silver S A, Tavassoli F A 2000 Glomus tumor arising in a mature teratoma of the ovary: report of a case simulating a metastasis from cervical squamous carcinoma. Arch Pathol Lab Med 124: 1373–1375
417. Beham A, Fletcher C D M 1991 Intravascular glomus tumour: a previously undescribed phenomenon. Virchow's Arch [A] 418: 175–177
418. Googe P B, Griffin W C 1993 Intravenous glomus tumor of the forearm. J Cutan Pathol 20: 359–363
419. Calonje E, Fletcher C D M 1995 Cutaneous intraneural glomus tumor. Am J Dermatopathol 17: 395–398
420. Sawada S, Honda M, Kamide R et al. 1995 Three cases of subungual glomus tumors with von Recklinghausen neurofibromatosis. J Am Acad Dermatol 32: 277–278

421. Okada O, Demitsu T, Manabe M et al. 1999 A case of multiple subungual glomus tumors associated with neurofibromatosis type 1. J Dermatol 26: 535–537
422. De Smet L, Sciot R, Legius E 2002 Multifocal glomus tumours of the fingers in two patients with neurofibromatosis type 1. J Med Genet 39: 45
423. Haque S, Modlin I M, West A B 1992 Multiple glomus tumors of the stomach with intravascular spread. Am J Surg Pathol 16: 291–299
424. Albrecht S, Zbieranowski J 1990 Incidental glomus coccygeum. When a normal structure looks like a tumor. Am J Surg Pathol 14: 922–924
425. Van Geertruyden J, Lorea P, Goldschmidt D et al. 1996 Glomus tumours of the hand. A retrospective study of 51 cases. J Hand Surg (Br) 21: 257–260
426. Brathwaite C D, Poppiti R J Jr 1996 Malignant glomus tumor. A case report of widespread metastases in a patient with multiple glomus body hamartomas. Am J Surg Pathol 20: 233–238
427. Watanabe K, Sugino T, Saito A et al. 1998 Glomangiosarcoma of the hip: report of a highly aggressive tumour with widespread distant metastases. Br J Dermatol 139: 1097–1101
428. Kayal J D, Hampton R W, Sheehan D J et al. 2001 Malignant glomus tumor: a case report and review of the literature. Dermatol Surg 27: 837–840
429. Park J H, Oh S H, Yang M H et al. 2003 Glomangiosarcoma of the hand: a case report and review of the literature. J Dermatol 30: 827–833
430. Folpe A L, Fanburgh-Smith J C, Miettinen M et al. 2001 Atypical and malignant glomus tumors: analysis of 52 cases, with a proposal for the reclassification of glomus tumors. Am J Surg Pathol 25: 1–12
431. Slater D N, Cotton D W K, Azzopardi J G 1987 Oncocytic glomus tumour: a new variant. Histopathology 11: 523–531
432. Pulitzer D R, Martin P C, Reed R J 1995 Epithelioid glomus tumor. Hum Pathol 26: 1022–1027
433. Jalali M, Netscher D T, Connelly J H 2002 Glomangiomatosis. Ann Diagn Pathol 6: 326–328.
434. Wood W S, Dimmiek J E 1977 Multiple infiltrating glomus tumours in children. Cancer 40: 1680–1685
435. Gould E W, Manivel J C, Albores-Saavedra J et al. 1990 Locally infiltrative glomus tumors and glomangiosarcoma. A clinical, ultrastructural and immunohistochemical study. Cancer 65: 310–318
436. Dervan P A, Tobbin I N, Casey M et al. 1989 Glomus tumours: an immunohistochemical profile of 11 cases. Histopathology 14: 483–491
437. Porter P L, Bigler S A, McNutt M et al. 1991 The immunophenotype of hemangiopericytomas and glomus tumors with special reference to muscle protein expression: an immunohistochemical study and review of the literature. Mod Pathol 4: 46–52
438. Liapi-Avgeri G, Karabela-Bouropoulou X, Agnanti N 1994 Glomus tumor. A histological, histochemical and immunohistochemical study of the various types. Pathol Res Pract 190: 2–10
439. Mentzel T, Hugel H, Kutzner H 2002 CD34-positive glomus tumor: clinicopathologic and immunohistochemical analysis of six cases with myxoid stromal changes. J Cutan Pathol 29: 421–425
440. Hiruta N, Kameda N, Tokudome T et al. 1997 Malignant glomus tumor: a case report and review of the literature. Am J Surg Pathol 21: 1096–1103
441. López-Rios F, Rodríguez-Peralto J L, Castaño E et al. 1997 Glomangiosarcoma of the lower limb: a case report with a literature review. J Cutan Pathol 24: 571–574
442. Stout A P, Murray M R 1942 Hemangiopericytoma: a vascular tumor featuring Zimmermann's pericytes. Ann Surg 116: 26–33
443. Battifora H 1973 Hemangiopericytoma: ultrastructural study of five cases. Cancer 31: 1418–1432
444. Nunnery E W, Khan L B, Reddick R L et al. 1981 Hemangiopericytoma: a light microscopic and ultrastructural study. Cancer 47: 906–914
445. Dardick I, Hammar S P, Scheithauer B W 1989 Ultrastructural spectrum of hemangiopericytoma: a comparative study of fetal, adult, and neoplastic pericytes. Ultrastruct Pathol 13: 111–154
446. Middleton L P, Duray P H, Merino M J 1998 The histologic spectrum of hemangiopericytoma: application of immunohistochemical analysis including proliferative markers to facilitate diagnosis and predict prognosis. Hum Pathol 29: 636–640
447. Schurch W, Skalli O, Lagace R et al. 1990 Intermediate filament proteins and actin isoforms as markers for soft tissue tumor differentiation and origin III. Hemangiopericytomas and glomus tumors. Am J Pathol 136: 771–786
448. Tsuneyoshi M, Daimaru Y, Enjoji M 1984 Malignant hemangiopericytoma and other sarcomas with hemangiopericytoma-like pattern. Pathol Res Pract 178: 446–453
449. Fletcher C D M 1994 Haemangiopericytoma – a dying breed? Reappraisal of an "entity" and its variants. Curr Diagn Pathol 1: 19–23
450. Nappi O, Ritter J H, Pettinato G et al. 1995 Hemangiopericytoma: histopathological pattern or clinicopathologic entity? Semin Diagn Pathol 12: 221–232
451. Stout A P 1949 Hemangiopericytoma. A study of twenty-five new cases. Cancer 2: 1027–1035
452. Granter S R, Badizadegan K, Fletcher C D M 1998 Myofibromatosis in adults, glomangiopericytoma and myopericytoma. A spectrum of tumors showing perivascular myoid differentiation. Am J Surg Pathol 22: 513–525
453. Enzinger F M, Smith B H 1976 Hemangiopericytoma. An analysis of 106 cases. Hum Pathol 7: 61–82
454. Angervall L, Kindblom L G, Moller Nielsen J M et al. 1978 Hemangiopericytoma, a clinicopathologic, angiographic and microangiographic study. Cancer 42: 2412–2427
455. Pavelic K, Cabrijan T, Hrascan R et al. 1998 Molecular pathology of hemangiopericytomas accompanied by severe hypoglycemia: oncogenes, tumor-suppressor genes and the insulin-like growth factor family. J Cancer Res Clin Oncol 124: 307–314
456. Guthrie B L, Ebersold M J, Scheithauer B W et al. 1989 Meningeal hemangiopericytoma: histopathological features, treatment and long-term follow-up of 44 cases. Neurosurgery 25: 514–522
457. Mena H, Ribas J L, Pezeshkpour G H et al. 1991 Hemangiopericytoma of the central nervous system: a review of 94 cases. Hum Pathol 22: 84–91
458. Compagno J, Hyams V J 1976 Hemangiopericytoma-like intranasal tumors. A clinicopathologic study of 23 cases. Am J Clin Pathol 66: 672–683
459. Eichhorn J H, Dickersin G R, Bhan A K et al. 1990 Sinonasal hemangiopericytoma. A reassessment with electron microscopy, immunohistochemistry, and long-term follow-up. Am J Surg Pathol 14: 856–866
460. Coffin C M, Dehner L P 1991 Fibroblastic-myofibroblastic tumors in children and adolescents: a clinicopathologic study of 108 examples in 103 patients. Pediatr Pathol 11: 569–588
461. Mentzel T, Calonje E, Nascimento A G et al. 1994 Infantile haemangiopericytoma versus infantile myofibromatosis: a study of a series suggesting a spectrum of infantile myofibroblastic lesions. Am J Surg Pathol 18: 922–930
462. Dictor M, Elner A, Andersson T et al. 1992 Myofibromatosis-like hemangiopericytoma metastasising as differentiated vascular smooth muscle and myosarcoma. Myopericytes as a subset of "myofibroblasts." Am J Surg Pathol 16: 1239–1247
463. Variend S, Bax N M, Van Gorp J 1995 Are infantile myofibromatosis, congenital fibrosarcoma and congenital haemangiopericytoma histogenetically related? Histopathology 26: 57–62
463a. Mentzel T, Dei Tos A P, Sapi Z, Kutzner H 2006 Myopericytoma of skin and soft tissues: clinicopathologic and immunohistochemical study of 54 cases. Am J Surg Pathol 30: 104–113
464. Requena L, Kutzner H, Hugel H et al. 1996 Cutaneous adult myofibroma: a vascular neoplasm. J Cutan Pathol 23: 445–457
465. Sakamoto A, Oda Y, Nagayoshi Y et al. 2001 Glomangiopericytoma causing oncogenic osteomalacia. A case report with immunohistochemical analysis. Arch Orthop Trauma Surg 121: 104–108
466. McMenamin M E, Fletcher C D M 2002 Malignant myopericytoma: expanding the spectrum of tumors with myopericytic differentiation. Histopathology 41: 450–460
467. Vallet-Decouvelaere A V, Dry S M, Fletcher C D M 1998 Atypical and malignant solitary fibrous tumors in extrathoracic locations: evidence of their comparability to intra-thoracic tumors. Am J Surg Pathol 22: 1501–1511
468. McMenamin M E, Calonje E 2002 Intravascular myopericytoma. J Cutan Pathol 29: 557–561

表4A.3	鼻窦部（鼻黏膜）乳头状瘤：临床病理学特征		
	中隔型	内翻型	嗜酸细胞型
百分率	20%～50%	47%～73%	3%～8%
性别、年龄	男>女；20～50岁	男>女；40～70岁	男=女；>50岁
部位	鼻中隔	鼻外侧壁中甲的位置，并扩展至鼻窦（上颌窦或筛窦）	鼻外侧壁和鼻窦（上颌窦或筛窦）
病灶	单侧	多为单侧，双侧罕见	单侧
组织学形态	乳头主要由鳞状（表皮样）上皮构成；也可有黏液细胞（杯状细胞）和上皮内黏液囊肿；纤细的纤维血管轴心	增厚的鳞状上皮呈内生性或"内翻性"生长，病变由鳞状、移行和柱状细胞组成（所有三种细胞可出现在同一病变中），伴有黏液细胞（杯状细胞）和上皮内黏液囊肿；表面上皮全层均可见混合的慢性炎细胞浸润是其特征	由含有丰富嗜酸性颗粒状胞浆的柱状细胞构成的复层上皮增生；增生上皮的表面可见纤毛；可见上皮内黏液囊肿，其中常含有多形核白细胞
HPV发生率	大约50%阳性；HPV 6和11；HPV 16和18少见；HPV 57罕见	大约38%阳性；HPV 6和11；HPV 16和18少见；HPV 57罕见	一般缺乏
恶变率	罕见	2%～27%	4%～17%

分子生物学分析［原位杂交和（或）聚合酶链反应］发现，在鼻中隔和内翻型乳头状瘤中有 HPV 6/11，HPV 16/18 少见，其他类型 HPV（例如 HPV 57）罕见[11-15]。Barnes 在一篇文献综述指出，38%（131/341）的内翻型乳头状瘤 HPV 阳性[16]。HPV 感染与鼻黏膜乳头状瘤的发生之间是否存在因果关系尚有待确定。迄今为止，分子生物学分析尚未发现嗜酸细胞型乳头状瘤存在 HPV。与上呼吸道其他部位乳头状瘤的发生无关。在内翻型乳头状瘤中还发现有 EB 病毒，可能意味着 EB 病毒与这些肿瘤的发生有关[17]；然而，其他研究未能证实 EB 病毒存在于肿瘤细胞中[18]。

鼻中隔乳头状瘤是乳头状外生性的疣状病变，呈粉红色至棕褐色不等，质地坚硬或呈橡皮硬度。常以基底部狭窄或较宽的蒂与黏膜相连。组织学上，可见乳头状结构，主要由增厚的鳞状（表皮样）上皮组成，呼吸型上皮不常见（图 4A.1）。表面角化少见。可见黏液细胞（杯

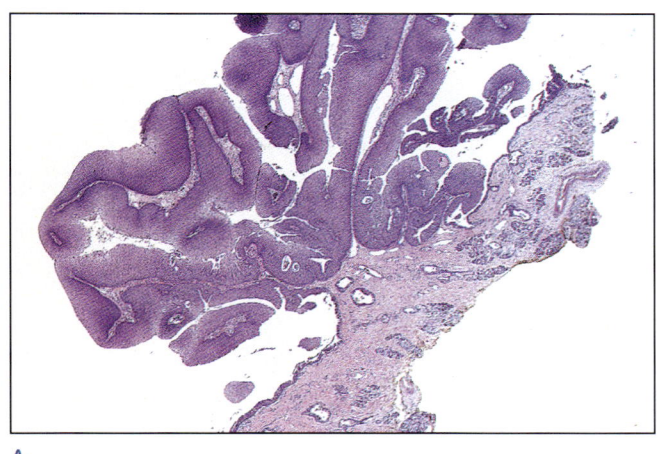

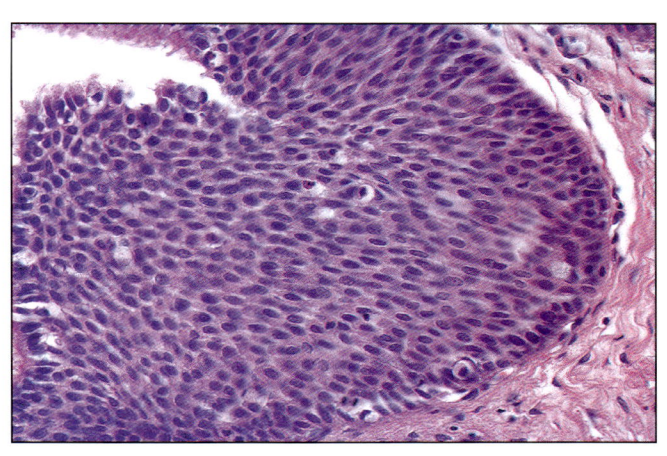

图4A.1 鼻黏膜乳头状瘤，外生（中隔）型。（A）肿瘤由表面呼吸性上皮向外呈乳头状生长，由增厚的非角化性鳞状（表皮样）上皮构成；注意黏膜下可见小涎腺成分，表明起源于黏膜而不是皮肤。（B）在较高放大倍数下，上皮呈良性，细胞保留极性，缺乏细胞学非典型性，可见散在的黏液性囊肿和上皮内炎细胞浸润；沿表面可见残留的非肿瘤性纤毛呼吸上皮。

状细胞）和上皮内黏液囊肿。纤细的纤维血管轴心构成基质成分。

内翻型乳头状瘤体积较大，灰红色半透明状，质地从硬韧到脆而易碎不等。组织学上，这些肿瘤具有内生性或"内翻性"生长方式，表现为明显增厚的鳞状上皮向下增生，进入其下的间质（图4A.2）。上皮细胞构成不同，包括鳞状、移行和柱状细胞（所有三种细胞可以出现在同一个病变中），伴有混合性黏液细胞（杯状细胞）和上皮内黏液囊肿。上皮全层出现混合性慢性炎细胞浸润是其特征。这些细胞通常呈良性表现，细胞核均匀一致，并不密集。然而，可以出现多形性和细胞非典型性。上皮成分可能具有广泛的透明细胞特征，说明含有大量糖原成分。上皮基底和副基底部可见核分裂象，但无非典型性核分裂象。表面可以出现角化。间质成分从黏液样到纤维性不等，伴有慢性炎症细胞和数量不等的血管成分。

嗜酸细胞型鼻黏膜乳头状瘤是暗红色至棕色的乳头状或息肉样病变。组织学上，有多层上皮增生，由具有丰富的嗜酸性颗粒状胞浆的柱状细胞构成（图4A.3）。细胞核从空泡状到深染不等，核仁常不清楚；增生上皮的表面可见纤毛。上皮内黏液囊肿常常含有多形核白细胞；黏膜下没有黏液囊肿。间质成分从黏液样到纤维化不等，伴有慢性炎症细胞和不同数量的血管成分。

鼻中隔乳头状瘤的鉴别诊断包括寻常疣和鳞状上皮乳头状瘤。与所有鼻窦性乳头状瘤不同，鼻前庭鳞状上皮乳头状瘤没有黏液细胞作为肿瘤性增生的一部分。内翻性乳头状瘤的鉴别诊断包括鼻窦炎性息肉、非角化性呼吸上皮（"移行上皮"）癌和疣状癌。嗜酸细胞型乳头状瘤的鉴别诊断包括鼻孢子菌病和（低级别）乳头状腺癌。

所有鼻窦型乳头状瘤的治疗都是包括邻近未受累黏膜在内的完全性手术切除；必须切除未受累黏膜，因为肿瘤可以沿着邻近鳞状化生的鼻窦黏膜生长和扩展[2,3]。充分手术切除包括侧鼻切除术或内上颌骨切除术，伴有肿瘤整块切除术[19]。这一组肿瘤如果未能完全切除，将会复发；复发可能是疾病持续，而不是肿瘤多中心生长。一般来说，完全手术切除后预后良好；然而，如果未能完全切除，这些肿瘤将有可能继续生长，沿着黏膜表面扩散，破坏骨质和侵蚀重要结构。没有发现辅助治疗（化学治疗和放射治疗）对于鼻窦乳头状瘤有效。然而，对于选择性的因局部晚期疾病而未能手术切除的患者，放射治疗可能有效[20]。

与鼻黏膜乳头状瘤有关的并发症包括复发和恶变。内翻型和嗜酸细胞型乳头状瘤可发生恶变。恶变的发生率取决于亚型：据报道内翻型乳头状瘤的恶变率为2%～27%[1,3,16,21-24]；嗜酸细胞型乳头状瘤的恶变率为4%～17%[1,3,17,20]；鼻中隔乳头状瘤如果曾发生恶变的话，也是十分罕见的。其发生与鼻黏膜乳头状瘤有关的恶性肿瘤多数是鳞状细胞癌（角化性和非角化性），分化程度高低不等。在少数情况下，可以发生其他类型的癌，包括疣状癌、黏液表皮样癌、小细胞癌、腺癌和鼻窦未分化癌（sinonasal undifferentiated carcinoma，SNUC）。癌与乳头状瘤可同时或异时发生；异时发生的癌从乳头状瘤发生到癌出现的平均时间间隔为63个

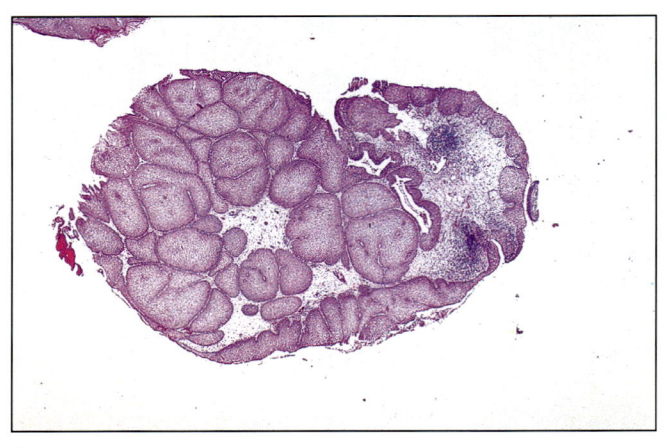

A

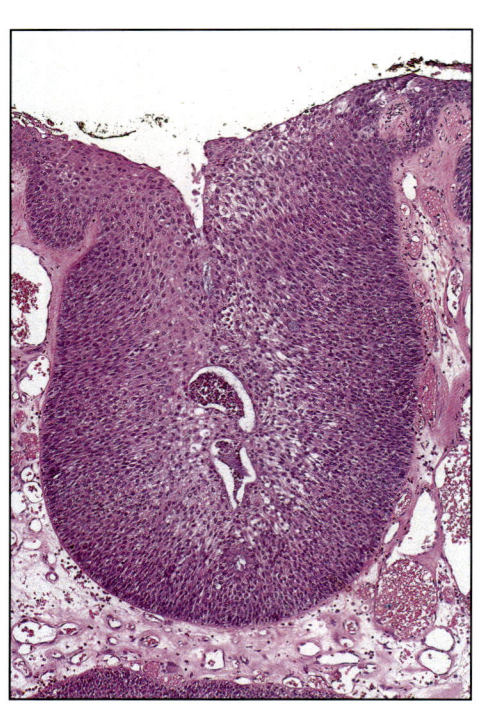

B

图4A.2 鼻黏膜乳头状瘤，内翻型。（A）与外生型不同，内翻型鳞状上皮向下增生，伸入水肿的间质。（B）来自内衬鼻黏膜正常呼吸上皮鳞状化生的良性上皮呈球状，向下（内翻）生长；可见伴有炎症细胞的上皮内囊肿。

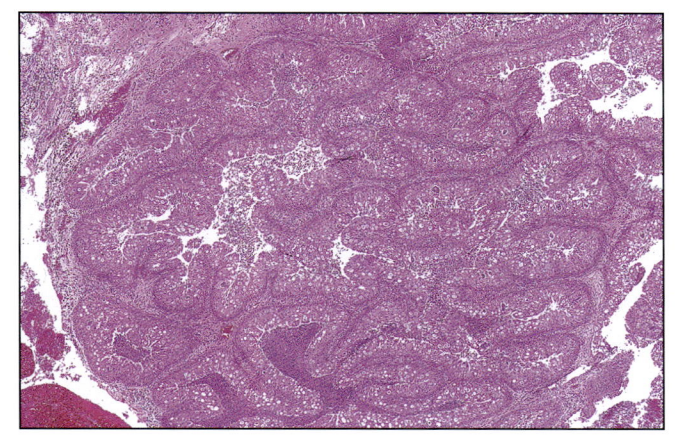
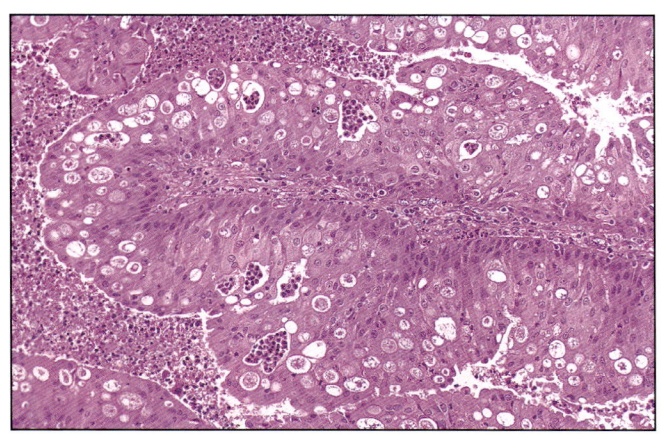
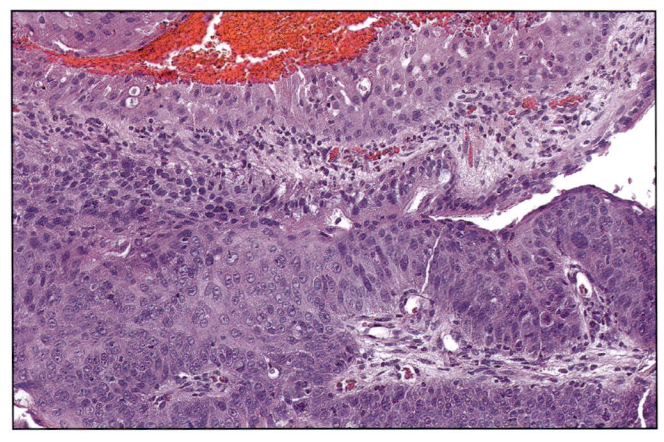

图4A.3 鼻黏膜乳头状瘤，嗜酸细胞型。（A）上皮外生性增生，伴有明显嗜酸性表现。（B）在较高放大倍数下，上皮为多层，由含有丰富的嗜酸性和颗粒状胞浆的柱状细胞组成；可见上皮内黏液囊肿，某些囊肿伴有多形核白细胞。（C）嗜酸细胞型乳头状瘤恶变，显示残留的良性上皮（上）原位癌区域（下）。本例有浸润性角化性鳞状细胞癌（未显示）。

月（从6个月到13年）[16]。癌灶可为局限性或广泛性，可以显示上皮异型增生以及原位癌或浸润癌。可能存在这样的肿瘤，肿瘤以良性（乳头状瘤）为主，仅仅伴有局限性的恶性病灶，或者肿瘤以癌为主，伴有非常有限的残留的乳头状瘤。某些病例可能没有先前存在的良性肿瘤的证据，而只是通过病史才知道患者从前患有良性鼻窦乳头状瘤。没有可靠的组织学特征能够预测哪一个乳头状瘤可能恶变。伴有细胞成分增加、多形性和核分裂活性增加的乳头状瘤，并不一定已恶变。出现中度到重度上皮异型增生可能是恶变的指征。同样，表面角化和角化不良也被认为可能是恶变的征兆。任何显示中度到重度异型增生或有表面角化的鼻窦乳头状瘤，均应及时对所有切除组织进行组织学检查，以除外恶性的可能。复发次数与癌的发生之间没有相关性。

鼻窦乳头状瘤恶变的治疗包括手术切除和放射治疗。预后不一。某些患者癌灶仅仅是局灶浸润，治疗之后预后较好；另外一些患者可能有广泛浸润，伴有重要结构受累和（或）转移性疾病；不论是否进行治疗，这些患者的临床结局一般均较差。

鳞状上皮乳头状瘤 Squamous papillomas

鳞状上皮乳头状瘤是上呼吸消化道黏膜最常见的良性肿瘤，常见于口腔和喉部。少数鳞状上皮乳头状瘤发生于鼻咽部和鼻前庭[25,26]。鼻前庭鳞状上皮乳头状瘤起源于皮肤。与鼻窦型乳头状瘤不同，皮肤鳞状上皮乳头状瘤缺乏上皮内黏液囊肿和软骨成分，它们来源于内胚层。鳞状上皮乳头状瘤为外生性、疣状或菜花样肿瘤，最大径从几毫米到3厘米不等。组织学上，这些肿瘤由良性鳞状上皮构成，排列成多发性指状突起，伴有明显的纤维血管轴心。鳞状上皮没有任何异型增生性改变。一般来说，这些肿瘤缺乏表面角化，但在任何肿瘤均可能有（过度）角化、角化不全和正常角化。出现表面角化并不具有发生癌的另外危险。尽管少见，鼻窦型（鼻黏膜）乳头状瘤可来源于与鼻窦部没有任何联系的鼻咽部位，可能是来源于错位的外胚层来源的鼻窦黏膜上皮残余[27]。可选择手术切除，并可以治愈。复发不常见，且与手术切除不完全有关[27]。不发生恶变。

小涎腺的良性肿瘤
Benign neoplasms of minor salivary glands

鼻窦和鼻咽的良性涎腺肿瘤并不常见。通常，小涎腺肿瘤最常发生于鼻腔，而很少发生于副鼻窦。多形性腺瘤（良性混合瘤）是主要的组织学类型[28]；单形性腺瘤不常发生，例如肌上皮瘤和嗜酸细胞瘤。

多形性腺瘤主要发生于鼻中隔（骨或软骨成分），比任何其他部位都要常见[28]。尽管这些肿瘤可发生于副鼻窦，但副鼻窦受累较常来源于鼻腔内病变的继发性蔓延。这些肿瘤表现为息肉样或呈外生性生长，表面通常被覆完整的黏膜，大小不同，从 1~7 cm 不一。如同所有上呼吸消化道小涎腺肿瘤（良性或恶性）一样，多形性腺瘤均无包膜。然而，与恶性小涎腺肿瘤不同，这些肿瘤界限相对清楚，而无浸润性生长；表面上皮受累并不等于浸润。组织学上，这些肿瘤与大涎腺肿瘤相同（见第 7 章），包括混合性导管或小管状结构，梭形肌上皮细胞和黏液软骨样间质。鼻腔多形性腺瘤倾向于富于细胞，显示突出的肌上皮成分。后者通常表现为浆细胞样（玻璃样细胞），而不是梭形肌上皮细胞（图 4A.4）。假设这些肿瘤出现导管或小管状结构以及黏液软骨样间质，就不应考虑为肌上皮瘤。肌上皮瘤是单形性腺瘤的一种类型，仅由肌上皮细胞构成。典型的肌上皮瘤是梭形细胞型肿瘤，在少数情况下，肿瘤细胞是浆细胞样细胞。肌上皮分化可由免疫反应显示，例如细胞角蛋白、S-100 蛋白和平滑肌肌动蛋白[29]，以及肌上皮分化的特异性标记物，包括 p63 和钙调理蛋白（图 4A.4）。所有类型的小涎腺良性肿瘤均选择手术治疗。手术通常可以治愈。局灶复发见于不到 10% 的病例[28]。

良性神经外胚层性肿瘤
Benign neuroectodermal tumors

垂体腺瘤　Pituitary adenoma

起源于蝶鞍的垂体肿瘤（见第 17 章）偶尔可以延伸到鼻窦或鼻咽部，而似乎表现为这些部位的原发性肿瘤。与蝶鞍没有任何连续性的异位垂体腺瘤可以起源于来自 Rathke 囊残余的上呼吸消化道的任何部位。这些部位的垂体腺瘤可能被误诊为其他神经内分泌肿瘤或恶性上皮肿瘤。异位垂体腺瘤发生在成人，无性别差异，表现为气道阻塞、慢性鼻窦炎、视野缺损、脑脊液漏出以及内分泌疾病的表现（如 Cushing 综合征、多毛症）[30,31]。异位垂体

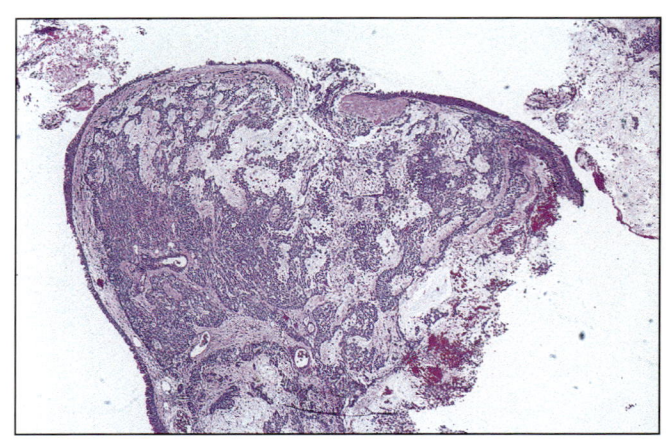

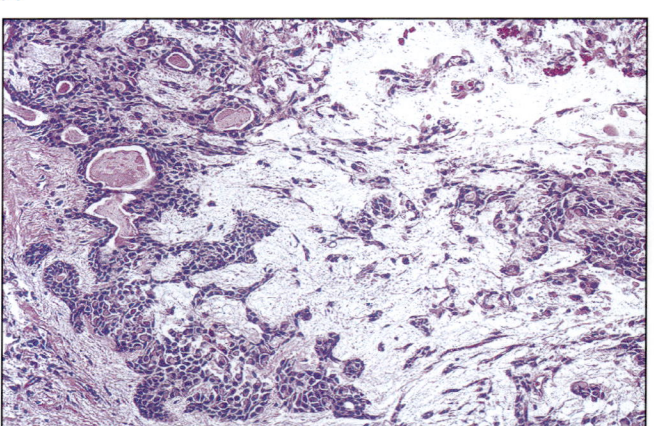

图 4A.4　鼻内以肌上皮为主的多形性腺瘤。（A）黏膜下丰富的肿瘤细胞增生，无包膜，伴有黏液软骨样间质。（B）腺体、黏液软骨样间质以及明显的浆细胞样肌上皮细胞混合存在；出现导管结构，腺体和黏液软骨样间质可归为多形性腺瘤，而以肌上皮为主，又不是肌上皮瘤，最好称为单形性腺瘤。（C）除了细胞角蛋白染色以外，肌上皮细胞 S-100 蛋白染色也有免疫反应（细胞核和胞浆）。

腺瘤最常发生于蝶窦，其次为鼻咽部。其他不常见的部位包括鼻腔和筛窦。肿瘤可以表现为息肉状。组织学上，黏膜下有增生的上皮样肿瘤细胞，伴有实性、器官样和小梁状生长方式（图4A.5）。上皮样细胞核呈圆形，染色质弥漫分布，胞浆为嗜酸性颗粒状。无多形性、坏死和核分裂活性。无腺体和鳞状上皮分化的证据。免疫表型和激素表达的差异类似于原发性垂体病变（见第17章）。治疗选择广泛手术切除；完全切除可以治愈，无复发或进行性肿瘤生长，而且内分泌疾病也得以消退[31]。少数情况下异位垂体腺瘤可以发生恶变[32]。

副神经节瘤　Paraganglioma

肾上腺外副神经节瘤见于全身各个部位，根据发生的解剖部位进行分类。发生于头颈部的副神经节瘤包括颈总动脉、颈静脉鼓室和迷走神经来源的肿瘤（见第28章）。在少数情况下，副神经节瘤可以发生于上呼吸消化道黏膜的其他部位，包括鼻腔，从而引起鼻塞和（或）鼻出血。副交感神经的副神经节遍布全身，上呼吸消化道的所有副神经节均可发生副神经节瘤[33]。这些部位的副神经节瘤多数为非功能性，但少数病例为促肾上腺皮质激素生成性鼻副神经节瘤，伴有Cushing综合征[34]。不管来源部位如何，所有肾上腺外副神经节瘤的组织学表现相同（见第28章）。如同其他部位一样，具有标志性的组织学特征是出现细胞巢或"细胞球"（Zellballen）结构，细胞球由不同数量的非典型性主细胞组成，其周围绕以支持细胞。该部位副神经节瘤的免疫组化所见也与其他部位副神经节瘤相同[35,36]。仅有少数病例表达细胞角蛋白[36]。治疗选择手术切除。完全切除后预后良好。虽然这些肿瘤多数为行为惰性的良性肿瘤，但是可以出现局部复发和浸润。少数肿瘤为恶性[37]。组织学所见不能可靠地预示恶性行为，任何恶性副神经节瘤都是通过出现转移性病变确定的。

脑膜瘤　Meningioma

脑膜瘤是脑膜细胞发生的良性肿瘤，占所有颅内肿瘤的13%～18%[38]。发生于中枢神经系统以外的被认为是异位脑膜瘤；这些脑膜瘤被分为与中枢神经系统没有联系（原发性）和与中枢神经系统有联系（继发性）的两种。头颈部异位脑膜瘤最常发生的部位包括中耳和颞骨、鼻窦、眼眶、口腔和腮腺[39]。鼻窦脑膜瘤最常发生于鼻腔，或鼻腔和副鼻窦均有发生[40]；孤立发生于鼻咽部、额窦或蝶窦不常见[40]。鼻窦脑膜瘤的症状包括鼻塞、鼻出血、头痛、局部疼痛、视力障碍和面部变形。肿瘤可侵蚀鼻窦骨组织，伴有周围软组织和眼眶受累，偶尔累及颅底[40]。这些肿瘤表现为息肉状肿块。肿瘤常常被刮出，收集到的是实性白色破碎组织。可能出现均匀沙粒质地。组织学表现类似于颅内脑膜瘤（见第26章）。在脑膜瘤的组织学亚型中，脑膜上皮瘤型（meningotheliomatous type）脑膜瘤在鼻窦腔中最为常见。组织学特征包括小叶状生长方式，伴有肿瘤细胞巢形成，肿瘤细胞巢之间有数量不等的纤维组织间隔（图4A.6）。特征性表现为核边缘呈凿孔状，这是由于细胞核内胞浆包涵体引起典型颅内脑膜上皮瘤性脑膜瘤可见许多沙粒体，但在异位脑膜瘤沙粒体并不常见。脑膜瘤的免疫组

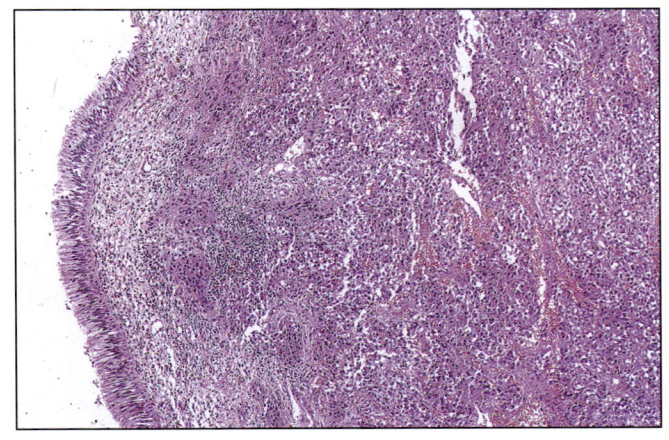

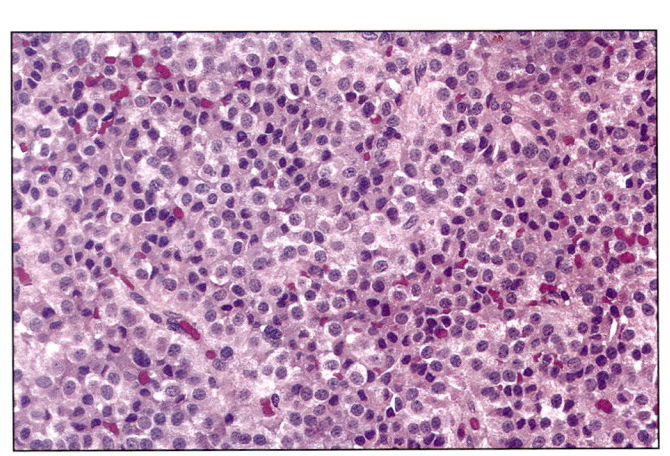

图4A.5　异位（鼻咽）垂体腺瘤。（A）肿瘤浸润黏膜下，由呈器官样生长方式的上皮样肿瘤细胞组成。（B）上皮样细胞核圆形，染色质弥漫分布，胞浆颗粒状，嗜酸性。免疫组化染色证实为垂体肿瘤。

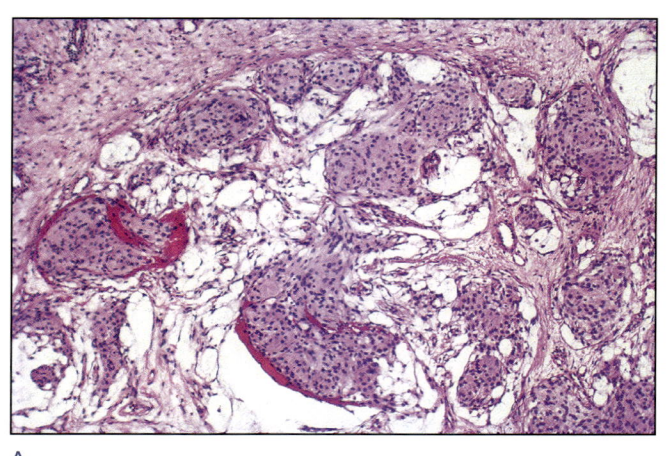
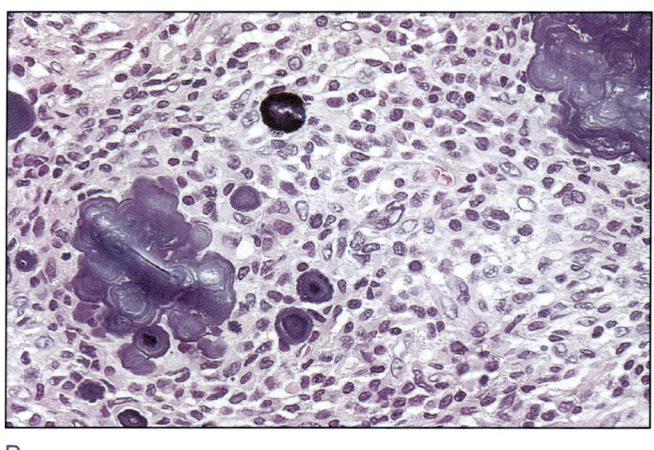

图4A.6 鼻窦（异位）脑膜瘤。（A）这个黏膜下富于细胞的增生性病变呈分叶状生长，肿瘤细胞巢被不同量的纤维结缔组织分开，呈漩涡状排列。（B）肿瘤细胞具有圆形到卵圆形的细胞核，胞浆淡染，细胞界限不清，由于核内有胞浆包涵体，可见凿孔状或中空表现；可见几个沙粒体。

化抗原谱包括具有上皮膜抗原（EMA）和波形蛋白的免疫反应，缺乏细胞角蛋白和神经内分泌标记（嗜铬素和突触素）。治疗选择手术切除，然而可能难以完全手术切除，因此容易复发，复发率可高达30%[39-41]。组织学诊断之后，重要的是要排除从颅内原发性肿瘤扩散而来的可能性。

良性间叶性肿瘤
Benign mesenchymal neoplasms

血管瘤　Hemangiomas

分叶状毛细血管瘤（lobular capillary hemangioma，LCH）是良性血管肿瘤，从前常常称为化脓性肉芽肿。肿瘤为息肉状毛细血管瘤，主要发生在皮肤和黏膜（见第3章）。除了分叶状毛细血管瘤，鼻窦和鼻咽其他类型的血管瘤十分少见[42,43]。鼻窦部血管瘤多发生于黏膜基底部，但也可发生于这个部位的骨组织内（骨内血管瘤，intraosseous hemangiomas）。

分叶状毛细血管瘤的发生没有性别差异。年龄分布广泛，但是这些病变最常见于30～50岁的患者，16岁以下少见。分叶状毛细血管瘤最常见于鼻中隔前部[42,44]称为Little区或Kisselbach三角的部位；第二个最常见的鼻窦部位是鼻甲[42,44]。最常见的临床表现是鼻出血；也可出现阻塞性无痛性肿块。

发病机制目前仍不清楚。少数病例可能与从前的外伤有关。分叶状毛细血管瘤的发生可能与妊娠以及口服避孕药有关，提示可能有激素因素参与。然而，Nichols等[45]对于21例分叶状毛细血管瘤进行了免疫组化研究，在这些肿瘤中并未发现雌激素或孕激素受体。妊娠相关性化脓性肉芽肿在分娩后偶尔消退，其机制仍不清楚。最近，Yuan和Lin评估了血管内皮生长因子（VEGF）和血管形成素2（angiopoietin-2，Ang-2）在妊娠相关性化脓性肉芽肿消退中的作用[46]。他们发现，VEGF的量在妊娠肉芽肿中升高，而在分娩之后几乎检测不到，结论是缺乏VEGF与内皮细胞凋亡和病变消退有关。他们发现，仅有Ang-2对于病变消退不起作用。

分叶状毛细血管瘤的大体表现是光滑的分叶状息肉样红色肿块，直径可达1.5 cm。组织学检查，其特征为黏膜下血管增生，排列成小叶或簇状，由中心毛细血管和较小的分支状血管组成（图4A.7）。中心毛细血管的

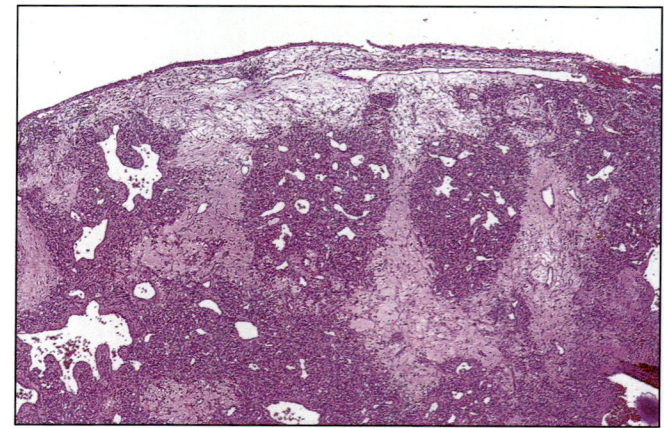

图4A.7 鼻窦分叶状毛细血管瘤。黏膜下血管呈分叶状增生，可见不同大小的血管，包括某些不规则到鹿角形的血管。

口径和形状不同，在较"成熟"的病变可见"鹿角状"改变。内衬的内皮细胞可能突出，而且可能出现内皮细胞簇和核分裂象。然而，没有见于血管肉瘤的血管间隙之间的交通，也没有真正的细胞学非典型性和非典型性核分裂象。周围与血管成分密切相关的是肉芽组织和混合性慢性炎细胞浸润。表面上皮常常有溃疡形成，伴有坏死。分叶状毛细血管瘤的诊断以及与其他病变的鉴别诊断通常光学显微镜检查即可明确，一般无需免疫组化染色。与 Kaposi 肉瘤不同，分叶状毛细血管瘤没有人疱疹病毒 -8（HHV-8）潜在核抗原 -1（LNA-1）免疫反应[47]。

分叶状毛细血管瘤的治疗是保守性的，不过需要完全手术切除。手术切除后预后很好。复发相对少见。

与毛细血管瘤相比，海绵状血管瘤不常发生于上呼吸道。一般来说，海绵状血管瘤与毛细血管瘤的临床表现相似，但较常见于鼻甲、鼻腔侧壁或骨内，而鼻中隔少见[48]。与其他部位的海绵状血管瘤（见第 3 章）类似，鼻窦部海绵状血管瘤由多个大小不一、内衬内皮细胞的扩张薄壁血管组成。手术切除可以治愈。

鼻咽血管纤维瘤
Nasopharyngeal angiofibroma

鼻咽血管纤维瘤是一相对少见的肿瘤，占所有头颈部肿瘤不到 1%[42,49-52]。这种肿瘤几乎全部发生于男性，有人认为它是一种局限于男性人群的肿瘤[53]。鼻咽血管纤维瘤发病年龄广泛，但最常见于 10～20 岁。25 岁以上少见。然而，这些肿瘤也可发生于老年人，因此否定了"幼年型"血管纤维瘤这一命名。最常见的临床症状是持续性鼻塞和鼻出血[50]。晚期症状和体征包括面部肿胀或变形（面颊肿胀）、流涕、眼球突出、复视、头痛、鼻窦炎、颅神经麻痹、嗅觉和听力缺失[50]。疼痛可以出现，但被认为是一种不常见表现。典型者在诊断之前症状已经出现 1 年以上。发生部位常为鼻顶蝶腭孔区域后外侧部分。大肿瘤可能向前扩展至鼻腔，引起鼻塞，并类似于原发性鼻内或副鼻窦肿瘤。向后延伸可能充满鼻咽并扩展至口咽部，导致软腭偏移。通过蝶腭孔扩展可累及翼突上腭窝和颞下窝，引起面部变形[54]。如果肿瘤侵入并破坏翼状突，则可扩展至颅中窝。

由于这种肿瘤主要发生于男性而被认为与激素有关，依赖于睾酮并受制于雌激素[55]。在这些肿瘤内发现有雄激素受体[56]，但是没有雌激素受体[55,57]。在家族性腺瘤性息肉病（FAP）患者具有发生鼻咽血管纤维瘤的家族倾向性[58,59]。家族性腺瘤性息肉病患者鼻咽血管纤维瘤发生率是同龄人的 25 倍[58,59]。研究提示，伴有 APC 基因突变的鼻咽血管纤维瘤患者存在 APC-β-连环蛋白通道的作用。据报道，在散发性鼻咽血管纤维瘤病例中存在无 APC 基因突变的活性 β-连环蛋白突变[60,61]。Zhang 等[62]经免疫组织化学研究支持 β-连环蛋白在鼻咽血管纤维瘤中的作用。他们发现 β-连环蛋白、c-kit（CD117）以及神经生长因子（NGF）在鼻咽血管纤维瘤间质细胞中的表达高于鼻息肉，而且比鼻息肉常见。极少数鼻咽血管纤维瘤患者可以并发消耗性凝血病，提示术前凝血检查可能有助于手术前后的止血[63]。

常规 X 线片显示上颌窦后壁特征性的弓形突出[64]以及翼状板变形向后偏移（Holman-Miller 征）。动脉造影所见通常具有诊断性[50,52]，显示肿瘤具有明显的血管肥大和动脉数目增加，而无串珠、扩张、节段性狭窄或动脉瘤样扩张。血供可为单侧或双侧，一般来自颈外动脉分支（上颌内侧支或咽升支）。如果颈内动脉为主要血供，应考虑肿瘤延伸至颅内。有人提出根据疾病的范围进行放射学分期[65-68]。

血管纤维瘤为无蒂或分叶状的肿块，偶尔呈息肉状或带蒂。组织学上，肿瘤无包膜，特征是纤维胶原间质增生，伴有大小不一的血管间隙（图 4A.8）。血管成分由薄壁血管构成，大小不一的血管由于明显受间质纤维组织挤压，所以呈星状或鹿角状，直到难以辨认。内皮细胞单层、扁平或肥胖。血管壁缺乏弹力纤维，特征是具有一层可能不完全或不连续的平滑肌，管壁厚度明显不同[69]。肿瘤中央区血管可能相对较少。间质由纤维组织组成，伴有纤细或粗大的胶原纤维，局部可呈黏液样。间质细胞为梭形和星形，细胞核肥胖，倾向于围绕血管呈放射状排列。可见核多形性和多核巨细胞。核分裂象罕见。常可见肥大细胞；然而，缺乏其他炎症细胞，除非接近表面溃疡的区域。在组织切片中可见术前栓塞的证据，表现为血管内含有异物的纤维素性血栓，而且肿瘤梗死。较长时间的肿瘤倾向于纤维化，而血管成分减少。免疫组化染色显示血管周围有平滑肌肌动蛋白阳性的细胞[69]。梭形和星形间质细胞波形蛋白阳性。另外，Hwang 及其同事[56]发现间质细胞睾酮受体强阳性。

对于没有合并症的病例（肿瘤局限于鼻咽部），治疗选择经由腭横切通路手术切除。为了控制出血，外科手术之前通常进行血管栓塞[70]。应用损伤性轻微的技术治疗已经取得成功，可使病情减轻，而且复发率也不增加[71]。也有人提出非手术治疗，包括雌激素疗法[57]、应用睾酮受体阻断剂 [如氟他胺（flutamide）][72]或者放射治疗[73-75]。这些治疗方法可以减少肿瘤的血管瘤成分，并且可以用于那些认为肿瘤不能切除的患者。与血管纤维瘤有关的并发症包括大量出血、肿瘤复发以及肿瘤向鼻咽外延伸，累及邻近的解剖学腔隙（鼻窦、口咽、

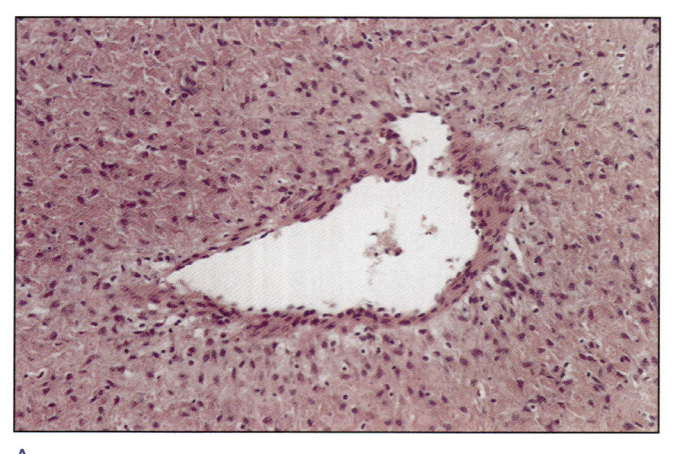
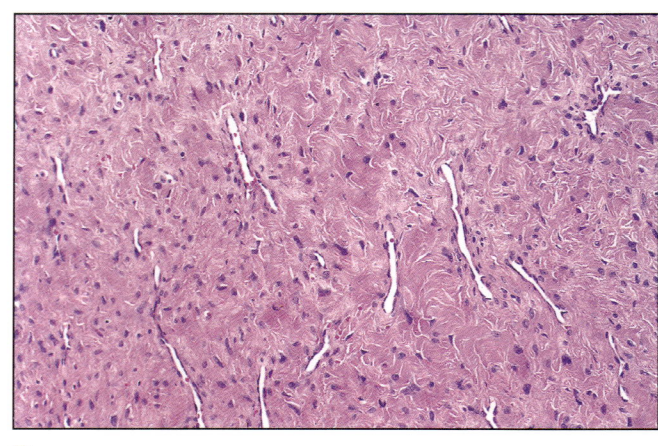

图4A.8 鼻咽血管纤维瘤。这些肿瘤由不同数量的纤维胶原间质和大小不一的血管间隙混合而成。血管成分包括不同表现的薄壁血管，从（A）容易辨认到（B）因受胶原纤维间质挤压而不甚明显。注意血管壁有不完整的平滑肌或缺乏平滑肌层。

翼突上颌窝、上颊沟、眼眶、颞下窝和颅腔）[54]。由于肿瘤容易出血，活检应当特别小心[76]。复发率从 6%～24% 不等[77]。累及颅底的鼻咽血管纤维瘤复发率高，且易早期复发；伴有颅内延伸的病例复发比较常见。没有颅内延伸的病例肿瘤复发通常发生在治疗之后 2 年以内。一般来说，手术切除后预后很好；死亡率为 3%[51]～9%[50]。在少数情况下，肿瘤可以自发性消退[78,79]。恶性（肉瘤性）转变很少发生，与放射治疗有关（放射后肉瘤，post-irradiation sarcoma）[80-83]。

孤立性纤维性肿瘤　Solitary fibrous tumor

孤立性纤维性肿瘤（SFT）是一种具有特色的肿瘤，由 CD34 阳性的纤维母细胞构成（见第 24 章）[84,85]。孤立性纤维性肿瘤罕见，但可发生于上呼吸消化道，主要累及鼻腔和副鼻窦[86-88]。该部位肿瘤患者表现为鼻塞。症状通常存在很长一段时间（1 年或更长）。

这些肿瘤一般呈息肉状。组织学上，肿瘤界限清楚，但无包膜，由细胞多少不等的良性增生的梭形细胞构成，缺少任何独特的生长方式，伴有瘢痕样胶原束和薄壁血管间隙（图 4A.9）。局部血管间隙可能突出，常常具有分支状血管外皮细胞瘤样表现。该部位的多数病例显示核分裂率低，而且没有坏死。免疫组化染色显示 CD34、bcl-2 和 CD99 阳性，而 S-100 蛋白、结蛋白或肌动蛋白阴性。

由于肿瘤倾向于呈息肉状，鼻窦部孤立性纤维性肿瘤易于完全手术切除，通常可以治愈[86,87]。鼻咽部孤立性纤维性肿瘤可能难以完全切除。

纤维瘤病（侵袭性纤维瘤病；腹壁外纤维瘤，纤维瘤型纤维瘤病）
Fibromatosis (aggressive fibromatosis; extra-abdominal desmoid, desmoid-type fibromatosis)

纤维瘤病是一种局限浸润性/侵袭性、非转移性、由良性纤维母细胞构成的肿瘤（见第 24 章）[89,90]。头颈部纤维瘤病主要发生于颈部软组织[91]。除颈部以外，常见的发生部位是鼻窦、鼻咽、舌和口腔[92,93]。在鼻窦部中，上颌窦是最常见的部位[94]。这种病变见于儿童和成人，但最常发生于 20～40 岁的患者。发病部位不同，症

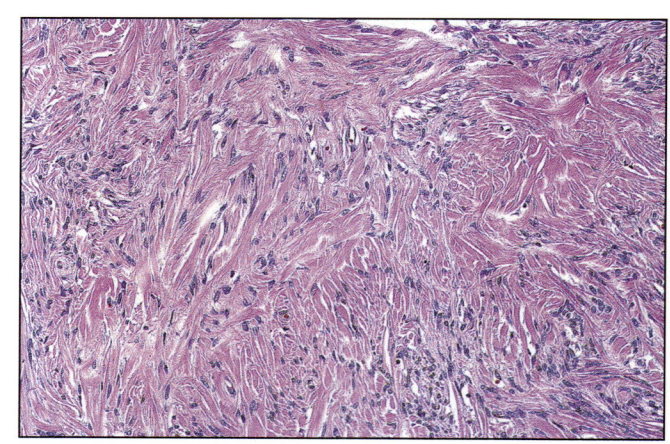

图4A.9 鼻窦部孤立性纤维性肿瘤。这个没有包膜的肿瘤由细胞多少不等、良性增生的梭形细胞构成，缺乏任何生长方式，伴有玻璃样变的胶原。

状也不相同。鼻窦部和鼻咽部纤维瘤病的临床表现包括无痛性增大的肿块或鼻塞[92,93]。随着病程进展，也可出现其他症状，例如鼻出血、面部变形、眼球突出和咽下困难。

大体和组织学表现与发生于常见部位的纤维瘤病相同（见第24章）。

鉴别诊断主要包括反应性纤维化和纤维肉瘤[93]。与纤维肉瘤不同的是，纤维瘤病缺乏人字形生长方式、细胞过多和核分裂率增多等纤维肉瘤具有的特征。其他鉴别诊断包括外周神经鞘肿瘤、黏液瘤和纤维黏液瘤、孤立性纤维性肿瘤、肌纤维瘤病、结节性筋膜炎、纤维骨性病变和肌纤维母细胞肿瘤（炎性肌纤维母细胞肿瘤、低级别肌纤维母细胞肉瘤）。

治疗选择广泛手术切除。一般来讲，预后较好[93]。然而，由于病变侵入邻近组织而无清楚界限，可能使这些病变的处理出现困难。由于完全切除病变困难，以致常常复发[94]。复发通常发生于手术后最初几年内。对于有肿瘤残留和（或）复发的患者，采用放射治疗可能获得一些成功[95,96]。应用激素治疗取得了不同的效果[97,98]。局灶性病变未能控制可能导致死亡，但这只是一种例外情况。

良性外周神经鞘肿瘤（良性神经鞘瘤和神经纤维瘤）
Benign peripheral nerve sheath tumors (benign schwannoma and neurofibroma)

头颈部良性外周神经鞘肿瘤常见，约占所有软组织病变的45%。然而，鼻窦和鼻咽的良性外周神经鞘肿瘤并不常见，所占不到4%[99-101]。在此部位，神经鞘瘤实际上比神经纤维瘤常见。成人最常发生，无性别差异。患者出现与鼻塞和鼻出血相关的症状。鼻咽部受累可导致单侧浆液性中耳炎[101]。在Hasegawa等[101]报道的2个病例中，患者由于肿瘤延伸到颅内而引起视力障碍。这些肿瘤可以引起骨的压迫性侵蚀[99,100]。

与发生在软组织的良性神经鞘瘤不同，上呼吸消化道的良性神经鞘瘤没有包膜（图4A.10）。除了这种表现以外，其组织学特征类似于其他部位的良性外周神经鞘肿瘤（见第27章）。这些肿瘤细胞可能非常丰富，但是多形性不显著。核分裂象通常少见，而且不出现非典型性核分裂象。S-100蛋白免疫组化染色呈弥漫强阳性反应（胞浆和胞核）。细胞角蛋白、肌动蛋白、结蛋白、CD34和上皮膜抗原染色阴性。细胞增殖率低（例如MIB-1染色），1%-5%的肿瘤细胞核阳性[102]。治疗选择手术切除，可以治愈。

该部位的神经纤维瘤位于黏膜下，肿瘤界限相对清

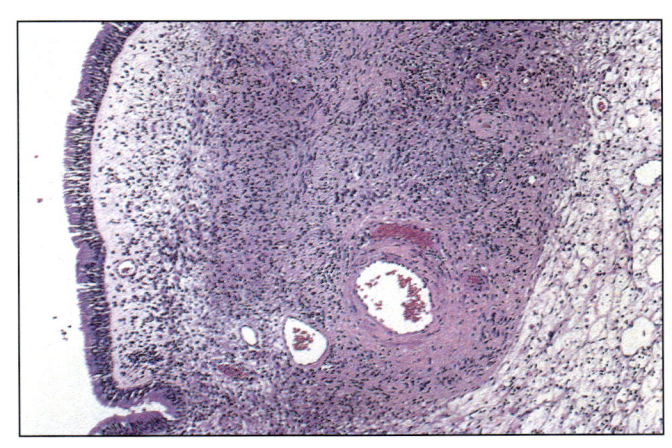

图4A.10　鼻窦良性外周神经鞘肿瘤（良性神经鞘瘤）。肿瘤位于黏膜下，无包膜，由良性增生的梭形细胞组成，细胞核呈波浪状或弯曲状，混有炎症细胞。血管周围玻璃样变性。

楚，由梭形细胞组成，细胞核呈"波浪状"或弯曲状，深染，胞浆不清。伴随的间质成分胶原化和（或）黏液样。肿瘤细胞S-100蛋白阳性，但是染色程度不如神经鞘瘤明显。手术切除可以治愈。

平滑肌瘤　Leiomyoma

一般来说，平滑肌瘤是头颈部最少见的间叶性肿瘤之一。最常发生于皮肤和口腔（唇、舌和腭）。在少数情况下，平滑肌瘤可以发生于鼻窦部，表现为引起鼻塞的无痛性肿块[103,104]。这种肿瘤好发于成人，高峰发病年龄为50～60岁。鼻窦部平滑肌瘤最常见于鼻甲。组织学上，肿瘤局限于黏膜下，境界非常清楚，特征为出现交错排列的细胞束，细胞核两端钝圆或呈"雪茄形"，胞浆丰富嗜酸性。细胞核也可呈圆形。肿瘤细胞与血管的关系往往十分密切。肿瘤可发生退变，包括间质纤维化和黏液样变。细胞过多的平滑肌瘤称为富于细胞性平滑肌瘤（cellular leiomyoma），其特征为细胞明显增多，但缺乏显著多形性、核分裂活性、坏死或侵袭性生长。在鼻窦部平滑肌肿瘤中提出的另外一种类型是所谓的恶性潜能不确定的平滑肌肿瘤（smooth muscle tumors of uncertain malignant potential, SMTUMP）[104]。SMTUMP的组织学特征为细胞增多、中度核多形性以及出现少于4个/10HPF的核分裂象[104]。SMTUMP可能出现局灶性浸润性生长（例如向骨内浸润）[104]。免疫组化染色显示，平滑肌瘤和SMTUMP的肿瘤细胞均为肌动蛋白（平滑肌肌动蛋白和肌肉特异性肌动蛋白）和结蛋白阳性；S-100阴性。两种平滑肌肿瘤的MIB-1指数均低（≤5%）[104]。单纯手术切除可以治愈。

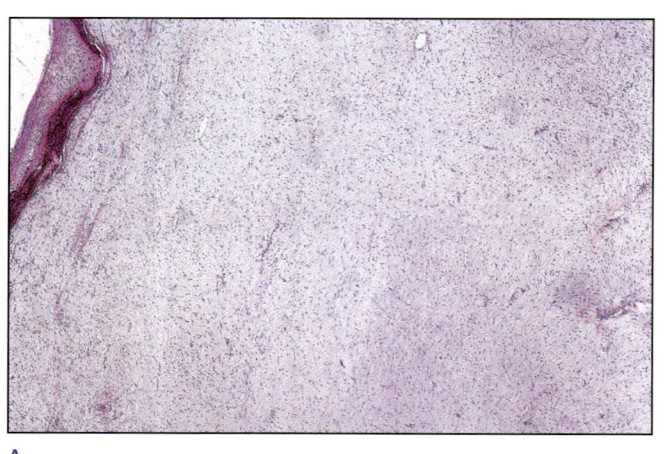
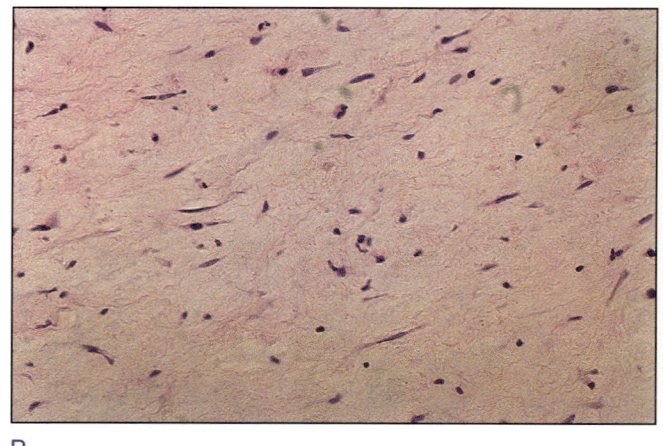

图4A.11 鼻窦黏液瘤。（A）黏膜下增生的细胞稀疏排列，血管受压但仍可辨认。（B）细胞呈梭形或星形；细胞核均匀一致，小而深染，位于丰富的黏液性间质内。

横纹肌瘤　Rhabdomyoma

在少数情况下，成人型或胎儿型横纹肌瘤（见第24章）可以发生于鼻窦或鼻咽部[105-107]。胎儿型横纹肌瘤的细胞特征为不同分化阶段的横纹肌母细胞，包括梭形细胞和带状细胞。这些表现令人担忧，可能会考虑横纹肌肉瘤（RMS）的诊断，然而与横纹肌肉瘤不同的是，胎儿型横纹肌瘤倾向于局限性生长，缺乏核的非典型性或核分裂活性[107]。

鼻窦黏液瘤和纤维性黏液瘤　Sinonasal myxoma and fibromyxoma

黏液瘤和纤维性黏液瘤是具有特征性组织学表现的不能确定组织来源的良性肿瘤，常具有侵袭性（浸润性）生物学行为。当间质出现较大量胶原时，即称纤维性黏液瘤（或黏液性纤维瘤，myxofibroma）。在鼻窦部，这些肿瘤似乎起源于骨。肿瘤发生无性别差异，发病年龄广泛，但多见于10～30岁[108,109]。一般来说，这些肿瘤是颌的肿瘤，下颌（后侧和髁突部位）受累比上颌（颧突和牙槽骨）常见。颌外肿瘤少见，主要累及鼻窦；特别是上颌窦最常受累，继而延伸到鼻腔。通常表现为病变区的无痛性肿胀。局限于颌骨的肿瘤曾被认为是起源于原始牙源性间充质或骨源性胚胎性结缔组织。

放射学检查表现为单房性或多房性X线透明的阴影，伴有"蜂房状"或"肥皂泡样"表现。大体上，这些病变境界清楚，但无包膜，为多结节状胶样表现。组织学上，增生的梭形或星形肿瘤细胞稀少而疏松，位于丰富的黏液性间质中（图4A.11）。细胞核小而深染。缺乏细胞多形性、核分裂象和坏死。不同病例之间胶原纤维含量不同，根据其程度可命名为"纤维性黏液瘤"（图4A.12）。肿瘤周围界限清楚，但可见局灶性浸润，并取代骨组织。血管成分易见，但数量有限。黏液性间质酸性黏多糖染色阳性。治疗采取保守性局部扩大切除。这些肿瘤生长缓慢，通常具有良性经过，但切除不充分可能导致局灶性破坏。复发或转移未见发生。推测是来自鼻窦黏液瘤或纤维黏液瘤转移的诊断应该引起高度怀疑，这种病变可能是某些类型的黏液肉瘤。

鉴别诊断包括牙乳头、鼻炎症性息肉、外周神经鞘肿瘤、低级别纤维黏液样肉瘤[110]、其他黏液样肉瘤和软骨肿瘤。

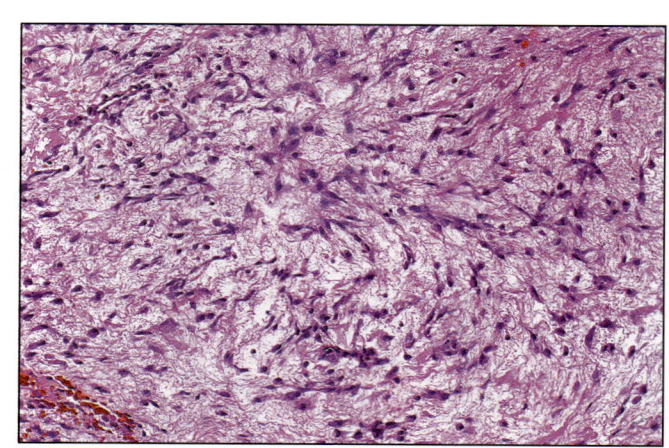

图4A.12 鼻窦纤维黏液瘤。与黏液瘤不同的是，其间质成分含有大量胶原纤维性物质，而且这种病变常常富于细胞。缺乏特异性免疫反应，需要排除其他病变方可诊断纤维性黏液瘤。

骨性、纤维骨性和软骨性病变
Osseous, fibro-osseous and cartilaginous lesions

骨瘤　Osteoma

骨瘤是形成骨的良性肿瘤，这种肿瘤几乎完全见于颅面骨。在鼻窦任何部位均能发生骨瘤，但最常见于额窦和筛窦[111-112]。这些肿瘤多无症状，仅在放射学检查时发现。与副鼻窦骨瘤有关的症状包括头痛、面颊肿胀或畸形以及眼的功能障碍[113]。鼻窦骨瘤最常见于男性，发病年龄广泛，但最常见于10～40岁。鼻窦骨瘤常以单一病变出现，但可能伴有Gardner综合征。Gardner综合征是一种常染色体显性遗传疾病，它以肠（结肠直肠）息肉病、软组织病变（纤维瘤病、皮肤表皮样囊肿、脂肪瘤、平滑肌瘤）和多发性颅面骨瘤为特征[114]。放射学表现为境界清楚的不透X线的病变，局限于骨或突入鼻窦。组织学上，骨瘤非常局限，主要由致密而成熟的板层骨组成，有时周围有成骨细胞包围。骨内间隙可由纤维、纤维血管或脂肪组织组成，而且可能存在造血成分。除非有症状，骨瘤一般不需治疗。完全手术切除可以治愈。

良性纤维骨性病变
Benign fibro-osseous lesions

骨化性纤维瘤　Ossifying fibroma

与（骨）纤维性结构不良（fibrous dysplasia）不同（见下：表4A.4），骨化性纤维瘤较常见于女性，而且倾向于发生在较大年龄组，最常见于20～40岁，但任何年龄均可受累[115]。据报道，更易发生于黑人妇女[116]。累及鼻窦者一般无症状，常在放射学检查时偶然诊断。有症状的肿瘤表现为牙齿移位或膨胀性肿块。放射学特征包括出现非常局限或境界清楚的病变，轮廓光滑。

骨化性纤维瘤为褐色/灰色到白色的沙粒样质硬肿物，大小不等，从0.5～10 cm。组织学上，骨化性纤维瘤由杂乱分布的成熟（板层）骨板组成，周围有成骨细胞包绕，混有纤维性间质（图4A.13）。虽然一般将骨的成分描述为成熟骨，但中心部分可为编织骨，在其外周为板层骨。完全成熟的骨少见。纤维性间质可能致密而富于细胞，核分裂象少见到缺乏。可出现继发性改变，包括出血、炎症和巨细胞。骨化性纤维瘤主要应与纤维性结构不良进行鉴别诊断（见下：表4A.4）。骨化性纤维瘤的治疗选择手术切除，由于病变非常局限，手术切

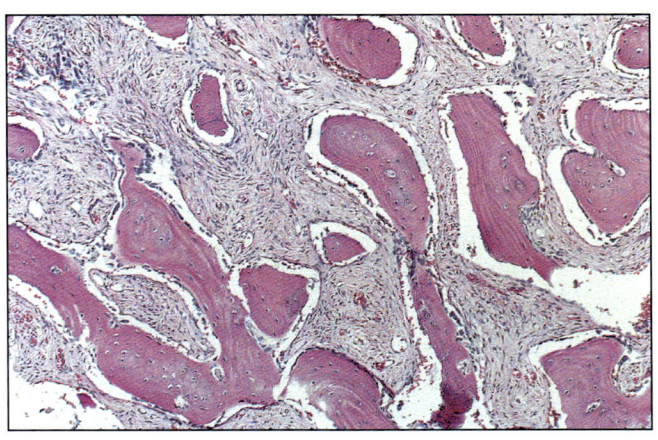

图4A.13　副鼻窦的骨化性纤维瘤，由成熟的（板层）骨板构成，边缘为成骨细胞，伴有混合性的纤维性间质。

除相对容易。完全切除后预后良好。复发罕见。

沙粒体样（活动性）骨化性纤维瘤（牙骨质化或牙骨质骨化性纤维瘤）
Psammomatoid (active) ossifying fibroma (cementifying or cemento-ossifying fibroma)

这是骨化性纤维瘤的一种变异型。典型病变发生于鼻窦部，可能具有侵袭性行为，伴有局部浸润和破坏的能力[117]。无性别差异，虽然一般发生于较年轻年龄组（20岁以下），但发病年龄可能广泛，包括老年个体[117]。出现的症状包括面部肿胀、鼻塞、疼痛、鼻窦炎、头痛和眼球突出。这些病变可发生于鼻窦任何部位，而以筛窦和眶上前额区域最为常见[117,118]。可能累及单个或多个鼻窦；也可累及眼眶。放射学表现是溶解性或溶解性/不透X线的混合性的骨和（或）软组织肿块，从境界清楚到伴骨侵蚀不一。有人提示骨化性纤维瘤来源于牙周韧带的间充质，因此其与牙骨质骨化性纤维瘤有关[118]。

组织学表现为良性纤维骨性增生，由骨板和骨球组成，混有纤维性间质。最具特征性的成分是矿化或钙化的"沙粒体样"小体或小骨片（图4A.14）。这些小骨片的数目从少数几个到无数密集成群的球形小体不等。小骨片界限清楚，中央为蓝色到黑色，其周边为粉红色，伴有同心圆性层状结构。小骨片大小不一，从小的圆形到卵圆形小体到较大的不规则小体不等，位于骨小梁内以及邻近富于细胞的间质内。与带有圆形或波浪形从较大到不规则形的小梁外形不同，小骨片内有破骨细胞，沿其表面可见成骨细胞。骨小梁表现不同，包括曲线形

表4A.4　良性纤维骨性病变：临床病理学比较

	骨化性纤维瘤	沙粒体样骨化性纤维瘤	纤维性结构不良
性别，年龄	女＞男；20~40岁	女＝男；较年轻年龄组（20岁以下），但也可出现在老人	女＝男；20岁以下
部位	无特殊部位	筛窦；眶上前额区域	无特殊部位
病灶	单一部位	单一部位或累及多个（连续）部位/鼻窦	单骨性（75%~80%）；多骨性（20%~25%）
放射学	局限性或界限清楚的病变，边缘光滑	溶解性或溶解性/不透X线的混合性骨和（或）软组织肿块，境界清楚或侵蚀骨组织	境界不清的膨胀性骨病变，伴有薄而完整的皮质；以纤维组织为主的病变透射线；以骨组织为主的病变不透射线；等量纤维和骨组织混合性病变具有毛玻璃样表现
组织学	杂乱分布的成熟（板层）小骨片，周围绕以成骨细胞，混合有纤维性间质；中心部分可为编织骨，其周围为板层骨	小骨片和特殊的矿化或钙化"沙粒体样"小体或小骨，混有纤维性间质；沙粒体样小体数目从少数几个到无数密集成群的球形小体不等；小骨内存在破骨细胞，其周围可见成骨细胞；骨小梁表现不同，包括曲线形、奇形怪状的骨小梁	纤维组织成分难以归类，细胞构成不同；骨的成分包括不规则形骨小梁和不成熟（编织）骨，方向紊乱，伴有奇形怪状的畸形骨小梁，包括"C"或"S"形结构；骨小梁周围一般缺乏成骨细胞
症状	没有已知的伴随症状	无已知的伴随症状	Albright综合征（1%~3%）
治疗	手术切除	手术切除	本病在青春期稳定，因此儿童期发病者如有可能应延至青春期后治疗；手术切除指征是功能损害、进行性变形、伴有病理性骨折或发生恶性的病例
预后	良好	完全切除后预后良好；切除不完全常常复发；可能有侵袭性行为，伴有局部破坏和侵犯重要结构	预后良好；复发率低，少数病例延伸到重要结构而发生死亡
恶性变	尚不知道发生恶变	尚不知道发生恶变	发生恶性变（骨肉瘤）不足1%

的奇形怪状的骨小梁。骨小梁由板层骨组成，伴有一圈破骨细胞和成骨细胞。可见球形小骨片和骨小梁之间的移行带。非骨性成分包括富于细胞的间质，伴有束状到席纹状排列方式，由圆形到多边形到梭形的细胞组成，细胞核明显嗜碱性，细胞边界不清。可见核分裂象，但核分裂活性并不明显，没有非典型性核分裂。在沙粒体样小骨或散在分布于整个非骨性间质成分中可见巨细胞。可局灶性出现骨样结构。

治疗选择完全手术切除。完全切除后预后良好，但是如果边缘受累，复发非常常见，而且肿瘤可能具有侵袭性行为，伴有局部破坏，而且可能侵犯重要结构[117]。

纤维性结构不良　　Fibrous dysplasia

纤维性结构不良是一种特发性的非肿瘤性骨疾病，其正常髓质骨被结构上薄的纤维性和骨组织所取代（见第25章）。纤维性结构不良可为单骨性（仅单一骨受累

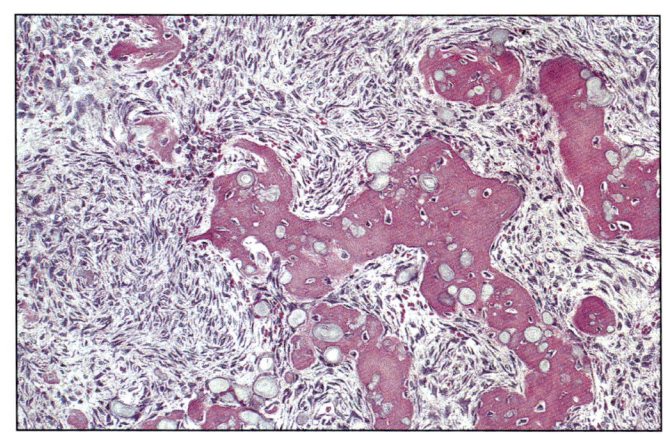
图4A.14 沙粒体样骨化性纤维瘤。最具特征性的成分是出现矿化或钙化的"沙粒体样"小体或小骨。

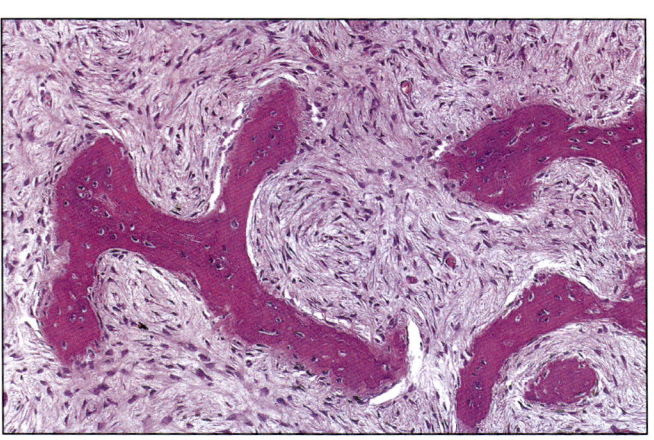
图4A.15 鼻窦纤维性结构不良，包括形状不规则的不成熟（编织）骨，周边一般缺乏成骨细胞，伴有难以归类的纤维组织成分。

或多骨性（两个或两个以上的骨受累）。多数纤维性结构不良患者在30岁以下，通常在20岁以下。纤维性结构不良的颅面部症状包括伴有功能障碍的无痛性、不对称性肿胀。鼻窦部纤维性结构不良的症状和体征包括头痛、眼球突出和鼻塞。颅面或颌部受累发生于多达50%的多骨性病变患者，多达25%患者伴有单骨性病变[119,120]。少数（1%～3%）纤维性结构不良病变与Albright综合征（或McCune-Albright综合征）有关，其特征为由多骨性纤维性结构不良、内分泌功能障碍[甲状腺功能亢进和(或)性早熟，后者主要见于女性]和皮肤色素沉着过多组成的三联征。

放射学表现为界限不清的膨胀性骨病变，伴有薄而完整的骨皮质。以纤维为主的病变可透X线，而以骨为主的病变不透X线。纤维和骨成分均等混合的病变呈毛玻璃样外观。组织学上，纤维组织成分难以归类，细胞成分多少不定。骨性成分包括不规则形的骨小梁和来源于纤维性间质的不成熟（编织）骨，畸形骨小梁方向不定，细胞成分增多，边缘不规则，而且形成奇特的几何图形，包括"C"或"S"构型（所谓的中国字构型）（图4A.15）。骨小梁边缘一般缺乏成骨细胞。可见多核巨细胞、巨噬细胞、血管成分增多和钙化。

颌的纤维骨性病变（纤维性结构不良和骨化性纤维瘤）在组织学上可能不易区别；因此，诊断和鉴别诊断需要依靠临床、放射学和组织病理学的相互关系。骨化性纤维瘤与纤维性结构不良的鉴别诊断非常重要，因为这些病变的治疗方案不同。对于纤维性结构不良来说，喜欢应用保守性的手术切除进行治疗，但仅适用于伴有功能损害、进行性畸形、疼痛、伴有病理性骨折或发生恶变的病例。本病在青春期可能稳定，因此儿童期发病患者治疗应尽可能延迟到青春期后[121]。复发率低，因延伸到重要结构而引起死亡的病例罕见。恶变率低于1%[122,123]，如果发生恶变，则最常见的是骨肉瘤。由于有引起恶变的危险，故不选择放射治疗[111]。

巨细胞修复性肉芽肿
Giant cell reparative granuloma

巨细胞修复性肉芽肿是一种良性反应性纤维骨性增生。巨细胞修复性肉芽肿与动脉瘤性骨囊肿具有许多共同特征，在许多情况下，这些病变可能无法区分[124]。在头颈部，最常发生于上颌骨和下颌骨。鼻窦部和鼻咽部受累少见。主要局限于骨内（例如颌骨）的病变称为中心性巨细胞修复性肉芽肿，而主要累及软组织（例如鼻窦部或口腔）的病变被称为周围性巨细胞修复性肉芽肿[125,126]。鼻窦受累伴有疼痛和肿胀。头颈部巨细胞修复性肉芽肿较常见于女性，且发生于30岁以下的患者（大多数在20岁以下）[127]。激素因素可能影响巨细胞修复性肉芽肿的生长[128,129]。

中心性和周围性巨细胞肉芽肿的组织学表现相同，是由富于细胞的纤维母细胞间质组成的，其中含有多核巨细胞。巨细胞多聚集于出血灶内和其周围。少数情况下，巨细胞弥散分布于纤维母细胞间质内。纤维母细胞可见核分裂象，但巨细胞没有核分裂象，可以出现囊肿结构和反应性新骨。周围性巨细胞修复性肉芽肿为黏膜下病变，位于完整而未被累及的呼吸道或鳞状上皮下方。治疗选择手术刮除。多达15%的颌病变可能复发[127]，而鼻窦部病变在刮除术后很少复发。由于巨细胞修复性肉芽肿的组织学表现与甲状旁腺功能亢进的棕色瘤（brown tumor）相同，所以慎重的处理应该包括对于甲状旁腺功能的实验室评估。

巨细胞瘤　Giant cell tumor

骨巨细胞瘤是具有潜在侵袭性的良性肿瘤，不常见于头颈部（见第 25 章）[125,130,131]。鼻窦部和鼻咽部受累罕见。与巨细胞修复性肉芽肿不同，巨细胞瘤的特征是具有大量多核巨细胞，这种多核巨细胞弥散分布，较大，有较多的细胞核（50～100），并且伴有单核细胞间质成分，而不是以纤维母细胞为背景。间质单核细胞可见核分裂象，但不出现非典型性核分裂象。认为出现非典型性核分裂象是恶性的标志[132]。端粒结合是最常见的染色体畸形[132]。据报道，发生于 Paget 病患者蝶骨的恶性巨细胞瘤已有报告[133]。

软骨瘤　Chondroma

鼻窦部和鼻咽部的软骨瘤少见。最常发生于鼻中隔和鼻咽部[134,135]。放射学研究显示鼻窦浑浊化或局限性X线通透性病变。鼻窦软骨瘤为息肉状、质硬、表面光滑的结节，大小通常在 0.5～2 cm 之间，少数情况下大于 3 cm。组织学上，软骨瘤为分叶状肿瘤，由组织学表现类似于正常软骨的软骨细胞组成。不出现细胞多形性、双核软骨细胞及核分裂活性增加。治疗方法是选择保守性的完全手术切除。复发少见。

造釉细胞瘤　Ameloblastoma

造釉细胞瘤是一种局部侵袭性的颌骨肿瘤，复发率高，认为来源于残余的牙源性上皮、牙源性囊肿的内衬以及其上口腔黏膜的基底层细胞（见第 6 章）[136]。造釉细胞瘤可以发生于任何年龄患者的上颌骨和下颌骨，但最常见于 20～50 岁，主要表现为下颌骨无痛性膨胀[137]。鼻窦部受累少见，通常是来自上颌骨病变的继发性蔓延。然而，与颌部没有联系的真正的原发性鼻窦造釉细胞瘤少见。Schafer 及其同事[138]报告了 24 例原发性鼻窦造釉细胞瘤。在这一组病例中男性占有明显优势，男女比例为 3.8:1，诊断时的中位年龄为 59.7 岁（比发生在颌骨的造釉细胞瘤大约晚 15～25 年）。患者多出现肿块性病变和鼻塞。症状持续时间从 1 个月到数年不等。受累部位或仅为鼻腔，或仅为副鼻窦，或两个部位同时受累。与颌骨造釉细胞瘤特征性的多房性X线通透性表现不同，鼻窦造釉细胞瘤的放射学表现是实性肿块或浑浊[138]，可出现骨破坏、腐蚀和骨再塑（残留骨鞘限制病变生长）。

组织学上，鼻窦造釉细胞瘤的表现类似于颌骨造釉细胞瘤。丛状结构（plexiform pattern）是主要的组织学结构，由长而相互吻合的牙源性上皮条索网组成（图 4A.16）[138]。上皮细胞条索周围有一层柱状细胞，柱状细胞核深染，呈栅栏状排列，核的极向保留，同时有核下胞浆空泡形成。在丛状组织学类型中，伴随造釉细胞瘤其他结构出现的星网状层样成分常常不甚明显[139]。还可见到棘皮瘤性结构（acanthomatous pattern），其特征是上皮岛的中心部分有鳞状化生和角质形成，但这仅限于继发性病变或为局灶性成分。造釉细胞瘤性增生可以发生在与完整的鼻窦表面黏膜上皮直接连续的部位。后一种表现，加上缺乏与颌骨部位的连续，支持这些鼻窦肿瘤的组织发生是来源于鼻窦黏膜上皮的全能细胞（totipotential cells）[138]。

对于所有病例治疗均选择手术切除。Schafer 及其同事[138]报道其复发率为 22%。肿瘤复发一般发生在初次手术后 1～2 年之内，但其中一例在初次手术后 13 年出现复发。总的治疗成功与结合详细的放射影像学所见积极进行完全手术切除有关。未见肿瘤引起死亡、转移或恶变的报道[138]。

颅咽管瘤　Craniopharyngioma

颅咽管瘤来源于脑垂体（蝶鞍）部位的 Rathke 囊，或沿着导致 Rathke 囊和脑垂体发生的通道（见第 17 章）。蝶鞍外颅咽管瘤可发生于鼻窦或鼻咽部，或由蝶鞍肿瘤直接扩展而来，或与蝶鞍受累无关[140-143]。症状包括鼻塞、鼻出血、头痛及视力损害。多数病例发生于 10 岁之前[140]。组织学上，颅咽管瘤是上皮性肿瘤，其组成成分是位于中心的核小、胞浆透明的星形细胞，周围围绕一层呈基底细胞样表现的柱状细胞，核有极性，排列成栅栏状。肿瘤中可见诸如鬼影细胞和钙化等退行性、渐进性坏死改变。这些特征非常类似于颌骨造釉细胞瘤的表现。然而，颅咽管瘤的临床特征明显不同于鼻窦部造釉细胞瘤，因此这些病变容易区分。治疗方法为完全手术切除，且一般可以治愈[140]。

良性畸胎瘤　Benign teratoma

上呼吸消化道的畸胎瘤是罕见的肿瘤，占所有畸胎瘤的 2% 以下[144]。发病无性别差异。畸胎瘤可见于成人，但多数发生于新生儿或婴儿，而且很少见于 1 岁以上（颈部畸胎瘤）和 2 岁以上（鼻咽部畸胎瘤）的小儿。见于上呼吸消化道黏膜的畸胎瘤的最常见部位是鼻咽部；其他不常见部位包括口腔（扁桃体、舌、腭）、鼻窦腔以及耳和颞骨。鼻咽部畸胎瘤表现为突入口腔或咽部的肿块，引起咽下困难和（或）气道阻塞。畸胎瘤的发生可能与母亲羊水过多和死产有关[145]。与发生在儿科年龄组的畸胎瘤不同，成人头颈部畸胎

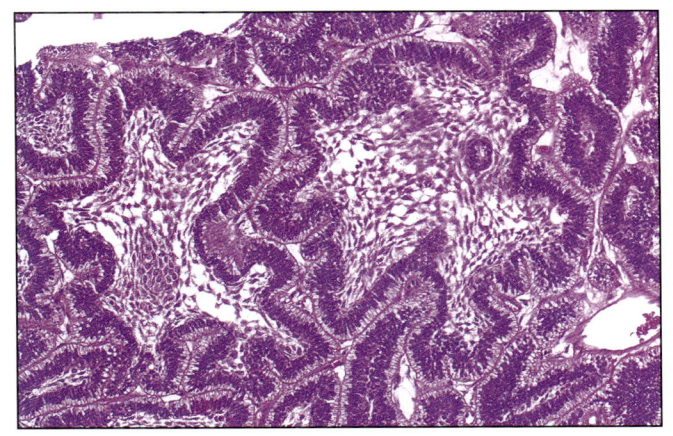

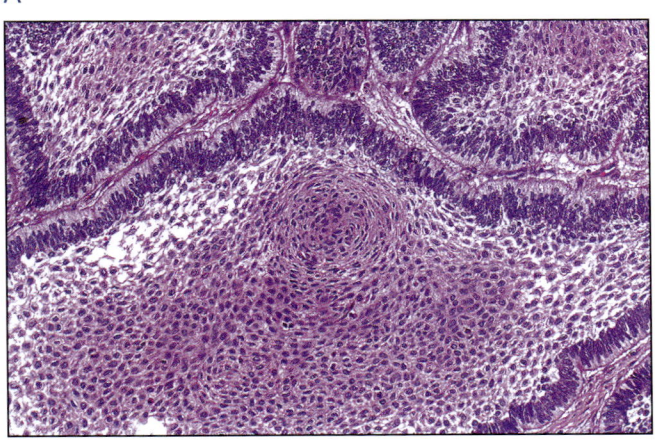

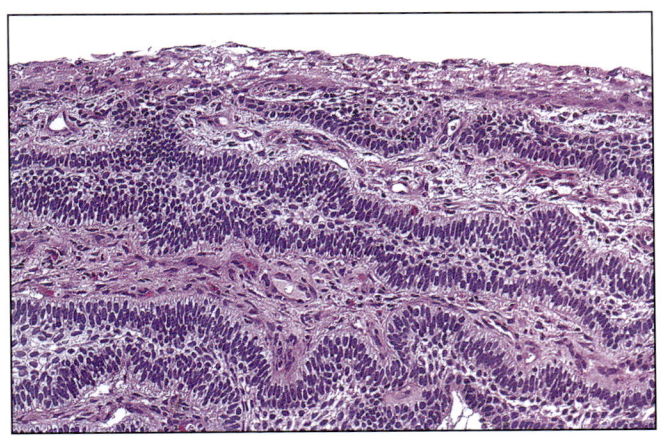

图4A.16 鼻窦造釉细胞瘤。（A）这个没有包膜的肿瘤由增生的牙源性上皮细胞巢或细胞岛组成，中心区域疏松排列的细胞类似釉质器的星网状层，周围区域是呈栅栏状排列的柱状或立方细胞，细胞核小而深染，远离基底膜排列（反向极性）。（B）可见棘皮瘤性变化，作为局灶性变化或突出的表现。（C）造釉细胞瘤性增生可以发生在与完整鼻窦表面黏膜上皮直接连续的部位。出现不与颌骨连续的孤立性鼻窦肿块，支持这些鼻窦肿瘤在组织发生上是来源于鼻窦黏膜上皮的全能细胞。

瘤非常少见，一旦出现绝大多数是恶性肿瘤。

畸胎瘤是有包膜的囊性、实性或多房性肿瘤，直径5～17 cm不等。畸胎瘤的组织学成分是来源于所有三个胚层的组织，包括上皮（角化性鳞状上皮、柱状上皮、纤毛性呼吸道上皮或胃肠型上皮）、皮肤附属器、小涎腺、神经外胚层和中枢神经系统组织、软骨、骨、脂肪组织和平滑肌组织。有突出的内衬上皮的囊性间隙。整个肿瘤中可见未成熟或胚胎组织成分，但这并不具有任何预后意义。在鼻咽畸胎瘤，神经外胚层和神经组织成分明显。可见坏死和出血。成人恶性畸胎瘤有明显的神经成分，而且伴有低分化癌和（或）肉瘤［见后，恶性畸胎瘤（畸胎癌肉瘤）项下］。

治疗选择完全手术切除。由于肿瘤大小和发生部位不同，本病的病况可能严重。如果在早期采取手术治疗，死亡率低；然而，在治疗不适当的病例则可能导致死亡，死亡通常是由于呼吸道梗阻并发症引起的。鼻咽畸胎瘤可向颅内扩散。在儿科年龄组，尚未见头颈部畸胎瘤恶变（或恶性行为）的报道。

鼻咽畸胎瘤的鉴别诊断包括鼻咽部皮样囊肿（所谓的毛息肉，hairy polyp）[146]。鼻咽皮样囊肿是一种发育性（先天性）异常，主要由皮肤（外胚层来源）组成，但也可包括分化好的软骨（中胚层来源）；缺乏内胚层衍化而来的结构，而且存在有限的异源性组织成分，不支持畸胎瘤这一诊断。实际上这种病变含有皮肤，而正常鼻咽部并未发现这一组织类型，提示最好将这种病变归入迷芽瘤（choristoma）而不是错构瘤（hamartoma），可能来源于第一鳃弓[147,148]。然而，某些作者认为最好将这些病变归类为良性畸胎瘤的亚型[149]。

恶性潜能不能确定的肿瘤
Tumors of indeterminant malignant potential

鼻窦型血管外皮细胞瘤
Sinonasal-type hemangiopericytoma

发生在许多部位的所谓的血管外皮细胞瘤（hemangiopericytoma，HPC）现在常被重新分类为孤立性纤维性肿瘤（solitary fibrous tumor，SFT）（见第3章）。鼻窦型血管外皮细胞瘤是一种非常少见的肿瘤，显示血管周围肌样分化，一般表现为良性生物学行为[150-153]。考虑到光镜和免疫组化检查具有肌样分化的证据，而且实际上光镜下鼻窦型血管外皮细胞瘤的特征也不同于软组织血管外皮细胞瘤,所以对于鼻窦部病变比较恰当的命名可能是肌外皮细胞瘤(myopericytoma)或球血管外皮细胞瘤(glomangiopericytoma)[151]。尽管这种鼻窦肿瘤通常具有惰性的行为,但最近的WHO鼻窦部肿瘤分类还是将鼻窦型血管外皮细胞瘤归为不能确定生物学潜能的肿瘤[154]。

鼻窦型血管外皮细胞瘤无性别差异;发病年龄广泛,最常见于50~70岁的患者[155]。这些病变实际上可发生于任何部位,但最常见的发生部位是鼻腔和副鼻窦。鼻窦型血管外皮细胞瘤典型的表现为单侧性鼻腔肿块,伴有鼻塞和鼻出血。可以扩展到邻近的副鼻窦,但是孤立性副鼻窦受累并不常见。鼻窦型血管外皮细胞瘤的放射学表现通常为鼻窦浑浊。由于压迫可能造成骨质侵蚀。动脉造影显示为富于血管的肿瘤。致病因素尚不清楚。

鼻窦型血管外皮细胞瘤大体表现为大小不等的息肉状肿块,肿块呈红到灰褐色,质软或质硬。组织学上,鼻窦型血管外皮细胞瘤为一黏膜下肿瘤,境界清楚但无包膜。与分叶状毛细血管瘤不同,鼻窦型血管外皮细胞瘤具有弥散性的生长方式,是由位于内衬内皮细胞的血管间隙周围的单一类型细胞组成的(图4A.17)。肿瘤细胞通常排列成短束状,少数病例可能显示席纹状、漩涡状、甚或栅栏状生长方式。肿瘤细胞均匀一致,核呈卵圆形,伴有圆形到卵圆形的细胞核,染色质呈空泡状到深染,并有模糊的嗜酸性胞浆;偶尔可见较多的梭形细胞。可见轻度核的多形性,偶见核分裂象,但核分裂活性通常没有明显增加,而且没有非典型性核分裂象。通常见不到坏死。血管腔从毛细血管大小到较大的窦状间隙,可呈"鹿角状"结构。一个特征性改变是血管周围出现透明变性,但不具有诊断意义(图4A.17)。细胞增生可以压迫血管,并引起较小血管结构不清。常见红细胞外渗。炎症细胞成分散在分布于整个肿瘤中,通常包括肥大细胞和嗜酸性细胞。少数病例可见多核瘤巨细胞[151]。可见纤维化或黏液样间质,尤其是在肿瘤发生退行性变时。偶尔可见异源性化生成分,包括骨和软骨。

在发生于比较常见部位的所谓软组织血管外皮细胞瘤,肿瘤细胞肌肉特异性肌动蛋白和结蛋白染色阴性[156,157],而鼻窦型血管外皮细胞瘤的免疫表型包括波形蛋白、平滑肌肌动蛋白、肌肉特异性肌动蛋白、Ⅷa因子以及血管内皮生长因子阳性[151,152,158]。细胞角蛋白、Ⅷ因子相关抗原、神经元特异性烯醇化酶、KP-1(CD68)、bcl-2、CD99和CD117(c-kit)免疫染色阴性。超微结构所见包括出现细胞周围基底膜、胞饮小泡、胞浆内细丝、致密小体和膜状附着斑[159,160]。

鉴别诊断包括分叶状毛细血管瘤、血管纤维瘤、血管球瘤(球血管瘤)、孤立性纤维性肿瘤、平滑肌肿瘤(平

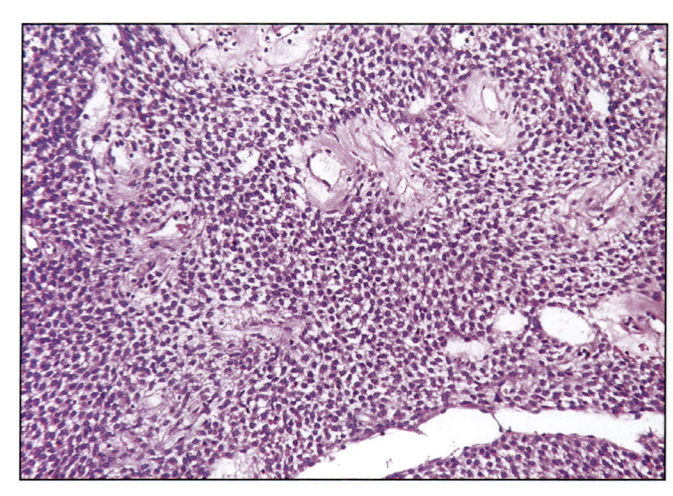

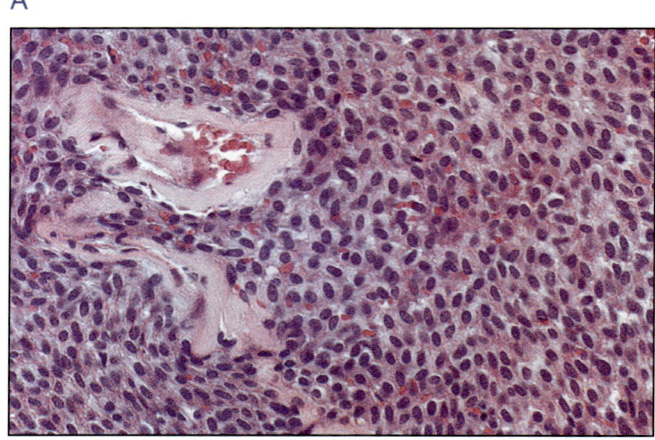

图4A.17 鼻窦型血管外皮细胞瘤。(A)肿瘤富于细胞,弥散生长,血管丰富。肿瘤细胞排列紧密,伴有深染的细胞核,位于内衬内皮细胞的血管腔隙周围。(B)与血管腔隙有关的特征性所见是血管周围出现透明变性,结合细胞形态学改变有助于辨认这种肿瘤。

滑肌瘤和平滑肌肉瘤)和滑膜肉瘤。鼻窦型血管外皮细胞瘤和孤立性纤维性肿瘤均可表达CD34;然而,CD34免疫反应范围不同。鼻窦型血管外皮细胞瘤CD34呈局限性表达,而孤立性纤维性肿瘤CD34倾向于弥散表达。另外,与孤立性纤维性肿瘤不同,鼻窦型血管外皮细胞瘤缺乏"绳索状"瘢痕疙瘩样胶原纤维或石棉样纤维,且不表达bcl-2。

治疗选择手术切除。血管外皮细胞瘤对放射治疗不敏感。鼻窦型血管外皮细胞瘤是行为惰性的肿瘤,5年总生存率高于90%[152,156]。局部复发出现于多达30%的病例,可能是因为手术切除不充分。Eichorn等[160]和El-Naggar等[161]报告,鼻窦型血管外皮细胞瘤在很长的随访期(10~20年)均可能复发。具有侵袭性行为的鼻

窦型血管外皮细胞瘤少见，包括局部破坏或转移性肿瘤[155]。与侵袭性行为可能有关的所见包括肿瘤较大（> 5 cm）、核多形性明显、核分裂活性增加、坏死、浸润性生长（例如骨）以及增殖指数 > 10%[152,162,163]。少数情况下肿瘤发生局部淋巴结和肺的转移，而且常常发生于局部复发之前[155]。

恶性上皮性和神经外胚层肿瘤
Malignant epithelial and neuroectodermal neoplasms

鼻前庭癌　Carcinoma of the nasal vestibule

鼻前庭癌少见，且被认为是皮肤癌而非黏膜癌[164]。在 Taxy[164] 报道的 5 个病例中，4 例男性，1 例女性；病人年龄分布从 52～82 岁。肿瘤位于鼻前庭或黏膜皮肤交界处。鳞状细胞癌为最常见的肿瘤类型。这些肿瘤大多数为高分化。可以发生基底细胞癌，但不常见[164]。鉴别诊断包括鳞状上皮乳头状瘤、鼻黏膜乳头状瘤和疣状癌（见下）。治疗包括局部切除和（或）放射治疗。多数病人预后很好。5 年生存率为 70%～80%[164]。可能侵犯下方邻近的鼻中隔软骨膜或骨。可以发生颈部淋巴结转移，但不常见。

鼻窦部和鼻咽部鳞状细胞癌
Squamous cell carcinoma of the sinonasal tract and nasopharynx

鼻窦和鼻咽内衬的上皮能沿不同细胞系分化，是发生于这些表面上皮的癌形态各异的原因。上呼吸消化道黏膜的鳞状细胞癌根据组织学亚型分类。最常见的鼻窦部鳞状细胞癌是普通型鳞状细胞癌，包括角化性和非角化性鳞状细胞癌。此外，普通型鳞状细胞癌尚有许多不同亚型，包括外生性或乳头状鳞状细胞癌、疣状癌、梭形细胞鳞状细胞癌、基底细胞样鳞状细胞癌和鳞腺癌，这些亚型具有不同的病理学特征，生物学行为和治疗方法，值得分别加以讨论。

鼻窦部鳞状细胞癌（普通类型）
Squamous cell carcinoma (conventional type) of the sinonasal tract

鳞状细胞癌是鼻窦部恶性上皮性肿瘤中最常见的类型。然而，它大约只占头颈部所有恶性肿瘤的 3% 以及所有恶性肿瘤的 1% 以下[165-167]。鼻窦鳞状细胞癌男性多于女性，最常见于 50～70 岁的病人，而且 95% 的病例发生在 40 岁以上的成人。按发生率递减的顺序，发生部位包括上颌窦、鼻腔、筛窦以及蝶窦和额窦[165-167]。虽然癌可能原发于额窦和蝶窦，但是累及额窦和蝶窦的多数肿瘤来源于筛窦或鼻咽部。临床表现包括面部不对称、一侧鼻塞、鼻出血、可触及的瘤块或在口腔或鼻腔内可见肿块、疼痛、持久的脓漏、经久不愈的溃疡和突眼。因为疾病早期阶段的临床症状和体征类似于慢性鼻窦炎，故副鼻窦癌的诊断常被延误。而鼻腔癌通常可以早期诊断，因为其症状可以促使早期临床检查[168]。与鼻窦部鳞状细胞癌有关的危险因素包括接触镍[169,170]、纺织粉尘、吸烟、从前应用胶体钍以及发生鼻黏膜乳头状瘤。后者可能发现人乳头状瘤病毒，但直接的因果关系还不清楚。鼻腔鳞状细胞癌患者处于患第二个恶性肿瘤的较高危险之中，或在上呼吸消化道黏膜的另外一个部位，或发生于肺、胃肠道或乳腺[171]。

鼻窦鳞状细胞癌的大体表现不同，包括外生性、息肉样、乳头状和蕈样结构，或为内翻性生长方式，可能境界清楚，伴有膨胀性生长和局灶性浸润，或坏死，而且脆而易碎，伴有出血表现和破坏性生长。

组织学上，鼻窦鳞状细胞癌被分为角化性和非角化性 2 种亚型。以角化性鳞状细胞癌最常见。肿瘤可以分为高分化、中分化和低分化癌。高分化鳞状细胞癌容易见到明显的角化，伴有角化珠形成或单个细胞角化（图 4A.18）。角化不良（异常角化）可能明显。可见细胞间桥。肿瘤细胞显示轻到中度的核非典型性，伴有核增大、深染，核分裂活性低。当鳞状细胞癌分化较差时（较高的组织学级别），显示肿瘤角化较少，核的非典型性比较明显，伴有核分裂活性增加，包括非典型性核分裂象。即使在低分化癌，通常也可出现局部角化的证据。间质浸润可能包括粘着的细胞巢或恶性细

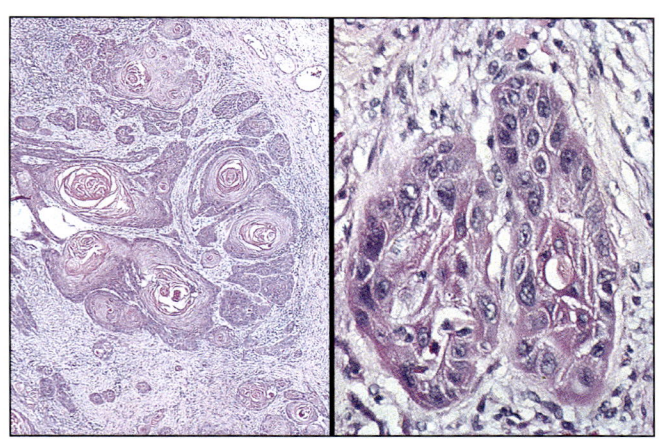

图 4A.18　鼻窦鳞状细胞癌，角化型。左：浸润性角化性鳞状细胞癌。右：可见单个细胞角化和细胞间桥。

胞条索，或可能是孤立的恶性细胞浸润。浸润癌的宿主反应（纤维组织增生）包括胶原沉积，伴或不伴慢性炎症细胞反应。

非角化性鳞状细胞癌也可呈乳头状或外生性生长方式，但常常显示向下（内翻性或内生性）生长，伴有宽的相互连接的肿瘤上皮细胞带或细胞巢（图4A.19）。肿瘤细胞巢可能具有圆形或光滑的边缘，或可见基底膜样物质包绕。这种生长方式与膀胱癌相似，因此这些肿瘤被命名为移行细胞型癌[172]。这种类型的肿瘤由细长的细胞组成，伴有圆柱状或柱状表现，垂直于表面生长，一般缺乏角化的证据。局部可能出现角化，但不是肿瘤的重要成分。一般说来，这些肿瘤细胞丰富，其特征为细胞核具有多形性，深染，核浆比例增高，细胞极性丧失以及核分裂活性增加，包括非典型性核分裂象（图4A.19）。由于肿瘤边缘光滑或周围有基底膜样物质，这些肿瘤可能不被认为是浸润性肿瘤，而被低诊断判为有重度异型增生的乳头状瘤或原位癌。邻近或其上方的表面上皮可见鳞状细胞癌和异型增生。异型增生可以从轻度到中重度（即原位癌）不等。鼻窦鳞状细胞癌的鉴别诊断包括鼻窦（鼻黏膜）乳头状瘤（见上）。

鼻窦鳞状细胞癌的治疗为完全手术切除并辅以放射治疗[173,174]。目前，手术方法改进，能够切除复杂的肿瘤并构建周围结构，使得功能和容貌得以改善[174]。对于晚期鼻窦鳞状细胞癌的处理，最近的趋势是拓宽了选择放射治疗和化学治疗的指征[174,175]。肿瘤局部复发常见，但是如果肿瘤局限于受累的鼻窦，则转移性疾病并不常见。肿瘤扩展至鼻窦壁外，将会导致局部淋巴结转移的发生率增高。一般来说，预后不良[168]。临床分期的预后意义比组织学类型重要。预后较差的因素包括疾病较高的临床分期，累及多个解剖学部位，扩展到鼻腔或副鼻窦外以及局部淋巴结转移。浸润方式可能也影响预后。具有"弥漫性扩散"或单个细胞浸润性生长方式的肿瘤，其生存率降至30%～40%，而具有粘着或"推挤性"浸润方式的肿瘤生存率为80%～90%[170]。Crissman和Zarbo讨论了肿瘤浸润方式的意义及其与预后的相关性[176]。这些作者指出，与较大的粘着性肿瘤细胞巢相比，伴有单个细胞或小的肿瘤细胞巢侵入宿主基质的浸润性癌更容易出现淋巴管浸润。

乳头状（外生性）鳞状细胞癌
Papillary (exophytic) squamous cell carcinoma

上呼吸消化道鳞状细胞癌（角化性和非角化性）以外生性或乳头状生长为特征，临床上类似良性乳头状或

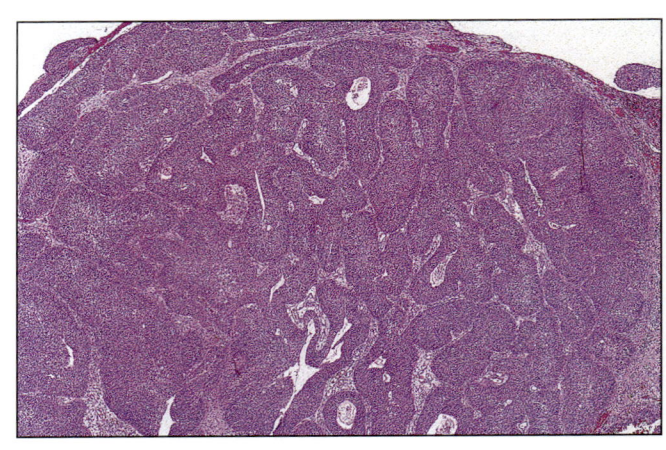

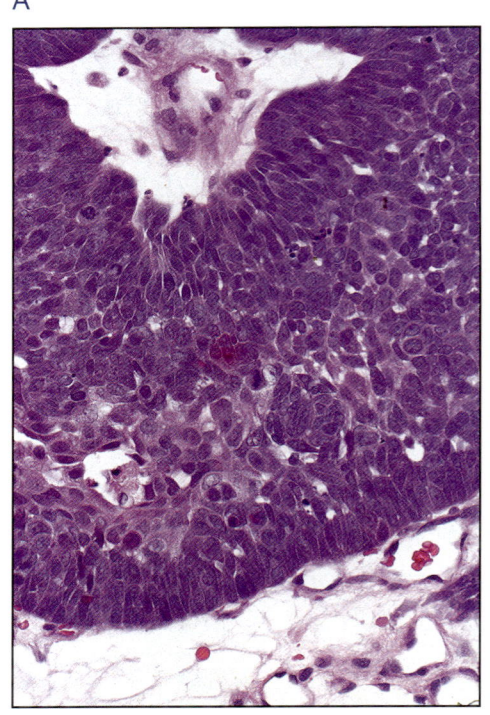

图4A.19 鼻窦鳞状细胞癌，非角化型。（A）肿瘤侵入黏膜下层，表现为相互连接的肿瘤上皮带，向下生长（"内翻"）进入间质。（B）显著的细胞多形性，伴有极性消失，核浆比例增高以及核分裂活性增加。

疣状癌的表现，但与良性乳头状瘤或疣状癌不同的是，外生性和乳头状鳞状细胞癌的肿瘤细胞均表现为恶性的细胞学特征[177-180]。乳头状（外生性）鳞状细胞癌是头颈部鳞状细胞癌的一种不常见的独特亚型。人口统计学资料显示与普通鳞状细胞癌相似，男性多于女性，倾向于发生在成人，中位年龄为60～70岁。乳头状鳞状细胞癌最常见于喉、口腔、口咽和下咽以及鼻窦部。喉是最常见的发生部位。由于受累部位不同，症状也各不相

同。在乳头状鳞状细胞癌和先前存在的乳头状瘤患者中，已经发现多达34%的患者有HPV（通过原位杂交和PCR）[180]。

乳头状鳞状细胞癌最常见表现为孤立性病变，伴有外生性或乳头状生长方式。肿瘤大小可以从2 mm到4 cm不等。组织学上，乳头状鳞状细胞癌具有丝状生长方式，伴有指状突起，并且可见纤维血管轴心，或为一个宽基底的球状到外生性肿物，伴有圆形突起，类似于菜花状生长结构，其中虽然可见纤维血管轴心，但是倾向于局限或缺如（图4A.20）。鳞状上皮在细胞学上表现为恶性，这种恶性上皮确定这些肿瘤是癌，而非乳头状瘤。表面角化一般有限，而且常常缺乏。在活检标本中可能难以确定明确的浸润，因为癌性上皮提示为原位病变，而不是浸润性癌。然而，临床上形成可以看得到的外生性肿块的生长范围已经超出了原位癌的一般概念。即使缺乏明显的间质浸润，也应考虑这些肿瘤具有浸润性。

乳头状鳞状细胞癌通常是新形成的肿瘤，没有共存的良性病变，例如乳头状瘤，但已有报道与前体病变乳头状瘤有关，或者患者发生乳头状鳞状细胞癌的部位从前有乳头状瘤的病史。

治疗选择外科手术；可以应用辅助治疗。多数乳头状鳞状细胞癌临床分期较低（T_2期）。总的来说，其生物学行为与类似分期的普通鳞状细胞癌相似，但某些作者报道T分期相同的乳头状鳞状细胞癌总的预后比普通鳞状细胞癌好。

乳头状或外生性鳞状细胞癌的鉴别诊断包括喉乳头状瘤病、普通的鳞状细胞癌和疣状癌。通过其具有良性的上皮增生可将喉乳头状瘤病鉴别开来。喉乳头状瘤病可见细胞学异常，但是趋向于局灶性，而且达不到见于乳头状鳞状细胞癌的异型增生的水平。疣状癌以外生性生长方式为特征，伴有明显角化，缺乏核非典型性、基底层外缺乏核分裂活性以及为挤推性，而不是浸润性的侵袭方式。这些特征不同于乳头状和外生性鳞状细胞癌。

疣状癌　Verrucous carcinoma（VC）

疣状癌是高度分化的鳞状细胞癌的一种变型，伴有局灶破坏能力，但不转移。疣状癌可以发生于上呼吸消化道的任何部位，最常见的部位依次为口腔、喉、鼻前庭、鼻窦部和鼻咽部[181-184]。在鼻窦部，上颌窦是最常受累的副鼻窦（93%）[185,186]。部位不同临床症状不同。在鼻窦部和鼻咽部，最常见的表现分别为呼吸道阻塞和咽下困难。疣状癌的病因仍在推测之中，包括使用烟草产品[184]。在疣状癌的发生中，病毒性诱因可能也是一个因素[187,188]。然而，文献中应用原位杂交技术检测HPV DNA的结果却不一致。一些研究者或在任何口腔疣状癌中均未证实有HPV DNA[189]，或仅在数量非常有限的病例中发现HPV DNA[190-193]。这些不一致性也许与原位杂交结果难以解释有关。非特异性染色或检测的敏感性低使得这一问题变得更加复杂[194]，而且还不清楚能否可靠区分疣状癌与普通鳞状细胞癌。对疣状癌进行HPV的PCR分析已证实有HPV DNA[195,196]。这些研究提示，HPV在发病机制中具有直接作用，而不是在疣状癌的发生过程中没有任何相关性。HPV的活性作用可能是作为上呼吸消化道鳞状细胞癌发生多步骤过程中的启动因子。Dyson等[197]研究显示，HPV蛋白产物可与视网膜母细胞瘤基因产物相结合，从而能够消除细胞周期从G_1期进入S期的调节阻断作用。

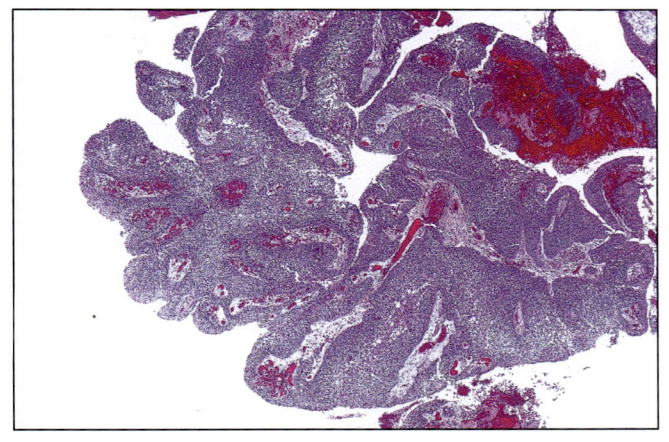

A

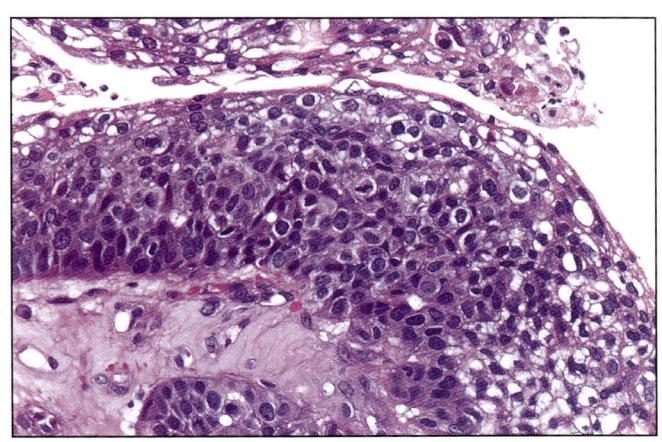

B

图4A.20　外生性（乳头状）鳞状细胞癌。（A）上皮呈明显的外生性和乳头状生长；（B）整个上皮成分均为恶性。

无论疣状癌发生于哪个部位，其病理学变化一般是相同的。疣状癌大体表现为褐色或白色的疣状、蕈样或外生性质硬肿物，直径可达 10 cm。一般来说，肿瘤具有宽基底。疣状癌的组织学表现是温和的鳞状细胞增生，细胞均匀一致，缺乏异型增生性特征（图 4A.21）。细胞有序成熟，保留极性。核浆比例、核的多形性或角化不良并不增加。基底部可见核分裂象，但是其他部位不出现核分裂象。除了温和的上皮细胞增生之外，还有明显的表面角化（"教堂塔尖样"角化，church-spire keratosis），特征性的宽或球状钉突推挤性向下伸入间质。向黏膜下浸润的生长方式不是其特征，例如成角的粘着性细胞巢或单个松散的肿瘤细胞。在间质中可见明显的淋巴细胞、浆细胞和组织细胞等慢性炎细胞浸润。可见病毒相关性细胞病变改变（挖空细胞）。疣状癌充分的组织学诊断需要有足够的上皮和其下的间质组织。在缺乏间质的情况下，应该认为活检不充分，不能做出疣状癌的明确诊断。

诊断疣状癌一般不需要任何特殊染色（即组织化学或免疫组化）。在某些情况下，显著而温和的上皮增生可能继发于真菌感染，例如念珠菌病。银染色是观察真菌的最好方法，例如 Gomori 乌洛托品银染色（GMS）。真菌应出现在增生上皮的深部，而不是局限于表面角化或最浅表的上皮。真菌可继发性存在于任何增生的鳞状上皮，而且也可伴随肿瘤性增生而出现，包括疣状癌。

疣状癌必须与"普通"型鳞状细胞癌相区别。从临床表现和病理组织学两个方面来看，这两种肿瘤之间均可能有重叠。疣状癌与普通鳞状细胞癌在组织学上的区别是根据是否出现细胞学异常。出现任何异型增生性改变均应除外疣状癌的诊断。轻度异型增生性改变局限于疣状癌的基底部。普通鳞状细胞癌可见角化不良，但这一般不是疣状癌的特征。疣状癌的病理诊断可能相当困难，在出现明显的诊断特征之前几年内，可能需要多次活检。临床医师和病理医师都需要了解这一事实。为了这个目的，最初活检材料充分是至关重要的，应该包括较好的上皮‐间质交界面。如没有见到病变与其下间质的相互关系，病理医师不应过度诊断像癌一样的疣样病变。同样，在出现异型增生性鳞状上皮改变的情况下，为了除外浸润癌需要有充分的上皮‐间质交界面。

对于疣状癌来说，手术切除是明确诊断的方式[182,198]。鼻窦部疣状癌常常表现为晚期疾病，最初就处于 T3 期或更高阶段[185]。可以出现颈部淋巴结肿大，但为反应性改变，而非转移性病变[183]。由于可诱导退行性转化的传说，某些文献支持放射治疗是治疗疣状癌禁忌证这一教条。然而，有许多理由怀疑放射治疗诱导疣状癌间变性转化的真实性。疣状癌类似的转化发生在手术、冷冻手术后，甚至在无任何治疗干预的情况下[183,199]。Batsakis 等[182]指出了反对放射与诱导转化有关的几个因素，其中包括放射治疗与高级别恶性肿瘤之间的间隔可能非常短（少于 8 个月）这一事实，以及大多数疣状癌"间变转化"的描述和图示并不充分。比较可能的情况是"宿主肿瘤"不是疣状癌，而是取样可能不够充分的普通鳞状细胞癌。因此，要排除低分化（"间变性"）病灶，那是肿瘤开始的一部分。治疗仍然选择手术，85% 的患者获得了局部控制[200]。放射治疗的局部控制率低于 50%[200]。Vidyasagar 等[201]报道了 107 例照射的病人，其中 31% 出现肿瘤复发。他们认为这些数字与手术后复发率比较是相似的。放射治疗可以选择性用于某些临床情况，例如局部进展性患者或不适合选择手术的患者[202]。

梭形细胞鳞状细胞癌（肉瘤样癌）
Spindle cell squamous carcinoma (sarcomatoid carcinoma)

主要由梭形细胞组成的鳞状细胞癌发生于鼻窦部和鼻咽部[202-204]。在这些解剖部位，梭形细胞鳞状细胞癌常常表现为蕈样、溃疡性肿块，而在较常见的上呼吸消化道部位（例如喉、口腔）则呈息肉样或外生性表现。

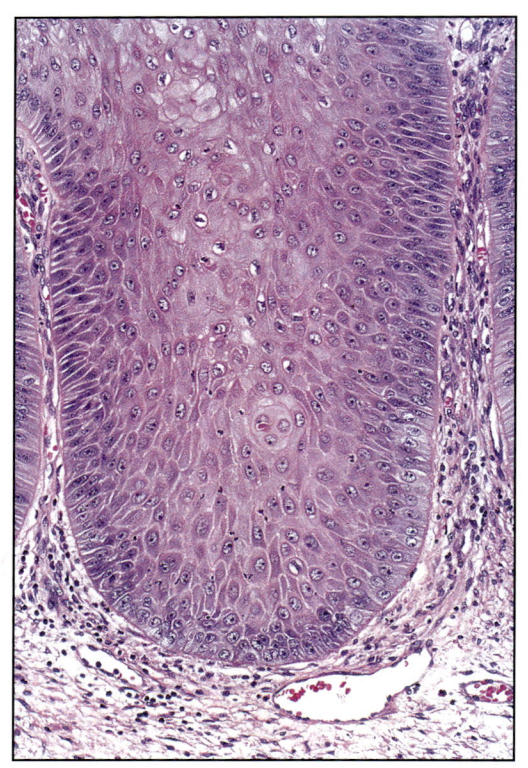

图 4A.21　疣状癌。上皮温和，缺乏细胞非典型性或核分裂活性。

诊断梭形细胞鳞状细胞癌的组织学特征包括在分化性鳞状细胞成分中出现恶性未分化性梭形细胞增生，分化性鳞状细胞成分包括重度异型增生、原位癌或明显的浸润性鳞状细胞癌（图4A.22）。然而，缺乏分化性成分而完全由梭形和多形性（未分化）成分组成的肿瘤并不少见。一般来说，这些肿瘤细胞丰富，由多形性表现的梭形细胞和上皮样细胞构成，伴有大而深染的细胞核、核浆比例增加，不显著到明显的嗜酸性核仁，不明显到充分的嗜酸性到双嗜色性胞浆，核分裂活性（典型性和非典型性）增多，并有坏死。梭形细胞鳞状细胞癌的生长方式可呈束状、席纹状或栅栏状，伴或不伴黏液瘤性间质。如果表面上皮完整，恶性梭形细胞成分不与表面分离，而且可能与表面上皮密切相关。完整的表面上皮可有或无异型增生。

在某些梭形细胞鳞状细胞癌，增生的梭形细胞稀疏，分布于明显纤维化或胶原化的间质中（图4A.23）。在这些细胞稀少的梭形细胞鳞状细胞癌中，表面上皮可能完整，没有异型增生或明确的鳞状细胞癌。在这种情况下，诊断恶性可能非常困难。细胞稀少的梭形细胞鳞状细胞癌也是息肉样病变，累及浅表的黏膜下层，而且增生的梭形或多形性细胞具有非典型性核的特征，核分裂活性增加，包括典型或非典型性核分裂象。肿瘤位置表浅和出现核的非典型性有助于将梭形细胞鳞状细胞癌与间叶性肿瘤或反应性增生区别开来，例如以肌纤维母细胞为主的病变。可见异源性成分，包括骨和软骨。这些成分可能显示恶性特征（软骨肉瘤和骨肉瘤灶）。

免疫组化评估可能有利于梭形细胞鳞状细胞癌的诊断（图4A.23）。多数病例梭形细胞角蛋白阳性，但是多达40%的病例可能缺乏细胞角蛋白[205]。其他作

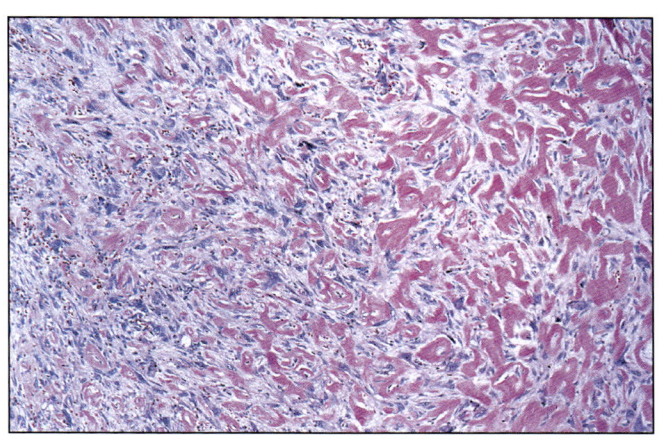

图4A.23　梭形细胞鳞状细胞癌。该病例具有明显的胶原性间质。

者发现具有类似的细胞角蛋白染色结果，阳性病例从30%～50%不等，取决于所用的抗体[203,206-210]。因此，缺乏细胞角蛋白染色不能除外梭形细胞鳞状细胞癌的诊断。p63作为鳞状细胞和肌上皮细胞的标记物，在标记梭形细胞鳞状细胞癌的梭形细胞时与细胞角蛋白同样有效，在梭形细胞鳞状细胞癌的诊断中应该联合应用p63和细胞角蛋白[211]。在缺乏细胞角蛋白反应时，通过缺乏对于其他诊断可能特异的免疫反应可以提示梭形细胞鳞状细胞癌的诊断，例如S-100蛋白对于黏膜恶性黑色素瘤，或间叶细胞标记物［结蛋白和肌细胞生成素（myogenin）］反应可以诊断为肉瘤。然而，某些对于传统上是间叶性分化的标记物呈现阳性反应的病例，可能出现复杂的诊断问题。已有报道，波形蛋白和各种肌源性标记物（结蛋白和肌动蛋白）存在于梭形细胞鳞状细胞癌中[204,206,210-214]。如同常常见于其他部位的梭形细

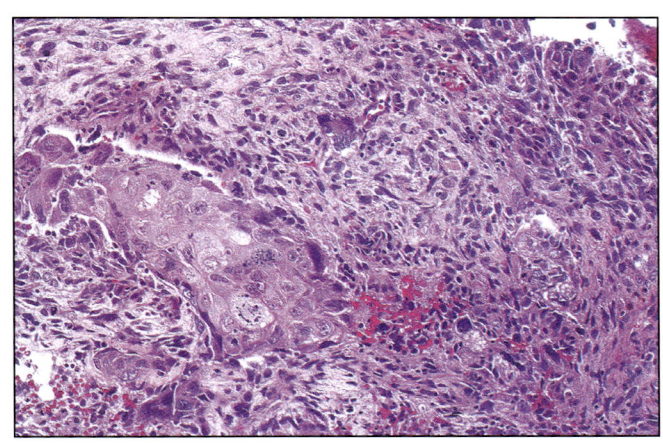

A

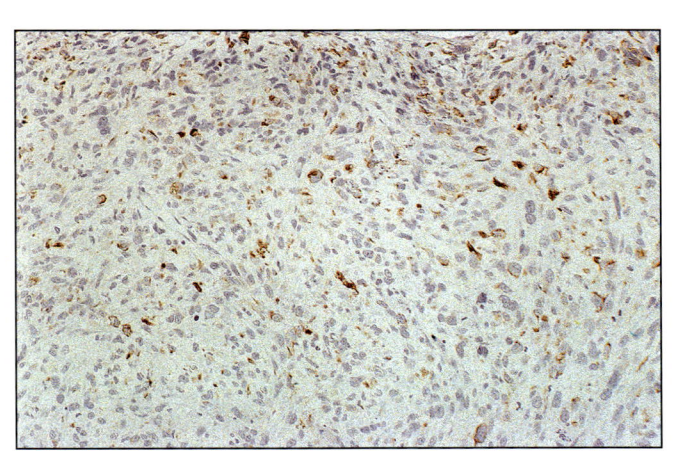

B

图4A.22　上颌窦梭形细胞鳞状细胞癌。（A）分化性鳞状上皮成分（在本图中为浸润性鳞状细胞癌）和与之密切相关的恶性梭形和多形性细胞浸润成分混合是诊断该瘤的特征。（B）细胞角蛋白免疫反应阳性，通常为局灶性，但是可以为阴性。

胞癌一样，一项26例来自上呼吸消化道不同部位的梭形细胞鳞状细胞癌的研究发现，42%的肿瘤表达细胞角蛋白，100%表达波形蛋白，42%表达肌源性标记物HHF-35（广谱肌动蛋白）和α-平滑肌肌动蛋白[209]。25%的病例共同表达细胞角蛋白和波形蛋白。超微结构检查，梭形细胞鳞状细胞癌通常出现上皮分化的证据，包括桥粒、张力丝和粘着斑，偶尔超微结构检查可能是做出诊断最可靠的手段[204,208,210]。

一般来说，梭形细胞鳞状细胞癌比普通鳞状细胞癌更具侵袭性，而且对于放射治疗更不敏感。鼻窦梭形细胞癌比上呼吸消化道其他部位的梭形细胞癌预后更差。在对于上呼吸消化道不同部位梭形细胞癌的对比研究中，Batsakis及其同事[215]报道鼻窦梭形细胞鳞状细胞癌死亡率为70%，而口腔梭形细胞鳞状细胞癌为60%，喉梭形细胞鳞状细胞癌为30%。另外，局部复发和转移性疾病常见。转移主要发生于颈部淋巴结和肺[216,217]。转移性病灶的组织学所见可能仅有普通鳞状细胞癌，仅有梭形细胞癌，或二者皆有[216]。与鼻窦或鼻咽梭形细胞鳞状细胞癌相关的病原学因素还未证实。一项有关口咽部梭形细胞鳞状细胞癌的研究未能发现HPV感染[215]。

基底细胞样鳞状细胞癌
Basaloid squamous cell carcinoma

基底细胞样鳞状细胞癌（BSCC）是鳞状细胞癌的一种高级别亚型，好发于下咽（梨状窦）、声门上喉、口腔、舌、扁桃体和腭[218-223]。在少数情况下，鼻窦部可能受累[222,224,225]。在鼻窦部表现为一个肿块性病变，伴有单侧鼻塞[225]。与非鼻窦部病变相关的病因学因素包括过多饮酒和（或）吸烟[223,226]，而鼻窦部肿瘤的特异性病因学因素尚未发现[225]。

基底细胞样鳞状细胞癌为坚硬的褐色-白色肿块，常伴有中心坏死，肿块最大径可达6.0 cm。可以呈外生性生长，但是少见。组织学表现为浸润性肿瘤，有多种生长方式，全都可能见于任何一个肿瘤内，包括实性、分叶状、细胞巢、筛状、条索状、小梁状以及腺样或囊性间隙。肿瘤来源于表面上皮，可以显示重度异型增生和（或）直接与浸润癌连续。肿瘤小叶中心通常可见粉刺样坏死。一个具有特色的细胞学特征是出现基底细胞样成分，由小而紧密排列的细胞组成，细胞核深染、胞浆稀少，核分裂活性显著；大细胞和多形性也可见（图4A.24）。另外一个重要细胞学特征是与鳞状分化灶密切相关，或为异型增生、原位癌，或为浸润癌。另外，肿瘤性梭形细胞癌的成分可能伴有基底细胞样鳞状成分。细胞间出现嗜酸性玻璃样或黏液玻璃样物质沉积，类似与小涎腺来源肿瘤有关的基底膜物质的再现。可见玫瑰花样结构[227]。基底细胞样鳞状细胞癌是浸润较深的肿瘤，常常浸润软组织并具有向神经性。

基底膜样物质PAS和阿辛蓝染色阳性。免疫组化染色显示，细胞角蛋白以及其他上皮标记物阳性，包括上皮膜抗原（EMA）和癌胚抗原（CEA）[224,225]。神经内分泌标记物嗜铬素和突触素一般阴性，但已有报道少数病例嗜铬素阳性[227]；神经胶质原纤维酸性蛋白（GFAP）和黑色素细胞标记物HMB-45均为阴性。波形蛋白、S-100蛋白和肌动蛋白免疫染色呈现不同程度的反应。电子显微镜检查显示基底细胞样成分含有桥粒、少数张力丝和松散的卫星状颗粒或囊腔内折转的基底层[218]。Hewan-Lowe和Dardick[228]发现超微结构特征有助于区分基底细胞样鳞状细胞癌和腺样囊性癌。这些作者比较了3例基底细胞样鳞状细胞癌和3例腺样囊性癌的超微结构特征，发现基底细胞样鳞状细胞癌具有鳞状细

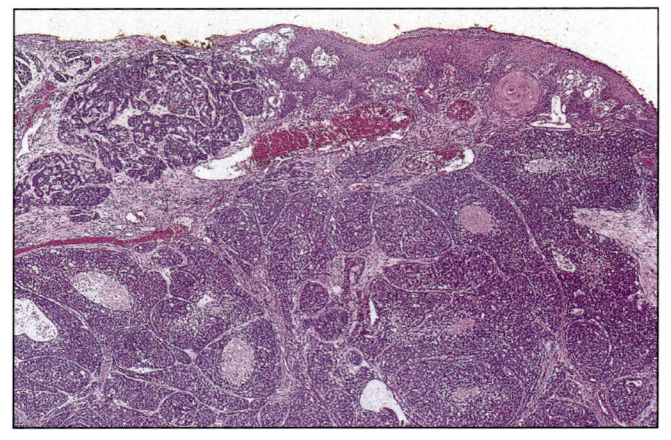

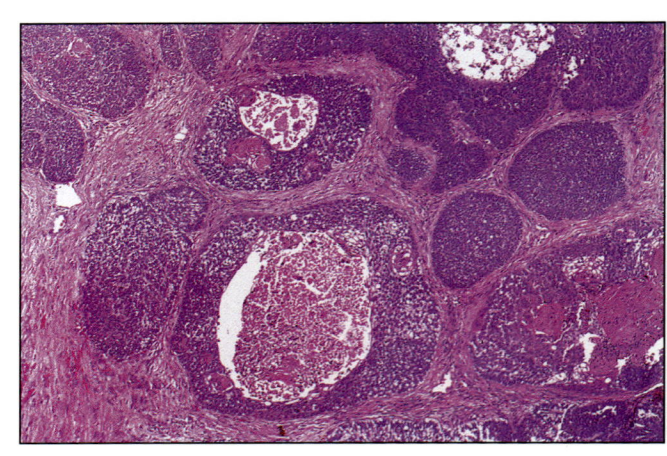

图4A.24 鼻窦部基底细胞样鳞状细胞癌。（A）浸润癌伴有小叶状生长方式和粉刺型坏死、小梁状生长灶（右上）以及突然出现的角化灶（左上）。（B）这种肿瘤主要由增生的基底细胞样细胞构成，伴有轻微但可以辨认的鳞状分化。

癌的特征，包括伴有许多明显张力丝束的细胞团、突出的桥粒和上皮珠。腺样囊性癌并不出现这些特征[228]。腺体分化的特征仅仅见于腺样囊性癌，而不见于基底细胞样鳞状细胞癌，后者缺少纤毛和腔隙（大腔和较小的受压的腔）。

由于容易早期转移到局部淋巴结和内脏，基底细胞样鳞状细胞癌的治疗选择多模式治疗，包括根治性手术切除、颈淋巴结清扫术、放射治疗和常采用的化学治疗[218,222,223,226]。

上呼吸消化道所有部位的基底细胞样鳞状细胞癌都是一种侵袭性的高级别肿瘤，倾向于呈多灶性生长，容易浸润深部和转移，甚至在早期就可发生[218]。表浅活检不能达到浸润的深度和范围，因而不能代表整个病变，容易导致错误分期。多灶性包括头颈部其他黏膜部位以及胃肠道受累[229]。可经由淋巴道和血道发生转移，尤其是转移到局部和远处淋巴结。大约64%患者具有（或将会发生）颈部淋巴结转移[227]，多达44%的病例发生远处转移[183]，累及肺、骨、皮肤和脑[218,222,226]。转移包括基底细胞样和鳞状细胞两种成分。

腺鳞癌
Adenosquamous carcinoma（ASC）

腺鳞癌是来源于表面上皮的鳞状细胞癌的另外一种高级别亚型，显示腺癌和鳞状细胞癌两种组织学特征。腺鳞癌是鳞状细胞癌的一种不常见亚型。实际上，这种肿瘤可以发生于上呼吸消化道的任何部位，但最常见于喉、下咽、口腔和鼻窦腔[230-235]。在鼻窦部，肿瘤表现为有痛或无痛性肿块，并引起气道阻塞。病因不明，可能与饮酒和（或）吸烟有关。

这些肿瘤可以是外生性或位于黏膜下，质脆，水肿，或呈颗粒状，表面溃疡可有可无，大小在0.6～5.0 cm。组织学表现为浸润性肿瘤，伴有实性和腺体结构。鳞状细胞癌成分从高分化到低分化分化程度不同；表面上皮常有原位癌，原位癌延伸到邻近的小涎腺，以及（或）发生于表面上皮的浸润癌。鳞状细胞分化明显，表现为单个细胞角化、细胞间桥、角化珠形成和（或）角化不良（图4A.25）。腺癌成分见于黏膜下层，通过存在腺体分化容易识别（图4A.25）。可能见不到黏液细胞分化，黏液细胞分化不是诊断的前提条件。鳞状细胞癌和腺癌可以混合存在，也可彼此分开单独存在。可有明显的细胞多形性、核分裂象增加、坏死灶和神经周围浸润。细胞内和管腔内的黏液卡红和抗淀粉酶PAS阳性物质与腺体成分有关。腺鳞癌中出现的上皮性黏液不同于腺样鳞状细胞癌。肿瘤细胞细胞角蛋白阳性。

腺鳞癌的鉴别诊断包括基底细胞样鳞状细胞癌（见上）和高级别（低分化）黏液表皮样癌。鉴别诊断非常重要，因为基底细胞样鳞状细胞癌的生物学行为和预后比低分化黏液表皮样癌差得多。腺鳞癌的治疗是选择根治性的手术切除，因为这种肿瘤易于出现早期局部淋巴结转移，所以作为整个治疗的一部分，最初治疗可能需要根治性颈淋巴结清扫。放射治疗的效果尚有争议。这种肿瘤是侵袭性强的高度恶性肿瘤，预后差[230]。即使是在疾病早期，腺鳞癌也倾向于多灶性、深部浸润和易于转移[234]。组织学上，转移性病变类似于原发性肿瘤，包括两种组织学成分。5年生存率大约为22%[234]。无论肿瘤大小，这些肿瘤均具有高度侵袭性的生物学行为。

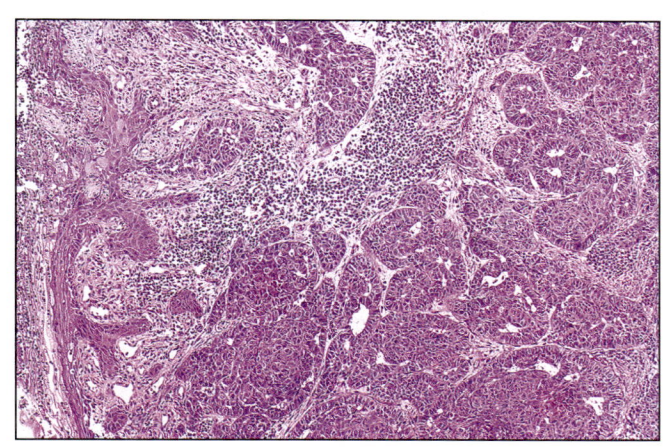 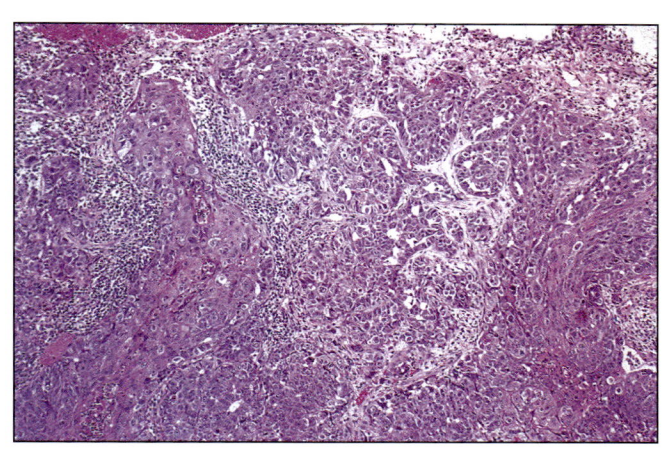

图4A.25 腺鳞癌。（A）此浸润癌来源于表面上皮（左），显示鳞状分化（表面）和腺体分化（浸润性成分）。（B）浸润癌中出现混合性鳞状和腺体分化。

淋巴上皮癌　Lymphoepithelial carcinoma

鼻窦部淋巴上皮癌在形态学上类似于最熟悉的鼻咽部淋巴上皮癌的组织学表现（见下）。这是一种少见的鼻窦部癌，主要发生于40～70岁的男性[236]。发生于鼻腔的鼻窦部淋巴上皮癌比副鼻窦常见。临床表现包括鼻塞、鼻出血以及在出现浸润性生长时引起眼球突出和颅神经麻痹[237,238]。与鼻咽部淋巴上皮癌相似，这种肿瘤与EB病毒密切相关[236-240]。

组织学所见与鼻咽癌相似（见下）。免疫组化染色各种细胞角蛋白阳性。在大多数病例，EB病毒编码的RNA强烈表达（EBER）[236-240]。

鉴别诊断包括鼻窦未分化癌、黏膜恶性黑色素瘤和非Hodgkin淋巴瘤（见下）。重要的是要排除鼻咽部原发性肿瘤累及鼻窦，为此，对于鼻咽部要进行详细的临床评估。

预后良好，由于局部放射治疗有效。在诊断时可能出现颈部淋巴结转移。即使在出现淋巴结转移的情况下，预后依然很好[236,237,240]。

关于鼻窦部鳞状细胞癌及其变型的总体考虑　General considerations for sinonasal tract squamous cell carcinoma and variants

前体病变　Precursor lesions

与上呼吸消化道其他部位（特别是口腔和喉）不同，鼻窦部的前体病变（即异型增生和原位癌）尚未确定。正如前面鼻窦型（鼻黏膜）乳头状瘤一节所述，鳞状细胞癌及其变型可从内翻型和嗜酸细胞型鼻黏膜乳头状瘤发展而来。因此，鼻黏膜乳头状瘤似乎是鼻窦鳞状细胞癌的前体病变。在这些类型的鼻黏膜乳头状瘤中可以发现人乳头瘤病毒（HPV），但HPV的存在与鼻窦鳞状细胞癌发生之间没有明确的联系。鼻窦上皮鳞状化生与鳞状细胞癌发生之间也无明确相关。

分子遗传学　Molecular genetics

多数头颈部鳞状细胞癌及其前体病变患者的9号染色体短臂存在基因改变[241]，特殊类型的鳞状细胞癌显示独特的分子改变[241]。这些发现支持这些染色体早期参与鳞状细胞癌的发生，而且支持其短暂的发生早于恶性表型的转化[241]。

鼻咽癌（表4A.5）
Nasopharyngeal carcinoma (NPC)

鼻咽癌是一种来源于表面上皮的鳞状细胞癌，根据WHO分类分为两种组织学亚型：角化性和非角化性[242]。非角化型进一步分为"分化性"和"未分化性"。目前的WHO分类保留了1991的分类术语，并增加了基底细胞样鳞状细胞癌的类型[243]。根据定义，鼻咽癌起源于鼻咽黏膜上皮，而且通过光镜、免疫组化或电子显微镜检查显示鳞状分化的证据。因此，应用该术语是为了排除可能发生于该部位的其他恶性肿瘤，包括腺癌（小涎腺来源和非涎腺来源）。鼻咽癌的同义词包括淋巴上皮瘤、Rigaud型淋巴上皮瘤和Schmincke型淋巴上皮瘤以及移行细胞癌。淋巴上皮瘤（lymphoepithelioma）这一命名是个误称。这是一个完全来源于上皮的肿瘤，伴有继发性的良性淋巴成分。应用淋巴上皮瘤这一术语可能导致与恶性淋巴瘤的诊断相混淆。从前WHO应用数字表示的命名，即1型（鳞状细胞癌）、2型（非角化性癌）和3型（未分化癌），已不再应用。应该注意的是，尽管它们都用"未分化"这一不合宜的称呼，但在鼻窦未分化癌（见下）和鼻咽未分化癌之间并不存在相关关系，它们的解剖部位不同，具有不同的治疗方法和生物学行为。

总的说来，鼻咽癌在美国是一种不常见的肿瘤，大约占所有癌症的0.25%[244,245]，在中国，占所有癌症的18%[246]，而且1/40的男性在72岁前会发生鼻咽癌[247]。鼻咽癌男性多于女性，发病年龄范围广泛，但最常见于30～60岁的病人。20%以下的病例发生在儿科年龄组。儿童鼻咽癌最常见于北非和中非，占所有病例的10%～20%，而在中国大约仅有2%的鼻咽癌发生于儿童[248-250]。不论组织学类型如何，临床表现都是相似的，包括出现无症状的颈部肿块，一般局限于颈后三角或颈上淋巴结链，其他临床症状和体征包括鼻塞、流涕、鼻出血、疼痛、浆液性中耳炎、耳痛、听力丧失和头痛[244-252]。症状和体征常常轻微，且不具有特异性，常常导致在疾病晚期才做出临床诊断。多达25%的患者可有颅神经受累[253]。最常见的发生部位为鼻咽侧壁（咽隐窝，fossa of Rosenmüller），其次是鼻咽后上壁[251]。

在估价局部病变范围和有无转移方面，放射影像为重要的辅助诊断[254,255]。除了其他影像学检查（例如普通X线片、超声检查和CT）之外，PET-CT（正电子发射体层摄影和计算机体层摄影，positron emission tomography and computed tomography）已被用于检测肿瘤的局部和远处播散。

鼻咽癌的发生与多种相互作用的病因因素有关。遗传和地理因素在鼻咽癌的发生中起重要作用。在中国鼻咽癌的发病率高，尤其是南方（广东省）和北方各省及中国台湾[246]。尽管移民到低发病率地区后的中国人发病率下降，但仍比非中国人群的发病率高[246,256]。人

表4A.5	鼻咽癌（NPC）		
	角化型[a]	非角化型[b]	未分化型[c]
百分数	约25%	最少见，<15%	最常见，>60%
性别，年龄	男＞女；30～60岁	男＞女；30～60岁	男＞女；30～60岁；也可见于儿童
组织学	角化，细胞间桥；普通型鳞状细胞癌，分为高、中和低分化；对于浸润有纤维组织增生性反应	几乎无角化，相互连接的条索状生长方式（类似移行细胞尿路上皮癌）；对于浸润几乎没有纤维组织增生性反应	缺乏角化，合体细胞性生长方式，细胞粘着或松散，伴有圆形细胞核、突出的嗜酸性核仁、少量胞浆和有限的核分裂象；明显的非肿瘤性淋巴细胞成分；一般缺乏对于浸润的纤维组织增生性反应
E-B病毒	弱相关	强相关	强相关
治疗	放射治疗效果不好	放射治疗有效	放射治疗有效
预后	5年生存率20%～40%	5年生存率65%	5年生存率65%

[a] WHO命名为鼻咽癌，角化性
[b] WHO命名为鼻咽癌，非角化性，分化性
[c] WHO命名为鼻咽癌，非角化性，未分化性

类白细胞抗原（HLA）-A_2、HLA-B_{17}、HLA-B_W46 和 HLA-B_W58 组织相容性基因座提示可以作为鼻咽癌遗传敏感性标记物[246]。EB病毒与鼻咽癌发生的联系或许最为重要[246,257,258]。某些鼻咽癌与EB病毒密切相关，提示EB病毒在鼻咽癌的发生中可能具有癌基因的作用[258]。非角化型和未分化型鼻咽鳞状细胞癌均与EB病毒DNA的存在有关。在鼻咽癌患者可见免疫球蛋白A（IgA）抗体[抗病毒衣壳抗原（VCA）]和IgG抗体[抗早期抗原（EA）]滴度升高[259-265]，其检出率可高达93%[243]；抗体滴度升高已被作为高危地区人群筛查的一种标记物，并可作为疾病复发的一种潜在标记物[260,261,265]。已有报道，90%的非角化型患者血清抗EB病毒阳性[266]。以重组EB病毒抗原[例如EB病毒核抗原（EBNA）、膜抗原（MA）及其他抗原]为基础的较新的抗体试验已用于鼻咽癌的诊断，同样，定量PCR可以检测血浆和血清中EB病毒DNA升高，据报道在鼻咽癌中的敏感率可达96%[267-270]。通过原位杂交（ISH）或PCR进行鼻咽癌的生物分子学分析发现，75%～100%的鼻咽癌有EB病毒DNA或RNA[271,272]。角化性鼻咽癌并非如此，其中，EB病毒基因组的检出率不同，如果存在，一般也是局限于散在的异型增生的上皮细胞内。Pathmanathan 等[273]报道，在鼻咽癌的发生中，EB病毒是一个早期启动事件。他们注意到，EB病毒出现在侵袭前（前体）鼻咽病变，这种EB病毒DNA是克隆性的，提示侵袭前病变来源于感染了EB病毒的单个细胞，而且这些侵袭前病变可在1年之内发展为浸润癌[273]。鼻咽癌中的EB病毒感染导致EB病毒核抗原-1（EBNA-1）和隐形膜蛋白-1（LMP-1）的表达，带有丰富的EBER[243]。Hording 等[274]对38例鼻咽癌的HPV状况进行了评估，发现15例角化性鳞状细胞癌中4例HPV为阳性，而非角化性或未分化性鼻咽癌患者中没有发现HPV。在某些鼻咽角化性鳞状细胞癌的发病机制中，HPV可能具有一定的作用，而在非角化性或未分化性鳞状细胞癌中HPV不起作用。提示与鼻咽癌有关的其他因素包括饮食（含高亚硝胺的腌鱼）、卫生条件不好以及非饮食性环境因素，包括大气因素，例如灰尘、烟尘、化学烟雾、来自燃烧木、草和香的家庭烟雾和吸入（主动或被动）香烟的烟雾，以及在治疗鼻疾病时使用中草药和吸入剂[246]。

在鼻咽癌中发现了3号染色体短臂始终一致的非随机性缺失和重排[275-278]。遗传不稳定性（缺失和获得）是鼻咽癌常见的分子事件，而且在鼻咽癌的发生和发展中具有重要作用。杂合性缺失（LOH）和比较基因组杂交（CGH）研究显示，常常出现染色体1p、3p、9p、9q、11q、13q、14q、16q和19q等位基因缺失[279-281]。CGH分析显示，染色体1q、8q、18q上获得，而9p缺失，这与鼻咽癌进展密切相关。杂合性缺失分析还显示，来自中国南方人群的正常鼻咽上皮（74%）和异型增生性病变（75%）常常出现3号染色体短臂杂合性缺失，提示3号染色体短臂杂合性缺失可能是鼻咽癌发生过程中

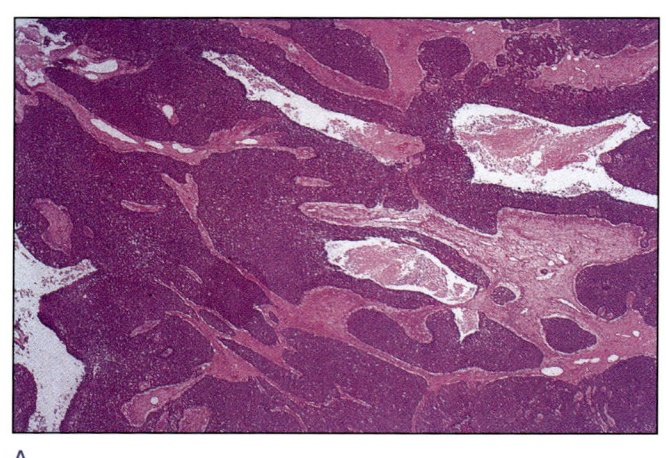 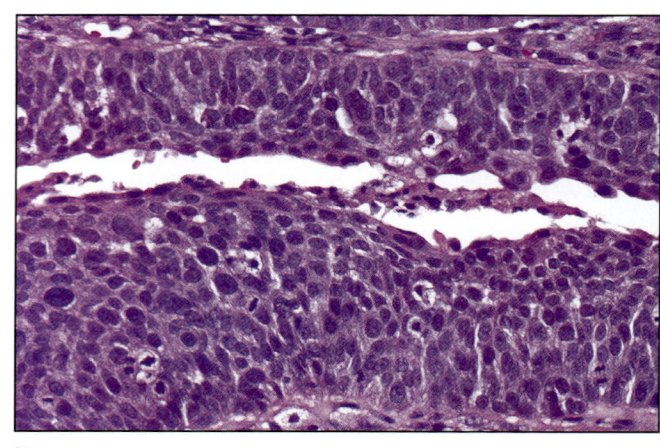

图4A.26 鼻咽非角化性癌，分化型。（A）肿瘤浸润，形成广泛吻合的条索和小梁。（B）肿瘤细胞具有多形性细胞核，伴有核分裂活性增加，缺乏角化。

的一个较早期的基因事件[280]。

连锁分析（linkage analysis）指出，HLA 基因和细胞色素 p4502E 基因可能是鼻咽癌的易感性基因。通过杂合性缺失、比较基因组杂交、连锁分析和 cDNA 微阵列分析，鼻咽癌的特异性生物学标记物可用于较早期诊断和预后的估计[280]。在有遗传和环境易感因素存在的情况下，鼻咽癌的发生可能涉及基因和外基因（epigenetic）改变的积累[282]。广泛基因组（genome-wide）研究证实，涉及特异性癌基因和肿瘤抑癌基因的多个染色体异常，包括位于染色体 9p21 上的 p16 肿瘤抑制基因的失活，这是鼻咽癌肿瘤发生过程中最常见的分子生物学改变[283,284]。诸如 Ras 相关功能区家族 1A（RASSF1A）、p16/INK4A、p14/ARF 等基因改变提示，鼻咽癌细胞有多细胞通路的功能障碍。癌前病变的研究显示，在鼻咽癌的发生中有早期基因改变，而且 EB 病毒潜在感染具有重要作用[243,282]。

鼻咽癌的大体表现不同，从伴有完整上皮的黏膜隆起，到伴有表面上皮广泛受累的明显浸润性肿块，到偶然发现的完全无法辨认的显微镜下病变。根据主要表现，可分为三种组织学类型[285]。普通角化性鳞状细胞癌的特征是出现角化和细胞间桥，具有低分化、中分化和高分化三种不同的分化程度。这种组织学类型鼻咽癌的浸润性生长一般可以引起反应性纤维组织增生。角化性鼻咽癌大约占全部鼻咽癌的 25%，罕见于 40 岁以下患者[286]。

非角化性癌几乎没有角化，其生长方式类似于膀胱移行细胞癌，包括细胞为复层，与周围间质界限分明（图4A.26），细胞边界清楚，可以出现模糊的细胞间桥。偶尔可见角化细胞。一般没有对于浸润性生长的纤维组织增生性反应。非角化性癌可有囊肿形成，伴有坏死，这种形态也可转移至颈淋巴结。此外，原发癌灶可能很小，位于黏膜下（例如隐窝上皮），表面上皮完整，难以归类，可能是一种潜隐的原发癌（图 4A.27）。这种类型的鼻咽癌最少见，约占所有鼻咽癌的 12%[286]。

未分化鼻咽癌约占所有鼻咽癌的 60%[274]，是儿科年龄组最常见的肿瘤类型[249]。肿瘤细胞特征为细胞核呈圆形，有突出的嗜酸性核仁，核染色质分散，胞浆稀少，嗜酸性到双嗜性（图 4A.28）。缺乏角化。核分裂象增加，包括非典型性核分裂象。伴随恶性上皮成分可见由成熟淋巴细胞和浆细胞组成的明显的非瘤性淋巴成分，但任何病例的淋巴浆细胞均可稀少或缺乏。可能出现其他类型炎症细胞，包括嗜酸性粒细胞和中性粒细胞，而且可

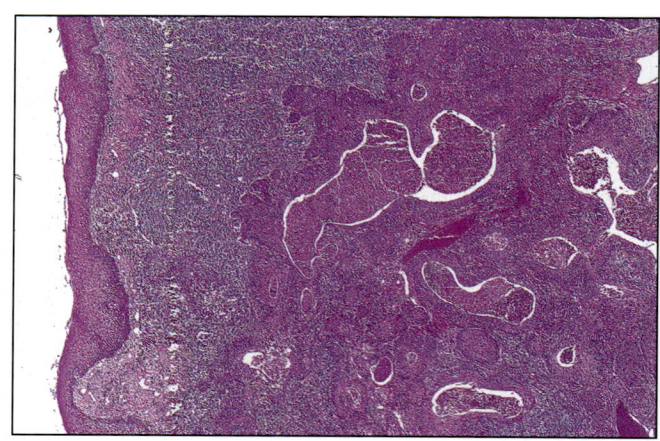

图4A.27 鼻咽非角化性癌，分化型，起源于隐窝上皮。表面上皮不显著。这可能是颈侧淋巴结转移癌的原发（隐匿）灶。因此，类似于腮裂囊肿或起源于腮裂囊肿的癌（所谓的腮裂癌）。

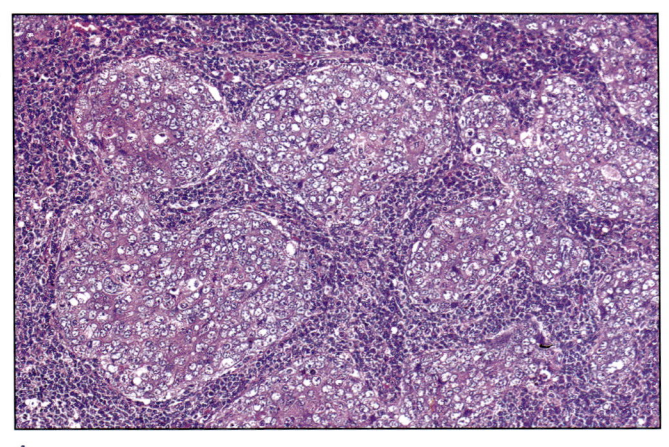
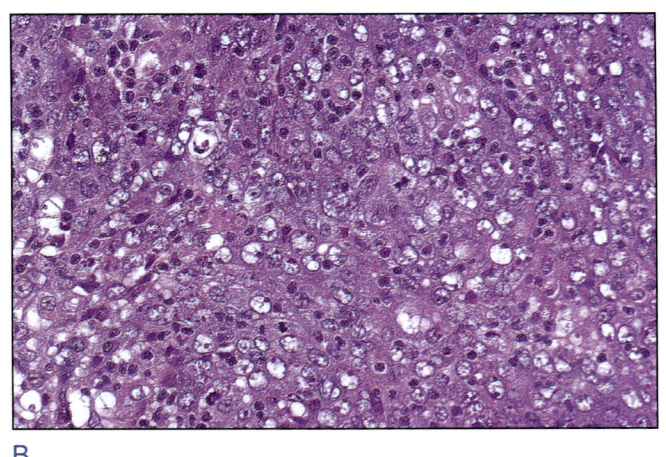

图4A.28 鼻咽非角化性癌，未分化型。（A）癌巢易见，与周围非肿瘤性淋巴细胞浸润界限分明。（B）肿瘤细胞的特征是具有大而圆的细胞核，染色质呈空泡状，有明显的嗜酸性核仁，而且有少量的嗜酸性和双嗜性胞浆。可见非肿瘤性淋巴成分。

能出现散在的上皮样肉芽肿。未分化鼻咽癌可能有合体细胞生长方式，伴有粘着或成巢的细胞，或由松散的细胞呈弥散性生长。弥漫性结构在光镜下与恶性淋巴瘤很难区分。Regaud 和 Schmincke 型鼻咽癌分别指伴有合体细胞和单个细胞生长方式的肿瘤。这些命名（及其相关的生长方式）与疾病的生物学行为无关。这种肿瘤的浸润性生长一般不引起宿主的纤维组织增生性反应。在活检标本中可能出现问题，因为良性淋巴组织细胞浸润可能超出肿瘤，从而容易造成漏诊（图4A.29）。同样，在有颈部淋巴结转移时，受累的淋巴结可能也不产生纤维组织增生性反应。

因为区分分化型非角化性和未分化型非角化性鼻咽癌没有临床或预后意义，所以不一定进行分化型和未分化型的再分类[243]。Shanmugaratnam 等[287]报道，26%的鼻咽癌具有一种以上肿瘤类型的特征。在这种情况下，应根据主要成分来分类。应该注意的是，这三种不同类型鼻咽癌之间的组织学差异并不总是清晰的，任一肿瘤均可出现重叠的组织学特征。

很少见到表现为上皮内异型增生或原位癌的前体病变。如果存在，其改变类似于上呼吸消化道其他部位肿瘤的表现，特征为出现不同程度的增厚的上皮，核深染，细胞极性消失，伴有核密集，核浆比例增高，核仁明显以及核分裂活性增加。这些改变可在上皮表面或隐窝内看见。

鼻咽癌所有三种组织学类型均可表达细胞角蛋白，包括广谱细胞角蛋白和高分子量细胞角蛋白；低分子量细胞角蛋白呈弱阳性表达（图4A.29）。不表达细胞角蛋白 7 和 20。Franchi 等估价了头颈部各种类型鳞

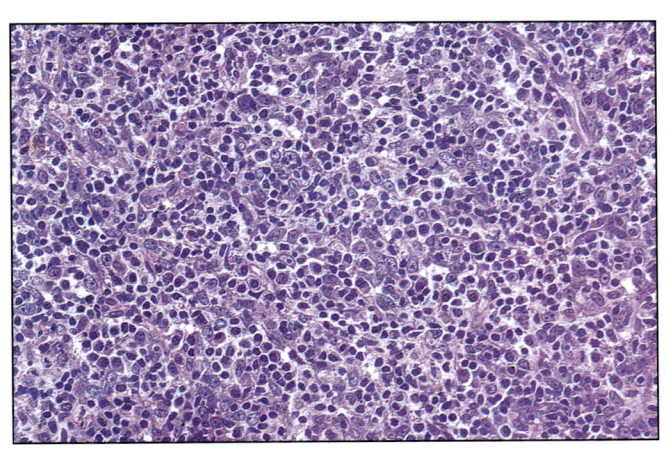
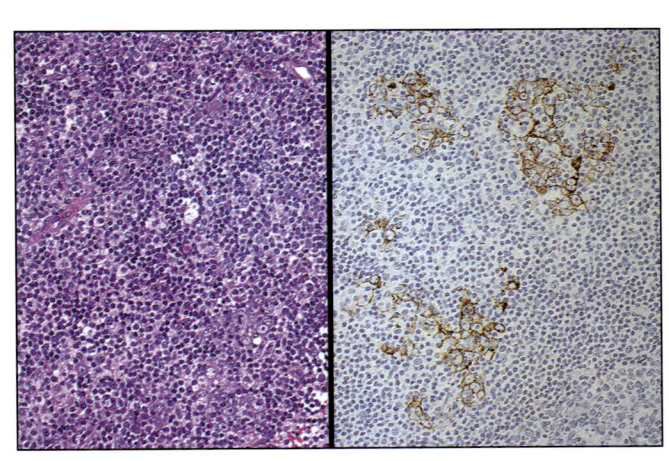

图4A.29 鼻咽非角化性癌，未分化型。（A）此病例缺乏纤维组织增生性反应，共存的非肿瘤性淋巴细胞浸润使得肿瘤细胞变得模糊，造成诊断困难。（B）细胞角蛋白染色（右）突显了肿瘤细胞的存在（左）。

状细胞癌不同的细胞角蛋白染色，发现鼻咽癌表达 CK 5/6、CK 8、CK 13 和 CK 18（表 4A.6）[288]。角化型和非角化型鼻咽癌的诊断通常容易。未分化型鼻咽癌可能难以与非 Hodgkin 恶性淋巴瘤鉴别，特别是当散在的肿瘤细胞呈弥漫性、浸润性生长时。通过免疫组化染色容易鉴别。鼻咽癌可表达细胞角蛋白，但无白细胞共同抗原（LCA）；而鼻咽部非 Hodgkin 淋巴瘤主要是 B 细胞系列，因此可表达 LCA 和 B 细胞系的标记物。

由于受鼻咽解剖学部位的限制，这些肿瘤倾向于在疾病晚期发现，因此，治疗考虑选择超高电压（65～70Gy 以上）放射治疗。角化性鳞状细胞癌总的 5 年生存率为 20%～40%，非角化性鳞状细胞癌（分化和未分化）总的 5 年生存率约为 65%[286]。诊断时的分期是最重要的预后因素。5 年疾病特异性生存率（disease-specific survival，DSS）如下：

- Ⅰ期，98%
- ⅡA-B 期，95%
- Ⅲ期，86%
- ⅣA-B 期，73%[243]

可能影响预后的因素包括：临床分期、患者的年龄和性别、角化的出现、淋巴结转移以及可能的遗传因素。临床分期较低、患者较年轻以及女性预后较好，而临床分期较高、老年患者和男性预后较差[246,287]。Reddy 等[289] 评估了 50 例鼻咽癌患者，发现角化型鼻咽癌局限进展的发生率较高，但淋巴管和（或）远处播散的发生率较低。尽管有这些发现，但角化型鼻咽癌患者的 5 年生存率还是比其他组织学亚型的鼻咽癌差，由于局部病变不能控制和淋巴结转移而引起较高的死亡率[289]。鼻咽癌常常转移到局部淋巴结，而且出现淋巴结转移使生存率大约降低 10%～20%[287]。同样，大部分鼻咽癌，特别是未分化型鼻咽癌，可转移到锁骨以下部位，包括肺、骨（肋骨和脊柱）和肝[290,291]。伴有 HLA-A_W33-C3-B58/DR3 单倍型鼻咽癌患者预后较差，而伴有 A2-C_W11-B_W46/DR9 单倍型鼻咽癌患者生存率较长[246]。对于鼻咽癌的 DNA 倍体已有研究，但结果各异[292,293]。研究提示，明显的肿瘤血管生成和 c-erbB2 表达是预后不好的指征[294]。

在鼻咽癌的治疗中，较新的治疗方法已被评估。Chua 等评估了应用诱导化学治疗和放射治疗以及单独应用放射治疗的鼻咽癌患者的长期结果。虽然他们报道应用以顺铂为基础的诱导化学治疗和放射治疗的晚期鼻咽癌患者，复发轻度（但有意义）减少，疾病特异性生存率有所改善，但总生存率无明显提高[295]。鼻咽癌患者同时或异时发生第二个原发性恶性肿瘤的危险性约为 4%[296]。第二个恶性肿瘤倾向于发生在上呼吸消化道。

鼻窦部未分化癌
Sinonasal undifferentiated carcinoma (SNUC)

鼻窦部未分化癌最初的定义由 Frierson 等[297] 报道，它是组织发生不明的鼻腔和副鼻窦的高级别恶性上皮性肿瘤，伴有或不伴有神经内分泌分化，但无鳞状或腺体分化的证据。随后，WHO 分类将鼻窦部未分化癌定义为组织发生不明的高度侵袭性、具有独特临床病理学特征的癌，一般表现为局灶广泛性的病变；它由多形性肿瘤细胞组成，常伴有坏死，应与淋巴上皮（和其他）癌或嗅神经母细胞瘤鉴别[298]。

鼻窦未分化癌是一种罕见肿瘤，已报道的病例不到 100 例。发病以男性为主（男女比为 2:1～3:1）[298,299]，发病年龄分布广泛，从 20～90 岁不等，诊断时的中位年龄为 50～60 岁[297,299]。一般来说，鼻窦未分化癌在诊断时是广泛的病变，累及多个部位，包括鼻腔、一个

表4A.6	鼻窦部和鼻咽部不同类型癌的细胞角蛋白表达						
	AE1/AE3	CK 5/6	CK 7	CK 8	CK 13	CK 14	CK 19
鳞状细胞癌	+	+ (9/10)	+ (6/10)	+ (9/10)	+ (9/10)	+ (8/10)	+ (9/10)
非角化性鳞状细胞癌	+	+ (9/10)	−	+ (9/10)	+ (9/10)	+ (8/10)	+ (9/10)
鼻窦部未分化癌	+	−	+ (3/6)	+ (6/6)	−	−	+ (3/6)
鼻咽癌，未分化型	+	+ (4/5)	−	+ (4/5)	+ (4/5)	−	+ (5/5)

Reproduced from Franchi et al.[288]

或多个副鼻窦、颅底、眼眶、颅底和脑[297,300]。多数患者为单侧性病变，但双侧性病变也可发生。典型的是，病人出现短期的多种症状，包括鼻塞、鼻出血、眼球突出、视力障碍（例如复视）、面部疼痛和颅神经受累的症状。放射学检查（CT扫描、MRI）常显示较大的（鼻窦）肿块，一般伴有局部浸润性生长，延伸到骨外，局限于眼眶和（或）颅骨受累[299]，也可向颅内延伸。

鼻窦未分化癌是一种组织学发生不明确的肿瘤。鼻窦未分化癌似来源于鼻黏膜上皮，因而是由外胚层衍化而来。然而，由于嗅神经母细胞瘤和神经内分泌癌具有重叠的临床、光镜、免疫组化和超微结构特征，因而推测细胞起源可能与鼻黏膜和嗅觉上皮均有关系。通过免疫组化和电镜显示的神经内分泌特征，Mills[301]提出鼻窦未分化癌可能是在分类上基本与肺大细胞（神经内分泌）癌相同的一种神经内分泌癌。已有报道，可有非常局限的鳞状上皮分化病灶出现，这种所见支持表面鼻黏膜上皮来源[302]。

鼻窦未分化癌病因不清。EB病毒检查一般阴性[303,304]，尽管已有报道在亚洲和意大利的鼻窦未分化癌患者发现有EB病毒RNA，但在其他西方国家的鼻窦未分化癌患者中却没有发现EB病毒RNA[305,306]。根据报道，某些病例发生于鼻咽癌患者放射治疗之后[303]。没有特异的病因与鼻窦未分化癌的发生相关，但在鼻窦未分化癌患者已证实与吸烟和接触镍有关[297]。视网膜母细胞瘤基因缺失也与鼻窦未分化癌的发生有关[307]。

鼻窦未分化癌通常为较大的肿瘤，典型者最大径可达4 cm以上，倾向于呈覃样生长，边缘不清，浸润邻近结构和（或）解剖部位，包括骨的破坏。组织学特征为增生的细胞丰富，伴有不同的生长方式，包括小梁状、片块样、带状、实性、小叶状和器官样结构（图4A.30）。可见表面受累，表现为重度异型增生/原位癌，但通常有溃疡形成，妨碍观察表面上皮来源的证据。浸润细胞由多形性细胞组成，细胞核中等到大，圆形到卵圆形，深染到空泡状，核仁不明显到显著，胞浆量不等，嗜酸性，细胞膜不清，但某些病例细胞边界可能清楚；偶尔可见胞浆透明的细胞。核浆比例高。核分裂活性增加，包括非典型性核分裂象，而且常有明显肿瘤坏死（汇合区域和单个细胞）和凋亡（图4A.30）。经常出现淋巴管浸润和亲神经性。鳞状或腺体分化不明显；然而，近来有证据显示，只要绝大部分肿瘤显示鼻窦未分化癌的形态学特征，鼻窦未分化癌出现非常局灶的鳞状分化是可以接受的[302]。见不到神经原纤维物质和真正的神经菊形团。

组织化学研究对于诊断鼻窦未分化癌没有帮助；上皮黏液染色阴性。不同病例的免疫组化抗原分布可能不同，但是鼻窦未分化癌对于上皮性标记物一直存在免疫反应，包括广谱角蛋白和单一的角蛋白（即CK 7、CK 8和CK 19）；广谱角蛋白反应常常强烈而弥漫。CK 4、CK 5/CK 6和CK 14染色为阴性（表4A.6）[288]。*p63*有不同的反应。已报道不到一半的病例表达EMA、NSE或*p53*[304]，仅有少数病例表达突触素、嗜铬素、S-100蛋白或Leu-7。通常缺乏波形蛋白、肌肉标记物（结蛋白、肌红蛋白、myf-4、肌动蛋白）、血液淋巴标记物（LCA、B和T细胞）、黑色素细胞标记物（HMB-45、melan-A）和CD99（Ewing标记物）。电镜观察可见少数有膜包绕的致密核心的神经分泌颗粒，偶见发育不良的桥粒[297,301,308]。

鼻窦未分化癌的鉴别诊断包括嗅神经母细胞瘤（高级别）、小细胞未分化神经内分泌癌、鼻咽型未分化癌[303]、淋巴上皮癌、黏膜恶性黑色素瘤、鼻型自然杀伤细胞（NK）/T细胞淋巴瘤、横纹肌肉瘤以及其他肿

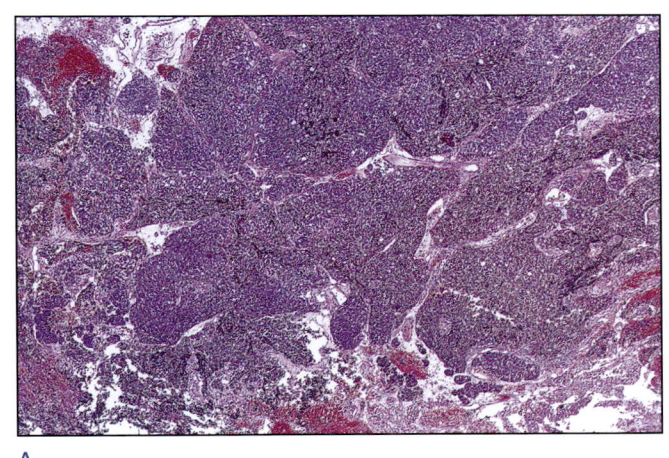
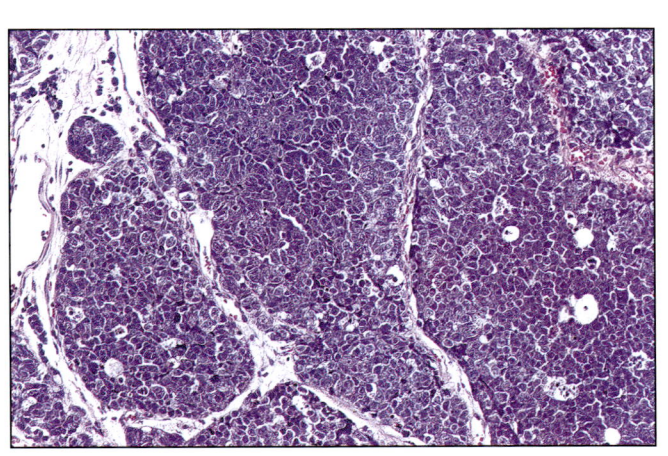

图4A.30 鼻窦未分化癌。（A）细胞丰富的浸润性肿瘤，显示小梁状和小叶状生长方式。（B）在较高放大倍数下，浸润细胞具有圆形到卵圆形、深染和多形性细胞核，核仁明显，核分裂活性增加，并有单个细胞坏死。

瘤。虽然通过光镜评估可以识别其差异，但对于一个假定的肿瘤的鉴别诊断常常需要依靠免疫组化染色。在鼻窦和鼻咽的上皮性恶性肿瘤中，据报道角化性鳞状细胞癌、非角化性鳞状细胞癌、鼻窦未分化癌以及鼻咽未分化癌的细胞角蛋白染色有所不同（表 4A.7）[288]。

鼻窦未分化癌需要进行强化的多学科治疗，包括手术切除和辅助性治疗（放射治疗，化学治疗）。然而，鼻窦未分化癌是一种高度侵袭性的肿瘤，手术不能完全根除，对于放射治疗也无反应。Frierson 等[297]报道带病患者的中位生存期为 4 个月，其他研究报道中位生存期低于 18 个月[254,258,259]，5 年生存率低于 20%[311]。Deutsch 等[312]报道，先放射治疗，再进行根治性手术切除，随后给予化学治疗（环磷酰胺、阿霉素和长春新碱）可以提高患者生存率。这些作者以及其他一些作者[313]推荐不管疾病的范围如何，均应用这种治疗方案，大剂量化学治疗和自体骨髓移植已应用[314]。对一般情况好、肿瘤局限于颅内或眶内的患者，提倡首先化学治疗，随后进行颅面部切除[315]。对于那些疾病处于晚期而不能手术的患者，单单进行放化疗可以明显减轻症状。最近发现，诱导化学治疗之后同时进行放化疗是鼻窦未分化癌的一种具有潜力的治疗策略[316]。局部复发常见，同时也是发病和死亡的主要原因[299]。可发生骨、脑、肝和颈部淋巴结的转移[304]。

嗅神经母细胞瘤
Olfactory neuroblastoma（ONB）

嗅神经母细胞瘤被认为是起源于鼻窦嗅膜的一种恶性神经外胚层肿瘤。这种肿瘤有不同名称，包括嗅基板肿瘤（olfactory placode tumor）、感觉神经母细胞瘤（esthesioneuroblastoma）、感觉神经细胞瘤（esthesioneurocytoma）、感觉神经上皮瘤（esthesioneuroepithelioma）和感觉神经瘤（esthesioneuroma）。嗅神经母细胞瘤好像来源于鼻中隔上 1/3～1/2、筛板和上鼻甲上内侧表面的嗅觉神经上皮[317]。随着年龄增长，嗅觉上皮退化并被呼吸上皮取代[317]。嗅觉神经上皮由双极感觉神经元、支持细胞和贮备（基底）细胞构成。后者具有核分裂活性，推测是嗅神经母细胞瘤的祖代细胞。

嗅神经母细胞瘤是一种不常见的恶性肿瘤，大约占鼻窦肿瘤的 2%～3%。无性别差异[318]。发病年龄分布广泛，从 3～90 岁不等，10～20 岁到 50～60 岁为两个发病年龄高峰[318-323]。主要症状为单侧鼻塞和鼻出血；不常见表现包括嗅觉丧失、头痛、疼痛、流泪以及眼功能障碍[320]。最常见发生部位是筛板区域的鼻腔上部；常有筛窦受累。"异位"起源于鼻腔下部，任何一个副鼻窦（例如上颌窦）和鼻咽部均可发生[324]。放射学检查显示，鼻窦肿块引起鼻窦浑浊，伴或不伴骨破坏。嗅神经母细胞瘤可能伴有钙化，X 线照片分析可见斑点状结构。MRI 研究证实有血管病变存在，注射钆（gadolinium）后加强扫描在 T1 加强图像上可以见到[325]。

尚无已知的病因学因素。投予二乙基亚硝胺给大田鼠[326,327]以及投予 N- 亚硝基哌啶给鼠[328]可引起组织学表现与嗅神经母细胞瘤相同的鼻肿瘤。关于嗅神经母细胞瘤包含在外周神经外胚层肿瘤（PNET）范畴内的资料是矛盾的。传统上，PNET 对于识别 Ewing 肉瘤细胞表面糖蛋白 p30/32^{MIC2} 的单克隆抗体有反应[329,330]，而且 t（11；12）染色体易位，伴有 EWS/FL1 基因融合[331]。根据嗅神经母细胞瘤有 t（11；12）染色体易位[332]和存在 EWS/FLI1 基因融合[333]的报道，这些资料支持嗅神经母细胞瘤属于与 Ewing 肉瘤有关的 PNET 的范畴。然而，应用免疫组化、荧光原位杂交和 RT-PCR 的其他研究未能发现这些 PNET 的"标记物"，也不能证实嗅神经母细胞瘤存在这种易位[334-338]。因此，至少在目前还是应该将嗅神经母细胞瘤看作与 PNET 和 Ewing 肉瘤家族肿瘤明显不同的肿瘤。

嗅神经母细胞瘤大体表现为软的息肉样肿块，表面光泽，有黏膜被覆，肿瘤大小不同，从直径不到 1 cm 的小结节到充满鼻腔的肿块，可扩展到邻近副鼻窦和鼻咽部。根据 Hyams 的定义，组织学表现分为四级（表 4A.8）[339]。Ⅰ级是高分化肿瘤；呈小叶状结构，小叶之间彼此连接。肿瘤细胞分化好，具有均一的圆形到空泡状细胞核，有或无核仁（图 4A.31），细胞边界不清。核被神经原纤维物质包绕。常可见假玫瑰花形（Homer Wright rosettes）。也能见到不同程度的钙化。小叶间纤维间质常含有多量血管。缺乏核分裂活性和坏死。Ⅱ级肿瘤与Ⅰ级病变有许多相同的组织学特征，但不易见到神经原纤维成分，肿瘤细胞核多形性明显。可见散在的核分裂象。Ⅲ级肿瘤可以保持小叶状结构，伴有富于血管的间质。与Ⅰ级或Ⅱ级肿瘤相比，这些肿瘤的特征是增生的肿瘤细胞丰富，细胞间变和深染，而且核分裂活性增加。可见坏死。局部可以出现神经原纤维成分，但与Ⅰ级或Ⅱ级肿瘤相比则不明显得多（图 4A.32）。可见真正的神经玫瑰花形（Flexner-Wintersteiner rosettes）（图 4A.33）；然而，一般来说这些结构并不常见。缺乏钙化。Ⅳ级肿瘤也可以保持总的小叶状结构，但在所有组织学分级中，Ⅳ肿瘤成分最不分化，间变最明显。在这些高级别肿瘤中，浸润细胞的特征是核具有多形性，常有明显的嗜酸性核仁，胞浆不清楚。常见坏死，核分裂活性增加，包括非典型性核分裂象。可见真正的神经菊形团，但是如同Ⅲ级嗅神经母细胞瘤一样，并不常见。一般缺乏神经原纤维成分。缺乏钙化。

表4A.7 鼻窦恶性肿瘤免疫组化(选择性)反应

	CK	NSE	嗜铬素	突触囊泡蛋白	S-100蛋白	HMB	LCA	CD56	CD99	波形蛋白	结蛋白	Myf4
鳞状细胞癌	+	−	−	−	−	−	−	−	−	−	−	−
鼻窦未分化癌	+	V	−	−	−	−	−	−	−	−	−	−
嗅神经母细胞瘤	−	+	V	V	+[a]	−	−	−	−	−	−	−
小"燕麦"细胞未分化神经内分泌癌	+	+	+	+	+	−	−	+	−	−	−	−
黏膜恶性黑色素瘤	−	−	−	−	+	+	−	−	−	+	−	−
鼻型NK/T细胞淋巴瘤	−	−	−	−	−	−	V	−	−	V	−	−
横纹肌肉瘤	−	−	−	−	−	−	−	−	−	+	+	+
原始(外周)神经外胚层肿瘤/骨外Ewing肉瘤(PNET)	R+	V	−	V	V	−	−	−	+	+	−	−

HMB: HMB-45(以及其他黑色素细胞标记物, Melan A); LCA: 白细胞共同抗原; CD99: Ewing标记物。
+, 阳性; −, 阴性; V, 阳性程度不定; R+, 阳性罕见
[a], 位于周围的支持细胞阳性。

表4A.8	嗅神经母细胞瘤的Hyam组织学分级方法[339] ©1982年美国临床病理医师学会			
组织学特征	I级	II级	III级	IV级
结构	小叶状	小叶状	小叶状±	小叶状±
多形性	缺乏到轻度	存在	明显	显著
神经原纤维基质	明显	存在	可能存在	缺乏
菊形团	存在[a]	存在[a]	可能存在[b]	可能存在[b]
核分裂象	缺乏	存在	明显	显著
坏死	缺乏	缺乏	存在	明显
腺体	可能存在	可能存在	可能存在	可能存在
钙化	不定	不定	缺乏	缺乏

[a]Homer Wright 玫瑰花形团（假玫瑰花形）
[b]Flexner-Wintersteiner 玫瑰花形（真正的神经玫瑰花形）

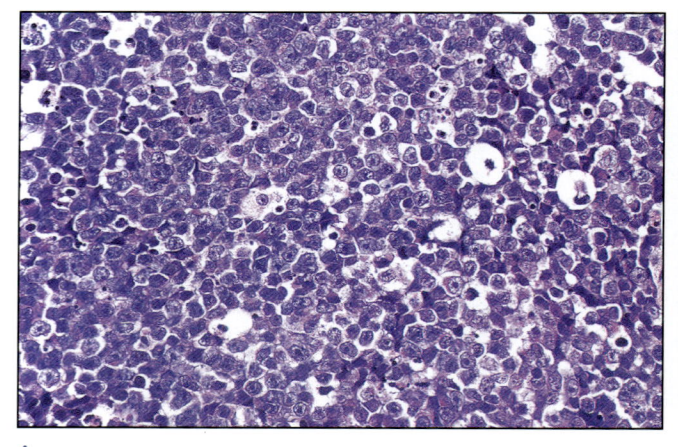

A

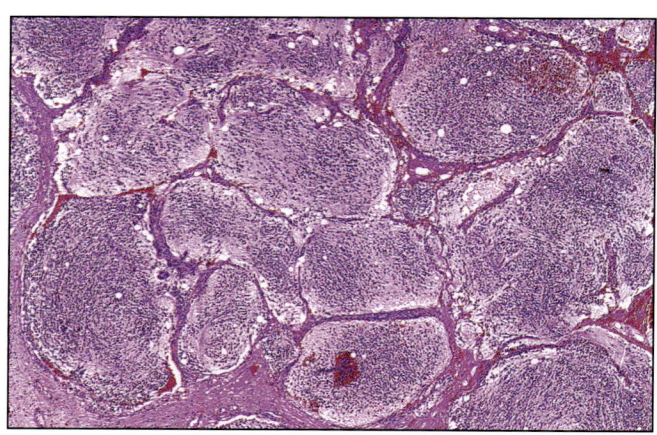

A

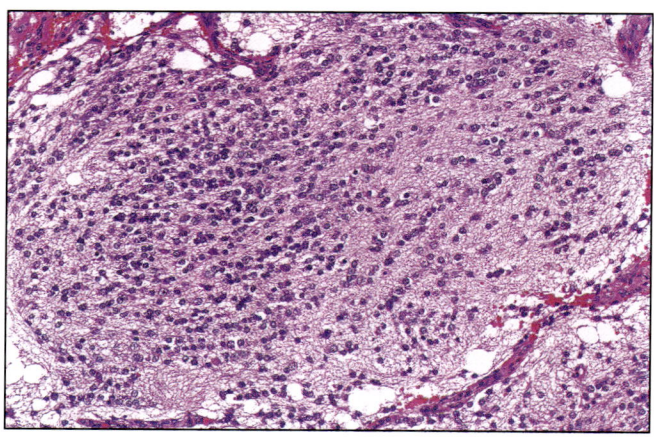

B

图4A.31 嗅神经母细胞瘤，I级。（A）典型的分叶状生长方式；（B）均一表现的圆形细胞周围有神经原纤维物质包绕。

图4A.32 嗅神经母细胞瘤，III级。（A）与较低级别的嗅神经母细胞瘤不同，这种高级别的肿瘤缺乏神经原纤维基质，是一种伴有核分裂活性增加的多形性细胞浸润。在这种情况下，免疫组化染色对于诊断和与其他恶性肿瘤的鉴别诊断尤为重要。（B）嗅神经母细胞瘤，不论组织学分级如何，神经元特异性烯醇化酶均呈阳性反应，且（C）显示S-100蛋白染色，通常局限于肿瘤细胞巢周围（支持细胞样排列）。

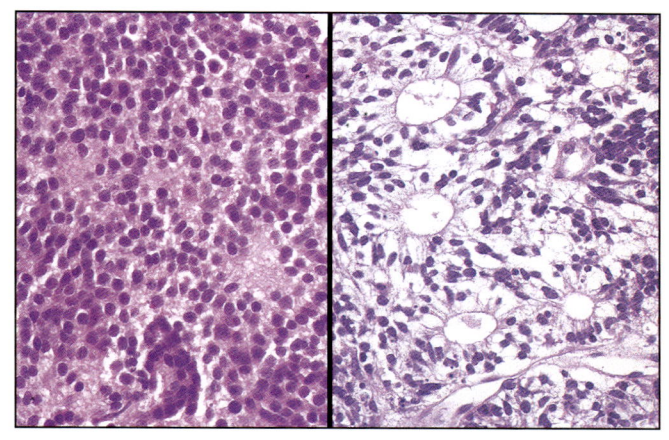

图4A.33 嗅神经母细胞瘤伴有玫瑰花形。本图比较见于Ⅰ级和Ⅱ级嗅神经母细胞瘤的Homer Wright假玫瑰花形（左）和Flexner-wintersteiner真正的神经玫瑰花形（右）。前者的特征为成群的细胞围绕神经原纤维基质成环状排列，但无明显的基底膜，而后者细胞排列成腺样结构，围绕着内衬清楚细胞膜的间隙。

极少数情况下，嗅神经母细胞瘤可与腺癌、鳞状细胞癌或未分化癌病灶共存，此时被称为混合性嗅神经母细胞瘤和癌[340]。Miller及其同事[340]提出，嗅觉上皮的基底细胞是这些混合性肿瘤的祖细胞。另外，这些混合性肿瘤也可来源于嗅上皮下的浆液黏液性腺体（Bowman腺）。这位作者曾见到少数这样的肿瘤，我们将其命名为嗅癌（olfactory carcinomas）。

一般情况下，通过光镜检查容易识别和诊断低级别的嗅神经母细胞瘤。辅助检查可能有助于诊断，特别是组织学分级较高的肿瘤。在嗅神经母细胞瘤诊断中，组织化学染色已被免疫组化所取代。

最一致的标记物是NSE（图4A.32）。S-100蛋白一般局限于沿肿瘤性小叶周边排列的支持细胞，但较高级别的嗅神经母细胞瘤这种细胞可能稀少（图4A.32）。多数病例还出现突触素、神经细丝蛋白、Ⅲ类β-微管蛋白和微管相关蛋白反应，而且可能出现不同程度的嗜铬素、GFAP和Leu-7免疫反应[341,342]。细胞角蛋白常为阴性；某些病例可以出现斑片状点状分布的阳性细胞，或少数情况下出现弥散性阳性反应。缺乏上皮性标记物，包括EMA和CEA。也不表达LCA、HMB-45、结蛋白和CD99。应用Ki-67和MIB-1进行增生标记研究显示，增生指数高达10%～50%，流式细胞分析显示多倍体/非整倍体比例增高[343,344]。电子显微镜检查是一种有用的辅助诊断工具，可以发现直径为80～250 nm的致密核心神经分泌颗粒[324,345,346]。此外，可见神经细丝和神经微管，偶尔可见神经鞘样细胞。

鉴别诊断包括本章讨论的各种鼻窦其他恶性肿瘤。

虽然通过光镜评估可以辨认其中的差异，但是一个肿瘤与所有这些类型的肿瘤的鉴别诊断常需依靠免疫组化染色（表4A.7）。

治疗选择完全手术切除（颅面切除术，包括切除筛板），随后进行全程放射治疗[321,322,347]。对于晚期不能切除的肿瘤和（或）有播散性疾病的患者，应用化学治疗取得成功的机会有限[348]。包括以铂为基础的大剂量化学治疗方案和自体骨髓移植可以取得长期生存的效果[349-351]。已有报道，总的5年、10年和15年生存率分别为78%、71%和68%[349]。最初采取多科性治疗，低级别肿瘤有80%的5年生存率，而高级别肿瘤的5年生存率为40%[347]。复发多数发生于最初2年以内[322]。最常见的是局部复发，复发率在30%左右。预后通常与Kadish确定的临床分期有关[352]（表4A.9），A、B、C期肿瘤患者的5年生存率分别是75%、68%、41%[320,352]。研究发现，完全切除肿瘤比临床分期具有更为重要的预后意义[323]。与预后有关的其他因素包括组织学分级、增生率和倍体。根据报告，组织学上较低级别（Ⅰ级和Ⅱ级）肿瘤的5年生存率高于较高级别（Ⅲ级和Ⅳ级）的肿瘤[353]。增生指数高和倍体/非整倍体比率高与发病率（即肿瘤复发和转移）以及死亡率（即生存率降低）增加有关[343,344]。多数肿瘤的行为表现为局部侵袭性病变，主要累及邻近结构（眼眶和颅腔）。在初次诊断后数年可以出现局部复发和远处转移。大约15～70%的患者有局部复发，10%～25%出现颈淋巴结转移，大约10%～60%发生远处转移[320,327,349,354]。较常见的转移部位包括淋巴结、肺和骨。所有组织学分级的肿瘤均能发生转移。

神经内分泌癌
Neuroendocrine carcinoma（NEC）

神经内分泌癌是一组异源性的恶性肿瘤，沿着上皮和神经内分泌细胞系呈现不同的分化。神经内分泌癌的

表4A.9	嗅神经母细胞瘤的临床分期	
分期	肿瘤范围	5年生存率
A	肿瘤局限于鼻腔	75%～91%
B	肿瘤累及鼻腔和一个或一个以上鼻窦	68%～71%
C	肿瘤延伸到鼻窦腔外	41%～47%

Modified from Elkon et al.[320] and Kadish et al.[352]

分类仍有争议。有些作者将这些肿瘤分成3种类型：（1）类癌；（2）非典型性类癌；和（3）小细胞癌[355,356]。其他作者根据分化程度分类：（1）高分化神经内分泌癌（相当于类癌）；（2）中分化神经内分泌癌（相当于非典型性类癌）；和（3）低分化神经内分泌癌[相当于小"燕麦"细胞未分化神经内分泌癌（SCUNC）][357]。少数作者将小细胞神经内分泌癌进一步分为小细胞亚型和大细胞亚型[358]。根据由来已久的术语和为了减少混淆，这一节中将应用WHO提出的类癌、非典型性类癌和小细胞癌分类[355,359]。然而应该记住，"非典型性"类癌完全是一种致死性肿瘤，而"非典型性"这个术语不应给临床医师造成安全的错误感觉，即认为这种肿瘤在生物学行为上与相对惰性的"典型"类癌仅有轻微差异。

一般来说，所有这3种亚型的神经内分泌癌在头颈部均不常见，在鼻窦部更是如此。头颈部最常见的神经内分泌癌亚型或许是小"燕麦"细胞未分化神经内分泌癌，其次为非典型性类癌，类癌最不常见。实际上，小"燕麦"细胞未分化神经内分泌癌可以发生于上呼吸消化道的任何部位，但特别容易累及喉、涎腺（腮腺）和鼻窦部[356-362]。鼻窦部小"燕麦"细胞未分化神经内分泌癌无性别差异，发病年龄范围广泛，从20～30岁到70～80岁不等，平均年龄为49岁[363]。鼻窦部小"燕麦"细胞未分化神经内分泌癌最常见于上鼻腔或下鼻腔，常扩展至邻近的副鼻窦（即上颌窦和筛窦）[363]。在缺乏鼻腔受累的情况下，可以发生原发性副鼻窦疾病。出现的症状和体征包括鼻塞、鼻出血和疼痛。局部浸润可能导致眼球突出。

不论发生部位，小"燕麦"细胞未分化神经内分泌癌的组织学表现相同。这些肿瘤细胞丰富，伴有不同的生长方式，包括片块状、条索状或带状。细胞小，深染，有卵圆形至梭形的细胞核，无核仁，胞浆稀少。容易见到明显的细胞多形性、核浆比例增高、核分裂活性增加、融合性坏死区域和单个细胞坏死。特征性表现是可见肿瘤细胞挤压假象。偶尔可以出现鳞状细胞灶；腺体或导管分化罕见。尽管少见，但小"燕麦"细胞未分化神经内分泌癌可见神经玫瑰花形[360,361]。小"燕麦"细胞未分化神经内分泌癌是浸润性肿瘤，常伴有淋巴血管和神经周围浸润。

小"燕麦"细胞未分化神经内分泌癌可有上皮性黏液[361,364]。可见嗜银，但缺乏亲银染色。由于分化低，小"燕麦"细胞未分化神经内分泌癌的免疫组化抗原表达可因病例不同而不同。对以下抗体可有不同程度的表达：细胞角蛋白、嗜铬素、突触素、NSE和S-100蛋白[361,364]。细胞角蛋白反应表现为核旁点状或球状阳性产物，类似于Merkel细胞癌的特征性表现。Chan等[365]比较了不同解剖学部位的小"燕麦"细胞未分化神经内分泌癌与Merkel细胞癌的CK20染色结果，发现CK20更易在Merkel细胞癌中出现。此外，那些被诊断为涎腺来源的小"燕麦"细胞未分化神经内分泌癌的肿瘤，包括细胞角蛋白核旁点状染色结构，CK20也呈阳性反应。这些结果提示被称为涎腺小"燕麦"细胞未分化神经内分泌癌的肿瘤实际上是Merkel细胞癌，或来源于皮肤部位，继发累及腮腺，或起源于腮腺内。少数情况下，小"燕麦"细胞未分化神经内分泌癌可以出现降钙素（calcitonin）反应，但LCA、CK 20、HMB-45和CD99阴性。超微结构检查可能显示50～200nm的神经分泌颗粒[361,364]。细胞连接复合体稀少，包括桥粒和张力丝，通常缺乏腔隙（细胞间和细胞内）。

鉴别诊断包括本章讨论过的各种其他鼻窦恶性肿瘤。虽然通过光镜检查可以辨别其间的差异，但对于假定的肿瘤，鉴别所有这些类型肿瘤常常需要依靠免疫组化染色（表4A.7）。

小"燕麦"细胞未分化神经内分泌癌最好采取多学科综合治疗，包括系统的化学治疗和放射治疗[361]。由于其转移率高，所以并不认为手术治疗恰当[361]。其为高度恶性的肿瘤；据报道，头颈部小"燕麦"细胞未分化神经内分泌癌的中位生存率是14.5个月[366]。常发生局部复发和远处转移，其发生率分别为45%和35%[363]。可转移至颈部淋巴结、肺、肝和骨。

黏膜恶性黑色素瘤
Mucosal malignant melanoma（MMM）

恶性黑色素瘤是神经嵴衍生的肿瘤，起源于黑色素细胞，并证实有黑色素细胞分化。所有恶性黑色素瘤大约15%～25%来源于头颈部[337]。在头颈部恶性黑色素瘤中，80%以上为皮肤来源。上呼吸消化道的黏膜恶性黑色素瘤占所有部位恶性黑色素瘤的0.5%～3%[368]。在头颈部非皮肤恶性黑色素瘤中，多数为眼睛来源，大约6%～8%起源于上呼吸消化道黏膜[367]。认为鼻窦部是黏膜恶性黑色素瘤不常见的发生部位，占所有鼻窦肿瘤的5%以下[369]。不论发生部位如何，上呼吸消化道的黏膜恶性黑色素瘤男性比女性常见。这是一种主要发生于成年人的疾病，其发病年龄广泛，但最常见于50～60岁和70～80岁的[367,370-372]。大多数上呼吸消化道黏膜恶性黑色素瘤病例发生在白人，但也可发生于黑人。症状不同，取决于发生部位，鼻窦和鼻咽部肿瘤的症状包括呼吸不畅、鼻出血、疼痛、不易愈合的溃疡和异型增生。在鼻窦部鼻腔受累比副鼻窦常见。在鼻腔，最常见的发生部位是鼻中隔（前部）（图4A.34）和鼻侧壁。在鼻窦，上颌窦是最常见部位，其次为筛骨、额窦和蝶窦。鼻腔和副鼻窦常同时发生黑色素瘤，或为直接

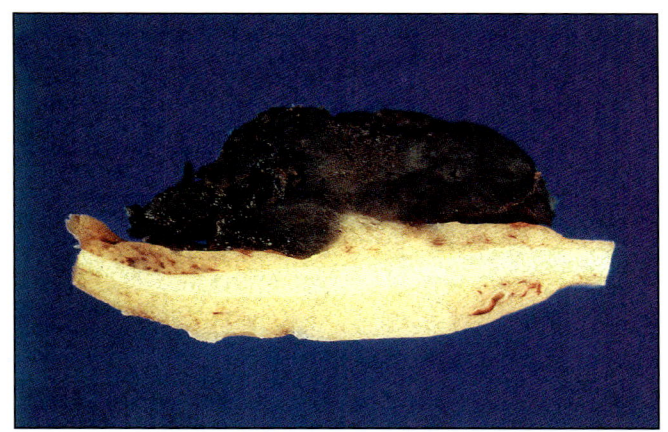

图4A.34 鼻中隔的黏膜恶性黑色素瘤。

扩展的结果，或为多中心性肿瘤。黏膜恶性黑色素瘤的病因不明。然而，Reuter 和 Woodruff[373] 推测吸烟在喉恶性黑色素瘤的发生中具有重要作用。

可见各种大体表现：肿瘤可以为息肉状或无蒂，表现为棕色、黑色、粉红色或白色的易碎到橡胶样硬度的肿块，大小从 1 cm 至更大，可引起阻塞的症状和体征。一般情况下，常见表面溃疡。在具有完整表面上皮的肿瘤中，通常可见肿瘤与表面上皮的连续性（交界性或 Paget 样改变）。交界性或原位成分的出现提示黏膜恶性黑色素瘤来源于表面上皮，但不是诊断黏膜恶性黑色素瘤的必要条件，因为黑色素细胞可出现于上呼吸消化道的浆液黏液腺和黏膜下层[374-376]。

黏膜恶性黑色素瘤的细胞形态学特征包括最常见的上皮样细胞和（或）梭形细胞（图 4A.35）。伴有小细胞形态学改变的肿瘤也相对常见[377]。以上皮样细胞为主或完全由上皮样细胞组成的黏膜恶性黑色素瘤的生长方式不同，可为实性、器官样、巢状、小梁状和腺泡状，或为这些结构的任意组合。细胞呈圆形到卵圆形，倾向于有明显的多形性，核浆比例增加，核呈空泡状到深染，有明显的嗜酸性核仁，胞浆嗜酸性到透明。可出现核内假包涵体和细胞核变形。上皮样细胞可能具有浆细胞样特征，表现为细胞核偏心和胞浆嗜酸性。然而，与浆细胞增生不同，核染色质致密深染，而且没有核旁透明带。以梭形细胞为主或完全由梭形细胞组成的黏膜恶性黑色素瘤，可以呈席纹状或束状生长方式。细胞卵圆形到雪茄形，具有明显的多形性，伴有大的空泡状到深染的细胞核，缺乏明显的核仁，具有少量嗜酸性胞浆。梭形细胞黏膜恶性黑色素瘤可以伴有黏液样间质。这两种细胞形态的黏膜恶性黑色素瘤均常常出现坏死和明显的核分裂象，伴有非典型性核分裂象。不常见的特征包括瘤巨细胞以及腺样或鳞状分化[368]。

光镜下，黏膜恶性黑色素瘤可有大量黑色素沉着，但是大约 1/3 的病例仅为局灶性微弱的色素沉着，或为无色素沉着的肿瘤[372,373]。组织化学和免疫组化染色有助于黏膜恶性黑色素瘤的诊断。组织化学染色在辨认黑色素方面可能具有很高的价值，表现为亲银和嗜银染色阳性；然而，免疫组化染色仍是诊断的金标准。选择的免疫组化诊断参数是上皮样细胞和梭形细胞出现 S-100 蛋白、HMB-45 和波形蛋白阳性染色[368,372]。S-100 蛋白和 HMB-45 染色均强，而且染色范围弥漫。例外的情况是纤维组织增生性黑色素瘤 HMB-45 染色可能没有反应。此外，黑色素瘤还表达 T311（抗酪氨酸酶）、A103 和 D5[378]。而不表达细胞角蛋白、EMA 或肌源性标记物。

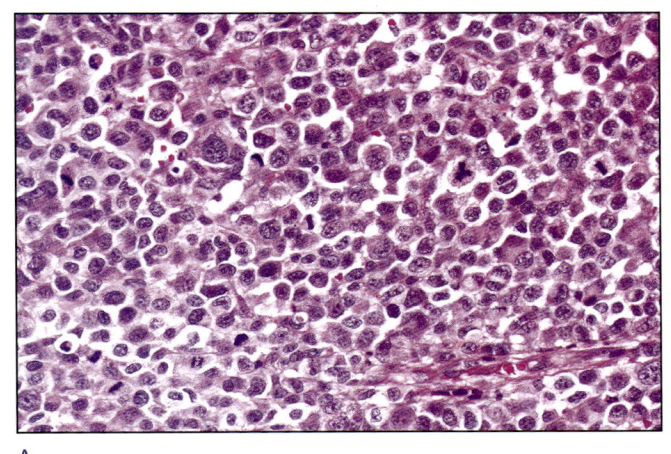

A

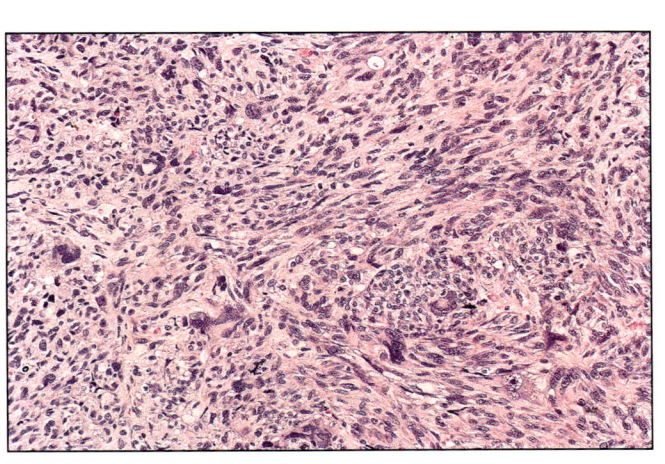

B

图4A.35 鼻窦黏膜恶性黑色素瘤。这些肿瘤可具有不均一的细胞形态，包括：（A）多形性的上皮样细胞，核大，核仁突出，核变形，核分裂活性增加。（B）多形性的梭形细胞，伴有席纹状的生长方式，类似于间叶性肿瘤。

超微结构检查可见黑色素小体和前黑色素小体[368]。

鉴别诊断包括本章已讨论过的各种其他鼻窦恶性肿瘤。虽然通过光镜观察可以辨别其间的差异，但是对于一个给定的肿瘤来说，鉴别所有这些类型的肿瘤常常需要依靠免疫组化染色（表4A.7）。

不论其组织来源如何，黏膜恶性黑色素瘤是一组侵袭性的高度致死性肿瘤。治疗选择根治性的手术切除。在黏膜恶性黑色素瘤的治疗中，放射治疗或化学治疗对于局部或转移性病变的作用似乎有限，现在用于辅助性治疗[379]。总之，所有上呼吸消化道部位发生的黏膜恶性黑色素瘤预后都差，5年生存率一般小于30%[380]。鼻窦部黏膜恶性黑色素瘤，其5年DSS从17%～46%不等[380]。患有黏膜恶性黑色素瘤的患者，没有被认为有治愈的期限。众所周知，恶性黑色素瘤在最初诊断后保持一段很长的休眠期，仅在数年到数十年后才有表现。在"治愈"数十年后，可以出现复发、转移和死亡。转移最常发生于肺、淋巴结和脑。在做出上呼吸消化道原发性黏膜恶性黑色素瘤的诊断之前，必须排除来自于表皮的原发性恶性黑色素瘤，甚或其他以黏膜为基础的恶性黑色素瘤的转移。皮肤恶性黑色素瘤可以自发性消退，休止多年以后重现为转移性病变（远离发生肿瘤的原发性皮肤部位）[381]。在缺乏从前或同时发生的其他部位恶性黑色素瘤的情况下，才可以将黏膜恶性黑色素瘤考虑为原发性肿瘤。

鼻窦（黏膜）腺癌
Sinonasal (mucosal) adenocarcinoma

鼻窦部腺癌占这个部位所有原发性恶性肿瘤的10%～20%[382]，但除了涎腺型肿瘤以外，它仅占所有鼻窦部恶性肿瘤的6.3%[383]。在鼻窦部可见两种主要类型的非涎腺型腺癌，即肠型腺癌（intestinal-type adenocarcinoma，ITAC）和非肠型腺癌。

肠型腺癌 Intestinal-type adenocarcinomas

肠型腺癌是鼻窦部的恶性上皮性腺体肿瘤，其组织学表现类似于肠的腺癌和腺瘤。肠型腺癌男性比女性常见，发病年龄分布广泛，但最常见于40～50岁和60～70岁的病人。肠型腺癌最常累及筛窦，其次为鼻腔（下鼻甲和中鼻甲）和上颌窦；然而，肠型腺癌可以发生于鼻窦部的任何部位[382]。本病早期症状无特异性，从鼻不通气到持久性鼻塞不同，可能伴有鼻出血，这是另外一个突出的临床表现。由于诊断延误，在有症状时肿瘤可能已经很大，而且伴有广泛的浸润。晚期肿瘤表现为疼痛、颅神经受损、视力障碍以及眼球突出。与肠型腺癌发生有关的病因因素包括接触硬木粉尘、皮革和软木；在木工和制鞋工人中腺癌的发病率增加[382,384-388]。与职业无关的散发性肠型腺癌女性多于男性，多数肿瘤累及上颌窦[382]。

这些肿瘤具有不同的表现；可有清楚的边界，或边界不清呈浸润性，肿瘤扁平到外生性或呈乳头状生长，褐色/白色至粉色，质地易脆到硬韧。黏液性或胶状特性易见。组织学上，肠型腺癌是伴有不同生长方式的侵袭性肿瘤，包括乳头-腺管状、腺泡-黏液样或腺泡-杯状细胞，印戒细胞以及混合性[382,384,389,390]。肠型腺癌有两种分类（表4A.10）。Barnes[382]将这些肿瘤分成5类：(1)乳头状；(2)结肠性；(3)实性；(4)黏液性；(5)混合性。Kleinsasser和Schroeder[384]将肠型腺癌分成4类：(1)乳头状管状圆柱细胞（PTCC）Ⅰ-Ⅲ型（Ⅰ型=高分化，Ⅱ型=中分化，Ⅲ型=低分化）；(2)腺泡杯状细胞型；(3)印戒细胞型；(4)转化型。Barnes分类中的乳头状、结肠性和实性型分别相当于Kleinsasser和Schroeder分类中的PTCC Ⅰ、PTCC Ⅱ和PTCC Ⅲ。两种分类法都可接受，但喜欢应用Barnes分类，因为简单，本文也应用这种分类。与木匠有关的以及散发性的病例最常见的组织学类型是乳头状型和结肠型[382,384]。

乳头状型（PTCC Ⅰ或高分化腺癌）约占病例的18%，出现明显的乳头状结构，偶尔伴有管状腺体，有轻度的细胞学非典型性，核分裂象少见（图4A.36A）。

结肠型（PTCC Ⅱ或中分化腺癌）主要为腺管状结构，乳头罕见，核多形性和分裂活性增加（图4A.36B）。

实性型（PTCC Ⅲ或低分化腺癌）分化丧失，以实性和小梁状生长为特征，并伴有孤立的小管状结构，

表4A.10	鼻窦肠型腺癌的分类		
Barnes[382]	Kleinsasser和Schroeder[384]	病例百分数	3年累积生存率[a]
乳头状型	PTCC Ⅰ	18%	82%
结肠型	PTCC Ⅱ	40%	54%
实体型	PTCC Ⅲ	20%	36%
黏液型	腺泡状杯状细胞	少见	48%
	胞印戒细胞	少见	0%
混合型	转化性	罕见	71%

PTCC，乳头状管状圆柱细胞。
[a]生存资料来自Klesinsasser & Schroder[384]。

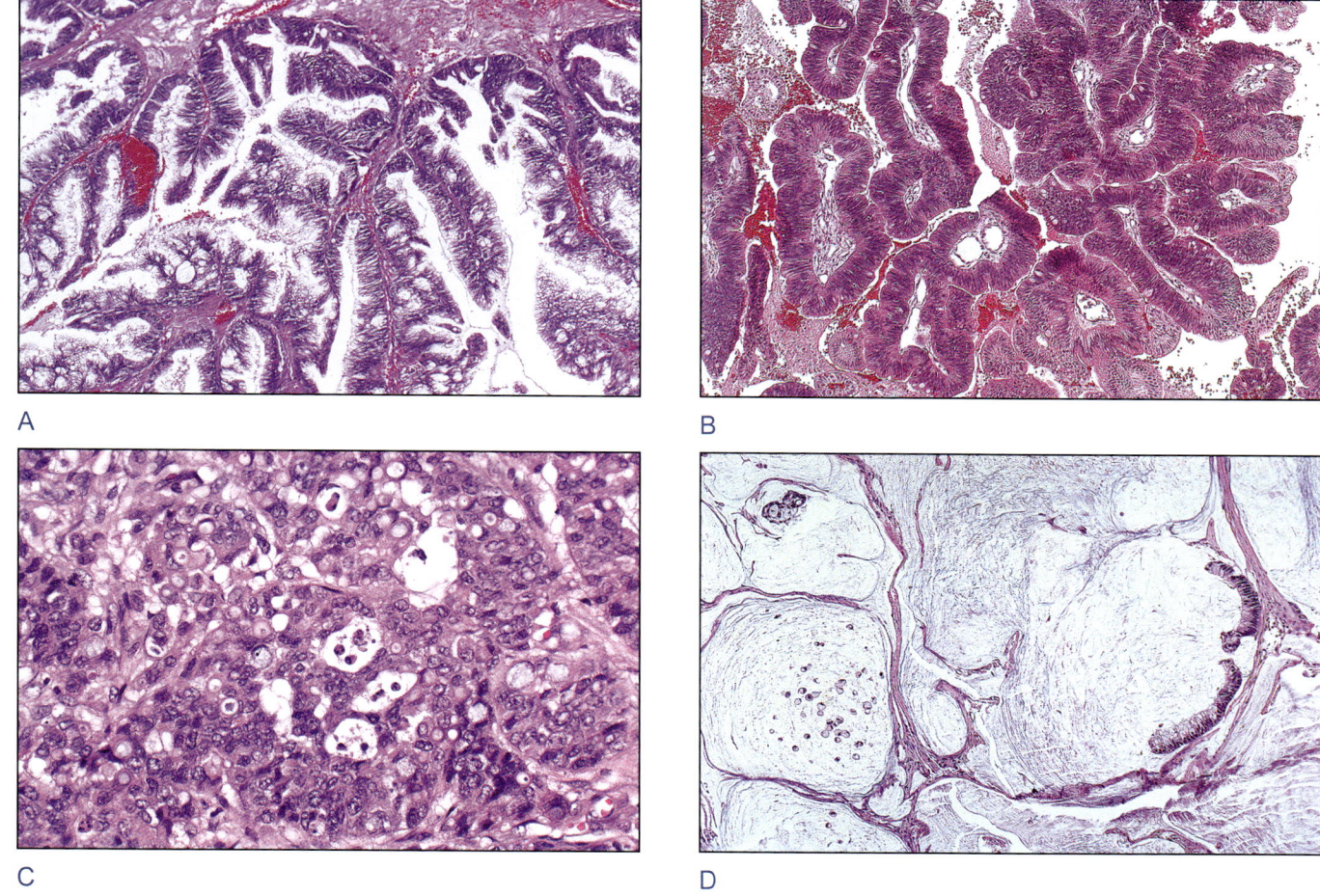

图4A.36 鼻窦肠型腺癌包括各种亚型：(A) 乳头状；(B) 结肠型；(C) 实性；(D) 黏液性。

伴有核多形性的较小的立方形细胞数目明显增加，核呈圆形空泡状，核仁明显，而且核分裂象增加（图4A.36C）。

与结肠腺癌相似，某些肠型腺癌主要由大量黏液组成，分类为黏液性肠型腺癌（图4A.36D）。黏液性肠型腺癌（腺泡状杯状细胞和印戒细胞）包括两种生长方式。一种生长方式为实性细胞簇、单个腺体、印戒细胞和伴或不伴纤维血管轴心的短乳头状结构；黏液主要在细胞内，而且可出现黏液样基质。另一种生长方式是出现大而形成完好的腺体，其内充满黏液，并有细胞外黏液池[384,390,391]。细胞外黏液池被薄结缔组织间隔分开，形成腺泡状结构。在黏液池周围主要是单层立方形或杯状肿瘤细胞，黏液外渗可引起炎症反应，可能包括多核巨细胞。那些以黏液成分为主的肿瘤（>50%）与胃肠道的对应肿瘤相似，可归为黏液腺癌[391]。

混合型（转化性）由两种或两种以上上述类型混合构成。

不论组织学类型如何，肠型腺癌在组织学上类似正常肠黏膜，可能包括绒毛、Paneth细胞、肠嗜铬细胞和黏膜肌层。少数病例的病变由形成完好的绒毛构成，被覆类似于吸收上皮的柱状细胞；在这种情况下，绒毛下方可见类似于黏膜肌层的平滑肌束[392]。

肠型腺癌上皮标记物弥漫阳性，包括EMA、B72.3、Ber-EP4、BRST-1、Leu-M1和人类乳脂小体（HMFG-2），对抗细胞角蛋白的鸡尾酒染色呈强阳性[394]。CEA染色不定，导致文献报道矛盾[393,394]。肠型腺癌显示CK20阳性（73%～86%），CK7反应不定（43%～93%的病例）[395-400]。CDX-2是一种涉及肠上皮细胞分化的核转录因子，弥漫表达于肠型腺癌，在肠型腺癌中也能发现[395,397-399]。也可出现claudins和绒毛蛋白（villin）的表达[397]。肿瘤细胞可以表达多种激素肽，包括5-羟色胺、胆囊收缩素、胃泌素、生长抑素和亮脑啡肽（leu-enkephalin）[401]。也可见嗜铬素和突触素阳性细胞[393,397]。

肠型腺癌的治疗是完全手术切除，一般通过鼻侧切开术；手术不同，从局部切除到根治性手术切除（上颌骨切除术、筛窦切除术和加脏器去除术），取决于肿瘤范围和组织学表现。放射治疗可以用于广泛扩展的患者或高级别肿瘤。

所有肠型腺癌都被认为是潜在侵袭性、致死性肿瘤。

颈部淋巴结转移和远处扩散并不常见，分别发生在约10%和20%的病例[384,386,390,391]。5年累积生存率约为40%，死亡多数发生在3年以内。死亡原因是未能控制伴有扩散的局部病变和侵犯重要结构，以及（或）有转移性疾病。鼻窦部肠型腺癌一般是局部侵袭性肿瘤，常伴有局部障碍（大约50%）。因为多数病人表现为晚期局部病变，所以临床分期一般没有区别。组织学亚型已被确认为临床行为的指征，乳头状型（Ⅰ级）病变的行为比其他亚型更为惰性（表4A.7）[382,384,390,391]。由职业因素引起的肠型腺癌和散发性肠型腺癌的生物学行为没有不同。

非肠（非涎腺）型腺癌
Non-intestinal (non-salivary gland) adenocarcinomas

非肠非涎腺型腺癌是那些不是小涎腺来源，也不具有鼻窦"肠型"腺癌组织病理学特征的鼻窦部肿瘤。这些腺癌分为低级别和高级别两种类型。

鼻窦非肠型腺癌主要发生于成人，但发病年龄广泛，从9～80岁不等[402]。低级别腺癌的平均发病年龄为53岁，而高级别腺癌的平均发病年龄为59岁[402]。低级别腺癌男性略占优势，而高级别腺癌男性的发生率要高得多[402]。低级别非"肠型"腺癌最常发生于筛窦（比"肠型"腺癌范围小）。高级别非"肠型"腺癌最常发生于上颌窦[402]。每一种类型的肿瘤均可来源于鼻腔，其他副鼻窦，或（并不少见）多个不同鼻窦部位同时发生[402]。低级别腺癌患者主要表现为鼻塞和鼻出血。疼痛是一种少见的特征[402]，症状持续的时间可从2个月到5年不等，平均为5.5个月。高级别腺癌患者出现的症状主要包括鼻塞、鼻出血、疼痛和面部畸形（例如眼球突出）。症状持续的时间可从2周到5年，平均为2.5个月[402]。

尚未发现职业或环境因素与非"肠型"腺癌有关。

这些肿瘤具有不同的表现，包括边界清楚到不清楚，以至浸润，从扁平到外生性或乳头状生长，从褐色/白色到粉红色，质地从脆而易碎到硬韧。

这些肿瘤不论级别高低均可限于黏膜下而不累及表面，或可以累及其上的纤毛呼吸上皮。低级别腺癌具有腺体或乳头状生长方式，界限可能清楚，但无包膜。可见许多均一的小腺体或腺泡，伴有背靠背的生长方式，其间没有间质（图4A.37）。偶尔可见大而不规则的囊性间隙。腺体内衬单层无纤毛的立方到柱状细胞，伴有均一圆形的细胞核，核可局限于细胞基底，或为复层伴有极性消失，胞浆嗜酸性。细胞多形性轻到中度，偶见核分裂象，但无非典型性核分裂和坏死。尽管组织学表现相对温和，但可根据复杂的生长方式、缺乏两层细胞、缺乏包膜以及出现黏膜下浸润诊断为腺癌。亚型包括乳头状、透明的细胞和嗜酸性细胞腺癌。任何一个肿瘤均可见多种形态学结构。

鼻窦高级别腺癌是一种侵袭性肿瘤，主要为实性生

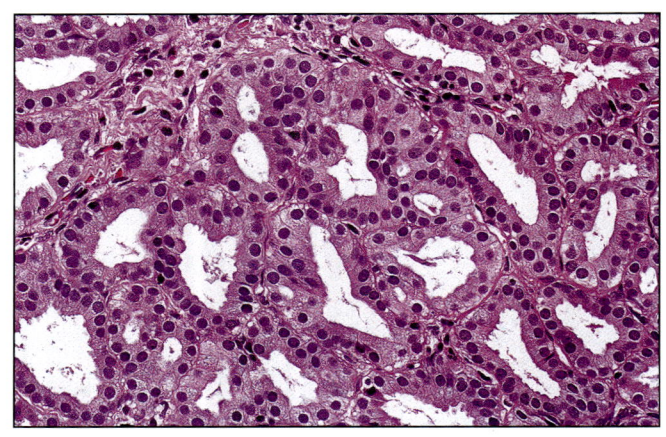 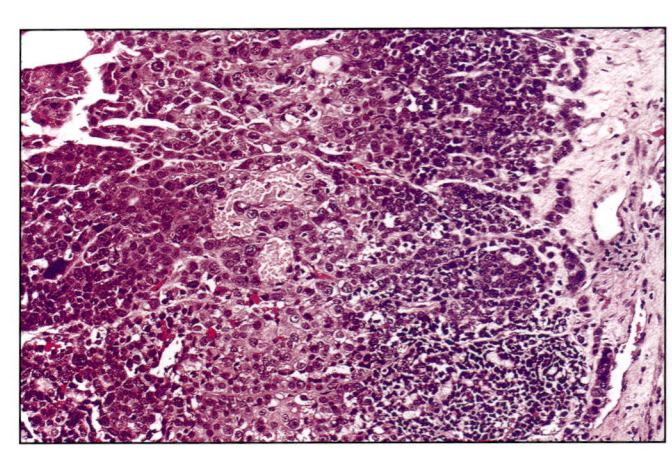

A　　　　　　　　　　　　　　　　　　　　　B

图4A.37　鼻窦非肠、非涎腺型腺癌包括浸润性低级别和高级别肿瘤。（A）低级别腺癌的特征是出现大量小腺体或腺泡，伴有背靠背生长方式，其间没有间质；腺体内衬无纤毛的单层立方到柱状细胞，伴有均匀一致的圆形细胞核。细胞多形性不明显。生长方式复杂，缺乏两层细胞，缺乏包膜以及侵入黏膜下是诊断腺癌的特征。（B）高级别腺癌的特征是出现中度到重度的细胞多形性，核分裂活性增加，包括非典型性核分裂象以及坏死。

长，但也可见腺体和乳头状生长方式。这些肿瘤的特征是出现中度到重度细胞多形性，核分裂活性增加，包括非典型性核分裂象，以及出现坏死（图 4A.37）。

非肠型腺癌对于 CK7 总是呈现强烈表达，但与肠型腺癌不同，不表达 CK20、CDX2、绒毛素（villin）、claudins、嗜铬素和突触素[395-397,399]。

对于所有组织学亚型的非肠、非涎腺型鼻窦腺癌的治疗均采取完全手术切除，一般通过鼻侧壁切开术；手术方法的选择取决于肿瘤范围和组织学特征，可从局部切除到根治性切除（上颌骨切除术、筛窦切除术以及另外加上内脏术）。放射治疗可用于有广泛性疾病或高级别肿瘤患者。低级别肿瘤患者预后好，而高级别肿瘤患者预后不良，3 年生存率大约为 20%[402]。

恶性涎腺肿瘤
Malignant salivary gland tumors

鼻窦部和鼻咽部最常见的恶性涎腺肿瘤是腺样囊性癌。大涎腺较常见的恶性肿瘤在鼻窦部和鼻咽部却不常见，包括黏液表皮样癌和腺泡细胞腺癌。读者可以参考第 7 章中有关各种类型涎腺恶性肿瘤的详细讨论。

腺样囊性癌
Adenoid cystic carcinoma（ACC）

腺样囊性癌的特征是具有独特的组织学表现，倾向于侵犯神经，具有漫长而温和的临床经过。所有腺样囊性癌大约 20% 发生于鼻窦部[403]。腺样囊性癌大约占鼻窦部恶性肿瘤的 5%[383,404]。

最常见的受累部位是上颌窦（57%），其次是鼻腔（24%）、筛窦（14%）和其他部位（5%）[403]。鼻窦部腺样囊性癌是一种发生于成人的肿瘤，很少见于 20 岁以下。症状可能包括呼吸不畅、鼻出血和疼痛。这些肿瘤在诊断时可能很大，伴有广泛的浸润性生长。

大体上，腺样囊性癌具有不同程度的包膜，为实性、橡胶硬度到质硬、褐白色到灰粉色的肿块，最大径可达 2～4 cm。腺样囊性癌组织学表现为无包膜的浸润性肿瘤，伴有包括筛状、腺管/导管状以及实性的不同结构。单个肿瘤可具有一种生长方式，但其特征是显示多种生长类型，而且可以任何一种生长方式为主。最常见的是筛状型（cribriform type），被认为是"经典"结构，表现为细胞以有许多卵圆形或环状间隙的细胞排列成"瑞士奶酪样"构型，伴有许多卵圆形到圆形的间隙。这些间隙内含有嗜碱性黏液样物质或玻璃样嗜酸性物质。管状型（tubular type）的细胞排列成导管或小管，其中含

有弱嗜酸性黏液样物质。筛状和小管状结构常常同时出现。最少见的类型是实性型（solid type），肿瘤细胞排列成大小和形状不同的片块状或巢状。几乎没有囊腔、小管或导管形成。不论生长方式如何，肿瘤均由大小相当、均匀一致的细胞构成，细胞核小，深染，圆形到卵圆形或多角形，胞浆稀少，双嗜性到透明，细胞边界不清。核浆比例大约为 1:1。多数肿瘤细胞为远离管腔型的肌上皮细胞。在筛状或经典性腺样囊性癌中见到的囊性间隙是假性囊肿，它们位于细胞外，内衬折转的基底膜。在这些远离管腔的细胞中散在有导管细胞，导管细胞围绕着真正的小腺腔。真正的导管样腔隙是腺样囊性癌的一种不常见特征，而最常见的是腺管状结构。在实性型腺样囊性癌，主要是由基底细胞样肌上皮细胞组成的。与上皮成分界限分明的间质从黏液样到玻璃样变表现不一。细胞及核多形性、坏死和核分裂活性局限于筛状和腺管状结构中。然而，这些特征更常见于实性结构。所有组织学亚型所共有的倾向是侵犯神经（趋神经性），包括神经周围和神经内的浸润。然而，腺样囊性癌并不是唯一显示趋神经性的涎腺肿瘤。

腺样囊性癌的组织化学特征包括在假囊肿中出现抗淀粉酶的 PAS 阳性和黏液卡红阳性物质。阿辛蓝染色也出现于假囊肿内。腺样囊性癌的免疫组化表现不同，取决于细胞类型。肌上皮细胞表达细胞角蛋白、S-100 蛋白、p63、钙结合蛋白（calponin）、波形蛋白和肌动蛋白，伴有不同程度的 GFAP 反应。导管细胞显示细胞角蛋白、EMA 和 CEA 阳性。超微结构研究显示有双向分化的细胞，包括管腔或导管细胞以及远离管腔或肌上皮/基底细胞[405]。

腺样囊性癌治疗选择广泛的局部切除和术后放射治疗。手术切除腺样囊性癌出现的问题与这些肿瘤的浸润性本质有关，由于它们倾向于沿着神经蔓延，而且靠不住的界限清楚的大体表现使这个问题更加复杂。复发率高，从 75%～90% 不等[403]，与手术切除不充分直接相关。腺样囊性癌放射敏感，放射治疗对于控制最初手术之后的微小病变，治疗局部复发性疾病或减轻不能手术切除肿瘤的症状特别有用。放射治疗不能治愈。鼻窦和鼻咽部腺样囊性癌的生物学行为与其他部位的腺样囊性癌相似。短期预后一般良好，因为肿瘤生长缓慢，但长期预后差。这些事实反映在所有头颈部腺样囊性癌的 5 年和 20 年生存率分别为 75% 和 13%[406]。肿瘤部位影响预后。位于大涎腺的腺样囊性癌的预后比小涎腺的好。在预测预后方面，腺样囊性癌的临床分期比组织学分级具有更加明显的作用[407,408]。Spiro 和 Huvos[407] 报告，Ⅰ期、Ⅱ期、Ⅲ期和Ⅳ期患者的 10 年累积生存率分别为 75%、43% 和 15%。

低级别鼻咽乳头状腺癌
Low-grade nasopharyngeal papillary adenocarcinoma

低级别鼻咽乳头状腺癌是一种不常见的鼻咽表面上皮来源的恶性肿瘤，它伴有腺癌性分化和惰性的生物学行为[409]。其发生无性别差异，发病年龄范围广泛，从10～0岁到60～70岁均可发生（中位数年龄为37岁）。肿瘤可发生于鼻咽任何部位，鼻咽后壁最常受累。最常见的症状为鼻塞。病因不明。

这些肿瘤为外生性，呈乳头状、结节状或菜花样生长，质软或有砂粒感，大小从数毫米至4.0厘米不等[410]。组织学上，肿瘤无包膜，呈乳头状及腺样生长。乳头结构复杂，伴有分支和透明变性的纤维血管轴心（图4A.38）。同样，腺样结构亦很复杂，其特征是背靠背和筛状结构。细胞从假复层柱状到立方细胞表现各异。核圆形至卵圆形，伴有空泡状到透明表现的染色质，核仁模糊，胞浆嗜酸性（图4A.38）。可见核轻到中度多形性，散在的核分裂象，但无非典型性核分裂象。可见局灶性坏死。可以出现沙粒体。在取样充分的标本中可见表面上皮衍化，表现为有从正常鼻咽表面上皮向肿瘤性增生的移行区域。

组织化学染色显示上皮黏液阳性（胞浆内抗淀粉酶PAS染色阳性，胞浆内和腺腔内黏液卡红阳性）。免疫组化方面，细胞角蛋白和EMA呈弥漫阳性。CEA局灶阳性。S-100蛋白或GFAP阴性。因其组织学特征与甲状腺乳头状癌相似，故应进行甲状腺球蛋白免疫组化染色。鼻咽乳头状腺癌不表达甲状腺球蛋白，但有表达甲状腺转录因子1（TTF-1）的报道[410a]。与EB病毒无关。

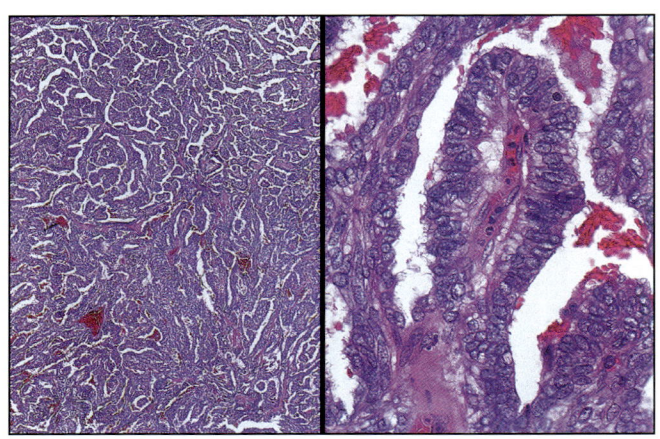

图4A.38 低级别鼻咽乳头状腺癌。左图：肿瘤无包膜，呈浸润性生长，而且具有复杂的乳头状结构，伴有纤维血管轴心。右图：乳头状小叶结构伴有纤维血管轴心，细胞核特征与甲状腺乳头状癌相似，但肿瘤标志物（例如甲状腺球蛋白）为阴性。

保守而又充分的手术切除可以治愈[409,410]。手术通常经由腭通路。辅助治疗（放射治疗）似乎无效。肿瘤生长缓慢，如切除不彻底，则有可能复发；不发生转移。

非上皮性恶性肿瘤
Non-epithelial malignant neoplasms

鼻窦部非Hodgkin淋巴瘤
Non-Hodgkin lymphomas of the sinonasal tract

鼻窦部非Hodgkin淋巴瘤（SNT-ML）是异质性肿瘤，临床上可能具有侵袭性[411]。虽然多年来应用多形性网状细胞增生症、致死性中线肉芽肿、中线恶性网状细胞增生症以及特发性中线破坏性疾病这些术语作为SNT-ML的同义词，但从分类学上讲是不正确的。发生在鼻窦部的非肿瘤性病变、炎症、感染性疾病以及许多良性和恶性肿瘤均可导致这个区域中线部位的破坏性病变。因此，特发性中线破坏性疾病并非专业术语，不应再用于表示一种恶性淋巴增生性肿瘤的诊断。这种病变的其他命名还有血管中心性免疫增生性病变和外周T细胞淋巴瘤，最通用的命名是鼻型血管中心性NK/T细胞淋巴瘤（angiocentric NK/T-cell lymphoma of nasal type）[412]。SNT-ML还包括B细胞系的淋巴瘤，其中最常见的类型是弥漫性大B细胞淋巴瘤（DLBCL）[413]。这个部位其他B细胞淋巴瘤还有Burkitt淋巴瘤，结外边缘区黏膜相关淋巴组织（MALT）B细胞淋巴瘤以及滤泡性淋巴瘤[415]。发生于鼻腔的淋巴瘤主要是NK/T细胞性淋巴瘤，而多数B细胞淋巴瘤发生于副鼻窦[411]。

在美国，SNT-ML并不常见，只占非Hodgkin淋巴瘤的1.5%[414,415]。然而，在亚洲及南美洲国家报道的发病率较高，这些地区鼻窦原发性非Hodgkin恶性淋巴瘤的发病率约占所有恶性淋巴瘤的6.7～8.0%[414,416,417]。实际上，可见淋巴瘤形态学类型的整个谱系（见第21章）。鼻窦部淋巴瘤最常见的类型是鼻型结外NK/T细胞淋巴瘤[411,418]。鼻型NK/T细胞淋巴瘤主要发生于男性，是一种成年人的疾病，发病中位年龄为50～60岁[418]。最常见于亚洲，据报道在南美和中美以及墨西哥也相当常见[419,420]。在这些人群中，本病主要见于具有美洲本地血统的个体。尽管少见，鼻型NK/T细胞淋巴瘤亦可发生在西方人群中，而且可以累及白种人[412]。鼻窦部弥漫性大B细胞淋巴瘤主要也是发生于男性，发病中位年龄为60～70岁[411,418]。发生部位可能包括鼻腔、一个或多个副鼻窦，或鼻窦部的多个区域同时受累[411]。

其临床表现不同，取决于组织学类型和（或）免疫表型。低级别淋巴瘤可能表现为鼻腔或副鼻窦的肿块，伴有气道阻塞的症状。高级别淋巴瘤多半表现为侵袭性的症状和体征，包括经久不愈的溃疡、颅神经症状、面部肿胀、鼻出血或疼痛。高级别 B 细胞淋巴瘤常常破坏骨和软组织，特别是眼眶，伴有眼球突出[411]。鼻型 NK/T 细胞淋巴瘤通常会破坏中面部的组织结构，伴有鼻中隔缺损、腭骨破坏、眼眶肿胀或出现与肿块有关的阻塞性症状。

不管种族背景如何，鼻型 NK/T 细胞淋巴瘤均与EB 病毒密切相关[413]。然而，鼻窦 B 细胞淋巴瘤与 EB 病毒仅为弱相关[413]。鼻窦淋巴瘤的危险性增加，主要是弥漫性大 B 细胞淋巴瘤，还有鼻型 NK/T 细胞淋巴瘤，也与包括移植后和人类免疫缺陷病毒（HIV）感染等免疫抑制有关[421-423]。

鼻型NK/T细胞淋巴瘤
NK/T-cell lymphoma of nasal type

鼻型 NK/T 细胞淋巴瘤可能显示广泛的组织学谱系，但在细胞学上通常出现非典型性细胞[412,424]。非典型性细胞大小可以不同，从小细胞、中等大小的细胞直到大细胞，细胞核深染。非典型性细胞可能有不规则和细长的细胞核，核仁明显，或有透明的胞浆（图 4A.39）。可出现趋上皮性和假上皮瘤样增生。可见明显的混合性炎症细胞浸润，包括浆细胞、组织细胞和嗜酸性细胞。多形态的细胞群可能会掩盖非典型性细胞，从而造成诊断困难。缺乏多核巨细胞和真正的肉芽肿。

在取样充分的标本中，低倍镜下几乎均可见地图样坏死，特征为淡蓝色或所谓的"砂粒样"坏死（图 4A.39）。带状坏死结构提示血管生成。非典型性细胞浸润并破坏血管（图 4A.40），因此破坏血管是命名为"血

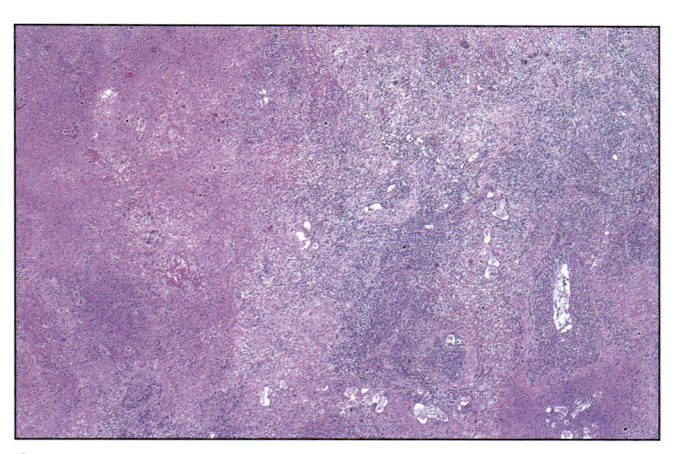 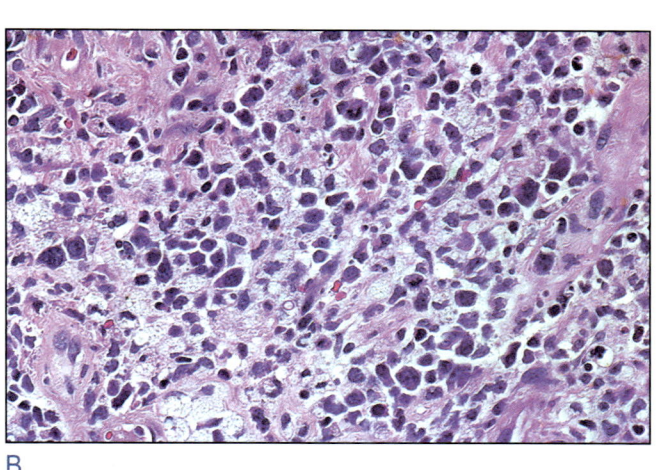

图4A.39 鼻型结外NK/T细胞淋巴瘤。（A）低倍镜下可见地图样坏死区域（左），伴有细胞丰富的浸润，局灶性围绕于血管周围（右）。（B）高倍镜下可见弥漫松散的细胞增生，细胞为中等大小到大细胞，伴有圆形到卵圆形到不规则和变长的细胞核，核呈空泡状到深染，并有不清楚的嗜酸性胞浆。

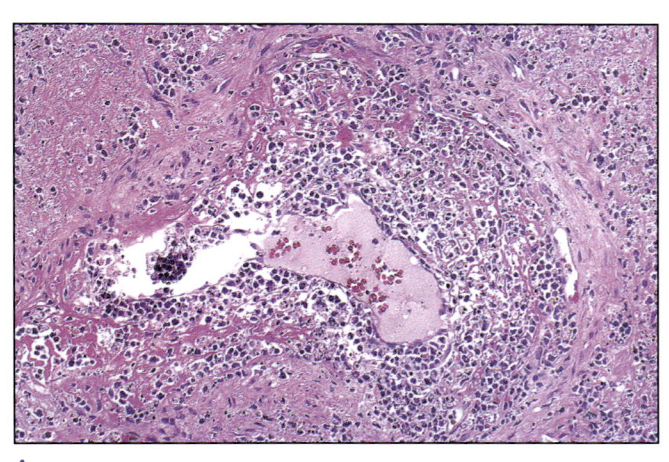 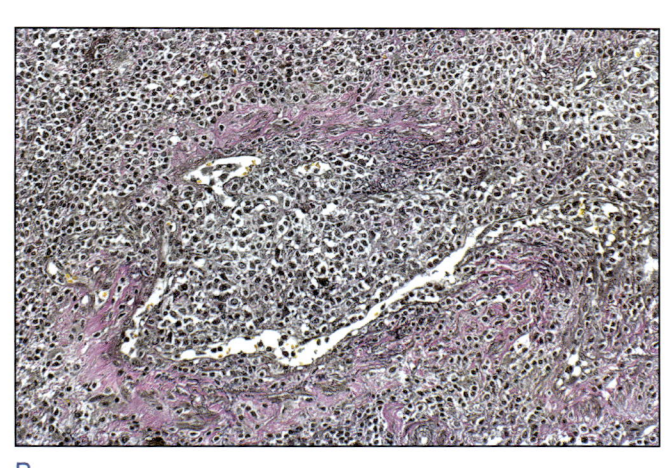

图4A.40 鼻型结外NK/T细胞淋巴瘤。（A）肿瘤细胞围绕并浸润血管腔隙（血管中心性）。（B）弹性纤维染色显示，肿瘤浸润造成整个血管壁弹性膜中断，并栓塞血管腔。

非上皮性恶性肿瘤

表4A.11 鼻窦恶性淋巴瘤、Wegener肉芽肿病以及过敏性肉芽肿病和血管炎（Churg-Strauss）的临床病理学比较

	血管中心性NK/T细胞淋巴瘤	弥漫性大B细胞淋巴瘤	Wegener肉芽肿病（WG）	过敏性肉芽肿病和血管炎[a]
性别，年龄	男＞女；50～60岁；最常见于亚洲人；也可发生于西方人群，但不常见	男＞女；60～70岁	男＞女；30～50岁；喉Wegener肉芽肿病女＞男	男＞女；年龄分布广泛（20～60岁）
部位	一般局限于鼻窦；发生鼻窦外疾病，代表分期较高的肿瘤	鼻腔和一个或一个以上副鼻窦	位于上呼吸消化道，鼻腔比副鼻窦常见；其他部位包括鼻咽、喉（声门下）、口腔、气管、耳、涎腺	多系统疾病，包括肺、鼻、肾、皮肤、心和神经系统受累
症状	中面部破坏性病变：鼻中隔穿孔，阻塞，腭破坏，眶肿胀	不易愈合的溃疡，鼻出血，面部肿胀，疼痛，颅神经表现	鼻窦：鼻窦炎，伴或不伴化脓性鼻溢、阻塞、疼痛、鼻出血、嗅觉丧失、头痛 喉：呼吸困难，声嘶，声音改变 口腔：溃疡性病变 耳：听力丧失，疼痛	哮喘，过敏性鼻炎，嗜酸性粒细胞、血清和组织（如嗜酸细胞性肺炎、嗜酸细胞性胃肠炎、其他）证据，血管炎证据
系统性受累	主要为局限性（IE/II/E期）；可能进展为播散性/系统性受累	主要为局限性（IE/II/E期）；可能进展为播散性/系统性受累	ELK分类： E：耳，鼻，咽喉 L：肺 K：肾 E，EL=局限性WG ELK=系统性 WG	一般为多系统受累，但存在局限性粒疾病
血清学	ANCA阴性；无特异性血清学标记物	ANCA阴性；无特异性血清学标记物	ANCA阳性： • 在原发性疾病和复发性疾病均有增加 • （C-ANCA比P-ANCA特异）	ANCA可有可无；外周血嗜酸性粒细胞增多

管中心性淋巴瘤"的原因。血管中心性的定义是血管周围和血管内出现肿瘤细胞，伴有血管壁浸润和破坏。位于血管周围并不足以说明是血管中心性。

免疫组化染色显示，肿瘤细胞通常呈CD2阳性，表面（膜）CD3阴性，胞浆CD3e阳性以及CD56（神经细胞粘附因子，NCAM）阳性[412]。T细胞标记物，包括CD43和UCHL1（CD45RO）为阳性。存在代表细胞毒性表型的穿孔素（perforin）、TIa1和粒酶B（granzyme B）的表达[413]。T细胞受体基因常表现为种系构型[412]。CD56阴性的肿瘤如果表达T细胞和细胞毒性标记物，而且EB病毒阳性，仍可归入NK/T细胞淋巴瘤[413]。

EBER原位杂交[425]发现95%以上的NK/T细胞淋巴瘤EB病毒阳性[413]。因为鼻腔黏膜或鼻腔炎性病变中一般缺乏EB病毒阳性细胞，所以原位杂交发现EB病毒结合显微镜观察可用来诊断鼻腔NK/T细胞淋巴瘤。

EB病毒可以诱导某些细胞因子的表达（例如肿瘤坏死因子α），从而导致肿瘤坏死，即使没有血管浸润的病例也是如此。NK/T细胞淋巴瘤常见Fas和Fas配体表达，这可能也是引起坏死的原因[425,426]。

鉴别诊断包括本章中讨论过的各种其他鼻窦部恶性肿瘤。虽然可以通过光镜评估来辨别肿瘤的差异，但是对于一个特定的肿瘤来说，鉴别所有这些类型的肿瘤常常需要依靠免疫组化染色（表4A.7）。鉴别诊断还包括鼻窦部感染性疾病和Wegener肉芽肿病（表4A.11）。通过特殊染色辨认微生物或进行微生物培养，均有助于确定感染性疾病的病因。Wegener肉芽肿病的组织学特征（见本章后一部分）结合抗中性白细胞胞浆抗体（antineutrophil cytoplasmic antibody，ANCA）升高，有助于确定Wegener肉芽肿病的诊断并与NK/T细胞淋巴瘤相鉴别。

表4A.11(续) 鼻窦恶性淋巴瘤、Wegener肉芽肿病以及过敏性肉芽肿病和血管炎（Churg-Strauss）的临床病理学比较

	血管中心性NK/T细胞淋巴瘤	弥漫性大B细胞淋巴瘤	Wegener肉芽肿病（WG）	过敏性肉芽肿病和血管炎[a]
组织学	明显恶性细胞浸润，但在早期恶性细胞可能不容易辨认；血管中心性和血管侵袭性；缺血性坏死；无巨细胞或肉芽肿；微生物培养和染色阴性	中等到大的非粘着细胞弥漫性增生，核大，圆形到卵圆形，空泡状（无核裂），核仁明显，核分裂活性增多，并有坏死	多形性（良性）细胞浸润；血管炎；缺血性坏死；孤立的多核巨细胞（非典型形态的肉芽肿）；微生物培养和染色阴性	多形性（良性）细胞浸润，主要为嗜酸性粒细胞，可表现为肉芽肿性血管炎（受累血管壁有多核巨细胞）；嗜酸性粒细胞微脓肿；微生物培养和染色阴性
免疫组化	CD56，CD2，胞浆CD3e阳性；T-细胞标记物（CD3，UCHL-1）阳性	白细胞共同抗原和B-细胞标记物（CD20，CD79）阳性	多形性和多克隆性	多形性和多克隆性
EB病毒	强相关	不相关或弱相关	阴性	阴性
治疗	放疗用于局限性病变；化疗用于播散性病变	放疗和（或）化疗	环磷酰胺和强的松	系统给予皮质类固醇
预后	总生存率30%～50%；局部复发和全身衰竭常见	取决于分期；生存率35%～60%	局限性疾病，预后很好，偶可自发性消退；死亡率与肺、肾并发症有关	5年生存率62%；由于心脏受累导致充血性心力衰竭或心梗而使发病率和死亡率增加

ANCA：抗中性白细胞胞浆抗体
[a] 亦称Churg-Strauss综合征

弥漫性大B细胞淋巴瘤
Diffuse large B-cell lymphoma

弥漫性大B细胞淋巴瘤（DLBCL），在黏膜下有弥漫性散在的中等至大细胞浸润，核大，圆形到卵圆形，呈空泡状（无核裂），可有多个有膜包绕的小核仁，或单个位于中心的突出的嗜酸性核仁。可见核分裂活性、坏死及凋亡。

免疫组化染色对于确定诊断以及恶性淋巴瘤和癌的鉴别诊断非常重要。DLBCL显示LCA（或CD45）和包括CD20及CD79a在内的全B细胞标记物染色阳性。

大部分鼻型NK/T细胞淋巴瘤在诊断时为局限性病变（ⅠE/ⅡE期）[366]。NK/T细胞淋巴瘤对放射治疗敏感，但一旦肿瘤出现播散则预后通常较差。对于播散性疾病采取积极的化学治疗。为了缓解症状（例如气道阻塞），有些患者可能需要手术切除。总生存率为30%～50%[418,427,428]。局部复发和全身衰竭常见[427,429]。全身衰竭表现为播散至皮肤、睾丸和胃肠道的危险增加[429]。见于某些鼻型NK/T细胞淋巴瘤病例的合并症

是噬血综合征，噬血综合征不利于患者生存[412,429]。其他不利于预后的因素还包括疾病处于晚期、全身状态不佳、B症候群以及肿瘤巨大[428]。

对于包括DLBCL在内的B细胞淋巴瘤，其预后与临床分期有关。鼻窦部DLBCL患者通常表现为低临床分期（ⅠE/ⅡE期）[413,418]。治疗主要有放射治疗和（或）化学治疗。必要时可采取手术切除以缓解症状。生存率从35%～60%不等[418,421]。全身衰竭表现为播散至淋巴结和膈下结外部位（例如主动脉旁淋巴结、胃肠道）的危险性增加[429]。

Waldeyer扁桃体组织恶性淋巴瘤
Malignant lymphomas of Waldeyer's tonsillar tissues

Waldeyer扁桃体环包括鼻咽、扁桃体及舌根的淋巴组织。它代表结外部位，而非淋巴外部位的病变。Waldeyer环淋巴瘤约占头颈部所有结外非Hodgkin淋巴瘤的50%，头颈部结外非Hodgkin淋巴瘤仅次于胃肠道[430,431]。在西方国家，Waldeyer扁桃体环淋巴瘤绝

大部分是 B 细胞淋巴瘤，最常见的亚型是 DLBCL。Waldeyer 扁桃体环 B 细胞淋巴瘤男性稍多于女性，最常见的年龄为 40～70 岁[432-435]。最常见发生部位（依发生率高低次序）是扁桃体、鼻咽和舌根。最常见症状包括气道阻塞、耳痛、听力下降、疼痛和咽喉痛。Waldeyer 环淋巴瘤与 EB 病毒之间无明确相关性[425]。

大体，黏膜下巨大肿块，伴或不伴表面溃疡形成。大多数病例累及单侧。通常情况下，浸润细胞呈松散排列，偶尔可能呈合体细胞性或粘着性生长，类似上皮性恶性肿瘤。大细胞性淋巴瘤细胞中等大小到较大，伴有大圆形到卵圆形的空泡状细胞核（无核裂），可见多个核仁，常位于核周。可出现许多巨噬细胞（呈"星空样"表现）或上皮样细胞。可见核分裂活性、坏死及凋亡现象。免疫母细胞淋巴瘤细胞较大，伴有圆形到卵圆形的细胞核和大而明显、常位于中央的核仁。坏死（单个细胞坏死或融合性坏死）以及伴有非典型性核分裂象的核分裂象活性增多是其常见特征。这些肿瘤可以显示浆细胞性分化。

免疫组化对于确诊以及恶性淋巴瘤与癌的鉴别诊断非常重要。几乎所有淋巴瘤 LCA（CD45）染色均呈阳性，而细胞角蛋白则呈阴性。绝大多数 Waldeyer 环淋巴瘤都是滤泡中心细胞起源，反映在它们表达 B 细胞系标记物（CD20）而缺乏 T 细胞标记物。

除了免疫组化特征外，与 DLBCL 有关的其他所见包括部分病例存在免疫球蛋白基因重排和 EB 病毒以及 I 型人类亲 T 淋巴细胞病毒（HTLV-1）；许多 B 细胞肿瘤有 t（14;18）染色体易位[436]。

Waldeyer 环淋巴瘤患者最重要的预后因素是临床分期[436,437]。治疗主要包括放射治疗和（或）化学治疗。为了缓解症状，可能需要手术切除。大部分患者为局部病变（IE/ⅡE 期）[413]。据报道，IE 期的 DLBCL 患者 5 年生存率从 58%～86% 不等[432,433,438]。处于ⅡE 期或更高分期患者的预后要差得多。

髓外浆细胞瘤
Extramedullary plasmacytoma（EMP）

EMP 约占所有浆细胞肿瘤的 3%～5%[439]。80% 的 EMP 发生于头颈部，多数病例主要累及上呼吸消化道，包括鼻窦部和鼻咽部[439-441]。80% 的 EMP 为原发性（孤立性）病变，其他部位无肿瘤的证据；20% 的 EMP 为与多发性骨髓瘤有关的全身表现的一部分[439]。EMP 男性多于女性；发病年龄范围广泛，但绝大多数发生在 40 岁以上的病人。EMP 好发于黏膜相关部位，包括鼻窦、鼻咽、咽（包括扁桃体）、喉、口腔、涎腺以及甲状腺。

临床表现取决于肿瘤发生部位，可包括软组织肿块、气道阻塞、鼻出血、疼痛、眼球突出或侵犯颅神经[441]。血清免疫电泳可能显示系统性及局限性病例均有单克隆异常；多达 25% 的 EMP 患者将罹患单克隆性 γ-球蛋白病（M 蛋白成分）[440]。M 成分消失可以作为治愈的指标[440]。EMP 的放射学特征包括软组织密度增高，可能出现骨质破坏，在原发性 EMP 患者骨骼检查可无异常[440]。

EMP 可表现为无蒂或有蒂的被覆黏膜的肿块，最大径 1～7.5 cm。质地从软到橡皮硬度到坚硬，伴不同颜色。活检时容易出血。EMP 一般位于黏膜下，呈弥漫性生长，并取代正常实质。浆细胞恶性肿瘤由具有不同成熟程度和非典型性浆细胞组成（见第 21 章）。浆细胞圆形到卵圆形，伴有偏心位圆形细胞核；细胞核具有特征性的表盘状染色质结构，但也可见弥散分布的核染色质；特征性的核旁空晕为 Golgi 体，Golgi 体分泌其加工和糖基化的免疫球蛋白[440]。胞浆丰富，嗜碱性。伴随浆细胞浸润可能出现淀粉样物沉积。组织化学（刚果红或结晶紫）和（或）免疫组化（AA 蛋白）染色有助于证实淀粉样物质的存在。组织化学评估包括胞浆嗜派洛宁（甲基绿派洛宁，MGP）；浆细胞染成红色。免疫组化染色，表现为单型性胞浆免疫球蛋白重链和（或）轻链限制性，如同浆细胞相关抗原（CD38，CD138，VS38）一样；浆细胞性恶性肿瘤 CD45 和 CD20 一般阴性[442]。

浆细胞瘤的间变亚型可以发生在上呼吸消化道部位，其特征是细胞具有增大的多形性的细胞核，嗜酸性的核仁模糊或明显，伴有多少不等的嗜酸性胞浆。可能出现瘤巨细胞，核分裂活性增多，包括非典型性核分裂象。在这些间变性的病变中，细胞可能有浆细胞样表现，但总的来说缺乏诊断浆细胞肿瘤的组织学特征。与大细胞性（免疫母细胞性）淋巴瘤鉴别或许非常困难。有助于鉴别的特征是浆细胞瘤既往史，伴有向低分化转化（即间变性病灶）的残余的浆细胞肿瘤的证据和（或）支持浆细胞肿瘤的免疫组化特征。

与非 Hodgkin 淋巴瘤一样，在开始治疗之前需要仔细分期，而且可能需要骨髓活检。治疗方法的选择视病变范围而定，包括采取单纯放射治疗，或对于较大肿瘤可局部切除后进行放射治疗。许多 EMP 病例病变局限，手术切除后采用放射治疗（30-50Gy）可以治愈[440]。70% 的 EMP 患者存活期达 10 年，中位存活期为 7-9 年[440,441]。头颈部受累可以是由多发性骨髓瘤扩散而来，或者原发性头颈部 EMP 亦可扩散至其他部位。预后明显受播散性疾病的影响，肿瘤播散之后的中位生存期不到 2 年[440,441]。

其他造血淋巴恶性肿瘤及相关病变
Other hematolymphoid malignancies and related lesions

发生在 Waldeyer 环的其他造血淋巴恶性肿瘤包括 NK/T 细胞淋巴瘤、间变性大细胞性淋巴瘤（anaplastic large-cell lymphoma，ALCL）、Burkitt 淋巴瘤以及 Hodgkin 淋巴瘤（HL）。

在亚洲人群中，Waldeyer 环恶性淋巴瘤以 B 细胞为主的说法并不正确，由于 NK/T 细胞淋巴瘤和外周 T 细胞淋巴瘤有较高的比例，那里 B 细胞淋巴瘤占 60%[416]。发生在 Waldeyer 环的鼻型结外 NK/T 细胞淋巴瘤男性比女性常见，中位年龄为 50～60 岁[416]。头颈部的结外 ALCL 罕见，但可见于 HIV 感染患者[442,443]。Burkitt 淋巴瘤是一种由 B 细胞组成的具有高度侵袭性的肿瘤，常发生于包括头颈部（如颌、鼻窦、鼻咽及其他部位）在内的结外部位，而且好发于儿童和年轻成人[444]。

原发于上呼吸消化道黏膜部位的 Hodgkin 淋巴瘤罕见，而且与 EB 病毒感染有关[445,446]。

滤泡性树突状细胞肿瘤（follicular dentritic cell tumor，FDCT）（肉瘤）是一种罕见的、显示滤泡性树突状细胞形态和表型特征的梭形至卵圆形细胞肿瘤。FDCT 一般发生于成年人，无性别差异。FDCT 表现为无痛性淋巴结肿大，最常见于颈部区域，少数可见于腋部。发生在结外部位的包括上呼吸消化道的黏膜组织，特别是扁桃体和咽部[447-451]；大约 10%FDCT 病例的发生与 Castleman 病有关，通常是透明血管型[452]。

发生在上呼吸消化道处黏膜组织的 FDCT 常呈息肉状，表面上皮完整。生长方式包括弥漫性、席纹状、束状和旋涡状。增生的细胞包括卵圆形到梭形的细胞，伴有圆形到卵圆形均一表现的长的细胞核，染色质呈空泡状或颗粒状，核仁不明显，胞浆淡染或微嗜酸性，细胞界限不清。可见散在的多核巨细胞；可能出现核内包涵体。核分裂象缺乏到散在(0～10 个核分裂象/高倍视野)，非典型性核分裂象、明显的多形性和坏死并不常见。整个肿瘤可见以淋巴细胞浸润为背景，或为单个细胞或成簇，常围绕在血管周围（袖套现象）；偶尔可见生长中心形成。

FDCT 一般表达 CD21、CD35、CD23 和波形蛋白。此外，其他滤泡性树突状细胞标记物（如 R4/23、Ki-M4P、Ki-FDRC1p）、fascin、HLA-DR 和 EMA 阳性少见，但事实上正常滤泡性树突状细胞 EMA 为阴性。S-100 蛋白、CD68、CD45、CD20 和 SMA 呈现不同程度的反应。FDCT 病人 EB 病毒和 HHV-8 均为阴性。最近发现，100% 的 FDCT 病例均呈丛生蛋白（clusterin）弥漫强阳性反应，包括传统标记物（CD21、CD23、CD35）阴性的病例，但是这些病例是根据超微结构特征分类的[453]。超微结构上，FDCT 细胞具有复杂的指状（绒毛）胞浆突起或延长，并通过许多细胞连接相互连接，包括发育完好的细胞间桥。治疗包括手术切除，伴有或不伴有辅助治疗（即放射治疗和化学治疗）。总的行为非常惰性，被比拟成低级别肉瘤[454]。

恶性间叶性肿瘤
Malignant mesenchymal neoplasms

恶性外周神经鞘肿瘤（神经源性肉瘤；神经纤维肉瘤）
Malignant peripheral nerve sheath tumor (neurogenic sarcoma; neurofibrosarcoma)

鼻窦和鼻咽部恶性外周神经鞘肿瘤（MPNST）是不常见的肿瘤。高达 14% 的恶性神经鞘瘤（见第 27 章）发生在头颈部，颈部是最常见的受累部位；所有部位均可受累，包括鼻腔和鼻咽部[455]。MPNST 可以是原发性的，也可以发生在 1 型神经纤维瘤病（NF1）基础上[456]。

组织学上，鼻窦部 MPNST 可为梭形细胞或上皮样细胞，表现为低级别或高级别。大部分鼻窦 MPNST 为低级别梭形细胞型，表现为难以归类的梭形细胞成束增生，围绕并在非肿瘤性腺体内[455]。细胞核外形不规则，常呈波纹状或弯曲状；胞浆不明显。与良性神经鞘瘤相比，其细胞更加丰富，核具有非典型性，核分裂活性增加。伴有黏液样间质的细胞稀少区可与细胞密集区交替出现。可见异源性成分，包括骨与软骨。与良性神经鞘瘤不同，低级别 MPNST S-100 蛋白反应呈局灶弱阳性，而高级别 MPNST 仅有程度不一的表达[457]。治疗选择完全手术切除。放疗可用于结合手术治疗，或有复发疾病的病例。鼻窦 MPNST 的预后一般相对较好。不良预后一般与发生于 NF1 背景下、男性患者和组织学分级较高有关[455,456]。

纤维肉瘤和所谓的恶性纤维组织细胞瘤
Fibrosarcoma and so-called malignant fibrous histiocytoma

鼻窦和鼻咽部的纤维肉瘤和所谓的恶性纤维组织细胞瘤（见第 24 章）少见[92,455,458]。最常见的发生部位为副鼻窦。患者表现为肿块性病变所引起的症状与体征，包括鼻塞、鼻出血、面部肿胀及疼痛。组织学上，纤维肉瘤由梭形细胞组成，排列成束或呈"人字形"生长方式，而且伴有胶原沉积。这种肿瘤在光镜下缺乏任何特异性分化，而且缺乏支持诊断其他类型肿瘤的免疫组织化学证据（如 S-100 支持 MPNST；CK 支持梭形细胞鳞状细胞癌或单向性滑膜肉瘤）。这些肿瘤的组织学分级包括低级别和高级别肿瘤[455]。低级别纤维肉瘤有轻度的细胞多形性，核分裂象易见（但不见非典型性核分裂象），而且保留成束的生长方式。与低级别肿瘤不同，高级别纤维肉瘤细胞束状排列不明显，显示明显的核非典型性，伴有核分裂活性显著增加，包括非典型性核分裂象，而且伴有出血和坏死。然而，这种肿瘤缺乏具有深染细胞核和明显核仁的奇异细胞或瘤巨细胞。出现奇异细胞或瘤巨细胞支持未分化多形性肉瘤的诊断，以前常被称为恶性纤维组织细胞瘤。纤维肉瘤和恶性纤维组织细胞瘤的免疫组化所见对于诊断没有帮助。由于许多恶性肿瘤的生长方式与纤维肉瘤和所谓的恶性纤维组织细胞瘤相似，所以重要的是要证实缺乏可能诊断其他类型肿瘤的标记物的免疫反应，例如各种细胞角蛋白、S-100 蛋白或 HMB-45。治疗采取手术切除。对于高级别肿瘤或累及手术缘的肿瘤，可辅以放疗。化疗适用于肿瘤广泛局部复发或发生转移的患者。肿瘤局部复发是这些患者最重要的死亡原因[455,459]。

横纹肌肉瘤　Rhabdomyosarcoma（RMS）

横纹肌肉瘤是一种显示骨骼肌分化的恶性间叶性肿瘤。头颈部横纹肌肉瘤主要发生于儿童，但并非仅见于儿童[460]。如将所有年龄考虑在内，横纹肌肉瘤占头颈部软组织肉瘤的 50%（见第 24 章）；局限于儿童年龄组的横纹肌肉瘤占头颈部所有软组织肉瘤的 75%[461,467]；在该年龄组，横纹肌肉瘤也是最常见的耳部恶性肿瘤。其发病无性别差异。头颈部横纹肌肉瘤最常见的发生部位（按发病率递减顺序）包括眼眶、鼻咽、中耳/颞骨和鼻窦[462-464]。如仅考虑成人，最常见的部位是鼻窦[465,466]。症状不同，取决于发生部位。鼻窦横纹肌肉瘤患者可出现鼻窦炎、鼻漏、鼻塞、鼻出血、疼痛、耳痛、面部肿胀和头痛等症状。与儿童患者不同，成人横纹肌肉瘤是侵袭较强的肿瘤[465-467]。在鼻窦部，疾病进展可能导致眼球突出、面部畸形、视觉障碍和（或）颅神经受损。

鼻窦横纹肌肉瘤最常表现为结节状、分叶状或息肉状肿块，伴有类似于鼻窦炎性息肉的外观。大约 25% 的鼻咽和鼻窦横纹肌肉瘤表现为葡萄状肉瘤的葡萄样、多结节状或息肉样外观。

头颈部横纹肌肉瘤多数是胚胎型，主要为葡萄状肉瘤（80%～85%），其次是腺泡状（10%～15%）（图 4A.41）[462]。其他组织学类型包括梭形细胞型（胚胎性横纹肌肉瘤的一种亚型）和多形性横纹肌肉瘤，也可发生于头颈部，但均不常见。这些肿瘤的细胞构成一般存在差异，伴有交替出现的细胞过多和细胞疏少区；细胞疏少区常伴有黏液样间质。肿瘤由处于肌生成不同阶段的原始间叶细胞组成。未分化的小细胞（原始表现）是圆形或梭形细胞，核深染，胞浆不清；可见轻度核多形性、核分裂活性增加和坏死。分化的细胞体积较大，圆形到卵圆形，伴有嗜酸性胞浆。少数胚胎型横纹肌肉瘤可能伴有明显的细胞多形性病灶，被称为间变性亚型。

葡萄状肉瘤（葡萄状横纹肌肉瘤）是胚胎型横纹肌肉瘤的一个大体变型。其大体表现的特征为息肉样和黏液样肿块。组织学上，表面上皮下方有一层致密的细胞聚集，称之为新生层（cambium layer）。

腺泡状横纹肌肉瘤的特征是边界不清的低分化，但相对均匀一致的小圆形至卵圆形肿瘤细胞集聚（图 4A.42）。中央区域细胞粘着常常丧失，导致"腺泡样"

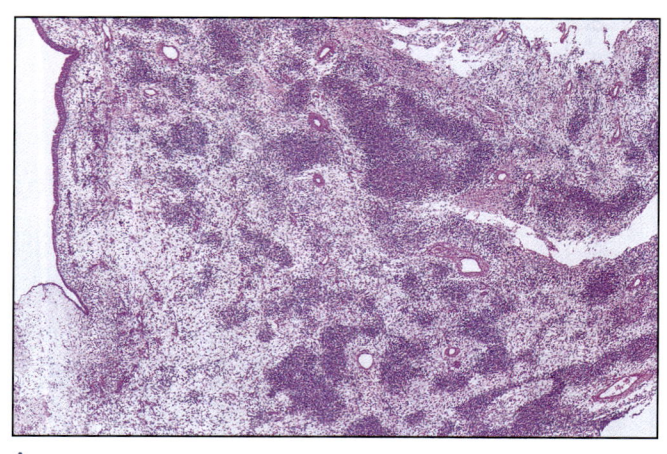
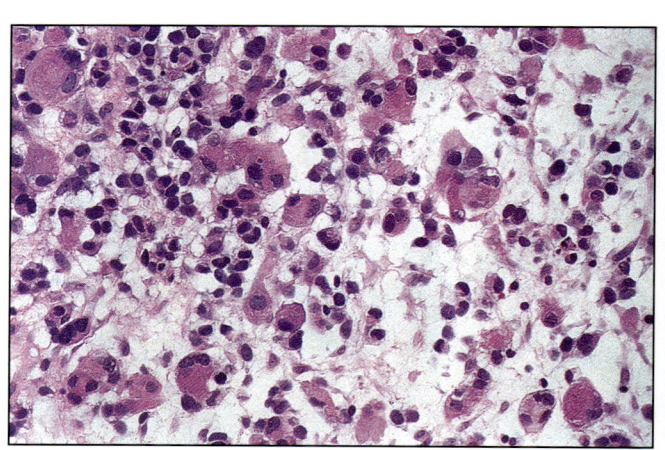

图 4A.41　鼻窦胚胎性横纹肌肉瘤。（A）低倍镜下显示黏膜下浸润为交替出现的富于细胞和黏液样区域。（B）高倍镜下出现具有嗜酸性胞浆的特征性的横纹肌母细胞。

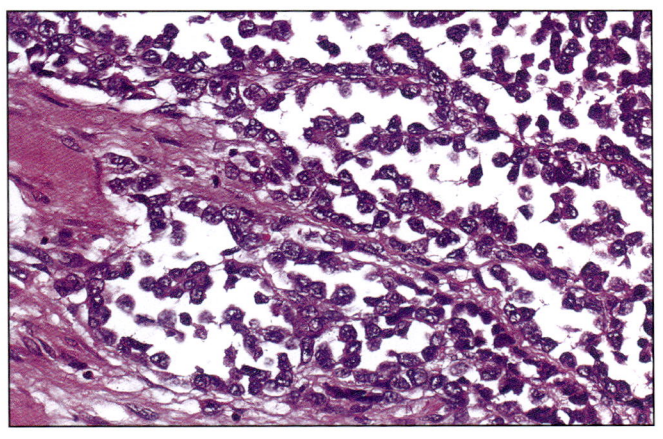

图4A.42 鼻咽部腺泡状横纹肌肉瘤。肿瘤细胞粘附到纤维间隔上，中心细胞粘着性丧失，形成腔隙或腺泡，呈"腺泡状"生长方式。

结构；但其他区域（或整个肿瘤）由实性肿瘤细胞集聚组成，有时排列成小梁状结构。部分肿瘤细胞被致密纤维结缔组织形成的间隔分开，并伴有明显的血管腔隙。腺泡状腔隙周围细胞保存得最好，常常粘附在纤维间隔上。伴有明显颗粒状嗜酸性胞浆的肿瘤性横纹肌母细胞在腺泡型横纹肌肉瘤中要比胚胎型横纹肌肉瘤少见。腺泡型横纹肌肉瘤常见核位于周围而形成的花环样多核细胞，这是一个重要的诊断线索。

对于缺乏横纹证据的低分化肿瘤，特殊染色对于确定横纹肌肉瘤的诊断非常重要。免疫组化是诊断横纹肌肉瘤的重要辅助方法，包括结蛋白、myf-4、肌动蛋白（肌肉特异性）和肌红蛋白的反应。

细胞遗传学分析对于横纹肌肉瘤的诊断及鉴别诊断可能具有重要意义（表4A.12；见第24章）[468,469]。

鉴别诊断包括本章所讨论过的其他各种鼻窦恶性肿瘤。尽管光镜能区分这些肿瘤的不同，但所有这些类型肿瘤的鉴别常常需要依靠免疫组化染色（表4A.7）。

在横纹肌肉瘤组间研究（Intergroup Rhabdomyosarcoma Study，IRS）的成果出来之前[460]，横纹肌肉瘤的治疗采取手术切除，头颈部横纹肌肉瘤的5年生存率不足20%。然而，IRS提出了横纹肌肉瘤的分期系统[460]，并发现多学科综合治疗，包括手术、放射治疗和化学治疗（长春新碱、更生霉素、环磷酰胺和阿霉素），比单一学科治疗生存率高。活检诊断之后，治疗选择取决于几个因素，包括肿瘤生长部位、临床症状以及疾病分期。

肿瘤分期是全面治疗本病的一个重要因素。根据临床分期总的5年生存率为：Ⅰ期和Ⅱ期为85%～88%；Ⅲ期为66%；Ⅳ期为26%[470]。为了统计目的，IRS将头颈部横纹肌肉瘤分为三类[471]，包括（1）眼眶横纹肌肉瘤，5年生存率92%；（2）脑膜旁横纹肌肉瘤，包括中耳-乳突、外耳道、鼻咽、鼻窦和颞下窝，5年生存率70%；（3）头颈其他部位，包括颈部、头皮、口咽、喉和腮腺，5年生存率55%。那些治疗后无瘤期达2年的患者可能已经治愈，但IRS的研究发现[460]，在他们无瘤生存2年的患者中有8%随后出现复发。除了临床分期以外，患者年龄和组织学类型也与预后相关[472]。横纹肌肉瘤有侵犯骨质的倾向，在头颈部这种倾向可能导致广泛的脑膜受累。未经充分治疗的肿瘤常有复发。转移最常累及肺、骨和淋巴结。

血管肉瘤　Angiosarcoma

鼻窦和鼻咽的血管肉瘤罕见，表现为肿块性病变，伴有或不伴有鼻出血气道阻塞[473,474]。血管肉瘤（见第3章）常呈结节状或形成溃疡，境界不清，呈略带浅蓝的红色。组织学上，多数为低级别肿瘤，包括增生的分支状和相互吻合的血管腔，将周围结构分隔开。内衬血管腔的内皮细胞肥胖，有非典型性，数量增多，并沿着血管腔集聚，形成乳头状结构。可见核分裂活性，包括非典型性核分裂象。内皮细胞可能为梭形、上皮样或多边形。免疫组化染色有助于诊断；Ⅷ-因子相关抗原、CD31或CD34阳性。上皮样血管肉瘤CK可能阳性，以致造成与癌的鉴别诊断存在困难。少数上皮样血管内皮细胞瘤病例可以发生在鼻窦[475]。治疗采取完全手术切除，特别是边界清楚和孤立性的肿瘤。对于多灶性边界不清的肿瘤，放射治疗和化学治疗可能有效。

Kaposi 肉瘤　Kaposi's sarcoma

Kaposi 肉瘤是一种恶性血管肿瘤，其发生主要有三

表4A.12	横纹肌肉瘤的细胞遗传学

胚胎性横纹肌肉瘤
染色体11p15.5杂合性缺失
11号染色体短臂异常
一般缺乏PAX3/FKHR和PAX7/FKHR融合转录物

梭形细胞横纹肌肉瘤
没有关于细胞遗传学异常的资料

腺泡状横纹肌肉瘤
多数病例t (2;13) (q36;q14) 易位
少数病例t (1;13) (p36;q14) 易位
*PAX3/FKHR*融合转录物（80%～90%的病例）
*PAX7/FKHR*融合转录物（10%～20%的病例）

种类型：(1) 经典性（地方性）；(2) 流行性；(3) 获得性免疫缺陷综合征（AIDS）相关性和移植相关性（见第 3 章）。发生于鼻窦及鼻咽的 Kaposi 肉瘤很少见，通常仅仅发生于 AIDS 病人[476-478]。这种类型的 Kaposi 肉瘤，肿瘤表现为蓝红色或青紫色的黏膜丘疹或结节，可能类似于良性血管增生的外观[479]。组织学上，肿瘤通常呈结节状，由均匀一致的嗜酸性梭形细胞组成，细胞排列成束状。可见散在的核分裂象。增生的梭形细胞被含有红细胞的裂隙所分隔。细胞内和细胞外可见抗淀粉酶的 PAS 阳性的玻璃样小体。通常出现 CD34 和 CD31 免疫反应。HHV-8 免疫组化阳性支持 Kaposi 肉瘤的诊断[480]。PCR 检测发现鼻分泌物和唾液中存在 HHV-8 提示其中常常有脱落的疱疹病毒，特别是在 Kaposi 肉瘤的患者[481,482]。除了出于诊断目的以外，一般不采取手术治疗。

平滑肌肉瘤　Leiomyosarcoma

多达 10% 的平滑肌肉瘤发生在头颈部[483]。鼻窦部的平滑肌肉瘤发生于成年人，无性别差异。表现为鼻塞、疼痛和鼻出血。鼻窦平滑肌肉瘤境界清楚，但无包膜，为息肉状或无蒂的肿块，直径通常大于 5 cm[484]。组织学上为富于细胞的肿瘤，类似于其他部位的平滑肌肉瘤（见第 24 章）。呈局部浸润性生长，核分裂活性增加（>4 核分裂象 / 每 10 个高倍视野），并有局灶性坏死[104]。肌动蛋白（平滑肌和肌肉特异性）、结蛋白和 h-钙调结合蛋白（h-caldesmon）免疫染色呈弥漫强阳性。可见上皮样形态和黏液瘤性改变，有时可能为主要表现[484]。治疗选择广泛手术切除。辅助疗法（放射治疗和化学治疗）疗效不确定。预后取决于肿瘤发生部位和范围，而不是组织学形态[484]。局限于鼻腔的肿瘤预后较好，完全切除可以治愈[104,484]。鼻腔和鼻窦均被累及的肿瘤往往具有侵袭性行为，复发率和死亡率较高[484]。

骨肉瘤（成骨肉瘤）
Osteosarcoma（osteogenic sarcoma）

多达 10% 的普通骨肉瘤发生在头颈部[485,486]。颅面部骨肉瘤（除了那些发生在 Paget 病的骨肉瘤）男女发病均等，其发病年龄比面部以外的骨肉瘤要晚 10～20 岁[487,488]。最常累及颌骨，且下颌骨比上颌骨常见[485-487]。最常见的临床主诉包括面部肿痛、出现牙的问题、鼻塞和鼻出血。放射学检查显示，骨肉瘤具有破坏性，境界不清，可见溶骨、骨质硬化，或为混合性病变。

骨肉瘤的大体表现取决于肿瘤矿化程度与间质成分的对比。因此，骨肉瘤的表现多样，从质硬韧和沙粒样到鱼肉样和纤维化。头颈部骨肉瘤的组织病理学特征类似于其他部位的骨肉瘤（见第 25 章）。骨肉瘤的预后与组织学亚型无关[489,490]。

头颈部骨肉瘤为侵袭性肿瘤，易于局部复发和远处转移[488]。与单纯手术相比，多科性治疗，包括完全手术切除并辅以放疗和化疗能为控制疾病提供最好的机会[488]。颅面部骨肉瘤比面部以外的骨肉瘤预后好[486,489]。这是由于这个部位的骨肉瘤倾向于局限性生长，转移扩散仅发生在病程晚期，而且其组织学分级较低。尽管颅面部骨肉瘤总体预后较好，但这些肿瘤仍然可能是致死性的肿瘤，需要从根本上治疗。其总的 5 年生存率不到 35%[486,489,491]。发生在 Paget 病的骨肉瘤呈高度恶性，5 年生存率几乎为零。

软骨肉瘤　Chondrosarcoma

发生在头颈部的软骨肉瘤所占比例从 5%～12% 不等[492,493]。在头颈部，软骨肉瘤男性稍多于女性，主要发生在 30～70 岁的患者。大约 2% 的软骨肉瘤发生在 20 岁以下人群[492-495]。头颈部最常见的发病部位是喉部；实际上，软骨肉瘤可发生在所有有软骨的其他部位，但主要见于颅面部，包括下颌骨、上颌骨、上面部的骨骼（鼻及鼻窦）以及颅底和鼻咽部[492,494,496,497]。症状随发生部位不同而不同。颅面部软骨肉瘤可引起鼻塞、鼻出血、牙的病变（牙齿松动或萌出）、眼球突出、视觉障碍以及因肿瘤长大而引起的疼痛、牙关紧闭、头痛和神经缺陷。颅面部软骨肉瘤放射学检查表现为一种破坏性病变，表现为单个或多个射线透明区、射线不透明区，或混合表现的区域，以及粗糙的钙化。放射学表现可能与组织学分级相关[498]。

软骨肉瘤的大体表现为光滑、分叶状、质硬的黏膜下肿块，直径大于 2cm。组织学上，软骨肉瘤是分叶状且细胞丰富的肿瘤；肿瘤细胞核深染、有多形性，常为双核或多核，核仁明显，核分裂活性增加。这种表现与其他部位的软骨肉瘤相似（见第 25 章），且 I 级病变最常见于头颈部。软骨肉瘤的组织学变型在鼻窦和鼻咽部罕见，包括去分化软骨肉瘤、间叶性软骨肉瘤和透明细胞性软骨肉瘤。

对于上颌面部的软骨肉瘤，需要根治性切除伴有足够的边缘[496]。这些部位的软骨肉瘤是一种缓慢生长但持续存在的肿瘤，以多次复发为特征。上颌面部软骨肉瘤比喉部软骨肉瘤更具致死性，这可能是因为它们的组织学分级往往较高[496]，但更可能是由于它们毗邻重要结构而难以做到切缘阴性。死亡一般是由于未能控制的局部疾病浸润并破坏重要结构，包括向颅内扩散。头颈部软骨肉瘤总的 5 年生存率大约为 70%[493,494]。

脊索瘤　Chordoma

脊索瘤（见第 25 章）发病男性多于女性，任何年龄均可发生，但 40 岁以下发病通常较少见。颅颈部脊索瘤最常见于鞍背区、斜坡和鼻咽部[499]。症状随肿瘤发生部位和范围不同而不同，包括复视、视野缺损、头痛、疼痛、鼻塞、鼻出血、鼻腔排液、软组织包块和内分泌疾病（继发于蝶鞍破坏）。放射学检查可见膨胀性及破坏性的溶骨性病变，常常伴有软组织肿块。

脊索瘤是境界清楚或有包膜，质软，呈黏液样或胶冻状的肿瘤，具有多彩的外观，包括实性和囊性区域。组织学上，形态与较常见的脊柱脊索瘤（见第 25 章）相似，常含有特征性的空泡细胞（physaliferous cell）（图 4A.43）。免疫组化表达 CK、EMA 和 S-100 蛋白（图 4A.43）[500,501]。治疗选择完全手术切除。40 岁以下患者的 5 年生存率可达 100%，而 40 岁以上的只有 22%[501]。

恶性畸胎瘤（畸胎癌肉瘤）
Malignant teratoma (teratocarcinosarcoma)

鼻窦恶性畸胎瘤是一种罕见的肿瘤，具有癌肉瘤和畸胎瘤的组织学特征[502,503]。这些肿瘤发生在成人，以男性为主，中位年龄在 60 岁。鼻窦恶性畸胎瘤生长迅速。最常见的受累部位是鼻腔；其他受累部位包括筛窦和上颌窦。症状包括鼻塞和鼻出血。这些肿瘤是质脆易碎到质地硬韧的红棕色包块。组织学上，恶性畸胎瘤的特征是具有上皮和间叶组织两种成分，生长方式差异很大[502]。上皮成分包括腺体或导管结构，内衬良性表现的部分有纤毛的柱状上皮，伴有向非角化鳞状上皮移行的区域，伴有或没有透明细胞。此外，可见鳞癌和腺癌区域。间叶成分可能包括不同程度良性或恶性表现的纤维母细胞或肌纤维母细胞、横纹肌肉瘤、伴不成熟表现的良性软骨以及软骨肉瘤或成骨组织。畸胎样成分包括"胎儿表现"的透明细胞鳞状上皮、器官样结构或表现为神经菊形团和神经原纤维基质的神经组织。"胎儿表现"的透明细胞鳞状上皮是本病特征性的组织学所见，同时也是支持这种肿瘤畸胎性本质的证据，这在其他器官系统的畸胎瘤也有描述[502]。这些肿瘤没有发现伴有精原细胞瘤、生殖细胞瘤、绒毛膜癌或胚胎性癌病灶。免疫组化染色取决于细胞类型：上皮成分 CK 和 EMA 阳性；神经成分 NSE、CD99、嗜铬素、突触素、GFAP 和 S-100 蛋白阳性；间叶成分波形蛋白阳性，而且根据细胞类型可能与肌源性标记或平滑肌肌动蛋白有反应[503,504]。鼻窦恶性畸胎瘤是高度恶性肿瘤，平均存活时间不足 2 年[502]。需要积极治疗，

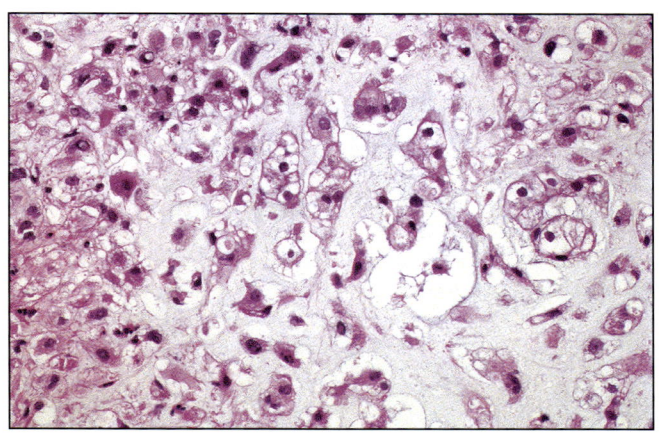

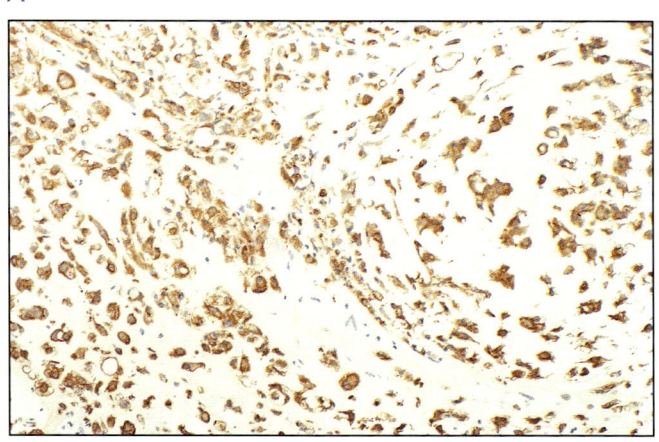

C

图 4A.43　鼻咽脊索瘤。（A）肿瘤细胞呈上皮样，伴有空泡状的细胞核和丰富的颗粒状到空泡状的胞浆。空泡形成相当于存在糖原或黏液；当糖原或黏液较多时，可产生肥皂泡样外观，细胞核受压，形成具有特征性的空泡细胞。肿瘤细胞免疫组化染色 CK（B）和 S-100（C）蛋白阳性。

包括根治性的手术治疗和放射治疗[505]。肿瘤复发常见，而且伴有广泛的局部浸润。转移主要发生在颈部淋巴结。

其他肿瘤　Miscellaneous tumors

可能发生于鼻窦和鼻咽部的其他恶性肿瘤包括脂肪来源的肿瘤[506,507]、滑膜肉瘤[508]、腺泡状软组织肉瘤[509]、外周（原始）神经外胚层肿瘤或 / 骨外 Ewing 肉瘤[510-513]和内胚窦瘤[514,515]。

继发性肿瘤　Secondary tumors

转移至鼻窦和鼻咽的肿瘤可能是疾病的最初表现，或是转移性肿瘤的第一个已知部位。转移至上呼吸消化道（UADT）常是肿瘤广泛转移的一部分。虽然实际上每一种恶性肿瘤均可转移至 UADT，但转移到此部位的最常见原发性肿瘤是肾细胞癌[516-518]。

假瘤性病变　Pseudoneoplastic lesions

鼻窦（炎性）息肉
Sinonasal (inflammatory) polyps

鼻窦炎性息肉是鼻窦黏膜的非肿瘤性炎性隆起。发病无性别差异；可发生于任何年龄，但多见于 20 岁以上的成人，而 5 岁以下的儿童罕见[519]。这个年龄限制的例外情况发生在囊性纤维化患者，他们可在 10～20 岁发生鼻息肉[520]。大多数息肉发生在鼻外侧壁或筛骨隐窝。鼻腔和鼻窦同时受累并不少见。息肉可为单侧性或双侧性，单发性或多发性。症状包括鼻塞、鼻漏和头痛。鼻息肉、哮喘和阿司匹林不耐受三联征已经得到公认[521]。病因与多种因素有关，包括过敏、囊性纤维化、感染、糖尿病和阿司匹林不耐受。

上颌窦后鼻孔息肉（antrochoanal polyps）是特指发生于上颌窦的鼻窦息肉[522]。它们大约占所有鼻窦息肉的 3%～6%[523]。上颌窦后鼻孔息肉男性多于女性，与鼻息肉相比，主要发生在较年轻的患者。大多数上颌窦后鼻孔息肉为伴有鼻塞的单个单侧性病变。从上颌窦向后扩展至鼻咽部可能导致鼻咽阻塞，临床常疑为鼻咽原发性肿瘤。上颌窦后鼻孔息肉常伴有双侧上颌窦炎，而且还可能伴有比较典型的鼻窦息肉。多达 40% 病例可能有过敏史[523,524]。

鼻窦炎性息肉的放射学表现包括软组织密度影、液气平面、黏膜增厚以及副鼻窦混浊。当病变广泛时，炎性息肉可膨胀，甚至破坏骨质。上颌窦后鼻孔息肉可表现为后鼻孔或鼻咽部的软组织密度影，伴有上颌窦模糊或混浊。

鼻窦息肉是质软的鱼肉样息肉样病变，呈黏液样外观。息肉大小不同，直径可达数个厘米。上颌窦后鼻孔息肉除了有一个蒂附着于上颌窦以外，与其他鼻息肉相同。组织学上，表面被覆以完整的呼吸道上皮，但可显示鳞状化生。基底膜可能增厚，呈嗜酸性表现。间质明显水肿，值得注意的是缺乏黏液浆液性腺体。有混合性慢性炎细胞浸润，主要由嗜酸性粒细胞、浆细胞和淋巴细胞组成。感染来源的息肉可能以中性粒细胞为主。间质含有良性表现的纤维母细胞和小至中等大小的血管。继发性改变包括表面溃疡形成、纤维化、梗死、肉芽组织、淀粉样间质沉着，骨和（或）软骨化生，腺体增生，肉芽肿形成以及非典型性间质细胞。肉芽肿来自黏液囊肿破裂、胆固醇肉芽肿或作为对鼻内注射药物（类固醇）或吸入剂的反应。非典型性间质细胞可见于鼻窦息肉和上颌窦后鼻孔息肉，但较常见于后者。这些非典型性细胞形态怪异，伴有增大而深染的多形性细胞核，核仁模糊或明显，胞浆嗜酸或嗜碱性（图 4A.44），这些细胞倾向于在受损组织（如在形成血栓的血管附近）附近成簇排列。非典型性间质细胞可与恶性细胞混淆（例如横纹肌母细胞），但它们局限于病变的部位，结合缺乏核浆比例和核分裂象增加，或缺乏横纹，可以排除恶性肿瘤的诊断。这些细胞是肌纤维母细胞来源，可能是创伤愈合的一种成分[524]。

一种分别被称为血管瘤性[525]或血管扩张性[526]的鼻息肉具有明显血管成分的，在临床上及组织学上均类似于恶性肿瘤，这些病变会发生梗死或伴有无细胞的嗜酸性物质，类似于淀粉样物沉积[526]。

确定和去除可能的致病因子是治疗鼻窦息肉的首要方法。对于鼻息肉进行息肉切除，而对于上颌

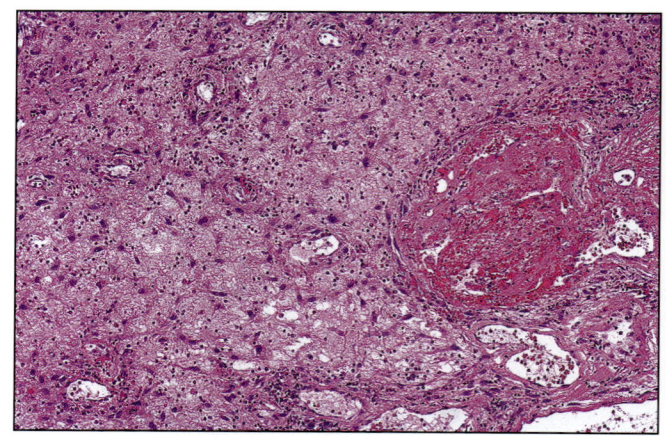

图 4A.44　伴有非典型性间质细胞的上颌窦后鼻孔息肉。非典型性间质细胞（即肌纤维母细胞）核大深染、多形性，核仁模糊或明显，原纤维表现的胞浆呈嗜酸性或嗜碱性。这些细胞通常在受损组织附近局灶排列成簇，包括在有血栓形成的血管周围，如本图最右侧所示。

窦后鼻孔息肉则进行包括息肉蒂在内的内侧上颌骨切除术（Caldwell-Luc 术式）。鼻息肉术后大约 50% 的患者复发；在阿司匹林耐受和哮喘的患者中复发率最高[519]。上颌窦后鼻孔息肉的复发率也高，特别是有过敏史的患者；内镜切除术可能导致较高的复发率[527]。手术切除息肉一并切除其蒂可以明显降低复发的可能性。

异位中枢神经系统组织（神经胶质异位、鼻神经胶质瘤）Heterotopic central nervous system tissue (glial heterotopias, nasal glioma)

异位中枢神经系统组织（HCNST）被认为是颅外部位神经胶质组织的非肿瘤性异位（见第 27 章）。神经胶质异位通常被视为是脑膨出的一种变型，其与中枢神经系统的交通已经关闭，尚未被发现，或已发生纤维化。尽管 HCNST 可发生于任何年龄，但通常出现于新生儿或生后最初几年[528]。在鼻窦及鼻咽部，HCNST 最常发生于鼻腔及鼻腔附近，但可累及筛窦、鼻咽及咽部[529]。皮下病变表现为沿着鼻梁的蓝色或红色包块。鼻内病变表现为鼻塞、呼吸困难、鼻出血、鼻中隔偏离、脑脊液鼻漏或脑膜炎。鼻内病变可能与鼻息肉混淆。可出现混合性鼻内和鼻外 HCNST，其发生是由于鼻骨缺损形成内外交通所致。Furstenberg 试验，即压迫同侧颈静脉后会出现一个隆起或搏动的病变，在脑膨出一般阳性，而 HCNST 为阴性。为了排除可能被看成是与颅腔相通（脑膨出）的骨质缺损，需要进行放射学研究，尤其是磁共振检查[530]。

组织学上，HCNST 由星形细胞和神经胶质纤维组成，伴有纤维性富于血管的结缔组织。可出现反应性星形细胞，包括多核或原浆性星形细胞。神经元稀疏或缺如。在长期未被临床发现的病例中，可有突出的纤维性间质，并掩盖了星形细胞和神经胶质纤维。与鼻部病变不同，鼻咽部病变可能出现室管膜成分以及胞浆内黑色素[529]。免疫组化染色 GFAP 和 S-100 蛋白阳性[531]。治疗选择外科手术，可以治愈。

呼吸上皮腺瘤样错构瘤 Respiratory epithelial adenomatoid hamartoma

呼吸上皮腺瘤样错构瘤是鼻腔、副鼻窦或鼻咽部固有腺体的一种不常见的良性非肿瘤性过度生长，起源于表面上皮，缺乏外胚层、神经外胚层和（或）中胚层的成分[532,533]。该部位的大多数错构瘤都是单纯性上皮性错构瘤[533]。可发生间叶性错构瘤或混合性上皮-间叶性错构瘤[532-534]。呼吸上皮腺瘤样错构瘤主要发生于成年患者，男性占明显优势，病人年龄从 20～90 岁不等，中位年龄为 50-60 岁[533]。多数呼吸上皮腺瘤样错构瘤发生在鼻腔，特别是后鼻中隔；鼻内其他部位受累不常发生，但可见于鼻侧壁、中鼻道和下鼻甲[533]。其他受累的部位包括鼻咽部、筛窦和额窦。病变大部分为单侧性，偶尔可以发生双侧性病变。患者表现为鼻塞或鼻阻塞、鼻中隔偏离、鼻出血及慢性（复发性）鼻窦炎。症状可能持续数月至数年。

这种错构瘤表现为息肉样肿块，质地比炎性息肉稍硬[532]。组织学检查，这些病变的特征为腺体明显增生，为被间质组织分开的间隔较宽的小至中等大小的腺体。某些区域可见腺体直接与内陷到黏膜下的表面上皮相连（图 4A.45）。这种腺体为圆形到卵圆形，由复层纤毛呼吸上皮组成。常常混合有分泌黏液的（杯状）细胞。其特征性表现是间质出现玻璃样变，腺体被增厚的嗜酸性基底膜包绕。可见小的呈分泌性表现的浆液黏液腺。间质水肿或纤维化，含有混合性的慢性炎细胞浸润。

可见于呼吸上皮腺瘤样错构瘤的其他所见包括炎性鼻窦息肉、增生和（或）与腺瘤样增生无关的表面上皮鳞状化生，骨化生，少数病例伴有内翻性乳头状瘤和 SFT[532]。

鉴别诊断包括内翻型乳头状瘤和腺癌。误诊可导致不恰当的外科治疗。局限但完全的手术切除可以治愈[532]。

畸胎样病变（鼻咽部皮样囊肿；鼻咽部"毛息肉"）Teratoid lesions (nasopharyngeal dermoid; nasopharyngeal "hairy polyp")

鼻咽部畸胎样病变是发育性（先天性）异常，而非肿瘤性病变；它们主要由外胚层成分组成（例如皮肤），也可包括中胚层结构（例如软骨），但无内胚层衍化而来的结构[535]。缺乏内胚层衍化而来的结构以及存在有限的异质性组织类型均不支持它是畸胎瘤。事实上，这些病变含有皮肤，一种正常鼻咽部不存在的组织类型，提示最好将其归为迷芽瘤（choristoma），而非错构瘤，可能起源于第一鳃弓[536-538]。一些作者认为最好将这些病变归为良性畸胎瘤的一个亚型[539]。

鼻咽部皮样囊肿呈息肉样，大部分为实性，但部分为囊性病变，可能有蒂或无蒂。组织学上，各种外胚层和中胚层组织混合存在，包括皮肤（角化性鳞状上皮）、皮肤附属器、软骨、骨、肌肉（横纹肌或平滑肌）、纤维组织或成熟的脂肪组织。这些病变呈息肉样，表面被覆带有毛囊和皮脂腺的皮肤组织。此外，可见

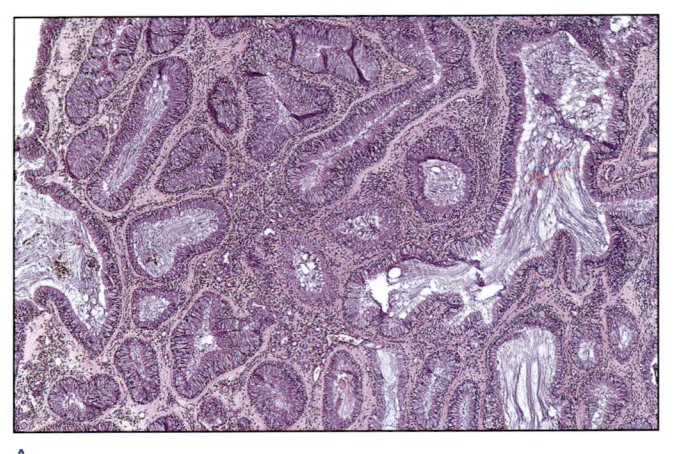 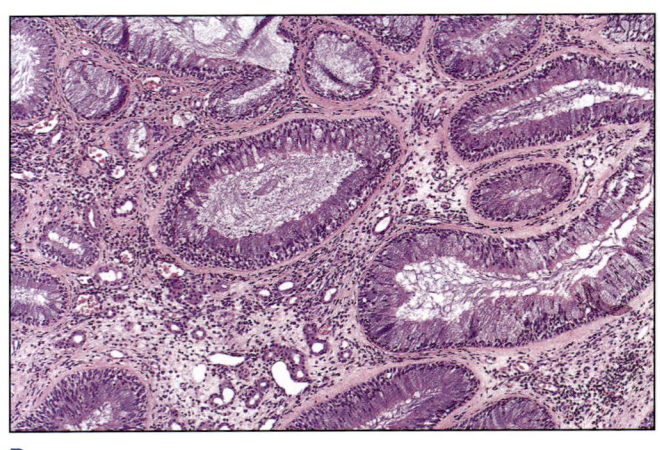

图4A.45 呼吸上皮腺瘤样错构瘤。（A）这些病变起源于表面上皮，黏膜下可见内陷和增生的腺体。（B）腺体内衬纤毛呼吸上皮，伴有间质玻璃样变，特征性的包围腺瘤性增生的腺体；在腺瘤样增生及其周围可见残余的小涎腺。

弹性软骨。在耳的病变中见到这些组织学成分提示某些作者这些病变来源于鳃裂，是先天性副耳廓，类似于副耳屏[537]。除了软骨以外，还可见不同程度的其他类型的组织，包括肌肉（平滑肌和横纹肌）、纤维脂肪组织和血管组织。

由于这些病变被定义为一种非肿瘤性发育性异常，故主要应与畸胎瘤进行鉴别诊断。缺乏内胚层衍化而来的组织，并缺乏通常见于畸胎瘤的各种类型的组织，可将这些病变鉴别开来。单纯手术切除可以治愈。

鼻软骨间叶性错构瘤
Nasal chondromesenchymal hamartoma

鼻软骨间叶性错构瘤是鼻窦的一种肿胀性病变，由软骨和间质成分混合组成，伴有囊性特征，类似于胸壁错构瘤[540]。这些病变形态学上与呼吸上皮腺瘤样错构瘤有某些相似之处，两者可归于同一类型病变谱系。然而，二者又有不同之处，与呼吸上皮腺瘤样错构瘤相比，本病多数发生于新生儿年龄组，病变倾向于较大，而且更具侵袭性[540]，迄今为止报道不到20例[540,541]。主要发生于男性。这些病变多数发生于3个月以内的新生儿，但亦可发生于10～20岁[539,539a]，甚或成年人[539a]。患者表现为呼吸困难和鼻内肿物，或有明显面部肿胀。其中某些肿瘤还可侵犯颅腔（通过筛板区），这种表现可能类似于脑膜脑膨出[542]。

组织学特征是出现大小、形状及轮廓各异的软骨结节。而且，软骨分化程度不一，某些结节的表现类似于软骨黏液样纤维瘤的软骨黏液瘤性结节，而另外一些结节则由分化好的软骨组成。软骨结节周围可见一些松散的梭形细胞间质，或突然转化为细胞稀少的纤维性间质。

其他结构包括黏液样到梭形细胞间质，纤维骨性增生伴有富于细胞的间质成分，以及小片骨或不成熟的（编织状）骨小梁。其他所见可能包括间质内局灶性的破骨细胞样巨细胞，以及类似于动脉瘤样骨囊肿的充满红细胞的间隙[540,543]。增生上皮成分不是明显特征。软骨间叶性成分相对富于细胞及"不成熟"，也许反映了患者未成熟的年龄。因此认为这些病变是鼻错构瘤的一个独特的临床病理亚型。

扁桃体淋巴管瘤性息肉（淋巴样息肉）
Lymphangiomatous polyp of the tonsil (lymphoid polyp)

淋巴管瘤性息肉是非肿瘤性发育性病变，由鼻咽部固有的组织成分组成，因此被归为错构瘤[544]。淋巴管瘤性息肉并不常见。男女发病相等；发病年龄广泛，从1～70岁均可发病，平均年龄25岁[544]。临床表现包括吞咽困难、咽喉疼痛以及咽喉部异物感。症状可出现数周至数年。这些病变为单侧性，左右侧发病率相当。大部分起源于腭扁桃体，但偶可起源于鼻咽部或鼻咽扁桃体（腺样体）[544]。

大部分病变呈息肉状或带蒂，表面光滑，质地呈海绵到实性。切面白色、褐色或黄色，最大径为0.5～3.8 cm。某些病变无蒂。息肉表面被覆鳞状上皮或呼吸上皮，黏膜下为增生扩张的淋巴管和数量不等的纤维结缔组织。脉管成分壁薄，通常含有蛋白性液体和成熟淋巴细胞。另外，在任何一个病变中均可见成熟脂肪组织和明显的纤维化。

其他改变包括上皮增生、角化过度以及不伴有异常增生的角化不全或上皮内淋巴细胞[544]。

诊断通常无需特殊染色。单纯手术切除可以治愈，通常采取单侧扁桃体切除术。鉴别诊断包括鼻咽部（青少年）血管纤维瘤、纤维上皮样息肉、乳头状瘤和淋巴管瘤。

鼻窦和鼻咽部感染性疾病
Sinonasal and nasopharyngeal infectious diseases

鼻窦和鼻咽部感染性疾病在临床上可能类似于肿瘤性疾病的表现。这些部位某些较常见的感染有真菌感染，例如曲菌病[545,546]、鼻孢子虫病[547]和毛真菌病[548]，细菌性疾病，例如鼻硬结病[549]和绿脓杆菌引起的细菌球（葡萄状菌病）[550]，以及分枝杆菌病，例如麻风和结核病。结节病是一种病因不明的非干酪性肉芽肿性疾病，可作为全身性疾病的一部分累及鼻腔，或作为一种孤立性疾病[551]。在免疫缺陷病人中，诸如单纯疱疹病毒、巨细胞病毒和HIV[552]等病毒感染以及诸如小孢子菌病[553]等原虫感染，可引起鼻窦和鼻咽部的溃疡性和（或）肿块性病变，临床上与肿瘤性病变相似（见下）。传染性单核细胞增多症是一种全身性、良性、自限性淋巴组织增生性疾病，可能导致鼻咽扁桃体（腺样体）或腭扁桃体增大，临床上及组织学检查均与肿瘤（例如恶性淋巴瘤）相似。传染性单核细胞增多症主要发生于青少年及年轻成人。传染性单核细胞增多症通常由EB病毒感染引起，但其他微生物感染亦可引起非常相似的病理学改变，包括兔弓形虫、风疹、A型肝炎病毒和腺病毒。

肌小球体病（myospherulosis）是一种假真菌性包块，是红细胞与外科包扎材料中凡士林软膏相互作用发生改变而形成的一种反应性现象[554]。

Waldeyer扁桃体组织的HIV感染
Human immunodeficiency virus infection of Waldeyer's tonsillar tissues

人免疫缺陷病毒（HIV）感染在临床上可能最先表现为Waldeyer环淋巴组织增大，包括扁桃体和腺样体[552]。这些淋巴组织是病毒复制的主要部位。最初的HIV感染导致一系列组织病理学改变，可能是无症状HIV感染患者的初始表现。临床上扁桃体肿大，特别是鼻咽部淋巴组织（腺样体）肿大，可能是HIV感染最早的临床表现[552]。扁桃体和腺样体肿大可为单侧性，引起临床关注并可能诊断为淋巴瘤。

这些组织感染HIV引起一系列的独特诊断特征，包括明显的滤泡增生、滤泡消散以及HIV感染出现的多核巨细胞。血清学检查可以证实HIV感染。HIV导致的扁桃体和腺样体肿大的组织形态学表现随着病情的发展而变化。在感染早期，组织形态学改变可能包括明显的滤泡增生，伴或不伴滤泡破碎，以及滤泡消散伴滤泡复旧的区域（图4A.46）。其他所见包括出现单核细胞样B细胞增生、副皮质区和滤泡间区由于免疫母细胞和浆细胞而增宽、滤泡间区出现成簇的有明显内皮细胞的小静脉、滤泡内出血以及出现多核巨细胞（图4A.46）。巨细胞特征是在腺样体表面上皮或扁桃体隐窝上皮内或其附近成簇排列。

本病较晚期患者的组织学特征与上述表现不同，而是与见于HIV感染末期或AIDS病人的淋巴组织消失有关。在这些病例，淋巴结结构消失，正常淋巴细胞群消失，被良性浆细胞浸润取代，而且血管成分增加。在较晚期阶段的HIV感染见不到本病早期和慢性阶段可见的特征

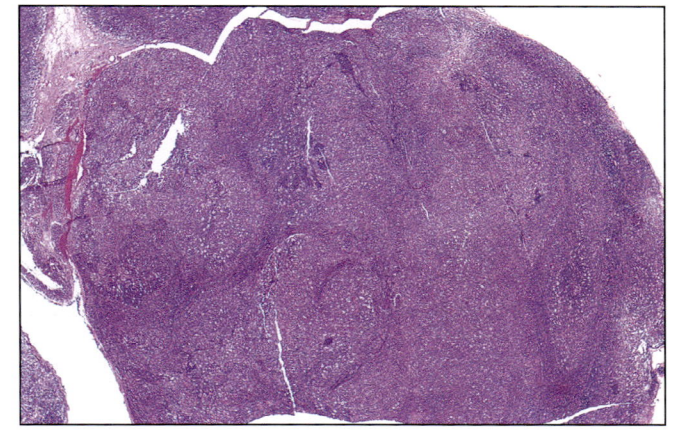

A

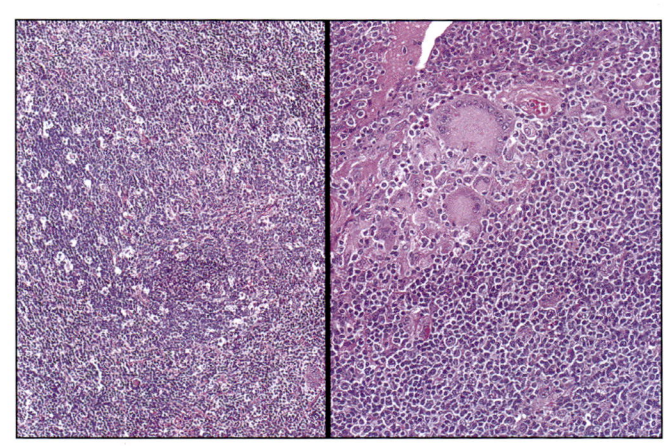

B

图4A.46 扁桃体HIV感染。（A）明显的滤泡增生；（B）左图：滤泡消散，伴有套区淋巴细胞减少和丧失；右图：在表面[和（或）隐窝上皮]上皮附近成簇的多核巨细胞。

性多核巨细胞。

HIV p24（gag protein）反应作为活动性 HIV 感染的标志，在本病早期和慢性阶段总是阳性。抗 HIV p24 反应见于生发中心的滤泡树突细胞网、滤泡间散在的淋巴细胞、多核巨细胞以及隐窝上皮的上皮内细胞。HIV p24 阳性的上皮内细胞 S-100 蛋白（树突状细胞的标记物）阳性，且形态学表现与树突状细胞一致。

Wegener 肉芽肿病（WG）
Wegener's granulomatosis（WG）

Wegener 肉芽肿病（WG）是一种系统性坏死性血管炎，典型者累及肾、肺和上呼吸消化道（UADT）。经典的 WG 定义包括头颈部、肺和肾受累[555,556]。需要注意的是，多数 WG 患者最初并不同时出现典型的临床三征。WG 可以表现为局限于鼻窦的一种孤立性疾病，而无系统性受累；鼻窦受累可以是系统性疾病的最初表现[557,558]。WG 的病因学仍不清楚。

WG 可以是系统性或局限性（局灶性）。疾病程度反映在临床表现上，局限性或局灶性疾病可无症状，而系统性疾病患者则总是呈现病态。WG 可从局限性进展为系统性受累，或局限性病变得以维持，甚或在治疗后消退。WG 的 ELK[555] 分类如下：

E = 耳、鼻和咽喉受累

L = 肺受累

K = 肾受累

E 或 EL 期患者被认为是局限性 WG，而 ELK 疾病则相当于系统性 WG。局限性 WG（limited WG）的发生率从 29%～58% 不等[555]。UADT 的局灶性 WG 男性多于女性（喉部 WG 除外，其主要发生于女性）。WG 发病年龄广泛，平均发病年龄为 40～50 岁，WG 不常发生于 10 岁以下个体。在上呼吸消化道，WG 最常见的发生部位是鼻窦部（依次为鼻腔、上颌窦、筛窦、额窦和蝶窦），其他受累部位可能包括鼻咽部、喉（声门下）、口腔、耳（外耳和中耳，包括乳突）和涎腺。鼻窦和鼻咽部 WG 可表现为鼻窦炎，伴或不伴鼻脓性排液、鼻塞、鼻中隔穿孔、疼痛、鼻出血、嗅觉丧失和头痛。WG 的一个重要实验室所见是 ANCA 水平升高。WG 的特征是伴有胞浆 ANCA（C-ANCA），只在少数情况下伴有核周 ANCA（P-ANCA）[557-559]。C-ANCA 比 P-ANCA 更具特异性。试验的敏感性随疾病范围而不同；50%～67% 局限性 WG 患者 C-ANCA 阳性，而系统性 WG 患者 60%～100%C-ANCA 阳性[558,560]。ANCA 试验阴性不能排除 WG。虽然在其他血管炎[561]和炎症性肠病以及肝胆疾病[562,563]可见 ANCA，但 ANCA 滴度在 WG 升高，而在感染性疾病或淋巴瘤并不升高。

头颈部 WG 主要表现为鼻腔和副鼻窦受累。临床表现为弥漫性黏膜肿胀伴有溃疡性和结痂性病变以及组织破坏；晚期病例可见鼻中隔穿孔，导致"鞍鼻"畸形。由于许多 WG 病变都具有破坏性本质，所以有时临床疑为恶性肿瘤。

组织学特征包括血管炎、组织坏死和肉芽肿性炎在内的典型三征（可能累及血管壁和支持组织）（图 4A.47）。然而，在一次活检甚或一系列的活检中发现所有 3 项"特征"的实际上非常少见[564]。血管炎累及小至中等大小的动脉，由多形性炎症细胞浸润构成，包括淋巴细胞和组织细胞，以及不常见的嗜酸性粒细胞和多形核白细胞。坏死为"缺血"型或"地图"型，伴有嗜碱性模糊的表现。上呼吸消化道的 WG 出现散在多核巨细胞的肉芽肿性炎是其典型表现，而结构完整的肉芽肿却不常见。WG 实质的炎细胞浸润一般为混合性，主要是由淋巴细胞、组织细胞、浆细胞和中性粒细胞组成的；嗜酸性粒细胞一般不常见，但在个别病例可有许多嗜酸性粒细胞。

弹性纤维染色可能有助于血管炎的诊断。需要考虑的主要组织学鉴别诊断是感染和肿瘤。必须排除感染性病变（例如真菌、分枝杆菌、寄生虫）引起的肉芽肿性反应。因此，通过组织染色和培养来排除感染性因子应该作为评估所有 WG 可疑患者的基本方法之一。同样，在某些活检中，可能需要考虑某些异物（例如肌小球病）引起的肉芽肿性反应，而且，建议对所有 WG 可疑病例均应对组织进行偏振光异物检查。

由于某些鼻窦 NK/T- 细胞淋巴瘤是血管中心性淋巴瘤，所以血管浸润会被误认为是 WG 的血管炎（表 4A.11）。淋巴细胞浸润的细胞学特征常可用于区分这两种疾病。一般来说，WG 的淋巴细胞浸润缺乏细胞学非典型性。非典型性是恶性淋巴瘤肿瘤细胞的特征。由于单凭光学显微镜特征辨认淋巴细胞非典型性可能具有某种程度的主观性，所以通过免疫组化和分子生物学研究证实单克隆性可能会有帮助。WG 的炎症浸润一般为多形性，而且显示 B 细胞系和 T- 细胞系标记物均可反应。鼻窦恶性淋巴瘤通常可见单形性浸润，谱系标记物一般会显示 B 或 T 细胞系专一性。另外，恶性淋巴瘤不会出现 WG 的微脓肿和散在的巨细胞以及 C-ANCA 水平升高。由于 WG 的炎症浸润可能包括相当数量的嗜酸性粒细胞，这就提出有无 Churg-Strauss 肉芽肿病的问题（表 4A.11）。Churg-Strauss 肉芽肿病（变应性肉芽肿病和血管炎）的特点是哮喘、系统性血管炎以及组织和外周嗜酸性粒细胞增多。这些所见应该有助于 WG 的鉴别诊断。因为有报道 Churg-Strauss 病 ANCA 水平升高[565,566]，所以 ANCA 升高不能用于 Churg-Strauss 病与 WG 的鉴别

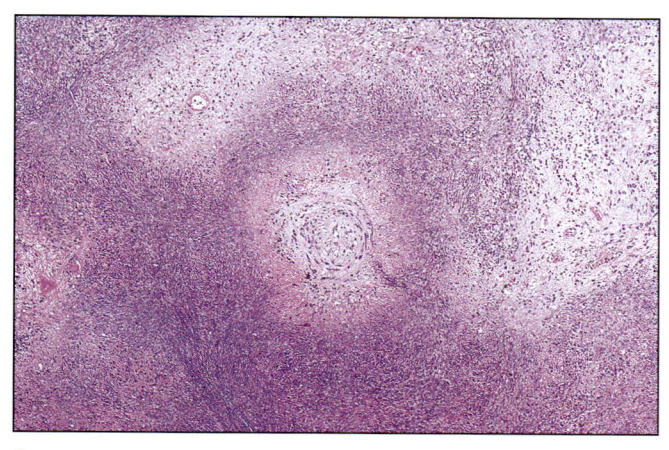

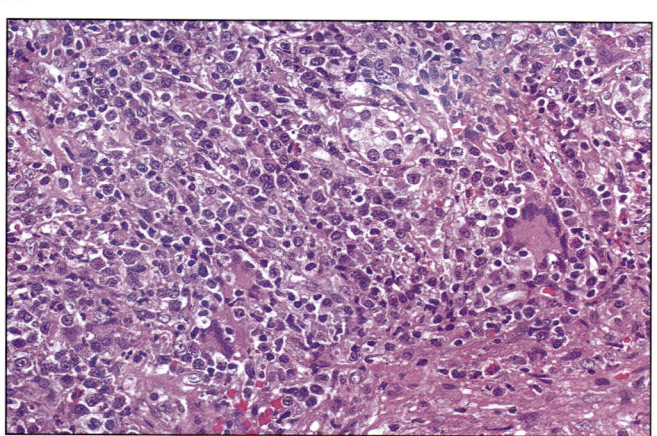

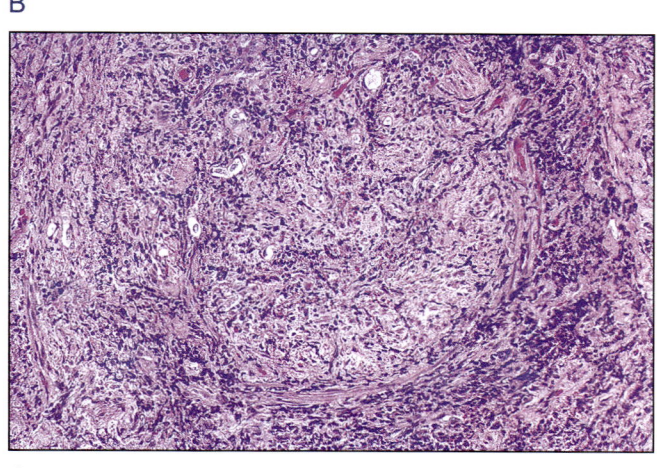

图4A.47 鼻窦Wegener肉芽肿病。（A）低倍镜下的改变包括出现多灶性坏死（"地图"或"缺血型"坏死），图中心闭塞血管的周围呈嗜碱性模糊的表现。（B）Wegener肉芽肿病炎症细胞浸润为多形性，由不同数量的成熟淋巴细胞、浆细胞、组织细胞、嗜酸性粒细胞和中性粒细胞混合而成，没有非典型性或明显恶性细胞的证据；在所有这些图中均有孤立的多核巨细胞，这是本病的肉芽肿成分（较差的肉芽肿），因为一般见不到结构完整的肉芽肿。（C）血管炎，在组织学检查时可能难以发现，这里所见血管炎伴有炎症细胞浸润，围绕在血管周围（血管中心性）并侵入血管壁（血管浸润），伴有管腔内衬内皮的闭塞性改变。

诊断。应该记住，不要期待Churg-Strauss病在临床上出现鼻窦部病变，发生这种病变的机会非常有限。

结外窦组织细胞增多症伴有巨大淋巴结病（Rosai-Dorfman病）
Extranodal sinus histiocytosis with massive lymphadenopathy (Rosai-Dorfman disease)

窦组织细胞增多症伴有巨大淋巴结病（SHML）是一种以淋巴结为基础的特发性组织细胞增生性疾病，通常可以自发性消退[567-569]。免疫表型研究支持SHML细胞是单核吞噬细胞和免疫调节效应器（M-PIRE）系统的一部分，属于巨噬细胞/组织细胞家族[570]。SHML可以作为累及淋巴结的全身性疾病的一部分，或可能累及结外部位，与淋巴结的状况无关[571]。头颈部是SHML较常累及的结外部位之一[569,571]。在头颈部，好发于鼻腔和副鼻窦[571]。鼻窦受累形成息肉样、结节状或外生性肿块，引起鼻塞而且酷似肿瘤。组织病理学特征包括黏膜下出现淋巴细胞集聚，与弥漫性累及黏膜下的由组织细胞、淋巴细胞和浆细胞带构成的淡染区域交替出现。特征性组织细胞（或SHML细胞）具有圆形至卵圆形、空泡状至深染的细胞核，伴有嗜双色性至嗜酸性、颗粒状、泡沫样至透明的细胞浆（图4A.48）。细胞核没有像Langerhans细胞组织细胞那样的分叶、切迹或纵沟。组织细胞具有吞噬功能（emperipolesis）。被吞噬的细胞通常是淋巴细胞，但在组织细胞胞浆内还可见被吞噬的浆细胞、红细胞和中性粒细胞。SHML细胞S-100蛋白弥漫阳性。另外，SHML细胞还可能表达CD68、溶菌酶和MAC-387[571-573]。无理想治疗方法[574]。治疗方法的选择要依据其临床表现。在气道受损的病例中，需要手术处理以直接减轻阻塞症状。死亡的报道少见[575]。SHML病因仍然不清。有人提出感染病因学[567,568]，但从未分离出感染因子。其他考虑有影响但从未得到证实的SHML原因包括免疫缺陷、自身免疫性疾病或肿瘤性病变[569]。

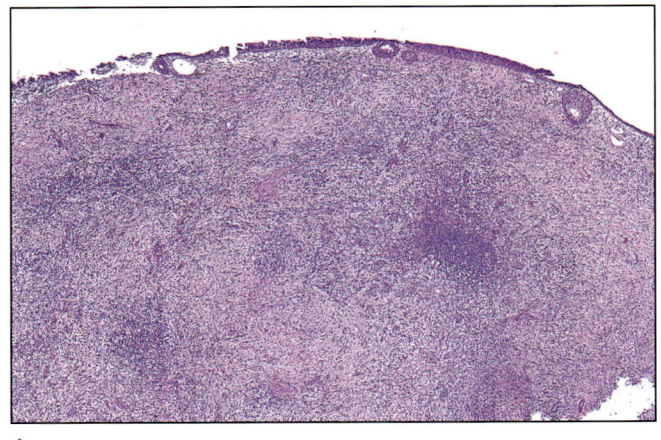 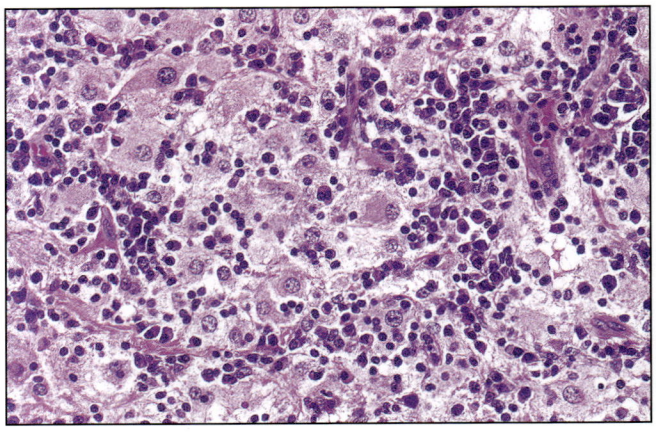

图4A.48 鼻窦结外窦组织细胞增多症伴有巨大淋巴结病。（A）黏膜下弥漫性炎症细胞浸润，伴有正常黏膜下结构消失；右侧中心可见良性淋巴细胞集聚，连同富于细胞的浸润一起使人想起这种结构表现类似于淋巴结实质。（B）在较高倍数下，浸润细胞包括成熟淋巴细胞和浆细胞，在某种程度上遮盖了浸润的组织细胞；后者具有吞噬单核细胞的作用。

参考文献

1. Lampertico P, Russel WO, MacComb WS 1963 Squamous papilloma of the upper respiratory epithelium. Arch Pathol 75: 293–302
2. Hyams V J 1971 Papillomas of the nasal cavity and paranasal sinuses: a clinicopathologic study of 315 cases. Ann Otol Rhinol Laryngol 80: 192–206
3. Hyams V J, Batsakis J G, Michaels L 1988 Papilloma of the sinonasal tract. In: Tumors of the upper respiratory tract and ear, series 2, fascicle 25. Armed Forces Institute of Pathology, Washington, DC, p 34–44
4. Joseph M, Carroll E, Goodman M L et al. 1980 Inverted papilloma of the nasal septum. Arch Otolaryngol 106: 767–771
5. Christensen W N, Smith R R L 1986 Schneiderian papillomas: a clinicopathologic study of 67 cases. Hum Pathol 17: 393–400
6. Lawson W, Le Benger J, Som P et al. 1989 Inverted papilloma: an analysis of 87 cases. Laryngoscope 99: 1117–1124
7. Siivonen L, Virolainen E 1989 Transitional papillomas of the nasal cavity and paranasal sinuses. ORL J Otorhinolaryngol Relat Spec 51: 262–267
8. Lawson W, Ho B T, Shaari C M et al. 1995 Inverted papilloma: A report of 112 cases. Laryngoscope 105: 282–288
9. Buchwald C, Franzmann M-B, Tos M 1995 Sinonasal papillomas: a report of 82 cases in Copenhagen county, including a longitudinal clinical study. Laryngoscope 105: 72–79
10. Peters BW, O'Reilly RC, Wilcox TO Jr et al. 1995 Inverted papilloma isolated to the sphenoid sinus. Otolaryngol Head Neck Surg 113: 771–781
11. Brandwein M, Steinberg B, Thung S et al. 1989 Human papillomavirus 6/11 and 16/18 in schneiderian inverted papillomas: in situ hybridization with human papillomavirus RNA probes. Cancer 63: 1708–1713
12. Judd R, Zaki S R, Coffield L M et al. 1991 Sinonasal papillomas and human papillomavirus: human papillomavirus 11 detected in fungiform Schneiderian papillomas by in situ hybridization and polymerase chain reaction. Hum Pathol 22: 550–556
13. Sarkar F H, Visscher D W, Kintanar E B et al. 1992 Sinonasal Schneiderian papillomas: human papillomavirus typing by polymerase chain reaction. Mod Pathol 5: 329–332
14. Buchwald C, Franzmann M-B, Jacobsen G K et al. 1995 Human papillomavirus (HPV) in sinonasal papillomas: a study of 78 cases using in situ hybridization and polymerase chain reaction. Laryngoscope 105: 66–71
15. Harris M O, Beck J C, Terrell J E et al. 1998 Expression of human papillomavirus 6 in inverted papilloma arising in a renal transplant patient. Laryngoscope 108: 115–119
16. Barnes L 2002. Schneiderian papillomas and nonsalivary glandular neoplasms of the head and neck. Mod Pathol 15: 279–297
17. Macdonald M R, Le K T, Freeman J et al. 1995 A majority of inverted sinonasal papillomas carries Epstein–Barr virus genomes. Cancer 75: 2307–2312
18. Gaffey M J, Frierson H F, Weiss L M et al. 1996 Human papillomavirus and Epstein–Barr virus in sinonasal Schneiderian papillomas. An in situ hybridization and polymerase chain reaction study. Am J Clin Pathol 106: 475–482
19. Myers E N, Fernau J L, Johnson J T et al. 1990 Management of inverted papilloma. Laryngoscope 100: 481–490
20. Mendenhall W M, Million R R, Cassisi N J et al. 1985 Biologically aggressive papillomas of the nasal cavity: the role of radiation therapy. Laryngoscope 134: 73–79
21. Klemi P J, Joensu H, Siivonen L et al. 1989 Association of DNA aneuploidy with human papillomavirus-induced malignant transformation of sinonasal transitional papillomas. Otolaryngol Head Neck Surg 100: 563–567
22. Ward B E, Fechner R E, Mills S E 1990 Carcinoma arising in oncocytic Schneiderian papilloma. Am J Surg Pathol 14: 364–369
23. Kapadia S B, Barnes L, Pelzman K et al. 1993 Carcinoma ex oncocytic Schneiderian (cylindrical cell) papilloma. Am J Clin Pathol 14: 1–7
24. Lesperanie M M, Esclamado R M 1995 Squamous cell carcinoma arising in inverted papilloma. Laryngoscope 105: 178–183
25. Norris H J 1962 Papillary lesions of the nasal cavity and paranasal sinuses. Part I: Exophytic (squamous) papillomas. A study of 28 cases. Laryngoscope 72: 1784–1797
26. Batsakis J G 1980 The pathology of head and neck tumors: nasal cavity and paranasal sinuses, part 5. Head Neck Surg 2: 410–419
27. Sulica R L, Wenig B M, Debo R F et al. 1999 Schneiderian papillomas of the pharynx. Ann Otol Rhinol Laryngol 108: 392–397
28. Compagno J, Wong R T 1977 Intranasal mixed tumors (pleomorphic adenomas). A clinicopathologic study of 40 cases. Am J Clin Pathol 68: 213–218
29. Begin L R, Rochon L, Frenkiel S 1991 Spindle cell myoepithelioma of the nasal cavity. Am J Surg Pathol 15: 184–190
30. Lloyd R V, Chandler W F, Kovacs K et al. 1986 Ectopic pituitary adenomas with normal anterior pituitary glands. Am J Surg Pathol 10: 546–552
31. Wenig B, Heffess C, Adair C et al. 1995 Ectopic pituitary adenomas: a clinicopathologic study of 15 cases. Mod Pathol 8: 56A (abstract)
32. Hosaka N, Kitajiri S, Hiraumi H et al. 2002 Ectopic pituitary adenoma with malignant transformation. Am J Surg Pathol 26: 1078–1082
33. Zak F G, Lawson W 1982 The paraganglionic chemoreceptor system: physiology, pathology and clinical medicine. Springer-Verlag, New York
34. Apple D, Kreines K 1982 Cushing's syndrome due to ectopic ACTH production by a nasal paraganglioma. Am J Med Sci 283: 32–35
35. Kliewer K E, Wen D-R, Cancilla P A et al. 1989 Paragangliomas: assessment of prognosis by histologic, immunohistochemical, and ultrastructural techniques. Hum Pathol 20: 29–39
36. Johnson T L, Zarbo R J, Lloyd R V et al. 1988 Paragangliomas of the head and neck: immunohistochemical neuroendocrine and intermediate filament typing. Mod Pathol 1: 216–223
37. Nguyen Q A, Gibbs P M, Rice D H 1995 Malignant nasal paraganglioma: a case report and review of the literature. Otolaryngol Head Neck Surg 113: 157–161
38. Burger P C, Scheithauer B W 1994 Tumors of meningiothelial cells. In: Rosai J, Sobin L H (eds) Tumors of the central nervous system, series 3, fascicle 10. Armed Forces Institute of Pathology, Washington, DC, p 259–286
39. Perzin K H, Pushparaj N 1984 Non-epithelial tumors of the nasal cavity, paranasal sinuses, and nasopharynx: a clinicopathologic study. XIII. Meningiomas. Cancer 54: 1860–1869
40. Thompson L D, Gyure K A 2000 Extracranial sinonasal tract meningiomas: a clinicopathologic study of 30 cases with a review of the literature. Am J Surg Pathol 24: 640–650
41. Ho K L 1980 Primary meningioma of the nasal cavity and paranasal sinuses. Cancer 46: 1442–1447

42. Fu Y S, Perzin K H 1974 Non-epithelial tumors of the nasal cavity, paranasal sinuses, and nasopharynx: a clinicopathologic study. I. General features and vascular tumors. Cancer 33: 1275–1288
43. Sheppard L M, Michaelson S A 1990 Hemangioma of the nasal septum and paranasal sinuses. Henry Ford Hosp Med J 38: 25–27
44. Mills S E, Cooper P H, Fechner R E 1980 Lobular capillary hemangioma: the underlying lesion of pyogenic granuloma. A study of 73 cases from the oral and nasal mucous membranes. Am J Surg Pathol 4: 471–479
45. Nichols G E, Gaffey M J, Mills S E et al. 1992 Lobular capillary hemangioma. An immunohistochemical study including steroid hormone receptor status. Am J Clin Pathol 97: 770–775
46. Yuan K, Lin M T 2004 The roles of vascular endothelial growth factor and angiopoietin-2 in the regression of pregnancy pyogenic granuloma. Oral Dis 10: 179–185
47. Cheuk W, Wong K O, Wong C S et al. 2004 Immunostaining for human herpesvirus 8 latent nuclear antigen-1 helps distinguish Kaposi sarcoma from its mimickers. Am J Clin Pathol 121: 335–342
48. Batsakis J G, Rice D H 1981 The pathology of head and neck tumors. Vasoformative tumors, part 9A. Head Neck Surg 3: 231–239
49. Apostol J V, Frazell E L 1965 Juvenile nasopharyngeal angiofibroma. A clinical study. Cancer 18: 869–878
50. Neel H B, Whicker J H, Devine K D et al. 1973 Nasopharyngeal angiofibroma. Review of 120 cases. Am J Surg 126: 547–556
51. McGavran M H, Dorfman R F, Davis D O et al. 1969 Nasopharyngeal angiofibroma. Arch Otolaryngol 90: 68–78
52. Amedee R, Klaeyle D, Mann W et al. 1989 Juvenile angiofibromas: a 40-year surgical experience. ORL J Otorhinolaryngol Relat Spec 51: 56–61
53. Hyams V J, Batsakis J G, Michaels L 1988 Angiofibroma. In: Tumors of the upper respiratory tract and ear, series 2, fascicle 25. Armed Forces Institute of Pathology, Washington, DC, p 130–134
54. Hazarika P, Nayak R G, Chandran M 1985 Extra-nasopharyngeal extension of juvenile angiofibroma. J Laryngol Otol 99: 813–817
55. Johnson S, Kloster J H, Schiff M 1966 The actions of hormones on juvenile angiofibroma. Acta Otolaryngol 61: 153–160
56. Hwang H C, Mills S E, Patterson K et al. 1998 Expression of androgen receptors in nasopharyngeal angiofibroma: an immunohistochemical study of 24 cases. Mod Pathol 11: 1122–1126
57. Johns M E, MacLeod R M, Cantrell R W 1980 Estrogen receptors in nasopharyngeal angiofibromas. Laryngoscope 90: 628–634
58. Giardello F M, Hamilton S R, Krush A J et al. 1993 Nasopharyngeal angiofibroma in patients with familial adenomatous polyposis. Gastroenterology 105: 1550–1552
59. Ferouz A S, Mohr R M, Paul P 1995 Juvenile nasopharyngeal angiofibroma and familial adenomatous polyposis: an association? Otolaryngol Head Neck Surg 113: 435–439
60. Abraham S C, Montgomery E A, Giardiello F M et al. 2001 Frequent β-catenin mutations in juvenile nasopharyngeal angiofibromas. Am J Pathol 158: 1073–1078
61. Guertl B, Beham A, Zachner R et al. 2000 Nasopharyngeal angiofibroma: an APC-gene-associated tumor? Hum Pathol 31: 1411–1413
62. Zhang P J, Weber R, Liang H-H et al. 2003 Growth factors and receptors in juvenile nasopharyngeal angiofibroma and nasal polyps: an immunohistochemical study. Arch Pathol Lab Med 127: 1480–1484
63. Baguley C, Sandhu G, O'Donnell J et al. 2004 Consumptive coagulopathy complicating juvenile angiofibroma. J Laryngol Otol 118: 835–839
64. Sessions R B, Wills P I, Alford B R et al. 1976 Juvenile angiofibroma: Radiographic aspects. Laryngoscope 86: 2–18
65. Sessions R B, Bryan R N, Naclerio R M et al. 1981 Radiographic staging of juvenile angiofibroma. Head Neck Surg 3: 279–283
66. Fisch U 1983 The infratemporal fossa approach for nasopharyngeal tumors. Laryngoscope 93: 36–44
67. Chandler J R, Goulding R, Moskowitz L et al. 1984 Nasopharyngeal angiofibromas: staging and management. Ann Otol Rhinol Laryngol 93: 322–329
68. Radkowski D, McGill T, Healy G B et al. 1996 Angiofibroma. Changes in staging and treatment. Arch Otolaryngol Head Neck Surg 122: 122–129
69. Beham A, Fletcher C D M, Kainz J et al. 1993 Nasopharyngeal angiofibroma in an immunohistochemical study of 32 cases. Virchows Archiv (A) Pathol Anat 423: 281–285
70. Garcia-Cervigon E, Bien S, Rufenacht D et al. 1988 Pre-operative embolization of nasopharyngeal angiofibromas. Report of 58 cases. Neuroradiology 30: 556–560
71. Mann W J, Jecker P, Amedee R G 2004 Juvenile angiofibromas: changing surgical concept over the last 20 years. Laryngoscope 114: 291–293
72. Gates G A, Rice D H, Koopman C F Jr et al. 1992 Flutamide-induced regression of angiofibroma. Laryngoscope 102: 641–644
73. Fields J N, Halverson K J, Devineni V R et al. 1990 Juvenile nasopharyngeal angiofibroma: efficacy of radiation therapy. Radiology 176: 263–265
74. Gudea F, Vega M, Canals E et al. 1990 Role of radiation therapy for juvenile angiofibroma. J Laryngol Otol 104: 725–726
75. Kaspar M E, Parsons J T, Mancuso A A et al. 1993 Radiation therapy for juvenile angiofibroma: evaluation by CT and MRI, analysis of tumor regression, and selection of patients. Int J Radiat Oncol Biol Phys 25: 689–694
76. Biller H F 1978 Juvenile nasopharyngeal angiofibroma. Ann Otol Rhinol Laryngol 87: 630–632
77. Gullane P J, Davidson J, O'Dwyer T et al. 1992 Juvenile nasopharyngeal angiofibroma: a review of the literature and a case series report. Laryngoscope 102: 928–933
78. Weprin L S, Siemers P 1991 Spontaneous regression of juvenile nasopharyngeal angiofibroma. Arch Otolaryngol Head Neck Surg 117: 796–799
79. Dohar J E, Duvall A J 1992 Spontaneous regression of juvenile nasopharyngeal angiofibroma. Ann Otol Rhinol Laryngol 101: 469–471
80. Batsakis J G, Klopp C T, Newman N 1958 Fibrosarcoma arising in a "juvenile" nasopharyngeal angiofibroma following extensive radiation therapy. Am Surg 21: 786–793
81. Gisselsson L, Lindgren M, Stenram U 1958 Sarcomatous transformation of juvenile nasopharyngeal angiofibroma. Acta Pathol Microbiol Scand 42: 305–312
82. Chen K T K, Bauer F W 1982 Sarcomatous transformation of nasopharyngeal angiofibroma. Cancer 49: 369–371
83. Spagnolo D V, Papadimitiou J M, Archer M 1984 Postirradiation malignant fibrous histiocytoma arising in juvenile nasopharyngeal angiofibroma producing alpha-1-antitrypsin. Histopathology 8: 339–352
84. Hasegawa T, Hirose T, Seki K et al. 1996 Solitary fibrous tumors of soft tissue. An immunohistochemical and ultrastructural study. Am J Clin Pathol 106: 325–331
85. Suster S, Nascimento A G, Miettinen M et al. 1995 Solitary fibrous tumors of soft tissue. A clinicopathologic and immunohistochemical study of 12 cases. Am J Surg Pathol 19: 1257–1266
86. Zukerberg L R, Rosenberg A E, Randolph G et al. 1991 Solitary fibrous tumor of the nasal cavity and paranasal sinuses. Am J Surg Pathol 15: 126–130
87. Witkin G B, Rosai J 1991 Solitary fibrous tumor of the upper respiratory tract. Am J Surg Pathol 15: 842–848
88. Fukunaga M, Ushigome S, Nomura K et al. 1995 Solitary fibrous tumor of the nasal cavity and orbit. Pathol Int 45: 952–957
89. Karlsson I, Mandahl N, Heim S et al. 1988 Complex chromosome rearrangements in an extraabdominal desmoid tumor. Cancer Genet Cytogen 32: 241–245
90. Bridge J A, Sreekantaiah C, Mouron B et al. 1992 Clonal chromosomal abnormalities in desmoid tumors: implications for histogenesis. Cancer 69: 430–436
91. Enzinger F M, Weiss S W 1995 Fibromatoses. In: Enzinger F M, Weiss S W (eds) Soft tissue tumors, 3rd edn. Mosby, St Louis, p 201–229
92. Fu Y S, Perzin K H 1976 Non-epithelial tumors of the nasal cavity, paranasal sinuses, and nasopharynx: a clinicopathologic study. VI. Fibrous tissue tumors (fibroma, fibromatosis, fibrosarcoma). Cancer 37: 2912–2928
93. Gnepp D R, Henley J, Weiss S et al. 1996 Desmoid fibromatosis of the sinonasal tract and nasopharynx. Cancer 78: 2572–2579
94. Batsakis J G, Raslan W 1994 Extra-abdominal desmoid fibromatosis. Ann Otol Rhinol Laryngol 103: 331–334
95. Sherman N E, Romsdahl M, Evans H et al. 1990 Desmoid tumors: a 20-year radiotherapy experience. Int J Radiat Oncol Biol Phys 19: 37–40
96. McCollough W M, Parsons J T, van der Griend R et al. 1991 Radiation therapy for aggressive fibromatosis: the experience of the University of Florida. J Bone Joint Surg 73: 717–725
97. Lanari A 1983 Effect of progesterone on desmoid tumors (aggressive fibromatosis). N Engl J Med 309: 1523
98. Easter D W, Halasz N A 1989 Recent trends in the management of desmoid tumors. Summary of 19 cases and review of the literature. Ann Surg 210: 765–769
99. Shugar J M A, Som P A, Biller H F et al. 1981 Peripheral nerve sheath tumors of the paranasal sinuses. Head Neck Surg 4: 72–76
100. Fu Y S, Perzin K H 1974 Non-epithelial tumors of the nasal cavity, paranasal sinuses, and nasopharynx: a clinicopathologic study. XII. Schwann cell tumors (neurilemmoma, neurofibroma, malignant schwannoma). Cancer 50: 65–69
101. Hasegawa S L, Mentzel T, Fletcher C D M 1997 Schwannomas of the sinonasal tract and nasopharynx. Mod Pathol 10: 777–784
102. Buob D, Wacrenier A, Chevalier D et al. 2003 Schwannoma of the sinonasal tract: a clinicopathologic and immunohistochemical study of 5 cases. Arch Pathol Lab Med 127: 1196–1199
103. Fu Y S, Perzin K H 1976 Non-epithelial tumors of the nasal cavity, paranasal sinuses, and nasopharynx: a clinicopathologic study. IV. Smooth muscle tumors (leiomyoma, leiomyosarcoma). Cancer 35: 1300–1308
104. Huang, H Y, Antonescu C R 2003 Sinonasal smooth muscle cell tumors: a clinicopathologic and immunohistochemical analysis of 12 cases with emphasis on the low-grade end of the spectrum. Arch Pathol Lab Med 127: 297–304
105. Fu Y S, Perzin K H 1976 Non-epithelial tumors of the nasal cavity, paranasal sinuses, and nasopharynx: a clinicopathologic study. V. Skeletal muscle tumors (rhabdomyoma, rhabdomyosarcoma). Cancer 37: 364–376
106. Gale N, Rott T, Kambic V 1984 Nasopharyngeal rhabdomyoma. Report of a case (light and electron microscopic studies) and review of the literature. Pathol Res Pract 178: 454–460
107. Kapadia S B, Meis J M, Frisman D M et al. 1993 Fetal rhabdomyoma of the head and neck: a clinicopathologic and immunophenotypic study of 24 cases. Hum Pathol 24: 754–765
108. Fu Y S, Perzin K H 1977 Non-epithelial tumors of the nasal cavity, paranasal sinuses, and nasopharynx: a clinicopathologic study. VII. Myxomas. Cancer 39: 195–203

109. Heffner D K 1993 Sinonasal myxomas and fibromyxomas in children. Ear Nose Throat J 72: 365–368
110. Evans H 1993 Low-grade fibromyxoid sarcoma. A report of 12 cases. Am J Surg Pathol 17: 595–600
111. Fu Y S, Perzin K H 1974 Non-epithelial tumors of the nasal cavity, paranasal sinuses, and nasopharynx: a clinicopathologic study. II. Osseous and fibro-osseous lesions, including osteoma, fibrous dysplasia, ossifying fibroma, osteoblastoma, giant cell tumor and osteosarcoma. Cancer 33: 1289–1305
112. Earwaker J 1993 Paranasal sinus osteomas: a review of 46 cases. Skeletal Radiol 22: 417–423
113. Atallah N, Jay M M 1981 Osteomas of the paranasal sinuses. J Laryngol Otol 95: 291–304
114. Bulow S, Sondergaard J O, Witt I et al. 1984 Mandibular osteomas in familial polyposis coli. Dis Col Rectum 27: 105–108
115. Waldron C A, Giansati J S 1973 Benign fibro-osseous lesions of the jaws: a clinico-pathologic-histologic review of sixty-five cases. II. Benign fibro-osseous lesions of peridontal ligament origin. Oral Surg 35: 340–350
116. Nevelle B W, Albenesius R J 1986 The prevalence of benign fibro-osseous lesions of the peridontal ligament origin in black women: a radiographic survey. Oral Surg 62: 340–344
117. Wenig B M, Vinh T N, Smirniotopoulos J G et al. 1995 Aggressive psammomatoid ossifying fibromas of the sinonasal region. A clinicopathologic study of a distinct group of fibro-osseous lesions. Cancer 76: 1155–1165
118. Johnson L C, Youssefi M, Vinh T N et al. 1991 Juvenile active ossifying fibroma. Its nature, dynamics and origin. Acta Otolaryngol Suppl 488: 1–40
119. Harris W H, Dudley H R Jr, Barry R J 1962 The natural history of fibrous dysplasia. An orthopedic, pathological and roentenographic study. J Bone Joint Surg (Am) 44A: 207–233
120. Gibson M J, Middlemiss J H 1971 Fibrous dysplasia of bone. Br J Radiol 44: 1–13
121. Henry A 1969 Monostotic fibrous dysplasia. J Bone Joint Surg (Br) 51: 300–306
122. Yabut S M Jr, Kenan S, Sissons H A et al. 1988 Malignant transformation of fibrous dysplasia. A case report and review of the literature. Clin Orthop 228: 281–289
123. Taconis W K 1988 Osteosarcoma in fibrous dysplasia. Skeletal Radiol 17: 1047–1056
124. Oda Y, Tsuneyoshi M, Shinohara N 1993 "Solid" variant of aneurysmal bone cyst (extragnathic giant cell reparative granuloma) in axial skeleton and long bones. A study of its morphologic spectrum and distinction from allied bone lesions. Cancer 70: 2642–2649
125. Smith G A, Ward P H 1978 Giant cell lesions of the facial skeleton. Arch Otolaryngol 7: 366–370
126. Hirsch I S, Katz A 1974 Giant cell reparative granuloma outside the jaw bone. Hum Pathol 5: 171–181
127. Waldron C A, Shafer W G 1966 The central giant cell reparative granuloma of the jaws. An analysis of 38 cases. Am J Clin Pathol 45: 437–447
128. McGowan D A 1969 Central giant cell tumours of the mandible in pregnancy. Br J Oral Med 7: 131–135
129. Littler B O 1979 Central giant cell granuloma of the jaw – a hormonal influence. Br J Oral Surg 17: 43–46
130. Bertoni F, Unni K K, Beabout J W et al. 1992 Giant cell tumor of the skull. Cancer 70: 1124–1132
131. Saleh E A, Taibh A K, Naguib M et al. 1994 Giant cell tumor of the lateral skull: a case report. Otolaryngol Head Neck Surg 111: 314–318
132. Bridge J A, Neff J R, Bhatia P S et al. 1990 Cytogenetic findings and biologic behavior of giant cell tumors of bone. Cancer 65: 2697–2703
133. Chan J, Gannon F H, Thompson L D 2003 Malignant giant cell tumor of the sphenoid. Ann Diagn Pathol 7: 100–105
134. Fu Y S, Perzin K H 1974 Non-epithelial tumors of the nasal cavity, paranasal sinuses, and nasopharynx: a clinicopathologic study. III. Cartilaginous tumor (chondroma, chondrosarcoma). Cancer 34: 453–463
135. Kilby D, Amegaokar A G 1977 The nasal chondroma. J Laryngol Otol 91: 415–426
136. Shafer W G, Hine M K, Levy B M 1983 A textbook of oral pathology, 4th edn. W B Saunders, Philadelphia, p 258–317
137. Waldron C A 1995 Odontogenic cysts and tumors. In: Neville D W, Damm D D, Allen C M et al. (eds) Oral and maxillofacial pathology. W B Saunders, Philadelphia, p 453–540
138. Schafer D R, Thompson L D R, Smith B C et al. 1998 Primary ameloblastoma of the sinonasal tract. A clinicopathologic study of 24 cases. Cancer 82: 667–674
139. Guilemany J M, Ballesteros F, Alos L et al. 2004 Plexiform ameloblastoma presenting as a sinonasal tumor. Eur Arch Otorhinolaryngol 261: 304–306
140. Bryne M N, Sessions D G 1990 Nasopharyngeal craniopharyngioma. Case report and literature review. Ann Otol Rhinol Laryngol 99: 633–639
141. Chakrabarty A, Mitchell P, Bridges LR 1998 Craniopharyngioma invading the nasal and paranasal spaces, and presenting as nasal obstruction. Br J Neurosurg 12: 361–363
142. Taguchi Y, Tanaka K, Miyakita Y et al. 2000 Recurrent craniopharyngioma with nasopharyngeal extension. Pediatr Neurosurg 32: 140–144
143. Buhl R, Nabavi A, Fritsch M 2004 Nasopharyngeal extension of a craniopharyngioma in a 4 year old girl. Acta Neurochir (Wien) 143: 1283–5128
144. Dehner L P 1983 Gonadal and extragonadal germ cell neoplasia of childhood. Hum Pathol 14: 493–511
145. Tharrington C L, Bosen E H 1992 Nasopharyngeal teratomas. Arch Pathol Lab Med 116: 165–167
146. Coppit G L, Perkins J A, Manning S 2000 Nasopharyngeal teratomas and dermoids: a review of the literature and case series. Int J Pediatr Otorhinolaryngol 52: 219–227
147. Heffner D K, Thompson L D R, Schall D G et al. 1996 Pharyngeal dermoids ("hairy polyps") as accessory auricles. Ann Otol Rhinol Laryngol 10: 819–824
148. Heffner D K 1983 Problems in pediatric otorhinolaryngic pathology, III. Teratoid and neural tumors of the nose, sinonasal tract, and nasopharynx. Int J Pediatr Otorhinolaryngol 6: 1–21
149. Ferlito A, Devaney K O 1995 Developmental lesions of the head and neck: terminology and biological behavior. Ann Otol Rhinol Laryngol 104: 913–918
150. Gorenstein A, Facer G W, Weiland L H 1978 Hemangiopericytoma of the nasal cavity. ORL J Otorhinolaryngol Relat Spec 86: 405–415
151. Thompson L D, Miettinen M, Wenig B M 2003 Sinonasal-type hemangiopericytoma: a clinicopathologic and immunophenotypic analysis of 104 cases showing perivascular myoid differentiation. Am J Surg Pathol 27: 737–749
152. Kuo F Y, Lin H C, Eng H L et al. 2005 Sinonasal hemangiopericytoma-like tumor with true pericytic myoid differentiation: a clinicopathologic and immunohistochemical study of five cases. Head Neck 27: 124–129
153. Fletcher C D M 1994 Haemangiopericytoma: a dying breed? Reappraisal of an "entity" and its variants. Curr Diagn Pathol 1: 19–23
154. Fanburg-Smith J, Thompson L D R, Wenig B M 2005 Borderline and LMP tumours of soft tissue. In: Barnes L, Eveson J, Reichart P et al. (eds) World Health Organization classification of tumours. Pathology and genetics of head and neck tumours. IARC Press, Lyon, France, p 44–45
155. Compagno J, Hyams V J 1976 Hemangiopericytoma-like intranasal tumors. A clinicopathologic study of 23 cases. Am J Clin Pathol 66: 672–683
156. Schürch W, Skalli O, Lagace R et al. 1990 Intermediate filament proteins and actin isoforms as markers for soft tissue differentiation and origin: III. Hemangiopericytomas and glomus tumors. Am J Pathol 136: 771–786
157. Porter P L, Bigler S A, McNutt M et al. 1991 The immunophenotype of hemangiopericytomas and glomus tumors, with special reference to muscle protein expression: an immunohistochemical study and review of the literature. Mod Pathol 4: 46–52
158. Kapadia S K, Meis J M, Wenig B M et al. 1993 Sinonasal hemangiopericytoma. Mod Pathol 6: 81A (abstract)
159. Dardick I, Hammar S P, Sheithauer B W 1989 Ultrastructural spectrum of hemangiopericytoma: a comparative study of fetal, adult and neoplastic pericytes. Ultrastruct Pathol 13: 111–154
160. Eichorn J H, Dickerson G R, Bhan A K et al. 1990 Sinonasal hemangiopericytoma: a reassessment with electron microscopy, immunohistochemistry and long term follow-up. Am J Surg Pathol 14: 856–866
161. El-Naggar A, Batsakis J G, Garcia G M et al. 1992 Sinonasal hemangiopericytomas. A clinicopathologic and DNA content study. Arch Otolaryngol Head Neck Surg 118: 134–137
162. Billings K R, Fu Y S, Calcaterra T C et al. 2000 Hemangiopericytoma of the head and neck. Am J Otolaryngol 21: 238–243
163. Kowalski P J, Paulino A F 2001 Proliferation index as a prognostic marker in hemangiopericytoma of the head and neck. Head Neck 23: 492–496
164. Taxy J B 1997 Squamous carcinoma of the nasal vestibule. An analysis of five cases and literature review. Am J Clin Pathol 107: 698–703
165. Bosch A, Vallecillo L, Frias Z 1976 Cancer of the nasal cavity. Cancer 37: 1458–1463
166. Jackson R T, Fitz-Hugh G S, Constable W C 1977 Malignant neoplasms of the nasal cavities and paranasal sinuses. Laryngoscope 87: 726–736
167. Hopkin N, McNicoll W, Dalley V M et al. 1984 Cancer of the paranasal sinuses and nasal cavities. Part I. Clinical features. J Laryngol Otol 98: 585–595
168. Batsakis J G, Rice D H, Solomon A R 1980 The pathology of head and neck tumors: squamous and mucous-gland carcinomas of the nasal cavity, paranasal sinuses, and larynx, part 6. Head Neck Surg 2: 497–508
169. Pedersen E A, Hogetreit A C, Andersen A 1973 Cancer of the respiratory organs among workers at a nickel refinery in Norway. Int J Cancer 12: 32–41
170. Trojussen W, Solberg L A, Hogetveit A C 1979 Histopathologic changes of nasal mucosa in nickel workers. A pilot study. Cancer 44: 963–974
171. Shibuya H, Amagasa T, Hanai A et al. 1986 Second primary carcinomas in patients with squamous cell carcinoma of the maxillary sinus. Cancer 58: 1122–1125
172. Osborn D A 1970 Nature and behavior of transitional tumors in the upper respiratory tract. Cancer 25: 50–60
173. Giri S P G, Reddy E K, Gemer L S et al. 1992 Management of advanced squamous cell carcinomas of the maxillary sinus. Cancer 69: 657–661
174. Day T A, Beas R A, Schlosser R J 2005 Management of paranasal sinus malignancy. Curr Treat Options Oncol 6: 3–18
175. Diaz E M Jr, Kies M S 2001 Chemotherapy for skull base cancers. Otolaryngol Clin North Am 34: 1079–1085
176. Crissman J D, Zarbo R J 1989 Dysplasia, in situ carcinoma, and progression to invasive squamous cell carcinoma of the upper aerodigestive tract. Am J Surg Pathol 13 (suppl. 1): 5–16
177. Crissman J D, Kessis T, Shah K V et al. 1988 Squamous papillary neoplasia of the adult upper aerodigestive tract. Hum Pathol 19: 1387–1396

178. Ishiyama A, Eversole L R, Ross D A et al. 1994 Papillary squamous neoplasms of the head and neck. Laryngoscope 104: 1446–1452
179. Thompson L D R, Wenig B M, Heffner D K et al. 1999 Exophytic and papillary squamous cell carcinoma of the larynx: a report of 104 cases. Otolaryngol-Head Neck Surg 120: 718–724
180. Suarez P A, Adler-Storthz K, Luna M A et al. 2000 Papillary squamous cell carcinomas of the upper aerodigestive tract: a clinicopathologic and molecular study. Head Neck 22: 360–368
181. Kraus F T, Perez-Mesa C 1966 Verrucous carcinoma. Clinical and pathologic study of 105 cases involving oral cavity, larynx and genitalia. Cancer 19: 26–38
182. Batsakis J G, Hybels R, Crissman J D et al. 1982 The pathology of head and neck tumors: verrucous carcinoma, part 15. Head Neck Surg 5: 29–38
183. Medina J E, Dichtel W, Luna M A 1984 Verrucous-squamous carcinomas of the oral cavity. A clinicopathologic study of 104 cases. Arch Otolaryngol 110: 437–440
184. Luna M A, Tortoledo M E 1988 Verrucous carcinoma. In: Gnepp D R (ed) Pathology of the head and neck. Churchill Livingstone, New York, p 497–515
185. Paleri V, Orvidas L J, Wight R G et al. 2004 Verrucous carcinoma of the paranasal sinuses: case report and clinical update. Head Neck 26: 184–189
186. Ram B, Saleh H A, Baird A R et al. 1998 Verrucous carcinoma of the maxillary antrum. J Laryngol Otol 112: 399–402
187. Abramson A L, Brandsma J L, Steinberg B M et al. 1985 Verrucous carcinoma of the larynx: possible human papillomavirus etiology. Arch Otolaryngol 111: 709–715
188. Brandsma J L, Steinberg B M, Abramson A L et al. 1986 Presence of HPV-16 related sequences in verrucous carcinoma of the larynx. Cancer Res 46: 2185–2188
189. Young K, Min K W 1991 In situ hybridization analysis of oral papillomas, leukoplakias, and carcinomas for human papillomavirus. Oral Surg Oral Med Oral Pathol 71: 726–729
190. Watts S L, Brewer E E, Fry T L 1991 Human papillomavirus DNA types in squamous cell carcinomas of the head and neck. Oral Surg Oral Med Oral Pathol 71: 701–707
191. Kashima H K, Kutcher M, Kessis T et al. 1990 Human papillomavirus in squamous cell carcinoma, leukoplakia, lichen planus, and clinically normal epithelium of the oral cavity. Ann Otol Rhinol Laryngol 99: 55–61
192. Löning T, Ikenberg H, Becker J et al. 1985 Analysis of oral papillomas, leukoplakias, and invasive carcinomas for human papillomavirus type related DNA. J Invest Dermatol 84: 417–420
193. Löning T 1986 Detection of papillomavirus DNA in oral papillomas and carcinomas: application of in situ hybridization with biotinylated HPV 16 probes. J Oral Path 15: 292–296
194. Shroyer K R, Greer R O, Fanhouser C A et al. 1993 Detection of human papillomavirus DNA in oral verrucous carcinoma by polymerase chain reaction. Mod Pathol 6: 669–772
195. Kasperbauer J L, O'Halloran G L, Espy M J et al. 1993 Polymerase chain reaction (PCR) identification of human papillomavirus (HPV) DNA in verrucous carcinoma of the larynx. Laryngoscope 103: 416–420
196. Fliss D M, Noble-Topham S E, McLachlin M et al. 1994 Laryngeal verrucous carcinoma: a clinicopathologic study and detection of human papillomavirus using polymerase chain reaction. Laryngoscope 104: 146–152
197. Dyson N, Howley P M, Münger K et al. 1989 The human papillomavirus-16 E7 oncoprotein is able to bind the retinoblastoma gene product. Science 243: 934–937
198. Hagen P, Lyons G D, Haindel C 1993 Verrucous carcinoma of the larynx: role of human papillomavirus, radiation, and surgery. Laryngoscope 103: 253–257
199. McDonald J S, Crissman J D, Gluckman J L 1982 Verrucous carcinoma of the oral cavity. Head Neck 5: 22–34
200. Tharp M E II, Shidnia H 1995 Radiotherapy in the treatment of verrucous carcinoma of the head and neck. Laryngoscope 105: 391–396
201. Vidyasagar M S, Fernandes D J, Pai Kasturi D et al. 1992 Radiotherapy and verrucous carcinoma of the oral cavity. A study of 107 cases. Acta Oncol 31: 43–47
202. Leventon G S, Evans H L 1981 Sarcomatoid squamous cell carcinoma of the mucous membranes of the head and neck: a clinicopathologic study of 20 cases. Cancer 48: 994–1003
203. Piscioli F, Aldovini D, Bondi A et al. 1984 Squamous cell carcinoma with sarcoma-like stroma of the nose and paranasal sinuses: report of two cases. Histopathology 8: 633–639
204. Zarbo R J, Crissman J D, Venkat H et al. 1986 Spindle-cell carcinoma of the aerodigestive tract mucosa: an immunohistologic and ultrastructural study of 18 biphasic tumors and comparison with seven monophasic spindle-cell tumors. Am J Surg Pathol 10: 741–753
205. Hyams V J, Batsakis J G, Michaels L 1988 Spindle cell carcinoma of the upper aerodigestive tract. In: Tumors of the upper respiratory tract and ear, series 2, fascicle 25. Armed Forces Institute of Pathology, Washington, DC, p 76–81
206. Ellis G L, Langloss J M, Heffner D K et al. 1987 Spindle-cell carcinoma of the aerodigestive tract: an immunohistochemical analysis of 21 cases. Am J Surg Pathol 11: 335–342
207. Huntington A C, Langloss J M, Hidayat H A 1990 Spindle cell carcinoma of the conjunctiva. An immunohistochemical and ultrastructural study of six cases. Am Acad Opthalmol 97: 711–717
208. Takata T, Ito H, Ogawa I et al. 1991 Spindle cell squamous carcinoma of the oral cavity. An immunohistochemical and ultrastructural study on the histogenesis and differential diagnosis with a clinicopathologic analysis of six cases. Virchows Arch (A) Pathol Anat 419: 177–182
209. Nakleh R E, Zarbo R J, Ewing S et al. 1993 Myogenic differentiation in spindle cell (sarcomatoid) carcinoma of the upper aerodigestive tract. Appl Immunohistochem 1: 58–68
210. Balercia G, Bhan A K, Dickersin G R 1995 Sarcomatoid carcinoma: an ultrastructural study with light microscopic and immunohistochemical correlation of 10 cases from various anatomic sites. Ultrastruct Pathol 19: 249–263
211. Krassilnik N, Gologan O, Ghali V et al. 2004 p63 and p16 expression in spindle cell squamous carcinoma of the head and neck (SCSCHN). Mod Pathol 17: 226A
212. Ellis G, Langloss J M, Enzinger F M 1985 Coexpression of keratin and desmin in a carcinosarcoma involving the maxillary alveolar ridge. Oral Surg Oral Med Oral Pathol 60: 410–416
213. Ophir D, Marshak G, Czernobilsky B 1987 Distinctive immunohistochemical labeling of epithelial and mesenchymal elements in laryngeal pseudosarcoma. Laryngoscope 97: 490–494
214. Smith K J, Skelton H G III, Morgan A M et al. 1992 Spindle cell neoplasms coexpressing cytokeratin and vimentin (metaplastic squamous cell carcinoma). J Cutan Pathol 19: 286–293
215. Batsakis J G, Rice D H, Howard D R 1982 The pathology of head and neck tumors: spindle cell lesions (sarcomatoid carcinomas, nodular fasciitis, and fibrosarcoma) of the upper aerodigestive tracts, part 14. Head Neck Surg 4: 499–513
216. Lambert P R, Ward P H, Berci G 1980 Pseudosarcoma of the larynx: a comprehensive analysis. Arch Otolaryngol 106: 700–708
217. Larsen E T, Duggan M A, Inoue M 1994 Absence of human papilloma virus DNA in oropharyngeal spindle-cell squamous carcinomas. Am J Clin Pathol 101: 514–518
218. Wain S L, Kier R, Vollmer R T et al. 1986 Basaloid-squamous carcinoma of the tongue, hypopharynx and larynx. Hum Pathol 17: 1158–1166
219. Batsakis J G, El Naggar A 1989 Basaloid-squamous carcinomas of the upper aerodigestive tracts. Ann Otol Rhinol Laryngol 98: 919–920
220. McKay M J, Bilous A M 1989 Basaloid-squamous carcinomas of the hypopharynx. Cancer 63: 2528–2531
221. Luna M A, El Naggar A, Parichatikanond P et al. 1990 Basaloid squamous cell carcinoma of the upper aerodigestive tract: clinicopathologic and DNA flow cytometric analysis. Cancer 66: 537–542
222. Banks E R, Frierson H F Jr, Mills S E et al. 1992 Basaloid squamous cell carcinoma of the head and neck: a clinicopathologic and immunohistochemical study of 40 cases. Am J Surg Pathol 16: 939–946
223. Barnes L, Ferlito A, Altavilla G et al. 1996 Basaloid squamous cell carcinoma of the head and neck: clinicopathological features and differential diagnosis. Ann Otol Rhinol Laryngol 105: 75–82
224. Wan S K, Chan J K C, Tse K C 1992 Basaloid-squamous cell carcinoma of the nasal cavity. J Laryngol Otol 106: 370–371
225. Wieneke J, Thompson L D R, Wenig B M 1999 Basaloid squamous cell carcinoma of the nasal cavity and paranasal sinuses. Cancer 85: 841–854
226. Raslan W F, Barnes L, Krause J R et al. 1994 Basaloid squamous cell carcinoma of the head and neck: a clinicopathologic and flow cytometric study of 10 new cases with review of the English literature. Am J Otolaryngol 15: 204–211
227. Morice W G, Ferreiro J A 1998 Distinction of basaloid squamous cell carcinoma from adenoid cystic and small cell undifferentiated carcinoma by immunohistochemistry. Hum Pathol 29: 609–612
228. Hewan-Lowe K, Dardick I 1995 Ultrastructural distinction of basaloid-squamous carcinoma and adenoid cystic carcinoma. Ultrastruct Pathol 19: 371–381
229. Seidman J, Berman J J, Yost B A et al. 1991 Basaloid squamous carcinoma of the hypopharynx and larynx associated with second primary tumors. Cancer 68: 1545–1549
230. Gerughty R M, Hennigar G R, Brown F M 1968 Adenosquamous carcinoma of the nasal, oral, and laryngeal cavities. Cancer 22: 1140–1155
231. Damiani J M, Damiani K K, Hauck K et al. 1981 Mucoepidermoid-adenosquamous carcinoma of the larynx and hypopharynx: a report of 21 cases and review of the literature. Otolaryngol Head Neck Surg 89: 235–243
232. Siar C H, Ng K H 1987 Adenosquamous carcinoma of the floor of the mouth and lower alveolus: a radiation-induced lesion? Oral Surg Oral Med Oral Pathol 63: 216–220
233. Aden K K, Adams G L, Niehans G et al. 1988 Adenosquamous carcinoma of the larynx and hypopharynx with five new case presentations. Trans Am Laryngol Assoc 109: 216–221
234. Fujino K, Ito J, Kanaji M et al. 1995 Adenosquamous carcinoma of the larynx. Am J Otolaryngol 16: 115–118
235. Napier S S, Gormley J S, Ramsay-Baggs P 1995 Adenosquamous carcinoma. A rare neoplasm with an aggressive course. Oral Surg Oral Med Oral Pathol 79: 607–611
236. Tsang W Y W, Chan J K C 2005 Lympoepithelial carcinoma. In: Barnes L, Eveson J, Reichart P et al. (eds) World Health Organization classification of tumours. Pathology and genetics of head and neck tumours. IARC Press, Lyon, France, p. 18
237. Jeng Y M, Sung M T, Fang C L et al. 2002 Sinonasal undifferentiated carcinoma and nasopharyngeal-type undifferentiated carcinoma: two

clinically, biologically, and histopathologically distinct entities. Am J Surg Pathol 26: 371–376

238. Leung S Y, Yuen S T, Chung L P et al. 1995 Epstein–Barr virus is present in a wide histological spectrum of sinonasal carcinomas. Am J Surg Pathol 19: 994–1001
239. Dubey P, Ha C S, Ang K K et al. 1998 Nonnasopharyngeal lymphoepithelioma of the head and neck. Cancer 82: 1556–1562
240. Zong Y, Liu K, Zhong B et al. 2001 Epstein–Barr virus infection of sinonasal lymphoepithelial carcinoma in Guangzhou. Chin Med J (Engl) 114: 132–136
241. Choi H R, Roberts D B, Johnigan R H et al. 2004 Molecular and clinicopathologic comparisons of head and neck squamous carcinoma variants: common and distinctive features of biological significance. Am J Surg Pathol 28: 1299–1310
242. Shanmugaratnam K, Sobin L H, Barnes L et al. 1991 World Health Organization histological classification of tumours. Histological typing of tumours of the upper respiratory tract and ear, 2nd edn. Springer-Verlag, Berlin, p 32–33
243. Chan J K C, Bray F, McCarron P et al. 2005 Nasopharyngeal carcinoma. In: Barnes L, Eveson J, Reichart P et al. (eds) World Health Organization classification of tumours. Pathology and genetics of head and neck tumours. Lyon, France, IARC Press, p 87–99
244. Easton J M, Levine P H, Hyams V J 1981 Nasopharyngeal carcinoma in the United States. A pathologic study of 177 US and 30 foreign cases. Arch Otolaryngol 106: 88–91
245. Dickson R I, Flores A D 1985 Nasopharyngeal carcinoma: an evaluation of 134 patients treated between 1971–1980. Laryngoscope 95: 276–283
246. Huang D P 1991 Epidemiology and aetiology. In: van Hasselt C A, Gibb A G (eds) Nasopharyngeal carcinoma. The Chinese Free Press, Hong Kong, p 23–35
247. Parkin D M, Whelan S L, Ferlay J et al. 2003 Cancer incidence in five continents, vol VIII. IARC Press, Lyon
248. Jenkin R D T, Anderson J R, Jereb B et al. 1981 Nasopharyngeal carcinoma– a retrospective review of patients less than thirty years of age: A report from children's cancer study group. Cancer 47: 360–366
249. Heffner D K 1983 Problems in pediatric otorhinolaryngic pathology. IV. Epithelial and lymphoid tumors of the sinonasal tract and nasopharynx. Int J Pediatr Otorhinolaryngol 6: 219–237
250. Hawkins E P, Krisher J P, Smith B E et al. 1990 Nasopharyngeal carcinoma in children – a retrospective review and demonstration of Epstein–Barr virus genomes in tumor cell cytoplasm: a report of the pediatric oncology group. Hum Pathol 21: 805–810
251. Batsakis J G, Solomon A R, Rice D H 1981 The pathology of head and neck tumors: carcinoma of the nasopharynx, part 11. Head Neck Surg 3: 511–524
252. Skinner D W, van Hasselt C A, Tsao S Y 1991 Nasopharyngeal carcinoma: a study of the modes of presentation. Ann Otol Rhinol Laryngol 100: 544–551
253. Wang C C, Little J B, Schulz M D 1962 Cancer of the nasopharynx. Its clinical and radiotherapeutic considerations. Cancer 15: 921–926
254. Chong V F, Fan Y F 1996 Skull base erosion in nasopharyngeal carcinoma: detection by CT and MRI. Clin Radiol 51: 625–631
255. Ng S H, Chang T C, Ko S F et al. 1997 Nasopharyngeal carcinoma: MRI and CT assessment. Neuroradiology 39:741–746
256. Buell P 1974 The effect of migration on the risk of nasopharyngeal cancer among Chinese. Cancer Res 34: 1189–1191
257. Vasef M A, Ferlito A, Weiss L M 1997 Nasopharyngeal carcinoma with emphasis on its relationship to Epstein–Barr virus. Ann Otol Rhinol Laryngol 106: 348–356
258. Raab-Traub N 2002 Epstein–Barr virus in the pathogenesis of NPC. Semin Cancer Biol 12: 431–441
259. Henderson B E, Louie E, Jing J S et al. 1976 Risk factors associated with nasopharyngeal carcinoma. N Engl J Med 295: 1101–1106
260. Zeng Y, Zhang L G, Li H Y et al. 1982 Serological mass survey for early detection of nasopharyngeal carcinoma in Wuzhou City, China. Int J Cancer 29: 139–141
261. de-Vaithaire F, Sancho-Garnier H, de-Thé H et al. 1988 Prognostic value of EBV markers in the clinical management of nasopharyngeal carcinoma (NPC): a multicenter follow-up study. Int J Cancer 42: 176–181
262. Young L S, Dawson C W, Clark D et al. 1988 Epstein–Barr virus gene expression in nasopharyngeal carcinoma. J Gen Virol 69: 1051–1065
263. Gasmi J, Bachouchi M, Cvitkovic E et al. 1990 Nasopharyngeal carcinoma: a medical oncology viewpoint: the Gustave Roussy experience. Ann Oncol 1: 245–253
264. Feinmesser R, Miyazaki I, Chueng R et al. 1992 Diagnosis of nasopharyngeal carcinoma by fine-needle aspiration. N Engl J Med 326: 17–21
265. Tam J S 1991 Epstein–Barr virus serologic markers. In: van Hasselt C A, Gibb A G (eds) Nasopharyngeal carcinoma. The Chinese Free Press, Hong Kong, p 147–156
266. Hadar T, Rahima M, Kahan E et al. 1986 Significance of specific Epstein–Barr virus IgA and elevated IgG antibodies to viral capsid antigens in nasopharyngeal carcinoma patients. J Med Virol 20: 329–339
267. Chan K C, Lo Y M 2002 Circulating EBV DNA as a tumor marker for nasopharyngeal carcinoma. Semin Cancer Biol 12: 489–496
268. Lin J C, Chen K Y, Wang W Y et al. 2001 Detection of Epstein–Barr virus DNA in the peripheral-blood cells of patients with nasopharyngeal carcinoma: relationship to distant metastasis and survival. J Clin Oncol 19: 2607–2615
269. Lo Y M, Chan L Y, Lo K W 1999 Quantitative analysis of cell-free Epstein–Barr virus DNA in plasma of patients with nasopharyngeal carcinoma. Cancer Res 59: 1188–1191
270. Shotelersuk K, Khorprasert C, Sakdikul S et al. 2000 Epstein–Barr virus DNA in serum/plasma as a tumor marker for nasopharyngeal cancer. Clin Cancer Res 6: 1046–1051
271. Akao I, Sato Y, Mukai K et al. 1991 Detection of Epstein–Barr virus DNA in formalin-fixed paraffin-embedded tissue of nasopharyngeal carcinoma using polymerase chain reaction and in-situ hybridization. Laryngoscope 101: 279–283
272. Tsai S-T, Jin Y-T, Su I-J 1996 Expression of EBER1 in primary and metastatic nasopharyngeal carcinoma tissues using in-situ hybridization. A correlation with WHO subtypes. Cancer 77: 231–236
273. Pathmanathan R, Prasad U, Sadler R et al. 1995 Clonal proliferation of cells infected with Epstein–Barr virus in preinvasive lesions related to nasopharyngeal carcinoma. N Engl J Med 333: 693–698
274. Hording U, Nielsen H W, Daugaard S et al. 1994 Human papillomavirus types 11 and 16 detected in nasopharyngeal carcinomas by polymerase chain reaction. Laryngoscope 204: 99–102
275. Huang D P, Ho J H, Chan W K et al. 1989 Cytogenetics of undifferentiated nasopharyngeal carcinoma xenografts from southern Chinese. Int J Cancer 43: 936–939
276. Waghray M, Parhar R S, Taibah K 1992 Rearrangements of chromosome arm 3q in poorly differentiated nasopharyngeal carcinoma. Genes Chromosomes Cancer 4: 326–330
277. Choi P H R, Suen M M, Huang D P et al. 1993 Nasopharyngeal carcinoma: genetic changes, Epstein–Barr virus infection, or both. A clinical and molecular study of 36 patients. Cancer 72: 2873–2878
278. Wong N, Hui A B, Fan B et al. 2003 Molecular cytogenetic characterization of nasopharyngeal carcinoma cell lines and xenografts by comparative genomic hybridization and spectral karyotyping. Cancer Genet Cytogenet 140: 124–132
279. Shao J Y, Zeng W F, Zeng Y X 2002 Molecular genetic progression on nasopharyngeal carcinoma. Ai Zheng 21: 1–10
280. Shao J Y, Huang X M, Yu X J et al. 2001 Loss of heterozygosity and its correlation with clinical outcome and Epstein–Barr virus infection in nasopharyngeal carcinoma. Anticancer Res 21: 3021–2039
281. Fang Y, Guan X, Guo Y et al. 2001 Analysis of genetic alterations in primary nasopharyngeal carcinoma by comparative genomic hybridization. Genes Chromosomes Cancer 30: 254–260
282. Lo K W, Huang D P 2002 Genetic and epigenetic changes in nasopharyngeal carcinoma. Semin Cancer Biol 12: 451–462
283. Lo K W, Huang D P, Lau K M 1995 p16 gene alterations in nasopharyngeal carcinoma. Cancer Res 55: 2039–2043
284. Lo K W, Cheung S T, Leung S F et al. 1996 Hypermethylation of the p16 gene in nasopharyngeal carcinoma. Cancer Res 56: 2721–2725
285. Nicholls J M 1997 Nasopharyngeal carcinoma: classification and histologic appearances. Adv Anat Pathol 4: 71–84
286. Barnes L 2001 Nasopharyngeal carcinoma. In: Barnes L (ed) Surgical pathology of the head and neck, 2nd edn. Marcel Dekker, New York, p 527–535
287. Shanmugaratnam K, Chan S H, de-The G et al. 1979 Histopathology of nasopharyngeal carcinoma: correlations with epidemiology, survival rates, and other biological characteristics. Cancer 44: 1029–1044
288. Franchi A, Moroni M, Massi D et al. 2002 Sinonasal undifferentiated carcinoma, nasopharyngeal-type undifferentiated carcinoma, and keratinizing and nonkeratinizing squamous cell carcinoma express different cytokeratin patterns. Am J Surg Pathol 26: 1597–1604
289. Reddy S P, Raslan W F, Gooneratne S et al. 1995 Prognostic significance of keratinization in nasopharyngeal carcinoma. Am J Otolaryngol 16: 103–108
290. Ahmad A, Stefani S 1986 Distant metastases of nasopharyngeal carcinoma: a study of 256 male patients. J Surg Oncol 33: 194–197
291. McGuire L J, Suen M W M 1991 Histopathology. In: van Hasselt C A, Gibb A G (eds) Nasopharyngeal carcinoma. The Chinese Free Press, Hong Kong, p 47–84
292. Cheng D S, Campbell B H, Clowry L J et al. 1990 DNA content in nasopharyngeal carcinoma. Am J Otolaryngol 11: 393–397
293. Costello F, Mason B R, Collins R J et al. 1990 A clinical and flow cytometric analysis of patients with nasopharyngeal carcinoma. Cancer 66: 1789–1795
294. Roychowdhury D F, Tseng A, Fu K K et al. 1996 New prognostic factors in nasopharyngeal carcinoma. Tumor angiogenesis and C-erbB2 expression. Cancer 77: 1419–1426
295. Chua D T, Ma J, Sham J S et al. 2005 Long-term survival after cisplatin-based induction chemotherapy and radiotherapy for nasopharyngeal carcinoma: a pooled data analysis of two phase III trials. J Clin Oncol 20: 1118–1124
296. Cooper J S, Scott C, Marcial V et al. 1991 The relationship of nasopharyngeal carcinomas and second independent malignancies based on radiation therapy oncology group experience. Cancer 67: 1673–1677
297. Frierson H F Jr, Mills S E, Fechner R E et al. 1986 Sinonasal undifferentiated carcinoma. An aggressive neoplasm derived from Schneiderian epithelium and distinct from olfactory neuroblastoma. Am J Surg Pathol 10: 771–779

298. Frierson H F 2005 Sinonasal undifferentiated carcinoma. In: Barnes L, Eveson J, Reichart P et al. (eds) World Health Organization classification of tumours. Pathology and genetics of head and neck tumours. IARC Press, Lyon, France, p 19
299. Righi P D, Francis F, Aron B S et al. 1996 Sinonasal undifferentiated carcinoma: a 10-year experience. Am J Otolaryngol 17: 167–171
300. Helliwell T R, Yeoh L H, Stell P M 1986 Anaplastic carcinoma of the nose and paranasal sinuses. Light microscopy, immunohistochemistry and clinical correlation. Cancer 58: 2038–2045
301. Mills S E 2002 Neuroectodermal neoplasms of the head and neck with emphasis on neuroendocrine carcinomas. Mod Pathol 15: 264–278
302. Ejaz A, Wenig B M 2005 Sinonasal undifferentiated carcinoma. Clinical and pathologic features and a discussion on classification, cellular differentiation, and differential diagnosis. Adv Anat Pathol 12: 134–143
303. Jeng Y M, Sung M T, Fang C L et al. 2002 Sinonasal undifferentiated carcinoma and nasopharyngeal-type undifferentiated carcinoma: two clinically, biologically, and histopathologically distinct entities. Am J Surg Pathol 26: 371–376
304. Cerilli L A, Holst V A, Brandwein M S et al. 2001 Sinonasal undifferentiated carcinoma: immunohistochemical profile and lack of EBV association. Am J Surg Pathol 25: 156–163
305. Lopategui J R, Gaffey M J, Frierson H F Jr et al. 1994 Detection of Epstein–Barr viral RNA in sinonasal undifferentiated carcinoma from western and Asian patients. Am J Surg Pathol 18: 391–398
306. Gallo O, Di Lollo S, Graziani P et al. 1995 Detection of Epstein–Barr virus genome in sinonasal undifferentiated carcinoma by use of in situ hybridization. Otolaryngol Head Neck Surg 112: 659–664
307. Greger V, Schirmacher P, Bohl J et al. 1990 Possible involvement of the retinoblastoma gene in undifferentiated sinonasal carcinoma. Cancer 66: 1954–1959
308. Mills S E, Fechner R E 1989 "Undifferentiated" neoplasms of the sinonasal tract: differential diagnosis based on clinical, light microscopic, immunohistochemical, and ultrastructural features. Semin Diagn Pathol 6: 316–328
309. Kramer D, Durham J S, Sheehan F et al. 2004 Sinonasal undifferentiated carcinoma: case series and systemic review of the literature. J Otolaryngol 33: 32–36
310. Kim B S, Vongtama R, Juillard G 2004 Sinonasal undifferentiated carcinoma: case series and literature review. Am J Otolaryngol 25: 162–166
311. Gallo O, Graziani P, Fini-Storchi O 1993 Undifferentiated carcinoma of the nose and paranasal sinuses. An immunohistochemical and clinical study. Ear Nose Throat J 72: 588–590, 593–595
312. Deutsch B D, Levine P A, Stewart F M et al. 1993 Sinonasal undifferentiated carcinoma: a ray of hope. Otolaryngol Head Neck Surg 108: 697–700
313. Pitman K T, Costantino P D, Lassen L F 1995 Sinonasal undifferentiated carcinoma: current trends in treatment. Skull Base Surg 5: 269–272
314. Stewart F M, Lazarus L M, Levine P A et al. 1989 High-dose chemotherapy and autologous marrow transplantation for esthesioneuroblastoma and sinonasal undifferentiated carcinoma. Am J Clin Oncol 12: 217–221
315. Musy P Y, Reibel J F, Levine P A 2002 Sinonasal undifferentiated carcinoma: the search for a better outcome. Laryngoscope 112: 1450–1455
316. Rischin D, Porceddu S, Peters L et al. 2004 Promising results with chemoradiation in patients with sinonasal undifferentiated carcinoma. Head Neck 26: 435–441
317. Nakashima T, Kimmelman C P, Snow J B Jr 1984 Structure of human fetal and adult olfactory neuroepithelium. Arch Otolaryngol 110: 641–646
318. Wenig B M, Dulguerov P, Kapadia S B et al. 2005 Neuroectodermal tumours. In: Barnes L, Eveson J, Reichart P et al. (eds) World Health Organization classification of tumours. IARC Press, Lyon, France, 66–76
319. Baker D C, Perzin N H, Conley J 1979 Olfactory neuroblastoma. Otolaryngol Head Neck Surg 87: 279–283
320. Elkon D, Hightower S I, Lim M L et al. 1979 Esthesioneuroblastoma. Cancer 44: 1087–1094
321. Dulguerov P, Calcaterra T 1992 Esthesioneuroblastoma: the UCLA experience 1970–1990. Laryngoscope 102: 843–849
322. Dulguerov P, Allal A S, Calcaterra T C 2001 Esthesioneuroblastoma: a meta-analysis and review. Lancet Oncol 2: 683–690
323. Mills S E, Frierson H F Jr 1985 Olfactory neuroblastoma. A clinicopathologic study of 21 cases. Am J Surg Pathol 9: 317–327
324. Hirose T, Scheithauer B W, Lopes M B S et al. 1995 Olfactory neuroblastoma. An immunohistochemical, ultrastructural, and flow cytometric study. Cancer 76: 4–19
325. Woodhead P, Lloyd G A 1988 Olfactory neuroblastoma: imaging by magnetic resonance, CT and conventional techniques. Clin Otolaryngol 13: 387–394
326. Herrold K M 1964 Induction of olfactory neuroepithelial tumors in Syrian hamsters by diethylnitrosamine. Cancer 17: 114–121
327. Bailey B J, Barton S 1975 Olfactory neuroblastoma: management and prognosis. Arch Otolaryngol 101: 1–5
328. Vollrath M, Altmannsberger M, Weber K et al. 1986 Chemically induced tumors of rat olfactory epithelium: a model for human esthesioneuroblastoma. JNCI 76: 1205–1216
329. Ambros I M, Ambros P F, Strehl S et al. 1991 MIC2 is a specific marker for Ewing's sarcoma and peripheral primitive neuroectodermal tumors. Evidence for a common histogenesis of Ewing's sarcoma and peripheral primitive neuroectodermal tumors from MIC2 expression and specific chromosome aberration. Cancer 67: 1886–1893
330. Fellinger E J, Garin-Chesa P, Triche T J et al. 1991 Immunohistochemical analysis of Ewing's sarcoma cell surface antigen p30/32^{MIC2}. Am J Pathol 139: 317–325
331. Ladanyi M 1995 The emerging molecular genetics of sarcoma translocations. Diagn Mol Pathol 4: 162–167
332. Whang-Peng J, Freier R E, Knutsen T 1987 Translocation t(11;22) in esthesioneuroblastoma. Cancer Genet Cytogenet 29: 155–157
333. Sorensen P H B, Wu J K, Berean K W et al. 1996 Olfactory neuroblastoma is a peripheral primitive neuroectodermal tumor related to Ewing sarcoma. Proc Natl Acad Sci USA 93: 1938–1943
334. Nelson R S, Perlman E J, Askin F B 1995 Is esthesioneuroblastoma a peripheral neuroectodermal tumor? Hum Pathol 26: 639–641
335. Devaney K, Wenig B M, Abbondanzo S L 1996 Olfactory neuroblastoma and other round cell lesions of the sinonasal cavity. Mod Pathol 9: 658–663
336. Argani P, Perez-Ordonez B, Xiao H et al. 1998 Olfactory neuroblastoma is not related to the Ewing family of tumors. Absence of EWS/FLI1 gene fusion and MIC2 expression. Am J Surg Pathol 22: 391–398
337. Kumar S, Perlman E, Pack S et al. 1999 Absence of EWS/FLI1 fusion in olfactory neuroblastomas indicates these tumors do not belong to the Ewing's sarcoma family. Hum Pathol 30: 1356–1360
338. Mezzelani A, Tornielli S, Minoletti F et al. 1999 Esthesioneuroblastoma is not a member of the primitive peripheral neuroectodermal tumour – Ewing's group. Br J Cancer 81: 586–591
339. Hyams V J 1982 Olfactory neuroblastoma (case 6). In: Batsakis J G, Hyams V J, Morales A R (eds) Special tumors of the head and neck. ASCP Press, Chicago, p 24–29
340. Miller D C, Goodman M L, Pilch B Z et al. 1984 Mixed olfactory neuroblastoma and carcinoma. A report of two cases. Cancer 54: 2019–2028
341. Frierson H F Jr, Ross G W, Mills S E et al. 1990 Olfactory neuroblastoma. Additional immunohistochemical characterization. Am J Clin Pathol 94: 547–553
342. Choi H S H, Anderson P J 1986 Olfactory neuroblastoma: an immunohistochemical and electron microscopic study of S-100-protein cells. J Neuropathol Exp Neurol 45: 576–587
343. Tatagiba M, Samii M, Dankoweit T et al. 1995 Esthesioneuroblastomas with intracranial extension. Proliferative potential and management. Arq Neuropsiquiatr 53: 577–586
344. Vartanian R K 1996 Olfactory neuroblastoma: an immunohistochemical, ultrastructural and flow cytometric study. Cancer 77: 1957–1959
345. Kahn L B 1974 Esthesioneuroblastoma. A light and electron microscopic study. Hum Pathol 5: 364–371
346. Taxy J B, Hidvegi D F 1977 Olfactory neuroblastoma. An ultrastructural study. Cancer 39: 131–138
347. Morita A, Ebersold M J, Olsen K D et al. 1993 Esthesioneuroblastoma: prognosis and management. Neurosurgery 32: 706–715
348. Wade P M Jr, Smith R E, Johns M E 1984 Response of esthesioneuroblastoma to chemotherapy. Report of five cases and review of the literature. Cancer 53: 1036–1041
349. Eden B V, Debo R F, Larner J M et al. 1994 Esthesioneuroblastoma. Long term follow-up and patterns of failure – the University of Virginia experience. Cancer 73: 2556–2562
350. O'Conor G T Jr, Drake C R, Johns M E et al. 1985 Treatment of advanced esthesioneuroblastoma with high-dose chemotherapy and autologus bone marrow transplanatation. A case report. Cancer 55: 347–349
351. Polin R S, Sheehan J P, Chenelle A G et al. 1998 The role of preoperative adjuvant treatment in the management of esthesioneuroblastoma: the University of Virginia experience. Neurosurgery 42: 1029–1037
352. Kadish S, Goodman M, Wang C C 1976 Olfactory neuroblastoma. A clinical analysis of 17 cases. Cancer 37: 1571–1576
353. Hyams V J, Batsakis J G, Michaels L 1988 Tumors of the upper respiratory tract and ear, 2nd edn. Armed Forces Institute of Pathology, Washington, DC
354. Kapadia S 2001 Olfactory neuroblastoma. In: Barnes L (ed) Surgical pathology of the head and neck. Marcel Dekker, New York, p 841–845
355. Shanmugaratnam K, Sobin L H, Barnes L et al. 1991 World Health Organization histological classification of tumours. Histological typing of tumours of the upper respiratory tract and ear, 2nd edn. Springer-Verlag, Berlin, p 32–33
356. Ferlito A, Rosai J 1991 Terminology and classification of neuroendocrine neoplasms of the larynx. ORL J Otorhinolaryngol Relat Spec 53: 185–187
357. Wenig B M, Hyams V J, Heffner D K 1988 Moderately differentiated neuroendocrine carcinoma of the larynx: A clinicopathologic study of 54 cases. Cancer 62: 2658–2676
358. Woodruff J M, Huvos A G, Erlandson R A et al. 1985 Neuroendocrine carcinomas of the larynx. A study of two types, one of which mimics thyroid medullary carcinoma. Am J Surg Pathol 9: 771–790
359. Ferlito A, Rinaldo A, Barnes L et al. 2005 Neuroendocrine neoplasms. In: Barnes L, Eveson J, Reichart P et al. (eds) World Health Organization classification of tumours. Pathology and genetics of head and neck tumours. IARC Press, Lyon, France, p 139–142
360. Huntrakoon M 1987 Neuroendocrine carcinoma of the parotid gland: a report of two cases with ultrastructural and immunohistochemical studies. Hum Pathol 18: 1212–1217
361. Gnepp D R 1991 Small cell neuroendocrine carcinoma of the larynx. ORL J Otorhinolaryngol Relat Spec 53: 210–219

362. Perez-Ordonez B, Caruana S, Huvos A G et al. 1998 Small cell neuroendocrine carcinoma of the nasal cavity and paranasal sinuses. Hum Pathol 29: 826–832
363. Perez-Ordonez B 2005 Neuroendocrine carcinomas. In: Barnes L, Eveson J, Reichart P et al. (eds) World Health Organization classification of tumours. Pathology and genetics of head and neck tumours. IARC Press, Lyon, France, p 26–27
364. Wenig B M, Gnepp D R 1989 The spectrum of neuroendocrine carcinomas of the larynx. Semin Diagn Pathol 6: 329–350
365. Chan J K C, Suster S, Wenig B M et al. 1997 Cytokeratin 20 immunoreactivity distinguishes Merkel cell (primary cutaneous) neuroendocrine carcinomas and salivary gland small cell carcinomas from small cell carcinomas of various sites. Am J Surg Pathol 21: 226–234
366. Galanis E, Frytak S, Lloyd R V 1997 Extrapulmonary small cell carcinoma. Cancer 79: 1729–1736
367. Barnes L 2001 Malignant melanoma of the nasal cavity and paranasal sinuses. In: Barnes L (ed) Surgical pathology of the head and neck, 2nd edn. Marcel Dekker, New York, p 523–527
368. Wenig B M 1995 Laryngeal mucosal malignant melanoma: a clinicopathologic, immunohistochemical and ultrastructural study of four cases and a review of the literature. Cancer 75: 1568–1575
369. Thompson L D, Wieneke J A, Miettinen M 2003 Sinonasal tract and nasopharyngeal melanomas: a clinicopathologic study of 115 cases with a proposed staging system. Am J Surg Pathol 27: 594–611
370. Panje W R, Moran W J 1986 Melanoma of the upper aerodigestive tract: a review of 21 cases. Head Neck Surg 8: 309–312
371. Trapp T K, Fu Y S, Calcaterra T C 1987 Melanoma of the nasal and paranasal sinus mucosa. Arch Otolaryngol Head Neck Surg 113: 1086–1089
372. Franquemont D W, Mills S E 1991 Sinonasal malignant melanoma: a clinicopathologic and immunohistochemical study of 14 cases. Am J Clin Pathol 96: 689–697
373. Reuter V E, Woodruff J M 1986 Melanoma of the larynx. Laryngoscope 94: 389–393
374. Goldman J L, Lawson W, Zak F G et al. 1972 The presence of melanocytes in the human larynx. Laryngoscope 82: 824–835
375. Busuttil A 1976 Dendritic pigmented cells within the human laryngeal mucosa. Arch Otolaryngol 102: 43–44
376. Taira K 1985 Endocrine-like cells in the laryngeal mucosa of adult rabbits demonstrated by electron microscopy and by the Grimelius silver-impregnation method. Biomed Res 6: 377–385
377. Reganer S, Anderhuber W, Richtig E et al. 1998 Primary mucosal melanomas of the nasal cavity and paranasal sinuses. A clinicopathological analysis of 14 cases. APMIS 106: 403–410
378. Prasad M L, Jungbluth A A, Iversen K et al. 2001 Expression of melanocytic differentiation in malignant melanomas of the oral and sinonasal mucosa. Am J Surg Pathol 25: 782–787
379. Harwood A, Stringer S P, Million R 1994 Melanoma of the head and neck. In: Million R R, Cassisi N J (eds) Management of head and neck cancer, 2nd edn. J B Lippincott, Philadelphia, p 705–709
380. Wenig B M, Dulguerov P, Kapadia S B et al. Mucosal malignant melanoma. In: Barnes L, Eveson J, Reichart P et al. (eds) World Health Organization classification of tumours. Pathology and genetics of head and neck tumours. IARC Press, Lyon, France, p 72–75
381. McGovern V J 1982 The nature of melanoma: a critical review. J Cutan Pathol 9: 61–81
382. Barnes L 1986 Intestinal-type adenocarcinoma of the nasal cavity and paranasal sinuses. Am J Surg Pathol 10: 192–202
383. Robin P E, Powell D J, Stansbie J M 1979 Carcinoma of the nasal cavity and paranasal sinuses: incidence and presentation of different histological types. Clin Otolaryngol 4: 432–456
384. Kleinsasser O, Schroeder H G 1988 Adenocarcinoma of the inner nose after exposure to wood dust: morphological findings and relationships between histopathology and clinical behavior in 79 cases. Arch Otorhinolaryngol 245: 1–15
385. Hadfield E H, Macbeth R G 1971 Adenocarcinoma of ethmoids in furniture workers. Ann Otol Rhinol Laryngol 80: 699–703
386. Hadfield E H 1970 A study of adenocarcinoma of the paranasal sinuses in woodworkers in the furniture industry. Ann R Coll Surg Engl 46: 302–319
387. Acheson E D, Cowdell R H, Hadfield E H et al. 1970 Nasal cancer in the Northamptonshire boot and shoe industry. Br Med J 1: 385–393
388. Cecchi F, Buiatti E, Kreibel D et al. 1980 Adenocarcinoma of the nose and paranasal sinuses in shoemakers and woodworkers in the province of Florence, Italy (1963–77). Br J Ind Med 37: 222–225
389. Batsakis J G, Holtz F, Sueper R H 1968 Adenocarcinoma of the nasal and paranasal cavities. Arch Otolaryngol 77: 625–633
390. Franquemont D W, Fechner R E, Mills S E 1991 Histologic classification of sinonasal intestinal-type adenocarcinoma. Am J Surg Pathol 15: 368–375
391. Franchi A, Gallo O, Santucci M 1999 Clinical relevance of the histological classification of sinonasal intestinal-type adenocarcinomas. Hum Pathol 30: 1140–1145
392. Mills S E, Fechner R E, Cantrell R W 1982 Aggressive sinonasal lesion resembling normal intestinal mucosa. Am J Surg Pathol 6: 803–809
393. McKinney C D, Mills S E, Franquemont D W 1995 Sinonasal intestinal-type adenocarcinoma: immunohistochemical profile and comparison with colonic adenocarcinoma. Mod Pathol 8: 421–426

394. Urso C, Ninu M B, Franchi A et al. 1993 Intestinal-type adenocarcinoma of the sinonasal tract: a clinicopathologic study of 18 cases. Tumori 79: 205–210
395. Franchi A, Massi D, Baroni G et al. 2003 CDX-2 homeobox gene expression. Am J Surg Pathol 27: 1390–1391
396. Bashir A A, Robinson R A, Benda J A et al. 2003 Sinonasal adenocarcinoma: immunohistochemical marking and expression of oncoproteins. Head Neck 25: 763–771
397. Amre R, Ghali V, Elmberger G et al. 2004 Sinonasal "intestinal type" adenocarcinoma (SNITAC): an immunohistochemical (IHC) study of 22 cases. Mod Pathol 17: 221A
398. Kennedy M T, Jordan R C, Berean K W et al. 2004 Expression pattern of CK7, CK20, CDX-2, and villin in intestinal-type sinonasal adenocarcinoma. J Clin Pathol 57: 932–937
399. Cathro H P, Mills S E 2004 Immunophenotypic differences between intestinal-type and low-grade papillary sinonasal adenocarcinomas: an immunohistochemical study of 22 cases utilizing CDX2 and MUC2. Am J Surg Pathol 28: 1026–1032
400. Franchi A, Massi D, Palomba A et al. 2004 CDX-2, cytokeratin 7 and cytokeratin 20 immunohistochemical expression in the differential diagnosis of primary adenocarcinomas of the sinonasal tract. Virchows Arch 445: 63–67
401. Batsakis J G, Mackay B, Ordonez N G 1984 Enteric-type adenocarcinoma of the nasal cavity. An electron microscopic and immunocytochemical study. Cancer 54: 855–860
402. Heffner D K, Hyams V J, Hauck K W et al. 1982 Low-grade adenocarcinoma of the nasal cavity and paranasal sinuses. Cancer 50: 312–322
403. Barnes L, Brandwein M 2001 Adenoid cystic carcinoma. In: Barnes L (ed.) Surgical pathology of the head and neck, 2nd edn. Marcel Dekker, New York, p 522–523
404. Eby L S, Johnson D S, Baker H W 1972 Adenoid cystic carcinomas of the head and neck. Cancer 29: 1160–1168
405. Orenstein J M, Dardick I, van Nostrand A W 1985 Ultrastructural similarities of adenoid cystic carcinoma and pleomorphic adenoma. Histopathology 9: 623–638
406. Tomich C E 1991 Adenoid cystic carcinoma. In: Ellis G L, Auclair P L, Gnepp D R (eds) Surgical pathology of the salivary glands. W B Saunders, Philadelphia, p 333–349
407. Spiro R H, Huvos A G 1992 Stage means more than grade in adenoid cystic carcinoma. Am J Surg 164: 623–628
408. Kadish S B, Goodman M L, Wang C C 1972 Treatment of minor salivary gland malignancies of upper food and air passage epithelium. Cancer 29: 1020–1026
409. Wenig B M, Hyams V J, Heffner D K 1988 Nasopharyngeal papillary adenocarcinoma. A clinicopathologic study of a low-grade carcinoma. Am J Surg Pathol 12: 946–953
410. Kuo T T, Chan J K C, Wenig B M et al. Nasopharyngeal papillary adenocarcinoma. In: Barnes L, Eveson J, Reichart P et al. (eds) World Health Organization classification of tumours. Pathology and genetics of head and neck tumours. IARC Press, Lyon, France, p 100
410a. Carrizo F, Luna M A 2005 Thyroid transcription factor-1 expression in thyroid-like nasopharyngeal papillary adenocarcinoma: report of 2 cases. Ann Diagn Pathol 9: 189–192
411. Abbondanzo S L, Wenig B M 1995 Non-Hodgkin's lymphoma of the sinonasal tract: a clinicopathologic and immunophenotypic study of 120 cases. Cancer 75: 1281–1291
412. Jaffe E S, Chan J K C, Su I-H et al. 1996 Report of the workshop on nasal and related extranodal angiocentric T/natural killer cell lymphomas. Definitions, differential diagnosis, and epidemiology. Am J Surg Pathol 20: 103–111
413. Chan A C L, Chan J K C, Cheung M M C et al. 2005 Hematolymphoid tumours. In: Barnes L, Eveson J, Reichart P et al. (eds) World Health Organization classification of tumours. Pathology and genetics of head and neck tumours. IARC Press, Lyon, France, p 59–65
414. Arber D A, Weiss L M, Albujar P F et al. 1993 Nasal lymphomas in Peru: high incidence of T-cell immunophenotype and Epstein–Barr virus infection. Am J Surg Pathol 17: 392–399
415. Fellbaum Chr, Hansmann M-L, Lennert K 1989 Malignant lymphomas of the nasal cavity and paranasal sinuses. Virchows Archiv (A) Pathol Anat 414: 399–405
416. Ho F C S, Loke S L, Ng R P et al. 1984 Clinico-pathological features of malignant lymphomas in 294 Hong Kong Chinese patients, retrospective study covering an eight-year period. Int J Cancer 34: 143–148
417. Ng C S, Chan J K C, Lo S T H et al. 1986 Immunophenotypic analysis of non-Hodgkin's lymphomas in Chinese. A study of 75 cases in Hong Kong. Pathology 18: 419–425
418. Cheung M M, Chan J K, Lau W H et al. 1998 Primary non-Hodgkin's lymphoma of the nose and nasopharynx: clinical features, tumor immunophenotype, and treatment outcome in 113 patients. J Clin Oncol 16: 70–77
419. Anderson J R, Armitage J O, Weisenburger D D 1998 Epidemiology of the non-Hodgkin's lymphomas: distributions of the major subtypes differ by geographic locations. Non-Hodgkin's Lymphoma Classification Project. Ann Oncol 9: 717–720
420. Quintanilla-Martinez L, Franklin J L, Guerrero I et al. 1999 Histological and immunophenotypic profile of nasal NK/T cell lymphomas from Peru: high prevalence of p53 overexpression. Hum Pathol 30: 849–855

421. Cuadra-Garcia I, Proulx G M, Wu C L et al. 1999 Sinonasal lymphoma: a clinicopathologic analysis of 58 cases from the Massachusetts General Hospital. Am J Surg Pathol 23: 1356–1369
422. Pomilla P V, Morris A B, Jaworek A 1995 Sinonasal non-Hodgkin's lymphoma in patients infected with human immunodeficiency virus: report of three cases and review. Clin Infect Dis 21: 137–149
423. Canioni D, Arnulf B, Asso-Bonnet M et al. 2001 Nasal natural killer lymphoma associated with Epstein–Barr virus in a patient infected with human immunodeficiency virus. Arch Pathol Lab Med 125: 660–662
424. Jaffe E S, Krenacs L, Kumar S et al. 1999 Extranodal peripheral T-cell and NK-cell neoplasms. Am J Clin Pathol 111: S46–S55
425. Chan J K C, Yip T T C, Tsang W Y W et al. 1994 Detection of Epstein–Barr viral RNA in malignant lymphomas of the upper aerodigestive tract. Am J Surg Pathol 18: 938–946
426. Ohshima K, Suzumiya J, Shimazaki K et al. 1997 Nasal T/NK cell lymphomas commonly express perforin and Fas ligand: important mediators of tissue damage. Histopathology 31: 444–450
427. Cheung M M, Chan J K, Lau W H et al. 2002 Early stage nasal NK/T-cell lymphoma: clinical outcome, prognostic factors, and the effect of treatment modality. Int J Radiat Oncol Biol Phys 54: 182–190
428. Cheung M M, Chan J K, Wong K F 2003. Natural killer cell neoplasms: a distinctive group of highly aggressive lymphoma/leukemia. Semin Hematol 40: 221–232
429. Kim G E, Koom W S, Yang W I 2004 Clinical relevance of three subtypes of primary sinonasal lymphoma characterized by immunophenotypic analysis. Head Neck 26: 584–593
430. Freeman C, Berg J W, Cutler S J 1972 Occurrence and prognosis of extranodal lymphomas. Cancer 29: 252–260
431. Otter R, Gerrits W B J, Sandt M M V D et al. 1989 Primary extranodal and nodal non-Hodgkin's lymphomas: survey of a population-based registry. Eur J Cancer Clin Oncol 25: 1203–1210
432. Hoppe R T, Burke J S, Glatstein E et al. 1978 Non-Hodgkin's lymphoma: involvement of Waldeyer's ring. Cancer 42: 1096–1104
433. Barton J H, Osborne B M, Butler J J et al. 1984 Non-Hodgkin's lymphoma of the tonsil: a clinicopathologic study of 65 cases. Cancer 53: 86–95
434. Saul S M, Kapadia S B 1985 Lymphoma of Waldeyer's ring: clinicopathologic study of 68 cases. Cancer 56: 157–166
435. Shima N, Kobashi Y, Tsutsui K et al. 1990 Extranodal non-Hodgkin's lymphoma of the head and neck: a clinicopathologic study in the Kyoto-Nara area of Japan. Cancer 66: 1190–1197
436. Medeiros L J, Bagg A, Cossman J 1992 Application of molecular genetics to the diagnosis of hematopoietic neoplasms. In: Knowles D M (ed) Neoplastic hematopathology. Williams & Wilkins, Baltimore, p 263–298
437. Carbone P P, Kaplan H S, Musshoff K et al. 1971 Report of the committee on Hodgkin's disease staging classification. Cancer Res 31: 1860–1861
438. Shimm D S, Dosoretz D E, Harris N L et al. 1984 Radiation therapy of Waldeyer's ring lymphoma. Cancer 54: 426–431
439. Kapadia S, Desai U, Cheng U 1982 Extramedullary plasmacytoma of the head and neck: a clinicopathologic study of 20 cases. Medicine 61: 317–329
440. Grogan T M, Spier C M 1991 The B cell immunoproliferative disorders, including multiple myeloma and amyloidosis. In: Knowles D (ed) Neoplastic hematopathology. Williams & Wilkins, Baltimore, p 1235
441. Kinney M C, Swerdlow S H 2001 Plasma cell neoplasms. In: Barnes L (ed) Surgical pathology of the head and neck. Marcel Dekker, New York, p 1323–1329
442. Carbone A, Vaccher E, Barzan L et al. 1995 Head and neck lymphomas associated with human immunodeficiency virus infection. Arch Otolaryngol Head Neck Surg 121: 210–218
443. Alexanian R 1985 Ten-year survival in multiple myeloma. Arch Intern Med 145: 2073–2074
444. Heffner D K 1983 Problems in pediatric otorhinolaryngic pathology. IV. Epithelial and lymphoid tumors of the sinonasal tract and nasopharynx. Int J Pediatr Otorhinolaryngol 6: 219–237
445. Kapadia S B, Roman L N, Kingma D W et al. 1995 Hodgkin's disease of Waldeyer's ring. Clinical and histoimmunophenotypic study and association with Epstein–Barr virus in 16 cases. Am J Surg Pathol 19: 1431–1439
446. Moghe G M, Borges A M, Soman C S et al. 2001. Hodgkin's disease involving Waldeyer's ring: a study of four cases. Leuk Lymphoma 41: 151–156
447. Perez-Ordonez B, Erlandson R A, Rosai J 1996 Follicular dendritic cell tumor: report of 13 additional cases of a distinctive entity. Am J Surg Pathol 20: 944–955
448. Perez-Ordonez B, Rosai J 1998 Follicular dendritic cell tumor: review of the entity. Semin Diagn Pathol 15: 144–154
449. Biddle D A, Ro J Y, Yoon G S et al. 2002 Extranodal follicular dendritic cell sarcoma of the head and neck region: three new cases, with a review of the literature. Mod Pathol 15: 50–58
450. Weiss L M, Grogan T M, Müller-Hermelink H-K et al. 2001 Follicular dendritic cell sarcoma/tumour. In: Jaffe ES, Harris NL, Stein H et al. (eds) World Health Classification of tumours. Pathology and genetics. Tumours of haematopoietic and lymphoid tissues. IARC Press, Lyon, p 288–289
451. Dominguez-Malagon H, Cano-Valdez A M, Mosqueda-Taylor A et al. 2004 Follicular dendritic cell sarcoma of the pharyngeal region: histologic, cytologic, immunohistochemical, and ultrastructural study of three cases. Ann Diagn Pathol 8: 325–332
452. Chan A C, Chan K W, Chan J K et al. 2001 Development of follicular dendritic cell sarcoma in hyaline-vascular Castleman's disease of the nasopharynx: tracing its evolution by sequential biopsies. Histopathology 38: 510–518
453. Grogg K L, Lae M E, Kurtin P J et al. 2004 Clusterin expression distinguishes follicular dendritic cell tumors from other dendritic cell neoplasms: report of a novel follicular dendritic cell marker and clinicopathologic data on 12 additional follicular dendritic cell tumors and 6 additional interdigitating dendritic cell tumors. Am J Surg Pathol 28: 988–998
454. Chan J K, Fletcher C D, Nayler S J et al. 1997 Follicular dendritic cell sarcoma. Clinicopathologic analysis of 17 cases suggesting a malignant potential higher than currently recognized. Cancer 79: 294–313
455. Heffner D K, Gnepp D R 1992 Sinonasal fibrosarcomas, malignant schwannomas, and "Triton" tumors. A clinicopathologic study of 67 cases. Cancer 70: 1089–1101
456. Loree T R, North J H Jr, Werness B A et al. 2000 Malignant peripheral nerve sheath tumors of the head and neck: analysis of prognostic factors. Otolaryngol Head Neck Surg 122: 667–672
457. Wick M R, Swanson P E, Scheithauer B W et al. 1987 Malignant peripheral nerve sheath tumor. An immunohistochemical study of 62 cases. Am J Clin Pathol 87: 425–433
458. Barnes L, Kanbour A 1988 Malignant fibrous histiocytoma of the head and neck. A report of 12 cases. Arch Otolaryngol Head Neck Surg 114: 1149–1156
459. Perzin K H, Fu Y S 1980 Non-epithelial tumors of the nasal cavity, paranasal sinuses, and nasopharynx: a clinicopathologic study. XI. Fibrous histiocytomas. Cancer 45: 2616–2626
460. Mauer H M, Beltangady M, Gehan E A et al. 1988 The Intergroup Rhabdomyosarcoma Study – I. A final report. Cancer 61: 209–220
461. Weiss S W, Goldblum J R 2001 Rhabdomyosarcoma. In: Weiss S W, Goldblum J R (eds) Enzinger and Weiss's soft tissue tumors, 4th edn. Mosby, St. Louis, p 785–835
462. Barnes L 2001 Rhabdomyosarcoma. In: Barnes L (ed) Surgical pathology of the head and neck, 2nd edn. Marcel Dekker, New York, p. 960–967
463. Anderson G J, Tom L W C, Womer R B et al. 1990 Rhabdomyosarcoma of the head and neck in children. Arch Otolaryngol Head Neck Surg 116: 428–431
464. Callender T A, Weber R S, JanJan N et al. 1995 Rhabdomyosarcoma of the nose and paranasal sinuses in adults and children. Head Neck Surg 112: 252–257
465. El-Naggar A K, Batsakis J G, Ordonez N G et al. Rhabdomyosarcoma of the adult head and neck: a clinicopathological study and DNA ploidy study. J Laryngol Otol 107: 716–720
466. Nakhleh R E, Swanson P E, Dehner L P 1991 Juvenile (embryonal and alveolar) rhabdomyosarcoma of the head and neck in adults. A clinical, pathologic, and immunohistochemical study of 12 cases. Cancer 67: 1019–1024
467. Nayar R C, Prudhomme F, Parise O Jr et al. 1993 Rhabdomyosarcoma of the head and neck in adults. A study of 26 patients. Laryngoscope 103: 1362–1366
468. Parham D M, Barr F G 2002 Embryonal rhabdomyosarcoma. In: Fletcher C D M, Unni K K, Mertens F (eds) In: World Health Organization classification of tumours. Pathology and genetics. Tumours of soft tissue and bone. IARC Press, Lyon, p 146–149
469. Parham D M, Barr F G 2002 Alveolar rhabdomyosarcoma. In: Fletcher C D M, Unni K K, Mertens F (eds) In: World Health Organization classification of tumours. Pathology and genetics. Tumours of soft tissue and bone. IARC Press, Lyon, p 150–152
470. Maurer H M, Gehan E A, Beltangady M et al. 1993 The Intergroup Rhabdomyosarcoma Study II. Cancer 71: 1904–1922
471. Newton W A Jr, Gehan E A, Webber B L et al. 1995 Classification of rhabdomyosarcoma and related sarcomas. Pathologic aspects and proposal for a new classification – an Intergroup Rhabdomyosarcoma study. Cancer 76: 1073–1085
472. Raney R B, Asmar L, Vassilopoulou-Sellin R et al. 1999 Late complications of therapy in 213 children with localized, nonorbital soft tissue sarcoma of the head and neck: a descriptive report from the Intergroup Rhabdomyosarcoma Studies (IRS)-II and -III. IRS Group of the Children's Cancer Group and the Pediatric Oncology Group. Med Pediatr Oncol 33: 362–371
473. Bankaci M, Myers E N, Barnes L et al. 1979 Angiosarcoma of the maxillary sinus. Head Neck Surg 1: 274–280
474. Panje W R, Moran W J, Bostwick D G et al. 1986 Angiosarcoma of the head and neck: review of 11 cases. Laryngoscope 96: 1381–1384
475. Di Girolamo A, Giacomini P G, Coli A et al. 2003 Epithelioid haemangioendothelioma arising in the nasal cavity. J Laryngol Otol 117: 75–77
476. Goldberg A N 1993 Kaposi's sarcoma of the head and neck in acquired immunodeficiency syndrome. Am J Otolaryngol 14: 5–14
477. Fliss D M, Parikh J, Freeman J L 1992 AIDS-related Kaposi's sarcoma of the sphenoid sinus. J Otolaryngol 21: 235–237
478. Moazzez A H, Alvi A 1998 Head and neck manifestations of AIDS in adults. Am Fam Physician 57: 1813–1822
479. Wyatt M E, Finlayson C J, Moore-Gillon V 1998 Kaposi's sarcoma masquerading as pyogenic granuloma of the nasal mucosa. J Laryngol Otol 112: 280–282

480. Cheuk W, Wong K O, Wong C S et al. 2004. Immunostaining for human herpesvirus 8 latest nuclear antigen-1 helps distinguish Kaposi sarcoma from its mimickers. Am J Clin Pathol 121: 335–342
481. Blackbourn D J, Lennette E T, Ambroziak J et al. 1998 Human herpesvirus 8 detection in nasal secretions and saliva. J Infect Dis 177: 213–216
482. Gandhi M, Koelle D M, Ameli N et al. 2004 Prevalence of human herpesvirus-8 salivary shedding in HIV increases with CD4 count. J Dent Res 83: 639–643
483. Barnes L 2001 Leiomyosarcoma. In: Barnes L (ed) Surgical pathology of the head and neck, 2nd edn. Marcel Dekker, New York, p 979–984
484. Kuruvilla A, Wenig B M, Humphrey D M et al. 1990 Leiomyosarcoma of the sinonasal tract. A clinicopathologic study of nine cases. Arch Otolaryngol Head Neck Surg 116: 1278–1286
485. Dahlin D C, Unni K K 1986 Bone tumors: general aspects and data on 8542 cases, 4th edn. Charles C Thomas, Springfield, p 227–259
486. Batsakis J G 1987 Osteogenic and chondrogenic sarcomas of jaws. Ann Otol Rhinol Laryngol 96: 474–475
487. Waldron C A 1985 Osteosarcoma. In: Neville B D, Damm D D, Allen C M, Bouquot J E (eds) Oral and maxillofacial pathology. W B Saunders, Philadelphia, p 482–485
488. Mark R J, Sercarz J A, Tran L et al. 1991 Osteogenic sarcoma of the head and neck. The UCLA experience. Arch Otolaryngol Head Neck Surg 117: 761–766
489. Garrington G E, Scofield H H, Coryn J et al. 1967 Osteosarcoma of the jaws. An analysis of 56 cases. Cancer 20: 377–391
490. Fechner R E, Mills S E 1993 Conventional intramedullary osteosarcoma. In: Rosai J, Mills S E (eds) Tumors of the bones and joints, series 3, fascicle 8. Armed Forces Institute of Pathology, Washington, DC, p 38–50
491. Caron A S, Hajdu S I, Strong E W 1971 Osteogenic sarcoma of the facial and cranial bones. A review of forty-three cases. Am J Surg 122: 719–725
492. Ruark D S, Schlehaider U K, Shah J P 1992 Chondrosarcomas of the head and neck. World J Surg 16: 1010–1016
493. Burkey B B, Hoffman H T, Baker S R et al. 1990 Chondrosarcoma of the head and neck. Laryngoscope 100: 1301–1305
494. Mark R J, Tran L M, Sercarz J et al. 1993 Chondrosarcoma of the head and neck. The UCLA experience, 1955–1988. Am J Clin Oncol (CCT) 16: 232–237
495. Huvos A G, Marcove A C 1987 Chondrosarcoma in the young. A clinicopathologic analysis of 79 patients younger than 21 years of age. Am J Surg Pathol 11: 930–942
496. Finn D G, Goepfert H, Batsakis J G 1984 Chondrosarcoma of the head and neck. Laryngoscope 94: 1539–1544
497. Webber P A, Hussain S S, Radcliffe G J 1986 Cartilaginous neoplasms of the head and neck. J Laryngol Otol 100: 615–619
498. Rosenthal D I, Schiller A L, Mankin H J 1984 Chondrosarcoma: correlation of radiological and histological grade. Radiology 150: 21–26
499. Perzin K H, Pushparaj N 1986 Non-epithelial tumors of the nasal cavity, paranasal sinuses, and nasopharynx: a clinicopathologic study. XIV. Chordomas. Cancer 57: 784–796
500. Meis J M, Giraldo A 1988 Chordoma. An immunohistochemical study of 20 cases. Arch Pathol Lab Med 112: 553–556
501. Mitchell A, Scheithauer B W, Unni K K et al. 1993 Chordoma and chondroid neoplasms of the spheno-occiput. An immunohistochemical study of 41 cases with prognostic and nosologic implications. Cancer 72: 2943–2949
502. Heffner D K, Hyams V J 1984 Teratocarcinosarcoma (malignant teratoma?) of the nasal cavity and paranasal sinuses. A clinicopathologic study of 20 cases. Cancer 53: 2140–2154
503. Pai S A, Naresh K N, Masih K et al. 1998 Teratocarcinosarcoma of the paranasal sinuses: a clinicopathologic and immunohistochemical study. Hum Pathol 29: 718–722
504. Shimazaki H, Aida S, Tamai S 2000 Sinonasal teratocarcinosarcoma: ultrastructural and immunohistochemical evidence of neuroectodermal origin. Ultrastruct Pathol 24: 115–122
505. Chao K K, Eng T Y, Barnes J et al. 2004 Sinonasal teratocarcinosarcoma. Am J Clin Oncol 27: 29–32
506. Fu Y S, Perzin K H 1977 Non-epithelial tumors of the nasal cavity, paranasal sinuses, and nasopharynx: a clinicopathologic study. VIII. Lipoma and liposarcoma. Cancer 40: 1314–1317
507. McCullough T M, Makielski K H, McNutt M A 1992 Head and neck liposarcoma. A histopathologic reevaluation of reported cases. Arch Otolaryngol Head Neck Surg 118: 1045–1049
508. Shmookler B M, Enzinger F M, Brannon R B 1982 Orofacial synovial sarcoma. A clinicopathologic study of 11 new cases and review of the literature. Cancer 50: 269–276
509. Simmons W B, Haggerty H S, Ngan B et al. 1989 Alveolar soft part sarcoma of the head and neck. A disease of children and young adults. Int J Pediatr Otorhinolaryngol 17: 139–153
510. Pontius K I, Sebek B A 1981 Extra-skeletal Ewing's sarcoma arising in the nasal fossa. Light- and electron-microscopic observations. Am J Clin Pathol 75: 410–415
511. Lane S, Ironside J W 1990 Extra-skeletal Ewing's sarcoma of the nasal fossa. J Laryngol Otol 104: 570–573
512. Toda T, Atari E, Sadi A M et al. 1999 Primitive neuroectodermal tumor in sinonasal region. Auris Nasus Larynx 26: 83–90
513. Windfuhr J P 2004 Primitive neuroectodermal tumor of the head and neck: incidence, diagnosis, and management. Ann Otol Rhinol Laryngol 113: 533–543
514. Lack E E 1985 Extragonadal germ cell tumors of the head and neck region: review of 16 cases. Hum Pathol 16: 56–64
515. Manivel C, Wick M R, Dehner L P 1986 Transitional (cylindric) cell carcinoma with endodermal sinus tumor-like features of the nasopharynx and paranasal sinuses. Clinicopathologic and immunohistochemical study of two cases. Arch Pathol Lab Med 110: 198–202
516. Bernstein J M, Montgomery W W, Balogh K Jr 1966 Metastatic tumors to the maxilla, nose, and paranasal sinuses. Laryngoscope 76: 621–650
517. Kent S E, Majumdar B 1985 Metastatic tumours in the maxillary sinus. A report of two cases and a review of the literature. J Laryngol Otol 99: 459–462
518. McClatchey K D, Lloyd R V, Schaldenbard J D 1985 Metastatic carcinoma to the sphenoid sinus. Case report and review of the literature. Arch Otorhinolaryngol 241: 219–224
519. Drake-Lee A B, Lowe D, Swanston A et al. 1984 Clinical profile and recurrence of nasal polyps. J Laryngol Otol 98: 783–793
520. Settipane G A, Chafee F H 1977 Nasal polyps in asthma and rhinitis. A review of 6037 patients. J Allergy Clin Immunol 59: 17–21
521. Patriarca G, Nucera E, Di Rienzo V et al. 1991 Nasal provocation test with lysine acetylsalicylate in aspirin-sensitive patients. Ann Allergy 67: 60–62
522. Killian G 1906 The origin of choanal polypi. Lancet 2: 81–82
523. Sirola R 1966 Choanal polyps. Acta Otolaryngol 61: 42–48
524. Nakayama M, Wenig B M, Heffner D K 1995 Atypical stromal cells in inflammatory nasal polyps: immunohistochemical and ultrastructural analysis in defining histogenesis. Laryngoscope 105: 127–134
525. Sheahan P, Crotty P L, Hamilton S et al. 2005 Infarcted angiomatous nasal polyps. Eur Arch Otorhinolaryngol 262: 225–230
526. Yfantis H G, Drachenberg C B, Gray W et al. 2000 Angiectatic nasal polyps that clinically simulate a malignant process: report of 2 cases and review of the literature. Arch Pathol Lab Med 124: 406–410
527. Orvidas L J, Beatty C W, Weaver A L 2001 Antrochoanal polyps in children. Am J Rhinol 15: 321–325
528. Theaker J M, Fletcher C D M 1991 Heterotopic glial nodules: a light microscopic and immunohistochemical study. Histopathology 18: 255–260
529. Heffner D K 1983 Problems in pediatric otorhinolaryngic pathology. III. Teratoid and neural tumors of the nose, sinonasal tract, and nasopharynx. Int J Pediatr Otorhinolaryngol 6: 1–21
530. Puppala B, Mangurten H H, McFadden J et al. 1990 Nasal glioma presenting as neonatal respiratory distress. Clin Pediatr 29: 49–52
531. Kapadia S B, Popek E J, Barnes L 1994 Pediatric otorhinolaryngic pathology: diagnosis of selected lesions. Pathol Annu 29: 159–209
532. Graeme-Cook F, Pilch B Z 1992 Hamartomas of the nose and nasopharynx. Head Neck 14: 321–327
533. Wenig B M, Heffner D K 1995 Respiratory epithelial adenomatous hamartomas of the sinonasal tract and nasopharynx: a clinicopathologic study of 31 cases. Ann Otol Rhinol Laryngol 104: 639–645
534. Baille E E, Batsakis J G 1974 Glandular (seromucinous) hamartoma of the nasopharynx. Oral Surg 38: 760–762
535. Kapadia S B, Popek E J, Barnes L 1994 Pediatric otorhinolaryngic pathology: diagnosis of selected lesions. Pathol Annu 29: 159–209
536. Burns B V, Axon P R, Pahade A 2001 'Hairy polyp' of the pharynx in association with an ipsilateral branchial sinus: evidence that the 'hairy polyp' is a second branchial arch malformation. J Laryngol Otol 115: 145–148
537. Heffner D K, Thompson L D R, Schall D G et al. 1996 Pharyngeal dermoids ("hairy polyps") as accessory auricles. Ann Otol Rhinol Laryngol 105: 819–824
538. Heffner D K 1983 Problems in pediatric otorhinolaryngic pathology. III. Teratoid and neural tumors of the nose, sinonasal tract, and nasopharynx. Int J Pediatr Otorhinolaryngol 6: 1–21
539. Ferlito A, Devaney K O 1995 Developmental lesions of the head and neck. Terminology and biologic behavior. Ann Otol Rhinol Laryngol 104: 913–918
539a. Ozolek J A, Carrau R, Barnes E L, Hunt J L 2005 Nasal chondromesenchymal hamartoma in older children and adults: series and immunohistochemical analysis. Arch Pathol Lab Med 129: 1444–1450
540. McDermott M B, Ponder T D, Dehner L P 1998 Nasal chondromesenchymal hamartoma: an upper respiratory tract analogue of the chest wall mesenchymal hamartoma. Am J Surg Pathol 22: 425–433
541. Norman E S, Bergman S, Trupiano J K 2004 Nasal chondromesenchymal hamartoma: report of a case and review of the literature. Pediatr Dev Pathol 7: 517–520
542. Kim B, Park S H, Min H S 2004 Nasal chondromesenchymal hamartoma of infancy clinically mimicking meningoencephalocele. Pediatr Neurosurg 40: 136–140
543. Shet T, Borges A, Nair C et al. 2004 Two unusual lesions in the nasal cavity of infants – a nasal chondromesenchymal hamartoma and an aneurysmal bone cyst like lesion. More closely related than we think? Int J Pediatr Otorhinolaryngol 68: 359–364
544. Kardon D E, Wenig B M, Heffner D K et al. 2000 Tonsillar lymphangiomatous polyps: a clinicopathologic series of 26 cases. Mod Pathol 13: 1128–1133
545. Friedman G C, Hartwick W J, Ro J Y et al. 1991 Allergic fungal sinusitis: report of three cases associated with dematiaceous fungi. Am J Clin Pathol 96: 368–372
546. Saeed S R, Brooks G B 1995 Aspergillosis of the paranasal sinuses. Rhinology 33: 46–51
547. Satyanarayana C 1960 Rhinosporidiosis with a record of 225 cases. Acta Otolaryngol 51: 348–356

548. Nussbaum E S, Hall W A 1994 Rhinocerebral mucormycosis: changing patterns of disease. Surg Neurol 41: 152–154
549. Hyams V J, Batsakis J G, Michaels L 1988 Rhinoscleroma. In: Tumors of the upper respiratory tract and ear, series 2, fascicle 25. Armed Forces Institute of Pathology, Washington, DC, p 24–26
550. Wenig B M, Smirniotopolous J, Heffner D K 1996 Botryomycosis of the sinonasal tract: a report of two cases. Arch Pathol Lab Med 120: 1123–1128
551. Gordon W W, Cohn A M, Greenberg S D et al. 1976 Nasal sarcoidosis. Arch Otolaryngol 102: 11–14
552. Wenig B M, Thompson L D R, Frankel S S et al. 1996 Lymphoid changes of the nasopharynx and tonsils that are indicative of human immunodeficiency virus infection: a clinicopathologic study of 12 cases with a discussion on the possibility of transmucosal infection. Am J Surg Pathol 20: 572–587
553. Moss R, Beaudet L M, Wenig B M et al. 1997 Microsporidium-associated sinusitis. Ear Nose Throat J 76: 95–101
554. Kyriakos M 1977 Myospherulosis of the paranasal sinuses, nose and middle ear. Am J Clin Pathol 67: 118–130
555. DeRemee R A, McDonald T J, Harrison E G et al. 1976 Wegener's granulomatosis, anatomic correlates, a proposed classification. Mayo Clin Proc 51: 777–781
556. DeRemee R A 1988 Extrapulmonary manifestations of Wegener's granulomatosis and other respiratory vasculitides. Semin Resp Med 9: 403–408
557. Specks U, Wheatley C L, McDonald T J et al. 1989 Anticytoplasmic autoantibodies in the diagnosis and follow-up of Wegener's granulomatosis. Mayo Clin Proc 64: 28–36
558. Nolle B, Specks U, Ludemann J et al. 1989 Anticytoplasmic autoantibodies: their immunodiagnostic value in Wegener's granulomatosis. Ann Intern Med 111: 28–40
559. Fienberg R, Mark E J, Goodman M et al. 1993 Correlation of antineutrophil cytoplasmic antibodies with the extrarenal histopathology of Wegener's (pathergic) granulomatosis and related forms of vasculitis. Hum Pathol 24: 160–168
560. DeRemee R A 1991 Antineutrophil cytoplasmic autoantibody-associated disease: a pulmonologist's perspective. Am J Kidney Dis 18: 180–183
561. Falk R J, Jennette J C 1988 Anti-neutrophil cytoplasmic autoantibodies with specificity for myeloperoxidase in patients with systemic vasculitis and idiopathic necrotizing and crescenteric glomerulonephritis. N Engl J Med 318: 1651–1657
562. Hardarson S, Labrecque D R, Mitros F A et al. 1993 Antineutrophil cytoplasmic antibody in inflammatory bowel and hepatobiliary diseases: high prevalence in ulcerative colitis, primary sclerosing cholangitis, and autoimmune hepatitis. Am J Clin Pathol 99: 221–223
563. Zholudev A, Zurakowski D, Young W et al. 2004 Serologic testing with ANCA, ASCA, and anti-OmpC in children and young adults with Crohn's disease and ulcerative colitis: diagnostic value and correlation with disease phenotype. Am J Gastoenterol 99: 2235–2241
564. Devaney K O, Travis W D, Hoffman G et al. 1990 Interpretation of head and neck biopsies in Wegener's granulomatosis. Am J Surg Pathol 14: 555–564
565. Keogh K A, Specks U 2003 Churg–Strauss syndrome: clinical presentation, antineutrophil cytoplasmic antibodies, and leukotriene receptor antagonists. Am J Med 115: 284–290
566. Barnes L 2001 Midfacial destructive diseases. In: Barnes L (ed) Surgical pathology of the head and neck, 2nd edn. Marcel-Dekker, New York, p 759–786
567. Rosai J, Dorfman R F 1969 Sinus histiocytosis with massive lymphadenopathy: a newly recognized benign clinicopathologic entity. Arch Pathol 87: 63–70
568. Rosai J, Dorfman R F 1972 Sinus histiocytosis with massive lymphadenopathy: a pseudolymphomatous benign disorder. Cancer 30: 1174–1188
569. Foucar E, Rosai J, Dorfman R 1990 Sinus histiocytosis with massive lymphadenopathy (Rosai–Dorfman disease): review of the entity. Semin Diagn Pathol 7: 19–73
570. Foucar K, Foucar E 1990 The mononuclear phagocyte and immunoregulatory effector (M-PIRE) system: evolving concepts. Semin Diagn Pathol 7: 4–18
571. Wenig B M, Abbondanzo S L, Childers E L 1993 Extranodal sinus histiocytosis with massive lymphadenopathy (Rosai–Dorfman disease) of the head and neck. Hum Pathol 24: 483–492
572. Eisen R N, Buckley P J, Rosai J 1990 Immunophenotypic characterization of sinus histiocytosis with massive lymphadenopathy (Rosai–Dorfman disease). Semin Diagn Pathol 7: 74–82
573. Paulli M, Rosso R, Kindl S et al. 1992 Immunophenotypic characterization of the cell infiltrate in five cases of sinus histiocytosis with massive lymphadenopathy (Rosai–Dorfman disease). Hum Pathol 23: 647–654
574. Komp D M 1990 The treatment of sinus histiocytosis with massive lymphadenopathy (Rosai–Dorfman disease). Semin Diagn Pathol 7: 83–86
575. Foucar E, Rosai J, Dorfman R F 1984 Sinus histiocytosis with massive lymphadenopathy: an analysis of 14 deaths occurring in a patient registry. Cancer 54: 1834–1840

第二部分

喉和气管 Larynx and trachea

Ben Z. Pilch 著

王芳 季语祝 沈勤 庄利萍 郭君 唐莹 卜亚军 译

喉和气管		疣状癌	161
良性肿瘤	150	梭形细胞癌（肉瘤样癌）	163
鳞状上皮乳头状瘤	150	基底细胞样鳞状细胞癌（基底细胞样鳞癌）	166
颗粒细胞瘤	152	淋巴上皮癌	167
副神经节瘤	152	腺样鳞状细胞癌	167
声门下血管瘤	153	乳头状鳞状细胞癌	167
其他良性间叶性肿瘤	154	腺鳞癌	167
非肿瘤性肿块性病变	154	神经内分泌癌	168
其他罕见病变	158	腺癌	172
恶性肿瘤	158	软骨性肿瘤	173
鳞状细胞癌	158	其他恶性肿瘤	174

良性肿瘤 Benign neoplasms

鳞状上皮乳头状瘤 Squamous papilloma

喉鳞状上皮乳头状瘤是儿童最常见的喉部肿瘤[1-4]。其临床特征是具有多样性和反复复发，偶尔伴有长的潜伏期[1,3]。喉鳞状上皮乳头状瘤传统上分为幼年性及成人性，但多发性乳头状瘤，不论是发生于儿童还是成人，现在一般都认为基本上是相同的疾病[5,6]，但临床上儿童病例倾向于比开始就发生于成人的病例具有更加明显的侵袭性[2]。这些息肉样外生性病变可能引起明显的气道阻塞，特别是在儿童，因其难治性，而成为极为棘手的挑战。复发性乳头状瘤病的标准疗法是用二氧化碳激光器或吸切器予以清除[2]。新近的技术，例如脉冲式染料激光器的使用[7]以及病变内注射抗病毒药物西多福韦[8,9]，显示出有某些治疗方面的潜力。真声带是喉乳头状瘤最常见的发生部位，但是亦可发生于声门下、声门上和气管等[1,5]。偶尔，鳞状上皮乳头状瘤病可能累及整个呼吸道，包括气管支气管树到肺实质的水平[5,10]。如不幸发生这种疾病容易引起阻塞性肺炎和肺脓肿，而且可能导致死亡。研究发现，气管造口术与声门下和气管乳头状瘤发生率增加有关[1,3]，因此，有些人不赞成应用气管造口术，除非是在绝对必要的情况下[2]。然而，

Shapiro等的回顾性研究提示，气管造口术与有害的结局并无显著相关性，对于受累儿童严重气道受损，气管造口术仍是一种可行的治疗选择[11]。从前的概念是，幼年性喉乳头状瘤倾向于在青春期消退，而现在普遍认为自发性消退可能是难以捉摸和不能预测的[4,12,13]。

喉鳞状上皮乳头状瘤与HPV感染明显相关，而且似乎由HPV感染引起[1,2,14-16]，尤其是6型和11型[14-18]。这些HPV亚型还常与肛门生殖器尖锐湿疣有关，实际上，在妊娠或分娩时被患有湿疣的母亲感染被认为是婴儿获得本病的主要方式[1,4,19,20]。所幸的是，在缺乏先前照射的情况下，喉鳞状上皮乳头状瘤恶性变非常罕见[5]。报道的一例伴有重度异型增生/原位癌（CIS）的喉鳞状上皮乳头状瘤除了与HPV 11有关外，还与HPV 16（宫颈的一种"高危险"HPV）有关[21]；然而，其他一些从乳头状瘤病进展为癌的病例实际上均与HPV6/11有关[22]。

大体上，鳞状上皮乳头状瘤一般为外生性、质脆的菜花样肿块，单发或成簇生长。组织学上，其特征为指状或叶状突起，被覆增厚的复层鳞状上皮，伴有纤维血管轴心（图4B.1）。乳头可有一些分枝。乳头表面一般为一薄层角化不全上皮或无角化层，一般并不出现明显角化，这是一个鉴别诊断的线索（见下文）。鳞状上皮细胞显示显著的成熟停止[1,2]，缺乏扁平细胞及表面成熟的鳞状细胞，虽然最上层可能是一薄层扁平细胞。常见单个细胞角化不良，细胞极性有时丧失，形成上皮细胞杂乱排列的现象。挖空细胞改变，如女性生殖道所见

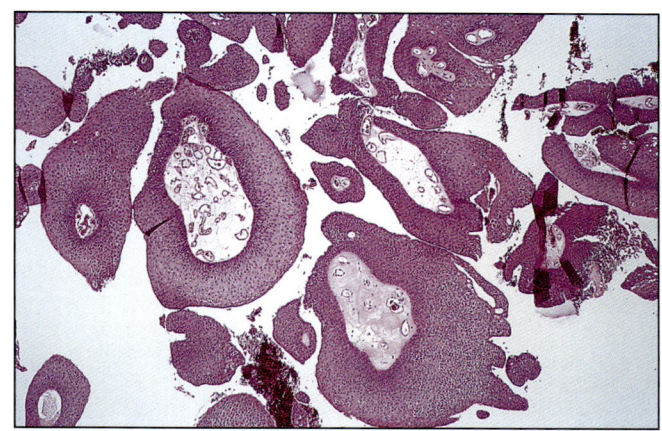

图4B.1 喉鳞状上皮乳头状瘤。增厚的鳞状上皮形成指状乳头，含有纤维血管轴心。

（深染皱缩的细胞核周围胞浆透明，偶尔伴有双核或三核细胞），并不少见（图 4B.2A），但一般不如宫颈明显[1,14,23]。由喉乳头状瘤病延伸至声门下或气管支气管树时，其被覆上皮可以是鳞状上皮或纤毛柱状上皮，而且可能含有所谓的"中间型细胞"，即表现介于鳞状上皮和立方/柱状上皮细胞之间的多角形细胞[24]。

有关乳头状瘤组织学"非典型性"及其伴随的侵袭性临床行为和局部复发仍有一些争论[25-27]。然而根据我的经验，"癌前"或异型增生性上皮改变，例如明显的核的多形性、核深染、核浆比例增大以及异常核分裂象等，很少见于 HPV 相关性喉鳞状上皮乳头状瘤。从前许多文献提到的"非典型性"变化可能与病毒相关性改变有关，例如成熟停止、角化不良和挖空细胞形成。某些研究显示，幼年性和成人性病毒相关性喉鳞状上皮乳头状瘤的组织病理学和临床行为之间均无相关性[1]，而另外一些研究提出，组织学"非典型性"增加与乳头状瘤的严重程度和（或）复发有关[25,26]；不过，尚未发现这些改变与随后发生癌相关[26]。应用常规免疫组化技术，偶尔可以发现乳头状瘤有 HPV 相关性抗原局灶性染色（图 4B.2B）；另外，应用诸如原位或 Southern 印迹杂交或 PCR 等较新的方法，能够更加一致地成功检测到病变中的 HPV DNA[1,14-18]。

鉴别诊断

见诸文献的所谓"孤立性成人乳头状瘤"或"角化性乳头状瘤"，都是用来描述发生于成人喉部的角化性乳头状孤立性病变[5]。它已被归入喉鳞状上皮乳头状瘤，但其与 HPV 无关，而是一种增生性角化性，偶尔伴有异型增生的喉部病变，具有乳头状结构，被认为是乳头状白斑性病变。它一般比病毒性乳头状瘤角化明显，通常为孤立性，没有挖空细胞形成。

与鳞状上皮乳头状瘤相比，疣状癌（verrucous

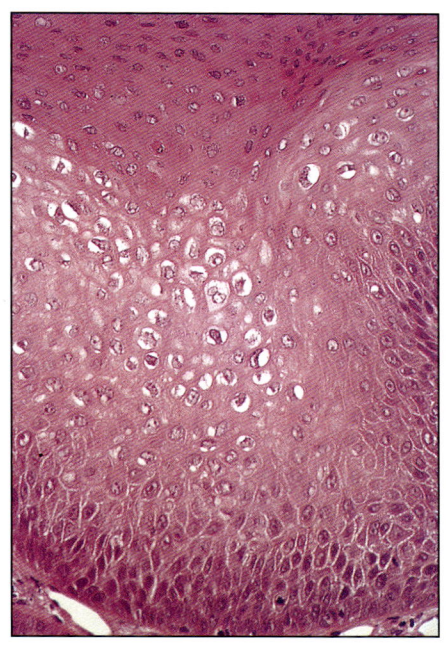

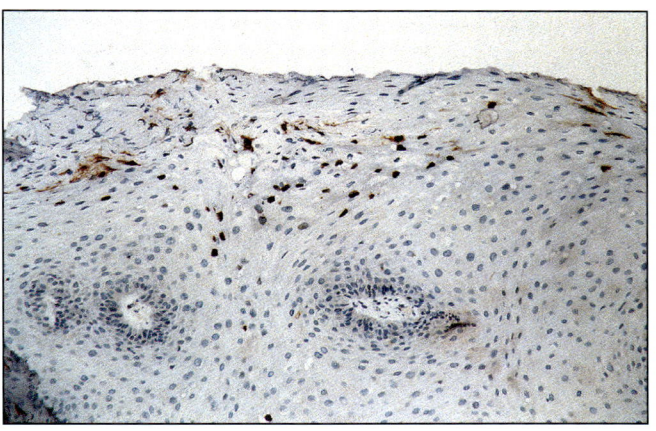

图4B.2 喉鳞状上皮乳头状瘤。（A）挖空细胞形成，表现为明显的核周透明，核外形不规则或"皱缩"，且在图的中央偏上可见一个双核细胞。（B）全HPV免疫组化染色显示多个细胞核呈阳性。

carcinoma）（见 161 页）是一种较大的广基病变，伴有增厚的鳞状上皮层，表面一般有明显的角化。这种病变倾向于以宽阔的推挤性方式浸润邻近的组织，其特征是在基底部有明显的慢性炎症浸润。喉部寻常疣（verruca vulgaris）罕有报道[28,29]。这种病变类似皮肤疣，伴有尖塔样乳头、丰富的角质形成和明显的颗粒细胞层，也与 HPV 感染有关。偶尔，"湿疣"一词被用于发生于上呼吸消化道的乳头状病变[14,23]。该术语用于伴有明显挖空细胞改变的部分鳞状上皮乳头状瘤可能是恰当的，反映它们与肛门生殖器部位的类似病变一样。乳头状鳞状细胞癌（papillary squamous cell carcinoma, PSCC）是一恶性病变，它缺乏鳞状上皮乳头状瘤良性的细胞核特征[26]。

在少数情况下，广泛的喉气管乳头状瘤虽然仍保持良性细胞学表现，而且与间质的交界分明，但却可能具有侵袭性并浸润周边组织。这种不常见的病变被称为"浸润性乳头状瘤病"（invasive papillomatosis）[10,24]。

涎腺型良性上皮性肿瘤
Benign epithelial neoplasms of salivary gland type

上呼吸道的浆液黏液腺可以视为与涎腺相同，因此预计涎腺型肿瘤可能出现于此（见第7章）。喉和气管的良性涎腺型肿瘤十分罕见。喉[30,31]和气管[32]的多形性腺瘤已有报道，其形态学和临床行为与涎腺多形性腺瘤相似。喉的嗜酸细胞性病变考虑为囊性腺体增生和（或）化生比较恰当，将在下面描述。喉气管涎腺型肿瘤多数是恶性肿瘤，将在恶性肿瘤中讨论。

颗粒细胞瘤　　Granular cell tumor

颗粒细胞瘤最常发生于皮肤和皮下组织，是一种其性质和组织发生尚有一些争议的相对少见的肿瘤（见第27章）[33,34]。口腔，特别是舌，也是常见的发生部位[33,35]，喉虽不常见，但也是公认的发生部位[36-38]。只有为数不多的几例报道发生于气管[39]。喉颗粒细胞瘤一般发生于30～40岁或40～50岁的患者，但5～82岁均见报道[38,40]。特征性的发生部位是声带[36,38]，尤其是声带后部[37]。主诉包括声嘶或咽喉痛，某些病变没有症状，为偶然发现[36]。这种病变通常较小，为境界不清的黏膜下圆形肿块[36]。几乎所有部位的颗粒细胞瘤都是良性的，喉部肿瘤少有复发[33,34,37,41,42]。曾报道一例"非典型性"喉部肿瘤伴有侵袭性临床行为（尽管没有转移）和组织学多形性[41]。

组织学上，颗粒细胞瘤的特征是由大的圆形、多角形，偶尔为纺锤形或梭形细胞构成的肿块，伴有丰富的嗜酸性颗粒状胞浆（图4B.3）。细胞界限可能不清，呈合体细胞样表现。肿瘤边界不清；颗粒细胞浸润邻近组织，并与之密切混合，包括神经和肌肉。细胞核通常小而规则，偶见大而深染的细胞核。核分裂象一般稀少或缺乏。

许多黏膜颗粒细胞瘤的一个独特而显著的组织学特征是肿瘤上方黏膜鳞状上皮出现假上皮瘤样增生（图4B.3）。这种改变有时可能非常明显，细胞学良性的表面上皮呈带状或舌状，向下延伸进入颗粒细胞病变。必须注意，不要将这种改变误诊为浸润性鳞状细胞癌。辨认原来的颗粒细胞瘤以及上皮细胞学的良性表现可以作为确定病变真正本质的线索。

虽然曾认为颗粒细胞瘤可能来源于组织细胞和原始

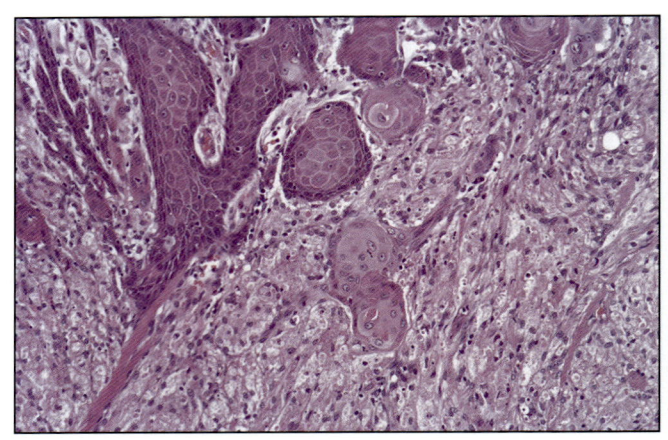

图4B.3　喉颗粒细胞瘤。呈片状分布的大细胞，胞浆丰富呈颗粒状，细胞境界不清，表面黏膜鳞状上皮呈假上皮瘤样增生。

间叶细胞，但现在的主要观点是多数颗粒细胞瘤是由神经衍化而来的，而且可能是schwann细胞来源[33,42,43]。

鉴别诊断

有关头颈部颗粒细胞瘤最重要的鉴别诊断问题可能是其伴随的表面假上皮瘤样增生与鳞状细胞癌的鉴别问题，这在上面已经做过讨论。曾有一例报道，舌部同时发生鳞状细胞癌和颗粒细胞瘤，这是非常罕见的病例，值得注意的是，在颗粒细胞瘤上方的假上皮瘤样黏膜增生细胞学是良性的，与癌不同[44]。成人型横纹肌瘤可能类似于颗粒细胞瘤，特别是在冰冻切片；然而，横纹肌瘤细胞含有丰富的糖原（淀粉酶敏感，非淀粉酶耐受），细胞境界清楚，常有特征性的"蜘蛛细胞"表现，胞浆丝从核的部位延伸至细胞膜，类似于蜘蛛网。嗜酸细胞瘤（oncocytoma）具有大的颗粒状嗜酸性细胞，但这些颗粒是由于大量的线粒体堆积而成，而非自噬溶酶体。如同横纹肌瘤细胞一样，嗜酸细胞瘤的细胞界限清楚，而非合体细胞表现，而且主要发生于上皮，通常是腺上皮，而非软组织。

副神经节瘤　　Paraganglioma

副神经节瘤（也见第28章）是发生于副神经节的不常见肿瘤，副神经节是小神经嵴衍化而来的分布于全身的神经外胚层结构，通常与自主神经、神经节和（或）血管结构密切相关[45,46]。颈动脉体瘤（carotid body tumors）是众所周知的最常见的副神经节瘤。喉部副神经节瘤十分罕见，但确有发生[46-49]，主要发生于位于假声带区域的喉上副神经节，或是较为少见的位于声门下环甲肌或环状软骨区的喉下副神经节，在少数病例还可位于甲状腺包膜（图4B.4）[46,47,50]。气管副神经节瘤就更为罕见了[51]。

大多数副神经节瘤（包括所有部位）为良性病变，但是仍有罕见的恶性副神经节瘤发生。仅靠形态学特征来准确地预测其临床行为十分困难，几乎不可能[46]。传统上报道，喉副神经节瘤中恶性肿瘤和疼痛的比例相对较高，是一种棘手的肿瘤。然而，新近的回顾性研究提示，报道的许多恶性喉副神经节瘤实际上可能是神经内分泌癌[46,48,49,52-54]，两者的组织学鉴别诊断偶尔可能遇到困难，应用免疫组化技术将有助于诊断（见下）[55]。这种解释使得多数喉副神经节瘤的生物学行为与其他部位的副神经节瘤一致（即主要为良性肿瘤）。

组织学上，喉和气管的副神经节瘤与其他部位的副神经节瘤相似（见第 28 章），肿瘤血管极其丰富，由主细胞巢构成，主细胞为圆形，偶为梭形，胞浆丰富，核位于中心。偶尔可见深染较小的成角支持细胞，通常位于主细胞巢周围。主细胞巢排列成特征性的细胞球（"balls of cell"，Zellballen）结构，有时呈肾小球样，与毛细血管密切相关（图 4B.5）。主细胞核从小到大不等，深染。核的多形性似乎与临床行为无关。喉部病变核分裂象一般稀少。

肿瘤细胞呈嗜银性，神经内分泌标记物免疫组化染色阳性，尤其是神经元特异性烯醇化酶和（或）嗜铬素[46,47]。支持细胞 S-100 蛋白阳性[47,49]。一个重要的

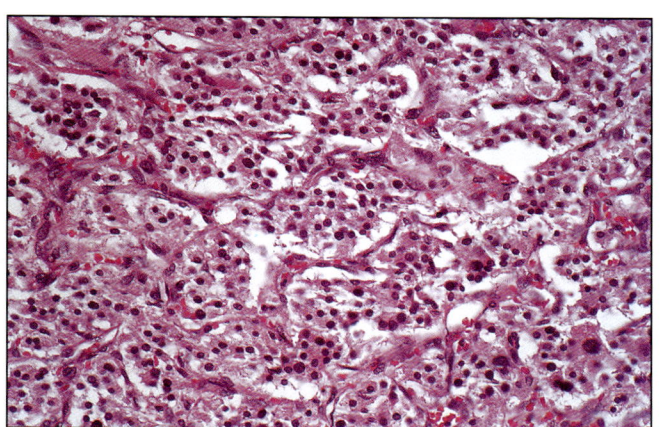

图 4B.5　喉副神经节瘤。主细胞特征性的"细胞球"（Zellballen）结构，与毛细血管密切相关。

鉴别诊断要点是副节瘤角蛋白一般阴性，而神经内分泌癌（类癌或"非典型性"类癌）角蛋白为阳性[47,54,55]。超微结构上，主细胞内可见特征性的伴有界膜的致密轴心神经分泌颗粒。

鉴别诊断包括癌，特别是类癌型的神经内分泌癌。典型的细胞球（Zellballen）结构将提示恰当的诊断。出现明显的嗜银性和嗜铬素阳性基本上可以排除非神经内分泌性肿瘤，缺乏角蛋白阳性细胞和出现 S-100 蛋白阳性的支持细胞倾向于排除神经内分泌癌。

声门下血管瘤　Subglottic hemangioma

喉的声门下血管瘤是一种发生于婴儿的血管增生性病变，尽管不常见，但有导致气道阻塞的潜在危险性[56,57]。尚未完全弄清这种病变是血管畸形还是真正的肿瘤[57]；无论怎样，为了方便起见，这里将其归为良性肿瘤。

声门下血管瘤常发生于 6 个月内的婴儿。临床上出现部分气道阻塞的症状预示着存在声门下血管瘤，例如喉气管炎样性质的喘鸣或哮吼[58]。约半数病例同时患有皮肤血管瘤[56-58]，呼吸道阻塞的程度可轻可重，在应急或感染时症状加重[57,59]，可能是病变内静脉压变化的结果[56,60]。头颈部幼年性（毛细血管）血管瘤，包括声门下血管瘤，经过几年之后常有自行消退的趋势[56-58]；不过，阻塞性病变常需立即进行治疗干预[57]。

内镜下表现具有特征性，病变表现为声门下质软的可压缩肿块，常带蓝色，偶为粉色，恰好位于声带下方，通常在偏后外侧的位置[56,57,59]。可出现明显的气道受损[56,59]。诊断常常无需活检；尽管某些学者担心手术操作后会引起广泛出血[59]，但另外一些学者则认为活检引起的重大并发症即便有也是非常少见的[57]。

组织学表现为婴儿型毛细血管瘤的形态（见第 3 章）[56,58]。许多血管，可能主要是中空和塌陷的血管，

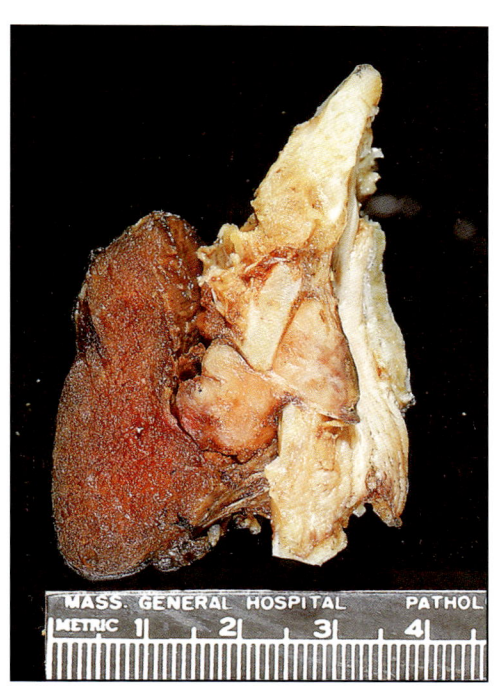

图 4B.4　喉下副神经节的副神经节瘤，在软骨和甲状腺毗邻组织之间突出，呈哑铃状。(Reproduced, with permission of the American Medical Association, from Googe R B, Ferry J A, Bhan A K et al. 1988 A comparison of paraganglioma, carcinoid tumor, and small cell carcinoma of the larynx. Arch Pathol Lab Med 112: 809-815.[47]) ©1998 American Medical Association. All rights reserved.

或为充满血液和扩张的血管，呈分叶状结构，在原有结构周围和其内浸润，例如浆液黏液腺体（图 4B.6）。病变具有浸润性，没有包膜[56]。血管内皮细胞肥胖，可见核分裂象。细胞成分可能丰富，以致血管腔部分阻塞[56]。组织形态学具有特征性，足以排除鉴别诊断的困难，例外的情况是，核分裂活跃的实性病变或许会提出有无血管肉瘤的可能性；然而，发生于婴儿的血管肉瘤实际上不存在这种可能。

其他良性间叶性肿瘤
Other benign mesenchymal neoplasms

良性神经鞘肿瘤可以发生于喉和气管，包括神经鞘瘤和神经纤维瘤，但很少见[60-64]。喉的神经纤维瘤可发生于Ⅰ型神经纤维瘤病和丛状神经纤维瘤患者[65]。曾报道一例发生于下咽部的富于细胞的神经鞘黏液瘤（cellular neurothekeoma）[66]。喉部神经鞘瘤的病理学表现与身体其他部位的相似。在少数情况下，良性肌肉肿瘤也可发生于喉部。普通平滑肌瘤[67]和血管平滑肌瘤[68]均有报道，同样，成人型[69]和胎儿型[70,71]横纹肌瘤也有报道。婴儿和儿童的喉部纤维瘤病罕见，儿童期纤维瘤病综合征就是一个例证[72,73]。喉和下咽脂肪瘤很少遇到[74]。报道的喉和气管罕见良性肿瘤病例包括纤维脂肪瘤[75]、所谓的血管外皮细胞瘤[76,77]、纤维组织细胞瘤[78-80]、纤维黏液瘤[81]、血管球瘤[82]、畸胎瘤[83]和良性透明细胞（"糖"）瘤[84]。

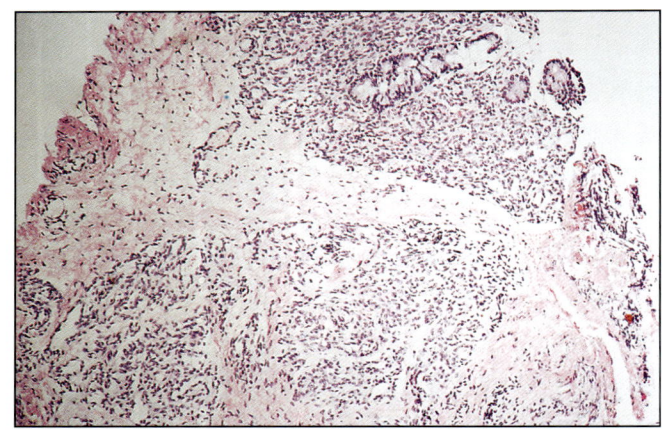

图 4B.6 发生于 9 个月婴儿的声门下血管瘤。许多管腔狭小的毛细血管结构，呈高度富于细胞表现，在原有组织内及其周围浸润，例如照片上方的腺体。（Reproduced from Shapshay S M and Aretz H T. Benign lesions of the larynx with permission of the American Academy of Otolaryngology-Head and Neck Surgery Foundation, copyright © 1984. All rights reserved）

非肿瘤性肿块性病变
Non-neoplastic tumorous lesions

声带息肉　Vocal cord polyps

声带息肉是局限性非肿瘤性隆起，被认为是由于滥用声带或"声带创伤"所致，也可能与空气中的刺激物有关[85,86]。尽管体积可能很小，但由于它们位于具有功能意义的真声带，所以可能引起声音嘶哑症状。息肉表现为局限性隆起，为单侧性或双侧性，可为灰白色半透明或带有蓝色，后一种类型类似于血管结构，过去临床上称为"声带静脉曲张"。组织学上，息肉疏松、水肿，上皮下结缔组织常有黏液样改变（图 4B.7A）。血管多样化，有明显内衬内皮细胞的血管间隙，伴有纤维蛋白沉积，纤维蛋白常很丰富，血管腔内外都存在（图 4B.7B）。息肉常常显示黏液样和血管结构混合存在。这种病变的组织发生被认为与声带创伤和（或）空气中刺激物的有害刺激所引起的血流和血管通透性增加有关。水肿液和纤维蛋白积聚在 Reinke 间隙（位于声带黏膜上皮与声带韧带之间的间隙）。纤维蛋白可以发生机化，类似于血栓机化。声带"小结"（vocal "nodule"）这一术语用于描述比典型息肉质硬或纤维化明显的隆起，但是有些学者仍然认为两者基本上是同一种病变[85]，这也是我们的观点。

接触性溃疡／"肉芽肿"
Contact ulcer / "granuloma"

接触性溃疡是发生于喉部的溃疡性病变，其特征是累及杓状软骨声带突上面的声带后部黏膜[87]。这种病变常常伴有增生的肉芽组织，导致被称为接触性"肉芽肿"的一个肿块性病变，但在病理学上它并不是一个真正的（组织细胞性）肉芽肿。病变可为单侧性或双侧性，缘于该部位菲薄黏膜的创伤性损害，或继发于插管所致的压迫性坏死[88]（插管术后"肉芽肿"）、胃内容物反流（"消化性肉芽肿"）[89,90]，或滥用声带，例如公共演讲者[91,92]。滥用声带或胃酸反流的病例主要发生于男性[93]。症状包括咽喉痛、声嘶、咽部异物感和吞咽困难[90-93]。检查发现为息肉样圆形、无蒂的肿块，常有溃疡形成，直径从数毫米到 3 cm 大小不等[93]。

组织学上，可见肉芽组织，毛细血管朝着黏膜表面方向呈放射状排列（图 4B.8）；表面黏膜或形成溃疡或被覆增生的再生性鳞状上皮。这种病变应与化脓性肉芽肿相鉴别，正常情况下化脓性肉芽肿并不发生于这个部位。化脓性肉芽肿是一种分叶状毛细血管瘤[94]，其毛细血管常围绕在中央较大血管周围，呈分叶状排列，而不

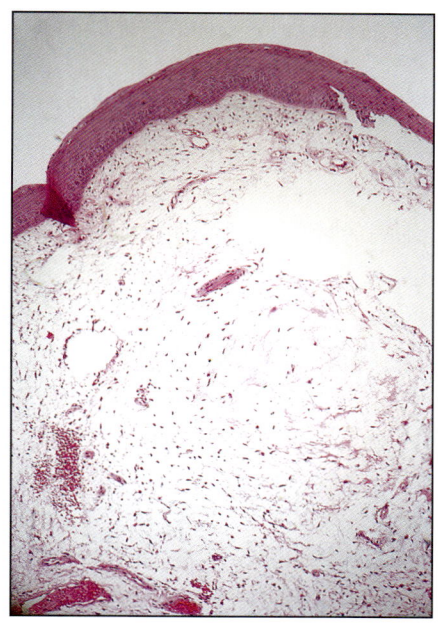

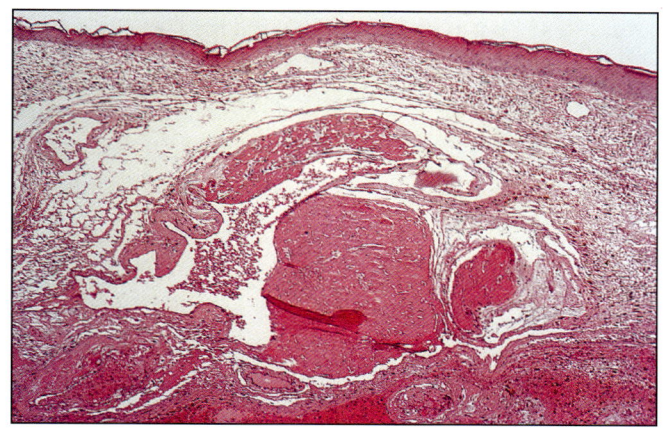

图4B.7　声带息肉。（A）黏液性息肉，伴有水肿黏液样间质。（B）血管性息肉，含有明显的血管腔和大量纤维蛋白性物质。

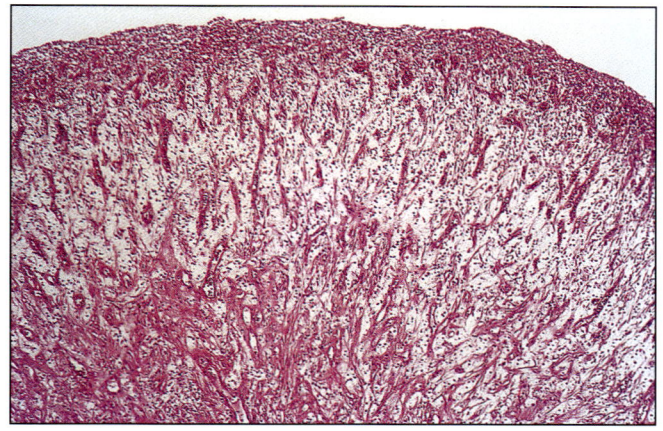

图4B.8　仪器操作后发生于前联合的接触性"肉芽肿"。溃疡性息肉样肉芽组织，毛细血管呈放射状向表面生长。

是接触性"肉芽肿"的放射状排列。在长时间插管损伤的病例，杓状软骨可能发生局灶性软骨炎和软骨坏死，常常伴有细菌感染。

特发性喉气管狭窄 Idiopathic laryngotracheal stenosis

虽然插管引起的损伤、以前的手术以及其他特异性感染和非感染性病变（例如淀粉样物沉积、Wegener 肉芽肿）均可引起明显的喉气管狭窄，但仍有一小部分病例表现为喉气管狭窄，通常累及喉的环状区域和气管最上部，却无已知的特殊病因。这种特发性喉气管狭窄疾病[95,96]主要发生于女性，年龄分布广泛。临床症状是进行性加重的呼吸困难；检查发现声门下气道狭窄，一般累及环状区域和气管最上部，是由于黏膜下常呈环状增厚所致。偶尔发生局灶性黏膜溃疡。

组织学上，这种病变的特征是瘢痕性致密纤维化，总的看来细胞稀少[95]。偶尔出现淋巴细胞和组织细胞，但通常并不丰富。这种病变倾向于非进行性，手术切除效果较好[95]。在某些声门下狭窄病例中，胃食管反流可能是一个致因因素[97]。

囊肿　Cysts

喉囊肿（laryngocele）是喉小囊（喉室前部一个狭窄的类似阑尾的外突）扩张形成的，它经由喉室与喉腔相通，其内充满空气[98-100]。可表现为声门下喉或杓会厌皱襞黏膜下的膨出物（内喉囊肿，internal laryngocele），或穿透甲状舌骨膜，通过含有喉上神经和血管的孔而表现为颈部囊性肿块（外喉囊肿，external laryngocele）。复合性喉囊肿（combined laryngocele）由两个部位的囊性肿块组成。喉囊肿在临床上可表现为声音嘶哑或颈部囊性肿块，由于囊性肿块与喉腔相通，故其大小可有波动。也可能没有症状。其发生可为先天性（例如先天性增大扩张的喉小囊）或后天性，由于喉小囊反复扩张而促成了喉囊肿的发生。这是由于声门上肌放松以对抗紧闭双唇造成的喉内压力升高引起，例如铜管乐器演奏者或吹玻璃的工人[98,101]。组织学上，喉囊肿是由固有的喉室小囊纤毛柱状黏膜囊性外突组成的。

喉小囊囊肿（saccular cysts）如同喉囊肿一样也是喉小囊扩张，但它们充满黏液，而且不与喉腔相通[99,102]，主要是由于狭窄的喉小囊开口阻塞引起，可为先天性或后天性。导致喉小囊囊肿/喉囊肿阻塞的可能原因包括炎症、创伤或肿瘤。事实上已经注意到了喉癌与喉囊肿的关系，而且喉小囊扩张可能由于喉室部位临床上不易觉察的癌引起。

小的喉导管囊肿（laryngeal ductal cysts）的发生可

由诸多喉的浆液黏液腺的任一导管阻塞而引起[102]。偶尔，导管或喉小囊来源的囊肿内衬嗜酸性细胞，常常形成乳头状皱襞，并且伴有细胞增生，类似于腮腺的Warthin瘤[103,104]（图4B.9）。这些病变有很多不同的名称，包括嗜酸细胞性囊腺瘤、乳头状囊腺瘤和嗜酸细胞性囊肿[105]。我们和其他一些学者认为，这种病变是由于嗜酸细胞化生/增生引起的，而非真正的肿瘤[103,104]。可以见到一系列的变化，从浆液黏液腺内孤立的嗜酸细胞化生灶（图4B.10）到全部或部分内衬嗜酸细胞的导管扩张，以至充分发展的乳头状囊性病变（图4B.9）均可见。它们主要发生于中老年人群，除非达到相当大小而引起症状，多数对于患者并无损害。对于这种化生性/增生性囊性病变，我们喜欢应用嗜酸细胞性囊肿（oncocytic cyst）这一术语。

慢性感染　Chronic infections

虽然喉结核病曾经作为晚期肺结核病相对常见的一个终末并发症，但在西方国家，仅有轻微或临床上不明显的胸部疾病的患者，喉结核病即可表现为类似于肿瘤的一个肿块性病变[106-108]。现在结核病比起20世纪早期少见得多；但近些年来结核病的发病率以惊人的速度上升，这部分是由于获得性免疫缺陷综合征（AIDS），部分是由于出现了耐药的分枝杆菌菌株，导致遇到喉结核病的机会增加[109]。本病的特征性表现是声音嘶哑和喉部的溃疡性或肿块性病变。组织学上，可见伴有巨细胞的典型坏死性肉芽肿性炎的形态学改变。在未经治疗患者的病变中通常可以发现少数抗酸杆菌。

在西方国家，比喉结核病更加少见的是喉部真菌感染，真菌感染在临床上也可能类似于肿瘤。喉部真菌感染包括组织胞浆菌病[110]、酵母菌病[111]、球孢子菌病[112]、类球孢子菌病[113]、孢子丝菌病[114]、曲菌病[115]和放线菌病（从学术上讲是一种细菌感染）[116]。喉念球菌病可能来自肺或播散性疾病，与慢性黏膜皮肤念球菌病有关[117]，或与抗生素治疗或免疫抑制状态或免疫抑制治疗有关[118]。有趣的是，某些喉真菌感染，包括念珠菌病，可伴有类似于癌的黏膜鳞状上皮增生[118]。

淀粉样物沉积　Amyloid deposition

全身性淀粉样变性累及喉和气管很少能达到具有临床意义的程度；然而，喉是公认的局限性淀粉样物沉积的部位[119-123]，而且根据报道是上呼吸消化道局限性淀粉样变性的最常见部位[122]。局限性病变也可能累及气管[124,125]。患者表现为声音嘶哑，少数伴有喘鸣、呼吸困难或咯血[124]。临床上，喉气管的淀粉样物可表现为散在的瘤样肿块或弥漫性黏膜下增厚[120,122,125]。两种类型的生长均倾向于非常缓慢。声门上喉/假声带区似乎最常受累[121,122]，但是声带和声门下区也可以是淀粉样物沉积的部位。在喉可以有多个部位受累[122]。孤立性的瘤样包块很少出现严重问题，而且预后也好。弥漫性黏膜下病变则比较麻烦，而且难以根除，非常罕见的弥漫性广泛气管支气管淀粉样变性可以致死，伴有阻塞和反复感染[124,125]。

组织学上，组织中的淀粉样物为无定形、同质性、嗜酸性细胞外沉积物（图4B.11A）。组织处理造成的人工假象常常形成一些小裂隙，将淀粉样物团块分开，呈"裂隙样"表现[119]。慢性炎症浸润常见，包括大量的浆细胞成分[122,123]。偶尔可见异物巨细胞，这是对于淀粉样物的反应。容易发生淀粉样物沉积的部位包括血管外膜、浆液黏液腺周围（图4B.11B），"挤入"腺体使其萎缩，偶尔围绕脂肪细胞呈"环状"结构[119,124]。淀粉样物有别于其他物质，应用刚果红染色在偏振光显微镜下观察时呈现独特的"苹果绿"双折射特性。研究发现，喉的局限性淀粉样物具有免疫球蛋白轻链衍化的特性[121-126]。

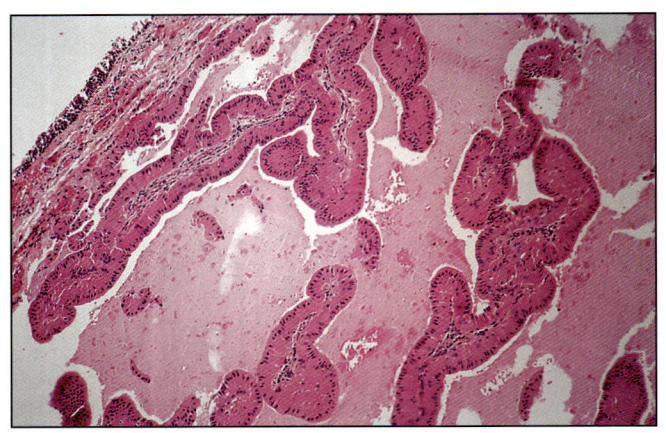

图4B.9　喉嗜酸细胞性囊肿。显示伴有局灶性内陷乳头状结构的大的多囊性病变，内衬嗜酸性细胞上皮。左上方为表面黏膜。

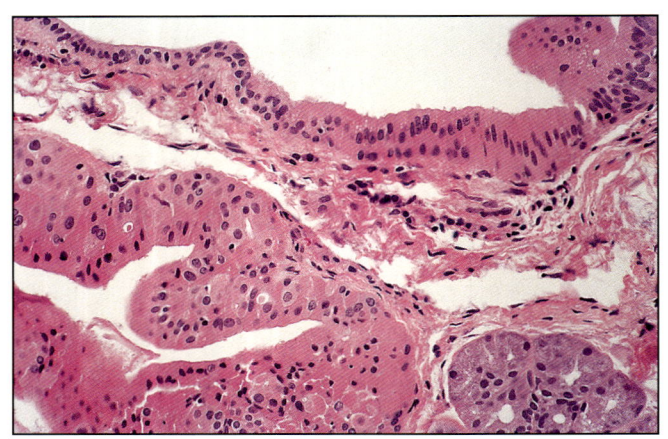

图4B.10　喉嗜酸细胞性囊肿，显示腺体导管嗜酸细胞化生。

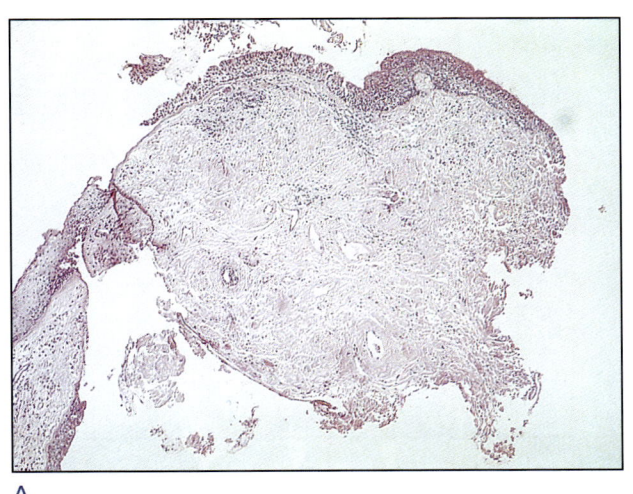
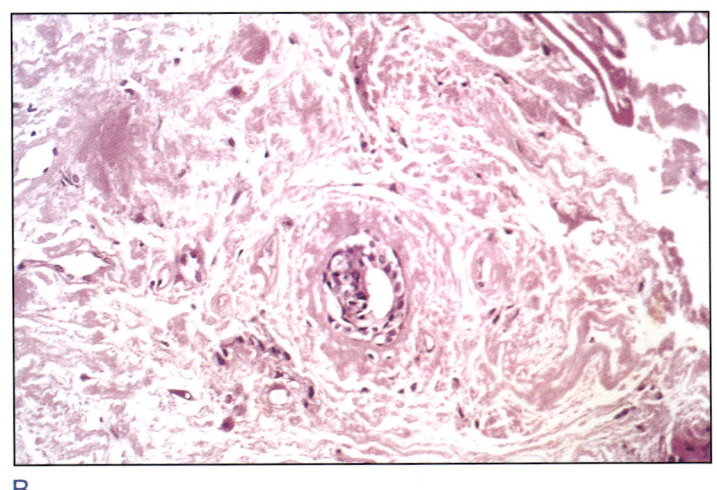

图4B.11 喉的淀粉样物沉积。（A）表面黏膜上皮深部可见无定形、同质性细胞外嗜酸性淀粉样物沉积。（B）淀粉样物沉积在一个孤立性小导管结构的周围。(Fig. 4B. 11B reproduced from Shapshay S M and Aretz H T. Benign lesions of the larynx with permission of the American Academy of Otolaryngology-Head and Neck Surgery Foundation, copyright © 1984. All rights reserved.)

需要考虑的两个鉴别诊断是血管性声带息肉和浆细胞瘤。声带息肉内的嗜酸性物质是纤维蛋白而非淀粉样物，因此应用刚果红染色不能产生特征性的双折射现象。此外，息肉常常出现黏液成分。浆细胞瘤可能伴有淀粉样物形成，但浆细胞瘤是肿瘤性病变，由相对单一的浆细胞群构成，免疫球蛋白轻链呈现单一类型的染色。Lewis 等[122]研究的伴有明显数量浆细胞的12例喉淀粉样物沉积病例中，浆细胞显示多克隆性免疫球蛋白轻链染色。然而，Berg 等[126]对于病例更进一步的研究发现，伴随淀粉样物的浆细胞免疫球蛋白 κ 轻链染色阳性，而 λ 轻链阴性，淀粉样物也是如此，提示虽然比典型的浆细胞瘤更加良性，而且好像不会进展为多发性骨髓瘤，但至少某些局限性淀粉样变性可能是浆细胞病的变型[126]。报道的另2例伴有单一类型淋巴浆细胞增生的肺局限性淀粉样变性倾向于支持这种看法[127]。另外，Thompson 等在检测的10例与喉淀粉样物沉积有关的浆细胞时发现，其中3例具有免疫球蛋白轻链限制性[123]。

骨质沉着性气管病
Tracheopathia osteoplastica

骨质沉着性气管病[128]（或骨软骨沉着性气管支气管病[129]）是一种以气管和支气管黏膜下出现多发性骨软骨结节为特征的病变。病情轻微的病例患者可能没有症状，病变是在尸检时诊断的[128]。然而，较为广泛受累的病例可能出现咳嗽、咯血、劳累性呼吸困难或喘息[129]。这种病变在常规前后位胸部 X 线照片中不易发现，但在侧位 X 线片、X 线断层照片和计算机断层扫描中则可显示出特征性的串珠状或贝壳样钙化[128,129]。内镜检查表现为黏膜下硬而韧的结节状肿块，有时类似于肿瘤，而且造成受累的气管段僵硬。病变好发于远端气管和近端支气管，但是气管上部[130]和喉亦可受累；少数情况下，喉可能是唯一受累的部位[131]。

组织学上，可见由透明软骨和板层骨构成的结节，有时含有造血的骨髓，位于黏膜下，向内（腔）达到内生性气管环（图4B.12）。在病变结节与气管环的内软骨膜之间常常可见胶原、软骨和（或）骨连接。这种病变不累及气管和支气管后部膜的部分。有关确切的病因和发病机制虽然尚无统一的说法，但是后一种所见倾向于支持是气管环的退化性外生软骨瘤（ecchondrosis）和外生骨疣（exostosis）的理论[128]。

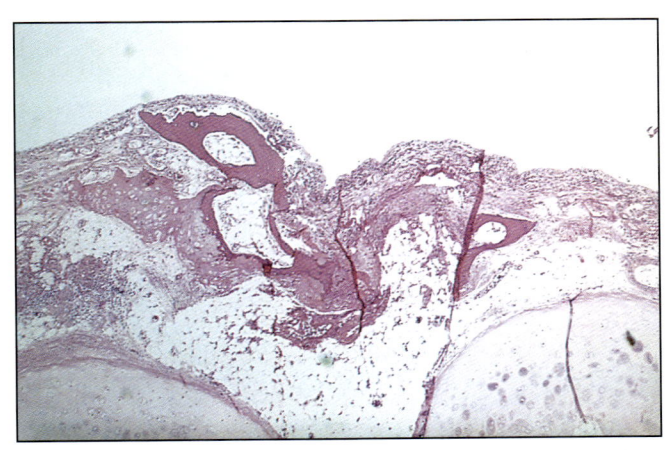

图4B.12 骨质沉着性气管病。骨质沉着恰好位于黏膜上皮深部，向内（腔）通往气管环。(Courtesy of Dr. E. Mark.)

其他罕见病变

在喉和（或）气管可能遇到的其他少见肿块性或肿瘤性病变包括 Wegener 肉芽肿病[132-134]、Rosai-Dorfman 病（窦组织细胞增多症伴巨大淋巴结病）[135-137]、结节病[133,138]、痛风[139]、声带 Teflon 肉芽肿[133,140,141]、错构瘤[142-145]、炎性假瘤[146]、软斑病[147]、疣状角化不良瘤[148]、血吸虫病[149]、动脉瘤样骨囊肿[150] 和 Kimura 病[151]。

恶性肿瘤 Malignant neoplasms

鳞状细胞癌 Squamous cell carcinoma

恶性前/浸润前病变（非典型性/原位癌、癌前病变）Premalignant/preinvasive lesions (atypicality/carcinoma in situ, precursor lesions)

上呼吸消化道黏膜的反应性改变包括增生、角化以及不同程度的结构和细胞学的非典型性。现在普遍认为，只有那些表现出明显非典型性或异型增生的黏膜病变才应被视为恶性前病变，具有发展为癌的较高倾向性[152-158]。

一般说来，喉和气管黏膜异型增生的程度随着细胞和（或）结构异常程度的增加以及这种变化向黏膜上皮表面的进展而增加（图 4B.13）。这与用于口腔和宫颈病变的研究方法类似。鳞状细胞原位癌（原位癌）传统上定义为非典型性占据黏膜上皮的全层[152]（图 4B.14）。

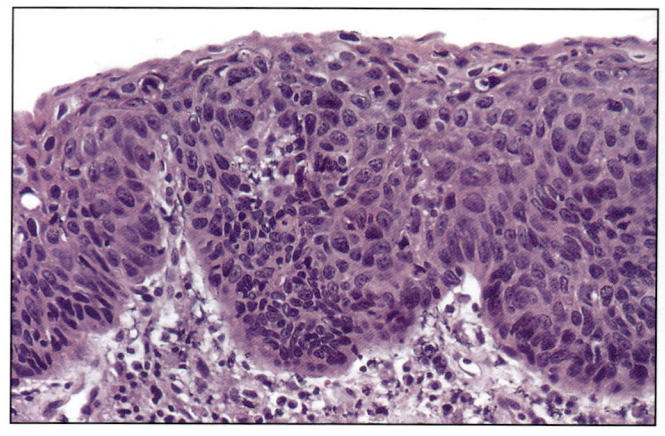

图4B.14 下咽部鳞状细胞原位癌。全层细胞均有非典型性；伴有增大细胞核和明显核仁的细胞的排列有些紊乱，而且占据整个黏膜上皮层。（Reproduced with permission from Fried M P 1996 The larynx: a multidisciplinary approach, 2nd edn. Mosby, New York, Fig. 40-60.）

已经提出了几种癌前病变的分类方案。现在应用最为普遍的三种方案是 WHO 分类系统、"鳞状上皮内肿瘤形成"（squamous intraepithelial neoplasia, SIN）以及在欧洲普遍采用的 Ljubljana 分类（表 4B.1）[153]。本章采用 WHO 分类系统。

表4B.1	前体和相关病变组织学分类图解	
2005WHO分类	鳞状上皮内肿瘤形成（SIN）	鳞状上皮内病变（SIL）Ljubljana 分类
鳞状细胞增生		鳞状细胞（单纯性）增生
轻度异型增生	SIN 1	基底/副基底细胞增生[a]
中度异型增生	SIN 2	非典型性增生[b]
重度异型增生	SIN 3[c]	非典型性增生[b]
原位癌	SIN 3[c]	原位癌

[a]基底/副基底细胞增生在组织学上可能类似于轻度异型增生，但前者在概念上为良性病变，后者则为低级别的前体病变。

[b]危险上皮。大约类似于中度和重度异型增生。

[c]提倡将重度异型增生和原位癌归在一起统称SIN 3。

Reproduced from Barnes L, Eveson J W, Reichart P et al[153].

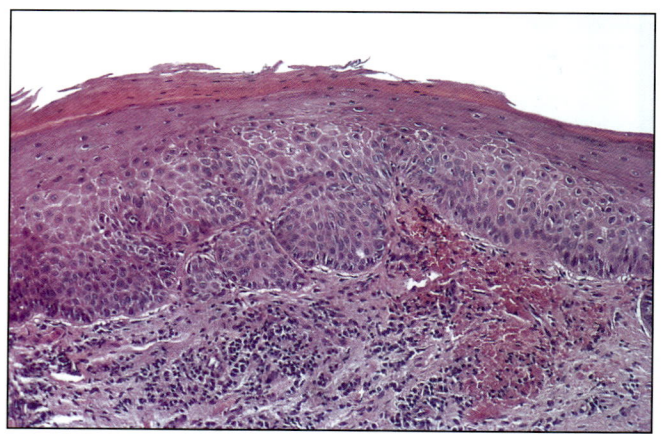

图4B.13 喉黏膜鳞状上皮中度非典型性。黏膜上皮增生，成熟障碍，伴有不成熟表现的细胞，某些细胞伴有增大而深染的细胞核，大约延伸至黏膜表面的1/2。

实际上，见于宫颈的原位癌的分类类型（即黏膜不成熟的基底细胞样细胞均一地增生，表面黏膜不成熟）并不常见于喉[157,158]。喉部最常见的是异型增生，其特征为细胞异常角化或角化不良，且出现具有嗜酸性胞浆的大的多形性细胞，而且经常出现表面角化[159]。这种改变被称为重度角化性异型增生（severe keratinizing dysplasia），并据报道与随后浸润癌的发生率增加相关[158]。此外，虽然许多人仍然应用异型增生和原位癌，但两者之间的差别轻微，常常难以区分，并带有主观性。一些学者（提倡SIN分类系统的）建议将这两者结合在一起并归为高级别上皮内肿瘤形成的范畴。这又与宫颈研究中的情况相类似[157-159]。

临床上，重度异型增生／原位癌可表现为红色黏膜斑（黏膜红斑病，erythroplakia）、增厚的白斑（黏膜白斑病，leukoplakia），或两者兼有（斑点状黏膜白斑病，speckled leukoplakia）。换句话说，它也可无明显临床表现。因此，其诊断和与较轻程度非典型性的鉴别诊断有赖于活体组织检查和组织学分析。

喉原位癌的临床意义及其自然病史难以准确判定，并且其进展为浸润性癌的几率各家报道也不一致，从3.5%～90%不等[160]。诊断标准和选择的病例不同或许是结果不一致的原因。另外，值得注意的是，原位癌常常不是一种孤立的病变，它可出现于明显的浸润癌附近。因此，恰当的临床和组织学样本采集显得十分重要。通常认为，重度异型增生／原位癌如果不经治疗，大多数病例将会发展为浸润癌，虽然不是每一个病例。因此，认为必须进行治疗；多数作者提倡对于局限性病变进行声带剥离或局部完全切除的保守治疗。同时也采用放射治疗[161]。

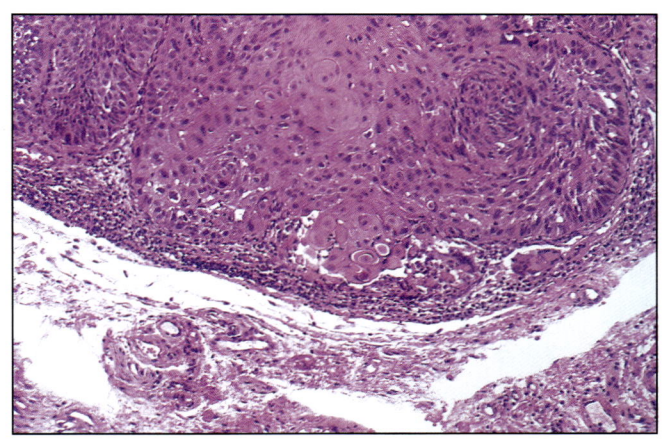

图4B.15 喉浅表浸润（微小浸润）性鳞状细胞癌。图中部的上皮灶边界不规则，似乎突入其下的结缔组织，而邻近的上皮基底圆形、均匀，与其下的组织分界清楚。微小浸润灶附近有数个多核巨细胞，符合对于穿过基底膜的角蛋白的异物反应。

正如宫颈中的情况一样[157-159,162,163]，浅表浸润或微小浸润鳞状细胞癌的概念在喉部也得到公认（图4B.15）。在以上皮内病变为主的病变中，辨认微小浸润灶（即穿透黏膜基底膜进入黏膜下间质）可能非常困难，尤其是在小的活检标本中。上皮内病变的基底膜可能会因炎症反应而变得模糊不清；另外，表现为圆形推挤边缘的癌巢可能具有基底膜成分，通过免疫组化染色（层粘连蛋白和Ⅳ型胶原）可以辨认[158,164]。诸如纤维组织增生性间质反应、间质内对于角蛋白的异物反应以及间质中出现孤立的微小肿瘤细胞簇（或单个肿瘤细胞）等特征，均是诊断浅表浸润有用的证据[165]。有人认为微小浸润的临床意义类似于原位癌／重度异型增生[157,166]，通过恰当的治疗预后甚佳[166]。

浸润性鳞状细胞癌
Invasive squamous cell carcinoma

鳞状细胞癌是迄今为止喉部最常见的恶性肿瘤。浸润性喉癌虽然不是一种最常见的恶性肿瘤，但并不罕见。据估计，2004年美国新增病例10 270例[167]。在美国，喉是头颈部发生原发性肿瘤的唯一的最常见的非表皮性器官[168]。喉癌男性明显多于女性，最常发生于40～70岁的病人[169]。估计2004年美国新增喉癌病例中8060例为男性，2210例为女性[167]。男女发病率的差异近来轻微下降，可能是由于女性吸烟率增加。吸烟和饮酒被认为是本病非常重要的病因学因素[165,170,171]。最近的一些证据提示，HPV感染、ras癌基因活化和胃食管反流也可能对喉癌发生有作用[165,166,170,172-174]。气管癌更为罕见，但鳞状细胞癌也是气管最常见的恶性肿瘤。其平均发病年龄为50岁左右[175]。声带或声门上喉癌的典型症状是声嘶、音调降低或声音改变。也可出现疼痛、咽下困难或咯血[161,176]。声门下喉癌容易引起喘鸣或气道梗阻，即便癌瘤不是很大，这是由于气流径直通过由环状软骨构成的声门下间隙所致，而环状软骨是呼吸道唯一的环形软骨[161]。不幸的是，梨状窦癌由于症状出现常较晚，故在发现时常常较大而且较晚。下咽部癌可能出现的症状有咽下困难、耳痛、继发于淋巴结病变的颈部包块或全身性营养不良[177]。当足以危及气道时，气管癌易产生喘鸣或喘息的症状。

喉分为声门上区、声门区和声门下区。声门上区由会厌、假声带、喉室、杓状会厌襞和杓状区组成；声门区包括真声带以及前连合和后连合。声门下区位于真声带与环状软骨下缘之间。声门与声门下区的分界线有不同的描述，大约位于真声带下方5 mm[178]以及喉室外侧缘下方1 cm[179]。较好的分界或许是弹性圆锥（因为它是以解剖结构来划界的），弹性圆锥是连接环状软骨上

鳞状细胞癌

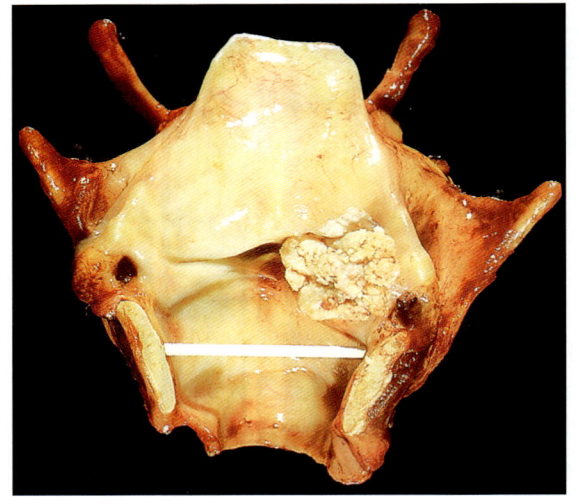

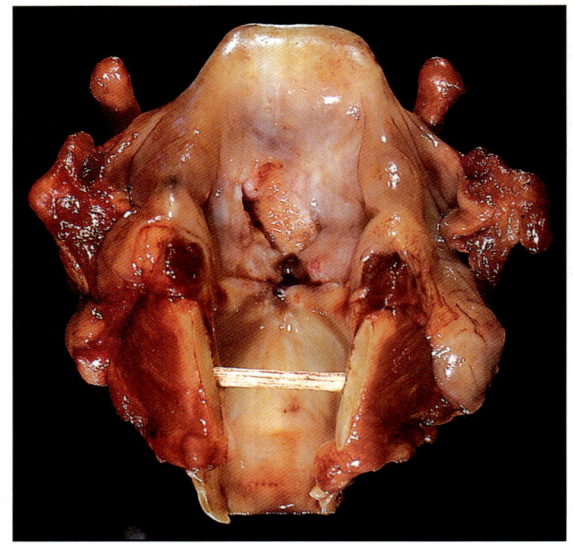

图4B.16 喉鳞状细胞癌。（A）外生性蕈样生长的肿瘤，侵犯右侧真声带。（B）隆起的斑块样声门上肿瘤，伴有灶性溃疡形成并越过中线。（C）溃疡浸润性声门上肿瘤。

面与声带韧带的膜性结构[165]。声门区位于弹性圆锥的外上侧，而声门下区位于其内下侧。声门癌是最常见的喉癌，其次是声门上癌。原发性声门下癌罕见[180]。声门上肿瘤比声门病变容易延伸越过中线。喉室似乎是癌在声门与声门上区之间扩散的屏障，从而使得声门上水平喉切除术成功用于治疗某些声门上癌。然而最新的报道指出，癌在这些腔隙之间存在扩散通道，值得注意的是从声门向喉室后杓状区的扩散、靠近甲状软骨的声门旁间隙侧向喉室的扩散以及向前连合区域的扩散，伴有前连合腱和（或）甲状软骨的浸润，并向下扩散[181-183]。因此，出现同时侵及声门及声门上区的跨声门的巨大肿瘤也就不足为奇了。这些肿瘤往往是侵袭性肿瘤，且预后不好。声门癌向声门下蔓延比向声门上蔓延更为常见；这是由于弹性圆锥对于肿瘤扩散的屏障作用并不完善。

下咽部，或喉咽部，有三个组成部分：（1）位于杓状会厌襞与甲状软骨板之间的梨状窦；（2）位于环状软骨后面的环状软骨后区；（3）位于咽后壁从会厌水平（与口咽交界处）至环状软骨下缘水平（与食管交界处）的下咽后区。大多数下咽部癌发生于梨状窦，咽后壁是第二个最常见的发生部位，而原发性环状软骨后癌是最少见的下咽部癌[184]。与喉癌的情况相似，下咽部癌也是男性罹患多于女性，而且根据报告90%的患者有吸烟史[184]。

喉鳞状细胞癌大体可表现为表面粗糙的外生性肿块，有或无表面溃疡形成，或表现为向深部生长的溃疡浸润性肿块，而表面没有明显肿块（图4B.16）。

喉、下咽部和气管鳞状细胞癌的组织学表现与其他部位（例如口腔、肺、食管、皮肤）鳞状细胞癌相类似[165]（图4B.17）。肿瘤可为角化性或非角化性，但多数肿瘤都产生细胞内或细胞外角蛋白，而且其分化程度

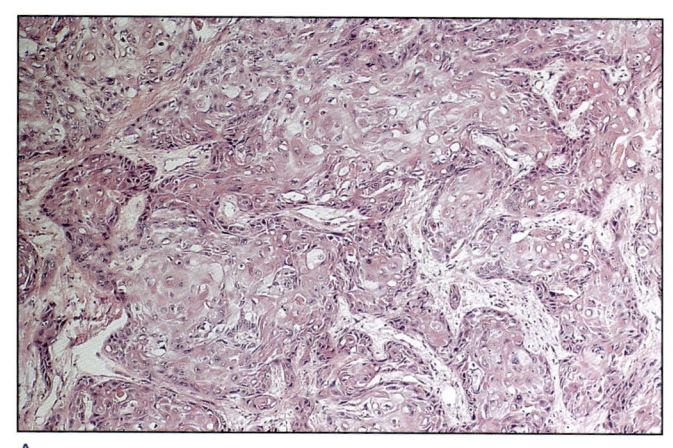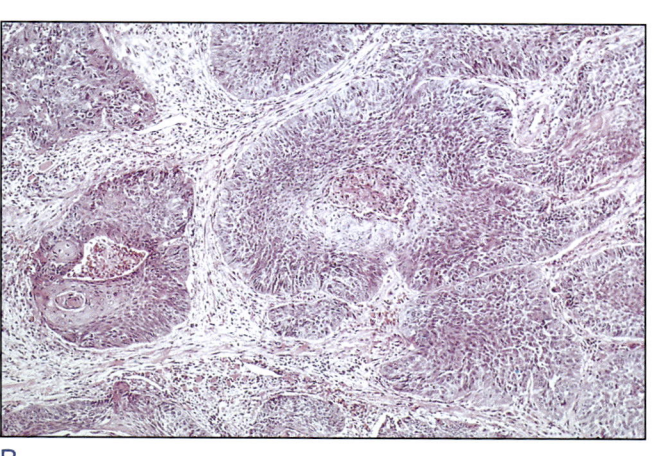

图4B.17 喉鳞状细胞癌。（A）高分化癌。（B）中分化癌。

从高分化到低分化不等。许多肿瘤在浸润灶附近可见原位癌。试图将预后意义与诸如分化程度之类的形态学特征联系起来的尝试都取得了不同程度的成功[185-191]。近来，有关进展期肿瘤的形态学结构、DNA分析、p53等癌基因和细胞周期素D1蛋白表达等资料显示，它们有望能够预测喉癌的临床行为[192-195]。基于诸如肿瘤分级、分期和大小、DNA和癌基因等因素以及患者一般情况等多因素的评价，似乎可以最准确地判断预后。

喉／下咽部鳞状细胞癌患者常常接受放射治疗；这会引起肿瘤和被照射组织发生形态学上可鉴别的改变。肿瘤纤维性消失和肿瘤角蛋白产物增加，以及对于角蛋白或其他肿瘤碎屑的异物巨细胞和（或）组织细胞反应，均可见于照射后；同时在宿主间质组织中还可见到淋巴管扩张和非典型性的间叶细胞核。照射区域内的非肿瘤性浆液黏液性腺体常常发生萎缩，同时伴有腺上皮细胞核增大。粗心的观察者可将这种现象误认为是残留的癌小岛。正确评价正常腺体的组织结构可能有助于辨认是萎缩的腺体，而不是肿瘤。

早期发现的小的喉鳞状细胞癌患者的预后良好。总的来说，在美国，60%以上的喉癌患者5年以后尚且生存[197]，T1期声带癌（小的局灶性癌）5年无病生存率高达90%[169]。正如所预期的一样，生存率随着病变进入进展期和发生淋巴结转移而下降，尤其当肿瘤向结外扩散时。美国癌症联合委员会推荐的分期系统列于表4B.2。声门下和下咽部肿瘤通常预后较差，可能与确诊时往往已处于晚期有关。单独或联合采用外科手术和放射治疗，应用或不应用辅助化学治疗已被作为喉癌和下咽部癌患者的治疗模式[180,184]。

鳞状细胞癌的各种亚型
Variants of squamous cell carcinoma

疣状癌　Verrucous carcinoma

疣状癌是一种鳞状上皮增生性病变，通常被认为是鳞状细胞癌的一种亚型。其临床和大体特征是基底部宽广的外生性疣状赘生物，组织学分化非常良好，生物学行为的特征是缓慢进行性、膨胀性和局灶破坏性生长，实际上不发生转移。最初被描述为一种口腔病变，发生于口腔的疣状癌最为常见[198]。据报道，喉是第二个最常见的好发部位。疣状癌也可发生于其他部位，例如肛门生殖器区域和肢体。这是一种仍有争论的疾病，以我们的观点，至今仍不完全清楚。这种病变在喉部罕见，其发病率大约占所有喉部恶性肿瘤的1%～3%[199-204]。它倾向于发生于50岁以上的个体，而且较常见于男性[203,204]。声带是喉部疣状癌最常见的部位[201,205]。临床上可见基底部宽广的表面肿物，肿物伴有角化，灰白色，呈外生性疣状生长（故此得名"疣状"）。如果不予治疗，它会广泛蔓延且向深部延伸，呈膨胀性、推挤性生长，边界清楚，侵犯并最终穿透其下结构，例如肌肉、软骨和骨。

组织学上，这种病变由棘层增厚的增生鳞状上皮组成，一般表现为被覆角化物的粗大乳头状皱襞，并呈球茎状突入其下组织，伴有推挤性、界限清楚的宽边缘（图4B.18和图4B.19）。鳞状上皮分化很好，仅有轻度非典型性（核分裂象、增大的核及核仁）[206]，且局限于基底层。仅靠病变底部有致密的慢性炎症细胞浸润为其特征（图4B.19）。角化物可深陷于相邻上皮皱襞之间，在组织中形成角质囊肿。在典型的"纯粹的"疣状癌，并不出现由单个细胞或小条索状或小簇状细胞造成的参差不齐的间质组织浸润。

鳞状细胞癌

表4B.2　喉癌的TNM分期

原发性肿瘤（T）

- TX　原发性肿瘤不能评估
- T0　无原发性肿瘤证据
- Tis　原位癌

声门上型

- T1　肿瘤局限于声门上的一个部位，声带活动正常
- T2　肿瘤侵犯声门上一个以上邻近部位的黏膜，或侵犯声门或侵犯声门上以外的区域（例如舌根、会厌谷和梨状窦内壁的黏膜），喉没有固定
- T3　肿瘤局限于喉，伴有声带固定和（或）侵犯任何下列部位：环状软骨后区、会厌前组织、声门旁间隙和（或）甲状软骨轻度侵蚀（例如内层）
- T4a　肿瘤侵透甲状软骨和（或）侵及喉外组织（例如气管和颈部软组织，包括深部舌外肌、颈部带状肌、甲状腺和食管）
- T4b　肿瘤侵及椎前间隙，包裹颈总动脉，或侵及纵隔结构

声门型

- T1　肿瘤局限于声带（可以侵及前连合或后连合），声带活动正常
- T1a　肿瘤局限于一侧声带
- T1b　肿瘤侵犯双侧声带
- T2　肿瘤延伸到声门上和（或）声门下，和（或）声带活动受损
- T3　肿瘤局限于喉，伴有声带固定，和（或）侵犯声门旁间隙，和（或）甲状软骨轻度侵蚀（例如内层）
- T4a　肿瘤侵透甲状软骨板和（或）侵及喉外组织（例如气管和颈部软组织，包括深部舌外肌、颈部带状肌、甲状腺和食管）
- T4b　肿瘤侵及椎前间隙，包裹颈动脉，或侵及纵隔结构

声门下型

- T1　肿瘤局限于声门下
- T2　肿瘤延伸到声带，声带活动正常或受损
- T3　肿瘤局限于喉，伴有声带固定
- T4a　肿瘤侵犯环状软骨或甲状软骨和（或）侵及喉外组织（例如气管和颈部软组织，包括深部舌外肌、颈部带状肌、甲状腺和食管）
- T4b　肿瘤侵及椎前间隙，包裹颈动脉，或侵及纵隔结构

区域淋巴结（N）

- NX　区域淋巴结不能评估
- N0　无区域淋巴结转移
- N1　同侧单个淋巴结转移，最大径≤3 cm
- N2　同侧单个淋巴结转移，最大径>3 cm，但≤6 cm，或同侧多个淋巴结转移，最大径≤6 cm，或双侧或对侧淋巴结转移，最大径≤6 cm
- N2a　同侧单个淋巴结转移，最大径>3 cm，但≤6 cm
- N2b　同侧多个淋巴结转移，最大径≤6 cm
- N2c　双侧或对侧淋巴结转移，最大径≤6 cm
- N3　转移淋巴结最大径>6 cm

远隔转移（M）

- MX　远隔转移不能评估
- M0　无远隔转移
- M1　有远隔转移

Reproduced with permission of the American Joint Committee on Cancer (AJCC), Chicago, Illinois. The original source for this material is the AJCC Cancer Staging Manual, Sixth Edition (2002). Published by Springer-Verlag, New York (www.springeronline.com).

这些组织学特征使得在小活检标本中作出疣状癌的诊断相当困难。在出现高分化而无间变的组织，以及缺乏明显的组织浸润时，人们不愿做出癌的诊断，这是可以理解的。外科医师和病理医师之间的通力合作与密切联系，可以引起对于这种广基外生性病变本质的关注，

最佳的活检标本可以显示病变范围深达邻近正常黏膜上皮的水平[202]。

疣状癌并不总是一种"单纯性"的病变，这一点越来越加清楚，已经发现在某些典型的疣状癌病例中出现普通的浸润性鳞状细胞癌病灶[205,207-210]。这种"杂合性"

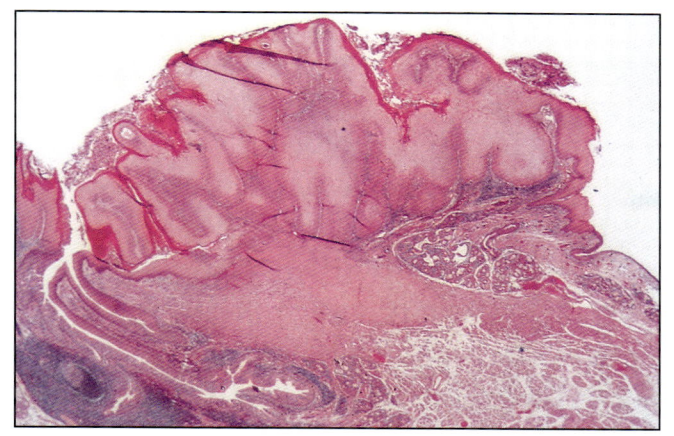

图4B.18 喉疣状癌。图示真声带肿瘤，广基，高分化，乳头状，棘层增厚。

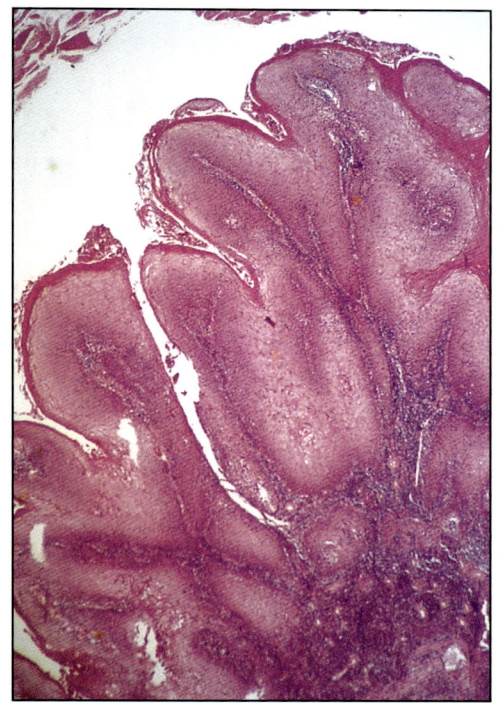

图4B.19 喉疣状癌。显示球茎状，伴有推挤性的边缘，相关致密慢性炎细胞浸润。

或混合性疣状鳞状细胞癌已见于口腔和喉。据称喉的混合性疣状鳞状细胞癌比"单纯性"疣状癌侵袭性强，其行为较类似于对应分期的普通鳞状细胞癌（因此值得治疗）[205]。显然，在疣状癌的标本中应该寻找并评估这样的病灶。

围绕这个具有兴趣病变的争论点之一是，有人认为照射有诱导疣状癌间变转化为侵袭性恶性肿瘤的趋势。虽然一些观察者报道了这种现象[199,210,211]，但仅肤浅的接受这一主张必须格外小心，因为如前所述，病变中较普通的鳞状细胞癌区域在活检时可能被遗漏掉。不过，在少数情况下这种特殊病例或许能反映这样的相关性。

疣状癌的治疗通常选择外科手术切除；并有报道"单纯性"疣状癌预后良好[205,211]。

鉴别诊断：疣状癌一般能通过增生程度并结合向其下组织延伸而与良性上皮增生性病变相鉴别。在口腔描述的一种疣状增生（verrucous hyperplasia）病变[212]类似于疣状癌，但它并不向下蔓延至邻近黏膜上皮层水平。Batsakis等[201]认为它是疣状癌的早期形式。与鳞状上皮乳头状瘤的鉴别前面已有描述（见151页）。喉的寻常疣（verruca vulgaris）十分罕见，但已有报道[28,29]。与典型疣状癌相比，这些病变被描述为具有比较突出的颗粒层和较为狭窄的乳头状结构，并且出现挖空细胞改变。应用免疫组化或分子生物学技术在喉部寻常疣病变中可以发现HPV感染的证据；然而，某些研究表明HPV也与某些疣状癌病例的发生有关，但疣状癌与HPV之间的关系并不明确[202,213]。通过较大程度的细胞学非典型性和浸润的性质，可与普通的鳞状细胞癌鉴别，但必须注意上面提到的"杂合性"或混合性病变。重要的是必须记住，某些喉鳞状细胞癌可呈乳头状或外生性[214,215]，而且这些病变在活检时可能并不显示明显的上皮下间质浸润。然而，这些肿瘤比疣状癌具有更加明显的细胞学非典型性，在活检中见到乳头状原位癌的表现时，不应做出疣状癌的诊断。

综上所述，我们应当意识到，疣状癌具备某些但并非所有普通恶性肿瘤的特性（表现为进行性的局部生长并扩展至其下组织，但缺乏显著的核的非典型性，而且可能缺乏转移潜能）。有些学者[216]主张"癌"是一种不太恰当的称谓，而应改称为"疣状棘皮病"（verrucous acanthosis）。在良性增生性黏膜上皮病变系列中，将疣状癌看作中间性病变或许是比较恰当的，即处于良性增生与明显普通转移性癌之间的位置[201]。

梭形细胞癌（肉瘤样癌）
Spindle cell carcinoma (sarcomatoid carcinoma)

梭形细胞癌是喉和下咽部的一种令人迷惑的肿瘤，引起了诸多争议和猜测。这主要是因为这种病变具有特征性的双相性的形态学本质，即同时兼有鳞状细胞癌病灶和（或）原位癌/重度异型增生，而且常常伴有类似于肉瘤的奇异梭形细胞/间叶性增生。这种形态学导致了应用几种术语并出现了几种相应的组织发生理论，包括梭形细胞癌[217-221]、癌肉瘤[222]、鳞状细胞癌伴有肉瘤样间质[223]、假肉瘤[224,225]、多形性癌、息肉样癌[226]以及肉瘤样癌[227-229]。正如目前所定义的那样，这种肿瘤通常被认为是鳞状细胞癌的一种变异型[221,230,231]。除了上呼吸道外，这种肿瘤也发生于食管[222,232]和口腔[233,234]，类

梭形细胞癌（肉瘤样癌）

似肿瘤还可发生于肺[235]。

多数喉肿瘤患者为老年男性[228,289]。多数病变位于声门[217,221]，表现为声音嘶哑，但下咽部、声门上及声门下也可发生肿瘤。有相当比例的患者曾接受过肿瘤放射治疗[228]。大多数肿瘤均表现为一种息肉样外生性结构，伴有宽广的基部或有相对狭窄的蒂[228,229]（图4B.20）。后一种类型的肿瘤可能发生整个或部分瘤体自动离断而被患者咳出[228]。无蒂肿瘤和溃疡浸润性肿瘤较少发生。

这种病变的预后及组织发生争议较大。目前，多数观点认为这种肿瘤具有潜在的致命性[228,229]。浅表息肉样肿瘤和位于真声带的肿瘤似乎比声门外和深部浸润性病变的预后好[223,227-229]。组织学表现和普通鳞状细胞癌所占的比例与临床结果之间似无明显相关性[223,227]，但有报道梭形细胞的角蛋白免疫组化染色阳性与生存率呈负相关[236]。

息肉样肿瘤常常出现广泛的溃疡，并伴有表面纤维蛋白沉积。特征性组织形态学改变是普通鳞状细胞癌混合有非典型性的梭形或间叶表现的细胞群（图4B.21）。鳞状细胞成分通常相当稀少，往往需要全面取材来证明。这种成分可为浸润性（常常只是浅表浸润）或原位癌，而且根据某些作者的报道[220]，在某些病例仅能见到重度异型增生的鳞状上皮。发现和确定鳞状成分的困难可能与常遇到表面广泛的溃疡形成有关。息肉样肿瘤的基底部已被建议作为寻找和定位普通癌组织的部位[217,229]。肉瘤样部分的特征是相当突出和广泛，其表现可能多样化。通常情况下，可出现一种类似于纤维肉瘤的非典型性梭形细胞成分（图4B.21A）。胶原一般稀少，但偶尔可能比较显著。肉瘤样成分可疏松或呈黏液样；可能出现富于血管的肉芽组织样成分，特别是在靠近表面的部分，伴有许多炎症细胞和（或）组织细胞。核分裂象常常丰富，并可出现非典型性核分裂象。常见奇异而深染的多核细胞。在我看来，诊断梭形细胞癌需要出现明确的上皮性成分。因而，如果依靠普通光学显微镜做出诊断，就必须识别出鳞状细胞癌或原位癌，或至少要能证明有重度鳞状上皮异型增生。在缺乏组织学上可识别的普通鳞状细胞癌成分的情况下，为了明确诊断就需要通过免疫组化标记和（或）超微结构检查来寻找上皮分化的证据。

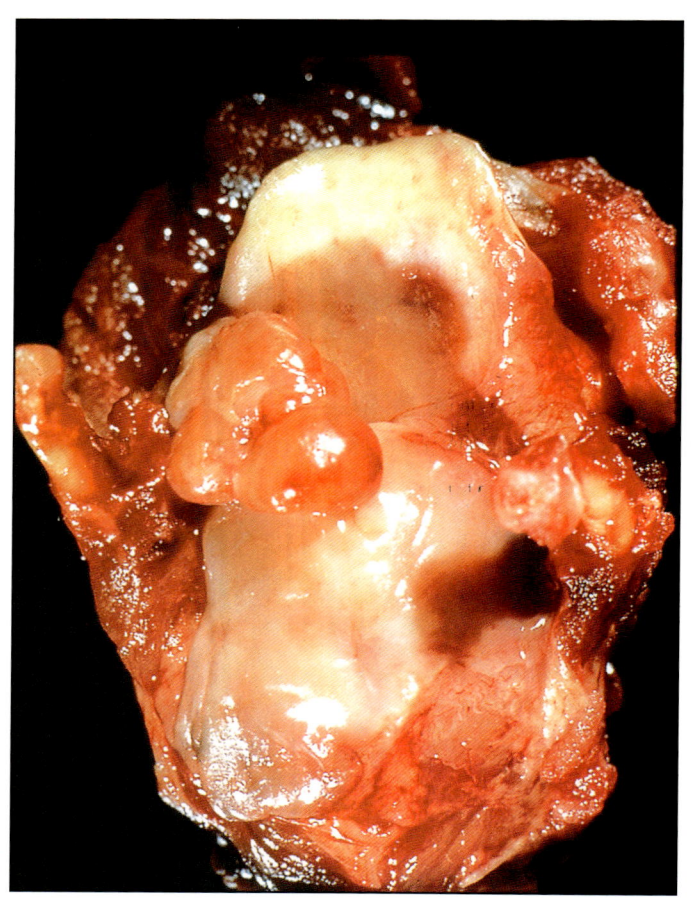

A

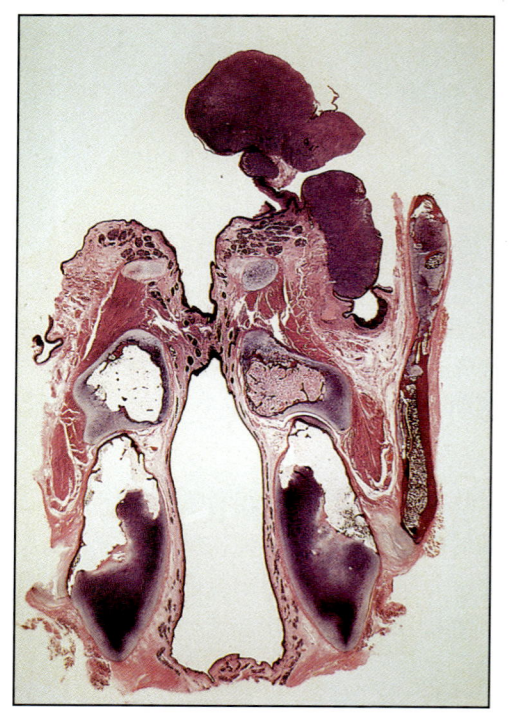

B

图4B.20 喉梭形细胞癌。（A）杓状区息肉状肿瘤的大体照片。（B）同一肿瘤的整个器官的切面，显示肿瘤大部分通过蒂与喉相连，部分肿瘤有宽广的基部。肿瘤无深部浸润。(Reproduced with permission from Fried M P 1996 The larynx: a multidisciplinary approach, 2nd edn. Mosby, New York, Fig. 40-30.)

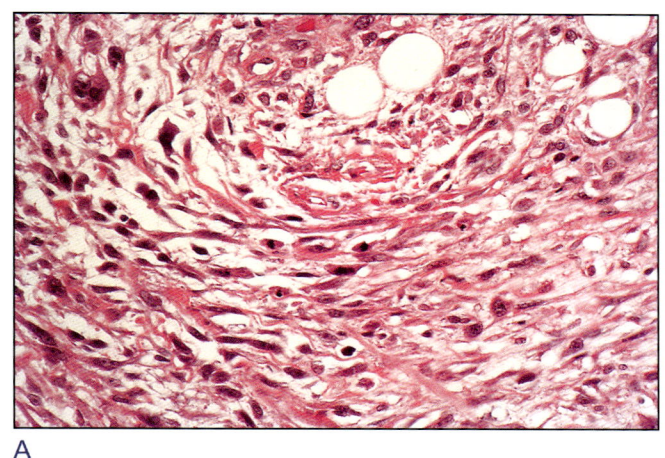 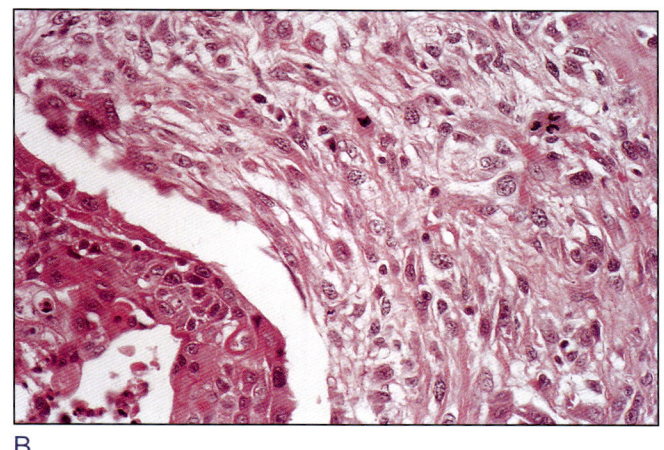

图4B.21 喉梭形细胞癌。（A）由多形性梭形细胞组成的梭形细胞成分，类似于肉瘤。（B）同一肿瘤，显示普通鳞状细胞癌（左下）与梭形细胞成分并存。

利用免疫组化方法，在肿瘤的梭形细胞成分中常常可以发现角蛋白阳性（图4B.22）；然而，并不是所有病例都能通过常规免疫组化技术来显示角蛋白阳性的梭形细胞[219,220]，并且角蛋白染色可仅呈局灶性。普通的癌的成分角蛋白染色几乎总是阳性。梭形细胞成分通常还表达波形蛋白，利用碱性磷酸酶双标记技术发现某些单个梭形肿瘤细胞角蛋白和波形蛋白染色均呈阳性[219]。此外，超微结构研究显示出完全不同的结果，有些梭形细胞显示间叶细胞的特征（丰富而扩张的粗面内质网），某些显示上皮细胞的特征（桥粒和张力丝），而另外一些兼有两种特征[218]。通过引用目前广为接受的肿瘤组织发生理论或许能够解释这些令人困惑的结果，即它是一种上皮性肿瘤，属于鳞状细胞癌的亚型，其中多数肿瘤性上皮细胞均经历了间叶性化生，在有些病例这种化生相当完全，以致丢失了绝大部分（若不是全部的话）的上皮性特征[218,227-229]。这种现象也可见于其他部位的肿瘤，并被称为"同源性假化生"（homologous neometaplasia）（Scully，个人交流）。这一情况类似于乳腺所谓的化生性癌或产生基质的乳腺癌。非典型性梭形细胞的概念是反应性非肿瘤性的间质成分，最初由Lane[224]提出，后又被Goellner等[225]重申；但转移性肿瘤中同时含有梭形成分和癌性成分，又与这种观点相矛盾[217]；免疫组化染色发现梭形细胞ras癌基因p21阳性[226]，进一步证明了这些细胞的肿瘤性本质。被描述为喉真性癌肉瘤的罕见病例偶见报道[237]，但也提出了一些疑问，这样的病例究竟是各自独立的两种祖细胞（一种上皮性，一种间叶性）同时发生恶性转化，还是这里描述过的化生性癌或"假化生"病例。普遍接受的是后一种观点。

鉴别诊断

需要考虑的三种主要鉴别诊断是肉瘤、奇异的照射后肉芽组织和所谓的炎性肌纤维母细胞瘤。通过梭形细胞癌中存在可识别的癌性成分常常可与肉瘤鉴别。滑膜肉瘤是个例外（见下）。在缺乏癌性成分的情况下，采用HE切片进行光学显微镜检查就会遇到诸多困难问题。对于这种病例，通过免疫组化和（或）超微结构检查证明上皮性分化有所帮助；然而，极少有肉瘤表达角蛋白。例如双相性滑膜肉瘤（罕见于头颈部，但偶见报道），除了有梭形细胞外，还可出现角蛋白阳性的癌性区域。后者通常表现为腺样，而非鳞状上皮形态；此外，梭形细胞成分的表现往往均匀一致，致密，富于细胞，而细胞多形性却不如典型的梭形细胞癌明显[229]。在所谓的恶性纤维组织细胞瘤中，很少有角蛋白阳性细胞描述[238]。这样的病例在HE切片光学显微镜检查中无癌性成分区域，超微结构检查也不出现上皮分化的特征，但考虑到可能存在的取样问题，其中有些病例很可能是

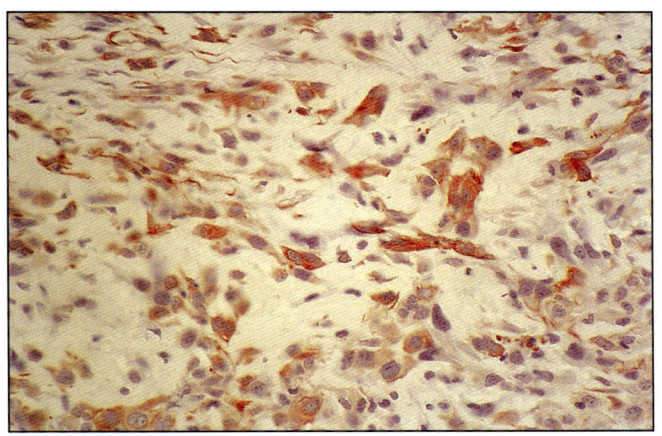

图4B.22 喉梭形细胞癌。免疫组化染色显示梭形细胞呈角蛋白阳性反应。

梭形细胞（肉瘤样）癌。在照射后可以发生奇异的高度非典型性增生的肉芽组织反应，并且可能十分类似于梭形细胞癌的肉瘤样成分[239]。这些病变缺乏癌性成分，而且已经提到这些病变的内皮细胞具有其他间叶细胞存在的非典型性[239]。少数喉炎性肌纤维母细胞瘤已有报道[240]。这些病变是梭形细胞和少数星形细胞的良性增生，细胞排列通常松散，常常伴有慢性炎性细胞浸润。肿瘤细胞温和到有轻度非典型性，并缺乏重度多形性和高核分裂率等特征，也不伴有普通鳞状细胞癌成分或角蛋白阳性的梭形细胞[240]。

基底细胞样鳞状细胞癌（基底细胞样鳞癌）
Basaloid squamous cell carcinoma（basaloid squamous carcinoma）

基底细胞样鳞状细胞癌是鳞状细胞癌的一种亚型，最近将其描述为一种独特的临床病理疾病[241-247]。据报道本病见于中年至老年患者的下咽部、喉和口腔，偶见于鼻腔[244,248]和鼻咽部，最近报道其也可发生于气管[249]。认识本病的重要性在于它是一种预后差的高级别的侵袭性肿瘤。在早期文献中，类似肿瘤在食管和宫颈已有报告，列在与腺样囊性癌有关的标题下[250-252]。最近，食管基底细胞样鳞状细胞癌作为一种独立的疾病已经得到公认[253]。

组织学上，基底细胞样鳞状细胞癌是一种高级别癌，由基底细胞样细胞和鳞状成分组成（图4B.23）。基底细胞样癌的成分排列呈巢状、团块状和条带状，由小的嗜碱性上皮细胞组成，伴有相对稀少的胞浆，核浆比例增高。细胞核常常深染，核仁一般不明显。细胞常常排列成分叶性巢状，恰恰深达黏膜上皮。外周细胞层呈栅栏状排列并不少见。基底细胞样细胞的特征是围成腺样或假腺样腔隙，有时呈筛状且含有阿辛蓝阳性的黏液样物质；然而，肿瘤细胞本身黏液染色却是阴性（图4B.23和4B.24）。肿瘤间质常可表现为玻璃样变和呈黏液样表现（图4B.24）。肿瘤细胞巢的中心常见粉刺样坏死。除了有基底细胞样肿瘤细胞以外，同时存在鳞状细胞癌的成分。这可能表现为肿瘤细胞巢内的鳞状分化、明显的鳞状细胞癌灶和（或）其上原位癌的区域（图4B.23和4B.25）。

鉴别诊断包括腺样囊性癌和腺鳞癌或黏液表皮样癌。基底细胞样鳞状细胞癌与腺样囊性癌具有一些共同特征，尤其是间变性变型，两者的基底细胞样细胞均呈筛状或假腺样排列。然而，腺样囊性癌的特征是缺乏鳞状成分。此外，多数腺样囊性癌的小管或腺管的外层肌上皮细胞成分，而基底细胞样鳞状细胞癌没有肌上皮成分。与基底细胞样鳞状细胞癌相比，腺样囊性癌的肿

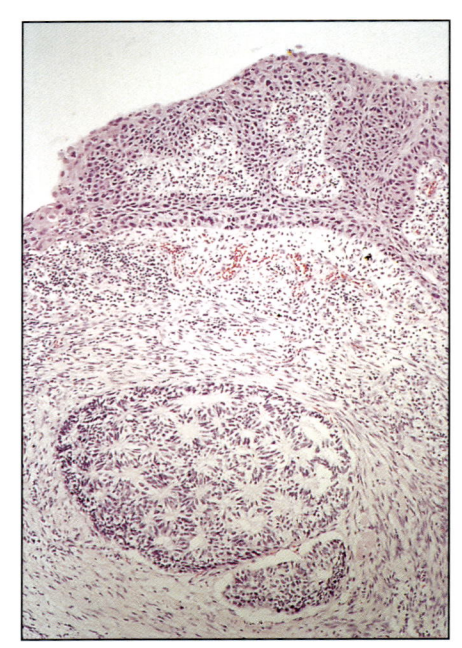

图4B.23 喉/下咽部基底细胞样鳞状细胞癌。图示基底细胞样癌巢伴有腺样间隙，类似于腺样囊性癌，位于黏膜鳞状细胞原位癌的下方。

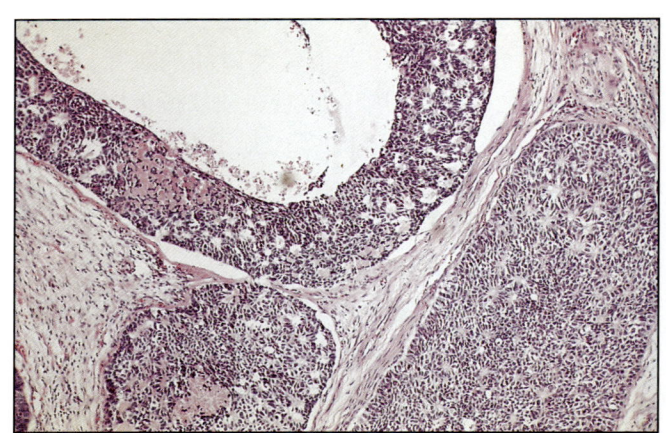

图4B.24 喉/咽下部基底细胞样鳞状细胞癌。基底细胞样癌巢伴有假腺腔，并见灶性无定形玻璃样物质。

瘤细胞通常较小，而且间变不明显。由Gerughty等[254]描述的腺鳞癌是一种与导管有关的肿瘤，可能含有导管腺体原位癌的区域和"玻璃样"大细胞；其特征是不伴有黏膜鳞状细胞原位癌。多数黏液表皮样癌的间变不如基底细胞样鳞状细胞癌明显，其中有些细胞含有胞浆内黏液。它们也可能是没有原发性表面黏膜成分的腺体病变。

淋巴上皮癌
Lymphoepithelial carcinoma

淋巴上皮瘤型未分化癌是鳞状细胞癌的一种亚型，

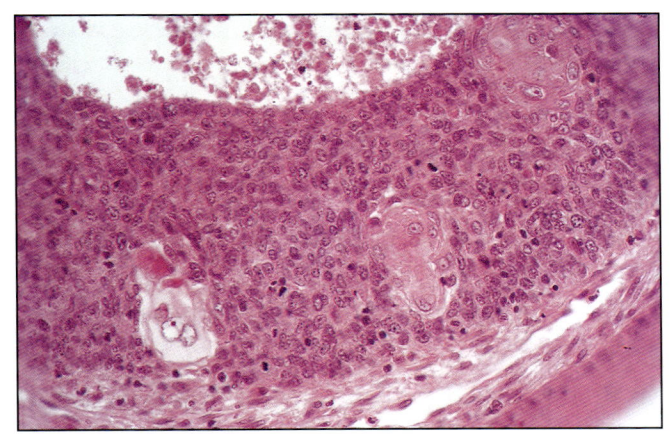

图4B.25 喉的基底细胞样鳞状细胞癌，显示基底细胞样细胞巢伴有灶状鳞状细胞珠。

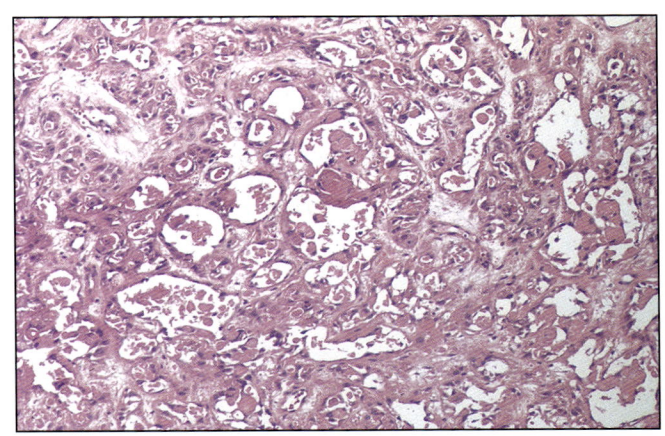

图4B.26 喉假血管腺样鳞状细胞癌。癌细胞巢棘层松解，形成类似于腺体或血管的腔隙。可见局灶性鳞状分化（图的中心）以及腔隙中变性的棘层松解的癌细胞。

典型的发生于鼻咽部（见第4A章）。它很少发生于腮腺[255]和胸腺[256]等其他部位。也有报道见于喉/下咽部的罕见病例[257-261]。这些位于喉/咽部肿瘤的形态学表现类似于鼻咽部的淋巴上皮癌。与鼻咽部病变一样，这类肿瘤与EB病毒有关的证据已在某些病例而不是所有病例中发现[260-262]。

腺样鳞状细胞癌（棘层松解性鳞状细胞癌、假血管性鳞状细胞癌） Adenoid squamous carcinoma (acantholytic squamous cell carcinoma, pseudovascular squamous cell carcinoma)

所谓的腺样或棘层松解性鳞状细胞癌好发于阳光暴露部位的皮肤[263]。它是鳞状细胞癌的一种变异型，其中肿瘤细胞巢中的鳞癌细胞棘层松解，形成腺样外观，棘层松解的细胞常常漂浮于这些腔隙中；然而，这些肿瘤黏液染色阴性。有时位于这些腔隙周围的癌细胞可能变扁，呈现血管外观，类似于血管肉瘤（假血管腺样鳞状细胞癌）[263]。虽然这些肿瘤特征性的报道发生于皮肤[263]，但我们在喉部也遇到了这样的肿瘤（图4B.26）。通过辨认这种病变棘层松解形成间隙的本质以及肿瘤细胞缺乏黏液，可与腺癌鉴别开来。通过发现普通鳞状细胞癌成分，以及缺乏诸如CD31、von Willebrand因子或CD34等血管标记物的免疫组化染色，并结合肿瘤细胞角蛋白阳性，可与血管肉瘤进行鉴别诊断[263]。

乳头状鳞状细胞癌 Papillary squamous cell carcinoma (PSCC)

在鳞状细胞癌中有一种类型的癌具有明显的乳头状结构，最近已经公认它是鳞状细胞癌的一种独特的临床病理学亚型[264,265]。这种肿瘤通常以恶性鳞状上皮包绕纤维血管轴心形成狭窄的乳头状或指状突起为特征（图4B.27）。肿瘤表面部分外观基本上是乳头状原位癌，也就是说，虽然细胞非典型性显著而且一般占据全层，但紧邻中央纤维血管轴心的上皮层基底部却常常是平坦的。在浅表的活检组织中常常见不到一般的浸润，但在深层组织可见。近来的一项研究显示，36%的头颈部乳头状鳞状细胞癌与HPV有关[265]。喉乳头状鳞状细胞癌在生物学上的侵袭性不如普通鳞状细胞癌，包括外生型鳞状细胞癌[264]，大约1/3的病例有复发，很少发生转移，生存率高，在Thompson等[264]报道的系列病例中，没有死于肿瘤者。因此，有必要认识鳞状细胞癌的这种亚型。

鉴别诊断包括喉部的其他乳头状鳞状上皮病变，包括鳞状上皮乳头状瘤、疣状癌、十分罕见的喉寻常疣以及外生型普通鳞状细胞癌。通过其温和的细胞学特征可与前三种病变鉴别，而乳头状鳞状细胞癌有显著的细胞学非典型性，类似于原位癌。与乳头状鳞状细胞癌相比，外生型鳞状细胞癌具有较宽的乳头状结构，而且指样突起不甚明显。

腺鳞癌 Adenosquamous carcinoma (ASC)

头颈部腺鳞癌最初被认为是黏液表皮样癌的一种类型（见下）。然而，近来公认ASC是一种独特的疾病，累及并可能起源于表面的鳞状黏膜上皮，伴有侵袭性生物学过程[266,267]。因此，这里考虑将其作为鳞状细胞癌的一种亚型。在头颈部，喉和口底是其最好发的部位[266]。男性受累明显多于女性。这种肿瘤是一种侵袭性肿瘤，常伴有局部复发和淋巴结转移，5年生存率仅约15%[266]。

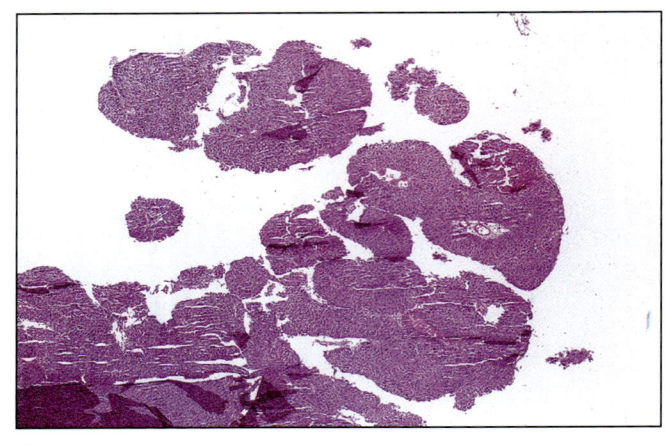

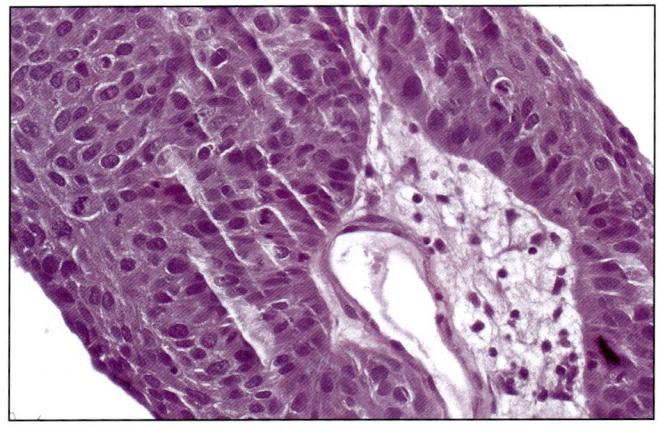

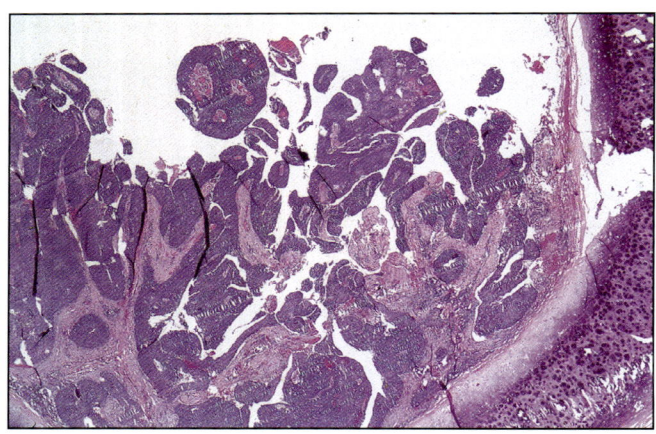

图4B.27 乳头状鳞状细胞癌。（A）喉：被覆鳞状上皮的多发性肿瘤性乳头包绕纤维血管轴心。（B）喉：高倍镜下显示被覆恶性鳞状上皮细胞，呈乳头状原位癌改变。（C）气管：乳头状鳞状细胞癌，显示侵及气管软骨膜水平。

组织学上，这种肿瘤由普通鳞状细胞癌区域和含有黏液的腺癌灶组成，前者有时伴有角化，后者通常排列成导管、小管或腺管状结构（图4B.28）。有表面黏膜鳞状细胞癌的成分，通常伴有黏膜重度异型增生/原位癌。几乎总是以鳞状成分为主[266,267]。腺癌成分一般主要见于肿瘤深部，常呈中分化或低分化。因为ASC更具侵袭性，所以应与黏液表皮样癌区分开来，即使是高级别的黏液表皮样癌。小涎腺/浆液黏液腺的黏液表皮样癌是一种腺体的肿瘤，而不是黏膜的肿瘤，见于黏膜下，累及表面的非常少见（一般仅为微小病变）。黏液表皮样癌在组织学上比ASC级别低，其特征为无角化产物，有明显的鳞状细胞癌成分，但呈"表皮样"，其实体区域一般主要由中间的细胞构成。基底细胞样鳞状细胞癌具有腔隙，但不是真正的恶性腺体。肿瘤细胞不含黏液，肿瘤内有大量具有基底细胞样特征的区域，不同于腺鳞癌中普通的鳞状细胞癌。

神经内分泌癌
Neuroendocrine carcinomas

喉的神经内分泌癌仅在近期才被描述为一种独特的分类。尽管不如支气管和肺的神经内分泌癌常见，但喉的神经内分泌癌正以不断增高的发生率而被认识。诸如免疫组化和电镜等辅助诊断技术的发展及其广泛应用，使人们已经认识到起初被归为其他类别（例如腺癌、未分化癌、副神经节瘤）的喉部肿瘤多半是神经内分泌癌。事实上，有些作者认为大多数非鳞状细胞喉癌均为神经内分泌癌[52]。

这类肿瘤的命名各异并且有些混乱，在文献中曾出现过这样一些术语，例如类癌、非典型性类癌、燕麦细胞癌、大细胞神经内分泌癌、小细胞癌、小细胞未分化癌以及嗜酸细胞/嗜酸细胞样类癌。随着对喉神经内分泌癌认识的增加，发现这些喉部肿瘤与肺部的同类肿瘤之间有诸多相似之处，并且由Gould等[268]推荐的针对肺神经内分泌肿瘤的命名法已被修改，并适用于喉的神经内分泌癌[53,54]。从而，这些肿瘤已被分类为高分化神经内分泌癌（类癌或典型类癌）、中分化神经内分泌癌（非典型类癌或大细胞神经内分泌癌）以及低分化神经内分泌癌（燕麦细胞癌、小细胞未分化癌、小细胞神经内分泌癌）。这一分类方案是将这些肿瘤认为具有神经内分泌特征（能产生肽类物质、"神经分泌"颗粒）的癌（恶性上皮肿瘤），在本病的连续谱系中，其组织学分化和生物学进展的程度有所不同。

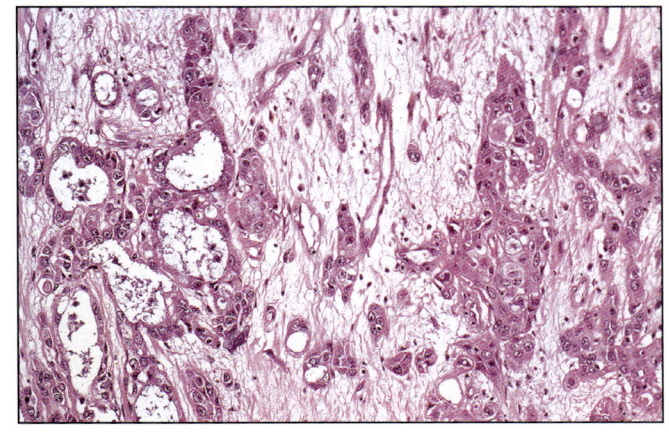
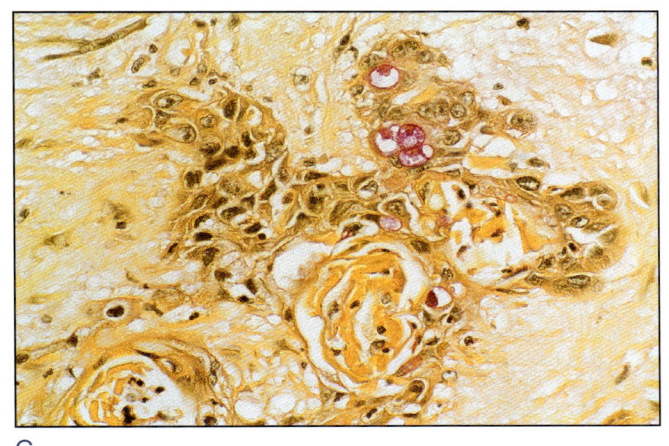
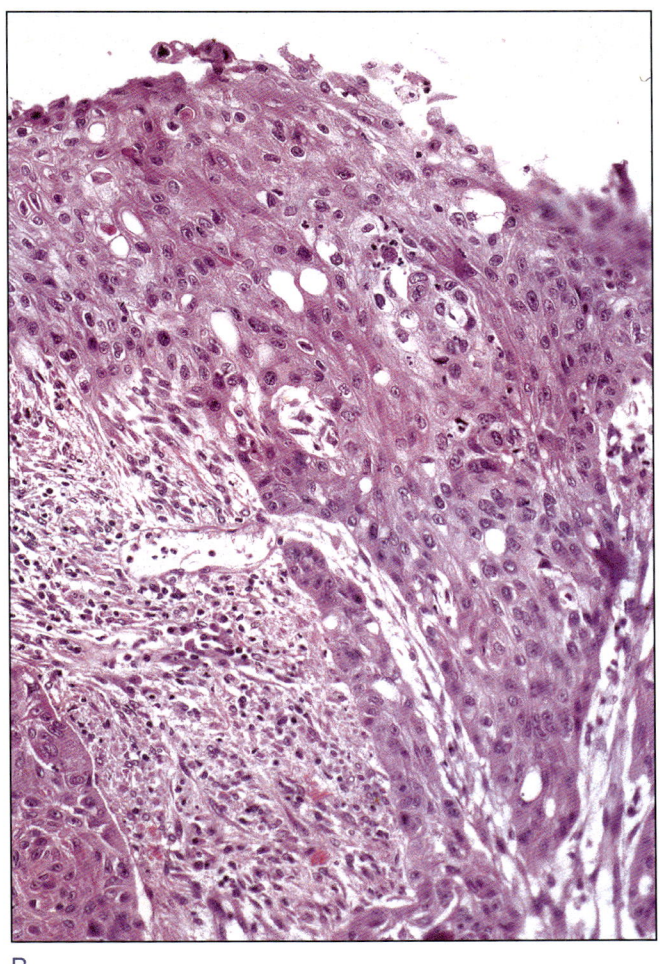

图4B.28 喉腺鳞癌。（A）图左侧为腺癌性腺体成分，右侧为鳞状细胞癌成分。（B）鳞状细胞癌成分累及表面。（C）黏液卡红染色显示具有腺样分化的癌内有黏液产物，邻近并累及伴有角化的鳞状细胞癌。

高分化神经内分泌癌（类癌，典型类癌）
Well-differentiated neuroendocrine carcinoma (carcinoid tumor, typical carcinoid tumor)

喉的高分化神经内分泌癌是一种非常罕见的肿瘤。文献中报告的许多喉类癌的病例极可能是中分化的神经内分泌癌或非典型类癌[54]。气管类癌也相当罕见[175,269]；而支气管类癌则较常见。在1991年El-Naggar和Batsakis的一篇综述中[270]，仅能搜集到13例能够接受的喉高分化神经内分泌癌的病例。患者主要是男性，年龄介于45～80岁之间。这些肿瘤主要位于声门上，常发生于杓状/杓状会厌皱襞区。尽管在少数情况下可能发生转移，但预后良好[54]。

组织学上，喉的高分化神经内分泌癌类似于其他部位的典型类癌。肿瘤界限清楚，一般由小而均一的细胞组成，排列成器官样结构，呈巢状，缎带样、小梁状和（或）腺泡状/腺样分布（图4B.29）。细胞核圆形至卵圆形，染色质点彩状，核仁不明显。核分裂象稀少。基本上没有核的多形性和肿瘤坏死。肿瘤嗜银染色阳性，例如Grimelius染色。

免疫组化方面，喉的高分化神经内分泌癌的神经内分泌标记物染色阳性，常用神经元特异性烯醇化酶（NSE）和嗜铬素标记。按理这类肿瘤的上皮性标记物免疫组化染色应该阳性，例如角蛋白，但是几乎未见有这种结果的报道[47]。电子显微镜检查可见特征性的具有致密核心的神经分泌颗粒。

鉴别诊断包括原发性副神经节瘤、中分化神经内分泌癌及高分化腺癌。高分化神经内分泌癌与副神经节瘤的鉴别要点已在有关副神经节瘤章节中讨论过（见152页）。中分化神经内分泌癌具有器官样神经内分泌形态，但与高分化神经内分泌癌相比，它是一个高级别肿瘤。因此，在形态学上可从核的非典型性和多形性、肿瘤浸润的特性以及坏死和核分裂活性来区分这两种病变（见

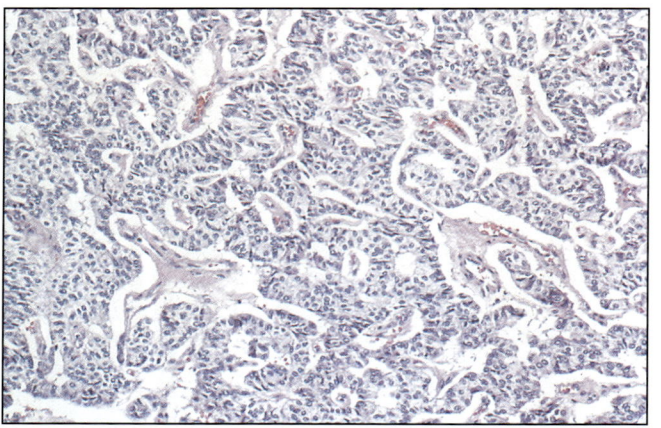

图4B.29 喉的高分化神经内分泌癌（类癌，典型类癌）。注意肿瘤细胞以小梁状排列成器官样结构。

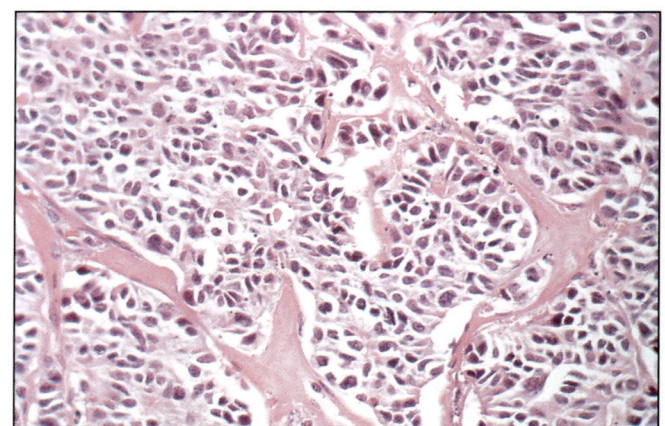

图4B.30 喉的中分化神经内分泌癌（非典型类癌），显示非典型性肿瘤细胞排列成器官样结构，但不如高分化神经内分泌癌明显。

下）。腺癌（非特异性）非嗜银性，免疫组化染色神经内分泌标记（例如嗜铬素）阴性，超微结构检查也不含有神经分泌颗粒。

中分化神经内分泌癌（非典型类癌）
Moderately differentiated neuroendocrine carcinoma（atypical carcinoid）

喉的中分化神经内分泌癌比高分化型常见。其中某些肿瘤在文献中作为类癌报道[271-273]。在1991年的一篇综述中[274]，Woodruff和Senie从文献中找出了大约200例中分化神经内分泌癌。本病特征性地发生于50~60岁或60~70岁的患者，且大多数病变位于声门上。在其中一组病例中[49]，大约1/3的患者出现严重疼痛。与喉的高分化神经内分泌癌不同，这些肿瘤具有侵袭性，报道的5年生存率为48%[274]。在Wenig和Gnepp系列研究中[54]，所有发生转移的患者均已死亡。有趣的是，这些肿瘤有向皮肤转移的倾向[274-276]。

组织学上，中分化神经内分泌癌是一种上皮性肿瘤，肿瘤细胞排列成巢状、片块状、腺体/腺泡状、小梁状和缎带状，表现出神经内分泌肿瘤特征性的"器官样"结构（图4B.30）。在一个单独的肿瘤内出现多种结构是其特征，而且几乎总是出现明显的腺样结构[53]。肿瘤细胞为圆形至多角形，伴有嗜酸性胞浆。偶尔描述存在具有嗜酸性细胞（oncocytic）特性的细胞[272]。核为圆形至卵圆形，染色质为点彩状，偶见多个核仁，但不明显，细胞核偶尔深染。常见核分裂象、细胞多形性以及浸润性的边缘，而且比高分化神经内分泌癌显著。典型的病例肿瘤细胞嗜银，而且角蛋白、嗜铬素NSE免疫染色阳性（图4B.31）。有趣的是，在许多喉的中分化神经内分泌癌中，降钙素免疫组化染色阳性[49,52,53,275]。超微结构检查可见神经分泌颗粒。

鉴别诊断主要是与高分化和低分化神经内分泌癌、腺癌、"未分化"癌以及甲状腺来源的髓样癌相鉴别。与高分化神经内分泌癌的鉴别前面已经讨论过。与低分化神经内分泌癌相比，中分化神经内分泌癌没有未分化癌的组织学结构，一般有较突出的神经内分泌标记物染色，而且具有较大数目的神经分泌颗粒。证实神经内分泌分化、组织化学、免疫组化和（或）超微结构检查，可以用来区分中分化神经内分泌癌和腺癌或非特异性癌。神经内分泌分化和降钙素阳性可能提出与甲状腺髓样癌鉴别的问题。多数中分化神经内分泌癌没有富含淀粉样物质的间质（尽管少数病例可能伴有淀粉样物质沉积）[49]，而且缺乏原发性甲状腺起源的肿瘤。此外，转移性甲状腺髓样癌患者血清降钙素水平常常升高。

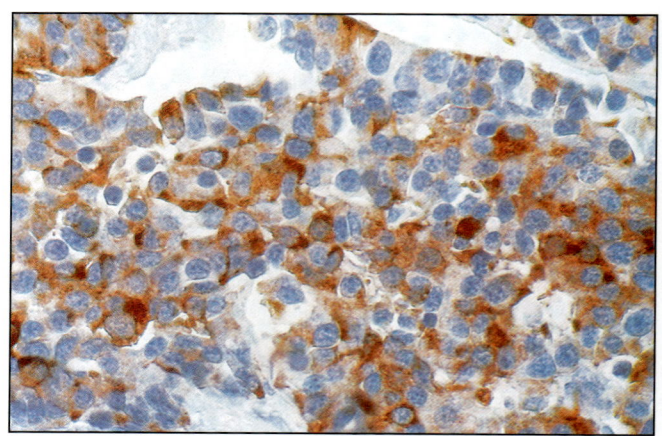

图4B.31 喉的中分化神经内分泌癌（非典型类癌）。嗜铬素免疫组化染色肿瘤细胞呈强阳性。

低分化神经内分泌癌（小细胞神经内分泌癌、小细胞癌、"燕麦细胞"癌）
Poorly differentiated neuroendocrine carcinoma (small cell neuroendocrine carcinoma, small cell carcinoma, "oat-cell" carcinoma)

虽然小细胞癌是一种常见的肺部肿瘤，但相似的低分化神经内分泌癌却少见于喉/下咽部[47,277-279]，非常罕见于气管[175,280]。喉的低分化神经内分泌癌主要为老年男性吸烟者。与其他喉的神经内分泌癌一样，绝大多数病变位于声门上部[54,279]。转移常见，大约半数患者有颈部转移[279]。偶有副肿瘤综合征报道[54,281]。预后极差，大约70%的患者死于本病[52,279]。与气管肿瘤[280]患者的情况相同，出现转移性疾病的患者预后更差[282]。

喉的低分化神经内分泌癌的组织形态学表现与肺部的相应肿瘤类似。肿瘤由小细胞构成，排列成未分化的片块状和巢状（图4B.32）。偶尔可见细胞排列成缎带状，同样可以形成罕见的玫瑰花样结构[279]。细胞为圆形，偶尔可呈梭形，胞浆非常稀少，胞核深染，核仁不明显（图4B.33A）。血管壁上可见核浸润（nuclear smearing）和DNA包壳（DNA encrustation）。还可见到稍大的细胞，伴有比较丰富的胞浆。尽管没有特别明显的核仁，但仍然可见。混合性小细胞癌是由低分化神经内分泌癌混有鳞状细胞癌和（或）腺癌组成的[283,284]（图4B.33B）。

低分化神经内分泌癌神经内分泌分化的证据不如高分化或中分化神经内分泌癌明显，而且可能难以找到这样的证据。肿瘤细胞仅偶尔嗜银，超微结构检查神经分泌颗粒稀少。诸如嗜铬素和NSE（后者对于神经内分泌

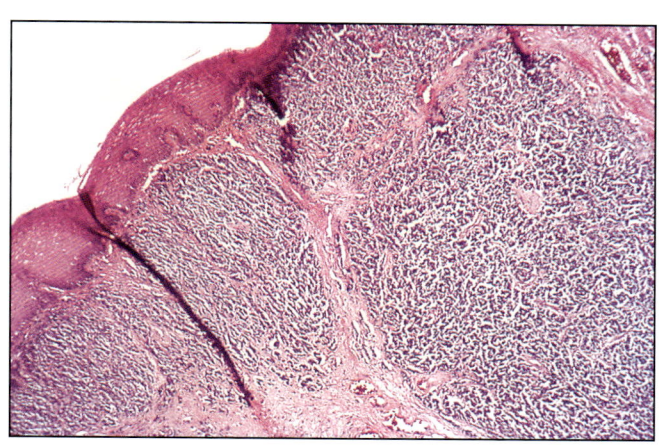

图4B.32 喉的低分化神经内分泌癌（小细胞癌）。小的未分化肿瘤细胞呈片块状排列，位于表面黏膜上皮的深部。

细胞并不完全特异）等神经内分泌标记物的免疫组化染色常显示阳性，但不是每个病例都容易得到证实[47]。Gnepp[279]断言，诊断喉的低分化神经内分泌癌必须要有神经内分泌分化的免疫组化或超微结构证据存在。Aguilar等[285]认为，喉小细胞癌可能显示、也可能不显示明确的神经内分泌分化证据。可以想像，分化最差的神经内分泌癌，有些低分化神经内分泌癌可能已经丢失了传统技术可以检出的神经内分泌的特征，或者某些伴有低分化神经内分泌癌组织学特征的原始喉部肿瘤，起源于具有神经内分泌和（或）非内分泌上皮分化能力的多潜能干细胞，其组成的肿瘤细胞具有表达上皮性而不是神经内分泌性的免疫组化和超微结构特征。总而言之，将这种伴有低分化神经内分泌癌特征的肿瘤和那些

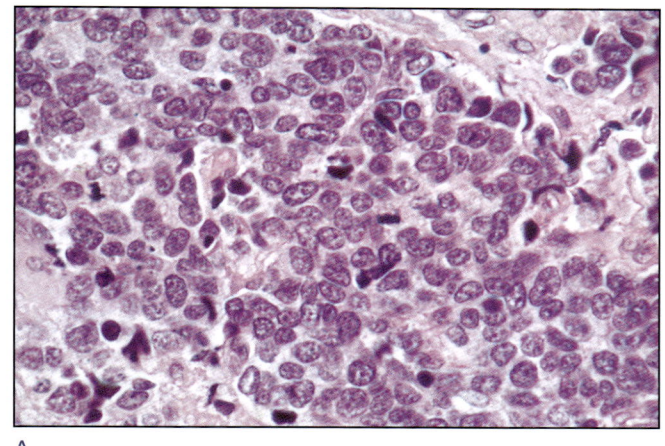
A

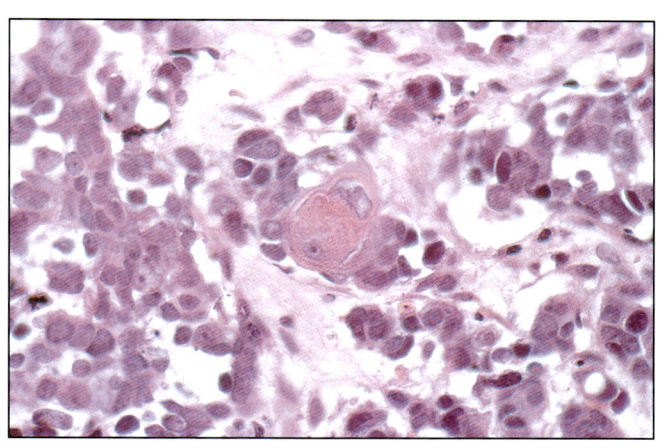
B

图4B.33 喉的低分化神经内分泌癌（小细胞癌）。（A）小的未分化肿瘤细胞，伴有少量不清楚的胞浆，核染色质细点彩状，核仁一般不明显。（B）局部鳞状分化（鳞状细胞珠）。

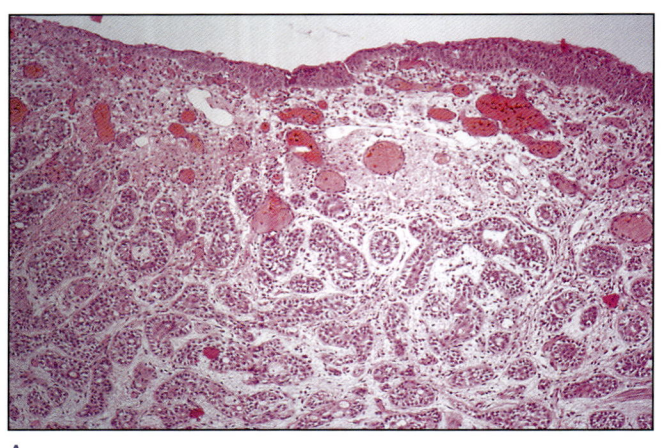
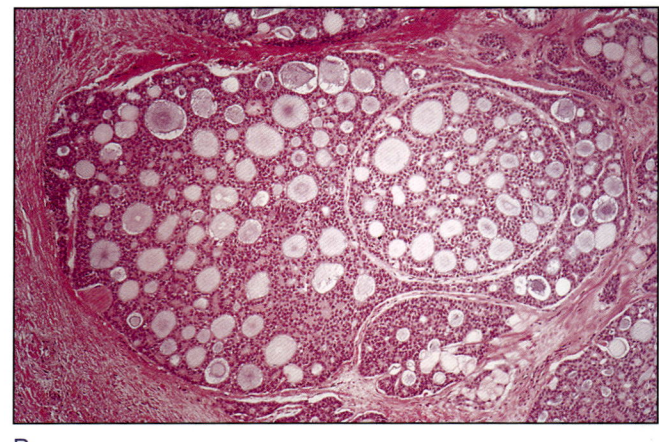

图4B.34　气管腺样囊性癌。（A）肿瘤主要呈腺管状结构，位于黏膜上皮深部。（B）腺样囊性癌典型的筛状结构。

没有神经内分泌分化证据的肿瘤称为小细胞癌应该慎重。

低分化神经内分泌癌与其他神经内分泌肿瘤的鉴别已在前面讨论过。与淋巴瘤/白血病的鉴别诊断可能存在问题。淋巴瘤/白血病血液学标记物染色应该阳性，例如白细胞共同抗原（CD45），低分化神经内分泌癌则为阴性，而上皮性标记物、角蛋白和（或）上皮膜抗原染色应为阳性。

关于喉的神经内分泌癌的组织发生存在争议。可能来源于Kulchitsky型的嗜银黏膜细胞（人类喉部可见非常少数的黏膜嗜银性细胞）[286]或多潜能上皮干细胞。混合性低分化神经内分泌癌的存在是支持后一假说的证据。

腺癌　Adenocarcinoma

喉和气管的原发性腺癌相当少见，据估计其发生率约占喉部肿瘤的1%[287-289]。正如所料，它们最常发生于浆液黏液腺最丰富的区域（即声门上区和声门下区）。大多数气管腺癌为腺样囊性癌（adenoid cystic carcinoma）[175,290]。传统上，喉腺癌最常见的组织学亚型通常为非特异性腺癌[287-289]；然而，就像涎腺肿瘤一样，因为比较特异的腺癌亚型已被认识，所以喉腺癌可能需要进一步分类。例如喉腺泡细胞癌[291]、涎腺导管癌[292]以及上皮-肌上皮癌[293]的病例均有报道，有些最初诊断为非特异性腺癌的病变可能是神经内分泌癌[53,289]。

喉和气管腺癌最常见的特殊亚型是腺样囊性癌[175,294-296]。腺样囊性癌比其他的喉腺癌更易于累及年轻人，常位于声门下。它与发生于涎腺的腺样囊性癌具有某些共同的临床特征，即表现为缓慢的进行性生长、广泛的浸润性特性、常常超出其临床大体范围、常常局部复发、特征性的进行性的临床过程持续多年，死亡常发生于诊断之后10年或10年以上。喉气管腺样囊性癌的组织形态学类似于大涎腺和口腔小涎腺等好发部位的表现（图4B.34）（见第7章）。

黏液表皮样癌（mucoepidermoid carcinoma，MEC）是另外一种发生于喉部的罕见的涎腺类型的肿瘤[297-300]。诊断时的平均年龄约为60岁[298-300]，好发于声门上区。这些肿瘤的形态学和临床行为类似于涎腺的黏液表皮样癌（图4B.35）（见第7章）。低级别肿瘤（显著的囊性结构、丰富的黏液、实性区稀少、几乎没有细胞的多形性）倾向于比高级别肿瘤的预后好；据报道，低级别肿瘤的5

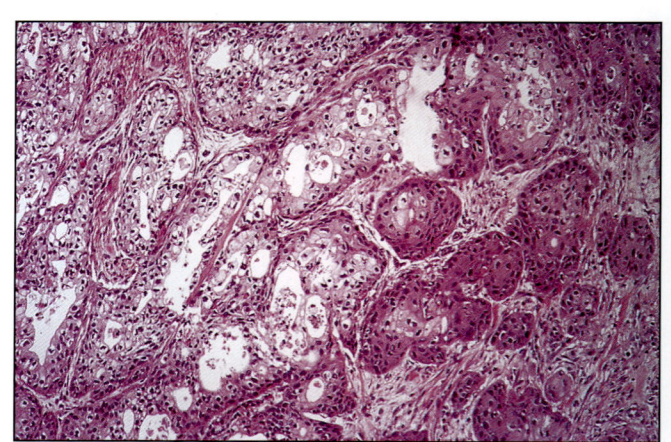

图4B.35　喉的黏液表皮样癌。图左侧肿瘤伴有腺体区域，而右侧为较实性的鳞状癌巢。

年生存率为90%～100%，而高级别肿瘤约为50%，喉的所有黏液表皮样癌的5年生存率为77%～80%[298-300]。高级别肿瘤一般缺乏显著的囊性结构，有比较明显的实性鳞状区域，而且核的非典型性和核分裂活性增加。Gerughty等[254]在"腺鳞癌"的标题下描述发生于鼻腔、口腔及喉部的一种肿瘤，这种肿瘤具有高度侵袭性的临床经过。由于存在单独的腺癌，鳞状细胞癌以及导管原位癌，因此将这种肿瘤从黏液表皮样癌中分离出来[253,301]。Damiani等[298]在他们的资料中将这种肿瘤并入高级别黏液表皮样癌，而且不像Gerughty等[254]报道的预后那么不好。最近，"腺鳞癌"这一术语指的是一种伴有鳞状和腺体成分的癌，并且具有明显的表面黏膜鳞状细胞癌的成分（见前）[302,303]。这些肿瘤通常为高级别病变。该作者将这些腺鳞癌基本上看作黏膜起源的伴有灶性腺性分化的鳞状细胞癌，类似于肺的腺鳞癌；并认为黏液表皮样癌是一种涎腺来源的肿瘤（或发生于喉气管的病例为浆液黏液腺来源）。

传统上归类为非特异性腺癌的肿瘤在诊断时常常已处于晚期，而且伴有侵袭性的行为以及不好的预后[287-289]。

软骨性肿瘤 Cartilaginous tumors

软骨性肿瘤是罕见的喉部病变，极少见于气管[304]。喉部肿瘤最常累及环状软骨，其次为甲状软骨[304-308]。会厌软骨和杓状软骨的肿瘤特别罕见。声带"软骨瘤"已有9例报道，与喉的软骨均不相连[309]，实际上可能是声带的软骨样化生[310]。喉软骨性肿瘤患者往往为男性，多数在50岁以上，中位年龄65岁左右[306-308]。其症状取决于肿瘤的部位，包括咽下困难、呼吸困难、喘鸣或颈部肿块。X线片可能显示肿瘤内有点状钙化，这实际上也是喉软骨性肿瘤的特异病症[304,307]。

这种肿瘤表现为质硬的光滑分叶状黏膜下肿块，分界清楚，切面呈灰色黏液样外观（图4B.36和4B.37）。组织学上，软骨细胞往往在蓝色软骨样和（或）黏液样基质中排列成簇。肿瘤细胞构成以及核的大小和多核软骨细胞出现的多少在同一肿瘤和不同肿瘤之间可能不同（图4B.38）[165,304,311]；然而，一般不出现明显的间变、坏死和非典型性。因而，应用小骨软骨性肿瘤的普通诊断标准，大多数喉的软骨性肿瘤都将归类于低级别软骨肉瘤（或者软骨肉瘤1级或2级）[306,308]。特别罕见的喉透明细胞软骨肉瘤病例已被报道[312]。尽管具有这种组织学表现，但喉的软骨性肿瘤的生物学行为不如其他部

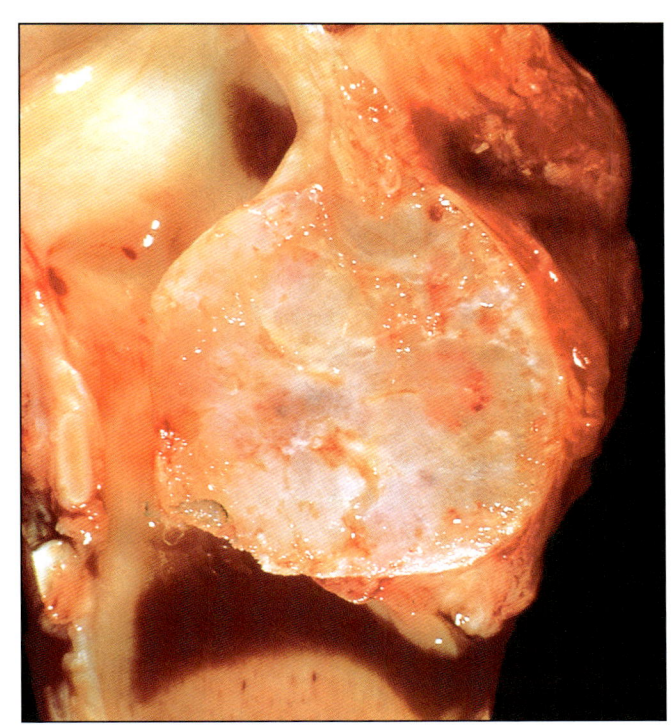

图4B.36 喉软骨性肿瘤。肿瘤发生于环状软骨，切面呈蓝灰色黏液样，且声门下腔明显狭窄。（Reproduced from shapshay S M and Aretz H T.Benign lesions of the larynx with permission of the American Academy of Otolaryngology-Head and Neck Surgery Foundation,copyright©1984.All rights reserved.）

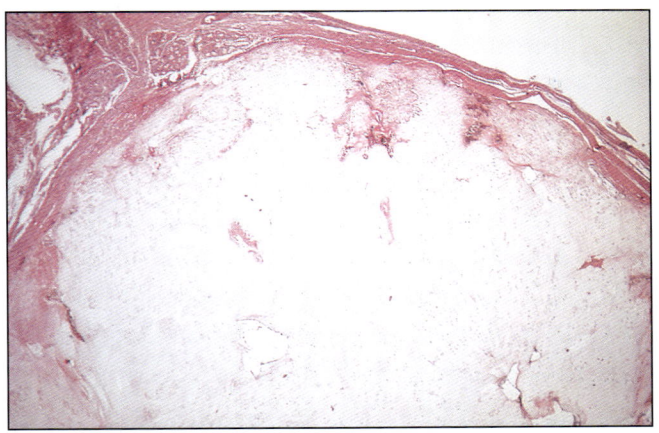

图4B.37 喉软骨性肿瘤。低倍照片显示位于喉黏膜下组织中的境界清楚的软骨性结节。

位软骨肉瘤的侵袭性强[307,313]。肿瘤生长缓慢，如未充分切除，则最后会局部复发，但极少转移[306,307]。喉的高级别软骨肉瘤（软骨肉瘤3级或去分化型软骨肉瘤）也可发生[308,314-316]，但非常罕见。由于有些肿瘤具有侵袭性而有些没有，因此，难以总结出它们的生物学行为[316]。

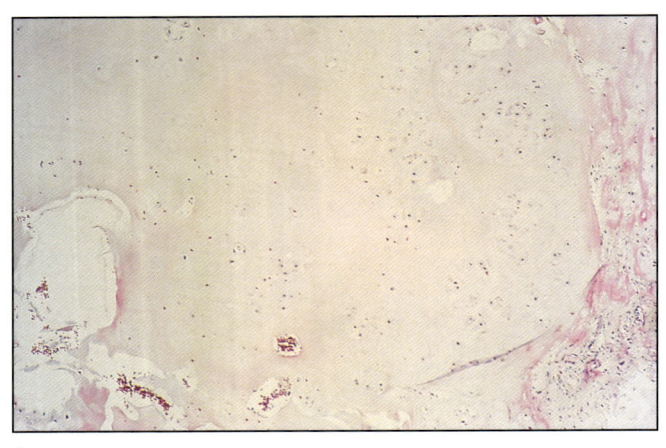
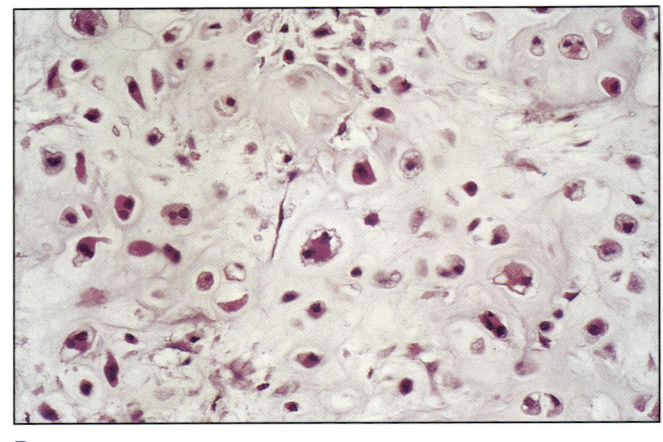

图4B.38 喉的软骨肿瘤。（A）"软骨"区，细胞稀疏，核小。（B）另一肿瘤的"肉瘤样"外观，示细胞增多，体积大，核大，并见大量双核软骨细胞。(Reproduced from Shapshay S M and Aretz H T. Benign lesions of the larynx with permission of the American Academy of Otolaryngology – Head and Neck Surgery Foundation, copyright © 1984. All rights reserved.)

其他恶性肿瘤
Other malignant neoplasms

除了原发性软骨性肿瘤以外，喉和气管的恶性间叶性肿瘤也十分罕见。纤维肉瘤最初被认为是最常见的喉的恶性间叶性肿瘤[317,318]；然而，现代诊断技术的发展使得喉纤维肉瘤的诊断率下降[318]。起初认为是纤维肉瘤的病变可能证明为其他病变，譬如梭形细胞癌、单相性滑膜肉瘤或纤维瘤病[318]。喉纤维肉瘤这一名称应该用于采用诸如免疫组化和电镜检查等现代诊断技术只能发现纤维母细胞的恶性间叶性肿瘤。

已经报道的喉的其他恶性间叶性肿瘤（均罕见发生）包括横纹肌肉瘤[317,319-321]、所谓的恶性纤维组织细胞瘤[322]、骨肉瘤[323,324]、滑膜肉瘤[318,325-327]、脂肪肉瘤（位于喉及下咽部的脂肪肉瘤一般为高分化，因而在组织学上常常难以与脂肪瘤相区分）[328,329]、恶性神经鞘瘤[330]、平滑肌肉瘤[318,331]、血管肉瘤[332]、恶性血管外皮细胞瘤[333]以及骨外 Ewing 肉瘤[334]。我们医院有一例尚未发表的喉 Kaposi 肉瘤[335]。气管平滑肌肉瘤也见报道[335]。恶性淋巴瘤可累及气管[175]，而喉部的淋巴瘤可为原发性，也可为全身性淋巴瘤的一部分[336-338]；蕈样肉芽肿病（mycosis fungoides）累及喉的病例已有描述[339,340]。发生于喉和气管的浆细胞瘤有时会进展为多发性骨髓瘤，或作为多发性骨髓瘤的一部分[175,341,342]。已有会厌粒细胞肉瘤[343]和喉肥大细胞肉瘤[344]的病例报道。恶性黑色素瘤可累及喉，但很少为原发性肿瘤，而是一种转移性病变[345-347]。Weber 和 Grillo[175] 报道了一例气管黑色素瘤。Eble 等[348] 报道了唯一 1 例喉胚细胞瘤（laryngeal blastoma）。

喉和气管的继发性恶性肿瘤可由邻近组织的肿瘤（例如甲状腺癌或食管癌）直接扩散而来，或由血行转移所致。有临床意义的远处转移到喉的情况很少发生。据报道，来源于黑色素瘤和肾细胞癌最常见，但其他部位（胰腺、结肠、卵巢）来源也有报道[349-351]。远处转移到气管的肿瘤包括子宫内膜癌、结肠癌、乳腺癌和子宫颈癌[175]。

参考文献

1. Abramson A L, Steinberg B M, Winkler B 1987 Laryngeal papillomatosis: clinical, histopathologic and molecular studies. Laryngoscope 97: 678–685
2. Derkay C S 2001 Recurrent respiratory papillomatosis. Laryngoscope 111: 57–69
3. Cohen S R, Seltzer S, Geller K A et al. 1980 Papilloma of the larynx and tracheobronchial tree in children. A retrospective study. Ann Otol Rhinol Laryngol 89: 497–503
4. Bauman N M, Smith R J H 1996 Recurrent respiratory papillomatosis. Pediatr Clin North Am 43: 1385–1401
5. Batsakis J G, Raymond A K, Rice D H 1983 The pathology of head and neck tumors. Papillomas of the upper aerodigestive tracts, part 18. Head Neck Surg 5: 332–344
6. Kleinsasser O, Oliveira E, Cruz G 1973 "Juvenile" und "adulte" Kehlkopfpapillome. HNO 21: 97–106
7. Franco R A, Zeitels S M, Farinelli W A et al. 2002 585-NM pulsed dye laser treatment of glottal papillomatosis. Ann Otol Rhinol Laryngol 111: 486–492
8. Naiman A N, Ceruse P, Coulombeau B et al. 2003 Intralesional cidofovir and surgical excision for laryngeal papillomatosis. Laryngoscope 113: 2174–2181
9. Pransky S M, Albright J T, Magit A E 2003 Long-term follow-up of pediatric recurrent respiratory papillomatosis managed with intralesional cidofovir. Laryngoscope 113: 1583–1587
10. Fechner R E, Goepfert H, Alford B R 1974 Invasive laryngeal papillomatosis. Arch Otolaryngol 99: 147–151
11. Shapiro A M, Rimell F L, Pou A et al. 1996 Tracheotomy in children with juvenile-onset recurrent respiratory papillomatosis: The Children's Hospital of Pittsburgh experience. Ann Otol Rhinol Laryngol 105: 1–5

12. Lindeberg H, Elbrond O 1989 Laryngeal papillomas: clinical aspects in a series of 231 patients. Clin Otolaryngol 14: 333–342
13. Doyle D J, Gianoli G J, Espinola T et al. 1994 Recurrent respiratory papillomatosis: juvenile versus adult forms. Laryngoscope 104: 523–527
14. Duggan M A, Lim M, Gill M J et al. 1990 HPV DNA typing of adult-onset respiratory papillomatosis. Laryngoscope 100: 639–642
15. Quiney R E, Wells M, Lewis F A et al. 1989 Laryngeal papillomatosis: correlation between severity of disease and presence of HPV 6 and 11 detected by in-situ DNA hybridisation. J Clin Pathol 42: 694–698
16. Terry R M, Lewis F A, Griffiths S et al. 1987 Demonstration of human papillomavirus types 6 and 11 in juvenile laryngeal papillomatosis by in-situ DNA hybridization. J Pathol 153: 245–248
17. Lie E S, Heyden A, Johannesen M K et al. 1996 Detection of human papillomavirus in routinely processed biopsy specimens from laryngeal papillomas: evaluation of reproducibility of polymerase chain reaction and DNA in situ hybridization procedures. Acta Otolaryngol (Stockh) 116: 627–632
18. Shen J, Tate J E, Crum C P et al. 1996 Prevalence of human papillomaviruses (HPV) in benign and malignant tumors of the upper respiratory tract. Mod Pathol 9: 15–20
19. Quick C A, Krzyzek R A, Watts S L et al. 1980 Relationship between condylomata and laryngeal papillomata. Clinical and molecular virological evidence. Ann Otol Rhinol Laryngol 89: 467–471
20. Kosko J R, Derkay C S 1996 Role of cesarean section in prevention of recurrent respiratory papillomatosis – is there one? Int J Pediatric Otorhinolaryngol 35: 31–38
21. Lin K-Y, Westra W H, Kashima H K et al. 1997 Coinfection of HPV-11 and HPV-16 in a case of laryngeal squamous papillomas with severe dysplasia. Laryngoscope 107: 942–947
22. Go C, Schwartz M R, Donovan D T 2003 Molecular transformation of recurrent respiratory papillomatosis: viral typing and p53 overexpression. Ann Otol Rhinol Laryngol 112:298–302
23. Nash M, Lucente F E, Srinivasan K et al. 1987 Condylomatous lesions of the upper aerodigestive tract. Laryngoscope 97: 1410–1416
24. Fechner R E, Fitz-Hugh G S 1980 Invasive tracheal papillomatosis. Am J Surg Pathol 4: 79–86
25. Quick C A, Foucar E, Dehner L P 1979 Frequency and significance of epithelial atypia in laryngeal papillomatosis. Laryngoscope 89: 550–560
26. Crissman J D, Kessis T, Shah K V et al. 1988 Squamous papillary neoplasia of the adult upper aerodigestive tract. Hum Pathol 19: 1387–1396
27. Heffner D K 1984 Problems in pediatric otorhinolaryngic pathology. V. Diseases of the larynx and trachea. Int J Pediatr Otorhinolaryngol 7: 203–219
28. Fechner R E, Mills S E 1982 Verruca vulgaris of the larynx. A distinctive lesion of probable viral origin confused with verrucous carcinoma. Am J Surg Pathol 6: 357–362
29. Barnes L, Yunis E J, Krebs F J III et al. 1991 Verruca vulgaris of the larynx. Demonstration of human papillomavirus types 6/11 by in-situ hybridization. Arch Pathol Lab Med 115: 895–899
30. MacMillan R H III, Fechner R E 1986 Pleomorphic adenoma of the larynx. Arch Pathol Lab Med 110: 245–247
31. Batsakis J G 1972 Neoplasms of the minor and lesser major salivary glands. Surg Gynecol Obstet 135: 289–298
32. Ma C K, Fine G, Lewis J et al. 1979 Benign mixed tumor of the trachea. Cancer 44: 2260–2266
33. Lack E E, Worsham G F, Callihan M D et al. 1980 Granular cell tumour: a clinicopathologic study of 110 patients. J Surg Oncol 13: 301–316
34. Morrison J G, Gray G F, Dao A H et al. 1987 Granular cell tumors. Am Surg 53: 156–160
35. Frable M A, Fischer R A 1976 Granular cell myoblastomas. Laryngoscope 86: 36–42
36. Compagno J, Hyams V J, Ste-Marie P 1975 Benign granular cell tumors of the larynx: a review of 36 cases with clinicopathologic data. Ann Otol 84: 308–314
37. Coates H L, Kevine K D, McDonald T J et al. 1976 Granular cell tumors of the larynx. Ann Otol 85: 504–507
38. Nolte E, Kleinsasser O 1982 Granularzelltumoren des Kehlkopfes. HNO 30: 333–339
39. Burton D M, Heffner D K, Patow C A 1992 Granular cell tumors of the trachea. Laryngoscope 102: 807–813
40. Garud O, Elverland H H, Bostad L et al. 1984 Granular cell tumor of the larynx in a 5-year-old child. Ann Otol Rhinol Laryngol 93: 45–47
41. Brandwein M, LeBenger J, Strauchen J et al. 1990 Atypical granular cell tumor of the larynx: an unusually aggressive tumor clinically and microscopically. Head Neck 12: 154–159
42. Mazur M T, Shultz J J, Myers J L 1990 Granular cell tumor. Immunohistochemical analysis of 21 benign tumors and one malignant tumor. Arch Pathol Lab Med 114: 692–696
43. Nathrath W B J, Remberger K 1986 Immunohistochemical study of granular cell tumours. Demonstration of neuron specific enolase, S100 protein, laminin and alpha-I-antichymotrypsin. Virchows Arch [A] 408: 421–434
44. Said-Al-Naief N, Brandwein M, Lawson W et al. 1997 Synchronous lingual granular cell tumor and squamous carcinoma. A case report and review of the literature. Arch Otolaryngol Head Neck Surg 123: 543–547
45. Lack E E 1997 Tumors of the adrenal gland and extra-adrenal paraganglia. Atlas of tumor pathology, series 3, fascicle 19. Armed Forces Institute of Pathology, Washington, DC
46. Barnes L 1991 Paraganglioma of the larynx. A critical review of the literature. ORL J Otorhinolaryngol Relat Spec 53: 220–234
47. Googe P B, Ferry J A, Bhan A K et al. 1988 A comparison of paraganglioma, carcinoid tumor, and small cell carcinoma of the larynx. Arch Pathol Lab Med 112: 809–815
48. Baugh R F, McClatchey K D, Sprik S A et al. 1987 Laryngeal paraganglioma. J Otolaryngol 16: 167–168
49. Milroy C M, Rode J, Moss E 1991 Laryngeal paragangliomas and neuroendocrine carcinomas. Histopathology 18: 201–209
50. Lawson W, Zak F G 1974 The glomus bodies ("paraganglia") of the human larynx. Laryngoscope 84: 98–111
51. Liew S H, Leong A S-Y, Tang H M K 1981 Tracheal paraganglioma: a case report with review of the literature. Cancer 47: 1387–1393
52. Woodruff J M, Huvos A G, Erlandson R A et al. 1985 Neuroendocrine carcinomas of the larynx. A study of two types, one of which mimics thyroid medullary carcinoma. Am J Surg Pathol 9: 771–790
53. Wenig B M, Hyams V J, Heffner D K 1988 Moderately differentiated neuroendocrine carcinoma of the larynx. A clinicopathologic study of 54 cases. Cancer 62: 2658–2676
54. Wenig B, Gnepp D R 1989 The spectrum of neuroendocrine carcinomas of the larynx. Semin Diagn Pathol 4: 329–350
55. Bosq M J, Micheau C, Nivet P et al. 1991 Paragangliomas of the head and neck. Immunohistochemical analysis of 16 cases in comparison with neuroendocrine carcinoma. Pathol Res Pract 187: 814–823
56. Brodsky L, Yoshpe N, Ruben R J 1983 Clinical pathological correlates of congenital subglottic haemangiomas. Ann Otol Rhinol Laryngol 92 (suppl 105): 4–18
57. Shikhani A H, Marsh B R, Jones M M et al. 1986 Infantile subglottic hemangiomas. An update. Ann Otol Rhinol Laryngol 95: 336–347
58. Meeuwis J, Bos C E, Hoeve L J et al. 1990 Subglottic hemangiomas in infants: treatment with intralesional corticosteroid injection and intubation. Int J Pediatr Otorhinolaryngol 19: 145–150
59. Cotton R T, Richardson M A 1981 Congenital laryngeal anomalies. Otolaryngol Clin North Am 14: 203–218
60. Batsakis J G, Fox J E 1970 Supporting tissue neoplasms of the larynx. Surg Gynecol Obstet 131: 989–997
61. Cummings C W, Montgomery W W, Balogh K Jr 1969 Neurogenic tumors of the larynx. Ann Otol Rhinol Laryngol 78: 76–95
62. Ma C K, Raju U, Fine G et al. 1981 Primary tracheal neurilemoma. Report of a case with ultrastructural examination. Arch Pathol Lab Med 105: 187–189
63. Schaeffer B T, Som P M, Biller H F et al. 1986 Schwannomas of the larynx: review and computed tomographic scan analysis. Head Neck Surg 8: 469–472
64. Al-Otieschan A T, Mahasin Z Z, Gangopadhyay K et al. 1996 Schwannoma of the larynx: Two case reports and review of the literature. J Otolaryngol 25: 412–415
65. Cohen S R, Landing B H, Isaacs H 1978 Neurofibroma of the larynx in a child. Ann Otol Rhinol Laryngol 87 (suppl 52): 29–31
66. Chow L T C, Ma T K F, Chow W H 1997 Cellular neurothekeoma of the hypopharynx. Histopathology 30: 192–194
67. Karma P, Hyrynkangas K, Rasanen O 1978 Laryngeal leiomyoma. J Laryngol Otol 92: 411–415
68. Shibata K, Komune S 1980 Laryngeal angiomyoma (vascular leiomyoma): clinicopathological findings. Laryngoscope 90: 1880–1886
69. Boedts D, Mestdagh J 1979 Adult rhabdomyoma of the larynx. Arch Otorhinolaryngol 224: 221–229
70. Di Sant'Agnese P A, Knowles D M 1980 Extracardiac rhabdomyoma: a clinicopathologic study and review of the literature. Cancer 46: 780–789
71. Granich M S, Pilch B Z, Nadol J B et al. 1983 Fetal rhabdomyoma of the larynx. Arch Otolaryngol 109: 821–826
72. Rosenberg H S, Vogler C, Close L G et al. 1981 Laryngeal fibromatosis in the neonate. Arch Otolaryngol 107: 513–517
73. McIntosh W A, Kassner G W, Murray J F 1985 Fibromatosis and fibrosarcoma of the larynx and pharynx in an infant. Arch Otolaryngol 111: 478–480
74. Wenig B M 1995 Lipomas of the larynx and hypopharynx: a review of the literature with the addition of three new cases. J Laryngol Otol 109: 353–357
75. Jesberg N 1982 Fibrolipoma of the pyriform sinuses: thirty-seven year follow-up. Laryngoscope 92: 1157–1159
76. Ballard R W, Yarington C T Jr 1981 Hemangiopericytoma of the tracheal wall. Arch Otolaryngol 107: 558–560
77. Schwartz M R, Donovan D T 1987 Hemangiopericytoma of the larynx: a case report and review of the literature. Otolaryngol Head Neck Surg 96: 369–372
78. Cohen S R, Landing B H, Isaacs H 1978 Fibrous histiocytoma of the trachea. Ann Otol Rhinol Laryngol 87 (suppl. 52): 2–4
79. Gonzalez-Campora R, Matilla A, Sanchez-Carrillo J J et al. 1981 "Benign" fibrous histiocytoma of the trachea. J Laryngol Otol 95: 1287–1292
80. Van Laer C, Hamans E, Neetens I et al. 1996 Benign fibrous histiocytoma of the larynx: presentation of a case and review of the literature. J Laryngol Otol 110: 474–477
81. Pollak E R, Naunheim K S, Little A G 1985 Fibromyxoma of the trachea. A review of benign tracheal tumors. Arch Pathol Lab Med 109: 926–929
82. Garcia-Prats M D, Sotelo-Rodriguez M T, Ballestin C et al. 1991 Glomus tumour of the trachea: report of a case with microscopic, ultrastructural

and immunohistochemical examination and review of the literature. Histopathology 19: 459–464
83. Cannon C R, Johns M E, Fechner R E 1987 Immature teratoma of the larynx. Otolaryngol Head Neck Surg 96: 366–368
84. Küng M, Landa J F, Lubin J 1984 Benign clear cell tumor ("sugar tumor") of the trachea. Cancer 54: 517–519
85. Kambic V, Radsel Z, Zargi M et al. 1981 Vocal cord polyps: incidence, histology and pathogenesis. J Laryngol Otol 95: 609–618
86. Kleinsasser O 1982 Pathogenesis of vocal cord polyps. Ann Otol Rhinol Laryngol 91: 378–381
87. Holinger P H, Johnston K C 1960 Contact ulcer of the larynx. JAMA 172: 511–515
88. Barton R T 1953 Observation of the pathogenesis of laryngeal granuloma due to endotracheal anesthesia. N Engl J Med 248: 1097–1099
89. Ward P H, Zwitman D, Hanson D et al. 1980 Contact ulcers and granulomas of the larynx: new insights into their etiology as a basis for more rational treatment. Otolaryngol Head Neck Surg 88: 262–269
90. Miko T L 1989 Peptic (contact ulcer) granuloma of the larynx. J Clin Pathol 42: 800–804
91. Al-Dousary S 1997 Vocal process granuloma. ENT – Ear Nose Throat J 76: 382–387
92. Thompson L D R 1997 Diagnostically challenging lesions in head and neck pathology. Eur Arch Otorhinolaryngol 254: 357–366
93. Wenig B M, Heffner D K 1990 Contact ulcers of the larynx. A reacquaintance with the pathology of an often underdiagnosed entity. Arch Pathol Lab Med 114: 825–828
94. Mills S E, Cooper P H, Fechner R E 1980 Lobular capillary hemangioma: the underlying lesion of pyogenic granuloma. A study of 73 cases from the oral and nasal mucous membranes. Am J Surg Pathol 4: 471–479
95. Grillo H C, Mark E J, Mathisen D J et al. 1993 Idiopathic laryngotracheal stenosis and its management. Ann Thorac Surg 56: 80–87
96. Park S S, Streitz J M, Rebeiz E E et al. 1995 Idiopathic subglottic stenosis. Arch Otolaryngol Head Neck Surg 121: 894–897
97. Jindal J R, Milbrath M M, Hogan W J et al. 1994 Gastroesophageal reflux disease as a likely cause of "idiopathic" subglottic stenosis. Ann Otol Rhinol Laryngol 103: 186–191
98. Canalis R F, Maxwell D S, Hemenway W G 1977 Laryngocele – an updated review. J Otolaryngol 6: 191–199
99. Holinger L D, Barnes D R, Smid L J et al. 1978 Laryngocele and saccular cysts. Ann Otol 87: 675–68
100. Baker H L, Baker S R, McClatchey K D 1982 Manifestations and management of laryngoceles. Head Neck Surg 4: 450–456
101. Macfie D D 1966 Asymptomatic laryngoceles in wind-instrument bandsmen. Arch Otolaryngol 83: 270–275
102. DeSanto L W, Devine K D, Weiland L H 1970 Cysts of the larynx – classification. Laryngoscope 80: 145–176
103. Yamase H T, Putman H C III 1979 Oncocytic papillary cystadenomatosis of the larynx. A clinicopathologic entity. Cancer 44: 2306–2311
104. Newman B H, Taxy J B, Laker H I 1984 Laryngeal cysts in adults: clinicopathologic study of 20 cases. Am J Clin Pathol 81: 715–720
105. Oliveira C A, Roth J A, Adams G L 1977 Oncocytic lesions of the larynx. Laryngoscope 87: 1718–1725
106. Hunter A M, Millar J W, Wightman A J A et al. 1981 The changing pattern of laryngeal tuberculosis. J Laryngol Otol 95: 393–398
107. Yarnal J R, Golish J A, Van der Kuypt F 1981 Laryngeal tuberculosis presenting as carcinoma. Arch Otolaryngol 107: 503–505
108. Thaller S R, Gross J R, Pilch B Z et al. 1987 Laryngeal tuberculosis as manifested in the decades 1963–1983. Laryngoscope 97: 848–850
109. Kandiloros D C, Nikolopoulos T P, Ferekidis E A et al. 1997 Laryngeal tuberculosis at the end of the 20th century. J Laryngol Otol 111: 619–621
110. Caldarelli D D, Friedberg S A, Harris A A 1979 Medical and surgical aspects of the granulomatous diseases of the larynx. Otolaryngol Clin North Am 12: 767–781
111. Blair P A, Gnepp D R, Riley R S et al. 1981 Blastomycosis of the larynx. South Med J 74: 880–882
112. Platt M A 1977 Laryngeal coccidioidomycosis. JAMA 237: 1234–1235
113. Maymo Arganaraz M, Luque A G, Tosello M E et al. 2003 Paracoccidioidomycosis and larynx carcinoma. Mycoses 46: 229–232
114. Khabie N, Boyce T G, Roberts G D et al. 2003 Laryngeal sporotrichosis causing stridor in a young child. Int J Pediatr Otorhinolaryngol 67: 819–823
115. Nakahira M, Matsumoto S, Mukushita N et al. 2002 Primary aspergillosis of the larynx associated with CD4+ T lymphocytopenia. J Laryngol Otol 116: 304–306
116. Brandenburg J H, Finch W W, Kirkham W R 1978 Actinomycosis of the larynx and pharynx. Trans Am Acad Ophthalmol Otolaryngol 86: 739–742
117. Kobayashi R H, Rosenblatt H M, Carney J M et al. 1980 Candida esophagitis and laryngitis in chronic mucocutaneous candidiasis. Pediatrics 66: 380–384
118. Pabuççuoglu U, Tuncer C, Sengiz S 2002 Histopathology of candidal hyperplastic lesions of the larynx. Path Res Pract 198: 675–678
119. Barnes E L Jr, Zafar T 1977 Laryngeal amyloidosis: clinicopathologic study of seven cases. Ann Otol Rhinol Laryngol 86: 856–863
120. Hellquist H, Olofsson J, Sokjer H et al. 1979 Amyloidosis of the larynx. Acta Otolaryngol 88: 443–450
121. Godbersen G S, Leh J F, Rudert H et al. 1992 Organ-limited laryngeal amyloid deposits: clinical, morphological, and immunohistochemical results of five cases. Ann Otol Rhinol Laryngol 101: 770–775
122. Lewis J E, Olsen K D, Kurtin P J et al. 1992 Laryngeal amyloidosis: a clinicopathologic and immunohistochemical review. Otolaryngol Head Neck Surg 106: 372–377
123. Thompson L D R, Derringer G A, Wenig B M 2000 Amyloidosis of the larynx: a clinopathologic study of 11 cases. Mod Pathol 13: 528–535
124. Michaels L, Hyams V J 1979 Amyloid in localised deposits and plasmacytomas of the respiratory tract. J Pathol 128: 29–38
125. Simpson G T II, Skinner M, Strong M S et al. 1984 Localized amyloidosis of the head and neck and upper aerodigestive and lower respiratory tracts. Ann Otol Rhinol Laryngol 93: 374–379
126. Berg A M, Troxler R F, Grillone G et al. 1993 Localized amyloidosis of the larynx: evidence for light chain composition. Ann Otol Rhinol Laryngol 102: 884–889
127. Weirich Ch IG, Gaa A, Schaefer H E 1996 Amyloid tumors of the lung – an immunocytoma? Pathol Res Pract 192: 446–452
128. Young R H, Sandstrom R E, Mark G J 1980 Tracheopathia osteoplastica. J Thorac Cardiovasc Surg 79: 537–541
129. Nienhuis D M, Prakash U B S, Edell E S 1990 Tracheobronchopathia osteochondroplastica. Ann Otol Rhinol Laryngol 99: 689–694
130. Birzgalis A R, Farrington W T, O'Keefe L et al. 1993 Localized tracheopathia osteoplastica of the subglottis. J Laryngol Otol 107: 352–353
131. Paaske P B, Tang E 1985 Tracheopathia osteoplastica in the larynx. J Laryngol Otol 99: 305–310
132. Thomas K 1970 Laryngeal manifestations of Wegener's granuloma. J Laryngol Otol 84: 101–106
133. Wenig B M, Devaney K L, Wenig B L 1995 Pseudoneoplastic lesions of the oropharynx and larynx simulating cancer. Pathol Annu 30: 143–187
134. Matt B H 1996 Wegener's granulomatosis, acute laryngotracheal airway obstruction and death in a 17-year-old female: case report and review of the literature. Int J Pediatr Otorhinolaryngol 37: 163–172
135. Carpenter R J III, Banks P M, McDonald T J et al. 1978 Sinus histiocytosis with massive lymphadenopathy (Rosai–Dorfman disease): report of a case with respiratory tract involvement. Laryngoscope 88: 1963–1969
136. Case records 1981 Case no. 52. N Engl J Med 305: 1572–1580
137. Wenig B M, Abbondanzo S L, Childers E L et al. 1993 Extranodal sinus histiocytosis with massive lymphadenopathy (Rosai–Dorfman disease) of the head and neck. Hum Pathol 24: 483–492
138. Weisman R A, Canalis R F, Powell W J 1980 Laryngeal sarcoidosis with airway obstruction. Ann Otol Rhinol Laryngol 89: 58–61
139. Marion R B, Alperin J E, Maloney W H 1972 Gouty tophus of the true vocal cord. Arch Otolaryngol 96: 161–162
140. Dedo H H, Carlsoo B 1982 Histologic evaluation of Teflon granulomas of human vocal cords. A light and electron microscopic study. Acta Otolaryngol 93: 475–484
141. Varvares M A, Montgomery W W, Hillman R E 1995 Teflon granuloma of the larynx: etiology, pathophysiology, and management. Ann Otol Rhinol Laryngol 104: 511–515
142. Wey W, Torhorst J 1974 Hamartom des Hypopharynx (Verlaufsbeobachtung eines Falles uber 11 Jahre). HNO 22: 217–219
143. Patterson H C, Pilch B Z, Dickersin G R et al. 1981 Hamartoma of the hypopharynx. Arch Otolaryngol 107: 767–772
144. Zapf B, Leymann W B, Snyder G G III 1981 Hamartoma of the larynx: an unusual cause of stridor in an infant. Otolaryngol Head Neck Surg 89: 797–799
145. Fine E D, Dahms B, Arnold J E 1995 Laryngeal hamartoma: a rare congenital abnormality. Ann Oto Rhinol Laryngol 104: 87–89
146. Manni J J, Mulder J J S, Schaafsma H E 1992 Inflammatory pseudotumor of the subglottis. Eur Arch Otorhinolaryngol 249: 16–19
147. Gabrielides C G, Karkavelas G, Triarides C et al. 1981 Malakoplakia of the larynx. Pathol Res Pract 172: 53–57
148. Kambic V, Gale N, Radsel Z 1982 Warty dyskeratoma of the vocal cord. First reported case. Arch Otolaryngol 108: 385–387
149. Manni H J, Lema P N, Van Raalte J A et al. 1983 Schistosomiasis in otorhinolaryngology: review of the literature and case report. J Laryngol Otol 97: 1177–1181
150. Libera D D, Redlich G, Bittesini L et al. 2001 Aneurysmal bone cyst of the larynx presenting with hypoglottic obstruction. A case report and review of the literature. Arch Pathol Lab Med 125: 673–676
151. Cho M S, Kim E S, Kim H J et al. 1997 Kimura's disease of the epiglottis. Histopathology 30: 592–594
152. Fechner R E 1974 Laryngeal keratosis and atypia. Can J Otolaryngol 3: 516–521
153. Barnes L, Eveson J W, Reichart P et al. (eds) 2005 WHO classification of tumors. Pathology and genetics of head and neck tumors, Lyon, France, IARC Press
154. Hellquist H, Olofsson J, Grontoft O 1981 Carcinoma in-situ and severe dysplasia of the vocal cords. A clinicopathologic and photometric investigation. Acta Otolaryngol 92: 543–555
155. Crissman J D 1982 Laryngeal keratosis preceding laryngeal carcinoma. A report of four cases. Arch Otolaryngol 108: 445–448
156. Crissman J D, Fu Y S 1986 Intraepithelial neoplasia of the larynx. A clinicopathologic study of six cases with DNA analysis. Arch Otolaryngol Head Neck Surg 112: 522–528
157. Crissman J D, Zarbo R J, Drozdowicz S et al. 1988 Carcinoma in-situ and microinvasive squamous carcinoma of the laryngeal glottis. Arch Otolaryngol Head Neck Surg 114: 299–307

158. Crissman J D, Zarbo R J 1989 Dysplasia, in situ carcinoma, and progression to invasive squamous cell carcinoma of the upper aerodigestive tract. Am J Surg Pathol 13 (suppl. 1): 5–16
159. Crissman J D 1985 Histopathologic diagnosis of early cancer. In: Chretien P B, Johns M E, Shedd D P et al. (eds) Head and neck cancer. Decker, Philadelphia, vol 1, p 134–140
160. Bouquot J E, Gnepp D R 1991 Laryngeal precancer: a review of the literature, commentary, and comparison with oral leukoplakia. Head Neck 13: 488–497
161. Fried M P, Gopal H 1996 Carcinoma of the glottis and subglottis. In: Fried M P (ed) The larynx: a multidisciplinary approach, 2nd edn. Mosby, St Louis, p 503–517
162. McGavran M H, Stutsman A C, Ogura J H 1974 Superficially invasive epidermoid carcinoma of the true vocal cord. Can J Otolaryngol 3: 526–527
163. Gillis T M, Incze J, Strong M S et al. 1983 Natural history and management of keratosis, atypia, carcinoma in-situ, and microinvasive cancer of the larynx. Am J Surg 146: 512–516
164. Sakr W A, Zarbo R J, Jacobs J R et al. 1987 Distribution of basement membrane in squamous cell carcinoma of the head and neck. Hum Pathol 18: 1043–1050
165. Pilch B Z, Dorfman D M, Brodsky G L et al. 1996 Pathology of laryngeal malignancies. In: Fried M P (ed) The larynx: a multidisciplinary approach, 2nd edn. Mosby, St Louis, p 461–485
166. Nguyen C, Naghibzadeh B, Black MJ et al. 1996 Glottic microinvasive carcinoma: is it different from carcinoma in situ? J Otolaryngol 25: 223–226
167. Jemal A, Tiwari R C, Murray T et al. 2004 Cancer statistics, 2004. CA Cancer J Clin 54: 8–29
168. Muir C, Weiland L 1995 Upper aerodigestive tract cancers. Cancer 75: 147–153
169. Wang C C 1983 Head and neck neoplasms. In: Mansfield C M (ed) Therapeutic radiology: new directions in therapy. Medical Examination Publishing, New Hyde Park, NY, p 144–169
170. Koufman J A, Burke A J 1997 The etiology and pathogenesis of laryngeal carcinoma. Otolaryngol Clin North Am 30: 1–19
171. Talamini R, Bosetti C, La Vecchia C et al. 2002 Combined effect of tobacco and alcohol on laryngeal risk: a case-control study. Cancer Causes Control 13: 957–964
172. McKaig R G, Baric R S, Olshan A F 1998 Human papillomavirus and head and neck cancer: epidemiology and molecular biology. Head Neck 20: 250–265
173. Fischer M, Von Winterfeld F 2003 Evaluation and application of a broad-spectrum polymerase chain reaction assay for human papillomaviruses in the screening of squamous cell tumours of the head and neck. Acta Otolaryngol 123: 752–758
174. Bacciu A, Mercante G, Ingegnoli A et al. 2003 Reflux esophagitis as a possible risk factor in the development of pharyngolaryngeal squamous cell carcinoma. Tumori 89: 485–487
175. Weber A L, Grillo H C 1978 Tracheal tumours. A radiological, clinical and pathological evaluation of 84 cases. Radiol Clin North Am 16: 227–246
176. Maisel R H, Cohen C J 1996 Carcinoma of the supraglottis. In: Fried M P (ed) The larynx: a multidisciplinary approach, 2nd edn. Mosby, St Louis, p 487–501
177. Fabian R L, Varvares M A 1996 Carcinoma of the laryngopharynx and cervical esophagus. In: Fried M P (ed) The larynx: a multidisciplinary approach, 2nd edn. Mosby, St Louis, p 549–560
178. Wang C C 1997 Radiation therapy for head and neck neoplasms, 3rd edn. Wiley-Liss, New York, p 224
179. American Joint Committee on Cancer 1997 AJCC cancer staging manual, 5th edn. Lippincott-Raven, Philadelphia, p 41–42
180. Shah J P, Karnell L H, Hoffman H T et al. 1997 Patterns of care for cancer of the larynx in the United States. Arch Otolaryngol Head Neck Surg 123: 475–483
181. Kirchner J A 1997 Glottic–supraglottic barrier: fact or fantasy? Ann Otol Rhinol Laryngol 106: 700–704
182. Ferlito A, Olofsson J, Rinaldo A 1997 Barrier between the supraglottis and the glottis: myth or reality? Ann Otol Rhinol Laryngol 106: 716–719
183. Weinstein G S, Laccourreye O, Brasnu D et al. 1995 Reconsidering a paradigm: the spread of supraglottic carcinoma of the glottis. Laryngoscope 105: 1129–1133
184. Hoffman H T, Karnell L H, Shah J P et al. 1997 Hypopharyngeal cancer patient care evaluation. Laryngoscope 107: 1005–1017
185. McGavran M H, Bauer W C, Ogura J H 1961 The incidence of cervical lymph node metastases from epidermoid carcinoma of the larynx and their relationship to certain characteristics of the primary tumor. A study based on the clinical and pathological findings for 96 patients treated by primary en bloc laryngectomy and radical neck dissection. Cancer 14: 55–66
186. Jakobsson P A, Eneroth C-M, Killander D et al. 1973 Histologic classification and grading of malignancy in carcinoma of the larynx. Acta Radiol Ther Phys Biol 12: 1–8
187. Fisher H R 1975 Grading of biopsies of laryngeal carcinomas by multiple criteria. Can J Otolaryngol 4: 881–884
188. Helweg-Larsen K, Graem N, Miestrup-Larsen K-I et al. 1978 Clinical relevance of histological grading of cancer of the larynx. Acta Pathol Microbiol Scand Sect A 86: 499–504
189. Jacobs J R, Sessions D G, Ogura J H 1980 Recurrent carcinoma of the larynx and the hypopharynx. Otolaryngol Head Neck Surg 88: 425–433
190. Glanz H K 1984 Carcinoma of the larynx. Growth, p-classification and grading of squamous cell carcinoma of the vocal cords. Adv Otorhinolaryngol 32: 1–123
191. Wiernik G, Millard P R, Haybittle J L 1991 The predictive value of histological classification into degrees of differentiation of squamous cell carcinoma of the larynx and hypopharynx compared with the survival of patients. Histopathology 19: 411–417
192. Cappellari J O 1997 Histopathology and pathologic prognostic indicators of laryngeal cancer. Otolaryngol Clin North Am 30: 251–268
193. Bryne M, Jenssen N, Boysen M 1995 Histological grading in the deep invasive front of T1 and T2 glottic squamous cell carcinomas has high prognostic value. Virchows Arch 427: 277–281
194. Welkoborsky H-J, Hinni M, Dienes H-P et al. 1995 Predicting recurrence and survival in patients with laryngeal cancer by means of DNA cytometry, tumor front grading, and proliferation markers. Ann Otol Rhinol Laryngol 104: 503–510
195. Capaccio P, Pruneri G, Carboni N et al. 1997 Cyclin D1 protein expression is related to clinical progression in laryngeal squamous cell carcinomas. J Laryngol Otol 111: 622–626
196. Narayana A, Vaughan A T M, Gunaratne S et al. 1998 Is p53 an independent prognostic factor in patients with laryngeal carcinoma? Cancer 82: 286–291
197. Cann C I, Rothman K J, Fried M P 1988 Epidemiology of laryngeal cancer. In: Fried M P (ed) The larynx: a multidisciplinary approach, 2nd edn. Mosby, St Louis, p 425–436
198. Ackerman L V 1948 Verrucous carcinoma of the oral cavity. Surgery 23: 670–678
199. Van Nostrand A W P, Olofsson J 1972 Verrucous carcinoma of the larynx. A clinical and pathologic study of 10 cases. Cancer 30: 691–702
200. Burns H P, van Nostrand A W P, Bryce D P 1976 Verrucous carcinoma of the larynx. Management by radiotherapy and surgery. Ann Otol 85: 538–543
201. Batsakis J G, Hybels R, Crissman J D et al. 1982 The pathology of head and neck tumors. Verrucous carcinoma, part 15. Head Neck Surg 5: 29–38
202. Ferlito A 1985 Diagnosis and treatment of verrucous squamous cell carcinoma of the larynx: a critical review. Ann Otol Rhinol Laryngol 94: 575–579
203. Lundgren J A V, van Nostrand A W P, Harwood A R et al. 1986 Verrucous carcinoma (Ackerman's tumor) of the larynx: diagnostic and therapeutic considerations. Head Neck Surg 9: 19–26
204. Ferlito A, Recher G 1980 Ackerman's tumor (verrucous carcinoma) of the larynx. A clinicopathologic study of 77 cases. Cancer 46: 1617–1630
205. Orvidas L J, Olsen K D, Lewis J E et al. 1998 Verrucous carcinoma of the larynx: a review of 53 patients. Head Neck 20: 197–203
206. Biller H F, Ogura J H, Bauer W C 1971 Verrucous cancer of the larynx. Laryngoscope 81: 1323–1329
207. Fisher H R 1975 Verrucous carcinoma of the larynx – a study of its pathologic anatomy. Can J Otolaryngol 4: 270–277
208. Medina J E, Dichtel W, Luna M A 1984 Verrucous-squamous carcinomas of the oral cavity. A clinicopathologic study of 104 cases. Arch Otolaryngol 110: 437–440
209. Niparko J K, Rubinstein M I, McClatchey K D 1988 Invasive squamous cell carcinoma within verrucous carcinoma. J Otolaryngol 17: 38–40
210. Smith R R L, Kuhajda F P, Harris A E 1985 Anaplastic transformation of verrucous carcinoma following radiotherapy. Am J Otolaryngol 6: 448–452
211. Maurizi M, Cadoni G, Ottaviani F et al. 1996 Verrucous squamous cell carcinoma of the larynx: diagnostic and therapeutic considerations. Eur Arch Otorhinolaryngol 253: 130–135
212. Shear M, Pindborg J J 1980 Verrucous hyperplasia of the oral mucosa. Cancer 46: 1855–1862
213. Lopez-Amado M, Garcia-Caballero T, Lozano-Ramirez A et al. 1996 Human papillomavirus and p53 oncoprotein in verrucous carcinoma of the larynx. J Laryngol Otol 110: 742–747
214. Crissman J D, Kessis T, Shaw K V et al. 1988 Squamous papillary neoplasia of the adult upper aerodigestive tract. Hum Pathol 19: 1387–1396
215. Thompson L D R, Wenig B M, Heffner D R et al. 1999 Exophytic and papillary squamous cell carcinomas of the larynx: a clinicopathologic series of 104 cases. Otolaryngol Head Neck Surg 120: 718–724
216. Glanz H, Kleinsasser O 1987 Verrucous carcinoma of the larynx – a misnomer. Arch Otorhinolaryngol 244: 108–111
217. Hyams V J 1975 Spindle cell carcinoma of the larynx. Can J Otolaryngol 4: 307–313
218. Battifora H 1976 Spindle cell carcinoma. Ultrastructural evidence of squamous origin and collagen production by tumor cells. Cancer 37: 2275–2282
219. Zarbo R J, Crissman J D, Venkat H et al. 1986 Spindle-cell carcinoma of the upper aerodigestive tract mucosa. An immunohistologic and ultrastructural study of 18 biphasic tumors and comparison with seven monophasic tumors. Am J Surg Pathol 10: 741–753
220. Ellis G L, Langloss J M, Heffner D K et al. 1987 Spindle-cell carcinoma of the aerodigestive tract. An immunohistochemical analysis of 21 cases. Am J Surg Pathol 11: 335–342
221. Lewis J E, Olsen K D, Sebo T J 1997 Spindle cell carcinoma of the larynx: review of 26 cases including DNA content and immunohistochemistry. Hum Pathol 28: 664–673
222. Miranda F J, Neto J A K, da Costa E A et al. 1980 Carcinosarcoma of the esophagus. Int Surg 65: 463–467

223. Appelman H D, Oberman H A 1965 Squamous cell carcinoma of the larynx with sarcoma-like stroma. A clinicopathologic assessment of spindle cell carcinoma and "pseudosarcoma." Am J Clin Pathol 44: 135–145
224. Lane N 1957 Pseudosarcoma (polypoid sarcoma-like masses) associated with squamous cell carcinoma of the mouth, fauces, and larynx. Report of ten cases. Cancer 10: 19–41
225. Goellner J R, Devine K D, Weiland L H 1973 Pseudosarcoma of the larynx. Am J Clin Pathol 59: 312–326
226. Toda S, Yonemitsu N, Miyabara S et al. 1989 Polypoid squamous cell carcinoma of the larynx. An immunohistochemical study for *ras* p21 and cytokeratin. Pathol Res Pract 185: 860–866
227. Leventon G S, Evans H L 1981 Sarcomatoid squamous cell carcinoma of the mucous membranes of the head and neck: a clinicopathologic study of 20 cases. Cancer 48: 994–1003
228. Batsakis J G, Rice D H, Howard D R 1982 The pathology of head and neck tumors. Spindle cell lesions (sarcomatoid carcinomas, nodular fasciitis, and fibrosarcoma) of the aerodigestive tracts, part 14. Head Neck Surg 4: 499–513
229. Weidner N 1987 Sarcomatoid carcinoma of the upper aerodigestive tract. Semin Diagn Pathol 4: 157–168
230. Mills SE, Gaffey MJ, Frierson HF Jr 2000 Tumors of the upper respiratory tract and ear. Atlas of tumor pathology, series 3, fascicle 26. Armed Forces Institute of Pathology, Washington, DC, p 98–106
231. Choi H R, Sturgis E M, Rosenthal D I et al. 2003 Sarcomatoid carcinoma of the head and neck. Molecular evidence for evolution and progression from conventional squamous cell carcinoma. Am J Surg Pathol 27: 1216–1220
232. Takubo K, Tsuchiya S, Nakagawa H et al. 1982 Pseudosarcoma of the esophagus. Hum Pathol 13: 503–505
233. Ellis G L, Corio R L 1980 Spindle cell carcinoma of the oral cavity. A clinicopathologic assessment of fifty-nine cases. Oral Surg 50: 523–534
234. Takata T, Ito H, Ogawa I et al. 1991 Spindle cell squamous carcinoma of the oral region. An immunohistochemical and ultrastructural study on the histogenesis and differential diagnosis with a clinicopathological analysis of six cases. Virchows Archiv [A] Pathol Anat 419: 177–182
235. Ro J Y, Chen J L, Lee J S et al. 1992 Sarcomatoid carcinoma of the lung. Immunohistochemical and ultrastructural studies of 14 cases. Cancer 69: 376–386
236. Olsen K D, Lewis J E, Suman V J 1997 Spindle cell carcinoma of the larynx and hypopharynx. Otolaryngol Head Neck Surg 116: 47–52
237. Klijanienko J, Vielh P, Duvillard P et al. 1992 True carcinosarcoma of the larynx. J Laryngol Otol 106: 58–60
238. Litzky L A, Brooks J J 1992 Cytokeratin immunoreactivity in malignant fibrous histiocytoma and spindle cell tumors: comparison between frozen and paraffin-embedded tissues. Mod Pathol 5: 30–34
239. Weidner N, Askin F B, Berthrong M et al. 1987 Bizarre (pseudomalignant) granulation-tissue reactions following ionizing-radiation exposure. A microscopic, immunohistochemical, and flow-cytometry study. Cancer 59: 1509–1514
240. Wenig B M, Devaney K, Bisceglia M 1995 Inflammatory myofibroblastic tumor of the larynx. A clinicopathologic study of eight cases simulating a malignant spindle cell neoplasm. Cancer 76: 2217–2229
241. Wain S L, Kier R, Vollmer R T et al. 1986 Basaloid-squamous carcinoma of the tongue, hypopharynx, and larynx: report of 10 cases. Hum Pathol 17: 1158–1166
242. Batsakis J G, El Naggar A 1989 Basaloid-squamous carcinomas of the upper aerodigestive tracts. Ann Otol Rhinol Laryngol 98: 919–920
243. Luna M A, El Naggar A, Parichatikanond P et al. 1990 Basaloid squamous carcinoma of the upper aerodigestive tract. Clinicopathologic and DNA flow cytometric analysis. Cancer 66: 537–542
244. Banks E R, Frierson H F Jr, Mills S E et al. 1992 Basaloid squamous cell carcinoma of the head and neck. A clinicopathologic and immunohistochemical study of 40 cases. Am J Surg Pathol 16: 939–946
245. Raslan W F, Barnes L, Krause J R et al. 1994 Basaloid squamous cell carcinoma of the head and neck: a clinicopathologic and flow cytometric study of 10 new cases with review of the English literature. Am J Otolaryngol 15: 204–211
246. Barnes L, Ferlito A, Altavilla G et al. 1996 Basaloid squamous cell carcinoma of the head and neck: clinicopathological features and differential diagnosis. Ann Otol Rhinol Laryngol 105: 75–82
247. Bahar G, Feinmesser R, Popovtzer A et al. 2003 Basaloid squamous carcinoma of the larynx. Am J Otolaryngol 24: 204–208
248. Wan S K, Chan J K C, Tse K C 1992 Basaloid-squamous carcinoma of the nasal cavity. J Laryngol Otol 106: 370–371
249. Saltarelli M G, Fleming M V, Wenig B M et al. 1995 Primary basaloid squamous cell carcinoma of the trachea. Am J Clin Pathol 104: 594–598
250. Epstein J I, Sears D L, Tucker R S et al. 1984 Carcinoma of the esophagus with adenoid cystic differentiation. Cancer 53: 1131–1136
251. Ferry J A, Scully R E 1988 "Adenoid cystic" carcinoma and adenoid basal carcinoma of the uterine cervix. A study of 28 cases. Am J Surg Pathol 12: 134–144
252. Tsang W Y W, Chan J K C, Lee K C et al. 1991 Basaloid-squamous carcinoma of the upper aerodigestive tract and so-called adenoid cystic carcinoma of the oesophagus: the same tumour type? Histopathology 19: 35–46
253. Abe K, Sasano H, Itakura Y et al. 1996 Basaloid-squamous carcinoma of the esophagus. A clinicopathologic, DNA ploidy, and immunohistochemical study of seven cases. Am J Surg Pathol 20: 453–461
254. Gerughty R M, Hennigar G R, Brown F M 1968 Adenosquamous carcinoma of the nasal, oral and laryngeal cavities. A clinicopathologic survey of ten cases. Cancer 22: 1140–1155
255. Kott E T, Goepfert H, Ayala A G et al. 1984 Lymphoepithelial carcinoma (malignant lymphoepithelial lesion) of the salivary glands. Arch Otolaryngol 110: 50–53
256. Suster S, Rosai J 1991 Thymic carcinoma. A clinicopathologic study of 60 cases. Cancer 67: 1025–1032
257. Micheau C, Luboinski B, Schwaab G et al. 1979 Lymphoepitheliomas of the larynx (undifferentiated carcinomas of nasopharyngeal type). Clin Otolaryngol 4: 42–48
258. Toker C, Peterson D W 1978 Lymphoepithelioma of the vocal cord. Arch Otolaryngol 104: 161–162
259. Ferlito A 1976 Histological classification of larynx and hypopharynx cancers and their clinical implications. Pathologic aspects of 2052 malignant neoplasms diagnosed at the ORL department of Padua University from 1966 to 1976. Acta Otolaryngol Suppl 342: 1–88
260. Andryk J, Freije J E, Schultz C J et al. 1996 Lymphoepithelioma of the larynx. Am J Otolaryngol 17: 61–63
261. Zbären P, Borisch B, Läng H et al. 1997 Undifferentiated carcinoma of nasopharyngeal type of the laryngopharyngeal region. Otolaryngol Head Neck Surg 117: 688–693
262. Marioni G, Mariuzzi L, Gaio E et al. 2002 Lymphoepithelial carcinoma of the larynx. Acta Otolaryngol 122: 429–434
263. Nappi O, Wick M R, Pettinato G et al. 1992 Pseudovascular adenoid squamous cell carcinoma of the skin. A neoplasm that may be mistaken for angiosarcoma. Am J Surg Pathol 16: 429–438
264. Thompson L D R, Wenig B M, Heffner D K et al. 1999 Exophytic and papillary squamous cell carcinoma of the larynx: a clinicopathologic series of 104 cases. Otolaryngol Head Neck Surg 120: 718–724
265. Suarez P A, Adler-Storthz K, Luna M A et al. 2000 Papillary squamous cell carcinoma of the upper aerodigestive tract: a clinicopathologic and molecular study. Head Neck 22: 360–368
266. Keelawat S, Liu C Z, Roehm P C et al. 2002 Adenosquamous carcinoma of the upper aerodigestive tract: a clinicopathologic study of 12 cases and review of the literature. Am J Otolaryngol 23: 160–168
267. Alos A, Castillo M, Nadal A et al. 2004 Adenosquamous carcinoma of the head and neck: criteria for diagnosis in a study of 12 cases. Histopathology 44: 570–579
268. Gould V E, Linnoila R I, Memoli V A et al. 1983 Neuroendocrine cells and neuroendocrine neoplasms of the lung. Pathol Ann 18: 287–330
269. Briselli M, Mark G J, Grillo H C 1978 Tracheal carcinoids. Cancer 42: 2870–2879
270. El-Naggar A K, Batsakis J G 1991 Carcinoid tumor of the larynx. A critical review of the literature. ORL J Otorhinolaryngol Relat Spec 53: 188–193
271. Tamai S, Iri H, Maruyama T et al. 1981 Laryngeal carcinoid tumor: light and electron microscopic studies. Cancer 48: 2256–2259
272. Stanley R J, DeSanto L W, Weiland L H 1986 Oncocytic and oncocytoid carcinoid tumors (well-differentiated neuroendocrine carcinomas) of the larynx. Arch Otolaryngol Head Neck Surg 112: 529–535
273. Baugh R F, Wolf G T, McClatchey K D et al. 1987 Carcinoid (neuroendocrine carcinoma) of the larynx. Ann Otol Rhinol Laryngol 96: 315–321
274. Woodruff J M, Senie R T 1991 Atypical carcinoid tumor of the larynx. A critical review of the literature. ORL J Otorhinolaryngol Relat Spec 53: 194–209
275. Ereno C, Lopez J I, Sanchez J M 1997 Atypical carcinoid of larynx: presentation with scalp metastases. J Laryngol Otol 111: 89–91
276. Ottinetti A, Colombo E, Dardano F et al. 2003 Cutaneous metastasis of neuroendocrine carcinoma of the larynx: report of a case. J Cutan Pathol 30: 512–515
277. Mills S E, Cooper P H, Garland T A et al. 1983 Small cell undifferentiated carcinoma of the larynx. Report of two patients and review of 13 additional cases. Cancer 51: 116–120
278. Gnepp D R, Ferlito A, Hyams V 1983 Primary anaplastic small cell (oat cell) carcinoma of the larynx. Review of the literature and report of 18 cases. Cancer 51: 1731–1745
279. Gnepp D R 1991 Small cell neuroendocrine carcinoma of the larynx. A critical review of the literature. ORL J Otorhinolaryngol Relat Spec 53: 210–219
280. Baugh R F, Wolf G T, McClatchey K D 1986 Small cell carcinoma of the head and neck. Head Neck Surg 8: 343–354
281. Medina J E, Moran M, Goepfert H 1984 Oat cell carcinoma of the larynx and Eaton–Lambert syndrome. Arch Otolaryngol 110: 123–126
282. Giddings N A, Kennedy T L, Vrabec D P 1987 Primary small cell carcinoma of the larynx: analysis of treatment. J Otolaryngol 16: 157–166
283. Ferlito A, Recher G, Caruso G 1985 Primary combined small cell carcinoma of the larynx. Am J Otolaryngol 6: 302–308
284. Chen D A, Mandell-Brown M, Moore S F et al. 1986 "Composite" tumor – mixed squamous cell and small cell anaplastic carcinoma of the larynx. Otolaryngol Head Neck Surg 95: 99–103
285. Aguilar E A III, Robbins K T, Stephens J et al. 1987 Primary oat cell carcinoma of the larynx. Am J Clin Oncol 10: 26–32
286. Pesce C, Tobia-Gallelli F, Toncini C 1984 APUD cells of the larynx. Acta Otolaryngol 98: 158–162
287. Whicker J H, Weiland L H, Neel H B III et al. 1974 Adenocarcinoma of the larynx. Ann Otol 83: 487–490

288. Fechner R E 1975 Adenocarcinoma of the larynx. Can J Otolaryngol 2: 284–289
289. Spiro R H, Hajdu S I, Lewis J S et al. 1976 Mucus gland tumors of the larynx and laryngopharynx. Ann Otol 85: 498–503
290. Hajdu S I, Huvos A G, Goodner J T et al. 1970 Carcinoma of the trachea. Clinicopathologic study of 41 cases. Cancer 25: 1448–1456
291. Crissman J D, Rosenblatt A 1978 Acinous cell carcinoma of the larynx. Arch Pathol Lab Med 102: 233–236
292. Ferlito A, Gale N, Hvala H 1981 Laryngeal salivary duct carcinoma: a light and electron microscopic study. J Laryngol Otol 95: 731–738
293. Mikaelian D O, Contrucci R B, Batsakis J G 1986 Epithelial-myoepithelial carcinoma of the subglottic region: a case presentation and review of the literature. Otolaryngol Head Neck Surg 95: 104–106
294. Pearson F G, Thompson D W, Weissberg D et al. 1974 Adenoid cystic carcinoma of the trachea. Experience with 16 patients managed by tracheal resection. Ann Thorac Surg 18: 16–29
295. Oloffsson J, van Nostrand A W P 1977 Adenoid cystic carcinoma of the larynx. A report of four cases and a review of the literature. Cancer 40: 1307–1313
296. Ferlito A, Caruso G 1983 Biological behaviour of laryngeal adenoid cystic carcinoma. Therapeutic considerations. ORL J Otorhinolaryngol Relat Spec 45: 245–256
297. Binder W J, Kaneko M, Som P et al. 1980 Mucoepidermoid carcinoma of the larynx. A case report and review of the literature. Ann Otol Rhinol Laryngol 89: 103–107
298. Damiani J M, Damiani K K, Hauck K et al. 1981 Mucoepidermoid-adenosquamous carcinoma of the larynx and hypopharynx: a report of 21 cases and a review of the literature. Otolaryngol Head Neck Surg 89: 235–243
299. Ferlito A, Recher G, Bottin R 1981 Mucoepidermoid carcinoma of the larynx. A clinicopathological study of 11 cases with review of the literature. ORL J Otorhinolaryngol Relat Spec 41: 280–299
300. Ho K-J, Jones J M, Herrera G A 1984 Mucoepidermoid carcinoma of the larynx: a light and electron microscopic study with emphasis on histogenesis. South Med J 77: 190–195
301. Ferlito A 1976 A pathologic and clinical study of adenosquamous carcinoma of the larynx. Report of four cases and review of the literature. Acta Otorhinolaryngol Belg 30: 379–389
302. Ellis G L, Auclair P L, Gnepp D R et al. 1991 Other malignant epithelial neoplasms. In: Ellis G L, Auclair P L, Gnepp D L (eds) Surgical pathology of the salivary glands. Saunders, Philadelphia, p 455–459
303. Heffner D K 1991 Sinonasal and laryngeal salivary gland lesions. In: Ellis G L, Auclair P L, Gnepp D L (eds) Surgical pathology of the salivary glands. Saunders, Philadelphia, p 554–557
304. Weber A L, Shortsleeve M, Goodman M et al. 1978 Cartilaginous tumors of the larynx and trachea. Radiol Clin North Am 16: 261–271
305. Cantrell R W, Jahrsdoerfer R A, Reibel J F et al. 1980 Conservative surgical treatment of chondrosarcoma of the larynx. Ann Otol Rhinol Laryngol 89: 567–571
306. Neel H B III, Unni K K 1982 Cartilaginous tumors of the larynx: a series of 33 patients. Otolaryngol Head Neck Surg 90: 201–207
307. Ferlito A, Nicolai P, Montaguti A et al. 1984 Chondrosarcoma of the larynx: review of the literature and report of three cases. Am J Otolaryngol 5: 350–359
308. Thompson L D R, Gannon F H 2002 Chondrosarcoma of the larynx, a clinicopathologic study of 111 cases with a review of the literature. Am J Surg Pathol 26: 836–851
309. Hyams V J, Rabuzzi D D 1970 Cartilaginous tumors of the larynx. Laryngoscope 80: 755–767
310. Burtner D, Goodman M, Montgomery W 1972 Elastic cartilaginous metaplasia of vocal cord nodules. Ann Otol Rhinol Laryngol 81: 844–847
311. Huizenga C, Balogh K 1970 Cartilaginous tumors of the larynx. A clinicopathologic study of 10 new cases and a review of the literature. Cancer 26: 201–210
312. Kleist B, Poetsch M, Lang C et al. 2002 Clear cell chondrosarcoma of the larynx. A case report of a rare histologic variant in an uncommon location. Am J Surg Pathol 26: 386–392
313. Goethals P L, Dahlin D C, Devine K D 1963 Cartilaginous tumors of the larynx. Surg Gynecol Obstet 117: 77–82
314. Bleiweiss I J, Kaneko M 1988 Chondrosarcoma of the larynx with additional malignant mesenchymal component (dedifferentiated chondrosarcoma). Am J Surg Pathol 12: 314–320
315. Brandwein M, Moore S, Som P et al. 1992 Laryngeal chondrosarcomas: a clinicopathologic study of 11 cases, including two "dedifferentiated" chondrosarcomas. Laryngoscope 102: 858–867
316. Rinaggio J, Duffey D, McGruff H S 2004 Dedifferentiated chondrosarcoma of the larynx. Oral Surg Oral Med Oral Pathol Oral Radiol Endod 97: 369–375
317. Gorenstein A, Neel H B III, Weiland L H et al. 1980 Sarcomas of the larynx. Arch Otolaryngol 106: 8–12
318. Ferlito A, Nicolai P, Barion U 1983 Critical comments on laryngeal fibrosarcoma. Acta Otorhinolaryngol Belg 37: 918–925
319. Winther L K, Lorentzen M 1978 Rhabdomyosarcoma of the larynx. Report of two cases and a review of the literature. J Laryngol Otol 92: 417–424
320. Balazs M, Egerszegi P 1989 Laryngeal botryoid rhabdomyosarcoma in an adult. Report of a case with electron microscopic study. Pathol Res Pract 184: 643–649
321. Libera D D, Falconieri G, Zanella M 1999 Embryonal "botryoid" rhabdomyosarcoma of the larynx: a clinicopathologic and immunohistochemical study of two cases. Ann Diagn Pathol 3: 341–349
322. Ferlito A, Nicolai P, Recher G et al. 1983 Primary laryngeal malignant fibrous histiocytoma: review of the literature and report of seven cases. Laryngoscope 93: 1351–1358
323. Dahm L J, Schaefer S D, Carder H M et al. 1978 Osteosarcoma of the soft tissue of the larynx. Report of a case with light and electron microscopic studies. Cancer 42: 2343–2351
324. Van Laer C G, Atkinson M W A, Helliwell T R et al. 1989 Osteosarcoma of the larynx. Ann Otol Rhinol Laryngol 98: 971–974
325. Quinn H J Jr 1984 Synovial sarcoma of the larynx treated by partial laryngectomy. Laryngoscope 94: 1158–1161
326. Pruszczynski M, Manni J J, Smedts F 1989 Endolaryngeal synovial sarcoma: case report with immunohistochemical studies. Head Neck 11: 76–80
327. Chew K K, Sethi D S, Stanley R E et al. 1992 View from beneath: pathology in focus. Synovial sarcoma of hypopharynx. J Laryngol Otol 106: 285–287
328. Wenig B M, Heffner D K 1995 Liposarcomas of the larynx and hypopharynx: a clinicopathologic study of eight new cases and a review of the literature. Laryngoscope 105: 747–756
329. Wenig B M, Weiss S W, Gnepp D R 1990 Laryngeal and hypopharyngeal liposarcoma: a clinicopathologic study of 10 cases with a comparison to soft tissue counterparts. Am J Surg Pathol 14: 134–141
330. DeLozier H L 1982 Intrinsic malignant schwannoma of the larynx. A case report. Ann Otol Rhinol Laryngol 91: 336–338
331. Paczona R, Jori J, Tiszlavicz L et al. 1999 Leiomyosarcoma of the larynx. Review of the literature and report of two cases. Ann Otol Rhinol Laryngol 108: 677–682
332. Ferlito A, Nicolai P, Caruso G 1985 Angiosarcoma of the larynx. Case report. Ann Otol Rhinol Laryngol 94: 93–95
333. Ferlito A 1978 Primary malignant haemangiopericytoma of the larynx. A case report with autopsy. J Laryngol Otol 92: 511–519
334. Abramowski C R, Witt W J 1983 Sarcoma of the larynx in the newborn. Cancer 51: 1726–1730
335. Pearson F G, Todd T R J, Cooper J D 1984 Experience with primary neoplasms of the trachea and carina. J Thorac Cardiovasc Surg 88: 511–518
336. Wang C C 1972 Malignant lymphoma of the larynx. Laryngoscope 82: 97–100
337. Ferlito A, Carbone A, Volpe R 1981 Diagnosis and assessment of non-Hodgkin's malignant lymphomas of the larynx. ORL J Otorhinolaryngol Relat Spec 43: 61–78
338. Swerdlow J B, Merl S A, Davey F R et al. 1984 Non-Hodgkin's lymphoma limited to the larynx. Cancer 53: 2546–2549
339. Gordon L J, Lee M, Conley J J et al. 1992 Mycosis fungoides of the larynx. Otolaryngol Head Neck Surg 107: 120–123
340. Kuhn J J, Wenig B M, Clark D A 1992 Mycosis fungoides of the larynx. Report of two cases and review of the literature. Arch Otolaryngol Head Neck Surg 118: 853–858
341. Bjelkenkrantz K, Lundgren J, Olosson J 1981 Extramedullary plasmacytoma of the larynx. J Otolaryngol 10: 28–34
342. Kost K M 1990 Plasmacytomas of the larynx. J Otolaryngol 19: 141–146
343. Ferguson J L, Maragos N E, Weiland L H 1987 Granulocytic sarcoma (chloroma) of the epiglottis. Otolaryngol Head Neck Surg 97: 588–590
344. Horny H-P, Parwaresch M R, Kaiserling E et al. 1986 Mast cell sarcoma of the larynx. J Clin Pathol 39: 596–602
345. El-Barbaray A E-S, Fouad H A, El-Sayed A F-I 1968 Malignant melanoma involving the larynx. Report of two cases. Ann Otol 77: 338–343
346. Reuter V E, Woodruff J M 1986 Melanoma of the larynx. Laryngoscope 96: 389–393
347. Wenig B M 1995 Laryngeal mucosal melanoma. A clinicopathologic, immunohistochemical, and ultrastructural study of four patients and a review of the literature. Cancer 75: 1568–1577
348. Eble J N, Hull M T, Bojrab D 1985 Laryngeal blastoma: a light and electron microscopic study of a novel entity analogous to pulmonary blastoma. Am J Clin Pathol 84: 378–385
349. Freeland A P, van Nostrand A W P, Jahn A F 1979 Metastases to the larynx. J Otolaryngol 8: 448–456
350. Oku T, Hasegawa M, Watanabe I et al. 1980 Pancreatic cancer with metastasis to the larynx. J Laryngol Otol 94: 1205–1209
351. Maung R, Burke R C, Hwang W S 1987 Metastatic renal carcinoma to larynx. J Otolaryngol 16: 16–18

肺和胸膜肿瘤
Tumors of the lung and pleura

Cesar A. Moran 和 Saul Suster 著

王功伟 译　回允中 校

引言	181
分类	181
支气管原性（"非小细胞"）癌	181
神经内分泌癌	187
涎腺型肿瘤	190
双相性上皮性/间叶性肿瘤	192
肺间叶性肿瘤	193
淋巴组织增生性疾病	197
来源于胚胎移位或异位组织的肿瘤	199
不能确定组织来源的肿瘤	201
其他良性肿瘤	203
肺转移性肿瘤	204
胸膜肿瘤	205

引言

目前，肺癌在许多发达国家是引起死亡的主要原因之一。已经明确这些肿瘤与吸烟有关，近年来观察到女性患者数量增加。然而，肺癌的病因似乎是多因素的，环境和遗传学状况均起到一定作用。其依据是这些肿瘤可以发生在儿童和非吸烟者。不过，绝大多数患者是伴有吸烟史的35岁以上的成人。不同组织学类型肺癌的发生频率有某种趋势。例如，目前在美国，腺癌是肺癌最常见的组织学类型；而在统计学上看，鳞状细胞癌是与吸烟关系最为密切的肿瘤。其他人口统计学趋势包括黑人男性肺癌发病率较白人高，而白人女性鳞状细胞癌发病率比黑人女性高。新近的观察显示，普通人群肺癌的发病率已经达到高峰，将来可能会下降[1-8]。无论这种假设正确与否，事实是肺癌仍然是一个严重的健康问题，而且是寻求医疗服务的主要原因。这些肿瘤的预后仍然很差，多数患者在诊断之后5年内死亡。因此，为了改善本病患者的预后，有必要进一步进行有关治疗和预防方面的研究。

分类

最被认可的肺肿瘤分类方法是世界卫生组织（WHO）提出的[9]。然而，目前这个分类正在评价之中，因为我们认识的这些肿瘤有许多新的进展，而且出现了一些新的组织病理学类型。因此，这些明显的变化将来有可能融入WHO的分类方案中。提出一个新的肺肿瘤的分类不在本章的范围之内。然而，为了便于研究，我们将遵循一种方案，试图概括我们理解的这些肿瘤目前的趋势，并且融入肺肿瘤病理学中最近描述的疾病（表5.1）。

支气管原性（"非小细胞"）癌
Bronchogenic（"non-small cell"）carcinomas

非小细胞性支气管原性癌是肺癌的最常见的形式；这些肿瘤通常累及50～60岁或60～70岁的个体[10]。很久以前已经证实，在这些肿瘤中有许多特异性的遗传学异常、生长因子异常的自分泌产物，以及促生长基因和肿瘤抑制基因的变化[11]。在肺癌中发现肿瘤抑制基因 *TP53* 的广泛突变。肺肿瘤中常见的事件是17p13一个等位基因的缺失，它是 *TP53* 所在的位点[12]。在体外应用烟草中的致癌物诱导出了肺癌的 *p53* 突变，支持这种突变可能直接与吸烟有关的观点[13]。肺癌的启动基因包括具有酪氨酸激酶受体功能的癌基因，例如表皮生长因

表5.1　肺肿瘤分类

I. 恶性上皮性肿瘤
    A. 支气管原性非小细胞癌
        腺癌
        亚型：细细支气管肺泡癌
            黏液性（所谓的"胶样"）癌
            乳头状癌
        鳞状细胞癌
        亚型：梭形细胞鳞癌
            基底细胞样癌
            淋巴上皮瘤样癌
        多形性癌（梭形/巨细胞癌）
        间变性大细胞癌
    B. 神经内分泌癌
        高分化神经内分泌癌（类癌）
        中分化神经内分泌癌（非典型性类癌）
        低分化神经内分泌癌
        亚型：小细胞癌
            混合性小细胞/大细胞癌
            大细胞神经内分泌癌
    C. 涎腺型肿瘤
        腺样囊性癌
        腺泡细胞癌（Fechner瘤）
        涎腺型混合瘤
        黏液表皮样癌
        上皮-肌上皮癌
        嗜酸细胞瘤
II. 双相性上皮性/间叶性肿瘤
    A. 癌肉瘤
    B. 肺母细胞瘤
III. 间叶性肿瘤
    良性间叶性肿瘤和肉瘤（所有类型）
IV. 淋巴增生性疾病
    非Hodgkin淋巴瘤
    淋巴瘤样肉芽肿病
    Hodgkin淋巴瘤
V. 来源于胚胎性移位或异位组织的肿瘤
    脑膜瘤
    胸腺瘤
    血管球瘤
    恶性黑色素瘤
    副神经节瘤
    神经节母细胞瘤
    生殖细胞肿瘤
VI. 不能确定组织来源的肿瘤
    支气管颗粒细胞瘤
    硬化性血管瘤
    透明细胞"糖"瘤
    炎性假瘤
VII. 其他良性肿瘤
    软骨性错构瘤
    支气管内脂肪瘤
    腺泡状腺瘤
    黏液腺腺瘤
    乳头状腺瘤
    纤维腺瘤
    肺微小化学感受器瘤
VIII. 肺转移性肿瘤

子受体以及myc和ras癌基因家族。ras癌基因家族的变化通常出现在非小细胞癌中，尤其是腺癌。肺肿瘤中最常见的突变性ras基因是K-ras；大约30%的肺腺癌显示K-ras 12号密码子突变。这种突变最常见于吸烟者，显示出吸烟与这些肿瘤发生之间的相互关系[14]。异常启动子甲基化是一种替代的通路，通过转录沉默基因缺失或突变造成其功能丧失[15]。在肺肿瘤和吸烟损伤的非恶性肺组织中，已经证实有多种基因的异常启动子的甲基化[16,17]。在癌症研究演化领域中进一步研究可以阐明肺癌发生分子特征中的其他重要的通路，例如最近的资料提示，存在EGFR突变可以预测对gefitinib（酪氨酸激酶靶向抑制剂）治疗有反应[18]。

支气管原性癌的症状取决于肿瘤的解剖学分布。位于中心的病变多半引起支气管阻塞的症状，包括咳嗽、咯血、呼吸困难、喘鸣或肺炎；位于周边的病变仅当肿瘤较大和侵犯周围结构时才发生症状。后一种肿瘤多半是在常规胸部X线检查时诊断的。在癌的某种亚型中，例如细支气管肺泡癌，患者可以表现为支气管漏（大量黏液性咳出物）[19]。肿瘤晚期可以侵犯周围结构，例如胸膜、胸壁和（或）纵隔，产生胸膜疼痛、Pancoast综合征或上腔静脉综合征的症状[10,19]。其他临床表现为副肿瘤综合征（paraneoplastic sydrome），例如抗利尿激素分泌障碍、Cushing综合征或肢端肥大症[10,19,20]。在某些情况下，腺癌可能伴有其他非肿瘤性肺病变，例如纤维化性肺疾病、结核、支气管扩张或肺炎[21-23]。鳞状细胞癌可伴有高钙血症。

在影像学研究中，腺癌可以表现为孤立性肺部肿物，边界清楚或不清[8,24]。在某些情况下，肿瘤可以沿着胸膜表面生长，类似于胸膜间皮瘤。当肿瘤位于周围并且较小时，薄层CT扫描可以有助诊断，因为在大约65%的病例中这种检查可以显示支气管含气造影图像和细支气管含气造影图像。这些特征可有助于区别癌和良性病变[25]。磁共振成像可能也有助于评价胸壁浸润，因为在T2加强成像中会有信号密度增加[26]。鳞状细胞癌常常是位于中心的生长在主支气管内的肿瘤。典型的X线表现是完全性或部分性支气管阻塞。这种临床表现可以导致阻塞性肺炎。对于成人的难治性肺炎应该密切注意存在潜在恶性肿瘤的可能性。

大体上，腺癌较常累及肺上叶，通常表现为胸膜下肿物或结节，伴有胸膜回缩。"瘢痕癌"（scar cancer）这个术语用于形容与瘢痕有关的胸膜下腺癌，它已经失去了临床意义，因为在多数病例中已经发现，"瘢痕"是对肿瘤本身继发的纤维组织增生性间质反应，而不是促成病变的原因。尽管鳞状细胞癌常常表现为阻塞支气管腔的中心性病变，但是在大约1/3的病例也可以表现为周围性肿物。大约10%鳞状细胞癌出现中心性空洞。

非小细胞癌一般采取手术切除治疗，并根据肿瘤分期辅以放疗或化疗。诊断时肿瘤的分期是评价预后的单一最重要的参数。分期越晚，预后越差。在某些类型的非小细胞癌中，例如多形性癌，肿瘤的侵袭性很强，平均生存期只有18个月。腺鳞癌也被认为是比普通鳞状细胞癌或腺癌侵袭性强的肿瘤。相反，细支气管肺泡癌和黏液性癌常常表现为低度恶性。然而，当细支气管肺泡癌弥漫累及肺大范围时，预后也是不容乐观的。

腺癌 Adenocarcinoma

原发性肺腺癌的定义是显示腺体分化特征的恶性上皮性肿瘤。根据腺体分化的程度和范围将腺癌分为高分化、中分化和低分化腺癌。高分化肿瘤的特征是形成完好的腺体增生，内衬非典型细胞，浸润周围间质；而低分化肿瘤细胞呈实性片块状生长，缺乏腺体或腺体结构形成不完整，是在有细胞内黏液产物的基础上被认定为腺癌的（图5.1）。高分化腺癌的腺体通常是由高柱状或黏液性上皮构成的，胞浆完全透明或嗜酸，细胞核位于基底部，核仁明显，核分裂象常见。在中分化腺癌中，腺体增生分布杂乱，其间有比较明显的间质反应和炎症，并且肿瘤细胞表现为比较明显的非典型性，核分裂象常见。这些

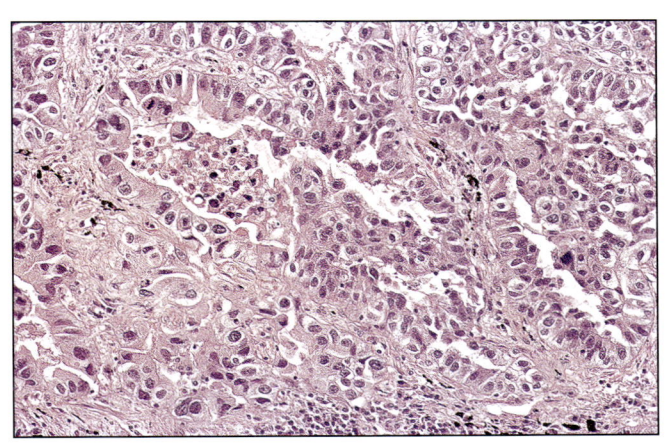

图5.1 肺中分化腺癌。

肿瘤的局部可以出现许多不常见的形态学表现。这些不常见的形态学特征中有些是确定肺腺癌组织学亚型的基础。在这方面，伴有广泛印戒细胞特征的肺腺癌特别具有侵袭性[27]。胎儿肺型腺癌在下文"肺母细胞瘤"标题下讨论。

细支气管肺泡癌
Bronchioloalveolar carcinoma

细支气管肺泡癌是一种独特类型的肿瘤，其特征是增生的肿瘤细胞完全沿着肺泡壁的内衬生长，称为"鳞屑性"（lepidic）生长方式[28]。细胞以轻度非典型性为特征，可以出现一些核分裂活性，但局限于肺泡壁，没有任何浸润到间质的证据（图5.2）。大体上，病变可

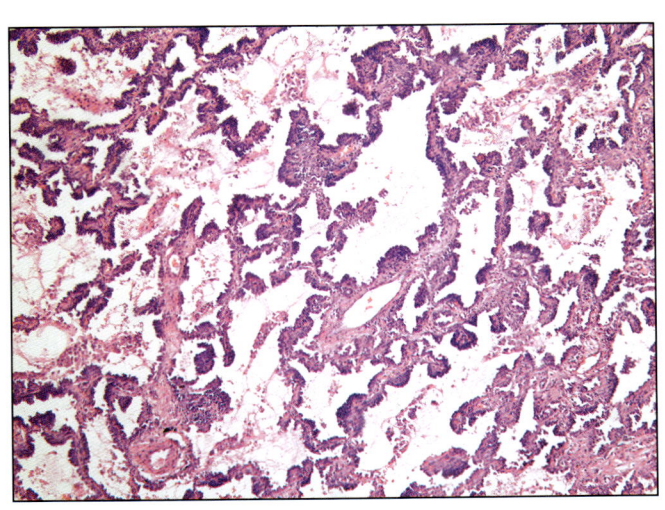

图5.2 细支气管肺泡癌。

以是单发性、多灶性或弥漫性。当肿瘤呈弥漫性生长时，大体和X线上病变的表现类似肺炎。有以下两种基本的组织学类型：（1）黏液型的特征是均匀一致的分泌黏液的柱状细胞增生，这些细胞完全取代了正常的肺泡内衬细胞；（2）非黏液型的特征是圆形或立方形细胞，胞浆稀少，核明显深染，常常形成"鞋钉样"结构。后者显示为Clara细胞或Ⅱ型肺泡细胞的超微结构特征。在某些病例，核内胞浆包涵体也是明显的特征。特别需要指出的是，许多普通腺癌病例可见局灶细支气管肺泡结构；这种肿瘤最好命名为"腺癌伴有细支气管肺泡特征"。细支气管肺泡癌的诊断不仅需要确定其独特的生长方式（包括缺乏形成完好的腺体），而且需要没有肿瘤浸润周围肺实质或间质的证据。同样值得注意的是，偶尔从其他器官转移到肺的腺癌也有细支气管肺泡生长方式，尤其是来自结肠、乳腺、胰腺、胃和肾的转移。

黏液性（所谓的"胶样"）癌 Mucinous (so-called "colloid") carcinoma

黏液性癌是最近描述的腺癌的亚型[29]。肺黏液性腺癌典型的生长方式是以大量黏液池集聚并破坏正常肺间质为特征（图5.3）。肺泡壁可以出现局灶性伴有非典型性的黏液上皮。这些肿瘤另外一个独特而又具有诊断意义的特征是黏液池内出现小簇状或单个散在的黏液性肿瘤细胞。过去，伴有同样组织学特征的肿瘤有几个诊断术语，其中包括黏液性囊腺瘤和交界恶性黏液性囊性肿瘤。因为它们具有向远处转移的能力和侵袭性的行为，我们喜欢将其通通命名为黏液性癌[29-31]。应该强调的是，黏液性癌的诊断是一种除外性诊断；除非临床和X线检查已经完全排除了其他部位（例如乳腺、结肠、胆囊和膀胱）存在原发性病变，否则不应作出黏液性腺癌的诊断。

乳头状癌 Papillary carcinoma

乳头状生长方式可以见于普通腺癌，伴有或不伴有明显的细支气管肺泡结构。然而，某些病例以乳头状生长方式为主，这种病变可以诊断为乳头状癌。在这样的病例中，肿瘤以出现大量伴有纤细的纤维结缔组织轴心的乳头为特征，乳头完全充满含气腔隙并且造成含气腔隙变形（图5.4）。间质中还可以出现沙粒体，类似于卵巢乳头状癌的表现。肺乳头状腺癌的发病率和死亡率明显高于细支气管肺泡癌也被证实[34]。肺乳头状癌还需要临床与病理密切联系，以排除从隐匿的或远处原发部位肿瘤转移而来的可能性。

鳞状细胞癌 Squamous cell carcinoma

肺鳞状细胞癌是指显示鳞状（表皮样）分化特征的恶性上皮性肿瘤。鳞状细胞癌分为高分化、中分化和低分化三种类型，取决于肿瘤内鳞状分化的程度，如是否存在细胞间桥和角化。高分化肿瘤的特征是片块状的肿瘤细胞形成砌砖样（pavement-like）结构，含有丰富的嗜酸性胞浆，细胞核圆形或卵圆形，有明显的核仁。细胞边界非常清楚，可见形成良好的细胞间桥（图5.5A）。在低分化肿瘤中，可能仅在局部见到上述特征，这些病变的特征是较明显的细胞非典型性，核分裂活性增加以及常常出现坏死和（或）出血区域。中心性粉刺样坏死通常见于较高分化的病变中（图5.5B）。有意思的是，

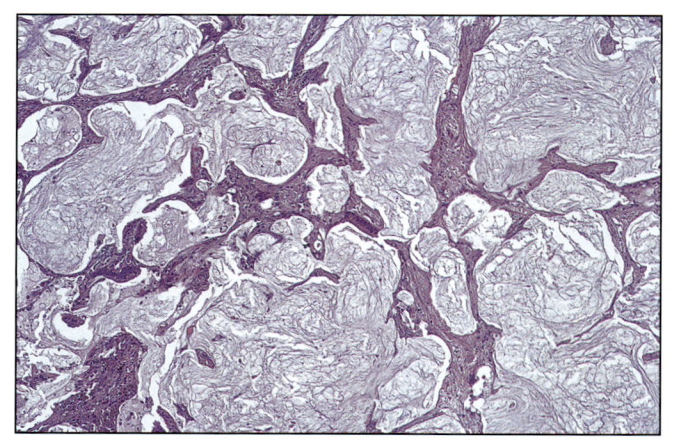

图5.3 黏液性（"胶样"）癌。

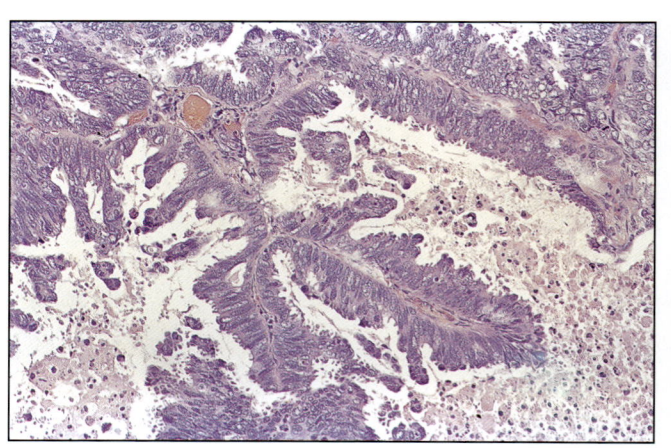

图5.4 肺的乳头状癌。

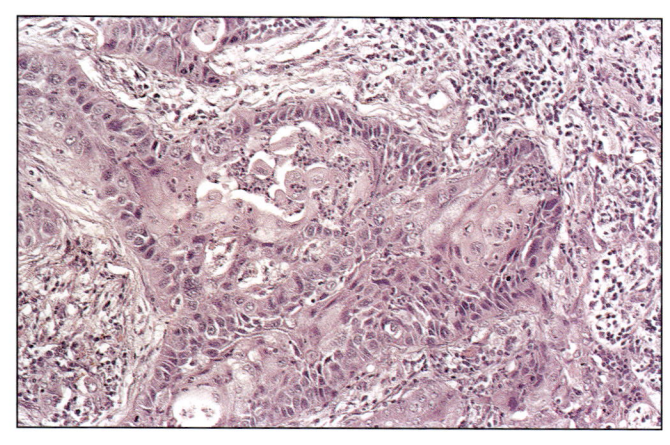
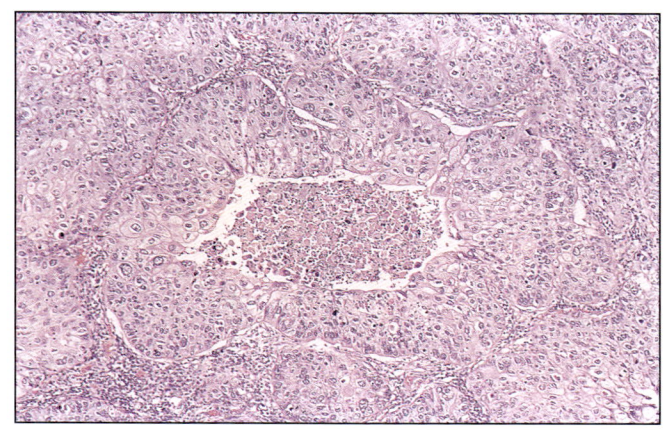

图5.5（A）高分化到中分化鳞状细胞癌；（B）低分化鳞状细胞癌伴有中心粉刺样坏死区域。

在鳞状细胞癌中可见原位癌，但不伴有肺腺癌。取自典型正常的支气管黏膜和典型鳞状细胞癌交界部位的切片常常表现出从鳞状化生到上皮内非典型增生（异型增生），再到原位癌的改变。由于糖原聚集，少数病变可能显示明显的胞浆透明。过去，这样的肿瘤被称为肺透明细胞癌，并被视为一个独立的分类。然而，伴有明显透明细胞改变的鳞状细胞癌与普通鳞状细胞癌具有相同的行为，因此它不需要作为一个单独的分类[35]。少数鳞状细胞癌可能形成支气管内息肉样肿物，有些类似于皮肤的角化棘皮瘤，这种病变有时称为外生性鳞状细胞癌[36]。这种肿瘤的分化通常很好，表现为其下固有层的轻微浸润。然而，其他三种少见的组织学类型也值得提及。

梭形细胞鳞状细胞癌
Spindle cell squamous carcinoma

梭形细胞鳞状细胞癌也叫肉瘤样癌（sarcomatoid carcinoma），它的特征是具有类似于肉瘤的表现[37,38]。这种肿瘤主要是由梭形细胞构成的，伴有细长的细胞核，中等量的胞浆以及突出的核仁。然而，局部区域通常可见梭形肿瘤细胞与普通的鳞状细胞癌混合存在（图5.6）。尽管某些肉瘤样癌病例可有明显的慢性炎症成分，并且酷似炎性假瘤，但其最重要的是与梭形细胞肉瘤鉴别[39]。梭形细胞鳞状细胞癌的特征是肿瘤细胞存在角蛋白反应，以及超微结构检查证实有张力丝和桥粒型细胞间连接[37]。梭形细胞鳞状细胞癌和多形性（梭形/巨细胞）癌之间存在某种程度的重叠（见第186页）。后者可能是同一肿瘤的一个分化较差的亚型，伴有较突出的细胞非典型性和多形性，多核肿瘤细胞以及相应较为明显的侵袭性行为。

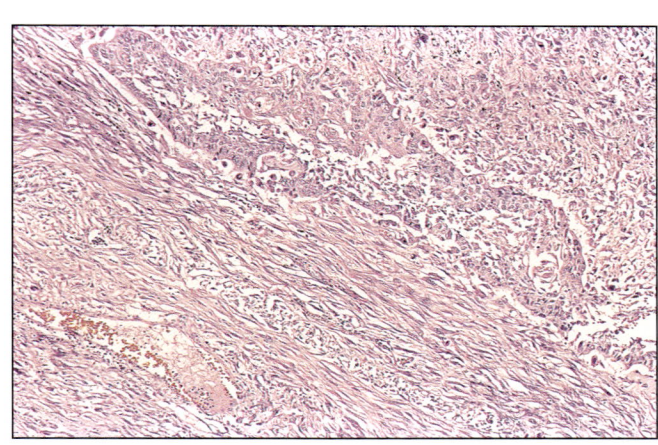

图5.6 来自鳞状细胞癌（上）的梭形细胞鳞状细胞癌。

基底细胞样癌　Basaloid carcinoma

基底细胞样癌是最近描述的一个支气管原性癌的亚型，其特征是相对大而深染的肿瘤细胞呈岛状增生，周围有明显栅栏状排列的细胞核（图5.7）。细胞常呈非典型性，核分裂象同样常见[40]。关于这个肿瘤是支气管原性癌的另外一个独特的亚型，还是仅为一种不常见而又非特异性的生长方式还有争论；然而，这种特征的病变好像比普通鳞状细胞癌具有更强的侵袭性的临床行为，因此将其视为一个独立的临床病理类型是有道理的[40]。

淋巴上皮瘤样癌
Lymphoepithelioma-like carcinoma

淋巴上皮瘤样癌[41,42]相当于低分化鳞状细胞癌伴有明显的淋巴细胞间质，类似于发生在鼻咽部的淋巴上皮瘤样癌。肿瘤细胞的特征是大的空泡状细

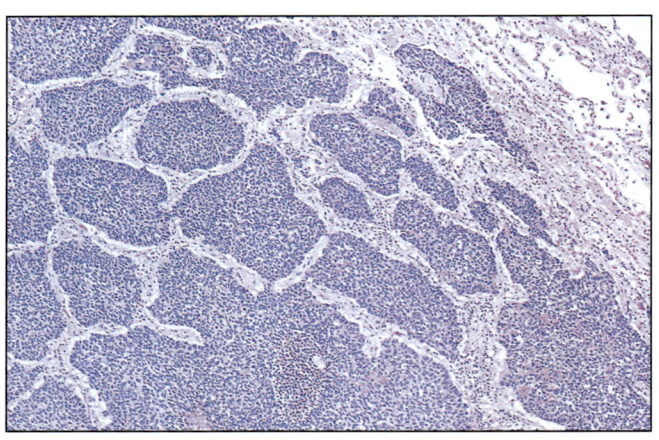

图5.7 基底细胞样癌中的实性肿瘤细胞岛,周围有栅栏状排列的细胞核。

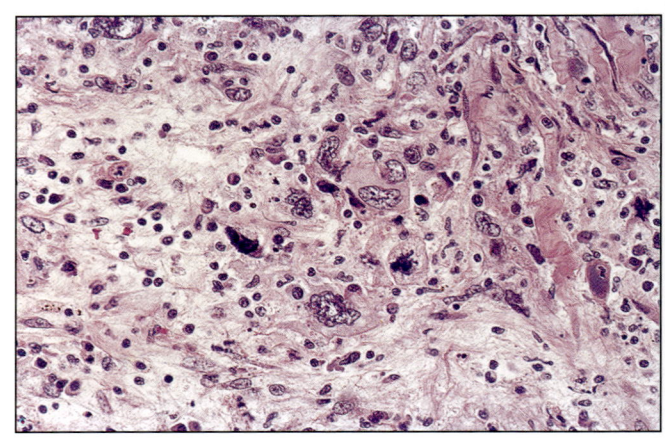

图5.9 肺大细胞癌。注意奇异的肿瘤细胞,周围有丰富的炎性浸润。

胞核,伴有明显的嗜酸性核仁,周围有一圈少量的胞浆。肿瘤细胞岛的特征是被明显的淋巴浆细胞宿主反应所围绕。仅在少数病例中证实 EB 病毒血清学阳性[41,42]。

多形性癌　Pleomorphic carcinoma

这种肿瘤以前被称为巨细胞癌或伴有假肉瘤性间质的癌[43,44]。这些肿瘤的特征是高度多形性,具有核分裂活跃的巨细胞和梭形肿瘤细胞团,通常伴有出血和(或)坏死区域(图5.8)。其主要的组织学成分是梭形细胞成分,通常混有高度多形性的恶性巨细胞成分。在某些病例中,可见局灶性普通腺癌或鳞状细胞癌区域,因此,有些作者把这种病变视为一个表型而不是一个独立病变[45]。然而,一般认为这种肿瘤是重新发生的,与任何普通类型的癌,例如腺癌或鳞状细胞癌没有任何关系[43,46]。正如它的名字所提示的一样,这种肿瘤不同于鳞状细胞癌的梭形细胞亚型,它有显著的多形性和突出的巨细胞成分。这种类型的病例似乎具有较差的预后[44]。

大细胞癌　Large cell carcinoma

也被称为未分化大细胞癌或间变性癌,是指由片块状低分化大细胞组成的肿瘤,它不显示任何明显向腺癌或鳞状细胞癌分化的组织学特征。旧的"未分化大细胞癌"的名称应该弃用,因为通过免疫组织化学和超微结构研究已经充分证实了肿瘤的上皮性本质;因此,较准确的命名应该是低分化间变性癌而不是未分化[9]。这一组肿瘤有别于多形性癌,它缺乏大细胞成分或非典型性多核细胞和瘤巨细胞。这些肿瘤的组织学特征是成片的肿瘤性大细胞,伴有圆形或卵圆形的细胞核,核仁明显,核分裂活性增加以及明显的细胞非典型性。某些病例的另外一个明显的特征是间质中存在大量的多形核白细胞,与间变的肿瘤细胞相混合(图5.9)。另外还有具有突出的"横纹样"特征的肿瘤病例,伴有丰富的偏心性强嗜酸性胞浆包涵体,由漩涡状的胞浆内中间丝组成,这种结构也可见于其他类型非小细胞癌[47]。

混合性肿瘤　Mixed tumors

显示上述几种类型特征的混合性肿瘤在临床实践中并不少见。在这个范畴中最常见的类型是腺鳞癌。如同名字的含义一样,这些肿瘤显示有普通腺癌和鳞状细胞癌两种表现的区域(图5.10)。有人提出,任何一种成分至少必须达到5%～10%才能作出这种诊断[48-50]。在少数病例中,两种成分之间可能有明显界限,而在另外一些病例中则可表现为两种成分密切混合。腺鳞癌不

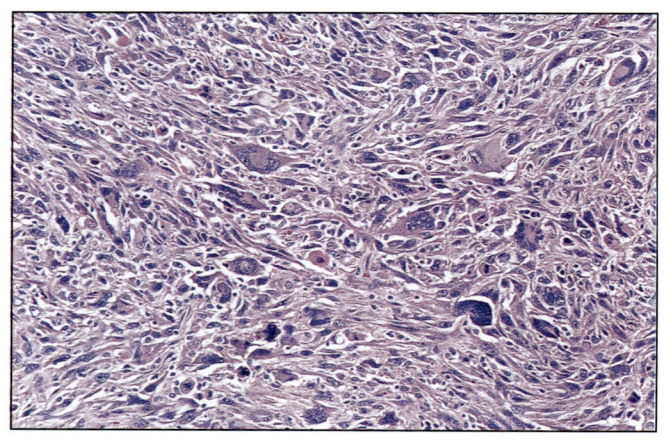

图5.8 多形性(梭形和巨细胞)癌。

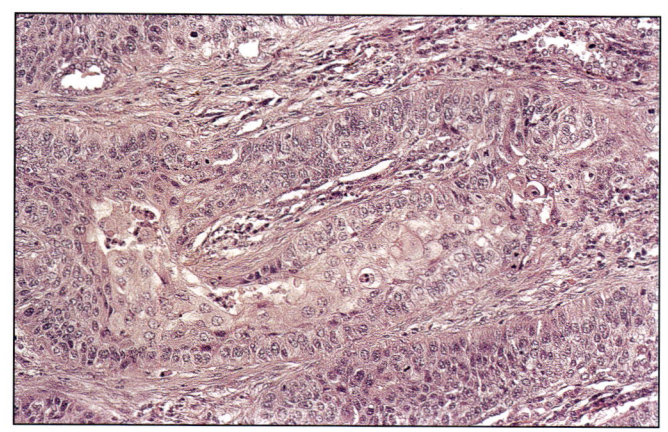

图5.10 腺鳞癌。

同于黏液表皮样癌,因为后者见不到完整的腺体结构。这种类型肿瘤的临床意义尚不明确;然而,腺鳞癌好像比普通的单纯性鳞状细胞癌或腺癌具有较强的侵袭性行为。

其他的组合也不少见,如腺癌或鳞状细胞癌伴有小细胞神经内分泌癌的区域(见下文)。这样的肿瘤在旧版WHO肺小细胞癌分类中被称为"混合性"癌("combined" carcinomas)。

神经内分泌癌
Neuroendocrine carcinoma

这一节中所应用的"神经内分泌"这个术语指的是肿瘤含有部分神经内分泌分化的证据,从非常高分化的神经内分泌肿瘤(传统上称为类癌)到伴有神经内分泌特征的低分化恶性肿瘤,典型的是小细胞癌。这些病变的亚分类有些争议;不过,目前通用的分类方法具有可重复性和临床意义[51]。神经内分泌分化在形态学水平上的定义是存在典型的器官样生长方式,在超微结构水平上有致密核心的神经分泌颗粒,而在免疫组化水平上存在神经内分泌标记物的免疫反应,例如嗜铬素A、突触素,或肽类激素,例如5-羟色胺、肾上腺皮质激素和蛙皮素(bombesin)[52]。最近,由于采用命名为大细胞神经内分泌癌的新的分类而引起了许多争议。还不能确定这样的肿瘤是独立的临床病理类型还是仅仅相当于显示假的或异常的神经内分泌分化的低分化癌。这个分类需要进一步研究,以便确定与非小细胞支气管原性癌相比,它们的预后和对治疗的反应是否存在差别[53-55]。

有些神经内分泌癌的一个重要的临床相关性是由于肽类激素异常表达而发生副肿瘤综合征,包括Cushing综合征和抗利尿激素分泌障碍综合征。大约10%的高分化神经内分泌癌病例伴有类癌综合征[56,57]。肺神经内分泌癌的临床症状取决于肿瘤大小、部位和生物学活性。这些肿瘤一般位于支气管内,从而引起哮喘、咳嗽、咯血等症状。X线检查显示,肿瘤可以部分或完全阻塞支气管腔。然而,高分化肿瘤(类癌)也可以位于肺的周边。这些肿瘤最常发生在于40~50岁和60~70岁的成人,没有性别差异。然而,这种肿瘤现在更常见于较年轻的患者。

高分化神经内分泌癌(类癌)
Well-differentiated neuroendocrine carcinoma (carcinoid tumor)

肺的高分化神经内分泌癌的标志是存在非常温和的单形性肿瘤细胞群,其特征是具有发育良好的"器官样"或神经内分泌生长方式,形成被纤细的纤维血管间隔分开的界限清楚的肿瘤细胞巢(细胞球,zellballen;图5.11A)。这些肿瘤其他常见的生长方式包括匍行性肿瘤细胞条索和条带,排列成缎带状或花边样结构,或形成小的玫瑰花环样微小腺泡状结构(图5.11B)。在细胞学形态上看,肿瘤细胞相对小,圆形或多角形,细胞核位于中心,有丰富的轻度嗜酸性的颗粒状胞浆。细胞核通常显示散在的粗糙点彩状染色质(椒盐状,salt-and-pepper),偶见小的核仁。通常缺乏核分裂活性,但偶尔可以出现(每10个高倍视野多达1~2个核分裂象)。坏死和出血不是这些肿瘤的特征。几种不常见的组织学亚型包括:主要由伴有明显的嗜酸性胞浆的细胞构成的肿瘤(嗜酸细胞性类癌,oncocytic carcinoid),色素沉着性黑色素性肿瘤(色素沉着性类癌,pigmented carcinoid),伴有化生性骨形成的类癌以及以腺体形成和丰富的间质黏液产物为特征的肿瘤[58-62]。另外一种少见的亚型是主要由排列成束的梭形细胞组成的肿瘤,类似于肉瘤或其他梭形细胞肿瘤;后者常常位于肺周围。然而,类癌出现梭形细胞生长方式不应被认为是"非典型性类癌"的同义语。这些肿瘤多数位于中心,并且表现为边界清楚的息肉样支气管内病变,表面被覆完整的支气管黏膜。这种肿瘤大约占肺肿瘤的1%~2%,可以发生在任何年龄组。在多数情况下非常容易诊断,而且可以通过应用组织化学染色(亲银反应阴性和嗜银反应阳性)、免疫组织化学染色(广谱和低分子量角蛋白、嗜铬素、突触素、神经元特异性烯醇化酶、5-羟色胺以及蛙皮素阳性)以及电子显微镜检查(证实神经分泌颗粒的密度)可协调诊断。绝大多数肿瘤可以通过手术切除治愈。然而,大约10%~15%的病例可以发

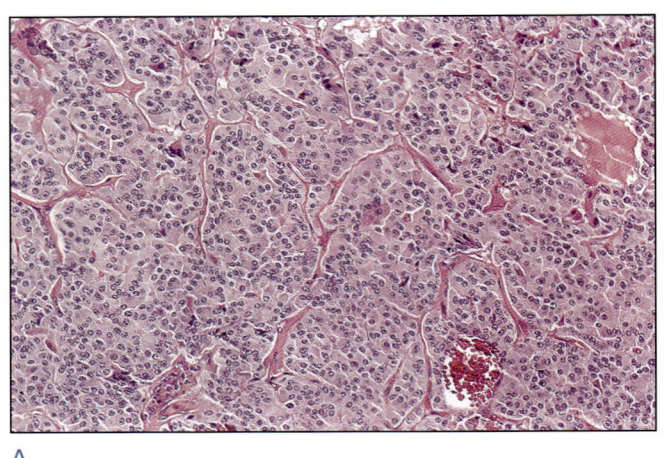 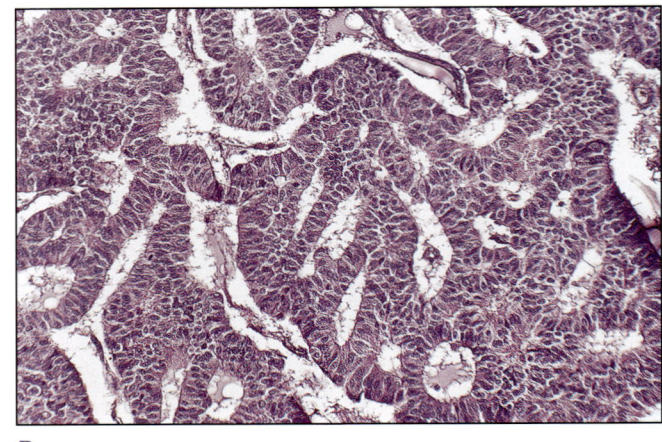

图5.11 （A）高分化神经内分泌癌（支气管类癌型）显示明显的神经内分泌（细胞球）生长方式；（B）高分化神经内分泌癌（支气管类癌型）伴有带状、小梁状生长方式。

生区域性转移，这就是最好把它们看做是低度恶性肿瘤的原因。与肺外类癌不同，这些病变以及非典型性类癌 TTF-1 染色总是阳性[63]。

中分化神经内分泌癌（非典型性类癌）
Moderately differentiated neuroendocrine carcinoma（atypical carcinoma）

肺中分化神经内分泌癌是 Arrigoni 等于 1972 年首次描述的[64]，作者注意到其与类癌具有许多共同特征，但又具有明显的细胞非典型性和核分裂活性的肺部病变，这些病变显示出具有较大的转移和侵袭性行为的倾向。这些肿瘤是中分化的病变，从概念上讲，它们在肺的神经内分泌肿瘤分化谱系中处于中间分化的位置。组织学上，这些肿瘤与普通的肺类癌具有许多共同的特征，不同之处在于前者具有明显的细胞非典型性，核分裂活性增加（每 10 个高倍视野大于 5 个核分裂象）以及常出现坏死灶[64-67]。肿瘤细胞通常显示较高的核浆比例、明显的核仁以及异常的核分裂象。通常可见中心粉刺样坏死区域（图 5.12）。这些肿瘤通常为浸润性，而且常常显示血管和淋巴管浸润灶。肿瘤大小和分期增加、高核分裂率、细胞非典型性程度以及坏死可能与预后不良有关[68]。

低分化神经内分泌癌
Poorly differentiated neuroendocrine carcinoma

这一组肿瘤处于肺神经内分泌肿瘤谱系中最不分化的一端，由高级别肿瘤构成，临床上具有高度侵袭性的行为。其中某些病例可能难以证实神经内分泌分化的特

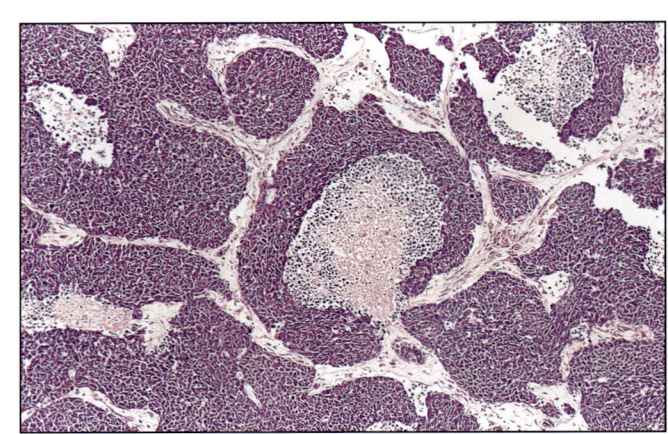

图5.12 中分化神经内分泌癌（非典型性类癌型）。

征，并且不是所有肿瘤对于神经内分泌标记物免疫组化染色都能给出期望的阳性反应。诊断基本依靠常规光镜检查，辨认出特征性的细胞学改变。旧的 WHO 术语分为三种形式：小细胞（燕麦细胞）、中等细胞以及混合性细胞。最近，一个新的低分化神经内分泌癌的亚型增加到了这个分类中，即大细胞神经内分泌癌[53,54]。后者是否真正代表独立的临床病理类型目前还有争议；然而，这一节中的低分化神经内秘癌包括这种病变，即承认这类肿瘤是伴有神经内分泌特征的高级别肺癌的一种新的亚型。

肺的低分化神经内分泌癌大约占支气管原性癌的 20%，最常发生在 50～70 岁的患者。这些肿瘤的特征是早期迅速播散[62,63]。然而，最近随着 X 线检查和化学治疗的进展，某些患者症状明显缓解、生存时间延长。临床上，这些肿瘤通常位于中心，表现为气道阻塞的症状。肿瘤常常早期播散到纵隔，引起上腔静脉综合

征、声嘶和吞咽困难。广泛的肺门和纵隔淋巴结转移是常见的转移模式。常见的胸腔外转移部位包括骨、骨髓、肝和脑。伴有副肿瘤综合征是小细胞肺癌的特征，例如 Cushing 综合征、抗利尿激素分泌障碍综合征以及 Eaton-Lambert 综合征。

小细胞癌　Small cell carcinoma

小细胞肺癌的特征是原始的圆形或卵圆形的肿瘤细胞增生，细胞平均大小是正常小淋巴细胞的 2～3 倍。在典型的燕麦细胞癌亚型中，肿瘤细胞形成杂乱排列的单形性肿瘤细胞片块，可以被纤细的纤维分隔，并可见大片坏死区域（图 5.13A）。细胞很小，伴有少量胞浆，核圆形或卵圆形，染色质致密，呈颗粒状。核仁通常不明显或缺乏，肿瘤细胞的特征是核分裂活跃。在血管壁内有嗜碱性 DNA 物质沉积，称为核的包壳（nuclear encrustation）或 Azzopardi 现象，它是这些肿瘤的另外一个特征。在小的内镜活检标本中，肿瘤细胞往往显示明显的变形和挤压，这个表现传统上认为与小细胞癌有关，但也可见于淋巴细胞肿瘤。梭形细胞核是其另外一个特征，偶尔可见（图 5.13B）。少数小细胞癌可见肿瘤细胞呈小梁状或缎带样排列，周围细胞核呈栅栏状，并且形成玫瑰花环样微腺泡结构，这些特征提示较高程度的分化（例如非典型性类癌）。然而，它们偶尔可以见于以低分化神经内分泌肿瘤为主的肿瘤，而且很有可能是代表同一肿瘤中高级别和中级别分化区域之间的转化。在"中间"亚型的小细胞癌中，细胞似乎较大，卵圆或多角形，伴有较明显的核多形性、少量点彩状染色质、较突出的核仁以及较丰富的胞浆（图 5.13C）。后面这些特征在固定良好的标本中容易识别。这样的病例 TTF-1 阳性，结合 p63 阴性，有助于与低分化鳞状细胞癌鉴别。

混合性小细胞/大细胞癌
Mixed small cell/large-cell carcinoma

混合性小细胞/大细胞癌的特征是在普通的肺小细胞癌中出现单个或小簇状大而未分化的肿瘤细胞亚群[71,72]。大细胞的大小通常是小细胞的两倍，细胞核大而深染，周围有少量双染性到轻度嗜酸性的胞浆（图 5.14）。通常可以见到连续的细胞类型，从典型的小细胞（燕麦细胞）到大细胞都有。在普通小细胞癌的转移部位，也常常可以见到大细胞成分与小细胞混合存在。混合性小细胞/大细胞癌与典型的小细胞癌相比，生存率似乎较差，而且对于治疗的反应也很有限[71,73]。

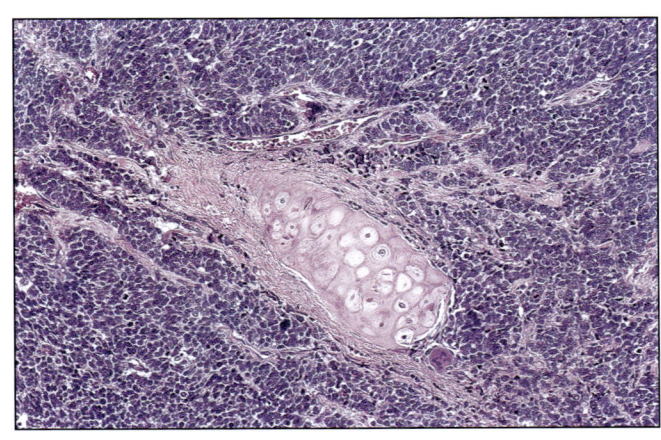

A

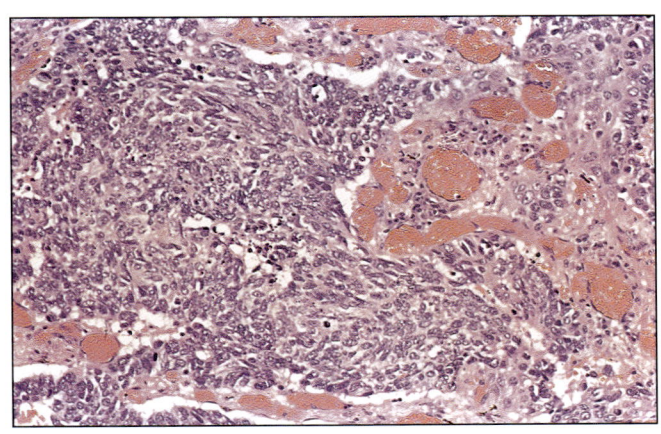

B

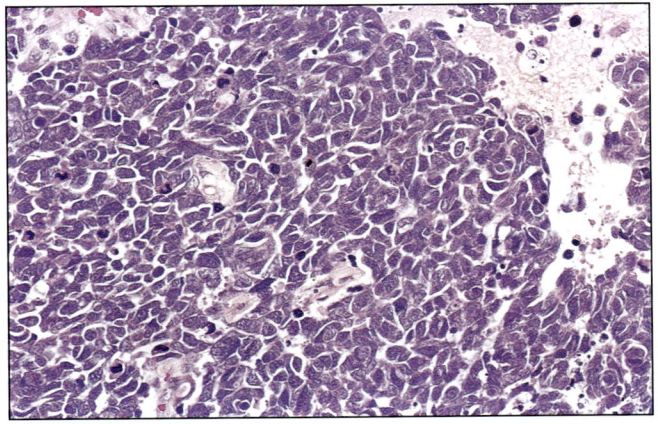

C

图 5.13　（A）肺的低分化神经内分泌癌，小细胞型；（B）小细胞癌伴有梭形细胞特征；（C）小细胞癌，中间细胞型。

大细胞神经内分泌癌
Large-cell neuoendocrine carcinoma

大细胞神经内分泌癌是一个有争议的分类，其真正的临床意义以及诊断的组织病理学标准仍未完全确定。

涎腺型肿瘤

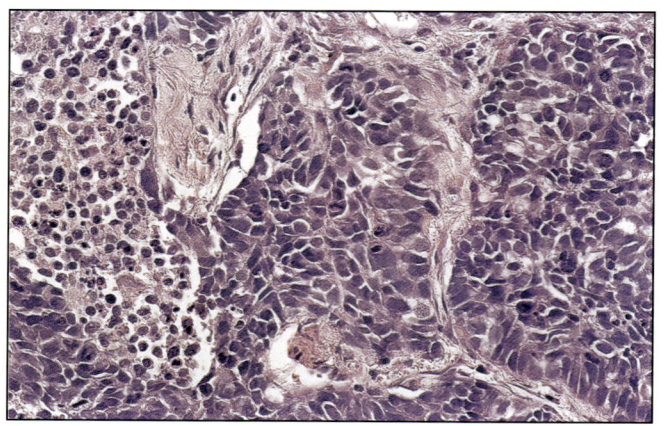

图5.14 肺的低分化神经内分泌癌，混合性小细胞/大细胞型。

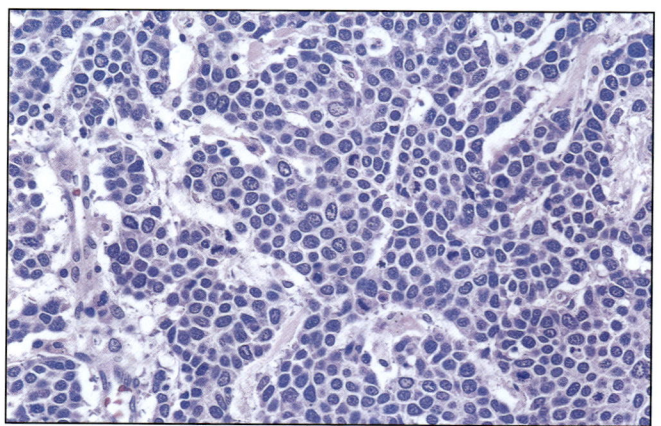

图5.15 大细胞神经内分泌癌。

概括说来，这种病变总的组织病理学表现是低分化非小细胞癌。然而，增生的细胞局灶性可以排列成缎带状或条索状，混有玫瑰花环样结构，赋予这种病变一种模糊的神经内分泌的表现（图5.15）。另外，肿瘤细胞可能显示神经内分泌标记物染色阳性，例如突触素或嗜铬素[53-55]。肿瘤中还可能见到的另外一种特征是存在"基底细胞样"表现的区域。后一种特征类似于基底细胞样癌，它是鳞状细胞癌的一个亚型。这两种肿瘤是否是同一种疾病还存在争议。是应该把大细胞神经内分泌癌看做是神经内分泌癌的独特亚型，还是仅仅应该看做是伴有神经内分泌标记物异常表达的非小细胞癌的亚型，这个问题还没有得到解决。

涎腺型肿瘤 Salivary gland-type tumors

这是一种少见的肺原发性肿瘤，组织学重现了涎腺肿瘤的表现（见第7章）。因为这些肿瘤的组织学特征与对应的涎腺肿瘤无法区分，故在肺中作出这种类型肿瘤诊断之前，必须获得全部病史以排除从头颈部原发肿瘤转移而来的可能性。这些肿瘤多半起源于支气管黏膜下腺体；不过，并不是所有肿瘤的发生都与支气管有关。在少数情况下，它们可以发生在肺实质内或肺的周围，与支气管结构没有直接联系。

一般来说，肺的原发性涎腺型肿瘤少见。然而，近些年来已有几个报道论述其生物学行为并提出组织病理学特征谱系[74-83]。尽管见于涎腺的多数肿瘤也可见于肺，当将这两个部位进行对比时，发现其发病率并不存在平行的关系。例如，混合瘤是涎腺最常见的肿瘤，而在肺却罕见。还有，这些病变的组织学特征和行为也存在着其他微小的差别。这些肿瘤可以发生在任何年龄组，没有性别差异。对于肺或肺段好像没有任何特别的好发部位。临床上，这些肿瘤最常表现为支气管内病变，导致与支气管阻塞有关的症状，包括咳嗽、呼吸困难和咯血。位于肺周围的病变多半没有症状，是在常规胸部X线检查中偶尔发现的。

作为一组肿瘤，当完全切除时，涎腺型肿瘤往往具有低级别肿瘤的行为，伴有良好的临床预后。尤其是涎腺型混合瘤、腺泡细胞癌、低级别黏液表皮样癌、上皮-肌上皮癌仅仅通过手术切除即可治愈。然而也有某些例外；例如腺样囊性癌可能具有侵袭性的经过，伴有远处播散和高死亡率，取决于最初诊断时的分期。诊断时处于晚期的肿瘤常常证明是致命性的，与组织学特征无关。低分化涎腺型混合瘤和高级别组织学表现的黏液表皮样癌也显示出高度侵袭性的行为，可因广泛转移而导致死亡。

腺样囊性癌 Adenoid cystic carcinoma

支气管的腺样囊性癌可有多种组织学生长方式：（1）筛状（圆柱瘤性）；（2）管状；（3）实性[75]。其中，筛状生长方式最常见，其特征是肿瘤细胞巢和细胞岛具有轮廓清楚的腔隙，其内常常充满黏液性物质（图5.16）。肿瘤细胞岛被纤维带分隔，组成细胞伴有轮廓清晰的圆形细胞核和少量嗜酸性胞浆。囊性区域由两排细胞构成，通常缺乏核分裂象。实性生长方式最不常见，其特征是类似的细胞形成弥漫性片块状结构。核分裂象较常见于后一种生长方式。神经周围浸润是腺样囊性癌另外一个常见的特征；然而，虽然在局部复发中可能具有一定作用，但这个特征与预后较差无关。预测这些肿瘤预后的唯一可靠参数是最初诊断时的分期。免疫组化染色可以识别腺体分泌和肌上皮成分。应用广谱角蛋白和癌胚抗原（CEA）染色腺体成

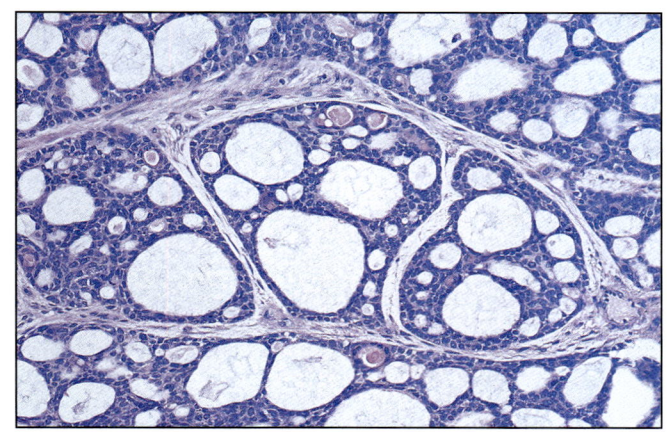

图5.16 腺样囊性癌,圆柱瘤性结构。

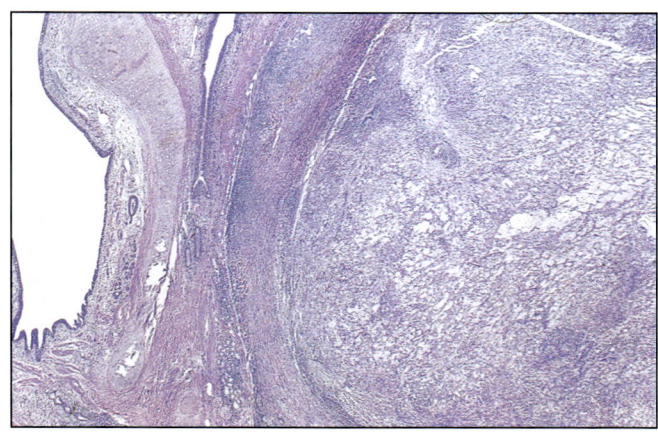

图5.17 支气管腺体涎腺型混合瘤。

分呈强阳性；肌上皮成分共同表达角蛋白和肌动蛋白中间丝，以及不同程度地表达波形蛋白（vimentin）、S-100蛋白和胶质纤维酸性蛋白（glial fibrillary acidic protein, GFAP）[75]。

腺泡细胞癌（Fechner瘤）
Acinic cell carcinoma（Fechner tumor）

这是少见的原发性低级别肺肿瘤，在儿童和成人均有报道[76,77]。转移似乎非常少见。这些肿瘤具有几种形态学生长方式，包括腺泡样、囊性或乳头囊性、巢状以及嗜酸细胞性。这些病变的特征是透明细胞的肿瘤性增生，细胞核向周围移位（类似于印戒细胞），含有丰富的颗粒状嗜酸性胞浆，PAS染色呈强阳性反应。肿瘤可以排列成巢，被纤细的纤维带分隔。在其他区域，肿瘤可以含有内衬肿瘤细胞的囊性间隙。有些肿瘤主要由嗜酸性细胞构成，表现为明显的巢状生长方式，因此非常类似于神经内分泌肿瘤。肿瘤细胞出现PAS阳性染色有助于诊断。然而，最重要的诊断特征是通过电镜检查发现600～800 nm有界膜的细胞内酶原颗粒[76,77]。在这些肿瘤中免疫组化染色价值有限，免疫表型基本符合分泌性上皮细胞。据报道，胰淀粉酶免疫染色对于涎腺腺泡细胞癌的诊断有所帮助，但是根据我们的经验，这个抗体在肺原发性肿瘤中很少呈阳性。

涎腺型混合瘤
Salivary gland-type mixed tumor

这类肿瘤的定义为间叶和上皮成分的双相性肿瘤。上皮成分通常形成导管、腺体和实性区域，由相当小的嗜酸性或透明细胞构成，细胞核圆形或卵圆形，核仁不明显。有些病例中实性细胞增生可以表现为浆细胞样外观。在多数病例中，主要成分是实性肌上皮细胞增生。免疫组化染色显示角蛋白和肌动蛋白共同表达，证实这些细胞本质上是肌上皮细胞。肌上皮性肿瘤细胞还强烈表达波形蛋白，而且S-100蛋白和GFAP可有不同程度的阳性。混合瘤中间叶性间质成分的特征是疏松的软骨黏液样组织，在少数情况下可以形成软骨基质（图5.17）。要注意的是，尽管腮腺混合瘤中最主要的间叶成分是成熟的软骨，但是这种分化在肺的涎腺型混合瘤中并不常见。这种肿瘤可以完全为实性，显示轻到中度核分裂活性，但其行为仍然是低级别方式，完全手术切除通常可以治愈。存在核分裂活动增加、坏死、血管浸润以及明显的细胞非典型性可以提示病理医师有恶性混合瘤的可能[80]。这种肿瘤的行为类似于高级别恶性肿瘤，具有广泛转移的能力和致命的后果。

黏液表皮样癌
Mucoepidermoid carcinoma

黏液表皮样癌是最常见的肺原发性涎腺型肿瘤，是儿童最常见的肺原发性肿瘤之一。这些肿瘤可以分成低级别肿瘤和高级别肿瘤。它们的特征是显示表皮样分化的细胞呈片块状分布，混合有含细胞内和细胞外黏液的黏液细胞（图5.18）。较实性的成分可以主要由透明细胞构成，位于纤维性间质中。在低级别肿瘤中，实性或表皮样成分缺乏明显的细胞非典型性或核分裂活性。出现明显的细胞非典型性和核分裂活性以及坏死和出血区域是高级别肿瘤的特征。在任何一个肿瘤中均可见低级别和高级别恶性之间的过渡区。在同一个肿瘤中如果缺乏高分化黏液表皮样癌成分，则无法区分高级别黏

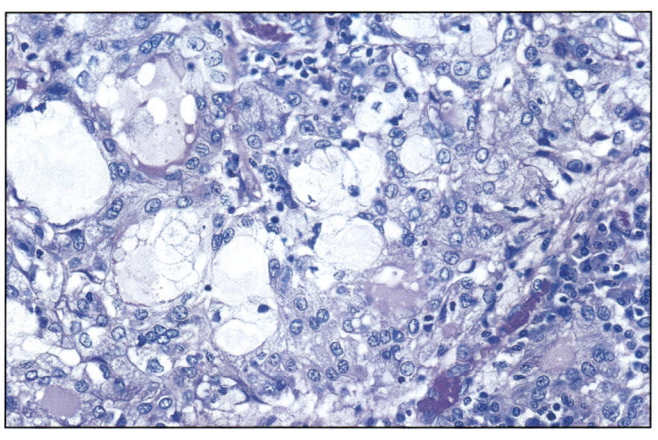

图5.18 支气管黏液表皮样癌。

液表皮样癌与低分化鳞状细胞癌[78]。免疫组化染色对于诊断价值有限。然而在分化较低的病例中，PAS 和黏液卡红染色有助于识别混在上皮样细胞中的散在的黏液细胞。

上皮性-肌上皮性癌
Epithelial-myoepithelial carcinoma

这是一种不常见的肿瘤，以腺体和腺管状结构为特征，组成细胞含有丰富的透明胞浆，细胞核的特征性改变是向周围移位[79]（图 5.19）。肿瘤细胞通常没有任何的细胞非典型性、多形性或核分裂活性。免疫组化染色证实透明细胞具有肌上皮本质；有角蛋白和肌动蛋白的同时表达以及波形蛋白和 S-100 蛋白局灶阳性。

嗜酸细胞瘤　Oncocytoma

嗜酸细胞瘤类似于涎腺的相应肿瘤，过去已有少数病例作为肺的原发性肿瘤报道[81-83]。这些肿瘤的特征是大圆形细胞的单一性增生，伴有小的位于中心的细胞核和丰富的嗜酸性胞浆。然而，在我们个人实践中还没有见到任何真正的这种类型的肿瘤。

双相性上皮性/间叶性肿瘤
Biphasic epithelial/mesenchymal neoplasams

这个术语包括一组肿瘤，以同一病变内上皮和间叶成分混合为特征[84-95]。它们少于所有肺原发性恶性肿瘤的 1%。在这个范畴中两个最重要的病变是癌肉瘤和肺母细胞瘤[84]。在这方面值得注意的是，肺母细胞瘤可以完全或主要由上皮组织构成。

癌肉瘤　Carcinosarcoma

这一节中应用的癌肉瘤这个术语是指由确切的上皮和间叶两种成分构成的肿瘤，而且两种成分在形态学上都显示为恶性特征[94,95]。这些肿瘤必须与伴有良性骨或软骨化生的癌相区别。为了诊断肺的癌肉瘤，在常规光镜检查中必须辨认上皮和间叶两种成分，该两种成分均为恶性成分（图 5.20）。癌肉瘤还必须与肉瘤样癌或梭形细胞癌相鉴别。后者完全由恶性增生的上皮细胞所构成，免疫组化或超微结构发现肉瘤样或梭形细胞成分具有上皮性分化的证据，通过光镜检查、免疫组化和超微结构研究发现，癌肉瘤中两种独立的成分显示出明确的或为上皮性或为间叶性分化的特征[37,91,93,95]。临床上，癌肉瘤可以表现为周围性或中心性（支气管内）病变。该病似乎是以男性发病为主，并且直接与吸烟相关。肿瘤好发于成人，平均年龄 60 岁。临床症状通常与肿瘤

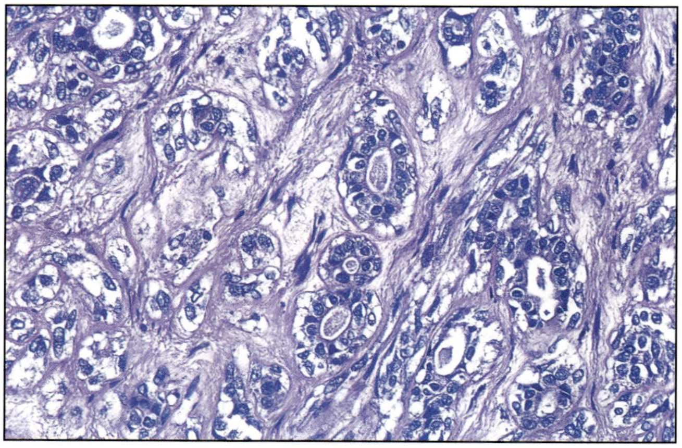

图5.19 上皮性-肌上皮性癌。注意腺体外层为透明的肌上皮细胞层。

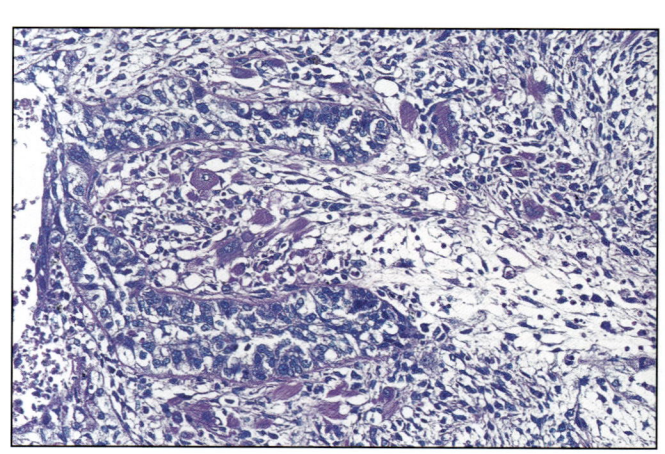

图5.20 肺癌肉瘤。腺体周围的间质成分由横纹肌母细胞构成。

发生的解剖位置有关；位于中心的肿瘤不仅较小而且由于支气管阻塞容易早期出现症状。另一方面，发生在肺周围的肿瘤在出现症状之前多半已经较大。因此，这些肿瘤的预后虽然不好，但是也与解剖位置有关。中心性病变最常见的临床症状是咳嗽、咯血和阻塞性肺炎，而周围性病变最常见的症状是胸痛[92,93]。大体上，肿瘤界限清楚，最大直径可从 1 cm 到 20 cm 以上不等。尽管肿瘤通常为孤立性，但在主要病变的附近可以见到卫星结节。

组织学上，上皮性成分可以是腺癌、鳞状细胞癌、小细胞癌或间变性大细胞癌。间叶成分通常相当于一种分化明确的软组织肉瘤，例如软骨肉瘤、骨肉瘤或横纹肌肉瘤。如前所述，通过常规光镜检查这些成分应该容易辨认；免疫组化染色的作用通常仅仅是证实诊断。

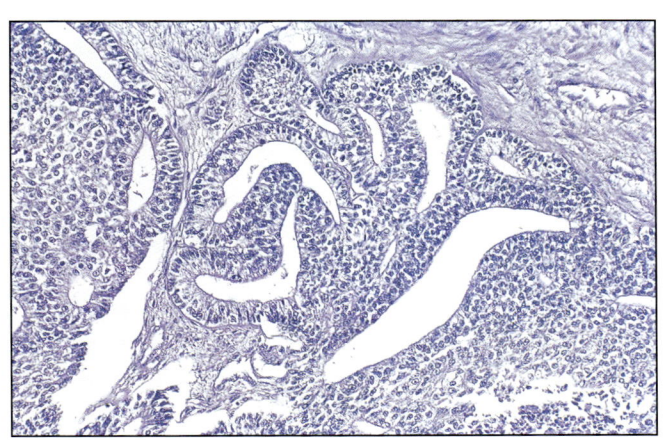

图5.21 肺母细胞瘤。注意位于基底的细胞核和丰富透明的胞浆。

肺母细胞瘤　Pulmonary blastoma

该类肿瘤相当于混合性上皮性/间叶性肿瘤，这两种成分提示胚胎性结构中不成熟或原始的腺体或间质成分[84]。它是完全不同于胸膜肺母细胞瘤（pleuropulmonary blastoma）的疾病，后者发生在儿童（见第 210 页）。肺母细胞瘤有两种组织学亚型：(1)以上皮为主性（单相性）；(2)混合性上皮性/间叶性（双相性母细胞瘤）。以上皮为主的肿瘤还有许多其他的名称，包括胎儿肺型腺癌、高分化胎儿性腺癌，类似于胎儿肺的内胚层肿瘤以及肺胚胎瘤[84,85,87-89]。这样的术语反映了这些肿瘤中组织的胎儿性表现，被认为是妊娠第 9 周到 11 周发育中的肺的再现。

临床上，这些肿瘤最常见于成人，平均年龄 35 岁。位于中心的肿瘤多半引起支气管阻塞的症状，而位于肺周围的肿瘤常常没有症状，直到肿瘤较大时才有症状。

大体上，肿瘤界限通常清楚，没有包膜，孤立性，直径可从 1cm 到 20 cm 以上不等。在切面上，这些病变质硬或橡皮样，大约 50% 的病例出现坏死区域。在某些病例中，肿瘤可以表现为息肉样支气管内肿物。

组织学上，双相性肿瘤的特征是不同大小腺管状结构构成的腺体增生，被致密的富于细胞的梭形细胞间质成分所分隔（图 5.21）。腺管状结构可以与子宫内膜腺体相似，或表现出透明细胞的特征，伴有明显的核下空泡，类似于胎儿肺。在单相性病变中，即高分化胎儿性腺癌，腺体增生表现出类似于双相肺母细胞瘤的组织学特征，但是通常伴有少量或不明显的间质梭形细胞成分。最近，有报道描述了单相性上皮型的高级别肺母细胞瘤[89]。肺母细胞瘤的另外一个明显的特征是腺体结构附近出现散在的卵圆形或梭形细胞团，这些细胞没有非典型性或核分裂活性。这些结构被称为"桑葚"（morules）。在双相性肿瘤中，梭形细胞成分可以完全未分化或显示普通肉瘤的特征。在肺母细胞瘤中偶尔可能遇到的其他成分包括软骨、骨和多核滋养细胞样巨细胞[84]。PAS 染色显示肿瘤细胞有中等量的糖原；然而，黏液卡红和 D-PAS 染色却显示细胞内黏液为阴性反应。不过，黏液卡红和 D-PAS 染色可以显示腺腔结构内的黏液沉积物。免疫组化染色一般显示上皮性标记物阳性，例如角蛋白和上皮膜抗原（EMA）。有趣的是，桑葚可以显示阳性嗜铬素染色。

肺母细胞瘤的预后与癌肉瘤一样不好。然而，单相性肿瘤比双相性肿瘤预后要好[90]。

肺间叶性肿瘤　Pulmonary mesenchymal neoplasms

肺实质内可以发生纯粹的间叶性肿瘤已获公认。理论上，累及软组织的任何类型的肿瘤都可以作为原发性肿瘤发生在肺[96]。肺的肉瘤可以累及儿童和成人，没有性别、肺叶或左右肺的特殊好发差异。因为肺是软组织肉瘤常见的转移部位，因此，在作出肺原发性肉瘤诊断之前，必须获得全部的临床病史和检查，以排除来自原发性软组织肿瘤转移的可能性。

平滑肌肉瘤　Leiomyosarcoma

平滑肌肉瘤是最常见的肺间叶性肿瘤之一，可以发生在所有年龄，包括儿童[97-99]。因为这些肿瘤可以发生

肺间叶性肿瘤

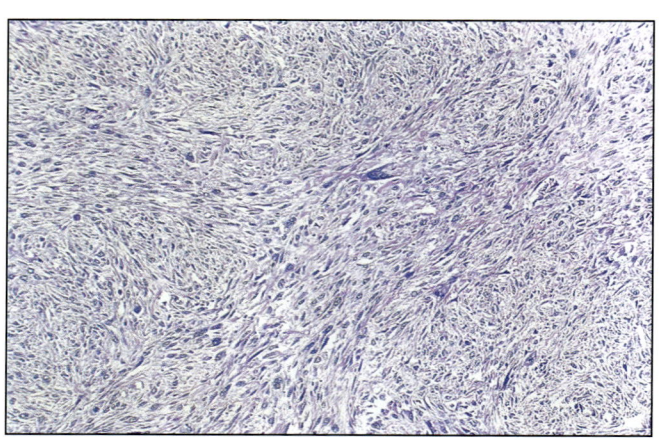

图5.22 肺的平滑肌肉瘤，由成束的非典型性梭形细胞构成，伴有雪茄形细胞核。

在支气管内，故患者可以出现肺阻塞的症状，例如咳嗽、咯血和呼吸困难。另一方面，当肿瘤位于周围时，患者可以完全没有症状。

这些肿瘤的形态学特征与软组织平滑肌肉瘤相同，即梭形细胞成束增生，伴有中等量的嗜酸性胞浆，核呈雪茄形，核仁不明显（图5.22）。肺平滑肌肉瘤可以显示广泛的分化谱系[96]。低级别肿瘤的特征是发育良好的肿瘤细胞成束排列，束与束间呈直角交叉，有少数核分裂象（< 3/10 HPF），而且细胞缺乏非典型性，无坏死和出血。中级别肿瘤的特征是细胞成分增加，伴有轻度到中度核的非典型性和明显的核分裂活性（3 ~ 8/10 HPF）。高级别肿瘤的病变细胞非常丰富，伴有细胞核的多形性和非典型性、高核分裂活性（平均8 ~ 12/10 HPF），并有大量坏死和出血。

免疫组化检查，低级别（高分化）肿瘤多半显示肌肉标记物的免疫反应，例如平滑肌肌动蛋白（SMA）和结蛋白（desmin），而分化较低（高级别）的肿瘤对所有的肌肉标记物均可阴性，可能需要通过超微结构检查来确定诊断。需要特别注意，有些平滑肌肉瘤可以表现为角蛋白阳性反应。因此，当评价肺的梭形细胞肿瘤时提倡应用一组标记物，以免误诊为梭形细胞癌。

这类肿瘤较好的治疗模式是手术切除肿瘤后给以放射或化疗。预后直接与肿瘤分级和分化程度相关。低级别肿瘤的侵袭性过程通常不如中级别或高级别肿瘤[96]。

横纹肌肉瘤　　Rhabdomyosarcoma

横纹肌肉瘤很少作为原发性肺肿瘤发生。这些肿瘤在儿童以及成人均可发生[100-104]。在儿童，横纹肌肉瘤最常见于肺囊性病变中[103,104]。横纹肌肉瘤可以表现为肺实质内的实性肿物，也可表现为支气管内病变，引起典型的肺阻塞症状。组织学上，多数原发性肺横纹肌肉瘤是腺泡状或胚胎性亚型。肿瘤的特征是小圆"蓝"细胞增生和散在的伴有丰富的强嗜酸性胞浆的横纹肌母细胞。尽管传统上认为胞浆横纹对于诊断非常重要，但是非常难于发现横纹，而且在多数病例中不出现横纹。免疫组化染色对于诊断具有重要价值，而且对于区分这些病变和其他小"蓝"细胞肿瘤非常有用。其中多数病变显示肌动蛋白，结蛋白和肌红蛋白呈某种程度的阳性反应[100]。不管是否进行手术和化疗这类肿瘤预后都差。这些肿瘤通常在胸腔内外广泛转移。

恶性外周神经鞘肿瘤　Malignant peripheral nerve sheath tumor

恶性外周神经鞘肿瘤（MPNST）是一种不常见的肺原发性肉瘤（见第27章）。在多数病例中，患者有神经纤维瘤病的病史[105]。然而，有些病例可以缺乏这样的病史而发生。这些肿瘤可以见于任何年龄或性别的患者；然而，好像较常见于年轻成人，很少累及儿童[105-107]。

大体上，肿瘤可以表现为支气管内肿物或肺实质内的实性结节，与支气管树没有任何联系。其大小可从几厘米到15厘米以上，常常出现出血和（或）坏死区域。

组织学上，这些肿瘤由成束的梭形细胞增生构成，取代肺的实质。梭形细胞增生可以显示模糊的席纹状结构，并且可有黏液样或水肿性间质，但最常见的特征是"人字形"结构，伴有长而弯曲的细胞束形成。肿瘤与肿瘤之间的细胞非典型性和核分裂活性不同，可以轻度或明显。在高级别病变中，肿瘤细胞围绕血管分布是一种常见的现象。在少数情况下，伴随这些肿瘤可以见到横纹肌分化的特征；如同在软组织一样，这样的肿瘤被命名为恶性"蝾螈"瘤（malignant "triton" tumors）[108]。

在缺乏其他标记物的情况下，这些肿瘤的免疫组化诊断依靠S-100蛋白阳性。可惜的是，仅仅在分化较好的肿瘤病例才能证实这种标记物的阳性反应；另外，S-100蛋白阳性不是神经源性肿瘤特有的标记物。在低分化的病例和缺乏神经纤维瘤病病史的病例，超微结构检查可能是确定诊断的唯一可靠手段。

单相性滑膜肉瘤　Monophasic synovial sarcoma

相对而言，单相性滑膜肉瘤是一种新近认识的肺疾病，可以累及相对年轻的个体以及年龄更大的患者；没有性别差异[109,110]。肿瘤最大直径可从1 cm到20cm不等，大体呈浅棕色，橡皮样，切面均匀一致。也可以存在出血和（或）坏死区域。

组织学上，这些肿瘤的特征是单一性的梭形细胞增生，常常呈"人字形"生长方式，而且常常显示明显的血管外皮细胞的血管结构。肿瘤细胞有卵圆形的细胞核，边缘有少量嗜酸性胞浆。在某些区域，肿瘤细胞可以有较明显的上皮样表现，伴有圆形细胞核和较丰富的胞浆。某病例中可见坏死、出血区域或化生骨的形成。每10个高倍视野核分裂象可以从2个到20个以上不等（图5.23）。免疫组化研究具有诊断价值；肿瘤细胞通常至少有一种上皮标记物阳性，例如EMA（它是最敏感的标记物）、广谱角蛋白和低分子量角蛋白抗体。肿瘤细胞中这些标记物一般与波形蛋白共同表达[109]。20%～30%肿瘤中也可见到S-100蛋白阳性。滑膜肉瘤中肿瘤细胞另外一种强阳性的标记物是bcl-2。即使当肿瘤细胞上皮标记物仅仅弱阳性或局灶阳性时，这个标记物也呈强阳性表达[111]。然而，这个抗原特异性有限。肺的单相性滑膜肉瘤的生物学行为类似于软组织的相似病变（见第24章）。肿瘤基本上呈现漫长的临床经过，也可以显示侵袭性的行为，以患者死亡而告终[109]。这类肿瘤尽管没有特异性的治疗，但手术完全切除是令人满意的选择。最近报道，相对缺乏双相性的病例很可能反映了其在罕见部位的总发病率较低。

纤维肉瘤，孤立性纤维性肿瘤（血管外皮细胞瘤）以及恶性纤维组织细胞瘤
Fibrosarcoma, solitary fibrous tumor (hemangiopericytoma), and malignant fibrous histiocytoma

这一组纤维和纤维组织细胞肿瘤，血管外皮细胞瘤（目前重新归类为肺内孤立性纤维性肿瘤）是其中一部分，基本上是除外性诊断[96]。过去，纤维肉瘤和恶性纤维组织细胞瘤（MFH）常常是肺最常诊断的肉瘤。然而，现在技术更加成熟，应用免疫组化染色、电镜和细胞遗传学检查已经能够比较准确地特化这样的病变。

纤维和纤维组织细胞肿瘤可以累及从儿童到成人的任何个体，没有性别差异、左右侧或肺段的差别。这些肿瘤可以发生在支气管内，引起支气管阻塞的症状[96,112-118]。目前对于血管外皮细胞瘤的诊断有很大的争议；有些作者仍然认为它是一个正确的诊断分类，但其他作者认为它仅仅是一种非特异性的生长方式，而不是真正的临床病理类型[96,118]。我们回顾过去诊断为肺血管外皮细胞瘤的一些病例，这些病例全部被重新分类为肺内孤立性纤维性肿瘤或滑膜肉瘤。区分孤立性纤维性肿瘤与纤维肉瘤，以及区分纤维肉瘤与恶性纤维组织细胞瘤的标准非常有限。大体上讲，我们形成一种概念，就是将所有这些肿瘤都作为分化连续过程和谱系的组成部分，孤立性纤维性肿瘤相当于谱系相对良性的一端，纤维肉瘤是中间类型，而恶性纤维组织细胞瘤则是低分化的组成部分[96]。

大体上，肿瘤可能小而界限清楚，或者可以较大，伴有中心空洞形成和坏死。支气管内亚型也有描述。组织学上，孤立性纤维性肿瘤（见第208页）的特征是温和表现的梭形细胞增生，可以伴有类似于其他软组织梭形细胞肿瘤的各种生长方式，包括纤维肉瘤、纤维组织细胞瘤、神经肿瘤、滑膜肉瘤和血管外皮细胞瘤[119,120]。实性梭形细胞团的特征是与弥漫性间质硬化区域相混合，并且含有明显的血管成分。这些肿瘤的显著特征是存在分隔梭形细胞的绳索样瘢痕瘤性胶原带（图5.24）。肿瘤界限通常清楚，周围往往有陷入的呼吸道上皮，表

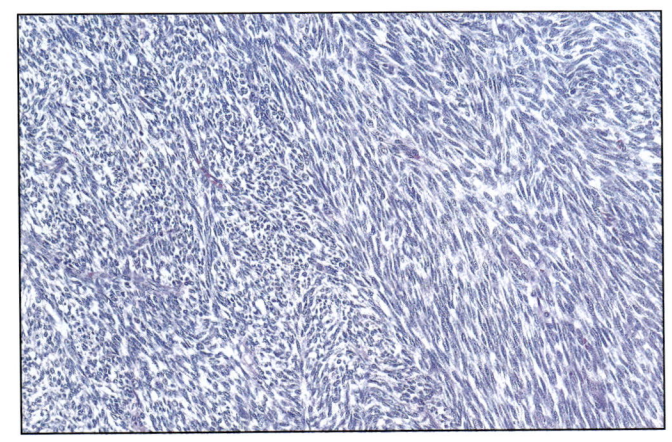

图5.23 肺的原发性滑膜肉瘤由成束单一的非典型性梭形细胞构成，伴有人字形结构。

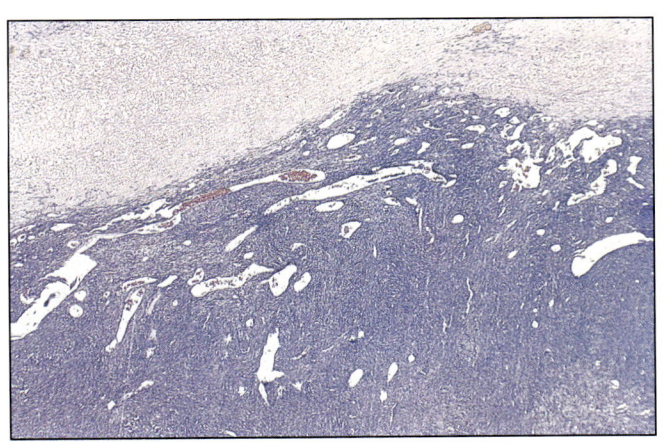

图5.24 肺内孤立性纤维性肿瘤。注意扩张的血管外皮细胞瘤样血管。

现为双相性（或"纤维腺瘤样"）的外观。免疫组化染色缺乏特异性标记物的免疫反应，例如角蛋白（keratin）、结蛋白（desmin）、肌动蛋白（actin）或 S-100 蛋白，但是肿瘤细胞 CD34 染色始终阳性[121,122]。我们最近发现这些肿瘤 bcl-2 染色呈弥漫强阳性，这个特征可能有助于诊断[111]。然而，因为 CD34 和 bcl-2 可见于多种梭形细胞增生，对于这些肿瘤均不特异，所以诊断还要依靠辨认组织病理学特征，以及肿瘤缺乏其他分化较特异标记物的免疫反应。肺纤维肉瘤的定义是具有成纤维细胞分化特征的细胞所构成的恶性梭形细胞增生。这些特征最好通过超微结构检查证实，但也可通过光学显微镜特征加以推断。这种肿瘤由两端变细的非典型性梭形细胞组成，细胞核细长，周围有少量双染性胞浆，间质中有明显的胶原基质沉积，并且缺乏任何特异性分化标记物的免疫反应，例如角蛋白、肌动蛋白、结蛋白和 S-100 蛋白[96]。虽然"人字形"结构是该肿瘤的特点，但是已经不再作为诊断标准，因为这种结构在滑膜肉瘤和恶性外周神经鞘肿瘤中同样常见。出现较显著的细胞非典型性、多核细胞、细胞核的多形性和奇异的核分裂象提示为不能分类的多形性肉瘤或所谓的恶性纤维组织细胞瘤。另外，这是除外性诊断，通过证实缺乏任何目前所能得到的特异性分化标记物的免疫反应可以支持这个诊断。鉴别诊断包括肉瘤样（梭形细胞）癌、多形性、转移性恶性黑色素瘤以及其他类型肉瘤的低分化亚型。

对于这类的肿瘤没有特异性的治疗。肺内孤立性纤维性肿瘤单独手术切除效果良好。然而，对于高级别肉瘤，完全手术切除后放疗和化疗具有一定价值[112,113,115,117]。

形成骨和软骨的肉瘤
Bone-and cartilage-forming sarcomas

这一组原发性肉瘤在肺中极其少见[123-127]。有少数记录完整的病例报道。无论如何，在任何一个肿瘤中出现恶性软骨或骨，病理医师均应警惕有双相性肿瘤（即癌肉瘤）的可能性，并应立即仔细寻找恶性上皮性成分。最好通过广泛而充分的标本取材来寻找上皮成分。文献中报告的属于这一组肿瘤的许多病例实际上可能就是癌肉瘤。这类肿瘤没有特殊治疗，预后一般不良，死亡通常在发病 12 个月内。

Kaposi 肉瘤和血管肉瘤
Kaposi's sarcoma and angiosarcoma

肺原发性血管肿瘤罕见[128-132]。Kaposi 肉瘤一般见于人类免疫缺陷病毒（HIV）感染的情况下[128-130]。另一方面，血管肉瘤常常是心脏原发性肿瘤或某些其他远隔部位原发性肿瘤转移的结果[132]。

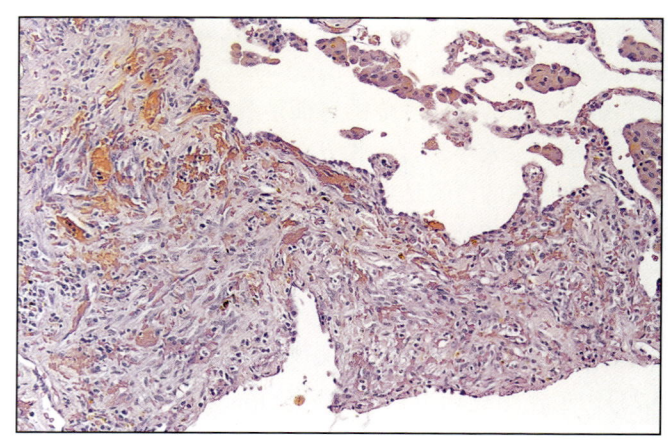

图5.25　肺Kaposi肉瘤。

Kaposi 肉瘤（见第 3 章）的特征是梭形细胞增生，伴有轻度核非典型性，核分裂活性低，可见血管裂隙，伴有红细胞外渗（图 5.25）。肿瘤往往围绕大血管和气道生长，在肺内常沿淋巴管分布，可能造成诊断困难。通常，肿瘤细胞 CD34、CD31 和 HHV-8 呈中等到弥漫阳性染色。偶尔有报道描述这些肿瘤 VIII 因子和肌动蛋白阳性，但是这种反应不稳定，不能依靠它进行诊断。

另外一方面，血管肉瘤的特征是内衬相互吻合的血管腔的非典型性细胞的增生，血管内皮标记物，例如 VIII 因子相关抗原、CD31 和 CD34 有强烈反应。当出现多发性结节而不是以单个肿块为主时，应该想到转移的可能性，并立即寻找肺外原发性病灶[132]。存在多发性血管内结节常常提示有心脏原发性肿瘤（尤其是右心房）。

上皮样血管内皮细胞瘤
Epithelioid hemangioendothelioma

上皮样血管内皮细胞瘤（见第 3 章）是少见类型的血管内皮肿瘤，形态学上被认为是中间型，其行为介于血管瘤和普通血管肉瘤之间。这个肿瘤最初被认为是肺的蜕膜病变，后来被解释为血管内细支气管肺泡肿瘤（IVBAT）[133,134]。随后免疫组化和超微结构研究证实瘤细胞具有血管内皮的本质[135,136]。临床上，该类肿瘤好发于 30~40 岁以及 40~50 岁的女性。典型的表现是多发性界限清楚的肺内结节。临床上可见肺阻塞的症状，例如咳嗽和呼吸困难。

组织学上，肿瘤特征是圆形或卵圆性上皮样细胞增生，伴有丰富的嗜酸性胞浆，细胞核卵圆形，核仁不明显，肿瘤细胞位于黏液样或玻璃样变的基质内（图 5.26）。一个显著的特征是肿瘤细胞出现大的胞浆内空泡。在早期病变中，舌状肿瘤组织往往呈息肉样充满肺泡，产生

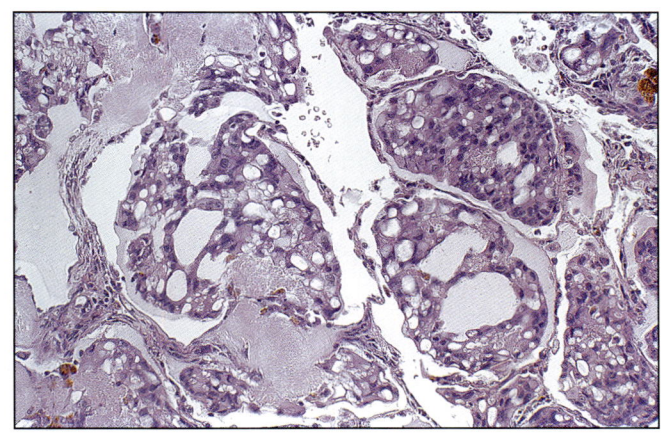
图5.26 肺上皮样血管内皮细胞瘤。注意充满肺泡腔的肾小球样上皮样细胞团。

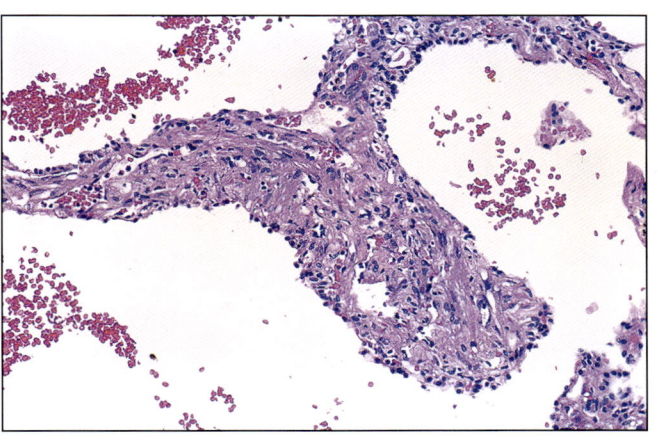
图5.27 淋巴管平滑肌瘤病的特征是由于平滑肌增生而造成肺泡间隔增厚。

明显的肾小球样表现。较陈旧的病变可以显示较明显的间质玻璃样变，仅残留少量肿瘤细胞。在这些肿瘤中通常见不到坏死、出血或核分裂活性。肿瘤细胞血管内皮标记物呈强阳性，包括Ⅷ因子相关抗原、CD31和CD34。有些病例也可以表现为角蛋白阳性。电镜检查显示血管内皮细胞的特征，包括紧密的细胞连接、基底膜物质、胞饮活动以及在少数情况下可见Weibel-Palade小体。

这些肿瘤没有特异性治疗，预后取决于肺实质受累的范围。因为存在双侧多发性肺结节，多数患者于10～15年后死于呼吸功能不全[134]。

淋巴管平滑肌瘤病（见第3章）
Lymphangioleiomyomatosis

这是一种累及生育年龄女性的少见的肺疾病，一般在发病10年内死于呼吸衰竭。少数病例伴有结节性硬化。大体上，肺显示弥漫性蜂窝状结构，在囊腔之间缺乏纤维组织沉积[137,138]。组织学上，这类病变的特征是良性表现的平滑肌细胞增生，沿着支气管淋巴管周围、小叶间间隔和胸膜分布（图5.27）。梭形细胞增生可以相当局限和不明显，而且不伴有可以辨认的肿瘤结节形成。平滑肌肌动蛋白（SMA）和HMB-45免疫组化染色对于证实淋巴管周围的梭形细胞增生可能十分有用。

淋巴组织增生性疾病
Lymphoproliferative disorders

肺淋巴组织增生性疾病相当少见，范围可从良性、可逆性病变到高级别恶性淋巴瘤。少见的浆细胞瘤病例也可发生[139]。由于引入了支气管相关淋巴组织（bronchus-associated lymphoid tissue，BALT）的概念，已经能够较好地理解肺的淋巴组织增生性疾病，结果是许多以前认为是假性淋巴瘤的病变现在确认是低级别单克隆性淋巴组织恶性肿瘤[140,141]。这一组疾病中三个最重要的分类是：(1)低级别B细胞淋巴瘤；(2)淋巴瘤样肉芽肿病；(3) Hodgkin病（HD）。

恶性非Hodgkin淋巴瘤
Malignant non-Hodgkin's lymphoma

绝大多数肺的恶性淋巴瘤是B细胞表型和低级别恶性淋巴瘤[142]。其中某些病变最近被诊断为"BALT淋巴瘤"（BALT lymphoma），其中代表是支气管相关淋巴组织淋巴瘤[140-143]。这些肿瘤最常见于50～60岁的成人。放射学上，肿瘤可以表现为肺部结节或弥漫性肺部浸润。临床上，患者可以完全没有症状，或表现为体质上的症状，例如体重减轻、发热和盗汗。有些病例可见肺门淋巴结肿大[143-148]。组织学上，这种病变的特征是单一性小淋巴细胞增生，细胞核轻度不规则，混合有散在的免疫母细胞。在小淋巴细胞中常常见到浆细胞样分化的特征，而且可以出现Russell或Dutcher小体。淋巴细胞团的一个显著特征是细胞核周围存在一圈透明的胞浆，类似于中心细胞性或单核细胞样（滤泡旁）B细胞。在多达70%的病例中可见伴有发育良好生发中心的反应性滤泡。另外一个重要的特征是存在所谓的"淋巴上皮病变"，其定义是小淋巴细胞浸润支气管上皮（图5.28）。BALT淋巴瘤的其他特征包括多核巨细胞或结节病样肉芽肿（sarcoid-like granulomas），见于多达50%的病例。有趣的是，骨髓受累和血清免疫球蛋白的尖峰信号仅见于大约20%的病例，而肺门淋巴结受累可以出现在多达30%的病例[147]。多数BALT淋巴瘤病例是Ⅰ期肿瘤，5年和10年生存率高到80%。

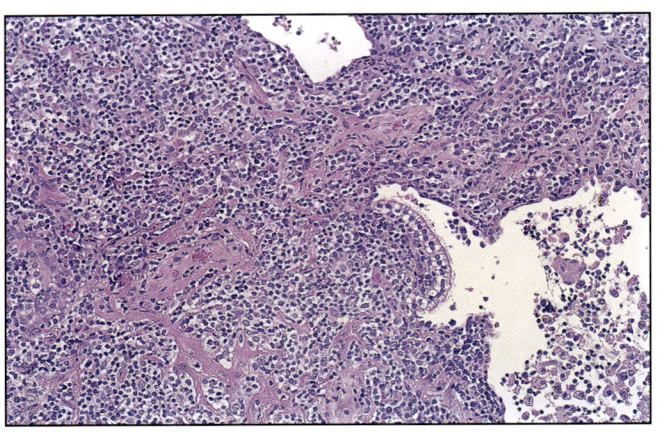

图5.28 支气管相关淋巴组织（BALT）淋巴瘤是由小淋巴细胞单一性增生构成,支气管黏膜局部受累。

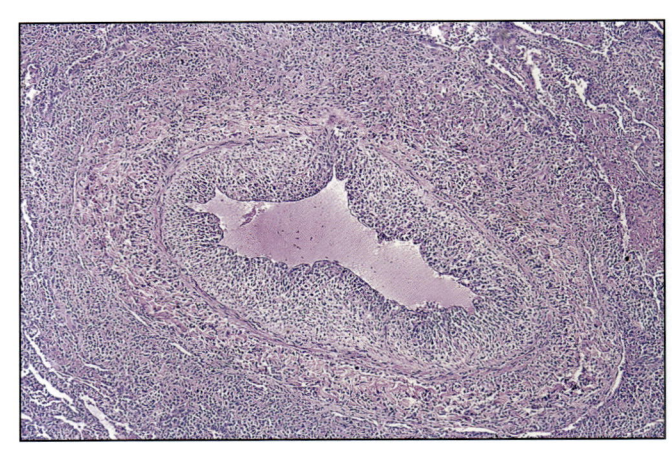

图5.29 肺的淋巴瘤样肉芽肿病。注意非典型性淋巴细胞浸润并破坏血管壁。

这类肿瘤的免疫组化诊断依靠单克隆性的证实。这可以通过应用石蜡切片的 kappa 和 lambda 轻链抗体染色、流式细胞检查免疫表型或进行基因重排分析来完成。

鉴别诊断包括假性淋巴瘤和淋巴细胞间质性肺炎[144]。肺假性淋巴瘤现在诊断为结节性 BALT 增生（nodular BALT hyperplasia），多半是 BALT 淋巴瘤的前期病变,其特征是多角形小淋巴细胞团,伴有明显的生发中心形成[145]。组织学上,结节性 BALT 增生与 BALT 淋巴瘤的区别在于淋巴细胞增生程度较轻,淋巴细胞缺乏"单核细胞样"特征,以及缺乏淋巴上皮病变。弥漫性 BALT 增生（diffuse form of BALT hyperplasia）与过去文献中的淋巴细胞间质性肺炎（lymphoid interstitial pneumonia，LIP）是同义词。这种类型的 BALT 增生可能与各种免疫疾病有关,包括获得性免疫缺陷综合征（AIDS）。放射学和组织学上这种病变的特征是伴有纤维化的弥漫性间质淋巴细胞浸润。浸润的细胞主要由小 B 淋巴细胞组成,混合有浆细胞,偶尔有组织细胞。淋巴滤泡常见,也可出现小的肉芽肿。有些病变可以进展为淋巴瘤;其他的仍然保留在局部或随着时间而消退。

肺的原发性淋巴瘤也可以罕见地表现出大 B 细胞淋巴瘤（large cell lymphoma of B-cell type）的特征。这样的病变通常表现为大的边界不清的肿瘤,伴有坏死区域并侵犯其上的胸膜,通常伴有支气管软骨和气道的广泛破坏[149]。其中某些病变可以保留在肺的局部一段时间,这个发现支持它们可能是低级别 BALT 淋巴瘤的高级别转化这一观点[143]。

淋巴瘤样肉芽肿病 / 血管免疫增生性病变 Lymphomatoid granulomatosis / angioimmunoproliferative lesion

另外一种不常见但非常具有特征的肺非 Hodgkin 大细胞淋巴瘤最初被 Liebow 等描述为淋巴瘤样肉芽肿病[150],现在也叫血管免疫增生性病变（AIL）[144]。虽然传统上认为它是肺的血管中心性 T 细胞淋巴瘤,但是现在重新评估这个病变,认为其有可能是富于 T 细胞的大 B 细胞淋巴瘤。男性受累似乎比女性常见,最常发生于 40～60 岁的个体。然而,发生于儿童的病例已有报道。放射学上,患者可以表现为多发性肺结节、网状结节性浸润或孤立性的肺肿瘤。可见皮肤受累,表现为皮肤结节、皮疹或溃疡[150-155]。组织学上,肿瘤的特征是伴有明显血管中心性的非典型性淋巴细胞浸润。常常可见类似于 Hodgkin 淋巴瘤的核仁明显嗜酸性的双核（Reed-Sternberg）细胞。肿瘤细胞常混有组织细胞,产生假肉芽肿性外观。这些病变通常伴有广泛坏死,并且显示肿瘤细胞明显浸润和破坏血管壁（图 5.29）。迄今为止,免疫组化研究似乎均表明非典型性肿瘤细胞为 T 细胞系,尽管关于这种病变的确切本质还有争议。少数研究提示其中某些病例可能是富于 T 细胞的大 B 细胞淋巴瘤。

Hodgkin病　Hodgkin's disease

严格定义的缺乏其他部位（包括肺门淋巴结）Hodgkin 淋巴瘤的原发性肺 Hodgkin 淋巴瘤极其少见[156-158]。这种病变大体上可以表现为单发或多发性界限清楚的肺内结节。组织学上,这些病变并不常见典型 Hodgkin 淋巴瘤的特征,并且可能难以诊断。一般可见混合性细胞浸润,其中含有小淋巴细胞、浆细胞、嗜酸性粒细胞以及散在的大淋巴细胞,大淋巴细胞有一个或多个细胞核以及明显的嗜酸性核仁（图 5.30）。免疫组化是诊断的关键,非典型性细胞 CD30 和 CD15 抗体染色显示细胞膜和核旁胞浆呈强阳性反应,而白细胞共同抗原以及 B 细胞、T 细胞标记物染色则为阴性。

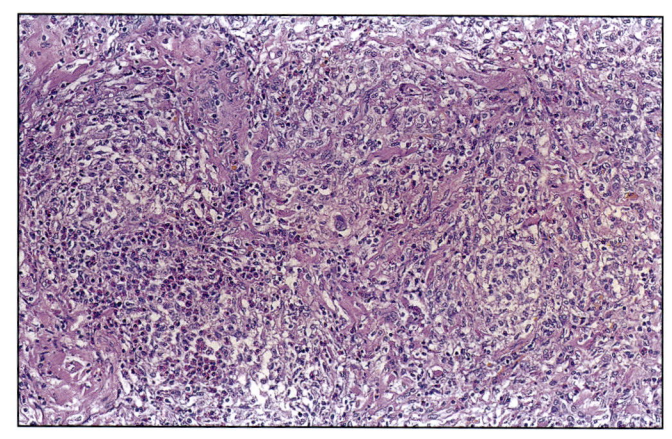

图5.30 肺Hodgkin淋巴瘤，显示在小淋巴细胞、浆细胞和嗜酸性粒细胞的背景中有非典型性增生的单核和多核细胞。

来源于胚胎移位或异位组织的肿瘤
Tumors derived from embryologically displaced or ectopic tissues

来源于胚胎移位或异位组织的肿瘤是见于人体其他部位的，但不常发生在肺。根据推测，这些肿瘤来源于胚胎移位或异位组织，例如脑膜上皮残留、胸腺上皮、血管球细胞以及神经外胚层起源[159]。

肺的脑膜瘤　Pulmonary meningioma

肺的脑膜瘤相对少见[160-163]。放射学上，它们表现为界限清楚的肺实质内肿物，最大直径可达10 cm。患者通常是成人；没有性别、好发肺或肺段的差异。肺的脑膜瘤的形态学特征与颅内脑膜瘤相同（见第26章）。过渡型和纤维型都有。这些肿瘤显示良性表现的梭形细胞增生，往往形成漩涡状结构（图5.31）。核分裂象罕见，细胞非典型性不明显。沙粒体的存在通常有助于诊断。肺的脑膜瘤中可以见到的少见特征包括化生性骨形成和泡沫样巨噬细胞集聚。支持诊断最重要的免疫组化染色是相同肿瘤细胞同时表达EMA和波形蛋白。这些肿瘤可能局灶阳性的其他标记物包括角蛋白、S-100蛋白和CD34。手术完全切除后的病例预后好像极好。颅内脑膜瘤晚期偶尔可能转移到肺，因此在诊断肺的原发性脑膜瘤之前必须获得全部的病史[160]。

肺内胸腺瘤　Intrapulmonary thymoma

肺内胸腺瘤极其少见。肺的肿物偶尔可以是纵隔胸腺瘤的最初表现，因此在诊断肺原发性胸腺瘤之前必须通过适当的影像学检查以排除纵隔肿瘤。放射学上，这些肿瘤表现为界限清楚的结节，直径可以达到10 cm。与位于纵隔的胸腺瘤不同，肺内胸腺瘤不伴有重症肌无力[164-166]。

组织学上，肿瘤具有与正常前纵隔的胸腺瘤相同的形态学特征（见第2章），也就是由上皮细胞与淋巴细胞混合构成的双相细胞群，伴有明显的小叶状结构和纤维化（图5.32）。某些病例的组织学表现可能是梭形细胞增生，伴有明显的束状或血管外皮细胞生长方式。核分裂活性通常非常低，仅有散在的核分裂象。胸腺瘤角蛋白抗体染色呈强阳性。然而，在这种情况下这种标记物是非特异性的，不能用于区分胸腺瘤与梭形细胞癌、滑膜肉瘤或其他上皮性肿瘤的转移。通过辨认双相性细胞群（上皮细胞/淋巴细胞），在低倍镜下观察到特征性的小叶状结构，以及识别胸腺分化的其他器官型特征，例如血管周围腔隙和"髓样"分化区域（见第21章），可能有助于诊断。肺内胸腺瘤是生长缓慢的肿瘤，可以

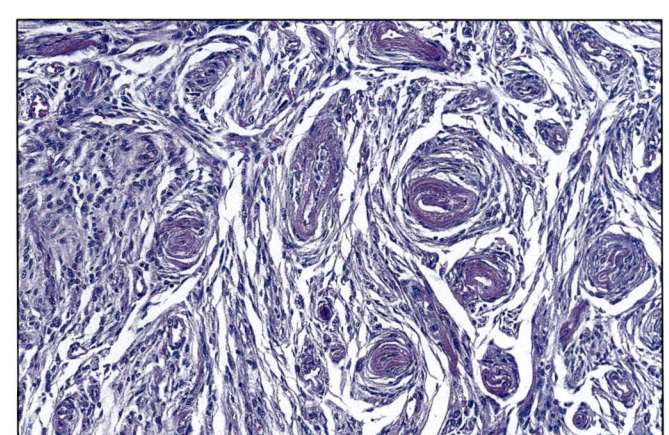

图5.31 肺的脑膜瘤。

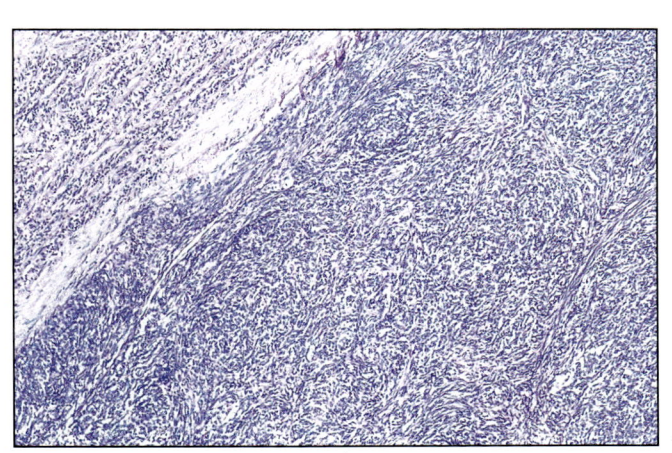

图5.32 肺内胸腺瘤。

血管球瘤　Glomus tumor

血管球瘤起源于血管球器或Sucquet-Hoyer管，这是一个特化的涉及血液和皮肤温度控制的动静脉吻合（见第3章）。有趣的是，虽然，血管球瘤在皮肤之外的其他几个器官也有描述，但在诸如肺等体内器官中并没有发现这样的结构。在肺仅有几例记录完整的病例报告[167,168]。肿瘤最常累及成人，没有性别和好发于哪一侧肺的差异。多数患者无症状，这种病变是在常规身体检查中偶尔发现的。大体上，肿瘤界限清楚，平均直径3～4 cm。组织学上，血管球瘤的特征是单一性圆形或卵圆形细胞增生，伴有一圈嗜酸性或透明的胞浆，细胞膜清楚，核位于中心，核仁不明显（图5.33）。坏死、出血或核分裂活性均不常见。肿瘤细胞往往呈片块状生长，并且常常围绕呈海绵状扩张的厚壁血管排列。在免疫组化水平上，血管球瘤的特征是SMA强阳性。其他例如角蛋白、结蛋白和S-100蛋白肿瘤分化的标记物阴性。完全手术切除肿瘤可以治愈，预后良好。

原发性支气管恶性黑色素瘤
Primary malignant melanoma of bronchus

这是另外一种不常见的肺的原发性肿瘤，文献中记录完整的病例报告不足30例。这些肿瘤发生在成人，正确诊断为原发性肿瘤最重要的是其他部位缺乏相似肿瘤（或病史）。多数病变位于肺中心，而且可以在支气管内生长，呈息肉样或外生性表现[169-173]。

组织学上，支气管恶性黑色素瘤可以显示如同或皮肤其他器官黑色素瘤同样广泛的生长方式。肿瘤细胞通常排列成明显的巢状结构，呈上皮样外观，细胞伴有中等量嗜酸性胞浆，核圆形，核仁明显，核分裂象常见。某些肿瘤可能主要由梭形细胞构成，伴有明显的细胞非典型性（图5.34）。某些病例可见黑色素，但不是所有病例。少数病例在支气管黏膜附近可见原位黑色素瘤。然而，当肿瘤侵蚀支气管上皮时，原位成分可能很难评价，但缺乏原位成分不应妨碍医师作出诊断[169]。与其他部位黑色素瘤一样，支气管黑色素瘤S-100蛋白和HMB-45呈强阳性反应。要特别注意的是，在完全由梭形细胞构成的肿瘤中HMB-45可以阴性。另一方面，这些肿瘤偶尔可有其他抗体异常表达，例如CEA、EMA、CD-99或bcl-2。

这些肿瘤没有特殊治疗，预后不良，通常在18个月内导致死亡。

肺的副神经节瘤
Pulmonary paraganglioma

肺的副神经节瘤（见第28章）是少见而有争议的肿瘤。有些作者认为所有这样的病例实际上都是不常见的类癌，因为在肺尚未证实有正常的副神经节。肿瘤的特征是圆形或卵圆形细胞增生，伴有大而常常深染的细胞核，染色质呈点彩状，胞浆丰富双染性。肿瘤细胞常具有典型神经内分泌肿瘤的巢状（细胞球）生长方式。玫瑰花结、缎带状、小梁状或花边样结构不是副神经瘤的特征，可以用于与支气管类癌的鉴别。另外一个有助于与类癌区分的显著特征是存在核的非典型性，伴有细长、偶尔呈分叶状和深染的细胞核。副神经节瘤的肿瘤细胞通常与神经内分泌标记物有反应，例如嗜铬素、突触素、NSE和间位脑啡肽（met-enkephalin），但是绝大多数病例角蛋白抗体阴性。另外一个显著特征是肿瘤细胞巢周围的支持细胞呈网状S-100蛋白阳性染色，尽管在类癌中也有这样细胞的描述。多数病例为良性，单

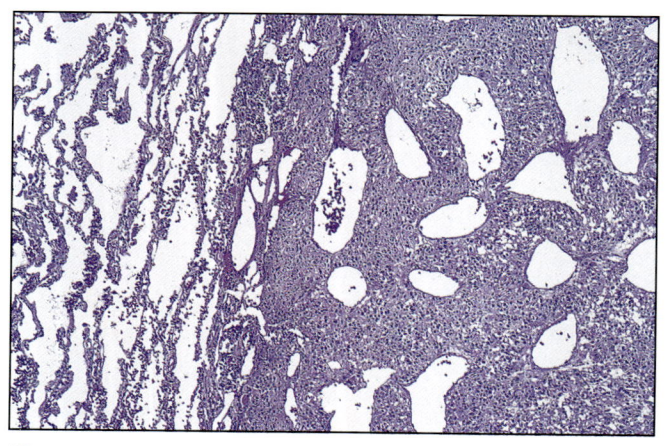

图5.33　肺内血管球瘤。

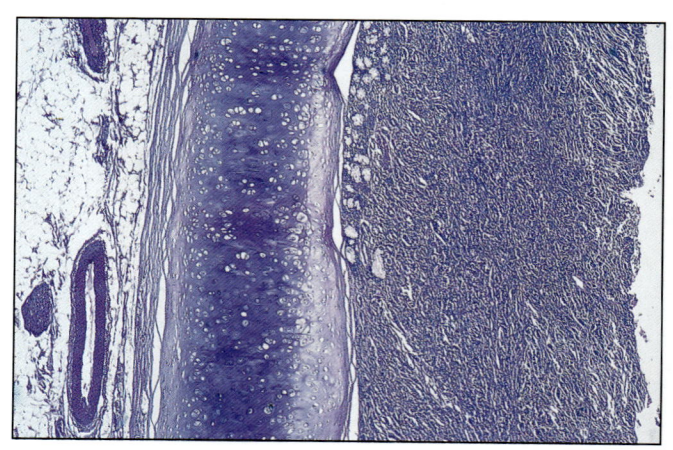

图5.34　支气管原发性黑色素瘤。

独手术切除就已足够[174,175]。

神经节母细胞瘤　Ganglioneuroblastoma

神经节母细胞瘤是肺极其少见的肿瘤（见第28章）。文献中仅有几例记录完整的病例报告[176,177]。成人肺神经节母细胞瘤已有描述，由于支气管内病变而表现出阻塞的症状。至少一个肿瘤病例伴有多发性内分泌肿瘤综合征，但这种发现可能是巧合。大体上，肿瘤界限清楚，直径可以达到5 cm。组织学上，神经节母细胞瘤的特征是具有细胞突起的小细胞增生，细胞边界不清，胞浆中等量嗜酸性，细胞核圆形或卵圆形，核仁不明显。较大的细胞含有丰富的胞浆和圆形细胞核，其中某些胞浆中还可见到Nissl物质，代表神经节分化。增生细胞成分的特征是包埋在富于神经纤维网（neuropil）的基质中。核分裂活性或明显细胞非典型性不是这些肿瘤的特征。肿瘤可以显示神经丝蛋白、S-100蛋白和GAFP不同程度的阳性反应。上皮标记物阴性，例如角蛋白和EMA。由于报道的病例稀少，很难确定这些肿瘤的临床行为。然而，它们有可能侵犯邻近的器官并转移到肺门淋巴结。

生殖细胞肿瘤　Germ-cell tumors

在少数情况下，良性和恶性畸胎瘤可以起源于肺[178,179]。肿瘤常常较大，囊性，左肺上叶好发。可以表现为咳嗽、咯血、胸痛，偶尔咳出毛发。它们的组织病理学特征与性腺的畸胎瘤相同（见第14章）。肺罕见的原发性绒毛膜癌也有报道[180]。

不能确定组织来源的肿瘤
Tumors of uncertain histogenesis

这一组肿瘤是指组织来源不能确定或有争议的肿瘤，包括支气管颗粒细胞瘤、硬化性血管瘤（肺细胞瘤）、透明细胞（糖）瘤和炎性肌纤维母细胞瘤。

支气管颗粒细胞瘤
Granular cell tumor of bronchus

肺的支气管颗粒细胞瘤是少见的病变。它主要累及成人，平均发病年龄45岁[181,182]。典型的病例，肿瘤出现在支气管内，大约50%的患者表现为与支气管阻塞有关的症状。孤立性肿瘤最常见，但有些病例为多发性。已有肺外颗粒细胞瘤伴有肺内颗粒细胞瘤的病例描述[183,184]。组织学上（见第27章），颗粒细胞瘤的特征是相对大的圆形或卵圆形细胞增生，细胞边界清楚，有丰富的颗粒状胞浆，细胞核小圆形，偏心，缺乏核仁。

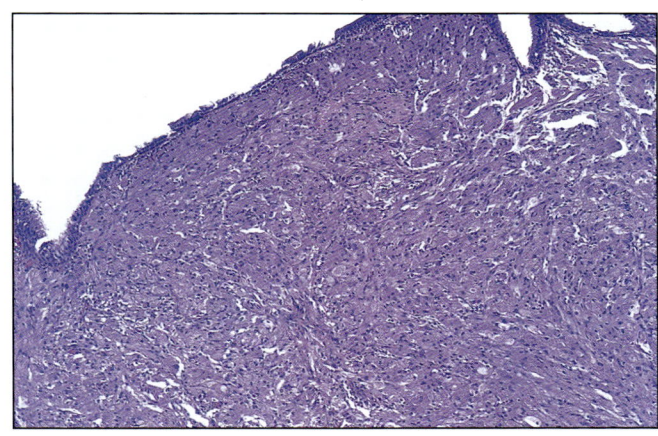

图5.35　支气管颗粒细胞瘤。

在有些病例中，细胞可以表现为印戒细胞结构。肿瘤可以非常局限，或有浸润性边界。一般看不到明显的细胞非典型性、坏死、出血和核分裂活性。被覆的支气管上皮可以表现为鳞状化生，但没有肿瘤细胞浸润的证据（图5.35）。这些肿瘤的免疫组化染色结果可以不同。一般来说，多数病变S-100蛋白强阳性。诸如角蛋白或EMA等上皮标记物以及神经内分泌标记物阴性。完全手术切除似乎可以治愈。

硬化性"血管瘤"（肺细胞瘤）
Sclerosing "hemangioma" (pneumocytoma)

硬化性血管瘤是肺少见的良性肿瘤，由Liebow和Hubbell于1956年首次描述[185]。肿瘤明显好发于女性，较常见于30~40岁或40~50岁的病人。在某些病例中，肿瘤是在常规胸部X线检查中偶尔发现的，但是某些患者可能表现为胸痛。大体上，这些肿瘤表现为相对较小的（直径5 cm）界限清楚的肺实质内肿物，与支气管结构无关，切面呈细颗粒状。

硬化性血管瘤的组织学特征是具有多种生长方式[186]，包括乳头状、实性、血管瘤性和硬化性结构。少数病例显示明显的肉芽肿性反应以及囊性表现[187]。肿瘤细胞群的特征是圆形或多角形良性表现的肿瘤细胞呈单一性增生，细胞核位于中心，没有核仁，胞浆丰富，透明或轻度嗜酸性（图5.36A）。在乳头状区域（图5.36B），乳头表面由单层小而模糊的立方细胞构成，细胞核大，深染，不成熟。在较实性的区域，肿瘤细胞可与泡沫样巨噬细胞相混合，而且常常含有陷入的肺泡结构。血管瘤性结构明显的区域可以类似于毛细血管瘤或海绵状血管瘤；血管周围玻璃样变伴有大量胶原基质沉积，导致

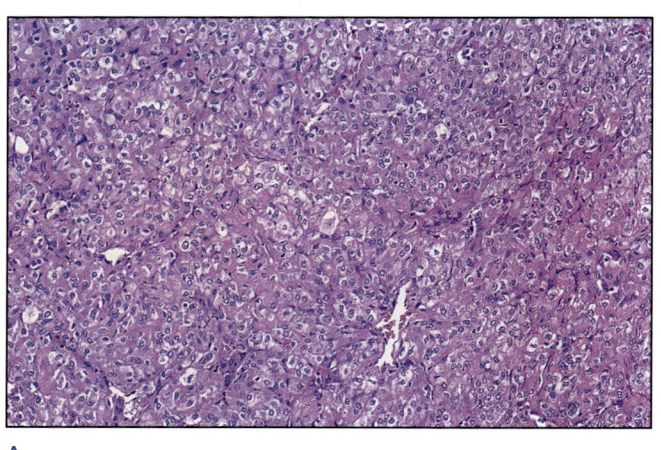
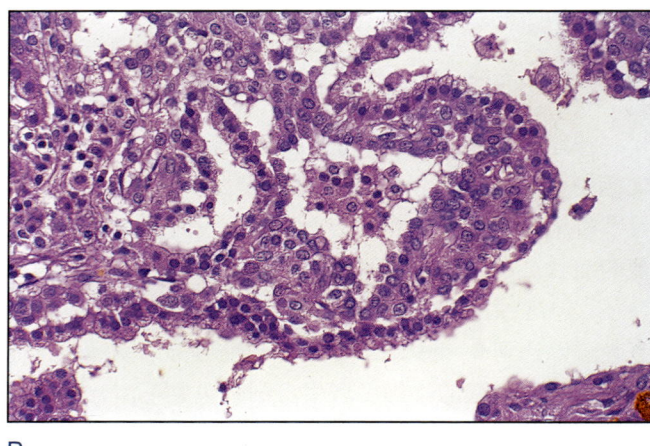

图5.36 肺硬化性血管瘤。（A）实性结构：注意伴有透明胞浆良性表现的细胞呈单一性增生；（B）乳头状结构。

"硬化"的特征性表现。坏死、出血和核分裂活性不是这些肿瘤的特征[185,188-190]。

最近的超微结构和免疫组化研究指出，肿瘤细胞是上皮性的，非常符合肺泡细胞[191-193]。多数研究显示，肿瘤细胞表面活性载体蛋白（surfactant apoprotein）免疫组化染色强阳性，但不是所有研究结果都是如此[193]。这些肿瘤一贯表达的标记物包括EMA和波形蛋白。有人报告角蛋白中间丝染色阳性，但是无人能重复取得这样的结果。一项免疫组化研究还显示神经内分泌标记物的阳性结果[194]。

硬化性血管瘤是良性肿瘤。可选择完全手术切除病变，并且可以治愈。然而，有一例肺硬化性血管瘤伴有淋巴结转移的病例报告[195]。

透明细胞（糖）瘤 Clear cell (sugar) tumor

透明细胞瘤是一种少见的肺部良性肿瘤，由于其组织发生至今尚未确定，所以是文献中争论颇多的肿瘤。肿瘤主要累及成人，没有性别差异，最常表现为孤立性的外周性"硬币样"病变[196,197]。

组织学上，其特征是大的圆形或卵圆形细胞增生，细胞核圆形，核仁不明显，周围有一圈明显的透明胞浆。肿瘤含有许多裂隙样血管，增生细胞之间结缔组织非常稀少（图5.37）。没有坏死、出血、细胞非典型性或核分裂活性。淀粉酶消化的PAS组织化学反应显示，肿瘤细胞有丰富的胞浆糖原。研究显示，这些肿瘤HMB-45和HMB-50抗体反应阳性[198,199]，这个发现被解释为黑色素细胞分化或推测是向独特的血管周上皮样细胞分化[199]。其他研究报道突触素、Leu-7、NSE、S-100蛋白和CD34阳性[198,200]。至于这些病变是否表达肌原性分化的标记物尚无完整的资料，而其他解剖部位有表达。

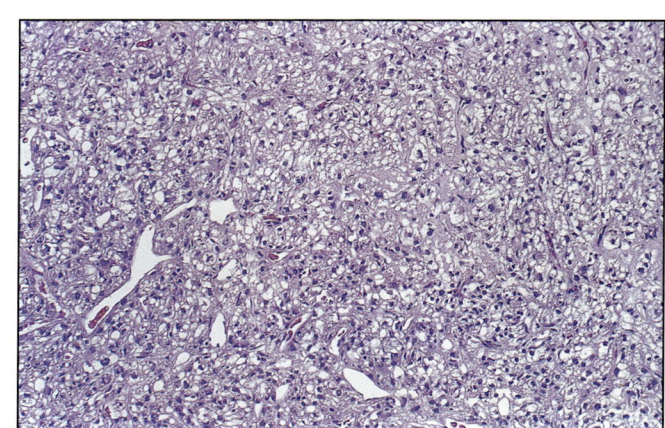

图5.37 肺透明细胞"糖"瘤。

超微结构上，肿瘤可能显示有致密轴心的神经分泌颗粒和（或）胞饮小泡，伴有胞浆内细丝。完全手术切除肿瘤可以治愈。

炎性肌纤维母细胞瘤 Inflammatory myofibroblastic tumors

炎性肌纤维母细胞瘤从前也叫炎性假瘤，通常是一种良性、生长缓慢的病变，病因不明。它主要累及年轻患者，性别分布无差异。过去用于这种病变的其他命名包括浆细胞性肉芽肿、组织细胞瘤和黄色纤维瘤[201-205]。当肿瘤发生在支气管内时，可以表现为继发性的阻塞症状，或者可以完全没有症状，常规检查发现孤立性硬币样病变。大体上，这些肿瘤通常界限清楚，较小，但偶尔可以较大并浸润纵隔。

该肿瘤分为两种主要的组织学亚型：(1)浆细胞肉芽肿亚型（plasma cell granuloma variant），其特征是出现含有不同数量肥大成纤维细胞的玻璃样变的纤

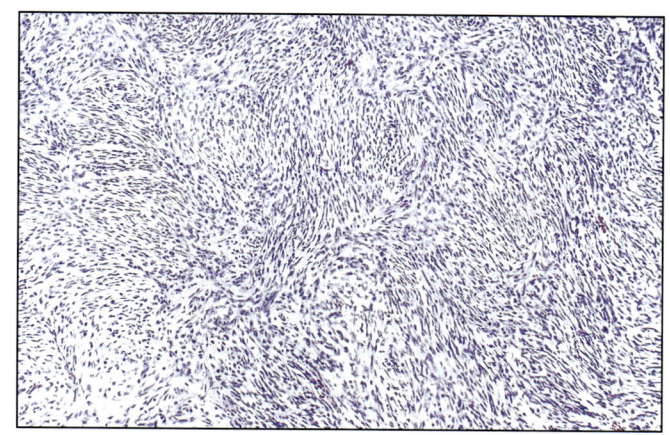

图5.38 炎性假瘤显示明显的席纹状结构。

维结缔组织区域，其中有成片的浆细胞浸润，混有组织细胞、肥大细胞和淋巴细胞；(2)纤维组织细胞亚型（fibrohistiocytic variant），是由密集的梭形细胞增生构成的，排列成漩涡状、束状或席纹状，可能类似于肉瘤（图5.38）。核分裂象可见，然而，核分裂活性低，而且不应该有异常核分裂象。在较晚期阶段，出现广泛纤维化和透明变性，产生中心瘢痕性病变，可能非常类似于终末阶段的间质纤维化。有些病例中可见钙化。在少数情况下，本病可能与感染性病变（例如曲菌病）同时存在，以致掩盖这种病变的真正本质。

可选择完全手术切除。然而，某些病例几年之后可以复发。复发较常见于纤维组织细胞亚型的病例，个别病例可以进展为真正的肉瘤。偶尔有复发和恶性的病例，实际上提示这种病变是肿瘤性的，而且可能与其他部位的炎性纤维母细胞瘤有关（见第24章），某些病例出现ALK基因重排也支持这一点[206]。

其他良性肿瘤
Miscellaneous benign tumors

软骨错构瘤　Cartilaginous hamartoma

软骨错构瘤是最常见的肺部良性肿瘤[207,208]。男性比女性常见，而且较常见于成人。然而，儿童错构瘤病例已有报道。肿瘤可以表现为支气管内病变或肺实质内结节。组织学上，该肿瘤的特征是上皮成分与间叶成分混合存在，伴有数量不等的成熟软骨和脂肪组织，其周围含有陷入的呼吸上皮。有趣的是，这些病变显示有独特的克隆性细胞遗传学异常，与脂肪瘤、子宫平滑肌瘤和其他良性肿瘤基本相同，导致高活动组（high-mobility group，HMG）基因重排[209,210]。治疗选择手术切除，而且可以治愈。

支气管内脂肪瘤　Endobronchial lipoma

支气管内脂肪瘤是少见病变，最常见于成人[211]。大体上，表现为有蒂或息肉样支气管内肿瘤，质软，黄色外观。组织学上，这些肿瘤由成熟脂肪组织构成。可选择手术切除，并且可以治愈。

肺泡性腺瘤　Alveolar adenoma

肺泡性腺瘤是罕见的肺肿瘤[212-214]，过去常被误诊为某一种形式的肺淋巴管瘤。肿瘤主要累及成人，通常无症状，仅为常规放射线检查的偶然发现。大体上，肿瘤界限清楚，伴出血以及有囊性区域，最大直径通常小于3 cm。

组织学上，低倍镜下肿瘤是血管性的，因为存在多发性囊性扩张的结构，其内充满血清样蛋白性物质（图5.39）。然而，扩张的结构内衬肺泡性肺细胞，有些细胞表现为鞋钉样外观。肿瘤是良性的，手术切除可以治愈。

支气管"黏液腺"腺瘤　Bronchial "mucous gland" adenoma

黏液腺腺瘤是不常见的良性肿瘤。它的发生是由于支气管浆液黏液腺体过度增大而造成的[215]。该肿瘤最常见于成人，没有任何特殊肺的部位或性别差异。因为这些肿瘤位于支气管内，患者通常表现为支气管阻塞的症状。

大体上，这些病变是外生性的，有蒂，界限清楚，质软，表面呈黏液样；最大径达可到6 cm。组织学上，由于正常支气管腺体充满黏液而造成扩张，所以低倍镜下肿瘤通常具有囊性表现（图5.40）。在肿瘤的其他区域可以显示乳头状结构与扩张的支气管腺体混合存在。仔细检查发现，肿瘤是由良性表现的细胞构成的，没有细胞非典型性或核分裂活性。有些细胞可以表现为细胞核向周围移位，而且具有丰富的颗粒状胞浆。D-PAS或

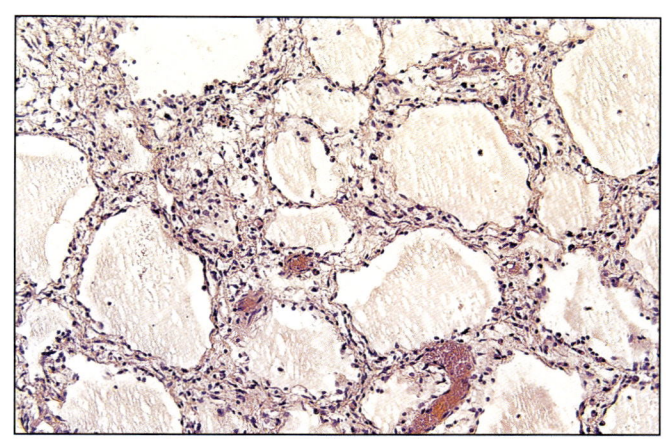

图5.39 肺泡性腺瘤。

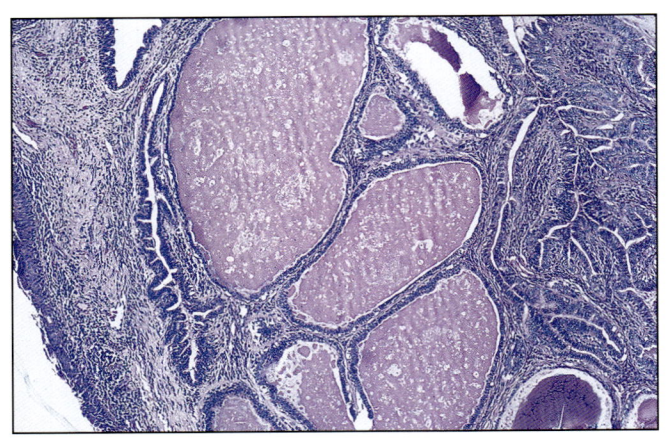

图5.40 黏液腺腺瘤显示囊性扩张的支气管腺体。

黏液卡红染色显示有丰富的细胞内黏液，而且PAS染色证实糖原成分稀少。可选择手术切除，并且可以治愈。

乳头状腺瘤 Papillary adenoma

乳头状腺瘤是极其少见的肿瘤[216,217]，可发生于各种年龄段。肿瘤通常小而没有症状，X线上表现为位于周围的孤立性硬币样病变。临床完全呈良性经过。组织学上，肿瘤是界限清楚的结节，有复杂的分支乳头状结构，乳头由纤维轴心被覆均匀一致的立方到柱状细胞构成。超微结构检查这些上皮细胞具有Ⅱ型肺泡细胞的特征。

肺腺纤维瘤 Pulmonary adenofibroma

肺腺纤维瘤是成人不常见的肺部病变[218]。这种病变通常小而界限清楚，与支气管结构无关。组织学上，这些肿瘤的特征是复杂分支的腺样间隙，内衬单层立方或柱状上皮，周围有丰富的梭形细胞纤维性间质。腺样间隙常常显示特征性的棒状乳头状结构，类似于卵巢的Müller腺纤维瘤（图5.41）。免疫组化检查示，上皮内衬细胞显示上皮性标记物染色阳性，例如角蛋白和EMA。病变的间质S-100蛋白、肌动蛋白、角蛋白、EMA、结蛋白和CD34均呈阴性反应。鉴别诊断主要是孤立性纤维性肿瘤。与孤立性纤维性肿瘤不同，肺腺纤维瘤的腺样区域均匀分布于整个病变，而在孤立性纤维性肿瘤中陷入的腺体结构通常仅见于病变周围。可选择手术切除治疗，并且可以治愈。

微小肺"化学感受器瘤"（脑膜样结节） Minute pulmonary "chemodectoma" (meningothelial–like nodule)

微小肺化感器瘤最初被误认为是副神经节残留，其最常见的特征是胸膜下多发性灰粉色的小结节，最大径大约2 mm，由圆形或卵圆形细胞集聚而成，细胞界限不清，有丰富的嗜酸性胞浆。这些细胞的特征是往往具有漩涡状的外观，类似于脑膜瘤[219,220]。通过免疫组化检查，这些细胞波形蛋白和EMA染色强阳性，而角蛋白、S-100蛋白、嗜铬素蛋白（chromogranin）、NSE和肌动蛋白染色阴性。超微结构观察显示，病变具有脑膜上皮细胞特征，包括由桥粒连接的交互排列的胞浆突起以及丰富的中间丝。因此，这些病变的免疫组化和超微结构特征非常接近于脑膜蛛网膜肉芽肿（meningeal arachnoid granulations），而不是真正的化学感受器瘤[220]。这样的病变往往是在尸检或因为其他原因而进行的肺切除术时的偶尔发现，因此几乎没有临床重要性。一般认为这些病变的本质是反应性的，与普通的脑膜瘤相比具有完全不同的分子发病机制[221]。

肺转移性肿瘤 Metastases to the lungs

肺是许多恶性肿瘤转移最常见的内脏之一。实际上，转移是肺肿瘤最常见的类型。有许多肿瘤可以转移到肺，所以评价肺病变时获得完整的临床病史总是很重要，以免将转移性肿瘤误诊为原发肿瘤。单单根据形态学来区分肺原发性病变和孤立性转移性肿瘤可能是困难的，需要多学科的方法，包括完整的临床和放射线检查，仔细询问临床病史以及应用特殊的病理学技术[222,223]。

肺的终末血管床是循环性肿瘤细胞最常见的停留部位之一；周围胸膜下肺组织是最初血行转移的部位。因此肺转移性肿瘤的典型表现是双侧多发性周围性结节形成。作为单个硬币样病变发生的孤立性转移非常

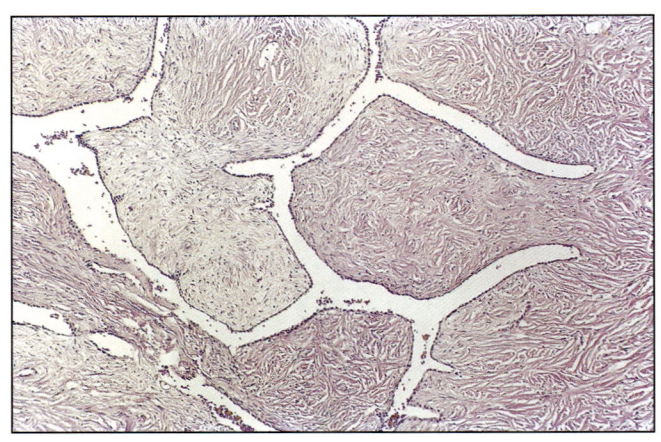

图5.41 肺的腺纤维瘤。注意类似于卵巢腺纤维瘤的棒样乳头。

少见，但是仍可以见于9%的病例[224]。支气管内转移类似于原发性支气管癌，是另外一种少见的生长方式，这种方式在结肠、直肠、胆道、胰腺、乳腺、子宫和肾已有描述。尤其是原发性支气管癌，通常表现为息肉样支气管内肿物。其他可能导致诊断困难的肺转移方式是以微小肿瘤结节的粟粒样扩散为特征，临床和放射学检查时与诸如结核等感染性病变和结节病十分相似。与肺转移性扩散相关的一种形式是癌性淋巴管炎（lymphangitis carcinomatosa），可见弥漫的瘤栓阻塞支气管的薄壁血管。这样的扩散方式常表现为双侧网状结节浸润，在影像学检查时可以导致与间质性肺病或血管栓塞性现象混淆。另一种少见的肺转移播散形式可能造成明显的诊断困难，其特征是肿瘤细胞沿着肺泡壁的内衬生长，产生与肺原发性细支气管肺泡癌极其类似的表现。这种特殊的播散方式在结肠、直肠、胆囊、乳腺、胰腺、胃、前列腺、甲状腺和肾已有描述。在这样的病例中，为了辨认失去细支气管肺泡样表现而显示较典型的原发性病变的区域，有必要检查深切的切片。

在肺部描述的另外一种少见的现象是推测为"良性"的肿瘤发生肺转移。这种病例的例子是"良性转移性平滑肌瘤"，指的是肺内出现单个，有时为多发性的细胞学良性的平滑肌肿瘤[225,226]。在多数病例中，患者是女性，伴有许多年前切除子宫平滑肌瘤或多发性良性平滑肌瘤切的病史。尽管这些病变的本质仍有争议，有些作者认为它们是非常低级别的高分化子宫平滑肌肉瘤的晚期转移[226]。相似改变可见于其他类型的"良性"肿瘤，包括脑膜瘤、胸腺瘤和骨巨细胞肿瘤（破骨细胞瘤）[223]。

胸膜肿瘤　Tumors of the pleura

胸膜可以为许多肿瘤性病变累及，包括良性和恶性病变。另外，胸膜也是一个常见的转移部位。最近，已经认识到胸膜是罕见的原发性脓胸相关性淋巴瘤（pyothorax-related lymphoma）的发病部位，它可能与EB病毒有关[227]。由于这个原因，正确解释胸膜活检结果不仅包括获得充足的检查材料，而且包括来自临床医师的临床和放射学相关信息。

恶性间皮瘤　Malignant mesothelioma

胸膜恶性间皮瘤发生年龄范围广，但是最常见于超过50岁的成年人，男性明显多于女性（男女之比为3:1）。多数胸膜间皮瘤与接触石棉有关，但必须记住，接触石棉更常见的并发症是肺癌而不是间皮瘤。肿瘤通常发生在接触石棉多年之后（>20年）；在有些病例中很难获得确切的石棉接触史[228,229]。潜伏期长是间皮瘤新增病例持续增加（以及在许多地方正在增加）的原因，尽管许多年前就已认识到石棉的危险性。接触石棉可以是职业性的，或是通过与工作无关的环境因素[230]。

间皮瘤的诊断依靠多种发现，包括石棉接触史，临床症状和体征，放射线发现，组织病理学特征，以及免疫组化和超微结构研究[231-234]。通常有隐匿发作的胸膜疼痛和气短的病史。常常出现胸膜渗出，可以为血性而且渗出量大。临床上，累及胸膜表面的间皮瘤和腺癌有重叠。而且，腺癌在组织学上可以与间皮瘤非常相似。由于这个原因，要获得满意的诊断结果需要多种手段，包括普通的组织学、特殊染色和电镜检查。另外，间皮瘤具有独特的核型异常，来自胸膜渗出的细胞遗传学分析可能具有鉴别诊断意义[235]。胸廓切开术仔细检查胸腔为诊断提供了最大的可能性；然而，可以观察胸膜表面并进行病变直接活检的胸腔镜检查也能获得可以接受的结果。

恶性间皮瘤的生物学行为令人担忧。症状发作和死亡之间的平均时间间隔是18个月，目前对于这种疾病的治疗通常无效，少数例外的病例可以进行根治性手术治疗[236]。影响预后的因素很少，但是某些组织学亚型可能与侵袭性的行为有关，例如肉瘤样型。临床上很少发现间皮瘤转移（尽管由于发病率增加，这样的病例变得比较常见），最常见的是在胸腔内局部扩散。肿瘤开始为胸膜表面小而隆起的区域，进而形成融合的结节，最终形成大的胸膜肿物。间皮瘤典型的大体表现是一层完全包裹肺的增厚的纤维胶原组织。鱼肉样肿瘤浸润其下的肺实质，与伴有假间皮瘤样生长方式的原发性肺腺癌可能特别难以鉴别[237]。近些年来，已经发现了少数局限性间皮瘤（localized mesothelioma），这些肿瘤常常可以手术切除，具有明显良好的预后[237a]。

恶性间皮瘤可以有三个基本的组织学类型：(1)上皮样；(2)肉瘤样；(3)混合性（双相性）。最常见的是，在同一个肿瘤内可能遇到这三种类型特征混合存在的区域。大约70%的间皮瘤以上皮样为主，25%以双相性为主，而只有5%以肉瘤样为主。也存在非常少见的高分化乳头状间皮瘤，这种肿瘤预后较好[238]。

上皮样间皮瘤（epithelioid mesothelioma）的特征是圆形或多角形肿瘤细胞增生，伴有丰富的深嗜酸性胞浆和温和的细胞核，常常缺乏核分裂象。肿瘤细胞可有多种生长方式，其中最常见的是管状乳头状

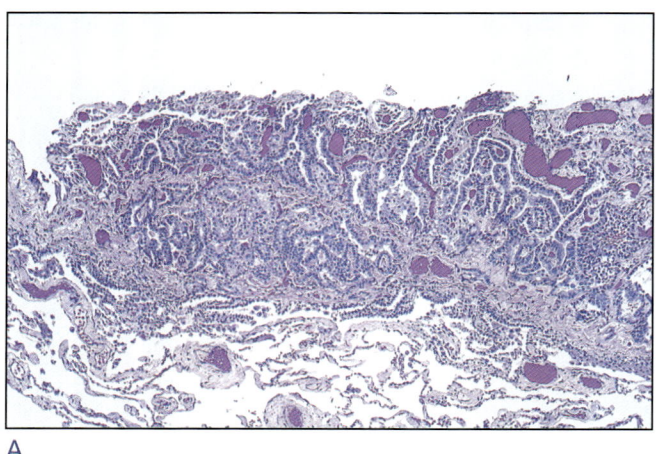
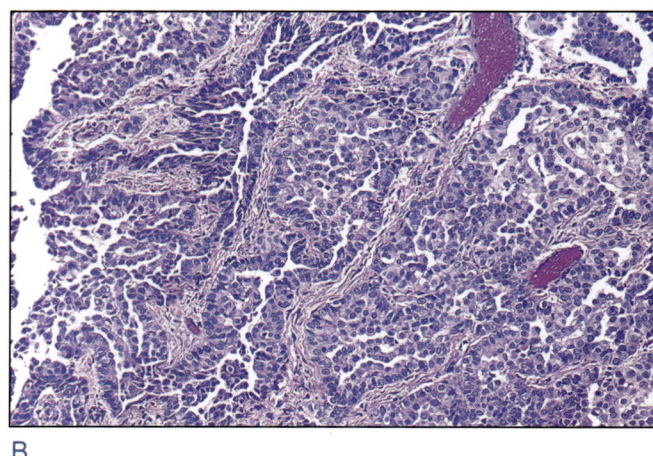

图5.42 （A）上皮样间皮瘤沿着胸膜表面呈斑片状生长；（B）高倍镜下显示管状乳头状生长方式。

型，以形成内衬立方细胞的腺管状结构混合含有纤细纤维血管轴心的乳头状结构为特征（图5.42）。这些区域中偶尔可见沙粒体，但是没有诊断意义。也可以见到微腺管状生长方式；其特征是内衬单层立方或柱状上皮的小腺样结构的增生。这种结构与腺癌转移性胸膜扩散可能很难区别。肿瘤细胞也可以是大的多角形细胞呈实性片块状生长，细胞核圆形，偶尔有明显的核仁。这种亚型被称为蜕膜样间皮瘤（deciduoid mesothelioma）[239]。其他不常见的生长方式包括主要由小而深染细胞构成的肿瘤，核浆比例高，类似于小细胞癌；伴有大而奇异细胞的肿瘤，包括多形性巨细胞，可能类似于肺间变性癌或转移性肉瘤；含有大量炎细胞与肿瘤性间皮成分混合的肿瘤（所谓的淋巴组织细胞样间皮瘤，lymphohistiocytoid mesothelioma）[240]；由透明细胞构成的肿瘤，可能类似于肾细胞癌[240a]；显示印戒细胞特征的肿瘤，类似于胃恶性肿瘤转移，以及伴有明显的横纹样胞浆包涵体的肿瘤，这些病例与特殊的侵袭性过程明显相关[204b]。含有丰富酸性黏多糖的明显的黏液样间质（透明质酸）虽然不常见，但却是上皮样间皮瘤另外一个明显的特征（图5.43），这种改变可能与预后较好有关[240c]。

肉瘤样间皮瘤（sarcomatoid mesothelioma）是由成束的梭形细胞增生构成的，伴有卵圆形细胞核，少量双染性胞浆，偶尔有突出的核仁。肿瘤细胞可以表现为纤维肉瘤样外观，伴有显示人字形结构的细长的细胞束和丰富的细胞间胶原沉积，或者可能具有明显的席纹状外观，与所谓的恶性纤维组织细胞瘤无法区别，但多形性通常不是显著的特征（图5.44）。当间质胶原化变得明显时，肿瘤具有明显的纤维组织增生性外观，在小的活检标本中无法与纤维性胸膜炎相鉴别（图

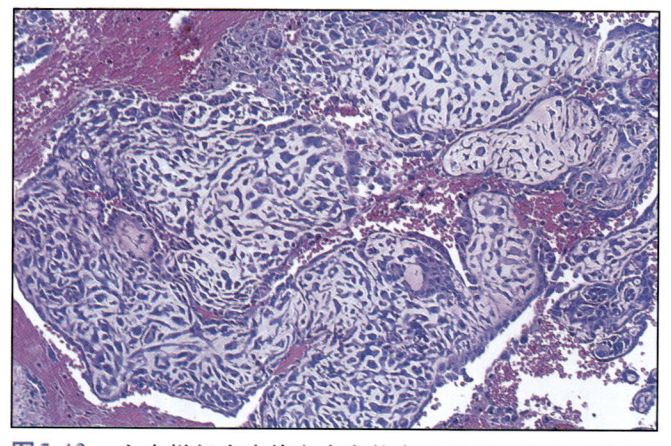

图5.43 上皮样间皮瘤伴有丰富的富于透明质酸的黏液样基质。

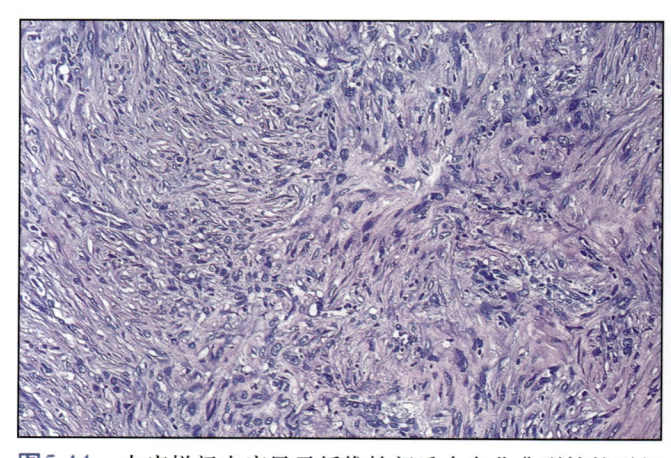

图5.44 肉瘤样间皮瘤显示纤维性间质内有非典型性梭形细胞群。

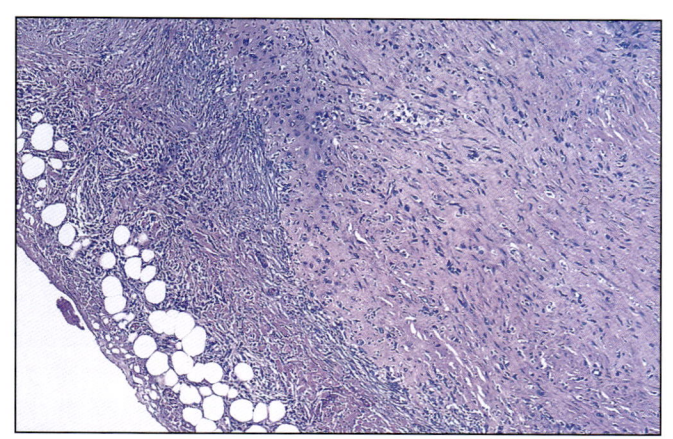

图5.45 纤维组织增生性间皮瘤。注意不规则的脂肪浸润。

5.45)。在这种情况下，浸润胸壁软组织（例如脂肪组织）是重要的诊断线索。一般来说，肉瘤样间皮瘤的非典型性比上皮样间皮瘤明显，而且常常显示核分裂活性和坏死灶。少数显示骨化生和软骨化生病例也有描述。

双相性间皮瘤（biphasic mesothelioma）的特征是容易识别的上皮样成分和肉瘤样成分以不同的比例混合存在。

因为间皮瘤可能具有多种形态学表现，而且许多胸膜转移性肿瘤在临床、放射学和大体表现上均类似于间皮瘤，所以许多病例都很难作出明确的诊断。即使与反应性间皮增生的区分通常也极其困难[241]，虽然坏死，细胞非典型性和EMA染色形态或许有助于诊断，但通常需要证实有令人信服的邻近胸膜下组织的浸润。通常需要应用多种技术才能作出诊断，包括组织化学、免疫组化和超微结构检查。最常应用的组织化学染色是淀粉酶消化的PAS；肿瘤细胞内存在淀粉消化后的PAS强阳性物质，提示有上皮性黏液，不支持恶性间皮瘤的诊断，虽然偶尔可见少数阳性细胞已经得到公认。阿利新蓝（Alcian blue）染色间皮瘤中的透明质酸阳性；通过透明质酸酶消化能够特征性地去除蓝色阳性反应。

免疫组化是目前确立间皮瘤诊断应用最广泛的技术。可惜的是，没有可靠的或特异性的标记物能够确立恶性间皮瘤的诊断，诊断是根据一组抗体的免疫反应形态进行的除外性诊断[231-233,242-244]。间皮瘤角蛋白和EMA染色普遍阳性；然而，因为这些标记物广泛分布于其他上皮性肿瘤，所以对于诊断的价值可能有限。目前推荐的恶性间皮瘤的免疫染色包括至少两种阳性和两种阴性抗体的组合。认为最有鉴别意义的间皮瘤"阴性"标记物的抗体包括CEA、MOC31、Ber-EP4以及B 72.3，最好的"阳性"标记物包括细胞角蛋白（cytokeratin）5/6和钙结合蛋白（calretinin）[243]。最近提出MUC4作为一个有价值的阴性鉴别标记物[245]，而D2-40和膜黏蛋白（podoplanin）被认为是非常特异的阳性标记物[245a]。然而，重要的是必须提到，许多"阴性"标记物在少数恶性间皮瘤病例中可能阳性，而且几个"阳性"标记物在非间皮来源的腺癌和其他需要鉴别诊断的病变已经证实为阳性[244,246]。重要的是，间皮瘤偶尔还可能表达平滑肌标记物，例如肌动蛋白和结蛋白，尤其是肉瘤样成分，可能导致与平滑肌肿瘤的混淆[247]。实际上，免疫组化染色在肉瘤样间皮瘤的鉴别诊断中往往没有意义[248]。许多年来，电镜检查被认为是诊断间皮瘤的"金标准"[231-233]。间皮瘤细胞（至少是伴有上皮样形态学的肿瘤细胞）的特征是表面有大量明显变长的微绒毛，缺乏分泌性胞浆颗粒。然而，当电镜检查所得到的材料固定不充分时，超微结构检查不是在所有的病例均有可能作出诊断，在低分化肿瘤或肉瘤样间皮瘤中，特征性的细长的微绒毛可能并不明显。近些年来，已经引入许多号称特异性的间皮标记物用于恶性间皮瘤的诊断，其中包括血栓调节蛋白（thrombomodulin）、钙结合蛋白、钙黏附蛋白（cadherins）、CD44、HBME-1、WT-1和角蛋白5/6[249-253]。然而，所有这些标记物与其他多种肿瘤均有交叉反应，尤其是转移癌，使得其应用有些局限性[244]。因此，间皮瘤的诊断依然需要依赖多种方法，包括临床特征、大体和显微镜下特征、免疫组化和电镜检查才能作出明确诊断[231,233]。

假间皮瘤性腺癌
Pseudomesotheliomatous adenocarcinoma

近些年来特别关注周围性肺腺癌的一种类型，它在临床、放射学和组织学上可能类似于弥漫性恶性间皮瘤。Harwood及其同事把这些病变命名为假间皮瘤性腺癌[254]。这里讨论这些肿瘤是因为它们可能与原发性恶性间皮瘤非常类似，而且它们主要累及胸膜部位。在近期发表的文献中，已有几项研究描述了这种病变[237,254-256]。

假间皮瘤性腺癌发生在老年患者，男性比女性常见。临床症状与恶性间皮瘤没有区别，包括胸痛、呼吸困难、咳嗽和浸润性胸膜肿瘤的征象。最常见的胸部X线发现是胸膜渗出，伴或不伴有胸膜肿块。在一项研究中，多达21%的患者有石棉接触史[255]。多达73%的病例有吸烟史。大体上，肿瘤表现为厚的鱼肉样胸膜斑片和肿块，沿着胸膜表面延伸并包裹肺脏。组织学上，成巢或成片的细胞浸润胸膜，局部形成腺体或管状乳头状结构（图

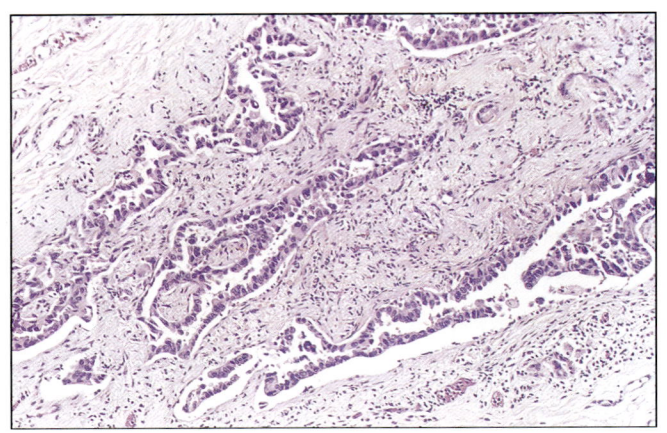

图5.46　假间皮瘤性腺癌累及胸膜，伴有局灶管状乳头状生长方式。

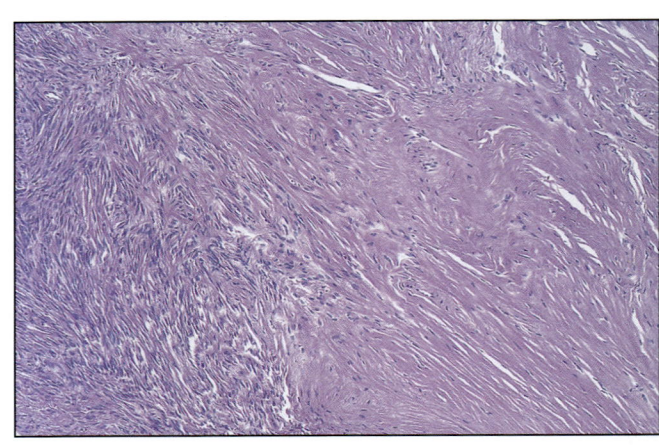

图5.47　胸膜孤立性纤维性肿瘤，显示实性梭形细胞区域和弥漫性硬化性区域之间的移行。

5.46）。也可以见到沙粒体，尤其是在乳头状区域。纤维性间质中常常发现孤立的腺体。腺腔常常充满PSA阳性抗淀粉酶消化的黏液或胞浆内空泡。免疫组化研究显示，在100%的病例中多克隆CEA和低分子量角蛋白强阳性，其次是BER-EP4（60%）、Leu-M1（53%）和B 72.3（47%）[255]。多数病例同时表达一种以上的抗体。

有人提出，类似于间皮瘤的腺癌可能来源于位于胸膜下的相对较小的腺癌。在文献报道的尸检病例中，镜下或大体检查已经发现了这样的肿瘤[254,255]。然而，在某些病例中，胸膜肿瘤的来源不能排除来自肺外隐匿部位转移的可能性。这些肿瘤预后非常不好，至少和间皮瘤一样差。鉴别这种类型腺癌和间皮瘤主要具有医学法律上的重要性，而不是预后或临床治疗反应上的差异。

胸膜间叶性肿瘤
Mesenchymal tumors of the pleura

胸膜原发性间叶性肿瘤相对少见。绝大多数肿瘤是良性的，其特征是界限清楚，息肉样和有蒂的病变，附着于壁层或脏层胸膜。原发性胸膜肉瘤极其少见，多数胸膜肉瘤样肿瘤或为转移性肿瘤，或为肉瘤样间皮瘤。

孤立性纤维性肿瘤（solitary fibrous tumor）是最常见的良性间叶性胸膜肿瘤。这些肿瘤最初被Klemperer和Rabin描述为局灶性纤维性间皮瘤[257]。随后Scharifker和Kaneko[258]以及其他作者的超微结构研究证实，肿瘤细胞没有间皮细胞的特征，而是显示出成纤维细胞的特征，因此命名为间皮下纤维瘤、局限性纤维性肿瘤或孤立性纤维性肿瘤[259,260]。这些肿瘤最常见于40～50岁和50～60岁的成人。多数患者无症状，但是胸痛、呼吸困难和发热等症状已有报道[261-263]。有些肿瘤特征性地伴有低血糖。肿瘤大体边界清楚，息肉样，有包膜，直径可以达到20 cm，通常以短蒂附着于胸膜。肿瘤通常压迫肺，因此，胸部X线检查可以发现类似于胸膜下肺肿物。

组织学上，这些肿瘤的特征是多变的形态学表现，这种特征常常导致误诊为其他间叶性肿瘤。通常可以遇到不同比例的两种基本成分：实性梭形细胞成分和弥漫性硬化性成分[120]（图5.47）。实性梭形细胞成分可以有多种生长方式，可误诊为其他确切类型的间叶性肿瘤，这些生长方式包括类似于纤维组织细胞瘤的短席纹状结构，血管外皮细胞性、血管纤维瘤性和人字形生长方式，显示波浪状神经结构的区域，伴有明显的神经型栅栏状排列，以及单相性滑膜肉瘤的交织成束的生长方式。另外，可能出现退行性间质改变，例

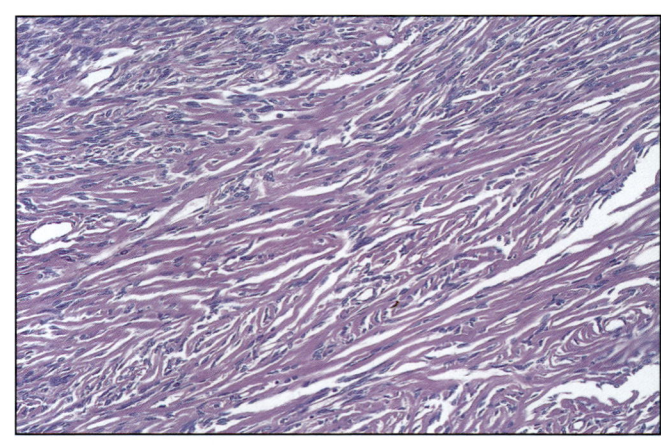

图5.48　胸膜孤立性纤维性肿瘤，实性梭形细胞区域，伴有纵形带状绳索样胶原的沉积。

如明显的黏液样基质沉积、胶原变性、化生性骨形成、"石棉样"纤维形成以及多核间质细胞，增加了诊断的困难。肿瘤细胞通常为卵圆形，细胞核温和，染色质散在，核仁不明显，核周有一圈不清楚的双染性胞浆。肿瘤细胞的胞浆常常具有树突状突起，最好应用特殊染色或电镜检查来评估。这些肿瘤非常独特的表现是平行于梭形细胞分布的条索状瘢痕样胶原带沉积（图5.48）。多数病例核分裂象缺乏或很少。弥漫性硬化性结构由细胞稀少的区域构成，显示明显的胶原纤维沉积和间质玻璃样变性，尤其是围绕在血管周围。弥漫性硬化和实性梭形细胞增生之间常见混合和移行。诊断依靠发现特征性的组织病理学表现，结合临床情况和病变的大体特征（例如以胸膜为基底的息肉样和带蒂的肿物）。

免疫组化在诊断中具有重要的辅助作用，它有助于排除其他的分化。肿瘤细胞波形蛋白染色一致阳性，但是角蛋白、EMA、肌动蛋白、结蛋白和S-100阴性。在多达80%的孤立性纤维性肿瘤病例中，梭形细胞CD34染色阳性[121,122]。在两项研究的所有病例中，肿瘤细胞bcl-2染色均匀一致的强阳性[111,264]。另外，CD99免疫染色阳性是相对一致的发现[265]。这些标记物中没有一个是特异性的，在许多其他梭形细胞肿瘤中它们均可阳性，因此，必须结合临床情况和组织学所见来解释这些标记物。

孤立性纤维性肿瘤是最常见的通过局部手术切除可以治愈的良性肿瘤。然而，5%～10%的肿瘤界限不清，浸润邻近结构，核分裂活性以及细胞核多形性明显，因此符合恶性诊断。从概念上讲，最好将恶性孤立性纤维性肿瘤看成是胸膜的纤维肉瘤[266]。良性孤立性纤维性肿瘤和恶性孤立性纤维性肿瘤的分界点尚不清楚。England等提出，出现细胞过多、多形性、坏死以及每10个高倍视野多于4个核分裂象作为这些肿瘤恶性的诊断标准[260]。然而，我们观察到这样一些病例，这是一些界限清楚的息肉样有被膜的肿瘤，虽然具有包括坏死、细胞过多、细胞核的多形性以及核分裂活跃等恶性的形态学特征，但其行为却是惰性的[120]。因此我们个人认为，除了细胞学非典型性以外，在对这些肿瘤作出恶性诊断之前必须存在边界不清和浸润邻近结构。

胸膜平滑肌肿瘤（smooth muscle tumors）最近已经得到认识[267,268]。这些肿瘤可以表现为位于胸膜的肿物或弥漫性胸膜增厚，类似于弥漫性恶性间质瘤。临床上，患者表现出胸痛咳嗽、呼吸困难和（或）发热的症状，没有其他部位的病史。组织学上，胸膜平滑肌肉瘤与软组织平滑肌肉瘤相似。这些肿瘤由增生的细长梭形细胞组成，伴有中等量的嗜酸性胞浆，雪茄形细胞核，伴有不同程度非典型性和核分裂活性。免疫组化研究证实平滑肌标记物和波形蛋白阳性，而上皮性标记物、CD34、以及 *bcl-2* 阴性。诊断取决于识别任何部位平滑肌肿瘤独特的组织病理学特征，免疫组化或超微结构证实平滑肌表型以及缺乏其他分化，而且通过充分的临床检查没有发现身体其他部位有类似的肿瘤。

胸膜滑膜肉瘤（synovial sarcomas）也已被认识[269]。这些肿瘤主要发生于儿童、青少年和年轻人。临床以多次复发和转移为特征，可以导致患者死亡。胸膜滑膜肉瘤与其他部位滑膜肉瘤具有相同的组织学、免疫组化和超微结构特征（见第24章）。这些肿瘤都相当于双相性滑膜肉瘤，虽然单相性滑膜肉瘤也可发生。主要应与双相性间皮瘤进行鉴别诊断。与恶性间皮瘤不同，胸膜滑膜肉瘤发生在比较年轻的患者，生长迅速并形成界限清楚的肿瘤结节，而不是弥漫性的浸润性肿物，并且比较容易治疗。

胸膜假间皮瘤样（上皮样）血管肉瘤[pseudomesotheliomatous (epithelioid) angiosarcoma]是最近描述的另外一种病变[270,271]。这些肿瘤的特征是大的上皮样血管内皮细胞增生，可能与上皮性肿瘤非常相似。临床上，肿瘤表现为弥漫性胸膜增厚和出血性渗出。组织学上，这种病变表现出的特征从上皮样血管内皮细胞瘤到明显的上皮样血管肉瘤都有。肿瘤的特征是肿瘤细胞成片或成簇，细胞核大呈空泡状，偶尔有明显的核仁，胞浆丰富，嗜酸性，常常含有胞浆空泡（图5.49A）。也可见到类似于间皮瘤的管状乳头状生长方式（图5.49B）。一项免疫组化研究显示波形蛋白强阳性，而角蛋白呈局灶弱阳性[270]。肿瘤细胞至少共同表达两种常见的内皮细胞标记物，包括CD31、CD34、VIII因子相关抗原和荆豆凝集素-I（Ulex europaeus agglutinin-I）。这些肿瘤的临床行为具有非常强侵袭性，在诊断时常常伴有播散性疾病，而且在诊断几个月内死亡。

胸膜罕见的肿瘤
Rare tumors of the pleura

胸膜胸腺瘤（pleural thymomas）是少见病变，可能表现为局灶性瘤块或弥漫性胸膜增厚，类似于恶性间皮瘤[272,273]。患者通常是成年人，表现为局灶性胸膜肿块，无纵隔受累。这些病例与重症肌无力无关。组织学上，肿瘤与发生在前纵隔的肿瘤基本相同（见第21章），其特征是由上皮细胞与淋巴细胞混合而构成的双相细胞团，排列成分叶状，并被粗大的纤维条带分隔。梭形细胞形态学也有描述。上皮性肿瘤细胞角蛋白抗体阳性，

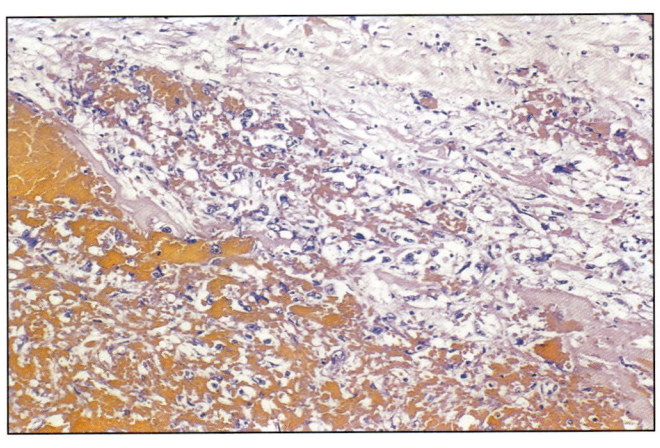 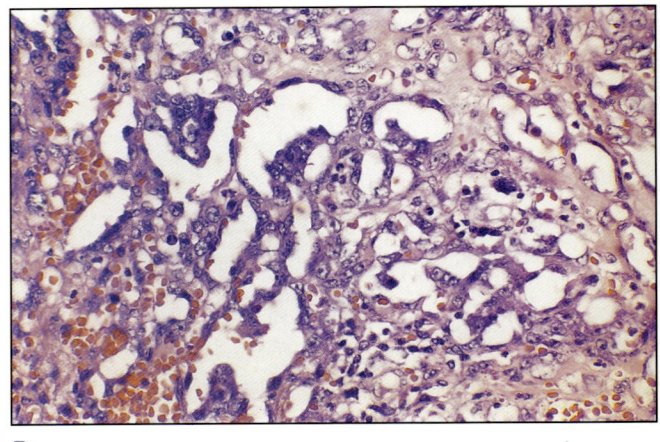

图5.49 （A）胸膜假间皮瘤样血管肉瘤；（B）胸膜假间皮瘤样血管肉瘤中的管状乳头状结构。

这个发现有利于诊断。在梭形细胞胸腺瘤病例中，可能需要与肉瘤样间皮瘤和孤立性纤维性肿瘤进行鉴别诊断。对于局限性肿瘤选择完全手术切除进行治疗。然而，伴有弥漫性胸膜受累的病例或当肿瘤切除不完全时，可能需要放疗。

发生在胸膜的腺瘤样瘤（adenomatoid tumors）已有描述[274]。这些病变表现为胸膜小结节，是在与其无关的肺内肿物手术时偶然发现的。肿瘤由增生的上皮样细胞构成，纤维性间质中有明显的空泡和管状间隙，类似于其他部位的腺瘤样瘤。角蛋白染色有助于证实这些病变中细胞的上皮性本质。

黏液表皮样癌（mucoepidermoid carcinoma）是另外一个最近描述的胸膜原发性恶性肿瘤[275]。这些肿瘤的特征是胸膜部位发生局限性肿物，组织学检查表现为岛屿状非典型性鳞状上皮与散在黏液细胞混合，黏液卡红染色黏液细胞呈强阳性。其中一例报道是以含有丰富的梭形成纤维细胞的明显的纤维性间隔为特征的，提出了需要考虑双相性间皮瘤诊断的问题。然而，肿瘤局限性的本质和存在明显显示黏液表皮样分化特征的肿瘤细胞岛，可以正确地诊断这种病变[275]。

胸膜肺母细胞瘤（pleuropulmonary blastomas）是一组主要发生在儿童的肿瘤，包括以前命名为发生在先天性囊性腺瘤样畸形或支气管原性囊肿的肉瘤的各种肿瘤，以及间叶性囊性错构瘤[276-279]。大体上，这些病变可以表现为囊性或实性肿瘤，大小差别可以很大，直径从几厘米到20 cm不等。单纯性囊性病变罕见。组织学上，与成人的肺母细胞瘤完全不同（见第193页），不成熟上皮性成分不是这个病变的一部分。婴儿胸膜肺母细胞瘤可有不同的组织学表现，伴有软骨肉瘤、骨肉瘤、平滑肌肉瘤、横纹肌肉瘤或未分化间质性成分的区域。当肿瘤是囊性时，可见未被累及的正常上皮内衬囊性结构。免疫组化染色仅对证实病变的间叶性本质以及排除上皮性或间皮性分化具有价值。这些患者的预后主要取决于诊断时的分期和肉瘤成分的分级，但是一般来说，这些肿瘤是侵袭性的肿瘤，伴有实性成分的病例5年生存率低于50%[277]。不常见的单纯性囊性病变预后较好。

参考文献

1. Garfinkel L, Silverberg E 1991 Lung cancer and smoking trends in the United States over the past 25 years. CA 41: 137–145
2. Rubin S A 1991 Lung cancer: past, present, and future. J Thorac Imaging 7: 1–8
3. Stanley K, Stjernsward J 1989 Lung cancer: a worldwide health problem. Chest 96 (suppl): 1s–5s
4. Gritz E R 1993 Lung cancer: now, more than ever, a feminist issue. CA 43: 197–199
5. Aronchick J M 1990 Clinical aspects of lung cancer. Semin Roentgenol 25: 5–11
6. Devesa S S, Shaw G L, Blot W J 1991 Changing patterns of lung carcinoma. Cancer Epidemiol Biomarkers Prev 1: 29–34
7. Travis W D, Travis L B, Devesa S S 1995 Lung cancer. Cancer 75: 191–202
8. Rosado-de-Christenson M L, Templeton P A, Moran C A 1994 Bronchogenic carcinoma: radiologic/pathologic correlation. Radiographics 14: 429–446
9. Sobin L, Yesner R 1981 Histologic typing of lung tumors. International histologic classification of tumors, 2nd edn. World Health Organization, Geneva, vol 1
10. Fraser R G, Pare J A P, Pare P D et al. 1989 Neoplastic diseases of the lung. In: Fraser R G, Pare J A P, Pare P D et al. (eds) Diagnosis of diseases of the chest, 3rd edn. Saunders, Philadelphia, PA, p 1327–1399
11. Viallet J, Minna J D 1990 Dominant oncogenes and tumor suppressor genes in the pathogenesis of lung cancer. Am J Respir Cell Mol Biol 2: 225–237
12. Takahashi T, Takahashi Y, Suzuki H et al. 1991 The *p53* gene is frequently mutated in small cell lung cancer with a distinctive nucleotide substitution pattern. Oncogene 6: 1775–1778

13. Harris C C, Hollstein M 1993 Clinical implications of the *p53* tumor-suppressor gene. N Engl J Med 329: 1318–1327
14. Rodenhuis S, Slebos R J C 1992 Significance of *ras* oncogene activation in human lung cancer. Cancer Res 52: 2665–2669
15. Baylin S B, Herman J G, Graaf J R et al. 1998 Alterations in DNA methylation. A fundamental aspect of neoplasia. Adv Cancer Res 72: 141–196
16. Zuchbauer-Muller S, Fong K M, Virmani A K et al. 2001 Aberrant promoter methylation in multiple genes in non-small cell cancers. Cancer Res 61: 249–255
17. Damman R, Li C, Yoon J-H et al. 2000 Epigenetic inactivation of a RAS associated domain family protein from the lung tumor suppressor locus 3p21.3. Nat Genet 25: 315–319
18. Paez J G, Janne P A, Lee J C et al. 2004. *EGFR* mutations in lung cancer: correlation with clinical reponse to gefitinib therapy. Science 304: 1497–1500
19. Grippi M A 1990 Clinical aspects of lung cancer. Semin Roentgenol 25: 12–24
20. Boyards M C 1991 Clinical manifestations of carcinoma of the lung. J Thorac Imaging 7: 21–28
21. Haque A K 1991 Pathology of carcinoma of the lung: an up-date on current concepts. J Thorac Imaging 7: 9–20
22. Pietra G G 1990 The pathology of carcinoma of the lung. Semin Roentgenol 25: 25–33
23. Yesner R 1988 Histopathology of lung cancer. Semin Ultrasound CT MR 9: 4–26
24. Wilson R W, Frazier A 1998 Pathological and radiological correlation of endobronchial neoplasms: part II, malignant tumors. Ann Diagn Pathol 2: 31–54
25. Kuriyama K, Tateishi R, Doi O et al. 1977 Prevalence of air bronchograms in small peripheral carcinomas of the lung on thin-section CT: comparison with benign lesions. AJR 128: 893–914
26. White C S, Templeton P A 1993 Radiologic manifestations of bronchogenic cancer. Clin Chest Med 14: 56–67
27. Tsuta K, Ishii G, Yoh K et al. 2004 Primary lung carcinoma with signet-ring cell carcinoma components. Clinicopathologic analysis of 39 cases. Am J Surg Pathol 28: 868–874
28. Liebow A A 1960 Bronchiolo-alveolar carcinoma. Advances in internal medicine. Year Book, Chicago, vol 10
29. Moran C A, Hochholzer L, Fishback N F et al. 1992 Mucinous (so-called colloid) carcinoma of lung. Mod Pathol 5: 634–638
30. Graeme-Cook F, Mark E J 1991 Pulmonary mucinous cystic tumors of borderline malignancy. Hum Pathol 22: 185–190
31. Kragel P J, Devaney K O, Meth B M et al. 1990 Mucinous cystadenoma of the lung: a report of two cases with immunohistochemical and ultrastructural analysis. Arch Pathol Lab Med 114: 1053–1056
32. Higashiyama M, Doi O, Kodama K et al. 1992 Cystic mucinous adenocarcinoma of the lung: two cases of cystic variant of mucinous-producing lung adenocarcinoma. Chest 101: 763–766
33. Moran C A 1995 Mucin-rich tumors of the lung. Adv Anat Pathol 2: 299–305
34. Silver S A, Askin F B 1997 True papillary carcinoma of the lung. A distinct clinicopathologic entity. Am J Surg Pathol 21: 43–51
35. Katzenstein A-L A, Prioleau P G, Askin F B 1980 The histologic spectrum and significance of clear cell change in lung carcinoma. Cancer 45: 943–947
36. Dulmet-Brender E, Jaubert F, Huchou G 1986 Exophytic endobronchial epidermoid carcinoma. Cancer 57: 1358–1364
37. Suster S, Huczar M, Herczeg E 1987 Spindle cell squamous carcinoma of lung. A light microscopic, immunohistochemical and ultrastructural study of a case. Histopathology 11: 871–878
38. Nappi O, Glasner S D, Swanson P E et al. 1994 Biphasic and monophasic sarcomatoid carcinomas of the lung. A reappraisal of "carcinosarcomas" and "spindle-cell carcinomas." Am J Clin Pathol 102: 331–340
39. Wick M R, Ritter J H, Nappi O 1995 Inflammatory sarcomatoid carcinoma of the lung. Hum Pathol 26: 1014–1021
40. Brambilla E, Moro D, Veale D et al. 1992 Basal cell (basaloid) carcinoma of the lung. A new morphologic and phenotypic entity with separate prognostic significance. Hum Pathol 23: 993–998
41. Chang Y L, Wu C T, Shih J Y et al. 2002. New aspects in clinicopathologic and oncogene studies of 23 pulmonary lymphoepithelioma-like carcinomas. Am J Surg Pathol 26: 715–723
42. Butler A E, Colby T V, Weiss L M et al. 1989 Lymphoepithelioma-like carcinoma of the lung. Am J Surg Pathol 13: 629–632
43. Fishback N F, Travis W D, Moran C A et al. 1994 Pleomorphic (spindle/giant cell) carcinoma of the lung. Cancer 73: 2936–2945
44. Rossi G, Cavazza A, Sturm N et al. 2003 Pulmonary carcinomas with pleomorphic, sarcomatoid, or sarcomatous elements. A clinicopathologic and immunohistochemical study of 75 cases. Am J Surg Pathol 27: 311–324
45. Attanoos R L, Papagiannis A, Suttinont P et al. 1998 Pulmonary giant cell carcinoma: pathological entity or morphological phenotype? Histopathology 32: 225–231
46. Przygodzki R M, Koss M N, Moran C A et al. 1996 Pleomorphic (giant and spindle cell) carcinoma is genetically distinct from adenocarcinoma and squamous cell carcinoma by K-*ras*-2 and *p53* analysis. Am J Clin Pathol 106: 487–492
47. Tamboli P, Toprani T H, Amin M B et al. 2004. Carcinoma of lung with rhabdoid features. Hum Pathol 35: 8–13
48. Sridhar K S, Bounassi M J, Raub W et al. 1990 Clinical features of adenosquamous lung carcinoma in 127 patients. Am Rev Respir Dis 142: 19–23
49. Naunheim K S, Taylor J R, Skosey C et al. 1987 Adenosquamous lung carcinoma: clinical characteristics, treatment and prognosis. Ann Thorac Surg 44: 462–469
50. Fitzgibbons P L, Kern W H 1985 Adenosquamous carcinoma of the lung: a clinical and pathological study of seven cases. Hum Pathol 16: 463–467
51. Travis W D, Gal A A, Colby T V et al. 1998 Reproducibility of neuroendocrine lung tumor classification. Hum Pathol 29: 272–279
52. Gould V E, Linnoila R I, Memoli V A et al. 1983 Neuroendocrine cells and neuroendocrine neoplasms of the lung. Pathol Annu 18: 287–305
53. Mooi W J, Dewar A, Springall D et al. 1988 Non-small cell lung carcinoma with neuroendocrine features. A light microscopic, immunohistochemical, and ultrastructural study of 11 cases. Histopathology 13: 329–334
54. Travis W D, Linnoila R I, Tsokos M G et al. 1991 Neuroendocrine tumors of the lung with proposed criteria for large cell neuroendocrine carcinomas. An ultrastructural, immunohistochemical, and flow cytometric study of 35 cases. Am J Surg Pathol 16: 529–553
55. Jiang S-X, Kameya T, Shoji M 1998 Large cell neuroendocrine carcinoma of the lung. A histologic and immunohistochemical study of 22 cases. Am J Surg Pathol 22: 526–537
56. Ricci C, Patrassi N, Massa R et al. 1973 Carcinoid syndrome in bronchial adenoma. Am J Surg 126: 671–675
57. Minna J D, Pass H I, Gladstein E et al. 1989 Cancer of the lung. In: DeVita V T, Hellman S, Rosenberg S A (eds) Cancer. Principles and practice of oncology, 3rd edn. J B Lippincott, Philadelphia, PA, p 591
58. Cebelin M S 1980 Melanocytic bronchial carcinoid tumor. Cancer 46: 1843–1848
59. Grazer R, Cohen S M, Jacobs J B 1982 Melanin-containing peripheral carcinoid of the lung. Am J Surg Pathol 6: 73–78
60. Gal A A, Koss M N, Hochholzer L et al. 1993 Pigmented pulmonary carcinoid tumor: an immunohistochemical and ultrastructural study. Arch Pathol Lab Med 117: 832–836
61. Sklar J L, Churg A, Bensch K G 1980 Oncocytic carcinoid tumor of the lung. Am J Surg Pathol 4: 287–292
62. Wise W S, Bonder D, Aikawa M et al. 1982 Carcinoid tumor of lung with varied histology. Am J Surg Pathol 6: 261–267
63. Du EZ, Goldstraw P, Zacharias J et al. 2004. TTF-1 expression is specific for lung primary in typical and atypical carcinoids: TTF-1-positive carcinoids are predominantly in peripheral location. Hum Pathol 35: 825–831
64. Arrigoni M G, Woolner L B, Bernatz P E 1985 Atypical carcinoid tumors of the lung. J Thorac Cardiovasc Surg 89: 8–15
65. Paladugu R R, Benfield J R, Pak H Y et al. 1989 Bronchopulmonary Kultchizky cell carcinomas. A new classification scheme for typical and atypical carcinoids. Cancer 64: 1304–1310
66. El-Naggar A K, Ballance W, Abdul-Karim F W et al. 1991 Typical and atypical bronchopulmonary carcinoids: a clinicopathologic and flow cytometric study. Am J Clin Pathol 95: 828–834
67. Travis W D, Rush W, Flieder D B et al. 1998 Survival analysis of 200 pulmonary neuroendocrine tumors with clarification of criteria for atypical carcinoid and its separation from typical carcinoid. Am J Surg Pathol 22: 934–944
68. Beasley M B, Thunnissen F B J M, Brambilla E et al. 2000 Pulmonary atypical carcinoid: predictors of survival in 106 cases. Hum Pathol 31: 1255–1265
69. Kato Y, Ferguson T B, Bennet D E et al. 1969 Oat cell carcinoma of the lung. A review of 138 cases. Cancer 23: 517–523
70. Spiegelman D, Maurer L H, Ware J H et al. 1989 Prognostic factors in small cell carcinoma of the lung. An analysis of 1521 patients. J Clin Oncol 7: 344–356
71. Adelstein D J, Tomashefski J F, Snow N J et al. 1986 Mixed small cell and non-small cell lung cancer. Chest 89: 699–708
72. Nicholson S A, Beasley M B, Brambilla E et al. 2002 Small cell lung carcinoma (SCLC). A clinicopathologic study of 100 cases with surgical specimens. Am J Surg Pathol 26: 1184–1197
73. Radice P A, Matthews M J, Inde D C et al. 1982 The clinical behavior of "mixed" small cell/large cell bronchogenic carcinoma compared to "pure" small cell subtype. Cancer 50: 2894–2903
74. Moran C A 1995 Primary salivary gland-type tumors of the lung. Semin Diagn Pathol 12: 106–122
75. Moran C A, Suster S, Koss M N 1994 Primary adenoid cystic carcinomas of the lung: a clinicopathologic and immunohistochemical study of 16 cases. Cancer 73: 1390–1397
76. Moran C A, Suster S, Koss M N 1992 Acinic cell carcinoma of the lung (Fechner tumor): a clinicopathologic, immunohistochemical, and ultrastructural study of five cases. Am J Surg Pathol 16: 1039–1050
77. Fechner R E, Bentnick B R, Askew J B Jr 1972 Acinic cell tumor of the lung. A histologic and ultrastructural study. Cancer 29: 501–508
78. Yousem S A, Hochholzer L 1987 Mucoepidermoid tumors of the lung. Cancer 60: 1346–1352
79. Wilson R W, Moran C A 1997 Epithelial-myoepithelial carcinoma of the lung: immunohistochemical and ultrastructural observations and review of the literature. Hum Pathol 28: 631–635
80. Moran C A, Suster S, Askin F B et al. 1994 Benign and malignant salivary gland-type mixed tumors of the lung: a clinicopathologic and immunohistochemical study of eight cases. Cancer 73: 2481–2490

81. Fechner R E, Bentnick B R 1973 Ultrastructure of bronchial oncocytoma. Cancer 31: 1451–1457
82. Nielsen A L 1985 Malignant bronchial oncocytoma: a case report and review of the literature. Hum Pathol 16: 852–854
83. Santos-Briz A, Jenron J, Sastre R et al. 1977 Oncocytoma of the lung. Cancer 40: 1330–1336
84. Berho M, Moran C A, Suster S 1995 Malignant mixed epithelial/mesenchymal neoplasms of the lung. Semin Diagn Pathol 12: 123–139
85. Barnard W G 1952 Embryoma of the lung. Thorax 7: 229–234
86. Spencer H 1961 Pulmonary blastomas. J Pathol Bacteriol 82: 161–165
87. Kodama T, Shimosato Y, Watanabe S et al. 1984 Six cases of well differentiated adenocarcinoma simulating fetal lung tubules in the pseudoglandular stage. Comparison with pulmonary blastoma. Am J Surg Pathol 8: 735–744
88. Nakatani Y, Dickersin R, Mark E 1990 Pulmonary endodermal tumor resembling fetal lung. A clinicopathologic study of five cases with immunohistochemical and ultrastructural characterization. Hum Pathol 21: 1095–1104
89. Nakatani Y, Kitamura H, Inayama Y et al. 1998 Pulmonary adenocarcinomas of the fetal lung type. Am J Surg Pathol 22: 399–411
90. Koss M N, Hochholzer L, O'Leary T 1991 Pulmonary blastomas. Cancer 67: 2368–2381
91. Nappi O, Wick M R 1993 Sarcomatoid neoplasms of the respiratory tract. Semin Diagn Pathol 10: 137–147
92. Ludwigsen E 1977 Endobronchial carcinosarcoma. Virchows Arch [A] Pathol Anat Histopathol 373: 293–302
93. Kakos G S, Williams T E, Assor D et al. 1971 Pulmonary carcinosarcoma: Etiologic, therapeutic, and prognostic considerations. J Thorac Cardiovasc Surg 61: 777–783
94. Davis M P, Eagan R T, Weiland L H et al. 1984 Carcinosarcoma of the lung: Mayo Clinic experience and response to chemotherapy. Mayo Clin Proc 59: 598–603
95. Koss M N, Hochholzer L, Frommelt R A 1999 Carcinosarcomas of the lung. A clinicopathologic study of 66 patients. Am J Surg Pathol 23: 1514–1526
96. Suster S 1995 Primary sarcomas of the lung. Semin Diagn Pathol 12: 140–157
97. Moran C A, Suster S, Abbondanzo S L et al. 1997 Primary leiomyosarcomas of the lung: a clinicopathologic and immunohistochemical study of 18 cases. Mod Pathol 10: 121–128
98. Guccion J G, Rosen S H 1972 Bronchopulmonary leiomyosarcoma and fibrosarcoma: a study of 32 cases and review of the literature. Cancer 30: 836–847
99. Wick M R, Scheithauer B W, Piehler J M et al. 1982 Primary pulmonary leiomyosarcoma: a light and electron microscopy study. Arch Pathol Lab Med 106: 510–514
100. Przygodzki R M, Moran C A, Suster S et al. 1995 Primary pulmonary rhabdomyosarcomas: a clinicopathologic and immunohistochemical study of three cases. Mod Pathol 8: 658–661
101. Drennan J M, McCormack R J M 1960 Primary rhabdomyosarcoma of the lung. J Pathol 79: 1960–1962
102. Lee S H, Rengachary S S, Paramesh J 1981 Primary pulmonary rhabdomyosarcoma. Hum Pathol 12: 92–94
103. Murphy J J, Blair G K, Fraser G C et al. 1992 Rhabdomyosarcoma arising within congenital pulmonary cyst. J Pediatr Surg 27: 1364–1366
104. Ueda K, Gruppo R, Unger F et al. 1977 Rhabdomyosarcoma of the lung arising in congenital cystic adenomatoid malformation. Cancer 40: 383–385
105. Roviaro G, Montorsi M, Varoli F et al. 1983 Primary pulmonary tumors of neurogenic origin. Thorax 38: 942–945
106. Malik S K, Behera D, Kalra A K 1987 Intrabronchial schwannoma. Scand J Thor Cardiovasc Surg 21: 281–282
107. Bartley T D, Arean V M 1965 Intrapulmonary neurogenic tumors. J Thorac Cardiovasc Surg 50: 114–123
108. Moran C A, Suster S, Koss M N 1997 Primary malignant "triton" tumour of the lung. Histopathology 30: 140-144
109. Zeren H, Moran C A, Suster S et al. 1995 Primary malignant spindle cell neoplasms of the lung with features of monophasic synovial sarcoma: clinicopathologic, immunohistochemical and ultrastructural study of 25 cases. Hum Pathol 26: 474–480
110. Essary L R, Vargas S O, Fletcher C D M 2002 Primary pleuropulmonary synovial sarcoma: reappraisal of a recently described anatomic subset. Cancer 94: 459–469
111. Suster S, Fisher C, Moran C A 1998 Expression of bcl-2 oncoprotein in benign and malignant spindle cell tumors of soft tissue, skin, serosal surfaces and gastrointestinal tract. Am J Surg Pathol 22: 863–872
112. Carswell J, Kraeft N H 1950 Fibrosarcoma of the bronchus. J Thorac Surg 19: 117–123
113. Nascimento A G, Unni K K, Bernatz P E 1982 Sarcomas of the lung. Mayo Clin Proc 57: 355–359
114. Meade J B, Whitwell F, Bickford J K B 1974 Primary hemangiopericytoma of lung. Thorax 29: 1–15
115. Kern W H, Hughes R K, Meyer B W et al. 1979 Malignant fibrous histiocytoma of the lung. Cancer 44: 1793–1801
116. Bedrossian C W M, Veroni R, Unger K M et al. 1979 Pulmonary malignant fibrous histiocytoma. Chest 75: 186–189
117. Lee J T, Shelburne J D, Linder J 1984 Primary malignant fibrous histiocytoma of the lung: a clinicopathologic and ultrastructural study of five cases. Cancer 53: 1124–1130
118. Yousem S A, Hochholzer L 1987 Primary pulmonary hemangiopericytoma. Cancer 59: 549–555
119. Yousem S A, Flynn S D 1988 Intrapulmonary localized fibrous tumor. Intraparenchymal so-called localized fibrous mesothelioma. Am J Clin Pathol 89: 365–369
120. Moran C A, Suster S, Koss M N 1992 The spectrum of histologic growth patterns in benign and malignant solitary fibrous tumors of the pleura. Semin Diagn Pathol 9: 109–180
121. Van de Rijn M, Rouse R V 1994 CD-34. A review. Appl Immunohistochem 2: 71–80
122. Westra W H, Gerald W L, Rosai J 1994 Solitary fibrous tumor. Consistent CD-34 immunoreactivity and occurrence in the orbit. Am J Surg Pathol 18: 992–998
123. Morgenroth A, Pfeuffer H P, Viereck H J et al. 1989 Primary chondrosarcoma of the left inferior lobar bronchus. Respiration 56: 241–244
124. Nosanchuck J S, Weatherbee L 1969 Primary osteogenic sarcoma of the lung. J Thorac Cardiovasc Surg 58: 242–248
125. Colby T V, Bilbao J E, Battifora H et al. 1989 Primary osteosarcoma of the lung. A reappraisal following immunohistologic study. Arch Pathol Lab Med 113: 1147–1150
126. Reingold I M, Amromin G D 1971 Extraosseous chondrosarcoma of the lung. Cancer 28: 491–498
127. Loose J H, El-Naggar A K, Ro J Y et al. 1990 Primary osteosarcoma of the lung. Report of two cases and review of the literature. J Thorac Cardiovasc Surg 100: 867–873
128. Ognibene F P, Steis R G, Macher A M et al. 1985 Kaposi's sarcoma causing pulmonary infiltrates and respiratory failure in the acquired immunodeficiency syndrome. Ann Intern Med 102: 471–475
129. Moran C A, Suster S, Pavlova Z et al. 1994 The spectrum of pathological changes in the lung in children with AIDS: an autopsy study of 36 cases. Hum Pathol 25: 877–882
130. Meduri G U, Stover D E, Lee M et al. 1986 Pulmonary Kaposi's sarcoma in the acquired immune deficiency syndrome: clinical, radiographic and pathological manifestation. Am J Med 81: 5–12
131. Spragg R G, Wolf P L, Haghighi P et al. 1983 Angiosarcoma of the lung with fatal pulmonary hemorrhage. Am J Med 74: 1072–1076
132. Yousem S A 1986 Angiosarcoma presenting in the lung. Arch Pathol Lab Med 110: 112–115
133. Farinacci C J, Blauw A S, Jennings E M 1973 Multifocal pulmonary lesions of possible decidual origin (so-called pulmonary deciduosis). Report of a case. Am J Clin Pathol 59: 508–514
134. Dail D H, Liebow A A, Gmelich J T et al. 1983 Intravascular bronchiolar and alveolar tumor of the lung (IVBAT). Cancer 51: 452–464
135. Bhagavan B S, Murthy M S N, Dorfman H D et al. 1982 Intravascular bronchioalveolar tumor (IVBAT). A low-grade sclerosing epithelioid angiosarcoma of lung. Am J Surg Pathol 6: 41–52
136. Azumi N, Churg A 1981 Intravascular and sclerosing bronchioloalveolar tumor. A pulmonary sarcoma of probable vascular origin. Am J Surg Pathol 5: 587–596
137. Corrin B, Liebow A A, Friedman P J et al. 1975 Pulmonary lymphangioleiomyomatosis. Am J Pathol 79: 348–368
138. Ramani P, Shah A 1993 Lymphangioleiomyomatosis. Histologic and immunohistochemical analysis of four cases. Am J Surg Pathol 17: 329–335
139. Koss M N, Hochholzer L, Moran C A et al. 1998 Pulmonary plasmacytomas: a clinicopathologic and immunohistochemical study of five cases. Ann Diagn Pathol 2: 1–11
140. Addis B J, Hyjek E, Isaacson P G 1988 Primary pulmonary lymphoma: a reappraisal of its histogenesis and its relationship to pseudolymphoma and lymphoid interstitial pneumonia. Histopathology 13: 1–17
141. Isaacson P G, Spencer J 1983 Malignant lymphoma of mucosa-associated lymphoid tissue. A distinctive type of B-cell lymphoma. Cancer 52: 1410–1417
142. Fiche M, Capron F, Berger F et al. 1995 Primary pulmonary non-Hodgkin's lymphomas. Histopathology 26: 529–537
143. Herbert A, Wright D H, Isaacson P G 1984 Primary malignant lymphoma of the lung. Hum Pathol 15: 415–422
144. Koss M N 1995 Pulmonary lymphoid disorders. Semin Diagn Pathol 12: 158–171
145. Abbondanzo S L, Rush W, Bijwaard K E et al. 2000 Nodular lymphoid hyperplasia of the lung. A clinicopathologic study of 14 cases. Am J Surg Pathol 24: 587–597
146. Nicholson A G, Wotherspoon A C, Diss T C et al. 1995 Pulmonary B-cell non-Hodgkin's lymphomas. Histopathology 26: 395–403
147. Li G, Hansmann M L, Zwingers T et al. 1990 Primary lymphoma of the lung: morphological, immunohistochemical and clinical features. Histopathology 16: 519–531
148. L'Hoste R J, Filippa D A, Lieberman P H et al. 1984 Primary pulmonary lymphomas: a clinicopathologic analysis of 36 cases. Cancer 54: 1397–1406
149. Koss M N, Hochholzer L, Nichols P W et al. 1983 Primary non-Hodgkin's lymphomas and pseudolymphomas of the lung: a study of 161 patients. Hum Pathol 14: 1024–1038
150. Liebow A A, Carrington C B, Friedman P J 1972 Lymphomatoid granulomatosis. Hum Pathol 3: 457–558
151. Fauci A S, Haynes B F, Costa J et al. 1982 Lymphomatoid granulomatosis – prospective clinical and therapeutic experience over 10 years. N Engl J Med 306: 68–74

152. Katzenstein A L, Carrington C B, Liebow A A 1979 Lymphomatoid granulomatosis – a clinicopathologic study of 152 cases. Cancer 43: 360–373
153. Koss M N, Hochholzer L, Langloss J M et al. 1986 Lymphomatoid granulomatosis: a clinicopathologic study of 42 patients. Pathology 18: 283–288
154. Jaffe E S 1988 Pulmonary lymphocytic angiitis: a nosologic quandary. Mayo Clin Proc 63: 411–413
155. Saldana A M, Patchefsky A S, Israel H I et al. 1977 Pulmonary angiitis and granulomatosis: the relationship between histological features, organ involvement, and response to treatment. Hum Pathol 8: 391–409
156. Kern W H, Crepean A G, Jones J L 1961 Primary Hodgkin's disease of the lung: report of four cases and review of the literature. Cancer 14: 1151–1165
157. Yousem S A, Weiss L M, Colby T V 1986 Primary pulmonary Hodgkin's disease: a clinicopathologic study of 15 cases. Cancer 57: 1217–1224
158. Radin A I 1990 Primary pulmonary Hodgkin's disease. Cancer 65: 550–563
159. Marchevsky A M 1995 Lung tumors derived from ectopic tissues. Semin Diagn Pathol 12: 172–184
160. Moran C A, Hochholzer L, Rush W et al. 1996 Primary intrapulmonary meningiomas: a clinicopathologic and immunohistochemical study of ten cases. Cancer 78: 2328–2333
161. Kodama K, Osamu D, Higashiyma M et al. 1991 Primary and metastatic pulmonary meningioma. Cancer 67: 1412–1417
162. Drlicek M, Grisold W, Lorber J et al. 1991 Pulmonary meningioma. Am J Surg Pathol 15: 455–459
163. Flynn S D, Yousem S A 1991 Pulmonary meningioma. Hum Pathol 22: 469–474
164. Moran C A, Suster S, Fishback N F et al. 1995 Primary intrapulmonary thymoma: a clinicopathologic and immunohistochemical study of eight cases. Am J Surg Pathol 19: 304–313
165. Yeoh C B, Ford J M, Lattes R et al. 1966 Intrapulmonary thymoma. J Thorac Cardiovasc Surg 51: 131–136
166. James C L, Iver P V, Leong A S 1992 Intrapulmonary thymoma. Histopathology 21: 175–177
167. Tang C, Toker C K, Foris N P et al. 1978 Glomangioma of the lung. Am J Surg Pathol 2: 103–109
168. Koss M N, Hochholzer L, Moran C A 1998 Primary pulmonary glomus tumor. A clinicopathologic and immunohistochemical study of three cases. Mod Pathol 11: 253–258
169. Wilson R W, Moran C A 1997 Primary melanoma of the lung: a clinicopathologic and immunohistochemical study of eight cases. Am J Surg Pathol 21: 1196–1202
170. Alghanem A A, Mehan J, Hassan A A 1987 Primary malignant melanoma of the lung. J Surg Oncol 34: 109–112
171. Cagle P, Mace M L, Judge D M et al. 1984 Pulmonary melanoma: primary vs metastatic. Chest 85: 125–126
172. Farrell D J, Kashyap A P, Ashcroft T et al. 1996 Primary malignant melanoma of the bronchus. Thorax 51: 223–224
173. Gephart G N 1981 Malignant melanoma of the bronchus. Hum Pathol 12: 671–673
174. Singh G, Lee R E, Brooks D H 1997 Primary pulmonary paraganglioma. Report of a case and review of the literature. Cancer 40: 2286–2289
175. Fawcett F J, Husband E M 1967 Chemodectoma of the lung. J Clin Pathol 20: 260–262
176. Cooney T P 1981 Primary pulmonary ganglioneuroblastoma in an adult: maturation, involution, and the immune response. Histopathology 5: 451–463
177. Hochholzer L, Moran C A, Koss M N 1998 Primary pulmonary ganglioneuroblastoma: a clinicopathologic and immunohistochemical study of two cases. Ann Diagn Pathol 2: 154–158
178. Jamieson M P G, McGowan A R 1982 Endobronchial teratoma. Thorax 37: 157–159
179. Day S W, Taylor S A 1975 An intrapulmonary teratoma associated with thymic tissue. Thorax 30: 582–587
180. Tanimura A, Natsuyama H, Kawano M et al. 1985 Primary choriocarcinoma of the lung. Hum Pathol 16: 1281–1284
181. Deavers M, Guinee D, Koss M N et al. 1995 Granular cell tumors of the lung: clinicopathologic study of 20 cases. Am J Surg Pathol 19: 627–635
182. Alvarez-Fernandez E, Carretero-Albinana L 1987 Bronchial granular cell tumor. Presentation of three cases with tissue culture and ultrastructural study. Arch Pathol Lab Med 111: 1065–1069
183. Roger C L 1965 Multicentric endobronchial myoblastoma. Arch Otolaryngol 82: 652–655
184. Seo I S, Azzarelli B, Warner T F et al. 1984 Multiple visceral and cutaneous granular cell tumors. Ultrastructural and immunohistochemical evidence of Schwann cell origin. Cancer 53: 2104–2110
185. Liebow A A, Hubbell D S 1972 Sclerosing hemangioma (histiocytoma, xanthoma) of the lung. Cancer 30: 512–518
186. Spencer H, Nambu S 1986 Sclerosing haemangiomas of the lung. Histopathology 10: 477–487
187. Moran C A, Zeren H, Koss M N 1994 Sclerosing hemangioma of the lung: granulomatous variant. Arch Pathol Lab Med 108: 128–130
188. Noguchi M, Kodama T, Morinaga S et al. 1986 Multiple sclerosing hemangiomas of the lung. Am J Surg Pathol 10: 429–435
189. Huszar M, Suster S, Herczer E et al. 1986 Sclerosing hemangioma of the lung: immunohistochemical demonstration of mesenchymal origin using antibodies to tissue-specific intermediate filaments. Cancer 58: 2422–2427
190. Yousem S A, Wick M R, Singh G et al. 1988 So-called sclerosing hemangioma of lung: an immunohistochemical study supporting a respiratory epithelial origin. Am J Surg Pathol 12: 582–590
191. Fukuyama M, Koike M 1988 So-called sclerosing hemangioma of the lung. An immunohistochemical, histochemical and ultrastructural study. Acta Pathol Jpn 38: 627–642
192. Shimosato Y 1995 Lung tumors of uncertain histogenesis. Semin Diagn Pathol 12: 185–192
193. Leong A S-Y, Chan K-W, Seneviratne H S K 1995 A morphological and immunohistochemical study of 25 cases of so-called sclerosing haemangioma of the lung. Histopathology 27: 121–128
194. Xu H M, Li W H, Hou N et al. 1997 Neuroendocrine differentiation in 32 cases of so-called sclerosing hemangioma of the lung: identified by immunohistochemical and ultrastructural study. Am J Surg Pathol 21: 1013–1022
195. Tanaka I, Inoue M, Matsui Y et al. 1986 A case of pneumocytoma (so-called sclerosing hemangioma) with lymph node metastasis. Jpn J Clin Oncol 16: 77–86
196. Liebow A A, Castleman B 1971 Benign clear cell (sugar) tumors of the lung. Yale J Biol Med 43: 213–222
197. Becker N H, Soifer I 1971 Benign clear cell tumor (sugar tumor) of the lung. Cancer 27: 712–719
198. Gaffey M J, Mills S E, Zambo R et al. 1991 Clear cell tumor of the lung. Immunohistochemical and ultrastructural evidence of melanogenesis. Am J Surg Pathol 15: 644–653
199. Bonetti F, Pea M, Martignoni G et al. 1994 Clear cell ("sugar") tumor of the lung is a lesion strictly related to angiomyolipoma. The concept of a family of lesions characterised by the presence of a perivascular epithelioid (PEC) cell. Pathology 26: 230–236
200. Lantuejoul S, Isaac S, Pinel N et al. 1997 Clear cell tumor of lung: an immunohistochemical and ultrastructural study supporting a pericytic differentiation. Mod Pathol 10: 1001–1008
201. Spencer H 1984 The pulmonary plasma cell/histiocytoma complex. Histopathology 8: 903–907
202. Buell R, Wang N S, Seemayer T A et al. 1976 Endobronchial plasma cell granuloma (inflammatory pseudotumor): a light and electron microscopic study. Hum Pathol 7: 411–415
203. Monzon C, Gilchrist G, Burgert E et al. 1982 Plasma cell granuloma of the lung in children. Pediatrics 70: 268–271
204. Berardi R, Lee S, Chen H et al. 1983 Inflammatory pseudotumor of the lung. Surg Gynecol Obstet 36: 108–110
205. Pettinato G, Manivel J C, De Rosa N et al. 1990 Inflammatory myofibroblastic tumor (plasma cell granuloma). Clinicopathologic study of 20 cases with immunohistochemical and ultrastructural observations. Am J Clin Pathol 94: 538–542
206. Coffin C M, Patel A, Perkins S et al. 2001 ALK1 and p80 expression and chromosomal rearrangements involving 2p23 in inflammatory myofibroblastic tumor. Mod Pathol 14: 569–576
207. Tomashevski J F Jr 1982 Benign endobronchial mesenchymal tumors. Am J Surg Pathol 6: 531–540
208. Van Den Bosch J M, Wagenaar S S, Corrin B et al. 1987 Mesenchymoma of the lung (so-called hamartoma): a review of 154 parenchymal and endobronchial cases. Thorax 42: 790–793
209. Dal Cin P, Kools P, de Jonge I et al. 1993 Rearrangement of 12q14-15 in pulmonary chondroid hamartoma. Genes Chromos Cancer 8: 131–133
210. Xiao S, Lux M L, Reeves R et al. 1997 HMG-I(Y) activation by chromosome 6p21 rearrangements in multilineage mesenchymal cells from pulmonary hamartoma. Am J Pathol 150: 901–910
211. Moran C A, Suster S, Koss M N 1994 Endobronchial lipomas: a clinicopathologic study of four cases. Mod Pathol 7: 212–214
212. Yousem S A, Hochholzer L 1986 Alveolar adenoma. Hum Pathol 17: 1066–1070
213. Oliveira P, Nunes J G M, Clode A L et al. 1996 Alveolar adenoma of the lung: further characterization of this uncommon tumor. Virchows Arch 429: 101–108
214. Burke L M, Rush W I, Khoor A et al. 1999 Alveolar adenoma: a histochemical, immunohistochemical and ultrastructural analysis of 17 cases. Hum Pathol 30: 158–167
215. England D M, Hochholzer L 1995 Truly benign "bronchial adenoma:" report of 10 cases of mucous gland adenoma with immunohistochemical and ultrastructural findings. Am J Surg Pathol 19: 887–899
216. Fantone J C, Geisinger K, Appelman H D 1982 Papillary adenoma of the lung with lamellar and electron dense granules. Cancer 50: 2839–2844
217. Hegg C A, Flint A, Singh G 1992 Papillary adenoma of the lung. Am J Clin Pathol 97: 393–397
218. Suster S, Moran C A 1993 Pulmonary adenofibroma: report of two cases of an unusual type of hamartomatous lesion of the lung. Histopathology 23: 547–551
219. Korn D, Bensch K, Liebow A A et al. 1960 Multiple minute pulmonary tumors resembling chemodectoma. Am J Pathol 37: 641–672
220. Gaffey M J, Mills S F, Askin F G 1988 Minute pulmonary meningothelial-like nodules. A clinicopathologic study of so-called pulmonary chemodectoma. Am J Surg Pathol 12: 167–175
221. Ionescu D N, Sasatomi E, Aldeeb D et al. 2004 Pulmonary meningothelial-like nodules: a genotypic comparison with meningiomas. Am J Surg Pathol 28: 207–214

222. Suster S 1994 Pulmonary metastases of extrapulmonary tumors. In: Saldana M J (ed) Pathology of pulmonary disease. J B Lippincott, Philadelphia, p 701–710
223. Suster S, Moran C A 1995 Unusual manifestations of metastatic tumors of the lungs. Semin Diagn Pathol 12: 193–206
224. Toomes H, Delphenial A, Manke H-G et al. 1983 The coin lesion of the lung. A review of 995 resected coin lesions. Cancer 51: 534–537
225. Abell M R, Littler E R 1975 Benign metastasizing uterine leiomyoma. Cancer 36: 2206–2213
226. Wolff M, Kaye G, Silva F 1979 Pulmonary metastases (with admixed epithelial elements) from smooth muscle neoplasms. Am J Surg Pathol 3: 325–342
227. Nakatsuka S, Yao M, Hoshida Y et al. 2002 Pyothorax-associated lymphoma: a review of 106 cases. J Clin Oncol 20: 4255–4260
228. Legha S S, Muggia F M 1977 Pleural mesothelioma: clinical features and therapeutic implications. Ann Intern Med 87: 613–617
229. Whitwell F, Scott J, Grimshaw M 1977 Relationship between occupation and asbestos fiber content of the lungs in patients with pleural mesothelioma, lung carcinoma, and other diseases. Thorax 32: 377–384
230. Selikoff I J, Churg J, Hammond E C 1965 Relation between exposure in asbestos and mesothelioma. N Eng J Med 272: 560–563
231. Bedrossian C M W, Bonsib S, Moran C A 1992 Differential diagnosis between mesothelioma and adenocarcinoma: a multimodal approach based on ultrastructure and immunohistochemistry. Semin Diagn Pathol 9: 124–135
232. Ordonez N G, Mackay B 1996 The role of immunohistochemistry and electron microscopy in distinguishing epithelial mesothelioma of pleura from adenocarcinoma. Adv Anat Pathol 5: 273–282
233. Moran C A, Wick M R, Suster S 2000 The role of immunohistochemistry in the diagnosis of malignant mesothelioma. Semin Diagn Pathol 17: 178–183
234. Bedrossian C W M 1994 Malignant mesothelioma and other pulmonary tumors. In: Saldana M J (ed) Pathology of pulmonary disease. J B Lippincott, Philadelphia, p 657–671
235. Granados R, Cibas E S, Fletcher J A 1994 Cytogenetic analysis of effusions in malignant mesothelioma. Acta Cytol 38: 711–717
236. Sugarbaker D J, Flores R M, Jaklitsch M T et al. 1999 Resection margins, extrapleural nodal status and cell type determine postoperative long-term survival in trimodality therapy of malignant pleural mesothelioma: results in 183 patients. J Thorac Cardiovasc Surg 117: 54–63
237. Koss M N, Hochholzer L, Moran C A et al. 1992 Pseudomesotheliomatous adenocarcinoma. Semin Diagn Pathol 9: 97–105
237a. Allen T C, Cagle P T, Churg A M et al. 2005 Localized malignant mesothelioma. Am J Surg Pathol 29: 866–873
238. Galateau-Salle F, Vigraud J M, Burke L et al. 2004 Well differentiated papillary mesothelioma of the pleura. A series of 24 cases. Am J Surg Pathol 28: 534–540
239. Ordonez N G 2000 Epithelial mesothelioma with deciduoid features. Report of four cases. Am J Surg Pathol 24: 816–823
240. Khalidi H S, Medeiros L J, Battifora H 2000 Lymphohistiocytoid mesothelioma. An often misdiagnosed variant of sarcomatoid malignant mesothelioma. Am J Clin Pathol 113: 649–654
240a. Ordonez N G 2005 Mesothelioma with clear cell features: an ultrastructural and immunohistochemical study of 20 cases. Hum Pathol 36: 465–473
240b. Ordonez N G 2006 Mesothelioma with rhabdoid features: an ultrastructural and immunohistochemical study of 10 cases. Mod Pathol 19: 373–383
240c. Shia J, Qin J, Erlandson R A et al. 2005 Malignant mesothelioma with a pronounced myxoid stroma: a clinical and pathological evaluation of 19 cases. Virchows Arch 447: 828–834
241. Henderson D W, Shilkin K B, Whitaker D 1998 Reactive mesothelial hyperplasia vs mesothelioma, including mesothelioma in situ. A brief review. Am J Clin Pathol 110: 397–404
242. Wick M R, Moran C A, Mills S E et al. 2001 Immunohistochemical differential diagnosis of pleural effusions, with emphasis on malignant mesotheliomas. Curr Opin Pulm Med 7: 187–192
243. Ordoñez N G 2003 The immunohistochemical diagnosis of mesothelioma: a comparative study of epithelioid mesothelioma and lung adenocarcinoma. Am J Surg Pathol 27: 1031–1051
244. Lugli A, Forster Y, Haas P et al. 2003 Calretinin expression in human normal and neoplastic tissue: a tissue microarray analysis of 5233 tissue samples. Hum Pathol 34: 994–1000
245. Llinares K, Escande F, Aubert S et al. 2004 Diagnostic value of MUC4 immunostaining in distinguishing epithelial mesothelioma and lung adenocarcinoma. Mod Pathol 17: 150–157
245a. Ordonez N G 2005 D2-40 and podoplanin are highly specific and sensitive immunohistochemical markers of epithelioid malignant mesothelioma. Hum Pathol 36: 372–380
246. Pan C-C, Paul C-H, Chou T-Y et al. 2003 Expression of calretinin and other mesothelioma-related markers in thymic carcinoma and thymoma. Hum Pathol 34: 1155–1162
247. Mayall F G, Goddard H, Gibbs A R 1992 Intermediate filament expression in mesotheliomas: leiomyoid mesotheliomas are not uncommon. Histopathology 21: 453–457
248. Lucas D R, Pass H I, Madan S K et al. 2003 Sarcomatoid mesothelioma and its histologic mimics: a comparative immunohistochemical study. Histopathology 42: 270–279
249. Ordoñez N G 1997 Value of antibodies 44-3AG, SM3, HBME-1 and thrombomodulin in differentiating epithelial pleural mesotheliomas from lung adenocarcinoma. A comparative study with other commonly used antibodies. Am J Surg Pathol 21: 1399–1408
250. Attanoos L L, Goddard H, Gibbs A R 1996 Mesothelioma-binding antibodies: thrombomodulin, OV 632, and HBME-1 and their use in the diagnosis of malignant mesothelioma. Histopathology 29: 209–215
251. Doglioni C, Dei Tos A P, Laurino L et al. 1996 Calretinin: a novel immunocytochemical marker for mesothelioma. Am J Surg Pathol 20: 1037–1046
252. Clover J, Oates J, Edwards C 1997 Anticytokeratin 5/6: A positive marker for epithelial mesothelioma. Histopathology 31: 140–143
253. Han A C, Peralta-Soler A, Knudsen K A et al. 1997 Differential expression of N-cadherin in pleural mesothelioma and E-cadherin in lung adenocarcinoma in formalin-fixed paraffin-embedded tissues. Hum Pathol 28: 641–645
254. Harwood T R, Gracey D R, Yokoo H 1976 Pseudomesotheliomatous carcinoma of the lung. A variant of peripheral lung cancer. Am J Clin Pathol 65: 159–167
255. Koss M N, Fleming M, Przygodzki R M et al. 1998 Adenocarcinoma simulating mesothelioma: a clinicopathologic and immunohistochemical study of 29 cases. Ann Diagn Pathol 2: 89–98
256. Attanoos R L, Gibbs A R 2003 "Pseudomesotheliomatous" carcinomas of the pleura: a 10-year analysis of cases from the Environmental Lung Disease Research Group, Cardiff. Histopathology 43: 444–452
257. Klemperer P, Rabin C B 1937 Primary neoplasms of the pleura. Report of five cases. Arch Pathol 11: 385–412
258. Scharifker D, Kaneko M 1979 Localized fibrous "mesothelioma" of pleura (submesothelial fibroma): a clinicopathologic study of 18 cases. Cancer 43: 627–635
259. Burrig K-F, Kastendieck H 1984 Ultrastructural observations on the histogenesis of localized fibrous tumors of the pleura (benign mesothelioma). Virchows Arch [A] 403: 413–424
260. Said J W, Nash B, Banks-Schlegel S et al. 1984 Localized fibrous mesothelioma: an immunohistochemical and electron microscopy study. Hum Pathol 15: 440–446
261. England D M, Hochholzer L, McCarthy M J 1989 Localized benign and malignant fibrous tumors of the pleura: a clinicopathologic review of 223 cases. Am J Surg Pathol 13: 640–648
262. Dalton W R, Zollicker A S, McCaughey M T E et al. 1979 Localized primary tumors of the pleura: an analysis of 40 cases. Cancer 44: 1465–1475
263. Briselli M, Mark E J, Dickersin G R 1981 Solitary fibrous tumor of the pleura: eight new cases and review of 360 cases in the literature. Cancer 47: 2678–2689
264. Chilosi M, Facchetti F, Dei Tos A P et al. 1997 Bcl-2 expression in pleural and extrapleural solitary fibrous tumors. J Pathol 181: 362–367
265. Renshaw A A 1995 O13 (CD99) in spindle cell tumors. Appl Immunohistochem 3: 250–256
266. Carter D, Otis C N 1988 Three types of spindle cell tumors of the pleura. Fibroma, sarcoma, and sarcomatoid mesothelioma. Am J Surg Pathol 12: 747–753
267. Moran C A, Suster S, Koss M N 1995 Smooth muscle tumors presenting as pleural neoplasms. Histopathology 27: 227–234
268. Proca D M, Ross P Jr, Pratt J et al. 2000 Smooth muscle tumor of the pleura: a case report and review of the literature. Arch Pathol Lab Med 124: 1688–1692
269. Gaertner E, Zeren H, Colby T V et al. 1996 Biphasic synovial sarcomas arising in the pleural cavity: a clinicopathologic study of five cases. Am J Surg Pathol 20: 36–45
270. Falconieri G, Bussani R, Mirra M et al. 1997 Pseudomesotheliomatous angiosarcoma: a pleuropulmonary lesion simulating malignant pleural mesothelioma. Histopathology 30: 419–424
271. Lin B T-Y, Colby T, Gown A M et al. 1996 Malignant vascular tumors of the serous membranes mimicking mesothelioma. Am J Surg Pathol 20: 1431–1439
272. Moran C A, Rosado-de-Christenson M L, Koss M N et al. 1992 Thymomas presenting as pleural tumors. Am J Surg Pathol 16: 138–142
273. Attanoos R L, Galateau-Salle F, Gibbs A R et al. 2002 Primary thymic epithelial tumors of the pleura mimicking malignant mesothelioma. Histopathology 41: 42–49
274. Kaplan M A, Tazelaar H D, Hayashi T et al. 1996 Adenomatoid tumors of the pleura. Am J Surg Pathol 20: 1219–1223
275. Moran C A, Suster S 2003 Primary mucoepidermoid carcinoma of the pleura: a clinicopathologic study of three cases. Am J Clin Pathol 120: 381–385
276. Manivel J C, Priest J, Watterson J et al. 1988 Pleuropulmonary blastoma. The so-called pulmonary blastoma of childhood. Cancer 62: 1516–1526
277. Priest J R, McDermott M B, Bhatia S et al. 1997 Pleuropulmonary blastoma. A clinicopathologic study of 50 cases. Cancer 80: 147–161
278. Hedlung G, Bisset G, Bove K 1989 Malignant neoplasms arising in cystic hamartomas of the lung in childhood. Radiology 173: 77–79
279. Hachitanda Y, Aoyama C, Sato J K et al. 1993 Pleuropulmonary blastoma in childhood. A tumor of divergent differentiation. Am J Surg Pathol 17: 382–391

口腔肿瘤
Tumors of the oral cavity

The late D. Gordon MacDonald 和 Paul M. Speight 著

王功伟 译 回允中 校

引言	215
口腔上皮肿瘤	215
间叶性肿瘤和瘤样病变	220
牙源性囊肿和肿瘤	223
不伴有牙源性间质的牙源性上皮性肿瘤	224
伴有牙源性外胚层间质的牙源性上皮性肿瘤	227
伴有或不伴有牙源性上皮的牙源性外胚层间质肿瘤	229
恶性牙源性肿瘤	231
牙源性囊肿	233

引言

口腔最常见的肿瘤来源于口腔复层鳞状上皮。这些肿瘤与发生在身体其他部位的复层鳞状上皮肿瘤十分相似，仅在少数情况下出现诊断上的问题。口腔间叶组织不常发生肿瘤，但是对于慢性刺激可以发生一些反应性过度生长，而且重要的是要区分这些病变和真正的肿瘤。颌的肿瘤也可能存在问题，因为许多肿瘤罕见，或可能显示部位特异性的特征。牙源性囊肿和肿瘤起源于牙齿组织，表现出可以重现牙齿发育各个阶段的不同特征。牙源性肿瘤少见，但常常给不熟悉牙齿组织的病理医师带来诊断问题；因此，在本章中会更多地强调这些病变。牙源性囊肿常见，尽管很少是肿瘤性的，但这些病变也被包括在内，因为分类可能混乱，并且常常引起诊断困难。

口腔上皮肿瘤
Tumors of oral epithelium

鳞状细胞乳头状瘤和相关病变
Squmous cell papilloma and related lesions

临床特征

分散的口腔上皮外生性乳头状肿物可以发生在口腔内的任何部位，主要累及成年人。尽管这些病变在临床和组织学表现上有重叠，但是可能有几个亚型存在。所有这些病变均生长缓慢，而且没有证据表明这些病变是癌前病变。诊断为鳞状细胞乳头状瘤或疣的病变在人类免疫缺陷病毒（HIV）感染的患者中发病率有所增加。

组织学表现

在典型的鳞状细胞乳头状瘤中，伴有不同程度角化或过度角化的上皮呈明显均匀一致的增厚，并被覆疏松的血管结缔组织轴心。上皮深层细胞可以存在某种程度的非典型性，而且核分裂活性常常增加。如果上皮浅层有白色念珠菌感染，上述改变可能更加明显。

在某些口腔病变中可见寻常疣（verruca vulgaris）的典型组织学表现，而且可能与手指的皮肤疣有明显的关系。口腔尖锐湿疣（condyloma acuminatum）也有报道，这种病变不能依靠组织学检查来确定诊断[1]。当散在的乳头状外生性生长显示棘层增厚，取代厚度相对均匀一致的上皮皱襞（图6.1），并且有核分裂象明显增多时，应该怀疑有尖锐湿疣。

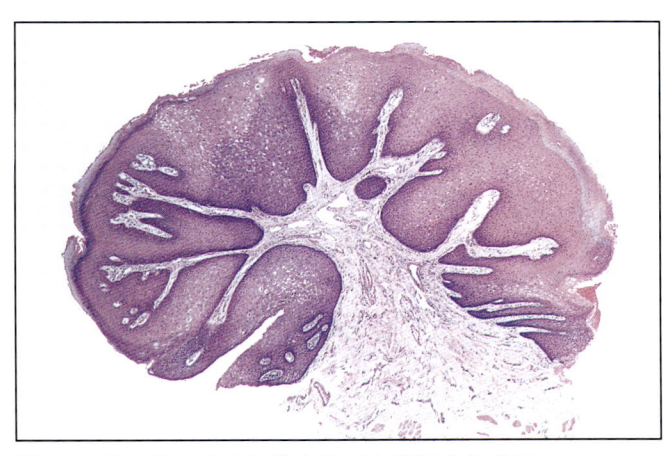

图6.1 外生性上皮生长伴有提示尖锐湿疣的特征。

局灶上皮增生
Focal epithelial hyperplasia

由人类乳头状瘤病毒（HPV）13 和 32[2]引起的局灶上皮增生（Heck 病）表现为多发性无蒂的隆起性结节。组织学上，纤维组织过度生长，被覆不规则增生的上皮（图 6.2）。在棘细胞层可以出现被描述为有丝分裂样细胞（mitosoid cell）的停滞的碎片状中期细胞分裂。

鳞状细胞癌　Squamous cell carcinoma

临床特征

鳞状细胞癌[3]是口腔最常见的恶性肿瘤。肿瘤起源于下唇，并发生在口腔内多个不同部位。多数教科书引述舌的侧缘是最常见的口腔内部位，但是针对小而无症状肿瘤的特殊研究提示，口底是小的推测为"早期"肿瘤的最常见的部位，尤其前部。另一个最常见的部位是由软腭，咽门前柱以及后磨牙区构成的"软腭复合体"（soft palate complex）。

世界上的某些地区口腔癌发病率高，例如印度，多数口腔癌发生在黏膜白斑病的区域。相反，在发达国家，小的口腔内癌几乎总是红色的或以红色为主[4]。后者多数发生在临床上明显正常的上皮内。

组织学表现

口腔鳞状细胞癌与其他部位鳞状细胞癌有相同的特征和亚型（见第 23 章），通常容易诊断。最早期的浸润可能难以确定，微小浸润的标准尚未完全确定。尤其是在疣状癌，高分化病变，这是一个诊断上的问题。所幸的是，当病变处于微小浸润这一阶段时，这样的病变不可能发生转移，适合于疣状病变的局部切除也适合于微小浸润癌的治疗。当存在白色念珠菌感染时，外生性疣状病变会产生特殊问题。这种情况常常伴有核分裂象明显增多，重要的是要认识到这些病变没有达到异型增生的程度。对于这种情况，明智的做法是推迟恶性的诊断，直到治愈真菌感染以及病变再次活检。

有多种方案试图从分析组织学特征来预测口腔癌的预后[5,6]，但是没有发现其中任何一个得到普遍认可。有些病理医师应用单个细胞或小的条索构成的肿瘤浸润作为转移扩散到淋巴结可能性增加的指征。血管和神经周围浸润也是重要的指征[7]。几项研究表明了肿瘤厚度的重要性。厚度应该从扁平病变的实际表面，或推测的外生性或溃疡病变最初的上皮表面进行测量。逐渐取得的一致意见是，肿瘤厚度超过 5 mm 时转移的危险性明显增加[8]。

鳞状细胞癌的亚型
Variants of squamous cell carcinoma

已有许多亚型描述[9,10]，其意义在于这些亚型具有不同的预后。有些肿瘤完全由亚型构成，但是在许多情况下，病变是由普通鳞状细胞癌和其他亚型混合而成的。在这种情况下，最好是报告为混合性肿瘤，并提示其行为可能是由最具侵袭性的亚型所决定的。

梭形细胞癌　Spindle cell carcinoma

梭形细胞癌是多形性梭形细胞肿瘤，最常见于头颈部[11]。所有类型的梭形细胞肿瘤在口腔都不常见，但是口腔可以发生整个谱系的软组织肉瘤（见第 24 章）。在任何这样的病例中，鉴别诊断应该考虑梭形细胞癌。这些肿瘤可以见到广泛的组织学表现（图 6.3 和图 6.4）。肿瘤细胞免疫组化染色证实细胞角蛋白阳性强烈支持该诊断。应用不同的角蛋白抗体可以获得不同的结果，但是根据我们的经验，应用 AE1/3 往往能够得到阳性结果。多数病例在作出梭形细胞癌的诊断之前，要求找到普通鳞状细胞癌或重度上皮异型增生的做法是明智的，普通鳞状细胞癌或重度异型增生通常位于肿瘤的边缘，尽管黏膜溃疡可能妨碍其辨认。

腺样（或棘层松解性）鳞状细胞癌以及腺鳞癌
Adenoid (or acantholytic) squamous cell carcinoma and adenosquamous carcinoma

腺样鳞状细胞癌这一术语所描述的病例是肿瘤细胞巢的中心细胞间的黏附性丧失，类似于腺样分化（图 6.5），这些肿瘤预后差[12,13]。腺鳞癌也是预后差的肿瘤[14]。

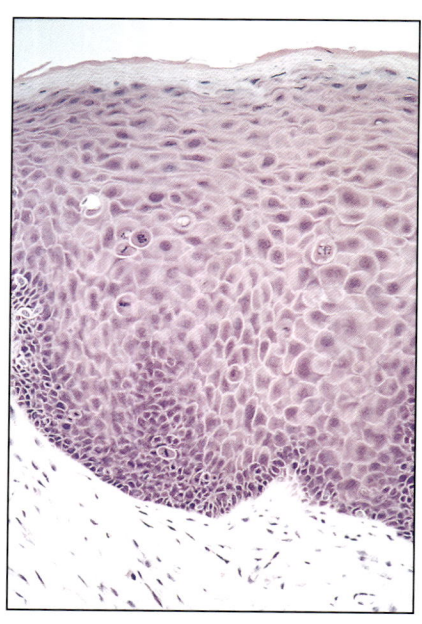

图 6.2　局灶上皮增生，显示棘层增厚的角化性上皮，棘细胞层内可见有丝分裂样细胞。

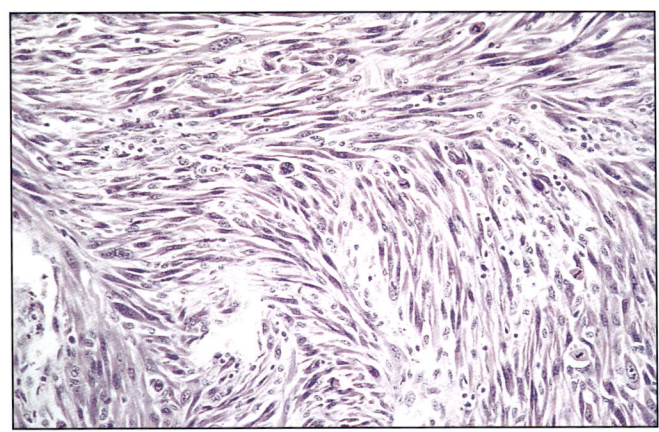

图6.3 梭形细胞癌完全呈间叶性肿瘤的外观。

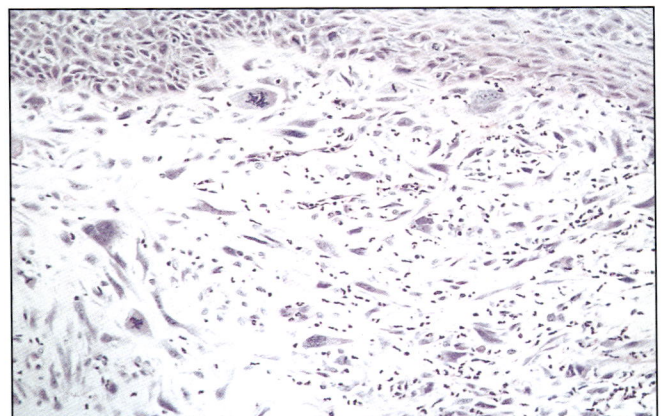

图6.4 梭形细胞癌分散的肿瘤细胞群中有奇异的细胞学表现。注意邻近异型增生的表面上皮。

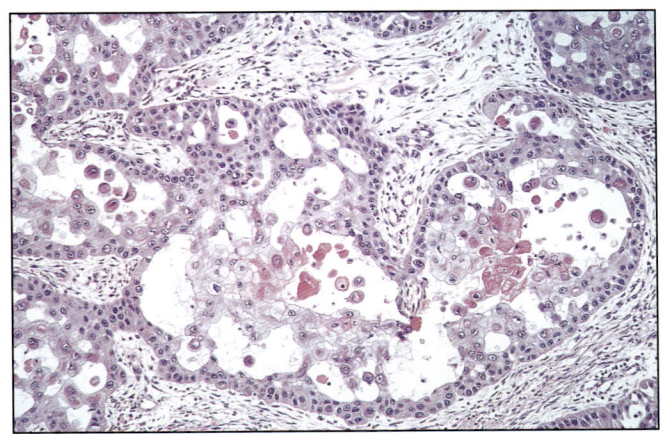

图6.5 腺样鳞状细胞癌的肿瘤细胞巢中细胞间黏附丧失,导致假腺样表现。

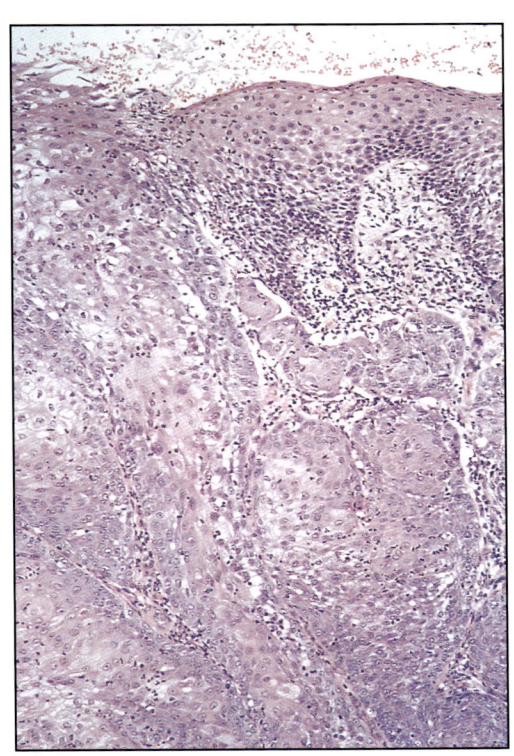

图6.6 腺鳞癌,显示起源于表面上皮的普通鳞状细胞癌的一个视野。

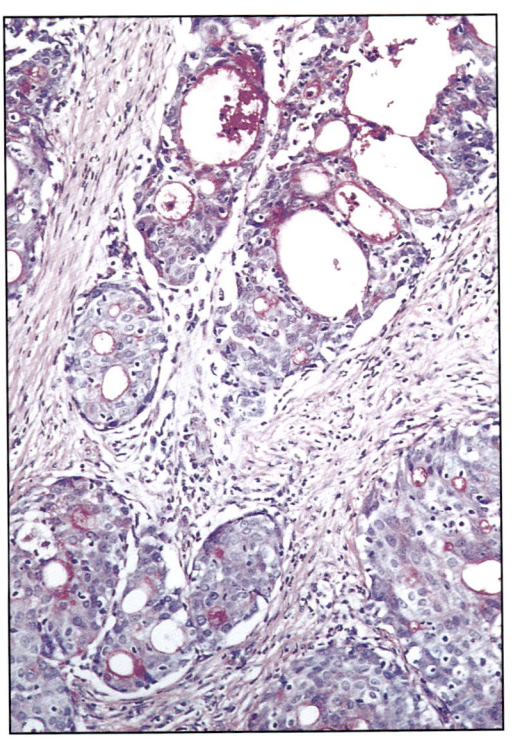

图6.7 腺鳞癌。图示与图6.6同一肿瘤的腺癌分化部分。D-PSA染色。

在这些病变中,有涎腺导管的受累,通常与起源于黏膜表面的肿瘤并发。主要的鉴别诊断是黏液表皮样癌,通过辨认散在的腺癌区域和起源于表面上皮的鳞状细胞癌的区域可以鉴别开来(图6.6和图6.7)。少部分普通鳞状细胞癌可以有少量分泌黏液的细胞,但在缺乏导管分化的情况下(图6.8),即使证实黏液细胞的存在也不足以诊断为腺鳞癌。同样重要的是,要正确认识有与鳞状细胞癌浸润涎腺相混淆的可能性(图6.9)。

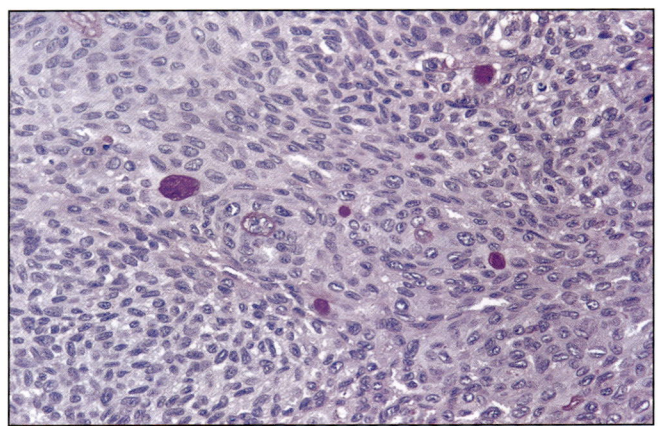

图6.8 鳞状细胞癌伴有少量分泌黏液的细胞。D-PSA染色。

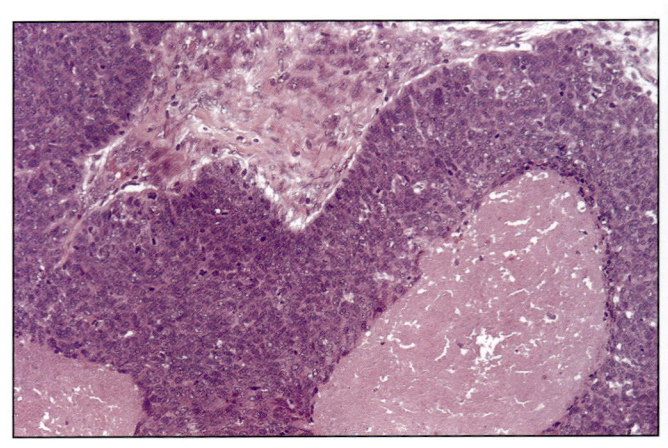

图6.10 基底细胞样鳞状细胞癌显示成团基底细胞伴有粉刺样坏死。

基底细胞样鳞状细胞[15,16]
Basaloid squamous cell carcinoma

这种不常见的鳞状细胞癌亚型（见第4章）通常与普通鳞状细胞癌混合存在。基底细胞样区域表现为界限清楚的细胞巢，周围细胞呈栅栏样排列，具有基底细胞的形态学改变以及许多核分裂象。粉刺样坏死常见（图6.10）。这些病变通常具有侵袭性，早期发生淋巴结转移。基底细胞样鳞状细胞最常见于舌的后方或舌底，必须与其他基底细胞样病变鉴别，尤其是实性腺样囊腺癌或涎腺导管癌。

疣状癌 Verrucous carcinoma

这个术语最初用于显示细胞轻度非典型性的外生性棘层显著增厚的病变，根据严格的组织学标准，不应将其诊断为癌。但随后这个术语已经被滥用。疣状癌的预后比普通鳞状细胞癌好。

临床特征：疣状癌是外生性角化性病变，表面呈白色乳头状或疣状。本病主要见于老年人，与吸烟有关。肿瘤表面的大小可达几个厘米，显示表面扩散性生长而不是向较深组织的浸润性生长。

组织学表现：有明显的棘层增厚，常常伴有粗大的球状突起，中心为角化柱（图6.11）。虽然为外生性，伴有高出邻近黏膜表面的角化柱，但也存在内生性成分。球状网突向深部"推挤"固有层，以致病变的基底部位

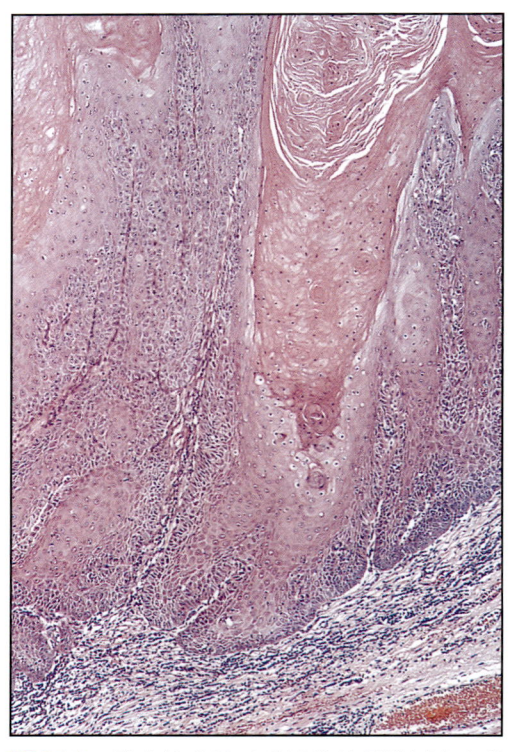

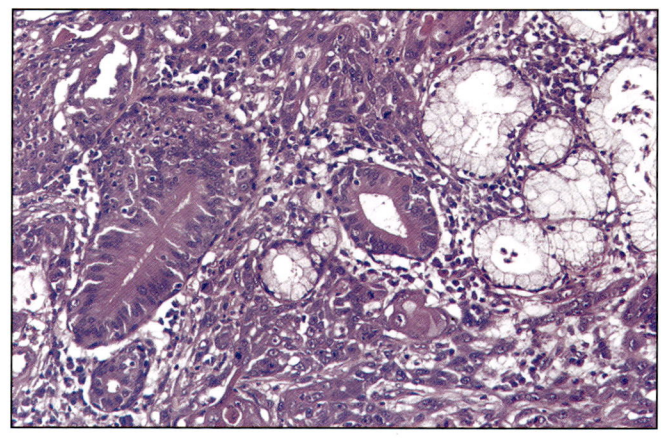

图6.9 鳞状细胞癌浸润舌的小涎腺。注意腺泡和导管是来自原来的腺体，而不是肿瘤的一部分，尽管一个导管表现为鳞状化生。

图6.11 外生性癌显示明显的棘层增厚和角化柱。肿瘤存在圆钝的推挤性边缘。许多病理医师会将这种类型的病变诊断为疣状癌，尽管存在异型增生。

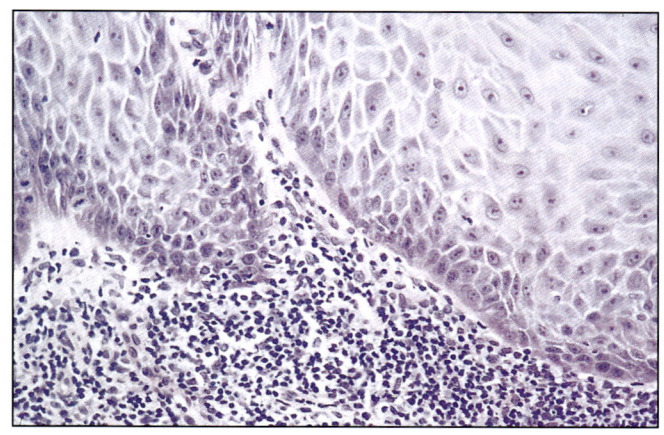

图6.12 外生性癌推进性边缘的高倍镜下所见。某些病理医师将这种类型的病变诊断为疣状癌,尽管其他病理医师可能提示,轻度异型增生的存在可以排除这个诊断。

于附近上皮基底膜的下方。没有恶性细胞学的证据。固有层内通常有明显的慢性炎细胞浸润(图6.12)。只有在将临床病理状况联系起来之后,才能作出这个部位疣状癌的诊断[17]。

鉴别诊断:主要应与普通的鳞状细胞癌进行鉴别。许多口腔癌是外生性的,并且高分化,但是表现出恶性的细胞学特征和浸润。尽管某些作者将这样的病变也称为疣状癌,但是这是不恰当的。有些肿瘤同时存在疣状癌和普通鳞状细胞癌的区域,重要的是在作出疣状癌的诊断之前,要寻找鳞状细胞癌的成分。

乳头状鳞状细胞癌
Papillary squamous carcinoma

当乳头状鳞状细胞癌这个术语用于口腔时,通常是指某些具有外生性乳头状表面的普通鳞状细胞癌。真正的口腔乳头状癌罕见,而最常见于喉和喉下部[9]。这些肿瘤由外生性乳头状上皮小叶构成,被覆于纤维血管轴心外。上皮具有相当明显的细胞非典型性,但是间质浸润可能并不明显。鉴别诊断是疣状癌和鳞状细胞乳头状瘤,乳头状癌是外生性的,显示上皮异型增生。与普通外生性癌的鉴别依靠间质浸润程度和明确的真正乳头状癌的乳头状结构。

口腔癌前病变 Oral premalignancy

临床上公认,白斑(leukoplakia)和红斑(erythroplakia)是潜在的恶性病变。这些病变活检的主要原因是排除已经出现癌的可能性。因此,要求病理医师对存在的任何异型增生进行评价和分级。其根据是假设异型增生是可能进展为恶性病变的一个指征。这种假设的理论基础是异型增生可能是由于上皮突变造成的。导致异型增生的突变与造成进展为恶性的突变不太可能是同一种突变。微阵列研究指出了异型增生主要的基因组改变[18],提示许多改变是附带现象,与恶性变并无直接联系。上皮异型增生越明显,越容易出现与恶性转化有关的关键性突变。因此,较严重的异型增生性病变进展为恶性的危险性较大。总的来说,仅有少数显示上皮异型增生的病变进展为恶性[19];然而,恶性肿瘤也可以发生在缺乏异型增生的上皮,其中通过倍体分析发现DNA异常可以预测癌的发生[20]。

新的WHO分类[9]认为,评价异型增生存在的问题是非常主观的,分级的差异不仅存在于不同的病理医师之间,而且也存在于在不同时间检查同一材料的同一个病理医师身上。如果存在角质层可以忽略,应在生存的细胞层评价异型增生。提倡从结构变化和细胞学变化两个方面来评价上皮(表6.1)。如果结构改变局限于上皮的下1/3,则为轻度异型增生(图6.13);延伸到中1/3提示中度异型增生(图6.14),而累及表面1/3则为重度异型增生(图6.15)。当将细胞学特征的严重性考虑在内时,可能需要修改根据结构变化程度作出的这些初步判断。在这个基础上,将图6.16中最初评价为中度异型增生的病变提升分级为重度异型增生。

表6.1	用于诊断异型增生的标准
结构	**细胞学**
不规则上皮复层	细胞核大小变化异常(核大小不一)
基底层细胞失去极向	核的形状变化异常(核的多形性)
滴状网嵴	细胞大小变化异常(细胞大小不一)
核分裂象数量增加	细胞形状变化异常(细胞多形性)
异常浅层核分裂象	核浆比例增加
单个细胞早熟角化	细胞核增大
网嵴内角化珠	异常核分裂象
细胞间连接丧失	核仁数量和大小增加 核深染

Based on the 2005 World Health Organization classification[9].

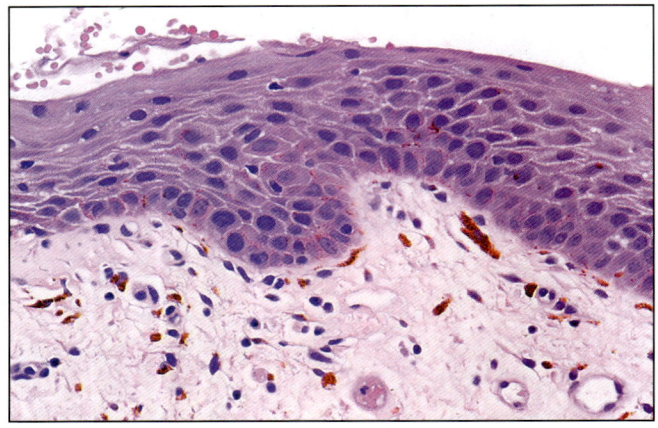

图6.13　轻度异型增生，其改变局限于上皮下1/3，仅有轻度细胞学改变。这个口底病变的色素沉着是与吸烟有关的反应性黑变病。

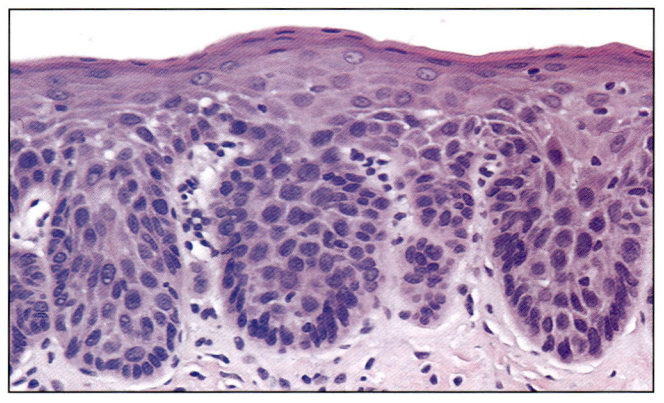

图6.14　中度异型增生。明显的滴状网嵴显示中度细胞学改变，延伸到上皮的中1/3。

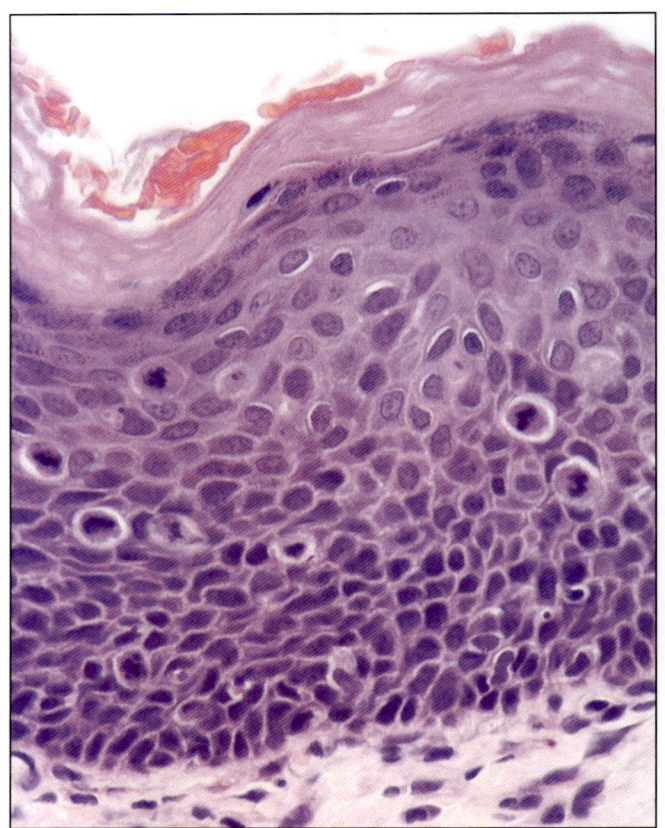

图6.15　重度异型增生。结构改变延伸到上皮表面1/3，浅层核分裂象增多，并见异常核分裂象。

在确定是否有异型增生存在时，重要的是要辨认可能与异型增生相似的其他病变。这些病变包括可能与炎症、溃疡和放射有关的再生性和修复性改变。诸如铁、叶酸盐或维生素 B_{12} 等营养缺乏也可能酷似异型增生。

原位癌的概念是上皮已经发生恶性转化，但是还没有发生浸润。累及上皮全层（或几乎全层）的异型增生，诊断原位癌是恰当的（图6.17）。

增生性疣状白斑（proliferative verrucous leukoplakia）[21,22]：是一种特别具有侵袭性的白斑，开始表现为单纯性过度角化，随后呈明显的恶性临床经过。临床特征[23]是诊断的关键，并且强调在适当的临床情况下需要作出组织病理学诊断。因此，根据多发性和复发性病变的病史和逐渐增加的侵袭性行为作出的是回顾性的诊断。

毛状白斑（hairy leukoplakia）：这个术语用于描述临床上特殊的过度角化，主要是局限于HIV阳性患者的舌侧面。这种病变是由EB病毒感染引起的，不常见于其他免疫抑制的个体。这种病变没有异型增生，也没有癌前病变的证据。

间叶性肿瘤和瘤样病变
Mesenchymal neoplasms and tumor-like lesions

口腔组织可以发生与身体其他部位相同的间叶性肿瘤（见第3章、第23章和第24章）。所有肿瘤都不常见，其中仅有少数是恶性肿瘤。最常见的是良性神经性肿瘤、脂肪瘤和肌纤维瘤。然而，提交进行组织病理学诊断的最常遇到的病变是各种非肿瘤性纤维性过度生长，通常与某些慢性刺激有关。

纤维性和血管性过度生长
Fibrous and vascular overgrowths

纤维性过度生长作为颊或舌的散在性病变并不少见，其发生与慢性刺激有关，通常来源于某些牙齿相关性的原因或慢性颊或舌的咬伤。

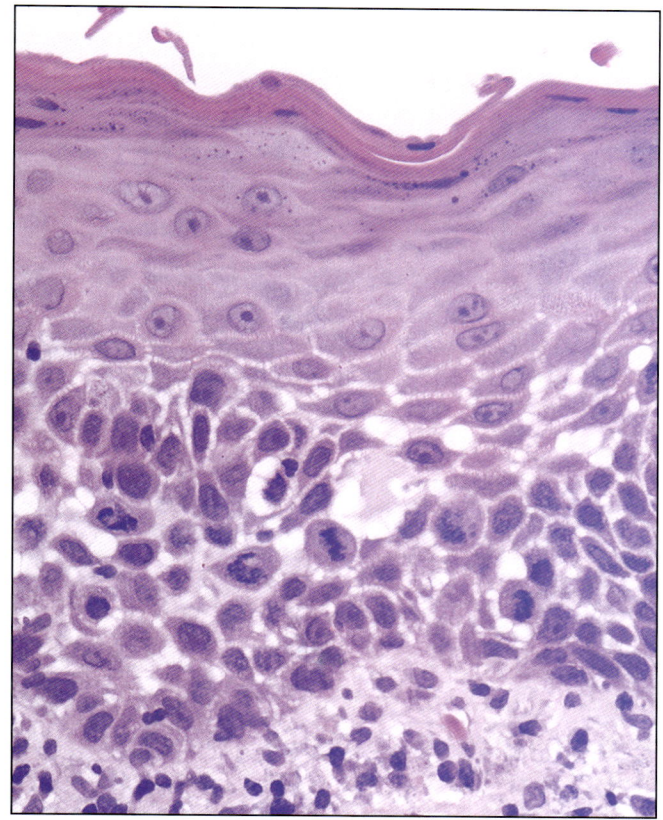

图6.16 中度上皮异型增生被重新划分为重度异型增生。虽然结构改变似乎局限于上皮下2/3，但是显著的细胞学改变有理由将这个病变重新划分为重度异型增生。

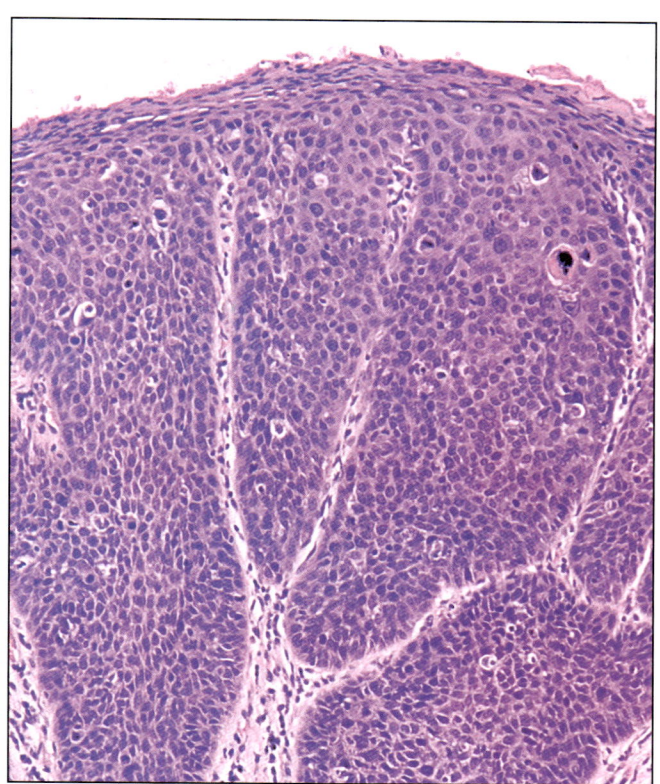

图6.17 原位癌。结构和细胞学改变涉及上皮全层。

组织学表现

这些病变通常有蒂，由相对富于细胞的胶原结缔组织构成，被覆的上皮可以增生或萎缩，但总出现角化。在某些病例中可见增大成角的纤维母细胞，偶尔可见多核纤维母细胞。某些作者将这样的病变称为巨细胞性纤维瘤（giant cell fibroma），但这似乎是不恰当的，因为这种病变没有肿瘤的证据。

化脓性肉芽肿　Pyogenic granuloma

虽然牙龈是这种病变的常见部位，但在下面牙龈瘤项下讨论的化脓性肉芽肿（见第3章）可以在口内任何部位过度生长。临床的鉴别诊断包括其他血管瘤和血管肉瘤，以及杆菌性血管瘤病和Kaposi肉瘤。

组织学表现

通常有表面上皮溃疡形成，这可以解释浅表肉芽组织带。大多数病变是由疏松结缔组织构成的，含有增生的分叶状毛细血管，核分裂可能活跃。

鉴别诊断

仅仅根据组织学检查不能鉴别血管性牙龈瘤和伴有表面溃疡的血管瘤。与比较罕见的血管性肿瘤的鉴别诊断可能需要专家会诊，尤其是因为这个部位的化脓性肉芽肿常见内皮细胞核的非典型性。

牙龈瘤　Epulides

牙龈瘤这个术语描述了牙龈的局部肿胀。这种病变常常与慢性刺激密切相关。有三种主要类型：(1) 纤维性牙龈瘤（fibrous epulis）；(2) 巨细胞性牙龈瘤（giant cell epulis）；(3) 血管性牙龈瘤（vascular epulis）。这些病变的临床表现相似。表面上皮的溃疡常见，导致病变表浅部位形成肉芽组织。所有的病变均容易复发，通常是因为刺激没有消除。

纤维性牙龈瘤　Fibrous epulis

组织学表现：病变的主体是无被膜的高度富于细胞的结缔组织区（图6.18），细胞学表现温和。常常出现无细胞的小圆形钙化灶。不同成熟程度的化生骨的形成十分常见。这样的病变往往被不恰当地诊断为"周围性骨化性纤维瘤"。可见少量多核巨细胞。纤维性牙龈瘤的区域可以类似于骨纤维性结构不良或骨化性纤维瘤，但是通过临床上纤维性牙龈瘤位于周围而不发生在骨内，容易与这些骨病变鉴别。

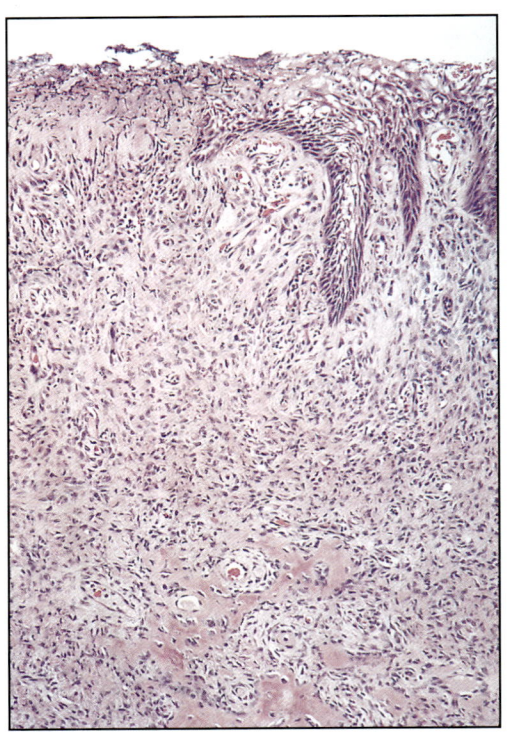

图6.18 纤维性牙龈瘤，显示高度富于细胞的纤维组织肿块和骨的形成。表面上皮通常存在溃疡，病变表浅部分由肉芽组织构成。

巨细胞性牙龈瘤（同义词：周围巨细胞性肉芽肿） Giant cell epulis (synonym: peripheral giant cell granuloma)

组织学表现：巨细胞性牙龈瘤的主要特征是没有包膜的肿物，由位于富于血管的间质中的密集排列的破骨细胞样多核巨细胞组成，其中含有肥大的单核细胞，推测其为巨细胞的单核前体细胞（图6.19）。这些细胞常有明显的核分裂活性。

鉴别诊断：主要的鉴别诊断是中心性巨细胞病变，这些病变从骨蔓延出来，表现为软组织病变。中心性巨细胞肉芽肿（central giant cell granuloma）的诊断是在排除甲状旁腺功能亢进后作出的[25]。囊性纤维性骨炎的棕色瘤（brown tumors of osteitis fibrosa cystica）通常是骨内病变，但是向周围蔓延时在组织学上无法与巨细胞牙龈瘤区分。在非常罕见的情况下，巨细胞牙龈瘤是甲状旁腺功能亢进的一种表现。当巨细胞性牙龈瘤为多发性或与妊娠有关时，应该考虑这个诊断，它可能是甲状旁腺功能亢进的突出表现。

血管性牙龈瘤 Vascular epulides

发生在牙龈的血管性牙龈瘤本质上是化脓性肉芽肿，这是最常见的口内部位（见第3章）。妊娠牙龈瘤（pregnancy epulis）是发生在妊娠期的病变；它生长可以十分旺盛，直径达到2 cm或3 cm。

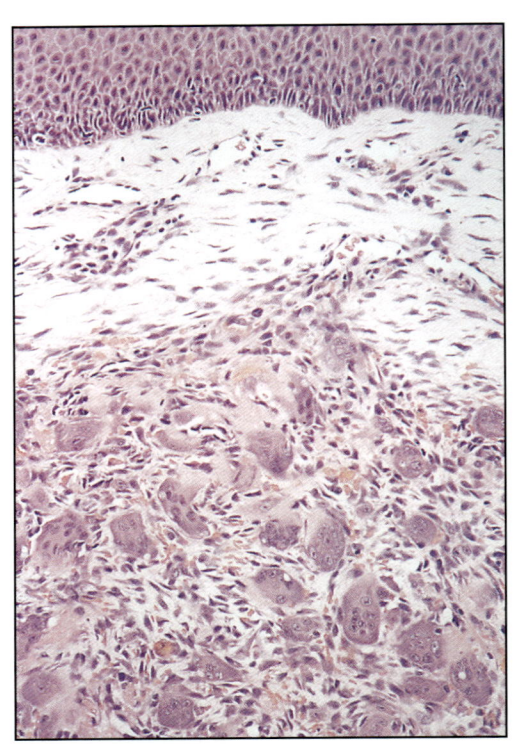

图6.19 巨细胞性牙龈瘤，在富于血管的间质内有许多多核巨细胞。

组织学表现：正如以上所描述的一样，这种病变与口内其他部位所见的化脓性肉芽肿相同。

先天性牙龈瘤（同义词：颗粒细胞牙龈瘤） Congenital epulis (synonym: granular cell epulis)

先天性牙龈瘤是一种罕见而又具有特征性的口腔病变，病因不明，见于新生儿的牙槽。几乎所有受累的患者均为女性。这种病变在组织学上类似于其他部位的颗粒细胞瘤，但是S-100阴性（见第27章）。免疫组化研究提示其具有原始周皮细胞或肌纤维母细胞分化[26]。

与义齿有关的纤维性过度生长 Fibrous overgrowths related to wearing of dentures

义齿是常见的刺激来源，尤其是陈旧的和不合适的义齿。义齿可以引起黏膜过度生长，对此应用不同的名称。如果没有去除病因，切除后可能存在复发问题。

义齿引起的增生（不好的同义词：义齿肉芽肿，缝龈瘤，刺激性纤维瘤） Denture-induced hyperplasia (poor synonyms: denture granuloma, epulis fissuratum, irritation fibroma)

这些过度生长通常见于义齿周围的唇沟或颊沟。少数发生在上颌义齿颚的后缘。"叶状纤维瘤"（leaf fibroma）是一个描述性术语，有时用于有蒂的扁平纤维性过度生长，可以发生于颚，占据不合适义齿和颚黏膜之间的间隙。这个术语是不恰当的，因为这个病变不是真正的肿瘤。

组织学表现：这种病变主要由胶原结缔组织构成。表面上皮从增生性改变到溃疡形成不一，在有溃疡形成的病例中，部分组织可能是肉芽组织。

颚的乳头状增生
Papillary hyperplasia of the palate

这个病变发生在颚穹隆部义齿的下方，表现为粗糙的颗粒状软组织肿物。

组织学表现：组织学可见中等量的血管结缔组织轴心，被覆不规则增生的上皮。在低倍镜下有时类似于浸润（图6.20），伴有上皮向下生长，有时有明显的角化珠形成。高倍镜下检查证实具有完全良性的细胞学特征。

牙源性囊肿和肿瘤
Odontogenic cysts and tumors

颌骨是人体骨内唯一可以见到上皮的部位。牙板上皮参与牙釉质的形成，并构成牙齿的形状。当牙齿形成结束时，在不同的区域仍有残留的上皮。这些上皮可以产生一系列的病变，包括肿瘤和错构瘤，当发现其与牙齿有关时，诊断不会出现问题，但在其他情况下可以引起诊断困难。最常见的上皮残留是Malassez上皮残余（the debris of Malassez），见于牙周韧带，表现为小簇状或条带状的非角化鳞状上皮，但是偶尔可为较大的细胞巢。在拔牙后这些上皮可以留在牙槽骨内。这些上皮最常引起牙源性上皮囊肿，即牙根端囊肿（radicular cyst），它是由牙髓炎蔓延而来的炎症性囊肿。上皮残留也可以见于与未萌出牙牙冠有关的滤泡内，它们可能被误诊为成釉细胞纤维瘤（ameloblastic fibroma）[27]。增生性滤泡内还可以发生钙化，有时是多发性的[28]。被覆于部分萌出的下颌第三磨牙的软组织常常含有牙源性上皮小的错构瘤性过度生长，可能类似于某些类型的牙源性肿瘤[29,30]。不常见的是，牙源性上皮性错构瘤表现为小的牙龈过度生长，不应该过诊断为周围性成釉细胞瘤。

牙源性病变的分类最近进行总结[9,31]，但是非常复杂。本章所应用的分类基本上是WHO较早提供的分类版本[32]。多数病变适用于这种分类，但是将牙源性肿瘤分为是具有肿瘤标记的多种明确病变的不同组别可能是恰当的。几种疾病可能显示重叠的特征，而且最好按照该分类来描述。分类的一个主要基本原则是归纳牙组织的相互作用，其中肿瘤发生类似于正常牙齿的发育。正常牙板上皮来自口腔上皮向下生长。成牙质细胞分化之后形成牙乳头结缔组织，开始形成牙，然后成釉细胞开始形成牙釉质。牙源性肿瘤可以完全由上皮或间叶成分构成，或者表现为上皮和间叶成分混合存在。硬组织结构可能不同，在牙瘤中可见从少量沉积的牙样物质到产生成形的牙样结构。起源于牙源性上皮肿瘤的组织病理学已有评估[33]，而且对于整个领域均有详细描述[31]。虽然可能引起明显的局部破坏和变形，但几乎所有的牙源性肿瘤都是良性非转移性的。

良性肿瘤分类列在表6.2中，并且指出了每个病变的相对发病率。

表6.2	良性牙源性肿瘤分类和相对发病率
	发病率（%）
牙源性上皮不伴有牙源性外胚层间质	
成釉细胞瘤	12
鳞状牙源性肿瘤	<1
钙化性上皮性牙源性肿瘤	<1
牙源性上皮伴有牙源性外胚层间质，伴或不伴牙硬组织结构	
成釉细胞纤维瘤	2
成釉细胞纤维性牙本质瘤和成釉纤维-牙瘤	2
牙成釉细胞瘤	<1
腺瘤样牙源性肿瘤	3
钙化性牙源性囊肿	2
复合性牙瘤	41
混合性牙瘤	33
牙源性外胚层间质伴或不伴有诱导性牙源性上皮	
牙源性纤维瘤	<1
牙源性黏液瘤	3
成牙骨质细胞瘤	<1

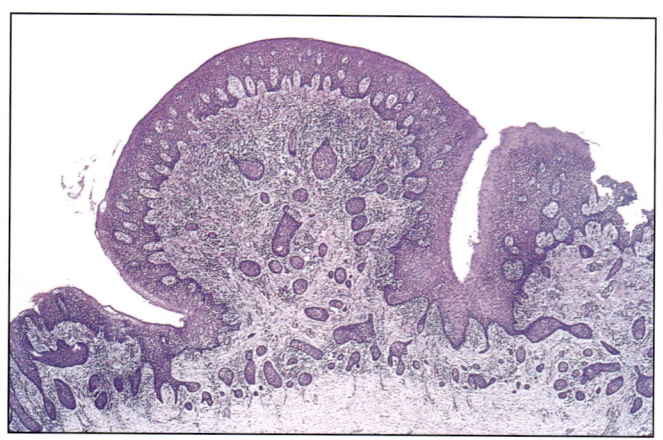

图6.20 颚乳头状增生伴有不规则上皮过度生长，低倍镜下给人一种浸润的印象。

不伴有牙源性外胚层间质的牙源性上皮性肿瘤
Tumor of odontogenic epithelium without odontogenic ectomesenchyme

成釉细胞瘤　Ameloblastoma

临床特征

成釉细胞瘤是最常见的牙源性肿瘤[34]，下颌骨最常见，尤其是后部。肿瘤可以发生在任何年龄，但是报道的发病高峰是30～40岁。下颌骨肿瘤是无痛性生长缓慢的肿物，可以产生特征性的多囊性或肥皂泡样放射线改变。也可以发生单房性亚型。肿物呈局部膨胀性生长，浸润并破坏邻近组织。未经治疗的病例肿瘤可以很大。肿瘤从骨蔓延到周围软组织是预后不良的迹象。

上颌骨成釉细胞瘤发生在较大年龄组，预后较差。手术后有较高的复发率，可能与上颌骨有不同的骨结构以及早期扩散到骨外软组织和鼻旁窦有关。

最常见的成釉细胞瘤类型是普通性或实性/多囊性成釉细胞瘤[31]。这种类型可以有许多组织学亚型，但这些亚型没有预后意义。也可见到周围性和单囊性成釉细胞瘤（表6.3）。

大体表现

成釉细胞瘤大体表现差异很大，从完全实性到不同程度的囊性病变都有。当检查任何颌的囊性病变时，重要的是要在组织学上检查任何增厚或向囊腔内生长的区域，看有无可能存在成釉细胞瘤。

组织学表现

成釉细胞瘤是由上皮构成的，缺乏任何分化为牙齿硬组织的证据。在普通性、实性/多囊性病变中，上皮可以显示滤泡或丛状结构，但在同一个肿瘤中可见混合性生长方式。最常见的结构是滤泡（图6.21），特征是形成上皮岛，其周围高柱状细胞呈栅栏状排列，极向

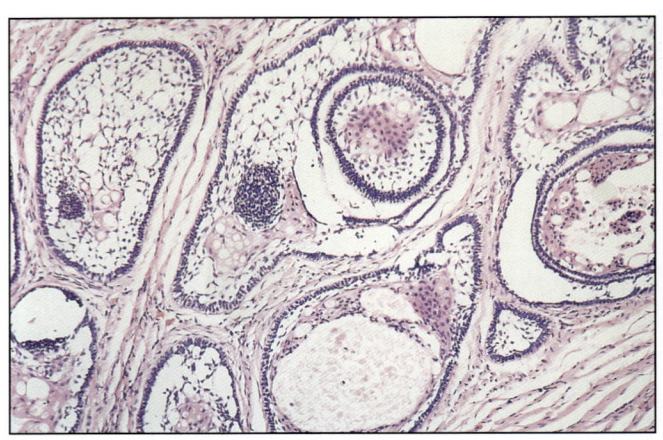

图6.21　滤泡性成釉细胞瘤，伴有明显的周围栅栏状和中心星状网区域。某些滤泡显示鳞状分化，而另外一些滤泡有囊性变。

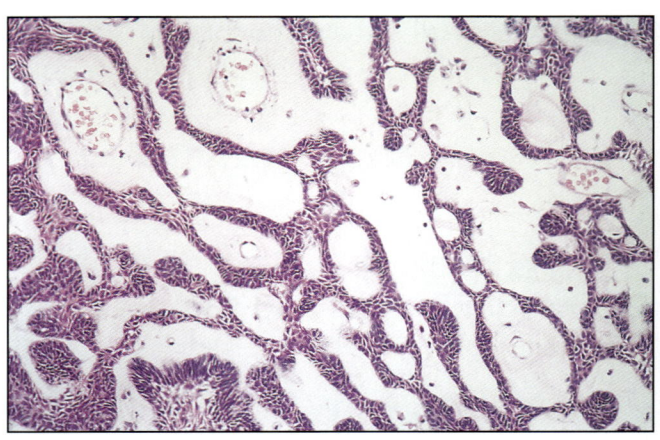

图6.22　丛状成釉细胞瘤。带状上皮交错排列，常常缺乏滤泡性成釉细胞瘤典型的周围栅栏状和星状网区域。

颠倒，细胞核远离基底膜排列。这些细胞与正常牙齿发育中的前成釉细胞相似。细胞岛的中心含有疏松排列的星形细胞，类似于牙胚的星网状组织。丛状结构由带状或条索状上皮构成（图6.22），通常相互连接。周围可见柱状成釉细胞样细胞，但是很难发现星状网区域。在这两种结构中，可以有富于细胞的亚型。棘皮瘤性成釉细胞瘤（acanthomatous ameloblastomas）在肿瘤性滤泡中有鳞状化生的证据，缺乏星网状表现，可见角化。少数肿瘤有嗜酸性颗粒细胞区域（图6.23），偶尔可能是

表6.3	成釉细胞瘤的类型，相对发病率和主要特征	
亚型	发病率（%）	特征
普通性成釉细胞瘤（实性/多囊性）	85	骨内病变，可为实性或多囊性。滤泡或丛状结构。最常见于下颌角。局灶侵袭性。
单囊性成釉细胞瘤	14	骨内大的单房性囊肿。可以有腔内突起。预后好，刮除后通常可以治愈。
周围性成釉细胞瘤	1	骨外，位于牙龈。滤泡或丛状结构。预后好，很少复发。

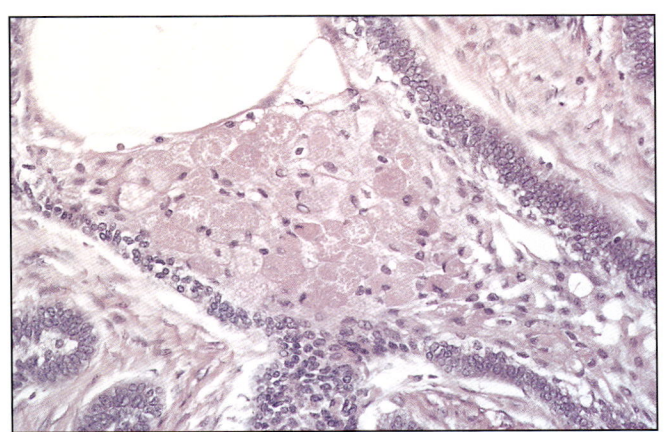

图6.23 滤泡性成釉细胞瘤的颗粒细胞区域。

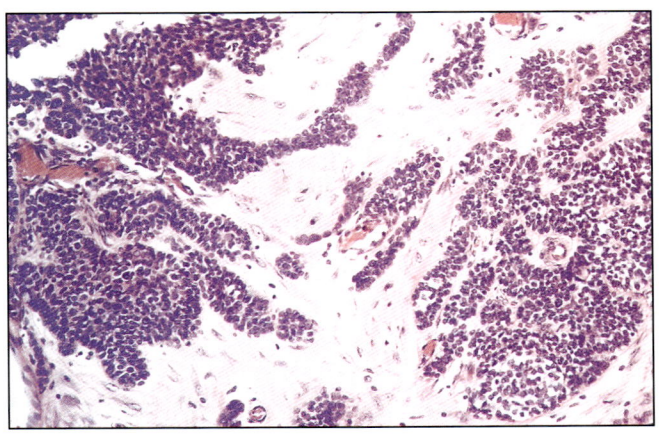

图6.25 成釉细胞瘤的基底细胞样结构。为了做出诊断，在这些病例中重要的是要寻找比较典型的成釉细胞瘤。

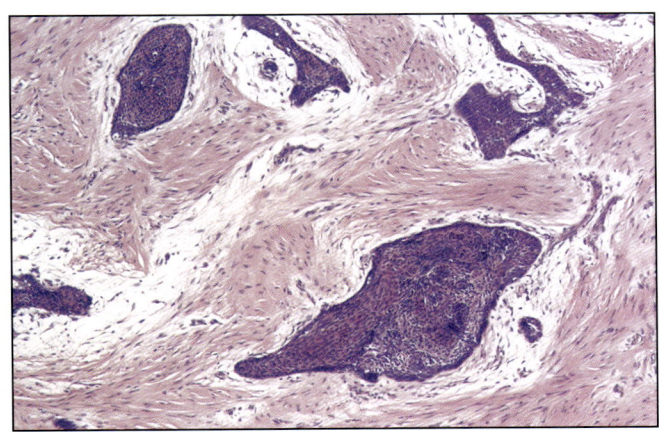

图6.24 纤维组织增生性成釉细胞瘤的上皮成分广泛分布于致密的胶原性间质中。最大的上皮岛显示棘皮瘤性成釉细胞瘤的特征，缺乏星形网结构。

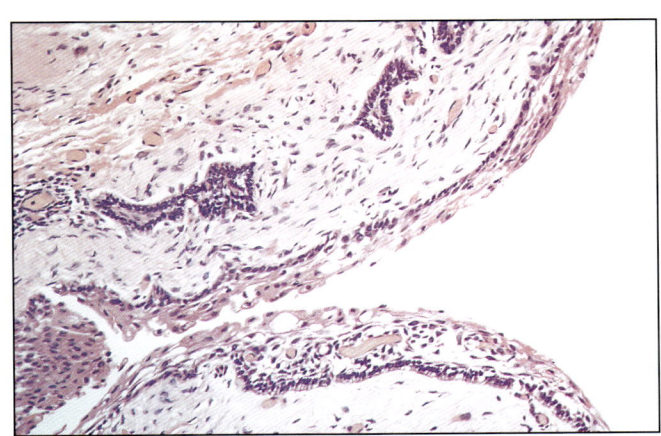

图6.26 囊性成釉细胞瘤。部分囊的内衬显示可辨认的成釉细胞瘤的特征，而其他区域是缺乏成釉细胞瘤特征的复层鳞状上皮。注意囊壁内的丛状成釉细胞瘤细胞巢。

非常突出的特征，以致难以作出成釉细胞瘤的诊断，尤其是在小的活检标本中。纤维组织增生性成釉细胞瘤（desmoplastic ameloblastomas）有广泛的间质纤维组织增生，其特征是密集的胶原纤维组织以及偶尔有骨的形成[35]。上皮成分可以减少变薄，相互吻合成带状，但通常可见周围呈栅栏状排列的典型的滤泡（图6.24）。其他不常见的亚型是基底细胞样（babaloid）（图6.25）和乳头状（papilliferous）成釉细胞瘤。透明细胞不常见，但是公认的是，透明细胞是与侵袭性和可能与恶性行为有关的一种不好的特征[36,37]（见下文恶性成釉细胞瘤）。

成釉细胞瘤常有囊肿形成。囊肿内衬上皮通常容易辨认出是成釉细胞瘤的上皮，但是囊肿偶尔可能内衬部分变薄的鳞状上皮，缺乏成釉细胞瘤的特征（图6.26）。这在某些病例可能造成诊断困难，尤其是在活检标本中，故应该鼓励外科医师在实性或多囊性区域而不是在大囊肿部分进行活检。

细胞学上，成釉细胞瘤表现温和。上皮细胞巢周围和中心细胞之间细胞核的形状不同，而细胞和细胞核的大小以及染色强度的变化有限。通常很难发现核分裂象。如果见到几个以上的核分裂象，应该考虑恶性成釉细胞瘤的可能（见下文）。

单囊性成釉细胞瘤
Unicystic ameloblastoma

少数成釉细胞瘤表现为单房性囊肿[31,38]。这些肿瘤术前常常不能诊断为成釉细胞瘤，而是诊断为其他类型的牙源性囊肿。这些囊肿常常通过剜除术治疗，随后由病理医师做出诊断。单房性成釉细胞瘤与普通性成釉细胞瘤发生部位相同，但发生在较年轻的年龄组，常常在10～20岁。三种亚型已有描述。第一个亚型为单纯性囊性病变，内衬成釉细胞瘤上皮，上皮可能变扁，类似于单纯性鳞状上皮。在第二个亚型中，囊腔内可能有增生的成釉细胞瘤上皮。腔内亚型通常是伴有带状上皮的丛状结构[39]（丛状单房性成釉细胞瘤，plexiform unicystic ameloblastoma），有时缺乏明显的成釉细胞瘤的特征。这种病变与非肿瘤性囊肿的增生可能难以鉴别，主要依靠增生的数量。这两种类型的病变预后较好，即使保守手术以后复发率也低。第三种亚型显示向结缔组织囊壁内生长，就是所谓的壁内增生。该亚型不是真正的单房性囊肿，可能是普通滤泡性成釉细胞瘤的囊性改变。它与普通性成釉细胞瘤预后相似，同样需要积极治疗。

周围性成釉细胞瘤
Peripheral ameloblastoma

在非常少见的情况下，成釉细胞瘤可以来源于牙龈或牙槽的口腔上皮而不是发生于骨内。这些病变可以用周围性成釉细胞瘤来命名[31,40]，其表面上类似于皮肤的基底细胞癌。周围性成釉细胞瘤的侵袭性不如骨内病变。

鳞状牙源性肿瘤
Squamous odontogenic tumor

临床特征

鳞状牙源性肿瘤起源于 Malassez 残留上皮，在1975年被描述为一个独立的疾病[41]，仅有少数病例报告。它表现为邻近牙根牙槽骨内明显的囊性病变，引起牙齿松动和移位。多中心和家族性的病例已有报告[42]。

组织学表现

肿瘤由位于胶原性间质中的良性表现的复层鳞状上皮岛和条带所组成。可见单个细胞角化和小灶状的角质；上皮岛内可以发生囊性退变。上皮内可能出现钙化和结晶样结构，但是没有发现牙齿的硬组织或淀粉样物。

鉴别诊断

与成釉细胞瘤的鉴别诊断是通过上皮岛周围缺乏栅栏状排列的细长细胞，而且缺乏星状网区域而做出的。与鳞状细胞癌的鉴别诊断非常重要，鉴别要点在于鳞状牙源性肿瘤缺乏任何的恶性细胞学特征。鳞状牙源性瘤样增生（squamous odontogenic tumor-like proliferations）也与某些牙源性囊肿有关[43]，但是这些病变似乎没有预后意义。

钙化性上皮性牙源性肿瘤
Calcifying epithelial odontogenic tumor

该肿瘤也被称为 Pindborg 瘤，1958 年由 Pindborg 最先报告[44]，后来又有较详细的描述[45]。

临床特征

已经报道的病例年龄范围广泛，但中年成人最常受累。上颌骨是最常见的部位。临床和放射学特征与成釉细胞瘤相似。肿瘤表现为边界不清的多房性或单房性射线通透区，但是常常有钙化物质，这可能与未萌出牙有关。偶尔发生骨外病变，但本质上是良性和非破坏性病变。钙化性上皮性牙源性肿瘤有 10%～15% 的局部复发率。

组织学表现

这种肿瘤的组织学表现多种多样（图 6.27），并不总是容易诊断。成片和带状多角形上皮细胞位于纤维性间质中，尤其是玻璃样变的间质，可以含有广泛的营养不良性或牙骨质样钙化。肿瘤常常含有圆形淀粉样物质团块，这种物质可以钙化。可以出现囊性结构。常见的一个显著特征是细胞核大小明显不一，核多形性以及细胞核深染（图 6.28）。这些会造成侵袭性的假象，但是缺乏或极少有核分裂活性。

鉴别诊断

这个病变容易与成釉细胞瘤鉴别。可以出现透明细胞区域[46]（图 6.28），当同时存在奇异性细胞核的特征时，

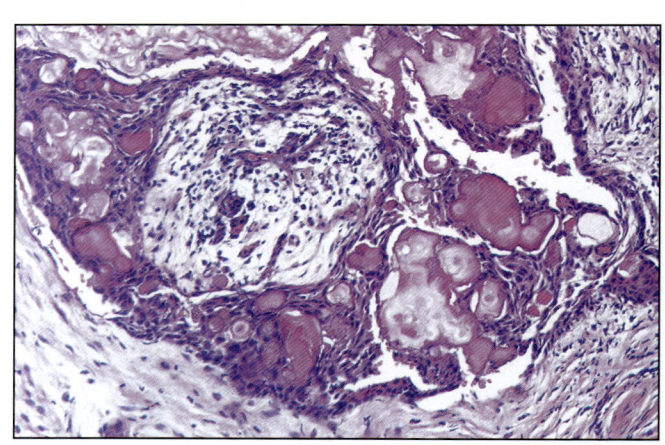

图6.27　钙化性上皮性牙源性肿瘤，类似于复层鳞状上皮，伴有淀粉样区域。

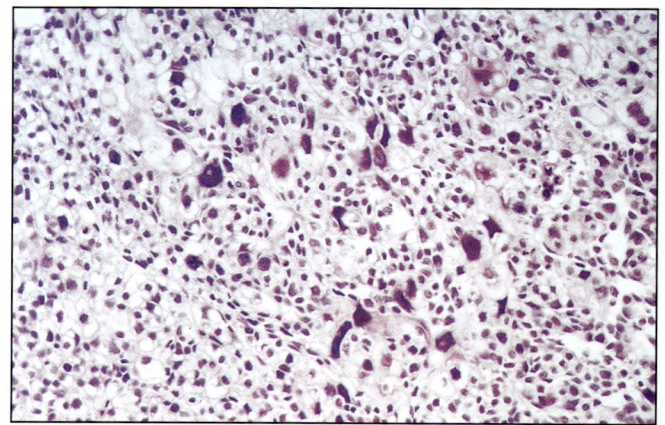

图6.28　钙化性上皮性牙源性肿瘤。局灶显示明显的细胞学非典型性，但在透明细胞亚型中没有分裂活性。

需要与黏液表皮样癌、转移性透明细胞肿瘤或透明细胞牙源性癌鉴别。

伴有牙源性外胚层间质的牙源性上皮性肿瘤
Tumors of odontogenic epithelium with odontogenic ectomesenchyme

成釉细胞纤维瘤、成釉细胞纤维性牙质瘤和成釉细胞纤维性牙瘤
Ameloblastic fibroma, ameloblastic fibrodentinoma, ameloblastic fibro-odontoma

有些作者把这些肿瘤作为混合性牙源性肿瘤归在同一组内[31,47]。这些肿瘤是少见病变，它们具有许多共同特征，但是钙化性牙组织成分不同。这些病变大约发生在20岁之前，是牙瘤发生谱系的一部分。然而，有些成釉细胞纤维瘤和成釉细胞纤维性牙质瘤超出这个年龄，表现为良性肿瘤。单单根据组织学检查不可能鉴别肿瘤性和错构瘤性亚型。

临床特征

这种病变最常见于20岁以下个体。表现可以类似于成釉细胞瘤，但其侵袭性弱，生长缓慢，诊断时通常小于4 cm。已有报道成釉细胞纤维瘤保守手术后复发[48]。

组织学表现

牙源性间质与上皮混合存在，前者常常是黏液瘤性并类似于原始的牙髓，或者呈条带状和小巢状分布。存在牙源性间叶成分和上皮的混合，间叶成分通常是黏液样，类似于原始牙髓（图6.29）。上皮的特征是类似于分支带状牙板，伴有类似于成釉器的小芽。另外，成釉

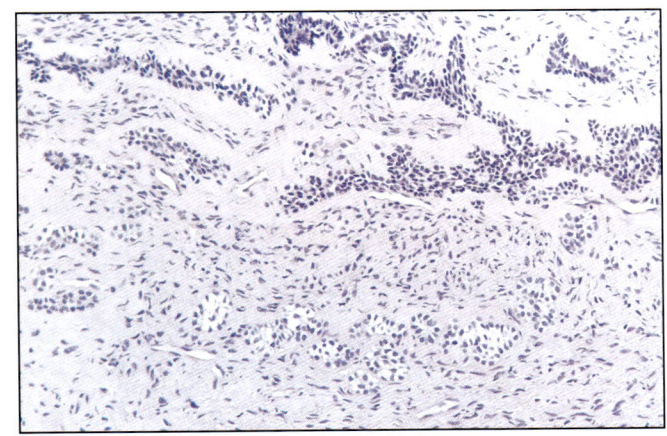

图6.29 成釉细胞纤维瘤伴有牙源性上皮和富于细胞的结缔组织。见于这个视野的透明细胞成分没有任何的预后意义。

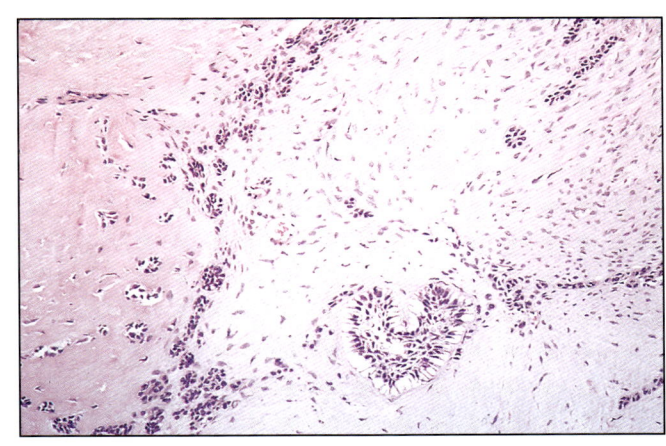

图6.30 成釉细胞纤维性牙质瘤显示异型增生的牙质，伴有牙源性上皮和间质增生。

细胞纤维性牙质瘤显示异型增生的牙质（图6.30），而成釉细胞纤维性牙瘤显示牙瘤形成（见下文）。组织学上，成釉细胞纤维瘤必须与成釉细胞瘤鉴别，以便预防对于年轻人作出不恰当的积极治疗的危险。成釉细胞瘤不含有牙板样条带，间质是胶原性纤维性组织，而不是见于典型的成釉细胞纤维瘤的疏松的牙源性间质。

成釉细胞牙瘤　Odontoameloblastoma

该肿瘤非常少见，表现为普通的成釉细胞瘤伴有牙瘤形成[49]。其行为与成釉细胞瘤相同。

腺瘤样牙源性肿瘤
Adenomatoid odontogenic tumor

腺瘤样牙源性肿瘤[50]是良性病变，过去称为腺成釉细胞瘤（adenoameloblastoma），但是应将这个病变归入错构瘤还是良性肿瘤还有争议。

临床特征

这些肿瘤最常发生在10～20岁的个体，上颌骨受累几乎是下颌骨的2倍。大约40%与未萌出的上颌尖牙牙冠有关。强烈提示牙源性肿瘤的特征是在囊腔内出现不透放射线的区域。腺瘤样牙源性肿瘤没有症状，生长缓慢；它们常常是在放射线检查中偶然发现的，但是病变可以大到足以引起肿胀。保守手术治疗通常可以治愈；即使是在不完全切除之后复发也非常罕见。

组织学表现

通常有界限清楚的上皮增生，其中可能有囊性成分。上皮主要是由几乎没有胞浆的多角形小细胞组成的，呈带状、片块状和漩涡状分布，没有特殊提示牙源性来源（图6.31）。腺瘤样成分（图6.32）是病变周围盲端内折

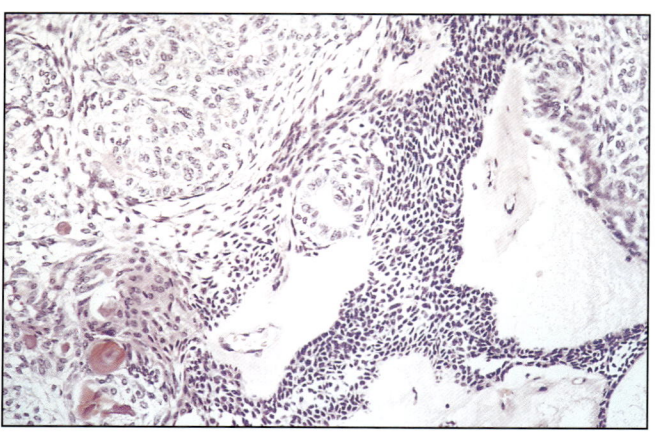

图6.31 腺瘤样成釉细胞瘤显示小而深染的细胞和呈漩涡状排列的较大的淡染细胞。

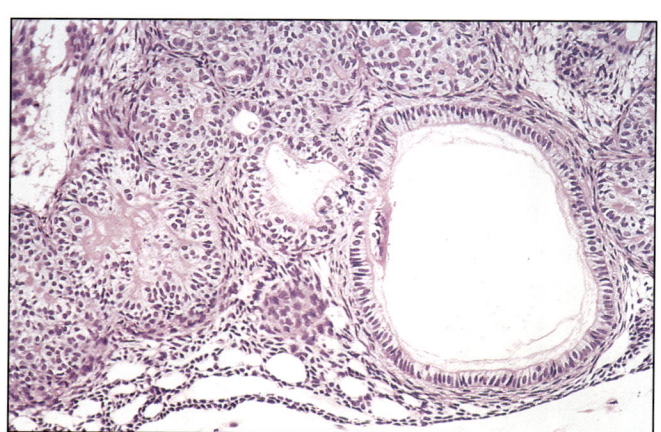

图6.32 腺瘤样牙源性肿瘤的腺瘤样成分伴有其他上皮结构。

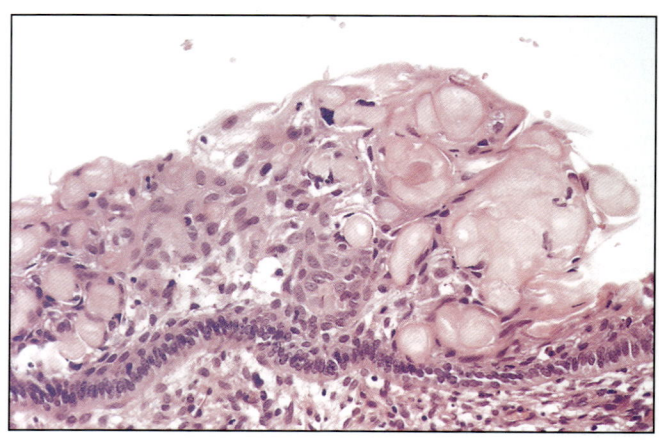

图6.33 钙化性牙源性囊肿的鬼影细胞。要注意基底细胞在周围呈栅栏样排列。

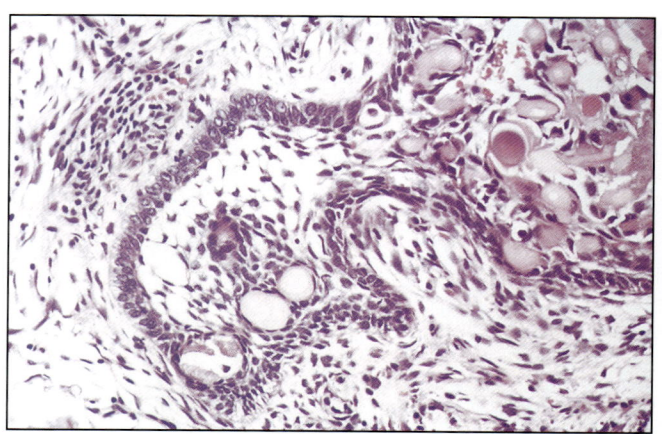

图6.34 实性牙源性鬼影细胞病变（牙源性鬼影细胞肿瘤）伴有非常类似于成釉细胞瘤的区域。

的横切面，内衬立方或柱状细胞，在任何已知的病例中腺瘤样成分出现的几率是不同的。另外一个易变的特征是基质形成，表现为小圆形无细胞的嗜酸性团块，可能是釉质蛋白的一种形式，或在少数情况下表现为较大的异型增生的牙本质区，可能伴有钙化。偶尔可以发现淀粉样物质[51]，在个别情况下出现黑色素沉着[52]。

牙源性鬼影细胞病变
Odontogenic ghost cell lesions

含有鬼影细胞的颌骨病变少见，但是很好辨认。然而，其分类复杂且有争议。为了详细讨论这个主题，读者可以参考专业教科书[9,31]。最常遇到的病变是钙化性牙源性囊肿，它是一种单纯的囊性病变。也可见到少数肿瘤亚型，分别被命名为钙化性囊性牙源性肿瘤（calcifying cystic odontogenic tumor）以及囊性和实性亚型的牙质生成性鬼影细胞肿瘤（dentinogenic ghost cell tumor）[9,31,53,54]。

临床特征

该病变通常表现为无症状的单房性囊肿。通常伴有未萌出牙或牙瘤[55]。中心性[31,56]和不常见的周围性病变[57]均有几种亚型。

组织学表现

这一组病变的特征是存在鬼影细胞（图6.33），类似于毛母质瘤的表现（见第23章）。这些细胞为嗜酸性，细胞界限清楚，其中许多细胞的细胞核染色呈不明显的鬼影状。存活的上皮通常出现周围核呈栅栏状排列和疏松的星网样区域。可以明显类似于成釉细胞瘤（图6.34）。可见鬼影细胞钙化的区域。邻近的上皮可以存在异型增生的牙质或牙瘤。实际上，在组织学上通常不可能区分单纯性钙化性牙源性囊肿和钙化性囊性牙源性肿瘤。必须根据临床行为、放射学和组织学表现做出判断。不管怎样，这两种病变都是良性的，保守性摘除通常可以治愈。实性亚型的牙质生成性鬼影细胞肿瘤可以发生在较大的年龄组，具有较强的侵袭性。这些肿瘤的处理方式与成釉细胞瘤相同。

鉴别诊断

报告显示，钙化性牙源性囊肿特征的病变与许多其他类型的牙源性肿瘤有关[56]。这个病变必须与囊肿或实性成釉细胞瘤鉴别，这种鉴别一般比较容易，除非鬼影细胞稀少。累及颚的病变必须与颅咽管瘤（craniopharyngioma）鉴别。

牙瘤 dontoma (odontome)

根据定义，牙瘤必须包括所有的钙化性牙组织。这些病变属于错构瘤，而且是最常见的牙源性肿瘤[47]（表6.2）。

临床表现

牙瘤见于青少年，多是放射线检查的偶然发现，或在少数情况下表现为缓慢生长的肿块。这些病变常常伴有未萌出牙，而且可以导致年轻人恒牙不能萌出。有时黏膜表面形成溃疡，口腔细菌进入引起感染导致疼痛表现。

组织学表现

确定的两种亚型具有不同的临床和组织学特征。复杂性牙瘤（complex odontoma）最常见于下颌骨后部，由与牙齿没有相似之处的牙硬组织混合而成。混合性牙瘤（compound odontoma）最常见的部位是上颌骨前部，由许多小的不规则形牙齿构成。主要的组织通常是牙质，通过存在小管可以辨认。牙釉质（图6.35）是无细胞的淡染物质，仅见明显的釉柱边缘。存在牙骨质和牙髓的疏松结缔组织。通常有牙源性上皮区域，伴牙釉质区域（图6.36），但是仅占整个肿块的一小部分。相关的牙质生成性囊肿并不少见。

鉴别诊断

牙瘤通常是单纯性的孤立性病变。然而，它们可以伴有其他牙源性肿瘤，例如钙化性牙源性囊肿[55]，或在

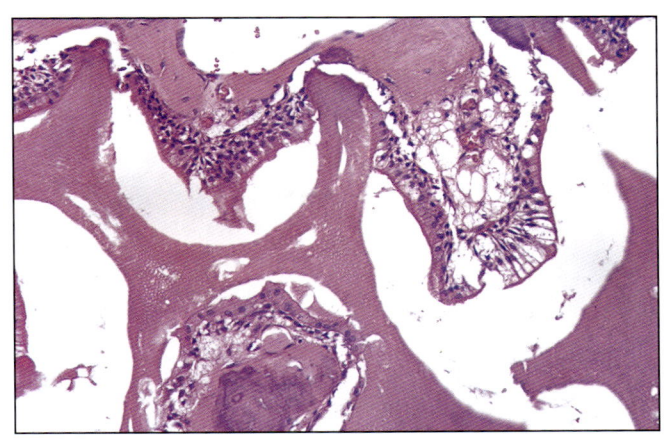

图6.36 牙瘤伴有活跃的牙质生成性上皮。

非常少见的情况下可以伴有成釉细胞瘤样增生，有理由诊断为牙成釉细胞瘤。不成熟或发生中的牙瘤可能无法与成釉细胞纤维瘤或其他混合性牙源性肿瘤区别。

伴有或不伴有牙源性上皮的牙源性外胚层间质肿瘤
Tumour of odontogenic ectomesenchyme with or without included ododntogenic epithelium

牙源性黏液瘤（同义词：颌骨黏液瘤） dontogenic myxoma (synonym: myxoma of jaw)

临床特征

牙源性黏液瘤可以发生在颌骨的任何部位，但最常见于下颌骨的磨牙前区。它们是生长缓慢的肿块，放射学上表现为多房性或肥皂泡样射线通透区。这些肿瘤可以为浸润性和局部侵袭性，保守手术治疗后常常复发[31,58]。

组织学表现

肿瘤是由散在的良性表现的星状或梭形纤维母细胞构成的，位于黏液瘤性基质中（图6.37）。可见小岛状牙源性上皮，但不是作出诊断的必要条件。可以见到胶原带，当出现胶原带时可以作出黏液纤维瘤（myxofibroma）的诊断。肿瘤界限不清，浸润到明显超出放射线学范围以外的骨髓间隙。

鉴别诊断

牙源性黏液瘤的诊断是在排除其他黏液性肿瘤的可能性之后做出的。这些肿瘤包括黏液样脂肪肉瘤、黏液样软骨肉瘤、软骨黏液样纤维瘤、黏液样神经纤维瘤和神经纤维肉瘤。

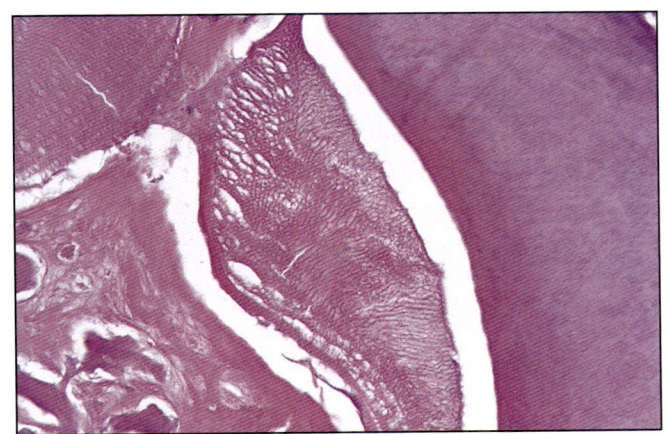

图6.35 牙瘤显示牙釉质基质和实性的牙质区。

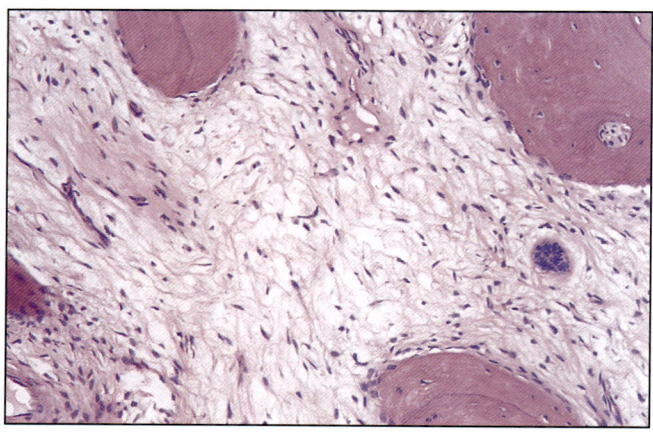

图6.37 牙源性黏液瘤浸润骨。可见不活跃的小巢状牙源性上皮。

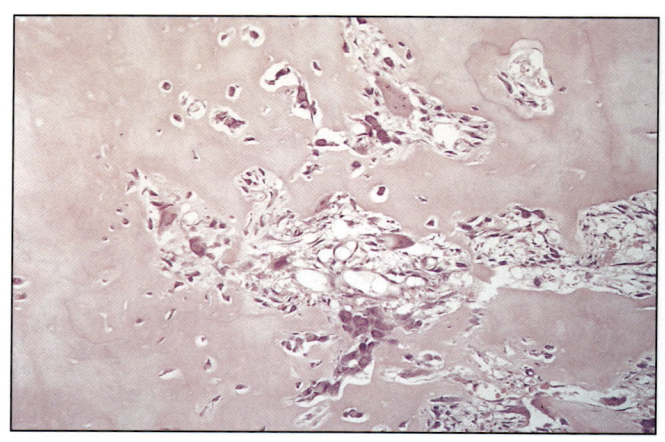

图6.38 成牙骨质细胞瘤。形成活跃的钙化组织,没有明显可辨认的牙骨质。可以出现明显的骨翻转线,有时伴有Paget样表现。

牙源性纤维瘤　Odontogenic fibroma

临床特征

这个术语用于一种以上的疾病[59]。与未萌出牙有关的增大滤泡可能表现出相对不成熟的结缔组织,伴有条带状增生的牙源性上皮。有些作者认为这种病变是牙源性纤维瘤,但是多数口腔病理医师将其诊断为增大的或增生性牙滤泡。除了这样的病变以外,还有牙源性纤维瘤的骨内(中心性)[59]和周围性病变。中心性病变表现为界限相对清楚的射线通透区,而较常见的周围性病变表现为牙龈瘤[60]。

组织学表现

中心性牙源性纤维瘤是界限清楚的非浸润性病变,由疏松的胶原纤维结缔组织构成,类似于牙滤泡。在整个病变中可见广泛散在分布的不活跃牙源性上皮岛。有些病变还含有钙化,类似于牙骨质、骨或牙质。周围性病变表现为相似的特征,但钙化比较常见[61]。

成牙骨质细胞瘤　Cementoblastoma

在以前命名为各种类型牙骨质肿瘤的病变中,现在仅把成牙骨质细胞瘤看作是牙源性肿瘤[9,31]。以前命名的牙骨质化纤维瘤现在分类为骨化性纤维瘤(见第25章)。根尖周牙骨质异型增生和巨大牙骨质瘤不再被认为是牙骨质肿瘤,而被认为是非肿瘤性病变,尽管有关它们的真正本质还有争议。成牙骨质细胞瘤与成骨细胞瘤相似,而且可能具有非常局灶的破坏性。

临床特征

成牙骨质细胞瘤通常表现为年轻人牙槽骨有触痛,有时是疼痛性的肿胀。放射学上,它表现为边界清楚的不透射线的牙根膨胀,最常见于下颌第一恒磨牙,具有射线通透性边缘。偶尔它表现为一种持续性的病变,直到相关牙齿拔牙后。

组织学表现

这个病变是由不规则的小梁状和岛状钙化组织构成,可以融合成肿块。成牙骨质细胞可以陷入组织内,可有明显的骨翻转线。在肿瘤的周围常常有大量基质形成。看上去非常活跃的肥胖的成牙骨质细胞可能是令人担忧的(图6.38)。

鉴别诊断

组织学上,这种病变可能与成骨细胞瘤相同,但与牙根明显相关可以做出诊断[63]。重要的是,不同的组织学特征不要过诊断为骨肉瘤,在作出这样的诊断之前总是需要考虑临床和放射学特征。

其他"牙骨质"病变[63]　Other "cemental" lesions

牙骨质是变异骨,它随着与牙齿的关系而改变。从前试图从组织学上区分牙骨质和骨样组织,现在认为这是没有根据的。从前命名为牙骨质化性纤维瘤的肿瘤现在被认为是骨化性纤维瘤谱系中的一部分(见第25章)。有许多其他颌骨病变是由钙化组织和富于细胞的结缔组织混合构成的,因此笼统分类为纤维-骨性病变。其中最常见的病变本质被认为是异型增生性而不是肿瘤性,牙骨质-骨性异型增生这个术语可以涵盖这一组病变。

牙骨质-骨性异型增生　Cemento-osseous dysplasias

目前认为3种疾病具有类似的组织学特征,表现为不同程度细胞构成的结缔组织和钙化组织(图6.39)。

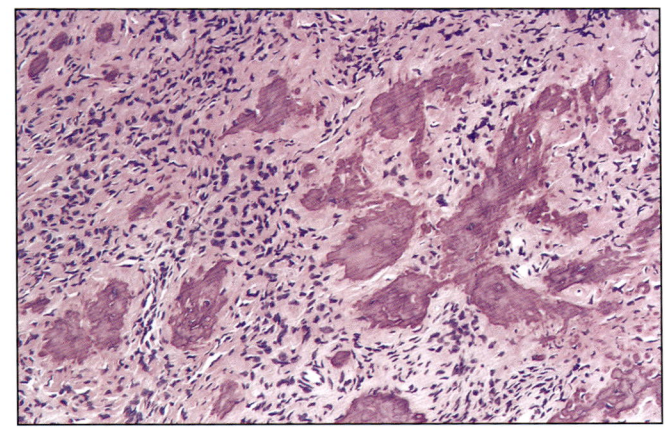

图6.39 牙骨质-骨性异型增生。这个伴有局限性钙化物质的富于细胞的视野来自根尖周围牙骨质异型增生。

实际上,并不容易把具体病例分类,最好把这些病变看成是形态学谱系的一部分,而不是独立的疾病。这些病变在组织学上无法鉴别。活髓牙根尖的根尖周围牙骨质异型增生一般表现为多发性射线通透区。这些改变在放射学上可能被误诊为根尖周围炎症性病变,但随时间改变而逐渐发生较明显的钙化。孤立性病变可能与牙齿无关,被命名为局灶性牙骨质-骨性异型增生[64],而多发性病变见于显著的牙骨质-骨性异型增生。

恶性牙源性肿瘤
Malignant odontogenic neoplasms

这些肿瘤均非常少见,这里不深入讨论。该分类列在表6.4中。该分类是以WHO分类为基础的[9]。牙源性癌起源于骨内,比口腔黏膜癌累及骨少见的多。当肿瘤较大,并且具有表面和骨内成分时,可能无法确定肿瘤的起源部位。一般来说,只有首先排除来自其他部位原发性病变的转移,才能作出牙源性癌的诊断。

恶性成釉细胞瘤
Malignant ameloblastoma

恶性成釉细胞瘤可能来源于已经存在的成釉细胞瘤,或者从一开始就可能为恶性。有两种类型:一种是组织学上类似于普通成釉细胞瘤,但发生转移;另一种是有恶性细胞学证据。后者已经被命名为成釉细胞癌(ameloblastic carcinoma)[9,31,65]。需要出现可辨认的成釉细胞瘤的区域,提示恶性的区域细胞比较密集(图6.40),具有恶性细胞学特征。肿瘤周围浸润性区域可以表现为未分化癌(图6.41)。复发常见,可见肺转移和局部淋巴结转移。

转移性成釉细胞瘤(metastasizing ameloblastomas)

表6.4	恶性牙源性肿瘤分类和主要特征
牙源性癌	
恶性成釉细胞瘤	成釉细胞瘤伴有转移的证据。原发性病变和转移性病变显示类似于普通成釉细胞瘤的组织学特征。
成釉细胞癌	成釉细胞瘤显示恶性细胞学证据。可以是新形成的肿瘤或者发生于先前存在的普通成釉细胞瘤。可以转移。
原发性骨内癌	由残留的牙源性上皮衍化而来的鳞状细胞癌。必须完全位于骨内,并且必须排除由黏膜病变蔓延而来或转移性肿瘤。
透明细胞牙源性癌	完全由透明细胞构成。侵袭性,可以转移。排除其他肿瘤的透明细胞亚型和转移。
牙质生成性鬼影细胞癌	牙质生成性鬼影细胞肿瘤的恶性亚型。特征鲜明,但非常少见。
其他牙源性上皮性肿瘤的恶性亚型	多数肿瘤很少描述有恶性亚型。主要特征是细胞学非典型性或有转移的证据。
牙源性囊肿恶变	在多种囊肿均有描述,但最多见于角化囊肿。恶性细胞学证据伴有良性囊肿残留的区域。
牙源性肉瘤	
成釉细胞纤维肉瘤	成釉细胞纤维瘤,但间叶性成分细胞密集,有细胞非典型性的证据。
成釉细胞纤维牙本质性肉瘤,成釉细胞纤维牙肉瘤	间叶性成分中有细胞学非典型性的证据。

非常罕见,其组织学特征是颌骨病变和转移病灶中均为普通性实性/多囊性成釉细胞瘤。许多成釉细胞瘤转移的最初报告是转移到经历多次口腔手术患者的肺。许多明显的转移现在已经被认为可能是医源性血管扩散,或者甚至可能是肿瘤的吸入。毫无疑问,可以发生真正的血管和淋巴管转移,证明这些肿瘤具有恶性本质。转移性成釉细胞瘤预后不良。

出现在成釉细胞瘤中的透明细胞(图6.42)与临床侵袭性有关,而且逐渐形成的一种观点,即将这些病变看成是低级别癌[36,37]。当除了透明细胞区域之外的肿瘤还显示有成釉细胞瘤区域时,应该能够做出诊断[66]。

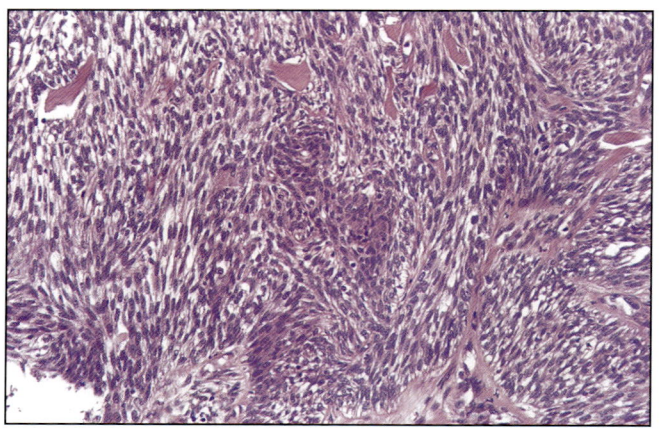

图6.40 成釉细胞瘤中密集的富于细胞的区域，但是没有显示成釉细胞瘤的显著特征。

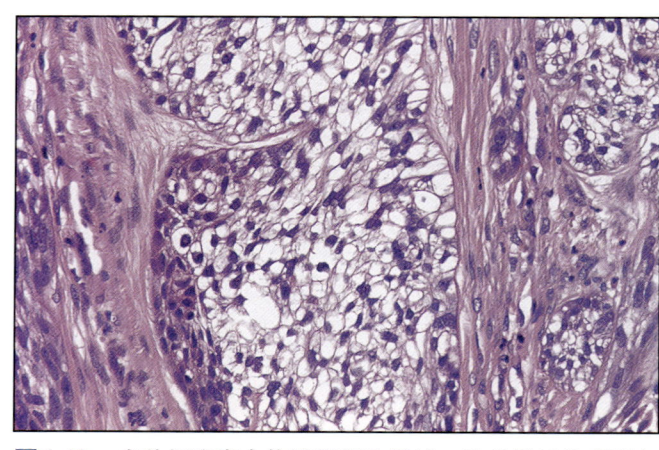

图6.42 成釉细胞瘤中的透明细胞区域。这些区域的表现与透明细胞牙源性癌非常类似。

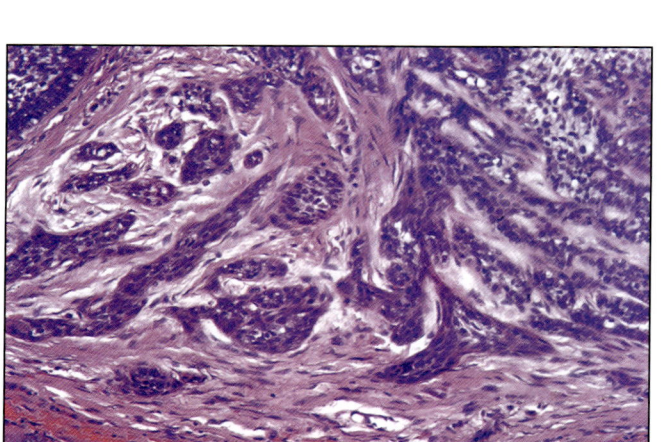

图6.41 恶性成釉细胞瘤边缘的未分化浸润性癌。

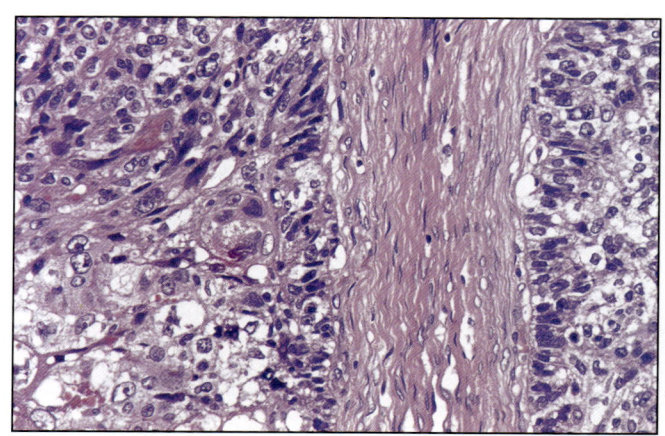

图6.43 原发性骨内癌伴有明显的恶性特征，一个区域显示局限性的栅栏状排列的基底细胞，提示牙源性来源。

原发性骨内癌
Primary intraosseous carcinoma

这些病变主要是发生在骨内的鳞状细胞癌，可能是起源于牙源性上皮巢（图6.43）。在排除了黏膜肿瘤侵犯骨、来源于牙源性囊肿的肿瘤或转移的可能性后可以做出诊断[67]。原发性骨内癌以男性为主，最常见于下颌磨牙区域。

透明细胞牙源性癌
Clear cell odontogenic carcinoma

这个肿瘤最初称为透明细胞牙源性肿瘤[32,68]，但是现在看来，这是明显的侵袭性病变，伴有转移的潜能。因此逐渐形成一种观点，即牙源性肿瘤中的透明细胞代表恶性，现在命名为癌是恰当的[9,31]。临床上这种病变最常表现为疼痛性颌骨肿胀，放射线显示为射线通透区，境界不清，伴牙齿松动和骨破坏。

组织学表现

多数细胞具有透明或模糊的颗粒状富于糖原的胞浆（图6.44）。细胞在胶原性间质中排列成簇或带状[69]，伴有广泛的髓腔浸润。部分肿瘤可以形成基底细胞样细胞团，但是当肿瘤显示具有其他类型牙源性肿瘤的特征性区域时，不要诊断为透明细胞牙源性癌。有些作者则不同意这个观点，建议将透明细胞牙源性癌和伴有透明细胞的成釉细胞瘤归为一组[70]。

鉴别诊断

主要的鉴别诊断是其他透明细胞肿瘤[71]，包括成釉细胞瘤的透明细胞亚型、钙化性上皮性牙源性肿瘤、诸如黏液表皮样癌和腺泡细胞癌等涎腺肿瘤。应该寻找这些肿瘤的其他比较典型的区域。需要除外转移性透明细胞肿瘤，尤其来源于肾脏的肿瘤。

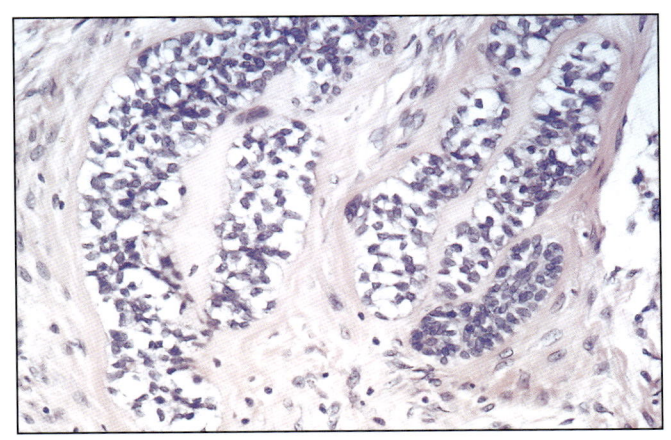

图6.44 透明细胞牙源性癌。细胞学特征各异,但是某些肿瘤温和的细胞学表现与侵袭性行为不符。

其他牙源性肿瘤的恶性亚型
Malignant variants of other odontogenic tumors

这些病例是个案报告,并且非常少见,其表现方式或行为尚不清楚。诊断依靠识别良性亚型的特征,并伴有可辨认的恶性肿瘤的细胞学特征或生物学行为[31]。

牙源性囊肿恶性变
Malignant change in odontogenic cysts

起源于牙源性囊肿的鳞状细胞癌是一种少见的并发症,但这仍然是最常见的恶性牙源性肿瘤。为了准确地作出这种诊断,必须确认非肿瘤性囊肿内衬的区域,而且排除邻近口腔黏膜肿瘤扩散偶尔累及囊肿。这样的癌通常发生在长期存在的囊肿,常常伴有感染和囊肿内衬的角化。有时可能表现为角化囊肿,但是其他病例可能是由于角化性化生。

牙源性肉瘤和癌肉瘤
Odontogenic sarcomas and carcinosarcomas

这些肿瘤非常罕见,但已有病例描述,主要是个案报告[72,73]。组织学特征类似于相应的良性肿瘤,恶性诊断是根据细胞学特征或行为做出的。这样看来,这些罕见的病变似乎最常发生在先前存在的良性病变中。

牙源性囊肿　Odontogenic cysts

牙源性囊肿是良性囊性病变,起源于颌骨内残留的牙源性上皮。它们的分类混乱,有些病变可能被误认为是肿瘤。因此,这里有必要简要描述一下常见而又重要的病变。某些病变因为其大小或有复发的潜能而特别容易与肿瘤混淆。其中包括牙源性角化囊肿、腺性牙源性囊肿和葡萄状牙源性囊肿。这些病变将做简要讨论,而较详细的内容可见专业性教科书[10,74]。表6.5中列出了牙源性囊肿的简单分类和主要特征。

根尖囊肿　Radicular cyst

这是一种最常见的牙源性囊肿,还有诸如牙囊肿、根尖囊肿或根尖周围囊肿等不同的命名。这些囊肿的发生是牙齿根尖炎症性改变的结果,因此与死髓牙有关,通常是龋齿的结果。囊肿是由于以前存在的慢性炎症性病变(根尖周围肉芽肿)中的 Malassez 残留上皮增生而形成。临床上病变表现为生长缓慢的肿胀,或者是偶尔发现的牙齿根尖界限清楚的放射线通透区。牙齿拔出后,囊肿偶尔仍然残留在无牙的颌骨中,称为残留囊肿。

组织学表现

根尖囊肿是由内衬非角化性复层鳞状上皮的炎症性纤维性囊壁构成的(图6.45)。不成熟囊肿的上皮是增生性的,而且可以形成明显的拱桥和细带,但是随着时间的变化,内衬上皮逐渐变薄乃至增厚。囊肿壁内通常可以发现胆固醇裂隙,上皮可以含有嗜酸性透明小体。黏液化生的区域并不少见。

含牙囊肿　Dentigerous cyst

含牙囊肿是发育性囊肿,起源于未萌出牙牙冠周围变薄的牙釉质上皮。该病变最常见于阻生的第三磨牙(智齿)或上尖牙,表现为围绕未萌出牙牙冠的界限清楚的射线通透区。萌出牙上面表浅的含牙囊肿有时称为萌牙囊肿(eruption cyst)。一种囊肿常常与含牙囊肿混淆,其发生与乳头状萌出牙牙冠有关,它来源于炎症而不是发育性病变,称为牙周囊肿(paradental cyst)[75]。

组织学表现

典型者,囊肿壁是由没有炎症的疏松胶原纤维结缔组织构成的,内衬薄而规则的复层鳞状上皮,小囊肿的内衬可能仍然类似于牙釉质上皮,包括一层立方或矮柱状上皮,可被认为是腺体上皮(图6.46)。根据定义,这种囊肿在牙骨质和牙釉质交界处附着于相关牙齿的颈部,大体标本检查有助于证实这一点。

牙源性囊肿

表6.5 牙源性囊肿的简单分类，相对发病率和主要特征

	发病率（%）	特征
炎症性牙源性囊肿		
根尖囊肿	65	发生在牙根尖端区域，为死髓牙。炎症性纤维性囊壁内衬增厚或增生的复层鳞状上皮。常见胆固醇裂隙。
牙周囊肿	<5	发生在活髓牙的附近，通常是部分萌出的第三磨牙。由于滤泡上皮的炎症性增生，组织学类似于根尖囊肿。
发育性牙源性囊肿		
含牙囊肿	20	发生于滤泡上皮并包围未萌出牙的牙冠。非炎症性囊壁内衬薄而规则的复层上皮。
牙源性角化囊肿	5	发生在骨内残留的牙板，可能与牙有关。下颌角多房性射线通透区。非炎症性囊壁内衬薄而规则的角化不全上皮。明显的基底层和内衬折叠。可伴有痣基底细胞癌综合征。角化性囊性牙源性肿瘤的肿瘤性类型已有描述。
侧牙周囊肿	<1	发生于邻近活髓牙的Malassez细胞残留区域。单纯性囊肿内衬薄而规则的复层上皮，伴有特征性的斑片状增厚。
葡萄状牙源性囊肿	<1	侧牙周囊肿的多房性亚型。可能复发，因为内衬上皮卷曲呈脑回状。
腺性牙源性囊肿	<1	多房性囊肿，发生于牙的附近。内衬显示腺体化生，伴有黏液细胞和导管样结构。可以复发。
牙龈囊肿	1	内衬复层鳞状上皮的小的单纯性囊肿（<1cm）。可以角化。见于成人的龈缘或婴儿的牙槽。

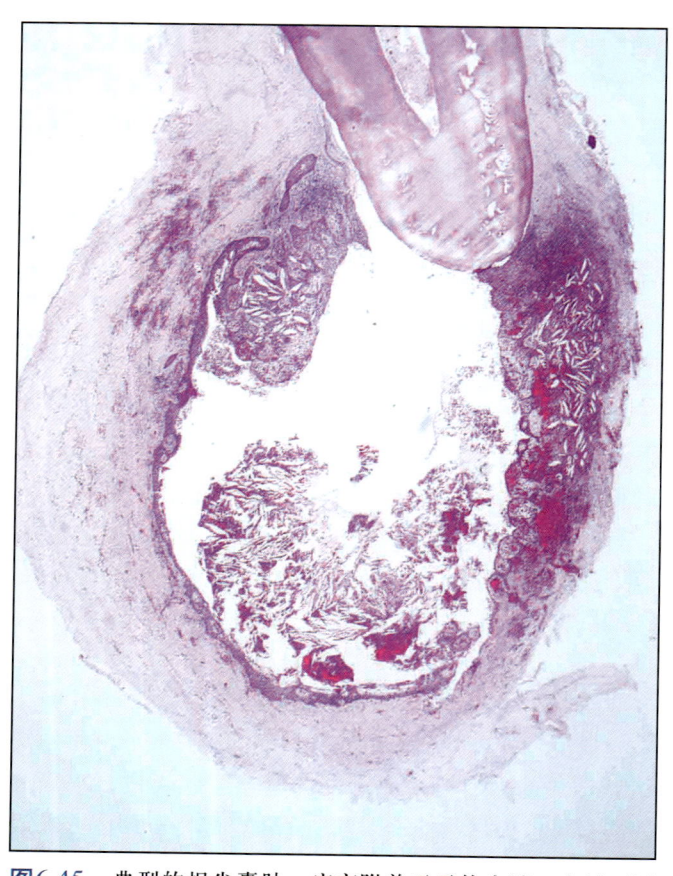

图6.45 典型的根尖囊肿。病变附着于牙的尖端，内衬不同程度增生的复层鳞状上皮。在炎症性纤维性囊壁中常见胆固醇裂隙。

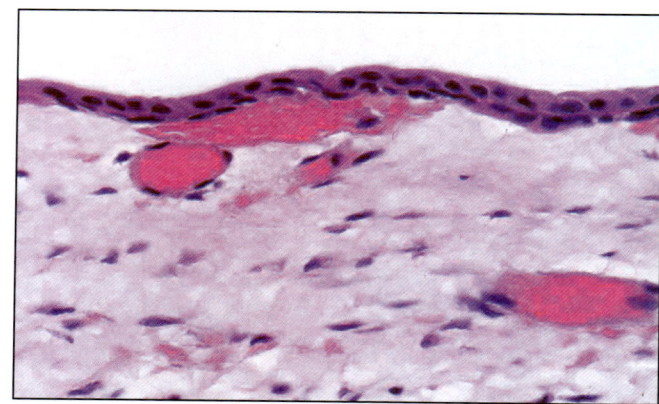

图6.46 含牙囊肿。这个小囊肿的内衬仅由两层细胞组成，类似于退化的牙釉质上皮。注意囊壁缺乏炎症。炎症性含牙囊肿可能类似于根尖囊肿。

牙源性角化囊肿 Odontogenic keratocyst

牙源性角化囊肿通常被认为是发育性囊肿，但是现在有证据表明，这种病变至少部分可能是良性囊性肿瘤。在最新的WHO分类中，已经提出了一种新的疾病，即角化性囊性牙源性肿瘤（keratinizing cystic odontogenic tumor）[9]。其根据是发现有些角化囊肿侵袭性行为，实性亚型已有描述[76]，以及有些病变伴有痣基底细胞癌综合征（Gorlin综合征）中的基底细

胞癌。Gorlin 综合征中的角化囊肿和少部分自发性病变具有与基底细胞癌类似的 *PTCH* 基因突变[77]，而且分子学研究显示其有克隆性和多个肿瘤抑制基因缺失的证据[78,79]。散发性病变也常常显示等位基因不平衡性[79a]。单纯性囊肿和肿瘤性亚型的组织学鉴别标准尚未确立。

临床特征

牙源性角化囊肿一般最常表现为无痛性的颌骨膨胀，伴有多房性射线通透区。下颌角是最常见的部位。病变通常为孤立性，而伴有痣样基底细胞癌综合征时可见多发性和复发性囊肿。角化囊肿可以包裹未萌出牙，放射线上表现为成牙，或者偶尔可以取代牙齿。这些肿瘤起源于残留的牙板，但是替代的名字"始基囊肿"（primordial cyst）却出自错误的概念，即认为这种囊肿是来源于钙化组织形成之前的退化的牙胚。

组织学表现

该囊肿的诊断特征是角化的内衬。上皮通常较薄，密集成折，伴有栅栏状排列的基底层以及表面薄层波浪状的不全角化层（图 6.47）。囊肿通常大而呈多房性，尤其是位于下颌骨后部的囊肿。少数病变为多囊性或实性，被认为是肿瘤性谱系的一端[76]。复发可能是因为囊肿切除不完全，或者是因为主要囊肿附近有子囊肿生长。角化囊肿壁内偶尔可见成釉细胞瘤样增生，不要过诊断。在炎症性区域角化可能被漏掉。某些角化囊肿的内衬具有正角化（orthokeratosis）的区域，完全内衬正角化上皮的囊肿的侵袭性是不明显的。

葡萄状牙源性囊肿[80]
Botryoid odontogenic cyst

该囊肿是侧牙周囊肿的多房性亚型，是起源于牙周韧带残留上皮的发育性囊肿。内衬非角化性复层鳞状上皮，其显著特征是出现上皮斑的增厚区（图 6.48）。尽管通常较小，本病的多房性本质可以导致术后病变残留和复发。

腺性牙源性囊肿（涎腺-牙源性囊肿）[81,82]
Glandular odontogenic cyst (sialo-odontogenic cyst)

这些罕见的多房性囊肿与葡萄状牙源性囊肿有许多共同的特征。另外的具有特征性的特点是存在腺上皮区域（图 6.49），常常伴有上皮内衬的腺腔并产生黏液。表面细胞可以是立方或柱状细胞，有时可见纤毛。重要的鉴别诊断是中心性黏液表皮样癌[83]。

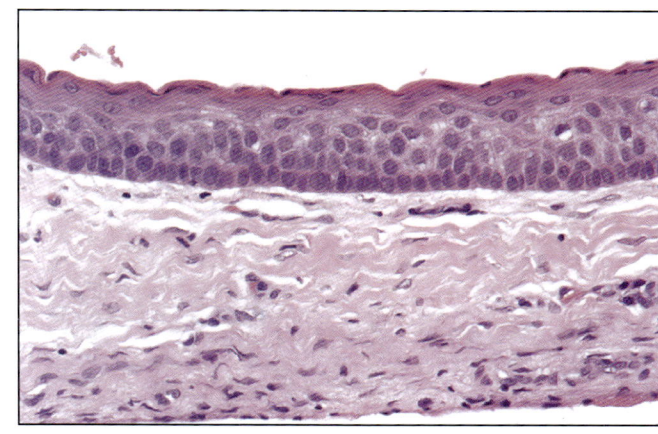

图 6.47　牙源性角化囊肿伴有表面薄层角化不全。基底层不同，从如同本例的呈直线排列的矮柱状细胞到较长的栅栏状排列的细胞都有。

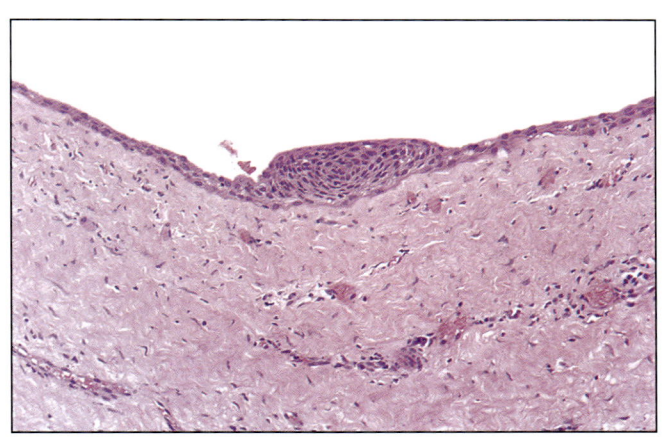

图 6.48　葡萄状牙源性囊肿内衬薄层非角化性复层鳞状上皮，伴有上皮斑的增厚区。

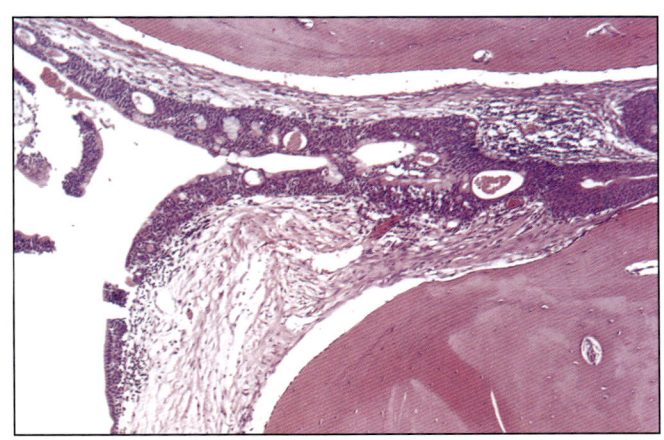

图 6.49　骨内复发性腺性牙源性囊肿。

参考文献

1. Henley J D, Summerlin D-J, Tomich C E 2004 Condyloma acuminatum and condyloma-like lesions of the oral cavity: a study of 11 cases with an intraductal component. Histopathology 44: 216–221
2. Henke R P, Guerin-Reverchon I, Milde-Langosch K et al. 1989 In situ detection of human papillomavirus types 13 and 32 in focal epithelial hyperplasia of the oral mucosa. J Oral Pathol Med 18: 419–421
3. Speight P M, Farthing P M, Bouquot J E 1996 The pathology of oral cancer and precancer. Curr Diagn Pathol 3: 165–176
4. Mashberg A, Feldman L J 1988 Clinical criteria for identifying early oral and oropharyngeal carcinoma: erythroplasia revisited. Am J Surg 156: 273–275
5. Anneroth G, Batsakis J, Luna M 1987 Review of the literature and a recommended system of malignancy grading in oral squamous cell carcinomas. Scand J Dent Res 95: 229–249
6. Bryne M, Koppang H, Lilleng R et al. 1992 Malignancy grading of the deep invasive margins of oral squamous cell carcinomas has high prognostic value. J Pathol 166: 375–381
7. Woolgar J A 1995 Prediction of cervical lymph node metastasis in squamous cell carcinoma of the tongue/floor of mouth. Head Neck 17: 463–472
8. Fukano H, Matsuura H, Hasegawa Y et al. 1997 Depth of invasion a predictive factor for cervical lymph node metastasis in tongue carcinoma. Head Neck 19: 205–210
9. Barnes L, Eveson J W, Reichart P, Sidransky D (eds) 2005 WHO classification of tumours. Pathology and genetics of head and neck tumours. IARC Press, Lyon
10. Odell E W, Morgan P R 1998 Biopsy pathology of the oral tissues. Chapman & Hall Medical, London, p 214–236
11. Ellis G L, Corio R L 1980 Spindle cell carcinoma of the oral cavity. Oral Surg Oral Med Oral Pathol 50: 523–534
12. Batsakis J G, Huser J 1990 Squamous carcinomas with gland-like (adenoid) features. Ann Otol Rhinol Laryngol 99: 87–88
13. Ferlito A, Devaney K O, Rinaldo A et al. 1996 Mucosal adenoid squamous cell carcinoma of the head and neck. Ann Otol Rhinol Laryngol 105: 409–413
14. Izumi K, Nakajima T, Maeda T et al. 1998 Adenosquamous carcinoma of the tongue. Oral Surg Oral Med Oral Pathol 85: 178–184
15. Banks E R, Frierson H F, Mills S E et al. 1992 Basaloid squamous cell carcinoma of the head and neck. Am J Surg Pathol 16: 939–946
16. Barnes L, Ferlito A, Altavilla G et al. 1996 Basaloid squamous cell carcinoma of the head and neck: clinicopathological features and differential diagnosis. Ann Otol Rhinol Laryngol 105: 75–82
17. Luna M A, Tortoledo M E 1988 Verrucous carcinoma. In: Gnepp D R (ed) Pathology of the head and neck. Churchill Livingstone, Edinburgh, p 497–515
18. Hunter K D, Parkinson E K, Harrison P R 2005 Profiling early head and neck cancer. Nat Rev Cancer 5: 127–135
19. Schepman K P, van der Meij E H, Smeele L E et al. 1998 Malignant transformation of oral leukoplakia: a follow-up study of a hospital-based population of 166 patients with oral leukoplakia from The Netherlands. Oral Oncol 34: 270–275
20. Sudbo J, Ried T, Bryne M et al. 2001 Abnormal DNA content predicts the occurrence of carcinomas in non-dysplastic oral white patches. Oral Oncol 37: 558–565
21. Hansen L S, Olson J A, Silverman S 1985 Proliferative verrucous leukoplakia: a long term study of thirty patients. Oral Surg Oral Med Oral Pathol 60: 285–298
22. Batsakis J G, Suarez P, El-Naggar A K 1999 Proliferative verrucous leukoplakia and its related lesions. Oral Oncol 35: 354–359
23. Zakrzewska J M, Lopes V, Speight P et al. 1996 Proliferative verrucous leukoplakia. Oral Surg Oral Med Oral Pathol 82: 396–401
24. Renshaw A A, Rosai J 1993 Benign atypical vascular lesions of the lip. A study of 12 cases. Am J Surg Pathol 17: 557–565
25. MacDonald D G, Boyle I T 1990 Skeletal diseases. In: Jones J H, Mason D K (eds) Oral manifestations of systemic disease, 2nd edn. Bailliere Tindall, London, p 616–659
26. Damm D D, Cibull M L, Geissler R H et al. 1993 Investigation into the histogenesis of congenital epulis of the newborn. Oral Surg Oral Med Oral Pathol 76: 205–212
27. Kim J, Ellis G L 1993 Dental follicular tissue: misinterpretation as odontogenic tumors. J Oral Maxillofac Surg 51: 762–767
28. Gardner D G, Radden B 1995 Multiple calcifying hyperplastic dental follicles. Oral Surg Oral Med Oral Pathol 79: 603–606
29. Philipsen H P, Thosaporn W, Reichart P A et al. 1992 Odontogenic lesions in opercula of permanent molars delayed in eruption. J Oral Pathol Med 21: 38–41
30. Yonemochi H, Noda T, Saku T 1998 Pericoronal hamartomatous lesions in the opercula of teeth delayed in eruption: an immunohistochemical study of the extracellular matrix. J Oral Pathol Med 27: 441–452
31. Reichart P A, Philipsen H P 2004 Odontogenic tumours and allied lesions. Quintessence Publishing, London
32. Kramer I R H, Pindborg J J, Shear M 1992 Histological typing of odontogenic tumors, 2nd edn. Springer-Verlag, Berlin
33. MacDonald D G, Browne R M 1997 Tumours of odontogenic epithelium. In: Anthony P P, MacSween R N M, Lowe D G (eds) Recent advances in histopathology 17. Churchill Livingstone, Edinburgh, p 139–166
34. Reichart P A, Philipsen H P, Sonner S 1995 Ameloblastoma: biological profile of 3677 cases. Eur J Cancer B Oral Oncol 31: 86–99
35. Philipsen H P, Ormiston I W, Reichart P A 1992 The desmo- and osteoplastic ameloblastoma. Int J Oral Maxillofac Surg 21: 352–357
36. Waldron C A, Small I A, Silverman H 1985 Clear cell ameloblastoma – an odontogenic carcinoma. J Oral Maxillofac Surg 43: 707–717
37. Muller H, Slootweg P 1986 Clear cell differentiation in an ameloblastoma. J Maxillofac Surg 14: 158–160
38. Philipsen H P, Reichert P A 1998 Unicystic ameloblastoma. A review of 193 cases from the literature. Oral Oncol 34: 317–325
39. Gardner D G, Corio R L 1984 Plexiform unicystic ameloblastoma. Cancer 53: 1730–1735
40. Gardner D G 1977 Peripheral ameloblastoma: a study of 21 cases including 5 reported as basal cell carcinoma of the gingiva. Cancer 39: 1625–1633
41. Pullon P A, Shafer W G, Elzay R P et al. 1975 Squamous odontogenic tumor. Oral Surg Oral Med Oral Pathol 40: 616–630
42. Leider A S, Jonker L A, Cook H E 1989 Multicentric familial squamous odontogenic tumor. Oral Surg Oral Med Oral Pathol 68: 175–181
43. Unal T, Gomel M, Gunel O 1987 Squamous odontogenic tumor-like islands in a radicular cyst. J Oral Maxillofac Surg 45: 346–349
44. Pindborg J J 1958 A calcifying epithelial odontogenic tumor. Cancer 11: 838–843
45. Franklin C D, Pindborg J J 1976 The calcifying epithelial odontogenic tumor. Oral Surg Oral Med Oral Pathol 42: 753–765
46. Hick M J, Flaitz C M, Wong M E K et al. 1994 Clear cell variant of calcifying epithelial odontogenic tumor: a case report and review of the literature. Head Neck 16: 272–277
47. Philipsen H P, Reichart P A, Praetorius F 1997 Mixed odontogenic tumours and odontomas. Considerations on interrelationship. Review of the literature and presentation of 134 new cases of odontomas. Oral Oncol 33: 86–99
48. Zallen R D, Preskar M H, McClary S A 1982 Ameloblastic fibroma. J Oral Maxillofac Surg 40: 513–517
49. La Briola J D, Steiner M, Bernstein M L et al. 1980 Odontoameloblastoma. J Oral Surg 38: 139–143
50. Philipsen H P, Reichart P A, Zhang K H et al. 1991 Adenomatoid odontogenic tumor: biologic profile based on 499 cases. J Oral Pathol Med 20: 149–158
51. Buchner A, David R 1976 Amyloid-like material in odontogenic tumors. J Oral Surg 34: 320–323
52. Takeda Y 1989 Pigmented adenomatoid odontogenic tumour. Virchows Arch [A] 415: 571–575
53. Hong S P, Ellis G L, Hartman K S 1991 Calcifying odontogenic cyst. Oral Surg Oral Med Oral Pathol 72: 56–64
54. Toida M 1998 So-called calcifying odontogenic cyst: review and discussion on the terminology and classification. J Oral Pathol Med 27: 49–52
55. Hirshberg A, Kaplan I, Buchner A 1994 Calcifying odontogenic cyst associated with odontoma. J Oral Maxillofac Surg 52: 555–558
56. Buchner A 1991 The central (intraosseous) calcifying odontogenic cyst: an analysis of 215 cases. J Oral Maxillofac Surg 49: 330–339
57. Buchner A, Merrill P W, Hansen L S et al. 1991 Peripheral (extraosseous) calcifying odontogenic cyst: a review of 45 cases. Oral Surg Oral Med Oral Pathol 72: 65–70
58. Baker B F 1999 Odontogenic myxoma. Semin Diagn Pathol 16: 297–301
59. Gardner D G 1996 Central odontogenic fibroma – current concepts. J Oral Pathol Med 25: 556–561
60. Buchner A, Ficarra G, Hansen L S 1987 Peripheral odontogenic fibroma. Oral Surg Oral Med Oral Pathol 64: 432–438
61. Slabbert H de V, Altini M 1991 Peripheral odontogenic fibroma: a clinicopathologic study. Oral Surg Oral Med Oral Pathol 72: 86–90
62. Slootweg P J 1992 Cementoblastoma and osteoblastoma: a comparison of histologic features. J Oral Pathol Med 21: 385–389
63. Waldron C A 1993 Fibro-osseous lesions of the jaws. J Oral Maxillofac Surg 51: 828–835
64. Su L, Weathers D R, Waldron C A 1997 Distinguishing features of focal cemento-osseous dysplasias and cemento-osseous fibromas. Oral Surg Oral Med Oral Pathol 84: 301–309
65. Simko E J, Brannon R B, Eibling D E 1998 Ameloblastic carcinoma of the mandible. Head Neck 20: 654–659
66. Mari A, Escutia E, Carrera M et al. 1995 Clear cell ameloblastoma or odontogenic carcinoma. J Cranio Maxillo-Fac Surg 23: 387–390
67. Suei Y, Tanimoto K, Taguchi A et al. 1994 Primary intraosseous carcinoma: review of the literature and diagnostic criteria. J Oral Maxillofac Surg 52: 580–583
68. Hansen L S, Eversole L R, Green T L et al. 1985 Clear cell odontogenic tumor – a new histologic variant with aggressive potential. Head Neck Surg 8: 115–123
69. Eversole L R, Duffey D C, Powell N B 1995 Clear-cell odontogenic carcinoma – a clinicopathologic analysis. Arch Otolaryngol Head Neck Surg 121: 685–689
70. Yamamoto H, Inui M, Mori A et al. 1998 Clear cell odontogenic carcinoma. Oral Surg Oral Med Oral Pathol 86: 86–89
71. Maiorano E, Altini M, Favia G 1997 Clear cell tumours of the salivary glands, jaws and oral mucosa. Semin Diagn Pathol 14: 203–212
72. Chomette G, Auriol M, Guilbert F et al. 1983 Ameloblastic fibrosarcoma of the jaws – report of three cases. Pathol Res Pract 178: 40–47

73. Wood R M, Markle T L, Barker B F et al. 1988 Ameloblastic fibrosarcoma. Oral Surg Oral Med Oral Pathol 66: 74–77
74. Cawson R A, Speight P, Binnie W H et al. (eds) 1998 Lucas's pathology of the tumors of the oral tissues, 5th edn. W B Saunders, Philadelphia
75. Craig G T 1976 The paradental cyst. A specific inflammatory odontogenic cyst. Br Dent J 141: 9–14
76. Vered M, Buchner A, Dayan D et al. 2004 Solid variant of odontogenic keratocyst. J Oral Pathol Med 33: 125–128
77. Barreto D C, Gomez R S, Bale A et al. 2000 PTCH gene mutations in odontogenic keratocysts. J Dent Res 79: 1418–1422
78. Shear M 2002 The aggressive nature of the odontogenic keratocyst: is it a benign cystic neoplasm? Part 2. Proliferation and genetic studies. Oral Oncol 38: 323–331
79. Agaram N P, Collins B M, Barnes L et al. 2004 Molecular analysis to demonstrate that odontogenic keratocysts are neoplastic. Arch Pathol Lab Med 128: 313–317
79a. Henley J, Summerlin D J, Tomich C et al. 2005 Molecular evidence supporting the neoplastic nature of odontogenic keratocyst: a laser capture microdissection study of 15 cases. Histopathology 47:582–586
80. Gurol M, Burkes E J, Jacoway J 1995 Botryoid odontogenic cyst: analysis of 33 cases. J Periodontol 66: 1069–1073
81. Hussain K, Edmondson H D, Browne R M 1995 Glandular odontogenic cysts. Oral Surg Oral Med Oral Pathol 79: 593–602
82. Koppang H S, Johannessen S, Haugen L K et al. 1998 Glandular odontogenic cyst (sialo-odontogenic cyst): report of two cases and literature review of 45 previously reported cases. J Oral Pathol Med 27: 455–462
83. Manojlovic S, Grgurvic J, Knezevic G et al. 1997 Glandular odontogenic cyst: a case report and clinicopathologic relationship to central mucoepidermoid carcinoma. Head Neck 19: 227–231

涎腺肿瘤
Salivary gland tumors

Wah Cheuk 和 John K.C. Chan 著

高松源 译　回允中 校

正常涎腺肿瘤	239	间叶性肿瘤和瘤样病变	303
涎腺肿瘤	240	血液淋巴肿瘤和瘤样病变	305
上皮性肿瘤和瘤样病变	244	涎腺上皮性肿瘤的诊断分析方法	310

正常涎腺肿瘤
The normal salivary glands

应用解剖学　Applied anatomy

涎腺系统由3对大腺体（腮腺，颌下腺和舌下腺）以及500～1000个分布在口腔黏膜下层的小涎腺小叶组成。根据定义，鼻腔、喉和支气管的浆液黏液腺虽然不能产生唾液，但是组织学上和小涎腺相似，并且其肿瘤具有与3大腺体肿瘤相似的模式。

正常成人腮腺重15～30g。面神经穿行于深叶和浅叶之间。多数涎腺肿瘤起源于浅叶并且表现为面部肿胀。发生在深叶的肿瘤常常扩展到咽旁间隙，表现为咽部肿胀[1]。腮腺副叶位于腮腺导管（Stenson's duct）附近，且与腮腺的主体相分离，见于21%的正常个体[2]。发生在副叶的肿瘤常常表现为面颊中部的肿块[3]。正常情况下，腮腺内大约有20个淋巴结和随意分布的淋巴细胞集聚。后一种成分是黏膜相关淋巴组织（mucosa-associated lymphoid tissue，MALT）[4]。发生在腮腺内淋巴结的普通类型的结内淋巴瘤可能表现为涎腺肿瘤。相反，在腮腺内，腮腺旁和颈部淋巴结中可能出现涎腺组织，并且可以引起淋巴结Warthin肿瘤以及其他的涎腺肿瘤，类似于转移性疾病[5]。

颌下腺和舌下腺大约分别重7～15g和2～4g。与腮腺不同，虽然在正常情况下颌下腺附近存在淋巴结，但是颌下腺实质内没有淋巴结以及大的神经穿过。

在舌的侧缘、唇、颊黏膜、腭和舌咽区域可以发现小涎腺。其中，腭是发生涎腺肿瘤的主要发病部位。

组织学

组织构成

除了舌下腺的包膜不完整外，大涎腺均被一层薄的纤维性包膜所包被。涎腺小叶由不同比例的浆液细胞和黏液细胞组成。腮腺完全是浆液腺，颌下腺是混合性浆液黏液腺，舌下腺则以黏液腺为主；小涎腺是浆液黏液腺或以黏液腺为主，取决于其部位。

腮腺是管泡状外分泌腺，腺泡是位于末端的分泌单位。分泌物通过导管单位到达口腔，导管单位由闰管、集合管（striated ducts）、小叶间导管、分泌导管和涎腺导管组成（图7.1）。小叶结构的保留是支持非肿瘤性病变的诊断而不是肿瘤的一个重要的特征。整个腺体

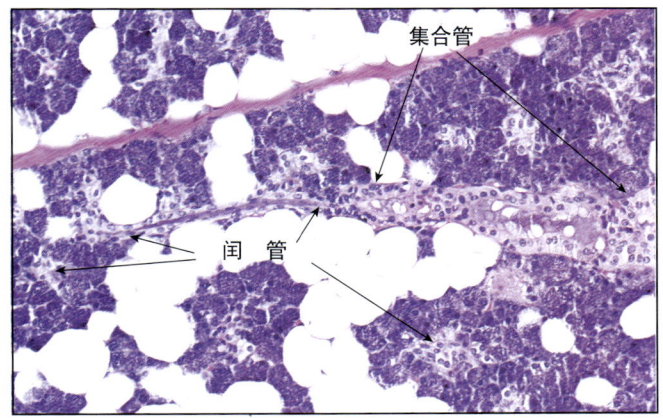

图7.1　正常腮腺。腺泡由锥体形的浆液细胞组成，核位于基底部，并有丰富的暗紫色酶原颗粒。它们引流到狭窄的内衬立方细胞的闰管。闰管与集合管连续，集合管具有比较宽大的管腔，内衬柱状嗜酸性粒细胞。

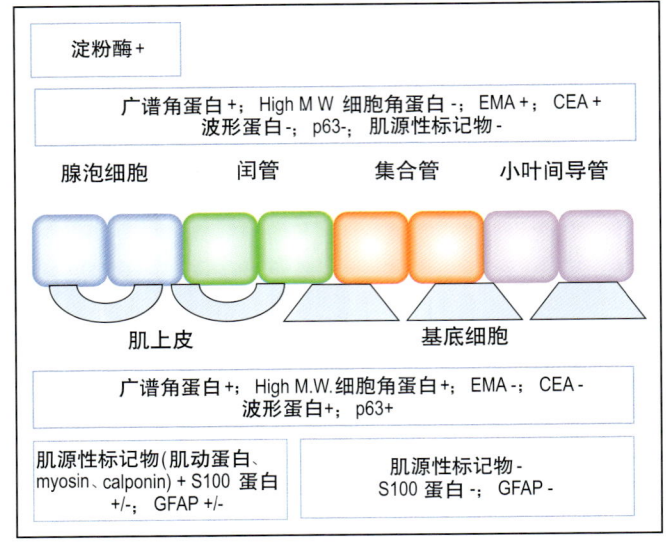

图7.2 构成浆液性分泌单位细胞类型的简图及其免疫表型谱。

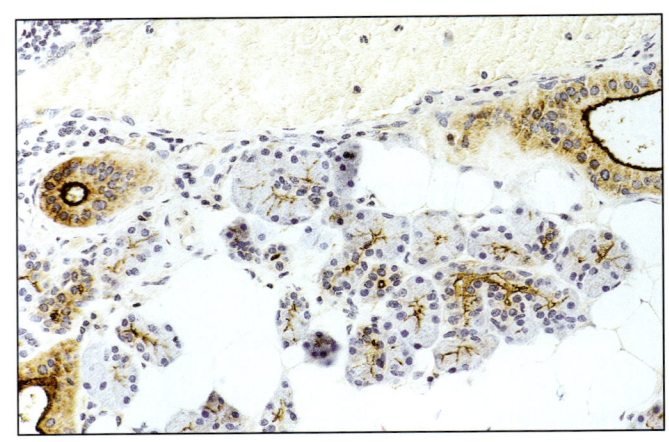

图7.3 正常腮腺上皮膜抗原（EMA）的免疫染色。分泌细胞的腔缘和导管明显阳性。

是一种双层结构，由腔面（腺泡和导管细胞）和腔外（肌上皮和基底细胞）两部分细胞组成。分泌性腺泡和闰管被肌上皮细胞包围（图7.2）。集合管和下游的导管单位内衬单层或假复层柱状上皮，在涎腺导管中逐渐转变成鳞状上皮，并且由基底细胞支持。

细胞形态学和免疫表型谱

浆液细胞呈锥体形，核位于基底部，含有大量富于酶原颗粒的嗜碱性胞浆，PAS染色阳性（抗淀粉酶），黏液卡红染色阴性。黏液细胞呈立方形或柱状，具有淡染的细小空泡状含涎黏蛋白的胞浆。它们PAS阳性（抗淀粉酶），而且黏液卡红也呈阳性反应。闰管的腔面细胞呈立方形，具有嗜酸性或两染性的胞浆，细胞核位于中心。集合管内衬柱状细胞，胞浆颗粒状（富于线粒体），由于细胞膜基底有突出的皱褶，核下出现垂直的条纹（图7.1）。通过细胞角蛋白（cytokeratin）、癌胚抗原（CEA）和上皮膜抗原（EMA）免疫染色，容易辨认腔面细胞（图7.2和图7.3）。正常涎腺细胞CD117/c-kit是阴性的，但有趣的是，在不同类型的涎腺肿瘤中腔缘（腺体）细胞常常阳性。

肌上皮细胞是生理上和功能上均已变异的上皮细胞，位于腔面细胞和基底膜之间。肌上皮细胞是伴有胞浆突起的包围腺泡的星形细胞，或为围绕闰管的梭形细胞。然而，在光镜下不易区分肌上皮细胞和基底细胞。超微结构检查显示，肌上皮细胞存在桥粒、中间丝、胞饮小泡和肌丝，具有上皮和平滑肌双重表型特征[6]。肌上皮细胞产生细胞外基质，例如基底膜物质和黏液样物质，这可能是各种涎腺肿瘤具有不同形态的原因。它们还可以通过促进上皮分化，分泌蛋白酶抑制剂和抑制血管生成而产生抗肿瘤浸润的作用[7]。最好通过p63、高分子量细胞角蛋白（包括CK 14）、钙调节蛋白（Calponin）、肌动蛋白（actin）和不同程度的GFAP免疫染色来显示肌上皮细胞（图7.2和图7.4）。

集合管、外分泌导管和涎腺导管的腔外细胞是基底细胞，在超微结构上，它们与肌上皮细胞的不同之处在于缺乏肌丝。它们保持多向分化的能力，且在再生和化生改变过程中起着重要作用[8]。基底细胞p63和高分子量细胞角蛋白免疫反应阳性（图7.2和7.4B），但肌样标记物阴性。

嗜酸细胞性细胞（oncocytic cells）的特征是由于线粒体的堆积而具有丰富的嗜酸性颗粒状胞浆，在50岁以前不常见，之后数量增加，直到70岁以后几乎普遍存在。在导管腺泡单位，正常细胞被嗜酸细胞不同程度地取代。嗜酸细胞化生已经参与了嗜酸细胞增生（oncocytic hyperplasia），结节性嗜酸细胞增生症（nodulaar oncocytosis），乃至嗜酸细胞瘤（oncocytoma）的发生[9]。

正常情况下，脂肪组织是腮腺的一种显著的部分，脂肪组织所占比例随着年龄的增加而增加。腮腺可能出现成群的皮脂腺，而且是涎腺皮脂腺肿瘤的正常对应成分（图7.5）。

涎腺肿瘤　Salivary gland neoplasms

一般特征

全世界涎腺肿瘤的年发生率为0.4～13.5例/每100 000人[10]。一般来说，涎腺肿瘤最常见于老年人，除了Warthin瘤和高级别的癌以外，女性比男性多见。

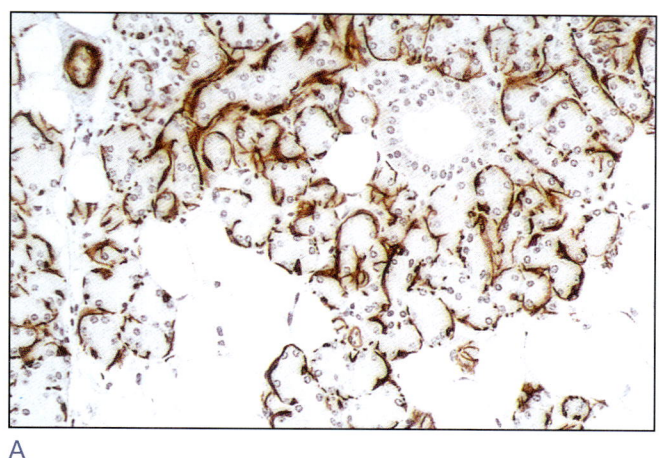
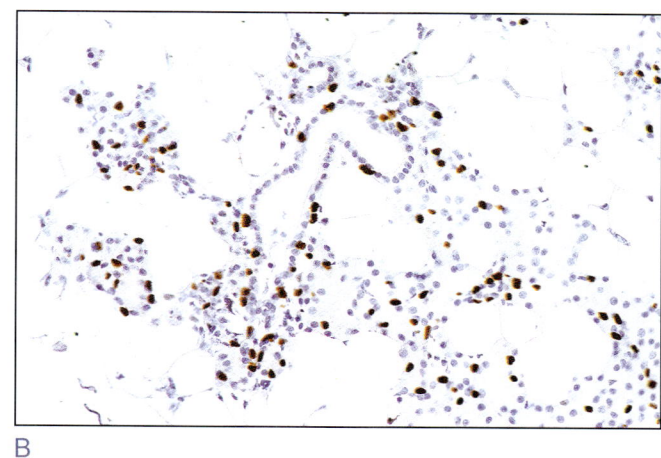

图7.4 正常涎腺肌上皮或基底细胞标记物的免疫染色。（A）肌上皮细胞（包被在腺泡和闰管周围的胞浆突起）表达钙调节蛋白，但集合管周围的基底细胞没有表达。（B）分泌导管单位周围的肌上皮细胞和基底细胞核均有p63表达。

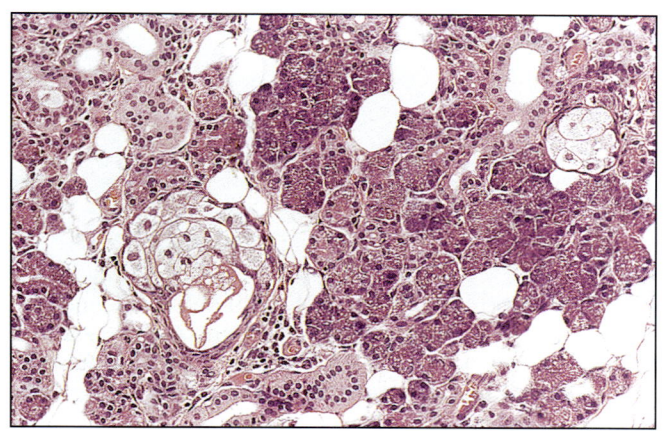

图7.5 正常腮腺。如果取材广泛，在浆液性腺泡和集合管中经常可以见到成团的皮脂腺细胞。注意腮腺中还有大量的脂肪细胞。

上皮性肿瘤占所有涎腺肿瘤的80%～90%，多数为良性肿瘤（75%），多形性腺瘤最常见（约占所有肿瘤的65%）（表7.1）。腮腺是发生涎腺肿瘤最常见的部位。某些类型的肿瘤或好发于大涎腺，或好发于小涎腺，因此，了解有关肿瘤的好发部位有助于诊断（表7.2）。

涎腺原发性癌少见，占所有癌症的0.3%不到。按照病例数目递减顺序，其发生部位是：腮腺、颌下腺、腭、颊和舌。然而，发生在磨牙后区（89.7%）、口底（88.2%）、舌（85.7%）和舌下腺（70.2%）的肿瘤，恶性的可能性最大[11]，但所有腮腺肿瘤大约只有20%为恶性。在涎腺癌中，按照递减顺序最常见的组织学类型依次为：黏液表皮样癌、腺样囊性癌、非特异性（not otherwise specified，NOS）腺癌和腺泡细胞癌，在小涎腺中，则是以多形性低级别腺癌（polymorphous low-grade adenocarcinoma，PLGA）取代非特异性腺癌[12,13]。

恶性肿瘤的发生年龄和良性肿瘤相似或略高于良性肿瘤。实际上，大多数的涎腺恶性肿瘤在临床上和良性肿瘤是不易区分的，除非肿瘤迅速增大、疼痛，固定于相邻的结构，形成溃疡或颈部淋巴结肿大。面神经麻痹是恶性肿瘤的一种较为一致的征象，常见于高级别的肿瘤，例如鳞状细胞癌和未分化癌，在少数情况下也可以发生于Warthin瘤和多形性腺瘤中[14]。

涎腺肿瘤一般罕见于儿童。在18岁以下的患者中，半数上皮性肿瘤是恶性的，其中低级别的黏液表皮样癌最常见[14-16]。在婴儿，间叶性肿瘤（血管瘤和淋巴管瘤）最常见，而且某些不常见的肿瘤，例如涎腺母细胞瘤（sialoblastoma）和涎腺始基瘤（salivary gland anlage tumor），几乎全部发生在这个年龄组。

涎腺癌的行为

某些涎腺癌在生物学上属于低级别（例如腺泡细胞癌，多形性低级别腺癌（PLGA），基底细胞腺癌，上皮-肌上皮癌，透明细胞癌，囊腺癌），而另外一些涎腺癌在生物学上则属于高级别（例如涎腺导管癌，多形性腺瘤中的癌的多数病例，未分化癌，嗜酸细胞癌），某些涎腺肿瘤（例如黏液表皮样癌，腺样囊性癌）具有一系列的生物学行为，取决于其分级。单个肿瘤类型的预后还受临床分期和肿瘤边缘状态的影响[12]。TNM分期列在表7.3中。

某些研究表明，增生指数（Ki-67指数）高、非整倍体DNA和p53蛋白表达与预后不良有关[17]。因为某些涎腺肿瘤具有非常漫长的临床经过，伴有晚期复发或转移，所以通常需要长期随访以确定是否真正治愈。图7.6中显示的3种主要类型涎腺癌的生存曲线是最有指示意义的[18]。在最初下降之后出现的曲线平高线表明，有相当比例的黏液表皮样癌患者能够治愈。

涎腺肿瘤

表7.1 涎腺上皮性肿瘤的组织学分类（修订自2005年WHO分类）

良性上皮性肿瘤	恶性上皮性肿瘤
多形性/单形性腺瘤家族 多形性腺瘤	**对应的恶性肿瘤** 多形性腺瘤中的癌 转移性多形性腺瘤 癌肉瘤
基底细胞腺瘤 肌上皮瘤	基底细胞腺癌 肌上皮癌
嗜酸细胞性肿瘤 Warthin瘤 嗜酸细胞肿瘤	**对应的恶性肿瘤** 发生在Warthin瘤的癌 嗜酸细胞癌
皮脂腺肿瘤 皮脂腺腺瘤 皮脂腺淋巴腺瘤	**对应的恶性肿瘤** 皮脂腺癌 皮脂腺淋巴腺癌
腺瘤伴有另外的间质成分 淋巴腺瘤 脂肪腺瘤（涎腺脂肪瘤） 腺纤维瘤	
导管乳头状瘤 内翻性导管乳头状瘤 导管内乳头状瘤 乳头状涎腺腺瘤	**对应的恶性肿瘤** 导管乳头状瘤恶性变
其他良性肿瘤 囊腺瘤 小管腺瘤 角化囊瘤 涎腺始基瘤 硬化性多囊性腺病	**对应的恶性肿瘤** 囊腺癌
	其他涎腺型癌 黏液表皮样癌 腺样囊性癌 腺泡细胞癌 多形性低级别腺癌 上皮-肌上皮癌 透明细胞癌（非特异性和玻璃样变变型） 涎腺导管癌 导管内癌 涎腺母细胞癌
	未分化癌 小细胞癌（Merkel型和肺型） 大细胞癌 淋巴上皮癌
	"非特异性"癌 非特异性腺癌 黏液性腺癌 印戒细胞腺癌 鳞状细胞癌

表7.2 支持大涎腺或小涎腺诊断的线索

完全或主要发生在大涎腺的肿瘤	完全或主要发生在小涎腺的肿瘤
• Warthin瘤 • 腺泡细胞癌 • 基底细胞腺瘤/腺癌 • 嗜酸细胞瘤/嗜酸细胞癌 • 上皮肌上皮癌 • 涎腺导管癌 • 淋巴上皮癌	• 小管腺瘤（唇，颊黏膜） • 多形性低级别腺癌（腭） • 囊腺瘤/囊腺癌（唇，颊黏膜） • 内翻性乳头状瘤（唇，颊黏膜） • 导管内乳头状瘤（唇，颊黏膜） • 乳头状涎腺腺瘤（腭）

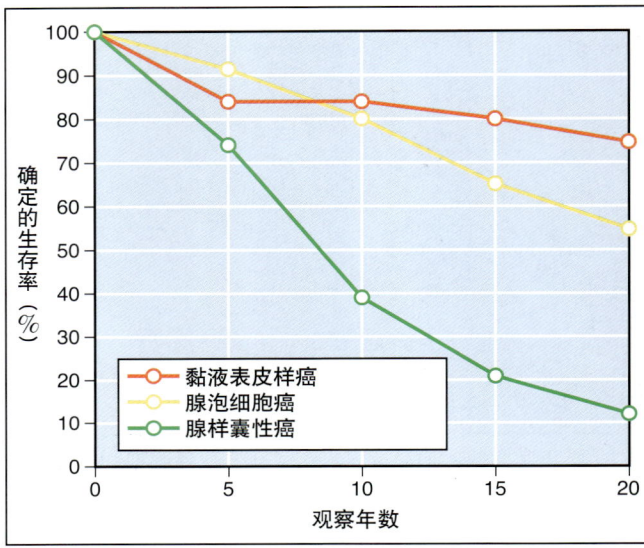

图7.6 涎腺黏液表皮样癌，腺泡细胞癌和腺样囊性癌患者的生存曲线。注意黏液表皮样癌生存曲线的平高线，以及腺样囊性癌不良的长期生存结果。（Adapted from Eneroth CM, Hamberger CA: Principles of treatment of different types of parotid tumors. Laryngoscope 84: 1732-40, 1974[18].）

腺泡细胞癌是一种惰性肿瘤，直到10年以后可能也不出现明显的不良事件。腺样囊性癌的短期生存是好的，但是长期结果却不乐观；也就是说，大部分患者最后死于肿瘤[13]。

诊断

由于涎腺肿瘤罕见，形态学范围广泛以及不同类型肿瘤的形态学有重叠，所以出现诊断难的问题并不少见。重要的是要了解每种类型肿瘤的基本细胞结构

表7.3　大涎腺肿瘤的TNM分期系统

原发性肿瘤（T）

- TX　原发性肿瘤不能评估
- T0　没有原发性肿瘤的证据
- T1　肿瘤最大径小于或等于2 cm，且没有实质外扩张*
- T2　肿瘤最大径大于2 cm但不超过4 cm，且没有实质外扩张*
- T3　肿瘤大于4 cm和（或）肿瘤有实质性扩张*
- T4a　肿瘤浸润皮肤、下颌骨、耳道和（或）面神经
- T4b　肿瘤浸润颅底和（或）翼状板，和（或）包围颈动脉

局部淋巴结（N）

- NX　局部淋巴结不能评估
- N0　没有局部淋巴结转移
- N1　单个同侧淋巴结转移，最大径小于或等于3 cm
- N2　单个同侧淋巴结转移，最大径大于3 cm但不超过6 cm，或多个同侧淋巴结转移，最大径均不大于6 cm，或双侧或对侧淋巴结转移，最大径均不大于6 cm。
- N2a　单个同侧淋巴结转移，最大径大于3 cm但不超过6 cm
- N2b　多个同侧淋巴结转移，最大径均不大于6 cm
- N2c　双侧或对侧淋巴结转移，最大径均不大于6 cm
- N3　淋巴结转移，最大径大于6 cm

远处转移（M）

- MX　远处转移不能评估
- M0　无远处转移
- M1　有远处转移

分期

分期	T	N	M
I期	T1	N0	M0
II期	T2	N0	M0
III期	T3	No	M0
	T1	N1	M0
	T2	N1	M0
	T3	N1	M0
IVA期	T4a	N0	M0
	T4a	N1	M0
	T1	N2	M0
	T2	N2	M0
	T3	N2	M0
	T4a	N2	M0
IVB期	T4b	任何N	M0
	任何T	N3	M0
IVC期	任何T	任何N	M1

*注意：实质外扩张是指临床或大体检查有侵犯软组织和神经的证据。为了分类的目的，仅有显微镜下证据不作为实质外扩张。

(Used with the permission of the American Joint Committee on Cancer (AJCC), Chicago, Illinois. The original source of the material is the AJCC Cancer Staging Manual, Sixth Edition (2002) published by Springer-Verlag New York, www.springeronline.com)

特征，尤其是肿瘤是否显示腺腔-腔外双重细胞分化（图7.7），以便通过分析细胞成分、细胞排列和细胞外成分，符合逻辑地作出诊断（见下文"诊断分析方法"一节）。

组织化学

组织化学研究对于涎腺肿瘤的诊断作用有限。虽然常常提到腺样囊性癌有黏液物质和基底膜物质染色，但是这种染色无助于腺样囊性癌的诊断。任何伴有腔面细胞分化的涎腺肿瘤的腔内都可能有上皮型黏液（PAS染色通常阳性，抗淀粉酶）。许多类型的肿瘤伴有基底膜样物质形成（PAS染色阳性，抗淀粉酶），尤其是那些显示肌上皮细胞或基底细胞分化的肿瘤。在许多类型的涎腺肿瘤中还可能发现不同量的酸性间质黏液（阿利新蓝染色阳性，但PAS阴性），例如多形性腺瘤和腺样囊性癌组织化学有限的应用包括：

1. PAS淀粉酶染色证实浆液细胞分化，有助于腺泡细胞癌的诊断。
2. 胞浆内存在黏液，有助于高级别黏液表皮样癌的诊断。低级别到中级别黏液表皮样癌的诊断常常不需要进行黏液染色，因为常规组织学切片常常有明显的黏液。
3. 在以基底细胞或肌上皮细胞为主的肿瘤中，PAS淀粉酶染色可能有助于发现局灶性腔面细胞分化，例如实性型的腺样囊性癌，或富于透明细胞的上皮-肌上皮癌。
4. 磷钨酸苏木素染色能够突现线粒体，有助于透明细胞亚型嗜酸细胞瘤的诊断。

		伴有内腔 - 腔外细胞双重分化的肿瘤
局限性	多形性腺瘤	增生的腔外细胞至少有局灶性与间质"融合";如果存在,软骨样基质和浆细胞样玻璃样细胞具有特征性
	基底细胞腺瘤	基底细胞样细胞为主;肿瘤岛和小梁与间质界限清楚;无软骨样基质或浆细胞样玻璃样细胞
	Warthin瘤	嗜酸细胞性内腔细胞和基底细胞;乳头状结构;突出的淋巴细胞间质
浸润性	腺样囊性癌	基底细胞样腔外细胞超过了内腔细胞;常见筛状结构;多数囊腔是内衬腔外细胞的假囊腔
	上皮 - 肌上皮癌	大而透明的腔外细胞;筛状结构非常罕见
	基底细胞腺癌	基底细胞样细胞为主;内腔细胞或腺体结构通常很少;肿瘤小叶经常显示拼图样结构

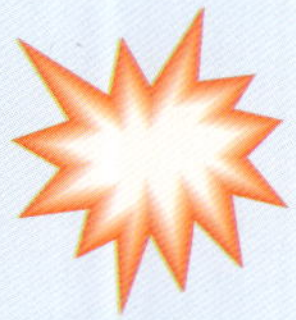

图7.7 图示有助于伴有腔面-腔外双重细胞分化的涎腺肿瘤鉴别诊断的一些特征。

免疫组织化学

目前,免疫组织化学染色在涎腺肿瘤的诊断中只能起到有限的作用。其主要应用是:

1. 确定结构复杂的肿瘤是否存在两种类型细胞的分化,但由于出现异常的免疫表型而结果可能令人失望。
2. 通过证实适当的免疫表型来确定肌上皮瘤/肌上皮癌的诊断。
3. Ki-67增生指数可以用于区分腺瘤和癌(Ki-67指数在腺瘤通常小于5%,而在癌通常大于10%)。

遗传学研究

遗传学研究已经发现,多形性腺瘤(染色体8q12和12q13-15重排),黏液表皮样癌(染色体11q21和19p13易位),腺样囊性癌(6q,8q和12q结构和分子改变)和涎腺导管癌(HER-2扩增)有几种经常发生的事件。应用微阵列基因表达谱研究还发现了能够区分良性涎腺组织和肿瘤的一些基因,并且证实多形性腺瘤、腺样囊性癌、黏液表皮样癌、透明细胞癌、腺泡细胞癌和涎腺导管癌具有不同的基因表达谱[19-23]。然而,目前尚未确立分子学研究在常规诊断中的作用。

杂交瘤　Hybrid tumor

少数涎腺肿瘤显示杂交瘤的特性。杂交瘤指的是在同一部位由两种或多种组织学不同的成分组成的肿瘤[24]。杂交癌最常见的成分是涎腺导管癌、上皮-肌上皮癌和腺样囊性癌[24-28]。其他的包括黏液表皮样癌、腺泡细胞癌、鳞状细胞癌、基底细胞腺癌和多形性低级别腺癌[24,26,29,30]。治疗最好根据具有较高级别恶性程度的组织学成分而定[28]。杂交腺瘤(hybrid adenomas)罕见,包括基底细胞腺瘤和小管腺瘤,Warthin瘤和皮脂腺腺瘤以及Warthin瘤和嗜酸细胞瘤的联合[24]。推测杂交瘤是起源于异向分化或两种类型肿瘤的碰撞。然而,至少文献中报道的某些杂交癌病例可以解释为去分化的病变(例如低级别癌和涎腺导管癌的联合)。

涎腺肿瘤的进展
Progression in salivary gland tumors

多数涎腺肿瘤为良性或低度恶性。因此,在长期存在的肿瘤中由于获得其他遗传学改变(例如p53突变和c-erbB2扩增)而发生生物学进展并不奇怪。肿瘤进展可以表现为恶性变,间质浸润,向高级别进展,过度生长和去分化(表7.4)。

上皮性肿瘤和瘤样病变
Epithelial tumors and tumor-like lesions

多形性腺瘤　Pleomorphic adenoma

定义

多形性腺瘤是一种良性肿瘤,由向上皮(腔面)和肌上皮(腔外)分化的细胞组成,伴有不同数量的特征性间质。细胞和间质成分的混合导致不同的形态学改变。上皮和间叶成分明显共同存在的情况产生了"混合瘤"(mixed tumor)这个同义词。现在

表7.4	涎腺肿瘤进展的不同模式	
现象	与组成成分的关系	例子
恶性变	良性肿瘤→恶性肿瘤	• 多形性腺瘤→多形性腺瘤中的癌 • 基底细胞腺瘤→癌（包括基底细胞腺癌） • 肌上皮瘤→肌上皮癌 • Warthin瘤→癌或淋巴瘤 • 嗜酸细胞瘤→嗜酸细胞癌
间质浸润	原位癌→浸润癌	• 导管内癌→涎腺导管癌 • 发生在多形性腺瘤中的原位癌→浸润性癌（包膜内，微小浸润和明显浸润的癌）
过度生长	伴有双重细胞分化的癌→伴有一种细胞分化的癌	• 上皮-肌上皮癌→肌上皮癌
高级别进展	同一类型肿瘤，低级别→高级别	• 腺样囊性癌（低级别→高级别） • 黏液表皮样癌（低级别→高级别）
去分化	癌→丧失原来细胞分化的高级别肿瘤	• 去分化腺泡细胞癌 • 去分化腺样囊性癌 • 去分化黏液表皮样癌 • 去分化上皮-肌上皮癌 • 去分化多形性低级别腺癌 • 去分化涎腺导管癌（肉瘤样变型）

普遍认为多形性腺瘤是一种伴有异向分化的纯粹的上皮性肿瘤，而不是上皮性肿瘤和间叶性肿瘤的混合。分子学分析也证明上皮和间叶成分均为单克隆来源[31]。

临床特征

多形性腺瘤女性比男性常见，且最常见于30～40岁到50～60岁个体，平均年龄为45岁。它通常表现为缓慢生长的无痛性肿物。当发生在小涎腺时，偶尔可见被覆黏膜溃疡形成或明显固定于周围组织。多形性腺瘤可能发生在不同的黏膜部位，例如鼻腔、支气管、皮肤（也叫软骨样汗腺腺瘤，chondroid syringoma）、乳腺和软组织[32-36]。

治疗可选择完整手术切除。完整切除后的5年和10年复发率分别是3.4%和6.3%[37]。单纯剜除肿瘤、在切除期间肿瘤破裂或散落、主要瘤体外出现突出物、丰富的软骨黏液样间质以及病人年轻都和复发率高有关[14,38-41]。在多数情况下，复发的肿瘤保持原来的组织学表现；然而，随着每一次复发，恶变的可能性会增加。与恶变危险性增加的相关因素是：高龄患者、长期的肿瘤、位于颌下、肿瘤较大、明显的玻璃样变区域以及至少有中等的核分裂活性[42]。

大体表现

肿瘤大小范围从几毫米到几厘米不等。肿瘤一般有薄的包膜，而且呈孤立性。口腔内的病例可能缺乏明确的包膜，尤其是发生在腭的肿瘤。切面可为橡皮样、鱼肉样、黏液的或有光泽，取决于肿瘤内间质的数量（图7.8）。在缺乏包膜的区域，肿瘤出芽可能直接进入邻近的涎腺组织[43]。复发性肿瘤一般表现为多结节状，散在分布于以前手术过的区域内（图7.9）。

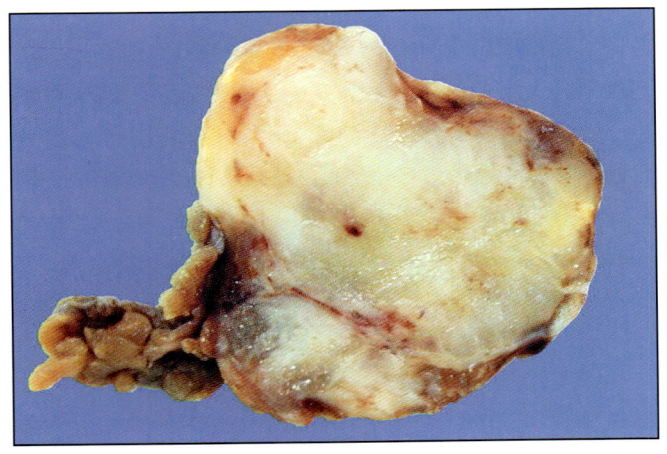

图7.8 多形性腺瘤大体标本。切面显示具有光泽的褐色实性肿瘤，有光泽可能与存在软骨黏液样基质有关。

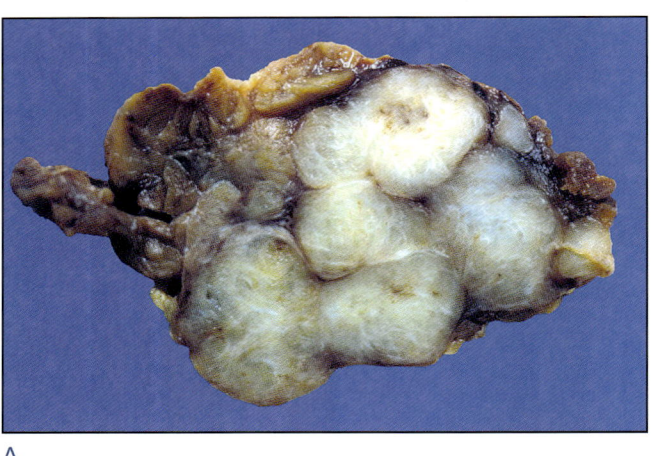
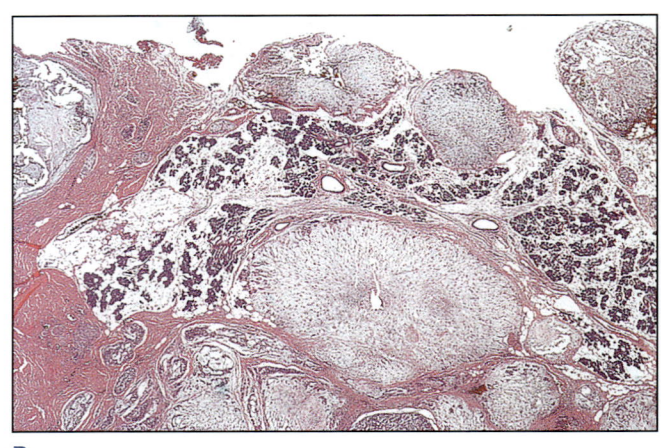

图7.9 腮腺复发性多形性腺瘤。注意典型的多结节状生长方式。如同本例一样，肿瘤呈黏液样非常常见。（A）大体标本。（B）相应的组织学特征。

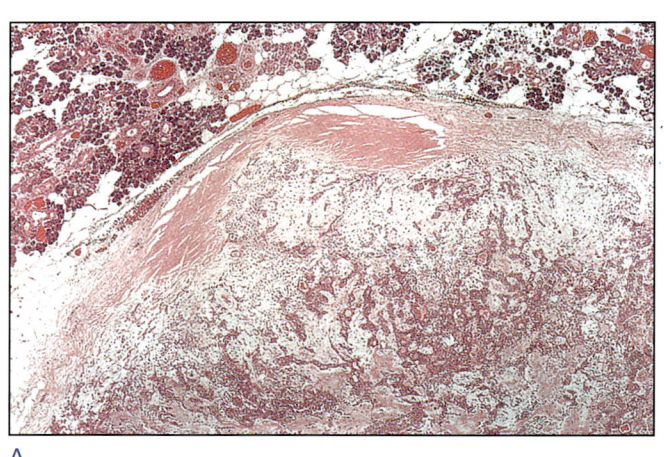
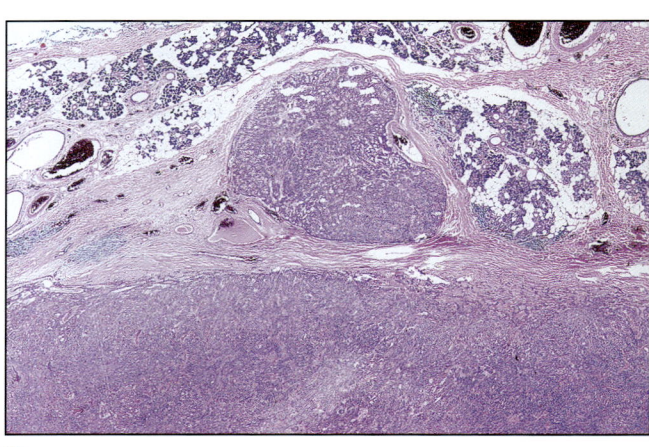

图7.10 多形性腺瘤低倍镜下所见。（A）肿瘤的特征是界限非常清楚。在这个放大倍数下可见明显的松散黏液样基质。（B）在肿瘤菲薄的包膜外有一个小的卫星结节。这是突出的肿瘤结节，在切片的这个平面上没有明显穿透包膜的部位。这种发现仍然符合良性多形性腺瘤的诊断。

显微镜下表现

生长方式：多形性腺瘤有薄的包膜包裹（图7.10A）。几个小而外形光滑的肿瘤芽（小的隆起物）可通过纤维性包膜向外突出。偶尔，肿瘤岛可能出现在包膜外，距离肿瘤主体有一小段距离（图7.10B），但是连续切片通常表明，这种卫星结节实际上与肿瘤主体连续，不应将其视为浸润。在极少数的情况下，多形性腺瘤可以完全生长在一个扩张的导管内。多形性腺瘤的特征是在同一个肿瘤的不同区域表现出高度可变的生长方式（图7.11）。

基本的细胞构成：原型的组织学表现是由位于软骨黏液样间质中的肌上皮套包被的管状结构组成的。肿瘤岛与间质之间的界限通常不甚清楚。肌上皮套呈离心性放射状排列，形成片块状、簇状、网格状结构，并有孤

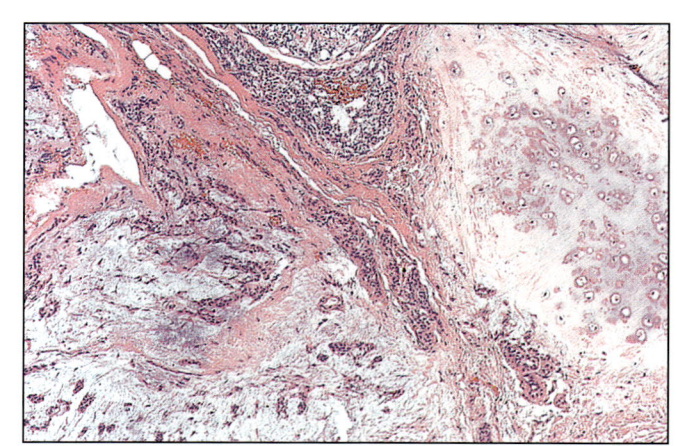

图7.11 多形性腺瘤。注意细胞构成、细胞排列和基质的量具有特征性的部位差异。视野右侧可见软骨样基质（透明软骨）。

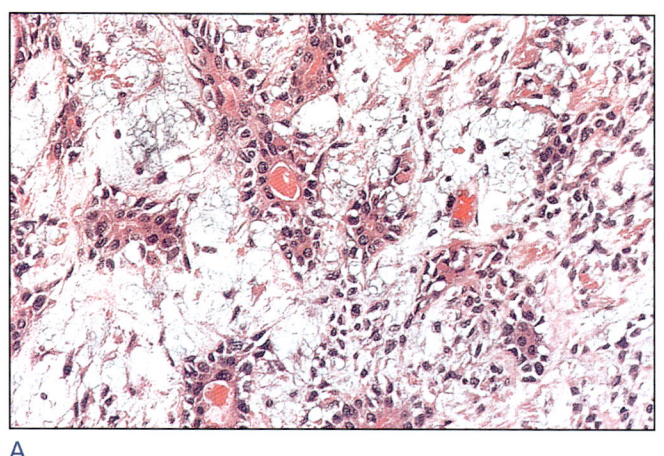 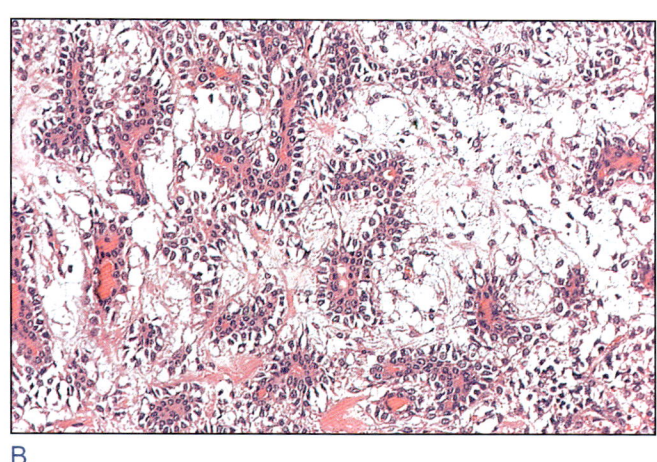

图7.12 多形性腺瘤，显示这种类型肿瘤的基本特征。小管内层内衬导管细胞，外层是不同厚度的变化了的肌上皮细胞。肌上皮细胞分散在黏液样基质中，以致难以确定单个小管的外形。在任何其他类型的涎腺肿瘤中见不到这种生长方式。（A）本例的小管腔内含有嗜酸性分泌物。（B）本例的肌上皮细胞与小管轴呈垂直排列，并且显示离心性分散分布于间质之中。

立的细胞出现，肌上皮似乎"融合"到由其产生的丰富的间质中（图7.12）。虽然这种"融合"现象具有特征性，但它可能是局灶性的，而且肿瘤的某些区域可能由位于间质中的小管或小梁组成（图7.13）。甚至可能出现类似于黏液表皮样癌或腺样囊性癌的灶状区域（图7.14），但是不应该诊断为多形性腺瘤中的癌，除非形成散在的膨胀性病变。

腔面细胞成分：腔面细胞成分形成相互吻合的小管、囊腔、带状和实性片块状结构（图7.15）。细胞可能是柱状、立方或扁平细胞。导管腔可能是空的或含有嗜酸性胶样物质，PAS阳性，抗淀粉酶，黏液卡红染色不同程度阳性（图7.12和图7.15）。在少数情况下，可能存在鳞状上皮、皮脂腺、嗜酸细胞或透明细胞等化生性改

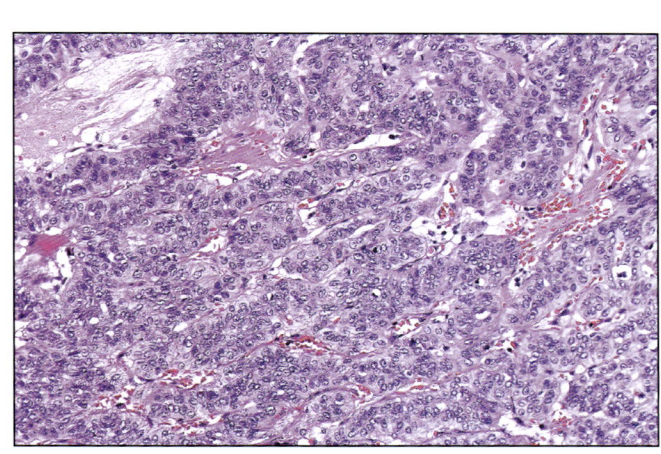

图7.13 富于细胞性多形性腺瘤。这种富于细胞的肿瘤显示明显的小梁状结构和少量的间质。

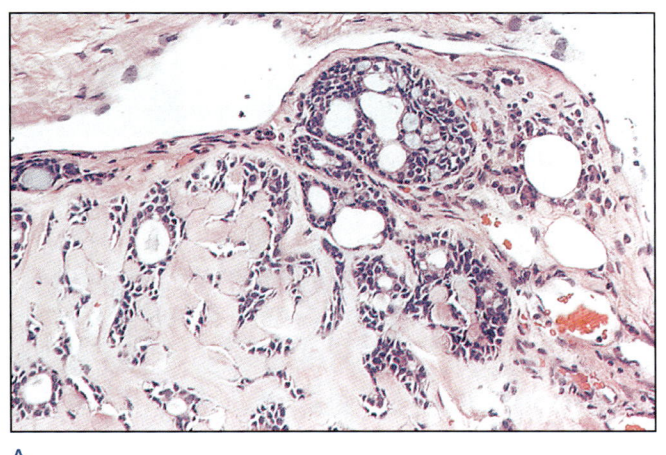 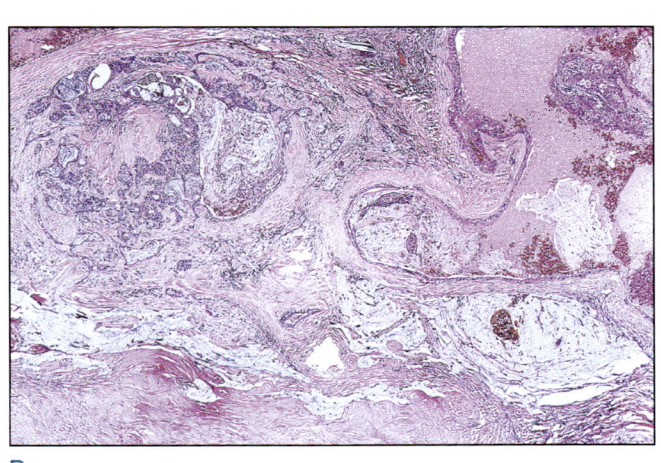

图7.14 伴有类似于腺样囊腺癌或黏液表皮样癌灶状区域的多形性腺瘤。（A）有一些筛状结构和小管，与间质界限分明，视野左侧显示间质广泛玻璃样变性。如果肿瘤为局限性，而且其他区域显示典型的细胞结构特征，上述特征依然符合多形性腺瘤的诊断。（B）出现充满黏液的腺体结构以及黏液外渗进入纤维性间质，导致肿瘤酷似低级别黏液表皮样癌。

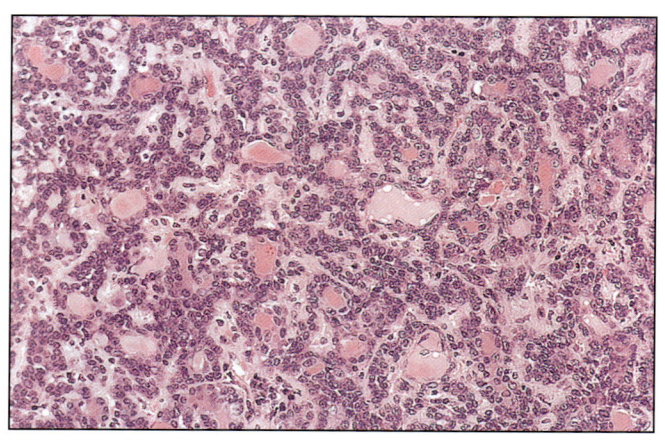

图7.15 富于细胞性多形性腺瘤。这种富于细胞和缺少间质的肿瘤是由相互吻合的小管构成的。虽然没有明显的"融合"结构,但其间质内含有散在的肥胖细胞。不过,这个视野与伴有肌上皮衍化而来的间质的基底细胞腺瘤不能区分。

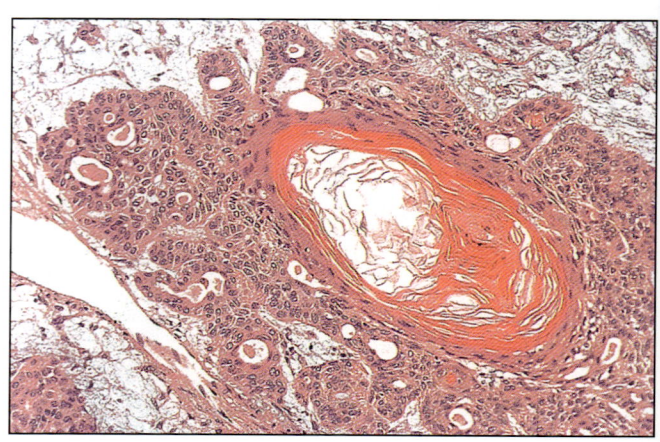

图7.17 多形性腺瘤。在复杂的腺体结构中可见伴有角化的灶状鳞状分化。在黏液表皮样癌中实际上从未见过这种明显程度的鳞状分化。

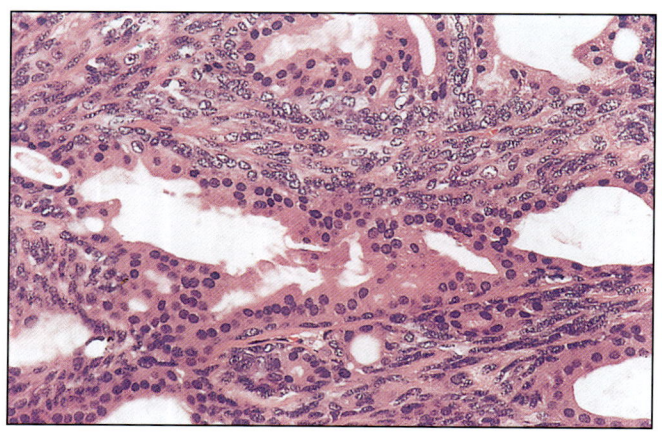

图7.16 多形性腺瘤。导管内层细胞显示嗜酸细胞改变。外层的多角形肌上皮细胞与成束的梭形细胞紧密混合。

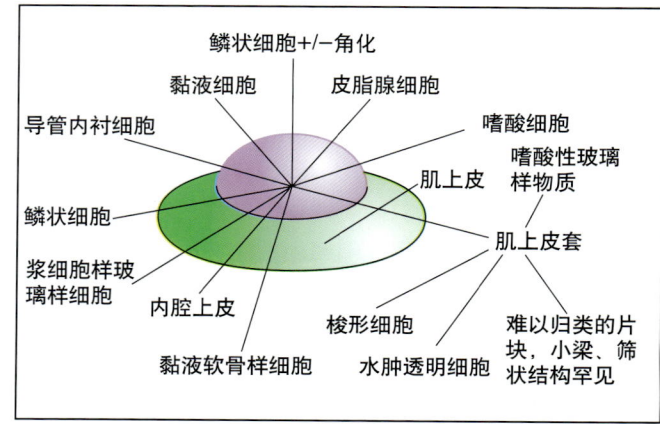

图7.18 多形性腺瘤(PA)多潜能的细胞分化。显示腔面导管细胞和腔外细胞(肌上皮细胞)可能的分化谱系和表现。

变(图7.16~图7.18)。在非常偶然的情况下,上皮可以形成杯状细胞或黏液细胞并且伴有鳞状上皮,可能导致黏液表皮样癌的错误诊断。

肌上皮成分:肌上皮细胞或变异的肌上皮细胞表现为立方形、梭形、星形的浆细胞样玻璃样细胞、难以归类的上皮样细胞和水肿透明细胞(图7.18)。梭形或立方形细胞环绕在导管的周围,排列成单层、厚套或放射冠状(图7.12,图7.16和图7.19)。它们可形成难以归类的片块状、小梁状甚至是筛状结构。

浆细胞样玻璃样细胞(plasmacytoid hyaline cells)是最独特的变异肌上皮细胞类型;这种细胞呈卵圆形,伴有同质性嗜酸性玻璃样胞浆(图7.20A)。细胞核圆形,偏心,致密的染色质倾向于集中在核的周缘。浆细胞样玻璃样细胞之所以这样命名是因为它们表面上类似于浆细胞,但是较大,粗块状染色质不明显,而且缺乏核周

Golgi带。它们通常排列成团或片块状,常常伴有疏松生长的灶状区域(图7.20)。由于浆细胞样玻璃样细胞的出现局限于多形性腺瘤和肌上皮瘤,所以辨认它们具有很大的诊断价值,尤其是在小的活检标本中。有一种过渡的类型,显示与其他类型的肌上皮细胞有相互重叠的特征。

星形或梭形肌上皮细胞单个出现或形成相互吻合的条带,漂浮在丰富的黏液样基质中(图7.21)。肌上皮细胞可以融入鳞状细胞巢或内衬充满角化物的囊性鳞状结构,提示具有向鳞状细胞系分化的能力,但并不常见。少数病例肿瘤以肌上皮细胞为主。在罕见的情况下,可以出现骨骼肌分化和散在的黑色素细胞,后者还赋予肿瘤一种色素沉着性的大体表现[44,45]。

间质:细胞外间质是多形性腺瘤明确的组成成分之一,间质可能稀少,也可能丰富。间质主要由变异的肌上皮细胞产生的酸性黏液物质组成,阿利新蓝(Alcian

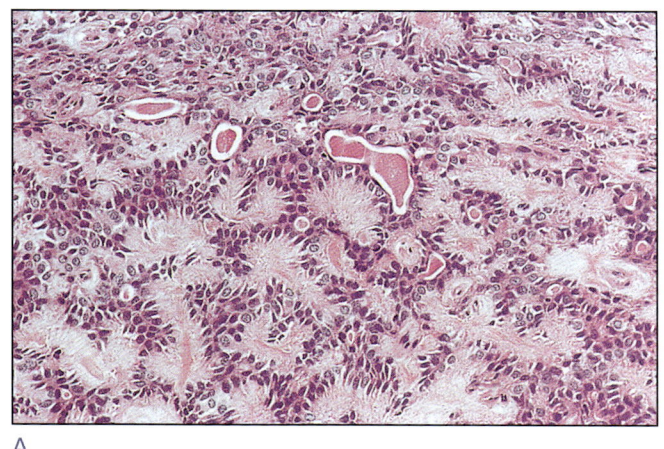
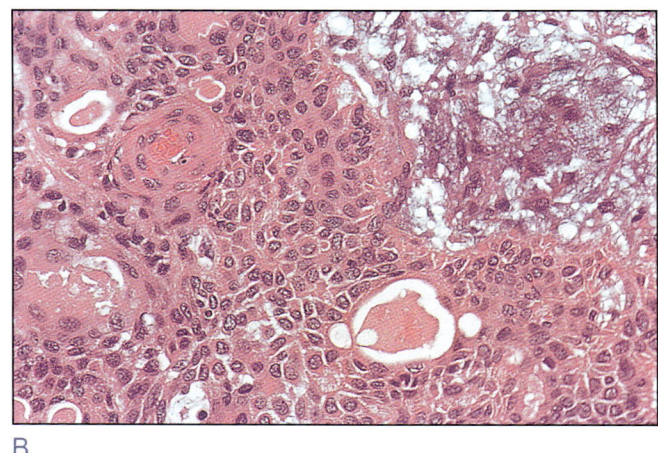

图7.19　多形性腺瘤。（A）相互吻合的小管被星形原纤维性胶原纤维分开。（B）导管广泛融合形成实性细胞片块，散在一些腺腔结构。这个视野可见许多多角形细胞，是变异的肌上皮细胞，在右上视野混入黏液样基质中。

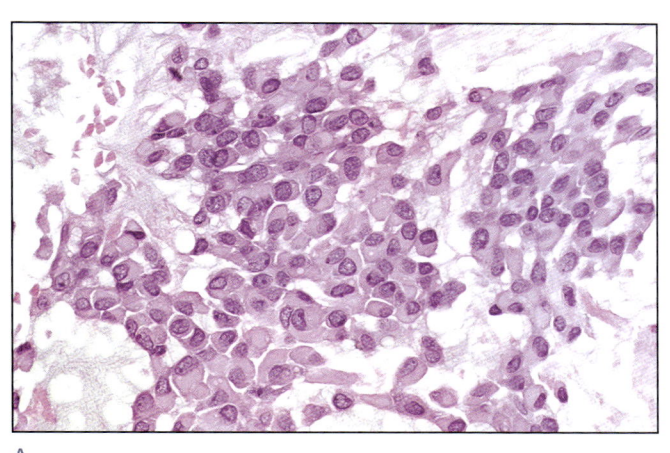
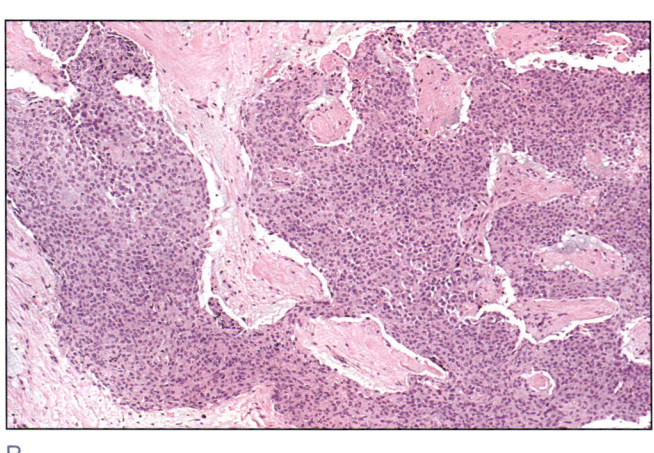

图7.20　富于浆细胞样玻璃样细胞的多形性腺瘤。（A）浆细胞样玻璃样细胞一般呈卵圆形，细胞核偏心，具有丰富的嗜酸性玻璃样胞浆。它们常常散在分布于黏液样间质中。（B）浆细胞样玻璃样细胞可以形成实性片块状结构。

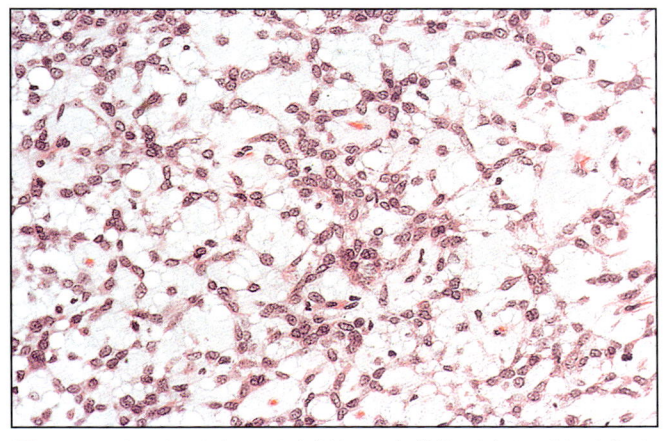

图7.21　多形性腺瘤。黏液样间质中的梭形和星形细胞倾向于排列成网格样结构。这些是变异的肌上皮细胞。肌上皮瘤可能显示类似的表现。

blue）染色阳性，而 PAS 染色不同程度阳性。间质表现为混合存在的软骨样（透明软骨）、黏液样、软骨黏液样和玻璃样物质，极少数为骨和脂肪组织（图7.11，图7.12和图7.21）[46]。有趣的是，除了皮肤部位以外，脂肪细胞分化并不常见[46a]。基质中可见孤立的或成群的星形、卵圆形或多角形细胞。在涎腺肿瘤中出现软骨黏液样间质几乎可以作出多形性腺瘤的诊断（图7.11）。在以软骨黏液样基质为主的肿瘤中，导管结构最有可能见于紧贴包膜下的周边区域。伴有非常稀少或没有细胞外间质的肿瘤经常被称为"富于细胞性多形性腺瘤"（cellular pleomorphic adenomas）（图7.13，图7.15和图7.22）；通过肌上皮套的局灶性"融合"可以辨认它们。有人提出，富于间质的肿瘤在手术过程中黏液样间质溢出的机会较高，肿瘤复发比较常见。另一方面，高度富于细胞的肿瘤可能比较容易恶变。

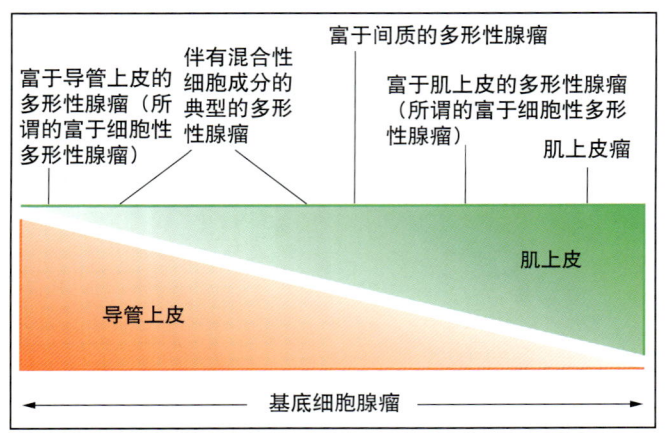

图7.22 多形性腺瘤—基底细胞腺瘤—肌上皮瘤家族的连续性。导管上皮和肌上皮细胞的相对比例以及与基质的相互作用决定肿瘤归入哪一种类型。

在上皮或肌上皮细胞中可能散在同质性的原纤维或放射状玻璃样物质（图7.14A和图7.19A）。在细胞或间质成分之间可能出现由胶原物质、酪氨酸和草酸盐组成的类晶体。黏液样间质中的酪氨酸结晶常常呈现"雏菊花头"结构。多数多形性腺瘤可有不同数量的弹力纤维，且在长期存在的病变中尤其丰富。弹力纤维染色呈现球状团块或不规则的带状结构，伴绒毛状的外形（图7.23）。这些粗大的弹力纤维有助于诊断，因为在其他涎腺肿瘤中并不常见。

细针吸取相关性改变：细针吸取常常导致出血和微小坏死，伴有不同的修复性改变（图7.24）。还可能发生完全性或不完全性梗死（图7.25）。可以有明显的肌

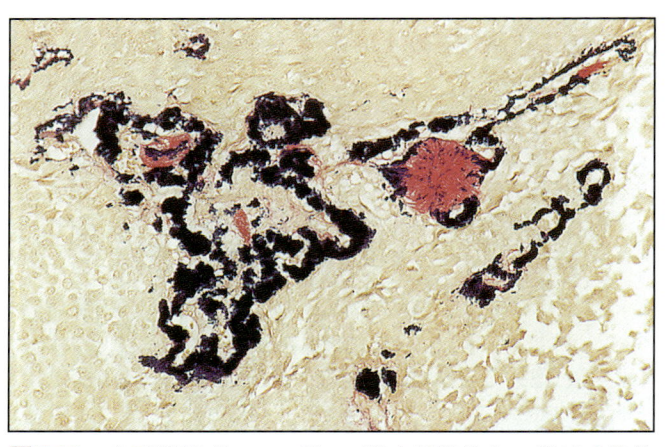

图7.23 多形性腺瘤，van Gieson弹力纤维染色。伴绒毛状外形的粗大弹力纤维是多形性腺瘤的特征，而且很少见于其他类型的涎腺肿瘤。

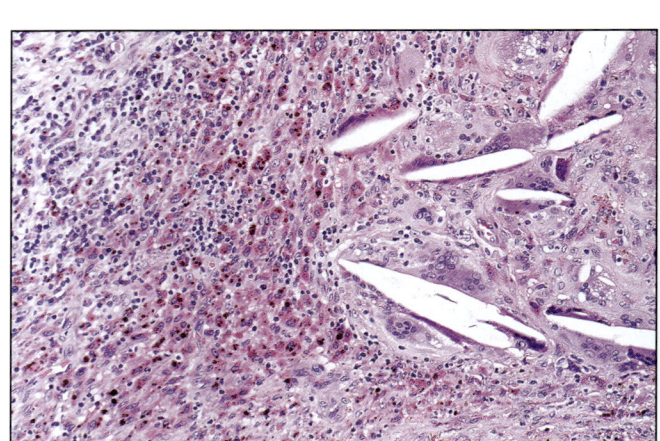

图7.24 多形性腺瘤，细针吸取活检后的变化。组织损伤的反应表现为慢性炎症细胞浸润，噬铁细胞集聚和胆固醇结晶引起的异物巨细胞反应。

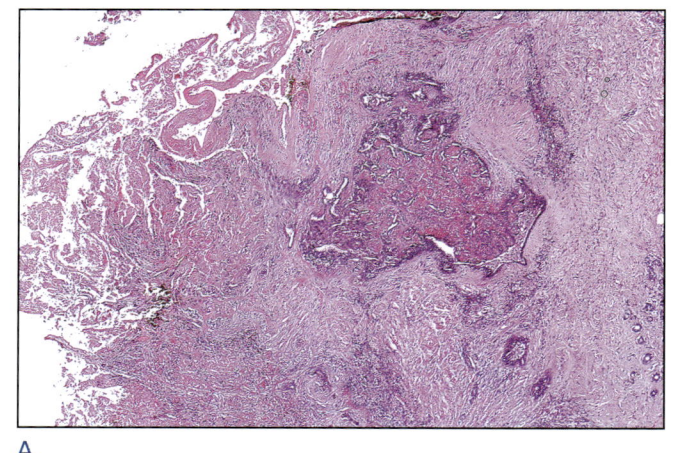

A

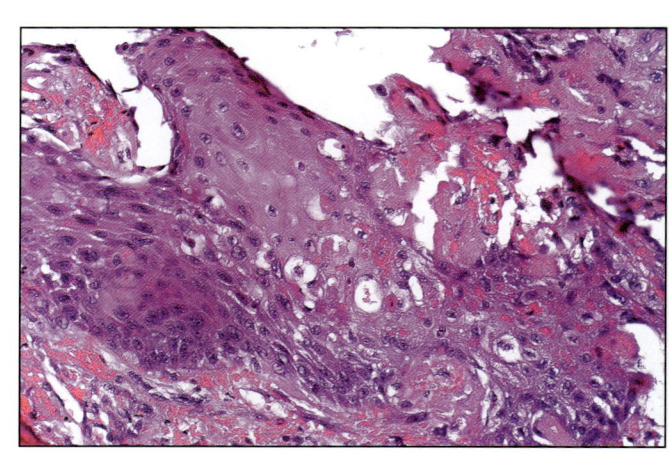

B

图7.25 多形性腺瘤，细针吸取后引起的梗死。（A）这个肿瘤几乎全部梗死。（B）存活的肿瘤细胞岛常常显示鳞状化生，伴有不同程度核的非典型性，酷似鳞状细胞癌或黏液表皮样腺癌。

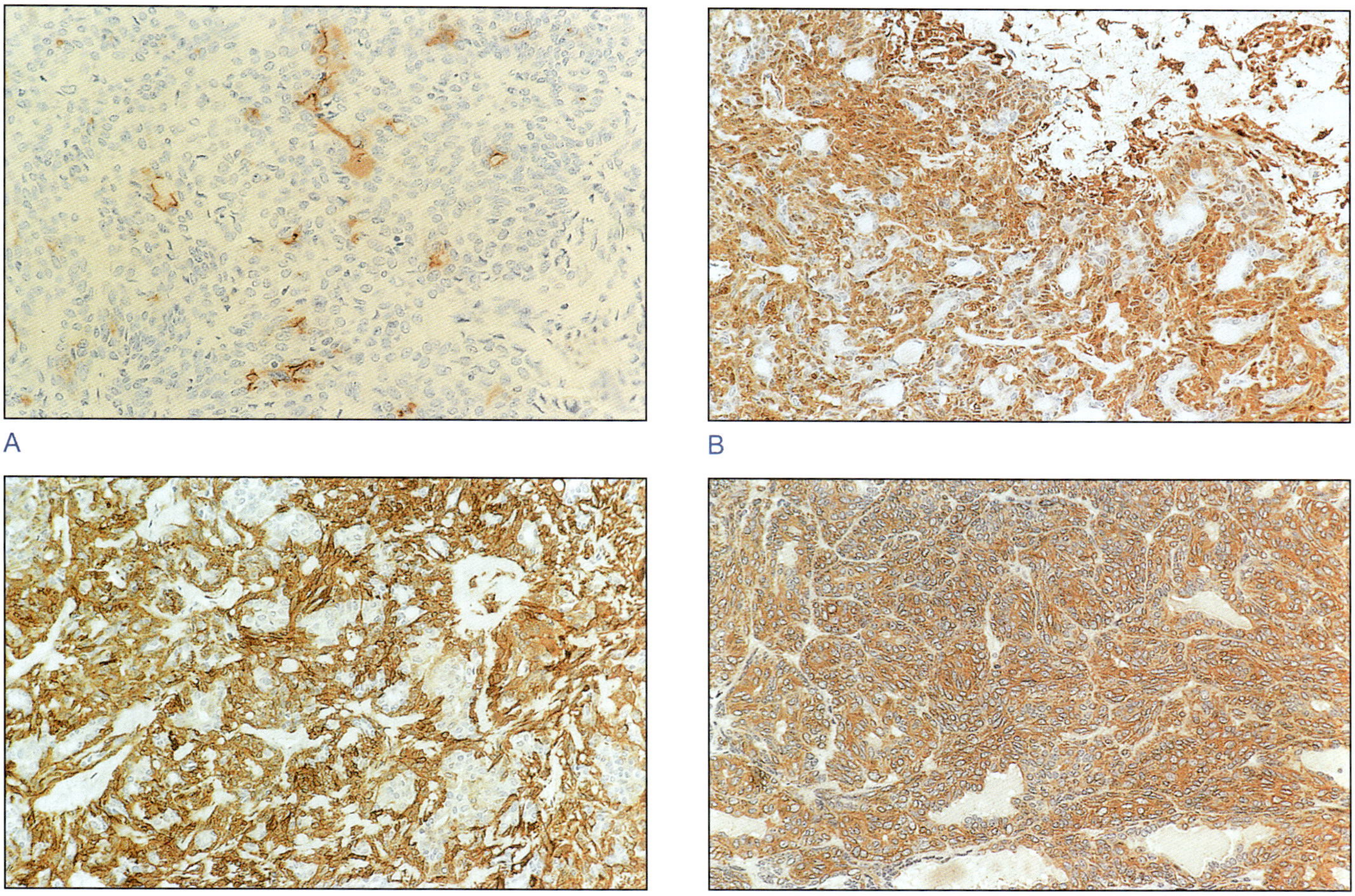

图7.26 多形性腺瘤免疫组织化学谱。（A）上皮膜抗原染色显示导管腔。（B）S-100蛋白染色常常显示腔外细胞以及位于基质内的细胞。本例导管细胞阴性，但在某些病例可呈不同程度的阳性。（C）钙调节蛋白染色显示肌上皮细胞和变异的肌上皮细胞。在某些病例中染色可能呈片块状。（D）本例细胞角蛋白14染色弥漫阳性。矛盾的是，与正常导管上皮阴性染色不同，该肿瘤的导管细胞染色较强。

上皮反应性增生，增生的肌上皮可能突入到纤维性包膜中，或在静脉内皮下呈现结节状出芽。非典型性鳞状化生也很常见（图7.25B）[47]。

免疫组织化学

免疫组织化学的主要应用是在不能确定诊断的时候，证实腺体成分和肌上皮成分共同存在。通过EMA、CEA和c-kit染色可以显示不明显的腺状成分（图7.26）。肌上皮和变异的肌上皮细胞细胞角蛋白染色阳性，但EMA和CEA阴性。虽然CK14和各种肌样标记物（例如肌动蛋白和肌浆球蛋白）可以清楚地标记正常肌上皮，但在肿瘤中的染色形态却是混乱的：肿瘤肌上皮的染色可呈片块状或完全阴性，而腔面细胞的染色则可能呈强阳性（图7.26D）。肌上皮成分S-100蛋白和GFAP常常阳性，但S-100免疫反应可以不同程度地见于腔面细胞（图7.26）。目前，肿瘤性肌上皮成分最可信的标记物是p63和钙调节蛋白（Calponin）（图7.27）[48]。

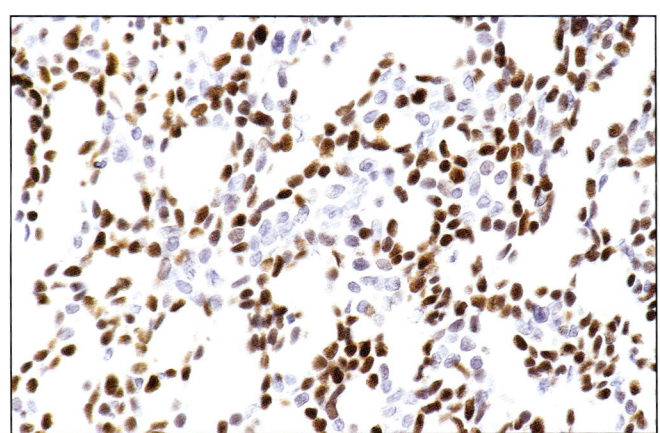

图7.27 多形性腺瘤p63的免疫染色。变异的肌上皮细胞（腔外细胞）明显阳性，而腔面细胞阴性。

多形性腺瘤Ki-67增生指数低（平均1.6%），p53蛋白免疫反应罕见（阳性细胞平均为1.2%）；BCL-2染色弱阳性。这些参数有助于与腺样囊性癌的鉴别，因为后者平均 Ki-67 指数为 20.5% ~ 54%，取决于肿瘤的分级，p53 蛋白阳性细胞平均为 4.3% ~ 24%，而且 BCL-2 染色呈强阳性[49,50]。

遗传学特征

细胞遗传学研究证实大约 70% 的多形性腺瘤有异常的发现，表现为以下 3 种模式之一[51]：

1. 8q12 重排（39%），例如 t (3;8) (p21;q12), t (5;8) (p13;q12) 或
2. 12q13-15 重排（8%），例如 t (9;12) (p24; q14-15)，ins (9;12) (p24;q12q15) 或
3. 偶尔发生的不涉及 8q21 或 12q13-15 的克隆性改变（23%）[52]。

在染色体 8q 和 12q 上的靶基因分别是 *PLAG1* 和 *HMGA2*（以前称作 *HMGIC*），这些靶基因编码转录因子[53,54]。推测易位导致的这些基因的过表达在发病机制上起着重要作用。在涎腺肿瘤中，因为仅有多形性腺瘤发现 *PLAG1* 或 *HMGA2* 基因易位，所以通过反转录聚合酶链反应（RT-PCR）或荧光原位杂交（FISH）发现这些基因易位有助于这种类型肿瘤的诊断。

主要的鉴别诊断（见"诊断分析方法"一节，第310页）

1. 单形性腺瘤，例如基底细胞腺瘤，肌上皮瘤
2. 腺样囊性癌
3. 多形性低级别腺癌
4. 上皮-肌上皮癌
5. 黏液表皮样癌
6. 各种间叶性细胞瘤，例如神经鞘肿瘤，平滑肌肿瘤

转移性多形性腺瘤
Metastasizing pleomorphic adenoma

转移性多形性腺瘤是多形性腺瘤的一种罕见的并发症。一般来说，转移发生在一个相对长的时期后（从 1.5 年到 51 年，平均 16.3 年），且可能同时或随后发生局部复发。在少数情况下，转移性肿瘤可能是涎腺隐匿性多形性腺瘤的最初表现[55]。

转移性肿瘤的特征是保留了多形性腺瘤的良性组织学特征。回顾性分析和流式细胞检查均未发现任何可以预示转移的特征[56]。最常见的转移部位是骨（50%）、肺（30%）和淋巴结（30%）；头皮、腹壁和肝转移也有报告[57]。尽管转移性病变在组织学上呈良性表现，但多达 37% 的患者死于本病。在免疫受损的宿主，本病具有更迅速的侵袭性经过[58]。转移性多形性腺瘤恶变的病例也有报告[59]。

除一个病例之外[55]，多数转移性多形性腺瘤均有一次或多次手术的历史。故发生转移的可能机制是血管浸润继发机械性种植[60]。治疗可选择局部切除原发性和转移性肿瘤。

多形性腺瘤中的癌
Carcinoma ex pleomorphic adenoma

定义

多形性腺瘤中的癌是先前存在的多形性腺瘤的恶变，通常发生在长期存在的多形性腺瘤或有肿瘤多次复发的情况下。不同的研究系列显示其发生率从 1.9% 到 23.3% 不等（平均 6.2%）[42]。恶变的危险性随着肿瘤持续时间的延长而增加，肿瘤出现不到 5 年恶变的发生率是 1.6%，而肿瘤出现超过 15 年恶变的发生率增加 9.5%[61]。恶变可能逐步发生（图 7.28），表现为[62]：

1. 原位癌（carcinoma in situ）：在最早阶段，癌细胞取代导管腔面细胞，而保留完整的肿瘤性但无非典型性的肌上皮层（图 7.29）。
2. 包膜内癌（intracapsular carcinoma）：癌进一步发展，出现间质浸润，但是没有侵犯原本多形性腺瘤的纤维性包膜（图 7.30）[63,64]。
3. 浸润癌（invasive carcinoma）：随后发生包膜外浸润（图 7.31）。

临床特征

长期存在的肿瘤大小变化不明显，而后迅速生长预示有恶变。恶性的征象还包括与周围组织固定，溃疡形成，面神经麻痹和局部淋巴结肿大。出现恶变的平均年龄是 61 岁，大约比多形性腺瘤大 10 岁[63,65]。多数患者处于疾病的 III/IV 期（65%）。大部分患者出现复发和转移，总的 5 年生存率仅为 30%[63]。

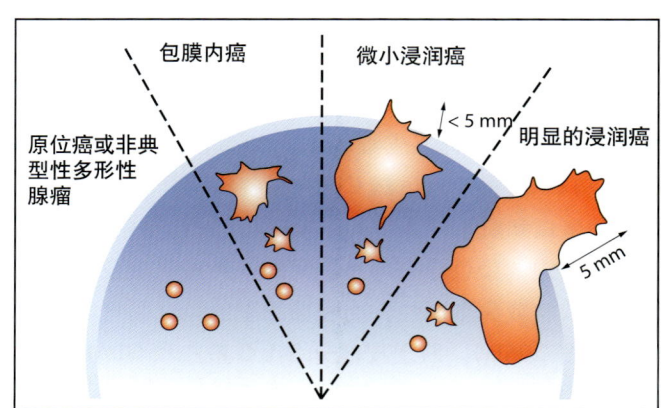

图7.28 图解显示多形性腺瘤中的癌的命名和演变步骤。深蓝色，多形性腺瘤；浅蓝色，纤维性包膜；红色，癌。

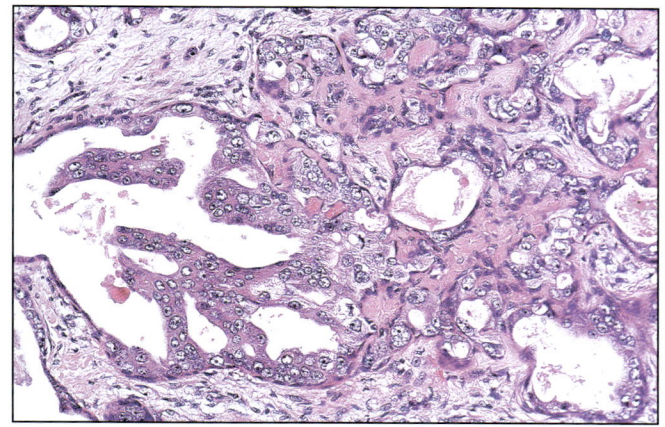

图7.29 多形性腺瘤中的原位癌。视野右侧可见先前存在的多形性腺瘤。视野左侧多形性腺瘤融合到原位癌中，表现为大的非典型性顶浆分泌样细胞取代了腔面细胞。其他部位，癌细胞穿破肌上皮层并侵入间质（没有显示）。

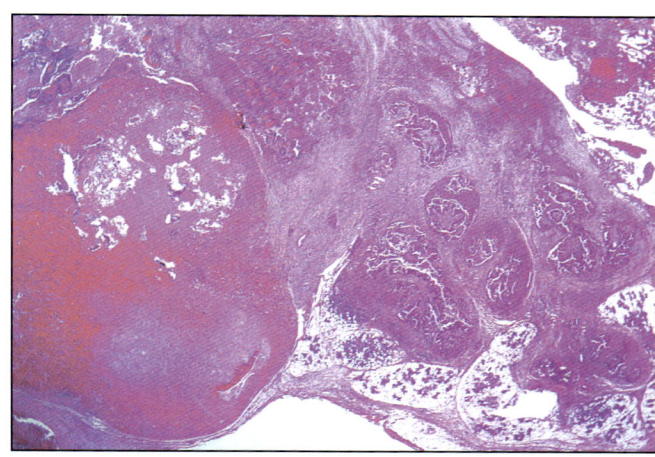

图7.31 多形性腺瘤中的明显的浸润癌。视野左侧的局限性结节是原有的多形性腺瘤。并发的癌浸润到原有的肿瘤以外，进入周围的腮腺实质。在这个病例中，浸润的肿瘤距离原有肿瘤8 mm。

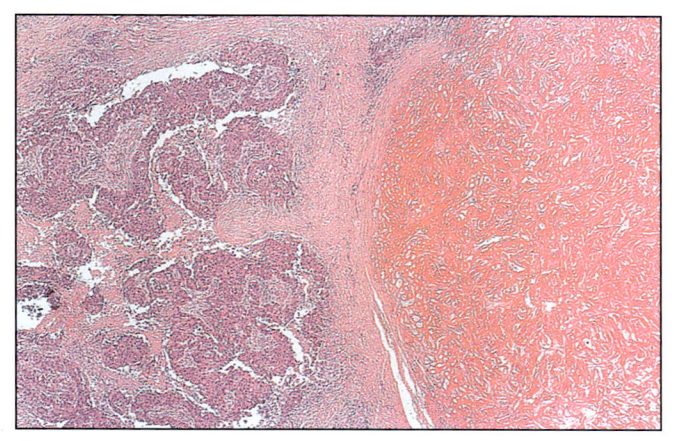

A

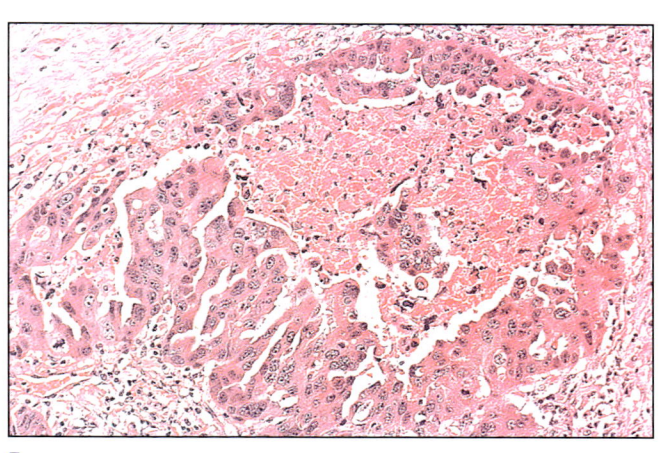

B

图7.30 多形性腺瘤中的包膜内癌。（A）视野右侧显示原有的多形性腺瘤，伴有广泛沉积的粗大弹力纤维。视野左侧显示并发的癌伴有坏死。（B）这种癌是一种高级别的浸润性腺癌，已经浸润到了原有的多形性腺瘤的间质。

病理学

肿瘤通常比其相应的良性肿瘤要大。多数病例有明显的浸润；坏死或出血区域常见。组织学上，恶性成分的特征是广泛而显著的细胞多形性，高核分裂计数，非典型性核分裂象，凝固性坏死以及在原有的腺瘤内出现膨胀性或浸润性结节（图7.30和图7.31）。

在多数情况下，肿瘤以恶性成分为主，且最常见的是高级别癌（85%的病例），例如非特异性腺癌或涎腺导管癌（图7.30B），但有时可能是腺鳞癌、未分化癌或肉瘤样癌。低级别的癌，例如多形性低级别腺癌、腺样囊性癌、黏液表皮样癌、上皮-肌上皮癌和肌上皮癌也偶有发生（图7.32）[62,63,65]。可能出现介于恶性和良性成

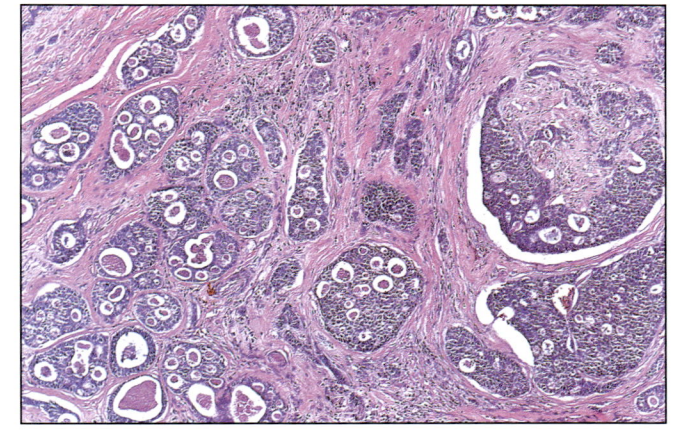

图7.32 多形性腺瘤中的癌。这个并发的浸润癌显示非常类似于腺样囊性癌的细胞结构特征。

分之间形态学特征的移行带。

残余的多形性腺瘤通常难以发现，且其可能表现为细胞减少或显著的玻璃样变。残余的多形性腺瘤存在的线索是：
1. 在癌中或癌的附近出现玻璃样变或钙化的结节
2. 结节中有S-100蛋白或肌动蛋白阳性的梭形细胞
3. 粗大的绒毛状弹力纤维（最好通过弹力纤维染色显示）
4. 复发性多形性腺瘤的临床病史或长期存在的肿块[63]

因此，当一个涎腺癌不易归类为一种公认的肿瘤时，应该认真考虑到多形性腺瘤中的癌的可能性。

预后

最重要的预后因素是包膜外浸润的范围。除了一例个案报告有颈淋巴结转移以外[66]，原位癌和包膜内癌没有转移的潜能[63,64]。几项大的系列研究发现，包膜外浸润分别小于 8 mm[67]、5 mm[63] 或 1.5 mm[68] 的肿瘤有极好的预后。换句话说，确定伴有最小转移潜能的多形性腺瘤中的癌的理想切点目前还未确立，而这些不同的发现可能反映出难以进行可重复性的测量。另外发现预后不良和以下因素有关：(1)恶性成分的组织学分级高（5 年生存率为 30%，而组织学分级低的 5 年生存率为 96%）；(2)病理学分期高；(3)癌的比例超过了肿瘤的 50%[63,67]。

遗传学研究

多形性腺瘤中的癌经常出现染色体 8q21 和 12q13-15 的变化或重排，类似于相应的良性肿瘤。另外，染色体 12q13-15 上的基因，包括 *CDK4*、*HMGIC* 和 *MDM2* 的扩增和过表达可能是恶变的重要遗传事件[69]。c-erbB2 过表达或基因扩增发生在 21% ~ 82% 的病例中[63,64,70-72]。有人提出，c-erbB2 染色可能有助于多形性腺瘤中的癌和非典型性多形性腺瘤的鉴别诊断[64]。*p53* 基因改变见于 29% ~ 67% 的病例，而 p53 蛋白过表达见于 41% ~ 75% 的病例，提示 p53 在转化中可能具有作用[63,73-76]。与原有的多形性腺瘤相比，Ki-67 增生指数增加（平均 35%）[64]。

非典型性多形性腺瘤
Atypical pleomorphic adenoma

包膜受累和血管瘤栓在良性多形性腺瘤中是可能出现的特征[77,78]。在看上去温和的细胞背景中出现孤立的增大的或多形性的细胞核也可以被忽略，因为它们不代表预后更差（图 7.33）。然而，少数肿瘤可能出现非典型性特征，例如核的弥漫性轻度非典型性和偶尔出现核分裂象，但没有凝固性肿瘤坏死或形成膨胀

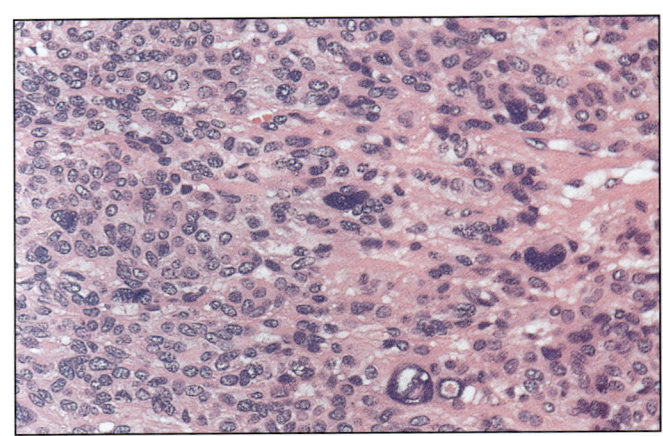

图 7.33 多形性腺瘤。在温和表现的细胞中偶尔出现增大深染甚至奇异的细胞核并不代表有较侵袭性的行为，尤其是当不伴有核分裂象时。

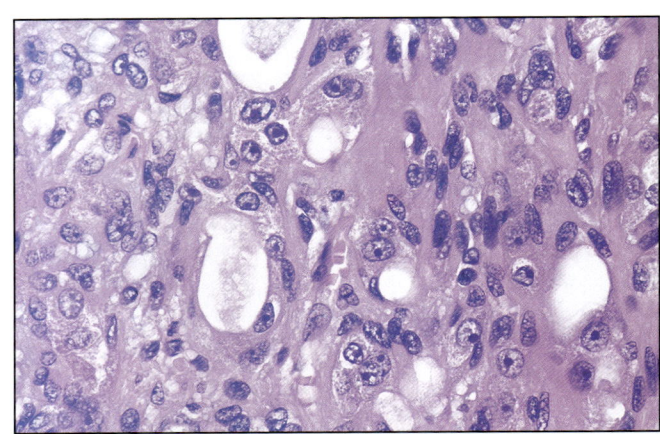

图 7.34 非典型性多形性腺瘤。这种肿瘤令人担忧，因为普遍存在核的非典型性，包括突出的核仁。然而，由于核分裂象罕见且没有浸润性生长，诊断为"非典型性多形性腺瘤"是恰当的。

的肿块（图 7.34）。在这种情况下，命名为"非典型性多形性腺瘤"可能是恰当的。这种保守的称谓是合理的，因为即使已经有了癌变，只要没有包膜外浸润，预后还是非常好的。

癌肉瘤　Carcinosarcoma

癌肉瘤，或真正的恶性混合瘤是非常罕见的[79]。平均发病年龄是 62 岁，且没有性别差异。肿瘤最常累及大涎腺。在三分之一的病例中，临床和组织学上有多形性腺瘤共存的证据[80]。组织学上，肿瘤由明显恶性的上皮和间叶成分组成。最常见的上皮成分是鳞状细胞癌或腺癌，而最常见的恶性间叶性成分是软骨肉瘤，其次是纤维肉瘤、平滑肌肉瘤、骨肉瘤、脂肪肉瘤和横纹肌肉

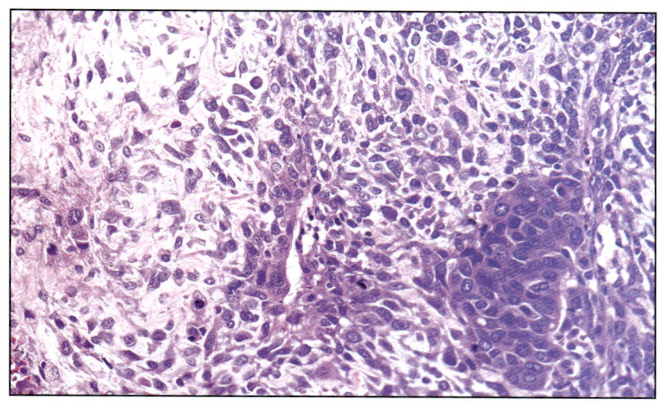

图7.35 癌肉瘤。癌的成分由黏着的多角形细胞组成（右下视野），而肉瘤成分由疏松散在的梭形到星形细胞组成。

瘤（图7.35）[80,81]。它是一种侵袭性的肿瘤，平均生存时间仅为29.3个月[81]。

基底细胞腺瘤　Basal cell adenoma

定义

基底细胞腺瘤是一种由基底细胞样细胞组成的良性肿瘤，通过基底膜样物质与间质截然分开。它通常表现为单一的实性、小梁状、管状或膜状生长方式。根据定义，其缺乏软骨黏液样间质。

临床特征

基底细胞腺瘤一般表现为孤立性，缓慢生长的无症状肿块。发病的年龄高峰是50～60岁和60～70岁之间，且女性多发。大约70%的基底细胞腺瘤发生在腮腺，10%～20%发生在上唇。

膜性基底细胞腺瘤（membranous basal cell adenoma）又称类皮肤肿瘤（dermal analogue tumor），是一种独特的亚型，可能伴有皮肤附件肿瘤。没有性别差异。

治疗选择手术切除。复发罕见，膜性基底细胞腺瘤是个例外，由于其为多灶性而有25%的复发率[82]，其他的基底细胞腺瘤均很少复发。在少数情况下，基底细胞腺瘤可能发生恶变（单形性腺瘤中的癌，4%），成为基底细胞腺癌、腺样囊性癌、涎腺导管癌或非特异性腺癌[83,84]。膜性亚型的恶变率更高一些，可达28%[82]。

病理学特征

基底细胞腺瘤是非常局限的肿瘤，伴有或没有纤维性包膜。切面均匀一致，颜色从淡褐色到棕色不等。缺乏多形性腺瘤特征性的软骨样或黏液样表现。膜性基底细胞腺瘤通常为多灶性（50%的病例）和多结节性。

组织学上，小的基底细胞样细胞具有圆形均匀一致的嗜碱性细胞核和少量胞浆（图7.36）。见不到细胞核的多形性和核分裂象。有时可以辨别出两种基底细胞样细胞，暗细胞和亮细胞。某些内衬伴有大量嗜酸性胞浆细胞的导管结构经常散布在基底细胞样细胞之中（图7.36B）。肿瘤通常以一种类型的结构为主（下文详述），但是有时也能见到混合性结构。

实性型：基底细胞样细胞形成宽带状、外形光滑的拼图样细胞岛和实性团块，周围细胞呈栅栏状排列，这种结构可能非常突出，以致类似于成釉细胞瘤（图7.36A）。基底细胞样细胞通过基底膜与疏松的常常是高度富于血管的间质截然分开。这种特征与多形性腺瘤的离心性或"融合性"生长方式形成对比。

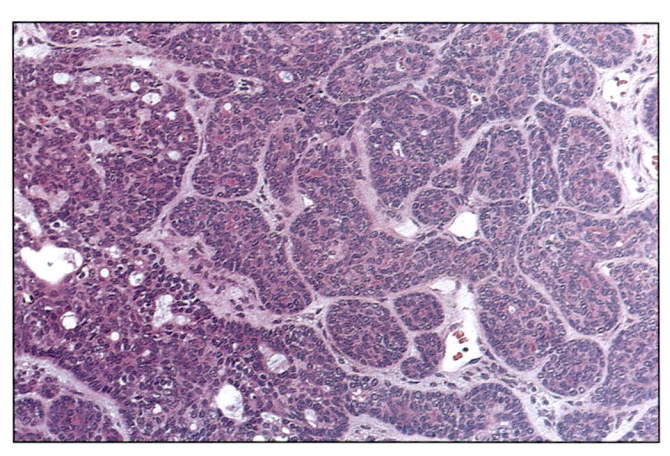

A

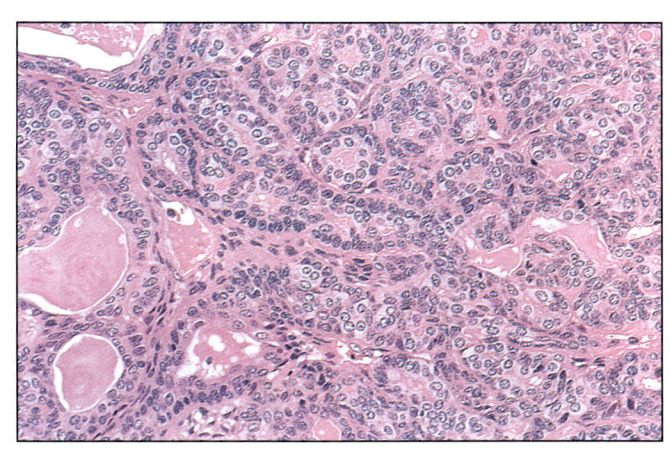

B

图7.36 基底细胞腺瘤。（A）该肿瘤的特征是基底细胞样细胞排列成岛状和宽阔的小梁状。有一些散在的小的腺体间隙。与多形性腺瘤不同，肿瘤细胞岛与间质的界限非常清楚。（B）管状型基底细胞腺瘤。导管腔面-腔外双重细胞清晰可见。这个视野与多形性腺瘤的某些病灶很难区分。

小梁型：小梁型由相互连接的或窄或宽的细胞小梁组成，形成一种网状结构（图7.37）。

管状型：管状型是最少见的一种类型，由散在的或相互吻合的小管构成，小管内衬两层不同的细胞，内层是立方形导管细胞，外层围绕着基底细胞样细胞（图7.36B）。腔内常常含有PAS-阳性的嗜酸性分泌物。少数肿瘤形成筛状结构，且为肿瘤的主要成分，酷似腺样囊性癌（图7.38）。

伴有肌上皮来源的间质的基底细胞腺瘤（Basal cell adenoma with myoepithelium-derived stroma）：这是一种不常见的亚型，其特征是基底细胞样细胞条索和细胞岛被富于梭形细胞的间质分开[85]（图7.39）。这些梭形细胞 S-100 蛋白强阳性，并且显示肌上皮的超微结构特征，但肌动蛋白和p63常常阴性。这种肿瘤腔外基底细胞样细胞与间质界限分明，不同于多形性腺瘤。

膜型：膜型的特征是外形光滑的肿瘤细胞岛周围出现大量浓厚的嗜酸性和PAS-阳性的玻璃样基底膜物质。单个细胞之间也有小滴状玻璃样物质。在肿瘤岛内可能有一些散在的腺腔（图7.40和图7.41）。可能发生灶状鳞状化生。因为膜型基底细胞腺瘤以多结节方式生长，而且正常的涎腺组织常常陷入肿瘤之中，所以可能被认为是恶性病变。

膜型基底细胞腺瘤在组织学上与皮肤圆柱瘤相同（图7.42）。伴有多发性圆柱瘤、毛发上皮瘤、小汗腺腺瘤和粟粒疹的家族性病例构成常染色体Brooke-Spriegler综合征（家族性圆柱瘤病或头巾样瘤综合征）。圆柱瘤

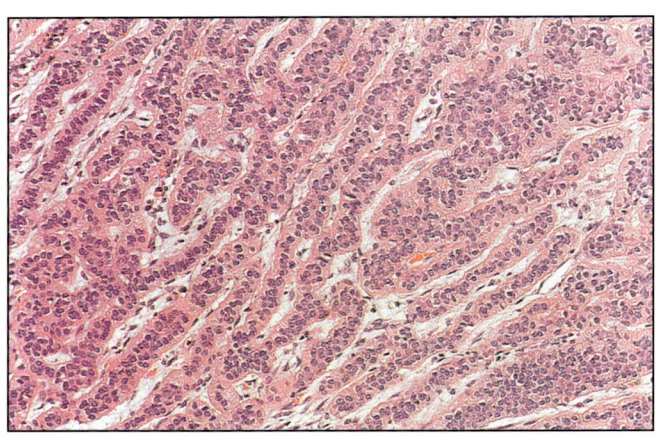

图7.37　基底细胞腺瘤，小梁状亚型。伴有温和细胞核的柱状或立方形细胞小梁被疏松的间质分开。

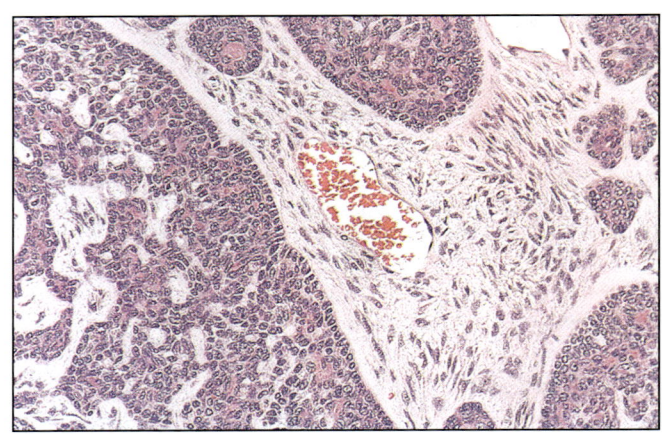

图7.39　伴有肌上皮来源间质的基底细胞腺瘤。肿瘤小梁和细胞岛之间的纤维性间质中有伴有肥胖细胞核的梭形细胞。这些梭形细胞S-100蛋白阳性（没有显示）。与多形性腺瘤不同，肿瘤小梁是分散的，周边细胞呈栅栏状排列，且不直接"融合"到间质中。

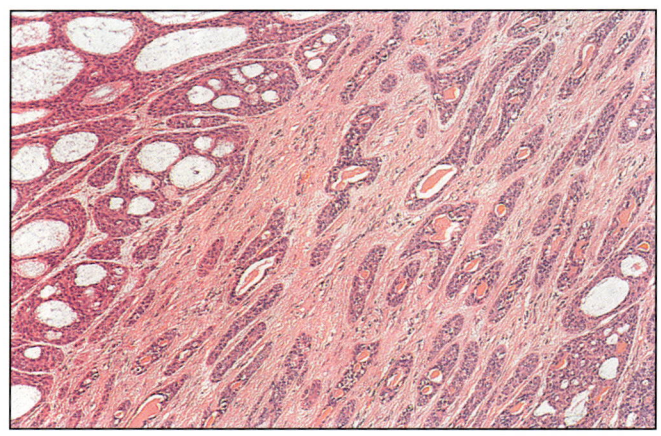

图7.38　基底细胞腺瘤。该肿瘤由小管和筛状结构组成，伴有致密的基质。不分析边缘状况就不能明确与腺样囊性癌鉴别开来。

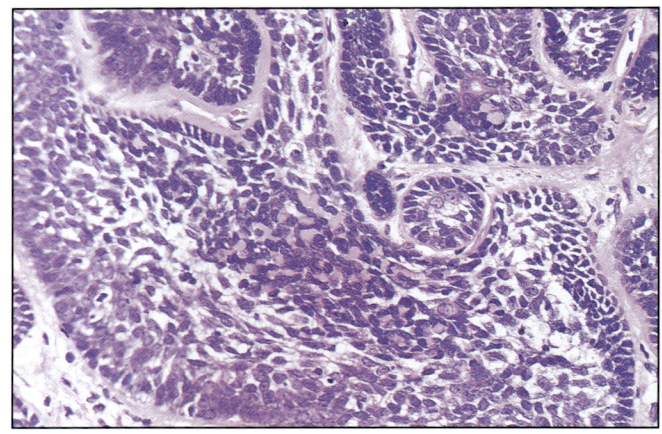

图7.40　基底细胞腺瘤，膜型。基底细胞样细胞岛通常被由基底膜物质构成的嗜酸性玻璃样鞘围绕。

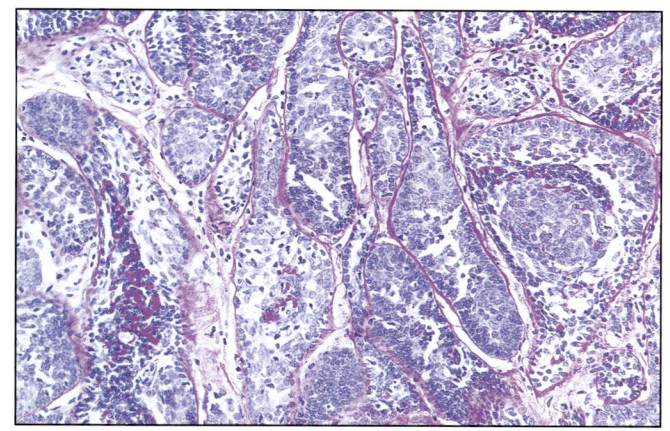

图7.41 基底细胞腺瘤，膜型。PAS淀粉酶染色显示肿瘤细胞岛周围有显著增厚的玻璃样鞘，肿瘤细胞之间有玻璃样物质。

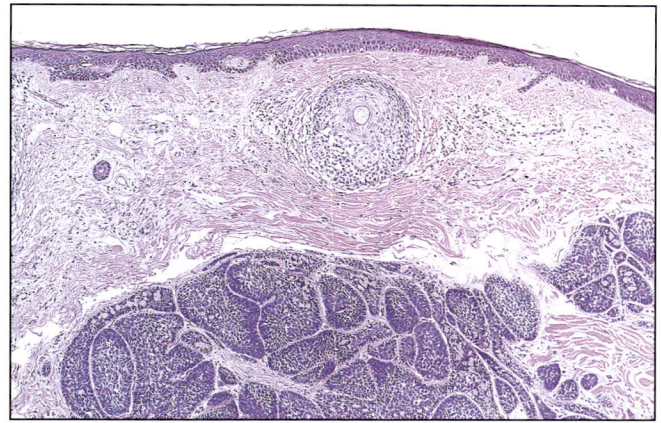

图7.42 膜型基底细胞腺瘤患者同时发生的皮肤圆柱瘤。注意两种类型肿瘤的组织学表现非常一致，这是膜型基底细胞腺瘤可用"类皮肤肿瘤"这一名词替代的原因。

病基因（CYLD）是位于染色体16q12-q13上的一种肿瘤抑制基因，其种系突变与这些家族性病例有关。这种基因的体细胞突变还常常见于散发性病例 [86,87]。

免疫组织化学

绝大多数基底细胞腺瘤显示导管腔面-腔外细胞双重分化。腔面细胞可以表达上皮标记物（细胞角蛋白，CEA，EMA）。位于周围的基底细胞样细胞可以不同程度地表达肌上皮标记物（p63，钙调节蛋白，肌动蛋白，GFAP，S100） [48,88,89]。

基底细胞腺癌 Basal cell adenocarcinoma

定义

基底细胞腺癌是一种低级别的恶性肿瘤，其细胞学改变类似于基底细胞腺瘤 [90]。恶性的诊断通常依靠证实有周围涎腺小叶、神经或血管的浸润。

临床特征

肿瘤发病的平均年龄是60岁，没有性别差异。多数肿瘤一开始就发生在腮腺、很少出现在颌下腺、口腔和上呼吸道 [92,93]。大约23%的病例肿瘤可能发生在先前存在的基底细胞腺瘤，尤其是膜型亚型或其他单形性腺瘤基础上 [91,94]。

基底细胞腺癌一般是伴有局部破坏和有复发倾向的低级别癌；不常发生局部淋巴结和远处转移。经过充分的外科治疗预后良好。然而，与发生在大涎腺的肿瘤相比，小涎腺肿瘤似乎具有较高的复发率（71%）、转移率（21%）和死亡率（29%）（大涎腺相应的数字为37%、11%和3%） [84,91,92,94-96]。

病理学特征

基底细胞腺癌以实性生长为主 [97]，特征为拼图样的基底细胞样细胞岛，周围细胞呈栅栏状排列，浸润边缘通常较宽（图7.43）。常常可见小面积的小梁状或膜性排列。在罕见的情况下，局部可见内衬两种类型细胞的明确的管状结构。如同基底细胞腺瘤一样，存在两种类型独特的基底细胞样细胞，即小的暗细胞和大的淡染细胞（图7.44A）。25%的病例可见局灶性的鳞状分化，而且某些肿瘤细胞可以呈梭形表现（图7.45） [92]。在基底细胞样细胞岛中，可能有少数散在分布的内衬立方细胞的腺体间隙。

显示核非典型性和易见核分裂象的病例容易辨别出是恶性肿瘤（图7.44B）。然而，多数病例具有相对温和的细胞学表现，只有发现浸润性生长才能诊断为恶性（图7.43）。25%~35%的病例可见神经周围浸润或血管侵犯 [95,97,98]。免疫组织学谱和基底细胞腺瘤相似（见上文） [99,100]。

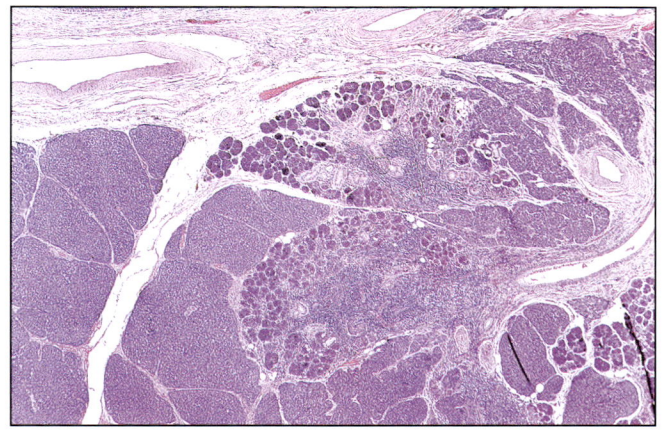

图7.43 基底细胞腺癌。这种基底细胞肿瘤具有明显的浸润性生长，可以将其明确的归入恶性的范畴。基底细胞腺癌一般呈小叶状生长，常常伴有拼图样结构。

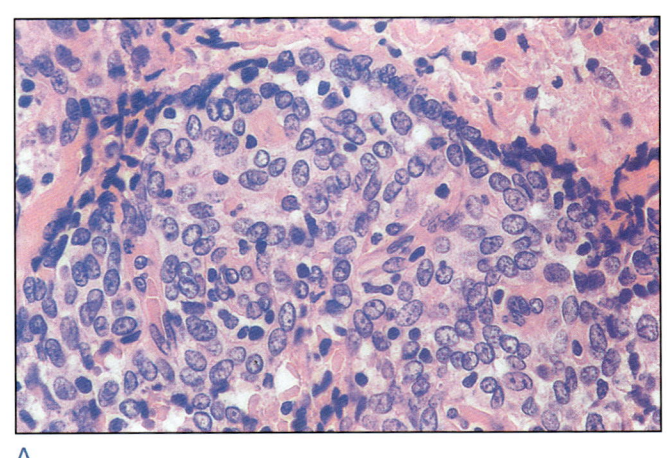
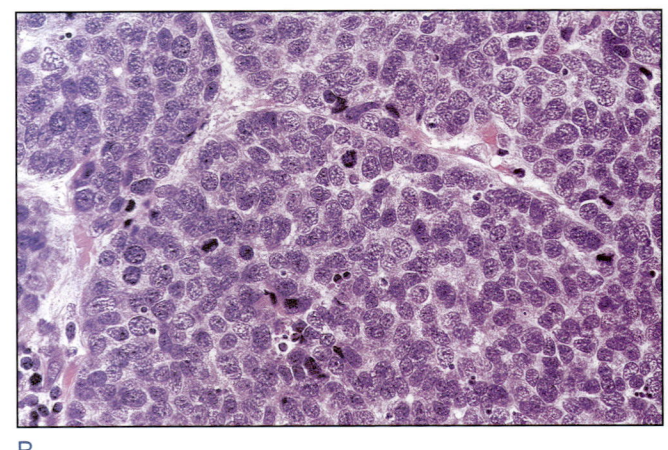

图7.44 基底细胞腺癌。（A）注意周围细胞呈特征性的栅栏状排列。本例细胞表现温和，与基底细胞腺瘤的区别是出现明显的浸润性生长。基底细胞腺癌的特征是，某些细胞有深染的细胞核，某些细胞有大而淡染的细胞核。（B）本例显示基底细胞样细胞有明显的核的非典型性和核分裂活性。

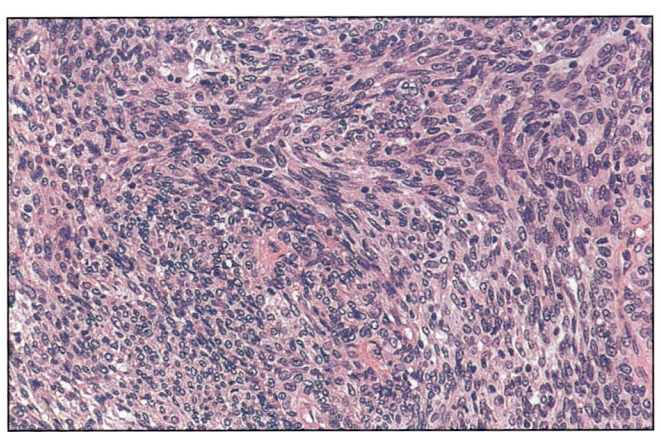

图7.45 基底细胞腺癌。某些病例肿瘤细胞岛的中心可能有梭形细胞。

主要的鉴别诊断（见"诊断的分析方法"和"腺样囊性癌"，第310页）

1. 基底细胞腺瘤
2. 腺样囊性癌，实性亚型
3. 未分化癌
4. 基底细胞样鳞状细胞癌
5. 肌上皮癌

肌上皮瘤　Myoepithilioma

定义

肌上皮瘤是一种良性肿瘤，完全或几乎完全由显示肌上皮分化的细胞组成。虽然某些作者要求这种肿瘤需要完全缺乏导管成分[65]，但多数作者认为可以有少量上皮成分（例如少于5%～10%）[101-103]。

多形性腺瘤、基底细胞腺瘤和肌上皮瘤可能是一个连续的谱系：肌上皮瘤可能是没有导管成分的基底细胞腺瘤的一种极端的形式，而基底细胞腺瘤是"失去特征性基质成分的多形性腺瘤"，多形性腺瘤则处于这个连续谱系的中间（图7.22）[104]。然而，既然所有这些病变的性质均为良性，命名的问题只不过是一个语义学上的问题。

临床特征

肌上皮瘤最常见于腮腺和腭。少数病例可能发生在皮肤、乳腺或软组织[35,105]。临床上表现为无痛性的肿块。发病高峰年龄从20～30岁到40～50岁，没有性别差异[65,104,106]。治疗选择手术切除。

预后极好，完全切除之后不再复发。不过，根据组织学检查可能难以预测肌上皮肿瘤的生物学行为，因为明显良性表现的病变可能意外地发生转移（图7.46）。

病理学特征

肌上皮瘤常常有薄的包膜，切面实性，褐色或黄色。肿瘤性肌上皮细胞可以是梭形细胞、浆细胞样玻璃样细胞、上皮样细胞、透明细胞或嗜酸细胞，前两种类型的细胞最常见。一个肿瘤内或以一种类型的细胞为主，或是几种类型细胞混合存在。小涎腺的肌上皮瘤常常由浆细胞样细胞组成，而腮腺的肌上皮瘤通常由梭形细胞或上皮样细胞组成。间质通常稀少，但是可能出现不同量的黏液样或玻璃样间质。可以出现不同量的放射状排列的胶原结晶和细胞间玻璃样物质（图7.47）[104,107]。

梭形细胞细长，中央有空泡状细胞核和嗜酸性胞浆（图7.48A）。它们形成不同程度的交错排列的细胞束。

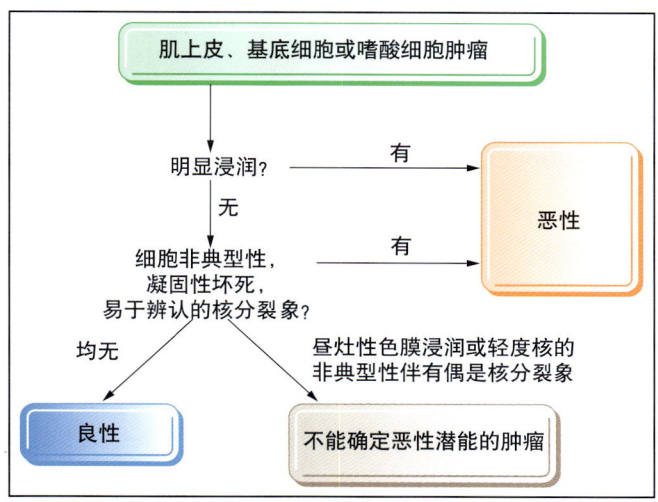

图7.46 评估涎腺肌上皮、基底细胞和嗜酸细胞肿瘤恶性潜能的实用方法。

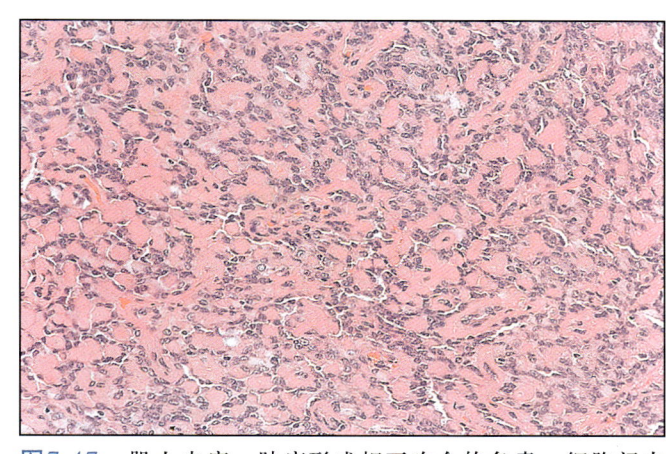

图7.47 肌上皮瘤。肿瘤形成相互吻合的条索。细胞间丰富的玻璃样物质和核呈模糊的栅栏状排列，产生神经鞘瘤样表现。

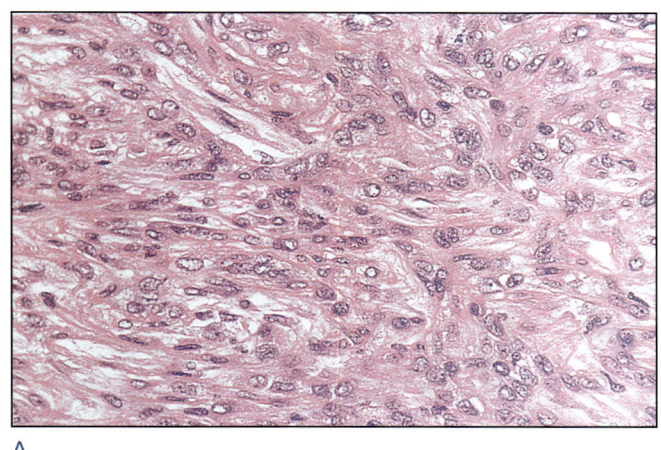

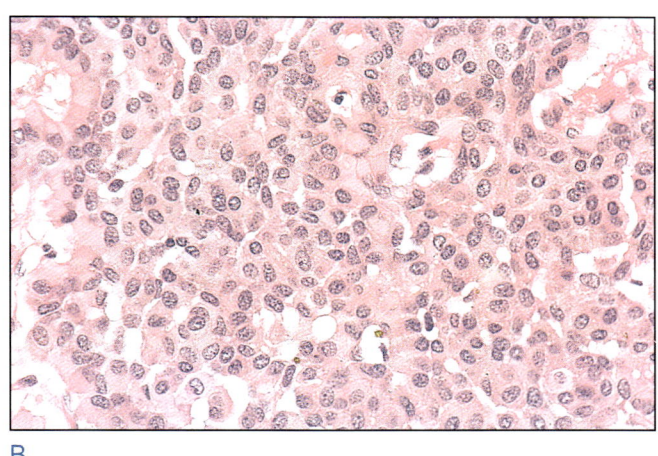

图7.48 肌上皮瘤。（A）该肿瘤是由伴有嗜酸性胞浆的肥胖的梭形细胞组成的。（B）该肿瘤主要是由浆细胞样玻璃样细胞组成的。这些细胞与多形性腺瘤中见到的细胞相同。

主要由梭形细胞组成的肌上皮瘤倾向于富于细胞，几乎无纤维性间质。然而，某些病例可能富于胶原，酷似孤立性纤维性肿瘤（图7.49）。

肌上皮瘤中的浆细胞样玻璃样细胞和在多形性腺瘤中见到的一样（图7.48B）；它们常常伴有疏松的黏液样间质。肿瘤形成不具特征性的细胞岛和片块，或表现为孤立的细胞、细胞条索或细胞团，散在分布于黏液样基质中，而且缺乏真正的软骨样分化。浆细胞样玻璃样细胞缺乏肌样分化的免疫组化和超微结构证据[108]，但是钙调节蛋白，肌动蛋白和p63染色阳性表明，这种细胞的确显示肌上皮分化[48,104,109,110]。

上皮样细胞是大的多角形细胞，伴有嗜酸性胞浆和位于中心的温和的细胞核。它们常常为网状、小梁状或实性生长方式（图7.50）。

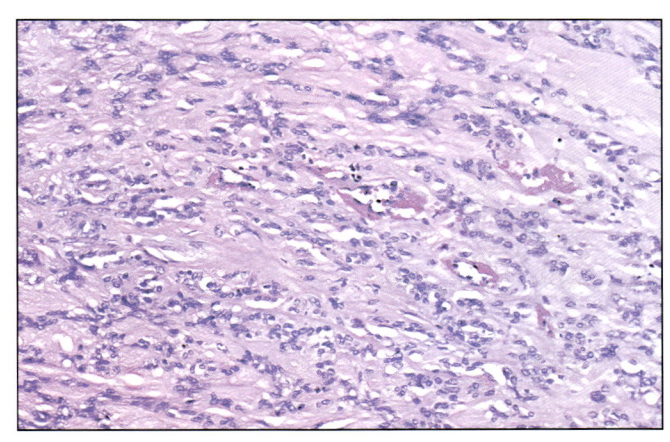

图7.49 肌上皮瘤。该梭形细胞肌上皮瘤伴有丰富的胶原性间质，酷似孤立性纤维性肿瘤。

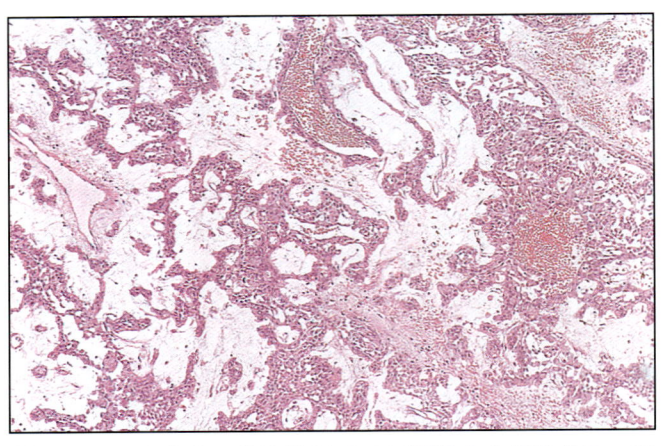

图7.50 肌上皮瘤。黏液样间质破坏了肌上皮细胞片块，形成小梁状或网状结构。根据定义，肿瘤缺乏软骨样基质。

透明细胞糖原含量多。它们通常仅出现在局部，但是偶尔可能非常突出，以致难以与其他透明细胞肿瘤鉴别。

该肿瘤无浸润性生长，无细胞多形性，核分裂象和凝固性坏死少见。然而，在良性表现的背景中，可以出现少数增大而深染的细胞核。

免疫组织化学和超微结构研究

广谱细胞角蛋白和肌上皮标记物（钙调节蛋白，S-100，GFAP，肌动蛋白，CK14，p63）一般阳性，但是每种标记物阳性的频率和阳性细胞的百分数差异很大。据报道，S-100是最有意义的标记物，但是缺乏特异性[104]。许多病例还表达EMA，但仅有少数表达CEA。超微结构检查时通过辨认上皮（半桥粒）和肌样特征（伴有局灶致密的肌丝，饮液小泡），对于确定肌上皮分化有一定作用。

鉴别诊断

1. 多形性腺瘤或基底细胞腺瘤
2. 肌上皮癌
3. 各种间叶性病变，例如神经鞘肿瘤，结节性筋膜炎，孤立性纤维性肿瘤

肌上皮癌（恶性肌上皮瘤）
Myoepithelial carcinoma (malignant myoepithelioma)

定义

肌上皮癌是一种具有细胞学非典型性和潜在侵袭性行为的肌上皮肿瘤[90]。可见良性肌上皮瘤和肌上皮癌之间所有级别的肿瘤，良性和恶性的鉴别取决于有无浸润性生长、细胞非典型性、核分裂象以及凝固性坏死。对于显示某些令人担忧的特征但是缺乏明确浸润性生长的肿瘤，应用"不能确定恶性潜能的肌上皮肿瘤"这一称谓可能是恰当的（图7.46）。

临床特征

发病高峰年龄是50～60岁，大约比相应的良性肿瘤要大10岁。大约有一半的病例发生于先前存在的多形性腺瘤和肌上皮瘤，尤其是复发的病例[111-113]。最常累及腮腺，但是其他大涎腺或小涎腺以及乳腺也可能受累[106,109,111,114,115]。肌上皮癌是一种中级别到高级别的癌。大约有三分之一的患者死亡，另外三分之一复发，主要是多发性的病例，其余三分之一无病生存[65,106,109,111]。最常见的转移部位是肺，其次是肝和椎骨[65]。不同的系列报道临床结果各异，可能反映了诊断恶性肌上皮瘤的标准不同。

病理学特征

肌上皮癌通常没有包膜，可以出现坏死和囊性变的区域，但是少数病例可有包膜。一项25个病例的报告显示，肿瘤大小从2.1 cm到5.5 cm不等[111]。多数肿瘤显示推挤性浸润（图7.51）。肿瘤细胞岛周围富于细胞，中心常常为坏死或黏液样区域。如同肌上皮瘤一样，它可能出现一种或多种以下类型的细胞：梭形细胞，上皮样细胞，浆细胞样玻璃样细胞和透明细胞。核的非典型性从轻微到明显（图7.52）。常见实性、束状、小梁状和花边样生长方式，但未见到腺体结构（图7.51～图7.53）。可能有不同量的黏液样、胶原性或玻璃样间质（图7.51）。也可能有化生性改变，例如鳞状化生（常常伴有角化）或皮脂腺化生的特征，这些细胞逐渐融合到周围的肿瘤细胞中。

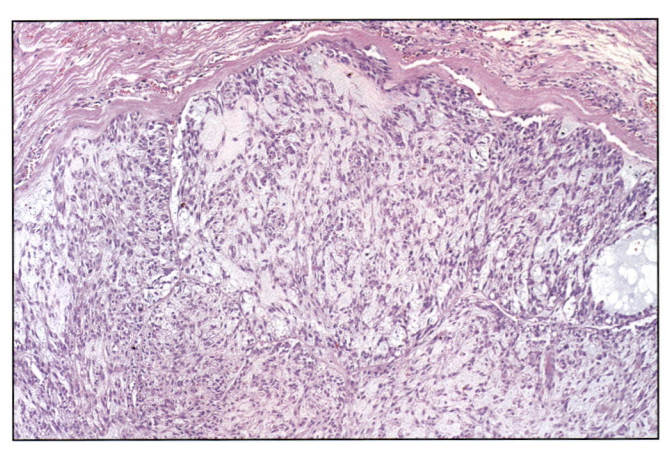

图7.51 肌上皮癌。肿瘤浸润腮腺实质，边缘宽广（视野上部）。这种浸润可将该肿瘤确定为恶性肿瘤。肿瘤呈现小梁状-网状结构，伴有不同量的黏液玻璃样间质。

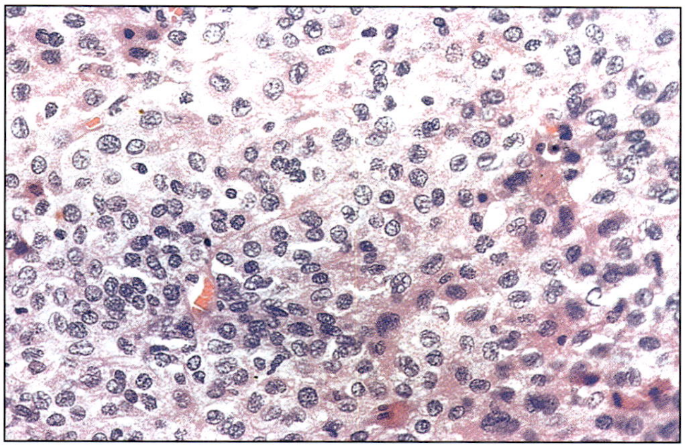

图7.52 肌上皮癌。（A）本例是由良性表现的伴有嗜酸性胞浆的多角形细胞片块组成的，诊断恶性是根据其出现明确的浸润性生长。（B）本例细胞学表现明显恶性。肥胖的梭形细胞具有多形性的细胞核和核分裂活性。胞浆嗜酸性是肌上皮肿瘤的特征。（C）本例纯粹由多角形细胞组成，核呈空泡状，核仁明显，胞浆嗜酸性。诊断恶性可能是因为细胞学非典型性和出现核分裂象。其他区域还有凝固性肿瘤坏死。问题是要证明肿瘤细胞具有肌上皮分化。（D）在某些肌上皮癌中透明细胞（视野左侧）可能占据相当比例。

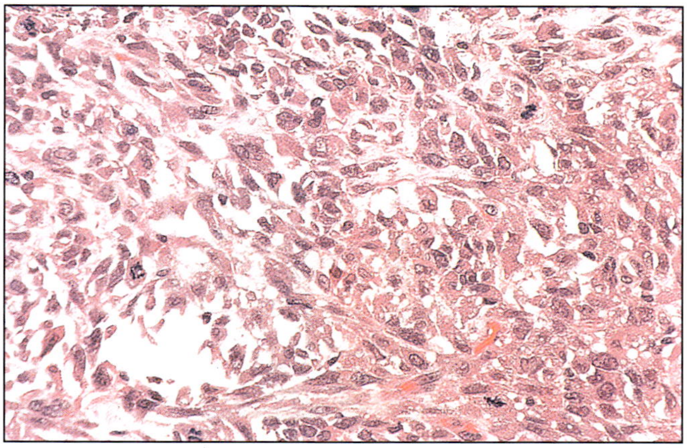

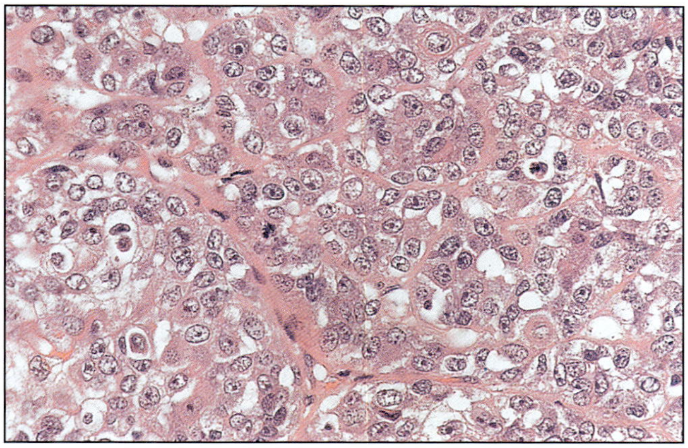

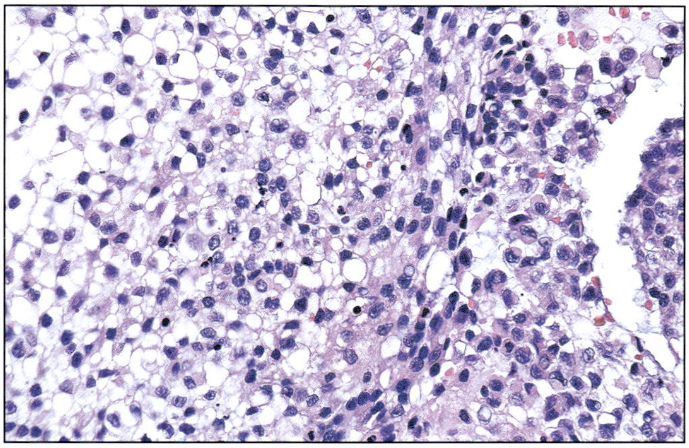

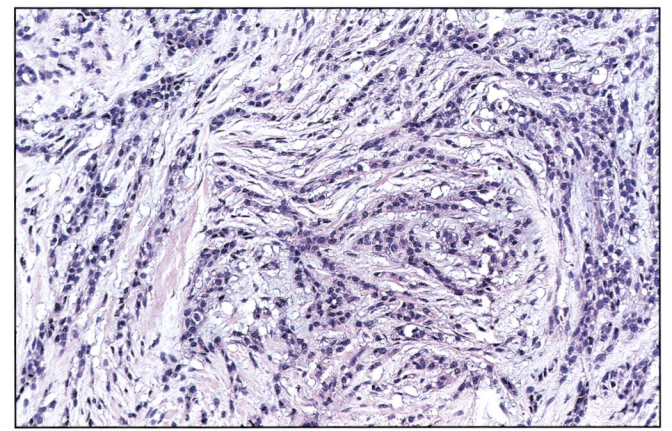

图7.53 肌上皮癌。肿瘤呈小梁状生长，被不同量的纤维黏液样间质分开，这是肌上皮癌特征性的结构之一。

Nagao等发现[109]，通过每10个高倍视野核分裂计数大于7或Ki-67指数大于10%，可将肌上皮癌和良性肌上皮瘤鉴别开来。而且，伴有明显细胞多形性、神经周围浸润、高核分裂计数（>61/10高倍视野）、高Ki-67指数（>50%）和p53蛋白过表达的肿瘤与预后不良有关[109]。另一方面，少数肌上皮癌病例可呈温和表现，而且核分裂计数低（图7.52A）；证实浸润生长对于确立其恶性本质是必要的。原位发生的肌上皮癌和那些起源于多形性腺瘤或肌上皮瘤的肌上皮癌的预后没有差异。去分化性肌上皮癌也有少数报告[116]。

免疫组织化学

为了作出肌上皮癌的诊断，必须通过免疫组织化学或电子显微镜检查证实肌上皮分化。免疫组织化学谱类

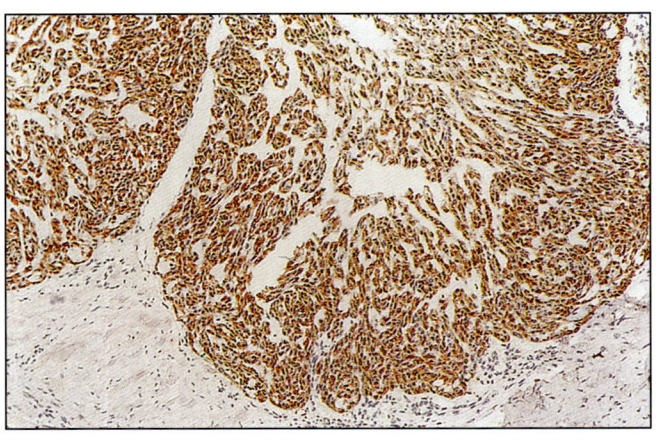

图7.54 肌上皮癌。该肿瘤显示S-100蛋白免疫反应强阳性。

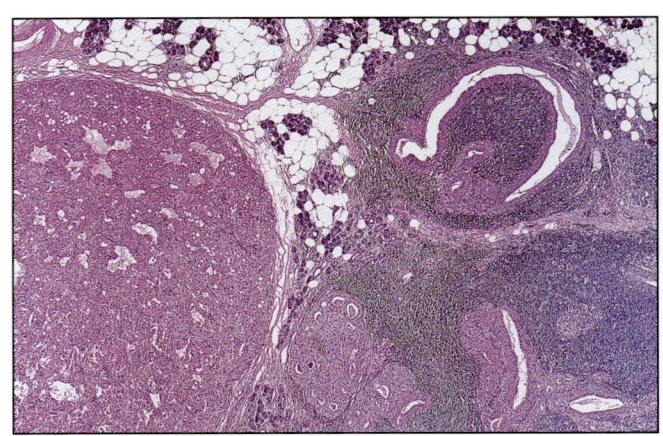

图7.55 显示嗜酸细胞瘤（视野左侧）和Warthin瘤（视野右侧）双重特征的少见的肿瘤。与Warthin瘤的实性腺体成分不同，嗜酸细胞瘤呈小梁状和成束的生长方式。

似于相应的良性肿瘤。肿瘤细胞表达p63、钙调节蛋白、S-100蛋白、CK 14、EMA和不同程度的表达细胞角蛋白（90%），肌动蛋白（70%～80%），GFAP（50%），但不表达CEA和HMB-45（图7.54）[48,109]。

鉴别诊断

鉴别诊断包括肌上皮瘤，各种肉瘤（平滑肌肉瘤，纤维肉瘤，所谓的恶性纤维组织细胞瘤，恶性外周神经鞘肿瘤），指突状树突细胞肉瘤和黑色素瘤。后两种肿瘤还表达S-100蛋白，但不表达细胞角蛋白和肌样标记物。

透明细胞肌上皮癌还存在与涎腺各种透明细胞肿瘤的鉴别诊断问题（表7.5）[101]。

嗜酸细胞瘤 Oncocytoma

定义和相关疾病

嗜酸细胞瘤是完全由嗜酸细胞组成的散在的有包膜的肿瘤，而且缺乏其他类型肿瘤的特征[117]。当嗜酸细胞瘤伴有淋巴细胞间质时，可能无法与Warthin瘤区分。另外，有关嗜酸细胞瘤可能是缺乏淋巴细胞间质的Warthin瘤这一观点尚有争论[118]。然而，由于两者均为良性肿瘤，所以并无鉴别意义。偶尔，嗜酸细胞瘤甚至可能与Warthin瘤共同存在（图7.55）。

嗜酸细胞增生症（oncocytosis）是涎腺的弥漫性嗜酸细胞化生性病变，常常伴有周围涎腺实质萎缩（图7.56）[119,120]。然而，小叶结构是保留的。结节性嗜酸细胞增生（nodular oncocytic hyperplasia）由密集排列的嗜酸细胞多结节性增生组成。与嗜酸细胞瘤相比，结节界限不清，而且缺乏纤维性包膜[120,121]。由于药物可以诱导鼠产生嗜酸细胞增生症，而且这些病变随后可以转化为嗜酸细胞瘤[9]，所以上述各种嗜酸细胞病变可能同属单一疾病谱系[122]。这3种病变的鉴别特征已有描述，

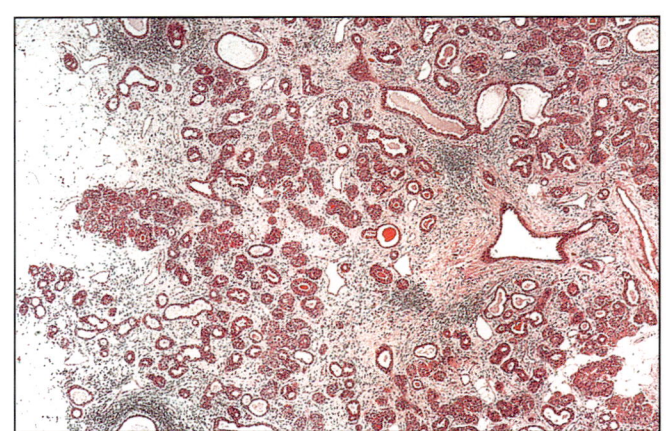

图7.56 颌下腺弥漫性嗜酸细胞增生症。导管细胞广泛嗜酸性化生，伴有腺泡单位丧失。注意小叶结构保留。

但是由于其具有相似的极好的预后和治疗方式，所以对于有争议的病例不值得花费时间去进一步加以鉴别。

临床特征

嗜酸细胞瘤最常发生在老年人的腮腺（平均年龄58～77岁），没有性别差异[65,120,123]，但是颌下腺也可能受累[117]。在大约20%的病例，其发病机制与头颈部接触放射线有关；这种危险因素引起的病变比没有放射史者要早20年[120]。治疗选择手术切除，复发少见（0～10%）[117,120,123]。

病理学特征和特殊研究

嗜酸细胞瘤是有菲薄包膜的红棕色实性病变（图7.57）。肿瘤细胞形成小梁，束状，弥漫性片块，在极少数情况下形成腺体，被薄的纤维性间隔或少量疏松的富于血管的间质分开（图7.57）。偶尔，增生的嗜酸细胞来源于已经有嗜酸细胞化生的导管上皮细胞。嗜酸细

表7.5 含有显著透明细胞的涎腺肿瘤的鉴别诊断

	透明细胞嗜酸细胞瘤	透明细胞癌	黏液表皮样癌	上皮-肌上皮癌	透明细胞肌上皮瘤和肌上皮癌	腺泡细胞癌	转移性肾细胞癌
透明细胞的性质	嗜酸细胞	导管细胞	中间性细胞，黏液细胞	肌上皮细胞	肌上皮细胞	腺泡细胞	肿瘤性肾上皮细胞
胞浆透明状的原因	糖原	糖原	分别为糖原和黏液	糖原	糖原	组织处理产生的假象	糖原和脂质
生长方式	有包膜或界限清楚；小梁状或成束	浸润性；实性或小梁状；硬化性或玻璃样变间质	浸润性，炎症性纤维性间质；上皮样、中间性和黏液细胞巢；某些囊性间隙	浸润性；导管结构，内层为立方细胞，外层为透明的肌上皮细胞	小叶、巢、小梁和束状；可能有胶原小体	浸润的边缘较宽；微囊性结构	突出的窦状隙；出血和含铁血黄素沉积；某些腺体结构
透明细胞的细胞学特征	细胞核圆形，位于中心；周围的一圈胞浆可能染成粉色颗粒状	伴有水样透明胞浆的多角形细胞；核位于中心或偏心	中间性透明细胞是大细胞，伴有水样透明的胞浆；黏液细胞有含絮状物的胞浆	多角形细胞，核位于基底或中心；水样透明的胞浆	细胞多角形或梭形；不同程度的核非典型性；经常混有一些伴有嗜酸性胞浆的细胞	核位于周边；某些细胞浆有稀少含嗜碱性颗粒	水样透明的胞浆；不同程度的核的非典型性
透明细胞的染色特性	PTAH+ 线粒体抗体+	CK+，EMA+，肌上皮标记物（肌动蛋白、钙调节蛋白、p63）−	中间性透明细胞PAS+，PASD+，黏液细胞；黏液PAS+，PASD+	S-100+，肌动蛋白+，钙调蛋白+，p63+	S-100+，肌动蛋白+，钙调蛋白+，p63+	PASD+颗粒，淀粉酶+	脂质+，PASD−，PAS+，CK+，EMA+，肌上皮标记物−

PTAH, 磷钨酸苏木精；CK, 细胞角蛋白；EMA, 上皮膜抗原；PAS, 过碘酸希夫反应；PAS-D, 应用淀粉酶预处理的过碘酸希夫反应。

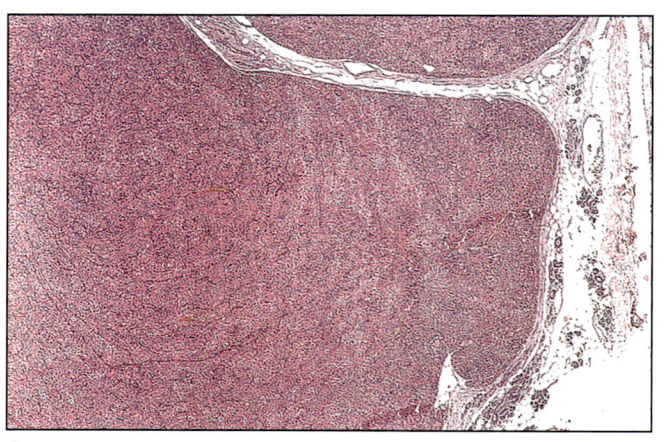

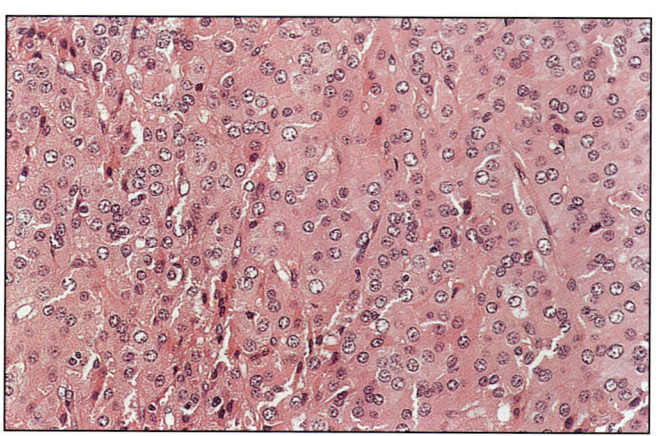

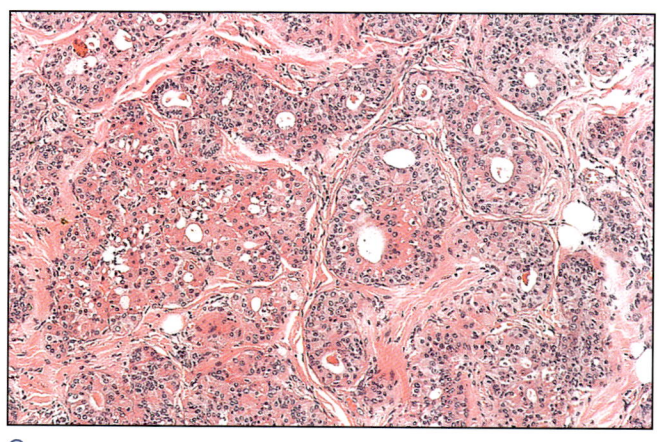

图7.57 嗜酸细胞瘤。（A）肿瘤界限清楚,本例由两个相邻的结节组成。（B）肿瘤由多形性细胞紧密排列的小梁组成,伴有丰富的嗜酸性颗粒状胞浆。（C）少数嗜酸细胞瘤可以形成腺体结构。

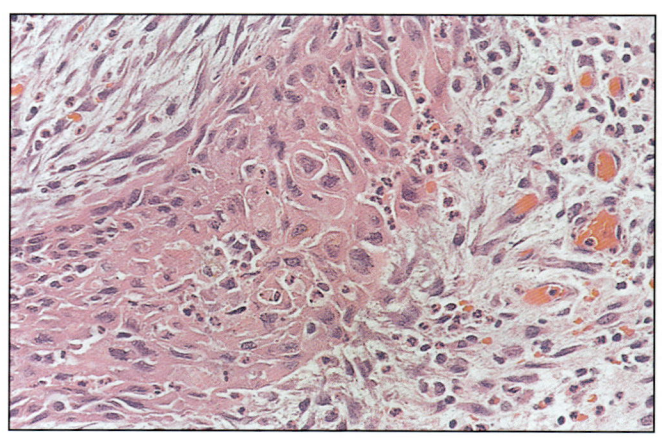

图7.58 嗜酸细胞瘤合并梗死。存活的肿瘤细胞岛中有鳞状化生。细胞非典型性可能导致鳞状细胞癌的错误诊断。注意特征性的修复性/炎症性背景。

是多角形或立方形细胞,伴有丰富的嗜酸性颗粒状胞浆,细胞核圆形,位于中心,常常有明显的核仁（图7.57）。胞浆充满线粒体,应用磷钨酸苏木精染色或抗线粒体抗体免疫染色可以显示出来[124]。可出现局灶性的皮质腺、杯状细胞或鳞状分化以及沙粒体。虽然许多研究质疑嗜酸细胞瘤中存在肌上皮细胞或基底细胞[48,89,125],但是通常p63或CK14免疫染色常常可以证实这样的细胞(伴有变薄的表现)。

在某些嗜酸细胞瘤和邻近的集合管中可能发现富于酪氨酸的结晶[126]。这些嗜酸性结晶呈针形或片状。它们见于细胞外以及嗜酸细胞内。这样的晶体也可以见于Warthin瘤和嗜酸细胞性囊腺瘤。

嗜酸细胞瘤容易发生梗死,或为自发性,或发生在细针穿刺吸取之后。坏死的细胞表现为鬼影或嗜酸性颗粒状物质。残留的存活肿瘤或邻近的涎腺上皮常常发生鳞状化生,核有(修复性)非典型性,酷似鳞状细胞癌(图7.58)(见"诊断的分析方法"一节,第310页)[47]。

亚型：透明细胞嗜酸细胞瘤 clear cell oncocytoma

透明细胞见于11%的嗜酸细胞瘤中,作为肿瘤的主要成分或部分成分。结构和普通的嗜酸细胞瘤相同[127-129]（图7.59）。胞浆透明是由于糖原积聚,但是仍然存在稀少的颗粒。常常可见透明细胞向典型的嗜酸细胞转化。与普通的嗜酸细胞瘤相比,透明细胞嗜酸细胞瘤似乎具有较高的双向肿瘤发病率和复发率[130]。

鉴别诊断

典型的嗜酸细胞瘤不难诊断。主要的诊断难点是嗜酸细胞瘤与伴有明显嗜酸细胞改变的涎腺肿瘤的鉴别,最显著的是Warthin瘤、多形性腺瘤、基底细胞腺瘤和黏液表皮样癌的嗜酸细胞亚型(见"诊断分析方法"一节,第310页)。有时,嗜酸细胞瘤可能被误诊为腺泡细胞癌,因为其细胞排列相似(细胞群或细胞索)和胞浆呈颗粒

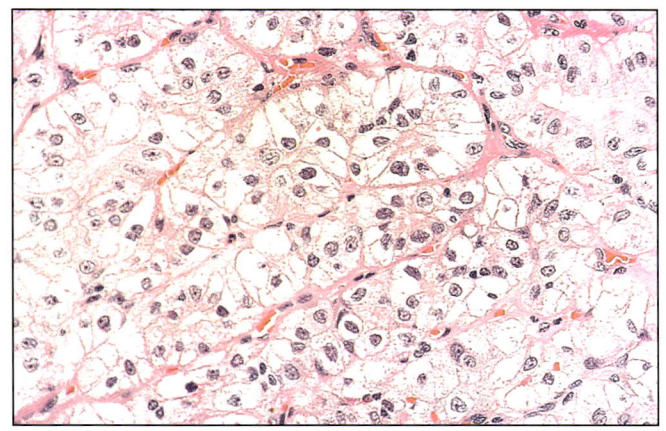

图7.59 透明细胞嗜酸细胞瘤。如同普通的嗜酸细胞瘤一样，多角形细胞紧密排列成小梁状，被纤细的血管结构分开。这个视野的多数细胞具有透明的胞浆，而在某些细胞的胞浆中仍有片块状颗粒。

状，尤其是在术中冰冻切片。然而，腺泡细胞癌的核位于周边，与嗜酸细胞瘤位于中心的圆形核不同[123,131]。透明细胞嗜酸细胞瘤还可能被误诊为其他透明细胞涎腺肿瘤（表7.5）。

嗜酸细胞癌（恶性嗜酸细胞瘤）
Oncocytic carcinoma (malignant oncocytoma)

临床特征

嗜酸细胞癌是一种具有恶性组织学特征的嗜酸细胞肿瘤。多数病例发生在60岁以上患者的腮腺[65]。某些病例可能来源于先前存在的嗜酸细胞瘤。与嗜酸细胞瘤不同，嗜酸细胞癌与从前接触放射线无关。它是一种高级别的肿瘤，伴有频繁的复发（56%）和转移（80%），最常转移到肺、肾、肝、甲状腺、纵隔和骨[65,132]。据报道，伴有转移的患者的平均生存时间是3.8年[123]。直径小于2 cm的肿瘤比较大的肿瘤预后要好[132]。

病理学特征

嗜酸细胞癌是一种没有包膜的孤立性或多结节性肿瘤。与相应的良性肿瘤相比，嗜酸细胞的大小和形状不同，核有多形性，虽然某些病例核的非典型性可能轻微。它们形成小梁状、片块状、巢状或导管结构，浸润涎腺实质和周围结缔组织（图7.60）。常见非典型性核分裂象，可见神经周围和血管浸润（图7.60A）。凝固性肿瘤坏死对于嗜酸细胞癌似乎比对于嗜酸细胞瘤更加特异，而且可能具有不良的预后[123]；千万不要与肿瘤梗死混淆，肿瘤梗死也可以见于嗜酸细胞瘤。

转移性嗜酸细胞瘤和不能确定恶性潜能的嗜酸细胞肿瘤
Metastasizing oncocytoma and oncocytic neoplasm of uncertain malignant potential

通过细胞核的多形性和浸润性边缘，多数嗜酸细胞癌的恶性本质容易辨认[65]。然而某些作者提出，嗜酸细胞瘤和嗜酸细胞癌可能没有明显的组织学差别，而且少数看似温和的肿瘤可能意外地发生转移[123,132,133]。Sugimoto报道一例伴有轻度核的非典型性和核分裂计数低的有包膜的嗜酸细胞瘤，就诊时有淋巴结转移。在7个月时发生多发性远处转移，患者在18个月时死亡[134]。这些肿瘤可能是转移性嗜酸细胞瘤，类似于转移性多形性腺瘤，两者均预示有不良的临床结果。

对于显示交界性非典型性特征的肿瘤，例如仅仅有细胞非典型性，偶尔出现核分裂象，或存在有限的局灶性浸润，应用"不能确定恶性潜能的嗜酸细胞肿瘤"的命名指出其行为的不确定性可能是恰当的（7.46）。

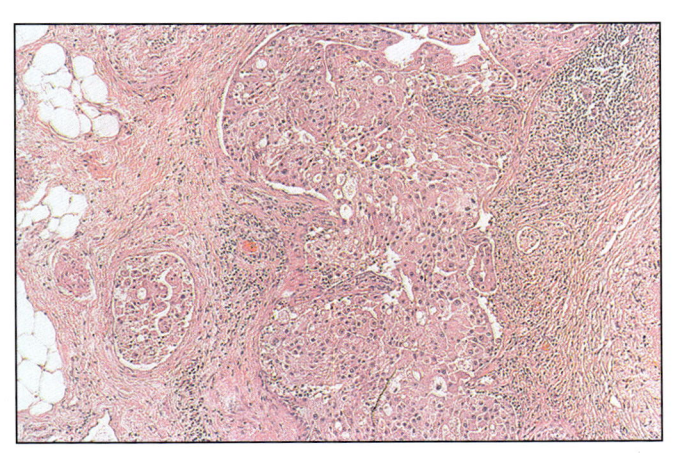
A

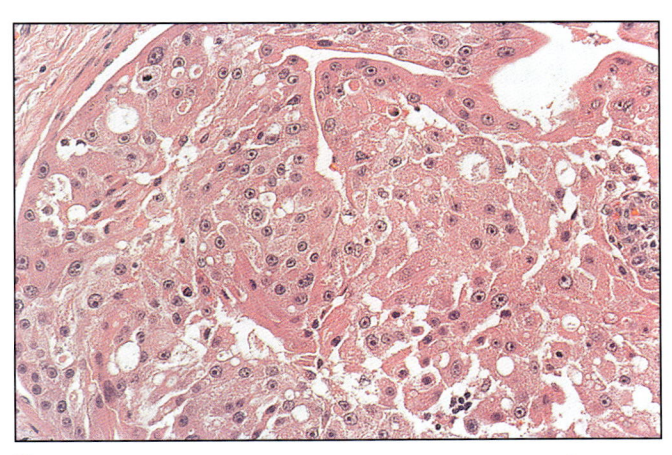
B

图7.60 嗜酸细胞癌。（A）这个肿瘤与嗜酸细胞瘤的区别是浸润性生长。视野左侧还有明显的淋巴管浸润。（B）嗜酸细胞性肿瘤细胞显示轻到中度细胞核的多形性和突出的核仁。

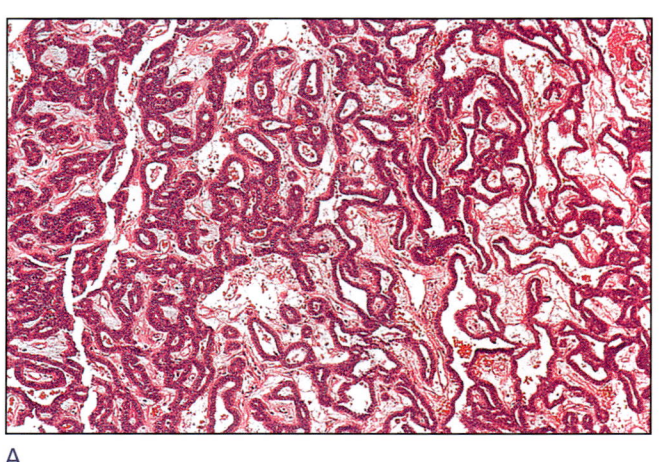
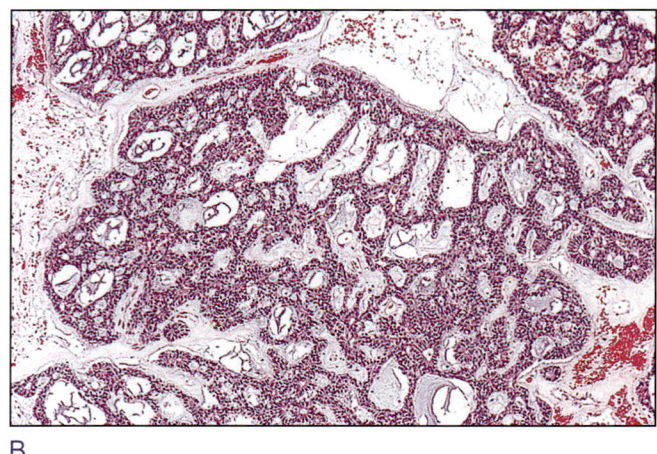

图7.61 小管腺瘤。（A）典型的低倍镜下表现，特征性的轨道样双排细胞平行排列，合并成某些小结，其他区域部分形成扩张的间隙。注意特征性的疏松间质。（B）这是一个不太典型的病例，显示双排细胞复杂的相互吻合的结构。

小管腺瘤　Canalicular adenoma

临床特征

小管腺瘤最常发生在老年人，平均年龄为65岁，女性略为好发[65]。它主要是一种口腔病变。上唇是好发部位，占所有病例的74%，其次是颊黏膜（12%）和腭，很少发生在大涎腺。患者表现为生长缓慢的非溃疡性无痛性肿块。少数病例可见多灶性结节，溃疡形成，坏死和骨破坏[135-137]。完全切除后不会复发[136,138]。

病理学特征

小管腺瘤通常较小（< 3 cm），界限清楚，有或没有包膜。多灶性病变并不少见[135]。它由两层细胞索组成，相互毗连和偶然分离，形成单排、串珠、小管和假乳头状结构（图7.61）。形成条索的上皮细胞为立方形或柱状，伴有中等量的两染性胞浆和规则的卵圆形细胞核（图7.62）。没有细胞的多形性和核分裂象。间质特征性的表现为水肿，伴有许多毛细血管和窦状隙；间质可能非常疏松，以致肿瘤细胞条索好像"漂浮在空气中"一样[65]。可能出现基底细胞样细胞灶，导致难以与基底细胞腺瘤鉴别，尤其是小梁状变型，但从治疗的目的来看这种鉴别并不重要。

免疫组织化学和电子显微镜检查

免疫组织化学和电子显微镜检查显示完全呈腔面细胞分化，没有肌上皮细胞或基底细胞参与。肿瘤细胞细胞角蛋白、波形蛋白、S-100蛋白阳性，EMA阳性少见[88,139,140]。

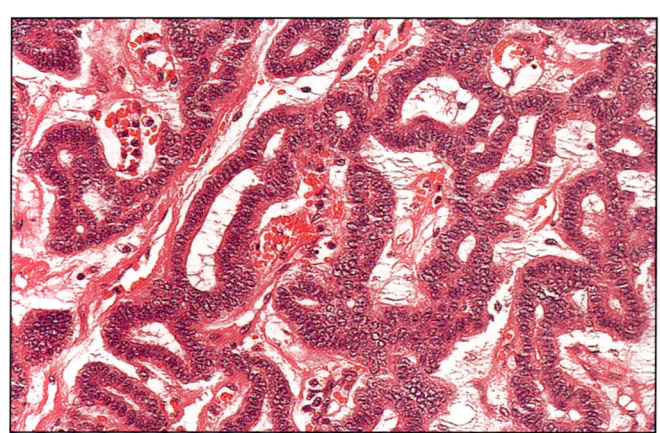

图7.62 小管腺瘤。间隙内衬温和表现的柱状导管细胞。未见肌上皮细胞。

Warthin瘤　Warthin tumor

定义

Warthin瘤又称腺淋巴瘤（adenolymphoma）或淋巴瘤性乳头状囊腺瘤（papillary cystadenoma lymphomatosum），是由嗜酸细胞和基底细胞样上皮两层细胞组成的，形成囊性结构、乳头和腺体，伴有致密淋巴细胞间质。近来的分子研究表明，上皮成分为多克隆性，且不显示克隆性的等位基因缺失，提示这种肿瘤不是一种真正的肿瘤[141-143]。

临床特征

Warthin瘤是第二常见的涎腺肿瘤[144-146]。几乎全部发生在腮腺和腮腺周围淋巴结。它常常发生在50～60岁和60～70岁的患者，40岁以下罕见。主要发生在男性（男女比为5～26:1）。有趣的是，近年来发现有男性发病率下降，同时女性发病率上升的趋势。这种变化可能是由于男性吸烟习惯下降而女性吸烟习惯上升造成的[148,149]，已经明确吸烟是这种肿瘤的危险因素[147]。对原子弹爆炸幸存者的研究提示，辐射可能也与肿瘤发生有关[150]。较早有人认为本病与 EB 病毒密切相关[151]，但是尚未得到证实[153,153]。

这种肿瘤一般表现为发生在腮腺下极的柔软囊性的肿块。与其他单形性腺瘤不同，Warthin 瘤可以出现各种症状。患者可以没有症状，或可能有疼痛、面部无力以及同侧耳部症状，例如耳痛、耳鸣和耳聋。肿物可以突然增大伴有急性疼痛（称为淋巴瘤性乳头状囊腺瘤综合征），可能是由于液体漏出流入周围组织以及经由口腔 Stensen 腮腺导管逆行感染引起的[154]。罕见的病例中，面神经麻痹可能见于并发炎性和纤维化的肿瘤，临床上和术中可能被误诊为癌。12%～20% 患者的 Warthin 瘤是多中心的（或为同时发生或为异时发生），而且 5%～14% 的病例是双向性的[155,156]。另外，连续切片可能发现 50% 的病例有另外的亚临床病变[157]。这种肿瘤有时伴有其他良性涎腺肿瘤，尤其是多形性腺瘤[158,159]。

该肿瘤经浅叶腮腺切除术或肿瘤剜出术可以治愈。复发（< 2%）被认为是第二个原发性肿瘤或者是多灶性肿瘤[160-164]。年老患者或那些手术危险高的患者，可以选择观察而不进行手术。

大体表现

Warthin 瘤是一种界限清楚的球形或卵圆形的病变。切面通常为实性肿瘤，散在含有透明、黏液样、棕色液体或"干酪样"半固体碎屑的囊性间隙，大体检查时，后者有时可能给人一种结核性淋巴结炎的假象。通常有纤细的乳头状突起突入囊性间隙（图 7.63A）。先前的细针吸取活检常常导致局部出血、坏死或纤维化（图 7.63B）。

显微镜下表现

Warthin 瘤由不规则的囊性结构组成，其内衬上皮突出形成乳头状皱襞（图 7.64A）。上皮也可以向下延伸，形成疏松排列或密集排列的管状腺体（图 7.64B）。上皮由两层构成，内层嗜酸性柱状细胞由一层不连续的嗜酸性基底细胞支撑（图 7.65）。腔面细胞的细胞核均匀一致，朝向游离面呈栅栏状排列。由于线粒体的积聚，胞浆呈鲜明的嗜酸性颗粒状[124]。基底细胞具有圆形或卵圆形的细胞核和小而突出的核仁。囊腔含有浓厚的蛋白分泌物、细胞碎屑和胆固醇结晶，有时含有类似于淀粉样体（corpora amylacea）的板层小体（laminated bodies）[165]。

囊肿内衬和淋巴样间质由一层清楚的基底膜分开，淋巴样间质由小淋巴细胞以及一些浆细胞、组织细胞和肥大细胞组成。某些病例可见生发中心和窦状隙。有时可能出现伴有 Langhans 型巨细胞的肉芽肿反应。这个肿瘤腺体结构和淋巴样间质之间关系密切，故有"腺淋巴瘤"（adenolymphoma）的称谓。淋巴细胞的来源仍有争议，可能是残留淋巴结的淋巴组织，或是肿瘤引起的反应性淋巴组织增生。发生在腮腺外淋巴结（例如颈淋巴结）的肿瘤有可能被误诊为转移性 Warthin 瘤。

上皮成分可能发生鳞状细胞、黏液细胞甚至纤毛细胞等化生性改变，尤其是在有炎症或梗死性反应时（图 7.66）。有时肿瘤发生梗死，或者为自发性，或者

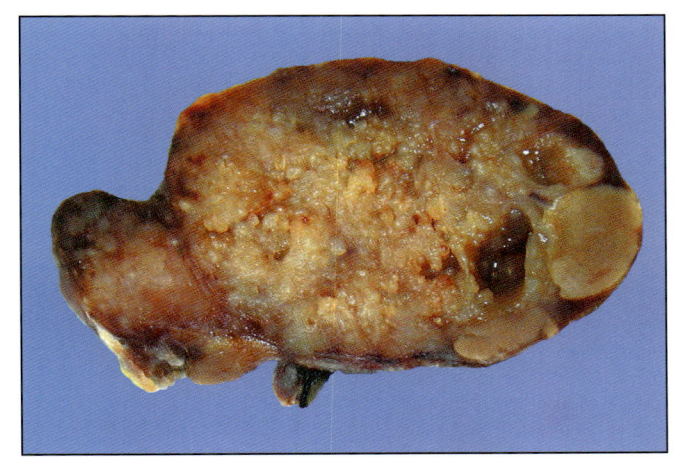

A

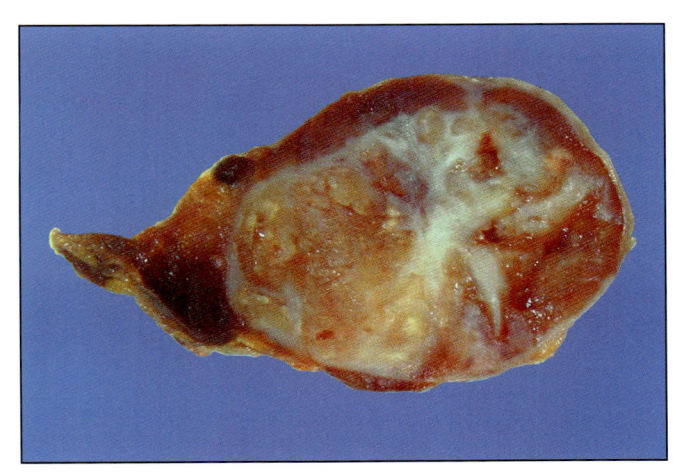

B

图 7.63　Warthin 瘤，大体表现。（A）切面显示肿瘤包膜完整，伴有一些囊肿和呈颗粒状质地的棕色实性区域。（B）本例显示明显的纤维化，是由从前细针穿刺吸取活检后修复引起的。

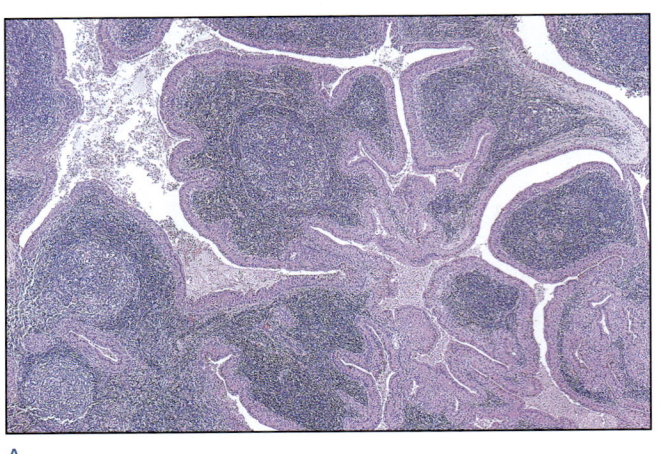
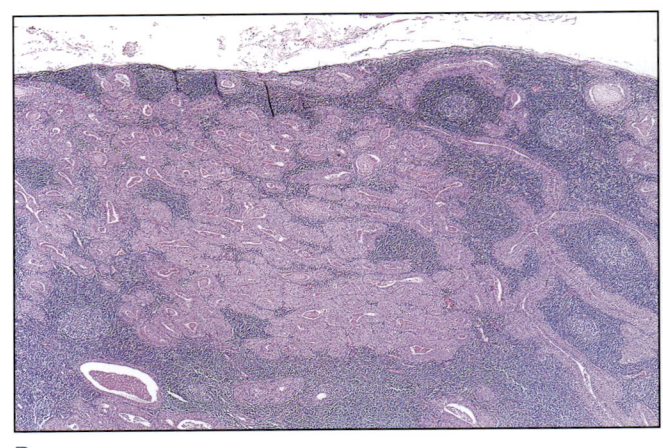

图7.64 Warthin瘤。（A）被覆粉色上皮和有致密的淋巴样细胞的乳头突入囊性间隙。淋巴滤泡明显。（B）嗜酸细胞性上皮可以增生形成密集排列的小管，但仍伴有淋巴样间质。

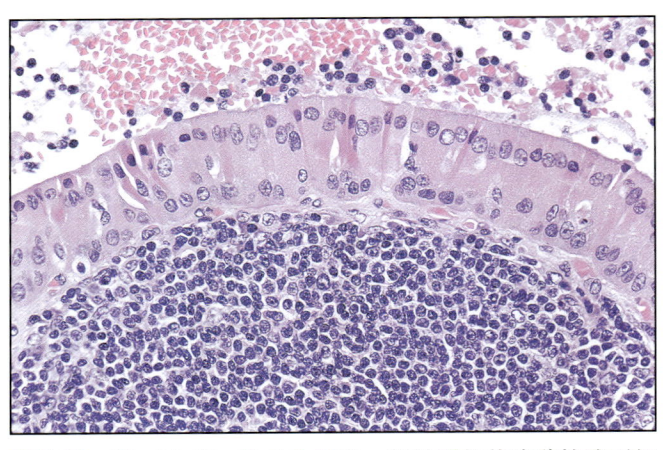

图7.65 Warthin瘤。乳头和腺体一般被覆柱状嗜酸性腔面细胞，核常有极性朝向腔内排列。腔面细胞下方是一层基底细胞，与其下的淋巴样间质界限分明。

发生在细针穿刺吸取活检之后，且肿瘤细胞可能被坏死、肉芽组织、炎症反应和纤维化掩盖。更加糟糕的是，残存肿瘤细胞的非典型性和化生鳞状上皮的假浸润性表现经常引起鳞状细胞癌或黏液表皮样癌的错误诊断[166]。缺乏向周围实质真正的浸润性生长，而且非典型性鳞状上皮岛和嗜酸细胞性上皮混合存在可以作出正确的诊断（图7.67）[47]。

Warthin瘤的上皮和淋巴样成分的相对比例不同。Seifert把Warthin瘤分成为4种亚型：1型（典型的Warthin瘤）上皮成分占50%（占所有Warthin瘤的77%）；2型（间质稀少）上皮成分占70%~80%（占所有病例的14%）；3型（间质丰富）上皮成分仅占20%~30%（2%）以及4型，其特征是广泛的鳞状化生[164]。2型在形态学上与嗜酸细胞瘤有重叠。实际上，Dardick认为，Warthin瘤和嗜酸细胞瘤是病变谱系的两个极端[6]。这种分类没有临床意义，但可用于提醒病理医师，这种表面上单调的肿瘤具有不同的表现。

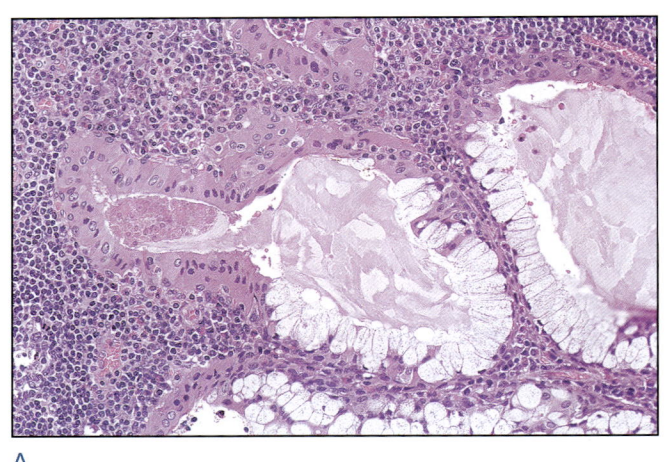
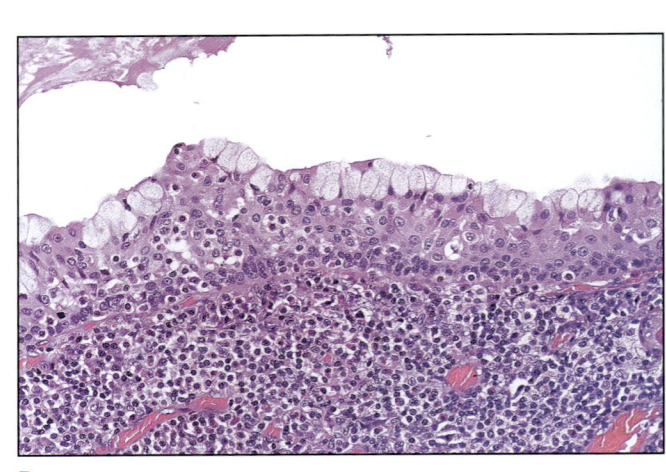

图7.66 伴有化生性上皮的Warthin瘤。（A）从嗜酸性上皮（左）到黏液上皮（右）有一个突然的转变。（B）嗜酸性上皮化生形成黏液和鳞状细胞，导致类似于黏液表皮样癌。

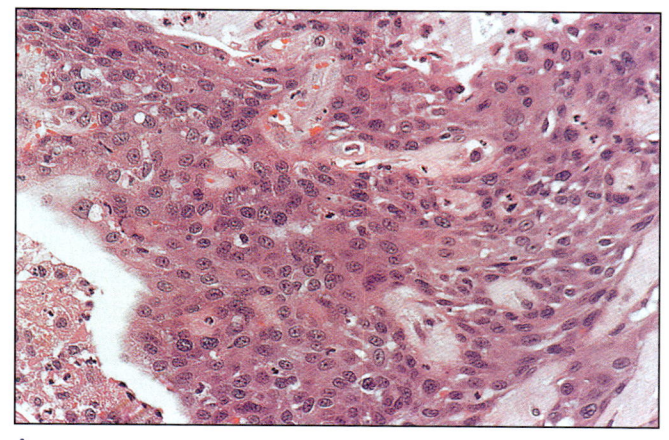

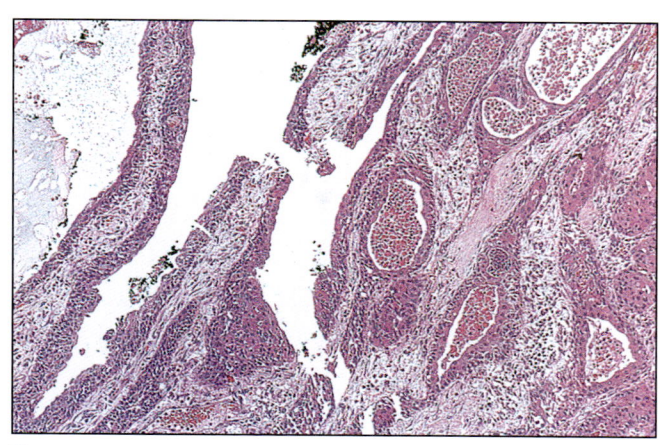

图7.67 Warthin瘤合并梗死和鳞状化生。（A）残留的肿瘤上皮发生鳞状化生。细胞非典型性的出现可能导致误诊为鳞状细胞癌或黏液表皮样癌。（B）辨认鳞状上皮和残存的嗜酸性上皮（视野右侧）的连续性可以确立鳞状增生的化生性本质。注意梗死病变引起的炎性反应。

Warthin 瘤恶变

在极少数的情况下，Warthin瘤的上皮或淋巴成分可以发生恶变[65]，估计其发生率少于0.1%[167]。按照发生顺序，最常见的癌是鳞状细胞癌、嗜酸细胞癌、腺癌、未分化癌、黏液表皮样癌和Merkel细胞癌[168-172]。根据文献报告，三分之一的患者有局部淋巴结转移，而且某些病例还可能发生远处转移。

发生于淋巴样间质的淋巴瘤的特征是相对单一形态的浸润，伴有上皮和淋巴结构变形。各种类型的非Hodgkin淋巴瘤和Hodgkin淋巴瘤均有报道[173-176]。

鉴别诊断

典型的Warthin瘤形态学表现非常特殊，不存在诊断问题。它与嗜酸细胞瘤的不同之处在于出现突出的淋巴成分、乳头和腺体，且不是小梁状或成束排列，而且有显而易见的基底细胞（嗜酸细胞瘤基底细胞不明显）。鳞状化生性Warthin瘤可能被误诊为鳞状细胞癌或黏液表皮样癌，尤其是在出现梗死时。Warthin瘤的鳞状化生通常缺乏角化，角化见于多数鳞状细胞癌。与低级别黏液表皮样癌不同，它没有明确的浸润性生长，而且肿瘤细胞表现出较明确的鳞状性质。

皮脂腺肿瘤　Sebaceous neoplasias

正常情况下，皮脂腺细胞可以见于腮腺、颌下腺和口腔的小涎腺。皮脂腺肿瘤是非常罕见的肿瘤，一般认为是来源于皮脂腺分化的细胞。应该注意的是，不同类型的腮腺肿瘤可以显示局灶性的皮脂腺分化，例如多形性腺瘤、Warthin瘤和黏液表皮样癌[177]。

皮脂腺腺瘤和淋巴腺瘤　Sebaceous adenoma and lymphadenoma

临床特征：受累的患者一般在50～60岁或60～70岁，男性发病率略高。这些肿瘤通常表现为无症状缓慢生长的肿块。腮腺是最常见的部位，与皮脂腺的自然发生状况相同。完全切除可以治愈。

皮脂腺腺瘤　Sebaceous adenoma

皮脂腺腺瘤是有包膜的肿瘤，由伴有纤维性间质的多发性不完全分化的皮脂腺小叶组成。每个小叶由成熟的皮脂腺细胞群组成，周围绕以基底细胞样细胞。某些细胞可能显示两种类型细胞过渡的特征。皮脂腺细胞含有多个小的蜂窝状脂质空泡，冰冻切片油红O染色可以显示脂质。常见局灶性的鳞状、黏液或嗜酸细胞化生。成熟的皮脂腺细胞崩解可能导致小叶中囊肿形成。也可能有内衬鳞状、柱状或立方形细胞的囊性结构，伴或不伴有皮脂腺细胞。纤维性间质中可以有大量炎症细胞浸润，包括脂肪肉芽肿形成，可能是对外渗皮脂产生的反应。

皮脂腺淋巴腺瘤　Sebaceous lymphadenoma

皮脂腺淋巴腺瘤与Warthin瘤非常相似。岛状皮脂腺小叶、导管样结构或囊肿紧密混合，伴有致密的淋巴样间质。淋巴样间质常常含有许多反应性的淋巴滤泡。常常出现与挤压出的皮脂有关的异物型肉芽肿（图7.68）。与Warthin瘤相似的皮脂腺淋巴腺瘤可能来源于腮腺淋巴结内异位的涎腺组织[90,178]。不过，与有关Warthin瘤的争议一样，淋巴样间质同样被解释为伴随肿瘤的反应[65]。

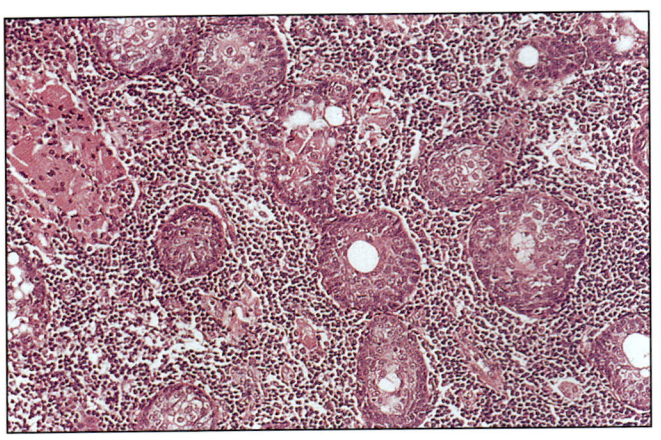

图7.68 皮脂腺淋巴腺瘤。在位于淋巴样背景的上皮岛中，基底细胞样细胞位于外周，而皮质腺细胞位于中心。视野最左侧有组织细胞积聚，可能是对于从肿瘤中挤出的皮脂的反应。

皮脂腺癌和淋巴腺癌
Sebaceous carcinoma and lymphadenocarcinoma

皮脂腺癌（Sebaceous carcinoma）：皮脂腺癌是一种罕见的中级别的恶性肿瘤。有两个年龄分布高峰，一个是20～30岁，另一个是60～80岁。没有性别差异。患者出现肿块性病变，疼痛或面神经麻痹。对于低分期的癌，治疗选择广泛手术切除。对于高分期和高级别的肿瘤，提倡辅助性放疗。总的5年生存率为62%[65,177]。

这些肿瘤部分界限清楚，但是至少有局灶性的浸润性边缘。基底细胞样细胞、鳞状细胞和皮脂腺细胞形成不同大小的细胞岛，片块和浸润性条索。常见导管样和囊性间隙。许多细胞是未分化细胞，但是多数或某些肿瘤细胞岛的中心出现伴有泡沫状胞浆的独特的皮脂腺细胞。所有的病例均有细胞多形性和核的非典型性，而且常见核分裂象。

肿瘤坏死常见，神经周围浸润见于20%的病例[170]。

皮脂腺淋巴腺癌（Sebaceous lymphadenocarcinoma）：皮脂腺淋巴腺癌是一种非常罕见的恶性肿瘤，是皮脂腺淋巴腺瘤的恶性转化。报告的所有3个病例均发生在年龄70岁以上的患者[177,180]。其中一名患者死于不相关的原因，另外两名患者在6年和14年时无病生存。肿瘤含有典型的皮脂腺淋巴腺瘤，与明显的恶性成分并列；后者缺乏特征性的淋巴样间质，而且可能是皮脂腺癌、未分化癌、腺样囊性癌或上皮-肌上皮癌[177,178]。

囊腺瘤 Cystadenoma

定义

囊腺瘤是一种罕见的非浸润性上皮性肿瘤，以囊性导管上皮囊性增生为特征[65,181]。

临床特征

大涎腺和小涎腺的发病情况相同（最常发生在唇、颊黏膜、腭和扁桃体）。平均年龄55岁，女性好发。肿瘤通常表现为无症状的、波动的、缓慢生长的囊肿[181]。完全切除可以治愈。少数病例可能发生恶变[182]。

病理学特征

肿瘤切面显示多囊性间隙或者单个大的囊肿，囊内可能有结节状突出。肿瘤界限清楚，伴或不伴纤维性包膜。显微镜下，有单个或多发性不同大小的囊肿，被致密的纤维性间质分开。囊肿内衬扁平、立方或柱状上皮细胞，可能形成乳头状皱襞（图7.69）。细胞核呈良性表现，核分裂象非常罕见。上皮细胞可能发生局灶性或

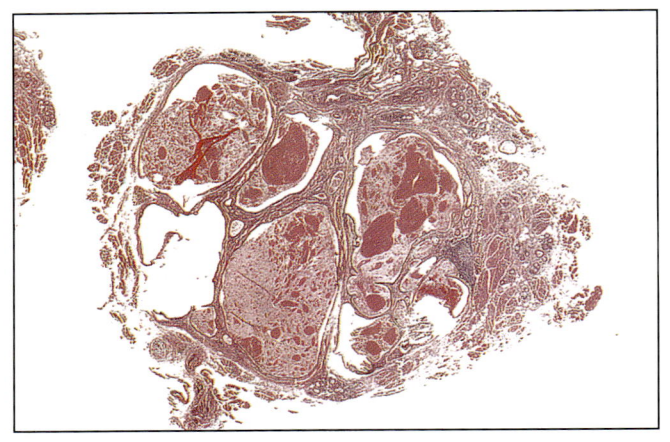

A

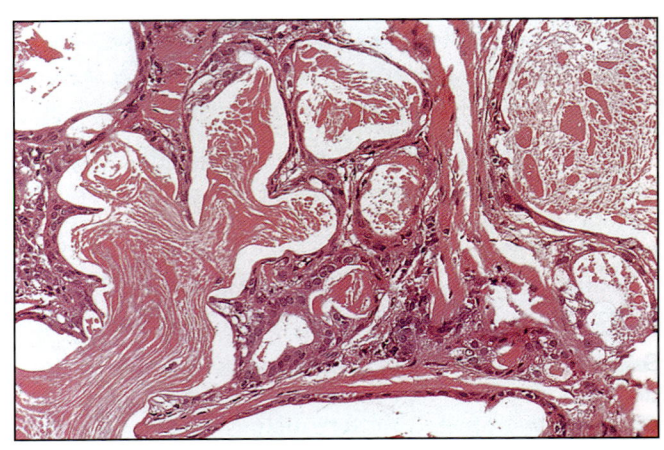

B

图7.69 舌的囊腺瘤。（A）这个界限清楚的肿瘤由不同大小的多发性囊肿组成，囊肿内含浓稠的分泌物。（B）囊肿内衬良性表现的扁平或立方细胞。缺乏低级别黏液表皮样癌特征性的细胞多样性。

广泛性的黏液和嗜酸细胞化生，少数病例发生鳞状化生。囊腔含有蛋白性液体。

因为乳头状结构几乎是一个恒定的特征，所以囊腺瘤有时叫做乳头状囊腺瘤[90]。当嗜酸细胞或黏液性化生明显时，可以应用诸如乳头状嗜酸细胞囊腺瘤或乳头状黏液性囊腺瘤的名称[178]。

鉴别诊断

主要的鉴别诊断包括低级别黏液表皮样癌（浸润性，出现某些实性细胞岛，混合性细胞类型），囊腺癌（出现明确的浸润），导管扩张，多囊性疾病和硬化性多囊性腺病。见"诊断分析方法"，第310页。

囊腺癌　Cystadenocarcinoma

临床特征

囊腺癌或乳头状囊腺癌是一种罕见的低级别恶性肿瘤，是囊腺瘤对应的恶性肿瘤。多数患者年龄在50岁以上（平均59岁）。没有性别差异。大约65%发生在大涎腺，其余的累及颊黏膜、唇和腭。它表现为缓慢生长的无症状肿块。腭的肿瘤可以侵犯到骨骼。局部复发和区域淋巴结转移率分别是7.5%和10%[183]。

病理学特征

与相应的良性肿瘤相似，肿瘤切面显示单个或多个内含透明或棕色液体的囊肿。肿瘤直径从0.4 cm到6 cm不等。显微镜下，肿瘤的恶性本质表现为侵犯周围的组织（图7.70）[180]。神经周围浸润发生在9%的病例。肿瘤由许多不同大小的囊肿组成，常常伴有腔内乳头状突起。某些病例有显而易见的实性生长灶和腔外延伸。囊肿内衬小的立方形细胞、大的立方形细胞或柱状细胞，或这些细胞混合存在。细胞非典型性通常为轻到中度，但核仁通常突出[65]。主要由假复层高柱状细胞组成的肿瘤似乎有较高的转移率[183]。间质呈纤维化、硬化、玻璃样变到纤维组织增生等。

低级别筛状囊腺癌　Low-grade cribriform cystadenocarcinoma

最近的WHO分类，将低级别筛状囊腺癌列在了囊腺癌的亚型中[184]。如同在随后一节中讨论的一样（见第295页），这个术语容易使人误解，而且这个肿瘤实际上是一种导管内的涎腺导管癌。

鉴别诊断

鉴别囊腺癌与乳头状囊性腺泡细胞癌和黏液表皮样癌是非常重要的，因为它不太需要根治性手术而且预后较好。囊腺癌和囊腺瘤的区别在于出现浸润、实性生长灶，以及某些病例有细胞非典型性。通过低级别的细胞核和缺乏粉刺样坏死可以与涎腺导管癌鉴别开来。

导管腺瘤　Dactal adenomas

乳头状涎腺腺瘤、内翻性导管乳头状瘤和导管内乳头状瘤属于一组罕见的良性涎腺肿瘤，由排泄管或导管与黏膜上皮交界处发生，且以乳头状生长为特征。明显好发于小涎腺。

乳头状涎腺腺瘤　sialadenoma papilliferum

患者的平均年龄是59岁，略好发于的男性。肿瘤从颊黏膜表面形成外生性乳头状或疣状肿物，伴有宽的或带蒂的基底。类似的皮肤病变是乳头状汗腺囊腺瘤（syringocystadenoma papilliferum）。组织学上，肿瘤由多个乳头状突起组成，其间有迂曲的裂缝和间隙。病变的表面部分被覆棘层增厚的复层鳞状上皮，与邻近的黏膜上皮连续。在病变的较深部位，移行到由一层腔面柱状细胞组成的导管上皮，并由一层立方形基底细胞支撑。在乳头蒂部下方的导管上皮增生，可能形成囊肿或导管样结构，伴有不规则的腔隙轮廓。间质以富含浆细胞为特征。

与其他类型的导管腺瘤相比，乳头状涎腺腺瘤切除以后具有较高的复发率（10%～15%）[185]。恶变为上皮-肌上皮癌和微乳头状癌的个案已有报道[186]。

内翻性导管乳头状瘤　Inverted ductal papilloma

该肿瘤表现为明显完整的表面黏膜下的结节状肿块。乳头状增生从黏膜表面的小凹开始，且向内生长进

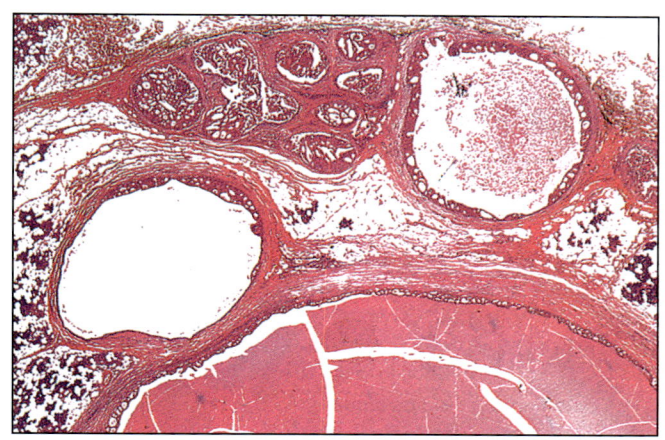

图7.70　囊腺癌。该囊状肿瘤被归类为恶性肿瘤是因为出现了腮腺实质的浸润（视野上部）。

入其下的间质。上皮岛外形光滑，与邻近的固有膜界限分明。被覆乳头的上皮主要是由非角化性鳞状上皮或移行上皮组成，偶尔伴有柱状细胞和杯状细胞。这种病变在形态学上类似于鼻窦内翻性乳头状瘤。完全切除以后不再复发[185]。

导管内乳头状瘤　Intraductal papilloma

导管内乳头状瘤发生于深在的涎腺导管内，常常表现为一个导管的单囊性扩张。可见复杂的乳头状增生突入到囊腔内。被覆上皮由单层、双层立方或柱状细胞组成，乳头轴心为纤细的纤维血管组织。没有囊壁浸润。在乳腺见到的一种类似的病变也被称为导管内乳头状瘤。伴有恶变的病例已有报道，其特征是具有细胞学非典型性，向导管内延伸，有微小浸润以及淋巴结转移[187]。

角化囊瘤　Keratocystoma

临床特征

角化囊瘤是一种罕见的良性肿瘤，由良性鳞状上皮增生形成的多发性囊性结构和实性细胞巢构成。仅有3例报道[188,189]。所有的病例均发生在儿童或年轻成人的腮腺（年龄为8岁到38岁），表现为无痛性肿块。完全切除之后没有复发。

病理学特征

大体上，肿瘤是一种充满角质样物质的多房性囊性病变。组织学上，为由鳞状细胞组成的杂乱排列的多发性囊性结构和实性细胞巢。囊性结构内衬非异型增生性复层鳞状上皮，伴有正常角化或角化不全，但缺乏颗粒层。囊腔充满分层的角质。基底层通过基底膜与间质限分明。间质纤维化，伴有中等量的慢性炎症细胞浸润。也可出现由囊肿破裂溢出的角质引起的异物反应。鳞状细胞表达广谱细胞角蛋白和CK 14，但不表达S-100蛋白或肌动蛋白。

涎腺始基瘤　Salivary gland anlage tumor

临床特征

鼻咽部涎腺始基瘤发生于新生儿或生后最初几周内，表现为呼吸窘迫[190]。特别好发于男性，男女比例为7:1。这种肿瘤可能是错构瘤，因为其组织学特征类似于胚胎的涎腺，虽然某些学者倾向于用畸胎瘤来解释[191]。手术切除之后尚无复发或转移的报道[192]。

病理学特征

这种肿瘤形成一个光滑的或结节状的鼻咽中线的肿块，有时带有狭窄的蒂。表面被覆非角化性复层鳞状上皮，向下延伸形成鳞状细胞巢、分支导管和囊性结构（图7.71A）。这些上皮结构之间散在有致密的富于细胞的结节，由肥胖的间叶细胞样梭形细胞组成，伴有局部漩涡状和发育不完全的导管腺体结构（图7.71B）。结节之间间质内的上皮单位（细胞角蛋白阳性）与富于细胞的结节（细胞对于细胞角蛋白、波形蛋白和肌动蛋白的免疫反应差异很大）混合存在。超微结构上，构成结节的细胞具有上皮、肌上皮和肌原性特征。没有发现软骨样或黏液软骨样组织，因此，从前命名为"先天性多形性腺瘤"是不恰当的[193]。

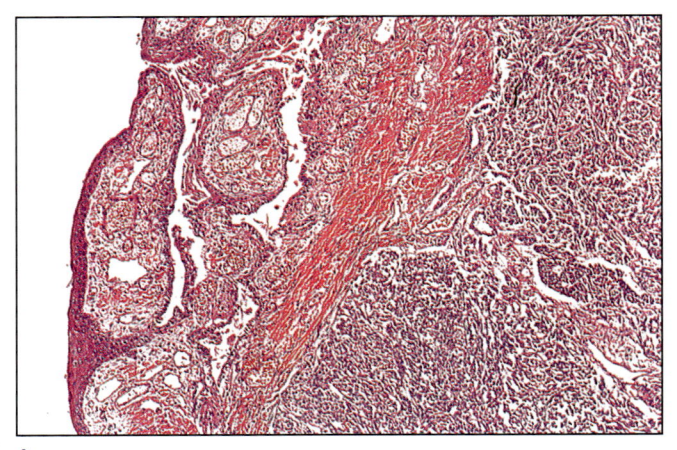

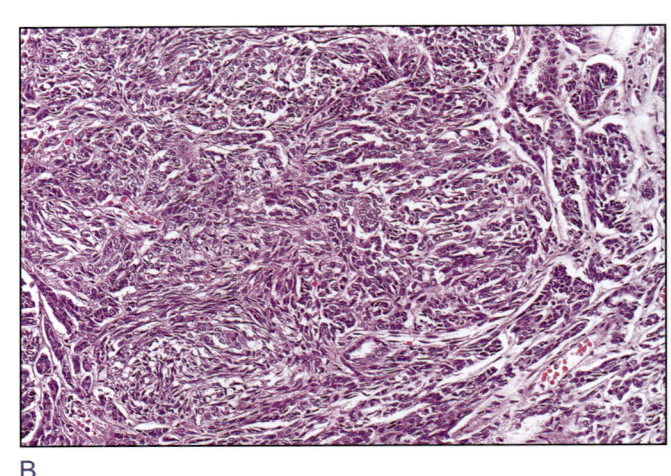

图7.71　鼻咽部涎腺始基瘤。（A）裂隙样腺体结构与表面上皮连续。漩涡状和束状的梭形细胞出现在深部。（B）腺体融入成束的良性表现的梭形细胞中。

硬化性多囊性腺病
Sclerosing polycystic adenosis

临床特征

硬化性多囊性腺病是一种性质不明的病变，其特征为形态学上与乳腺纤维囊性改变非常相似[194-199a]。它发生于从9岁到80岁的病人（平均年龄为33～44.5岁），女性与男性比例为22：15。多数病例起源于大涎腺，但口腔内的小腺体也可受累。病人表现为缓慢生长的肿块。几乎三分之一的病例出现复发，但多半为多灶性疾病。至今未见转移或死亡的病例报道。

病理学特征

这种病变界限清楚，且有部分包膜。多数有导管、腺体和腺泡排列成小叶状结构（图7.72）。硬化性间质内有局灶性淋巴细胞浸润。腺上皮细胞显示一系列的泡沫状、顶浆分泌样腺体和黏液性表现。某些细胞含有大而鲜亮的嗜酸性颗粒（图7.73A）。可有不同程度的上皮增生，形成实性细胞巢和筛状结构。还有类似于硬化性腺病的缩窄的小管（图7.73B）。40%～75%的病例可见导管上皮非典型性，从轻度异型增生到原位癌均有报道[194-199a]。

免疫组织化学显示，腺腔上皮细胞表达CEA、BRST-2、雌激素受体（20%）和孕激素受体（80%），但不表达c-erbB2[199]。在导管和腺泡周围可见一层连续的肌上皮细胞[199a]。

腮腺多囊性疾病
Polycystic disease of parotid gland

腮腺多囊性（发育不全性）疾病是一种发育上的畸形，可能是闰管缺陷和扩张的结果[200-202]。多数患者表现为儿童期反复发生的腮腺肿胀。组织学上，小叶结构保留。小叶与小叶之间受累范围不同。病变由不同大小和形状的蜂窝状格子样囊肿组成，内衬扁平立方到矮柱状或顶浆分泌样细胞。偶尔腺泡单位的分泌导管与囊肿交通。囊腔内常常含有絮状分泌物，有时含有分层的细石。纤维间隔常见轻度慢性炎症浸润（图7.74）。

伴有另外间质成分的腺瘤
Adenoma with additional stromal components

淋巴腺瘤　Lymphadenoma

淋巴腺瘤是一种罕见的肿瘤，表现为腺瘤伴有致密的淋巴细胞浸润。与没有皮脂腺成分的皮脂腺淋巴瘤相

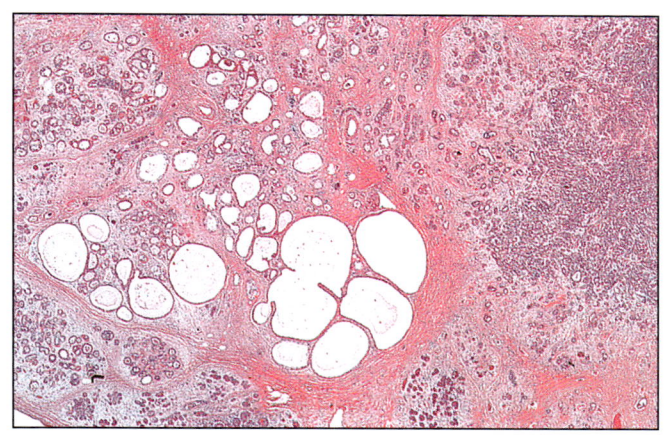

图7.72　硬化性多囊性腺病。这种病变一般与正常涎腺实质（没有显示）界限分明。小叶结构尚存。间质硬化，且有囊肿集聚。视野右侧显示细胞比较丰富。

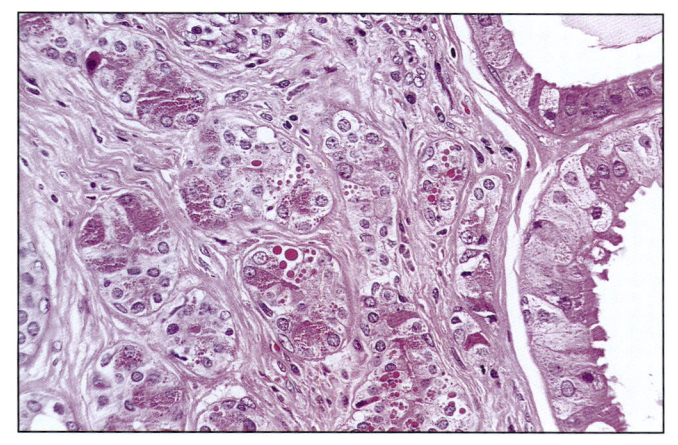

A

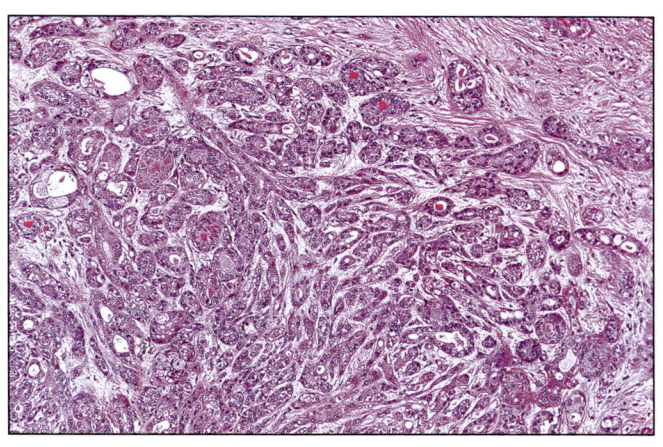

B

图7.73　硬化性多囊性腺病。（A）某些管泡状单位内衬顶浆分泌腺样细胞，其内充满鲜亮的嗜酸性透明小体。（B）富于细胞的区域由密集排列的狭窄小管构成，类似于乳腺的硬化性腺病。

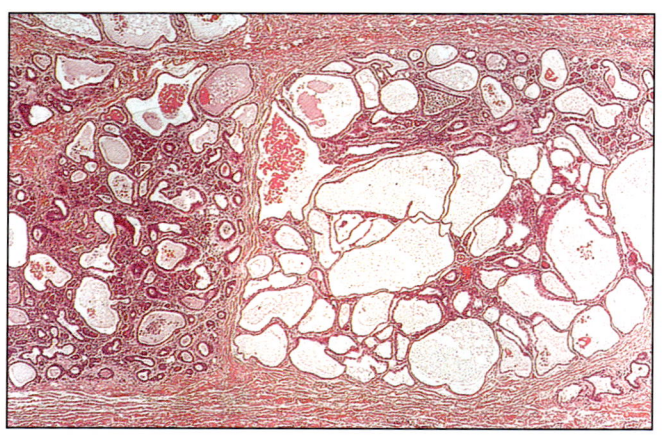

图7.74 腮腺多囊性（发育不全性）疾病。小叶结构尚存，但不同大小的囊肿取代了正常的小叶导管单位。由扩张导管形成的囊肿内衬扁平上皮细胞。

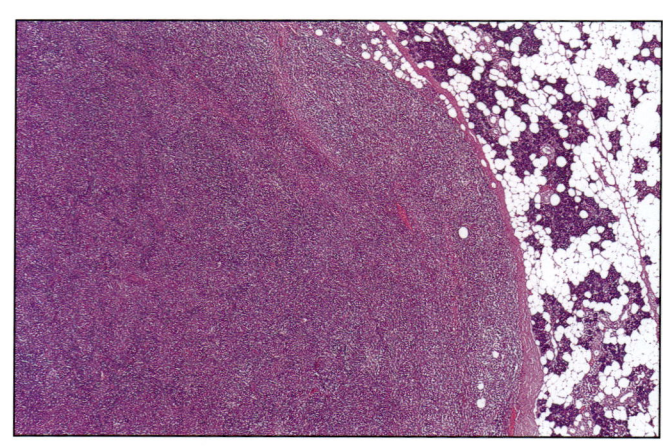

图7.75 淋巴腺瘤。肿瘤一般局限，并有大量淋巴细胞浆细胞浸润。

似。淋巴腺瘤很可能不是一种独特的肿瘤类型，而只不过是一种伴有重度淋巴细胞浸润的基底细胞腺瘤或囊腺瘤[203,204]。所有病例均见于男性患者的腮腺，年龄从17岁到57岁。完全手术切除可以治愈。

病理学特征：肿瘤为腺瘤性增生，伴有致密的淋巴细胞浸润（图7.75）。一般认为后者是肿瘤相关性淋巴组织增生，因此可以排除发生在淋巴结内的普通的涎腺腺瘤。上皮成分可以表现为相互吻合的小梁、岛屿、实性小管、充满蛋白性物质的囊性扩张的腺体，或乳头状结构。内衬囊肿或腺体的细胞为立方形或柱状细胞，没有显著的细胞学非典型性。小梁由基底细胞样细胞组成。在某些病例，上皮成分可被淋巴细胞掩盖，PAS-淀粉酶可以用来标记上皮岛周围的基底膜样物质（图7.76）。

淋巴腺瘤可与淋巴上皮癌鉴别，它缺乏浸润性生长，缺乏明确的核非典型性或显著的核分裂活性，至少有局灶性的导管分化，并且缺乏EB病毒相关性。简而言之，淋巴腺瘤是腺体肿瘤，而淋巴上皮癌是鳞状上皮相关性肿瘤。淋巴腺瘤可与淋巴上皮性涎腺炎(lymphoepithelial sialadenitis，LESA)鉴别，前者边界清楚，并有增生的上皮成分。

脂肪腺瘤（涎腺脂肪瘤） Lipoadenoma（sialolipoma）

脂肪腺瘤，也称涎腺脂肪瘤，是一种主要由脂肪组织组成的良性肿瘤，混有数量不等的腺瘤性成分。

受累患者年龄范围广泛（20～75岁，平均54.5岁），且男性好发。临床一般表现为缓慢生长的无症状的腮腺肿块，或偶尔发生在腭部。完全手术切除之后不再复发。

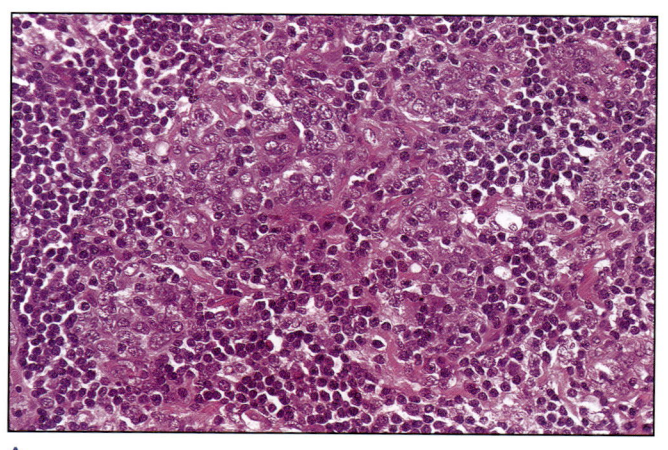

A

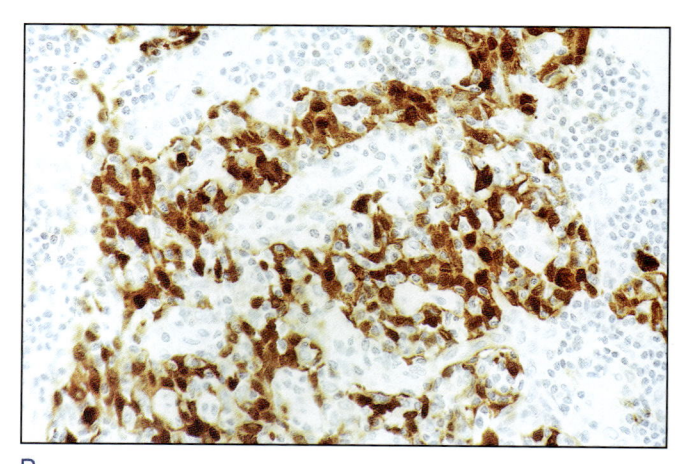

B

图7.76 淋巴腺瘤。（A）表现为实性小管和小梁结构的上皮成分被淋巴成分掩盖。（B）S-100蛋白免疫染色显示管腔外的上皮成分明显阳性。

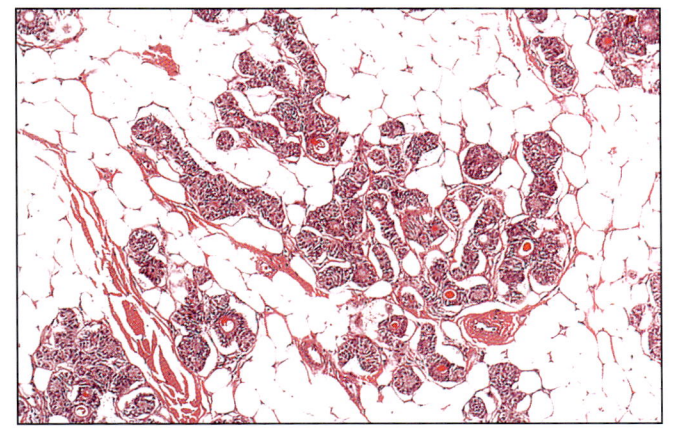

图7.77 脂肪腺瘤。在这个局限性的肿瘤中，"Sertroli形"狭窄的小管与丰富的成熟脂肪细胞混合存在。

病理学上，脂肪腺瘤有薄的被膜包被或为局限性，由成熟的脂肪组织和良性的涎腺组织组成，前者通常占肿瘤组织的90%以上。腺体成分与脂肪界限分明，由正常的导管-腺泡单位组成，没有细胞非典型性或增生活性，或表现出腺瘤性特征，形成Sertoli形小管。可见局灶性的嗜酸细胞改变，导管扩张伴有纤维化以及皮脂腺或鳞状化生（图7.77）[205,208]。目前还不清楚腺体成分是陷入的涎腺组织还是肿瘤的一部分。

腺纤维瘤 Adenofibroma

腺纤维瘤是一种非常罕见的肿瘤，由增生的腺瘤性腺体混有显著的富于细胞的间质组成，间质中纤细的梭形细胞CD34阳性，但缺乏肌上皮特征（S-100、肌动蛋白和p63阴性）。

黏液表皮样癌 Mucoepidermoid carcinoma

定义

黏液表皮样癌，以前叫做"黏液表皮样肿瘤"，是一种浸润性的恶性肿瘤，由分泌黏液的细胞、表皮样细胞和中间性细胞以不同比例组合而成，形成囊肿和实性细胞岛。这是成人和儿童最常见的涎腺恶性肿瘤[65]。

临床特征

这种肿瘤一般表现为缓慢生长的无痛性肿块。大约三分之一的患者有触痛、疼痛、同侧耳内排液、吞咽困难和牙关紧闭。除了高分级的肿瘤以外，面瘫不常见[14]。发病年龄从10岁之前到80～90岁，高峰年龄在30～40岁。有轻微的女性好发倾向。腮腺（45%）和腭（21%）是最常见的发病部位[65]。

黏液表皮样癌是广岛和长崎原子能爆炸幸存者中放射相关性涎腺癌主要的组织学类型[150]。这种肿瘤在接受高剂量和低剂量放射治疗的儿童白血病和头癣患者中的发病率也有增加[209,210]。

黏液表皮样癌在鼻腔、鼻旁窦、鼻咽、乳腺、支气管、胸腺和皮肤中已有描述[211-216]。颌骨中心性黏液表皮样癌可能来源于牙源性囊肿内衬上皮的恶性转化。这种肿瘤一般表现为无症状的可透射线的病变。它通常显示低级别的恶性行为和组织学改变。

大体表现

黏液表皮样癌表现为界限不清的肿块，可有部分包膜，质地硬韧。可能有散在的囊肿，其内含有黏液或血性液体。

显微镜下表现

大多数病例表现为不规则的浸润性边缘，至少为局灶性（图7.78）。肿瘤由不规则分布的充满黏液的囊肿和肿瘤细胞巢组成，肿瘤细胞巢由不同比例的黏液细胞、鳞状（表皮样）细胞和不能归类的中间性细胞构成（图7.79）。间质的特征是硬化而且丰富，伴有慢性炎性细胞浸润，偶尔有外渗的黏液池（图7.78和图7.80）。这种间质改变最常见于低级别和中级别的黏液表皮样癌。极少情况下，可能有致密的淋巴浆细胞样浸润，混有肿瘤细胞岛，间质中散在多核巨细胞，或黑色素沉积[203,217,218]。

低级别黏液表皮样癌（Low-grade mucoepidermoid carcinoma）：肿瘤的大部分是由不同大小的、充满黏液的囊性结构组成的，且有丰富的黏液细胞（图7.81A）。然而，几乎总是存在不规则形状的上皮细胞岛（图7.79）。肿瘤

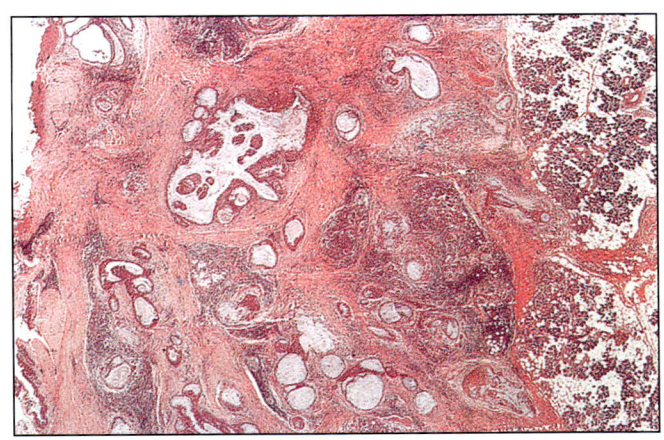

图7.78 低级别黏液表皮样癌。本图显示该肿瘤原型的低倍镜下表现：浸润性的边界（视野右侧为残留的腮腺组织），致密的纤维化背景伴有慢性炎性细胞集聚，囊肿和实性肿瘤细胞岛，以及黏液出现。

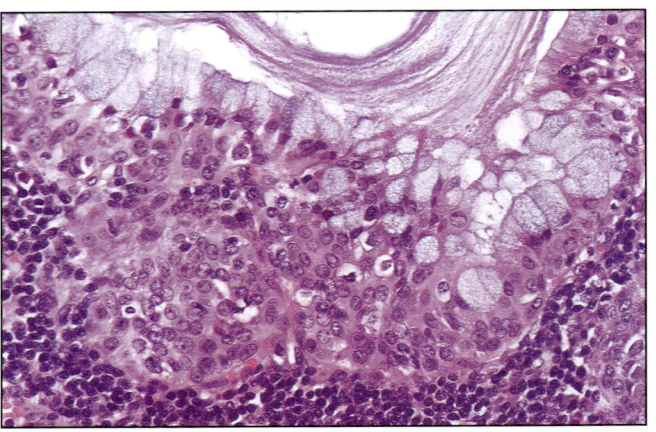

图7.79 黏液表皮样癌，低级别。组成细胞包括黏液细胞、中间性细胞和鳞片状细胞。细胞核一般呈良性表现。

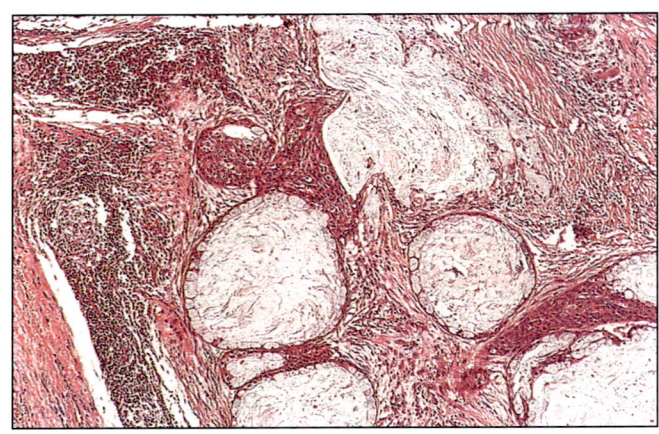

图7.80 黏液表皮样癌，低级别。其特征为囊性肿瘤岛位于慢性炎性纤维性间质中。有外渗到间质中的黏液（右上视野）；炎症和纤维化可能是由外渗的黏液引起的。

细胞有良性表现的细胞核，且很少见到核分裂象（图7.79）。

黏液细胞大，为柱状、杯状或伴有丰富黏液的多角形细胞，胞浆呈毛玻璃样表现（图7.81B）。通过黏液卡红或淀粉酶-PAS染色容易发现细胞内的黏液。黏液细胞可以形成密集排列的细胞巢，内衬囊肿结构，或散在分布于鳞状细胞巢中。

另外一种主要类型的细胞是中间性细胞，为小到中等大小的多角形细胞，具有不能归类的表现（图7.79）。推测它是黏液细胞和表皮样细胞共同的前体细胞[219]。中间性细胞形成细胞巢和成片分布，而且常常混合在其他类型的细胞中。

鳞片状（表皮样）细胞出现在细胞巢中或内衬囊性间隙。它们具有分层的表现，但细胞间桥常常并不明显（图7.79）。尤其是从来没有角化或角珠形成。

含有黏液的囊肿可以破裂，黏液进入间质，引起炎症反应，随后出现硬化。淋巴细胞浸润可能明显，伴有淋巴滤泡形成,类似于淋巴结内的转移性病变（图7.80）。

高级别黏液表皮样癌（High-grade mucoepidermoid carcinoma）：高级别黏液表皮样癌含有较多的实性区域，几乎没有囊性间隙，且常见神经周围和血管浸润。实性区域是由伴有淡染到嗜酸性胞浆和明显细胞边缘的大的多角形鳞片状（表皮样）细胞和不能归类的中间性细胞组成的（图7.82）。与低级别黏液表皮样癌相比，鳞状特征常常更加明显，可能有细胞间桥甚至单个细胞角化，但是角珠罕见。细胞多形性，细胞核深染以及核分裂象显著，而且可以出现凝固性坏死区域。黏液细胞通常稀少，可能需要进行黏液染色辨认它们。一般来说，高级

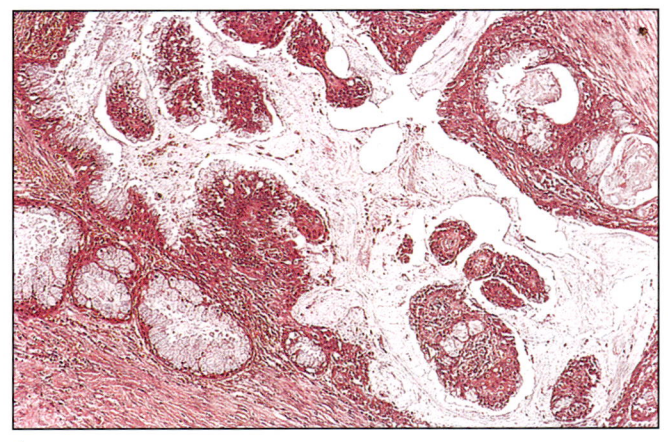

A

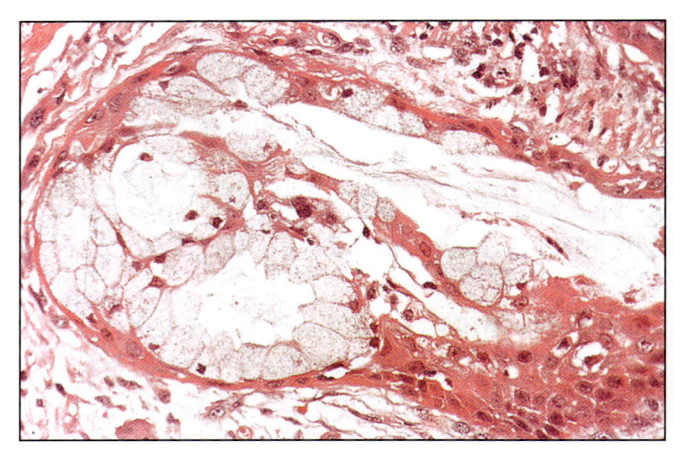

B

图7.81 黏液表皮样癌，低级别。（A）囊性肿瘤岛腔内可以形成乳头状皱褶。内衬囊性间隙的细胞常常是黏液细胞，伴有轻度嗜碱性的胞浆。（B）这个囊性肿瘤岛是由黏液细胞和鳞片状细胞混合组成的。在鳞片状细胞中有模糊的细胞间桥。如同低级别黏液表皮样癌的特征一样，肿瘤细胞也呈良性表现。

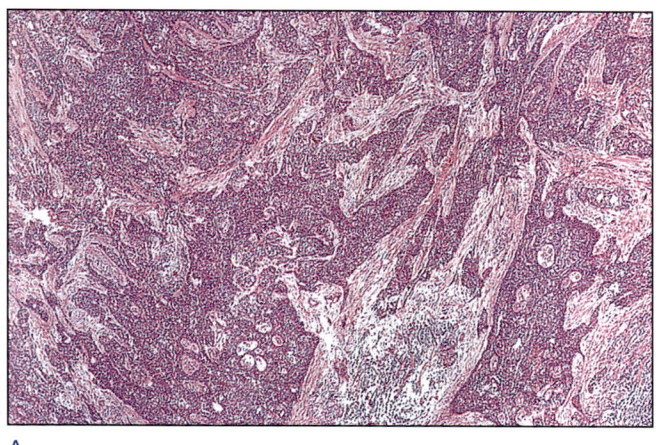
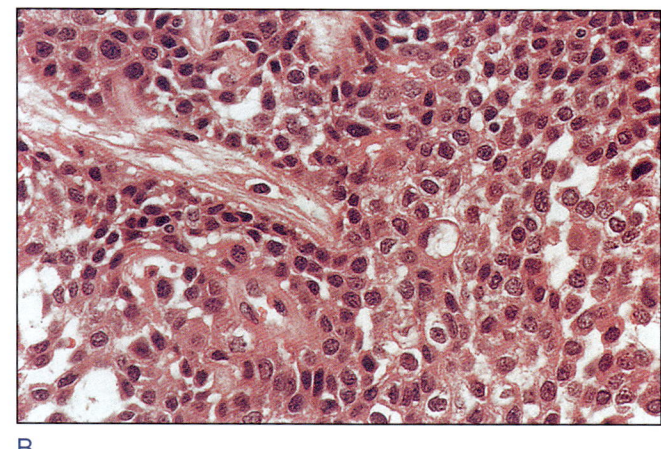

图7.82 黏液表皮样癌，高级别。（A）肿瘤生长成相互吻合的不规则的实性细胞岛，缺乏散在的囊性间隙。（B）高倍镜下显示表皮样细胞伴有细胞间桥，细胞核有中度多形性。有少数散布的空泡状细胞。

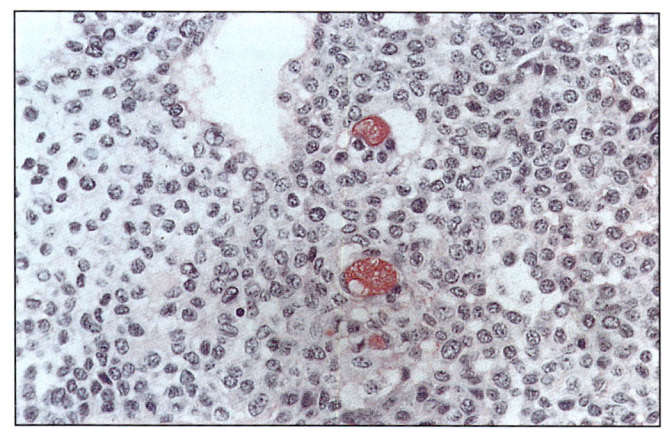

图7.83 黏液表皮样癌，高级别，黏液卡红染色（与图7.82为同一病例）。在这个以鳞片状肿瘤为主的病例中，常常需要黏液染色证实存在分泌黏液的细胞。

别肿瘤的纤维性间质或慢性炎症浸润不如低级别肿瘤明显。极少情况下，出现低级别黏液表皮样癌成分，提示高级别肿瘤是通过分化进行性丧失而发生的。

中级别黏液表皮样癌（Intermediate-grade mucoepidermoid carcinoma）：中级别肿瘤的组织学表现处于低级别肿瘤和高级别肿瘤之间。囊性间隙不是肿瘤的主要组成部分。肿瘤细胞具有某种程度的细胞核多形性（图7.84）。中级别肿瘤的表皮样特征一般比低分级肿瘤明显。

黏液表皮样癌的变型（Variants of mucoepidermoid carcinoma）：伴有不连续细胞膜，丰富的透明胞浆和偏心细胞核的大的多角形透明细胞是大多数黏液表皮样癌的次要成分（图7.85A）。胞浆透明是由于糖原集聚造成的。偶尔，这些细胞构成肿瘤的主要成分，因此，它需要与其他透明细胞肿瘤鉴别。位于透明细胞岛周围部分的细胞常常较小，伴有嗜酸性胞浆，呈鳞片状表现。透

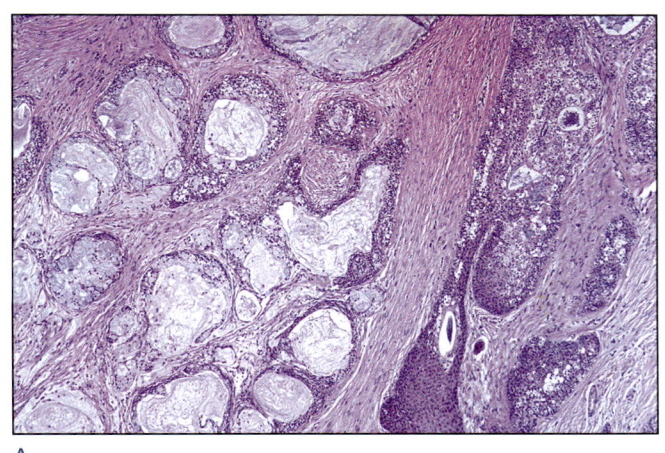
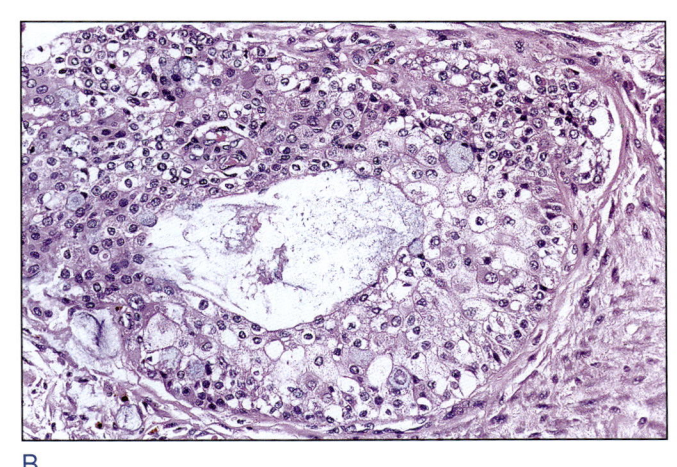

图7.84 黏液表皮样癌，中级别。（A）实性和囊性肿瘤岛浸润纤维性间质。与低级别肿瘤相比，囊性间隙不是突出成分。（B）以中间性细胞和鳞片状细胞为主，偶尔伴有散在的黏液细胞。有轻到中度细胞核的非典型性。

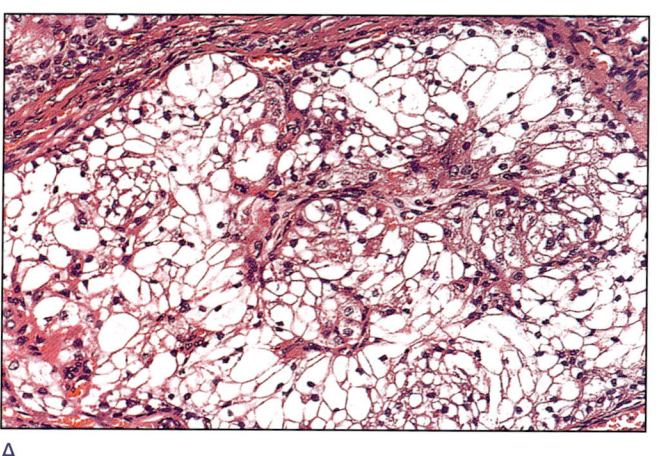
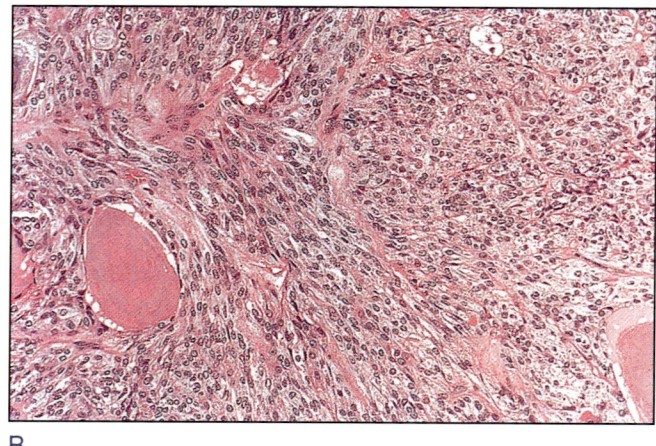

图7.85 黏液表皮样癌变型。（A）透明细胞具有清楚的细胞膜和水样透明的胞浆。（B）梭形细胞束（视野左侧）位于多角形细胞之间。

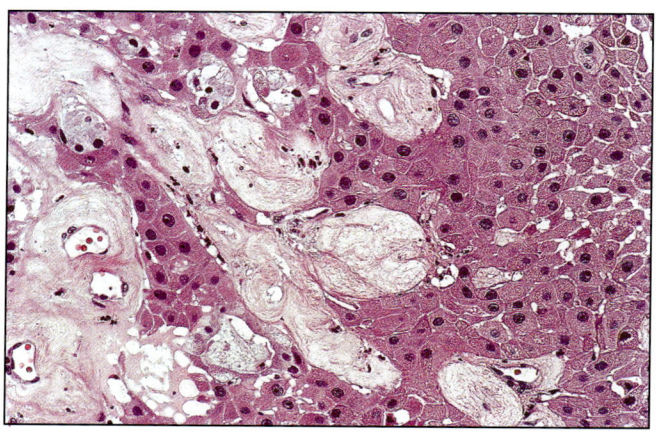

图7.86 黏液表皮样癌的嗜酸细胞变型。这种变型可能被误诊为嗜酸细胞瘤。

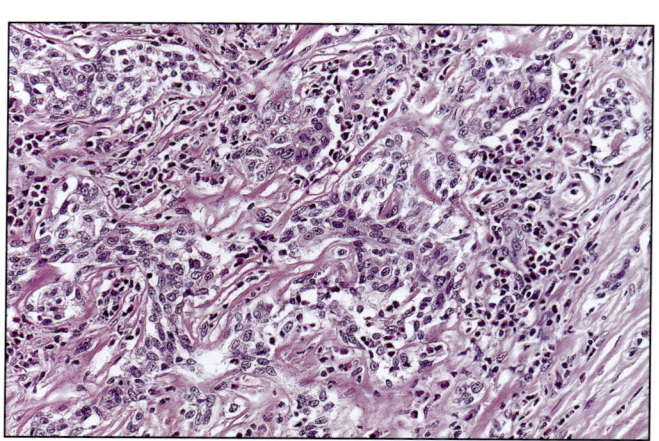

图7.87 伴有嗜酸细胞增多的硬化性黏液表皮样癌。这种腮腺肿瘤由鳞片状细胞岛和小梁组成，浸润富于淋巴细胞和嗜酸性细胞的硬化性间质。黏液细胞散布在某些肿瘤细胞岛中（没有显示）。

明细胞变型似乎较常见于腭部。

在某些黏液表皮样癌中可见少数局灶性的梭形和嗜酸细胞改变（图7.85B）。罕见的嗜酸细胞变型（嗜酸细胞占所有细胞的60％以上）可能与嗜酸细胞瘤混淆（图7.86）[220,221]。

硬化性变型表现为中央显著的瘢痕样硬化和周围的淋巴细胞浸润。由于肿瘤细胞岛稀少，且常常局限于周边部位，因此这种变型可能被误诊为炎症性病变[222-225]。

伴有嗜酸细胞增多的硬化性黏液表皮样癌的特征是肿瘤细胞岛散布在硬化性的间质中，伴有致密的慢性炎性细胞和嗜酸细胞浸润（图7.87）[226]。它与相应的同样命名的甲状腺肿瘤以及普通的涎腺黏液表皮样癌的关系还不清楚[227]。

免疫组织化学

肿瘤细胞细胞角蛋白染色阳性。EMA、CEA 和 S-100 可能有不同程度的染色。中间性细胞、鳞片状细胞和透明细胞 p63 免疫反应可能阳性[48]，但肌上皮标记物阴性，例如肌动蛋白和钙调节蛋白[228]。与鳞状细胞癌不同，黏液表皮样癌 CK7 通常阳性[229]。

遗传学特征

分别涉及位于19号和11号染色体的黏液表皮样癌易位1（MECT1）和策划样基因家族（MAML2）的易位，是黏液表皮样癌最常见的遗传学改变[230]，而且使 Notch 信号通路中断[231]。通过原位杂交和 RT-PCR 检测在多达70％的病例中可以发现基因融合，可以用于黏液表皮样癌的辅助诊断[232]。在 Warthin 瘤中没有发现这种改变，虽然以往曾那样认为[233,234]。

预后因子

黏液表皮样癌的行为与临床分期和组织学分级密切

表7.6　黏液表皮样癌：标准的三级分级系统

分级的组织学参数	低级别	中级别	高级别
囊肿	许多大囊和小囊	有一些囊肿	极少有囊肿
黏液细胞	许多	有些	很少
核分裂象	很少	很少或有些	许多
细胞学	普通	有些非典型性	显著的细胞多形性
生物学潜能	局灶性浸润；缓慢生长	中间性	高度浸润；迅速生长
复发	0～6%	20%～39%	61%～78%
转移	非常少见	某些病例（淋巴结22%）	常见（44%～72%；常常见于淋巴结；远处转移33%）
5年生存率	92%	70%～83%	22%～42%

表7.7　黏液表皮样癌：AFIP分级系统（仅应用于口腔内和腮腺肿瘤）[237,238]

参数	评分
囊内成分<20%	+2
神经浸润	+2
坏死	+3
核分裂象≥4/10高倍视野	+3
间变（核的多形性，核-浆比例增加，核仁大，色素不均，核深染）	+4

总评分	说明	在所有黏液表皮样癌中出现的频率	复发率	局部淋巴结转移	死于肿瘤
0～4	低级别	84%	7.5%	2.5%	0%
5～6	中级别	9%	8.3%	0%	8.3%
7～14	高级别	7%	40%	70%	60%

相关。这种肿瘤可以治愈，尤其是低级别和中级别的肿瘤（图7.6）。几种二级或三级的分级系统正在应用（表7.6和图7.7）[223,235-241]。最近，一种应用5种组织病理学特征的新的分级系统已经显示出具有可重复性和预后意义[237,242,243]。不过，最新的Mayo Clinic研究表明，如果实行了根治性手术，则分级和分期并不重要[244]。

颌下腺黏液表皮样癌具有显著的转移潜能，不管组织学分级如何。例如，13%的低级别肿瘤患者死于肿瘤[237,238]。增生指数高（核分裂象>2/10 HPF，或MIB1指数大于10%）、MUC1的表达、血管浸润、边缘受累以及非整倍体也和预后不良有关[239,245-248]。

鉴别诊断

大涎腺黏液囊肿非常罕见。当大涎腺出现伴有纤维化和慢性炎症的不能解释的黏液池时，最有可能的诊断就是低级别黏液表皮样癌。广泛取材通常会显示诊断性的肿瘤细胞岛。

应该考虑在鉴别诊断中的肿瘤（见"诊断分析方法"一节，第310页）是：

1. 伴有鳞状/黏液化生的Warthin瘤
2. 伴有鳞状分化的多形性腺瘤
3. 囊腺瘤或囊腺癌
4. 低分化腺癌（与高级别黏液表皮样癌）
5. 鳞状细胞癌。支持黏液表皮样癌诊断而不是鳞状细胞癌的特征包括：可见散在的黏液性肿瘤细胞（例如通过组织化学染色）、显著的硬化性而不是纤维组织增生性间质、出现低级别黏液表皮样癌成分、CK7免疫反应以及MUC5AC免疫反应[248]。

腺样囊性癌　Adenoid cystic carcinoma

定义

腺样囊性癌是一种侵袭性肿瘤，主要由伴有肌上皮/基底细胞分化的基底细胞样细胞组成，伴有散在的导管结构。它的特征是表现为筛状、管状和（或）实性生长方式，并具有黏液玻璃样间质[249]。

临床特征

腺样囊性癌最常出现在 30～40 岁到 50～60 岁的患者，有轻微的女性好发的趋势（男女之比为 2：3）。腮腺、颌下腺和腭是最常受累。该肿瘤也可以发生在泪腺、耳道、上呼吸道、肺、消化道、皮肤、乳腺、前列腺和女性下生殖道[250-255]。

临床上，最常见的主诉是缓慢生长的肿块。大的肿瘤常常固定于皮肤或较深部的组织。由于肿瘤有显著的浸润神经的倾向，所以也可能出现触痛、疼痛和面神经麻痹[256]。腭的肿瘤常常有溃疡形成。可能发生骨的浸润而没有影像学上的改变，因为肿瘤通过骨髓间隙浸润。肿瘤常常侵犯到临床上明显的边界以外[249,257,264]。

虽然腺样囊性癌一般呈惰性表现，但是长期预后不良（图7.4）。5 年生存率大约是 60%～75%，但 10 年生存率却降至 30%～54%[12,14,37]。多数受累患者（80%～95%）经过长期的临床过程最终死于本病，其特征为反复的局部复发和转移[249,265]。远处转移（最常见于肺、骨和软组织）比局部淋巴结转移常见[266]，而且经常发生在最初治疗以后 5～10 年[267]。治疗选择根治性手术切除，放射治疗的作用尚未得到证实[256,268]。

病理学

大体，肿瘤为褐色、鱼肉样、硬韧的浸润性肿块。组织学检查通常可见明显的浸润性生长，神经周围浸润非常常见（图 7.88）。在同一个病例中可以出现不同比例的 3 种特征性的生长方式（筛状、管状和实性）。与多形性腺瘤不同，没有基底细胞样细胞"融入"间质的现象（图 7.89）。间质是纤维性的，伴有不同量的黏液玻璃样物质而不是纤维组织增生性间质，没有软骨形成。有时广泛的玻璃样变性导致肿瘤细胞岛"缩窄"，以致只有少数肿瘤细胞残留，或产生缎带样结构（图 7.90）。

筛状结构：筛状结构是腺样囊性癌最具特征的表现。筛状结构几乎总是存在，但有时非常局灶。筛状结构是大小不同、外形光滑的散在或融合的细胞岛，由小而一致的基底细胞样细胞组成，并有圆形间隙，导致"瑞士干酪样"表现。大多数间隙不是腺腔，而是间质内陷（假

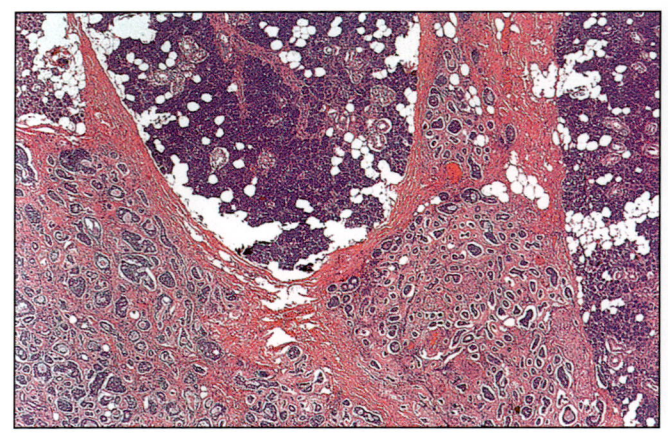

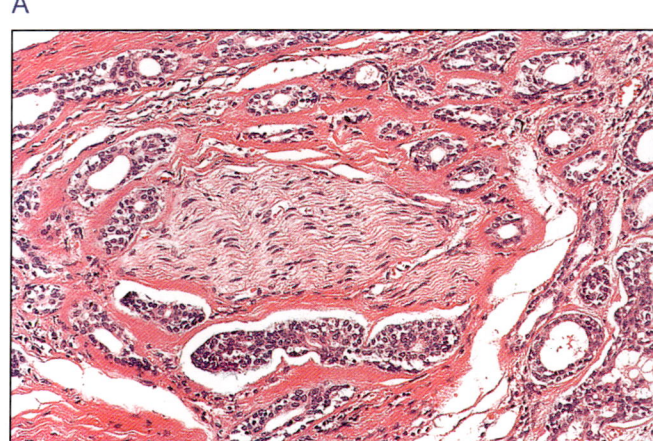

图7.88　腺样囊性癌。（A）本图描绘该肿瘤原型的低倍镜下表现：浸润性边缘，管状和筛状结构以及硬化性或玻璃样变的间质。（B）神经周围浸润是常见的特征。

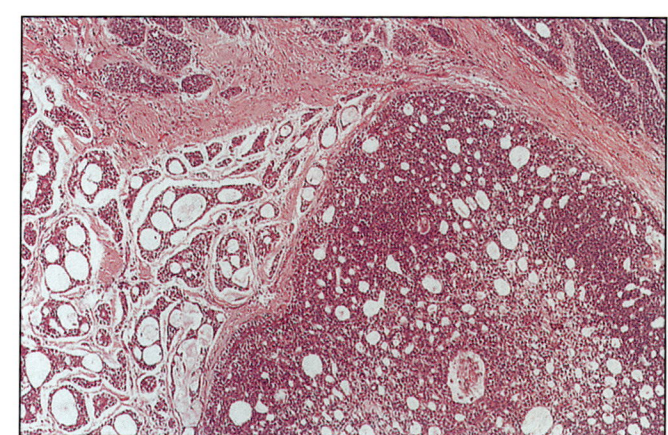

图7.89　腺样囊性癌。这种肿瘤常常显示不同部位形态差异很大。视野左侧以小的筛状结构为主，而视野右侧被大的筛状结构占据。视野上部显示某些实性细胞岛。

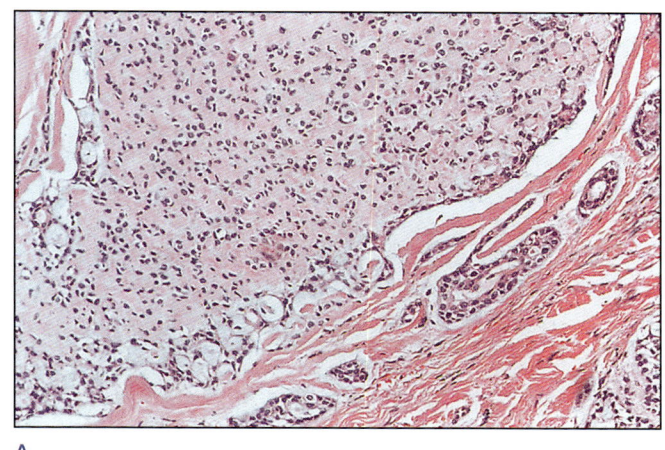
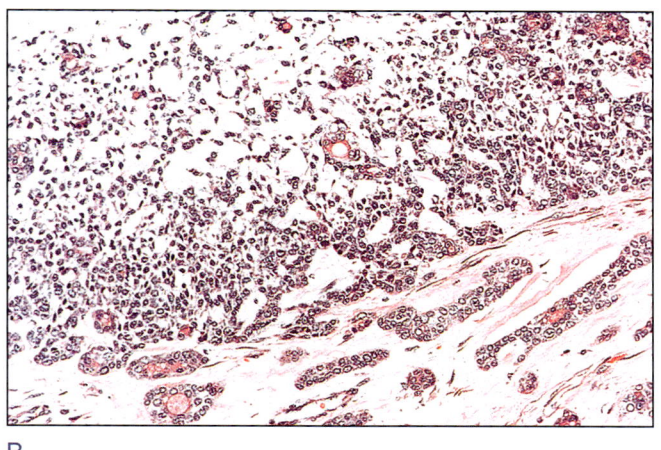

图7.90 腺样囊性癌，伴有玻璃样变性或黏液样改变，类似于多形性腺瘤。（A）筛状岛（视野上部和左侧）显示丰富的玻璃样物质沉淀，伴有肿瘤细胞"缩窄"。如果腺样囊性癌显示如同本例一样广泛的玻璃样变，可能难以作出诊断。这种形态不同于多形性腺瘤的玻璃样变，后者玻璃样变局限于细胞岛中，与纤维性间质界限分明。（B）筛状岛（视野上部）显示黏液样改变，类似于见于多形性腺瘤的"融合"结构。与后者不同，这种改变局限于大的细胞岛，而细胞岛本身与间质界限分明。

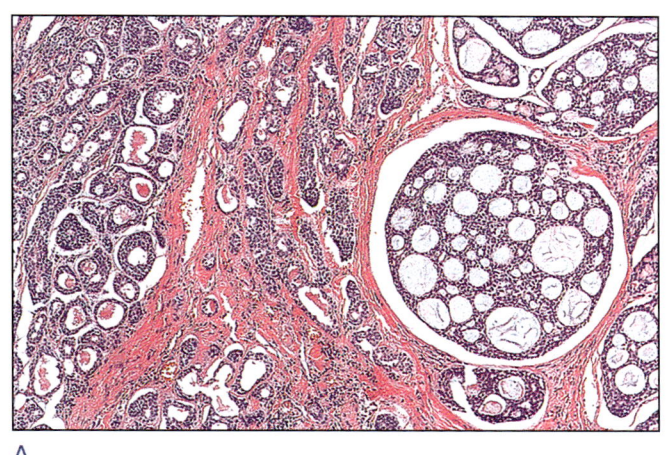
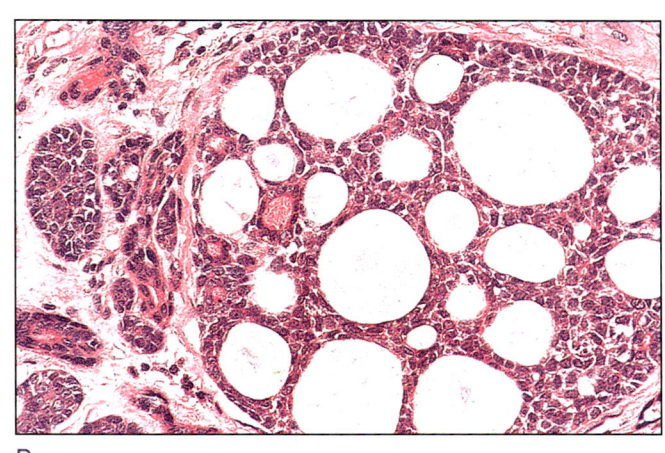

图7.91 腺样囊性癌，筛状型。（A）可见筛状结构（视野右侧）和某些管状结构（视野左侧）。单单这个视野与多形性腺瘤或基底细胞腺瘤不能区分。（B）在这个筛状结构中，实际上所有的间隙均为假囊肿，周围绕以基底细胞样（改变了的肌上皮）细胞。间隙中充满弱嗜碱性的黏液。左侧出现少数小的真正的腺体间隙。

囊肿）；有时可以与间质连续。这些间隙充满嗜酸性玻璃样物质（PAS阳性，抗淀粉酶）和（或）轻微嗜碱性的黏液样物质（阿尔辛蓝阳性）（图7.89，图7.91和图7.92）。超微结构上，这些物质是糖胺聚糖和重复的基底膜。这些筛状岛内偶尔可见真正狭窄的腺体，内衬伴有嗜酸性胞浆的矮立方细胞（图7.91A）。沿着腔缘可以出现嗜酸性薄膜，而腺腔内可能含有PAS阳性抗淀粉酶的嗜酸性分泌物。偶尔，腺体结构发育不全，表现为伴有嗜酸性胞浆的空泡状细胞的小的集聚（图7.93A）。少数情况下，腺腔细胞可能表现出嗜酸细胞改变（图7.93B）。

肿瘤性基底细胞样细胞组成了主要的细胞群。它们具有圆形或成角的细胞核，胞浆稀少，细胞边界不清（图7.93A）。某些细胞可有淡染或透明的胞浆。细胞核的多

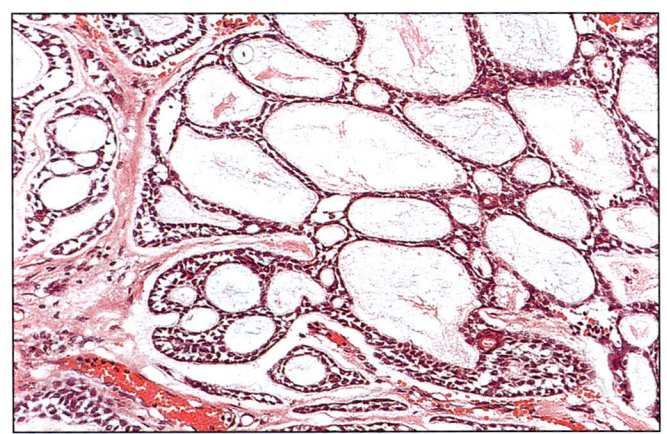

图7.92 腺样囊性癌。大的筛状结构，其间隙内充满了嗜酸性玻璃样物质或轻微嗜碱性的黏液物质。注意这种间隙与周围的间质连续（左侧）。

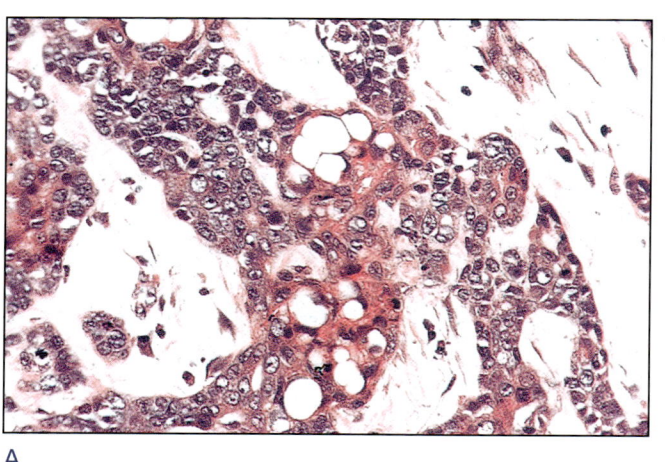 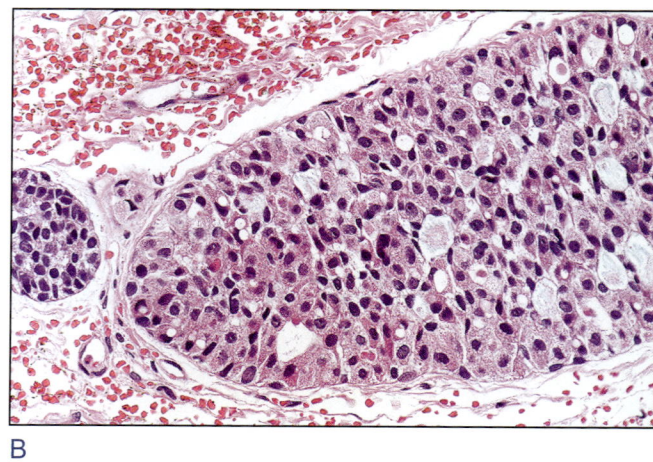

图7.93 腺样囊性癌，不常见的表现。（A）基底细胞样细胞岛中的管状结构发育不全，被描述为伴有嗜酸性胞浆的空泡状细胞团。（B）腺腔细胞呈嗜酸细胞改变。

形性一般轻微，核分裂象通常稀少或缺乏。

管状结构：细长的管状结构内衬单层导管上皮细胞，周围绕以单层或多层基底细胞样细胞。这种结构形态最容易发现腺腔。腺腔中空或含有分泌物。少数情况下腺腔可能扩张（图7.94）。管状结构可能明显地沿着自身盘绕，产生项圈样表现。管状结构常常位于丰富的玻璃样变的间质中，以致达到可能出现腺腔狭窄的程度。

实性结构：实性结构的特征是外形光滑或局灶凹凸不平的密集排列的基底细胞样细胞片块和细胞岛（图7.95）。几乎没有散在的假囊肿。与基底细胞腺癌不同，缺乏细胞核栅栏状排列。基底细胞样细胞与那些见于筛状或管状结构的细胞不同，通常具有较显著的细胞核多形性和核分裂活性。凝固性肿瘤坏死并不少见。通常几乎没有真正的腺腔（图7.88）。实性生长方式很少表现为单纯形式，如果出现单纯性结构，诊断可能非常困难[269]。

去分化腺样囊性癌
Dedifferentiated adenoid cystic carcinoma

腺样囊性癌去分化伴有巨大肿块，常常局部复发和转移，而且迅速致死[270,271]。它可以发生在原发性或复发性肿瘤。去分化成分通常是低分化腺癌，肉瘤样癌或未分化癌（图7.96）。与原来的腺样囊性癌不同，去分化成分具有不同程度的p53基因突变、Her2/neu过表达、周期蛋白D1过表达和Rb表达的缺失[27,272]。

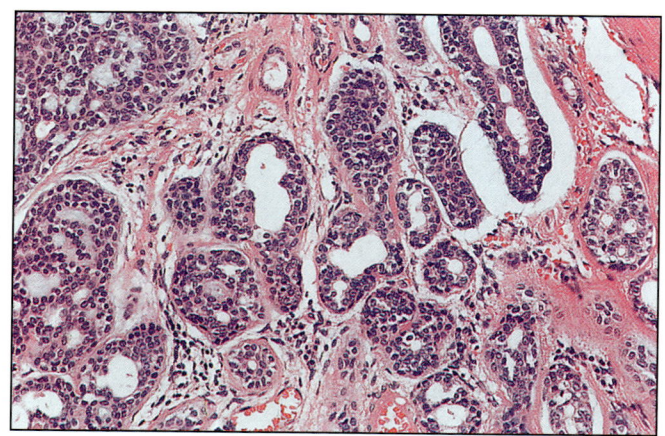 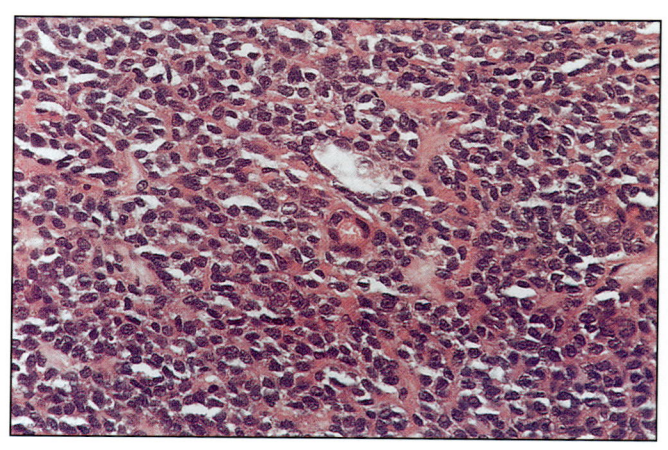

图7.94 腺样囊性癌，管状型。纤维性间质中可见散在的单管或较复杂的管状结构。腺管有一层具有嗜酸性胞浆的内层细胞和一层基底细胞样的外层细胞。单单这个视野不能与基底细胞腺瘤（管状变型）或多形性腺瘤鉴别。

图7.95 腺样囊性癌，实性变型。肿瘤主要为大的实性基底细胞样细胞岛。在基底细胞样细胞中，仅仅有少数管状结构散在分布（视野中心）。注意实性变型中的基底细胞样细胞显示比普通的腺样囊性癌具有较大程度的核非典型性。

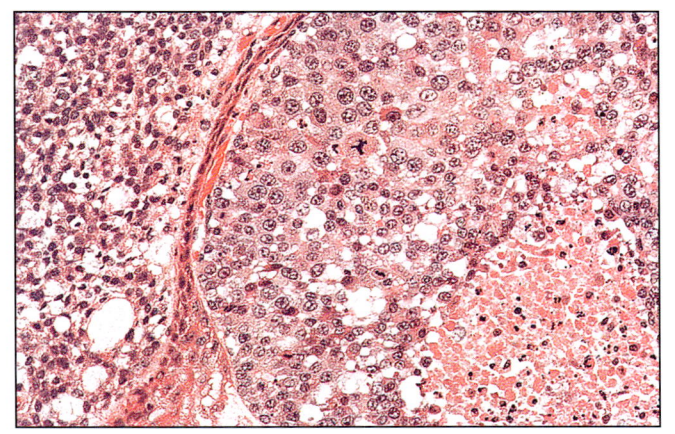

图7.96 去分化腺样囊性癌。视野左侧显示先前存在的腺样囊性癌，由基底细胞样细胞组成，伴有散布的假囊性间隙。视野右侧显示低分化（去分化）实性肿瘤，由大的多形性和核分裂活跃的细胞组成，伴有凝固性坏死。

免疫组织化学

免疫组织化学染色证实基底细胞样细胞主要为肌上皮分化。这些细胞表达细胞角蛋白、波形蛋白、S-100蛋白（通常呈片块状染色）、肌动蛋白（不同程度）、钙调节蛋白和p63[273]，而散在的导管上皮细胞表达细胞角蛋白（强阳性）、CEA、EMA和c-kit（CD117）（图7.97）。Ⅳ型胶原和层黏连蛋白染色可以显示间质玻璃样变物质。虽然导管细胞表达c-kit[274,276]，但是应用特异性酪氨酸激酶受体抑制剂（Imatinib）进行临床试验显示没有治疗效果[276]，这种结果是可以预料的，因为这些病变缺乏c-kit基因活性突变。

遗传学特征

涉及6p、9p、17p12-13的最常见的细胞遗传学畸变以及t（6；9）（q21-24；p13-23）易位在几种肿瘤中已有报告，认为这些改变至少是少数腺样囊性癌的原发性事件[274,277-280]。微卫星标记物分析显示6q23-qter、12q、13q21-q22和19q常常缺失[280]。p16启动子甲基化见于20%的病例[281]。一项25个病例的研究发现，该肿瘤常常出现6q23-25杂合性缺失，而且这种改变与临床结果不良有关[282,283]。

预后因素

组织学分级对于预后有显著的影响，这主要是由不同的生长方式决定的（表7.8）[269,284,285]。显示管状和筛状结构的肿瘤是低级别的肿瘤[269,284,285]。实性结构与肿瘤大、较早复发和常常复发、较高的转移发生率以及较早的致命性结果有关[263,265]。Yamamoto等提出假设，即实性区域是由管状和筛状区域转化而来的，伴有p53和Rb基因突变[286]，而且实性成分也较常伴有DNA非整倍体[287]。在对79例腺样囊性癌长期生存率的分析中，Szanto等发现，具有显著实性区域的癌（大于肿瘤面积的30%）累积的5年和15年生存率分别只有14%和5%，而没有显著实性成分的肿瘤分别为92%和39%[285]。

根据报道，临床分期晚、位于小涎腺、肿瘤大（大于2～4 cm）、骨浸润、切缘阳性、非二倍体DNA成分、高S期分数以及高Ki-67指数是预后不良的因素[256,263,265,268,288,289]。

鉴别诊断

由于具有重叠的形态学特征，腺样囊性癌可能难以与其他伴有明显肌上皮/基底细胞成分的涎腺肿瘤区别，例如基底细胞腺瘤/腺癌和多形性腺瘤（图7.7）（见"诊断分析方法"一节，第310页）。与上皮-肌上皮癌

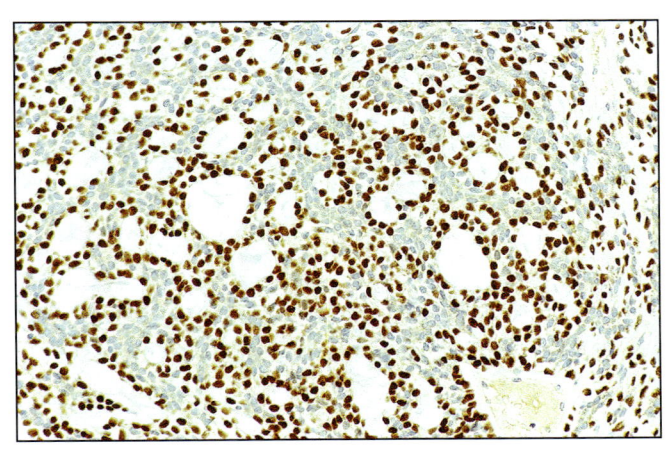
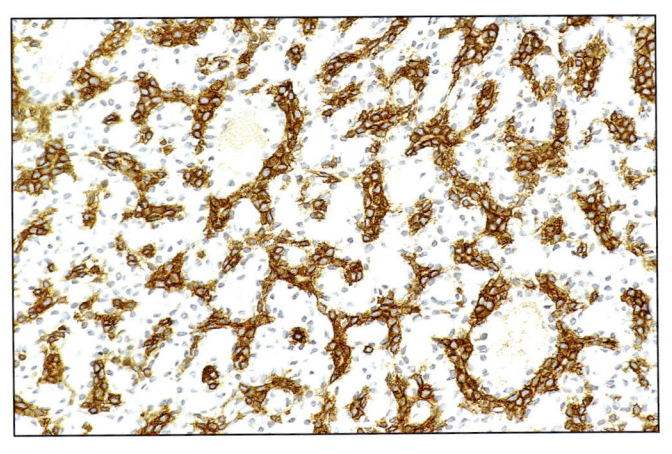

图7.97 腺样囊性癌，免疫组织化学特征。（A）腔外细胞的细胞核p63蛋白染色阳性。腔面细胞完全阴性。（B）相反，腔面细胞c-kit（CD117）免疫染色阳性。

表7.8	腺样囊性癌：分级系统（MD Anderson癌症中心和Batsakis等[284]）		
	I 级	II 级	III 级
分级标准	管状和筛状结构，没有实性区域；细胞学温和；几乎没有核分裂象	单纯性筛状结构，或混合性结构，但实性区域小于30%；与I级相比，细胞学有非典型性	实性区大于30%；通常伴有坏死；细胞非典型性和核分裂较明显
肿瘤行为	肿瘤通常小，甚至可能有包膜；可以完全切除，具有长期的临床经过	中间行为	肿瘤较大，难以完全切除；常常早期复发；常常在4年内导致死亡
15年生存率	39%	26%	5%

和多形性低级别腺癌的鉴别在其相应的章节讨论。新近研究尚未证实c-kit免疫反应对于诊断腺样囊性癌具有价值[274,275]。

通过浸润周围实质或神经以及通常以筛状结构为主，可以将腺样囊性癌与基底细胞腺瘤和多形性腺瘤鉴别开来。腺样囊性癌缺乏多形性腺瘤的"融合的"肌上皮结构和软骨样基质；在腺样囊性癌较大的肿瘤细胞岛中偶尔可以出现玻璃样变和黏液样改变，不要将其误认为"融合"现象（图7.90）。实性腺样囊性癌在与基底细胞癌和基底细胞样鳞状细胞癌的鉴别诊断中可能会出现一些特殊问题（表7.9）。

腺泡细胞癌　Acinic cell carcinoma

定义

腺泡细胞癌，以前称为"腺泡细胞肿瘤"，是一种至少具有局灶性向浆液性腺泡细胞分化的肿瘤。这种肿瘤不显示肌上皮成分。

临床特征

最常见的发生部位是腮腺（84%）和颌下腺（4%），其次为颊黏膜、上唇和上腭[65]。它是最常见的可能双侧发生的肿瘤（3%）[290]。有轻微的女性好发趋势，平

表7.9	主要由基底细胞样细胞组成的恶性肿瘤的特征对比：腺样囊性癌（实性类型），基底细胞腺癌和基底细胞样鳞状细胞癌		
	腺样囊性癌，实性变型	基底细胞腺癌	基底细胞样鳞状细胞癌
发生部位	大涎腺或小涎腺	大涎腺或小涎腺	黏膜部位，例如喉、下咽部、舌底
结构形态	虽然主要为细胞岛和弥漫性片块，但是几乎总是出现筛状结构；在某些大的实性细胞岛中可以出现粉刺样坏死	散在的拼图样细胞岛；少数可能显示小梁状或管状结构；缺乏筛状结构或非常局限；粉刺样坏死罕见	伴有花彩状的小叶和小梁状结构以及粉刺样坏死
细胞间玻璃样小滴	非常少见	常见	偶尔见到
间质或空隙内嗜碱性黏液物质	常见	少见	常见
肿瘤岛周围细胞栅栏状排列	通常不明显	常常为突出的特征	通常不明显
主要细胞类型	大部分是具有深染细胞核和单一表现的基底细胞样细胞；腔面细胞非常稀少	基底细胞样细胞包括小而深染的细胞和较大的淡染细胞；腔面细胞非常稀少	基底细胞样细胞伴有淡染和非典型性细胞核，核分裂多见；真正的腺体细胞少见
鳞状分化	少见	有时出现在细胞岛的中心	常常出现（常常表现为明显的鳞状细胞癌或原位癌）

均发病年龄是 44 岁。腺泡细胞癌在上颌窦[291]、喉[292]、下颌骨[156]、乳腺[293]、肺[294]和胰[295]也有报道。

腺泡细胞癌一般表现为缓慢生长的肿块，伴有或不伴有疼痛。面神经麻痹少见（5%～10%）[296,297]。这种惰性的肿瘤具有漫长的临床经过（图 7.4）[297-299]。在包括 65 位患者随访长达 45 年的 Mayo Clinic 系列研究中，44% 的患者有局部复发，19% 转移，25% 的患者死于本病[300]。局部复发和转移常常延缓，有时发生在最初发现 30 年后。总的 5 年生存率大概是 90%，10 年生存率 83%，20 年生存率 67%。因此，终生随访是绝对必要的，即使是在明显完全切除以后[300]。发生在小涎腺的腺泡细胞癌好像具有较好的预后[65]。治疗选择完全手术切除，如果切缘受累，则辅以术后放射治疗。

大体表现

腺泡细胞癌常常为局限性，伴有不完全的包膜，但是它可能为多结节状或浸润性。切面实性，伴有或不伴有囊性区域。

显微镜下表现

腺泡细胞癌一般形成实性肿块或多发性结节，呈宽舌状浸润。肿瘤细胞密集排列，除了偶尔有纤维性条带穿越以外，几乎没有硬化性间质（图 7.98）。可能出现淋巴细胞集聚，伴有或不伴有淋巴滤泡形成。肿瘤经常显示混合性生长方式，由重现腺泡-闰管单位的许多细胞类型组成。一般来说，细胞核呈温和表现，核分裂象罕见。

肿瘤细胞最常排列成有分支状纤细血管穿过的器官样片块，由微囊性间隙、条索、缠绕的实性或接近实性小管组成的片块以及融合的腺泡（图 7.99 和图 7.100）。缺乏正常涎腺小叶结构。

微囊性结构是最具特征性的生长方式，虽然它并不一定出现。有多发性小而空的间隙，产生花边状现象（图 7.100）。认为这些微囊性结构的形成是由于缺乏排除分泌物和破坏产物的导管，引起细胞之间液体集聚。偶尔微囊融合形成较大的囊腔。微囊性间隙不同于微腺体间隙，其周围的细胞并不围绕间隙排列。

腺泡细胞癌与其对应的良性肿瘤相似，肿瘤性腺泡细胞具有嗜碱性颗粒状胞浆和位于基底的细胞核。胞浆颗粒 PAS 阳性且抗淀粉酶，但是黏液卡红染色呈阴性反应。与正常腺泡细胞不同，这些细胞是多角形而不是三角形，细胞大小和细胞核深染差异很大，它们常常显示有不同的颗粒，即使是在同一个镜下视野内，某些细胞颗粒稀少以致难以辨认（图 7.101）。某些细胞胞浆可能呈网状或泡沫状（图 7.99）。细胞核常常排列成具有特

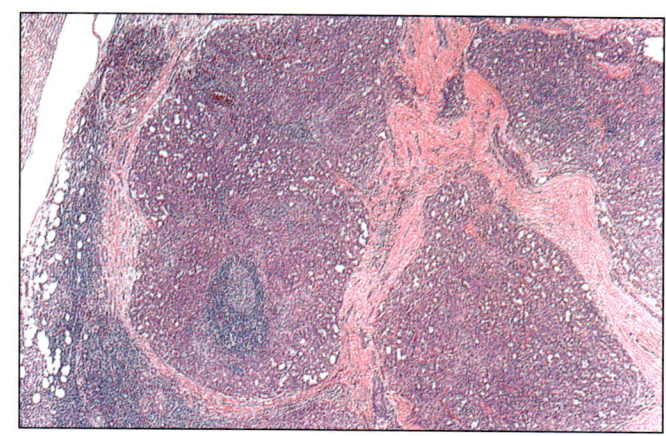

图7.98　腺泡细胞癌。本图显示这种类型肿瘤的原型表现：推挤性舌状浸润，除了肿瘤结节之间以外缺乏间质，肿瘤细胞呈紫罗兰色，微囊性间隙以及散在的淋巴细胞集聚。

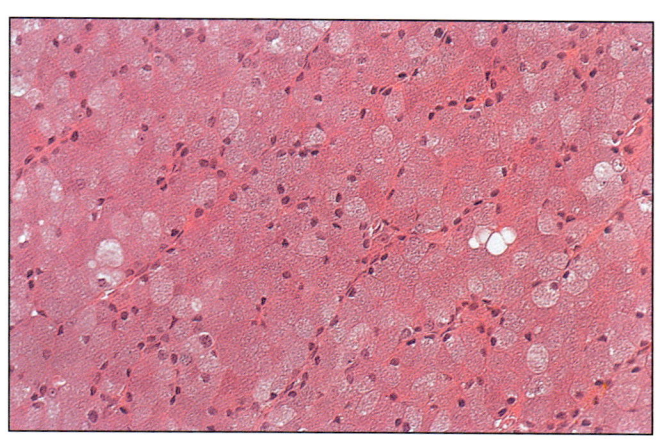

图7.99　腺泡细胞癌。多角形细胞呈实性生长，有非常纤细的血管穿过。肿瘤细胞含有非常细的嗜碱性颗粒，使胞浆呈泡沫状表现。注意细胞核成排排列。

征性的 "成排" 结构（图 7.99）[131]。胞浆内发现不同大小的空泡是这种肿瘤的重要特征。

某些肿瘤细胞类似于闰管细胞，呈立方形，细胞核位于中心，胞浆粉染。它们经常形成小的、密集排列的腺体结构（图 7.101）。还有一些非特异性腺体细胞，一般较小，胞浆嗜酸性或双染性，经常形成片状（图 7.101）。不常见的细胞类型包括伴有孤立性或多发性透明空泡的空泡细胞（图 7.102）[128]以及透明细胞（胞浆透明可能是由于组织处理造成的人工假象或细胞器的改变，而不是糖原集聚）（图 7.103）[301]。

腺泡细胞癌具有特殊的自我破坏的特性。肿瘤可以自发性或在细针穿刺吸取后发生缺血和梗死，导致继发性出血，脂肪肉芽肿性反应和（或）囊性退变[47]。在纤

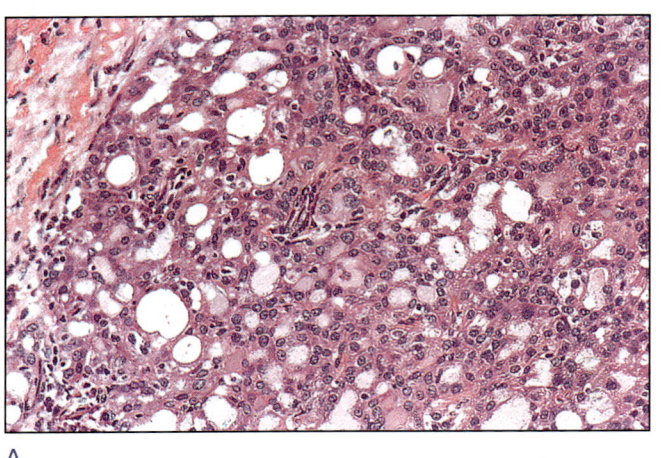
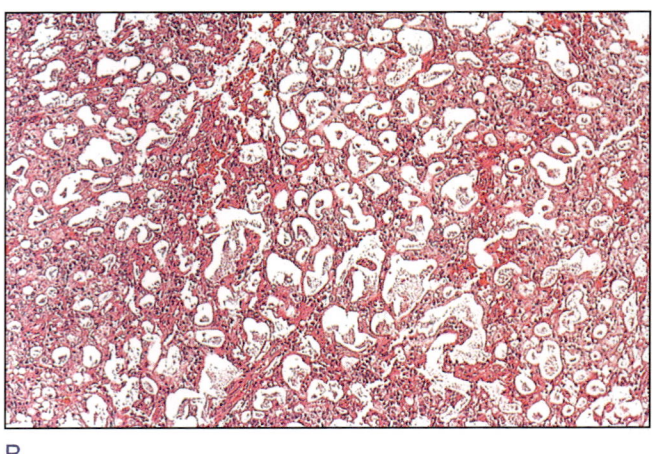

A
B

图7.100 腺泡细胞癌，显示特征性的微囊性结构。（A）实性肿瘤岛中有不规则形状的小的囊性间隙。间隙周围的细胞并不显示围绕间隙有特殊的排列；这种特征可将微囊性结构和微腺体结构区分开来。还要注意胞浆呈紫罗兰色，这在腺泡细胞常常见到。（B）本例可见较大的微囊性间隙。

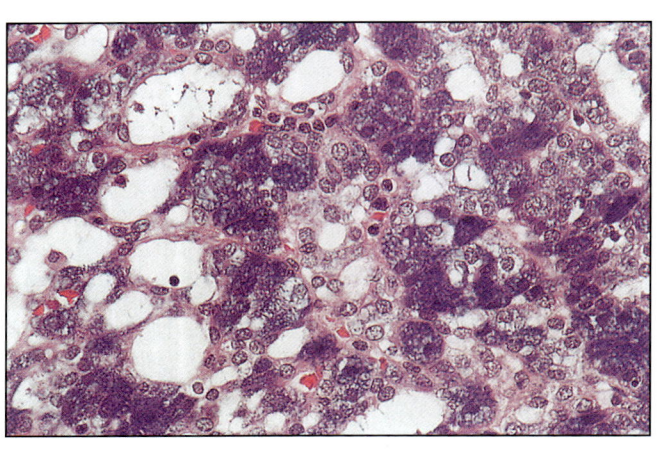
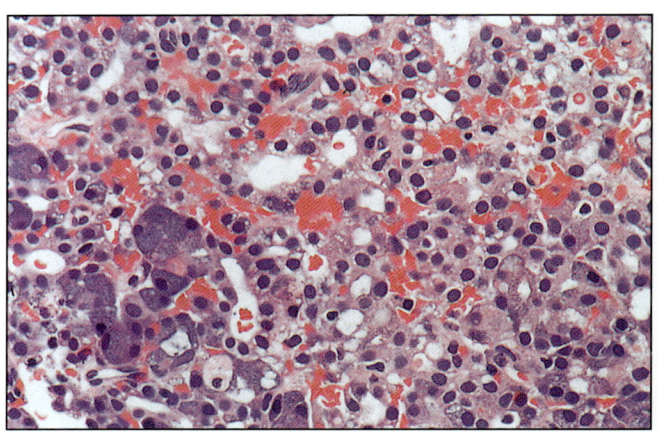

A
B

图7.101 腺泡细胞癌。即使是在同一个镜下视野中，肿瘤细胞常常出现各种胞浆颗粒。常常混合不同于腺泡细胞类型的细胞。（A）某些细胞有较多的颗粒，而其他细胞颗粒稀少或者没有颗粒。在视野中心，有明显的闰管分化，伴有小的管腔。（B）某些肿瘤细胞含有嗜碱性颗粒（左下视野）。大部分细胞为多角形，许多细胞类似于闰管细胞。注意细胞核表现温和。

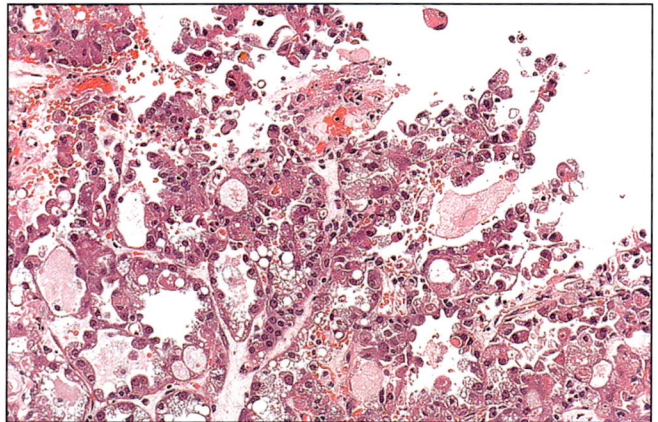

图7.102 腺泡细胞癌。有许多鞋钉细胞和一些空泡细胞。这样的细胞最常见于乳头状囊性变型。

维性间质中甚至在肿瘤细胞内常常发现含铁血黄素沉积。

乳头状囊性变型（Papillary-cystic variant）：这种罕见变型的特征是内衬单层或复层立方上皮的囊性间隙，伴有一些乳头状突起（图7.104）。乳头被覆鞋钉细胞、闰管样细胞、空泡细胞、非特异性腺体细胞以及不能归类的细胞，这种细胞具有嗜酸性或两染性胞浆，细胞核位于中心，细胞边界不清（图7.102）。可能发现也可能没有纤维血管轴心。

滤泡性变型（Follicular variant）：这种罕见的变型是由密集排列的圆形囊性间隙组成的，囊内充满均质嗜酸性胶样物质，与甲状腺滤泡非常相似（图7.105）。

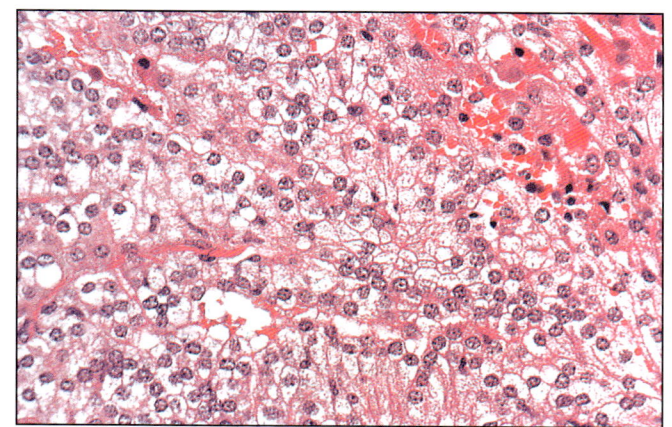

图7.103 伴有透明细胞的腺泡细胞癌。仅仅根据这个视野很难与其他透明细胞肿瘤鉴别；检查肿瘤其他部位会显示较多的诊断性形态结构。

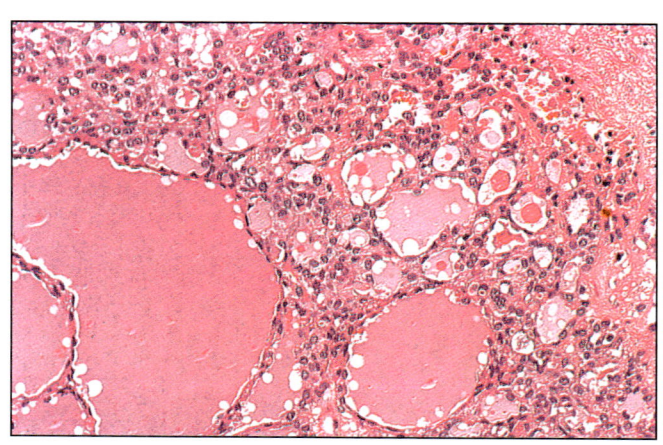

图7.105 腺泡细胞癌，滤泡性变型。这种罕见变型的特征是出现含有嗜酸性胶样物质的滤泡。与甲状腺滤泡非常相似。

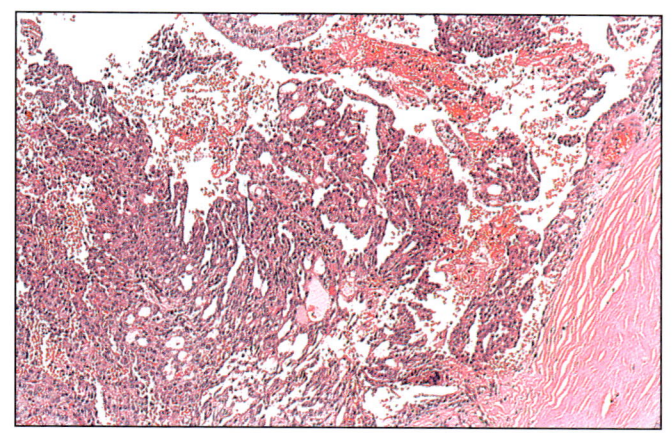

图7.104 腺泡细胞癌，乳头状囊性变型。这种变型的特征是囊腔内有乳头和假乳头状突起。

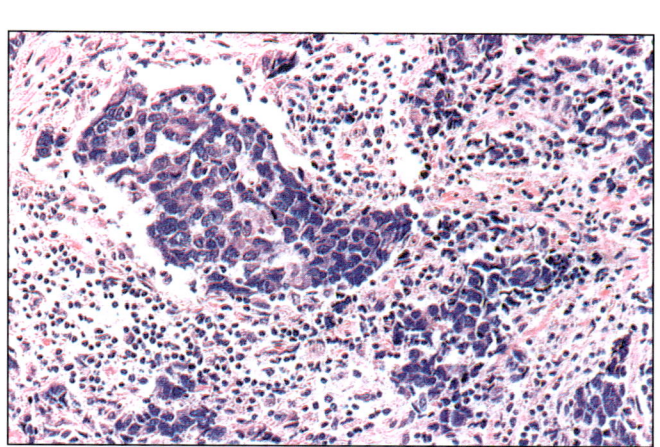

图7.106 去分化性腺泡细胞癌。这个视野显示低分化癌，辨认不出是腺泡细胞癌。肿瘤其他区域表现出典型的腺泡细胞癌（没有显示）。

胶样物质 PAS 染色强阳性且抗淀粉酶。滤泡内衬闰管样细胞和非特异性腺体细胞。甲状腺球蛋白免疫染色有助于排除甲状腺滤泡性肿瘤。

去分化性腺泡细胞癌（Dedifferentiated acinic cell carcinoma）：在少数情况下，原发性或复发性腺泡细胞癌可以去分化，成为高级别腺癌、低分化癌或未分化癌（图 7.106）。两种成分通常并列，彼此没有移行。去分化腺泡细胞癌伴有肿瘤迅速生长、明显疼痛、面神经麻痹、肿瘤巨大和预后非常不好[296,302-304]。

免疫组织化学和电镜检查

大多数肿瘤细胞表现出向腺泡细胞和导管细胞分化的免疫组织化学证据，例如细胞角蛋白（尤其是低分子量细胞角蛋白）、CEA 和淀粉酶阳性。然而，淀粉酶染色价值有限，因为只有 15% 的病例阳性[305]。没有肌上皮 / 基底细胞分化的免疫组织化学证据[48,125]。超微结构研究显示，至少某些肿瘤细胞中有酶原颗粒。

预后因子

最重要的预后指征是临床分期和切缘状况。虽然核分裂象常见或高增生指数（MIB1 指数大于 5%）、局灶坏死、神经浸润、大体浸润、纤维组织增生、非典型性和间质淋巴细胞消失与复发和转移有关，但是没有发现组织学分级是一个可靠的预后因素[65,265,297,299,300,306]。一项研究提示，间质有致密淋巴细胞，伴有明显生发中心形成的肿瘤，以及普遍显示微囊性生长的肿瘤具有非常好的预后(随访 19 个月到 14 年没有复发或转移)（图 7.107）[307]。

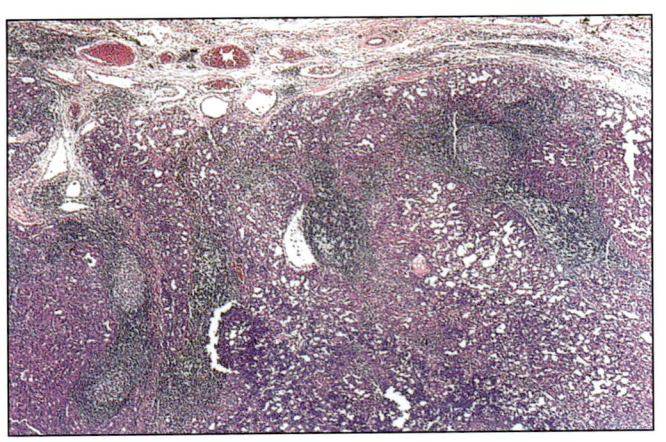

图7.107 腺泡细胞癌，"预后良性"变型。这种肿瘤的特征为局限性，有显著的淋巴细胞成分，包括许多淋巴滤泡，而且整个肿瘤全部为微囊性结构。

鉴别诊断

1. 嗜酸细胞瘤
2. 腺样囊性癌
3. 非特异性腺癌或囊腺癌
4. 正常涎腺组织，尤其是活检
5. 转移性甲状腺癌
6. 颗粒细胞瘤

多形性低级别腺癌
Polymorphous low-grade adenocarcinoma（PLGA）

定义

多形性低级别腺癌是一种以浸润性生长，形态学多样性和细胞学一致性为特征的恶性肿瘤。其他名称包括小叶癌[308]、终末导管癌[309]和低级别乳头状腺癌。

临床特征

多形性低级别腺癌几乎全发生在小涎腺。仅仅有极少的病例发生在大涎腺，在这种情况下，最常见的是多形性腺瘤中的癌的恶性成分[65,310-312]。最常见的发生部位是上腭（60%～70%），其次是颊黏膜（16%）、上唇（12%）、磨牙后区、舌根[65,313,314]，以及在罕见的情况下发生于泪腺[315]。多形性低级别腺癌发生在鼻咽部[316]、外阴和阴道[317]、上颌（骨内）[318]和肺[319]也有报告。发病的高峰年龄是40～50岁和50～60岁，但是儿童也可能受累[320]。女性较男性好发。临床上，肿瘤表现为无症状的肿块，伴有或不伴有溃疡形成。

多形性低级别腺癌是一种低级别的肿瘤，95%以上的患者在平均随访10年以后仍然存活[314]。局部复发和局部转移率分别是9%～17%和9%～15%，可能发生在最初治疗之后长达14年的时候（平均7年）[314,321,322]。据报告，伴有明显乳头状结构的肿瘤颈部淋巴结转移的发生率较高[322]。治疗选择完全手术切除。

大体和镜下表现

大体，多数肿瘤为局限性，但是没有包膜。切面浅褐色到灰色光泽。尽管大体界限清楚，但是组织学检查有明显的浸润性生长，伴有涎腺小叶，邻近脂肪组织或肌肉的浸润（图7.108）。常见神经周围浸润（76%）[313]。

生长方式呈多样性，包括单纯的腺管，复合或融合的腺管、小梁状、单个细胞排列、靶样漩涡、实性巢、束状，以及筛状、乳头状或乳头状-囊状结构（图7.109）。最常见的3种生长方式是：(1)管状；(2)小梁状；(3)实性巢（图7.110）[313]。生长方式的可变性是这种肿瘤最一致的特征。

管状结构倾向于成小叶状或流水样成排排列。常常见到复杂的融合性管状腺体结构（图7.110）。筛状结构表现为被稀疏的圆形间隙分隔的肿瘤细胞岛，间隙中空或充满黏液样物质。多形性低级别腺癌相对的诊断性特

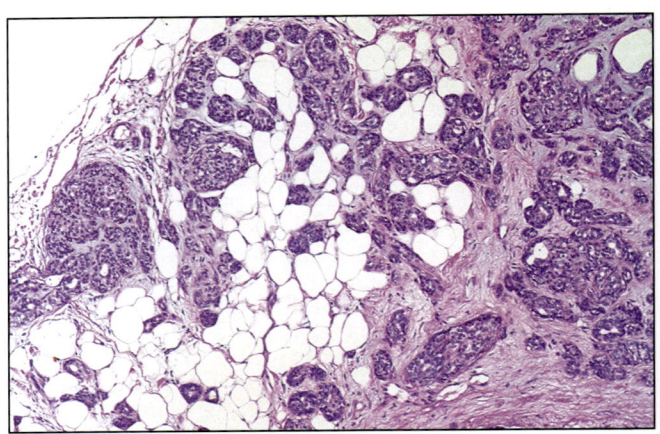

图7.108 多形性低级别腺癌。肿瘤一般浸润到相邻的组织。

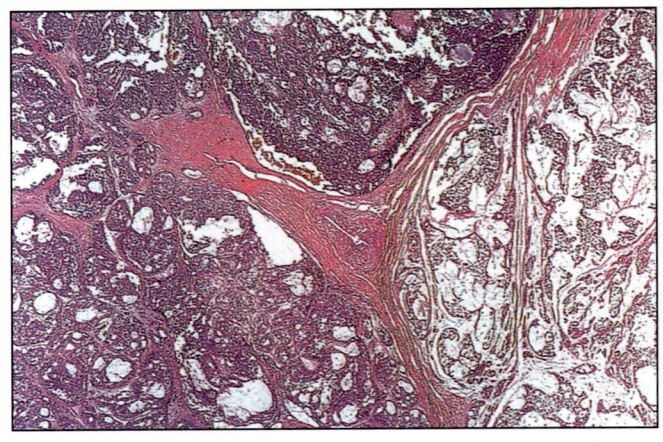

图7.109 多形性低级别腺癌。在肿瘤的不同区域有非常不同的生长方式。

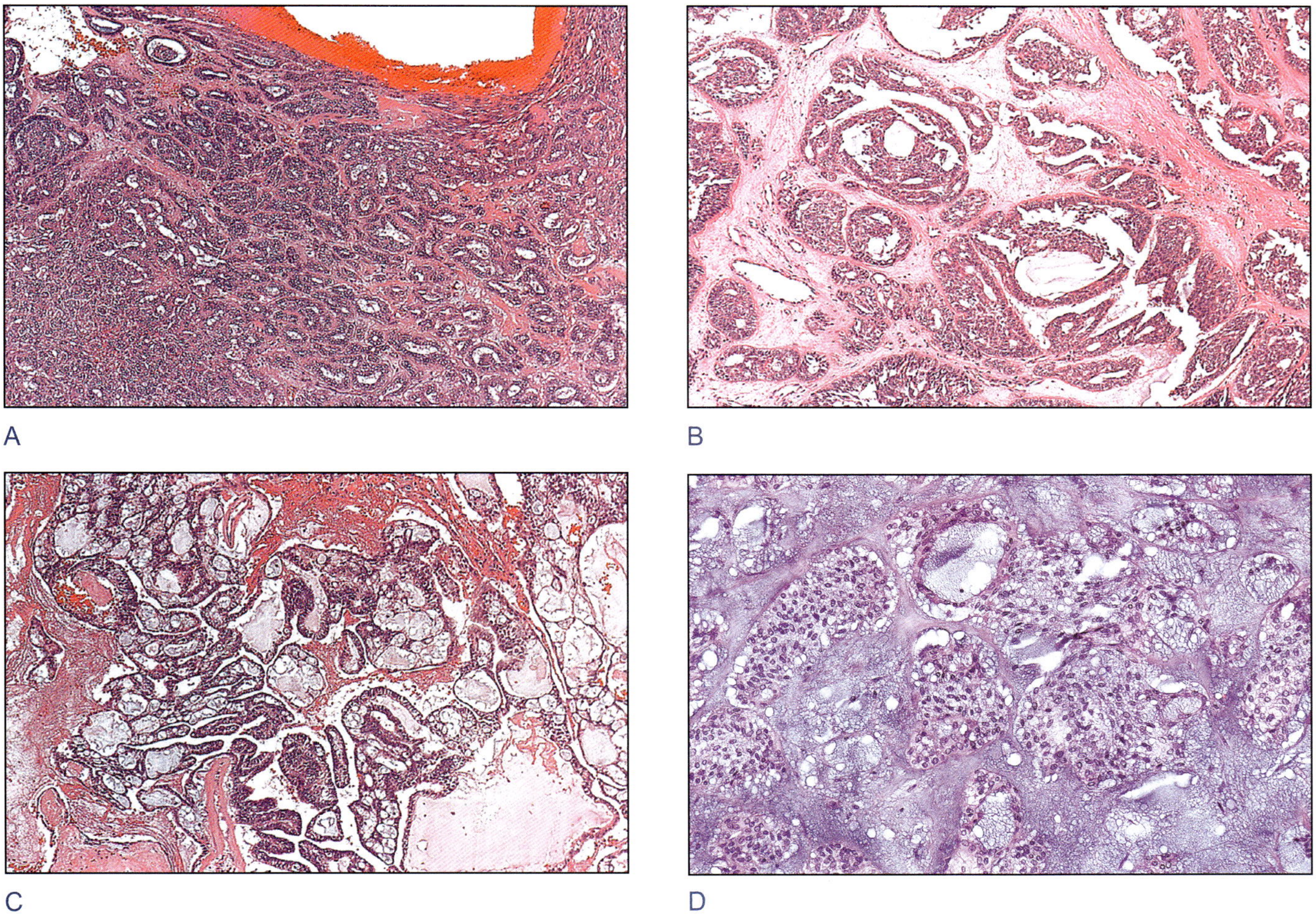

图7.110 多形性低级别腺癌,显示肿瘤中有多种生长方式。(A) 单纯的导管以及较复杂的腺体融合在左下视野的实性区域内。(B) 复杂管状乳头状结构。(C) 以乳头状结构为主。(D) 肿瘤岛可能淹没在黏液性间质中,酷似多形性腺瘤。

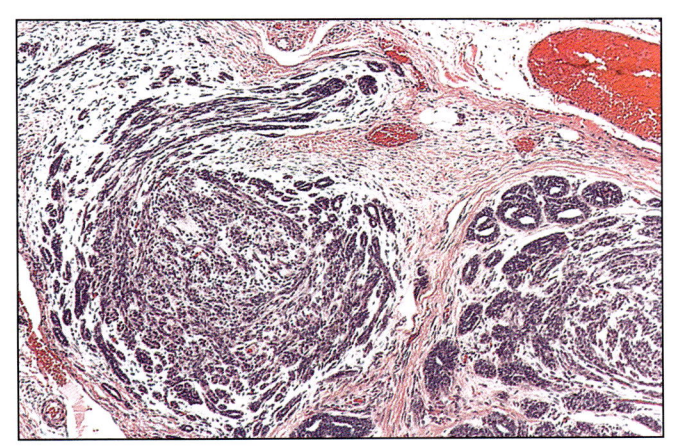
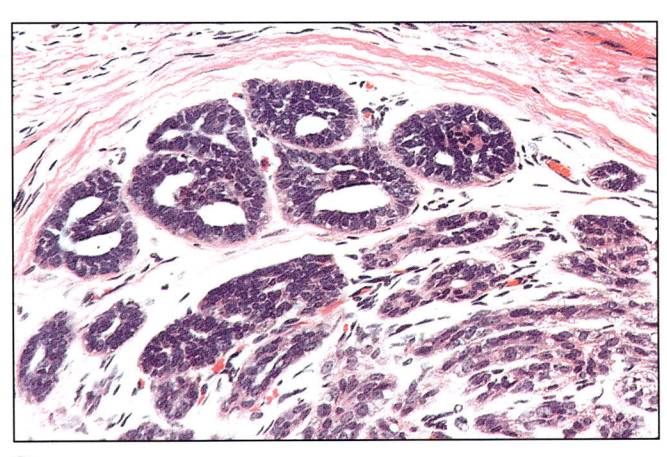

图7.111 多形性低级别腺癌。(A) 显示非常特征性的水流样结构,类似于乳腺硬化性腺病。(B) 伴有开放管腔的小管和缩窄的小管呈水流样生长方式。小管内衬单一细胞类型,没有肌上皮细胞。

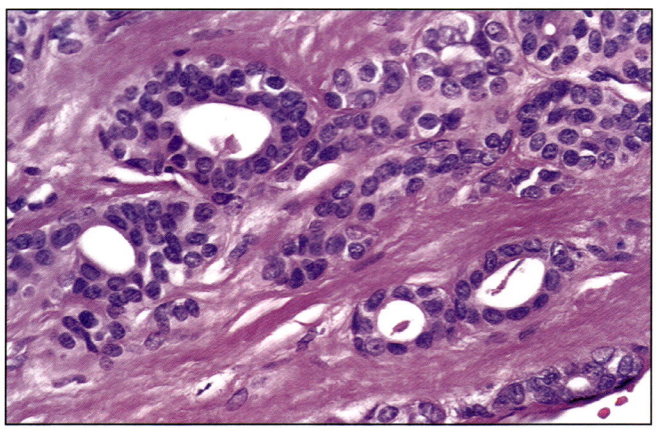

图7.112 多形性低级别腺癌。小管仅仅内衬导管细胞。细胞核一般淡染，呈良性表现。

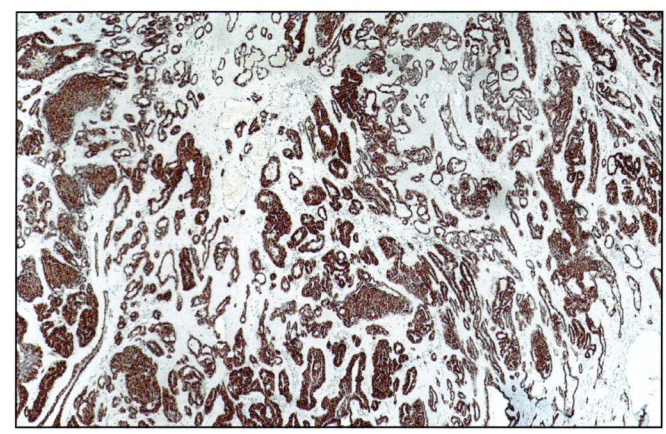

图7.113 多形性低级别腺癌。这种肿瘤一般显示S-100蛋白呈弥散强阳性免疫反应。

征是，由同心圆排列的细胞索和狭窄的小管形成的靶样结构，类似于乳腺的硬化性腺病（图7.111）。乳头状或乳头状-囊状结构是由伴有小的囊腔内乳头状突起的扩张的囊肿组成的（图7.110）。乳头被覆单层肿瘤细胞。

一般只有一种单一的细胞类型（导管细胞），形成所有上述结构。肿瘤细胞有圆形淡染的细胞核，染色质细，分布均匀，核仁不明显（图7.112）。有中等量的轻度嗜酸性胞浆。肿瘤细胞可能是立方形、柱状、梭形或多角形，但总是保持温和的细胞学特征。偶尔能够见到黏液细胞或透明细胞。坏死或核分裂象非常罕见。虽然某些作者认为肌上皮是这种肿瘤类型的组成成分[269,323]，但在光学显微镜水平缺乏肌上皮细胞，或最多是非常局灶性地出现肌上皮细胞[324]。肿瘤细胞被玻璃样变的嗜酸性间质所围绕，间质偶尔出现黏液样改变。暗蓝灰色的间质具有特征性[325]（图7.110D）。在某些病例中可以发现沙粒体胶原性或酪氨酸型结晶。

在最初诊断或有症状之后多年，少数病例可能形成去分化多形性低级别腺癌。这样的病变常常类似于涎腺导管癌[326,327]，伴有显著的实性或囊性结构、高级别的细胞核以及明显的肿瘤坏死。

免疫组织化学和特异性研究

肿瘤细胞显示细胞角蛋白、EMA 和 S-100 蛋白的免疫反应（图7.113）。GFAP 染色一般阴性，某些病例偶尔出现阳性细胞[49,111,313,314,328-332]。部分肿瘤细胞可能表达 p63，杂乱分布[48,88]；肌上皮分化标记物（平滑肌肌动蛋白，平滑肌肌球蛋白重链，钙调节蛋白）阴性[125]。电子显微镜检查显示，多数肿瘤细胞向腔面细胞方向分化，但可能有一小部分细胞显示腔外细胞或移行性特征[333]。

已经证实多形性低级别腺癌总是有 bcl-2 蛋白过度表达。与光镜下观察到的核分裂计数低一致，多形性低级别腺癌的增生指数也低（平均 Ki-67 指数 1.56% ~ 7%）[49,50,313]，这可能有助于与腺样囊性癌（平均 Ki-67 指数大于 20%，范围从 11% 到 57%）的鉴别诊断[50]。核分裂计数低结合 bcl-2 过度表达提示，在肿瘤发生过程中不良凋亡可能具有作用[49]。

鉴别诊断

多形性腺瘤和腺样囊性癌是最重要的鉴别诊断。

多形性腺瘤可以通过以下特征与多形性低级别腺癌鉴别：

1. 非浸润性
2. 腔面和腔外细胞双重分化
3. 软骨样基质，如果出现的话
4. 浆细胞样玻璃样细胞，如果出现的话
5. 肌上皮层"融合到"周围的间质
6. 邻近上皮巢的间叶样细胞群 GFAP 染色阳性，这常常是多形性腺瘤而不是多形性低级别腺癌的特征[328]

腺样囊腺癌可以通过以下特征与多形性低级别腺癌鉴别：

1. 肿瘤细胞显示高核/浆比率以及较深染的细胞核
2. 显著的腔外细胞成分
3. 筛状结构更为常见
4. EMA 染色局限于腺腔而不是弥散性分布；S-100蛋白染色常常呈片块状，染色不强；且增生指数较高[49,50,313]
5. p63 免疫染色可以显示位于肿瘤岛周边的细胞呈"团块状"分布，与多形性低级别腺癌中杂乱分布的阳性细胞不同

舌的筛状腺癌
Cribriform adenocarcinoma of the tongue

在 WHO 分类中，认为舌的筛状腺癌可能是多形性

低级别腺癌的变型,由于它们的形态学、免疫表型和临床行为相似[334,335]。然而,与后者不同,这种肿瘤全部发生在舌根,而且所有的患者在诊断时均有颈淋巴结转移。组织学上,这种浸润性肿瘤表现为不同的生长方式,包括实性、微囊性、滤泡状、筛状和乳头状。肿瘤细胞表现温和,具有均匀一致的常常是重叠的细胞核,伴有空泡状或"毛玻璃状"染色质,类似于乳头状甲状腺癌。没有显著的核分裂活性、坏死或出血。肿瘤细胞表达细胞角蛋白和不同程度的表达S-100蛋白。肌上皮标记物阴性或者仅仅局部阳性。

上皮-肌上皮癌
Epithelial-myoepithelial carcinoma

定义

上皮-肌上皮癌是一种由导管结构组成的恶性肿瘤,导管结构内衬单层导管细胞,周围绕以单层或多层透明肌上皮细胞。其在乳腺的对应肿瘤是腺肌上皮瘤[114,336,337]。

临床特征

发病的高峰年龄是50岁至70岁之间,有轻微的女性好发趋势。大约60%的病例发生在腮腺,而其余的发生在颌下腺以及口腔内的小涎腺。大多数的患者表现为无症状的肿块,一小部分患者出现疼痛和面神经麻痹。这种肿瘤也有发生在泪腺、肺、支气管、气管、鼻腔、鼻咽和肝脏的报道[338-345]。

上皮-肌上皮癌是一种相对低级别的恶性肿瘤。根据报道,30%~40%的病例复发,可以发生在最初手术后长达28年之久[346-350]。10%~20%的病例发生局部淋巴结转移,但是远处转移(肺、肾和脑)少见(9%)[346]。肿瘤相关性死亡率低(0~9%)[346,347]。Fonseca和Soares报道,伴有超过20%细胞显示核非典型性的肿瘤与预后不良有关[351]。

大体和镜下表现

大体,肿瘤一般为多结节性,界限清楚。切面褐色,质硬。组织学上,肿瘤呈舌状侵犯周围实质,形成由硬化性间质分隔的多发性肿瘤结节(图7.114)。有时可见神经周围和血管侵犯。肿瘤结节内的间质可能稀少、疏松、黏液样、玻璃样变或为纤维性。

标准的双细胞结构由内衬导管细胞的导管构成,周围有一层或几层透明细胞,其外由界限清晰的基底膜包裹(图7.115)。管腔细胞立方形,伴有圆形良性表现的细胞核以及中等量的粉色胞浆,类似于闰管细胞。极少数情况下可能有鳞状分化。透明细胞是相当大的多角形细胞,具有丰富的水样透明胞浆。胞浆透明是因为糖原积聚。这些细胞具有肌上皮的免疫表型和超微结构特征。

在某些肿瘤中,散在的导管被融合的导管、复杂的腺体结构、乳头状-囊状结构、小梁状结构以及由厚的基底膜包裹的透明细胞片块所替代(图7.114B和7.115B)。在以透明细胞为主的区域,可能难以发现小导管细胞,因此与透明细胞癌的鉴别可能是困难的(图7.115C)[65,346]。极少数情况下,可以形成梭形透明细胞(肌上皮细胞)束。

在多数情况下,细胞非典型性轻微,核分裂计数低(图7.115)。然而,极少数病例可以显示向较大程度核的非典型性,比较明显的实性结构以及常见核分裂的区

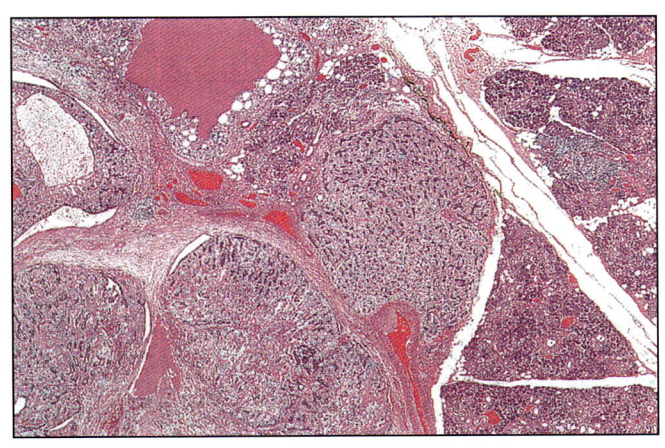

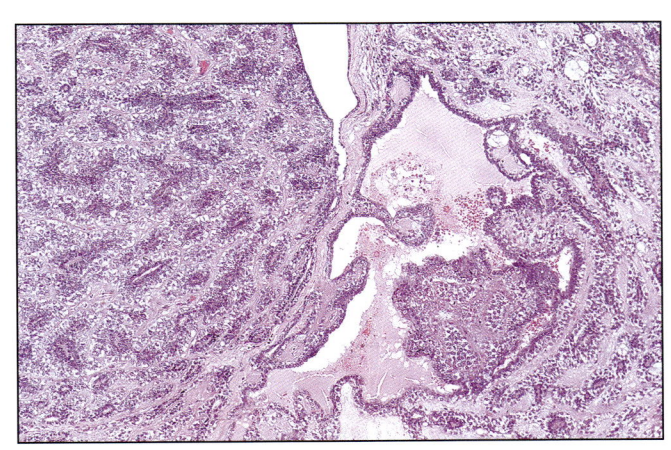

图7.114 上皮-肌上皮癌。(A)肿瘤的特征是呈舌状浸润(视野右侧可见正常涎腺组织)。肿瘤结节之间可见纤维性间质。(B)某些腺体结构具有扩张的腺腔,并有乳头状皱褶(视野右侧)。腺样囊性癌实际上从未见过这种特征。

域转化，提示肿瘤可以发展为高级别的上皮-肌上皮癌。这种现象伴有明显的比较侵袭性的行为[65,342,349,350]。根据报道，极少数病例去分化形成低分化癌，不再被认为是上皮-肌上皮癌[352-354]。

免疫组织化学和特异性研究

导管细胞广谱细胞角蛋白强阳性，S-100蛋白不同程度阳性，但是肌上皮标记物阴性。透明细胞广谱细胞角蛋白（通常弱）、高分子量细胞角蛋白、p63、S-100蛋白、钙调节蛋白和肌动蛋白阳性（图7.116）。增生（Ki-67）指数低：导管细胞少于1%，肌上皮透明细胞少于3%[349,352]。倍体分析显示大部分肿瘤（>80%）为二倍体[349]。

主要的鉴别诊断

该肿瘤必须与其他透明细胞肿瘤鉴别，尤其是那些显示融合性透明细胞岛和透明细胞片块的肿瘤（表7.5）。为了发现诊断性的双细胞结构，可能需要仔细检查和广泛取材。上皮-肌上皮癌中的透明细胞显示肌上皮分化，而透明细胞癌中的透明细胞则没有。

上皮-肌上皮癌和腺样性囊癌均为浸润性肿瘤，伴有导管-肌上皮双重分化。以下特征支持前者而不是后者的诊断：

1. 腔外细胞更大，伴有透明胞浆和淡染的细胞核（腺样囊性癌如果出现透明细胞，则非常局限）
2. 筛状结构罕见（图7.117）
3. 微囊性间隙内淡嗜碱性黏液物质稀少
4. 不规则的分支状腺腔，如果存在
5. 增生指数（Ki-67）较低

涎腺导管癌　Salivary duct carcinoma

定义

涎腺导管癌是一种侵袭性的恶性肿瘤，形态学上和乳腺导管癌相似。它可以是新生成的肿瘤，或作为多形性腺瘤中癌的恶性成分[346,355,359]。

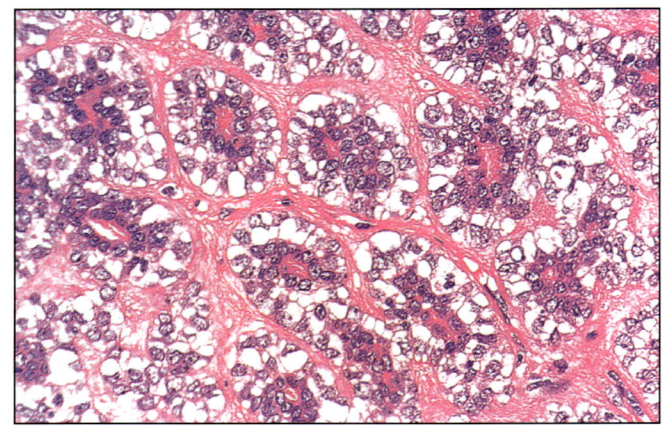

A

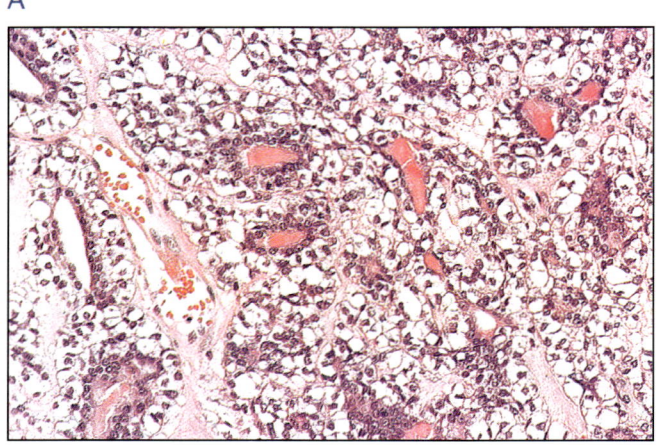

B

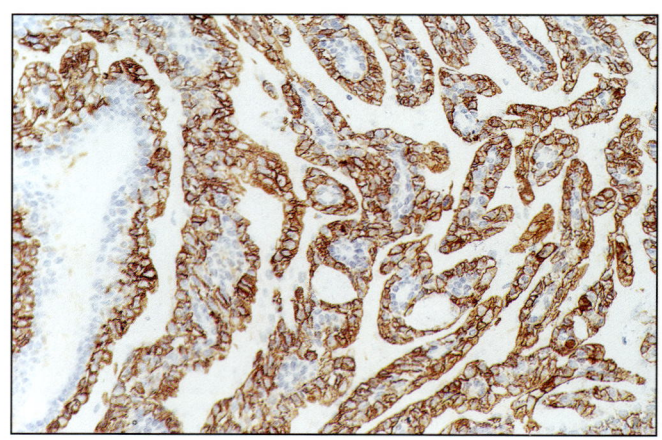

图7.116　上皮-肌上皮癌。透明肌上皮细胞肌动蛋白免疫反应阳性。

C

图7.115　上皮-肌上皮癌。（A）基本的肿瘤单位由散在的小管组成，小管内层内衬伴有嗜酸性胞浆的导管细胞，外层为大的透明肌上皮细胞。小管被玻璃样变间质分隔。（B）小管可能被厚的透明细胞套包围，彼此融合形成较大的细胞岛。（C）显著的融合形成大的细胞岛，主要由透明细胞组成。仅有少数散在的小管结构，内衬伴有嗜酸性胞浆的细胞。

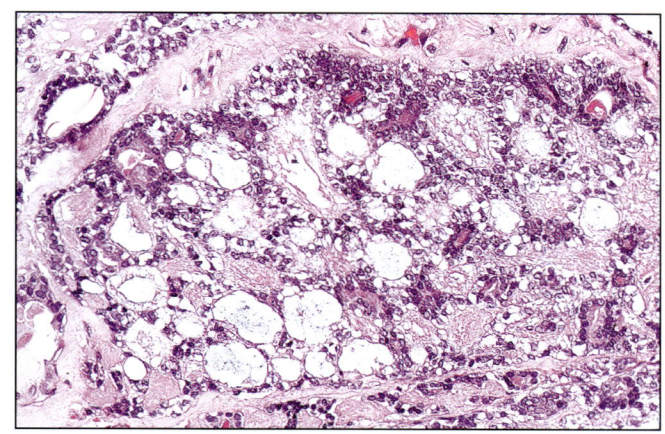

图7.117 上皮-肌上皮癌。少数情况下,小管融合形成筛状结构,类似于腺样囊性癌。

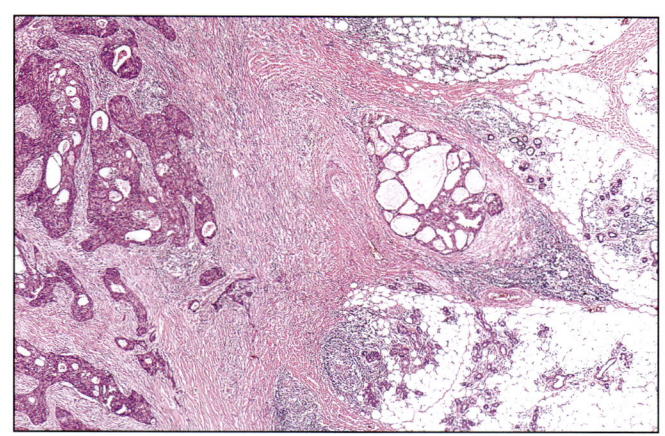

图7.118 涎腺导管癌。肿瘤(视野左侧)浸润腮腺实质(视野右侧),且伴有纤维组织增生性间质。这个肿瘤呈筛状生长方式。

临床特征

涎腺导管癌最常发生在老年人(发病高峰年龄在50～70岁之间),男女发病比例是3～6:1。腮腺占所有病例的80%,其余的发生在颌下腺,极少数发生在口腔内的小涎腺。患者通常表现为迅速增大的腮腺肿块,伴有面神经麻痹(42%)、疼痛(23%)以及颈部淋巴腺肿大(35%)[356]。

这是一种最具有浸润性的涎腺癌。平均随访3年发现这种肿瘤的死亡率可以高达77%[356]。35%～66%的患者发生局部复发,66%淋巴结转移,50%～70%远处转移[346,356,360]。最常见的远处转移部位是肺、骨和脑。推荐的治疗包括完全手术切除、颈部清扫以及术后放疗。

病理学特征

肿瘤界限不清,主要为实性,呈褐色。经常有局灶性坏死。大体检查,肿瘤延伸到涎腺外发生在大约70%的病例[356]。组织学上,浸润性肿瘤类似于乳腺导管内癌和浸润性导管癌(图7.118)。导管内样成分显示筛状、乳头状-囊状或实性结构,经常伴有显著的粉刺状坏死(图7.119)。然而,其中多数没有真正的导管内增生,因为缺乏肌上皮层,而且在转移性病变中可以看见相似的结构。明显的浸润性成分由条索状、巢状、小腺体以及单个细胞组成(图7.120)。两种成分的肿瘤性细胞具有类似的形态学改变,其特征为伴有丰富嗜酸性胞浆的顶浆分泌表现、大的多形性空泡状细胞核以及显著的核仁(图7.121)。胞浆内偶尔出现黏液。容易发现核分裂象。间质为致密的纤维性或纤维组织增生性间质。通常可见血管浸润、周围神经浸润、血管内瘤栓以及浸润邻近结构[357]。

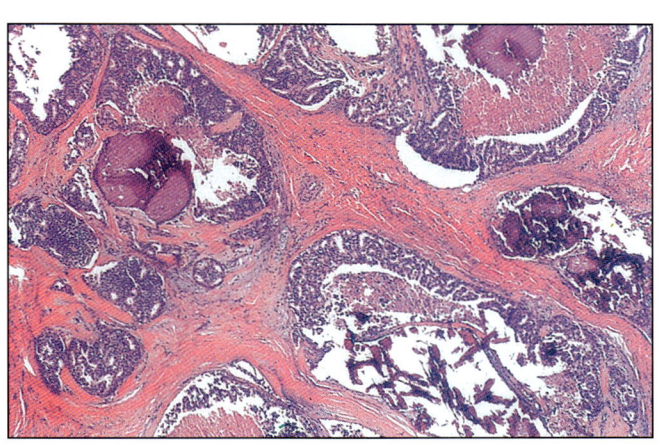

A

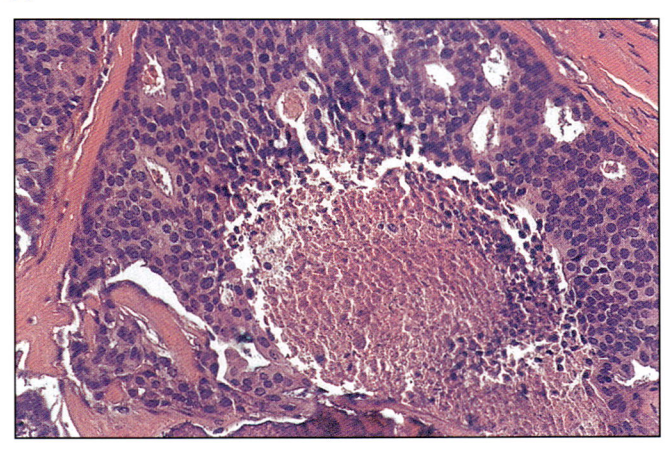

B

图7.119 涎腺导管癌。(A)这是一种浸润性的肿瘤,但是伴有粉刺状坏死的大的筛状肿瘤单位,类似于乳腺导管内癌。(B)显示由中度多形性细胞组成的筛状结构和中心粉刺状坏死。

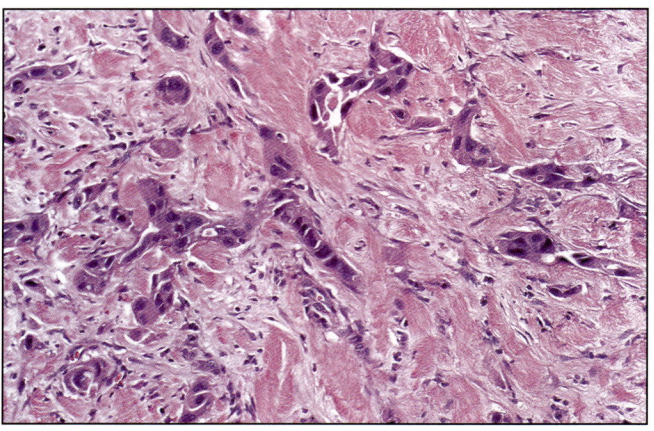

图7.120 涎腺导管癌。在这些区域中，肿瘤细胞呈条索状浸润纤维性间质，类似于普通的乳腺浸润性导管癌。

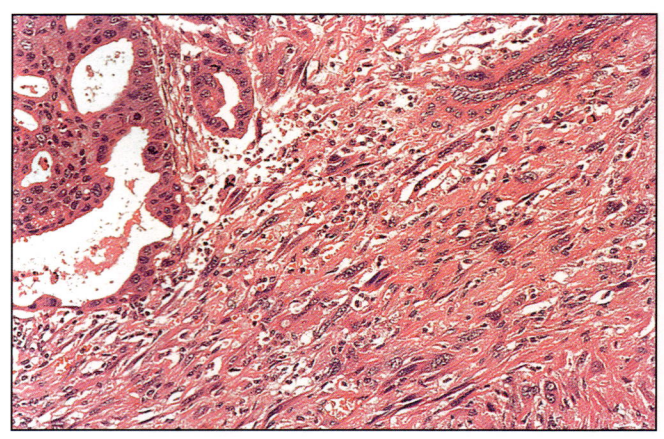

图7.122 涎腺导管癌，肉瘤样（去分化）变型。视野左上可见普通的涎腺导管癌成分。肉瘤性成分由伴有多形性细胞核的梭形和星形细胞组成。

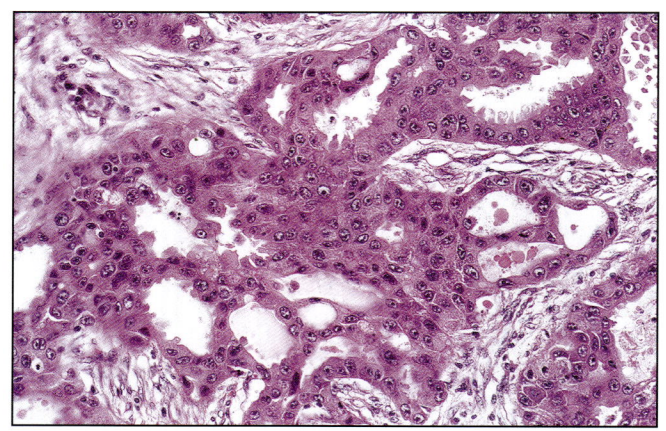

图7.121 涎腺导管癌。这个病例显示筛状生长方式。组成肿瘤的细胞具有顶浆分泌样特性，细胞核有显著的多形性。

涎腺导管癌的几种组织学变型已有描述[361-363]。本质上，它们是由典型的涎腺导管癌成分和另外一种组织学上独特的成分组成的。在两种成分之间常常可见过渡区域。

肉瘤样变型（去分化涎腺导管癌）[Sarcomatoid variant (dedifferentiated salivary duct carcinoma)]：肉瘤样成分由间变的梭形细胞、奇异形多核巨细胞、横纹肌样细胞以及极少数情况下的骨肉瘤性细胞组成（图7.122）[361,361]。这些细胞通常证明有局灶性上皮分化的免疫组织化学和超微结构证据。我们认为这种变型是涎腺导管癌去分化的一种形式。

富于黏液的变型（Mucin-rich variant）：这种变型的特征是具有黏液性/胶样癌的区域，黏液池中漂浮着伴或不伴胞浆黏液的成簇的癌细胞。

浸润性微乳头状变型（Invasive micropapillary variant）：这种变型的特征是不伴有纤维血管轴心的桑葚样肿瘤细胞簇，周围绕以透明间隙，在形态学上类似于乳腺或尿路上皮癌的微乳头状变型。

预后因素

以前的研究提示，肿瘤小于3 cm有较好的预后[367,368]，但是这一点没有得到 Mayo Clinic 的研究所证实[356]。似乎没有一种组织学参数具有预后意义[356,357,369]，尽管微乳头状变型可能具有较强的侵袭性[363]。

免疫组织化学

免疫组织化学和超微结构研究证实，肿瘤细胞具有腺腔上皮的特性，伴有细胞角蛋白、EMA 和 CEA 弥漫强阳性反应。几乎所有的病例均表达雄激素受体，虽然不具有特异性，但这是涎腺癌的一种特征[370,371]。雌激素和孕激素受体通常阴性[372]。大多数病例 c-erbB2 过表达。肿瘤细胞大囊肿病液体蛋白-15（GCDFP-15 或 BRST-2）通常局灶阳性[373]，而 S-100 蛋白和肌上皮标记物一般阴性。某些病例可能表达前列腺酸性磷酸酶、前列腺特异性抗原、或 CK 20[229,374]。Ki-67 指数较高（平均21.3%）[375]。伴有神经内分泌分化的涎腺导管癌已有个案报告[376]。肌上皮标记物染色显示，真正的以周围有一圈变扁的肌上皮为特征的原位（导管内）成分通常较少。

遗传学特征

已经发现染色体 9p21，6q，16q，17p 和 17q 部位常有杂合性缺失[377,378]。TP53 基因和蛋白突变和过表达是经常发生的[25,377,379]。HER-2/nue 基因扩增发生在36%

的病例，而蛋白过表达发生在50%～100%的病例[359,380]，根据报道，这与较侵袭性的行为有关。基因表达谱显示，凋亡相关基因 CASP10 和 MMP11 有过表达[23]。CDKN2A/p16 基因失活与肿瘤进展相关[378]。

主要的鉴别诊断

除了转移性乳腺癌或前列腺癌外，主要的鉴别诊断包括高级别黏液表皮样癌、嗜酸细胞癌、囊腺癌和导管内癌。

乳腺癌的临床病史、雌激素/孕激素受体阳性以及雄激素受体阴性强烈支持转移性乳腺癌的诊断。GCDFP-15（BRST-2）免疫染色没有意义，因为多数涎腺导管癌也呈阳性反应[356,373,381]。

高级别黏液表皮样癌可能类似于涎腺导管癌，尤其是在冰冻切片时。然而，在涎腺导管癌中见不到混合性细胞类型，例如上皮样细胞和杯状细胞。

嗜酸细胞癌（oncocytic carcinoma）的特征是伴有充满线粒体的颗粒状嗜酸性胞浆的大的肿瘤细胞。嗜酸细胞癌和囊腺癌均缺乏通常见于涎腺导管癌的粉刺状坏死和导管内样结构。

罕见的导管内癌一定不要误诊为涎腺导管癌，因为其预后要好得多（见下文）。

导管内癌（所谓的低级别涎腺导管癌或低级别筛状囊腺癌）
Intraductal carcinoma (so-called low-grade salivary duct carcinoma or low-grade cribriform cystadenocarcinoma)

涎腺导管内癌的概念和命名问题

导管内癌最初于1983年描述，在2005年WHO分类中不是一种公认的疾病。其特征为纯粹的肿瘤细胞导管内增生，可能是涎腺导管癌的原位成分。导管内癌的概念还没有得到广泛的接受，因为某些伴有明显的纯粹导管内样生长的涎腺导管癌仍然具有侵袭性的经过，而且导管内样成分有时可以在转移癌中出现。这些观察可以归因于不加区别地应用"导管内"这一术语，根据定义，该术语应该要求存在完整的肌上皮层，如同乳腺导管内癌一样。按照严格的定义，导管内癌是一种具有低度恶性潜能的肿瘤，其行为类似于乳腺导管内癌[382]。

导管内癌在文献中常常在"低级别涎腺导管癌"的名称下报告[283,384]。然而，"导管内癌"这个术语比较恰当，因为它强调了基本特征，而且避免了与较侵袭性涎腺导管癌可能存在的混淆。新版WHO分类所采用的"低级别筛状囊腺癌"这一术语甚至更容易混淆[181]。

临床特征

与涎腺导管癌相似，这种肿瘤最常累及老年人的腮腺（平均年龄62岁），伴有轻微的女性好发趋势。小涎腺（例如舌、腭、口腔）也可以受累[382]。完全切除以后，预后很好，在随访2～12年时没有转移和死亡，不论核的分级如何。切除不完全可能导致复发。

病理学特征

这种肿瘤的特征是多发性伴有上皮细胞增生的外形光滑的导管，形成筛状、有孔的、实性粉刺状、微乳头状或罗马桥（Roman bridge）结构，类似于乳腺非典型性导管增生或导管内癌的结构形态（图7.123和7.124A）。组成细胞一般显示低到中级别，但有时是高级别的细胞学非典型性（图7.124A）。某些细胞可以显示顶浆分泌。细胞岛周围变薄的肌上皮细胞层在光镜下可能明显或不明显。间质硬化，可以出现继发性改变，例如出血、慢性炎症浸润以及营养不良性钙化。

少数情况下显微镜下有浸润成分，在形态学上与涎腺导管癌相同，或者出现在原发病变或者出现在复发时[383,385]。微小浸润的临床意义还不清楚，但是预后良好。

诊断的必要条件

只有当充分取材以后排除了浸润性成分时，才可以明确地作出导管内癌的诊断。进行免疫染色来确定每一个肿瘤岛周围的完整的肌上皮层也是绝对必要的（图7.124B），因为鉴别原位癌和浸润性导管癌非常困难。必须慎重作出这种诊断，因为可供选择的解释是涎腺导管癌，它是高度侵袭性的肿瘤。

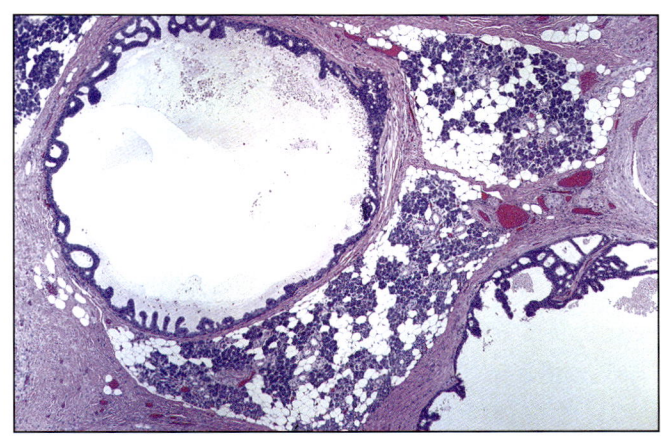

图7.123　腮腺导管内癌。扩张的导管显示细胞增生呈微乳头状和罗马桥结构，类似于乳腺导管内癌。

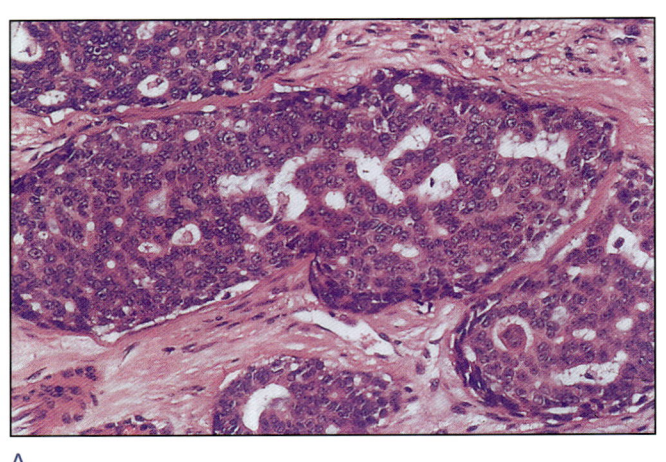 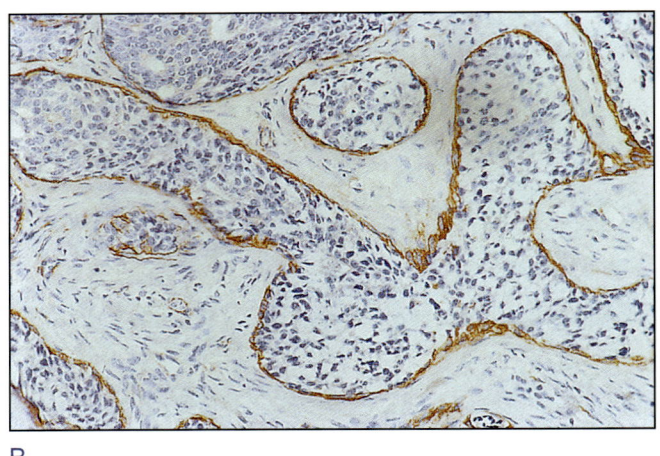

图7.124 口腔黏膜导管内癌。（A）散在的增生细胞岛类似于乳腺非典型性导管增生或导管内癌。在这个病例中，细胞非典型增生并不显著。（B）肌肉特异性肌动蛋白免疫染色显示细胞岛周围有完整的肌上皮细胞，证明肿瘤病变的原位特性。

透明细胞癌，非特异性
Clear cell carcinoma, not otherwise specified

定义

非特异性透明细胞癌也叫透明细胞腺癌，是由单一形态的伴有水样透明胞浆的上皮细胞组成的，没有肌上皮分化的证据。它是一种排除性的诊断，应该缺乏其他肿瘤的特征，最值得注意的是上皮-肌上皮、透明细胞嗜酸细胞瘤、黏液表皮样癌、腺泡细胞癌、透明细胞肌上皮肿瘤、皮脂腺癌以及转移性肾细胞癌[128]。

临床特征

透明细胞癌最常发生在40～50岁和60～70岁的患者，没有性别差异。报道的病例多数来自于口腔小涎腺，表现为无痛性缓慢生长的肿块，某些病变可以形成溃疡或固定于周围组织。它是一种低级别的局部浸润性肿瘤，容易局部复发[386]。颈部淋巴结转移仅仅发生在极少数的病例，由这种肿瘤引起死亡是特殊情况[65]。治疗选择广泛切除；辅助性放疗的作用还不清楚。

病理学

肿瘤境界不清，切面颜色为带白色的褐色。它是由片块状、水流样柱状、巢状、大的单形性透明细胞条索组成的，其大小有轻微的变异（图7.115）。细胞具有断续的细胞膜和由于糖原（PAS阳性以及淀粉酶敏感，黏液卡红染色阴性）积累而形成的丰富的透明胞浆。细胞核位于中心或偏心，染色质细颗粒状，核仁不显著。细胞核的非典型性范围从轻度到中度。部分肿瘤细胞可能有嗜酸性胞浆（图7.116）。核分裂象罕见。没有导管形成。可以出现不同数量的纤维性间质。见表7.5的鉴别诊断。

免疫组织化学和特异性研究

这些肿瘤对于细胞角蛋白有局灶性到弥散性的免疫反应。与转移性肾细胞癌不同，这种肿瘤表达高分子量细胞角蛋白和CEA[387]。肌上皮标记物应该阴性。超微结构和免疫组织化学研究已经表明仅仅有导管但没有肌上皮分化[65,386]。

变型：玻璃样变透明细胞癌
Variant: hyalinizing clear cell carcinoma

玻璃样变透明细胞癌是由Milchgrub等描述的透明细胞癌的一个亚群[388]。大多数病例来自于小涎腺，但是大涎腺也可以受累。口腔是最常见的部位，尤其是舌根和腭[388-391]。据报道，少数病例发生在喉、鼻咽、下咽部、下颌和上颌[388,392-394]。肿瘤通常表现为缓慢生长和无痛性的黏膜下肿块。临床上呈惰性经过。不过，某些病例在多年内可以出现多次复发，而且在少数情况下可以发生颈部淋巴结转移和肺转移[388,392,394]。具有广泛转移且在一年之内死亡的个案报告显示，肿瘤具有局灶性的核分裂活性、坏死和间变，因此可以认为是去分化的玻璃样变透明细胞癌[395]。治疗选择广泛的局部切除，伴有或不伴有放射治疗。

如上所述，组织学上浸润性的肿瘤是由一致的透明细胞和伴有嗜酸性胞浆的细胞组成的（图7.125），形成实性细胞巢、小梁状、条索状以及一个到两个细胞宽度的水流样柱状结构[388,392,396]。间质以丰富的、粗大平行的纤维组织带为特征，伴有玻璃样变和黏液样物质，并且混合有富于细胞的纤维（纤维组织增生性）组织。

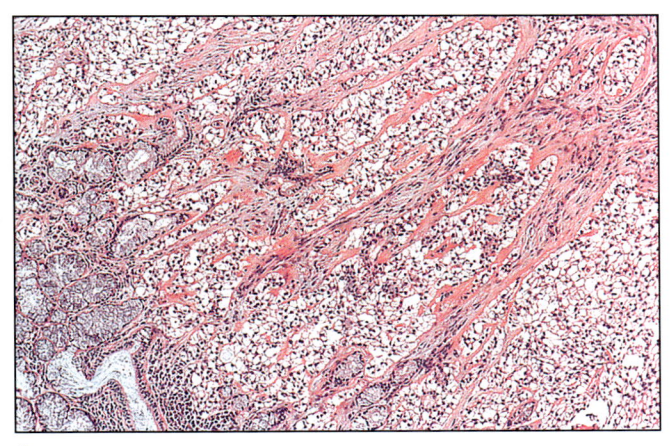
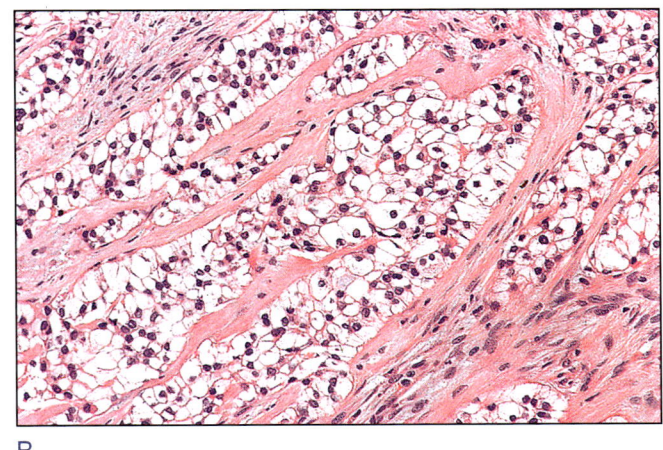

图7.125 腭的玻璃样变透明细胞癌。（A）肿瘤是浸润性的，视野左下可见残留的涎腺小叶。注意明显的透明细胞和玻璃样物质。（B）多角形透明细胞的宽阔的小梁被同质性的嗜酸性玻璃样物质和富于细胞的纤维组织增生性间质分开。

玻璃样变的间质类似于淀粉样物，但是PAS染色阳性而刚果红染色阴性。

免疫组织化学染色显示，肿瘤细胞细胞角蛋白和EMA染色弥漫阳性，而CEA局灶阳性。肌上皮标记物（S-100蛋白，钙调节蛋白和平滑肌肌动蛋白）总是阴性。电子显微镜检查显示张力丝、发育良好的桥粒和半桥粒，证实肿瘤具有纯粹的上皮性本质。

未分化癌 Undifferentiated carcinoma

涎腺未分化癌是一种少见的高级别的恶性肿瘤，光镜下显示肿瘤具有分化极差的特征，不能放在任何一种特殊类型癌的范畴之内。局部孤立的腺体结构或鳞状分化不能排除这种诊断，超微结构证实这些特征也不能排除这种诊断。总的来说，这些肿瘤可以分为小细胞型和大细胞型。淋巴上皮癌是未分化癌的一种特殊亚型，具有相对良好的预后。

小细胞癌 Small cell carcinoma

定义：小细胞癌的特征是由小的上皮细胞（<30 μm）组成的肿瘤，胞浆稀少，染色质细，而且核仁不明显。根据超微结构和免疫组织化学特征[397-399]，可以将其分为：

1. 神经内分泌型
   (a) Merkel 细胞亚型
   (b) 肺的亚型
2. 导管型

临床特征：小细胞癌最常发生在腮腺，少数发生在颌下腺和舌下腺。患者年龄从40～50岁到60～70岁（平均年龄54～56岁），有男性好发的趋势。肿瘤表现为迅速增长的肿块，伴有或不伴有并发的颈部淋巴结肿大。60%的患者发生面神经麻痹[14]。疼痛仅仅偶尔出现。

这是一种侵袭性的恶性肿瘤。根据报道，在诊断以后2～26个月50%以上的患者局部复发和远处转移[400]。总的生存率是40%～50%[397,401-403]。这个数字可与皮肤的Merkel细胞癌相比，而且远远高于肺或肺外其他部位的小细胞癌。已经发现，Merkel细胞亚型，肿瘤小（小于3～4 cm）以及表达较多的神经内分泌标记物与预后较好有关[400,404]。

病理学特征：大体，这种肿瘤是广泛浸润的肿块，质地硬韧，白色到黄色。组织学上，肿瘤呈弥漫性或条索样生长方式（图7.126）。肿瘤细胞比淋巴细胞稍大，染色质细腻，点彩状，而且核仁不明显。细胞核容易出现挤压人工假象，导致核变形和凝聚以及染色质物质弥散。通常可见坏死。血管和神经周围侵犯常见。肿

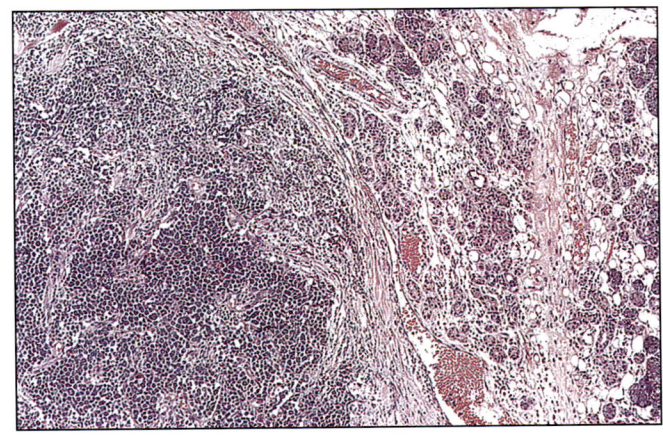

图7.126 腮腺小细胞癌，Merkel细胞型。肿瘤在涎腺内表现为广泛的，弥散性破坏性生长。

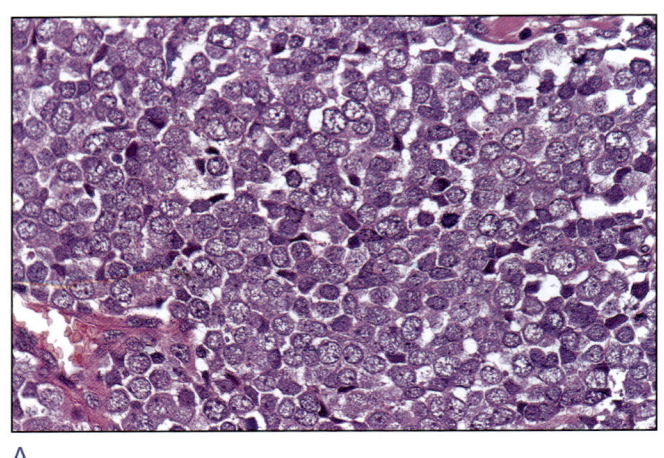
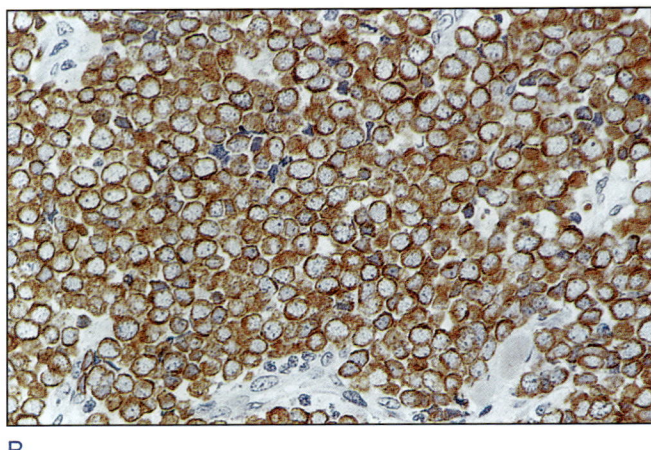

图7.127 腮腺小细胞癌，Merkel细胞型。（A）肿瘤细胞呈片块状生长。作为Merkel细胞癌的特征，细胞核类似于吹胀的气球，具有淡染的"褪色的"染色质。细胞核变形轻微。（B）CK20免疫反应具有特征性。

瘤经常有纤细的纤维血管间隔通过。

在Merkel细胞亚型中，细胞核通常呈圆形，没有变形，类似于吹胀的气球，伴有淡染和"褪色的"染色质（图7.127）。在肺的亚型中，肿瘤细胞通常是短梭形，伴有细胞核变形；可能有假菊形团形成（图7.128）[402]。然而，这两种亚型的形态学特征有重叠，单独根据组织学检查可能不能明确区分两者。最近一项大的系列研究显示[404]，73%的涎腺小细胞癌表达CK20（Merkel细胞亚型；图7.127B）；已经证实这些病例比CK20阴性组（肺的亚型）总体生存期长。两种亚型均表达神经内分泌标记物，例如嗜铬素、突触素以及CD56。Merkel细胞亚型还表达神经细丝，但不表达甲状腺转录因子-1[404,405]。

孤立性导管分化和伴有角化的鳞状分化在少数病例已有描述，这些肿瘤称为导管型小细胞癌（ductal-type small cell carcinoma）[397,406,407]。

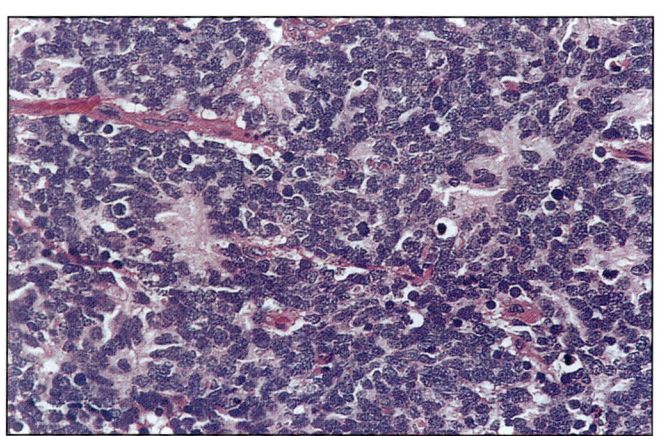

图7.128 腮腺小细胞癌，肺型。与Merkel细胞型不同，细胞核通常较长，染色质丰富，变形。本例还可见由原纤维性胞浆形成的假菊形团。

鉴别诊断：鉴别诊断包括淋巴瘤、实性腺样囊性癌以及转移性皮肤Merkel细胞癌。小细胞癌和恶性淋巴瘤在组织学上可能很难区别。淋巴瘤细胞的生长方式比较弥散，通常伴有持久的腺体结构的残留，即使在广泛受累区域。这不同于小细胞癌的腺体结构广泛破坏和常被完全取代。淋巴瘤细胞常常具有较不规则的折叠的细胞核和致密的染色质，而且它们不形成相互吻合的条索或细胞巢。通过免疫染色（例如白细胞共同抗原和细胞角蛋白）可以很容易地将这两种肿瘤明确区分开来。

实性腺样囊性癌，伴有大的同形性基底细胞样细胞岛和片状结构，可能与小细胞癌混淆，但是仔细观察之后，常常可以发现筛状结构。某些肿瘤细胞S-100蛋白、肌动蛋白和钙调节蛋白阳性，而局灶性导管结构显示CEA和EMA的免疫反应。除了EMA以外，小细胞癌这些标记物免疫染色均为阴性。

在作出原发性涎腺小细胞癌的诊断之前，必须排除转移性小细胞或Merkel细胞癌。临床病史和临床检查对于这种鉴别诊断都是必要的。

大细胞癌 Large-cell carcinoma

定义：大细胞癌是一种高级别的恶性肿瘤，由大的胞浆丰富的多形性细胞组成，缺乏其他特异性肿瘤类型的特征。

临床特征：大细胞癌是一种罕见的肿瘤，主要发生在腮腺和颌下腺。发病高峰年龄是60~80岁，而且没有性别差异。没有种族差异，与EB病毒无关[408]。

患者最常表现为迅速生长的质硬的肿块，与邻近组织固定。颈部淋巴结肿大常见，即多数患者处于晚期阶段（75%为Ⅳ期）[408]。它是一种高度侵袭性的肿瘤，

2年生存率仅为36%。预后不良的因素包括年龄大于50岁,肿瘤大于4 cm以及颈部淋巴结转移[400,408,409]。

病理学特征:大体,大细胞癌形成实性褐色浸润性肿块。形态学上类似于肺、甲状腺或胰腺的间变性癌。它们由片状和不规则岛状的大的多形性细胞组成,细胞界限清楚,有丰富的双染性到嗜酸性胞浆以及含有明显核仁的大的细胞核(图7.129)。偶尔出现多核瘤巨细胞。核分裂象、肿瘤坏死以及淋巴管和血管浸润常见。间质为纤维组织增生性,伴有不同数量的淋巴细胞和浆细胞浸润。还可能有散在的反应性破骨细胞巨细胞。超微结构检查可以显示腺体、鳞状或神经内分泌特征,这些特征在光镜下并不不明显。

大细胞神经内分泌癌
Large-cell neuroendocrine carcinoma

少数大细胞癌具有神经内分泌特征,包括菊形团样结构和伴有周围栅栏状排列的器官样生长。肿瘤细胞表达神经内分泌标记物,例如嗜铬素和突触素,但不是CK20。广谱细胞角蛋白和EMA也有表达。电镜检查发现有致密轴心颗粒[400,410,411]。大细胞神经内分泌癌的临床行为与普通的大细胞癌没有不同。

鉴别诊断:大细胞癌应该与淋巴上皮癌、转移癌、间变性大细胞淋巴瘤以及恶性黑色素瘤鉴别。另外,必须考虑与转移性肿瘤以及去分化涎腺肿瘤的鉴别。

淋巴上皮癌　Lymphoepithelial carcinoma

淋巴上皮癌,以前称做恶性淋巴上皮病变或淋巴上皮瘤样癌,是一种罕见的癌,在爱斯基摩人和中国南部远远比在白种人中流行[412,413]。在爱斯基摩人、中国人和日本人中,这种肿瘤几乎总是伴有EB病毒感染[152,414-419]。相反,在白种人中常常缺乏EB病毒感染,但不总是缺乏[415,420-422]。

临床特征:通常为成年人受累,平均年龄44.5岁,伴有不明确的或者轻微的女性好发趋势[408]。这种肿瘤最常发生在腮腺和颌下腺,表现为无症状的肿胀,伴有或不伴有疼痛[413];小涎腺也可以受累[423]。与Sjögren综合征无关。面神经麻痹少见,但在晚期病例与其下组织或皮肤固定。在诊断时大约40%的患者发生局部淋巴结转移[416,419,424,425]。

在疾病过程中可以出现局部复发和远处转移。在未分化癌中,淋巴上皮癌的预后最好[408]。虽然以前的研究报告预后不良(生存率低至17%),但是最近通过对手术和放射联合治疗患者的研究,报告生存数字为75%~86%[408,416,419,425]。

与淋巴上皮性涎腺炎(良性淋巴上皮病变)的关系 [Relationship with lymphoepithelial sialadenitis (begign lymphoepithelial lesion)]:过去认为淋巴上皮癌来自于淋巴上皮性涎腺炎(LESA)的恶性转化(见第305页)。这种论点现在已被多数研究者反对[413,416,419]。以前报告的邻近淋巴上皮癌的良性淋巴上皮病变,可能是残留涎腺实质的反应性改变,或者将伴有散在淀粉样小体的多形性不明显的肿瘤误认为是淋巴上皮病变(上皮肌上皮岛,epimyoepithelial islands)。

病理学特征:涎腺淋巴上皮癌在形态学上与发生在身体其他部位的淋巴上皮癌相同,尤其是鼻咽部未分化癌。这种浸润性肿瘤呈弥散性片块状,相互吻合的岛状、巢状或条索状生长,被纤维组织增生性间质分开(图7.130)。肿瘤细胞一般较大,胞浆嗜酸性,细胞边界不清。它们具有空泡状的细胞核和突出的核仁。在某些情况下,细胞核较小,核仁不明显,造成难以辨认这种病变的恶性本质。可能发生局灶性的鳞状分化(图7.131)。肿瘤细胞有时可能呈梭形[426]。在肿瘤细胞中可以出现淀粉样小体[419]。肿瘤坏死和核分裂象通常明显。肿瘤的特征是有致密的淋巴细胞和浆细胞浸润,伴有淋巴滤泡形成。组织细胞有时浸润肿瘤岛,形成星空现象[413]。某些病例可见伴有或不伴有多核巨细胞的非干酪坏死性肉芽肿[419]。神经周围和淋巴血管浸润可能出现(图7.132)[413]。

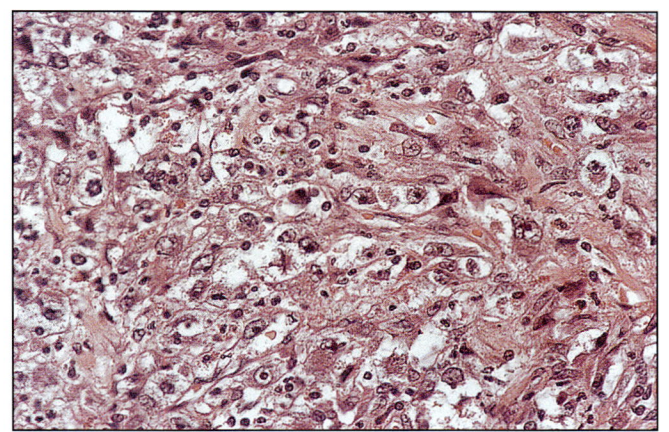

图7.129　大细胞未分化癌。大的多角形细胞片块,伴有这种肿瘤细胞特征性的高度多形性的细胞核。常常有散在的炎症细胞。

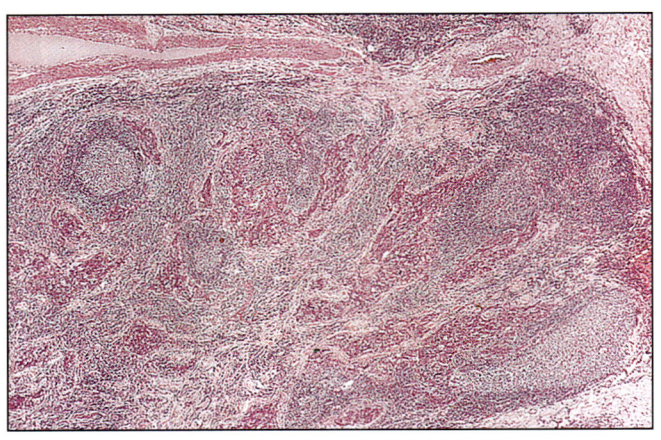

图7.130 淋巴上皮癌。大而不规则的肿瘤岛浸润伴有大量淋巴细胞的纤维性间质。淋巴滤泡也可以出现。

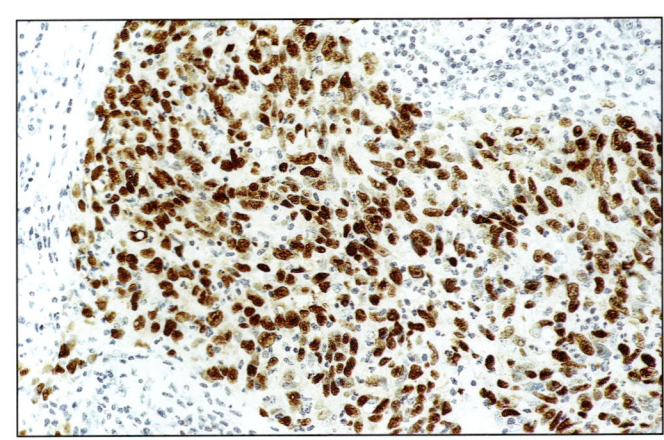

图7.132 淋巴上皮癌。EB病毒编码的RNA（EBER）原位杂交，肿瘤细胞的细胞核选择性阳性。

免疫组织化学和特异性研究：肿瘤细胞细胞角蛋白和EMA免疫反应阳性。超微结构检查一般显示鳞状特征，例如桥粒和张力丝。在所有来自爱斯基摩、中国东南部和日本的病例中，EB病毒原位杂交均呈阳性，在其他人种仅有少数阳性（图7.132）[421,427,428]。

鉴别诊断：淋巴上皮癌在组织学、免疫组织化学以及超微结构上均不能与鼻咽部未分化癌相区别。因为鼻咽癌很常见，所以在作出涎腺淋巴上皮癌的诊断之前，应该进行临床检查和内镜查并作活检，以排除这种可能性[425]。为了预后的原因，淋巴上皮癌应该与大细胞癌鉴别。

在淋巴上皮癌中见到的肿瘤细胞岛明显不同于淋巴上皮性涎腺炎的淋巴上皮病变；后者缺乏上皮非典型性，而且常常伴有基底膜样物质。除了少数散在的淋巴细胞以外，淋巴上皮性涎腺炎的上皮岛EB病毒编码的RNAs（EBER）原位杂交总是阴性[417]，然而，淋巴上皮癌的上皮细胞EB病毒通常阳性。

鳞状细胞癌　Squamous cell carcinoma

定义

原发性涎腺鳞状细胞癌是一种非常少见的恶性肿瘤，应该排除来自邻近鳞状细胞癌的浸润或转移。这种疾病很少能在小涎腺作出诊断，因为不可能排除黏膜鳞状细胞癌。一般来说，涎腺转移性鳞状细胞癌多于原发性鳞状细胞癌。

临床特征

这种肿瘤主要发生在老年男性，平均年龄64岁。从前由于痤疮、良性和恶性肿瘤、胸腺、甲状腺和扁桃体肿大而进行放疗被认为是某些病例的好发因素[65]。三分

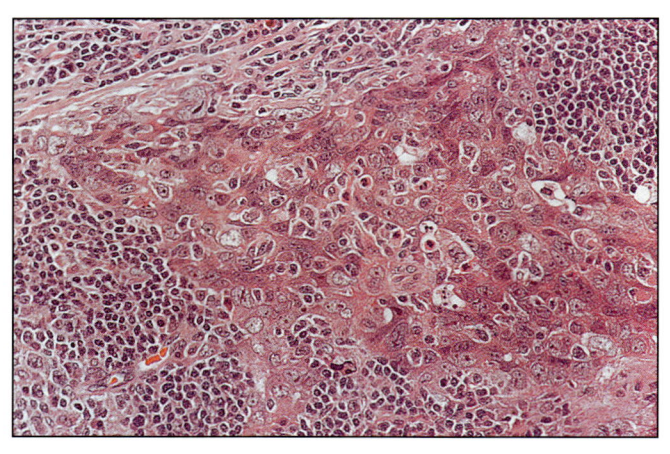

A　　　　　　　　　　　　　　　　　　　　B

图7.131 淋巴上皮癌。（A）肿瘤细胞边界一般不清，核大淡染。淋巴细胞浸润肿瘤岛和间质。（B）有时，肿瘤内淋巴细胞浸润非常突出，以致肿瘤的上皮性本质不易辨认。本例有孤立的伴有嗜酸性胞浆的细胞，符合局灶性鳞状分化。

之二的肿瘤发生在腮腺，其余的发生在颌下腺。多数患者出现迅速生长的坚硬而固定的肿块。局部淋巴结受累以及面神经麻痹常见。

鳞状细胞癌倾向于浸润和迅速扩展。因为颈淋巴结转移常见，所以常规根治性颈部清扫是可取的。5年生存率大约只有30%。溃疡形成、固定、患者年龄大、肿瘤分期高以及面神经麻痹是预后不良的因素[429,430]。

病理学

肿瘤通常为浸润性、褐色、质硬。它通常是中到高分化鳞状细胞癌，由鳞状细胞片块和细胞岛组成，容易辨认角质形成和细胞间桥。间质纤维组织增生。虽然有些细胞可能水肿，但是细胞内缺乏黏液，否则应该考虑黏液表皮样癌的诊断。偶尔，在大的排泄管中可见异型增生的鳞状上皮。

鉴别诊断

除了高级别黏液表皮样癌和转移癌以外，原发性涎腺鳞状细胞癌必须与Warthin瘤、嗜酸细胞瘤、伴有与梗死和炎症有关的明显非典型性鳞状化生的多形性腺瘤，以及坏死性涎腺化生相鉴别（见"诊断分析方法"，第310页）。

黏液性腺癌　Mucinous adenocarcinoma

这种肿瘤在组织学上相当于胃肠道、乳腺和皮肤的黏液性癌或胶样癌。其特征为成簇的肿瘤细胞漂浮在细胞外黏液池中[431]。偶尔，肿瘤细胞可以形成导管、乳头、囊肿以及筛状结构。文献中仅有几个病例报告。所有受累的患者均是成人，没有性别差异。黏液性腺癌可能是一种低级别的肿瘤，治疗选择完全切除。

小涎腺印戒细胞（产生黏液）腺癌　Signet-ring cell (mucin-producing) adenocarcinoma of minor salivary gland

定义

这是一种小涎腺低级别恶性肿瘤，其特征为有含有黏液的印戒细胞。

临床特征

患者平均年龄是56.4岁，有女性好发的趋势，女性与男性发病比为2.5:1[432]。报告的所有病例均发生在口腔小涎腺，表现为可能是固定的外生性结节或肿块。手术切除之后没有复发或转移。

病理学特征

浸润性肿瘤，由狭窄平行的条带、随机分布的散在的小巢或孤立的细胞组成。印戒细胞的特征是有单个或几个胞浆黏液空泡，细胞核偏心，有凹陷。与这些印戒细胞混合的是少数伴有嗜酸性或透明胞浆的肿瘤细胞。总的来说，细胞学非典型性非常轻微，几乎没有核分裂象，而且没有坏死。在报告的7个病例中仅有1例有细胞外黏液池[432]。神经周围浸润并不少见。肿瘤细胞强烈表达CAM5.2（低分子量细胞角蛋白）和p63，不同程度表达肌动蛋白、S-100和GFAP。钙调节蛋白阴性。

腺癌，非特异性　Adenocarcinoma, not otherwise specified

定义

几乎所有的来源于涎腺本身的癌均为腺癌。非特异性腺癌（adenocarcinoma NOS）指的是涎腺原发性癌，显示腺体分化但缺乏其他明确的肿瘤类型的诊断标准。由于越来越多的涎腺肿瘤性疾病是有特征性的（比如PLGA），故非特异性腺癌成了一个逐渐缩小的诊断废纸篓（表7.10）。

临床特征

非特异性腺癌最常发生在老年人，高峰年龄在50～60岁和70～80岁之间，伴有男性好发的趋势[431,433]。最常见的部位依次是腮腺、颌下腺、腭和颊黏膜。患者表现为无症状或生长迅速的疼痛性肿块，伴有溃疡形成并固定于邻近的结构。面神经麻痹常见。Spiro等发现[434]，低级别、中级别和高级别腺癌的15年生存率分别为54%、31%和3%，但是其他研究没有发现分级具有意义[435]。分期也很重要，因为不管分级如何，I期肿瘤的10年治愈率是75%。有报告称，累及口腔的肿瘤比腮腺和颌下腺肿瘤预后要好[435,436]。

病理学

大体上，肿瘤表现出不规则的浸润性边缘。切面褐色实性，伴有出血或坏死区域。

肿瘤以不同组成的腺体或导管结构为特征（图7.133）。生长方式变化不定，包括腺体、乳头状、囊性、筛状、实性、小叶状、巢状以及带样，伴有单一的特征，缺乏可以辨认的诊断其他特异性肿瘤的形态（图7.133）[433]。肿瘤小部分区域可能类似于特异性肿瘤，例如腺泡细胞癌或上皮-肌上皮癌，但是如果总的图像

表7.10	根据细胞学分级将各种涎腺腺癌的统一特征分组（除外黏液表皮样癌、腺泡细胞癌和腺样囊性癌）	
	低级别腺癌	高级别腺癌
包括的肿瘤	• 多形性低级别腺癌 • 上皮-肌上皮癌 • 基底细胞腺癌 • 囊腺癌 • 低级别腺癌，非特异性	• 涎腺导管癌 • 嗜酸细胞癌 • 高级别腺癌，非特异性
统一的组织学特征	• 浸润性生长 • 最小或轻度核的非典型性 • 核分裂象不常见 • 凝固性坏死不常见	• 浸润性生长 • 核的分级高 • 核分裂象常见 • 凝固性坏死常见
行为	• 缓慢生长，惰性 • 如果切除不完全可能复发 • 局部淋巴结转移5%～15% • 远处转移非常少见 • 预后良好	• 迅速生长 • 早期和常常转移到淋巴结或远处 • 预后不良

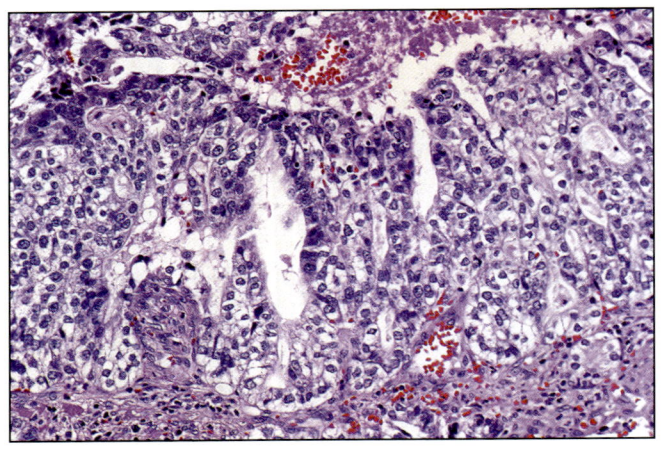

A

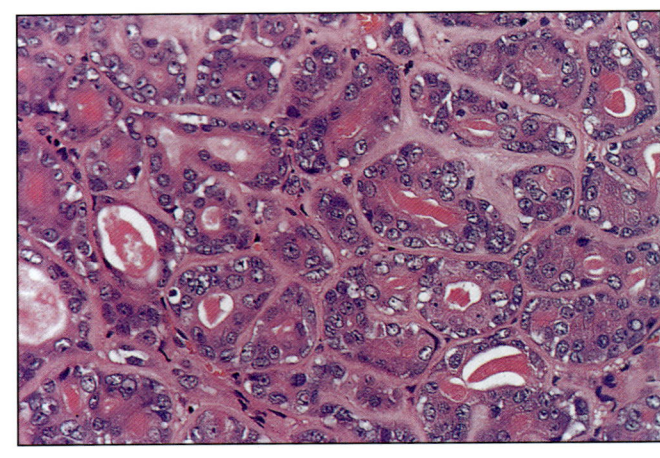

B

图7.133 非特异性腺癌，中级别。（A）肿瘤以大的岛屿状的形式生长，偶尔可见腺体间隙。（B）肿瘤由没有特征的管状结构组成，内衬中度非典型性细胞，缺乏各种已知肿瘤类型的诊断结构。

与已知肿瘤的组成成分不一致，非特异性腺癌的诊断仍然是适用的。

肿瘤细胞可以是嗜酸性、透明、黑色素瘤样、黏液性、皮脂腺或浆细胞样[433]。腺体结构是由单一类型细胞组成的（仅仅有腔面细胞），或者在极少数情况下有两种类型的细胞（腔面细胞和基底/肌上皮细胞）。常见正常实质、神经和血管的浸润。

有人试图对于非特异性腺癌进行再分类，但是迄今为止尚未发现与预后有关的亚类。管状型显示突出的导管结构[431]。硬化型以明显的纤维组织增生为特征，肿瘤成分可能被掩盖[431]。多数非特异性腺癌在组织学上是高级别的，但是分级是一种相对主观的评价，没有明确的标准。

涎腺母细胞瘤 Sialoblastoma

定义

涎腺母细胞瘤，也叫胚组织瘤（embryoma）[437]、先天性癌[15]或先天性基底细胞腺瘤[438]，是一种新生儿或婴儿的肿瘤，由原始表现的细胞组成，偶尔伴有导管形成，重现了胚胎涎腺组织结构。偶尔在涎腺母细胞瘤附近发现胎儿或胚胎期发育不良的涎腺组织，可能是这种病变的前身[439]。

临床特征

肿瘤发生在大涎腺，最常见于腮腺。它们发生在出生时或出生后第一年或第二年内，表现为无症状的肿块。少数病例可能伴有皮肤溃疡、面神经麻痹、分娩障碍、先天性痣以及伴发的肝母细胞瘤。

临床行为变化很大。大约三分之一的病例发生局部复发，6%发生局部淋巴结转移[443]。有一例报告还发生了大脑内扩散和肺部转移[444]。根据报告，在多次复发的病例，间变和增生活性增加[443]。治疗选择完全手术切除[445]；复发和不完全切除的病例可以进行辅助性放射治疗。

病理学

这种肿瘤可能非常局限，或为浸润性，由被纤维性间质分开的密集排列或疏松散在的细胞岛组成。多数细胞看上去原始，呈基底细胞样，具有大的卵圆形空泡状细胞核和少量胞浆（图7.134）。肿瘤细胞形成细胞丰富的小管和实性器官样细胞巢，肿瘤岛周围有模糊的栅栏状排列的细胞核。细胞核有轻度的非典型性，并有不同程度的核分裂活性。局部可见内衬伴有嗜酸性胞浆的较大的多角形到立方形细胞的导管，导管腔内经常含有分泌产物[438,442,446]。局部可以出现类似于腺样囊性癌的筛状结构。不同病例之间可有不同程度的细胞学非典型性、坏死以及神经或血管浸润，而且提示与临床结果相关[446,447]。细胞角蛋白免疫染色可以突显导管结构。位于周围的基底细胞样细胞显示S-100蛋白和肌动蛋白染色阳性。

间叶性肿瘤和瘤样病变
Mesenchymal neoplasms and tumor-like lesions

间叶性肿瘤大约占所有涎腺肿瘤的2%～5%[11,14,448]，其中95%以上的病例累及大涎腺。良性肿瘤数目超过恶性肿瘤，根据不同的研究结果，其比例从2.4:1到18:1不等[11,14]。血管瘤和淋巴管瘤最常见，占Hamburg涎腺肿瘤登记处（1965—1981年）所有间叶性肿瘤的50%[14]，其次是脂肪瘤（19.2%）、神经鞘肿瘤（神经纤维瘤，神经鞘瘤：15.8%）以及肉瘤（7.5%）。血管瘤也是儿童最常见的涎腺肿瘤[449]。根据Luna等复习的85个病例，涎腺最常见的肉瘤类型是横纹肌肉瘤和所谓的恶性纤维组织细胞瘤[450]。间叶性肿瘤与见于身体其他部分那些肿瘤具有相同的组织学特征和行为（见第3章，第24章和第27章）。

血管肿瘤和瘤样病变
Vascular tumors and tumor-like lesions

毛细血管瘤　Capillary hemangioma

临床特征：毛细血管瘤，常常称为细胞性血管瘤、幼年性血管内皮瘤或婴儿血管内皮瘤，倾向于发生于两

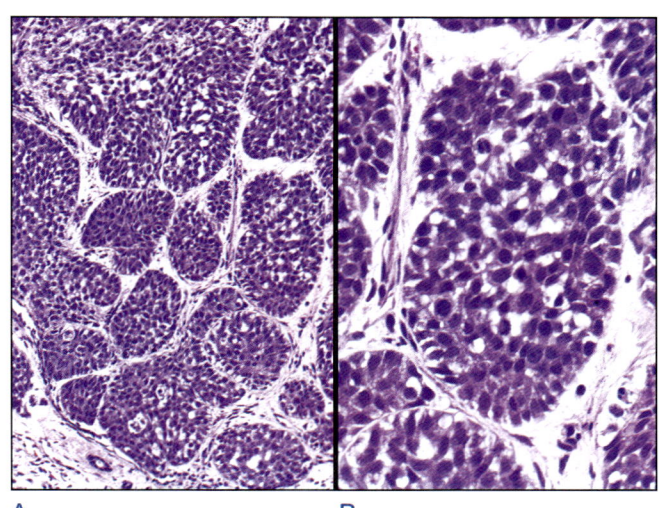

图7.134　涎腺母细胞瘤。（A）肿瘤由基底细胞样小叶组成。（B）与基底细胞腺瘤或基底细胞腺癌不同，细胞核空泡状较明显，看上去较活跃，周围部分细胞核栅栏状排列不显著。

性的婴儿[15,65,451,452]。其表现不同，从出生时或生后不久发现的无症状的肿块到迅速增大的病变。多数病变见于腮腺[65,452]，表面皮肤可能表现出淡蓝色的变色。缺乏疼痛和面神经麻痹，但是少病例可能合并消耗性凝血病（Kasabach-Merritt综合征）。到了7岁时，75%～90%的病例有望自发性消退[65,453]。少数病例呈现进行性生长，甚至可能转化为血管肉瘤[454,455]。

病理学：大体检查，肿瘤呈暗红色、分叶状，没有包膜，大小从直径1 cm到直径8 cm。某些病例可以表现为延伸到周围的组织。

在未成熟的形式（细胞性血管瘤）中，肿瘤性内皮细胞肥胖，伴有大而规则的细胞核，核分裂象常见。血管腔通常不明显，被梭形的外皮细胞形成的袖套所包围（图7.135）。实性的表现和活跃的核分裂象可能导致错误地诊断为肉瘤。随着病变的成熟，通常从周围开始向内形成完好的血管腔，毛细血管内衬扁平的内皮细胞（图7.135）。涎腺小叶结构保存完好，即使在受累的区域，这种特征表明这种肿瘤具有非侵袭性本质（图7.135A）。残留的涎腺导管和腺泡"舒适的"散布在增生的血管中（图7.135A）。偶尔能够发现神经的浸润，但这并不意味是恶性。肿瘤退化与进行性弥漫性间质纤维化有关。

海绵状血管瘤　Cavernous hemangioma

涎腺海绵状血管瘤罕见，主要发生于成人[65]。没有自发性消退的倾向。组织学上，扩张的薄壁血管内衬扁平内皮细胞。机化血栓中常见营养不良性钙化。

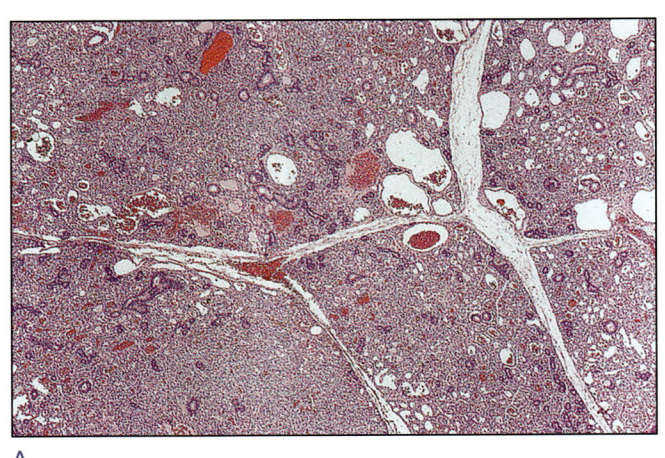
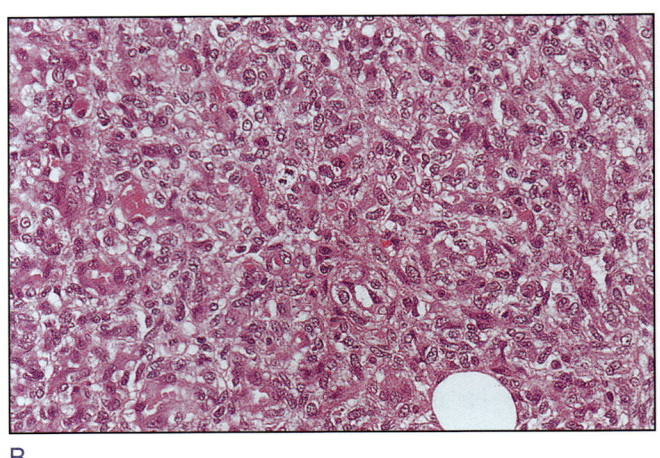

图7.135 腮腺细胞性血管瘤。（A）涎腺小叶结构保留是其特征。（B）在某些小叶中，可见形成完好的毛细血管。其他视野显示不成熟的毛细血管，表现为实性生长方式，结合轻度细胞核的非典型性以及散在的核分裂象，可能错误地解释为恶性肿瘤。

上皮样血管瘤 Epithelioid hemangioma

上皮样血管瘤，也叫伴有嗜酸性粒细胞增多的血管淋巴组织增生（angiolymphoid hyperplasia with eosinophilia）[456]，在少数情况下可以累及腮腺或其他大涎腺。它可能伴有外周血嗜酸性粒细胞增多。在手术切除以后，大约三分之一的病例复发[453]。

上皮样血管瘤的特征是毛细血管到中等大小的血管呈小叶状增生，内衬立方性或多角性内皮细胞，伴有丰富的常常呈空泡状的嗜酸性玻璃样胞浆（图 7.136）。可能有明显的类似于腺体的结构。血管常常伴有许多嗜酸性细胞、淋巴细胞、肥大细胞以及浆细胞。在病变的周围部分淋巴组织成分常常致密。

恶性血管肿瘤 Malignant vascular tumors

涎腺原发性血管肉瘤非常罕见。其主要发生在大

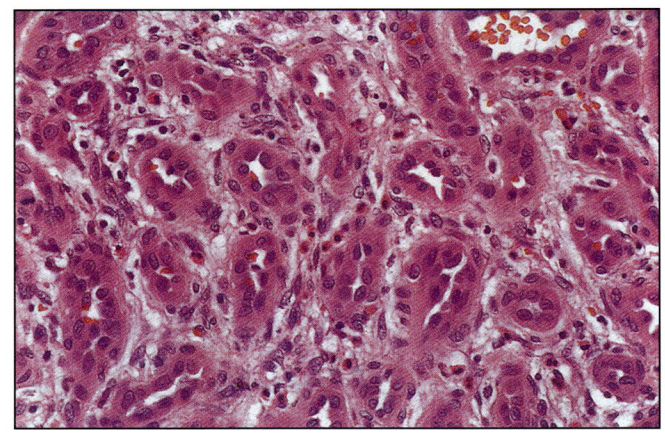

图7.136 腮腺上皮样血管瘤。小管（血管）内衬伴有嗜酸性胞浆的上皮样内皮细胞，这是这种肿瘤的特征，可能被误诊为上皮性肿瘤。血管之间有一些嗜酸性粒细胞。

涎腺，发病高峰是在50～60岁之间[457]。肿瘤通常表现为肿块性病变，伴有新近增大和出血。形态学上，可见具有高度代表性的上皮样变型（多达三分之一的病例）[457-460]。治疗选择外科手术。尚未证实放疗和化疗有效。

腮腺上皮样血管内皮瘤也有少数报道[461]。

Kimura病 Kimura disease

临床特征

Kimura病常常与上皮样血管瘤混淆，它是一种与之完全不相关的病变[462]。人们认为本病起因于过敏性或自身免疫性免疫反应。Kimura病一般表现为皮下肿块，淋巴结肿大和（或）腮腺、颌下腺的肿胀，发生于年轻的东方男性，但是非东方人也可受累。肿块为硬结或橡皮硬度，边界不清，生长缓慢。外周血嗜酸性粒细胞总是增多，常常伴有红细胞沉降率和血清免疫球蛋白E（IgE）升高。病变经常持续多年不变，但是可能发生新的病变。手术后通常复发。

病理学

涎腺通常片块状受累，伴有致密的炎症细胞浸润、萎缩、腺泡丧失以及导管周围和小叶间硬化。炎性浸润包括淋巴细胞、浆细胞和嗜酸性粒细胞。有突出的淋巴滤泡，经常伴有生发中心血管化、坏死、嗜酸性粒细胞浸润甚或脓肿形成。滤泡间区显示血管增生，但是这些血管是高内皮的小静脉，内衬伴有淡染胞浆的立方形到扁平状的内皮（图 7.137）。这样，增生的血管不同于上皮样血管瘤，缺乏玻璃样改变和丰满的胞浆，而且缺乏胞浆空泡。

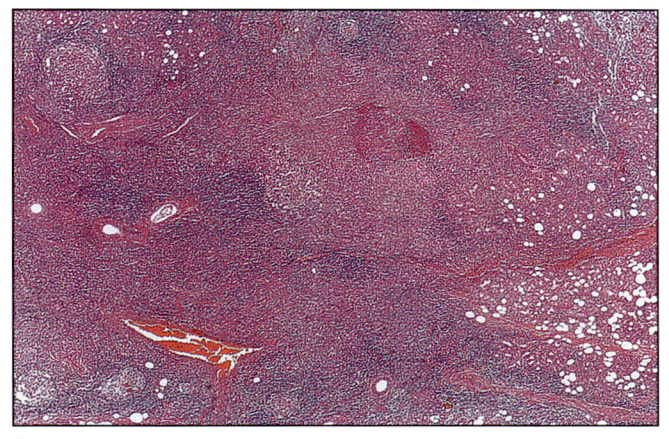
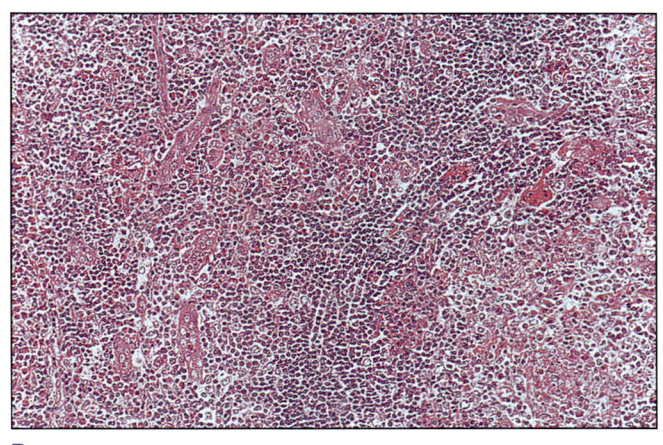

图7.137 Kimura病累及腮腺。（A）这种病变边界不清，以淋巴细胞和嗜酸性粒细胞浸润为特征，伴有涎腺实质破坏。可见淋巴滤泡（视野左上）。还可见到嗜酸性粒细胞脓肿（视野中上部）。（B）视野右下可见反应性淋巴滤泡，其生发中心有嗜酸性粒细胞浸润。滤泡间区的淋巴细胞中嗜酸性粒细胞增多。增生的血管是高内皮的小静脉。

孤立性纤维性肿瘤　Solitary fibrous tumor

孤立性纤维性肿瘤（见第24章）是一种纤维母细胞或肌纤维母细胞肿瘤，最初描述发生于胸膜，但现在公认，人体几乎所有的部位均可发生[463,464]。某些病例报告发生在大涎腺[465-472]。通常表现为无痛性的肿块。多数病例呈现良性经过。

孤立性纤维性肿瘤一般为卵圆形或圆形，而且非常局限。切面灰白色或呈漩涡状。显微镜下，肿瘤特征为伴有少量胞浆的短梭形或肥胖细胞随意生长，混有不同程度的玻璃样变的胶原。典型的病变有细胞减少（富于胶原）和细胞增多（富于肿瘤细胞）区域交替出现。经常可见外皮细胞瘤性血管。肿瘤细胞CD34弥漫强阳性表达。

炎性假瘤　Inflammatory pseudotumor

炎性假瘤是一种形成肿块的纤维炎症性病变（不同于炎症性肌纤维母细胞性肿瘤），可以累及涎腺，尤其是腮腺。其表现为质硬的结节状肿块，男性和女性发病相同，平均年龄为70岁[65,473-476]。手术切除可以治愈。大体检查显示为局限性的肿块，切面呈灰白色漩涡状。这种病变由梭形细胞（纤维母细胞和肌纤维母细胞）组成，混有胶原纤维和不同量的浆细胞、淋巴细胞、多形核白细胞以及泡沫状组织细胞。梭形细胞可以形成模糊的束状或席纹状结构。常见多核组织细胞性巨细胞和钙化。某些梭形细胞CD68和肌动蛋白免疫染色阳性，但是细胞角蛋白阴性。

结节性筋膜炎　Nodular fasciitis

涎腺结节性筋膜炎常常表现为儿童或婴儿的孤立性、迅速生长的疼痛性的肿块[477,478]。它是一种自限性的病变，复发罕见。结节性筋膜炎是局限性的，没有被膜的卵圆形肿块，由反应性的纤维母细胞或肌纤维母细胞组成[479]。梭形细胞排列成短而宽的细胞束，伴有局灶性席纹状结构。细胞稀少的区域具有黏液样，羽毛样表现，散布有小的黏液池。梭形细胞具有空泡状的细胞核，有时有突出的核仁。容易发现核分裂象，但是没有非典型性核分裂象。病变中散布的是淋巴细胞和外渗的红细胞。

巨细胞瘤　Giant cell tumor

在大涎腺中有少数巨细胞瘤报告[480,481]。半数病例伴有癌，通常是涎腺导管癌和多形性腺瘤中的癌。巨细胞成分包括在单核细胞背景中均匀一致分布的破骨细胞性巨细胞。虽然在形态学上类似于骨巨细胞瘤，但是单核细胞经常表达上皮性标记物和雄激素受体，并且显示微卫星结构，比较类似于癌，而且具有比较侵袭性的行为[481]。少数高级别的癌伴有散在的破骨细胞性巨细胞，不要将其看成是巨细胞瘤的一种形式[482]。

血液淋巴肿瘤和瘤样病变
Hematolymphoid tumors and tumor-like lesions

淋巴上皮涎腺炎
Lymphoepithelial sialadenitis

定义

淋巴上皮性涎腺炎（LESA）以前称为肌上皮性涎腺炎或良性淋巴上皮病变[65,483-486]，其特征是涎腺实质

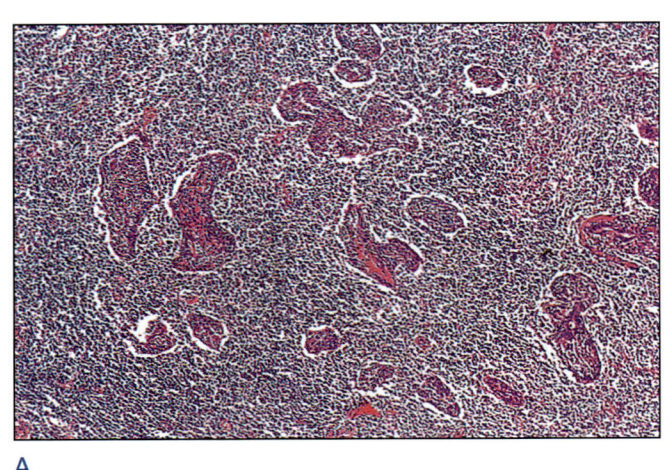 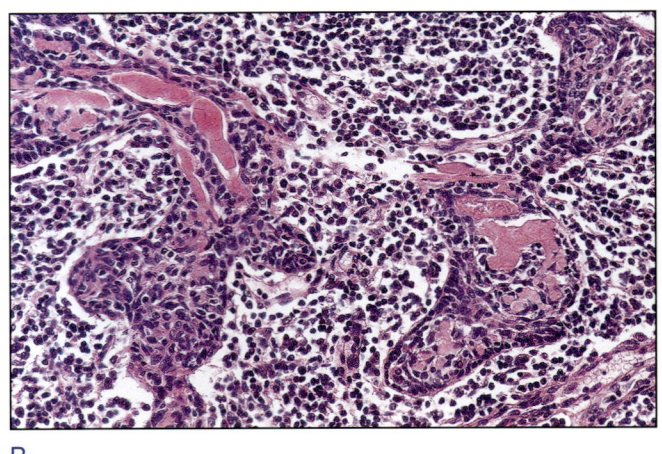

图 7.138 淋巴上皮性涎腺炎。（A）不规则的上皮岛散布在致密的淋巴细胞间质中。（B）淋巴上皮岛，也叫上皮肌上皮岛，是以先前存在的导管上皮增生为特征，最初的管腔常常消失。细胞间常常发现玻璃样基底膜样物质。上皮肌上皮岛被小的淋巴细胞浸润。

淋巴细胞浸润，腺泡萎缩以及导管增生，伴有淋巴上皮病变（从前称为上皮肌上皮岛）形成。"肌上皮性涎腺炎"这个名词属于误解，因为没有充分的证据表明肌上皮参与淋巴上皮病变的形成。

临床特征

LESA 主要累及腮腺（80%～85%）以及颌下腺（10%～15%）[65,477]，表现为反复发生的、弥漫性质硬的肿块。20%的患者发生于两侧，40%的病例出现疼痛[477]。大部分（50%～84%）受累的患者具有 Sjögren 综合征的临床和实验室的证据[487,488]。有女性好发的趋势（男女比例为 1∶3），高峰年龄为 30～40 岁和 60～70 岁。

LESA 是发生涎腺淋巴瘤的危险因素，尤其是当伴有 Sjögren 综合征或其他相关结缔组织疾病时，例如类风湿性关节炎[489]。估计危险增加 44 倍，且 80% 的淋巴瘤是结外边缘区 B 细胞（MALT）淋巴瘤[486,490-492]。尚未发现诸如 EB 病毒、人类疱疹病毒 8、人类亲淋巴病毒-1 以及丙种肝炎病毒等病毒在淋巴瘤的转化中具有作用[493,494]。应该注意的是，以前报告为 LESA 的某些病变实际上是 MALT 淋巴瘤或 LESA 合并 MALT 淋巴瘤[495,496]。根据报告，LESA 中淋巴瘤的发病率从 20%至 28%不等[497,498]。

根据形态学可能难以辨认 LESA 中早期的淋巴瘤性改变。某些研究者应用检测单克隆 B 细胞增多来提示"前淋巴瘤性"改变或诊断淋巴瘤[496,499-503]。Jordan 等通过联合应用免疫组织化学，PCR 以及原位杂交技术能够在 77% 的 LESA 中鉴别出单克隆群体[504]。虽然某些病例最后确实发生淋巴瘤[491]，但伴有单克隆群体的多数病例具有平常的经过[505]。这样，在缺乏淋巴瘤形态学证据的情况下，LESA 中的克隆性群体的意义尚有争议[496,502,506-508]。

因为发生淋巴瘤的危险性增加以及在小的活检或细针吸取标本中难以排除淋巴瘤的存在，所以腮腺切除术是选择性的治疗。术后仍然需要长期随访伴随的自身免疫性疾病和淋巴增生性疾病。

病理学特征

LESA 病变散在或边界不清，但是涎腺小叶结构保留。淋巴细胞浸润明显开始于周围区域，且逐渐取代涎腺小叶。病变包括小淋巴细胞和浆细胞，伴有或不伴有生发中心形成。腺泡组织明显萎缩或丧失，但残留的导管上皮增生，而且淋巴细胞潜入上皮，形成了特征性的淋巴上皮病变（上皮肌上皮岛）（图7.138）[509-512]。淋巴上皮病变由圆形或不规则的实性细胞岛组成，其中可有小的残留的导管腔。上皮细胞肥胖，为梭形、多角形或合体细胞，具有均匀一致的卵圆形的细胞核，伴有细腻的染色质，类似于乳腺导管内上皮增生（图7.138B）。在细胞中间常常见到玻璃样基底膜样物质。增生的细胞被认为是混合性导管和肌上皮细胞，但是，最近的研究没有发现有肌上皮参与的证据[513]。在极少数的情况下，可以发生鳞状化生和角化[506,514,515]。

免疫染色显示，淋巴上皮病变的上皮细胞细胞角蛋白免疫反应阳性。淋巴上皮病变的淋巴细胞主要是B细胞。B细胞和T细胞混合存在，前者的数目多于后者[484]。提示LESA中存在淋巴瘤的特征列在表7.11中。

原发性涎腺淋巴瘤
Primary lymphoma of salivary gland

原发性涎腺淋巴瘤罕见，仅占涎腺肿瘤的 2.4%～4.5%[14,477,516]，多数的病例发生在腮腺（50%～93%）和

表7.11	支持MALT淋巴瘤或MALT淋巴瘤合并LESA而不是LESA的形态学和免疫组化特征
形态学特征	免疫组化特征
• 上皮岛周围出现透明细胞（单核细胞样B细胞样）环；Hyjek等（1988）[514]和Diss等（1995）[506]认为这是并发淋巴瘤最早期的证据 • 由大的淋巴细胞簇形成的上皮岛"腔洞" • 浸润纤细的小叶间隔或神经	• 证实轻链限制性 • 证实弥漫性B细胞片块 • 异常的B细胞免疫表型，例如CD43的共同表达

颌下腺[14,477,517]。诊断原发性涎腺淋巴瘤要求疾病的绝大部分位于涎腺内。然而，根据临床或组织学检查，通常很难区分发生于涎腺本身的淋巴瘤（原发性涎腺淋巴瘤）和发生于包埋在涎腺中的淋巴结的淋巴瘤（普通的淋巴结淋巴瘤）。后一种类型的淋巴瘤在形态学和预后上与那些发生在其他淋巴结的淋巴瘤没有不同。最常见的类型是Hodgkin淋巴瘤、滤泡性淋巴瘤和弥漫性大B细胞淋巴瘤，但是任何类型的淋巴结淋巴瘤均可发生[65,486,497,500]。

MALT淋巴瘤是最常见的原发性涎腺淋巴瘤，其次为弥漫性大B细胞淋巴瘤和滤泡性淋巴瘤[486,490,518]。在获得性免疫缺陷综合征（AIDS）的患者，发生高级别B细胞淋巴瘤的危险有所增加，而且其中某些淋巴瘤与EB病毒相关[519,520]。在极少数的情况下，外周T细胞淋巴瘤、间变性大细胞淋巴瘤以及自然杀伤/T细胞淋巴瘤可以作为原发性涎腺淋巴瘤而发生，而且它们经常具有侵袭性的过程[521]。

MALT淋巴瘤（MALT型结外边缘区B细胞淋巴瘤）
MALT lymphoma (extranodal marginal zone B-cell lymphoma of MALT type)

MALT淋巴瘤的临床、组织学和免疫遗传学所见在第21章详细描述。这一节仅仅讨论与涎腺有关的特征。

临床特征：涎腺MALT淋巴瘤最明确的好发因素是LESA或Sjögren综合征以及丙种肝炎感染[490-492]。在一组33例的研究中，46%的病例和LESA相关，29%的病例伴有丙种肝炎病毒感染[491]。平均年龄是61岁（年龄范围是55岁至65岁），伴有女性好发的趋势。患者通常表现为涎腺缓慢生长的肿块。诊断时大约30%的患者可见颈部淋巴结受累。25%的病例发现血清单克隆成分（IgG和IgM）[491]。总体预后极好，5年生存率为85%～90%[491,492]。局部治疗似乎已经足够，例如手术或放射治疗。预后不良的因素包括转化为弥漫性大B细胞淋巴瘤（发生率12%）以及年龄较大。

病理学：大体上，肿瘤为非局限性，质硬，褐色。经常发现由于导管扩张而形成的散在的囊肿（图7.139）。组织学特征与发生在其他部位的MALT淋巴瘤相似，经常表现为混合性细胞类型（通常包括类似于单核细胞样B细胞的透明细胞）、反应性淋巴滤泡以及许多淋巴上皮病变。受累的涎腺可能广泛破坏，或者可能仍然保留小叶结构（图7.140）。正如Isaacson和Norton强调的一样[518]，直接生成的MALT淋巴瘤或由LESA进展而来的MALT淋巴瘤的最早的证据是淋巴上皮病变周围出

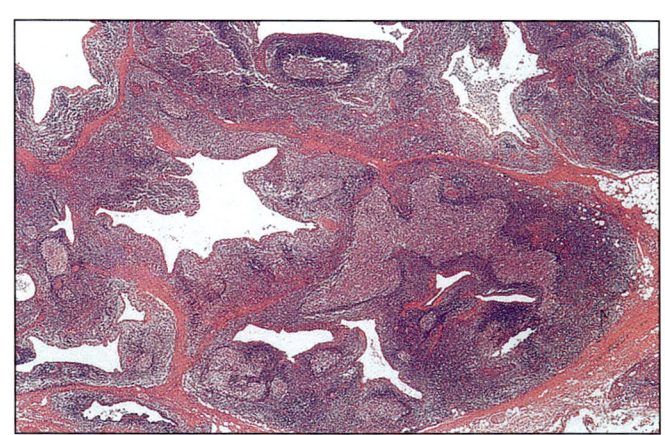

图7.139 低级别B细胞MALT淋巴瘤。常常出现由于导管扩张而形成的多发性囊肿。在致密的淋巴细胞浸润中，出现特征性的反应性淋巴滤泡。

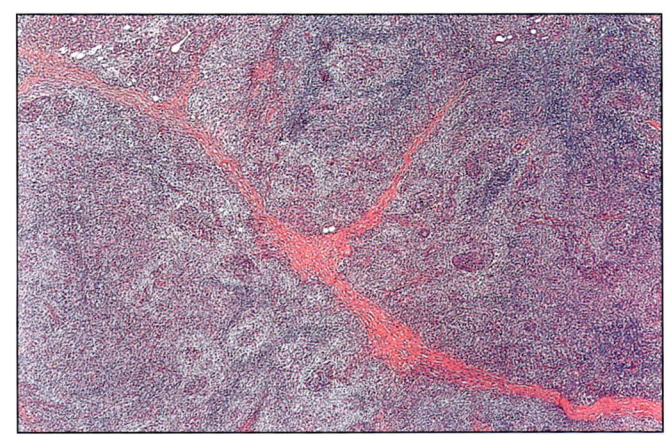

图7.140 低级别B细胞MALT淋巴瘤。在这个致密增生的淋巴细胞中，上皮岛（淋巴上皮病变）周围淡染的细胞环为诊断MALT淋巴瘤而不是良性淋巴上皮病变提供了一个最有意义的线索。散布有许多反应性的淋巴滤泡。

现宽大的透明细胞环（图 7.140 和 7.141）。淋巴上皮病变是肿瘤性淋巴细胞引起的导管显著膨胀和扭曲变形，而且在增生的上皮内可能形成"脓肿"。导管内和导管周围的淋巴细胞一般比其余的肿瘤细胞大，伴有卵圆形或有凹陷的细胞核，以及丰富的淡染或透明的胞浆，类似于单核细胞样 B 细胞（图 7.141B）。其他的淋巴细胞类似于小淋巴细胞，或有折叠的细胞核（中心细胞样）。常常有不同数目的浆细胞，其通常成簇排列；浆细胞可能显示轻微的非典型性，而且可能含有 Dutcher 小体。经常出现孤立散在的大淋巴细胞，伴有圆形细胞核以及清晰的核仁（图 7.142）。在偶然情况下，淋巴上皮病变周围可见上皮样组织细胞环。

免疫染色显示，有致密的 B 细胞片块（CD20+）（图 7.143），而且常常可能证实轻链限制性。CD5、CD10 和周期素 D1（cyclin D1）阴性。B 细胞可能显示异常的 CD43 共同表达，这种特征可能有助于诊断不典型的淋巴瘤病例。

遗传学特征：在部分病例已经证实有 t（14；18），伴有 IgH/MALT 融合以及 3 号和 18 号染色体三体，而 t（11；18）非常罕见，它最常见于胃和肺的 MALT 淋巴瘤[522,523]。

发生在MALT淋巴瘤的弥漫性大B细胞淋巴瘤
Diffuse large B-cell lymphoma arising in MALT lymphoma

MALT 淋巴瘤可以转化为弥漫性大 B 细胞淋巴瘤，此时其行为变得更加具有侵袭性。然而，在如何定义大细胞转化这个问题上，还没有普遍被接受的最低标准。当有致密的大细胞片块或相当大的细胞簇时，可以明确诊断为并发大 B 细胞淋巴瘤。最大的问题是，当大细胞数增加时，也密集混进一些小细胞。在这种情况下，作出诸如"MALT 淋巴瘤伴有大细胞增加"这样的诊断是有道理的。最近有证据表明，与普通的 MALT 淋巴瘤相

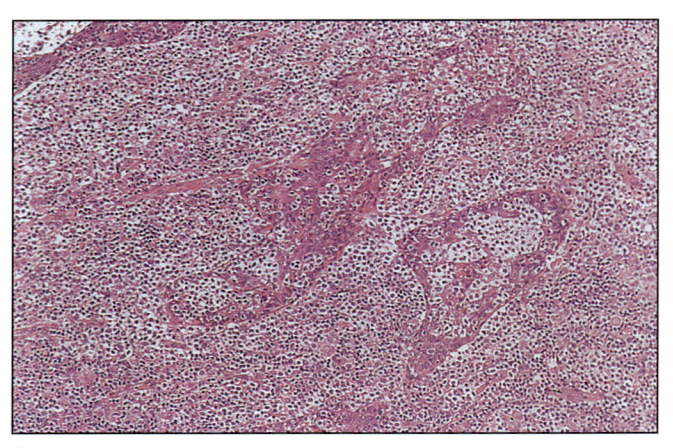

A

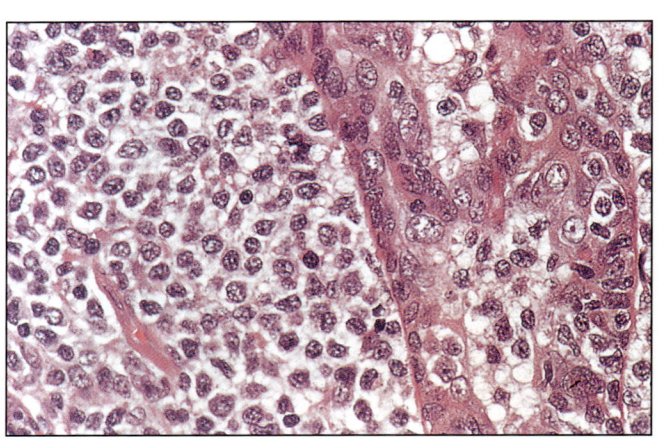

B

图 7.141 低级别MALT淋巴瘤。（A）特征性的淋巴上皮病变广泛浸润，并被淡染的细胞包绕。（B）高倍放大显示淡染的细胞类似于单核细胞样B细胞。许多这样的细胞也浸润导管上皮（视野右侧），形成淋巴上皮病变。

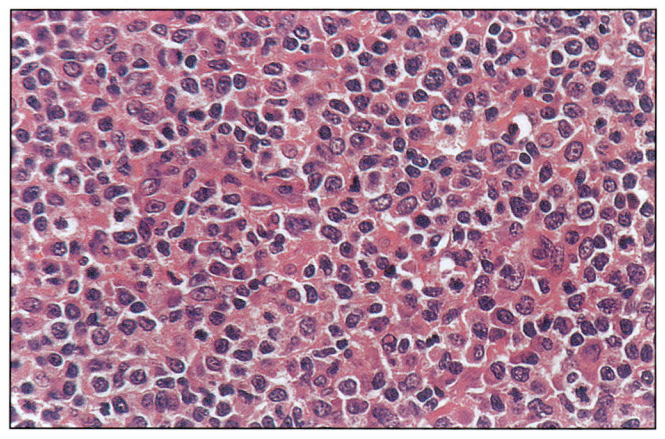

图 7.142 低级别B细胞MALT淋巴瘤。主要的淋巴细胞是小淋巴细胞，混有浆细胞以及偶见大而活化的细胞。

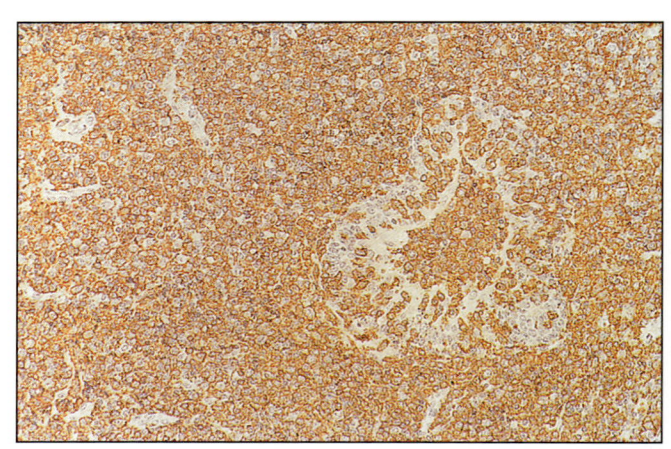

图 7.143 低级别B细胞MALT淋巴瘤。L26（CD20）免疫染色显示弥漫性B细胞片块，这种特征强烈支持淋巴瘤的诊断。构成淋巴上皮病变（视野右侧）的淋巴细胞也显示为B细胞。

比，大细胞超过 5% 有较不好的结果[524]。

淋巴上皮囊肿　Lymphoepithlial cyst

涎腺淋巴上皮囊肿的特征是内衬上皮，囊壁上伴有致密的淋巴细胞间质。有人提出它来自于腮腺内淋巴结涎腺包含物的囊性增生。在过去的 20 年中其发病率大大增加，与人类免疫缺陷病毒（HIV）感染相关[5]。

临床特征

与 HIV 无关的淋巴上皮囊肿，一般发生于成年人（平均年龄 45 岁），且有男性好发的趋势。它通常表现为腮腺肿块，手术切除可以治愈。

HIV 相关性淋巴上皮囊肿（也叫囊性淋巴组织增生），通常表现为两侧腮腺肿块，伴有颈淋巴结肿大。肿块缓慢生长且为无痛性。男性受累比女性常见（7 : 1），高峰年龄为 10～20 岁和 30～40 岁。这种囊肿可能是 HIV 感染的第一个临床表现，同时发生持续性全身淋巴结肿大综合征。缺乏 Sjögren 综合征特征性的口腔干燥和眼球干燥的症状。通过腮腺切除术、切除术、刮除术或放射治疗主要是为了整容的目的，并不影响 HIV 感染的过程[525-527]。

病理学

与 HIV 感染无关的淋巴上皮囊肿几乎都是孤立的，而 HIV 相关性淋巴上皮囊肿通常由多发性不同大小的囊肿组成（图 7.144）。囊肿腔面通常呈波浪形，内衬复层鳞状上皮，虽然可以内衬立方、柱状、或呼吸道上皮。上皮下有增厚的淋巴组织带，其基底常常与周围的涎腺实质界限分明。经常出现淋巴滤泡，而且小淋巴细胞可以浸润上皮。

在 HIV 相关性淋巴上皮囊肿，淋巴组织增生明显，类似于持续性全身淋巴结肿大的淋巴结（图 7.144）。有非常明显的滤泡增生、滤泡溶解、单核细胞样 B 细胞增加、血管结构增加以及浆细胞浸润。可以发现一些淋巴上皮病变。主要的鉴别诊断是 MALT 淋巴瘤。

慢性硬化性涎腺炎（Kuttner 瘤）　Chronic scleraosing sialadenitis（Kuttner tumor）

临床特征

慢性硬化性涎腺炎是一种慢性炎症性疾病，是由浓缩的分泌物、结石或微小结石引起的，由于上行感染而使病变继续存在[528-530]。近来证实，病变中有丰富的 IgG4 阳性的浆细胞，提出可能与 IgG4 相关性硬化性淋巴浆细胞性胰腺炎/胆管炎综合征有关[531]。本病几乎完全累及颌下腺，在其晚期阶段称为 Kuttner 瘤，因为临床上表现为坚硬的肿物，与肿瘤不能区分[533]。本病可能为双侧性。患者的平均年龄是 42～44 岁，有轻微的男性好发趋势[528,530]。

病理学

组织学特征各异，取决于发展的阶段和炎性的严重程度[528,530]。小叶结构保存，小叶与小叶之间受累程度不同。在早期阶段，淋巴浆细胞浸润开始围绕涎腺导管，随后导管周围纤维化（图 7.145）。接下来是局灶鳞状和黏液状化生以及导管上皮增生，但是几乎没有淋巴上皮病变。导管可能含有浓缩的分泌物。淋巴细胞浸润和纤维化加剧并逐渐累及整个小叶，伴有腺泡萎缩。经常出

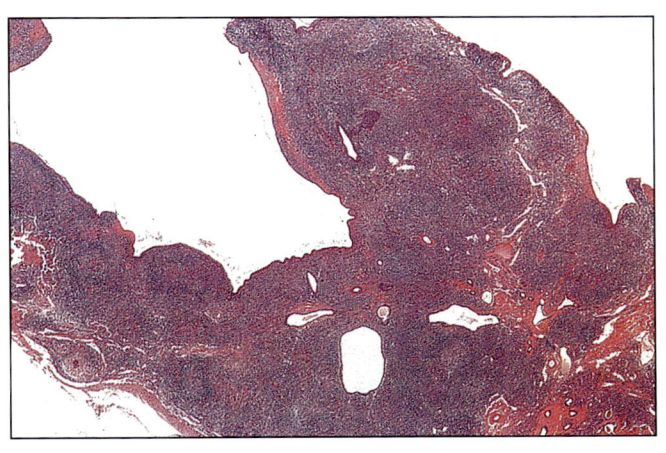
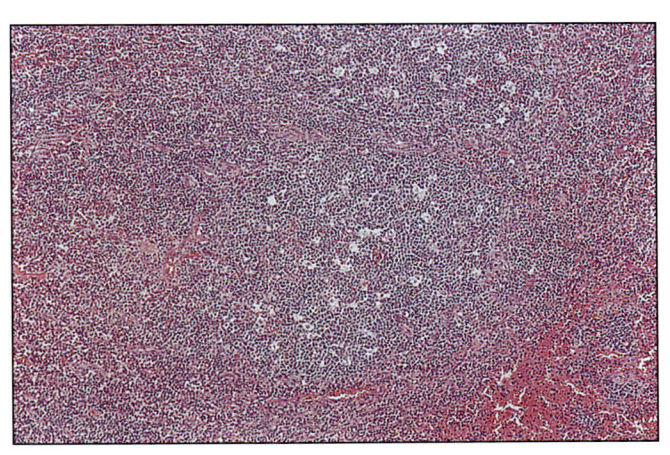

图 7.144　接受治疗的 HIV 血清阳性患者的囊性淋巴组织增生（淋巴上皮囊肿）。（A）出现多发性内衬上皮的囊肿。囊腔波浪状的表现是由于凸出的淋巴组织结节产生的。（B）淋巴组织表现为"裸露的"反应性滤泡，这常常见于 HIV 相关性淋巴结的显著增生的滤泡中。

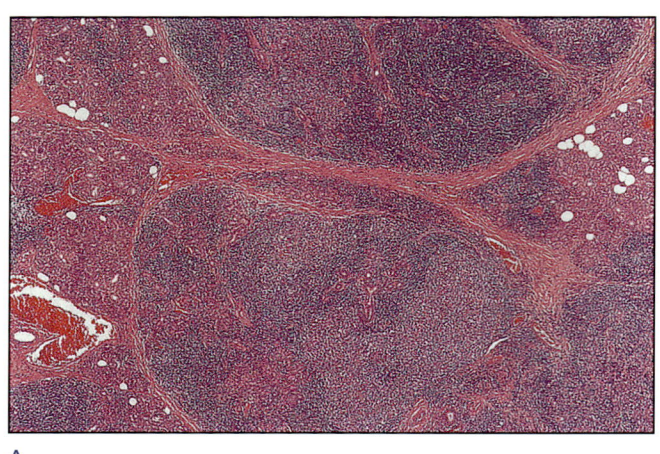
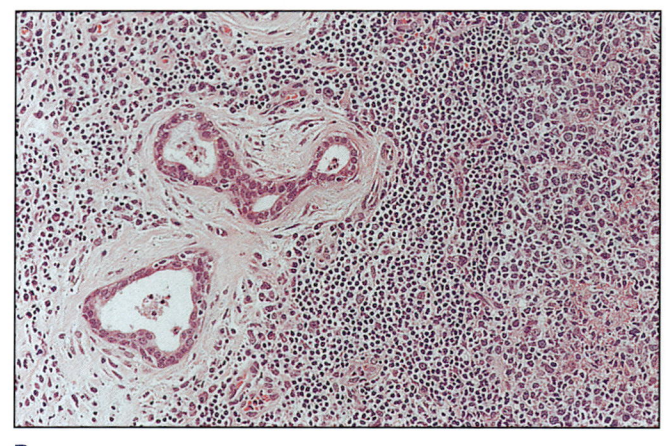

图 7.145 颌下腺慢性硬化性涎腺炎（Kuttner瘤）。（A）小叶结构保留，间隔显示硬化。有淋巴细胞浸润，伴有淋巴滤泡形成，腺泡和导管丧失。（B）经常发现导管周围硬化。与淋巴上皮性涎腺炎不同，淋巴上皮病变罕见。

现反应性的淋巴滤泡。在晚期阶段，有明显的纤维化和实质丧失，类似于肝硬化[14]。免疫染色显示以T细胞为主，并且显示与导管和腺泡密切相关。B细胞主要局限于淋巴滤泡中[533]。

对于Kuttner瘤的认识不足，常常被误诊为LESA；通过其缺乏淋巴上皮病变以及通常有较突出的硬化可以与后者相鉴别[528]。另一方面，酷似Kuttner瘤的硬化性滤泡性淋巴瘤，以及在少数情况下MALT淋巴瘤合并Kuttner瘤也有报道[534,535]。

涎腺上皮性肿瘤的诊断分析方法

诊断问题

Warthin瘤常常有定型的表现，很少出现诊断上的问题。多数多形性腺瘤也不存在诊断上的问题，因为有特征性的软骨黏液样间质。然而，从不同类型涎腺肿瘤的描述可以看出，每个肿瘤的组织学范围可能非常广泛，而且各种肿瘤之间有相当程度的形态学的重叠。例如，虽然筛状结构是腺样囊性癌的主要特征，但它也可以局灶性出现在多形性腺瘤、基底细胞腺瘤、PLGA、涎腺导管癌和上皮-肌上皮癌，这些肿瘤具有非常不同的预后（图7.14 A，图7.38，图7.91和图7.117）。腺样囊性癌可能有少量透明细胞成分，局部类似于上皮-上皮肌上皮癌。

因此，在简洁陈述的诊断中，不能仅仅依靠肿瘤孤立的镜下所见，而是应该考虑所有的特征，其中最重要的是[131]：

1. 肿瘤边界
2. 细胞构成
3. 结构排列
4. 细胞学特征
5. 间质成分

如果形态为非诊断性，对于肿瘤进行充分取材常常是有益的，因为常常可以发现一些比较具有诊断意义的病灶。诊断中的主要陷阱列在表7.12和表7.13中。

评估基底细胞、肌上皮细胞以及嗜酸性细胞肿瘤的恶性潜能尤其困难。对于这个问题的图解方法见图7.46。表7.10显示低级别和高级别腺癌的统一特征。

形态学评价

浸润还是没有浸润？

无论是在大体还是在镜下水平，评价肿瘤与邻近组织的交界面极为重要。良性肿瘤界限清楚，而恶性肿瘤具有浸润性的边界。伴有以下例外情况：某些腺泡细胞癌和多形性腺瘤中的癌可以有局限性的边界，而Warthin瘤并发梗死或炎症可能导致许多与周围组织黏连，在临床上或大体上类似于恶性肿瘤。不同类型癌的浸润方式也有不同，上皮-肌上皮癌、基底细胞腺癌、肌上皮癌（除了高级别癌）以及腺泡细胞癌倾向于推挤性生长（图7.43，图7.51和图7.98）；而其他的癌通常表现为不规则的舌样浸润性生长（图7.78，图7.108和图7.118）。

不能过分强调辨认浸润的重要性。如果没有发现组织浸润，则腺样囊性癌的假定诊断一定是错误的；同样，如果肿瘤广泛取材未能显示神经周围浸润，对于这个诊断也应持怀疑态度。因为腺样囊性癌在形态学上可能与

表7.12 涎腺上皮性肿瘤常见的误诊（过诊断）

过诊断为恶性		
良性肿瘤	误诊为…	支持正确诊断的线索和特征
Warthin瘤或嗜酸细胞瘤伴有鳞状和（或）黏液化生	鳞状细胞癌或黏液表皮样癌	• 原发性鳞状细胞癌非常罕见 • 缺乏浸润性生长 • Warthin瘤的卷曲的囊状结构 • 低级别黏液表皮样癌从无明显的鳞状表现 • 非典型性鳞状细胞与残留的嗜酸细胞混合 • 明显的修复性特征
多形性腺瘤伴有鳞状或黏液化生（常常在细针穿刺吸取后发生）	黏液表皮样癌	• 缺乏浸润性生长 • 低级别黏液表皮样癌从来没有明显的鳞状或角化 • 出现粗大的弹性纤维 • 出现具有两种细胞的导管肌上皮结构的区域 • 浆细胞样玻璃样细胞，如果出现 • 软骨黏液样间质，如果出现
多形性腺瘤或基底细胞腺瘤伴有筛状结构	腺样囊性癌	• 缺乏浸润性生长 • 肌上皮细胞至少灶性的"融合"在间质中
嗜酸细胞瘤的透明细胞变型	透明细胞癌或黏液表皮样癌	• 缺乏浸润性生长 • 至少局灶性出现典型的嗜酸细胞 • PTAH和抗线粒体抗体染色阳性
非皮脂腺淋巴腺瘤	淋巴上皮癌	• 缺乏显著的核的非典型性（轻度核的非典型性可以接受） • 至少局灶性出现腺体分化（形态学或免疫组织化学） • EB病毒阴性

PTAH，磷钨酸苏木素

基底细胞腺瘤，有时与多形性腺瘤重叠，所以辨认浸润是作出诊断的一个最重要的参数。对于某些肿瘤来说，仅仅出现明显的浸润性特征就能自动地将一个良性肿瘤归入恶性肿瘤的范畴，即使肿瘤在形态学上表现温和，例如肌上皮、基底细胞和嗜酸细胞肿瘤（图 7.46）。其含义在于肿瘤边缘必须充分取材进行检查。在某些情况下，没有机会评价肿瘤边缘，也就不可能作出明确的诊断，例如穿刺或切开活检的标本。

肿瘤显示双重细胞群还是仅有单一细胞分化？

图 7.7 列出了伴有腔面和腔外两种细胞分化的不同的涎腺肿瘤。辨认这种特征可以大大缩小鉴别诊断范围。例如，腺样囊性癌可能难以与多形性低级别腺癌（PLGA）鉴别，但是前者显示两种细胞分化，而后者却没有（图 7.146）。小管腺瘤可以通过缺乏腔外细胞成分而与基底细胞腺瘤相区别。在某些肿瘤中，为了辨认两种细胞类型的分化需要仔细寻找和详细的形态学分析，有时需要借助于恰当的免疫组织化学检查。少数非特异性腺癌可能显示两重细胞分化，但是根据定义，应该缺乏腺样囊性癌和基底细胞腺瘤的诊断性特征。某些 PLGA 也能够显示非常局灶性的两重细胞分化。虽然在光镜水平嗜酸细胞瘤的基底细胞（腔外细胞）并不显著，但是免疫染色基底细胞常常明显，表现为扁平细胞。

结构排列

某些肿瘤显示可以提供重要诊断线索的结构特征（表 7.14）。当在纤维性间质中见到外渗的黏液，伴有慢性炎症细胞浸润时，最可能的诊断是低级别黏液表皮样癌（图 7.147）。对于任何"难于分类"的癌来说，必须考虑多形性腺瘤中的癌的可能性。

常常部分或完全呈囊性的某些肿瘤是 Warthin 瘤、囊腺瘤、囊腺癌、黏液表皮样癌以及腺泡细胞癌的乳头

涎腺上皮性肿瘤的诊断分析方法

表7.13 涎腺上皮性肿瘤常见的误诊（诊断不足）

恶性肿瘤诊断不足		
恶性肿瘤	误诊为…	支持正确诊断的线索或特征
囊性黏液表皮样癌	良性囊肿或囊腺瘤	• 至少在某些区域囊肿内衬细胞为多层 • 细胞形成腔内结节 • 多种细胞类型 • 纤维性囊壁或囊外上皮岛
黏液表皮样癌伴有大量黏液外渗	黏液囊肿	• 大涎腺中出现外渗的黏液池时，要求仔细寻找低级别黏液表皮样癌，因为外渗性黏液囊肿非常罕见
多形性低级别腺癌	多形性或基底细胞腺瘤	• 浸润性边界 • 常见神经浸润 • 缺乏两重细胞分化 • 缺乏软骨黏液样间质 • 不同的生长方式 • 细胞核淡染
黏膜部位的腺样囊性癌	多形性或基底细胞腺瘤	• 浸润性生长，如果在活检中见到 • 玻璃样变间质挤压小管 • 局部筛状结构
黏液表皮样癌嗜酸细胞变型	嗜酸细胞瘤	• 浸润性生长 • 某些病灶出现其他类型细胞（例如表皮样、中间性和黏液细胞） • 炎症性纤维性间质
腺泡细胞癌的囊性或乳头状囊性变型	良性囊肿	• 内衬鞋钉样细胞 • 内衬空泡状细胞 • 局灶性细胞丛突入囊腔内 • 内衬细胞有腺泡细胞分化（PAS阳性的颗粒状胞浆） • 纤维性囊壁上有局灶性肿瘤岛
上皮-肌上皮癌	多形性或基底细胞腺瘤	• 浸润性生长 • 小管或细胞岛的外层为突出的透明细胞
淋巴上皮癌	淋巴腺瘤	• 浸润性生长经常出现 • 明确的核的非典型性（虽然有时轻微） • 在形态学和免疫组织化学水平上，肿瘤细胞显示鳞片状/鳞状，而不是腺体特征 • 存在肿瘤细胞的EB病毒

状-囊性变型（图7.148）。许多反应性囊性病变也能形成瘤样肿块，例如淋巴上皮囊肿、角化囊肿、黏液囊肿、涎腺导管囊肿以及硬化性多囊性腺病（图7.72和图7.74）。

细胞学特征

当在涎腺肿瘤中发现某种细胞类型时，这些类型的细胞可能提供重要的分类线索（图7.15）。出现空泡状细胞应该考虑腺泡细胞癌和皮脂腺肿瘤的可能性。有助于鉴别不同肿瘤中的透明细胞的特征列在表7.5中。为了实用的目的，应将大多数透明细胞涎腺肿瘤看成是恶性肿瘤（图7.149）。

伴有或不伴有角化的鳞状细胞巢可以见于各种肿瘤。重要的是，在低级别到中级别黏液表皮样癌中几乎从未见过明显的鳞状特征，例如细胞间桥和角化；正确的诊断或许是多形性腺瘤或伴有鳞状化生的Warthin瘤（图7.17和图7.67）。诸如在Warthin瘤、嗜酸细胞瘤以及嗜酸细胞癌中见到的肿瘤性嗜酸细胞也容易发生鳞状化生，这是对于缺血或炎症造成的损伤的反应；这种化生的鳞状细胞常常显示不同程度的非典型性，导致误诊为鳞状细胞癌（图7.58；表7.12）。

坏死性涎腺化生（necrotizing sialometaplasia）是需要与鳞状细胞癌鉴别诊断的反应性病变。它几乎全

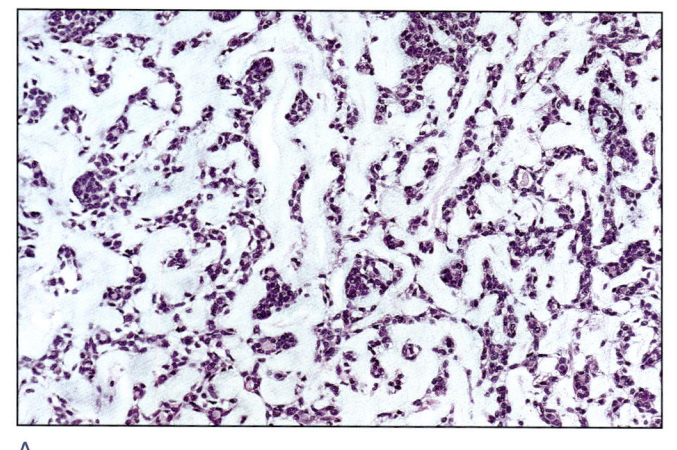 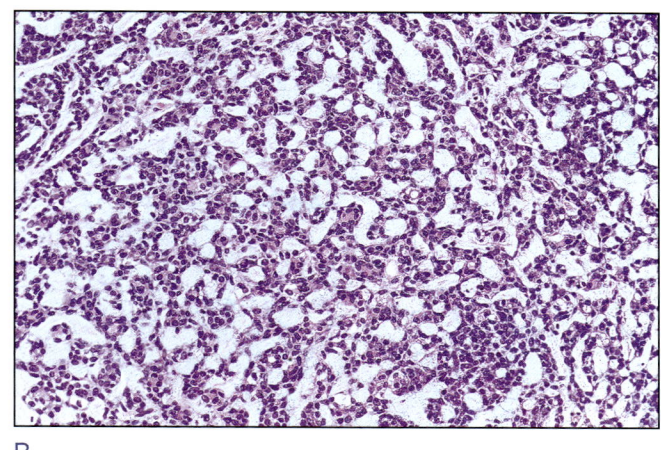

图7.146 鼻腔腺样囊性癌。（A）黏液玻璃样物质造成腺管狭窄是常见的特征。（B）由于有明显的相互吻合的由两种类型细胞组成的腺管，如果没有发现明确的浸润性生长的话，与富于细胞性多形性腺瘤或基底细胞腺瘤的鉴别诊断是困难的。

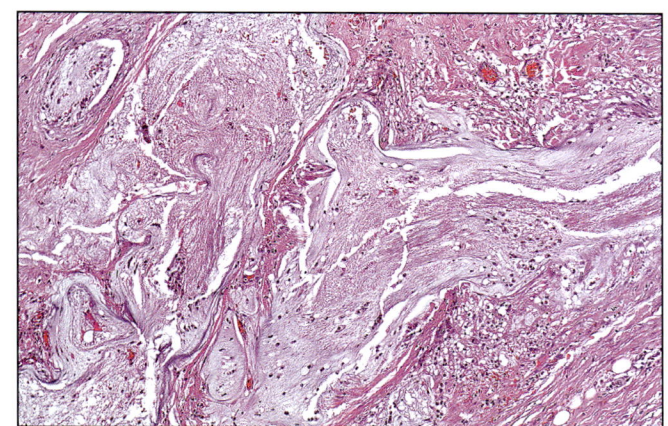 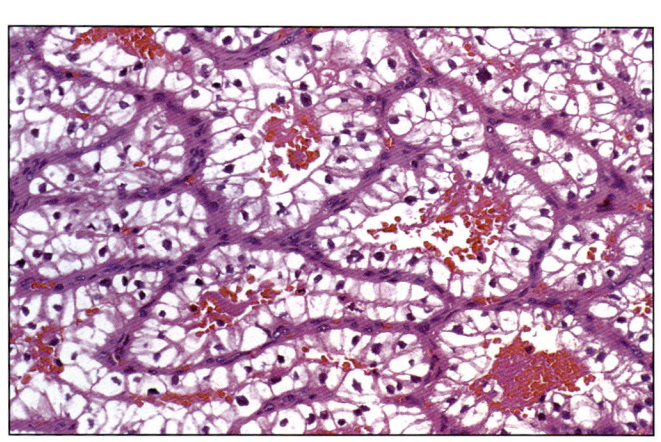

图7.147 大涎腺"黏液囊肿"。大涎腺间质出现外渗的黏液池实际上与低级别黏液表皮样癌的诊断是同义的。本例仔细寻找的确发现了黏液表皮样癌（没有显示）。

图7.149 腮腺转移性肾细胞癌。支持这种诊断而不是涎腺原发性透明细胞癌的特征包括：纤细的纤维血管间隔，真正腺体结构以及腔内出血。

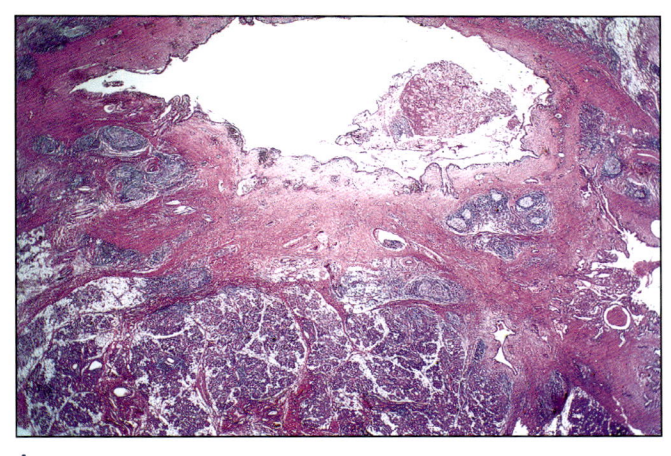 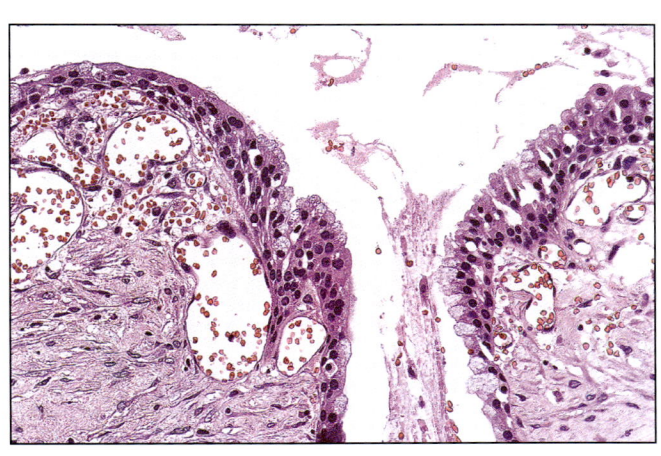

图7.148 囊性黏液表皮样癌酷似单纯性囊肿。（A）腮腺具有单个的囊肿。纤维性囊壁上出现淋巴滤泡。（B）虽然许多区域囊肿内衬扁平上皮，但是至少局部存在黏液表皮样上皮。

表7.14　提供涎腺肿瘤诊断线索的结构性特征

结构形态	考虑的诊断	评论
微囊性	• 腺泡细胞癌 • 多形性低级别腺癌（局灶性） • 肌上皮瘤（某些病例）	每当微囊性结构突出时均应首先考虑腺泡细胞癌，尤其是当伴有淋巴细胞浸润时
筛状	• 腺样囊性癌 • 涎腺导管癌 • 导管内癌 • 多形性/基底细胞腺瘤（局灶性） • 多形性低级别腺癌（局灶性） • 舌的筛状腺癌	在腺样囊性癌中，筛状结构非常具有特征性，但不具有诊断性。腺样囊性癌筛状结构的多数间隙与间质连续而不是真正的腺体间隙。然而，涎腺导管癌和导管内癌的筛状结构是真正的腺体间隙
管状	• 腺样囊性癌 • 多形性低级别腺癌 • 上皮-肌上皮癌 • 腺癌，非特异性 • 多形性/基底细胞腺瘤（局灶性） • 囊腺瘤和囊腺癌（某些病例） • 涎腺导管癌（某些病例） • 嗜酸细胞瘤和嗜酸细胞癌（少数病例）	涎腺肿瘤常见管状结构。评价肿瘤与周围组织的交界，细胞组成和分化，以及肿瘤细胞的细胞形态学对于诊断是有帮助的
束状	• 肌上皮瘤和肌上皮癌 • 基底细胞腺瘤伴有肌上皮衍化的间质 • 多形性腺瘤（局灶性） • 多形性低级别腺癌（局灶性） • 上皮-肌上皮癌（局灶性） • 各种间叶性肿瘤	除了间叶性肿瘤以外，梭形细胞成束出现通常代表具有肌上皮分化，除多形性低级别腺癌
乳头状	• Warthin瘤 • 囊腺瘤和囊腺癌 • 导管乳头状瘤 • 腺泡细胞癌，乳头状-囊性变型 • 腺癌，非特异性（某些病例） • 多形性低级别腺癌（某些病例） • 上皮-肌上皮癌（非常局灶）	分析被覆乳头的肿瘤细胞有助于诊断。双重细胞分化见于Warthin瘤和上皮-肌上皮癌，乳头状涎腺腺瘤，以及导管内乳头状瘤
网格状	• 肌上皮瘤和肌上皮癌 • 多形性腺瘤（局灶性） • 腺样囊性癌（局灶性，在广泛玻璃样变的区域）	网格状结构是某些肌上皮肿瘤的突出特征，而在其他涎腺肿瘤中罕见。 舌的外胚层间质性软骨黏液样肿瘤（不是涎腺肿瘤）也表现为突出的网格状生长方式

部发生于小涎腺，最常表现为腭部的溃疡性病变[536,537]。缺血最可能是这种病变的病因，例如血管炎，动脉粥样硬化性栓子以及长期的插管[536,538,539]。某些病例与疱疹感染[540]，外伤性损伤或以前手术有关。这种病变与癌鉴别的最重要的组织学特征是小叶结构保留。涎腺小叶局部坏死伴有邻近导管和腺泡明显的鳞状化生，类似于见于前列腺梗死周围区域的现象（图7.150）。经常出现炎性浸润。表面鳞状上皮通常表现为假上皮瘤性增生。

当在涎腺中遇见以下肿瘤时，在诊断其为原发性肿瘤之前，应该考虑转移性肿瘤的可能性。这些肿瘤包括鳞状细胞癌、透明细胞癌、小细胞癌、淋巴上皮癌和神经内分泌癌。

间质成分

嗜酸性玻璃样或基底膜样物质一般代表存在肌上皮或基底细胞分化（图7.14A，图7.41，图7.47，图7.90，图7.92和图7.115），玻璃样透明细胞癌（其表现为单纯的腔面细胞分化；图7.125）是个例外。实际上，对于发生在大涎腺以外的肿瘤来说，间质玻璃样物质可能是

表7.15 特殊细胞类型作为诊断涎腺肿瘤的线索

	嗜酸细胞	鳞状细胞	基底细胞样细胞	梭形细胞	皮脂腺细胞	透明细胞	大汗腺或大汗腺样细胞
构成主要成分	• Warthin瘤 • 嗜酸细胞瘤 • 嗜酸细胞癌 • 嗜酸细胞囊腺瘤	• Warthin瘤或嗜酸细胞肿瘤伴有鳞状化生 • 鳞状细胞癌(原发性、转移性,或从邻近部位浸润而来) • 腺鳞癌 • 高级别黏液表皮样癌 • 角化囊瘤	• 基底细胞腺瘤 • 基底细胞腺癌 • 多形性腺瘤(某些病例) • 腺样囊性癌 • 淋巴腺瘤 • 基底细胞样鳞状细胞癌 • 涎腺母细胞瘤	• 肌上皮瘤 • 肌上皮癌 • 涎腺原基瘤 • 多形性腺瘤(某些病例) • 各种良性和恶性的间叶性肿瘤	• 皮脂腺瘤淋巴腺瘤 • 皮脂腺癌淋巴腺癌	• 透明细胞癌 • 上皮-肌上皮癌 • 透明细胞嗜酸细胞瘤 • 皮脂腺腺瘤或腺癌 • 透明细胞肌上皮瘤或肌上皮癌 • 黏液表皮样癌,透明变型 • 转移性肾细胞癌	• 涎腺导管癌 • 导管内癌
局部出现	• 许多不同的肿瘤类型,例如多形性腺瘤,腺泡细胞癌,黏液表皮样癌,腺样囊性癌,多形性低级别腺癌 • 非特异性腺癌	• 多形性腺瘤 • 基底细胞腺瘤或腺癌(细胞岛的中心) • 皮脂腺腺瘤或腺癌 • 上皮-肌上皮癌	• 上皮-肌上皮癌 • 多形性低级别腺癌 • 小管腺瘤	• 基底细胞腺瘤或腺癌(某些病例) • 上皮-肌上皮癌(某些病例) • 淋巴上皮癌(某些病例)	• Warthin瘤(很少) • 多形性腺瘤(很少) • 黏液表皮样癌(很少) • 腺样囊性癌(很少)	• 黏液腺癌 • 腺泡细胞癌 • 多形性腺癌 • 鳞状细胞癌(很少) • 腺样囊性癌(很少) • 多形性低级别腺癌(很少) • 非特异性腺癌 • 透明细胞嗜酸细胞增生	• 多形性腺瘤(很少) • 多形性腺瘤中的癌
可能误诊为肿瘤的非肿瘤性病变	• 嗜酸细胞化生 • 嗜酸细胞增多症 • 结节性嗜酸细胞增生	• 坏死性涎腺化生 • 角化性囊肿	• 淋巴上皮性涎腺炎	• 炎性假瘤 • 结节性筋膜炎		• 透明细胞嗜酸细胞增生	• 硬化性多囊性腺病

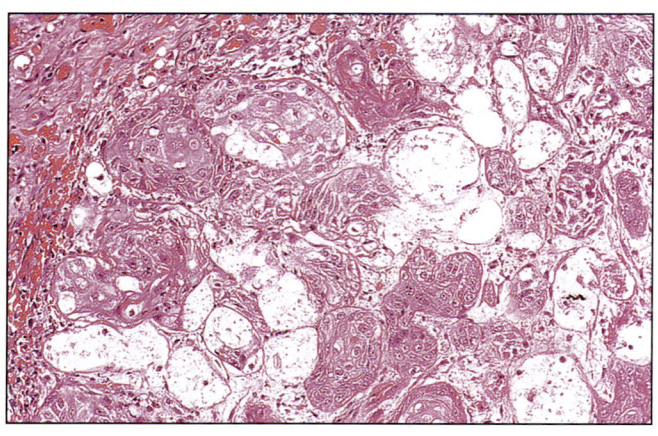

图7.150 腭坏死性涎腺化生。某些腺泡"消失"，留下稀疏的空间。其他腺泡充满鳞状细胞，伴有轻度核的非典型性。常常有散在的慢性炎症细胞。鉴别这种病变与鳞状细胞癌的最重要的特征是小叶结构保留（没有显示）。

诊断涎腺型肿瘤的首要线索。玻璃样物质见于细胞岛的周围，假腺体的间隙，或在肿瘤细胞中呈散在的带状（例如多形性腺瘤和肌上皮瘤）或小滴状（例如膜性基底细胞腺瘤和基底细胞腺瘤）分布。

在长期的多形性腺瘤中常常出现丰富的弹性纤维，通常形成粗大的或松散的分支状纤维（图7.23）。在多形性腺瘤的癌中，它们能够提供存在这种肿瘤的线索。

间质黏液是涎腺肿瘤一种常见的表现，在HE染色切片中呈微嗜碱性，在肿瘤分类中它不具有特别的价值（图7.21和图7.110D）。不过，当出现丰富的黏液时，最有可能的诊断是多形性腺瘤。

在涎腺肿瘤中出现软骨实际上是诊断多形性腺瘤的同义词（图7.11）。偶尔，软骨也可能出现在癌肉瘤和多形性腺瘤的癌中。

涎腺肿瘤切除的外科病理学报告

外科病理学报告应该提供以下信息[541]：

1. 肿瘤部位和诊断（和变型，如果适用的话）
2. 所有的预后因素，例如肿瘤大小，肿瘤分级，核分裂计数，浸润范围，血管浸润，神经浸润，淋巴结状况
3. 切缘状况。为了避免切缘变形，在切开之前最好完整固定组织。切缘应该适当的用墨水标记

涎腺肿瘤穿刺或切开活检的解释

涎腺肿瘤穿刺或切开活检的诊断有时是容易的。例如，当见到典型的软骨黏液样样基质或出现特征性的浆细胞样玻璃样细胞时，容易确认为多形性腺瘤（图7.20）。然而，不是总能作出明确的诊断，甚至不能确定肿瘤是良性或恶性。困难来自于不同肿瘤类型之间形态学重叠，而且活检标本难以适当评估肿瘤边缘。例如，一个活检标本显示腺管具有腔外和腔面两种细胞分化，它可能是多形性腺瘤、基底细胞腺瘤、腺样囊性癌、上皮-肌上皮癌甚或者非特异性腺癌（图7.151）。在缺乏较明确的诊断性特征时，可能只能做出"涎腺肿瘤"这一描述性的诊断，为了明确诊断，需要完全切除或较大的活检。

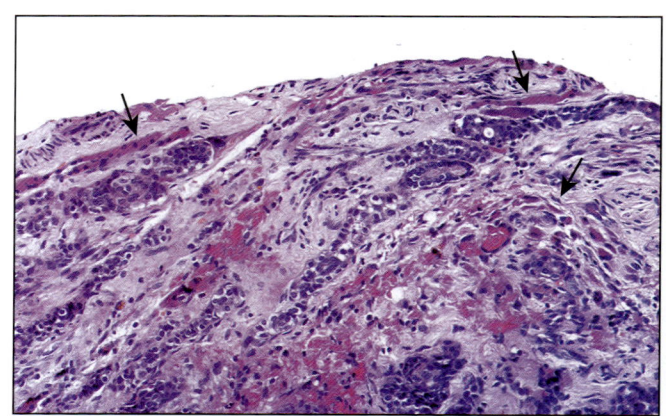

图7.151 舌腺样囊性癌的穿刺活检所见。在这个活检标本中，硬化的间质中可见由腔面-腔外两层细胞内衬的腺管。这种结构可能见于多形性腺瘤、管状型的基底细胞腺瘤以及腺样囊性癌。在考虑的鉴别诊断中，骨骼肌纤维浸润（箭头）支持将这个肿瘤诊断为腺样囊性癌。

参考文献

1. Kaplan M, Johns M 1993 Malignant neoplasms. In: Cummings C, Fredrickson J, Harker L et al. (eds) Otolaryngology – head and neck surgery, 2nd edn. C V Mosby, St. Louis, p 1043–1078
2. Frommer J 1977 The human accessory parotid gland: its incidence, nature, and significance. Oral Surg Oral Med Oral Pathol 43: 671–676
3. Lin D T, Coppit G L, Burkey B B et al. 2004 Tumors of the accessory lobe of the parotid gland: a 10-year experience. Laryngoscope 114: 1652–1655
4. Harris N 1991 Extranodal lymphoid infiltrates and mucosa-associated lymphoid tissue (MALT). A unifying concept. Am J Surg Pathol 15: 879–884
5. Cleary K R, Batsakis J G 1990 Lymphoepithelial cysts of the parotid region: a new face on an old lesion. Ann Otol Rhnol Laryngol 99:162–164
6. Dardick I 1996 Color atlas/text of salivary gland tumor pathology. Igaku-Shoin, New York
7. Savera A T, Zarbo R J 2004 Defining the role of myoepithelium in salivary gland neoplasia. Adv Anat Pathol 11: 69–85
8. Ihrler S, Zietz C, Sendelhofert A et al. 2002 A morphogenetic concept of salivary duct regeneration and metaplasia. Virchows Arch 440: 519–526
9. Krech R, Zerban H, Bannasch P 1981 Mitochondrial anomalies in renal oncocytes induced in rat by N-nitrosomorpholine. Eur J Cell Biol 25: 331–339
10. Auclair P L, Ellis G L, Gnepp D R et al. 1991 Salivary gland neoplasms: general considerations. In: Ellis G L, Auclair P L, Gnepp D R (eds) Surgical pathology of the salivary glands. Major problems in pathology. W B Saunders, Philadelphia, PA, p 135–164
11. Ellis G L, Auclair P L, Gnepp D R 1991 Surgical pathology of the salivary glands. In: LiVolsi V (ed.) Major problems in pathology. Saunders, Philadelphia, PA
12. Kokemueller H, Swennen G, Brueggemann N et al. 2004 Epithelial malignancies of the salivary glands: clinical experience of a single institution– a review. Int J Oral Maxillofac Surg 33: 423–432
13. Wahlberg P, Anderson H, Biorklund A et al. 2002 Carcinoma of the parotid and submandibular glands – a study of survival in 2465 patients. Oral Oncol 38: 706–713
14. Seifert G, Miehlke A, Haubrich J et al. 1986 Diseases of the salivary glands. Georg Thieme, Stuttgart
15. Lack E E, Upton M P 1988 Histopathologic review of salivary gland tumors in childhood. Arch Otolaryngol Head Neck Surg 114: 898–906
16. da Cruz Perez D E, Pires F R, Alves F A et al. 2004 Salivary gland tumors in children and adolescents: a clinicopathologic and immunohistochemical study of fifty-three cases. Int J Pediatr Otorhinolaryngol 68: 895–902
17. Nagao T, Sugano I, Ishida Y et al. 1998 Basal cell adenocarcinoma of the salivary glands: comparison with basal cell adenoma through assessment of cell proliferation, apoptosis, and expression of p53 and bcl-2. Cancer 82: 439–447
18. Eneroth C M, Hamberger C A 1974 Principles of treatment of different types of parotid tumors. Laryngoscope 84: 1732–1740
19. Maruya S, Kim H W, Weber R S et al. 2004 Gene expression screening of salivary gland neoplasms: molecular markers of potential histogenetic and clinical significance. J Mol Diagn 6: 180–190
20. Francioso F, Carinci F, Tosi L et al. 2002 Identification of differentially expressed genes in human salivary gland tumors by DNA microarrays. Mol Cancer Ther 1: 533–538
21. Frierson H F Jr, El-Naggar A K, Welsh J B et al. 2002 Large scale molecular analysis identifies genes with altered expression in salivary adenoid cystic carcinoma. Am J Pathol 161: 1315–1323
22. Gibbons M D, Manne U, Carroll W R et al. 2001 Molecular differences in mucoepidermoid carcinoma and adenoid cystic carcinoma of the major salivary glands. Laryngoscope 111: 1373–1378
23. Leivo I, Jee K J, Heikinheimo K et al. 2005 Characterization of gene expression in major types of salivary gland carcinomas with epithelial differentiation. Cancer Genet Cytogenet 156: 104–113
24. Seifert G, Donath K 1996 Hybrid tumours of salivary glands. Definition and classification of five rare cases. Eur J Cancer B Oral Oncol 32B: 251–259
25. Nagao T, Sugano I, Ishida Y et al. 2002 Hybrid carcinomas of the salivary glands: report of nine cases with a clinicopathologic, immunohistochemical, and p53 gene alteration analysis. Mod Pathol 15: 724–733
26. Croitoru C M, Suarez P A, Luna M A 1999 Hybrid carcinomas of salivary glands. Report of 4 cases and review of the literature. Arch Pathol Lab Med 123: 698–702
27. Grenko R T, Abendroth C S, Davis A T et al. 1998 Hybrid tumors or salivary gland tumors sharing common differentiation pathways? Reexamining adenoid cystic and epithelial-myoepithelial carcinomas. Oral Surg Oral Med Oral Pathol Oral Radiol Endod 86: 188–195
28. Ruiz-Godoy L M, Mosqueda-Taylor A, Suarez-Roa L et al. 2003 Hybrid tumours of the salivary glands. A report of two cases involving the palate and a review of the literature. Eur Arch Otorhinolaryngol 260: 312–315
29. Chetty R 2000 Intercalated duct hyperplasia: possible relationship to epithelial-myoepithelial carcinoma and hybrid tumours of salivary gland. Histopathology 37: 260–263
30. Zardawi I M 2000 Hybrid carcinoma of the salivary gland. Histopathology 37: 283–284
31. Noguchi S, Aihara T, Yoshino K et al. 1996 Demonstration of monoclonal origin of human parotid gland pleomorphic adenoma. Cancer 77: 431–435
32. Sweeney E C, McDermott M 1996 Pleomorphic adenoma of the bronchus. J Clin Pathol 49: 87–89
33. Badia L, Weir J N, Robinson A C 1996 Heterotopic pleomorphic adenoma of the external nose. J Laryngol Otol 110: 376–378
34. Tyagi N, Abdi U, Tyagi S P et al. Pleomorphic adenoma of skin (chondroid syringoma) involving the eyelid. J Postgrad Med 42: 125–126
35. Kilpatrick S E, Hitchcock M G, Kraus M D et al. Mixed tumors and myoepitheliomas of soft tissue: a clinicopathologic study of 19 cases with a unifying concept. Am J Surg Pathol 21: 13–22
36. Agnantis N J, Maounis N, Priovolou-Papavangelou M et al. 1992 Pleomorphic adenoma of the human female breast. Pathol Res Pract 188: 235–240; discussion 240–241
37. Hickman R E, Cawson R A, Duffy S W 1984 The prognosis of specific types of salivary gland tumors. Cancer 54: 1620–1654
38. Jackson S R, Roland N J, Clarke R W et al. Recurrent pleomorphic adenoma. J Laryngol Otol 107: 546–549
39. Laskawi R, Schott T, Schroder M 1998 Recurrent pleomorphic adenomas of the parotid gland: clinical evaluation and long-term follow-up. Br J Oral Maxillofac Surg 36: 48–51
40. Henriksson G, Westrin K M, Carlsoo B et al. 1998 Recurrent primary pleomorphic adenomas of salivary gland origin: intrasurgical rupture, histopathologic features, and pseudopodia. Cancer 82: 617–620
41. McGregor A D, Burgoyne M, Tan K C 1988 Recurrent pleomorphic salivary adenoma – the relevance of age at first presentation. Br J Plast Surg 41: 177–181
42. Auclair P L, Ellis G L 1996 Atypical features in salivary gland mixed tumors: their relationship to malignant transformation. Mod Pathol 9: 652–657
43. Lam K H, Wei W I, Ho H C et al. 1990 Whole organ sectioning of mixed parotid tumors. Am J Surg 160: 377–381
44. Lam P W, Chan J K, Sin V C 1997 Nasal pleomorphic adenoma with skeletal muscle differentiation: potential misdiagnosis as rhabdomyosarcoma. Hum Pathol 28: 1299–1302
45. Takeda Y, Satoh M, Nakamura S 2004 Pigmented pleomorphic adenoma, a novel melanin-pigmented benign salivary gland tumor. Virchows Arch 445: 199–202
46. Lee K C, Chan J K, Chong Y W 1992 Ossifying pleomorphic adenoma of the maxillary antrum. J Laryngol Otol 106: 50–52
46a. Haskell H D, Butt K M, Woo S B 2005 Pleomorphic adenoma with extensive lipometaplasia. Report of three cases. Am J Surg Pathol 29: 1389–1393.
47. Chan J K, Tang S K, Tsang W Y et al. 1996 Histologic changes induced by fine-needle aspiration. Adv Anat Pathol 3: 71–90
48. Bilal H, Handra-Luca A, Bertrand J C et al. 2003 p63 is expressed in basal and myoepithelial cells of human normal and tumor salivary gland tissues. J Histochem Cytochem 51: 133–139
49. Vargas H, Sudilovsky D, Kaplan M J et al. 1997 Mixed tumor, polymorphous low grade adenocarcinoma and adenoid cystic carcinoma of the salivary gland: pathogenic implications and differential diagnosis by Ki67 (MIB1), BCL2 and S100 immunohistochemistry. Appl Immunohistochem 5: 8–16
50. Skalova A, Simpson R H, Lehtonen H et al. 1997 Assessment of proliferative activity using the MIB1 antibody help to distinguish polymorphous low grade adenocarcinoma from adenoid cystic carcinoma of salivary glands. Pathol Res Pract 193: 695–703
51. Eveson J W, Kusafuka K, Stenman G et al. 2005 Pleomorphic adenoma. In: Barnes L, Eveson J W, Reichart P et al. (eds) World Health Organization classification of tumours. Pathology and genetics: head and neck tumours. IARC, Lyon, p 254–258
52. Bullerdiek J, Wobst G, Meyer-Bolte K et al. 1993 Cytogenetic subtyping of 220 salivary gland pleomorphic adenomas: correlation to occurrence, histological subtype, and in vitro cellular behavior. Cancer Genet Cytogenet 65: 27–31
53. Voz M L, Agten N S, Van de Ven W J et al. 2000 PLAG1, the main translocation target in pleomorphic adenoma of the salivary glands, is a positive regulator of IGF-II. Cancer Res 60: 106–113
54. Geurts J M, Schoenmakers E F, Roijer E et al. 1998 Identification of NFIB as recurrent translocation partner gene of HMGIC in pleomorphic adenomas. Oncogene 16: 865–872
55. Czader M, Eberhart C G, Bhatti N et al. 2000 Metastasizing mixed tumor of the parotid: initial presentation as a solitary kidney tumor and ultimate carcinomatous transformation at the primary site. Am J Surg Pathol 24: 1159–1164
56. Wenig B M, Hitchcock C L, Ellis G L et al. 1992 Metastasizing mixed tumor of salivary glands. a clinicopathologic and flow cytometric analysis. Am J Surg Pathol 16: 845–858
57. Qureshi A A, Gitelis S, Templeton A A et al. 1994 "Benign" metastasizing pleomorphic adenoma. A case report and review of literature. Clin Orthop Rel Res 308: 192–198
58. Sampson B A, Jarcho J A, Winters G L 1998 Metastasizing mixed tumor of the parotid gland: a rare tumor with unusually rapid progression in a cardiac transplant patient. Mod Pathol 11: 1142–1145
59. Fujimura N, Sugawara T, Seki H et al. 1997 Carcinomatous change in the cranial metastasis from a metastasizing mixed tumor of the salivary gland – case report. Neurol Med Chir (Tokyo) 37: 546–550

60. Hoorweg J J, Hilgers F J, Keus R B et al. 1998 Metastasizing pleomorphic adenoma: a report of three cases. Eur J Surg Oncol 24: 452–455
61. Eneroth C M, Zetterberg A 1974 Malignancy in pleomorphic adenoma. A clinical and microspectrophotometric study. Acta Otolaryngol (Stockh) 77: 426–432
62. Altemani A, Martins M T, Freitas L et al. 2005 Carcinoma ex pleomorphic adenoma (CXPA): immunoprofile of the cells involved in carcinomatous progression. Histopathology 46: 635–641
63. Lewis J E, Olsen K D, Sebo T J 2001 Carcinoma ex pleomorphic adenoma: pathologic analysis of 73 cases. Hum Pathol 32: 596–604
64. Di Palma S, Skalova A, Vanieek T et al. 2005 Non-invasive (intracapsular) carcinoma ex pleomorphic adenoma: recognition of focal carcinoma by HER-2/neu and MIB1 immunohistochemistry. Histopathology 46: 144–152
65. Ellis G L, Auclair P L 1996 Tumors of the salivary glands. Atlas of tumor pathology, 3rd series, fascicle 17. Armed Forces Institute of Pathology, Washington, DC
66. Felix A, Rosa-Santos J, Mendonca M E et al. 2002 Intracapsular carcinoma ex pleomorphic adenoma. Report of a case with unusual metastatic behaviour. Oral Oncol 38: 107–110
67. Tortoledo M E, Luna M A, Batsakis J G 1984 Carcinomas ex pleomorphic adenoma and malignant mixed tumors. Histomorphologic indexes. Arch Otolaryngol 110: 172–176
68. Brandwein M, Huvos A G, Dardick I et al. 1996 Noninvasive and minimally invasive carcinoma ex mixed tumor: a clinicopathologic and ploidy study of 12 patients with major salivary tumors of low (or no?) malignant potential. Oral Surg Oral Med Oral Pathol Oral Radiol Endod 81: 655–664
69. Roijer E, Nordkvist A, Strom A K et al. 2002 Translocation, deletion/amplification, and expression of HMGIC and MDM2 in a carcinoma ex pleomorphic adenoma. Am J Pathol 160: 433–440
70. Sugano S, Mukai K, Tsuda H et al. 1992 Immunohistochemical study of c-erbB-2 oncoprotein overexpression in human major salivary gland carcinoma: an indicator of aggressiveness. Laryngoscope 102: 923–927
71. Muller S, Vigneswaran N, Gansler T et al. 1994 c-erbB-2 oncoprotein expression and amplification in pleomorphic adenoma and carcinoma ex pleomorphic adenoma: relationship to prognosis. Mod Pathol 7: 628–632
72. Rosa J C, Fonseca I, Felix A et al. 1996 Immunohistochemical study of c-erbB-2 expression in carcinoma ex-pleomorphic adenoma. Histopathology 28: 247–252
73. Nordkvist A, Roijer E, Bang G et al. 2000 Expression and mutation patterns of p53 in benign and malignant salivary gland tumors. Int J Oncol 16: 477–483
74. Karja V J, Syrjanen K J, Kurvinen A K et al. 1997 Expression and mutations of p53 in salivary gland tumours. J Oral Pathol Med 1997 26: 217–223
75. Li X, Tsuji T, Wen S et al. 1997 Detection of numeric abnormalities of chromosome 17 and p53 deletions by fluorescence in situ hybridization in pleomorphic adenomas and carcinomas in pleomorphic adenomas. Correlation with p53 expression. Cancer 79: 2314–2319
76. Deguchi H, Hamano H, Hayashi Y 1993 c-myc, ras p21 and p53 expression in pleomorphic adenoma and its malignant form of the human salivary glands. Acta Pathol Jpn 43: 413–422
77. Coleman H, Altini M 1999 Intravascular tumour in intra-oral pleomorphic adenomas: a diagnostic and therapeutic dilemma. Histopathology 35: 439–444
78. Altini M, Coleman H, Kienle F 1997 Intra-vascular tumour in pleomorphic adenomas – a report of four cases. Histopathology 31: 55–59
79. Talmi Y, Halpern M, Finkelstein Y et al. 1990 View from beneath: pathology in focus. True malignant mixed tumour of the parotid gland. J Larngol Otol 104: 360–361
80. Kwon M Y, Gu M 2001 True malignant mixed tumor (carcinosarcoma) of parotid gland with unusual mesenchymal component. A case report and review of the literature. Arch Pathol Lab Med 125: 812–815
81. Gnepp D R 1993 Malignant mixed tumors of the salivary glands: a review. Pathol Annu 28: 279–328
82. Batsakis J G, Luna M A, el-Naggar A K 1991 Basaloid monomorphic adenomas. Ann Otol Rhinol Laryngol 100: 687–690
83. Nagao T, Sugano I, Ishida Y et al. 1997 Carcinoma in basal cell adenoma of the parotid gland. Pathol Res Pract 193: 171–178
84. Gallimore A P, Spraggs P D, Allen J P et al. Basaloid carcinomas of salivary glands. Histopathology 24: 139–144
85. Dardick I, Daley T D, van Nostrand A W 1986 Basal cell adenoma with myoepithelial cell-derived "stroma": a new major salivary gland tumor entity. Head Neck Surg 8: 257–267
86. Biggs P J, Wooster R, Ford D et al. 1995 Familial cylindromatosis (turban tumour syndrome) gene localised to chromosome 16q12-q13: evidence for its role as a tumour suppressor gene. Nat Genet 11: 441–443
87. Choi H R, Batsakis J G, Callender D L et al. 2002 Molecular analysis of chromosome 16q regions in dermal analogue tumors of salivary glands: a genetic link to dermal cylindroma? Am J Surg Pathol 26: 778–783
88. Edwards P C, Bhuiya T, Kelsch R D 2004 Assessment of p63 expression in the salivary gland neoplasms adenoid cystic carcinoma, polymorphous low-grade adenocarcinoma, and basal cell and canalicular adenomas. Oral Surg Oral Med Oral Pathol Oral Radiol Endod 97: 613–619
89. Weber A, Langhanki L, Schutz A et al. 2002 Expression profiles of p53, p63, and p73 in benign salivary gland tumors. Virchows Arch 441: 428–436
90. Seifert G, Sobin L H 1991 Histological typing of salivary gland tumours. World Health Organization international histological classification of tumours, 2nd edn. Springer-Verlag, New York

91. Muller S, Barnes L 1996 Basal cell adenocarcinoma of the salivary glands. Report of seven cases and review of the literature. Cancer 78: 2471–2477
92. Fonseca I, Soares J 1996 Basal cell adenocarcinoma of minor salivary and seromucous glands of the head and neck region. Semin Diagn Pathol 13: 128–137
93. Jayakrishnan A, Elmalah I, Hussain K et al. 2003 Basal cell adenocarcinoma in minor salivary glands. Histopathology 42: 610–614
94. Luna M A, Batsakis J G, Tortoledo M E et al. 1989 Carcinomas ex monomorphic adenoma of salivary glands. J Laryngol Otol 103: 756–759
95. Ellis G L, Wiscovitch J G 1990 Basal cell adenocarcinomas of the major salivary glands. Oral Surg Oral Med Oral Pathol 69: 461–469
96. Atula T, Klemi P J, Donath K et al. 1993 Basal cell adenocarcinoma of the parotid gland: a case report and review of the literature. J Laryngol Otol 107: 862–864
97. Ellis G L, Auclair P L 1991 Basal cell adenocarcinoma. In: Ellis G L, Auclair P L, Gnepp D R (eds): Surgical pathology of the salivary glands. W B Saunders, Philadelphia, PA, p 585–661
98. Murty G T, Welch A, Soames J V 1990 Basal cell adenocarcinoma of the parotid gland. J Laryngol Otol 104: 150–151
99. Williams S B, Ellis G L, Auclair P L 1993 Immunohistochemical analysis of basal cell adenocarcinoma. Oral Surg Oral Med Oral Pathol 75: 64–69
100. Quddus M R, Henley J D, Affify A M et al. 1999 Basal cell adenocarcinoma of the salivary gland: an ultrastructural and immunohistochemical study. Oral Surg Oral Med Oral Pathol Oral Radiol Endod 87: 485–492
101. Dardick I, Thomas M J, van Nostrand A W 1989 Myoepithelioma – new concepts of histology and classification: a light and electron micropic study. Ultrastruct Pathol 13: 187–224
102. Dardick I, Cavell S, Boivin M et al. 1989 Salivary gland myoepithelioma variants. Histological, ultrastructural, and immunocytological features. Virchows Arch A Pathol Anat Histopathol 416: 25–42
103. Dardick I 1995 Myoepithelioma: definitions and diagnostic criteria. Ultrastruct Pathol 19: 335–345
104. Simpson R H, Jones H, Beasley P 1995 Benign myoepithelioma of the salivary glands: a true entity? Histopathology 27: 1–9
105. Hornick J L, Fletcher C D 2003 Myoepithelial tumors of soft tissue: a clinicopathologic and immunohistochemical study of 101 cases with evaluation of prognostic parameters. Am J Surg Pathol 27: 1183–1196
106. Alos L, Cardesa A, Bombi J et al. 1996 Myoepithelial tumors of salivary glands: a clinicopathologic, immunohistochemical, ultrastructural, and flow-cytometric study. Semin Diagn Pathol 13: 138–147
107. Skalova A, Leivo I, Michal M et al. 1992 Analysis of collagen isotypes in crystalloid structures of salivary gland tumors. Hum Pathol 23: 748–754
108. Franquemont D W, Mills S E 1993 Plasmacytoid monomorphic adenoma of salivary glands. Absence of myogenous differentiation and comparison to spindle cell myoepithelioma. Am J Surg Pathol 17: 146–153
109. Nagao T, Sugano I, Ishida Y et al. 1998 Salivary gland malignant myoepithelioma: a clinicopathological and immunohistochemical study of ten cases. Cancer 83: 1292–1299
110. Savera A T, Gown A M, Zarbo R J 1997 Immunolocalization of three novel smooth muscle-specific proteins in salivary gland pleomorphic adenoma: assessment of the morphogenetic role of myoepithelium. Mod Pathol 10: 1093–1100
111. Savera A T, Sloman A, Huvos A G et al. 2000 Myoepithelial carcinoma of the salivary glands: a clinicopathologic study of 25 patients. Am J Surg Pathol 24: 761–774
112. Di Palma S, Guzzo M 1993 Malignant myoepithelioma of salivary glands: clinicopathological features of ten cases. Virchows Arch A Pathol Anat Histopathol 423: 389–396
113. Nagao K, Matsuzaki O, Saiga H et al. 1981 Histopathologic studies on carcinoma in pleomorphic adenoma of the parotid gland. Cancer 48: 113–121
114. Tavassoli F A 1991 Myoepithelial lesions of the breast. Myoepitheliosis, adenomyoepithelioma, and myoepithelial carcinoma. Am J Surg Pathol 15: 554–568
115. Lakhani S R, O'Hare M J, Monaghan P et al. 1995 Malignant myoepithelioma (myoepithelial carcinoma) of the breast: a detailed cytokeratin study. J Clin Pathol 48: 164–167
116. Ogawa I, Nishida T, Miyauchi M et al. 2003 Dedifferentiated malignant myoepithelioma of the parotid gland. Pathol Int 53: 704–709
117. Thompson L D, Wenig B M, Ellis G L 1996 Oncocytomas of the submandibular gland. A series of 22 cases and a review of the literature. Cancer 78: 2281–2287
118. Pecorella I, Garner A 1997 Ostensible oncocytoma of accessory lacrimal glands. Histopathology 30: 264–270
119. Takeda Y 1986 Diffuse oncocytosis of the parotid gland. Int J Oral Maxillofac Surg 15: 765–768
120. Palmer T J, Gleeson M J, Eveson J W et al. 1990 Oncocytic adenomas and oncocytic hyperplasia of salivary glands: a clinicopathological study of 26 cases. Histopathology 16: 487–493
121. Hartwick R W, Batsakis J G 1990 Non-Warthin's tumor oncocytic lesions. Ann Otol Rhinol Laryngol 99: 674–677
122. Capone R B, Ha P K, Westra W H et al. 2002 Oncocytic neoplasms of the parotid gland: a 16-year institutional review. Otolaryngol Head Neck Surg 126: 657–662
123. Brandwein M S, Huvos A G 1991 Oncocytic tumors of major salivary glands. A study of 68 cases with follow-up of 44 patients. Am J Surg Pathol 15: 514–528

124. Shintaku M, Honda T 1997 Identification of oncocytic lesions of salivary glands by anti-mitochondrial immunohistochemistry. Histopathology 31: 408–411
125. Prasad A R, Savera A T, Regezi J A et al. 1999 Immunohistochemical demonstration of myoepithelial cell participation in salivary gland basal cell and canalicular adenomas. Mod Pathol 12: 130A (abstract)
126. Gilcrease M Z, Nelson F S, Guzman-Paz M 1998 Tyrosine-rich crystals associated with oncocytic salivary gland neoplasms. Arch Pathol Lab Med 122: 644–649
127. Ellis G L 1988 "Clear cell" oncocytoma of salivary gland. Hum Pathol 19: 862–867
128. Ellis G L 1998 Clear cell neoplasms in salivary glands: clearly a diagnostic challenge. Ann Diagn Pathol 2: 61–78
129. Maiorano E, Altini M, Favia G 1997 Clear cell tumors of the salivary glands, jaws, and oral mucosa. Semin Diagn Pathol 14: 203–212
130. Huvos A G 2005 Oncocytoma. In: Barnes L, Eveson J W, Reichart P et al. (eds) World Health Organization classification of tumours. Pathology and genetics: head and neck tumours. IARC, Lyon, France, p 273
131. Perzin K H 1982 A systematic approach to the diagnosis of salivary gland tumors. In: Fenoglio C M, Wolff M (eds) Progress in surgical pathology. Masson, New York, vol 4, p 137–180
132. Goode R R, Corio R L 1988 Oncocytic adenocarcinoma of salivary glands. Oral Surg Oral Med Oral Pathol 65: 61–66
133. Batsakis J 1979 Tumors of the head and neck. Clinical and pathological considerations, 2nd edn. Williams & Wilkins, Baltimore
134. Sugimoto T, Wakizono S, Uemura T et al. 1993 Malignant oncocytoma of the parotid gland: a case with an immunohistochemical and ultrastructural study. J Laryngol Otol 107: 69–74
135. Rousseau A, Mock D, Dover D G et al. 1999 Multiple canalicular adenomas: a case report and review of the literature. Oral Surg Oral Med Oral Pathol 57: 181–188
136. Suarez P, Hammong H L, Luna M A et al. 1998 Palatal canalicular adenoma: report of 12 cases and review of the literature. Ann Diagn Pathol 2: 224–228
137. Smullin S E, Fielding A F, Sausarla S M et al. 2004 Canalicular adenoma of the palate: case report and literature review. Oral Surg Oral Radiol Endod 98: 32–36
138. Batsakis J 1991 Oral monomorphic adenomas. Ann Otol Rhinol Laryngol 100: 348–350
139. McMillan M D, Smith C J, Smillie A C 1993 Canalicular adenoma: report of five cases with ultrastructural observations. J Oral Pathol Med 22: 368–373
140. Zarbo R J, Prasad A R, Regezi J A et al. 2000 Salivary gland basal cell and canalicular adenomas: immunohistochemical demonstration of myoepithelial cell participation and morphogenetic considerations. Arch Pathol Lab Med 124: 401–405
141. Arida M, Barnes E L, Hunt J L 2005 Molecular assessment of allelic loss in Warthin tumors. Mod Pathol 18: 964–968
142. Honda K, Kashuma K, Daa T et al. 2000 Clonal analysis of the epithelial component of Warthin's tumor. Hum Pathol 31: 1377–1380
143. Teymoortash A, Werner J A 2005 Tissue that has lost its track: Warthin's tumor. Virchows Arch 446: 585–588
144. Eneroth C 1971 Salivary gland tumors in the parotid gland, submandibular gland, and the palate region. Cancer 27: 1415–1418
145. Eveson J W, Cawson R A 1989 Infarcted ('infected') adenolymphomas. A clinicopathological study of 20 cases. Clin Otolaryngol 14: 205–210
146. Spiro R H 1986 Salivary neoplasms: overview of a 35-year experience with 2807 patients. Head Neck Surg 8: 177–184
147. Kotwell C 1992 Smoking as an etiologic factor in the development of Warthin's tumor of the parotid gland. Am J Surg 164: 646–647
148. Monk J J, Church J 1992 Warthin's tumor. A high incidence and no sex predominance on central Pennsylvania. Arch Otolaryngol Head Neck Surg 118: 477–478
149. Yoo G H, Eisele D W, Askin F B et al. 1994 Warthin's tumor: a 40-year experience at the Johns Hopkins Hospital. Laryngoscope 104: 799–803
150. Saku T, Hayashi Y, Takahara O et al. 1997 Salivary gland tumors among atomic bomb survivors, 1950–1987. Cancer 79: 1465–1475
151. Santucci M, Gallo O, Calzolari A et al. 1993 Detection of Epstein–Barr viral genome in tumor cells of Warthin's tumor of parotid gland. Am J Clin Pathol 100: 662–665
152. Chan J K, Yip T T, Tsang W Y et al. 1994 Specific association of Epstein–Barr virus with lymphoepithelial carcinoma among tumors and tumorlike lesions of the salivary gland. Arch Pathol Lab Med 118: 994–997
153. Ogata T, Hongfang Y, Kayano T et al. 1997 No significant role of Epstein–Barr virus in the tumorigenesis of Warthin tumor. J Med Dent Sci 44: 45–52
154. Chapnik J 1983 The controversy of Warthin's tumor. Laryngoscope 93: 695–716
155. Maiorano E, Lo Muzio L, Favia G et al. 2002 Warthin's tumour: a study of 78 cases with emphasis on bilaterality, multifocality and association with other malignancies. Oral Oncol 38: 35–40
156. Gnepp D R 2001 Diagnostic surgical pathology of the head and neck. Saunders, Philadelphia
157. Lam K H, Ho H C, Ho C M et al. 1994 Multifocal nature of adenolymphoma of the parotid. Br J Surg 81: 1612–1614
158. Shikhani A H, Shikhani L T, Kuhajda F P et al. 1993 Warthin's tumor-associated neoplasms: report of two cases and review of the literature. Ear Nose Throat J 72: 264–269, 272–273
159. Lefor A T, Ord R A 1993 Multiple synchronous bilateral Warthin's tumors of the parotid glands with pleomorphic adenoma. Case report and review of the literature. Oral Surg Oral Med Oral Pathol 76: 319–324
160. Dykun R, Deitel M, Borowy Z 1980 Treatment of parotid neoplasms. Can J Surg 23: 14–19
161. Ebbs S, Webb A 1986 Adenolymphoma of the parotid: aetiology, diagnosis and treatment. Br J Surg 73: 627–630
162. Eveson J, Cawson R 1985 Salivary gland tumors, A review of 2410 cases with particular reference to histological types, site, age and sex distribution. J Pathol 146: 51–58
163. Heller K S, Attie J N 1988 Treatment of Warthin's tumor by enucleation. Am J Surg 156: 294–296
164. Seifert G, Bull H G, Donath K 1980 Histologic subclassification of the cystadenolymphoma of the parotid gland. Analysis of 275 cases. Virchows Arch [Pathol Anat] 388: 13–38
165. David R, Buchner A 1978 Corpora amylacea in adenolymphoma (Warthin's tumor). Am J Clin Pathol 69: 173–175
166. Taxy J B 1992 Necrotizing squamous/mucinous metaplasia in oncocytic salivary gland tumors. A potential diagnostic problem. Am J Clin Pathol 97: 40–45
167. Nagao T, Sugano I, Ishida Y et al. 1998 Mucoepidermoid carcinoma arising in Warthin's tumor of the parotid gland: report of two cases with histopathological, ultrastructural and immunohistochemical studies. Histopathology 33: 379–386
168. Kessler E, Koznicky I L, Schinderl J 1977 Malignant Warthin's tumor. Oral Surg Oral Med Oral Pathol 43: 111–115
169. Therkildsen M, Christensen N, Andersen L et al. 1992 Malignant Warthin's tumor: a case study. Histopathology 21: 167–171
170. Bolat F, Kayaselcuk F, Erkan A N et al. 2004 Epidermoid carcinoma arising in Warthin's tumor. Pathol Oncol Res 10: 240–242
171. Foschini M P, Malvi D, Betts C M 2005 Oncocytic carcinoma arising in Warthin tumour. Virchows Arch 446: 88–90
172. Fornelli A, Eusebi V, Pasquinelli G et al. 2001 Merkel cell carcinoma of the parotid gland associated with Warthin tumour: report of two cases. Histopathology 39: 342–346
173. Medeiros L J, Rizzi R, Lardelli P et al. 1990 Malignant lymphoma involving a Warthin's tumor: a case with immunophenotypic and gene rearrangement analysis. Hum Pathol 21: 974–977
174. Bunker M L, Locker J 1989 Warthin's tumor with malignant lymphoma. DNA analysis of paraffin-embedded tissue. Am J Clin Pathol 91: 341–344
175. Melato M, Falconieri G, Fanin R et al. 1986 Hodgkin's disease occurring in a Warthin's tumor: first case report. Pathol Res Pract 181: 615–620
176. Park C K, Manning J T Jr, Battifora H et al. 2000 Follicle center lymphoma and Warthin tumor involving the same anatomic site. Report of two cases and review of the literature. Am J Clin Pathol 113: 113–119
177. Gnepp D R 1983 Sebaceous neoplasms of salivary gland origin: a review. Pathol Annu 18: 71–102
178. Gnepp D R, Brannon R 1984 Sebaceous neoplasms of salivary gland origin. Report of 21 cases. Cancer 53: 2155–2170
179. Ellis G L, Auclair P L, Gnepp D R et al. 1991 Other malignant epithelial neoplasms. In: Ellis G L, Auclair P L, Gnepp D R (eds) Surgical pathology of the salivary glands. W B Saunders, Philadelphia, PA, p 455–488
180. Linhartova A 1974 Sebaceous glands in salivary gland tissue. Arch Pathol 98: 320–324
181. Auclair P L, Ellis G L, Gnepp D R 1991 Other benign epithelial neoplasms. In Ellis G L, Auclair P L, Gnepp D R (eds) Surgical pathology of the salivary glands. Major problems in pathology. Saunders, Philadelphia, PA, p 252–268
182. Michal M, Skalova A, Mukensnabl P 2000 Micropapillary carcinoma of the parotid gland arising in mucinous cystadenoma. Virchows Arch 437: 465–468
183. Foss R D, Ellis G L, Auclair P L 1996 Salivary gland cystadenocarcinomas. A clinicopathologic study of 57 cases. Am J Surg Pathol 20: 1440–1447
184. Brandwein-Genster M, Gnepp D R 2005 Low-grade cribriform cystadenocarcinoma. In: Barnes L, Eveson J W, Reichart P et al. (eds) World Health Organization classification of tumours. Pathology and genetics: head and neck tumours. IARC, Lyon, France, p 241
185. Brannon R B, Sciubba J J, Giulani M 2001 Ductal papillomas of salivary gland origin: a report of 19 cases and a review of the literature. Oral Surg Oral Med Oral Pathol Oral Radiol Endod 92: 68–77
186. Shimoda M, Kameyama K, Morinaga S et al. 2004 Malignant transformation of sialadenoma papilliferum of the palate: a case report. Virchows Arch 445: 641–646
187. Nagao T, Sugano I, Matsuzaki O et al. 2000 Intraductal papillary tumors of the major salivary glands. Case reports of benign and malignant variants. Arch Pathol Lab Med 124: 291–295
188. Seifert G, Donath K, Jautzke G 1999 Unusual choristoma of the parotid gland in a girl. A possible trichoadenoma. Virchows Arch 434: 355–359
189. Nagao T, Serizawa H, Iwaya K et al. 2002 Keratocystoma of the parotid gland: a report of two cases of an unusual pathologic entity. Mod Pathol 15: 1005–1010
190. Dehner L P, Valbuena L, Perez-Atayde A et al. 1994 Salivary gland anlage tumor ("congenital pleomorphic adenoma"). A clinicopathologic, immunohistochemical and ultrastructural study of nine cases. Am J Surg Pathol 18: 25–36
191. Buchino J 1995 Salivary gland anlage tumor: a newly recognized clinicopathologic entity of uncertain histogenesis. Adv Anat Pathol 2: 94–98

192. Cohen E G, Yoder M, Thomas R M et al. 2003 Congenital salivary gland anlage tumor of the nasopharynx. Pediatrics 112: e66–e69
193. Har-El G, Zirkin H Y, Tovi F et al. 1985 Congenital pleomorphic adenoma of the nasopharynx (report of a case). J Laryngol Otol 99: 1281–1287
194. Gnepp D R 2003 Sclerosing polycystic adenosis of the salivary gland: a lesion that may be associated with dysplasia and carcinoma in situ. Adv Anat Pathol 10: 218–222
195. Smith B C, Ellis G L, Slater L J et al. 1996 Sclerosing polycystic adenosis of major salivary glands. A clinicopathologic analysis of nine cases. Am J Surg Pathol 20: 161–170
196. Batsakis J G 1996 Sclerosing polycystic adenosis: newly recognized salivary gland lesion – a form of chronic sialadenitis. Adv Anat Pathol 3: 298–304
197. Donath K, Seifert G 1997 [Sclerosing polycystic sialadenopathy. A rare non-tumorous disease.] Pathologe 18: 368–373
198. Kabani S, Gallagher G 2002 Sclerosing polycystic adenosis (SPCA) of minor salivary glands. Oral Surg Oral Med Oral Pathol Radiol Endod 94: 187
199. Skalova A, Michal M, Simpson R H W et al. 2002 Sclerosing polycystic adenosis of parotid gland with dysplasia and ductal carcinoma in situ. Report of three cases with immunohistochemical and ultrastructural examination. Virchows Arch 440: 29–35
199a. Gnepp D R, Wang L J, Brandwein-Gensler M et al. 2006 Sclerosing polycystic adenosis of the salivary gland: a report of 16 cases. Am J Surg Pathol 30: 154–164
200. Batsakis J G, Bruner J M, Luna M A 1988 Polycystic (dysgenetic) disease of the parotid glands. Arch Otolaryngol Head Neck Surg 114: 1146–1148
201. Dobson C M, Ellis H A 1987 Polycystic disease of the parotid glands: case report of a rare entity and review of the literature. Histopathology 11: 953–961
202. Seifert G, Thomsen S, Donath K 1981 Bilateral dysgenetic polycystic parotid glands. Morphological analysis and differential diagnosis of a rare disease of the salivary glands. Virchows Arch [Pathol Anat] 390: 273–288
203. Auclair P L 1994 Tumor-associated lymphoid proliferation in the parotid gland. A potential diagnostic pitfall. Oral Surg Oral Med Oral Pathol 77: 19–26
204. Ma J, Chan J K, Chow C W et al. 2002 Lymphadenoma: a report of three cases of an uncommon salivary gland neoplasm. Histopathology 41: 342–350
205. Yau K C, Tsang W Y, Chan J K 1997 Lipoadenoma of the parotid gland with probable striated duct differentiation. Mod Pathol 10: 242–246
206. Hirokawa M, Shimizu M, Manabe T et al. 1998 Oncocytic lipoadenoma of the submandibular gland. Hum Pathol 29: 410–412
207. Hornigold R, Morgan P R, Pearce A et al. 2005 Congenital sialolipoma of the parotid: first reported case and review of the literature. Int J Pediatr Otorhinolaryngol 69: 429–434
208. Nagao T, Sugano I, Ishida Y et al. 2001 Sialolipoma: a report of seven cases of a new variant of salivary gland lipoma. Histopathology 38: 30–36
209. Loy T, McLaughlin R, Odom L et al. 1989 Mucoepidermoid carcinoma of the parotid as a second malignant neoplasm in children. Cancer 64: 2174–2177
210. Modan B, Chetrit A, Alfandary E et al. 1998 Increased risk of salivary gland tumors after low-dose irradiation. Laryngoscope 108: 1095–1097
211. Nonaka D, Klimstra D, Rosai J 2004 Thymic mucoepidermoid carcinomas: a clinicopathologic study of 10 cases and review of the literature. Am J Surg Pathol 28: 1526–1531
212. Shilo K, Foss R D, Franks T J et al. 2005 Pulmonary mucoepidermoid carcinoma with prominent tumor-associated lymphoid proliferation. Am J Surg Pathol 29: 407–411
213. Riedlinger W F, Hurley M Y, Dehner L P et al. 2005 Mucoepidermoid carcinoma of the skin: a distinct entity from adenosquamous carcinoma: a case study with a review of the literature. Am J Surg Pathol 29: 131–135
214. Simpson R J, Hoang K G, Hyams V J et al. 1988 Mucoepidermoid carcinoma of the maxillary sinus. Otolaryngol Head Neck Surg 99: 419–423
215. Pia-Foschini M, Reis-Filho J S, Eusebi V et al. 2003 Salivary gland-like tumours of the breast: surgical and molecular pathology. J Clin Pathol 56: 497–506
216. Kuo T, Tsang N M 2001 Salivary gland type nasopharyngeal carcinoma: a histologic, immunohistochemical, and Epstein–Barr virus study of 15 cases including a psammomatous mucoepidermoid carcinoma. Am J Surg Pathol 25: 80–86
217. Sekine J, Anami M, Fujita S et al. 2005 A case of mucoepidermoid carcinoma with melanin pigmentation manifested in the palate. Virchows Arch 446: 460–462
218. Donath K, Seifert G, Roser K 1997 The spectrum of giant cells in tumours of the salivary glands: an analysis of 11 cases. J Oral Pathol Med 26: 431–436
219. Ross J, Huaman J, Barsky S 1992 A study of the heterogeneity of the mucoepidermoid tumor and the implication for future therapies. Arch Otol Head Neck Surg 118: 1172–1178
220. Jahan-Parwar B, Huberman R M, Donovan D T et al. 1999 Oncocytic mucoepidermoid carcinoma of the salivary glands. Am J Surg Pathol 23: 523–529
221. Brannon R B, Willard C C 2003 Oncocytic mucoepidermoid carcinoma of parotid gland origin. Oral Surg Oral Med Oral Pathol Oral Radiol Endod 96: 727–733
222. Chan J K, Saw D 1987 Sclerosing mucoepidermoid tumour of the parotid gland: report of a case. Histopathology 11: 203–207
223. Batsakis J G, Luna M A 1990 Histopathologic grading of salivary gland neoplasms: I. Mucoepidermoid carcinomas. Ann Otol Rhinol Laryngol 99: 835–838
224. Muller S, Barnes L, Goodurn W J Jr 1997 Sclerosing mucoepidermoid carcinoma of the parotid. Oral Surg Oral Med Oral Pathol Oral Radiol Endod 83: 685–690
225. Fadare O, Hileeto D, Gruddin Y L et al. 2004 Sclerosing mucoepidermoid carcinoma of the parotid gland. Arch Pathol Lab Med 128: 1046–1049
226. Urano M, Abe M, Horibe Y et al. 2002 Sclerosing mucoepidermoid carcinoma with eosinophilia of the salivary glands. Pathol Res Pract 198: 305–310
227. Baloch Z W, Solomon A C, LiVolsi V A 2000 Primary mucoepidermoid carcinoma and sclerosing mucoepidermoid carcinoma with eosinophilia of the thyroid gland: a report of nine cases. Mod Pathol 13: 802–807
228. Prasad A R, Savera A T, Gown A M et al. 1999 The myoepithelial immunophenotype in 135 benign and malignant salivary gland tumors other than pleomorphic adenoma. Arch Pathol Lab Med 123: 801–806
229. Nikitakis N G, Tosios K I, Papanikolaou V S et al. 2004 Immunohistochemical expression of cytokeratins 7 and 20 in malignant salivary gland tumors. Mod Pathol 17: 407–415
230. Nordkvist A, Gustafsson H, Juberg-Ode M et al. 1994 Recurrent rearrangements of 11q14-22 in mucoepidermoid carcinoma. Cancer Genet Cytogenet 74: 77–83
231. Tonon G, Modi S, Wu L et al. 2003 t(11;19)(q21;p13) translocation in mucoepidermoid carcinoma creates a novel fusion product that disrupts a Notch signaling pathway. Nat Genet 33: 208–213
232. Martins C, Cavaco B, Tonon G et al. 2004 A study of MECT1-MAML2 in mucoepidermoid carcinoma and Warthin's tumor of salivary glands. J Mol Diagn 6: 205–210
233. Bullerdiek J, Haubrich J, Meyer K et al. 1988 Translocation t(11;19)(q21;p13.1) as the sole chromosome abnormality in a cystadenolymphoma (Warthin's tumor) of the parotid gland. Cancer Genet Cytogenet 35: 129–132
234. Mark J, Dahlenfors R, Stenman G et al. 1989 A human adenolymphoma showing the chromosomal aberrations del (7)(p12p14-15) and t(11;19)(q21;p12-13). Anticancer Res 9: 1565–1566
235. Evans H L 1984 Mucoepidermoid carcinoma of salivary glands: a study of 69 cases with special attention to histologic grading. Am J Clin Pathol 81: 696–701
236. Hicks M J, el-Naggar A K, Flaitz C M et al. 1995 Histocytologic grading of mucoepidermoid carcinoma of major salivary glands in prognosis and survival: a clinicopathologic and flow cytometric investigation. Head Neck 17: 89–95
237. Auclair P L, Goode R K, Ellis G L 1992 Mucoepidermoid carcinoma of intraoral salivary glands. Evaluation and application of grading criteria in 143 cases. Cancer 69: 2021–2030
238. Goode R K, Auclair P L, Ellis G L 1998 Mucoepidermoid carcinoma of the major salivary glands: clinical and histopathologic analysis of 234 cases with evaluation of grading criteria. Cancer 82: 1217–1224
239. Fonseca I, Clode A L, Soares J 1993 Mucoepidermoid carcinoma of major and minor salivary glands, a survey of 43 cases with study of prognostic indicators. Int J Surg Pathol 1: 3–12
240. Jensen O J, Poulsen T, Schiodt T 1988 Mucoepidermoid tumors of salivary glands. A long term follow-up study. APMIS 96: 421–427
241. Eversole L R, Rovin S, Sabes W R 1972 Mucoepidermoid carcinoma of minor salivary glands: report of 17 cases with follow-up. J Oral Surg 30: 107–112
242. Guzzo M, Andreola S, Sirizzotti G et al. 2002 Mucoepidermoid carcinoma of the salivary glands: clinicopathologic review of 108 patients treated at the National Cancer Institute of Milan. Ann Surg Oncol 9: 688–695
243. Monoo K, Sageshima M, Ito E et al. 2003 Histopathological grading and clinical features of patients with mucoepidermoid carcinoma of the salivary glands. Nippon Jibiinkoka Gakkai Kaiho 106: 304–308
244. Boahene D K, Olsen K D, Lewis J E et al. 2004 Mucoepidermoid carcinoma of the parotid gland: the Mayo clinic experience. Arch Otolaryngol Head Neck Surg 130: 849–856
245. Skalova A, Lehtonen H, von Boguslawsky K et al. 1994 Prognostic significance of cell proliferation in mucoepidermoid carcinomas of the salivary gland: clinicopathological study using MIB 1 antibody in paraffin sections. Hum Pathol 25: 929–935
246. Kokemueller H, Brueggemann N, Swennen G et al. 2005 Mucoepidermoid carcinoma of the salivary glands – clinical review of 42 cases. Oral Oncol 41: 3–10
247. Pires F R, de Almeida O P, de Araujo V C et al. 2004 Prognostic factors in head and neck mucoepidermoid carcinoma. Arch Otolaryngol Head Neck Surg 130: 174–180
248. Handra-Luca A, Lamas G, Bertrand J C et al. 2005 MUC1, MUC2, MUC4, and MUC5AC expression in salivary gland mucoepidermoid carcinoma: diagnostic and prognostic implications. Am J Surg Pathol 29: 881–889
249. Perzin K H, Gullane P, Clairmont A C 1978 Adenoid cystic carcinomas arising in salivary glands: a correlation of histologic features and clinical course. Cancer 42: 265–282
250. Huvos A G, Strong E W 1973 Epithelial tumors of the lacrimal gland (abstract). Lab Invest 28: 386
251. Hajdu S I, Huvos A G, Goodner J T et al. 1970 Carcinoma of the trachea, a clinicopathologic study of 41 cases. Cancer 25: 1448
252. Nelms D, Luna M 1972 Primary adenocystic carcinoma (cylindromatous carcinoma) of the esophagus. Cancer 29: 440

253. Gray H R, Helwig E B 1963 Epithelioma adenoides cysticum and solitary trichoepithelioma. Arch Dermatol 87: 102
254. Weltzer S 1970 Adenoid cystic carcinoma of the breast. Am Surg 36: 271
255. Lassaletta L, Patron M, Oloriz J et al. 2003 Avoiding misdiagnosis in ceruminous gland tumours. Auris Nasus Larynx 30: 287–290
256. Friedrich R E, Bleckmann V 2003 Adenoid cystic carcinoma of salivary and lacrimal gland origin: localization, classification, clinical pathological correlation, treatment results and long-term follow-up control in 84 patients. Anticancer Res 23: 931–940
257. Chomette G, Auriol M, Tranbaloc P et al. 1982 Adenoid cystic carcinoma of minor salivary glands. Analysis of 86 cases. Clinico-pathological, histoenzymological and ultrastructural studies. Virchows Arch [Pathol Anat] 395: 289–301
258. Conley J, Dingman D L 1974 Adenoid cystic carcinoma in the head and neck (cylindroma). Arch Otolaryngol 100: 81–90
259. Eby L S, Johnson D S, Baker H W 1972 Adenoid cystic carcinoma of the head and neck. Cancer 29: 1160–1168
260. Eneroth C M, Zajicek J 1969 Aspiration biopsy of salivary gland tumors. IV. Morphologic studies on smears and histologic sections from 45 cases of adenoid cystic carcinoma. Acta Cytol 13: 59–63
261. Leafstedt S W, Gaeta J F, Sako K et al. 1971 Adenoid cystic carcinoma of major and minor salivary glands. Am J Surg 122: 756–762
262. Matsuba H M, Simpson J R, Mauney M et al. 1986 Adenoid cystic salivary gland carcinoma: a clinicopathologic correlation. Head Neck Surg 8: 200–204
263. Nascimento A G, Amaral A L, Prado L A et al. 1986 Adenoid cystic carcinoma of salivary glands. A study of 61 cases with clinicopathologic correlation. Cancer 57: 312–319
264. Spiro R H, Huvos A G, Strong E W 1974 Adenoid cystic carcinoma of salivary origin. A clinicopathologic study of 242 cases. Am J Surg 128: 512–520
265. Hamper K, Lazar F, Dietel M et al. 1990 Prognostic factors for adenoid cystic carcinoma of the head and neck: a retrospective evaluation of 96 cases. J Oral Pathol Med 19: 101–107
266. Chilla R, Schroth R, Eysholdt U et al. 1980 Adenoid cystic carcinoma of the head and neck. Controllable and uncontrollable factors in treatment and prognosis. ORL J Otorhinolaryngol Relat Spec 42: 346–367
267. Rapidis A D, Givalos N, Gakiopoulou H et al. 2005 Adenoid cystic carcinoma of the head and neck. Clinicopathological analysis of 23 patients and review of the literature. Oral Oncol 41: 328–335
268. Kokemueller H, Eckardt A, Brachvogel P et al. 2004 Adenoid cystic carcinoma of the head and neck – a 20 years experience. Int J Oral Maxillofac Surg 33: 25–31
269. Batsakis J G, El-Naggar A K 1999 Myoepithelium in salivary and mammary neoplasms is host-friendly. Adv Anat Pathol 6: 218–226
270. Cheuk W, Chan J K C, Ngan R K C 1999 Dedifferentiation in adenoid cystic carcinoma of salivary gland: an uncommon complication associated with an accelerated clinical course. Am J Surg Pathol 23: 465–472
271. Nagao T, Gaffey T A, Serizawa H et al. 2003 Dedifferentiated adenoid cystic carcinoma: a clinicopathologic study of 6 cases. Mod Pathol 16: 1265–1272
272. Chau Y, Hongyo T, Aozasa K et al. 2001 Dedifferentiation of adenoid cystic carcinoma: report of a case implicating *p53* gene mutation. Hum Pathol 32: 1403–1407
273. Emanuel P, Wang B, Wu M et al. 2005 p63 immunohistochemistry in the distinction of adenoid cystic carcinoma from basaloid squamous cell carcinoma. Mod Pathol 18: 645–650
274. Edwards P C, Bhuiya T, Kelsch R D 2003 *C-kit* expression in the salivary gland neoplasms adenoid cystic carcinoma, polymorphous low-grade adenocarcinoma, and monomorphic adenoma. Oral Surg Oral Med Oral Pathol Oral Radiol Endod 95: 586–593
275. Mino M, Pilch B Z, Faquin W C 2003 Expression of *KIT* (CD117) in neoplasms of the head and neck: an ancillary marker for adenoid cystic carcinoma. Mod Pathol 16: 1224–1231
276. Hotte S J, Winquist E W, Lamont E et al. 2005 Imatinib mesylate in patients with adenoid cystic cancers of the salivary glands expressing *c-kit*: a Princess Margaret Hospital phase II consortium study. J Clin Oncol 23: 585–590
277. Nordkvist A, Mark J, Gustafsson H et al. 1994 Non-random chromosome rearrangements in adenoid cystic carcinoma of the salivary glands. Genes Chromos Cancer 10: 115–121
278. Sandros J, Mark J, Happonen R P et al. 1988 Specificity of 6q- markers and other recurrent deviations in human malignant salivary gland tumors. Anticancer Res 8: 637–643
279. Jin C, Martins C, Jin Y et al. 2001 Characterization of chromosome aberrations in salivary gland tumors by FISH, including multicolor COBRA-FISH. Genes Chromos Cancer 30: 161–167
280. El-Rifai W, Rutherford S, Knuutila S et al. 2001 Novel DNA copy number losses in chromosome 12q12-q13 in adenoid cystic carcinoma. Neoplasia 3: 173–178
281. Maruya S, Kurotaki H, Shimoyama N et al. 2003 Expression of p16 protein and hypermethylation status of its promoter gene in adenoid cystic carcinoma of the head and neck. ORL J Otorhinolaryngol Relat Spec 65: 26–32
282. Stallmach I, Zenklusen P, Komminoth P et al. 2002 Loss of heterozygosity at chromosome 6q23-25 correlates with clinical and histologic parameters in salivary gland adenoid cystic carcinoma. Virchows Arch 440: 77–84
283. Queimado L, Reis A, Fonseca I et al. 1998 A refined localization of two deleted regions in chromosome 6q associated with salivary gland carcinomas. Oncogene 16: 83–88
284. Batsakis J G, Luna M A, el-Naggar A 1990 Histopathologic grading of salivary gland neoplasms: III. Adenoid cystic carcinomas. Ann Otol Rhinol Laryngol 99: 1007–1009
285. Szanto P A, Luna M A, Tortoledo M E et al. 1984 Histologic grading of adenoid cystic carcinoma of the salivary glands. Cancer 54: 1062–1069
286. Yamamoto Y, Virmani A K, Wistuba I I et al. 1996 Loss of heterozygosity and microsatellite alterations in *p53* and *RB* genes in adenoid cystic carcinoma of the salivary glands. Hum Pathol 27: 1204–1210
287. Enamorado I, Lakhani R, Korkmaz H et al. 2004 Correlation of histopathological variants, cellular DNA content, and clinical outcome in adenoid cystic carcinoma of the salivary glands. Otolaryngol Head Neck Surg 131: 646–650
288. Greiner T C, Robinson R A, Maves M D 1989 Adenoid cystic carcinoma. A clinicopathologic study with flow cytometric analysis. Am J Clin Pathol 92: 711–720
289. Nordgard S, Franzen G, Boysen M et al. 1997 *Ki-67* as a prognostic marker in adenoid cystic carcinoma assessed with the monoclonal antibody MIB1 in paraffin sections. Laryngoscope 107: 531–536
290. Gnepp D R, Schroeder W, Heffner D 1989 Synchronous tumors arising in a single major salivary gland. Cancer 63: 1219–1224
291. Von Biberstein S E, Spiro J D, Mancoll W 1999 Acinic cell carcinoma of the nasal cavity. Otolaryngol Head Neck Surg 121: 759–762
292. Crissman J D, Rosenblatt A 1978 Acinous cell carcinoma of the larynx. Arch Pathol Lab Med 102: 233–236
293. Schmitt F C, Ribeiro C A, Alvarenga S et al. 2000 Primary acinic cell-like carcinoma of the breast: a variant with a good prognosis? Histopathology 36: 286–289
294. Lee H Y, Mancer K, Koong H N 2003 Primary acinic cell carcinoma of the lung with lymph node metastasis. Arch Pathol Lab Med 127: e216–e219
295. Ohike N, Kosmahl M, Kloppel G 2004 Mixed acinar-endocrine carcinoma of the pancreas. A clinicopathological study and comparison with acinar-cell carcinoma. Virchows Arch 445: 231–235
296. Colmenero C, Patron M, Sierra I 1991 Acinic cell carcinoma of the salivary glands. A review of 20 new cases. J Craniomaxillofac Surg 19: 260–266
297. Ellis G L, Corio R L 1983 Acinic cell adenocarcinoma. A clinicopathologic analysis of 294 cases. Cancer 52: 542–549
298. Abrams A M, Melrose R J 1978 Acinic cell tumors of minor salivary gland origin. Oral Surg Oral Med Oral Pathol 46: 220–233
299. Abrams A, Cornyn J, Scofield H et al. Acinic cell adenocarcinoma of the major salivary glands: a clinicopathologic study of 77 cases. Cancer 18: 1145–1162
300. Lewis J, Olsen K, Weiland L 1991 Acinic cell carcinoma. Clinicopathological review. Cancer 67: 172–179
301. Chaudhry A, Cutler L, Leifer C et al. 1986 Histogenesis of acinic cell carcinoma of the major and minor salivary glands. An ultrastructural study. J Pathol 148: 307–320
302. Stanley R J, Weiland L H, Olsen K D et al. 1988 Dedifferentiated acinic cell (acinous) carcinoma of the parotid gland. Otolaryngol Head Neck Surg 98: 155–161
303. Henley J D, Geary W A, Jackson C L et al. 1997 Dedifferentiated acinic cell carcinoma of the parotid gland: a distinct rarely described entity. Hum Pathol 28: 869–873
304. Timon C I, Dardick I 2001 The importance of dedifferentiation in recurrent acinic cell carcinoma. J Laryngol Otol 115: 639–644
305. Childers E L, Ellis G L, Auclair P L 1996 An immunohistochemical analysis of anti-amylase antibody reactivity in acinic cell adenocarcinoma. Oral Surg Oral Med Oral Pathol Oral Radiol Endod 81: 691–694
306. Skalova A, Leivo I, Von Boguslawsky K et al. 1994 Cell proliferation correlates with prognosis in acinic cell carcinomas of salivary gland origin. Immunohistochemical study of 30 cases using the MIB 1 antibody in formalin-fixed paraffin sections. J Pathol 173: 13–21
307. Michal M, Skalova A, Simpson R H et al. 1997 Well-differentiated acinic cell carcinoma of salivary glands associated with lymphoid stroma. Hum Pathol 28: 595–600
308. Freedman P D, Lumerman H 1983 Lobular carcinoma of intraoral minor salivary gland origin. Report of twelve cases. Oral Surg Oral Med Oral Pathol 56: 157–166
309. Batsakis J G, Pinkston G R, Luna M A et al. 1983 Adenocarcinomas of the oral cavity: a clinicopathologic study of terminal duct carcinomas. J Laryngol Otol 97: 825–835
310. George M K, Mansour P, Pahor A L 1991 Terminal parotid duct carcinoma. J Laryngol Otol 105: 780–781
311. Ritland F, Lubensky I, LiVolsi V A 1993 Polymorphous low-grade adenocarcinoma of the parotid salivary gland. Arch Pathol Lab Med 117: 1261–1263
312. Nagao T, Gaffey T A, Kay P A et al. 2004 Polymorphous low-grade adenocarcinoma of the major salivary glands: report of three cases in an unusual location. Histopathology 44: 164–171
313. Perez-Ordonez B, Linkov I, Huvos A G 1998 Polymorphous low-grade adenocarcinoma of minor salivary glands: a study of 17 cases with emphasis on cell differentiation. Histopathology 32: 521–529
314. Castle J T, Thompson L D, Frommelt R A et al. 1999 Polymorphous low grade adenocarcinoma: a clinicopathologic study of 164 cases. Cancer 86: 207–219

315. Selva D, Davis G J, Dodd T et al. 2004 Polymorphous low-grade adenocarcinoma of the lacrimal gland. Arch Ophthalmol 122: 915–917
316. Lengyel E, Somogyi A, Godeny M et al. 2000 Polymorphous low-grade adenocarcinoma of the nasopharynx. Case report and review of the literature. Strahlenther Onkol 176: 40–42
317. Young S, Leon M, Talerman A et al. 2003 Polymorphous low-grade adenocarcinoma of the vulva and vagina: a tumor resembling adenoid cystic carcinoma. Int J Surg Pathol 11: 43–49
318. Sato T, Indo H, Takasaki T et al. 2001 A rare case of intraosseous polymorphous low-grade adenocarcinoma (PLGA) of the maxilla. Dentomaxillofac Radiol 30: 184–187
319. Lee V K, McCaughan B C, Scolyer R A 2004 Polymorphous low-grade adenocarcinoma in the lung: a case report. Int J Surg Pathol 12: 287–292
320. Tsang Y W, Tung Y, Chan J K 1991 Polymorphous low grade adenocarcinoma of the palate in a child. J Laryngol Otol 105: 309–311
321. Vincent S D, Hammond H L, Finkelstein M W 1994 Clinical and therapeutic features of polymorphous low-grade adenocarcinoma. Oral Surg Oral Med Oral Pathol 77: 41–47
322. Evans H L, Luna M A 2000 Polymorphous low-grade adenocarcinoma: a study of 40 cases with long-term follow up and an evaluation of the importance of papillary areas. Am J Surg Pathol 24: 1319–1328
323. Fonseca I, Felix A, Soares J 1997 Cell proliferation in salivary gland adenocarcinomas with myoepithelial participation. A study of 78 cases. Virchows Arch 430: 227–232
324. Araujo V, Sousa S, Jaeger M et al. 1999 Characterization of the cellular component of polymorphous low-grade adenocarcinoma by immunohistochemistry and electron microscopy. Oral Oncol 35: 164–172
325. Thompson L D 2004 Polymorphous low-grade adenocarcinoma. Pathol Case Rev 9: 259–263
326. Pelkey T J, Mills S E 1999 Histologic transformation of polymorphous low-grade adenocarcinoma of salivary gland. Am J Clin Pathol 111: 785–791
327. Simpson R H, Pereira E M, Ribeiro A C et al. 2002 Polymorphous low-grade adenocarcinoma of the salivary glands with transformation to high-grade carcinoma. Histopathology 41: 250–259
328. Gnepp D R, el-Mofty S 1997 Polymorphous low-grade adenocarcinoma: glial fibrillary acidic protein staining in the differential diagnosis with cellular mixed tumors. Oral Surg Oral Med Oral Pathol Oral Radiol Endod 83: 691–695
329. Anderson C, Krutchkoff D, Pedersen C et al. 1990 Polymorphous low grade adenocarcinoma of minor salivary gland: a clinicopathological and comparative immunohistochemical study. Mod Pathol 3: 76–82
330. Regezi J A, Zarbo R J, Stewart J C et al. 1991 Polymorphous low-grade adenocarcinoma of minor salivary gland. A comparative histologic and immunohistochemical study. Oral Surg Oral Med Oral Pathol 71: 469–475
331. Simpson R H, Clarke T J, Sarsfield P T et al. 1991 Polymorphous low-grade adenocarcinoma of the salivary glands: a clinicopathological comparison with adenoid cystic carcinoma. Histopathology 19: 121–129
332. Curran A E, White D K, Damm D D et al. 2001 Polymorphous low-grade adenocarcinoma versus pleomorphic adenoma of minor salivary glands: resolution of a diagnostic dilemma by immunohistochemical analysis with glial fibrillary acidic protein. Oral Surg Oral Med Oral Pathol Oral Radiol Endod 91: 194–199
333. Dardick I, Burford-Mason A P 1994 Pathology of the salivary glands: the contribution of electron microscopy. Microsc Res Tech 27: 46–60
334. Michal M, Skalova A, Simpson R H et al. 1999 Cribriform adenocarcinoma of the tongue: a hitherto unrecognized type of adenocarcinoma characteristically occurring in the tongue. Histopathology 35: 495–501
335. Luna M A, Wenig B M 2005 Polymorphous low-grade adenocarcinoma. In: Barnes L, Eveson J W, Reichart P et al. (eds) World Health Organization classification of tumours. Pathology and genetics: head and neck tumours. IARC, Lyon, p 231–232
336. Seifert G 1998 Are adenomyoepithelioma of the breast and epithelial-myoepithelial carcinoma of the salivary glands identical tumours? Virchows Arch 433: 285–288
337. Loose J H, Patchefsky A S, Hollander I J et al. 1992 Adenomyoepithelioma of the breast. A spectrum of biologic behavior. Am J Surg Pathol 16: 868–876
338. Fulford L G, Kamata Y, Okudera K et al. 2001 Epithelial-myoepithelial carcinomas of the bronchus. Am J Surg Pathol 25: 1508–1514
339. Chan W M, Liu D T, Lam L Y et al. 2004 Primary epithelial-myoepithelial carcinoma of the lacrimal gland. Arch Ophthalmol 122: 1714–1717
340. Ru K, Srivastava A, Tischler A S 2004 Bronchial epithelial-myoepithelial carcinoma. Arch Pathol Lab Med 128: 92–94
341. Doganay L, Bilgi S, Ozdil A et al. 2003 Epithelial-myoepithelial carcinoma of the lung. A case report and review of the literature. Arch Pathol Lab Med 127: e177–e180
342. Lee H M, Kim A R, Lee S H 2000 Epithelial-myoepithelial carcinoma of the nasal cavity. Eur Arch Otorhinolaryngol 257: 376–378
343. Imate Y, Yamashita T, Endo S et al. 2000 Epithelial-myoepithelial carcinoma of the nasopharynx. ORL J Otorhinolaryngol Relat Spec 62: 282–285
344. Horinouchi H, Ishihara T, Kawamura M et al. 1993 Epithelial myoepithelial tumour of the tracheal gland. J Clin Pathol 46: 185–187
345. Tsuneyama K, Hoso M, Kono N et al. 1999 An unusual case of epithelial-myoepithelial carcinoma of the liver. Am J Surg Pathol 23: 349–353
346. Luna M A, Batsakis J G, Ordonez N G et al. 1987 Salivary gland adenocarcinomas: a clinicopathologic analysis of three distinctive types. Semin Diagn Pathol 4: 117–135
347. Hamper K, Brugmann M, Koppermann R et al. 1989 Epithelial-myoepithelial duct carcinoma of salivary glands: a follow-up and cytophotometric study of 21 cases. J Oral Pathol Med 18: 299–304
348. Corio R L, Sciubba J J, Brannon R B et al. 1982 Epithelial-myoepithelial carcinoma of intercalated duct origin. A clinicopathologic and ultrastructural assessment of sixteen cases. Oral Surg Oral Med Oral Pathol 53: 280–287
349. Cho K J, el-Naggar A K, Ordonez N G et al. 1995 Epithelial-myoepithelial carcinoma of salivary glands. A clinicopathologic, DNA flow cytometric, and immunohistochemical study of Ki-67 and HER-2/neu oncogene. Am J Clin Pathol 103: 432–437
350. Fonseca I, Soares J 1993 Proliferating cell nuclear antigen immunohistochemistry in epithelial-myoepithelial carcinoma of the salivary glands. Arch Pathol Lab Med 117: 993–995
351. Fonseca I, Soares J 1993 Epithelial-myoepithelial carcinoma of the salivary glands. A study of 22 cases. Virchows Arch A Pathol Anat Histopathol 422: 389–396
352. Alos L, Carrillo R, Ramos J et al. 1999 High-grade carcinoma component in epithelial-myoepithelial carcinoma of salivary glands: clinicopathological, immunohistochemical and flow-cytometric study of three cases. Virchows Arch 434: 291–299
353. Simpson R H, Clarke T J, Sarsfield P T et al. 1991 Epithelial-myoepithelial carcinoma of salivary glands. J Clin Pathol 44: 419–423
354. Manuel S, Mathews A, Chandramohan K et al. 2002 Carcinosarcoma of the parotid gland with epithelial-myoepithelial carcinoma and pleomorphic sarcoma components. Br J Oral Maxillofac Surg 40: 480–483
355. Delgado R, Vuitch F, Albores-Saavedra J 1993 Salivary duct carcinoma. Cancer 72: 1503–1512
356. Lewis J E, McKinney B C, Weiland L H et al. 1996 Salivary duct carcinoma. Clinicopathologic and immunohistochemical review of 26 cases. Cancer 77: 223–230
357. Barnes L, Rao U, Krause J et al. 1994 Salivary duct carcinoma. Part I. A clinicopathologic evaluation and DNA image analysis of 13 cases with review of the literature. Oral Surg Oral Med Oral Pathol 78: 64–73
358. Barnes L, Rao U, Contis L et al. 1994 Salivary duct carcinoma. Part II. Immunohistochemical evaluation of 13 cases for estrogen and progesterone receptors, cathepsin D, and c-erbB-2 protein. Oral Surg Oral Med Oral Pathol 78: 74–80
359. Jaehne M, Roeser K, Jaekel T et al. 2005 Clinical and immunohistologic typing of salivary duct carcinoma. A report of 50 cases. Cancer 103: 2526–2533
360. Guzzo M, Di Palma S, Grandi C et al. 1997 Salivary duct carcinoma: clinical characteristics and treatment strategies. Head Neck 19: 126–133
361. Nagao T, Gaffey T A, Serizawa H et al. 2004 Sarcomatoid variant of salivary duct carcinoma: clinicopathologic and immunohistochemical study of eight cases with review of the literature. Am J Clin Pathol 122: 222–231
362. Simpson R H, Prasad A R, Lewis J E et al. 2003 Mucin-rich variant of salivary duct carcinoma: a clinicopathologic and immunohistochemical study of four cases. Am J Surg Pathol 27: 1070–1079
363. Nagao T, Gaffey T A, Visscher D W et al. 2004 Invasive micropapillary salivary duct carcinoma: a distinct histologic variant with biologic significance. Am J Surg Pathol 28: 319–326
364. Ide F, Mishima K, Saito I 2003 Sarcomatoid salivary duct carcinoma of the oral cavity. Virchows Arch 443: 686–689
365. Henley J D, Seo I S, Dayan D et al. 2000 Sarcomatoid salivary duct carcinoma of the parotid gland. Hum Pathol 31: 208–213
366. Padberg B C, Sasse B, Huber A et al. 2005 Sarcomatoid salivary duct carcinoma. Ann Diagn Pathol 9: 86–92
367. Hui K K, Batsakis J G, Luna M A et al. 1986 Salivary duct adenocarcinoma: a high grade malignancy. J Laryngol Otol 100: 105–114
368. Brandwein M S, Jagirdar J, Patil J et al. 1990 Salivary duct carcinoma (cribriform salivary carcinoma of excretory ducts). A clinicopathologic and immunohistochemical study of 12 cases. Cancer 65: 2307–2314
369. Grenko R T, Gemryd P, Tytor M et al. 1995 Salivary duct carcinoma. Histopathology 26: 261–266
370. Nasser S M, Faquin W C, Dayal Y 2003 Expression of androgen, estrogen, and progesterone receptors in salivary gland tumors. Frequent expression of androgen receptor in a subset of malignant salivary gland tumors. Am J Clin Pathol 119: 801–806
371. Moriki T, Ueta S, Takahashi T et al. 2001 Salivary duct carcinoma: cytologic characteristics and application of androgen receptor immunostaining for diagnosis. Cancer 93: 344–350
372. Fan C Y, Wang J, Barnes E L 2000 Expression of androgen receptor and prostatic specific markers in salivary duct carcinoma: an immunohistochemical analysis of 13 cases and review of the literature. Am J Surg Pathol 24: 579–586
373. Kapadia S B, Barnes L 1998 Expression of androgen receptor, gross cystic disease fluid protein, and CD44 in salivary duct carcinoma. Mod Pathol 11: 1033–1038
374. James G K, Pudek M, Berean K W et al. 1996 Salivary duct carcinoma secreting prostate-specific antigen. Am J Clin Pathol 106: 242–247
375. Martinez-Barba E, Cortes-Guardiola J A, Minguela-Puras A et al. 1997 Salivary duct carcinoma: clinicopathological and immunohistochemical studies. J Craniomaxillofac Surg 25: 328–334
376. Laforga J B 2004 Salivary duct carcinoma with neuroendocrine features. Virchows Arch 444: 473–476
377. Hoang M P, Callender D L, Sola Gallego J J et al. 2001 Molecular and biomarker analyses of salivary duct carcinomas: comparison with mammary duct carcinoma. Int J Oncol 19: 865–871

378. Cerilli L A, Swartzbaugh J R, Saadut R et al. 1999 Analysis of chromosome 9p21 deletion and *p16* gene mutation in salivary gland carcinomas. Hum Pathol 30: 1242–1246
379. Mutoh H, Nagata H, Ohno K et al. 2001 Analysis of the *p53* gene in parotid gland cancers: a relatively high frequency of mutations in low-grade mucoepidermoid carcinomas. Int J Oncol 18: 781–786
380. Skalova A, Starek I, Vanecek T et al. 2003 Expression of HER-2/neu gene and protein in salivary duct carcinomas of parotid gland as revealed by fluorescence in-situ hybridization and immunohistochemistry. Histopathology 42: 348–356
381. Wick M R, Ockner D M, Mills S E et al. 1998 Homologous carcinomas of the breasts, skin, and salivary glands. A histologic and immunohistochemical comparison of ductal mammary carcinoma, ductal sweat gland carcinoma, and salivary duct carcinoma. Am J Clin Pathol 109: 75–84
382. Cheuk W, Miliauskas J R, Chan J K 2004 Intraductal carcinoma of the oral cavity: a case report and a reappraisal of the concept of pure ductal carcinoma in situ in salivary duct carcinoma. Am J Surg Pathol 28: 266–270
383. Delgado R, Klimstra D, Albores-Saavedra J 1996 Low grade salivary duct carcinoma. A distinctive variant with a low grade histology and a predominant intraductal growth pattern. Cancer 78: 958–967
384. Brandwein-Gensler M, Hille J, Wang B Y et al. 2004 Low-grade salivary duct carcinoma. Description of 16 cases. Am J Surg Pathol 28: 1040–1044
385. Anderson C, Muller R, Piorkowski R et al. 1992 Intraductal carcinoma of major salivary gland. Cancer 69: 609–614
386. Wang B, Brandwein M, Gordon R et al. 2002 Primary salivary clear cell tumors – a diagnostic approach: a clinicopathologic and immunohistochemical study of 20 patients with clear cell carcinoma, clear cell myoepithelial carcinoma, and epithelial-myoepithelial carcinoma. Arch Pathol Lab Med 126: 676–685
387. Rezende R B, Drachenberg C B, Kumar D et al. 1999 Differential diagnosis between monomorphic clear cell adenocarcinoma of salivary glands and renal (clear) cell carcinoma. Am J Surg Pathol 23: 1532–1538
388. Milchgrub S, Gnepp D R, Vuitch F et al. 1994 Hyalinizing clear cell carcinoma of salivary gland. Am J Surg Pathol 18: 74–82
389. Urban S D, Keith D A, Goodman M 1996 Hyalinizing clear cell carcinoma: report of a case. J Oral Pathol Med 25: 562–564
390. Balakrishnan R, Nayak D R, Pillai S et al. 2002 Hyalinizing clear cell carcinoma of the base of the tongue. J Laryngol Otol 116: 851–853
391. Chao T K, Tsai C C, Yeh S Y et al. Hyalinizing clear cell carcinoma of the hard palate. J Laryngol Otol 118: 382–384
392. Tang S K, Wan S K, Chan J K 1995 Hyalinizing clear cell carcinoma of salivary gland: report of a case with multiple recurrences over 12 years. Am J Surg Pathol 19: 240–241
393. Berho M, Huvos A G 1999 Central hyalinizing clear cell carcinoma of the mandible and the maxilla: a clinicopathologic study of two cases with an analysis of the literature. Hum Pathol 30: 101–105
394. Ereno C, Grande J, Alija V et al. 2000 Hyalinizing clear cell carcinoma of the hypopharynx metastasizing to the lung: a case report. Histopathology 37: 89–91
395. O'Regan E, Shandilya M, Gnepp D R et al. 2004 Hyalinizing clear cell carcinoma of salivary gland: an aggressive variant. Oral Oncol 40: 348–352
396. Simpson R H, Sarsfield P T, Clarke T et al. 1990 Clear cell carcinoma of minor salivary glands. Histopathology 17: 433–438
397. Gnepp D R, Wick M R 1990 Small cell carcinoma of the major salivary glands. An immunohistochemical study. Cancer 66: 185–192
398. Toyosawa S, Ohnishi A, Ito R et al. 1999 Small cell undifferentiated carcinoma of the submandibular gland: immunohistochemical evidence of myoepithelial, basal and luminal cell features. Pathol Int 49: 887–892
399. Chan J K, Suster S, Wenig B M et al. 1997 Cytokeratin 20 immunoreactivity distinguishes Merkel cell (primary cutaneous neuroendocrine) carcinomas and salivary gland small cell carcinomas from small cell carcinomas of various sites. Am J Surg Pathol 21: 226–234
400. Hui K K, Luna M A, Batsakis J G et al. 1990 Undifferentiated carcinomas of the major salivary glands. Oral Surg Oral Med Oral Pathol 69: 76–83
401. Gnepp D R, Corio R L, Brannon R B 1986 Small cell carcinoma of the major salivary glands. Cancer 58: 705–714
402. Huntrakoon M 1987 Neuroendocrine carcinoma of the parotid gland: a report of two cases with ultrastructural and immunohistochemical studies. Hum Pathol 18: 1212–1217
403. Kraemer B B, Mackay B, Batsakis J G 1983 Small cell carcinomas of the parotid gland. A clinicopathologic study of three cases. Cancer 52: 2115–2121
404. Nagao T, Gaffey T A, Olsen K D et al. 2004 Small cell carcinoma of the major salivary glands: clinicopathologic study with emphasis on cytokeratin 20 immunoreactivity and clinical outcome. Am J Surg Pathol 28: 762–770
405. Cheuk W, Kwan M Y, Suster S et al. 2001 Immunostaining for thyroid transcription factor 1 and cytokeratin 20 aids the distinction of small cell carcinoma from Merkel cell carcinoma, but not pulmonary from extrapulmonary small cell carcinomas. Arch Pathol Lab Med 125: 228–231
406. Koss L G, Spiro R H, Hajdu S 1972 Small cell (oat cell) carcinoma of minor salivary gland origin. Cancer 30: 737–741
407. Hayashi Y, Nagamine S, Yanagawa T et al. 1987 Small cell undifferentiated carcinoma of the minor salivary gland containing exocrine, neuroendocrine, and squamous cells. Cancer 60: 1583–1588
408. Wang C P, Chang Y L, Ko J Y et al. 2004 Lymphoepithelial carcinoma versus large cell undifferentiated carcinoma of the major salivary glands. Cancer 101: 2020–2027
409. Batsakis J G, Luna M A 1991 Undifferentiated carcinomas of salivary glands. Ann Otol Rhinol Laryngol 100: 82–84
410. Larsson L G, Donner L R 1999 Large cell neuroendocrine carcinoma of the parotid gland: fine needle aspiration, and light microscopic and ultrastructural study. Acta Cytol 43: 534–536
411. Nagao T, Sugano I, Ishida Y et al. 2000 Primary large-cell neuroendocrine carcinoma of the parotid gland: immunohistochemical and molecular analysis of two cases. Mod Pathol 13: 554–561
412. Eversole L R, Gnepp D R, Eversole G M 1991 Undifferentiated carcinoma. In: Ellis G L, Auclair P L, Gnepp D R (eds) Surgical pathology of the salivary glands. W B Saunders, Philadelphia, PA, p 422–440
413. Saw D, Lau W H, Ho J H et al. 1986 Malignant lymphoepithelial lesion of the salivary gland. Hum Pathol 17: 914–923
414. Huang D P, Ng H K, Ho Y H et al. 1988 Epstein–Barr virus (EBV)-associated undifferentiated carcinoma of the parotid gland. Histopathology 13: 509–517
415. Hamilton-Dutoit S J, Therkildsen M H, Neilsen N H et al. 1991 Undifferentiated carcinoma of the salivary gland in Greenlandic Eskimos: demonstration of Epstein–Barr virus DNA by in situ nucleic acid hybridization. Hum Pathol 22: 811–815
416. Tsai C H, Chen C L, Hsu H C et al. 1996 Expression of Epstein–Barr virus in carcinomas of major salivary glands: a strong association with lymphoepithelioma-like carcinoma. Hum Pathol 27: 258–262
417. Nagao T, Ishida Y, Sugano I et al. 1996 Epstein–Barr virus-associated undifferentiated carcinoma with lymphoid stroma of the salivary gland in Japanese patients. Comparison with benign lymphoepithelial lesion. Cancer 78: 695–703
418. Leung S Y, Chung L P, Yuen S T et al. 1995 Lymphoepithelial carcinoma of the salivary gland: in situ detection of Epstein–Barr virus. J Clin Pathol 48: 1022–1027
419. Kuo T, Hsueh C 1997 Lymphoepithelioma-like salivary gland carcinoma in Taiwan: a clinicopathological study of nine cases demonstrating a strong association with Epstein–Barr virus. Histopathology 31: 75–82
420. Gallo O, Santucci M, Calzolari A et al. 1994 Epstein–Barr virus (EBV) infection and undifferentiated carcinoma of the parotid glands in Caucasian patients. Acta Otolaryngol 114: 572–575
421. Kotsianti A, Costopoulos J, Morgello S et al. 1996 Undifferentiated carcinoma of the parotid gland in a white patient: detection of Epstein–Barr virus by in situ hybridization. Hum Pathol 27: 87–90
422. Mrad K, Ben Brahim E, Driss M et al. 2004 Lymphoepithelioma-like carcinoma of the submandibular salivary gland associated with Epstein–Barr virus in a North African woman. Virchows Arch 445: 419–420
423. Worley N K, Daroca P J Jr 1997 Lymphoepithelial carcinoma of the minor salivary gland. Arch Otolaryngol Head Neck Surg 123: 638–640
424. Hanji D, Gohao L 1983 Malignant lymphoepithelial lesions of the salivary glands with anaplastic carcinomatous change. Report of nine cases and review of literature. Cancer 52: 2245–2252
425. Saw D, Ho J H, Lau W H et al. 1986 Parotid swelling as the first manifestation of nasopharyngeal carcinoma: a report of two cases. Eur J Surg Oncol 12: 71–75
426. Christiansen M S, Mourad W A, Hales M L et al. 1995 Spindle cell malignant lymphoepithelial lesion of the parotid gland: clinical, light microscopic, ultrastructural, and in situ hybridization findings in one case. Mod Pathol 8: 711–715
427. Squillaci S, Bertalot G, Vago L et al. 2000 Lymphoepithelioma-like carcinoma of the parotid gland. Description of a case with detection of EBV by in situ hybridization. Pathologica 92: 89–194
428. Bialas M, Sinczak A, Choinska-Stefanska A et al. 2002 EBV-positive lymphoepithelial carcinoma of salivary gland in a woman of a non-endemic area – a case report. Pol J Pathol 53: 235–238
429. Shemen L J, Huvos A G, Spiro R H 1987 Squamous cell carcinoma of salivary gland origin. Head Neck Surg 9: 235–240
430. Gaughan R, Olsen K, Lewis J 1992 Primary squamous cell carcinoma of the parotid gland. Arch Otolaryngol Head Neck Surg 118: 798–801
431. Cawson R A, Gleeson M J, Eveson J W 1997 Carcinomas of salivary glands. pathology and surgery of the salivary glands. ISIS Medical Media, Oxford, p 167–169
432. Ghannoum J E, Freedman P D 2004 Signet-ring cell (mucin-producing) adenocarcinomas of minor salivary glands. Am J Surg Pathol 28: 89–93
433. Li J, Wang B Y, Nelson M et al. 2004 Salivary adenocarcinoma, not otherwise specified: a collection of orphans. Arch Pathol Lab Med 128: 1385–1394
434. Spiro R H, Huvos A G, Strong E W 1982 Adenocarcinoma of salivary origin. Clinicopathologic study of 204 patients. Am J Surg 144: 423–431
435. Matsuba H M, Mauney M, Simpson J R et al. 1988 Adenocarcinomas of major and minor salivary gland origin: a histopathologic review of treatment failure patterns. Laryngoscope 98: 784–788
436. Spiro R H, Koss L G, Hajdu S I et al. 1973 Tumors of minor salivary origin. A clinicopathologic study of 492 cases. Cancer 31: 117–129
437. Vawter G, Tefft M 1966 Congenital tumors of the parotid gland. Arch Pathol 82: 242–245
438. Canalis R F, Mok M W, Fishman S M et al. 1980 Congenital basal cell adenoma of the submandibular gland. Arch Otolaryngol 106: 284–286
439. Ortiz-Hidalgo C, de Leon-Bojorge B, Fernandez-Sobrino G et al. 2001 Sialoblastoma: report of a congenital case with dysembryogenic alterations of the adjacent parotid gland. Histopathology 38: 79–84

440. Simpson P R, Rutledge J C, Schaefer S D et al. 1986 Congenital hybrid basal cell adenoma – adenoid cystic carcinoma of the salivary gland. Pediatr Pathol 6: 199–208
441. Siddiqi S H, Solomon M P, Haller J O 2000 Sialoblastoma and hepatoblastoma in a neonate. Pediatr Radiol 30: 349–351
442. Harris M D, McKeever P, Robertson J M 1990 Congenital tumours of the salivary gland: a case report and review. Histopathology 17: 155–157
443. Brandwein M, Al-Naeif N, Manwani D et al. 1999 Sialoblastoma: clinicopathological/immunohistochemical study. Am J Surg Pathol 23: 342–348
444. McKnight H A 1939 Malignant parotid tumor in the newborn. Am J Surg 45: 128–130
445. Hsueh C, Gonzalez-Crussi F 1992 Sialoblastoma: a case report and review of the literature on congenital epithelial tumors of salivary gland origin. Pediatr Pathol 12: 205–214
446. Batsakis J G, Frankenthaler R 1992 Embryoma (sialoblastoma) of salivary glands. Ann Otol Rhinol Laryngol 101: 958–960
447. Batsakis J G, Mackay B, Ryka A F et al. 1988 Perinatal salivary gland tumours (embryomas). J Laryngol Otol 102: 1007–1011
448. Cawson R A, Gleeson M J, Eveson J W 1997 Pathology and surgery of the salivary glands. ISIS Medical Media, Oxford
449. Kane W, McCaffrey T, Olsen K et al. 1991 Primary parotid malignancies. Arch Otolaryngol Head Neck Surg 117: 307–315
450. Luna M, Tortoledo M, Ordonez N et al. 1991 Primary sarcomas of the major salivary glands. Arch Otolaryngol Head Neck Surg 117: 302–306
451. Mantravadi J, Roth L, Kafrawy A 1993 Vascular neoplasms of the parotid gland. Oral Surg Oral Med Oral Pathol 75: 70–75
452. Childers E L B, Furlong M A, Fanburg-Smith J C 2002 Hemangioma of the salivary gland: a study of ten cases of a rarely biopsied/excised lesion. Ann Diagn Pathol 6: 339–344
453. Enzinger F M, Weiss S W 1995 Soft tissue tumors, 3rd edn. C V Mosby, St. Louis
454. Robertson J S, Wiegand D A, Schaitkin B M 1991 Life-threatening hemangioma arising from the parotid gland. Otolaryngol Head Neck Surg 104: 858–862
455. Damiani S, Corti B, Neri F et al. 2003 Primary angiosarcoma of the parotid gland arising from benign congenital hemangioma. Oral Surg Oral Med Oral Pathol Oral Radiol Endod 96: 66–69
456. Wells G, Whimster I 1969 Subcutaneous angiolymphoid hyperplasia with eosinophilia. Br J Dermatol 81: 1–14
457. Fanburg-Smith J C, Furlong M A, Childers E L 2003 Oral and salivary gland angiosarcoma: a clinicopathologic study of 29 cases. Mod Pathol 16: 263–271
458. Piscioli F, Leonardi E, Scappini P et al. 1986 Primary angiosarcoma of the gingiva. Case report with immunohistochemical study. Am J Dermatopathol 8: 430–435
459. Tomec R, Ahmad I, Fu Y S et al. Malignant hemangioendothelioma (angiosarcoma) of the salivary gland: an ultrastructural study. Cancer 43: 1664–1671
460. Wesley R K, Mintz S M, Wertheimer F W 1975 Primary malignant hemangioendothelioma of the gingiva. Report of a case and review of the literature. Oral Surg Oral Med Oral Pathol 39: 103–112
461. Falvo L, Marzullo A, Catania A et al. 2004 Epithelioid haemangioendothelioma of the parotid salivary gland: a case report. Chir Ital 56: 457–462
462. Chan J K C, Hui P K, Ng C S et al. 1989 Epithelioid hemangioma and Kimura's disease in Chinese. Histopathology 15: 557–574
463. Chan J K C 1997 Solitary fibrous tumor – everywhere, and a diagnosis in vogue. Histopathology 31: 568–576
464. Nascimento A G 1996 Solitary fibrous tumor: a ubiquitous neoplasm of mesenchymal differentiation. Adv Anat Pathol 3: 388–395
465. Hanau C, Miettinen M 1995 Solitary fibrous tumor: histological and immunohistochemical spectrum of benign and malignant variants presenting at different sites. Hum Pathol 26: 440–449
466. Brunnemann R, Ro J, Ordonez N et al. 1997 Extrathoracic localized fibrous tumor: a clinicopathologic study of 24 cases. Mod Pathol 12: 1034–1042
467. Ferreiro J A, Nascimento A G 1996 Solitary fibrous tumour of the major salivary glands. Histopathology 28: 261–264
468. Guarino M, Giordano F, Pallotti F et al. 1998 Solitary fibrous tumor of the submandibular gland. Histopathology 32: 571–572
469. Gunhan O, Yildiz F R, Celasun B et al. 1994 Solitary fibrous tumour arising from sublingual gland: report of a case. J Laryngol Otol 108: 998–1000
470. Sato J, Asakura K, Yokoyama Y et al. 1998 Solitary fibrous tumor of the parotid gland extending to the parapharyngeal space. Eur Arch Otorhinolaryngol 255: 18–21
471. Hofmann T, Braun H, Kole K W et al. 2002 Solitary fibrous tumor of the submandibular gland. Eur Arch Otorhinolaryngol 259: 470–473
472. Ogawa I, Sato S, Kudo Y et al. 2003 Solitary fibrous tumor with malignant potential arising in sublingual gland. Pathol Int 53: 40–45
473. Williams S B, Foss R D, Ellis G L 1992 Inflammatory pseudotumors of the major salivary glands. Clinicopathologic and immunohistochemical analysis of six cases. Am J Surg Pathol 16: 896–902
474. Inui M, Tagawa T, Mori A et al. 1993 Inflammatory pseudotumor in the submandibular region. Oral Surg Oral Med Oral Pathol 76: 333–337
475. Rahimi S, Mafera B, Vigili M G 2004 Inflammatory pseudotumor of the parotid gland: report of a case with fine needle aspiration cytology. Acta Cytol 48: 574–576
476. Kojima M, Nakamura S, Itoh H et al. 2001 Inflammatory pseudotumor of the submandibular gland: report of a case presenting with autoimmune disease-like clinical manifestations. Arch Pathol Lab Med 125: 1095–1097
477. Cawson R, Gleeson M, Eveson J 1997 Mesenchymal, lymphoreticular, metastatic and periglandular tumours and other uncommon types of salivary gland tumours. In: Cawson R, Gleeson M, Eveson J (eds) The pathology and surgery of the salivary glands. ISIS Medical Media, Oxford, p 170–190
478. Carr M M, Fraser R B, Clarke K D 1998 Nodular fasciitis in the parotid gland of a child. Head Neck 20: 645–648
479. Fischer J R, Abdul-Karim F W, Robinson R A 1989 Intraparotid nodular fasciitis. Arch Pathol Lab Med 113: 1276–1278
480. Eusebi V, Martin S A, Govoni E et al. 1984 Giant cell tumor of major salivary glands: report of three cases, one occurring in association with a malignant mixed tumor. Am J Clin Pathol 81: 666–675
481. Tse L L, Finkelstein S D, Siegler R W et al. 2004 Osteoclast-type giant cell neoplasm of salivary gland. A microdissection-based comparative genotyping assay and literature review: extraskeletal "giant cell tumor of bone" or osteoclast-type giant cell "carcinoma"? Am J Surg Pathol 28: 953–961
482. Balogh K, Wolbarsht R, Federman M et al. 1985 Carcinoma of the parotid gland with osteoclast-like giant cells, immunohistochemical and ultrastructural observations. Arch Pathol Lab Med 109: 756–761
483. Kondratowicz G, Smallman L, Morgan D 1988 Clinicopathological study of myoepithelial sialadenitis and chronic sialadenitis (sialolithiasis). J Clin Pathol 41: 403–409
484. Metwaly H, Cheng J, Ida-Yonemochi H et al. 2003 Vascular endothelial cell participation in formation of lymphoepithelial lesions (epi-myoepithelial islands) in lymphoepithelial sialadenitis (benign lymphoepithelial lesion). Virchows Arch 443: 17–27
485. Carbone A, Gloghini A, Ferlito A 2000 Pathological features of lymphoid proliferations of the salivary glands: lymphoepithelial sialadenitis versus low-grade B-cell lymphoma of the MALT type. Ann Otol Rhinol Laryngol 109: 1170–1175
486. Harris N L 1999 Lymphoid proliferation of the salivary glands. Am J Clin Pathol 111: S94–S103
487. Ostberg Y 1983 The clinical picture of benign lympho-epithelial lesion. Clin Otolaryngol 8: 381–390
488. Gleeson M J, Cawson R A, Bennett M H 1986 Benign lymphoepithelial lesion: a less than benign disease. Clin Otolaryngol 11: 47–51
489. Barnes L, Myers E N, Prokopakis E P 1998 Primary malignant lymphomas of the parotid gland. Arch Otolaryngol Head Neck Surg 124: 573–577
490. Dunn P, Kuo T T, Shih L Y et al. 2004 Primary salivary gland lymphoma: a clinicopathologic study of 23 cases in Taiwan. Acta Hematol 112: 203–208
491. Ambrosetti A, Zanotti R, Pattaro C et al. 2004 Most cases of primary salivary mucosa-associated lymphoid tissue are associated with Sjögren syndrome or hepatitis C virus infection. Br J Hematol 126: 43–49
492. Zucca E, Conconi A, Pedrinis E et al. 2003 Nongastric marginal zone B-cell lymphoma of mucosa-associated lymphoid tissue. Blood 101: 2489–2495
493. Royer B, Cazals-Hatem D, Sibilia J et al. 1997 Lymphomas in patients with Sjögren's syndrome are marginal zone B-cell neoplasms, arise in diverse extranodal and nodal sites, and are not associated with viruses. Blood 90: 766–775
494. Mariette X 1999 Lymphomas in patients with Sjögren's syndrome: review of the literature and physiopathologic hypothesis. Leuk Lymphoma 33: 93–99
495. Bridges A J, England D M 1989 Benign lymphoepithelial lesion: relationship to Sjögren's syndrome and evolving malignant lymphoma. Semin Arthritis Rheum 19: 201–208
496. Falzon M, Isaacson P G 1991 The natural history of benign lymphoepithelial lesion of the salivary gland in which there is a monoclonal population of B cells. A report of two cases. Am J Surg Pathol 15: 59–65
497. Gleeson M J, Bennett M H, Cawson R A 1986 Lymphomas of salivary glands. Cancer 58: 699–704
498. Takahashi H, Cheng J, Fujita F et al. 1992 Primary malignant lymphoma of the salivary gland: a tumor of mucosa-associated lymphoid tissue. J Oral Pathol Med 21: 318–325
499. Schmid U, Lennert K, Gloor F 1989 Immunosialadenitis (Sjögren's syndrome) and lymphoproliferation. Clin Exp Rheumatol 7: 175–180
500. Schmid U, Helbron D, Lennert K 1982 Primary malignant lymphomas localized in salivary glands. Histopathology 6: 673–677
501. Fishleder A, Tubbs R, Hesse B et al. Uniform detection of immunoglobulin-gene rearrangement in benign lymphoepithelial lesions. N Engl J Med 316: 1118–1121
502. Freimark B, Fantozzi R, Bone R et al. 1989 Detection of clonally expanded salivary gland lymphocytes in Sjögren's syndrome. Arthritis Rheum 32: 859–869
503. Speight P M, Jordan R, Colloby P et al. 1994 Early detection of lymphomas in Sjögren's syndrome by in situ hybridization for kappa and lambda light chain mRNA in labial salivary glands. Oral Oncol Eur J Cancer 30: 244–247
504. Jordan R, Pringle J, Speight P 1995 High frequency of light chain restriction in labial salivary gland biopsies of Sjögren's syndrome detected by in situ hybridisation. J Pathol 177: 35–40
505. Pablos J L, Carreira P E, Morillas L et al. 1994 Clonally expanded lymphocytes in the minor glands of Sjögren's syndrome patients without lymphoproliferative disease. Arthritis Rheum 37: 1441–1444

506. Diss T C, Wotherspoon A C, Speight P et al. 1995 B-cell monoclonality, Epstein Barr virus, and t(14;18) in myoepithelial sialadenitis and low-grade B-cell MALT lymphoma of the parotid gland. Am J Surg Pathol 19: 531–536
507. Bahler D W, Swerdlow S H 1998 Clonal salivary gland infiltrates associated with myoepithelial sialadenitis (Sjögren's syndrome) begin as nonmalignant antigen-selected expansions. Blood 91: 1864–1872
508. Quintana P G, Kapadia S B, Bahler D W et al. 1997 Salivary gland lymphoid infiltrates associated with lymphoepithelial lesions: a clinicopathologic, immunophenotypic, and genotypic study. Hum Pathol 28: 850–861
509. Palmer R M, Eveson J W, Gusterson B A 1986 'Epimyoepithelial' islands in lymphoepithelial lesions: an immunocytochemical study. Virchows Arch [Pathol Anat] 408: 603–609
510. Chaudhry A P, Cutler L S, Yamane G M et al. 1986 Light and ultrastructural features of lymphoepithelial lesions of the salivary glands in Mikulicz's disease. J Pathol 146: 239–250
511. Caselitz J, Osborn M, Wustrow J et al. 1986 Immunohistochemical investigations on the epimyoepithelial islands in lymphoepithelial lesions. Lab Invest 55: 427–432
512. Dardick I, van Nostrand A W P, Rippstein P et al. 1988 Characterization of epimyoepithelial islands in benign lymphoepithelial lesions of major salivary gland: an immunohistochemical and ultrastructural study. Head Neck Surg 10: 168–178
513. Ihrler S, Zietz C, Sendelhofert A et al. 1999 Lymphoepithelial duct lesions in Sjögren-type sialadenitis. Virchows Arch 434: 315–323
514. Hyjek E, Smith W J, Isaacson P G 1988 Primary B-cell lymphoma of salivary glands and its relationship to myoepithelial sialadenitis. Hum Pathol 19: 766–776
515. Hsi E D, Zukerberg L R, Schnitzer B et al. 1995 Development of extrasalivary gland lymphoma in myoepithelial sialadenitis. Mod Pathol 8: 817–824
516. Abbondanzo S L 2001 Extranodal marginal-zone B-cell lymphoma of the salivary gland. Ann Diagn Pathol 5: 246–254
517. Takahashi H, Tsuda N, Tezuka F et al. 1990 Non-Hodgkin's lymphoma of the major salivary gland: a morphologic and immunohistochemical study of 15 cases. J Oral Pathol Med 19: 306–312
518. Isaacson P G, Norton A J 1994 Extranodal lymphomas. Churchill Livingstone, Edinburgh, p 67–83
519. Egerter D A, Beckstead J H 1988 Malignant lymphomas in the acquired immunodeficiency syndrome. Additional evidence for B-cell origin. Arch Pathol Lab Med 112: 602–608
520. Ioachim H L, Antonescu C, Giancotti F et al. 1998 EBV-associated primary lymphomas in salivary glands of HIV-infected patients. Pathol Res Pract 194: 87–95
521. Chan J K, Tsang W Y, Hui P K et al. 1997 T- and T/natural killer-cell lymphomas of the salivary gland: a clinicopathologic, immunohistochemical and molecular study of six cases. Hum Pathol 28: 238–245
522. Ye H, Liu H, Attygalle A et al. 2003 Variable frequencies of t(11;18)(q21;q21) in MALT lymphomas of different sites: significant association with CagA strains of *H. pylori* in gastric MALT lymphoma. Blood 102: 1012–1018
523. Streubel B, Simonitsch-Klupp I, Mullauer L et al. 2004 Variable frequencies of MALT lymphoma-associated genetic aberrations in MALT lymphomas of different sites. Leukemia 18: 1722–1726
524. Harris N L, Jaffe E S, Diebold J et al. 1999 World Health Organization classification of neoplastic diseases of the hematopoietic and lymphoid tissues: report of the Clinical Advisory Committee meeting, Airlie House, Virginia, November 1997. J Clin Oncol 17: 3835–3849
525. Ferraro F J, Rush B J, Ruark D et al. 1993 Enucleation of parotid lymphoepithelial cyst in patients who are human immunodeficiency virus positive. Surg Gynecol Obstet 177: 524–526
526. Goldstein J, Rubin J, Silver C et al. 1992 Radiation therapy as a treatment for benign lymphoepithelial parotid cysts in patients infected with human immunodeficiency virus-1. Int J Radiat Oncol Biol Phys 23: 1045–1050
527. Huang R, Pearlman S, Friedman W et al. 1991 Benign cystic vs solid lesions of the parotid gland in HIV patients. Head Neck 13: 522–527
528. Chan J K C 1998 Kuttner tumor (chronic sclerosing sialadenitis) of the submandibular gland: an underrecognized entity. Adv Anat Pathol 5: 239–251
529. Isaacson G, Lundquist P G 1982 Salivary calculi as an aetiological factor in chronic sialadenitis of the submandibular gland. Clin Otolaryngol 7: 231–236
530. Seifert G 1992 Tumour-like lesions of the salivary glands. The new WHO classification. Pathol Res Pract 188: 836–846
531. Kitagawa S, Zen Y, Harada K et al. 2005 Abundant IgG4-positive plasma cell infiltration characterizes chronic sclerosing sialadenitis (Kuttner's tumor). Am J Surg Pathol 29: 783–791
532. Yoshihara T, Kanda T, Yaku Y et al. 1983 Chronic sialadenitis of the submandibular gland (so-called Kuttner tumor). Auris Nasus Larynx 10: 117–123
533. Tiemann M, Teymoortash A, Schrader C et al. 2002 Chronic sclerosing sialadenitis of the submandibular gland is mainly due to a T lymphocyte immune reaction. Mod Pathol 15: 845–852
534. Kojima M, Nakamura S, Itoh H et al. 2003 Sclerosing variant of follicular lymphoma arising from submandibular glands and resembling "Kuttner tumor": a report of 3 patients. Int J Surg Pathol 11: 303–307
535. Ochoa E R, Harris N L, Pilch B Z 2001 Marginal zone B-cell lymphoma of the salivary gland arising in chronic sclerosing sialadenitis (Kuttner tumor). Am J Surg Pathol 25: 1546–1550
536. Brannon R B, Fowler C B, Hartman K S 1991 Necrotizing sialometaplasia, a clinicopathologic study of 69 cases and review of the literature. Oral Surg Oral Med Oral Pathol 72: 317–325
537. Abrams A M, Melrose R J, Howell F V 1973 Necrotizing sialometaplasia. A disease simulating malignancy. Cancer 32: 130–135
538. Walker G, Fehner R, Johns M et al. 1982 Necrotizing sialometaplasia of the larynx secondary to atheromatous embolism. Am J Clin Pathol 77: 221–223
539. Wenig B M 1995 Necrotizing sialometaplasia of the larynx, a report of cases and a review of the literature. Am J Clin Pathol 103: 609–613
540. Ben-Izhak O, Ben-Arieh Y 1993 Necrotizing squamous metaplasia in herpetic tracheitis following prolonged intubation: a lesion similar to necrotizing sialometaplasia. Histopathology 22: 265–269
541. Min K W, Houck J R Jr 1998 Protocol for the examination of specimens removed from patients with carcinomas of the upper aerodigestive tract: carcinomas of the oral cavity including lip and tongue, nasal and paranasal sinuses, pharynx, larynx, salivary glands, hypopharynx, oropharynx, and nasopharynx. Cancer Committee, College of American Pathologists. Arch Pathol Lab Med 122: 222–230

食管和胃肿瘤
Tumors of the esophagus and stomach

Fiona Campbell、Gregory Y. Lauwers 和 Geraint T. Williamas 著

杜金荣　韩丽姝　陈英准 译

食管	327	胃	340
上皮性肿瘤	327	上皮性肿瘤	340
非上皮性肿瘤	337	非上皮性肿瘤	356
瘤样病变	339	瘤样病变	364

食管　Esophagus

上皮性肿瘤　Epithelial tumors

鳞状细胞乳头状瘤和乳头状瘤病 Squamous cell papilloma and papillomatosis

临床特征：鳞状细胞乳头状瘤可发生于食管的任何部位，但最常见于下1/3，为单发性边界清楚的管腔内无蒂肿瘤，向食管腔内生长，直径一般小于1.5 cm[1]。巨大乳头状瘤[2]和多发性病变[3]也有报道，有时可伴Goltz综合征（局灶性皮肤发育不全，focal dermal hypoplasia）[4]。尽管有些病例与慢性刺激有关[3]，有些病例与人乳头状瘤病毒（HPV）感染有关[5,6]，但是这种病变的病因尚不清楚。

组织学表现：组织学上，鳞状细胞乳头状瘤具有乳头状结构，伴有血管结缔组织轴心，表面被覆增生的正常成熟的鳞状上皮（图8.1）。可有乳头状瘤病毒相关性改变，包括挖空细胞和多核细胞形成。尚未发现这种病变具有潜在恶性。

鉴别诊断：在活检标本中，鳞状细胞乳头状瘤必须与高分化的疣状鳞状细胞癌相鉴别（见下文）。

腺瘤　Adenoma

腺瘤罕见，通常为息肉状，组织学上与胃腺瘤不能区别（见第340页），常常是柱状（Barrett）食管异型增生隆起的一种表现[7]。已有多发性腺瘤性息肉同时伴发腺癌的报道[8]。

多形性腺瘤　Pleomorphic adenoma

食管的多形性腺瘤只有少数几例报道，其起源于黏膜下层的黏液腺，与起源于涎腺的多形性腺瘤（见第7章）相类似[9]。

上皮异型增生（上皮内肿瘤形成） Epithelial dysplasia (intraepithelial neoplasia)

发生在鳞状上皮或柱状上皮的上皮异型增生被看作是一种癌前病变，即可以进展成癌的异常组织学表现。上皮异型增生的特征是细胞非典型性、异常分化和结构紊乱，所有这些特征在重度或高级别异型增生时更为显著。相反，所有这些细胞学和结构异常在轻度或低级别异型增生时相对较轻。因为高级别异型增生在组织学上与上皮内癌或原位癌无法区别，所以上皮内肿瘤形成常常作为异型增生的同义词使用。

鳞状细胞异型增生　Squamous cell dysplasia

食管鳞状细胞异型增生，在形态学上与诸如宫颈等

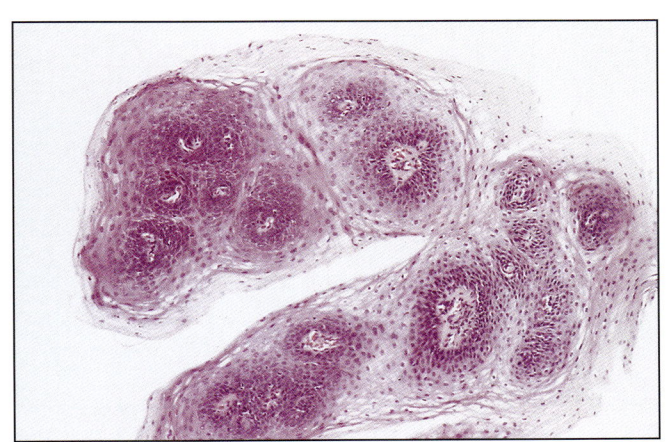

图8.1　食管良性鳞状细胞乳头状瘤。

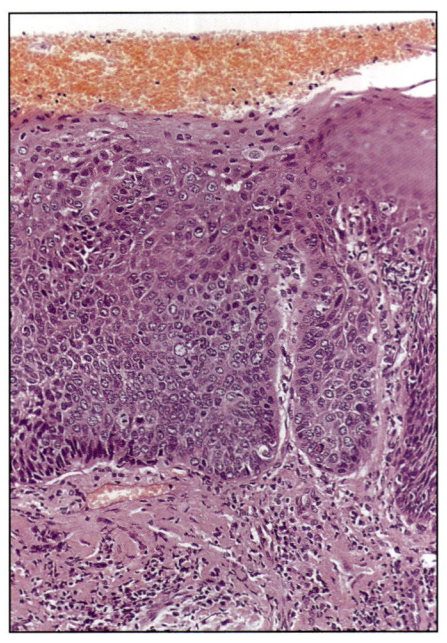

图8.2 邻近浸润性鳞状细胞癌的食管鳞状上皮重度异型增生。

其他部位的鳞状黏膜异型增生无法区分，经常出现在浸润性鳞状细胞癌发生之前或与其同时存在。仔细检查非放射因素引起的食管鳞状细胞癌的切除标本，发现多数病例邻近癌的黏膜中有各种级别的鳞状上皮异型增生性病变（图8.2）[10]，而且前瞻性研究表明，随着异型增生级别的增加，发生恶性的危险性相对增加[11]。在食管癌的高危人群中，例如中国北方，内窥镜下检查可见组织学诊断明确的食管鳞状上皮异型增生[12]。这些发现支持从食管鳞状细胞异型增生进展为浸润性鳞状细胞癌是一个连续的病变过程这一观点。确认的鳞状细胞异型增生有两种组织学变型：一种是异常细胞局限于基底层的基底鳞状细胞异型增生[13]，另一种是异型增生细胞仅占据上皮中层的Paget样鳞状细胞异型增生[14]。

腺上皮异型增生 Glandular dysplasia

食管腺上皮异型增生被认为是Barrett食管发生腺癌的前驱病变；腺上皮异型增生性病变可以弥漫或局限，内窥镜下检查可有异常或无异常表现。腺上皮异型增生还可以与腺癌一起出现，可以邻近肿瘤组织，也可以远离肿瘤组织[15]。如同鳞状细胞异型增生一样，腺上皮异型增生也可以根据结构或细胞异常的程度区分为低级别或高级别异型增生[16]。

"早期癌" "Early cancer"

所谓的食管"早期癌"是一个临床概念，就病理学而论，相当于严格地局限于黏膜层或黏膜下层的浸润性癌，伴有或不伴有淋巴结转移。最好称为"浅表性癌" (superficial carcinoma)。食管浅表性癌大多数是普通的鳞状细胞癌[17]，但是发生于Barrett食管的腺癌也可以表现为浅表性癌[18]。

鳞状细胞癌 Squamous cell carcinoma

临床特征：鳞状细胞癌是食管最常见的恶性肿瘤，男性多于女性。其发病率随着年龄的增加而增加，中位发病年龄为65岁。发病率存在明显的地域差异，中亚、中国和南非发病率高，而欧洲和北美发病率低。推测病因因素包括吸烟、酗酒、饮食缺陷、食品被真菌污染以及摄入碱液；并与Paterson-Kelly（Plummer-Vinson）综合征、贲门失弛缓症、食管憩室以及乳糜泻（celiac disease）有关[19]。上述多数病变有慢性食管炎，多无症状，但其发生率和组织学诊断仍有争议，特别是在高危人群中[20,21]。尽管食管癌的发病率似乎存在地域差异[24]，但研究显示，人乳头状瘤病毒在某些食管癌的发生机制中具有促进作用，尤其是HPV 16和18[22,23]。除了罕见的常染色体遗传性胼胝形成（autosomally inherited tylosis）（非表皮松解性掌跖皮肤角化病）患者食管癌的发病率非常高之外[25]（图8.3），尚无充分证据表明遗传在食管癌发生中起重要作用。对于食管癌分子异常的研究显示，经由表皮生长因子和转化生长因子-α的表皮生长因子受体过表达的，周期蛋白D1(cyclin D1)扩增，$p53$和$MTS1$基因突变，$p53$、Rb和APC基因等位缺失，以及染色体3p、9q、10p、17q、18q、19q和21q位点的杂合性缺失具有自泌性刺激作用[26,27]。特别有意思的是，大约70%的散发性食管鳞状细胞癌有染色体17q的杂合性缺失，因为它通常是参与遗传性胼胝症的基因位点，表明它具有食管癌肿瘤抑癌基因的作用[28]。

鳞状细胞癌通常发生于食管的中部下1/3，临床上表现为进行性吞咽困难、体重下降、贫血，或在罕见情况下可发生食管穿孔。肿瘤可在纵隔内局部扩散，或

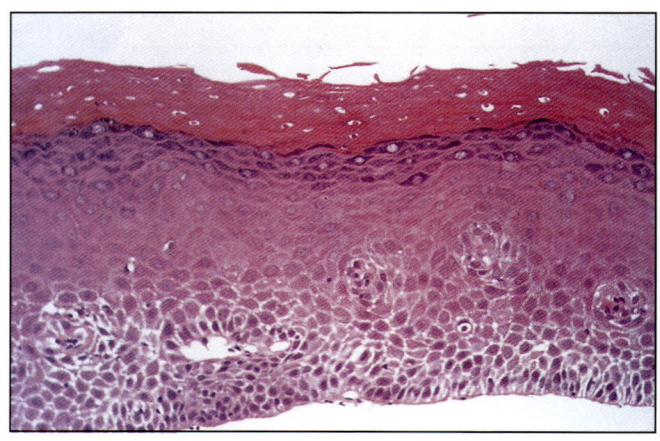

图8.3 胼胝形成患者的食管活检，显示食管鳞状上皮角化不良和颗粒层增厚。

在侵犯淋巴管后发生更广泛的扩散，出现扩散通常已是晚期，总的预后较差[29,30]。然而，所谓的浅表性（早期）鳞状细胞癌的病例，即病变局限于黏膜和黏膜下层者预后要好得多[17]，遗憾的是，这种肿瘤绝大多数没有症状，是在内窥镜下检查或着色内窥镜下检查（chromoendoscoy）时偶然诊断的。大约10%的食管鳞状细胞癌病人，不管是浅表性癌还是进展期癌，会同时或不同时出现口咽环的鳞状细胞癌[31]。

鳞状细胞癌的疣状亚型（verrucous variant）不常见，尽管分化很好，生长缓慢，而且极少转移，但是引起死亡的并不少见，因为在广泛局部扩散发生之前不能作出诊断[32]。这是因为内窥镜活检常常显示为非典型性不明显的高分化鳞状上皮碎片，而被病理医师误诊为反应性上皮增生，即使是在内窥镜下检查有显著异常时也会如此。因此，为了作出正确诊断，将临床、内窥镜、放射学及组织学特征结合起来是非常重要的。

大体表现：鳞状细胞癌通常为环形，部分为外生性，部分为溃疡性病变，导致食管狭窄（图8.4）。早期（浅表性）肿瘤常为灰白色斑块样结节，表面偶尔糜烂，给人以类似于食管炎的外观，或在大体检查时实际上无法确认（图8.5）。高分化疣状鳞状细胞癌通常为大的疣状病变（图8.6），切面显示边界清楚，边缘呈推进状。另一方面，某些广泛浸润的低分化病变可能引起食管壁弥漫性增厚，边界不清，类似于皮革胃。Paterson-Kelly综合征的环状软骨后癌无特殊大体特征；与其相伴随的食管蹼可以表现为一层薄的结缔组织隔。

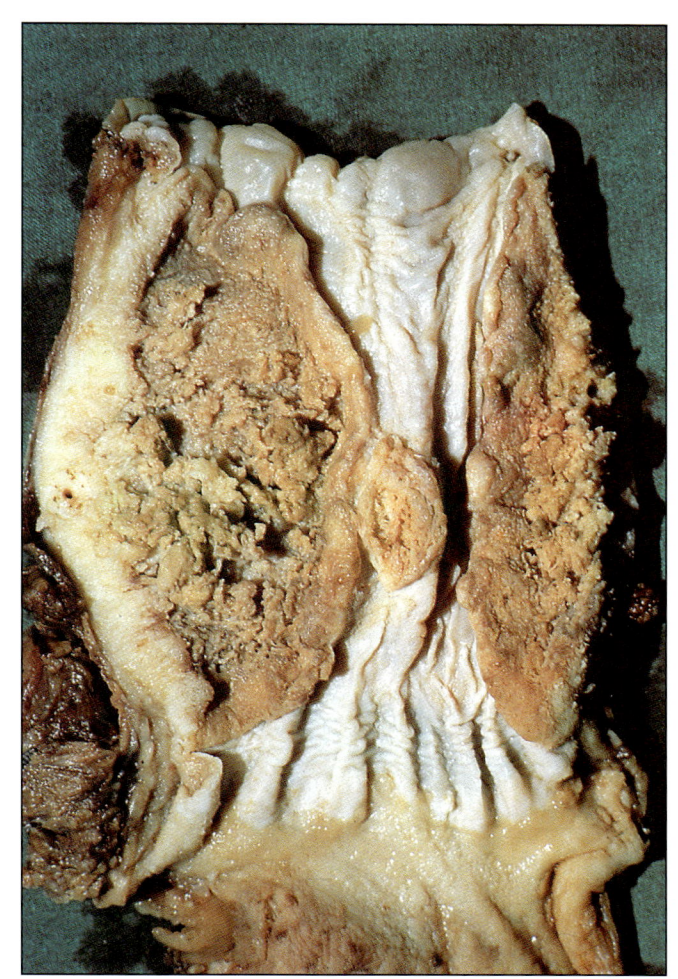

图8.4 晚期溃疡型鳞状细胞癌，肿瘤环绕食管腔一周。

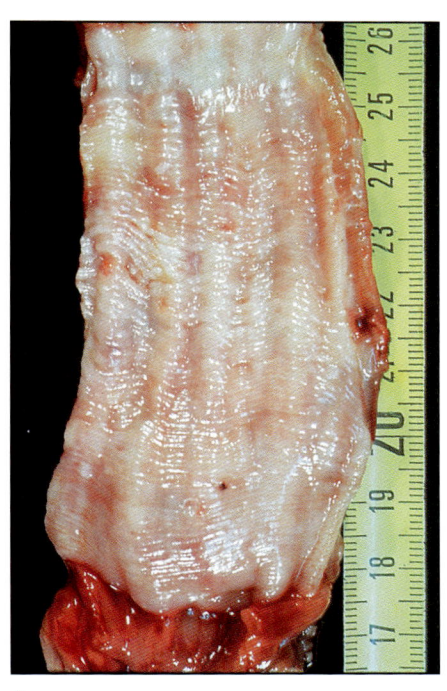 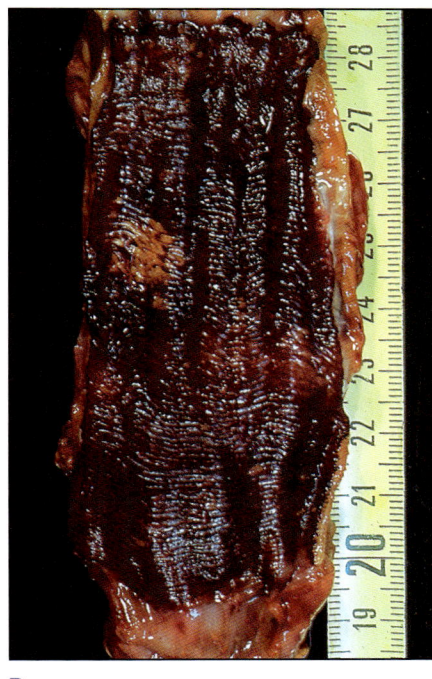

A B

图8.5 Lugol液应用前（A）和应用后（B）的浅表性鳞状细胞癌。在新鲜标本中肿瘤不明显，但经Lugol液处理后，因相对缺乏碘染色而被突现出来。(Reproduced with permission from Bogomoletz WV, Molas G, Gayet B et al. 1989 Superficial squamous cell carcinoma of the esophagus. Am J Surg Pathol 13:535-546.)

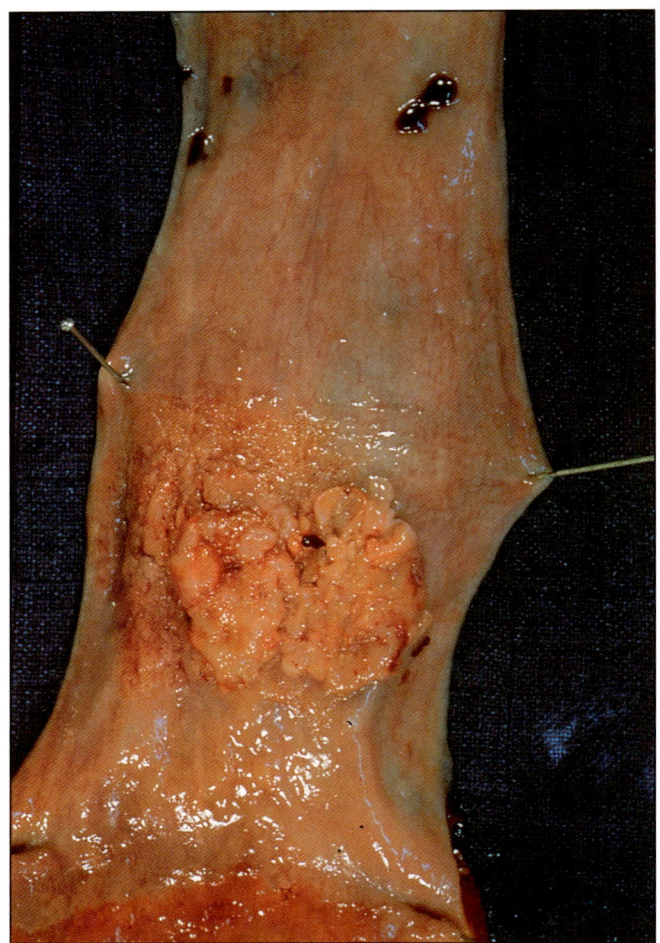

图8.6 早期（浅表性）疣状型鳞状细胞癌。(Reproduced with permission from Bogomoletz WV, Molas G, Gayet B et al. 1989 Superficial squamous cell carcinoma of the esophagus. Am J Surg Pathol 13:535-546.)

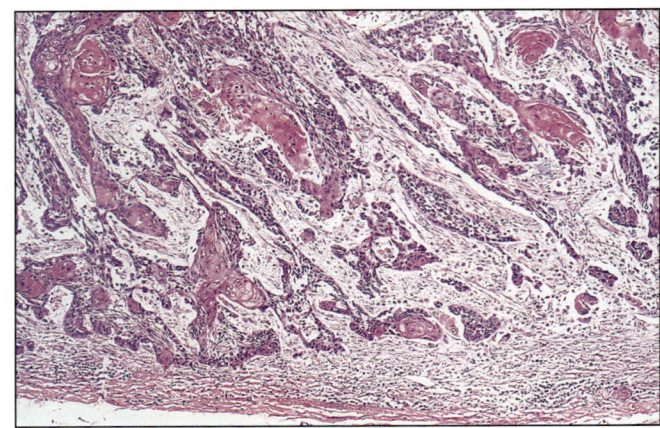

图8.7 食管的浸润性高分化角化性鳞状细胞癌。

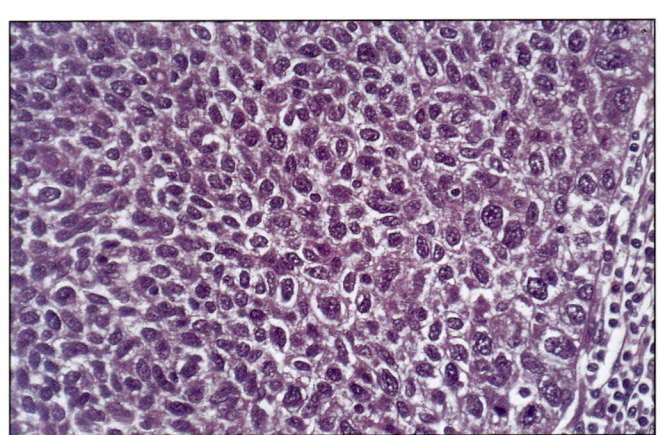

图8.8 低分化鳞状细胞癌。

多中心性食管鳞状细胞癌的确可以发生，但是罕见，有关其发生率和发病机制的资料相互矛盾。多中心性病变可能是由于几个共存的异型增生性病变同时发生恶变[33]，或单个原发性肿瘤沿黏膜下层扩散而形成卫星结节[34]。这种隐匿性管壁内扩散可能导致手术切除不充分，因此，对于切缘应该进行组织学检查，以便检查是否有隐匿性病变[35]。

镜下表现：食管鳞状细胞癌显示不同的分化程度，从显著角化并含有明显细胞间桥的高分化病变（图8.7）到低分化性实际为间变的大细胞或小细胞肿瘤不等，后者只有仔细寻找才能发现鳞状分化的形态学证据（图8.8）。有时，同一病变的不同区域分化程度亦不同。偶尔，鳞状细胞癌伴有少量第二种肿瘤成分，或为腺癌[36]或为小细胞癌成分[37]（见下文）。在切除标本中，常可见肿瘤侵犯肌层，或穿透肌层，发生不同程度的管壁外纵隔组织浸润；其局部扩散的范围是重要的预后因素[38]。许多病例显示在食管壁内广泛浸润，特别是黏膜下层和淋巴管，加上沿着食管腺体的导管扩散[39]，可能导致肿瘤在食管壁内向近端和远端广泛播散，并出现一些卫星病灶。肿瘤中出现明显的纤维组织增生性反应或显著的淋巴细胞反应[40]均为预后好的标志[38]，这些反应如果出现在肿瘤的边缘则造成大体上判断浸润范围非常困难，组织学评估深（周缘）切缘对于分析切除是否彻底十分重要。侵袭性行为的其他组织学指征包括低分化、肿瘤坏死以及侵犯淋巴管或血管[38]。流式细胞DNA分析发现鳞状细胞癌常常为非整倍体；但这好像不是判断预后的有用指标[41]。

浅表扩散性癌（superficial spreading carcinoma）是浅表鳞状细胞癌的一个组织学亚型，其特征是局限于黏膜或黏膜下层的原位癌或浸润性癌的范围达到20 mm或20 mm以上[42]。据报道，其具有特别高的淋巴管侵犯和淋巴结转移率，并且预后较差。

鳞状细胞癌疣状亚型（verrucous variant）[32]的特征是具有高分化角化鳞状上皮构成的宽乳头，细胞异型性很小；病变浸润下方组织形成宽阔的浸润边缘，表

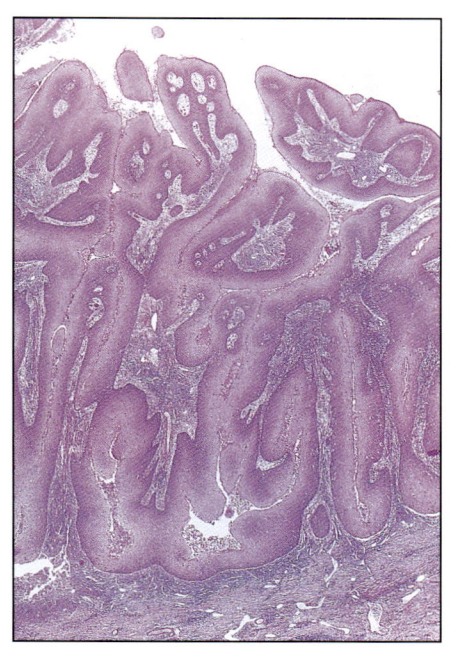

图8.9 食管疣状癌。

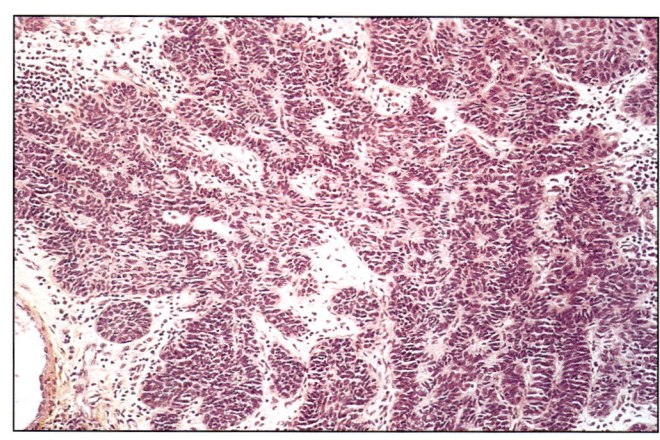

图8.10 基底细胞样型鳞状细胞癌。

现为界限清楚的球形上皮脚（图8.9）。上文已着重指出了诊断中的因难。

浅表性基底细胞癌（superficial basal cell carcinoma）非常少见，在形态上类似于皮肤的基底细胞癌，预后特别好[43]。本病需与另外一种尚未完全认识的癌，即所谓的基底细胞样鳞状细胞癌（basaloid squamous cell carcinoma）相鉴别，基底细胞样鳞状细胞癌为典型的浸润性和（或）原位鳞状细胞癌伴有基底细胞样成分，基底细胞样成分构成实性、散在的细胞巢或小叶，细胞小，核分裂活跃，具有淡染的核和小的核仁（图8.10），有时伴有含嗜碱性物质的微囊性间腔或中央坏死灶，但无明显的周边细胞栅栏状排列[44,45,46]。这种肿瘤最常见于老年男性，并有侵袭性行为和显著的转移能力。有些病例显示明显的间质玻璃样变，给人以类似于腺样囊性癌的表现；实际上，文献中报道的多数食管腺样囊性癌的侵袭性比相应的涎腺腺样囊性癌强得多，有人认为前者是被误诊了的基底细胞样鳞状细胞癌[45]。

鉴别诊断：食管鳞状细胞癌的组织学诊断一般并不因难。在活检标本中主要需与良性溃疡边缘的再生鳞状上皮相鉴别，后者可出现膨胀的基底细胞增生带，核分裂活跃。支持其为良性反应性增生的最有价值的特征为表层上皮细胞成熟，缺乏核的多形性和非典型性核分裂象。当这些上皮改变伴有与肉芽组织有关的奇异的反应性间质细胞时，诊断特别困难（图8.11），因为这些细胞核可能深染，具有多形性和大的核仁，容易被误诊为浸润性癌[47,48]。不过，这些间质细胞大多几乎没有核分裂活性，而且相互之间缺乏黏着力，提示其为非上皮性

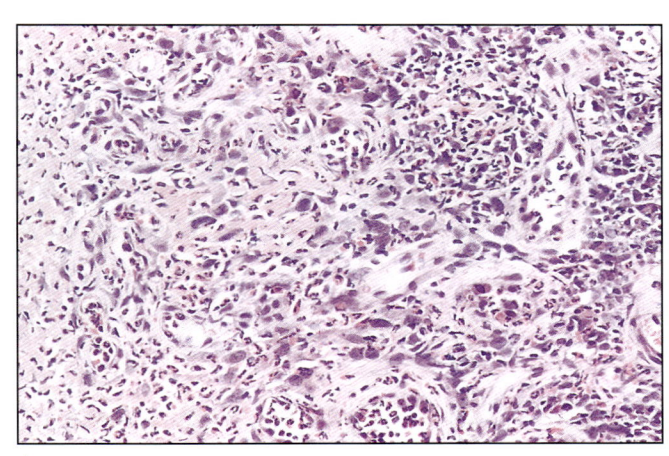

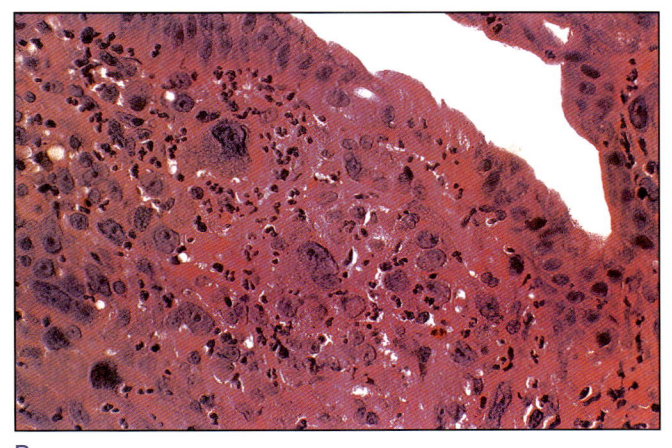

图8.11 肉芽组织中的多形性梭形细胞和内皮细胞（A），来自食管下段良性溃疡的活检标本，以及（B）胃食管交界处的小的炎性息肉。

本质。造成诊断困难的另外一个原因是，放疗后鳞状上皮细胞出现核的非典型性[10]，可能导致放疗后恶性肿瘤复发的错误诊断。对于西方病理医师来说，只有当明确的肿瘤性上皮细胞成团浸润时才能确诊为浸润性鳞状细胞癌，但是日本病理医师诊断癌仅仅依据细胞核和组织结构的改变[49]。这可能与日本的食管浅表鳞状细胞癌的发生率较高而且预后较好有关。在疣状癌的病例，浅表的活检标本很少能够证实明确的浸润，因此临床与病理相结合对于作出正确诊断非常关键。

梭形细胞（肉瘤样）癌（同义词：息肉样癌、癌肉瘤和假肉瘤）
Spindle cell (sarcomatoid) carcinoma (syn.: polypoid carcinoma, carcinosarcoma and pseudosarcoma)

临床特征：现已公认，梭形细胞癌、息肉样癌、癌肉瘤和假肉瘤是同义词，它是一种不常见的食管上皮性肿瘤，具有独特的大体和镜下表现[50-52]。这种肿瘤通常出现吞咽困难和体重减轻的短期病史，最常见于中老年男性。多数报道显示它的预后好于典型的鳞状细胞癌[53]。转移与否与肿瘤侵犯食管壁的范围及肿瘤的大小有关很好理解；直径大于 8 cm 的肿瘤几乎全部发生扩散，而较小的病变大约只有 40% 发生扩散[53]。

大体表现：肿瘤几乎均为大块息肉状，向食管腔内生长，有时有很细的蒂（图 8.12），位于食管的中部或下部 1/3，长度可达 15 cm[52]。

镜下表现：这些肿瘤的特征是由两种成分构成，一种是恶性梭形细胞肉瘤样成分，另一种是原位或浸润性癌成分，通常为鳞状细胞癌（图 8.13），但是偶尔可以显示腺体分化[51]。尽管肉瘤样成分常占优势，但是两种成分的比例在不同病例差别很大。实际上，癌组织常局限于肿瘤的最表层，易于形成溃疡。肉瘤样成分通常由杂乱无章或交织成束排列的梭形细胞构成，核分裂活跃，其间混有多少不等的奇异巨细胞，偶有异源性成分，包括肿瘤性骨、软骨或横纹肌[54]。有趣的是，肉瘤样成分的增生指数通常高于上皮样成分，而且常常为非整倍体[55]。间质可能含有大量胶原，或呈黏液样外观。尽管肿瘤体积较大且有间变表现，但对食管壁的浸润有时却仅限于表层，已报告的病例中相当数量局限于黏膜和黏膜下层。当发生转移时，转移灶可能包含癌的成分、梭形细胞成分，或两者都有。尽管对于这种肿瘤确切的组织发生尚无清楚的认识，但对肉瘤样成分最普遍的解释是梭形细胞分化或浸润性鳞状细胞癌中所谓的间

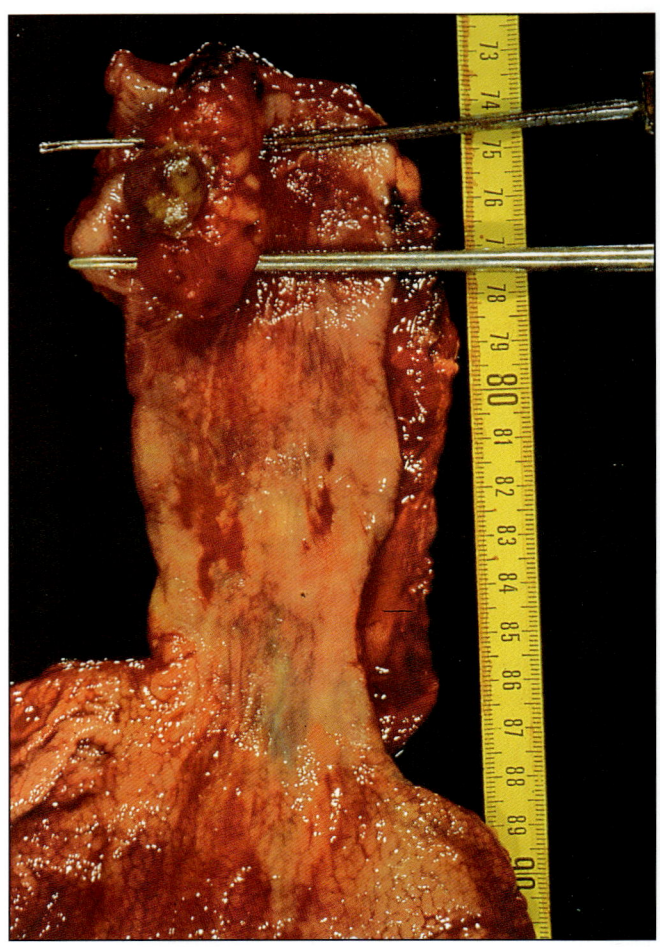

图 8.12 典型的食管梭形细胞癌表现为具有细蒂的息肉状肿物。

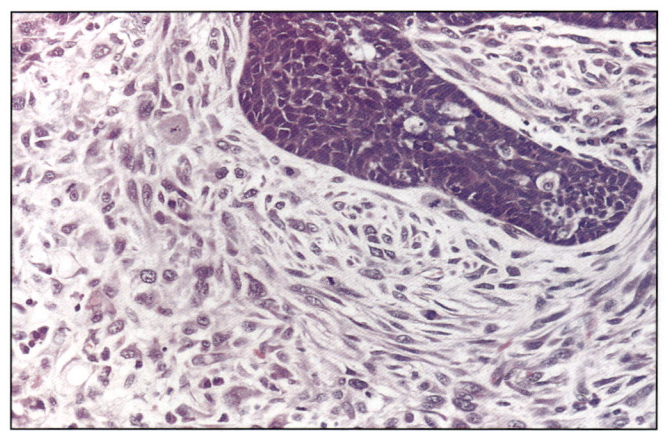

图 8.13 梭形细胞癌，上皮和梭形细胞成分均显示恶性细胞学的特征。

叶化生。大部分病例中至少部分梭形细胞成分保留角蛋白（keratin）免疫组化染色局灶阳性。最近的杂合性缺失研究结果也支持这一观点[56]，然而，其临床和病理学特征是很特别的，值得将其列为一种特殊类型。

鉴别诊断：在活检标本，甚至在切除标本中，如果仅能见到肿瘤的梭形细胞成分则诊断困难，此时主要应与息肉样平滑肌肉瘤鉴别。胃肠道间质瘤（GIST）在鉴别诊断时需要考虑，但它很少发生于食管，而且细胞学一般趋于良性（见下文）。多做切片，仔细寻找癌的成分，一般可以作出正确诊断。对于活检标本，组织块应该深切；对于切除标本，在无溃疡的肿瘤表面或肿瘤邻近的黏膜仔细取材，多半可以奏效，若仍失败，检查局部淋巴结有时可发现转移灶内具有上皮分化。如果梭形细胞角蛋白免疫组化染色明确阳性，则支持梭形细胞癌的诊断。结蛋白（Desmin）和平滑肌肌动蛋白（smooth muscle actin）阳性提示为平滑肌肉瘤，而 KIT 免疫阳性则支持为 GIST。然而，也有报告认为 KIT 表达可以见于癌肉瘤[57]，不过这可能是抗原修复造成的人工假象。在良性食管糜烂或溃疡的边缘发现显著的反应性上皮改变和奇异的间质细胞（见上文）[47,48]，给人的第一印象就是具有癌肉瘤的可能性，与内窥镜表现结合起来一般可以作出正确诊断。

腺癌　Adenocarcinoma

临床特征：绝大多数原发性食管腺癌发生于食管下段，有 Barrett 食管的腺体（柱状）化生背景，因此，大多数病例与慢性胃食管反流有关[15]。然而，尽管化生区域的长度可能比较重要[58]，但发生于 Barrett 食管的癌与患食管炎的时间和严重程度的关系并不清楚。越来越多的证据表明，体质指数（body mass index）增加与腺癌有关[59]，松弛胃食管扩约肌的药物诸如抗胆碱类和 β-受体阻断剂等，也可能增加恶变的危险性[60]。目前尚不清楚抗返流手术是否可以降低癌变的危险性。食管腺癌的流行病学与胃贲门癌非常相似[61]，男性远比女性常见，与吸烟、酗酒及新鲜水果摄入量减少有关，且有证据表明，西方人群的发病率呈上升趋势[62]。在 Barrett 食管腺癌中，已报道有许多遗传性改变。p53 基因突变、伴 17 号染色体长臂等位缺失、c-erbB-2 过表达、p16 的杂合性缺失和甲基化在肿瘤的发病机制中具有重要的作用[63-65]，而且在异型增生和非肿瘤性化生性 Barrett 黏膜也有以上改变[64]。在化生—异型增生—癌这一病变序列中，COX-2（环加氧酶-2）表达上调，它对于化疗耐受可能具有重要意义[66]。

大多数食管腺癌是在先前没有作出 Barrett 食管临床诊断的患者中诊断的，而且处于晚期，由于广泛浸润食管壁而造成进行性吞咽困难和体重降低。这些有症状的患者预后不良。一项研究显示，可手术的病例只有 34% 存活 2 年，15% 存活 5 年[67]。然而，增加对于 Barrett 食管患者的内窥镜监测可以发现早期肿瘤，预后得以改善[68]。

发生于缺乏 Barrett 食管组织学证据的食管腺癌少见，这些病例可能是原来化生的黏膜已被肿瘤破坏[69]。在少数情况下，腺癌也可能发生于异位的胃黏膜，例如发生在颈部入口斑（cervical inlet patch）处[70]。

大体表现：大多数腺癌为扁平、有溃疡形成的浸润性病变，导致食管腔狭窄。某些病例有外生性息肉状成分，而在少数病例则整个肿瘤均为外生性。化生性 Barrett 黏膜背景呈红色细颗粒状外观，可能容易与灰白色光滑的食管鳞状上皮区分开来。

镜下表现：大多数病例为"肠型"管状或乳头状腺癌，分化程度不一，其形态学表现与胃贲门腺癌非常相似（图 8.14）[71]。背景为 Barrett 型化生性腺上皮的高级别异型增生非常常见（图 8.15）[72]。某些肿瘤具有黏液性腺癌结构，产生明显的细胞外黏液，但是弥漫性印戒细胞癌非常少见[73]。虽然在 Barrett 食管化生和异型增生中经常见到神经内分泌细胞，但仅约 20% 的食管腺癌可见神经内分泌细胞[74]。然而，在食管已有腺癌混有类癌的报道[71]。也有少数报道称肿瘤中有鳞状分化区域[71]，一例癌肉瘤的上皮成分是腺癌[75]。有症状的（非普查发现的）肿瘤预后不好，即使可以切除，但因为 80% 以上的肿瘤已侵透食管肌层，故常常伴有明显的神经周围浸润；并常有淋巴结转移，流式细胞分析显示 DNA 为非整倍体。所有这些都是预后差的指标[15]。

鉴别诊断：组织学上诊断困难的大部分是食管活检标本，主要是要鉴别腺上皮反应性增生、异型增生和肯

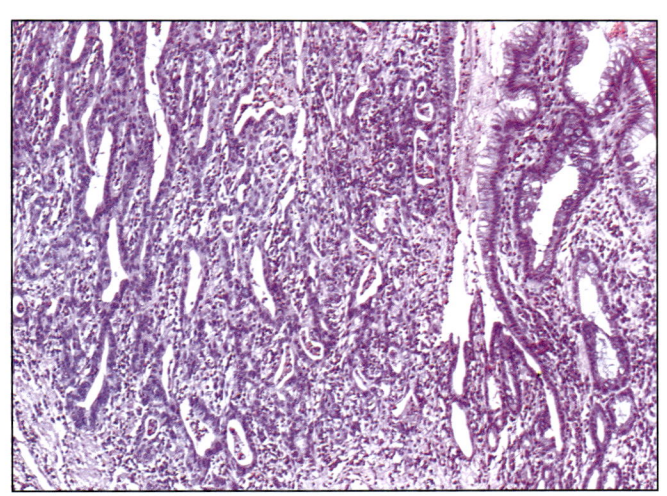

图8.14　发生于Barrett食管的腺癌。视野右侧可见化生的肠型上皮。

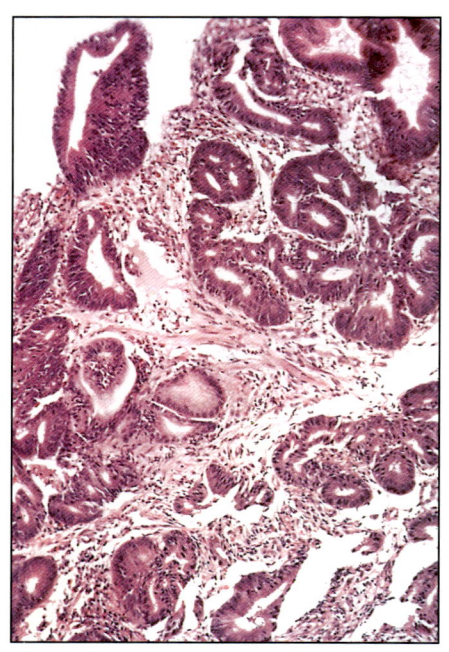

图8.15 Barrett食管化生腺上皮呈高级别异型增生。

定无疑的浸润性腺癌。鉴别诊断的原则与胃腺癌活检诊断原则相同，与Vienna癌前病变分类一起在第344页有详细的阐述（表8.2）[.6]。在活检标本中常常难以区分Barrett黏膜高级别异型增生和腺癌，主要根据是否有明确的浸润来判断，但这一标准并不总是那么准确，因为约20%活检诊断为高级别异型增生的病例，在随后的切除标本中却有浸润性癌[76]。因此，有权威专家建议，将明确诊断的高级别异型增生作为手术的指征。由于这样的病例淋巴结转移非常少见，故另外有人主张应用各种不同的局部内窥镜疗法，包括内窥镜黏膜切除（endoscopic mucosal resection，EMR）、光动力学疗法（photodynamic therapy）和氩血浆凝固（argon plasma coagulation）。对于内窥镜黏膜切除标本需要进行仔细的病理学检查，以评估切除是否充分（一项研究显示，切除常常不完全[77]）。在光动力学疗法治疗随访患者的活检标本中，可以见到残留的肿瘤，表面被覆再生的鳞状上皮[78]。

黏液表皮样癌和腺样囊性癌 Mucoepidermoid and adenoid cystic carcinoma

文献中有关这两种食管肿瘤的命名、定义和组织发生的说法非常混乱，因此很难对已发表的报道进行评价。如果应用涎腺肿瘤的标准（见第7章）严格加以定义的话，发生在食管黏膜下腺体的"经典性黏液表皮样癌和腺样囊性癌"均极为少见[79,80]。它们通常为小的管壁内病变，表面覆盖完整的非肿瘤性鳞状上皮，并伴有相对较好的预后。

然而，大多数已报道的食管黏液表皮样癌或腺样囊性癌却是完全不同的；它们为大的侵袭性肿瘤，其中黏液表皮样[79,81]或腺样囊性[82,83]区域混有其他成分，通常为典型的鳞状细胞癌或未分化癌。这些肿瘤常常广泛转移，其预后类似于单纯的鳞状细胞癌。与经典的涎腺型相应肿瘤不同的是，它们常常累及表面上皮（有时为典型的原位癌）[83]；核分裂活跃，但是几乎没有神经周围侵犯的倾向。此外，所谓的黏液表皮样成分常有角化，这不是经典肿瘤的特征，而且腺样囊性区域常有坏死。某些作者在选择名称时反映了这些非典型的特征；例如，应用"癌伴有腺样囊性分化"取代腺样囊性癌[83]；另外一些作者强调，这种肿瘤与上面描述的所谓的基底细胞样鳞状细胞癌相似，后者可能含有间质玻璃样变区域和微囊结构。而且，多达21%的食管鳞状细胞癌可见腺体、分泌黏液和筛状成分，这些成分通常构成肿瘤表面区域的一小部分[36]，提示最好将这个肿瘤的整个谱系看作是具有双向分化的鳞状细胞癌的亚型。

腺鳞癌 Adenosquamous carcinoma

除了上文描述的黏液表皮样癌和腺样囊性癌以外，尚有许多所谓的腺鳞癌的报告，它是由浸润性腺癌和浸润性鳞癌组成的，后者常有角化[84]。多数腺鳞癌病例发生在食管下段，伴有Barrett食管[71]。还有腺鳞癌混有梭形细胞癌的报告[85]。

小细胞癌 Small cell carcinoma

临床特征：这种罕见的高度恶性的神经内分泌肿瘤的临床和病理学所见与肺的小细胞癌相似[37,86,87]。较常见于男性，通常发生于中老年人，表现为吞咽困难和体重减轻。虽然应用免疫细胞化学方法偶尔可以发现肿瘤细胞中有这样的肽类存在[89]。但仅在罕见的情况下症状与异位激素分泌有关[88]。由于肿瘤早期广泛转移，预后很差。

大体表现：大多数已报道的病例为大的外生性和浸润性肿块（图8.16A），位于食管中或下1/3。偶尔可以表现为多灶性肿瘤。

镜下表现：肿瘤由小的间变细胞构成，胞浆稀少，核卵圆形或圆形，深染，常常变形，核仁不明显，核分裂象常见（图8.16B）。细胞通常形成片块，常常伴有坏死区域；偶可排列成巢状、条索状、带状或形成玫瑰花结。血管侵犯和淋巴结转移常见。不同病例之间

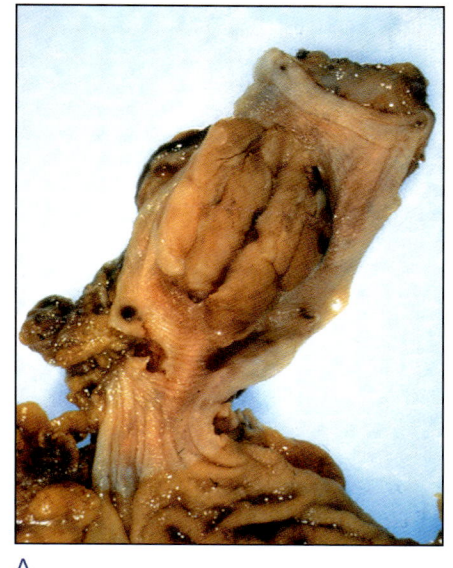

绒毛膜癌 Choriocarcinoma

食管绒毛膜癌已有报道，其中包括纯粹的绒毛膜癌[91]、伴有食管下段腺癌[92]，以及由纵隔绒毛膜癌直接扩散而形成的继发性病变[93]。

Paget 病 Paget't disease

来自食管腺鳞癌[94]或黏液腺癌（mucous gland carcinoma）[95]的鳞状上皮 Paget 样浸润已有报道。类似的扩散方式可以发生在食管恶性黑色素瘤；在活检标本中，应用黏液组织化学染色、癌胚抗原和 S-100 蛋白免疫组织化学染色有助于这些病变的鉴别诊断。

食管癌的病理学分期

食管癌不管其组织学类型如何，通常都可用 TNM 系统进行分期[96]。这要考虑肿瘤直接浸润的深度（pT）、局部淋巴结有无转移（pN）以及有无远处转移（pM）；详见表 8.1。病理报告还应该说明近切缘、远切缘以及周缘切除是否彻底[97]。

在检查和报告术前经过化疗和放疗的食管癌切除标本时需要格外小心。实际上，肿瘤表面和深部退变达到了一定的程度，在肉眼上有可能看不到黏膜病变。只有应用放大显微镜检查黏膜表面和仔细触摸食管

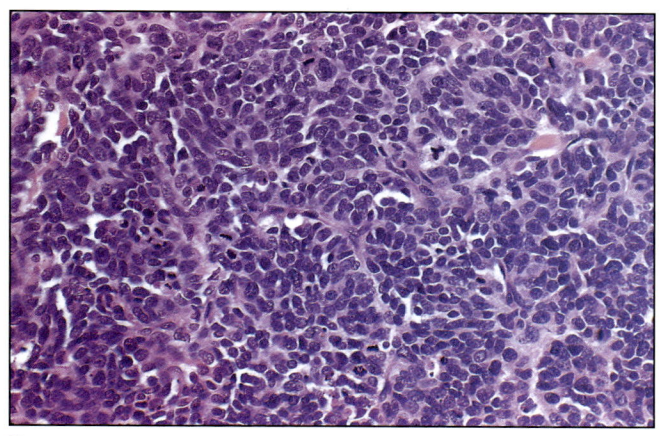

图 8.16（A, B）食管小细胞癌。大体标本（A）显示这是一个食管下 1/3 的外生性肿瘤。

和同一病例内可以显示不同程度的内分泌分化的证据，包括嗜银性胞浆、内分泌标记物 [嗜铬素、PGP（protein gene product，蛋白基因产物）9.5、突触素或 Leu-7] 免疫反应阳性，或超微结构下证实有神经分泌颗粒。可有内分泌型淀粉样物质沉积[37]。相当多的食管小细胞癌伴有原位或浸润性鳞状细胞癌[37,86]和（或）腺癌，反映肿瘤有多方向的分化[37,90]。

鉴别诊断：食管小细胞癌需与扩散至食管的肺原发性小细胞癌、低分化鳞状细胞癌、基底细胞样鳞状细胞癌以及恶性淋巴瘤相鉴别。嗜银染色、免疫细胞化学和电子显微镜下检查均具有诊断价值。

表8.1	食管癌的病理学TNM分期[96]
T－原发性肿瘤	
pT1	肿瘤浸润固有膜或黏膜下层
pT2	肿瘤浸润固有肌层
pT3	肿瘤浸润外膜
pT4	肿瘤浸润邻近组织
N－局部淋巴结	
pN0	没有局部淋巴结转移
pN1	有局部淋巴结转移
M－远处转移[a]	
M0	没有远处转移
M1	有远处转移

[a] 病理学分期通常不能确定有无远处转移，除非提交远处器官的活检标本进行组织学检查。

壁才能发现瘢痕或增厚的区域。食管壁必须完整取材进行组织学检查。有学者提出了有关肿瘤退变分级的方法,它是根据对于残存的癌组织和纤维化进行半定量分析作出的[98]。应用这种方法的困难是,无法弄清放化疗前肿瘤相关性纤维化的程度。更为重要的是,对治疗后切除标本残余肿瘤的范围进行病理学分期,这是判断预后的最好指标[99]。

恶性黑色素瘤 Malignant melanoma

临床特征:原发性食管恶性黑色素瘤罕见,但确有文献记载,最常发生于中老年人食管的中下段。患者表现为吞咽困难[100]。据报道,日本人发病率较高,尤其是女性[101]。发生于较年轻的患者罕见。该类肿瘤预后差[100,102],而且与皮肤黑色素瘤不同,预后似乎与原发病变的厚度无关[101]。继发转移至食管的黑色素瘤比较常见,但总体上看仍属罕见;3.2%的播散性黑色素瘤尸解病例可见食管转移[100]。

大体表现:虽然许多报告描述食管恶性黑色素瘤为息肉状管腔内生长方式,但是多数病例的大体特征与其他原发性食管恶性肿瘤难以区别。只有少数肿瘤产生足够的黑色素,伴有色素沉着(图 8.17)。如同皮肤黑色素瘤一样,原发性肿瘤周围可见所谓的卫星病灶。

镜下表现:食管恶性黑色素瘤与发生于皮肤或其他黏膜表面的恶性黑色素瘤相比,并无特殊的组织学特征;它们显示同样的从上皮样到梭形细胞类型的变化(图 8.18)。大多数为无黑色素性黑色素瘤。虽然许多肿瘤具有溃疡性或结节状生长方式,但是有些肿瘤为表浅扩散型,伴有明显的 Paget 样或色素斑样肿瘤性黑色素细胞巢侵入邻近的鳞状上皮(图 8.19)。邻近上皮的交界活性改变也很常见[104],且有伴较广泛的局限性或弥漫性食管黑变病(图 8.17)和黑色素细胞非典型性[105]的病例报告。相反,虽然在慢性炎症时黑色素细胞数量可能增加,黑色素细胞仅见于大约 4% 的没有食管疾病的个体[106],在食管癌中也有类似现象出现[107]。原发性食管黑色素瘤的组织学特征不能预示其生物学行为。

鉴别诊断:无黑色素性恶性黑色素瘤必须与低分化癌和肉瘤鉴别。当邻近上皮出现黑色素细胞非典型性或 Paget 样浸润时(在除外真正的 Paget 病之后,见上文),免疫组织化学检测 S-100 和黑色素细胞标志物(例如 HMB-45)非常重要。后一改变也有助于鉴别原发性和转移性黑色素瘤。知道恶性黑色素瘤有时可能表达 KIT 也非常重要。尽管实际上几乎所有的食管黑色素细胞肿

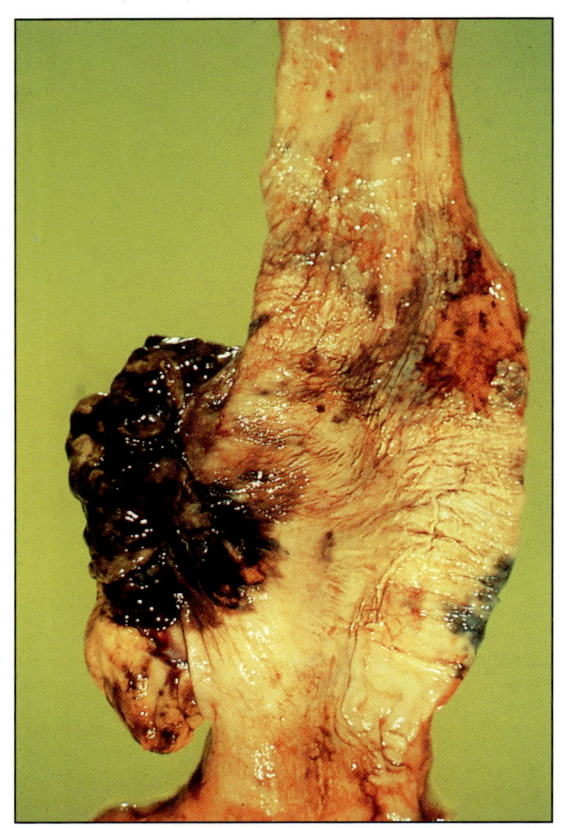

图8.17 色素性食管恶性黑色素瘤伴有黏膜黑变病背景。
(Reproduced with permission from Bogomoletz W V 1989 Rare and secondary (metastasis) tumors [of esophagus]. In: Whitehead R (ed) Gastrointestinal and esophageal pathology. Churchill Livingstone, Edinburgh, p701-710.)

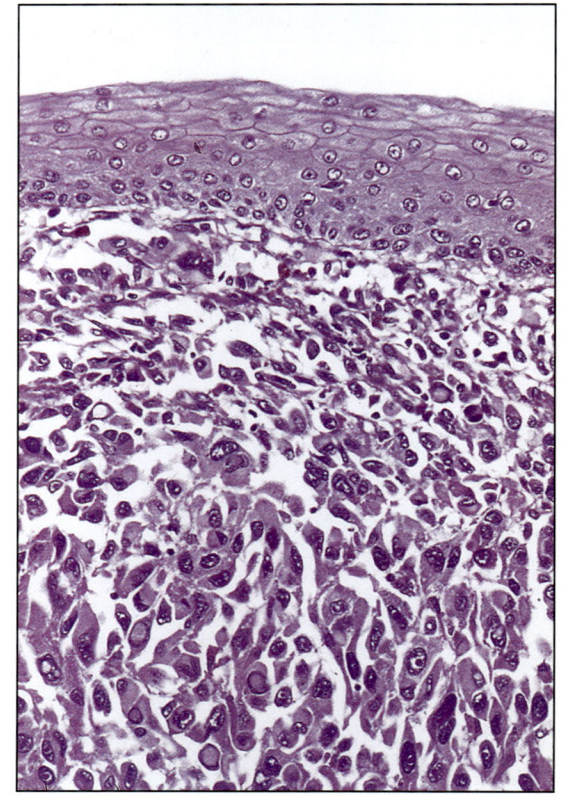

图8.18 食管恶性黑色素瘤。

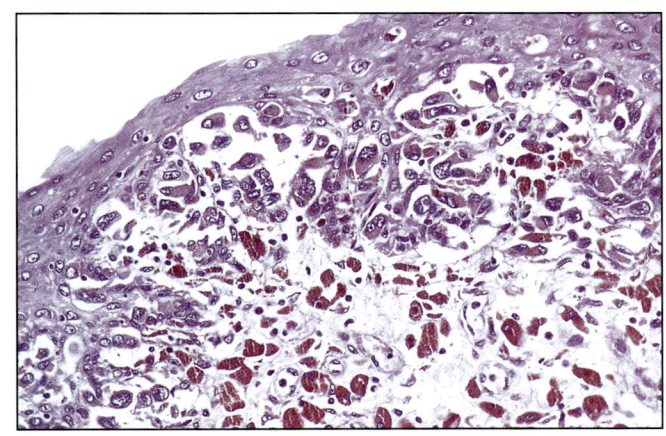

图8.19 图8.18中恶性黑色素瘤附近的放射状色素斑性成分。

瘤都是恶性黑色素瘤，但是我们知道有1例良性黑色素细胞病变的报道，其组织学来源不能确定，可能是蓝痣[108]。

非上皮性肿瘤　Non-epithelial Tumors

平滑肌肿瘤　Smooth muscle tumors

临床特征：平滑肌肿瘤少见，最常见于中年人，表现为吞咽困难和烧心。许多患者无症状，少部分可有出血。男性略多见，其发病率沿着食管长度增加而增加（即食管远端发生率高）[109,110]。平滑肌瘤是最常见的食管间叶性肿瘤，其数量远远多于平滑肌肉瘤，后者一般见于老年人。两种病变通常均为单发性，虽然发生于Ⅰ型多发性内分泌肿瘤患者的多发性平滑肌瘤也有报道[111]，且有时伴发所谓的"食管弥漫性平滑肌瘤病"（diffuse leiomyosarcoma of the esophagus）（见第339页）。获得食管平滑肌肉瘤可靠的预后信息是不可能的，因为它十分罕见，而且，已报道的某些病例可能是误诊的梭形细胞癌。不过，其临床行为似乎与诊断时局部扩散的范围有关；可以切除的肿瘤具有较好的预后，只有少数导致播散性血行转移[112,113]。

大体表现：肿瘤可发生于食管平滑肌层的任何部位[109]，通常形成大的息肉状管腔内肿块，表面被覆黏膜（图8.20），黏膜可继发形成溃疡；较少见的为边界清楚、分叶状、向管壁外生长的纵隔内肿瘤。临床症状明显的局限于食管壁内的肿瘤罕见，尽管在尸检或切除标本中偶尔发现位于食管贲门交界处的固有肌层甚或黏膜肌层的微小平滑肌瘤并不少见，这种肿瘤即所谓的"秧苗平滑肌瘤"（sedling leiomyomas）[114]。典型的平滑肌肿瘤切面隆起，呈灰白色漩涡状，有时伴有斑点状钙化，而平

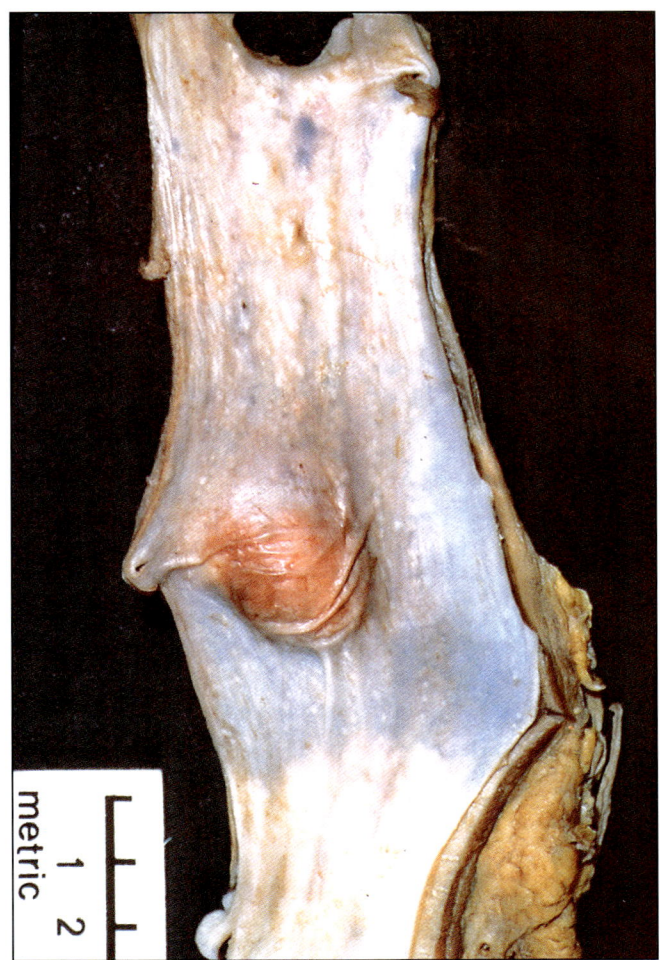

图8.20 息肉样食管平滑肌瘤。

滑肌肉瘤则常常呈鱼肉状，伴有坏死区域和浸润性生长方式（图8.21）。

镜下表现：大多数食管平滑肌肿瘤与发生于身体其他部位者相似，由交织排列的平滑肌细胞束构成，其间混有多少不等的胶原。细胞具有两端圆钝雪茄形的细胞核和含有肌原纤维的嗜酸性胞浆（图8.22），结蛋白（desmin）或平滑肌肌动蛋白（smooth muscle actin，SMA）免疫染色阳性，KIT和CD34阴性。尽管仅仅根据组织学图像常常难以明确区分平滑肌瘤与平滑肌肉瘤，但是平滑肌肉瘤可能显示明显的间变特征，伴有显著的核多形性、瘤巨细胞以及异常核分裂象。支持恶性的特征包括肿瘤体积大（直径大于5 cm），肿瘤内坏死或出血，以及每10个标准高倍视野核分裂象超过5个。

鉴别诊断：需要鉴别的肿瘤包括神经鞘肿瘤、GIST、梭形细胞癌（见上文）和无色素性恶性黑色素瘤。

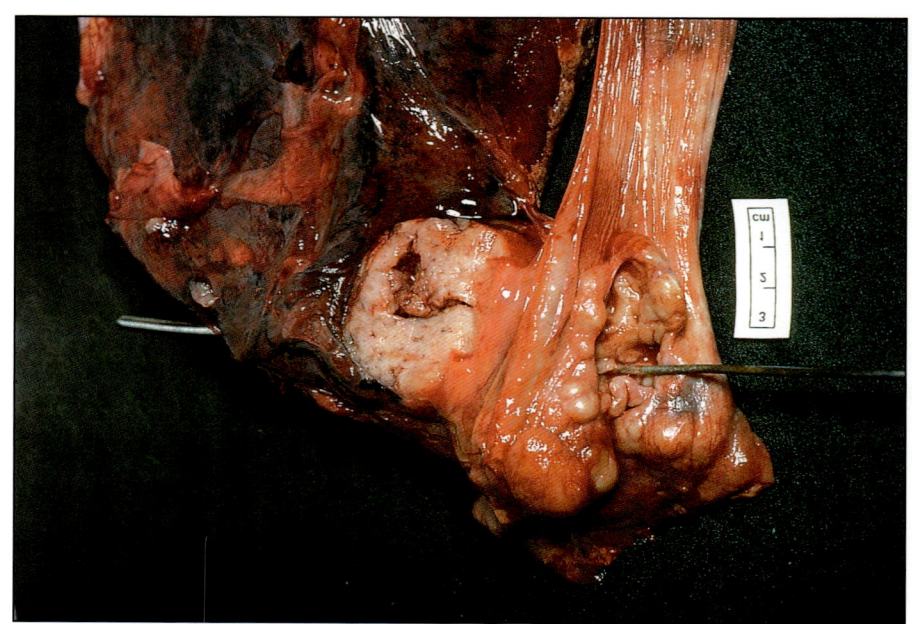

图8.21 食管平滑肌肉瘤侵犯纵隔及邻近的肺组织。

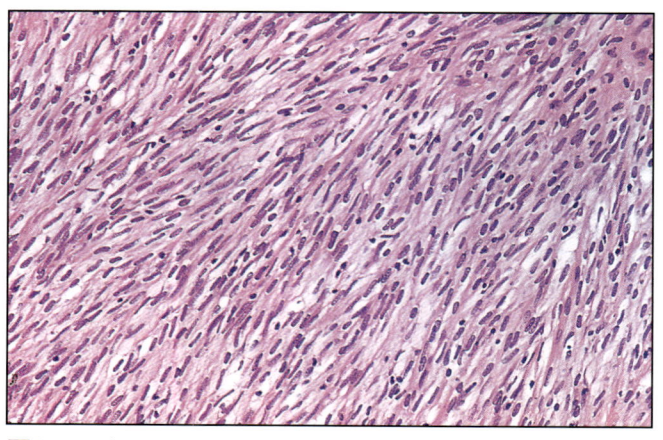

图8.22 富于细胞性食管平滑肌瘤。

胃肠道间质瘤（GIST）
Gastrointestinal stromal tumor (GIST)

发生于食管的胃肠道间质瘤（GISTs）并不常见，但是在临床上经常为恶性，而且常有肝转移[113,115]。发生于老年人，一般表现为吞咽困难。大多数为梭形细胞肿瘤，其形态学与免疫组织化学特征与胃的间质瘤相同（见第356页）。

颗粒细胞瘤　Granular cell tumor

尽管不常见，而且通常仅为尸检时的偶然发现，但颗粒细胞瘤发生在食管比其他部位常见[116]。多数位于食管下1/3，形成孤立的界限清楚的黏膜下结节，高起黏膜面1～2 cm，质硬、淡黄色；偶为多发性[117]。较大的肿瘤可致食管环形狭窄，并产生吞咽困难的症状[118]。组织学上，与其他部位的颗粒细胞瘤无法区别（参见第27章），其由梭形或多边形细胞集聚而成，细胞核形态规则，胞浆嗜酸性颗粒状，PAS染色阳性，含有免疫反应的S-100蛋白；被覆的鳞状上皮可呈假上皮瘤样增生。虽然一般为良性肿瘤，但也有少数恶性的报道[119]。

其他结缔组织肿瘤
Other connective tissue tumors

从良性到恶性的各种食管结缔组织肿瘤都有病例报道。良性病变包括丛状神经鞘瘤[120]和神经纤维瘤[121]、食管近端横纹肌的横纹肌瘤[122]、血管瘤和淋巴管瘤[123,124]、血管球瘤[13]、脂肪瘤[125,126]、软骨瘤和骨软骨瘤[127]。其中有些病变可能是错构瘤而并非真性肿瘤[128]。

原发性食管肉瘤的报道包括儿童胚胎性横纹肌瘤[129]、恶性横纹肌样肿瘤[130]、免疫缺陷患者的Kaposi肉瘤[131]、脂肪肉瘤[132]、血管外皮细胞瘤[133]、恶性间叶瘤[134]、所谓的恶性纤维组织细胞瘤[135]、骨肉瘤[136]和滑膜肉瘤[137]。在作出这样的诊断之前，必须广泛取材以排除梭形细胞癌特殊的肉瘤性分化（见上文）；在已经发表的许多病例报道中，难以确认是否真正做到了这一点。

淋巴瘤和白血病　Lymphoma and leukemia

淋巴瘤累及食管非常少见[138]。肿瘤可为溃疡性或息肉状，通常表现为出血或吞咽困难。原发性Hodgkin[139]和非Hodgkin淋巴瘤均有报道，后者包括T细胞肿瘤[140]和具有B细胞[141]表型的黏膜相关淋巴组织（MALT）淋巴瘤[141,142]、弥漫性大B细胞淋巴瘤和套细胞淋巴瘤[141,142]。一例局灶性食管淋巴组织增生的病例报告报道了其具有提示局限性Castleman病的某些特征[143]。食管髓外浆细胞瘤也有报道[144]。血液淋巴组织恶性肿瘤继发累及食管可能较为常见，包括来自原发性胃恶性淋巴瘤的直接蔓延[145]、受累的纵隔淋巴结的扩散，或作为全身性淋巴瘤或白血病一部分的食管黏膜下层的多发性病灶；后者可能发生坏死和溃疡[146]。

继发性肿瘤　Secondary tumors

食管不是转移性疾病的常见部位。然而，来自胃、甲状腺、咽喉部、支气管和肺的肿瘤的直接蔓延已有报告，同样也有来自食管旁淋巴结的直接浸润。食管转移性肿瘤最常来自乳腺癌和恶性黑色素瘤，其他包括胃、胰腺、肺、前列腺、睾丸、肾、子宫颈以及子宫内膜的原发性癌。

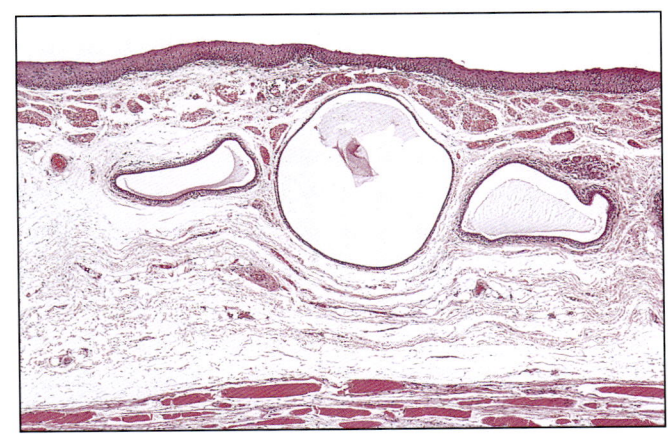

图8.23　食管黏膜下包涵囊肿。

瘤样病变　Tumor-like lesions

纤维血管性（纤维性）息肉　Fibrovascular (fibrous) polyp

纤维血管性息肉最常见于食管上1/3，在环状软骨水平。典型的纤维血管性息肉为孤立性有蒂的病变，常有一长蒂，其体积可相当大，引起吞咽困难。有时可以反入口腔，有嵌顿于喉而引起死亡的报道。正如其命名所提示的一样，纤维血管性息肉是由水肿的黏膜、黏膜下层纤维或纤维脂肪组织和血管轴心构成的，被覆增厚的或有溃疡形成的鳞状上皮[147]。病因尚不清楚，某些病例可能为对损伤或慢性刺激的过度反应，而另外一些可能为错构瘤。有少数纤维血管性息肉内发生鳞状细胞癌的病例报告[148]。

炎性纤维性息肉　Inflammatory fibroid polyp

与纤维血管性息肉相比，炎性纤维性息肉更常见于中段和下段食管，不常有蒂，较易发生溃疡，并可累及食管壁全层，有时替代肌层，甚至明显"浸润"邻近组织。可有出血或梗阻症状。与发生于消化道其他部位的炎性纤维性息肉一样（见第9章），它们是由疏松水肿的肉芽样组织构成的，含有数量不等的单核细胞、浆细胞、中性粒细胞、嗜酸性粒细胞、肥大细胞以及肥胖的梭形的纤维母细胞，纤维母细胞有围绕一明显血管呈同心圆状排列的倾向[149]。这种病变是真正的炎性病变还是不常见的结缔组织肿瘤仍有争议，但其临床行为总是良性的。

囊肿　Cysts

先天性食管囊肿分为两种类型。单房性壁内包涵囊肿(unilocular intramural inclusion cysts)见于食管下段(图8.23)[150]，内衬一层平滑的柱状、纤毛柱状或鳞状上皮，偶可形成乳头状突起。多次复发的支气管源性和神经肠管源性囊肿（bronchogenic and neurenteric cysts）是由比较复杂的前肠发育异常引起的[151]，可累及食管壁或孤立地位于后纵隔，此时可能伴有脊柱异常。囊肿内衬食管、支气管或胃型上皮，通常被覆在明显的固有肌层之上。也可含有软骨或胰腺组织[152]。已有食管壁内囊肿内衬鳞状上皮发生鳞状细胞癌的报道[153]。

获得性潴留囊肿（acquired retention cysts）有时被错误地称为假憩室，它是由于黏膜下层食管腺体外分泌导管炎症后囊性扩张而形成的。通常见于食管下段，内衬可为立方或鳞状上皮。

淀粉样物　Amyloid

已知有1例食管壁内淀粉样瘤（amyloid tumor）的报道[154]。系统性淀粉样变累及食管黏膜下层但不形成肿块的比较常见。

糖原棘皮症　Glycogenic acanthosis

这种病变病因不明，最常见于食管下1/3，由多数白色散在的隆起性黏膜斑块构成，斑块直径通常只有几毫米，主要发生在食管纵行皱襞嵴的部位[155]。显微镜下，鳞状上皮表层由于富含糖原空泡细胞而变厚（图8.24）。基底层一般并不增生，也无任何非典型性的证据或角化过度。这种病变没有恶性潜能。据报道，弥漫性或广泛的糖原棘皮症是Cowden综合征的一个特征[156]。

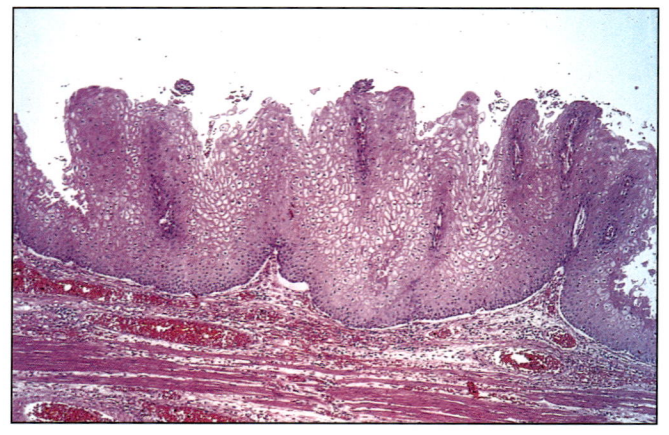

图8.24 糖原棘皮症。

弥漫性平滑肌瘤病　Diffuse leiomyomatosis

这是一种病因不明的罕见病变,食管肌层弥漫性增厚,有时局部病变突出,形成融合性结节甚至明显的平滑肌瘤。尽管有些病例为老年人尸检时偶然发现,多数病例报道为儿童或年轻成人,表现为吞咽困难。显微镜下,环行和纵行平滑肌层弥漫性增生,正常肌纤维结构被杂乱而不规则的漩涡状交织排列的肌纤维代替[157]。可以发生变性和营养不良性钙化[158],也可有慢性炎症和神经增粗。这些病变有时累及黏膜肌层,或者可能扩展累及到胃的近端肌层[158]。尽管本病通常为散发性,但是常染色体显性遗传性食管平滑肌瘤病可能伴有贲门失弛缓症[159]、Alport 样肾病[158]、气管支气管或女性生殖系统(尤其是外阴)平滑肌瘤[158,160]、肠平滑肌瘤、神经纤维瘤、色素性荨麻疹、系统性肥大细胞病等[159]临床特征。

异位　Heterotopias

所谓的颈部入口斑(cervical inlet patch),传统上被认为是发生于食管环状软骨后区的异位胃黏膜,内窥镜下在正常的灰白色黏膜中可见1个或多个边界清楚的粉红色斑片,直径可达4 cm。胃样腺体可能取代正常鳞状上皮或位于上皮下组织内。多数病例没有症状,是内窥镜检查时偶然发现的没有临床意义的病变,但有少数报道会发生消化道溃疡进而导致食管气管瘘,并可发生腺癌[161]。最近发现,异位胃黏膜与Barrett食管黏膜的表型类似,这对所有病例都是真正的胃黏膜异位的观点提出了挑战[162]。异位胰腺组织少见;有发生于食管上段[163]和重复囊肿[152]的报道。

其他已报道的各种异位包括内窥镜下表现为隆起黄色斑块的位于食管黏膜下层的皮脂腺[164]和呼吸道型纤毛上皮[165]。然而,严格地说,后者并非真正的异位而是发育残件,因为它是正常胎儿食管的组成部分。

胃食管交界处的增生性息肉　Hyperplastic polyps at the gastroesophageal junction

胃食管交界处长期黏膜损害,伴有糜烂性食管炎,(食管与胃)"交界部位炎"(junctitis)和与胃食管反流有关的溃疡形成,都与胃食管交界处黏膜的炎症和息肉样增生有关[166]。这样的炎性或增生性息肉通常是由再生的贲门黏膜构成的,有时混有鳞状上皮。肉芽组织中的上皮或间质细胞可以出现明显的非典型性(见第331页和图8.11B),千万不要过诊断为异型增生或癌[48]。当然,发生真正异型增生的病例也有报道[166]。

胃

上皮性肿瘤　Epithelial tumors
腺瘤　Adenoma

临床特征:胃腺瘤通常发生于伴有肠上皮化生的萎缩性胃炎的情况下[167,168]。多数表现为孤立性大的(3～4 cm)无蒂或有蒂息肉[169,170],直到出血、溃疡形成或引起胃的流出道梗阻时才有症状。这些病变的发病率随年龄而增加,而且可以发生于患有家族性腺瘤性息肉病的患者[171]。因其为侵袭前的肿瘤,具有发展为癌的可能[168,169,172],所以必须通过局部切除治疗,通常进行内窥镜下息肉切除术或内窥镜下黏膜切除术。除了其本身为癌前病变外,腺瘤还可与胃内其他部位的癌共存;这种现象原因不明,在男性尤为多见[168,173]。

大体表现:腺瘤为无蒂或有蒂的黏膜病变,表面光滑柔软,呈分叶状(图8.25)。邻近的胃黏膜可能平坦和萎缩。

镜下表现:根据定义,胃腺瘤是由异型增生的上皮组成的,由于常常发生于肠上皮化生的背景中,所以通常显示某种程度的肠型分化,分化为吸收细胞、杯状细胞、内分泌细胞甚至 Paneth 细胞。因此,许多胃腺瘤实际上无法与结肠、直肠腺瘤区分,它们显示同样的结构、分化和细胞增生异常,根据结构不同将其进一步分成管状、管状绒毛状和绒毛状型,而且根据核密集的程度、核深染、层次的多少、核分裂象、胞浆分化以及结构异常等分为低级别或高级别上皮异型增生(图8.26、8.27)[172,174]。然而,少数胃腺瘤在形态学和黏液组

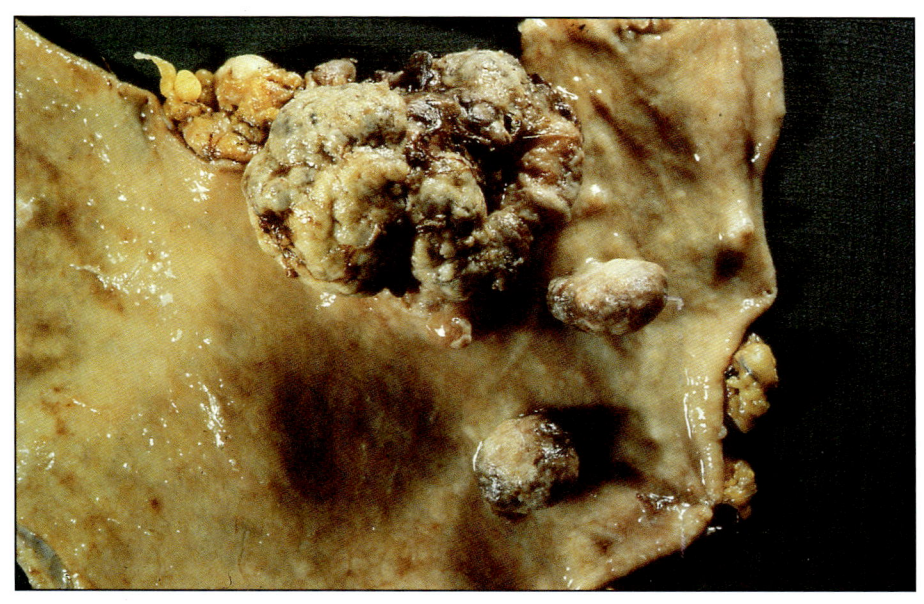

图8.25 部分切除的胃标本,含有1个大的息肉样腺癌(上)和2个较小的有蒂腺瘤(下和右)。

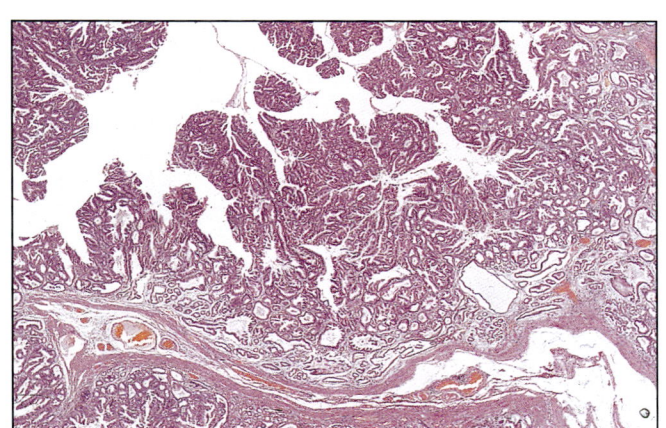

图8.26 胃的无蒂管状绒毛状腺瘤。

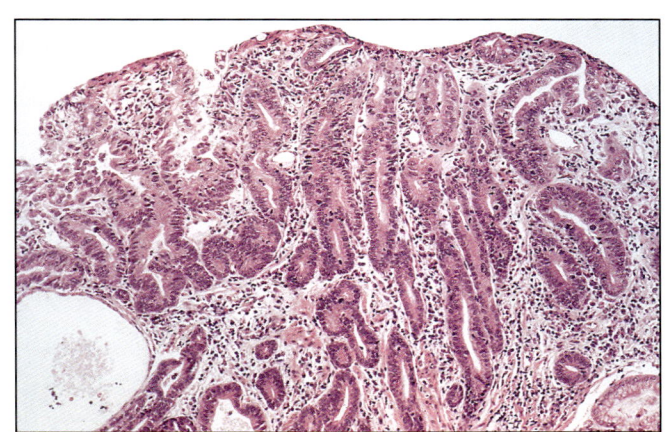

图8.28 胃无蒂腺瘤,伴有黏膜上半部分高级别异型增生和胃窦腺体囊性扩张(左下)。在日本文献中,这种类型腺瘤被称为"交界性病变"。

织化学染色上显示胃小凹或幽门腺上皮的特征[170,175,176](见下文Ⅱ型异型增生),其他则具有胃和肠两型上皮的特征[177]。另一种罕见的亚型是所谓的Paneth细胞腺瘤[178],其中Peneth细胞是其主要细胞类型。

尽管大多数胃腺瘤具有外生性生长方式,形成隆起的无蒂或比较少见的有蒂的肿块,但少数病例可能是"平坦"的甚至是低于周围黏膜轮廓的凹陷性病变[179],支持可以将腺瘤和扁平黏膜异型增生看作是单一疾病这种观点。无蒂腺瘤通常为低级别的异型增生的管状腺体局限于黏膜上半部分,而其深层被变形和囊状扩张的非肿瘤性腺体占据,内衬胃窦型黏液细胞或有肠上皮化生(图8.28)[172]。

如同结肠腺瘤一样,胃腺瘤恶变的危险性与其大小、异型增生程度以及绒毛状生长方式有关。因此,直

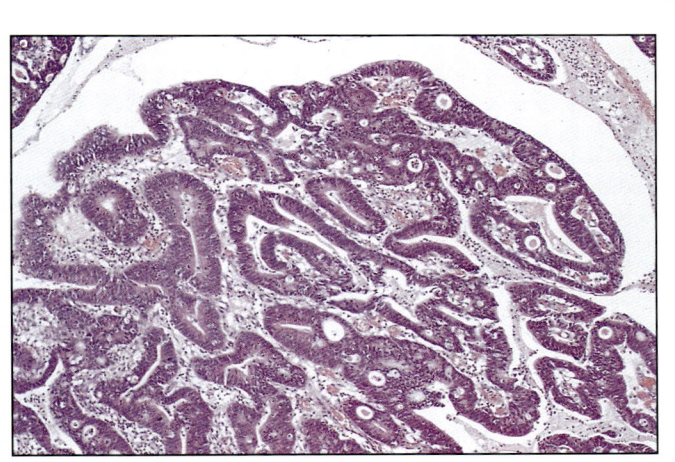

图8.27 管状腺瘤伴有高级别异型增生。视野上方伴有背靠背腺体的结构,非典型性程度相当于早期浸润性黏膜内腺癌。

表8.2	胃肠道上皮性肿瘤的Vienna分类[16] Reproduced with permission from the BMJ Publishing Group.
1型	没有肿瘤/异型增生
2型	肿瘤/异型增生不确定
3型	非浸润性低级别肿瘤 （低级别腺瘤/异型增生）
4型	非浸润性高级别肿瘤 　4.1 高级别腺瘤/异型增生 　4.2 非浸润性癌（原位癌）[a] 　4.3 可疑浸润性癌
5型	浸润性肿瘤 　5.1 黏膜内癌[b] 　5.2 黏膜下癌或超出黏膜下的癌

[a] 非浸润是指缺乏浸润证据
[b] 黏膜内是指侵入固有层或黏膜肌层

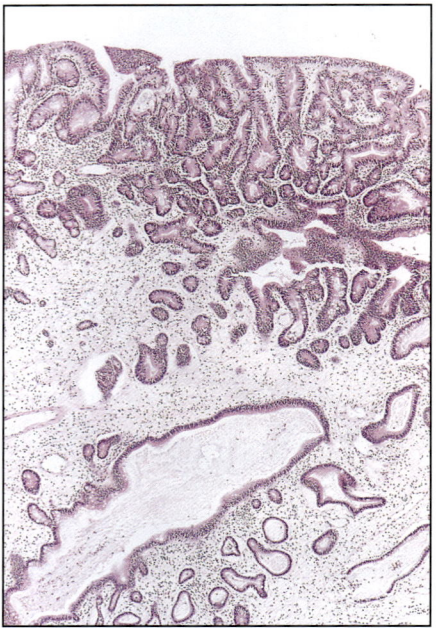

图8.29　发生于增生性（再生性）息肉表浅部分的高分化黏膜内腺癌。

径小于1 cm的有蒂腺瘤通常为伴低级别异型增生的管状病变，癌的发生率低，异型增生局限于表浅区域的无蒂腺瘤也是如此。较大的有蒂腺瘤多为伴高级别异型增生的绒毛状腺瘤，其中相当一部分含有浸润型癌；这在40%～50%的肿瘤直径大于2 cm的病例中可以见到[177]。诊断黏膜内腺癌意味着出现肿瘤性上皮侵入固有层或深达黏膜下层。有时这种现象可能明显表现为肿瘤性上皮呈不规则锯齿状突入周围疏松结缔组织中。在另外一种情况下，只能根据严重的结构异常进行推断，例如实性生长方式、背靠背腺体集聚形成筛状结构或不伴有明显纤维组织增生的小的浸润性发育不全的腺体（见图8.27）。西方病理医师通常根据前者（即浸润）诊断为癌，而日本病理医师一般采用后者；这种诊断上的地域性差异可能是东西方之间报道胃癌发病率明显不同的原因[180,181]。为了使这两种意见取得一致，提出了胃肠道癌前病变的Vienna分类[16]（表8.2）。从某些方面来说，区分腺瘤和息肉内的腺癌是属于学术性的，因为实际上可以忽略经过息肉完全切除后的黏膜内息肉样腺癌发生转移扩散的危险性。因此，病理医师的主要责任是通过检查足够的切片来判断病变切除是否彻底。

鉴别诊断：息肉样胃腺瘤必须与较为常见的胃上皮性息肉相鉴别，包括增生性息肉（hyperplastic polyps）、胃底腺息肉（fundic gland polyps）、错构瘤性息肉（hamartomatous polyps）、异位（heterotopias）以及息肉样Ménétrier病，所有这些病变将在下文描述[168,169]。区分腺瘤与这些病变的主要标准为是否存在异型增生，但有时可能难以区别，尤其是糜烂性或炎性增生性息肉，此时炎性胃小凹上皮的再生性改变可能非常类似于异型增生。诊断异型增生的标准包括缺乏上皮细胞表面成熟和出现肠型分化，在非肿瘤性息肉中肠型分化常不明显。另一方面，"洋葱皮样"腺体排列（见第364页）是增生性息肉的诊断性特征。

罕见情况下，大的增生性息肉可以发生真正的异型增生甚至明显的腺癌，通常在其尖端，这就使得情况变得更为复杂（图8.29）[169,182]。这种病变的命名尚有争议，但一般不认为它们是腺瘤，不过其临床处理原则与腺瘤相似。

平坦胃黏膜异型增生
Dysplasia in flat gastric mucosa

临床特征：胃黏膜异型增生并不总是表现为肉眼可见的胃内隆起性病变或腺瘤。实际上，异型增生较常见于平坦的黏膜或正常或外观仅有轻微异常的黏膜[183]。因此，胃的异型增生本身引起的症状是不可靠的，诊断常常是通过胃黏膜随机活检作出的，内窥镜下所见仅有轻微的异常。有时，易碎的肿瘤性上皮似乎更常见于消化性溃疡，从浅表溃疡的边缘活检可以作出诊断。胃异型增生通常是一种老年性疾病；最常见于50～60岁以上的老人，通常发生在长期慢性胃炎的情况下。显然，其主要临床意义与胃癌有关；一旦诊断异型增生，慎重的做法是对患者进行再次内窥镜检查，以期发现原来活检部位附近的隐匿性胃癌。

现在常规将胃的异型增生分为高级别（以前为重度）

和低级别（以前为轻度和中度）两种[16,183-187]。有证据表明，低级别异型增生进展为癌的相对少见（＜20%）而且缓慢，实际上可能并不一定能进展为癌[188-190]。对于这些病例，建议立即重新做内窥镜检查并多处活检以排除同时发生的癌，随后定期随访检查（每年2次），直到两次内窥镜下检查结果阴性后放宽为每年检查1次。

高级别异型增生伴发胃癌的相当多见（至少70%），以致许多人认为恰当的处理是立即进行胃切除术[187-189]，术前最好通过多处活检确定病变范围，以决定手术的近切缘。然而，随着内窥镜技术的进步，包括内窥镜超声检查，应用活体染料喷涂显色技术和内窥镜下黏膜切除术，现在可以避免进行胃切除术。对于这样切除的标本需要进行仔细的病理学检查，以证实切除是否完全，如果有浸润性肿瘤，还要判定不利的预后指标[191,192]。

大体表现：根据定义，"平坦"胃黏膜异型增生是一种大体检查不明显的病变。它可能完全没有特殊表现，或可能表现为黏膜轻度隆起、增厚、充血，边界不清的结节，或为轻度凹陷的病变，周围绕以放射状的黏膜皱襞[193]。在内窥镜检查时应用活体染料喷涂显色技术（成色内窥镜，chromoendoscopy）和放大内窥镜，可以突出显示胃黏膜的不规则性。高级别异型增生倾向于表现为凹陷性病变，而低级别异型增生则常为轻微隆起性病变。某些病变，尤其是高级别异型增生，可能发生浅表糜烂甚至明显的溃疡形成。胃窦黏膜比胃体黏膜更易受累，尤其是小弯侧。有时累及贲门黏膜，此时病变可能与Barrett食管混合。

镜下表现：胃异型增生的主要特征包括细胞学、分化和结构的异常，这在腺瘤一节已经描述[174,183-190]。这些异常可以累及胃小凹的浅层和腺颈部水平（图8.30），常常伴有其下方特化腺体的囊状扩张，或累及黏膜全层（图8.31）。常有肠上皮化生的背景，出现特征性的分泌III型硫酸黏蛋白的不成熟性变型，发生在这种情况下的异型增生常常显示肠型分化，伴有杯状细胞形成，有时显示极向紊乱（图8.32）。非化生性小凹上皮的异型增生[170]（图8.30）有时被称为II型异型增生，此种异型增生少见得多，可能是弥漫型胃癌的前驱病变[184]。异型增生的分级主观，但是一般来说，当核深染，多形性和复层化的程度有限，缺乏非典型性核分裂象，而且腺体结构相对保留时，诊断为低级别异型增生。相反，高级别异型增生显示较明显的细胞学非典型性，伴有大而不规则的核仁，腺体结构更加复杂，包括出现背靠背的腺体，可与原位癌混合存在[174,183-188]。人们曾经尝试过

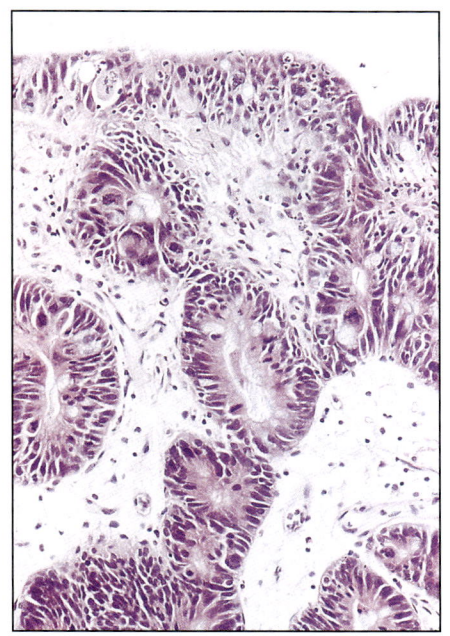

图8.30　非化生性胃小凹上皮呈高级别异型增生。

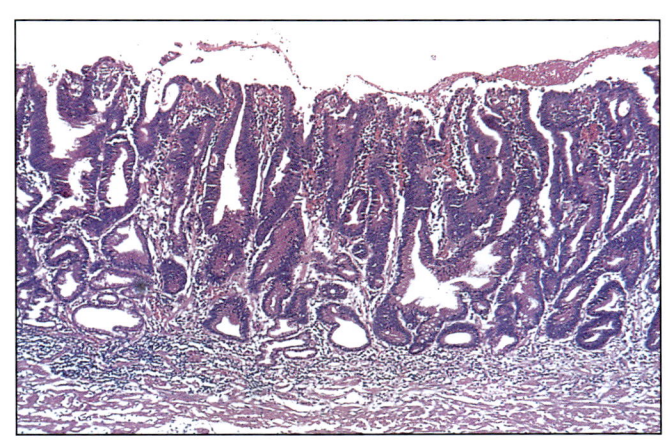

图8.31　发生于化生性上皮的高级别异型增生，累及黏膜全层。

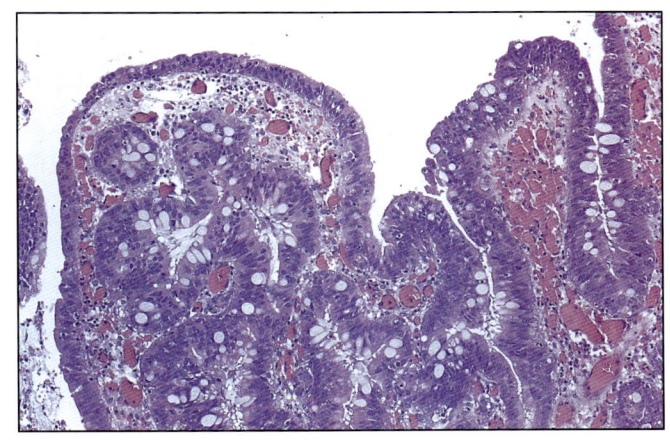

图8.32　化生性上皮显示低级别异型增生，伴有明显的杯状细胞，其中有些细胞极向紊乱或"营养不良"。

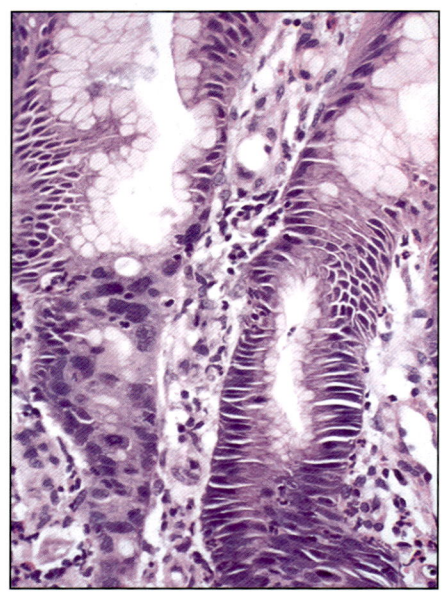

图8.33 在活动性胃炎中再生性胃小凹上皮增生并有非典型性。注意，右侧腺体中可见明显的上皮内中性粒细胞，左侧腺体上部的上皮分化成熟。

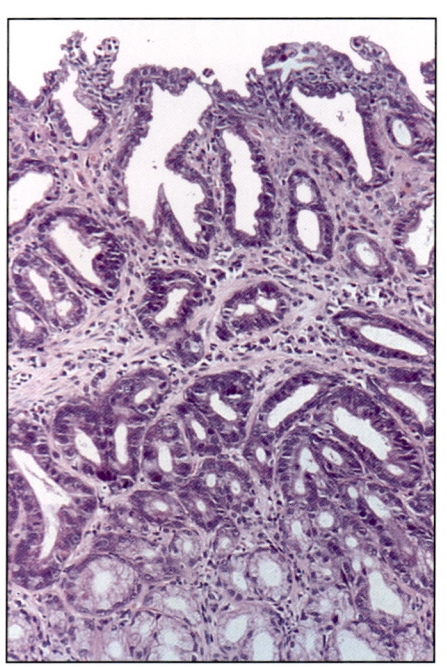

图8.34 反应性胃炎伴有明显的小凹上皮增生。尽管视野中央部分上皮细胞核有明显的非典型性，但在胃小凹上部和黏膜表面细胞成熟，这不是异型增生。

很多方法以协助确定胃异型增生的分类，以消除分级的主观性。这些方法包括黏液组织化学、免疫细胞化学检测分化或细胞增殖标记物，以及癌基因产物和形态测量分析。遗憾的是，至今尚无一种方法比传统的形态学分析更具有明显的优势。

鉴别诊断：异型增生主要的鉴别诊断包括与胃炎、糜烂或溃疡有关的再生性上皮增生/非典型性的鉴别。胃炎几乎总是伴有小凹上皮增生，但仅在极少数情况下，其所伴有的非典型性可以达到需要处理的程度。首先是急性重度炎症（图8.33）；避免误诊的最佳方法是，当上皮内有大量中性粒细胞时，慎作高级别异型增生的诊断。其次是反应性（化学性或反流性）胃炎，其特征是黏膜水肿、血管扩张、纤维化、平滑肌增生和小凹上皮增生，但炎细胞相当少见[194]。此时，由于缺少中性粒细胞，再生上皮的非典型性非常明显，以致过诊断为异型增生。在这两种胃炎中，支持是再生而非异型增生性改变的有用指标是腺体结构相对保存完整，增生的上皮存在某种程度向黏膜表面的成熟分化。另外，再生性增生的细胞核虽然浓染，但通常为圆形，位于基底，核仁明显但小而规则。再次，在胃糜烂或溃疡的附近，再生性增生伴有变性腺体的肿胀和核的非典型性，引起令人警觉的现象，它不仅提示异型增生甚至如同明显的癌（图8.35）[47]。最具特征的是非典型性的腺体常被包埋于嗜酸性纤维素、肉芽组织或溃疡坏死组织中，而不是位于

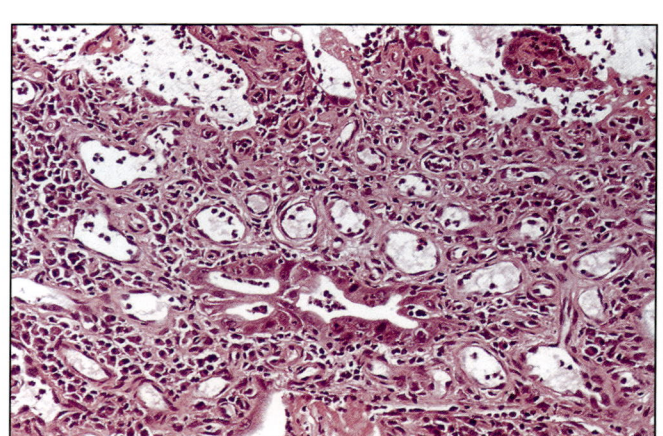

图8.35 在良性消化性溃疡边缘的肉芽组织中，可见奇异的、细胞学上呈现非典型性的腺体。

正常的固有层内。最后是与放化疗有关的上皮非典型性。此时，非典型性的程度可能特别明显，但是不同于真正的异型增生，它既累及胃小凹又累及黏膜深层特化的区域，并且伴有胞浆嗜酸性变和胞浆内空泡形成，有时腺体出现微囊性改变。与真正的异型增生不同，放化疗所致的增生活性局限于深部胃小凹区，非典型性核分裂象少见，并且细胞向腺腔表面成熟分化[195]。

腺癌 Adenocarcinoma

临床特征：腺癌是胃最常见的恶性肿瘤。男性多于

女性，男女之比在年轻成人为1，而在60岁成人则为2或2以上。胃腺癌在儿童和青少年极为罕见。在日本、中美和南美、北欧和东欧的部分地区，胃腺癌的发病率较高[196]，但是第二代移民的发病率与居住国相似。在北欧和美国，胃内肿瘤的分布正在发生变化，贲门部肿瘤增加，而胃远侧的肿瘤减少。同样，肠型肿瘤进行性减少，而弥漫型肿瘤却不断增加[197]。尽管总的发病率在下降，但在世界范围内，胃腺癌仍是恶性疾病所致死亡的第二个最常见的病因[196]。

从流行病学观点看，与胃癌有关的环境因素包括社会经济状况低下、摄入高盐饮食和干燥或腌渍的食物、吸烟和酗酒；新鲜水果和蔬菜中的维生素C、类胡萝卜素和绿茶具有保护作用[196]。某些病例有明显的遗传倾向；在弥漫型家族性胃癌和早期发作的胃癌中，可见E-cadherin基因（CDH1）的种系突变[198]，而肠型胃癌可能见于其他癌的家族综合征，特别是遗传性非息肉病性结直肠癌综合征[199]。癌前病变包括伴有萎缩和肠上皮化生（尤其是"不完全性"化生[200]）的慢性胃炎、胃切除术后残胃、胃腺瘤和Ménétrier病[201]。胃慢性幽门螺杆菌感染在胃癌发生的早期阶段起主要作用（贲门癌除外），尤其是携带有细胞毒素相关基因（CagA）菌株的感染[202,203]。宿主对于这种感染的反应也很重要，因为不同个体对胃萎缩和胃癌的敏感性不同，这与前炎症性白介素-1基因多态性有关[204]。幽门螺杆菌胃炎（Helicobacter pylori gastritis）患者病变分布广泛，主要累及胃体，比较迅速地发展为胃萎缩，处于高度危险之中；许多宿主和环境因素似乎能够减缓这一进程[205]。贲门癌具有不同的流行病学特征，类似于食道下段腺癌。在伴有淋巴细胞间质的胃癌（以及少部分"普通"胃癌）

中，应用聚合酶链反应（PCR）和原位杂交法可以检出高比例的Epstein-Barr病毒（EBV）[206]，但是其在癌发生过程中的作用还不清楚。

分子生物学和免疫细胞化学检查发现胃癌具有诸多方面的异常，包括微卫星不稳定性，体细胞突变，K-ras、K-sam、APC、c-met、c-erbB-2、p53、TGFα、TGFβ、CD44、bcl-2、cyclin E、E-cadherin和nm23的异常表达或放大，染色体1p、1q、3p、5q（APC位点），7q、13q、17p（p53位点）、18q（DCC位点）的等位基因缺失，以及端粒酶表达[27]。其中某些改变可能与胃癌特定的组织学类型有关（比如肠型胃癌有p53突变或微卫星不稳定性[207]，而弥漫型胃癌有K-sam扩增[27]），而其他改变（比如c-erbB-2扩增和7q缺失）则与疾病进展有关，而且可能具有预后意义[27]。

腺癌常常发生于胃窦或胃小弯，较少见于胃体。然而，近年来注意到，贲门部腺癌所占比例逐渐增加（占28%），反映出来源于Barrett食管的食管腺癌有所增加[15,61,208]。实际上，整个胃弥漫受累也不少见。临床症状或体征包括消化不良、厌食、体重下降、出血、胃的流入或流出道梗阻，但是除非肿瘤进入晚期，很少出现明显的症状和体征，因此总的预后很差。不过，早期胃癌的诊断比较常见，通常是在有提示消化性溃疡症状的患者，或是通过对于无症状的人群进行普查时发现肿块，因为日本提倡进行普查。事实上，现在日本的早期胃癌多数都是新诊断的病例。

大体表现：进展期胃癌可为息肉型（见图8.25）、蕈伞型、溃疡型或弥漫浸润型（图8.36），后者即所谓的皮革胃（linitis plastica），或几种形态混合存在。溃疡

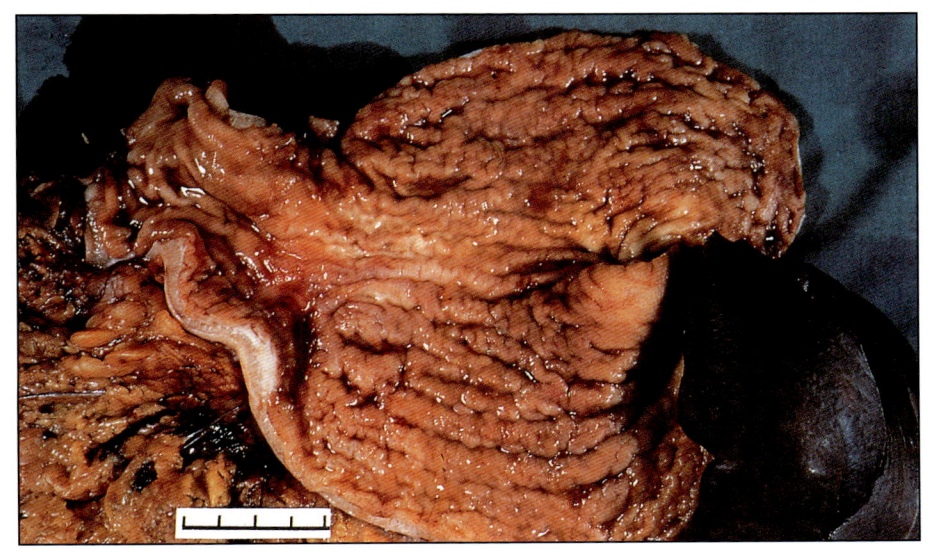

图8.36 弥漫浸润型胃腺癌，皮革胃。

型胃癌最常见于胃窦部小弯侧，与典型消化性溃疡的不同之处在于其轮廓不规则、边缘隆起、卷曲。然而，准确无误地作出这种区分是不可能的，重要的是在临床处理之前，应在溃疡所有边缘多处活检以明确诊断。息肉型和蕈伞型胃癌较常见于胃体，多位于大弯侧，而弥漫浸润型胃癌可表现为边界不清、具有浅表溃疡的斑块，其下方胃壁明显增厚，或者在少数情况下，整个胃壁弥漫性增厚，即"革袋胃"（leather bottle stomach）。遗传性弥漫型胃癌时，多灶性胃壁内印戒细胞癌常累及胃窦胃体交界区[209]。各种大体类型中均有部分肿瘤可以产生许多细胞外黏液，大体出现胶样癌的胶冻样外观。

镜下表现：总的来说，胃腺癌可由腺管状、腺泡状或乳头状结构构成，也可以由不相黏着的单个细胞构成，肿瘤细胞广泛浸润，隐匿的散在于胃壁各层。细胞学上，肿瘤细胞可以显示胃型或肠型特征，包括向壁细胞[210]和嗜银性内分泌细胞[211,212]，甚至 Paneth 细胞分化[213]。肿瘤细胞通常产生黏液，淀粉酶-PAS 或阿利新蓝(Alcian blue) 染色阳性，可含有硫酸涎糖蛋白，而且大多数病例癌胚抗原（CEA）和 CA19-9 免疫染色阳性。胃癌的组织学形态和分化程度常常具有显著的差异。已提出多种组织学分类方法。

WHO 分类[177]将胃腺癌分为4个主要类型：乳头状、腺管状、黏液性以及印戒细胞腺癌。腺癌也可分为高、中、低分化。乳头状腺癌以多数具有纤维血管轴心的乳头状突起为特征（图 8.37）；腺管状腺癌主要由肿瘤性腺管构成，腺管常有不规则的分支和相互吻合（图 8.38）；黏液性腺癌（胶样或黏液样癌）的特征为有多量细胞外黏液（占肿瘤的 50% 以上）（图 8.39）；而印戒细胞癌主要是由含有胞浆内黏液空泡的单个或成簇的细胞构成，这种细胞应占肿瘤的 50% 以上（图 8.40）。印戒细胞癌易于弥散性浸润胃壁，常常伴有明显的纤维化，形成皮革胃的大体表现。腺管状、乳头状和黏液性腺癌常为局限性胃癌，大体类型既可为息肉型、蕈伞型，也可为溃疡型。腺管状腺癌的嗜酸细胞亚型已有报道[214]。WHO 分类中胃癌的其他类型包括许多不常见的特殊亚型（下文描述）和未分化癌，未分化癌缺乏明显的腺管状结构或任何其他特征的分化。

Laurén 组织学分类方法[215]是将胃腺癌分为两种主要类型：肠型和弥漫型。肠型胃腺癌有清楚的腺体结构，伴有乳头状、腺管状甚至实性的区域（见图 8.37，图 8.38）。内衬的肿瘤性管腔上皮由肠型高柱状细胞构成，常常伴有明显的刷状缘及散在的分泌黏液的杯状细胞。然而，丰富的细胞内黏液产物并非其特征。肿瘤常有界限清楚的"推进性"边缘，并且常见间质炎细胞浸润。邻近的胃黏膜常常显示为慢性胃炎，伴有广泛的肠上皮化生，而且也可显示异型增生。相反，弥漫型胃腺癌主要由散在的单个细胞或成簇的细胞构成。虽然可以出现在肿瘤较表浅的部位，但腺管状分化少见。多数细胞小而一致，

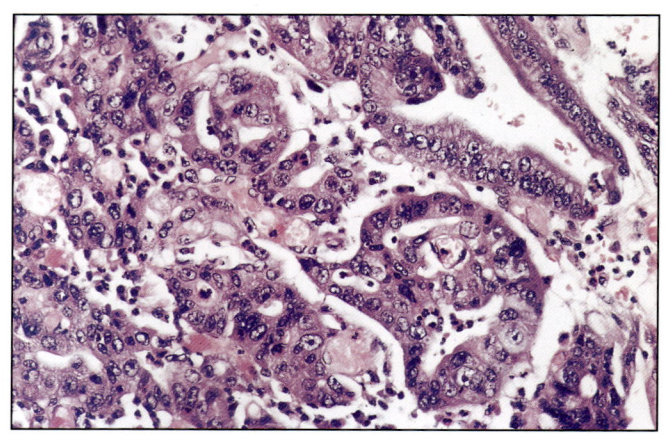

图 8.38 中分化胃腺癌，腺管状结构（肠型）。

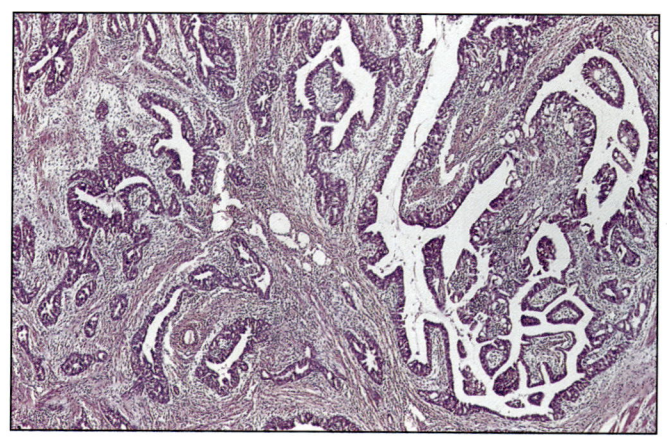

图 8.37 高分化胃腺癌，由乳头和腺管混合组成。

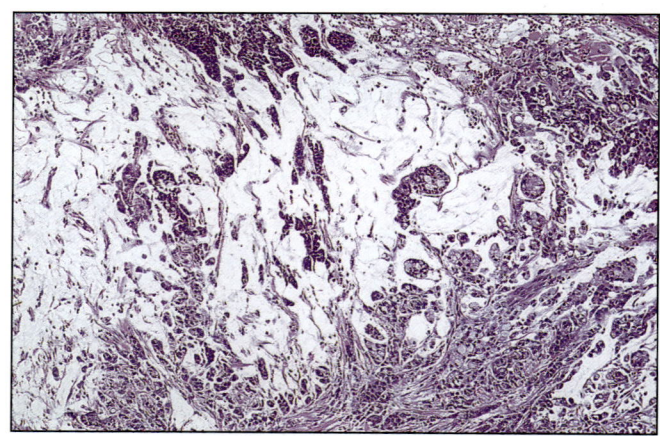

图 8.39 胃黏液性腺癌。

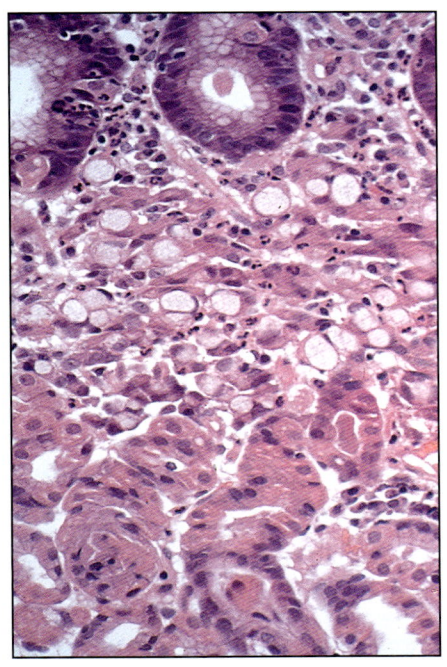

图8.40 早期印戒细胞胃腺癌，浸润黏膜固有层的肿瘤细胞局限于胃小凹区（上）和特殊分化的腺体区（下）之间的上皮细胞增生区。

细胞之间黏着性较差，某些细胞具有印戒细胞的形态学表现。肿瘤边界不清，广泛浸润（图8.41）。邻近胃黏膜肠上皮化生相当少见，异型增生同样少见；如果出现异型增生，为胃小凹型增生[184]。实际上，肿瘤细胞通常起源于形态学正常胃腺的胃小凹，是为原位的印戒癌细胞，而后直接侵犯固有层（见图8.40），或表现为局部胃小凹和腺体内衬上皮下的Paget样浸润[216]。相当一部分病例（高达15%）显示肠型和弥漫型两种组织学形态，被归入中间型。

Laurén分类的有用之处在于描述了病因学和组织发生可能根本不同的两大类型的肿瘤。肠型胃癌与慢性胃炎和肠上皮化生密切相关，流行病学调查显示其与"环境"因素关系比较密切；胃癌发病率地域上的不同主要是由于肠型胃癌的差异造成的。没有发现弥漫型胃癌与这些因素有关。两种类型胃癌的扩散方式也不同。肠型胃癌通常为远处血行传播，而典型的弥漫型胃癌则是腹膜内广泛播散[217]。

Ming[218]的分类将胃腺癌分为两型，即膨胀型和浸润型；而Mulligan和Rember[219]将Laurén分类进一步扩展，增加了第三种类型，即幽门贲门腺癌（pylorocardiac gland carcinoma）。这种类型胃癌发生于胃窦或贲门，常常表现为边界清楚的蕈伞状肿物。组织学上为高分化腺管状或乳头状结构，显著特征是细胞胞浆透亮和空泡化，类似于特化的胃窦或贲门腺的正常细胞（图8.42）。

事实上，胃腺癌有多种组织学分类，但没有一种分类是完全令人满意的。观察者的可重复性差是主要问题，但是Ming的分类可能是个例外[220]，虽然各种不同的亚型也无法进行一致的预后分组。一般来说，在进展期胃癌中，弥漫型、浸润型、印戒细胞和未分化癌预后不佳，但矛盾的是，浅表性肿瘤并不如此[221]。最近，Goseki等[222]根据腺管状分化程度和细胞内黏液的多少将胃癌分为4种组织学类型。他们认为这4种类型能够预示肿瘤不同的扩散方式，是直接蔓延还是经淋巴管或血行扩散。几项独立的研究证明，这种分类具有实用性和可重复性[223]。Carneiro等提出了更加简单的（可能具有高度可重复性）分类系统，把胃癌分成（a）孤立细胞型、（b）

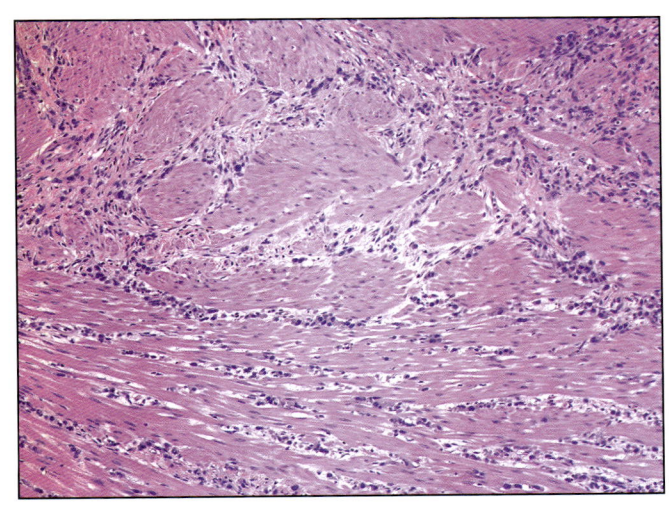

图8.41 进展期弥漫型胃癌，肿瘤细胞在胃壁平滑肌束内浸润。

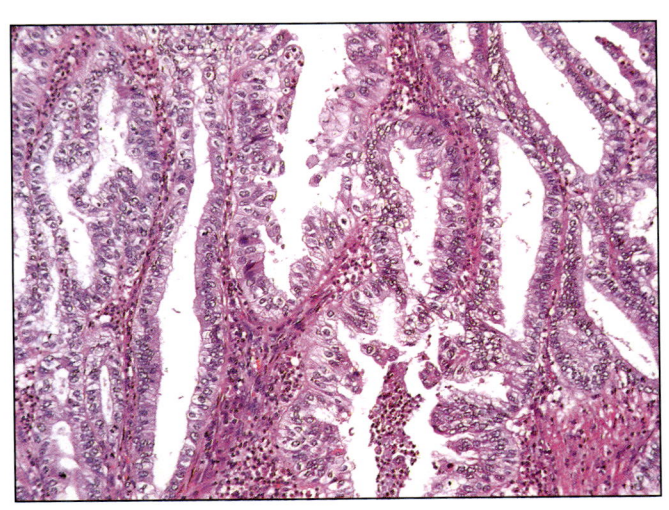

图8.42 幽门贲门型胃腺癌。

腺管型、(c) 实性型和 (d) 混合型[224]。后者是指既有孤立细胞成分，又有腺管或实性成分者（腺管和实性成分混合的肿瘤根据其主要成分分别归入腺管型或实性型）。他们发现，占所研究病例 38.5% 的混合型胃癌比其他单纯型胃癌预后要差，而且多因素分析表明，这种分型具有独立的预后意义，仅次于 TNM 分期系统。混合型胃癌是预后差的独立因素已得到证实，这与单纯型胃癌具有不同的分子生物学表现有关[225]。

检测胃癌其他潜在的预后标志物作用不大。检测有关分化的组织化学标志物也是令人失望的，包括是否存在内分泌细胞[211]，尽管有人认为壁细胞分化与预后较好有关，壁细胞分化表现为肿瘤细胞含有丰富的嗜酸性颗粒状胞浆，磷钨酸苏木精（PTAH）和 Luxol fast blue 染色阳性[210,226]。细胞增殖[227,228] 和 DNA 倍体[228-230] 的研究结果矛盾，现在尚不能作为常规应用。尽管血管[223,231] 或者神经[232] 侵犯具有独立的预后意义，但是迄今最有用的预后因素仍是确诊时肿瘤的临床病理学分期。有趣的是，EBV 阳性的肠型胃癌似乎具有特别好的预后[233]。

临床病理学分期：西方国家广泛应用 TNM 分期系统[96]，见表 8.3；它是最好的预测预后的分类方法[231]，因而被推荐使用。考虑到尚未穿透胃壁肌层的胃癌具有较好的预后（5 年生存率大于 50%），最近把 pT2 期胃癌分成 pT2a 和 pT2b[234]。肿瘤累及的淋巴结数目也有重要的预后意义[235]，根据规定，正确的"N"分期要求至少检查 15 个淋巴结。此外，通过免疫组化法检查淋巴结内隐匿的肿瘤细胞可能也有预后意义[236]。遗憾的是，TNM 分期系统没有在世界范围内被广泛应用（比如，日本采用自己的分期系统）[237]，这样，很难对临床研究进行国际性的比较分析。

胃和食管交界处肿瘤的分期也出现困难，因为食道癌和胃癌的 TNM 分期系统不同（对比表 8.1 和表 8.3），导致对于个别病例无法确定应用哪一种分期系统。Siewert 等[238] 提出的交界部肿瘤的分期方法如下：Ⅰ型癌发生在食道远端三分之一，通常在 Barrett 食管区，可能直接累及或不累及胃食管交界部；Ⅱ型癌跨越胃食管交界部，可能是真正发生在胃和食管交界处的肿瘤；Ⅲ型癌是贲门下方的胃癌向近端生长，累及胃食管交界部。他们的结论是：Ⅱ型交界部癌淋巴结播散的方式与胃癌相似，应该根据胃癌原则进行分期。

在未接受普查的西方人群，由于临床症状出现太晚，75% 以上的病例发现时病变已达晚期，只能行姑息性手术[239]。肿瘤常直接蔓延至食管，较少浸润至十二指肠。淋巴转移也常见，累及小弯侧和大弯侧或腹腔和腹主动脉旁淋巴结。膈上甚至纵隔淋巴结也可有转移灶，虽然通过胸导管转移至左锁骨上淋巴结（Virchow 淋巴结）已经得到公认，但并不常见。在无淋巴转移的情况下，也可经血行转移至远处器官。肝转移最为常见，但亦可见于其他部位，包括肺、骨、皮肤和脑。双侧卵巢广泛受累（Krukenberg 瘤）可能是经腹膜或血行转移的结果。即使进行了彻底的淋巴结清扫（即所谓的 D2 胃切除术），"根治性"胃切除术患者的预后依然不好，并发症的发生率较高，某些研究显示 5 年生存率为 50%[240]。迄今为止，辅助化疗尚未取得显著疗效。尽管如此，确诊时肿瘤局限于胃壁内的病例预后仍较好，并且可以将这种肿瘤分为两期，即所谓的"早期"（pT1）胃癌和"固有肌层"（pT2a）胃癌（PM gastric cancer）。

早期胃癌（Early gastric cancer）：也称表面或浅表性胃癌，其定义是癌局限于黏膜或黏膜下层，不管淋巴有无受累，相当于 pT1 期胃癌。"早期"这一术语与肿瘤的大小、形状或病程长短无关，而是指肿瘤处于可能治愈的阶段。实际上，早期胃癌手术切除后的 5 年生存率平均为 80%～95%[221,241]。

早期胃癌分为 3 种主要的大体类型。Ⅰ型（隆起型）

表8.3	胃癌的TNM病理学分期[96]

T－原发肿瘤

pT1　肿瘤侵入固有层或黏膜下层
pT2　肿瘤侵入固有肌层或浆膜下层
　　　pT2a　肿瘤侵入固有肌层
　　　pT2b　肿瘤侵入浆膜下层
pT3　肿瘤穿透浆膜（脏层腹膜），未侵犯邻近器官
pT4　肿瘤侵犯邻近器官

N－区域淋巴结

pN0　无区域淋巴结转移
pN1　1～6个区域淋巴结转移
pN2　7～15个区域淋巴结转移
pN3　15个以上区域淋巴结转移

M－远处转移[a]

M0　无远处转移
M1　有远处转移

[a] 除非对远处器官活检进行组织学检查，否则病理分期一般不能判断有无远处转移。

肿瘤突入胃腔，可为息肉状、结节状或绒毛状。Ⅱ型（浅表型）的特征为黏膜表面不平，又可进一步分为隆起型（Ⅱa）（图8.43）、平坦型（Ⅱb）和凹陷型（Ⅱc）（图8.44）。Ⅲ型（深凿型）表现为深浅不一的溃疡，溃疡边缘伴有腺癌。这3种类型常常混合存在。

早期胃癌的镜下特征基本与进展期胃癌相同，各种组织学形态都可存在。Ⅰ型和Ⅱa型肿瘤几乎都是高分化腺管状或乳头状腺癌（图8.45），而Ⅱc和Ⅲ型肿瘤多为低分化腺癌或为印戒细胞腺癌。不难理解，早期胃癌的预后与浸润深度有关，大多数发生淋巴结转移的病例有黏膜下层浸润[221,241]。但矛盾的是，向黏膜下层广泛浸润的隆起型高分化肠型胃癌的侵袭性似乎较强，早期胃癌中发生远处转移的那一小部分通常为这种类型[242]。这类肿瘤也多为非整倍体[243,244]。大约10%的早期胃癌患者同时或不同时发生第二个胃癌。因此，在对早期胃癌行部分胃切除术前检查是否存在第二个肿瘤至关重要，并要确保对治疗后的残胃进行长期监测。黏膜内早期胃癌淋巴结转移的发生率很低（可达7%），因此，对于小的非溃疡性肿瘤，尤其是那些分化较好的肿瘤，内窥镜下黏膜切除是首选的治疗方法[192]。对于切除标本要进行仔细的组织学检查，以除外进一步手术的3个指征，即黏膜下浸润、切除不完全和淋巴管浸润[192]。

固有肌层胃癌（PM gastric cancer）：日本学者用此术语描述侵入但没有穿透固有肌层（proper muscle，PM）的胃癌，不管是否有淋巴结转移[234]，相当于T2a期胃癌。切除的肿瘤中约15%属于这种类型，其预后明显好于较晚期的胃癌；在大多数日本系列研究和一项英国的研究中，其5年生存率大于60%[228,234]。固有肌

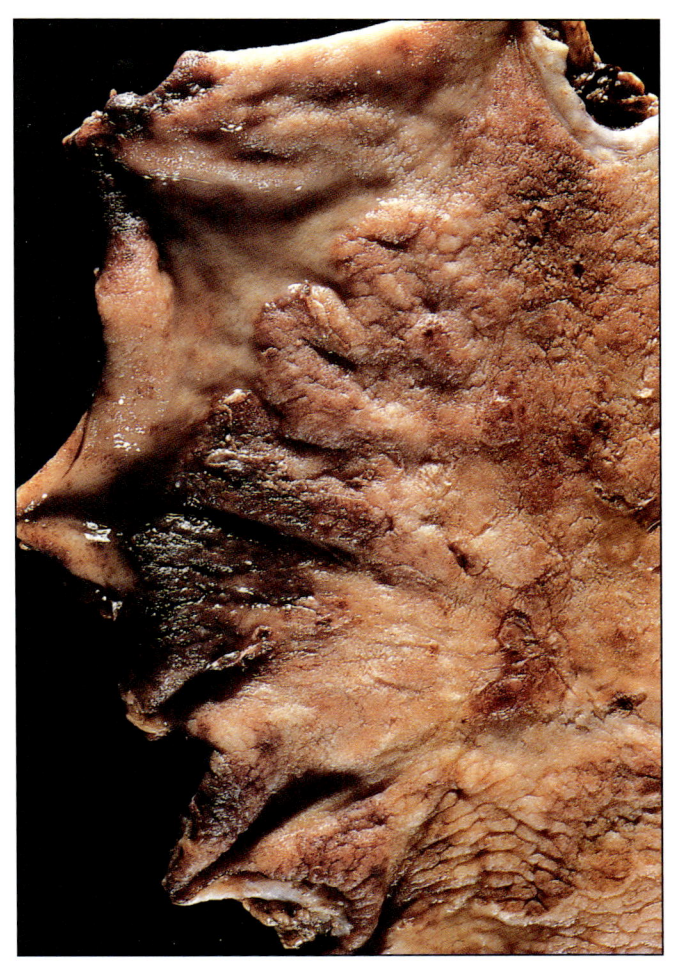

图8.43 隆起型早期（T1）胃癌，实际上几乎累及全胃；只有胃体部小片区域（左上）未受累。

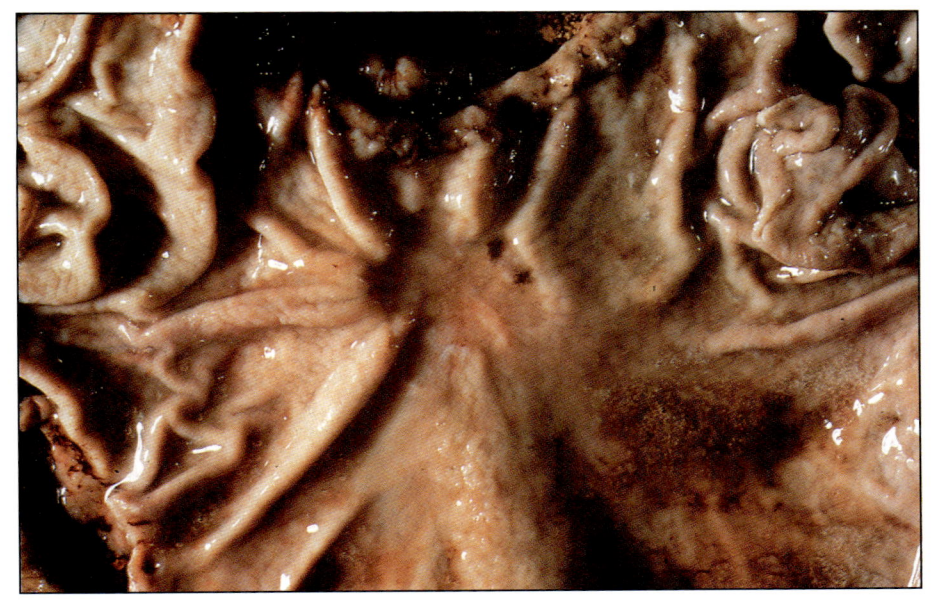

图8.44 凹陷型早期（T1）胃癌，周边可见放射状黏膜皱襞。

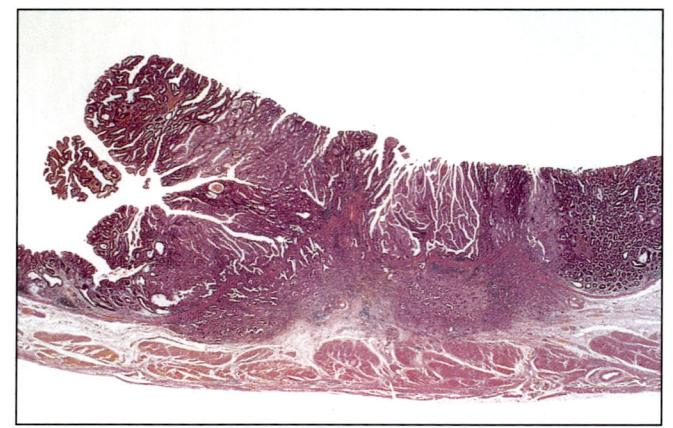

图8.45 腺管状和乳头状高分化早期（T1）胃癌，累及黏膜和黏膜下层。

层胃癌进一步分为侵犯固有肌层浅层和侵犯固有肌层深层两种，两者相比，前者5年生存率与早期胃癌相似，明显好于后者[234]。因此，有理由认为固有肌层胃癌是一组预后较好的肿瘤。

溃疡癌　Ulcer-cancer

溃疡癌的定义是发生于先前存在的消化性溃疡的腺癌，癌组织局限于溃疡边缘。这个定义意味着只能在早期诊断溃疡癌，此时组织学上仍可区分炎性和肿瘤性病变。溃疡癌约占胃癌的1%。

大体上看，溃疡癌一般较大。通常表现为僵硬、苍白而倾斜的边缘，与良性消化性溃疡柔软、充血、界限清楚的深凿状边缘形成对比。显微镜下，癌的成分局限于溃疡边缘的黏膜；作出诊断之前必须与再生性改变仔细鉴别。也可见到慢性消化性溃疡的特征性改变，特别是致密的瘢痕组织中有淋巴细胞聚集，基底部有闭塞性动脉内膜炎，溃疡边缘可见黏膜肌层和肌层融合。尽管认为溃疡癌是由原有的消化性溃疡恶变而来的观点具有一定的说服力，但这并不是对于这种表现的唯一解释。有些黏膜内胃癌是生长缓慢的病变，经过数月甚至数年也不发生深部浸润，这已得到公认[245]。因此，也有理由认为溃疡癌是大的黏膜内腺癌，继发消化性溃疡。

残胃癌　Gastric stump carcinoma

残胃癌是公认的部分胃切除的长期并发症，通常发生在原来手术后20年或20年以上。早期文献对其总的危险性可能有所夸大，近期大宗研究提示，术后25年的危险性大约为3～5倍[246]。大体上看，残胃癌发生于吻合线的胃的一侧，通常紧靠吻合线。胃癌的各种大体和镜下改变在残胃癌中均可见到。

残胃癌的发病机制尚不明确。残胃可发生许多病理改变，改变部位通常紧靠吻合口，包括慢性萎缩性胃炎、肠化生、异型增生、腺瘤性息肉以及炎性息肉等；后者可能特别明显，表现为所谓的"囊性息肉状胃炎"（gastritis cystica polyposa）（见下文）[247]。不过，在对残胃活检标本作异型增生的诊断时必须非常小心，因为小肠内容物常常通过吻合口发生反流，引起反应性（反流性或化学性）胃炎[194]，伴有显著的小凹上皮增生，可能酷似异型增生（见上文）。

鉴别诊断：诊断困难仅见于胃活检标本，此时主要的问题是对小而变形的碎片诊断过度，碎片通常来自胃糜烂或溃疡，显示明显的反应性上皮增生、腺体肿胀和变性，而且在纤维素性渗出物或肉芽组织中有陷入的腺体（见图8.35）。Isaacson曾对这个问题进行详细论述[47]。在肉芽组织中，如果反应性纤维母细胞和内皮细胞出现异样的表现，伴有明显的颗粒状胞浆，核深染或为多形性，并有明显的核仁，则可能被误诊为弥漫型癌；这种改变在放疗后明显，在消化性溃疡也不少见[47]。这些细胞（即反应性纤维母细胞和内皮细胞）黏液染色或CK免疫组化染色阴性，核虽有明显的多形性，却难以见到核分裂象，因此通常可以推断出其真正的本质。良性胃息肉表面发生浅表糜烂时可有类似改变[248]。

印戒细胞和未分化的癌细胞必须与固有层内含有脂质或黏液的巨噬细胞鉴别。最好是通过仔细观察细胞核的形态来鉴别；巨噬细胞核呈明显的空泡状，有一个或多个小核仁，异染色质细，而印戒细胞癌的细胞核较大，深染，多形性，染色质粗而分散，偶见分裂象（图8.46）。淀粉酶-PAS染色对于鉴别诊断价值不大，因为嗜黏液细胞（muciphages）和印戒细胞的胞浆都为阳性，但在诊断困难的病例，应用上皮和巨噬细胞标记物进行免疫细胞化学检查可能有所帮助。实际上，嗜黏液细胞在胃活检标本中并不常见，这一点不同于结直肠活检，而且固有层内发现可疑细胞的多数病例进一步检查证明有癌。其他罕见而又重要的类似病变是见于急性糜烂性胃炎变性上皮细胞的印戒改变[249]、恶性黑色素瘤以及"印戒细胞"性间质肿瘤和恶性淋巴瘤（见下文）；适当的黏液染色和免疫组化方法通常有助于鉴别诊断。另外，与转移性乳腺小叶癌相混淆的也不少见，在没有恰当的临床病史时，这个问题可能特别突出。不同的细胞角蛋白染色对鉴别诊断有一定帮助：多数乳腺小叶癌CK7+，CK20-，而具有这种表型的胃癌不到20%。另一方面，50%～

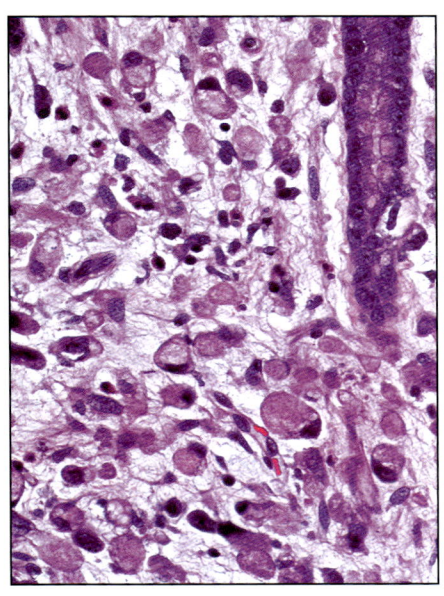

图8.46 低分化黏膜内腺癌,肿瘤细胞核呈多形性,可与充满黏液的组织细胞鉴别。

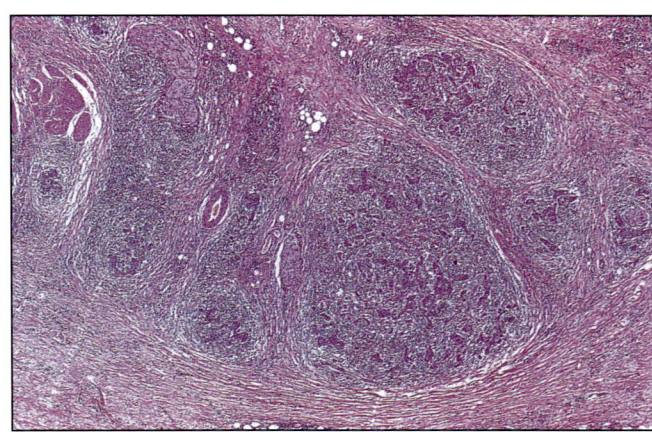

图8.47 伴有淋巴细胞间质的胃髓样癌,常有界限清楚的推进性生长边缘。

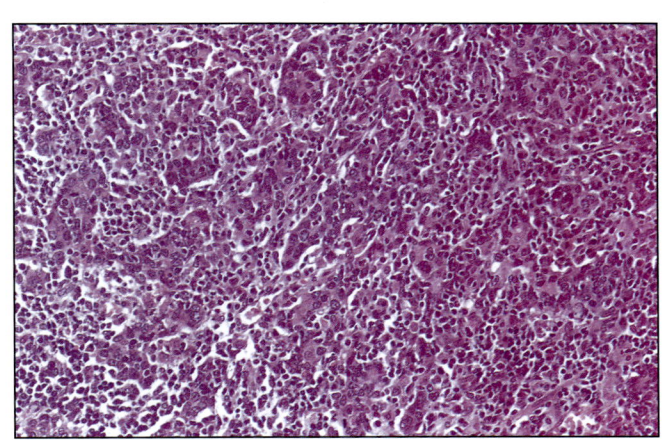

图8.48 伴有淋巴细胞间质的胃髓样癌。偶尔淋巴细胞浸润非常致密,以致可能需用免疫组织化学方法识别癌细胞。

65%的弥漫型胃癌CK20+,虽然有时是局灶性的[250]。在特定情况下,雌激素受体阳性几乎均代表是来自乳腺原发性肿瘤的转移[250a]。

胃癌不常见的亚型
Uncommon varieties of gastric carcinoma

伴有淋巴细胞间质的胃癌(髓样癌)[Gastric carcinoma with lymphoid stroma (medullary carcinoma)]:这种富于细胞的肿瘤主要是由大的嗜酸性癌细胞形成的实性巢构成的,腺管状分化相对不明显或者缺乏,肿瘤中混杂有密集、弥漫浸润的成熟淋巴细胞和浆细胞,有时形成淋巴滤泡和少数巨细胞(图8.47,图8.48)[251,252]。注意避免与恶性淋巴瘤或组织细胞肉瘤相混淆(必要时可做细胞角蛋白和淋巴细胞标记物的免疫染色)。免疫表型通常显示,在反应性的淋巴细胞成分中CD8+的T细胞明显多于B细胞。网状纤维染色显示间质中网状纤维呈细网状分布,但无纤维组织增生性反应。肿瘤边界一般清楚(见图8.47),呈膨胀性生长。有趣的是,髓样癌中超过80%的病例肿瘤细胞含有Epstein-Barr病毒,通过原位杂交法可以显示编码非多聚腺苷酸RNA-1的EBV在核内表达[206]。有些研究提示髓样癌比普通腺癌预后更好,其5年生存率高达77%[251],特别是在那些伴有高频率微卫星不稳定性的患者[252]。

伴有广泛中性粒细胞浸润的胃癌(Gastric carcinoma with extensive neutrophilic infiltration):最近报道了5例由高度多形性、无黏附性的恶性细胞组成的间变性胃癌,伴有间质内致密的中性粒细胞浸润[253]。作者推测中性粒细胞浸润是对肿瘤细胞产生的白介素-8产物的反应。随后的研究提示,这种癌的预后较好,尤其是在女性[254]。

腺鳞癌和鳞状细胞癌(Adenosquamous and squamous cell carcinoma):胃的腺鳞癌罕见,肿瘤中不同比例的腺癌和鳞癌共存(图8.49)[255]。大多数已报道的病例发生于胃窦部,诊断时已是晚期,预后差。鳞状分化和角化的程度各异,但有时可见明显的细胞间桥和角化珠。推测这种肿瘤由起源于腺体的肿瘤细胞双向分化而形成;偶尔在单个肿瘤细胞内可见鳞状和腺体两种分化特征的超微结构证据[256]。单纯的胃鳞

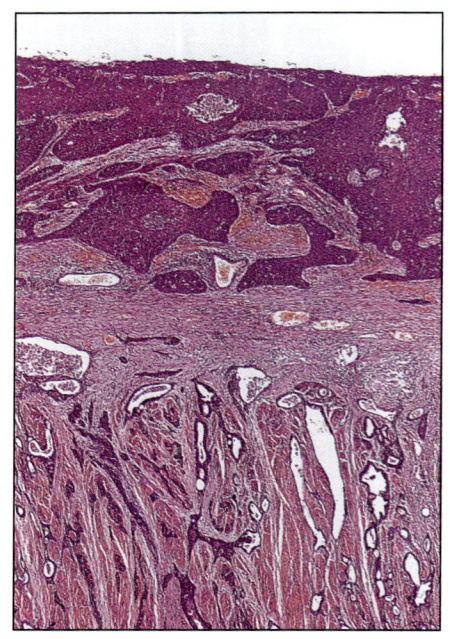

图8.49 腺鳞癌。视野中鳞状成分（上）和腺体成分（下）分界清楚，但在其他区域，两种成分混合存在。

状细胞癌极为罕见，对有疑问的病例进行仔细的组织学取样常可发现小的腺癌病灶[257]。发生于贲门部的单纯鳞状细胞癌可能是由食管原发性肿瘤扩散而来的。

波形蛋白阳性的伴有横纹肌样特征的胃癌（"恶性横纹肌样瘤"）[Vimentin-positive gastric carcinoma with rhabdoid features ("malignant rhabdoid tumor")]：波形蛋白阳性免疫反应在胃癌中极为少见。表达波形蛋白这种中间丝的罕见病例通常具有特征性的形态学表现，是一种呈弥漫性或腺泡状方式生长的实性肿瘤，由黏附性差或无黏附性的多形性、多角形细胞构成，核呈空泡状、核仁明显，胞浆丰富，强嗜酸性[258]。大部分病例有大的核旁玻璃样胞浆内包涵体；包涵体波形蛋白免疫染色强阳性，这一特征相当于所谓的"肾外恶性横纹肌样瘤"，除非不再将后者看作一种特殊类型的成人疾病（见第24章）。肿瘤细胞还常常表达细胞角蛋白和神经元特异性烯醇化酶，但不表达癌胚抗原。这种形态学结构可以单独存在，也可与普通类型胃癌共存。预后非常差。

肝样和产生甲胎蛋白的癌（Hepatoid and alpha-fetoprotein-producing carcinoma）：少数原发性胃癌含有免疫反应阳性的甲胎蛋白，还常表达癌胚抗原[259]，有时表达白蛋白和a-1-抗糜蛋白酶。其中某些肿瘤在形态学上与肝细胞癌相似，有些具有透明细胞腺管乳头状腺癌结构，另外一些显示这两种结构混合存在。这些不同的结构可能是消化系统胚胎内胚层分别向胎儿肝和肠分化发育的重复。一例报道还含有胎儿软骨[260]。这种癌预后差。

绒毛膜癌（Choriocarcinoma）：正常胃腺体颈部存在人绒毛膜促性腺激素免疫反应阳性细胞[261]。因此，已有50余例没有其他部位原发性肿瘤的胃绒毛膜癌的报道也许并不令人奇怪[262]。男女皆可发病。组织学上，多数肿瘤由典型的绒毛膜癌（由恶性合体滋养细胞和细胞滋养细胞构成）和不同分化程度的一般腺癌成分组成。偶尔混有胚胎性癌[263]或卵黄囊[264]成分。某些病例伴有血清绒毛膜促性腺激素水平升高，用免疫组化方法在滋养细胞中也可以检测到绒毛膜促性腺激素。常见播散性血行和淋巴转移。

小细胞癌（Small cell carcinoma）：胃小细胞癌是一种形态、组织化学和临床特征均与支气管小细胞癌相似的恶性肿瘤，并被认为是低分化内分泌细胞肿瘤[265-267]。这种类型的癌不到胃癌的1%；偶尔可能混有一般腺癌或类癌成分。

组织学上，肿瘤呈实性或片块状生长方式（图8.50），偶尔伴有腺泡状或小梁状结构，基底呈栅栏状排列，有时可见较普通的类癌结构。间质血管丰富，坏死十分常见。细胞小或中等大小，圆形或梭形，胞浆稀少，核形态相当规则，深染，核仁不明显，常有明显的核分裂和凋亡活性。部分肿瘤细胞胞浆有嗜银性，电镜显示偶见神经分泌颗粒。免疫细胞化学通常显示嗜铬素A或PGP 9.5阳性。在少数情况下，可见一种或多种肽类激素的表达，例如5-羟色胺、YY肽

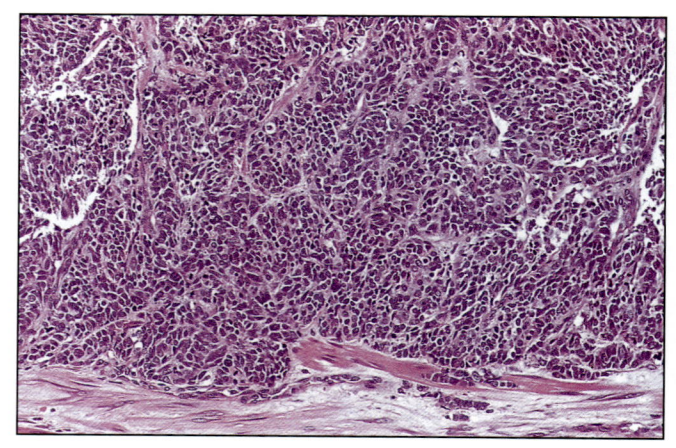

图8.50 胃小细胞癌常有清楚的边界。肿瘤细胞的细胞学特征与食管小细胞癌相似（见图8.16）。

生长抑素或胃泌素，但是由这些激素分泌所致的临床综合征非常少见。小细胞癌诊断时通常已是晚期，预后差，平均生存期不到1年。

癌肉瘤（Carcinosarcoma）：胃的癌肉瘤罕见[268,269]。男性常见，一般比普通胃腺癌患者年轻。多数病例发生于幽门，常为息肉状、浸润性的肿瘤，预后差。组织学上，可见腺癌的腺体成分与梭形细胞肉瘤样区域混合存在，肉瘤样区域可有骨肉瘤性、横纹肌肉瘤性、平滑肌肉瘤性[270]或软骨肉瘤性分化。曾报道了一例胃腺肉瘤，双向分化的肿瘤是由细胞学良性的腺体结构和散在的平滑肌肉瘤性间质成分组成的[271]。

类癌 Carcinoid tumors

临床特征：类癌是不常见的胃肿瘤，通常发生于中年人，表现为无症状的胃息肉[265,266,272]。大部分类癌为多发性无症状的胃体病变，发生在引起高胃泌素血症的内分泌细胞增生背景之上。与高胃泌素血症无关的散发性类癌少见，可发生于胃体或胃窦，一般较大，为侵袭性较强的病变，可以产生提示胃癌的临床症状[265,266]。

基于临床病理特征，WHO分类系统将胃的内分泌肿瘤分为3型[177]，此外，最近又提出第4种类型[273]。这4种类型胃内分泌肿瘤的主要特征总结在表8.4中。病变主要是根据发病机理而非病理学表现划分的，事实上，4种类型肿瘤的显微镜下特征通常是相似的。大多数肿瘤是低级别的肠嗜铬样（enterochromaffin-like, ECL）细胞肿瘤，正常情况下这种细胞位于胃体，在胃酸分泌中起主要作用。这些肠嗜铬样细胞的增生以及随之发生的肿瘤转化是由高胃泌素血症诱导的，高胃泌素血症是发生Ⅰ型、Ⅱ型和Ⅳ型类癌的根本原因，而且在这些病例中，也能见到发生于ECL细胞增生和异型增生背景之上的多发性肿瘤。在Ⅰ型类癌中，高胃泌素血症是由胃体慢性萎缩性胃炎，通常为自身免疫性胃炎，以及伴随的胃酸减少引起的[272,274,275]。在Ⅱ型类癌中，

表8.4　胃类癌的WHO分型（经Abraham等修正后[273]）

	Ⅰ型	Ⅱ型	Ⅲ型	Ⅳ型[a]（暂定）
先前存在的病变	胃体胃炎（通常为自身免疫性）	Zollinger-Ellison综合征（通常伴有MEN1）	无（散发的）	胃壁细胞盐酸分泌机能障碍
高胃泌素血症	存在	存在	没有	存在
类癌	小（<1.5 cm），常常多发，无非典型性	常小（但20%>15cm），通常多发，无非典型性	大，单发，可能有细胞学非典型性	小，多发，无非典型性
远处（肝）转移	2%～5%	10%	22%～75%	不清楚[b]
结局	不致命	很少致命	死亡率为25%	不清楚[b]
ECL细胞增生/异型增生	存在	存在	没有	存在
背景黏膜	慢性萎缩性胃炎和肠化生	肥大的泌酸腺体，增生的壁细胞	正常	肥大而扩张的泌酸腺体，增生的空泡状的壁细胞
临床处理	保守的内窥镜息肉切除；少数大的或明显恶性的肿瘤行胃切除	保守的内窥镜息肉切除；少数大的或明显恶性的肿瘤行胃切除	胃切除；息肉切除仅用于小的可以完全切除的组织学良性的肿瘤	不确定[b]

ECL：肠嗜铬样
[a] 假设的
[b] 报告的病例不充分，但是可能与Ⅰ型相似

高胃泌素血症是由 Zollinger-Ellison 综合征引起的，几乎总是发生在多发性内分泌肿瘤 I 型（而不是散发的胃泌素瘤）的背景之上，并且伴有胃酸过多症[276]。在 IV 型类癌中，高胃泌素血症是继发于原发性壁细胞分泌胃酸缺陷所致的胃酸缺乏，泌酸黏膜中的这些壁细胞组织学上呈现显著的增生和空泡变性[272,277]。III 型类癌是完全不同的一种类癌。尽管常常显示 ECL 细胞分化，但它们是散发的，通常为孤立性的肿瘤，没有高胃泌素血症或内分泌细胞增生的背景，体积较大，恶性度高，通常表现为出血，梗阻或转移[266,272,278]。在 ECL 细胞肿瘤中，因为肽类激素过度分泌而导致的临床症状非常少见，一般局限于非典型性类癌综合征[279]。罕见的原发性胃类癌可能显示伴有胃泌素产物的 G 细胞分化（位于胃窦），或伴有 5-羟色胺产物的 ECL 细胞分化[265]。异位促肾上腺皮质激素分泌导致的 Cushing 综合征也有报道[280]。

大多数类癌体积小，生长缓慢，尽管有局部浸润，但一般为低度恶性。局限于黏膜或黏膜下，而且显微镜下没有血管侵犯的直径小于 1 cm 的肿瘤极少转移，但随着肿瘤的增大，会出现脉管或固有肌层浸润，细胞学非典型性和核分裂活跃（所谓的非典型性类癌[265,266,278]），肿瘤易扩散，通常转移至局部淋巴结或肝[278]。然而，出现转移并不意味着患者不可以长期存活。导致临床高分泌综合征的功能性胃肿瘤几乎总是恶性的，但是相当少见。表 8.5 总结了有助于预测生物学行为的病理学特征[278,281]。发生高胃泌素血症的 I 型、II 型和 IV 型类癌通常较小（< 1 cm），转移少见[265,266]，II 型类癌体积常大于 I 型和 IV 型病变。有些 I 型类癌随着时间的推移可能消退[282]。因此，对于本组肿瘤的临床治疗措施是保守的，目的在于完全切除可见的病变，或者通过局部切除或进行内窥镜息肉切除术，此后进行内窥镜随访，并切除可能出现的新生病变[283]。少数 I 型类癌病例应用这种方法难以控制，胃窦切除术（切除引起高胃泌素血症的胃窦 G 细胞）可能有效。只有在肿瘤体积很大或数目较多，或显示明确的恶性特征时，才考虑胃切除术。另一方面，散发性 III 型类癌通常是一种伴有细胞学非典型性的核分裂比较活跃的肿瘤，具有潜在的侵袭性[265,266,272,278]，这类肿瘤最好应用与胃癌外科处理同样的原则进行部分或全胃切除术，除非肿瘤较小，可行息肉切除术，而切除的标本上显示良性的组织学特征（见表 8.5）。

大体表现：多数类癌表现为黏膜和黏膜下层的息肉状隆起，病变小而光滑，质硬，边界清楚。较大的肿瘤可能累及胃壁全层，偶有中心溃疡，切面呈灰黄色。周围胃体黏膜在 I 型 ECL 细胞类癌中呈现萎缩性改变，而在 II 型和 IV 型类癌黏膜可能肥大，伴有突出的黏膜皱褶，反映壁细胞增生。

镜下表现：典型的类癌是由小而一致的多边性或立方形细胞构成的，胞浆微嗜酸性，细颗粒状，细胞核规则，圆形或卵圆形，染色质点彩状，核分裂象罕见，核有轻

表8.5	胃类癌临床行为的病理学指征（after Capella et al.[281] With kind permission of Springer Science and Business Media.）

良性

< 1 cm，局限于黏膜和黏膜下层，没有血管浸润

交界性

局限于黏膜和黏膜下层
< 1 cm，出现血管浸润者
1～2 cm，没有血管浸润者

低级别恶性

任何功能性肿瘤
浸润超出黏膜下层
1～2 cm，出现血管浸润者
> 2 cm，没有血管浸润者

高级别恶性

非典型性类癌或小细胞癌

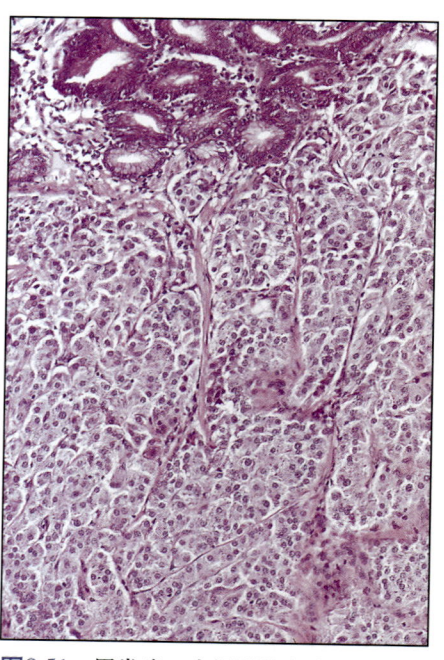

图8.51 胃类癌，由规则的内分泌细胞巢组成，胞浆嗜双色性。

度多形性（图 8.51）。一种透明细胞亚型曾被描述[284]。类癌细胞常为混合性生长方式，细胞排列成巢状或小梁状，由疏松的结缔组织间质分隔（图 8.52）。偶尔肿瘤细胞形成玫瑰花形团、小管状或腺泡状结构。肿瘤发生于胃黏膜，常常浸润黏膜下层，但很少有更深层的浸润。肿瘤细胞团周围收缩造成的人为假象，可能给人以淋巴血管浸润的印象。必须与具有预后意义的真正的脉管浸润鉴别（见表 8.5）。神经周围浸润可以发生，但不常见，其临床意义尚未确定。

多数胃类癌是嗜银性的，Grimelius（图 8.53）和 Sevier-Munger 染色均可呈阳性反应[272-276]，几乎没有亲银阳性反应的病例。免疫细胞化学染色显示嗜铬素 A、突触素、Leu-7 和 PGP（prprotein gene product，，蛋白基因产物）9.5 始终阳性，多数病例癌胚抗原阳性[262]。VMAT-2（vesicular monoamine transporter type 2，2 型小泡状单胺转运子）免疫染色是 ECL 细胞的特异标记物[285]，另外，虽然肿瘤还可能含有组胺[286]和组胺酸脱羧酶，但它难以在常规固定的切片上得到证实。电镜检查可见特征性的神经分泌小泡和实性颗粒（图 8.54）[265]。其他肽类激素也有少量存在, 例如 5- 羟色胺、胃泌素、生长抑素、胰多肽、高血糖素、降钙素和人绒毛膜促性腺激素（HCG）[265,272]。散发性肿瘤多半含有具这些内分泌颗粒的细胞。

I 型、II 型和 IV 型类癌周围胃体黏膜表现出显著的 ECL 细胞增生。这使胃腺体内的内分泌细胞数目增多，既可散在也可形成线状链索，扩展入胃固有膜和（或）黏膜肌层，形成结节或小巢（图 8.55）[274-276,287]。当这些结节或小巢不断扩大，融合并且开始浸润诱导间质生成时，称为异型增生[288]，当它们的直径超过 0.5 mm 或浸润黏膜下层时，就被定义为类癌。在 I 型类癌中还有慢性萎缩性胃炎的改变，并伴有显著的肠上皮化生，而在 II 型类癌，胃体黏膜常常由于泌酸腺体伸长、增生以及 Zollinger-Ellison 综合征的典型壁细胞增生，而引起黏膜皱襞肥大。壁细胞增生和肥大在两例 IV 型类癌的个案中也有描述[272,277]，不过这种壁细胞呈空泡状，其胞浆突入到扩张的泌酸性腺体中，腺腔内含有浓缩的嗜酸性物质，这与细支气管上皮（纤毛状）化生有关。

对病理医师来说，正确区分有细胞学非典型性的类癌和比较常见的"典型性"类癌非常重要，因为这一点具有重要的预后和治疗意义。非典型性类癌[278]的特征是，具有浸润性的生长方式，可能含有明显的血管侵犯

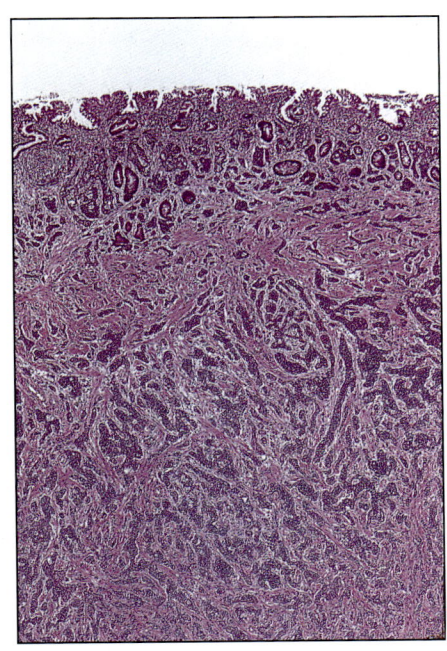

图 8.52 胃底类癌，伴有明显的小梁状生长方式，浸润黏膜和黏膜下层。散在显示肠上皮化生的残存腺体，提示背景存在与恶性贫血有关的慢性萎缩性胃炎。

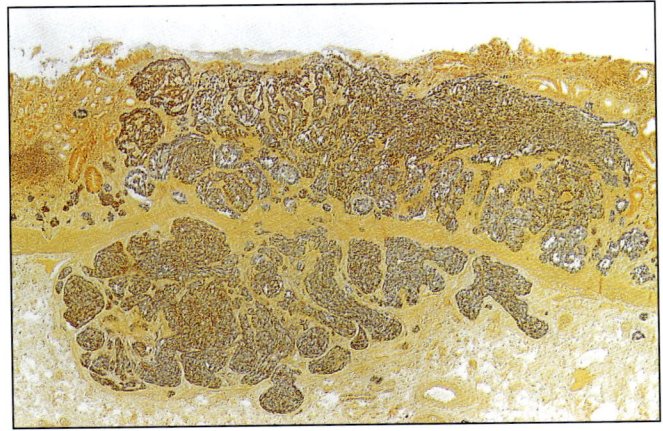

图 8.53 恶性贫血患者的肠嗜铬样细胞型胃类癌的嗜银细胞（Grimelius阳性），注意该视野左侧背景黏膜中的微小内分泌细胞巢（与图8.54对比）。

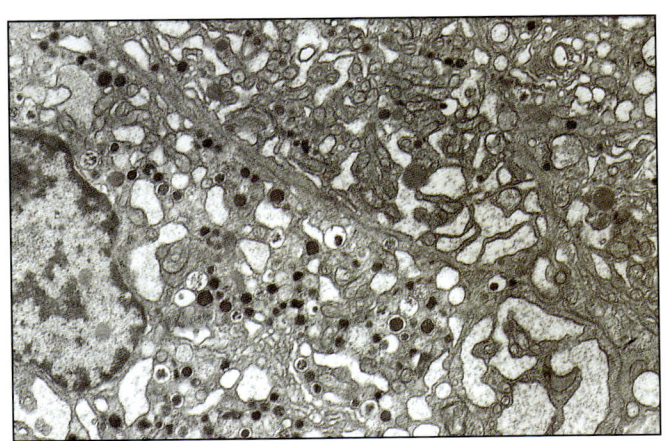

图 8.54 图 8.53中肿瘤细胞的超微结构，显示肠嗜铬样细胞的内分泌细胞颗粒。

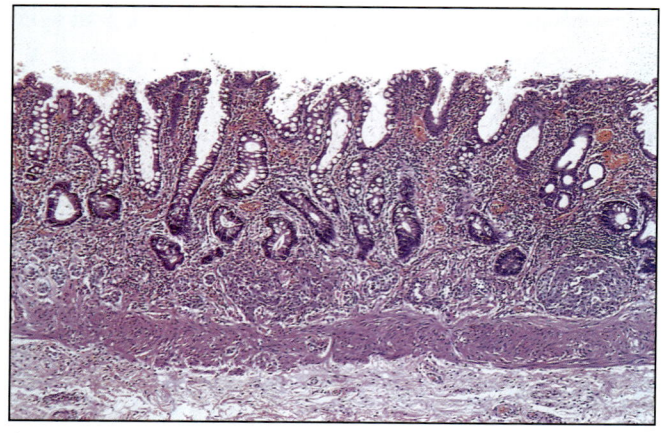

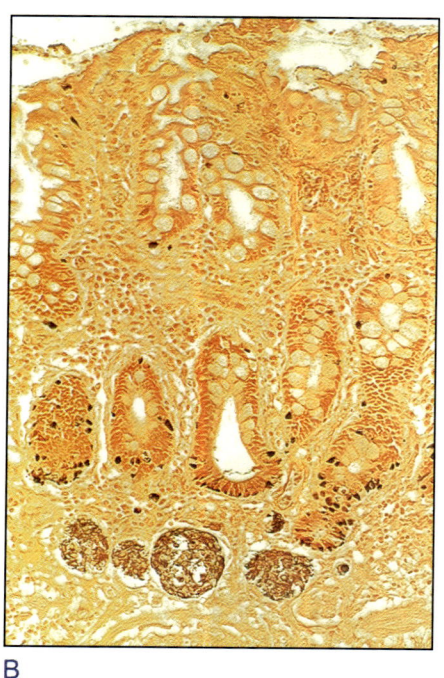

图8.55　H.E.染色切片（A）慢性萎缩性胃炎病变中肠嗜铬样细胞增生。在黏膜肌上方的黏膜基底部，清楚可见内分泌细胞呈结节状聚集。Grimelius 嗜银反应（B）也可显示胃腺体内分泌细胞增加。

和出现坏死区域。细胞学非典型性表现为核深染和核的多形性，常有明显的核仁，每10个高倍视野核分裂象多于两个[265]，以及表达 p53[278]。当这些特征特别明显时，某些作者使用大细胞神经内分泌癌这一术语[267]，因此，他们是与不良预后相关的。非典型性类癌的这些特征一方面可与普通类癌共存，另一方面，也可与显著恶性的小细胞癌共存（见第352页）。少数类癌，通常是具有非典型特征的类癌，也可与普通胃腺癌共存，即所谓的混合性肿瘤(composite tumors)、腺类癌(adenocarcinoids)或类癌腺癌（carcinoid adenocarcinomas）[289]。它们的预后类似于单纯性腺癌。

胃非上皮性肿瘤　Non-epithelial tumors

胃肠间质瘤
Gastrointestinal stromal tumors（GIST）

现在已经知道，绝大多数胃的间叶组织肿瘤不是以往所认为的平滑肌或神经鞘的肿瘤，而是一种显示 Cajal 间质细胞（肠的起搏细胞）分化特征的独特的肿瘤[290-292]。最显著的特征是免疫组化示酪氨酸激酶生长因子受体 KIT（CD117）的过度表达，并且已发现了阻断这种受体和类似受体的抑制剂，例如伊马替尼（imatinib），对于 GIST 的临床治疗可能具有显著而良好的作用[293]。因此，将 GIST 从其他少见的胃间质肿瘤中区分出来具有深远的临床意义。

临床特征：GIST 可发生于胃的任何部位。多见于30岁以上的成人，男女发病率相等，但也有儿童发病的记载。仅见于少数病例的公认的易感病变包括 I 型神经纤维瘤病[294] 和 Carney 等描述的两个综合征[295,296]。其中 GIST 与肺软骨瘤和（或）肾上腺外副神经节瘤共存，以及在罕见情况下，遗传性生长因子受体基因的种系突变，这种情况在散发性肿瘤的发病机制中可能起作用[297,298]。

小的胃间质肿瘤为无症状的胃壁内病变，常在其他无关疾病行剖腹术时偶然发现。较大的肿瘤常出现出血或腹痛，或偶然发生肿瘤破裂。肿瘤可以直接扩散到邻近器官，腹膜播散，以及经血行扩散到肝和肺[299,300]。

大体表现：胃间质瘤可单发或多发，大小不等，从微型壁内显微镜下可见的病变[301] 到巨大肿块都有。发生于胃近端的肿瘤比胃窦常见，而且可能更具侵袭性[299]。多数肿瘤为外生性浆膜下病变，突出于胃壁外表面。另一些肿瘤突入胃腔，表现为内生性息肉状黏膜下肿物，表面易发生溃疡和出血；少数肿瘤可向两个方向生长，形成哑铃状外观。肿瘤通常有清楚的边界，为结节状或有圆形凸起的肿块，缺乏真正的包膜。切面呈灰白色或粉红色，硬如橡皮或质地较软（图 8.56）。较大的肿瘤常发生囊性变、梗死、出血和坏死。除了明显侵犯邻近器官外，提示恶性的唯一大体特征是肿瘤的大小；小于5 cm 肿瘤的转移比大于10 cm 的肿瘤相对少见，而后者占绝大多数[299,302,303]。

镜下表现：胃间质瘤的组织学表现范围较宽，但是总的来说可见两种基本的细胞类型，即梭形细胞和上皮样细胞。典型的梭形细胞肿瘤（图 8.57）由交织成束状或漩涡状排列的均匀一致的梭形细胞构成，细胞核卵圆

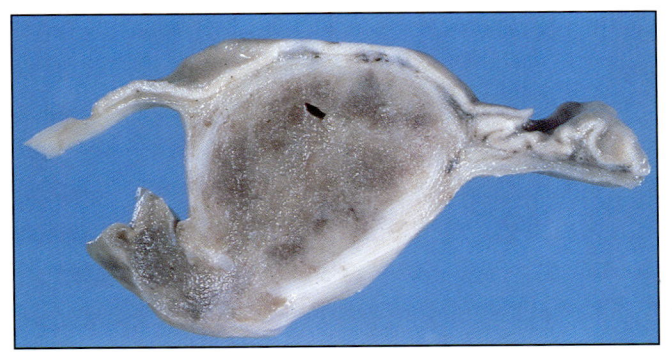

图8.56　主要呈外生性生长的胃间质瘤的横切面。

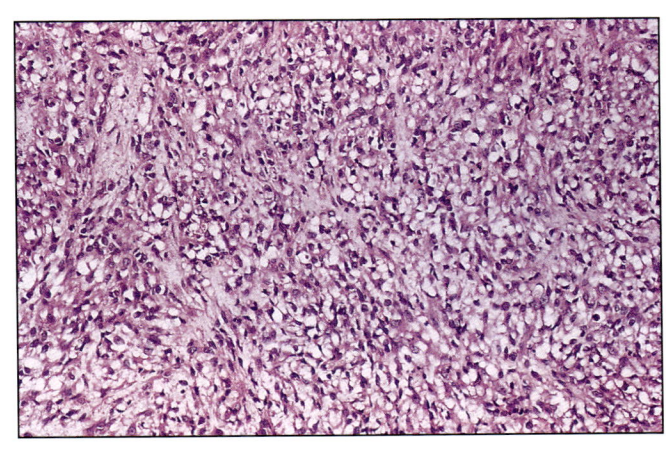

图8.58　伴有明显胞浆内空泡的上皮样胃间质瘤。

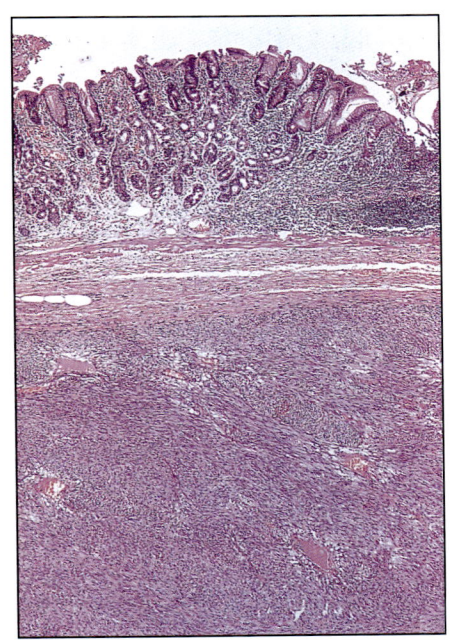

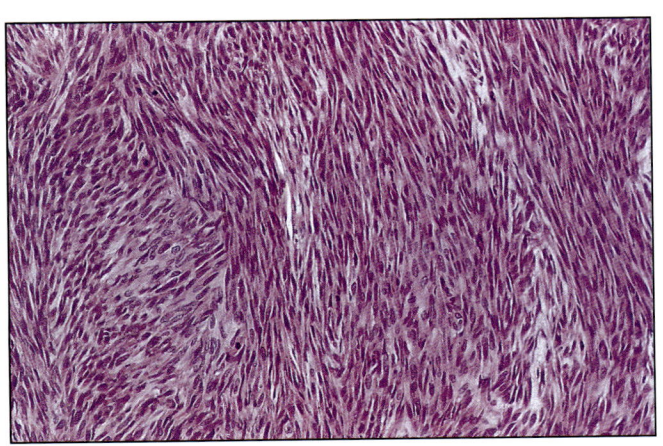

图8.57　梭形细胞胃间质瘤伴有清楚的边界（A）。有些区域细胞丰富，核深染，核分裂象常见（B），预示恶性临床行为。

形或细长，两端钝圆，纤维原性嗜酸性胞浆，其中可能含有一个清楚的核周空泡。有些肿瘤血管非常丰富，另一些肿瘤则显示神经分化，包括核呈栅栏状排列或丛状生长方式。少数病例含有"丝球样"（skeinoid）纤维，是散在分布于肿瘤细胞之间的小的球形或曲线形嗜酸性丝状物质的集聚[114]。细胞基质可能硬化、玻璃样变甚至钙化，一些病例有丰富的、富于透明质酸的黏液样结缔组织成分，其中散在分布圆形、星形或含有"花环样"核的多核肿瘤细胞[304]。胃梭形细胞性间质瘤（spindle celled GISTs）的细胞密集程度在同一肿瘤内部及不同肿瘤之间差异很大；多形性少见，而且通常与恶性潜能有关，但偶尔也可见于良性肿瘤变性区域的附近。Miettinen等[299]描述了一系列的形态学改变，他们将其称为硬化性、栅栏-空泡性、富于细胞性和肉瘤性，反映预后不良的频率依次增加。在明显恶性的梭形细胞肿瘤中，偶尔可见灶状脂肪肉瘤性、软骨肉瘤性、甚至横纹肌肉瘤性分化[305]，但是根据现今的标准，应怀疑这些肿瘤是否为真正的GIST。罕见情况下，可以见到具有这些表现的单相性肿瘤（见下文）。

上皮样间质瘤（epitheliod GISTs），以前称作"平滑肌母细胞瘤"或"奇异性平滑肌肿瘤"，多发生于胃窦，主要由圆形空泡状或透明细胞构成，一般排列成紧密连接的片块或细胞巢,形似上皮样结构（图8.58）[303]。胞浆内空泡可部分或全部包绕细胞核，偶尔似"印戒"细胞形态[306]，不要与脂肪母细胞瘤混淆。某些肿瘤是由连接松散或含丰富的嗜酸性胞浆的细胞组成的（图8.59）。这些细胞偶尔可具有显著的浆细胞样外观[114]。细胞核的特征不同，从伴有散在分布的细染色质和小核仁的圆形或卵圆形细胞核，到具有大的嗜酸性核仁的多形性细胞核，后者有时在多核瘤巨细胞中更为明显（图8.60）。同样，核分裂的多少也有较大差异，以致在谱系的另一端呈现明显的肉瘤性组织学图像。大约10%

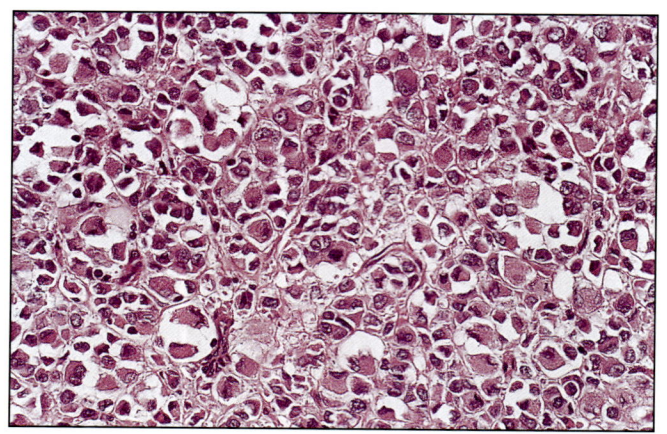

图8.59 恶性上皮样胃间质瘤，由单形性细胞组成，胞浆嗜酸性，核分裂象常见。

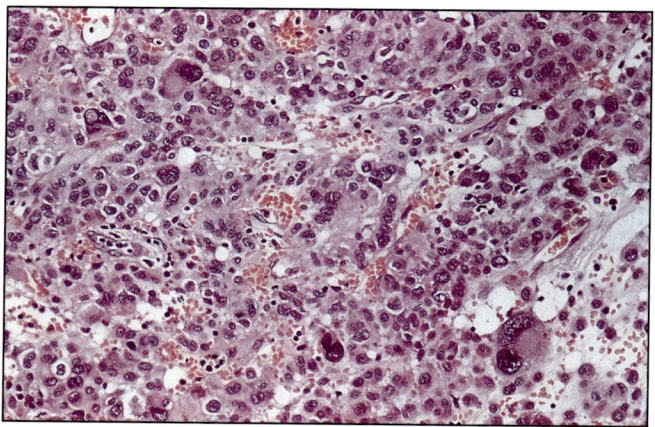

图8.60 上皮样胃间质瘤，显示明显的多形性和瘤巨细胞。

的胃 GIST 在不同区域显示梭形和上皮样两种细胞形态[299]。

在20世纪80年代和90年代，许多文献描述电镜下显示肠神经丛分化特征的胃间质瘤，即所谓的胃肠自主神经肿瘤（gastrointestinal autonomic nerve tumors, GANT）[307,308]，GANT 比其他的胃间质瘤具有更大的恶性潜能。发生在腹部器官或腹膜后者尤其易于复发和转移。然而近期研究指出，多数 GANT 具有与 GIST[309] 同样的光镜、免疫组化及分子特征，尤其是上皮样 GIST，故一般不再支持将 GANT 作为一个独立病种了。

GIST 最重要的免疫组化标记物是 KIT（CD117）的表达。KIT 见于绝大多数 GIST（>90%）[115,299,302,310]。染色显示通常较强而广泛，可以弥漫性分布于整个胞浆，局限于核旁呈点状分布或定位于细胞膜。然而，在某些病例中，KIT 染色可以是片块状或微弱的。多数胃 GIST（超过 80%）还表达 CD34，有些病例依然为片块状，约 25% 表达 SMA，约 5% 表达结蛋白，不到 1% 的病例表达 S100 蛋白[299]。常常报道的 GIST 的其他标记物包括波形蛋白、蛋白激酶 C（theta）、巢蛋白（nestin）、bcl-2 以及钙调结合蛋白（caldesmon），而某些病例表达 p53、PGP 9.5、神经元特异性烯醇化酶、Leu-7 和突触素[302,311]。

多数 GIST 病例 KIT 过表达的分子基础是 KIT 基因激活突变[310]，最常发生在 11 号或 9 号外显子，或为缺失或为点突变。这种突变在梭形细胞 GIST 比上皮样细胞 GIST 更为常见。越来越多的证据表明，KIT 突变的位点和特征影响肿瘤的生物学行为和对治疗的反应，即外显子缺失的肿瘤似乎比点突变的肿瘤更具侵袭性，9 号外显子突变的肿瘤对伊马替尼治疗的反应不如 11 号外显子突变的肿瘤[312]。然而，少数 GIST 却是另外一个生长因子受体基因，即血小板驱动的生长因子受体 α（platelet drived growth factor receptor alpha，PDGFRA）发生突变[313]。这些肿瘤常常具有上皮样的形态学表现，而且可能具有良好的预后[314]。虽然 KIT 免疫组化过表达也可见于许多 PDGFRA 突变的肿瘤[299]，但那决不是普遍的。同样，尽管具有典型的形态学（以及其他的免疫组化）特征[315,316]，某些 GIST 可以是"KIT 阴性"的（"KIT-negative"），另一方面，由于某些 KIT 阴性的肿瘤对包括伊马替尼在内的酪氨酸激酶受体抑制剂可能有反应，所以必须认识到 KIT 免疫阳性不是诊断 GIST 的必要条件。有人发现，伊马替尼治疗后的患者，KIT（和 CD34）免疫阳性缺失，同时伴随着从梭形细胞到上皮样表型的转变，这会引起诊断的混淆[317]。与伊马替尼治疗后有关的其他组织学特征包括细胞密度降低、间质玻璃样变性或黏液样改变，以及出现伴囊性变的液化坏死区域。然而，广泛取材可以发现富于细胞的肿瘤区域，这也许是已经获得了新的突变的肿瘤病灶，是造成抗药的原因。

预测行为：发生于胃的 GIST 多数呈现良性经过[299]。然而，病理学评估 GIST 的良恶性是相当困难的，除非有明显的邻近器官浸润或有明确的转移[318]。有人发现，诸如细胞密集和核的多形性等支持恶性的一般组织学指征有助诊断[318]，但是另外一些病例的结果却令人失望，尤其是上皮样肿瘤，上述指征似乎显示为良性行为；据报道，核的多形性意味着良性行为，而恶性肿瘤则为容易使人误诊的单形性细胞[53,303]。一般来讲，上皮样肿瘤比梭形细胞肿瘤恶性的危险性更大，虽然血管浸润或非典型性核分裂象是提示恶性的较好指标，但却并不常见[305]。当组织学检查证实有明确的固有膜浸润时，高度提示为恶性[53,299]，而且凝固性坏死（而不是伴有囊性变的液化性坏死）也与不良预后有关。然而迄今为止，最有用的参数是肿瘤的大小[302,303,319]和核分裂数[13,300,302,305]（或 Ki-67 标记的增殖指数[302,320]）。表 8.6 显示预测发生在胃肠道所有部位 GIST 生物学行为的统一方法[292]。现将

表8.6	确定任何解剖部位GISTs侵袭性行为危险性的NIH统一标准（Fletcher 等[292]）	
	大小（cm）（最大径）	核分裂计数（每50 HPF）
非常低度危险	<2	<5
低度危险	2～5	≤5
中度危险	≤5 5～10	6～10 ≤5
高度危险	>5 >10 任何大小	≥5 任何核分裂计数 >10

这种方法复制于此，因为它已广泛用于病人治疗和临床研究。因为即使是小的、形态学上温和的 GIST 在少见情况下也可转移，所以应该避免将任何的间质瘤明确地称为良性间质瘤。最近对于在新的疗法出现以前诊断的，有长期随访资料的 1765 例单纯性胃 GIST 的研究发现[299]，基本支持这一统一的预测方法，但也发现一些差异。在这一研究中，"非常低度危险"（very low risk）组中，没有病例发生肿瘤相关性死亡，而少于 3% 的"低度危险"（low risk）肿瘤病人疾病进行性进展，作者分别将其称为良性和可能良性（probably benign）。然而，按这种方法划分为"中度危险"（intermediate risk）的两组肿瘤却存在差异。最大径 5～10 cm，伴有低核分裂率（<5/50 HPF）的肿瘤其行为表现为"低度危险"，而最大径 2～5 cm，核分裂性象 >5/50 HPF 的肿瘤侵袭性较强，肿瘤相关性死亡率是 12%～15%。按这种方法分类为"高度危险"（high risk）的肿瘤中，核分裂率似乎比肿瘤大小更为重要，以致所有最大径大于 5 cm、伴有核分裂数 >5/50 HPF 的肿瘤均具有高度恶性潜能，伴有 49%～86% 的肿瘤相关死亡率。而 >10 cm、核分裂数少的肿瘤被认为具有相对低的侵袭性。这项研究提出的评价单纯性胃 GIST 恶性潜能的标准总结在表 8.7 中。

许多研究试图将 DNA 倍体和分化标志物的免疫组化表达与肿瘤恶性潜能联系起来。不出意料，尽管只有少数恶性肿瘤为二倍体，但非整倍体与预后不好明显相关[319,321]。对于应用其他标准认为是交界性的肿瘤，DNA 倍体分析可能具有重要价值；一项研究显示，所有非整倍体的交界性肿瘤均被证实为致死性的[318]。另一研究提示，纯粹的交界性梭形细胞肿瘤有平滑肌标记物的表达是预后良好的一个指征，正如任何一种类型的肿瘤出现神经标记物的表达也是如此[311]。

鉴别诊断：除了下面所描述的真正的平滑肌和神经鞘瘤以外，胃 GIST 的鉴别诊断包括炎性纤维性息肉（inflammatory fibroid polyp）（见第 366 页）以及少数非常罕见的梭形细胞增生性病变。这些病变包括胃炎性肌纤维母细胞瘤（gastric inflammatory myofibroblastic tumor），这是几乎只发生于儿童[322]和年轻成人的病变；还有发生于胃浆膜的孤立性纤维瘤（solitary fibrous tumor）[323]、所谓的胃壁钙化性纤维瘤（calcifying fibrous tumor）[324]，以及累及胃的韧带样纤维瘤病（desmoid fibromatosis）（见第 24 章）。KIT、CD34、结蛋白、S-100、bcl-2、CD99、Alk-1 以及 β-连环蛋白（β-catenin）的免疫染色有助于解决多数病例的诊断问题。虽然病理医师在任何少见胃肿瘤的鉴别诊断中考虑 GIST 是明智的，但重要的是要认识到不是所有 KIT 阳性的（KIT-positive）胃肿瘤都是 GIST。表达 KIT 这种标记物的其他病变包括骨髓肿瘤、小细胞癌、转移性黑色素瘤、精原细胞瘤、乳腺癌、炎性肌纤维母细胞瘤，以及纤维瘤病也可以有 KIT 表达。

平滑肌瘤 Smooth muscle tumors

真正的平滑肌肿瘤在形态学上与发生于食管的一样（见第 337 页），的确有少数病例发生在胃贲门部[13,291]。肿瘤强烈表达结蛋白和 SMA，而不表达 KIT。

神经鞘瘤 Schwannomas

约 2% 的胃间叶性肿瘤是良性神经鞘瘤[325,326]。这些肿瘤与神经纤维瘤病无关，一般表现为结节状或多结节状、息肉样或胃壁内肿瘤，几乎无出血、坏死或囊性变。肿瘤由在纤维背景上排列成束的细长的 S100 蛋白阳性的细胞组成；可以有核的多形性，但核分裂象非常少见。Verocay 小体、血管玻璃样变性、Antoni A 和 Antoni B 区很少见，其表现与软组织神经鞘瘤不同[326]。

表8.7	评价胃GISTs恶性潜能的推荐标准（参照Miettinen 等[299]）	
	大小（cm）（最大径）	核分裂计数（每50 HPF）
良性	<2	<5
可能良性	2～10	<5
不确定或可能低度恶性	<2	>5
可能低到中度恶性	2～5 >10	>5 <5
可能高度恶性	>5	>5

肿瘤边缘特征性地被显著的淋巴细胞袖套所包绕，可以有生发中心形成。胃神经鞘瘤通常 GFAP 阳性，偶尔含有 CD34 阳性细胞。然而，KIT、结蛋白和 SMA 阴性。

脉管肿瘤　Vascular tumors

发生于胃壁内的脉管肿瘤包括血管瘤[327]、淋巴管瘤[328]、血管内皮细胞瘤[329]（包括上皮样型血管内皮细胞瘤[330]），Kaposi 肉瘤（可为发生于 AIDS 患者的原发性胃肿瘤[331]或为全身性疾病的一部分[332]），以及血管肉瘤[333]（包括上皮样血管肉瘤[334]）。血管球瘤发生在胃窦部为仅次于皮肤的第二个最常见的部位，常在胃壁内形成结节，可以形成溃疡并引起出血[335]。其较常见于女性，极少数的病例发生转移。组织学及免疫表型检查示胃血管球瘤与皮肤的血管球瘤的病变相同（图 8.61）

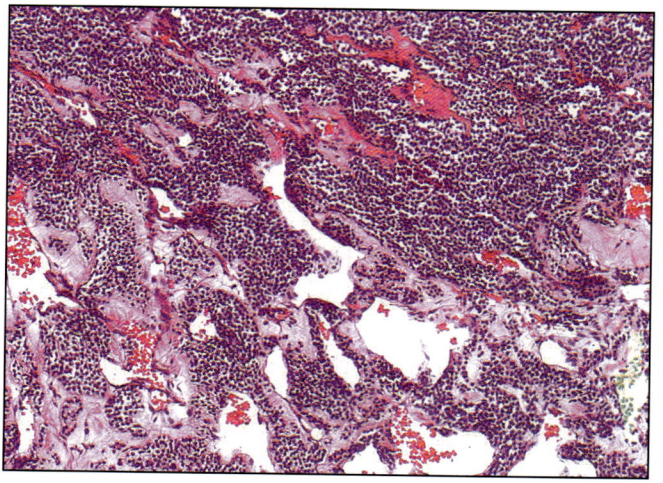

图 8.61　胃血管球瘤。

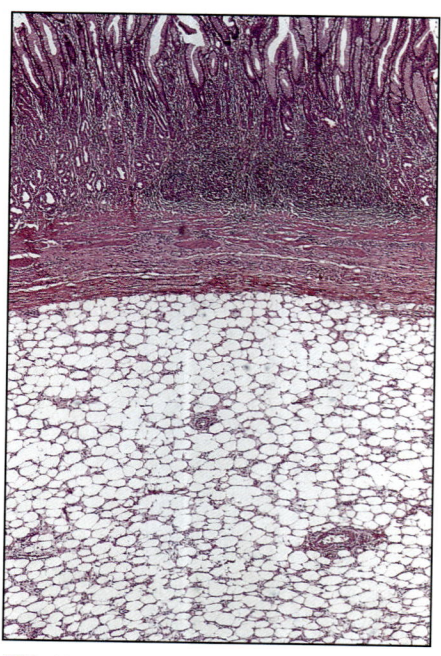

图 8.62　胃黏膜下脂肪瘤。

（见第 3 章），但如果不注意，可与上皮样间质瘤、类癌、其他血管肿瘤甚至恶性淋巴瘤混淆。

其他结缔组织肿瘤　Other connective tissue tumors

胃的很多良性和恶性结缔组织肿瘤已有记载，常为个案报道。这些肿瘤包括横纹肌瘤[336]和横纹肌肉瘤[337]，黏膜下[338]（图 8.62）或浆膜下脂肪瘤、血管脂肪瘤[339]、脂肪肉瘤[340]、良性纤维组织细胞瘤[341]、滑膜肉瘤[342]、透明细胞肉瘤[343]、副神经节瘤[344]、神经节细胞瘤和神经节母细胞瘤[345,346]、单发或多发性颗粒细胞瘤[116]、良性间叶瘤[347]和畸胎瘤[348]。

胃恶性淋巴瘤　Malignant lymphoma of the stomach

近年来对胃肠道黏膜相关淋巴组织（mucosa-associated lymphoid tissue，MALT）的认识已有很大进展（见第 21 章）。对于细胞系细致的形态学、免疫组织化学和分子生物学研究，让人们对于胃的淋巴组织肿瘤进行重新评价，并正确认识不同类型的肿瘤[349,350]。

胃恶性淋巴瘤可为原发性，也可继发于全身性淋巴瘤[350]。支持原发性肿瘤的特征为肿瘤主体位于胃和(或)局部淋巴结，不累及浅表或纵隔淋巴结、肝、脾、骨髓或外周血液。然而，这种区分多少存在人为因素，有时并不能识别少见的细胞表型，尽管其强烈提示是来源于胃肠道的播散性淋巴瘤。

免疫表型显示绝大部分原发性胃淋巴瘤为 B 细胞系，大部分来自 MALT，少数是套细胞淋巴瘤[350]。T 细胞和无标记细胞（null cell）肿瘤非常少见[351]。胃原发性 Hodgkin 淋巴瘤从未见报道，尽管播散性 Hodgkin 淋巴瘤可以累及胃。至于以累及小肠为特征的淋巴瘤，即肠病相关性 T 细胞淋巴瘤(enteropathy-associated T-cell lymphoma)，并非胃的原发性肿瘤，而免疫增生性小肠疾病（地中海淋巴瘤，α-链病）累及胃非常罕见；有一例浸润性胃印戒细胞淋巴瘤的报道[352]。

"MALT"的原发性胃B细胞淋巴瘤　Primary gastric B-cell lymphoma "of MALT"

临床特征：这是迄今为止西方人群中最常见的胃淋巴瘤。多数患者为中年或老年人，表现为消化性溃疡或胃癌的特征，取决于病变的程度[353]。实际上，90%以上的肿瘤均发生在慢性幽门螺杆菌相关性胃炎的基础上[354,355]。流行病学研究提示，幽门螺杆菌在本病的发病机制中具有重要作用[350]，而且低级别胃 MALT 淋巴瘤（MALT lymphoma）患者在根除幽门螺杆菌后肿瘤

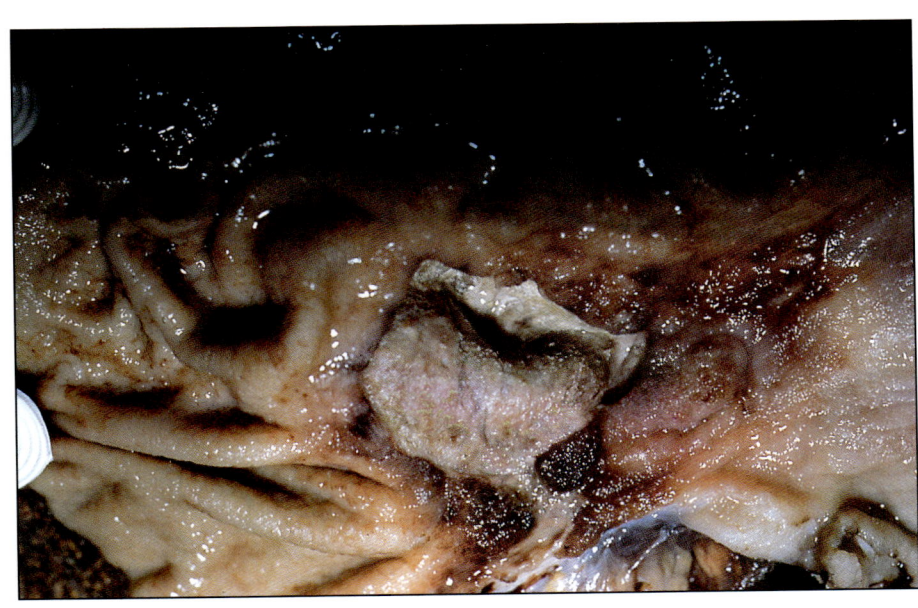

图8.63 溃疡型高级别胃恶性淋巴瘤。

常常消退,这就进一步证实了上述观点[356]。部分但不是全部显示弥漫性大 B 细胞淋巴瘤(diffuse large B-cell lymphoma,DLBCL)形态的高级别淋巴瘤是从这种低级别淋巴瘤转化而来的[349,354,357]。幽门螺杆菌阴性的胃黏膜相关淋巴组织淋巴瘤(MALToma)与丙型肝炎病毒感染以及某些自身免疫疾病有关[355]。根据报道,少数胃 MALT 淋巴瘤发生于免疫抑制的 AIDS 或器官移植术后的患者[358];后一组病例的高级别淋巴瘤可能与幽门螺杆菌无关,而通常与 EB 病毒有关[359]。还有同时发生胃原发性腺癌和 MALT 淋巴瘤的报道,但罕见[360]。

胃 MALT 淋巴瘤的预后与诊断时的疾病分期和肿瘤分级有关[361]。修正的 Ann Arbor 结外淋巴瘤分期系统已广泛应用[362],在发现时绝大多数患者病变局限于胃或区域淋巴结(I_E 期和 II_E 期)。最近提出的以 TNM 分期原则为基础的 Paris 分期系统更有临床意义[363]。局限于胃黏膜和黏膜下层的低级别淋巴瘤可以首先通过根除幽门螺杆菌予以治疗,治疗失败的患者通常需要手术切除。较晚期的低级别肿瘤或高级别肿瘤患者采用手术治疗,辅以化疗和放疗。一项大的系列研究显示,低级别肿瘤总的 5 年生存率是 91%,而高级别为 56 %[361]。由于本病常在胃内多灶发生,经过治疗的患者需要在内窥镜下随访以确定有无局部复发[364]。应该注意的是,有些肿瘤容易转移至其他有 MALT 的器官,包括肠的其他区域、涎腺、甲状腺和肺[365]。

大体特征:许多胃 B 细胞淋巴瘤大体与胃癌相似,可为息肉样、蕈伞状或溃疡性肿瘤(图 8.63),最常位于胃窦部。另外一些肿瘤与消化性溃疡难于区分,某些早期低级别肿瘤大体表现相对没有特征性,内窥镜医师可能将其描述为重度胃炎,有时黏膜呈结节和鹅卵石状,伴有糜烂或浅表溃疡形成[353]。可有局部淋巴结肿大。

镜下特征:胃黏膜内有大量弥漫分布的低级别 MALT 淋巴瘤(边缘带 B 细胞淋巴瘤,marginal zone B-cell lymphoma),通常为多形性的细胞浸润,这些细胞具有边缘带 B 细胞免疫表型(CD20+CD21+CD35+IgM+IgD-)[349,353,355,361,366,367],具有活跃生发中心的反应性滤泡(可能是幽门螺杆菌感染的宿主反应)被成片的小到中等大小的不规则的肿瘤性淋巴细胞包绕,这些细胞具有不规

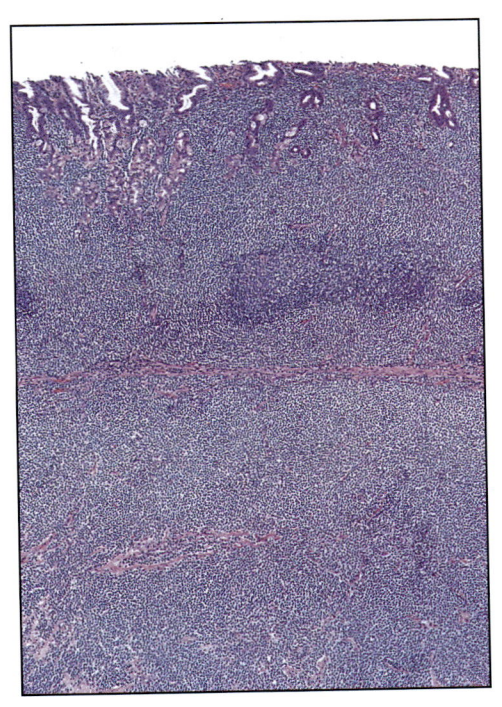

图8.64 原发性低级别胃B细胞淋巴瘤。成片的小到中等大小的淋巴细胞浸润黏膜和黏膜下层,包绕反应性的黏膜淋巴滤泡,固有的黏膜腺体消失。

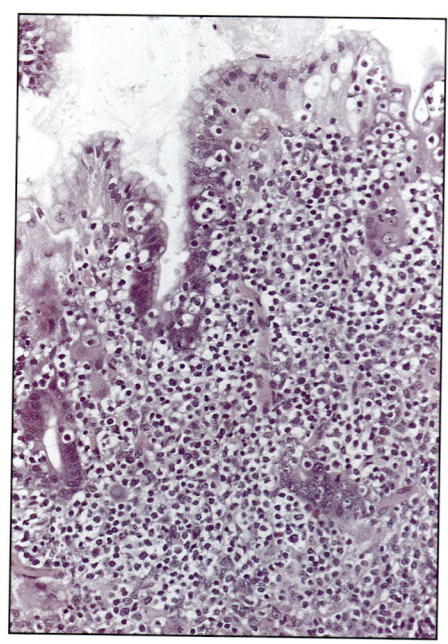

图8.65 原发性低级别B细胞淋巴瘤的淋巴上皮病变。本例固有层内的中心细胞样细胞胞浆透亮，类似于单核细胞样B细胞。

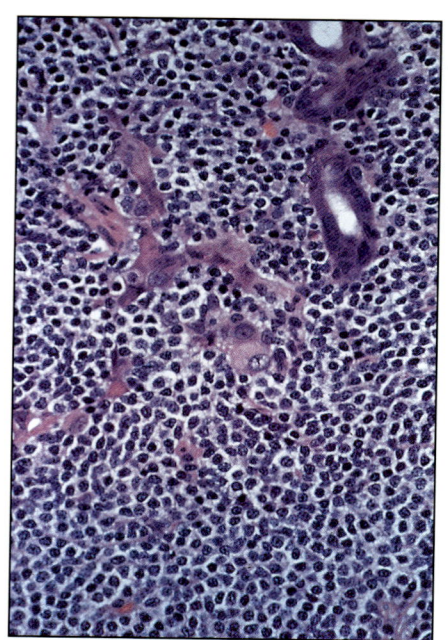

图8.66 原发性低级别B细胞淋巴瘤。固有的腺体实际上已被肿瘤性淋巴细胞破坏，仅仅偶见残存的嗜酸性上皮细胞簇。

则的细胞核（图8.64），即所谓的"中心细胞样细胞"(centrocyte-like cells)。中心细胞样细胞弥漫扩散进入周围的胃黏膜，并且特征性地侵犯胃腺体上皮，形成淋巴上皮病变（图8.65）。这些腺体的显著破坏常常导致在大片的中等大小淋巴细胞中出现孤立残存的嗜酸性上皮细胞（图8.66）；偶尔这些细胞具有印戒样特征，必须小心不要误诊为癌[368]。肿瘤细胞并非总像中心细胞，有时它们更像小淋巴细胞或有丰富淡染胞浆的单核细胞样B细胞[366]。肿瘤通常存在散在的母细胞，而且常有明显的浆细胞分化，特别是在黏膜的表浅部分，浆细胞可在表面上皮下方形成带状结构[353]。中心细胞样细胞

可浸润或"蔓延"至反应性的B细胞滤泡，或选择性地"进入"生发中心，不损害套区。当局部淋巴结受累时，首先显示在滤泡边缘周围有同样的浸润，酷似所谓的"单核细胞样B细胞淋巴瘤"(monocytoid B-cell lymphoma)，可能与完全不同的T区淋巴瘤的滤泡旁浸润相混淆[367]。免疫表型显示，肿瘤细胞B细胞标记物（CD20，CD79a）染色阳性，但肿瘤细胞CD5，CD10，CD23，bcl-6或周期蛋白（cyclin）D1阴性[349,350,355]。胃MALT淋巴瘤的分子病理学和细胞生物学是复杂的[349,355]，不能在这里一一详述。然而，具有特殊临床意义的是，具有染色体易位 t（11;18）(q21;q21) 的肿瘤导致融合蛋白 AP12-

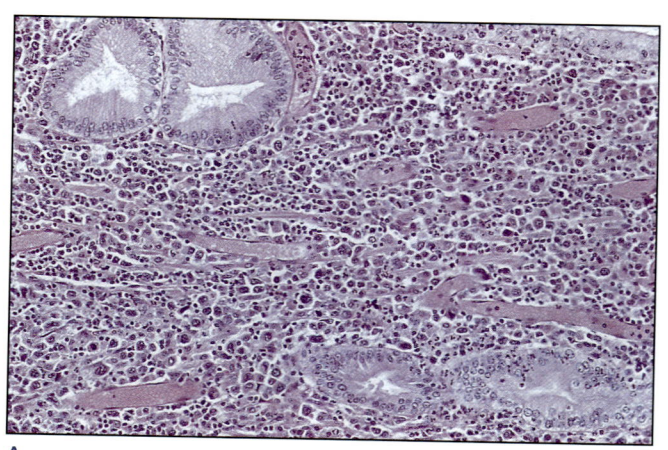

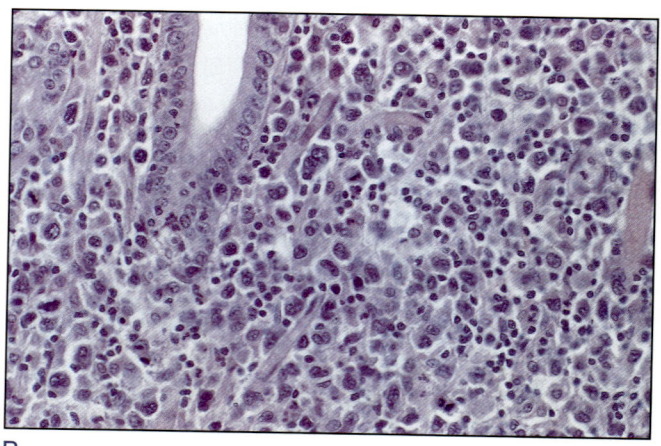

图8.67 (A, B) 原发性高级别胃B细胞淋巴瘤。浸润的肿瘤细胞为多形性，有大量核分裂活跃的母细胞，不同于低级别淋巴瘤的中心细胞样细胞，不形成淋巴上皮病变。

MALT1表达，而伴有 bcl-10 细胞核表达的肿瘤通常对幽门螺杆菌根除疗法无反应，并且更容易播散到胃外[349,369-372]。

胃的高级别B细胞淋巴瘤或原发的胃DLBCL（图8.67）以成片的转化母细胞为特征，通常类似于中心母细胞，但有时类似免疫母细胞，常使胃腺体和原有的淋巴滤泡消失。这些细胞可与低级别肿瘤中相似的多种形态的细胞或反应性的小T细胞混合存在；只有少数病例形成淋巴上皮病变[354]。可见肿瘤坏死。仔细观察广泛取材的高级别淋巴瘤将会发现，25%以上的病例伴有典型的低级别肿瘤的特征[357]，有分子遗传学证据表明，这代表后者的高级别转化[372]。高级别肿瘤不会随幽门螺杆菌的根除而消退[356]，因此，在内窥镜活检组织中通过识别融合成片或成簇的母细胞来确定高级别成分的存在是非常重要的（数量较少的弥漫散在的母细胞在低级别肿瘤中是常见的）[354]。根据母细胞的相对比例和分布特征的内窥镜活检分级系统具有很强的临床实用性[373]。

鉴别诊断：过去习惯上认为，最重要的鉴别诊断是假淋巴瘤，这是一种成熟淋巴组织的反应性增生，可累及胃壁全层，常伴有溃疡形成。然而，最近的研究，尤其是应用克隆性标志物的研究表明，大多数假淋巴瘤实际上是低度恶性的真正的淋巴瘤[353,367,374,375]。仔细研究发现，特征性存在中心细胞样细胞、淋巴上皮病变和限制性轻链。假淋巴瘤行部分胃切除术后表现出明显的良性行为，只不过是反映了对于低级别B细胞淋巴瘤手术治疗取得成功。因此，有人提议应该废除假淋巴瘤这一名称。这并不是说胃壁从不发生显著的良性淋巴细胞浸润；偶尔，其可见于胃的炎性病变，例如消化性溃疡或Crohn病，但在这种情况下，通常形成淋巴细胞聚集而不是淋巴瘤的中心细胞样细胞的片状浸润。

主要的诊断难点在于区分MALT低级别B细胞淋巴瘤与有时发生在慢性胃炎的重度慢性炎症细胞浸润，尤其是在内窥镜活检时。实际上，这种鉴别也许是不可能的，尤其是在小块活检组织中，可能需要重复取样或密切内窥镜随访以鉴别这种情况。如果淋巴细胞浸润严重而伴有弥漫胃腺消失，那么淋巴瘤的诊断是明确的。另一方面，如果浸润呈片状而并没有将腺体推挤开，则很可能是反应性的[350]。出现明显的淋巴上皮病变可以考虑诊断为淋巴瘤，前者定义是腺体结构被三个以上成群的淋巴细胞浸润破坏[374]；尽管在极少数情况下，严重的幽门螺杆菌胃炎也可见到上皮内成簇的B淋巴细胞，但他们并不伴具有胞浆嗜酸性变的上皮细胞破坏[354]。应该强调的是，淋巴上皮病变明显不同于淋巴细胞性胃炎散在的上皮内淋巴细胞增多，后者通常在表面上皮特别明显，实际上从不成群，由T细胞组成[376]。免疫染色证实，浸润的细胞为克隆性免疫球蛋白轻链限制，如果确定的话，支持恶性诊断，但由于混合的反应性淋巴细胞及背景染色的存在，明确判定常常是困难的。PCR克隆性免疫球蛋白基因重排检测既不敏感也不特异；仅有大约75%的淋巴瘤呈现阳性结果，而且11%的慢性幽门螺杆菌胃炎的活检也呈阳性反应[377]。

低级别MALT淋巴瘤必须与其他少见类型的累及胃的小细胞恶性淋巴瘤相鉴别（见下文）。除了形态学以外，应用一系列的抗体进行的免疫组化染色有助于解决诊断问题，包括CD5、CD23、CD10、bcl-6和周期蛋白D1。高级别淋巴瘤可能与非淋巴类型的恶性肿瘤混淆。弥漫型胃癌最为相似，尤其当淋巴上皮病变破坏腺体，出现孤立的印戒样形态的上皮细胞时[367]（必须牢记，两种病变偶尔共同存在[360]）。容易混淆的其他病变包括髓细胞白血病浸润（绿色瘤，chloroma）、胃肉瘤和转移性恶性黑色素瘤；一例报告[378]强调了黑色素瘤细胞浸润上皮非常类似于淋巴上皮病变。黏液组织化学和免疫细胞化学染色对于做出正确诊断是非常重要的。

恶性淋巴瘤性息肉病（Malignant lymphomatous polyposis）：胃黏膜和黏膜下广泛受累有时表现为多发性息肉，或更常见的是胃黏膜弥漫性增厚、黏膜皱襞苍白粗大，形成了一种脑回样的大体表现。这些肿瘤不是MALT淋巴瘤，基本上都是套细胞淋巴瘤；在这些病例中，胃的病变几乎都是播散性系统性疾病的一部分，在循环血液中通常可以检测到肿瘤细胞。显微镜下显示形态单一的小淋巴细胞弥漫性浸润，细胞核常为不规则折叠状，围绕但不进入残留的非肿瘤性生发中心，有时散在有透明变性的胶原带[379]。常可见散在的上皮样组织细胞[350,380]。与MALT B细胞淋巴瘤不同，该肿瘤细胞很少形成淋巴上皮病变，肿瘤细胞显示CD5、IgD和核内周期蛋白D1阳性，后者反映了t(11;14)染色体易位，这是套细胞淋巴瘤的特征。这种肿瘤预后不好，中位生存期为2～3年[350]。

尽管曾经有人认为恶性淋巴瘤性息肉病表现套细胞淋巴瘤的特征，但现在认为同样的大体表现在少数情况下可以见于其他类型的淋巴瘤，包括滤泡中心细胞淋巴瘤[350]和T细胞淋巴瘤[381]。

其他淋巴瘤（Other lymphomas）：任何不同类型的发生于外周淋巴结的低级别或高级别的B细胞或T细胞淋巴瘤，均可发生于胃（见第21章）。不过，经仔细检查排除原发性MALT型B细胞淋巴瘤后，这类肿瘤并不多见，多数证明原来是继发性胃肿瘤[382]。4种淋巴瘤

(见第21章）值得提出：滤泡性淋巴瘤（follicular lymphoma），其中肿瘤性滤泡必须与发生在低级别MALT淋巴瘤中的肿瘤性中心细胞样细胞植入的反应性滤泡相鉴别[350]；淋巴细胞性淋巴瘤（lymphocytic lymphoma，又称为慢性淋巴细胞性白血病，chronic lymphocytic leukemia），以表达CD5、CD23但核不表达周期蛋白D1的小圆形淋巴细胞为特征；Burkitt淋巴瘤（Burkitt's lymphoma），通常见于儿童及年轻成人，其组织学表现与发生在其他部位者相同；以及罕见的孤立性浆细胞瘤（solitary plasmacytomas）[383]，本病必须与更为罕见的反应性病变（浆细胞肉芽肿[384]）相鉴别，通过检测免疫球蛋白轻链限制来判定。

胃的T细胞淋巴瘤是罕见的侵袭性淋巴瘤，多数报道来自远东地区，通常与HTLV-1感染有关[385,386]。他们主要是成人T细胞白血病/淋巴瘤或外周T淋巴瘤的胃侵袭病灶，肿瘤由小、中等到大多形性细胞组成，其细胞谱系只能通过免疫细胞化学或克隆性T细胞受体基因重排证实。很少病例表现上皮内T细胞表型，与肠内发生的T细胞淋巴瘤相似（见第384页）[387]。

朗汉斯细胞组织细胞增生症（组织细胞增生症X）
Langerhans cell histiocytosis (histiocytosis X)

胃可作为朗汉斯细胞组织细胞增生症的一部分而受累（见第21章），亦可作为局限性病变部位，有时形成黏膜小结或息肉[388]。需借助免疫细胞化学，有时还需电子显微镜与其他类型的胃单核细胞浸润相鉴别。

髓细胞增生性疾病
Myeloproliferative diseases

髓细胞性白血病累及胃壁可形成黏膜小结或斑块，罕见情况下形成息肉状或弥漫性浸润肿块（所谓的粒细胞肉瘤或绿色瘤）[389,390]。髓细胞样化生浸润胃窦部胃壁而导致幽门梗阻也有报道[391]。髓细胞增生性病变的诊断是根据细胞形态、氯乙酸酯酶组织化学和免疫细胞化学，并借助临床和血液学发现对其进行解释（见第22章）。

继发性肿瘤　Secondary tumors

转移至胃的肿瘤罕见。尽管有些转移性肿瘤可以引起幽门或贲门梗阻、出血或穿孔，但多数无症状。肺、胰腺、结肠、乳腺、甲状腺和前列腺癌，恶性黑色素瘤以及肝细胞癌是最常见的原发肿瘤[392,393]。转移性肿瘤可为单发或多发，转移性乳腺小叶癌可弥漫性浸润胃壁，酷似皮革胃（图8.68）[394]。

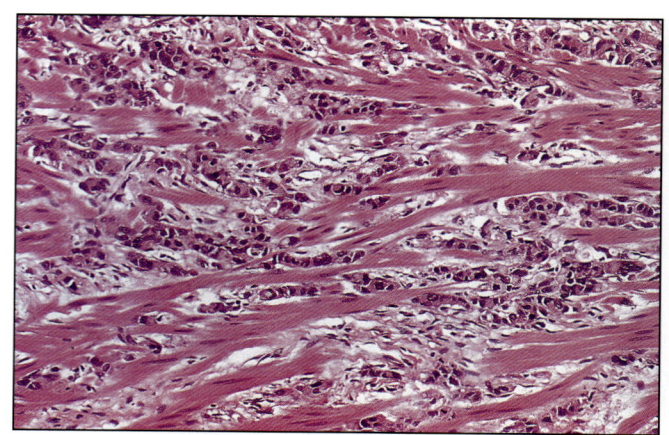

图8.68　胃壁内转移的乳腺小叶癌。

瘤样病变　Tumor-like lesions

胃增生性（再生性）息肉
Hyperplastic (regenerative or hyperplasiogenous) polyps of stomach

临床特征：增生性息肉是胃息肉中最常见的类型[168,169,172,782]。Nakamura将其分为两型（I型和II型）[172]。这种病变被认为是黏膜损伤后过度再生所致，例如慢性螺杆菌相关性胃炎[395]、恶性贫血，可发生在溃疡和糜烂边缘部，或位于胃肠吻合口处，常常发生在伴有肠化生的萎缩性胃炎的背景上[396]。Nakamura I型增生性息肉通常为单发性，位于胃窦部；而II型息肉通常为多发性，分布于胃底黏膜远端，常常在大致相当于胃体胃窦交界的部位成行排列。

增生性息肉随着时间的增长数目可能增多，也可消退，或为自行消退，或比较常见的是在根除幽门螺杆菌后消退[396]。少数（可以达到3%）息肉，通常是直径超过2cm的息肉显示异型增生或黏膜内癌（见图8.29）[182,201]，而且同时伴有胃其他部位癌的病例也有报告[169,172,182]；因此，对于所有的增生性息肉患者的背景黏膜进行仔细的内窥镜下检查非常重要。2cm或2cm以上的病变应该完全切除，并进行组织学检查以除外肿瘤。

大体表现：增生性息肉可无蒂或有蒂，表面光滑或分叶状，直径一般小于2cm。Nakamura II型息肉常有中央凹陷，相当于乳头状表面上皮的内折（图8.69）。常常发生表浅糜烂。

镜下表现：组织学上，两种类型的息肉均有胃小凹上皮增生，导致腺体变长扭曲，显示囊性改变和不规则分支（图8.70）[397]。另外，在Nakamura II型息肉，息

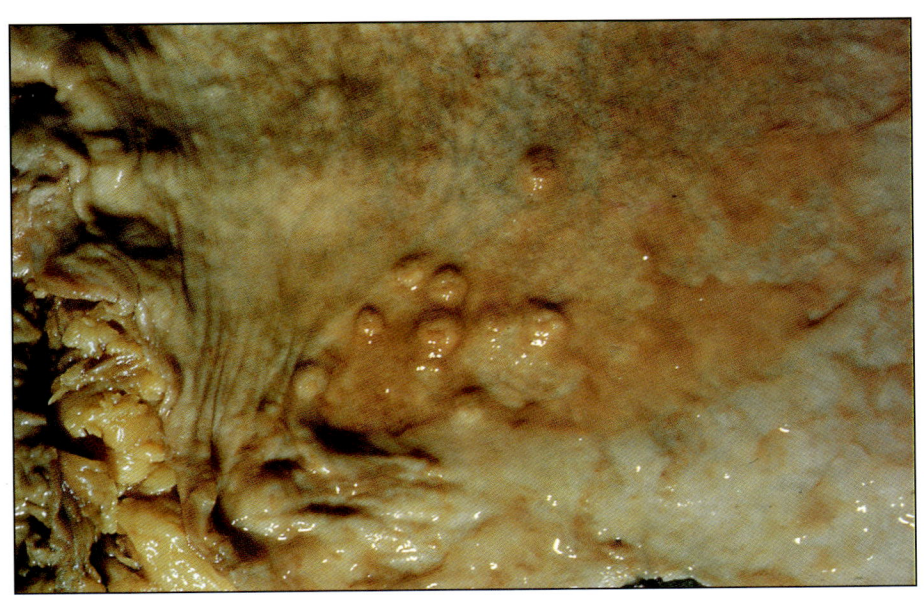

图8.69 胃多发性无蒂增生性息肉，伴有中央凹陷。

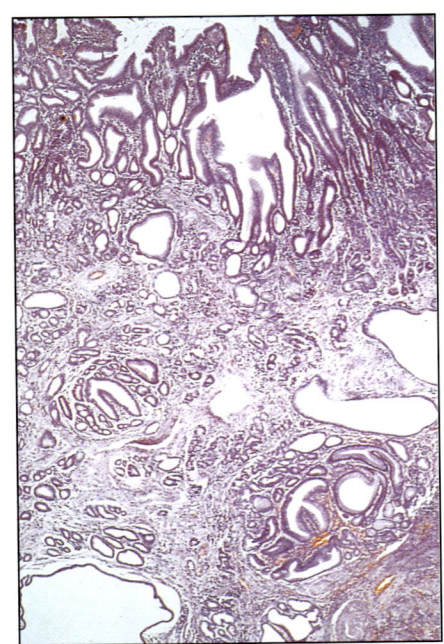

图8.70 胃增生性息肉。

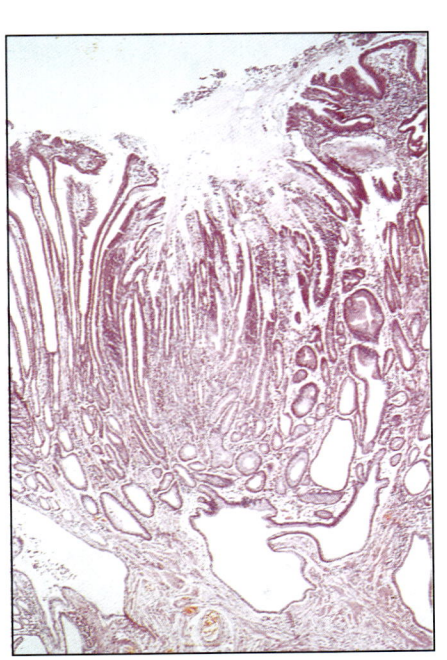

图8.71 胃增生性息肉，表面浅表腺体呈洋葱皮样排列，相当于大体所见的凹陷（图8.69）。

肉中央部分的腺体呈洋葱皮样外观（图8.71）[172]。腺体内衬单层增生的小凹型上皮，也可以见到幽门型腺体、主细胞、壁细胞以及肠化生灶，特别是在深层。息肉表面可见溃疡和急性炎症，上皮和间质细胞显示变性和再生性非典型性；这一点可能造成诊断混淆，因为在增生性息肉中（见上文）可以见到真正的癌（见图8.29）[182]和假浸润[248]。息肉间质水肿，有浆细胞和淋巴细胞（包括伴有生发中心的滤泡）以及嗜酸性粒细胞浸润，而且基底部胃腺体之间可见由黏膜肌层延伸而来的平滑肌纤维。

鉴别诊断：与腺瘤性息肉的鉴别在第342页已经讨论过。增生性息肉可能难以与局限性 Ménétrier 病（见第368页）、幼年性错构瘤性息肉、或 Cronkhite-Canada 综合征（见下文）鉴别。综合考虑临床、内窥镜和大体表现通常有助于诊断。

胃底腺息肉 Fundic gland polyps

胃底腺息肉可为散发性[168,398,399]，也可发生于家族性腺瘤性息肉病（familial adenomatous polyposis, FAP）患者[171]，或为局限于胃的家族性病变[400]。以往认为本病常见于长期接受质子泵抑制剂治疗的病人[398]，这种观点已经受到质疑[401]。胃底腺息肉一般为多发性，可以见于任何年龄的男性或女性。大体表现为玻璃样透明的无蒂息肉，直径小于1 cm，局限于胃体-胃底部黏膜。

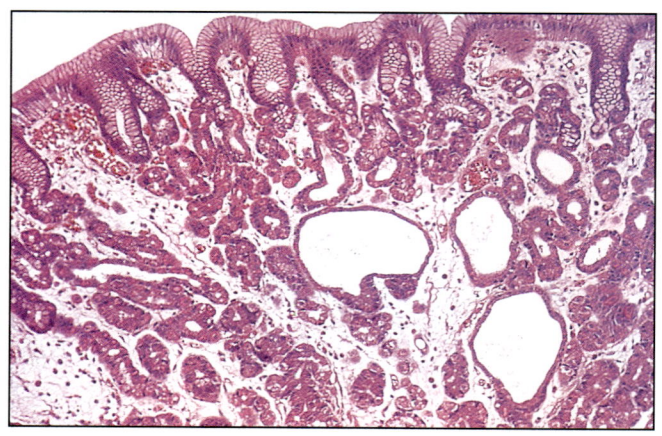

图8.72 发生于胃体的胃底腺息肉。

组织学上，息肉由囊状扩张的腺体构成，腺体内衬增生的胃底腺上皮，包括壁细胞和主细胞，混有正常的腺体（图8.72）[398]。其上方的小凹缩小，一般无炎症和非典型性的证据[402]。在囊性腺体周围可能有不规则的紊乱分布的平滑肌纤维[398]。接受质子泵抑制剂治疗的患者伴有壁细胞肥大和增生，这些细胞突入胃小凹腔内，产生锯齿样结构（图8.73）[403]。

最近，偶有伴异型性增生的胃底腺息肉的病例报告，或为散发性，或发生于家族性腺瘤性息肉病的背景上，伴有APC基因体细胞突变[404]。这一发现加之在无异型增生的胃底腺息肉发现的β-catinin突变[405]，提出一种可能性，即某些病变（即使不是所有的）可能是真正的肿瘤，而不是以前所认为的错构瘤性或增生性病变。另一方面，自发性消退也有报道[399]。病人治疗的意义目前还不明确。虽然多发性异型增生性胃底腺息肉患者可以进行内窥镜监测，尤其是发生在FAP背景之上者，但是目前并不提倡用于散发性无异型增生的病例。然而，在年青患者发现胃底腺息肉，需要考虑存在FAP的可能性。

炎性纤维性息肉
Inflammatory fibroid polyp

这是一种不常见的良性病变，原因不明，见于任何年龄的男性或女性成人，而且某些病例伴有胃酸过低或缺乏[406,407]。通常见于胃窦部，可为偶然发现，或表现为胃出血或出现胃流出道梗阻的症状。

该息肉大体检查为小的，边界清楚的，孤立性，无蒂或有蒂的病变，常有溃疡形成（图8.74），有时确诊困难。组织学上，病变通常以黏膜下层为中心（尽管单纯的黏膜内病变曾被描述），类似于水肿的肉芽组织（图8.75），病变由小的薄壁血管周围环绕具有长的胞浆突起的梭形细胞构成，这些细胞在较大血管的周围可能排列成"洋葱皮"结构。有时可见具有深染核的"花环"样多核巨细胞。有慢性炎细胞浸润，常以嗜酸性粒细胞为主，但

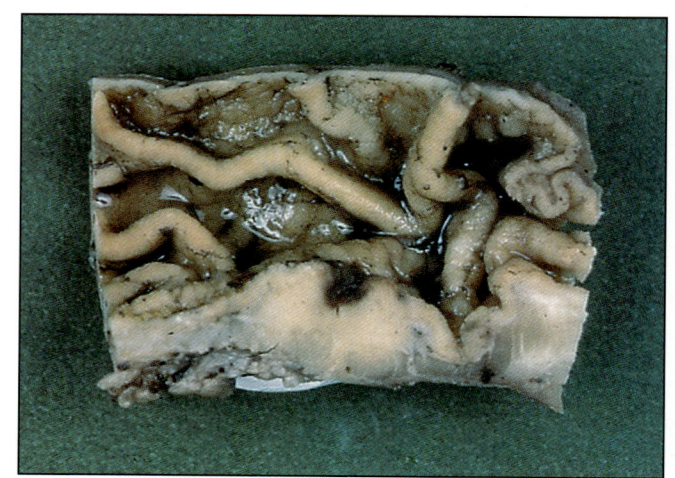

图8.74 伴有表面溃疡的胃炎性纤维性息肉的横切面。

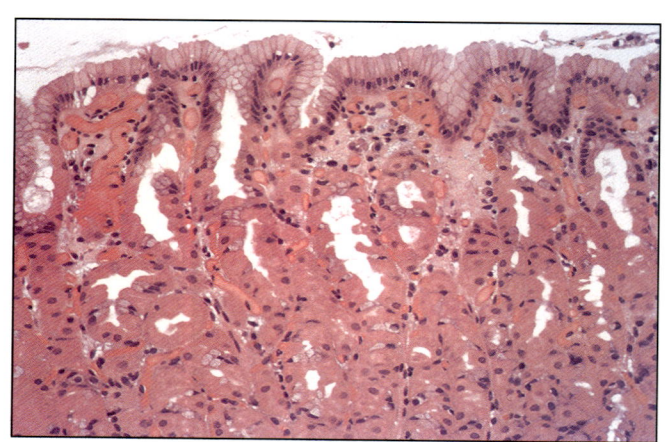

图8.73 接受质子泵抑制剂治疗的患者胃底腺壁细胞增生。

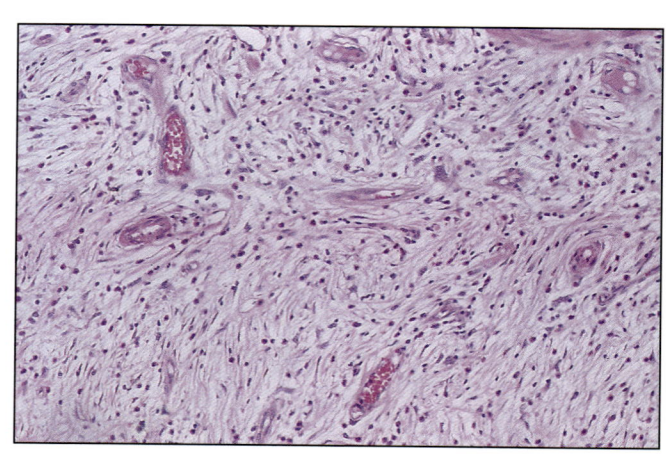

图8.75 炎性纤维性息肉含有大量嗜酸性粒细胞。

与嗜酸性粒细胞性胃炎（eosinophilic gastritis）不同，后者发生于儿童或年轻成人，表现为胃窦弥漫性增厚和变形，从而造成幽门狭窄，炎性纤维性息肉不伴有循环血中嗜酸性粒细胞增加，也无特异性反应性病史。梭形细胞显示 CD34、fascin 以及（通常）钙调节蛋白（calponin）免疫染色阳性，提示本病或为树突状细胞或为肌纤维母细胞系起源[407]。KIT（以及钙调结合蛋白）染色常为阴性，可以用于与胃间质瘤鉴别。炎性纤维性息肉还应该与罕见的与寄生虫感染有关的嗜酸细胞性肉芽肿鉴别。

其他黏膜息肉　Other mucosal polyps

Peutz-Jegher 息肉病[408]可以累及胃，但远比累及小肠和结肠少见。这些错构瘤性息肉由增生的腺体构成，腺体内衬小凹型上皮，被分枝状的平滑肌束分隔，伴有深部腺体成分萎缩（图 8.76）。有 Peutz-Jegher 息肉病伴胃癌的罕见报道[409]，但原先存在的息肉发生癌变的几率如何，还远不清楚。然而，有报道称，在一例胃 Peutz-Jegher 息肉中发现异型增生[410]。

胃的幼年性息肉（juvenile polyps）罕见，常常发生在幼年性息肉病的基础上，或仅发生于胃[411]，或发生于整个胃肠道（伴有或不伴有家族史）。可以在任何年龄发生，通常伴有贫血和低蛋白血症，最常见于胃窦。幼年性息肉病与患胃肠道癌的危险性增高有关，尤其是在结直肠，但胃也处于危险之中，胃幼年性息肉病发生异型增生和癌已有描述[411]。组织学上，胃幼年性

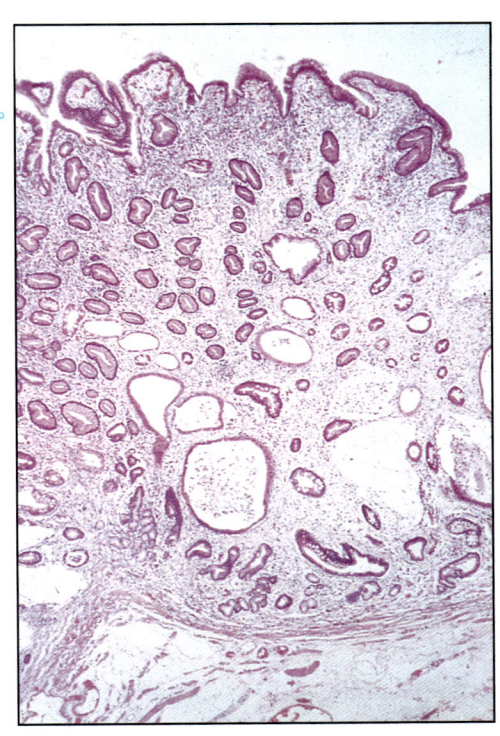

图 8.77　胃幼年性息肉。其表现难以与 Cronkhite-Canada 综合征鉴别，也可以非常类似于增生性息肉。

息肉是由水肿和发炎的黏膜构成，伴有小凹明显伸长、扭曲和囊状扩张（图 8.77）。其大小比具有更明显的小凹上皮增生的囊性胃底腺息肉要大。幼年性息肉不具有 Peutz-Jegher 息肉中的平滑肌纤维，但可与增生性息肉相混淆。

胃息肉也可以发生在 Cowden 病，由上皮和（或）结缔组织（平滑肌或神经）组成。文献中有关其组织学描述很少，但有一个病例报告，息肉是由增大变长的小凹腺体和基底部伴有乳头状内折的囊性扩张的腺体组成的。平滑肌纤维与黏膜成分相混杂，囊状结构有时延伸到黏膜下层[412]。

Cronkhite-Canada 综合征的息肉发生在胃已被认识[168]，通常连带有胃肠道其他部分的病变。组织学上与幼年性息肉无法区别，只有在出现脱发、指（趾）甲萎缩或色素沉着过多等临床表现时才可诊断[413,414]。

异位　Heterotopias

胰腺异位[415]是胃先天性异位最常见的类型，表现为胃部肿块，伴有幽门梗阻或消化性溃疡的症状，或为内窥镜检查、剖腹术或尸检时的偶然发现。通常见于幽门部或胃窦，为位于胃壁内的半圆形、圆锥形或短圆柱状的肿块。最具特征性的表现是黏膜表面中央凹陷，表示 1 个或多个残留的胰腺导管的开口。切面类似于正常胰腺。组织学上，肿块由正常胰腺腺泡和导管构成（图

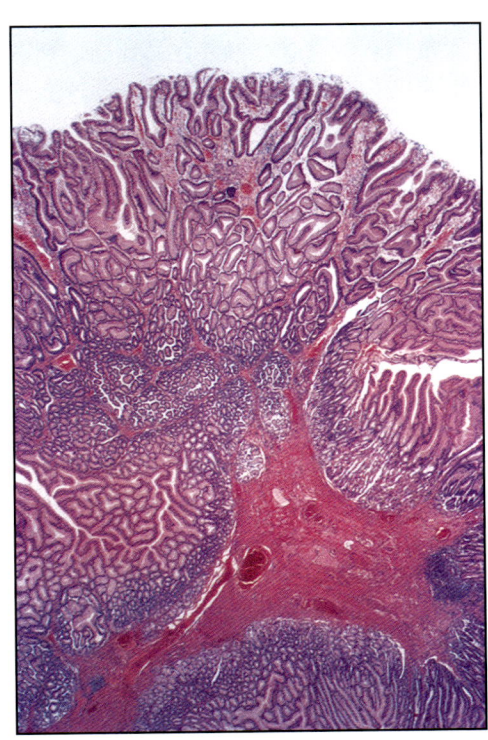

图 8.76　胃 Peutz-Jeghers 息肉。

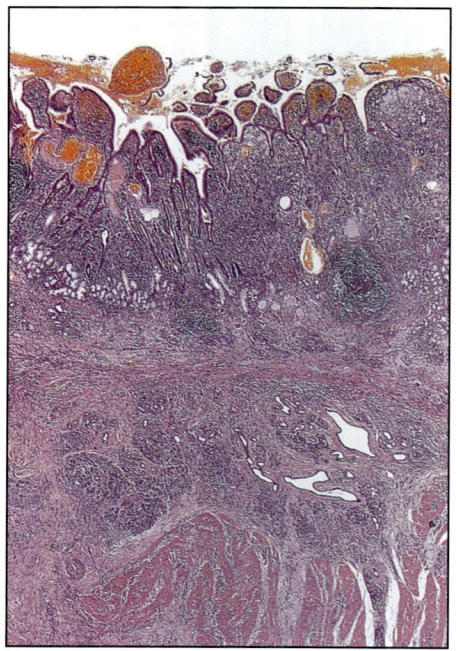

图8.78 胃与十二指肠交界处的胰腺异位，黏膜下层可见胰腺腺泡和导管，深达肌层。

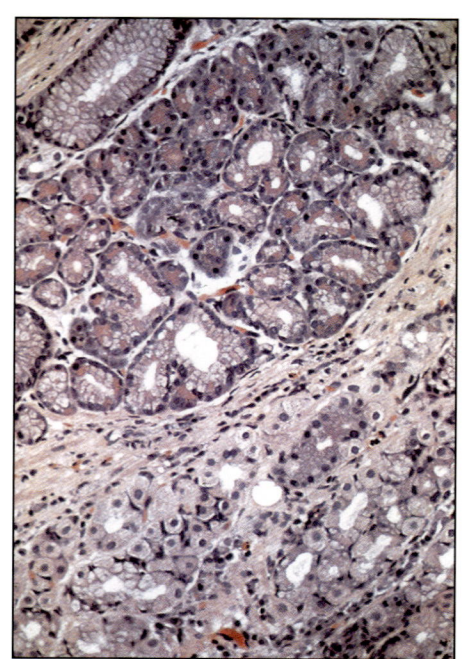

图8.80 贲门的胰腺腺泡化生。

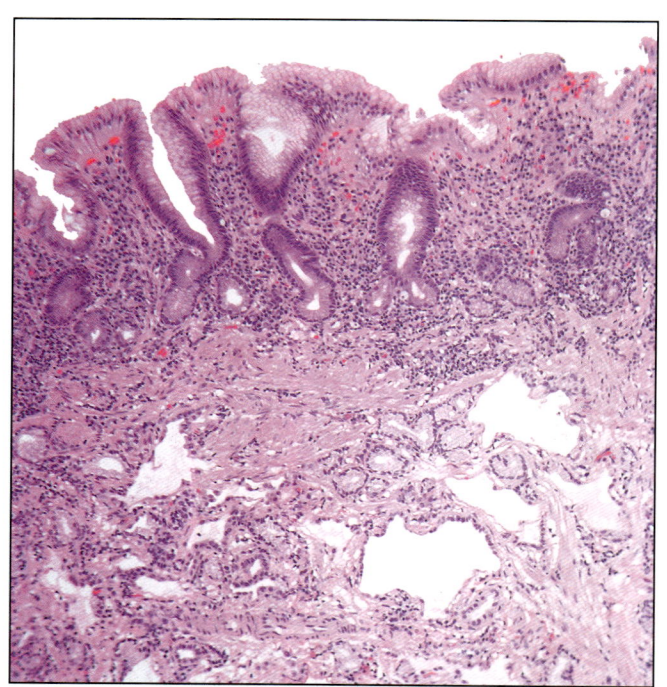

图8.79 胃腺肌瘤的活检。

8.78），其中许多导管和腺泡发生囊性扩张，偶见胰岛和十二指肠型腺体（Brunner-type glands）。当平滑肌和导管样结构(伴有或不伴有 Brunner 腺）为仅有的成分时(图8.79），称为腺肌瘤（肌上皮性错构瘤）[416]。有罕见的腺肌瘤[417]或异位胰腺[418]发生腺癌的记载。局限于黏膜的局灶性胰腺型腺泡和导管被称为胰腺腺泡化生（图8.80）[419]，特别是在贲门部，尽管其来源可能是先天性而不是获得性的[420]。

胃内可能发生的其他类型的异位包括局限性十二指肠腺聚集，可能形成所谓的"息肉样黏膜十二指肠腺瘤"（polypoid mucosal Brunner's adenoma）[421]，内衬纤毛上皮的胃壁内囊肿[422]，或伴有致密的淋巴细胞间质（"淋巴上皮囊肿"，lymphoepithelial cyst）[423]以及黏膜中的灶状鳞状上皮。还有1例累及整个胃后壁和小弯的鳞状上皮乳头状瘤病的报道[424]，其中胃黏膜被成熟的过度角化的鳞状上皮取代，没有非典型性的证据。在黏膜下层存在大片的鳞状包涵体，并且有乳头状瘤性鳞状上皮突出于浆膜面。可以想象，这种病变是化生性甚或肿瘤性的。

Ménétrier 病（增生性或肥大性胃病、巨大胃皱襞肥大）
Ménétrier's disease (hyperplastic or hypertrophic gastropathy, giant rugal hypertrophy)

临床特征：Ménétrier 病是一种病因不明的少见病变，少数病例有家族史[425]，与其他疾病没有明确关系[426]。好发于男性，尽管也有儿童发病的报道，但主要见于中年成人[427]。患者可无症状，或出现消化性溃疡病的症状，伴胃酸过低、低蛋白血症和贫血。本病可自行消退，也可发展为慢性萎缩性胃炎[428,429]。据报道，其与发生胃癌的危险性增加有关（图8.81），但是这种危险性的大小很难量化[201,426]。

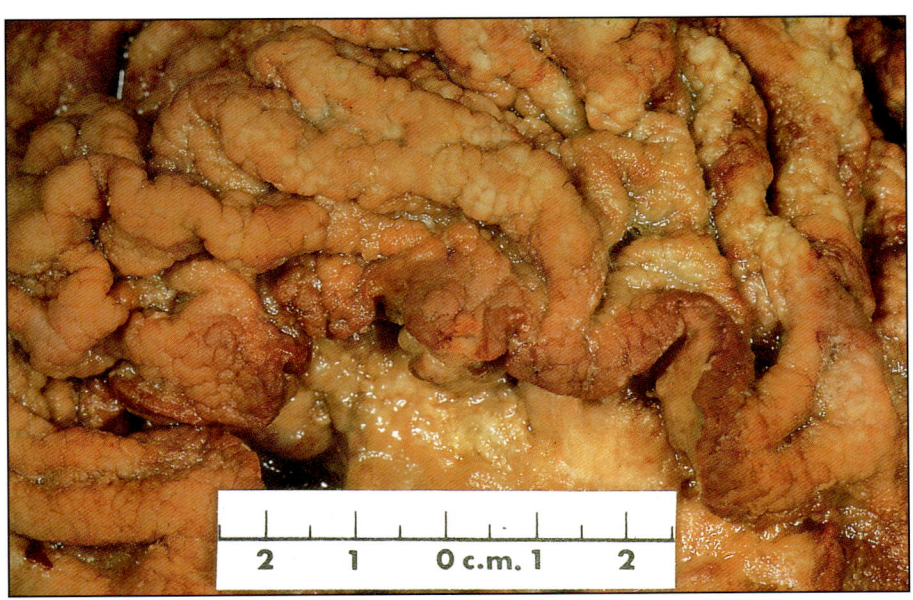

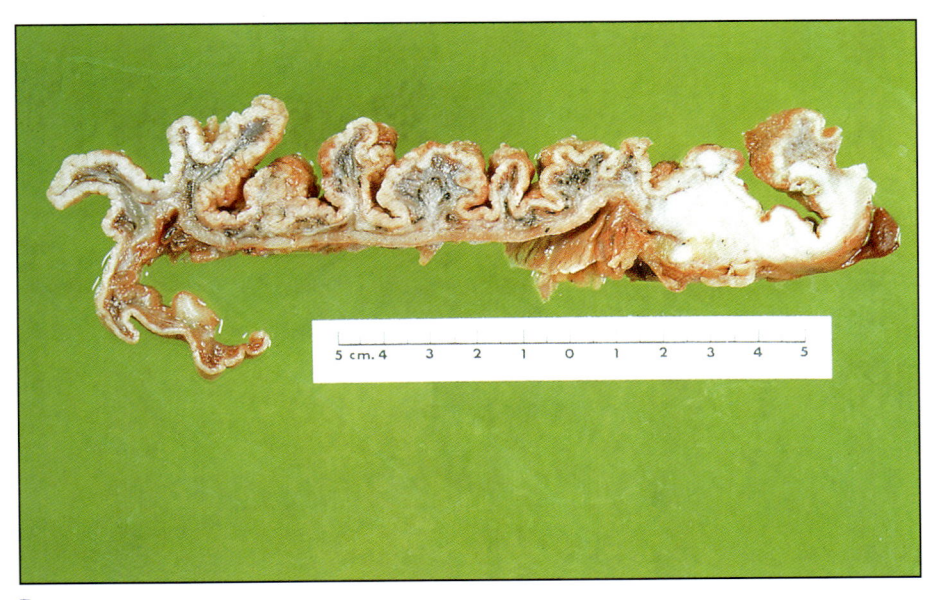

图8.81 (A, B) Ménétrier病合并溃疡性胃腺癌。增厚的胃黏膜显示明显的脑回状迂曲。

大体表现：Ménétrier病的特征性表现为黏膜皱襞肥大，可达1~3 cm高，类似于脑回状（图8.81），或为高低不平的结节状，似息肉病。病变可局限于胃大弯近端或泛发于胃体和胃底部。胃窦部极少受累（尽管可以显示组织学改变），正常和病变的黏膜间常有突然的分界。

镜下表现：典型病例显示明显的小凹增生，小凹变长、扭曲、扩张，内衬大量分泌黏液的细胞，其下方为囊性扩张、萎缩、特化的腺体，伴有黏膜深部壁细胞和主细胞数量减少。有时这些囊性腺体也衬有黏液细胞，并可向下进入黏膜下层。黏膜固有层明显水肿，可能有来自黏膜肌层的平滑肌纤维浸润。一般没有炎症浸润，但当出现炎症时，可能是突出的嗜酸性粒细胞浸润[430]。

鉴别诊断：大体表现可与恶性淋巴瘤、癌、胃息肉病或Zollinger-Ellison综合征混淆（见上文）。Ménétrier病的病理改变还需与état mammeloné鉴别，后者为一种正常变异，其特征为在排空的胃壁出现明显的纵行黏膜皱襞。组织学上，Ménétrier病的基本特征与增生性息肉相似；因此，临床病史和大体描述对于做出正确诊断至关重要。大体表现与Ménétrier病相像的某些病例（显微镜下显示明显的小凹增生和囊性腺体）具有重度的黏膜炎症，水肿相对较轻，并有明显的上皮内T淋巴细胞增多，提示他们可能是慢性淋巴细胞性胃炎临床病

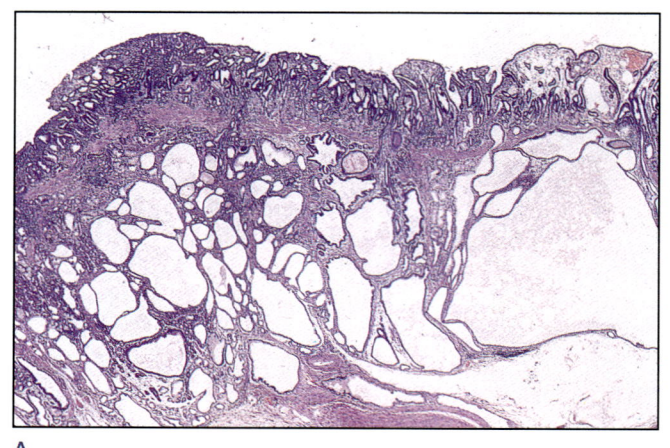

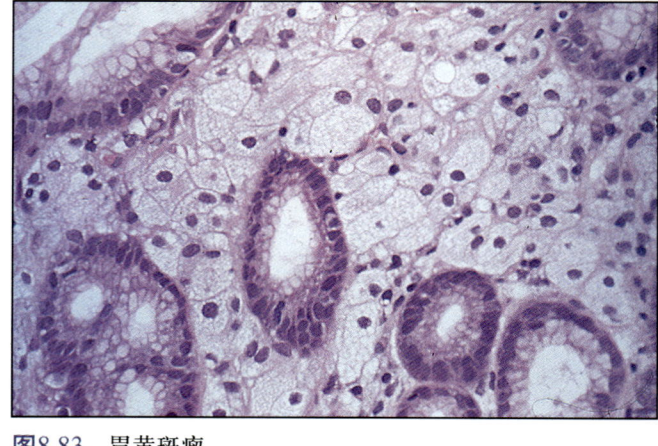

图8.83 胃黄斑瘤。

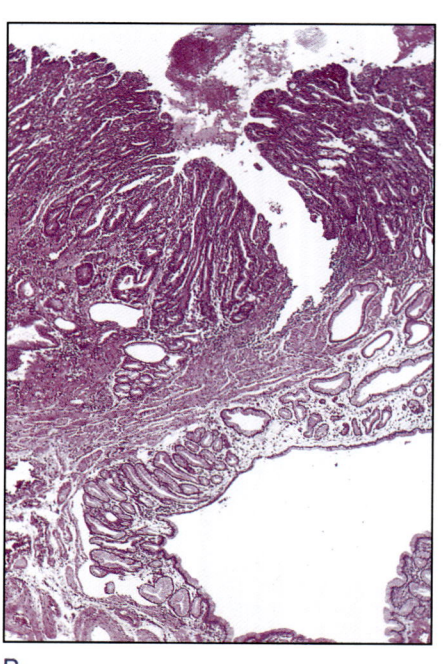

图8.82 囊性息肉状胃炎发生在胃肠吻合口部位（A）。共存的黏膜内腺癌（残胃癌）(B)。

理谱系的"肥大"的一端；有人提出应将这种情况与真正的 Ménétrier 病分开[430]。对于巨细胞病毒感染相关性 Ménétrier 样病存在同样的情况，本病发生于儿童及成年人，伴有胃肠道蛋白丢失[431]。

囊性息肉状或深在性胃炎
Gastritis cystica polyposa or profunda

这种病变通常见于胃肠吻合口[247,432]，但消化性溃疡边缘也可有类似的改变[396]。它与残胃癌的发生也有关系（图8.82）[247]。囊性息肉状胃炎以多发性无蒂息肉样病变为特征，息肉可环绕吻合口一周。组织学上类似于具有显著腺体囊性扩张的增生性息肉，但是与增生性息肉不同，这些扩张的腺体穿过增厚的或破损的黏膜肌层进入黏膜下层（见图8.82），可能伴有黏液外渗。可以出现肠上皮化生，被覆黏膜常常发生糜烂。由于与原先手术有关的局部缺血和慢性炎症，腺体可能误植于黏膜下层，这些腺体呈良性表现，细胞无非典型性，可与高分化腺癌鉴别。

黄色瘤/黄斑瘤 Xanthoma/xanthelasma

这类无临床意义的病变随年龄增长而增多，男性多于女性，常常伴有慢性胃炎和胃黏膜肠上皮化生，以及胆汁反流性胃病[433,434]。本病与高胆固醇血症无关，可能伴有增生性息肉。大体上，可为单发或多发，直径1~2cm，圆形或卵圆形，边界清楚，黄色，斑点状或结节状。病变最常沿着小弯分布。组织学上，病变位于固有膜，由成熟的充满脂质的巨噬细胞聚集而成，巨噬细胞中含有胆固醇和中性脂肪（图8.83）。在活检标本中与癌的鉴别已经在第350页讨论。其他的鉴别诊断包括鸟胞内分支杆菌（mycobacterium avium-intracellulare）感染、噬黏液细胞（muciphages）和颗粒细胞瘤。

淀粉样瘤 Amyloid tumors

胃黏膜或胃壁中的淀粉样瘤样肿块（图8.84）可为全身性淀粉样变的一部分[435]，或为原发性病变[436]。罕见情况下他们可与胃原发性淋巴瘤同时发生[437]。

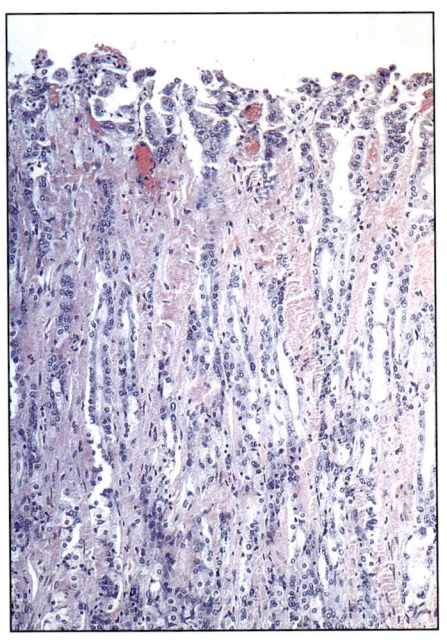
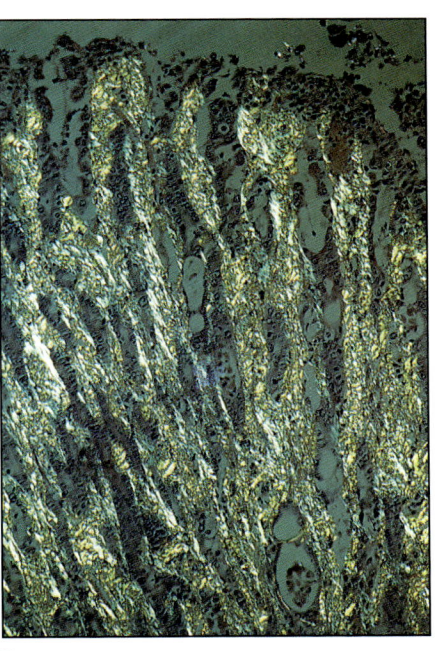

图8.84 长期类风湿性关节炎患者的胃黏膜淀粉样物斑块（A）。刚果红染色/偏振光显微镜（B）。

参考文献

1. Quitadamo M, Benson J 1988 Squamous papilloma of the esophagus: a case report and review of the literature. Am J Gastroenterol 83: 194–201
2. Walker J H 1978 Giant papilloma of the thoracic esophagus. Am J Roentgenol 131: 519–520
3. Parnell S A C, Peppercorn M A, Antonioli D A et al. 1978 Squamous cell papilloma of the esophagus. Report of a case after peptic esophagitis and repeated bougienage with review of the literature. Gastroenterology 74: 910–913
4. Brinson R R, Schuman B M, Mills L R et al. 1987 Multiple squamous papillomas of the esophagus associated with Goltz syndrome. Am J Gastroenterol 82: 1177–1179
5. Odze R, Antonioli D, Shocket D et al. 1993 Esophageal squamous papillomas. A clinicopathologic study of 38 lesions and analysis for human papillomavirus by the polymerase chain reaction. Am J Surg Pathol 17: 803–812
6. Carr N J, Bratthauer G L, Lichy J H et al. 1994 Squamous cell papillomas of the esophagus. A study of 23 lesions for human papillomavirus by in situ hybridization and the polymerase chain reaction. Hum Pathol 25: 536–540
7. Paraf F, Fléjou J-F, Potet F et al. 1992 Adenomas arising in Barrett's esophagus with adenocarcinoma. Report of 3 cases. Pathol Res Pract 188: 1028–1032
8. McDonald G B, Brand D L, Thorning D R 1977 Multiple adenomatous neoplasms arising in columnar lined (Barrett's) esophagus. Gastroenterology 72: 1317–1321
9. Banducci D, Rees R, Bluett M K et al. 1987 Pleomorphic adenoma of the cervical esophagus: a rare tumor. Ann Thorac Surg 44: 653–655
10. Mandard A M, Marnay J, Gignoux M et al. 1984 Cancer of the esophagus and associated lesions: detailed pathologic study of 100 esophagectomy specimens. Hum Pathol 15: 660–669
11. Wang G Q, Abnet C C, Shen Q et al. 2005 Histological precursors of oesophageal squamous cell carcinoma: results from a 13 year prospective follow up study in a high risk population. Gut 54: 187–192
12. Dawsey S M, Wang G Q, Weinstein W M et al. 1993 Squamous dysplasia and early esophageal cancer in the Minxian region of China: distinctive endoscopic lesions. Gastroenterology 105: 1330–1340
13. Lewin K J, Appelman H D 1996 Tumors of the esophagus and stomach. Atlas of tumor pathology. Armed Forces Institute of Pathology, Washington, DC, series 3, fascicle 18
14. Chu P, Stagias J, West B A et al. 1997 Diffuse pagetoid squamous cell carcinoma in situ of the esophagus. A case report. Cancer 79: 1865–1870
15. Potet F, Fléjou J-F, Gervaz H et al. 1991 Adenocarcinoma of the lower esophagus and esophagogastric junction. Semin Diagn Pathol 8: 126–136
16. Schlemper RJ, Riddell RH, Kato Y et al. 2000 The Vienna classification of gastrointestinal epithelial neoplasia. Gut 47: 251–255
17. Bogomoletz W V 1994 Early squamous carcinoma of esophagus. Curr Diagn Pathol 1: 212–215
18. De Baecque C, Potet F, Molas G et al. 1990 Superficial adenocarcinoma of the esophagus in Barrett's mucosa with dysplasia: clinicopathologic study of 12 patients. Histopathology 16: 213–220
19. Ribeiro U, Posner M C, Safatle-Ribeiro A V et al. 1996 Risk factors for squamous cell carcinoma of the oesophagus. Br J Surg 83: 1174–1185
20. Chang-Claude J C, Wahrendorf J, Liang Q S et al. 1990 An epidemiologic study of precursor lesions of esophageal cancer among young persons in a high-risk population in Hunxian, China. Cancer Res 50: 2268–2274
21. Dawsey S M, Lewin K J, Liu F S et al. 1994 Esophageal morphology from Linxian, China. Squamous histologic findings in 754 patients. Cancer 73: 2027–2037
22. Togawa K, Jaskiewicz K, Takahashi H et al. 1994 Human papillomavirus DNA sequences in esophagus squamous cell carcinoma. Gastroenterology 107: 128–136
23. Fidalgo P O, Cravo M L, Chaves P P et al. 1995 High prevalence of human papillomavirus in squamous cell carcinoma and matched normal esophageal mucosa. Cancer 76: 1522–1528
24. Poljak M, Cerar A, Seme K 1998 Human papillomavirus infection in esophageal carcinomas. Hum Pathol 29: 266–271
25. Marger R S, Marger D 1993 Carcinoma of the esophagus and tylosis: a lethal genetic combination. Cancer 72: 17–19
26. Stemmermann G, Heffelfinger S C, Noffsinger A et al. 1995 The molecular biology of esophageal and gastric cancer and their precursors: oncogenes, tumor suppressor genes, growth factors. Hum Pathol 25: 968–981
27. Tahara E (ed) 1997 Molecular pathology of gastroenterological cancer. Springer, Tokyo
28. Iwaya T, Maesawa C, Ogasawara S et al. 1998 Tylosis esophageal cancer locus on chromosome 17q25.1 is commonly deleted in sporadic human esophageal cancer. Gastroenterology 114: 1206–1210
29. Earlam R, Cunha-Melo J R 1980 Oesophageal squamous cell carcinoma: I. A critical review of surgery. Br J Surg 67: 381–390
30. Anderson L L, Lad T E 1982 Autopsy findings in squamous cell carcinoma of the esophagus. Cancer 50: 1587–1590
31. Fogel T D, Harrison L B, Son S H 1985 Subsequent aerodigestive malignancies following treatment of esophageal cancer. Cancer 55: 1882–1885
32. Jasim K A, Bateson M C 1990 Verrucous carcinoma of the oesophagus – a diagnostic problem. Histopathology 17: 473–475
33. Morita M, Kuwano H, Yasuda M et al. 1994 The multicentric occurrence of squamous epithelial dysplasia and squamous cell carcinoma in the esophagus. Cancer 74: 2889–2895
34. Pesko P, Rakic S, Milicevic M et al. 1994 Prevalence and clinicopathologic features of multiple squamous cell carcinoma of the esophagus. Cancer 73: 2687–2690
35. Lam K Y, Ma L T, Wong J 1996 Measurement of extent of spread of oesophageal squamous carcinoma by serial sectioning. J Clin Pathol 49: 124–129
36. Kuwano H, Ueo H, Sugimachi K et al. 1985 Glandular or mucus-secreting components in squamous cell carcinoma of the esophagus. Cancer 56: 514–518
37. Briggs J C, Ibrahim N B N 1983 Oat cell carcinoma of the oesophagus: a clinicopathologic study of 23 cases. Histopathology 7: 261–277

38. Edwards J M, Hillier V F, Lawson R A M et al. 1989 Squamous carcinoma of the oesophagus: histologic criteria and their prognostic significance. Br J Cancer 59: 429–433
39. Takubo K, Takai A, Takayama S et al. 1987 Intraductal spread of esophageal squamous cell carcinoma. Cancer 59: 1751–1757
40. Mori M, Matsuda H, Kuwano H et al. 1989 Oesophageal squamous cell carcinoma with lymphoid stroma. A case report. Virchow's Arch [A] 415: 473–479
41. Ruol A, Segalin A, Panozzo M et al. 1990 Flow cytometric DNA analysis of squamous cell carcinoma of the esophagus. Cancer 65: 1185–1188
42. Soga J, Tanaka O, Sasaki K et al. 1982 Superficial spreading carcinoma of the esophagus. Cancer 50: 1641–1645
43. Rubio C A, Liu F S 1990 The histogenesis of the microinvasive basal cell carcinoma of the esophagus. Pathol Res Pract 186: 223–227
44. Abe K, Sasano H, Itakura Y et al. 1996 Basaloid-squamous carcinoma of the esophagus. A clinicopathologic, DNA ploidy, and immunohistochemical study of seven cases. Am J Surg Pathol 20: 453–461
45. Sarbia M, Vereet P, Bittinger F et al. 1997 Basaloid squamous cell carcinoma of the esophagus: diagnosis and prognosis. Cancer 79: 1871–1878
46. Lam KY, Law S, Luk J M et al. 2001 Oesophageal basaloid squamous cell carcinoma: a unique clinicopathologic entity with telomerase activity as a prognostic indicator. J Pathol 195: 435–442
47. Isaacson P 1982 Biopsy appearances easily mistaken for malignancy in gastrointestinal endoscopy. Histopathology 6: 377–389
48. Gill P, Piris J, Warren B F 2003 Bizarre stromal cells in the oesophagus. Histopathology 42: 88–90
49. Schlemper R J, Dawsey S M, Itabashi M et al. 2000 Differences in diagnostic criteria for esophageal squamous cell carcinoma between Japanese and Western pathologists. Cancer 88: 996–1006
50. Osamura R Y, Shimamura K, Hata J et al. 1978 Polypoid carcinoma of the esophagus. A unifying concept for "carcinosarcoma" and "pseudosarcoma". Am J Surg Pathol 2: 201–208
51. du Boulay C E H, Isaacson P 1981 Carcinoma of the oesophagus with spindle cell features. Histopathology 5: 403–414
52. Cho S R, Henry D A, Schneider V et al. 1983 Polypoid carcinoma of the esophagus: a distinct radiologic and histopathologic entity. Am J Gastroenterol 78: 476–480
53. Appelman H D (ed) 1984 Stromal tumors of the esophagus, stomach and duodenum. In: Pathology of the esophagus, stomach and duodenum. Churchill Livingstone, Edinburgh, p 195–242
54. Guarino M, Reale D, Micoli G et al. 1993 Carcinosarcoma of the oesophagus with rhabdomyoblastic differentiation. Histopathology 22: 493–498
55. Lauwers G Y, Grant L D, Scott G V et al. 1998 Spindle cell squamous carcinoma of the esophagus: analysis of ploidy and tumor proliferative activity in a series of 13 cases. Hum Pathol 29: 863–868
56. Matsumoto T, Fujii H, Arakawa A et al. 2004 Loss of heterozygosity analysis shows monoclonal evolution with frequent genetic progression and divergence in esophageal carcinosarcoma. Hum Pathol 35: 322–327
57. Martland GT, Goodman AJ, Shepherd NA 2004 CD117 expression in esophageal carcinosarcoma: a potential diagnostic pitfall. Histopathology 44: 77–80
58. Iftikhar S Y, James P D, Steele R J C et al. 1992 Length of Barrett's oesophagus: an important factor in the development of dysplasia and adenocarcinoma. Gut 33: 1155–1158
59. Lagergren J, Bergstrom R, Nyren O 1999 Association between body mass and adenocarcinoma of the esophagus and gastric cardia. Ann Intern Med 130: 883–890
60. Lagergren J, Bergstrom R, Adami H O et al. 2000 Association between medications that relax the lower esophageal sphincter and risk for esophageal adenocarcinoma. Ann Intern Med 133: 165–175
61. Wang H H, Antonioli D A, Goldman H 1986 Comparative features of esophageal and gastric adenocarcinomas: recent changes in type and frequency. Hum Pathol 17: 482–487
62. Pera M, Cameron A J, Trastek V F et al. 1993 Increasing incidence of adenocarcinoma of the esophagus and esophagogastric junction. Gastroenterology 104: 510–513
63. Blount P L, Ramel S, Raskind W H et al. 1991 17p allelic deletions and p53 protein overexpression in Barrett's adenocarcinoma. Cancer Res 51: 5482–5486
64. Fléjou J-F, Paraf F, Muzeau F et al. 1994 Expression of c-erbB-2 oncogene product in Barrett's adenocarcinoma: pathologic and prognostic correlations. J Clin Pathol 47: 23–26
65. Klump B, Hsieh C J, Holzmann K 1998 Hypermethylation of the CDKN2/p16 promoter during neoplastic progression in Barrett's esophagus. Gastroenterology 115: 1381–1386
66. Shirvani VN, Ouatu-Lascar R, Kaur B S et al. 2000 Cyclooxygenase 2 expression in Barrett's esophagus and adenocarcinoma: ex vivo induction by bile salts and acid exposure. Gastroenterology 118: 487–496
67. Sanfey H, Hamilton S R, Smith R R L et al. 1985 Carcinoma arising in Barrett's esophagus. Surg Gynecol Obstet 161: 570–574
68. Corley D A, Levin T R, Habel L A et al. 2002 Surveillance and survival in Barrett's adenocarcinomas: a population-based study. Gastroenterology 122: 633–640
69. Cameron A J, Lomboy C T, Pera M et al. 1995 Adenocarcinoma of the esophagogastric junction and Barrett's esophagus. Gastroenterology 109: 1541–1546
70. Chatelain D, de Lajarte-Thirouard AS, Tiret E et al. 2002 Adenocarcinoma of the upper esophagus arising in heterotopic gastric mucosa: common pathogenesis with Barrett's adenocarcinoma? Virchow's Arch 441: 406–411
71. Smith R R L, Hamilton S R, Boitnott J K et al. 1984 The spectrum of carcinoma arising in Barrett's esophagus. A clinicopathologic study of 26 patients. Am J Surg Pathol 8: 563–573
72. Hamilton S R, Smith R R L 1987 The relationship between columnar epithelial dysplasia and invasive adenocarcinoma arising in Barrett's esophagus. Am J Clin Pathol 87: 301–312
73. Chejfec G, Jablokow V R, Gould V E 1983 Linitis plastica carcinoma of the esophagus. Cancer 51: 2139–2143
74. Hamilton K, Chiappori A, Olson S et al. 2000 Prevalence and prognostic significance of neuroendocrine cells in esophageal adenocarcinoma. Mod Pathol 13: 475–481
75. Dworak O, Koerfgen H P 1993 Carcinosarcoma in Barrett's oesophagus: a case report with immunohistologic examination. Virchows Arch [A] 422: 423–426
76. Falk G W 1999 Endoscopic surveillance of Barrett's esophagus: risk stratification and cancer risk. Gastrointest Endosc 49: S29–S34
77. Mino-Kenudson M, Brugge W R, Puricelli W P et al. 2005 Management of superficial Barrett's epithelium-related neoplasms by endoscopic mucosal resection: clinicopathologic analysis of 27 cases. Am J Surg Pathol 29: 680–686
78. Ban S, Mino M, Nishioka N S et al. 2004 Histopathologic aspects of photodynamic therapy for dysplasia and early adenocarcinoma arising in Barrett's esophagus. Am J Surg Pathol 28: 1466–1473
79. Bell-Thomson J, Haggitt R C, Ellis F H Jr 1980 Mucoepidermoid and adenoid cystic carcinomas of the esophagus. J Thorac Cardiovasc Surg 79: 438–446
80. Kabuto T, Taniguchi K, Iwanaga T et al. 1979 Primary adenoid cystic carcinoma of the esophagus. Report of a case. Cancer 43: 2452–2456
81. Woodard B H, Shelburne J D, Vollmer R T et al. 1978 Mucoepidermoid carcinoma of the esophagus: a case report. Hum Pathol 9: 352–354
82. Sweeney E C, Cooney T 1980 Adenoid cystic carcinoma of the esophagus. A light and electron microscopic study. Cancer 45: 1516–1525
83. Epstein J I, Sears D L, Tucker R S et al. 1984 Carcinoma of the esophagus with adenoid cystic differentiation. Cancer 53: 1131–1136
84. Yachida S, Nakanishi Y, Shimoda T et al. 2004 Adenosquamous carcinoma of the esophagus. Clinicopathologic study of 18 cases. Oncology 66: 218–225
85. Orsatti G, Corvalan A H, Sakurai H et al. 1993 Polypoid adenosquamous carcinoma of the esophagus with prominent spindle cells. Report of a case with immunohistochemical and ultrastructural studies. Arch Pathol Lab Med 117: 544–547
86. Mori M, Matsukuma A, Adachi Y 1989 Small cell carcinoma of the esophagus. Cancer 63: 564–573
87. Casas F, Ferrer F, Farrus B et al. 1997 Primary small cell carcinoma of the esophagus. A review of the literature with emphasis on therapy and prognosis. Cancer 80: 1366–1372
88. Watson K J R, Shulkes A, Smallwood R A et al. 1985 Watery diarrhea-hypokalemia-achlorhydria syndrome and carcinoma of the esophagus. Gastroenterology 88: 798–803
89. Johnson F E, Clawson M C, Bashiti H M et al. 1984 Small cell undifferentiated carcinoma of the esophagus. Case report with hormonal studies. Cancer 53: 1746–1751
90. Ho K J, Herrera G A, Jones J M et al. 1984 Small cell carcinoma of the esophagus: evidence for a unified histogenesis. Hum Pathol 15: 460–468
91. Trillo A A, Accettullo L M, Yeiter T L 1979 Choriocarcinoma of the esophagus: histologic and cytologic findings: a case report. Acta Cytol 23: 69–74
92. McKechnie J C, Fechner R E 1971 Choriocarcinoma and adenocarcinoma of the esophagus with gonadotropin secretion. Cancer 27: 694–702
93. Fine G, Smith R W Jr, Pachter M R 1962 Primary extragenital choriocarcinoma in the male subject. Am J Med 32: 776–794
94. Norihisa Y, Kakudo K, Tsutsumi Y et al. 1988 Paget's extension of esophageal carcinoma. Immunohistochemical and mucin histochemical evidence of Paget's cells in the esophageal mucosa. Acta Pathol Jpn 38: 651–658
95. Haleem A, Kfoury H, Al Juboury M et al. 2003 Paget's disease of the esophagus associated with mucous gland carcinoma of the lower esophagus. Histopathology 42: 61–65
96. Sobin L H, Wittekind Ch (eds) 2002 UICC: TNM classification of malignant tumours, 6th edn. John Wiley, New York
97. Dexter S P, Sue-Ling H, McMahon M J et al. 2001 Circumferential resection margin involvement: an independent predictor of survival following surgery for oesophageal cancer. Gut 48: 667–670
98. Mandard A M, Dalibard F, Mandard J C et al. 1994 Pathologic assessment of tumor regression after preoperative chemoradiotherapy of esophageal carcinoma: clinicopathologic correlations. Cancer 73: 2680–2686
99. Chirieac L R, Swisher S G, Ajani J A et al. 2005 Post-therapy pathologic stage predicts survival in patients with esophageal carcinoma receiving preoperative chemoradiation. Cancer 103: 1347–1355
100. Ludwig M E, Shaw R, DeSuto-Nagy G 1981 Primary malignant melanoma of the esophagus. Cancer 48: 2528–2534
101. Kato T, Takematsu H, Tomita Y et al. 1987 Malignant melanoma of mucous membranes. Arch Dermatol 123: 216–220
102. DiCostanzo D P, Urmacher C 1987 Primary malignant melanoma of the esophagus. Am J Surg Pathol 11: 46–52

103. de Mik J I, Kooijman C D, Hoekstra J B L et al. 1992 Primary malignant melanoma of the oesophagus. Histopathology 20: 77–79
104. Raven R W, Dawson I 1964 Malignant melanoma of the oesophagus. Br J Surg 51: 551–555
105. Guzman R P, Wightman R, Ravinsky E et al. 1989 Primary malignant melanoma of the esophagus with diffuse melanocytic atypia and melanoma in situ. Am J Clin Pathol 92: 802–804
106. De La Pava S, Nigogosyan G, Pickren J W et al. 1963 Melanosis of the esophagus. Cancer 16: 48–50
107. Ohashi K, Kato Y, Kanno J et al. 1990 Melanocytes and melanosis of the oesophagus in Japanese subjects – analysis of factors effecting their increase. Virchows Arch [A] 417: 137–143
108. Assor D 1975 A melanocytic tumor of the esophagus. Cancer 35: 1438–1443
109. Seremetis M G, Lyons W S, de Guzman V C et al. 1976 Leiomyomata of the esophagus: an analysis of 838 cases. Cancer 38: 2166–2177
110. Bourque M D, Spigland N, Bensoussan A L et al. 1989 Esophageal leiomyoma in children: two case reports and review of the literature. J Pediatr Surg 24: 1103–1107
111. McKeeby J L, Li X, Zhuang Z et al. 2001 Multiple leiomyomas of the esophagus, lung, and uterus in multiple endocrine neoplasia type 1. Am J Pathol 159: 1121–1127
112. Rocco G, Trastek V F, Deschamps C et al. 1998 Leiomyosarcoma of the esophagus: results of surgical treatment. Ann Thorac Surg 66: 894–896
113. Miettinen M, Sarlomo-Rikala M, Sobin L H et al. 2000 Esophageal stromal tumors: a clinicopathologic, immunohistochemical and molecular genetic study of 17 cases and comparison with esophageal leiomyomas and leiomyosarcomas. Am J Surg Pathol 24: 211–222
114. Takubo K, Nakagawa H, Tsuchiya S et al. 1981 Seedling leiomyoma of the esophagus and esophagogastric junction zone. Hum Pathol 12: 1006–1010
115. Suster S 1996 Gastrointestinal stromal tumors. Semin Diagn Pathol 13: 297–313
116. Johnston J, Helwig E B 1981 Granular cell tumors of the gastrointestinal tract and perianal region. A study of 74 cases. Dig Dis Sci 26: 807–816
117. Goldblum J R, Rice T W, Zuccaro G et al. 1996 Granular cell tumors of the esophagus: a clinical and pathologic study of 13 cases. Ann Thorac Surg 62: 860–865
118. Vuyk H D, Snow G B, Tiwari R M et al. 1985 Granular cell tumor of the proximal esophagus. A rare disease. Cancer 55: 445–449
119. Yoshizawa A, Ota H, Sakaguchi N et al. 2004 Malignant granular cell tumor of the esophagus. Virchow's Arch 444: 304–306
120. Cokelaere K, Sciot R, Geboes K 2000 Esophageal plexiform schwannoma. Int J Surg Pathol 8: 353–357
121. Saitoh K, Nasu M, Kamiyama R et al. 1985 Solitary neurofibroma of the esophagus. Acta Pathol Jpn 35: 527–531
122. Roberts F, Kirk A J, More I A et al. 2000 Oesophageal rhabdomyoma. J Clin Pathol 53: 554–557
123. Gilbert H W, Weston M J, Thompson M H 1990 Cavernous haemangioma of the oesophagus. Br J Surg 77: 106
124. Yoshida Y, Okamura T, Ezaki T et al. 1994 Lymphangioma of the oesophagus: a case report and review of the literature. Thorax 49: 1267–1268
125. Wolf B C, Khettry U, Leonardi H K et al. 1988 Benign lesions mimicking malignant tumors of the esophagus. Hum Pathol 19: 148–154
126. Akiyama S, Kataoka M, Horisawa M et al. 1990 Lipoma of the esophagus – report of a case and review of the literature. Jpn J Surg 20: 458–462
127. Mahour G H, Harrison E G Jr 1967 Osteochondroma (tracheobronchial choristoma) of the esophagus. Report of a case. Cancer 20: 1489–1493
128. Saitoh Y, Inomata Y, Tadaki N et al. 1990 Pedunculated intraluminal osteochondromatous hamartoma of the esophagus. J Otolaryngol 19: 339–342
129. Willen R, Lillo-Gil R, Willen H et al. 1989 Embryonal rhabdomyosarcoma of the oesophagus: case report. Acta Chir Scand 155: 59–64
130. Ng W C, Leong H T, Ma K F et al. 2003 Malignant rhabdoid tumour of the esophagus: a case report. J Clin Pathol 56: 713–714
131. Laine L, Amerian J, Rarick M et al. 1990 The response of symptomatic gastrointestinal Kaposi's sarcoma to chemotherapy: a prospective evaluation using an endoscopic method of disease quantification. Am J Gastroenterol 85: 959–961
132. Mansour K A, Fritz R C, Jacobs D M et al. 1983 Pedunculated liposarcoma of the esophagus: a first case report. J Thorac Cardiovasc Surg 86: 447–450
133. Burke J S, Ranchod M 1981 Hemangiopericytoma of the esophagus. Hum Pathol 12: 96–100
134. Haratake J, Jimi A, Horie A et al. 1984 Malignant mesenchymoma of the esophagus. Acta Pathol Jpn 34: 925–933
135. Naganuma H, Ohtani H, Sayama J et al. 1996 Malignant fibrous histiocytoma of the esophagus. Pathol Int 46: 462–466
136. McIntyre M, Webb J N, Browning G C P 1982 Osteosarcoma of the esophagus. Hum Pathol 13: 680–682
137. Anton-Pacheco J, Cano I, Cuadros J et al. 1996 Synovial sarcoma of the esophagus. J Ped Surg 31: 1703–1705
138. Okerbloom J A, Armitage J O, Zetterman R et al. 1984 Esophageal involvement by non-Hodgkin's lymphoma. Am J Med 77: 359–361
139. Stein H A, Murray R, Warner H A 1981 Primary Hodgkin's disease of the esophagus. Dig Dis Sci 26: 457–461
140. Bolondi L, de Giorgio R, Santi V et al. 1990 Primary non-Hodgkin's T-cell lymphoma of the esophagus: a case with peculiar endoscopic ultrasonographic pattern. Dig Dis Sci 35: 1426–1430
141. Hosaka S, Nakamura N, Akamatsu T et al. 2002 A case of primary low grade mucosa associated lymphoid tissue (MALT) lymphoma of the esophagus. Gut 51: 281–284
142. Remes-Troche J M, De-Anda J, Ochoa V et al. 2003 A rare case of multiple lymphomatous polyposis with widespread involvement of the gastrointestinal tract. Arch Pathol Lab Med 127: 1028–1030
143. Gervaz E, Potet F, Mahé R et al. 1992 Focal lymphoid hyperplasia of the oesophagus: report of a case. Histopathology 21: 187–189
144. Chetty R, Bramder A, Reddy A D 2003 Primary plasmacytoma of the esophagus. Ann Diagn Pathol 7: 174–179
145. Agha F P, Schnitzer B 1985 Esophageal involvement in lymphoma. Am J Gastroenterol 80: 412–416
146. Thompson B C, Feczko P J, Mezwa D G 1990 Dysphagia caused by acute leukemic infiltration of the esophagus. Am J Roentgenol 155: 654
147. Penagini R, Ranzi T, Velio P et al. 1989 Giant fibrovascular polyp of the oesophagus: report of a case and effects on oesophageal function. Gut 30: 1624–1629
148. Cokelaere K, Geboes K 2001 Squamous cell carcinoma in a giant esophageal fibrovascular polyp. Histopathology 38: 586–589
149. LiVolsi V A, Perzin K H 1975 Inflammatory pseudotumors (inflammatory fibrous polyps) of the esophagus: a clinicopathologic study. Dig Dis 20: 475–481
150. Arbona J L, Fazzi J G F, Mayoral J 1984 Congenital esophageal cysts: case report and review of literature. Am J Gastroenterol 79: 177–182
151. Kirwan W O, Walbaum P R, McCormack R J M 1973 Cystic intrathoracic derivatives of the foregut and their complications. Thorax 28: 424–428
152. Qazi F M, Geisinger K R, Nelson J B et al. 1990 Symptomatic congenital gastroenteric duplication cyst of the esophagus containing exocrine and endocrine pancreatic tissues. Am J Gastroenterol 85: 65–67
153. McGregor D H, Mills G, Boudet R A 1976 Intramural squamous cell carcinoma of the esophagus. Cancer 37: 1556–1561
154. Solanke T F, Olurin E O, Nwakonobi F et al. 1967 Primary amyloid tumour of the oesophagus treated by colon transplant. Br J Surg 54: 943–946
155. Bender M D, Allison J, Cuartas F et al. 1973 Glycogenic acanthosis of the esophagus: a form of benign epithelial hyperplasia. Gastroenterology 65: 373–380
156. Kay P S, Soetikno R M, Mindelzun R et al. 1997 Diffuse esophageal glycogenic acanthosis: an endoscopic marker of Cowden's disease. Am J Gastroenterol 92: 1038–1040
157. Heald J, Moussalli H, Hasleton P S 1986 Diffuse leiomyomatosis of the oesophagus. Histopathology 10: 755–759
158. Lonsdale R N, Roberts P F, Vaughan R et al. 1992 Familial oesophageal leiomyomatosis and nephropathy. Histopathology 20: 127–133
159. Marshall J B, Diaz-Arias A A, Bochna G S et al. 1990 Achalasia due to diffuse esophageal leiomyomatosis and inherited as an autosomal dominant disorder: report of a family study. Gastroenterology 98: 1358–1365
160. Wahlen T, Astedt B 1965 Familial coexistence of leiomyoma of vulva and oesophagus. Acta Obstet Gynecol Scand 44: 197–203
161. von Rahden BHA, Stein HJ, Becker K et al. 2004 Heterotopic gastric mucosa of the esophagus: literature review and proposal of a clinicopathological classification. Am J Gastroenterology 99: 543–551
162. Lauwers G Y, Mino M, Ban S et al. 2005 Cytokeratins 7 and 20 and mucin core protein expression in esophageal cervical inlet patch. Am J Surg Pathol 29: 437–442
163. Razi M D 1966 Ectopic pancreatic tissue of esophagus with massive upper gastrointestinal bleeding. Arch Surg 92: 101–104
164. Merino M J, Brand M, LiVolsi V A et al. 1982 Sebaceous glands in the esophagus diagnosed in a clinical setting. Arch Pathol Lab Med 106: 47–48
165. Raeburn C 1951 Columnar ciliated epithelium in the adult oesophagus. J Pathol Bacteriol 63: 157–158
166. Abraham S C, Singh V K, Yardley J H et al. 2001 Hyperplastic polyps of the esophagus and esophagogastric junction: histologic and clinicopathologic findings. Am J Surg Pathol 25: 1180–1187
167. Ito H, Hata J, Yokozaki H et al. 1986 Tubular adenoma of the human stomach. An immunohistochemical analysis of gut hormones, serotonin, carcinoembryonic antigen, secretory component and lysozyme. Cancer 58: 2264–2272
168. Oberhuber G, Stolte M 2000 Gastric polyps: an update of their pathology and biological significance. Virchow's Arch 437: 581–590
169. Laxén F, Sipponen P, Ihamäki T et al. 1982 Gastric polyps: their morphological and endoscopical characteristics and relation to gastric carcinoma. Acta Pathol Microbiol Scand Sect A 90: 221–228
170. Abraham, S C, Park S J, Lee J H et al. 2003 Genetic alterations in gastric adenomas of intestinal and foveolar phenotypes. Hum Pathol 16: 786–795
171. Domizio P, Talbot I C, Spigelman A D et al. 1990 Upper gastrointestinal pathology in familial adenomatous polyposis: results from a prospective study of 102 patients. J Clin Pathol 43: 738–743
172. Nakamura T, Nakano G I 1985 Histopathologic classification and malignant change in gastric polyps. J Clin Pathol 38: 754–764
173. Fieber S S, Boden R E 1977 Polypoid villous adenoma of the stomach. Am J Gastroenterol 68: 286–289
174. Morson B C, Sobin L H, Grundmann E et al. 1980 Pre-cancerous conditions and epithelial dysplasia in the stomach. J Clin Pathol 33: 711–721
175. Kushima R, Muller W, Stolte M et al. 1996 Differential p53 protein expression in stomach adenomas of gastric and intestinal phenotypes: possible sequences of p53 alteration in gastric carcinogenesis. Virchow's Arch 428: 223–227

176. Vieth M, Kushima R, Borchard F et al. 2003 Pyloric gland adenoma: a clinicopathological analysis of 90 cases. Virchow's Arch 442: 317–321
177. Hamilton S R, Aaltonen L A 2000 Pathology and genetics of tumours of the digestive system. World Health Organization Cassification of Tumours. Vol 2. IARC Press, Lyon
178. Rubio C A 1989 Paneth cell adenoma of the stomach. Am J Surg Pathol 13: 325–328
179. Ito H, Yasui W, Yoshida K et al. 1990 Depressed tubular adenoma of the stomach: pathologic and immunohistochemical features. Histopathology 17: 419–426
180. Schlemper R J, Itabashi M, Kato Y et al. 1997 Differences in diagnostic criteria for gastric carcinoma between Japanese and Western pathologists. Lancet 349: 1725–1729
181. Lauwers G Y, Shimizu M, Correa P et al. 1999 Evaluation of gastric biopsies for neoplasia – differences between Japanese and Western pathologists. Am J Surg Path 23: 511–518
182. Hattori T 1985 Morphologic range of hyperplastic polyps and carcinomas arising in hyperplastic polyps of the stomach. J Clin Pathol 38: 622–630
183. Lauwers G Y, Riddell R H 1999 Gastric epithelial dysplasia. Gut 45: 784–790
184. Ghandur-Mnaymneh L, Paz J, Roldan E et al. 1988 Dysplasia of nonmetaplastic gastric mucosa: a proposal for its classification and its possible relationship to diffuse-type gastric carcinoma. Am J Surg Pathol 12: 96–114
185. Tosi P, Baak J P A, Luzi P et al. 1989 Morphometric distinction of low- and high-grade dysplasias in gastric biopsies. Hum Pathol 20: 839–844
186. Lansdown M, Quirke P, Dixon M F et al. 1990 High-grade dysplasia of the gastric mucosa: a marker for gastric carcinoma. Gut 31: 977–983
187. Saraga E-P, Gardiol D, Costa J 1987 Gastric dysplasia: a histologic follow-up study. Am J Surg Pathol 11: 788–796
188. Ming S-C, Bajtai A, Correa P et al. 1984 Gastric dysplasia: significance and pathologic criteria. Cancer 54: 1794–1801
189. Kokkola A, Haapiainen R, Laxén F et al. 1996 Risk of gastric carcinoma in patients with mucosal dysplasia associated with atrophic gastritis: a follow-up study. J Clin Pathol 49: 979–984
190. Rugge M, Cassaro M, Di Mario F et al. 2003 The long term outcome of gastric non-invasive neoplasia. Gut 52: 1111–1116
191. Lauwers G Y, Ban S, Mino M et al. 2004 Endoscopic mucosal resection for gastric epithelial neoplasms: a study of 39 cases with emphasis on the evaluation of specimens and recommendations for optimal pathologic analysis. Mod Pathol 17: 2–8
192. Ono H, Kondo H, Gotoda T et al. 2001 Endoscopic mucosal resection for treatment of early gastric cancer. Gut 48: 225–229
193. Nagayo T 1986 Histopathology of gastric dysplasia. In: Filipe M I, Jass J R (eds) Gastric carcinoma. Churchill Livingstone, Edinburgh, p 116–131
194. Dixon M F, O'Connor H J, Axon A T et al. 1986 Reflux gastritis: a distinct histopathologic entity? J Clin Pathol 39: 524–530
195. Brien T P, Farraye F A, Odze R D 2001 Gastric dysplasia-like epithelial atypia associated with chemoradiotherapy for esophageal cancer: a clinicopathologic and immunohistochemical study of 15 cases. Mod Pathol 14: 389–396
196. Stewart B W, Kleihues P 2003 World Cancer Report. IARC Press, Lyon
197. Henson D E, Dittus C, Younes M et al. 2004 Differential trends in the intestinal and diffuse types of gastric carcinoma in the United States, 1973–2000. Arch Pathol Lab Med 128: 765–770
198. Guildford P, Hopkins J, Grady W et al. 1999 E-cadherin germline mutations define an inherited cancer syndrome dominated by diffuse gastric cancer. Hum Mutat 14: 249–255
199. Aarnio M, Salovaara R, Aaltonen L A et al. 1997 Features of gastric cancer in hereditary non-polyposis colorectal cancer syndrome. Int J Cancer 74: 551–555
200. Cassaro M, Rugge M, Gutierrez O et al. 2000 Topographic patterns of intestinal metaplasia and gastric cancer. Am J Gastroenterol 95: 1431–1438
201. Antonioli D A 1994 Precursors of gastric carcinoma. Hum Pathol 25: 994–1005.
202. Huang J-Q, Sridhar S, Chen Y et al. 1998 Meta-analysis of the relationship between Helicobacter pylori seropositivity and gastric cancer. Gastroenterology 114: 1169–1179
203. Parsonnet J, Friedman G D, Orentreich N et al. 1997 Risk for gastric cancer in people with CagA positive or CagA negative Helicobacter pylori infection. Gut 40: 297–301
204. El-Omar E M, Carrington M, Chow W H et al. 2000 Interleukin-1 polymorphisms associated with increased risk of gastric cancer. Nature 404: 398–402
205. Kuipers E J 1997 Helicobacter pylori and the risk and management of associated diseases: gastritis, ulcer disease, atrophic gastritis and gastric cancer. Aliment Pharmacol Ther 11 (suppl 1): 71–88
206. Oda K, Tamaru J, Takenouchi T et al. 1993 Association of Epstein–Barr virus with gastric carcinoma with lymphoid stroma. Am J Pathol 143: 1063–1071
207. Luinetti O, Fiocca R, Villani L et al. 1998 Genetic pattern, histologic structure and cellular phenotype in early and advanced gastric cancers. Hum Pathol 29: 702–709
208. Locke G R, Talley N J, Carpenter H A et al. 1995 Changes in the site- and histology-specific incidence of gastric cancer during a 50 year period. Gastroenterology 109: 1750–1756

209. Charlton A, Blair V, Shaw D et al. 2004 Hereditary diffuse gastric cancer: predominance of multiple foci of signet-ring cell carcinoma in distal stomach and transitional zone Gut 53: 814–820
210. Capella C, Frigerio B, Cornaggia M et al. 1984 Gastric parietal cell carcinoma – a newly recognized entity: light microscopic and ultrastructural features. Histopathology 8: 813–824
211. Bonar S F, Sweeney E C 1986 The prevalence, prognostic significance and hormonal content of endocrine cells in gastric cancer. Histopathology 10: 53–63
212. Tahara E, Ito H, Nakagami K et al. 1982 Scirrhous argyrophil carcinoma of the stomach with multiple production of polypeptide hormones, amine, CEA, lysozyme, and HCG. Cancer 49: 1904–1915
213. Ooi A, Nakanishi I, Itoh T et al. 1991 Predominant Paneth cell differentiation in an intestinal type gastric cancer. Pathol Res Pract 187: 220–225
214. Takubo K, Honma N, Sawabe M et al. 2002 Oncocytic adenocarcinoma of the stomach: parietal cell carcinoma. Am J Surg Pathol 26: 458–465
215. Laurén P 1965 The two histologic main types of gastric carcinoma: diffuse and so-called intestinal-type carcinoma. Acta Pathol Microbiol Scand 64: 31–49
216. Carneiro F, Huntsman D G, Smyrk T C et al. 2004 Model of the early development of diffuse gastric cancer in E-cadherin mutation carriers and its implications for patient screening. J Pathol 203: 681–687
217. Mori M, Sakaguchi H, Akazawa K et al. 1995 Correlation between metastatic site, histologic type, and serum tumor markers of gastric carcinoma. Hum Pathol 26: 504–508
218. Ming S-C 1977 Gastric carcinoma: a pathobiological classification. Cancer 39: 2475–2485
219. Mulligan R M 1972 Histogenesis and biological behavior of gastric carcinoma. Pathol Annual 7: 349–415
220. Roy P, Piard F, Dusserre-Guion L et al. 1998 Prognostic comparison of the pathological classifications of gastric cancer: a population-based study. Histopathology 33: 304–310
221. Williams G T 1986 Early gastric cancer. In: Filipe MI, Jass JR (eds) Gastric carcinoma. Churchill Livingstone, Edinburgh, p 172–196
222. Goseki N, Takizawa T, Koike M 1992 Differences in the mode of the extension of gastric cancer classified by histologic type: new histologic classification of gastric carcinoma. Gut 33: 606–612
223. McLaren K M, Burnett R A, Goodlad J R et al. 2003 Observer variability in the Goseki grouping of gastric adenocarcinoma in resection and biopsy specimens. Histopathology 42: 472–475
224. Carneiro F, Seixas M, Sobrinho-Simoes M 1995 New elements for an updated classification of the carcinoma of the stomach. Pathol Res Pract 191: 571–584
225. Kozuki T, Yao T, Nakamura S et al. 2002 Differences in p53 and cadherin-catenin complex expression between histological subtypes in diffusely infiltrating gastric carcinoma. Histopathology 41: 56–64
226. Byrne D, Holley M P, Cuschieri A 1988 Parietal cell carcinoma of the stomach: association with long-term survival after curative resection. Br J Cancer 58: 85–87
227. Jain S, Filipe M I, Hall P A et al. 1991 Prognostic value of proliferating cell nuclear antigen in gastric cancer. J Clin Pathol 44: 655–659
228. Filipe M I, Rosa J, Sandey A et al. 1991 Is DNA ploidy and proliferative activity of prognostic value in advanced gastric carcinoma? Hum Pathol 22: 373–378
229. Korenaga D, Okamura T, Saito A et al. 1988 DNA ploidy is closely linked to tumor invasion, lymph node metastasis and prognosis in clinical gastric cancer. Cancer 62: 309–313
230. Baretton G, Carstensen O, Schardey M et al. 1991 DNA-ploidy and survival in gastric carcinomas: a flow-cytometric study. Virchow's Arch [A] 418: 301–309
231. Setälä L P, Kosma V-M, Marin S et al. 1996 Prognostic factors in gastric cancer: the value of vascular invasion, mitotic rate and lymphoplasmacytic infiltration. Br J Cancer 74: 766–772
232. Tanaka A, Watanabe T, Okuno K et al. 1994 Perineural invasion as a predictor of recurrence of gastric cancer. Cancer 73: 550–555
233. Van Beek J, zur Hausen A, Kranenbarg E K et al. 2004 EBV-positive gastric adenocarcinomas: a distinct clinicopathological entity with a low frequency of lymph node involvement. J Clin Oncol 22: 664–670
234. Ishigami S, Natsugoe S, Miyazono F et al. 2004 Clinical merit of subdividing gastric cancer according to invasion of the muscularis propria. Hepatogastroenterology 51: 869–871
235. Wu C W, Hsiech M C, Lo S S et al. 1996 Relation of number of positive lymph nodes to the prognosis of patients with primary gastric adenocarcinoma. Gut 38: 525–527
236. Doekhie F S, Mesker W E, van Krieken J H J M et al. 2005 Clinical relevance of occult tumor cells in lymph nodes from gastric cancer patients. Am J Surg Pathol 29: 1135–1144
237. Japanese Research Society for Gastric Cancer 1995 Japanese classification of gastric carcinoma. Kanehara, Tokyo
238. Siewert R J, Feith M, Werner M et al. 2000 Adenocarcinoma of the esophagogastric junction: results of surgical therapy based on anatomical/topographical classification in 1002 consecutive patients. Ann Surg 232: 353–361
239. Fielding J W L, Roginski C, Ellis D J et al. 1984 Clinicopathologic staging of gastric cancer. Br J Surg 71: 677–680
240. Kappas A M, Fatouros M, Roukos D H 2004 Is it time to change surgical strategy for gastric cancer in the United States? Ann Surg Oncol 11: 727–730

241. Bogomoletz W V 1984 Early gastric cancer. Am J Surg Pathol 8: 381–391
242. Kodama Y, Inokuchi K, Soejima K et al. 1983 Growth patterns and prognosis in early gastric carcinoma: superficially spreading and penetrating growth types. Cancer 51: 320–326
243. Inokuchi K, Kodama Y, Sasaki O et al. 1983 Differentiation of growth patterns of early gastric carcinoma determined by cytophotometric DNA analysis. Cancer 51: 1138–1141
244. Brito M J, Filipe M I, Williams G T et al. 1993 DNA ploidy in early (T1) gastric cancer: a flow cytometric study of 100 European cases. Gut 34: 230–234
245. Eckardt V F, Willems D, Kanzler G et al. 1984 Eighty months persistence of poorly differentiated early gastric cancer. Gastroenterology 87: 719–724
246. Offerhaus G J A, Tersmette A C, Huibregtse K et al. 1988 Mortality caused by stomach cancer after remote partial gastrectomy for benign conditions: 40 years of follow-up of an Amsterdam cohort of 2633 postgastrectomy patients. Gut 29: 1588–1590
247. Bogomoletz W V, Potet F, Barge J et al. 1985 Pathologic features and mucin histochemistry of primary gastric stump carcinoma associated with gastritis cystica polyposa: a study of six cases. Am J Surg Pathol 9: 401–410
248. Dirschmid K, Walser J, Hügel H 1984 Pseudomalignant erosion in hyperplastic gastric polyps. Cancer 54: 2290–2293
249. Dimet S, Lazure T, Bedossa P 2004 Signet-ring cell change in acute erosive gastropathy. Am J Surg Pathol 28: 1111–1112
250. Chu P G, Weiss L M 2002 Keratin expression in human tissues and neoplasms. Histopathology 40: 403–439
250a. van Velthuysen M L, Taal B G, van der Hoevon J J, Peterse J L 2005 Expression of oestrogen receptor and loss of E-cadherin are diagnostic for gastric metastasis of breast carcinoma. Histopathology 46:153–157
251. Minamoto T, Mai M, Watanabe K et al. 1990 Medullary carcinoma with lymphocytic infiltration of the stomach. Cancer 66: 945–952
252. Lu B-J, Lai M, Cheng L et al. 2004 Gastric medullary carcinoma, a distinct entity with microsatellite instability-H, prominent intraepithelial lymphocytes and improved prognosis. Histopathology 45: 485–492
253. Griffiths A P, Rice A, Dixon M F 1998 Anaplastic gastric adenocarcinoma with extensive neutrophilic infiltration. Histopathology 33: 392–393
254. Caruso R A, Bellocco R, Pagano M et al. 2002 Prognostic value of intratumoral neutrophils in advanced gastric carcinoma in a high-risk area in northern Italy. Mod Pathol 15: 831–837
255. Mori M, Iwashita A, Enjoji M 1986 Adenosquamous carcinoma of the stomach: a clinicopathologic analysis of 28 cases. Cancer 57: 333–339
256. Mori M, Kukuda T, Enjoji M 1987 Adenosquamous carcinoma of the stomach: histogenetic and ultrastructural studies. Gastroenterology 92: 1078–1082
257. Volpe C M, Hameer H R, Masetti P et al. 1995 Squamous cell carcinoma of the stomach. Am Surg 61: 1076–1078
258. Ueyama T, Nagai E, Yao T et al. 1993 Vimentin-positive gastric carcinoma with rhabdoid features. Am J Surg Pathol 17: 813–819
259. Petrella T, Montagnon J, Roignot P et al. 1995 Alphafetoprotein-producing gastric adenocarcinoma. Histopathology 26: 171–175
260. Matsunou H, Konishi F, Jala R E A et al. 1994 Alpha-fetoprotein-producing gastric carcinoma with enteroblastic differentiation. Cancer 73: 534–540
261. Yakeishi Y, Mori M, Enjoji M 1990 Distribution of beta human chorionic gonadotrophin positive cells in non-cancerous gastric mucosa and in malignant gastric tumors. Cancer 66: 695–701
262. Ramponi A, Angeli G, Arcezi F et al. 1986 Gastric choriocarcinoma: an immunohistochemical study. Pathol Res Pract 181: 390–396
263. Krulewski T, Cohen L B 1988 Choriocarcinoma of the stomach: pathogenesis and clinical characteristics. Am J Gastroenterol 83: 1172–1175
264. Garcia R L, Ghali V S 1985 Gastric choriocarcinoma and yolk sac tumor in a man. Observations about its possible origin. Hum Pathol 16: 955–958
265. Rindi G, Luinetti O, Cornaggia M et al. 1993 Three subtypes of gastric argyrophil carcinoid and the neuroendocrine carcinoma: a clinicopathologic study. Gastroenterology 104: 994–1006
266. Rindi G, Bordi C, Rappel S et al. 1996 Gastric carcinoids and neuroendocrine carcinomas: pathogenesis, pathology, and behavior. World J Surg 20: 168–17
267. Matsui K, Jin X M, Kitagawa M et al. 1998 Clinicopathologic features of neuroendocrine carcinomas of the stomach: appraisal of small cell and large cell variants. Arch Pathol Lab Med 122: 1010–1017
268. Robey-Cafferty S S, Grignon D, Ro J Y et al. 1990 Sarcomatoid carcinoma of the stomach. A report of three cases with immunohistochemical and ultrastructural observations. Cancer 65: 1601–1606
269. Aiba M, Hirayama A, Suzuki T et al. 1991 Carcinosarcoma of the stomach: report of a case with review of the literature of gastrectomized patients. Surg Pathol 4: 75–83
270. Dundas S A C, Slater D N, Wagner B E et al. 1988 Gastric adenocarcinoleiomyosarcoma: a light and electron microscopic and immunohistochemical study. Histopathology 13: 347–350
271. Kallakury B V S, Bui H X, del Rosario A et al. 1993 Primary gastric adenosarcoma. Arch Pathol Lab Med 117: 299–301
272. Thomas R M, Baybick J H, Elsayed A M et al. 1994 Gastric carcinoids: an immunohistochemical and clinicopathologic study of 104 patients. Cancer 73: 2053–2058
273. Abraham S C, Carney J A, Ooi A et al. 2005 Achlorhydria, parietal cell hyperplasia, and multiple gastric carcinoids: a new disorder. Am J Surg Pathol 29: 969–975
274. Carney J A, Go V L W, Fairbanks V F et al. 1983 The syndrome of gastric argyrophil carcinoid tumors and nonantral gastric atrophy. Ann Int Med 99: 761–766
275. Borch K, Renvall H, Kullman E et al. 1987 Gastric carcinoid associated with the syndrome of hypergastrinaemic atrophic gastritis. Am J Surg Pathol 11: 435–444
276. Solcia E, Capella C, Fiocca R et al. 1990 Gastric argyrophil carcinoidosis in patients with Zollinger–Ellison syndrome due to type 1 multiple endocrine neoplasia. Am J Surg Pathol 14: 503–513
277. Ooi A, Ota M, Katsuda S et al. 1995 An unusual case of multiple gastric carcinoids associated with diffuse endocrine cell hyperplasia and parietal cell hypertrophy. Endocr Pathol 3: 229–237
278. Rindi G, Azzoni C, Larosa S et al. 1999 ECL cell tumor and poorly differentiated endocrine carcinoma of the stomach: prognostic evaluation by pathological analysis. Gastroenterology 116: 532–542
279. Christodoulopoulos J B, Klotz A P 1961 Carcinoid syndrome with primary carcinoid tumor of the stomach. Gastroenterology 40: 429–440
280. Marcus F S, Friedman M A, Callen P W et al. 1980 Successful therapy of an ACTH-producing gastric carcinoid APUD tumor: report of a case and review of the literature. Cancer 46: 1263–1269
281. Capella C, Heitz P, Hofler H et al. 1995 Revised classification of neuroendocrine tumours of the lung, pancreas and gut. Virchow's Arch 425: 547–560
282. Harvey R F 1988 Spontaneous resolution of multifocal gastric enterochromaffin-like cell carcinoid tumours. Lancet i: 821
283. Borch K, Ahren B, Ahlman H et al. 2005 Gastric carcinoids: biologic behavior and prognosis after differentiated treatment in relation to type. Ann Surg 242: 64–73
284. Ordonez N, Mackay B, El-Naggar A et al. 1993 Clear cell carcinoid tumour of the stomach. Histopathology 22: 190–193
285. Rindi G, Paolotti D, Fiocca R et al. 2000 Vesicular monoamine transporter 2 as a marker of gastric enterochromaffin-like cell tumors. Virchow's Arch 436: 217–223
286. Sundler F, Eriksson B, Grimelius L et al. 1992 Histamine in gastric carcinoid tumors: immunocytochemical evidence. Endocr Pathol 3: 23–27
287. Müller J, Kirchner R, Müller-Hermelink H K 1987 Gastric endocrine cell hyperplasia and carcinoid tumors in atrophic gastritis type A. Am J Surg Pathol 11: 909–917
288. Solcia E, Fiocca R, Villani L et al. 1995 Hyperplastic, dysplastic and neoplastic enterochromaffin-like cell proliferations of the gastric mucosa: classification and histogenesis. Am J Surg Pathol 19 (suppl 1): S1–S7
289. Ali M H, Davidson A, Azzopardi J G A 1984 Composite gastric carcinoid and adenocarcinoma. Histopathology 8: 529–536
290. Kindblom L-G, Remotti M E, Aldenborg F et al. 1998 Gastrointestinal pacemaker cell tumor (GIPACT): gastrointestinal stromal tumors show phenotypic characteristics of the interstitial cells of Cajal. Am J Pathol 152: 1259–1269
291. Miettinen M, Lasota J 2001 Gastrointestinal stromal tumors – definition, clinical, histological, immunohistochemical, and molecular genetic features and differential diagnosis. Virchow's Arch 438: 1–12
292. Fletcher C D M, Berman J J, Corless C et al. 2002 Diagnosis of gastrointestinal stromal tumors: a consensus approach. Hum Pathol 33: 459–465
293. Verweij J, Casali P G, Zalcberg J et al. 2004 Progression-free survival in gastrointestinal stromal tumours with high-dose imatinib: randomised trial. Lancet 364: 1127–1134
294. Fuller C E, Williams G T 1991 Gastrointestinal manifestations of type I neurofibromatosis (von Recklinghausen's disease). Histopathology 19: 1–11
295. Carney J A 1983 The triad of gastric epithelioid leiomyosarcoma, pulmonary chondroma and functioning extra-adrenal paraganglioma: a 5-year review. Medicine 62: 159–169
296. Carney J A, Stratakis C A 2002 Familial paraganglioma and gastric stromal sarcoma: a new syndrome distinct from the Carney triad. Am J Med Genet 108: 132–139
297. Hirota S, Nishida T, Isozaki K et al. 1998 Familial gastrointestinal stromal tumors with germline mutation of KIT gene. Nat Genet 19: 323–324
298. Chompret A, Kannengiesser C, Barrois M 2004 PDGFRA germline mutation in a family with multiple cases of gastrointestinal stromal tumor. Gastroenterology 126: 318–321
299. Miettinen M, Sobin LH, Lasota J 2005 Gastrointestinal stromal tumors of the stomach: a clinicopathologic, immunohistochemical, and molecular genetic study of 1765 cases with long-term follow-up. Am J Surg Pathol 29: 52–68
300. Evans H L 1985 Smooth muscle tumors of the gastrointestinal tract: a study of 56 cases followed for a minimum of 10 years. Cancer 56: 2242–2250
301. Yamada Y, Kato Y, Yanagisawa A et al. 1988 Microleiomyomas of human stomach. Hum Pathol 19: 569–572
302. Wong N A S, Young R, Malcomson R D et al. 2003 Prognostic indicators for gastrointestinal stromal tumours: a clinicopathological and immunohistochemical study of 108 resected cases of the stomach. Histopathology 43: 118–126
303. Appelman H D, Helwig E B 1976 Gastric epithelioid leiomyoma and leiomyosarcoma (leiomyoblastoma). Cancer 38: 708–728
304. Suster S, Sorace D, Moran C A 1995 Gastrointestinal stromal tumors with prominent myxoid matrix. Am J Surg Pathol 19: 59–70
305. Appelman H D, Helwig E B 1977 Sarcomas of the stomach. Am J Clin Pathol 67: 2–10

306. Suster S, Fletcher C D M 1996 Gastrointestinal stromal tumors with prominent signet-ring cell forms. Mod Pathol 9: 609–613
307. Lauwers G Y, Erlandson R A, Casper E S et al. 1993 Gastrointestinal autonomic nerve tumors: a clinicopathologic, immunohistochemical, and ultrastructural study of 12 cases. Am J Surg Pathol 17: 887–897
308. Shanks J H, Harris M, Banerjee S S et al. 1996 Gastrointestinal autonomic nerve tumours: a report of nine cases. Histopathology 29: 111–121
309. Lee J R, Joshi V, Griffin J W et al. 2001 Gastrointestinal autonomic nerve tumor: immunohistochemical and molecular identity with gastrointestinal stromal tumor. Am J Surg Pathol 25: 979–987
310. Hirota S, Isozaki K, Moriyama Y et al. 1998 Gain-of-function mutations of c-kit in human gastrointestinal stromal tumors. Science 279: 577–580
311. Newman P L, Wadden C, Fletcher C D M 1991 Gastrointestinal stromal tumours: correlation of immunophenotype with clinicopathologic features. J Pathol 164: 107–117
312. Heinrich M C, Corless C L, Demetri G D et al. 2003 Kinase mutations and imatinib response in patients with metastatic gastrointestinal stromal tumor. J Clin Oncol 21: 4342–4349
313. Heinrich M C, Corless C L, Duensing A et al. 2003 PDGFRA activating mutations in gastrointestinal stromal tumors. Science 299: 708–710
314. Lasota J, Dansonka-Mieszkowska A, Sobin L H et al. 2004 A great majority of GISTs with PDGFRA mutations represent gastric tumors of low or no malignant potential. Lab Invest 84: 874–883
315. Debiec-Rychter M, Wasag B, Stul M et al. 2004 Gastrointestinal stromal tumors (GISTs) negative for KIT (CD117 antigen) immunoreactivity. J Pathol 202: 430–438
316. Medeiros F, Corless C L, Duensing A et al. 2004 KIT-negative gastrointestinal stromal tumors. Am J Surg Pathol 28: 889–894.
317. Pauwels P, Debiec-Rychter M, Stul M et al. 2005 Changing phenotype of gastrointestinal stromal tumours under imatinib mesylate treatment: a potential diagnostic pitfall. Histopathology 47: 41–47
318. Cooper P N, Quirke P, Hardy G J et al. 1992 A flow cytometric, clinical and histologic study of stromal neoplasms of the gastrointestinal tract. Am J Surg Pathol 16: 163–170
319. Trupiano J K, Stewart R E, Misick C et al. 2002 Gastric stromal tumors: a clinicopathologic study of 77 cases with correlation of features with nonaggressive and aggressive clinical behaviors. Am J Surg Pathol 26: 705–714
320. Rudolph P, Gloeckner K, Parwaresch R et al. 1998 Immunophenotype, proliferation, DNA ploidy, and biological behavior of gastrointestinal stromal tumors: a multivariate clinicopathologic study. Hum Pathol 29: 791–800
321. Kiyabu M T, Bishop P C, Parker J W et al. 1988 Smooth muscle tumors of the gastrointestinal tract: flow cytometric quantitation of DNA and nuclear antigen content and correlation with histologic grade. Am J Surg Pathol 12: 954–960
322. Lazure T, Ferlicot S, Gauthier F 2002 Gastric inflammatory myofibroblastic tumors in children: an unpredictable course. J Pediatr Gastroenterol Nutr 34: 319–322
323. Lee W A, Lee M K, Jeen Y M 2004 Solitary fibrous tumor arising in gastric serosa. Pathol Int 54: 436–439
324. Delbecque K, Legrand M, Boniver J et al. 2004 Calcifying fibrous tumour of the gastric wall. Histopathology 44: 399–400
325. Sarlomo-Rikala M, Miettinen M 1995 Gastric schwannoma – a clinicopathologic analysis of six cases. Histopathology 27: 355–360
326. Hou Y, Tan Y, Xu J et al. 2006 Schwannoma of the digestive tract: a clinicopathologic, immunohistochemical and ultrastructural study of 33 cases. Histopathology 48 536–545
327. Palmer E D 1951 Benign intramural tumors of the stomach: a review with special reference to gross pathology. Medicine 30: 81–181
328. Chodack P, Hurwitz A 1964 Lymphangiectasis of stomach simulating polypoid neoplasm. Arch Intern Med 113: 225–229
329. Sawyer K C, Lubchenco A E 1951 Haemangioendothelioma of the stomach. Surgery 30: 383–387
330. Lee K C, Ng W F, Chan J K C 1988 Epithelioid haemangioendothelioma presenting as a gastric polyp. Histopathology 12: 335–337
331. Lustbader I, Sherman A 1987 Primary gastrointestinal Kaposi's sarcoma in a patient with acquired immune deficiency syndrome. Am J Gastroenterol 82: 894–895
332. Fay D E, Nisbeth H 1990 Massive gastrointestinal hemorrhage in an immunosuppressed man due to gastric Kaposi's sarcoma. Am J Gastroenterol 85: 607–609
333. Taxy J B, Battifora H 1988 Angiosarcoma of the gastrointestinal tract. A report of three cases. Cancer 62: 210–216
334. Amy C, Lazure T, Sales J P et al. 2001 Gastric epithelioid angiosarcoma, a biopsy diagnostic pitfall. Ann Pathol 21: 439–441
335. Miettinen M, Paal E, Lasota J et al. 2002 Gastrointestinal glomus tumors: a clinicopathologic, immunohistochemical, and molecular genetic study of 32 cases. Am J Surg Pathol 26: 301–311
336. Tuazon R 1969 Rhabdomyoma of the stomach. Report of a case. Am J Clin Pathol 52: 37–41
337. Fox K R, Moussa S M, Mitre R J et al. 1990 Clinical and pathologic features of primary gastric rhabdomyosarcoma. Cancer 66: 772–778
338. Maderal F, Hunter F, Fuselier G et al. 1984 Gastric lipomas: an update of clinical presentation, diagnosis and treatment. Am J Gastroenterol 79: 964–967
339. McGregor D H, Kerley S W, McGregor M S 1993 Gastric angiolipoma with chronic hemorrhage and severe anemia. Am J Med Sci 305: 229–235
340. Shokouh-Amiri M H, Hansen C P, Moesgaard F 1986 Liposarcoma of the stomach: a case report. Acta Chir Scand 152: 389–391
341. Alerte F 1963 Xanthofibroma of the stomach. Report of a case with severe secondary hypochromic anemia. Arch Pathol 75: 99–104
342. Billings S D, Meisner L F, Cummings O W et al. 2000 Synovial sarcoma of the upper digestive tract. Mod Pathol 13: 68–76.
343. Pauwels P, Debiec-Rychter M, Sciot R et al. 2002 Clear cell sarcoma of the stomach. Histopathology 41: 526–530
344. Schmid C, Beham A, Steindorfer P et al. 1990 Non functional malignant paraganglioma of the stomach. Virchow's Arch [A] 417: 261–264
345. Pack G T 1964 Unusual tumors of the stomach. Ann NY Acad Sci 114: 985–1011
346. Tapp E 1964 Ganglioneuroblastoma of the stomach. J Pathol Bacteriol 88: 79–82
347. Haqqani M T, Krasner N, Ashworth M 1983 Benign mesenchymoma of the stomach. J Clin Pathol 36: 504–507
348. Matsukuma S, Wada R, Daibou M et al. 1995 Adenocarcinoma arising from gastric immature teratoma. Cancer 75: 2663–2668
349. Isaacson P G, Du M Q 2005 Gastrointestinal lymphoma – where morphology meets molecular biology. J Pathol 205: 255–274
350. Chan J K C 1996 Gastrointestinal lymphomas: an overview with emphasis on new findings and diagnostic problems. Semin Diagn Pathol 13: 260–296
351. Mori N, Yatabe Y, Narita M et al. 1995 Primary gastric Hodgkin's disease: morphologic, immunohistochemical and immunogenetic analyses. Arch Pathol Lab Med 119: 163–166
352. Tungekar M F 1986 Gastric signet-ring cell lymphoma with alpha heavy chains. Histopathology 10: 725–733
353. Isaacson P G, Spencer J, Finn T 1986 Primary B-cell gastric lymphoma. Hum Pathol 17: 72–82
354. Isaacson P G 1996 Recent developments in our understanding of gastric lymphomas. Am J Surg Pathol 20 (suppl 1): S1–S7
355. Farinha P, Gascoyne R D 2005 Helicobacter pylori and MALT lymphoma. Gastroenterology 128: 1579–1605
356. Bayerdörffer E, Neubauer A, Rudolph B et al. 1995 Regression of primary gastric lymphoma of mucosa-associated lymphoid tissue type after cure of Helicobacter pylori infection. Lancet 345: 1591–1594
357. Chan J K C, Ng C S, Isaacson P G 1990 Relationship between high-grade lymphoma and low-grade B-cell mucosa-associated lymphoid tissue lymphoma (MALToma) of the stomach. Am J Pathol 136: 1153–1164
358. Wotherspoon A C, Diss T C, Pan L et al. 1996 Low-grade gastric B-cell lymphoma of mucosa-associated lymphoid tissue in immunocompromised patients. Histopathology 28: 129–134
359. Guettier C, Hamilton-Dutoit S, Guillemain R et al. 1992 Primary gastrointestinal malignant lymphomas associated with Epstein–Barr virus after heart transplantation. Histopathology 20: 21–28
360. Wotherspoon A C, Isaacson P G 1995 Synchronous adenocarcinoma and low-grade B-cell lymphoma of mucosa-associated lymphoid tissue (MALT) of the stomach. Histopathology 27: 325–331
361. Cogliatti S B, Schmid U, Schumacher U et al. 1991 Primary B-cell gastric lymphoma: a clinicopathologic study of 145 patients. Gastroenterology 101: 1159–1170
362. Musshoff K, Schmidt-Vollmer H 1975 Prognosis of non-Hodgkin's lymphomas with special emphasis on the staging classification. Z Krebsforsch 83: 323–341
363. Ruskone-Fourmestraux A, Dragosics B, Morgner A et al. 2003 Paris staging system for primary gastrointestinal lymphomas. Gut 52: 912–913
364. Wotherspoon A C, Doglioni C, Isaacson P G 1992 Low-grade gastric B-cell lymphoma of mucosa-associated lymphoid tissue (MALT): a multifocal disease. Histopathology 20: 29–34
365. Stephen M R, Farquharson M A, Sharp R A et al. 1998 Sequential MALT lymphomas of the stomach, small intestine, and gall bladder. J Clin Pathol 51: 77–79
366. Isaacson P G, Spencer J 1987 Malignant lymphoma of mucosa-associated lymphoid tissue. Histopathology 11: 445–462
367. Isaacson P G 1990 Lymphomas of mucosa-associated lymphoid tissue. Histopathology 16: 617–619
368. Zamboni G, Franzin G, Scarpa A et al. 1996 Carcinoma-like signet-ring cells in gastric mucosa-associated lymphoid tissue (MALT) lymphoma. Am J Surg Pathol 20: 588–598
369. Liu H, Ye H, Dogan A et al. 2001 T(11;18)(q21;q21) is associated with advanced mucosa-associated lymphoid tissue lymphoma that expresses nuclear BCL10. Blood 98: 1182–1187
370. Liu H, Ye H, Ruskone-Fourmestraux A et al. 2002 T(11;18) is a marker for all stage gastric MALT lymphomas that will not respond to H. pylori eradication. Gastroenterology 122: 1286–1294
371. Inagaki H, Nakamura T, Li C et al. 2004 Gastric MALT lymphomas are divided into three groups based on responsiveness to Helicobacter pylori eradication and detection of API2-MALT1 fusion. Am J Surg Pathol 28: 1560–1567
372. Peng H, Du M, Diss T C et al. 1997 Genetic evidence for a clonal link between low and high-grade components in gastric MALT B-cell lymphoma. Histopathology 30: 425–429
373. de Jong D, Boot H, van Heerde P et al. 1997 Histological grading in gastric lymphoma: pretreatment criteria and clinical relevance. Gastroenterology 112: 1466–1474
374. Zukerberg L R, Ferry J A, Southern J F et al. 1990 Lymphoid infiltrates of the stomach. Evaluation of histologic criteria for the diagnosis of low-grade

gastric lymphoma on endoscopic biopsy specimens. Am J Surg Pathol 14: 1087–1099
375. Abbondanzo S L, Sobin L H 1997 Gastric "pseudolymphoma". A retrospective morphologic and immunophenotypic study of 97 cases. Cancer 79: 1656–1663
376. Lynch D A F, Sobala G M, Dixon M F et al. 1995 Lymphocytic gastritis and associated small bowel disease: a diffuse lymphocytic gastroenteropathy? J Clin Pathol 48: 939–945
377. Calvert R J, Evans P A S, Randerson J A et al. 1996 The significance of B-cell clonality in gastric lymphoid infiltrates. J Pathol 180: 26–32
378. Attanoos R, Griffiths D F R 1992 Metastatic small cell melanoma to the stomach mimicking primary gastric lymphoma. Histopathology 21: 173–175
379. Isaacson P G, MacLennan K A, Subbuswamy S G 1984 Multiple lymphomatous polyposis of the gastrointestinal tract. Histopathology 8: 641–656
380. Fraga M, Lloret E, Sanchez-Verde L et al. 1995 Mucosal mantle cell (centrocytic) lymphomas. Histopathology 26: 413–422
381. Hirakawa K, Fuchigami T, Nakamura S et al. 1996 Primary gastrointestinal T-cell lymphoma resembling multiple lymphomatous polyposis. Gastroenterology 111: 778–782
382. Nakamura S, Iida M, Matsui T et al. 1991 Adult T-cell leukemia/lymphoma with gastric lesions. Report of three cases. J Clin Gastroenterol 13: 390–394
383. Nakanishi I, Kajikawa K, Migita S et al. 1982 Gastric plasmacytoma: an immunologic and immunohistochemical study. Cancer 49: 2025–2028
384. Isaacson P G, Buchanan R, Mepham B L 1978 Plasma cell granuloma of the stomach. Hum Pathol 9: 355–358
385. Hatano B, Ohshima K, Katoh A et al. 2002 Non-HTLV-1-associated primary gastric T-cell lymphomas show cytotoxic activity: clinicopathological, immunohistochemical characteristics and TIA-1 expression in 31 cases. Histopathology 41: 421–436
386. Iwamizu-Watanabe S, Yamashita Y, Yatabe Y et al. 2004 Frequent expression of CD30 antigen in the primary gastric non-B, non-Hodgkin lymphomas. Pathol Int 54: 503–509
387. Foss H D, Schmitt G A, Daum S et al. 1999 Origin of primary gastric T-cell lymphomas from intraepithelial T-lymphocytes: report of two cases. Histopathology 35: 9–15
388. Groisman G M, Rosh J R, Harpaz N 1994 Langerhans cell histiocytosis of the stomach: a cause of granulomatous gastritis and gastric polyposis. Arch Pathol Lab Med 118: 1232–1235
389. Brugo E A, Marshall R B, Riberi A M et al. 1977 Preleukemic granulocytic sarcomas of the gastrointestinal tract. Am J Clin Pathol 68: 616–621
390. Wong K F, Yuen R W S, Lok A S F et al. 1989 Granulocytic sarcoma presenting as bleeding gastric polyp. Pathology 21: 62–64
391. Ismail S M, Myers K 1989 Infiltrative myeloid metaplasia: an unusual cause of gastric outlet obstruction. J Clin Pathol 42: 1112–1113
392. Green L K 1990 Hematogenous metastases to the stomach. A review of 67 cases. Cancer 65: 1596–1600
393. Telerman A, Gerard B, van den Heule B et al. 1985 Gastrointestinal metastases from abdominal tumors. Endoscopy 17: 99–101
394. Taal B G, Peterse H, Boot H 2000 Clinical presentation, endoscopic features, and treatment of gastric metastases from breast carcinoma. Cancer 89: 2214–2221
395. Wauters G V, Ferrell L, Ostroff J W et al. 1990 Hyperplastic gastric polyps associated with persistent *Helicobacter pylori* infection and active gastritis. Am J Gastroenterol 85: 1395–1397
396. Ohkusa T, Takashimizu I, Fujiki K et al. 1998 Disappearance of hyperplastic polyps in the stomach after eradication of *Helicobacter pylori*. A randomized, clinical trial. Ann Int Med 129: 712–715
397. Muller-Lissner S A, Wiebecke B 1982 Investigations on hyperplasiogenous gastric polyps by partial reconstruction. Pathol Res Pract 174: 368–378
398. Odze R D, Marcial M A, Antonioli D 1996 Gastric fundic polyps: a morphologic study using mucin histochemistry, stereometry, and MIB-1 immunohistochemistry. Hum Pathol 27: 896–903
399. Iida M, Yao T, Watanabe H et al. 1980 Spontaneous disappearance of fundic gland polyposis: report of three cases. Gastroenterology 79: 725–728
400. Tsuchikame N, Ishimaru Y, Ohshima S et al. 1993 Three familial cases of fundic gland polyposis without polyposis coli. Virchow's Arch [A] 422: 337–340
401. Vieth M, Stolte M 2001 Fundic gland polyps are not induced by proton pump inhibitor therapy. Am J Clin Pathol 116: 716–720
402. Lee R G, Burt R W 1986 The histopathology of fundic gland polyps of the stomach. Am J Clin Pathol 86: 498–503
403. Riddell R H 1996 The biopsy diagnosis of gastroesophageal reflux disease, "carditis," and Barrett's esophagus, and sequelae of therapy. Am J Surg Pathol 20 (suppl 1): S31–S51
404. Abraham S C 2002 Sporadic fundic gland polyps with epithelial dysplasia: evidence for preferential targeting for mutations in the adenomatous polyposis coli gene. Am J Pathol 161:1735–1742
405. Torbenson M, Lee J H, Cruz-Correa M et al. 2002 Sporadic fundic gland polyposis: a clinical, histological, and molecular analysis. Mod Pathol 15: 718–23
406. Kolodziejczyk P, Yao T, Tsuneyoshi M 1993 Inflammatory fibroid polyp of the stomach: a special reference to an immunohistochemical profile of 42 cases. Am J Surg Pathol 17: 1159–1168
407. Pantanowitz L, Antonioli D A, Pinkus G S et al. 2004 Inflammatory fibroid polyps of the gastrointestinal tract: evidence for a dendritic cell origin. Am J Surg Pathol 28: 107–114
408. Bartholomew L G, Moore C E, Dahlin D C et al. 1962 Intestinal polyposis associated with mucocutaneous pigmentation. Surg Gynecol Obstet 115: 1–11
409. Shinmura K, Goto M, Tao H et al. 2005 A novel STK11 germline mutation in two siblings with Peutz–Jeghers syndrome complicated by primary gastric cancer. Clin Genet 67: 81–86
410. Cochet B, Carrel J, Desbaillets L et al. 1979 Peutz–Jeghers syndrome associated with gastrointestinal carcinoma. Gut 20: 169–175
411. Hizawa K, Iida M, Yao T et al. 1997 Juvenile polyposis of the stomach: clinicopathologic features and its malignant potential. J Clin Pathol 50: 771–774
412. Weinstein J V, Kawanishi H 1978 Gastrointestinal polyposis with orocutaneous hamartomas (Cowden's disease). Gastroenterology 74: 890–895
413. Kindblom L G, Angervall L, Santesson B et al. 1977 Cronkhite-Canada syndrome. Cancer 39: 2651–2657
414. Lipper S, Kahn L B 1977 Superficial cystic gastritis with alopecia. A forme fruste of the Cronkhite-Canada syndrome. Arch Pathol Lab Med 101: 432–436
415. Barrocas A, Fontenelle L, Williams M J 1973 Gastric heterotopic pancreas: a case report and review of the literature. Am Surg 39: 361–365
416. Yun-Zhong H, Guo Q-X 1990 Adenomyoma of the stomach presenting as an antral polyp. Histopathology 16: 99–101
417. Kneafsey P D, Demetrick D J 1992 Malignant transformation in a pyloric adenomyoma: a case report. Histopathology 20: 433–435
418. Goldfarb W B, Bennett D, Monafo W 1963 Carcinoma in heterotopic gastric pancreas. Ann Surg 158: 56–58
419. Doglioni C, Laurino L, Dei Tos A P et al. 1993 Pancreatic (acinar) metaplasia of the gastric mucosa. Am J Surg Pathol 17: 1134–1143
420. Wang H H, Zeroogian J M, Spechler S J et al. 1996 Prevalence and significance of pancreatic acinar metaplasia at the gastroesophageal junction. Am J Surg Pathol 20: 1507–1510
421. William S A W, Michie W 1957 Adenomatosis of the stomach of Brunner gland type. Br J Surg 45: 259–263
422. Gensler S, Seidenberg B, Rifkin H et al. 1966 Ciliated lined intramural cyst of the stomach: case report and suggested embryogenesis. Ann Surg 163: 954–956
423. Delvaux S, Ectors N, Begoes K et al. 1996 Gastric gland heterotopia with extensive lymphoid stroma: a gastric lymphoepithelial cyst. Am J Gastroenterol 91: 599–601
424. Carr G L, Squires C 1962 Squamous papillomatosis of the stomach. A new pathologic entity: report of a case. Am Surg 28: 790–793
425. Catanzaro C, Weeks C B, Kafka R M 1962 Chronic hypertrophic gastritis. Report of two cases in siblings. Am J Gastroenterol 37: 525–536
426. Scharschmidt B F 1977 The natural history of hypertrophic gastropathy (Ménétrier's disease). Am J Med 63: 644–652
427. Kraut J R, Powell R, Hruby M A et al. 1981 Ménétrier's disease in childhood: report of two cases and a review of the literature. J Pediatr Surg 16: 707–711
428. Frank B W, Kern F Jr 1967 Ménétrier's disease: spontaneous metamorphosis of giant hypertrophy of the gastric mucosa to atrophic gastritis. Gastroenterology 53: 953–960
429. Berenson M M, Sannella J, Freston J W 1976 Ménétrier's disease: serial morphologic, secretory and serological observations. Gastroenterology 70: 257–263
430. Wolfsen H C, Carpenter H A, Talley N J 1993 Menetrier's disease: a form of hypertrophic gastropathy or gastritis? Gastroenterology 1993: 1310–1319
431. Xiao S Y, Hart J 2001 Marked gastric foveolar hyperplasia associated with active cytomegalovirus infection. Am J Gastroenterol 96: 223–226
432. Franzin G, Novelli P 1981 Gastritis cystica profunda. Histopathology 5: 535–547
433. Lin P Y, Brown D B, Deppisch L M 1989 Gastric xanthelasma in hyperplastic gastric polyposis. Arch Pathol Lab Med 113: 428–430
434. Kimura K, Hiramoto T, Buncher C R 1969 Gastric xanthelasma. Arch Pathol 87: 110–117
435. Jensen K, Raynor S, Rose S G et al. 1985 Amyloid tumors of the gastrointestinal tract: a report of two cases and review of the literature. Am J Gastroenterol 80: 784–786
436. Bjornsson S, Johansson J H, Sigurjonsson F 1987 Localised primary amyloidosis of the stomach presenting with gastric haemorrhage. Acta Med Scand 221: 115–119
437. Goteri G, Ranaldi R, Pileri S A et al. 1998 Localised amyloidosis and gastrointestinal lymphoma: a rare association. Histopathology 32: 348–355

小肠和大肠（包括肛门部）肿瘤
Tumors of the small and large intestines (including the anal region)

Jeremy R. Jass 著

杜金荣 陈英淮 韩丽姝 译

小肠	379	大肠	393
上皮性肿瘤	379	上皮性肿瘤	393
非上皮性肿瘤（间叶性和脉管性）	381	非上皮性肿瘤	404
淋巴组织肿瘤	384	淋巴组织肿瘤	405
继发性肿瘤	387	继发性肿瘤	405
瘤样病变	387	瘤样病变	405
阑尾	390	肛管	409
上皮性肿瘤	390	上皮性肿瘤	409
内分泌肿瘤	391	肛缘肿瘤	411
瘤样病变	392	表皮和附属器肿瘤	411

小肠 Small intestine

上皮性肿瘤 Epithelial tumors

腺瘤 Adenoma

临床特征

小肠腺瘤少见[1]。大多见于壶腹周围区。患者年龄范围在 30～90 岁，60～70 岁为发病高峰。没有性别差异。临床表现与肿瘤的大小和部位有关。小的腺瘤通常没有症状，但若发生在壶腹部，可能会阻碍胆汁的流出。大的腺瘤常为绒毛状，可能引起肠梗阻、肠出血或肠套叠。多数小肠癌可能来自先前存在的腺瘤。研究证实，大的绒毛状腺瘤容易恶变。十二指肠多发性腺瘤常常是家族性腺瘤性息肉病的并发症（图 9.1），但体积通常较小[2]。

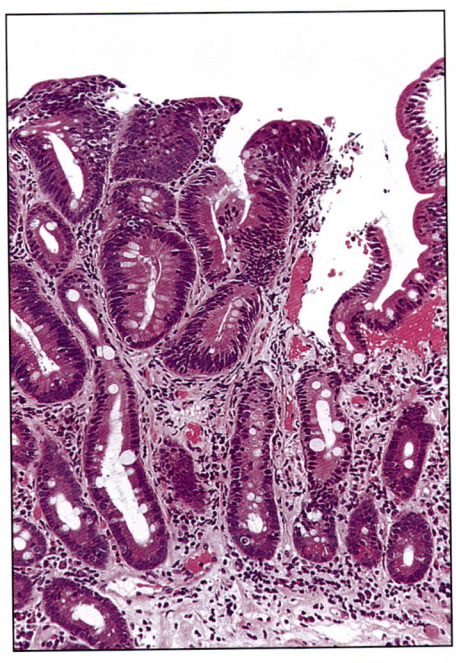

图 9.1 家族性腺瘤性息肉病患者的十二指肠管状腺瘤。内衬黏膜表面部分腺管的上皮显示轻度异型增生，伴有细胞核密集和增大。

大体表现

小肠和壶腹部的腺瘤具有与大肠腺瘤同样的大体特征，同样可以分为管状腺瘤、管状绒毛状腺瘤和绒毛状腺瘤。然而，与大肠不同，小肠腺瘤大部分是无蒂的绒毛状腺瘤[3]。

组织学表现

尽管吸收型的柱状细胞可能比较明显，小肠腺瘤的组织学表现类似于大肠腺瘤（见 393 页）。

鉴别诊断

鉴别壶腹部腺瘤与邻近乳头开口的发生在十二指肠黏膜的腺瘤十分重要。对后者通常采用保守性切除，而对于选择性的有症状的壶腹部腺瘤（具有很高的恶性危险）则采用根治性的手术治疗。壶腹部炎性息肉在临床和组织学上都与肿瘤相似。上皮异型增生是诊断腺瘤的先决条件。中至重度异型增生的腺瘤可能与低级别腺癌相似，发生在壶腹部通常代表其下有恶性肿瘤。

腺癌　Adenocarcinoma

临床特征

与胃或大肠癌相比，小肠腺癌少见得多，通常累及老年成人[4,5]。小肠内分泌肿瘤比较常见。因为小肠内容呈液体状态，所以梗阻出现较晚，在诊断时小肠腺癌通常处在晚期，而且预后不良[6]。大多数小肠癌发生在先前存在的腺瘤内。十二指肠壶腹周围是最常见的发病部位，患者常表现为无痛性黄疸和出血。少数经过根治性手术治疗的壶腹癌伴有良好的预后，故认为这些癌是早期和低级别的癌[7]。小肠癌可能发生在乳糜泻[8,9]、Crohn 病[10,11]以及遗传性（Lynch 综合征）非息肉病性结直肠癌（HNPCC）[12]的背景上。发生在壶腹周围的腺癌是家族性腺瘤性息肉病（FAP）的重要并发症[13]。

大体表现

壶腹癌为息肉样或溃疡性肿瘤；低级别腺癌附近经常能看到共存的腺瘤[7]。其余部位的癌通常呈环形生长。

组织学表现

多数为高分化或中分化腺癌，也可为黏液性腺癌，但印戒细胞癌罕见，应与来自其他部位特别是胃的印戒细胞癌的扩散仔细鉴别。壶腹部腺癌主要是肠型腺癌，正常壶腹部的反应性或再生性改变及其本身复杂的腺体结构应与恶性肿瘤仔细鉴别。

内分泌肿瘤　Endocrine tumors

临床特征

类癌（carcinoid tumor）一词用于描述由内分泌细胞组成的肿瘤。类癌大约占小肠肿瘤的1/3。典型的类癌发生于十二指肠或回肠，好发年龄为 40～60 岁，女性略为常见[14]。少数病例与炎症性肠病有关[15]。类癌生长缓慢，但可浸润肠壁引起狭窄。类癌可以转移到肝脏和肠系膜淋巴结。多发性类癌患者往往比较年轻而且预后不良[16]。肿瘤分泌 5-羟色胺（5-HT）和其他血管活性胺。当肝的转移性肿瘤长到足够大时，5-羟色胺释放到肝静脉而导致类癌综合征。类癌综合征具有三个组成部分：(1)腹泻；(2)面部潮红；(3)心脏病变，包括肺动脉瓣和三尖瓣狭窄。十二指肠类癌往往比空肠和回肠类癌小，侵袭性差，而空肠和回肠类癌常常发生浸润和转移[17]。类癌可以产生各种多肽激素，包括胃泌素、生长抑素、缩胆囊素（cholecystokinin）、胰多肽、胰高血糖素、蛙皮素、胃动素（motilin）和降钙素。某些内分泌肿瘤依其分泌的激素命名。例如，胃泌素瘤可使胃酸过度分泌，并引起胃、空肠和十二指肠多发性消化性溃疡（即 Zollinger-Ellison 综合征）。胃泌素瘤可以发生在十二指肠，但更常见于胰腺和胃（见第 8 章）。

大体表现

浸润性生长的类癌常常伴有纤维化和平滑肌增生，可导致肠腔狭窄。福尔马林固定后的类癌一般呈黄色（图9.2）。类癌常为多发性，并可同时伴有胃肠道的非内分泌性肿瘤。

组织学表现

类癌可能起源于肠隐窝基底部的内分泌细胞，首先浸润黏膜表层直到黏膜肌层，之后侵犯黏膜下层。肿瘤表面上皮隆起，可形成溃疡。镜下，类癌由小细胞组成，细胞核均匀一致，圆形，核分裂象非常少见。典型的类癌由排列成岛屿状的细胞组成，周围的细胞可能显示栅栏状结构（图9.3）。位于周围的细胞中最显著的是肠嗜

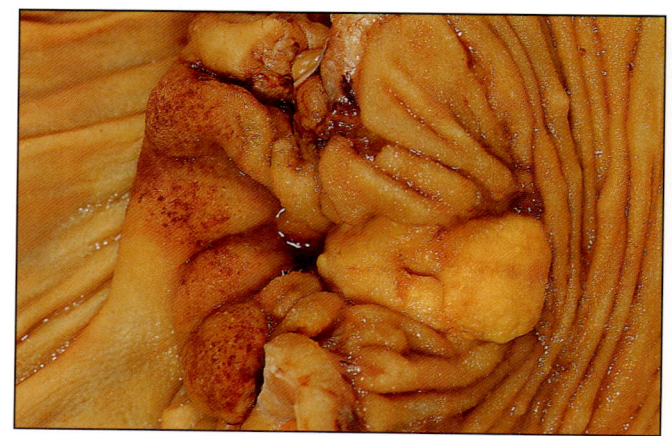

图9.2　回肠末端接近回盲瓣处的类癌。肿瘤呈结节状，黄色，不伴有溃疡形成。

铬细胞，胞浆含有明显的嗜酸性核下颗粒。其他的组织学结构包括小梁状、弥漫片块状、腺样结构，以及各种中间类型和混合性结构[18]。有时，腺样结构腔内可见少量黏液。预后与组织学特点无关。尽管被认为是恶性肿瘤，但是与腺癌相比，类癌生长缓慢，侵袭性小。体积大、显示广泛局部扩展伴有溃疡形成和坏死的类癌侵袭性较强。该部位极少数的高级别神经内分泌肿瘤具有小细胞癌的形态，临床上具有侵袭性[18a]。局限于肠壁的类癌5年生存率85%[19]。当肿瘤穿透浆膜时，5年生存率降至5%。特殊染色有助于证明肠嗜铬细胞存在。肠嗜铬细胞亲银反应呈黑色，重氮基染色呈砖红色，而铅苏木素（lead hematoxylin）染色呈蓝色。不产生5-羟色胺的内分泌细胞可用嗜银染色（例如Grimelius染色）和免疫组化（见下文）染色来证实。十二指肠类癌中侵袭性较小的一种肿瘤的特征是：出现PAS染色阳性的砂粒体并产生生长抑素（图9.4）[20]。这种生长抑素瘤（somatostatinomas）相对常见于壶腹周围[21]。

免疫组化检查

嗜铬素、突触素、NSE、PGP9.5（蛋白基因产物，protein gene product）阳性支持类癌的诊断。此外，应用抗多肽类激素抗体可以做到功能分类。应用原位杂交检测mRNA可以增加功能分类的敏感性。

电镜检查

可以证明特征性的电子密度的神经分泌颗粒，但很少用于诊断。

非上皮性肿瘤（间叶性和脉管性）
Non-epithelial tumors（mesenchymal and vascular）

胃肠道间质瘤
Gastrointestinal stromal tumors

小肠的大多数间质肿瘤属于现在所谓的胃肠道间质瘤（gastrointestinal stromal tumor，GIST）的范畴。和发生在胃的胃肠道间质瘤一样，这些病变最初被认为是平滑肌肿瘤[22]，但现在认为这种肿瘤是起源于间质Cajal细胞或向间质Cajal细胞分化的肿瘤[23,24]。间质Cajal细胞是起搏细胞，插在肠壁自主神经系统和平滑肌之间。假设Cajal细胞与介于神经元和平滑肌之间的细胞有关，就能理解文献中记录的经免疫组化和电镜证实的混合性神经和平滑肌表型的细胞。另外，60%～70%的GISTs表达普遍存在的中胚层标记物CD34[25]。然而，单一最重要的生物学标记物是跨膜酪氨酸激酶受体KIT（CD117）的过度表达[26,27]。这反过来可以用KIT基因体细胞突变来解释，KIT基因体细胞突变见于80%以上GISTs[28]。由于KIT过度表达，GISTs可用酪氨酸激酶抑制剂伊马替尼（STI-571）或甲磺酸伊马替尼（Gleevec）做特异性的靶向治疗，使得这些以前不被人们注意的肿瘤成为实体瘤靶向化疗的重要模型[29]。

与胃GISTs相比，小肠GISTs在超微结构水平具有更多向神经分化的证据。因此，文献中将少数小肠间质肿瘤称为丛状肉瘤（plexosarcoma）或胃肠道自主神经瘤（gastrointestinal autonomic nerve tumor，GANT）[30-34]。然而，现在似乎没有理由把GANTs作为一个独立的疾病从GISTs中分离出来，因为它们具有同样的KIT突变基因[35]。

临床特征

小的肿瘤可能在手术或尸检时偶然发现，而较大的肿瘤可能表现为出血或腹部不适。发病没有性别和种族

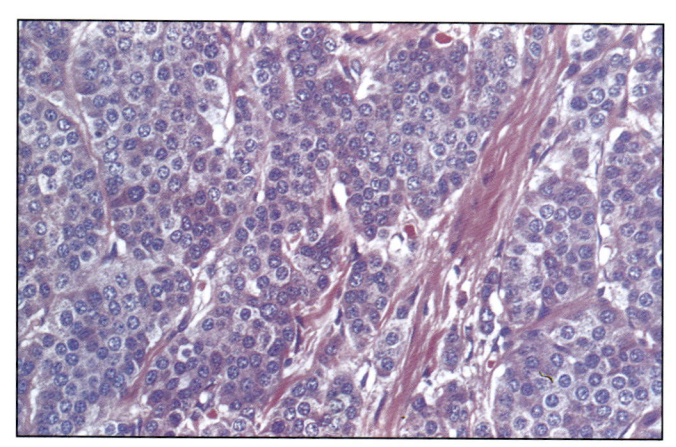

图9.3　回肠类癌，由排列成巢的均匀一致的细胞组成。

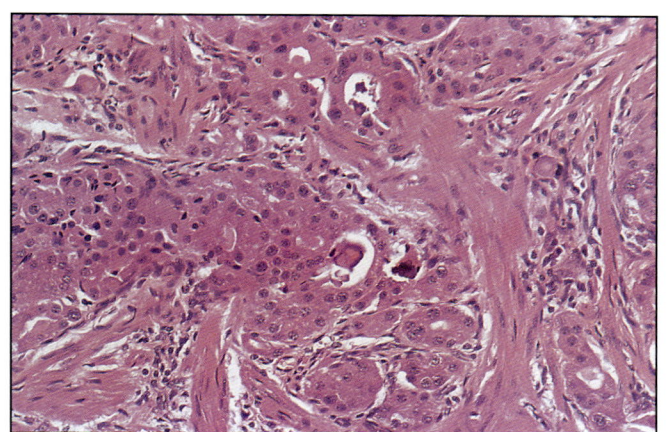

图9.4　分泌生长抑素的十二指肠类癌。肿瘤细胞排列成腺泡状，部分腺泡状结构内含有沙粒体。

差异，任何年龄成人均可发病；诊断时的中位年龄大约在50岁。GISTs在神经纤维瘤病中已有描述[36]。大约20%的GISTs发生在十二指肠，这个好发部位的长度相对有限。

大体表现

肿瘤可以突向肠腔，也可以向浆膜面突出，或者向两个方向生长，形成哑铃状结构。肿瘤可以延伸到肠系膜或腹膜后[37]。少数情况下，可能为多发性[38]。具有临床意义的肿瘤大小从直径2 cm到20 cm不等。肿瘤切面局限，缺乏真正的包膜。粉红色或灰色，质地如橡皮。某些肿瘤质软，伴有出血区域[34]。恶性GISTs可能较大，切面白色，有坏死区域。较大肿瘤不管是否具有恶性潜能，其特征是囊性退变（图9.5）。

组织学表现

肿瘤细胞可以为梭形（图9.6）和上皮样，胞浆淡染或嗜酸性，或两种细胞混合存在。肿瘤或浸润到周围正常结构中，或形成假包膜。常常具有发育良好的微血管结构，因而易于局部出血。少数GISTs以出现嗜酸性丝团样纤维为特征（图9.7）[34,37]。核的栅栏状排列可以很明显。伴有显著炎症成分的GISTs（类似于炎性假瘤）已有报道[39]。

免疫组化

最一致的表现是胞浆KIT（CD117）弥漫性阳性表达，有时与点状阳性并存。大约4%具有GISTs临床病理学特征的肿瘤不表达KIT。KIT阴性可能是由于技术失败、样本选择错误或经过克隆演化抗原丢失，以及与GISTs不能区别的真正缺乏KIT的肿瘤。KIT阴性的GISTs（KIT-negative GISTs）常常具有上皮样细胞形态，发生在网膜/腹膜表面以及具有血小板衍化生长因子受体α (platelet-derived growth factor receptor-alpha, PDGFRA) 突变，而不是KIT突变[40]。其中某些KIT阴性GISTs仍然具有PDGFRA或KIT突变，使它们对伊马替尼敏感[40]。

多达70%的GISTs病例CD34阳性，40%的病例平滑肌肌动蛋白（SMA）阳性。与真正平滑肌肿瘤不同，其结蛋白（Desmin）阳性染色非常少见。一般来说，神经标记物只有局灶阳性，例如S-100、突触素和神经微丝蛋白[23]。

预后标志

两种最常见的复发类型是腹腔内局部复发或肝转移。最重要的预后标志是肿瘤大小和每50个高倍视野的核分裂数。某些研究强调有些特征与预后有关，例如细胞构成、坏死和黏膜浸润，但是难以重复。小肠这个解剖部位与预后不好有关。预后的4个危险因素见表9.1。然而，即使是极低危险的GISTs有时也能复发，因此，

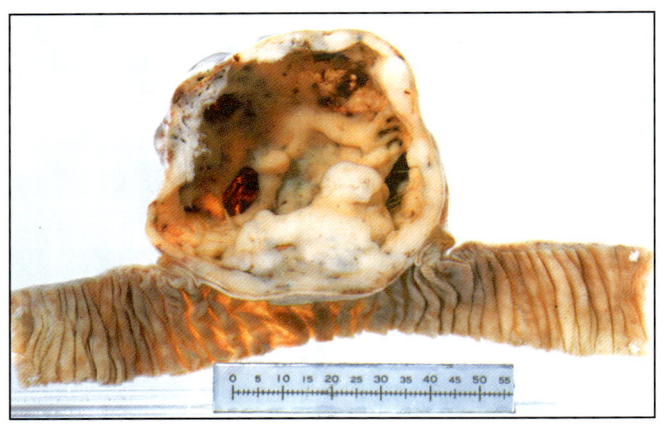

图9.5 发生在空肠的胃肠道间质瘤，显示囊性退变。患者男性，23岁，临床表现为黑粪症。囊腔充满血液，与溃疡表面相交通。

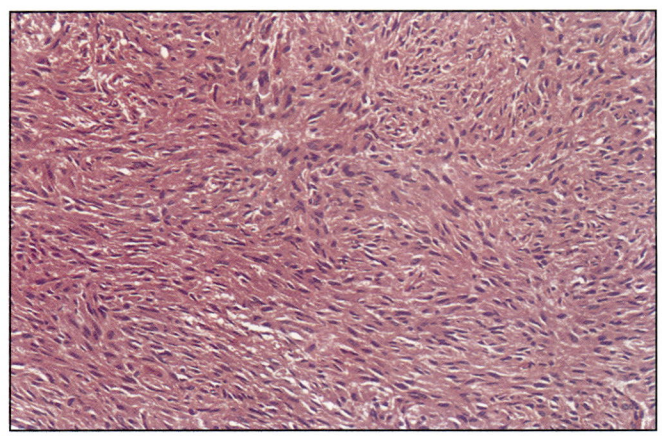

图9.6 胃肠道间质瘤，由胞浆淡嗜酸性的肥大的梭形细胞构成，排列成席纹状结构（与图9.5是同一病例）。

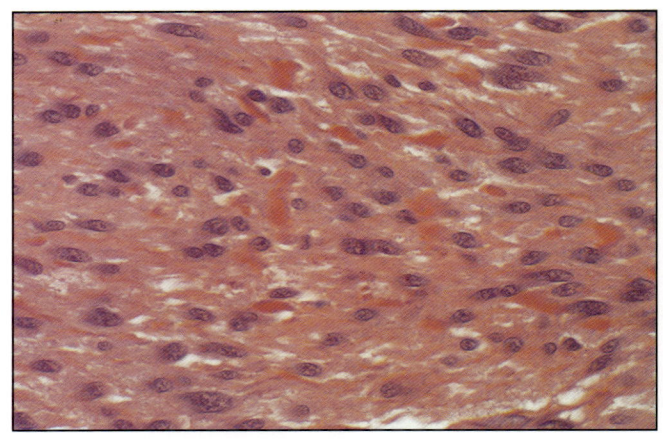

图9.7 胃肠道间质瘤，显示嗜酸性丝团样纤维。肿瘤发生在66岁男性患者的空肠，大小为90×80×70 mm。（Courtesy of Dr D.V.Spagnolo，Western Australia.）

表 9.1	胃肠道间质瘤侵袭性生物学行为的危险因素 (adapted from ref. 23)	
危险程度	大小（cm）	核分裂数/50 HPF
极低	<2	≤5
低	2~5	≤5
中	≤5 5~10	6~10 ≤5
高	>5 >10 任何	>5 任何 >10

即使是偶然发现的非常小的病变，某些病理医师也避免应用良性 GIST 这一术语[23]。存在 11 号外显子 KIT 突变的 GISTs 比存在 9 号外显子突变或没有检测到突变的 GISTs 对于伊马替尼的反应可能更好[41]。

脂肪瘤　Lipoma

脂肪瘤是罕见的肿瘤，男女发病率相等，多无症状[42]。肿瘤起源于黏膜下层，并向肠腔突出，可能有蒂。偶尔可能引起肠梗阻、肠套叠或溃疡形成伴有出血。组织学形态与其他部位的脂肪瘤相同。

脉管肿瘤　Vascular tumors

血管瘤　Hemangioma

来自血管的小肠肿瘤非常少见，且大多数为良性肿瘤[43]。血管瘤可以没有症状，但部分表现为肠梗阻、肠套叠，或更为常见的是出血和贫血。小肠血管瘤多见于男性，发病年龄从 6 个月至 70 多岁不等，但以青年人多见。

大体表现

有 5 种独特的组织学类型：
1. 弥漫浸润性海绵状血管瘤，主要见于小肠或直肠[44]。病变累及整个血液供应系统，包括肠系膜血管（图 9.8）。黏膜呈葡萄色外观，但是通常完整。
2. 局限性息肉样海绵状血管瘤，多为单个，发生于黏膜下层。
3. 单纯性毛细血管瘤，可为单发或多发。
4. 多发性静脉扩张，是小的病变，与海绵状血管瘤相似，但是位于黏膜下层，并与正常血管直接相通。通常没有症状。
5. 血管瘤病，可以伴有其他部位的多发性血管瘤。本病通常没有症状。

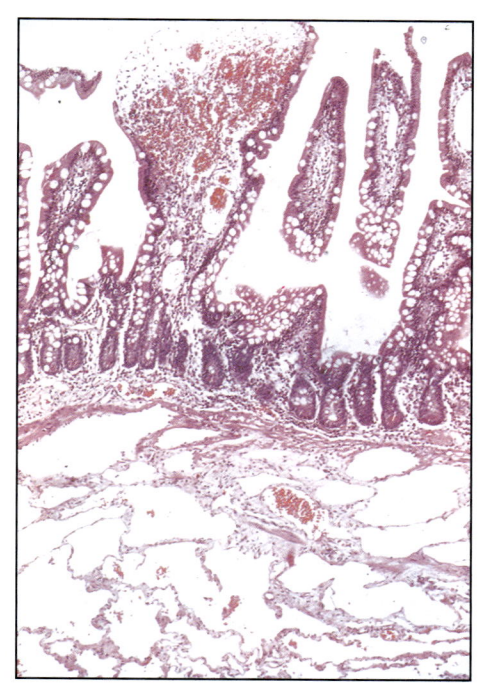

图9.8　小肠血管瘤。海绵状血管腔隙取代了黏膜下层。

组织学表现

组织学图像与其他组织内的血管瘤相似（图 9.8；也可见第 3 章）。

鉴别诊断

毛细血管瘤应与血管发育异常（angiodysplasia）鉴别[45]。后者主要发生于盲肠和升结肠，见于老年人，是一种退变性血管异常。小肠的血管球瘤罕见[46]。

血管肉瘤　Angiosarcoma

胃肠道血管肉瘤十分少见。具有高度侵袭性，可能是多中心的，偶尔与长期透析有关[47]。诊断小肠血管肉瘤时，首先应该排除播散转移的可能性，例如来自头皮。

淋巴管瘤　Lymphangioma

肠的淋巴管瘤十分罕见，通常为孤立性[48]。

神经源性肿瘤　Neurogenic tumors

小肠的神经源性肿瘤少见，并可难以与平滑肌肿瘤、错构瘤和反应性神经增生鉴别。一组起源于肌层的间质瘤电镜下显示有神经元分化，被称为胃肠道自主神经瘤（见上文，胃肠道间质瘤项下），但不再被认为是一种独立的疾病。

神经鞘瘤 Schwann 细胞瘤
Neurilemmoma (schwannoma)

尽管有胃神经鞘瘤的报道[49]，但小肠神经鞘瘤很少见。

神经纤维瘤和神经纤维瘤病
Neurofibroma and neurofibromatosis

von Recklinghausen 病患者如有胃肠道出血，提示有肠道受累的可能性。神经纤维瘤病伴有十二指肠类癌[50]和十二指肠节细胞性副神经节瘤[51]的病例已有报道（见下文）。有一神经纤维瘤病患者，同时伴有节细胞性副神经节瘤以及富于生长抑素的腺样类癌的病例报告[52]。提示这三种病变的组织起源可能有一定的联系。

节细胞性副神经节瘤
Gangliocytic paraganglioma[53,54]

该肿瘤罕见，多见于十二指肠。无性别差异，发病年龄在 50 岁左右，表现为胃肠道出血或腹痛。病变表现为息肉，表面可有溃疡。组织学上，肿瘤由内分泌细胞、S-100 蛋白阳性的梭形细胞和神经节细胞构成（图 9.9）。如果取材不全面或某一成分明显占优势时，它有可能被误诊为类癌或神经节瘤。报道中的孤立性十二指肠神经节瘤或许就是属于这种病变。

节细胞性神经瘤病 Ganglioneuromatosis

弥漫性肠道节细胞性神经瘤病与甲状腺髓样癌、嗜铬细胞瘤以及多发性神经瘤有关。所有这些病变组成了一种叫做 II B 型多发性内分泌腺瘤病（multiple endocrine adenomatosis type II B）的遗传综合征[55]。弥漫性节细胞性神经瘤病累及肠肌神经丛及黏膜下神经丛。这种病变应与息肉样节细胞性神经瘤病相鉴别，后者发生在大肠，以黏膜固有层内神经增生为特征[56]。

淋巴组织肿瘤
Tumors of lymphoid tissue

淋巴组织增生、淋巴组织息肉和息肉病
Lymphoid hyperplasia, lymphoid polyps, and polyposis

淋巴组织增生见于婴儿和儿童，临床表现为右髂窝疼痛、肠梗阻、有时发生肠套叠[57]。大约 20% 的成人原发性低丙种球蛋白血症病例合并弥漫性结节状淋巴组织增生[58]。这些患者发生肠癌和淋巴瘤的危险性增加[59]。

淋巴瘤 Lymphoma

临床特征

小肠原发性淋巴瘤少见，但大约占小肠恶性肿瘤的 30% 左右[60]。Burkitt 淋巴瘤经常发生在儿童，而其他类型大多发生在 40 岁以上的成人，临床表现为腹部疼痛、肠梗阻、肠穿孔、肠套叠、胃肠道出血、腹泻以及右髂窝肿块。男性多于女性。某些淋巴瘤发生在慢性疾病的基础上，包括获得性免疫缺陷综合征（AIDS）、伴有淋巴组织增生的低丙种球蛋白血症（见上文）、α-链病和乳糜泻[61]。预后一般较差，但随肿瘤类型和扩散程度而不同[60]。

胃肠道和其他结外淋巴瘤的分类不同于淋巴结的淋巴瘤（见第 8 章和第 21 章）。这反映了黏膜相关淋巴组织（MALT）特殊的生物学和胃肠道特有的病原学机制。胃肠道淋巴瘤的详细研究经常受到缺乏新鲜组织和组织固定不好的限制。尽管存在这些困难，胃肠道淋

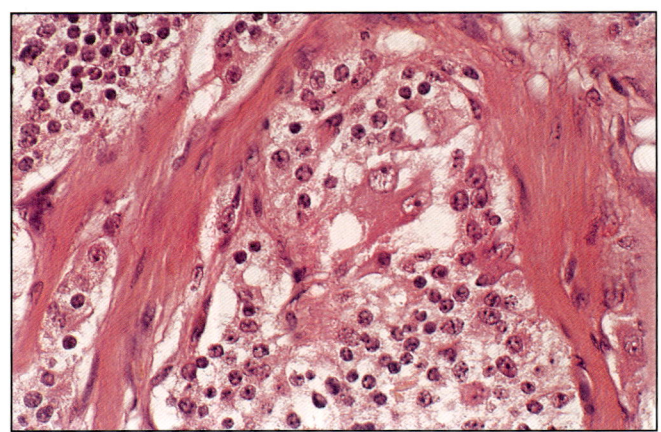

图 9.9 节细胞性副神经节瘤。肿瘤由神经节细胞和内分泌细胞混合而成。

表9.2	胃肠淋巴瘤的主要类型
B细胞	黏膜相关淋巴组织淋巴瘤（较常见于胃） 免疫增生性小肠病和地中海淋巴瘤 Burkitt 淋巴瘤 套细胞淋巴瘤（不是原发的） 滤泡性淋巴瘤（不常见） 浆细胞瘤（非常少见） 其他B细胞淋巴瘤（通常为高级别的）
T细胞	乳糜泻（肠病）相关性 伴有组织嗜酸细胞增多的T细胞淋巴瘤 其他T细胞淋巴瘤
真正的组织细胞性	非常少见
Hodgkin 淋巴瘤	十分罕见

巴瘤还是能够被合理地归入独特的分类中（表9.2）。一个重要的亚型是黏膜相关淋巴组织（MALT）淋巴瘤。它是一种低级别B细胞淋巴瘤，是在长期接触抗原的基础上发生的。以胃黏膜相关淋巴组织（MALT）淋巴瘤为例，其发生在幽门螺旋杆菌胃炎（Helicobacter pylori gastritis）基础上（第8章）。肠道没有明确相同的致病菌，但是小肠特有的两种类型淋巴瘤与长期接触抗原有关。第一种类型是包括免疫增生性小肠病（immunoproliferative small intestinal disease，IPSID）和地中海淋巴瘤（mediterranean lymphoma）在内的一种B细胞淋巴瘤[62]。第二种类型是与乳糜泻（celiac disease）相关的T细胞淋巴瘤[63]。后者十分容易引起肠穿孔，预后非常不好。Burkitt淋巴瘤是又一种类型的结外淋巴瘤；它是由类似于淋巴母细胞的B细胞构成的。回盲部是散发性Burkitt淋巴瘤的好发部位。EB病毒只与15%的病例有关（见第21章）。正确诊断这种侵袭性肿瘤十分重要，因为需要手术和化疗。其他肠道淋巴瘤有相应的淋巴结病变，恶性淋巴细胞和（或）结构形态与相应的淋巴结病变相似。这个部位发生滤泡性淋巴瘤十分少见[64]。弥漫性B细胞淋巴瘤通常是高级别的肿瘤，形成一个相当大的尚未被完全了解的亚群。尽管肿瘤性淋巴细胞与大的滤泡中心细胞（大的中心细胞、中心母细胞或免疫母细胞）相似，但这种肿瘤可能是由低级别MALT淋巴瘤转化而来的。套细胞淋巴瘤发病年龄较大（65岁左右），不同于前面提到的类型，而是一种与白血病播散有关的系统性疾病。不过，套细胞淋巴瘤可以出现在胃肠道，其一种特别的表现是所谓的淋巴瘤性息肉病（lymphomatous polyposis）。淋巴瘤性息肉病将在大肠部分（见第405页）讨论，但是它可以发生在整个胃肠道，并且易与MALT淋巴瘤混淆。

大体特征

大B细胞淋巴瘤一般形成巨大的突向肠腔的肿块，表面可有溃疡，多发生于小肠末端（图9.10）。地中海淋巴瘤常发生于小肠近端，并弥漫性浸润肠壁。Burkitt淋巴瘤表现为回盲部肿块，常常引起肠套叠。T细胞淋巴瘤常表现为近端小肠多发性溃疡，很少形成明显的肿块（图9.11）。这种病变最初被称为溃疡性空肠炎，随后证明了它的肿瘤性本质，称为恶性组织细胞增生症[65]。应该强调的是，小肠T细胞淋巴瘤的肿瘤性本质经常不明显，正确诊断往往取决于从前对于本病的了解。大多数淋巴瘤的切面均质灰白、质软，呈鱼肉状（图9.12）。

组织学表现

地中海淋巴瘤发生在α-链病或免疫增生性小肠病

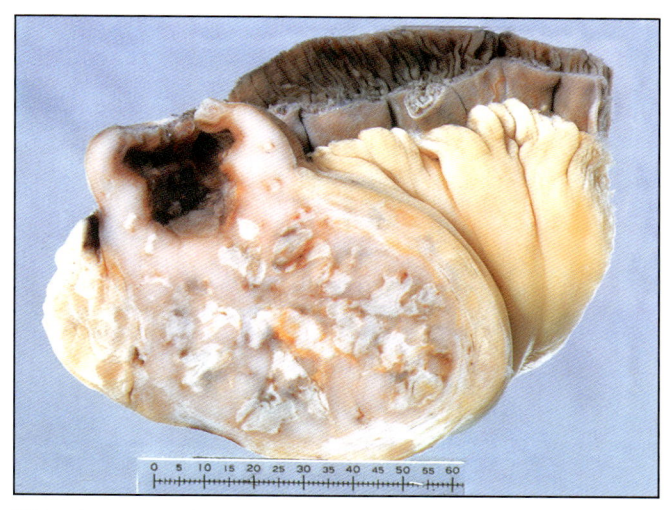

图9.10 回肠巨大局限性溃疡型淋巴瘤（B细胞型）。女性，61岁。

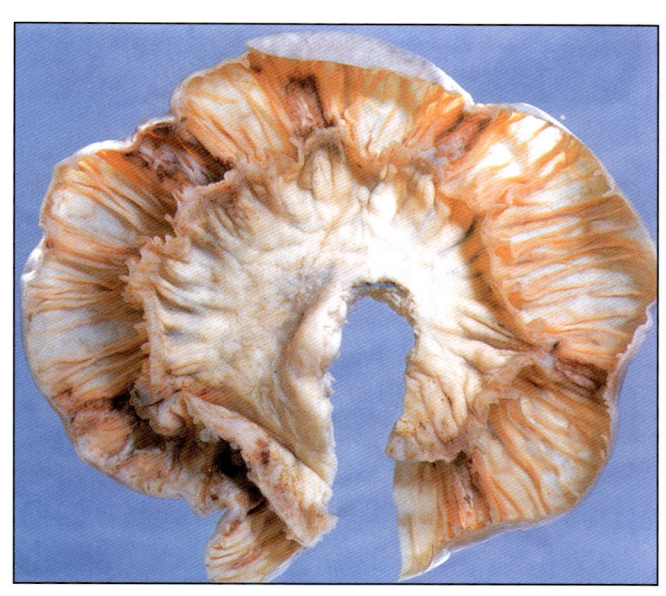

图9.11 空肠T细胞淋巴瘤，伴有多发性横向溃疡，临床表现为反复出血。男性，60岁。

的基础上[62]。这种病变显示黏膜内浆细胞、淋巴浆细胞样细胞浸润，伴有广泛的肠隐窝分离以及绒毛变宽和变短，但表面的上皮完整（图9.13）。有人将这个阶段看成是早期淋巴瘤，浸润的浆细胞的克隆性本质也支持这一观点[66]。如同胃的MALT淋巴瘤一样，在此阶段应用抗生素治疗常使病变消退。未经治疗的病例进一步发展转化为高级别B细胞淋巴瘤。

Burkitt淋巴瘤由淋巴母细胞样细胞组成，显示高核分裂率和由散在的含有细胞凋亡物质的可染小体巨噬细胞形成的"星空"（starry-sky）现象（图9.14）。肿瘤细胞浸润明显，在原有结构之间穿行生长而不破坏原有结构，并且围绕区域淋巴结而并不浸润至淋巴结内。肠套

淋巴组织肿瘤

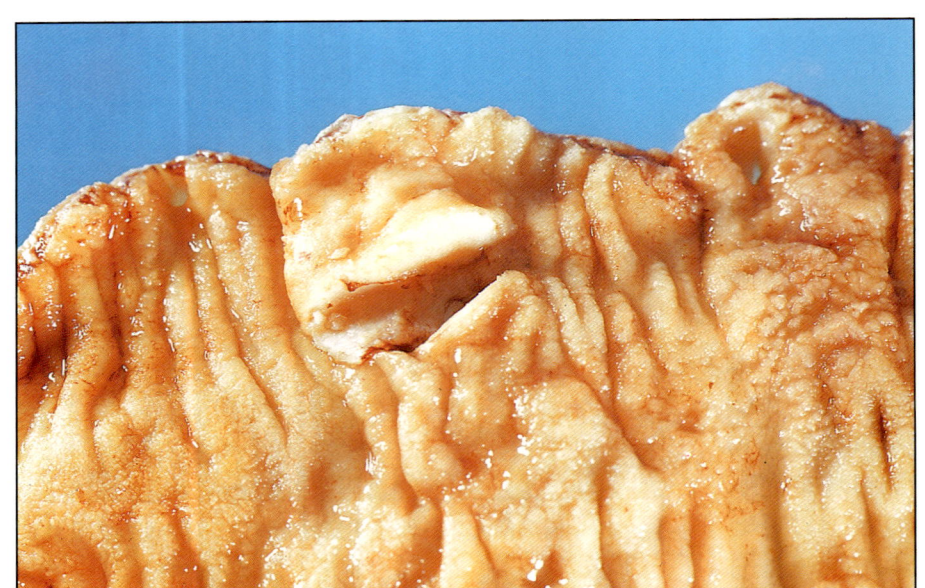

图9.12　低级别B细胞淋巴瘤引起小肠斑块样增厚。切面灰白，质地均匀，呈鱼肉状。

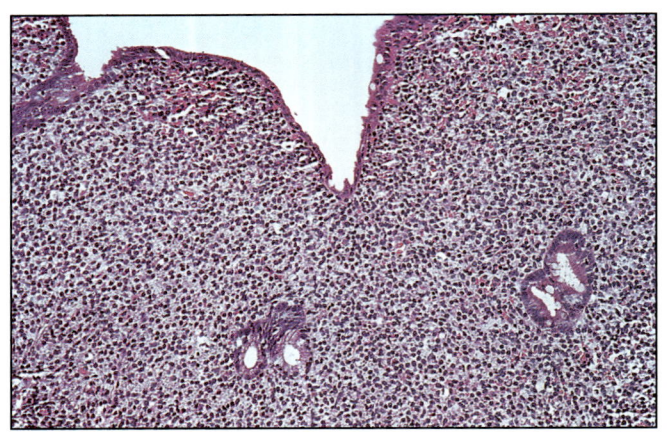

图9.13　免疫增生性小肠病或α-链病。绒毛萎缩，固有层内充满大量的淋巴浆细胞样细胞。

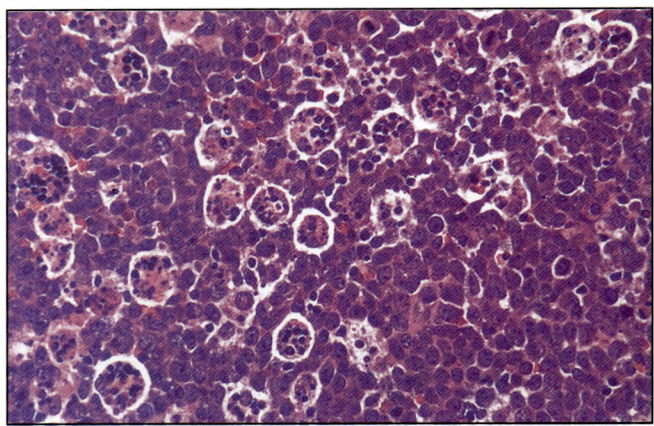

图9.14　小肠Burkitt淋巴瘤。肿瘤性淋巴细胞之间是大量的可染小体巨噬细胞，呈"星空状"改变。

叠可能伴有缺血性坏死，因而使淋巴瘤不易辨认。然而，即使是有坏死的病例，出现成群淋巴细胞穿过肌层仍是有利于辨认Burkitt淋巴瘤的依据。Burkitt淋巴瘤的典型免疫表型是CD10、CD20（L26）、CD79a和bcl-6阳性，但bcl-2阴性。分子遗传学研究显示c-myc癌基因重排。

其他B细胞淋巴瘤或者是低级别的，或者是比较常见的高级别MALT淋巴瘤，由类似于滤泡中心细胞（中心细胞、中心母细胞和免疫母细胞；图9.15）的细胞组成。可以见到不同程度的浆细胞分化。孤立性浆细胞瘤十分少见。在石蜡切片中可以得到证实的B细胞表型包括CD10、CD20（L26）、CD79a、kappa或lambda轻链以及bcl-10。罕见的滤泡性淋巴瘤表达CD10、CD20和bcl-2。

T细胞淋巴瘤的一个重要特征是与Crohn病相似的裂隙状溃疡。需要细致的组织学检查来辨认恶性淋巴细

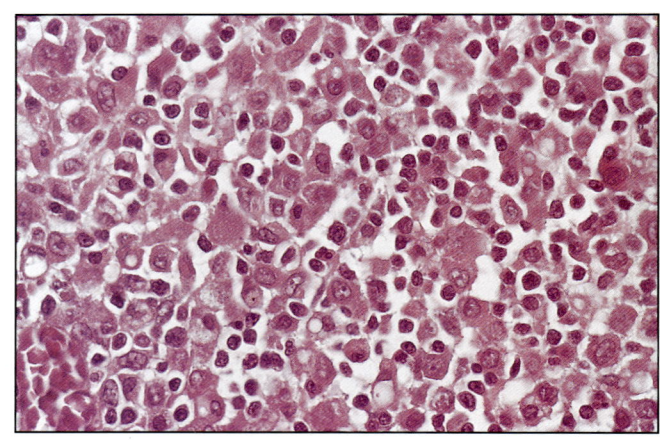

图9.15　由大B细胞（免疫母细胞）构成的B细胞淋巴瘤，其间为反应性的小淋巴细胞。

胞，恶性淋巴细胞可能稀少，并被反应性炎细胞掩盖。尤其是伴有乳糜泻的淋巴瘤[63]，通常是T细胞型[67]。有一种罕见的伴有明显组织嗜酸性细胞增多的T细胞淋巴瘤，可以发生在无乳糜泻的病例[68]。恶性T细胞形态学变化可能很大（图9.16）。福尔马林固定组织表达的T细胞表型包括CD3、CD43和UCHLI（CD45RO）。伴有乳糜泻的T细胞淋巴瘤，邻近的黏膜显示绒毛萎缩和隐窝增生。隐窝上皮可能被T淋巴细胞浸润，出现明显的上皮浸润可能是淋巴瘤前病变或早期淋巴瘤病变（图9.17）。另外，某些成人"乳糜泻"病例可能是上皮内低级别T细胞淋巴瘤的继发性表现[69]。不管先前是否存在乳糜泻，有研究认为，所有T细胞淋巴瘤都是来自少数上皮内肠T细胞的恶性肿瘤，伴随的免疫表型是CD3+、CD4－、CD8+/－、CD103+（后者只在冰冻切片可以得到证实）[70]。根据细胞大小、肿瘤细胞分布、溃疡的存在、肿瘤的大小以及绒毛萎缩程度，将T细胞淋巴瘤分成了四种类型[70]。

鉴别诊断

原发性淋巴瘤与反应性淋巴组织增生、继发性淋巴瘤、白血病浸润、小细胞癌和未分化癌鉴别十分重要。形态学上难以鉴别的病例，通过基因重排研究或免疫组化染色证实克隆性，常常可以作出鉴别诊断。胞浆内免疫球蛋白的聚集还可能造成肿瘤细胞在形态上与印戒细胞癌相似。

继发性肿瘤　Secondary tumors

小肠继发性肿瘤少见，但小肠是胃肠道转移性肿瘤的主要发生部位[71,72]。其原发部位包括支气管、乳腺、肾上腺、卵巢、胃、大肠及皮肤黑色素瘤。由大肠转移而来的肿瘤可以侵犯小肠黏膜形成息肉样肿块，因此类似于小肠原发性淋巴瘤。胃弥漫型腺癌可以播散累及到不同长度的小肠或大肠，形成肠腔狭窄，可能类似于Crohn病[73]。

瘤样病变　Tumor-like lesions

十二指肠腺错构瘤
Brunner gland hamartoma

这是指发生于十二指肠第一部分的无蒂肿块，由增生的但是外观正常的十二指肠腺（Brunner's gland）构成，伴有导管和间质。病变可有溃疡和出血，或者可能引起肠梗阻（图9.18和图9.19）[74]。

Peutz-Jeghers息肉和息肉病
Peutz-Jeghers polyp and polyposis

临床特征

Peutz-Jeghers综合征以胃肠道息肉病、口腔黏膜色素沉着为特征，为常染色体显性遗传性疾病[75]。多数有19号染色体短臂 *LKB1* 基因突变，在肿瘤发生中似乎具有重要的致病作用[76]。小肠是息肉最好发的部位，表现为腹部疼痛，有时出现肠套叠。Peutz-Jeghers息肉和息肉病患者发生胃肠道或其他部位恶性肿瘤的危险性增加，包括胰腺和乳腺[77,78]。特别值得注意的是，与伴有卵巢环状小管的性索间质肿瘤有关（见第13章A）[79]。

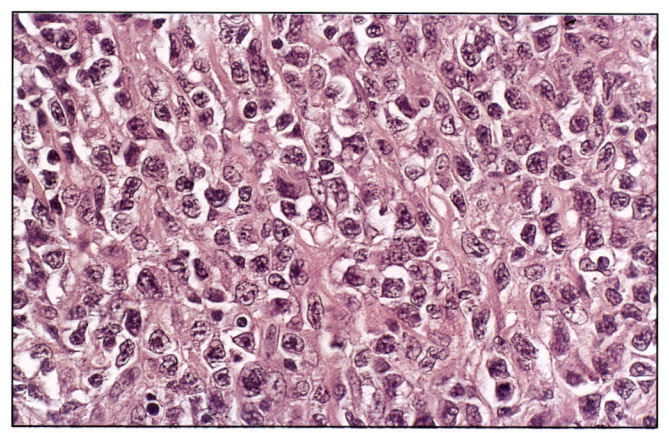

图9.16　小肠多形性T细胞淋巴瘤，由大的淋巴样细胞构成，细胞核扭曲、形状不规则，有明显的核仁。

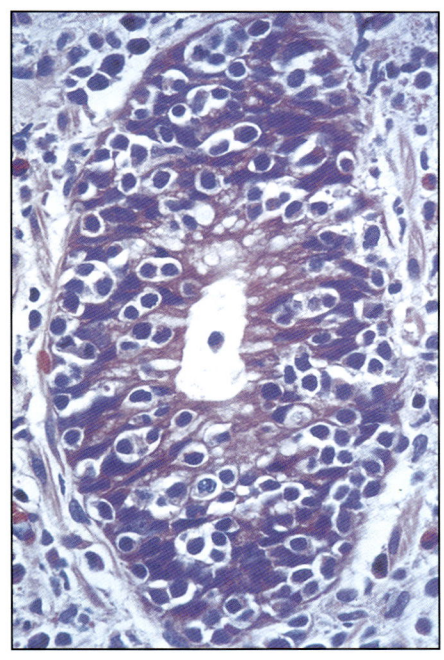

图9.17　邻近T细胞淋巴瘤的上皮内淋巴细胞增多。

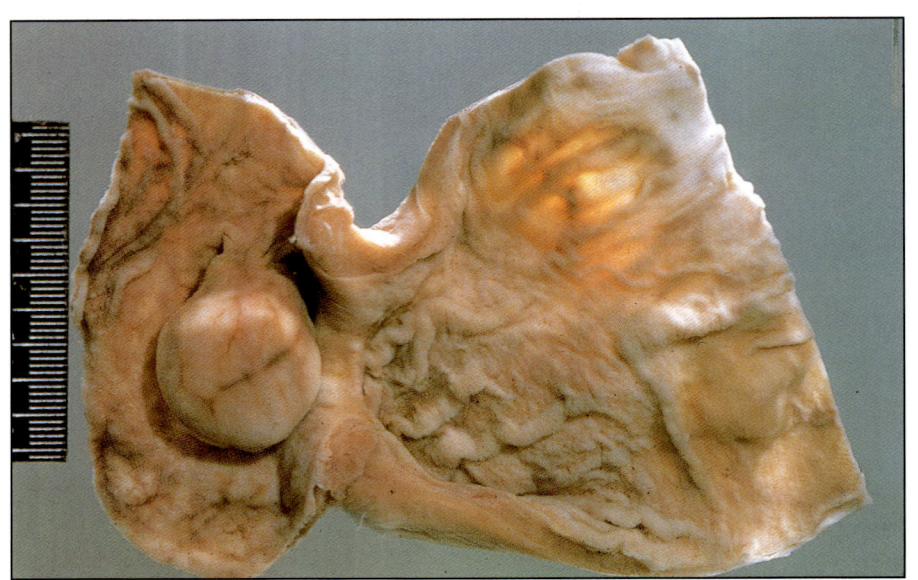

图9.18 十二指肠腺错构瘤，表现为十二指肠第一部分的黏膜下肿块，恰好位于幽门远端。

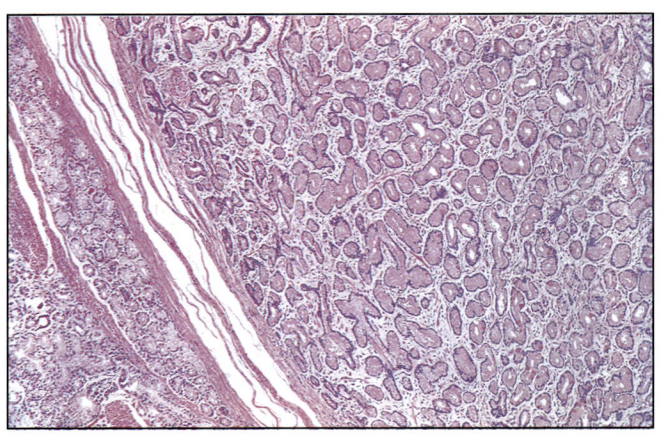

图9.19 错构瘤内的增生性十二指肠腺。

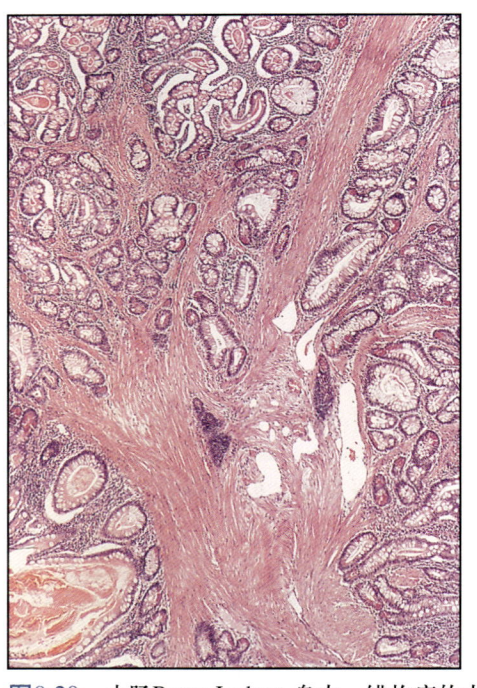

图9.20 小肠Peutz-Jeghers息肉。错构瘤的中心含有粗大的平滑肌束。

大体表现

Peutz-Jeghers息肉可以无蒂或有短而宽的蒂。息肉头部与腺瘤相似。

组织学表现

Peutz-Jeghers息肉是由粗大分支的平滑肌束被覆正常外观的腺上皮组成的错构瘤（图9.20）。黏膜上皮移位到黏膜下层、肌层，有时移位到浆膜，这种情况并不少见，而且可能与恶性浸润混淆（图9.21）[80]。异型增生和恶变非常少见，但是可以发生。孤立性Peutz-Jeghers息肉可以见于缺乏典型Peutz-Jeghers综合征的患者。

幼年性息肉和息肉病
Juvenile polyps and polyposis

见大肠部分。

胰腺异位　Panceatic heterotopia[81,82]

胰腺异位最常发生于十二指肠，表现为黏膜下或肠壁内结节，可以包括内分泌和外分泌两种成分，或仅有胰腺导管，其内混有平滑肌。胰腺异位偶尔见于整个胃肠道的其他部位，包括Meckel憩室[82]。

炎性纤维性息肉
Inflammatory fibroid polyp

临床特征

炎性纤维性息肉可见于整个胃肠道，小肠是好发部

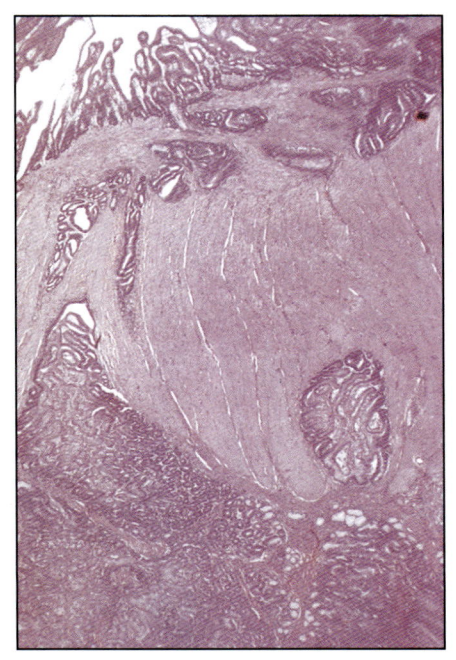

图9.21 Peutz-Jeghers息肉，上皮移位到小肠壁。

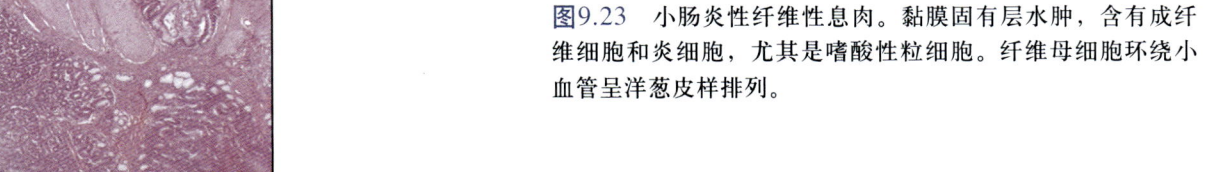

图9.23 小肠炎性纤维性息肉。黏膜固有层水肿，含有成纤维细胞和炎细胞，尤其是嗜酸性粒细胞。纤维母细胞环绕小血管呈洋葱皮样排列。

位，其次是胃。常为单发。可见于任何年龄，但以成人为主。临床表现为肠梗阻或肠套叠（图9.22）[83]。

大体表现

息肉多为单发性，开始生长时无蒂，但是随着体积的增大可以有蒂。直径常为2～5 cm，表面黏膜常有溃疡形成。病变穿透固有肌层时可以形成哑铃形肿块。

组织学表现

病变发生于黏膜下层，由疏松的或透明变性的纤维结缔组织构成，其内有嗜酸性粒细胞及浆细胞浸润。溃疡表面由肉芽组织覆盖。特征性的改变是，病变内的星状或梭形纤维母细胞围绕着小动脉呈同心圆性排列（图9.23）。虽然新近提出来源于树突状细胞，但其组织发生尚不能肯定[84]。

回盲瓣脂肪增生
Lipohyperplasia of the ileocecal valve

表现为回盲瓣黏膜下层有过多的脂肪组织，使之扭曲变形并突向盲肠[85]。

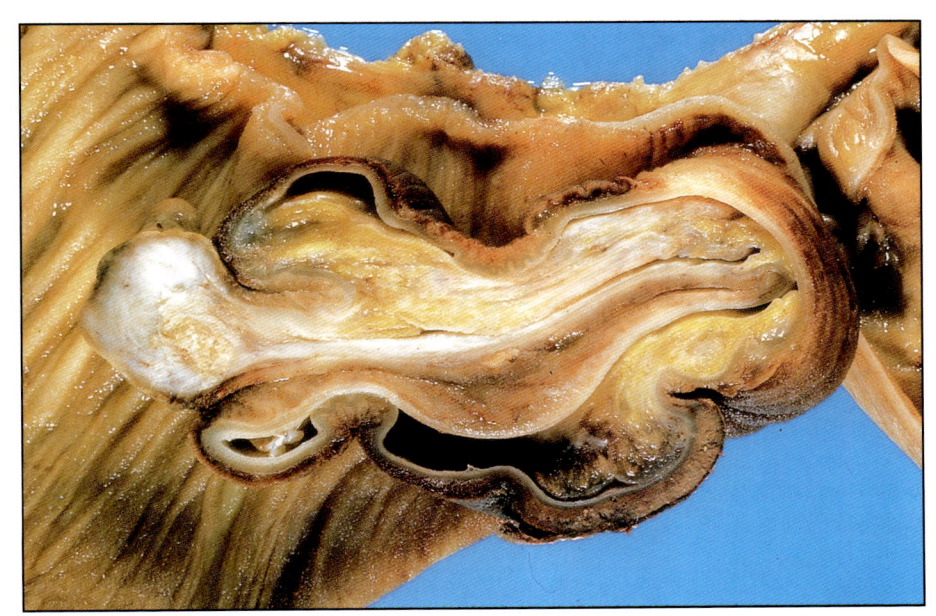

图9.22 炎性纤维性息肉引起肠套叠。

阑尾 Appendix

上皮性肿瘤 (Epithelial tumors)

腺瘤 (Adenoma)

临床特征

阑尾腺瘤少见。多为偶然发现，但黏液性（囊）腺瘤可能并发阑尾炎。

大体表现

腺瘤性改变通常弥漫累及黏膜。肿瘤性上皮分泌的黏液充满阑尾腔，可能形成香肠形肿块[86,87]。这样的肿瘤被称为黏液性囊腺瘤，有时可伴有腹膜假黏液瘤。阑尾腺瘤也可小而局限。家族性腺瘤性息肉病患者的阑尾出现小的管状腺瘤并不少见。

组织学表现

小而局限的腺瘤常为管状腺瘤（见大肠项下），显示低级别异型增生。黏液性囊腺瘤多可见到管状绒毛状或绒毛状结构，而且可有高级别异型增生。高级别异型增生在黏膜基底部较为明显。令人不解的是覆盖绒毛上半部分的上皮常常温和(图9.24)。黏液积聚在阑尾腔内，形成黏液囊肿，可使上皮变扁，以致可能妨碍异型增生的辨认。然而，这种扁平上皮常较局限，如果多做切片检查可以避免误诊。

如同胃肠道其他部位腺瘤一样，阑尾腺瘤也易于恶变。真正的恶性浸润可能类似于腺瘤性上皮移位和黏液池突入阑尾壁内。这可能是继发于黏液积聚造成阑尾腔内压力增大，或继发于炎症。移位的上皮类似于覆盖腺瘤表面的上皮，有急性炎症表现或脓肿形成，以及缺乏纤维组织增生性反应，有助于与恶性肿瘤的鉴别诊断。

偶尔，阑尾腺瘤的上皮呈锯齿状，类似于增生性息肉的改变（图9.25）。实际上，如同腺瘤一样，增生性息肉也可以广泛弥漫累及阑尾黏膜，可能造成鉴别十分困难。支持锯齿状腺瘤诊断的特征包括：腺体呈分支状和背靠背状、表面出现核分裂象、核增大和复层排列以及黏液囊肿形成。

腺癌 Adenocarcinoma

临床特征

阑尾腺癌罕见，可以表现为急性阑尾炎或右髂窝肿块，见于中年或老年患者。预后取决于恶性程度和扩散范围。阑尾腺癌可经淋巴管转移至局部淋巴结，并经门静脉转移至肝。一篇病例分析报道，其5年生存率为60%，但另外一些报道患者预后较差，特别是表现为肿瘤穿孔的患者[87-90]。

阑尾黏液性腺癌可伴有腹膜假黏液瘤（见第15章）。

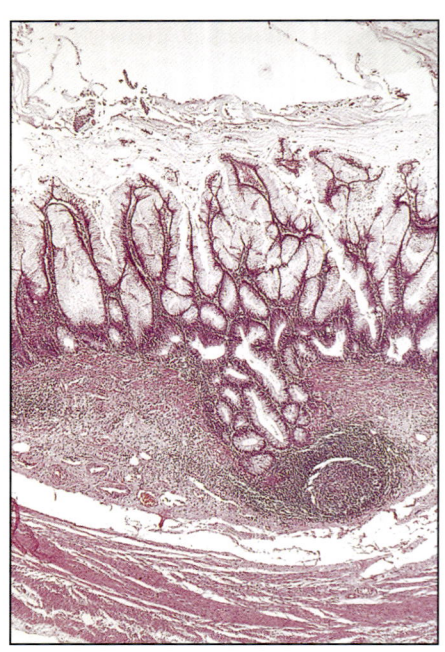

图9.24 阑尾腺瘤。黏膜增厚，由被覆分泌黏液细胞的绒毛取代。难以理解的是，细胞表现温和，只有隐窝底部细胞显示异型增生的特征。在一个淋巴滤泡附近可见上皮移位突破黏膜肌层。应与可能伴发腺瘤的真正的恶性浸润鉴别。

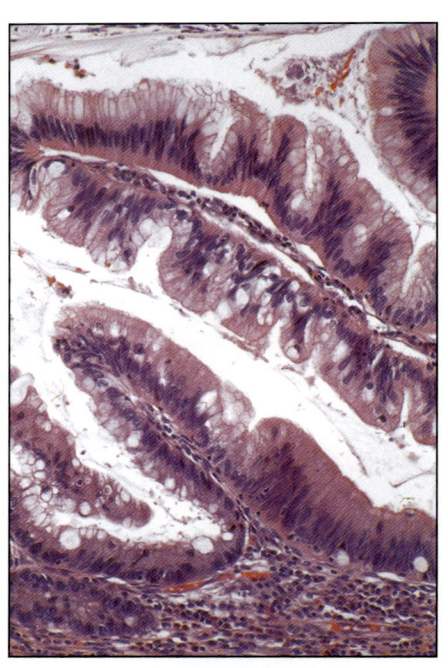

图9.25 阑尾腺瘤伴有锯齿状结构。

这是由于分泌黏液的肿瘤细胞从阑尾壁穿出进入腹腔所致。腹膜受累通常呈广泛性、进行性，最终危及患者生命。而阑尾腺瘤通过管壁溢出的移位黏液通常为局限性，且在切除阑尾病变之后消退[91]。

大体表现

最常见的是黏液性腺癌，其内产生大量黏液，常常形成黏液囊肿。

组织学表现

阑尾黏液性腺癌通常为高分化或中分化。没有大量黏液分泌的主要是中分化腺癌。腺癌附近常有腺瘤存在。典型的腺癌出现内分泌细胞并不能改变腺癌的诊断。在这些病变中微卫星不稳性（MSI）似乎不常出现[92]。

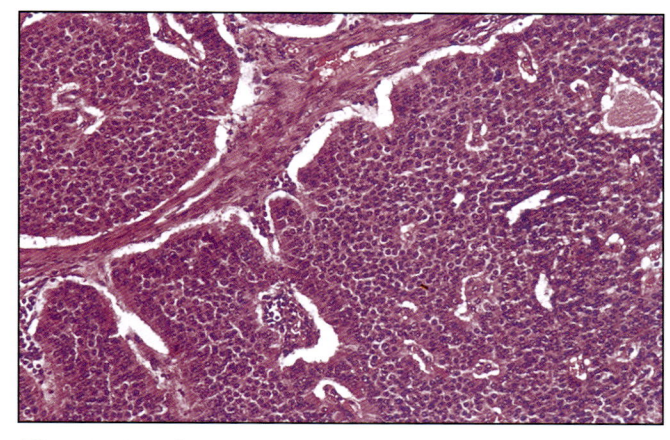

图9.26　阑尾类癌，显示细胞排成实性团块，周围有栅栏状排列的嗜酸性粒细胞。

内分泌肿瘤　Endocrine tumors

类癌　Carcinoid tumors

类癌是阑尾最常见的肿瘤。可以见于任何年龄，但以20～50岁多见。女性比男性常见。多数类癌是在因为某些不相关疾病剖腹手术切除阑尾或在急性阑尾炎切除标本中偶然发现的。类癌通常与阑尾炎同时发现。多数肿瘤较小，转移非常罕见，因此不产生类癌综合征。在个别情况下，类癌可以表现出恶性行为，在剖腹手术一般明显可见[93]。

大体表现

大多数类癌接近阑尾尖端，经福尔马林固定后呈黄色。多数直径小于1 cm，许多病例仅在显微镜下检查才能发现。肿瘤一般呈圆形，界限清楚，但也能见到弥漫性生长的病例。

组织学表现

正常情况下，内分泌细胞存在于隐窝底部以及单个或呈小团分布于固有层内，形成神经内分泌复合体[94]。这两个部位的内分泌细胞似乎均可发生类癌，但大多数类癌可能起源于固有层内的神经内分泌细胞[95]。典型的亲银性类癌（argentaffin carcinoids）与回肠的相应病变相同（见第380页）。肿瘤扩展累及固有肌层并常达阑尾系膜。由于组织收缩常常造成淋巴管浸润的假象；然而，也可以见到真正的淋巴管和神经周围侵犯。大多数亲银性类癌细胞呈实性巢状排列（图9.26），而侵入肌层的部分可呈条索状或缎带状排列。某些类癌有腺泡成分，腺泡状结构可以是主要的组织学表现。这样的病例肿瘤细胞可以形成实性细胞簇或小的腺泡，其内含有少量黏液。

非亲银性类癌（non-argentaffin carcinoids）通常很小，常在组织学检查时偶然发现。其结构与直肠或后肠类癌相似（见下文），由带状或小的腺体结构构成。胞浆内颗粒常为亲银性。

免疫组化

亲银性及非亲银性类癌均可分泌一种或多种肽类激素，包括生长抑素（somatostatin）、神经降压素（neurotensin）、胃动素（motilin）、胰多肽（pancreatic polypeptide）、胰高血糖素（glucagons）和胃泌素（gastrin）。

杯状细胞类癌　Goblet cell carcinoid

临床特征

最初报道认为，这种肿瘤的生物学行为与普通类癌相似，但近期的一些报道提示它具有较强的侵袭性[96-98]。患者通常为50～60岁，无明显性别差异。最常见的表现是急性阑尾炎或阑尾肿块。多数肿瘤在诊断时仍局限在阑尾，预后好。然而，肿瘤可以经淋巴管扩散至局部淋巴结，经淋巴管或血管浸润转移至肝，以及经腹腔蔓延至卵巢或腹膜表面。肿瘤扩散至阑尾外或切除不完全是进一步治疗的主要指征。大约20%的病例发生阑尾以外的扩散。

大体表现

杯状细胞类癌的大体形态及其在阑尾中的分布与阑尾的其他类癌相似。

组织学表现

肿瘤由团块状、条索状或腺样集聚的细胞组成，细胞学形态与杯状细胞或印戒细胞相似，其内充满黏液（图9.27）。黏液可以溢出进入阑尾深层形成黏液湖。肿瘤内有内分泌细胞，但数量远远少于典型的类癌。Paneth细胞也可散在出现。内分泌细胞常为嗜银性，而不是亲银性（图9.28）。与印戒细胞癌不同，这些黏液细胞呈簇状或花环状排列，通常缺乏核的多形性或核分裂活性。有些病例几乎见不到神经内分泌细胞，但仍将之称为杯状细胞类癌。

由于其组织学表现与典型的类癌不同，所以这种肿瘤曾被提出其他名称，包括黏液性类癌（mucinous carcinoid）[99]、腺类癌（adenocarcinoid）[100]和隐窝细胞癌（crypt cell carcinoma）[101]。

内分泌细胞成分的多少一般与恶性行为无关，如同普通类癌一样，神经周围浸润和淋巴管扩散是不可靠的预后特征。有报道认为，这种肿瘤的侵袭性与核的多形性和核分裂象多有关，但尚未被完全接受[97]。一些作者认为，不常见的混合性类癌-腺癌（mixed carcinoid-adenocarcinomas）具有大量癌的成分，侵袭性更强[102]。

免疫组化

几乎所有杯状细胞类癌都至少显示一种内分泌肿瘤标记物染色阳性，例如NSE、嗜铬素或PGP 9.5。这些内分泌细胞不分泌5-羟色胺，但有报告生长抑素和胰多肽染色阳性[97]。

电镜检查

目前仍不清楚内分泌颗粒和黏液小滴是否在同一个细胞内。这个问题对于研究组织起源更有意义，而与诊断无关。

鉴别诊断

杯状细胞类癌的鉴别诊断十分重要，特别是在缺乏内分泌细胞的情况下与阑尾普通的黏液性腺癌鉴别。后者侵袭性较强，需要根治手术治疗。

瘤样病变　Tumor-like lesions

错构瘤　Hamartomas

Pautz-Jephers息肉和幼年性息肉均可发生在阑尾。这些病变分别在小肠和大肠相关章节中描述。

增生性息肉　Hyperplastic polyp

增生性息肉在大肠一节中描述（第407页）。作为散在的病变，可以发生在阑尾，但是如同阑尾腺瘤一样，常呈弥漫性改变而广泛累及阑尾黏膜（图9.29）。这种增生样改变的本质尚不清楚。将其中某些病变称为轻度异型增生性锯齿状腺瘤（mildly dysplastic serrated adenomas）可能比较恰当。增生性息肉可以伴有典型的绒毛状腺瘤，或融入绒毛状腺瘤。

单纯性（阻塞性）黏液囊肿 Simple (obstructive) mucocele

黏液囊肿这一术语用于临床和大体检查时所见的由于黏液聚集而引起阑尾扩张的任何病变。因其非肿瘤性病变，形成的黏液囊肿通常较小，可作为炎症的结局。

神经鞘增生 Nerve sheath proliferations

神经纤维瘤病通常发生在von Recklinghausen病的基础上。有一例阑尾神经节瘤的报道[103]。在阑尾切除标本

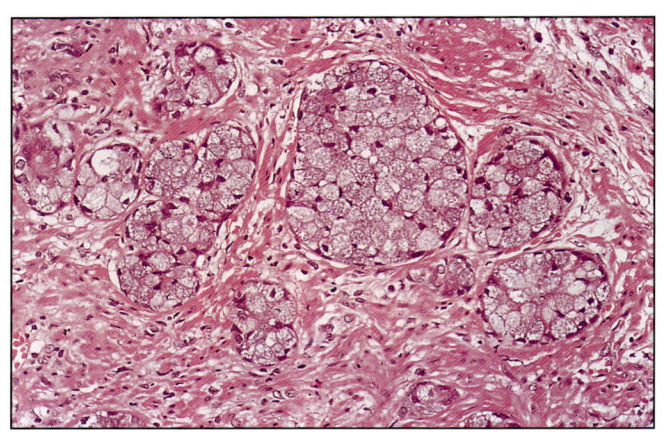

图9.27　阑尾杯状细胞类癌。充满黏液的细胞排列成岛屿状，周围的内分泌细胞具有颗粒状嗜酸性胞浆。

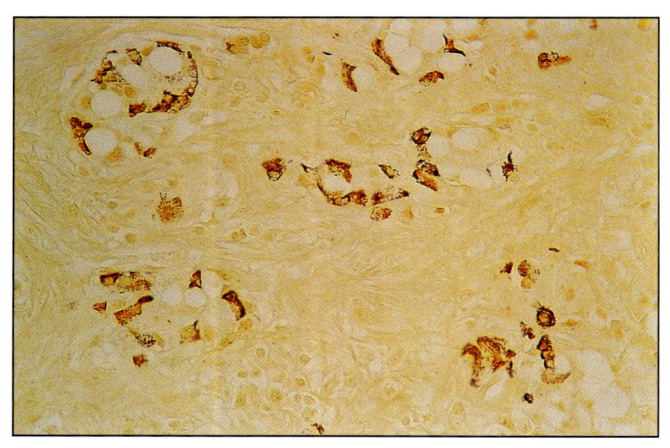

图9.28　阑尾杯状细胞类癌，显示嗜银细胞（棕色）散在分布于杯状细胞之间。Grimelius染色。

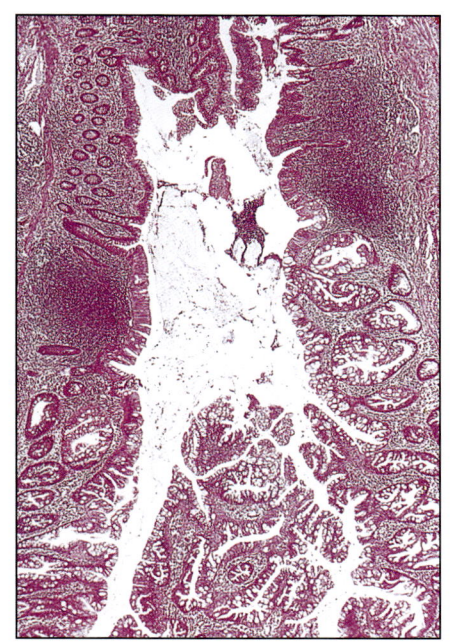

图9.29 阑尾的弥漫性增生性改变。

中，发现伴有内分泌细胞的弥漫性神经瘤性增生并不少见，特别是在阑尾末端腔内有纤维性阻塞的病例[104]。其发病率随年龄而增加。这种增生的组织发生尚未确定，但通常认为是炎症早期的继发性增生性改变。

子宫内膜异位　Endometriosis

子宫内膜异位常累及阑尾。异位的子宫内膜组织位于阑尾外层，可能类似于腺癌。

大肠　Large intestine

上皮性肿瘤　Epithelial tumors

腺瘤　Adenoma

临床表现

大肠腺瘤是界限清楚的良性上皮性肿瘤，但有恶变潜能。尸检发现，大肠腺瘤在结直肠癌高发区域比较常见，例如北美和欧洲[105,106]。结肠和直肠所有部位的腺瘤均多见于男性，而女性患者右半结肠癌高发。这种反常现象可能是由于女性的腺瘤通常较大且异型增生较为明显[105,107,108]。因此，女性腺瘤的发病率虽低，但转变为癌的几率却高。

腺瘤在40岁以下发病少见，但随着年龄的增长，发病率逐渐增高。高发区人群的尸检发现，老年组中接近50%的人患有腺瘤。此外，腺瘤大小与多发程度和年龄有关[109]。尸检研究还发现，腺瘤相对均匀地分布于整个大肠。然而，腺瘤多半发生在升结肠，且随年龄增长，这种趋势更加明显[106]。腺瘤的部位分布不同于腺癌，腺癌最常见于直肠和远端结肠。这可以解释为可能是因为远端结肠和直肠腺瘤的癌变率更高[106,109]。事实上，直肠和远端结肠腺瘤相对较大，而且比其他部位腺瘤异型增生明显，支持上述观点[110]。

腺瘤通常没有症状。较大的腺瘤可以出血，患者本人或通过便潜血试验可以发现。少数绒毛状腺瘤可以产生大量黏液，从而导致水和电解质丢失。

腺瘤通常具有家族倾向（且不说家族性腺瘤样息肉病），而且可能是由于常染色体显性遗传而引起的[111,112]。腺瘤的主要临床意义在于这些病变是大多数结直肠癌的前体病变。不过，腺瘤的发病率大约是结直肠癌的30倍，表明只有非常少的一部分腺瘤发生恶变[113]。

大体表现

小的腺瘤无蒂，颜色与周围黏膜相似。此时，不易与增生性息肉鉴别。随着腺瘤逐渐增大，常有蒂的形成；头部颜色较深，呈分叶状，外观如菜花样（图9.30）。大的腺瘤有时可能无蒂，或略微隆起于黏膜，形成绒毯样外观，或形成较明显的突出物。绒毛状腺瘤一般表现为质软的无蒂肿块，表面凹凸不平（图9.31）。与有蒂腺瘤相比，无蒂腺瘤界限常常不清。由于边界模糊不清，因此容易导致术后复发。一些最早来自于日本的报道表明，存在平坦型[114]甚至凹陷型[115]的腺瘤，这可能反映了胃肠道筛查内窥镜检查可以起到很大的作用。

组织学所见

腺瘤由内衬异型增生上皮的管状和（或）绒毛状结构构成。异型增生上皮不同于正常上皮，表现为含有增大、深染和复层细胞核的不成熟细胞的比例增高。核分裂活性不仅局限于基底部，而且上部腺体和表面上皮也有明显的核分裂活性。腺体结构不规则，可以卷曲，分支或密集。Paneth细胞和内分泌细胞可以杂乱散在分布于上皮中。

镜下，根据组织学结构可将腺瘤分为管状、管状绒毛状和绒毛状腺瘤。管状腺瘤（tubular adenoma）由位于固有膜内的分支管状腺体构成，而且分支管状腺体至少占肿瘤的80%以上。管状腺瘤通常有蒂，但也可以无蒂或平坦。绒毛状腺瘤（villous adenoma）是一种至少80%是由被覆上皮的固有膜分叶状或指状突起组成的肿瘤（图9.32）。绒毛状腺瘤通常无蒂，直径约数厘米。管状绒毛状腺瘤（tubulovillous adenoma）是由管状和绒毛状两种结构构成的，每种成分均不超过肿瘤的80%。

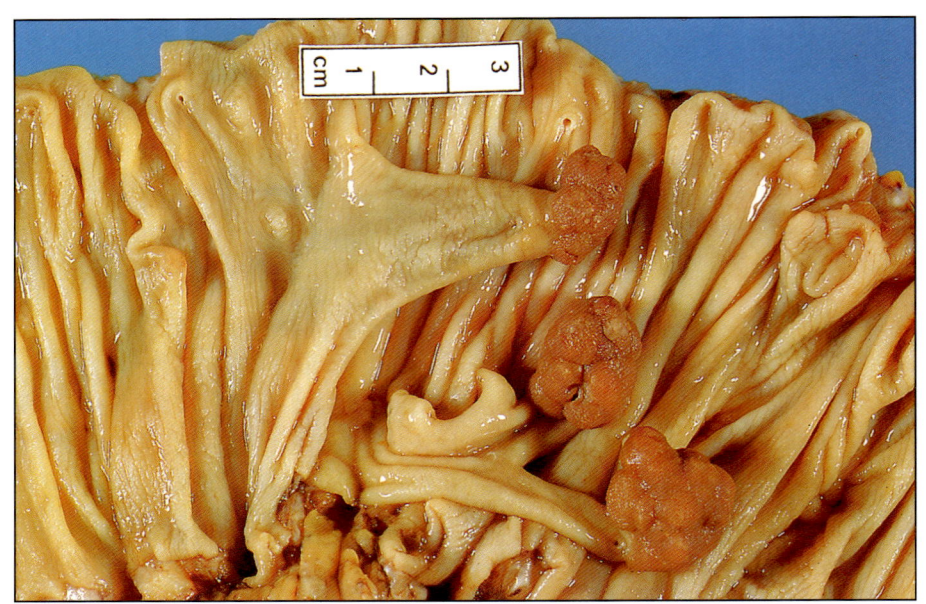

图9.30 发生于乙状结肠的3个管状腺瘤。长蒂是发生于这个部位的腺瘤的特征。

根据上皮异型增生的程度,可将大肠腺瘤分为轻度、中度或重度异型增生[110]。而分为低级别(包括轻度和中度)与高级别的两级分类方法可能更好。轻度异型增生(mild dysplasia),核浆比例较低,核细长,密集,复层(图9.33)。腺瘤黏液分泌通常保留,但可以减少甚至缺乏,上皮内的吸收细胞比例较高。重度异型增生

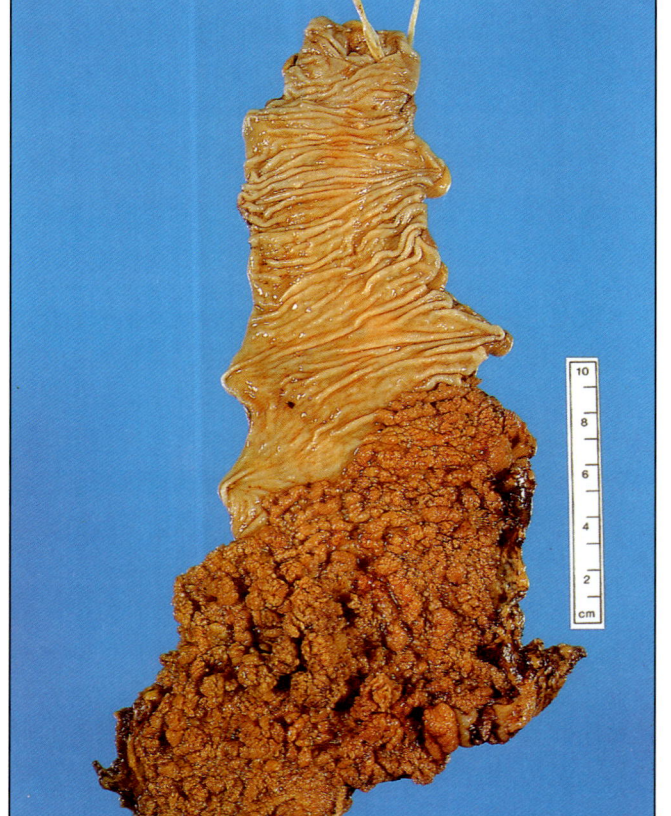

图9.31 直肠大而无蒂的绒毛状腺瘤。肿瘤累及上端直肠全周。

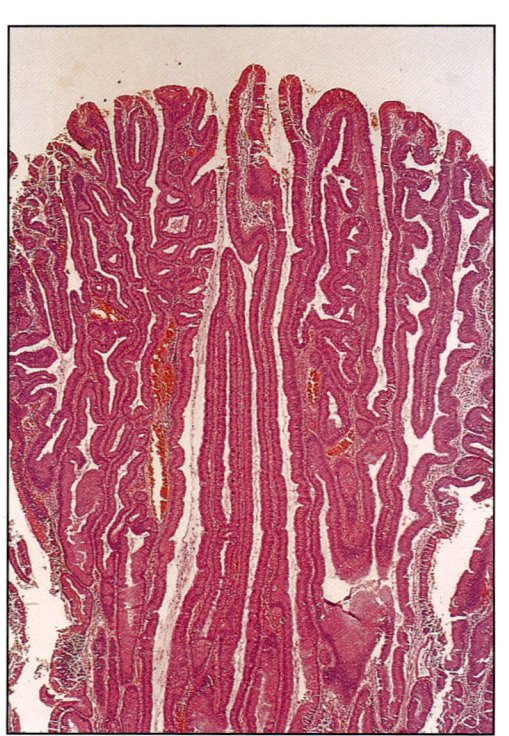

图9.32 大肠的绒毛状腺瘤,指状突起的表面被覆轻度异型增生的上皮。

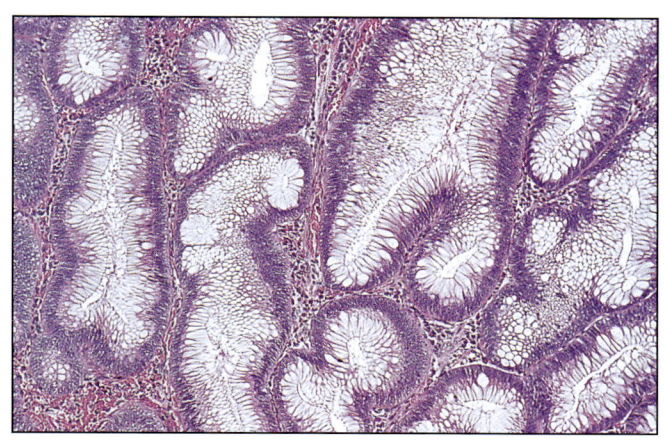

图9.33　管状腺瘤，上皮轻度异型增生。

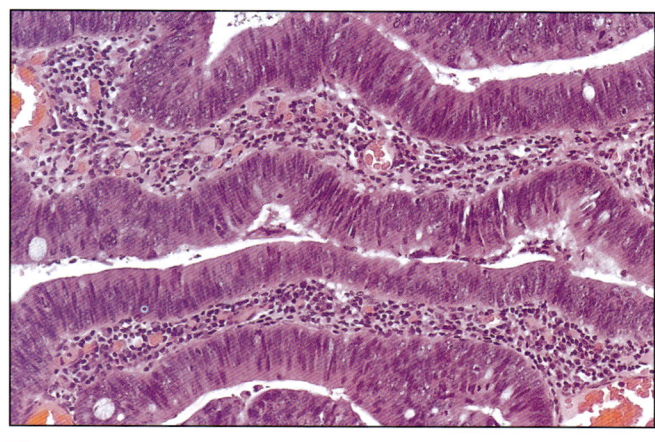

图9.35　大肠腺瘤，上皮中度异型增生。核增大，深染，假复层排列；仅见少数杯状细胞。

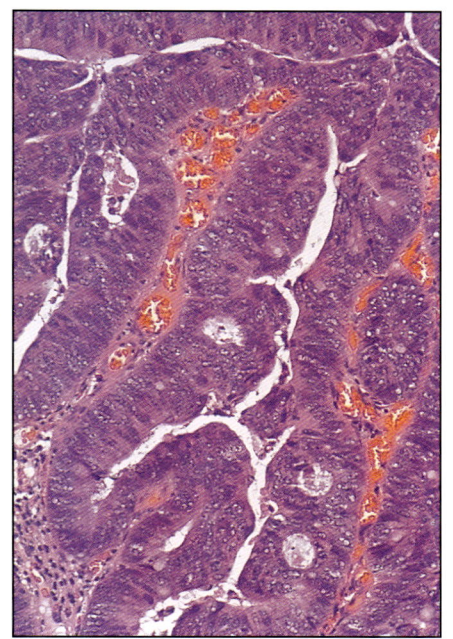

图9.34　管状腺瘤，上皮重度异型增生。

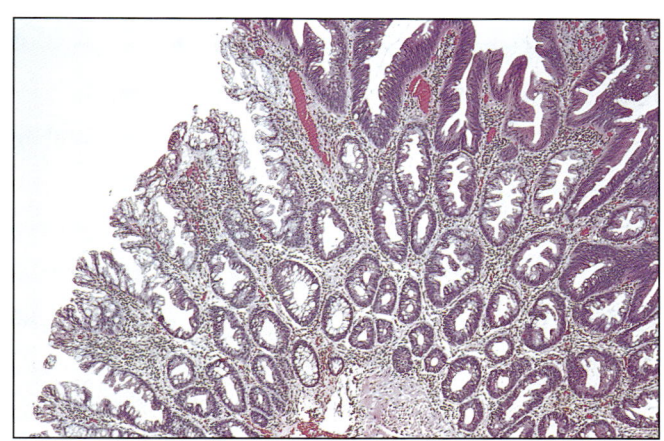

图9.36　混合性增生性息肉-腺瘤。推测腺瘤成分（右上）起源于增生性息肉。

(severe dyaplasia）的核增大，卵圆形或圆形，核深染，常有明显的核仁（图 9.34）。上皮细胞好像未分化，结构明显紊乱，腺体密集或背靠背。中度异型增生(moderate dysplasia) 表现介于两者之间（图 9.35）。多数腺瘤显示轻度异型增生，伴有重度异型增生的最不常见。原位癌（carconoma in situ）一词是指细胞学和组织结构表现基本上属于恶性，但尚未发生黏膜肌层浸润。证实黏膜肌层浸润是诊断浸润癌的重要先决条件。良性的上皮移位（假浸润）可以通过黏膜肌层进入黏膜下层，必须仔细与恶性浸润鉴别[116]。支持良性上皮移位的特征包括出血含铁血黄素沉积、移位腺体周围仍保留有固有膜、缺乏纤维组织增生，以及移位的上皮与其上的腺瘤性上皮相似。腺瘤恶变的危险与其大小、是否存在绒毛以及上皮异型增生的分级有关[117]。

混合性息肉和锯齿状腺瘤
Mixed polyps and serrated adenomas

传统上，腺瘤或肿瘤性息肉（neoplastic polyps）从根本上不同于增生性息肉（见第 407 页）[118]。这两种中间类型息肉的区别不是非常明显。混合性息肉是由典型的增生性息肉和腺瘤混合组成（图 9.36），而锯齿状腺瘤的上皮具有锯齿状结构特征，伴有腺瘤异型增生的细胞学改变（图 9.37）。很明显，锯齿状腺瘤和增生性息肉在组织学发生上是相关的。混合性息肉的腺瘤成分通常呈锯齿状，可能与增生性成分具有克隆相关性[119]。此外，增生性息肉和锯齿状腺瘤具有共同的某种表型的改变，例如胃和肠型黏液的产生，具有类似的致病遗传改变，包括 K-ras 或 *BRAF* 突变和 DNA 甲基化，造成

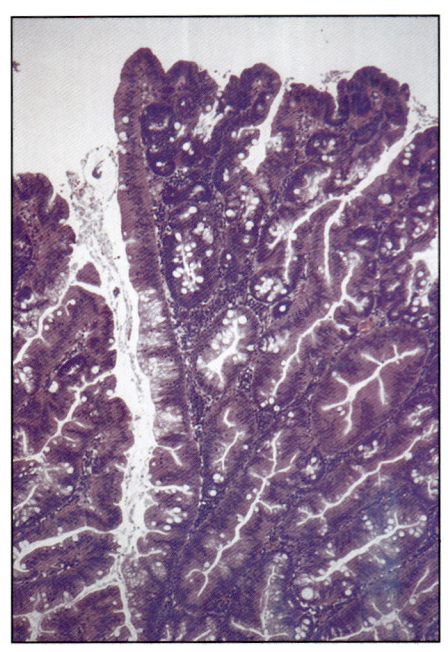

图9.37 锯齿状腺瘤。锯齿状结构伴有细胞非典型性。

诸如 hMLH1 基因的沉默[120]。

锯齿状腺瘤可以发生于整个结肠和直肠，但不同解剖部位也有差异[121]。远端结直肠的锯齿状腺瘤通常表现为隆起性病变，具有管状绒毛状或绒毛状结构，上皮呈强嗜酸性。锯齿状腺瘤可被误诊为腺瘤。不同于大多数腺瘤，锯齿状腺瘤的增生性部分依旧位于基底，通过基底可以异常地延伸达到隐窝上层[122]。近端结肠锯齿状腺瘤经常无蒂，黏液分泌亢进，几乎与增生性息肉相同。对于右半结肠息肉和增生性息肉病，可能很难区分是增生性息肉还是锯齿状腺瘤[123]。已经提出无蒂锯齿状腺瘤（sessile serrated adenoma）这一新的术语，用于诊断非常类似于增生性息肉的少数锯齿状息肉[124,125]。无蒂锯齿状腺瘤较常见于近端结肠，相对较大，由扩张的腺体组成，显示明显的锯齿状结构，具有扩大的增生区，但是缺乏明显的腺瘤性异型增生[124,125a]。这种类型的锯齿状息肉与少数散发性结直肠癌有关，以 DNA 甲基化、BRAF 突变和 DNA MSI（DNA 微卫星不稳定性）为特征[125,126]。

家族性腺瘤性息肉病
Familial adenomatous polyposis, FAP

临床表现

这种病变表现为成百上千的腺瘤遍布于整个大肠[127]（图9.38）。常染色体显性遗传是本病的发病基础，应答基因（APC）位于5号染色体长臂而且克隆化[128-130]。罕见的染色体隐性息肉病与 DNA 修复基因 MYH 的两个突变复制的遗传特性有关[131]。家族性腺瘤性息肉病的腺瘤通常在10～20岁发病，但也可能后来发生。有人提示，诊断本病至少需要见到100个腺瘤。对于有家族史的处于危险状态的青年人（即青春期前），腺瘤数目较少时也可以作出诊断，但一定要将几个息肉送检进行组织学诊断。APC 基因3号和4号外显子突变与腺瘤相对较少的轻微性疾病有关，这种类型的腺瘤一般是发生在右半结肠的扁平腺瘤。癌也可发生在右侧，而且比典型的腺瘤癌变出现得晚[132]。这种轻微性家族性腺瘤性息肉病（FAP）常被误诊为 HNPCC（见下文）。

现在知道，腺瘤不只局限于大肠，也可发生在十二指肠、回肠及胃窦部[2]。壶腹周围的腺瘤体积较大，有显著的恶性倾向[133]。伴有多种结肠外病变的病例已有

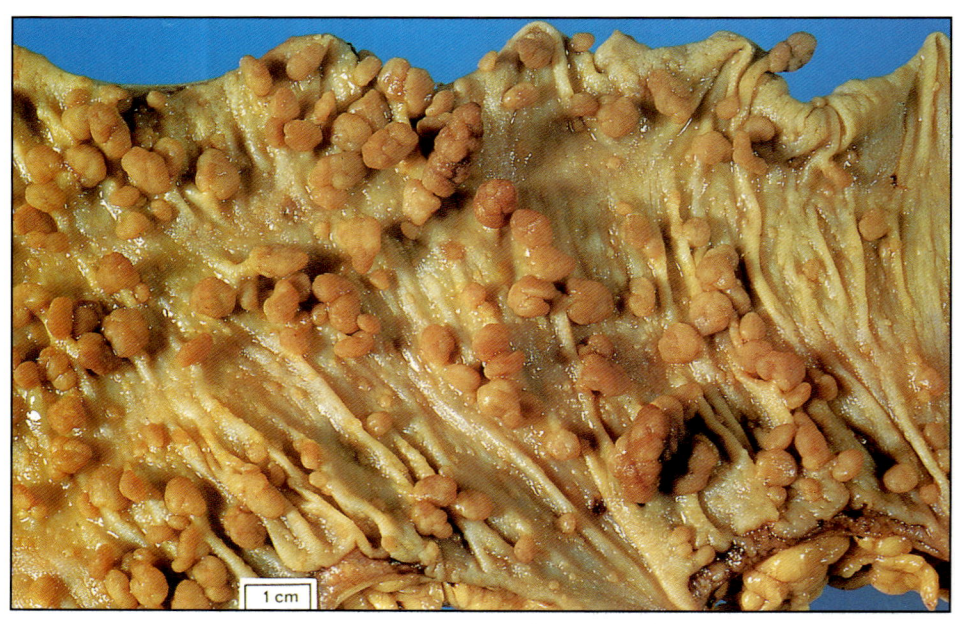

图9.38 家族性腺瘤样息肉病。大肠黏膜上遍布无数的管状腺瘤。

报道。伴有颅骨和下颌骨多发性骨瘤以及多发性皮肤表皮囊肿的病变称为 Gardner 综合征[134]。除了 Gardener 综合征患者 APC 基因 3'端有突变以外，家族性腺瘤性息肉病与 Gardner 综合征之间并没有重要的或遗传的差异[135]。其他的结肠外病变有腹壁及肠系膜纤维瘤病[136]（图9.39和图9.40）、特征性的软组织纤维瘤（见第24章）、牙源性囊肿[137]、视网膜色素沉着[138]、肝母细胞瘤[139]、甲状腺癌[140]以及髓母细胞瘤[141,142]。Turcot 综合征的病例原来是 FAP 或 HNPCC（见下）[142]。伴有晚期癌的综合征通常出现新的突变（一例可有 4 种突变），未做过检查的处于危险的亲属也是如此。癌可以发生在所有受累的患者，如果不进行治疗，癌的发生早于普通人群，通常在 40 岁左右。

大体表现

腺瘤的大小和数量受患者年龄及其分布的影响，可以呈现出一种对于特别种系突变具有特征性的形态结构。除了腺瘤相对较少的轻微性 FAP 以外（见上文），特别严重的疾病与 APC 基因 15 号外显子的特异性突变有关[143]。

组织学表现

多为管状腺瘤，也可发生管状绒毛状和绒毛状腺瘤。检查发现，明显正常的黏膜可能出现微小腺瘤（microadenomas），由一个或少数异型增生的腺体组成（图 9.41）。

癌　Carcinoma

临床特征

结肠与直肠癌是西北欧、北美及澳大利亚最常见的恶性肿瘤之一。非洲、亚洲及南美洲发病率低。然而，在一些生活方式西化的国家，其发病率在增加，例如在日本[144]。而原来发病率高的一些地区，例如北美，随着时间的推移，其死亡率逐渐下降，可能是由于饮食习惯的改变和筛查的结果。流行病学调查表明，散发性结直肠癌的发病与环境因素密切相关，与遗传因素有重要关系，但不是非常显著的关系[145]。环境因素中最主要

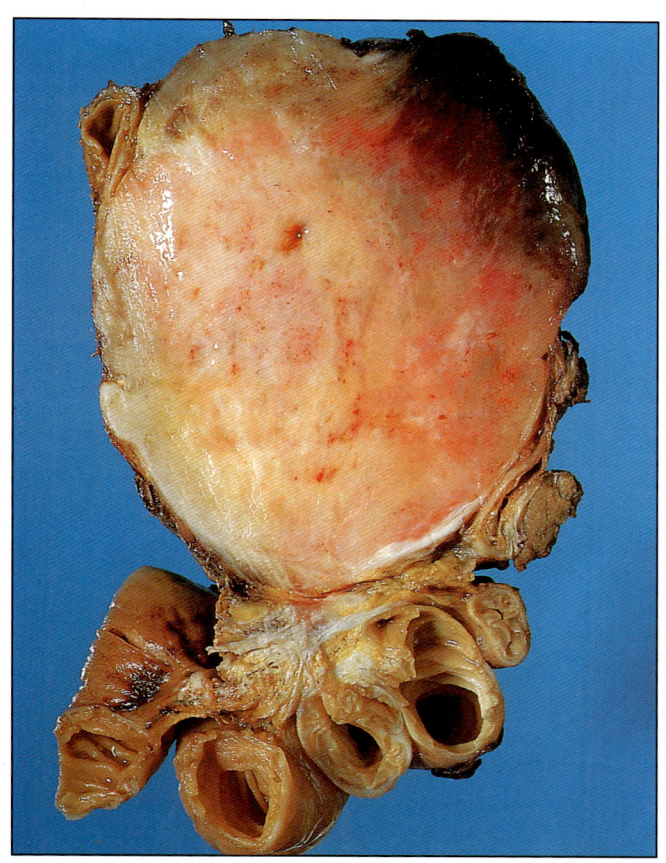

图9.39　家族性腺瘤性息肉病患者，发生在肠系膜的纤维瘤病（硬纤维瘤）。

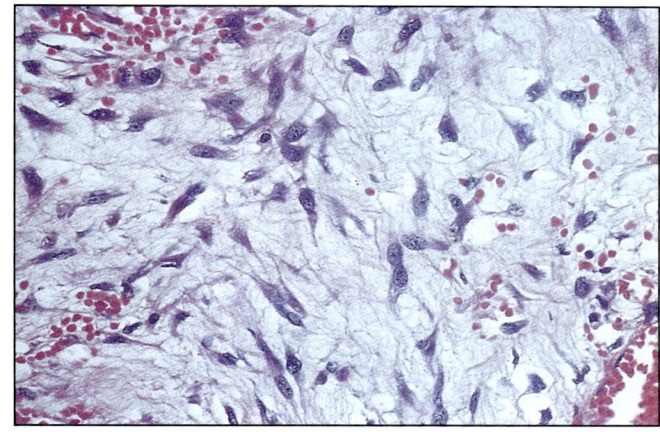

图9.40　腹腔内纤维瘤病，生长活跃的纤维母细胞位于黏液样的间质内，几乎不含胶原，类似于筋膜炎。

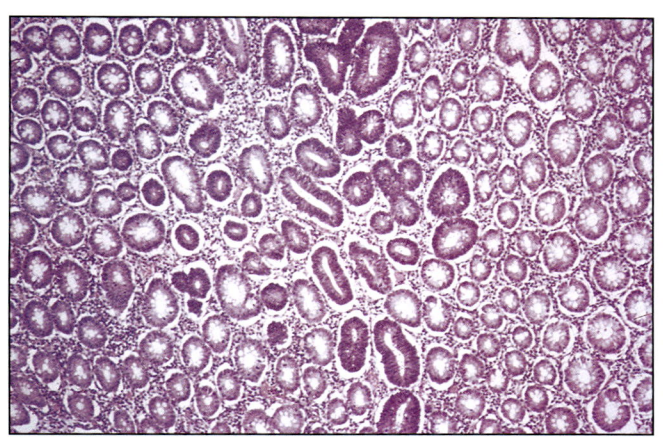

图9.41　家族性腺瘤性息肉病患者微小腺瘤的水平切面。

的是饮食；肉类的消耗量与大肠癌的发病率关系密切，而且酒精也是重要的危险因素[145,146]。其他食物，特别是蔬菜纤维，可以降低大肠癌的发生[147]。散发性结直肠癌的发病原因显然是多因素的。已有证据表明，遗传因素可决定腺瘤的易感性[111]。大肠癌高发地区的发病高峰年龄在65岁左右。癌与年龄明显相关。随着年龄增长癌的发病率进行性增加。

高危险地区大约8%的患者在50岁以下发病[148]。年轻患者与老年患者的预后几乎没有差别[149]。即使年轻人浸润性肿瘤的发生有所增加，但其手术风险降低，故死亡率较老年患者无明显差别。

大肠癌的发病率男性略多于女性。然而，如果将大肠按部位进行比较，会出现更有意义的结果[148]。右半结肠癌常见于各个年龄段的女性，左半结肠癌常见于50岁以下的女性以及70岁以上的男性。直肠癌常见于男性，而且随着年龄增长，其性别差异更加突出。男性大肠癌患者中，40%发生在直肠，30%在左半结肠，30%在右半结肠；而女性40%在右半结肠，30%在左半结肠，30%在直肠。这种分布随年龄而变化，年长的男女患者，均为右半结肠多见。年龄、性别和部位间复杂的相互作用提示大肠癌的进展可能是在多种因素作用下缓慢形成的。例如50岁以下的人以右半结肠癌多见，一种可能的解释是由于HNPCC发生在年轻人，并且好发于右半结肠[148]。此外，少数具有MSI和（或）DNA甲基化的散发性癌与女性、位于近端和年龄有关[150]。

毫无疑问，相当大一部分癌来自于先前存在的腺瘤[151]。也有一些报道描述，在小的溃疡性或非溃疡性癌中没有残存的腺瘤性组织[152-154]。这些病变已被命名为直接生成的癌（de novo carcinomas）。对于这种病变的组织发生，应用平坦腺瘤的概念可能更合乎逻辑。来自日本的报道表明，小而平坦的腺瘤可能具有重要的临床意义，因为难以发现而且转变为癌的倾向增加[114]。以DNA甲基化和DNA MSI为特征的少数结直肠癌与锯齿状前期病变有关，包括无蒂锯齿状腺瘤[124,125]、混合性息肉和锯齿状腺瘤[120,155]。结直肠癌也可发生在癌前病变的基础上，例如家族性腺瘤样息肉病（见上文），包括溃疡性结肠炎[156]、血吸虫病[157]和Crohn病[158]在内的慢性炎症性肠病，幼年性息肉病[159]以及盆腔照射之后[160]。然而，绝大多数癌并不发生在具有这些病变的患者。Lynch综合征或HNPCC，肿瘤发生于相对年轻的患者，并有常染色体显性遗传倾向[12]。HNPCC是造成1%～5%结直肠癌的原因[161]，是由种系突变引起的，这种种系突变可以是DNA错配修复基因家族中的一种突变，例如MSH2、MSH6、MLH1和PMS2[162]。癌多见于右半结肠且为多发性。也发生于其他部位，特别是子宫、卵巢、胃、小肠和脑。HNPCC患者癌发生于先前存在的腺瘤，这种腺瘤常有绒毛状成分[163]。目前认为Muir-Torre综合征（皮肤皮脂腺肿瘤伴结直肠癌）是HNPCC的同义词[164]。

结直肠癌的临床表现受肿瘤部位的影响。直肠癌常表现为出血或里急后重。左半结肠癌可导致排便习惯的改变，最终导致肠梗阻。肠穿孔可出现在肿瘤生长部位或发生癌性梗阻的近端肠管。右半结肠癌患者常因慢性失血而导致贫血，检查可以发现右髂窝部肿块。

癌可在肠壁中直接蔓延，或通过淋巴管转移至局部淋巴结，通过静脉形成肝转移，如肿瘤穿透浆膜可经腹腔发生扩散。只有得到相关的临床资料，才能对大肠癌作出完整的病理学诊断。非根治性（non-curative）手术的病例预后非常差。病理医师也可以通过观察手术切除标本的横切面，特别是深切缘或周缘来确定病例是否获得根治[165,167]。深切缘或周缘可以显示手术切除是否彻底。不幸的是，对于"治愈的"（curative）病例并不能保证具有好的前景，治愈率仅50%。这可以解释为已有肝内微小转移，但手术时未能发现[168]。然而，检查手术标本仍能提供与预后密切相关的病理学资料（见下文）。

大体表现

多数结直肠癌是溃疡性肿物，边缘隆起、外翻（图9.42）。肠壁环状受累可能引起狭窄和梗阻（图9.43）。有时肿块相对较小也会出现这种改变。环形生长的肿瘤有时称为"绳捆癌"（string carcinoma），因为其表现就像一条绳子紧紧系住了肠管。隆起型癌少见，其侵袭性相对较弱。隆起性肿瘤多见于右半结肠。大约10%的肿瘤切面呈黏液状，这是由于肿瘤细胞产生大量黏液所致。应将收到的新鲜手术标本打开，用墨水标记直肠癌的深切缘后，将标本用大头针固定在适宜的板上，然后浸泡在福尔马林中。24小时以后，可将大头针去掉，如果可能，应再固定24小时后再取材。应该通过肿瘤做多个水平切面，包括深切缘。如果展开并检查这些切面，就可以找到肿瘤浸润的最深处并且取材。随后的组织学检查可以证实肿瘤是否被切净。可疑浆膜穿透的部位应取材做组织学检查[169]。大体检查还包括肿瘤呈非常局限或呈弥漫性浸润的生长方式。肿瘤深部脂肪内的所有淋巴结都应取材，还包括自血管结扎处的淋巴结及所有有关的淋巴结。应该仔细检查静脉，并进行组织学检查，以观察血管腔内是否有肿瘤的证据。

多数大肠癌界限相对清楚，少有肉眼界限以外的黏膜下或肠壁内的扩散。因此，即使切缘靠近肿瘤，在远切缘上发现肿瘤的情况也很少见。远端切缘一般无需取材，除非肿瘤距离切缘在 2 cm 之内[170,171]。

组织学表现

大约 90% 的结直肠癌为腺癌，其中易见腺管状分化（图 9.44）。散在的 Paneth 细胞和内分泌细胞并不少见，但是出现这些细胞不影响诊断，而且没有预测预后的意义。某些肿瘤有明显的绒毛状结构，似乎具有较好的预后[172]。大约 10% 的大肠癌分泌大量的黏液。当肿瘤 50% 以上由黏液组成时，可以诊断为黏液性腺癌（图 9.45）。多数研究指出，黏液性腺癌预后较差，但这种

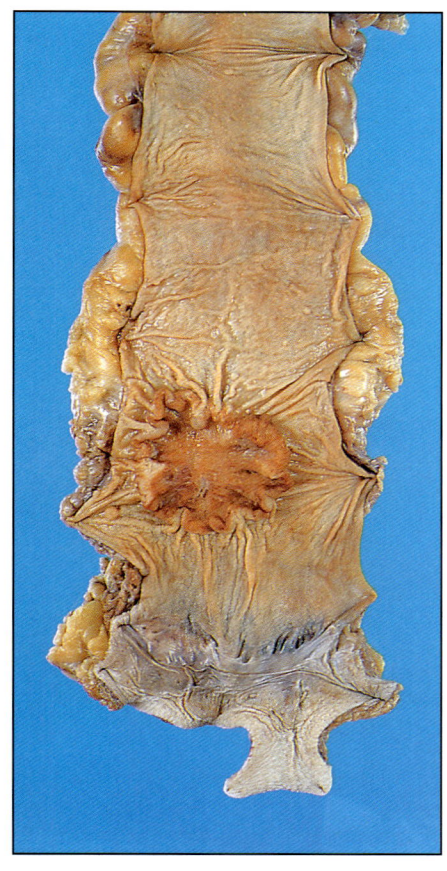

图9.42 直肠中段溃疡性腺癌，边缘隆起外翻。

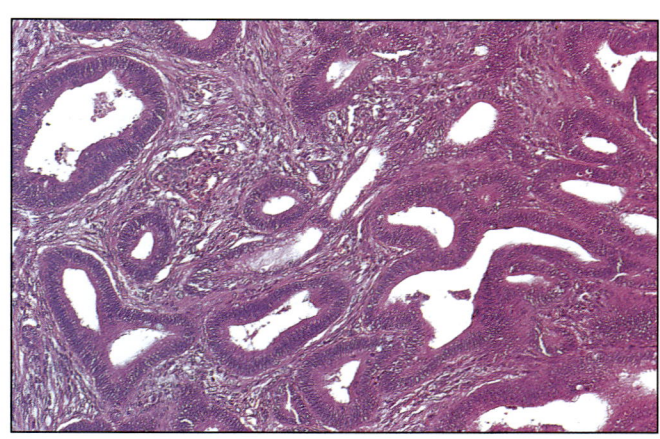

图9.44 大肠高分化腺癌。腺体形成良好，与腺瘤上皮非常相似。

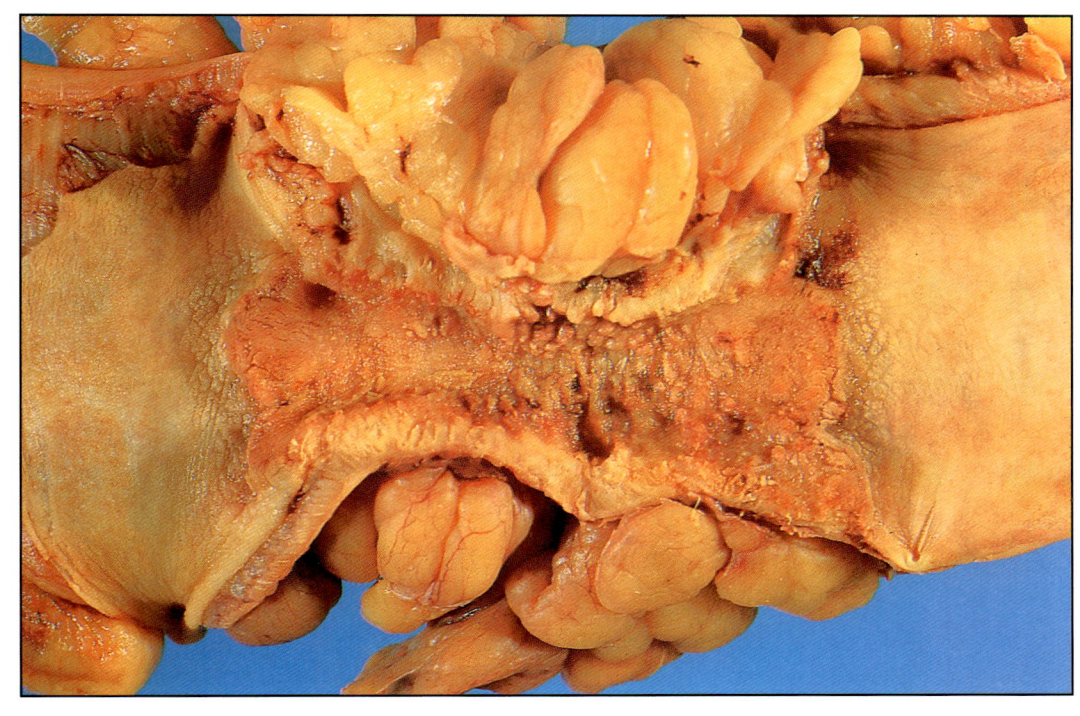

图9.43 结肠绳捆性腺癌，发生在长期溃疡性结肠炎的患者。肿瘤近端和远端黏膜萎缩。

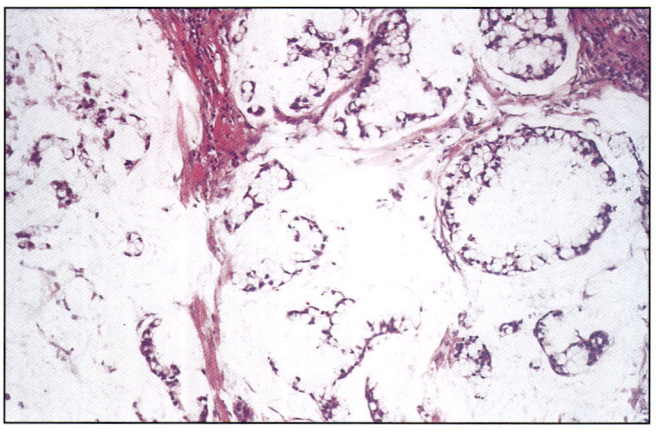

图9.45 大肠中分化黏液性腺癌。分泌黏液的细胞排列成链条状，周围有大量的细胞外黏液。

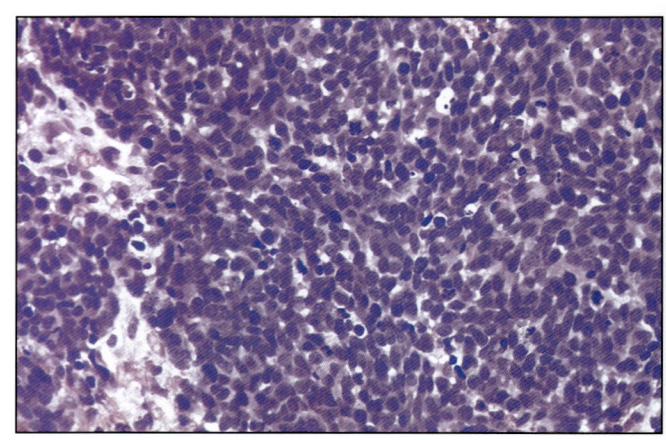

图9.47 直肠小细胞癌。

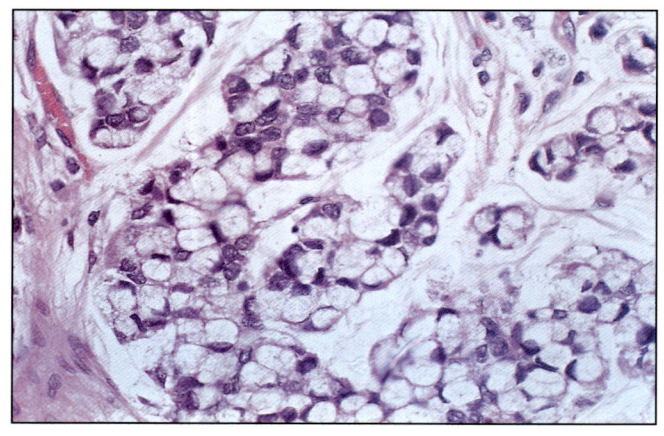

图9.46 大肠印戒细胞癌。深染的细胞核被胞浆内的黏液挤到周边部。

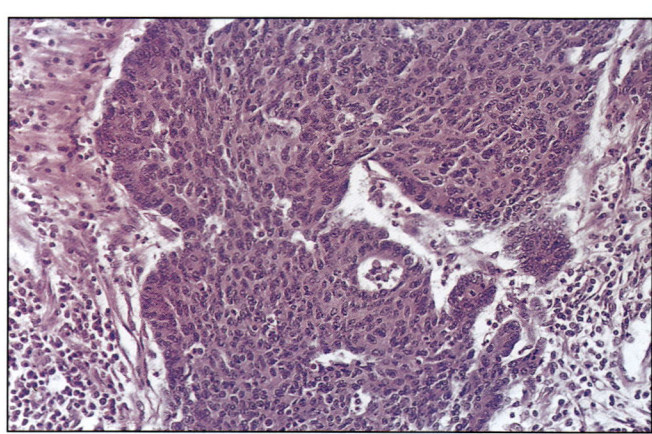

图9.48 大肠未分化（"髓样"）癌。肿瘤细胞形成实性团。这种类型的癌常常出现在遗传性非息肉病结直肠癌和散发性微卫星高度不稳定的癌。

差别较小并且与分期有关[173]。印戒细胞癌仅占原发性大肠癌的1%，预后不好（图9.46）[173]。印戒细胞癌是一种主要由孤立的含有胞浆内黏液的恶性细胞（>50%）组成的肿瘤。所有的大肠印戒细胞癌均应排除从胃印戒细胞癌扩散而来的可能。呈外生性生长的印戒细胞癌预后较好[174]。外生性或非常局限的印戒细胞癌伴有HNPCC和显示DNA MSI的散发性结直肠癌的发病率上升[175,176]。鳞状细胞癌和腺鳞状细胞癌极其少见。小细胞癌（燕麦细胞癌）少见，其组织学、生物学行为和组织化学均与肺的小细胞癌相似（图9.47）[177]。这种癌在发现时通常广泛播散，因此禁忌手术治疗。未分化癌无腺样结构及其他提示直接向腺体分化的特征（图9.48）。肿瘤可能相对均一，中等大小和大的细胞形成界限清楚的细胞团。可能类似于乳腺髓样癌，包括肿瘤内有致密

的淋巴细胞浸润以及肿瘤周围的炎症。这种类型的未分化癌常常显示DNA MSI，而且常常具有相对好的预后[178-180]。镜下有可能误诊为典型的类癌，但是未分化癌有核分裂象和核的多形性，而且缺乏内分泌细胞或内分泌细胞稀少，据此可以作出正确的诊断。未分化癌也可表现为高度多形性和浸润性，此时预后非常不好。通过应用特殊染色，包括免疫组化检查，容易与小细胞癌、淋巴瘤和白血病浸润鉴别开来。

大肠腺癌根据分化程度可分为高分化、中分化及低分化。高分化腺癌（20%）由完好的腺体组成，核的大小和形状均匀一致，而且保持在基底部位（图9.44）。常常有非常类似于腺瘤的上皮。中分化腺癌（60%）腺体不太规则，但仍然容易辨认。核大且不在基底部。低分化腺癌（20%）腺体高度不规则或难以辨认（图9.49）。

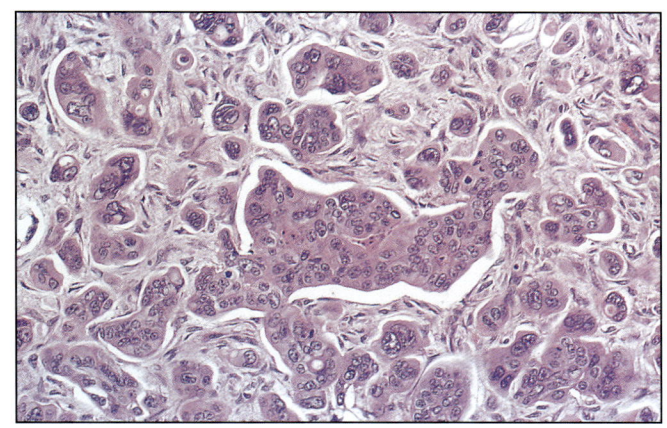

图9.49 大肠低分化腺癌。细胞成簇状不规则排列，几乎没有腺体分化的证据。

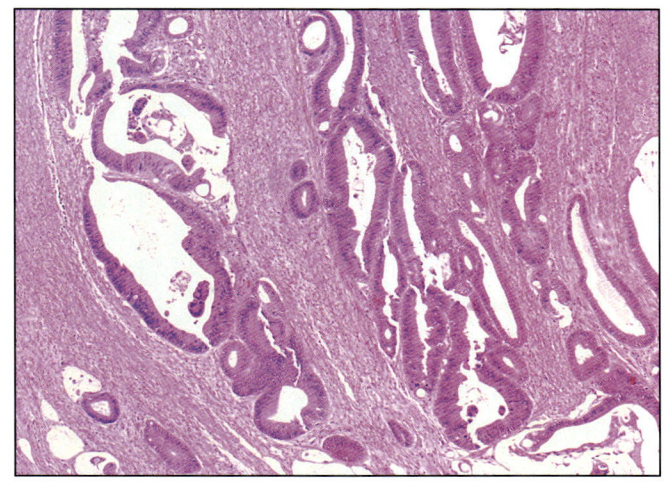

图9.50 大肠腺癌的弥漫浸润性生长方式。

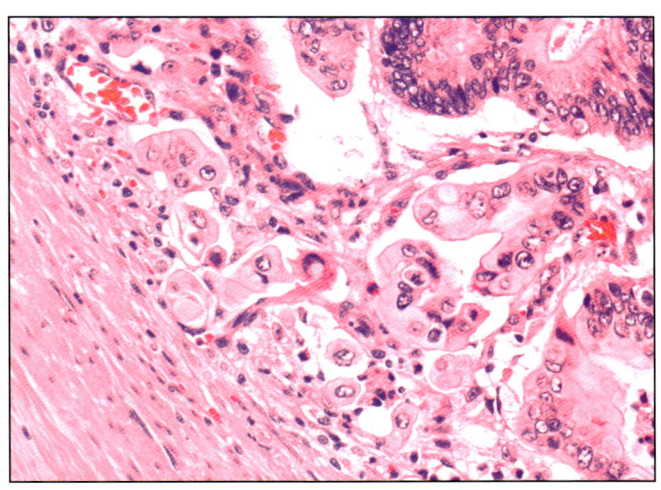

图9.51 浸润边缘的结直肠癌可见肿瘤出芽。其特征是腺体分化丧失，细胞分散，表现为单个细胞或小簇状细胞。

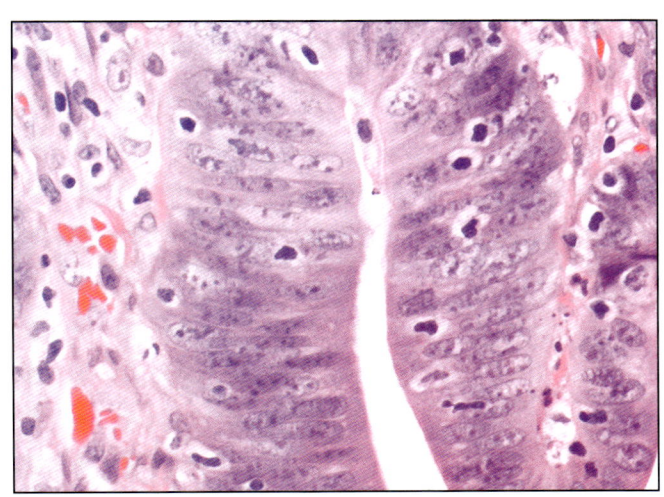

图9.52 肿瘤内浸润或上皮内淋巴细胞。这是诊断遗传性非息肉病结直肠癌和散发性微卫星高度不稳定性结直肠癌最重要的特征。

显示两个或两个以上分化级别的腺癌，应以分化最差的级别来分类。黏液性腺癌出现分泌黏液的柱状上皮代表高分化肿瘤。如上皮由条索状或不规则细胞簇组成，其周围绕以黏液，这种肿瘤可以称为中分化肿瘤（图9.45）。由小而不规则的细胞簇或含有相当数量的印戒细胞构成的黏液性腺癌，归入低分化肿瘤。肿瘤分级与预后有关，但是不如分期重要，而且多数多变量研究显示，分级不能作为一个独立的预后因素[181,182]。诊断低分化腺癌和早期结直肠癌的处理方式相关（见下文）。

肿瘤生长的边缘分为膨胀性或浸润性，多变量研究显示其与预后有关[181-183]。浸润性癌边缘的特征是腺体或舌状结构广泛散布于正常组织中（图9.50）。"浸润"（infiltrating）发生在大约20%～25%的病例，这一术语并不是指见于弥漫性胃癌的明显的壁内播散。在浸润的边缘，肿瘤出芽或去分化伴有浸润性生长方式和血管侵犯，是一个独立的预后不良因素（图9.51）[184]。出现淋巴细胞提示预后较好，不管是在肿瘤生长边缘的炎症细胞套内，还是在肿瘤内（上皮内）有淋巴细胞浸润（图9.52），或是表现为黏膜下或浆膜的Crohn病样淋巴细胞聚集[181, 183, 185]。肿瘤内淋巴细胞浸润也可以作为伴有DNA MSI的结直肠癌的敏感指标[186]。出现明显的纤维组织增生性反应（肿瘤间质由纤维母细胞和胶原构成）与预后不良有关，但也与临床分期有关[181]。纤维组织增生性间质是恶性肿瘤的特征，它的出现对于活检标本的诊断可能有所帮助。

显示广泛DNA MSI的癌多半是黏液性癌、低分化腺癌或未分化癌，但是，不管是发生于HNPCC情况下或是散发性结直肠癌的病例，其预后要好些[187]。部分原因可能是这些癌往往非常局限，缺乏肿瘤出芽，而且伴有肿瘤内淋巴细胞浸润[150,174,175]。根据肿瘤部位（近端结肠）和组织学特征可以怀疑 MSI 的存在，而当患者年龄小于 60 岁时，可以怀疑为 HNPCC 综合征。

扩散和分期

组织学检查的中心环节是判定肿瘤扩散的范围：
1. 肿瘤在直肠壁各层内的直接扩散；
2. 淋巴结转移；
3. 注意任何的血管或神经周围的扩散。

直接扩散的记载依照 TNM 系统的编码：肿瘤在原位或仅限于黏膜（Tis），浸润黏膜下层（T1），浸润固有肌层（T2），扩散到固有肌层外（T3）以及或浸润游离（浆膜）面或邻近器官（T4）[188]。

淋巴结转移可能是最重要的单一的病理学预后指标。随着阳性淋巴结数量的增多、沿着叫得上名的血管干分布的淋巴结受累[189]、阳性淋巴结在血管蒂的顶端[190]以及有逆行淋巴扩散的淋巴结受累者治愈率降低。据报道，出现微小转移（通过 RT-PCR 检测）也是预示预后不良的一种标志[191]。在 TNM 系统中，N0 表示无淋巴结转移，N1 表示有 1～3 个淋巴结转移，而 N2 则为 4 个或 4 个以上淋巴结转移。

Dukes 分期包括 A 期（肿瘤浸润黏膜下层或固有肌层），B 期（肿瘤延伸到固有肌层外），C1 期为有淋巴结转移，C2 期为有血管蒂顶端淋巴结转移[190]。A 期、B 期、C1 期和 C2 期的 5 年生存率分别为约 100%、75%、50% 和 25%[190]。

人们越来越赞成应用临床病理的方法进行分期，包括无（M0）或有（M1）远处转移。TNM 分类与分期的转换见表 9.3。存在残留疾病，例如切缘存在肿瘤，也应予以记录。

已经得到公认的是，静脉侵犯的发生率随着分期进展而增加，且与肿瘤远处扩散有关[192]。一些学者认为，可将其作为一个估计预后的独立指标，但也有人不支持这一观点[181]。不过，肿瘤浸润肠壁外厚壁静脉应当记录下来。虽然有人提出淋巴管浸润和神经周围扩散是有意义的预后因素[193]，但这些观察在早期结直肠癌中可能具有更大的价值（见下文）。

早期结直肠癌　Early colorectal cancer

组织学上（推测在生物学上）类似于癌的肿瘤性上皮可以局限于黏膜层。这种情况可见于腺瘤和结肠炎的黏膜。尽管黏膜中也有小血管，但事实上，在肿瘤突破黏膜肌层并侵入黏膜下层之前，不会发生淋巴结或远距离扩散。因此，一些作者将这种病变（更客观）称为重度异型增生（severe dysplasia）或高级别上皮内肿瘤形成（high-grade intraepithelial neoplasia），而不用原位癌（carcinoma in situ）这一术语[117]。早期结直肠癌（early colorectal cancer）这一术语是指肿瘤延伸到黏膜下层但未超出黏膜下层。即使这样，淋巴结转移的危险性依然很低，大约仅为 4%，其前提条件为非低分化的肿瘤[194]。不管肿瘤是发生在管状腺瘤（图 9.53）还是大而无蒂的绒毛状腺瘤，判定早期结直肠癌的病理学原则是相同的。早期结直肠癌只要切除完全，而且不是低分化肿瘤，局部切除就已足够[195]。另外的先决条件是没有小静脉或淋巴管侵犯[196]，尽管一项研究显示静脉侵犯没有预后意义[197]。类似的处理已经用于直肠下段小的溃疡性癌，即使肿瘤已经浸润固有肌层，也可通过局部盘状切除予以治疗，但是前提是肿瘤不能超出肌层[198]。

表9.3	结直肠癌的TNM分期系统		
0期	Tis	N0	M0
Ⅰ期	T1	N0	M0
	T2	N0	M0
Ⅱ期	T3	N0	M0
	T4	N0	M0
Ⅲ期	任何T	N1	M0
	任何T	N2	M0
Ⅳ期	任何T	任何N	M1

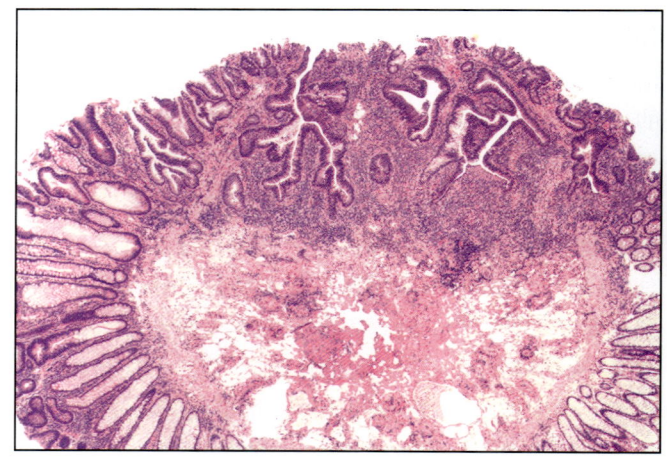

图9.53　管状腺瘤（左）伴有穿过黏膜肌层的小灶状高分化腺癌。切缘未见癌。癌伴有明显的淋巴细胞浸润，患者为43岁女性，患有遗传性非息肉病结直肠癌（HNPCC：hMLH1 种系突变）。腺瘤微小，仅有低级别异型增生。然而，发生在 HNPCC 患者的腺瘤具有侵袭性（迅速和早期转变为癌的可能性高）。

免疫表型和分子病理

根据 CEA、核的 β-连环蛋白 (beta-catenin) 和 CK20 阳性表达,以及 CK7 不表达,可以将原发性和转移性结直肠癌与其他上皮性恶性肿瘤鉴别开来。CDX2 也可以用来区分非肠源性腺癌[199]。过去 20 年间,结直肠癌的分子或遗传学改变已经得到深入研究,对于发病机制、分类、诊断和预后均有了新的见解。结直肠腺瘤进展为癌的过程中逐步发生的遗传学突变,已经成为实体肿瘤发病机制的重要范例。众所周知,在结直肠肿瘤形成的分子模型中,发现 *APC*、*K-ras* 和 *TP53* 改变是结直肠腺瘤启动、进展和转变过程的关键因素[200]。然而,最近发现结直肠癌不是通过单一突变途径进展的,事实上,只有 7% 的结直肠癌以 *APC*、*K-ras* 和 *TP53* 突变为特征[201]。

HNPCC 作为一种独立的临床病理疾病已经得到公认,并且采用结肠镜进行检测,这已提高了患者的存活率。根据诸如肿瘤内淋巴细胞浸润等组织学所见,病理医师可以根据组织学所见怀疑 HNPCC 的诊断,例如肿瘤内淋巴细胞浸润[202]。DNA 错配修复蛋白 MLH1、MSH2、MSH6 和 PMS2 免疫染色可以表明基因表达和定位的丧失,可能具有种系突变的发病机制[202]。伴 DNA MSI 的散发性结直肠癌主要是由于 DNA 修复基因 *MLH1* 启动子部位甲基化导致基因沉默引起的[203]。尽管伴 MSI 的散发性结直肠癌对标准化疗不太敏感,但预后可能较好[204]。这种类型也可以作为多发性或不同时发生的肿瘤的标志。因此,散发性 MSI 结直肠癌的分子学诊断变得越来越加重要。值得注意的是,散发性 MSI 结直肠癌可以既不表达 CK20 也不表达核的 β-连环蛋白。进一步研究结直肠癌分子遗传学的异质性,在未来几年内将会发现具有临床重要性的其他分子标记物。从这个角度看,最近的资料提示,结直肠癌的肿瘤核型可能具有预后意义[205]。

鉴别诊断

鉴别诊断中重要的是不要将移位上皮和(或)异型增生上皮过诊断为恶性肿瘤(见腺瘤一节)。诊断癌的标准是依据适当的细胞学和结构特征,出现纤维组织增生性的肿瘤间质以及浸润突破黏膜肌层(图 9.54)。要防止过诊断,尤其是对于具有息肉样病变的病例。取自腺瘤表面的挤压活检标本可能被误诊为癌,导致不必要的手术。发生在腺瘤、孤立性直肠溃疡综合征和炎症性肠病的异位上皮可能有囊状扩张。移位上皮显著囊性扩张的病例有时被描述为深在性囊性结肠炎 (colitis cystica profunda)[206],应与高分化黏液性腺癌相鉴别。

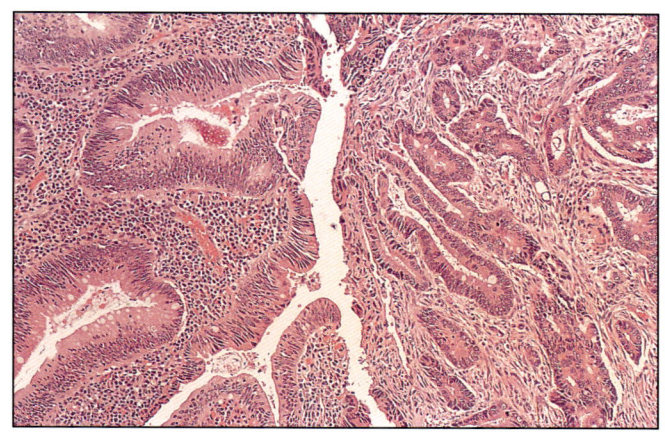

图 9.54 切片显示相邻的腺瘤(左)和腺癌(右)。腺癌的腺体小而不规则,位于纤维组织增生的间质内。腺瘤区域间质类似于正常的黏膜固有层。

内分泌肿瘤　Endocrine tumors

大肠的类癌少见,直肠是最常见的部位[207, 208]。直肠类癌通常表现为偶然发现的黏膜结节,直径小于 1cm,但在少数情况下可以呈浸润性的生长方式,表现为广泛扩散、坏死、核的多形性以及核分裂活性增高。某些报道显示恶性类癌的发生率明显增高,这是由于包括了小细胞癌和混合性腺癌-类癌。后肠类癌最常见的组织学形态是呈缎带状排列(图 9.55),其次是混合性岛屿状和小管状结构。一项研究显示,28% 的直肠类癌亲银反应阳性,而 55% 是嗜银性的[207]。肿瘤可以分泌各种多肽类激素。长期患溃疡性结肠炎的患者肠道活检标本可以出现内分泌细胞增生和肿瘤[209]。

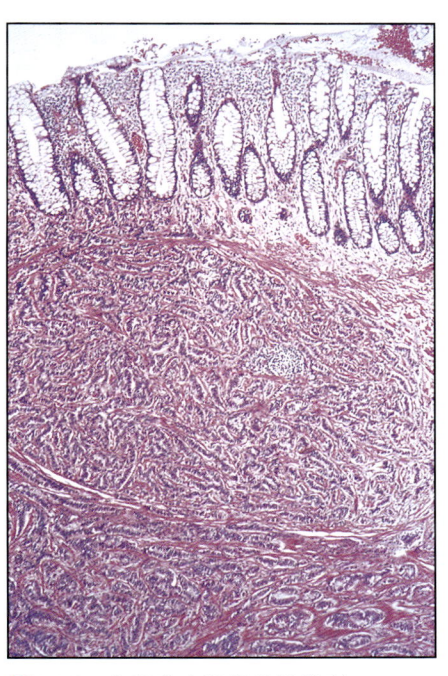

图 9.55 大肠类癌呈缎带样排列。

非上皮性肿瘤　Non-epithelial tumors

平滑肌和间质肿瘤（Smooth muscle and stromal tumors）

　　与发生在小肠的间质肿瘤不同，多数大肠良性间质肿瘤均具有平滑肌分化的免疫组化证据[210, 211]。直肠是好发部位[212]。小的平滑肌肿瘤起源于黏膜肌层，表现为偶尔发现的无蒂息肉（图 9.56）。临床经过为良性。起源于固有肌层或直肠内括约肌的较大的肿瘤并不能预测其转移行为；大小与核分裂数可能是预后的最好指标；大于 5 cm 的肿瘤应该被看作是恶性肿瘤[210, 213]。在恶性病变中，GIST 似乎比平滑肌肉瘤常见[214]。

脂肪瘤和脂肪瘤病　Lipoma and lipomatosis

　　小的脂肪瘤通常为偶然发现，而较大的病变可能表现为出血[215]。肠脂肪瘤病极其罕见。

良性血管性肿瘤　Benign vascular tumors

　　见小肠一节。

神经鞘肿瘤　Nerve shealth tumors

　　作为孤立性病变的神经纤维瘤和神经鞘瘤极其罕见，而多发性神经纤维瘤发生在 von Recklinghausen 病。肠的神经束膜瘤（perineurioma）新近已有描述，结肠镜下最常见的表现是小的息肉样黏膜内病变[215a]。

神经节瘤[216]　Ganglioneuroma

　　神经节瘤罕见，可以表现为孤立性病变或多发性病变[56]。孤立性神经节瘤可能伴有其他病理学改变，但这也可能是一种巧合[216]。在幼年性息肉病患者中已有神经节瘤性息肉病（ganglioneuromatous polyposis）的描述[217]。孤立性神经节瘤男女发病率均等，而多发性神经节瘤病可能较常见于男性。所有年龄的成人均可受累。肿瘤为息肉样或结节状，直径从几毫米到 2 厘米不等。可以发生于整个大肠，偶见于末端回肠。组织学上，神经节瘤由神经细丝蛋白和 NSE 染色阳性的神经节细胞、神经纤维和 S-100 阳性的梭形细胞（通常主要是神经鞘细胞）构成（图 9.57）。过度生长的神经可能局限于黏膜，引起固有膜膨胀，伴有腺体扭曲（低倍镜下与幼年性息肉相似），或累及黏膜和黏膜下层。神经节瘤最好被看做是迷芽瘤（choristomas）（因为正常黏膜内没有神经节细胞），且无恶性潜能。

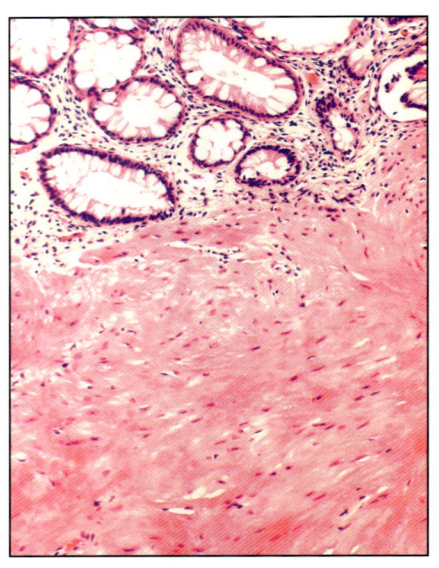

图9.56　发生在直肠黏膜肌层的良性平滑肌肿瘤或平滑肌瘤。

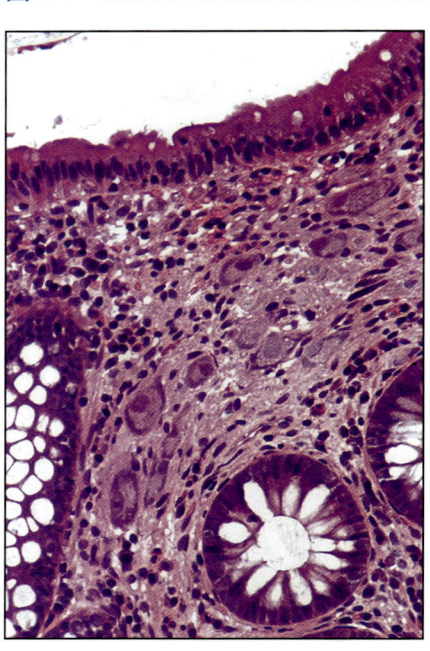

图9.57　直肠孤立性神经节瘤。边界不清，常呈息肉样，累及固有层是其特征。

弥漫性神经节瘤病[216, 218]　Diffuse ganglioneuromatosis

　　临床上，弥漫性神经节瘤病似乎不同于神经节瘤；可以发生于婴儿、儿童或成人。婴儿和儿童常有慢性便秘史，类似于 Hirschsprung 病。在成人，常伴有 IIb 型多发性内分泌肿瘤（MEN）[55]和 von Recklinghausen 病[218]。大体表现为缩窄或结节状肿块，可以累及长达 20 cm 的肠段。神经节瘤性增生主要以肠肌神经丛为中心，并延伸到邻近肠壁各层。这种现象被描述为"神经元性肠发育不良"（neuronal intestinal dysplasia），是肠神经丛的异常增生。通过临床病史和炎症性肠病的其他组织学特征，可与晚期 Crohn 病的神经元增生（也被描述为神经肌肉和血管错构瘤）区别开来[219]。

Kaposi 肉瘤和血管肉瘤
Kaposi's sarcoma and angiosarcoma

大肠 Kaposi 肉瘤可以是 AIDS 病人全身病变的一部分。病变为多灶性，累及黏膜和黏膜下层[220]。血管肉瘤偶尔表现为肠的转移性疾病，原发部位在皮肤。

淋巴组织肿瘤
Tumors of lymphoid tissue

良性淋巴组织息肉和息肉病
Benign lymphoid polyp and polyposis

良性淋巴组织息肉是小的黏膜下肿瘤，由增生的淋巴组织构成，推测其是对局部炎症的反应（图 9.58）。多数病变发生于直肠下段。临床上为小而局限的病变，借此可与低级别淋巴瘤相区别。良性淋巴组织息肉病见于儿童，发生于病毒感染之后[57]。这种病变也可以是家族性的，见于免疫缺陷的患者[58]。本病应与恶性淋巴瘤性息肉病鉴别（见下文）。

淋巴瘤　Lymphoma

大肠原发性恶性淋巴瘤罕见[221]。局限性淋巴瘤主要发生在盲肠或直肠。可以合并溃疡性结肠炎[222]和AIDS。绝大多数病例为高级别的 B 细胞淋巴瘤。套细胞淋巴瘤（见第 21 章）仅见于 60 岁到 70 岁的成人，通常表现为腹泻[221, 223]；肠道其他部位也常被累及，这种肿瘤应与原发性低级别 B 细胞淋巴瘤（MALToma）相鉴别。本病不适于手术治疗，因为它的本质是全身性疾病。肠黏膜散布多个息肉，因此最初被命名为恶性淋巴瘤性息肉病（malignant lymphomatous pylopsis）。组织学检查可见，肠黏膜层和表浅黏膜下层有淋巴细胞浸润，形成明显的结节状结构（图 9.59）。高倍镜下显示弥漫浸润的细胞几乎完全是小的生发中心样细胞。90%以上的病例肿瘤细胞 Cyclin D1（bcl-1）阳性。此外，这些细胞 CD20（L26）和 CD79a 也呈阳性反应，而 CD10 和 bcl-6 阴性。本病生长缓慢，但预后不良，最终出现全身淋巴结肿大并累及骨髓。

继发性肿瘤　Secondary tumors

大肠的继发性肿瘤罕见。偶尔前列腺癌可以直接蔓延至直肠。

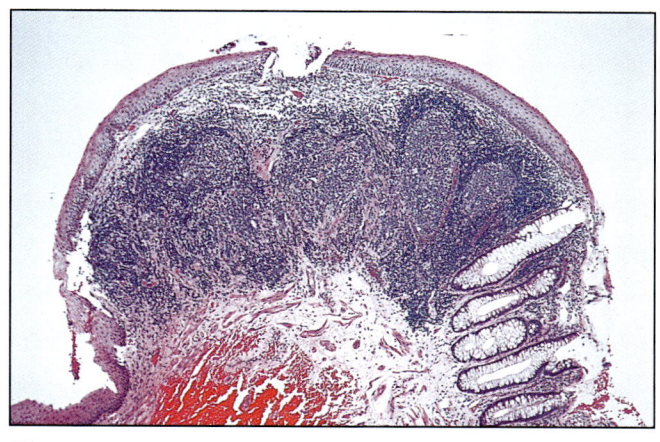

图9.58　肛门直肠交界处的良性淋巴组织息肉。

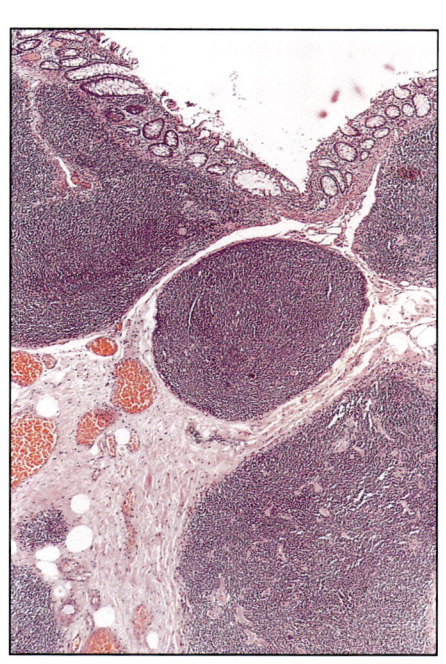

图9.59　大肠恶性淋巴瘤性息肉病（套细胞淋巴瘤）。黏膜下层生发中心细胞呈结节状集聚。

瘤样病变　Tumor-like lesions

Peutz-Jeghers 息肉和息肉病
Peutz-Jeghers polyps and polyposis

详见小肠一节。孤立性 Peutz-Jeghers 息肉可以发生于大肠，而不出现综合征。

幼年性息肉和息肉病
Juvenile polyps and polyposis

幼年性息肉常见于儿童，表现为直肠出血。本病可以发生在多达 1% 的儿童。过去认为幼年性息肉是一种孤立性病变，但是结肠镜检查显示，超过半数的儿童可以见到一个以上的息肉，而且息肉可以均匀分布于整个大肠[224]。幼年性息肉有蒂，头部呈球状。息肉头部主

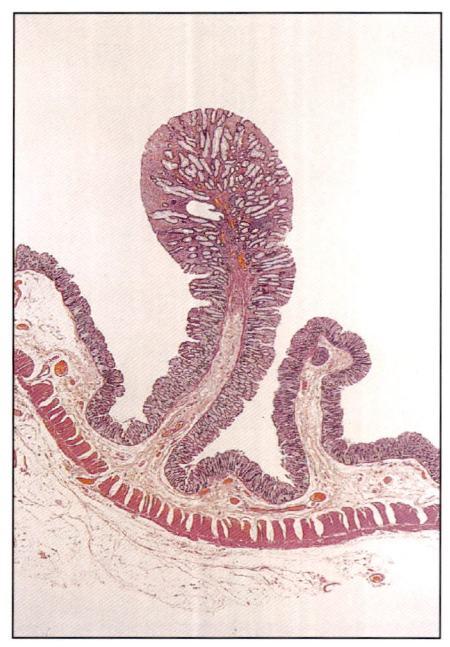

图9.60 大肠小的幼年性息肉。息肉头部呈球形，由丰富的固有膜组成，伴有显示囊性扩张的分支腺体。

要是由内衬腺管的正常上皮组成，腺体可呈囊状扩张（图9.60）。黏膜固有膜明显水肿。息肉表面可有溃疡形成，伴随的炎症可能导致上皮反应性增生，不要误认为是异型增生。幼年性息肉发生异型增生和癌的病例均极其少见。

幼年性息肉病是一种少见的病变，表现为两种类型。一种罕见的类型发生于婴儿，伴有腹泻、出血、蛋白丢失性肠病和肠套叠。于幼年时即可死亡。无家族史。其余的病例发病年龄不同，典型的表现是发生在 10~20 岁患者的直肠出血。息肉或者局限于结直肠（图9.61），或者分布于整个胃肠道。常有提示常染色体显性遗传的家族史，在几例儿童证实有染色体 18q 的 *SMAD4/DPC4* 突变[225]。可伴有心脏和颅的异常，并可伴腭裂、多指（趾）畸形和旋转不良。普遍认为幼年性息肉病是一种癌前病变，大约有 20% 的危险性[143]。息肉常为多分叶状（图9.62），伴有乳头状外观；固有层过多，所以孤立性息肉的特征可能不太明显。此外，上皮可能显示异型增生性改变。

发生于 Cowden 综合征的错构瘤
Hamartomas in Cowden's syndrome

Cowden 综合征是一种罕见的常染色体显性遗传性疾病，其特征包括皮肤、口腔黏膜、甲状腺和乳腺肿瘤，伴有胃肠道错构瘤性息肉[226]。这些息肉显示腺体结构扭曲和黏膜纤维组织增多。研究证实与染色体 10q 的 *PTEN* 有关[227, 228]。

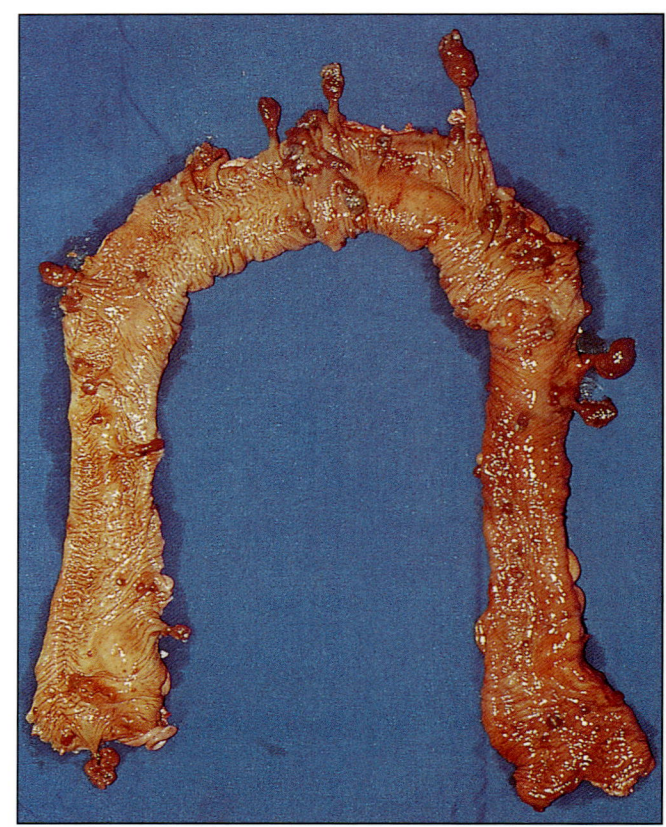

图9.61 大肠幼年性息肉病。

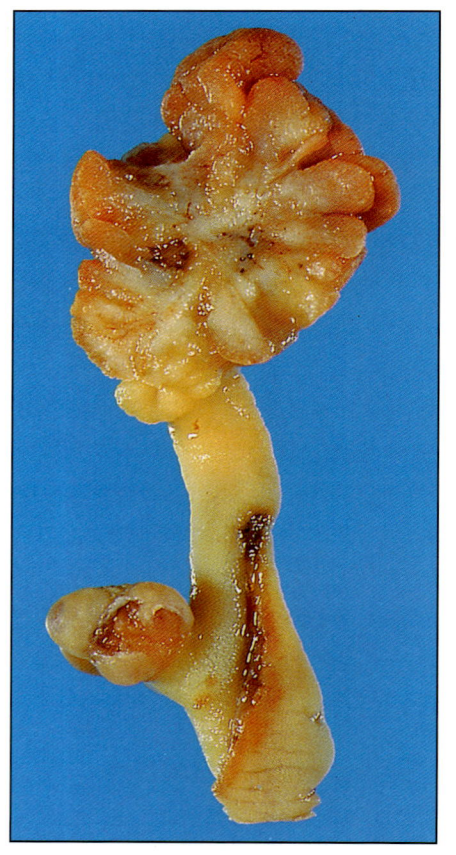

图9.62 典型的幼年性息肉的切面，取自幼年性息肉病的患者。

胃的异位 [229] Gastric heterotopia

胃的异位组织少见,其发生常常伴有消化道畸形。它可以表现为出血,或为偶然发现。其既可以表现为黏膜的一个界限清楚的颗粒状区,也可以表现为息肉样病变。

增生性息肉和息肉病
Hyperplastic polyp and polyposis

增生性息肉为小而无症状的黏膜息肉,常为内窥镜下或手术标本的偶然发现[230]。绝大多数发生于直肠和乙状结肠远端。可以大量成簇围绕着癌或与腺瘤伴发[231]。通常认为增生性息肉既不是肿瘤也不是癌前病变,但是最近细胞遗传学和分子学研究显示,这些病变具有克隆性改变,涉及到肿瘤相关的位点和基因[232, 233]。发生在结肠近端的大的增生性息肉与少数显示DNA甲基化和(或)DNA MSI的结直肠癌有关[120]。大部分息肉小于5 mm。组织学检查显示腺体变长,呈锯齿状结构(图9.63)。杯状细胞数目减少,柱状细胞嗜酸性,顶端充满分泌的黏液。核圆形,空泡状,伴有明显的核仁。核分裂象局限于隐窝基底部,内分泌细胞可能位于隐窝下部。黏膜固有层内平滑肌细胞增多,而淋巴细胞和浆细胞常减少[234]。偶尔,上皮可穿破黏膜肌层发生移位(图9.64),不要与癌混淆[235]。

有发生于相对年轻的患者的多发性增生性息肉的报告。这些息肉通常较大,遍布大肠[236]。可能存在锯齿状腺瘤(图9.37)和混有增生性和腺瘤性成分的息肉(图9.36),这些病变发生大肠癌的危险性增高[237]。许多增生性息肉病的病例实际上可能是锯齿状腺瘤性息肉病,有关这一问题尚有争论[123]。然而,增生性息肉和锯齿状腺瘤的鉴别诊断并不总是容易作出的(见第395页)。增生性息肉病可能具有家族性,而且与结直肠癌有关[233]。

Cronkhite-Canada 综合征
Cronkhite-Canada syndrome

Cronkhite-Canada 综合征是一种弥漫性胃肠道息肉病,伴有蛋白丢失性肠病、秃发、指甲萎缩和皮肤色素沉着。多发性无蒂的息肉样病变累及整个胃肠道。组织学检查显示腺体囊性扩张,位于水肿的固有层内(图9.65)[238]。

炎性息肉　Inflammatory polyp

炎性息肉可能是炎症性肠病、输尿管乙状结肠吻合术(图9.66)或黏膜脱垂的并发症。表现为黏膜间质因水肿和炎细胞浸润而膨大,隐窝分支,扩张或再生性增生。息肉表面可有溃疡及肉芽组织形成。

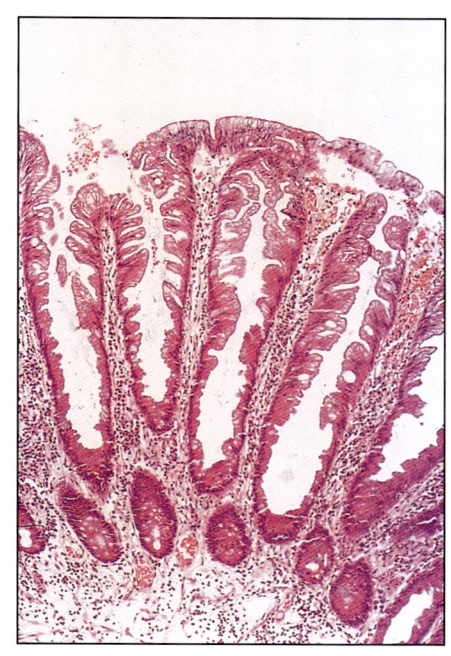

图9.63　大肠增生性息肉,显示隐窝不分支,伴有锯齿状外观。

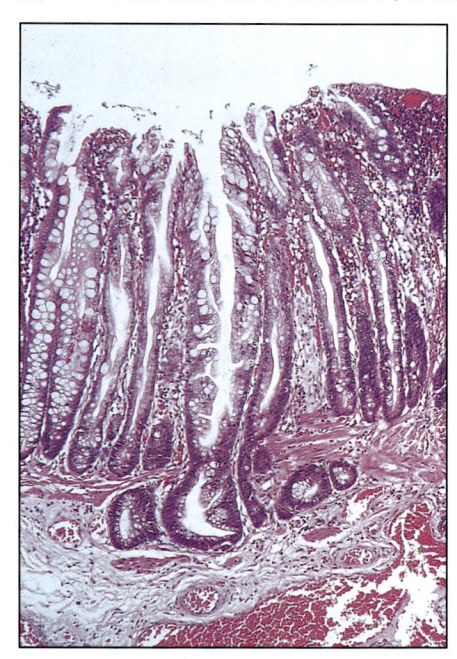

图9.64　增生性息肉的上皮移位。

黏膜脱垂的继发病变
Lesions secondary to mucosal prolapse

黏膜脱垂可见于结肠各个节段、直肠或肛门直肠部,是肠道运动功能障碍的结果。临床背景包括孤立性直肠溃疡综合征、脱垂性痔、完全性直肠脱垂、脱垂性直肠造口术、结肠造口术以及憩室性疾病[239]。脱垂的黏膜病变可因局部缺血、创伤或炎症而改变,导致它们的大体或镜下表现各不相同。孤立性直肠溃疡综合征可以为一个大的孤立性溃疡或多发性小溃疡。特征性的改变是固有层被平滑肌性的间质所代替,上皮呈增生性改变以及隐窝结构扭曲(图9.67)[240]。上皮可以通过黏膜肌

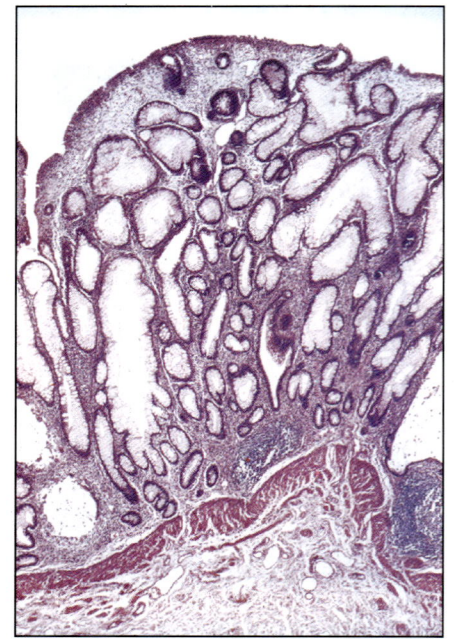

图9.65 Cronkhite-Canada综合征。

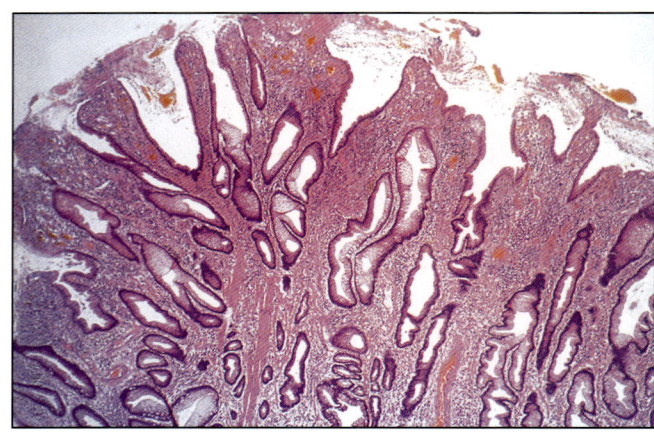

图9.67 孤立性直肠溃疡综合征,特征性的改变是增生性隐窝被平滑肌束分隔。

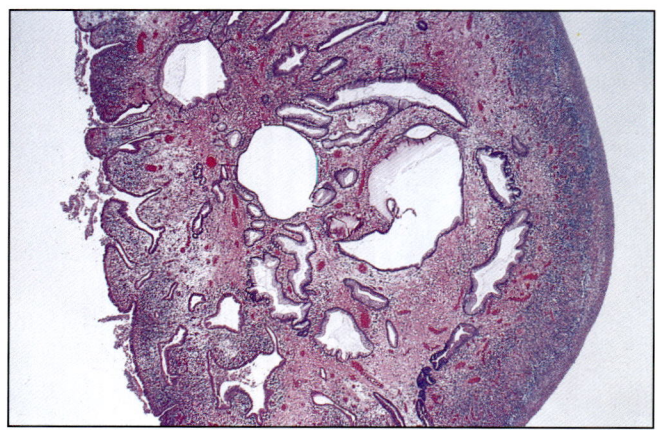

图9.66 发生在输尿管乙状结肠吻合口部的炎性息肉。

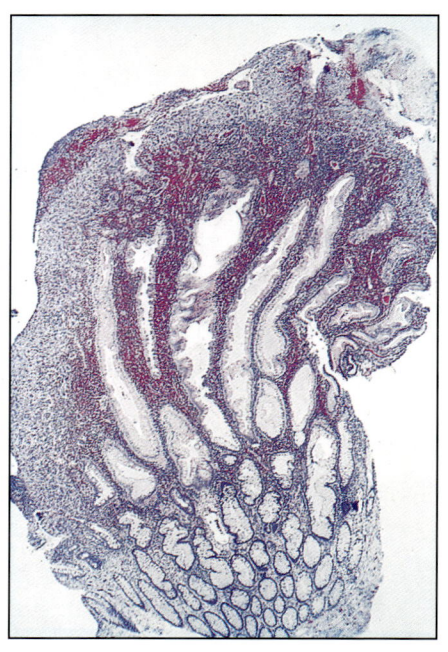

图9.68 炎性或"帽状"息肉,表面为肉芽组织形成的帽状结构。

层发生移位,移位显著的病例可能酷似癌。其他类型的黏膜脱垂可以导致形成单个或多发性炎性息肉,其表面常有肉芽组织形成的帽状结构(图9.68)[241]。类似的病变被描述为炎性腺肌性息肉(inflammatory myoglandular polyp)[242]。伴有表面乳头状上皮增生的孤立性息肉可以发生于肛门直肠交界部,这种病变被描述为炎性泄殖腔源性息肉(inflammatory cloacogenic polyp),可能类似于管状绒毛状腺瘤[243]或锯齿状腺瘤。

子宫内膜异位症　Endometriosis

子宫内膜异位症可以累及大肠,但通常无症状。乙状结肠和直肠是发生子宫内膜异位的主要部位。肠壁广泛受累可以导致排便习惯的改变,使肠壁变厚或形成硬结,可能类似于恶性肿瘤[244]。

软斑病[245]　Malakoplakia

胃肠道是软斑病第二常见的部位(仅次于泌尿道),通常发生于乙状结肠和直肠。病变呈息肉样或斑片状,镜下由大的嗜酸性组织细胞构成,其内含有特征性的钙化Michaelis-Gutmann小体(图9.69)。软斑病可以合并大肠化脓性癌。

癌前上皮性病变
Precancerous epithelial lesions

大肠异型增生已在腺瘤中讨论(见第393页)。异型增生发生于慢性溃疡性结肠炎(图9.70)和Crohn病患者的扁平黏膜。异型增生也可发生于隆起的病变或肿块,表面常呈乳头状(图9.71)。异型增生与炎性或再

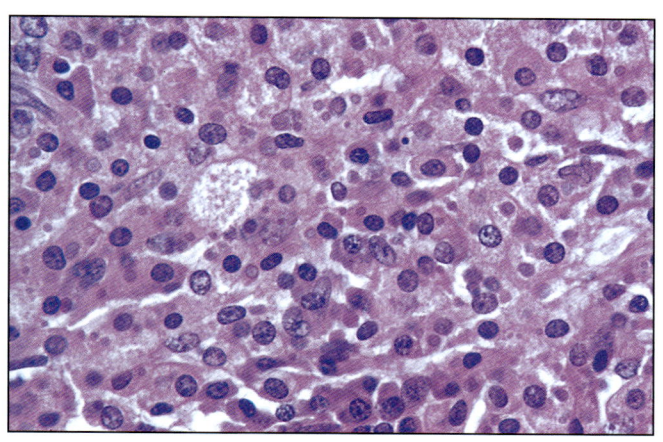

图9.69 大肠软斑病,其发生与腺癌有关(未显示)。

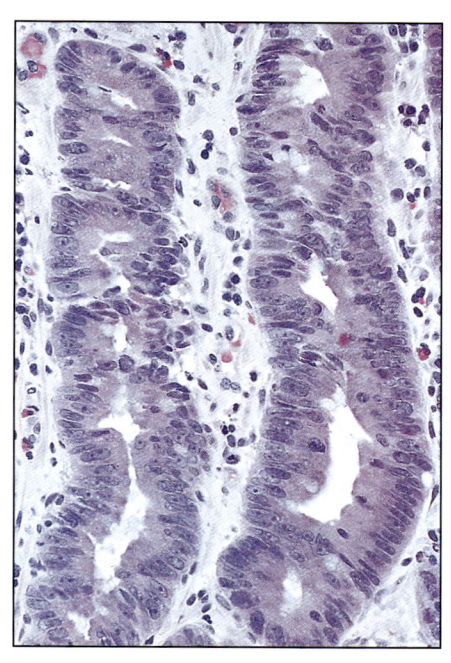

图9.70 溃疡性结肠炎的高级别上皮异型增生。核增大,伴有明显的核仁,胞浆不成熟。

生性改变可能难以区别。一般来说,在有活动性炎症的情况下,诊断异型增生是不明智的。鉴于评估有无异型增生并对其分级具有主观性,提倡将活检标本分为无异型增生、不能确定或有异型增生[156]。有异型增生者再进一步分为低级别或高级别异型增生,高级别异型增生接近于原位癌。诊断高级别异型增生可能导致直肠结肠切除术,因此提倡应该由两位有经验的病理医师取得一致的意见。

肛管 Anal canal

上皮性肿瘤 Epithelial tumors

肛管上皮性肿瘤相对少见,而良性肿瘤更为罕见。

鳞状细胞癌 Squamous cell carcinoma

临床特征

肛管鳞状细胞癌的发病率好像在增加,特别是在男性同性恋的个体中,不论有无AIDS[246]。人乳头状瘤病毒(HPV)16型和18型与本病的发生有关[247]。多数癌发生在齿状线上方的移行带(其上皮类似于尿道上皮)。肿瘤常向上直接蔓延。因此,多数肛管癌表现为直肠下段的溃疡型肿物[248]。

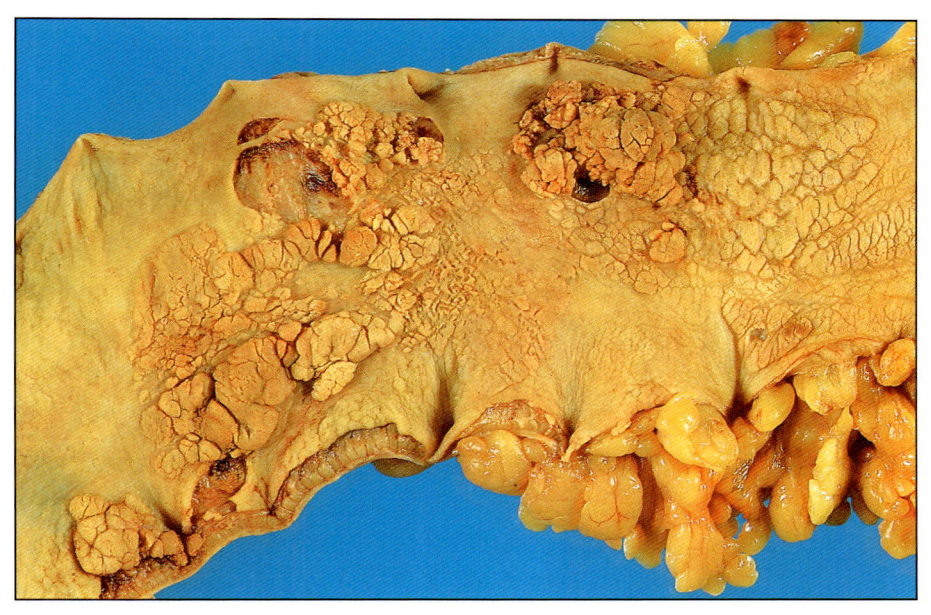

图9.71 长期溃疡性结肠炎病人的异型增生相关性病变或肿块。黏膜隆起,呈鹅卵石状的区域显示上皮异型增生。

组织学表现

肛管鳞状细胞癌分为大细胞角化性、大细胞非角化性以及基底细胞样癌（从前称为泄殖腔原癌）。基底细胞样癌大约占所有肛管鳞状细胞癌的50%，肿瘤由小细胞实性片块组成，周边细胞常呈栅栏状排列，中心突然转变为嗜酸性坏死或角化（图9.72）。应与肛周皮肤的基底细胞癌鉴别。鳞状细胞癌的分级是人为的，而且由于肿瘤类型多样化而变得十分复杂。高级别癌是由小簇状细胞组成的，常常显示边缘组织弥漫性浸润。核的大小和形状差别很大，而且有明显的核分裂活性。几乎没有角化。鳞状细胞癌可以含有充满黏液的微小囊腔。小细胞癌是肛管部位的罕见肿瘤[249]，应与淋巴瘤和黑色素瘤鉴别。检查邻近的鳞状上皮常常能够发现不同程度的异型增生直至原位癌[250]。其组织学改变（图9.73）与宫颈上皮内肿瘤形成一样。肛缘鳞状细胞癌通常发生于肛周皮肤与下段肛管鳞状上皮黏膜的交界处。肿瘤常为典型的大细胞角化性鳞状细胞癌，其分化相对较好。

预后受肿瘤大小、浸润深度以及有无淋巴结扩散等影响[251]。可以累及沿上痔静脉分布的淋巴结，盆腔侧壁淋巴结以及腹股沟淋巴结。然而，现在因为处理原则发生改变，故根治性手术标本中很少见到淋巴结。目前，直径不大于2 cm的肿瘤采用局部切除术（不包括高级别的恶性肿瘤），而比较大的肿瘤一般采用放化疗[252]。

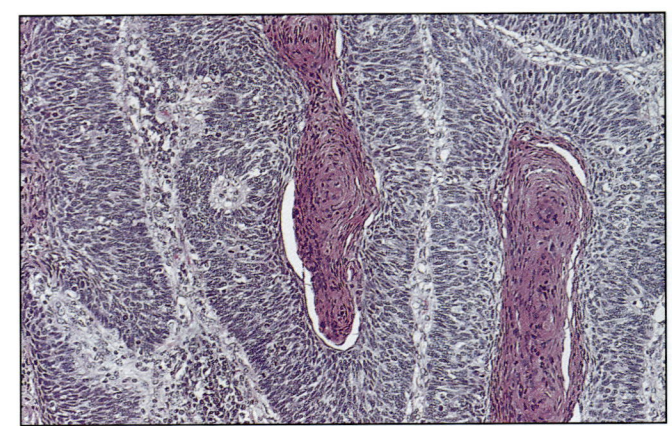

图9.72 肛管基底细胞样型鳞状细胞癌。细胞排列成巢，周边呈栅栏状排列，中心角化。

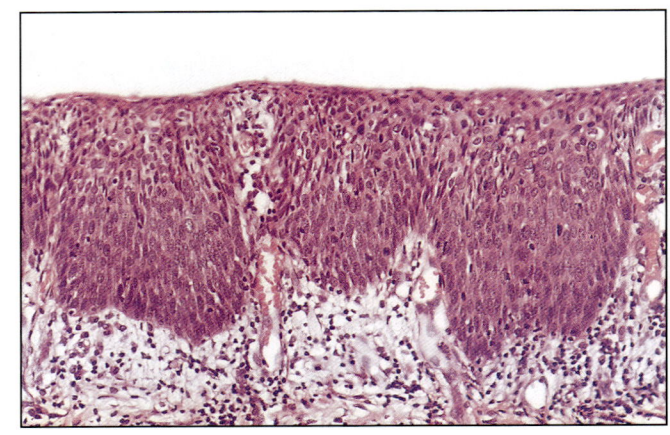

图9.73 肛管移行区黏膜的重度异型增生或肛门上皮内肿瘤形成，Ⅲ级。

巨大湿疣和疣状癌 [253]
Giant condyloma and verrucous carcinoma

一般认为巨大湿疣和疣状癌是同一种疾病，因为其病因、病理和临床特征都有诸多共同之处。尖锐湿疣主要局限于肛周皮肤，但组织学上相似的更为罕见的巨大湿疣常常表现为肛管直肠区的巨大肿块，而且广泛侵入肛门周围软组织、坐骨窝、直肠周围组织，甚至盆腔组织。尽管具有局部浸润性行为，但几乎没有侵犯淋巴管的倾向。这种病变与累及男性和女性生殖系统的Buschke-Lowenstein巨大湿疣相同（见第13章和第14章）。

腺癌 Adenocarcinoma

发生在肛管上端结直肠型黏膜的腺癌无法与直肠癌区别，因此被归入直肠癌。高分化黏液性腺癌偶尔可以发生在伴有肛门直肠瘘的情况下[254]。也可能有潜在的肠道病变，包括后肠下端或肛周反复发作的Crohn病。诊断常常延迟到临床上考虑有癌的可能性时。腺癌也可以起源于肛门部位的导管和腺体，但非常罕见[255]。这种起源的证据可能来源于肛管腺的异型增生。

恶性黑色素瘤 [256-258] Malignant melanoma

恶性黑色素瘤可以占到肛门原发性恶性肿瘤的15%。表现为大的隆起型或溃疡型肿块，常常延伸到直肠下段。肿瘤来源于齿状线上方移行带内正常存在的黑色素细胞。这一部位的恶性黑色素瘤有高度浸润性，局部广泛浸润至肛周和直肠周围组织，累及痔静脉淋巴结，并在早期发生血行转移至肝和肺。其组织学形态与其他部位黏膜的黑色素瘤一样，主要有两种组织学亚型，即上皮样黑色素瘤和梭形细胞黑色素瘤。主要应与淋巴瘤、直肠未分化癌和肛管低分化鳞状细胞癌以及小细胞癌相鉴别。肿瘤常常缺乏大量色素形成，但如果仔细寻找，大约50%的病例可发现黑色素。应注意观察邻近黏膜出现的交界性改变，但这些改变常被溃疡所破坏。

囊性错构瘤[259] Cystic hamartoma

囊性错构瘤是直肠后的病变，可以表现为肛门部肿瘤，伴有复发性瘘管和脓肿，并有疼痛和里急后重的病史。有两种病因：(1)炎症后肛门腺体上皮误植；(2)尾肠的先天性缺陷。病变由多房性囊肿构成，内衬鳞状上皮、移形上皮和柱状上皮（图9.74）。鉴别诊断包括单纯性肛门腺囊肿、畸胎瘤、皮样囊肿、直肠重复囊肿以及肛门腺高分化腺癌。已有恶性变的报道[260]。

肛缘肿瘤 Anal margin tumors

表皮和附属器肿瘤 Epidermal and adnexal neoplasms

肛缘皮肤肿瘤基本上与其他皮肤肿瘤一样（见第23章）。然而，肛周皮肤易于发生多种生长紊乱。这可能反映了皮肤黏膜交界处普遍存在的不稳定性，交界处是指肛管鳞状黏膜和肛周皮肤之间的交界。此外，几种病变是由特殊类型HPV感染（或伴有不同程度的感染）引起的[261]。这些病变包括尖锐湿疣、Bowen病、Bowen样丘疹病、上皮异型增生和鳞状细胞癌。需要强调的是，在这个部位HPV与肿瘤形成间的确切关系仍不清楚。角化棘皮瘤[262]和基底细胞癌[263]可以发生于肛周皮肤。基底细胞癌应与肛管基底细胞样癌（见上文）鉴别。乳头状汗腺瘤（hidradenoma papilliferum）（图9.75）是肛周皮肤最常见的汗腺肿瘤[264]。

肛管黏膜白斑是累及肛缘及肛管鳞状上皮的一种罕见病变[265]。需与炎症造成的单纯性角化过度加以鉴别，因为前者有恶性倾向。组织学检查显示过度角化、棘层增厚，表皮真皮交界处呈明显的锯齿状结构，并有条带状苔藓样的慢性炎细胞浸润（图9.76）。

Paget病也可见于肛周皮肤[266]，应当与向下扩展的

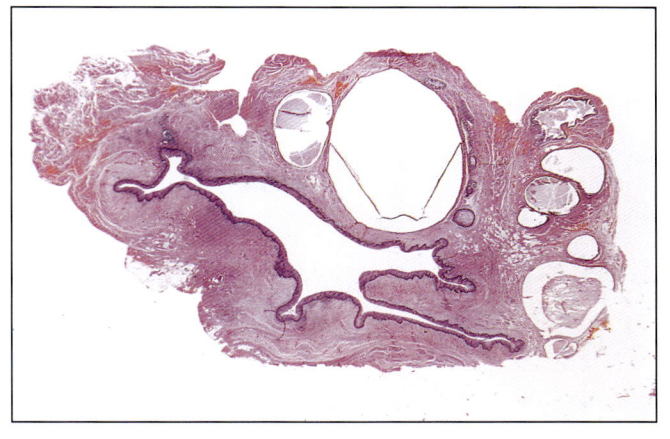

图9.74 直肠后囊性错构瘤，病变由内衬移行上皮的囊腔构成。周围间质内有排列紊乱的平滑肌。

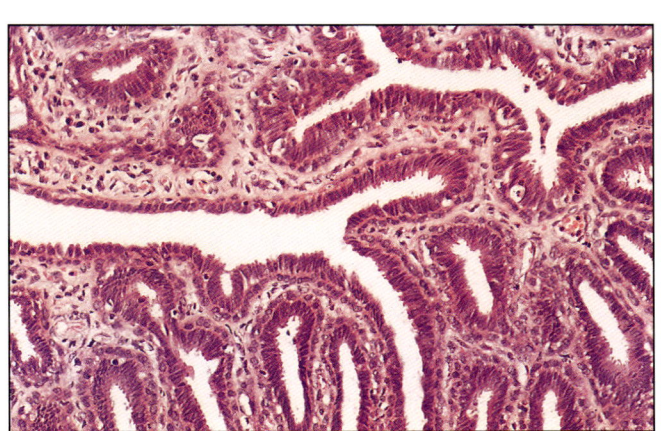

图9.75 肛缘乳头状汗腺瘤，显示具有独特的两层细胞内衬的腺体结构。

印戒细胞癌（伴有肛门直肠部位腺癌）相鉴别。与印戒细胞相比，Paget细胞含有少量黏液，核呈空泡状，且集中在表皮的基底部位（图9.77）。Paget细胞具有顶浆分泌的本质，通过大囊肿病液体蛋白（GCDFP）染色可以证实[266]。其他重要的鉴别诊断包括Bowen病和恶性黑色素瘤的Paget样扩散。与乳腺不同，肛周Paget病极少与皮肤下面的癌有关。

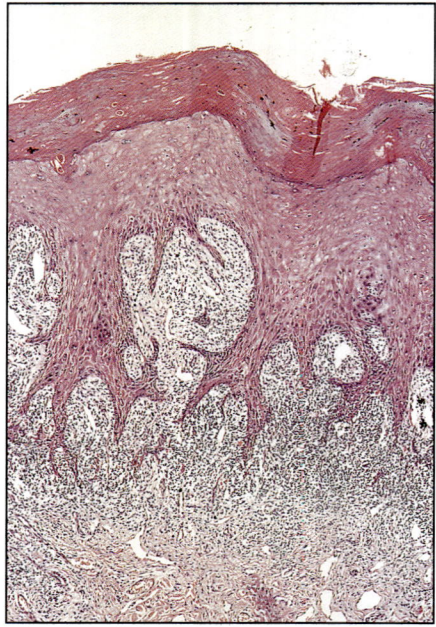

图9.76 肛周部位黏膜白斑，表现为角化过度，"钉突状"棘层增厚以及表皮真皮交界处带状慢性炎细胞浸润。

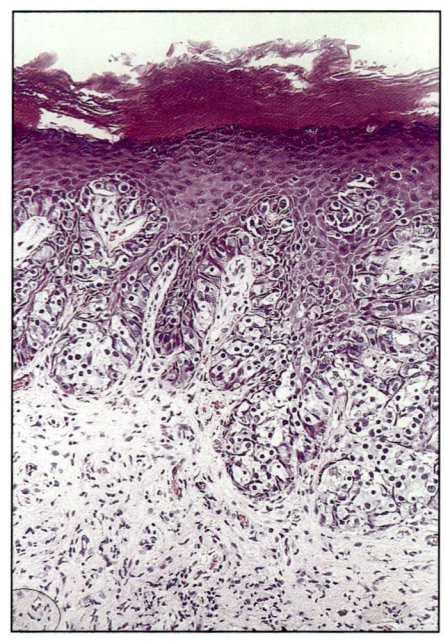

图9.77 肛周Paget病。Paget细胞核圆形，位于中心，胞浆透明，其内充满黏液，浸润鳞状上皮基底层。

参考文献

1. Perzin K H, Bridge M F 1981 Adenomas of the small intestine: a clinicopathologic review of 51 cases and a study of their relationship to carcinoma. Cancer 48: 799–819
2. Domizio P, Talbot I C, Spigelman A D et al. 1990 Upper gastrointestinal pathology in familial adenomatous polyposis: results from a prospective study of 102 patients. J Clin Pathol 43: 738–743
3. Komorowski R A, Cohen E B 1981 Villous tumors of the duodenum: a clinicopathologic study. Cancer 47: 1377–1386
4. Barclay T H, Schapira D V 1983 Malignant tumors of the small intestine. Cancer 51: 878–881
5. Howe J R, Karnell L H, Menck H R et al. 1999 The American College of Surgeons Commission on Cancer and the American Cancer Society. Adenocarcinoma of the small bowel: review of the National Cancer Data Base, 1985–1995. Cancer 86: 2693–2706
6. Dabaja B S, Suki D, Pro B et al. 2004 Adenocarcinoma of the small bowel. Presentation, prognostic factors and outcome of 217 patients. Cancer 101: 518–526
7. Talbot I C, Neoptolemos J P, Shaw D E et al. 1988 The histopathology and staging of carcinoma of the ampulla of Vater. Histopathology 12: 155–165
8. Holmes G K, Dunn G I, Cockel R et al. 1980 Adenocarcinoma of the upper small bowel complicating coeliac disease. Gut 21: 1010–1016
9. Farrell D J, Shrimankar J, Griffin S M 1991 Duodenal adenocarcinoma complicating coeliac disease. Histopathology 19: 285–287
10. Perzin K H, Peterson M, Castiglione C L et al. 1984 Intramucosal carcinoma of the small intestine arising in regional enteritis (Crohn's disease). Report of a case studied for carcinoembryonic antigen and review of the literature. Cancer 54: 151–162
11. Gyde S N, Prior P, Macartney J C et al. 1980 Malignancy in Crohn's disease. Gut 21: 1024–1029
12. Lynch H T, Smyrk T C, Watson P et al. 1993 Genetics, natural history, tumor spectrum, and pathology of hereditary nonpolyposis colorectal cancer: An updated review. Gastroenterology 104: 1535–1549
13. Sugihara K, Muto T, Kamiya J et al. 1982 Gardner's syndrome associated with periampullary carcinoma, duodenal and gastric adenomatosis. Report of a case. Dis Colon Rectum 25: 766–771
14. Godwin JD 2nd. 1975 Carcinoid tumors. An analysis of 2837 cases. Cancer 36: 560–569
15. Sigel J E, Goldblum J R 1998 Neuroendocrine neoplasms arising in inflammatory bowel disease: a report of 14 cases. Mod Pathol 11: 537–542
16. Yantiss R K, Odze R D, Farraye F A et al. 2003 Solitary versus multiple carcinoid tumors of the ileum. A clinical and pathologic review of 68 cases. Am J Surg Pathol 27: 811–817
17. Burke A P, Thomas R M, Elsayed A M et al. 1997 Carcinoids of the jejunum and ileum: an immunohistochemical and clinicopathologic study of 167 cases. Cancer 79: 1086–1093
18. Soga J, Tazawa K 1971 Pathologic analysis of carcinoids. Histologic reevaluation of 62 cases. Cancer 28: 990–998
18a. Nassar H, Albores-Saavedra J, Klimstra D S 2005 High grade neuroendocrine carcinoma of the ampulla of vater. A clinicopathologic and immunohistochemical analysis of 14 cases. Am J Surg Pathol 29: 588–594
19. Zakariai Y M, Quan S H, Hajdu S I 1975 Carcinoid tumors of the gastrointestinal tract. Cancer 35: 588–591
20. Griffiths D F, Jasani B, Newman G R et al. 1984 Glandular duodenal carcinoid – a somatostatin rich tumour with neuroendocrine associations. J Clin Pathol 37: 163–169
21. Makhlouf H R, Burke A P, Sobin L H 1999 Carcinoid tumors of the ampulla of Vater: a comparison with duodenal carcinoid tumors. Cancer 85: 1241–1249
22. Appelman H D 1986 Smooth muscle tumors of the gastrointestinal tract. What we know now that Stout didn't know. Am J Surg Pathol 10 (suppl. 1): 83–99
23. Fletcher C D, Berman J J, Corless C et al. 2002 Diagnosis of gastrointestinal stromal tumors: a consensus approach. Hum Pathol 33: 459–465
24. Sircar K, Hewlett B R, Huizinga J D et al. 1999 Interstitial cells of Cajal as precursors of gastrointestinal stromal tumors. Am J Surg Pathol 23: 377–389
25. Miettinen M, Virolainen M, Sarlomo-Rikala M 1995 Gastrointestinal stromal tumors – value of CD34 antigen in their identification and separation from true leiomyomas and schwannomas. Am J Surg Pathol 19: 207–216
26. Rubin B P 2006 Gastrointestinal stromal tumors: an update. Histopathology 48: 83–96
27. Miettinen M, Sarlomo-Rikala M, Lasota J 1999 Gastrointestinal stromal tumors: recent advances in understanding of their biology. Hum Pathol 30: 1213–1220
28. Corless C L, Fletcher J A, Heinrich M C 2004 Biology of gastrointestinal stromal tumors. J Clin Oncol 22: 3813–3825
29. Dematteo R P, Heinrich M C, El-Rifai W M et al. 2002 Clinical management of gastrointestinal stromal tumors: before and after STI-571. Hum Pathol 33: 466–477
30. Herrera G A, Pinto de Moraes H, Grizzle W E et al. 1984 Malignant small bowel neoplasm of enteric plexus derivation (plexosarcoma). Light and electron microscopic study confirming the origin of the neoplasm. Dig Dis Sci 29: 275–284
31. Walker P, Dvorak A M 1986 Gastrointestinal autonomic nerve (GAN) tumor. Ultrastructural evidence for a newly recognized entity. Arch Pathol Lab Med 110: 309–316
32. Lauwers G Y, Erlandson R A, Casper E S et al. 1993 Gastrointestinal autonomic nerve tumors. A clinicopathological, immunohistochemical, and ultrastructural study of 12 cases. Am J Surg Pathol 17: 887–897

33. Min K W 1992 Small intestinal stromal tumors with skeinoid fibers. Clinicopathological, immunohistochemical, and ultrastructural investigations. Am J Surg Pathol 16: 145–155
34. Ojanguren I, Ariza A, Navas-Palacios J J 1996 Gastrointestinal autonomic nerve tumor: further observations regarding an ultrastructural and immunohistochemical analysis of six cases. Hum Pathol 27: 1311–1318
35. Lee J R, Joshi V, Griffin J W Jr et al. 2001 Gastrointestinal autonomic nerve tumor: immunohistochemical and molecular identity with gastrointestinal stromal tumor. Am J Surg Pathol 25: 979–987
36. Schaldenbrand J D, Appelman H D 1984 Solitary solid stromal gastrointestinal tumors in von Recklinghausen's disease with minimal smooth muscle differentiation. Hum Pathol 15: 229–232
37. Segal A, Carello S, Caterina P et al. 1994 Gastrointestinal autonomic nerve tumors: a clinicopathological, immunohistochemical and ultrastructural study of 10 cases. Pathology 26: 439–447
38. Gall J A, Chetty R, Kemp A J et al. 1993 Multiple benign stromal cell tumours of the small bowel. J Clin Pathol 46: 869–871
39. Shek T W, Luk I S, Loong F et al. 1996 Inflammatory cell-rich gastrointestinal autonomic nerve tumor. An expansion of its histologic spectrum. Am J Surg Pathol 20: 325–331
40. Medeiros F, Corless C L, Duensing A et al. 2004 KIT-negative gastrointestinal stromal tumors. Proof of concept and therapeutic implications. Am J Surg Pathol 28: 889–894
41. Heinrich M C, Corless C L, Demetri G D et al. 2003 Kinase mutations and Imatinib response in patients with metastatic gastrointestinal stromal tumor. J Clin Oncol 21: 4342–4349
42. Furste W, Solt R Jr, Briggs W 1963 The gastrointestinal submucosal lipoma, a cause of bleeding and pain. Am J Surg 106: 903–909
43. Shepherd J A 1953 Angiomatous conditions of the gastro-intestinal tract. Br J Surg 40: 409–421
44. Parker G W, Murney J A, Kenoyer W L 1960 Cavernous hemangioma of the rectum and rectosigmoid: a case report and review. Dis Colon Rectum 3: 358–363
45. Pounder D J, Rowland R, Pieterse A S et al. 1982 Angiodysplasias of the colon. J Clin Pathol 35: 824–829
46. Geraghty J M, Everitt N J, Blundell J W 1991 Glomus tumour of the small bowel. Histopathology 19: 287–289
47. Usuda H, Naito M 1997 Multicentric angiosarcoma of the gastrointestinal tract. Pathol Int 47: 553–556
48. Elliott R L, Williams R D, Bayles D et al. 1966 Lymphangioma of the duodenum: case report with light and electron microscopic observation. Ann Surg 163: 86–92
49. Sarlomo-Rikala M, Miettinen M 1995 Gastric schwannoma – a clinicopathological analysis of six cases. Histopathology 27: 355–360
50. Arnesjo B, Idvall I, Ihse I et al. 1973 Concomitant occurrence of neurofibromatosis and carcinoid of the intestine. Scand J Gastroenterol 8: 637–643
51. Kheir S M, Halpern N B 1984 Paraganglioma of the duodenum in association with congenital neurofibromatosis. Possible relationship. Cancer 53: 2491–2496
52. Stephens M, Williams G T, Jasani B et al. 1987 Synchronous duodenal neuroendocrine tumours in von Recklinghausen's disease – a case report of co-existing gangliocytic paraganglioma and somatostatin-rich glandular carcinoid. Histopathology 11: 1331–1340
53. Perrone T, Sibley R K, Rosai J 1985 Duodenal gangliocytic paraganglioma. An immunohistochemical and ultrastructural study and a hypothesis concerning its origin. Am J Surg Pathol 9: 31–41
54. Burke A P, Helwig E B 1989 Gangliocytic paraganglioma. Am J Clin Pathol 92: 1–9
55. Williams E D, Pollock D J 1966 Multiple mucosal neuromata with endocrine tumours: a syndrome allied to von Recklinghausen's disease. J Pathol Bacteriol 90: 71–80
56. Weidner N, Flanders D J, Mitros F A 1984 Mucosal ganglioneuromatosis associated with multiple colonic polyps. Am J Surg Pathol 8: 779–786
57. Atwell J D, Burge D, Wright D 1985 Nodular lymphoid hyperplasia of the intestinal tract in infancy and childhood. J Pediatr Surg 20: 25–29
58. Webster A D, Kenwright S, Ballard J et al. 1977 Nodular lymphoid hyperplasia of the bowel in primary hypogammaglobulinaemia: study of in vivo and in vitro lymphocyte function. Gut 18: 364–372
59. Matuchansky C, Touchard G, Lemaire M et al. 1985 Malignant lymphoma of the small bowel associated with diffuse nodular lymphoid hyperplasia. N Engl J Med 313: 166–171
60. Domizio P, Owen R A, Shepherd N A et al. 1993 Primary lymphoma of the small intestine. A clinicopathological study of 119 cases. Am J Surg Pathol 17: 429–442
61. Levison D A, Hall P A, Blackshaw A J 1990 The gut-associated lymphoid tissue and its tumours. Curr Top Pathol 81: 133–175
62. Rambaud J C, Galian A, Matuchansky C et al. 1978 Natural history of alpha-chain disease and the so-called Mediterranean lymphoma. Recent Results Cancer Res 64: 271–276
63. Swinson C M, Slavin G, Coles E C et al. 1983 Coeliac disease and malignancy. Lancet 1: 111–115
64. Shia J, Ternya-Feldstein J, Pai D et al. 2002 Primary follicular lymphoma of the gastrointestinal tract. A clinical and pathologic study of 26 cases. Am J Surg Pathol 26: 216–224
65. Isaacson P, Wright D H 1978 Malignant histiocytosis of the intestine. Its relationship to malabsorption and ulcerative jejunitis. Hum Pathol 9: 661–677
66. Smith W J, Price S K, Isaacson P G 1987 Immunoglobulin gene rearrangement in immunoproliferative small intestinal disease (IPSID). J Clin Pathol 40: 1291–1297
67. Isaacson P G, O'Connor N T, Spencer J et al. 1985 Malignant histiocytosis of the intestine: a T-cell lymphoma. Lancet 2(8457): 688–691
68. Shepherd N A, Blackshaw A J, Hall P A et al. 1987 Malignant lymphoma with eosinophilia of the gastrointestinal tract. Histopathology 11: 115–130
69. Wright D H, Jones D B, Clark H et al. 1991 Is adult-onset coeliac disease due to a low-grade lymphoma of intraepithelial T lymphocytes? Lancet 337: 1373–1374
70. Schmitt-Graff A, Hummel M, Zemlin M et al. 1996 Intestinal T-cell lymphoma: a reassessment of cytomorphological and phenotypic features in relation to patterns of small bowel remodelling. Virchows Arch 429: 27–36
71. De Castro C A, Dockerty M B, Mayo C W 1957 Metastatic tumors of the small intestines. Surg Gynecol Obstet 105: 159–165
72. Washington K, McDonagh D 1995 Secondary tumors of the gastrointestinal tract: surgical pathologic findings and comparison with autopsy survey. Mod Pathol 8: 427–433
73. Correia J P, Baptista A S, Antonio J F 1968 Slowly evolving widespread diffuse alimentary tract carcinoma (linitis plastica). Gut 9: 485–488
74. ReMine W H, Brown P W Jr, Gomes M M et al. 1970 Polypoid hamartomas of Brunner's glands. Report of six surgical cases. Arch Surg 100: 313–316
75. Burdick D, Prior J T 1982 Peutz–Jeghers syndrome. A clinicopathologic study of a large family with a 27-year follow-up. Cancer 50: 2139–2146
76. Wang Z J, Ellis I, Zauber P et al. 1999 Allelic imbalance at the LKB1 (STK11) locus in tumours from patients with Peutz–Jeghers' syndrome provides evidence for a hamartoma-(adenoma)-carcinoma sequence. J Pathol 188: 9–13
77. Hsu S D, Zaharopoulos P, May J T et al. 1979 Peutz–Jeghers syndrome with intestinal carcinoma: report of the association in one family. Cancer 44: 1527–1532
78. Riley E, Swift M 1980 A family with Peutz–Jeghers syndrome and bilateral breast cancer. Cancer 46: 815–817
79. Young R H, Welch W R, Dickersin G R et al. 1982 Ovarian sex cord tumor with annular tubules: review of 74 cases including 27 with Peutz–Jeghers syndrome and four with adenoma malignum of the cervix. Cancer 50: 1384–1402
80. Shepherd N A, Bussey H J, Jass J R 1987 Epithelial misplacement in Peutz–Jeghers polyps. A diagnostic pitfall. Am J Surg Pathol 11: 743–749
81. Barbosa J D C, Dockerty M, Waugh J 1946 Pancreatic heterotopia. Surg Gynecol Obstet 82: 527–542
82. Lai E C, Tompkins R K 1986 Heterotopic pancreas. Review of a 26 year experience. Am J Surg 151: 697–700
83. Johnstone J M, Morson B C 1978 Inflammatory fibroid polyp of the gastrointestinal tract. Histopathology 2: 349–361
84. Pantanowitz L, Antonioli D, Pinkus G A et al. 2004 Inflammatory fibroid polyps of the gastrointestinal tract: evidence for a dendritic cell origin. Am J Surg Pathol 28: 107–114
85. Elliott G B, Sandy J T, Elliott K A et al. 1968 Lipohyperplasia of the ileocecal valve. Can J Surg 11: 179–187
86. Qizilbash A H 1975 Mucoceles of the appendix. Their relationship to hyperplastic polyps, mucinous cystadenomas, and cystadenocarcinomas. Arch Pathol 99: 548–555
87. Wolff M, Ahmed N 1976 Epithelial neoplasms of the vermiform appendix (exclusive of carcinoid). II. Cystadenomas, papillary adenomas, and adenomatous polyps of the appendix. Cancer 37: 2511–2522
88. Qizilbash A H 1975 Primary adenocarcinoma of the appendix. A clinicopathological study of 11 cases. Arch Pathol 99: 556–562
89. Gilhome R W, Johnston D H, Clark J et al. 1984 Primary adenocarcinoma of the vermiform appendix: report of a series of ten cases, and review of the literature. Br J Surg 71: 553–555
90. Misdraji J, Yantiss R K, Graeme-Cook F M et al. 2003 Appendiceal mucinous neoplasms. A clinicopathologic analysis of 107 cases. Am J Surg Pathol 27: 1089–1103
91. Ronnett B M, Kurman R J, Zahn C M et al. 1995 Pseudomyxoma peritonei in women: a clinicopathologic analysis of 30 cases with emphasis on site of origin, prognosis, and relationship to ovarian mucinous tumors of low malignant potential. Hum Pathol 26: 509–524
92. Kabbani W, Houlihan P S, Luthra R et al. 2002 Mucinous and nonmucinous appendiceal adenocarcinomas: different clinicopathological features but similar genetic alterations. Mod Pathol 15: 599–605
93. Moertel C G, Weiland L H, Nagorney D M et al. 1987 Carcinoid tumor of the appendix: treatment and prognosis. N Engl J Med 317: 1699–1701
94. Lundqvist M, Wilander E 1987 A study of the histopathogenesis of carcinoid tumors of the small intestine and appendix. Cancer 60: 201–206
95. Shaw P A 1991 The topographical and age distributions of neuroendocrine cells in the normal human appendix. J Pathol 164: 235–239
96. Park K, Blessing K, Kerr K et al. 1990 Goblet cell carcinoid of the appendix. Gut 31: 322–324.
97. Anderson N H, Somerville J E, Johnston C F et al. 1991 Appendiceal goblet cell carcinoids: a clinicopathological and immunohistochemical study. Histopathology 18: 61–65
98. Berardi R S, Lee S S, Chen H P 1988 Goblet cell carcinoids of the appendix. Surg Gynecol Obstet 167: 81–86
99. Subbuswamy S G, Gibbs N M, Ross C F et al. 1974 Goblet cell carcinoid of the appendix. Cancer 34: 338–344

100. Warkel R L, Cooper P H, Helwig E B 1978 Adenocarcinoid, a mucin-producing carcinoid tumor of the appendix: a study of 39 cases. Cancer 42: 2781–2793
101. Isaacson P 1981 Crypt cell carcinoma of the appendix (so-called adenocarcinoid tumor). Am J Surg Pathol 5: 213–224
102. Burke A P, Sobin L H, Federspiel B H et al. 1990 Goblet cell carcinoids and related tumors of the vermiform appendix. Am J Clin Pathol 94: 27–35
103. Zarabi M, LaBach J P 1982 Ganglioneuroma causing acute appendicitis. Hum Pathol 13: 1143–1146
104. Olsen B S, Holck S 1987 Neurogenous hyperplasia leading to appendiceal obliteration: an immunohistochemical study of 237 cases. Histopathology 11: 843–849
105. Clark J C, Collan Y, Eide T J et al. 1985 Prevalence of polyps in an autopsy series from areas with varying incidence of large-bowel cancer. Int J Cancer 36: 179–186
106. Johannsen L G, Momsen O, Jacobsen N O 1989 Polyps of the large intestine in Aarhus, Denmark. An autopsy study. Scand J Gastroenterol 24: 799–806
107. Hoff G, Foerster A, Vatn M H et al. 1985 Epidemiology of polyps in the rectum and sigmoid colon. Histological examination of resected polyps. Scand J Gastroenterol 20: 677–683
108. Jass J R, Young P J, Robinson E M 1992 Predictors of presence, multiplicity, size and dysplasia of colorectal adenomas. A necropsy study in New Zealand. Gut 33: 1508–1514
109. Williams A R, Balasooriya B A, Day D W 1982 Polyps and cancer of the large bowel: a necropsy study in Liverpool. Gut 23: 835–842
110. Konishi F, Morson B C 1982 Pathology of colorectal adenomas: a colonoscopic survey. J Clin Pathol 35: 830–841
111. Burt R W, Bishop T, Cannon L A et al. 1985 Dominant inheritance of adenomatous colonic polyps and colorectal cancer. N Engl J Med 312: 540
112. Aitken J F, Bain C J, Ward M et al. 1996 Risk of colorectal adenomas in patients with a family history of colorectal cancer: some implications for screening programmes. Gut 39: 105–108
113. Pollock A M, Quirke P 1991 Adenoma screening and colorectal cancer. The need for screening and polypectomy is unproved. Br J Med 303: 3–4
114. Muto T, Kamiya J, Sawada T et al. 1985 Small "flat adenoma" of the large bowel with special reference to its clinicopathologic features. Dis Colon Rectum 28: 847–851
115. Kuramoto S, Ihara O, Sakai S et al. 1990 Depressed adenoma in the large intestine. Endoscopic features. Dis Colon Rectum 33: 108–112
116. Muto T, Bussey H J, Morson B C 1973 Pseudo-carcinomatous invasion in adenomatous polyps of the colon and rectum. J Clin Pathol 26: 25–31
117. Muto T, Bussey H J, Morson B C 1975 The evolution of cancer of the colon and rectum. Cancer 36: 2251–2270
118. Longacre T A, Fenoglio-Preiser C M 1990 Mixed hyperplastic adenomatous polyps/serrated adenomas. A distinct form of colorectal neoplasia. Am J Surg Pathol 14: 524–537
119. Iino H, Jass J R, Simms L A et al. 1999 DNA microsatellite instability in hyperplastic polyps, serrated adenomas, and mixed polyps: a mild mutator pathway for colorectal cancer? J Clin Pathol 52: 5–9
120. Jass J R 2004 Hyperplastic polyps and colorectal cancer: is there a link? Clin Gastroenterol Hepatol 2: 1–8
121. Jass J R 2002 Serrated adenoma of the colorectum. Curr Diagn Pathol 8: 42–49
122. Kang M, Mitomi H, Sada M et al. 1997 Ki-67, p53, and Bcl-2 expression of serrated adenomas of the colon. Am J Surg Pathol 21: 417–423
123. Torlakovic E, Snover D C 1996 Serrated adenomatous polyposis in humans. Gastroenterology 110: 748–755
124. Torlakovic E, Skovlund E, Snover D C et al. 2003 Morphologic reappraisal of serrated colorectal polyps. Am J Surg Pathol 27: 65–81
125. Goldstein N S, Bhanot P, Odish E et al. 2003 Hyperplastic-like colon polyps that preceded microsatellite unstable adenocarcinomas. Am J Clin Pathol 119: 778–796
125a. Higuchi T, Sugihara K, Jass J R 2005 Demographic and pathological characteristics of serrated polyps of colorectum. Histopathology 47: 32–40
126. Kambara T, Simms L A, Whitehall V L J et al. 2004 BRAF mutation and CpG island methylation: an alternative pathway to colorectal cancer. Gut 53: 1137–1144
127. Bussey H J R 1975 Familial polyposis coli. Johns Hopkins Press, Baltimore
128. Bodmer W F, Bailey C J, Bodmer J et al. 1987 Localization of the gene for familial adenomatous polyposis on chromosome 5. Nature 328: 614–616
129. Groden J, Thliveris A, Samowitz W et al. 1991 Identification and characterization of the familial adenomatous polyposis gene. Cell 66: 589–600
130. Nishisho I, Nakamura Y, Miyoshi Y et al. 1991 Mutations of chromosome 5q21 genes in FAP and colorectal cancer patients. Science 253: 665–669
131. Al-Tassan N, Chmiel N H, Maynard J et al. 2002 Inherited variants of MYH associated with somatic G:C – T:A mutations in colorectal tumors. Nature Genet 30: 227–232
132. Spirio L, Olschwang S, Groden J et al. 1993 Alleles of the APC gene: an attenuated form of familial polyposis. Cell 75: 951–957
133. Jagelman D G, DeCosse J J, Bussey H J R 1988 Upper gastrointestinal cancer in familial adenomatous polyposis. Lancet 1: 1149–1151
134. Gardner E J 1962 Follow-up study of a family group exhibiting dominant inheritance for a syndrome including intestinal polyps, osteomas, fibromas and epidermal cysts. Am J Hum Genet 14: 376–390
135. Gebert J F, Dupon C, Kadmon M et al. 1999 Combined molecular and clinical approaches for the identification of families with familial adenomatous polyposis coli Ann Surg 229: 350–361
136. Simpson R D, Harrison E G Jr, Mayo C W 1964 Mesenteric fibromatosis in familial polyposis. A variant of Gardner's syndrome. Cancer 17: 526–534
137. Utsunomiya J, Nakamura T 1975 The occult osteomatous changes in the mandible in patients with familial polyposis coli. Br J Surg 62: 45–51
138. Heyen F, Jagelman D G, Romania A et al. 1990 Predictive value of congenital hypertrophy of the retinal pigment epithelium as a clinical marker for familial adenomatous polyposis. Dis Colon Rectum 33: 1003–1008
139. Kingston J E, Herbert A, Draper G J et al. 1983 Association between hepatoblastoma and polyposis coli. Arch Dis Child 58: 959–962
140. Thompson J S, Harned R K, Anderson J C et al. 1983 Papillary carcinoma of the thyroid and familial polyposis coli. Dis Colon Rectum 26: 583–585
141. Turcot J, Despré J-P, St Pierre F 1959 Malignant tumors of the central nervous system associated with familial polyposis of the colon: report of two cases. Dis Colon Rectum 2: 465–468
142. Hamilton S R, Liu B, Parsons R E et al. 1995 The molecular basis of Turcot's syndrome. N Engl J Med 332: 839–847
143. Vasen H F A, van der Luijt R B, Slors J F M et al. 1996 Molecular genetic tests as a guide to surgical management of familial adenomatous polyposis. Lancet 348: 433–435
144. Boyle P, Zaridze D G, Smans M 1985 Descriptive epidemiology of colorectal cancer. Int J Cancer 36: 9–18
145. Kune G 1996 Causes and control of colorectal cancer. A model for cancer prevention. Kluwer, Boston
146. Wynder E L, Reddy B S 1974 The epidemiology of cancer of the large bowel. Am J Dig Dis 19: 937–946
147. Burkitt D P 1971 Epidemiology of cancer of the colon and rectum. Cancer 28: 3–13
148. Jass J R 1991 Subsite distribution and incidence of colorectal cancer in New Zealand 1974–1983. Dis Colon Rectum 34: 56–59
149. Isbister W H, Fraser J 1990 Large-bowel cancer in the young: a national survival study. Dis Colon Rectum 33: 363–366
150. Jass J R, Do K-A, Simms L A et al. 1998 Morphology of sporadic colorectal cancer with DNA replication errors. Gut 42: 673–679
151. Jass J R 1989 Do all colorectal carcinomas arise in preexisting adenomas? World J Surg 13: 45–51
152. Lee Y S 1988 Early malignant lesions of the colorectum at autopsy. Dis Colon Rectum 31: 291–297
153. Hunt D R, Cherian M 1990 Endoscopic diagnosis of small flat carcinoma of the colon: report of three cases. Dis Colon Rectum 33: 143–147
154. Shimoda T, Ikegami M, Fujisaki J et al. 1989 Early colorectal carcinoma with special reference to its development de novo. Cancer 64: 1138–1146
155. Jass J R, Whitehall V L J, Young J et al. 2002 Emerging concepts in colorectal neoplasia. Gastroenterology 123: 862–876
156. Riddell R H, Goldman H, Ransohoff D F et al. 1983 Dysplasia in inflammatory bowel disease: standardized classification with provisional clinical applications. Hum Pathol 14: 931–968
157. Ming-Chai C, Chi-Yuan C, Pei-Yu C et al. 1980 Evolution of colorectal cancer in schistosomiasis: transitional mucosal changes adjacent to large intestinal carcinoma in colectomy specimens. Cancer 46: 1661–1675
158. Hamilton S R 1985 Colorectal carcinoma in patients with Crohn's disease. Gastroenterology 89: 398–407
159. Jass J R, Williams C B, Bussey H J R 1988 Juvenile polyposis – a precancerous condition. Histopathology 13: 619–630
160. Qizilbash A H 1974 Radiation-induced carcinoma of the rectum. A late complication of pelvic irradiation. Arch Pathol 98: 118–121
161. Mecklin J-P 1987 Frequency of hereditary colorectal carcinoma. Gastroenterology 93: 1021–1025
162. Kinzler K W, Vogelstein B 1996 Lessons from hereditary colorectal cancer. Cell 87: 159–170
163. Jass J R, Stewart S M 1992 Evolution of hereditary non-polyposis colorectal cancer. Gut 33: 783–786
164. Weitzer M, Pokos V, Jeevaratnam P et al. 1995 Isolated expression of the Muir–Torre phenotype in a member of a family with hereditary non-polyposis colorectal cancer. Histopathology 27: 573–575
165. Quirke P, Durdey P, Dixon M F et al. 1986 Local recurrence of rectal adenocarcinoma due to inadequate surgical resection. Histopathological study of lateral tumour spread and surgical excision. Lancet 2(8514): 996–999
166. Newland R C, Chapuis P H, Smyth E J 1987 The prognostic value of substaging colorectal carcinoma. A prospective study of 1117 cases with standardized pathology. Cancer 60: 852–857
167. Adam I J, Mohamdee M O, Martin I G et al. 1994 Role of circumferential margin involvement in the local recurrence of rectal cancer. Lancet 344: 707–711
168. Finlay I, McArdle C S 1986 Occult hepatic metastases in colorectal carcinoma. Br J Surg 73: 732–735
169. Shepherd N A, Baxter K R, Love S B 1997 The prognostic importance of peritoneal involvement in colonic cancer: a prospective evaluation. Gastroenterology 112: 1096–1102
170. Kirwan W O, Drumm J, Hogan J M et al. 1988 Determining safe margin of resection in low anterior resection for rectal cancer. Br J Surg 75: 720
171. Cross S S, Bull A D, Smith J H 1989 Is there any justification for the routine examination of bowel resection margins in colorectal adenocarcinoma? J Clin Pathol 42: 1040–1042
172. Loy T S, Kaplan P A 2004 Villous adenocarcinoma of the colon and rectum: a clinicopathologic study of 36 cases. Am J Surg Pathol 28: 1460–1465

173. Sasaki P, Atkin W S, Jass J R 1987 Mucinous carcinoma of the rectum. Histopathology 11: 259–272
174. Connelly J H, Robey-Cafferty S S, el-Naggar A K et al. 1991 Exophytic signet-ring cell carcinoma of the colorectum. Arch Pathol Lab Med 115: 134–136
175. Jass J R, Smyrk T C, Stewart S M et al. 1994 Pathology of hereditary non-polyposis colorectal cancer. Anticancer Res 14: 1631–1634
176. Kim H, Jen J, Vogelstein B et al. 1994 Clinical and pathological characteristics of sporadic colorectal carcinomas with DNA replication errors in microsatellite sequences. Am J Pathol 145: 148–156
177. Gaffey M J, Mills S E, Lack E E 1990 Neuroendocrine carcinoma of the colon and rectum. A clinicopathologic, ultrastructural, and immunohistochemical study of 24 cases. Am J Surg Pathol 14: 1010–1023
178. Gibbs N M 1977 Undifferentiated carcinoma of the large intestine. Histopathology 1: 77–84
179. Jessurun J, Romero-Guadarrama M, Manivel J C 1999 Medullary adenocarcinoma of the colon: clinicopathologic study of 11 cases. Hum Pathol 30: 843–848
180. Wick M R, Vitsky J L, Ritter J H et al. 2005 Sporadic medullary carcinoma of the colon. Am J Clin Pathol 123: 56–65
181. Jass J R, Atkin W S, Cuzick J et al. 1986 The grading of rectal cancer: historical perspectives and a multivariate analysis of 447 cases. Histopathology 10: 437–459
182. Quirke P, Dixon M F, Clayden A D et al. 1987 Prognostic significance of DNA aneuploidy and cell proliferation in rectal adenocarcinomas. J Pathol 151: 285–291
183. Jass J R, Ajioka Y, Allen J P et al. 1996 Assessment of invasive growth pattern and lymphocytic infiltration in colorectal cancer. Histopathology 28: 543–548
184. Ueno H, Murphy J, Jass J R et al. 2002 Tumour 'budding' as an index to estimate the potential of aggressiveness in rectal cancer. Histopathology 40: 127–132
185. Halvorsen T B, Seim E 1989 Association between invasiveness, inflammatory reaction, desmoplasia and survival in colorectal cancer. J Clin Pathol 42: 162–166
186. Greenson J K, Bonner J D, Ben-Yzhak O et al. 2003 Phenotype of microsatellite unstable colorectal carcinomas. Am J Surg Pathol 27: 563–570
187. Wright C M, Dent O F, Barker M et al. 2000 The prognostic significance of extensive microsatellite instability in sporadic clinicopathological stage C colorectal cancer. Br J Surg 87: 1197–1202
188. Hermanek P, Sobin L 1987 UICC TNM classification of malignant tulours, 4th edn. Springer-Verlag, Berlin
189. Hermanek P, Gall F P, Altendorf A 1980 Prognostic groups in colorectal carcinoma. J Cancer Res Clin Oncol 98: 185–193
190. Dukes C E, Bussey H J 1958 The spread of rectal cancer and its effect on prognosis. Br J Cancer 12: 309–320
191. Liefers G-J, Cleton-Jansen A-M, van de Velde C J H et al. 1998 Micrometastases and survival in stage II colorectal cancer. N Engl J Med 339: 223–228
192. Talbot I C, Ritchie S, Leighton M et al. 1981 Invasion of veins by carcinoma of rectum: method of detection, histological features and significance. Histopathology 5: 141–163
193. Knudsen J B, Nilsson T, Sprechler M et al. 1983 Venous and nerve invasion as prognostic factors in postoperative survival of patients with resectable cancer of the rectum. Dis Colon Rectum 26: 613–617
194. Morson B C 1966 Factors influencing the prognosis of early cancer of the rectum. Proc R Soc Med 59: 607–608
195. Morson B C, Whiteway J E, Jones E A et al. 1984 Histopathology and prognosis of malignant colorectal polyps treated by endoscopic polypectomy. Gut 25: 437–444
196. Muller S, Chesner I M, Egan M J et al. 1989 Significance of venous and lymphatic invasion in malignant polyps of the colon and rectum. Gut 30: 1385–1391
197. Geraghty J M, Williams C B, Talbot I C 1991 Malignant colorectal polyps: venous invasion and successful treatment by endoscopic polypectomy. Gut 32: 774–778
198. Whiteway J, Nicholls R J, Morson B C 1985 The role of surgical local excision in the treatment of rectal cancer. Br J Surg 72: 694–697
199. Werling R W, Yaziji H, Bacchi G E et al. 2003 CDX2, a highly sensitive and specific marker of adenocarcinomas of intestinal origin: an immunohistochemical survey of 476 primary and metastatic carcinomas. Am J Surg Pathol 27: 303–310
200. Vogelstein B, Fearon E R, Hamilton S R et al. 1988 Genetic alterations during colorectal-tumor development. N Engl J Med 319: 525–532
201. Smith G, Carey F A, Beattie J et al. 2002 Mutations in APC, Kirsten-ras, and p53 – alternative genetic pathways to colorectal cancer. Proc Natl Acad Sci (USA) 99: 9433–9438
202. Young J, Simms L A, Biden K G et al. 2001 Features of colorectal cancers with high-level microsatellite instability occurring in familial and sporadic settings: parallel pathways of tumorigenesis. Am J Pathol 159: 2107–2116
203. Kane M F, Loda M, Gaida G M et al. 1997 Methylation of the hMLH1 promoter correlates with lack of expression of hMLH1 in sporadic colon tumors and mismatch repair-defective human tumor cell lines. Cancer Res 57: 808–811
204. Ribic C M, Sargent D J, Moore M J et al. 2003 Tumor microsatellite instability status as a predictor of benefit from fluorouracil-based adjuvant chemotherapy for colon cancer. N Engl J Med 349: 247–257
205. Bardi G, Fenger C, Johansson B et al. 2004 Tumor karyotype predicts clinical outcome in colorectal cancer patients. J Clin Oncol 22: 2623–2634
206. Epstein S E, Ascari W Q, Ablow R C et al. 1966 Colitis cystica profunda. Am J Clin Pathol 45: 186–201
207. Federspiel B H, Burke A P, Sobin L H et al. 1990 Rectal and colonic carcinoids. A clinicopathologic study of 84 cases. Cancer 65: 135–140
208. Koura A N, Giacco G G, Curley S A et al. 1997 Carcinoid tumors of the rectum: effect of size, histopathology, and surgical treatment on metastasis free survival. Cancer 79: 1294–1298
209. Gledhill A, Hall P A, Cruse J P et al. 1986 Enteroendocrine cell hyperplasia, carcinoid tumours and adenocarcinoma in long-standing ulcerative colitis. Histopathology 10: 501–508
210. Moyana T N, Friesen R, Tan L K 1991 Colorectal smooth muscle tumors. A pathobiologic study with immunohistochemistry and histomorphometry. Arch Pathol Lab Med 115: 1016–1021
211. Tworek J A, Goldblum J R, Weiss S W et al. 1999 Stromal tumors of the abdominal colon: a clinicopathologic study of 20 cases. Am J Surg Pathol 23: 937–945
212. Walsh T H, Mann C V 1984 Smooth muscle neoplasms of the rectum and anal canal. Br J Surg 71: 597–599
213. Tworek J A, Goldblum J R, Weiss S W et al. 1999 Stromal tumors of the anorectum: a clinicopathologic study of 22 cases. Am J Surg Pathol 23: 946–954
214. Miettinen M, Sarlomo-Rikala M, Sobin L H et al. 2000 Gastrointestinal stromal tumors and leiomyosarcomas in the colon: a clinicopathologic, immunohistochemical and molecular genetic study of 44 cases. Am J Surg Pathol 24: 1339–1352
215. Michowitz M, Lazebnik N, Noy S et al. 1985 Lipoma of the colon. A report of 22 cases. Am J Surg 51: 449–454
215a. Hornick J L, Fletcher C D 2005 Intestinal perineuriomas: clinicopathologic definition of a new anatomic subset in a series of 10 cases. Am J Surg Pathol 29: 859–865
216. Shekitka K M, Sobin L H 1994 Ganglioneuromas of the gastrointestinal tract. Relation to Von Recklinghausen disease and other multiple tumor syndromes. Am J Surg Pathol 18: 250–257
217. Mendelsohn G, Diamond M P 1984 Familial ganglioneuromatous polyposis of the large bowel. Report of a family with associated juvenile polyposis. Am J Surg Pathol 8: 515–520
218. d'Amore E S, Manivel J C, Pettinato G et al. 1991 Intestinal ganglioneuromatosis: mucosal and transmural types. A clinicopathologic and immunohistochemical study of six cases. Hum Pathol 22: 276–286
219. Shepherd N A, Jass J R 1987 Neuromuscular and vascular hamartoma of the small intestine: is it Crohn's disease? Gut 28: 1663–1668
220. Friedman S L, Wright T L, Altman D F 1985 Gastrointestinal Kaposi's sarcoma in patients with acquired immunodeficiency syndrome. Endoscopic and autopsy findings. Gastroenterology 89: 102–108
221. Shepherd N A, Hall P A, Coates P J et al. 1988 Primary malignant lymphoma of the colon and rectum. A histopathological and immunohistochemical analysis of 45 cases with clinicopathological correlations. Histopathology 12: 235–252
222. Shepherd N A, Hall P A, Williams G T et al. 1989 Primary malignant lymphoma of the large intestine complicating chronic inflammatory bowel disease. Histopathology 15: 325–337
223. Isaacson P G, MacLennan K A, Subbuswamy S G 1984 Multiple lymphomatous polyposis of the gastrointestinal tract. Histopathology 8: 641–656
224. Mestre J R 1986 The changing pattern of juvenile polyps. Am J Gastroenterol 81: 312–314
225. Roth S, Sistonen P, Salovaara R et al. 1999 SMAD genes in juvenile polyposis. Genes Chromosomes Cancer 26: 54–61
226. Haggitt R C, Reid B J 1986 Hereditary gastrointestinal polyposis syndromes. Am J Surg Pathol 10: 871–887
227. Nelen M R, Padberg G W, Peeters E A J et al. 1996 Localization of the gene for Cowden disease to chromosome 10q22-23. Nature Genet 13: 114–116
228. Eng C 1998 Genetics of Cowden syndrome: through the looking glass of oncology. Int J Oncol 12: 701–710
229. Wolff M 1971 Heterotopic gastric epithelium in the rectum: a report of three new cases with a review of 87 cases of gastric heterotopia in the alimentary canal. Am J Clin Pathol 55: 604–616
230. Arthur J F 1968 Structure and significance of metaplastic nodules in the rectal mucosa. J Clin Pathol 21: 735–743
231. Cappell M S, Forde K A 1989 Spatial clustering of multiple hyperplastic, adenomatous, and malignant colonic polyps in individual patients. Dis Colon Rectum 32: 641–652
232. Williams G T 1997 Metaplastic (hyperplastic) polyps of the large bowel: benign neoplasms after all? Gut 40: 691–692
233. Jeevaratnam P, Cottier D S, Browett P J et al. 1996 Familial giant hyperplastic polyposis predisposing to colorectal cancer: a new hereditary bowel cancer syndrome. J Pathol 179: 20–25
234. Jass J R, Faludy J 1985 Immunohistochemical demonstration of IgA and secretory component in relation to epithelial cell differentiation in normal colorectal mucosa and metaplastic polyp: a semiquantitative study. Histochem J 17: 373–380
235. Sobin L H 1985 Inverted hyperplastic polyps of the colon. Am J Surg Pathol 9: 265–272
236. Williams G T, Arthur J F, Bussey H J R et al. 1980 Metaplastic polyps and polyposis of the colorectum. Histopathology 4: 155–170

237. Bengoechea O, Martinez-Penuela J M, Larrinaga B et al. 1987 Hyperplastic polyposis of the colorectum and adenocarcinoma in a 24 year old man. Am J Surg Pathol 11: 323–327
238. Kindblom L G, Angervall L, Santesson B et al. 1977 Cronkhite–Canada syndrome. Case report. Cancer 39: 2651–2657
239. du Boulay C E, Fairbrother J, Isaacson P G 1983 Mucosal prolapse syndrome – a unifying concept for solitary ulcer syndrome and related disorders. J Clin Pathol 36: 1264–1268
240. Madigan M R, Morson B C 1969 Solitary ulcer of the rectum. Gut 10: 871–881
241. Burke A P, Sobin L H 1990 Eroded polypoid hyperplasia of the rectosigmoid. Am J Gastroenterol 85: 975–980
242. Nakamura S, Kino I, Akagi T 1992 Inflammatory myoglandular polyps of the colon and rectum. A clinicopathological study of 32 pedunculated polyps, distinct from other types of polyps. Am J Surg Pathol 16: 772–779
243. Lobert P F, Appelman H D 1981 Inflammatory cloacogenic polyp. A unique inflammatory lesion of the anal transitional zone. Am J Surg Pathol 5: 761–766
244. Rowland R, Langman J M 1989 Endometriosis of the large bowel: a report of 11 cases. Pathology 21: 259–265
245. Sanusi I D, Tio F O 1974 Gastrointestinal malacoplakia. Report of a case and a review of the literature. Am J Gastroenterol 62: 356–366
246. Croxson T, Chabon A B, Rorat E et al. 1984 Intraepithelial carcinoma of the anus in homosexual men. Dis Colon Rectum 27: 325–330
247. Palmer J G, Shepherd N A, Jass J R et al. 1987 Human papillomavirus type 16 DNA in anal squamous cell carcinoma. Lancet 2(8549): 42
248. Morson B C, Pang L S 1968 Pathology of anal cancer. Proc R Soc Med 61: 623–624
249. Wick M R, Weatherby R P, Weiland L H 1987 Small cell neuroendocrine carcinoma of the colon and rectum: clinical, histologic, and ultrastructural study and immunohistochemical comparison with cloacogenic carcinoma. Hum Pathol 18: 9–21
250. Fenger C, Nielsen V T 1986 Precancerous changes in the anal canal epithelium in resection specimens. Acta Pathol Microbiol Immunol Scand [A] 94: 63–69
251. Shepherd N A, Schofield J H, Love S B et al. 1990 Prognostic factors in anal squamous carcinoma: a multivariate analysis of clinical, pathological and flow cytometric parameters in 235 cases. Histopathology 16: 545–555
252. Boman B M, Moertel C G, O'Connell M J et al. 1984 Carcinoma of the anal canal. A clinical and pathologic study of 188 cases. Cancer 54: 114–125
253. Bogomoletz W V, Potet F, Molas G 1985 Condylomata acuminata, giant condyloma acuminatum (Buschke–Loewenstein tumour) and verrucous squamous carcinoma of the perianal and anorectal region: a continuous precancerous spectrum? Histopathology 9: 155–169
254. Jones E A, Morson B C 1984 Mucinous adenocarcinoma in anorectal fistulae. Histopathology 8: 279–292
255. Hobbs C M, Lowry M A, Owen D et al. 2001 Anal gland carcinoma. Cancer 92: 2045–2049
256. Goldman S, Glimelius B, Pahlman L 1990 Anorectal malignant melanoma in Sweden. Report of 49 patients. Dis Colon Rectum 33: 874–877
257. Brady M S, Kavolius J P, Quan S H 1995 Anorectal melanoma. A 64-year experience at Memorial Sloan-Kettering Cancer Center. Dis Colon Rectum 38: 146–151
258. Ben-Izhak O, Levy R, Weill S et al. 1997 Anorectal malignant melanoma. A clinicopathologic study, including immunohistochemistry and DNA flow cytometry. Cancer 79: 18–25
259. Mills S E, Walker A N, Stallings R G et al. 1984 Retrorectal cystic hamartoma. Report of three cases, including one with a perirenal component. Arch Pathol Lab Med 108: 737–740
260. Marco V, Autonell J, Farre J et al. 1982 Retrorectal cyst-hamartomas. Report of two cases with adenocarcinoma developing in one. Am J Surg Pathol 6: 707–714
261. Ikenberg H, Gissmann L, Gross G et al. 1983 Human papillomavirus type-16-related DNA in genital Bowen's disease and in Bowenoid papulosis. Int J Cancer 32: 563–565
262. Elliott G B, Fisher B K 1967 Perianal keratoacanthoma. Arch Dermatol 95: 81–82
263. Nielsen O V, Jensen S L 1981 Basal cell carcinoma of the anus – a clinical study of 34 cases. Br J Surg 68: 856–857
264. Meeker J H, Neubecker R D, Helwig E B 1962 Hidradenoma papilliferum. Am J Clin Pathol 37: 182–195
265. Donaldson D, Jass J, Mann C 1987 Anal leukoplakia. Gut 28: A1368
266. Armitage N C, Jass J R, Richman P I et al. 1989 Paget's disease of the anus: a clinicopathological study. Br J Surg 76: 60–63

肝、胆囊和胆管肿瘤
Tumors of the liver, gallbladder, and biliary tree

10

Linda Ferrell 和 Sanjay Kakar 著

钱利华 译　回允中 校

非硬化性肝组织中的良性肝细胞病变	417
硬化性肝组织中的良性/癌前性肝细胞病变	421
恶性肝细胞病变	425
肝：良性间叶性肿瘤	435
肝：恶性间叶性肿瘤	439
胆囊：良性肿瘤	443
胆囊：化生和异型增生	444
胆囊：恶性肿瘤	445
瘤样病变	448
良性胆管肿瘤	449
恶性胆管肿瘤	451
胆管内前体病变	454
其他恶性肿瘤	455

非硬化性肝组织中的良性肝细胞病变
Benign hepatocellular lesions in non-cirrhotic liver

肝细胞腺瘤　Hepatic adenoma

临床特征

肝细胞腺瘤（HA）少见，几乎完全（95%）见于育龄期的年轻女性，极少见于男性[1,2]或儿童[3]。肝细胞腺瘤为肝组织内孤立性病变，其组织学表现为正常或接近正常。极少数"肝细胞腺瘤病"（liver cell adenomatosis）已有报告，描述的结节数量"超过10个"或"许多"，常常较小[4-6]。目前尚不清楚这些肿瘤是否代表一种特殊病变。过去认为与女性性别和性腺合成类固醇无关[4]，但后来的报道发现，74%的病人为女性，并且46%服用过口服避孕药[7]。这项研究还显示所有腺瘤病病例均与糖尿病有关，10%的病人有家族史。

临床通常表现为腹部肿块，但有些病人也可出现腹痛、不适或恶心。较大肿瘤可发生破裂和出血，伴有腹腔积血[8]。血清碱性磷酸酶可能升高，但血清甲胎蛋白（AFP）水平一般正常或有轻微升高。肝细胞腺瘤的CT表现为高密度非均质性肿瘤，偶尔可见中央出血，锝（Tc）-闪烁扫描检测无摄取表现。然而，即使结合新的影像技术往往也不可能进行精确诊断[9,10]。

肝细胞腺瘤被认为是服用口服避孕药所致：多数病人在诊断之前已服用5年以上[11-13]。然而，现在随着低剂量片剂的广泛应用，肝细胞腺瘤的发生率可能会减少。其他相关因素，如合成代谢类固醇、氯米芬（clomiphene）、达那唑（danazol）和卡马西平也与肝细胞腺瘤有关[14-17]。其他危险因素包括Klinefelter综合征以及代谢性疾病，尤其是I型和IV型糖原贮积病、半乳糖血症、家族性糖尿病以及高酪氨酸血症[18,19]。其他罕见的相关因素包括重度复合性免疫缺陷以及家族性腺瘤性息肉病[18,20]。胎盘原发性肝细胞腺瘤已有两例报告[21]。在没有激素或代谢性病因情况下，诊断肝细胞腺瘤应当小心，因为可能为高分化肝细胞癌（HCC）。有人建议，对于这些病人应当进行性腺类固醇异常分泌的检测[22]。国际工作组一致认为，对于硬化性肝组织内发生的病变不应诊断为腺瘤，除非去除刺激因素以后，病变出现消退表现，或者存在上述的一种危险因素时[23]。

病理学特征

大体病理学：肝细胞腺瘤切面一般隆起，质软，其颜色常比周围肝组织淡，但如果出现坏死或出血，其表现可能多样。大小差异很大，但多数肿瘤超过10 cm。肿瘤可有或无包膜。如有包膜，常为不完全性，与之毗邻的肝实质内可混有肿瘤细胞灶。肝细胞腺瘤常缺乏显著的纤维化或结节形成，但极少数情况下也可出现这些特征[24]。少数情况下，腺瘤可呈胆汁着色或由于出现大量脂褐素而呈暗蓝灰色至黑色，即所谓的黑色腺瘤（black adenoma）[19]。所有肿瘤血管丰富，那些与合成代谢/雄激素性类固醇相关的肿瘤也可出现大体可见的紫癜。瘢痕区域代表先前梗死灶。

显微镜下特征：肝细胞腺瘤由形态一致的肝细胞组成，排列成 1～3 个细胞厚度的肝细胞板结构（图 10.1）。与正常肝组织相比，腺瘤的肝细胞板常较不规则和非线性。关键特征是肝细胞板的网织纤维框架完整，类似于正常肝组织，或仅有局灶减少。肿瘤细胞常与正常肝细胞等大，核-浆比例正常。胞浆可为嗜酸性或透明（图 10.2），并含有脂肪、胆汁或脂褐素。可见抗淀粉酶消化的 PAS 阳性小体、巨大线粒体以及 Mallory 小体，但并不显著。细胞形态学其他少见的差异包括多核形成、局灶非典型性和核的多形性。不管细胞形态学如何，没有或极少有核分裂象。常见结构变异，例如腺泡形成（由肝细胞构成的假腺体或腺样结构）；这种腺泡可能含有胆汁。肝窦也可出现改变；可表现为肝窦受挤压，导致肿瘤呈均匀一致的实性表现，或出现肝窦扩张及肝紫癜病。大血管常非常显著。常出现梗死和出血区域。这些病灶机化可导致纤维瘢痕形成。可见 Kupffer 细胞，但数量少于正常肝组织。合成代谢类固醇相关性腺瘤容易出现细胞核的非典型性、明显的核仁、肝紫癜或显著的腺泡（假腺体）结构[19,23]。根据定义，腺瘤缺乏汇管区成分，并且出现小胆管就可以除外腺瘤的诊断。出现没有胆管伴行的小动脉成分，并且周围围绕少量结缔组织是肝细胞腺瘤的特征性表现（"裸露"小动脉）。

肝细胞腺瘤表达普通的肝细胞标记物，包括细胞角蛋白 CAM5.2 和多克隆性癌胚抗原（CEA）小管标记物。肝细胞腺瘤中肝细胞板的内衬细胞常出现 CD34 阳性（图 10.3），类似于局灶结节性增生（FNH）和肝细胞癌（HCC）。因此，CD34 对于这些病变没有鉴别意义[25]。甲胎蛋白（AFP）在肝细胞腺瘤呈阴性。

鉴别诊断

诊断问题常出现在肝细胞腺瘤与局灶结节性增生、高分化肝细胞癌、胚胎或巨梁型肝母细胞瘤以及单形性血管肌脂肪瘤（AML）的鉴别上。与肝细胞癌相比，肝细胞腺瘤的肿瘤细胞相对一致，类似于正常肝组织，肝细胞板厚度为 3 个细胞或者更少，无核分裂象，肝细胞板衬有完整的网织纤维框架。应用类固醇的病史以及缺少肝硬化也支持肝细胞腺瘤的诊断（表 10.1）。免疫组织化学在鉴别诊断中没有意义。肝细胞癌出现一致性的染色体改变，例如 1q、7q、8q 的增加和 16q 的丢失。这些改变即使在小的高分化病变也能观察到。与之相反，肝细胞腺瘤常缺乏明显的染色体异常。通过比较基因组杂交或荧光原位杂交证实这些染色体增加和丢失可能有助于鉴别诊断[26,27]；其他鉴别诊断在后面章节中讨论。

预后和结局

有些口服避孕药相关性肝细胞腺瘤撤药后会消退，但多数并非如此。偶尔，肝细胞癌可发生于腺瘤内[12,24]。腺瘤发生肝细胞癌的危险性可能较低[28]，鉴于存在瘤体破裂和腹腔积血等致命合并症的潜在可能，所有病例都

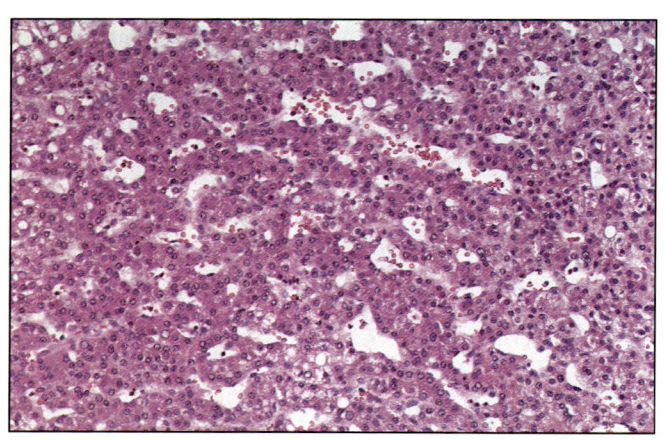

图 10.1　肝细胞腺瘤。1～2 个细胞厚的规则性肝板结构，核-浆比例较低，缺少汇管区。

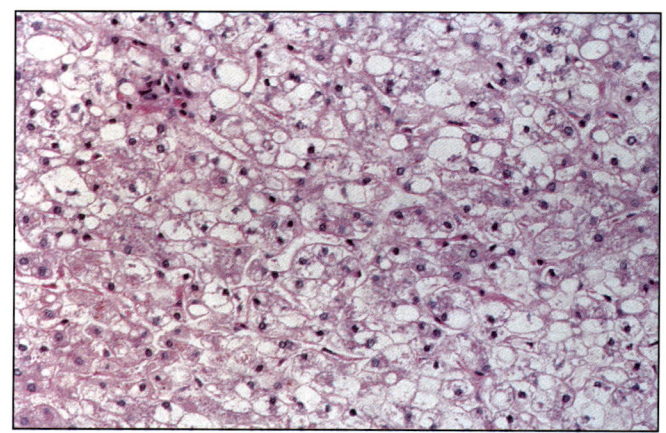

图 10.2　肝细胞腺瘤伴透明细胞特征。

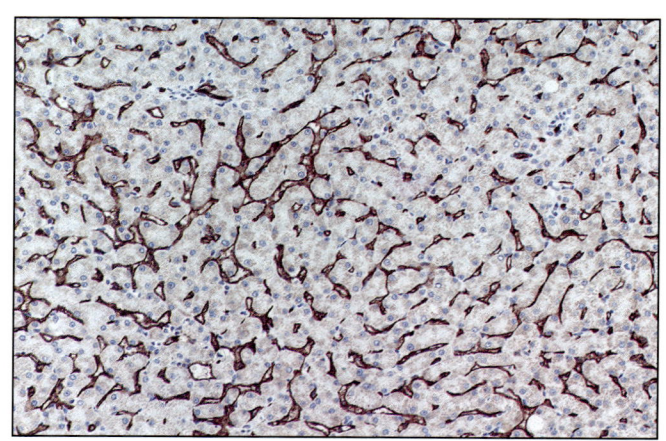

图 10.3　肝细胞腺瘤。CD34 染色肝窦呈阳性。

表10.1　局灶结节性增生、肝细胞腺瘤和肝细胞癌的鉴别

	局灶结节性增生	肝细胞腺瘤	肝细胞癌
临床特征			
年龄/性别	所有年龄；年轻女性多见	几乎所有女性，20~40岁	较多见于男性（3倍）
服用类固醇	偶尔	几乎都是	一般没有
肝组织背景	正常	正常	肝硬化（>80%）
甲胎蛋白（AFP）	正常	正常	常有升高；小肿瘤可能正常
放射学	CT和MRI呈均匀性增强。闪烁扫描检测摄取正常或增加。血管造影血管少	CT和MRI呈非均一性肿块。闪烁扫描检测摄取减少。血管造影血管多	CT对比检查动脉相增强。血管造影检查高度富于血管
形态学特征			
被膜	无	可有	可有
数量	可多个	常为单个	单个或多个
中央瘢痕	有	无	无，除了某些纤维板层型肝细胞癌
出血/坏死	极少	常见	较大肿瘤常见
实质	结节状	均质性	结节状或均质性
胆汁	无	可有	可有
胆管增生	有	无	无
小叶间胆管	无	无	无
血管	纤维性间质内的异常小动脉，伴肌内膜增厚	"裸露"小动脉，无胆管伴行，伴少量间质	"裸露"小动脉，无胆管伴行，伴少量间质
肝细胞板	1~3个细胞厚	1~3个细胞厚	常大于3个细胞厚
Kupffer细胞	可见	减少/无	无
核的非典型性	无	无/轻度	常见
核浆比例	正常	正常	增加
核仁	不定	不定	常显著
核分裂象	无	无	常可见
网状纤维	正常	正常	常减少或缺失
免疫组织化学			
肝窦CD34染色	可阳性	常阳性	阳性
分子学技术			
克隆性	多克隆（有些可为单克隆）	单克隆	单克隆
FISH，CGH	未知	正常或轻度异常	特征性的染色体改变（1q、7q、8q增加，16q丢失）

CT：计算机体层摄影术；MRI：磁共振成像；FISH：荧光原位杂交；CGH：比较基因组杂交

提倡手术切除。腺瘤病的治疗可能有些棘手，因为出血的危险性较高，实质内病灶较多不能切除时，可能有必要进行肝移植[7,29]。

局灶结节性增生　Focal nodular hyperplasia

临床特征

局灶结节性增生（FNH）为良性非肿瘤性病变，多见于20~40岁的年轻女性[2,8]。大约5%~15%的病变发生于男性，比例高于肝细胞腺瘤。典型局灶结节性增生常于手术或由于其他不相关疾病进行放射学检测时偶然发现，但也可出现上腹部疼痛，或极少数由于病变较大而出现类似出血的合并症[30]。肝功能检测一般正常，但有些病人可出现γ-谷氨酸转肽酶活性升高[30]。局灶结节性增生一般长期保持不变，但也有生长迅速和复发的病例报告，称为进展型局灶结节性增生[31]。

典型的局灶结节性增生常为孤立性病变；根据报告，20%~30%的病例为多灶性病变[30,32]。有局灶结节性

增生邻近血管瘤的描述，这种伴随情况较常见于多发性局灶结节性增生。某些所谓的多发性局灶结节性增生综合征病人至少具有两个局灶结节性增生病变，而且伴有一个或多个病变，如肝血管瘤、像 Klippel-Trenaunay-Weber 综合征的系统性动脉结构缺陷，以及大脑动脉瘤、脑膜瘤和星形细胞瘤等病变[32,33]。局灶结节性增生的一种少见亚型为毛细血管扩张型，常伴有多发性局灶结节性增生综合征[19]。

与肝细胞腺瘤不同，局灶结节性增生的发生并非由于口服避孕药的使用，但许多人推测，使用口服避孕药可使其增大，停药可使其缩小。目前得到支持的假设是，局灶结节性增生是一种增生，先前存在的动脉畸形周围的肝实质由于血流改变而出现反应性生长改变[34]。出现许多异常的肌性血管、伴发血管瘤以及 Budd-Chiari 综合征都支持这一理论。局灶结节性增生出现血管生成素基因（angiopoietin gene）异常表达，在增生性及营养不良性血管的形成过程中可能具有一定作用[35]。国际工作小组建议，对于伴有 Budd-Chiari 综合征和 Osler-Weber-Rendu 病的局灶结节性增生样病变不应命名为局灶结节性增生，最好称为再生性结节（regenerative nodules）（"局灶结节性增生样"结节）[23]。有关局灶结节性增生的克隆性本质尚有争议，但是近来资料显示局灶结节性增生为多克隆性，支持其为反应性病变而非肿瘤性病变[36,37]。

病理学特征

大体病理学：局灶结节性增生呈结节状表现（可提示大结节性肝硬化表现），与周围的肝组织相比，病变呈淡棕色（图 10.4）。这些病变一般位于靠近肝被膜的部位，偶尔可有蒂。局灶结节性增生由于呈结节状，边缘与周围正常肝实质分界清楚，没有纤维性包膜。多数病变较小，不足 5 cm，但大小差异较大，个别病例可累及整个肝叶。多数病变有"中央纤维瘢痕"，由纤维血管组织构成，而不是致密胶原成分。在不足 1 cm 的病变中可无中央瘢痕[23]。毛细血管扩张型为一少见类型，无中央纤维化区，大体上可类似于血管瘤或肝紫癜。

显微镜下特征：经典型局灶结节性增生由正常形态的肝细胞组成，肝细胞呈不完全性结节状排列，部分被纤维组织分隔，当存在中央纤维化区域时，这些纤维组织倾向于从中延伸而来。肝细胞板结构具有完整的网织纤维框架，类似正常肝组织，但肝细胞板一般较宽（2～3 个细胞厚），与再生性结节相同。肝细胞可能显示胞浆内糖原增加、局灶脂肪变性、瘀胆、脂褐素、铁色素、铜相关性蛋白以及 Mallory 小体[23]。可能出现局灶性非典型性肝细胞、细胞核大、轻度深染以及核仁明显。大细胞型的细胞学非典型性鲜有报告。一个重要特征是结节周边的纤维间质内可见数量不等的小胆管结构（图 10.5）。另外一个重要的诊断特征是出现中等至较大的厚壁肌性血管，常出现肌内膜黏液变或纤维肌性增生性改变。这些血管并不是汇管区成分，因为没有管径与之相似的门静脉或小叶间胆管伴行。病变内没有正常汇管区结构，但极少数病变的中央纤维化区内可见中等或较大的胆管成分[30]。肝窦稍有扩张，可见 Kupffer 细胞。炎症细胞相对较常见，一般为淋巴细胞，但也可见中性粒细胞和嗜酸性粒细胞，尤其是小胆管周围。极少数情况下可以见到肉芽肿结构。

毛细血管扩张型含有扩张的充满血液的血管腔，替代中央纤维化区。与典型的局灶结节性增生相比，这种类型病变中的动脉较小，数量较多，纤维间隔不甚明显[23,30]。另一种少见类型称为混合性增生性和腺瘤性病变，具有局灶结节性增生和腺瘤两者的特征。这种病变大体上类似于腺瘤，而且缺乏中央纤维化区。镜下可见类似于腺瘤的区域，与显示局灶结节性增生样特征的区域交替出现，常毛细血管扩张型。总是出现小胆管增生，但呈局灶性，且并不显著[30]。有人提议应将这些毛细血管型病变重新划分

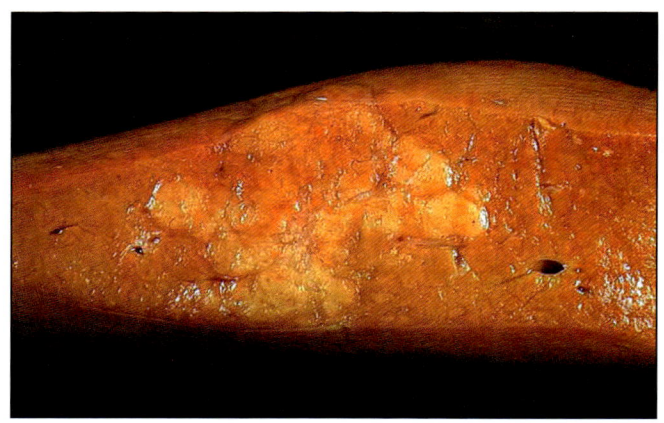

图10.4　局灶结节性增生，肿瘤境界清楚，呈结节状，中央瘢痕，实质呈褐色至淡棕色。

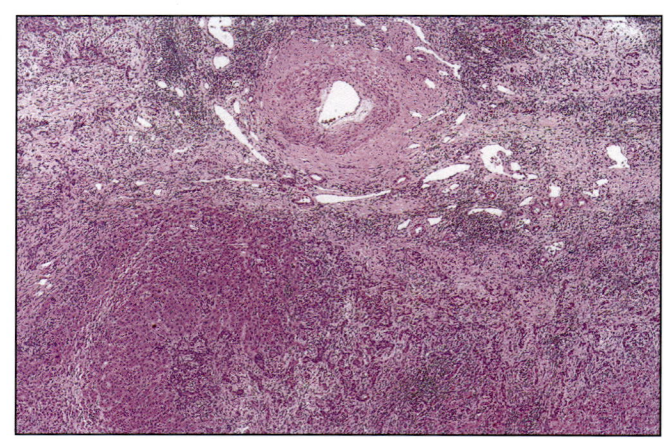

图10.5　局灶结节性增生，结节状肝细胞成分，纤维血管间质中伴有厚壁动脉和小胆管增生。

为腺瘤的一个亚型，但有关这一问题尚存争议[37]。

与肝细胞腺瘤一样，局灶结节性增生的肝细胞表达肝细胞标记物，如 Hep Par 1、CAM5.2 和多克隆 CEA。被覆肝细胞板的内皮细胞 CD34 一般呈阳性[25]。AFP 总是阴性。

鉴别诊断

局灶结节性增生需要与正常肝组织、肝细胞腺瘤、再生结节和肝细胞癌鉴别（表 10.1）。局灶结节性增生在 CT 及 MRI 上呈均匀性增强，伴中央瘢痕，而腺瘤表现为高密度非均一性肿块。局灶结节性增生锝硫胶体闪烁扫描（Tc-sulfur-colloid scintigraphy）检测正常或摄取增加，而腺瘤是一种没有摄取的病变[10]。即使结合了新影像学技术，术前诊断准确率也仅为 70%～85%[10]。组织学上，腺瘤与局灶结节性增生之间差异不大，穿刺活检时一般不易区分开。出现小胆管结构是局灶结节性增生最重要的鉴别特征，可以除外腺瘤诊断，但重要的是要记住，正常汇管区可能陷入局灶结节性增生、腺瘤以及肝细胞癌中。如同中央纤维化区域一样，伴有异常增生特征的大血管被结缔组织包绕支持局灶结节性增生的诊断。腺瘤大血管倾向于具有较正常的结构，并且血管周围缺乏明显的结缔组织间质。腺瘤的假腺样分化可误诊为小胆管。与 Budd-Chiari 综合征和血管畸形有关的再生结节类似局灶结节性增生，但是根据定义不能诊断为局灶结节性增生，因为周围肝组织并非正常。局灶结节性增生和纤维板层型肝细胞癌均可出现中央瘢痕，在放射学检测时容易相互混淆。瘢痕中出现钙化支持纤维板层型肝细胞癌，但局灶结节性增生偶有钙化的报告[38]。局灶结节性增生的某些典型特征，例如结节状结构伴有纤维化、小胆管增生以及缺乏小叶间胆管，可能非常类似于慢性胆管缺乏性疾病（chronic ductopenic biliary disease），尤其是在有限的活检标本中。在这种情况下，正常肝酶学检查的临床资料和放射学检查发现的一块局灶性肿块有助于局灶结节性增生的诊断。

预后和结局

局灶结节性增生为良性病变，与腺瘤不同，实际上并不存在合并出血及恶性变的危险性。尽管极少数病例伴有纤维板层型肝细胞癌[39]，但尚没有局灶结节性增生进展为癌的确切证据。根据推测，伴发的局灶结节性增生可能是由于癌组织血管成分增加，造成邻近肝实质的一种增生性反应。如果根据放射学检查可以明确诊断，可以采用保守治疗而不进行手术切除。对于所有可疑病例，均应经过病理学诊断得以证实。由于小的活检标本无助于腺瘤和局灶结节性增生的鉴别，因此提倡进行手术中活检或切除以取代经皮活检[10]。

其他良性肿瘤和瘤样病变
Other benign tumors and tumor-like lesions

局灶脂肪变（Focal fatty change，FFC）为局部区域的肝细胞含有大量脂肪，病变常位于被膜下，在大体或放射影像学上可能与肿瘤相混淆。局灶脂肪变可能伴有糖尿病或酒精性肝炎[40]。

假脂肪瘤（Pseudolipoma）为有包膜的成熟脂肪组织肿块，常出现坏死或钙化，一般发生于被膜下[41]。被认为是腹膜或结肠周围脂肪分离而附着于肝被膜。

孤立性坏死性结节（Solitary necrotic nodule）为极少见的非肿瘤性病变，其中央区为无定形嗜酸性碎片，周边为含有明显弹力纤维的玻璃样变的纤维性被膜。临床上可能将这些病变误诊为转移性病变。本病可能是良性病变的终末期表现，例如硬化性血管瘤[42]。有极少数病例伴有寄生虫感染[43]。

结节性再生性增生（Nodular regenerative hyperplasia，NRH）特征为多发性再生结节遍布整个肝组织，缺少纤维性间隔[23]。结节性再生性增生常与门静脉阻塞有关，而且可能伴有真性红细胞增多症、原因不明的骨髓化生、类风湿关节炎、Budd-Chiari 综合征、恶性淋巴瘤以及各种其他病变[2]。结节直径一般为 0.1～1.0 cm，但偶尔可能较大（达 10 cm），并可类似于肿瘤。在某些病例中，结节并不累及整个肝组织，而是局限于肝门区（部分结节性转化，partial nodular transformation）[44]。组织学上，结节由排列成 2～3 个细胞厚的肝细胞板组成。结节周边的肝细胞萎缩，网织纤维框架凝聚，最好应用网织纤维染色观察。没有纤维间隔，但常出现灶状肝窦纤维化。结节性再生性增生没有任何肿瘤潜能。本病很少与肿瘤混淆，除非当结节较大而且类似肝细胞腺瘤时。

硬化性肝组织中的良性/癌前性肝细胞病变
Benign/Premalignant hepatocellular lesions in cirrhotic liver

大再生（巨大再生）结节
Large regenerative (macroregenerative) nodule

在肝硬化中，大于典型肝硬化结节的良性结节有多种名称，包括大再生结节、巨大再生结节或腺瘤性增生。类似的结节可发生于 Budd-Chiari 综合征和门静脉血栓形成的非硬化性肝组织中，或为坏死后伴再生的后遗症，国际工作小组建议将其命名为多腺泡再生性结节 (multiacinar regenerative nodules)[23]。大再生结节和多腺泡再生性结节被认为是反应性病变，而非克隆性肿瘤前病变。

临床特征

大再生结节发生于肝硬化患者，在个别例外情况下，可见于没有完全硬化的慢性肝疾病[45]。常在尸检或肝移植时偶然发现，但在放射影像学检查时可以见到。血清 AFP 正常或处于慢性肝病或肝硬化范围之内。这些结节一般见于因乙型肝炎、丙型肝炎、酒精性肝炎以及血色素沉着症所致的肝硬化，但在原发性胆汁性肝硬化中不常见。

病理学特征

大体特征：大再生结节比典型的肝硬化结节大。普遍接受的大小下限为 1 cm，这些病变的最大径几乎总是小于 3 cm。结节倾向于从切面上膨出，边缘较圆，境界清楚，可呈胆汁着色，或与其他硬化性结节相比呈淡黄至褐色。

显微镜下特征：这些结节组织学上类似于肝硬化结节。大再生结节具有类似于正常肝组织的完整的网织纤维框架，肝细胞板为 1～2 个细胞厚。肝细胞的细胞学一般正常，但可出现局灶性细胞大小改变，尤其类似于其他肝硬化结节中可以见到的散在的大细胞改变。可出现 Mallory 小体、胆汁淤积、透明细胞胞浆改变、铁或铜沉积、细胞大小轻度减小以及局灶或弥漫性脂肪变[23,46]。结节内通常存在汇管区，小胆管增生可较为显著（图 10.6），但也可出现缺乏完整胆管、静脉和动脉的肝三联的纤维性间隔[47]。

大再生结节一般出现动脉数量增加，而缺少其他汇管区成分，即所谓的"无伴行动脉"(unpaired artery)。

然而，将诸如 CD34 或 CD31 等血管标记物作为肝窦毛细血管化标记物进行染色，显示结节周边阳性，类似肝硬化结节表现[48,49]。结节 AFP 染色为阴性[50]。细胞角蛋白和多克隆 CEA 着色方式类似于正常肝组织。

鉴别诊断

根据结节的大小可将其与其他肝硬化性结节鉴别开来。偶尔，巨大再生结节可以缺乏汇管区，但在硬化性的肝组织内，这一表现并不能成为诊断腺瘤的依据，除非有前面讨论的危险因素存在。与异型增生结节和高分化肝细胞癌鉴别的特征列于表 10.2。

重要性

一般认为这些结节是良性病变，为无克隆性增生的大再生性病灶。大再生结节伴有肝细胞癌的发生率在增加[51]。然而，这些研究将巨大再生结节在组织学上定义为缺乏高级别异型增生结节或肝细胞癌的特征。由于尚无克隆性研究用来区分巨大再生结节和低级别异型增生结节，因而尚不清楚癌危险性增加是与多克隆性大再生结节有关，还是与克隆性低级别异型增生结节有关，或与两者均有关。

异型增生　Dysplasia

肝硬化结节可出现两种不同类型的肝细胞非典型性，即大细胞异型增生和小细胞异型增生。由于有关其恶性潜能尚有争议，因此国际工作小组建议采用大细胞改变和小细胞改变这样的术语[23]。大细胞改变 (large cell change) 的特征为细胞核增大、深染、核仁明显，但胞浆丰富，因而核-浆比正常（图 10.7）。有些细胞可呈多核。尽管大细胞改变与肝细胞癌关系密切[52]，但在硬化性肝组织中过于常见，不能作为癌前病变[53]。与肝细胞癌不同，大细胞改变的核-浆比例

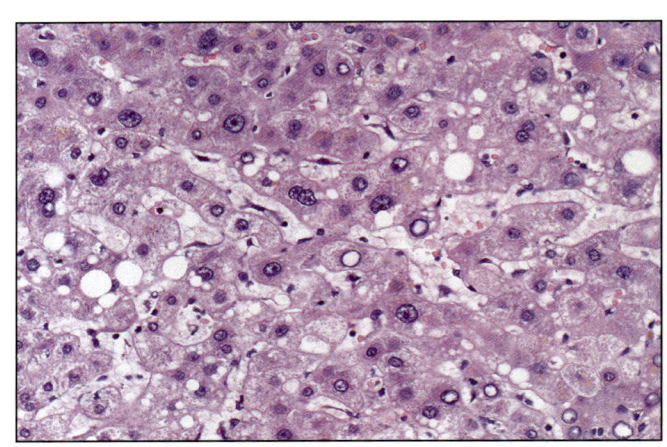

图 10.6　大再生结节伴有明显的小胆管增生。　　　　　图 10.7　大细胞改变。非典型性大细胞核，核-浆比正常。

表10.2	诊断特征：大再生结节、异型增生结节和高分化肝细胞癌			
形态学	大（巨大）再生结节	低级别异型增生结节	高级别异型增生结节	高分化肝细胞癌
肝细胞大小	类似于肝硬化结节	肝细胞一致，细胞学正常，提示克隆性增生	大小不一，一般接近正常大小或略缩小	与正常比较或大或小
小细胞改变或核密度大于正常2倍	没有，或仅见于散在细胞	没有，或仅见于散在细胞	个别较小病灶，可弥漫且显著；大结节内可出现结节状表现	常见
大细胞改变	散在细胞	无	散在细胞，大细胞不可能成团，除非在异型增生病灶内	可出现
梁状肝细胞板≥3个细胞厚	无	无	肝细胞板偶尔≥3个细胞厚	常见
汇管区	几乎总是存在；局灶胆管增生	常见	大的异型增生结节内常见	没有，除非从肿瘤边缘陷入
结节周围	境界清楚	境界清楚	有些可出现边缘不规则	常见浸润性边缘
网织纤维框架	完整；无网织纤维减少或缺失灶	完整	可出现局灶性缺失	常广泛缺失；增厚的索带可分隔肝细胞板
铁含量增加	可见	不明	可见	几乎总是缺失，即使是在铁质沉着的肝组织内

Adapted with permission from Ferrell L D 2004 Benign and malignant tumors of the liver. In: Odze R D, Goldblum J R, Crawford J M et al. (eds) Surgical Pathology of the GI tract, liver, biliary tract and pancreas. Saunders, Philadelphia, Table 42-3, p999-1026.

正常，无核分裂象，增殖率低，没有 p53 突变[54]。依据近期研究，大细胞改变对于肝细胞癌的预测值不足 20%[55]。可能为再生性或变性表现[56]，或是对长期胆汁郁积的反应[57]。小细胞改变（small cell change）的特征为其细胞小于正常肝细胞，核-浆比高于正常，细胞核深染。如果小细胞改变发生于膨胀性小病灶中，则其与肝细胞癌的关系可能比大细胞改变更为密切[52]。高增殖活性和 p53 过度表达已有报道[54,56]。然而，境界不清或弥漫分布的无结节状结构的小细胞改变可能为再生性表现，可见于慢性胆管病变，不太可能是肿瘤前驱病变[52,56]。

异型增生一词用来描述显示异常生长组织学特征的细胞，推测可能是由于遗传学改变引起，但不符合恶性确诊标准[23]。由于诊断异型增生的遗传学标准尚未建立，因此采用异常细胞的形态学特征以及分布情况来进行异型增生的诊断及分类。直径不足 1 mm 的小团异型增生肝细胞称作异型增生灶（dysplastic focus），而 1 mm 或更大的病变则称为异型增生结节（dysplastic nodule）。细胞学特征用来划分低级别和高级别异型增生结节。

异型增生灶见于多种疾病，例如慢性乙型和丙型肝炎、α_1-抗胰蛋白酶缺乏以及高酪氨酸血症[23]。病变边缘清楚，但不规则。细胞通常均匀一致，但细胞核有非典型性，而且胞浆染色也不同于周围肝细胞。细胞核非典型性的程度从轻度至重度不等。胞浆内脂肪或糖原含量可与相邻肝组织有所不同。

低级别异型增生结节
Low-grade dysplastic nodule

硬化性肝组织内的低级别异型增生结节被认为是肝细胞克隆性增生，但其大体及标准显微镜下特征与大再生结节不能区分。因此，低级别异型增生结节与上面描述的巨大再生结节具有共同的临床和病理学特征。低级别异型增生结节的本质是克隆性增生，其中的肝细胞较为均匀一致，但这种类型克隆性结节的特殊形态学特征尚未确立。在缺少克隆性研究的情况下，巨大再生结节和低级别异型增生结节这两个术语可以交换使用，用于描述缺乏高级别异型增生细胞或结构特征的结节。

高级别异型增生结节
High-grade dysplastic nodule

临床特征：高级别异型增生结节也称为交界性结节、II型巨大再生结节、非典型性腺瘤性增生以及非典型性巨大再生结节，几乎均发生于硬化性肝组织[23,46,47]。血清 AFP 正常或在慢性肝病或肝硬化范围之内。由于这些病变被认为是癌前病变，因此建议手术切除或采用消融疗法。

病理学特征

大体病理学：这些结节的大体病理学表现与大再生结节和低级别异型增生结节基本相同，例外的情况是某些结节境界不清或者边缘不规则。

显微镜下特征：结节的异型增生性改变可呈一致性，或在一个结节内出现一个或多个异型增生灶（图10.8）。非典型性特征不足以诊断肝细胞癌。通过核-浆比例增加的小细胞改变区常可辨认出这种结节。与正常肝组织相比，其细胞核密度（估计镜下每个视野肝细胞核的数量）增加（图10.9）[46]。大细胞改变极少为高级别异型增生结节的特征，但如果出现大细胞改变，必须为散在的非典型性细胞灶，而非结节内散在分布的单个增大的细胞核。其他常见特征为局灶区域肝细胞板达到3个细胞厚、网织纤维框架呈局灶性减少以及肝窦轻度扩张。这些结节也可出现灶状腺泡（假腺体）结构、Mallory小体、脂肪、透明细胞改变、胞浆嗜碱、胆汁以及汇管区。高级别异型增生性病变一般缺乏铁沉积，相比之下，再生性或低级别异型增生结节的铁沉积较为常见。

鉴别诊断：与明显的肝细胞癌的鉴别见表10.2。对于诊断肝细胞癌可能最有帮助的特征为小梁出现超过3个细胞厚的肝细胞板、中等量的核分裂象、细胞核密度大于正常的两倍、网织纤维框架显著减少、多数无伴行性动脉以及缺少汇管区。

异型增生：遗传学改变和结局
Dysplasia：genetic changes and outcome

进行性遗传学改变在大再生结节、异型增生结节以及肝细胞癌中已经得到证实，支持癌发生呈多步骤进展。等位基因失衡见于16%的巨大再生结节和50%的低级别异型增生结节[58]。高比例的等位基因缺失见于高级别异型增生结节，与肝细胞癌类似。4q、8p和Xq缺失见于大再生结节和低级别异型增生结节，而1p、13q、16q和17p缺失见于高级别异型增生[59]。

目前临床治疗中，大再生结节和低级别异型增生结节可通过影像学和血清学标记物进行随诊，而高级别异型增生性结节的治疗则比较积极，采用手术切除或消融疗法（ablative therapy）[46,58]。

其他癌前病变　Other premalignant lesions

缺铁灶（iron-free foci）为缺铁或铁含量比周围肝组织显著减少的肝细胞灶。常见于遗传性血色素沉着症合并肝细胞癌病人肝汇管区的周围。值率增高，可能为肿瘤前驱病变[60]。改变了的肝细胞灶（foci of altered hepatocytes）为肿瘤前驱病变，最初见于动物模型。也有报道见于硬化性肝组织内，表现为局灶性肝细胞糖原贮积病（由于糖原过剩而呈透明细胞灶）、嗜双色或嗜酸性细胞灶（富于线粒体）、混合性嗜双色和透明细胞灶[61,62]。这些病灶的确切意义尚不明确。

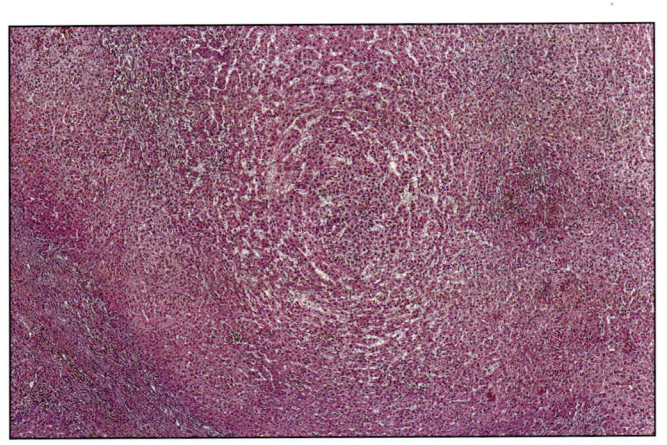

图10.8　高级别异型增生，呈结节内结节表现。

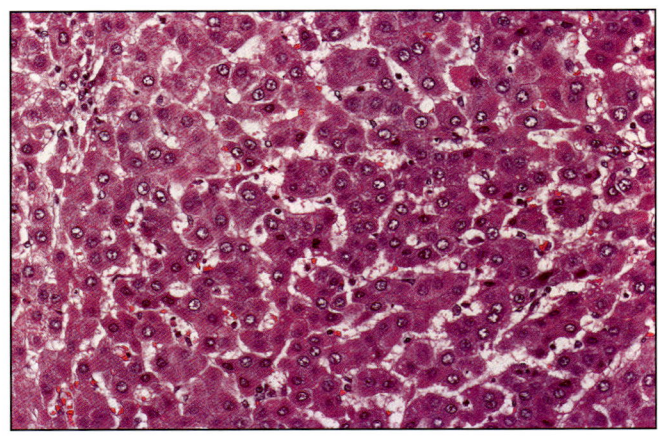

图10.9　高级别异型增生结节，核-浆比例高，细胞核密度增加。

恶性肝细胞病变
Malignant hepatocellular lesions

肝细胞癌及其亚型
Hepatocellular carcinoma and variants

临床特征

肝细胞癌是肝组织最常见的原发性恶性肿瘤。在世界范围内，它是男性第5位、女性第8位常见的恶性肿瘤。每年报告的病例超过500 000例。不同地域的发病率有所差异，欧洲和北美为每10万2~7例；中国台湾、中国东南部和非洲撒哈拉每10万30多例。在过去的25年中，美国肝细胞癌的发病率超过2倍[63]。男性为女性的3倍。

多数病人无症状或出现腹痛；不足10%的病人出现体重减轻、不适、发热、黄疸以及腹水[64]。通过放射影像学技术或AFP升高筛查而确诊的肝硬化病人日渐增加。肿瘤较大的病例中几乎2/3出现血清AFP水平升高（>1000ng/ml）[65]；肿瘤大小不足2~3 cm时不可能出现血清AFP升高[45]。血清AFP水平升高至500ng/ml可见于许多肝组织疾病，500~1000ng/ml为可疑肝细胞癌，但不完全特异。AFP也有助于监测治疗效果以及发现复发病例。影像学技术对于诊断具有重要作用。小肿瘤在超声检查中表现为低回声，而较大的肿瘤可呈高回声。由于肝细胞癌接受来自动脉的血供，而非门脉血供，因此在CT检查时它在较早的动脉相增强，而其余的肝组织对比显影后在较晚的门脉相增强。从前应用血管造影通过显示其丰富的血管成分来检测肝细胞癌，但现已大多被CT和MRI所替代。放射学技术的敏感性和特异性分别为70%和80%，但对于较小的肿瘤则显著减低[66]。

绝大多数肝细胞癌（>80%）发生于硬化性肝组织内；下列疾病可引起肝硬化，从而增加患肝细胞癌危险性[67]：

1. 乙型肝炎病毒（HBV）：为世界范围内最常见的肝细胞癌的主要病因，尤其是在肝细胞癌高发地区。对于HBV阳性男性，终生发生肝细胞癌的危险性为50%，女性为20%[67]。在这种情况下，肝细胞癌发生于年轻人，一般为20~30岁。个别病例发生于不伴有肝硬化的慢性病毒携带者[68]。

2. 丙型肝炎病毒（HCV）：为欧洲及北美地区发生肝细胞癌的主要病因。HCV阳性病人发生肝细胞癌的危险性为阴性对照组的17倍[69]。几乎所有肿瘤均发生于硬化性肝组织内。发生肝细胞癌的危险因素包括感染HCV时年龄较大、男性、肥胖、糖尿病、重度酗酒、共存HBV或HIV感染以及HCV感染时间较长[68]。

3. 酒精：长期酗酒（>50g/d）可导致肝硬化，为肝细胞癌的危险因素之一。伴有HBV、HCV感染以及糖尿病者危险性更高[68]。

4. 代谢性疾病：肝细胞癌在遗传性血色素沉着症中极为常见（有些系列报告其终生危险为45%）。在遗传性高酪氨酸血症中，存活两年以上的病人超过1/3发生肝细胞癌[67]。也有报道肝细胞癌伴有其他代谢性疾病，诸如α_1-抗胰蛋白酶缺乏以及Wilson病。尽管肝腺瘤在I型糖原贮积病中常见，但极少发生肝细胞癌[70]。

5. 药物及毒素：接触二氧化钍、黄曲霉毒素、雄性类固醇以及促孕药物与肝细胞癌有关[112]。黄曲霉毒素为黄曲霉菌的真菌性毒素，可能污染贮存于潮湿环境下的食物。接触黄曲霉素在HBV流行地区较常见[67]。

病理学特征

大体病理学：多数病例有肝硬化背景。分类时，肿瘤为孤立性大肿块称为大块型；肿瘤为多发散在结节时称结节型；肿瘤为多数不甚清晰的小结节时称弥漫型[65]。直径小于2 cm的肿瘤称为小肝细胞癌；这些小肿瘤一般缺少显著的血管浸润、坏死或出血。肿瘤一般较软，与周围肝组织相比，其颜色较淡或者胆汁着色（图10.10）。边界不规则，可见卫星结节。肝细胞癌容易出现血管浸润。门静脉和肝静脉可能受累，肿瘤可蔓延至下腔静脉。胆管受累并不常见，但可以见到。有些肝细胞癌形成多结节、巨大结节，并可类似于肝硬化（图10.11）。

显微镜下所见：WHO列举了肝细胞癌的一些典型组织学类型[1,71]。最常见的为梁状型（trabecular pattern），亦称肝窦型（sinusoidal pattern）（图10.12）。

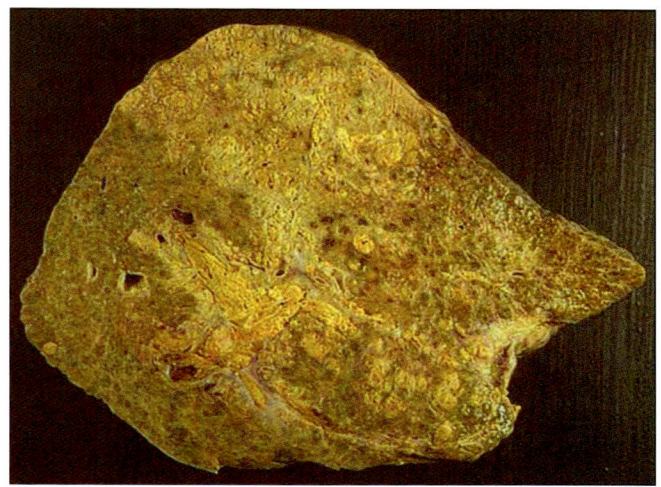

图10.10 发生于肝硬化的肝细胞癌。肿瘤呈黄褐色，边界不清，出现静脉浸润（中央靠左）。非肿瘤性肝组织呈硬化改变及胆汁着色（左）。

恶性肝细胞病变

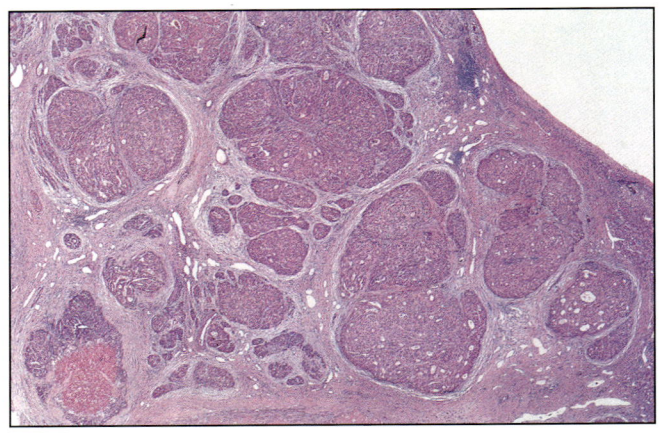

图10.11　肝细胞癌，多结节型。低倍镜下表现类似于大结节性肝硬化。

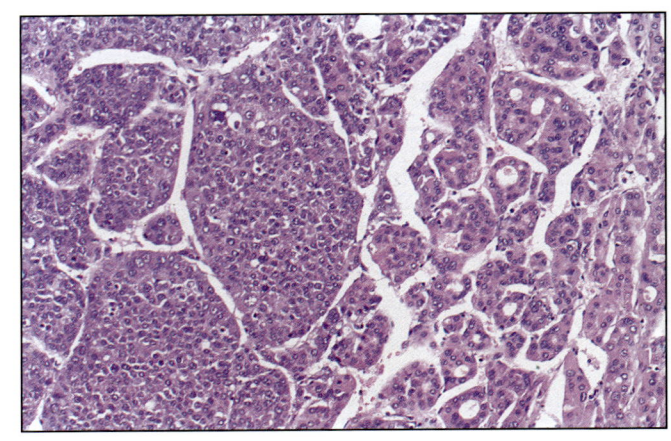

图10.14　肝细胞癌，梁状型（左）和假腺样型（右）。

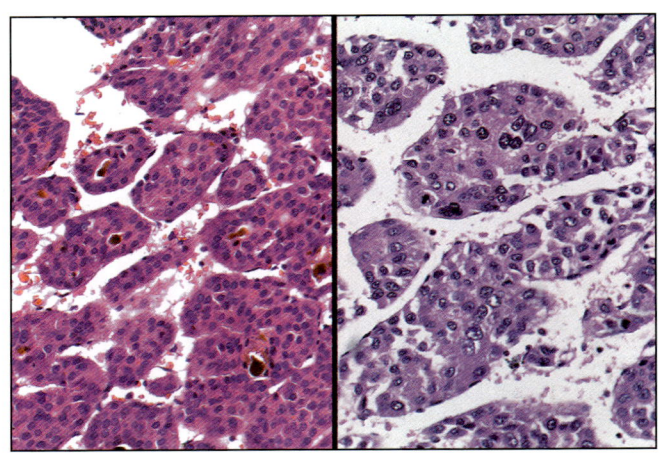

图10.12　肝细胞癌，梁状型，伴有大细胞改变（左）和小细胞改变（右）。注意肿瘤细胞产生的胆栓。

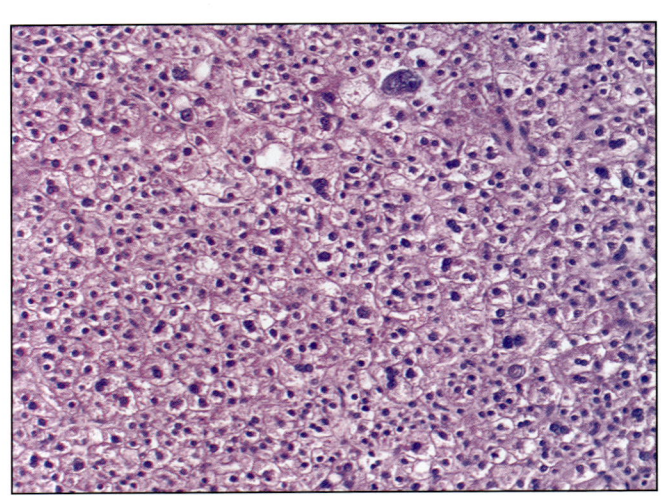

图10.15　肝细胞癌，实性（致密）型，缺少明确的肝细胞板结构。

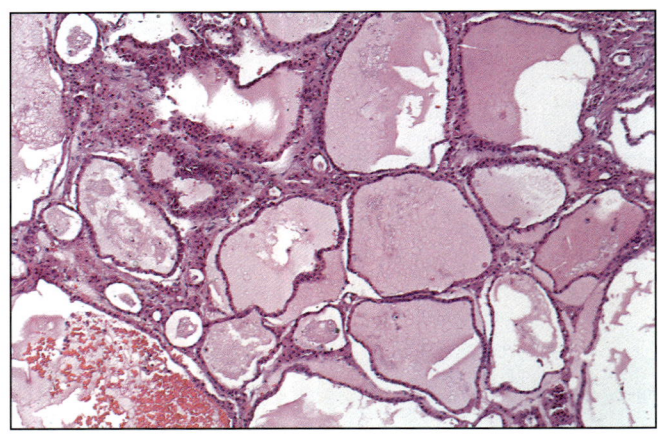

图10.13　肝细胞癌，假腺样型。

这种类型肿瘤的形态类似于正常肝组织的肝板结构，但肝细胞板厚度为3个细胞厚或更多，而正常或再生性肝组织为1~2个细胞厚。肿瘤性肝细胞板衬以内皮细胞，与正常肝组织类似，但网织纤维常常缺乏，显著减少或扭曲，伴有肝梁边缘网织纤维染色不规则或者缺乏。肿瘤细胞常具有小细胞改变的特征。大细胞改变也可见，

但并不常见，除非是高级别肿瘤。小细胞改变和大细胞改变病灶可混合出现。一般见不到Kupffer细胞。

腺泡性、假腺样或腺样型（acinar、pseudoglandular or adenoid pattern）肝细胞癌比梁状型少见。其特征为出现腺样腔隙或腺泡，内衬肿瘤性肝细胞（图10.13）。这些腺泡结构是由于胆小管扩张或膨胀形成的，常含有胆汁。少数情况下，腔隙是由中央坏死所致，并且可含蛋白、细胞碎片或吞噬细胞。由于形成腺样腔隙，可被误认为腺癌。腺泡型肝细胞癌常混有梁状型结构（图10.14）。

实性或致密型（solid or compact pattern）肝细胞癌相对少见，特征为肿瘤细胞密集成团，似乎缺少衬覆内皮细胞的肝小梁或者肝细胞板（图10.15）；然而，通过内皮细胞标记物标记仔细观察一般可显示受压的肝梁。在实性和密集区域，一般缺乏网织纤维框架。

硬化型（scirrhous pattern）含有局灶性或弥漫性纤维化区域，可伴有上述任何一种类型（图10.16）。可常与胆管癌或纤维板层癌混淆。类似的纤维化改变可发生于放疗或化疗后，不应认为是硬化型癌。硬化型肝细

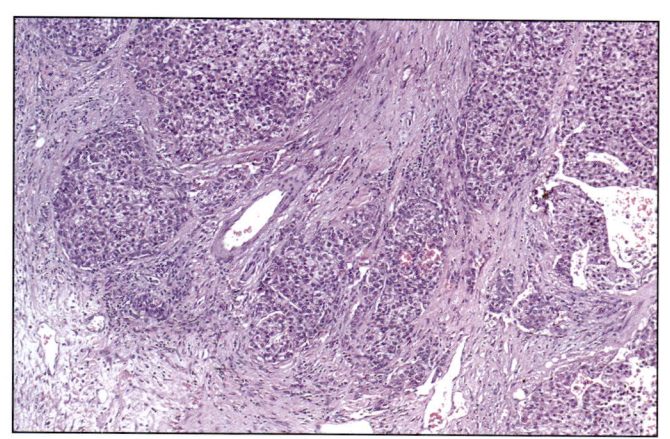

图10.16 肝细胞癌,硬化型;出现显著间质纤维化。

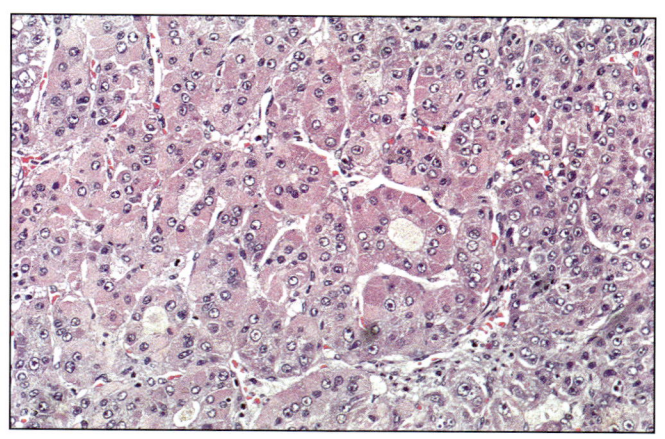

图10.18 肝细胞癌伴有明显的颗粒状(嗜酸性)胞浆。

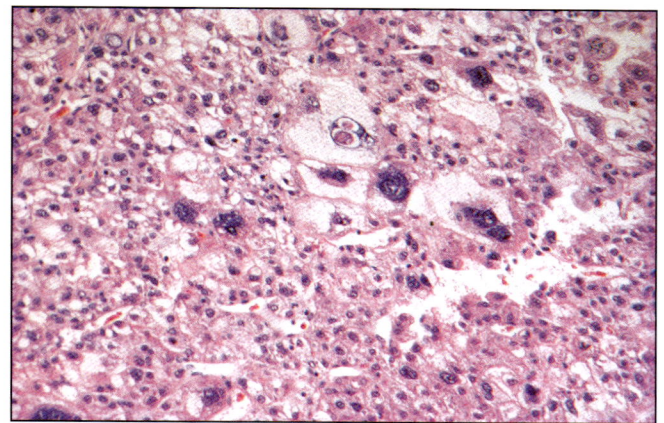

图10.17 肝细胞癌,可见多形性细胞灶。

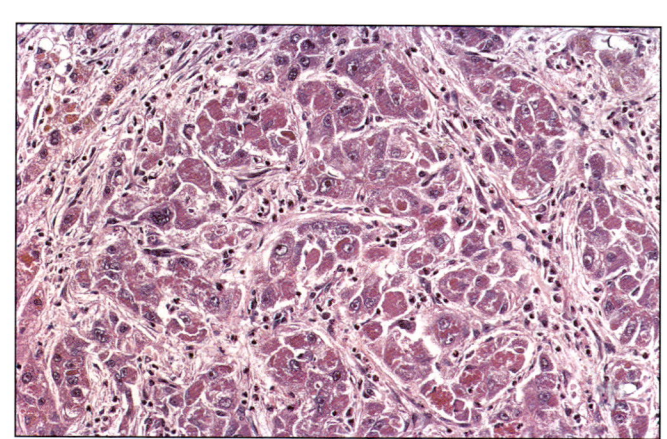

图10.19 肝细胞癌,可见Mallory小体。

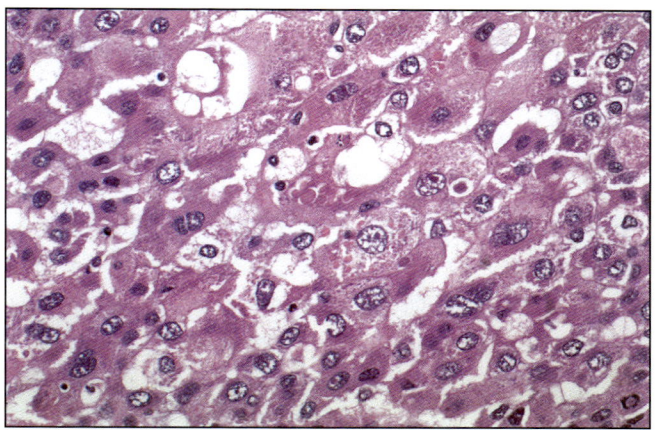

图10.20 肝细胞癌,胞浆内可见嗜酸性小体,这些小体一般为α_1-抗胰蛋白酶。

癌(sclerosing HCC)用来描述以高钙血症和显著间质纤维化为特征的一种肝细胞癌亚型[72]。有人认为硬化型肝细胞癌并非是特殊型病变,其中多数为肝内胆管癌[65]。

肝细胞癌的细胞学特征在这些类型当中也存在较大差异。肿瘤细胞一般保持多角形,具有圆形空泡状细胞核和明显的核仁。核内空泡(为胞浆内陷)以及核的糖原形成极为常见。小细胞改变(上面提到的)可能是最为常见的细胞学改变,但也可出现弥漫性或局灶性的大细胞改变以及巨细胞和(或)多形性细胞(图10.17)。胞浆的多少可能不同,与正常肝细胞相比常略呈嗜碱性。由于大量线粒体的出现,胞浆也可呈颗粒状或嗜酸性表现(图10.18)。也可见由包括白蛋白、纤维蛋白原、α_1-抗胰蛋白酶或铁蛋白组成的胞浆包涵体,诸如Mallory小体(图10.19)或球状嗜酸性小体(图10.20)。脂肪、糖原甚或水的成分可以较为明显,使得细胞呈"透明细胞"表现,被称为透明细胞型(clear cell variant)肝细胞癌(图10.21)。如果整个肿瘤表现为透明细胞变,并且发生于非硬化性肝组织内,则与转

移性透明细胞肿瘤可能难以鉴别,例如肾细胞癌。可见脂肪变性,在不足2 cm的小肿瘤中最为明显(图10.22)。随着肿瘤体积增大,脂肪成分呈减少趋势。淡染小体(pale bodies)呈圆形到卵圆形,为含有纤维蛋白原的轻度嗜酸性或透明胞浆。最多见于纤维板层型

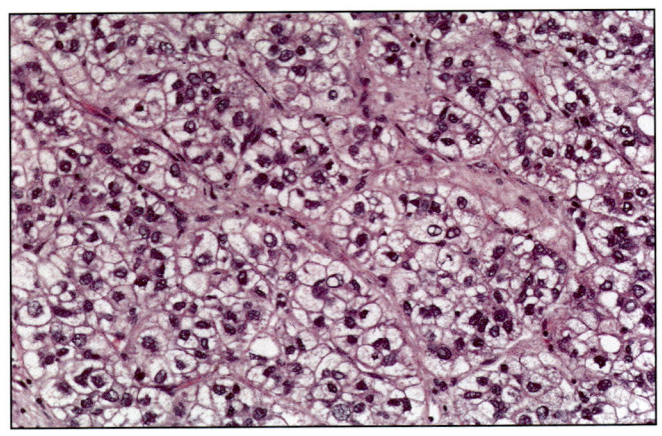

图10.21 肝细胞癌，透明细胞型，伴有丰富的胞浆内糖原。

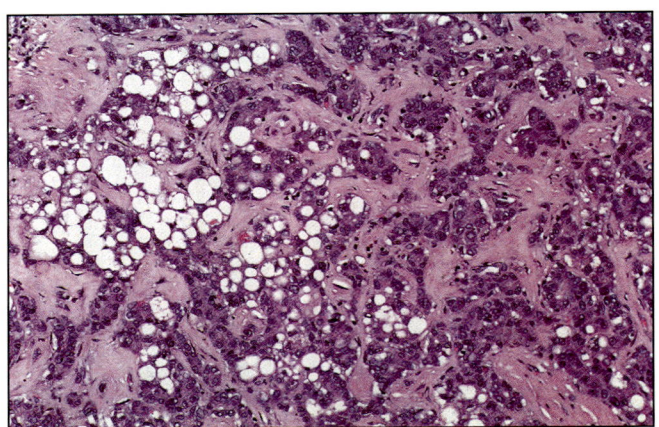

图10.22 肝细胞癌，伴有脂肪空泡。

肝细胞癌（见下纤维板层型肝细胞癌），但也可见于普通肝细胞癌，尤其是硬化型肝细胞癌。其他不大常见的胞浆变化包括见于某些HBV感染病人的含有乙型肝炎表面抗原（HBsAg）的毛玻璃细胞[73]，可能是陷入其中的HBsAg肝细胞，而并非肿瘤细胞。可见类似于Dubin-Johnson综合征中所见的棕黑色至黑色色素。肿瘤细胞中一般见不到铁，但在间质内的间叶性细胞中可以出现。少数类型的肝细胞癌，包括小细胞型和肉瘤样肝细胞癌可出现明显的梭形细胞成分。后者与肉瘤鉴别可能比较困难，但常可见与典型肝细胞癌相移行的区域。

肝细胞癌的其他特殊组织学类型包括包膜型肝细胞癌（encapsulated HCC）、带蒂型肝细胞癌（pedunculated HCC）、小的肝细胞癌（small HCC）、紫癜样肝细胞癌（pelioid HCC）以及伴有淋巴细胞间质的肝细胞癌（HCC with lymphoid stroma）。根据报告，3%～10%的肝细胞癌有包膜形成。包膜型肝细胞癌一般较小，境界清楚，切除后预后较好[74]。带蒂型肝细胞癌中，肿瘤经蒂与肝相连，可能来源于副叶。这些肿瘤生长缓慢，因位于肝外，所以预后较好[75]。小的肝细胞癌的定义为不足2 cm的肝细胞癌。这些肿瘤常为多灶性，分化好，发生于硬化性肝组织。除了大小以外，这些肿瘤与其他肝细胞癌相类似[65]。肝细胞癌中可出现大的血管腔隙，类似于肝紫癜，称为紫癜样肝细胞癌。肝细胞癌伴有淋巴细胞间质为少见亚型，可见致密的淋巴细胞和浆细胞浸润，并形成淋巴滤泡。多数病人为男性，AFP正常，淋巴细胞数量超过肿瘤细胞[76]。这些病人肝移植后预后较好。

肝细胞癌的分级依据Edmondson和Steiner1954年提出的分级系统，传统上分为三级或四级[77]。最初依据核浆比例增加、细胞核形状不同、核深染以及肝细胞板结构的丧失从低级别到高级别分为四级。这种分级方法经过一些修改目前仍用于低级别肿瘤的分级[1]。某些仅有轻度细胞学非典型性和结构异常的Edmondson和Steiner I级肿瘤，只是因为伴有高级别肝细胞癌区域或出现转移性病灶才被确认为恶性[65,7]。目前依据国际工作小组确定的标准，有些I级病变将划分为异型增生结节[23]。II级肿瘤也为高分化，但比I级肿瘤的细胞核大。II级病变出现假腺泡或梁状结构，并可见胆汁。III级肿瘤为中等分化，与II级病变相比，细胞学和结构出现更为明显的差异。比II级病变更容易见到局灶性分布的多核肿瘤细胞及瘤巨细胞，一般见不到胆汁。出现梁状结构时，一般比II级肿瘤的梁要宽，结构变化更为显著。IV级肿瘤由分化较差或间变性肿瘤组成，没有相应的临床资料例如肝硬化或血清AFP显著升高，很难确认为肝细胞癌。IV级病变可包含肉瘤样及小细胞成分。常应用替代的三级系统，I级为高分化肿瘤（上述的I级和II级混合）；II级为中分化肿瘤；III级为低分化肿瘤。

鉴别诊断

1. 肝细胞肿瘤：诊断中最多见的问题在于高分化肝细胞癌与非硬化性肝组织中的腺瘤或局灶结节性增生以及硬化性肝组织中的再生性/异型增生结节的鉴别上（表10.1和10.2）。网织纤维染色对于确认肝细胞癌有帮助，表现为网织纤维框架破碎或缺失（图10.23）。偶尔，高分化肝细胞癌可有完整的网织纤维框架。免疫过氧化物酶检测无助于良恶性肝细胞肿瘤的区分。CD34染色衬覆肝细胞癌肝梁的内皮细胞一般阳性，突出了血管成分的增加，但局灶结节性增生和腺瘤也常为阳性[25]。

2. 腺癌（胆管癌或转移性腺癌）（表10.3）：存在肝硬化、AFP水平升高以及呈梁状生长结构支持肝细胞癌。在硬化性肝组织中，胆管癌不多见，转移性腺癌极为少见。出现致密的纤维性间质支持腺癌，但硬化型肝细胞癌也有纤维性间质。腺泡状结构常见于肝细胞癌，因此并非是诊断腺癌的特征。同样，多发性病变在转移癌中较多见，而肝

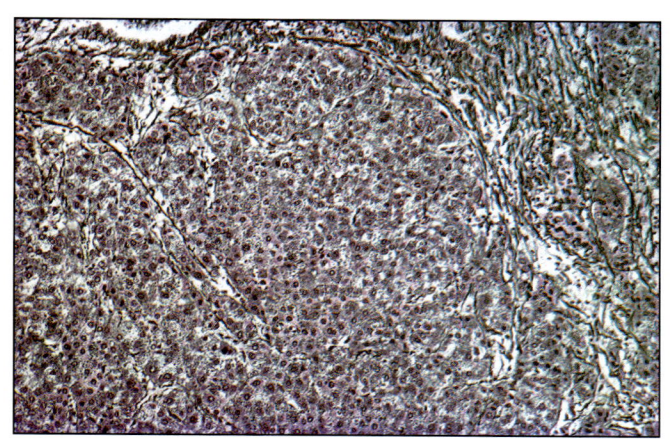

图10.23 肝细胞癌，网织纤维广泛缺失。

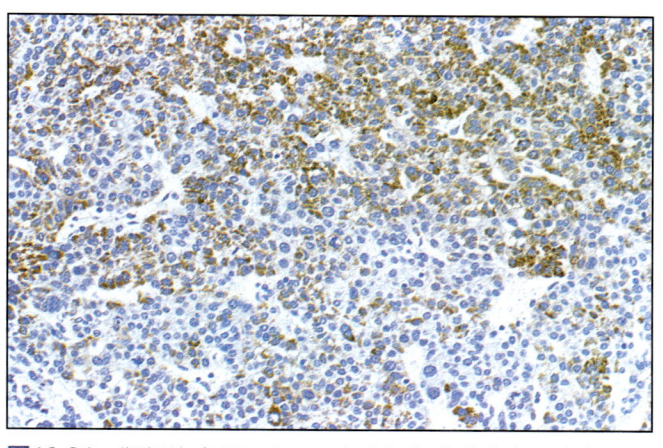

图10.24 肝细胞癌 Hep Par 1 免疫组织化学染色。大部分肿瘤（＞80%）出现弥漫性着色，但也可如本图中显示的片块状着色。

细胞癌也可为多灶性。

常规组织化学染色，例如黏液卡红或 PAS-淀粉酶染色可显示腺癌中的黏液。肝细胞癌中没有黏液，除非肝细胞癌与胆管癌混合以及某些纤维板层型肝细胞癌。PAS-淀粉酶染色可突出肝细胞癌胞浆内的糖蛋白，导致假阳性诊断。

免疫组织化学染色及白蛋白原位杂交有助于鉴别诊断。Hep Par 1 是肝细胞癌最敏感（＞90%）和特异性的免疫组织化学标记物（图 10.24）[78-82]。在

低分化和硬化性肝细胞癌中可呈阴性。在需要与肝细胞癌鉴别的肿瘤中，Hep Par 1 一般呈阴性，包括胆管癌、神经内分泌肿瘤、肾细胞癌、恶性黑色素瘤以及血管肌脂肪瘤。胰腺及结直肠的腺癌一般为阴性。然而，胃、食管以及肺的腺癌可呈强阳性反应[82]。多克隆 CEA 由于与胆汁糖蛋白呈交叉反应，所以90%以上的肝细胞癌出现特征性小管样着色（图 10.25）[80,83]。单克隆 CEA 在肝细胞癌为阴性。腺癌多克隆及单克隆 CEA 均呈胞浆着色。肝细胞癌

表10.3 肝细胞癌和腺癌（胆管癌或转移性腺癌）的鉴别诊断

	肝细胞癌	腺癌
临床特征		
肝硬化	常见（＞80%）	一般无
数量	一般单发；可见多结节	常为多灶
AFP	升高；肿瘤<2 cm时可为正常	正常
形态学		
结构	一般呈梁状；可出现假腺样结构	腺样；少数为实性或乳头状
纤维化	一般不明显，除非是硬化型或纤维板层型	一般较明显
黏液	无，除非是纤维板层型	可见
胆汁	常见	无
免疫组织化学		
Hep Par 1	高度敏感和特异；低分化肝细胞癌可呈阴性	阴性或弱阳性；胃、食管和肺的腺癌可呈强阳性
多克隆CEA	小管样着色	胞浆着色
AFP	特异，但敏感性低（30%~50%）	阴性
MOC-31	阴性	多数腺癌为膜的强阳性染色，临床应用为极好的标记物
细胞角蛋白	CAM5.2阳性；CK19及CK20一般为阴性	CK7/CK20染色依据部位；胆管癌CK19呈强阳性
白蛋白原位杂交	对肝细胞分化特异；敏感性>90%	阴性

的小管样着色可能难以判断；有类似着色在腺癌中局灶出现的报道。低分化肝细胞癌可呈阴性。CD10染色呈小管样结构，类似于肝细胞癌的多克隆CEA染色[80]。尽管CD10在腺癌中极少阳性，但由于敏感性较低（大约50%），使其不能成为有价值的多克隆CEA的替代品（或附加品）。如能除外卵黄囊瘤，AFP对于肝细胞癌是特异性标记物。然而其着色一般呈片块状分布，且敏感性较低（30%～50%），尤其对于小的高分化肝细胞癌[79]。白蛋白原位杂交（albumin in-situ hybridization）对于肝细胞分化是特异的（图10.26），且敏感性高（>90%）[84,85]。卵巢透明细胞腺癌可为弱阳性，原因尚不明确[85]。将白蛋白原位杂交与Hep Par 1结合起来，诊断肝细胞癌的敏感性可达100%[82]。

MOC-31为抗细胞表面糖蛋白的抗体，最初用于区分转移性腺癌和间皮瘤。在肝细胞肿瘤诊断中的价值近来才明确。胆管癌以及来自多个部位的腺癌呈一致的（80%～90%）阳性反应，例如结直肠、胰腺、胃、肺、乳腺以及卵巢。在腺癌中表现为弥漫性胞膜着色，容易判断[80,3]。肝细胞癌MOC-31染色几乎均为阴性。CK7、CK19及CK20有助于转移性腺癌的诊断以及确定其来源[86-88]。CK19在胆管癌基本上均为阳性。肝细胞癌一般呈阴性，但少数病例可呈局灶阳性[87,9]。CK8及CK18（CAM5.2抗体）一般在肝细胞癌中有表达。Leu-M1、B-72.3及Lex在腺癌一般呈阳性，肝细胞癌呈阴性[90]。与Hep Par 1和多克隆CEA联合应用时可能有助于诊断。[86-88]

其他标记物可用来诊断转移性腺癌，取决于临床状况，例如肺腺癌TTF-1胞核阳性，而前列腺腺癌前列腺特异性抗原（PSA）阳性。然而必须记住，非肿瘤性肝细胞以及许多肝细胞癌出现TTF-1胞浆阳性[91]。雌激素受体（ER）和孕激素受体（PR）与其他抗体联合应用可能有助于辨认乳腺来源的腺癌。但必须注意，肝细胞癌ER和PR可呈阳性。

3. 神经内分泌肿瘤：肝细胞癌与神经内分泌肿瘤的鉴别诊断也会出现困难，由于两者均可形成腺泡或梁状结构，而且可能由伴有多量嗜酸性胞浆和圆形细胞核的较大细胞组成。支持神经内分泌肿瘤的特征为突出的血管或毛细血管网和（或）间质玻璃样变。神经内分泌肿瘤几乎均为转移性，但有极少数原发于肝[65]。应用多种标记物染色发现包括纤维板层型在内的肝细胞癌以及肝母细胞瘤有局灶性神经内分泌分化，例如神经元特异性烯醇化酶、蛋白基因产物9.5、血管活性肠肽、降钙素及S-100染色[92-94]。然而，嗜铬素或突触素弥漫阳性强烈支持为神经内分泌肿瘤。

4. 血管肌脂肪瘤（AML）：上皮样型血管肌脂肪瘤与高分化肝细胞癌尤其难以鉴别。多数肝血管肌脂肪瘤并不伴有结节性硬化，且常缺少脂肪成分。出现胆汁或Mallory透明小体有助于鉴别，因为血管肌脂肪瘤没有这些特征。一旦怀疑到这种诊断，通过免疫组织化学染色容易得到证实，因为具有特征性染色所见。血管肌脂肪瘤共同表达诸如平滑肌肌动蛋白（SMA）或结蛋白等平滑肌标记物，以及诸如HMB-45、melan A和小眼相关因子等黑色素瘤标记物[95]。局灶S-100表达可见于血管肌脂肪瘤，一般位于上皮样细胞和脂肪细胞。Hep Par 1以及多克隆CEA没有表达。

5. 其他肿瘤：发生于没有AFP显著升高的非硬化性肝组织的透明细胞性肝细胞癌可出现诊断困难。

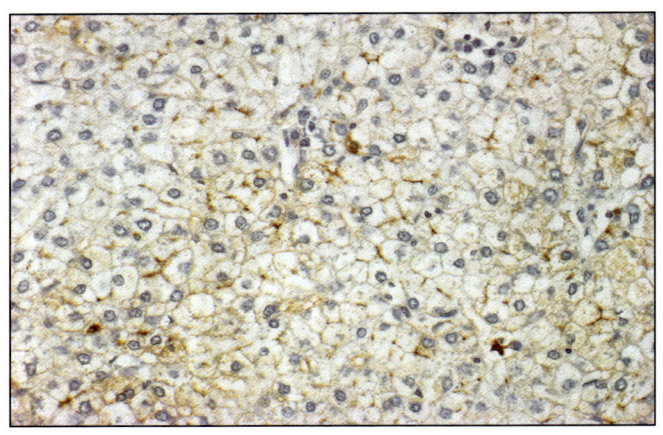

图10.25 肝细胞癌中多克隆癌胚抗原的小管样着色。

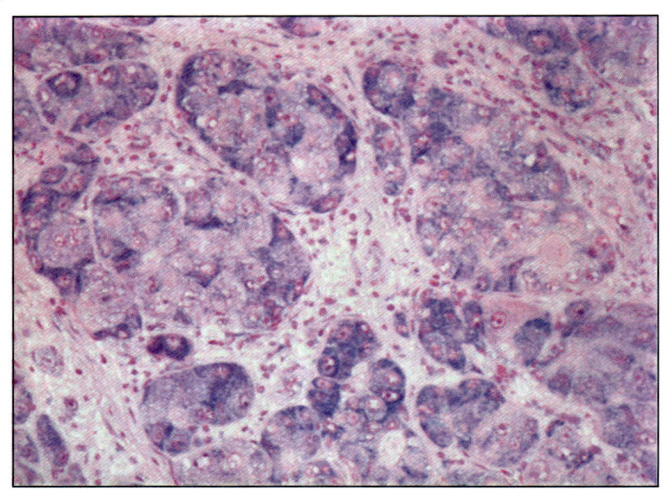

图10.26 肝细胞癌的白蛋白原位杂交，显示肿瘤细胞胞浆内的白蛋白（蓝色产物）。

主要应与转移性肾透明细胞癌相鉴别[96]。Hep Par 1及白蛋白原位杂交在透明细胞性肝细胞癌中均为阳性[82,85]。多克隆CEA呈小管型染色也支持肝细胞癌。上皮膜抗原（EMA）以及波形蛋白在肾细胞癌中有表达，但肝细胞癌阴性。角蛋白染色没有帮助，因为两者均为CAM5.2阳性，CK7及CK20为阴性。

黑色素瘤也可类似于肝细胞癌，但S-100及HMB-45在肝细胞肿瘤中呈阴性。黑色素瘤不表达Hep Par 1或多克隆CEA。个别情况下，肾上腺皮质肿瘤可能需要与原发性肝细胞肿瘤鉴别。肾上腺皮质肿瘤抑制素染色呈阳性，但肝细胞癌阴性，有助于诊断[97]。此外，肝细胞标记物如Hep Par 1和多克隆CEA在肾上腺皮质癌中不表达。

分子遗传学特征：与慢性肝疾病和肝硬化有关的低级别坏死性炎症活动产生细胞因子及其他细胞毒性物质，例如一氧化氮以及氧自由基，导致DNA损伤。坏死和再生的循环往复使得细胞容易出现突变，由于细胞的迅速转变使其没有足够时间来修复损伤的DNA[98]。肿瘤形成前期特点为转化生长因子-α（TGF-α）以及胰岛素样生长因子-2（IGF-2）过度表达，导致肝细胞增生加快[99]。

比较基因组杂交检测显示，肝细胞癌具有完全一致的染色体增加和缺失。最为明显的改变是8q（49%～81%）、1q（60%～79%）以及7q（40%～64%）染色体臂部分或整体增加以及16q（36%～65%）缺失[100-102]。其他常见异常包括Xq和5p过度表达，以及4q、8p、13q、16q及17p缺失。某些临床病理表现与特异性异常具有相关性。8q和20q增加与肿瘤较大有关[100]。8q增加和13q缺失多见于发生在非硬化性肝组织中的肝细胞癌[100]。据报道，9p和6q染色体缺失为预后不良的独立预测因子[101]。

p53基因突变在肝细胞癌中常见，多数报道中占30%～50%[103,104]。不同地区p53突变率差异较大，澳大利亚较低或没有，而塞内加尔为67%[104]。接触有黄曲霉毒素的饮食与p53基因249号密码子特异性G→T易位有关[105]。乙型肝炎中，由HBV X区编码的HBx蛋白与p53蛋白功能失活有关[106]。由HCV基因组编码的病毒蛋白，例如NS3和NS5A蛋白也可干扰p53活性[107,108]。作为Wnt信号通路重要成分的β-连环蛋白突变见于大约20%的肝细胞癌。在丙型肝炎相关性肝细胞癌中，突变率可高达40%[109]。有人提出肝癌发生主要有两个途径：一种出现β-连环蛋白突变和限制性遗传学改变，例如8p缺失；另一种为多数染色体广泛性等位基因缺失和p53突变，但是没有β-连环蛋白突变[101]。后一种肿瘤一般分化较差，行为更具侵袭性。细胞周期调节异常常见于肝细胞癌。大约40%的肝细胞癌p16由于启动子区过度甲基化而失活或视网膜母细胞瘤蛋白Rb由于基因突变而缺失[110,111]。据报道，细胞周期依赖激酶抑制剂p21和p27分别在38%和52%的肝细胞癌中表达有所减低[112,113]。HCV产生的核心蛋白也可抑制p21启动子[114]。

已经明确多种分子学异常为潜在的预后标记物。据报道，伴有p53、Rb和p16基因失活以及9p、6q和14q等位基因缺失的肿瘤结局不良[101,110,111,115]。免疫组织化学染色，肿瘤细胞表达p53则预后不良[116]。β-连环蛋白突变以及p27高表达则有较高生存率[101,117]，而细胞周期蛋白D过度表达是早期复发的标志[115]。高增生率、E-钙黏蛋白低表达以及细胞核表达β-连环蛋白可预测移植后复发[118]。然而大宗病例研究显示，这些表现尚无一项有足够的特异性能够用于临床。

治疗和预后：对于无肝硬化以及血管浸润或肝外疾病的病人，选择手术切除。无肝硬化病人的5年和10年生存率分别为40%和26%[119]。肝硬化病人的生存率较低，但肿瘤不足5cm、无血管或肝外受累以及功能状态良好（Child-Pugh分级A）的病人，5年存活率可达33%～44%。对于有肝硬化的肝细胞癌病人，治疗的最佳选择是肝移植。肿瘤大于5cm、超过3个肿瘤、多发性肿瘤其中之一大于3cm以及有肝外播散是肝移植的禁忌证。遵循这些标准，5年生存率可达到75%以上[120]。有人提出，孤立性肿瘤入选治疗的标准是大小应当增至6.5cm[121]。可在超声或CT引导下采用乙醇或射频消融治疗肝细胞癌。消融技术常用于由于部位关系而不能切除的小肿瘤，或并存晚期肝病以及等待肝移植的病人[122]。

肝细胞癌总体预后仍然较差，5年生存率为10%。生存率较差的相关因素包括男性、年龄较大、分化差以及存在肝硬化[123-126]。肿瘤有包膜、较小以及肿瘤内有明显炎细胞浸润时预后较好[123,126]。认为组织学结构预后意义不大，但根据报道梁状型与侵袭性行为有关，而紫癜样型预后可能较好[125]。血管浸润、淋巴结转移以及手术切缘呈阳性与切除后复发有关[123,126,127]。

纤维板层型肝细胞癌
Fibrolamellar variant of HCC

临床特征：纤维板层型肝细胞癌（FLM）发生于年轻成人（平均年龄26岁，女性多于男性）的非硬化性肝组织[128-130]。临床表现包括腹痛或腹胀、厌食、体重减轻、黄疸，以及在少数情况下出现腹腔积血。尚未发现明确的危险因素。局灶结节性增生样结节偶见于 FLM 的周边[131,132]，可能为局部灌注异常的结果[133]，而非纤维板层型肝细胞癌的癌前病变[134]。血清 AFP 水平一般正常；但也有报道在极少数肿瘤中 AFP 水平较高[128,129]。

病理学特征

大体特征：FLM 质硬，褐白色至棕色，境界清楚，但无包膜，呈分叶状，发生在背景正常的肝组织（图 10.27）。多数肿瘤较大，可达 17 cm。较大肿瘤可出现出血和坏死灶。60%～70% 的肿瘤为单发，也可多发，一般呈卫星灶表现。已经注意到有少数病例累及左叶。可出现明显的中央星状瘢痕，类似局灶结节性增生[128]。瘢痕见于少数肿瘤，也可见于淋巴结转移。

显微镜下特征：FLM 的标志性特征为大的多角形肿瘤细胞，伴有多量嗜酸性颗粒状胞浆、明显的巨大核仁以及板层状纤维化带（图 10.28）。胶原板层由厚薄不一的板状结缔组织堆积而成。以胶原 I、III 和 V 为主，由间质中纤维母细胞产生。板层结构并不是均匀一致地分布于整个肿瘤，多数病例常占肿瘤成分的一半。肿瘤细胞一般排列成条索状或呈巢状。除了核仁明显以外，细胞核可见胞浆向核内内陷以及染色质边集。颗粒样胞浆是由于出现大量线粒体成分。胞浆的其他特征包括"淡染小体"，可能含有纤维蛋白原和（或）白蛋白；也可见 PAS-D 阳性小体，可能为糖蛋白分泌物。胆栓常见，但一般没有脂肪。偶见的其他特征包括腺泡结构、黏液分泌、多核肿瘤细胞、铜、上皮样肉芽肿以及肝紫癜。也可见与梁状肝细胞癌类似的区域[135]；尚不清楚是 FLM 的一个亚型，还是 FLM 与普通肝细胞癌的混合。

免疫组织化学染色，FLM 类似普通肝细胞癌，表达 Hep Par 1、多克隆 CEA 以及低分子量角蛋白。AFP 免疫反应均为阴性。据报道，神经内分泌标记物（见上）可呈局灶阳性，但无明确临床意义[94]。白蛋白原位杂交在多数病例中呈阳性[82]。

治疗和预后：FLM 为侵袭性肿瘤，5 年生存率不足 50%。目前治疗方法为完整切除受累肝叶。如果由于肿瘤部位或者范围不能进行手术切除，可进行肝移植，但结局不良。一些研究显示，FLM 预后比普通肝细胞癌好。然而，FLM 与发生于非硬化性肝组织的普通肝细胞癌两者的预后类似[136,137]。FLM 的预后较好可能与没有肝硬化以及较高的切除率有关，而不是由于其具有独特的临床病理特征。

混合性肝细胞癌-胆管癌
Combined hepatocellular-cholangiocarcinoma (HCC-CC)

临床特征：这是一种少见肿瘤，在原发性肝肿瘤中所占不足 5%。因有证据表明它常伴有 HBV 或 HCV 感染及肝硬化，故与肝细胞癌密切相关[138,139]。然而，这种信息主要是根据亚洲的研究，而美国一项大型病例研究显示，混合性肝细胞癌-胆管癌中，乙型或丙型肝炎血清学阳性及肝硬化的发生率小于 15%，类似胆管癌[140]。

病理学特征：诊断是根据出现肝细胞和腺体分化（图 10.29）。按照 WHO 标准，通过出现梁状结构、产生胆汁或细胞间小胆管来辨认肝细胞成分。而胆管癌成分是通过明确的腺体结构或黏液产物来确定。可

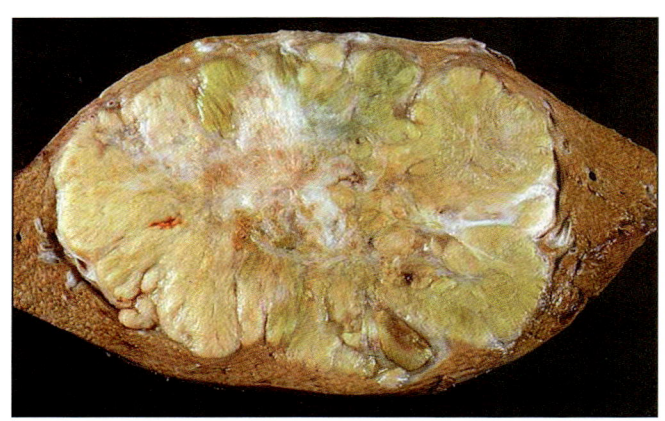

图 10.27 纤维板层型肝细胞癌，为褐-白色至棕色的无包膜分叶状肿物，伴有中央瘢痕。

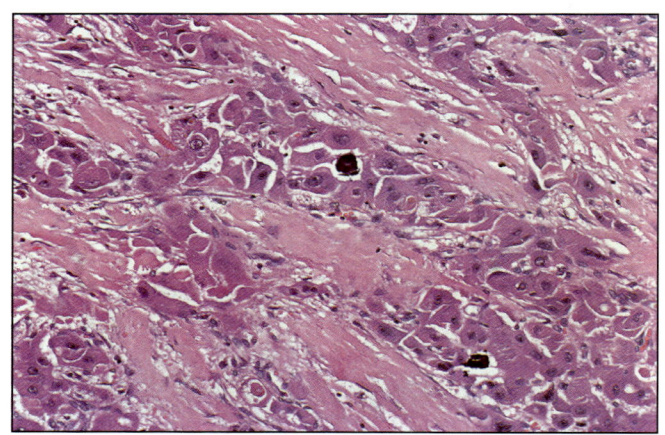

图 10.28 纤维板层型肝细胞癌显示大的多角形肿瘤细胞，伴有丰富的嗜酸性颗粒状胞浆、明显的巨大核仁以及板层带状纤维化。

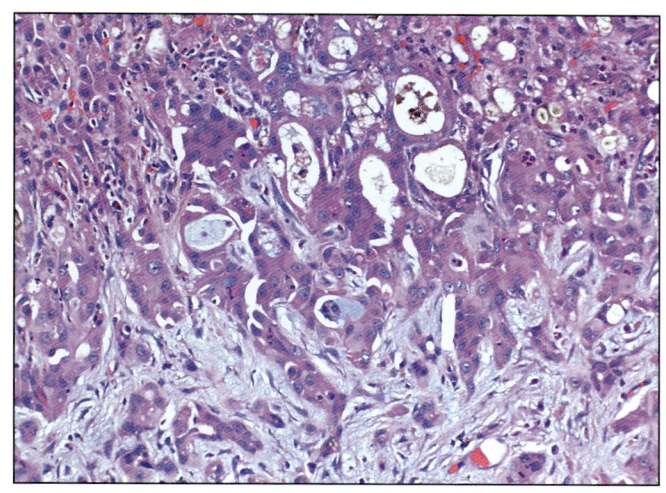

图10.29 混合性肝细胞癌-胆管癌。肿瘤出现肝细胞癌样多角形细胞的特征,具有丰富的胞浆和梁状结构,但是也可见含有碱性黏液或胆汁的腺样腔隙。还可出现胆管癌典型的间质纤维组织增生。

通过免疫组织化学染色来证实诊断,肝细胞癌成分表达 Hep Par 1、AFP 以及小管型多克隆 CEA;胆管癌成分表达 MOC31、CK7 和 CK19。常可出现肝细胞癌与胆管癌移行区域,原位杂交检测常显示两种成分均有白蛋白表达[141]。有些肿瘤可完全由细胞特征介于肝细胞癌与胆管癌之间的细胞构成,称为中间型癌(intermediate carcinomas)[142]。混合性肝细胞癌-胆管癌的组织发生尚不清楚,可能是肝细胞癌和胆管癌意外碰撞,或可能为单一肿瘤出现不同的分化[139,143]。前一种情况下,肿瘤可能为双克隆性,肝细胞癌和胆管癌成分没有紧密混杂。后一种情况下,肿瘤最初可能为肝细胞癌或胆管癌单克隆发生,然后向另一方面转化,或起源于伴有不同分化的中间型细胞。伴有中间型表型的混合性肝细胞癌-胆管癌 c-kit 常常阳性,支持其起源于祖细胞(progenitor cells)[142]。遗传学研究显示,多数混合型肝细胞癌-胆管癌起源于同一克隆,与普通肝细胞癌具有共同的异常改变,例如 4q、8p、17p 和 13q 等位基因缺失[143]。

预后和治疗:预后较差,本病比普通肝细胞癌或胆管癌更具侵袭性。切除之后,5 年生存率为 24%。对于未能切除的病例,几乎所有病人均在 2 年内死亡[140]。

肝母细胞瘤 Hepatoblastoma

临床特征

肝母细胞瘤为儿童最常见的恶性肝肿瘤,约占儿童恶性肿瘤的 1%。接近 90% 的病例发病时年龄在 6 个月至 5 岁之间。偶发于大龄儿童[144,145],极个别发生于成人[146]。病变较多见于男性,男女之比几乎为 2:1,但老年病例两性发病率相似。1/3 的病例伴有其他先天性病变,如 Beckwith-Wiedemann 综合征[145]、腭裂、膈疝[146]、Down 综合征、家族性结肠息肉病[148]、偏身肥大、肾畸形以及其他染色体异常[149]。多数病人表现为无症状性腹部肿块。体重减轻、厌食以及迅速增大的腹部肿块为常见症状。不常见的症状包括呕吐、腹泻或黄疸。少数情况下可出现诸如男性化等青春期早熟表现,这与肿瘤产生人绒毛膜促性腺激素(hCG)有关[150]。血清 AFP 几乎总是升高,是治疗后肿瘤复发或转移的有用标记物。

病理学特征

大体病理学:肝母细胞瘤发生于非硬化性肝组织,一般为大的孤立性肿物。大体表现可以多样,但肿瘤常呈多结节状,伴有出血和坏死灶(图 10.30)。由于肿瘤内不同结节或区域可能代表不同的组织成分,而

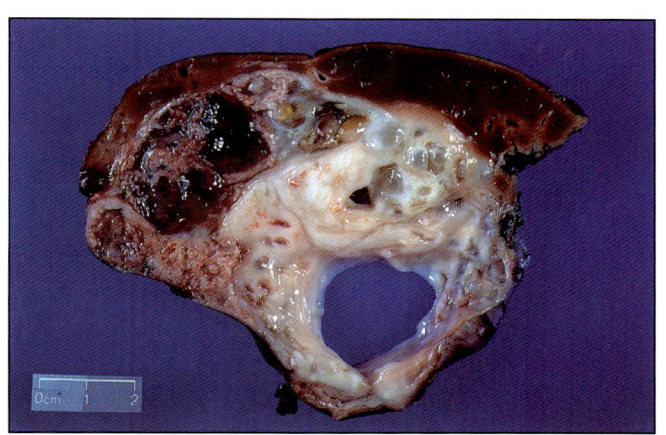

图10.30 肝母细胞瘤,肿瘤呈灰白色,多结节状,伴有出血及坏死区域。

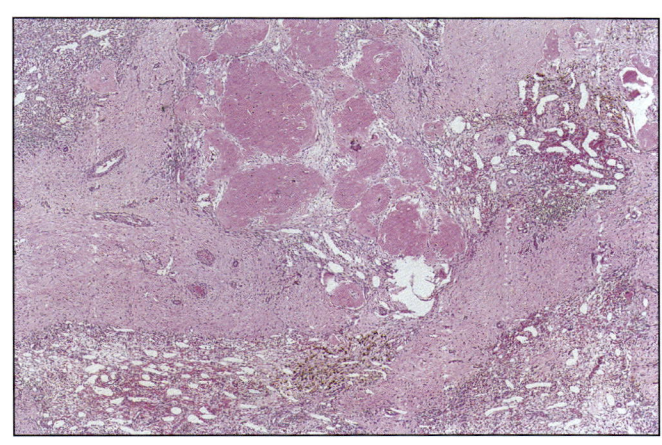

图10.31 肝母细胞瘤化疗后出现明显骨样成分。

组织成分又与预后相关,因而不同区域都应充分取材。化疗后肿瘤可明显坏死,而间质成分常较显著,尤其是骨样组织(图10.31)[151]。

显微镜下特征:肝母细胞瘤的两种形态学亚型为上皮型(55%)和上皮-间叶混合型(45%)。上皮型可出现胚胎型,胎儿型结构(图10.32),或两者混合存在(图10.33)。上皮-间叶混合型则由上皮和间叶成分混合构成。

胚胎型为较"不成熟"型,肿瘤细胞较小,排列成条索状、带状、花环样结构或小管状。细胞核呈圆形、卵圆形或细长形,并有少量嗜碱性胞浆。胎儿型较为"成熟",与胎儿肝极为类似,肿瘤细胞排列成板状或索条状。胎儿型的肿瘤细胞一般小于正常肝细胞,但比胚胎型的肿瘤细胞稍大,含有中等量的嗜碱性和(或)透明胞浆。透明细胞改变是由于含有脂质和(或)糖原。嗜酸性和透明胞浆的特征常出现于同一肿瘤中,导致极具特征性的粉色和苍白色交替出现的现象。胎儿型中的细胞核一般较小且圆,类似正常胎儿肝细胞。两种类型中核分裂象均极少见。髓外造血常可出现,常伴胎儿成分。

肝母细胞瘤不常见的上皮性亚型包括小细胞未分化型和巨梁型,总共约占5%。小细胞型由片块状肿瘤细胞构成,胞浆较少,类似于其他小蓝细胞肿瘤,例如神经母细胞瘤、Ewing肉瘤、淋巴瘤以及胚胎性横纹肌肉瘤。无肝细胞分化表现。识别肝母细胞瘤其他典型表现有助于明确诊断。巨梁型肝母细胞瘤形成大于10个细胞厚的较宽的梁状结构(图10.34)。胎儿型和(或)胚胎性肿瘤细胞一般构成这些梁状结构,但偶可见一种罕见的伴较多胞浆的大细胞类型,组织学上可能类似于肝细胞癌。出现其他肝母细胞瘤结构以及发生于非硬化性肝组织可能有助于区分这种巨梁型肝母细胞瘤和肝细胞癌。伴有有限巨梁成分的肿瘤应当依照其他主要结构来分类[152]。

几乎在半数病例中,上皮成分(胚胎型、胎儿型或两者)伴有间叶成分。在80%的混合性肿瘤中,间叶成分为不成熟的纤维组织、骨样组织和(或)软骨。剩余20%为肝母细胞瘤混有畸胎样特征,并出现其他组织类型,例如肠型腺体成分、鳞状上皮、黏液上皮、黑色素、骨骼肌或神经组织。

肝母细胞瘤胚胎型和胎儿型成分的肿瘤细胞表达AFP[153]。包括Hep Par 1以及多克隆CEA在内的肝细胞标记物上皮成分呈阳性,尤其是胎儿型上皮[154]。肝细胞型细胞角蛋白(8和18)以及胆管型细胞角蛋白(7和19)可呈不同程度阳性。有报道,胚胎型、胎儿型以及骨样成分呈嗜铬素A局灶阳性[153]。

鉴别诊断:单纯性胎儿型肝母细胞瘤组织学上可类似于腺瘤。肝母细胞瘤中的肿瘤细胞一般比腺瘤细胞小。肝母细胞瘤交替出现的粉色和苍白色胞浆染色一般在腺瘤中并不存在。临床资料对于区分这两种病变可能非常有用,因为5岁以前基本上不会发生肝细胞腺瘤,除非伴有代谢性疾病,例如糖原贮积病,并且腺瘤血清AFP

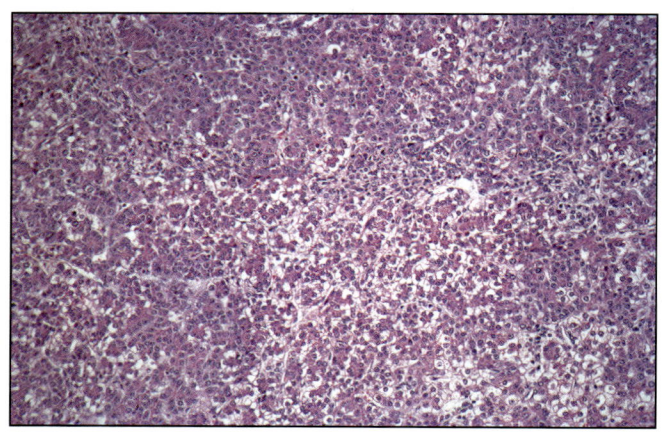

图10.32 肝母细胞瘤,胎儿型结构。

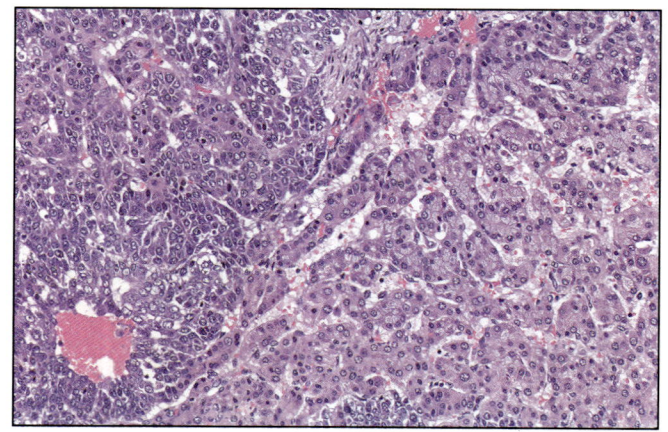

图10.33 肝母细胞瘤,胚胎型(左)及胎儿型(右)结构。

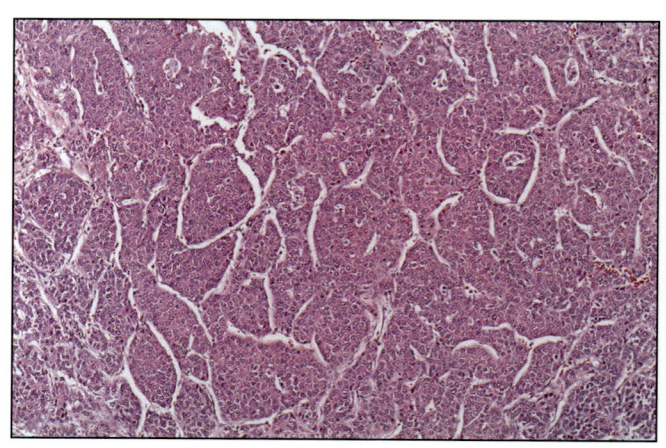

图10.34 肝母细胞瘤,巨梁型结构。小梁超过10个细胞厚。

不升高。临床检查在巨梁型肝母细胞瘤和肝细胞癌的鉴别方面也起重要作用，因为肝细胞癌也可发生于先前存在肝病或代谢性异常的年轻病人，通常为有肝硬化等情况下。出现肝母细胞瘤其他结构有助于诸如小细胞未分化及巨梁型等少见类型的诊断。伴有畸胎样特征的混合性肝母细胞瘤应当与畸胎瘤鉴别。后者缺乏肝母细胞瘤的胎儿型和胚胎型上皮成分。

分子遗传学改变：肝母细胞瘤细胞一般为二倍体或超倍体，而且出现限制性细胞遗传学改变，常累及1、2、8和20号染色体。最常见的改变为2及20号染色三体[155]。重排涉及1q和2q染色体，X染色体增加也有报道[156]。母系11p15杂合性缺失见于1/3的肝母细胞瘤。这是Beckwith-Wiedemann综合征病人的特征性改变，其发生肝母细胞瘤的危险性增加。11p15上的印记基因，例如IGF-2，在肝母细胞瘤中起重要作用[157]。Wnt/β-连环蛋白信号通路活化通过稳定性β-连环蛋白突变在肝母细胞瘤的发生过程中起重要作用。通过免疫组织化学染色可证实β-连环蛋白异常定位于多数肝母细胞瘤的细胞核。有些研究认为，上述改变在胚胎型及未分化肝母细胞瘤中比胎儿型更为常见，存活率低[157,158]，但其他研究并非如此[155]。APC突变见于散发性肝母细胞瘤以及伴有家族性腺瘤性息肉病的病例。p16基因由于过度甲基化而失活，导致细胞周期调节异常，与本病的发生有关[159]。

预后和治疗：预后与完整手术切除以及肿瘤分期直接相关[152]。5年存活率大约为75%[157]。治疗选择完整手术切除，但术前常采用化疗以缩小肿瘤，也用于残留肿瘤以及不能切除肿瘤的治疗。伴有无肝外扩散的多灶性、双叶性或复发性肝母细胞瘤的儿童，可选择肝移植治疗[160,161]。有些组织学亚型，如单纯性胎儿型，在完整切除后预后较好[144]。其他亚型，如小细胞及巨梁型预后较差[152]。切缘没有肿瘤极为重要，而血管浸润对于预后影响不大[144]。其他与预后不良相关的因素为年龄在1岁以下、肿瘤较大以及重要结构受累。

肝：良性间叶性肿瘤
Liver: benign mesenchymal tumors

海绵状血管瘤　Cavernous hemangioma
临床特征

海绵状血管瘤是肝最常见的原发性肿瘤，这种良性血管瘤一般在手术或尸检时偶然发现，可由于出血或体积较大而进行手术切除[162,163]。有人提出，雌激素疗法可导致肿瘤增大[162]。肝内这些肿瘤偶尔可为多发性，并可伴有其他部位血管瘤，成为von Hippel-Lindau病或骨骼/系统性血管瘤病综合征的一部分[164]。小血管瘤无症状，无需治疗。巨大血管瘤定义为4 cm或更大，可伴腹围增加、疼痛、恶心、黄疸或胆道出血，极少数可出现破裂[165,166]。较大血管瘤也可导致血小板减少或消耗性凝血病（Kasabach-Merritt综合征）[163,166]。

病理学特征

大体病理学：血管瘤为境界清楚的棕红色肿瘤，呈海绵样结构，表面为蜂窝状海绵样血管组织。许多肿瘤有血栓形成和硬化，使之质地较硬，呈白色至褐色外观（图10.35）。

显微镜下特征：这个肿瘤的标志是内衬单层扁平内皮细胞的海绵状血管腔隙，无细胞学非典型性或核分裂活性（图10.36）。这些血管腔隙的管壁由纤细的纤维性间质构成。扩张血管腔的分布常超出血管瘤主体的范围，类似于血管瘤病（图10.37）[167]。血管可出现血栓形成。可见硬化性区域，如硬化广泛，可类似局部瘢痕。

婴儿血管内皮细胞瘤
Infantile hemangioendothelioma

临床特征

婴儿血管内皮细胞瘤为3岁以下儿童第二个最常见肿瘤，仅次于肝母细胞瘤，几乎所有病例报道均发生于不到6个月大的婴儿。女孩发病率几乎为男孩的2倍[168,169]。10%~15%的病人其他器官出现血管瘤[163]。

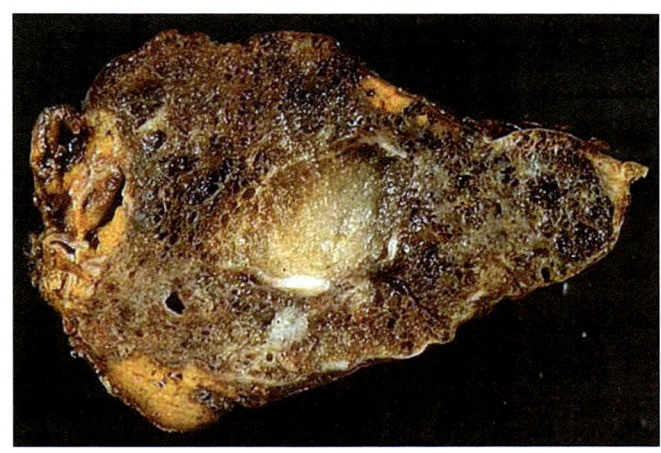

图10.35　海绵状血管瘤。大小不一的囊状出血性腔隙使之呈蜂窝状表现。中央白褐色区域为血栓形成和机化的结果。

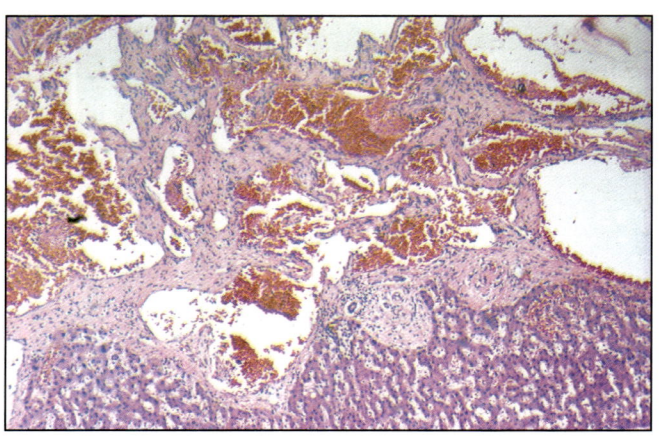

图10.36 海绵状血管瘤,肿瘤由被纤维组织分隔的较大血管腔隙构成,衬以扁平内皮细胞。

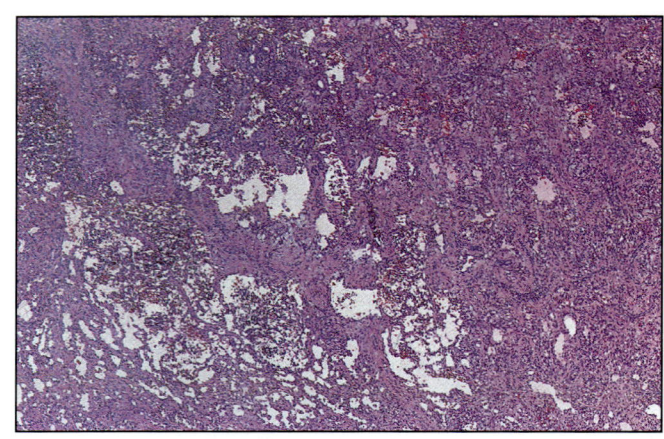

图10.38 婴儿血管内皮细胞瘤1型。不规则且大小不一的血管腔衬以一致的内皮细胞,被黏液样间质所包围。

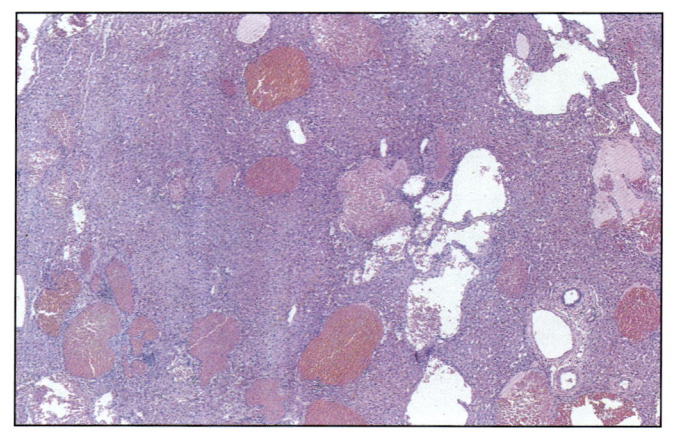

图10.37 海绵状血管瘤,扩张的血管腔常超出血管瘤主体范围,类似血管瘤病。

这种肿瘤也可伴有先天性异常,诸如双肾发育不全、Beckwith-Wiedemann 综合征、21 号染色体三体、偏身肥大或脊髓脊膜膨出[163,168]。婴儿血管内皮细胞瘤和间叶性错构瘤同时发生已有报道[170]。其临床特征为腹部肿物或腹胀,伴肝大、黄疸、腹泻、便秘、呕吐、充血性心力衰竭或发育不良[168]。其他少见表现包括肿瘤内血小板隔离造成的血小板减少症,或肿瘤破裂伴腹腔积血[8]。可出现 AFP 升高,但一般轻微[171]。

病理学特征

大体病理学:婴儿血管内皮细胞瘤常是一种境界不清的病变,可为实性和囊性,伴有大小不一的出血灶。几乎一半的肿瘤为多灶性,大小从不足 1 cm 至 15 cm 不等。

显微镜下特征:多数肿瘤由大量小血管腔和极少数较大的呈海绵样表现的不规则腔隙混合而成,周围以不成熟的含有散在胶原或网织纤维的纤维黏液瘤性间质(图10.38)。血管腔衬以单层内皮细胞。可有较多的核分裂象,但对预后没有影响。间质内可见小胆管和肝细胞,一般常接近肿瘤的周边。常可见局灶性坏死、出血、纤维化以及钙化。在一项综合性回顾中,Dehner 和 Ishak 将本病分为两种组织学类型[168]。上面提到的改变相当于 1 型病变。2 型病变为管腔结构不甚明显的相互吻合的腔隙,伴有乳头以及复杂的出芽或分支状结构。这些血管腔内衬以非典型性内皮细胞,细胞核较大、深染、细胞核边界不规则以及显著的核分裂活性[172,173]。2 型病变可为局灶性,建议肿瘤取材要充分。有些研究显示 2 型病变的肿瘤存在低度但明确侵袭性行为的危险性。如不考虑 2 型病变,多数病例的临床预后为良性。所有预后差的肿瘤均有 2 型病变。有些作者认为 2 型病变为侵袭性行为的标志,但并不等同于恶性肿瘤。然而,其他作者认为 2 型婴儿血管内皮细胞瘤为儿童血管肉瘤。支持这一观点的是有些病例出现实性病灶以及 Kaposi 样区域。这些病灶由成束梭形细胞构成,其间散布有 PAS 阳性抗淀粉酶小体。免疫组织化学染色,内皮细胞呈 CD34、CD31 以及 VIII 因子相关抗原阳性。间质细胞表达 α-SMA 和波形蛋白,缺乏结蛋白,这种染色结果与血管周细胞一致[174]。

预后和治疗:有关 2 型病变的意义尚有争议:有些人认为对预后没有影响[173],而其他人将 2 型婴儿血管内皮细胞瘤视为低级别血管肉瘤[163]。整体存活率为 70%,绝大多数死亡病例发生在诊断后第一个月内[163,173]。死亡率与肿瘤局限以及没有转移有关。出现心力衰竭、黄疸、多发性结节、浸润性边缘以及缺乏海绵样腔隙为预后不良的特征[172,173]。极少数伴有真性血管肉瘤病例已有报道[175]。肿瘤可自然消退，或者采用类固醇及α-干扰素治疗后消退。如果药物治疗失败，可考虑切除、肝移植、肝动脉结扎或栓塞[173,176]。

间叶性错构瘤　Mesenchymal hamartoma

临床特征

间叶性错构瘤不常见，几乎均发生于儿童，超过50%的病例在1岁以内确诊[177]。它是该年龄组第三种最常见的肝肿瘤，次于肝母细胞瘤和婴儿血管内皮细胞瘤[178]。仅有少数成人病例报告，最常见于女性[179]。病人常表现为可触及的肝肿物、腹部膨大或由于肿瘤压迫而出现呼吸窘迫。尚无已知的恶变危险。

病理学特征

大体病理学：肿瘤可为实性或囊性，伴有实性区域，一般呈褐色。有囊肿存在时常含有半透明液体或胶样物质[145,178]。这些囊肿的形成是由于肿瘤疏松间叶组织变性所致。这些囊肿内液体持续性聚集导致肿瘤体积增大。

显微镜下特征：间叶性错构瘤具有上皮及间质两种成分。前者由表现相对正常的肝细胞及胆管组成，均围以数量不等的黏液样或纤维化间质（图10.39）。肝细胞排列成大小不等的细胞簇，而且保留肝细胞板结构，如同正常肝组织。胆管结构一般呈分支状排列，胆管壁内或周围常有急性炎症细胞浸润。当囊腔存在时，内衬扁平至立方上皮细胞，并且围以疏松或致密纤维组织。囊肿也可没有任何内衬细胞。间质一般含有多量小血管、梭形细胞以及炎症细胞。见不到正常汇管区。常可出现髓外造血。在成人，间质显著纤维化且致密玻璃样变，仅有局灶黏液性区域[177]。某些病例中，间叶性成分可为病变的主要特征，伴有少量胆管成分。免疫组织化学染色，胆管成分表达CK7，无CK20表达。间质细胞SMA和波形蛋白呈阳性。涉及11、17和19号染色体的复杂染色体易位已有报道[180]。

预后和治疗

间叶性错构瘤为良性肿瘤，如完全切除预后良好[181]。由于间叶性错构瘤与von Meyenburg综合征的组织学类似，因而被认为是胆管板发育异常。然而，细胞遗传学异常以及偶尔出现非整倍体支持肿瘤性发病机制。有人根据其临床病理学特征存在交叉重叠，假设间叶性错构瘤与未分化胚胎性肉瘤之间有一定关系，而且已有胚胎性肉瘤发生于间叶性错构瘤的报道[182]。涉及19p染色体的类似遗传学异常可发生于间叶性错构瘤和胚胎性肉瘤。

血管肌脂肪瘤　Angiomyolipoma

临床特征

血管肌脂肪瘤在肝极为少见。肿瘤多见于30～40岁年龄段，女性占明显优势[95,183]。多数肝血管肌脂肪瘤并不伴有结节性硬化[95,183]。大约10%的病例发生于结节性硬化，并常伴有肾的血管肌脂肪瘤。已有超过15个肿瘤的多发性肝血管肌脂肪瘤报道[184]。肿瘤被认为向所谓的血管周围上皮样细胞（perivascular epithelioid cell, PEC）分化，其他器官的相关病变包括透明细胞"糖"瘤和淋巴管平滑肌瘤病[185]。

病理学特征

大体病理学：血管肌脂肪瘤可以较大，由于脂肪、坏死及出血而造成颜色各异（图10.40）[95,183]。

显微镜下特征：血管肌脂肪瘤由不同比例的平滑肌样细胞、血管和脂肪组成，常伴有造血细胞。平滑肌样分化在肝脏病变中常最为显著，由上皮样或梭形细胞构成，常围绕或"伴随"（spin off）血管（图10.41）。上皮样细胞呈圆形或多角形，伴有多量嗜酸性胞浆（图10.42）。细胞核一般较大，核仁明显，但其表现可以不同。胞浆成分可呈嗜酸性，而且细胞核周围的胞浆可能浓聚，靠近胞膜处有一透亮区，呈"蜘蛛网"（spider web）表现[95]。梭形细胞具有嗜酸性胞浆和小的卵圆形细胞核。以上皮样细胞为主要成分的小梁状结构也可见。可以上皮样或梭形细胞成分为主，而无其他成分。血管成分一般由厚壁动脉或静脉样管

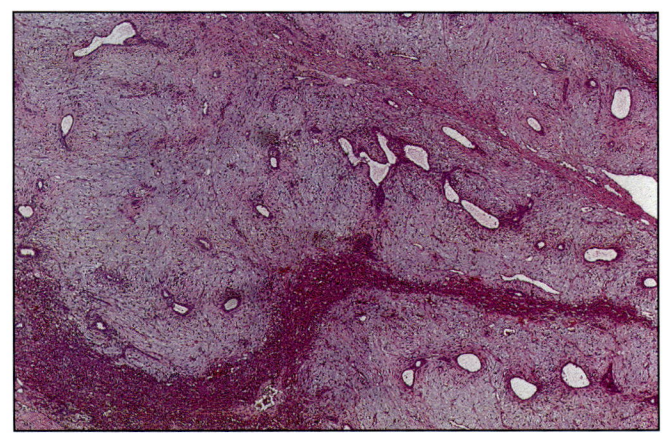

图10.39　间叶性错构瘤。导管成分位于纤维黏液样间质中。

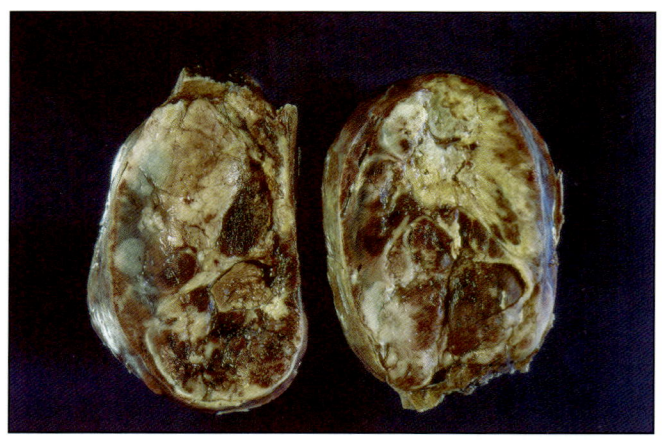

图10.40 血管肌脂肪瘤，肿瘤可以较大，伴有出血和坏死灶，类似于恶性病变。(Reproduced with permission from Ferrell L D 2003 Liver. In: Weidner N, Cote R J, Suster S, Weiss L M (eds) Modern surgical pathology. Saunders, Philadelphia, Fig.27-21, CD, p919–979.)

腔混合薄壁静脉样腔隙组成。脂肪组织由成熟脂肪细胞组成，单个、成簇或成片块状散布于整个肿瘤。肝的血管肌脂肪瘤，尤其是伴有单纯性窦状隙小梁状结构的单一型上皮样亚型，脂肪成分可能稀少或者缺乏[186]。含有细小脂滴的泡沫样细胞也常可见。可出现与出血区域密切相关的紫癜性腔隙。这些腔隙大多缺少内皮细胞衬覆。还可见由T细胞和B细胞混合而成的较为致密淋巴细胞聚集。极少数情况下，炎症细胞可伴有肿瘤间质的梭形细胞成分，类似于炎性假瘤。含铁血黄素和黑色素可见。在间质中常可见数量不等的造血成分，包括巨核细胞、红细胞系和髓细胞系的前体细胞。

多数诊断问题在于完全由上皮样平滑肌样细胞构成的单一型肿瘤，其细胞核大且圆，伴有明显的核仁和丰富的嗜酸性胞浆，类似于肝细胞癌、肝细胞腺瘤或转移性黑色素瘤。伴有梁状结构的上皮样亚型常缺少脂肪，更类似于肝细胞肿瘤。组织学上，肿瘤中出现胆汁和Mallory透明小体倾向于肝细胞癌。免疫组织化学染色，血管肌脂肪瘤一致性表达黑色素细胞标记物，诸如HMB-45（图10.43）、Melan A、酪氨酸酶以及小眼转录因子。另外，95%以上病例中，平滑肌样成分SMA呈阳性。梭形细胞成分SMA染色阳性常明显，而上皮样细胞HMB-45阳性较强[95]。有半数病例超微结构检查可见黑色素小体[187]。梭形细胞也可呈结蛋白阳性[95]。细胞角蛋白和Hep Par 1染色呈阴性。局灶S-100表达可见于血管肌脂肪瘤，一般位于上皮样细胞和脂肪细胞[95]。已有报道，血管肌脂肪瘤一致表达c-kit（CD117）[188]；其意义尚不明确，而且尚无影响治疗的证据。

预后和治疗：血管肌脂肪瘤为良性病变，切除可以治愈。目前尚无复发报道[189,190]。

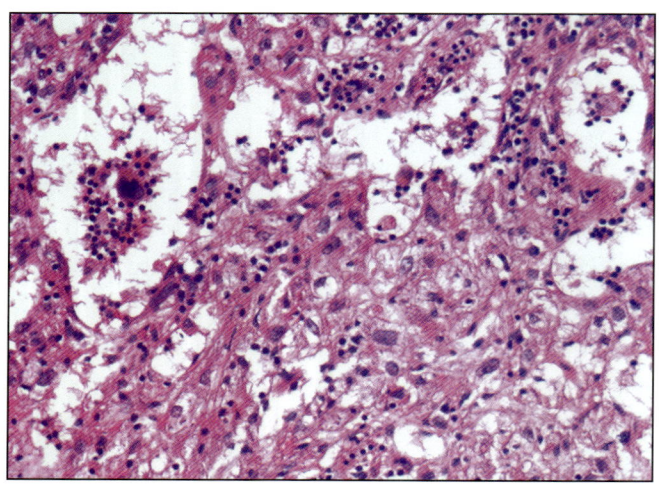

图10.41 血管肌脂肪瘤。梭形至多角形的肌样肿瘤细胞，伴有明显的血管成分和髓外造血。

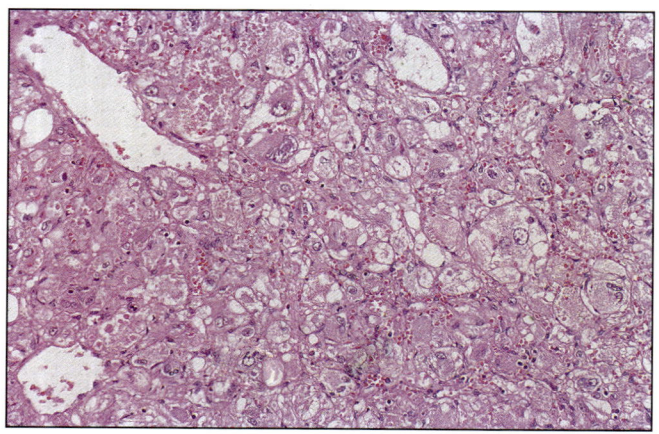

图10.42 伴有上皮样肿瘤细胞的单一型血管肌脂肪瘤。易被误诊为肝细胞肿瘤。

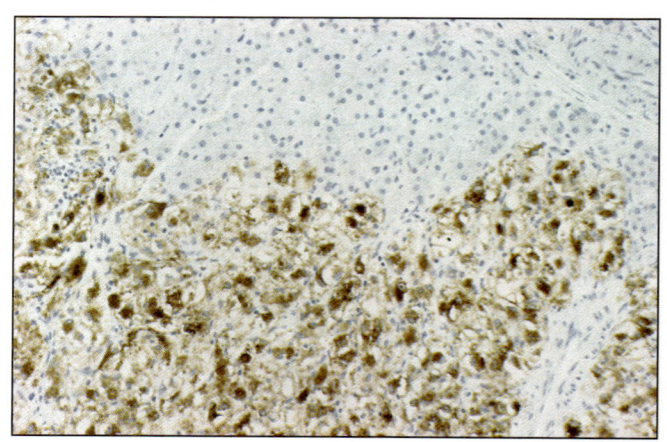

图10.43 血管肌脂肪瘤。HMB-45染色上皮样肿瘤细胞呈阳性（下部），而肝细胞呈阴性（上部）。

炎性假瘤 Inflammatory pseudotumor

临床特征

炎性假瘤是一种炎症性和纤维化性病变，多发生于肺及纵隔，极少数发生于肝[191-193]。本病的同义词包括炎症性肌纤维母细胞瘤和浆细胞肉芽肿。占所有局灶性肝脏病变的0.4%[194]。从目前看，肝炎性假瘤名下的病变好像具有异源性本质。病人可表现为腹痛、发热、寒战、黄疸、呕吐和体重减轻。伴有原发性硬化性胆管炎[193]、炎症性肠病、胆石症、儿童Papillon-Lefevre综合征、Kostmann病、白血病以及HIV的病例已有报道[195]。如果位于肝门部，临床上可被误认为是胆管癌。其发病机制尚不清楚，但感染、自身免疫以及实质内出血与其有关。Epstein-Barr病毒在多个部位已有发现，包括肝[196]。有些人提出后一种肝细胞病变实际上为滤泡性树突状细胞（follicular dendritic cell，FDC）肉瘤[196,197]。

病理学特征

大体病理学：病变表现差异较大，尤其是较大的病变，伴有灶状纤维化、出血和坏死[192]。肿瘤大小差别很大，可为孤立性或多发性。孤立性病变一般较大（2～15 cm）且位于肝门。病变为多发时一般较小，两叶均受累，可能类似于转移性病变[192,198]。

显微镜下特征：炎性假瘤由炎症及纤维组织混合而成，但这些成分的相对比例存在差异（图10.44）。可分为透明硬化性、黄色肉芽肿性以及浆细胞肉芽肿等几种类型，但在单个病变中可出现各种类型表现，因此这种分类作用不大[199]。病变的炎症成分一般含有多克隆性浆细胞，但常可见数量不等的中性粒细胞、嗜酸性细胞、淋巴细胞（主要为T细胞）以及巨噬细胞（通常为黄色肉芽肿性）[191,193]。梭形细胞成分由（肌）纤维母细胞构成，一般呈束状结构，常可见硬化性病灶。核分裂象可以见到，但不应过多，且无异常核分裂象[192]。偶尔也可见肉芽肿或静脉炎[191,193]。

鉴别诊断包括肝脓肿以及恶性间叶性肿瘤，例如血管肉瘤、平滑肌肉瘤以及转移性胃肠间质肉瘤。这些肉瘤出现细胞学非典型性，核分裂象多见，且常缺少多量炎症细胞。免疫组织化学染色可能有所帮助，血管肉瘤表达VIII因子相关抗原和其他血管内皮标记物，平滑肌肉瘤表达结蛋白，而转移性胃肠道间质肉瘤表达CD117。与滤泡性树突状细胞肿瘤鉴别可能比较困难，但缺乏浆细胞、出现多形性肿瘤细胞以及表达滤泡性树突状细胞肿瘤特异性标记物，例如CD21、CD35和R4/23，均支持为滤泡性树突状细胞肿瘤[197,199]。

预后和治疗

炎性假瘤为良性病变，但根据其发生部位以及在手术前与恶性病变不能准确鉴别情况下，可能需要切除大部肝组织。多数病人切除后完全康复，没有复发。内科治疗一般无效[200]。多发性小病变似乎比较复杂，可能无需任何特殊治疗[198]。

其他良性肿瘤和瘤样病变 Other benign tumors and tumor-like lesions

已经发现的肝良性肿瘤包括软骨瘤[201]、神经鞘瘤[202]、孤立性纤维性肿瘤[203]、纤维瘤、平滑肌瘤、脂肪瘤、淋巴管瘤病、黏液瘤以及肾上腺和胰腺残留[163]。

肝：恶性间叶性肿瘤 Liver: malignant mesenchymal tumors

血管肉瘤 Angiosarcoma

临床特征

血管肉瘤为罕见的原发性恶性肿瘤，占所有原发性肝脏肿瘤的2%，是肝最常见的恶性间叶性肿瘤，一般发生于中年成人，但在少数情况下可见于儿童[204]，偶发于婴儿血管内皮细胞瘤[173]。危险因素包括接触胶体钍、砷和乙烯基氯化物[205]。与之相关的其他物质如环磷酰胺以及合成代谢类固醇已有报道，但75%以上的病例没有明显的危险因素[205]。临床表现可能包括肝大、腹水、黄疸、血小板减少、腹腔积血和肝衰竭。

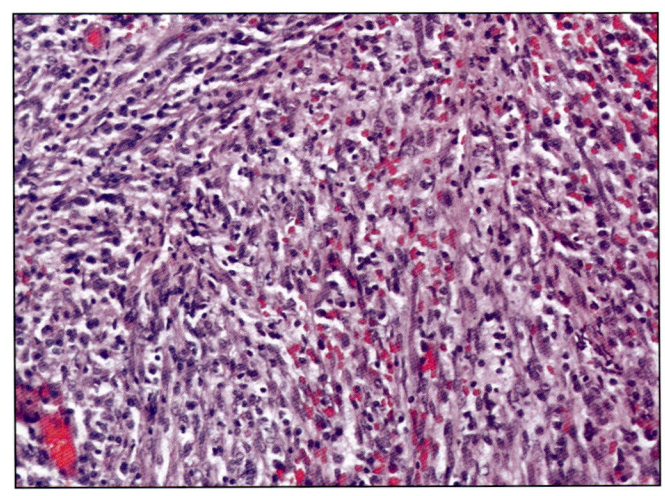

图10.44 炎性假瘤。一致的梭形细胞成分伴有致密淋巴细胞和浆细胞浸润。

病理学特征

大体病理学　血管肉瘤一般为较大的出血性肿瘤，境界不清，伴有程度不一的实性或囊性区域，囊性区域常含有血液成分（图10.45）。肿瘤大小一般在 4～20 cm 之间不等。可见卫星结节。

显微镜下特征　肿瘤在组织学上一般具有混合性窦隙状、实性、乳头状及海绵状生长结构。窦隙状结构最具特点，内皮细胞衬覆于肝细胞板两侧，呈支架样排列，将肝细胞板分开，常导致窦状隙扩张（图10.46）。衬覆于肝细胞板的肿瘤细胞量多，深染，而且大于正常内皮细胞。这种窦隙状结构多半位于肿瘤周边部，可能为早期生长结构，后来转变为实性或乳头状结构。实性结构可为梭形细胞束或呈漩涡状表现。乳头状结构由被覆肿瘤细胞的向腔内突出间质结节组成（图10.47）。海绵状结构由大的充血腔隙构成，常伴有其他结构类型。肿瘤细胞可以为梭形或上皮样。可出现细胞核多形性、奇异

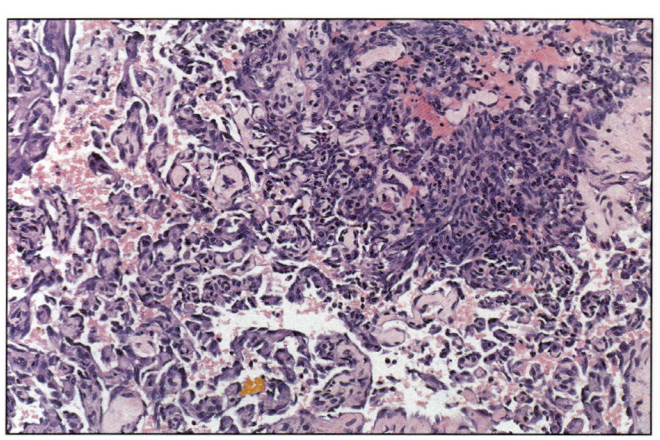

图10.47　血管肉瘤。肿瘤呈乳头状结构，伴有被覆肿瘤细胞的纤维组织结节状赘生物。

性细胞核、多核细胞以及较多核分裂象。常见侵犯肝小静脉和门静脉分支，可能是由于出血和坏死的缘故。显著的门静脉周围以及包膜纤维化见于乙烯基氯化物和胶体钍相关性病例。在 Kupffer 细胞、汇管区结缔组织以及静脉壁中可见胶体钍沉积，表现为颗粒状折光的粉棕色沉积物[206]。

肿瘤细胞表达内皮细胞标记物，例如 VIII 因子相关抗原、CD31 和 CD34，但所有肿瘤细胞着色并非均匀一致。这有助于与肝细胞癌、转移癌和其他间叶性肿瘤的鉴别。

遗传学改变

肝血管肉瘤的特征为 *p53* 突变、*K-ras-2* 突变以及由于过度甲基化引起的 *p16* 失活[207]。乙烯基氯化物相关性肿瘤具有高频率 *K-ras-2* 基因 G → A 转换以及 *p53* 基因 A:T → T:A 易位。

预后和治疗

肿瘤根治性切除为最佳的治疗方式，但鉴于病变范围广泛，并非总是可行。诊断后平均存活 6 个月[209]。

上皮样血管内皮细胞瘤
Epithelioid hemangioendothelioma

临床特征

上皮样血管内皮细胞瘤（EHE）为罕见的低级别恶性肿瘤，主要累及成人（30～40 岁），较常见于女性[210,211]，儿童罕见[212]。尚无已知的危险因素，有报道与口服避孕药有关，但尚未得到证实。许多病变为偶然发现，症状可能包括上腹部肿物或不适。多发性病变极为常见，可能类似于转移性疾病。血清碱性磷酸酶水平可能升高。

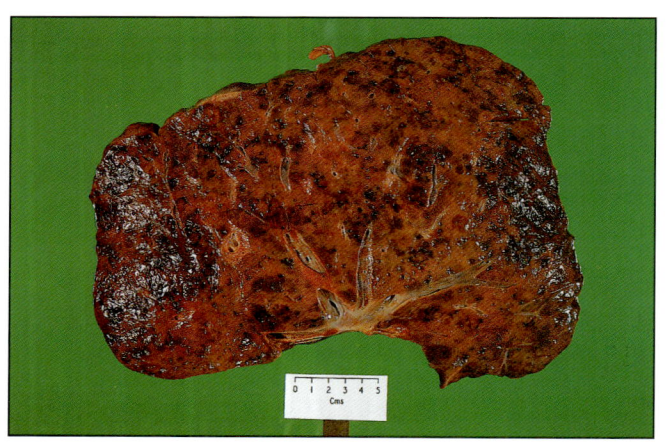

图10.45　血管肉瘤。肿瘤为出血性，伴有坏死区，而且边界不规则。（Courtesy of Dr. P. Anthony.）

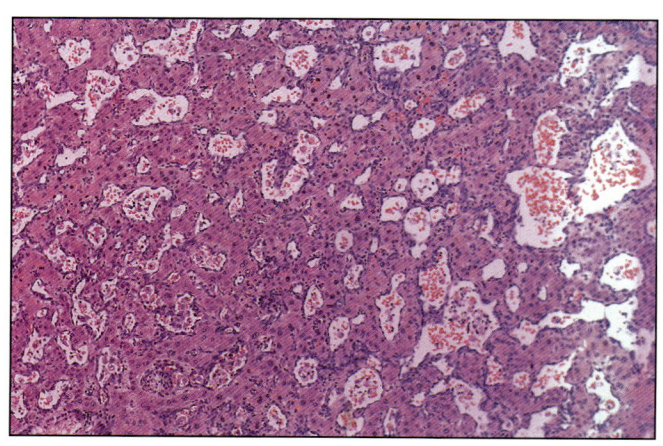

图10.46　血管肉瘤，窦隙状结构。

病理学特征

大体病理学：上皮样血管内皮细胞瘤为质硬的白色至黄色肿瘤，境界常常不清（图10.48）。分为两种不同类型：结节型为病变早期，见于大约10%的病例；弥漫型被认为是晚期病变，由多发性病变融合而成。肿瘤可为多灶性，累及左右两个肝叶。可见局灶钙化，使其质地有些呈沙粒样。

显微镜下特征：上皮样血管内皮细胞瘤的中心常为纤维性，细胞稀少，而周边部分细胞丰富（图10.49）。肿瘤倾向于环绕性生长，并完整保留原有的结构，例如汇管区和终末肝小静脉。肿瘤还特别容易侵犯血管结构，例如门静脉和中央静脉，可能类似于血管血栓形成的组织学表现。薄壁血管腔内可见小的乳头状突起或细胞簇。肿瘤内可见残留的肝细胞或胆管，尤其是靠近周边的区

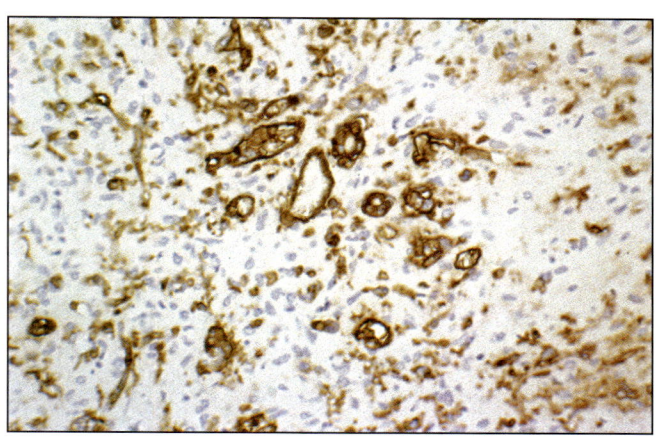

图10.50　上皮样血管内皮细胞瘤。CD34染色显示肿瘤细胞的内皮细胞属性。

域。肿瘤细胞可呈树突状或上皮样表现。树突状细胞形状不规则，细长或为星状，伴有分支状突起。胞质内可含有空泡，认为是细胞内腔隙，其中可含有红细胞。上皮样肿瘤细胞呈圆形，伴有较丰富的嗜酸性胞浆。上皮样细胞可见细胞核的非典型性和核分裂象。两种类型的细胞均被黏液样到纤维性间质包绕。较为致密的间质可以出现钙化。常可出现散在的炎症细胞，例如淋巴细胞和中性粒细胞。

主要鉴别诊断为腺癌（包括胆管癌）、血管肉瘤和肝细胞癌。可能有助于诊断的特征包括年轻、多发性病变、病变周边肿瘤浸润的特征性结构以及偶见钙化等表现。然而，需要应用免疫组织化学检测内皮细胞标记物，例如CD34（图10.50）、CD31和（或）VIII因子相关抗原来证实诊断。血管肉瘤也表达上皮细胞标记物，但其破坏性较强，而且常出现较大程度的细胞核非典型性和核分裂象。肿瘤角蛋白局灶阳性是由于有陷入的肝细胞和胆管，而且有些病例的肿瘤细胞也呈阳性表达，可被误认为癌[213]。另一个偶尔可遇到的诊断问题是上皮样血管内皮细胞瘤与静脉血栓形成/静脉阻塞性疾病的鉴别，因为肿瘤生长于大血管腔内，可能类似于血栓机化。

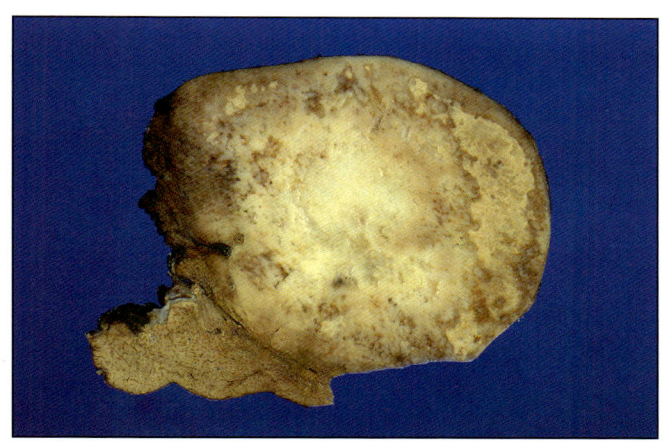

图10.48　上皮样血管内皮细胞瘤。肿瘤质硬，白色。
(Reproduced with permission from Ferrell L D 2003 Liver. In: Weidner N, Cote R J, Suster S, Weiss L M (eds) Modern surgical pathology. Saunders, Philadelphia, Fig.27-25, CD, p919-979.)

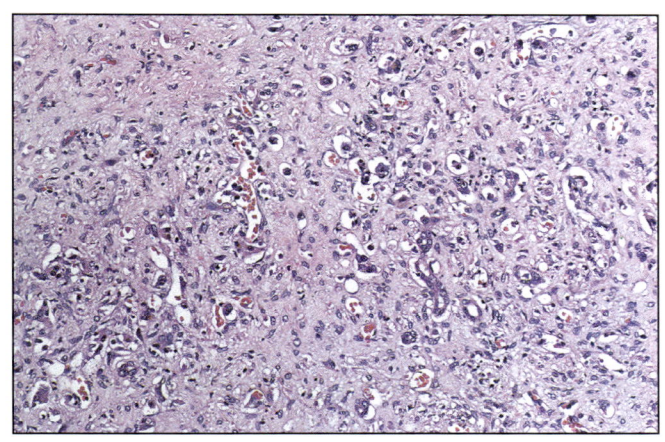

图10.49　上皮样血管内皮细胞瘤。分化较差的血管结构衬以上皮样肿瘤细胞，位于纤维性间质中。

预后和治疗

肿瘤的自然病程差异很大，有些病例未经治疗或未能完整切除也可长期存活，而另外一些病例尽管进行了完整切除和辅助治疗，但预后较差[211,214]。主要治疗方法为肝切除。对于不能切除的病例，肝移植已经取得成功[215]，然而，尚未得到长期生存的相关资料。肝外病变不是肝移植的禁忌证[216]。分化较差的肿瘤表达p53，而且血管内皮生长因子的表达减少[217]。总预后好于血管肉瘤，即使是未能完整切除或出现肝外转移。放疗或化疗对于上皮样血管内皮细胞瘤一般无反应，尽管偶有

报道，个别肿瘤采用干扰素 2-α 和动脉内 5-氟尿嘧啶治疗使瘤体减小[218]。

未分化胚胎性肉瘤
Undifferentiated embryonal sarcoma

临床特征

未分化胚胎性肉瘤为少见肿瘤，一般发生于 6～10 岁的儿童[219]。它是儿童最常见的肝恶性间叶性肿瘤。从前分别称为肝的恶性间叶瘤、纤维黏液肉瘤以及横纹肌肉瘤。腹部肿物和腹痛为常表现[219,220]。

病理学特征

大体病理学：胚胎性肉瘤一般较大，质软，伴有程度不一的囊性和实性区域，表面呈白色，有光泽，呈胶样或黏液样表现。常见坏死和出血区域。

显微镜下特征：肿瘤境界可能清楚，但常浸润到假包膜以外的肝组织中。肿瘤由梭形细胞和星状细胞混合而成，包裹于黏液样间质中（图 10.51）。肿瘤细胞具有颗粒状至泡沫状的淡粉色胞质，而且可能含有不同大小的胞质内小体，抗淀粉酶 PAS 染色呈阳性。这些小体也可见于间质中。其他特征包括较大的非典型性肿瘤细胞，伴有深染的细胞核、多核肿瘤细胞以及活跃的核分裂象。间质一般呈黏液样，但可见一些致密的胶原。髓外造血常见，周边部位可见陷入其中的肝细胞和（或）小胆管。波形蛋白和 bcl-2 为仅有的表达较为一致的免疫组织化学标记物，但是均不具有特异性[221]。常出现局灶阳性结果的标记物包括角蛋白、结蛋白和 α1-抗胰蛋白酶[220,222]。Hep Par 1、S-100、成肌素（myogenin）和 CD34 为阴性[221]。

遗传学改变

多发性染色体扩增及缺失已有报道，没有任何特征性改变[223]。19q13 染色体易位在胚胎性肉瘤和间叶性错构瘤中均可见[222]。其他间叶性肿瘤的 19q 部位也有改变，例如骨肉瘤和脂肪肉瘤。

预后和治疗

预后较差，大宗病例研究显示，长期存活率仅为 20%[219]。完整手术切除一般具有最好的结果[220,222]。由于在诊断时肿瘤一般较大，因而完整切除可能具有挑战性。现已有报道，采用术前和术后辅助性治疗可以改善预后[222]。

Kaposi 肉瘤　Kaposi sarcoma

临床特征

Kaposi 肉瘤常发生于免疫抑制情况下的肝组织，如获得性免疫缺陷综合征（AIDS）和肝移植。在免疫抑制病人中，人类疱疹病毒-8 与 Kaposi 肉瘤的发生有关[224]。

病理学特征

肝 Kaposi 肉瘤的多数表现与其他部位类似。肿瘤为纤维性到出血性，通常为多灶性，而且常以汇管区为中心。肿瘤由成束梭形细胞组成，伴有裂隙样腔隙。与其他部位的肿瘤相同，细胞多形性和核分裂活性程度较轻，典型者出现红细胞外渗、含铁血黄素沉积和小的嗜酸性小体。一般仅见于肝的一种结构是梭形肿瘤细胞在窦状隙内或沿窦状隙生长，大多位于肿瘤结节的周边部分（图 10.52）。这种生长结构导致扩张的

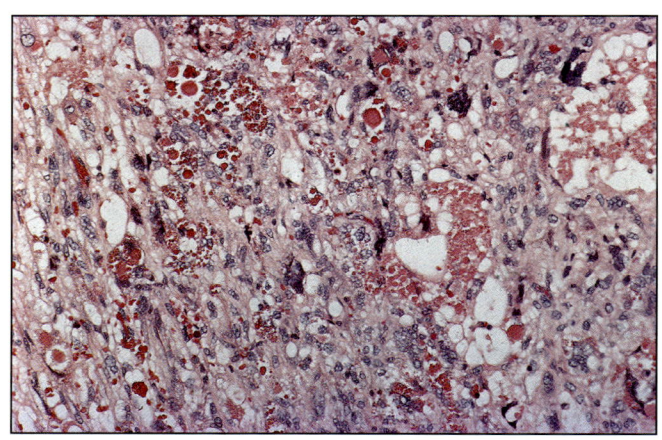

图 10.51　未分化胚胎性肉瘤，较大的非典型性肿瘤细胞位于黏液样间质中。注意细胞核深染和明显的胞质内小体。

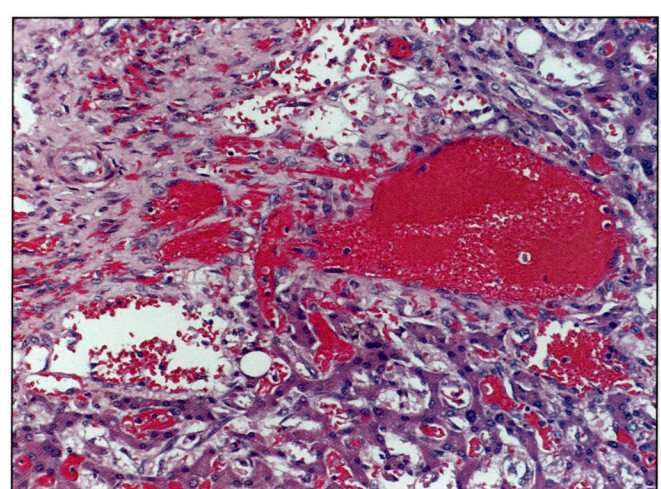

图 10.52　Kaposi 肉瘤。肿瘤常以汇管区为中心，向邻近肝实质扩展。肿瘤细胞沿窦状隙生长，导致窦状隙扩张和肝紫癜样表现。

含有红细胞的管腔取代了正常窦状隙，这种形态具有紫癜样表现。肿瘤也容易环绕或浸润汇管区，常保持肝动脉和小叶间胆管的完整性。免疫组织化学染色，肿瘤细胞内皮标记物 CD31 和 CD34 呈阳性，人类疱疹病毒 -8 也呈阳性，可能有助于 Kaposi 肉瘤与纤维母细胞增生的鉴别。

预后和治疗

Kaposi 肉瘤对于 HIV 阳性病人的预后是否有明显影响尚不清楚。致死性播散性 Kaposi 肉瘤发生于肝移植受者已有报道[225]。

造血细胞恶性肿瘤
Hematopoietic malignancies

各种类型的白血病和淋巴瘤（Hodgkin 和非 -Hodgkin）均可累及肝[225]。白血病累及肝时一般呈弥漫性，伴有白血细胞浸润肝窦，但慢性淋巴细胞性和急性淋巴母细胞性白血病例外，常累及汇管区，类似于淋巴瘤性浸润的结构。毛细胞性白血病还可形成肝紫癜样病变，由内衬肿瘤细胞的扩张窦隙所组成。

Hodgkin 淋巴瘤累及肝常呈结节状肿物，位于汇管区内。应当找到 Reed-Sternberg 细胞才能明确诊断，但如其他部位已经确诊为 Hodgkin 淋巴瘤，出现淋巴细胞浸润且混有浆细胞、嗜酸性细胞和一些非典型性细胞也可以诊断。偶尔，上皮样肉芽肿可见于肝实质或汇管区内，但仅有肉芽肿而没有上述其他特征情况下则不足以诊断。极少数情况下可出现肝内胆汁淤积，偶可伴有胆管缺失[226]。

非 -Hodgkin 淋巴瘤累及肝常作为播散性病变的一部分，在门管处形成结节状肿物。有些淋巴瘤可出现肿瘤细胞浸润窦状隙，类似于白血病所见[227]。肝组织受累特别常见于外周 T 细胞淋巴瘤，发生于多达 50% 的病人[228]。肝内胆汁淤积和上皮样肉芽肿等类似于 Hodgkin 淋巴瘤的所见也有报道。

肝原发性淋巴瘤罕见，占所有结外淋巴瘤的 0.4%。可能会有邻近淋巴结受累和肝外播散，但肝组织受累为主要临床表现。已有报道与 AIDS、乙型和丙型肝炎、免疫抑制治疗、自身免疫性疾病以及原发性胆汁性肝硬化有关[229]。这些肿瘤表现为孤立性或多发性肿物，偶可弥漫性浸润肝组织。多数淋巴瘤为弥漫性大 B 细胞型，其他像 Burkitt 淋巴瘤和低级别黏膜相关性 B 细胞淋巴瘤已有报道。能够切除的肿瘤选择手术切除，尽管早期病变目前选择化疗后放疗的治疗方法。5 年无复发存活率已达到 70%[230]。肝脾 T 细胞淋巴瘤起源于细胞毒性 γδ T 细胞，常累及肝，伴有窦状隙浸润和不同程度的汇管区受累[231]。脾和骨髓伴发受累常见。这些肿瘤具有高度侵袭性，平均存活 1 年。

其他恶性肿瘤

类癌、纤维肉瘤、所谓的恶性纤维组织细胞瘤、滤泡性树突状细胞肿瘤、平滑肌肉瘤、脂肪肉瘤、恶性间叶瘤、骨肉瘤、嗜铬细胞瘤、浆细胞瘤、恶性横纹肌样肿瘤、横纹肌肉瘤、恶性神经鞘瘤、鳞状细胞癌、恶性滋养细胞肿瘤、畸胎瘤和卵黄囊瘤等均可为肝原发性恶性肿瘤[232-240]。混合有上皮和间质成分的恶性肿瘤已有报道，可能是一种异源性肿瘤，例如混合性肝母细胞瘤和肉瘤样癌。有些病例出现骨化，称为骨化性间质 - 上皮肿瘤（ossifying stromal-epithelial tumor）[232,241]。

转移性肿瘤中，肺、乳腺、结肠和胰腺是最常见的原发部位，但任何部位的肿瘤均可播散至肝。黑色素瘤和神经内分泌肿瘤经常转移至肝，可能与肝细胞癌混淆。也可出现类似于肝硬化的弥漫性结节性肝浸润，最常见于转移性乳腺癌[242]。肝内胆管播散可见于转移性结肠腺癌，可能类似于胆管癌[243]。平滑肌肉瘤和胃肠道间质肉瘤为转移至肝的最常见间叶性肿瘤[232]。

胆囊：良性肿瘤
Gallbladder: benign neoplasms

腺瘤　Adenoma
临床特征

腺瘤不常见，但依然是胆囊最常见的良性肿瘤[244]。在成人，女性明显容易受累。症状类似于慢性胆囊炎，但常不伴有炎症或结石。已经发现胆囊腺瘤与 Gardner 综合征有关[245]。

病理学特征

大体病理学：腺瘤直径一般为 0.5 ~ 2 cm，大约 30% 的病例为多发性[244,246]。肿瘤一般有蒂，但有些可能无蒂。

显微镜下特征：病变可呈管状、乳头状或管状乳头状。管状腺瘤最为常见，由小而密集的腺体构成，被纤维性间质分开。间质一般稀少，但也可以比较明显，水肿性或玻璃样变。管状腺瘤可为幽门型或肠型（图 10.53）。幽门型管状腺瘤最常见，可有局灶鳞状梭形细胞化生[247]。乳头状腺瘤具有分支状树样结构，伴有纤维血管结缔组织轴心。轴心被覆单层立方到柱状上皮。

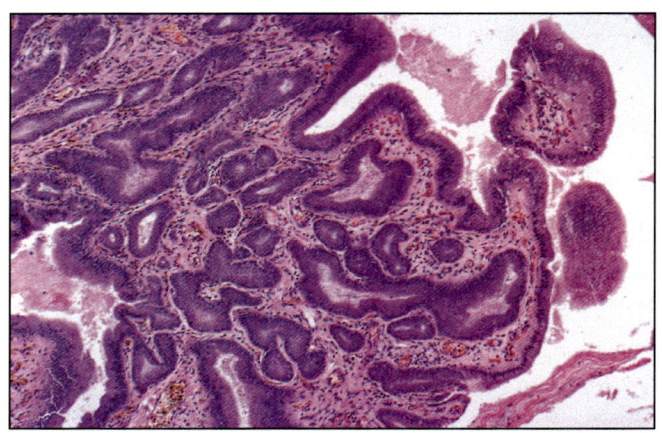

图10.53　胆囊：管状腺瘤，幽门型。

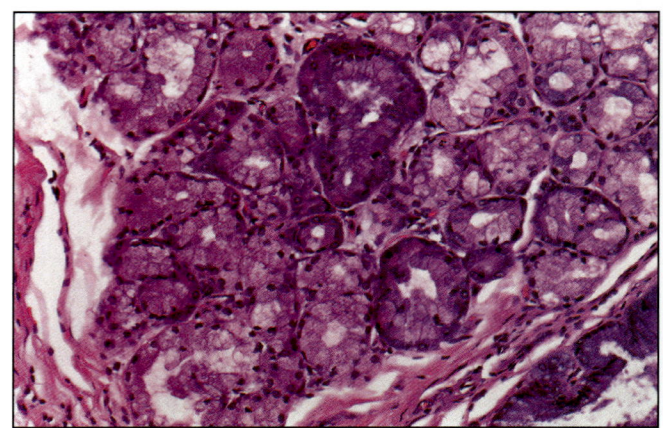

图10.54　胆囊：化生，幽门型。

较大的病变常有明显的异型增生，有些病例可出现原位癌灶[245]。

预后和治疗

腺瘤为良性病变，胆囊切除可以治愈。早期腺癌见于13.7%～39%的腺瘤[248]。较大的腺瘤（>12 mm）多半隐匿有腺癌灶[249]。有症状的息肉病人应当进行胆囊切除。对于无症状的病人，如果息肉无蒂、多发或大于1 cm时也应当考虑手术切除[250]。有人提出腺瘤-癌序列，与结肠肿瘤类似[251]，但腺瘤在胆囊癌发生中的作用尚有争议（见下）。

其他罕见良性肿瘤
Other rare benign tumors

颗粒细胞瘤极少发生于胆囊，但较多见于肝外胆管。发生于胆囊的良性间叶性肿瘤，例如脂肪瘤、平滑肌瘤、血管瘤以及淋巴管瘤均有报道。少数情况下，副神经节瘤可发生于胆囊，呈良性过程[252]。

胆囊：化生和异型增生
Gallbladder: metaplasia and dysplasia

总的来说，腺癌的发生机制被认为是由异型增生（非典型性增生）进展到癌[253,254]，或从腺瘤到癌[251]。化生性改变可能是或不是癌前病变[253-258]，但胆囊化生伴有腺癌的发生率较高，尤其是伴有肠型分化的腺癌[255,258]。

化生　Metaplasia

胆囊化生性上皮主要有两种类型：胃化生和肠化生，两者均容易发生在慢性胆囊炎基础上[258]，并与异型增生或腺癌有关[259,260]。

胃化生（gastric metaplasia）重现胃幽门或胃窦黏膜。局灶性胃化生见于大约50%有慢性炎症的胆囊。这种病变开始于隐窝基底，呈分支或出芽改变；这些腺体呈分叶状表现，类似于胃窦或幽门的结构（图10.54）。

肠化生（intestinal metaplasia）一般由局灶性杯状细胞组成，但也可见伴有刷状缘的柱状细胞和Paneth细胞[258]。杯状细胞最初容易发生于绒毛状结构（黏膜皱襞）尖端，而不是隐窝基底部。这些病变随后向下发展，并可见于Rokitansky-Aschoff窦。如果有神经内分泌细胞存在，其数量差异较大且随机分布。

鳞状上皮化生罕见，多半与有胆石有关，并可伴有异型增生或鳞状细胞癌[258]。

异型增生和原位癌
Dysplasia and carcinoma in situ

临床特征

异型增生，或非典型增生，和原位癌被认为是腺癌的前期病变。在切除的胆囊中，3.3%～13.5%有异型增生，1.6%～3.5%有原位癌[253,254]，而在伴有腺癌的胆囊中多达40%～88%[248,261]。在一组墨西哥人病例当中，异型增生病人比原位癌病人年轻5岁，而原位癌病人比浸润性腺癌病人年轻10岁。浸润癌诊断时的平均年龄为50多岁[253]。在另一项研究中，前期病变的平均年龄为69岁，与浸润性腺癌的发生时间类似[254]。基于这些数据，从异型增生到浸润性腺癌的进展期限大约为15年。这些研究还提示，异型增生在某些人群中发生年龄较早，女性比男性更容易受累。目前尚不能确定有慢性病变的胆囊是否更可能含有浸润前病变。密切监测这

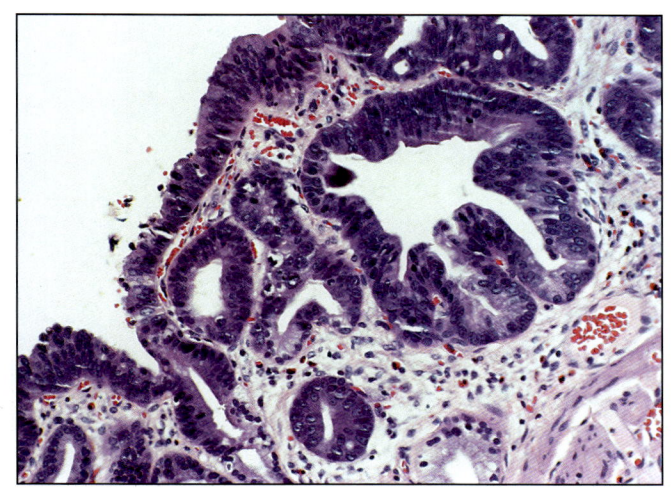

图10.55 胆囊高级别异型增生/原位癌。细胞核变长，密集，呈假复层结构。

些病变可以大大改善病人的预后，但如见微小浸润，则转移和死亡就有可能发生[253,262]。

病理学特征

异型增生可为单发性或多发性，片块状或广泛性，在不到1/3的病例中，随意取一张组织学切片即可发现异型增生性病变。建议常规检查应当取3个以上的纵切面[248]。异型增生和原位癌的组织学定义为上皮呈假复层、细胞核排列拥挤、细胞核非典型性以及上皮结构破坏，伴有严重改变时诊断为原位癌（图10.55）[253,254]。重度异型增生和原位癌并非总能鉴别，因为鉴别这两种病变的诊断标准不具有可重复性。与异型增生比较，原位癌细胞核较大，核仁数量常常增加，而且核仁更为明显。假复层或多层常出现，这种变化可能非常类似于结肠腺瘤性改变。可能出现的其他特征是巨细胞、细胞极性丧失和非典型性核分裂象。原位癌的细胞学改变可向下扩展至Rokitansky-Aschoff窦。此时应当小心不要与浸润性腺癌混淆[264]。一种极为少见类型的原位腺癌是印戒细胞型；原位鳞状细胞癌罕见[265]。

胆囊：恶性肿瘤
Gallbladder: malignant neoplasms

腺癌 Adenocarcinoma
临床特征

胆囊原发癌在常见的胃肠道恶性肿瘤中占第五位。腺癌占病例的75%~85%。这是老年性疾病，70~79岁为高发年龄，女性与男性比为3:1。在美国土著人、墨西哥人、墨西哥裔美国人、日本人以及中欧和东欧人的发病率高于非洲人和非裔美国人。以色列、智利和墨西哥发病率最高[265]。某些国家从1975—1985年发病率加倍，可能与胆囊切除病人数量减少有关[266]。胆囊癌通常在病程晚期已经转移或局部播散之后才被发现。多数病变无特殊特征性表现，常出现类似于慢性胆囊炎的症状。疼痛可能为最常见的症状；黄疸、右上腹部肿物、恶心、呕吐、厌食和体重减轻也可出现[267]。实验室所见也是非诊断性的，包括高胆红素血症、血清碱性磷酸酶升高以及血清CEA或CA19-9水平升高[268]。后者并非恶性肿瘤的特异性所见，因为在阻塞性胆道疾病以及其他部位腺癌也可升高。

胆石见于80%以上的胆囊癌病人[268-270]，胆囊癌和结石均多见于女性和美国土著人，进一步提示两者具有真正的因果关系。结石对胆道黏膜的慢性刺激被认为可以促进肿瘤性转化。弥漫性钙化或瓷状胆囊为另一种与腺癌密切相关的病变（10%~25%）[271]。异常胰胆管连接（anomalous pancreaticobiliary ductal junction，APBDJ）多发生于日本和中国（0.9%~8.7%），且与胆囊癌发生率（12.5%~65%）高有关[248]。异常胰胆管连接的病人，胆总管在十二指肠壁外与胰管连接，缺少正常括约肌结构，导致胰腺分泌物向上反流至胆道。另外有些证据表明，胆囊慢性伤寒杆菌感染[272]以及接触橡胶、汽车、纺织以及金属制作工业应用的化学物质均可增加患癌的危险性[267]。其他可能的危险因子包括溃疡性结肠炎/原发性硬化性胆管炎和遗传学疾病，例如家族性腺瘤性息肉病和Peutz-Jeghers综合征[273,274]。

病理学特征

大体病理学：腺癌常导致胆囊壁局部增厚并突向囊腔。少数情况下可导致胆囊壁弥漫性增厚或腔内乳头状生长（图10.56）。小的浸润性肿瘤可能被忽略或误认为慢性胆囊炎。绝大多数病例有胆石。大约90%的癌发生于胆囊体部或底部，其余发生于胆囊颈部[245]。多达70%的病例可浸润邻近肝实质。极少数情况下癌发生于胆囊部分切除后残余的胆囊[275]。胆囊可出现肿胀或狭窄，取决于肿瘤浸润胆囊的部位和范围。

显微镜下特征：最常见的肿瘤为腺癌，可呈中-高分化（40%~50%）、低分化（30%）、乳头状（12%）或黏液性（12%）。腺鳞癌和鳞状细胞癌不常见（7%）[267]。在高分化肿瘤中，腺体衬以柱状或立方性肿瘤细胞，类似于正常胆囊腺体。肿瘤细胞排列成片状、索条状、腺

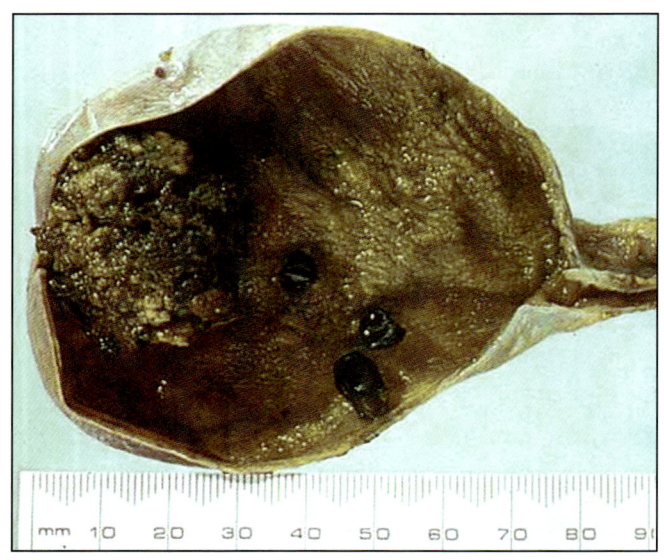

图10.56　胆囊腺癌。外生性肿瘤伴有乳头状分支和胆红素型结石。

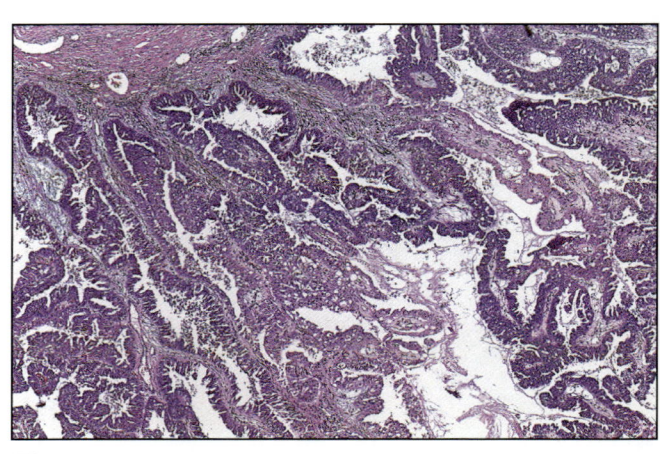

图10.58　胆囊腺癌,乳头状结构。腺癌的乳头状分支被覆非典型性柱状细胞。

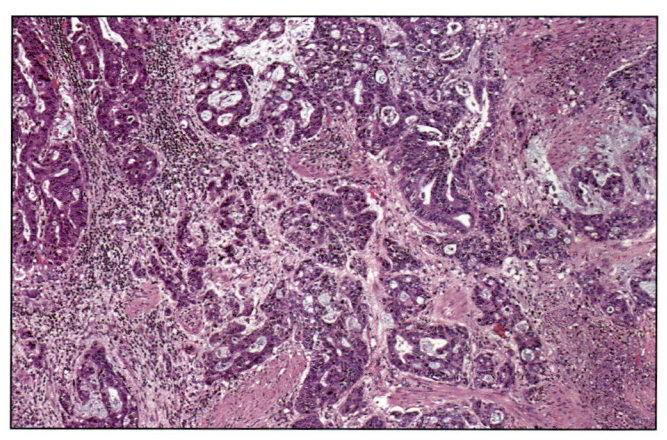

图10.57　胆囊腺癌,筛状结构。恶性腺体呈筛状侵犯胆囊壁。

体或筛状结构(图10.57)。细胞核一般呈圆形或卵圆形,多位于基底或中央。胞浆呈嗜酸性、轻度颗粒状、淡染、透明或黏液样。偶可见杯状细胞、Paneth细胞或内分泌细胞。核分裂象数量不等。腔内或细胞内的黏液量也可能有很大差异。许多恶性腺体中很可能找不到黏液成分,而且诊断高分化腺癌可能并不需要出现显著黏液产物。腺体周围纤维组织增生的数量多少不等,常可见炎症细胞浸润。

乳头状腺癌为高分化病变,向胆囊腔内生长(图10.58)。肿瘤细胞增生位于纤维血管轴心表面。这些肿瘤在浸润胆囊壁前可能充满囊腔,可能具有较好的预后[276]。相反,一旦出现浸润,则极具侵袭性[276a]。黏液性或胶样腺癌,大体上一般呈胶状、灰白色,由于黏液聚集胆囊可能扩张。肿瘤细胞常排列成小簇状,周围绕以较大的嗜碱性黏液湖。诊断黏液腺癌时,组织学上要以黏液成分为主。预后与其他常见的高分化腺癌病人相似。

透明细胞癌由排列成片状、巢状、小梁状、腺样或小乳头状结构的胞质透明的肿瘤细胞组成[277]。胞质酸性黏液及中性黏液染色均呈阴性,且含有淀粉酶消化的PAS阳性物质。电子显微镜检查,这些细胞含有糖原、明显的粗面内质网以及中等数量的线粒体。这些肿瘤多数为腺癌,并且含有典型的腺癌区域,所占比例不足肿瘤的一半。极少数可出现鳞状细胞癌的透明细胞亚型,相应的可以显示局灶性角化。肿瘤细胞免疫组织化学染色呈细胞角蛋白、上皮膜抗原以及红细胞生成相关抗原(erythropoiesis-associated antigen)阳性;这种病变容易被误诊为转移性肾细胞癌。CEA仅在极少数病例中呈阳性,神经内分泌标记物阴性。

其他腺癌亚型包括肠型、印戒细胞型及筛状型。肠型腺癌的特征或为明显的杯状细胞分化,或具有类似于结肠腺癌的表现[259]。结肠型腺癌腺体衬以高柱状细胞,只有少数杯状细胞。印戒细胞腺癌主要由印戒细胞构成。筛状型腺癌主要由伴有筛孔状腔隙的肿瘤细胞团构成,内衬细胞形态相当一致,细胞核深染。总的结构类似于乳腺筛状癌[264],在胆囊见到这种病变时应当除外来自乳腺原发癌的转移。

多形性巨细胞癌(pleomorphic giant cell carcinoma)为罕见类型,特征为数量不等的多核巨细胞以及多角形、圆形或梭形细胞成分,无明显腺体形成或黏液产生[264]。分化好的腺癌区域见于大约2/3的病例,这些肿瘤中

10%～20% 可能出现灶状鳞状细胞癌成分。多形性巨细胞癌一词应该用于以巨细胞为主要成分的肿瘤。常伴随的所见是广泛坏死和混合性炎症细胞浸润。在梭形细胞和巨细胞中有时可见黏液。这种肿瘤大约 70% 细胞角蛋白呈局灶阳性，75% 波形蛋白阳性，20% CEA 阳性。类似于骨巨细胞瘤的伴有破骨细胞样多核巨细胞并被梭形细胞包绕的癌已有报告[264]。需要与类似于骨巨细胞瘤的少见良性组织细胞病变鉴别，这些病变可发生于胆囊或胆道[277a]。

腺鳞癌（Adenosquamous carcinoma）由腺体和鳞状成分混合而成。肿瘤中这两种成分的组织学分化一般为中等程度，并非间变性或低分化。腺鳞癌伴有人绒毛膜促性腺激素产生[278]、梭形细胞灶[279]、神经内分泌分化[280]以及胃小凹型分化[281]已有报道。鳞状成分可较为显著，需要多切片来显示腺体成分。单纯性鳞状细胞癌的发生常与鳞状化生有关[264]。

小细胞（燕麦细胞）癌 [Small cell (oat cell) carcinoma] 占胆囊癌的不足 3%[282]。同腺癌一样，肿瘤发生于老年人（平均年龄 62.7 岁），女性多见。绝大多数病例伴有胆石。极少数病人出现瘤外综合征（paraneoplastic syndrome），例如由于肿瘤分泌肾上腺皮质激素而导致的 Cushing 综合征[264]。这些肿瘤侵袭性强，常见转移，死亡率高。对化疗药物敏感，包括阿霉素、长春新碱、环磷酰胺以及亚硝基脲，需要与其他未分化癌鉴别。大体上，肿瘤一般为大的灰白色肿块，伴有广泛坏死、黏膜溃疡以及上皮下播散。组织学与肺小细胞（燕麦细胞）癌类似。肿瘤细胞具有形状不规则的圆形至梭形，深染的细胞核，核仁不明显。胞质少，境界不清。肿瘤细胞可能排列成巢状、片状或条索状。小管状结构或假花环结构少见。伴有腺癌、鳞状细胞癌、非典型性类癌以及癌肉瘤区域的混合性癌已有报道，但这些成分并不影响预后[264,280,283,284]。多数呈神经内分泌标记物阳性，例如神经元特异性烯醇化酶（75%）、突触素（50%）以及嗜铬素（40%）。绝大多数角蛋白也呈阳性[264]。电镜下常可见少数神经分泌颗粒[264,283]。

梭形细胞肉瘤样癌（Spindle cell sarcomatoid carcinoma）是未分化癌的少见类型[285]。常出现小灶状鳞状或腺体分化的混合性病灶，有助于与肉瘤鉴别。

遗传学改变

p53 基因突变在胆囊腺癌中常见。尽管文献中报道范围较为广泛（35%～92%），而多数研究显示发生率在 50% 以上[286,287]。免疫组织化学染色 p53 过度表达与点突变的发生密切相关，多数发生于 5～8 号外显子。p53 过表达与预后无关[288]。9p21-22 上 CDKN2 基因由于突变或等位基因缺失而失活在胆囊腺癌中常见，发生于 50%～80% 的病例。CDKN2 为肿瘤抑制基因，编码的 p16 为一种蛋白质，通过抑制细胞周期依赖性激酶 4 来调节细胞周期[289,290]。其他常见的遗传学改变包括 8p22（44%）和 18q21 上 DCC 基因位点（31%）缺失[287]。与发生于肝外胆管的腺癌不同，K-ras 突变并不常见，发生于 5%～17% 的病例，尽管有些日本研究报道高达 59%[287]。方法学或地理分布方面的不同可能是导致 K-ras 突变发生率不一致的原因。发生于异常胰胆管连接的胆囊癌，K-ras 突变较常见，见于 50%～83% 的病例[287]。位于 5q 的 APC 基因和 RB 基因杂合性缺失在胆囊癌中并不常见。近来研究显示脆性组氨酸三联体 [fragile histidine triad (F-HIT)] 基因缺失普遍见于胆囊癌早期，它是位于 3p 上的候补肿瘤抑制基因，在胆囊癌的发生机制中可能具有重要作用[291]。

异型增生和原位癌也可出现 TP53 基因 17q13、CDNK 基因 9p21 和 DCC 基因 18q21 的等位缺失，提示这些改变是癌发生过程中的早期事件[248]。K-ras 突变在癌前病变中并不常见，除非是发生于异常胰胆管连接的癌，据报告其发生率高达 41%～83%[248]。

腺瘤在胆囊肿瘤形成中的作用尚有争议。有些作者已经提出腺瘤-癌序列，但其他人认为多数癌是由扁平异型增生/原位癌发展而来。腺瘤缺少胆囊异型增生和浸润性癌常见的分子学改变。K-ras 突变相对常见，而 5～8 号外显子的 TP53 突变以及 9p21 的杂合性缺失在 16 例胆囊腺瘤中均未发现[292]。p53 突变在发生于腺瘤的癌（尤其是幽门腺型）中发生率较低，提示这种腺癌可能具有特殊遗传学背景[248]。

预后和结果

胆囊腺癌预后一般很差，且与诊断时疾病的分期有关。胆囊癌分期取决于胆囊壁的浸润深度。诊断时肿瘤范围是存活率的最佳指标。在胆囊切除时偶然发现原位癌或限于胆囊壁的肿瘤（T1），只要切缘阴性，则预后极好，几乎 100% 存活[293]。如果肿瘤浸润浆膜（T2），应当进一步切除，包括肝切除和局部淋巴结切除。T2 肿瘤根治性切除的 5 年存活率为 61%～70%[294,295]。呈息肉样生长的肿瘤预后好于浸润性肿瘤[296]。一旦肿瘤播散至胆囊以外（T3 和 T4），预后较差，5 年存活率为 0%～28%。术后无残留病变的中位存活时间为 67.2 个月，而大体或镜下有残留病变时不足 10 个月[297]。遗憾的是，多数肿瘤处于此期。出现局部或远处转移时平均存活一般仅为 5.2 个月[245]。淋巴结状况为强有力的预后指标，在一些多变量分析研究中是唯一有意义的因素[293]。淋巴结阳性而长期存活的病例极为少见[298]。诊断时局部淋巴结播散见于大约 50% 的病例。受累淋巴结一般靠近胆囊管及肝门或为胆囊周围淋巴结，随后为胰腺周围及主动脉旁淋巴结。胆囊癌一般容易直接扩展至肝；少数侵犯胃、十二指肠或结肠。腹膜表面种植可导致腹腔内癌病和腹水，并可侵犯邻近空腔脏器，导致胆 - 肠瘘。最严重的合并症之一为胆囊穿孔，可导致腹膜炎、脓肿或瘘管形成。极少数病例可能播散至两侧卵巢，导致 Krukenberg 瘤[245]。

类癌　Carcinoid tumor

临床特征

胆囊类癌占胃肠道类癌的不足 1%，可能伴有类癌综合征[245]。

病理学特征

大体病理学：肿瘤一般较小，为黄色至灰白色的黏膜下病变。

显微镜下特征：肿瘤细胞一般排列成巢状或小梁状结构，间隔以纤细的胶原纤维带。肿瘤细胞可形成腺样结构或外周呈栅栏状排列[299]。细胞较小，伴有中等量淡染至轻度嗜酸性胞质。细胞核为圆形到卵圆形，核仁不明显，染色质点彩状。有些病变可类似腺类癌[245]、印戒细胞类癌[300] 或与腺癌混合[301]。如果出现核分裂象（每高倍视野大于 2 个）和坏死，应考虑诊断为非典型类癌。多数肿瘤细胞呈嗜银性，嗜铬素 A、神经元特异性烯醇化酶、生长抑素（somatostatin）、5- 羟色胺（serotonin）或溶菌酶染色呈阳性[300-302]。亲银染色也可呈阳性。

其他恶性肿瘤

发生于胆囊的其他少见恶性肿瘤为多种肉瘤，包括 Kaposi 肉瘤（与 AIDS 有关）、横纹肌肉瘤、平滑肌肉瘤、所谓的恶性纤维组织细胞瘤以及血管肉瘤。其他少见原发性肿瘤包括癌肉瘤、黑色素瘤以及非 Hodgkin 淋巴瘤。胆囊的转移性肿瘤包括来自于胃肠道其他部位的腺癌、肾细胞癌、黑色素瘤、气管源性的癌以及极其少见的 Hodgkin 淋巴瘤和骨髓瘤。

瘤样病变　Tumor-like lesions

腺肌瘤/腺肌瘤病
Adenomyoma/adenomyomatosis

临床特征

最常诊断的增生类型是腺肌瘤病[303]，一般被认为是与慢性炎症有关的反应性改变，但也可发生在无慢性炎症的情况下。常在因胆囊炎进行胆囊切除时偶然发现。尚无令人信服的证据表明其为肿瘤前期病变。影像学检查可识别出病变所致胆囊壁增厚。

病理学特征

大体病理学：胆囊壁出现弥漫性（腺肌瘤病）或局灶性（腺肌瘤）增厚改变。多数病变位于胆囊底部[304]，常局限于被称为倒圆锥形帽（phrygian cap）的胆囊隔[305]，但有些病变可呈环状生长，引起狭窄。胆囊壁内大体上可见囊腔，囊腔内可有胆石。囊性腔隙常见于胆囊壁肌层周围（外侧）的结缔组织。

显微镜下特征：上皮向下延伸，表现为黏膜内折进入增生的平滑肌肌束，形成分支状导管、腺样腔隙或较大囊肿（图 10.59）。内折黏膜内衬单层高柱状上皮细胞，类似胆囊黏膜表面的上皮。这些腔内可含有胆汁、结石或黏液。可出现局灶性慢性炎症表现。

胆囊壁显著增厚可被误认为腺癌，但仔细检查常可发现腺肌瘤/腺肌瘤病的囊性改变。增生的平滑肌成分有助于与慢性胆囊炎 Rokitansky-Aschoff 窦的鉴别。

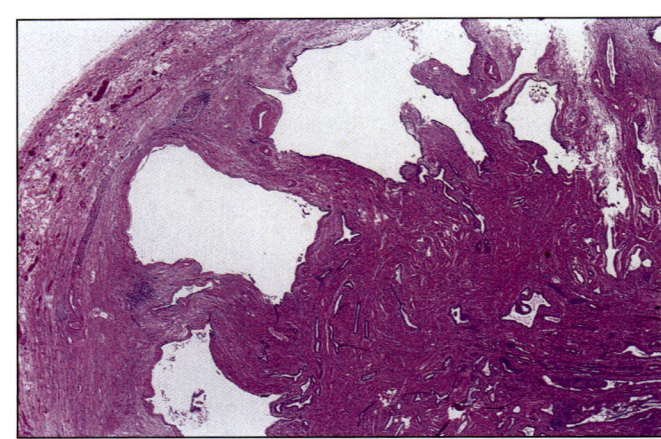

图 10.59　腺肌瘤。增生平滑肌肌束之中杂乱排列的腺样结构。

炎性息肉　Inflammatory polyp

这是瘤样病变相对少见的原因，一般认为是对慢性胆囊炎损伤的显著性炎症性反应[244,299]。息肉可为单发或多发，大小从 0.3～1.0 cm 不等。组织学上，息肉由炎性肉芽组织和纤维组织组成。有些息肉也可含有残留的腺上皮成分。常见溃疡形成、慢性炎症细胞浸润以及出血。

胆固醇性息肉　Cholesterol polyp

胆固醇性息肉是胆囊最常见的非肿瘤性息肉样病变，可占腔内息肉的 60%～90%[306-308]。常出现某种程度的胆固醇沉积症。通常是一较小的有蒂病变，直径不足 1 cm，常为多发性。较小病变呈亮黄色，但较大病变可呈褐色或胆汁着色。病变通过纤细的蒂与黏膜相连，可能容易剥离。也可被误认为粘附于胆囊壁的小胆石。组织学上，病变特征为表面呈绒毛状结构，并有结缔组织蒂，其内充满泡沫样巨噬细胞，类似胆固醇沉积症（图 10.60）。

异位　Heterotopias

胃、胰腺、肝、肾上腺和甲状腺组织在胆囊均有报道，并可在胆囊壁内形成肿物，临床上可与癌混淆。胰腺组织可出现内分泌和外分泌两种成分，极少数情况下，可发生急性胰腺炎，伴有出血和脂肪坏死[309,310]。伴有壁细胞和主细胞的发育好的胃底型黏膜需要区分是胃异位还是胃窦型增生[299]。胃异位多见于胆囊颈和胆囊底[244,311]。

良性胆管肿瘤　Benign biliary tumors

胆管错构瘤　Biliary hamartoma

临床特征

胆管错构瘤，或 von Meyenburg 综合征，被认为是胆管板畸形而非肿瘤，可散发或为多囊性肝疾病的一部分。

病理学特征

胆管错构瘤小（一般 < 0.5 cm），灰白色，形状不规则，常为多灶性。一般在肝活检或尸检时偶然发现。胆管错构瘤由多数小至中等大小、形状不规则的扩张小胆管组成，包裹于致密纤维组织中（图 10.61）。病变位于门管区或接近汇管区的边缘。小胆管衬以立方到扁平上皮，并可含有嗜酸性碎片或浓缩的胆汁，但与胆管系统并不相通。

预后

胆管错构瘤不是癌前病变，但已有极少数发生于胆管错构瘤的胆管癌的报道[312]。

胆管腺瘤　Bile duct adenoma

临床特征

胆管腺瘤比胆管错构瘤少见，"腺瘤"这一命名可能为用词不当，因为它可能不是真正的肿瘤，而是先前受损部位的局限性胆管增生[313]或胆管周围腺体的错构瘤[314]。常在手术或尸检时偶然发现，可能被送检进行冰冻切片以除外转移癌。

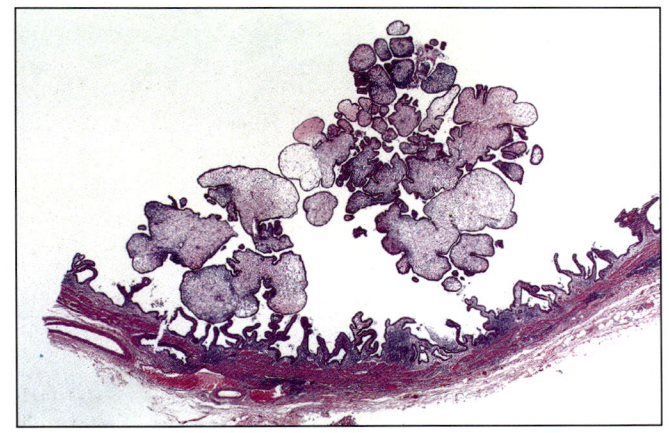

图 10.60　胆固醇性息肉。息肉呈绒毛状结构，间质充满泡沫样吞噬细胞。还有慢性胆囊炎。

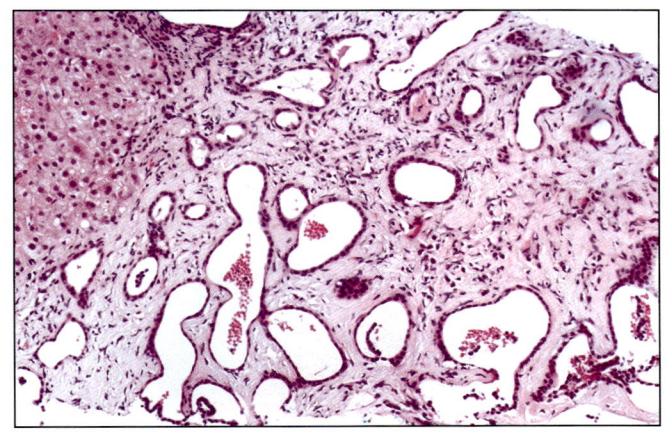

图 10.61　胆管错构瘤。形状不规则的扩张小胆管包裹于致密的纤维性间质中。

病理学特征

胆管腺瘤一般较小（<2 cm），质硬，灰白色，境界清楚，常位于被膜下，可为单发或多发。胆管大小均等，与错构瘤相比，其间隔的纤维组织较少（图10.62）。肿瘤中心部位的间质一般比外周部位丰富。病变的胆管呈圆形，内衬良性立方上皮，没有核分裂象。没有胆汁成分，而且小胆管与胆道不相通。可出现黏液性上皮化生、α_1-抗胰蛋白酶小体以及神经内分泌分化。内分泌细胞巢不应与转移性类癌或胰岛细胞肿瘤混淆[315]。一种少见的伴有透明细胞成分的亚型已有报道，可被误认为原发性或转移性透明细胞癌[316]。免疫组织化学染色，胆管腺瘤表达1F6和D10（从胆管细胞培养提取的抗原），类似小胆管和Hering管的免疫表达[314]。

鉴别诊断

与腺癌不同，胆管腺瘤无细胞核非典型性、核分裂象以及血管浸润。腺腔形态均一、呈圆形、间质相对较少、缺乏胆汁、无囊性改变，而且缺乏伴随的多囊性肝疾病等，均与胆管错构瘤不同。与胆管腺瘤不同，胆管错构瘤表达D10，但不表达1F6[314]。

预后

胆管腺瘤为良性病变，尚无令人信服的恶性变报道。

胆管（肝胆管）囊腺瘤和囊腺癌
Biliary (hepatobiliary) cystadenoma and cystadenocarcinoma

临床特征

胆管囊腺瘤为发生于肝的少见病变，女性发病率较高，组织学上相当于胰腺和卵巢的对应病变。可能与囊腺癌的发生有关，男性和女性发生率相等。发生囊腺癌的平均年龄（59岁）高于囊腺瘤（45岁）[317]。少数发生于肝外胆管和胆囊的病例已有报道[318]。多数病人出现疼痛、不适或可触及的肿物，但也可能发生黄疸、破裂或感染。血清CA19-9水平可有升高[319,320]。

病理学特征

大体病理学：囊腺瘤为5～5 cm的多房性囊肿，内面光滑或有些呈小梁状。这有助于与一般为单房性的发育性囊肿鉴别。囊肿数量相对较少（少囊的），一般较大（巨囊性），而且含有不同表现的液体，包括浆液性、黏液性、胶样，偶尔为出血性甚或化脓性。囊肿与胆管不相通。囊壁内出现较大的息肉样突起或实性肿物为囊腺癌的特征性表现。

显微镜下特征：囊肿衬以单层黏液性上皮细胞，可出现小的乳头状突起（图10.63）。上皮细胞核呈良性，位于基底部，没有核分裂活性。对于女性，囊肿几乎总是伴有富于细胞的间叶性成分，类似于卵巢间质。致密的玻璃样变间质常将卵巢样间质与相邻肝组织分隔开。囊肿壁也可局灶性衬以吞噬细胞，出现钙化或瘢痕样组织。

发生于这种情况下的囊腺癌常呈管状乳头状、实性或腺鳞状分化的组织学结构[317]。出现显著的细胞核多形性、极性消失、核分裂象以及上皮多层等特征提示恶性变，可诊断为原位腺癌，而诊断囊腺癌必须有间质浸润[317]。由于恶性变可呈局灶性，因此建议广泛取材[321]。多达1/3的囊腺癌出现良性上皮成分，支持至少某些囊腺癌是由囊腺瘤发展而来的观点。免疫组织化学染色，囊腺瘤和囊腺癌表达一致，CK、CEA和EMA呈阳性。偶可见散在嗜铬素阳性细胞。间叶性间质的免疫组织化学表达类似肌纤维母细胞，似乎不同于卵巢间质的表型[322]。

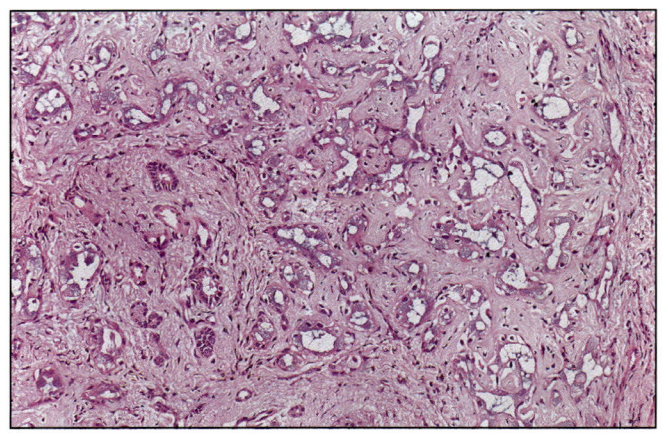

图10.62 胆管腺瘤。少量纤维性间质中可见形态一致的圆形胆管。

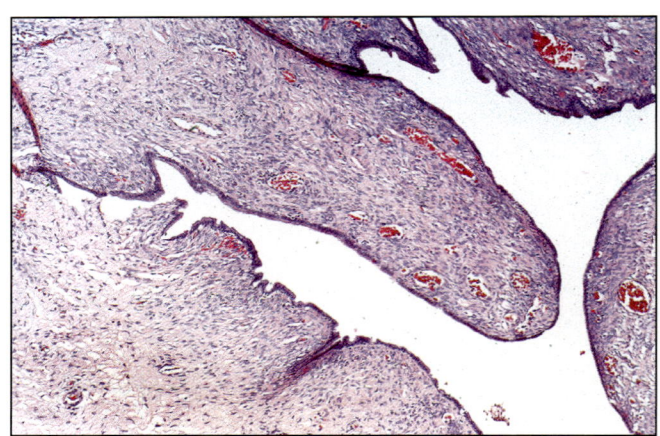

图10.63 黏液性囊腺瘤。多囊性肿瘤内衬良性柱状至立方黏液性上皮。梭形细胞间质富于细胞，类似于卵巢间质。

预后

囊腺瘤为良性肿瘤，完全切除可以治愈。囊腺癌可侵犯邻近脏器，偶尔可播散至局部淋巴结、腹膜和肺[323]。伴有间叶性间质成分的囊腺癌几乎全部发生于女性，具有惰性生物学行为。对于男性，这些肿瘤缺乏卵巢样间质，生物学行为较具侵袭性[317]。

其他良性胆管肿瘤或瘤样病变
Other benign biliary tumors or tumor-like condition

胆管腺纤维瘤（Biliary adenofibroma）为罕见病变，文献中只有3例报道[324]。由伴有微囊性扩张的扭曲及分支状小胆管成分构成，衬以立方形至扁平上皮，腺体之间可见突出的纤维母细胞间质，免疫组织化学染色表达D10，1F6为阴性[325]。因此，它与胆管错构瘤极为类似，但肿瘤一般较大且无任何典型von Meyenburg综合征表现。它与胆管腺瘤不同，后者通常缺少囊状结构，间质较少，1F6和D10均有表达。有一例报道出现22单体[326]。胆管腺纤维瘤为良性病变，未见有恶变。然而，肿瘤体积越大，越容易出现p53阳性免疫表达和4倍体，提示它可能是癌前病变。

浆液性囊腺瘤（Serous cystadenoma）在肝极少见，与胰腺同种病变类似，由多发性微囊肿构成，内衬富于糖原的良性立方上皮（图10.64）[317]。这种囊肿缺乏黏液性囊腺瘤富于细胞的特征性间叶性间质。

神经瘤（Neuromas）肝外胆管的神经瘤可引起梗阻性黄疸。常来源于创伤，典型者发生于胆囊切除术后[327]。组织学检查可见不规则的扭曲神经纤维束，混合以神经鞘细胞和纤维组织，散在分布于胆管黏膜下（图10.65）。

腺肌瘤（Adenomyoma）为错构瘤性病变，极少发生于肝外胆管[328]，较常见于壶腹部。其特征为腺体结构伴有交错的平滑肌束。

孤立性或多发性囊肿（Solitary or multiple cysts）可见于肝内大胆管周围，可能来源于胆管周围的腺体[329]。囊肿内衬柱状或立方上皮，与胆管不相通。胆管周围囊肿可发生于慢性晚期肝疾病和正常肝组织，但一般与多囊性肾或肝病无关。

肝纤毛性前肠囊肿（Ciliated hepatic foregut cyst）为极少见的良性孤立性囊肿，常在影像学检查或手术中偶然发现。较常见于男性以及肝左叶中段。一般为单房性，内衬假复层柱状上皮，上皮下为结缔组织、平滑肌以及外层纤维性包膜[330]。肝纤毛性前肠囊肿发生鳞状细胞癌的病例已有报道[331]。

颗粒细胞瘤 Granular cell tumors 可累及肝外胆管，多见于年轻人，尤其是黑人女性[332]。临床上可能类似于原发性硬化性胆管炎或胆管癌。组织学所见与其他部位的颗粒细胞瘤类似（见27章），切除可以治愈。

恶性胆管肿瘤
Malignant biliary tumors

胆管癌 Cholangiocarcinoma

胆管癌包括发生于肝内胆管（肝内、外周或胆管细胞性胆管癌）以及肝门周围和肝外胆管的恶性肿瘤。近来流行病学研究显示胆管癌的发生率在增加。导致发病率增加的原因尚不清楚，但是好像并不能完全用对疾病的识别增加来解释[333]。在美国，发病率大约为每百万

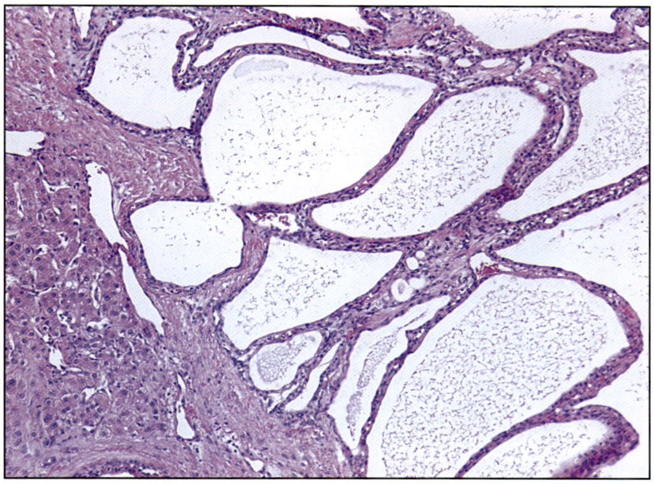

图10.64 浆液性囊腺瘤。多发性小囊肿内衬良性立方上皮。无卵巢样间质。

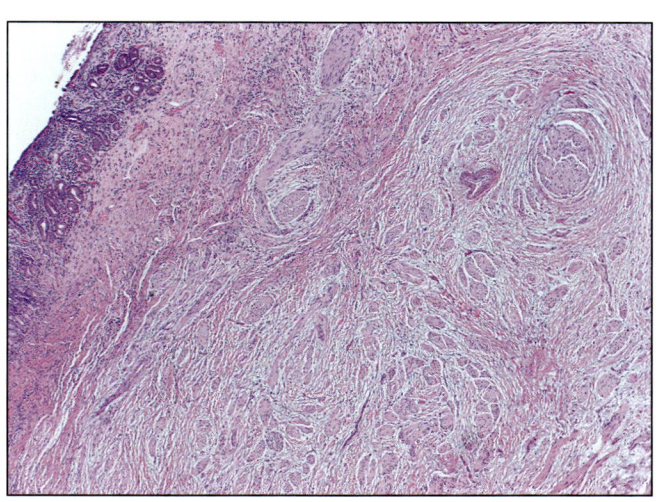

图10.65 肝外胆管神经瘤。肿瘤由增生的神经束组成。

人 8 例；其中 20%～30% 的病例为肝内胆管癌，其余发生于肝外部分[334]。肿瘤一般发生于年龄在 65 岁以上的病人，男性和女性均等受累。

肝内胆管癌
Intrahepatic cholangiocarcinoma

临床特征

病人常直到肿瘤晚期依旧无症状，或出现非特异性症状，例如腹痛、厌食和体重减轻。黄疸并不常见，但碱性磷酸酶常有升高。肿瘤标记物如 CA19-9、CEA 和 CA-125 可有升高。然而，这些标记物均属非特异性，它们在诊断中的作用尚不明确。CA19-9 在高达 85% 的胆管癌病人中有升高，但在胃癌、胰腺癌以及非肿瘤性病变例如梗阻性黄疸中也可升高。CA19-9 持续性升高提示为恶性，甚至在胆道减压之后，并可作为原发性硬化性胆管炎病人的筛查工具[335]。

已经明确的一些胆管癌危险因素包括：

1. 胆管疾病：原发性硬化性胆管炎是已知的最常见的易感因子，每年发生胆管癌的危险性为 1.5%[336-338]。吸烟可增加原发性硬化性胆管炎病人患癌的危险性，肝结石在西方并不常见，但在远东部分地区流行，远东地区 50% 以上的肝结石病人可能患有肝内胆管癌[339]。极少数病例报道伴 von Meyenburg 综合征、胆总管囊肿以及 Caroli 病[340-342]。

2. 寄生虫：胆管癌与两种肝吸虫有关，华支睾吸虫和麝猫后睾吸虫[342,343]。两者均在东南亚流行：华支睾吸虫流行于中国香港、中国南部以及朝鲜；麝猫后睾吸虫流行于泰国和老挝。

3. 其他：胶体钍是一种对比剂，在 20 世纪 50 年代被禁用，但相关危险性可持续数十年[344]。胆管癌可能与遗传性非息肉病性结肠癌（HNPCC）伴随发生[345]。吸烟和酗酒可作为辅助因素[346]。在日本和远东地区，乙型肝炎（大约 10%）和丙型肝炎（大约 25%）常与胆管癌共存，怀疑其在癌的发生中可能具有一定作用。尽管胆管癌一般发生于非硬化性肝组织，但日本的一项研究认为这一概念可能需要修正，他们发现非胆汁性肝硬化近 5% 伴有胆管癌[347]。

病理学特征

大体病理学：肝癌研究小组提出三种大体类型：肿块形成、胆管周围浸润和胆管内肿瘤[348]。肿块形成（mass-forming）是肝内胆管癌最常见的表现，特征为局限性肿瘤，边界清楚，生长迅速，无胆管周围或胆管内播散（图 10.66）。胆管周围浸润型（periductal-infiltrating type）沿胆管浸润，常伴有狭窄和胆管周围结缔组织受累。这两种类型病变由于有致密的纤维性间质而常常质硬，呈白色至褐色。晚期病例可出现混合性生长结构。胆管内型（intraductal type）的讨论见下。

显微镜下特征：绝大多数（>95%）肿瘤为腺癌。高分化肿瘤出现管状、乳头状及索条样结构，细胞学非典型性可以轻微（图 10.67）。细胞浆内空腔、局灶筛状结构、多层细胞核以及腔内细胞碎片支持癌的诊断，而非良性病变。与肝细胞癌相比，胆管癌细胞的核仁一般不甚明显。多数病例中可见黏液。显著的纤维组织增生性间质为胆管癌的一个特征。偶尔，肿瘤细胞形成小而狭窄的小管状结构，类似胆小管或 Hering 小管，这种形态称为胆管细胞癌（cholangiocellular carcinoma）。其他不常见的组织学亚型包括透明细胞癌、腺鳞癌、黏液性

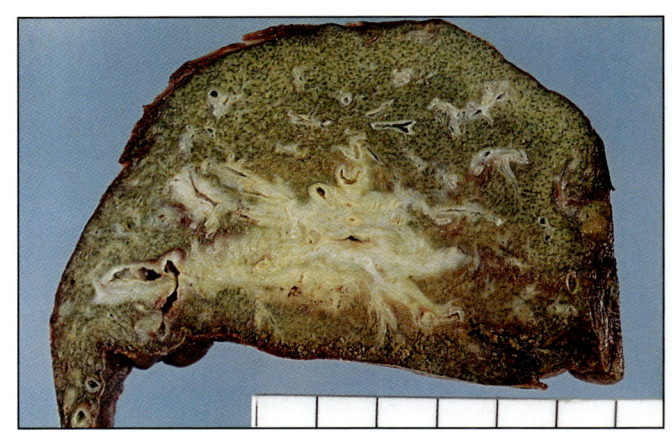

图 10.66 肝内胆管癌。肿块形成结构呈放射状生长，边界清楚，并且没有胆管周围或胆管内播散。非肿瘤性肝组织可见胆汁着色。（Courtesy of Dr. P. Anthony.）

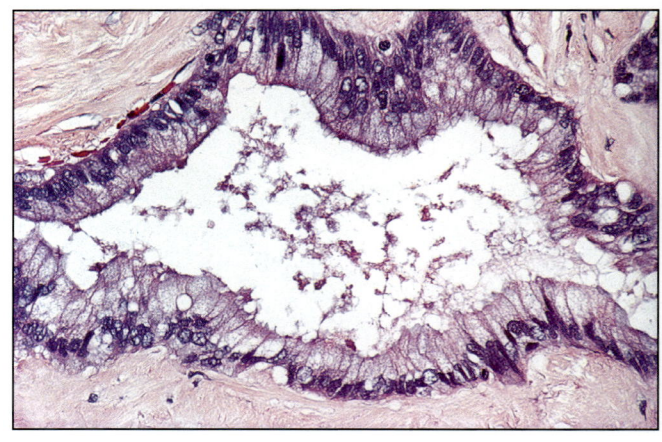

图 10.67 胆管癌，伴高分化黏液性肿瘤细胞。细胞核小，位于基底部。

癌、印戒细胞癌、肉瘤样癌、小细胞癌以及EB病毒相关性淋巴上皮样癌[342]。

鉴别诊断

1. 肝细胞癌：见上面肝细胞癌部分。
2. 转移性腺癌：来自胰腺、结肠、胃、肺和乳腺原发性肿瘤的肝转移性病变可能与胆管癌极为类似。形态学上与转移性腺癌很难区分。出现高柱状细胞和腔内坏死碎片支持转移性结肠癌。部位特异性免疫组织化学标记物可能有助于诊断，例如TTF-1对于肺癌，ER和PR对于乳腺癌，PSA对于前列腺癌，以及uroplakin对于膀胱癌。非部位特异性标记物，例如细胞角蛋白系列可以提供有用的信息。胆管癌一般为CK7+/CK20-，而90%以上的转移性结直肠腺癌病例为CK7-/CK20+ [86,87]。有人提出Lewis(x)、Leu-M1和B72.3免疫组织化学染色可能有助于区分胆管癌和转移性腺癌。Lewis(x)在胆管癌呈胞质和胞膜阳性，但在转移性腺癌仅为胞浆阳性。与之相反，Leu-M1和B72.3在胆管癌多为胞质阳性，而在转移性腺癌胞质和胞膜均呈阳性[90]。目前我们尚未常规应用Leu-M1、B72.3或Lewis(x)。

发病机制和遗传学异常

胆管癌的危险因素，例如原发性硬化性胆管炎以及寄生虫感染中，慢性炎症和胆汁淤积为其共同的相关病变。慢性炎症导致产生细胞因子，例如白细胞介素（interleukin）-1和6，以及干扰素（interferon）-γ，其中有些对于胆管上皮细胞产生显著的促有丝分裂效应。前炎症性细胞因子也可导致一氧化氮诱导合成酶（iNOS）的表达，从而产生一氧化氮和活化性氧基，其不可逆性损伤上皮细胞DNA。一氧化氮也可通过亚硝酰基化来灭活关键DNA修复蛋白，导致潜在癌基因突变的集聚[335,349]。Caspase蛋白酶亚硝酰基化可能造成Caspase 9失活，伴有凋亡抑制[350]。胆酸可增加胆管细胞环加氧酶（cyclooxygenase）-2和髓细胞白血病蛋白1水平；这两种分子可能具有显著的抗凋亡效应[351]。在慢性淤胆中胆汁成分有所改变，还原性谷胱甘肽水平减低。细胞内抗氧化损伤的基本性防护受到损害。因此，慢性炎症和胆汁淤积对于胆管上皮产生显著的增生和诱变影响。

p53缺失和K-ras突变是胆管癌最常见的分子学改变。据报告，p53缺失见于多达50%的肝内肿块形成性肿瘤，可以通过突变、17p杂合性缺失或MDM2基因扩增[349]。p53失活导致bcl-2下调，而且可能引起抵抗凋亡。bcl-2缺失与淋巴结转移、血管浸润以及p53表达异常有关[349]。K-ras突变常常累及12号密码子，而且依据地理分布和肿瘤部位的不同存在很大差异。发生率在英格兰高达100%，日本为50%~56%，而泰国为0%~8%，可能代表了潜在的病因学差异。K-ras突变在肝外胆管的胆管周围浸润性肿瘤比肿块形成性肝内胆管癌常见，而p53突变较常见于后者[352]。p16基因改变也较常见，过度甲基化的启动可能是肝内胆管癌p16失活最常见的原因。p16缺失可能是诊断原发性硬化性胆管炎相关性肿瘤的有用试验[353]。常见的人类端粒酶反转录酶（hTERT）过度表达见于异性增生和浸润性癌，提示它可能为癌发生的早期事件。在活检标本中检测端粒酶梯度被认为是极佳的诊断方法[354]。肝细胞生长因子c-met在胆管癌中呈过度表达，并且与肿瘤分化有关。其他改变包括E-钙黏蛋白、β-连环蛋白和DPC-4基因突变，HER-2/neu基因扩增以及微卫星不稳定性。

预后和治疗

手术切除受累肝组织是治愈的唯一希望，但只有少数病例获得成功，5年生存率为0%~43%[349,55]。对于肝内胆管癌，辅助化疗和放疗的作用尚不明确。并不提倡进行肝移植，其5年生存率不足20%[349]。淋巴结转移和手术切缘是影响预后的最常见因素。淋巴结受累见于50%以上的病人[334]。淋巴管或神经周围浸润、肝内卫星结节以及肝两叶均有肿瘤分布预示存活率较差[356]。肿块形成性肿瘤比导管周围浸润性肿瘤预后好[348]。伴有明显纤维组织增生性反应的肿瘤，其淋巴管浸润的发生率可能较高，并且具有较高的增生活性，存活率较差[342]。分化较差的肿瘤及其亚型侵袭性较强，例如印戒细胞癌和肉瘤样癌。

累及肝外胆管的癌
Carcinoma affecting the extrahepatic biliary tree

临床特征

肝外胆管癌可分为发生于肝门附近（肝门周围胆管癌）或发生于胆管远端部分的癌（远端胆管癌）。肝门周围的肿瘤（a.k.a. Klatskin 肿瘤）几乎占所有胆管癌的2/3。病人表现为梗阻性黄疸、反复发作的胆管炎以及胆汁淤积性生化检查改变。在无胆管炎的情况下，肿瘤标记物，例如CA19-9持续性升高可能有助于诊断。

病理学特征

肿瘤表现为浸润性（70%~80%）、结节状（20%）或导管内（<5%）生长结构。浸润性和结节状肿瘤一般分化较差，容易沿黏膜和黏膜下播散，并且伴有明显的

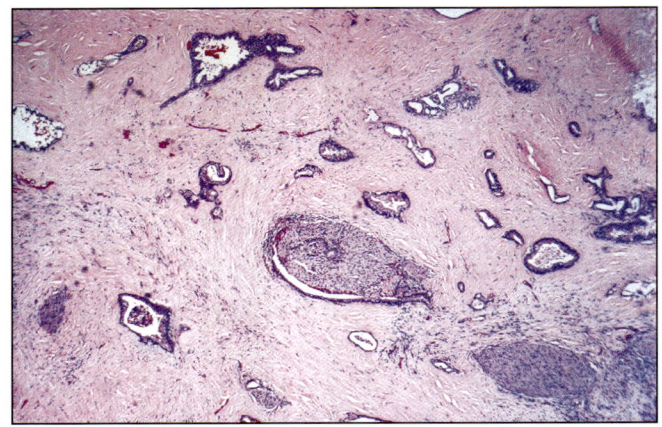

图10.68 胆管癌伴显著纤维组织增生性反应间质和神经周围浸润。

纤维组织增生性反应。肿瘤包绕左侧或右侧门静脉见于1/3的病人，导致同侧肝叶萎缩。个别病例具有乳头状生长方式[357]。淋巴结转移在手术切除病人中占30%～50%；肝门和胆总管周围淋巴结最易受累。发生于原发性硬化性胆管炎的肿瘤可为多灶性，并且伴有多部位的异型增生和原位癌。由于有明显的间质纤维组织增生（图10.68），病理学诊断常不甚明确，因而需要内镜多处活检和刷片。仅有40%～70%的活检病例可做出病理学诊断。应用辅助性技术，包括数字影像分析和荧光原位杂交来检测刷片或活检标本中的非整倍体细胞，可显著提高诊断敏感性[358]。

治疗和预后

手术治疗肝门周围胆管癌常需要切除部分肝组织以确保切缘阴性。由于尾叶单独引流，因此也提倡尾叶切除。远端病变采用Whipple手术治疗。在肿瘤可以切除且边缘为阴性的病例中5年生存率为20%～40%，手术死亡率为10%[359]。对于手术切除的病例，切缘阴性和T1病变为主要预后因素。肿瘤出现双侧胆管分支受累、肝叶萎缩伴肿瘤包绕门静脉以及转移至N2淋巴结或远隔部位者认为不能手术切除。不能手术切除者或晚期病人生存期不足1年。发生于原发性硬化性胆管炎的肿瘤预后特别不好，5年存活率小于10%。有些研究显示放疗和化疗有益于病痛的减轻，并可作为手术辅助方法，但效果尚有争议[359]。胆管癌被认为是肝移植禁忌证，因为可迅速复发。然而近来研究显示，应用新辅助性化疗和放疗的早期病变，其5年生存率为80%，并且对于选择性病人，肝移植可能有益[335]。

胆管内前体病变
Precursor intraductal biliary lesions

胆管异型增生（上皮内肿瘤形成/非典型性增生）
Biliary dysplasia (intraepithelial neoplasia/atypical hyperplasia)

胆管癌的肿瘤形成过程几乎总是沿着增生 - 异型增生 - 癌的顺序。胆管异型增生在肝活检中极为少见，但与在原发性硬化性胆管炎中出现胆管癌密切相关[338,360]。组织学上，其特征为细胞核多层、微乳头状和筛状结构、极性丧失、细胞核增大和深染以及细胞核形状不规则（图10.69）。胆管异型增生的活性高于胆管增生，但低于癌，支持肿瘤进行性发展的序列表现。如同胆管癌一样，异型增生的上皮常表达CEA、CA19-9和DUPAN-2，但表达可呈局灶性[361]。

肝内胆管有结石或肝吸虫常出现慢性炎症、上皮增生、肝内胆管周围腺体增生和纤维化。黏液性腺泡增生常见，并可出现假幽门腺化生。这些表现被称为慢性增生性胆管炎（chronic proliferative cholangitis）[361]。在出现肝吸虫时，肝内大导管壁内腺体显著增生被称为"胆管腺瘤性增生"。这些增生性病变可能发生多灶性胆管异型增生和胆管癌。

胆管内乳头状肿瘤形成
Intraductal papillary neoplasia

临床特征

胆管乳头状肿瘤的特征为胆管内乳头状肿物，伴有

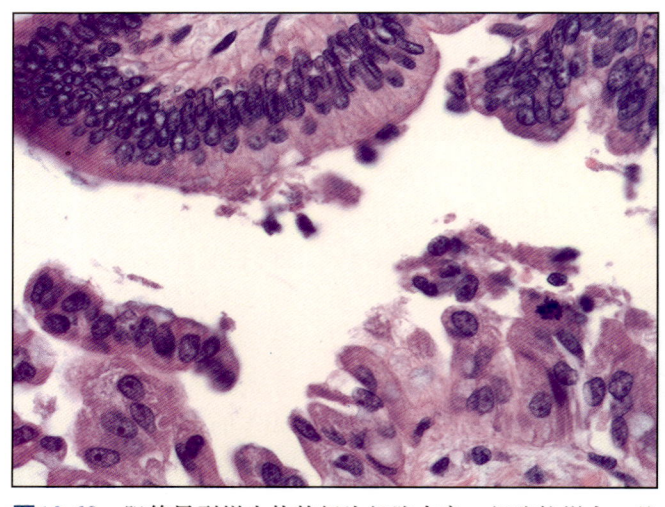

图10.69 胆管异型增生的特征为细胞丰富，细胞核增大、丛状、极性丧失以及核仁显著。与上部正常胆管上皮形成对比。

纤细的纤维血管轴心，而且包括胆管（胆管内）乳头状瘤病以及伴有胆管内生长结构的胆管癌。胆管内乳头状瘤病常广泛累及肝内和（或）肝外胆管，尤其是后者。病人常出现急性胆管炎反复发作和梗阻性黄疸[362]。

病理学特征

胆管乳头状瘤病（biliary papillomatosis）为癌前肿瘤性增生，特点为胆管内衬细胞呈多灶性或者弥漫性乳头状增生，无浸润或转移。肿瘤由纤细乳头构成，被覆高柱状细胞，细胞核位于基底部，并伴有轻度多形性表现（图10.70）。多数病例组织学上为良性，但可出现局灶性胆管上皮异型增生。诊断胆管癌必须要见到明显的乳头轴心及其下方小胆管周围组织的浸润。肝胆管内乳头状肿瘤另一种类型的特点为高度分泌黏液以及肿瘤性和非肿瘤性胆管呈节段性扩张。这种类型胆管内肿瘤的临床和病理学特征与胰腺导管内黏液性肿瘤极为类似[342,363,364]。扩张的胆管充满黏液和衬以黏液性上皮的乳头状赘生物。可出现嗜酸性及透明细胞改变。伴有杯状细胞成分的胃肠化生也较为常见。常累及胆管周围腺体。上皮可出现异型增生或原位癌，一般为多灶性。出现浸润性成分时常具有黏液性癌的特征。

分子遗传学异常

K-ras突变在胆管乳头状瘤病中可以见到，恶性变可能伴有MUC1和Tn抗原表达增加[365]。胆管内乳头状黏液性肿瘤常出现CK 7表达减少，以及CK 20和黏蛋白表达异常，例如MUC2、MUC5AC和MUC6[364]。不到1/3的病例有p53表达，但在伴有异型增生和癌的病例中较高。

预后

尽管多数病例在组织学上呈良性，但这些病变不仅是癌前病变，而且本身具有危害性，因为病变呈多中心性、容易复发以及诸如反复发作的胆管炎和败血症等合并症。然而，即使出现浸润，其预后也比典型的胆管癌

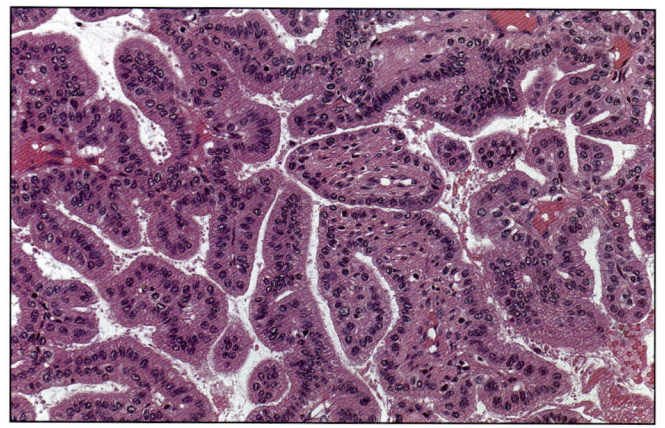

图10.70 胆管内乳头状瘤病：乳头被覆柱状细胞，细胞核呈轻度多形性。

好[362,64,66]。没有浸润时不发生淋巴结转移。约10%的胆管内乳头状肿瘤切除之后复发。

其他恶性肿瘤

类癌[367]、副神经节瘤[368]以及原发性恶性黑色素瘤[369]偶可发生于肝外胆管。在诊断原发性恶性黑色素瘤之前，要除外从其他原发部位转移而来的可能性。白血病和恶性淋巴瘤可累及肝外胆管，极少数情况下可为首发表现。胚胎性（葡萄状）横纹肌肉瘤为胆管少见肿瘤，但在儿童却是这个部位最常见的恶性肿瘤[370]。有极少数成人病例的报道。临床上，这些肿瘤表现为梗阻性黄疸、发热、体重减轻以及肝大。大体上，肿瘤突入胆管，呈质软的息肉样肿物。镜下，肿瘤细胞圆形至梭形，富于细胞与疏松黏液样区域呈不同程度混合排列。肿瘤细胞常密集分布于上皮下（新生层）。可见嗜酸性胞浆和横纹结构，其为横纹肌母细胞分化的证据。免疫组织化学肌肉标记物染色，例如结蛋白和肌形成蛋白可以证实诊断。手术切除结合放化疗可以长期存活，但大多数病例预后较差[370]。

参考文献

1. Ishak K, Anthony P, Sobin L H 1994 Histological typing of tumours of the liver, 2nd edn. Springer-Verlag, Berlin
2. Ishak K G, Goodman Z D, Stocker J T 2001 Tumors of the liver and intrahepatic bile ducts. Armed Forces Institute of Pathology, Washington, DC, p 9–48
3. Wheeler D, Edmondson H, Reynolds T 1986 Spontaneous liver cell adenoma in children. Am J Clin Pathol 85: 6–12
4. Flejou J F, Barge J, Menu Y et al. 1985 Liver adenomatosis: an entity distinct from liver adenoma? Gastroenterology 89: 1132–1138
5. Le Bail B, Jouhanole H, Deugnier Y et al. 1992 Liver adenomatosis in two patients on long-term oral contraceptives. Am J Surg Pathol 16: 982–987
6. Gokhele R, Whitington P F 1996 Hepatic adenomatosis in an adolescent. J Pediatr Gastroenterol Nutr 23: 482–486
7. Chiche L, Dao T, Salame E et al. 2000 Liver adenomatosis: reappraisal, diagnosis, and surgical management: eight new cases and review of the literature. Ann Surg 231: 74–81
8. Ishak K, Rabin L 1975 Benign tumors of the liver. Med Clin North Am 59: 995–1013
9. De Carlis L, Pirotta V, Rondinara G F et al. 1997 Hepatic adenoma and focal nodular hyperplasia: diagnosis and criteria for treatment. Liver Transpl Surg 3: 160–165
10. Herman P, Pugliese V, Machado M A et al. 2000 Hepatic adenoma and focal nodular hyperplasia: differential diagnosis and treatment. World J Surg 24: 372–376
11. Edmondson H A, Henderson B, Benton B 1976 Liver cell adenomas associated with use of oral contraceptives. N Engl J Med 294: 470–472
12. Tao L 1991 Oral contraceptive-associated liver cell adenoma and hepatocellular carcinoma: cytomorphology and mechanism of malignant transformation. Cancer 68: 341–347
13. Lindgren A, Olsson R 1993 Liver damage from low-dose oral contraceptives. J Intern Med 234: 287–292
14. Klava A, Super P, Aldridge M et al. 1994 Body builder's liver. J Roy Soc Med 87: 43–44
15. Carrasco D, Barrachina M, Prieto M et al. 1984 Clomiphene citrate and liver cell adenoma. N Engl J Med 310: 1120–1121
16. Bork K, Pitton M, Harten P et al. 1999 Hepatocellular adenomas in patients taking danazol for hereditary angio-oedema. Lancet 353: 1066–1067
17. Tazawa K, Yasuda M, Ohtani Y et al. 1999 Multiple hepatocellular adenomas associated with long-term carbamezapine. Histopathology 35: 92–94
18. Resnick M B, Kozakewich H P W, Perez-Atayde A R 1995 Hepatic adenoma in the pediatric age group. Am J Surg Pathol 19: 1181–1190
19. Hytiroglou P, Theise N 1998 Differential diagnosis of hepatocellular nodular lesions. Semin Diagn Pathol 15: 285–299
20. Bala S, Wunsch P H, Ballhausen W G 1997 Childhood hepatocellular adenoma in familial adenomatous polyposis: mutations in adenomatous polyposis coli gene and p53. Gastroenterology 112: 919–922
21. Vesoulis Z, Agamanolis D 1998 Benign hepatocellular adenoma of the placenta. Am J Surg Pathol 22: 355–359
22. Grange J D, Guechot J, Legendre C et al. 1987 Liver adenoma and focal nodular hyperplasia in a man with high endogenous sex steroids. Gastroenterology 93: 1409–1413
23. Wanless I, Callea F, Craig J et al. 1995 Terminology of nodular lesions of the liver. Hepatology 25: 983–993
24. Ferrell L 1993 Hepatocellular carcinoma arising in a focus of multilobular adenoma. Am J Surg Pathol 17: 525–529
25. Kong C, Appenzeller M, Ferrell L 2000 Utility of CD34 reactivity in evaluating focal nodular hepatocellular lesions sampled by fine needle aspiration biopsy. Acta Cytol 44: 218–222
26. Wilkens L, Bredt M, Flemming P et al. 2001 Differentiation of liver cell adenomas from well-differentiated hepatocellular carcinomas by comparative genomic hybridization. J Pathol 193: 476–482
27. Wilkens L, Bredt M, Flemming P et al. 2001 Diagnostic impact of fluorescence in situ hybridization in the differentiation of hepatocellular adenoma and well-differentiated hepatocellular carcinoma. J Mol Diagn 3: 68–73
28. Foster J H, Berman M M 1994 The malignant transformation of liver cell adenomas. Arch Surg 129: 712–717
29. Ribeiro A, Burgart L J, Nagorney D M et al. 1998 Management of liver adenomatosis: results with a conservative surgical approach. Liver Transpl Surg 4: 388–398
30. Nguyen B, Flejou J, Terris B et al. 1999 Focal nodular hyperplasia of the liver: a comprehensive pathologic study of 305 lesions and recognition of new histologic forms. Am J Surg Pathol 23: 1441–1454
31. Sadowski D C, Lee S S, Wanless I R et al. 1995 Progressive type of focal nodular hyperplasia characterized by multiple tumors and recurrence. Hepatology 21: 970–975
32. Wanless I R, Albrecht S, Bilbao J et al. 1989 Multiple focal nodular hyperplasia of the liver associated with vascular malformations of various organs and neoplasia of the brain: a new syndrome. Mod Pathol 2: 456–462
33. Haber M, Reuben A, Burrell M et al. 1995 Multiple focal nodular hyperplasia of the liver associated with hemihypertrophy and vascular malformations. Gastroenterology 108: 1256–1262
34. Wanless I, Mawdsley C, Adams R 1985 On the pathogenesis of focal nodular hyperplasia of the liver. Hepatology 5: 1194–1200
35. Paradis V, Bieche I, Dargere D et al. 2003 A quantitative gene expression study suggests a role for angiopoietins in focal nodular hyperplasia. Gastroenterology 124: 651–659
36. Paradis V, Laurent A, Flejou J F et al. 1997 Evidence for the polyclonal nature of focal nodular hyperplasia of the liver by the study of X-chromosome inactivation. Hepatology 26: 891–895
37. Paradis V, Benzekri A, Dargere D et al. 2004 Telangiectatic focal nodular hyperplasia: a variant of hepatocellular adenoma. Gastroenterology 126: 1323–1329
38. Caseiro-Alves F, Zins M, Mahfouz A-E et al. 1996 Calcification in focal nodular hyperplasia: a new problem for differentiation from fibrolamellar hepatocellular carcinoma. Radiology 198: 889–892
39. Berman M M, Libbey N P, Foster J H 1980 Hepatocellular carcinoma. Polygonal cell type with fibrous stroma – an atypical variant with a favorable prognosis. Cancer 46: 1448–1455
40. Kudo M, Ikekubo K, Yamamoto K et al. 1989 Focal fatty infiltration of the liver in acute alcoholic liver injury: hot spots with radiocolloid SPECT scan. Am J Gastroenterol 84: 948–952
41. Sasaki M, Harada K, Nakanuma Y et al. 1994 Pseudolipoma of Glisson's capsule. Report of six cases and review of the literature. J Clin Gastroenterol 19: 75–78
42. Sundaresan M, Lyons B, Akosa A B 1991 'Solitary' necrotic nodules of the liver: an aetiology reaffirmed. Gut 32: 1378–1380
43. Tsui W, Yuen R, Chow L et al. 1992 Solitary necrotic nodule of the liver: parasitic origin? J Clin Pathol 45: 975–978
44. Terayama N, Terada T, Hoso M 1995 Partial nodular transformation of the liver with portal vein thrombosis. J Clin Gastroenterol 20: 71–76
45. Theise N, Lopook J, Thung S 1993 A macroregenerative nodule containing multiple foci of hepatocellular carcinoma in a noncirrhotic liver. Hepatology 17: 993–996
46. Ferrell L, Crawford J, Dhillon A et al. 1993 Proposal for standardized criteria for the diagnosis of benign, borderline, and malignant hepatocellular lesions arising in chronic advanced liver disease. Am J Surg Pathol 17: 1113–1123
47. Ferrell L 1994 Hepatocellular nodules in the cirrhotic liver: diagnostic features and proposed nomenclature. In: Ferrell L (ed) Diagnostic problems in liver pathology. Pathology: state of the art reviews. Hanley & Belfus, Philadelphia, p 105–117
48. Park Y, Yang C-T, Fernandez G et al. 1998 Neoangiogenesis and sinusoidal "capillarization" in dysplastic nodules of the liver. Am J Surg Pathol 22: 656–662
49. Roncalli M, Roz E, Goggi G et al. 1999 The vascular profile of regenerative and dysplastic nodules of the cirrhotic liver: implications for diagnosis and classification. Hepatology 30: 1174–1178
50. Theise N, Fiel I, Hytiroglou P et al. 1995 Macroregenerative nodules in cirrhosis are not associated with elevated serum or stainable tissue alpha-fetoprotein. Liver 15: 30–34
51. Nakanuma Y, Terada T, Ueda K et al. 1993 Adenomatous hyperplasia of the liver as a precancerous lesion. Liver 13: 1–9
52. Le Bail B, Bernard P H, Carles J et al. 1997 Prevalence of liver cell dysplasia and association with HCC in a series of 100 cirrhotic liver explants. J Hepatol 27: 835–842
53. Crawford J 1990 Pathologic assessment of liver cell dysplasia and benign liver tumors: differentiation from malignant tumors. Semin Diagn Pathol 7: 115–128
54. Zhao M, Zhang N X, Laissue J A et al. 1994 Immunohistochemical analysis of p53 protein overexpression in liver cell dysplasia and in hepatocellular carcinoma. Virchows Arch 424: 613–621
55. Lee R G, Tsamandas A C, Demetris A J 1997 Large cell change (liver cell dysplasia) and hepatocellular carcinoma in cirrhosis: matched case-control study, pathological analysis, and pathogenetic hypothesis. Hepatology 26: 1415–1422
56. Su Q, Benner A, Hofmann W J et al. 1997 Human hepatic preneoplasia: phenotypes and proliferation kinetics of foci and nodules of altered hepatocytes and their relationship to liver cell dysplasia. Virchows Arch 431: 391–406
57. Natarajan S, Theise N D, Thung S N et al. 1997 Large-cell change of hepatocytes in cirrhosis may represent a reaction to prolonged cholestasis. Am J Surg Pathol 21: 312–318
58. Maggioni M, Coggi G, Cassani B et al. 2000 Molecular changes in hepatocellular dysplastic nodules on microdissected liver biopsies. Hepatology 32: 942–946
59. Yeh S H, Chen P J, Shau W Y et al. 2001 Chromosomal allelic imbalance evolving from liver cirrhosis to hepatocellular carcinoma. Gastroenterology 121: 699–709
60. Deugnier Y M, Charalambous P, Le Quilleuc D et al. 1993 Preneoplastic significance of hepatic iron-free foci in genetic hemochromatosis: a study of 185 patients. Hepatology 18: 1363–1369
61. Bannasch P, Klimek F, Mayer D 1997 Early bioenergetic changes in hepatocarcinogenesis: preneoplastic phenotypes mimic responses to insulin and thyroid hormone. J Bioenerg Biomembr 29: 303–313

62. Su Q, Benner A, Hofmann W J et al. 1997 Human hepatic preneoplasia: phenotypes and proliferation kinetics of foci and nodules of altered hepatocytes and their relationship to liver cell dysplasia. Virchows Arch 431: 391–406
63. El-Serag H B, Mason A C 1999 Rising incidence of hepatocellular carcinoma in the United States. N Engl J Med 340: 745–750
64. Trevisani F, D'Intino P E, Grazi G L et al. 1996 Clinical and pathologic features of hepatocellular carcinoma in young and older Italian patients. Cancer 77: 2223–2232
65. Ishak K G, Goodman Z D, Stocker J T 2001 Tumors of the liver and intrahepatic bile ducts. Armed Forces Institute of Pathology, Washington, DC, p 199–230
66. Befeler A S, Di Bisceglie A M 2002 Hepatocellular carcinoma: diagnosis and treatment. Gastroenterology 122: 1609–1619
67. Monto A, Wright T L 2001 The epidemiology and prevention of hepatocellular carcinoma. Semin Oncol 28: 441–449
68. El-Serag H B 2002 Hepatocellular carcinoma: an epidemiologic view. J Clin Gastroenterol 35 (5 suppl 2): S72–S78
69. Donato F, Boffetta P, Puoti M 1998 A meta-analysis of epidemiological studies on the combined effect of hepatitis B and C virus infections in causing hepatocellular carcinoma. Int J Cancer 75: 347–354
70. Talente G M, Coleman R A, Alter C et al. 1994 Glycogen storage disease in adults. Ann Intern Med 120: 218–226
71. Hamilton S R, Aaltonen L A 2000 WHO classification of tumors. Pathology and genetics of tumors of the digestive system. IARC Press, Lyon, p 157–202
72. Omata M, Peters R, Tatters D 1981 Sclerosing hepatic carcinoma: relationship to hypercalcemia. Liver 1: 33–49
73. Stromeyer F, Ishak K, Gerber M et al. 1980 Ground-glass cells in hepatocellular carcinoma. Am J Clin Pathol 74: 254–258
74. Okuda K, Musha H, Nakajima Y et al. 1977 Clinicopathologic features of encapsulated hepatocellular carcinoma: a study of 26 cases. Cancer 40: 1240–1245
75. Anthony P P, James K 1987 Pedunculated hepatocellular carcinoma. Is it an entity? Histopathology 11: 403–414
76. Emile J F, Adam R, Sebagh M et al. 2000 Hepatocellular carcinoma with lymphoid stroma: a tumour with good prognosis after liver transplantation. Histopathology 37: 523–529
77. Edmondson H, Steiner P 1954 Primary carcinoma of the liver: a study of 100 cases among 48 900 necropsies. Cancer 1: 462–503
78. Wennerberg A E, Nalesnik M A, Coleman W B 1993 Hepatocyte paraffin 1: a monoclonal antibody that reacts with hepatocytes and can be used for differential diagnosis of hepatic tumors. Am J Pathol 143: 1050–1054
79. Minervini M, Demetris A, Lee R et al. 1997 Utilization of hepatocyte-specific antibody in the immunocytochemical evaluation of liver tumors. Mod Pathol 10: 686–692
80. Morrison C, Marsh W Jr, Frankel W L 2002 A comparison of CD10 to pCEA, MOC-31 and hepatocyte for the distinction of malignant tumors in the liver. Mod Pathol 15: 1279–1287
81. Fan Z, van de Rijn M, Montgomery K et al. 2003 Hep Par 1 antibody stain for the differential diagnosis of hepatocellular carcinoma: 676 tumors tested using tissue microarrays and conventional tissue sections. Mod Pathol 16: 137–144
82. Kakar S, Muir T, Murphy L M et al. 2003 Immunoreactivity of Hep Par 1 in hepatic and extrahepatic tumors and its correlation with albumin in situ hybridization in hepatocellular carcinoma. Am J Clin Pathol 119: 361–366
83. Lau S K, Prakash S, Geller S A et al. 2002 Comparative immunohistochemical profile of hepatocellular carcinoma, cholangiocarcinoma, and metastatic adenocarcinoma. Hum Pathol 33: 1175–1181
84. Krishna M, Lloyd R V, Batts K P 1997 Detection of albumin messenger RNA in hepatic and extrahepatic neoplasms. A marker of hepatocellular differentiation. Am J Surg Pathol 21: 147–152
85. Oliveira A M, Erickson L A, Burgart L J et al. 2000 Differentiation of primary and metastatic clear cell tumors in the liver by in situ hybridization for albumin messenger RNA. Am J Surg Pathol 24: 177–182
86. Maeda T, Kajiyama K, Adachi E et al. 1996 The expression of cytokeratins 7, 19, 20 in primary and metastatic carcinomas of the liver. Mod Pathol 9: 901–909
87. Wang N, Zee S, Zarbo R et al. 1995 Coordinate expression of cytokeratins 7 and 20 defines unique subsets of carcinomas. Appl Immunohistochem 3: 99–107
88. Rullier A, Le Bail B, Fawaz R et al. 2000 Cytokeratin 7 and 20 expression in cholangiocarcinomas varies along the biliary tract but still differs from that in colorectal carcinoma metastases. Am J Surg Pathol 24: 870–876
89. Chu P, Wu E, Weiss L 2000 Cytokeratin 7 and cytokeratin 20 expression in epithelial neoplasms: a survey of 435 cases. Mod Pathol 13: 962–972
90. Fucich L, Cheles M, Thung S et al. 1994 Primary versus metastatic hepatic carcinoma: an immunohistochemical study of 34 cases. Arch Pathol Lab Med 118: 927–930
91. Wieczorek T J, Pinkus J L, Glickman J N et al. 2002 Comparison of thyroid transcription factor-1 and hepatocyte antigen immunohistochemical analysis in the differential diagnosis of hepatocellular carcinoma, metastatic adenocarcinoma, renal cell carcinoma and adrenal cortical carcinoma. Am J Clin Pathol 118: 911–921
92. Garcia de Davila M, Gonzalez-Crussi F, Mangkornkanok M 1987 Fibrolamellar carcinoma of the liver in a child: ultrastructural and immunohistologic aspects. Pediatr Pathol 7: 319–331
93. Ruck P, Harms D, Kaiserling E 1990 Neuroendocrine differentiation in hepatoblastoma: an immunohistochemical investigation. Am J Surg Pathol 14: 847–855
94. Wang J, Dhillon A, Sankey E et al. 1991 Neuroendocrine differentiation in primary neoplasms of the liver. J Pathol 163: 61–67
95. Tsui W, Colombari R, Bonetti F et al. 1999 Hepatic angiomyolipoma: a clinicopathologic study of 30 cases and delineation of unusual morphological variants. Am J Surg Pathol 23: 34–48
96. Murakata L, Ishak K, Nzeako U 2000 Clear cell carcinoma of the liver: a comparative immunohistochemical study with renal clear cell carcinoma. Mod Pathol 13: 874–881
97. Renshaw A, Granter S 1998 A comparison of A103 and inhibin reactivity in adrenal cortical tumors: distinction from hepatocellular carcinoma and renal tumors. Mod Pathol 11: 1160–1164
98. Idilman R, De Maria N, Colantoni A et al. 1998 Pathogenesis of hepatitis B and C-induced hepatocellular carcinoma. J Viral Hepat 5: 285–299
99. Thorgeirsson S S, Grisham J W 2002 Molecular pathogenesis of human hepatocellular carcinoma. Nat Genet 31: 339–346
100. Wong N, Lai P, Lee S W et al. 1999 Assessment of genetic changes in hepatocellular carcinoma by comparative genomic hybridization analysis: relationship to disease stage, tumor size, and cirrhosis. Am J Pathol 154: 37–43
101. Laurent-Puig P, Legoix P, Bluteau O et al. 2001 Genetic alterations associated with hepatocellular carcinomas define distinct pathways of hepatocarcinogenesis. Gastroenterology 120: 1763–1773
102. Balsara B R, Pei J, De Rienzo A et al. 2001 Human hepatocellular carcinoma is characterized by a highly consistent pattern of genomic imbalances, including frequent loss of 16q23.1–24.1. Genes Chromosomes Cancer 30: 245–253
103. Qin L X, Tang Z Y, Ma Z C et al. 2002 P53 immunohistochemical scoring: an independent prognostic marker for patients after hepatocellular carcinoma resection. World J Gastroenterol 8: 459–463
104. Kazachkov Y, Khaoustov V, Yoffe B et al. 1996 p53 abnormalities in hepatocellular carcinoma from United States patients: analysis of all 11 exons. Carcinogenesis 17: 2207–2212
105. Aguilar F, Hussain S P, Cerutti P 1993 Aflatoxin B1 induces the transversion of G→T in codon 249 of the p53 tumor suppressor gene in human hepatocytes. Proc Natl Acad Sci USA 90: 8586–8590
106. Elmore L W, Hancock A R, Chang S F et al. 1997 Hepatitis B virus X protein and p53 tumor suppressor interactions in the modulation of apoptosis. Proc Natl Acad Sci USA 94: 14707–14712
107. Ishido S, Hotta H 1998 Complex formation of the nonstructural protein 3 of hepatitis C virus with the p53 tumor suppressor. FEBS Lett 438: 258–262
108. Lan K H, Sheu M L, Hwang S J et al. 2002 HCV NS5A interacts with p53 and inhibits p53-mediated apoptosis. Oncogene 21: 4801–4811
109. Huang H, Fujii H, Sankila A et al. 1999 Beta-catenin mutations are frequent in human hepatocellular carcinomas associated with hepatitis C virus infection. Am J Pathol 155: 1795–1801
110. Hui A M, Li X, Makuuchi M et al. 1999 Over-expression and lack of retinoblastoma protein are associated with tumor progression and metastasis in hepatocellular carcinoma. Int J Cancer 84: 604–608
111. Matsuda Y, Ichida T, Matsuzawa J et al. 1999 p16(INK4) is inactivated by extensive CpG methylation in human hepatocellular carcinoma. Gastroenterology 116: 394–400
112. Hui A M, Kanai Y, Sakamoto M et al. 1997 Reduced p21(WAF1/CIP1) expression and p53 mutation in hepatocellular carcinomas. Hepatology 25: 575–579
113. Hui A M, Sun L, Kanai Y et al. 1998 Reduced p27Kip1 expression in hepatocellular carcinomas. Cancer Lett 132: 67–73
114. Lee M N, Jung E Y, Kwun H J et al. 2002 Hepatitis C virus core protein represses the p21 promoter through inhibition of a TGF-beta pathway. J Gen Virol 83: 2145–2151
115. Qin L X, Tang Z Y 2002 The prognostic molecular markers in hepatocellular carcinoma. World J Gastroenterol 8: 385–392
116. Qin L X, Tang Z Y, Ma Z C et al. 2002 P53 immunohistochemical scoring: an independent prognostic marker for patients after hepatocellular carcinoma resection. World J Gastroenterol 8: 459–463
117. Fiorentino M, Altimari A, D'Errico A et al. 2000 Acquired expression of p27 is a favorable prognostic indicator in patients with hepatocellular carcinoma. Clin Cancer Res 6: 3966–3972
118. Fiorentino M, Altimari A, Ravaioli M et al. 2004 Predictive value of biological markers for hepatocellular carcinoma patients treated with orthotopic liver transplantation. Clin Cancer Res 10: 1789–1795
119. Bismuth H, Chiche L, Castaing D 1995 Surgical treatment of hepatocellular carcinomas in noncirrhotic liver: experience with 68 liver resections. World J Surg 19: 35–41
120. Figueras J, Jaurrieta E, Valls C et al. 1997 Survival after liver transplantation in cirrhotic patients with and without hepatocellular carcinoma: a comparative study. Hepatology 25: 1485–1489
121. Yao F Y, Ferrell L, Bass N M et al. 2001 Liver transplantation for hepatocellular carcinoma: expansion of the tumor size limits does not adversely impact survival. Hepatology 33: 1394–1403
122. Befeler A S, Di Bisceglie A M 2002 Hepatocellular carcinoma: diagnosis and treatment. Gastroenterology 122: 1609–1619
123. Ng I O, Lai E C, Fan S T et al. 1995 Prognostic significance of pathologic features of hepatocellular carcinoma. A multivariate analysis of 278 patients. Cancer 76: 2443–2448

124. Nzeako U C, Goodman Z D, Ishak K G 1996 Hepatocellular carcinoma in cirrhotic and noncirrhotic livers. A clinico-histopathologic study of 804 North American patients. Am J Clin Pathol 105: 65–75
125. Chedid A, Ryan L M, Dayal Y et al. 1999 Morphology and other prognostic factors of hepatocellular carcinoma. Arch Pathol Lab Med 123: 524–528
126. Quaglia A, Bhattacharjya S, Dhillon A P 2001 Limitations of the histopathological diagnosis and prognostic assessment of hepatocellular carcinoma. Histopathology 38: 167–174
127. Lauwers G Y, Terris B, Balis U K et al. 2002 Prognostic histologic indicators of curatively resected hepatocellular carcinomas. A multi-institutional analysis of 425 patients with definition of a histologic prognostic index. Am J Surg Pathol 26: 25–34
128. Craig J, Peters R, Edmondson H et al. 1980 Fibrolamellar carcinoma of the liver: a tumor of adolescents and young adults with distinctive clinicopathologic features. Cancer 46: 372–379
129. Berman M, Libbey N, Foster J 1980 Hepatocellular carcinoma: polygonal cell type with fibrous stroma – an atypical variant with a favorable prognosis. Cancer 46: 1448–1455
130. Berman M, Sheahan D 1988 Fibrolamellar carcinoma of the liver: an immunohistochemical study of nineteen cases and a review of the literature. Hum Pathol 19: 784–794
131. Saul S, Titelbaum D, Gansler T et al. 1987 The fibrolamellar variant of hepatocellular carcinoma; its association with focal nodular hyperplasia. Cancer 60: 3049–3055
132. Saxena R, Humphreys S, Williams R et al. 1994 Nodular hyperplasia surrounding fibrolamellar carcinoma: a zone of arterialized liver parenchyma. Histopathology 25: 275–278
133. Hodgson H J 1987 Fibrolamellar cancer of the liver. J Hepatol 5: 241–247
134. Vecchio F M, Fabiano A, Ghirlanda G et al. 1984 Fibrolamellar carcinoma of the liver: the malignant counterpart of focal nodular hyperplasia with oncocytic change. Am J Clin Pathol 81: 521–526
135. Goodman Z, Ishak K, Langloss J et al. 1985 Combined hepatocellular–cholangiocarcinoma: a histologic and immunohistochemical study. Cancer 55: 124–135
136. Nagorney D M, Adson M A, Weiland L H et al. 1985 Fibrolamellar hepatoma. Am J Surg 149: 113–119
137. Kakar S, Burgart L J, Batts K P et al. 2005 Clinicopathologic features and survival in fibrolamellar carcinoma: comparison with conventional hepatocellular carcinoma with and without cirrhosis. Mod Pathol 18: 1417–1423
138. Ng I O, Shek T W, Nicholls J et al. 1998 Combined hepatocellular–cholangiocarcinoma: a clinicopathological study. J Gastroenterol Hepatol 13: 34–40
139. Yano Y, Yamamoto J, Kosuge T et al. 2003 Combined hepatocellular and cholangiocarcinoma: a clinicopathologic study of 26 resected cases. Jpn J Clin Oncol 33: 283–287
140. Jarnagin W R, Weber S, Tickoo S K et al. 2002 Combined hepatocellular and cholangiocarcinoma: demographic, clinical, and prognostic factors. Cancer 94: 2040–2046
141. Tickoo S K, Zee S Y, Obiekwe S et al. 2002 Combined hepatocellular–cholangiocarcinoma, a histopathologic, immunohistochemical and in situ hybridization study. Am J Surg Pathol 26: 989–997
142. Kim H, Park C, Han K H et al. 2004 Primary liver carcinoma of intermediate (hepatocyte–cholangiocyte) phenotype. J Hepatol 40: 298–304
143. Fujii H, Zhu X G, Matsumoto T et al. 2000 Genetic classification of combined hepatocellular–cholangiocarcinoma. Hum Pathol 31: 1011–1017
144. Haas J, Muczynski K, Krailo M et al. 1989 Histopathology and prognosis in childhood hepatoblastoma and hepatocarcinoma. Cancer 64: 1082–1095
145. Weinberg A, Finegold M 1983 Primary hepatic tumors of childhood. Hum Pathol 14: 512–537
146. Altmann H 1992 Epthelial and mixed hepatoblastoma in the adult. Pathol Res Pract 188: 16–26
147. Anthony P 1994 Tumours and tumour-like lesions of the liver and biliary tract. In: MacSween R, Anthony P, Scheuer P et al. (eds) Pathology of the liver, 3rd edn. Churchill Livingstone, Edinburgh, p 635–711
148. Haggitt R, Reid B 1986 Hereditary gastrointestinal polyposis syndromes. Am J Surg Pathol 10: 871–887
149. Stocker J 1994 Hepatoblastoma. Semin Diagn Pathol 11: 136–143
150. Arshad R R, Woo S Y, Abbassi V et al. 1982 Virilizing hepatoblastoma: precocious sexual development and partial response of pulmonary metastases to cis-platinum. CA Cancer J Clin 32: 293–300
151. Saxena R, Leake J, Shafford E et al. 1993 Chemotherapy effects on hepatoblastoma: a histological study. Am J Surg Pathol 17: 1266–1271
152. Conran R, Hitchcock C, Waclawiw M et al. 1992 Hepatoblastoma: the prognostic significance of histologic type. Pediatr Pathol 12: 167–183
153. Ruck P, Kaiserling E 1993 Melanin-containing hepatoblastoma with endocrine differentiation: an immunohistochemical and ultrastructural study. Cancer 72: 361–368
154. Murakata L, Ishak K, Nzeako U 2000 Clear cell carcinoma of the liver: a comparative immunohistochemical study with renal clear cell carcinoma. Mod Pathol 13: 874–881
155. Buendia M A 2002 Genetic alterations in hepatoblastoma and hepatocellular carcinoma: common and distinctive aspects. Med Pediatr Oncol 39: 530–535
156. Terracciano L M, Bernasconi B, Ruck P et al. 2003 Comparative genomic hybridization analysis of hepatoblastoma reveals high frequency of X-chromosome gains and similarities between epithelial and stromal components. Hum Pathol 34: 864–871
157. Schnater J M, Kohler S E, Lamers W H et al. 2003 Where do we stand with hepatoblastoma? Cancer 98: 668–678
158. Park W S, Oh R R, Park J Y et al. 2001 Nuclear localization of beta-catenin is an important prognostic factor in hepatoblastoma. J Pathol 193: 483–490
159. Shim Y H, Park H J, Choi M S et al. 2003 Hypermethylation of the p16 gene and lack of p16 expression in hepatoblastoma. Mod Pathol 16: 430–436
160. Cillo U, Ciarleglio F A, Bassanello M et al. 2003 Liver transplantation for the management of hepatoblastoma. Transplant Proc 35: 2983–2985
161. Otte J B, Pritchard J, Aronson D C et al. 2004 Liver transplantation for hepatoblastoma: results from the International Society of Pediatric Oncology (SIOP) study SIOPEL-1 and review of the world experience. Pediatr Blood Cancer 42: 74–83
162. Hobbs K 1990 Hepatic hemangiomas. World J Surg 14: 468–471
163. Ishak K G, Goodman Z D, Stocker J T 2001 Tumors of the liver and intrahepatic bile ducts. Armed Forces Institute of Pathology, Washington, DC, p 71–146
164. Kane R, Newman A 1973 Diffuse skeletal and hepatic hemangiomatosis. Calif Med 118: 41–44
165. Adam Y G, Huvos A G, Fortner J G 1970 Giant hemangiomas of the liver. Ann Surg 172: 239–245
166. Mikami T, Hirata K, Oikawa I et al. 1998 Hemobilia caused by a giant benign hemangioma of the liver: report of a case. Surg Today 28: 948–952
167. Kim G E, Thung S N, Tsui W M et al. 2003 Cavernous hemangioma: what have we been missing? (abstract) Mod Pathol 16: 279a
168. Dehner L, Ishak K 1971 Vascular tumors of the liver in infants and children: a study of 30 cases and review of the literature. Arch Pathol 92: 101–111
169. Stanley P, Geer G, Miller J et al. 1989 Infantile hepatic hemangiomas: clinical features, radiologic investigations and treatment of 20 patients. Cancer 64: 936–949
170. Bejarano P A, Serrano M F, Casillas J et al. 2003 Concurrent infantile hemangioendothelioma and mesenchymal hamartoma in a developmentally arrested liver of an infant requiring hepatic transplantation. Pediatr Dev Pathol 6: 552–557
171. Han S J, Tsai C C, Tsai H M et al. 1998 Infantile hemangioendothelioma with a highly elevated serum alpha-fetoprotein level. Hepatogastroenterology 45: 459–461
172. Amonkar P, Desai S, Deb R et al. 1999 Infantile hemangioendothelioma of the liver. Med Pediatr Oncol 32: 392–394
173. Selby D M, Stocker J T, Waclawiw M A et al. 1994 Infantile hemangioendothelioma of the liver. Hepatology 20: 39–45
174. Cerar A, Dolenc-Strazar Z, Bartenjev D 1996 Infantile hemangioendothelioma of the liver in a neonate: immunohistochemical observations. Am J Surg Pathol 20: 871–876
175. Selby D, Stocker J, Ishak K 1992 Angiosarcoma of the liver in childhood: a clinicopathologic and follow-up study of 10 cases. Pediatr Pathol 12: 485–498
176. Daller J A, Bueno J, Gutierrez J et al. 1999 Hepatic hemangioendothelioma: clinical experience and management strategy. J Pediatr Surg 34: 98–106
177. Stocker J T 2001 Hepatic tumors in children. Clin Liver Dis 5: 259–281
178. Stocker J, Ishak K 1983 Mesenchymal hamartoma of the liver: report of 30 cases and review of the literature. Pediatr Pathol 1: 245–267
179. Cook J R, Pfeifer J D, Dehner L P 2002 Mesenchymal hamartoma of the liver in the adult: association with distinct clinical features and histological changes. Hum Pathol 33: 893–898
180. Murthi G V, Paterson L, Azmy A 2003 Chromosomal translocation in mesenchymal hamartoma of liver: what is its significance? J Pediatr Surg 2003; 38: 1543–1545
181. Yen J B, Kong M S, Lin J N 2003 Hepatic mesenchymal hamartoma. J Paediatr Child Health 39: 632–634
182. O'Sullivan M J, Swanson P E, Knoll J et al. 2001 Undifferentiated embryonal sarcoma with unusual features arising within mesenchymal hamartoma of the liver: report of a case and review of the literature. Pediatr Dev Pathol 4: 482–489
183. Goodman Z, Ishak K 1984 Angiomyolipomas of the liver. Am J Surg Pathol 8: 745–750
184. Tang H, Hui P, Garcia-Tsao G et al. 2002 Multiple angiomyolipomata of the liver: a case report. Mod Pathol 15: 167–171
185. Hornick J L, Fletcher C D M 2006 PEComa: what do we know so far? Histopathology 48: 75–82
186. Yamasaki S, Tanaka S, Fujii H et al. 2000 Monotypic epithelioid angiomyolipoma of the liver. Histopathology 36: 451–456
187. Barnard M, Lajoie G 2001 Angiomyolipoma: immunohistochemical and ultrastructural study of 14 cases. Ultrastruct Pathol 25: 21–29
188. Makhlouf H R, Remotti H E, Ishak K G 2002 Expression of KIT (CD117) in angiomyolipoma. Am J Surg Pathol 26: 493–497
189. Ji Y, Zhu X, Xu J et al. 2001 Hepatic angiomyolipoma: a clinicopathologic study of 10 cases. Chin Med J (Engl) 114: 280–285
190. Ren N, Qin L X, Tang Z Y et al. 2003 Diagnosis and treatment of hepatic angiomyolipoma in 26 cases. World J Gastroenterol 9: 1856–1858
191. Anthony P, Telesinghe P 1986 Inflammatory pseudotumor of the liver. J Clin Pathol 39: 761–768
192. Shek T, Ng I, Chan K 1993 Inflammatory pseudotumor of the liver: report of four cases and review of the literature. Am J Surg Pathol 17: 231–238

193. Nakanuma Y, Tsuneyama K, Masuda S et al. 1994 Hepatic inflammatory pseudotumor associated with chronic cholangitis: report of three cases. Hum Pathol 25: 86–91
194. Torzilli G, Inoue K, Midorikawa Y et al. 2001 Inflammatory pseudotumors of the liver: prevalence and clinical impact in surgical patients. Hepatogastroenterology 48: 1118–1123
195. Amankonah T D, Strom C B, Vierling J M et al. 2001 Inflammatory pseudotumor of the liver as the first manifestation of Crohn's disease. Am J Gastroenterol 96: 2520–2522
196. Selves J, Meggetto F, Brousset P et al. 1996 Inflammatory pseudotumor of the liver: evidence for follicular dendritic reticulum cell proliferation associated with clonal Epstein–Barr virus. Am J Surg Pathol 20: 747–753
197. Cheuk W, Chan J K, Shek T W et al. 2001 Inflammatory pseudotumor-like follicular dendritic cell tumor: a distinctive low grade malignant abdominal neoplasm with consistent Epstein–Barr virus association. Am J Surg Pathol 25: 721–731
198. Lee S L, DuBois J J 2001 Hepatic inflammatory pseudotumor: case report, review of the literature, and a proposal for morphologic classification. Pediatr Surg Int 17: 555–559
199. Shek T, Ho F, Ng I et al. 1996 Follicular dendritic cell tumor of the liver: evidence for an Epstein–Barr virus-related clonal proliferation of follicular dendritic cells. Am J Surg Pathol 20: 313–324
200. Pokorny C S, Painter D M, Waugh R C et al. 1991 Inflammatory pseudotumor of the liver causing biliary obstruction. Treatment by biliary stenting with 5-year follow-up. J Clin Gastroenterol 13: 338–341
201. Fried R, Wardzala A, Willson R et al. 1992 Benign cartilaginous tumor (chondroma) of the liver. Gastroenterology 103: 678–680
202. Hytiroglou P, Linton P, Klion F et al. 1993 Benign schwannoma of the liver. Arch Pathol Lab Med 117: 216–218
203. Moran C A, Ishak K G, Goodman Z D 1998 Solitary fibrous tumor of the liver: a clinicopathologic and immunohistochemical study of nine cases. Ann Diagn Pathol 2: 19–24
204. Awan S, Davenport M, Portmann B et al. 1996 Angiosarcoma of the liver in children. J Pediatr Surg 31: 1729–1732
205. Zocchetti C 2001 Liver angiosarcoma in humans: epidemiologic considerations. Med Lav 92: 39–53
206. Ishak K G, Anthony P P, Niederau C et al. 2000 Mesenchymal tumors of the liver. In: Hamilton S R, Aaltonen L (eds) Tumors of the digestive system. IARC Press, Lyon, p 191–198
207. Tannapfel A, Weihrauch M, Benicke M et al. 2001 p16INK4A-alterations in primary angiosarcoma of the liver. J Hepatol 35: 62–67
208. Weihrauch M, Markwarth A, Lehnert E et al. 2002 Abnormalities of the ARF-p53 pathway in primary angiosarcomas of the liver. Hum Pathol 33: 884–892
209. Timaran C H, Grandas O H, Bell J L 2000 Hepatic angiosarcoma: long-term survival after complete surgical removal. Am Surg 66: 1153–1157
210. Ishak K, Sesterhenn I, Goodman Z et al. 1984 Epithelioid hemangioendothelioma of the liver: a clinicopathologic and follow-up study of 32 cases. Hum Pathol 15: 839–852
211. d'Annibale M, Piovanello P, Carlini P et al. 2002 Epithelioid hemangioendothelioma of the liver: case report and review of the literature. Transplant Proc 34: 1248–1251
212. Taege C, Holzhausen H, Gunter G et al. 1999 Malignant epithelioid hemangioendothelioma of the liver – a very rare tumor in children. Pathologe 20: 345–350
213. Gray M, Rosenberg A, Dickersin G et al. 1990 Cytokeratin expression in epithelioid vascular neoplasms. Hum Pathol 21: 212–217
214. Uchimura K, Nakamuta M, Osoegawa M et al. 2001 Hepatic epithelioid hemangioendothelioma. J Clin Gastroenterol 32: 431–434
215. Madariaga J, Marino I, Karavias D et al. 1995 Long-term results after liver transplantation for primary hepatic epithelioid hemangioendothelioma. Ann Surg Oncol 2: 483–487
216. Ben-Haim M, Roayaie S, Ye M Q et al. 1999 Hepatic epithelioid hemangioendothelioma: resection or transplantation, which and when? Liver Transpl Surg 5: 526–531
217. Theurillat J P, Vavricka S R, Went P et al. 2003 Morphologic changes and altered gene expression in an epithelioid hemangioendothelioma during a ten-year course of disease. Pathol Res Pract 199: 165–170
218. Kayler L K, Merion R M, Arenas J D et al. 2002 Epithelioid hemangioendothelioma of the liver disseminated to the peritoneum treated with liver transplantation and interferon alpha-2B. Transplantation 74: 128–130
219. Stocker J, Ishak K 1978 Undifferentiated (embryonal) sarcoma of the liver: report of 31 cases. Cancer 42: 336–348
220. Lack E, Schloo B, Azumi N et al. 1991 Undifferentiated (embryonal) sarcoma of the liver: Clinical and pathologic study of 16 cases with emphasis on immunohistochemical features. Am J Surg Pathol 15: 1–16
221. Frankel W L, Kiani B, Ferrell L D et al. 2003 Immunohistochemical analysis of embryonal sarcoma of the liver (abstract). Mod Pathol 16: 272a
222. Webber E M, Morrison K B, Pritchard S L et al. 1999 Undifferentiated embryonal sarcoma of the liver: results of clinical management in one center. J Pediatr Surg 34: 1641–1644
223. Sowery R D, Jensen C, Morrison K B et al. 2001 Comparative genomic hybridization detects multiple chromosomal amplifications and deletions in undifferentiated embryonal sarcoma of the liver. Cancer Genet Cytogenet 126: 128–133
224. Noel J C, Hermans P, Andre J et al. 1996 Herpesvirus-like DNA sequences and Kaposi's sarcoma: relationship with epidemiology, clinical spectrum, and histologic features. Cancer 77: 2132–2136
225. Marcelin A G, Roque-Afonso A M, Hurtova M et al. 2004 Fatal disseminated Kaposi's sarcoma following human herpesvirus 8 primary infections in liver-transplant recipients. Liver Transpl 10: 295–300
226. Hubscher S, Lumley M, Elias E 1993 Vanishing bile duct syndrome: a possible mechanism for intrahepatic cholestasis in Hodgkin's lymphoma. Hepatology 17: 70–77
227. Scheimberg I, Pollock D, Collins P et al. 1995 Pathology of the liver in leukaemia and lymphoma. Histopathology 26: 311–321
228. Jaffe E 1987 Malignant lymphomas: pathology of liver involvement. Semin Liver Dis 7: 257–268
229. Santos E S, Raez L E, Salvatierra J et al. 2003 Primary hepatic non-Hodgkin's lymphomas: case report and review of the literature. Am J Gastroenterol 98: 2789–2793
230. Page R D, Romaguera J E, Osborne B et al. 2001 Primary hepatic lymphoma: favorable outcome after combination chemotherapy. Cancer 92: 2023–2029
231. Cooke C B, Krenacs L, Stetler-Stevenson M et al. 1996 Hepatosplenic T-cell lymphoma: a distinct clinicopathologic entity of cytotoxic gamma delta T-cell origin. Blood 88: 4265–4274
232. Ishak K G, Goodman Z D, Stocker J T 2001 Tumors of the liver and intrahepatic bile ducts. Armed Forces Institute of Pathology, Washington, DC, p 271–280
233. Shek T, Ho F, Ng I et al. 1996 Follicular dendritic cell tumor of the liver: evidence for an Epstein–Barr virus-related clonal proliferation of follicular dendritic cells. Am J Surg Pathol 20: 313–324
234. Nelson V, Fernandes N F, Woolf G M et al. 2001 Primary liposarcoma of the liver: a case report and review of literature. Arch Pathol Lab Med 125: 410–412
235. Cozzutto C, Bernardi B, Comelli A et al. 1981 Malignant mesenchymoma of the liver in children: a clinicopathologic and ultrastructural study. Hum Pathol 12: 481–485
236. Kawarada Y, Uehara S, Noda M et al. 1985 Nonhepatocytic malignant mixed tumor primary in the liver: report of two cases. Cancer 55: 1790–1798
237. Demirhan B, Sokmensuer C, Karakayali H et al. 1997 Primary extramedullary plasmacytoma of the liver. J Clin Pathol 50: 74–76
238. Parham D, Peiper S, Robicheaux G et al. 1988 Malignant rhabdoid tumor of the liver: evidence for epithelial differentiation. Arch Pathol Lab Med 112: 61–64
239. Gresham G, Rue L 1985 Squamous cell carcinoma of the liver. Hum Pathol 16: 413–416
240. Heaton G, Matthews T, Christopherson W 1986 Malignant trophoblastic tumors with massive hemorrhage presenting as liver primary: a report of two cases. Am J Surg Pathol 10: 342–347
241. Heywood G, Burgart L J, Nagorney D M 2002 Ossifying malignant mixed epithelial and stromal tumor of the liver: a case report of a previously undescribed tumor. Cancer 94: 1018–1022
242. Borja E R, Hori J M, Pugh R P 1975 Metastatic carcinomatosis of the liver mimicking cirrhosis: case report and review of the literature. Cancer 35: 445–449
243. Riopel M A, Klimstra D S, Godellas C V et al. 1997 Intrabiliary growth of metastatic colonic adenocarcinoma: a pattern of intrahepatic spread easily confused with primary neoplasia of the biliary tract. Am J Surg Pathol 21: 1030–1036
244. Christensen A, Ishak K 1970 Benign tumors and pseudotumors of the gallbladder: report of 180 cases. Arch Pathol Lab Med 90: 423–432
245. Albores-Saavedra J, Henson D E, Klimstra D S 2000 Tumors of the gallbladder, extrahepatic bile ducts and ampulla of Vater. Armed Forces Institute of Pathology, Washington, DC, p 21–36
246. Melson G, Reiter F, Evens R 1976 Tumorous conditions of the gallbladder. Semin Roentgenol 11: 260–282
247. Nishihara K, Yamaguchi K, Hashimoto H et al. 1991 Tubular adenoma of the gallbladder with squamoid spindle cell metaplasia. Report of three cases with immunohistochemical study. Acta Pathol Jpn 41: 41–45
248. Sasatomi E, Tokunaga O, Miyazaki K 2000 Precancerous conditions of gallbladder carcinoma: overview of histopathologic characteristics and molecular genetic findings. J Hepatobiliary Pancreat Surg 7: 556–567
249. Kozuka S, Tsubone N, Yasui A et al. 1982 Relation of adenoma to carcinoma in the gallbladder. Cancer 50: 2226–2234
250. Shinkai H, Kimura W, Muto T 1998 Surgical indications for small polypoid lesions of the gallbladder. Am J Surg 175: 114–117
251. Nakajo S, Yamamoto M, Tahara E 1990 Morphometrical analysis of gall-bladder adenoma and adenocarcinoma with reference to histogenesis and adenoma–carcinoma sequence. Virchows Arch A Pathol Anat Histopathol 417: 49–56
252. Miller T, Weber T, Appelman H 1972 Paraganglioma of the gallbladder. Arch Surg 105: 637–639
253. Albores-Saavedra J, Alcantara-Vazquez A, Cruz-Ortiz H et al. 1980 The precursor lesions of invasive gallbladder carcinoma: hyperplasia, atypical hyperplasia and carcinoma. Cancer 45: 919–927
254. Ojeda V, Shilkin K, Walters M 1985 Premalignant epithelial lesions of the gallbladder: a prospective study of 120 cholecystectomy specimens. Pathology 17: 451–454
255. Yamamoto M, Nakajo S, Tahara E 1989 Histogenesis of well-differentiated adenocarcinoma of the gallbladder. Pathol Res Pract 184: 279–286

256. Kijima H, Watanabe H, Iwafuchi M et al. 1989 Histogenesis of gallbladder carcinoma from investigation of early carcinoma and microcarcinoma. Acta Pathol Jpn 39: 235–244
257. Hisatomi K, Haratake J, Horie A et al. 1990 Relation of histopathological features to prognosis of gallbladder cancer. Am J Gastroenterol 85: 567–572
258. Albores-Saavedra J, Nadji M, Henson D et al. 1986 Intestinal metaplasia of the gallbladder; a morphologic and immunocytochemical study. Hum Pathol 17: 614–620
259. Albores-Saavedra J, Nadji M, Henson D 1986 Intestinal-type adenocarcinoma of the gallbladder: a clinicopathologic and immunocytochemical study of seven cases. Am J Surg Pathol 10: 19–25
260. Yamamoto M, Nakajo S, Tahara E 1989 Dysplasia of the gallbladder. Its histogenesis and correlation to gallbladder adenocarcinoma. Pathol Res Pract 185: 454–460
261. Yamagiwa H 1989 Mucosal dysplasia of gallbladder: isolated and adjacent lesions to carcinoma. Jpn J Cancer Res 80: 238–243
262. Bivins B, Meeker W, Weiss D et al. 1975 Carcinoma in situ of the gallbladder: a dilemma. South Med J 68: 297–300
263. Albores-Saavedra J, Shukla D, Carrick K et al. 2001 In situ and invasive adenocarcinomas of the gallbladder extending into or arising from Rokitansky–Aschoff sinuses. Am J Surg Pathol 28: 621–628
264. Albores-Saavedra J, Molberg K, Henson D 1996 Unusual malignant epithelial tumors of the gallbladder. Semin Diagn Pathol 13: 326–338
265. Ligoury C, Canard J M 1983 Tumours of the biliary system. Clin Gastroenterol 12: 269–295
266. Serra I, Calvo A, Maturana M et al. 1990 Biliary tract cancer in Chile. Int J Cancer 46: 965–971
267. Brandt-Rauf P, Pincus M, Adelson S 1982 Cancer of the gallbladder: a review of forty-three cases. Hum Pathol 13: 48–53
268. Strom B L, Iliopoulos D, Atkinson B et al. 1989 Pathophysiology of tumor progression in human gallbladder: flow cytometry, CEA, and CA 19-9 levels in bile and serum in different stages of gallbladder disease. J Natl Cancer Inst 81: 1575–1580
269. Anderson J B, Cooper M J, Williamson R C N 1985 Adenocarcinoma of the extrahepatic biliary tree. Ann R Coll Surg Engl 67: 139–143
270. Kimura W, Shimada H, Kuroda A et al. 1989 Carcinoma of the gallbladder and extrahepatic bile ducts in autopsy cases of the aged, with special reference to its relationship to gallstones. Am J Gastroenterol 84: 386–390
271. Shimizu M, Miura J, Tanaka T et al. 1989 Porcelain gallbladder: relation between its type by ultrasound and incidence of cancer. J Clin Gastroenterol 11: 471–476
272. Welton J, Marr J, Friedman S 1979 Association between hepatobiliary cancer and typhoid carrier state. Lancet 1: 791–794
273. Sameshima Y, Uchimura M, Muto Y et al. 1987 Coexistent carcinoma in congenital dilatation of the bile duct and anomalous arrangement of the pancreatico-bile duct. Carcinogenesis of coexistent gall bladder carcinoma. Cancer 60: 1883–1890
274. Ozmen V, Martin P C, Igci A et al. 1991 Adenocarcinoma of the gallbladder associated with congenital choledochal cyst and anomalous pancreaticobiliary ductal junction. Eur J Surg 157: 549–551
275. Cowley L, Wood V 1964 Carcinoma developing in a remnant of the gallbladder. Ann Surg 159: 466–468
276. Albores-Saavedra J, Henson D E, Klimstra D S 2000 Tumors of the gallbladder, extrahepatic bile ducts and ampulla of Vater. Armed Forces Institute of Pathology, Washington, DC, p 61–104
276a. Albores-Saavedra J, Tuck M, McLaren B K et al. 2005 Papillary carcinomas of the gallbladder: analysis of noninvasive and invasive types. Arch Pathol Lab Med 129: 905–909
277. Vardaman C, Albores-Saavedra J 1995 Clear cell carcinomas of the gallbladder and extrahepatic bile ducts. Am J Surg Pathol 19: 91–99
277a. Albores-Saavedra J, Grider D J, Wu J et al. 2006 Giant cell tumor of the extrahepatic biliary tree: a clinicopathologic study of 4 cases and comparison with anaplastic spindle and giant cell carcinoma with osteoclast-like giant cells. Am J Surg Pathol 30: 495–500
278. Fukuda T, Ohnishi Y 1990 Gallbladder carcinoma producing human chorionic gonadotropin. Am J Gastroenterol 85: 1403–1406
279. Suster S, Huszar M, Herczeg E et al. 1987 Adenosquamous carcinoma of the gallbladder with spindle cell features. A light microscopic and immunocytochemical study of a case. Histopathology 11: 209–214
280. Iida Y, Tsutsumi Y 1992 Small cell (endocrine cell) carcinoma of the gallbladder with squamous and adenocarcinomatous components. Acta Pathol Jpn 42: 119–125
281. Nishihara K, Takashima K, Furuta T et al. 1995 Adenosquamous carcinoma of the gall-bladder with gastric foveolar-type epithelium. Pathol Int 45: 250–256
282. Albores-Saavedra J, Soriano J, Larraza-Hernandez O et al. 1984 Oat cell carcinoma of the gallbladder. Hum Pathol 15: 639–646
283. Cavazzana A, Fassina A, Tollot M et al. 1991 Small-cell carcinoma of the gallbladder. An immunocytochemical and ultrastructural study. Pathol Res Pract 187: 472–476
284. Duan H J, Ishigame H, Ishii Z et al. 1991 Small cell carcinoma of the gallbladder combined with adenocarcinoma. Acta Pathol Jpn 41: 841–846
285. Nishihara K, Tsuneyoshi M 1993 Undifferentiated spindle cell carcinoma of the gallbladder. Hum Pathol 24: 1298–1305
286. Fujii K, Yokozaki H, Yasui W et al. 1996 High frequency of p53 gene mutation in adenocarcinomas of the gallbladder. Cancer Epidemiol Biomarkers Prev 5: 461–466
287. Wistuba I I, Albores-Saavedra J 1999 Genetic abnormalities involved in the pathogenesis of gallbladder carcinoma. J Hepatobiliary Pancreat Surg 6: 237–244
288. Ajiki T, Onoyama H, Yamamoto M et al. 1996 p53 protein expression and prognosis in gallbladder carcinoma and premalignant lesions. Hepatogastroenterology 43: 521–526
289. Wistuba I I, Sugio K, Hung J et al. 1995 Allele-specific mutations involved in the pathogenesis of endemic gallbladder carcinoma in Chile. Cancer Res 55: 2511–2515
290. Yoshida S, Todoroki T, Ichikawa Y et al. 1995 Mutations of p16Ink4/CDKN2 and p15Ink4B/MTS2 genes in biliary tract cancers. Cancer Res 55: 2756–2760
291. Wistuba I I, Ashfaq R, Maitra A et al. 2002 Fragile histidine triad gene abnormalities in the pathogenesis of gallbladder carcinoma. Am J Pathol 160: 2073–2079
292. Wistuba I I, Miquel J F, Gazdar A F et al. 1999 Gallbladder adenomas have molecular abnormalities different from those present in gallbladder carcinomas. Hum Pathol 30: 21–25
293. Arnaud J P, Casa C, Georgeac C et al. 1995 Primary carcinoma of the gallbladder – review of 143 cases. Hepatogastroenterology 42: 811–815
294. Shoup M, Fong Y 2002 Surgical indications and extent of resection in gallbladder cancer. Surg Oncol Clin North Am 11: 985–994
295. Malats N, Porta M, Pinol J L et al. 1995 Ki-ras mutations as a prognostic factor in extrahepatic bile system cancer. J Clin Oncol 13: 1679–1686
296. Ouchi K, Owada Y, Matsuno S et al. 1987 Prognostic factors in the surgical treatment of gallbladder carcinoma. Surgery 101: 731–737
297. North J H Jr, Pack M S, Hong C et al. 1998 Prognostic factors for adenocarcinoma of the gallbladder: an analysis of 162 cases. Am Surg 64: 437–440
298. Bartlett D L, Fong Y, Fortner J G et al. 1996 Long-term results after resection for gallbladder cancer. Implications for staging and management. Ann Surg 224: 639–646
299. Weedon D 1984 Other primary tumors (melanoma, carcinoid). In: Weedon D (ed) Pathology of the gallbladder. Year Book Medical Publishers, Chicago, p 251–254
300. Papotti M, Galliano D, Monga G 1990 Signet-ring cell carcinoid of the gallbladder. Histopathology 17: 255–259
301. Yamamoto M, Nakajo S, Miyoshi N et al. 1989 Endocrine cell carcinoma (carcinoid) of the gallbladder. Am J Surg Pathol 13: 292–302
302. Noda M, Miwa A, Kitagawa M 1989 Carcinoid tumors of the gallbladder with adenocarcinomatous differentiation: a morphologic and immunohistochemical study. Am J Gastroenterol 84: 953–957
303. Bricker D, Halpert B 1963 Adenomyoma of the gallbladder. Surgery 53: 615–620
304. Shepard V, Walters W, Dockerty M 1942 Benign neoplasms of the gallbladder. Arch Surg 45: 1–18
305. Aguirre J, Boher R, Guraieb S 1969 Hyperplastic cholecystoses: a new contribution to the unitarian theory. Am J Roentgenol 107: 1–13
306. Ochsner S 1966 Solitary polypoid lesions of the gallbladder. Radiol Clin North Am 4: 501–510
307. Carrera G, Ochsner S 1958 Polypoid mucosal lesions of the gallbladder. JAMA 166: 888–892
308. MacBeth W 1964 Papillomas of the gallbladder. A technical consideration as illustrated by three cases. Am J Surg 108: 8–12
309. Qizilbash A 1976 Acute pancreatitis occurring in heterotopic pancreatic tissue in the gallbladder. Cancer J Surg 19: 413–414
310. Vidgoff I, Lewis A 1961 Acute hemorrhage from aberrant pancreatic tissue in the gallbladder. Calif Med 94: 317–319
311. Bentivegna S, Hirschl S 1972 Heterotopic gastric mucosa in the gallbladder presenting as a symptom-producing tumor. Am J Gastroenterol 57: 423–428
312. Jain D, Sarode V R, Abdul-Karim F W et al. 2000 Evidence for the neoplastic transformation of Von-Meyenburg complexes. Am J Surg Pathol 24: 1131–1139
313. Allaire G S, Rabin L, Ishak K G et al. 1988 Bile duct adenoma. A study of 152 cases. Am J Surg Pathol 12: 708–715
314. Bhathal P S, Hughes N R, Goodman Z D 1996 The so-called bile duct adenoma is a peribiliary gland hamartoma. Am J Surg Pathol 20: 858–864
315. O'Hara B J, McCue P A, Miettinen M 1992 Bile duct adenomas with endocrine component. Immunohistochemical study and comparison with conventional bile duct adenomas. Am J Surg Pathol 16: 21–25
316. Albores-Saavedra J, Hoang M P, Murakata L A et al. 2001 Atypical bile duct adenoma, clear cell type: a previously undescribed tumor of the liver. Am J Surg Pathol 25: 956–960
317. Devaney K, Goodman Z D, Ishak K G 1994 Hepatobiliary cystadenoma and cystadenocarcinoma. A light microscopic and immunohistochemical study of 70 patients. Am J Surg Pathol 18: 1078–1091
318. Davies W, Chow M, Nagorney D 1995 Extrahepatic biliary cystadenomas and cystadenocarcinoma. Ann Surg 222: 619–625
319. Thomas J A, Scriven M W, Puntis M C A et al. 1992 Elevated serum CA 19-9 levels in hepatobiliary cystadenoma with mesenchymal stroma. Cancer 70: 1841–1846
320. Lee J H, Chen D R, Pang S C et al. 1996 Mucinous biliary cystadenoma with mesenchymal stroma: expression of CA 19-9 and carcinoembryonic antigen in serum and cystic fluid. J Gastroenterol 31: 732–736
321. Shimada M, Kajiyama K, Saitoh A et al. 1996 Cystic neoplasms of the liver: a report of two cases with special reference to cystadenocarcinoma. Hepatogastroenterology 43: 249–254

322. Gourley W K, Kumar D, Bouton M S et al. 1992 Cystadenoma and cystadenocarcinoma with mesenchymal stroma of the liver. Immunohistochemical analysis. Arch Pathol Lab Med 116: 1047–1050
323. Ishak K G, Willis G W, Cummins S D et al. 1977 Biliary cystadenoma and cystadenocarcinoma: report of 14 cases and review of the literature. Cancer 39: 322–338
324. Tsui W M, Loo K T, Chow L T et al. 1993 Biliary adenofibroma. A heretofore unrecognized benign biliary tumor of the liver. Am J Surg Pathol 17: 186–192
325. Varnholt H, Vauthey J N, Cin P D et al. 2003 Biliary adenofibroma: a rare neoplasm of bile duct origin with an indolent behavior. Am J Surg Pathol 27: 693–698
326. Parada L A, Bardi G, Hallen M et al. 1997 Monosomy 22 in a case of biliary adenofibroma. Cancer Genet Cytogenet 93: 183–184
327. Wysocki A, Papla B, Budzynski P 2002 Neuromas of the extrahepatic bile ducts as a cause of obstructive jaundice. Eur J Gastroenterol Hepatol 14: 573–576
328. Ojima H, Takenoshita S, Nagamachi Y 2000 Adenomyoma of the common bile duct: report of a case. Hepatogastroenterology 47: 132–134
329. Nakanuma Y, Kurumaya H, Ohta G 1984 Multiple cysts in the hepatic hilum and their pathogenesis. A suggestion of periductal gland origin. Virchows Arch A Pathol Anat Histopathol 404: 341–350
330. Vick D J, Goodman Z D, Deavers M T et al. 1999 Ciliated hepatic foregut cyst: a study of six cases and review of the literature. Am J Surg Pathol 23: 671–677
331. Vick D J, Goodman Z D, Ishak K G 1999 Squamous cell carcinoma arising in a ciliated hepatic foregut cyst. Arch Pathol Lab Med 123: 1115–1117
332. Eisen R, Kirby W, O'Quinn J 1991 Granular cell tumor of the biliary tree. A report of two cases and a review of the literature. Am J Surg Pathol 15: 460–465
333. Davila J A, El-Serag H B 2002 Cholangiocarcinoma: the "other" liver cancer on the rise. Am J Gastroenterol 97: 3199–3200
334. Khan S A, Davidson B R, Goldin R et al. 2002 Guidelines for the diagnosis and treatment of cholangiocarcinoma: consensus document. Gut 51 (suppl 6): VI1–9
335. Gores G J 2003 Cholangiocarcinoma: current concepts and insights. Hepatology 37: 961–969
336. Wee A, Ludwig J, Coffey R et al. 1985 Hepatobiliary carcinoma associated with primary sclerosing cholangitis and chronic ulcerative colitis. Hum Pathol 16: 719–726
337. Chalasani N, Baluyut A, Ismail A et al. 2000 Cholangiocarcinoma in patients with primary sclerosing cholangitis: a multicenter case-control study. Hepatology 31: 7–11
338. Fleming K A, Boberg K M, Glaumann H et al. 2001 Biliary dysplasia as a marker of cholangiocarcinoma in primary sclerosing cholangitis. J Hepatol 34: 360–365
339. Koga A, Ichimiya H, Yamaguchi K et al. 1985 Hepatolithiasis associated with cholangiocarcinoma. Cancer 55: 2826–2829
340. Chauduri P, Chauduri B, Schuler J et al. 1982 Carcinoma associated with congenital cystic dilatation of bile ducts. Arch Surg 117: 1349–1351
341. Orii T, Ohkohchi N, Sasaki K et al. 2003 Cholangiocarcinoma arising from preexisting biliary hamartoma of liver – report of a case. Hepatogastroenterology 50: 333–336
342. Nakanuma Y, Harada K, Ishikawa A et al. 2003 Anatomic and molecular pathology of intrahepatic cholangiocarcinoma. J Hepatobiliary Pancreat Surg 10: 265–281
343. Okuda K, Nakanuma Y, Miyazaki M 2002 Cholangiocarcinoma: recent progress. Part 1: epidemiology and etiology. J Gastroenterol Hepatol 17: 1049–1055
344. Rubel L, Ishak K 1982 Thorotrast-associated cholangiocarcinoma. Cancer 50: 1408–1415
345. Mecklin J P, Jarvinen H J, Virolainen M 1992 The association between cholangiocarcinoma and hereditary nonpolyposis colorectal carcinoma. Cancer 69: 1112–1114
346. Altaee M Y, Johnson P J, Farrant J M et al. 1991 Etiologic and clinical characteristics of peripheral and hilar cholangiocarcinoma. Cancer 68: 2051–2055
347. Terada T, Kida T, Nakanuma Y et al. 1994 Intrahepatic cholangiocarcinomas associated with nonbiliary cirrhosis. A clinicopathologic study. J Clin Gastroenterol 18: 335–342
348. Shirabe K, Shimada M, Harimoto N et al. 2002 Intrahepatic cholangiocarcinoma: its mode of spreading and therapeutic modalities. Surgery 131 (1 suppl): S159–S164
349. Okuda K, Nakanuma Y, Miyazaki M 2002 Cholangiocarcinoma: recent progress. Part 2: molecular pathology and treatment. J Gastroenterol Hepatol 17: 1056–1063
350. Torok N J, Higuchi H, Bronk S et al. 2002 Nitric oxide inhibits apoptosis downstream of cytochrome C release by nitrosylating caspase 9. Cancer Res 62: 1648–1653
351. Yoon J H, Werneburg N W, Higuchi H et al. 2002 Bile acids inhibit Mcl-1 protein turnover via an epidermal growth factor receptor/Raf-1-dependent mechanism. Cancer Res 62: 6500–6505
352. Ohashi K, Nakajima Y, Kanehiro H et al. 1995 Ki-ras mutations and p53 protein expressions in intrahepatic cholangiocarcinomas: relation to gross tumor morphology. Gastroenterology 109: 1612–1617
353. Ahrendt S A, Eisenberger C F, Yip L et al. 1999 Chromosome 9p21 loss and p16 inactivation in primary sclerosing cholangitis-associated cholangiocarcinoma. J Surg Res 84: 88–93
354. Niiyama H, Mizumoto K, Kusumoto M et al. 1999 Activation of telomerase and its diagnostic application in biopsy specimens from biliary tract neoplasms. Cancer 85: 2138–2143
355. Hanazaki K, Kajikawa S, Shimozawa N et al. 2002 Prognostic factors of intrahepatic cholangiocarcinoma after hepatic resection: univariate and multivariate analysis. Hepatogastroenterology 49: 311–316
356. Kokudo N, Makuuchi M 2002 Extent of resection and outcome after curative resection for intrahepatic cholangiocarcinoma. Surg Oncol Clin North Am 11: 969–983
357. Hoang M P, Murakata L A, Katabi N et al. 2002 Invasive papillary carcinomas of the extrahepatic bile dicts: a clinicopathologic and immunohistochemical study of 13 cases. Mod Pathol 15: 1251–1258
358. Rumalla A, Baron T H, Leontovich O et al. 2001 Improved diagnostic yield of endoscopic biliary brush cytology by digital image analysis. Mayo Clin Proc 76: 29–33
359. Sarmiento J M, Nagorney D M 2002 Hepatic resection in the treatment of perihilar cholangiocarcinoma. Surg Oncol Clin North Am 11: 893–908
360. Bergquist A, Glaumann H, Stal P et al. 2001 Biliary dysplasia, cell proliferation and nuclear DNA-fragmentation in primary sclerosing cholangitis with and without cholangiocarcinoma. J Intern Med 249: 69–75
361. Shimonishi T, Sasaki M, Nakanuma Y 2000 Precancerous lesions of intrahepatic cholangiocarcinoma. J Hepatobiliary Pancreat Surg 7: 542–550
362. Lee S S, Kin M-H, Lee S K et al. 2004 Clinicopathologic review of 58 patients with biliary papillomatosis. Cancer 100: 783–793
363. Kim H J, Kim M H, Lee S K et al. 2000 Mucin-hypersecreting bile duct tumor characterized by a striking homology with an intraductal papillary mucinous tumor (IPMT) of the pancreas. Endoscopy 32: 389–393
364. Shimonishi T, Zen Y, Chen T C et al. 2002 Increasing expression of gastrointestinal phenotypes and p53 along with histologic progression of intraductal papillary neoplasia of the liver. Hum Pathol 33: 503–511
365. Amaya S, Sasaki M, Watanabe Y et al. 2001 Expression of MUC1 and MUC2 and carbohydrate antigen Tn change during malignant transformation of biliary papillomatosis. Histopathology 38: 550–560
366. Suh K S, Roh H R, Koh Y T et al. 2000 Clinicopathologic features of the intraductal growth type of peripheral cholangiocarcinoma. Hepatology 31: 12–17
367. Maitra A, Krueger J E, Tascilar M et al. 2000 Carcinoid tumors of the extrahepatic bile ducts. A study of seven cases. Am J Surg Pathol 11: 1501–1510
368. Caceres M, Mosquera L F, Shih J A et al. 2001 Paraganglioma of the bile duct. South Med J 94: 515–518
369. Wagner M S, Shoup M, Pickleman J et al. 2000 Primary malignant melanoma of the common bile duct: a case report and review of the literature. Arch Pathol Lab Med 124: 419–422
370. Ruymann F B, Raney R B Jr, Crist W M et al. 1985 Rhabdomyosarcoma of the biliary tree in childhood. A report from the Intergroup Rhabdomyosarcoma Study. Cancer 56: 575–581

胰腺外分泌肿瘤
Tumors of the exocrine pancreas

11

Günter Klöppel 和 David S. Klimstra 著

钱利华 译　回允中 校

分类和一般特征	463
导管腺癌	463
导管腺癌亚型	468
导管内乳头状黏液性肿瘤	470
黏液性囊性肿瘤	473
浆液性囊性肿瘤	474
腺泡细胞癌	476
胰母细胞瘤	478
实性假乳头状肿瘤	478
其他癌	479
婴儿和儿童肿瘤	480
非上皮性肿瘤和继发性肿瘤	480
瘤样病变	480

分类和一般特征

本章所采用的分类和命名是依据世界卫生组织（WHO）所提出的分类和命名并稍加修改[1]。其前提是胰腺肿瘤细胞表型与胰腺的三种主要上皮谱系（即导管细胞、腺泡细胞和内分泌细胞）中的一种类似。多数胰腺外分泌肿瘤属于显示导管细胞表型肿瘤的范畴，因而称为导管腺癌。当讨论"胰腺癌"或"胰腺腺癌"时，即指这种肿瘤及其亚型、腺鳞癌以及未分化癌等[2-7]。导管腺癌及其亚型为"实性"癌，一般发生于胰头部。胰腺其他"实性"肿瘤包括腺泡细胞癌、胰母细胞瘤和内分泌肿瘤。这些肿瘤特别少见，仅占4%（表11.1）。与大部分"实性"肿瘤相比，"囊性"胰腺肿瘤的特征是预后极好，不仅是交界类肿瘤，恶性肿瘤的预后也好。浆液性和黏液性囊性肿瘤以及实性假乳头状肿瘤和导管内乳头状黏液性肿瘤约占所有外分泌上皮性肿瘤的6%（表11.1）[4,8,9]。黏液性囊性肿瘤和导管内乳头状黏液性肿瘤均可依据其生物学行为分为良性肿瘤、交界性肿瘤（或不能确定恶性潜能的肿瘤）和恶性肿瘤。胰腺原发性非上皮性外分泌肿瘤极为少见，例如肉瘤和恶性淋巴瘤。胰腺内分泌肿瘤在第20章讨论。

导管腺癌　Ductal adenocarcinoma

流行病学和临床特征

导管腺癌的特征为局限于胰头部，在高度纤维组织增生性间质中可见浸润性导管样和管状结构。其发

表11.1　胰腺肿瘤的一般特征

类型	发生率（%）	预后
"实性肿瘤"		
导管腺癌及亚型	90	不良
腺泡细胞癌	1	不良[a]
胰母细胞瘤	<1	不良[a]
内分泌肿瘤	2	中等[b]
非上皮性肿瘤	极少	中等[b]
"囊性肿瘤"		
导管内乳头状黏液性肿瘤	2	好
黏液性囊性肿瘤	1	好
浆液性囊性肿瘤	1	好
实性假乳头状肿瘤	<1	好
其他囊性肿瘤	1	中等[b]
非上皮性病变和肿瘤	极少	中等[b]

[a] 治疗（手术，化疗）和在儿童病人预后可有改善
[b] 取决于亚型

病原因远未明确。已经提出的少数几种危险因素是吸烟、饮食中脂肪摄取过量和慢性胰腺炎,尤其是遗传性胰腺炎(hereditary pancreatitis)[10]。家族性病例罕见,但胰腺导管腺癌可发生于所谓的"癌症家族"(cancer families)[11]。一般情况下,伴有明显胰腺癌家族史的病人,其危险性明显提高[12]。近来,在大约20%的家族性导管腺癌中可以检测出BRCA2种系突变,并且常染色体显性遗传性导管腺癌的一个新的易感位点定位于染色体4q32-34[13]。在伴有后一种遗传学异常的家系中,胰腺病理学上可见肿瘤前导管内改变[14]。与胰腺癌有关的其他遗传综合征包括家族性非典型性多发性痣/黑色素瘤综合征、毛细血管扩张性共济失调以及Peutz-Jeghers综合征[15]。

在工业化国家,经过年龄校准的导管腺癌的年发病率为每10万人在3.1~20.8例之间[15]。两性受累几乎均等,发病高峰年龄在50~70岁,40岁以前极为少见[16,17]。大约2/3的病人肿瘤累及胰头部,引起胆管和胰腺导管的梗阻。病人表现为黄疸和体重减轻,而且由于早期侵犯后腹膜组织中的神经而常常伴有疼痛。另外,有些病人可有新近发生的糖尿病和急性胰腺炎。1/3的病人肿瘤位于胰体和(或)胰尾,少数位于钩状突。这些病人常出现疼痛和体重减轻或有来自"隐匿性"原发灶的肝转移,由于癌的生长几乎不受任何解剖学边界的阻碍,因而迅速累及胰腺外组织。随后受累的组织是腹膜后、腹膜、胃、结肠、脾和左侧肾上腺。

大体表现

不论位于胰头还是位于胰腺其余部分,导管腺癌一般为境界不清的"实性"肿瘤,质地较硬,黄白色至灰色,直径一般介于2~5 cm之间(图11.1)。出血、坏死、囊性变或在整个胰腺实质内弥漫性生长并不常见[18]。在少数情况下,导管腺癌可发生于异位胰腺组织[19]。

显微镜下表现

多数导管腺癌为高分化到中分化腺癌,由分泌黏液的柱状细胞所形成的管状和导管样结构构成(图11.2)。肿瘤性管状结构衬以高度不同的单层细胞,偶尔出现乳头状突起。个别情况下肿瘤出现所谓泡沫样腺体结构[20]、大导管型形态改变[18]、微乳头状结构[21]或透明细胞表型[22](参见479页其他癌部分)(图11.3)。肿瘤性腺体浸润胰腺实质使得非肿瘤性导管、腺泡和胰岛散布于癌性结构之间。这种生长方式通常伴有显著的纤维组织增生性反应。细胞核一般呈极性分布,

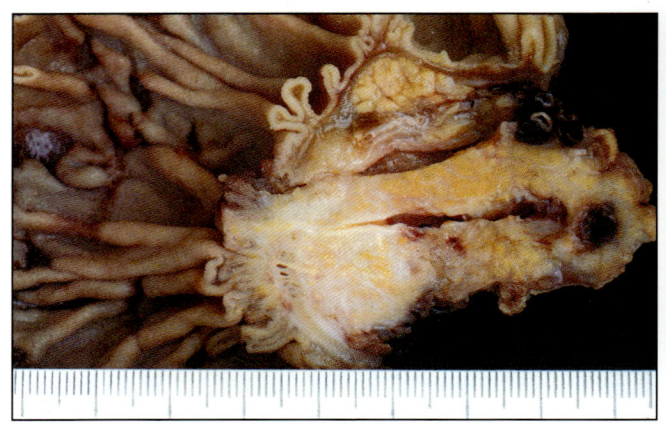

图11.1　胰头导管腺癌的大体标本,显示侵犯壶腹及十二指肠壁,伴有胆总管和胰腺导管梗阻。

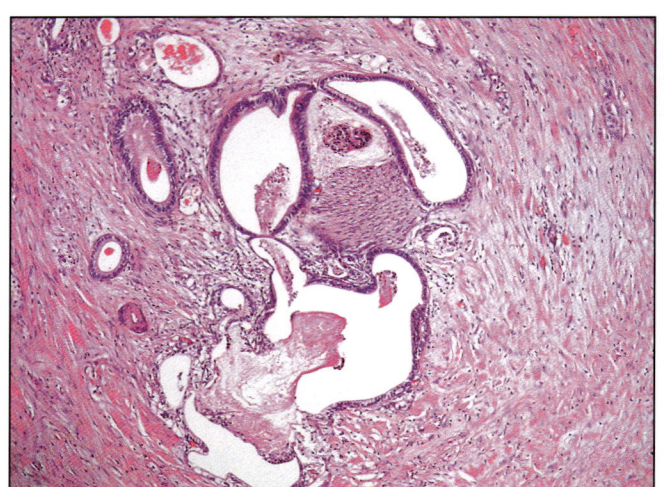

图11.2　导管腺癌伴有形成完好的管状和腺体结构。

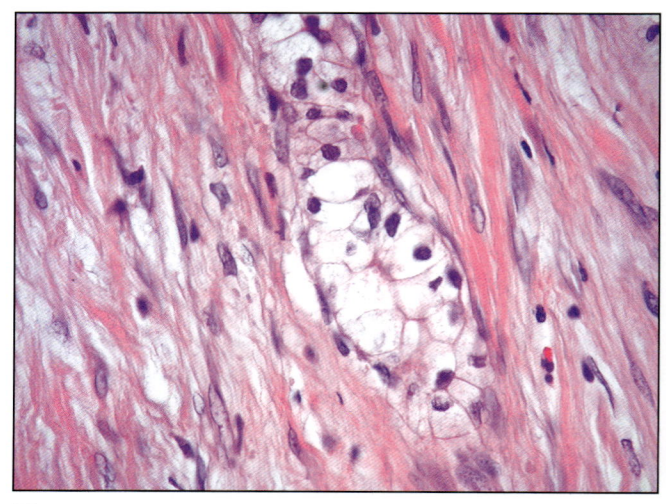

图11.3　导管腺癌伴有由透明细胞构成的管状结构。

核仁明显。

在中分化和低分化肿瘤中，组织学结构变得较不规则，腺体形成较差，黏液分泌减少（图 11.4）。细胞以及细胞核的大小差异加大。核分裂象显著。

诊断时这些肿瘤极少仅限于胰腺。几乎总是可见胰腺周围脂肪组织播散及神经周围浸润。此外，可能浸润淋巴管和静脉。因为呈导管梗阻性生长，肿瘤周围胰腺组织甚至整个残留的胰腺均可出现或轻或重的梗阻性慢性胰腺炎改变。

肿瘤周围组织中中等大小的导管常显示导管上皮被高柱状黏液细胞取代，而且常伴有乳头形成。这些病变并非肿瘤特异性改变，但与没有导管腺癌的病例相比，导管腺癌较常伴有这些改变[23-26]。由于这种相关性以及这些病变与浸润性腺癌具有相同的多种遗传学异常，因此这些导管改变被认为是癌前病变，并被称为胰腺上皮内肿瘤（pancreatic intraepithelial neoplasia，PanIN）1 至 3 级（表 11.2 和图 11.5）[27,28]。关于 PanIN-3，即原位癌，很难准确区分是与浸润癌相邻但不相连的 PanIN-3，还是肿瘤的导管内播散（"导管癌变"，duct cancerization）。除了 PanIN 病变以外，还可出现鳞状化生（图 11.6）。胰腺内出现鳞状化生似与导管腺癌或其他肿瘤无关，但可见于慢性胰腺炎的胰腺大导管长期放置支架之后。

胰腺活检和冰冻切片

胰腺活检为创伤性诊断方法，仅用于所有其他用来确诊胰腺肿瘤的诊断方法均告失败的病例。由于现代影像学技术的进步，通过超声、CT 或超声内镜检查引导

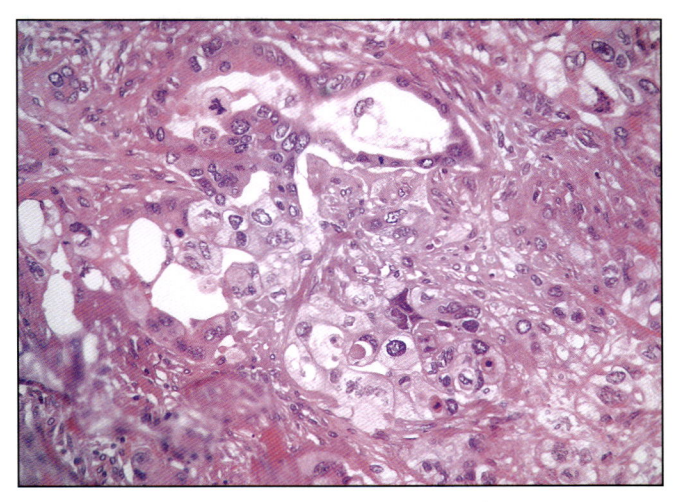

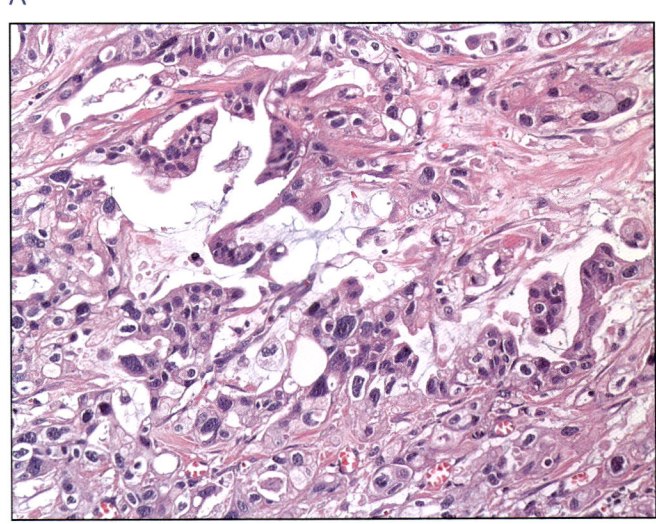

图 11.4　低分化导管腺癌（A），显示不规则腺体和多形性细胞（B）。

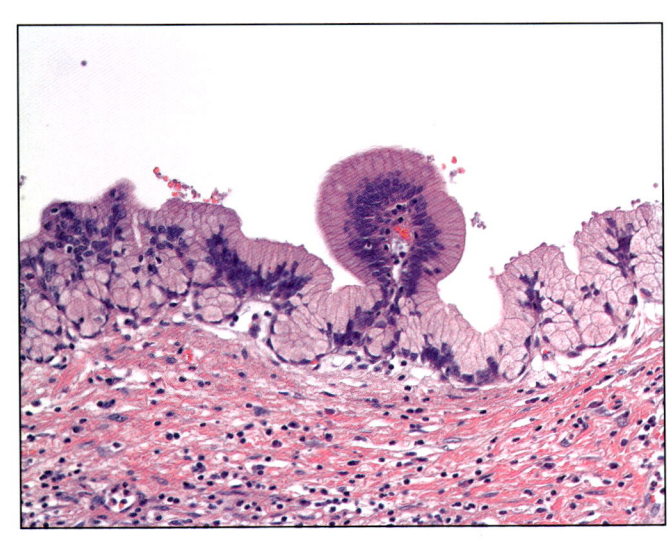

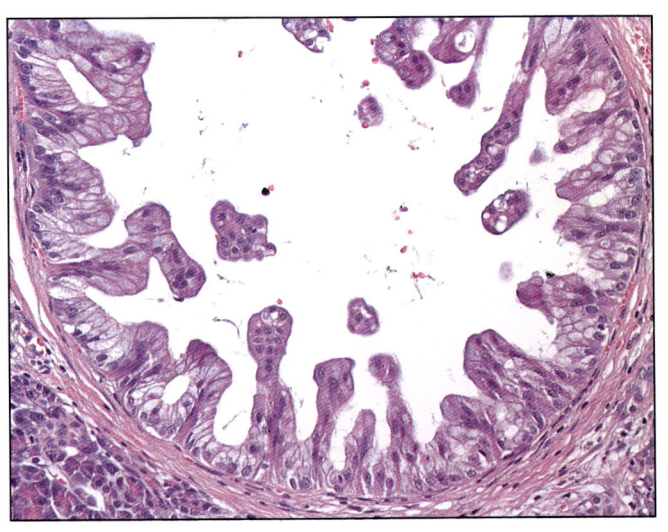

图 11.5　胰腺上皮内肿瘤形成，1级（A）和3级（B）。

表 11.2	胰腺上皮内肿瘤的分类

PanIN-1A（胰腺上皮内肿瘤1-A）：由高柱状细胞组成的扁平上皮病变，细胞核位于基底部，核上有多量黏液。由于许多PanIN-1A病例的肿瘤性质尚未得到肯定，因此这些导管改变可以应用"病变"这一修饰术语进行命名（"PanIN/L-1A"）。

PanIN-1B（胰腺上皮内肿瘤1-B）：上皮病变具有乳头状、微乳头状或基底部假复层结构，但其他方面与PanIN/L-1A相同。

PanIN-2（胰腺上皮内肿瘤2）：黏液性上皮病变可为扁平状，但多数呈乳头状。根据定义，这些病变必须具有某种程度的细胞核异常，但是达不到PanIN-3的程度。

PanIN-3（胰腺上皮内肿瘤3）：通常为乳头状或微乳头状病变，伴有重度细胞非典型性。这些病变的细胞核表现与癌相似，但是缺乏穿透基底膜的浸润。

下的胰腺细针活检已经成为可靠的方法，使得导管腺癌或任何其他比较少见的胰腺肿瘤的诊断具有高度敏感性和特异性。合并症极为少见，尤其是应用超声内镜检查引导下的活检。一个新的活检适应证是证明有某些标记物或基因突变而需要启动特殊治疗时，例如出现表皮生长因子受体（EGFR）则应用西妥昔单抗治疗。在活检标本中遇到的诊断问题集中在胰腺癌与慢性胰腺炎的鉴别诊断（见鉴别诊断）以及不同类型胰腺肿瘤的区分上（表 11.3）。术中冰冻切片评估胰腺病变的重点也是集中在导管癌和慢性胰腺炎的鉴别上。尽管冰冻切片诊断对于某个病例可能仍然存在困难，但据报告其诊断准确率可高达98%[29]。

免疫组织学

导管腺癌免疫染色显示 CK 7、8、18 和 19，上皮膜抗原（EMA），癌胚抗原（CEA）[30] 以及 CA19-9 或 DUPAN-2[31,32] 呈阳性表达。此外，脱辅基黏蛋白（apomucin）MUC1 也呈阳性（图 11.7）。另一方面，应用抗 MUC2、胰酶（例如胰蛋白酶）以及神经内分泌标记物抗体染色，肿瘤一般呈阴性（表 11.4）。

遗传学

多数导管腺癌出现 K-ras 癌基因活化突变和 CDKN2S/p16 肿瘤抑制基因失活突变。大约 50%~60% 的病例出现肿瘤抑制基因 p53 和 smad4/dpc4 失活突变[15,33,34]。发生率较低的基因改变包括 MKK4 基因、TGF-β 受体 R1 和 R2 基因、BRCA2 基因和 KLB/STK11 基因。

生长因子

在各种生长因子及其受体中，已经发现导管腺癌

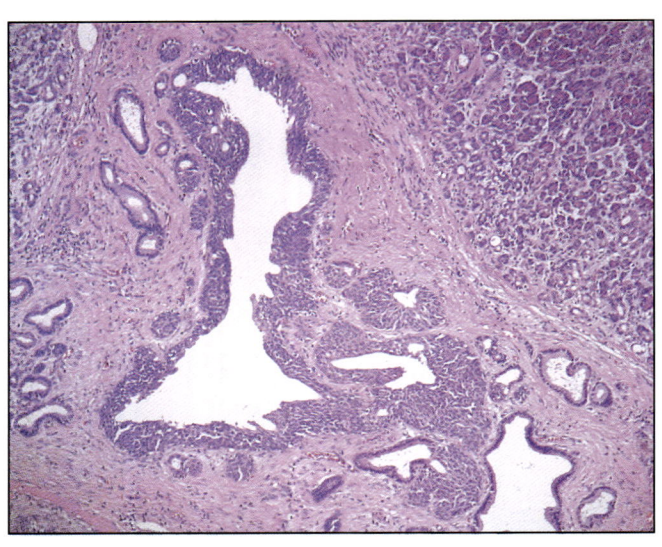

图 11.6 胰腺导管伴有鳞状化生。

表 11.3	诊断性胰腺活检的主要适应证	
影像学	鉴别诊断	
	良性	恶性
生物学不确定的实性肿物	常见：酒精性慢性胰腺炎 少见：自身免疫性胰腺炎 　　　　内分泌肿瘤	导管腺癌 内分泌癌 腺泡细胞癌 恶性间叶性肿瘤 淋巴瘤 转移性肿瘤
囊性肿物	假性囊肿 浆液性囊腺瘤 各种非肿瘤性囊肿	黏液性囊腺瘤 导管内乳头状黏液性肿瘤

表 11.4	最重要的胰腺肿瘤免疫组织学鉴别诊断											
肿瘤类型	CK7, 19	CK8, 18	VIM	MUC1	MUC2	TRYP	SYN	CG	NSE	CEA	AFP
导管腺癌	+	+	−	+	−	−	−	−	−	+	−
导管内乳头状黏液性肿瘤	+	+	−	+a	+b	−	(+)	(+)	−	+	−
黏液性囊性肿瘤	+	+	−	(+)	−	−	(+)	(+)	−	+	−
浆液性囊腺瘤	+	+	−	−	−	−	−	−	+	−	−
腺泡细胞癌	(+)/−	+	−	−	−	+	(+)	(+)	(+)	−	−
胰母细胞瘤	+	+	−	−	−	+	(+)	(+)	(+)	−	(+)
实性假乳头状肿瘤	−	−	+	−	−	−	−	−	+	−	−
内分泌肿瘤	(+)/−	+	−	−	−	−	+	+	+	−	−

(+)少数细胞；+多数细胞；CEA：癌胚抗原；TRYP：胰蛋白酶和其他胰酶；SYN：突触素；CG：嗜铬素 A；AFP：甲胎蛋白；CK：细胞角蛋白；VIM：波形蛋白；NSE：神经元特异性烯醇化酶；MUC：MUC核心蛋白。
a 胰胆管型
b 肠型

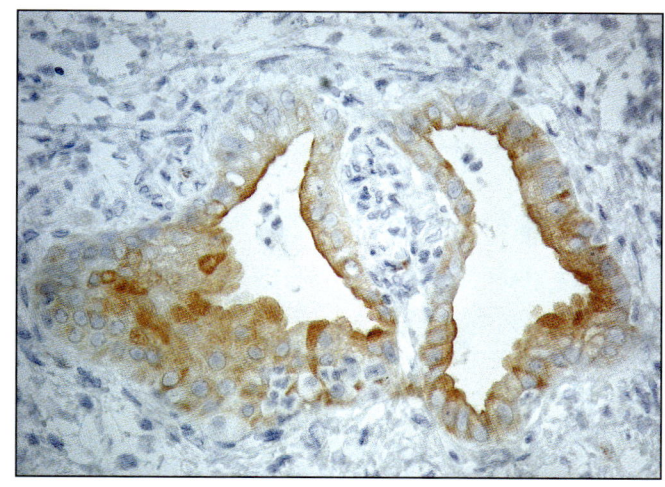

图11.7 高分化导管腺癌，分化良好，MUC1染色。

表达 *EGFR* 和 *HER2/neu*（*c-erb B2*）[35]。这两种因子分别具有促有丝分裂和生长因子信号转导功能，在导管腺癌中常有过度表达。血管生成因子 VEGF（vascular endothelial growth factor，血管内皮生长因子）在导管腺癌中有不同程度的表达[36]。

鉴别诊断

主要问题在于高分化导管腺癌与慢性胰腺炎的鉴别[37]。大体上，这两种病变表现极为相似。然而，如果在胰腺导管中见到结石，最可能的诊断为晚期慢性胰腺炎。镜下，活检标本（包括冰冻切片）和大块组织标本所采用的诊断标准相同（表 11.5）。低倍镜下，导管腺癌出现杂乱排列的浸润性管状及导管样结构，缺乏任何分叶状排列。有些肿瘤性导管可有破裂，出现乳头状上皮结构，并被纤维组织增生性间质包绕（图 11.8）。慢性胰腺炎

表 11.5	导管腺癌与慢性胰腺炎鉴别诊断的组织病理学标准	
	导管腺癌	慢性胰腺炎
导管特征		
分布	不规则，杂乱	排列规则，分叶状
部位	神经周围，血管内，胰腺外（脂肪组织中"裸露的导管"）	胰腺内
形状	破裂	导管完整
内容物	中性粒细胞，坏死碎片	结石，分泌物栓子
细胞学特征		
细胞核	多形性	一致，圆形-卵圆形
	核分裂象	无核分裂象
	核仁明显	无核仁或较小
细胞核极性	常常丧失	保留

中残留的小导管、单个腺泡和胰岛常保留小叶状排列。有些导管可出现扩张并含有结石。高倍镜下，导管腺癌出现不同程度的上皮非典型增生，并且常见核分裂象。另外，至少有局灶性细胞核极向紊乱，并可见明显的核仁。慢性胰腺炎的导管上皮可有萎缩或偶有增生，但一般无非典型性增生和核分裂象。免疫组织化学染色无特异性标记物，但 CEA、MUC1、*p53* 和（或）MIB1（图

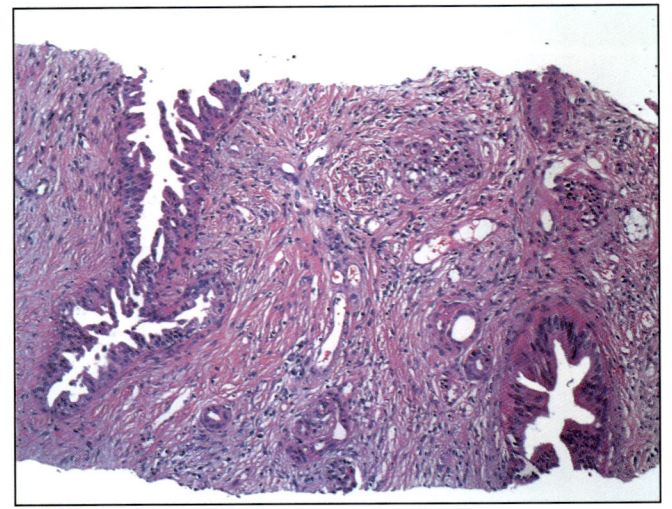

图11.8　高分化导管腺癌穿刺活检标本显示腺上皮呈乳头状。

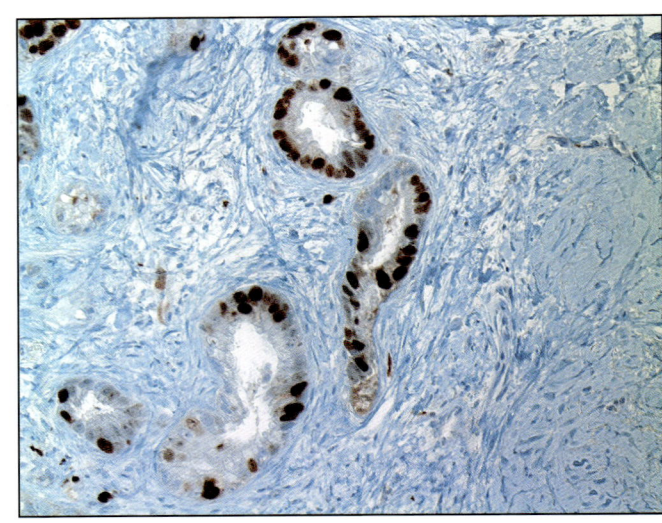

图11.9　高分化导管腺癌，细胞核MIB1染色。

11.9）阳性高度提示导管腺癌，如同 SMAD4/DPC4 表达完全缺失一样。有关导管腺癌与其他胰腺肿瘤，如导管内乳头状黏液性肿瘤、腺泡细胞癌或神经内分泌肿瘤的鉴别诊断，请参阅表11.4。

肿瘤播散、分期和分级

有关切除胰腺癌的标准化处理和准确分期有一些建议[38,39]。导管腺癌早期播散至腹膜后组织以及不同的"局部"（local）胰腺周围淋巴结，其精确的局部解剖取决于原发灶肿瘤的部位。"区域"（regional）淋巴结（即肝十二指肠韧带上至腹腔干）受累见于大约50%的病例，并且累及"区域旁"（juxtaregional），主要为主动脉旁淋巴结，大约占10%[40]。肝血行转移常见。肺、胸膜及骨转移仅见于晚期肿瘤，尤其胰体或胰尾部肿瘤；脑转移不常见。

导管腺癌现有的分级方案均按照三级系统（表11.6）[15,41]。分级资料显示，最具相关性的生物学差异在于G1/G2和G3之间的差异。肿瘤分级可能比增生指数更有意义[42]。

导管腺癌的病理学分期依据TNM分类[43]。它考虑到原发性肿瘤的大小和浸润范围（pT1-pT4）和有无区域淋巴结转移（如果多处区域淋巴结受累为pN1a或pN1b）以及远处转移（pM）（表11.7）。

预后

多数（80%～90%）导管腺癌诊断时已不能切除，病人极少能存活6个月以上。在可以切除肿瘤的病人中，大约80%～90%存活不足3年。术后5年存活率约为15%[44]。然而，近来来自日本、美国以及欧洲的病例报道其生存率有所改善[45-48]。手术切除后常有局部肿瘤复发，并且是决定预后的因素之一。

导管腺癌亚型
Variants of ductal adenocarcinoma

与导管腺癌密切相关的胰腺癌为腺鳞癌、所谓的未分化癌（包括破骨细胞样巨细胞瘤）以及混合性导管-内

表11.6	胰腺导管腺癌的分级方案		
分级[a]	腺体结构	核分裂象[b]	细胞核结构
I	高分化导管状，管状	<5	轻度多形性，核仁小
II	导管状、管状和微小腺体混合	6～10	明显多形性，核仁明显
III	腺样到未分化	>10	突出的多形性，伴有细胞核增大和突出的核仁

[a]肿瘤为异质性，应当给出最高的肿瘤分级
[b]随机选择10个高倍视野（×40）的核分裂计数

表11.7	胰腺导管腺癌的TNM分类

原发性肿瘤（T）

TX	原发性肿瘤不能评估
T0	无原发性肿瘤证据
Tis	原位癌
T1	肿瘤局限于胰腺，最大径2 cm或小于2 cm
T2	肿瘤局限于胰腺，最大径超过2 cm
T3	肿瘤延伸到胰腺以外，但未累及腹腔干或肠系膜上动脉
T4	肿瘤累及腹腔干或肠系膜上动脉

区域淋巴结（N）

NX	区域淋巴结不能评估
N0	无区域淋巴结转移
N1	区域淋巴结转移

远处转移（M）

MX	远处转移不能评估
M0	无远处转移
M1	远处转移

分组分期#

0期	Tis	N0	M0
IA期	T1	N0	M0
IB期	T2	N0	M0
IIA期	T3	N0	M0
IIB期	T1，T2，T3	N1	M0
III期	T4	任何N	M0
IV期	任何T	任何N	M1

pN0要求切除区域淋巴结，而且正常组织学检查10个或10个以上的淋巴结。

#肿瘤切除后R0期（无肿瘤残留证据）不同于R1或R2期（R1期镜下可见肿瘤残留证据；R2期大体可见肿瘤残留证据）。
Sobin LH, Wittekind C. International Union Against Cancer (UICC)© 2002 TNM Classification of Malignant Tumors, 6th edition. John Wiley & Sons, Inc., New York, USA. Reprinted with permission of John Wiley & Sons, Inc.

常能发现腺体成分。腺鳞癌也可含有间变或梭形细胞灶[52]。在转移癌中，常以腺癌成分为主，甚或仅出现腺癌成分。

未分化癌　Undifferentiated carcinoma

胰腺未分化癌（同义词：间变性癌、多形性大细胞癌、多形性巨细胞癌以及肉瘤样癌）占胰腺外分泌癌的2%～5%[2,53,54]。其性别和年龄分布一般与导管腺癌相似，但临床上更具侵袭性行为[54]。肿瘤一般较大，质软，伴有明显出血、坏死和（或）囊性变（图11.10）。

镜下，肿瘤常由位于少量间质中的单核多形性细胞组成（图11.11）。偶尔可出现奇异性多核巨细胞或梭形细胞，另外伴有鳞状成分。无特异性结构，细胞呈松散的片块状或肉瘤样排列。核分裂象常见。广泛组织取材常可发现普通的导管腺癌病灶。含有独特恶性腺体成分的未分化癌导致双相性表现，可能诊断为癌肉瘤，尤其

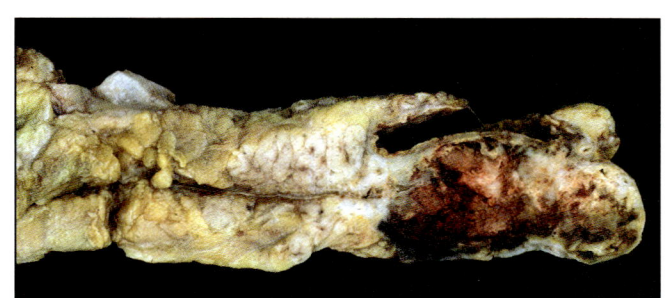

图11.10　胰尾部未分化癌，可见出血性坏死。

分泌癌[15]。黏液性非囊性（胶样）癌也曾被认为是导管腺癌的亚型[49]，近来被确认是一种与导管内乳头状黏液性肿瘤有关的特殊肿瘤类型[50]（见下）。

腺鳞癌　Adenosquamous carcinoma

腺鳞癌的性别分布、所处胰腺部位以及大体表现均与导管腺癌类似[15,51]。其特征为肿瘤性腺管与鳞状成分成不同比例混合。鳞状成分可很明显，并且几乎总是掩盖腺体成分，这种状况可能导致诊断为"鳞状细胞癌"。然而，即使在这样的病例，广泛组织取材

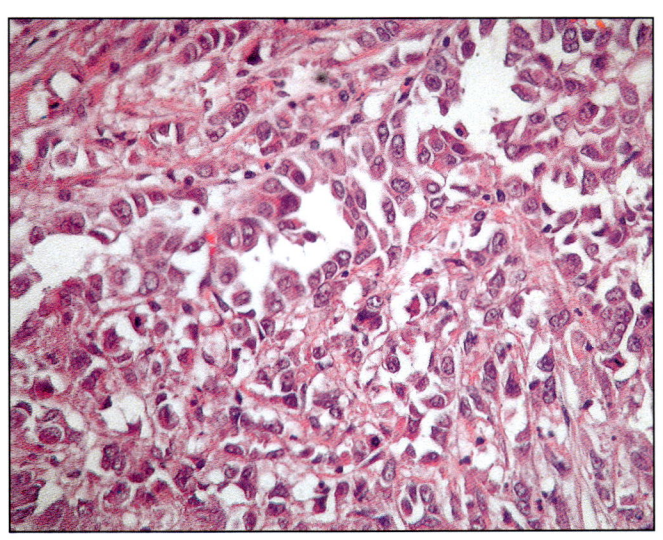

图11.11　由大的多形性细胞构成的未分化癌。

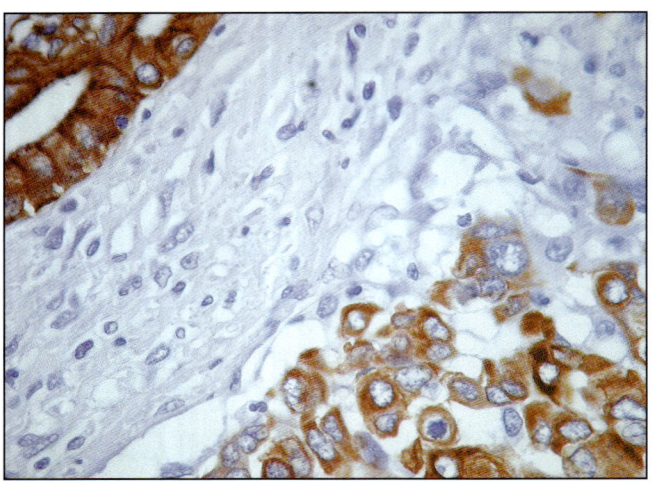

图11.12 未分化癌。多形性细胞和邻近的导管成分CK 7染色阳性。

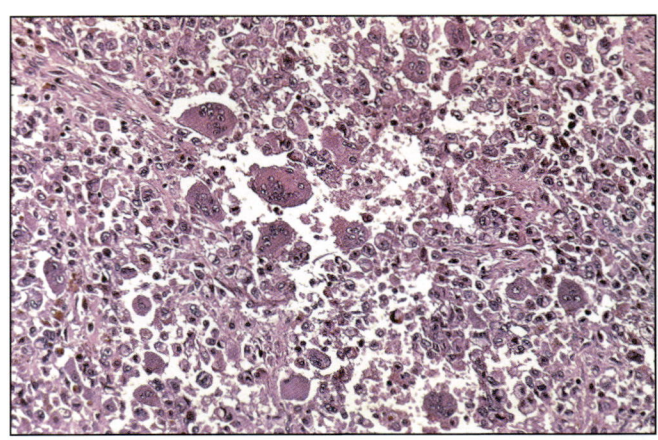

图11.13 未分化癌伴有多形性单核细胞和大量破骨细胞样多核巨细胞。

是当梭形细胞成分呈现异原性分化，伴有软骨样、骨样或骨骼肌成分时。多形性或梭形细胞的上皮性本质可通过细胞角蛋白免疫染色阳性来证实（图11.12）。然而，同一细胞波形蛋白也常呈阳性[55]。未分化癌常出现广泛淋巴管和血管侵犯。出现 K-ras 突变为导管起源提供了证据[54,55]。

伴有破骨细胞样巨细胞的未分化癌（同义词：破骨细胞型巨细胞瘤，破骨细胞样巨细胞瘤）
Undifferentiated carcinoma with osteoclast-like giant cells (synonym: giant cell tumor of the osteoclastic type, osteoclast-like giant cell tumor)

伴有破骨细胞样巨细胞的未分化癌的特征为具有单核多形性梭形和多角形细胞以及破骨细胞样多核巨细胞双重成分。类似肿瘤在其他器官也有描述，例如甲状腺和肺。多形性成分与未分化癌相同，显示高核分裂活性。破骨细胞样细胞的表现类似于正常破骨细胞（图11.13），没有核分裂活性，具有组织细胞特征，一般认为并非肿瘤性成分，并且缺乏在单核细胞成分中可检测到的 K-ras 突变[56]。它们常集中在出血区域附近。可出现腺样和实性结构。单核多形性细胞角蛋白免疫染色阳性，提示上皮性起源，但并非总是阳性[55,57,58]。破骨细胞样细胞免疫染色显示波形蛋白、白细胞共同抗原（CD45）以及组织细胞标记物 CD68 阳性。以前认为破骨细胞样巨细胞肿瘤的预后优于导管腺癌，但近来的一些报道否认这一观点，提出多数病人在一年内死亡[58]。

混合性导管-内分泌癌
Mixed ductal-endocrine carcinoma

在普通导管癌中偶尔见到并且很可能是非肿瘤性内分泌细胞的情况并非少见。在高分化导管腺癌尤其如此[59]。另一方面，伴有明显外分泌和内分泌成分的混合性癌极为少见。这种少见类型的癌由混有内分泌细胞的腺管状结构组成，内分泌细胞至少占所有肿瘤细胞的30%[59,60]。

印戒细胞癌　Signet-ring cell carcinoma

印戒细胞癌几乎完全（至少超过肿瘤的50%）由单个排列的印戒细胞构成，胞浆内含有黏液空泡，核有凹痕并呈扇贝状。肿瘤细胞呈弥漫性浸润。免疫组织学染色，肿瘤细胞 CEA 强阳性。鉴别诊断包括来自弥漫型胃腺癌或乳腺小叶癌的转移。印戒细胞癌的预后差，至少与普通导管腺癌一样。

导管内乳头状黏液性肿瘤
Intraductal papillary mucinous neoplasms

导管内乳头状黏液性肿瘤为大体可见的产生黏液的上皮性肿瘤，在胰腺导管内生长，而且常出现乳头状结构，但并非都是如此。导管内乳头状黏液性肿瘤常分泌大量黏液，并且伴有导管明显扩张，导致放射学及大体上呈囊性表现。有些病例中，黏液从 Vater 壶腹溢出。导管内乳头状黏液性肿瘤主要累及男性（平均60岁）。

多数肿瘤发生于胰头部。病人容易出现多年的胰腺炎样症状。导管内乳头状黏液性肿瘤约占胰腺外分泌肿瘤的3%～5%，由于放射影像学技术的广泛应用，随着较小导管内乳头状黏液性肿瘤检出的增加，其所占比例也在增加[61]。在所有类型的胰腺囊性肿瘤中（表11.8），导管内乳头状黏液性肿瘤占24%，而且是目前最常见的囊性肿瘤类型[61]。

过去，导管内乳头状黏液性肿瘤有多种名称，主要依据其主要特征是乳头状增生还是分泌大量黏液。这些名称包括导管内乳头状瘤、绒毛性腺瘤、导管内乳头状腺癌、产黏液性肿瘤、导管扩张性黏液性囊性肿瘤、黏液性导管扩张以及导管内黏液高分泌性肿瘤；现已不再主张应用这些名称。导管内乳头状黏液性肿瘤可出现不同程度的细胞结构非典型性，即使是在一个肿瘤内。根据导管内乳头状黏液性肿瘤非典型性最严重的区域进行分级，可将其分为伴有低度异型性的导管内乳头状黏液性肿瘤（或导管内乳头状黏液性腺瘤）、伴有中度异型性的导管内乳头状黏液性肿瘤（或交界性导管内乳头状黏液性肿瘤）以及伴有高度异型性的导管内乳头状黏液性肿瘤（或导管内乳头状黏液性原位癌）。导管内乳头状黏液性肿瘤相关浸润癌约占35%，任何浸润成分的大小和类型都应分别报告。因此，导管内乳头状黏液性肿瘤提供了一个肿瘤进展模式，即从良性导管内肿瘤开始异型性逐级增加，直到浸润癌[62-67]。

大体上，依据肿瘤主要累及大胰腺导管还是周围二级导管，导管内乳头状黏液性肿瘤可分为大导管型和分支导管型。整个胰腺导管系统（包括Vater壶腹）都可发生弥漫性受累。大导管型多位于胰头部，常含有黏稠的黏液（图11.14）。分支导管型导管内乳头状黏液性肿瘤较小（图11.15），多半不含有浸润癌，与大导管型相比，

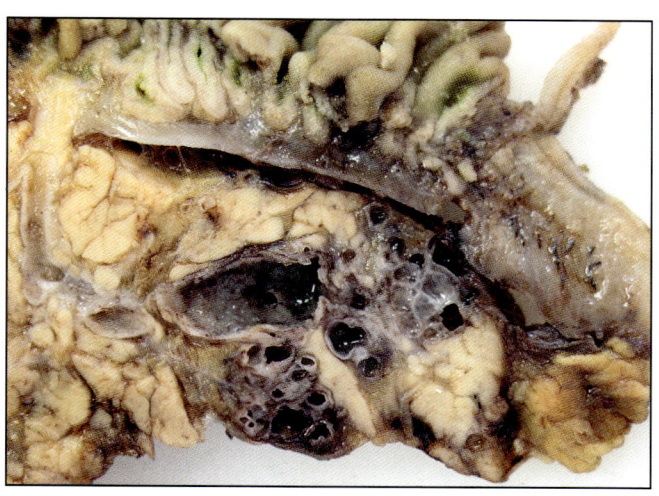

图11.15　导管内乳头状黏液性肿瘤切除标本，分支导管型。切除标本显示胰腺实质内可见一个大囊腔和多个小囊腔。（Courtesy of Dr. Hartmut Arps, Fulda, Germany）。

它主要累及胰腺局部区域[68]。肿瘤性乳头状生长结构的数量、分泌的黏液量以及导管扩张或囊肿形成的程度在每个病例之间各有不同。

组织学上，导管内乳头状黏液性肿瘤显示分泌黏液的柱状上皮细胞呈乳头状增生，取代正常导管上皮。伴有低度异型性的导管内乳头状黏液性肿瘤可见相对简单一致的乳头或伴有扁平上皮区域，细胞核均匀一致，位于基底部，缺少多形性或核分裂活性。伴有中度异型性者出现较为复杂的乳头，被覆细胞的细胞核呈假复层状分布，其形状及大小有中等程度的差异。伴有高度异型性者的特征是有非常复杂的乳头和微乳头结构，极性完全丧失，细胞核明显不规则，并且核分裂象易见。近来，已经确认四种不同形态学类型的乳头结构：肠型、胰胆管型、嗜酸细胞型（亦称导管内嗜酸细胞乳头状肿瘤，intraductal oncocytic papillary neoplasm）以及胃型[69,70]。肠型显示绒毛状生长结构，类似肠绒毛性腺瘤，并且产生MUC2和CDX2，但不产生MUC1（图11.16）[71,72]。伴随的浸润癌多为胶样（黏液性非囊性）亚型[49]，这种肿瘤至少80%是由细胞外黏液湖组成，其中漂浮有肿瘤性腺上皮细胞团或条索，甚或有少量印戒细胞成分（图11.17）。胰胆管乳头表型显示复杂的分支状乳头（图11.18），并且缺乏MUC2和CDX2表达，但MUC1染色阳性。其浸润性成分常类似于普通导管腺癌。嗜酸细胞型可见复杂乳头（图11.19），被覆伴有颗粒性嗜酸性胞浆的大细胞，不同程度表达MUC1或MUC2。胃型则常与其他类型共存，表现为乳头状突起，被覆类似于胃小凹细胞的黏液性细胞。这种细胞MUC5染色阳性（图11.20），而MUC1、MUC2和CDX2不表达。

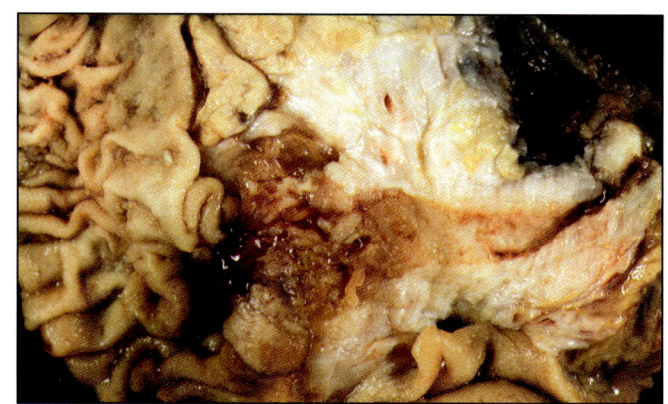

图11.14　导管内乳头状黏液性肿瘤切除标本，大导管型。切除标本显示Vater壶腹和胰腺大导管明显扩张，其内充满黏稠黏液。其余胰腺组织重度纤维化。

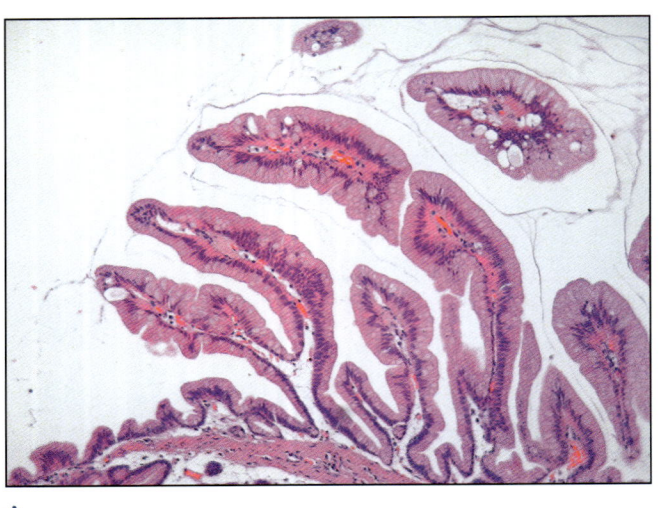 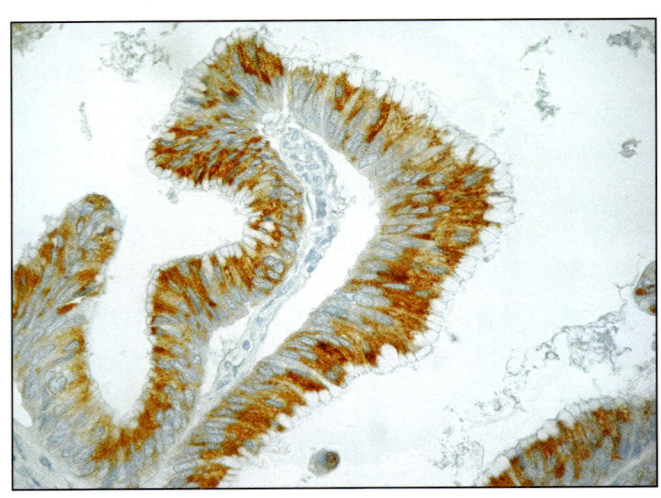

图11.16 导管内乳头状黏液性肿瘤,肠型,伴有导管内高分化柱状上皮乳头状增生(A)。肿瘤细胞MUC2染色(B)。

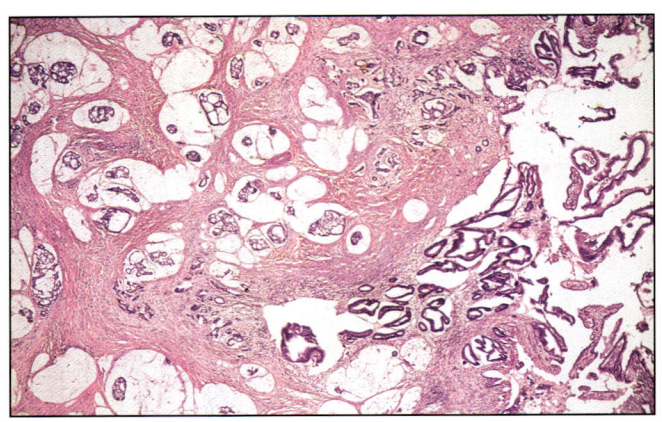 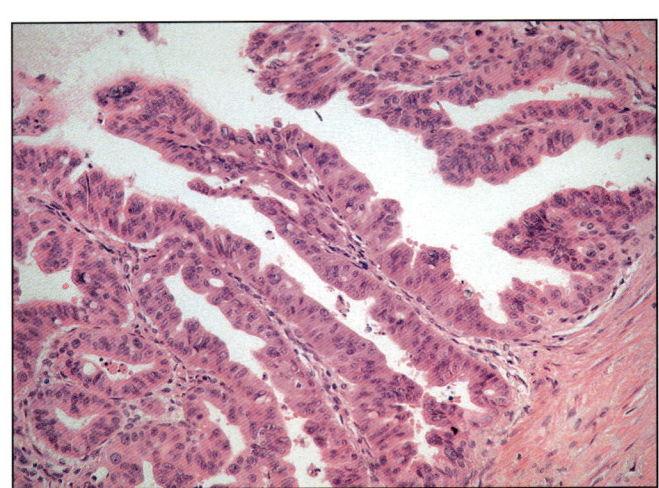

图11.17 导管内乳头状黏液性肿瘤,肠型,伴有导管内乳头状增生(右)并浸润周围胰腺组织(左)。浸润性成分显示胶样(黏液性非囊性)癌特征。

图11.18 导管内乳头状黏液性肿瘤,胰胆管型,可见分支状乳头和立方上皮。

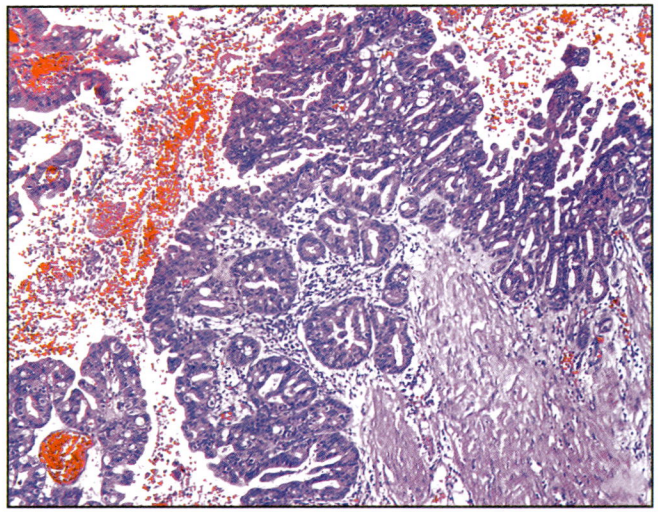 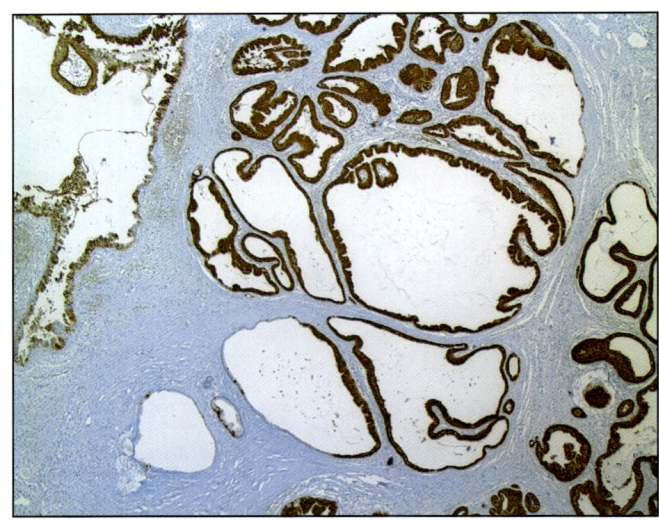

图11.19 导管内乳头状黏液性肿瘤,嗜酸细胞型,可见复杂乳头和多层上皮细胞。

图11.20 导管内乳头状黏液性肿瘤,胃肠型,MUC5免疫染色。

所有类型的导管内乳头状黏液性肿瘤均可扩展至萎缩性胰腺炎区域较小的导管，这种生长方式可能难以与浸润癌区分。肠型导管内乳头状黏液性肿瘤常出现导管中的黏液漏出，聚集形成无细胞的间质内黏液湖，类似于胶样癌。

导管内乳头状黏液性肿瘤的预后主要取决于浸润癌的出现、范围以及组织学类型[67]。完整切除导管内乳头状黏液性肿瘤（即使是伴有高度异型性的肿瘤）常可以治愈，但也有个别胰腺导管内局部复发的报道。浸润癌的发生常与胰胆管型肿瘤有关，其次为肠型；极少数情况下与胃型肿瘤有关。如果浸润性成分为范围较广的普通导管腺癌，则预后较差，与其他导管腺癌接近。然而，胶样癌侵袭性稍低，切除后5年生存率为55%[49]。

导管内乳头状黏液性肿瘤的鉴别诊断包括黏液性囊性肿瘤（表11.8），与导管内乳头状黏液性肿瘤不同，其与导管系统并不相通，好发于女性患者胰尾部，具有富于细胞成分的上皮下"卵巢样"间质，这种所见实际上具有特征性[73]。伴有胃型乳头的小分支导管的导管内乳头状黏液性肿瘤可能类似于导管潴留囊肿，但缺少明显的黏液性上皮或乳头状结构。区别小的胃型导管内乳头状黏液性肿瘤与大的胰腺上皮内肿瘤（PanIN）灶几乎是不可能的，尤其是0.5～1.0 cm的病变。近来发布的一项共识试图提出一些有用的标准[74]。

近来提出了胰腺导管内管状肿瘤（intraductal tubular neoplasms），包括幽门型导管内管状腺瘤以及其他迄今尚未完全特化的肿瘤[75,76]。虽然幽门型导管内管状腺瘤呈良性经过[77]，但已证实其他导管内管状肿瘤为癌[75]。

黏液性囊性肿瘤
Mucinous cystic neoplasms

一般认为，胰腺黏液性囊性肿瘤是由显示不同生物学行为的一系列病变组成的。如同导管内乳头状黏液性肿瘤一样，这些肿瘤依照细胞结构复杂程度分为伴有低度异型性的黏液性囊性肿瘤（黏液性囊腺瘤）、伴有中度异型性的黏液性囊性肿瘤（交界性黏液性囊性肿瘤）以及伴有高度异型性的黏液性囊性肿瘤（黏液性原位囊腺癌）[7-9,73]。浸润癌也可发生，包括多种不同组织学类型。黏液性囊性肿瘤几乎完全发生于女性（多数为中年妇女），多数病例发生在胰体尾部，最常见的表现是缓慢增大的腹部肿物。乏力、厌食和体重减轻是提示有浸润癌成分的特征。多数缺少浸润成分的黏液性囊性肿瘤病人完整切除可以治愈。浸润性黏液性囊腺癌的预后取决于浸润癌的范围；那些癌播散到囊壁外的病例预后较差[73,78]。有趣的是，明显良性的黏液性囊性肿瘤如果仅仅引流的话，可以复发，并伴有明显恶性特征，强调黏液性囊性肿瘤有肿瘤进展的潜能，即使是良性也应当完全切除。已有个例报道黏液性囊性肿瘤伴有胃泌素分泌以及Zollinger-Ellison综合征，可能是其中产生胃泌素的内分泌细胞所致。

大体上，黏液性囊性肿瘤境界清楚，有包膜，为单房或更常见的多房性囊肿，大小从2～30 cm不等（图11.21）。单个囊腔相对较大（与浆液性微囊性腺瘤相比，见下），多数病例每个囊腔大小为1～10 cm。囊腔内面光滑或出现乳头状突起和（或）囊壁小结节，尤其是那些伴有高度异型性或浸润癌的肿瘤。内容物为黏液性，偶尔可见出血。囊肿与导管系统不相通。

表11.8 胰腺囊性肿瘤最为重要的临床病理学特征

病变	平均年龄	男性（%）	女性（%）	大小（平均）(cm)	部位	与导管交通
IPMN	50～70	60	40	1～13（5）	胰头（80%）	是
MCN	40～60	1	99	3～23（10）	胰体-尾（90%）	否
SMA	60～80	10	90	2.5～16（6）	胰体-尾>胰头	否
SOIA	50～70	60	40	3～14（7）	胰头>胰体-尾	否
SPN	10～40	5	95	2～17（7）	整个胰腺	否
DAC，囊性	50～70	50	50	1～19（6）	胰头（70%）	否
NET，囊性	20～70	30	70	1.2～15（6）	整个胰腺	否

IPMN：导管内乳头状黏液性肿瘤；MCN：黏液性囊性肿瘤；SMA：浆液性微囊性腺瘤；SOIA：浆液性少囊性境界不清的腺瘤；SPN：实性假乳头状肿瘤；DAC：导管腺癌；NET：神经内分泌肿瘤。

黏液性囊性肿瘤

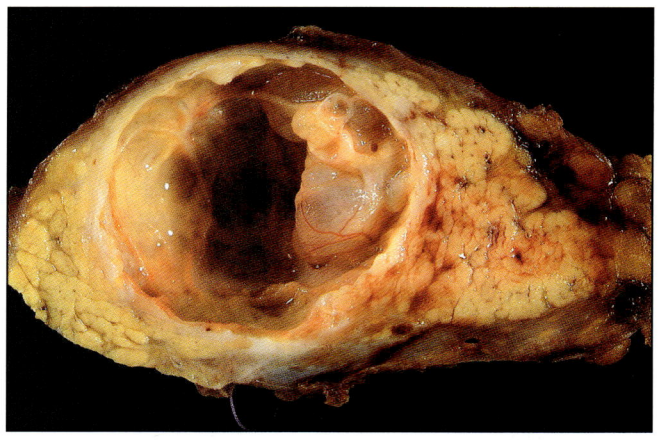

图11.21　黏液性囊性肿瘤切除标本，切面显示为多房性，内容物呈黏液样（Courtesy of Dr. J. Brenecke, Hannover, Germany）。

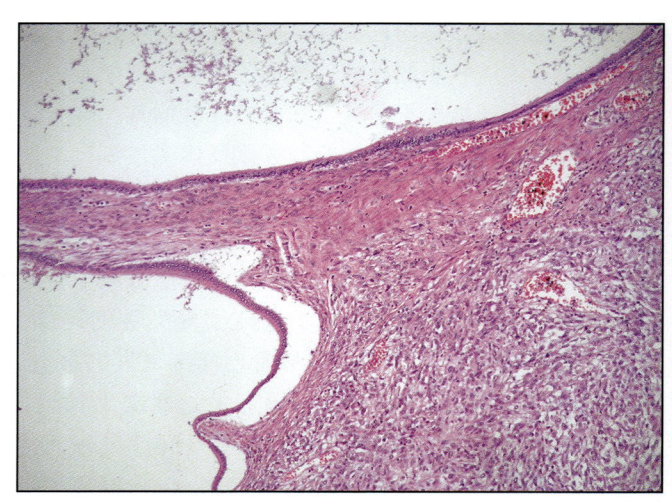

图11.23　黏液性囊性肿瘤伴有未分化（肉瘤样）多形性癌成分（右下方）。

组织学上，囊肿内衬分泌黏液的柱状上皮细胞，偶尔伴有一些内分泌细胞、Paneth细胞或杯状细胞。没有糖原。其他复杂结构也可见，例如细胞多层化、乳头或腺体结构以及腺管内陷，并有较大程度的非典型性，对应于上面列出的黏液性囊性肿瘤分级。伴有低度异型性的黏液性囊性肿瘤倾向于呈单纯性结构，细胞学呈良性表现。中度异型性的特征为乳头状内折，细胞呈假复层，细胞核不规则和密集。高度异型性包括重度非典型性上皮。许多黏液性囊性肿瘤具有不同级别程度的异型性区域（图11.22）。内衬上皮下可见致密的富于细胞性（"卵巢样"）间质，类似卵巢或胆管树的黏液性囊性肿瘤所见（图11.22）。这些间质细胞表达雌激素和孕激素受体以及CD10、抑制素和A103[73]。黏液性囊性肿瘤区域常见上皮剥脱，伴随的出血和炎症可能类似假性囊肿表现。出现浸润性成分时，常类似普通导管腺癌或其亚型。极少数情况下，囊肿壁出现假肉瘤样[80]或明显肉瘤性[81]区域，后者可能为丧失上皮分化的肉瘤样未分化癌（图11.23）。除了较为良性的区域外，任何黏液性囊性肿瘤均可含有高度异型性甚或浸润性的区域；因此建议即使不能全部取材，也要广泛取材。

多数黏液性囊性肿瘤上皮性抗原（细胞角蛋白7、8、18和19以及EMA）和CEA免疫反应阳性。有些肿瘤内分泌标记物免疫染色局灶阳性，特别是5-羟色胺。出现假肉瘤样或明显肉瘤性区域时，后者"间叶性"标记物（波形蛋白或平滑肌肌动蛋白）免疫染色可有不同程度的表达。

黏液性囊性肿瘤必须与导管内乳头状黏液性肿瘤（与导管系统相通，并非女性多见，无卵巢样间质）、包括浆液性囊腺瘤、实性假乳头状肿瘤、腺泡细胞囊腺癌、囊性内分泌肿瘤和淋巴上皮囊肿等在内的其他囊性肿瘤以及假性囊肿（无上皮内衬，伴有慢性胰腺炎，男性多见）相鉴别（见表11.8）。

浆液性囊性肿瘤
Serous cystic neoplasms

浆液性囊性肿瘤一般为良性[7-9,61,82]。常出现腹部膨大性肿物引起的症状和体征。极少有黄疸。无症状病例可在影像学检查或剖腹手术时偶然发现。

浆液性肿瘤包括浆液性微囊性腺瘤（微囊性浆液性囊腺瘤或富于糖原的腺瘤）[83]、浆液性少囊及界限不清的腺瘤（SOIA；或巨囊性浆液性囊腺瘤）[84,85]、von

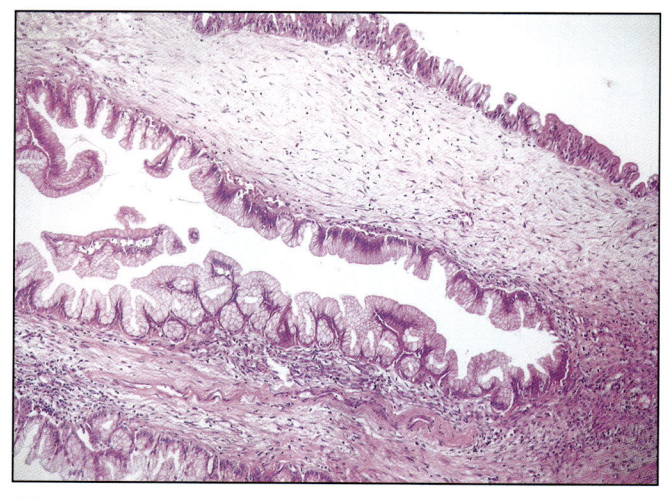

图11.22　黏液性囊性肿瘤显示分泌黏液的高分化单层柱状上皮细胞，其下方为富于细胞的"卵巢样"间质（下半部分），邻近非典型性上皮（上半部分）。

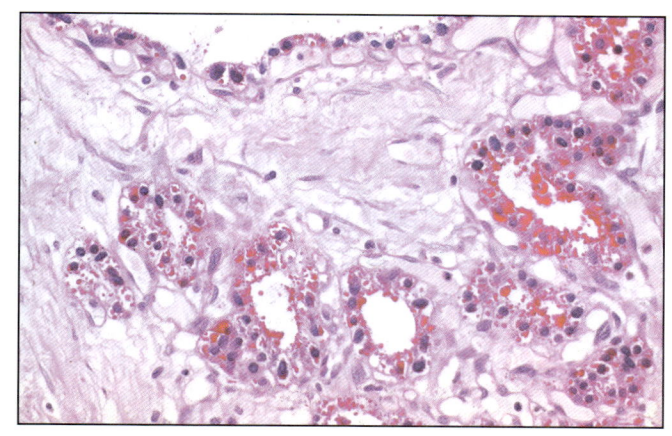

图11.24　浆液性囊性肿瘤伴有内衬立方细胞的小囊，胞浆呈空泡状或过PAS染色阳性。

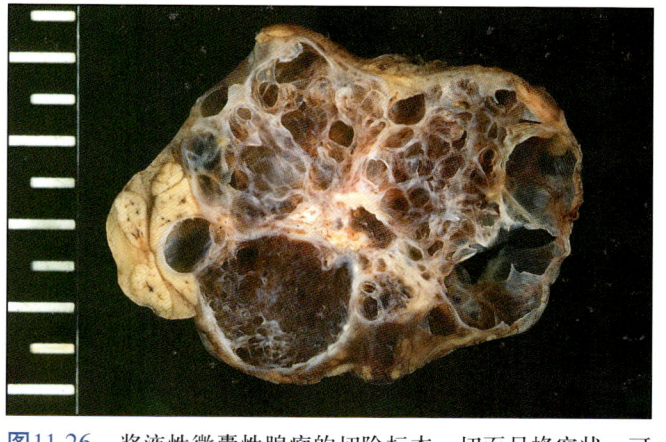

图11.26　浆液性微囊性腺瘤的切除标本，切面呈蜂窝状，可见中心纤维瘢痕。

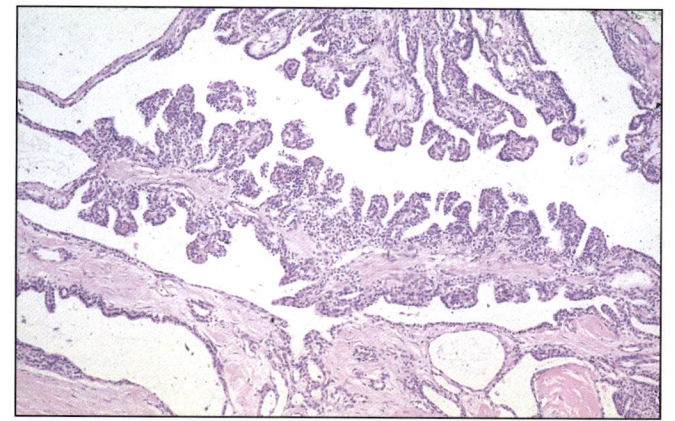

图11.25　浆液性微囊性腺瘤伴囊内乳头状结构。

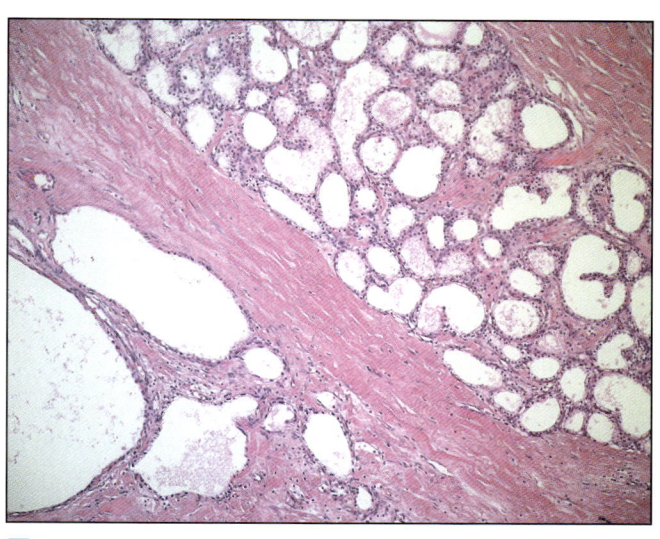

图11.27　浆液性微囊性腺瘤的小囊被玻璃样变的间质分隔。

Hippel-Lindau相关性囊性肿瘤（VHL-CN）、实性浆液性腺瘤（浆液性囊性腺瘤的实性亚型）[86]以及浆液性囊腺癌。所有这些类型的肿瘤都由同样的细胞组成。细胞扁平或立方形，核圆形并且规则，胞浆由于有过碘酸Schiff（PAS）阳性的糖原成分，而呈透明表现（图11.24），并有导管免疫表达。它可形成微乳头，被覆上皮细胞学呈良性表现（图11.25）[84,87-89]。然而，尽管这些细胞学相似，但浆液性囊性肿瘤在胰腺内的分布、大体表现、性别分布以及遗传学改变等方面均有差异[90]，提示它们是不同的疾病。实性浆液性腺瘤[86]和浆液性囊腺癌[91]在浆液性囊性肿瘤谱系中所处的位置尚不清楚，主要是由于迄今所报道病例数量较少[84,88,92]。

浆液性微囊性腺瘤最为常见，占所有浆液性囊性肿瘤的60%[61]。它表现为境界清楚、稍有凸起的单发圆形肿瘤，直径从2.5～16 cm不等。切面可见许多小囊（蜂窝状，直径仅为几毫米）排列在（近）中心星状瘢痕周围（图11.26），其中可含有钙化灶，并有纤细的纤维间隔向周边放射状分布。囊腔之间可见纤维组织，常呈玻璃样变性（图11.27），并可能含有陷入的胰岛。大约2/3的浆液性微囊性腺瘤发生于体尾部，并且几乎均发生于女性（平均年龄66岁）。常为偶然发现。

SOIA占浆液性囊性肿瘤的30%，由极少数相对较大的囊腔组成（由此也称为巨囊性浆液性囊腺瘤）[85]（图11.28），缺乏星状瘢痕和圆形外形，主要发生于胰头部，可阻塞胆总管并引起黄疸[84,88]。无性别差异。

VHL-CN常为多灶性发生，疾病晚期出现融合并累及整个胰腺[93,94]。由于VHL-CN可弥漫性累及胰腺，因而大体上与浆液性微囊性腺瘤和SOIA存在明显不同。生物学上值得注意的是，VHL-CN与SOIA一样并非以女性为主，不同于浆液性微囊性腺瘤。由此提示浆液性微囊性腺瘤在其发生机制上与VHL-CN和SOIA有所不同。近来报道的分子学资料支持这一假设。虽然发现

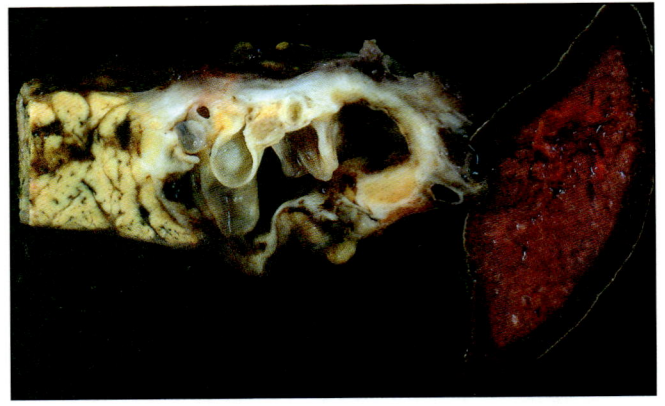

图11.28 浆液性少囊性及境界不清的腺瘤：胰腺切除标本左侧可见多房性囊性肿瘤，位于胰腺和脾之间。

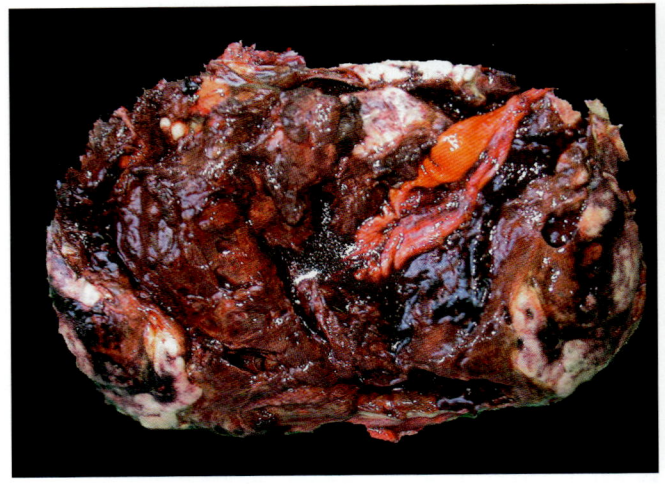

图11.29 腺泡细胞癌切除标本显示切面出血，呈鱼肉状。

VHL-CN 的特征是 3p 染色体上（含有 VHL 基因）出现杂合性缺失和一个 VHL 基因种系突变，但仅有 40% 的浆液性微囊性腺瘤在 3p 染色体上出现杂合性缺失，只有 2 例（22%）出现体细胞 VHL 基因突变[94]。值得注意的是，50% 以上的浆液性微囊性腺瘤在 10q 染色体上出现杂合性缺失。因此，VHL 基因改变在浆液性微囊性腺瘤中似乎并不十分重要，而 10q 上的基因改变可能具有重要作用。VHL 基因是否参与 SOIA 发病机制还有待说明。对于极少见的浆液性囊腺癌也同样如此[95]。

浆液性微囊性腺瘤的鉴别诊断主要是多灶性黏液性囊性肿瘤（见表 11.8），尽管其蜂窝状表现以及星状瘢痕使其极具特征性。区别 SOIA 与其他囊性病变比较困难，因为其大体表现差异较大。免疫组织化学染色，CEA 在浆液性囊性肿瘤中为阴性；不同于黏液性囊性肿瘤，而抑制素在浆液性囊性肿瘤中有表达，但在黏液性囊性肿瘤的内衬上皮中没有表达[73,89]。

胰腺实性浆液性腺瘤为浆液性囊性肿瘤的明显非囊性亚型[86]。这种病变由透明细胞小管构成，组织学上与发生于浆液性囊性肿瘤的病变难以区别。

浆液性囊腺癌是极为少见的恶性肿瘤；大体上及镜下所见类似于浆液性囊腺瘤，但可出现邻近结构和血管的浸润或者转移[95]。

腺泡细胞癌 Acinar cell carcinoma

腺泡细胞癌为伴有实性和腺泡结构的恶性上皮性肿瘤，证实其肿瘤细胞有产生酶的证据。腺泡细胞癌大约占胰腺外分泌肿瘤的 1%~2%。多数发生于成人，主要为男性，但也有极个别儿童和青少年病例报道[4,96]。成人腺泡细胞癌的行为与导管腺癌相同，伴有区域淋巴结、肝和肺的广泛转移；然而，临床经过并非迅速致死，平均存活 18 个月[96,97]。另一方面，儿童腺泡细胞癌的预后似乎较好。据报道，个别病人伴有多灶性脂肪坏死（皮下组织、骨髓和腹部）、多关节痛（由于大量分泌酯酶）[96]或非细菌性血栓性心内膜炎。

大体上，腺泡细胞癌可发生于胰腺任何部位，较大（直径 2~15 cm），境界清楚，质软，呈分叶状肿物，肉色至黄色。坏死或出血可以明显，可出现囊性退变（图 11.29）。手术时常见侵犯邻近结构（十二指肠、胃或脾）。

显微镜下，尽管肿瘤似乎境界清楚，但可局灶或弥漫性浸润周围胰腺组织。肿瘤明显富于细胞，大的肿瘤性小叶之间有少量玻璃样变性的带状纤维性间质（图 11.30）。肿瘤的生长方式多样，可为腺泡状（"微腺性"）（图 11.31）、实性或混合性；极少数肿瘤呈小梁状结构。有丰富的薄壁血管网。分化最好的细胞呈圆形，单一形

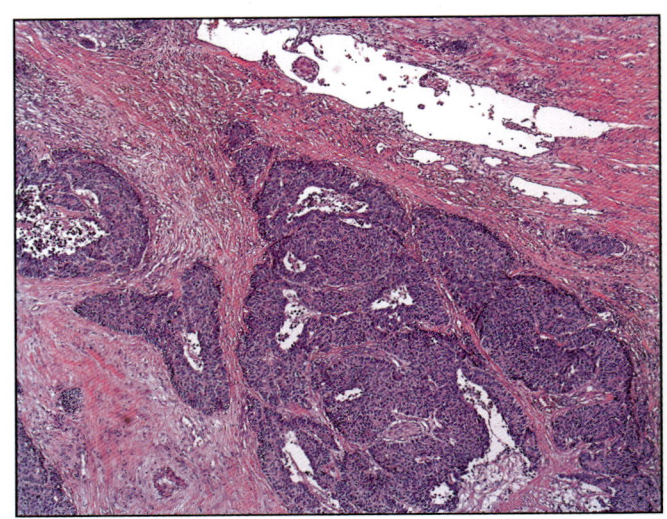

图11.30 腺泡细胞癌，显示位于纤维性间质中的单形性实性细胞巢。

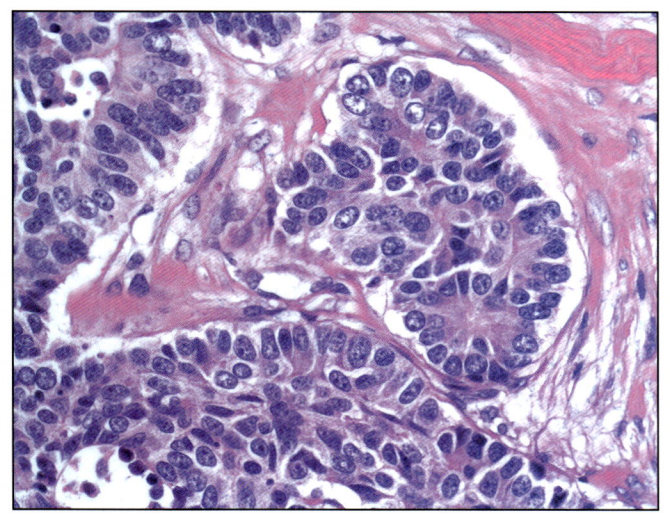

图11.31　腺泡细胞癌呈腺泡状及小梁状生长方式。

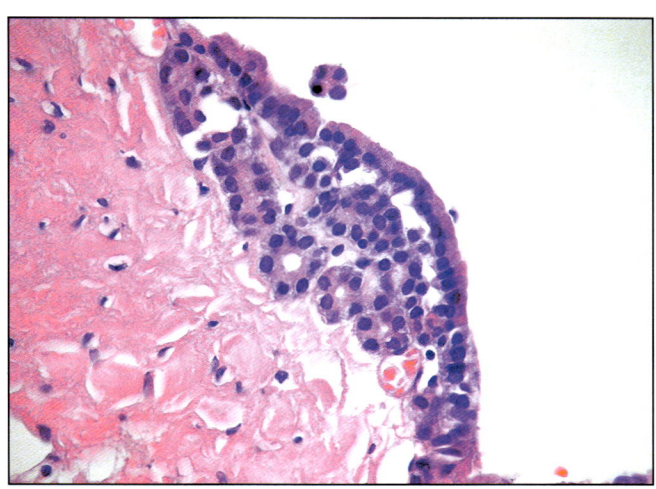

图11.33　腺泡细胞囊腺瘤可见单层上皮，并伴有腺泡成分。

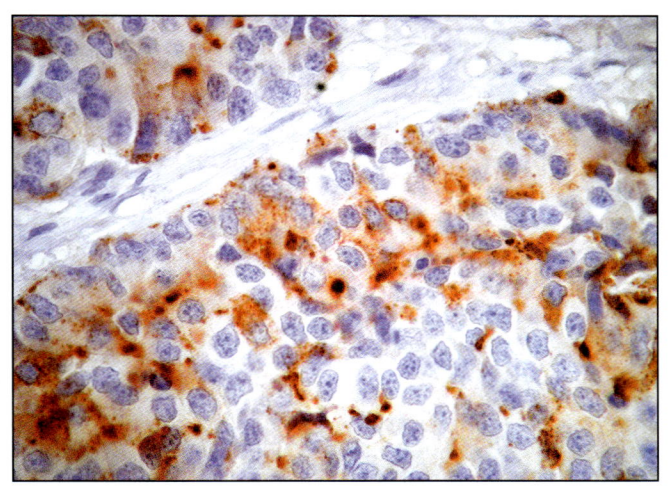

图11.32　腺泡细胞癌胰蛋白酶免疫染色。

态，中等大小至较大。胞浆相对丰富，嗜酸性细颗粒状，含有PAS阳性抗淀粉消化的酶原颗粒。细胞核均匀一致，圆形且较大，核仁明显。核分裂象常见。分化不良的细胞较小，细胞核特征不明显，缺乏嗜酸性颗粒状胞浆。

腺泡细胞癌免疫染色显示脂酶、胰蛋白酶和糜蛋白酶阳性（图11.32）[96,98]。相反，淀粉酶染色一般阴性。超微结构上，肿瘤细胞内可见酶原颗粒。分子遗传学所见包括偶见APC/β-连环蛋白通路异常[99]，但涉及导管腺癌的基因（p53、p16、K-ras或smad4/dpc4）没有异常。

腺泡细胞癌嗜铬素和突触素染色一般阴性，但30%～40%的病例含有散在的单个内分泌细胞，通过免疫组织学染色可以证实。极少数情况下，肿瘤可出现明显的一种以上的分化成分。伴有25%以上腺泡及内分泌细胞成分（由免疫组织学确定）的癌称为混合性腺泡内分泌癌（mixed acinar endocrine carcinomas）[59,100]，而伴有腺泡和导管成分混合的肿瘤（通过有黏液产物或诸如CEA或CA19.9等糖蛋白免疫表达确定）命名为混合性腺泡导管癌（mixed acinar ductal carcinomas）。极其少见的混合性腺泡内分泌导管癌（mixed acinar endocrine ductal carcinomas）具有明显的所有三种细胞系成分[101]。在多数情况下，这些混合性癌主要由腺泡成分组成，现有临床资料提示其生物学行为与单纯性腺泡细胞癌相似。

腺泡细胞囊腺癌（acinar cell cystadenocarcinoma）为腺泡细胞癌的一种罕见的囊性亚型[102]。虽然单个囊肿可衬以分化好的腺泡上皮，但也有实性区域，并且肿瘤浸润胰腺周围组织。腺泡细胞囊腺癌的侵袭性与实性腺泡细胞癌相同。

近来提出了一种特殊的腺泡细胞病变，称为腺泡细胞囊腺瘤（acinar cell cystadenoma）[103]。这些病变主要为囊性，每个囊腔衬以一层连续性的成熟腺泡细胞，胰酶染色阳性，并常混有正常腺泡（图11.33）。腺泡细胞囊腺瘤为良性病变，出现大小不等的囊腔，并混有正常胰腺实质成分。有些病变只是镜下偶然发现的几个囊腔，而另外一些病变可达10 cm，并累及整个胰腺。

腺泡细胞癌应与胰腺内分泌肿瘤鉴别，二者组织学表现相似。一般来说，内分泌肿瘤细胞学表现比较一致，并且PAS染色为阴性。它们弥漫性表达嗜铬素和突触素，而胰酶染色仅局限于散在的单个细胞。实性腺泡细胞腺瘤尚没有令人信服的病例报告，但在手术标本及尸检当中常可见腺泡细胞结节（局灶性腺泡细胞异型增生）[104]。在大多数情况下，这些境界清楚的有细胞学改变的腺泡细胞结节可能是变性改变，并非肿瘤前期病变。

胰母细胞瘤
Pancreatoblastoma

胰母细胞瘤（同义词：胰管母细胞瘤 pancreaticoblastoma，婴儿胰腺癌）是极为少见的恶性肿瘤，几乎均发生于婴儿和10岁以内的儿童[105]。但有少数较大儿童和成人的病例报道[106,107]。胰母细胞瘤男孩比女孩多见。肿瘤发生于胰头或胰体部，是较大、质软、境界清楚而又有（完全或部分性）包膜的肿瘤，直径为5～20 cm。切面呈分叶状，褐色，伴有出血、坏死，偶尔可有囊性变。

显微镜下，胰母细胞瘤主要由上皮成分组成，在极少数病例中也可有间叶性成分。上皮成分特征是形态单一的多角形细胞，胞质或腺腔内可见PAS阳性物质。这些细胞排列成实性、小梁状或腺泡性结构。核分裂象常见。形成的鳞状细胞巢或"小体"极具特征性，但不是能够确定诊断的特征（图11.34）。如果有间叶性成分出现，可由梭形细胞构成，伴有间质玻璃样变、纤维血管带以及黏液样或软骨样改变。胰腺母细胞瘤基本上是腺泡细胞肿瘤，呈现脂酶、胰蛋白酶和糜蛋白酶免疫染色阳性[105]。另外，可见内分泌或甲胎蛋白阳性细胞，同样导管型糖蛋白（CEA或Ca19.9）也可能阳性。超微结构上，肿瘤也表现为腺泡特征，许多上皮细胞内可见酶原颗粒。胰母细胞瘤缺乏导管腺癌典型的遗传学异常，代之以β-连环蛋白/APC通路异常[108]。如果胰母细胞瘤为局灶性，完整手术切除后预后常很好，至少在儿童病人如此；极少累及成人的病例常发生转移并导致死亡[105,106]。

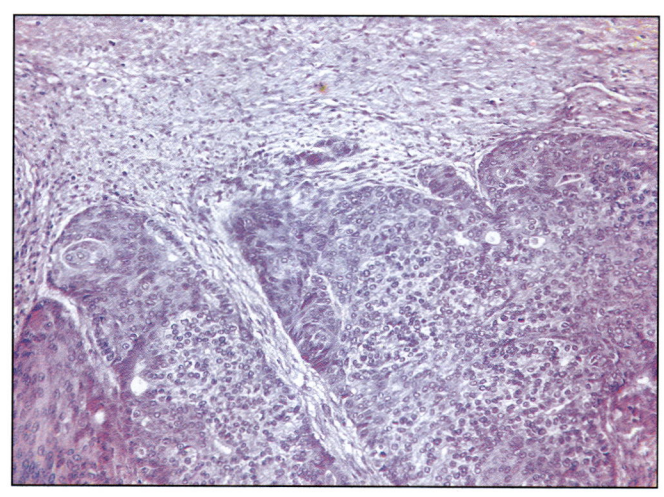

图11.34 胰母细胞瘤，出现分叶状的实性及腺泡状生长结构，左侧可见典型鳞状小体。

实性假乳头状肿瘤
Solid pseudopapillary neoplasm

实性假乳头状肿瘤（同义词：实性囊性或乳头状囊性肿瘤，实性和乳头状上皮性肿瘤）是一种不常见的肿瘤，常包括在胰腺"囊性"外分泌肿瘤内。肿瘤主要发生于青春期女孩和年轻女性，平均年龄为26岁。大约10%的病例发生于男性[109]。病人常出现腹部肿大和疼痛性肿物，但也有在腹部探查或影像学检查时偶然发现的无症状性病例。有些病例发现于腹部创伤后，引起肿瘤或腹腔内出血。认为实性假乳头状肿瘤是恶性肿瘤，但生物学分级极低，并且完全切除肿瘤后多数病人可无瘤存活多年。大约15%的病例伴有转移，基本上局限于肝和腹膜，并且通常出现在最初诊断时[7,110]。即使是转移性病例也有长期存活的报道。

肿瘤可发生于胰腺任何部位，大体上表现为圆形，貌似境界清楚的病变，直径大小为2～17 cm（平均8 cm）。切面为实性肿物，伴有囊性区域；并且常见有出血（图11.35）。

显微镜下，实性部分含有呈片块状、索条状和小梁状排列的均匀一致的小圆形细胞；这种器官样表现可类似于内分泌肿瘤。胞浆嗜酸性或空泡状，含有成簇的PAS阳性的玻璃样小体。细胞核为圆形到卵圆形，染色质细而散在，核仁不明显。有些细胞核可见核沟或有内陷。核分裂象极少见。实性部分也出现丰富而纤细的特征性血管网。远离血管的许多细胞出现变性，使得围绕血管的细胞残留下来而形成假花环或假乳头状结构（图11.36）。囊性区域是广泛变性的结果（图11.37），可有明显出血，并伴有胆固醇肉芽肿以及泡沫样组织细胞聚集。浸润性生长极为常见，并且出现向周围的胰腺、胰腺周围组织甚至血管内播散。然而，这些特征均没有预后意义。

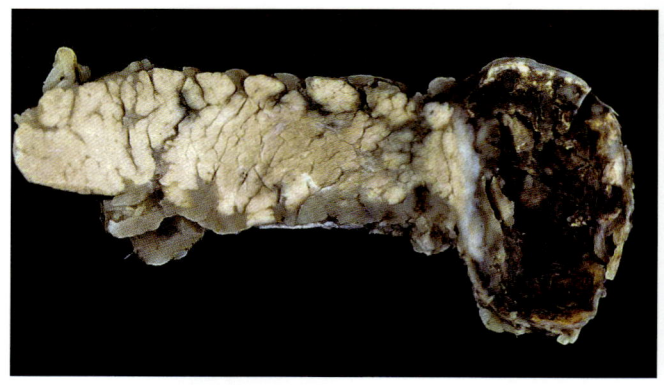

图11.35 实性假乳头状肿瘤的切除标本，几乎完全出血坏死。

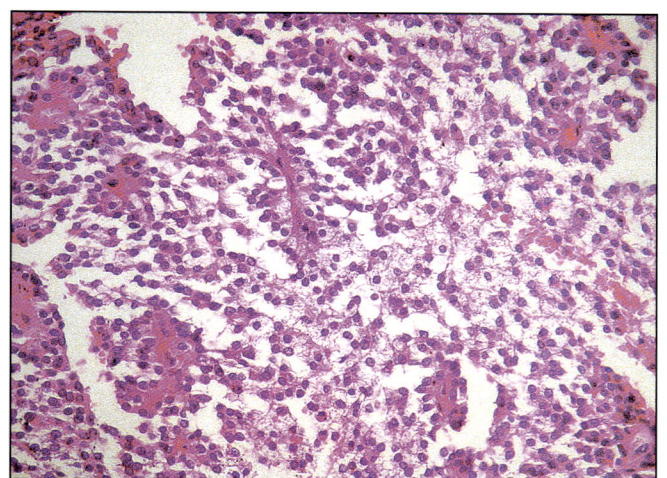

图11.36 实性假乳头状肿瘤由假乳头状结构组成。

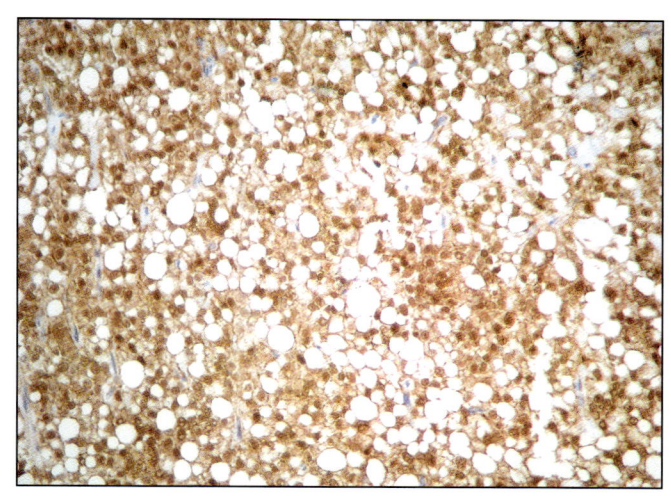

图11.38 实性假乳头状肿瘤β-连环蛋白免疫染色，注意细胞核阳性。

其他癌 Miscellaneous carcinomas

伴有髓样改变的癌
Carcinoma with medullary changes

新近报道了一种髓样型胰腺癌[119]。与结直肠髓样癌一样，这些肿瘤显示不同于导管腺癌的形态学特征。这些肿瘤由相当多形性的细胞组成，伴有合体细胞生长方式，核分裂率高，偶尔可见肿瘤内有淋巴细胞浸润。这些癌在本质上似乎属于异源性。与结直肠髓样癌不同的是，胰腺髓样癌仅有极个别伴有错配修复基因的突变[120]，并且其预后并不明显好于导管腺癌[120]。迄今为止，仅有一例报道出现遗传性非息肉病性结直肠癌（HNPCC）综合征表现[120]。

伴有淋巴上皮性改变的癌
Carcinoma with lymphoepithelial changes

胰体淋巴上皮性癌已有一例报道[121]。它表达EB病毒基因组成分。

伴有微乳头状改变的癌
Carcinoma with micropapillary changes

这种类型的癌最先在乳腺描述，也可见于胰腺[21]。

伴有嗜酸细胞改变的癌
Carcinoma with oncocytic changes

已有几例嗜酸细胞癌报告，发生于胰头或胰尾部，常伴有转移[122,123]。显微镜下，这些癌由成片或成巢的伴有丰富颗粒状嗜酸性胞浆的细胞构成。磷钨酸苏木素（PTAH）染色显示胞浆颗粒呈阳性，超微结构研究发现胞浆内有许多线粒体[123]。目前尚无令人信服的证据支

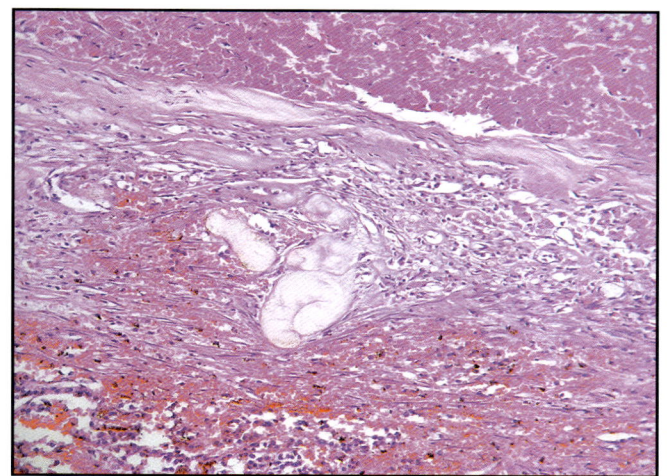

图11.37 实性假乳头状肿瘤，图片上半部分出现广泛坏死。

免疫组织化学及电镜检查研究发现，实性假乳头状肿瘤出现与肿瘤细胞表型相矛盾的结果[111-113]。肿瘤免疫染色显示α₁-抗胰蛋白酶、神经元特异性烯醇化酶、CD56、CD10、孕激素受体和波形蛋白阳性，有些病例表达突触素[114]。然而，嗜铬素和胰酶染色从无表达。细胞角蛋白仅有极少数表达。因此，实性假乳头状肿瘤的细胞系分化目前尚有争议。比较一致的异常表现为β-连环蛋白基因[115,116]，免疫组织化学染色出现β-连环蛋白异常细胞核定位被认为有助于诊断（图11.38）。值得注意的是，有一例出现特殊的13和17号染色体非平衡性易位[117]。

极少数实性假乳头状肿瘤出现由弥漫性成片细胞构成的高级别成分，伴有核-浆比率增高、坏死以及核分裂活性升高，提示有低分化癌发生[118]。这些肿瘤伴有进展迅速和致死性的临床经过。

伴有基底细胞样改变的癌
Carcinoma with basaloid changes

近来报道了一种由实性("基底细胞样")细胞巢所构成的伴有鳞状分化的小灶癌[124]。

伴有透明细胞变的癌
Carcinoma with clear cell changes

胰腺的透明细胞癌已有记载[22],出现胞浆空泡,其中含有糖原和数量不等的黏液,但没有脂肪。有一例含有导管内乳头状黏液性肿瘤(intraductal papillary-mucinous neoplasm, IPMN)成分[22]。其他病例似乎是导管腺癌亚型[125]。胰腺透明细胞癌必须与转移性肾细胞癌或肾上腺皮质癌鉴别。

伴有微腺体改变的癌
Carcinoma with microglandular changes

含有小或中等大小细胞曾被称为微腺体腺癌的肿瘤,以前被认为是导管腺癌的亚型或为伴有导管和神经内分泌双重分化的恶性肿瘤。这种肿瘤较大,出现广泛坏死,伴有侵袭性生物学行为。新近Cubilla和Fitzgerald对其微腺体癌病例再度进行了免疫组织化学染色评估,发现这些肿瘤本身并非为一种独立疾病,而是组织学特征及免疫染色表达各异的一组肿瘤[126]。其中包括一些应被划分为普通导管腺癌的肿瘤以及另外一些出现神经内分泌、腺泡或混合性免疫组织化学表型的肿瘤。

伴有小细胞癌特征的癌
Carcinoma with features of small cell carcinoma

胰腺小细胞癌极为少见,曾被认为是胰腺外分泌瘤和未分化癌的一个亚型。然而,由于小细胞癌常表达神经内分泌标记物,例如突触素或CD56,目前这些肿瘤被归入低分化神经内分泌癌(见第20章)。

婴儿和儿童肿瘤
Tumors in infants and children

胰腺外分泌肿瘤有极少数发生于婴儿和儿童。除了胰母细胞瘤以外(见478页),腺泡细胞癌、内分泌肿瘤以及实性假乳头状肿瘤也可发生[127],而导管腺癌实际上从不发生[17]。胰母细胞瘤为婴儿和较小儿童最常见的肿瘤,而实性假乳头状肿瘤、内分泌肿瘤以及腺泡细胞癌多见于较大儿童[128,129]。胰腺原始神经外胚层肿瘤(PNET)也可发生于儿童和年轻人[130]。这些肿瘤可能与胰腺内分泌肿瘤(常常同样表达CD99免疫活性)混淆。通过发现t(11;22)(q24;q12)或相关染色体易位可以证实诊断。

非上皮性肿瘤和继发性肿瘤
Non-epithelial tumors and secondary tumors

与比较常见的上皮起源的肿瘤不同,胰腺非上皮性肿瘤极为少见[131]。已经报道的肿瘤几乎包括所有已知组织学类型的良性恶性软组织肿瘤。最常见的是平滑肌肉瘤[132,133]和恶性外周神经鞘瘤,其次为脂肪肉瘤和所谓的恶性纤维组织细胞瘤。胰腺的恶性纤维组织细胞瘤多为去分化脂肪肉瘤,否则就是间变性癌。近来,透明细胞"糖"瘤(或血管肌脂肪瘤)[134,135]、纤维组织增生性小细胞肿瘤[136]、外周神经外胚层肿瘤[131]、孤立性纤维性肿瘤[137]以及胃肠道间质瘤[138]已有报道。与许多报道中所描述的胰腺炎症性肌纤维母细胞瘤有所不同的是,在多数情况下,这种"肿瘤"似乎是自身免疫性胰腺炎的一种假瘤性表现(见瘤样病变)。恶性淋巴瘤和白血病浸润偶尔可见于胰腺[139,140]。胰腺原发性淋巴瘤绝大多数为B细胞表型。转移癌累及胰腺并不常见,包括来自肾细胞癌、乳腺癌、小细胞肺癌以及黑色素瘤的转移[141,142]。

瘤样病变　Tumors-like lesions

胰腺非肿瘤性瘤样病变可类似实性或囊性胰腺外分泌肿瘤。实性非肿瘤性病变包括"炎性假瘤"和错构瘤[143];而囊性病变为假性囊肿、淋巴上皮囊肿以及先天性、潴留性和寄生虫性囊肿[61]。

炎性假瘤(inflammatory pseudotumors)临床和大体上类似于胰腺癌,一般由近来才有详细描述的两种类型的慢性胰腺炎所致[144]。包括自身免疫性胰腺炎(同义词:淋巴浆细胞性硬化性胰腺炎[145,146]、导管破坏性慢性胰腺炎)和十二指肠壁旁胰腺炎(同义词:十二指肠壁囊性营养不良、壶腹旁十二指肠壁囊肿以及沟槽状胰腺炎)[147]。自身免疫性胰腺炎(autoimmune pancreatitis）是一种慢性炎症性疾病，其病因和发病机制不清。病人常出现血清IgG4升高，这种表现在临床上可能有助于炎性假瘤与胰腺导管腺癌的鉴别[146]。自身免疫性胰腺炎主要发生于胰头部，包括远端胆管，形成炎症性包块，常常引发黄疸。镜下特征为致密淋巴浆细胞浸润，也可含有嗜酸性细胞和中性粒细胞。这种浸润最初围绕中等大小的导管，随后也可扩展至腺泡小叶。浸润扩展至腺泡小叶时出现致密纤维化，几乎可替代腺泡组织，偶尔出现多量呈席纹状排列的肌纤维母细胞。如果席纹状改变明显，自身免疫性胰腺炎可类似于炎症性肌纤维母细胞肿瘤（从前称为炎性假瘤）。闭塞性小静脉炎是另外一个特征性表现。近些年来，似乎许多自身免疫性胰腺炎病例是以这种诊断报道的[148-150]。本病可发生于所有年龄，但最多见于50～60岁之间。男性受累是女性的2倍。临床上常误诊为胰腺癌的第二种类型的慢性胰腺炎为十二指肠壁旁胰腺炎（paraduodenal wall pancreatitis）（同义词见上）[147]。这种慢性胰腺炎似乎发生于位于副乳头区域十二指肠黏膜下的异位胰腺组织[157]。一般情况下，有囊性和（或）假囊性改变，伴有富于细胞成分的纤维性组织，常穿过十二指肠壁扩展至附近胆管周围的胰腺组织。这可以导致十二指肠和（或）胆管狭窄。最常累及年龄为40～60岁的男性酗酒者。

近来发现，各种错构瘤均可产生胰腺实性或囊性瘤样病变[143,144,152]。其组成包括埋于纤维组织中的随意排列的成熟腺泡、导管和内分泌细胞，与周围正常胰腺实质分界清楚。其中有些病变因为也表达CD117，故与胃肠道间质瘤很难区分[152]。胰腺局灶性淋巴组织增生（focal lymphoid hyperplasia）（同义词：假淋巴瘤）的特

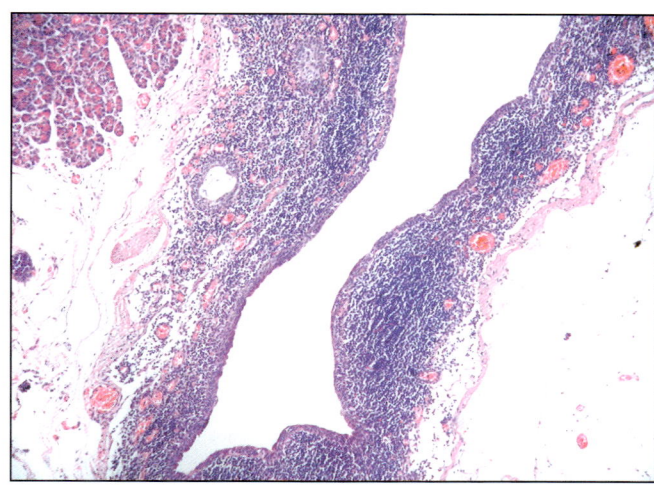

图11.39 胰腺淋巴上皮囊肿可见鳞状上皮，下方为淋巴细胞间质。

征为伴有生发中心的淋巴滤泡增生，不要误诊为结节性恶性淋巴瘤[61,153]。

在瘤样囊性病变中最常见的为假性囊肿（pseudocyst）。作为一个必要条件，它们的发生必须与胰腺炎有关[154]，一般为酗酒者，极少数为遗传性发病[155]。胰腺的良性淋巴上皮囊肿（benign lymphoepithelial cyst）为单房性囊肿，内衬成熟鳞状上皮，上皮周围是滤泡性淋巴组织（图11.39）[156,157]。与组织学表现类似的涎腺病变不同，没有证据表明与HIV感染有关。在鉴别诊断中偶尔提到的其他囊性非肿瘤性病变包括黏液性非肿瘤性囊肿[90]，一些罕见的诸如前肠纤毛囊肿等先天性囊肿，最后是潴留性囊肿和寄生虫囊肿[154]。

参考文献

1. Hamilton S R, Aaltonen L A 2000 Pathology and genetics of tumours of the digestive system. WHO classification of tumours. IARC Press, Lyon
2. Cubilla A L, Fitzgerald P J 1984 Tumors of the exocrine pancreas. AFIP Atlas of tumor pathology, series 2, fascicle 19. Armed Forces Institute of Pathology, Washington, DC
3. Solcia E, Capella C, Klöppel G 1997 Tumors of the pancreas. AFIP Atlas of tumor pathology, series 3, fascicle 20. Armed Forces Institute of Pathology, Washington, DC
4. Lack E E 1989 Primary tumors of the exocrine pancreas. Classification, overview, and recent contributions by immunohistochemistry and electron microscopy. Am J Surg Pathol 13, Suppl 1: 66–88
5. Oertel J E, Heffess C S, Oertel Y C 1996 Pancreas. In: Sternberg SS (ed) Diagnostic surgical pathology. Raven Press, New York, p 1419–1457
6. Klöppel G 1997 Pathology and classification of tumours of the exocrine pancreas. In: Trede M, Carter DC (eds) Surgery of the pancreas, 2nd edn. Churchill Livingstone, Edinburgh, p 447–462
7. Klöppel G, Solcia E, Longnecker D S 1996 Histological typing of tumours of the exocrine pancreas, 2nd edn. WHO International Histological Classification of Tumours. Springer, Berlin
8. Albores-Saavedra J, Gould E W, Angeles-Angeles A et al. 1990 Cystic tumors of the pancreas. In: Rosen PP, Fechner RE (eds) Pathology annual. Appleton & Lange, East Norwalk, vol 25, part 2, p 19–50
9. Bogomoletz W V 1991 Cystic tumours of the exocrine pancreas. In: Anthony PP, MacSween RNM (eds) Recent advances in histopathology. Churchill Livingstone, Edinburgh, p 141–155
10. Lowenfels A B, Maisonneuve P, Cavallini G et al. 1993 Pancreatitis and the risk of pancreatic cancer. N Engl J Med 328: 1433–1437
11. Lumadue J A, Griffin C A, Osman M et al. 1995 Familial pancreatic cancer and the genetics of pancreatic cancer. Surg Clin North Am 75: 845–855
12. Klein A P, Brune K A, Petersen G M et al. 2004. Prospective risk of pancreatic cancer in familial pancreatic cancer kindreds. Cancer Res 64: 2634–2638.
13. Eberle M A, Pfützer R, Pogue-Geile K L et al. 2002 A new susceptibility locus for autosomal dominant pancreatic cancer maps to chromosome 4q32–34. Am J Hum Genet 70: 1044–1048
14. Meckler K A, Brentnall T A, Haggitt R C et al. 2001 Familial fibrocystic pancreatic atrophy with endocrine cell hyperplasia and pancreatic carcinoma. Am J Surg Pathol 25: 1047–1053
15. Klöppel G, Hruban R H, Longnecker D S et al. 2000 Ductal adenocarcinoma of the pancreas. In: Hamilton SR, Aaltonen LA (eds) Pathology and genetics of tumours of the digestive system. WHO classification of tumours. IARC Press, Lyon, p 221–230
16. Blackbourne L H, Jones R S, Catalano C J et al. 1997 Pancreatic adenocarcinoma in the pregnant patient: case report and review of the literature. Cancer 79: 1776–1779
17. Lüttges J, Stigge C, Pacena M et al. 2004 Rare ductal adenocarcinoma of the pancreas in patients younger than age 40 years. An analysis of its features and a literature review. Cancer 100: 173–182
18. Kosmahl M, Pauser U, Anlauf M et al. 2005 Pancreatic ductal adenocarcinomas with cystic features: neither rare nor uniform. Mod Pathol 18: 1157–1164
19. Makhlouf H R, Almeida J L, Sobin L H 1999 Carcinoma in jejunal pancreatic heterotopia. Arch Pathol Lab Med 123: 707–711

20. Adsay V, Logani S, Sarkar F et al. 2000 Foamy gland pattern of pancreatic ductal adenocarcinoma. A deceptively benign-appearing variant. Am J Surg Pathol 24: 493–504
21. Nassar H, Pansare V, Zhang H et al. 2004 Pathogenesis of invasive micropapillary carcinoma: role of MUC1 glycoprotein. Mod Pathol 17: 1045–1050
22. Lüttges J, Vogel I, Menke M A O H et al. 1998 Clear cell carcinoma of the pancreas: an adenocarcinoma with ductal phenotype. Histopathology 32: 444–448
23. Cubilla A L, Fitzgerald P J 1976 Morphological lesions associated with human primary invasive nonendocrine pancreas cancer. Cancer Res 36: 2690–2698
24. Klöppel G, Bommer G, Rückert K et al. 1980 Intraductal proliferation in the pancreas and its relationship to human and experimental carcinogenesis. Virchow's Arch [A] Pathol Anat 387: 221–233
25. Lüttges J, Reinecke-Lüthge A, Mööllmann B et al. 1999 Duct changes and K-*ras* mutations in the disease-free pancreas: analysis of type, age relation and spatial distribution. Virchow's Arch 435: 461–468
26. Andea A, Sarkar F, Adsay N V 2003 Clinicopathological correlates of pancreatic intraepithelial neoplasia: a comparative analysis of 82 cases with and 152 cases without pancreatic ductal adenocarcinoma. Mod Pathol 16: 996–1006
27. Brat D J, Lillemoe K D, Yeo C J et al. 1998 Progression of pancreatic intraductal neoplasias to infiltrating adenocarcinoma of the pancreas. Am J Surg Pathol 22: 163–169
28. Hruban R H, Adsay N V, Albores-Saavedra J et al. 2001 Pancreatic intraepithelial neoplasia. A new nomenclature and classification system for pancreatic duct lesions. Am J Surg Pathol 25: 579–586
29. Cioc A M, Ellison E C, Proca D M et al. 2002 Frozen section diagnosis of pancreatic lesions. Arch Pathol Lab Med 126: 1169–1173
30. Bätge B, Bosslet K, Sedlacek H H et al. 1986 Monoclonal antibodies against CEA-related components discriminate between pancreatic duct type carcinomas and nonneoplastic duct lesions as well as nonduct type neoplasias. Virchow's Arch [A] Pathol Anat 408: 361–374
31. Atkinson B F, Ernst C, Herlyn M et al. 1982 Gastrointestinal cancer-associated antigen in immunoperoxidase assay. Cancer Res 42: 4820–4823
32. Takeda S, Nakao A, Ichihara T et al. 1991 Serum concentration and immunohistochemical localization of SPan-1 antigen in pancreatic cancer: a comparison with CA 19-9 antigen. Hepatogastroenterology 38: 143–148
33. Pellegata N S, Sessa F, Renault B et al. 1994 K-*ras* and *p53* gene mutations in pancreatic cancer: ductal and nonductal tumors progress through different genetic lesions. Cancer Res 54: 1556–1560
34. Hruban R H, Iacobuzio-Donahue C, Wilentz R E et al. 2001 Molecular pathology of pancreatic cancer. Cancer J 7: 251–258
35. Wirtz M, Nyarangi J, Köninger J et al. 2005 Molecular basis of pancreatic carcinogenesis: which concepts may be clinically relevant? In: Domínguez-Muñoz JE (ed) Clinical pancreatology for practising gastroenterologists and surgeons. Blackwell, Malden, MA, p 351–358
36. Sipos B, Weber D, Ungefroren H et al. 2002 Vascular endothelial growth factor mediated angiogenic potential of pancreatic ductal carcinomas enhanced by hypoxia: an in vitro and in vivo study. Int J Cancer 102: 592–600
37. Adsay N V, Bandyopadhyay S, Basturk O et al. 2004 Chronic pancreatitis or pancreatic ductal adenocarcinoma? Semin Diagn Pathol 21: 268–276
38. Lüttges J, Zamboni G, Klöppel G 1999 Recommendation for the examination of pancreaticoduodenectomy specimens removed from patients with carcinoma of the exocrine pancreas. A proposal for a standardized pathological staging of pancreaticoduodenectomy specimens including a checklist. Dig Surg 16: 291–296
39. Albores-Saavedra J, Heffess C, Hruban R H et al. 1999 Association of Directors of Anatomic and Surgical Pathology. Recommendations for the reporting of pancreatic specimens containing malignant tumors. Am J Clin Pathol 111: 304–307
40. Lüttges J, Vogel I, Menke M et al. 1998 The retroperitoneal resection margin and vessel involvement are important factors determining survival after pancreaticoduodenectomy for ductal adenocarcinoma of the head of the pancreas. Virchow's Arch 433: 237–242
41. Adsay N V, Basturk O, Bonnett M et al. 2005 A proposal for a new and more practical grading scheme for pancreatic ductal adenocarcinoma. Am J Surg Pathol 29: 724–733
42. Lüttges J, Schemm S, Vogel I et al. 2000 The grade of pancreatic ductal carcinoma is an independent prognostic factor and is superior to the immunohistochemical assessment of proliferation. J Pathol 191: 154–161
43. International Union Against Cancer (UICC) 2002 TNM. Classification of malignant tumours, 6th edn. Wiley-Liss, New York
44. Carpelan-Holmström M, Nordling S, Pukkala E et al. 2005 Does anyone survive pancreatic ductal adenocarcinoma? A nationwide study re-evaluating the data of the Finnish Cancer Registry. Gut 54: 385–387
45. Trede M, Schwall G, Saeger H D 1990 Survival after pancreatoduodenectomy. 118 consecutive resections without an operative mortality. Ann Surg 211: 447–458
46. Nagakawa T, Nagamori M, Futakami F et al. 1996 Results of extensive surgery for pancreatic carcinoma. Cancer 77: 640–645
47. Conlon K C, Klimstra D S, Brennan M F 1996 Long-term survival after curative resection for pancreatic ductal adenocarcinoma. Clinicopathologic analysis of 5-year survivors. Ann Surg 223: 273–279
48. Neoptolemos J P, Stocken D D, Friess H et al. 2004 A randomized trial of chemoradiotherapy and chemotherapy after resection of pancreatic cancer. N Engl J Med 350: 1200–1210
49. Adsay N V, Pierson C, Sarkar F et al. 2001 Colloid (mucinous noncystic) carcinoma of the pancreas. Am J Surg Pathol 25: 26–42
50. Seidel G, Zaharuk M, Iacobuzio-Donahue C et al. 2002 Almost all infiltrating colloid carcinomas of the pancreas and periampullary region arise from in situ papillary neoplasms. A study of 39 cases. Am J Surg Pathol 26: 56–63
51. Kardon D E, Thompson L D, Przygodzki R M et al. 2001 Adenosquamous carcinoma of the pancreas: a clinicopathologic series of 25 cases. Mod Pathol 14: 443–451
52. Bralet M P, Terris B, Brégeaud L et al. 1999 Squamous cell carcinoma and lipomatous pseudohypertrophy of the pancreas. Virchow's Arch 434: 569–572
53. Klöppel G 1984 Pancreatic, non-endocrine tumours. In: Klöppel G, Heitz PU (eds). Pancreatic pathology. Churchill Livingstone, Edinburgh, p 79–113
54. Paal E, Thompson L D R, Frommelt R A et al. 2001 A clinicpathologic and immunohistochemical study of 35 anaplastic carcinomas of the pancreas with a review of the literature. Ann Diagn Pathol 5: 129–140
55. Hoorens A, Prenzel K, Lemoine N R et al. 1998 Undifferentiated carcinoma of the pancreas: analysis of intermediate filament profile and Ki-ras mutations provides evidence of a ductal origin. J Pathol 185: 53–60
56. Westra W H, Sturm P, Drillenburg P et al. 1998 K-*ras* oncogene mutations in osteoclast-like giant cell tumors of the pancreas and liver. Genetic evidence to support origin from the duct epithelium. Am J Surg Pathol 22: 1247–1254
57. Newbould M J, Benbow E W, Sene A et al. 1992 Adenocarcinoma of the pancreas with osteoclast-like giant cells: A case report with immunocytochemistry. Pancreas 7: 611–615
58. Molberg K H, Heffess C, Delgado R et al. 1998 Undifferentiated carcinoma with osteoclast-like giant cells of the pancreas and periampullary region. Cancer 82: 1279–1287
59. Ohike N, Kosmahl M, Klöppel G 2004 Mixed acinar-endocrine carcinoma of the pancreas. A clinicopathological study and comparison with acinar-cell carcinoma. Virchow's Arch 445: 231–235
60. Permert J, Mogaki M, Andrén-Sandberg A et al. 1992 Pancreatic mixed ductal-islet tumors. Is this an entity? Int J Pancreatol 11: 23–29
61. Kosmahl M, Pauser U, Peters K et al. 2004 Cystic neoplasms of the pancreas and tumor-like lesions with cystic features: a review of 418 cases and a classification proposal. Virchow's Arch 445: 168–178
62. Sessa F, Solcia E, Capella C et al. 1994 Intraductal papillary-mucinous tumours represent a distinct group of pancreatic neoplasms: an investigation of tumour cell differentiation and K-*ras*, p53, and *c-erb*B-2 abnormalities in 26 patients. Virchow's Arch 425: 357–367
63. Santini D, Campione O, Salerno A et al. 1995 Intraductal papillary-mucinous neoplasm of the pancreas. A clinicopathologic entity. Arch Pathol Lab Med 119: 209–213
64. Nagai E, Ueki T, Chijiiwa K et al. 1995 Intraductal papillary mucinous neoplasms of the pancreas associated with so-called "mucinous ductal ectasia". Histochemical and immunohistochemical analysis of 29 cases. Am J Surg Pathol 19: 576–589
65. Paal E, Thompson L D, Przygodzki R M et al. 1999 A clinicopathologic and immunohistochemical study of 22 intraductal papillary mucinous neoplasms of the pancreas, with a review of the literature. Mod Pathol 12: 518–528
66. Adsay N V, Conlon K C, Zee S Y et al. 2002 Intraductal papillary-mucinous neoplasms of the pancreas. An analysis of in situ and invasive carcinomas in 28 patients. Cancer 94: 62–77
67. D'Angelica M, Brennan M F, Suriawinata A A et al. 2004 Intraductal papillary mucinous neoplasms of the pancreas: an analysis of clinicopathologic features and outcome. Ann Surg 239: 400–408
68. Terris B, Ponsot T, Paye F et al. 2000 Intraductal papillary mucinous tumors of the pancreas confined to secondary ducts show less aggressive pathologic features as compared with those involving the main pancreatic duct. Am J Surg Pathol 24: 1372–1377
69. Adsay N V, Adair C F, Heffess C S et al. 1996 Intraductal oncocytic papillary neoplasms of the pancreas. Am J Surg Pathol 20: 980–994
70. Furukawa T, Klöppel G, Adsay VN et al. 2005 Classification of types of intraductal papillary-mucinous neoplasm of the pancreas: a consensus study. Virchow's Arch 447: 794–799
71. Adsay N V, Merati K, Basturk O et al. 2004 Pathologically and biologically distinct types of epithelium in intraductal papillary mucinous neoplasms. Delineation of an "intestinal" pathway of carcinogenesis in the pancreas. Am J Surg Pathol 28: 839–848
72. Lüttges J, Zamboni G, Longnecker D et al. 2001 The immunohistochemical mucin expression pattern distinguishes different types of intraductal papillary mucinous neoplasms of the pancreas and determines their relationship to mucinous noncystic carcinoma and ductal adenocarcinoma. Am J Surg Pathol 25: 942–948
73. Zamboni G, Scarpa A, Bogina G et al. 1999 Mucinous cystic tumors of the pancreas. Clinicopathological features, prognosis and relationship to other mucinous cystic tumors. Am J Surg Pathol 23: 410–422
74. Hruban R H, Takaori K, Klimstra D S et al. 2004 An illustrated consensus on the classification of pancreatic intraepithelial neoplasia and intraductal papillary mucinous neoplasms. Am J Surg Pathol 28: 977–987

75. Albores-Saavedra J, Sheahan K, O'Riain C et al. 2004 Intraductal tubular adenoma, pyloric type, of the pancreas. Additional observations on a new type of pancreatic neoplasm. Am J Surg Pathol 28: 233–238
76. Tajiri T, Tate G, Inagaki T et al. 2005 Intraductal tubular neoplasms of the pancreas. Histogenesis and differentiation. Pancreas 30: 115–121
77. Nakayama Y, Inoue H, Hamada Y et al. 2005 Intraductal tubular adenoma of the pancreas, pyloric gland type. A clinicopathologic and imunohistochemical study of 6 cases. Am J Surg Pathol 29: 607–616
78. Wilentz R E, Albores-Saavedra J, Zahurak M et al. 1999 Pathologic examination accurately predicts prognosis in mucinous cystic neoplasms of the pancreas. Am J Surg Pathol 23: 1320–1327
79. Margolis R M, Jang N 1984 Zollinger–Ellison syndrome associated with pancreatic cystadenocarcinoma. N Engl J Med 311: 1380–1381
80. Garcia Rego J A, Valbuena Ruvira L, Alvarez Garcia A et al. 1991 Pancreatic mucinous cystadenocarcinoma with pseudosarcomatous mural nodules. A report of a case with immunohistochemical study. Cancer 67: 494–498
81. Wenig B M, Albores-Saavedra J, Buetow P C et al. 1997 Pancreatic mucinous cystic neoplasm with sarcomatous stroma. A report of three cases. Am J Surg Pathol 21: 70–80
82. Alpert L C, Truong L D, Bossart M I et al. 1988 Microcystic adenoma (serous cystadenoma) of the pancreas. A study of 14 cases with immunohistochemical and electron-microscopic correlation. Am J Surg Pathol 12: 251–263
83. Compagno J, Oertel J E 1978 Microcystic adenomas of the pancreas (glycogen-rich cystadenomas): a clinicopathologic study of 34 cases. Am J Clin Pathol 69: 289–298
84. Egawa N, Maillet B, Schröder S et al. 1994 Serous oligocystic and ill-demarcated adenoma of the pancreas: a variant of serous cystic adenoma. Virchow's Arch 424: 13–17
85. Lewandrowski K, Warshaw A, Compton C 1992 Macrocystic serous cystadenoma of the pancreas: a morphologic variant differing from microcystic adenoma. Hum Pathol 23: 871–875
86. Perez-Ordonez B, Naseem A, Lieberman P H et al. 1996 Solid serous adenoma of the pancreas. The solid variant of serous cystadenoma? Am J Surg Pathol 20: 1401–1405
87. Compagno J, Oertel J E 1978 Mucinous cystic neoplasms of the pancreas with overt and latent malignancy (cystadenocarcinoma and cystadenoma). A clinicopathologic study of 41 cases. Am J Clin Pathol 69: 573–580
88. Capella C, Solcia E, Klöppel G et al. 2000 Serous cystic neoplasms of the pancreas. In: Hamilton SR, Aaltonen LA (eds). Pathology and genetics. Tumours of the digestive system. WHO Classification of Tumours. IARC Press, Lyon, p 231–233
89. Kosmahl M, Wagner J, Peters K et al. 2004 Serous cystic neoplasms of the pancreas: an immunohistochemical analysis revealing alpha-inhibin, neuron-specific enolase, and MUC6 as new markers. Am J Surg Pathol 28: 339–346
90. Kosmahl M, Klöppel G 2003 Pancreatic tumours with cystic features. Cesk Patol 39: 155–162
91. George D H, Murphy F, Michalski R et al. 1989 Serous cystadenocarcinoma of the pancreas: a new entity? Am J Surg Pathol 13: 61–66
92. Compton C C 2000 Serous cystic tumors of the pancreas. Semin Diagn Pathol 17: 43–55
93. Lee W Y, Tzeng C C, Jin Y T et al. 1993 Papillary cystic tumor of the pancreas: a case indistinguishable from oncocytic carcinoma. Pancreas 8: 127–132
94. Mohr V H, Vortmeyer A O, Zhuang Z et al. 2000 Histopathology and molecular genetics of multiple cysts and microcystic (serous) adenomas of the pancreas in von Hippel-Lindau patients. Am J Pathol 157: 1615–1621
95. Yoshimi N, Sugie S, Tanaka T et al. 1992 A rare case of serous cystadenocarcinoma of the pancreas. Cancer 69: 2449–2453
96. Klimstra D S, Heffess C S, Oertel J E et al. 1992 Acinar cell carcinoma of the pancreas: a clinicopathologic study of 28 cases. Am J Surg Pathol 16: 815–837
97. Holen K D, Klimstra D S, Hummer A et al. 2002 Clinical characteristics and outcomes from an institutional series of acinar cell carcinomas of the pancreas and related tumors. J Clin Oncol 20: 4673–4678
98. Hoorens A, Lemoine N R, McLellan E E et al. 1993 Pancreatic acinar cell carcinoma. An analysis of cell lineage markers, p53 expression, and Ki-ras mutation. Am J Pathol 143: 685–698
99. Abraham S C, Wu T T, Hruban R H et al. 2002 Genetic and immunohistochemical analysis of pancreatic acinar cell carcinoma. Frequent allelic loss on chromosome 11p and alterations in the APC/β-catenin pathway. Am J Pathol 160: 953–962
100. Klimstra D S, Rosai J, Heffess C S 1994 Mixed acinar-endocrine carcinomas of the pancreas. Am J Surg Pathol 18: 765–778
101. Schron D S, Mendelsohn G 1984 Pancreatic carcinoma with duct, endocrine, and acinar differentiation. A histologic, immunocytochemical, and ultrastructural study. Cancer 54: 1766–1770
102. Stamm B, Burger H, Hollinger A 1987 Acinar cell cystadenocarcinoma of the pancreas. Cancer 60: 2542–2547
103. Zamboni G, Terris B, Scarpa A et al. 2002 Acinar cell cystadenoma of the pancreas. A new entity? Am J Surg Pathol 26: 698–704
104. Kishi K, Nakamura K, Yoshimori M et al. 1992 Morphology and pathological significance of focal acinar cell dysplasia of the human pancreas. Pancreas 7: 177–182
105. Klimstra D S, Wenig B M, Adair C F et al. 1995 Pancreatoblastoma. A clinicopathologic study and review of the literature. Am J Surg Pathol 19: 1371–1389
106. Hoorens A, Gebhard F, Kraft K et al. 1994 Pancreatoblastoma in an adult: its separation from acinar cell carcinoma. Virchow's Arch 424: 485–490
107. Dunn J L, Longnecker D S 1995 Pancreatoblastoma in an older adult. Arch Pathol Lab Med 119: 547–551
108. Abraham S C, Wu T T, Klimstra D S et al. 2001 Distinctive molecular genetic alterations in sporadic and familial adenomatous polyposis-associated pancreatoblastomas. Frequent alterations in the APC/β-catenin pathway and chromosome 11p. Am J Pathol 159: 1619–1627
109. Klöppel G, Maurer R, Hofmann E et al. 1991 Solid-cystic (papillary-cystic) tumours within and outside the pancreas in men: report of two patients. Virchow's Arch [A] Pathol Anat 418: 179–183
110. Klimstra D S, Wenig B M, Heffess C S 2000 Solid-pseudopapillary tumor of the pancreas: A typically cystic carcinoma of low malignant potential. Semin Diagn Pathol 17: 66–80
111. Stömmer P, Kraus J, Stolte M et al. 1991 Solid and cystic pancreatic tumors. Clinical, histochemical, and electron microscopic features in ten cases. Cancer 67: 1635–1641
112. Pettinato G, Manivel J C, Ravetto C et al. 1992 Papillary cystic tumor of the pancreas. A clinicopathologic study of 20 cases with cytologic, immunohistochemical, ultrastructural, and flow cytometric observations, and a review of the literature. Am J Clin Pathol 98: 478–488
113. Zamboni G, Bonetti F, Scarpa A et al. 1993 Expression of progesterone receptors in solid-cystic tumour of the pancreas: a clinicopathological and immunohistochemical study of ten cases. Virchow's Arch [A] Pathol Anat 423: 425–431
114. Kosmahl M, Seada L S, Janig U et al. 2000. Solid-pseudopapillary tumor of the pancreas: its origin revisited. Virchow's Arch 436: 473–480
115. Abraham S C, Klimstra D S, Wilentz R E et al. 2002 Solid-pseudopapillary tumors of the pancreas are genetically distinct from pancreatic ductal adenocarcinomas and almost always harbor β-catenin mutations. Am J Pathol 160: 1361–1369
116. Tanaka Y, Kato K, Notohara K et al. 2001 Frequent β-catenin mutation and cytoplasmic/nuclear accumulation in pancreatic solid-pseudopapillary neoplasm. Cancer Res 61: 8401–8404
117. Grant L D, Lauwers G Y, Meloni A M et al. 1996 Unbalanced chromosomal translocation, der(17)t(13;17)(q14;p11) in a solid and cystic papillary epithelial neoplasm of the pancreas. Am J Surg Pathol 20: 339–345
118. Tang L H, Aydin H, Brennan M F et al. 2005 Clinically aggressive solid pseudopapillary tumors of the pancreas. A report of two cases with components of undifferentiated carcinoma and a comparative clinicopathologic analysis of 34 conventional cases. Am J Surg Pathol 29: 512–519
119. Goggins M, Offerhaus G J, Hilgers W et al. 1998 Pancreatic adenocarcinomas with DNA replication errors (RER+) are associated with wild-type K-ras and characteristic histopathology. Poor differentiation, a syncytial growth pattern, and pushing borders suggest RER+. Am J Pathol 152: 1501–1507
120. Wilentz R E, Goggins M, Redston M et al. 2000 Genetic, immunohistochemical, and clinical features of medullary carcinoma of the pancreas: A newly described and characterized entity. Am J Pathol 156: 1641–1651
121. Kekis P B, Murtin C, Künzli B M et al. 2004 Epstein–Barr virus-associated lymphoepithelial carcinoma in the pancreas. Pancreas 28: 98–102
122. Bondeson L, Bondeson A G, Grimelius L et al. 1990 Oncocytic tumor of the pancreas. Report of a case with aspiration cytology. Acta Cytol 34: 425–428
123. Zerbi A, De Nardi P, Braga M et al. 1993 An oncocytic carcinoma of the pancreas with pulmonary and subcutaneous metastases. Pancreas 8: 116–119
124. Marucci G, Betts C M, Liguori L et al. 2005 Basaloid carcinoma of the pancreas. Virchow's Arch 446: 322–324
125. Ray B, New N E, Wedgwood K R 2005 Clear cell carcinoma of exocrine pancreas: a rare tumor with an unusual presentation. Pancreas 30: 184–185
126. Lonardo F, Cubilla A L, Klimstra D S 1996 Microadenocarcinoma of the pancreas – Morphologic pattern or pathologic entity? Am J Surg Pathol 20: 1385–1393
127. Lack E E, Cassady J R, Levey R et al. 1983 Tumors of the exocrine pancreas in children and adolescents. A clinical and pathologic study of eight cases. Am J Surg Pathol 7: 319–327
128. Klöppel G, Kosmahl M, Jänig U et al. 2004 Pancreatoblastoma: one of the rarest among the rare pancreatic neoplasms. Pancreatology 4: 441–453
129. Shorter N A, Glick R D, Klimstra D S et al. 2002 Malignant pancreatic tumors in childhood and adolescence: the Memorial Sloan-Kettering experience, 1967 to present. J Pediatr Surg 37: 887–892
130. Movahedi-Lankarani S, Hruban R H, Westra W H et al. 2002 Primitive neuroectodermal tumors of the pancreas. A report of seven cases of a rare neoplasm. Am J Surg Pathol 26: 1040–1047
131. Lüttges J, Pierré E, Zamboni G et al. 1997 Maligne nicht-epitheliale Tumoren des Pankreas. Pathologe 18: 233–237
132. de Alava E, Torramade J, Vazquez J J 1993 Leiomyosarcoma of the pancreas. Virchow's Arch [A] Pathol Anat 422: 419–422
133. Ishikawa O, Matsui Y, Aoki Y et al. 1981 Leiomyosarcoma of the pancreas. Report of a case and review of the literature. Am J Surg Pathol 5: 597–602

134. Zamboni G, Pea M, Martignoni G et al. 1996 Clear cell "sugar" tumor of the pancreas. A novel member of the family of lesions characterized by the presence of perivascular epithelioid cells. Am J Surg Pathol 20: 722–730
135. Ramuz O, Lelong B, Giovannini M et al. 2005 "Sugar" tumor of the pancreas: a rare entity that is diagnosable on preoperative fine-needle biopsies. Virchow's Arch 446: 555–559
136. Bismar T A, Basturk O, Gerald W L et al. 2004 Desmoplastic small cell tumor in the pancreas. Am J Surg Pathol 28: 808–812
137. Lüttges J, Mentzel T, Hübner G et al. 1999 Solitary fibrous tumour of the pancreas: a new member of the small group of mesenchymal pancreatic tumours. Virchow's Arch 435:37–42
138. Daum O, Klecka J, Ferda J et al. 2005 Gastrointestinal stromal tumor of the pancreas: case report with documentation of KIT gene mutation. Virchow's Arch 446: 470–472
139. Ezzat A, Jamshed A, Khafaga Y et al. 1996 Primary pancreatic non-Hodgkin's lymphomas. J Clin Gastroenterol 23: 109–112
140. Volmar K E, Routbort M J, Jones C K et al. 2004 Primary pancreatic lymphoma evaluated by fine-needle aspiration: findings in 14 cases. Am J Clin Pathol 121: 898–903
141. Thompson L D R, Heffess C S 2000 Renal cell carcinoma to the pancreas in surgical pathology material. A clinicopathologic study of 21 cases with a review of the literature. Cancer 89: 1076–1088
142. Adsay N V, Andea A, Basturk O et al. 2004 Secondary tumors of the pancreas: an analysis of a surgical and autopsy database and review of the literature. Virchow's Arch 444: 527–535
143. Pauser U, Kosmahl M, Kruslin B et al. 2005 Pancreatic solid and cystic hamartoma in adults: characterization of a new tumorous lesion. Am J Surg Pathol 29: 797–800
144. Adsay N V, Basturk O, Klimstra D S et al. 2004 Pancreatic pseudotumors: non-neoplastic solid lesions of the pancreas that clinically mimic pancreas cancer. Semin Diagn Pathol 21: 260–267
145. Notohara K, Burgart L J, Yadav D et al. 2003 Idiopathic chronic pancreatitis with periductal lymphoplasmacytic infiltration: clinicopathologic features of 35 cases. Am J Surg Pathol 27: 1119–1127
146. Klimstra D S, Adsay N V 2004 Lymphoplasmacytic sclerosing (autoimmune) pancreatitis. Semin Diagn Pathol 21: 237–246
147. Adsay N V, Zamboni G 2004 Paraduodenal pancreatitis: A clinicopathologically distinct entity unifying "cystic dystrophy of heterotopic pancreas", "para-duodenal wall cyst", and "groove pancreatitis". Semin Diagn Pathol 21: 247–254
148. Kroft S H, Stryker S J, Winter J N et al. 1995 Inflammatory pseudotumor of the pancreas. Int J Pancreatol 18: 277–283
149. Klöppel G, Lüttges J, Löhr M et al. 2003 Autoimmune pancreatitis: pathological, clinical, and immunological features. Pancreas 27: 14–19
150. Zamboni G, Lüttges J, Capelli P et al. 2004 Histopathological features of diagnostic and clinical relevance in autoimmune pancreatitis: a study on 53 resection specimens and 9 biopsy specimens. Virchow's Arch 445: 552–563
151. Fléjou J F, Potet F, Molas G et al. 1993 Cystic dystrophy of the gastric and duodenal wall developing in heterotopic pancreas: an unrecognized entity. Gut 34: 343–347
152. Pauser U, da Silva M T S, Placke J et al. 2005 Cellular hamartoma resembling gastrointestinal stromal tumor: a solid tumor of the pancreas expressing c-kit (CD117). Mod Pathol 18: 1211–1216
153. Nakashiro H, Tokunaga O, Watanabe T et al. 1991 Localized lymphoid hyperplasia (pseudolymphoma) of the pancreas presenting with obstructive jaundice. Hum Pathol 22: 724–726
154. Klöppel G 2000 Pseudocysts and other non-neoplastic cysts of the pancreas. Semin Diagn Pathol 17: 7–15
155. Klöppel G 2004 Chronic pancreatitis of alcoholic and nonalcoholic origin. Semin Diagn Pathol 21: 227–236
156. Iacono C, Cracco N, Zamboni G et al. 1996 Lymphoepithelial cyst of the pancreas. Report of two cases and review of the literature. Int J Pancreatol 19: 71–76
157. Adsay N V, Hasteh F, Cheng J D et al. 2002 Lymphoepithelial cysts of the pancreas: a report of 12 cases and a review of the literature. Mod Pathol 15: 492–501

泌尿道肿瘤
Tumors of the urinary tract

12

John N. Eble 和 Robert H. Young 著

刘毅强　时云飞　薛卫成 译

肾肿瘤	485
肾上皮性肿瘤	485
肾神经内分泌和神经外胚层肿瘤	502
肾间叶性肿瘤	502
肾转移性肿瘤	510
儿童肾肿瘤	510
肾盂及输尿管肿瘤	519
良性肿瘤及瘤样病变	519
移行细胞癌	520
膀胱肿瘤	523
良性上皮性肿瘤	523
移行细胞癌	526

鳞状细胞癌	537
腺癌	539
未分化癌	544
含有一种以上组织学类型的癌	545
间叶性肿瘤	545
混合性肿瘤	547
淋巴瘤与白血病	548
其他原发性肿瘤	549
膀胱继发性肿瘤	551
尿道肿瘤	552
良性肿瘤及瘤样病变	552
恶性肿瘤	554

肾肿瘤　Tumors of the Kidney

三十年前肾细胞癌和Wilms肿瘤这两个诊断涵盖了绝大多数肾肿瘤，但从那以后，肾肿瘤的分类越来越复杂[1]。以下关于上皮性肿瘤、间叶性肿瘤、儿童肾肿瘤以及新近认识的少见疾病的有关章节，将介绍肾肿瘤的诊断和预后等方面的内容，重点在于大体病理学及组织学检查。肾盂及输尿管肿瘤将在肾实质肿瘤以后的各自章节中介绍。

肾上皮性肿瘤
Epithelial tumors of the kidney

乳头状腺瘤　Papillary adenoma

尽管有历史及手术问题，根据现有资料，我们认为目前乳头状腺瘤的诊断标准是可靠、合理的（表12.1）。第一条诊断标准是乳头状腺瘤的显微镜下组织形态与乳头状肾细胞癌相似，包括1型和2型病变[2]。第二条诊断标准是生长能力有限，这包括了95%以上的肾小管乳头状肿瘤[3]。体积较大的肿瘤需更多关注，因为这些

表12.1	肾乳头状腺瘤的诊断标准
乳头状或管状乳头状结构	
直径≤5mm	
组织形态不同于透明细胞、嫌色细胞或集合管肾细胞癌	

肿瘤生长能力更强，可有远处转移的潜能。第三条诊断标准尚无令人信服的证据，即其他细胞类型的微小肿瘤可能不是微小癌。早在1938年，Bell[4]已经意识到区分乳头状肿瘤与那些组织学类似透明细胞肾癌的小肿瘤是重要的，并且在后者中"肿瘤的体积并不是一个有关其恶性程度的可靠诊断标准"。随后的研究和病例报告发现微小的透明细胞肾癌可以发生转移，从而证实了这一结论[5,6]。类似的乳头状腺瘤诊断标准已经在德国海德堡和美国明尼苏达州罗彻斯特召开的共识会以及最近的WHO共识会中被采纳[1,7]。

在尸检病例，根据尸检人群和研究方法的不同，肾皮质微小上皮性肿瘤的发生率也不同，最高可达37%[8-12]。微小乳头状肿瘤的发生率随年龄上升，在年龄大于65岁的人群中可升至40%。类似的病变常常

发生于接受长期血液透析和后天性肾囊性疾病的患者，有研究报道在后者发生率可高达33%[13]。人们很早就认识到了动脉硬化性肾血管病与乳头状腺瘤之间存在相关性[4]。Budin 和 McDonnell[14] 对尸检材料进行了研究，发现在血管硬化性肾血管病患者中，乳头状腺瘤发生率不仅显著升高，而且与年龄无关。Xipell[9] 发现乳头状腺瘤的发生与吸烟显著相关，Bennington[15] 也得到了同样的结论。

与正常肾相比，患肾细胞癌或嗜酸细胞瘤的肾罹患乳头状腺瘤的可能性更大，这一现象很早就为学者所知[16]。有时在肾细胞癌或嗜酸细胞瘤附近会发现多个腺瘤，表明某些局部因子可能促进腺瘤的发生。

大体表现 乳头状腺瘤肉眼所见表现为边界清楚、黄色或灰白色的肾皮质区结节。大多数位于肾包膜下，然而从皮质表面无法看到的肿物也不少见。小的病变通常呈圆形，较大的病变有时略呈圆锥形，在垂直于肾皮质表面的切面上呈楔形外观。有学者认为病变与肾皮质瘢痕有关，但此观点尚存在争论[10,14]。在大多数患者，腺瘤单发[10]，偶尔，乳头状腺瘤可以多发和双侧发生，罕见粟粒样病变；后者被称为"肾腺瘤病"[17]，与肾嗜酸细胞瘤病相似[18,19]。

组织学表现 乳头状腺瘤表现为管状、乳头状或管状乳头状结构（图 12.1），通常与 Thoenes 等[20,21] 所描述的嗜碱性细胞非常相似。有些肿瘤具有薄的纤维性假包膜，其余则没有。细胞核圆形或卵圆形，染色质可呈点彩状或粗大块状，核仁不明显。有时可见核沟。核分裂象常常缺如。绝大部分的乳头状腺瘤细胞胞浆稀少、淡染、嗜双色性或嗜碱性。有时可见瘤细胞胞浆较丰富，

透明或充满微小空泡。有时胞浆丰富且呈嗜酸性，类似于 2 型乳头状肾细胞癌，但比较少见[2]。常见沙粒体和泡沫状巨噬细胞。

免疫组化、超微结构及特殊检查 Cohen 等[22] 发现几乎所有的乳头状腺瘤表达上皮膜抗原和低分子量细胞角蛋白，大部分病例表达高分子量细胞角蛋白。有时可表达神经元特异性烯醇化酶和 α_1- 抗胰蛋白酶，而不表达癌胚抗原[22]。Hiasa 等[11] 研究了65例直径 1～5mm 的腺瘤，发现 52 例呈花生凝集素和上皮膜抗原阳性，而 Leu M1 和 Lotus tetragonolobus 凝集素均为阴性，这种表达方式与正常远曲小管相似。13 例具有相反的表型，与正常近曲小管衬覆的细胞相似[11]。

肾嗜酸细胞瘤 Renal oncocytoma

肾嗜酸细胞瘤是肾皮质肿瘤，常由于其他原因进行肾影像学检查偶然发现，也可以表现为临床可触及的肿物或出现血尿[23,24]。1976 年，Klein 和 Valensi[25] 注意到以往被认为是肾细胞癌的肾嗜酸细胞瘤，具有自身独特的病理学特征及良性临床过程。男女发病比例为 2:1，几乎所有患者均为成年人，年龄大部分为 50～80 岁。切除肿瘤可以治愈。最初认为影像学表现为显著的轮辐状就可以诊断嗜酸细胞瘤，但大量的临床经验认为这种表现并不特异，因为肾细胞癌也可有类似的表现。术前影像学检查或活检并不能准确地将这种肿瘤与肾细胞癌区分。因此，根治性肾切除是常见的术式。然而一些患者可以多中心或双侧发生[26]，因此而进行的保守性手术已经获得成功。

大体表现 肾嗜酸细胞瘤最具特征性的表现是其桃花心木样褐色外观（图 12.2），与肾透明细胞癌典型的亮黄色形成鲜明对比。许多嗜酸细胞瘤中心可见灰白色纤维间质并与周边相连（图 12.3），使被膜下切面形成浮雕样外观。有时肿瘤可见灶状出血，但坏死罕见，而且通常与外部因素有关。一般来说，出现明显的坏死或出血时，诊断嗜酸细胞瘤需要格外谨慎。大约 4% 病例可呈双侧或单侧多中心性，此现象比肾细胞癌更为常见。一种罕见的情况是双侧肾皮质中出现大量的微小嗜酸细胞瘤，这样的病变被命名为嗜酸细胞瘤病（oncocytomatosis）或嗜酸细胞增生症（oncocytosis）[18,27]。

组织学表现 肿瘤细胞通常弥漫成片或呈巢状分布，纤维间质背景疏松、水肿（图 12.4）。轻度扩张的小管状排列也很常见。罕见的情况下，细胞团含有玻璃

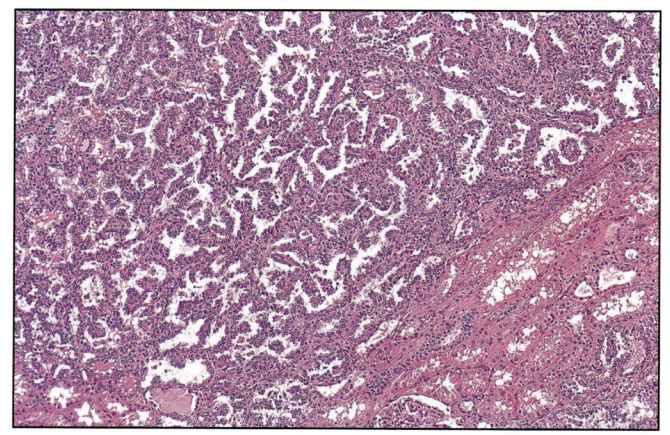

图12.1 乳头状腺瘤由被覆小细胞的复杂乳头构成。

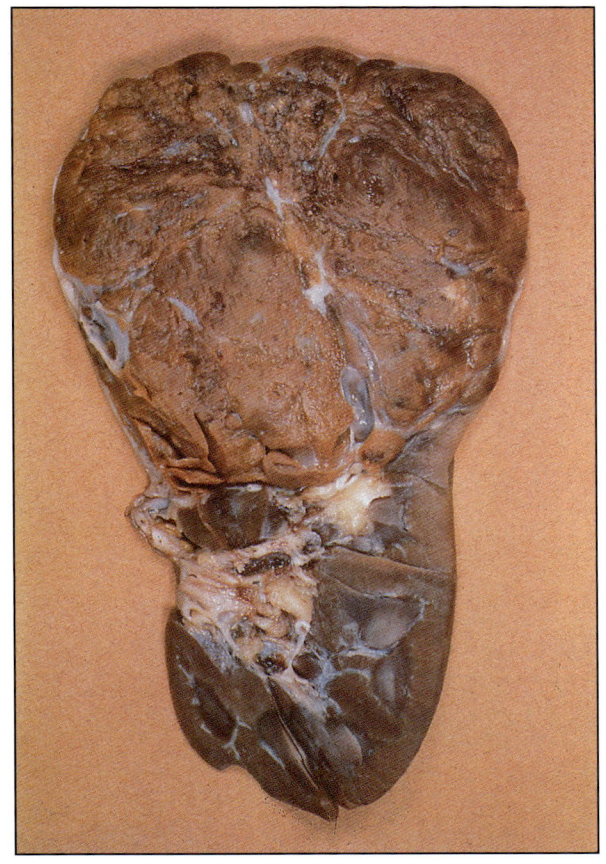

图12.2 肾嗜酸细胞瘤。膨胀性的大肿瘤呈均匀的红褐色。

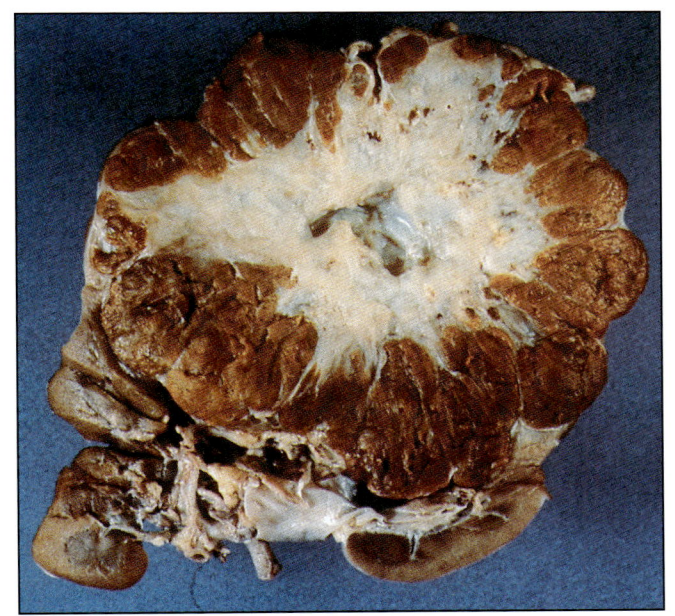

图12.3 肾嗜酸细胞瘤。这些肿瘤，尤其是体积较大者，中心常常可见灰白色纤维间质，可以发生空洞变性。

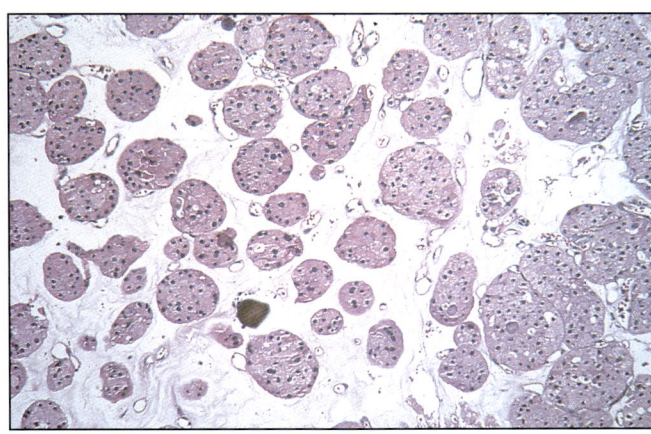

图12.4 肾嗜酸细胞瘤。肿瘤细胞含有丰富的嗜酸性胞浆，在水肿的间质中排列成岛状。

样Ⅳ型胶原蛋白沉积物，使之呈圆柱瘤样表现[28]。在HE染色的切片上，胞浆强嗜酸性、细颗粒状。无论胞浆中等量或丰富，其染色性质不变。核圆形，染色质呈微小块状，在10×的物镜下观察可见到核仁[29]。偶尔可出现增大的、含胞浆内陷的奇异核（图12.5）。嗜酸细胞瘤的核分裂象缺如或非常罕见。由于是良性病变，嗜酸细胞瘤没有分级。电镜下，胞浆充满线粒体，其他细胞器少见（图12.6）。微绒毛稀疏，完整的刷状缘并不常见[30]。

略多于5%的病例显微镜下可见向小静脉内蔓延，此现象似乎并无不良预后意义。近10%的病例可出现肾周脂肪组织微小侵犯，此现象似乎亦无不良影响。

鉴别诊断 主要的鉴别对象是嫌色细胞肾癌的嗜酸细胞变型。在大多数病例，严格遵循表12.2所列的标准

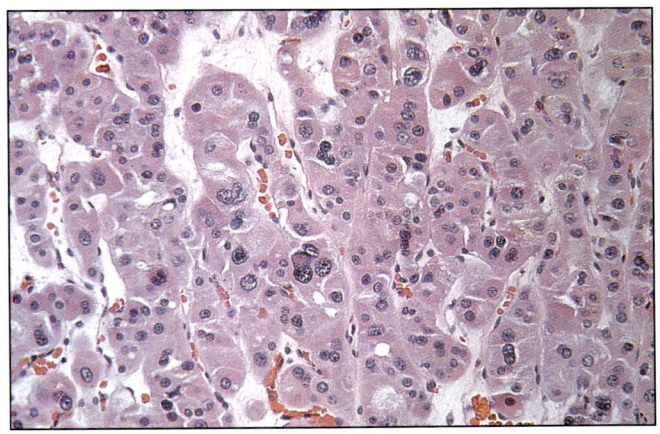

图12.5 肾嗜酸细胞瘤。某些嗜酸细胞瘤可出现灶状增大的退变细胞核，有时可见胞浆内陷。

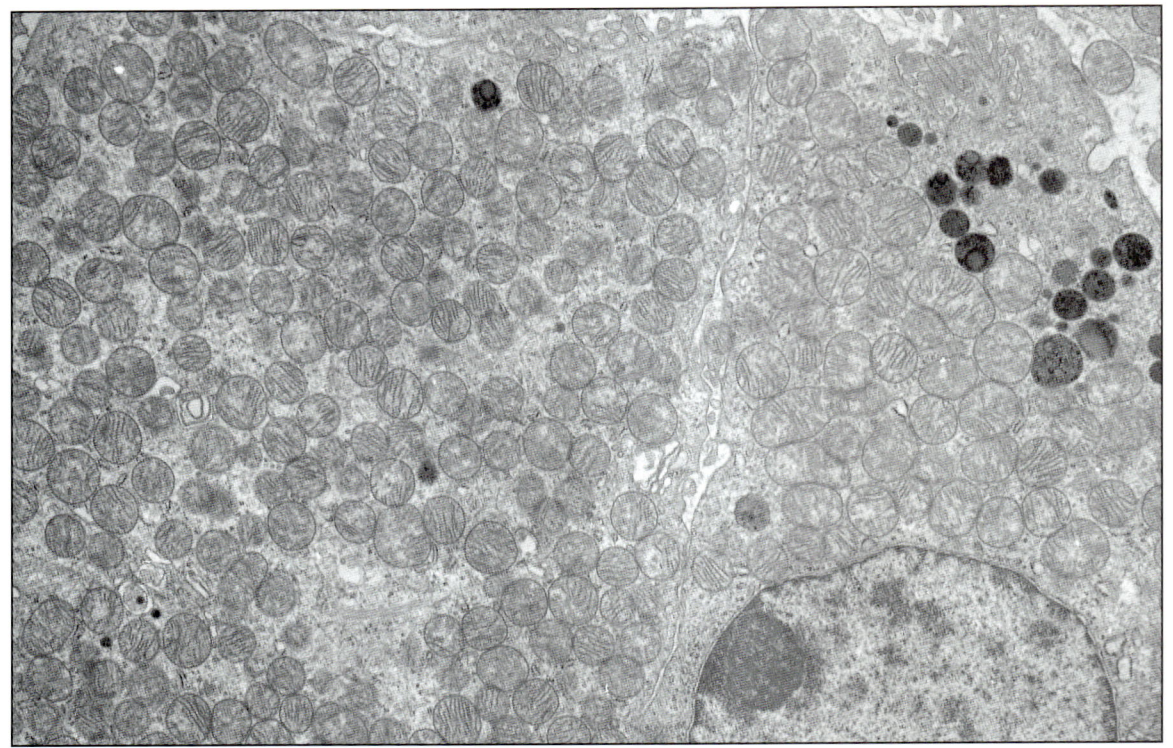

图12.6　肾嗜酸细胞瘤。超微结构显示嗜酸细胞瘤的胞浆充满线粒体，其他细胞器少见。

可以将两者区分开来。免疫组化有助于鉴别，在嗜酸细胞瘤中，细胞角蛋白7的典型表达方式是散在单个细胞或小团细胞着色，而在嫌色细胞肾癌中，几乎所有肿瘤细胞均表达细胞角蛋白7，而且主要为胞膜染色强阳性[31]。

表12.2	肾嗜酸细胞瘤的诊断特征
肾嗜酸细胞瘤的特征	
细颗粒状强嗜酸性胞浆 片状、岛状或管泡状结构 胞浆中充满线粒体，其他细胞器和微绒毛稀少	
肾嗜酸细胞瘤的少见特征	
显微镜下所见为血管侵犯 显微镜下所见为肾周脂肪侵犯	
肾嗜酸细胞瘤罕见或不具备的特征	
核分裂象 乳头状结构 透明或梭形细胞 胶体铁染色阳性或电镜下可见的嫌色细胞型囊泡 明显的血管侵犯 明显的肾周脂肪侵犯	

后肾腺瘤和后肾腺纤维瘤
Metanephric adenoma and metanephric adenofibroma

1980年，一种此前未曾认识的肾肿瘤引起了Pages和Granier[32]的注意，他们将其命名为"肾源性肾瘤（nephronogenic nephroma）"，认为这是一种起源于残存胚芽成分的纯上皮性肿瘤。从那以后，已经有超过100例的个案和综合研究报道，后肾腺瘤这个名称开始被认可[1,21]。

1992年，Hennigar和Beckwith[33]报道了5例混合性肿瘤，其上皮性成分与后肾腺瘤完全相同，同时含有增生的梭形细胞成分；他们提出了肾源性腺纤维瘤（nephrogenic adenofibroma）这一名称。现在Beckwith更赞同采用后肾腺纤维瘤这一名称来命名这类肿瘤，以强调它们与后肾腺瘤的密切关系。

后肾腺瘤可以发生于任何年龄，多见于40～60岁患者，女性多见，男女患病比例为1:2[34]。后肾腺瘤是儿童肾肿瘤中最常见的上皮性肿瘤[35]。50%患者是偶然发现，其他患者可出现红细胞增多、腹部或肋腹部疼痛、肿物或血尿等临床表现。红细胞增多常常在肿瘤切除后消退。迄今为止尚无复发或转移的病例报道。Davis等[34]所报道的50例患者中，4例同时患有肾细胞癌。

后肾腺纤维瘤患者年龄从13个月到36岁不等（中位年龄28个月）[36]。因病例数较少，性别倾向尚不明显。超过50%的患者患有红细胞增多症。其他的症状包括血尿[33]和高血压[33]。有些病例是偶然发现的。Hennigar和Beckwith[33]所报道的5例患者中，3例同时发现肾盂附近存在孤立的微小乳头状上皮性肿瘤，被认为是低度恶性的集合管癌。

大体表现　后肾腺瘤大小相差很大，最大者直径可达150mm，大部分直径为30～60mm[34]。Davis等[34]在50例患者中未发现双肾发生者，只有两例存在单肾多发病灶。肿瘤通常边界清楚，但大部分无包膜。薄的不连续的假包膜比真正的包膜更常见。切面灰色、褐色或黄色，质地可软可硬。大约20%的病例可出现钙化，少数钙化浓密。10%的肿瘤出现小囊腔，仅有一例完全囊性变[34]。常见出血和坏死灶[34,37]。典型的后肾腺纤维瘤是孤立的、质硬的、膨胀性肿物，没有包膜，边界不清[33,36]。切面灰色、褐色或黄色，实性，某些肿瘤偶尔可见囊腔。

组织学表现　组织形态上，典型的后肾腺瘤细胞丰富，排列成密集、形态一致的小圆腺泡结构（图12.7）。这些腺泡及其腺腔极小，以致于在低倍镜下会被误认为实性细胞团。长分支状和鹿角样腺管结构也很常见。间质不明显或表现为细胞稀少、疏松、水肿。10%～20%的肿瘤可出现玻璃样瘢痕或局灶骨化生[34]。大约50%的肿瘤含有乳头状结构，由小囊腔组成，内含类似未成熟肾小球的短粗小乳头。大部分乳头未见到血管。沙粒体很常见，有时数量很多。与正常肾组织分界明显，但缺乏假包膜。

后肾腺瘤细胞核小而一致，无核仁或核仁不明显。

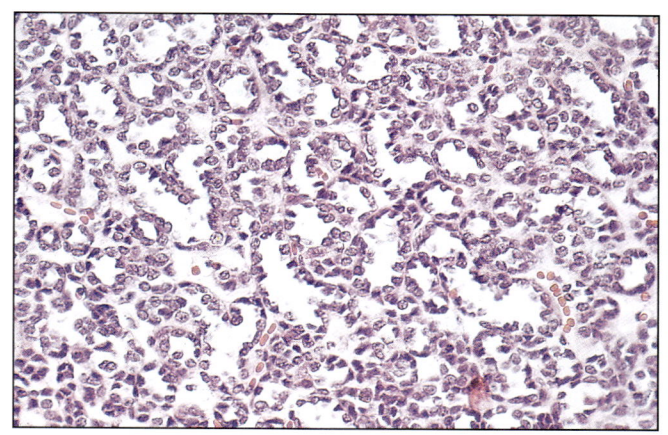

图12.7　后肾腺瘤。胞浆稀少、形态柔和的细胞排列成小管状结构。

细胞核比淋巴细胞稍大，圆形或卵圆形，染色质纤细。胞浆稀少、淡染或粉染。核分裂象罕见或缺如。

后肾腺纤维瘤是一种混合性肿瘤，表现为后肾腺瘤样的上皮结节被中等丰富的片状梭形细胞所包绕。梭形细胞由成纤维细胞样细胞组成（图12.8）[33,36]。胞浆嗜酸性但染色较浅，核卵圆形或纺锤形。核仁不明显，核分裂象缺如或罕见。可见多少不等的玻璃样变或黏液样变区域。肿瘤中梭形细胞和上皮成分相对含量多少不一，可以梭形细胞为主，也可仅有少量梭形细胞。肿瘤与正常肾组织分界不规则，梭形细胞向周围生长延伸时可将部分正常肾组织包绕于其中。正如上文后肾腺瘤所描述的那样，上皮成分由小的腺泡、小管和乳头状结构组成。沙粒体很常见，有时数量很多。后肾腺瘤及后肾腺纤

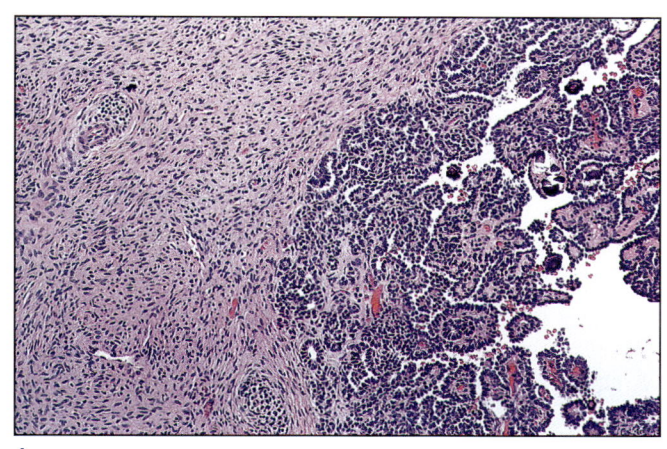
A

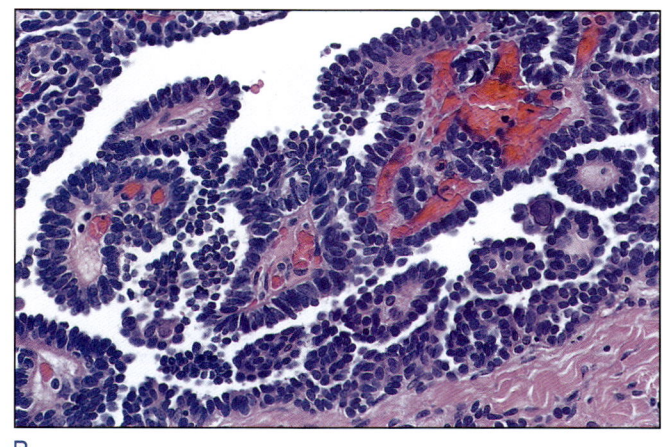
B

图12.8　后肾腺纤维瘤。胞浆中等丰富的梭形细胞组成的纤维瘤成分直接过渡为一个含沙粒体的上皮结节（A）。上皮成分由被覆小而一致的立方或柱状细胞的锯齿状乳头所构成（B）。(Courtesy of Dr. B. Beckwith and the National Wilms' Tumor Study Pathology Center.)

维瘤均未见胚芽成分，而且与肾源性残余无关。仅由间质成分组成的结节状、上皮样病变，被称为后肾间质肿瘤[38]。

免疫组织化学及外源凝集素组织化学研究在不同的实验室结果有所不同，因此它们在后肾腺瘤的鉴别诊断中意义不大[21]。

鉴别诊断 初次遇到后肾腺瘤时，紧密排列的小蓝染细胞和上皮分化会使人想到Wilms瘤。但是，后肾腺瘤细胞核较小，而且缺乏Wilms瘤中上皮细胞那种细长而且末端逐渐变细的细胞核形态。此外，后肾腺瘤中核分裂象罕见而且缺乏胚芽成分。后肾腺纤维瘤的纤维成分可能会被误认为是Wilms瘤的间质成分，但是在细胞学形态上，这些成分是良性的，而且缺乏Wilms瘤间质中常见的多向分化表现。

另一个重要的鉴别诊断是1型乳头状肾细胞癌。后肾腺瘤细胞胞浆稀少、乳头状结构以及沙粒体的存在会让人想到1型乳头状肾细胞癌。但是，大部分后肾腺瘤主要由横切面类似肾小管的一致性组织结构组成。乳头状肾细胞癌不具备此类典型表现。此外，后肾腺瘤经常含有被覆上皮细胞的细长而尖锐的分支管状结构。这些特点在乳头状肾细胞癌以及Wilms瘤中并不存在。乳头状肾细胞癌中常见的乳头轴心水肿以及间质泡沫细胞的聚集不是后肾腺瘤的典型表现。后肾腺瘤常常表达WT1蛋白，这一点有助于与乳头状肾细胞癌鉴别，利用荧光原位杂交检测乳头状肾细胞癌中常见的染色体扩增也有助于两者的鉴别[39,40]。

肾细胞癌 Renal cell carcinoma

目前，肾细胞癌被认为是一组起源于肾小管上皮的恶性肿瘤[1]。这些肿瘤具有独特的形态学特征，通过不同系列的基因改变而发生[7,41-43]。表12.3列出了目前的肾细胞癌分类。

由于新近才认识到肾细胞癌是通过不同基因改变而发生的一组疾病，因此目前所能获得的绝大部分临床及流行病学资料仍来自将所有类型肾细胞癌合并在一起而进行的研究，以下是主要结论。肾细胞癌是一种主要发生于成年人的肿瘤，在美国每年大约有30 000例新发病例，而且发病率逐渐上升[44]。60岁之前每十年其发病率随年龄而升高，男性发病率比女性高2～3倍[45]。20岁之前肾细胞癌罕见，只占儿童肾肿瘤的2%[35]。虽然肥胖[46]、吸烟[47]以及接触工业化学物质[48]被认为是肾细胞癌发生的危险因素，但大部分病例发病机制仍然不清楚。某些偶发病例与von Hippel-Lindau病有关，这些患者中，33%～50%可发生肾细胞癌[49,50]。结节性硬化症[51,52]和常染色体显性遗传多囊性肾病[53-55]与肾细胞癌的发生也有关系。慢性肾衰竭患者发生的获得性肾囊肿病也与肾细胞癌密切相关[56-58]。血尿、肋腹部疼痛和肿块被认为是肾癌典型的三联症[59]，但许多患者缺乏这些症状而表现为发热、身体不适或贫血等系统症状[60,61]。偶尔肾癌患者也会出现高血钙[62]、红细胞增多[63]、高血压[64]和淀粉样变[65]等副肿瘤综合征[63,66,67]。众所周知，肾癌还可以表现为原发部位不明的转移癌。同侧多中心肾癌发生率为7%～13%[68]，而双侧肾癌的发生率大约为1%[69]。

肾癌的临床过程因其不可预测而闻名，部分病例显示肾癌转移灶可以自发消退[70-72]。生存期较长的患者，大约10%的患者在肾切除术后10年甚至更长的时间才出现复发[73]。有证据表明孤立性转移灶的切除可以提高生存率[74]，而多发性转移则意味着预后不良[75]。但是，肾癌对放疗和化疗的不敏感使大部分出现远处转移的患者预后极差[76]。骨转移很常见，超过1/3转移至肩胛骨[77]。

透明细胞肾细胞癌 Clear cell renal cell carcinoma

所有肾细胞癌中，大约2/3至3/4是透明细胞肾细胞癌。这些肿瘤之所以如此命名是因为它们大部分或全部由富含透明胞浆的肿瘤细胞构成。但是，"透明细胞肾

表12.3	肾细胞肿瘤的分类
良性	
乳头状腺瘤	
嗜酸细胞瘤	
恶性	
透明细胞肾细胞癌	
乳头状肾细胞癌	
• 1型	
• 2型	
嫌色细胞肾细胞癌	
• 经典型	
• 嗜酸型	
集合管癌	
• 肾髓质癌	
Xp11易位癌	
神经母细胞瘤相关性肾癌	
黏液小管和梭形细胞癌	
未分类肾细胞癌	

细胞癌"仅仅是一个病名，其中许多肿瘤含有大量胞浆嗜酸的癌细胞，极少见的病例全部由胞浆嗜酸的肿瘤细胞构成。

透明细胞肾细胞癌的一个特征性表现是 3 号染色体短臂 (3p) 遗传物质的丢失。这种遗传物质的丢失表现为从整段染色体的丢失到高甲基化导致的功能丧失[78-80]。其他遗传学异常也很常见，有证据表明 14、8 和 9 号染色体的改变可以影响患者预后[81,82]。

总体上，透明细胞肾细胞癌的预后较其他常见类型肾细胞癌稍差[83,84]。透明细胞肾细胞癌对目前的化疗和放射治疗不敏感。免疫治疗效果也不理想。手术切除是主要治疗手段，因此肿瘤分期是最重要的预后因素[85,86]。同一分期病例中，肿瘤分级更加有助于预后的判断。肿瘤分级在下文讨论。

大体表现　典型的透明细胞肾细胞癌表现为肾皮质区圆形肿物（图 12.9），可起源于皮质区的任何区域，而且经常突出于正常肾轮廓之外。但有时可表现为内生性或弥漫浸润性生长。切面通常为五彩状（图 12.10），由质地较软的鲜黄色肿瘤实质以及灰白色的水肿性间质、出血区、坏死区以及囊性区构成。囊腔内充满黄色清亮液体或血性液体。透明细胞肾细胞癌可侵犯肾静脉系统，有时形成肾静脉内瘤栓并延伸至下腔静脉甚至右心房。大约 5% 的透明细胞肾细胞癌出现肉瘤样变。这些肿瘤大体上多表现为灰白色质地偏硬的实性肿物（图 12.11）。

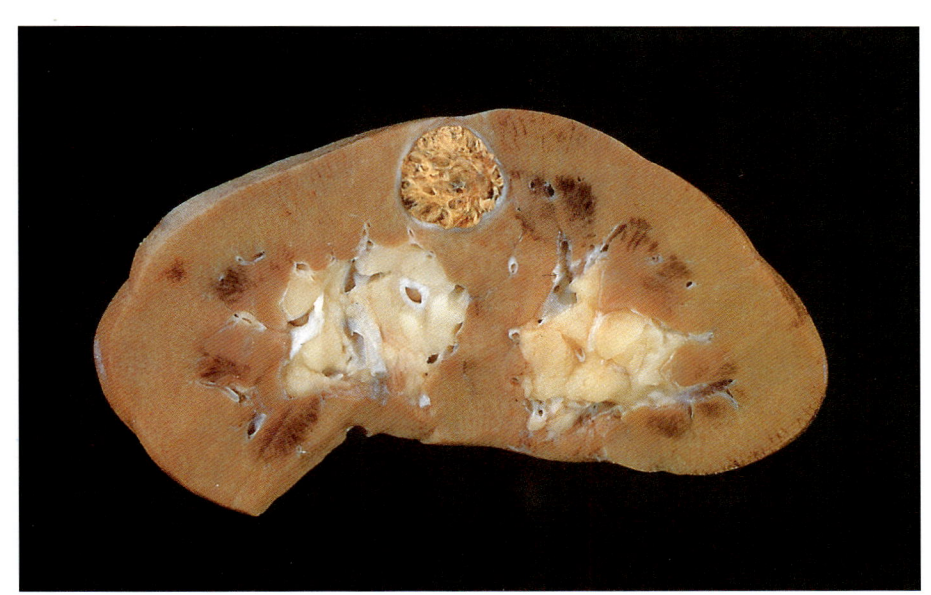

图 12.9　透明细胞肾细胞癌。肿瘤直径 1cm，切面黄色，球形，边界清楚。

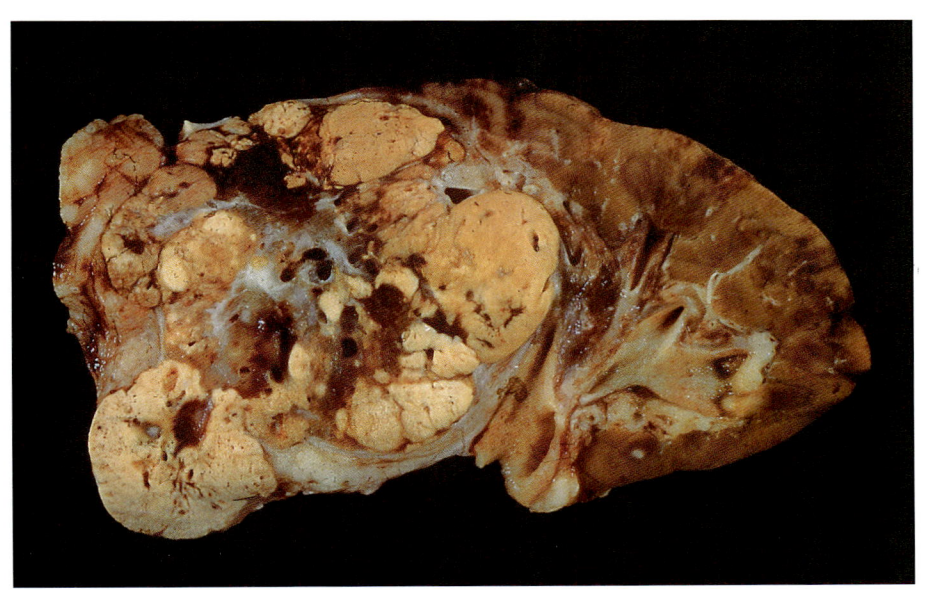

图 12.10　透明细胞肾细胞癌。这个体积巨大、膨胀性的肿瘤切面为典型的五彩状，包括黄色、土黄色、褐色，以及黑色的出血区和灰白色的富含间质区。

肾上皮性肿瘤

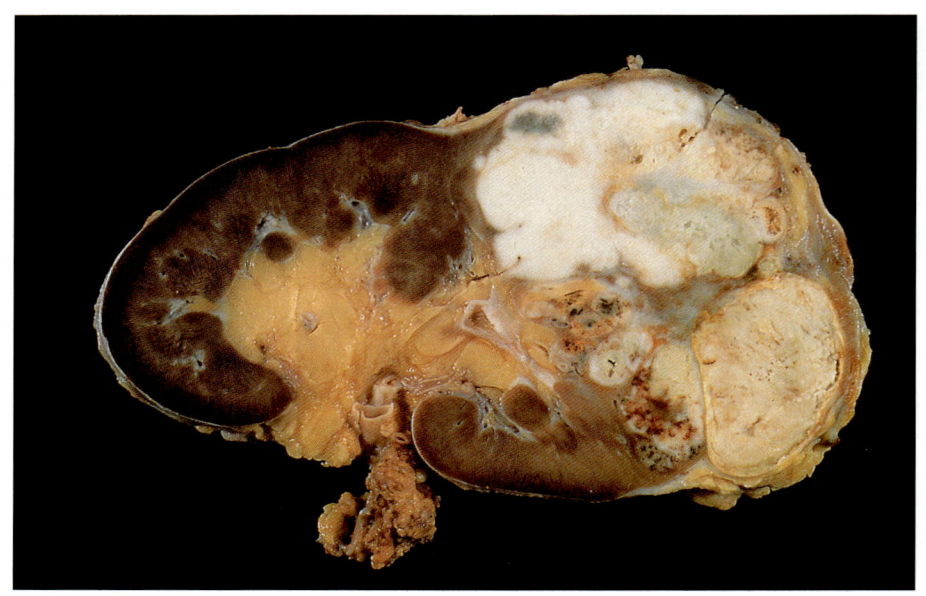

图12.11 透明细胞肾细胞癌。这个肿瘤中白色区域组织学上表现为肉瘤样结构。

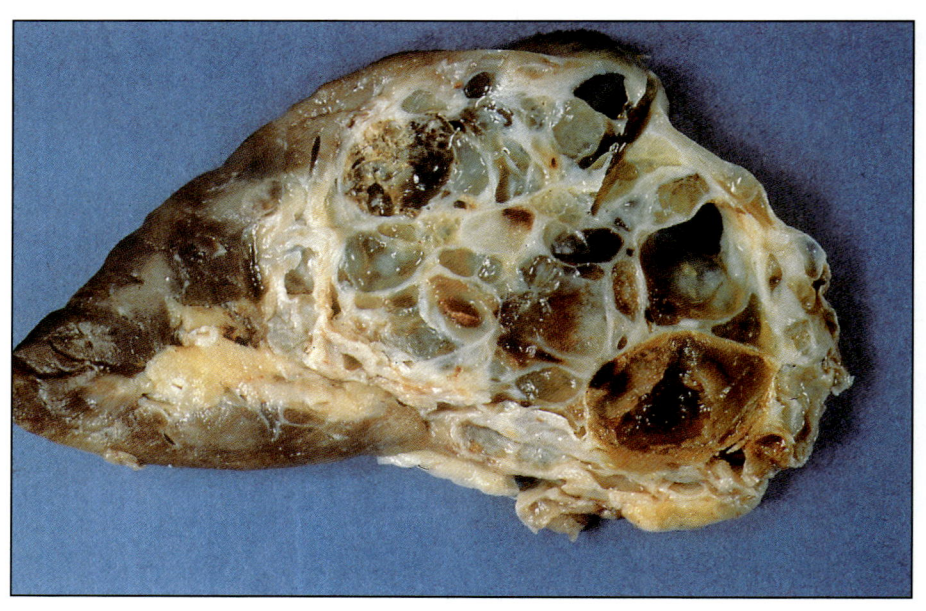

图12.12 多房性囊性肾细胞癌。肿瘤由多个大小不一的薄壁小囊腔构成。

少数情况下，大体表现类似囊性肾瘤并且符合表12.4中所列诊断标准的囊性肿物（图12.12），其纤维间隔中含有透明细胞团[87]。这些细胞常常具有小而深染的细胞核，组织形态与核分级1级的透明细胞肾细胞癌相同。尽管少有或没有证据表明这些肿瘤具有恶性生物学行为，但目前依照惯例诊断为"多房性囊性透明细胞肾细胞癌"。

组织学表现 透明细胞肾细胞癌通常具有小血管网状结构，其中充满腺泡状、片状的癌细胞（图12.13）。这些血管非常纤细，管径小而一致。这种血管组织结构对于诊断帮助很大，因为它是透明细胞肾细胞癌所特有

表12.4	Eble 和Bonsib提出的多房性囊性肾细胞癌诊断标准[87]
有纤维假包膜包绕的膨胀性肿物	
肿瘤内部完全由囊腔及间隔组成，未见膨胀性实性结节	
间隔中含有胞浆透明的上皮细胞团	

的，而不存在于其他类型的肾细胞癌中。

虽然实性片状的腺泡结构是常见的生长方式，但腺泡中央常存在内含渗出的新鲜红细胞的管腔。某些管腔较大，形成大小不一的镜下囊腔（图12.14）。在肾细

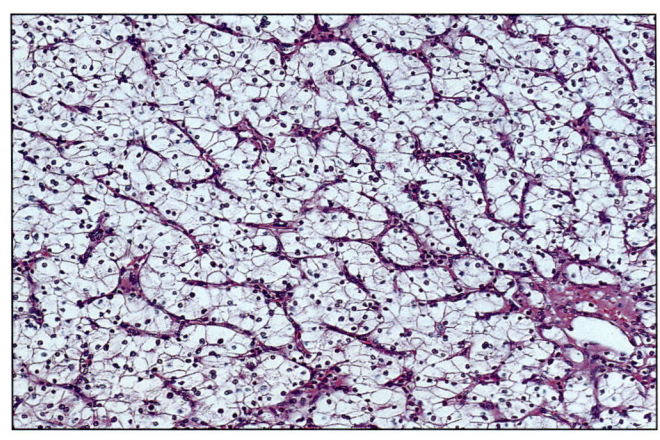

图12.13 透明细胞肾细胞癌。明显、纤细的血管结构围绕腺泡状排列的肿瘤细胞是透明细胞肾细胞癌的典型特征。

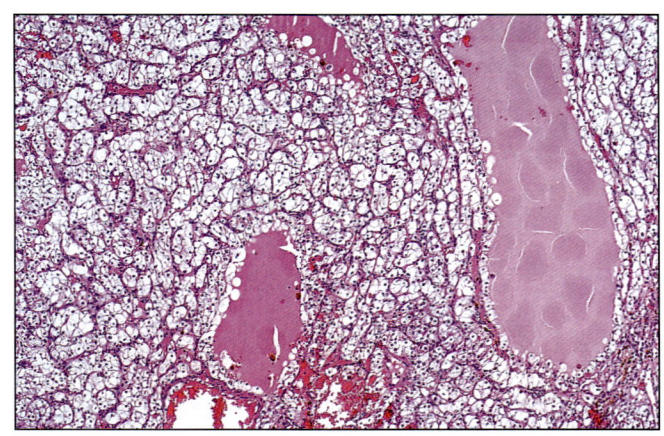

图12.14 透明细胞肾细胞癌。充满嗜酸性蛋白样液体和新鲜红细胞的小管和囊腔是透明细胞肾细胞癌的典型特征。

癌各种组织类型中，透明细胞癌是最倾向于形成或大或小囊腔的肿瘤，这种表现对诊断很有帮助。

透明细胞肾细胞癌的胞浆多少不一，从中等到丰富，但其特征是肿瘤的同一区域中细胞大小相似。这种大小相同肿瘤细胞的区域性分布与嫌色细胞肾细胞癌的混杂性分布是截然不同的。胞浆透明是标本处理过程中大量的脂质及糖原被溶解的缘故（图12.15）。少数病例可出现局灶含有玻璃样胞浆包涵体的横纹肌样肿瘤细胞[88]。

在透明细胞肾细胞癌中，乳头状结构非常少见，而且存在争议。病理科医师在诊断一个具有明显乳头状结构的肿瘤为透明细胞肾细胞癌之前应三思而行。乳头状肾细胞癌中常见的沙粒体及泡沫样巨噬细胞，很少见于透明细胞肾细胞癌。透明细胞肾细胞癌中极少出现黏液，一些学者认为含黏液者应该归类为未分类肾细胞癌。

鉴别诊断 典型透明细胞肾细胞癌的诊断通常并不困难。约5%透明细胞肾细胞癌可出现肉瘤样变，因类似肉瘤而造成诊断困难[89,90]。这个问题众所周知，但由

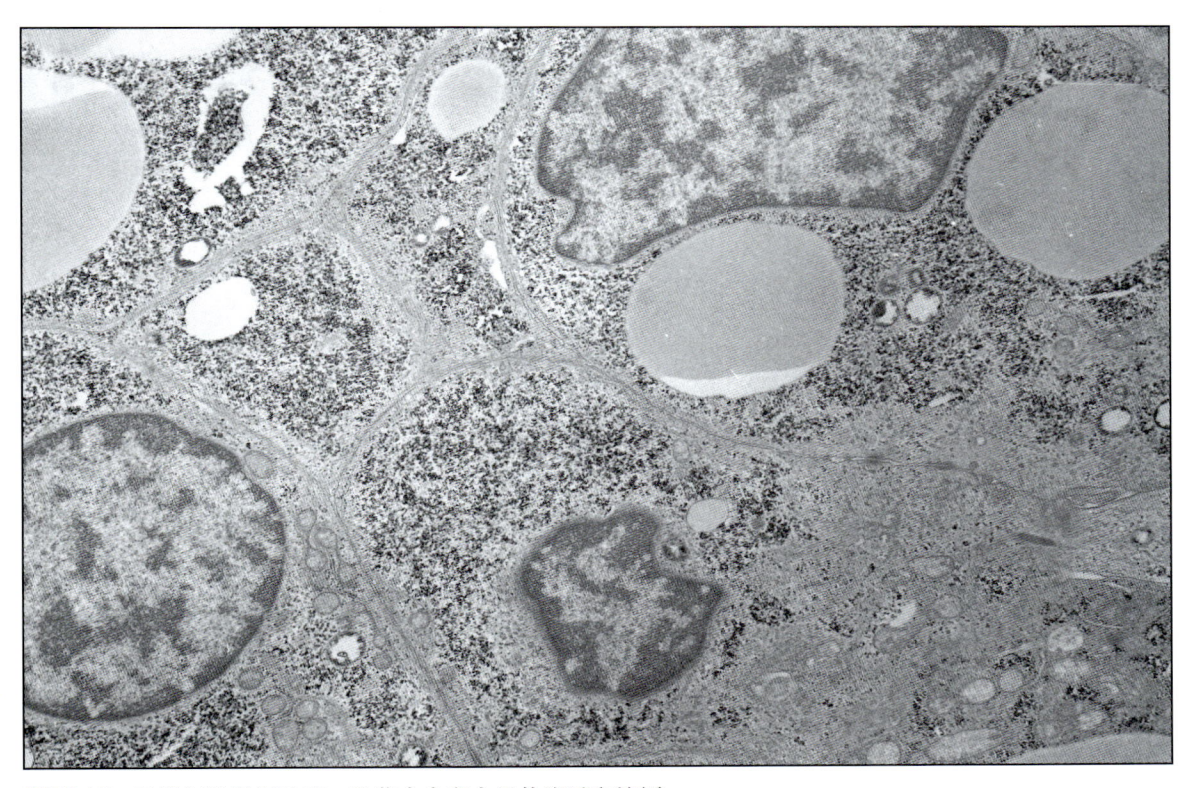

图12.15 透明细胞肾细胞癌。胞浆内含有大量的脂质和糖原。

于肾的肉瘤较罕见，因此诊断时应谨慎。广泛取材有助于诊断，因为这些肿瘤经常存在灶状、典型的肾细胞癌，从而能得出正确的诊断，尽管这些病灶有时非常微小。上皮标志物的免疫组化染色常常显示那些在 HE 染色切片中表现为肉瘤的肿瘤细胞具有上皮样特征。肉瘤样肾细胞癌预后通常比较差[89,90]。

在成年人，肾盂尿路上皮癌可能会被误诊为肾细胞癌，特别是当肿瘤体积很大并且广泛侵犯肾实质时。镜下诊断有时会比较困难，尤其是当肾盂肿瘤主要为肉瘤样成分时，这一点在上文已有论述[91]。有必要进行广泛取材，目的在于发现局部典型的移行细胞癌（即使是原位癌）或肾细胞癌。免疫组化染色高分子量角蛋白或癌胚抗原的表达可表明这种肿瘤是移行细胞起源[92]。

黄色肉芽肿性肾盂肾炎是一种不常见的炎症性病变，在临床及病理学表现上都有可能与肾细胞癌混淆[93,94]。临床症状与肾细胞癌相似，大部分患者的症状包括肋腹部疼痛、发热、不适、体重减轻和血尿[95,96]。肋腹部肿块的出现使术前诊断更加困难。大体检查同样使人迷惑，因为炎症会形成黄色的肿瘤样包块并侵犯肾周脂肪组织（图12.16）。尿路梗阻很常见，通常是由结石造成，有时是由于输尿管肾盂连接处变形所造成[97]。黄色肉芽肿性肾盂肾炎的镜下表现也会造成诊断困难，其中最主要的原因是病灶中大量的泡沫状组织细胞可能会被误认为是肾细胞癌中的透明细胞[98]（图12.17）。仔细观察可发现这些细胞胞浆呈泡沫样，与透明细胞肾细胞癌有所不同，不具有透明细胞肾细胞癌中特征性的血管结构，而其他炎症细胞，主要是淋巴细胞和浆细胞的存在可进一步有助于病变的诊断。软斑病 (malakoplakia) 是另一种类似于原发性肾肿瘤的炎症性病变[99]，大体上表现为体积较大的黄色肿块，有时可见肾周脂肪组织浸润，镜下软斑病所特有的大而嗜酸的组织细胞（von Hansemann 细胞）可能会与肾细胞癌的嗜酸细胞相混淆。Michaelis-Gutmann 小体的存在是正确诊断的重要指标，缺乏细胞非典型性且不具有肾细胞癌特征性的组织结构也是软斑病的诊断指标。

临床上，表现为远处转移而原发灶不明的隐匿性肾细胞癌以及成功进行根治性肾切除术后多年才出现复发的病例可能会引起诊断困难。大部分透明细胞肾细胞癌同时表达细胞角蛋白及波形蛋白[100]，此现象在肿瘤中并不常见，因此当原发部位不明的转移癌出现这一现象时则提示可能原发于肾[92]。超微结构上，细胞间及腺腔表面致密排列的微绒毛以及胞浆内大量糖原的存在提示可能为肾细胞癌[101]。向对侧肾上腺的孤立性转移性肾细胞癌可能类似于原发性肾上腺皮质癌。在这种情况下，上皮膜抗原和细胞角蛋白的免疫组化染色对于诊断很有帮助，因为肾细胞癌常常表达上皮膜抗原或细胞角蛋白，或两者同时表达，而肾上腺皮质癌并不表达上皮膜抗原[102]而且仅微弱表达细胞角蛋白。进一步行抑制素（inhibin）和 melanA 免疫组化染色也有助于诊断[103]。甲状腺的转移性肾细胞癌可与甲状腺透明细胞癌相似[104]；甲状腺球蛋白免疫组化染色和超微

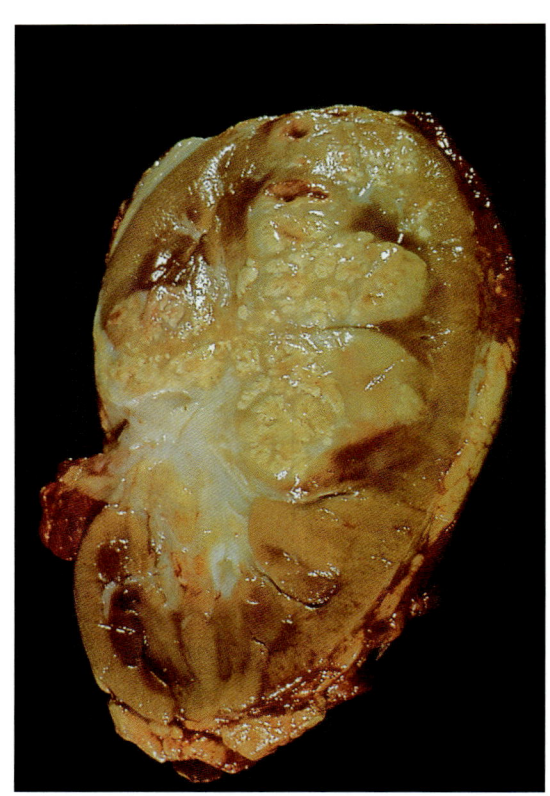

图12.16 黄色肉芽肿性肾盂肾炎。泡沫状组织细胞构成的黄色肿物，与肾细胞癌相似。

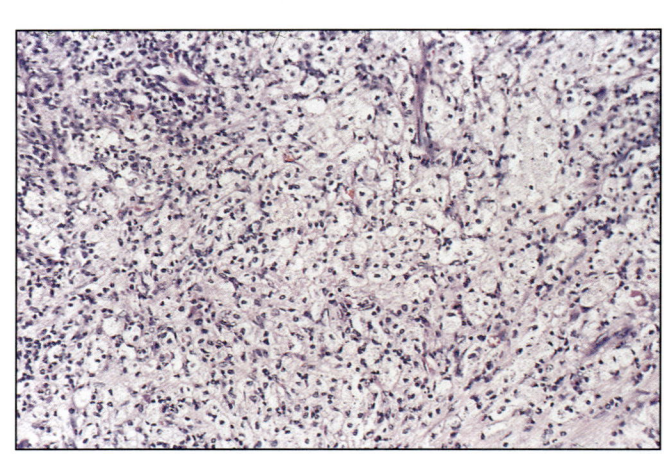

图12.17 黄色肉芽肿性肾盂肾炎。尽管泡沫状组织细胞表面上与透明细胞肾细胞癌相似，但淋巴细胞和浆细胞的浸润以及缺乏典型的血管结构可以明确诊断。

结构下胞浆内糖原的检测（甲状腺原发透明细胞癌不存在糖原）有助于两者的区分。卵巢的转移性肾细胞癌可与卵巢原发透明细胞癌混淆[105]。中枢神经系统的毛细血管母细胞瘤（capillary hemangioblastoma）与透明细胞肾细胞癌在 HE 染色切片上非常相似，而且两者均与 von Hippel-Lindau 病相关，也使它们的鉴别更加困难。上皮膜抗原免疫组化染色可以解决这一困难，因为毛细血管母细胞瘤不表达[106]而肾细胞癌表达这一标志物。

乳头状肾细胞癌
Papillary renal cell carcinoma

手术切除的肾细胞癌中，大约 10% ~ 15% 是乳头状肾细胞癌[41,83,84,107]。男性多见，性别比例约为 2∶1。发病年龄范围从年轻人到老年人，平均年龄 50 ~ 55 岁。该类型预后远好于透明细胞癌[83,84]，但 10 年死亡率不低于 16%[108]，有时以远处转移为首发症状[109]。

乳头状肾细胞癌具有特征性的、与其他类型肾细胞肿瘤不同的遗传学异常。表现为某条染色体增多，最常见的是出现 7 号和 17 号染色体三体或四体[110-112]。大部分发生于男性的乳头状肾细胞癌表现为 Y 染色体丢失[111]。这些研究结果已被多个实验室所证实[79,112-114]。

大体表现 乳头状肾细胞癌大体通常表现为边界清楚的淡褐色或棕褐色球形肿物。大约 2/3 的病例具有明显的出血和坏死，使之在影像学上表现为低血供[107,115]。许多肿瘤体积较大。切面质脆或颗粒状，是镜下乳头状结构的反映。体积较大的肿瘤周围常常为致密纤维组织所包绕[116]。大约 1/3 病例出现钙化[107,115]。

组织学表现 超过 90% 的乳头状肾细胞癌主要由乳头状或管状乳头状结构组成[41,117]。紧密排列的乳头使一些肿瘤表现为实性生长方式。这些乳头通常含有纤细的纤维血管轴心，表面被覆单层细胞。乳头的形状多样，从复杂的分支状到细长平行排列的条索[118]。乳头轴心有时因为泡沫状巨噬细胞的浸润（图 12.18）或水肿而膨胀。偶尔可见沙粒体的存在。宽大而富含胶原的乳头轴心罕见[118]。管状结构由小管构成，被覆单层细胞，与乳头被覆细胞形态相同。

乳头状肾细胞癌可分为两种类型，Delahunt 和 Eble 将其命名为 1 型和 2 型[2,119]。1 型远比 2 型常见。1 型乳头状肾细胞癌中，肿瘤细胞小，胞浆浅染而不明显（图 12.19），细胞核非常一致，小而近圆形，核仁小或无法见到。2 型乳头状肾细胞癌中，肿瘤细胞较大，通常含有丰富的嗜酸性胞浆，细胞核排列成假复层结构，体积大，圆形，常见明显的核仁（图 12.20）。

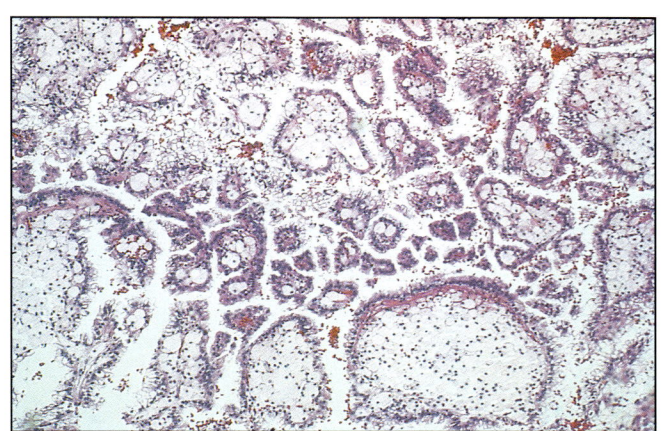

图12.18 乳头状肾细胞癌。乳头的间质轴心因为泡沫状的组织细胞聚集而膨胀。

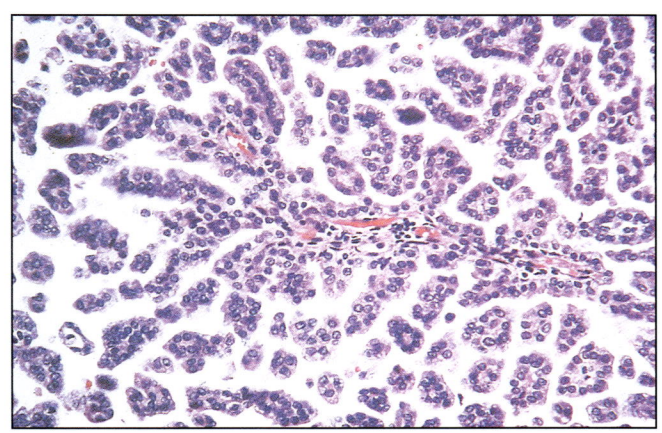

图12.19 乳头状肾细胞癌。1型乳头状肾细胞癌的乳头被覆肿瘤细胞小，胞浆淡染、不明显。

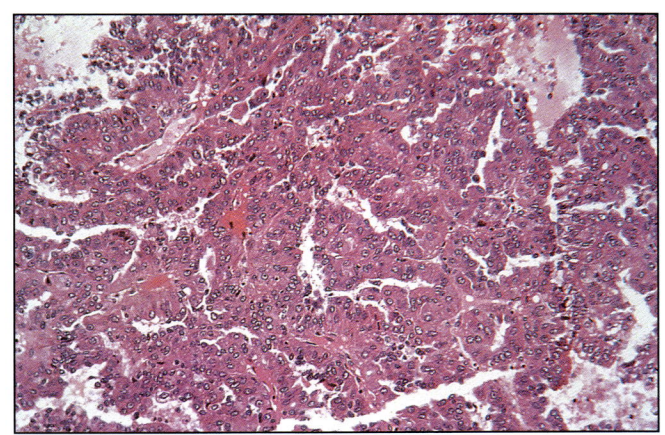

图12.20 乳头状肾细胞癌。2型乳头状肾细胞癌的乳头被覆肿瘤细胞胞浆丰富，细胞核呈假复层排列。

在一项 39 例病例的研究中，肿瘤细胞核形态与分期及预后有关[109]。因此，推荐使用核分级系统[120]。

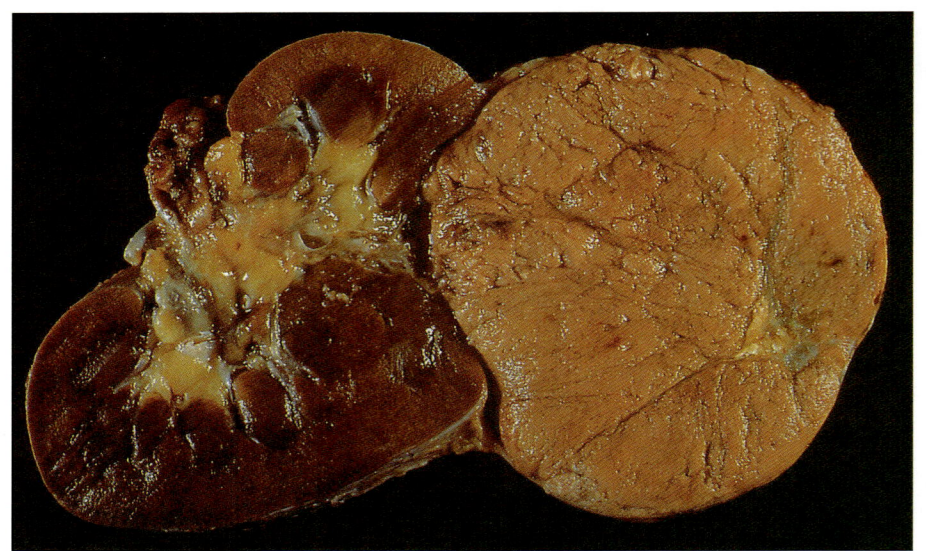

图12.21 嫌色细胞肾细胞癌。边界清楚的浅褐色或棕褐色圆形肿物。

鉴别诊断 在儿童及青少年，乳头状肾细胞癌必须与以上皮成分为主的 Wilms 瘤区分开。Beckwith[121] 强调指出，某些 Wilms 瘤与典型的肾细胞癌相似。对这些肿瘤充分取材，常常会发现胚芽成分以及分化的间质（如骨骼肌），这时做出 Wilms 瘤的诊断并不困难。细胞核的形状对于诊断也有帮助，Wilms 瘤中上皮成分细胞核细长，末端逐渐变细，而肾细胞癌细胞核呈圆形。对于年轻患者，只有在排除以上皮成分为主的 Wilms 瘤后才可以做出乳头状肾细胞癌的诊断。

嫌色细胞肾细胞癌
Chromophobe renal cell carcinoma

1985 年，Thoenes 等[122] 首先描述并命名了嫌色细胞肾细胞癌。从那以后，越来越多的证据表明大约 5% 的肾细胞癌是嫌色细胞肾细胞癌[84,123-126]。嫌色细胞肾细胞癌的遗传学标志是多条染色体的丢失[127-129]。

因嫌色细胞肾细胞癌而死亡的病例已有报道，证据表明该类型肿瘤是常见肾细胞癌中侵袭性最低的[83,84]。肉瘤样变在嫌色细胞癌中出现的频率与在其他类型的肾细胞癌中相同，而且似乎是引起死亡的重要因素[90,130]。

大体表现 嫌色细胞肾细胞癌通常表现为边界清楚的、圆形、实性、棕褐色或褐色肿瘤（图 12.21）。甲醛固定可能会使肿瘤褪色为灰白色。嫌色细胞肾细胞癌不易出现大的囊性变。

组织学表现 嫌色细胞肾细胞癌的组织学特征是肿瘤细胞胞浆内含有大量微小囊泡，在苏木素 - 伊红染色的切片上表现为淡染、网状或絮状胞浆（图 12.22）。这些囊泡在电镜下可以显示出来（图 12.23）。Hale 胶体铁染色将胞浆染成蓝色（图 12.24）[123]。最初的描述[122] 强调肿瘤细胞细胞膜厚且边界清楚，胞浆浅染、絮状，该类型现称为经典型嫌色细胞肾细胞癌。经典型还具有厚壁血管。肿瘤细胞大小相差很大，大小细胞镶嵌排列。随后，又发现了嫌色细胞肾细胞癌嗜酸细胞亚型[123]。这种亚型的超微结构和胶体铁染色结果与经典型相同，但在苏木素 - 伊红染色切片上常常类似于肾嗜酸细胞瘤（图 12.25）。因此，有必要常规收集各种肾肿瘤标本进行电镜检查，特别是那些缺乏透明细胞肾细胞癌典型黄色色泽的肿瘤。对任何需要与肾嗜酸细胞瘤和嫌色细胞肾细胞癌进行鉴别的肿瘤应行胶体铁染色加以判断。是

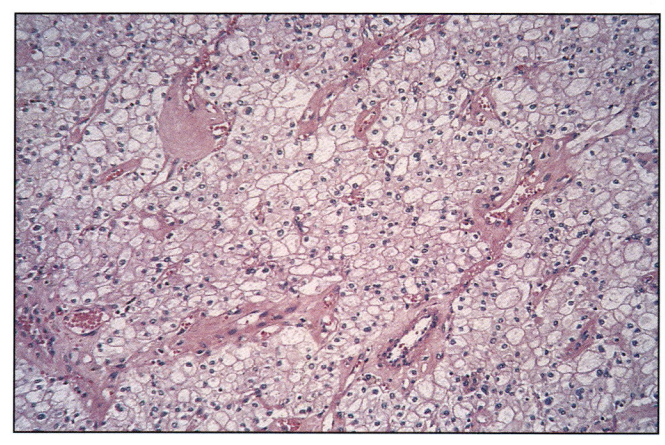

图12.22 嫌色细胞肾细胞癌。在HE切片上，典型嫌色细胞肾细胞癌胞浆呈絮状、浅粉色。

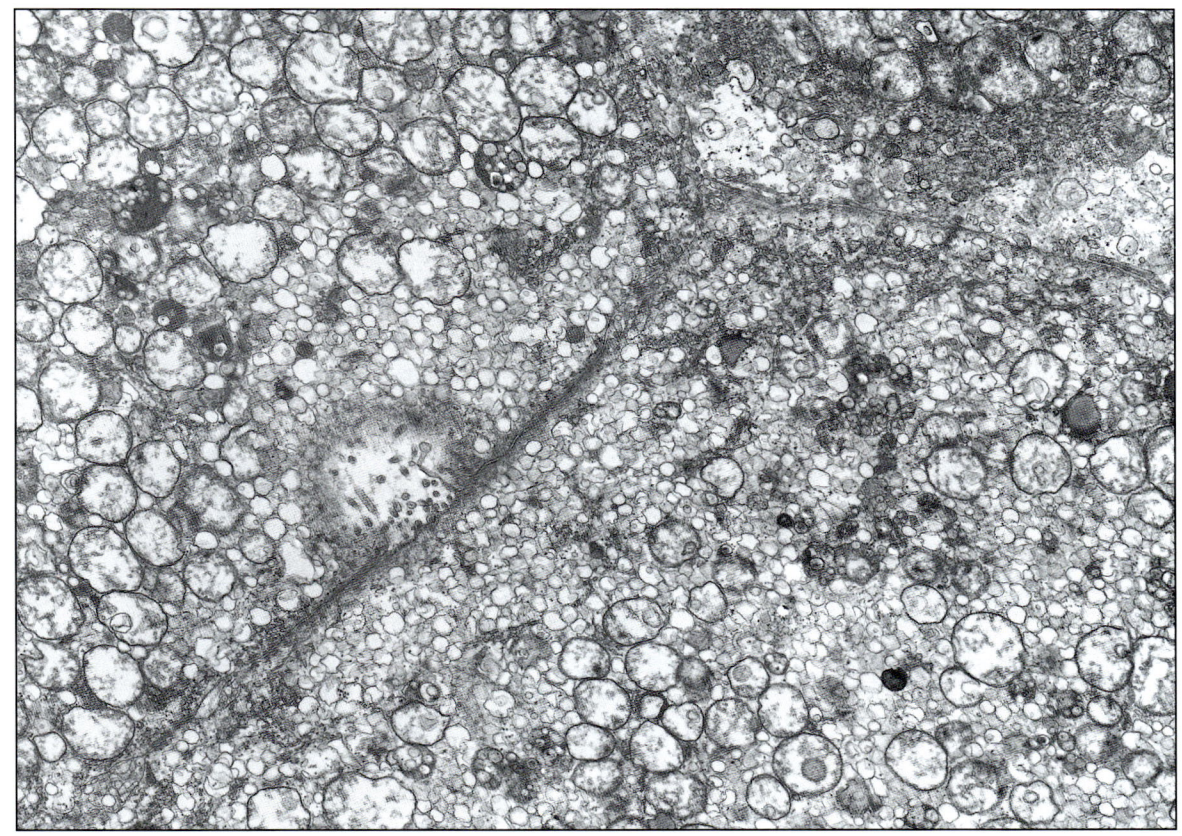

图12.23 嫌色细胞肾细胞癌。超微结构显示嫌色细胞胞浆内充满小囊泡。

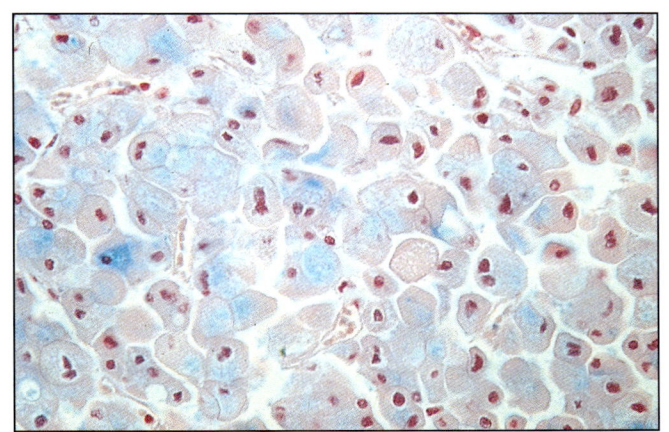

图12.24 嫌色细胞肾细胞癌。Hale染色显示嫌色细胞胞浆呈蓝色。

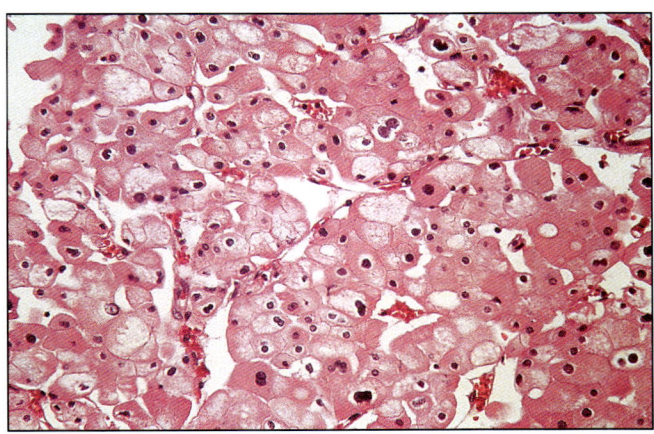

图12.25 嫌色细胞肾细胞癌。嗜酸细胞型嫌色细胞肾细胞癌由具有强嗜酸性、细颗粒状胞浆的肿瘤细胞组成。

否使用免疫组化染色对肾细胞癌进一步分类仍存在争议，因为在这方面常存在表型重叠[131,132]。

鉴别诊断 血管结构、大小不一镶嵌排列的肿瘤细胞和胞浆的特点构成了嫌色细胞肾细胞癌的典型特征，在常规切片上容易得出诊断。因为与嗜酸细胞瘤非常相似，嗜酸细胞亚型的诊断稍微困难一点。在苏木素-伊红染色切片上，核周空晕、皱缩而不规则的细胞核以及微小囊泡结构的存在支持嗜酸细胞型嫌色细胞肾细胞癌的诊断。Hale胶体铁组织化学染色有助于诊断，弥漫性胞浆着色支持嫌色细胞肾细胞癌的诊断，而阴性反应则支持嗜酸细胞瘤的诊断。

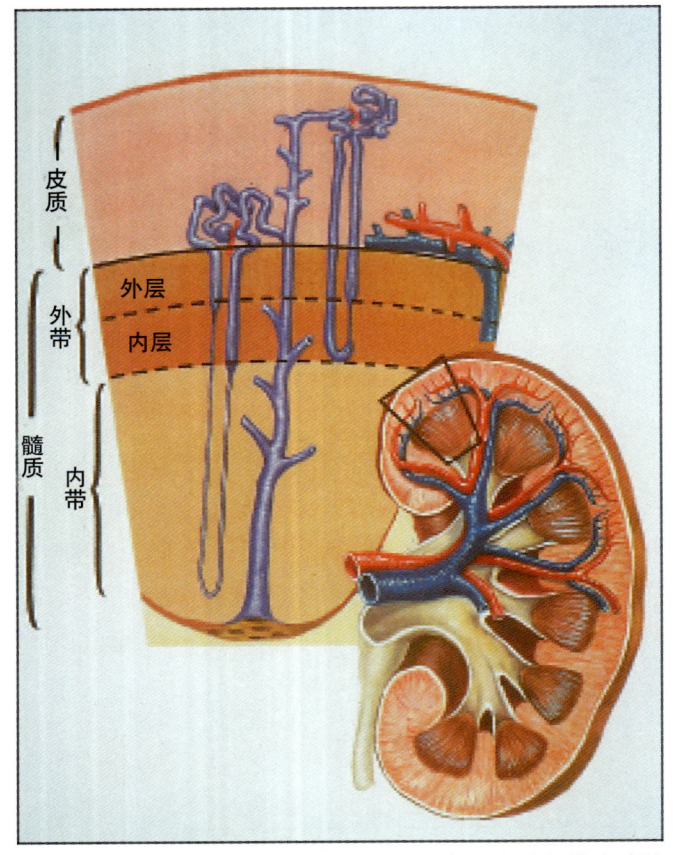

图12.26 肾集合管始于外层皮质,它们穿过皮质和髓质时通过连接小管的汇集而变粗。位于髓质乳头末段的是Bellini管。

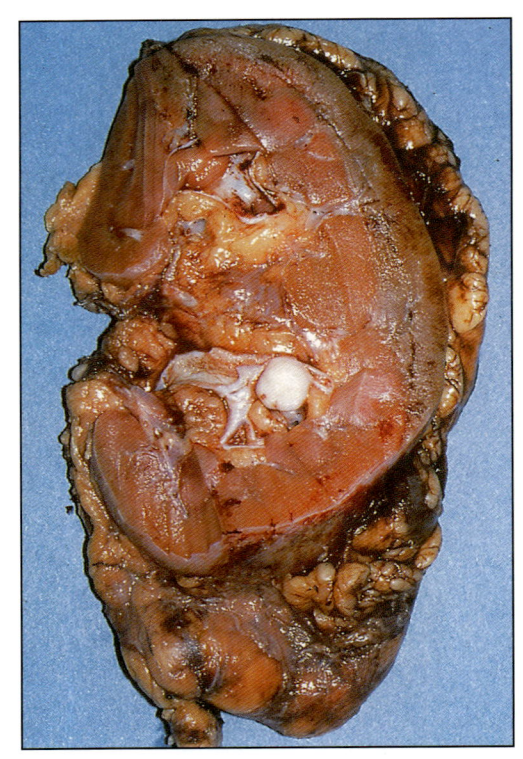

图12.27 集合管癌。体积较小的白色肿物发生于肾髓质。(Courtesy of Dr. Wei-Li Huang.)

集合管癌 Collecting duct carcinoma

集合管始于肾皮质,通过髓质下降至肾乳头(图12.26);位于乳头开口上方的短节段称为Bellini管[133]。有证据表明集合管的闰细胞(intercalated cell)可能是肾嗜酸细胞瘤[134]和嫌色细胞肾细胞癌[135]的起源细胞。然而,"集合管癌"这一诊断仅适用于被认为起源于肾髓质锥体Bellini管的一组高度恶性的上皮性肿瘤[136,137]。

总体而言,集合管癌预后差[137]。一种发生于患镰状红细胞病年轻患者的集合管癌亚型被称为"肾髓质癌"[138-140]。这些患者的预后非常差。

大体表现 尽管集合管位于肾皮质和髓质,肿瘤则主要位于内层髓质(图12.27),这里很少存在肾小管系统的其他部分,可作为诊断要点[141]。不幸的是,只有体积较小的肿瘤才有可能明确它位于髓质,而许多肿瘤在切除时体积已经非常大,因此很难确定它们在肾中的发生部位。肿瘤通常中部位于肾髓质,常常扩展至肾皮质和肾门组织[142,143];典型表现是边缘呈浸润性且切面灰白伴中央坏死[144];常与肾盂相连。

组织学表现 集合管癌是组织病理学独特的癌,兼有腺癌和移行细胞癌的特征[137,144]。显微镜下表现为轻度嗜碱性的丰富疏松间质中分布着高度不规则的腺管样结构和肿瘤细胞巢索(图12.28)。被覆管腔的癌细胞胞浆稀少或中等量,细胞核多形性,核膜厚。一个特别有

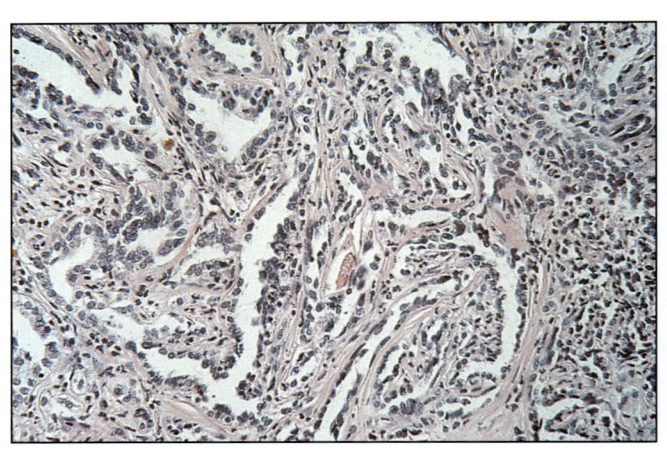

图12.28 集合管癌。位于丰富间质中的不规则分支的小管,管腔衬覆胞浆稀少的肿瘤细胞,这是集合管癌的典型表现。

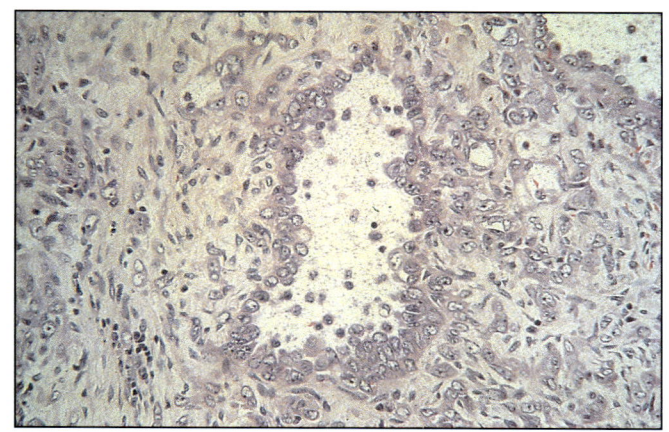

图12.29 集合管癌。胞浆轻度嗜碱性类似于肾髓质，小管和囊腔衬覆鞋钉样肿瘤细胞，这些是集合管癌的组织学特征。

助于诊断的组织学特点是有时被覆管腔的肿瘤细胞出现鞋钉样外观（图12.29），这一特点在肾细胞癌中罕见，且不存在于移行细胞癌中。某些病例癌组织附近的髓质肾小管可见非典型性上皮[143]。

鉴别诊断 知道集合管癌的存在并且充分认识上述不同于其他肾恶性肿瘤的组织学特点，就可以对大多数病例做出诊断。Rumpelt等[144]发现集合管癌呈细胞角蛋白19和荆豆凝集素染色强阳性，波形蛋白中等阳性，但不表达细胞角蛋白13。其他集合管癌免疫组化染色研究得出的结果各不相同[145,146]。目前，尚无公认的集合管癌特异性免疫组化染色谱，因此集合管癌这一诊断最好限于那些病理大体检查表明起源于集合管或具有上文所描述和图12.28及12.29所显示的组织学特征的那些肿瘤。交界性病例应该诊断为未分类肾细胞癌。

Xp11易位癌 Xp11 translocation carcinomas

近年来，一组涉及Xp11.2染色体易位的肾癌被确认[147]。所有这些易位均导致包含 TFE3 在内的基因融合。在2004年WHO肿瘤分类中将其分类为Xp11易位癌[1]。随后含有t(6;11)的肾癌也被确认，该易位导致 TFEB 与其他基因融合。TFE3 和 TFEB 基因都是 MiTF/TFE 转录因子基因家族的成员，将来可能会发现更多由该家族其他基因融合产生的肾癌[147]。尽管儿童肾肿瘤中肾癌所占比例不足5%，但易位癌在儿童肾癌中的比例至少达20%[35]。易位癌也可发生于成年人，但其发病率尚不清楚。不少患者是高分期病例但却表现为惰性临床过程。由于目前所研究的病例数较少，因此对这类肿瘤临床特征和预后的了解还比较肤浅。女性发病率可能比男性高，但尚无定论。有些患者发生了转移却长期生存。某些患者有其他疾病化疗史[147a]。

大体表现 易位癌通常表现为实性、黄褐色肿物；常见局部出血和坏死。

组织学表现 Xp11.2易位癌常常含有大片乳头状结构，被覆胞浆透明或淡染的肿瘤细胞（图12.30）。但是，也可有腺泡及巢状结构，常见嗜酸性肿瘤细胞。沙粒体常见，有时数量众多。Xp11易位癌随易位类型不同而在形态学上也存在细微差别。

t(6;11)易位癌由实性细胞巢和微囊构成，肿瘤细胞呈多角形，胞浆浅染或嗜酸性。乳头并不常见。还有一种比较特殊的结构，表现为胞浆稀少、染色质致密的肿瘤细胞围绕大腺泡中的玻璃样物结节，低倍镜下类似于菊形团。

与 TFE3 基因融合有关的易位癌特征性地表达核阳性的TFE3蛋白[148]。而与 TFEB 基因融合有关的易位癌特征性地表达核阳性的TFEB蛋白。Xp11易位癌不表达或弱表达上皮标志物，如上皮膜抗原和细胞角蛋白。t(6;11)癌常常表达HMB45、melan A以及TFEB蛋白[149]。

神经母细胞瘤相关性肾癌
Carcinoma associated with neuroblastoma

2岁前诊断为神经母细胞瘤的生存患者中，已知大约有20多例在儿童及青少年期诊断出患有肾细胞癌。

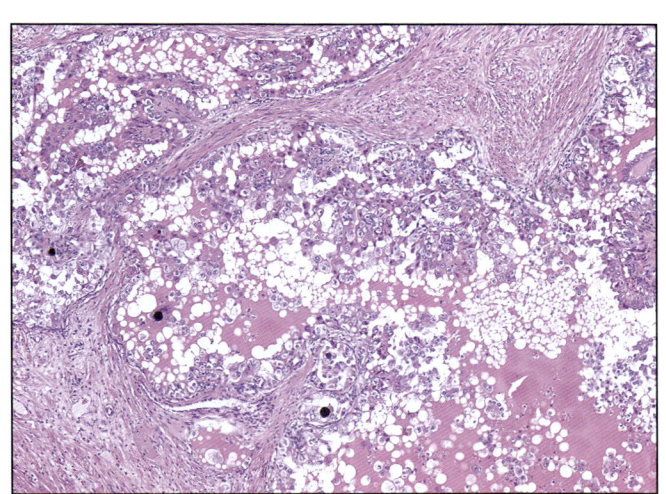

图12.30 Xp11易位癌。大的含嗜酸性胞浆的肿瘤细胞以及沙粒体构成乳头状和实性癌巢结构。

1999年，Medeiros等报道了4例幸存的神经母细胞瘤患者患有特殊组织类型的肾细胞癌，认为这是一种独立的临床病理学疾病；随后，第二篇小规模病例研究发表[150,151]。2004年版WHO肿瘤分类承认了这种独立疾病，并将其分类为"神经母细胞瘤相关性肾细胞癌"[1]。所有患者均在通常年龄发生神经母细胞瘤，他们中的两例既未行化学治疗，也未行放射治疗。诊断肾细胞癌的年龄从5岁到14岁不等。一例患者发生了肾细胞癌的肝和淋巴结转移。

大体表现 肿瘤主体直径为35～80mm；多发性和双侧性肾癌患者中20个体积较小的肿瘤直径1～24mm。两例癌组织侵犯肾被膜、肾血管系统或肾周淋巴系统。

组织学表现 最典型的神经母细胞瘤相关性肾细胞癌主要由含丰富细颗粒状嗜酸性胞浆的肿瘤细胞构成，呈乳头状或实性生长。有时可见沙粒体和小团泡沫状组织细胞。细胞核中等大，形态不规则。核仁易见，相当于3级核。可见核分裂象，但数量不多。所有研究病例均表达上皮膜抗原、波形蛋白和细胞角蛋白Cam5.2[152]。

黏液小管和梭形细胞癌
Mucinous tubular and spindle cell carcinoma

1998年以来，多篇个案和小规模病例研究报道了一种组织学特殊的、由立方形和梭形肿瘤细胞以及黏液样细胞外间质组成的肾肿瘤[152,153]。作者们对这些肿瘤提出过多个命名，通常因其类似于肾单位下段肾小管或Henle环，具有低级别癌细胞核以及存在部分梭形肿瘤细胞而进行命名。2002年12月举行的WHO共识会上采纳了"黏液小管和梭形细胞癌"这一名称[1]。所有患者均为成年人（中位年龄58岁）。女性多见，男女比例大约为1:3。Hes等[154]所报道的3例病例同时患有肾结石。大约50%的肿瘤体积较大（pT2期）；1例侵犯肾周脂肪组织，其他2例有淋巴结转移。所有患者均只进行了手术切除，尚未有复发的报道。

大体表现 黏液小管和梭形细胞癌直径22～130mm。切面实性、灰色、棕褐色或粉红色。一些肿瘤可见灶状出血或坏死。一例体积较小的肿瘤位于肾髓质。除1例外，其余所有肿瘤边界清楚，位于肾被膜内。

组织学表现 黏液小管和梭形细胞癌具有独特的组织学表现，由立方形肿瘤细胞排列成的细胞条索、小管和突然转化成的梭形细胞构成（图12.31）。这些上皮

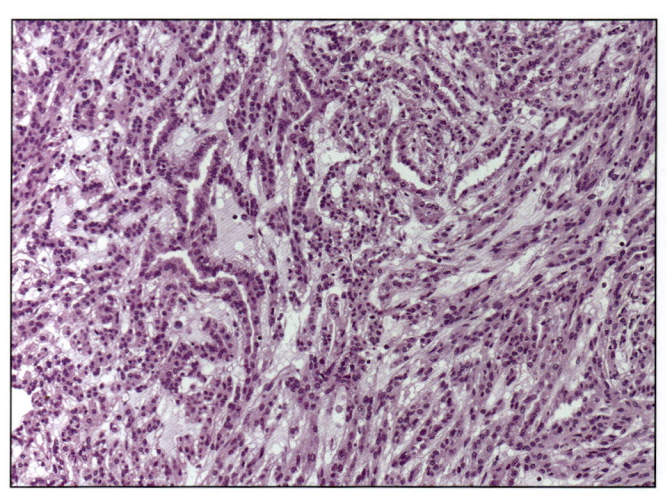

图12.31 黏液小管和梭形细胞癌。立方形和梭形细胞分布于黏液样细胞外间质中。

结构分布于轻度嗜碱性的黏液或黏液样背景中。细胞核圆形或卵圆形，含有少许染色质团块和小核仁。核分裂象并不常见。梭形细胞成分可呈片状分布。部分区域以黏液间质为主，而上皮成分形成小的细胞条索漂浮于黏液物质中。这些黏液物质卡红（mucicarmine）染色阴性，而阿辛蓝（alcian blue）染色强阳性[155]。有时可见浆细胞、肥大细胞和成团的泡沫样组织细胞[155,156]。免疫组化结果在不同的研究中有所不同[154,155-157]。波形蛋白和上皮膜抗原阳性表达是最常见的。在两项研究中，14例病例中有10例表达广谱细胞角蛋白AE1/AE3[154,155]。与集合管上皮发生反应的荆豆凝集素在各项研究中均未发现与黏液小管和梭形细胞癌的肿瘤细胞结合。这类肿瘤缺乏乳头状肾细胞癌中常见的细胞遗传学异常[157a]。

未分类肾细胞癌
Renal cell carcinoma, unclassified

当一种肾细胞癌无法明确归类于其他各个类型时，称为未分类肾细胞癌[1]。在手术病例中，这类肿瘤约占4%～5%。因为该类肿瘤形态学表现和遗传学特点多样，因此很难准确定义。提示应划归为这一类型的特征有：已知类型的混合型；没有可识别上皮成分的肉瘤样癌；产生黏液的癌；上皮和间质成分混合性癌；以及不能识别的细胞类型。这组肿瘤具有高度异质性，因此很难对它们的特征进行概括[158]。有趣的是，在这一类型肿瘤中，进一步的亚型分类是可能的，例如继发于获得性肾囊肿病的肾癌具有独特的形态学表现[158a]。

表12.5	肾细胞癌的分期
Robson分期[160,161]	TNM分期[162]
1期 局限于肾被膜内	T1局限于肾被膜内且≤70mm T1a≤40mm T1b≥40mm但≤70mm T2局限于肾被膜内且>70mm
2期 局限于Gerota筋膜内	T3a侵犯肾上腺或Gerota筋膜内脂肪组织 T3b大体可见侵犯肾静脉或横膈以下腔静脉
3期 A 大体可见侵犯肾静脉或腔静脉 B 有淋巴结转移 C 同时有血管侵犯和淋巴结转移	T3c血管内瘤栓扩散至横膈以上腔静脉或侵犯腔静脉壁 N1仅有一个区域淋巴结转移 N2一个以上区域淋巴结转移
4期 侵及邻近器官（肾上腺除外） 血行转移	肿瘤已超出Gerota筋膜 M1

肾细胞癌的分期和分级

肾细胞癌的扩散范围是主要的预后因素[159]。目前广泛应用的肾细胞癌分期体系有2种，包括Robson等提出的分期体系[160,161]以及肿瘤、淋巴结、远处转移（TNM）分期体系[162]，表12.5列出了两者之间的异同。这些组合大致类似，两者之间的各比较项目用水平线分开。手术切除是肾细胞癌的主要治疗手段，基于这个原因，两个体系都将局限于肾被膜内的肿瘤作为最好的一组。TNM分期体系考虑了肿瘤大小与生存期的相关性，因此根据肿瘤大小对其进一步分组。两个体系都将出现Gerota筋膜内肾周脂肪组织侵犯的肿瘤划分为下一分期。3期肿瘤的分期标准更加复杂和有争议；肾细胞癌经常侵犯肾静脉系统，这是3A期的划分标准。侵犯常常是通过肾窦的静脉实现[163,164]。静脉侵犯的预后意义很难确定，因为存在静脉侵犯的肿瘤常常具有其他高分期的表现，如转移。Medeiros等[165,166]比较了1期肿瘤和如果没有静脉侵犯便划分为1期的3期肿瘤，发现静脉侵犯在高级别肿瘤中是一个独立的预后因素，但对低级别肿瘤预后并无影响。肿瘤主体内的小静脉侵犯并不足以将其划分为3期，确切地说，要么必须是肉眼可见的侵犯，要么是镜下可见的位于肿瘤边缘或之外的具有平滑肌的大静脉侵犯。10%~15%的病例发生区域淋巴结转移但无远处转移[167,168]，50%肿大的区域淋巴结仅表现为炎症或增生性改变[169]。辅以区域淋巴结清扫的根治性肾切除作为肾细胞癌标准术式已经沿用了30多年[160]，但淋巴结清扫的治疗效果尚存在争议[170,171]。有时，经过输尿管旁静脉和淋巴管可发生转移[172]，基于这一原因，输尿管末端及其外膜组织便成为相关的手术切缘，在根治性肾切除标本中应该对其进行组织病理学检查。影像学技术的提高使许多患者无需切除肾上腺[173,174]。肾部分切除和腹腔镜下肾切除已经成为肾细胞癌标准的治疗方法[175,176]。

自从1932年Hand和Broders[177]引进了肾细胞癌的分级体系以来，研究者们提出了几种不同的分级体系，获得了一定的肯定。除了关注细胞核特征外，研究者还把胞浆和组织结构的特征也包括在内，导致了外科病理医师长时间的争论和相当大的困扰。1971年，Skinner等[178]重新对细胞核形态学特征与生存率的相关性进行了研究。这些研究结果为Fuhrman等[120]所证实并重新制定了一个临床可操作的分级体系。Fuhrman分级体系根据细胞核大小、形态以及核仁的明显与否分为四个级别（表12.6）。Medeiros等[165]证实在一个大规模肾细胞癌研究病例和另一个较小规模的1期肾细胞癌研究病例中，Fuhrman分级体系与生存率具有高度的相关性。

表12.6	肾细胞癌核分级体系
1级	核圆形，大小一致，直径约10μm，无核仁或核仁很小
2级	核外形轻微不规则，直径约15μm，400×镜下可见核仁
3级	核外形中度或显著不规则，直径约20μm，核仁大，100×镜下可见
4级	细胞核与3级相似，但还可见到分叶核、多核或奇异核，染色质粗大块状

患者的生存率从1级癌的86%降到4级癌的24%。核分级根据所发现的最高级别确定，无论其分布范围大小[179]。Green 等[180]研究了55例1期肾细胞癌患者，发现核分级4级患者的5年生存率显著下降。Helpap 等[181]同样证实了核仁形态学特征的重要性。但是各个观察者之间及观察者本人的诊断可重复性并不理想[182]。这个分级体系并不包括核分裂象，但1级和2级癌通常罕见核分裂象，如果每10个高倍视野超过1个核分裂象则意味着预后不好[179]。分级体系同样没有纳入肉瘤样变及凝固性坏死，这两种组织学特征同样意味着预后不佳[183]。

肾神经内分泌和神经外胚层肿瘤
Neuroendocrine and neuroectodermal neoplasms of the kidney

肾亦可发生类癌、小细胞癌和原始神经外胚瘤等神经内分泌和神经外胚层肿瘤[184-186]。男性及女性发病率相同，青少年至90多岁老年人均可发生，平均发病年龄约50岁。许多神经内分泌异常症状已有报道，包括类癌综合征[187]和胰高血糖素分泌过多[188]。转移常见，甚至在诊断为类癌的病例中。

发生于肾窦并压迫肾动脉的嗜铬细胞瘤似乎比发生在肾被膜内的嗜铬细胞瘤更为常见[189]，肾实质内也可发生嗜铬细胞瘤[190]而且与高血压有关。成年人很少发生肾神经母细胞瘤[184]。

大体表现 类癌常具有清楚的边界[191-193]，切面红褐色，可见出血[194]及坏死[195]。已有2例含有异常畸胎样成分的肾类癌报道[196,197]，有学者认为与马蹄肾有关[198]。肾小细胞癌通常体积巨大，并侵犯后腹膜软组织；区域淋巴结转移常见[199,200]。肾神经母细胞瘤通常体积较大，实性，切面红中带黄，可见出血[201]。

组织学表现 组织病理学上，这些肿瘤涵盖了类癌、小细胞癌和原始神经上皮肿瘤[184]。类癌由具有类癌细胞学特征的肿瘤细胞条索和细胞巢构成（图12.32）。在肿瘤分化谱的另一端是小细胞癌，由片状、核深染且胞浆不明显的低分化肿瘤细胞构成。坏死很常见，有2项研究[199,200]发现了Azzopardi现象（血管壁上DNA物质沉积）。原发于肾的原始神经外胚层肿瘤，其组织学表现与原发于骨与软组织的肿瘤相同[185]（见第25和27章），并且具有相同的涉及 EWS 基因的染色体易位。神经母细胞瘤的诊断标准与肾上腺同名肿瘤相同，神经毡

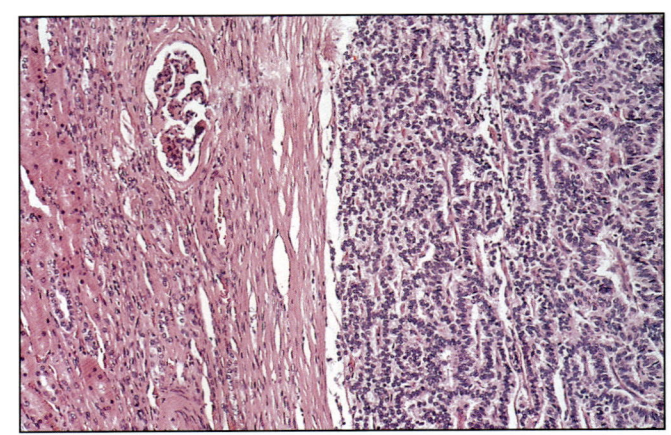

图12.32　肾类癌。细胞排列成缎带样，肿瘤边界清楚。

（neuropil）或 Homer Wright 菊形团的存在有助于与小细胞癌的鉴别。肾内嗜铬细胞瘤组织学表现与发生于肾上腺者类似。

肾间叶性肿瘤
Mesenchymal tumors of the kidney

血管平滑肌脂肪瘤　Angiomyolipoma

这种肾良性肿瘤由不同比例的脂肪、平滑肌和厚壁血管构成[202]。在成年人，血管平滑肌脂肪瘤与肾细胞癌一样常见[203]。在手术病例中，大约一半病例与结节性硬化病有关，另一半为散发病例。结节性硬化病相关患者常常无临床症状，肿瘤表现为多发性、双侧性、体积较小（图12.33）；而普通人群患者常常出现临床症状，肿瘤单发、体积大（图12.34）。普通人群中该疾病并不常见，而超过50%的结节性硬化病患者会发生此类肿瘤[204]。同与其密切相关的上皮样血管平滑肌脂肪瘤不同，血管平滑肌脂肪瘤是良性的，进展为肉瘤的可能性非常小[205]。

大体表现 血管平滑肌脂肪瘤直径从<1cm到≥20cm。大于4cm的肿瘤出现临床症状的可能性增加，出现临床症状的肿瘤平均直径为9cm[206]。肿瘤通常为金黄色，但颜色随着平滑肌和血管含量的不同而变化。肿瘤无包膜但界限清楚，有时可见局部浸润。肿瘤切面可类似于脂肪瘤。

组织学表现 肿瘤的组织学表现因脂肪、平滑肌和血管的相对含量（变化可以很大）而异（图12.35）[207]。平滑肌亦可表现出多种组织学形态。最为常见的是平滑肌细胞沿血管壁辐射状分布，也可表现为平滑肌束或散

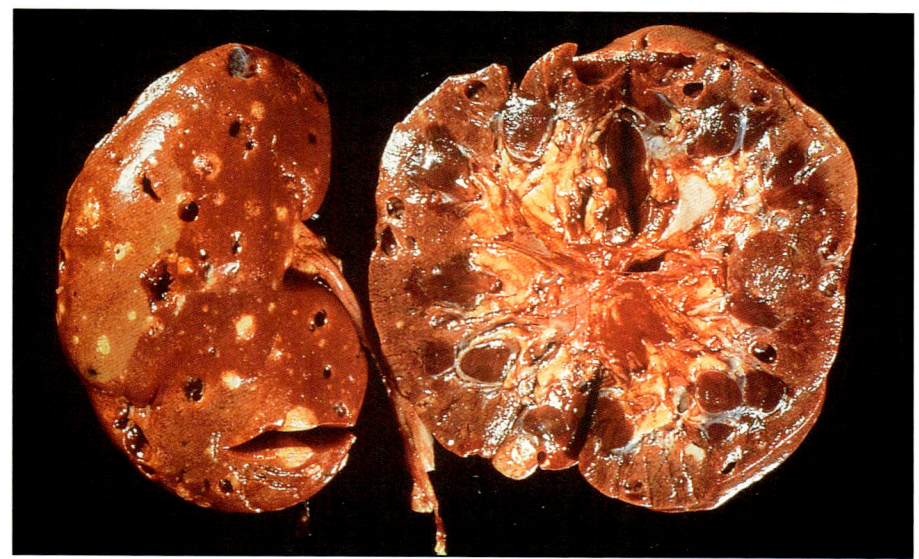

图12.33 血管平滑肌脂肪瘤。结节性硬化病患者肾可见多发性小的黄色肿物，是该病相关性血管平滑肌脂肪瘤的典型表现。

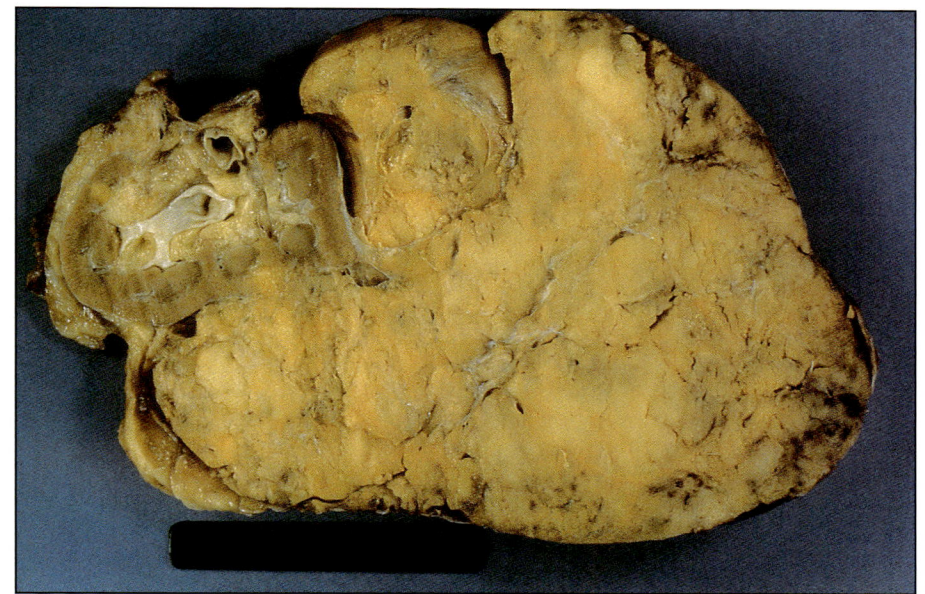

图12.34 血管平滑肌脂肪瘤。由分叶状黄色组织构成的体积巨大的单发性肿物是散发性血管平滑肌脂肪瘤的典型表现。

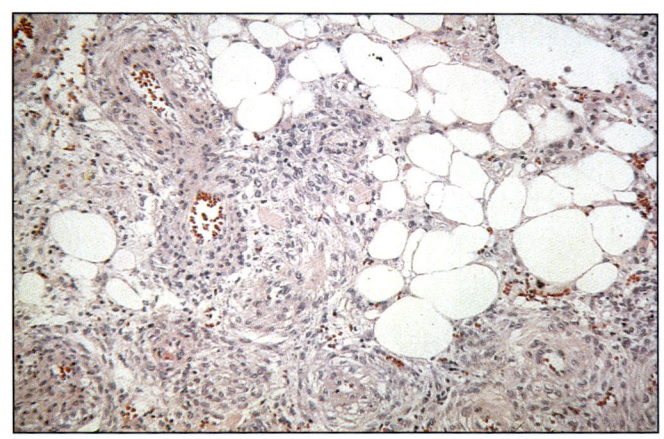

图12.35 血管平滑肌脂肪瘤。肿瘤由平滑肌、脂肪及厚壁血管组成。

在的肌纤维（图12.36）。平滑肌细胞通常为梭形，但有时表现为多角形或圆形，呈上皮细胞样形态，含有丰富的、颗粒状嗜酸性胞浆（图12.37）。血管形态异常，管壁厚，类似动脉壁，但管腔偏心或非常细小。核多形性可以非常显著，有时可见核分裂象。脂肪成分中可出现与脂肪母细胞无法区分的脂肪细胞。在大部分病例中，这些形态学表现并不意味着预后不佳。少数血管平滑肌脂肪瘤可出现大体和镜下可见的显著的囊腔，被覆形态温和的上皮组织[207a]。一些病例的区域淋巴结[208-210]和脾[211]可出现血管平滑肌脂肪瘤组织。不要将其误认为转移性肉瘤。偶尔，血管平滑肌脂肪瘤可侵犯肾静脉或

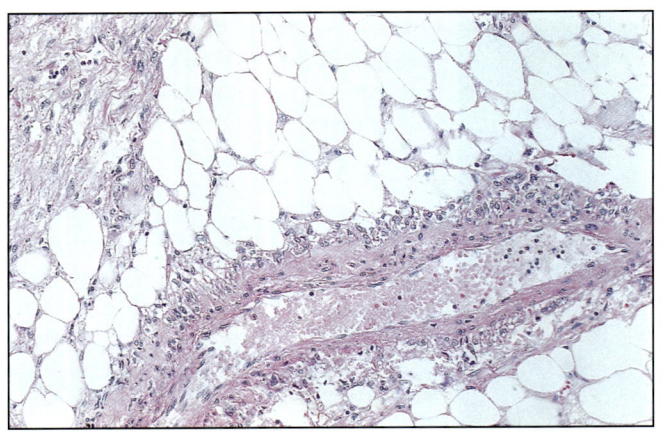

图12.36 血管平滑肌脂肪瘤。厚壁血管周围放射状分布的平滑肌纤维是常见表现。

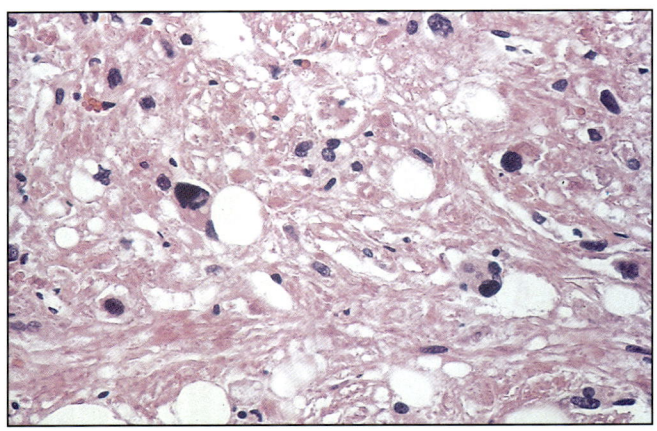

图12.37 血管平滑肌脂肪瘤。偶尔可见上皮样平滑肌细胞，细胞核可有非典型性。

下腔静脉，所有这些病例均可经手术治愈，因此并不提示恶性[202]。

最近被认识并命名为"上皮样血管平滑肌脂肪瘤"是血管平滑肌脂肪瘤的变异型，极易被误认为癌[1,212-214]。这种肿瘤由富含嗜酸性胞浆的多角形大细胞（类似神经节细胞）和短梭形细胞组成。肿瘤常常出现广泛出血和水肿。这种肿瘤的诊断有非常重要的临床意义，因为相当一部分可以进展并可致死。

免疫组化上，传统型和上皮样血管平滑肌脂肪瘤均表达平滑肌肌动蛋白和（或）结蛋白，同时表达HMB45和（或）Melan-A，与PEComa家族其他肿瘤相同。上皮性标志物阴性。

鉴别诊断 以脂肪为主的血管平滑肌脂肪瘤可与脂肪瘤甚至脂肪肉瘤混淆，需要广泛取材以发现肿瘤性血管及平滑肌成分。脂肪稀少的肿瘤可能会与其他间叶性肿瘤，如平滑肌瘤或平滑肌肉瘤混淆。具有上皮样形态学表现的血管平滑肌脂肪瘤可以类似于肾的上皮性肿瘤，因此遇到难以分类的上皮样肾肿瘤应当考虑到这种可能，特别是当患者患有结节性硬化病时。

在冰冻切片、细针穿刺涂片或常规标本切片中，上皮样血管平滑肌脂肪瘤常常被误诊为癌。遇到特殊的、由黏着性很差的嗜酸性多角形细胞构成的肾肿瘤时应考虑到这个诊断。

血管瘤　Hemangioma

肾血管瘤主要发生在成年人，男性和女性发病率相仿[215,216]。孤立性病变最为常见，但超过10%病例为多发性和双侧性。罕见情况下，与Klippel-Trenaunay和Sturge-Weber综合征有关[217]。多数病例无症状，仅在尸检时发现。在有症状的患者中，反复血尿是常见的主诉症状，并常常伴随贫血[218]。

大体表现 多数肿瘤直径小于1cm，肉眼很难发现。大的病灶直径可达18cm，表现为红色的海绵状外观。血管瘤可发生于肾任何部位，但大部分引起症状的病灶位于肾髓质和肾乳头[218]。

组织学表现 显微镜下，这些病变由大小不一的血管腔隙组成，其中一些管壁含有平滑肌和弹力组织。血栓和机化常见。肿瘤边界常不规则并与周围肾实质融合，但因缺乏内皮细胞核不典型性和多层排列，大部分病例很容易看出其良性本质。依据软组织肿瘤相同的诊断标准可以将它们与血管肉瘤区分开来（见第3章）；这也适用于本章所讨论的其他良性间叶性肿瘤。

淋巴管瘤　Lymphangioma

肾淋巴管瘤远比肾血管瘤少见，只有数十例报道，发病年龄从婴幼儿[219]到老年人不等，1/3为儿童，2/3为成年人[220]。大体上多表现为由含清亮液体小囊腔构成的孤立性、有包膜的肿物。显微镜下表现为被覆良性内皮细胞的腔隙，其间可见主要由纤维组织构成但也可含有平滑肌组织的间隔。位于肾窦的病变可以浸润肾髓质[221]，引起尿路阻塞。

平滑肌瘤　Leiomyoma

有症状的肾平滑肌瘤很少见[222]，可以表现为重达37kg的巨大肿物[223]；小的病灶常常由尸检偶然发现（图12.38）。大多数发生于成年人[224]。大体表现为边界清楚、实性、有弹性、切面编织状的肿物。与发生于子宫的平滑肌瘤一样，肿瘤由平滑肌束组成，局灶可见钙化和其他退行性变。出现坏死、细胞核非典型性或较多核分裂象则高度提示平滑肌肉瘤。

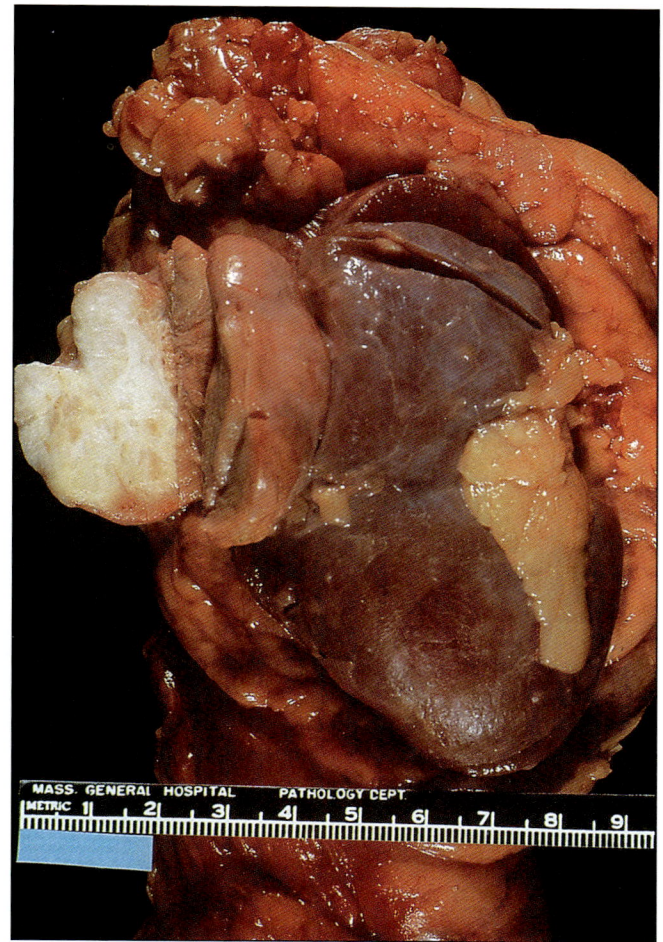

图12.38 肾平滑肌瘤。肿瘤实性,突出肾皮质表面,由白色组织构成。

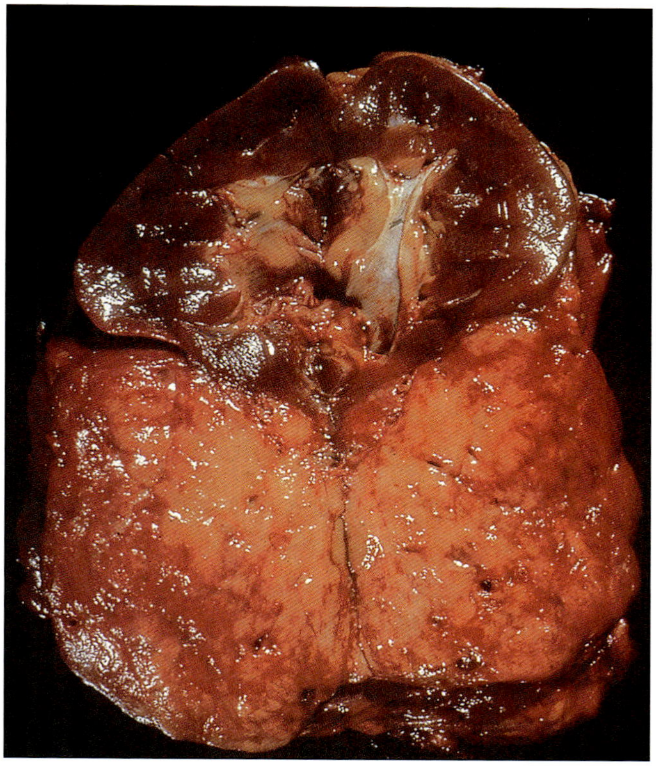

图12.39 肾平滑肌肉瘤。肿瘤体积大,由质地较软的棕褐色组织构成,伴出血。还可见局灶坏死及空洞形成。

脂肪瘤　Lipoma

有症状的肾脂肪瘤罕见[225]。患者常常表现为腹部或肋腹部疼痛。几乎所有病例均发生于中年妇女。与血管平滑肌脂肪瘤不同,它们与结节性硬化病无关。大体表现为黄色有包膜的肿物,组织学上完全由成熟的脂肪组织组成。正如上文提到的,血管平滑肌脂肪瘤可以脂肪成分为主,仔细切开寻找平滑肌和血管成分以便与脂肪瘤区分是必需的,因此充分取材是必要的。少见情况下,肾盂周围肾窦中的脂肪组织高度增生,类似肿瘤[226]。

平滑肌肉瘤　Leiomyosarcoma

这是最常见的肾原发性肉瘤,已有超过100例的病例报道[227]。患者从儿童到80多岁的老年人,大多发生在40岁以上,高峰为40～60岁。女性发病大约是男性的2倍。肋腹部肿物和疼痛是最常见的临床表现。

大体表现　大体表现常常类似于平滑肌瘤:质硬、实性、边界清楚、切面编织状,但坏死及出血更为常见(图12.39)[228]。平滑肌肉瘤可以起源于肾被膜[228]和肾静脉,而肿瘤的主体也可位于肾窦[229]。肾实质和肾周组织的浸润常见。

组织学表现　显微镜下,肿瘤由形态类似平滑肌的嗜酸性梭形细胞束组成。细胞核的多形性和分裂象的数量变化范围很大,目前尚无公认且明确的最低恶性诊断标准。肾平滑肌肿瘤中,坏死、核的多形性或较多核分裂象应作为平滑肌肉瘤的诊断指标。尤其是大的平滑肌肿瘤,应高度怀疑平滑肌肉瘤的可能性,因为它们即使核分裂象非常少,有时也会发生转移及导致患者死亡[230]。HMB45和Melan-A染色有助于除外平滑肌为主的血管平滑肌脂肪瘤。

脂肪肉瘤　Liposarcoma

脂肪肉瘤在后腹膜软组织中常见,但在肾非常罕见[231,232]。仔细的大体检查对于确定肿瘤起源于肾非常重要,因为后腹膜脂肪肉瘤侵犯或压迫肾远比肾脂肪肉瘤侵犯后腹膜软组织常见[228]。对于来源不明的病例（那些体积巨大而且侵犯范围广的肿瘤），应倾向于后腹膜软组织来源。回顾已报道的病例中，有一些应该是大的孤立性血管平滑肌脂肪瘤，并因此得出肾脂肪肉瘤预后较好这一结论。大体上，肿瘤呈黄色分叶状，边界相对清楚。组织病理学上，肾脂肪肉瘤与其他部位同类肿瘤表现相同；Farrow 等[228]报道的该类肿瘤中超过 80% 为黏液型。

所谓的恶性纤维性组织细胞瘤 So-called malignant fibrous histiocytoma

所谓的恶性纤维性组织细胞瘤（MFH）可发生于肾实质或肾被膜[233,234]。因为后腹膜软组织是恶性纤维性组织细胞瘤发生的常见部位，因此上文有关脂肪肉瘤原发部位的讨论和建议也适用于该肿瘤。临床上，肾恶性纤维性组织细胞瘤主要发生于成年人，男性占绝大多数。大部分病例为大的浸润性肿物，组织学类型以席纹状-多形性和炎症型为主。前者可能与肉瘤样肾细胞癌难以区分，而后者可类似于黄色肉芽肿性肾盂肾炎。目前认为发生在该部位的此类肿瘤实际上大部分是去分化脂肪肉瘤。

横纹肌肉瘤 Rhabdomyosarcoma

肾横纹肌肉瘤罕见[235-237]；Grignon 等回顾了有关文献，只发现了 8 例令人信服的病例，男女各半，发病年龄从 36 到 70 岁不等[238]。4 例在 14 个月内死于肉瘤，其余 4 例随访时间小于 12 个月。大多数形态学类似横纹肌肉瘤的肾肿瘤被证实为其他类型肿瘤，因此诊断横纹肌肉瘤应慎重。在儿童，Wilms 瘤可含有骨骼肌成分，因此在儿童患者中是否存在与 Wilms 瘤无关的横纹肌肉瘤尚存疑问。肾横纹肌样瘤（见下文）和肉瘤样肾细胞癌也可类似于横纹肌肉瘤。

其他肉瘤 Other sarcomas

滑膜肉瘤偶尔可原发于肾，可伴广泛的囊性变[239,240]。原发于肾的孤立性纤维瘤罕见[241,242]，而且与上文关于脂肪肉瘤的讨论一样，不易确定肾内或肾外来源[223,243]。这些肿瘤以前常被认为是血管外皮细胞瘤[244-246]。肿瘤通常体积大，常见囊腔和局部出血。骨源性肉瘤很少发生在肾实质或肾盂[247,248]，一些软骨肉瘤[249]和血管肉瘤[250,251]已有报道。它们的组织形态学特征与其他部位的同类肿瘤相同。

球旁细胞瘤 Juxtaglomerular cell tumor

球旁细胞瘤亦称为肾素瘤（reninomas），1967 年由 Robertson 和 Kihara 分别报道[252,253]。个案和小规模病例共报道了大约 100 例[254]。虽然绝大多数患者患有高血压，但 Corvol 及其同事[255]在 30 000 例新发高血压患者中只发现了 7 例该类型肿瘤患者。血清肾素水平升高是这些患者典型的临床表现，选择性肾静脉导管插入术是体积较小肿瘤切除的重要定位手段[256]。多数患者是年轻人和青少年，手术切除病例平均年龄为 27 岁[254]。但许多患者在手术切除前已有多年的高血压病史。高血压病的平均年龄仅为 22 岁。女性患者是男性的 2 倍。大多数病例经手术切除可治愈高血压，而且保守性手术切除对某些患者有效。已知有一例球旁细胞瘤病例发生了转移[257]。目前尚无局部浸润或复发、多灶性或双侧性病例的报道。

大体表现 多数病灶小于 3cm，某些病例在肾被膜剥离后未发现病灶。因此，当怀疑球旁细胞瘤时，必须对标本进行仔细的切开检查，任何异常的病灶都应取材进行组织病理学检查。肿瘤边界非常清楚，切面灰白、有弹性，有时可见内壁光滑的空洞（图 12.40）。

组织学表现 病变的组织病理学表现多样。常见的表现是多角形肿瘤细胞组成的不规则条索分布于疏松黏液样间质中（图 12.41）。小管状及小囊腔结构常见。血管常常很丰富，有时可见淋巴细胞浸润（图 12.42）。改良的 Bowie 染色可显示胞浆内颗粒，而免疫组化染色可发现胞浆内肾素的表达[258]。电镜检查有助于发现球旁细胞瘤内典型的菱形颗粒（图 12.43）[259]。

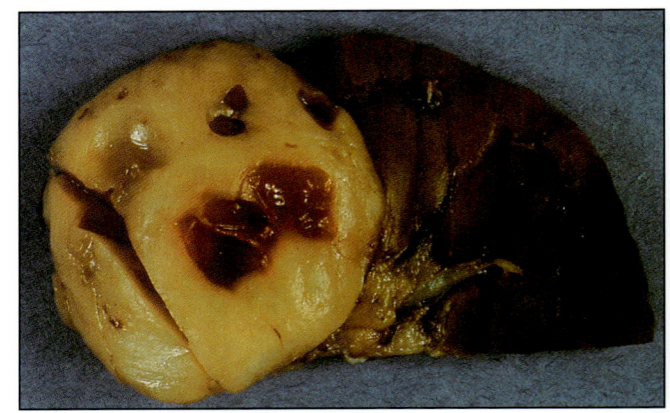

图12.40 球旁细胞瘤。肿瘤为边界清楚的球形肿物，切面黄色-棕褐色，有弹性，可见几个内壁光滑的空洞及局部出血。

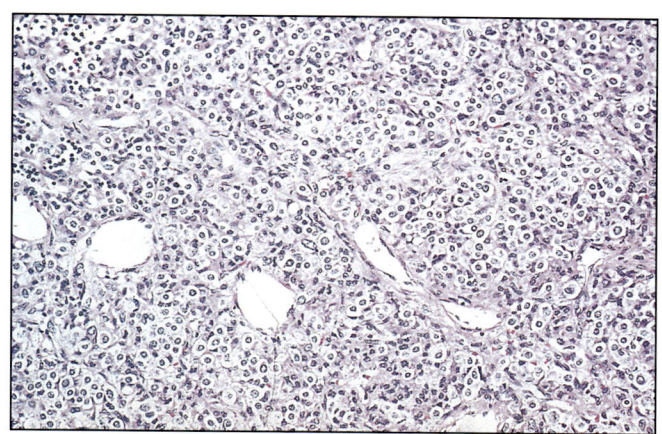
图12.41 球旁细胞瘤。胞浆浅染或透明的多角形肿瘤细胞分布于富含血管的间质中。

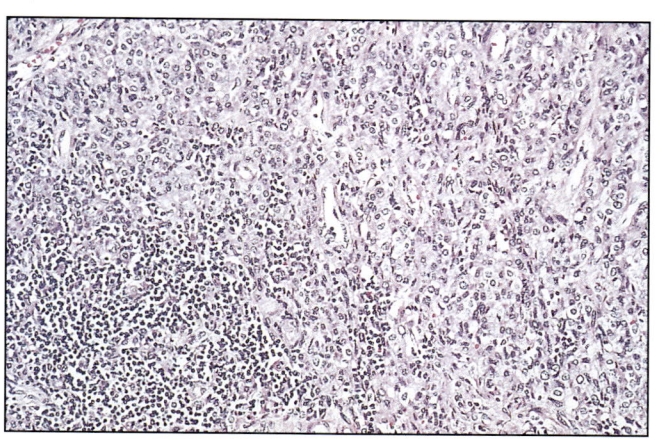
图12.42 球旁细胞瘤。肿瘤细胞呈片状排列，细胞核大小、形状不一，细胞浆呈不同程度嗜酸性，其间可见灶状的淋巴细胞浸润。

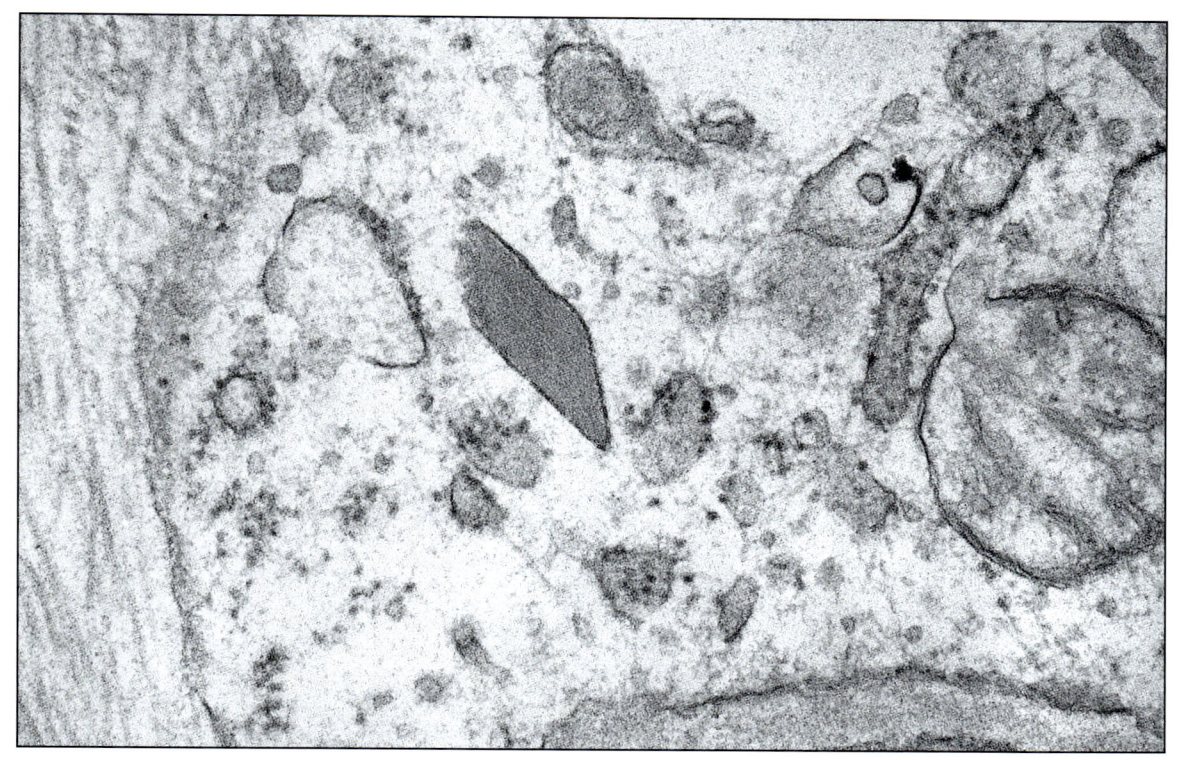
图12.43 球旁细胞瘤。超微结构下，含肾素的颗粒常常呈明显的菱形。

鉴别诊断 这种肿瘤几乎都是在检查高血压过程中发现的，因此其肿瘤的本质在术前常常会引起怀疑。大体检查发现体积小、颜色光亮、有弹性的肿瘤缩小了其鉴别诊断范围，而其组织学表现很有特征性。尽管已有研究发现肾细胞癌和Wilms瘤也表达肾素[260-262]，而且某些病例也可引起高血压，但通常不会导致诊断困难。

肾髓质间质细胞瘤
Renomedullary interstitial cell tumor

这种体积小的肾髓质肿瘤经常在尸检时偶然发现，有时在外科病理标本中也可见到[263]。超微结构和其他研究发现，这些病变由肾髓质间质细胞组成，这些细胞含对血压调节具有重要作用的血管活性物质。这些病变是真正的肿瘤还是对高血压反应产生的增生性结节尚存在争议。20岁以下年轻人罕见，而在一项对尸检肾进行仔细切开检查的大规模病例研究中发现，将近50%的20岁以上患者至少存在一个病灶，57%的肾髓质间质细胞瘤患者存在一个以上的病灶[264]。

由于多数肿瘤体积小，它们很少出现症状，也不会引起外科病理诊断上的困难。多数棘手的情况是在其他原因如肾移植而切除的肾标本中意外发现这类病变（图

肾间叶性肿瘤

12.44）。少数引起症状的病例常常是位于肾盂的带蒂肿物，早期文献将其称为肾盂纤维瘤[265]。

大体表现　肿瘤表现为白色结节，可以发生在肾髓质的任何部位（图12.45）。边界清楚，常为球形，大部分直径小于5mm。

组织学表现　显微镜下，小的星形细胞分布于弱嗜碱性疏松间质中，与肾髓质的间质相似。交错分布的疏松网状纤维束常见（图12.46）。结节周围常可见陷于间质基质中的肾髓质小管。"纤维瘤"是一个不准确的名称，

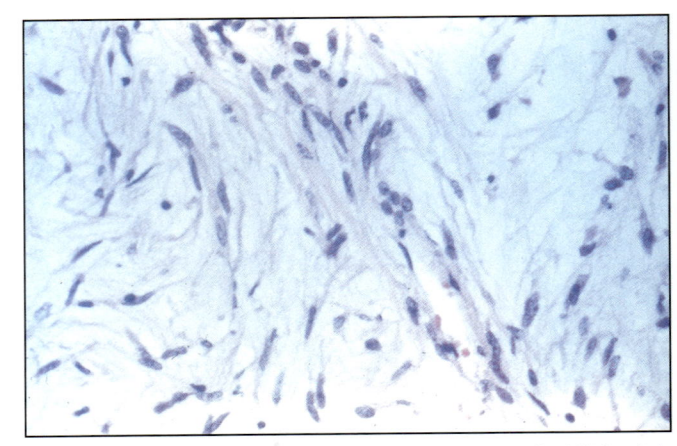

图12.46　肾髓质间质细胞瘤。肿瘤由分布于弱嗜碱性间质中的星形和梭形肿瘤细胞组成。

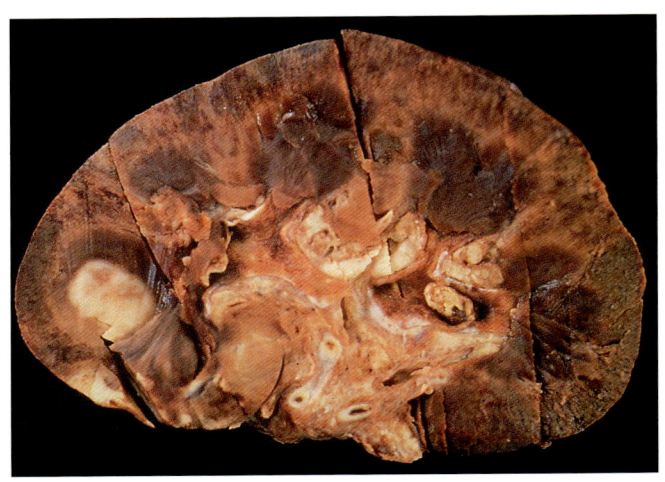

图12.44　肾髓质间质细胞瘤。因急性排斥反应而切除的肾标本中发现一个直径15mm、亮黄色、边界清楚的髓质内肿瘤。

因为大部分病变只含有很少胶原。某些病变确实因含有呈不规则块状沉积的淀粉样物质[266]，使稀薄疏松间质的特征不明显。

囊性肾瘤　Cystic nephroma

囊性肾瘤也称为多房性囊肿[267]和多房性囊性肾瘤[268]，是一种发生于成年人、不常见的肾良性肿瘤[87,269]。女性多于男性，发病比例大约为7:1。一些囊性肾瘤患者可发生肉瘤[87]。保守性手术通常可以治愈，但有一例患者在不完全切除后复发[87,270]。囊性肾瘤的诊断标准见表12.7。

大体表现　病变为有纤维包膜的边界清楚的球形肿物，由许多互不相通、内壁光滑的囊腔构成。囊内充满黄色清亮液体（图12.47）。未见实性区域，间隔厚度可薄如纸或厚达数毫米。大体上，囊性肾瘤无法与多房性囊性肾细胞癌以及囊性分化型肾母细胞瘤区分。

组织学表现　显微镜下，间隔由纤维组织构成，有

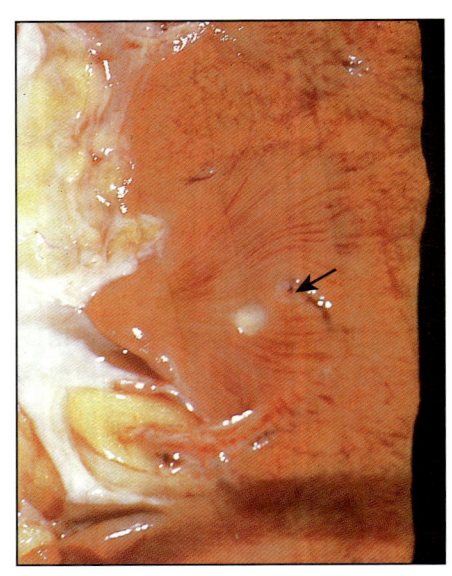

图12.45　肾髓质间质细胞瘤。略突出于肾切面的白色髓质内小结节是肾髓质间质细胞瘤的典型表现。

表12.7	Eble和Bonsib关于囊性肾瘤的诊断标准[87]

成年患者
有纤维假包膜的膨胀性肿物
内部完全由囊腔和间隔构成，无实性结节
囊腔被覆扁平、鞋钉样或立方上皮细胞
间隔中可见成熟肾小管样上皮结构
间隔中未见透明胞浆的上皮细胞
间隔中未见骨骼肌纤维

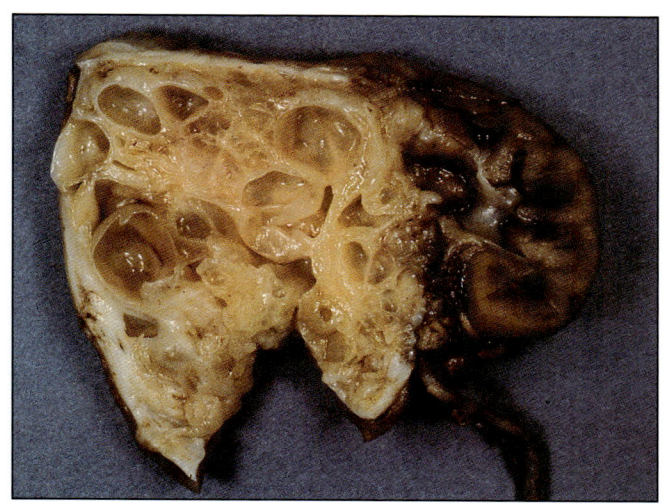

图12.47 囊性肾瘤。致密纤维组织包裹的多个、大小不同、内壁光滑的囊腔。

时可见灶状钙化。间隔中可见类似分化成熟的肾小管样结构（与Wilms瘤中特征性的小管形态不同）、炎症细胞和反应性纤维母细胞（图12.48）[271]。间隔的细胞组成变化很大，可以是细胞稀少的玻璃样变成分，也可以是富于梭形细胞的间质，类似于卵巢间质。囊腔被覆胞浆较少的扁平或矮立方上皮细胞；有时这些被覆细胞呈鞋钉样。胞浆嗜酸性或透明。

鉴别诊断 无论在临床、影像学还是病理学方面，主要与囊性Wilms瘤和囊性肾细胞癌鉴别。表12.7列出的诊断标准有助于这几种肿瘤的鉴别。关键的鉴别点

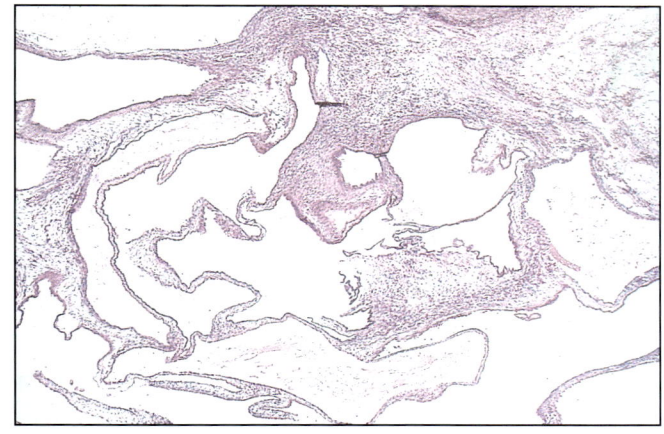

图12.48 囊性肾瘤。纤维组织构成的间隔厚薄不一，被覆立方或扁平上皮细胞。

是囊性肾瘤没有Wilms瘤中的胚芽等其他成分，间隔中也缺少簇状分布、含透明胞浆的上皮细胞。

肾混合性上皮和间质肿瘤
Mixed epithelial and stromal tumor of kidney

近年来，一种明显由肿瘤性间质和上皮成分混合构成的罕见而独特的肾肿瘤逐渐被认识[87]。这种肿瘤有很多名称[272-274]，但最能体现其特点的名称是混合性上皮和间质肿瘤，WHO分类也采纳了这个命名[1,275]。到目前为止，实际上所有的此类肿瘤都可以通过手术切除而治愈，除了近来描述的一些间质细胞具有非典型性并发生了转移的病例，但对这些病例尚存争议[276]。

大体上，肿瘤由大小不一的囊腔和实性区域构成[277]。一些病例广泛囊性变，很像囊性肾瘤。这些肿瘤发生于肾实质，可能是髓质起源，常突入肾盂。

显微镜下，包含细胞成分多少不等的间质，可以是玻璃样变的纤维组织，也可以是平滑肌[277]。某些病例出现脂肪组织。间质内含有复杂的上皮成分，形成囊腔和管状结构。管状结构可表现为类似于肾源性腺瘤那样的小管，也可为长的分支状小管。被覆立方、柱状、扁平上皮或尿路上皮。一些病例可类似于双相型滑膜肉瘤。免疫组化染色常常发现平滑肌分化。雌激素和孕激素受体常有表达，不表达HMB45。

淋巴瘤 Lymphoma

50%的播散性恶性淋巴瘤可继发累及肾。但淋巴瘤是否能原发于肾尚有争议[278,279]。少数表现为肾肿物的淋巴瘤已有报道，但大部分很快就发现了肾外淋巴瘤的存在。这些病例若出现临床症状，也类似于肾细胞癌[280]。

大体表现 肾淋巴瘤的大体表现变化多样。主要形成肾实质肿块性病变，边界清楚；而弥漫性病变不常见[281]。前者由肾内白色结节构成，从肾皮质表面可以看到（图12.49）；后者肾体积增大，皮质和髓质呈苍白色，它们之间的界限由于肿瘤细胞的浸润而模糊不清（图12.50）。表现为肾肿物的淋巴瘤常位于肾窦，包围和侵犯肾门组织[281]。

组织学表现 大体表现不同的不同类型淋巴瘤，其组织学表现也不同。由边界清楚的结节构成的淋巴瘤，病变几乎完全由淋巴瘤细胞组成。在弥漫浸润的病例中，肾间质中可见单形性的异型淋巴样细胞浸润，有时可见保存完好的肾小球和肾小管。肾原发瘤中，大细胞性淋巴瘤比小细胞性淋巴瘤更常见[280,281]，而Hodgkin淋巴瘤并不常见[281]。肾也可发生浆细胞瘤[282,283]。

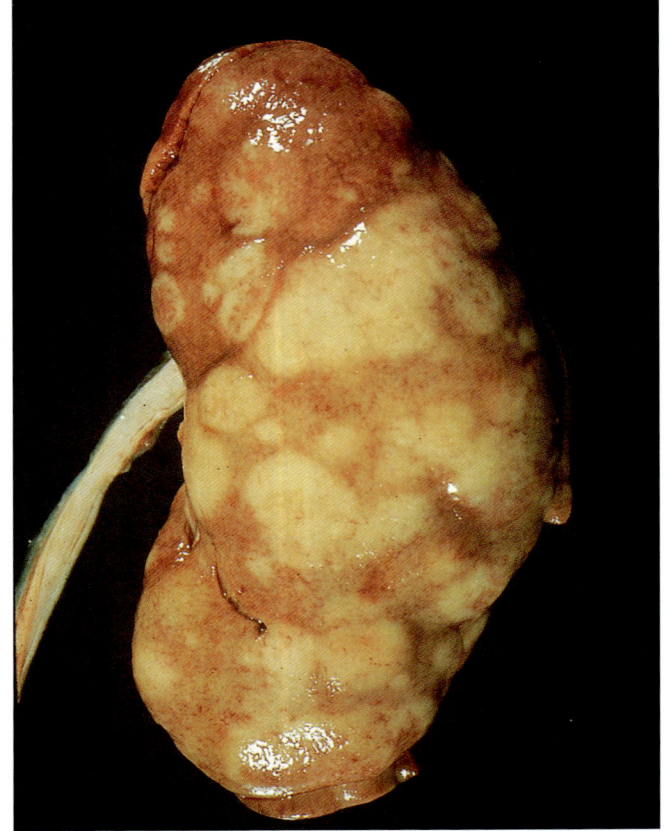

图12.49 肾恶性淋巴瘤。多个淋巴瘤结节取代了大部分肾实质。

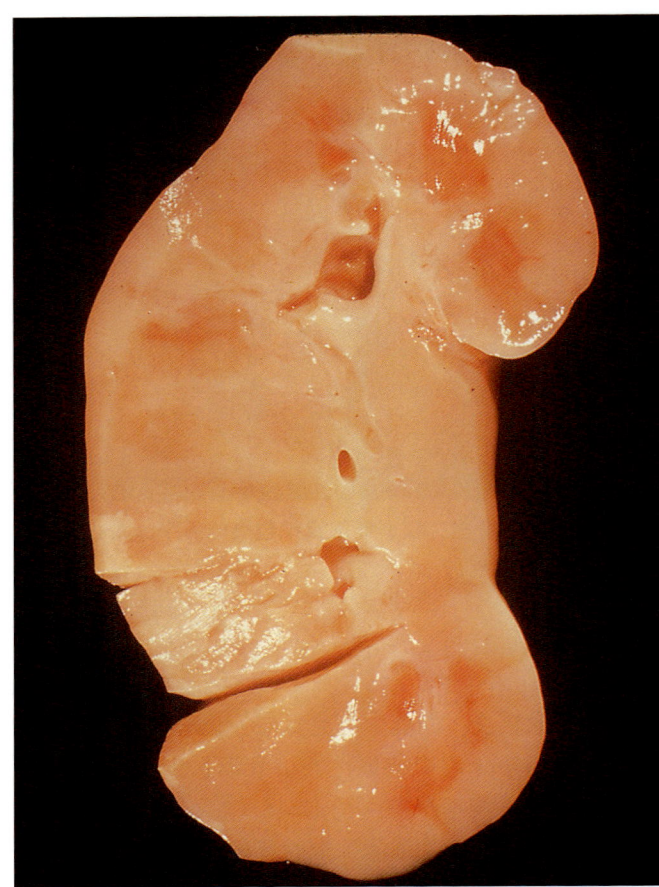

图12.50 肾恶性淋巴瘤。淋巴瘤弥漫浸润,肾总体轮廓保存,但体积增大,皮髓质界限不清。

肾转移性肿瘤
Secondary neoplasms of the kidney

在一项11 328例癌症患者的尸检研究中,Bracken等[284]发现7.2%的患者出现肾转移。这些发现为其他研究所证实[285-288]。支气管肺癌是转移癌最常见的来源[284,287]。肾转移性癌很少出现原发性肾肿瘤的临床症状,但可能会因为误诊而行手术治疗[286]。虽然孤立性转移灶大体上很像原发性肾肿瘤,但组织学发现非肾脏原发病变的形态特征时通常可以明确诊断。有时,转移癌仅表现为肾小球内广泛微转移(图12.51)[289],或肾淋巴管内弥漫浸润[290]。

儿童肾肿瘤
Renal tumors in children

儿童原发性肾肿瘤并不常见;在美国每年大约有500例新发病例。在常见的儿科恶性肿瘤和儿童腹部恶性肿瘤中分别居第五位和第二位。虽然绝对数量并非很多,但是随着Wilms瘤治疗的进展以及又确认了两种不同于Wilms瘤的高度恶性肿瘤,使得儿童肾肿瘤的正确诊断和分期具有重大临床价值[291-293]。肿瘤的形态学多样、彼此交叉重叠且病例稀少,使得这一组病变的诊断成为外科病理医师需要面对的特殊挑战。

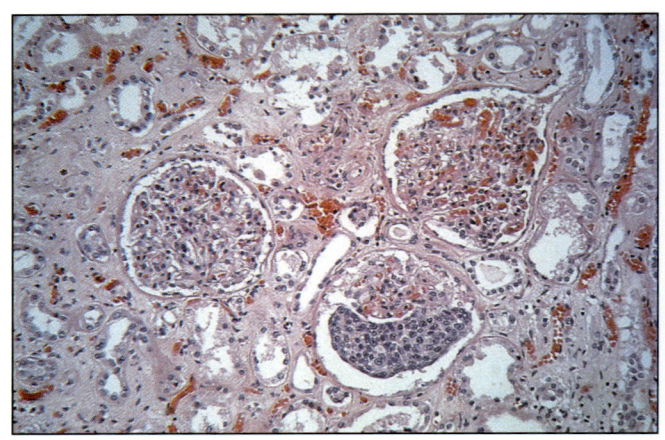

图12.51 肾转移癌。肺类癌转移至一个肾小球。

这组病变中最常见的是 Wilms 瘤（肾母细胞瘤）。透明细胞肉瘤和横纹肌样瘤在临床上很重要，因为它们对治疗不敏感，而且致残率和致死率颇高。3 个月内的幼儿中，中胚层肾瘤是最常见的肾肿瘤，通常预后很好。另一种少见的肿瘤是婴儿骨化性肾瘤，将在本章节简要介绍。通常发生于成年人的肾肿瘤，如肾细胞癌、淋巴瘤、各种肉瘤、神经内分泌肿瘤和血管平滑肌脂肪瘤在儿童罕见，但绝大部分儿童病例其病理学与成年人相同（见上文）。

目前我们所了解的儿童肾肿瘤病理学知识大多是来自 Bruce Beckwith 领导的国家 Wilms 瘤研究中心（NWTS）及其病理中心的成果。

Wilms 瘤　Wilms' tumor

Wilms 瘤占儿童肾肿瘤的 80% 以上[294]。大部分发生于 2~4 岁的儿童（男女平均年龄分别为 37 和 43 个月）[295]；6 个月以内的幼儿和 6 岁以上的儿童相对少见[296]。Wilms 瘤罕见于新生儿[297]。全世界不同地区人群发病率大致相同[298]。女性略多见[295]。4.4% 病例[299]为双侧发生，这些病例的平均年龄比单侧发生病例小一岁多[295]。它与一些遗传性疾病，特别是隐睾、尿道下裂、其他生殖器异常、偏身肥大以及无虹膜有关[300]。5% 的 Beckwith-Wiedemann 综合征患者可发生 Wilms 瘤[301]。Drash 综合征患者发生 Wilms 瘤的危险性也升高[302]。其他许多发育畸形与 Wilms 瘤发生关系不大[296,303]。家族性 Wilms 瘤并不常见[295]。Wilms 瘤罕见于成年人，发病时其临床分期和出现间变的几率均高于儿童患者，而且对治疗的敏感性较差[304,305]。

肾源性残余和肾母细胞瘤病（Nephrogenic rests and nephroblastomatosis）　数十年前研究者就发现儿童尸检病例及 Wilms 瘤患者手术切除的肾中存在类似胚芽的组织[306]。Bove 和 McAdams 研究了 69 例因 Wilms 瘤切除的肾标本，镜下发现 1/3 病例存在由胚芽样细胞构成的结节[307]。基于这些观察，根据组织学特征，他们对这些疾病进行了分类，包括结节性肾胚芽（nodular renal blastema）、后肾错构瘤（metanephric hamartoma）以及其他类型[307]。随后，研究者提出了另外一些命名系统，造成诊断术语的混乱[294]。1990 年，Beckwith 等[308]根据 NWTS 的大量研究结果提出了一个新的分类，下文的讨论即基于此。

肾源性残余指持续存在的类似于发育中的肾组织的肾源性细胞团（图 12.52）。可分为两种类型：叶周型肾源性残余，位于肾叶周边（皮质表面，Bertin 柱的中央，肾窦旁组织）；以及叶内型肾源性残余，位于肾叶皮质或髓质内。除了位置外，两者的不同之处还在于叶周型肾源性残余边界清楚，以胚基成分为主，常多灶或弥漫存在。叶内型肾源性残余常为单灶，与周围肾实质分界不清，并以间质成分为主。根据组织形态学的不同，肾源性残余还可进一步分为以下几种：静止型（dormant）或新生型（nascent）；成熟硬化型（maturing sclerosing）和退化型（obsolescent）；增生型（hyperplastic）；肿瘤型（neoplastic）。第一种类型通常由胚芽成分构成，显微镜下可见，核分裂象罕见。在成熟硬化型和退化型，存在分化的间质和上皮细胞，伴间质玻璃样变（图 12.53）。增生型肾源性残余大体可见，含有胚芽、胚胎或硬化性成分。少数情况下，增生型肾源性残余弥漫分布，取代大部分肾实质（图 12.54）。肿瘤型肾源性残余根据细胞

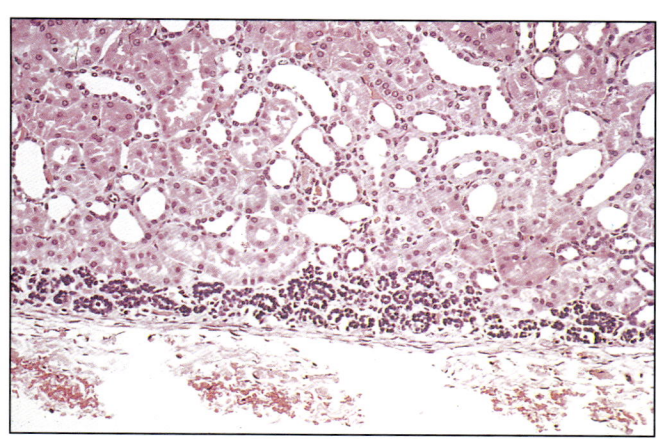

图 12.52　叶周型肾源性残余。由核深染的立方上皮构成的小管状结构呈线状排列于肾被膜下。（Courtesy of Dr. B.Beckwith and the National Wilms' Tumor Study Pathology Center.）

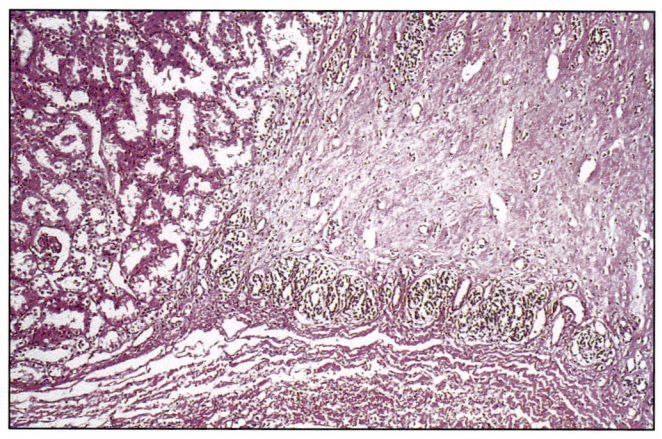

图 12.53　叶周型肾源性残余。退化型肾源性残余，主要由纤维组织构成，仅见少量未成熟的肾小管。（Courtesy of Dr. B.Beckwith and the National Wilms' Tumor Study Pathology Center.）

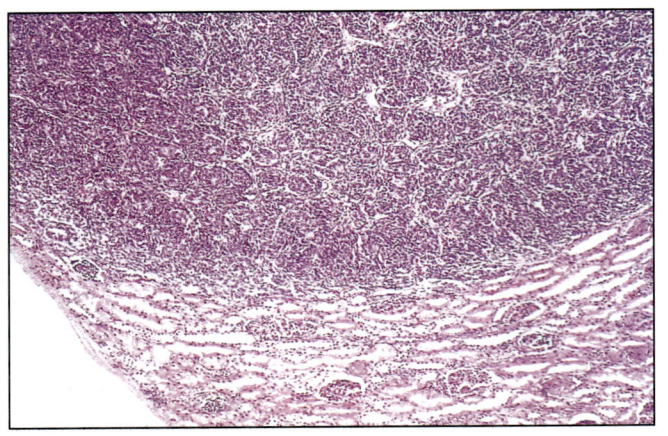

图12.54 叶周型肾源性残余。增生型肾源性残余，呈结节性生长，细胞密集。(Courtesy of Dr. B.Beckwith and the National Wilms' Tumor Study Pathology Center)

因为肾源性残余的存在提示双侧发生 Wilms 瘤的可能性很大，无论是同时或是异时。

大体表现 Wilms 瘤直径常常大于 5cm，1/3 以上病例可达 10cm[296]。重量常超过 500g。切面常为实性，质软，灰色或粉红色，很像脑组织（图 12.56）。灶状出血、坏死以及囊性变常见。罕见情况下肿瘤完全呈囊性。肿瘤常见明显的假包膜，由受压的肾组织和肾周组织形成，使肿物边界清楚或似有真正的包膜（图 12.57）。在肾盂内呈息肉状生长的大体类似葡萄状肉瘤的 Wilms 瘤，伴

密集程度和核分裂象的多少可以分为腺瘤型和肾母细胞瘤型。腺瘤型肾源性残余核分裂象不常见，而肾母细胞瘤型（早期 Wilms 瘤）核分裂象很常见。肿瘤型肾源性残余常呈肉眼可见的膨胀性球形病灶，发生于肾源性残余并压迫原先病灶。肾母细胞瘤病是指弥漫、多灶性肾源性残余，或多中心、双侧性 Wilms 瘤（图 12.55）。

叶周型肾源性残余在小于 3 个月的婴儿中发生率大约为 1%[69]，远高于 Wilms 瘤（1/10 000）；而叶内型肾源性残余除了伴随 Wilms 瘤发生外，几乎从不发生。肾源性残余极罕见于成年人[309]。NWTS 发现在单侧 Wilms 瘤患者中，叶周型和叶内型肾源性残余几率大致相同，均为 41%。在同时或异时双侧性 Wilms 肿瘤患者，肾源性残余的发生率高达 95%。因此，在 Wilms 瘤病例，对大体未见异常的肾标本进行仔细的检查很重要。

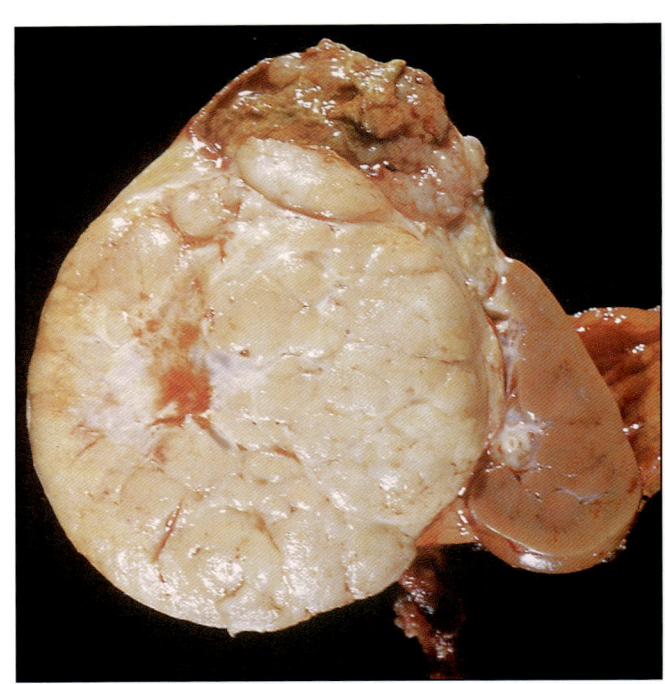

图12.56 Wilms瘤。肿瘤体积大，质地软，在颜色和质地上都与脑皮质相似，挤压正常肾组织。肿瘤上方可见褐色坏死区。

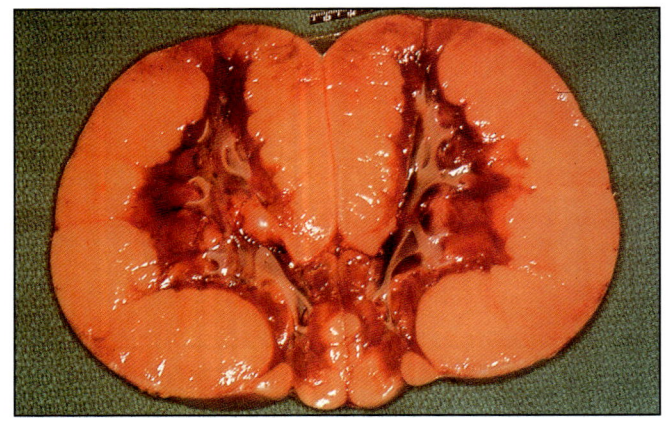

图12.55 肾母细胞瘤病。肾体积增大，被弥漫性质地较软的棕褐色组织取代。

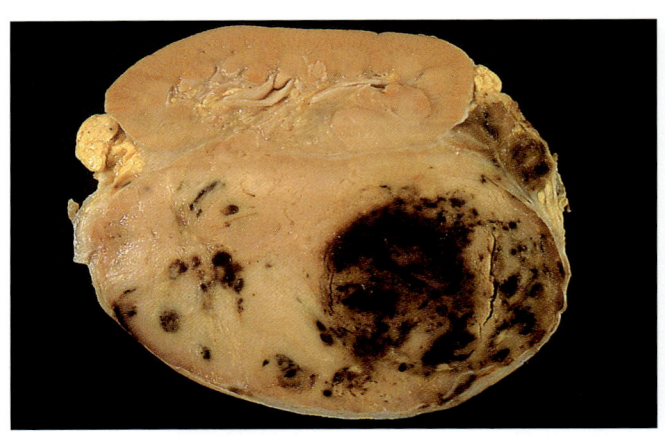

图12.57 Wilms瘤。肿瘤体积大，伴明显的炎性假包膜，并可见两个肿瘤浸润结。

广泛骨骼肌分化[310,311]，可能会被误诊为横纹肌肉瘤。

组织学表现 典型的Wilms瘤由多少不等的未分化胚芽组织、上皮和间质组成，然而某些病例只含两种甚至一种成分。胚芽细胞体积小，核深染，片状或不规则密集排列，核分裂象常见，胞浆稀少（图12.58），某些程度上类似于儿童其他类型的"小蓝细胞肿瘤"。胚芽成分常见三种排列方式：蜿蜒型、结节型和弥漫型。蜿蜒型和结节型最常见而且具有诊断意义。胚芽细胞形成相互吻合的蜿蜒型或圆形细胞团，与周围间质成分界限清楚（图12.59）。

上皮成分常呈小管或囊性结构，被覆原始的柱状或立方形细胞（图12.60）。细胞核细长呈楔形（图12.61）。Wilms瘤的上皮成分也可形成肾小球样结构，或向肾外组织分化，形成黏液上皮、鳞状上皮、神经上皮[312]或内分泌上皮[313]。以囊性为主的Wilms瘤间隔中含有胚芽组织及其他Wilms瘤组织成分（图12.62），这种类型被命名为部分囊性分化的肾母细胞瘤。

Wilms瘤的间质可以向任何类型的软组织分化。疏松黏液样和纤维母细胞性梭形细胞间质最为常见（图12.63），也可见向平滑肌、骨骼肌（图12.64）、脂肪、软骨、骨组织以及神经组织的分化[121]。偶尔，主要向较成熟的软组织类型弥漫分化，这些肿瘤被赋予特殊的名称，如胎儿横纹肌瘤样肾母细胞瘤[314]，而由分化性上皮和间质成分混合构成的肿瘤被称为畸胎瘤样Wilms瘤[315,316]。

鉴别诊断 部分囊性分化的肾母细胞瘤大体上可类似于囊性肾瘤，而且由于典型的Wilms瘤成分可能不明

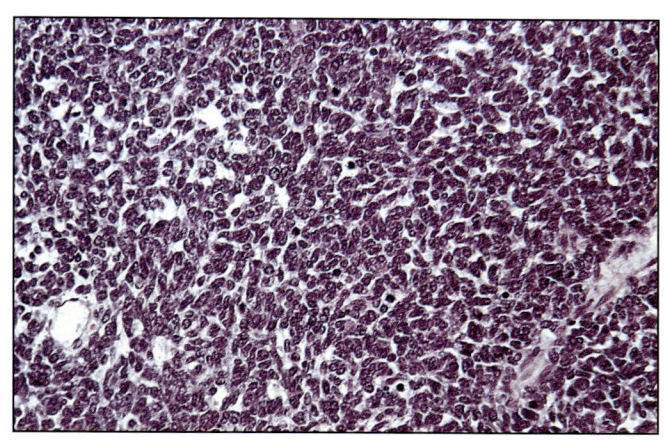

图12.58 Wilms瘤。胚芽成分由成片的小细胞组成，胞浆不明显，核深染，核分裂象常见。

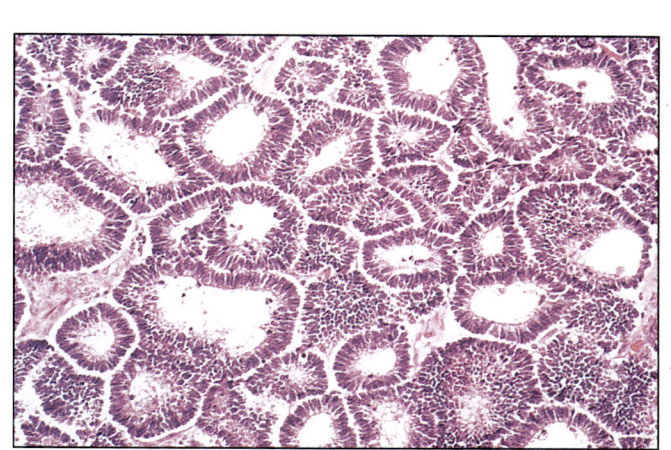

图12.60 Wilms瘤。上皮细胞柱状，形成管状结构。

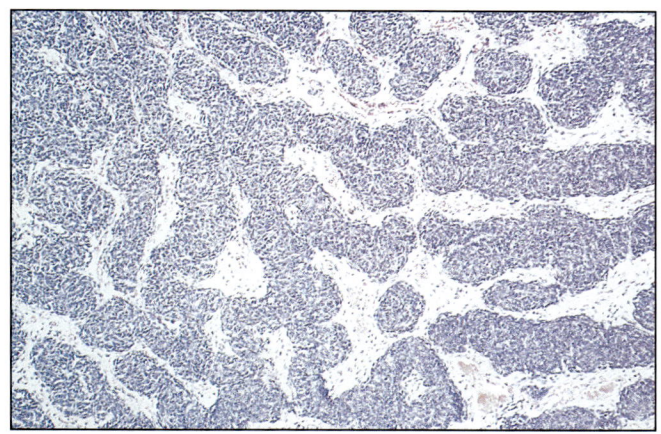

图12.59 Wilms瘤。胚芽成分蜿蜒排列。（Courtesy of Dr. B.Beckwith and the National Wilms' Tumor Study Pathology Center.）

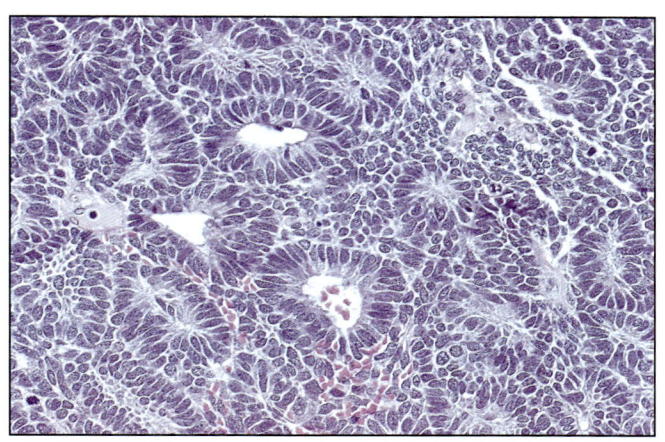

图12.61 Wilms瘤。上皮细胞核呈细长楔形，排列紧密。

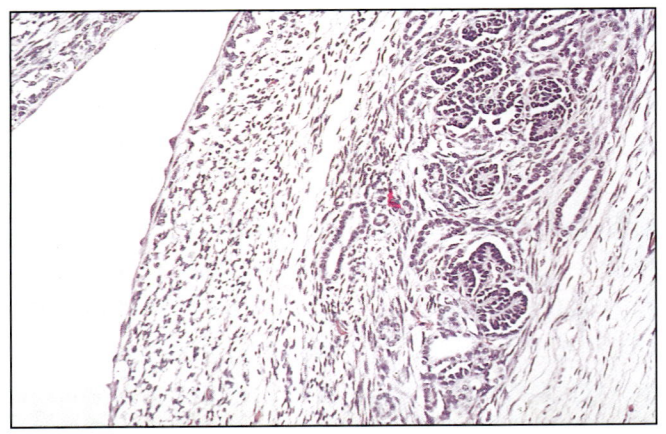

图12.62　Wilms瘤。部分囊性分化的肾母细胞瘤间隔中含有原始成分，此例出现不成熟的肾小管和肾小球。囊壁被覆扁平上皮。（Courtesy of Dr. B.Beckwith and the National Wilms' Tumor Study Pathology Center.）

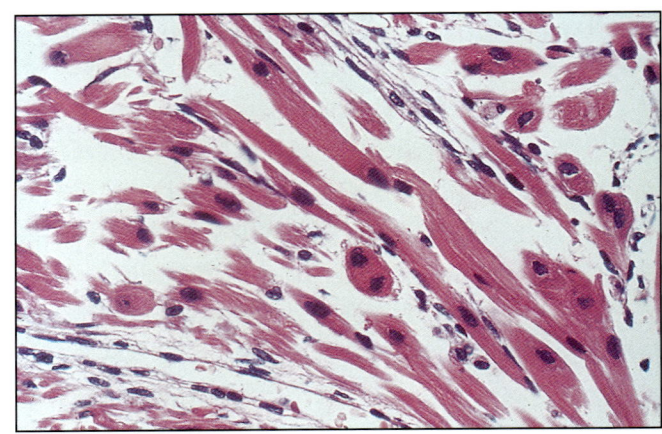

图12.64　Wilms瘤。一些病例的间质主要由骨骼肌构成。

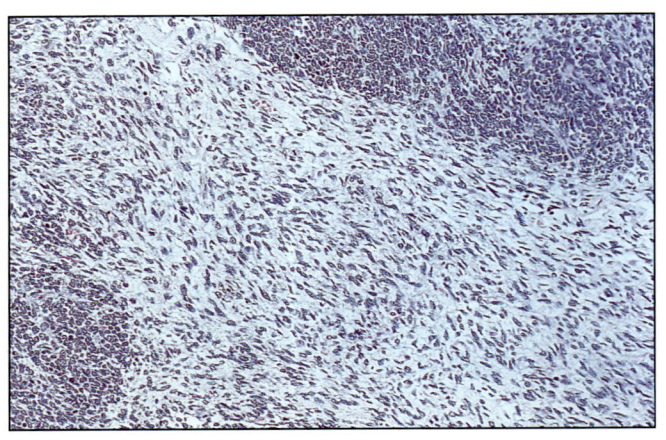

图12.63　Wilms瘤。尽管Wilms瘤的间质可以向很多组织类型分化，但最为常见的是由分布于弱嗜碱性基质中的梭形细胞组成。

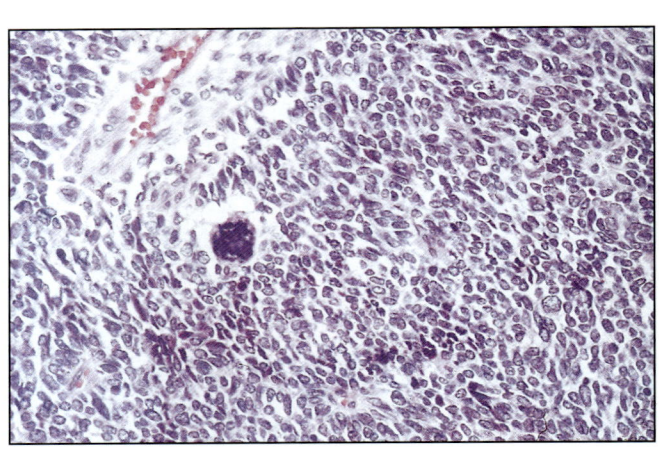

图12.65　Wilms瘤。体积大而深染的细胞核是诊断分化差组织类型（间变）的必要指标。（Courtesy of Dr. B.Beckwith and the National Wilms' Tumor Study Pathology Center.）

显，因此儿童囊性肾肿瘤应该充分取材，才能除外部分囊性分化的肾母细胞瘤。

胎儿横纹肌瘤样肾母细胞瘤不应与横纹肌肉瘤混淆，因为前者总体预后相当好。这种肿瘤含有大量相对成熟的骨骼肌组织，但缺乏恶性小细胞成分以及横纹肌肉瘤中的横纹肌母细胞。

一些Wilms瘤表现为单形上皮成分，可能会导致诊断困难，特别是在青少年和成年人，需要与肾细胞癌区分。掌握Wilms瘤上皮细胞典型的细胞核特征常常有助于将Wilms瘤与肾细胞癌区分开来。Wilms瘤上皮细胞核常常为细长或卵圆形，排列紧密，有时呈楔形（图12.61），这些形态学特征有助于单相型管状Wilms瘤与肾细胞癌的鉴别，后者细胞核通常为圆形。

Wilms瘤与横纹肌样瘤以及透明细胞肉瘤的鉴别将在下文讨论。

Wilms瘤的分级、分期及预后因素　根据NWTS的研究结果，Wilms瘤分为两种类型：根据有无间变的存在，分为分化好的组织学类型和分化差的组织学类型。约有6%的Wilms瘤可发生间变；很少发生在小于1岁的患者，80%以上发生于2岁以上[317]。NWTS早期研究发现，间变的存在使患者治疗失败和死亡的危险性明显升高[318]。间变的临床意义依赖于其发生范围；间变比较局限时治愈的可能性很高[319,320]。

NWTS将间变定义为出现细胞核增大、染色质增多以及多极核分裂象。间变的准确识别有赖于良好的组织学处理：恰当固定、切片和染色非常关键。间变细胞核的长度和宽度均至少是典型胚芽细胞核的3倍，而且核深染程度必须很明显（图12.65）。除了细胞核增大外，必须存在病理性多极核分裂象。评价一例Wilms瘤是否存在间变时必须牢记以下几点。首先，Wilms瘤间质中骨骼肌纤维增大的细胞核并不是间变的证据；其次，异常多极核分裂象的诊断标准非常严格，不仅要求核分裂象存在结构上的异常，还同时存在体积的增大。有时，由于人工假象，正常2倍体核分裂象也可类似多极现象，但其体积明显小于间变的多极核分裂象；与肿瘤其他部位胚芽组织正常大小的核分裂象进行比较有助于两者的区分。当间变只是灶状存在时，手术切除仍然是有可能治愈的[321]。

NWTS制定了一个Wilms瘤和其他儿童恶性肾肿瘤的分期标准（表12.8）[322]。但下文所列的表并不足以使外科病理医师应对在肿瘤分期上面临的挑战。I期和II期要求评估肾窦和肾被膜情况。肾窦是肾门深入肾实质所围成的腔隙，包含肾动脉和肾静脉主要分支以及大部分肾盂。在NWTS 5中，肾窦血管的侵犯被认为肿瘤扩散的证据，划分为II期。一般将肾窦软组织的侵犯划分为I期，但存在肿瘤侵犯切缘的情况则划分为III期。I期肿瘤的划分同样需要对肾被膜情况进行评价，这种判断常常比较困难，因为随着肿瘤的生长，依次被肾内假包膜、肾被膜、肾外假包膜、Gerota筋膜以及标本最外侧组织所包绕。各层组织常常融合，使人难以辨认真正的肾被膜。实际上，当Wilms瘤侵犯肾周脂肪组织时，脂肪细胞被破坏，纤维组织反应性增生，造成肾被膜内I期肿瘤的表现。如果肾被膜可以确认，则将其作为分期的标准。当肾被膜与Gerota筋膜软组织融合，则需将这一层结构作为分期的标准。肾被膜外炎性假包膜的形成目前并不适合作为划分II期的指标，但已有证据表明与复发率的升高有关[323]。表12.8所列的II期和IV期的划分标准比较明确。对于V期肿瘤，应对每个肾最高级别进展期的肿瘤依据上述分期标准单独进行亚分期，如V期，I亚期。

肾透明细胞肉瘤
Clear cell sarcoma of kidney

最初被英国学者Marsden等[324]称为儿童骨转移性肾肿瘤的透明细胞肉瘤[325]是一种高度恶性的肿瘤，传统的Wilms瘤治疗方案对其无效，但常常对含阿霉素的化疗方案敏感[326]。因此，透明细胞肉瘤的正确诊断具有相当重要的临床意义。透明细胞肉瘤的发生年龄段与Wilms瘤相同，约占儿童肾肿瘤的6%[327]；大部分确诊的患者年龄在12～36个月之间。透明细胞肉瘤罕见于成年人[328]。约66%的患者为男性。具有明显的骨转移倾向，其转移发生率至少是其他儿童肾恶性肿瘤的10倍。认识到这种病变与软组织透明细胞肉瘤无关这一点很重要（见第27章）。

大体表现 肿瘤切面表现多样：可以表现为均质状、灰白分叶状或多彩状，包括质硬的灰白色漩涡状和质软粉红色区域（图12.66）[329]。有时肿瘤产生大量的黏液使之呈胶冻样外观。大部分边界清楚。大约1/3病例可出现数毫米到数厘米的囊腔[330]。肿瘤重量常常超过500g[329]。未见双侧发生的报道[294]。

组织学表现 大部分肾透明细胞肉瘤由形态一致的肿瘤细胞构成，胞浆浅染或空泡状，边界不清。核染色质细颗粒状，核仁小（图12.67）。这种细胞核特征有助于透明细胞肉瘤与横纹肌样瘤的鉴别。在典型的病例，肿瘤细胞呈片状排列，具有明显的分支状小血管（图12.68）[330]。另一个特征性的组织学表现是肿瘤与周围肾实质之间的浸润性边界；经常可以见到被肉瘤细胞

	表12.8 美国Wilms瘤研究中心关于儿童肾肿瘤的分期[322]。（With kind permission of Springer Science and Business Media.）
I期	肿瘤局限于肾内，完整切除 具体诊断标准： 肿瘤未穿透肾被膜 肾窦静脉和淋巴管未受累 无淋巴结或血行转移
II期	肿瘤局部扩散至肾外，但可完整切除 具体诊断标准： 肾被膜被肿瘤穿透 肾窦静脉和淋巴管受累 肾静脉内可见肿瘤 局部污染或活检仅涉及肋腹部 标本切缘未见肿瘤，手术切除后无肿瘤残留 无转移
III期	局限于腹部的肿瘤残留，无血行转移 具体诊断标准： 腹部肉眼可见肿瘤残留 腹膜表面可见肿瘤种植 标本切缘可见肿瘤 腹部淋巴结可见肿瘤转移
IV期	血行转移或腹部外扩散
V期	肿瘤累及双侧肾

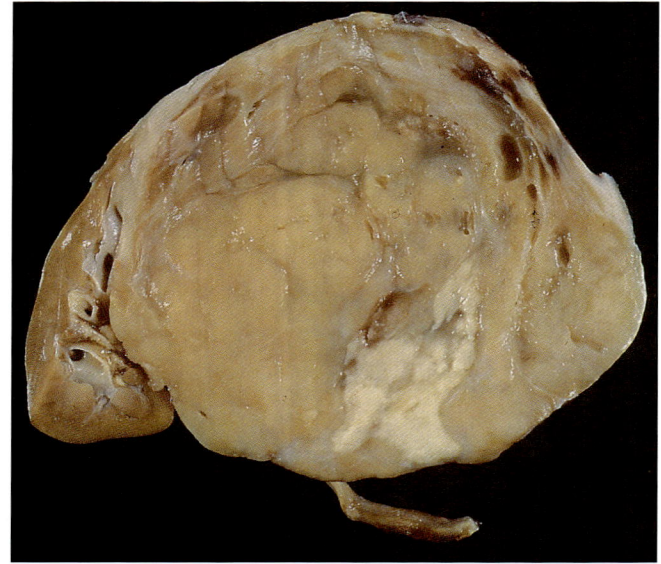

图12.66 肾透明细胞肉瘤。肿瘤灰褐色，体积大，质地软，局部见囊性变和坏死。

包裹的残存肾小管[329]。尽管被称为透明细胞肉瘤，但许多肿瘤细胞胞浆远不如透明细胞肾细胞癌显得透明，因此胞浆的透明度并不能作为诊断的可靠标准。典型的组织学表现外可出现另外一些令人迷惑的变型，包括梭形细胞增生、囊性变（图12.69）、玻璃样硬化以及栅栏状排列[121]。肿瘤应该充分取材，以便发现特征性的血管结构和细颗粒状染色质及小核仁等有助于正确诊断的指标。

鉴别诊断　透明细胞肉瘤与Wilms瘤的鉴别诊断中一些相关的阴性指标非常重要：透明细胞肉瘤无胚芽组织；非肾脏成分如软骨或肌肉不会出现在透明细胞肉瘤中；透明细胞肉瘤是单侧发生、单中心病灶，而未经治疗的Wilms瘤很少出现硬化性间质。透明细胞肉瘤中的典型血管结构有助于与Wilms瘤鉴别。透明细胞肉瘤与肾组织的边界经常是浸润性的，而Wilms瘤常常是"推挤性"边界。少数肾透明细胞肉瘤出现灶状核仁明显的肿瘤细胞，类似于肾横纹肌样瘤，但其他区域的典型组织学表现可以明确诊断。

肾横纹肌样瘤　Rhabdoid tumor of kidney

横纹肌样瘤是儿童肾肿瘤中恶性程度最高的，常发生广泛转移，并在确诊12个月内导致患者死亡[331]。患者确诊时年龄通常很小（NWTS研究发现年龄中值为11个月，3岁以后罕见），男女比例为1.5:1[331]。2岁以上患者预后明显要好[332]。研究发现与中枢神经系统胚胎性肿瘤[333]及副肿瘤性高血钙症[334]有关，有学者提出存在一种横纹肌样瘤易感综合征[335]。

大体表现　横纹肌样瘤缺少Wilms瘤和透明细胞瘤常见的包膜。肿瘤常位于肾中央部位[331]，肾窦和肾

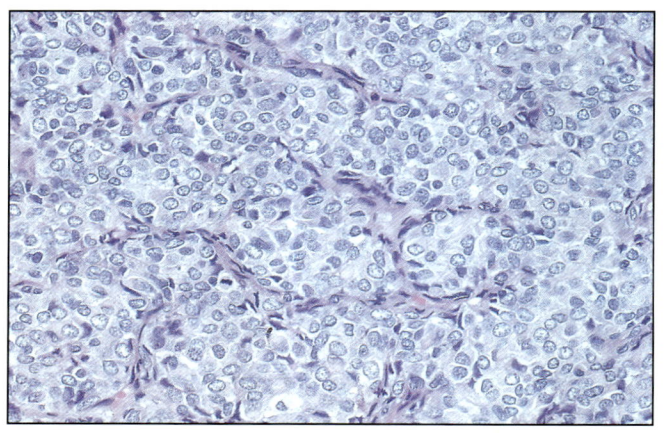

图12.67 肾透明细胞肉瘤。细胞核染色质细颗粒状，有时呈泡状核，核仁不明显，这是透明细胞肉瘤的典型表现。

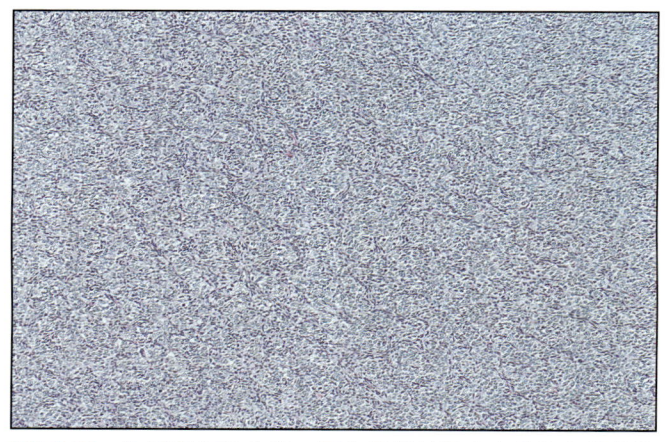

图12.68 肾透明细胞肉瘤。图中显著且呈分支状的血管结构是透明细胞肉瘤的特征性表现。

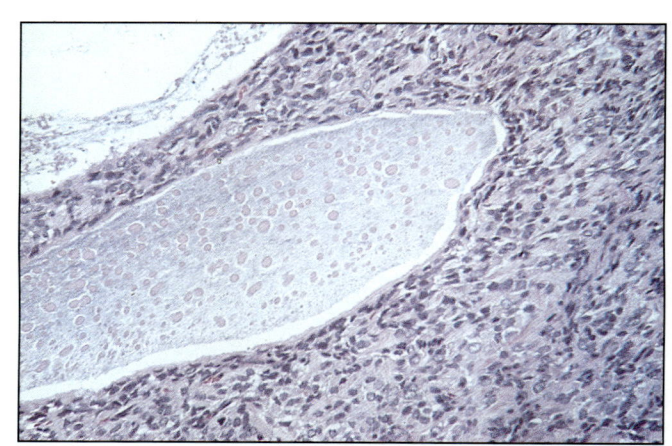

图12.69 肾透明细胞肉瘤。被覆扁平细胞的囊腔，内含蛋白质样及黏液样液体。

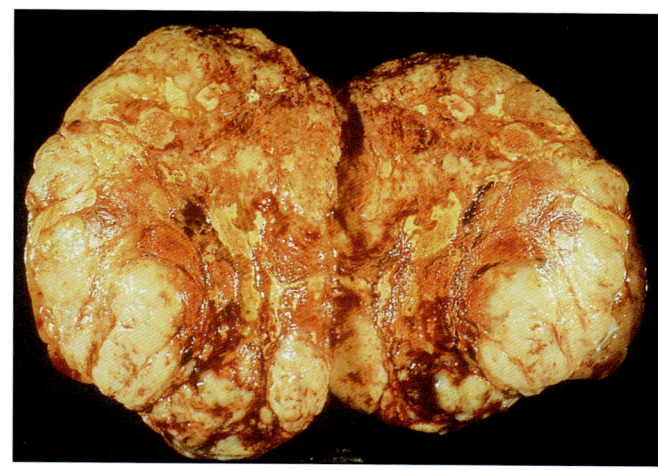

图12.70 肾横纹肌样瘤。大体表现为体积巨大的黄褐色肿物，伴出血及坏死。

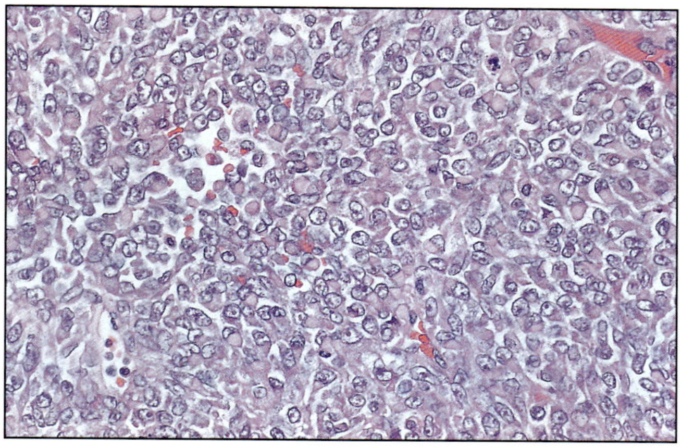

盂常被肿瘤侵犯。肿瘤通常为灰黄色或浅褐色，质脆易碎，边界不清（图12.70）。坏死和出血常见。

组织学表现 显微镜下，肾横纹肌样瘤的典型表现是形态一致的多角形肿瘤细胞弥漫分布，这些细胞中等或偏大，富含嗜酸性胞浆，核圆形，核膜厚，核仁明显（图12.71）。这类肿瘤由于其细胞浆形态类似于分化中的横纹肌母细胞而得名[325]。实际上，这类肿瘤仅仅是细胞形态与骨骼肌相似而已，如果存在骨骼肌分化的确凿证据，该肿瘤就不应诊断为横纹肌样瘤。肿瘤细胞胞浆内常可见到大的嗜酸性包涵体，将细胞核挤向外侧（图12.72）。电镜发现这些包涵体由互相缠结的微丝构成（图12.73）[336]。随着NWTS收集的病例越来越多，其他类型的组织学结构也得到确认，包括硬化性、上皮样、梭形细胞性、淋巴瘤样、血管性、假乳头状和囊性等[331]。

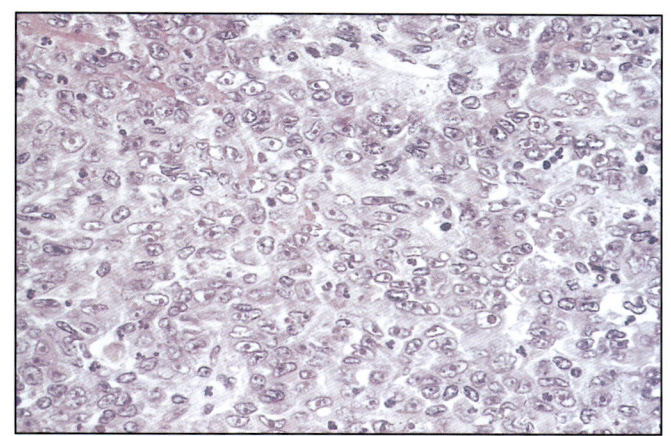

图12.71 肾横纹肌样瘤。显著的大核仁是肾横纹肌样瘤的特点。（Courtesy of Dr. B.Beckwith and the National Wilms' Tumor Study Pathology Center.）

图12.72 肾横纹肌样瘤。胞浆中常可见到球形的嗜酸性包涵体。

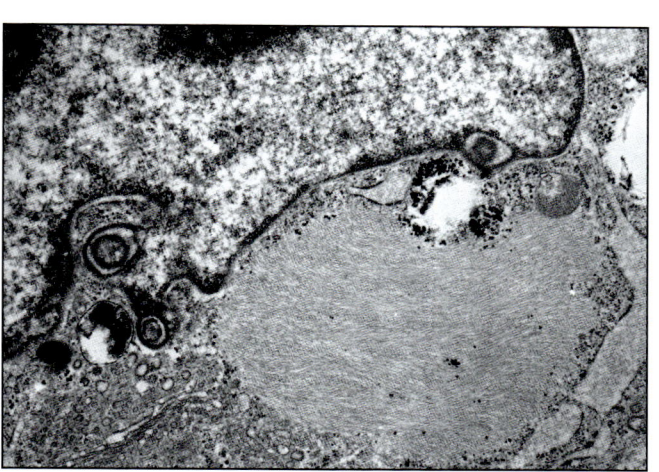

图12.73 肾横纹肌样瘤。电镜下，胞浆包涵体由致密的微丝构成。

这些组织学结构常常与典型的或其他类型的结构混合存在。核仁大而居中以及核膜厚等典型的细胞核特征仍然存在。免疫组化表型存在一定差异，但大部分病例表达波形蛋白（vimentin）和上皮膜抗原（EMA）。

在分子水平，横纹肌样瘤存在22号染色体长臂丢失或片段缺失，导致 *hSNF5/INI1* 基因缺失。这种异常导致INI1蛋白表达的缺失，可以作为一个非常有益的免疫组化标记[337]。

鉴别诊断 横纹肌样瘤的诊断中存在一个很重要的问题，就是很多肾及肾外肿瘤在苏木素-伊红染色切片中与该肿瘤很相似。NWTS研究指出Wilms瘤、先天性中胚层肾瘤、肾细胞癌、移行细胞癌、集合管癌、嗜酸细胞瘤、横纹肌肉瘤、神经内分泌癌以及淋巴瘤都可与肾横纹肌样瘤混淆[338]。在多数病例中，微丝构成的胞浆包涵体或显著的大核仁等特征常导致误诊。传统的光镜检查可以区分大部分病例，而一些组织学表现相似的病例需要借助电镜及免疫组化检查以除外肾横纹肌样瘤。胚芽细胞很少含有提示横纹肌样瘤的包涵体，因此特征性的胚芽组织结构，如结节或蜿蜒形排列，有助于明确诊断。

先天性中胚层肾瘤
Congenital mesoblastic nephroma

尽管所占比例不足儿童原发肾肿瘤的3%，但先天性中胚层肾瘤是3个月内婴幼儿最常见的肾肿瘤，并且几乎不发生于24个月以上的儿童[297,339,340]。有报道称此类肿瘤与羊水过多和早产有关[341,342]。几乎所有病例都表现为腹部肿块。1966年[343]首先认识此病，随后的研究[344]发现这是一种具有独特形态学表现的肿瘤，预后良好。绝大部分患者可经手术切除治愈[345-347]。少数复发及预后不良的病例也有报道，主要是发病年龄超过3个月的婴幼儿[348,349]。这种肿瘤在成年人非常罕见[350,351]。临床特点上，先天性中胚层肾瘤具有浸润性边界，外科病理医师必须认真检查其切缘，因为复发的危险性与切除不完全有关[352,353]。细胞型中胚层肾瘤具有与婴儿纤维肉瘤相同的遗传学改变（见第24章）[354]。

大体表现 相对于婴儿肾来说，多数中胚层肾瘤体积大。肿瘤和肾表面光滑，肾被膜和肾盏因肿瘤挤压而延长。表面膨隆。切面与平滑肌瘤很像：质地坚硬，编织状或小梁状，色泽明亮（图12.74）。肿瘤无包膜，常与周围肾组织交错，并可以延伸至周围组织。少部分病例可出现囊腔、出血以及坏死，尤其是镜下表现为细胞型的病例[355]。

组织学表现 Bolande等[344]描述的组织学类型表现为细胞中等程度增生，由粗大束状交错排列的梭形细胞组成，细胞核细长，肿瘤细胞常常显著侵入肾及肾周组织（图12.75），常见肾小球和肾小管嵌入。随后发现了另外一种更为常见的组织学亚型，表现为更加密集的多角形细胞增生，核分裂象易见，肿瘤边界呈推进式（图12.76）。这种亚型被称为细胞型中胚层肾瘤。这两种组织学亚型常常在同一个肿瘤中混合存在。组织学上，细胞型与后肾间质瘤相似，但后者很少呈浸润性边界，常呈结节状[38]。一些报道认为细胞型容易复发，但正如上文所述，年龄以及切除的完全性与否是预后不好的主要危险因素。鉴于中胚层肾瘤患者总体预后好，而且细胞

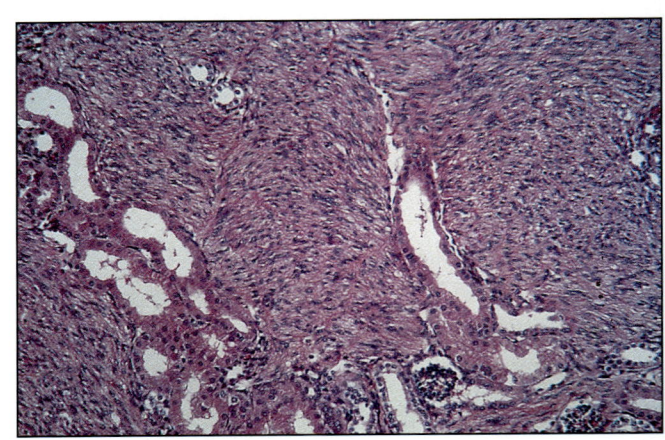

图12.75 中胚层肾瘤。肿瘤与肾组织交界处可见梭形肿瘤细胞浸润肾小管和肾小球之间的间质。

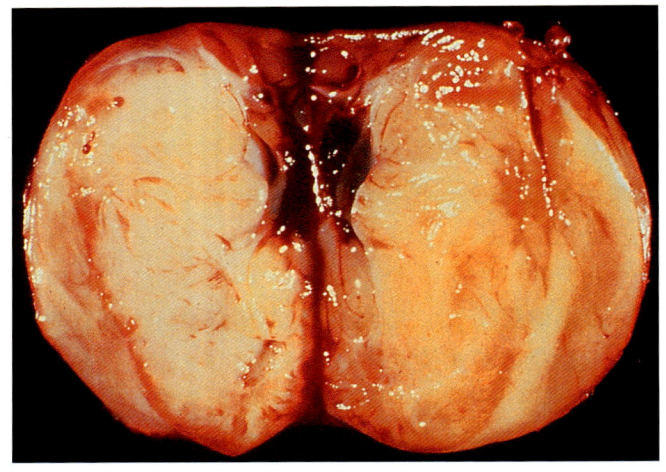

图12.74 中胚层肾瘤。肿瘤由黄褐色、有弹性的分叶状组织构成。

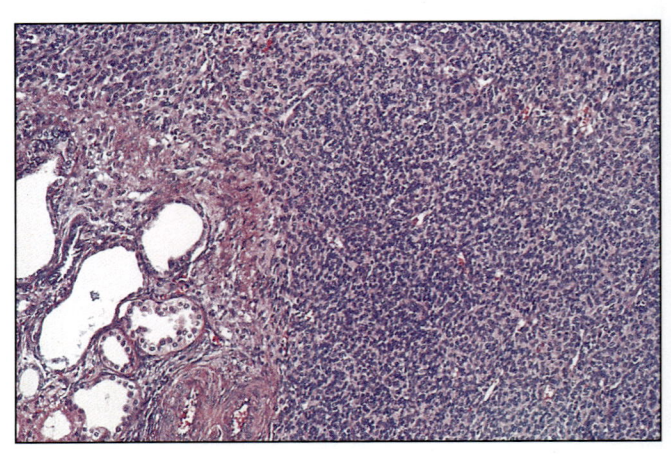

图12.76 中胚层肾瘤，细胞型。肿瘤细胞丰富，细胞呈圆形而不是梭形。

型占多数,因此与手术切除的充分性相比,组织学类型并不是制订治疗方案的主要参考因素。

鉴别诊断 充分考虑形态学表现以及患者的年龄,中胚层肾瘤通常很容易诊断。以间质成分为主的 Wilms 瘤可能会与中胚层肾瘤混淆,尤其是那些术前接受过治疗的病例。记住中胚层肾瘤不存在胚芽组织;Wilms 瘤边界清楚而中胚层肾瘤边界呈浸润性这些特点有助于解决这一难题。发病年龄有助于正确诊断,双侧发生者倾向于 Wilms 瘤。尽管发病年龄组相同,但中胚层肾瘤(即使是细胞型病例)与横纹肌样瘤的区别还是很明显的。

幼儿骨化性肾肿瘤 Ossifying renal tumor of infancy

这种罕见肿瘤的组织学来源不明,文献报道不足 20 例,所有患者年龄均小于 6 个月[356]。男性明显多见,血尿是最常见的症状。影像学检查常表现为集合管系统或肾盂钙化性肿块。尽管边界不规则并呈浸润性,但目前所了解的病例均呈良性临床过程。

大体上,肿瘤质地坚硬如石,突向肾盂腔内,与周边髓质边界不清。显微镜下,肿瘤主要由细胞成分稀少的骨样组织构成,其间可见含小卵圆形泡状核的细胞巢(图 12.77)。这些肥胖细胞比骨细胞大,在病变周边更为多见[357]。核分裂象少见。没有破骨细胞及软骨样组织。

生殖细胞肿瘤 Germ cell neoplasm

肾原发性畸胎瘤罕见且存在争议,因含有原始肾小球和肾小管等不成熟肾组织而难以与 Wilms 瘤区分[358]。所有三个胚层各种组织类型的存在对于诊断非常重要。在 Wilms 瘤并不常见的结构,如淋巴结、含有平滑肌及上皮的胃肠道样组织[359]或毛囊及汗腺[360]等的存在对诊断非常有帮助[359]。但大部分同时含有各种上皮及间质成分的肾肿瘤是 Wilms 瘤。

已有肾原发绒毛膜癌的报道[361]。因为一些高级别移行细胞癌可伴有绒毛膜癌的分化[362],因此这些病例都应该充分检查,以发现明确的移行细胞癌成分。

肾盂及输尿管肿瘤 Tumors of the renal pelvis and ureter

考虑到肾盂、输尿管和膀胱等器官在解剖结构以及接触尿源性致癌因素的相似性,大部分发生于膀胱的肿瘤都可以在其上游尿路各部位出现。下文着重介绍上游泌尿道肿瘤比较独特的表现,如读者需要了解关于这些肿瘤更加全面而详尽的内容,请参考关于膀胱肿瘤的章节。

输尿管原发肿瘤并不常见,且在一篇全面的综述中,Abeshouse[363]发现在此部位的癌比良性肿瘤更为常见。

良性肿瘤及瘤样病变 Benign tumors and tumor-like lesions

肾源性腺瘤 Nephrogenic adenoma

肾源性腺瘤在输尿管罕见,更常见于膀胱(见第 543 页),表现为外生性病变,大体上很像移行细胞癌,组织学上由被覆立方形或鞋钉样上皮细胞的良性乳头状和管状结构组成[364,365]。

内翻性乳头状瘤 Inverted papilloma

内翻性乳头状瘤是一种良性移行细胞肿瘤,在肾盂和输尿管比膀胱少见(见第 524 页)[366,367]。发生在输尿管的病例是肾盂的 2 倍[368]。男性多见,平均发病年龄为 65 岁[368]。在上泌尿道,这些肿瘤都是通过静脉肾盂造影[367]或因血尿偶然发现[369,370]。病变可以多发,并与其他部位尿路上皮癌同时存在[371]。大体表现为广基的半球形病变(图 12.78)。肿瘤由被覆典型移行上皮的乳头状结构组成,某些病例可出现被覆化生性黏液上皮的腺样结构[372]。有关这些肿瘤更加详细的组织学特征将在膀胱肿瘤相关章节介绍(见第 524 页)。少数情况下,移行细胞癌可起源于输尿管内翻性乳头状瘤[373,374]。

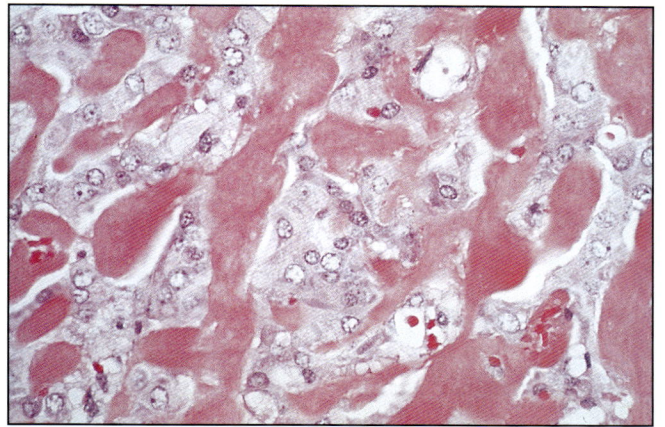

图 12.77 幼儿骨化性肾肿瘤。肿瘤细胞核规则,圆形或卵圆形,染色质粗,胞浆浅,量多少不一,分布于致密骨样基质中。(Courtesy of Dr. B.Beckwith and the National Wilms' Tumor Study Pathology Center.)

肾盂及输尿管肿瘤

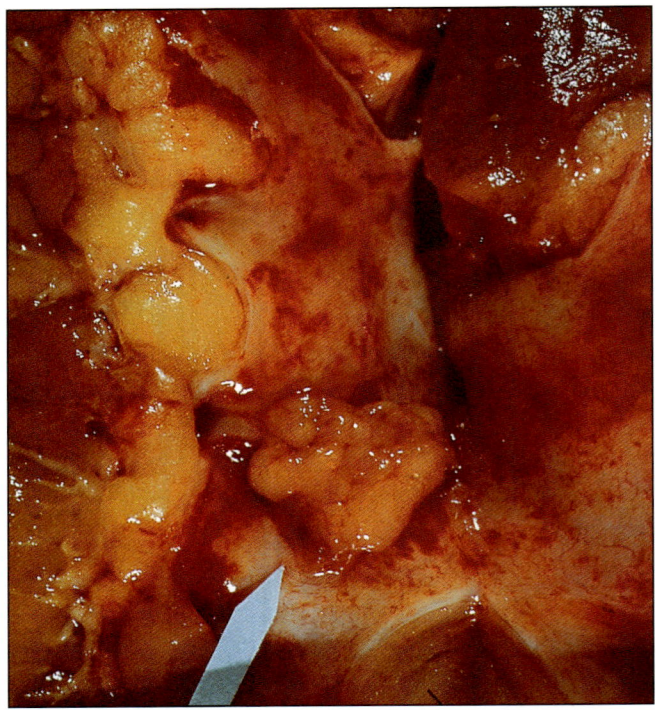

图12.78 肾盂内翻性乳头状瘤。肿瘤基底宽，分叶状，棕褐色。

纤维上皮性息肉　Fibroepithelial polyp

这是一种在肾盂[375]和输尿管[376]不常见的良性间叶性肿瘤。多见于青年和中年人，但儿童[377,378]和老年人[379]也可发生。Macksood等认为这是儿童输尿管最为常见的良性息肉状病变[378]。大部分（70%）患者是男性[380]。肋腹部绞痛和血尿是最常见的症状。大体上，肿瘤由单个或多个起源于黏膜、紧靠在一起且表面光滑而柔软的分叶状组织构成（图12.79）。最常见的发生部位是输尿管肾盂连接处和上段输尿管[381]。病因不明确[381]。

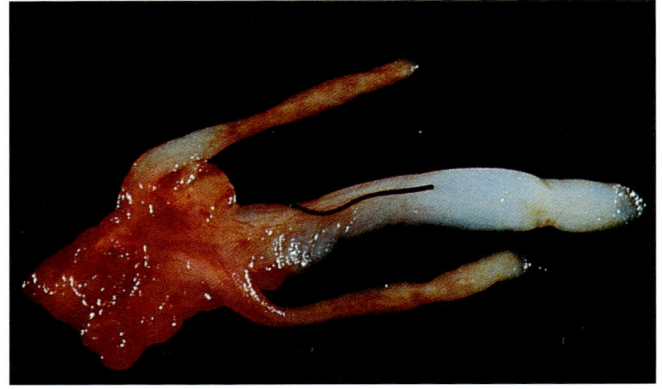

图12.79 输尿管纤维上皮性息肉。三个紧靠一起的位于黏膜表面的细长分叶状肿物。

组织学上，肿瘤具有疏松水肿的纤维血管轴心，可伴有数量不等的炎细胞，被覆正常的尿路上皮，有时可见局灶鳞状上皮化生或溃疡形成。

血管瘤　Hemangioma

发生于输尿管和肾盂的血管瘤是少见的息肉状肿物，由被覆正常移行上皮和富含血管的纤维间质构成[382,383]。发生于儿童和成年人，可以多发，常引起尿路梗阻。

移行细胞癌　Transitional cell carcinoma

上泌尿道移行细胞癌（也称为尿路上皮癌）的流行病学特点与发生于膀胱者相似[384]：男性多见[385]，常见于老年人，吸烟[386]和接触工业致癌物是危险因素。非那西汀的滥用[387,388]在某些人群中是最重要的危险因素，占肾盂肿瘤的近1/4，输尿管肿瘤的10%以上。Balkan肾病以及含钍的造影增强剂[389]是上泌尿道而不是膀胱移行细胞癌的危险因素。肾盂和肾盏肿瘤大约是输尿管肿瘤的两倍[385]。血尿是主要的临床症状，而肋腹部疼痛也很常见[390]。多灶性发生是上泌尿道肿瘤的显著特点[385,391]。近50%的患者有膀胱、输尿管移行细胞癌的病史或后来发生移行细胞癌[392,393]。在输尿管，最常见的发生部位是远端[394]。分级和分期是上泌尿道移行细胞癌最重要的预后指标，而肿瘤的多灶性也有一定的影响[391]。大约75%的病例是低级别和1期肿瘤[395]。分级系统与膀胱肿瘤相同，而分期系统与膀胱肿瘤相似。AJCC分期系统如表12.9所示[396]。手术切除时为1级和1期的肿瘤对患者的生存几乎没有影响[397]。肌层的侵犯是肿瘤进展的重要指标，它的出现使患者生存期显著下降[393]。肺是最常见的转移部位[398]。鉴于肿瘤远端输尿管的高复发率（>15%），包括部分膀胱袖口状切除在内的肾输尿管切除是首选术式[399]。

大体表现　大体表现与膀胱肿瘤相似，而那些体积较大的乳头状肿瘤常常充满肾盂腔或输尿管腔（图12.80），导致梗阻而引起肾积水（图12.81）。大的肾盂肿瘤可呈浸润性生长，广泛侵犯肾实质，甚至扩散至皮质外脂肪组织，表现为边界不清、质地非常坚硬的肿物（图12.82）。有时这些肿瘤几乎见不到肾盂黏膜起源的证据，需要广泛取材来证实。

组织学表现　上泌尿道移行细胞癌组织病理学改变与膀胱肿瘤相同，包括向鳞状上皮或腺样分化以及肉瘤样（图12.83）[91,400]和小细胞亚型[401]。罕见类型，如滋养层细胞分化（图12.84）和破骨细胞型巨细胞样肿瘤[402,402a]已有报道。当以肉瘤样成分为主，而上皮成

表12.9 肾盂及输尿管癌的病理TNM分期[396]

原发肿瘤（T）

- TX　原发肿瘤不能评估
- T0　无原发肿瘤证据
- Ta　非浸润性乳头状癌
- Tis　原位癌
- T1　肿瘤浸润到上皮下结缔组织
- T2　肿瘤浸润到肌层
- T3　（肾盂）肿瘤浸润超过肌层，浸润肾盂周围脂肪或肾实质
- T3　（输尿管）肿瘤浸润超过肌层，浸润输尿管周围脂肪组织
- T4　肿瘤浸润邻近器官或穿透肾浸润肾周脂肪

局部淋巴结（N）*

- NX　局部淋巴结不能评估
- N0　无局部淋巴结转移
- N1　单个淋巴结转移，最大直径≤2cm
- N2　单个淋巴结转移，直径2~5cm；或多个淋巴结转移，最大直径≤5cm
- N3　淋巴结转移，直径>5cm

* 注：同侧或对侧淋巴结转移的N分期没有差别

远处转移（M）

- MX　远处转移不能评估
- M0　无远处转移
- M1　远处转移

分组分期

分期	T	N	M
0a 期	Ta	N0	M0
0is 期	Tis	N0	M0
I 期	T1	N0	M0
II 期	T2	N0	M0
III 期	T3	N0	M0
IV 期	T4	N0	M0
	任何T	N1	M0
	任何T	N2	M0
	任何T	N3	M0
	任何T	任何N	M1

组织病理学类型

组织类型如下

尿路上皮(移行细胞)癌
鳞状细胞癌
表皮样癌
腺癌

组织学分级

- GX　分级不能评估
- G1　高分化
- G2　中分化
- G3-4　低分化或未分化

Used with permission of the American Joint Committee on Cancer (AJCC®), Chicago, Illinois. The original source for this material is the AJCC® Cancer Staging Manual, 5th Edition (1997) published by Lippincott-Raven Publishers, Philadelphia, Pennsylvania.

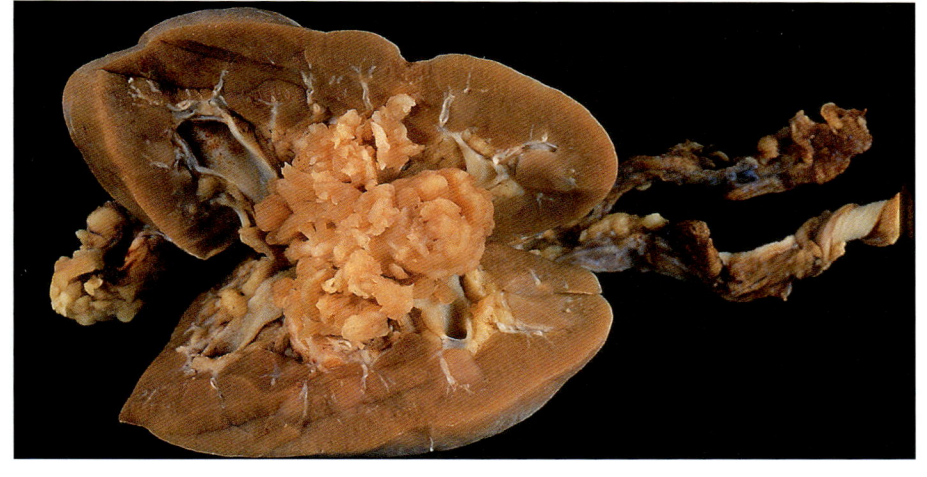

图12.80　肾盂移行细胞癌。乳头状肿物充满肾盂腔。

分不明显时，免疫组化和电镜检查有助于诊断[91,400]。基因图谱研究发现，所有肾盂和输尿管移行细胞癌都与标本其他部位黏膜中从增生到原位癌的各种病变有关[403]。

有研究发现肾盂和输尿管固有层毛细血管周基底膜的增厚是过度服用止痛剂的组织学标志，被称为毛细血管硬化病[387]。

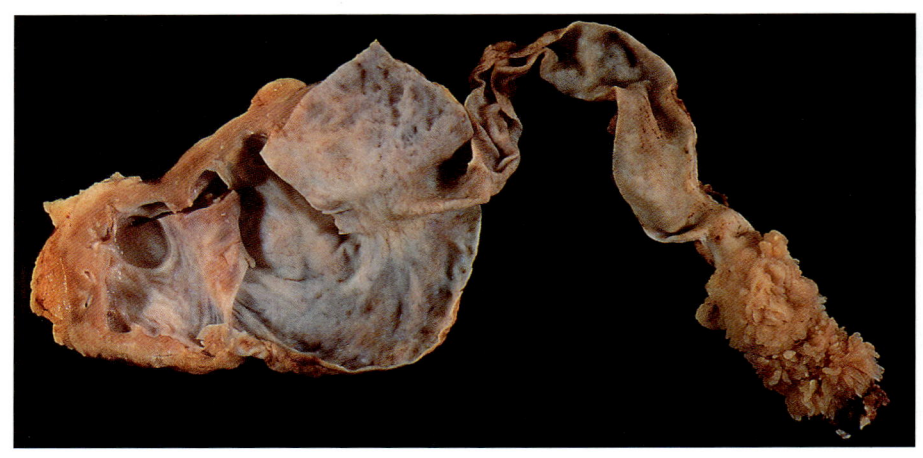

图12.81 输尿管移行细胞癌。乳头状肿物阻塞尿道，导致输尿管和肾积水。

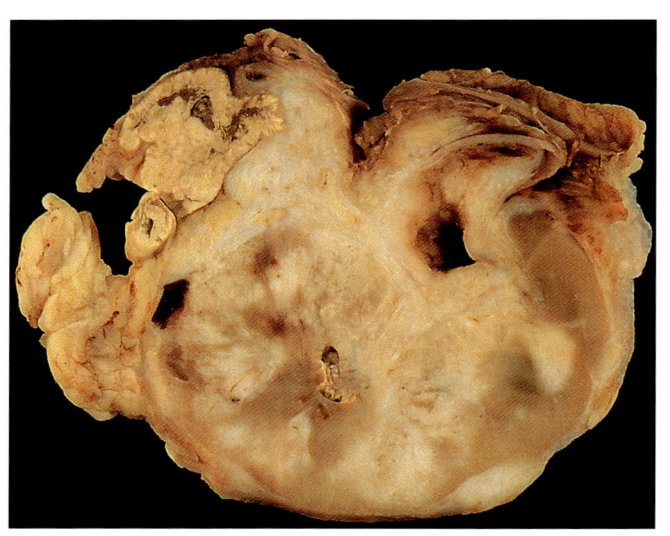

图12.82 肾盂移行细胞癌。高级别癌广泛浸润肾实质，无法分辨是否为肾盂起源。

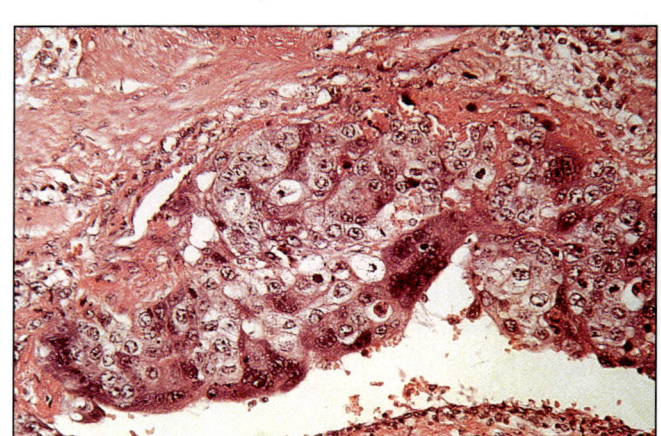

图12.84 肾盂移行细胞癌。肾盂癌出现滋养细胞分化。(Courtesy of Dr. D. Grignon.)

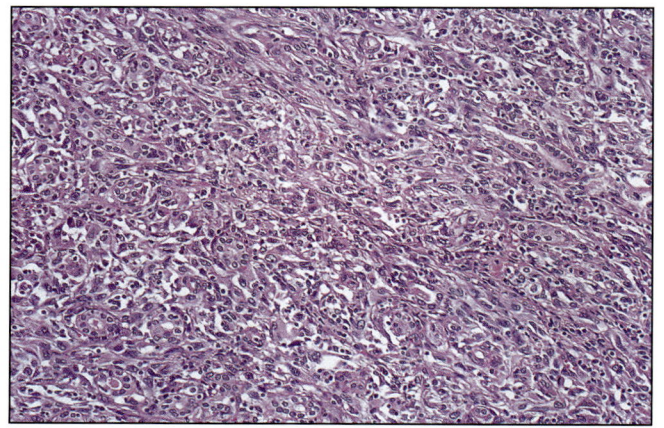

图12.83 肾盂移行细胞癌。肉瘤样癌的多形性梭形肿瘤细胞浸润肾，其中可见少许残存的肾小管。

腺癌　Adenocarcinoma

上泌尿道原发性腺癌罕见，主要是个案和小规模病例报道[404-409]。多数患者是成年人，但儿童也可发生[410]。结石、慢性炎症和感染似乎都是易感因素。腺样化生[411,412]可能是前驱病变，有时在肿瘤附近可以见到非浸润癌的存在。常见乳头状结构和类似于结肠黏液腺癌的病变（图12.85）。一个病例出现肝细胞样分化并含有胆色素[408]。

鳞状细胞癌　Squamous cell carcinoma

大约10%的肾盂肿瘤是鳞状细胞癌[413]，而输尿管鳞状细胞癌所占比例更小。结石和慢性感染常与鳞状细胞癌有关。与鳞状上皮化生的关系存在很大争议，一些

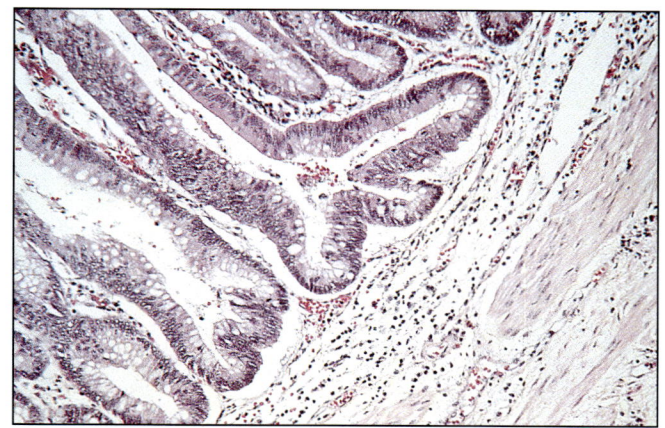

图12.85 肾盂腺癌。肿瘤由核异型性明显的柱状细胞组成，很像结肠腺癌。

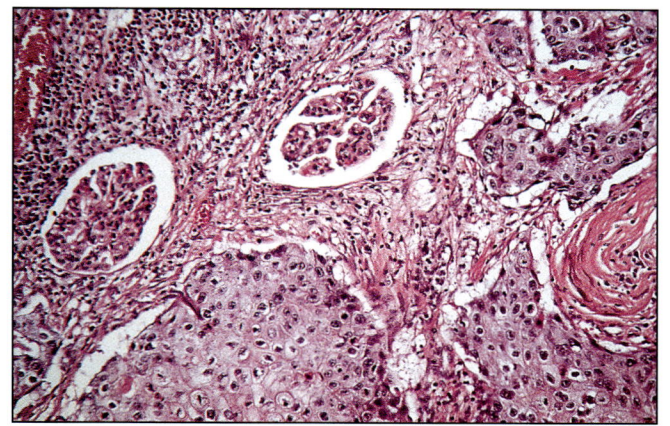

图12.86 肾盂鳞状细胞癌。角化性癌细胞浸润肾实质。

研究发现两者存在显著的相关性[414]，而另外的研究则未发现它们之间的相关性[415]。这些不同的结果可能是由于上泌尿道鳞状细胞癌比较罕见的原因。晚期肿瘤常见[416]，因此总体预后不佳[414]。这些肿瘤的组织病理学表现与发生于膀胱者相同（图12.86）。肾实质的广泛浸润很常见，5年生存率很低[414]。需要与转移性鳞状细胞癌鉴别，充分考虑临床和病理学特点后常比较容易诊断。罕见的无移行细胞癌成分的肾盂腺鳞癌已有报道，其发生与鹿角样结石有关[417]。

其他肿瘤　Other tumors

平滑肌肿瘤是肾盂和输尿管最常见的间叶来源肿瘤，平滑肌瘤[418,419]和平滑肌肉瘤[420,421]都已有报道。其他类型的肉瘤，如骨源性肉瘤[422]和恶性外周神经鞘瘤[423]非常罕见。肾盂黏膜也可以发生恶性黑色素瘤[424]。大约16%播散性淋巴瘤可浸润上游尿路，引起尿路梗阻[425]。

膀胱肿瘤　Tumors of the bladder

在以下关于膀胱和尿道的章节中，讨论的方法与前一节相似，主要关注常规切片中所涉及的鉴别诊断方面的实际问题。主要讨论各种肿瘤之间的鉴别，但在膀胱和尿道可遇到很多在大体和(或)显微镜下类似肿瘤的非肿瘤性病变[426]，因此这些病变也会谈及。表12.10列出了膀胱肿瘤的分类。

良性上皮性肿瘤　Benign epithelial tumors

乳头状瘤　Papillomas

膀胱乳头状瘤可以分为经典型和内翻性[427]；偶尔一种类型可混有少部分另一类型成分，但明显存在两种类型成分的病例罕见。在以前的文献中，乳头状瘤这一术语被广泛应用于如今通常称为1级乳头状移行细胞癌或低度恶性潜能肿瘤。由于大多数低级别乳头状移行细胞癌的预后很好，有学者建议恢复使用以前的命名[428]，但最近的研究[429,430]更加明确存在一种良性的乳头状移行细胞肿瘤，因此将乳头状瘤这一术语应用于这些肿瘤。

经典型乳头状瘤　Typical papilloma

这种病变罕见，按严格的诊断标准，占乳头状尿路上皮病变的比例不足1%。主要见于中年人，男性稍多见。大体表现为小的赘生物或纤细的分叶状病变。显微镜下，由单个或簇状乳头构成，被覆非常类似于正常的尿路上皮，盖细胞（umbrella cell）明显（图12.87）[429,430]。与典型的乳头状癌相比，乳头常常短而宽，但有时也可见细长的乳头结构。细胞层次通常少于7层，细胞缺乏或仅有轻微非典型性，核分裂象缺如或罕见，即使存在也位于基底层。上皮细胞可伴有一系列改变如空泡样变、退行性非典型性和大汗腺样胞浆[430]。

鉴别诊断　典型乳头状瘤的乳头可有分支，但无乳头状癌那样的复杂分支。此外，乳头被覆的尿路上皮细胞层次常少于7层，少于乳头状癌的细胞层次。即使细胞不超过7层，乳头状癌被覆细胞的非典型性仍很明显。乳头状瘤的盖细胞比乳头状癌更为常见。最后，尽管分裂象罕见并不是除外乳头状瘤的必要条件，但大量核分裂象的存在强烈支持癌的诊断。

良性上皮性肿瘤

表12.10　膀胱肿瘤组织学分类

良性上皮肿瘤
经典型乳头状瘤
内翻性乳头状瘤
绒毛状腺瘤
脐尿管黏液性囊腺瘤
鳞状细胞乳头状瘤

恶性上皮肿瘤
移行细胞癌
乳头状　　　　　　非乳头状
　（i）非浸润性　　　（i）移行细胞原位癌
　（ii）浸润性　　　　（ii）浸润性移行细胞癌
亚型：
- 伴鳞状分化和/或腺性分化
- 肉瘤样癌
- 微囊状癌
- 伴滋养叶分化
- 伴假肉瘤样间质
- 伴间质骨样或软骨样化生
- 伴破骨细胞样巨细胞

鳞状细胞癌
亚型：
- 疣状癌

腺癌
亚型：
- 经典肠型
- 黏液型（包括胶样）
- 印戒细胞型
- 透明细胞型
- 非特指型

未分化癌
亚型：
- 小细胞癌
- 巨细胞癌
- 淋巴上皮瘤样癌
- 非特指型

含有一种以上组织学类型的癌

间叶肿瘤
良性
恶性：
- 平滑肌肉瘤
- 横纹肌肉瘤
- 其他

混合性肿瘤
腺纤维瘤和腺肉瘤
癌肉瘤

淋巴造血肿瘤
淋巴瘤
白血病
浆细胞瘤

其他原发性肿瘤
副神经节瘤
类癌
恶性黑色素瘤
皮样囊肿
卵黄囊瘤

转移性肿瘤

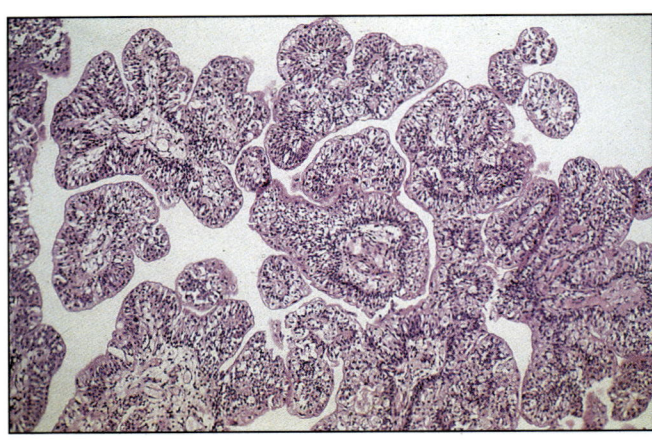

图12.87　膀胱经典型乳头状瘤。许多小而短粗的乳头，未见尿路上皮增生，可见大量盖细胞。

内翻性乳头状瘤　Inverted papilloma

内翻性乳头状瘤大约占肾盂、输尿管、膀胱和尿道所有肿瘤的2%[431,432]。大部分发生于膀胱。男女比率为9:1。患者平均年龄57岁[431]，最常见的症状是尿路梗阻和血尿。约80%的病变发生于三角区或膀胱颈。大体检查可见孤立、表面光滑程度不同或分叶状的息肉样肿物。常见宽大的基底部，但也可以有蒂。较小的病灶常常是结节状而不是息肉状。

根据镜下表现的不同，内翻性乳头状瘤可以分为梁状型和腺管型两种类型[431]。在一项对40位患者进行的研究中，25例为腺管型而15例为梁状型[431]。而我们的资料显示，梁状型更为常见。肿瘤细胞丰富，由相互吻合的小梁和细胞巢构成，被覆正常的尿路上皮（图12.88）。周围的细胞栅栏状排列与皮肤基底细胞癌相似（图12.89）。漩涡状结构的存在提示不完全的鳞状上皮化生，但明显的角化性鳞状细胞化生罕见。小梁和细胞巢中常常掺杂有囊状区（图12.90），腔内含有嗜酸性分泌物，囊壁被覆扁平上皮细胞。相反，腺管型由被覆黏液上皮的腺管样结构组成（图12.91）。罕见的情况下，被覆内翻性乳头状瘤的尿路上皮表面呈小的乳头状突起，很像经典型乳头状瘤。内翻性乳头状瘤常出现轻度细胞非典型性和极低的核分裂活性，然而一项研究发现15%病变"具有不同程度的核异常和核分裂活性增高"[431]。另一项新近的文献报道了其他各种不常见的组织学表现：明显的核仁；鳞状上皮化生，有时伴异型增生；移行细胞异型增生；可见巨细胞[432]。

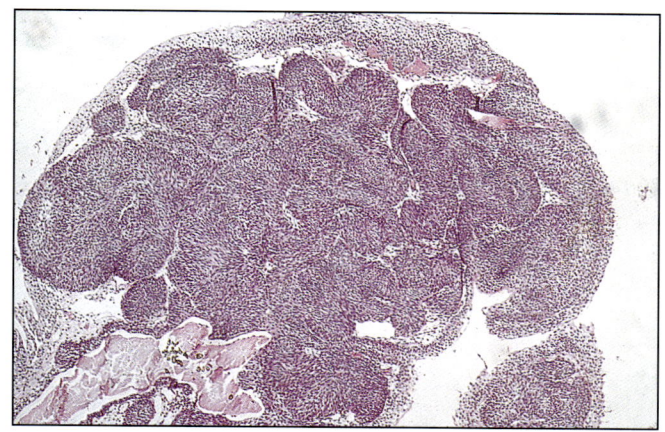

图12.88 膀胱内翻性乳头状瘤。息肉样结节被覆正常的尿路上皮,其下是基底细胞样细胞构成的相互吻合的小梁。

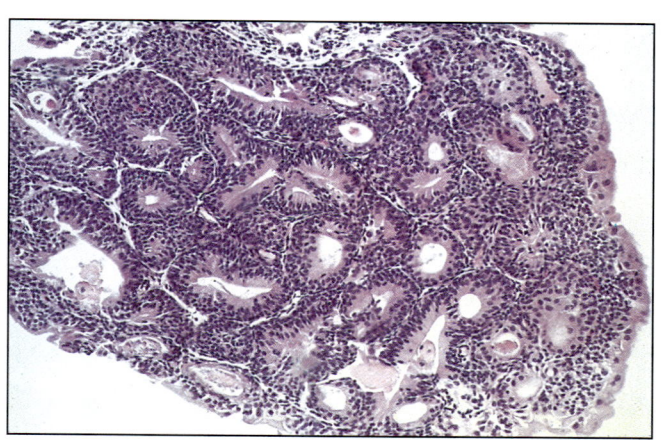

图12.91 膀胱内翻性乳头状瘤,腺管型。

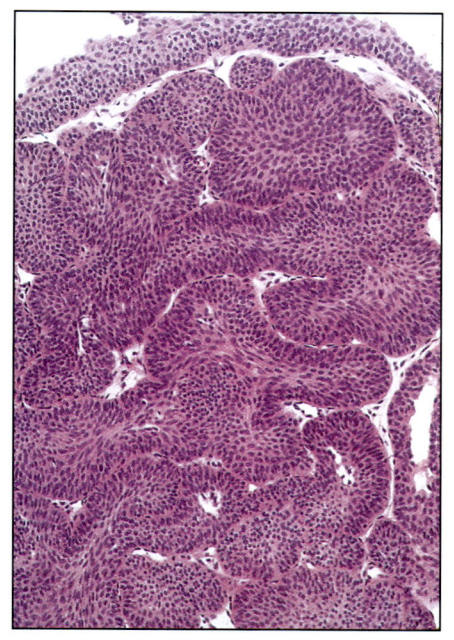

图12.89 梁状内翻性乳头状瘤。外周细胞呈栅栏状排列。

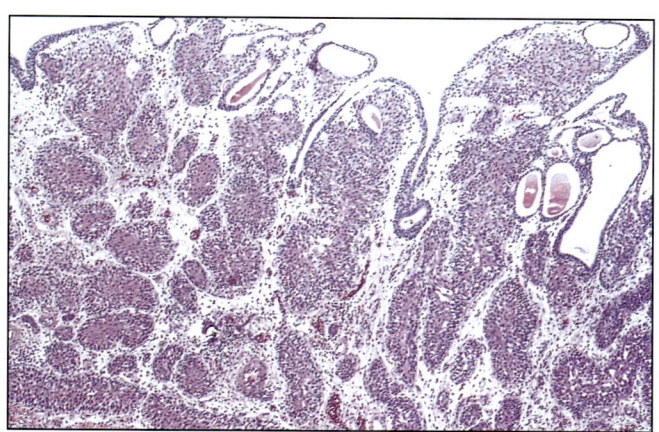

图12.92 内翻性生长的移行细胞癌。癌细胞不规则浸润深部组织,其表浅部分呈相对规则的小梁状和巢状。

鉴别诊断 内翻性乳头状瘤必须与相对罕见的呈内翻性生长的浸润性移行细胞癌鉴别(图12.92)[433]。后者呈较大的、界限清楚的圆形及卵圆形细胞巢推进式地浸润间质,而不是如下文所描述的更为常见的不规则或触须状浸润方式。与内翻性乳头状瘤生长方式相似的浸润性癌的细胞非典型性及分裂活性与前者不同,而且常常可以看到更为典型的浸润性癌的区域。角化性鳞状上皮化生在内翻性乳头状瘤很罕见,它的出现提示病变是癌的可能性大。此外,内翻性乳头状瘤只有很少的外生性成分,呈内翻性生长方式的肿瘤中显著乳头状结构的存在也提示癌。在一项对20例最初诊断为内翻性乳头状瘤的病例进行的回顾研究中,2例被修正为低级别移行细胞癌[434]。患者可能会同时患有内翻性乳头状瘤和移行细胞癌,上述研究中20%的患者就属于这种情况。有时候高度增生型von Brunn巢与发育中的小内翻性乳头状瘤很难区分,尽管两者的鉴别在临床上并不重要。

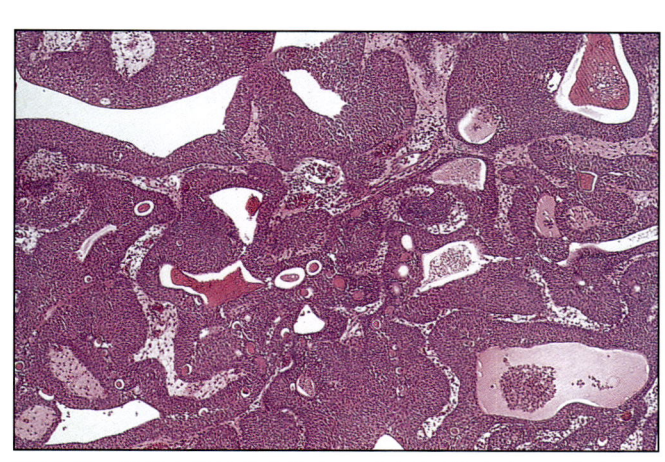

图12.90 膀胱内翻性乳头状瘤。可见明显的大小不一的囊腔。

鳞状细胞乳头状瘤　Squamous papilloma

鳞状细胞乳头状瘤罕见[434a]。做出这个诊断应该慎重，因为很多膀胱鳞状细胞癌可出现轻微异型性区域和乳头状结构，因此在小活检标本中出现错误诊断是可能的。

绒毛状腺瘤　Villous adenoma

从膀胱腺性病变总体来看，膀胱绒毛状腺瘤可以是脐尿管来源[435]或非脐尿管来源[436-438]。组织学表现（图12.93）类似于肠道绒毛状腺瘤。这种良性腺性病变主要与腺癌鉴别，两者可以同时存在[437,438]。绒毛状腺瘤规则的组织结构、位置表浅以及缺乏浸润和恶性细胞核特征都与腺癌不同。需要强调的是乳头状腺癌表浅部分可以类似于绒毛状腺瘤，因此后者的诊断需要慎重。

由于所提供的资料较少，一些文献报道的脐尿管良性腺性肿瘤很难证实。然而这些病变有些很像肠道绒毛状腺瘤[435]。一旦确定了脐尿管起源，即使在肌层出现腺管成分也不是恶性的征象，而只是脐尿管正常解剖学管道。除了位于膀胱顶这一点外，这些病变与非脐尿管源性绒毛状腺瘤并无显著差异。

黏液性囊腺瘤　Mucinous cystadenoma

虽然大部分脐尿管多房状囊性肿瘤常是高分化腺癌，但 Eble 等回顾总结文献发现脐尿管也可以发生黏液性囊腺瘤[435]。脐尿管黏液性囊腺瘤的诊断需要慎重，因为很多脐尿管囊腺癌可以存在局灶相对分化较好的成分。囊腺瘤的诊断只有在对病变充分取材确定不存在浸润和明显细胞异型性的情况下才能做出。膀胱也可以发生类似于卵巢那样的黏液性肿瘤谱系中的肿瘤[439]。

移行细胞癌　Transitional cell carcinoma

膀胱移行细胞癌（也称为尿路上皮癌）是全世界肿瘤发病和死亡的主要原因之一。常见于 50 岁以上患者，有时年轻人也可以发生，但儿童罕见。男性大约是女性的 3 倍。移行细胞癌的流行病学很有特点，因为它的发生与接触苯胺染料[440-442]和吸烟有关，并已经得到了证实。与肾细胞癌不同，膀胱癌很少出现全身症状、副肿瘤综合征或转移等。大多数患者表现为血尿，尽管排尿困难也很常见，但主要发生在高级别肿瘤患者[443]。

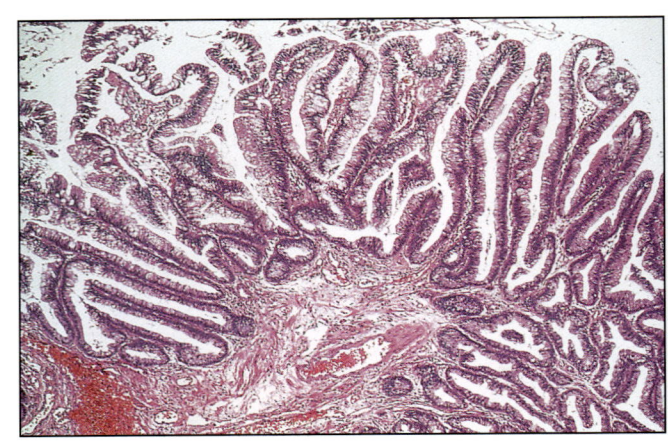

图 12.93　膀胱绒毛状腺瘤。

移行细胞癌传统上分为两种类型：乳头状和非乳头状（扁平广基型）。非浸润性乳头状癌约占原发性膀胱移行细胞癌的 25%。然而其中 10%~20% 患者可以发展为浸润性癌。从另外一个角度来看，大约 20% 浸润性膀胱癌患者先前存在非浸润性乳头状病变[444-446]。乳头状肿瘤患者临床病程可以很长，多年后才发展为浸润性癌。2 级乳头状肿瘤，特别是相对少见的 3 级肿瘤，发病时已存在浸润性癌的可能性更高。

乳头状移行细胞癌　Papillary transitional cell carcinoma

大体表现　这种病变绝大部分经膀胱镜检查发现，而较少见于膀胱切除标本，其大体表现多种多样（图12.94 和 12.95）。某些仅表现为小的乳头状赘生物，另一些可表现为体积巨大的融合乳头状肿物，呈"菜花样"外观，充满或几乎充满整个膀胱。肿瘤质地软、纤细、易碎，呈白色、棕褐色、粉红色或红色。常呈多灶性（图12.94）。常规切片中非浸润性肿瘤基底部与正常膀胱组织分界明显（图12.95）。

组织学表现　乳头状移行细胞癌由多个细长（图12.96）且常有分支的乳头构成。乳头可以相互分离或融合，特别是在基底部（图12.97）。乳头被覆细胞常超过

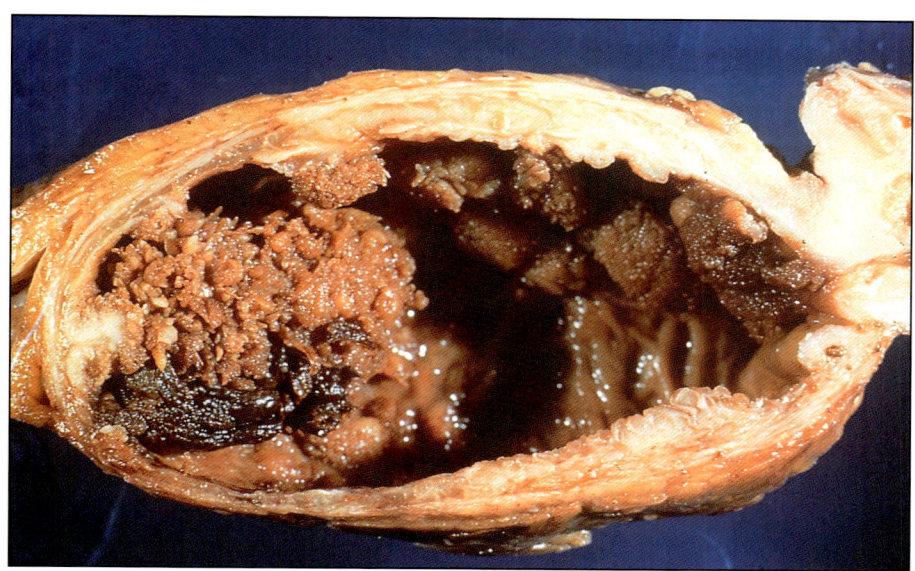

图12.94　膀胱乳头状移行细胞癌。切开的膀胱标本左侧壁可见巨大的乳头状肿瘤，右侧壁及顶部可见一些较小的肿瘤。

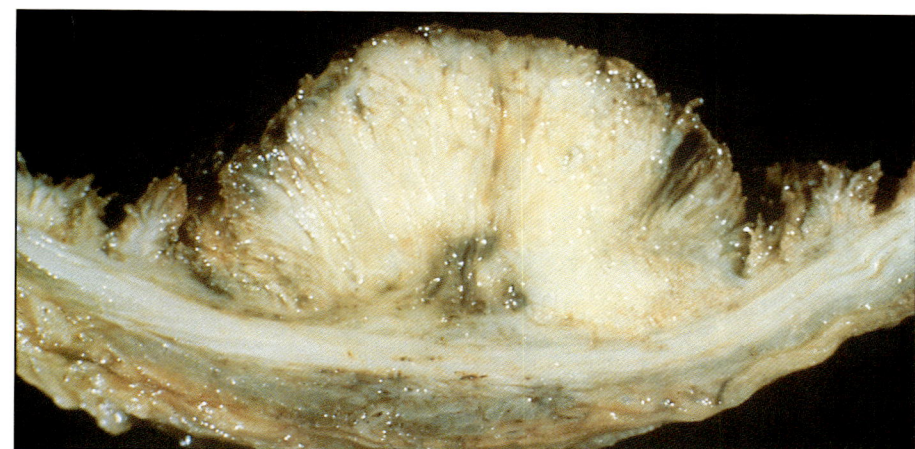

图12.95　膀胱乳头状移行细胞癌。肿瘤与其下的间质分界很明显。

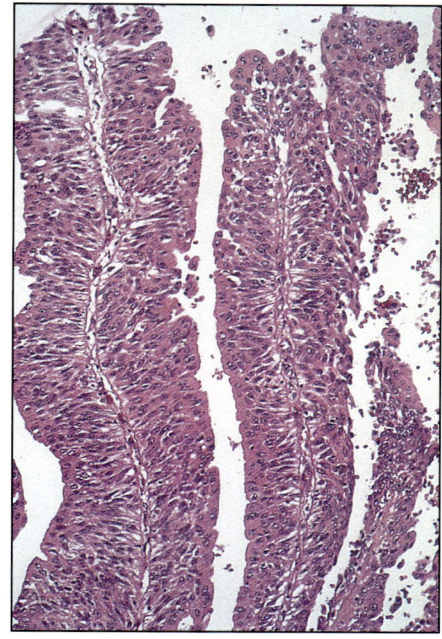

图12.96　膀胱乳头状移行细胞癌。细长的指状乳头是这种肿瘤的特点。

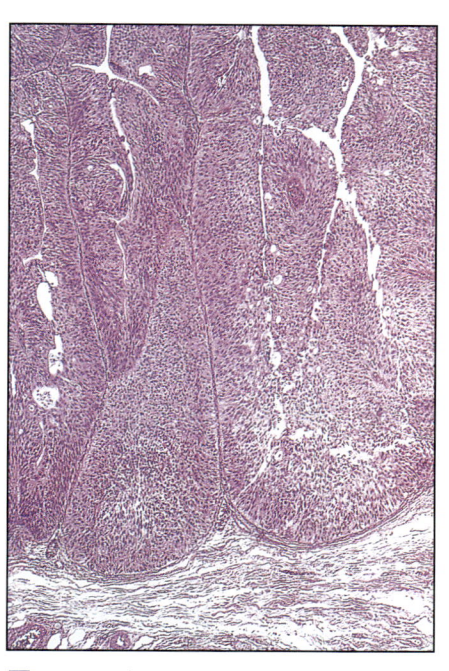

图12.97　膀胱乳头状移行细胞癌。在基底部乳头紧密相连。

移行细胞癌

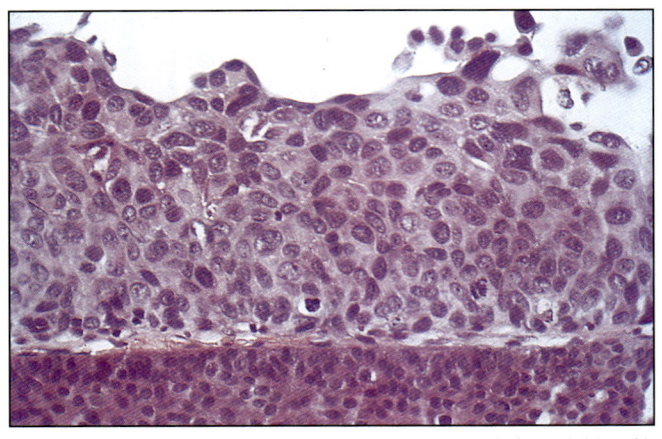

图12.98 膀胱乳头状移行细胞癌，2/3级。肿瘤细胞异型性中等，核分裂象易见。

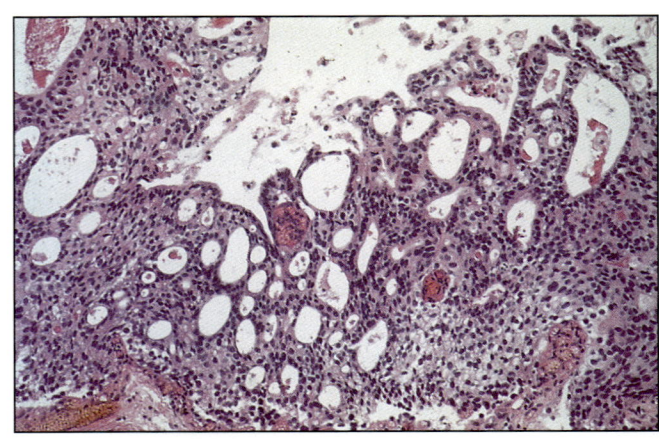

图12.99 伴腺性分化的膀胱乳头状移行细胞癌。

7层，细胞形态从接近正常到高度异型（图12.98）。胞浆常为中等量、弱嗜酸性，但有时胞浆丰富、强嗜酸性。乳头状癌根据细胞学标准进行分级，而且这种分级具有重要的预后意义。常用的是3级分级体系。1级病变尿路上皮细胞层次增加，细胞异型性较小，核分裂象罕见。2级病变细胞异型性中等，核分裂象可见。3级病变至少局部可见明显异型的肿瘤细胞，核分裂象易见。最近，有学者建议对分类和分级体系进行修订（表12.11）[447]。

表12.11	1998年世界卫生组织/国际泌尿病理协会公认的尿路上皮肿瘤分类

正常，包括以前诊断为轻度异型增生的病变
增生，扁平和乳头状
伴非典型性的扁平病变
反应性非典型性
意义不明的非典型性
异型增生
原位癌，包括以前诊断为重度异型增生的病变
乳头状肿瘤
乳头状瘤，经典型和内翻性
低度恶性潜能的乳头状肿瘤
乳头状癌，低级别
乳头状癌，高级别
浸润性肿瘤
浸润固有层
浸润肌层

因为目前有学者认为低级别乳头状移行细胞肿瘤是良性肿瘤，而有些学者则认为它们是低级别癌，这种对分类和分级体系进行修订的建议就是希望在一定程度上解决这种争议。腺性或鳞状上皮化生主要发生于中分化及低分化浸润性移行细胞癌，而在非浸润性乳头状癌并不常见，但有时可非常显著（图12.99）。腺性或鳞状上皮成分的分化程度与移行细胞癌相似。乳头轴心纤细，含有中等量的血管，偶尔结缔组织中出现炎细胞。它们并不表现为浸润性癌那样的间质，但有时水肿很明显，使病变呈息肉样而不是乳头状。一些病例的间质玻璃样变很明显，常伴血管壁的玻璃样变。罕见情况下，乳头出现梗死及钙化。

乳头状浸润癌的肿瘤形态与下文描述的非乳头状癌相似。间质浸润罕见于1级乳头状癌，除非非常明确，否则不应诊断。评判乳头状癌的浸润可能非常困难。乳头基底部横断面会给人固有层出现游离细胞巢的印象，酷似浸润。这些区域中血管的存在提示可能是乳头的边缘。乳头状癌可伴有von Brunn巢等非浸润癌成分，因此类似浸润（图12.100）。这些病变边界清楚，圆形或卵圆形，有助于它们与真正浸润的区分。乳头状癌的乳头基底部偶尔膨胀性生长，呈推进式突向间质，有时会挤压固有层使之紧邻固有肌层。浸润通常见于乳头基底部，但罕见的情况下也可以出现在乳头轴心。

鉴别诊断 乳头状癌与尿路上皮增生的鉴别通常并不困难，但由于乳头状癌由尿路上皮增生发展而来[448,449]，因此对乳头状尿路上皮增生和乳头状癌诊断的分界点存在争议并不意外。这些情况常常发生在有乳

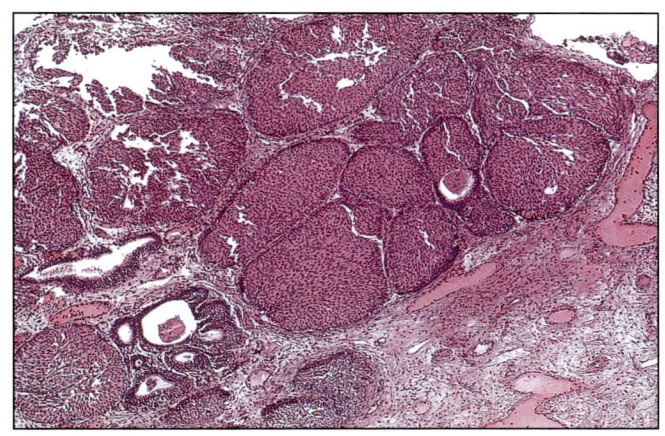

图12.100 累及 von Brunn 巢的低级别乳头状移行细胞癌，病灶膨胀生长酷似浸润。注意膨大的von Brunn 巢轮廓光滑。

头状癌病史的患者；既然这些患者仍然处于临床观察之下，因此这个问题通常不会引起临床困境。乳头状癌与乳头状瘤的鉴别已在上文讨论。

将乳头状癌与乳头状或息肉状膀胱炎区分开来很重要（图12.101）[450]。乳头状膀胱炎的乳头被覆正常的尿路上皮，盖细胞通常很明显，这一特征罕见于乳头状癌。乳头状癌中粗大的乳头常常出现小的乳头分支，这一现象在乳头状或息肉状膀胱炎中并不出现。尽管存在这些区别，乳头状膀胱炎和1级乳头状癌有可能还是难以区分。息肉状膀胱炎宽大的乳头比大部分乳头状癌的乳头粗大。与乳头状癌相比，乳头状和息肉状膀胱炎的纤维间质轴心通常具有更多的炎细胞和血管成分；尽管不能决定诊断，但却是一个诊断线索。患者的临床情况（如内置导管的留置或膀胱窦道的存在），都可能与乳头状或息肉状膀胱炎有关，对诊断很有帮助[450]。

移行细胞癌（非乳头状）
Transitional cell carcinoma (non-papillary)

移行细胞原位癌 Transitional cell carcinoma in situ

膀胱尿路上皮可出现一系列非典型病变，从细胞学不明显的轻度异型增生到明显恶性的移行细胞原位癌。正如身体其他部位发生的上皮癌前病变一样，对膀胱这些病变的理解也有很大的主观性。从外科病理医师的角度，在这方面最重要的是确定没有漏诊那些高级别的病变，包括重度异型增生或移行细胞原位癌（两者的处理手段常常相同）。尽管应对存在的轻度或中度异型增生做出诊断，但将其漏诊或误诊为反应性增生不会引起严重的不良后果。诊断为重度异型增生或移行细胞原位癌的病变必须出现与3级浸润性癌形态相同的肿瘤细胞。需要进一步了解膀胱癌前病变的读者可以参考早期经典的文献和其他更新的文献和综述[451-462]，其中两篇还讨论了起源于原位癌的早期浸润癌[461,462]。

大体检查，膀胱黏膜发生移行细胞原位癌的部位通常发红，也可以表现为细颗粒状，或常常由于水肿而呈球状隆起。镜下，异常尿路上皮的厚度相差很大，表现为单层、正常或增生。即使只有一层细胞，根据重度细胞非典型性也可诊断原位癌。病变细胞常常出现多形性，但有时形态相对一致。细胞连接的缺失（图12.102）以及与基底膜的分离，导致尿路上皮脱落。常常造成只有单层肿瘤细胞残留，有些病例可出现大范围的黏膜完全脱落。遇到这种活检标本时，病理医师必须仔细检查，不能漏过哪怕一小团高度不典型细胞。这些病例常需要进行深切，同时要紧密结合尿液细胞学的检查结果，因为原位癌的细胞学标本常常可以见到恶性细胞。过去，存在

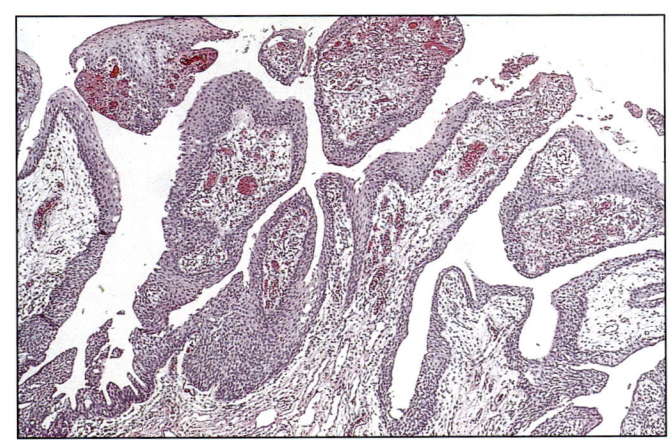

图12.101 乳头状/息肉状膀胱炎。儿童膀胱中出现乳头状及息肉状结构，它们的纤维轴心可见明显的炎症和血管。

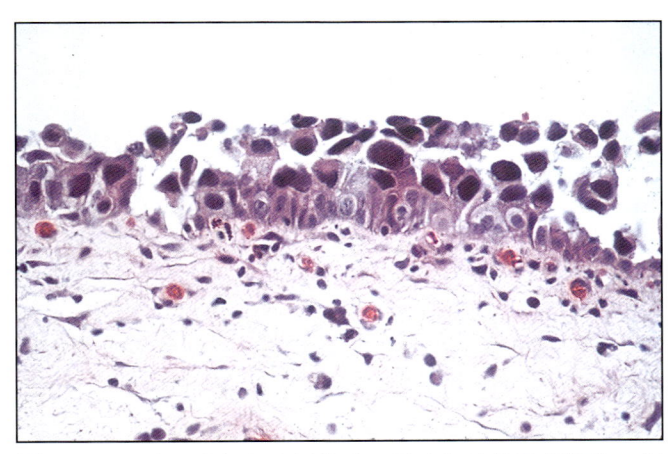

图12.102 膀胱移行细胞原位癌。肿瘤细胞核显著深染。细胞间缺乏粘连。

原位癌和显著尿路上皮脱落的患者有时被诊断为非特异的脱落性或间质性膀胱炎而进行长时期的随访[453,454]。在很多病例，低倍镜下移行细胞原位癌的诊断线索是固有层水肿、炎症显著以及血管丰富。一些移行细胞原位癌病例可以出现被覆非典型性细胞的息肉状小颗粒。这些病变需要与3级乳头状癌区分。移行细胞原位癌偶尔可表现为Paget病样生长方式[462,463]。

浸润性移行细胞癌
Invasive transitional cell carcinoma

大体表现 浸润性移行细胞癌可以由乳头状或广基型癌前病变发展而来，因此它的大体表现变化相当大（图12.103和12.104）。肿瘤可以呈明显的乳头状或息肉状，广基或溃疡型，在某些病例膀胱黏膜仅出现轻微异常，表现为细颗粒状或天鹅绒样；罕见情况下，特别是术前经过治疗的病例，切开膀胱壁之前可能几乎看不到肿瘤，甚至在切片中也观察不到明显的肿瘤组织。病变的大小变化也很大，从直径几毫米到肿物充满整个膀胱腔。肿瘤常为白色，但也可以是红色或棕褐色。可以出现出血或坏死，但通常不明显。肿瘤下面膀胱壁的大体表现明显与浸润程度有关，在浸润很深的肿瘤，膀胱壁常常被白色质硬的肿瘤组织取代。

组织学表现 浸润性移行细胞癌的镜下表现比大体表现更为多样。讨论了常见类型的浸润性移行细胞癌后，我们将会对几种特殊的组织学亚型进行描述，同时将关注与浸润深度评估有关等方面的问题。最常见的组织学表现是大而不规则的细胞巢（图12.105）、小的细胞条索（图12.106），以及单个肿瘤细胞不规则分布于黏膜固有层和固有肌层内（如后者被肿瘤细胞所浸润）。事实上，上皮性肿瘤的任何组织结构包括条索和孤立性的细胞巢（后者下文论述）均可出现。肿瘤有时可以出现弥漫生长方式，但即使在这些病例，也常常可见局灶的细胞巢和细胞条索。弥漫一致的生长方式很罕见。有时

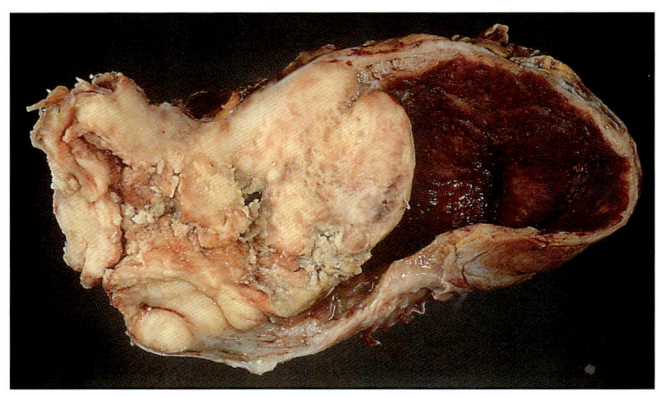

图12.103 非乳头状膀胱移行细胞癌。切面白色、局部结节状的巨大肿物突向膀胱腔内。

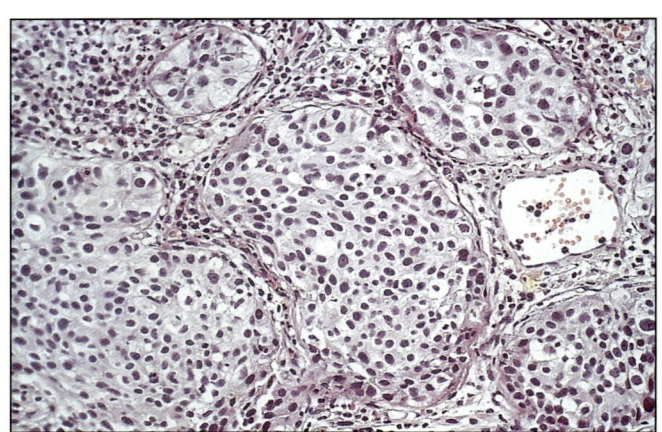

图12.105 膀胱移行细胞癌，2/3级。浸润性肿瘤由肿瘤细胞巢构成，肿瘤细胞胞浆中等量，弱嗜酸性，细胞核轻至中度非典型性。

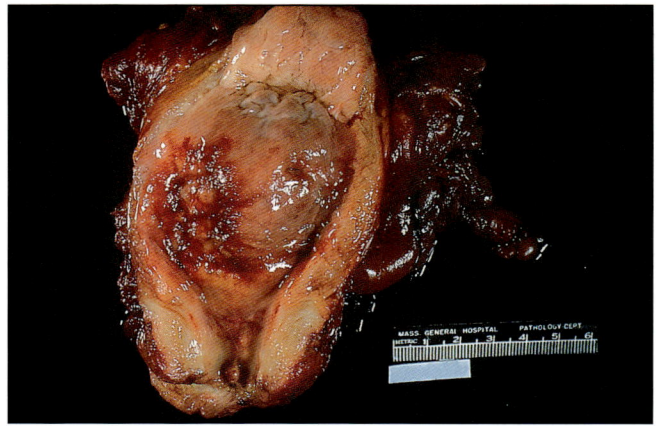

图12.104 非乳头状膀胱移行细胞癌。棕褐色的肿物稍高于相邻的黏膜。

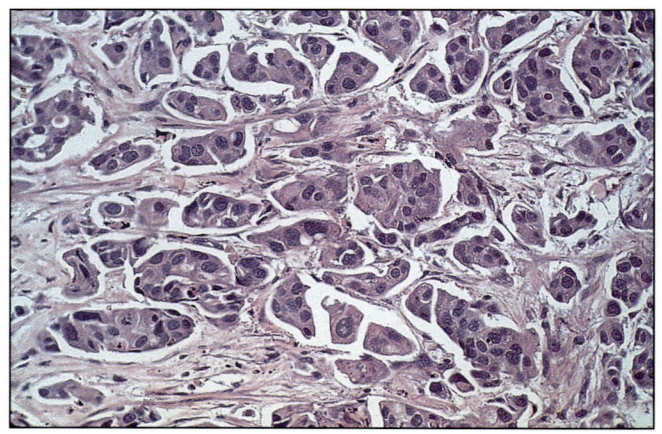

图12.106 膀胱移行细胞癌。肿瘤细胞排列成小的不规则条索。

肿瘤组织中可见显著的慢性炎细胞浸润，某些病例可能出现大量的嗜酸性粒细胞而使肿瘤细胞难以分辨，此时利用细胞角蛋白染色可使肿瘤细胞凸显（图 12.107）。

表现为上述组织学形态的移行细胞癌，肿瘤细胞通常中等大小，胞浆较丰富，淡染或轻度嗜酸性。一些病例肿瘤细胞胞浆非常丰富，透明或强嗜酸性（图 12.108）。细胞非典型性很显著，至少是中等程度，但有时也表现为轻度的非典型性。经过放射治疗的病例可能会出现形态奇异、核深染的肿瘤细胞（图 12.109）。核分裂象多少不等，与肿瘤的分级有关。高级别肿瘤中局部坏死很常见；出血并不常见。

病理医师在膀胱癌的分期中起着重要的作用，他们不仅仅要判断浸润的存在与否，还要对浸润的深度进行评估（表 12.12）。在大部分病例，肿瘤浸润非常明显，但偶尔浸润却很轻微，事实上有时仅限于几个细胞（图 12.110）或一小团肿瘤细胞的浸润（图 12.111）。Farrow 和 Utz[4611] 将这些病例命名为微小浸润移行细胞癌。他们在 70 例移行细胞原位癌中发现了 24 例存在小灶状浸润。他们将这种类型的肿瘤限制于浸润深度不超过 5mm 的病例。我们认为对于微浸润这一定义来说，这个深度太过于笼统，因此最好将此命名用于那些只有一小团甚至

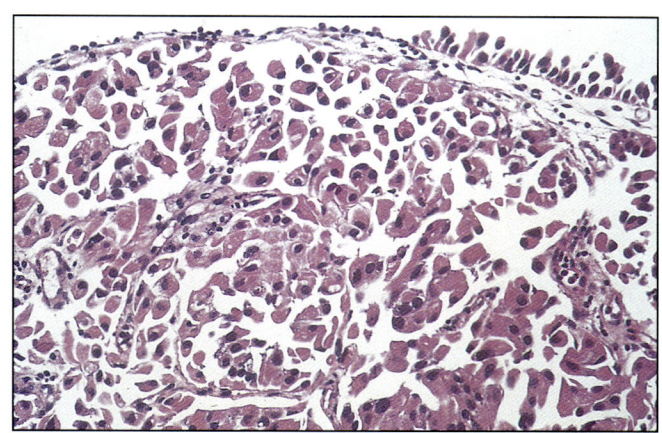

图 12.108　具有丰富嗜酸性胞浆的膀胱移行细胞癌。

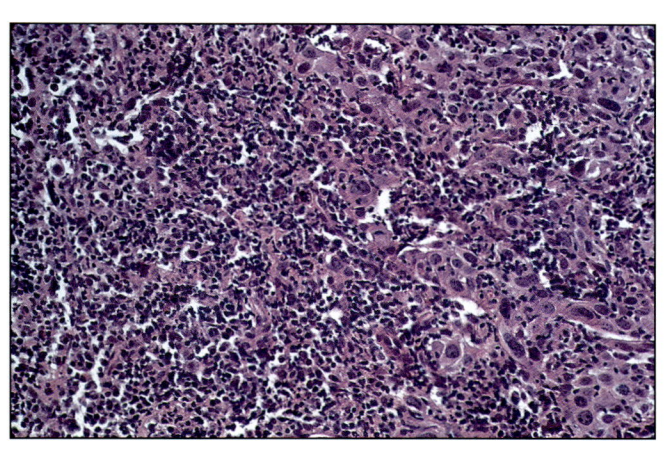

A

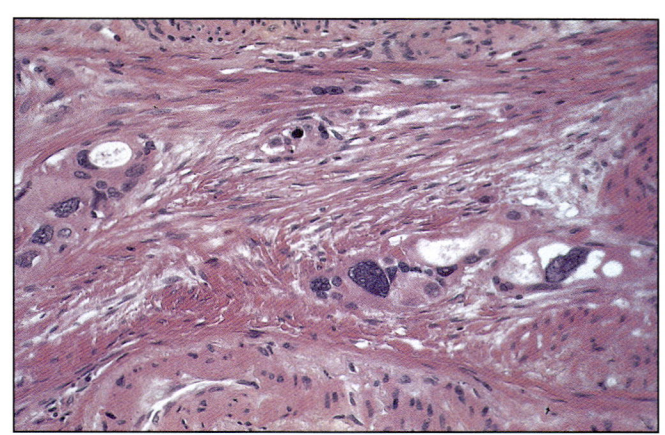

图 12.109　放射治疗后的膀胱移行细胞癌，出现怪异的细胞核。

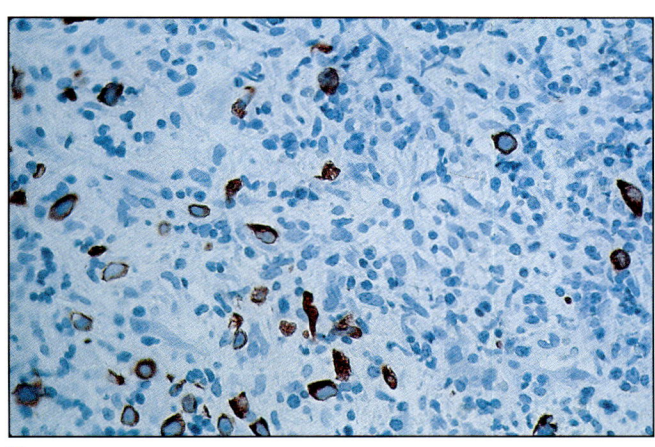

B

图 12.107　膀胱移行细胞癌伴有显著炎细胞浸润，部分区域癌细胞不容易辨认，图右侧较明显（A）。细胞角蛋白染色可以清楚地显示散在的癌细胞（B）。

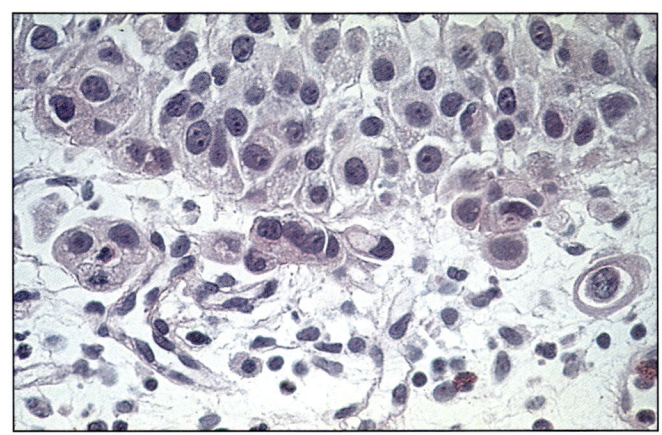

图 12.110　微浸润性移行细胞癌。小团和单个肿瘤细胞浸润至固有层浅层。

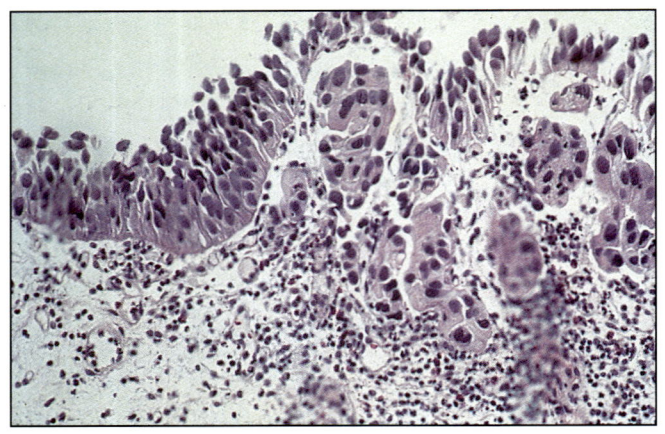

图12.111 微浸润性移行细胞癌。小团肿瘤细胞浸润至固有层浅层。

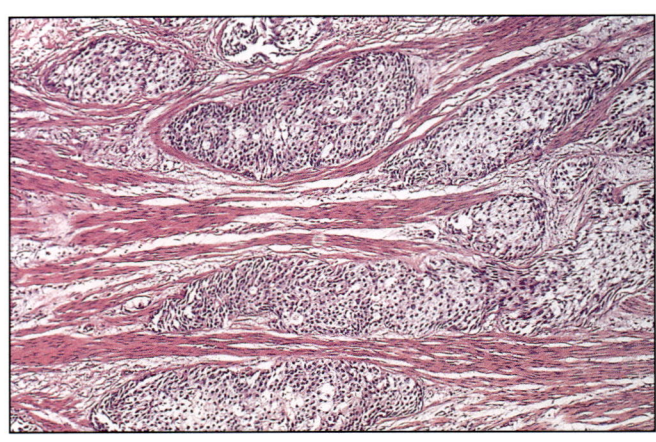

图12.112 移行细胞癌浸润至固有肌层。

表12.12	膀胱癌分期	
AJCC-TNM系统	JSM系统	
T0	—	无肿瘤存在
Tis	O	扁平原位癌
Ta	O	乳头状肿瘤,无浸润
T1	A	固有层浸润
T2	B1	浸润至浅肌层
T3a	B2	浸润至深肌层
T3b	C	浸润膀胱周围脂肪组织
T4a	D1	浸润相邻脏器
T4b	D2	固定于盆腔壁或腹壁
N0	—	无淋巴结转移
N1	D1	同侧单个淋巴结转移
N2	D1	对侧、双侧或多个淋巴结转移
N3	D1	固定于盆壁、与原发肿瘤分离的肿物
N4	D2	相邻区域淋巴结转移
M	D2	远处转移

AJCC = American Joint Commission on Cancer; JSM=Jewett-Strong (Marshall 修订)

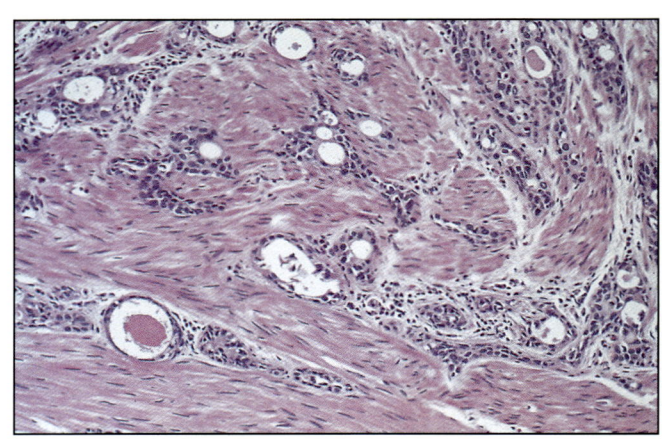

图12.113 伴腺性分化的移行细胞癌浸润肌层。

单个肿瘤细胞浸润至固有层浅层的病例[462]。明显的浸润通常表现为易于识别的不规则细胞团（图12.112 和 12.113），但正如上文关于乳头状瘤章节所提及的那样，有时组织结构完整的内翻性生长方式（图12.114）会造成诊断的困难[433]。

总体来说，对于预后最为重要的是是否存在固有肌层浸润（图12.112 和 12.113）。固有肌层浸润的判断常常比较容易，但有时电切造成的人工假象、显著的炎症和标本的不完整会造成困难。膀胱黏膜有一层薄的由平滑肌纤维构成的黏膜肌层，这一点非常重要（图12.115）[464-467]。一项研究显示71%的病例黏膜肌层中的肌纤维散在分布，20%的病例很显著但不连续，3%的病例形成明显的连续的一层，而6%的病例不存在[464]。

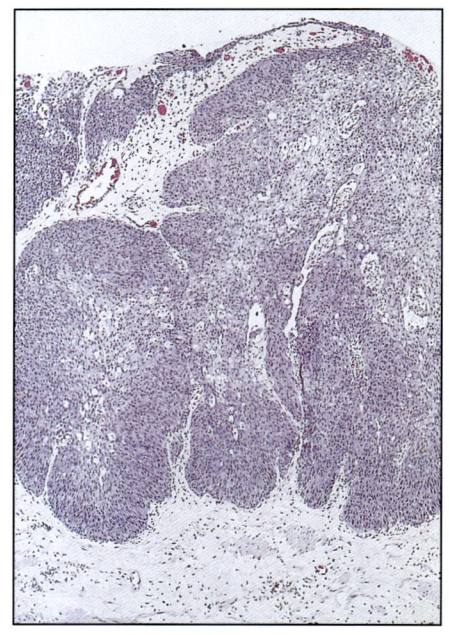

图12.114 膀胱移行细胞癌。这种浸润性癌并不常见，肿瘤细胞排列成边界清楚、形态规则的大细胞巢（所谓的内翻性生长）。

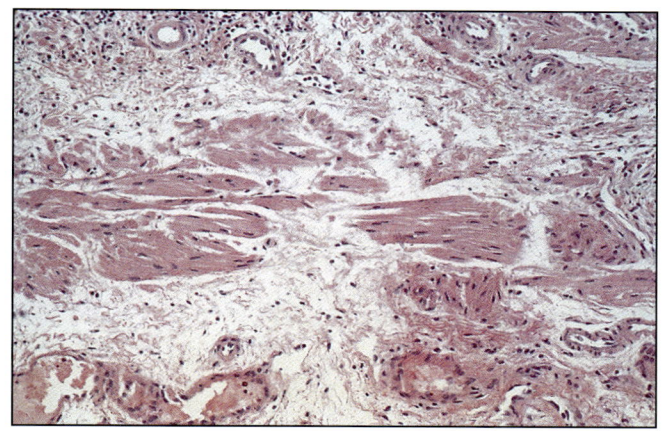

图12.115 黏膜肌层纤细、不连续的肌纤维。

而另一项研究发现只有35%的病例存在黏膜肌层,此现象在女性更为常见[467]。这一层纤薄的肌纤维与固有肌层肥厚的肌纤维束明显不同。另外,它们相对表浅的位置以及常常与血管关系密切这两点有助于辨认,它们的受侵不能错误诊断为固有肌层侵犯,后者被称为"肌层侵犯"并对泌尿科医师具有重要的临床意义。病理医师同样应该说明浸润癌中有无血管和淋巴管侵犯(图12.116),但是因为黏膜下组织常被完全破坏,所以在许多高级别浸润癌中很难发现脉管侵犯。

移行细胞癌亚型
Variants of transitional cell carcinoma

伴腺性或鳞状分化(With glandular or squamous differentiation) 大约10%的移行细胞癌具有局灶的腺性(图12.113)或鳞状分化。腺性分化的表现多种多样,从小的分布相对均一的腺管到紧密排列、不规则的中等和大的腺管不等。组织形态可以类似于肠型腺癌、苗勒管型腺癌,甚至包括透明细胞癌(见下文)等。腺性分化多见于中至高级别间质浸润较深的肿瘤,但有时也可见于高分化、间质浸润较表浅的肿瘤。鳞状分化没有特殊的形态学表现,从低分化癌到含大量角化物的高分化癌都可以出现。传统上这些原发肿瘤仍诊断为移行细胞癌,但应注明鳞状或腺性分化,因为它们可能有助于解释肿瘤的转移。

巢状癌(Nested carcinoma) 近期有学者强调浸润性移行细胞癌偶尔可以表现为相当整齐的巢状结构(图12.117至12.119)[468-471]。这些浸润性癌间质浸润通常较深,但细胞异型性不十分明显,可以使人误认为是增生的von Brunn巢[472]。

微囊性癌 Microcystic carcinoma

罕见情况下,移行细胞癌中的细胞巢可以形成腔隙[471,473-474]。这些腔隙可以增大形成囊腔,当这些囊腔

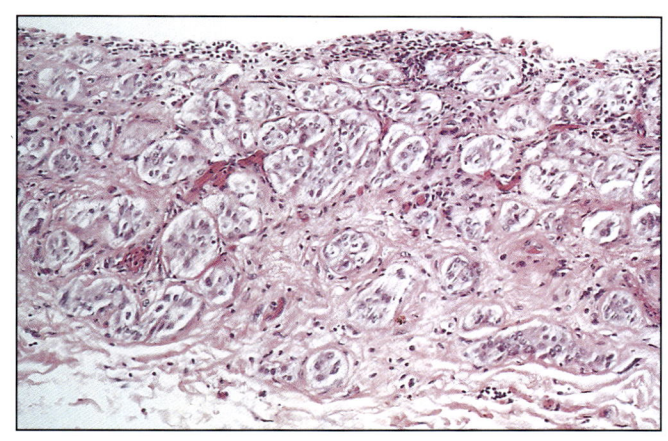

图12.117 膀胱移行细胞癌,1/3级。呈明显的小巢状结构。

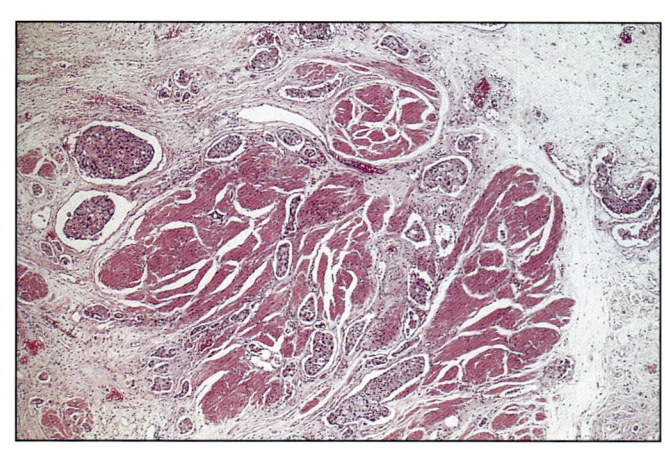

图12.116 伴明显淋巴管侵犯的移行细胞癌。

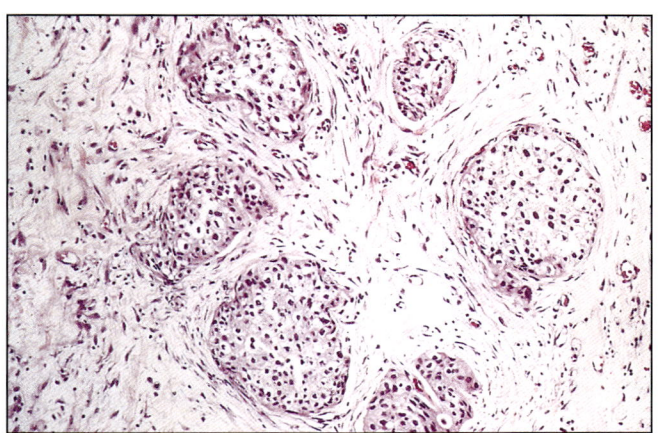

图12.118 膀胱移行细胞癌,1/3级。取材表浅的活检标本,细胞异型性不明显,呈巢状排列的浸润癌有时会误诊为良性病变。

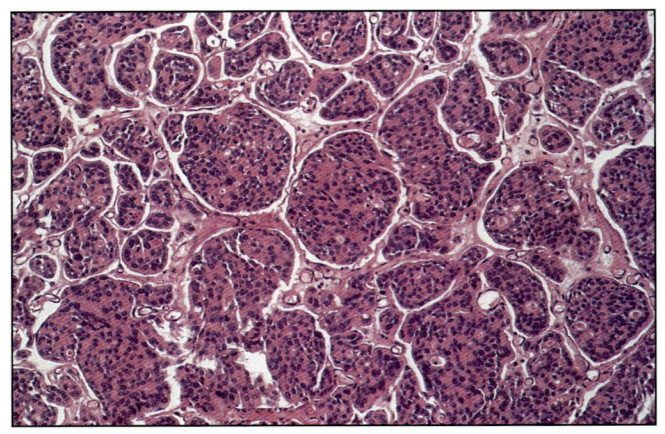

图12.119 膀胱移行细胞癌。肿瘤细胞排列成相对规则的圆形或卵圆形细胞巢。这种形态首先使人想到类癌。

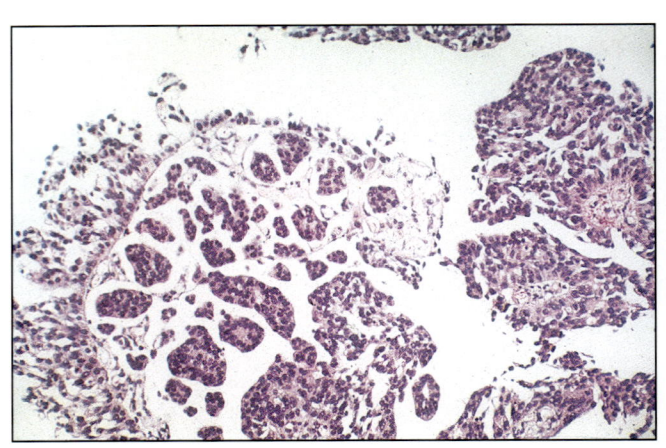

图12.121 微乳头状移行细胞癌。

很明显时便形成了相当显著的微囊性结构（图12.120）。这种结构通常散在分布，或紧邻典型的移行细胞癌，但有时几乎整个肿瘤都表现为这种结构。这些囊腔常常为圆形或卵圆形，可以表现为狭窄、细长和分支状的腔隙。在一些病例会形成一种很显著的组织结构，即大的囊腔周围分布着许多内含靶环样嗜酸性分泌物的小囊腔[471]。这些囊腔的中心常常充满粉红色黏液样分泌物，腔内有时出现脱落的细胞条索和坏死物。囊壁常常被覆数层尿路上皮细胞，但也可被覆腺上皮细胞；大的囊腔有时被覆形态相对温和的扁平上皮细胞，被覆上皮可完全脱落。在小的活检标本这些肿瘤完全有可能误诊为腺性膀胱炎或囊性膀胱炎。囊腔存在于相对较深的部位，不规则的形状和显著的细胞异型性有助于肿瘤与腺性膀胱炎或囊性膀胱炎的鉴别。

微乳头状癌（Micropapillary carcinoma） 少数情况下，移行细胞癌可以表现为类似卵巢浆液性乳头状癌的组织形态（图12.121）[475-477]。这种生长方式在固有肌层浸润灶和转移灶中仍然保留。尽管核异型性可能不显著，但这种微乳头状生长方式与预后不良相关。

肉瘤样癌（Sarcomatoid carcinoma） 一些高级别移行细胞癌具有数量不等的非典型梭形细胞区，可以称为肉瘤样癌[478-487]。这些肿瘤通常呈息肉样，体积很大（图12.122）。肿瘤细胞可表现为各种各样的组织结构。最为常见的是排列成束状，很像平滑肌肉瘤（图12.123）。有时可表现为漩涡状，与所谓的恶性纤维组织细胞瘤相似（图12.124）。当肿瘤类似横纹肌肉瘤时，会出现显著多形性的圆形或细长、富含嗜酸性胞浆的肿瘤细胞；有时肿瘤甚至可以很像血管肉瘤[487]。细胞核异型性通常比较明显，但有时不明显。典型区域核分裂象很常见，但某些区域并不显著。梭形肿瘤细胞常常紧密排列，但在某些病例它们被胶原纤维束分隔或分布于疏松、黏液样间质中（图12.125）[485]。肉瘤样成分常常与浸润性或原位移行细胞癌共同存在（图12.126），但有时也可以与其他变异型如鳞状细胞癌同时出现。充分的取材通常可以明确这些肿瘤的泌尿上皮来源，免疫组化有时也有助于诊断，因为这些梭形细胞表达细胞角蛋白（CK）、上皮膜抗原（EMA）和波形蛋白，而通常不表达结蛋白（Desmin）和肌源性抗原[488]。然而，我们曾经遇到过几例在常规苏木素-伊红染色（H&E）切片上明确为肉瘤样癌的病例不表达CK；因此，H&E染色仍然是诊断这些肿瘤的基础。

伴滋养叶细胞分化的癌（Carcinomas with trophoblastic differentiation） 免疫组化研究已经发现组织形态很典型的移行细胞癌，无论是浸润性癌和原位癌都可以表达人类绒毛膜促性腺激素（hCG）及其β亚单位，这种现

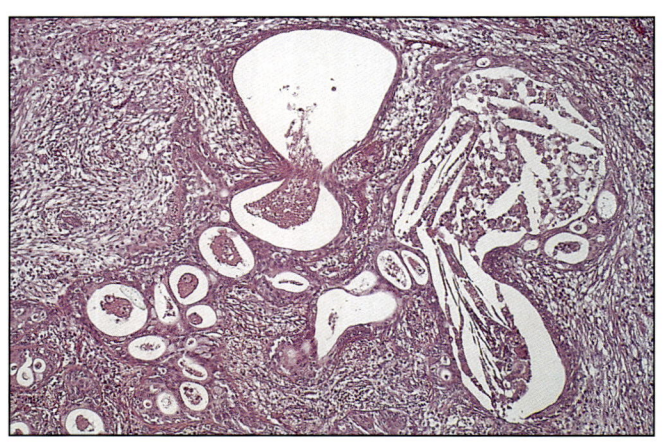

图12.120 膀胱微囊性移行细胞癌。注意大的囊腔周围的卫星小囊。

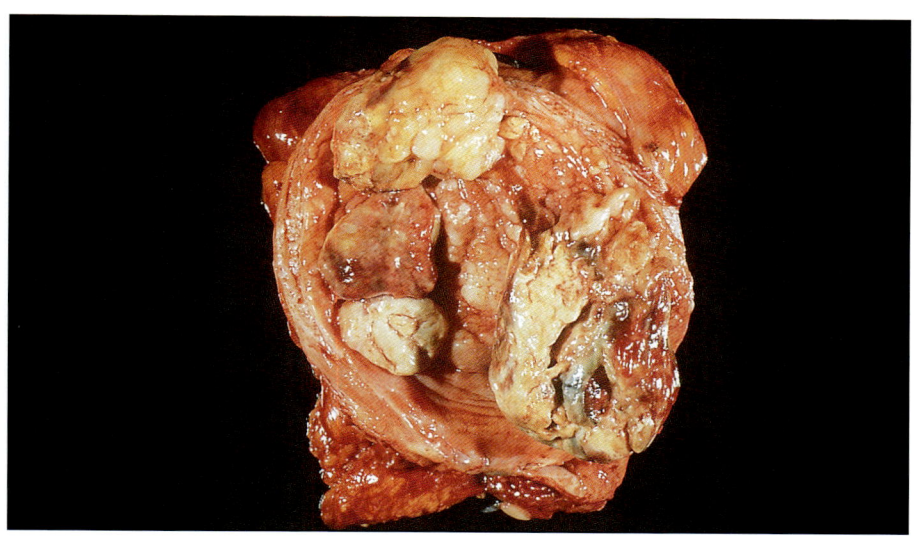

图12.122 膀胱肉瘤样癌。肿瘤呈多结节状,其中一些结节呈息肉样突向膀胱腔内。

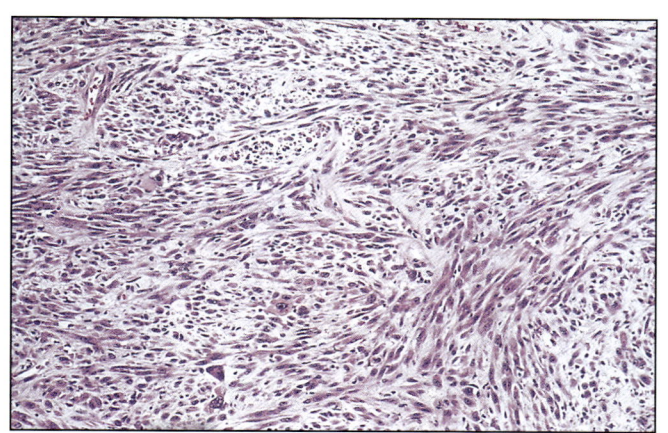

图12.123 膀胱肉瘤样癌。这个病例在形态学上很像平滑肌肉瘤。

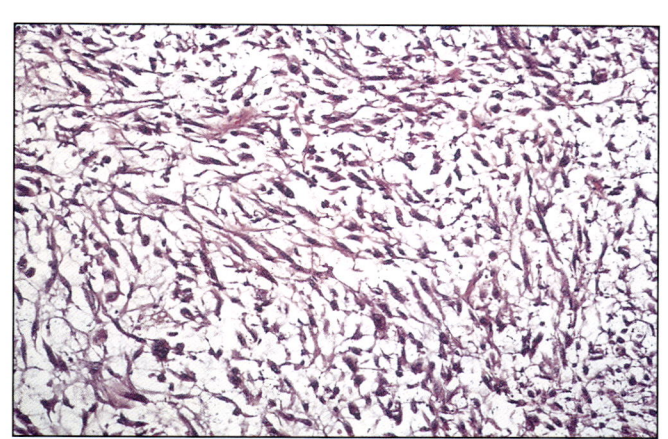

图12.125 膀胱肉瘤样癌。肿瘤局部具有显著的黏液样间质。

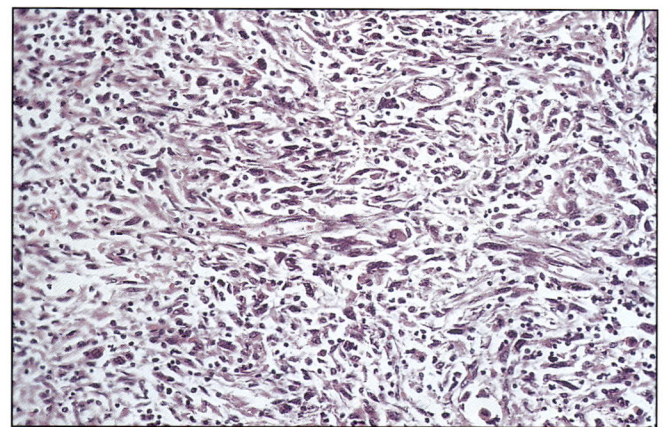

图12.124 漩涡状排列的膀胱肉瘤样癌,类似于所谓的恶性纤维组织细胞瘤。

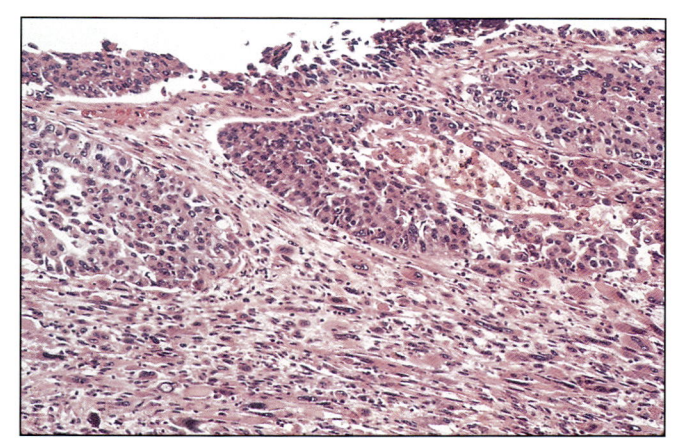

图12.126 肉瘤样癌(底部)与位于肿瘤表浅部位更为典型的移行细胞癌同时存在。

移行细胞癌

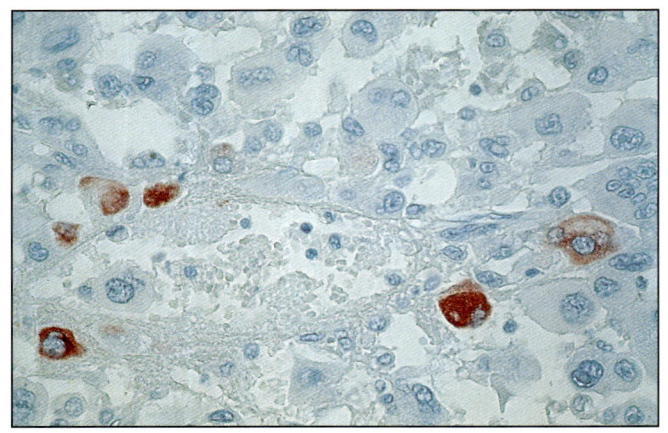

图12.127 移行细胞癌，3/3级，免疫组化染色显示一些肿瘤细胞表达人绒毛膜促性腺激素。

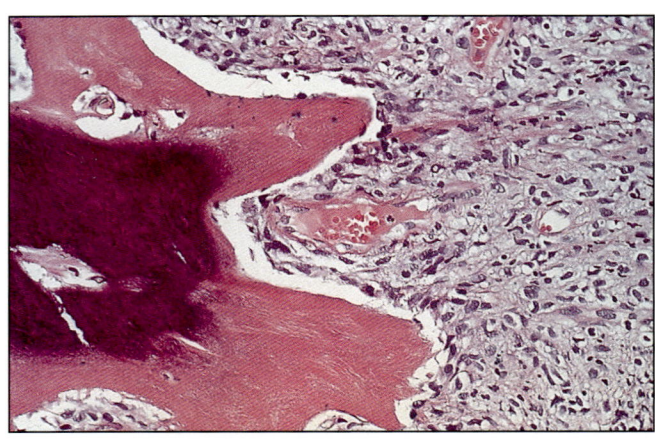

图12.129 伴间质骨化的移行细胞癌。

象发生于大约30%的3级癌[489]。高级别移行细胞癌常表达hCG及其产物（图12.127），以及那些明确的由尿路上皮癌衍生或并发的绒毛膜癌的存在，提示大部分（即使不是全部）伴滋养叶成分的膀胱肿瘤实际上是伴滋养叶细胞分化的移行细胞癌，而不是生殖细胞来源的绒毛膜癌[490,491]。

伴特殊间质改变的移行细胞癌（Transitional cell carcinomas with unusual stromal changes） 移行细胞癌可以出现与其他器官肿瘤相似的各种间质改变，只是常常不明显。可以表现为不同程度的纤维增生，但特别显著的纤维化并不常见。其他病例间质疏松或水肿，罕见情况下出现黏液样间质。有时间质中可见大量具有非典型性却是良性的间叶细胞，很像所谓巨细胞膀胱炎中见到的那种类型的细胞（图12.128）。当这些细胞位于癌细胞巢附近时，很容易被误认为是梭形癌细胞，即肉瘤样

癌。这些细胞的退行性表现、缺乏核分裂活性以及与明显的上皮细胞无移行现象都有助于它们的识别。免疫组化染色对于复杂病例的鉴别有帮助，与大部分肉瘤样癌不同，这些细胞不表达上皮性标志。这些伴有非典型性、非肿瘤性间质细胞的癌被称为伴假肉瘤性间质的移行细胞癌[492,493]。

移行细胞癌的间质很少发生骨化（图12.129）；软骨化生也很罕见[494]。这些肿瘤组织中的骨组织和软骨组织在细胞学表现上是良性的；这点对于将它们与含有恶性骨组织和软骨组织的癌肉瘤和骨肉瘤区别开来非常重要。

伴明显破骨细胞样巨细胞的移行细胞癌已有报道（图12.130）[402a,495]。如果这些破骨细胞样巨细胞大量存在而掩盖癌组织会造成诊断困难。这些破骨细胞样巨细胞在移行细胞癌中似乎并不常见，很有可能是机体反应的结果。

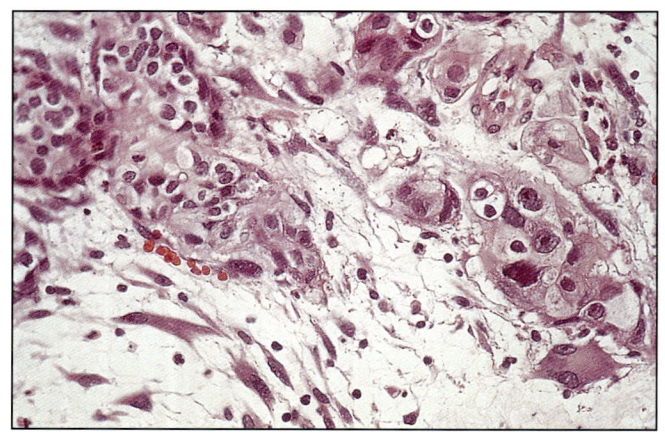

图12.128 伴假肉瘤样间质的移行细胞癌。浸润癌附近的固有层中存在不典型的间叶细胞。

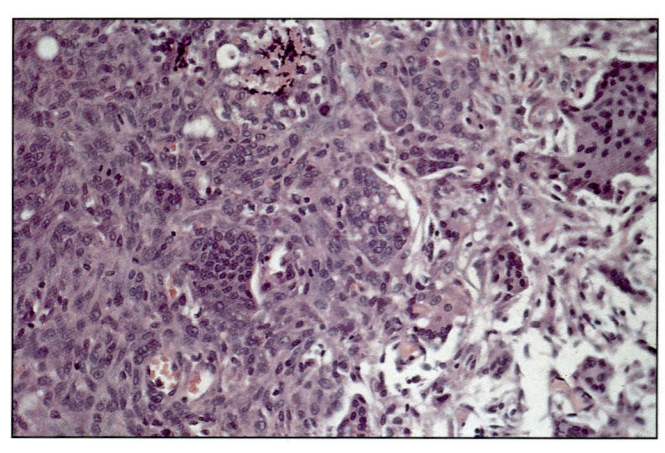

图12.130 伴间质内破骨细胞样巨细胞的移行细胞癌。

鉴别诊断　常见的浸润性移行细胞癌通常不会造成诊断困难。偶尔有小部分 1 级肿瘤（不超过全部病例的 5%）组织学表现很像 von Brunn 巢，可能会造成诊断困难[472]。这些所谓的巢状癌中的高分化癌细胞巢常密集排列，大小和形状较不规则，而 von Brunn 巢常为规则的圆形或卵圆形，分布较均匀（图 12.131），而大部分癌至少在局部存在不规则的组织结构，这一点有助于它们之间的鉴别。此外，深部生长的 von Brunn 巢边缘比较整齐，而巢状癌的浸润性边缘较不规则[472]。另一个需要与巢状移行细胞癌，甚至非巢状癌鉴别的是副神经节瘤，这个问题将在有关副神经节瘤的章节进行讨论（见第 549 页）。

伴鳞状和（或）腺性分化的移行细胞癌常为 2 级或 3 级癌，与非肿瘤病变的鉴别通常容易。少数肿瘤会含有小而规则的腺性成分，很像肾源性腺瘤中的小管。与这些小管结构同时存在的局灶移行细胞癌成分很容易帮助做出正确的诊断，但需要充分取材。肾源性腺瘤的小管周围并不存在移行细胞，而周围有移行细胞包绕正是移行细胞癌小管结构的典型特征。辨认出哪怕是非常少的移行细胞癌成分，是区分伴鳞状或腺性分化的移行细胞癌与纯粹的鳞状细胞癌或腺癌的关键。这一点在与膀胱转移癌的鉴别中非常重要。

单从组织形态表现来看，3 级移行细胞癌不具特征性表现而与其他类型的低分化癌很难鉴别。除非有明确的证据表明一个低分化膀胱癌是其他类型的癌时，否则要考虑它是移行细胞癌。男性膀胱发生的低分化肿瘤还应考虑前列腺癌的可能，特别是取自膀胱三角或膀胱颈的标本。对于这些病例，免疫组化对于诊断非常有帮助，因为大部分前列腺癌表达前列腺特异抗原（PSA）。有时缺乏明显上皮特征的移行细胞癌形态上很像恶性淋巴瘤[496]，但是小灶状的上皮分化以及高倍镜下肿瘤细胞并无典型淋巴瘤细胞特征这两点有助于鉴别。上皮和淋巴组织标志物的免疫组化染色有助于鉴别那些常规染色很难区分的病例。

需要与肉瘤样癌鉴别的肿瘤有肉瘤（平滑肌肉瘤、"恶性纤维组织细胞瘤"、多形性横纹肌肉瘤和罕见的血管肉瘤）、癌肉瘤和伴假肉瘤样间质的移行细胞癌。尽管肉瘤样癌和肉瘤的鉴别有时相当困难，但对常规切片中它们各自的形态学特点进行仔细的观察常常可以将它们区分开来。前者有诊断意义的病理学特点是肉瘤样成分与其他类型的浸润性移行细胞癌成分有形态学上的移行现象。但小的活检标本可能只有肉瘤样成分。

肉瘤样癌与癌肉瘤的不同之处在于前者的上皮成分渐进式地融合到梭形细胞成分中，两者的分布相对独立。而癌肉瘤则相反，明显的癌和肉瘤成分密切混合存在，在肉瘤样背景中癌的成分常常很明显（见第 548 页）。两种成分之间的移行有时可以见到，但并不如肉瘤样癌那么明显。癌肉瘤的肉瘤样成分还常常出现异源性分化，包括骨骼肌、软骨和骨组织的出现，这可以排除肉瘤样癌的诊断。

最后一个需要与肉瘤样癌鉴别的是恶性黑色素瘤，无论是膀胱原发还是转移，因为黑色素瘤细胞可以明显呈梭形。黑色素颗粒（有时存在）是一个重要的诊断指标；免疫组化染色也有帮助，特别是大部分黑色素瘤 S-100 和 HMB45 蛋白阳性，而细胞角蛋白和上皮膜抗原常常为阴性。

伴破骨细胞样巨细胞的移行细胞癌需要与巨细胞癌鉴别（见下文）。与破骨细胞样巨细胞相比，巨细胞癌的巨细胞异型性更加明显；另外，破骨细胞样巨细胞酸性磷酸酶染色是能够抵抗酒石酸，而巨细胞癌则无此特点。另一方面，巨细胞癌细胞角蛋白染色阳性，而破骨细胞样巨细胞则为阴性。

鳞状细胞癌　Squamous cell carcinoma

在非血吸虫病流行地区，鳞状细胞癌大约占所有膀胱癌的 5%[497]，但有些研究报道这一比例可高达

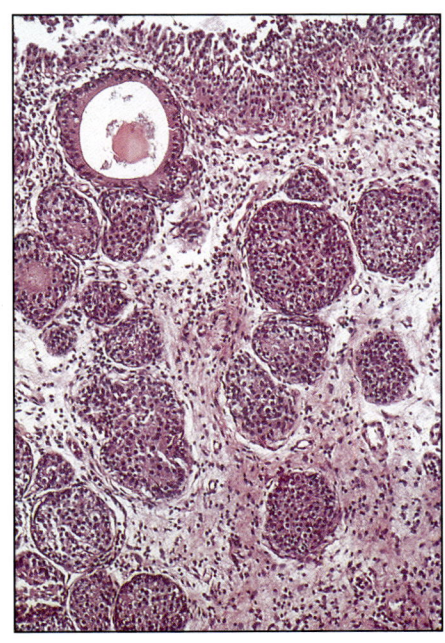

图 12.131　von Brunn 巢。位于固有层深部的细胞巢，这种形态学表现有时会使人误诊为癌。注意这些细胞巢呈非常规则的圆形或卵圆形。

10%~15%。然而，在血吸虫病流行地区，鳞状细胞癌可占膀胱肿瘤的75%左右。男：女发病比例比移行细胞癌低，但年龄分布大致相同。非疣状鳞状细胞癌预后很差[498-506]。

鳞状细胞癌的发生与膀胱慢性炎症有关，血吸虫病是典型病例。其他存在膀胱慢性炎症的状况也存在这种相关性。某项研究显示结石患者中大约15%的病例，尿道狭窄中20%病例，发生膀胱癌[502]。另外，20%的肿瘤发生于有膀胱憩室的病例，50%发生于无功能性膀胱，15%曾行肾移植。膀胱鳞状细胞癌患者与移行细胞癌患者的临床表现唯一不同的是尿路刺激症状相对常见，有时尿液中出现角蛋白样物质。

一项研究报道了19例膀胱疣状癌[507]。在鳞状细胞癌常见的埃及地区，当地两个研究机构的数据显示，这种类型占全部鳞状细胞癌病例的4.6%。患者平均年龄45岁，男女发病比例为6:1。在非血吸虫病流行地区只有3例膀胱疣状癌的报道[508-510]。两例为老年男性，一例为中年女性。其中一例可能来源于已经存在的尖锐湿疣[508]。尚无疣状癌发生扩散的报道。

大体和组织学表现 鳞状细胞癌的大体表现可以是广基、溃疡、乳头状、息肉样（图12.132）或结节状。它们的体积通常较大，浸润较深（约90%以上的病例），即使是分化好的肿瘤也是如此。组织病理学表现与其他部位的鳞状细胞癌相似（图12.133）。大部分为中-高分化，常常可见大量角化成分。对一例伴有外阴和尿道尖锐湿疣的肾移植患者发生的鳞状细胞癌进行DNA杂交研究发现，肿瘤组织中存在11型人乳头状瘤病毒基因[511]。疣状癌与其他部位的同类型肿瘤表现一致（见第4章）。

鉴别诊断 这种类型肿瘤常常伴发附近黏膜角化型鳞状上皮化生（所谓的黏膜白斑）[434a,512-514]，可通过观察细胞非典型程度和(或)有无间质浸润而区分开来。许多膀胱鳞状细胞癌分化好，肿瘤细胞只有轻-中度非典型性。膀胱其他良性鳞状上皮病变，如鳞状上皮乳头状瘤和湿疣相当罕见。这些病变缺乏细胞非典型性和间质浸润，可以与癌区分，同时湿疣中可见挖空细胞以及其他病毒感染的形态学特征。然而，如同在女性生殖道中所见到的一样，膀胱湿疣可以同时伴有鳞状细胞癌。

与较常见的生殖道疣状癌一样，膀胱疣状癌首先必须与尖锐湿疣和局部呈疣状癌结构的浸润性鳞状细胞癌（所谓的疣样癌）相鉴别。有助于将典型鳞状细胞癌与湿疣区分的组织学特点在此同样适用。疣状癌的诊断必

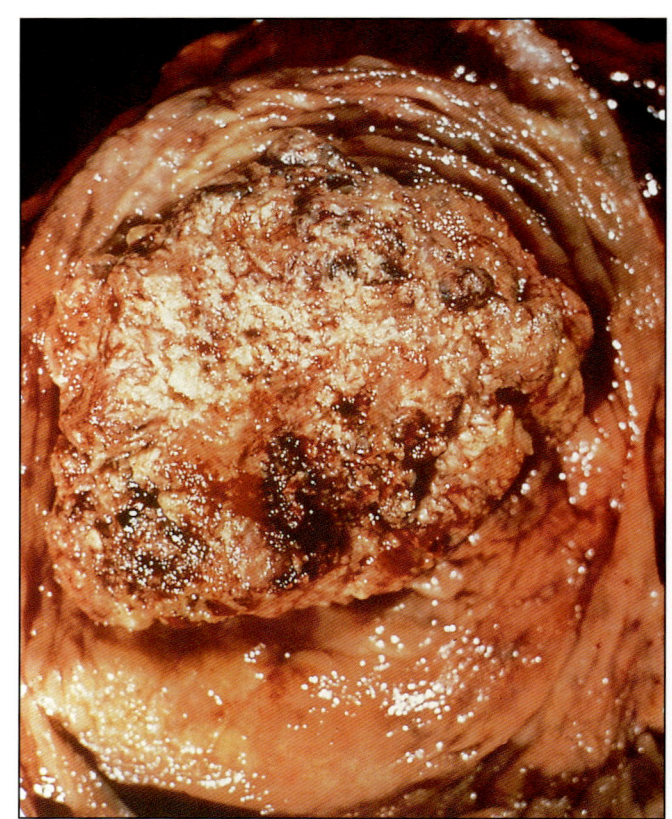

图12.132 膀胱鳞状细胞癌。突向膀胱腔内的体积巨大的息肉样肿物。患者有长期的慢性膀胱炎病史，肿瘤附近的膀胱黏膜可见角化型鳞状上皮化生。

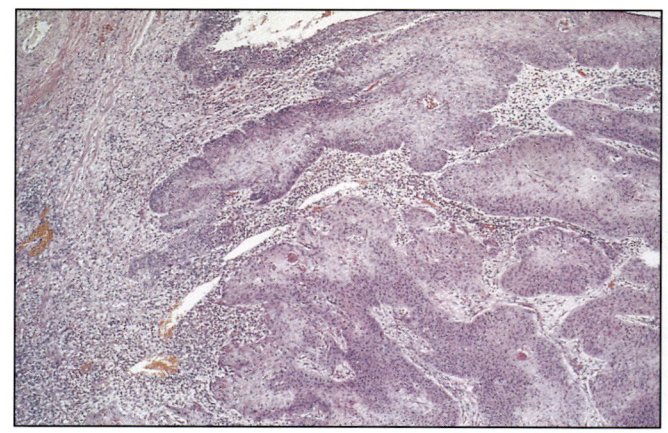

图12.133 膀胱鳞状细胞癌。

须严格用于那些全部呈疣状的肿瘤。例如，上文所提到的来源于埃及的那些资料中[507]，有3例呈疣状结构和典型浸润性鳞状细胞癌混合，另一篇报道也指出了这一

点[515]。因此，疣状癌的诊断只有在完整切除、充分取材的情况下才能做出。

腺癌　Adenocarcinoma

腺癌占膀胱癌的0.5%～2%[516-533]。它可以起源于脐尿管[534]，可能与膀胱外翻[535]、子宫内膜异位症有关[536,537]，也有可能与上述任何一种情况无关；最后一种情况最为常见。在一项大规模的病例研究中，1/3的肿瘤是脐尿管来源[533]。

腺癌的年龄分布以及男女比例与移行细胞癌相似，它们通常发生于>50岁的男性。临床表现很像移行细胞癌，但偶尔可出现黏液尿（mucusuria）。腺癌与鳞状细胞癌一样，在某些特殊情况下发生的膀胱癌中占相当大的比例，大约15%的病例发生于无功能膀胱患者，85%的病例与膀胱外翻相关[538]。膀胱腺癌的预后通常不佳，五年生存率从18%[527]到47%[533]。印戒细胞癌发现时常常已到晚期，预后比其他类型腺癌更差。脐尿管源性肿瘤预后比非脐尿管源性肿瘤好，可能与许多脐尿管腺癌是囊性低级别肿瘤有关[533]。

大体表现　腺癌的大体表现相当多样，与是否来源于脐尿管（图12.134），是否伴有膀胱外翻（图12.135）有关，或与这些情况没有任何关系。最后一种情况时肿瘤可以位于黏膜任何部位。可以呈乳头状、息肉样、结节状，可以广基及形成溃疡。肿瘤组织质地常常较软、黏液样（图12.136）；局灶出血和坏死常见。印戒细胞癌占膀胱腺癌的3%～5%[539-541]，黏膜常出现水肿，大部分病例出现溃疡，但有时大致正常[542]。一些病例膀胱弥漫纤维化，膀胱壁增厚呈皮革样（图12.137）。约20%的印戒细胞癌来源于脐尿管[542]。

脐尿管来源腺癌常常表现为膀胱顶部的黏膜下肿物，分为两大类型：呈外生性生长的囊性肿瘤[439]和侵袭性更强的非囊性肿瘤。一些肿瘤显著地沿上方的Retzius腔隙扩散至脐部。被覆黏膜常常呈不同程度的溃疡或异常，但并不一定。实性肿瘤切面常为胶冻样（图12.134）。伴有膀胱外翻的肿瘤主要位于前腹壁（图12.135）；这些肿瘤现在相当罕见。

组织学表现　膀胱腺癌主要有以下几种组织学亚型，并根据一项大规模的病例研究[533]，列出其所占比例：非特殊类型腺癌（28%）；黏液腺癌（24%）；肠型腺癌（19%）；印戒细胞癌（17%）；以及混合性腺癌（13%）。

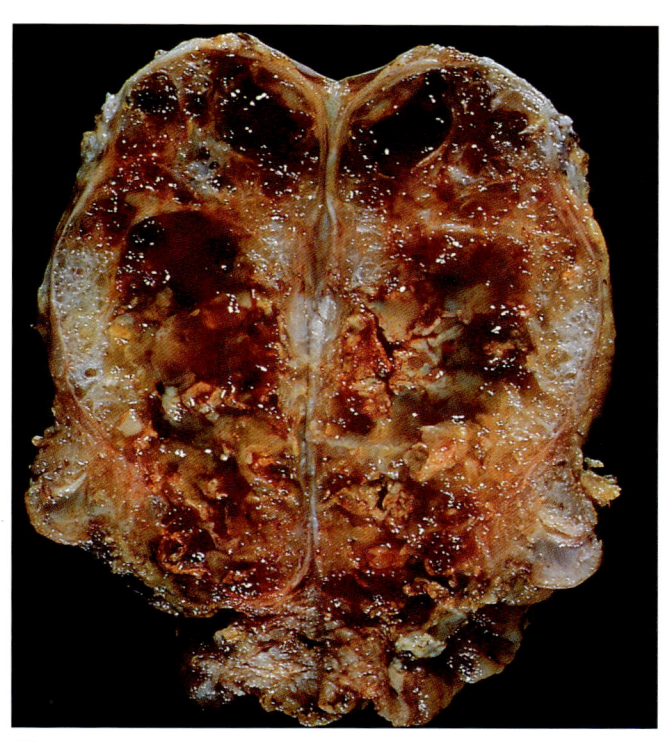

图12.134　脐尿管腺癌。侵及Retzius腔隙的巨大肿物切除标本，很像香肠，切面胶冻样。

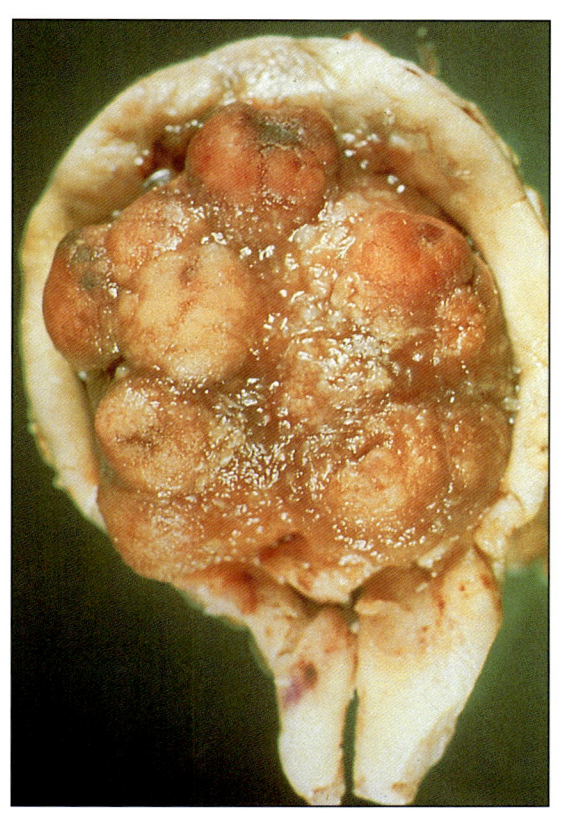

图12.135　发生于外翻性膀胱的腺癌。腹壁上巨大的结节状肿物。（Courtesy of Dr. Fred Askin.）

腺癌

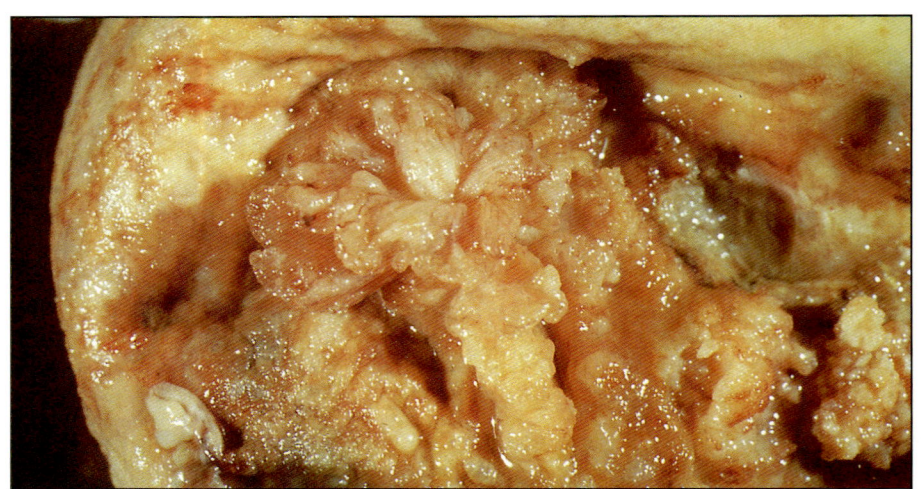

图12.136 截瘫患者发生的膀胱腺癌。肿瘤呈乳头状，部分胶冻样。

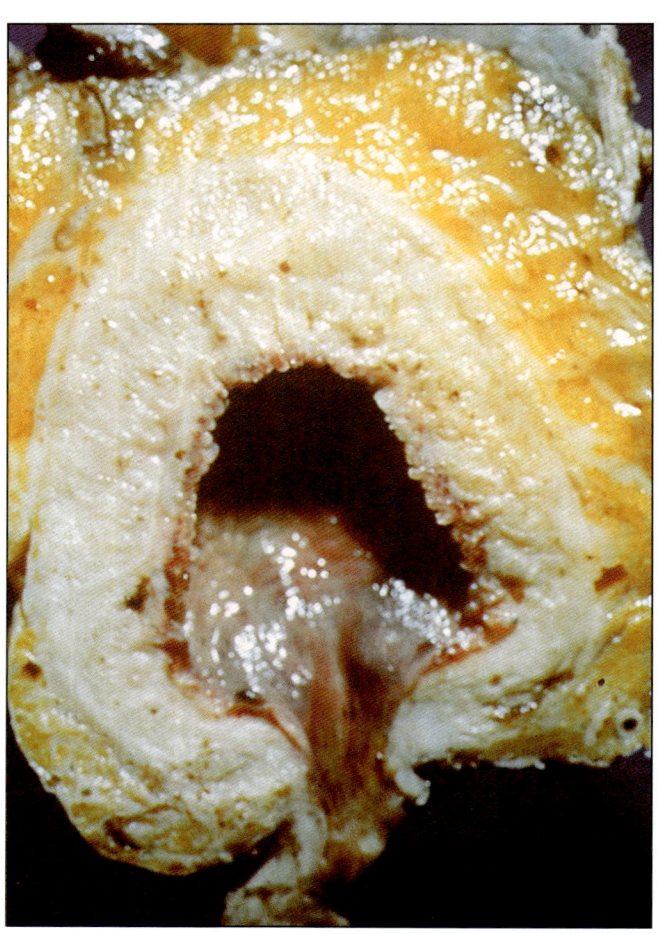

图12.137 膀胱印戒细胞癌。膀胱壁弥漫增厚，膀胱腔变小。

表12.13	脐尿管与非脐尿管腺癌亚型的发生率(%)[533]	
	脐尿管源性	非脐尿管源性
黏液性	50	10
肠型	29	15
混合性	17	10
印戒细胞癌	4	23
非特殊类型	0	42

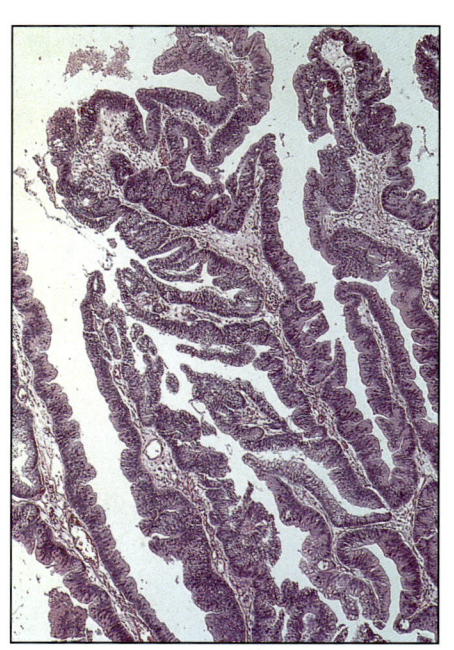

图12.138 膀胱乳头状腺癌。

这些组织学亚型在脐尿管源性与非脐尿管源性肿瘤中的发生频率不同（表12.13）。

　　显微镜下主要表现为管状和乳头状结构（图12.138），分化差的肿瘤可以见到实性生长区域。腺体形态并无特殊，通常类似典型的结肠腺癌或胶样腺癌（图12.139）。可以出现黏液或嗜酸性坏死物。被覆上皮具有显著的黏液分泌特征。潘氏细胞（Paneth cell）很罕见[531]。研究发现8%的肿瘤部分或全部由乳头状结构组成[527]，

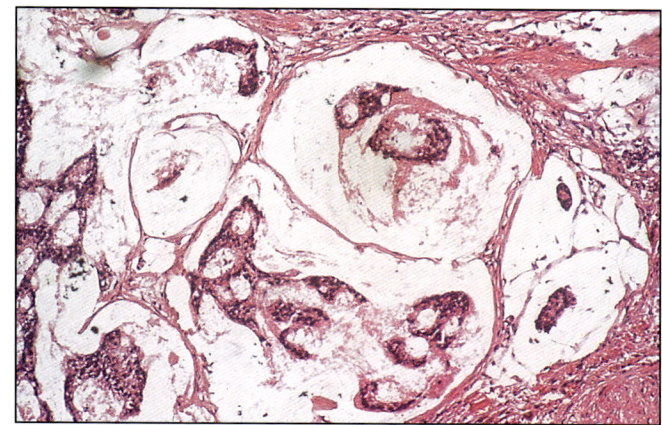

图12.139　膀胱胶样腺癌。

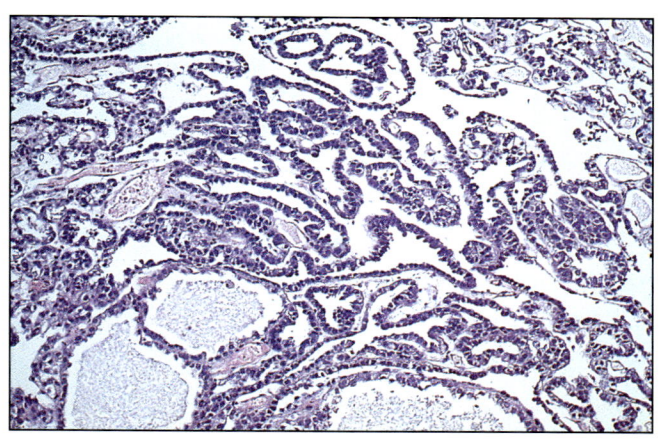

图12.141　膀胱透明细胞癌，可见囊状腺管结构和鞋钉样细胞。

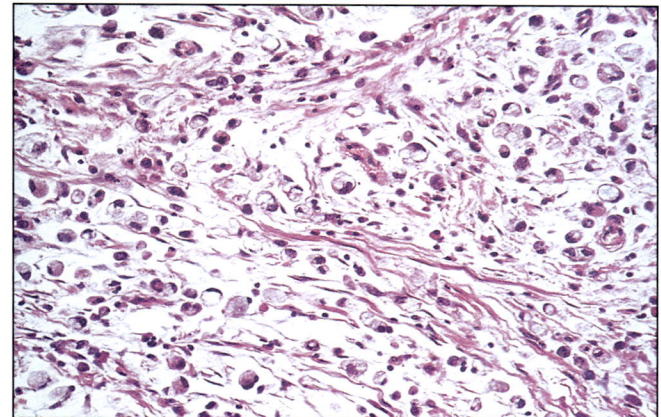

图12.140　膀胱印戒细胞癌。

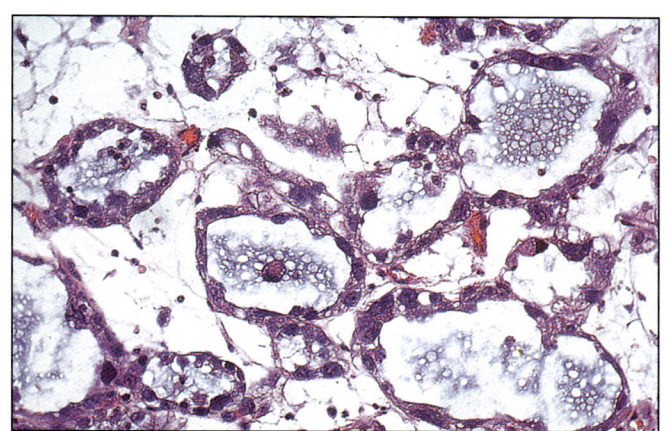

图12.142　与子宫内膜异位症有关的膀胱透明细胞腺癌。注意管腔内的黏液。

常常与腺性膀胱炎有关，通常是肠型，14%～66%的病例表面上皮发生黏液细胞化生[518,530]。脐尿管肿瘤中囊性更为常见，可以全部为囊内型或局限于被覆上皮内；这类肿瘤与卵巢低级别囊腺癌有一系列的相似点[439]。

膀胱印戒细胞癌形态学与其他部位的同类肿瘤一致（图12.140），印戒细胞可以漂浮于细胞外黏液池中，有时混有其他类型的腺癌成分。全部由印戒细胞构成的肿瘤预后比混有其他成分者更差。

透明细胞腺癌[537]可以单独表现为管状、囊性、乳头状及弥漫成片，也可以多种结构混合存在（图12.141和12.142）。大部分病例以腺管结构为主。尽管胞浆中常常富含透明糖原（图12.143），但并非诊断所必需，一些病例主要或全部由扁平或鞋钉样细胞组成。与子宫内膜异位症有关提示它们可能是苗勒管起源，但一些病例与之无关，可能是移行细胞源性肿瘤的腺性成分[537]。有一例发

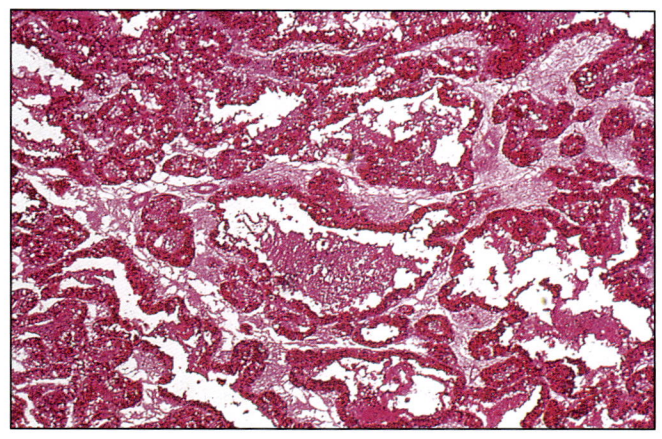

图12.143　膀胱透明细胞腺癌。肿瘤细胞含有丰富的胞浆内糖原（PAS染色）。

生于苗勒管囊肿的透明细胞癌表现为膀胱肿瘤[543]。然而，大多数膀胱透明细胞癌可能并不起源于苗勒管。

鉴别诊断　膀胱腺癌与原发单纯性移行细胞癌的鉴别并不困难，然而少数移行细胞癌巢中心会出现坏死，

形成假腺管样结构。正如上文所述，一些移行细胞癌会出现显著的腺性分化而引起诊断困难，此时很大程度上依靠充分取材。

腺癌与腺性膀胱炎的鉴别通常比较容易，因为后者腺体的位置表浅，结构规则，细胞无异型性。一些腺癌分化非常好，对于这些病例腺癌诊断的确定，组织结构特征比细胞形态学更有帮助。与肠型腺性膀胱炎的鉴别尤其困难[544]；后者缺乏细胞非典型性或肌层侵犯是诊断的关键。腺癌可伴有肠型腺性膀胱炎背景，有些病例同时存在正常、非典型性以及腺上皮癌变。腺癌还应与罕见膀胱绒毛状腺瘤鉴别。绒毛状腺瘤缺乏间质浸润，但在取材表浅的标本，这一现象可能不明显。建议对这些病变完整切除，以正确评估有无间质浸润。

腺癌还应与其他三种非肿瘤性病变，包括子宫内膜异位症[545]、宫颈内膜异位症[546]和输卵管内膜异位症[547]相鉴别。大部分的子宫内膜异位症很容易鉴别，因为这些病变中腺体周围可见子宫内膜间质。需要注意的是，在绝经期或经激素治疗的患者，子宫内膜间质可能出现萎缩，故在腺体周围并不明显。子宫内膜异位症和宫颈内膜异位症中腺上皮细胞的良性表现也有助于与腺癌的区分。由于缺乏子宫内膜间质以及存在黏液上皮，宫颈内膜异位症可能会造成诊断困难（图12.144和12.145）。同时由于异位宫颈内膜常常不规则分布于膀胱固有肌层中，不熟悉这种病变的医师有可能将其误诊为高分化黏液腺癌的深部浸润。与腺癌不同，输卵管内膜异位症细胞形态温和并且有纤毛。

膀胱原发性腺癌必须与其他器官腺癌的膀胱局部侵犯和转移区分。这种情况最常见于前列腺腺癌直接侵犯膀胱。对于大部分前列腺腺癌，常规染色切片显示特征性的小腺泡和筛状结构，这种形态表现与大多数膀胱腺癌不同。然而，有些病例的常规切片很难将两者区分；前列腺特异抗原（PSA）和前列腺酸性磷酸酶（PSAP）免疫组化染色可以明确诊断。即使前列腺腺癌出现特殊组织形态，也会表达其中一种抗原。需要记住的是，已有研究显示某些膀胱腺癌PSAP染色也出现阳性[548]，但PSA染色阴性，提示PSA和PSAP同时染色阳性的重要性。对于转移性肠癌，根据形态学很难鉴别，因为许多原发性膀胱腺癌很像肠癌。然而，当膀胱外部出现广泛浸润，而黏膜和固有层相对正常时，强烈提示肠道或其他器官腺癌侵犯。然而，晚期的转移性腺癌可以侵犯膀胱黏膜，目前已有明确的、具有这种形态表现的结肠或阑尾腺癌的报道[538]。因此，只有当临床排除肠道肿瘤继发侵犯膀胱后，才能明确做出膀胱原发性肠型腺癌的诊断。笔者曾遇到过临床表现以膀胱病变为首发的

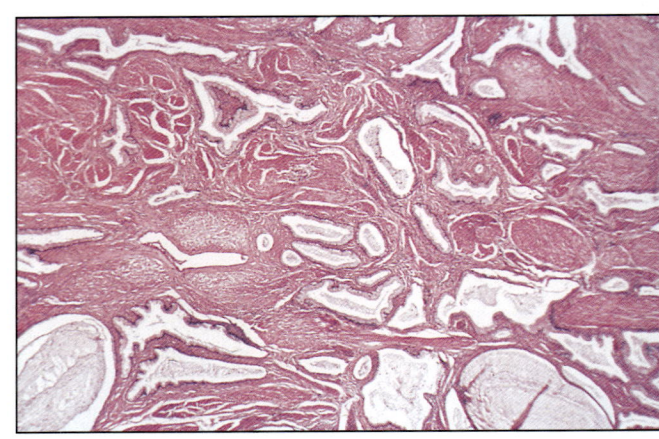

图12.144　膀胱宫颈内膜异位症。良性腺体杂乱地分布于固有肌层中，很像腺癌。

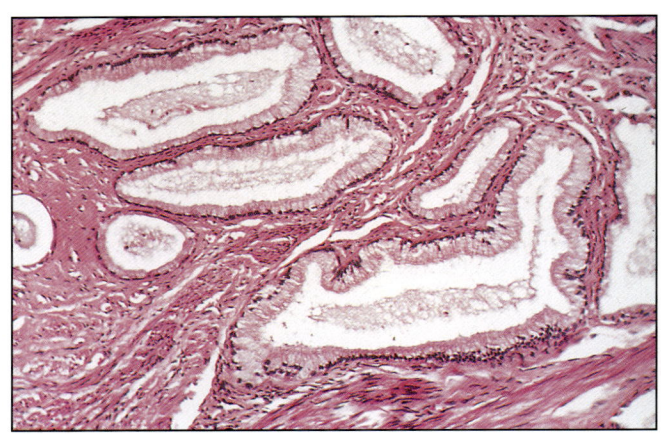

图12.145　膀胱宫颈内膜异位症。腺体被覆良性外观的黏液柱状上皮。

阑尾腺癌。

印戒细胞癌的主要鉴别诊断是转移性印戒细胞癌。形态学不能可靠区分。最终诊断依靠临床检查除外其他部位肿瘤的存在。印戒细胞癌与良性病变的鉴别一般并不困难，虽然有时肾源性腺瘤中的微小腺管可能类似于印戒细胞，但很少与印戒细胞癌混淆[549]。

肾源性腺瘤的其他独特形态（见下文）通常有助于诊断。

与透明细胞腺癌最难鉴别的是肾源性腺瘤（图12.146至12.148）[549]。肾源性腺瘤的临床特征与透明细胞腺癌截然不同。许多肾源性腺瘤患者<30岁（包括一些儿童），而最年轻的膀胱透明细胞腺癌患者年龄为43岁。肾源性腺瘤常常与泌尿生殖道手术史、创伤或结石有关，而透明细胞腺癌则缺乏这种病史。透明细胞腺癌比肾源性腺瘤体积大；前者不表现为显微镜下偶然发现的病灶，而肾源性腺瘤通常是镜下病灶，尽管直径达7cm的病例已有报道。有些病例在组织学上很难鉴别，因为二者均表现为腺管状、囊状和乳头状，一些肾源性腺瘤也可以出现细胞非典型性[550]。两种病变的被覆上皮也很相似，从柱状上皮细胞到扁平或鞋钉样上皮细胞（图12.147）。但有一些组织学特征支持癌的诊断：包括细胞弥漫分布，富含透明胞浆，胞浆内有大量糖原，核仁明显，核多形性和分裂象常见。但有些罕见的透明细胞腺癌形态温和，与肾源性腺瘤很难鉴别。对于这些病例，结合临床病史、体积大小并再次实施活检将有助于诊断。对于被认为是肾源性腺瘤而临床或病理学特征较特殊的病例，需要进行密切随访。需要了解的是肾源性腺瘤可以复发，因此在缺乏明确的恶性组织学证据时，出现复发并不能草率地诊断为癌。有学者认为透明细胞腺癌是与肾源性腺瘤相对应的恶性肿瘤，但两者临床表现不同且很少同时存在都不支持这种解释。此外，如果肾源性腺瘤是透明细胞腺癌的前驱病变，那么后者的发生应该是男性比女性多，膀胱比尿道多，但实际情况恰恰相反。

透明细胞腺癌特殊的组织学表现使之很容易与膀胱其他类型的原发性腺癌区分开。与从女性生殖道或肾转移而来的透明细胞癌的鉴别有时很困难。发病年龄轻以及围生期有己烯雌酚接触史，应该首先考虑女性生殖道转移的可能，但只有通过临床检查才能排除。在实际工作中这种情况非常罕见，因为在生殖道腺癌原发灶被发现之前就已经发生膀胱转移者几乎不可能出现，但有一例子宫内膜乳头状浆液性癌恰恰出现了这种情况[551]。弥漫生长的膀胱透明细胞腺癌可能与转移性肾细胞癌很难区分，但许多肾细胞癌中显著的纤细血管结构并不是少数已经确认的膀胱透明细胞腺癌的组织学特征。此外，与膀胱肿瘤不同，肾肿瘤不存在鞋钉样细胞以及胞浆内黏液。即使是晚期肿瘤，肾细胞癌也很少扩散至膀胱，这一点有助于诊断。

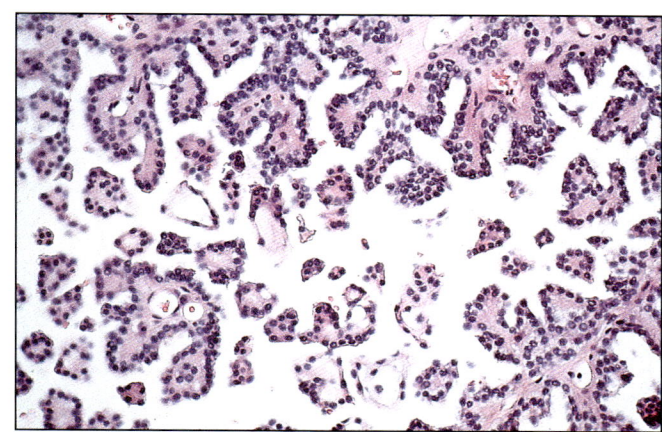

图12.146　具有明显乳头状结构的肾源性腺瘤。

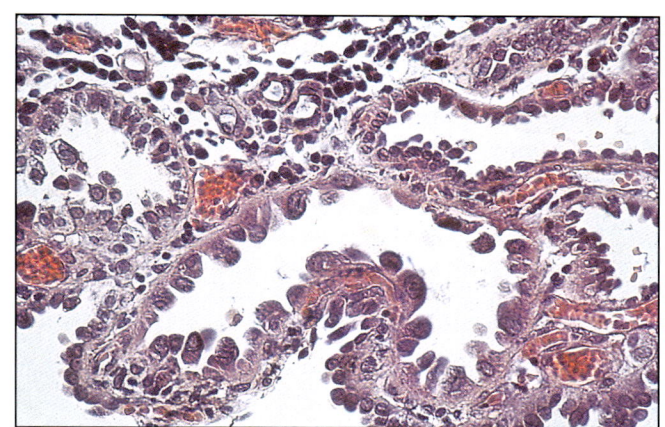

图12.147　肾源性腺瘤的鞋钉样细胞。

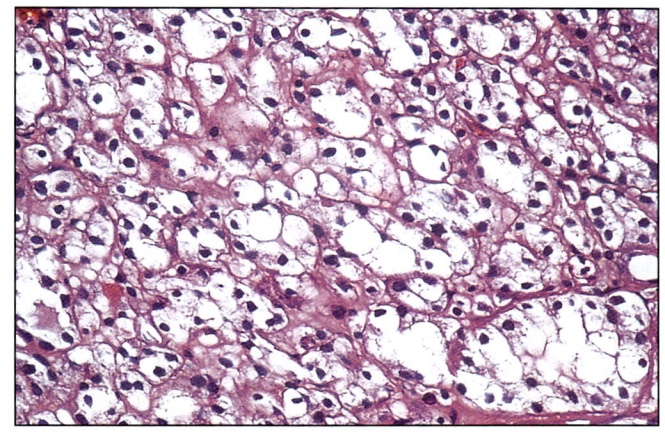

图12.148　肾源性腺瘤。肿瘤细胞具有丰富透明的胞浆。这只是局部表现，其他区域呈典型的肾源性腺瘤表现。

未分化癌 Undifferentiated carcinoma

正如其他器官中低分化癌和未分化癌分别代表不同的肿瘤类型一样，膀胱未分化癌名称的使用常常带有主观性。真正的膀胱未分化癌相对罕见，组织学表现常常与其他部位的未分化癌相似。主要从鉴别诊断的角度考虑，在此只讨论三种特殊的具有独特重要性的组织学亚型。

小细胞癌 Small cell carcinoma

组织学形态类似于肺同名肿瘤的膀胱小细胞未分化癌并不常见[552-559]。有一篇综述报道它们大约占膀胱恶性肿瘤的0.5%[556]。大约85%是男性。常为老年人，平均年龄69岁[553]，症状与其他类型的膀胱癌相似；肉眼血尿是最常见的主诉。至少有一例出现高血钙[555]，而另一例则产生异位促肾上腺皮质激素[557]。许多患者具有移行细胞癌病史或伴发移行细胞癌。这些肿瘤常为晚期，在一项研究中，22例患者中16例为C期或D期[553]。预后普遍很差，但有时根治性膀胱切除和高强度的辅助化疗可以使生存期延长几年[558]。

大体与组织学表现 肿瘤体积较大，呈息肉状，表面常有溃疡，组织学由成片的燕麦样小细胞构成，核深染；也可以由体积较大且核染色质多变的肿瘤细胞组成，与中间细胞型肺小细胞癌相似，或者由上述两种细胞混合构成（图12.149）。肿瘤可含有小的假菊形团，或偶尔出现癌巨细胞。常与其他类型的肿瘤混合存在，最常见的是原位或浸润性移行细胞癌，偶尔也出现鳞状细胞癌或腺癌。肿瘤浸润很深，常见广泛坏死。神经内分泌标志物免疫组化染色常为阳性。重要的是一部分病例表达TTF-1[560]，造成与肺癌转移鉴别的困难。电镜检查可以发现大部分病例含有直径150～250nm的致密核心颗粒。

鉴别诊断 小细胞癌可能会与淋巴瘤混淆，特别是在小的活检标本。淋巴和上皮标志物免疫组化染色有助于鉴别。膀胱原发性小细胞癌需要与转移癌区分开。临床检查排除了其他部位（特别是肺）的原发病灶，以及移行细胞癌（即使只有原位癌）的出现，强烈支持膀胱原发。

巨细胞癌 Giant cell carcinoma

有时膀胱未分化癌全部或主要由嗜酸性和嗜双色性胞浆的多形性大细胞构成，出现明显恶性的多核巨细胞（图12.150）[561]。这些肿瘤很像其他器官发生的巨细胞癌。不要将它们与上文提及的伴有破骨样巨细胞的肿瘤混淆（见536页）。这两种类型的巨细胞可以同时出现在一个肿瘤中。

淋巴上皮瘤样癌 Lymphoepithelioma-like carcinoma

近年来已有淋巴上皮瘤样癌的报道[562-564]。镜下由小淋巴细胞、浆细胞、嗜酸性粒细胞和类似大细胞淋巴瘤的非典型大细胞混合组成。在一些病例，非典型细胞的细胞角蛋白免疫组化染色对于明确它们的上皮来源非常重要。该部位肿瘤的发生似乎与Epstein-Barr病毒的感染无关[564]。与头颈部发生者相同，肿瘤主要与恶性淋巴瘤鉴别。只有在排除了淋巴上皮瘤样癌之后，才考

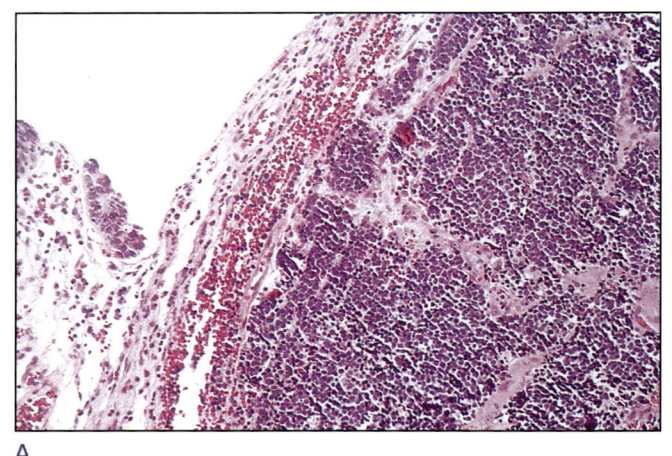

A

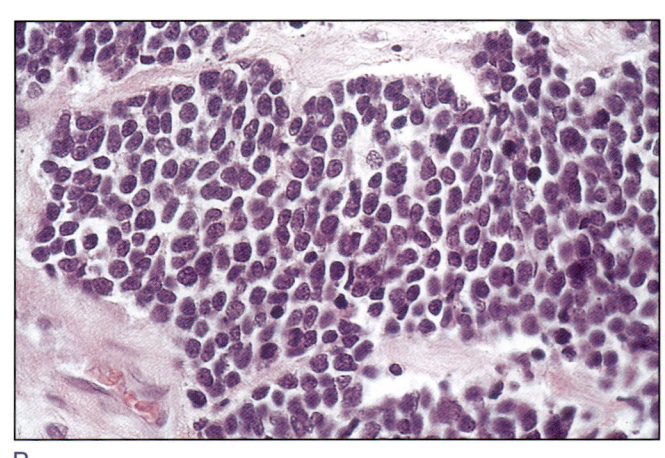

B

图12.149 膀胱小细胞未分化癌。巨大的息肉样肿物占据了大部分膀胱腔。

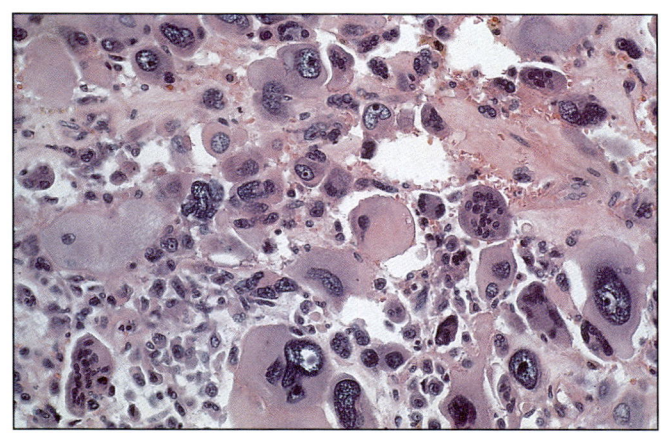

图12.150 膀胱巨细胞癌。

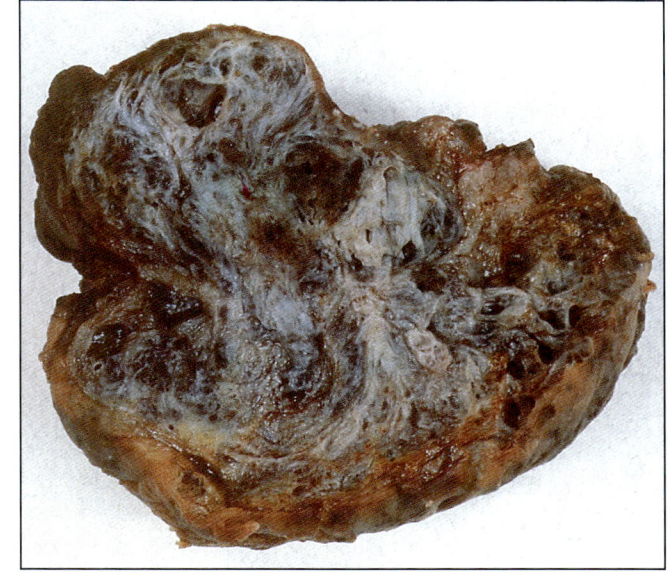

图12.151 膀胱血管瘤。肿瘤切面呈囊性、深蓝色。

虑膀胱恶性淋巴瘤的诊断。浸润细胞的不均一性是一条诊断线索，但是需要进行免疫组化染色来证实诊断。

含有一种以上组织学类型的癌
Carcinomas of more than one histologic type

这组病例之所以被列入膀胱肿瘤的分类中，目的在于引起大家注意：含两种或多种组织学类型的肿瘤并不少见。在诊断中要注明每一种类型，至少在备注中写明；其中一些类型，如典型移行细胞癌中出现的小细胞癌成分具有预后和治疗指导意义。

间叶性肿瘤 Mesenchymal tumors

良性间叶性肿瘤
Benign mesenchymal tumors

所有膀胱良性间叶性肿瘤都很罕见[565]，其中平滑肌瘤占多数[566-568]。目前已报道了大约150例，许多是比较老的文献，所用的名称也不同[569]。根据现有的报道，女性好发。肿瘤发生的部位不同，大体表现也不同，位于黏膜固有层者形成突向腔内的隆起型大肿物，而其他则形成膀胱壁间肿物或附着于浆膜的肿物。大体及镜下表现与较常见的子宫平滑肌瘤相似。少见类型，如上皮样平滑肌瘤可以发生但很罕见。同样，伴有细胞非典型性但无明显恶性表现的肿瘤在膀胱也很罕见。因此，与子宫不同，很少需要鉴别伴非典型性的平滑肌瘤与平滑肌肉瘤。

其他良性间叶性肿瘤，包括血管瘤（图12.151）、淋巴管瘤、神经纤维瘤、神经鞘瘤、颗粒细胞瘤、良性纤维组织细胞瘤以及脂肪瘤，也有文献报道[570-577]；尽管由于发生部位特殊而引起研究者的兴趣，但与常见部位的同类型肿瘤相比，并无任何特殊之处。正如预期的那样，血管瘤可以出现血尿。当患者确定患有von Recklinghausen病时，尤其应当考虑神经源性肿瘤。

恶性间叶性肿瘤
Malignant mesenchymal tumors

平滑肌肉瘤 Leiomyosarcoma

平滑肌肉瘤是成年人最常见的膀胱肉瘤[578-580]。膀胱平滑肌肉瘤偶尔可以发生于青少年，但在儿童罕见。这种年龄分布与膀胱横纹肌肉瘤截然不同，后者主要发生于儿童。膀胱平滑肌肉瘤患者临床表现与移行细胞癌相似。有些病例发生于环磷酰胺治疗后[581,582]。与平滑肌瘤一样，平滑肌肉瘤外观变化较大，但大部分呈明显息肉状，形成突向膀胱腔内的巨大肿物。肿瘤表面常有溃疡。切面白色，质软，可见灶状出血。有些肿瘤大体呈黏液样。组织学表现与其他部位的同类肿瘤差别不大（见第24章）。偶尔可出现黏液样平滑肌肉瘤[583]。

鉴别诊断 平滑肌肉瘤与肉瘤样移行细胞癌的鉴别在上文已经讨论过。另外需要重点与平滑肌肉瘤相鉴别的是两种非肿瘤性病变，即术后梭形细胞结节（图12.152）[584]和假肉瘤样反应性肌纤维母细胞增生（有时也称为炎性假瘤），后者最常见于年轻人[585-590]。近期膀胱手术史是诊断术后梭形细胞结节的关键线索，该病变比自发性反应性肌纤维母细胞增生更像平滑肌肉瘤。提

间叶性肿瘤

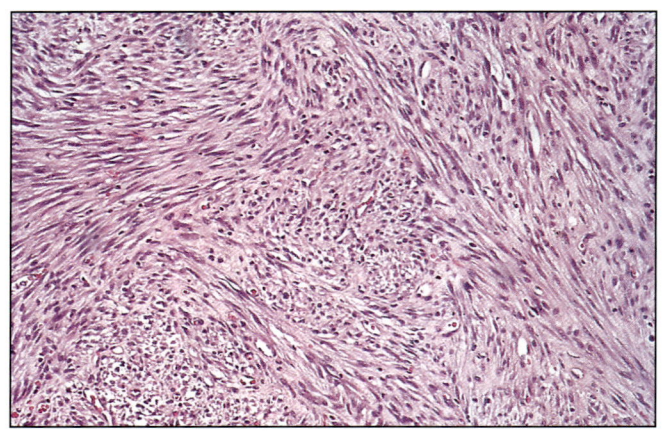

图12.152 膀胱术后梭形细胞结节。组织学表现很像平滑肌肉瘤。

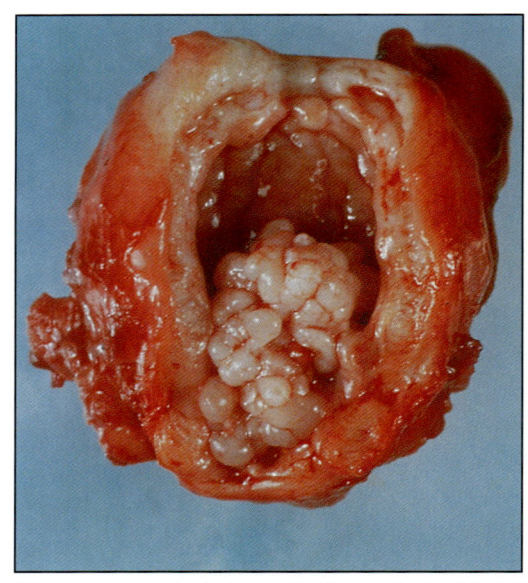

图12.153 儿童膀胱胚胎性横纹肌肉瘤（葡萄状肉瘤）。突向膀胱腔内一簇水肿的息肉状肿物，这是葡萄状肉瘤的典型表现。（Courtesy of Dr. Glenn Taylor.）

示术后梭形细胞结节的组织学特征是显著的血管增生，尽管这一表现并不总是出现。术后梭形细胞结节可以出现大量的核分裂象，但缺乏显著的细胞非典型性。自发性反应性肌纤维母细胞增生与平滑肌肉瘤的重要鉴别特征是前者出现明显水肿。这种病变常发生于年轻人，血管也很丰富，此外，它们常常含有很多炎症细胞。某些区域类似肉芽组织，梭形细胞与筋膜炎中的很像；缺乏深染细胞核和显著的细胞非典型性是重要的诊断线索。超微结构下，这两种非肿瘤性病变都含有典型肌纤维母细胞特征，不同于平滑肌肉瘤的平滑肌细胞，有助于鉴别诊断。免疫组化染色帮助不大，因为平滑肌肌动蛋白（SMA）、结蛋白（desmin）和角蛋白常为阳性[589]。一些病例也表达ALK-1，但缺乏*ALK*基因重排，提示它们可能与炎性肌纤维母细胞瘤无关[590]。

横纹肌肉瘤 Rhabdomyosarcoma

膀胱横纹肌肉瘤最常见于儿童，发病平均年龄大约是5岁[591-596]。然而，大部分患者年龄小于5岁，只是由于少部分患者要到青少年才发病致使平均年龄有所升高[595]。偶尔成年人也可以发生[597-601]。男女比例为3:2[601]。

大体表现 典型的横纹肌肉瘤呈息肉样，很像一串葡萄，这是葡萄状横纹肌肉瘤的典型表现（图12.153）。但也可见到其他特征性不强、与膀胱其他类型恶性肿瘤相似的大体表现。

组织学表现 显微镜下，膀胱横纹肌肉瘤呈分叶息肉状，由间质水肿的细胞稀疏区（图12.154）和深染的

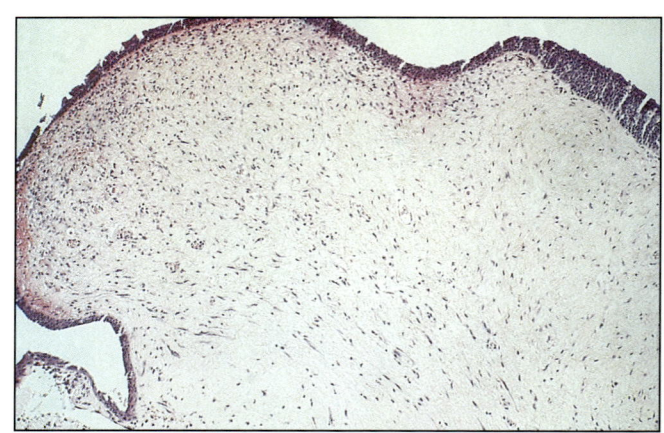

图12.154 膀胱胚胎性横纹肌肉瘤（葡萄状肉瘤）。注意这张插图中肿瘤组织显著水肿。

小细胞区构成，紧贴黏膜下可见一层致密的肿瘤细胞，这就是众所周知的新生层（见第24章）。在细胞丰富区，大部分肿瘤细胞较小，无明显特征，但散在的富于嗜酸性胞浆、偶尔可见横纹的肿瘤细胞则有助于做出诊断。这些小细胞常常具有明显的恶性表现，然而在某些肿瘤可以出现较成熟的骨骼肌细胞区。

鉴别诊断 一些其他类型的儿童膀胱肿瘤[602-604]，如罕见的错构瘤（图12.155和12.156），在大体上可以类似于横纹肌肉瘤，但组织病理学上无相像之处。组织学检查最常见的错误是低估病变程度，将其诊断为良性病变。这种情况通常发生于只含有少量肿瘤组织的活检标本；而对于完整切除的肿瘤标本则几乎不会出现这样

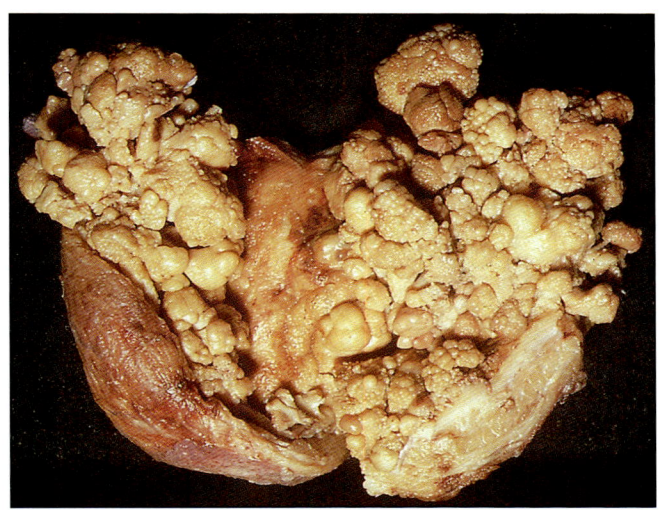

图12.155 儿童膀胱错构瘤。肿物体积巨大，呈明显的息肉样外观，很像葡萄状肉瘤。（Courtesy of Dr. Athanase Billis.）

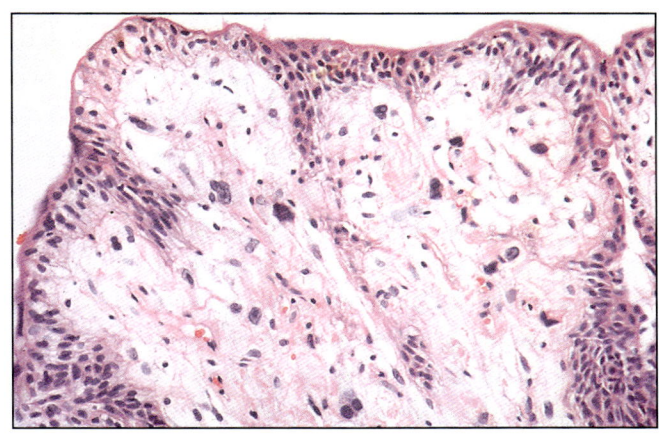

图12.157 伴非典型间质细胞的纤维上皮性息肉。非典型细胞具有深染的退变细胞核，无核分裂象。这种病变缺少新生层，而且发生于成年人，而需要与之鉴别的胚胎性横纹肌肉瘤很少发生于这个年龄段。

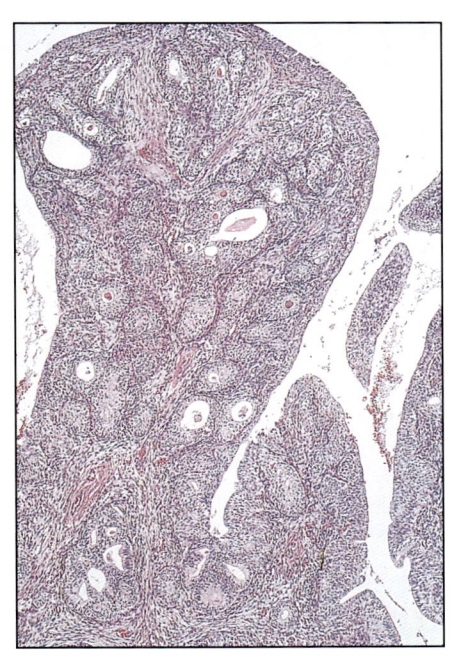

图12.156 儿童膀胱错构瘤。图12.155中肿物的组织学表现，息肉由类似于von Brunn巢、腺性膀胱炎以及囊性膀胱炎中的上皮细胞巢构成。（Courtesy of Dr. Athanase Billis.）

的问题，但是由于这种肿瘤的主要治疗手段是化疗，因此切除标本越来越少。对于儿童膀胱息肉样活检标本，应该高度怀疑横纹肌肉瘤。一个重要的鉴别诊断是反应性肌纤维母细胞增生[605]，因为后者好发于年轻患者，而实际上发病年龄经常要比大部分横纹肌肉瘤患者稍大。这种病变与横纹肌肉瘤的区分相对容易，因为前者具有均一的梭形细胞和明显的炎性细胞成分。尽管一些横纹肌肉瘤存在局灶分化很成熟的区域，提示横纹肌瘤的可能，但目前尚无膀胱横纹肌瘤的报道。了解横纹肌肉瘤可以出现分化较成熟的骨骼肌细胞这一事实可以避免误诊。含有非典型间质细胞的膀胱纤维上皮性息肉会使人考虑横纹肌肉瘤的可能[604]，但这种病变易发生于成年人而且细胞缺乏核分裂活性（图12.157）。

其他肉瘤　Other sarcomas

其他类型的肉瘤，如纤维肉瘤、所谓的恶性纤维组织细胞瘤以及骨肉瘤很少发生于膀胱[606-609]。它们与其他部位同类肿瘤相同。前两种肿瘤只有在小心除外肉瘤样癌之后才能诊断。骨肉瘤的鉴别诊断包括含骨组织的其他膀胱肿瘤，包括癌肉瘤（见下文）和伴间质骨化生的移行细胞癌（见上文）。

混合性肿瘤　Mixed tumors

良性混合性肿瘤　Benign mixed tumors

文献已有一例良性混合性肿瘤的报道。此例被命名为"腺纤维瘤"的肿瘤发生于一位46岁男性，临床出现血尿[610]，肿瘤大小3cm×2cm，位于膀胱前壁。大体上，肿瘤呈菜花样外观，可见囊腔形成。组织学上可见腺管样结构分布于局灶黏液样的纤维平滑肌组织中。一些管腔内可见乳头状突起，一些管腔囊性扩张并含有无结构的粉红色物质。

低级别恶性混合性肿瘤（腺肉瘤）　Low-grade malignant mixed tumors (adenosarcoma)

文献已有一例膀胱腺肉瘤的报道[611]，而许多年前

混合性肿瘤

所报道的一例"腺平滑肌瘤"有可能也是同一种病变[612]。确诊病例发生于一位62岁女性,伴血尿。肿瘤位于膀胱侧壁,呈蕈伞样,表面可见息肉状突起。显微镜下可见非典型性子宫内膜样间质包绕腺体,并浸透膀胱壁达周围脂肪组织。此患者伴有子宫内膜异位症,被认为是肿瘤的起源。

恶性混合性肿瘤
Malignant mixed tumors

目前已有大约50例证据可靠的膀胱癌肉瘤的报道[613-616]。大部分发生于老年人,平均年龄62岁。仅约10%的患者年龄小于50岁。临床症状与其他体积较大的膀胱肿瘤相似,大多数肿瘤体积巨大,外生性。显微镜下,表现为癌和肉瘤成分共同存在,两者紧密混合,这是该肿瘤的特征性表现(图12.158)。上皮成分通常类似高级别移行细胞癌,但1/3的病例可出现腺性或鳞状分化,偶尔为未分化癌。间质成分类似于高级别纤维肉瘤、平滑肌肉瘤或非特异性梭形细胞肉瘤。一半病例出现软骨肉瘤分化(图12.159),1/3出现骨分化,1/4出现骨骼肌分化;有一例肿瘤可见局部的脂肪肉瘤成分[615]。尽管大部分患者都进行了积极治疗,但其预后仍然很差。

鉴别诊断 膀胱癌肉瘤的鉴别诊断包括肉瘤样癌、伴间质骨或软骨化生的癌、膀胱原发性骨肉瘤或软骨肉瘤,以及伴假肉瘤样间质的癌。在肉瘤样癌,上皮成分不知不觉地融合于梭形细胞区,无异源性分化区域,而且梭形细胞至少局部表达细胞角蛋白。相反,在癌肉瘤

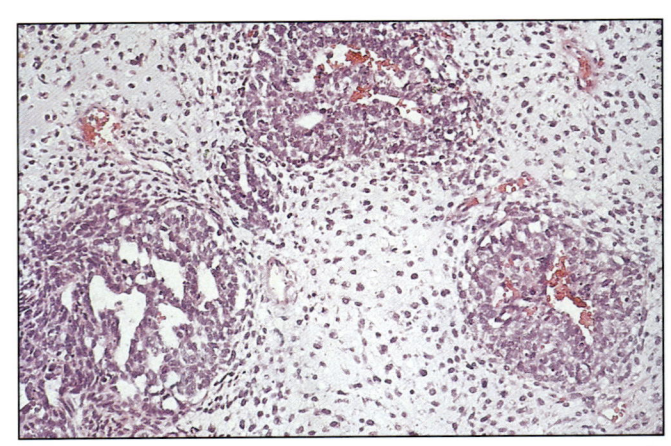

图12.159 膀胱癌肉瘤。三个癌细胞团被伴软骨分化的肿瘤性间质所包绕。

中,上皮成分与肉瘤背景形成对比,二者的转化更加突然。此外,癌肉瘤中的肉瘤成分和癌成分会出现多个区域的紧密混合,而肉瘤样癌中两种成分的这种相互交错并不常见。伴有化生性骨和软骨的癌与伴骨软骨成分的癌肉瘤之间的不同在于,前者的骨与软骨是良性的。膀胱骨肉瘤和软骨肉瘤缺少诊断癌肉瘤所必需的上皮性成分。伴假肉瘤样间质的癌,其非典型间质细胞缺少癌肉瘤中梭形肿瘤细胞典型的恶性特征。

淋巴瘤与白血病
Lymphoma and leukemia

非Hodgkin淋巴瘤患者的尸检发现大约10%~20%的病例膀胱可见淋巴瘤浸润[617];而Hodgkin淋巴瘤累及膀胱者只占4%。只有少数膀胱继发性淋巴瘤患者出现膀胱症状,而且几乎没有因此作为临床首发症状的患者(图12.160)[618]。膀胱原发性非Hodgkin淋巴瘤罕见。大部分文献只是很少的一些病例报道。多数肿瘤是低度或中度恶性,但偶尔也有高度恶性病例的报道[619-625]。最近的数据表明最常见的低度恶性淋巴瘤是B细胞来源的黏膜相关型(MALT型)(见第21章)[62]。T细胞淋巴瘤也有文献报道[624],其中少数表现为肉瘤样形态的病例,其诊断相当困难[625]。膀胱淋巴瘤的大体表现多样。一些病例的大体表现很有特征性,呈大的白色鱼肉样肿物,但有时也会出现并不典型的广基息肉样病变,伴膀胱壁增厚。肿瘤常常体积较大,表面被覆完整的黏膜,但有时也会出现局灶溃疡。目前只有一例

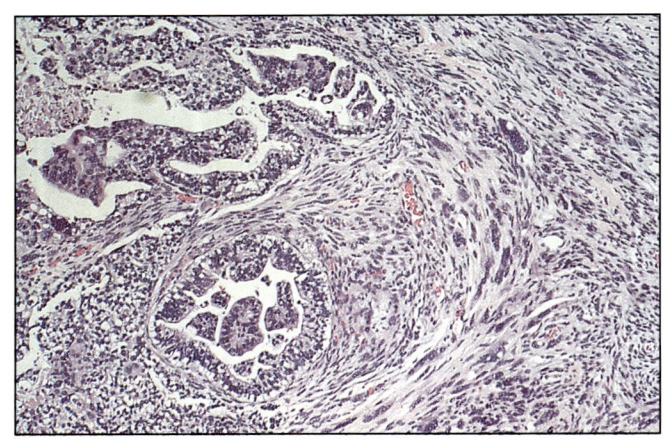

图12.158 膀胱癌肉瘤。恶性腺体被肉瘤性间质分隔开。

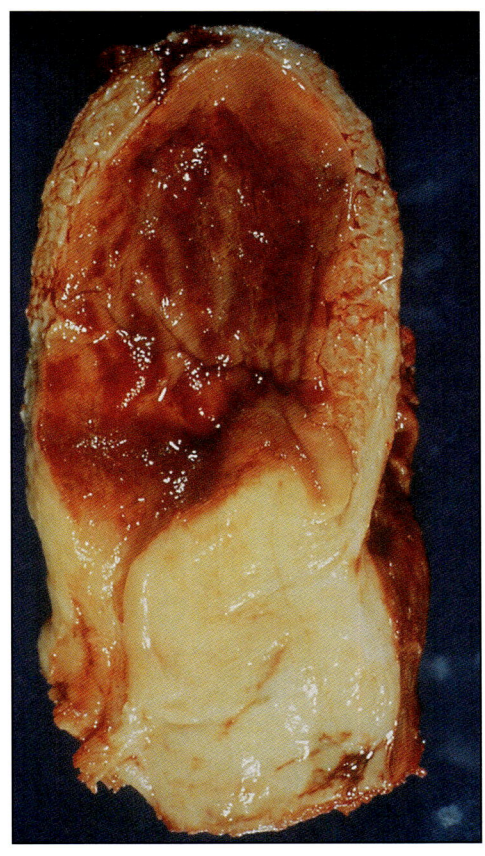

图12.160　膀胱恶性淋巴瘤。一个白色鱼肉状肿物占据了部分膀胱壁，并侵犯周围组织。（Courtesy of Dr. Fred Askin.）

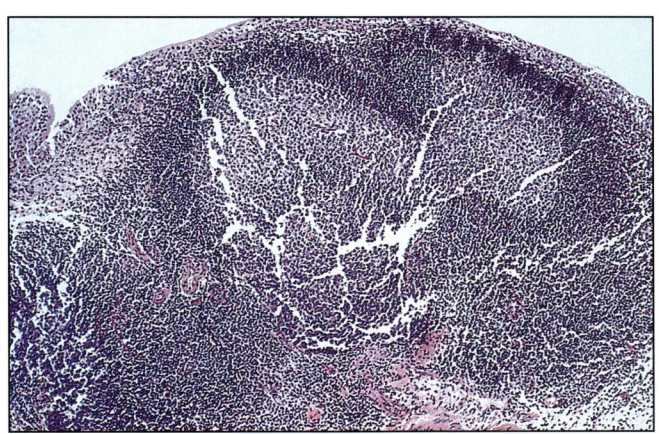

图12.161　滤泡性膀胱炎。这种病变可以形成肉眼可见的白色结节。此病例中的淋巴滤泡具有典型的增生性滤泡表现。

证据可信的膀胱原发性Hodgkin淋巴瘤的报道[626]。患者为56岁女性，膀胱镜检查发现多个突向膀胱腔的肿物。肿瘤的组织学表现最符合淋巴细胞为主型。

多发性骨髓瘤可以累及膀胱[627]，但对于已知病史的患者，诊断并不困难。无骨髓侵犯的浆细胞瘤或广义的骨髓瘤很少起源于膀胱[628]。所有患者均为成年人。大体表现与其他淋巴瘤相似，镜下检查显示浆细胞瘤的特征。

尸检发现大约25%的急性白血病和15%的慢性白血病患者出现膀胱受累[629]。文献报道一位29岁的女性出现膀胱粒细胞肉瘤，伴排尿困难和血尿，但在确诊时外周血及骨髓检查正常。膀胱镜检查发现一个8cm的息肉状黏膜下肿物。患者在出现症状3年后仍然健在[630]。

正如其他部位发生的恶性淋巴瘤一样，膀胱淋巴瘤需要与没有明显上皮分化证据的低分化癌鉴别。高倍镜下仔细观察淋巴细胞特有的组织学特征就可以解决这一问题，但在某些罕见的病例需要免疫组化帮助。应当记住的是，在常见的滤泡性膀胱炎（图12.161），膀胱黏膜也可以出现小的白色结节。但是，这种病变中的淋巴组织，包括可能会出现的生发中心，具有典型的反应性淋巴组织病变特征。

其他原发性肿瘤
Miscellaneous primary tumors

副神经节瘤　Paraganglioma

副神经节瘤（也见第28章）是膀胱非移行细胞肿瘤中比较重要的一种，尽管并不常见，但也并非罕见[631,632]。大约2/3的肿瘤可以产生激素，导致患者出现高血压。半数患者具有药物无效的头痛、心悸、高血压、视力模糊和（或）流汗等症状。约半数患者临床表现为血尿。患者年龄跨度很大，男女发病比例大致相同。少数患者同时患有神经纤维瘤病。

大体和组织学表现　肿瘤通常表现为分叶状实性肿物（图12.162），位于黏膜下或肌壁内，表面被覆完整的尿路上皮。这些肿瘤直径可达10cm，但多数最大直径只有几厘米。镜下检查常显示肿瘤细胞排列成特征性的球团状（Zellballen）结构（图12.163），但这种组织学表现并非一定出现，某些肿瘤呈弥漫性生长。固有肌层侵犯常常很明显（图12.164）。不同病例或同一肿瘤不同区域的核分裂活性和多形性均有变化。大约10%的肿瘤是恶性，这可以很准确地从膀胱壁的侵犯深度预测出来[632]。有时在膀胱外扩散前局部复发会持续很长时间。远处器官转移罕见。

鉴别诊断　当肿瘤的球团状结构很明显时，应当想到该病的诊断；但是，正如上文所述，这种结构并非总能见到。一个膀胱肿瘤含有丰富的嗜酸性胞浆时，应该

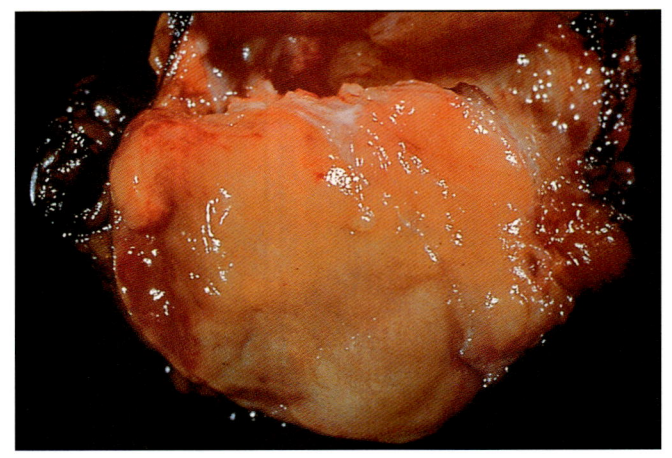

图12.162　膀胱副神经节瘤。肿瘤分叶状，棕褐色。

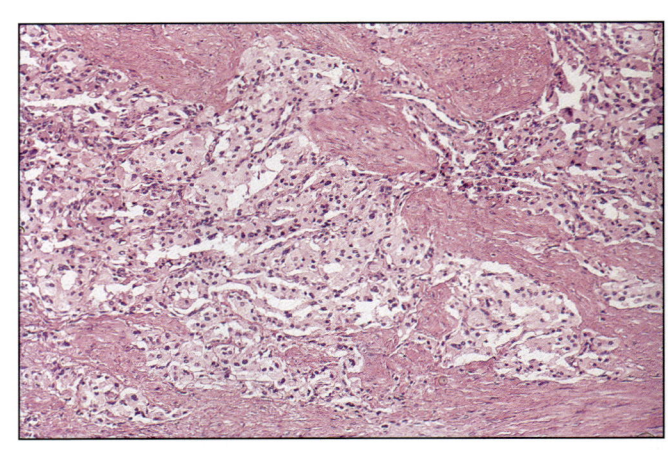

图12.164　膀胱副神经节瘤。肌层侵犯很明显。

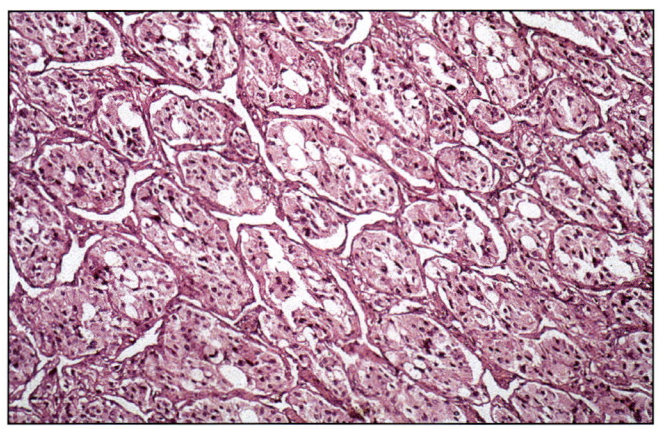

图12.163　膀胱副神经节瘤。球团状（Zellballen）结构。

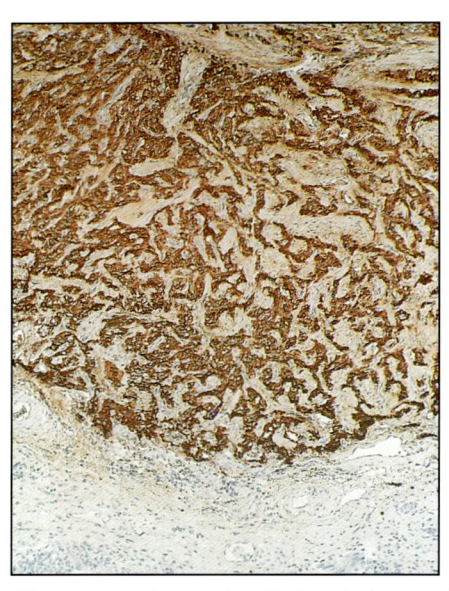

图12.165　膀胱副神经节瘤。免疫组化染色显示肿瘤细胞嗜铬素强阳性。

考虑到这种肿瘤的可能并进行适当的特殊染色来帮助诊断（见第28章）（图12.165）。临床病史以及不呈现膀胱癌常见的大体表现这两点更加支持该病诊断。最为困难的鉴别诊断是移行细胞癌，最近的一篇文献强调[631]，20%的肿瘤最初被误诊为癌。可能最具有欺骗性的表现是巢状的肿瘤细胞侵犯肌层，会使人认为是浸润性巢状移行细胞癌。经尿道切除标本常常会出现人工假象，而且这些肿瘤常常为初诊病例，使其诊断更加困难。当出现细胞非典型性以及核分裂象时，就更容易误诊为癌。因此这是膀胱病理学中非常需要免疫组化帮助的领域，当然，只有当病理学家能够怀疑副神经节瘤时才可能进行染色。

类癌　Carcinoid tumors

成人膀胱类癌的发病年龄为30～75岁[633]，没有一例出现类癌综合征。肿瘤最大径可达5cm，均位于黏膜下。镜下检查发现3例肿瘤呈典型的类癌表现，但有一例细胞非典型性很明显，提示小细胞癌的可能；此例肿瘤在临床上表现为恶性[634]。

鉴别诊断　膀胱类癌非常罕见，这意味着只有当其他类似于类癌的肿瘤被排除后才能做出诊断。例如，有些移行细胞癌会出现巢状生长方式，很像类癌。移行细胞癌和类癌细胞学特征的不同，以及银染、免疫组化或电镜检查有助于诊断。

恶性黑色素瘤　Malignant melanoma

膀胱恶性黑色素瘤非常罕见。在1984年发表的一篇重要综述中，只有3例已报道的病例被认为是可以承认的[635]。随后报道了另外一例病例[636]。患者年龄48～65岁。大体检查发现3例肿瘤呈棕褐色或黑色。其表现类似于皮肤黑色素瘤（见第23章）。

鉴别诊断　与转移性黑色素瘤的鉴别可能比较困难，因为原发性皮肤黑色素瘤可以发生消退。事实上，有学者认为要证明黑色素瘤原发于膀胱几乎是不可能的。与诸如肉瘤等其他类型肿瘤鉴别时，黑色素颗粒的存在以及S-100和HMB45蛋白的免疫组化染色阳性很有帮助。

皮样囊肿　Dermoid cysts

已有4例发生于30～49岁女性的膀胱皮样囊肿报道，这些患者有症状的时间很长。这些病变是囊性肿物，含有毛发和钙化物质[637,638]。应该记住的是卵巢皮样囊肿偶尔可以穿透膀胱壁进入膀胱腔内[637]。因为卵巢皮样囊肿远比膀胱发生者常见，因此在诊断膀胱原发皮样囊肿之前必须除外卵巢皮样囊肿继发性累及膀胱的可能。

绒毛膜癌　Choriocarcinoma

正如前文所述，移行细胞癌可以伴有滋养叶细胞分化，而且在某些病例，这种分化非常广泛，取材不充分时可能只发现绒毛膜癌成分。在缺少可辨认的移行细胞癌成分的情况下，要想知道肿瘤是起源于体细胞还是真正的生殖细胞肿瘤是不可能的。已报道的那个病例即使不存在移行细胞癌成分，也很难确定它不是体细胞来源的肿瘤。绒毛膜癌的形态学表现很有特征，容易做出诊断。除了区分纯粹的生殖细胞来源绒毛膜癌与体细胞来源绒毛膜癌外，并无其他方面的诊断问题。

卵黄囊瘤　Yolk sac tumor

有文献报道了一例发生于一个1岁男童的膀胱卵黄囊瘤，患者出现血尿，血清α-甲胎蛋白水平显著升高，肿瘤呈息肉样，红褐色，胶冻样，可见局灶出血和坏死[639]。患者接受了部分膀胱切除和化疗，术后14个月仍然状况良好。当遇到一例发生于儿童的膀胱肿瘤，如果肿瘤形态符合卵黄囊瘤，而且明显不是其他类型的肿瘤时，应考虑该诊断的可能。

膀胱继发性肿瘤
Secondary tumors of the bladder

邻近器官（通常是生殖道或结肠）发生的肿瘤有时可以侵犯膀胱（图12.166，12.167），少数情况下远处器官诸如乳腺等的肿瘤也可以转移至膀胱[275,640-643]。在一项研究中，排除淋巴瘤和白血病后，其他的继发性肿瘤大约占膀胱恶性肿瘤的15%[643]。这些肿瘤来源于女性生殖道(30%)、前列腺和精囊腺(26%)、下消化道(24%)，以及远处器官(20%)。大部分侵犯膀胱的肠道肿瘤来自直肠和乙状结肠[645,646]。亦有阑尾癌扩散至膀胱的报道[647]。

鉴别诊断　对于继发性肿瘤，诊断难易程度与原发瘤的形态有关[648,653]。在大部分病例，如果膀胱肿瘤的形态不足以明确诊断，了解原发瘤病史对于诊断很有帮助。在一些病例，原发瘤已经在多年前治疗过，而病史中没有提供。更为困难的是那些同时或先于原发瘤被发

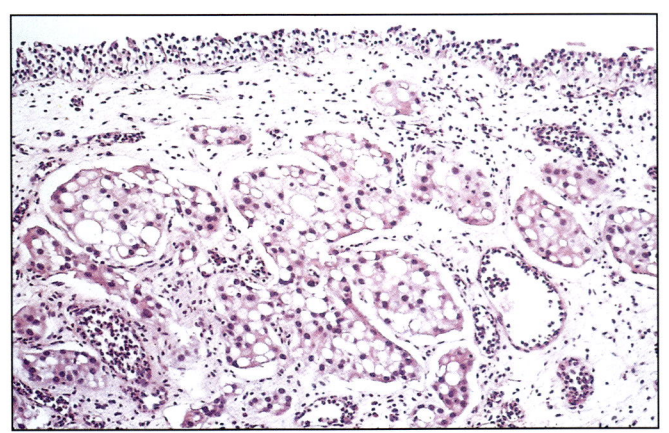

图12.166　前列腺腺癌转移至膀胱。表面可见尿路上皮。

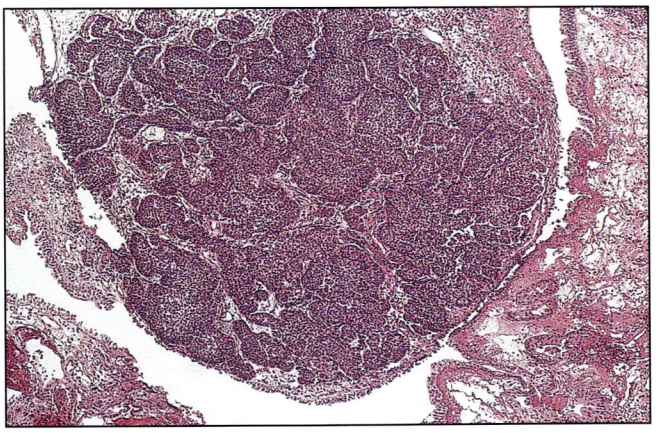

图12.167　宫颈鳞状细胞癌转移至膀胱。在某些区域肿瘤呈圆形细胞巢，低倍镜下很像内翻性乳头状瘤。

现的病例。大部分侵犯膀胱的女性生殖道原发肿瘤，其组织学表现均有特点，不同于任何类型的原发性膀胱癌。但是，对于那些阴道或宫颈鳞状细胞癌，单纯依靠形态表现不能与原发膀胱肿瘤区别开来。当肿瘤形态不是典型的膀胱癌，而且肿瘤主要广泛侵犯膀胱外层以及出现大量的血管和淋巴管癌栓时，应考虑转移癌的可能。

尿道肿瘤　　Tumors of the urethra

良性肿瘤及瘤样病变
Benign tumors and tumor-like lesions

目前为止，最常见的尿道肿物是尿道肉阜[654,655]，一项研究显示大约占尿道"肿瘤"的90%[655]。这种病变常常发生于绝经后女性的尿道口内侧。常为红色，质软，易出血。这种病变最重要的临床意义是某些肿瘤偶尔会被临床误诊为肉阜。例如，一项包括14例尿道癌的研究中，6例被临床医师诊断为肉阜[655]。显微镜下，肉阜和肿瘤的区分并不困难。其形态学表现多样，但常常为明确的良性表现。与它们红色的外观相吻合的是镜下检查常常会发现显著的血管；一些病例几乎全部由肉芽组织构成。另外一些病例间质水肿很明显而炎症并不显著。少数情况下，间质可出现间叶来源的非典型细胞，它们属于反应性增生细胞，可被误诊为肿瘤细胞（图12.168）[587]。有时病变表面可呈乳头状，这些乳头被覆增生的尿路上皮或鳞状上皮。

纤维上皮性息肉可发生于尿道，但比输尿管少见。报道病例多为小于10岁的男孩，但有一些发生于成年人[656,657]。它们常发生于邻近精阜的尿道后壁，但有报道称也可发生于尿道前壁[656]。大体和镜下表现与发生于输尿管者相似（见第520页）。

生殖道和肛周尖锐湿疣可以累及尿道[658]。通常只累及远端尿道[659]，但偶尔病变可扩散至近端尿道；膀胱和输尿管受累罕见[660,661]。这些病变在大体和镜下表现都与发生于生殖道黏膜者相似。应该仔细检查这些病变中的癌前改变。尿道口或其附近偶尔可以发生缺乏人乳头状瘤病毒感染特征性表现的良性乳头状鳞状上皮病变，对这些病变使用"鳞状上皮乳头状瘤"来命名[662]。

在一位女性患者，我们发现了类似于肠道腺瘤性息肉的尿道病变。文献已有三例绝经后妇女远端尿道绒毛状腺瘤的报道，它们与胃肠道发生的同名病变很像[663-665]。其中一例与腺癌伴发[663]。尿道腺癌可以表现为乳头状，因此任何伴有显著细胞非典型性的尿道乳头状腺体病变应该怀疑为癌，诊断绒毛状腺瘤应该慎重。有时显微镜下会意外发现尿道黏膜出现肠上皮化生[669]，这可以解释一部分尿道腺癌的组织来源问题，尽管大部分腺癌可能起源于尿道旁腺。

一种在文献中引起关注的尿道前列腺部良性病变现在被称为前列腺型息肉[667]。顾名思义，它们是由前列腺型上皮构成的乳头状病变[667-675]。大部分发生于年轻男性，特征性的临床表现是血尿或血精。一项包括25例患者的研究发现其发病年龄18~40岁[673]；而另外一项研究中患者平均年龄为31岁[667]。这种病变也可以发生于老年患者，一项研究显示其发病年龄39~70岁[675]。镜下检查显示病变由纤细的乳头或个别分叶状息肉构成，被覆类似前列腺腺泡内衬上皮的立方或矮柱状上皮细胞（图12.169和12.170）；也可出现移行细胞成分，特别是在病变的表面[667]。前列腺型腺体可以出

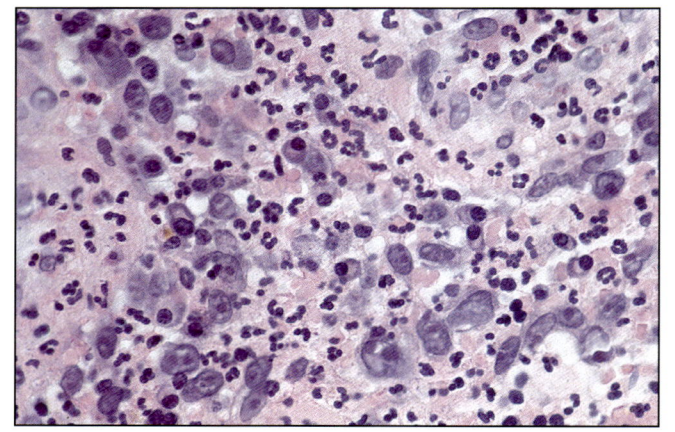

图12.168　尿道肉阜间质中的非典型细胞，被认为是间叶来源。

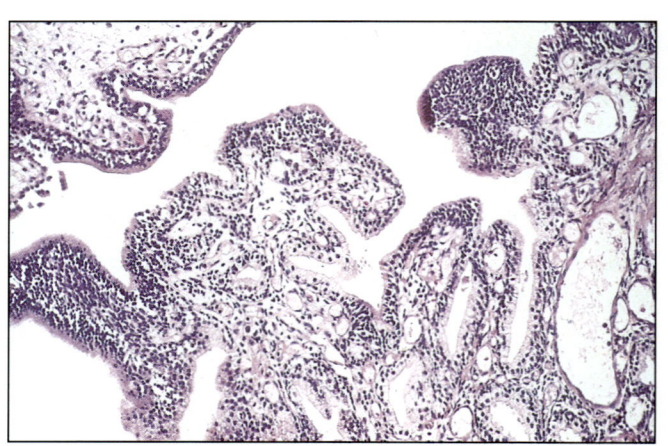

图12.169　尿道前列腺型息肉。

现在间质中。进行前列腺特异抗原和前列腺酸性磷酸酶的免疫组化染色可以明确这些上皮的前列腺源性。对于发生于年轻男性的前列腺型息肉,与息肉样突向尿道的前列腺腺癌的鉴别并不困难,但在老年患者存在困难,因为两者的临床表现相似(图12.171)[630,671]。因此,在老年患者,只有排除癌之后,才能做出前列腺型息肉的诊断。前列腺型息肉几乎不出现非典型性,但其中一些病例可以发生恶性转化[674,676]。

一种类似于肿瘤的重要尿道病变是肾源性腺瘤[677-685]。男女均可发生,但女性更常见。在女性患者,病变常常发生于尿道憩室内(图12.172),说明肾源性腺瘤和慢性炎症有关。在男性患者,一部分肾源性腺瘤发生于尿道球部,另外一部分发生于尿道前列腺部。尿道病变具有肾源性腺瘤的特征性组织学表现,与发生于膀胱者相同。病变通常局限于黏膜(或紧邻黏膜下方一个相对狭窄的区域),偶尔这些小腺管可向下延伸至较深的部位,在一些男性患者,病变可累及前列腺,有时与前列腺癌的鉴别困难[680,685]。

与乳头状或息肉样膀胱炎类似的息肉样、乳头样炎性病变可以发生于尿道任何位置[686]。

尿道经典型和内翻性尿路上皮乳头状瘤远比膀胱少见。在Kunze等的详尽综述中[431],只有3.5%的内翻性乳头状瘤发生于尿道,且全部位于尿道前列腺部。一个发生于尿道阴茎部的单发病灶已见报道[687]。这些病变的诊断标准与发生于膀胱者相同(见第523页)。与膀胱一样,尿道也可以出现混合性乳头状瘤(图12.173和12.174)。

尿道良性间叶性肿瘤(如平滑肌瘤[688,689])非常罕见,较常见于女性,但目前认为该病变与其他部位发生的同类肿瘤不存在病理学差异。其中一例特殊的尿道良性肿瘤,组织学类似于乳腺纤维腺瘤[690]。

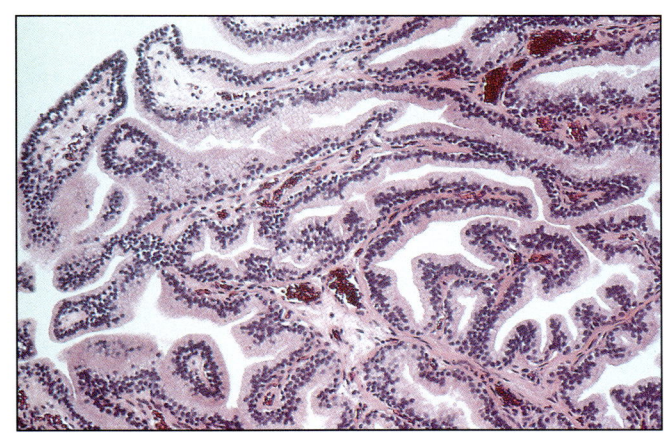

图12.170 尿道前列腺型息肉。注意基底细胞层、温和的细胞形态以及腺体之间的间质成分。

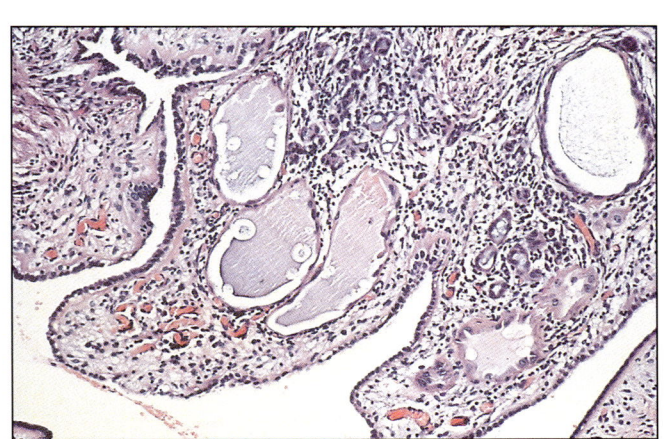

图12.172 发生于尿道憩室的肾源性腺瘤。高倍镜下可见肾源性腺瘤典型的小腺管和小囊结构。

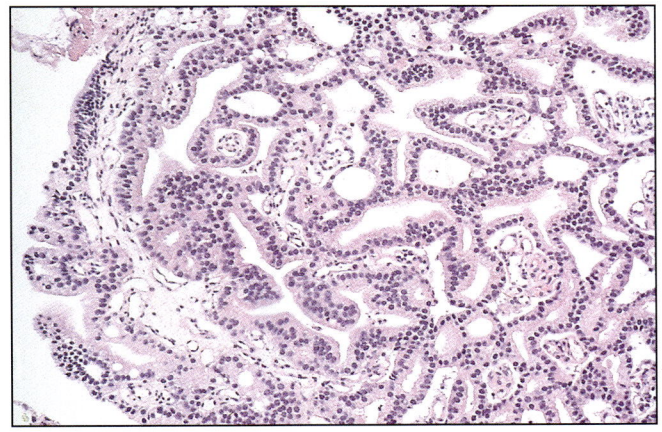

图12.171 形成息肉样尿道内肿块的前列腺腺癌。与图12.169和12.170中的良性病变相似。基底细胞缺如。

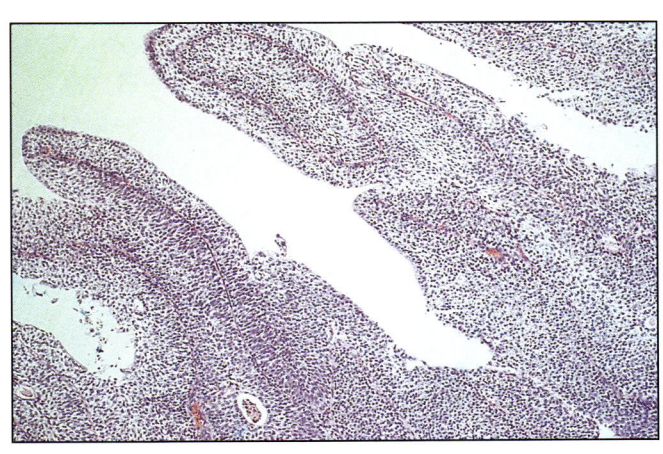

图12.173 尿道混合性乳头状瘤。此插图显示的是外生性成分。

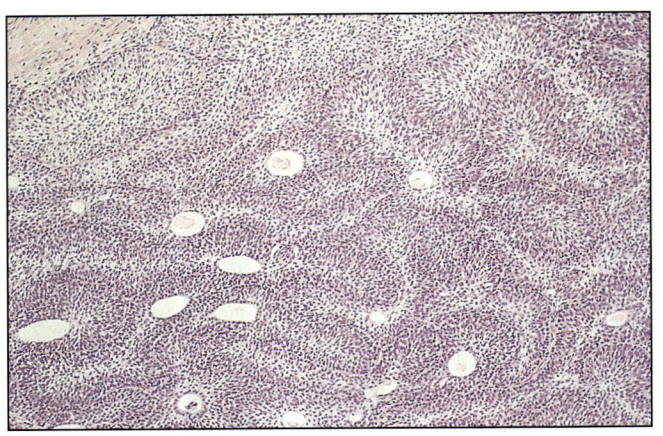

图12.174 尿道混合性乳头状瘤。此插图显示的是图12.173中病变的内翻性成分。

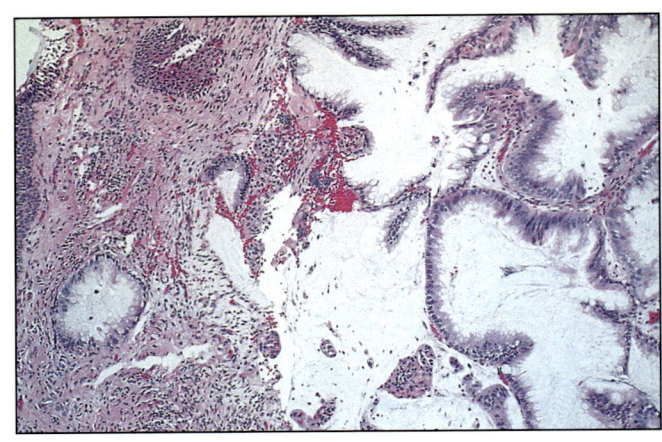

图12.175 尿道低级别黏液腺癌。

恶性肿瘤　Malignant tumors

癌　Carcinoma

大部分尿道恶性肿瘤是癌[691-715]。许多资料显示，与泌尿道其他器官不同，尿道癌在女性远比男性常见。在一篇综述中，女性发病率是男性的3倍稍多[692]。在男性和女性，鳞状细胞癌均占肿瘤的60%～70%。其余类型的肿瘤是移行细胞癌和腺癌，以及少量未分化癌。在一篇关于20岁以上该肿瘤女性患者的综述中[694]，腺癌病例是移行细胞癌的2倍。相反，一篇关于男性尿道肿瘤的综述发现，移行细胞癌的发病是腺癌的2倍稍多[715]。膀胱癌的相对发生率与尿道移行细胞癌（通常发生于尿道前列腺部）具有显著的相关性[716-719]。尿道移行细胞原位癌在有膀胱癌病史或同时伴有膀胱癌的患者中远比单独发生者常见。偶尔移行细胞癌以Paget病样生长方式侵犯尿道，有时可累及尿道旁腺或扩散至尿道口[720,721]。任何类型的膀胱恶性肿瘤都可以通过直接扩散的方式累及尿道；偶尔会出现极其罕见的膀胱肿瘤尿道复发。

尿道癌通常发生于50～70岁的老年患者，偶尔可发生于年轻人，而且至少已有一例青少年男性的个例报道[715]。男性及女性患者均发现与尿道狭窄有关；一篇综述认为大约1/3的男性患者与之有关[715]。男性及女性患者均具有尿道不适症状，众所周知，临床上这种情况的出现与疾病诊断困难有关。其他伴随症状少见，但至少已有3例高钙血症[711,722]、1例弥散性血管内凝血[723]和1例类甲状旁腺功能亢进[724]的报道。大约40例女性尿道肿瘤发生于尿道憩室[725,726]。超过一半为腺癌，其中大部分是透明细胞型。

尽管在尿道前列腺部常见，偶尔移行细胞癌也可出现在前段尿道，其中一例发生于舟状窝[727-729]。人类乳头状瘤病毒6型与一些男性低级别移行细胞癌和一例男性鳞状细胞癌有关[730,731]。与发生于膀胱者相同，一些肿瘤同时具有移行细胞癌和鳞状细胞癌的特征，偶尔会出现类似于直肠肛门区的泄殖腔癌[732,733]。腺鳞癌也有文献报道，其中一例还伴有高钙血症[722]。

男女患者腺癌的大体和组织学表现多样。一些肿瘤呈胶冻样，但大部分没有特殊的大体表现。组织学上通常具有非特异的腺管结构，但类似于结肠腺癌的形态学表现也很常见（图12.175）。后者中的一些病例为胶样癌[734]，局灶及弥漫分布的印戒细胞癌罕见[705,706,713]。肿瘤可能与附近的腺性尿道炎有关[700,713]，后者可出现癌前改变[734]。边界清楚的囊内乳头状囊腺癌偶尔可见[707]，可能来源于尿道旁腺。

透明细胞腺癌是一种重要的尿道腺癌亚型（图12.176）[735]。一篇包括22例女性尿道腺癌的病例报道中，9例是透明细胞型，其余13例是黏液腺癌[704]。大部分尿道透明细胞腺癌发生于女性。与女性生殖道的透明细胞腺癌很像，因此必须排除肿瘤扩散至尿道的可能。只有2例透明细胞腺癌发生于男性[736,737]。一种要与透明细胞腺癌进行鉴别诊断的重要病变是肾源性腺瘤，这个问题在第543页已经讨论。两种肿瘤中大约1/3发生于尿道憩室，在此处它们的鉴别诊断尤其困难，但在膀胱肿瘤章节所列出的诊断标准同样有帮助。

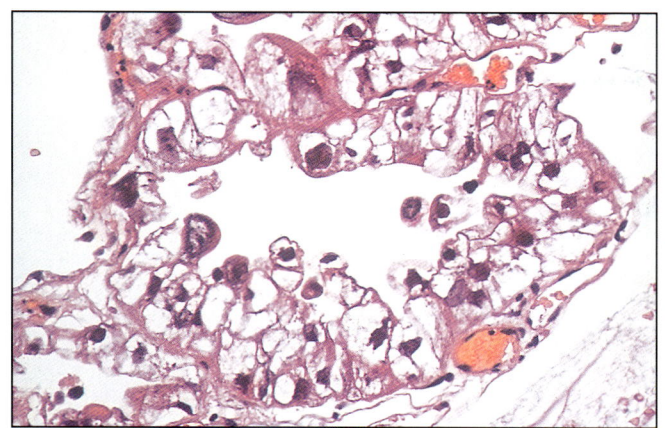

图12.176 尿道透明细胞腺癌。注意丰富的透明胞浆和少量的鞋钉样细胞。

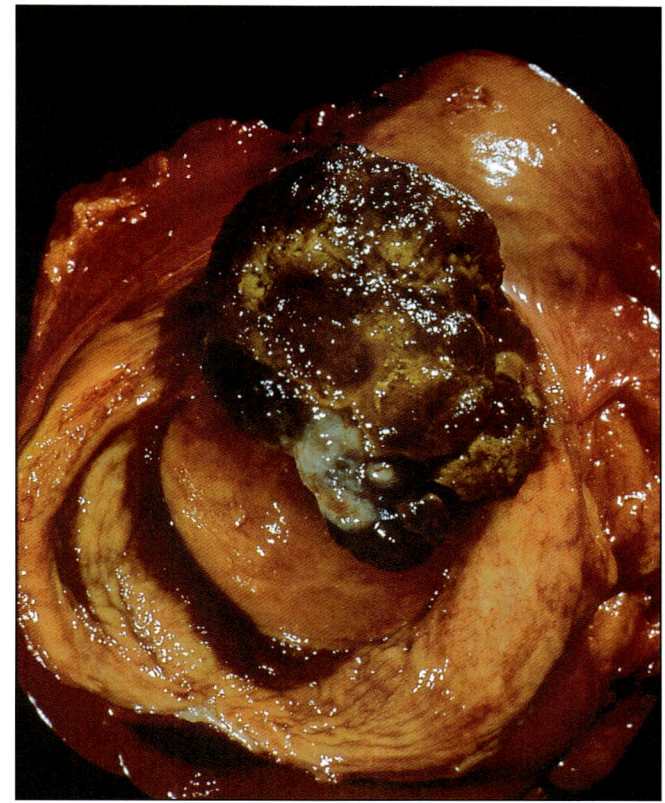

图12.177 尿道恶性黑色素瘤。肿瘤体积大，息肉样，局部呈黑色，提示其诊断。

有一种不常见的女性尿道腺癌在组织学上类似于前列腺腺癌，而且免疫组化显示前列腺特异抗原和前列腺酸性磷酸酶阳性[708]。另外一种特殊的女性尿道腺癌局灶甲胎蛋白免疫组化染色阳性[709]。

仅仅依靠组织学形态，尿道原发癌和转移癌的鉴别诊断常常比较困难，但疾病的临床过程和病灶的分布通常会有帮助。偶尔仍然会遇到一些困难的病例，例如原发结肠癌治疗6年后出现尿道复发[711]。

其他少见肿瘤 Other rare tumors

除癌之外，恶性黑色素瘤是尿道其他类型恶性肿瘤中最常见的一种（图12.177）[635,737-742]。尽管这种肿瘤并不常见，但一项研究[707]发现它们占尿道癌的4%，而且只考虑泌尿生殖道的话，尿道是黑色素瘤相对好发的部位。在一篇发表于1984年的详尽的文献综述中，Stein 和 Kendall[635]发现了23例男性以及40例女性原发性尿道黑色素瘤，从那时起又陆续报道了其他一些病例[740-742]。肿瘤常发生于50岁以上的患者。临床症状与其他尿道癌相似。男性患者大部分发生于舟状窝（55%），但尿道前列腺部（15%）、尿道球部（10%）、尿道悬垂部（15%）和尿道口（5%）也可以发生。在女性，尿道远端常见。与其他部位的黑色素瘤一样，由于其黑色的外观，病变的大体表现常常引人注意，明显提示其诊断（图12.177）。组织学上，这些病变与发生于皮肤者类似（见第23章）。黑色素颗粒多少不等，它的缺如可能会造成诊断困难[742]。同样，病变以梭形肿瘤细胞成分为主时也会造成诊断困难。一项对3例尿道黑色素瘤患者的研究发现，由于上述原因，一例最初误诊为肉瘤，另一例则误诊为尿路上皮癌[740]。即使采用大剂量的治疗，患者的预后也很差，少数患者可存活5年[739]。做出原发性恶性黑色素瘤诊断之前，应该取得详细的临床病史以除外尿道转移性肿瘤的可能。

尿道其他类型的恶性肿瘤并不常见，大部分通过个例报道为人所知。非Hodgkin淋巴瘤很少明确累及尿道，偶尔有Hodgkin淋巴瘤[697]和浆细胞瘤的报道[743-746]。有一例发生于AIDS患者的T细胞淋巴瘤，以尿道首发而被报道[747]。原发于尿道的卵黄囊瘤[748]、副神经节瘤[749]以及类癌[750]的个案已有报道，偶尔在有关尿道肿瘤的综述中涵盖了各种类型肉瘤的散发病例。

参考文献

1. Eble J N, Sauter G, Epstein J I et al. 2005 World Health Organization classification of tumours. Pathology and genetics of tumours of the urinary system and male genital organs. IARC Press, Lyon
2. Delahunt B, Eble J N 1997 Papillary renal cell carcinoma: a clinicopathologic and immunohistochemical study of 105 tumors. Mod Pathol 10: 537–544
3. Eble J N, Warfel K 1991 Early human renal cortical epithelial neoplasia. Mod Pathol 4: 45A
4. Bell E T 1938 A classification of renal tumors with observations on the frequency of the various types. J Urol 39: 238–243
5. Talamo T S, Shonnard J W 1980 Small renal adenocarcinoma with metastases. J Urol 124: 132–134
6. Eschwege P, Saussine C, Steichen G et al. 1996 Radical nephrectomy for renal cell carcinoma 30 mm or less: long-term followup results. J Urol 155: 1196–1199
7. Störkel S, Eble J N, Adlakha K et al. 1997 Classification of renal cell carcinoma, workgroup 1. Cancer 80: 987–989
8. Newcomb W D 1936 The search for truth, with special reference to the frequency of gastric ulcer-cancer and the origin of Grawitz tumours of the kidney. Proc R Soc Med 30: 113–136
9. Xipell J M 1971 The incidence of benign renal nodules (a clinicopathologic study). J Urol 106: 503–506
10. Reis M, Faria V, Lindoro J et al. 1988 The small cystic and noncystic noninflammatory renal nodules: a postmortem study. J Urol 140: 721–724
11. Hiasa Y, Kitamura M, Nakaoka S et al. 1995 Antigen immunohistochemistry of renal cell adenomas in autopsy cases: relevance to histogenesis. Oncology 52: 97–105
12. Hashine K, Sumiyoshi Y, Kagawa S 1996 A morphological study of renal adenoma and latent renal cell carcinoma in autopsy cases. Nippon Hinyokika Gakkai Zasshi 87: 667–675
13. Hughson M D, Buchwald D, Fox M 1986 Renal neoplasia and acquired cystic kidney disease in patients receiving long-term dialysis. Arch Pathol Lab Med 110: 592–601
14. Budin R E, McDonnell P J 1984 Renal cell neoplasms, their relationship to arteriolonephrosclerosis. Arch Pathol Lab Med 108: 138–140
15. Bennington J L 1973 Cancer of the kidney – etiology, epidemiology, and pathology. Cancer 32: 1017–1029
16. Cristol D S, McDonald J R, Emmett J L 1946 Renal adenomas in hypernephromatous kidneys: a study of their incidence, nature and relationship. J Urol 55: 18–27
17. Syrjänen K J 1979 Renal adenomatosis, report of an autopsy case. Scand J Urol Nephrol 13: 329–334
18. Warfel K A, Eble J N 1982 Renal oncocytomatosis. J Urol 127: 1179–1180
19. Katz D S, Gharagozloo A M, Peebles T R et al. 1996 Renal oncocytomatosis. Am J Kidney Dis 27: 579–582
20. Thoenes W, Störkel S, Rumpelt H-J 1986 Histopathology and classification of renal cell tumors (adenomas, oncocytomas and carcinomas) the basic cytological and histopathological elements and their use for diagnostics. Pathol Res Pract 181: 125–143
21. Grignon D J, Eble J N 1998 Papillary and metanephric adenomas of the kidney. Semin Diagn Pathol 15: 41–53
22. Cohen C, McCue P A, DeRose P B 1995 Immunohistochemistry of renal adenomas and carcinomas. J Urol Pathol 3: 61–71
23. Perez-Ordonez B, Hamed G, Campbell S et al. 1997 Renal oncocytoma: a clinicopathologic study of 70 cases. Am J Surg Pathol 21: 871–883
24. Dechet C B, Bostwick D G, Blute M L et al. 1999 Renal oncocytoma: multifocality, bilateralism, metachronous tumor development and coexistent renal cell carcinoma. J Urol 162: 40–42
25. Klein M J, Valensi Q J 1976 Proximal tubular adenomas of kidney with so-called oncocytic features, a clinicopathologic study of 13 cases of a rarely reported neoplasm. Cancer 38: 906–914
26. Mead G O, Thomas L R J, Jackson J G 1990 Renal oncocytoma: report of a case with bilateral multifocal oncocytomas. Clin Imaging 14: 231–234
27. Tickoo S K, Reuter V E, Amin M B et al. 1999 Renal oncocytosis: a morphologic study of fourteen cases. Am J Surg Pathol 23: 1094–1101
28. Kragel P J, Williams J, Emory T S et al. 1990 Renal oncocytoma with cylindromatous changes: pathologic features and histogenetic significance. Mod Pathol 3: 277–281
29. Tickoo S K, Amin M B 1998 Discriminant nuclear features of renal oncocytoma and chromophobe renal cell carcinoma: analysis of their potential utility in the differential diagnosis. Am J Clin Pathol 110: 782–787
30. Eble J N, Hull M T 1984 Morphologic features of renal oncocytoma: a light and electron microscopic study. Hum Pathol 15: 1054–1061
31. Mathers M E, Pollock A M et al. 2002 Cytokeratin 7: a useful adjunct in the diagnosis of chromophobe renal cell carcinoma. Histopathology 40: 563–567
32. Pages A, Granier M 1980 Le néphrome néphronogène. Arch Anat Cytol Pathol 28: 99–103
33. Hennigar R A, Beckwith J B 1992 Nephrogenic adenofibroma, a novel kidney tumor of young people. Am J Surg Pathol 16: 325–334
34. Davis C J Jr, Barton J H, Sesterhenn I A et al. 1995 Metanephric adenoma, clinicopathological study of fifty patients. Am J Surg Pathol 19: 1101–1114
35. Bruder E, Passera O, Harms D et al. 2004 Morphologic and molecular characterization of renal cell carcinoma in children and young adults. Am J Surg Pathol 28: 1117–1132
36. Arroyo M R, Green D M, Perlman E J et al. 2001 The spectrum of metanephric adenofibroma and related lesions: clinicopathologic study of 25 cases from the National Wilms Tumors Study Group Pathology Center. Am J Surg Pathol 25: 433–444
37. Jones E C, Pins M, Dickersin G R et al. 1995 Metanephric adenoma of the kidney, a clinicopathological, immunohistochemical, flow cytometric, cytogenetic, and electron microscopic study of seven cases. Am J Surg Pathol 19: 615–626
38. Argani P, Beckwith J B 2000 Metanephric stromal tumor. Report of 31 cases of a distinctive pediatric renal neoplasm. Am J Surg Pathol 24: 917–926
39. Muir T E, Cheville J C, Lager D J 2001 Metanephric adenoma, nephrogenic rests, and Wilms' tumor: a histologic and immunophenotypic comparison. Am J Surg Pathol 25: 1290–1296
40. Brunelli M, Eble J N, Zhang S et al. 2003 Metanephric adenoma lacks the gains of chromosomes 7 and 17 and loss of Y that are typical of papillary renal cell carcinoma and papillary adenoma. Mod Pathol 16: 1060–1063
41. Thoenes W, Störkel S, Rumpelt H J et al. 1990 Cytomorphological typing of renal cell carcinoma – a new approach. Eur Urol 18 (suppl): 6–9
42. Kovacs G, Akhtar M, Beckwith J B et al. 1997 The Heidelberg classification of renal cell tumours. J Pathol 183: 131–133
43. Linehan W M, Walther M M, Zbar B 2003 The genetic basis of cancer of the kidney. J Urol 170: 2163–2172
44. Hock L M, Lynch J, Balaji K C 2002 Increasing incidence of all stages of kidney cancer in the last 2 decades in the United States: an analysis of surveillance, epidemiology and end results program data. J Urol 167: 57–60
45. Dayal H H, Wilkinson G S 1989 Epidemiology of renal cell cancer. Semin Urol 7: 139–143
46. Maclure M, Willett W 1990 A case-control study of diet and risk of renal adenocarcinoma. Epidemiology 1: 430–440
47. La Vecchia C, Negri E, D'Avanzo B et al. 1990 Smoking and renal cell carcinoma. Cancer Res 50: 5231–5233
48. Sharpe C R, Rochon J E, Adam J M et al. 1989 Case-control study of hydrocarbon exposures in patients with renal cell carcinoma. Can Med Assoc J 140: 1309–1318
49. Solomon D, Schwartz A 1988 Renal pathology in von Hippel-Lindau disease. Hum Pathol 19: 1072–1079
50. Maher E R, Yates J R W, Harries R et al. 1990 Clinical features and natural history of von Hippel-Lindau disease. Q J Med 77: 1151–1163
51. Bernstein J, Robbins T O 1991 Renal involvement in tuberous sclerosis. Ann NY Acad Sci 615: 36–49
52. Washecka R, Hanna M 1991 Malignant renal tumors in tuberous sclerosis. Urology 37: 340–343
53. Gregoire J R, Torres V E, Holley K E et al. 1987 Renal epithelial hyperplasia and neoplastic proliferation in autosomal dominant polycystic kidney disease. Am J Kidney Dis 9: 27–38
54. Bernstein J, Evan A P, Gardner K D Jr 1987 Epithelial hyperplasia in human polycystic kidney diseases, its role in pathogenesis and risk of neoplasia. Am J Pathol 129: 92–101
55. Bonacina R, Di Natale G, Zois G et al. 1986 Adenocarcinoma renale associato a rene policistico (presentazione di un caso e revisone della letteratura). Chir Ital 38: 406–411
56. Fallon B, Williams R D 1989 Renal cancer associated with acquired cystic disease of the kidney and chronic renal failure. Semin Urol 7: 228–236
57. Matson M A, Cohen E P 1990 Acquired cystic kidney disease: occurrence, prevalence and renal cancers. Medicine 69: 217–226
58. Ishikawa I 1987 Development of adenocarcinoma and acquired cystic disease of the kidney in hemodialysis patients. Int Symp Princess Takamatsu Cancer Res Fund 18: 77–86
59. Gibbons R P, Montie J E, Correa R J Jr et al. 1976 Manifestations of renal cell carcinoma. Urology 8: 201–206
60. Cronin R E, Kaehny W D, Miller P D et al. 1976 Renal cell carcinoma: unusual systemic manifestations. Medicine 555: 291–311
61. Kiely J M 1966 Hypernephroma – the internist's tumor. Med Clin N Am 50: 1067–1083
62. Fahn H-J, Lee Y-H, Chen M-T et al. 1991 The incidence and prognostic significance of humoral hypercalcemia in renal cell carcinoma. J Urol 145: 248–250
63. Sufrin G, Chasan S, Golio A et al. 1989 Paraneoplastic and serologic syndromes of renal adenocarcinoma. Semin Urol 7: 158–171
64. Moran A 1990 Malignant hypertension due to renal carcinoma. Br J Urol 65: 299–299
65. Somer T P, Törnroth T S 1985 Renal adenocarcinoma and systemic amyloidosis, immunohistochemical and histochemical studies. Arch Pathol Lab Med 109: 571–574
66. Althaffer L F III, Chenault O W Jr 1979 Paraneoplastic endocrinopathies associated with renal tumors. J Urol 122: 573–577
67. Rosenblum S L 1987 Paraneoplastic syndromes associated with renal cell carcinoma. J S C Med Assoc 83: 375–378
68. Cheng W S, Farrow G M, Zincke H 1991 The incidence of multicentricity in renal cell carcinoma. J Urol 146: 1221–1223

69. Bennington J L, Beckwith J B 1975 Tumors of the kidney, renal pelvis, and ureter. Atlas of tumor pathology, series 2, fascicle 12. Armed Forces Institute of Pathology, Bethesda
70. Katz S E, Schapira H E 1982 Spontaneous regression of genitourinary cancer – an update. J Urol 128: 1–4
71. Kavoussi L R, Levine S R, Kadmon D et al. 1986 Regression of metastatic renal cell carcinoma: a case report and literature review. J Urol 135: 1005–1007
72. De Riese W, Goldenberg K, Allhoff E et al. 1991 Metastatic renal cell carcinoma (RCC): spontaneous regression, long-term survival and late recurrence. Int Urol Nephrol 23: 13–25
73. McNichols D W, Segura J W, DeWeerd J H 1981 Renal cell carcinoma: long-term survival and late recurrence. J Urol 126: 17–23
74. Hienert G, Latal D, Rummelhardt S 1988 Urological aspects of surgical management for metastatic renal cell cancer. Semin Surg Oncol 4: 137–138
75. Neves R J, Zincke H, Taylor W F 1988 Metastatic renal cell cancer and radical nephrectomy: identification of prognostic factors and patient survival. J Urol 139: 1173–1176
76. Elson P J, Witte R S, Trump D L 1988 Prognostic factors for survival in patients with recurrent or metastatic renal cell carcinoma. Cancer Res 48: 7310–7313
77. Gurney H, Larcos G, McKay M et al. 1989 Bone metastases in hypernephroma, frequency of scapular involvement. Cancer 64: 1429–1431
78. Gnarra J R, Duan D R, Weng Y et al. 1996 Molecular cloning of the von Hippel-Lindau tumor suppressor gene and its role in renal carcinoma. Biochim Biophys Acta 1242: 201–210
79. van der Hout A H, van den Berg E, van der Vlies P et al. 1993 Loss of heterozygosity at the short arm of chromosome 3 in renal-cell cancer correlates with the cytological tumour type. Int J Cancer 53: 353–357
80. Zbar B, Lerman M 1998 Inherited carcinomas of the kidney: histology. Adv Cancer Res 75: 164–201
81. Schullerus D, Herbers J, Chudek J et al. 1997 Loss of heterozygosity at chromosomes 8p, 9p, and 14q is associated with stage and grade of non-papillary renal cell carcinomas. J Pathol 183: 151–155
82. Presti J C Jr, Wilhelm M, Reuter V et al. 2002 Allelic loss on chromosomes 8 and 9 correlates with clinical outcome in locally advanced clear cell carcinoma of the kidney. J Urol 167: 1464–1468
83. Amin M B, Amin M B, Tamboli P et al. 2002 Prognostic impact of histologic subtyping of adult renal epithelial neoplasms, an experience of 405 cases. Am J Surg Pathol 26: 281–291
84. Cheville J C, Lohse C M, Zincke H et al. 2003 Comparisons of outcome and prognostic features among histologic subtypes of renal cell carcinoma. Am J Surg Pathol 27: 612–624
85. Delahunt B 1998 Histopathologic prognostic indicators for renal cell carcinoma. Semin Diagn Pathol 15: 68–76
86. Leibovich B C, Blute M L, Cheville J C et al. 2003 Prediction of progression after radical nephrectomy for patients with clear cell renal cell carcinoma, a stratification tool for prospective clinical trials. Cancer 97: 1663–1671
87. Eble J N, Bonsib S M 1998 Extensively cystic renal neoplasms: cystic nephroma, cystic partially differentiated nephroblastoma, multilocular cystic renal cell carcinoma, and cystic hamartoma of renal pelvis. Semin Diagn Pathol 15: 2–20
88. Gokden N, Nappi O, Swanson P E et al. 2000 Renal cell carcinoma with rhabdoid features. Am J Surg Pathol 24: 1329–1338.
89. de Peralta-Venturina M, Moch H, Amin M et al. 2001 Sarcomatoid differentiation in renal cell carcinoma; a study of 101 cases. Am J Surg Pathol 25: 275–284
90. Cheville J C, Lohse C M, Zincke H et al. 2004 Sarcomatoid renal cell carcinoma, an examination of underlying histologic subtype and an analysis of associations with patient outcome. Am J Surg Pathol 28: 435–441
91. Wick M R, Perrone T L, Burke B A 1985 Sarcomatoid transitional cell carcinoma of the renal pelvis, an ultrastructural and immunohistochemical study. Arch Pathol Lab Med 109: 55–58
92. Wick M R, Cherwitz D L, Manivel J C et al. 1990 Immunohistochemical findings in tumors of the kidney. In: Eble JN (ed) Tumors and tumor-like conditions of the kidneys and ureters. Churchill Livingstone, New York, p 207–247
93. Kimura I, Takahashi N, Okumura R et al. 1989 Perinephric xanthogranulomatous pyelonephritis simulating a renal or retroperitoneal tumor on x-ray CT and angiography. Radiat Med 7: 111–117
94. Malek R S, Greene L F, DeWeerd J H et al. 1972 Xanthogranulomatous pyelonephritis. Br J Urol 44: 296–308
95. Goodman M, Curry T, Russell T 1979 Xanthogranulomatous pyelonephritis (XGP): a local disease with systemic manifestations, report of 23 patients and review of the literature. Medicine 58: 171–181
96. Rosi P, Selli C, Carini M et al. 1986 Xanthogranulomatous pyelonephritis: clinical experience with 62 cases. Eur Urol 12: 96–100
97. Chuang C-K, Lai M-K, Chang P-L et al. 1992 Xanthogranulomatous pyelonephritis: experience in 36 cases. J Urol 147: 333–336
98. Parsons M A, Harris S C, Longstaff A J et al. 1983 Xanthogranulomatous pyelonephritis: a pathological, clinical and aetiological analysis of 87 cases. Diagn Histopathol 6: 203–219
99. Esparza A R, McKay D B, Cronan J J et al. 1989 Renal parenchymal malakoplakia, histologic spectrum and its relationship to megalocytic interstitial nephritis and xanthogranulomatous pyelonephritis. Am J Surg Pathol 13: 225–236
100. Waldherr R, Schwechheimer K 1985 Co-expression of cytokeratin and vimentin intermediate-sized filaments in renal cell carcinoma, a comparative study of the intermediate-sized filaments in renal cell carcinoma and normal human kidney. Virchow's Arch A Pathol Anat Histopathol 408: 15–27
101. Taxy J B 1981 Renal adenocarcinoma presenting as a solitary metastasis: contribution of electron microscopy to diagnosis. Cancer 48: 2056–2062
102. Wick M R, Cherwitz D L, McGlennen R C et al. 1986 Adrenocortical carcinoma, an immunohistochemical comparison with renal cell carcinoma. Am J Pathol 122: 343–352
103. Renshaw A A, Granter S R 1998 A comparison of A103 and inhibin reactivity in adrenal cortical tumors: distinction from hepatocellular carcinoma and renal tumors. Mod Pathol 11: 1160–1164
104. Green L K, Ro J Y, Mackay B et al. 1989 Renal cell carcinoma metastatic to the thyroid. Cancer 63: 1810–1815
105. Young R H, Hart W R 1992 Renal cell carcinoma metastatic to the ovary: a report of three cases emphasizing possible confusion with ovarian clear cell carcinoma. Int J Gynecol Pathol 11: 96–104
106. Hufnagel T J, Kim J H, True L D et al. 1989 Immunohistochemistry of capillary hemangioblastoma, immunoperoxidase-labeled antibody staining resolves the differential diagnosis with metastatic renal cell carcinoma, but does not explain the histogenesis of the capillary hemangioblastoma. Am J Surg Pathol 13: 207–216
107. Mancilla-Jimenez R, Stanley R J, Blath R A 1976 Papillary renal cell carcinoma, a clinical, radiologic, and pathologic study of 34 cases. Cancer 38: 2469–2480
108. Thoenes W, Störkel S 1991 Die Pathologie der benignen und malignen Nierenzelltumoren. Urologe [A] 30: W41–W50
109. Lager D J, Huston B J, Timmerman T G et al. 1995 Papillary renal tumors, morphologic, cytochemical, and genotypic features. Cancer 76: 669–673
110. Kovacs G 1989 Papillary renal cell carcinoma, a morphologic and cytogenetic study in 11 cases. Am J Pathol 134: 27–34
111. Kovacs G, Fuzesi L, Emanuel A et al. 1991 Cytogenetics of papillary renal cell tumors. Genes Chromosom Cancer 3: 249–255
112. Brunelli M, Eble J N, Zhang S et al. 2003 Gains of chromosomes 7, 17, 12, 16, and 20 and loss of Y occur early in the evolution of papillary renal cell neoplasia: a fluorescence in situ hybridization study. Mod Pathol 16: 1053–1059
113. Presti J C Jr, Rao P H, Chen Q et al. 1991 Histopathological, cytogenetic, and molecular characterization of renal cortical tumors. Cancer Res 51: 1544–1552
114. van den Berg E, van der Hout A H, Oosterhuis J W et al. 1993 Cytogenetic analysis of epithelial renal-cell tumors: relationship with a new histopathological classification. Int J Cancer 55: 223–227
115. Bard R H, Lord B, Fromowitz F 1982 Papillary adenocarcinoma of kidney, II. Radiographic and biologic characteristics. Urology 19: 16–20
116. Reznicek S B, Narayana A S, Culp D A 1985 Cystadenocarcinoma of the kidney: a profile of 13 cases. J Urol 134: 256–259
117. Amin M B, Corless C L, Renshaw A A et al. 1997 Papillary (chromophil) renal cell carcinoma: histomorphologic characteristics and evaluation of conventional pathologic prognostic parameters in 62 cases. Am J Surg Pathol 21: 621–635
118. Renshaw A A, Corless C L 1995 Papillary renal cell carcinoma, histology and immunohistochemistry. Am J Surg Pathol 19: 842–849
119. Delahunt B, Eble J N, McCredie M R E et al. 2001 Morphologic typing of papillary renal cell carcinoma: comparison of growth kinetics and patient survival in 66 cases. Hum Pathol 32: 590–595
120. Fuhrman S A, Lasky L C, Limas C 1982 Prognostic significance of morphologic parameters in renal cell carcinoma. Am J Surg Pathol 6: 655–663
121. Beckwith J B 1983 Wilms' tumor and other renal tumors of childhood: a selective review from the National Wilms' Tumor Study Pathology Center. Hum Pathol 14: 481–492
122. Thoenes W, Störkel S, Rumpelt H-J 1985 Human chromophobe cell renal carcinoma. Virchow's Arch [B] 48: 207–217
123. Thoenes W, Störkel S, Rumpelt H-J et al. 1988 Chromophobe cell renal carcinoma and its variants – a report on 32 cases. J Pathol 155: 277–287
124. Crotty T B, Farrow G M, Lieber M M 1995 Chromophobe renal cell carcinoma: clinicopathologic features of 50 cases. J Urol 154: 964–967
125. Durham J R, Keohane M, Amin M B 1996 Chromophobe renal cell carcinoma. Adv Anat Pathol 3: 336–342
126. Peyromaure M, Misrai V, Thiounn N et al. 2004 Chromophobe renal cell carcinoma, analysis of 61 cases. Cancer 100: 1406–1410
127. Kovacs A, Kovacs G 1992 Low chromosome number in chromophobe renal cell carcinomas. Genes Chromosom Cancer 4: 267–268
128. Bugert P, Gaul C, Weber K et al. 1997 Specific genetic changes of diagnostic importance in chromophobe renal cell carcinoma. Lab Invest 76: 203–208
129. Brunelli M, Eble J N, Zhang S et al. 2005 Eosinophilic and classic chromophobe renal cell carcinomas have similar frequent losses of multiple chromosomes from among chromosomes 1, 2, 6, 10, and 17, and this pattern of genetic abnormality is not present in renal oncocytoma. Mod Pathol 18: 161–169
130. Akhtar M, Tulbah A, Kardar A H et al. 1997 Sarcomatoid renal cell carcinoma: the chromophobe connection. Am J Surg Pathol 21: 1188–1195
131. Pan C-C, Chen P C, Ho D M 2004 The diagnostic utility of MOC31, BerEP4, RCC marker and CD10 in the classification of renal cell carcinoma and renal oncocytoma: an immunohistochemical analysis of 328 cases. Histopathology 45: 452–459

132. Martignoni G, Pea M, Brunelli M et al. 2004 CD10 is expressed in a subset of chromophobe renal cell carcinomas. Mod Pathol 17: 1455–1463
133. Kriz W, Bankir L 1988 A standard nomenclature for structures of the kidney. Kidney Int 33: 1–7
134. Störkel S, Pannen B, Thoenes W et al. 1988 Intercalated cells as a probable source for the development of renal oncocytoma. Virchow's Arch [B] 56: 185–189
135. Störkel S, Steart P V, Drenckhahn D et al. 1989 The human chromophobe cell renal carcinoma: its probable relation to intercalated cells of the collecting duct. Virchow's Arch [B] 56: 237–245
136. Amin M B, Varma M D, Tickoo S K et al. 1997 Collecting duct carcinoma of the kidney. Adv Anat Pathol 4: 85–94
137. Srigley J R, Eble J N 1998 Collecting duct carcinoma of kidney. Semin Diagn Pathol 15: 54–67
138. Davis C J Jr, Mostofi F K, Sesterhenn I A 1995 Renal medullary carcinoma: the seventh sickle cell nephropathy. Am J Surg Pathol 19: 1–11
139. Swartz M, Karth J, Schneider D T et al. 2002 Renal medullary carcinoma: clinical, pathologic, immunohistochemical, and genetic analysis with pathogenetic implications. Urology 60: 1083–1089
140. Simpson L, He X, Pins M et al. 2005 Renal medullary carcinoma and ABL gene amplification. J Urol 173: 1883–1888
141. Aizawa S, Kikuchi Y, Suzuki M et al.1987 Renal cell carcinoma of lower nephron origin. Acta Pathol Jpn 37: 567–574
142. Fleming S, Lewi H J E 1986 Collecting duct carcinoma of the kidney. Histopathology 10: 1131–1141
143. Kennedy S M, Merino M J, Linehan W M et al. 1990 Collecting duct carcinoma of the kidney. Hum Pathol 21: 449–456
144. Rumpelt H J, Störkel S, Moll R et al. 1991 Bellini duct carcinoma: further evidence for this rare variant of renal cell carcinoma. Histopathology 18: 115–122
145. Kuroda N, Naruse K, Miyazaki E et al. 2000 Vinculin: its possible use as a marker of normal collecting ducts and renal neoplasms with collecting duct system phenotype. Mod Pathol 13: 1109–1114
146. Vecchione A, Galetti T P, Gardiman M et al. 2004 Collecting duct carcinoma of the kidney: an immunohistochemical study of 11 cases. BMC Urol 4: 11–12
147. Argani P, Ladanyi M 2005 Translocation carcinomas of the kidney. Clin Lab Med 25: 363–378
147a. Argani P, Lae M, Ballard E T et al. 2006 Translocation carcinomas of the kidney after chemotherapy in childhood. J Clin Oncol 24: 1529–1534
148. Argani P, Lal P, Hutchinson B et al. 2003 Aberrant nuclear immunoreactivity for TFE3 in neoplasm with TFE3 gene fusions, a sensitive and specific immunohistochemical assay. Am J Surg Pathol 27: 750–761
149. Argani P, Lae M, Hutchinson B et al. 2005 Renal carcinomas with the t(6;11)(p21;q12). Clinicopathologic features and demonstration of the specific Alpha-TFEB gene fusion by immunohistochemistry, RT-PCR and DNA PCR. Am J Surg Pathol 29: 230–240
150. Medeiros L J, Palmedo G, Krigman H R et al. 1999 Oncocytoid renal cell carcinoma after neuroblastoma: a report of four cases of a distinct clinicopathologic entity. Am J Surg Pathol 23: 772–780
151. Koyle M A, Hatch D A, Furness P D et al. 2001 Long-term urologic complications in survivors younger than 15 months of advanced stage abdominal neuroblastoma. J Urol 166: 1455–1458
152. Eble J N 2003 Mucinous tubular and spindle cell carcinoma and post-neuroblastoma carcinoma: newly recognised entities in the renal cell carcinoma family. Pathology 35: 499–504
153. Ferlicot S, Allory Y, Compérat E et al. 2005 Mucinous tubular and spindle cell carcinoma, a report of 15 cases with a review of the literature. Virchow's Arch 447: 978–983
154. Hes O, Hora M, Perez-Montiel D M et al 2002 Spindle and cuboidal renal cell carcinoma, a tumour having frequent association with nephrolithiasis: report of 11 cases including a case with hybrid conventional renal cell carcinoma/spindle and cuboidal renal cell carcinoma components. Histopathology 41: 549–555
155. Parwani A V, Husain A N, Epstein J I et al. 2001 Low-grade myxoid renal epithelial neoplasms with distal nephron differentiation. Hum Pathol 32: 506–512
156. Rakozy C, Schmahl G E, Bogner S et al. 2002 Low-grade tubular-mucinous renal neoplasms: morphologic, immunohistochemical, and genetic features. Mod Pathol 15: 1162–1171
157. Srigley J R, Eble J N, Grignon D J et al. 1999 Unusual renal cell carcinoma (RCC) with prominent spindle cell change possibly related to the loop of Henle. Mod Pathol 12: 107A
157a. Cossu-Rocca P, Eble J N, Delahunt B et al. 2006 Renal mucinous tubular and spindle carcinoma lacks the gains of chromosomes 7 and 17 and losses of chromosome Y that are prevalent in papillary renal cell carcinoma. Mod Pathol 19: 488–493
158. Zisman A, Chao D H, Pantuck A J et al. 2002 Unclassified renal cell carcinoma: clinical features and prognostic impact of a new histological subtype. J Urol 168: 950–955
158a. Tickoo S K, dePeralta-Venturina M N, Harik L R et al. 2006 Spectrum of epithelial neoplasms in end-stage renal disease: an experience from 66 tumor-bearing kidneys with emphasis on histologic patterns distinct from those in sporadic adult renal neoplasia. Am J Surg Pathol 30: 141–153
159. Schouman M, Warter A, Roos M et al. 1984 Renal cell carcinoma: statistical study of survival based on pathological criteria. World J Urol 2: 109–113
160. Robson C J 1963 Radical nephrectomy for renal cell carcinoma. J Urol 89: 37–42
161. Robson C J, Churchill B M, Anderson W 1969 The results of radical nephrectomy for renal cell carcinoma. J Urol 101: 297–301
162. American Joint Committee on Cancer 2002 Kidney (sarcomas and adenomas are not included). AJCC Cancer Staging Manual, 6th Ed. Springer, New York, p 323–328
163. Bonsib S M 2004 The renal sinus is the principal invasive pathway, a prospective study of 100 renal cell carcinomas. Am J Surg Pathol 28: 1594–1600
164. Bonsib S M 2005 T2 clear cell renal cell carcinoma is a rare entity: a study of 120 clear cell renal cell carcinomas. J Urol 174: 1199–1202
165. Medeiros L J, Gelb A B, Weiss L M 1988 Renal cell carcinoma, prognostic significance of morphologic parameters in 121 cases. Cancer 61: 1639–1651
166. Medeiros L J, Gelb A B, Weiss L M 1987 Low-grade renal cell carcinoma, a clinicopathologic study of 53 cases. Am J Surg Pathol 11: 633–642
167. Giuliani L, Giberti C, Martorana G et al. 1990 Radical extensive surgery for renal cell carcinoma: long-term results and prognostic factors. J Urol 143: 468–474
168. Herrlinger A, Schrott K M, Sigel A et al. 1984 Results of 381 transabdominal radical nephrectomies for renal cell carcinoma with partial and complete en-bloc lymph-node dissection. World J Urol 2: 114–121
169. Studer U E, Scherz S, Scheidegger J et al. 1990 Enlargement of regional lymph nodes in renal cell carcinoma is often not due to metastases. J Urol 144: 243–245
170. Blute M L, Leibovich B C, Cheville J C et al. 2004 A protocol for performing extended lymph node dissection using primary tumor pathological features for patients treated with radical nephrectomy for clear cell renal cell carcinoma. J Urol 172: 465–469
171. Pantuck A J, Zisman A, Dorey F et al. 2003 Renal cell carcinoma with retroperitoneal lymph nodes, impact on survival and benefits of immunotherapy. Cancer 97: 2995–3002
172. Mitty H A, Droller M J, Dikman S H 1987 Ureteral and renal pelvic metastases from renal cell carcinoma. Urol Radiol 9: 16–20
173. Ito A, Satoh M, Ohyama C et al. 2002 Adrenal metastasis from renal cell carcinoma: significance of adrenalectomy. Int J Urol 9: 125–128
174. Han K R, Bui M H, Pantuck A J et al. 2003 TNM T3a renal cell carcinoma: adrenal gland involvement is not the same as renal fat invasion. J Urol 169: 899–903
175. McKiernan J, Yossepowitch O, Kattan M W et al. 2002 Partial nephrectomy for renal cortical tumors: pathologic findings and impact on outcome. Urology 60: 1003–1009
176. Gill I S, Desai M M, Kaouk J H et al. 2002 Laparoscopic partial nephrectomy for renal tumor: duplicating open surgical techniques. J Urol 167: 469–476
177. Hand J R, Broders A C 1932 Carcinoma of the kidney: the degree of malignancy in relation to factors bearing on prognosis. J Urol 28: 199–216
178. Skinner D G, Colvin R B, Vermillion C D et al. 1971 Diagnosis and management of renal cell carcinoma, a clinical and pathological study of 309 cases. Cancer 28: 1165–1177
179. Grignon D J, Ayala A G, El-Naggar A et al. 1989 Renal cell carcinoma, a clinicopathologic and DNA flow cytometric analysis of 103 cases. Cancer 64: 2133–2140
180. Green L K, Ayala A G, Ro J Y et al. 1989 Role of nuclear grading in stage I renal cell carcinoma. Urology 34: 310–315
181. Helpap B, Knüpffer J, Essmann S 1990 Nucleolar grading of renal cancer, correlation of frequency and localization of nucleoli to histologic and cytologic grading and stage of renal cell carcinomas. Mod Pathol 3: 671–678
182. Al-Aynati M, Chen V, Salama S et al. 2003 Interobserver and intraobserver variability using the Fuhrman grading system for renal cell carcinoma. Arch Pathol Lab Med 127: 593–596
183. Sengupta S, Lohse C M, Frank I et al. 2005 Histologic coagulative necrosis as a prognostic indicator of renal cell carcinoma aggressiveness. Cancer 104: 511–520
184. Parham D M, Roloson G J, Feely M et al. 2001 Primary malignant neuroepithelial tumors of the kidney: a clinicopathologic analysis of 146 adult and pediatric cases from the National Wilms' Tumor Study Group Pathology Center. Am J Surg Pathol 25: 133–146
185. Jimenez R E, Folpe A L, Lapham R L et al. 2002 Primary Ewing's sarcoma/primitive neuroectodermal tumor of the kidney, a clinicopathologic and immunohistochemical analysis of 11 cases. Am J Surg Pathol 26: 320–327
186. Majhail N S, Elson P, Bukowski R M 2003 Therapy and outcome of small cell carcinoma of the kidney, report of two cases and a systematic review of the literature. Cancer 97: 1436–1441
187. Resnick M E, Unterberger H, McLoughlin P T 1966 Renal carcinoid producing the carcinoid syndrome. Med Times 94: 895–896
188. Gleeson M H, Bloom S R, Polak J M et al. 1971 Endocrine tumour in kidney affecting small bowel structure, motility, and absorptive function. Gut 12: 773–782
189. Raghavaiah N V, Singh S M 1976 Extra-adrenal pheochromocytoma producing renal artery stenosis. J Urol 116: 243–245
190. Takahashi M, Yang X J, McWhinney S et al. 2005 cDNA microarray analysis assists in diagnosis of malignant intrarenal pheochromocytoma originally masquerading as a renal cell carcinoma. J Med Genet 42: e48
191. Zak F G, Jindrak K, Capozzi F 1983 Carcinoidal tumor of the kidney. Ultrastruct Pathol 4: 51–59

192. Ghazi M R, Brown J S, Warner R S 1979 Carcinoid tumor of kidney. Urology 14: 610–612
193. Acconcia A, Miracco C, Mattei F M et al. 1988 Primary carcinoid tumor of kidney, light and electron microscopy, and immunohistochemical study. Urology 31: 517–520
194. Cauley J E, Almagro U A, Jacobs S C 1988 Primary renal carcinoid tumor. Urology 32: 564–566
195. Huettner P C, Bird D J, Chang Y C et al. 1991 Carcinoid tumor of the kidney with morphologic and immunohistochemical profile of a hindgut endocrine tumor: report of a case. Ultrastruct Pathol 15: 655–661
196. Kojiro M, Ohishi H, Isobe H 1976 Carcinoid tumor occurring in cystic teratoma of the kidney, a case report. Cancer 38: 1636–1640
197. Fetissof F, Benatre A, Dubois M P et al. 1984 Carcinoid tumor occurring in a teratoid malformation of the kidney, an immunohistochemical study. Cancer 54: 2305–2308
198. Bégin L R, Guy L, Jacobson S A et al. 1998 Renal carcinoid and horseshoe kidney: a frequent association of two rare entities – a case report and review of the literature. J Surg Oncol 68: 113–119
199. Capella C, Eusebi V, Rosai J 1984 Primary oat cell carcinoma of the kidney. Am J Surg Pathol 8: 855–861
200. Tetu B, Ro J Y, Ayala A G et al. 1987 Small cell carcinoma of the kidney, a clinicopathologic, immunohistochemical, and ultrastructural study. Cancer 60: 1809–1814
201. Gohji K, Nakanishi T, Hara I et al. 1987 Two cases of primary neuroblastoma of the kidney in adults. J Urol 137: 966–968
202. Eble J N 1998 Angiomyolipoma of kidney. Semin Diagn Pathol 15: 21–40
203. Filipas D, Spix C, Schulz-Lampel D et al. 2003 Screening for renal cell carcinoma using ultrasonography: a feasibility study. BJU Int 91: 595–599
204. O'Callaghan F J, Noakes M J, Martyns C N et al. 2004 An epidemiological study of renal pathology in tuberous sclerosis complex. BJU Int 94: 853–857
205. Ferry J A, Malt R A, Young R H 1991 Renal angiomyolipoma with sarcomatous transformation and pulmonary metastases. Am J Surg Pathol 15: 1083–1088
206. Oesterling J E, Fishman E K, Goldman S M et al. 1986 The management of renal angiomyolipoma. J Urol 135: 1121–1124
207. L'Hostis H, Deminiere C, Ferriere J-M et al. 1999 Renal angiomyolipoma: a clinicopathologic, immunohistochemical, and follow-up study of 46 cases. Am J Surg Pathol 23: 1011–1020
207a. Davis C J, Barton J H, Sesterhenn I A 2006 Cystic angiomyolipoma of the kidney: a clincopathologic description of 11 cases. Mod Pathol 19: 669–674
208. Taylor R S, Joseph D B, Kohaut E C et al. 1989 Renal angiomyolipoma associated with lymph node involvement and renal cell carcinoma in patients with tuberous sclerosis. J Urol 141: 930–932
209. McIntosh G S, Hamilton Dutoit S, Chronos N V et al. 1989 Multiple unilateral renal angiomyolipomas with regional lymphangioleiomyomatosis. J Urol 142: 1305–1307
210. Ro J Y, Ayala A G, El-Naggar A et al. 1990 Angiomyolipoma of kidney with lymph node involvement, DNA flow cytometric analysis. Arch Pathol Lab Med 114: 65–67
211. Hulbert J C, Graf R 1983 Involvement of the spleen by renal angiomyolipoma: metastasis or multicentricity. J Urol 130: 328–329
212. Mai K T, Perkins D G, Collins J P 1996 Epithelioid variant of renal angiomyolipoma. Histopathology 28: 277–280
213. Eble J N, Amin M B, Young R H 1997 Epithelioid angiomyolipoma of the kidney, a report of five cases with a prominent and diagnostically confusing epithelioid smooth muscle component. Am J Surg Pathol 21: 1123–1130
214. Pea M, Bonetti F, Martignoni G et al. 1998 Apparent renal cell carcinomas in tuberous sclerosis are heterogeneous: the identification of malignant epithelioid angiomyolipoma. Am J Surg Pathol 22: 180–187
215. Peterson N E, Thompson H T 1971 Renal hemangioma. J Urol 105: 27–31
216. Edward N C, DeWeerd J H, Woolner L B 1962 Renal hemangiomas. Mayo Clin Proc 37: 545–566
217. Schofield D, Zaatari G S, Gay B B 1986 Klippel-Trenaunay and Sturge-Weber syndromes with renal hemangioma and double inferior vena cava. J Urol 136: 442–445
218. Moros Garcia M, Martinez Tello D, Ramon y Cajal Junquera S et al. 1988 Multiple cavernous hemangioma of the kidney. Eur Urol 14: 90–92
219. Caduff R F, Schwöbel M G, Willi U V et al. 1997 Lymphangioma of the right kidney in an infant boy. Pediatr Pathol Lab Med 17: 631–637
220. Honma I, Takagi Y, Shigyo M et al. 2002 Lymphangioma of the kidney. Int J Urol 9: 178–182
221. Pickering S P, Fletcher B D, Bryan P J et al. 1984 Renal lymphangioma: a cause of neonatal nephromegaly. Pediatr Radiol 14: 445–448
222. Di Palma S, Giardini R 1988 Leiomyoma of the kidney. Tumori 74: 489–493
223. Clinton-Thomas C L 1956 A giant leiomyoma of the kidney. Br J Surg 43: 497–501
224. Zollikofer C, Castaneda-Zuniga W, Nath H P et al. 1980 The angiographic appearance of intrarenal leiomyoma. Radiology 136: 47–49
225. Dineen M K, Venable D D, Misra R P 1984 Pure intrarenal lipoma – report of a case and review of the literature. J Urol 132: 104–107
226. Hurwitz R S, Benjamin J A, Cooper J F 1978 Excessive proliferation of peripelvic fat of the kidney. Urology 11: 448–456
227. Deyrup A T, Montgomery E, Fisher C 2004 Leiomyosarcoma of the kidney, a clinicopathologic study. Am J Surg Pathol 28: 178–182
228. Farrow G M, Harrison E G Jr, Utz D C et al. 1968 Sarcomas and sarcomatoid and mixed malignant tumors of the kidney in adults – part I. Cancer 22: 545–550
229. Grignon D J, Ro J Y, Papadopoulos N E et al. 1991 Leiomyosarcoma of renal vein. Urology 38: 255–258
230. Grignon D J, Ayala A G, Ro J Y et al. 1990 Primary sarcomas of the kidney, a clinicopathologic and DNA flow cytometric study of 17 cases. Cancer 65: 1611–1618
231. Mayes D C, Fechner R E, Gillenwater J Y 1990 Renal liposarcoma. Am J Surg Pathol 14: 268–273
232. Cano J Y, D'Altorio R A 1976 Renal liposarcoma: case report. J Urol 115: 747–749
233. Takashi M, Murase T, Kato K et al. 1987 Malignant fibrous histiocytoma arising from the renal capsule: report of a case. Urol Int 42: 227–230
234. Joseph T J, Becker D I, Turton A F 1991 Renal malignant fibrous histiocytoma. Urology 37: 483–489
235. Srinivas V, Sogani P C, Hajdu S I et al. 1984 Sarcomas of the kidney. J Urol 132: 13–16
236. Penchansky L, Gallo G 1979 Rhabdomyosarcoma of the kidney in children. Cancer 44: 285–292
237. Gonzalez-Crussi F, Baum E S 1983 Renal sarcomas of childhood, a clinicopathologic and ultrastructural study. Cancer 51: 898–912
238. Grignon D J, McIsaac G P, Armstrong R F et al. 1988 Primary rhabdomyosarcoma of the kidney, a light microscopic, immunohistochemical, and electron microscopic study. Cancer 62: 2027–2032
239. Argani P, Faria P A, Epstein J I et al. 2000 Primary renal synovial sarcoma: molecular and morphologic delineation of an entity previously included among embryonal sarcomas of the kidney. Am J Surg Pathol 24: 1087–1096
240. Kim D-H, Sohn J H, Lee M C et al. 2000 Primary synovial sarcoma of the kidney. Am J Surg Pathol 24: 1097–1104
241. Magro G, Cavallaro V, Torrisi A et al. 2002 Intrarenal solitary fibrous tumor of the kidney, report of a case with emphasis on the differential diagnosis in the wide spectrum of monomorphous spindle cell tumors of the kidney. Pathol Res Pract 198: 37–43
242. Wang J, Arber D A, Frankel K et al. 2001 Large solitary fibrous tumor of the kidney: report of two cases and review of the literature. Am J Surg Pathol 25: 1194–1199
243. Weiss J P, Pollack H M, McCormick J F et al. 1984 Renal hemangiopericytoma: surgical, radiological and pathological implications. J Urol 132: 337–339
244. Bowers D L, Te A, Hibshoosh H et al. 1995 Renal hemangiopericytoma, case report and review of the literature. Urol Int 55: 162–166
245. Richard G K, Freeborn W A, Zaatari G S 1996 Hemangiopericytoma of the renal capsule. J Urol Pathol 4: 85–98
246. Siniluoto T M J, Päivänsalo M, Hellström P A et al. 1988 Hemangiopericytoma of the kidney: A case with preoperative ethanol embolization. J Urol 140: 137–138
247. O'Malley F P, Grignon D J, Shepherd R R et al. 1991 Primary osteosarcoma of the kidney, report of a case studied by immunohistochemistry, electron microscopy, and DNA flow cytometry. Arch Pathol Lab Med 115: 1262–1265
248. Leventis A K, Stathopoulos G P, Boussiotou A C et al. 1997 Primary osteogenic sarcoma of the kidney, a case report and review of the literature. Acta Oncol 36: 775–777
249. Gomez-Brouchet A, Soulie M, Delisle M B et al. 2001 Mesenchymal chondrosarcoma of the kidney. J Urol 166: 2305–2305
250. Tsuda N, Chowdhury P R, Hayashi T et al. 1997 Primary renal angiosarcoma: a case report and review of the literature. Pathol Int 47: 778–783
251. Cerilli L A, Huffman H T, Anand A 1998 Primary renal angiosarcoma: a case report with immunohistochemical, ultrastructural, and cytogenetic features and review of the literature. Arch Pathol Lab Med 122: 929–935
252. Robertson P W, Klidjian A, Harding L K et al. 1967 Hypertension due to a renin-secreting renal tumour. Am J Med 43: 963–976
253. Kihara I, Kitamura S, Hoshino T et al. 1968 A hitherto unreported vascular tumor of the kidney: a proposal of "juxtaglomerular cell tumor." Acta Pathol Jpn 18: 197–206
254. Martin S A, Mynderse L A, Lager D J et al. 2001 Juxtaglomerular cell tumor, a clinicopathologic study of four cases and review of the literature. Am J Clin Pathol 116: 854–863
255. Corvol P, Pinet F, Galen F X et al. 1988 Seven lessons from seven renin secreting tumors. Kidney Int Suppl 34, Suppl. 25: S-38–S-44
256. Valdés G, Lopez J M, Martinez P et al. 1980 Renin-secreting tumor, case report. Hypertension 2: 714–718
257. Duan X, Bruneval P, Hammadeh R et al. 2004 Metastatic juxtaglomerular cell tumor in a 52-year-old man. Am J Surg Pathol 28: 1098–1102
258. Camilleri J-P, Hinglais N, Bruneval P et al. 1984 Renin storage and cell differentiation in juxtaglomerular cell tumors: an immunohistochemical and ultrastructural study of three cases. Hum Pathol 15: 1069–1079
259. Lindop G B M, Stewart J A, Downie T T 1983 The immunocytochemical demonstration of renin in a juxtaglomerular cell tumour by light and electron microscopy. Histopathology 7: 421–431
260. Lindop G B M, Fleming S 1984 Renin in renal cell carcinoma – an immunocytochemical study using an antibody to pure human renin. J Clin Pathol 37: 27–31
261. Steffens J, Bock R, Braedel H U et al. 1990 Renin-producing renal cell carcinoma. Eur Urol 18: 56–60
262. Lindop G B M, Fleming S, Gibson A A M 1984 Immunocytochemical localisation of renin in nephroblastoma. J Clin Pathol 37: 738–742

263. Horita Y, Tadokoro M, Taura K et al. 2004 Incidental detection of renomedullary interstitial cell tumour in a renal biopsy specimen. Nephrol Dial Transplant 19: 1007–1008
264. Warfel K A, Eble J N 1985 Renomedullary interstitial cell tumors. Am J Clin Pathol 83: 262–262
265. Eble J N 1990 Unusual renal tumors and tumor-like conditions. In: Eble JN (ed) Tumors and tumor-like conditions of the kidneys and ureters. Churchill Livingstone, New York, p 145–176
266. Zimmermann A, Luscieti P, Flury B et al. 1981 Amyloid-containing renal interstitial cell nodules (RICNs) associated with chronic arterial hypertension in older age groups. Am J Pathol 105: 288–294
267. Taxy J B, Marshall F F 1983 Multilocular renal cysts in adults, possible relationship to renal adenocarcinoma. Arch Pathol Lab Med 107: 633–637
268. Boggs L K, Kimmelstiel P 1956 Benign multilocular cystic nephroma: report of two cases of so-called multilocular cyst of the kidney. J Urol 76: 530–541
269. Kanomata N, Halling K, Eble J N 1997 Non-random X chromosome inactivation in cystic nephroma demonstrates its neoplastic nature. J Urol Pathol 7: 81–87
270. Castillo O A, Boyle E T Jr, Kramer S A 1991 Multilocular cysts of kidney, a study of 29 patients and review of the literature. Urology 37: 156–162
271. Joshi V V, Beckwith J B 1989 Multilocular cyst of the kidney (cystic nephroma) and cystic, partially differentiated nephroblastoma, terminology and criteria for diagnosis. Cancer 64: 466–479
272. Pawade J, Soosay G N, Delprado W et al. 1993 Cystic hamartoma of the renal pelvis. Am J Surg Pathol 17: 1169–1175
273. Durham J R, Bostwick D G, Farrow G M et al. 1993 Mesoblastic nephroma of adulthood, report of three cases. Am J Surg Pathol 17: 1029–1038
274. Truong L D, Williams R, Ngo T et al. 1998 Adult mesoblastic nephroma; expansion of the morphologic spectrum and review of the literature. Am J Surg Pathol 22: 827–839
275. Michal M, Syrucek M 1998 Benign mixed epithelial and stromal tumor of the kidney. Pathol Res Pract 194: 445–448
276. Nakagawa T, Kanai Y, Fujimoto H et al. 2004. Malignant mixed epithelial and stromal tumours of the kidney: a report of the first two cases with a fatal clinical outcome. Histopathology 44: 302–304
277. Adsay N V, Eble J N, Srigley J et al. 2000 Mixed epithelial and stromal tumor of the kidney. Am J Surg Pathol 24: 958–970
278. Ferry J A, Harris N L, Papanicolaou N et al. 1995 Lymphoma of the kidney, a report of 11 cases. Am J Surg Pathol 19: 134–144
279. Ferry J A, Young R H 1997 Malignant lymphoma of the genitourinary tract. Curr Diagn Pathol 4: 145–169
280. Osborne B M, Brenner M, Weitzner S et al. 1987 Malignant lymphoma presenting as a renal mass: four cases. Am J Surg Pathol 11: 375–382
281. Farrow G M, Harrison E G Jr, Utz D C 1968 Sarcomas and sarcomatoid and mixed malignant tumors of the kidney in adults – part II. Cancer 22: 551–555
282. Rebelakos A G, Papanastasiou K, Apostolikas N 1995 Renal plasmacytoma. Br J Urol 75: 562–562
283. Igel T C, Engen D E, Banks P M et al. 1991 Renal plasmacytoma: Mayo Clinic experience and review of the literature. Urology 37: 385–389
284. Bracken R B, Chica G, Johnson D E et al. 1979 Secondary renal neoplasms: An autopsy study. South Med J 72: 806–807
285. Klinger M E 1951 Secondary tumors of the genito-urinary tract. J Urol 65: 144–153
286. Payne R A 1960 Metastatic renal tumours. Br J Surg 48: 310–315
287. Wagle D G, Moore R H, Murphy G P 1975 Secondary carcinomas of the kidney. J Urol 114: 30–32
288. Pascal R R 1980 Renal manifestations of extrarenal neoplasms. Hum Pathol 11: 7–17
289. Melato M, Laurino L, Bianchi P et al. 1991 Intraglomerular metastases. A possibly maldiagnosed entity. Zentralbl Allg Pathol 137: 90–92
290. Naryshkin S, Tomaszewski J E 1991 Acute renal failure secondary to carcinomatous lymphatic metastases to kidneys. J Urol 146: 1610–1612
291. Mierau G W, Beckwith J B, Weeks D A 1987 Ultrastructure and histogenesis of the renal tumors of childhood: an overview. Ultrastruct Pathol 11: 313–333
292. Webber B L, Parham D M, Drake L G et al. 1992 Renal tumors in childhood. Pathol Annu 27, part 1: 191–232
293. Beckwith J B 1997 New developments in the pathology of Wilms tumor. Cancer Invest 15: 153–162
294. Sotelo-Avila C 1990 Nephroblastoma and other pediatric renal cancers. In: Eble JN (ed) Tumors and tumor-like conditions of the kidneys and ureters. Churchill Livingstone, New York, p 71–121
295. Breslow N, Beckwith J B, Ciol M et al. 1988 Age distribution of Wilms' tumor: report from the National Wilms' Tumor Study. Cancer Res 48: 1653–1657
296. Lemerle J, Tournade M-F, Gerard-Marchant R et al. 1976 Wilms' tumor: natural history and prognostic factors, a retrospective study of 248 cases treated at the Institut Gustave-Roussy 1952–1967. Cancer 37: 2557–2566
297. Hrabovsky E E, Othersen H B Jr, deLorimier A et al. 1986 Wilms' tumor in the neonate: a report from the National Wilms' Tumor Study. J Pediatr Surg 21: 385–387
298. Innis M D 1973 Nephroblastoma: index cancer of childhood. Med J Aust 2: 322–323
299. Blute M L, Kelalis P P, Offord K P et al. 1987 Bilateral Wilms tumor. J Urol 138: 968–973
300. Breslow N E, Beckwith J B 1982 Epidemiological features of Wilms' tumor: results of the National Wilms' Tumor Study. J Natl Cancer Inst 68: 429–436
301. Sotelo-Avila C, Gonzalez-Crussi F, Fowler J W 1980 Complete and incomplete forms of Beckwith-Wiedemann syndrome: their oncogenic potential. J Pediatr 96: 47–50
302. Heppe R K, Koyle M A, Beckwith J B 1991 Nephrogenic rests in Wilms tumor patients with Drash syndrome. J Urol 145: 1225–1228
303. Miller R W, Fraumeni JF Jr, Manning M D 1964 Association of Wilms's tumor with aniridia, hemihypertrophy and other congenital malformations. N Engl J Med 270: 922–927
304. Huser J, Grignon D J, Ro J Y et al. 1990 Adult Wilms' tumor: a clinicopathologic study of 11 cases. Mod Pathol 3: 321–326
305. Arrigo S, Beckwith J B, Sharples K et al. 1990 Better survival after combined modality care for adults with Wilms' tumor, a report from the National Wilms' Tumor Study. Cancer 66: 827–830
306. Bove K E, Koffler H, McAdams A J 1969 Nodular renal blastema, definition and possible significance. Cancer 24: 323–332
307. Bove K E, McAdams A J 1976 The nephroblastomatosis complex and its relationship to Wilms' tumor: a clinicopathologic treatise. Perspect Pediatr Pathol 3: 185–223
308. Beckwith J B, Kiviat N B, Bonadio J F 1990 Nephrogenic rests, nephroblastomatosis, and the pathogenesis of Wilms' tumor. Pediatr Pathol 10: 1–36
309. Scharfenberg J C, Beckman E N 1984 Persistent renal blastema in an adult. Hum Pathol 15: 791–793
310. Eble J N 1983 Fetal rhabdomyomatous nephroblastoma. J Urol 130: 541–543
311. Gonzalez-Crussi F, Hsueh W, Ugarte N 1981 Rhabdomyogenesis in renal neoplasia of childhood. Am J Surg Pathol 5: 525–532
312. Grimes M M, Wolff M, Wolff J A et al. 1982 Ganglion cells in metastatic Wilms' tumor, review of a histogenetic controversy. Am J Surg Pathol 6: 565–571
313. Cummins G E, Cohen D 1974 Cushing's syndrome secondary to ACTH-secreting Wilms' tumor. J Pediatr Surg 9: 535–539
314. Wigger H J 1976 Fetal rhabdomyomatous nephroblastoma – a variant of Wilms' tumor. Hum Pathol 7: 613–623
315. Fernandes E T, Parham D M, Ribeiro R C et al. 1988 Teratoid Wilms' tumor: The St Jude experience. J Pediatr Surg 23: 1131–1134
316. Variend S, Spicer R D, MacKinnon A E 1984 Teratoid Wilms' tumor. Cancer 53: 1936–1942
317. Bonadio J F, Storer B, Norkool P et al. 1985 Anaplastic Wilms' tumor: clinical and pathologic studies. J Clin Oncol 3: 513–520
318. Breslow N E, Palmer N F, Hill L R et al. 1978 Wilms' tumor: prognostic factors for patients without metastases at diagnosis, results of the National Wilms' Tumor Study. Cancer 41: 1577–1589
319. Beckwith B 1996 Focal versus diffuse anaplasia in nephroblastoma. Arch Anat Cytol Pathol 44: 53–53
320. Vujanic G M, Harms D, Sandstedt B et al. 1999 New definitions of focal and diffuse anaplasia in Wilms tumor: the International Society of Paediatric Oncology (SIOP) experience. Med Pediatr Oncol 32: 317–323
321. Faria P, Beckwith J B, Mishra K et al. 1996 Focal versus diffuse anaplasia in Wilms tumor – new definitions with prognostic significance, a report from the National Wilms Tumor Study Group. Am J Surg Pathol 20: 909–920
322. Perlman E J 2005 Pediatric renal tumors: practical updates for the pathologist. Pediatr Dev Pathol 8: 320–338
323. Weeks D A, Beckwith J B, Luckey D W 1987 Relapse-associated variables in stage I favorable histology Wilms' tumor, a report of the National Wilms' Tumor Study. Cancer 60: 1204–1212
324. Marsden H B, Lawler W 1978 Bone-metastasizing renal tumour of childhood. Br J Cancer 38: 437–441
325. Beckwith J B, Palmer N F 1978 Histopathology and prognosis of Wilms tumor, results from the First National Wilms' Tumor Study. Cancer 41: 1937–1948
326. Argani P, Perlman E J, Breslow N E et al. 2000 Clear cell sarcoma of the kidney, a review of 351 cases from the National Wilms' Tumor Study Group Pathology Center. Am J Surg Pathol 24: 4–18
327. Mierau G W, Weeks D A, Beckwith J B 1989 Anaplastic Wilms' tumor and other clinically aggressive childhood renal neoplasms: Ultrastructural and immunocytochemical features. Ultrastruct Pathol 13: 225–248
328. Amin M B, de Peralta-Venturina M N, Ro J Y et al. 1999 Clear cell sarcoma of kidney in an adolescent and in young adults: a report of four cases with ultrastructural, immunohistochemical, and DNA flow cytometric analysis. Am J Surg Pathol 23: 1455–1463
329. Sotelo-Avila C, Gonzalez-Crussi F, Sadowinski S et al. 1986 Clear cell sarcoma of the kidney: a clinicopathologic study of 21 patients with long-term follow-up evaluation. Hum Pathol 16: 1219–1230
330. Marsden H B, Lawler W 1980 Bone metastasizing renal tumour of childhood, histopathological and clinical review of 38 cases. Virchow's Arch [A] 387: 341–351
331. Weeks D A, Beckwith J B, Mierau G W et al. 1989 Rhabdoid tumor of kidney, a report of 111 cases from the National Wilms' Tumor Study Pathology Center. Am J Surg Pathol 13: 439–458
332. Tomlinson G E, Breslow N E, Dome J et al. 2005. Rhabdoid tumor of the kidney in the National Wilms' Tumor Study: age at diagnosis as a prognostic factor. J Clin Oncol 23: 7641–7645
333. Bonnin J M, Rubinstein L J, Palmer N F et al. 1984 The association of embryonal tumors originating in the kidney and in the brain, a report of seven cases. Cancer 54: 2137–2146

334. Mayes L C, Kasselberg A G, Roloff J S et al. 1984 Hypercalcemia associated with immunoreactive parathyroid hormone in a malignant rhabdoid tumor of the kidney (rhabdoid Wilms' tumor). Cancer 54: 882–884
335. Lee H-Y, Yoon C-S, Sevenet N et al. 2002 Rhabdoid tumor of the kidney is a component of the rhabdoid predisposition syndrome. Pediatr Dev Pathol 5: 395–399
336. Haas J E, Palmer N F, Weinberg A G et al. 1981 Ultrastructure of malignant rhabdoid tumor of the kidney, a distinctive renal tumor of children. Hum Pathol 12: 646–657
337. Hoot A C, Russo P, Judkins A R et al. 2004. Immunohistochemical analysis of hSNF5/INI1 distinguishes renal and extra-renal malignant rhabdoid tumors from other pediatric soft tissue tumors. Am J Surg Pathol 28: 1485–1491
338. Weeks D A, Beckwith J B, Mierau G W et al. 1991 Renal neoplasms mimicking rhabdoid tumor of kidney, a report from the National Wilms' Tumor Study Pathology Center. Am J Surg Pathol 15: 1042–1054
339. Marsden H B, Lawler W 1983 Primary renal tumours in the first year of life. A population based review. Virchow's Arch [A] 399: 1–9
340. Argani P, Beckwith J B 2000 Metanephric stromal tumor, report of 31 cases of a distinctive pediatric renal neoplasm. Am J Surg Pathol 24: 917–926
341. Blank E, Neerhout R C, Burry K A 1978 Congenital mesoblastic nephroma and polyhydramnios. JAMA 240: 1504–1505
342. Favara B E, Johnson W, Ito J 1968 Renal tumors in the neonatal period. Cancer 22: 845–855
343. Kay S, Pratt C B, Salzberg A M 1966 Hamartoma (leiomyomatous type) of the kidney. Cancer 19: 1825–1832
344. Bolande R P 1973 Congenital mesoblastic nephroma of infancy. Perspect Pediatr Pathol 1: 227–250
345. Howell C G, Othersen H B, Kiviat N E et al. 1982 Therapy and outcome in 51 children with mesoblastic nephroma: a report of the National Wilms' Tumor Study. J Pediatr Surg 17: 826–831
346. Chan H S L, Cheng M-Y, Mancer K et al. 1987 Congenital mesoblastic nephroma: a clinicoradiologic study of 17 cases representing the pathologic spectrum of the disease. J Pediatr 111: 64–70
347. Furtwaengler R, Reinhard H, Leuschner I et al. 2006 Mesoblastic nephroma – a report from the Gesellschaft fur Paediatrische Onkologie und Hamatologie (GPOH). Cancer 106: 2275–2283
348. Joshi V V, Kasznica J, Walters T R 1986 Atypical mesoblastic nephroma. Arch Pathol Lab Med 110: 100–106
349. Gonzalez-Crussi F, Sotelo-Avila C, Kidd J M 1980 Malignant mesenchymal nephroma of infancy, report of a case with pulmonary metastases. Am J Surg Pathol 4: 185–190
350. Trillo A A 1990 Adult variant of congenital mesoblastic nephroma. Arch Pathol Lab Med 114: 533–535
351. Van Velden D J J, Schneider J W, Allen F J 1990 A case of adult mesoblastic nephroma: ultrastructure and discussion of histogenesis. J Urol 143: 1216–1219
352. Beckwith J B, Weeks D A 1986 Congenital mesoblastic nephroma, when should we worry? Arch Pathol Lab Med 110: 98–99
353. Gormley T S, Skoog S J, Jones R V et al. 1989 Cellular congenital mesoblastic nephroma: what are the options. J Urol 142: 479–483
354. Rubin B P, Chen C-J, Morgan T W et al 1998 Congenital mesoblastic nephroma t(12;15) is associated with ETV6-NTRK3 gene fusion; cytogenetic and molecular relationship to congenital (infantile) fibrosarcoma. Am J Pathol 153: 1451–1458
355. Pettinato G, Manivel J C, Wick M R et al. 1989 Classical and cellular (atypical) congenital mesoblastic nephroma: a clinicopathologic, ultrastructural, immunohistochemical, and flow cytometric study. Hum Pathol 20: 682–690
356. Sotelo-Avila C, Beckwith J B, Johnson J E 1995 Ossifying renal tumor of infancy: a clinicopathologic study of nine cases. Pediatr Pathol 15: 745–762
357. Chatten J, Cromie W J, Duckett J W 1980 Ossifying tumor of infantile kidney, report of two cases. Cancer 45: 609–612
358. Dehner L P 1973 Intrarenal teratoma occurring in infancy: Report of a case with discussion of extragonadal germ cell tumors in infancy. J Pediatr Surg 8: 369–378
359. Aubert J, Casamayou J, Denis P et al. 1978 Intrarenal teratoma in a newborn child. Eur Urol 4: 306–308
360. Aaronson I A, Sinclair-Smith C 1980 Multiple cystic teratomas of the kidney. Arch Pathol Lab Med 104: 614–614
361. Mihatsch M J, Bleisch A, Six P et al. 1972 Primary choriocarcinoma of the kidney in a 49-year-old woman. J Urol 108: 537–539
362. Young R H, Eble J N 1991 Unusual forms of carcinoma of the urinary bladder. Hum Pathol 22: 948–965
363. Abeshouse B S 1956 Primary benign and malignant tumors of the ureter, a review of the literature and report of one benign and twelve malignant tumors. Am J Surg 91: 237–271
364. Satodate R, Koike H, Sasou S et al. 1984 Nephrogenic adenoma of the ureter. J Urol 131: 332–334
365. Lugo M, Petersen R O, Elfenbein I B et al. 1983 Nephrogenic metaplasia of the ureter. Am J Clin Pathol 80: 92–97
366. Naito S, Minoda M, Hirata H 1983 Inverted papilloma of ureter. Urology 22: 290–291
367. Lausten G S, Anagnostaki L, Thomsen O F 1984 Inverted papilloma of the upper urinary tract. Eur Urol 10: 67–70
368. Kyriakos M, Royce R K 1989 Multiple simultaneous inverted papillomas of the upper urinary tract. A case report with a review of ureteral and renal pelvic inverted papillomas. Cancer 63: 368–380
369. Embon O M, Saghi N, Bechar L 1984 Inverted papilloma of ureter. Eur Urol 10: 139–140
370. Arrufat J M, Vera-Román J M, Casas V et al. 1983 Papiloma invertido de uréter. Actas Urol Esp 7: 225–228
371. Palvio D H B 1985 Inverted papillomas of the urinary tract, a case of multiple, recurring inverted papillomas of the renal pelvis, ureter and bladder associated with malignant change. Scand J Urol Nephrol 19: 299–302
372. Kunze E, Schauer A, Schmitt M 1983 Histology and histogenesis of two different types of inverted urothelial papillomas. Cancer 51: 348–358
373. Kimura G, Tsuboi N, Nakajima H et al. 1987 Inverted papilloma of the ureter with malignant transformation: a case report and review of the literature. Urol Int 42: 30–36
374. Grainger R, Gikas P W, Grossman H B 1990 Urothelial carcinoma occurring within an inverted papilloma of the ureter. J Urol 143: 802–804
375. Wolgel C D, Parris A C, Mitty H A et al. 1982 Fibroepithelial polyp of renal pelvis. Urology 19: 436–439
376. Goldman S M, Bohlman M E, Gatewood O M B 1987 Neoplasms of the renal collecting system. Semin Roentgenol 22: 284–291
377. Bartone F F, Johansson S L, Markin R J et al. 1990 Bilateral fibroepithelial polyps of ureter in a child. Urology 35: 519–522
378. Macksood M J, Roth D R, Chang C-H et al. 1985 Benign fibroepithelial polyps as a cause of intermittent ureteropelvic junction obstruction in a child: a case report and review of the literature. J Urol 134: 951–952
379. van Poppel H, Nuttin B, Oyen R et al. 1986 Fibroepithelial polyps of the ureter, etiology, diagnosis, treatment and pathology. Eur Urol 12: 174–179
380. Williams P R, Feggeter J, Miller R A et al. 1980 The diagnosis and management of benign fibrous ureteric polyps. Br J Urol 52: 253–256
381. Stuppler S A, Kandzari S J 1975 Fibroepithelial polyps of ureter, a benign ureteral tumor. Urology 5: 553–558
382. Uhlir K 1973 Hemangioma of the ureter. J Urol 110: 647–649
383. Jansen T T H, van deWeyer F P H, deVries H R 1982 Angiomatous ureteral polyp. Urology 20: 426–427
384. Kvist E, Lauritzen A F, Bredesen J et al. 1988 A comparative study of transitional cell tumors of the bladder and upper urinary tract. Cancer 61: 2109–2112
385. Mazeman E 1976 Tumours of the upper urinary tract calyces, renal pelvis and ureter. Eur Urol 2: 120–128
386. McLaughlin J K, Blot W J, Mandel J S et al. 1983 Etiology of cancer of the renal pelvis. J Natl Cancer Inst 71: 287–291
387. Palvio D H B, Andersen J C, Falk E 1987 Transitional cell tumors of the renal pelvis and ureter associated with capillarosclerosis indicating analgesic abuse. Cancer 59: 972–976
388. Steffens J, Nagel R 1988 Tumours of the renal pelvis and ureter, observations in 170 patients. Br J Urol 61: 277–283
389. Verhaak R L O M, Harmsen A E, van Unnik A J M 1974 On the frequency of tumor induction in a thorotrast kidney. Cancer 34: 2061–2068
390. Nielsen K, Ostri P 1988 Primary tumors of the renal pelvis: evaluation of clinical and pathological features in a consecutive series of 10 years. J Urol 140: 19–21
391. Corrado F, Ferri C, Mannini D et al. 1991 Transitional cell carcinoma of the upper urinary tract: Evaluation of prognostic factors by histopathology and flow cytometric analysis. J Urol 145: 1159–1163
392. Bonsib S M 1990 Pathology of the renal pelvis and ureter. In: Eble JN (ed) Tumors and tumor-like conditions of the kidneys and ureters. Churchill Livingstone, New York, p 177–205
393. Olgac S, Mazumdar M, Dalbagni G et al. 2004. Urothelial carcinoma of the renal pelvis. A clinicopathologic study of 130 cases. Am J Surg Pathol 28: 1545–1552
394. Anderström C, Johansson S L, Pettersson S et al. 1989 Carcinoma of the ureter: a clinicopathologic study of 49 cases. J Urol 142: 280–283
395. Blute M L, Tsushima K, Farrow G M et al. 1988 Transitional cell carcinoma of the renal pelvis: nuclear deoxyribonucleic acid ploidy studied by flow cytometry. J Urol 140: 944–949
396. American Joint Committee on Cancer 1997 Renal pelvis and ureter. AJCC Cancer Staging Manual. Lippincott-Raven, Philadelphia, p 235–239
397. Murphy D M, Zincke H, Furlow W J 1980 Primary grade 1 transitional cell carcinoma of the renal pelvis and ureter. J Urol 123: 629–631
398. Huben R P, Mounzer A M, Murphy G P 1988 Tumor grade and stage as prognostic variables in upper tract urothelial tumors. Cancer 62: 2016–2020
399. Nocks B N, Heney N M, Daly J J et al. 1982 Transitional cell carcinoma of renal pelvis. Urology 19: 472–477
400. Piscioli F, Bondi A, Scappini P et al. 1984 "True" sarcomatoid carcinoma of the renal pelvis. Eur Urol 10: 350–355
401. Essenfeld H, Manivel J C, Benedetto P et al. 1990 Small cell carcinoma of the renal pelvis: A clinicopathological, morphological and immunohistochemical study of 2 cases. J Urol 144: 344–347
402. Kenney R M, Prat J, Tabernero M 1984 Giant-cell tumor-like proliferation associated with a papillary transitional cell carcinoma of the renal pelvis. Am J Surg Pathol 8: 139–144
402a. Baydar D, Amin M B, Epstein J I 2006 Osteoclast-rich indifferentiated carcinomas of the urinary tract. Mod Pathol 19: 161–171
403. Mahadevia P S, Karwa G L, Koss L G 1983 Mapping of urothelium in carcinomas of the renal pelvis and ureter. Cancer 51: 890–897

404. Martínez García R, Boronat Tormo F, Domínguez Hinarejos C et al. 1989 Adenocarcinoma de pelvis renal. Actas Urol Esp 13: 470–472
405. Takezawa Y, Saruki K, Jinbo S et al. 1990 A case of adenocarcinoma of the renal pelvis. Acta Urol Jpn 36: 841–845
406. Stein A, Sova Y, Lurie M et al. 1988 Adenocarcinoma of the renal pelvis, report of two cases, one with simultaneous transitional cell carcinoma of the bladder. Urol Int 43: 299–301
407. Kim Y I, Yoon D H, Lee S W et al. 1988 Multicentric papillary adenocarcinoma of the renal pelvis and ureter: report of a case with ultrastructural study. Cancer 62: 2402–2407
408. Ishikura H, Ishiguro T, Enatsu C et al. 1991 Hepatoid adenocarcinoma of the renal pelvis producing alpha-fetoprotein of hepatic type and bile pigment. Cancer 67: 3051–3056
409. Brawer M K, Waisman J 1982 Papillary adenocarcinoma of ureter. Urology 19: 205–209
410. Moncino M D, Friedman H S, Kurtzberg J et al. 1990 Papillary adenocarcinoma of the renal pelvis in a child: case report and brief review of the literature. Med Pediatr Oncol 18: 81–86
411. Bullock P S, Thoni D E, Murphy W M 1987 The significance of colonic mucosa (intestinal metaplasia) involving the urinary tract. Cancer 59: 2086–2090
412. Gordon A 1963 Intestinal metaplasia of the urinary tract epithelium. J Pathol Bacteriol 85: 441–444
413. Utz D C, McDonald J R 1957 Squamous cell carcinoma of the kidney. J Urol 78: 540–552
414. Blacher E J, Johnson D E, Abdul-Karim F W et al. 1985 Squamous cell carcinoma of renal pelvis. Urology 25: 124–125
415. Hertle L, Androulakakis P 1982 Keratinizing desquamative squamous metaplasia of the upper urinary tract: leukoplakia-cholesteatoma. J Urol 127: 631–635
416. Strobel S L, Jasper W S, Gogate S A et al. 1984 Primary carcinoma of the renal pelvis and ureter, evaluation of clinical and pathologic features. Arch Pathol Lab Med 108: 697–700
417. Howat A J, Scott E, Mackie B et al. 1983 Adenosquamous carcinoma of the renal pelvis. Am J Clin Pathol 79: 731–733
418. Kao V C T, Graff P W, Rappaport H 1969 Leiomyoma of the ureter, a histologically problematic rare tumor confirmed by immunohistochemical studies. Cancer 24: 535–542
419. Zaitoon M M 1986 Leiomyoma of ureter. Urology 28: 50–51
420. Gislason T, Arnarson O O 1984 Primary ureteral leiomyosarcoma. Scand J Urol Nephrol 18: 253–254
421. Rushton H G, Sens M A, Garvin A J et al. 1983 Primary leiomyosarcoma of the ureter: a case report with electron microscopy. J Urol 129: 1045–1046
422. Eble J N, Young R H, Störkel S et al. 1991 Primary osteosarcoma of the kidney: a report of three cases. J Urogenital Pathol 1: 83–88
423. Fein R L, Hamm F C 1965 Malignant schwannoma of the renal pelvis: A review of the literature and a case report. J Urol 94: 356–361
424. Frasier B L, Wachs B H, Watson L R et al. 1988 Malignant melanoma of the renal pelvis presenting as a primary tumor. J Urol 140: 812–813
425. Scharifker D, Chalasani A 1978 Ureteral involvement by malignant lymphoma, ten years' experience. Arch Pathol Lab Med 102: 541–542
426. Young R H 1989 Non-neoplastic epithelial abnormalities and tumorlike lesions. In: Young RH (ed) Pathology of the urinary bladder. Churchill Livingstone, New York, p 1–63
427. Eble J N, Young R H 1989 Benign and low-grade papillary lesions of the urinary bladder: a review of the papilloma-papillary carcinoma controversy, and a report of five typical papillomas. Semin Diagn Pathol 6: 351–371
428. Jordan A M, Weingarten J, Murphy W M 1987 Transitional cell neoplasms of the urinary bladder, can biological potential be predicted from histologic grading? Cancer 60: 2766–2774
429. McKenney J K, Amin M B, Young R H 2003 Urothelial (transitional cell) papilloma of the urinary bladder: A clinicopathologic study of 26 cases. Mod Pathol 16:623–629
430. Magi-Galluzzi C, Epstein J I 2004 Urothelial papilloma of the bladder. A review of 34 de novo cases. Am J Surg Pathol 28:1615–1620
431. Kunze E, Schauer A, Schmitt M 1983 Histology and histogenesis of two different types of inverted urothelial papillomas. Cancer 51: 348–358
432. Broussard J N, Tan P H, Epstein J I. 2004 Atypia in inverted urothelial papillomas: pathology and prognostic significance. Hum Pathol 35: 1499–1504
433. Amin M B, Gomez J A, Young R H 1997 Urothelial transitional cell carcinoma with endophytic growth patterns. Am J Surg Pathol 21: 1057–1068
434. Mattelaer J, Leonard A, Goddeeris P et al. 1988 Inverted papilloma of bladder: clinical significance. Urology 32: 192–197
434a. Guo C C, Fine S W, Epstein J I 2006 Noninvasive squamous lesions in the urinary bladder: a clinicopathologic analysis of 29 cases. Am J Surg Pathol 30: 883-891
435. Eble J N, Hull M T, Rowland R G et al. 1986 Villous adenoma of the urachus with mucusuria: a light and electron microscopic study. J Urol 135: 1240–1244
436. Adegboyega P A, Adesokan A. 1999 Tubulovillous adenoma of the urinary bladder. Mod Pathol 12:735–738
437. Cheng L, Montironi R, Bostwick D G 1999 Villous adenoma of the urinary tract: a report of 23 cases, including 8 with coexistent adenocarcinoma. Am J Surg Pathol 23: 764–771
438. Seibel J L, Prasad S, Weiss R E et al. 2002 Villous adenoma of the urinary tract: a lesion frequently associated with malignancy. Hum Pathol 33: 236–241
439. Choi W W L, Amin M B, Tamboli P et al. 2005 Glandular neoplasms of the urachus: clinicopathological and immunohistochemical analysis of 43 cases with special emphasis on low-grade mucinous cystic tumors. Mod Pathol 18 (suppl): 134A
440. Oyasu R, Hopp M L 1974 The etiology of cancer of the bladder. Surg Gynecol Obstet 138: 97–108
441. Morrison A S 1984 Advances in the etiology of urothelial cancer. Urol Clin North Am 11: 557–566
442. Wallace D M A 1988 Occupational urothelial cancer. Br J Urol 61: 175–182
443. Royce R K, Ackerman L V 1951 Carcinoma of the bladder: therapeutic and pathologic aspects of 135 cases. J Urol 65: 66–86
444. Kaye K W, Lange P H 1982 Mode of presentation of invasive bladder cancer: reassessment of the problem. J Urol 128: 31–33
445. Brawn P N 1982 The origin of invasive carcinoma of the bladder. Cancer 50: 515–519
446. Newman L H, Tannenbaum M, Droller M J 1988 Muscle-invasive bladder cancer: Does it arise de novo or from pre-existing superficial disease? Urology 32: 58–62
447. Epstein J I, Amin M B, Reuter V E et al. Bladder Consensus Conference Committee 1998 The World Health Organization/International Society of Urological Pathology consensus classification of urothelial (transitional cell) neoplasms of the urinary bladder. Am J Surg Pathol 22: 1435–1438
448. Sarma K P 1981 Genesis of papillary tumours: histological and microangiographic study. Br J Urol 53: 228–236
449. Taylor D C, Bhagavan B S, Larsen M P et al. 1996 Papillary urothelial hyperplasia. A precursor to papillary neoplasms. Am J Surg Pathol 20:1481–1488
450. Young R H 1988 Papillary and polypoid cystitis, a report of eight cases. Am J Surg Pathol 12: 542–546
451. Melicow M M 1952 Histological study of vesical urothelium intervening between gross neoplasms in total cystectomy. J Urol 68: 261–278
452. Melamed M R, Voutsa N G, Grabstald H 1964 Natural history and clinical behavior of in situ carcinoma of the human urinary bladder. Cancer 17: 1533–1545
453. Elliott G B, Moloney P J, Anderson G H 1973 "Denuding cystitis" and in situ urothelial carcinoma. Arch Pathol 96: 91–94
454. Utz D C, Zincke H 1974 The masquerade of bladder cancer as interstitial cystitis. J Urol 111: 160–161
455. Koss L G, Nakanishi I, Freed S Z 1977 Nonpapillary carcinoma in situ and atypical hyperplasia in cancerous bladders: further studies of surgically-removed bladders by mapping. Urology 9: 442–455
456. Utz D C, Farrow G M, Rife C C et al. 1980 Carcinoma in situ of the bladder. Cancer 45: 1842–1848
457. Prout G R Jr, Griffin P P, Daly J J et al. 1983 Carcinoma in situ of the urinary bladder with and without associated vesical neoplasms. Cancer 52: 524–532
458. Kakizoe T, Matumoto K, Nishio Y et al. 1985 Significance of carcinoma in situ and dysplasia in association with bladder cancer. J Urol 133: 395–398
459. Nagy G K, Frable W J, Murphy W M 1982 Classification of premalignant urothelial abnormalities, a Delphi study of the National Bladder Cancer Collaborative Group A. Pathol Annu 17: 219–233
460. Murphy W M, Soloway M S 1982 Developing carcinoma (dysplasia) of the urinary bladder. Pathol Annu 17 (Pt1): 197–217
461. Farrow G M, Utz D C 1982 Observations on microinvasive transitional cell carcinoma of the urinary bladder. Clin Oncol 1: 609–615
462. McKenney J K, Gomes J A, Desai S et al. 2001 Morphologic expression of urothelial carcinoma in situ. A detailed evaluation of its histologic patterns with emphasis on carcinoma in situ with microinvasion. Am J Surg Pathol 25:356–362
463. Lopez-Beltran A, Luque R J, Moreno A et al. 2002. The pagetoid variant of bladder urothelial carcinoma in situ. A clinicopathological study of 11 cases. Virchow's Arch 441: 148–153
464. Ro J Y, Ayala A G, El-Naggar A 1987 Muscularis mucosa of urinary bladder, importance for staging and treatment. Am J Surg Pathol 11: 668–673
465. Keep J C, Piehl M, Miller A et al. 1989 Invasive carcinomas of the urinary bladder, evaluation of tunica muscularis mucosae involvement. Am J Clin Pathol 91: 575–579
466. Younes M, Sussman J, True L D 1990 The usefulness of the level of the muscularis mucosae in the staging of invasive transitional cell carcinoma of the urinary bladder. Cancer 66: 543–548
467. Weaver M G, Abdul-Karim F W 1990 The prevalence and character of the muscularis mucosae of the human urinary bladder. Histopathology 17: 563–566
468. Talbert M L, Young R H 1989 Carcinomas of the urinary bladder with deceptively benign-appearing foci, a report of three cases. Am J Surg Pathol 13: 374–381
469. Drew P A, Furman J, Civantos F et al. 1996 The nested variant of transitional cell carcinoma: An aggressive neoplasm with innocuous histology. Mod Pathol 9: 989–994
470. Lin O, Cardillo M, Dalbagni G et al. 2003 Nested variant of urothelial carcinoma: A clinicopathologic and immunohistochemical study of 12 cases. Mod Pathol 16: 1289–1298

471. Young R H, Oliva E 1996 Transitional cell carcinomas of the urinary bladder that may be underdiagnosed: a report of four invasive cases exemplifying the homology between neoplastic and non-neoplastic transitional cell lesions. Am J Surg Pathol 20: 1448–1454
472. Volmar K E, Chan T Y, DeMarzo A M et al. 2003 Florid von Brunn nests mimicking urothelial carcinoma. A morphologic and immunohistochemical comparison to the nested variant of urothelial carcinoma. Am J Surg Pathol 27: 1243–1252
473. Young R H, Zukerberg L R 1990 Microcystic transitional cell carcinomas of the urinary bladder, a report of four cases. Am J Clin Pathol 96: 635–639
474. Paz A, Rath-Wolfson L, Lask D et al. 1997 The clinical and histological features of transitional cell carcinoma of the bladder with microcysts: analysis of 12 cases. Br J Urol 79: 772–725
475. Amin M B, Ro J Y, El-Sharkawy T et al. 1994 Micropapillary variant of transitional cell carcinoma of the urinary bladder, histologic pattern resembling ovarian papillary serous carcinoma. Am J Surg Pathol 18: 1224–1232
476. Samaratunga H, Khoo K 2004 Micropapillary variant of urothelial carcinoma of the urinary bladder; a clinicopathological and immunohistochemical study. Histopathology 45: 55–64
477. Alvarado-Cabrero I, Sierra-Santiesteban F I, Mantilla-Morales A et al. 2005 Micropapillary carcinoma of the urothelial tract. A clinicopathologic study of 38 cases. Ann Diag Pathol 9: 1–5
478. Young R H, Wick M R, Mills S E 1988 Sarcomatoid carcinoma of the urinary bladder, a clinicopathologic analysis of 12 cases and review of the literature. Am J Clin Pathol 90: 653–661
479. Pearson J M, Banerjee S S, Haboubi N Y 1989 Two cases of pseudosarcomatous invasive transitional cell carcinoma of the urinary bladder mimicking malignant fibrous histiocytoma. Histopathology 15: 93–99
480. Ro J Y, Wishnow K I, Ayala A G et al. 1988 Sarcomatoid bladder carcinoma: clinicopathologic and immunohistochemical study on 44 cases. Surg Pathol 1: 359–374
481. Ikegami H, Iwasaki H, Ohjimi Y et al. 2000 Sarcomatoid carcinoma of the urinary bladder: A clinicopathologic and immunohistochemical analysis of 14 patients. Hum Pathol 31: 332–340
482. Murata T, Soga T, Tajima K et al. 1994 Sarcomatoid carcinoma of the urinary tract. Pathol Int 44: 138–144
483. Torenbeek R, Blomjous C E M, deBruin P C 1994 Sarcomatoid carcinoma of the urinary bladder. Clinicopathologic analysis of 18 cases with immunohistochemical and electron microscopic findings. Am J Surg Pathol 18:241–249.
484. Serio G, Zampatti C, Ceppi M. 1995 Spindle and giant cell carcinoma of the urinary bladder: a clinicopathological light microscopic and immunohistochemical study. Br J Urol 75: 167–172
485. Jones E C, Young R H 1997 Myxoid and sclerosing sarcomatoid transitional cell carcinoma of the urinary bladder: a clinicopathologic and immunohistochemical study of 25 cases. Mod Pathol 10: 908–916
486. Perret L, Chaubert P, Hessler D et al. 1998 Primary heterologous carcinosarcoma (metaplastic carcinoma) of the urinary bladder. A clinicopathologic, immunohistochemical, and ultrastructural analysis of eight cases and a review of the literature. Cancer 82: 1535–1549.
487. Pitt M A, Morphopoulos G, Wells S et al. 1995 Pseudoangiosarcomatous carcinoma of the genitourinary tract. J Clin Pathol 48: 1059–1061
488. Wick M R, Brown B A, Young R H et al. 1988 Spindle-cell proliferations of the urinary tract: an immunohistochemical study. Am J Surg Pathol 12: 379–389
489. Martin J E, Jenkins B J, Zuk R J et al. 1989 Human chorionic gonadotropin expression and histological findings as predictors of response to radiotherapy in carcinoma of the bladder. Virchow's Arch [A] 414: 273–277
490. Burry A F, Munn S R, Arnold E P et al. 1986 Trophoblastic metaplasia in urothelial carcinoma of the bladder. Br J Urol 58: 143–146
491. Morton K D, Burnett R A 1988 Choriocarcinoma arising in transitional cell carcinoma of the bladder: a case report. Histopathology 12: 325–328
492. Young R H, Wick M R 1988 Transitional cell carcinoma of the urinary bladder with pseudosarcomatous stroma. Am J Clin Pathol 90: 216–219
493. Mahadevia P S, Alexander J E, Rojas-Corona R et al. 1989 Pseudosarcomatous stromal reaction in primary and metastatic urothelial carcinoma, a source of diagnostic difficulty. Am J Surg Pathol 13: 782–790
494. Eble J N, Young R H 1991 Stromal osseous metaplasia in carcinoma of the urinary bladder. J Urol 145: 823–825
495. Zukerberg L R, Armin A-R, Pisharodi L et al. 1990 Transitional cell carcinoma of the urinary bladder with osteoclast-type giant-cells: a report of two cases and review of the literature. Histopathology 17: 407–411
496. Zukerberg L R, Harris N L, Young R H 1991 Carcinomas of the urinary bladder simulating malignant lymphoma: a report of five cases. Am J Surg Pathol 15: 569–576
497. Friedell G H, Bell J R, Burney S W et al. 1976 Histopathology and classification of urinary bladder carcinoma. Urol Clin North Am 3: 53–70
498. Sakkas J L 1966 Clinical pattern and treatment of squamous cell carcinoma of the bladder. Int Surg 45: 71–76
499. Rous S N 1978 Squamous cell carcinoma of the bladder. J Urol 120: 561–562
500. Faysal M H 1981 Squamous cell carcinoma of the bladder. J Urol 120: 598–599
501. Newman D M, Brown J R, Jay A C et al. 1968 Squamous cell carcinoma of the bladder. J Urol 100: 470–473
502. Bessette P L, Abell M R, Herwig K R 1974 A clinicopathologic study of squamous cell carcinoma of the bladder. J Urol 112: 66–67
503. Rundle J S H, Hart A J L, McGeorge A et al. 1982 Squamous cell carcinoma of bladder. A review of 114 patients. Br J Urol 54: 522–526
504. Costello A J, Tiptaft R C, England H R et al. 1984 Squamous cell carcinoma of bladder. Urology 23: 234–236
505. Richie J P, Waisman J, Skinner D G et al. 1976 Squamous carcinoma of the bladder: treatment by radical cystectomy. J Urol 115: 670–672
506. Johnson D E, Schoenwald M B, Ayala A G et al. 1976 Squamous cell carcinoma of the bladder. J Urol 115: 542–544
507. El Sebai I, Sherif M, El Bolkainy M et al. 1974 Verrucose squamous carcinoma of bladder. Urology 4: 407–410
508. Walther M, O'Brien D P, Birch H W 1986 Condyloma acuminata and verrucous carcinoma of the bladder: case report and literature review. J Urol 135: 362–365
509. Wyatt J K, Craig I 1980 Verrucous carcinoma of urinary bladder. Urology 16: 97–99
510. Holck S, Jørgensen L 1983 Verrucous carcinoma of urinary bladder. Urology 22: 435–437
511. Querci Della Rovere G, Oliver R T D, McCance D J et al. 1988 Development of bladder tumour containing HPV type 11 DNA after renal transplantation. Br J Urol 62: 36–38
512. Rabson S M 1936 Leukoplakia and carcinoma of the urinary bladder, report of a case with a review of the literature. J Urol 35: 321–341
513. Connery D B 1953 Leukoplakia of the urinary bladder and its association with carcinoma. J Urol 69: 121–127
514. Benson R C Jr, Swanson S K, Farrow G M 1984 Relationship of leukoplakia to urothelial malignancy. J Urol 131: 507–511
515. Melamed M R, Farrow G M, Haggitt R C 1987 Case 19 in Urologic neoplasms, Proceedings of the 50th Annual Anatomic Slide Seminar of the American Society of Clinical Pathologists. ASCP 98–103
516. Wheeler J D, Hill W T 1954 Adenocarcinoma involving the urinary bladder. Cancer 7: 119–135
517. Mostofi F K, Thomson R V, Dean A L Jr 1955 Mucous adenocarcinoma of the urinary bladder. Cancer 8: 741–758
518. Thomas D G, Ward A M, Williams J L 1971 A study of 52 cases of adenocarcinoma of the bladder. Br J Urol 43: 4–15
519. Johnson D E, Hogan J M, Ayala A G 1972 Primary adenocarcinoma of the urinary bladder. South Med J 65: 527–530
520. Daroca P J Jr, MacKenzie F, Reed R J et al. 1976 Primary adenovillous carcinoma of the bladder. J Urol 115: 41–45
521. Jacobo E, Loening S, Schmidt J D et al. 1977 Primary adenocarcinoma of the bladder: a retrospective study of 20 patients. J Urol 117: 54–56
522. Fuselier H A Jr, Brannan W, Ochsner M G et al. 1978 Adenocarcinoma of the bladder as seen at Ochsner Medical Institutions. South Med J 71: 804–806
523. Kramer S A, Bredael J, Croker B P et al. 1979 Primary non-urachal adenocarcinoma of the bladder. J Urol 121: 278–281
524. Jones W A, Gibbons R P, Correa R J Jr et al. 1980 Primary adenocarcinoma of bladder. Urology 15: 119–121
525. Nocks B N, Heney N M, Daly J J 1983 Primary adenocarcinoma of urinary bladder. Urology 21: 26–29
526. Malek R S, Rosen J S, O'Dea M J 1983 Adenocarcinoma of bladder. Urology 21: 357–359
527. Anderström C, Johansson S, von Schultz L 1983 Primary adenocarcinoma of the urinary bladder, a clinicopathologic and prognostic study. Cancer 52: 1273–1280
528. Bennett J K, Wheatley J K, Walton K N 1984 10-year experience with adenocarcinoma of the bladder. J Urol 131: 262–263
529. O'Brien A M E, Urbanski S J 1985 Papillary adenocarcinoma in situ of bladder. J Urol 134: 544–546
530. Abenoza P, Manivel C, Fraley E E 1987 Primary adenocarcinoma of urinary bladder, clinicopathologic study of 16 cases. Urology 29: 9–14
531. Pallesen G 1981 Neoplastic Paneth cells in adenocarcinoma of the urinary bladder: a first case report. Cancer 47: 1834–1837
532. Young R H, Parkhurst E C 1984 Mucinous adenocarcinoma of bladder. Case associated with extensive intestinal metaplasia of urothelium in patient with nonfunctioning bladder for twelve years. Urology 24: 192–195
533. Grignon D J, Ro J Y, Ayala A G et al. 1991 Primary adenocarcinoma of the urinary bladder: a clinicopathologic analysis of 72 cases. Cancer 67: 2165–2172
534. Sheldon C A, Clayman R V, Gonzalez R et al. 1984 Malignant urachal lesions. J Urol 131: 1–8
535. O'Kane H O J, Megaw J M 1968 Carcinoma in the exstrophic bladder. Br J Surg 55: 631–635
536. Al-Izzi M S, Horton L W L, Kelleher J et al. 1989 Malignant transformation in endometriosis of the urinary bladder. Histopathology 14: 191–198
537. Oliva E, Amin M, Jimenez R et al. 2002 Clear cell carcinoma of the urinary bladder. A report and comparison of four tumors of mullerian origin and nine of probable urothelial origin with discussion of histogenesis and diagnostic problems. Am J Surg Pathol 26:190–197
538. Young R H 1989 Unusual variants of primary bladder carcinoma and secondary tumors of the bladder. In: Young RH (ed) Pathology of the urinary bladder. Churchill Livingstone, New York, p 103–139
539. Saphir O 1955 Signet-ring cell carcinoma of the urinary bladder. Am J Pathol 31: 223–231

540. Rosas-Uribe A, Luna M A 1969 Primary signet ring cell carcinoma of the urinary bladder. Report of two cases. Arch Pathol 88: 294–297
541. Grignon D J, Ro J Y, Ayala A G et al. 1991 Primary signet-ring cell carcinoma of the urinary bladder. Am J Clin Pathol 95: 13–20
542. Torenbeck R, Koot R A C, Blomjous C E M et al 1996 Primary signet-ring cell carcinoma of the urinary bladder. Histopathology 28: 33–40
543. Novak R W, Raines R B, Sollee A N 1981 Clear cell carcinoma in a Müllerian duct cyst. Am J Clin Pathol 76: 339–341
544. Young R H, Bostwick D H 1996 Florid cystitis glandularis of intestinal type with mucin extravasation: a mimic of adenocarcinoma. Am J Surg Pathol 20: 1462–1468
545. Clement P B 1990 Pathology of endometriosis. Pathol Annu 25: 245–295
546. Clement P B, Young R H 1992 Endocervicosis of the urinary bladder, a report of six cases of a benign müllerian lesion that may mimic adenocarcinoma. Am J Surg Pathol 16: 533–542
547. Young R H, Clement P B 1996 Mullerianosis of the urinary bladder. Mod Pathol 9:731–737
548. Epstein J I, Kuhajda F P, Lieberman P H 1986 Prostate-specific acid phosphatase immunoreactivity in adenocarcinomas of the urinary bladder. Hum Pathol 17: 939–942
549. Oliva E, Young R H 1995 Nephrogenic adenoma of the urinary tract: A review of the microscopic appearance of 80 cases with emphasis on unusual features. Mod Pathol 8: 722–730
550. Cheng L, Cheville J C, Selo T J et al. 2000 Atypical nephrogenic metaplasia of the urinary tract. A precursor lesion? Cancer 88: 853–861
551. Young R H, Johnston W H 1990 Serous adenocarcinoma of the uterus metastatic to the urinary bladder mimicking primary bladder neoplasia, a report of a case. Am J Surg Pathol 14: 877–880
552. Mills S E, Wolfe J T III, Weiss M A et al. 1987 Small cell undifferentiated carcinoma of the urinary bladder, a light-microscopic, immunocytochemical, and ultrastructural study of 12 cases. Am J Surg Pathol 11: 606–617
553. Grignon D J, Ro J Y, Ayala A G et al. 1992 Small cell carcinoma of the urinary bladder, a clinicopathologic analysis of 22 cases. Cancer 69: 527–536
554. Abrahams N A, Moran C, Reyes A O et al. 2005 Small cell carcinoma of the bladder: a contemporary clinicopathological study of 51 cases. Histopathology 46: 57–63
555. Reyes C V, Soneru I 1985 Small cell carcinoma of the urinary bladder with hypercalcemia. Cancer 56: 2530–2533
556. Blomjous C E M, Vos W, De Voogt H J et al. 1989 Small cell carcinoma of the urinary bladder, a clinicopathologic, morphometric, immunohistochemical, and ultrastructural study of 18 cases. Cancer 64: 1347–1357
557. Partanen S, Asikainen U 1985 Oat cell carcinoma of the urinary bladder with ectopic adrenocorticotropic hormone production. Hum Pathol 16: 313–315
558. Davis M P, Murthy M S N, Simon J et al. 1989 Successful management of small cell carcinoma of the bladder with cisplatin and etoposide. J Urol 142: 817–818
559. Holmäng S, Borghede G, Johansson S L 1995 Primary small cell carcinoma of the bladder: a report of 25 cases. J Urol 153: 1820–1822
560. Jones T D, Kernek K M, Yang X J et al. 2005 Thyroid transcription factor 1 expression in small cell carcinoma of the urinary bladder: an immunohistochemical profile of 44 cases. Hum Pathol 36: 718–723
561. Komatsu H, Kinoshita K, Mikata N et al. 1985 Spindle and giant cell carcinoma of the bladder: report of 3 cases. Eur Urol 11: 141–144
562. Young R H, Eble J N 1993 Lymphoepithelioma-like carcinoma of the urinary bladder. J Urol Pathol 1: 63–67
563. Amin M B, Ro J Y, Lee K M et al. 1994 Lymphoepithelioma-like carcinoma of the urinary bladder. Am J Surg Pathol 18: 466–473
564. Lopez-Beltran A, Luque R J, Vicioso L et al. 2001. Lymphoepithelioma-like carcinoma of the urinary bladder: a clinicopathologic study of 13 cases. Virchow's Arch 438: 552–557
565. Walker A N, Mills S E, Young R H 1989 Mesenchymal and miscellaneous other primary tumors of the urinary bladder. In: Young RH (ed) Pathology of the urinary bladder. Churchill Livingstone, New York, p 139–178
566. Knoll L D, Segura J W, Scheithauer B W 1986 Leiomyoma of the bladder. J Urol 136: 906–908
567. Belis J A, Post G J, Rochman S C et al. 1979 Genitourinary leiomyomas. Urology 13: 424–429
568. Bramwell S P, Pitts J, Goudie S E et al. 1987 Giant leiomyoma of the bladder. Br J Urol 60: 178
569. Munsie W J, Foster E A 1968 Unsuspected very small foci of carcinoma of the prostate in transurethral resection specimens. Cancer 21: 692–698
570. Cheng L, Nascimento A G, Neumann R M et al. 1999 Hemangioma of the urinary bladder. Cancer 86: 498–504
571. Sarma D P, Weiner M 1983 Hemangioma of the urinary bladder. J Surg Oncol 24: 142–144
572. Bolkier M, Ginesin Y, Lichtig C et al. 1983 Lymphangioma of bladder. J Urol 129: 1049–1050
573. Brooks P T, Scally J K 1985 Case report: bladder neurofibromas causing ureteric obstruction in von Recklinghausen's disease. Clin Radiol 36: 537–538
574. Blum M D, Bahnson R R, Carter M F 1985 Urologic manifestations of von Recklinghausen neurofibromatosis. Urology 26: 209–217
575. Mouradian J A, Coleman J W, McGovern J H et al. 1974 Granular cell tumor (myoblastoma) of the bladder. J Urol 112: 343–345
576. Karol J B, Eason A A, Tanagho E A 1977 Fibrous histiocytoma of bladder. Urology 10: 593–595
577. Cheng L, Scheithauer B W, Leibovich B C et al. 1999 Neurofibroma of the urinary bladder. Cancer 86: 505–513
578. McCrea L E, Post E A 1955 Sarcoma of the bladder. Urol Surv 5: 307–356
579. Sen S E, Malek R S, Farrow G M, Lieber M M 1985 Sarcoma and carcinosarcoma of the bladder in adults. J Urol 133: 29–30
580. Mills S E, Bova G S, Wick M R et al. 1989 Leiomyosarcoma of the urinary bladder, a clinicopathologic and immunohistochemical study of 15 cases. Am J Surg Pathol 13: 480–489
581. Rowland R G, Eble J N 1983 Bladder leiomyosarcoma and pelvic fibroblastic tumor following cyclophosphamide therapy. J Urol 130: 344–346
582. Sigal S H, Tomaszewski J E, Brooks J J et al. 1991 Carcinosarcoma of bladder following long-term cyclophosphamide therapy. Arch Pathol Lab Med 115: 1049–1051
583. Young R H, Proppe K H, Dickersin G R et al. 1987 Myxoid leiomyosarcoma of the urinary bladder. Arch Pathol Lab Med 111: 359–362
584. Proppe K H, Scully R E, Rosai J 1984 Postoperative spindle cell nodules of the genitourinary tract resembling sarcomas, a report of eight cases. Am J Surg Pathol 8: 101–108
585. Nochomovitz L E, Orenstein J M 1985 Inflammatory pseudotumor of the urinary bladder – possible relationship to nodular fasciitis, two case reports, cytologic observations, and ultrastructural observations. Am J Surg Pathol 9: 366–373
586. Ro J Y, Ayala A G, Ordóñez N G et al. 1986 Pseudosarcomatous fibromyxoid tumor of the urinary bladder. Am J Clin Pathol 86: 583–590
587. Young R H, Scully R E 1987 Pseudosarcomatous lesions of the urinary bladder, prostate gland, and urethra, a report of three cases and review of the literature. Arch Pathol Lab Med 111: 354–358
588. Albores-Saavedra J, Manivel J C, Essenfeld H et al. 1990 Pseudosarcomatous myofibroblastic proliferations in the urinary bladder of children. Cancer 66: 1234–1241
589. Lundgren L, Aldenberg F, Angervall L et al. 1994 Pseudomalignant spindle cell proliferations of the urinary bladder. Hum Pathol 25: 181–191
590. Hirsch M S, Dal Cin P, Fletcher C D M 2006 ALK expression in pseudosarcomatous myofibroblastic proliferations of the genitourinary tract. Histopathology 48: 569–578
591. Dehner L P 1989 Pathology of the urinary bladder in children. In: Young RH (ed) Pathology of the urinary bladder. Churchill Livingstone, New York, p 179–211
592. Mostofi F K, Morse W H 1952 Polypoid rhabdomyosarcoma (sarcoma botryoides) of bladder in children. J Urol 67: 681–687
593. Ober W B, Edgcomb J H 1954 Sarcoma botryoides in the female urogenital tract. Cancer 7: 75–91
594. Ghazali S 1973 Embryonic rhabdomyosarcoma of the urogenital tract. Br J Surg 60: 124–128
595. Hays D M, Raney R B Jr, Lawrence W Jr et al. 1982 Bladder and prostatic tumors in the intergroup rhabdomyosarcoma study (IRS-I). Results of therapy. Cancer 50: 1472–1482
596. Williams D I, Schistad G 1964 Lower urinary tract tumours in children. Br J Urol 36: 51–65
597. Hellstrom H R, Fisher E R 1961 Embryonal rhabdomyosarcoma of the bladder in the aged. J Urol 86: 336–339
598. Joshi D P, Wessely Z, Seery W H et al. 1966 Rhabdomyosarcoma of the bladder in an adult: case report and review of the literature. J Urol 96: 214–217
599. Henriksson C, Zetterlund C G, Boiesen P et al. 1986 Large rhabdomyosarcoma of the urinary bladder in an adult: case report. J Urol Nephrol 19: 237–239
600. Tripathi V N P, Dick V S 1969 Primary sarcoma of the urogenital system in adults. J Urol 101: 898–904
601. Narayana A S, Loening S, Weimar G W et al. 1978 Sarcoma of the bladder and prostate. J Urol 119: 72–76
602. Keating M A, Young R H, Lillehei C W et al. 1987 Hamartoma of the bladder in a 4-year-old with hamartomatous polyps of the gastrointestinal tract. J Urol 138: 366–369
603. Billis A, Queiroz L S, Oliveira E R et al. 1980 Adenoma of bladder in siblings with renal dysplasia. Urology 16: 299–302
604. Young R H 1986 Fibroepithelial polyp of the bladder with atypical stromal cells. Arch Pathol Lab Med 110: 241–242
605. Hojo H, Newton W A, Hamoudi A B et al. 1995 Pseudosarcomatous myofibroblastic tumors of the urinary bladder in children: a study of 11 cases with a review of the literature. Hum Pathol 19: 1224–1236
606. Keenan R A, Buchanan J D 1979 Fibrosarcoma of bladder exhibiting endocrine characteristics of phaeochromocytoma. J R Soc Med 72: 618–620
607. Harrison G S M 1986 Malignant fibrous histiocytoma of the bladder. Br J Urol 58: 457–458
608. Stroup R M, Chang Y C 1987 Angiosarcoma of the bladder: a case report J Urol 137: 984–985
609. Young R H, Rosenberg A E 1987 Osteosarcoma of the urinary bladder, report of a case and review of the literature. Cancer 59: 174–178
610. Levi M, Soloman C 1953 Adenofibroma of urinary bladder: a case report. J Urol 70: 898–899
611. Vara A R, Ruzics E P, Moussabeck O et al. 1990 Endometrioid adenosarcoma of the bladder arising from endometriosis. J Urol 143: 813–815

612. Judd E S 1921 Adenomyoma presenting as a tumor of the bladder. Surg Clin North Am 1: 1271–1278
613. Young R H 1987 Carcinosarcoma of the urinary bladder. Cancer 59: 1333–1339
614. Cross P A, Eyden B P, Joglekar V M 1989 Carcinosarcoma of the urinary bladder, a light, immunohistochemical, and electron microscopical case report. Virchow's Arch [A] 415: 91–95
615. Bloxham C A, Bennett M K, Robinson M C 1990 Bladder carcinosarcomas: three cases with diverse histogenesis. Histopathology 16: 63–67
616. Vieillefond A, Sinico M, Tighilt M et al. 1988 Carcinosarcomes de vessie, 3 cas avec étude immunohistochimique. Ann Pathol 8: 223–227
617. Sufrin G, Keogh B, Moore R H et al. 1977 Secondary involvement of the bladder in malignant lymphoma. J Urol 118: 251–253
618. Chaitin B, Manning J T, Ordóñez N G 1984 Hematologic neoplasms with initial manifestations in lower urinary tract. Urology 23: 35–42
619. Tremann J A, Norris H T, McRoberts J W 1971 Lymphoproliferative disease of the bladder. J Urol 106: 687–691
620. Siegelbaum M H, Edmonds P, Seidmon E J 1986 Use of immunohistochemistry for identification of primary lymphoma of the bladder. J Urol 136: 1074–1076
621. Aigen A B, Phillips M 1986 Primary malignant lymphoma of urinary bladder. Urology 28: 235–237
622. Forrest J B, Saypol D C, Mills S E et al. 1983 Immunoblastic sarcoma of the bladder. J Urol 130: 350–351
623. Kempton C L, Kurtin P J, Inwards D et al. 1997 Malignant lymphoma of the bladder: evidence from 36 cases that low-grade lymphoma of the MALT-type is the most common primary bladder lymphoma. Am J Surg Pathol 21: 1324–1333
624. Mourad W A, Khalil S, Radwi A et al. 1998 Primary T-cell lymphoma of the urinary bladder. Am J Surg Pathol 22: 373–377
625. Allory Y, Merabet Z, Copie-Bergman et al. 2005 Sarcomatoid variant of anaplastic large cell lymphomas mimics ALK-1-positive inflammatory myofibroblastic tumor in bladder. Am J Surg Pathol 29:838 (Letter to the Editor)
626. Marconis J T 1959 Primary Hodgkin's (paragranulomatous type) disease of the bladder. J Urol 81: 275–281
627. Neal M H, Swearingen M L, Gawronski L et al. 1985 Myeloma cells in the urine. Arch Pathol Lab Med 109: 870–872
628. Yang C, Motteram R, Sanderman T F 1982 Extramedullary plasmacytoma of the bladder. A case report and review of literature. Cancer 50: 146–149
629. Givler R L 1971 Involvement of the bladder in leukemia and lymphoma. J Urol 105: 667–670
630. Meis J M, Butler J J, Osborne B M et al. 1986 Granulocytic sarcoma in nonleukemic patients. Cancer 58: 2697–2709
631. Zhou M, Epstein J I, Young R H 2004 Paraganglioma of the urinary bladder. A lesion that may be misdiagnosed as urothelial carcinoma in transurethral resection specimens. Am J Surg Pathol 28: 94–100
632. Cheng L, Leibovich B C, Cheville J C et al 2000 Paraganglioma of the urinary bladder. Can biologic potential be predicted? Cancer 88: 844–852
633. Colby T V 1980 Carcinoid tumor of the bladder. Arch Pathol Lab Med 104: 199–200
634. Aoyama H, Yoshida K, Kondo T et al. 1978 Primary carcinoid tumor of the urinary bladder (report of a case). Nippon Hinyokika Gakkai Zasshi 69: 124–133
635. Stein B S, Kendall A R 1984 Malignant melanoma of the genitourinary tract. J Urol 132: 859–868
636. Ironside J W, Timperley W R, Madden J W et al. 1985 Primary melanoma of the urinary bladder presenting with intracerebral metastases. Br J Urol 57: 593–594
637. Cauffield E W 1956 Dermoid cysts of the bladder. J Urol 75: 801–804
638. Lazebnik J, Kamhi D 1961 A case of vesical teratoma associated with vesical stones and diverticulum. J Urol 85: 796–799
639. Taylor G, Jordan M, Churchill B et al. 1983 Yolk sac tumor of the bladder. J Urol 129: 591–594
640. Ganem E J, Batal J T 1956 Secondary malignant tumors of the urinary bladder metastatic from primary foci in distant organs. J Urol 75: 965–972
641. Sheehan E E, Greenberg S D, Scott R J Jr 1963 Metastatic neoplasms of the bladder. J Urol 90: 281–284
642. Goldstein A G 1967 Metastatic carcinoma to the bladder. J Urol 98: 209–215
643. Bates A W, Baithun S I 2000 Secondary neoplasms of the bladder are histological mimics of nontransitional cell primary tumours: clinicopathological and histological features of 282 cases. Histopathology 36: 32–40
644. Melicow M M 1955 Tumors of the urinary bladder: a clinicopathological analysis of over 2500 specimens and biopsies. J Urol 74: 498–521
645. Majnarich G, Malament M 1958 Urinary tract metastases by cancers of large bowel. Surgery 44: 520–528
646. Hermann H B 1929 Metastatic tumors of the urinary bladder originating from the carcinomata of the gastro-intestinal tract. J Urol 22: 257–273
647. Dalton D P, Dalkin B L, Sener S F et al. 1987 Enterovesical fistula secondary to mucinous adenocarcinoma of appendix. J Urol 138: 617–618
648. Haid M, Ignatoff J, Khandekar J D et al. 1980 Urinary bladder metastases from breast carcinoma. Cancer 46: 229–232
649. Silverstein L I, Plaine L, Davis J E et al. 1987 Breast carcinoma metastatic to bladder. Urology 29: 544–547
650. Coltart R S, Stewart S, Brown C H 1985 Small cell carcinoma of the bronchus: a rare cause of haematuria from a metastasis in the urinary bladder. J R Soc Med 78: 1053–1054
651. Remis R E, Halverstadt D B 1986 Metastatic renal cell carcinoma to the bladder: case report and review of the literature. J Urol 136: 1294–1296
652. Meyer J E 1974 Metastatic melanoma of the urinary bladder. Cancer 34: 1822–1824
653. Edson M, Colmenares E 1983 Transitional cell carcinoma of bladder originating from transitional cell carcinoma of anus. Urology 22: 198–199
654. Palmer J K, Emmett J L, McDonald J R 1948 Urethral caruncle. Surg Gynecol Obstet 87: 611–620
655. Marshall F C, Uson A C, Melicow M M 1960 Neoplasms and caruncles of the female urethra. Surg Gynecol Obstet 110: 723–733
656. Foster R S, Garrett R A 1986 Congenital posterior urethral polyps. J Urol 136: 670–672
657. Tsuzuki T, Epstein J I 2005 Fibroepithelial polyp of the lower urinary tract in adults. Am J Surg Pathol 29: 460–466
658. Debenedictis T J, Marmar J L, Praiss D E 1977 Intraurethral condylomas acuminata: management and review of the literature. J Urol 118: 767–769
659. Gartman E 1956 Intraurethral verruca acuminata in men. J Urol 75: 717–718
660. Bissada N K, Cole A T, Fried F A 1974 Extensive condylomas acuminata of the entire male urethra and the bladder. J Urol 112: 201–203
661. Keating M A, Young R H, Carr C P et al. 1985 Condyloma acuminatum of the bladder and ureter: case report and review of the literature. J Urol 133: 465–467
662. Huvos A G, Grabstald H 1973 Urethral meatal and parameatal tumors in young men: a clinicopathologic and electron microscopic study. J Urol 110: 688–692
663. Powell I, Cartwright H, Jano F 1981 Villous adenoma and adenocarcinoma of female urethra. Urology 18: 612–614
664. Howells M R, Baylis M S, Howell S 1985 Benign urethral villous adenoma. Case report. Br J Obstet Gynaecol 92: 1070–1071
665. Raju G C, Roopnarinesingh A, Woo J 1987 Villous adenoma of female urethra. Urology 29: 446–447
666. Maung R, Kelly J K, Grace D A 1988 Intestinal metaplasia and dysplasia of prostatic urethra secondary to stricture. Urology 32: 361–363
667. Chan J K C, Chow T C, Tsui M S 1987 Prostatic-type polyps of the lower urinary tract: three histologic types? Histopathology 11: 789–801
668. Nesbit R M 1962 The genesis of benign polyps in the prostatic urethra. J Urol 87: 416–418
669. Butterick J D, Schnitzer B, Abell M R 1971 Ectopic prostatic tissue in urethra: a clinicopathological entity and a significant cause of hematuria. J Urol 105: 97–104
670. Craig J R, Hart W R 1975 Benign polyps with prostatic-type epithelium of the urethra. Am J Clin Pathol 63: 343–347
671. Stein A J, Prioleau P G, Catalona W J 1980 Adenomatous polyps of the prostatic urethra: a cause of hematospermia. J Urol 124: 298–299
672. Walker A N, Mills S E, Fechner R E et al. 1983 Epithelial polyps of the prostatic urethra, a light-microscopic and immunohistochemical study. Am J Surg Pathol 7: 351–356
673. Baroudy A C, O'Connell J P 1984 Papillary adenoma of the prostatic urethra. J Urol 132: 120–122
674. Glancy R J, Gaman A J, Rippey J J 1983 Polyps and papillary lesions of the prostatic urethra. Pathology 15: 153–157
675. Zeid M, Gaeta J F, Asirwatham J E et al. 1986 Papillary adenoma of the prostatic urethra. Prostate 9: 9–14
676. Walker A N, Mills S E, Fechner R E et al. 1982 "Endometrial" adenocarcinoma of the prostatic urethra arising in a villous polyp, a light microscopic and immunoperoxidase study. Arch Pathol Lab Med 106: 624–627
677. Ford T F, Watson G M, Cameron K M 1985 Adenomatous metaplasia (nephrogenic adenoma) of urothelium, an analysis of 70 cases. Br J Urol 57: 427–433
678. Odze R, Bégin L R 1989 Tubular adenomatous metaplasia (nephrogenic adenoma) of the female urethra. Int J Gynecol Pathol 8: 374–380
679. Bhagavan B S, Tiamson E M, Wenk R E et al. 1981 Nephrogenic adenoma of the urinary bladder and urethra. Hum Pathol 12: 907–916
680. Allan C H, Epstein J I 2001 Nephrogenic adenoma of the prostatic urethra. A mimicker of prostatic adenocarcinoma. Am J Surg Pathol 25: 802–808
681. Peterson L J, Matsumoto L M 1978 Nephrogenic adenoma in urethral diverticulum. Urology 11: 193–195
682. Piazza R, Aragona F, Pizzarella M et al. 1987 Nephrogenic adenoma in urethral diverticulum: an unusual finding. Urol Int 42: 69–70
683. Martin S A, Santa Cruz D J 1981 Adenomatoid metaplasia of the prostatic urethra. Am J Clin Pathol 75: 185–189
684. Medeiros L J, Young R H 1989 Nephrogenic adenoma arising in urethral diverticula, a report of five cases. Arch Pathol Lab Med 113: 125–128
685. Young R H 1992 Nephrogenic adenomas of the urethra involving the prostate gland: a report of two cases of a lesion that may be confused with prostatic adenocarcinoma. Mod Pathol 5: 617–620
686. Schinella R, Thurm J, Feiner H 1974 Papillary pseudotumor of the prostatic urethra: proliferative papillary urethritis. J Urol 111: 38–40
687. Heaton N D, Kadow C, Yates-Bell A J 1990 Inverted papilloma of the penile urethra. Br J Urol 66: 661–662
688. Noto L 1983 Obstructive urethral leiomyoma in a female. Br J Urol 55: 239

689. Saad A G, Kaouk J H, Kaspar H G et al. 2003 Leoimyoma of the urethra: report of 3 cases of a rare entity. Int J Surg Pathol 11: 123–126
690. Bertrand G, Deroide J P, Bidabe M C 1984 Fibroadénome des glandes para-uréthrales: une nouvelle entite tumorale? Ann Pathol 4: 147–150
691. Young R H, Srigley J R, Amin M B et al. 2000 Tumors of the prostate gland, seminal vesicles, male urethra and penis. Atlas of tumor pathology, Series 3, fascicle 28. American Registry of Pathology, Washington, DC
692. Levine R L 1980 Urethral cancer. Cancer 45: 1965–1972
693. Roberts T W, Melicow M M 1977 Pathology and natural history of urethral tumors in females. Urology 10: 583–589
694. Zeigerman J H, Gordon S F 1970 Cancer of the female urethra: a curable disease. Obstet Gynecol 36: 785–788
695. Monaco A P, Murphy G B, Dowling W 1958 Primary cancer of the female urethra. Cancer 11: 1215–1221
696. Grabstald H, Hilaris B, Henschke U et al. 1966 Cancer of the female urethra. JAMA 197: 835–842
697. Turner A G, Hendry W F 1980 Primary carcinoma of the female urethra. Br J Urol 52: 549–554
698. Bracken R B, Johnson D E, Miller L S et al. 1976 Primary carcinoma of the female urethra. J Urol 117: 188–192
699. Desai S, Libertino J A, Zinman L 1973 Primary carcinoma of the female urethra. J Urol 110: 693–695
700. Tiltman A J 1974 Primary adenocarcinoma of the female urethra. J Pathol 117: 97–99
701. Schnitzer B 1964 Primary adenocarcinoma of the female urethra: a review and report of two cases. J Urol 92: 135–139
702. Knoblich R 1960 Primary adenocarcinoma of the female urethra: a review and report of 3 cases. Am J Obstet Gynecol 80: 353–364
703. Ampil F L 1975 Primary malignant neoplasm of the female urethra. Obstet Gynecol 66: 799–804
704. Meis J M, Ayala A G, Johnson D E 1987 Adenocarcinoma of the urethra in women, a clinicopathologic study. Cancer 60: 1038–1052
705. Menville J G, Counseller V S 1935 Mucoid carcinoma of the female urethra. J Urol 33: 76–81
706. Peterson D T, Dockerty M B, Utz D C et al. 1973 The peril of primary carcinoma of the urethra in women. J Urol 110: 72–75
707. Teoh T B 1960 Papillary adenocarcinoma of the female urethra: a case report. Br J Surg 48: 151–152
708. Svanholm H, Andersen O P, Røhl H 1987 Tumour of female paraurethral duct. Immunohistochemical similarity with prostatic carcinoma. Virchow's Arch [A] 411: 395–398
709. Hanai J, Lin M 1990 Primary adenocarcinoma of the female urethra with three histologic patterns and partial AFP positivity. Acta Pathol Jpn 40: 838–844
710. Kreutzmann H A R, Colloff B 1939 Primary carcinoma of the male urethra. Arch Surg 39: 513–529
711. Grabstald H 1973 Tumors of the urethra in men and women. Cancer 32: 1236–1255
712. Melicow M M, Roberts T W 1978 Pathology and natural history of urethral tumors in males, review of 142 cases. Urology 11: 83–89
713. Posso M A, Berg G A, Murphy A I et al. 1961 Mucinous adenocarcinoma of the urethra: report of a case associated with urethritis glandularis. J Urol 85: 944–948
714. Mandler J I, Pool T L 1966 Primary carcinoma of the male urethra. J Urol 96: 67–72
715. Kaplan G W, Bulkley G J, Grayhack J T 1967 Carcinoma of the male urethra. J Urol 98: 365–371
716. Gowing N F C 1960 Urethral carcinoma associated with cancer of the bladder. Br J Urol 32: 428–438
717. Coutts A G, Grigor K M, Fowler J W 1985 Urethral dysplasia and bladder cancer in cystectomy specimens. Br J Urol 57: 535–541
718. Tobisu K-I, Tanaka Y, Mizutani T et al. 1991 Transitional cell carcinoma of the urethra in men following cystectomy for bladder cancer: multivariate analysis for risk factors. J Urol 146: 1551–1554
719. De Paepe M E, André R, Mahadevia P 1990 Urethral involvement in female patients with bladder cancer, a study of 22 cystectomy specimens. Cancer 65: 1237–1241
720. Tomaszewski J E, Korat O C, Livolsi V A et al. 1986 Paget's disease of the urethral meatus following transitional cell carcinoma of the bladder. J Urol 135: 368–370
721. Bégin L R, Deschênes J, Mitmaker B 1991 Pagetoid carcinomatous involvement of the penile urethra in association with high-grade transitional cell carcinoma of the urinary bladder. Arch Pathol Lab Med 115: 632–635
722. Saito R 1982 An adenosquamous carcinoma of the male urethra with hypercalcemia. Hum Pathol 23: 383–385
723. Taylor R N, Lacey C G, Shuman M A 1985 Adenocarcinoma of Skene's duct associated with a systemic coagulopathy. Gynecol Oncol 22: 250–256
724. Colapinto V, Evans D H 1977 Primary carcinoma of the male urethra developing after urethroplasty for stricture. J Urol 118: 581–584
725. Hamilton J D, Leach W B 1951 Adenocarcinoma arising in a diverticulum of the female urethra. Arch Pathol 51: 90–97
726. Gonzalez M O, Harrison M L, Boileau M A 1985 Carcinoma in diverticulum of female urethra. Urology 26: 328–332
727. Maltby C C, Johnston S R 1988 Transitional cell carcinoma of the male anterior urethra. Br J Urol 62: 489
728. Fernando J J R, Wanas T M 1991 Primary transitional cell carcinoma of the anterior urethra: a rare presentation. Genitourin Med 67: 244–246
729. Bans L L, Eble J N, Lingeman J E et al. 1983 Transitional cell carcinoma of the fossa navicularis of the male urethra. J Urol 129: 1055–1056
730. Mevorach R A, Cos L R, di Sant'Agnese P A et al. 1990 Human papillomavirus type 6 in grade I transitional cell carcinoma of the urethra. J Urol 143: 126–128
731. Grussendorf-Conen E-I, Deutz F J, De Villiers E M 1987 Detection of human papillomavirus-6 in primary carcinoma of the urethra in men. Cancer 60: 1832–1835
732. Lucman L, Vadas G 1973 Transitional cloacogenic carcinoma of the urethra. Cancer 31: 1508–1510
733. Díaz-Cano S J, Ríos I J, Rivera-Hueto F et al. 1992 Mixed cloacogenic carcinoma of male urethra. Histopathology 20: 82–84
734. Bostwick D G, Lo R, Stamey T A 1984 Papillary adenocarcinoma of the male urethra, case report and review of the literature. Cancer 54: 2556–2563
735. Oliva E, Young R H 1996 Clear cell adenocarcinoma of the urethra: a clinicopathologic analysis of 19 cases. Mod Pathol 9: 513–520
736. Cantrell B B, Leifer G, DeKlerk D P et al. 1981 Papillary adenocarcinoma of the prostatic urethra with clear-cell appearance. Cancer 48: 2661–2667
737. Ingram E A, DePauw P 1985 Adenocarcinoma of the male urethra with associated nephrogenic metaplasia, case report and review of the literature. Cancer 55: 160–164
738. Gupta T D, Grabstald H 1965 Melanoma of the genitourinary tract. J Urol 93: 607–614
739. Block N L, Hotchkiss R S 1971 Malignant melanoma of the female urethra: report of a case with 5-year survival and review of the literature. J Urol 105: 251–255
740. Oldbring J, Mikulowski P 1987 Malignant melanoma of the penis and male urethra, report of nine cases and review of the literature. Cancer 59: 581–587
741. Manivel J C, Fraley E E 1988 Malignant melanoma of the penis and male urethra: 4 case reports and literature review. J Urol 139: 813–816
742. Oliva E, Quinn T R, Amin M B et al. 2000 Primary malignant melanoma of the urethra. A clinicopathologic analysis of 15 cases. Am J Surg Pathol 24: 785–796
743. Melicow M M, Lattes R, Pierre-Louis C 1972 Lymphoma of the female urethra masquerading as a caruncle. J Urol 108: 748–749
744. Touhami H, Brahimi S, Kubisz P et al. 1987 Non-Hodgkin's lymphoma of the female urethra. J Urol 137: 991–992
745. Nabholtz J M, Friedman S, Tremeaux J C et al. 1989 Non-Hodgkin's lymphoma of the urethra: a rare extranodal entity. Gynecol Oncol 35: 110–111
746. Mark J A, Pais V M, Chong F K 1990 Plasmacytoma of the urethra treated with transurethral resection and radiotherapy. J Urol 143: 1010–1011
747. Kahn D G, Rothman P J, Weisman J D 1991 Urethral T-cell lymphoma as the initial manifestation of the acquired immune deficiency syndrome. Arch Pathol Lab Med 115: 1169–1170
748. Ro J, Dexeus F, Logothetis C et al. 1991 Pure yolk sac tumors in adults: A clinicopathologic study in 18 patients. Mod Pathol 4: 50a (abstract)
749. Cholhan H J, Caglar H, Kremzier J E 1991 Suburethral paraganglioma. Obstet Gynecol 78: 555–558
750. Sylora H O, Diamond H M, Kaufman M et al. 1975 Primary carcinoid tumor of the urethra. J Urol 114: 150–153

女性生殖道肿瘤
Tumors of the female genital tract

13

第一部分

卵巢、输卵管以及阔韧带和圆韧带
Ovary, fallopian tube, and broad and round ligaments

Charles F. Zaloudek 著

刘芳芳 译　回允中 校

卵巢、输卵管以及阔韧带和圆韧带	
卵巢的肿瘤	567
卵巢上皮性肿瘤	567
性索-间质肿瘤	588
非特异性间叶性肿瘤	603
恶性淋巴瘤/白血病	603
生殖细胞肿瘤	604
其他罕见的卵巢肿瘤	616
卵巢转移性肿瘤	618
卵巢良性瘤样病变	622
输卵管肿瘤	624
阔韧带和圆韧带肿瘤	628

卵巢的肿瘤
Tumors of the ovary

原发性卵巢肿瘤有三种主要的类型。它们是：

1. 上皮性肿瘤，起源于卵巢的表面上皮、上皮包涵物或者子宫内膜异位；
2. 性索-间质肿瘤，起源于卵巢间质、性索衍生物或两者；
3. 生殖细胞肿瘤，起源于生殖细胞。

另外，一些卵巢非特异性肿瘤，例如软组织肿瘤和淋巴瘤，可以在卵巢这个部位发生，还有从卵巢外原发部位转移至卵巢的肿瘤。

在三种主要的类型中，上皮性肿瘤是最常见的，占所有卵巢肿瘤的58%（表13A.1）[1-5]。浆液性和黏液性囊腺瘤是最常见的上皮性肿瘤，总共占卵巢肿瘤的30%。各种类型的癌都有一定的发生率，但浆液性和黏液性交界性肿瘤是比较常见的。性索-间质肿瘤中的纤维卵泡膜细胞瘤占卵巢肿瘤的9%。最常见的恶性性索-间质肿瘤是颗粒细胞瘤，仅占卵巢肿瘤的1%。其他性索-间质肿瘤罕见。单一最常见的卵巢肿瘤是生殖细胞肿瘤，良性囊性畸胎瘤占卵巢肿瘤的32%。包括所有恶性生殖细胞肿瘤在内的各种其他类型生殖细胞肿瘤都是罕见的。

表13A.1	常见的卵巢肿瘤
肿瘤名称	占卵巢肿瘤的百分比(%)
良性囊性畸胎瘤	32
浆液性囊腺瘤	16
黏液性囊腺瘤	14
浆液性癌	9
纤维-卵泡膜细胞瘤	9
交界性浆液性肿瘤	4
子宫内膜样癌	3
交界性黏液性肿瘤	1
透明细胞癌	1
黏液性癌	1

卵巢上皮性肿瘤
Epithelial tumors of the ovary

上皮性肿瘤占所有卵巢肿瘤的58%，并且90%以上为恶性肿瘤。根据它们主要的分化方式，多数肿瘤可被分

表13A.2 卵巢上皮性肿瘤的类型

浆液性	Brenner／移行细胞
黏液性	未分化
子宫内膜样	罕见类型
混合性中胚层	混合性
透明细胞	不能分类

表13A.3 上皮性肿瘤的分类

良性	中间类型	恶性
囊腺瘤	交界性肿瘤（也叫具有低度恶性潜能的肿瘤、非典型性增生性肿瘤）	癌
表面乳头状瘤		
腺纤维瘤		
囊腺纤维瘤（伴有局灶性低级别增生或非典型性）		

为浆液性、黏液性、子宫内膜样、混合性中胚层、透明细胞、Brenner／移行细胞或未分化的肿瘤（表13A.2）。混合性细胞类型多见。不是主要细胞类型的小灶状细胞可以忽略，但是当出现相当数量（多于10%）的几种细胞类型时，最好将其归入混合性上皮性肿瘤。不能归入特殊类型的上皮性肿瘤罕见，可以命名为未分化的肿瘤。

上皮性肿瘤依据它们的病理学特征，可分为良性、恶性或中间类型（表13A.3）。依据肿瘤在卵巢中的位置、囊肿形成的程度和间质的数量，又可将良性上皮性肿瘤分为囊腺瘤、表面乳头状瘤、囊腺纤维瘤或腺纤维瘤。恶性上皮性肿瘤主要是腺癌。尽管非常少见，移行细胞癌和鳞状细胞癌也可发生于卵巢。混合性中胚层肿瘤具有恶性上皮成分，临床行为与癌相似，因此它们通常被归为上皮性肿瘤。

对于中间类型肿瘤的恰当命名存有争论。自从世界卫生组织（WHO）于1973年批准这些命名以来[6]，这些肿瘤被称为交界性肿瘤，或者具有低度恶性潜能的肿瘤。它们具有良好的预后，而且很少进展成癌。也有人提出应将这些肿瘤命名为非典型增生性上皮性肿瘤[7]。然而，这些称谓并没有被普遍接受。在这一章中，中间类型的上皮性肿瘤被称作交界性肿瘤，以便和目前的WHO分类取得一致[8,9]。这种命名包括了一系列的肿瘤，从增生和非典型性程度相当于单纯性增生的 I 级交界性肿瘤，到显示明显增生和（或）重度细胞学非典型性相当于原位癌的 III 级交界性肿瘤，但是缺乏浸润或融合性生长[10]。具有明显细胞学非典型性的交界性上皮性肿瘤，被称为交界性肿瘤伴有上皮内癌。病理医师应该使用可被清楚理解的命名来做出他们的诊断。其他广泛使用的诊断名词可以恰当引用，以确保每个阅读病理报告的人能够清楚地理解这一诊断[11]。

临床特征 几乎没有例外，在一定的类别内，所有类型上皮性肿瘤的临床表现、治疗和治疗结果都是类似的。

上皮性肿瘤主要发生于成人，在儿童和少年并不常见[12-16]。良性和交界性肿瘤发生在任何年龄，但经常发生于绝经前的妇女[17]。癌主要发生于围绝经期和绝经后的妇女。卵巢癌很少发生于妊娠妇女，如果发生，最可能是浆液性或黏液性癌[18]。超过70%的卵巢癌妇女在诊断时已有广泛的卵巢外肿瘤播散。部分原因可能是由于上皮性肿瘤引起的症状是模糊和非特异性的，不能及时做出早期诊断。最常见的症状是盆腔不适或疼痛、腹部胀满或压迫感、胃肠紊乱、尿频和偶有月经异常[19]。肿瘤扭转或破裂可以导致急腹症。直径大于15 cm的肿瘤，由于体积太大而不适于在盆腔生长，肿瘤可能膨胀生长进入腹部，可被患者触及。腹水是患有卵巢肿瘤妇女腹部膨胀的另外一个原因。腹水很少由良性肿瘤引起，它是癌的最好提示。腹水干扰胃肠功能，导致恶心和呕吐。任何程度的卵巢增大，特别是在超过45岁的妇女，都应怀疑有无卵巢癌的问题，并需要进一步评估。通过超声或一些其他影像学技术来鉴定实性或复杂的卵巢肿块是特别令人担忧的。

CA-125单克隆抗体血液试验能够检测高分子量糖蛋白抗原[20-22]。在患有晚期交界性和恶性上皮性肿瘤以及某些伴有局灶性病变的妇女，CA-125试验通常为阳性。CA-125试验对卵巢癌并不是特异的，因为这种抗原血清浓度增加还可见于其他癌症，并与良性病变有关，例如妊娠、子宫内膜异位、骨盆炎症性疾病、平滑肌瘤、肝脏疾病和某些胶原-血管疾病[23]。

卵巢肿瘤的治疗主要是手术治疗。良性肿瘤通过囊肿切除术或单侧输卵管卵巢切除术可以治愈。

交界性肿瘤预后较好，即使在晚期阶段[24]。大约80%的病例肿瘤局限于卵巢。其余20%的患者有盆腔或腹膜种植。淋巴结受累不常见[25]，同样，播散到实质器官或腹腔外也不常见[26]。所有各期病人的长期生存率超过90%[17,24,27-32]。肿瘤局限于卵巢的患者生存率达到100%[32-35]。肿瘤相关死亡归入三个范畴：

1. 患者死于癌症；
2. 患者发生了交界性肿瘤的致命并发症，例如纤维性粘连伴有肠梗阻；
3. 患者死于治疗的并发症[36]。

交界性肿瘤适于保守治疗，除了少数妇女出现与侵袭性行为或癌相关的特征之外。这些特征包括浸润性腹膜种植或复发，如同低级别浆液性癌[36]。

交界性肿瘤标准的手术治疗是全子宫切除、双侧输卵管-卵巢切除、网膜切除以及切除种植于卵巢外的肿瘤。许多患有交界性肿瘤的妇女处在生育年龄，希望保留其生育能力。在某些情况下，单侧输卵管-卵巢切除术，甚或膀胱切除术可以考虑作为一种治疗选择，尽管以这种方式治疗患者大约会有25%的对侧卵巢复发的危险性[31,35,37-42]。腹腔镜治疗已经开展，即使在有小的腹膜种植的妇女，也在尝试保留生育能力[43,44]。在某些情况下，采用保守手术以保存生育能力好像是可能的，甚至对于有卵巢外肿瘤播散的患者[45]。微乳头状交界性浆液性肿瘤患者似乎比典型的交界性浆液性肿瘤更易播散于卵巢外。然而，当分期和种植类型得到矫正时，证实其生存率并无差异[46]。对于初次手术分期不当的妇女进行手术再次分期是有争议的。大约15%的经过手术再次分期的妇女，肿瘤分期发生改变，但是复发的危险性对于是否进行手术再次分期的妇女来说是相似的[47,48]。再次分期对于患有微乳头状交界性浆液性肿瘤的妇女最有价值，因为她们发生浸润性腹腔种植的危险性更大[49]。复发一般出现在初次治疗多年之后，复发性疾病可能缓慢进展。复发性肿瘤可以是交界性浆液性肿瘤、低级别浆液性癌[36,50]，或在较少见的情况下，可以是高级别浆液性癌[51]。某些作者注意到，当复发表现为低级别浆液性癌时，疾病进展速率增高[31]，但是其他作者没有发现这一现象。手术切除对侧或卵巢外肿瘤是对于进行性或复发性肿瘤最有效的治疗方式[36,52]。肿瘤医师并不完全同意这一做法，面对经不住手术切除的进行性疾病，多数肿瘤医师仅仅采取化疗或放疗[41,52-55]。生存率高，即使是处于晚期肿瘤的妇女[56]。

浸润性卵巢癌直接侵犯邻近器官或经由腹膜的液体播散至网膜、腹膜、腹腔内脏的浆膜表面和膈膜。淋巴结转移常见，并且偶尔可以远处转移至肺、胸膜和心包。临床分期（图13A.4）是最重要的预后因素。

卵巢癌的治疗通常包括手术和化疗[57,58]。标准的手术治疗是子宫切除术、双侧输卵管-卵巢切除术、网膜切除术、盆腔和主动脉旁淋巴结清扫。有必要的话进行分期活检和阑尾切除术。为了加强后续的化疗或放疗，妇科肿瘤医师倾向于切除尽可能多的卵巢外肿瘤（"细胞减灭手术"）[59-62]。早期（I-II期）疾病预后最好[63]。患有IA期高分化腺癌的年轻妇女可以通过单侧输卵管-卵巢切除术、网膜切除术进行治疗，如果患者希望保留其生育能力可以进行彻底分期操作[64,65]。某些晚期卵巢癌妇女在手术之前应该进行化疗，以便随后易于手术切

表13A.4 卵巢癌的FIGO分期。(Reprinted from International Journal of Gynecology and Obstetrics. Benedet JL, Pecorelli S. Staging classification and clinical practice guidelines of gynaecologic cancers. p94, ©2000. With permission from International Federation of Gynecology and Obstetrics.)

分期	疾病范围
I	肿瘤局限于卵巢内
IA	肿瘤局限于一侧卵巢；包膜完整；卵巢表面没有肿瘤；腹水或腹腔冲洗液中无恶性细胞
IB	肿瘤局限于双侧卵巢；包膜完整；卵巢表面没有肿瘤；腹水或腹腔冲洗液中无恶性细胞
IC	肿瘤局限于一侧或双侧卵巢内，伴有以下任何一种特征：包膜破裂；卵巢表面可见肿瘤；腹水或腹腔冲洗液中可见恶性细胞
II	肿瘤累及一侧或双侧卵巢，伴有盆腔扩散
IIA	扩散和(或)种植到子宫和(或)输卵管；腹水或腹腔冲洗液中无恶性细胞
IIB	扩散至其他盆腔组织；腹水或腹腔冲洗液中无恶性细胞
IIC	盆腔扩散，腹水或腹腔冲洗液中有恶性细胞
III	肿瘤累及一侧或双侧卵巢，伴有显微镜下检查证实的盆腔外腹膜转移和(或)局部淋巴结转移
IIIA	镜下腹膜转移超出盆腔
IIIB	大体可见的腹膜转移超出盆腔，最大径≤2 cm
IIIC	腹膜转移超出盆腔，最大径≥2 cm和(或)局部淋巴结转移
IV	远处转移

除[66]。以铂为基础的联合化疗方案一般用于高级别IA期癌和那些有卵巢外播散或腹水细胞学阳性的妇女[67-75]。在大约85%的晚期卵巢癌妇女中，化疗可以导致临床症状部分或完全消失，但是多数患者在2~3年内复发，远期生存率小于20%~30%[76]。有时用于卵巢癌其他类型的治疗包括腹腔内化疗[77,78]、腹膜内放射性胶体[79]以及外部的光束放疗[80,81]。

浆液性肿瘤 Serous tumors

浆液性肿瘤在所有卵巢肿瘤中大约占30%，是唯一一组最常见的肿瘤。其中包括22%的卵巢良性肿瘤和接近50%的卵巢恶性原发性肿瘤。在所有的浆液性肿瘤中，50%为良性，15%为交界性，以及35%是浸润性癌[5]。

良性浆液性肿瘤　Benign serous tumors

浆液性囊腺瘤（serous cystadenoma）可以是单房性或多房性。囊肿薄壁，内含清亮液体。囊壁内、外表面通常是光滑的，但是在囊壁内衬偶尔可见小的乳头状赘生物。浆液性腺纤维瘤（serous adenofibroma）是实性肿瘤，具有质硬的白色或褐色纤维性切面。可见散在的小囊，或者由于出现许多小囊而肿瘤呈海绵状外观。浆液性囊腺纤维瘤（serous cystadenofibroma）比腺纤维瘤常见[82]；它是单房性或多房性囊性肿瘤，肿瘤的囊壁内伴有实性腺纤维瘤的区域。浆液性表面乳头瘤（serous surface papilloma）是不常见的肿瘤，在卵巢表面呈乳头状赘生物性生长。大约20%良性浆液性肿瘤是双侧的。

显微镜下，良性浆液性肿瘤内衬纤毛性和非纤毛性柱状细胞，具有温和的卵圆形细胞核，位于基底（图13A.1）。如果囊肿具有张力，上皮将变得扁平。在腺纤维瘤和囊腺纤维瘤中，丰富的纤维间质围绕着腺体和囊肿（图13A.2）。最近的一项研究发现，仅仅14%的浆液性囊腺瘤是单细胞性的，通常为较大的肿瘤[83]。因此有人提出，只有那些显示上皮增生证据的肿瘤，例如细胞呈复层或呈乳头状，应该称为囊腺瘤或囊腺纤维瘤[84]，但这个观点还没有被广泛地接受。少数良性浆液性肿瘤可有小灶状的轻到中度核的非典型性，或有分支乳头状生长。对于具有小灶状交界样生长方式肿瘤的行为，尚未充分研究[85]，但是，当仅仅在少数低倍视野下观察到这些特征时（≤肿瘤的5%～10%），临床经过一般是良性的，而且这样的肿瘤通常被归类为浆液性囊腺瘤、囊性腺纤维瘤或腺纤维瘤，伴有局灶性低级别非典型性或增生[86]。在某些患者，交界性浆液性肿瘤含有增生活性较低的区域，或者对侧卵巢包含有局灶增生活跃的浆液性肿瘤，这就提出了一种可能性，即伴有局灶增生的浆液性肿瘤可能不完全是无关紧要的，而且在少数情况下肿瘤可能有所进展[31]。

交界性浆液性肿瘤　Borderline serous tumors

交界性浆液性肿瘤是大的，通常为多房性的囊性肿瘤，35%～40%的病例为双侧性[42]。囊壁内衬可见粗乳头状赘生物。在某些肿瘤中乳头生长是局灶性的，另外一些有融合，而且40%～50%的病例出现在卵巢的外表面。除了腺纤维瘤性交界性肿瘤外，实性生长区域少见。出血和坏死区域也少见[87]。

低倍镜下，从囊肿内衬到囊腔（图13A.3）或从卵巢表面[86]，乳头呈多分支状的方式生长。复杂的乳头状和腺体结构以及继发性囊肿形成是典型的表现。乳头具有显著的纤维血管轴心，即使在较小的分支内也很明显，乳头被覆增生的柱状细胞，可分数层（图13A.4）。可以出现纤毛细胞。局部细胞成丛，由此成簇或单个细胞脱落进入囊腔。有不同程度但通常是低级别的核非典型性，可见散在的核分裂象。在柱状肿瘤细胞中，可见单个散在或呈小簇状排列的具有丰富嗜酸性胞浆的细胞，即"未分化"或"化生性"的细胞；这种细胞在乳头尖端最为明显。在交界性浆液性肿瘤中，偶尔可见含有腺

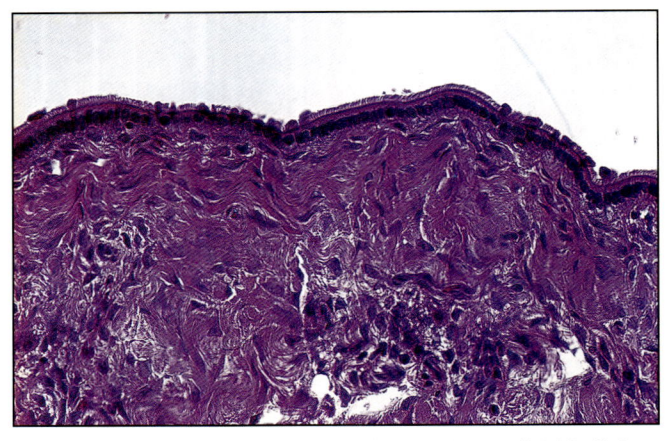

图13A.1　浆液性囊腺瘤。囊肿内衬具有纤毛的矮柱状细胞，细胞核温和，位于基底。

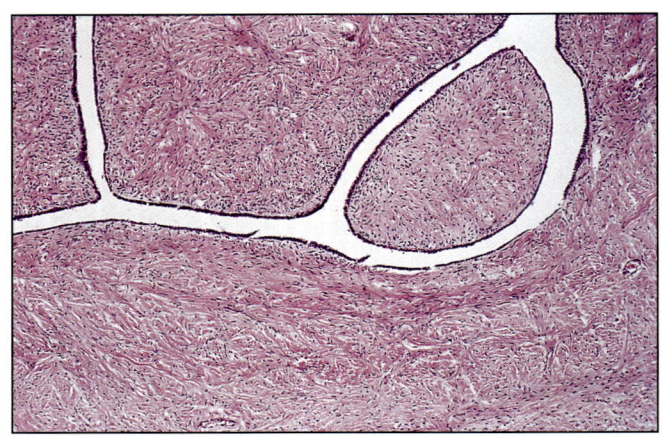

图13A.2　浆液性囊腺纤维瘤。上皮成分被丰富的纤维间质围绕。

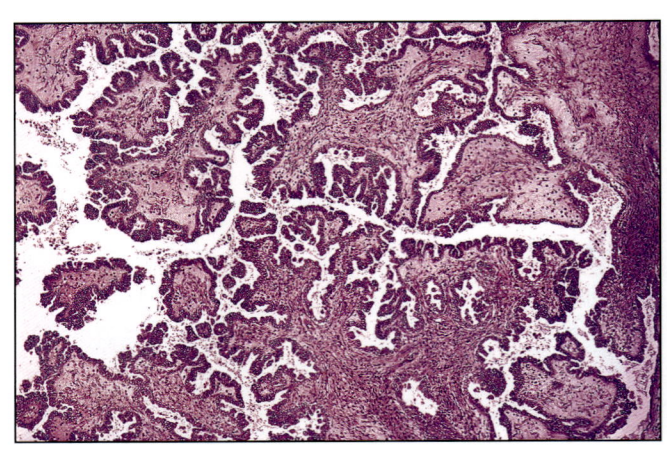

图13A.3　交界性浆液性肿瘤。分支状乳头被覆增生的柱状细胞，其中一些细胞脱落进入囊腔。

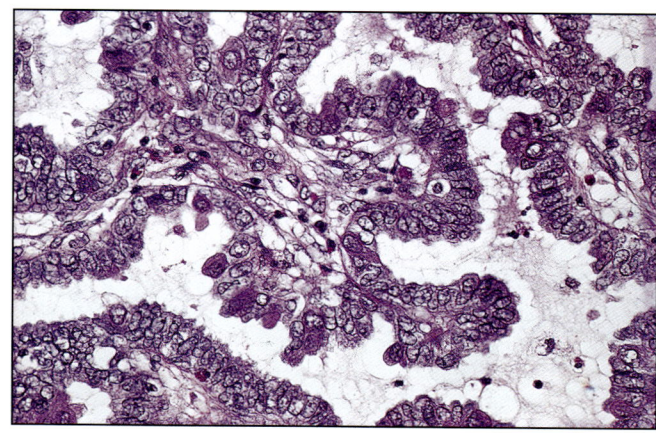

图13A.4 交界性浆液性肿瘤。乳头被覆柱状细胞，这些细胞具有大的空泡状核。与浆液性囊腺瘤相比，核浆比例增高，局灶可见复层核的结构。注意散在的未分化细胞具有显著的嗜酸性胞浆。

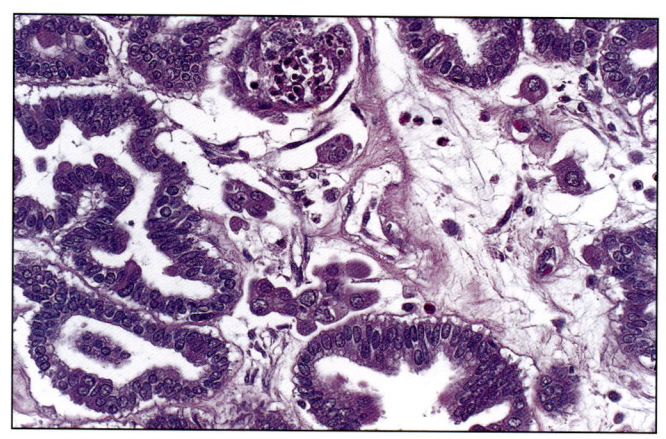

图13A.5 交界性浆液性肿瘤的间质微小浸润。腺体之间的间质中出现具有丰富嗜酸性胞浆的单个和成团的细胞。微小浸润的细胞具有增大的空泡状核，其中某些含有核仁。许多细胞团被透明间隙围绕。

体和乳头的疏松纤维组织斑块或小结。这些改变类似于纤维组织增生性腹膜种植（见下），并被称为"自体种植"（autoimplants）。自体种植易在分期高的肿瘤内见到，但好像并不具有预后意义[31]。交界性浆液性肿瘤的囊壁通常比囊腺瘤厚，而且某些肿瘤具有足够的间质，可以归入交界性浆液性腺纤维瘤或囊腺纤维瘤。鉴别浆液性交界性肿瘤与浆液性癌的显微镜下特征是前者缺乏弥漫性间质浸润。在交界性肿瘤，出现在间质内的乳头和腺体是人工假象，是由正切囊肿内衬上皮的复杂内折造成的。这样的腺体并不是浸润，而且其周围没有间质纤维母细胞或炎症性反应。

交界性浆液性肿瘤偶尔可见间质的微小浸润[88-90]。为了确定微小浸润，浸润灶必须小于3mm[86]。这样的病例一般会出现多灶性微小浸润[91]。两种形式的微小浸润已被描述。首先，也是最常见的一种微小浸润是，囊壁或乳头的纤维间质中杂乱分布有小簇状和条索状的细胞，这些细胞胞浆嗜酸性，核圆形呈空泡状，核仁明显（图13A.5）。这些细胞的周围通常看不到间质反应。偶尔于淋巴管内可见这些细胞，但其临床意义还不清楚[89]。第二种微小浸润的形态是，间质中有乳头、小的腺体、上皮条索或融合的上皮细胞巢浸润[89]。肿瘤细胞被炎症性或黏液样纤维间质围绕，或位于小的透明间隙内。当出现这种形式的微小浸润时，必须充分评估以除外比较广泛的浸润区域。在低倍镜下很难辨认间质的微小浸润；细胞角蛋白或上皮膜抗原的免疫染色可能有助于突显间质中微小浸润的上皮细胞[91]。多数具有间质微小浸润的患者具有平淡的经过，少数患者预后不好是因为其他因素，例如浸润性种植和不完全分期[17,33,40,88-93]。新近研究发现，少数伴有微小浸润的患者具有进展性疾病[33,94]，而且最近一项大宗交界性浆液性肿瘤的研究显示微小浸润是一个明显不利的发现[31]。出现微小浸润应该在病理报告中注明，尽管它的临床意义仍然未予充分肯定。被覆交界性浆液性肿瘤的上皮包括嗜酸性"化生性"和"未分化"的细胞。在具有间质微小浸润的肿瘤中这些细胞数量更多，并且在从妊娠患者切除的肿瘤中更加显著。一项研究显示，相当数量伴有微小浸润的妇女是妊娠妇女[93]。在从妊娠妇女切除的肿瘤中，还可看到黏蛋白分泌和间质蜕膜反应[89,93]。与伴有小面积微小浸润的交界性浆液性肿瘤不同，伴有较大面积浸润的肿瘤如果播散到卵巢外，则有明显进展的危险[95]。

15%～30%的交界性浆液性肿瘤患者可见腹膜或网膜的肿瘤种植。尽管偶尔可见较大的实性或囊性种植，但通常是小而浅表的结节性赘生物，直径仅仅几个毫米。这些种植物究竟是来自卵巢肿瘤的转移还是同时发生在腹膜部位的肿瘤尚有争议[96]，虽然越来越多的研究显示，卵巢和卵巢外肿瘤具有相似的基因表达谱[97-102]。有三种类型的种植发生：

1. 非浸润性上皮型
2. 非浸润性纤维组织增生型
3. 浸润型[10,86,103]。

在非浸润性上皮型内，乳头状交界性浆液性肿瘤生长在腹膜表面或恰在腹膜下囊肿间隙内（图13A.6）。生长局限，并不浸润其下的间质。非浸润性纤维组织增生性种植是血管纤维间质斑块，其中含有少数上皮细胞、小簇细胞，或者内衬温和上皮细胞的散在的小腺体（图13A.7）。这种种植好像是贴附在腹膜表面，并不向下浸润间质。非浸润性乳头的生长可以位于这些纤维组织增生性种植的表面。非浸润性种植患者倾向于具有良好的预后，但其中少数疾病进展并死于肿瘤[31,104-106]。

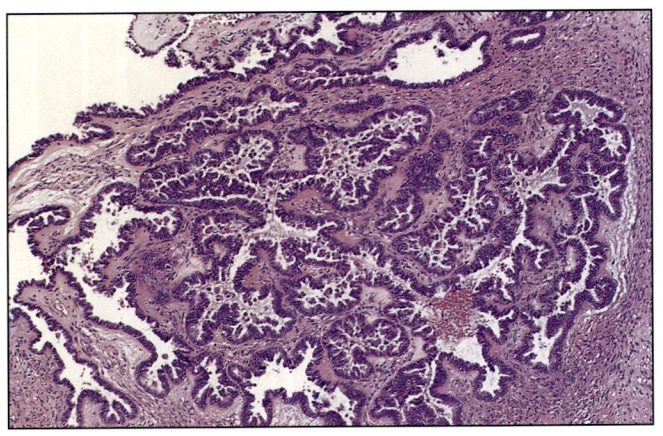

图13A.6 交界性浆液性肿瘤的非浸润性乳头状种植。乳头状种植类似于原发的卵巢交界性浆液性肿瘤。它正好位于腹膜表面。（腹膜间隙在左侧，腹膜表面在右侧。）

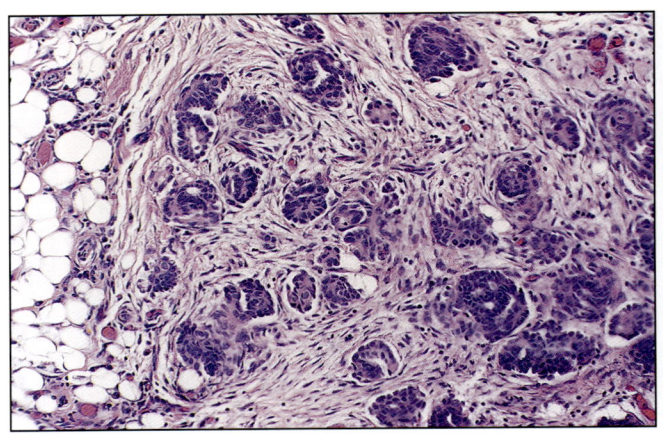

图13A.8 交界性浆液性肿瘤的浸润性种植。多数小的上皮细胞巢，某些上皮巢周围绕以裂隙，侵犯纤维间质。注意，这个浸润性种植有丰富的上皮，与图13A.7的纤维组织增生性非浸润性种植形成对比。

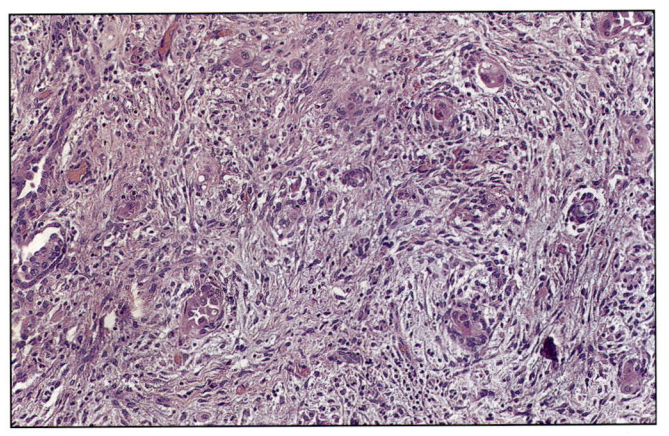

图13A.7 交界性浆液性肿瘤的非浸润性纤维组织增生性种植。散在的温和上皮细胞小巢被丰富的纤维间质围绕。

浸润性种植罕见（5%～10%），但是与肿瘤分期较晚一起，似乎是交界性浆液性肿瘤患者最有意义的不利预后表现[31-33,46,103,107]。某些研究难于评估，因为作者没有应用浸润性种植的标准定义[108]。一项不包括任何会诊病例，而且没有发现浸润性种植的57例患者的研究指出，从业病理医师很少能见到这种类型的种植[34]。浸润性种植的上皮比纤维组织增生性种植丰富，并且有浸润到腹膜下组织或周围网膜的生长方式（图13A.8）。扩大的浸润性种植的标准已被提出，但仍有争议[109]。其中包括微乳头状生长方式、肿瘤细胞簇周围的透明间隙或裂隙，以及没有扩散到其下组织的浸润性腺体。

多达1/3的晚期交界性肿瘤患者，肿瘤可以出现在盆腔或主动脉旁淋巴结[25,110,111,111a]。淋巴结受累主要有两种形态。一种，肿瘤呈分支乳头状生长，类似于原发性肿瘤。另外一种，单个或小巢状肿瘤细胞出现在包膜下窦内。在少数情况下，增生的间皮细胞累及淋巴结，类似于后一种形态[112]。伴随的腹膜间皮增生、细胞的形态，以及间皮标记物免疫染色阳性，例如钙视网膜蛋白（calretinin）、血栓调节蛋白（thrombomodulin）和CK5/6，可用于鉴别增生的间皮细胞和肿瘤细胞[113]。少数交界性浆液性肿瘤患者，在最初手术时或随后发现腹部外淋巴结有肿瘤[26,114]。在因子宫癌而进行手术的患者中，5%～25%可见盆腔或主动脉旁淋巴结内有上皮包涵囊肿，内衬矮柱状细胞，其中多数为纤毛细胞[115]。这些包涵囊肿，定义为良性上皮包涵囊肿或输卵管内膜异位症，较常见于交界性浆液性肿瘤患者[25,116]。有人提出，它们可能是交界性浆液性肿瘤累及淋巴结的一种类型[116]。然而，多数妇科病理医师并不接受这种观点，而将其看作是良性包涵囊肿。有人认为，交界性浆液性肿瘤累及淋巴结可能是同时发生在上皮包涵囊肿中的肿瘤，而不是来自卵巢肿瘤的转移。然而，在缺乏卵巢肿瘤的情况下，原发性卵巢外浆液性肿瘤很少起因于良性上皮包涵囊肿[117]。不管它的起源如何，多数研究认为交界性浆液性肿瘤累及淋巴结好像并不是一种预后不良的表现[25,31,32,118]，尽管新近的资料提示，结节性聚集的肿瘤细胞超过1mm可能与生存期下降有关[111a]。

微乳头状浆液性癌（micropapillary serous carcinoma）这一术语用于一组增生性浆液性肿瘤，其形态学谱系包括某些高级别交界性非浸润性肿瘤以及某些低级别浸润性浆液性癌[107,119]。临床随访提示，多数微乳头状浆液性肿瘤患者处于Ⅰ期，可以通过手术治愈[49,120]。微乳头状浆液性肿瘤多半双侧发生，呈现表面乳头状生长，卵巢外疾病，在某些研究中尚有浸润性种植[49,104]。一旦校正了分期和种植类型，生存率似乎类似于普通的交界性浆液性肿瘤[31,33,46,49,104,121]。尽管这是一种仍有争论的疾病，但是现在多数妇科病理医师将非浸润性微乳头状浆液性肿瘤看作是交界性浆液性肿瘤的增生性变型而不是浆液性癌。

大体检查，微乳头状交界性浆液性肿瘤是囊实性肿瘤，直径平均 8～9 cm。肿瘤倾向于双侧发生，典型的病例具有囊内和表面乳头状肿瘤生长。显微镜下，微乳头状交界性浆液性肿瘤发生在典型的交界性浆液性肿瘤的背景中，而且人为规定局灶性微乳头状生长大于 0.5cm[120]。几乎没有纤维性间质支持的长丛状上皮细胞，从球状的纤维血管间质乳头处长出（图 13A.9），从囊肿壁长出，或者当正切时，与具有较多间质的较大乳头包裹在一起。乳头长度是其宽度的 5 倍或者 5 倍以上[49]。沿着乳头表面呈局灶性筛状生长的肿瘤，也可归入微乳头状交界性浆液性肿瘤[49,104]。肿瘤细胞为立方形、鞋钉形或柱状，具有均匀一致的细胞核，仅有轻或中度非典型性（图 13A.10）。核分裂象不常见。微乳头状浆液性肿瘤中的纤毛细胞比典型的交界性浆液性肿瘤少见。

浆液性癌　Serous carcinoma

浆液性癌较大，经常双侧发生，其中有囊性、乳头状和实性混合的生长方式。实性区呈褐色或白色，伴有局灶出血和坏死。癌常常穿透卵巢被膜，并在卵巢表面生长。浆液性表面乳头状癌（serous surface papillary carcinona）主要生长在卵巢表面，伴有轻微的实质浸润，不向囊内生长[122-125]。当广泛的卵巢外浆液性癌仅仅伴有卵巢表面局灶性（≤0.5cm）生长时，这种病变可被看作是原发性腹膜浆液性癌卵巢受累（见第 15 章）[126]。显微镜下，浆液性癌弥漫浸润纤维性间质。经常出现乳头状结构，至少是局灶性的（图 13A.11）。乳头被覆复层矮柱状细胞。肿瘤细胞也可内衬腺样或呈实性条索状生长。在高级别肿瘤中，有实性细胞巢和片块状肿瘤细胞。实性生长灶内出现细长的裂隙样腺体是高级别浆液性癌的一个特征性发现。偶尔出现局灶性微囊性生长，有时混有印戒细胞[127]。细胞学非典型性和核分裂活性程度不同，但是多数浆液性癌是高级别的，伴有显著的核非典型性，核分裂象常见（图 13A.12）。显微镜下可见的浆液性癌（microscopic serous carcinomas）已有报告，但数量有限[128]。这些肿瘤倾向于是高级别的肿瘤，尽管它们的体积较小，提示典型的浆液性癌开始就是高级别的肿瘤。

免疫组化研究显示，浆液性癌 CK7 阳性，CK20 阴性（表 13A.5）[129]。大多数高级别浆液性癌显示 OC-125 膜染色[130,131]，以及 WT-1[132-136] 和 p53 蛋白[137-142] 核染色。WT-1 染色对于鉴别卵巢浆液性癌和子宫内膜浆液性癌是有帮助的，后者具有类似的组织学表现，但

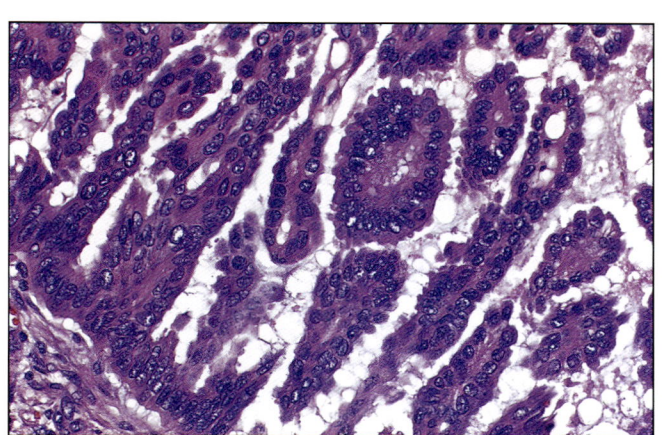

图13A.10　交界性浆液性肿瘤具有微乳头状特征。注意细长的微乳头状突起被覆立方或矮柱状细胞，仅有轻到中度核的非典型性。

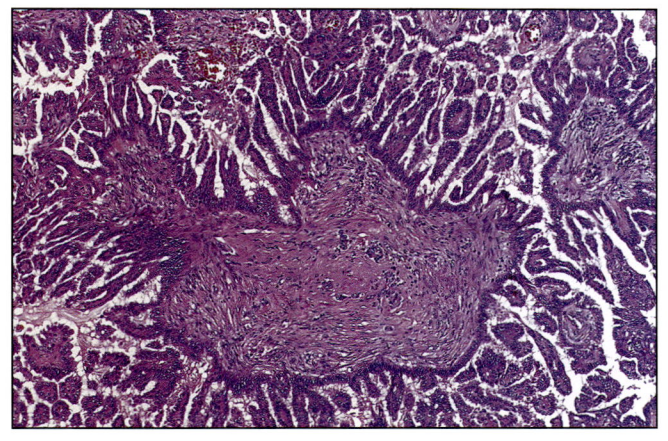

图13A.9　交界性浆液性肿瘤具有微乳头状特征。细长的微乳头，多数缺乏纤维血管轴心，从粗大乳头表面长出。

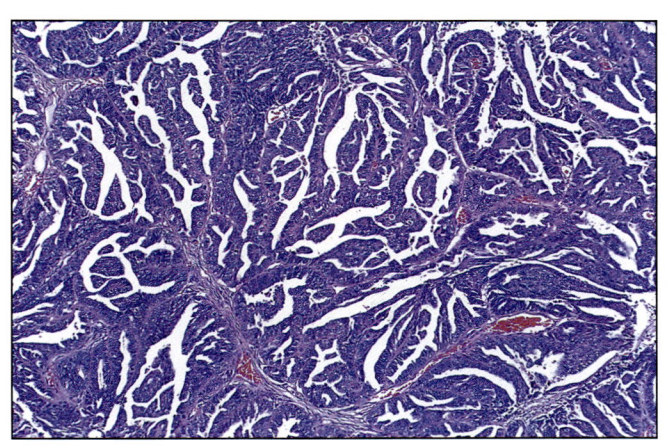

图13A.11　浆液性癌。融合性的乳头状生长方式是浆液性癌的特征。

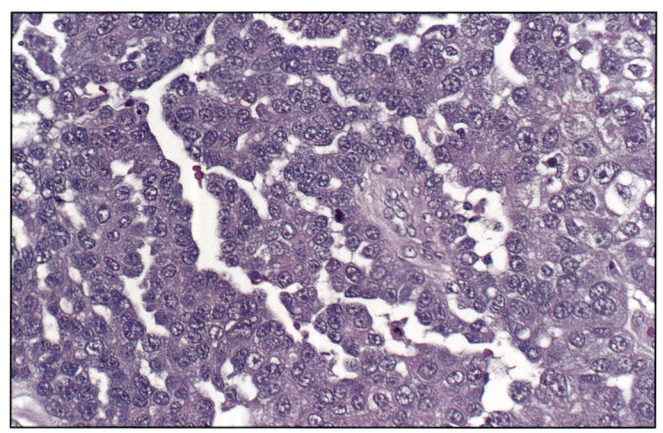

图13A.12 浆液性癌。肿瘤细胞覆盖乳头，呈片状生长。它们具有大的空泡状细胞核，染色质粗糙，某些细胞具有显著的核仁。

图13A.13 低级别浆液性癌。叶状微乳头，多数周围绕以透明间隙，浸润卵巢间质。核的非典型性是低级别的，核分裂象数目稀少。

表13A.5	卵巢癌的免疫组化检查						
	CK 7	CK 20	WT1	CA125	CEA	CDX2	VIM
浆液性癌	+	−	+	+	−	−	−
TCC	+	−	+	+	−	−	−
子宫内膜样癌	+	−	−	+	−	−	V
黏液性癌，肠型	+	V	−	−	+	V	−
透明细胞癌	+	−	−	+	−	−	−
转移性结直肠癌	−	+	−	−	+	+	−

"V"=不定阳性；"+"=阳性；"−"=阴性；
CK 7=细胞角蛋白7；CK 20=细胞角蛋白20；CEA=癌胚抗原；
VIM=波形蛋白；TCC=移行细胞癌

表13A.6	卵巢癌通用的分级系统
1. 结构评分	
腺体为主	1分
乳头为主	2分
实性为主	3分
2. 核的评分	
轻度非典型性	1分
中度非典型性	2分
重度非典型性	3分
3. 核分裂象评分	
0~10个 核分裂象/10 高倍视野	1分
11~25个核分裂象/10 高倍视野	2分
>25个核分裂象/10 高倍视野	3分
4. 肿瘤分级	
3~5分	1级
6~7分	2级
8~9分	3级

很少有 WT-1 染色[143,144]。

少数浆液性癌是低级别癌；其发生机制可能不同于高级别浆液性癌[120,145-151]。在低级别浆液性癌中，具有轻度核非典型性的腺体、微乳头或肿瘤细胞巢浸润纤维性间质（图 13A.13）[120]。肿瘤细胞簇或微乳头经常被裂隙或透明间隙围绕，浸润性癌的区域可以混有典型的或微乳头状浆液性交界性肿瘤[95]。某些或所有的低级别浆液性癌均可从交界性肿瘤进展而来。卵巢低级别浆液性癌的远处转移可能难以诊断，例如淋巴结、乳腺或纵隔转移[152,153]。

卵巢癌的分级尚未标准化，但是由 Silverberg 及其同事提出的针对所有类型卵巢癌的"通用的"分级系统已被广泛应用[154]。应用这种系统，浆液性癌的分级是由核的非典型性程度、核分裂象出现的频率，以及肿瘤细胞形成乳头或腺体的范围决定的（表 13A.6）[155,156]。

具有 BRCA1 和 BRCA2 突变的妇女发生卵巢癌的危险增加。大约 10% 的卵巢癌发生在具有 BRCA1 或 BRCA2 种系突变的妇女。多数发生在 BRCA 突变妇女的癌是浆液性癌；其他常见类型的卵巢癌，例如透明细胞癌和黏液性癌，在这一组患者中少见[157]。许多具有 BRCA 突变或卵巢癌家族史患者的治疗是，通过双侧输卵管-卵巢切除术来减低危险，已经发现这种治疗能够降低患者发生癌的危险性[158-160]。但癌的危险并没有完全消除，因为这些患者仍然处于患腹膜浆液性癌和乳腺癌的危险之中[159,161,162]。已经发现 2%~18% 的无症状妇女有显微镜下可见的局灶性原位癌或浸润癌，甚至有肉眼可见的癌[158,159,163-166]。在预防性输卵管-卵

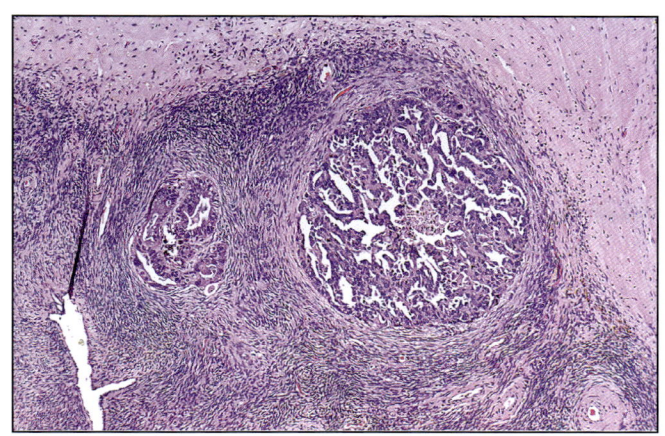

图13A.14 显微镜下可见的卵巢高级别浆液性癌,见于伴有 BRCA 突变妇女的为降低危险的卵巢切除标本中,肿瘤直径小于1mm。

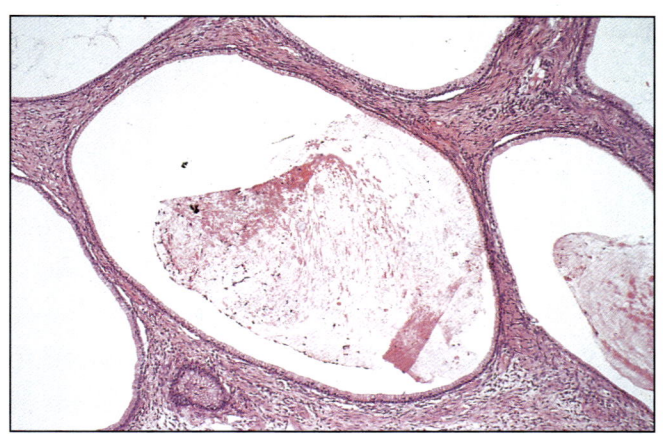

图13A.15 黏液性囊腺瘤。这个多房性囊性肿瘤内衬单层柱状黏液细胞。

巢切除标本中发现的癌多数是浆液性癌,直径仅仅几个毫米,而且是高级别癌(图 13A.14)[147,166]。肿瘤或发生于卵巢,或发生于输卵管,或两个部位均有[164]。为了发现小灶状肿瘤,必须对于双侧卵巢和输卵管切除标本充分切片[167,168]。p53 蛋白免疫组化染色可能有助于辨认小灶状肿瘤。临床发现的 BRCA 突变携带者的肿瘤主要是高级别浆液性癌,尽管偶尔也可发生其他类型肿瘤[157,169-171]。与对照人群相比,BRCA 突变患者患原发性输卵管癌也有增加,主要是浆液性癌[157]。

沙粒体是层状钙化小体,是细胞变性形成的圆形产物[172]。浆液性肿瘤常常出现沙粒体,特别是浆液性癌,偶尔有许多沙粒体。在罕见的低级别浸润性浆液性癌中沙粒体的数量可以很多,以至造成肿瘤的上皮成分变得模糊,这样的癌称为浆液性沙粒体癌(serous psammocarcinomas),当肿瘤能被完全切除时,可有非常好的预后[173-175]。腹膜可以发生类似的原发性肿瘤[176]。伴有多量沙粒体的高级别浆液性癌预后不好,并且被排除在"沙粒体癌"分类之外。沙粒体虽然提示浆液性肿瘤,但是它们还可能与非肿瘤性病变有关,例如上皮包涵囊肿和输卵管内膜异位症。

黏液性肿瘤 Mucinous tumors

黏液性囊腺瘤是最常见的卵巢黏液性肿瘤,其发生率大约与浆液性囊腺瘤相同。交界性和恶性黏液性肿瘤比交界性和恶性浆液性肿瘤少,而交界性黏液性肿瘤的数目超出黏液性癌。

良性黏液性肿瘤 Benign mucinous tumors

黏液性囊腺瘤一般为单侧性。平均直径大约10cm,但是巨大的肿瘤也有报告[177]。切面显示为单房性或不同大小的多房性充满黏液的囊肿。黏液性腺纤维瘤是以实性为主,白色或褐色的纤维性肿瘤,含有小的充满黏液的囊肿。黏液性囊腺纤维瘤是一种囊性肿瘤,具有类似于黏液性腺纤维瘤的实性纤维性区域。

显微镜下,良性黏液性肿瘤可见一层柱状细胞被覆囊肿、乳头和隐窝样结构(图 13A.15)。多数肿瘤细胞是宫颈内膜样或胃样,核圆形或卵圆形,均匀一致,位于基底,胞浆透明或双染性(图 13A.16)。胞浆酸性黏液染色阳性,中性黏液染色程度较弱。许多黏液性囊腺瘤中出现伴有杯状细胞或 Paneth 细胞的肠型上皮。组织化学和免疫组织化学研究显示含有不同肽类激素的嗜银细胞。多数黏液性肿瘤的柱状细胞表达胃和胰胆管的抗原和黏蛋白[178,179],而肠抗原主要在肠型上皮细胞中表达[180,181]。黏液性囊腺瘤的周围偶尔可见黄素化的间质细胞或 Leydig 细胞[182]。这个发现可能与临床类固醇激素分泌有关。黏液性腺纤维瘤或囊腺纤维瘤有丰富的纤维间质围绕腺体,这是主要的组织学结构[183,184]。少

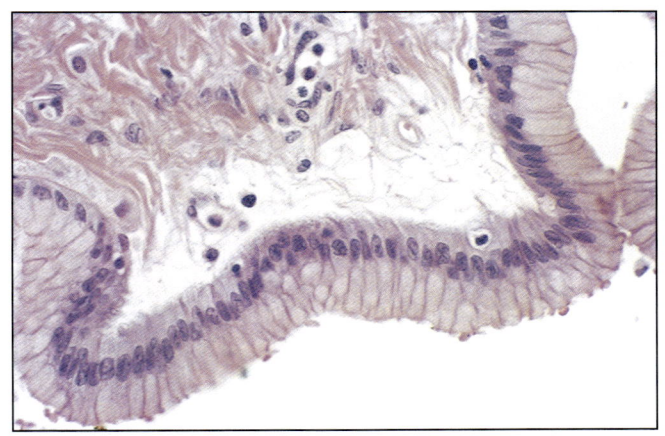

图13A.16 黏液性囊腺瘤。囊肿内衬高柱状细胞,伴有透明胞浆和温和的位于基底的细胞核。

数黏液性囊腺瘤或腺纤维瘤具有小灶状轻到中度核的非典型性或核的复层结构。当这些改变仅仅占据几个低倍视野时（≤肿瘤的5%～10%），临床经过总是良性的。这样的肿瘤最好归入伴有局灶性低级别非典型性的黏液性囊腺瘤、囊腺纤维瘤或腺纤维瘤。

交界性黏液性肿瘤
Borderline mucinous tumors

交界性黏液性肿瘤通常为单侧性[42,185,186]。双侧性交界性肿瘤占5%，主要是宫颈内膜样的（也称Müller性或浆液黏液性）交界性黏液性肿瘤[5]。交界性黏液肿瘤较大，平均直径大约15cm。多数为多房性肿瘤，尽管少数肿瘤为单房性或少囊性[185]。囊内充满黏液，具有光滑或天鹅绒般的内衬。在肠型交界性黏液性肿瘤中，囊内乳头并不常见，但是可以见于Müller性或宫颈内膜样交界性黏液性肿瘤。囊肿周围有数量不等的纤维间质。

显微镜下，可见两种类型的交界性黏液性肿瘤[187]。肠型交界性黏液性肿瘤（intestinal-type borderline mucinous tumors，IBMT）是迄今为止最常见的类型[10]。生长方式比较复杂，腺体密集，并形成继发性囊肿、复杂的腺体和由纤细纤维血管结缔组织轴心支持的乳头（图13A.17）[188,189]。可以出现宫颈内膜样的细胞，但以杯状细胞和类似于肠吸收细胞的细胞更为显著（图13A.18）。有增生活跃的证据，部分细胞分为2或3层[29,186]。肿瘤细胞核圆形至卵圆形，呈空泡状，通常有轻到中度的非典型性[24]。可有显著的核仁，偶见核分裂象。伴有显著核非典型性的非浸润性黏液性肿瘤，被称为伴有上皮内癌的交界性黏液性肿瘤（borderline mucinous tumors with intraepithelial carcinoma）[190,191]。充分研究显示，非浸润性黏液性肿瘤复发和转移的危险较低[190-193]。确实发生转移的少数肿瘤倾向于是伴有上皮内癌的交界性黏液性肿瘤[191]。转移很可能是反映了在一个大的以交界性肿瘤为主的肿瘤中，存在小的未被发现的浸润性癌灶。

直径小于3mm的间质微小浸润灶发生于5%～10%的肠型交界性黏液性肿瘤[90,194]。微小浸润的肿瘤细胞簇或小而复杂的腺体被炎性或水肿性间质、纤维组织增生性间质反应或透明的间隙围绕。多数伴有微小浸润的患者有着良好的预后[90,190,191,194]，但是少数患者发生转移[195]。

无细胞性卵巢假黏液瘤（acellular pseudomyxoma ovarii）是囊肿和腺体破裂，无细胞黏液释放到周围卵巢间质的一种病变（图13A.19）。外渗的黏液池常常被组织细胞和多核异物巨细胞围绕，黏液可以机化，伴有纤维母细胞和血管向内生长。细胞性卵巢假黏液瘤（cellular pseudomyxoma ovarii）的黏液池中含有成簇的和带状上皮细胞，主要见于腹膜假黏液瘤（pseudomyxoma peritonei）患者，是预后不良的表现[186,196]。

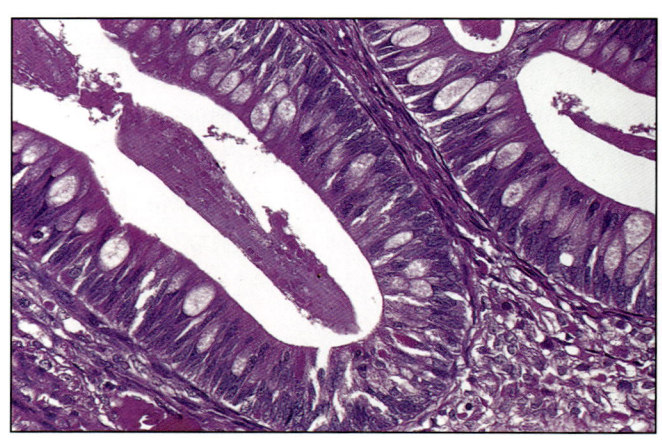

图13A.18 交界性黏液性肿瘤，肠型。某些肿瘤细胞有致密的嗜酸性胞浆，类似于肠的吸收细胞，而另外一些是杯状细胞，伴有显著的胞浆黏液空泡。核深染，分为两到三层。

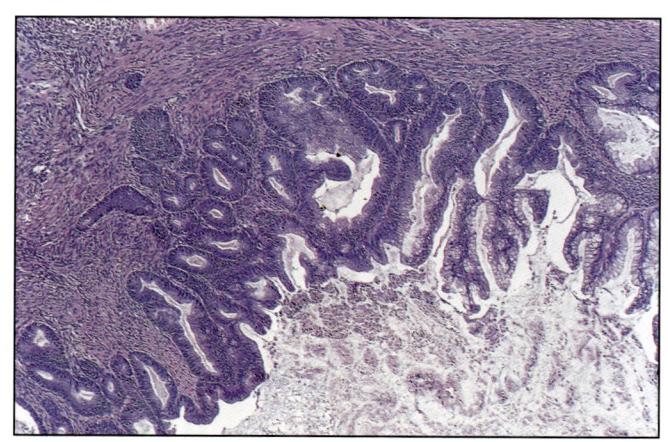

图13A.17 交界性黏液性肿瘤，肠型。黏液上皮被覆复杂的腺体和乳头。注意缺乏间质浸润。

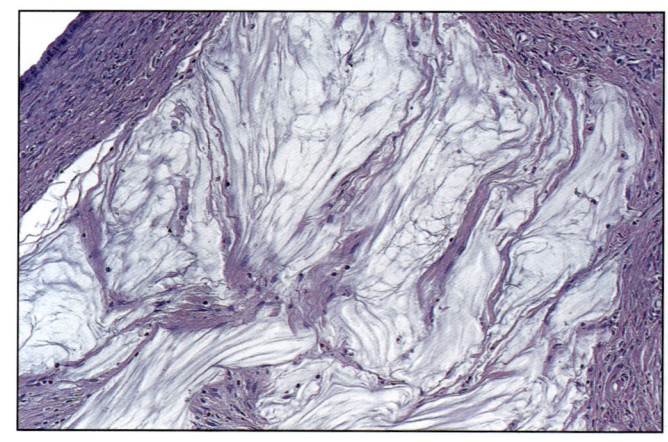

图13A.19 无细胞性卵巢假黏液瘤。间质中出现无细胞的黏液池。

有卵巢外肿瘤扩散的患者预后不好。少数患者有腹膜或网膜浸润性腺体种植，但典型的卵巢外肿瘤表现为腹膜假黏液瘤。腹膜假黏液瘤是一种进行性的病变，这种病变表现为含有温和上皮条索的黏液沉积物发生纤维性机化、粘连和进入网膜和腹膜，最后充满腹腔。具有 IBMT 肿瘤表现的黏液性肿瘤常常伴有腹膜假黏液瘤，但是目前的观点是，见于这种情况的几乎所有卵巢肿瘤都是继发于原发性阑尾或结肠肿瘤。腹膜假黏液瘤在转移性肿瘤一节中将做详细讨论。

宫颈内膜样交界性黏液性肿瘤（endocervical-like borderline mucinous tumors，EBMT），也叫 Müller 黏液性或浆液黏液性交界性肿瘤，占交界性黏液性肿瘤的 5%～15%[29,186,197-200]。它们具有分支乳头状生长方式，类似于交界性浆液性肿瘤（图 13A.20）[200,201]。囊肿和乳头被覆柱状黏液性宫颈内膜细胞和数量不等的具有嗜酸性胞浆的细胞（图 13A.21）。常见局灶性子宫内膜样和浆液性分化，乳头尖端常常出现具有丰富嗜酸性胞浆的多角形未分化细胞丛，由此成簇的细胞脱落进入囊腔内。既不出现杯状细胞也不出现肠吸收细胞。多数肿瘤核分裂象少见，通常有轻度的核非典型性。少数宫颈内膜样交界性黏液性肿瘤有明显的核非典型性和核分裂活性，这些肿瘤被称为显示上皮内癌的宫颈内膜样交界性黏液性肿瘤[199-201]。腔内黏液、上皮和间质有多形核白细胞浸润。在 30% 或更多的病例发现邻近肿瘤的卵巢组织内有子宫内膜异位[197]。宫颈内膜样交界性黏液性肿瘤偶尔出现最大径小于 3mm 的间质微小浸润[199-201]。

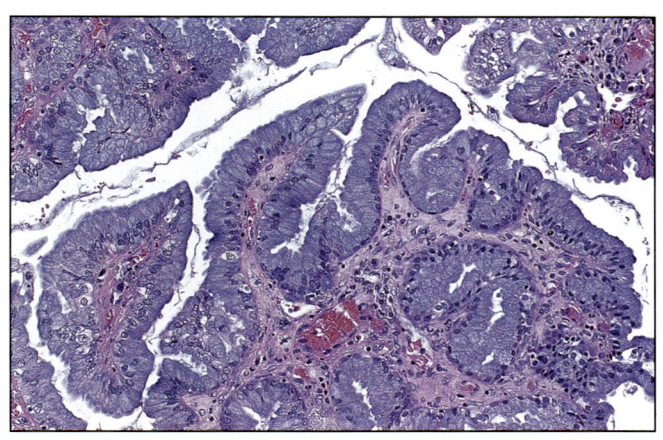

图13A.21　交界性黏液性肿瘤，宫颈内膜样。乳头被覆柱状细胞，核位于基底，胞浆丰富，充满黏液。

在 15%～30% 的宫颈内膜样交界性黏液性肿瘤的间质中，可见成簇的嗜酸性或浅染的细胞，周围通常没有反应[90,194,199,200]。宫颈内膜样交界性黏液性肿瘤常常为双侧性，而且 20%～30% 的病例出现腹膜种植。种植一般为非浸润性上皮类型，常常被纤维组织增生性间质围绕。预后与交界性浆液性肿瘤相似，即使出现非浸润性卵巢外肿瘤种植也伴有良性的进展[29,197,201]。上皮内癌和间质微小浸润均与预后不良无关[199,200]。

宫颈内膜样交界性黏液性肿瘤的免疫表型与肠型交界性黏液性肿瘤不同。两种类型的交界性黏液性肿瘤 CK7 染色均呈阳性反应，但是仅有肠型交界性黏液性肿瘤显示 CK20 阳性染色[202]，而且大约 40% 的病例 CDX-2 阳性。肠型交界性黏液性肿瘤癌胚抗原免疫染色常常弥漫强阳性。宫颈内膜样交界性黏液性肿瘤很少有癌胚抗原表达，但当癌胚抗原有表达时，经常仅仅是嗜酸细胞有反应[203]。宫颈内膜样交界性黏液性肿瘤表达雌激素和孕激素受体，而肠型交界性黏液性肿瘤缺乏雌激素和孕激素受体表达[204]。50% 以上的肠型交界性黏液性肿瘤可见嗜银细胞，免疫组织化学染色显示其中含有肽类，例如 5-羟色胺、ACTH、突触素、胰高血糖素、胃泌素和嗜铬素[178,180,198,205-209]。

黏液性癌　Mucinous carcinoma

黏液性癌是大的多房性肿瘤，平均直径 15～20cm[188,210]。可见质硬的鱼肉样白色或褐色的实性区域，常常伴有局灶性出血或坏死，特别是在大的肿瘤。双侧性和表面生长见于不到 10% 的病例[185]，因为肿瘤较大以及这些肿瘤的黏液性内容物，往往造成被膜破裂。双侧性或小的（≤10 cm）黏液性癌可能是转移的，而大的单侧性黏液性癌则有可能是原发性肿瘤[211]。

显微镜下，腺体和囊肿密集而复杂，伴有不规则的内折和突入周围间质（图 13A.22）。多数黏液性癌以肠

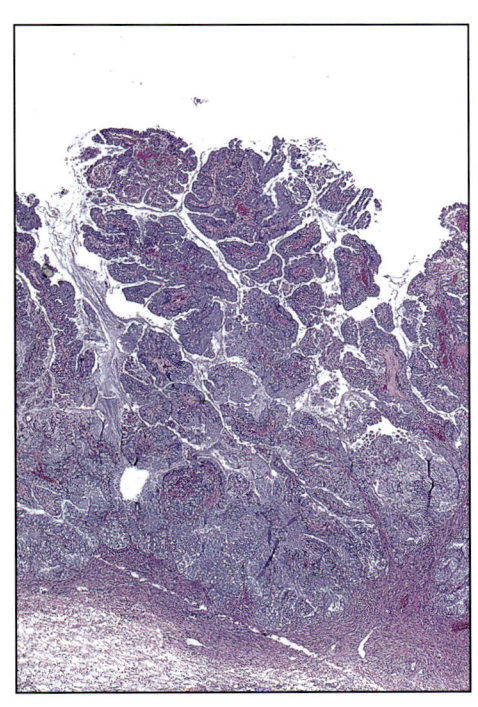

图13A.20　交界性黏液性肿瘤，宫颈内膜样。复杂的分支状乳头长入囊腔。

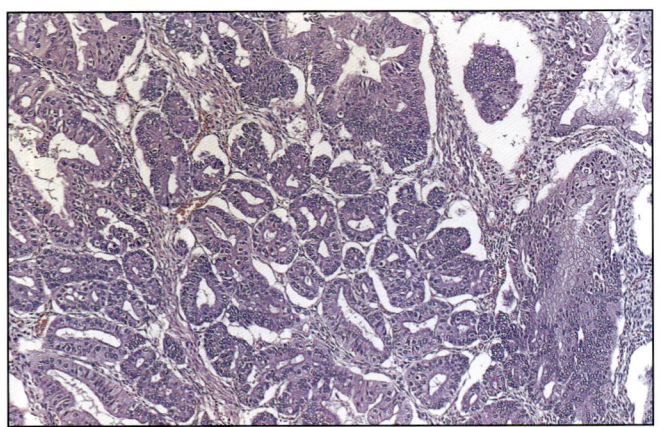

图13A.22　黏液性癌。融合性生长方式伴有背靠背的腺体。某些腺体绕以透明间隙。

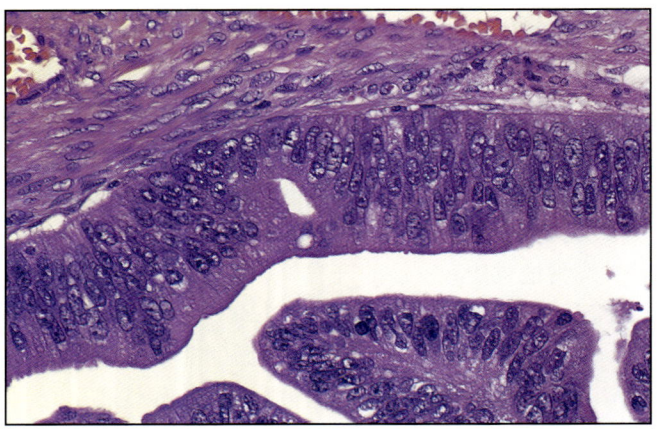

图13A.23　黏液性癌。多数细胞具有致密的嗜酸性胞浆。核大而呈空泡状，复层，染色质粗，某些细胞核含有突出的核仁。

型细胞为主。细胞呈柱状，有嗜酸性胞浆，倾向于分成两层或更多的层次（图13A.23）。核大，空泡状，染色质粗，核仁明显。核分裂象从少到多不等，常见非典型性核分裂象。可以出现杯状细胞和嗜银细胞。在黏液性癌中常常出现交界性和良性表现的黏液上皮，最常见于低级别癌中。某些黏液性癌缺乏肠分化，而是含有突出的宫颈内膜样细胞成分[200,201,212]。这些肿瘤是宫颈内膜样交界性黏液性肿瘤的对应恶性肿瘤。肿瘤细胞内衬腺体、囊肿，并被覆乳头。类似于宫颈内膜的具有黏液性胞浆的柱状细胞是主要成分，尽管还可以出现其他类型的分化，特别是子宫内膜样分化[212]。免疫表型与宫颈内膜样交界性黏液性肿瘤相似，CK7以及雌激素和孕激素受体强阳性，而CK20染色阴性或很弱[212]。这些肿瘤的侵袭性可能低于以肠型细胞为主的肿瘤，虽然研究的病例太少以致无法得以确定，但死于肿瘤的病例已有报告[200,213]。

诊断黏液性癌以及有关鉴别高分化黏液性癌和交界性黏液性肿瘤的标准过去一直存在争议，但是现在诊断黏液性癌的标准取得一致，即不规则的肿瘤细胞条索或细胞巢，或融合膨胀的背靠背腺体或乳头结节浸润间质 ["破坏性间质浸润" (destructive stromal invasion)][8,191]。病理医师在病理报告中应该注明存在哪一种类型的浸润，因为如果出现破坏性间质浸润，复发的危险性较大[187,190,214]。然而，仅有融合性的浸润方式并不能保证不会复发[195]。在复杂的黏液性肿瘤中可能难以辨认破坏性间质浸润，而且有人提出在缺乏间质浸润的情况下诊断癌的其他标准[188,215]。提示一个肿瘤可能是癌的特征包括，细胞分为四层或四层以上、局限性的筛状结构、没有间质轴心的乳头以及显著的核非典型性，但这些都不是独立的诊断标准。如果在没有见到浸润的肿瘤中出现这样的特征，那就需要进行比较充分的显微镜下检查。目前，间质浸润是将卵巢黏液肿瘤归类为癌的唯一标准。没有明确浸润的肿瘤最好归类为交界性肿瘤，并注意有无上皮内癌的特征。应该通知临床医师，这样的病例具有低度复发和转移的危险性，特别是在肿瘤取材不充分的情况下[29]。

如同其他原发性卵巢上皮性肿瘤一样，黏液性癌CK7一般阳性（见表13A.5）[129,216,217]。多数肿瘤CK20染色阳性，但是倾向于斑片状弱至中等强度的染色[218,219]，和转移性结直肠腺癌的弥漫性强阳性染色形成对比。黏液性癌CDX-2染色可能阳性[218]，但是这种抗体在卵巢黏液性肿瘤中的染色仍有待于评估。某些原发性黏液性癌没有CDX-2染色[220]，而另外一些染色范围和强度不如转移性结直肠腺癌[216,221,222]。

黏液性癌的几种不常见亚型已有描述。"肉瘤样"结缔组织附壁结节（mural nodule）、肉瘤或间变性癌偶尔发生于黏液性肿瘤，通常是交界性肿瘤或癌[223,224]。反应性附壁结节倾向于界限清楚，大小可至5cm，可以是单发性，但比较常见的是多发性结节。这些结节由梭形的纤维母细胞、肌纤维母细胞和可能的间皮下细胞、组织细胞、炎症细胞和偶尔的多核细胞组成。已经描述有三个亚型：龈瘤样型（epulis-like type），由单核间质细胞和多核巨细胞组成；多形性型（pleomorphic type），由梭形细胞和巨细胞组成；以及组织细胞型（histiocytic type）[225]。间质通常水肿伴有局灶状出血和坏死。Vimentin和CD68免疫染色阳性。细胞角蛋白弱表达，并且是局灶阳性，不同于典型癌的弥漫性强阳性染色[225-227]。间变性癌的附壁结节可以为单发性或多发性，直径从小于1cm到大于10cm不等。结节具有浸润性的边界，由成巢和成片的未分化多角形上皮细胞，或成片和成束的恶性梭形细胞组成（图13A.24）[190,228-232]。核分裂象多见，而且可能是异常核分裂象。细胞角蛋白或上皮膜抗原的免疫反应是重要的诊断线索。罕见的癌肉瘤样结节也有报告[233]。肉瘤附壁结节是由恶性梭形

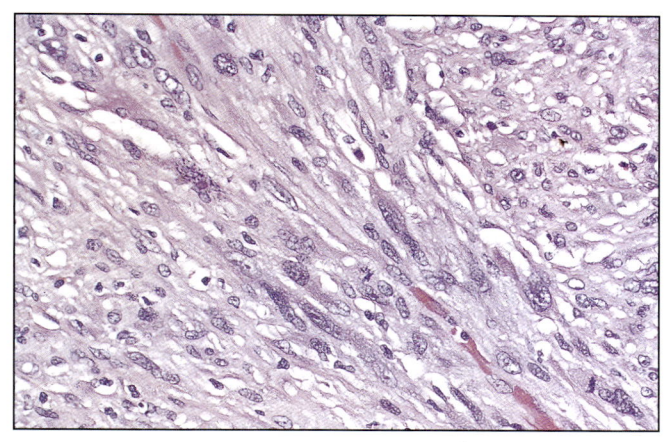

图13A.24 黏液性肿瘤壁上的肉瘤样癌附壁结节。这种梭形细胞肿瘤来自于黏液性癌。肿瘤细胞显示细胞角蛋白强阳性表达,代表这是肉瘤样癌的区域,而不是真正的肉瘤。

细胞构成的,通常类似于纤维肉瘤或未分化肉瘤[234,235]。肿瘤细胞细胞角蛋白阴性,但Vimentin阳性,而且诸如actin和desmin等其他中间丝也可能阳性,取决于肉瘤的类型。

局灶性神经内分泌癌偶尔出现于黏液性肿瘤,最常见的是黏液性癌[236-240]。肿瘤细胞可能较小,核深染,染色质细,而且胞浆稀少,类似于肺的小细胞癌;肿瘤细胞也可能较大,伴有大而深染或空泡状的细胞核以及显著的核仁和较为丰富的细胞浆,类似于肺的大细胞神经内分泌癌。神经元特异性烯醇化酶、嗜铬素、突触素或其他神经内分泌分化标记物免疫组化染色可能有助于正确分类小细胞成分。电子显微镜检查可以用于证实肿瘤细胞胞浆中的神经内分泌颗粒。黏液性肿瘤的腺体或间质中出现的个别神经内分泌细胞或显微镜下可见的神经内分泌细胞巢,可能是这种神经内分泌癌起源的部位[241]。少数的病例报告显示,在临床上神经内分泌癌好像具有侵袭性。

子宫内膜样肿瘤　Endometrioid tumors

卵巢的子宫内膜样肿瘤具有类似于增殖期、增生性或恶性子宫内膜的上皮成分。良性或交界性子宫内膜样肿瘤罕见。根据报告,罕见的交界性子宫内膜样肿瘤病例的肿瘤细胞可以脱落进入腹膜腔,或播散到卵巢外,但是具有同样较好的临床结果[27,184,242-244]。一项报告引起注意,少数经过单侧卵巢-输卵管切除术治疗的患者,对侧卵巢发生了子宫内膜样癌[27]。子宫内膜样癌在组织学上类似于子宫内膜腺癌,是第二个最常见的卵巢腺癌类型,占所有卵巢恶性上皮性肿瘤的12%~30%[5,245,246]。相对于其他类型的卵巢腺癌来讲,子宫内膜样癌有较好的预后[245,247]。具有融合性浸润性生长方式的低级别I期子宫内膜样癌很少进展,尽管那些具有破坏性浸润方式的肿瘤侵袭性可能更强,因为是高级别的肿瘤[214,243]。子宫内膜样癌通常发生于具有子宫内膜异位症的患者,多达1/3的子宫内膜样癌发生在子宫内膜异位症或其附近,非典型性子宫内膜异位症患者可能具有较大的危险性[245,248-251]。子宫内膜异位症相关性肿瘤发生于年轻妇女,出现在较早阶段,其侵袭性可能不如表面上皮起源的子宫内膜样癌[248,249,252-254]。

良性子宫内膜样肿瘤
Benign endometrioid tumors

所有良性子宫内膜样肿瘤都是腺纤维瘤,它们大约占卵巢腺纤维瘤的10%[184,255]。它们是实性的纤维性肿瘤,平均直径8～10 cm。切面呈褐色或白色,而且含有直径从几个毫米到几个厘米的小囊。显微镜下,腺管状的或囊性腺体被纤维性间质包绕或分开(图13A.25)。腺体内衬单层子宫内膜型细胞。这些细胞呈柱状,胞浆嗜碱性或双染性,核均匀一致,圆形或卵圆形。细胞核可是假复层的,如同增生期子宫内膜,但核分裂象通常罕见或缺乏。鳞状化生可以出现,在极少数肿瘤中,腺体内衬纤毛细胞[255,256]。在一个少见的病例中,卵巢子宫内膜样腺纤维瘤手术切除之后6周发现阴道复发,是手术种植的结果[184]。

交界性子宫内膜样肿瘤
Borderline endometrioid tumors

过去,交界性子宫内膜样肿瘤有各种命名,造成文献中有关这个题目存在诸多的混淆。Russell和Roth等应用"增生性(proliferating)"子宫内膜样肿瘤这一命名[27,255];Kao和Norris报告的肿瘤称为"腺纤维瘤伴有上皮非典型性"[257];Bell和Scully将他们研究的交界性子宫内膜样腺纤维瘤分为两组,称为"非典型性"和"交界性"[258];Snyder等和Norris将交界性子宫内膜样肿

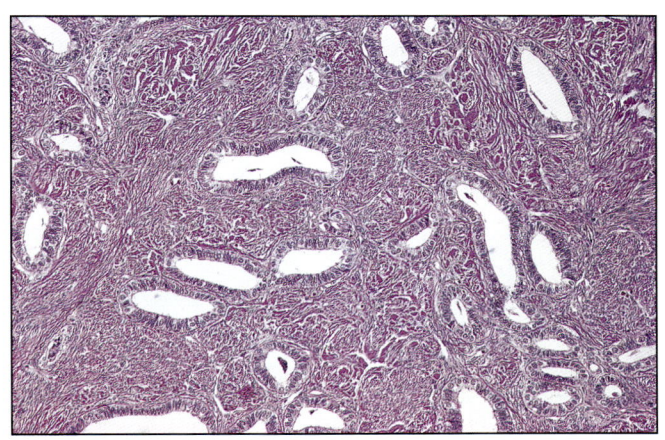

图13A.25 子宫内膜样腺纤维瘤。内衬单层良性子宫内膜型细胞的腺体生长在致密的纤维间质中。

瘤分为"增生性（proliferative）"和"潜在低度恶性（low malignant potential）"两类[242,259]。本书作者希望将所有这些肿瘤均归入交界性子宫内膜样肿瘤，新近的WHO分类已经做到了这一点[8]。交界性子宫内膜样肿瘤谱系中的低级别病变是腺体成分类似于子宫内膜单纯性增生的腺纤维瘤。中间类型是腺体密集而又不规则的腺纤维瘤，如同子宫内膜复合性增生。最高级别的交界性子宫内膜肿瘤的上皮，显示与子宫内膜复合性非典型性增生同样程度的增生活性和核非典型性。

交界性子宫内膜样肿瘤通常为单侧性（新近一项研究发现仅8%为双侧性），多数表现为腺纤维瘤或囊腺纤维瘤[243]，肿瘤一般以实性为主，但是有些肿瘤含有囊腔，特别是高级别肿瘤。平均直径6～10cm，切面为褐色或白色。在某些肿瘤的囊腔中，肉眼可见乳头状赘生物。显微镜下，低级别交界性子宫内膜样肿瘤是伴有腺体密度增加的腺纤维瘤，相当于良性子宫内膜样肿瘤，显示不同的结构和局灶性密集[260]。可有小灶状的筛状结构，或者腺体密集排列的区域。上皮细胞核为假复层或复层，核有轻至中度非典型性，偶见核分裂象（≤3/10HPF）。高级别交界性子宫内膜样肿瘤显示两种主要的生长方式[27,242,258,260]。某些肿瘤是伴有腺体密度增加的腺纤维瘤；显著的腺体拥挤区域（图13A.26），直径通常超过5mm；局灶性筛状结构；以及显著的核非典型性、复层和核分裂活性。第二种生长方式是有乳头伸入囊性间隙。乳头常常有绒毛腺管状表现，伴有宽的纤维血管轴心。被覆乳头的细胞显示不同程度的复层和非典型性。核分裂活性通常较低（≤3/10HPF），但是有些肿瘤核分裂象比较常见。交界性子宫内膜肿瘤的增生活性可能显著，但是腺体的密集程度通常不如子宫内膜样癌，并且增生的细胞巢具有光滑的轮廓并被间质包绕。鳞状和黏液化生常见，特别是在腺纤维瘤性肿瘤中[243]，而且少数肿瘤含有许多纤毛细胞[256]。子宫内膜异位症常常出现在受累的卵巢和盆腔其他部位，而且在少数病例可以证实来源于子宫内膜异位症[242,243,255]。间质微小浸润见于5%～15%的交界性子宫内膜样肿瘤，其中小而不规则的腺体浸润间质，或有灶状融合性腺体生长区域，直径小于3mm[242,243,258,260]。具有微小浸润的患者中没有发现复发的病例。

子宫内膜样癌　Endometrioid carcinoma

子宫内膜样癌是一种囊性和实性或完全实体的肿瘤，典型者直径可达10～20cm[245,261,262]。实体区域可能质硬或质软，灰白色或褐色。常见出血和坏死区。只有10%～20%的病例为双侧性[5]。

子宫内膜样癌是一种腺样或乳头状的肿瘤，类似于子宫内膜腺癌。生长方式是腺样、乳头状或两者混合，浸润的方式可以是偶然浸润间质或融合性生长[243]。腺体倾向于较小，大小和形状相对一致（图13A.27）。乳头常常有绒毛腺管状形态，具有显著的纤维血管支持轴心。腺体和乳头被覆柱状细胞，具有双染性到嗜碱性胞浆。核位于基底部，圆形或卵圆形，可以见到核仁（图13A.28）。当肿瘤级别增加时，非典型性程度、核复层的范围以及腺体融合成实性病灶的程度也增加。子宫内膜样癌可以应用子宫内膜腺癌同样的标准进行分级[263]。I级肿瘤呈现腺样或乳头状生长方式，实性结构<5%。II级肿瘤实性结构占5%～50%，而III级肿瘤实性结构超过50%。在确定实性结构的百分比时，鳞状或梭形细胞分化区域不计在内。如果核是III级，而生长方式是I或II级，

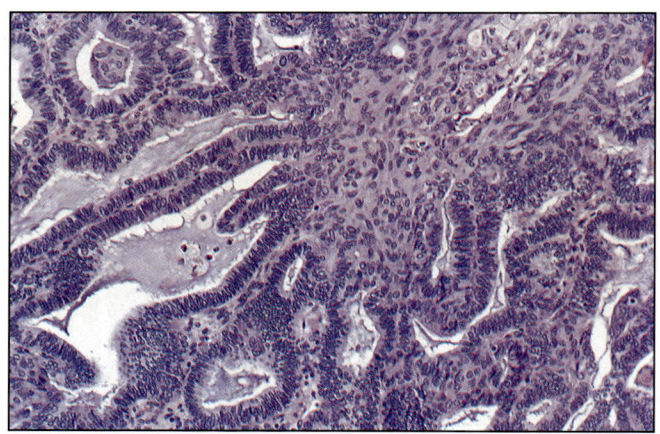

图13A.26　交界性子宫内膜肿瘤。腺体结构类似于子宫内膜复合性增生。肿瘤细胞核仅显示轻度非典型性。注意视野中心不成熟的鳞状化生。

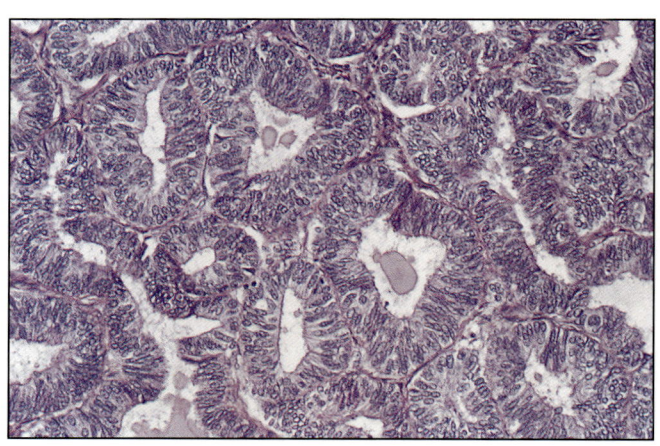

图13A.27　子宫内膜样癌。背靠背的腺体内衬复层柱状细胞，细胞核深染。

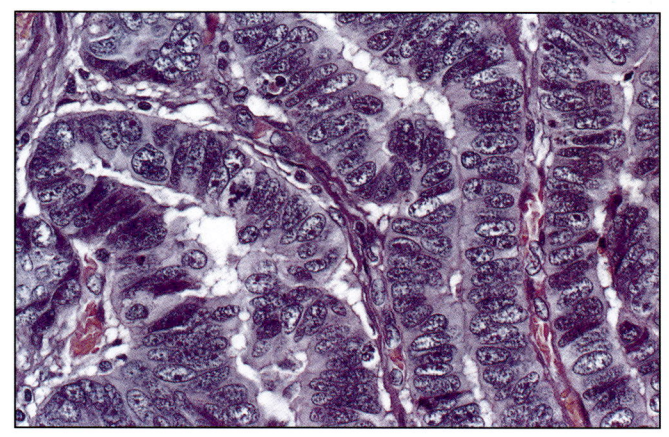

图13A.28 子宫内膜样癌。这个中分化腺癌腺体内衬细胞核浆比例增大。核圆形或卵圆形，染色质粗糙。某些核含有一个或多个显著的核仁。注意视野左侧中心的非典型性核分裂象。

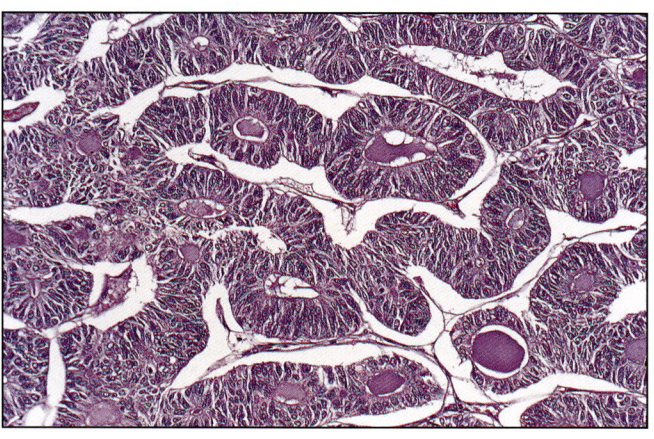

图13A.29 Sertoli型子宫内膜样癌。肿瘤细胞形成小梁并内衬小的腺体。显微镜下表现类似于Sertoli细胞瘤，但与典型的Sertoli细胞瘤相比，细胞核复层和非典型性均较明显。

最后的分级要提高一个水平。子宫内膜样癌也可以应用以前讨论过的用于卵巢癌的"通用分级方法"来分级（见表13A.6）[154]。

局灶鳞状分化出现在25%～50%的子宫内膜样癌中，细胞学表现可是良性的，也可以是恶性的。角蛋白肉芽肿（keratin granulomas）偶尔见于这些患者的腹膜中，外科医师可能将其误认为肿瘤种植[264]。有人报告伴有混合的透明细胞癌成分的子宫内膜样癌预后不好[261,265]，如同子宫内膜样癌混有浆液性或未分化癌一样[266]。因此，病理医师报告子宫内膜样癌是单纯性的还是混合有其他类型表面上皮性肿瘤是很重要的。

有几种不常见的、可能引起混淆的子宫内膜样癌亚型，其中某些类似于性索间质肿瘤。微腺管性结构（microglandular pattern）在子宫内膜样癌中不常见，但是当出现这种形态时，有可能被误诊为颗粒细胞瘤[267]。Sertoli型（Sertoliform）子宫内膜样癌具有显著的肿瘤细胞生长成长形、分支状、管状腺体或小梁状的区域（图13A.29）[267-269]。这种亚型类似于Sertoli或Sertoli-Leydig细胞瘤，特别是当间质丰富，或出现纤维性和黄素化间质细胞时。子宫内膜样癌的嗜酸性亚型（oxyphilic variant）具有显著的大的多角形肿瘤细胞成分，细胞具有丰富的嗜酸性胞浆和位于中心的圆形细胞核，含有大的核仁[270]。肿瘤细胞成巢或片块状生长或内衬管状腺体。梭形细胞亚型（spindle cell variant）具有突出的温和梭形细胞成分。带状和条索状肿瘤细胞混有分叶状的梭形细胞巢，可能类似于性索-间质肿瘤[271]。临床上，显微镜下以及免疫组化特征均可用于这些亚型子宫内膜样癌与性索-间质肿瘤的鉴别。它们发生于围绝经期和绝经后的妇女，很少伴有类固醇激素产物的临床证据。

大体检查，它们的切面缺乏代表性索-间质肿瘤特征的金黄色或黄色外观。可以是双侧发生。显微镜下，仔细寻找可能发现典型的子宫内膜样癌灶以及鳞状化生或腺纤维瘤的区域。子宫内膜样癌CK和EMA强阳性[272,273]，多数病例抑制素（inhibin, I）和calretinin（CR）染色阴性[269,274]，虽然也有少数inhibin或calretinin阳性的子宫内膜样癌的报告[275]。Sertoli和Sertoli-Leydig细胞瘤细胞角蛋白阳性，大约1/3的颗粒细胞瘤细胞角蛋白也呈阳性反应，而性索-间质肿瘤上皮膜抗原几乎总是阴性，而inhibin和calretinin强阳性[274]。因此，CK$^+$、EMA$^+$、I$^-$、CR$^-$这种免疫表型支持子宫内膜样癌的诊断，而免疫表型CK$^+$、EMA$^-$、I$^+$、CR$^+$支持性索-间质肿瘤的诊断。

少数子宫内膜样癌和卵黄囊瘤混合存在的病例已有描述[276,277]。这些肿瘤与子宫内膜样癌发生于同一年龄组，肿瘤较大，预后不好。卵黄囊瘤成分甲胎蛋白免疫染色强阳性，结合组织学表现可以确认。

10%～20%患有卵巢子宫内膜样癌妇女的子宫内膜可见子宫内膜样癌（图13A.30）[245,248,261,278,279]。子宫内膜癌通常为表浅的高分化癌，当癌局限于子宫和卵巢时，生存率高[279-283]。在这种情况下，卵巢和子宫内膜癌可能是单独的、同时发生的原发性肿瘤，而不是晚期子宫内膜腺癌伴有卵巢转移，或晚期卵巢癌伴有子宫内膜转移。然而，在某些同时发生肿瘤的患者，卵巢肿瘤是从子宫内膜癌转移而来的。提示卵巢癌可能是转移而来的特征包括：子宫内膜癌为高级别或浸润较深；有子宫肌层或卵巢门的淋巴管浸润；癌出现在输卵管管腔内；卵巢肿瘤小；卵巢肿瘤多结节状或实性；卵巢肿瘤是双侧性；出现卵巢表面种植；而且卵巢外转移出现在子宫

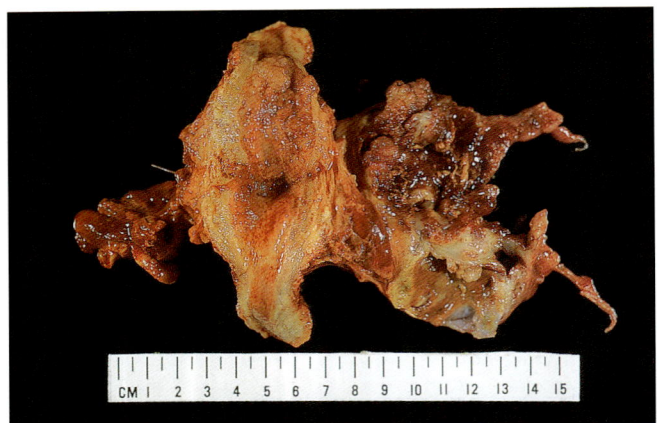

图13A.30 同时发生的卵巢子宫内膜样癌（右）和子宫内膜腺癌。

内膜腺癌特征性的分布部位（例如淋巴结转移可能比腹膜转移常见）[280,284]。分子诊断技术可能提供较明确的信息，但是目前尚不适于常规临床使用[285-290]。需要解决的问题包括，某些病例的分子和临床病理学所见不一致，而且偶尔缺乏有用的结果。

混合性中胚层肿瘤、腺肉瘤和子宫内膜样间质肉瘤
Mixed mesodermal tumor, adenosarcoma, and endometrioid stromal sarcoma

混和性中胚层肿瘤或腺肉瘤，以及子宫内膜样间质肉瘤来自于子宫内膜异位症或化生。腺肉瘤可以直接来自于卵巢上皮或间质，或者子宫内膜异位症。这些肿瘤的临床行为类似于比较常见的子宫对应肿瘤。

混合性中胚层肿瘤和腺肉瘤
Mixed mesodermal tumor and adenosarcoma

混合性中胚层肿瘤（MMT），也叫癌肉瘤，主要发生于低产次的绝经后妇女[291-293]。最常见症状是盆腔或腹部疼痛，腹部膨胀，肠道症状和体重降低[294,295]。血清CA125浓度通常升高。多数患者有可触及的附件肿块，许多患者有腹水。70%以上的MMT在诊断时已经播散至卵巢外[296]。播散的方式如同卵巢癌一样，主要是播散至腹膜、网膜和局灶淋巴结[292,294,297,298]。治疗是通过子宫切除术、双侧输卵管卵巢切除术，并且尽可能多地切除卵巢外的肿瘤。具有局限性疾病的患者应该彻底分期。预后不好；在超过400例患者的研究中，中位生存率仅为6～12个月，而且70%以上的患者一年内死亡[293,299,300]。多数研究显示化疗反应不好，而且比类似分期的癌预后更差[300,301]，虽然有些作者报告对于化疗效果较好[302,303]。几乎所有的患者最后都会复发，某些研究的5年生存率小于10%[295,296,304]。分期是最重要的预后参数[305,306]。组织学参数，例如癌和肉瘤成分的类型和分级，似乎没有预后意义[292,295,296,306]。少数患者表现为早期肿瘤（I-II期）；她们具有较长的生存期，而且很可能已经治愈[291,295,304,306,307]。

混合性中胚层肿瘤倾向于较大，平均直径15cm[308]。肿瘤或为囊性和实性，或者完全为实性。实性的部分呈灰白色或褐色，通常有显著的出血和坏死。显微镜下，MMT是双相性肿瘤，具有混合性的上皮和间叶成分（图13A.31）。上皮成分可以是任何类型的表面上皮性癌，但是浆液性、子宫内膜样和未分化癌最常见[292]。间叶性成分是单纯性肉瘤或不同类型的混合性肉瘤。同源性肉瘤成分包括纤维肉瘤、平滑肌肉瘤和未分化肉瘤。异源性成分出现在多数的卵巢MMT中，例如横纹肌肉瘤、软骨肉瘤或骨肉瘤（图13A.32）[291,308,309]。嗜酸性透明小体经常出现在MMT中，散在分散于上皮或间叶

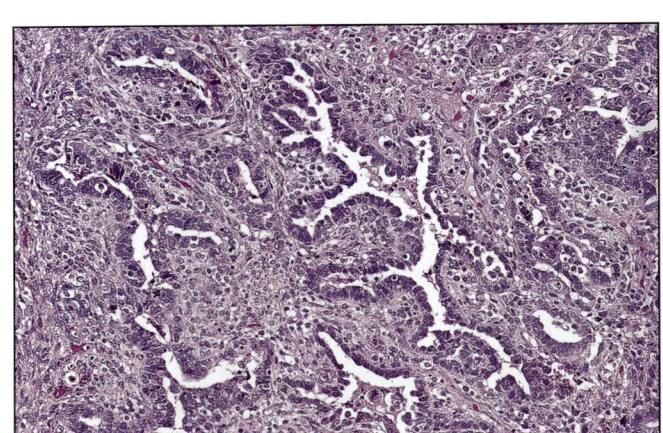

图13A.31 混合性中胚层肿瘤（癌肉瘤）。不规则的恶性腺体被肉瘤样间质包绕。

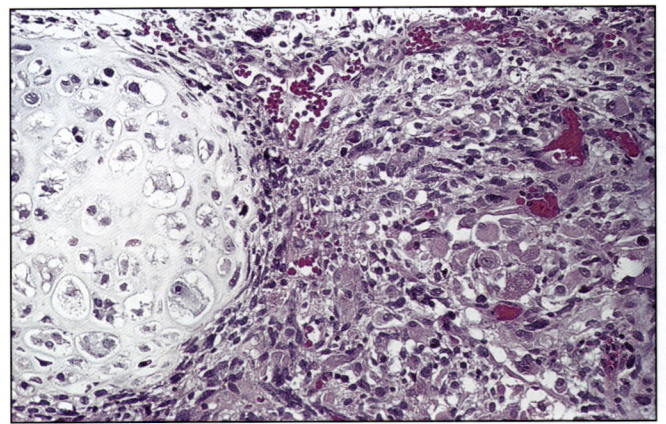

图13A.32 混合性中胚层肿瘤（癌肉瘤）。出现在本例的肉瘤性成分包括软骨肉瘤和横纹肌肉瘤。左侧，非典型性软骨细胞位于恶性软骨的陷窝中；右侧，有伴有丰富嗜酸性胞浆的圆形横纹肌母细胞。

细胞中[292,310]。这些透明小体 PAS 染色阳性，而且少数透明小体 α₁- 抗胰蛋白酶免疫反应阳性。据报道个别的MMT 病例显示滋养细胞或神经外胚层分化，或者表达甲胎蛋白[311-313]。在诊断时腹膜或网膜转移的显微镜下研究一般显示癌和肉瘤混合存在，而淋巴结转移通常是单纯的癌[291,298]。据报道，晚期转移肉瘤性成分比例增加，或者完全是肉瘤成分[310,314-316]。

免疫组化染色可能有助于鉴别上皮和间叶成分[314,317,318]。上皮成分细胞角蛋白和上皮膜抗原阳性，而间叶成分 vimentin 阳性[319,320]。Desmin 和肌细胞生成素（myogenin）免疫染色有助于辨认横纹肌母细胞[314,317,318,321]。

腺肉瘤发生在比 MMT 患者更年轻的妇女，平均年龄是 50 多岁[322]。症状不具有特异性，多数肿瘤是单侧性的。与混合性中胚层肿瘤相反，多数患者表现为早期阶段肿瘤[322]。腺肉瘤易在盆腔和腹部复发，而且多数患者最终死于肿瘤[322,323]，术后放疗和化疗的作用还不完全清楚。

腺肉瘤是大的部分囊性的肿瘤，直径 10～15cm。显微镜下，腺肉瘤是一种混合性的肿瘤，其中的间叶成分为恶性，而上皮成分为良性[322,323]。上皮内衬囊肿，被覆囊肿内的乳头或息肉样的间质赘生物，并内衬肿瘤实性成分的长的裂隙和单管状腺体。上皮从未分化的立方细胞到柱状的子宫内膜样细胞或纤毛性输卵管型细胞。某些肿瘤出现局灶性鳞状或黏液性化生。间叶成分通常是纤维肉瘤或子宫内膜样间质肉瘤，虽然偶尔出现异源性的肉瘤成分，例如横纹肌肉瘤或软骨肉瘤。囊肿内衬上皮下方和腺体周围间质细胞丰富，而远离囊肿和腺体的部位细胞稀少，胶原较多。核非典型性的程度通常为轻或中度。核分裂象总是出现，每 10 个高倍视野通常为 4 个或 4 个以上。间质偶尔出现性索样分化，而且多数腺肉瘤显示肉瘤过度生长，其中上皮缺失，富于细胞的恶性间质弥散生长。复发性肿瘤可以是单纯的肉瘤或为腺肉瘤。不良的预后因素包括诊断时年龄较轻、肿瘤破裂、高级别的肉瘤成分，以及肉瘤过度生长[322]。

子宫内膜样间质肉瘤
Endometrioid stromal sarcoma

子宫通常是间质肉瘤的原发部位，但它也可以发生于包括卵巢在内的子宫外部位[324]。患者年龄平均 50～55 岁，表现为腹胀或腹痛[325-328]。诊断时常常出现卵巢外播散。患有低级别间质肉瘤的妇女具有相对较好的短期预后，但是有相当比例的肿瘤复发，包括相当数量的诊断后 5 年以上复发的病例，某些患者死于肿

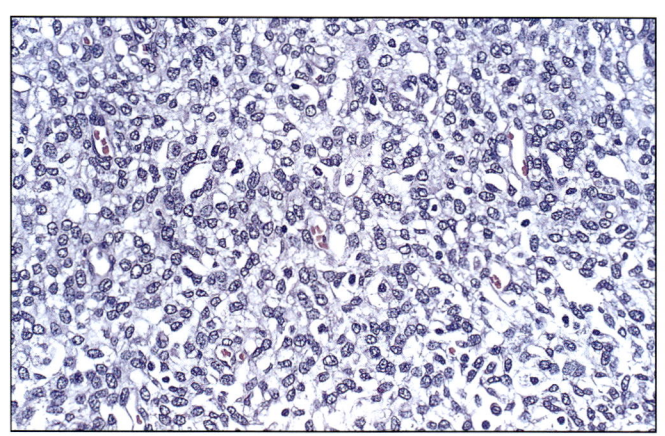

图13A.33　低级别子宫内膜样间质肉瘤。肿瘤细胞具有均匀一致的小而温和的细胞核，细胞界限不清。

瘤[327,328]。临床进展分析困难，因为随访资料有限。黄体酮、化疗或放疗的治疗价值并不清楚，尽管有对黄体酮治疗反应良好的个别报告[329]。高级别间质肉瘤似乎更具有侵袭性的临床经过。

间质肉瘤直径平均 11cm。多数肿瘤是实性或囊实性的，切面褐色、黄色或白色，伴有局灶出血或坏死。显微镜下，低级别间质肉瘤由小细胞组成，类似于增生期子宫内膜间质细胞[326-328,330,331]。它们具有均匀一致的圆形、卵圆形或梭形的深染细胞核，核染色质细，核仁不明显（图 13A.33）。胞浆稀少，细胞界限不清。细胞学非典型性轻微，核分裂象少见。偶尔可见局灶性上皮样分化[328]。一旦肿瘤侵袭到卵巢外，就有显著的肿瘤细胞巢和细胞条索浸润卵巢实质并有淋巴管浸润。偶尔可以证实来源于（或伴有）卵巢子宫内膜异位症。高级别间质肉瘤是由非典型性较为显著或核分裂活性增高（≥10/10HPF）的细胞组成的[327]。

主要的鉴别诊断是子宫的子宫内膜间质肉瘤转移到卵巢和卵泡膜细胞瘤。子宫内膜间质肉瘤常常侵犯附件和扩展至卵巢。任何患有卵巢间质肉瘤的妇女都应该仔细检查子宫，子宫切除术应该作为手术治疗的一部分[327]。低级别间质肉瘤可能含有类似于卵泡膜细胞瘤的纤维性区域。彻底的组织学评估通常可以发现典型的间质肉瘤区域，抑制素（inhibin）免疫组化染色阴性，而在卵泡膜细胞瘤通常阳性。

透明细胞肿瘤　Clear cell tumors

最初认为透明细胞肿瘤起源于中肾，但 Scully 和 Barlow 发现透明细胞肿瘤来源于子宫内膜异位症或表面上皮[332]。多数透明细胞肿瘤是癌，但是良性和交界性的透明细胞肿瘤也可发生[27,184,257,333,334]。患有交界性透明细

胞肿瘤的妇女通常具有良好的预后，但也有个别患者发生转移或死于肿瘤[42,334]。90%以上的透明细胞肿瘤是癌。这种类型的癌占所有卵巢癌的5%～10%[261,335-337]。有关透明细胞癌的许多研究显示，本病存活率好，或至少相当于其他上皮性肿瘤[261,337-343]。新近的报告倾向于将透明细胞癌看作是一种不好的组织学类型，与其他常见的上皮性肿瘤相比，晚期预后较差，而且对以铂为基础的化疗效果不佳[247,344-349]。有人提示，与以往单纯应用以铂为基础的治疗方案相比，紫杉醇（paclitaxel）和铂（platinum）联合应用可以改善预后[350]。透明细胞癌可以发生几种副肿瘤综合征（paraneoplastic syndrome）[351]。透明细胞癌与高钙血症的关系可能比其他类型的上皮性癌更为密切[344]，患有透明细胞癌的妇女还多半出现血栓栓塞，例如深静脉血栓形成和肺栓子[345,346]。有一例患有由转移性透明细胞癌引起高钙血症的患者，其血清中发现甲状旁腺激素相关蛋白，原发性卵巢癌和转移可以解释高钙血症的原因[352]。

良性透明细胞肿瘤 Benign clear cell tumors

良性透明细胞肿瘤是单侧实性肿瘤，直径在3～15cm。仔细检查白色或褐色切面通常可见小的囊肿。显微镜下，所有的良性透明细胞肿瘤都是腺纤维瘤[184,333,334]。小管或囊肿内衬立方形或鞋钉样细胞，具有透明或颗粒状嗜酸性胞浆（图13A.34）。间质由梭形纤维母细胞和胶原束组成。没有细胞非典型性或核分裂活性。

交界性透明细胞肿瘤 Borderline clear cell tumors

交界性透明细胞肿瘤是单侧性以实性为主的肿瘤。典型者直径在10～15 cm。切面白色、灰白色或褐色，含有小到中等大小的囊肿。显微镜下，交界性透明细胞肿瘤是腺纤维瘤[27,333,334]。小管和囊肿内衬立方形或鞋钉样细胞，具有透明或嗜酸的胞浆，不规则的分布于纤维性间质中。偶尔，上皮复层或成簇，或表现为小而界限清楚的实性巢。出现轻到中度核的非典型性和散在的核分裂象（通常≤1/10HPF）可将交界性透明细胞肿瘤与良性透明细胞肿瘤区分开来。少数透明细胞肿瘤以微房性（parvilocular）方式生长，其中内衬透明细胞的囊肿被间质包绕。这些病例多数具有足够的非典型性或核分裂活性，可以将其归为交界性肿瘤。缺乏间质浸润可将透明细胞腺纤维瘤和透明细胞癌鉴别开来。如果将这种分类理解为包括具有上皮内癌的肿瘤的话，那么伴有显著核非典型性或核分裂象常见的非浸润性透明细胞腺纤维瘤就可以归入交界性肿瘤。只有在充分的组织学检查之后才能做出良性或交界性透明细胞肿瘤的诊断，因为透明细胞癌经常见到良性表现的区域。

透明细胞癌 Clear cell carcinoma

多数透明细胞癌是大的肿瘤，直径为10～30 cm不等。肿瘤呈实性，或较为常见的是部分囊性，其囊壁上具有灰-褐色结节状实性区域。切面质软，褐色或灰白色。局限于卵巢内（I期）的肿瘤通常为单侧性，但当将所有分期的肿瘤都考虑在内时，大约30%为双侧性。

显微镜下，可见不同的细胞类型，包括透明细胞、具有颗粒状嗜酸性胞浆的细胞，以及伴有透明或嗜酸性胞浆的鞋钉样细胞（图13A.35）[261,332,335,336,338,340]。通常可出现混合类型的细胞。透明细胞是立方形、矮柱状或多角形细胞，胞浆丰富而透明，核位于中央，呈空泡状，通常有显著的核仁。PAS染色和电子显微镜检查显示，它们具有丰富的胞浆内糖原。除了具有颗粒状嗜酸性胞

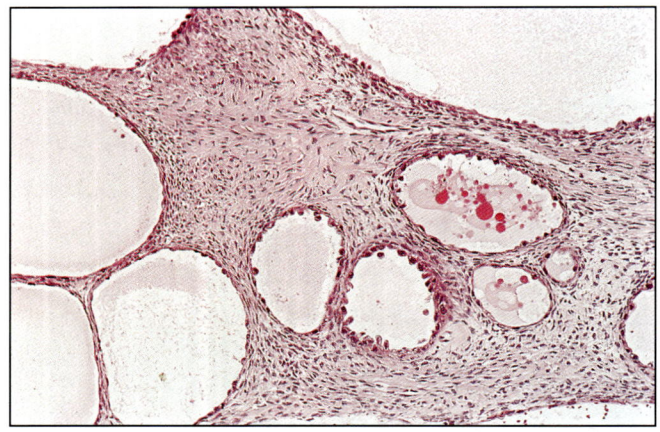

图13A.34 透明细胞腺纤维瘤。小管和囊肿内衬伴有透明胞浆的立方形到矮柱状细胞，周围绕以纤维性间质。注意"鞋钉样"核突入囊腔。

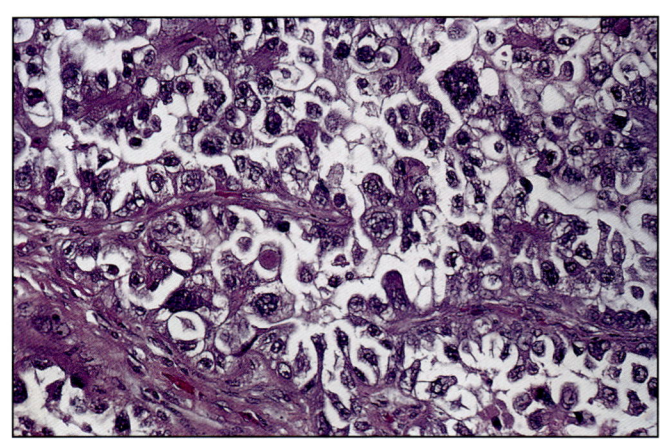

图13A.35 透明细胞癌。肿瘤细胞呈立方形或柱状。某些细胞具有透明胞浆，而另外一些细胞是双染性和颗粒状胞浆。核具有非典型性和多形性。某些细胞是"鞋钉"样细胞，核位于顶端并突入囊腔。注意左侧中央部位的嗜酸性透明小体。

浆以外，伴有嗜酸性胞浆的细胞的大小、形状以及核的特征均与透明细胞相似。鞋钉样细胞呈柱状，并且有颗粒状嗜酸性或透明胞浆。细胞核深染，位于顶端并突入囊腔。透明细胞癌的核分裂活性一般比其他类型的卵巢癌低；有人提出细胞增生比率低可能是化疗效果不佳的一个原因[349]。一组研究发现，具有高核分裂象比率的肿瘤预后不好[338]。

透明细胞癌的肿瘤细胞具有不同的方式生长，多数肿瘤显示混合性生长方式。在某些区域，肿瘤细胞内衬腺体、小管（图13A.36）或囊肿，或形成乳头。印戒样小管内衬具有透明胞浆的立方形细胞，其内充满嗜酸性分泌物，非常具有特征性。在其他部位，有由具有透明或嗜酸性胞浆的多角形细胞组成的实性生长区域（图13A.37）。嗜酸性透明小体常常散在分布于肿瘤细胞中[353]，间质或乳头的结缔组织轴心中常见无定形的嗜酸性透明物质。根据超微结构表现以及IV型胶原及层粘连蛋白的免疫组化染色，认为透明物质可能是基底膜样物质[343,354,355]。少见的嗜酸性透明细胞癌（oxyphilic clear cell carcinoma）主要是由大的多角形细胞组成，具有丰富的嗜酸性胞浆[356]。充分取材对于显示更加典型的透明细胞癌的区域是必要的，而且由此可以做出诊断。某些透明细胞癌混合有少量子宫内膜样癌或其他类型表面上皮性癌。透明细胞癌可以应用普通的分级方法（表13A.6）分级，但是多数研究显示，组织学分级没有预后意义[357]。

透明细胞癌与子宫内膜异位症密切相关，或在受累的卵巢内，或在盆腔其他部位[253,261,344,346,350]，而且偶尔有透明细胞癌直接来源于子宫内膜异位症的例子[332,358]。在某些系列中，伴有子宫内膜异位症的百分比超过50%，包括非典型性子宫内膜异位症[249,359]。

诊断透明细胞癌通常并不需要免疫组化染色。透明细胞癌CK7（表13A.5）和高分子量角蛋白染色阳性，而CK20阴性，雌激素受体可以阳性[360-362]。相反，转移性肾透明细胞癌CK7和高分子量角蛋白阴性，CD10和肾细胞癌抗原阳性，后两者在卵巢透明细胞癌均为阴性[360,363]。卵黄囊瘤偶尔也可出现鉴别诊断问题，尽管临床背景足够将其与透明细胞癌鉴别开来（见605页）。卵黄囊瘤CK7或上皮膜抗原（EMA）染色阴性，但甲胎蛋白染色呈片块状，通常是弱染色[364]。

Brenner瘤和移行细胞癌
Brenner tumor and transitional cell carcinoma

良性Brenner瘤　Benign Brenner tumor

Brenner瘤是腺纤维瘤的一种类型，其中移行上皮巢生长在纤维性间质中[365-371]。Brenner瘤占所有卵巢肿瘤的大约2%[366]。多数肿瘤较小并偶然发现[371]。大约20%与黏液性或浆液性囊腺瘤、良性囊性畸胎瘤或某些其他类型的良性畸胎瘤，例如卵巢甲状腺肿一起发生[367,372-374]。

大体检查，Brenner瘤是局限性的、质硬、淡黄或灰白色的实性纤维性肿瘤。多数Brenner瘤可有局灶钙化。少数Brenner瘤呈部分囊性，大约5%为双侧性[371,375]。大小从显微镜下可见到大于10cm不等，但是一般较小；肿瘤平均大小只有1~2cm。显微镜下，卵圆形或多角形上皮细胞巢或条索在纤维性间质中生长，类似于膀胱的泌尿道上皮细胞（图13A.38）。核圆形或卵圆形，有小的核仁。经常可见纵行的核沟，这是Brenner瘤的特征。胞浆从透明至致密和嗜酸性。微囊内衬移行细胞，或在细胞巢中偶尔出现化生的柱状宫颈内膜样黏液细胞，偶尔有局灶性鳞状上皮化生。间质由梭形纤维母细胞和不同比例的胶原组成。10%~15%的Brenner瘤间

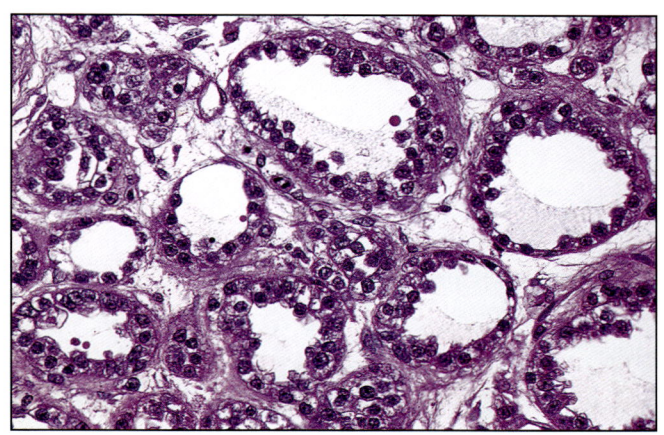

图13A.36　透明细胞癌，管囊型。小管内衬立方形细胞，具有透明胞浆和非典型性深染的细胞核。

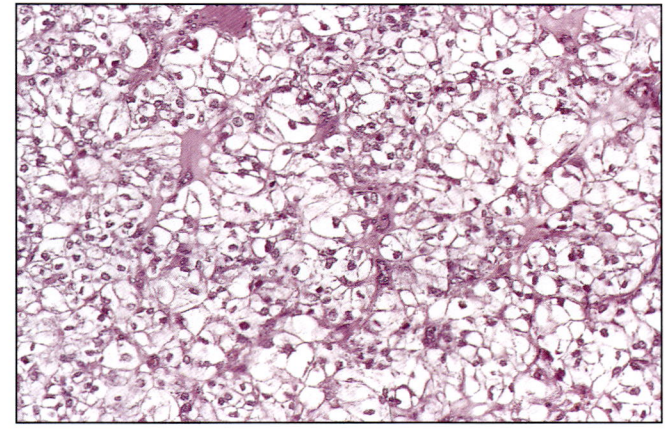

图13A.37　透明细胞癌。弥漫生长的多角形细胞具有丰富的透明胞浆。

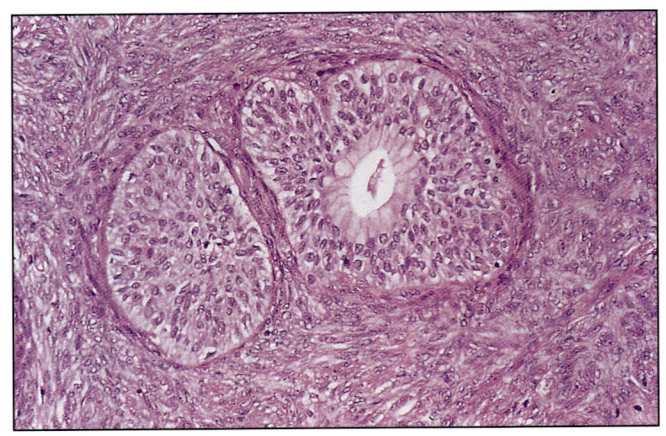

图13A.38　良性Brenner瘤。移行上皮细胞巢由纤维性间质围绕。在右侧细胞巢中，微囊内衬化生的柱状宫颈内膜样黏液细胞。

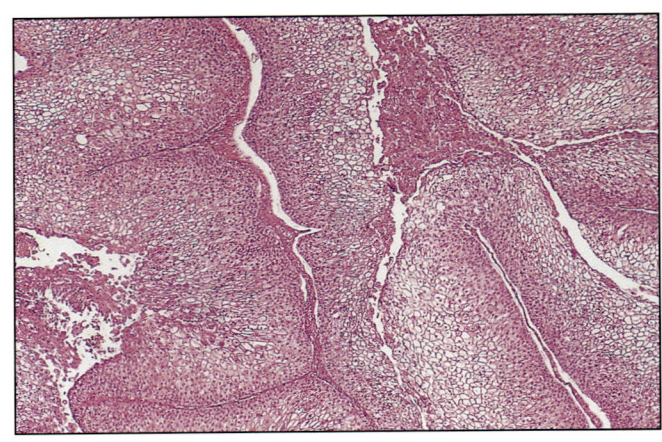

图13A.39　交界性（增生性）Brenner瘤。乳头被覆多层移行上皮。

质中出现黄素化细胞，在某些病例伴有类固醇激素分泌的证据，例如子宫内膜增生[367]。

交界性（增生性）Brenner瘤
Borderline (proliferating) Brenner tumor

交界性Brenner瘤传统上被称为"增生性"Brenner瘤，因为它们具有良性临床经过[376-381]。Roth等提出，交界性或中间型Brenner瘤可再分为增生性和潜在低度恶性两种类型，根据后者具有较大程度的核非典型性[377,382]。这一组中所有肿瘤的临床行为好像都是相似的，作者的观点是，它们只不过是低级别和高级别的交界性Brenner瘤。

交界性Brenner瘤通常为单侧性[378,381]。它们是局限性的白色或褐色肿瘤，明显大于良性Brenner瘤。直径为8～30cm不等，平均14cm。多数肿瘤部分或大部分为囊性，伴有息肉或易碎的乳头突向囊腔。显微镜下，上皮增生，类似于泌尿道的低级别乳头状移行细胞癌[377,378,380,381]。囊肿内衬大部分是由具有纤维血管轴心的宽的乳头组成，乳头被覆多层移行细胞（图13A.39）。囊肿的非乳头部分内衬相似的上皮。由纤维性间质围绕的低级别移行细胞巢可能出现在肿瘤壁上。肿瘤细胞具有均匀一致的轻度非典型的细胞核，核浆比例轻度增加。核分裂象一般不多，虽然某些肿瘤可能常见核分裂象[378]。某些增生性Brenner瘤中可见鳞状分化[381]。高级别交界性Brenner瘤不同于低级别的主要特征是具有较大程度核的非典型性[377]。如果在非浸润性Brenner瘤中见到明显的核非典型性和核分裂活性，可以诊断上皮内癌[383]。交界性Brenner瘤可能有较显著的上皮增生，但它完全是局限性的，通常在囊内，没有间质浸润。多数交界性Brenner瘤混有灶状良性Brenner瘤，或与其相邻。

恶性Brenner瘤和移行细胞癌
Malignant Brenner tumor and transitional cell carcinoma

恶性Brenner瘤是一种癌，其特征是移行细胞癌、鳞状细胞癌或未分化癌伴有灶状的良性或交界性Brenner瘤[382,384,385]。不伴有良性Brenner瘤的移行细胞类型的癌叫做移行细胞癌[382,386,387]。区分恶性Brenner瘤和移行细胞癌很重要，因为后者侵袭性较强，但是化疗可能有效[384]。近年来的倾向是较常诊断移行细胞癌。它占原发性卵巢癌的5%～10%[388]，某些研究显示在高分期的癌中甚至占有更大的比例[386,389]。有人报道，移行细胞癌化疗很可能有效，而且比其他高级别晚期卵巢癌有更好的生存率[386,388,390,391]，但并非所有的作者都能证实这一点[389,392]。

恶性Brenner瘤是单侧性的，直径为5～25cm不等。多数为大的部分囊性的肿瘤，平均直径15cm[378,384]。实性区域灰白色、黄色或褐色，经常有钙化。显微镜下，恶性Brenner瘤类似于泌尿道高级别移行细胞癌[376,380,384,385,393,394]。肿瘤细胞多角形，伴有中等量的双染性胞浆和多形性非典型性细胞核（图13A.40）。没有核沟，核分裂象多见。移行上皮内衬囊肿，被覆宽的乳头并浸润间质，表现为融合的肿块或不规则的细胞条索和细胞巢。鳞状或腺体分化常见[384]。在诊断恶性Brenner瘤时，必须有混合存在的良性或交界性肿瘤，或在癌的附近见到良性或交界性肿瘤[385]。

移行细胞癌是部分囊性的肿瘤，平均直径10cm，当局限于卵巢时通常为单侧性[386,387]。显微镜下，除了不能发现良性或增生性Brenner瘤外，移行细胞癌类似于恶性Brenner瘤的表现[384]。常常混有其他类型的表面上皮性肿瘤，包括浆液性、子宫内膜样和未分化

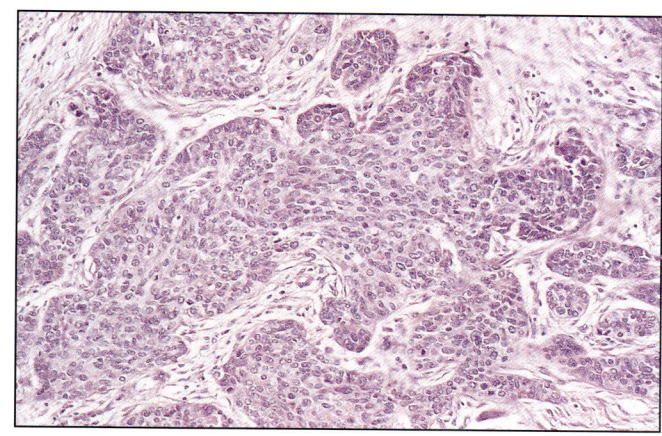

图13A.40 移行细胞癌。恶性移行细胞巢或细胞岛浸润纤维组织增生性间质。当移行细胞癌附近发现良性或增生性Brenner瘤时，诊断为恶性Brenner瘤。

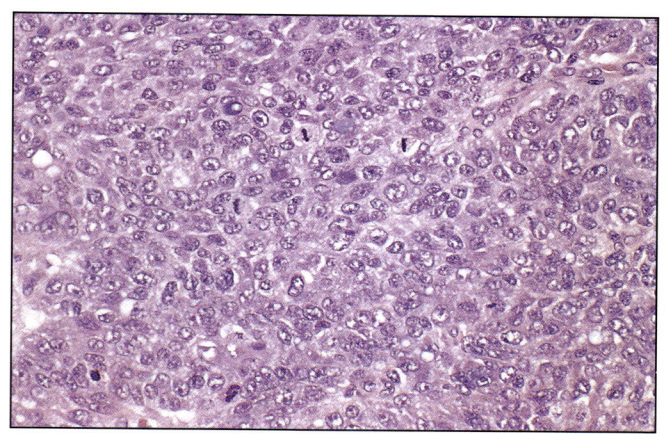

图13A.41 未分化癌。实性片块状间变性恶性细胞，伴有大的细胞核、显著的核仁和多数核分裂象。

癌[386]，但是必须以移行细胞癌为主时（即≥50%）才能做出诊断。两种显微镜下形态已被描述。最常见的形态是乳头状结构，具有显著纤维血管轴心和光滑腔面的粗乳头长入囊性间隙[386,389,390,395]。乳头和囊肿被覆复层恶性移行细胞，这些细胞具有中等量的嗜酸性胞浆和非典型性核，伴有一个或多个核仁。核分裂象较多。肿瘤实性部分有成巢或成片的恶性移行细胞浸润间质。肿瘤细胞中常常出现微小间隙和裂隙样窗孔，既可出现在乳头状区域也可出现在实性生长区域。可见局灶黏液性或鳞状分化、梭形细胞分化和不规则的腺体结构。多数移行细胞癌分化差，常见坏死灶。其次，少见的形态是"恶性Brenner型"移行细胞癌，主要为实性生长，伴有恶性移行细胞巢或条索浸润突出的纤维性间质（图13A.40）[382,387]。在移行细胞癌中，转移性肿瘤的镜下表现可能是重要的。一项研究显示，类似于移行细胞癌转移的患者比类似于其他类型卵巢癌（通常为浆液性癌）转移的患者生存率高[386]。

卵巢Brenner瘤和移行细胞癌的免疫组化研究显示，癌胚抗原、CA19-9抗原、细胞角蛋白、上皮膜抗原、细胞角蛋白7阳性（见表13A.5）[394,396,397]。良性Brenner瘤的免疫染色结果提示向泌尿道上皮分化，包括Uroplakin III、血栓调节素（thrombomodulin）和细胞角蛋白20阳性[398-400]。另一方面，移行细胞癌的免疫组化染色类似于卵巢其他类型的表面上皮性癌；没有提示泌尿道上皮分化的染色结果。移行细胞癌Uroplakin III、血栓调节素和细胞角蛋白20染色阴性[396,401]，而雌激素受体、WT-1和CA-125通常阳性[398,399,402]。卵巢与膀胱移行细胞癌之间的免疫表型差异可以用于病理医师关心的那些罕见病例，也就是看卵巢肿瘤是否是由泌尿道移行细胞癌转移而来[396,403-405]。

未分化癌 Undifferentiated carcinoma

大约5%的卵巢癌由于分化太差而难以归类，被称为"未分化癌"[262,406]。多数未分化癌病例在诊断时已播散到卵巢以外，而且多数患者不能被最佳地减缩肿块体积[406]。在任何类型的表面上皮性癌中，未分化癌的预后最差。一项研究显示，35例未分化癌患者，有29例在3年内死于肿瘤。6例存活超过3年的患者，5例最终死于肿瘤[406]。

未分化癌是一种大的以实性为主的肿瘤，伴有局灶出血和坏死。多数为双侧性[406]。显微镜下，癌呈片块状生长，多形性上皮细胞具有大的空泡状核、显著的核仁和不同量的胞浆（图13A.41）[262,406]。核非典型性显著，核分裂象多见，并且可能出现异常的奇异瘤巨细胞。某些肿瘤可见结构不甚清楚的腺体，具有模糊鳞状或移行特征的区域，或恶性细胞巢和条索。可能需要免疫组化染色显示细胞角蛋白或上皮膜抗原阳性，以证实肿瘤是癌。多数病例B72.3免疫染色阳性，大约50%的病例OC125染色阳性[406]。

罕见类型的癌 Rare types of carcinoma

卵巢癌通常可以归类为一种常见的类型。不常见类型的癌仅占少数，包括神经内分泌癌、鳞状细胞癌、肝样癌和伴有局灶恶性生殖细胞肿瘤分化的癌。

最常见的卵巢神经内分泌癌是小细胞癌（small cell carcinoma），形态上与肺和其他部位的小细胞癌相似[237,330,407]。这种类型的癌常常是指"肺"型小细胞癌，不同于仅发生在卵巢的血钙过高性小细胞癌（见

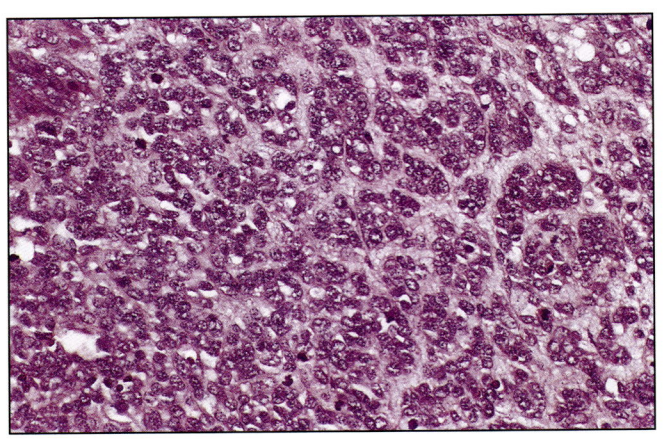

图13A.42 神经内分泌型小细胞癌。肿瘤发生于黏液性癌附近。肿瘤细胞胞浆稀少，核均匀一致，深染，圆形，有许多核分裂象。

616页）。神经内分泌性小细胞癌由成巢或片块状分布的小到中等大小的细胞组成，细胞核深染，圆形到卵圆形，核染色质细颗粒状，核仁不明显或缺乏（图13A.42）。邻近细胞的细胞核经常彼此挤压变形。胞浆稀少淡染，细胞界限不清。免疫表型不定。大约半数病例细胞角蛋白或上皮膜抗原阳性。神经元特异性烯醇化酶或CD56染色一般阳性，但嗜铬素或突触素染色仅见于少数肿瘤。由较大或较多形性细胞组成的神经内分泌癌也可发生于卵巢[240,407]。这些肿瘤称为大细胞神经内分泌癌，组成肿瘤的细胞具有空泡状核、核仁大，胞浆丰富，或者由具有粗染色质的深染核的细胞组成，有多个核仁和中等量的双染性胞浆。细胞成巢状、片块状或小梁状生长，并可形成结构不清的腺体。在大细胞神经内分泌癌中，上皮和神经内分泌标志物一般阳性。多数神经内分泌癌与表面上皮类型的肿瘤密切相关，最典型的或为子宫内膜样癌或为黏液性癌，而且可能来源于上皮性肿瘤内的神经内分泌细胞[236-240,408,409]。卵巢神经内分泌癌的临床表现和转移方式类似于其他类型的卵巢癌，预后不好。卵巢神经内分泌癌患者偶可发生副肿瘤综合征（paraneoplastic syndrome），例如由肿瘤细胞分泌甲状旁腺激素而引起的高钙血症[410]。在鉴别诊断中必须考虑来自肺和其他部位的转移性神经内分泌癌[411-413]。甲状腺转录因子1（TTF-1）的表达并不一定代表小细胞癌是来自于肺的转移，因为相当数量的非肺小细胞癌也表达TTF-1[414-416]。

鳞状细胞癌不常发生于卵巢。多数病例是发生于良性囊性畸胎瘤的继发性肿瘤；这种类型的卵巢鳞状细胞癌在畸胎瘤一节中讨论（见612页）。卵巢鳞状细胞癌可从宫颈或其他原发部位转移而来，它可以发生于混合性表面上皮性肿瘤、恶性Brenner瘤，或原发性或转移性子宫内膜样型腺鳞癌，因此，在做出纯粹的原发性卵巢鳞状细胞癌诊断之前，必须仔细寻找其他成分。卵巢非畸胎瘤性鳞状细胞癌起源于子宫内膜异位症、表皮样囊肿或者表面上皮[417,418]。它倾向于是一个以实性为主的肿瘤，伴有小的囊肿。恶性鳞状细胞呈实性片块状生长，浸润间质，被覆囊肿或乳头，某些肿瘤为梭形细胞生长方式。预后与分期和分级紧密相关，因为多数卵巢鳞状细胞癌被发现时已是晚期，所以整体预后很差。

某些罕见的、显然是原发性的卵巢癌，发生于老年妇女，组织学上类似于肝细胞癌。这些肿瘤被称为肝样癌（hepatoid carcinoma），由具有空泡状核和丰富的嗜酸或透明胞浆的多角形细胞组成[419]。见于某些或所有这种肿瘤中的另外一些肝样分化的特征包括：肿瘤细胞和间质中的玻璃样小体，抗肝细胞抗体、甲胎蛋白和白蛋白的免疫反应，多克隆癌胚抗原染色的小管状形态，以及胆汁染色阳性[420-423]。需要考虑的主要鉴别诊断是卵黄囊瘤的肝样亚型和转移性肝细胞癌[419,424,425]。所有这些肿瘤抗肝细胞抗体和甲胎蛋白免疫反应均为阳性，因此鉴别诊断必须结合组织学和临床表现[420]。某些肝样癌与其他类型的表面上皮性癌混合存在，表明它是起源于卵巢[421]。

如同其他器官的腺癌一样，卵巢表面上皮性癌偶尔也可以局灶分化成恶性生殖细胞成分。少数癌分泌人绒毛膜促性腺激素（HCG）或含有散在的滋养细胞[312,426,427]，但是伴有绒毛膜分化的癌（carcinoma with differentiation into choriocarcinoma）仅有少数报道[428]。除了原来的癌以外，这些患者的肿瘤含有出血性结节，结节内具有典型的绒毛膜癌的双相性结构，即出现细胞滋养细胞和合体滋养细胞。合体滋养细胞HCG免疫组化染色阳性。伴有绒毛膜癌分化的癌具有侵袭性的生物学行为，易于血行播散，具有绒毛膜癌的特征。少数起源于恶性上皮性肿瘤的卵黄囊瘤（yolk sac tumor arising from a malignant epithelial tumor）病例已有报告，通常是起源于子宫内膜样癌[276,277,429]。这些肿瘤具有卵黄囊瘤典型的组织学结构，甲胎蛋白免疫反应阳性，并分泌甲胎蛋白进入血液。这种肿瘤的预后似乎较差。

性索-间质肿瘤
Sex cord-stromal tumors

来源于性索或卵巢间叶的肿瘤占所有卵巢肿瘤的5%～12%（表13A.7）[1,3]。在纤维瘤-卵泡膜细胞瘤组的

表13A.7	卵巢性索-间质肿瘤

性索-间质肿瘤

颗粒细胞瘤
　　成年型
　　幼年型
卵泡膜细胞瘤
　　典型性
　　黄素化性
纤维卵泡膜细胞瘤
纤维瘤
　　典型性
　　富于细胞性
纤维肉瘤
伴有少量性索成分的纤维瘤或卵泡膜细胞瘤
Sertoli-Leydig细胞瘤
　　高分化
　　中分化
　　低分化
　　网状型（伴有异源性成分）
Sertoli细胞瘤
伴有环状小管的性索肿瘤（SCTAT）
Leydig细胞瘤
类固醇细胞瘤（脂质细胞瘤）
两性母细胞瘤
硬化性间质瘤
间质黄体瘤
卵巢非特异性软组织肿瘤
淋巴瘤和白血病
未分类肿瘤

良性肿瘤相对常见。其他性索-间质肿瘤和间叶肿瘤罕见。

颗粒细胞瘤　Granulosa cell tumor

颗粒细胞瘤占所有卵巢肿瘤的1%～2%，是最常见的恶性性索-间质肿瘤[1,430]。有两种类型的颗粒细胞瘤：一种是成年型，主要发生于绝经后妇女，一种是幼年型，主要发生于儿童。

成年型颗粒细胞瘤
Adult granulosa cell tumor

临床表现　成年型颗粒细胞瘤最常见于绝经后妇女[431-435]。这些肿瘤发生的年龄范围广泛，从青少年到老年。平均年龄50～55岁。典型的颗粒细胞瘤分泌雌激素，刺激子宫内膜增生。常见的症状是老年妇女绝经后出血以及绝经前妇女月经过多、子宫不规则出血或闭经[436]。子宫内膜的活检显示30%～40%的患者子宫内膜增生，5%～10%的患者有子宫内膜腺癌[433,437-441]。少数成年型颗粒细胞瘤分泌雄激素并引起男性化，大多发生于15～35岁的年轻妇女[442-446]。典型的症状包括多毛症、阴蒂肥大、声音变粗和闭经[442]。大约25%的颗粒细胞瘤患者具有非特异性症状，例如腹胀、腹痛或者可触及的肿块。肿瘤破裂或扭转，以及肿瘤内出血可以引起急腹症。少数颗粒细胞瘤发生于妊娠妇女[447]。

多数颗粒细胞瘤患者有可触及的单侧附件肿块；双侧性肿瘤少见。在诊断时，80%～90%病例的肿瘤局限于卵巢（FIGO I期）[433,434,437,448]。标准的治疗是腹式全子宫切除术和双侧输卵管卵巢切除术。对于希望保留生育力的IA期年轻妇女，单侧输卵管卵巢切除术是恰当的治疗。所有的颗粒细胞瘤均具有恶性潜能，虽然多数并不复发或转移。IA期肿瘤的复发率在10%～15%，总的复发率在20%～30%[432-434,438,449,450]。卵巢外播散到腹膜和网膜，偶尔播散到肝或肺[451,452]。当诊断时出现腹腔内播散（III期）或肿瘤复发时，多达2/3的患者死于肿瘤[432,435,439]。颗粒细胞瘤生长缓慢，转移常常见于首次治疗5年以后[433,435,439,441]。无病生存超过20年的病例已有报告[453]。某些晚期或复发性颗粒细胞瘤患者对包括顺铂在内的联合化疗有反应[436,454-456]，但是这种反应很少持久。放疗的价值还不清楚[431]。

在颗粒细胞瘤患者的血清中已经发现了几种潜在的肿瘤标记物，包括雌二醇、Müller抑制物（Müllerian inhibiting substance）[457]、滤泡调节蛋白[458]和抑制素[459]。抑制素（inhibin）已成为应用最广泛的肿瘤标志物，因为几乎所有的原发性或复发性颗粒细胞瘤患者血清中抑制素的水平均有所提高[460,461]。抑制素对颗粒细胞瘤并不特异，因为抑制素血清浓度增高在卵巢其他类型肿瘤中也可见到[462,463]，不过一旦诊断确定，它可用于监测治疗和检测复发。

病理学　颗粒细胞瘤从小的直径仅有几个毫米的偶然发现的结节，到直径超过30cm的巨大肿瘤不等。平均直径大约10cm。某些肿瘤完全实性，但是多数为部分囊性。实性部分粉红色、褐色、棕色或浅黄色，质地不同，从软到硬。少数颗粒细胞瘤表现为大的囊肿，囊壁厚度仅有几毫米。与其他颗粒细胞瘤相比，这些肿瘤可能更具男性化特征[443,450]。

显微镜下，肿瘤细胞类似于正常颗粒细胞。细胞小、圆形、立方形或梭形，胞浆浅淡，细胞界限不清。核圆形或卵圆形，染色质细，伴有单个小的核仁（图13A.43）。许多细胞核内可见纵向核的皱褶或核沟，这是成年型颗粒细胞瘤的特征。这些肿瘤可以出现核分裂象以及核的多形性和非典型性，但不常见。某些肿瘤可见伴有奇异核的细

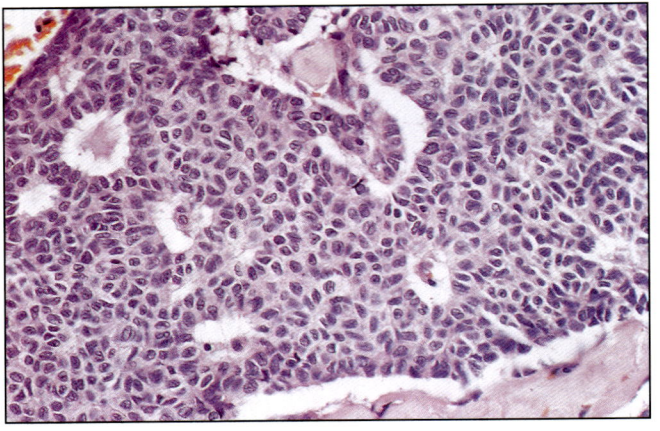

图13A.43　成年型颗粒细胞瘤。细胞形态单一，具有一致的核沟。注意Call-Exner小体。Call-Exner小体是微囊性间隙，含有嗜酸性分泌物或细胞碎屑，内衬栅栏状排列的颗粒细胞。

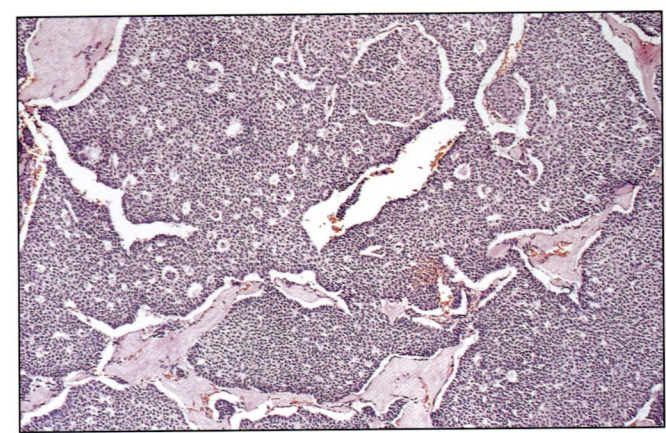

图13A.45　成年型颗粒细胞瘤。微滤泡结构，在弥漫性增生的肿瘤性颗粒细胞内可见较多Call-Exner小体。

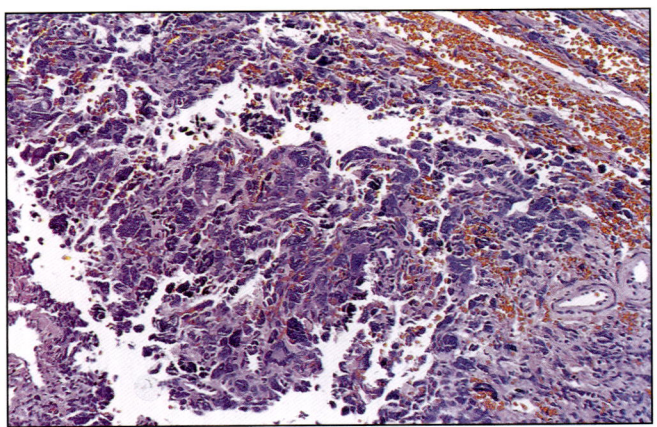

图13A.44　成年型颗粒细胞瘤。肿瘤细胞具有局灶奇异性核。

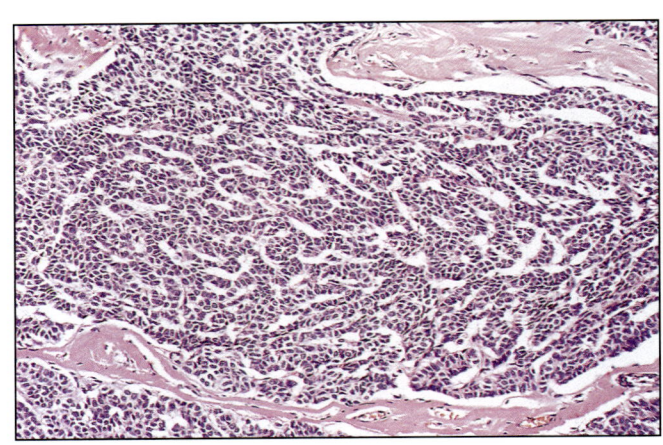

图13A.46　成年型颗粒细胞瘤。小梁状结构，由带状和条索状的肿瘤性颗粒细胞组成。

胞（图13A.44），但对预后并无不良影响[464-466]。大约1%的成年型颗粒细胞瘤的细胞有广泛的黄素化。黄素化的颗粒细胞具有丰富的嗜酸性胞浆，细胞界限清楚，核位于中央，类似于黄体的黄素化颗粒细胞。黄素化颗粒细胞瘤（luteinized granulosa cell tumor）发生在妊娠[447]、产生男性性征肿瘤患者[442]或是特发性的表现[467]。

几种组织学形态已有描述。这些形态常常是混合存在的，但是没有预后意义。微滤泡结构（microfollicular pattern）最具有特征性，由具有小的腔隙的成巢或成片的颗粒细胞组成，腔隙内含有嗜酸性分泌物和细胞碎屑（图13A.45）。这种腔隙类似于发育中滤泡的Call-Exner小体。巨滤泡结构（macrofollicular pattern）是一种内衬复层颗粒细胞的大的常常是不规则形状的滤泡。小梁状结构（trabecular pattern），颗粒细胞排列成相互吻合的带状和条索状结构（图13A.46）；脑回状或水绸样结构（gyriform or watered-silk pattern），是不规则的波浪形带状结构；以及岛屿状结构（insular pattern），为局限性的细胞巢或细胞岛。实性或弥漫性结构（solid or diffuse pattern），细胞呈大而不规则的片块状生长，没有组织结构。许多颗粒细胞瘤含有大的囊肿，内衬单层或几层颗粒细胞。这些囊肿常常含有血液，而且囊肿和囊壁内常常出现充满含铁血黄素的巨噬细胞。罕见的囊性颗粒细胞瘤（cystic granulosa cell tumor）表现为大的单房性囊肿，内衬复层颗粒细胞，其中是微滤泡或小梁状生长区域。

颗粒细胞瘤含有不定量的纤维或卵泡膜细胞瘤性间质。具有明显的纤维-卵泡膜细胞瘤性间质的肿瘤从前被称为颗粒细胞卵泡膜细胞瘤（granulosa-theca cell tumor）。实际上，现在认为任何颗粒细胞成分占到10%以上的肿瘤均可归为颗粒细胞瘤。仅有少量颗粒细胞成分的肿瘤最好归入卵泡膜细胞瘤或伴有少量性索成分的纤维瘤[468]。少数颗粒细胞瘤含有异源性黏液上皮或为伴有黏液成分的混合性肿瘤[469-472]。据报道，少数颗粒细胞瘤伴有局灶性肝细胞分化[473,474]。

通过病理学检查难以预测颗粒细胞瘤的预后，尽管某些病理学表现与临床结果相关[432,433,475]。直径超过15cm的较大肿瘤、双侧性肿瘤，以及已经破裂或播散到卵巢外的肿瘤（例如，超过 FIGO IA 期）预后较差。分期是最有力的单一预后指征[476]。具有弥漫性中到重度核非典型性或高核分裂率（>2 或 4/10HPF）的肿瘤，似乎更易复发[434,435,448,449,477]。组织学结构与临床结果无相关性。

小的非肿瘤性颗粒细胞增生，可能类似于小的成年型颗粒细胞瘤，偶尔可发生于妊娠或产后妇女的卵巢[478]。与颗粒细胞瘤不同，这些增生的颗粒细胞较小，呈多灶性，局限于闭锁卵泡腔。它们不具有妊娠期颗粒细胞瘤的表现[447]。在血管腔内偶尔可以见到成条或成簇的非肿瘤性颗粒细胞，可能是手术期间或排卵时造成的误植[479]。这些小的良性颗粒细胞聚集，常常见于卵泡附近的血管间隙中，可能是一种人工假象，不应误认为是肿瘤细胞。

免疫组化染色对于诊断颗粒细胞瘤有用。几乎所有的颗粒细胞瘤 vimentin 阳性[480,481]。角蛋白染色结果取决于所用的抗体和组织是如何预处理的。多克隆性角蛋白抗体染色通常为阴性结果[482,483]，但是应用抗低分子量角蛋白 8 和 18 的单克隆性抗体（例如 Cam 5.2，AE1/3）有 30%～60% 的颗粒细胞瘤阳性[480,484,485]。点样或球样核周染色特别提示是颗粒细胞瘤，但某些肿瘤可见广泛的核周或弥漫性胞浆染色。在大约半数的阳性病例中，整个肿瘤细胞均呈阳性，而在其余的阳性病例，仅有少数细胞阳性。多数肿瘤平滑肌肌动蛋白（SMA）阳性，但颗粒细胞 desmin 一般阴性[485,486]。大约 50% 的颗粒细胞瘤显示 S-100 蛋白核或胞浆染色阳性[485]。大约 70% 的颗粒细胞瘤显示 CD99（MIC2 基因产物）膜的染色[487,488]。最有意义的阴性染色反应是上皮膜抗原（EMA），EMA 在颗粒细胞瘤中一致缺失[482,485,489]。最重要的阳性染色反应是 inhibin[490,491]。几乎所有的颗粒细胞瘤均显示 inhibin 胞浆阳性反应(图 13A.47)[275,492-498]。染色常常呈斑片状，染色强度不一，阳性反应对于颗粒细胞瘤并不特异，因为其他类型的性索-间质肿瘤也有阳性反应。多数上皮性肿瘤 inhibin 阴性，但是偶尔可以发现局灶性或弥漫性 inhibin 阳性染色[275,496,499]。Calretinin 是颗粒细胞瘤更加敏感的标志物，但是如同 inhibin 一样，它不特异，因为其他类型性索-间质肿瘤也阳性[497,500,501]。Calretinin 胞核和胞浆染色均呈阳性。上皮性肿瘤 Inhibin 偶尔染色阳性，间皮瘤 Inhibin 呈弥漫性强阳性染色[497]。用于诊断颗粒细胞瘤的免疫组化染色标志物应该包括 inhibin、calretinin、cytokeratin（包括 cytokeratin 8 和 18）、EMA，以及在某些情况下应用 LCA 和嗜铬素（chromogranin）（表 13A.8）。

幼年型颗粒细胞瘤
Juvenile granulosa cell tumor

少于 5% 的颗粒细胞瘤发生在儿童和青少年。其中多数具有特征性的临床病理学特征，已被称为幼年型颗粒细胞瘤[502-506]。

临床表现 幼年型颗粒细胞瘤可以发生于任何年龄，从婴儿到老年，但是多数发生在儿童[502,503,507,508]。患者平均年龄 15 岁。但在儿科肿瘤登记处的一项局限于儿童的研究中，平均年龄仅为 7.1 岁[509]。

症状经常由肿瘤分泌的雌激素引起[502,503,507,508,510]。月经前的女孩经常（50%～75%）有同性早熟假青春期，伴有乳腺发育、耻毛和腋毛生长、阴道出血以及骨龄增加。雌激素的影响可在阴道涂片中见到。大龄儿童和绝经前妇女有月经异常，包括闭经。1/3～1/2 的患者出现非特异性症状，例如腹胀、腹痛或可以触及的腹部肿块。少数患者由于肿瘤扭转或破裂而发生急腹症。

表 13A.8	卵巢肿瘤的免疫表型				
肿瘤	Inhibin	Cytokeratin	EMA	LCA	Chromogranin
颗粒细胞瘤	+	−/+	−	−	−
小细胞癌	−	+/−	+/−	−	+/−
Sertoli-Leydig 细胞瘤	+	+	−	−	−
癌	−	+	+	−	−
类癌	−	+	+	−	+
淋巴瘤	−	−	−	+	−

＋＝通常阳性；−＝通常阴性；＋/−＝可能阳性或阴性；EMA＝上皮膜抗原；LCA＝白细胞共同抗原

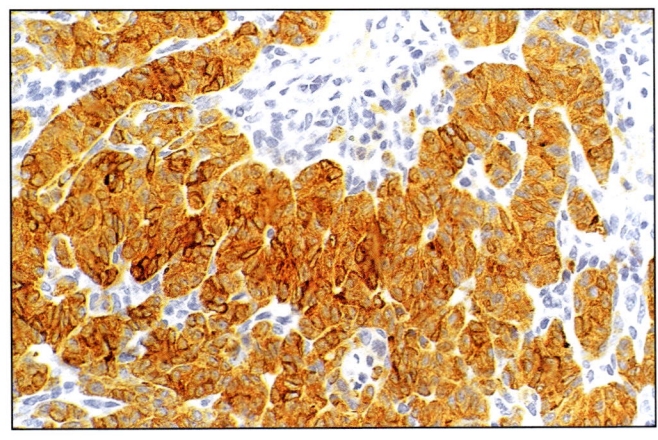

图 13A.47 成年型颗粒细胞瘤。肿瘤细胞 inhibin 免疫反应强阳性。

70%以上的患者有可触及的附件肿块。有极少数例外[509]，幼年型颗粒细胞瘤单侧发生，其中95%以上的肿瘤局限于卵巢（I期）。IC期肿瘤患者预后似乎较差，因此收集腹腔冲洗液用于细胞学评价十分重要。幼年型颗粒细胞瘤与Ollier（内生性软骨瘤病）和Mafucci（内生性软骨瘤病和多发性皮下血管瘤）综合征有关[502,505,510-513]。

幼年型颗粒细胞瘤在诊断时一般可见包膜，局限于一个卵巢（IA期），通过单侧输卵管-卵巢切除术来治疗已经足够[508]。因为多数患者年轻，子宫切除术和双侧输卵管-卵巢切除术应该用于少数晚期疾病（II、III或IV期）患者。长期生存率较高，但是出现肿瘤破裂、或显示阳性腹膜细胞学、或有卵巢外肿瘤播散的患者，具有明显复发的危险[502,503,506,514]。如果出现复发，通常在诊断后的3年内发现。晚期复发的病例少有报告[515]。某些具有晚期、持续性或复发性疾病的患者对以铂为基础的联合化疗有反应[516,517]。作为肿瘤标记物，inhibin和müller抑制物质对于发现和随访幼年型颗粒细胞瘤患者有用[518,519]。

病理学　幼年型颗粒细胞瘤直径为2.5～30cm不等，平均大约12cm。多数肿瘤具有混合性囊实性外观，但是有些完全为实性，而另外一些主要为囊性。实性区域黄色或褐色。出血常见，但坏死不常见。

显微镜下，肿瘤由混合性囊性和实性的小叶状或结节性区域组成（图13A.48）。巨滤泡、实性和囊性生长方式是幼年型颗粒细胞瘤的特征。在某些肿瘤，巨滤泡呈圆形且大小相对一致，而在另外一些肿瘤，滤泡大小明显不同，而且形状不规则（图13A.49）。巨滤泡含有黏液性物质，内衬一层或多层颗粒细胞，而且可能有一圈卵泡膜细胞围绕。实性区域由成片的颗粒细胞组成，混有不同量的梭形卵泡膜细胞或纤维母细胞性间质细胞。通常不出现成年型颗粒细胞瘤典型的生长方式，例如微滤泡和岛屿状结构，虽然有些肿瘤的颗粒细胞呈局灶性小梁状或小管样结构。这些肿瘤的颗粒细胞不同于成年型颗粒细胞瘤的颗粒细胞。其形状为多角形到梭形，具有数量不等、但通常是充分的双染性或粉红色胞浆。局灶性或广泛的黄素化是典型所见。肿瘤细胞核大，圆形，通常深染（图13A.50）。缺少核沟，可有显著的核仁。某些细胞有明显增大的多形性细胞核，而另外一些为多核细胞。核分裂象平均大约6个/10HPF。

有关幼年型颗粒细胞瘤的免疫组化研究很少。肿瘤细胞vimentin和inhibin阳性，低分子量细胞角蛋白染色大约半数病例阳性，calretinin染色胞核和胞浆阳性，CD99染色胞膜阳性[274,275,489,492-494,506,509,520]。Inhibin阳性染色有助于鉴别幼年型颗粒细胞瘤和高钙血症型小细胞癌以及卵黄囊瘤。后两者inhibin阴性[493]。最有帮助的

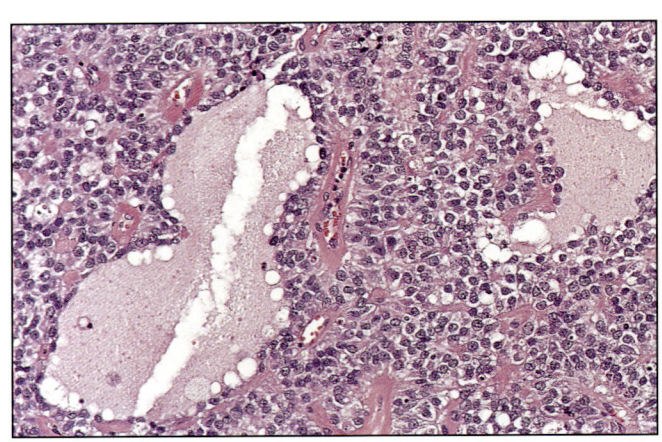

图13A.49　幼年型颗粒细胞瘤。不规则的巨滤泡内充满嗜酸性分泌物，周边围绕着弥漫性增生的肿瘤性颗粒细胞。

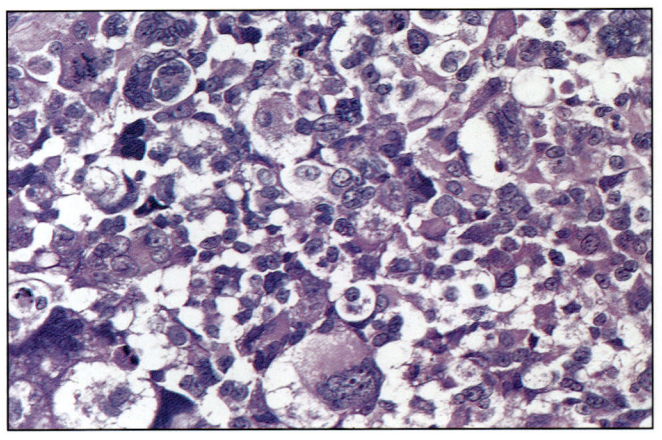

图13A.48　幼年型颗粒细胞瘤。典型的多结节状生长方式，伴有不规则的巨滤泡腔隙。

图13A.50　幼年型颗粒细胞瘤。肿瘤细胞黄素化并有嗜酸性胞浆。具有大而圆的细胞核，某些细胞具有明显非典型性。

阳性染色是 inhibin、calretinin 和 CD99，而最有帮助的阴性染色是 EMA。

卵泡膜细胞瘤 Thecoma

卵泡膜细胞瘤是性腺间质肿瘤，其细胞类似于卵泡内膜（theca interna）细胞。卵泡膜细胞瘤少见，占性索-间质肿瘤的7%[2]。

临床表现 卵泡膜细胞瘤发生于所有年龄的患者，但是多数发生在围绝经期或绝经后的妇女。患者平均年龄在50～55岁之间[2,430,431,437,439]。卵泡膜细胞瘤很少发生在儿童[509]。黄素化型卵泡膜细胞瘤发生年龄较轻，主要累及20多岁或30多岁的妇女[521]。老年患者通常表现为绝经后出血，但是多达25%的患者具有非特异性症状，例如盆腔或腹部疼痛或腹胀。后者可由大的肿瘤或由腹水引起。某些患者具有 Meigs 样综合征，伴有腹水和胸腔积液。绝经前妇女或者具有内分泌相关性症状，例如不规则出血或闭经，或者有不太特异的主诉，例如盆腔或腹部疼痛或腹胀。某些患者有男性化的表现，通常是黄素化的卵泡膜细胞瘤患者[521-523]。大约15%的患者，肿瘤分泌雌激素引起子宫内膜增生，其中多达30%的患者患有子宫内膜腺癌[437,439]。卵泡膜细胞瘤几乎都是良性的，手术切除是恰当的治疗方法[439]。实际上，并不发生卵巢外播散，但是大约5%的患者有双侧性肿瘤[430,431]。因为许多卵泡膜细胞瘤伴有子宫内膜增生或子宫内膜癌，所以子宫切除术伴有双侧输卵管-卵巢切除术是标准的治疗方法。对于年轻妇女，只要子宫内膜正常，单侧输卵管-卵巢切除术是足够的治疗。罕见的伴有明确的卵泡膜细胞瘤性分化的恶性肿瘤已有报告[521,523-525]。然而，已经证实报告为"恶性卵泡膜细胞瘤"的多数肿瘤是肉瘤样或黄素化的颗粒细胞瘤、纤维肉瘤，或其他类型的恶性间叶性肿瘤。

在少数情况下，硬化性腹膜炎（sclerosing peritonitis）发生在患有少见类型的黄素化卵泡膜细胞瘤的年轻妇女[526-530]。临床表现为腹胀，伴有慢性肠梗阻的症状或急腹症。多数患者有腹水，某些患者有胸腔积液。网膜、肠系膜和小肠的浆膜显示纤维性增厚和结节，常常伴有粘连和肠梗阻。这种病变好像是自限性的，通过切除卵巢肿瘤和局部腹部手术治疗已经足够，包括松解粘连、网膜切除术以及当需要缓解梗阻时进行肠切除术。某些病例核分裂率高，但是至今尚无复发和转移的报道，尽管几个患者死于肠梗阻和与腹膜病变有关的脓毒症。

病理学 卵泡膜细胞瘤是一种质硬的肿瘤。大小不同，从偶然发现的直径小于1cm的结节到直径大于20cm的肿块。平均直径大约7cm。切面灰色或褐色，通常伴有局灶性到广泛性的黄色区域。可能出现变性改变，例如囊肿和钙化。

显微镜下，肿瘤是由成束或成片的肥胖、梭形或卵圆形间质细胞组成的，类似于卵泡内膜细胞（图13A.51）。间质细胞具有淡染的圆形或梭形细胞核，伴有细致而弥散的染色质。胞浆双染性或轻度嗜酸性。某些细胞胞浆透明或含有空泡，最好应用未固定的冰冻切片进行脂肪染色加以证实（图13A.52）。在卵泡膜样细胞中混有不同数量的纤维母细胞。网状纤维染色显示单个肿瘤细胞周围有网状的原纤维围绕。玻璃样变的结缔组织斑块和微小钙化常见，而且在累及年轻妇女的卵泡膜细胞瘤中偶尔可见广泛的钙化[531]。邻近卵泡膜细胞瘤的卵巢皮质常常增生。

电子显微镜研究提示，纤维瘤和卵泡膜细胞瘤是由同样类型的细胞衍生而来的，它们的不同仅仅表现在形成胶原以及形成类固醇的细胞的比例上[532,533]。因此，发现难以归类为纤维瘤或卵泡膜细胞瘤的中间

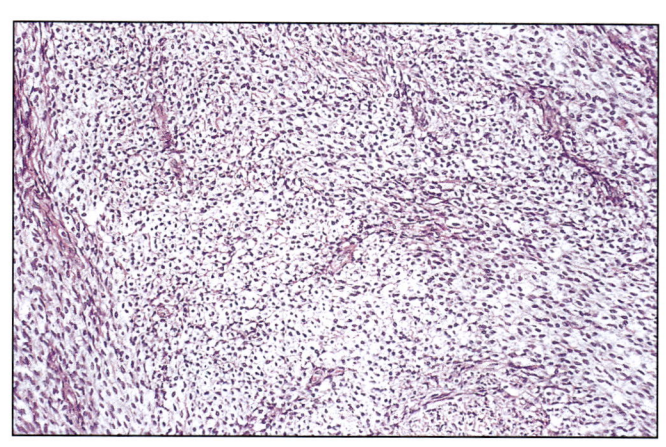

图13A.51 卵泡膜细胞瘤。浅淡的空泡状梭形细胞巢，细胞核小，位于中央。

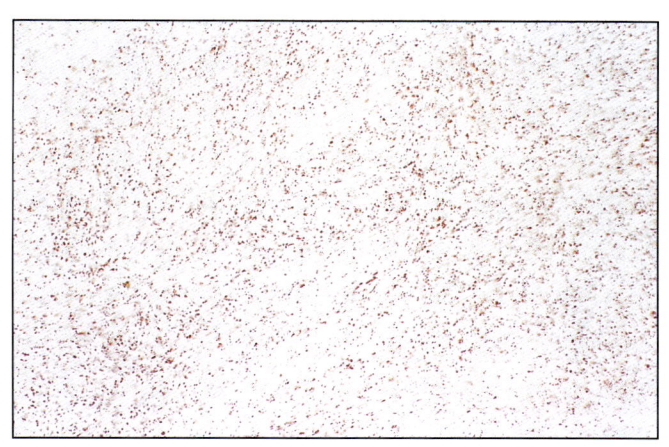

图13A.52 卵泡膜细胞瘤。油红O染色证明肿瘤细胞中有脂质。

类型并不奇怪。这些肿瘤被命名为纤维卵泡膜细胞瘤（fibrothecoma）。纤维卵泡膜细胞瘤和卵泡膜细胞瘤的不同之处在于，具有透明胞浆或胞浆脂质空泡的肿瘤细胞数目较少，而且通常是非功能性肿瘤（图 13A.53）。与纤维瘤不同，纤维卵泡膜细胞瘤细胞比较丰富，具有少量胶原、肥胖的肿瘤细胞，而且至少有少量的卵泡膜细胞。从实用的观点来看，卵泡膜细胞瘤的诊断应该限制在显示类固醇激素分泌证据的、或具有显著的伴有透明或空泡状胞浆的细胞成分的、或含有黄素化细胞的肿瘤，这将在下面讨论。含有许多 inhibin 免疫反应细胞的肿瘤也可以诊断为卵泡膜细胞瘤。在日常工作中，卵泡膜细胞瘤是一种不常见的诊断，而纤维瘤和纤维卵泡膜细胞瘤相对常见。

在卵泡膜细胞瘤-纤维瘤组中的某些肿瘤中，可以发现成簇、成巢或成片的黄素化细胞（图 13A.54）。不管肿瘤是卵泡膜细胞瘤、纤维卵泡膜细胞瘤还是纤维瘤，如果出现黄素化的肿瘤细胞，就可以诊断为黄素化的卵泡膜细胞瘤（luteinized thecoma）[521,522]。黄素化的卵泡膜细胞瘤可是雌激素性的（50%）、雄激素性的（11%）或为非功能性的（39%）[521]。几乎所有的雄激素性卵泡膜细胞瘤都是黄素化的卵泡膜细胞瘤。黄素化的卵泡膜细胞瘤与间质 Leydig 细胞瘤的唯一区别是后者出现胞浆内 Reinke 结晶。

少数含有卵泡膜细胞或黄素化细胞的性腺间质肿瘤在临床上是恶性的。可能提示恶性的特征包括肿瘤大、细胞丰富、核的非典型性和常见核分裂象（≥4/10HPF）[521,524,534]，但是恶性卵泡膜细胞瘤明确的组织学诊断标准还未建立。

卵泡膜细胞瘤 vimentin、inhibin 和 calretinin 免疫组化染色阳性，而 cytokeratin 阴性[275,484,492-495,497,500,520,535]。某些卵泡膜细胞瘤可以发现细胞遗传学异常，12 号染色体三体[536-539]。

伴有硬化性腹膜炎的卵巢肿瘤可以分为两类。某些患者具有大的纤维瘤性或卵泡膜细胞瘤性肿瘤，其间可见黄素化细胞（即它们是黄素化卵泡膜细胞瘤）[526,528]。这些肿瘤与普通的黄素化卵泡膜细胞瘤的不同之处在于它们倾向于双侧发生，而且黄素化细胞出现在小而界限不甚清楚的细胞簇中。另外，某些肿瘤仅仅部分黄素化。某些肿瘤有轻度的核非典型性，但核分裂象多（15～50个/10HPF）（图 13A.55）。其他一些具有双侧性结节状卵巢皮质梭形细胞增生的患者，可见不同但可能是相关的卵巢异常，表现为息肉样的外形，但并不形成分散的肿瘤团块[526,527,540,541]。这种病变可能是一种早期形式的间质瘤或少见类型的间质增生。在增生的间质细胞中可见散在分布的小簇状部分或完全黄素化的细胞。未见显著的核非典型性，但核分裂象可能较多。尽管核分裂活性令人担忧，但数量有限的随访病例没有转移性播散发生。高核分裂率是否是恶性潜能的指征目前尚不清楚。硬化性腹膜炎累及网膜、腹膜和肠的浆膜。浆膜增厚，伴有

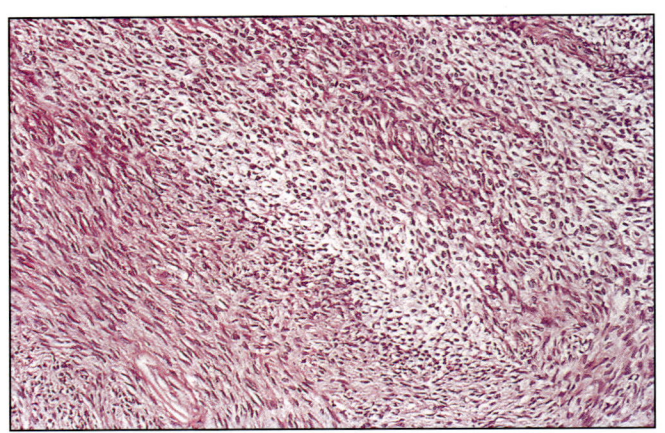

图13A.53 纤维卵泡膜细胞瘤。淡染的含有脂质的卵泡膜细胞混有纤维瘤特征性的梭形细胞区域。

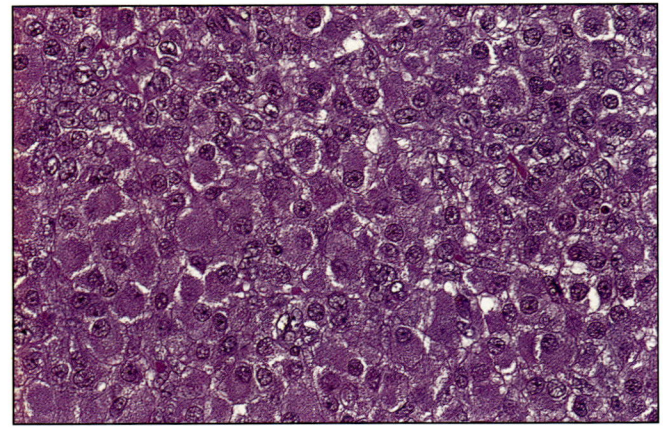

图13A.54 黄素化卵泡膜细胞瘤。弥漫性片块状黄素化卵泡膜细胞，具有丰富的嗜酸性胞浆。

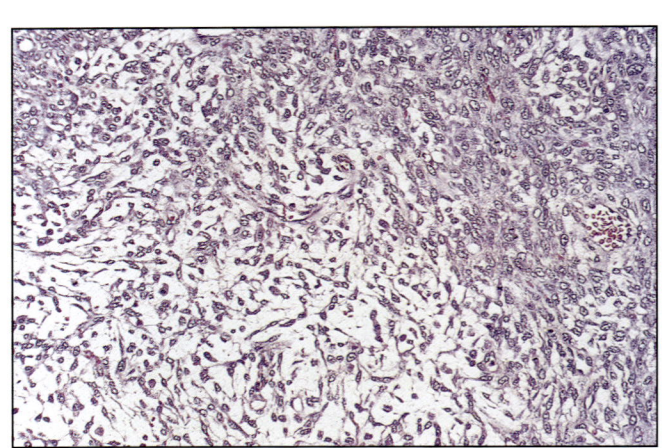

图13A.55 卵泡膜细胞瘤伴有硬化性腹膜炎。有明显的水肿。卵泡膜细胞肥胖，多数细胞具有明显的粉红色胞浆。可见多数核分裂象。

纤维母细胞和肌纤维母细胞增生、胶原沉积和局灶性炎症、间皮增生以及纤维蛋白沉积。

纤维瘤 Fibroma

卵巢纤维瘤是一种良性肿瘤，由纤维母细胞和胶原纤维组成。它是至今为止最常见的性索-间质肿瘤，占所有卵巢肿瘤的1%～5%[2,542,543]。纤维肉瘤可以发生于卵巢，但是罕见[544]。

临床特征 临床表现为非特异性。纤维瘤发生于20～80岁的患者，平均年龄50岁或者更大一些[2,543,545]。肿瘤常常较小，没有症状，只有当患者由于某些其他疾病手术时才能发现。大的纤维瘤、富于细胞性纤维瘤以及纤维肉瘤引起腹痛或腹胀，30%的患者有腹水[543]。Meigs综合征是不常见的情况，表现为卵巢纤维瘤伴有腹水和胸腔积液[546]。大约17%的痣样基底细胞癌综合征（nevoid basal cell carcinoma syndrome，表现为多发性皮肤基底细胞癌、牙源性角化囊肿以及其他异常）患者患有卵巢纤维瘤，可能是双侧性的[547]。

纤维瘤通过手术切除治疗已经足够。富于细胞性纤维瘤是一种不能确定恶性潜能的肿瘤。如果切除不完全，它具有局部侵袭性生长的能力，而且偶尔发生转移，说明鉴别富于细胞性纤维瘤和纤维肉瘤的标准尚不完善。纤维肉瘤是恶性间叶性肿瘤，预后不良。治疗方式是完整切除，随后化疗[544,548]。

病理学 纤维瘤是质硬的肿瘤，具有光滑的分叶状表面。大小从小于1 cm到大于10 cm不等，切面实性，白色或褐色。5%～10%的病例为双侧性。富于细胞性纤维瘤和纤维肉瘤大而质软，可有出血和坏死区。

纤维瘤由细长的梭形细胞组成，呈漩涡状和相互吻合的束状生长方式（图13A.56）。细胞核梭形，均匀一致。胞浆稀少，淡嗜酸性。肿瘤细胞周围有不等量的胶原间质。

纤维瘤中偶尔可见不规则的性索细胞小巢或小管。性索细胞呈多角形，具有均匀一致的细胞核和少量的胞浆；它们类似于未分化的性索细胞或颗粒细胞。当它们的数量少于肿瘤的10%时，性索细胞好像没有任何预后意义。含有性索细胞的肿瘤被称为伴有性索成分的纤维瘤（fibromas with sex cord elements）[468]。

少数纤维母细胞性肿瘤细胞丰富，细胞间几乎没有胶原。梭形肿瘤细胞排列成人字形、十字缝和席纹状结构。可以出现坏死，而且有时比较广泛。当核的非典型性为轻至中度，而且核分裂象≤3个/10HPF时，这样的肿瘤被称为富于细胞性纤维瘤（cellular fibromas）（图13A.57），而当核有中到重度非典型性，而且核分裂象≥4个/10HPF时，称为纤维肉瘤（fibrosarcoma）[544,548]。具有交界性核分裂计数的肿瘤难于精确分类，而且少数分类为富于细胞性纤维瘤的肿瘤可以复发或转移。增生指数和原位杂交研究（检测8号染色体三体）可能有助于这些肿瘤的分类[548,549]，但是并未得到广泛应用。将具有重于轻度核非典型性和核分裂象2～3个/10HPF的富于细胞性纤维瘤报告为不能确定恶性潜能的肿瘤，应取慎重态度。纤维肉瘤偶尔伴有另外一种类型的肿瘤，例如良性囊性畸胎瘤，而且还有一例纤维卵泡膜细胞瘤性肿瘤伴有少量性索成分的报告[550,551]。

12号染色体三体是卵巢纤维瘤一贯的细胞遗传学表现[536,537,552]。

Sertoli-Leydig细胞瘤 Sertoli-Leydig cell tumor

Sertoli-Leydig细胞瘤占卵巢肿瘤的不到1%[553]。有两种主要的临床病理学类型：

1. 高分化Sertoli-Leydig细胞瘤，占所有这类肿瘤的10%；

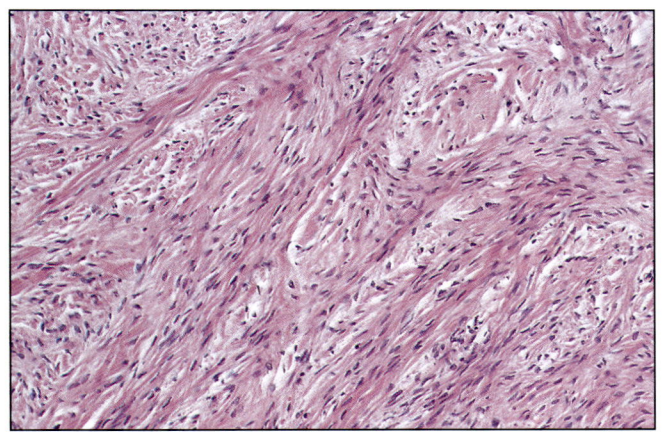

图13A.56 纤维瘤。温和的梭形纤维母细胞被丰富的嗜酸性胶原分开。

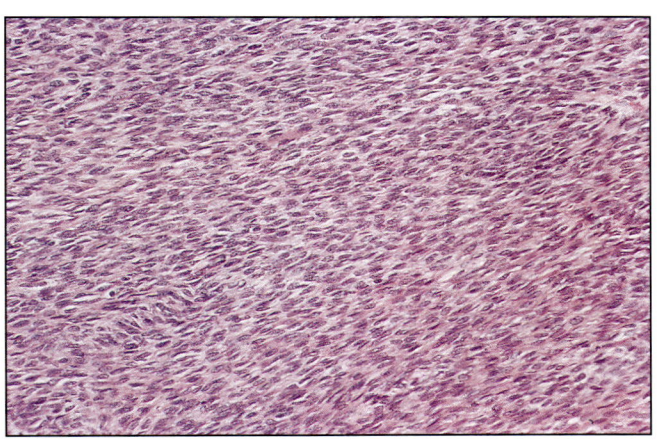

图13A.57 富于细胞性纤维瘤。肿瘤细胞丰富，但无核的非典型性或核分裂活性。

2. 中分化和低分化Sertoli-Leydig细胞瘤，构成其余的90%。

临床表现　Sertoli-Leydig细胞瘤主要发生于年轻妇女，偶尔发生于儿童和绝经后妇女[509]。平均年龄24岁，75%的患者在30岁以下[554-556]。高分化Sertoli-Leydig细胞瘤的妇女平均年龄40岁，比中分化和分化差肿瘤患者年龄高出10～15岁[554-556]。据报道，网状Sertoli-Leydig细胞瘤主要发生于较年轻的患者，平均年龄16岁[557-559]。然而，新近一组报告显示患者的平均年龄是31岁，说明除了年轻人以外，网状Sertoli-Leydig细胞瘤也可以发生于成年甚至老年妇女[560]。

大约50%的Sertoli-Leydig细胞瘤分泌类固醇激素，其分泌量足以引起症状，40%患者男性化[554-556]。男性化患者具有不同的症状，包括闭经、嗓音变粗、多毛症、暂时性脱发、阴蒂肥大和痤疮。男性化患者血清睾酮水平和尿17-酮类固醇水平增高。

非男性化患者表现为非特异性症状，例如异常阴道出血、腹胀、腹部肿块或者腹部或盆腔疼痛。5%～10%的患者由于肿瘤扭转或破裂而引起急腹症。偶尔，Sertoli-Leydig细胞瘤是在无症状的妇女中发现的。

Sertoli-Leydig细胞瘤倾向于单侧发生，在诊断时常局限于卵巢内（IA期）。诊断时少于5%的病例有卵巢外肿瘤播散，但是5%～15%的病例，肿瘤破裂或腹膜液体中有肿瘤细胞(FIGO Ic期)[554]。对于多数患者来说，单侧卵巢-输卵管切除术已经足够。对于老年患者，腹式全子宫切除术和双侧卵巢-输卵管切除术是恰当的治疗方式，对于出现不良预后因素的年轻患者来说也可考虑这种治疗方式，例如肿瘤破裂、卵巢外播散、低分化肿瘤伴有频现的间质细胞核分裂象，或有异源性间叶分化（软骨或骨骼肌，或局灶性神经母细胞瘤）[554,555]。肿瘤切除之后，男性化消退，月经恢复正常。少数Sertoli-Leydig细胞瘤分泌甲胎蛋白，但是准确的发生率尚不清楚，因为通常并不进行这种检测[557,559,561-566]。

高分化Sertoli-Leydig细胞瘤临床上表现良性，在完全切除后不再复发[555,567]。中分化和低分化Sertoli-Leydig细胞瘤的预后通常较好。一项研究发现仅有18%的患者复发[554]，另外一项研究发现5年生存率为92%[555]。与所有的肿瘤相比，网状Sertoli-Leydig细胞瘤预后略差[557,559]。复发一般出现在治疗之后最初几年。接受化疗的患者大约一半有效[454,554,568]。

病理学　高分化Sertoli-Leydig细胞瘤是实性、单侧性、有包膜的肿瘤，直径从1.5cm至10cm不等[567]。平均大小为5cm。切面黄色或黄褐色。中分化和低分化肿瘤较大，平均直径15cm。低分化肿瘤倾向于比中分化肿瘤更大，但有相当多的重叠。Sertoli-Leydig细胞瘤通常部分实性，部分囊性，但是以实性或以囊性为主的肿瘤并不少见。实性区域质硬或质软，呈灰粉色、黄色或桔黄色。伴有网状分化的肿瘤有时可见乳头。

显微镜下，在高分化Sertoli-Leydig细胞瘤中，可见内衬柱状Sertoli细胞的完全发育的中空或闭合的小管，周围绕以纤维性间质（图13A.58）。间质中还可出现Leydig细胞聚集，Leydig细胞具有丰富的嗜酸性胞浆和位于中央的圆形或卵圆形细胞核。Leydig细胞中偶尔可见Reinke结晶。一例少见的肿瘤有中心骨化[569]。细胞的非典型性和核分裂活性没有意义，而且缺乏不成熟的未分化性腺间质、网状小管和异源性成分。

中分化和低分化Sertoli-Leydig细胞瘤中，可见成熟和不成熟的Sertoli细胞被覆结构完好的小管、界限不清的小管和小梁，以及类似于胚胎性索的条索样结构（图13A.59）。10%～25%的中分化和低分化肿瘤的小管具有网状表现，偶尔成为占据优势的组织学图像，以致达到难以辨认肿瘤是否为Sertoli-Leydig细胞瘤的程

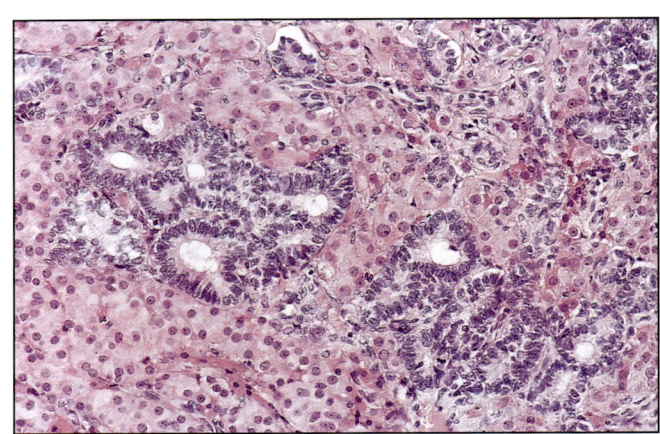

图13A.58　高分化Sertoli-Leydig细胞瘤。内衬Sertoli细胞的结构完好的小管，周围绕以含有肥胖的Leydig细胞的间质，Leydig细胞具有丰富的嗜酸性胞浆。

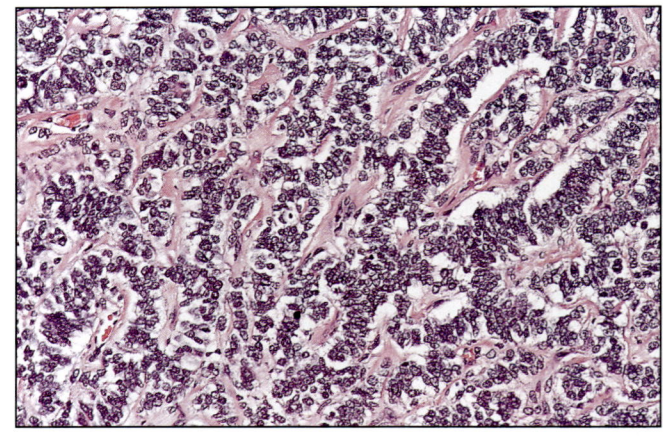

图13A.59　中分化Sertoli-Leydig细胞瘤。Sertoli细胞排列成小梁状结构。

度[560]。网状小管长而分支，而且可能扩张，伴有突出的乳头状生长区域（图 13A.60）[570]。网状小管内衬矮柱状到立方形细胞，胞浆稀少，细胞核深染，卵圆形。Sertoli 细胞核分裂象少见，但内衬网状小管的细胞偶尔可见许多核分裂象。在某些肿瘤中，出现具有奇异性非典型性细胞核的 Sertoli 细胞，但这似乎并不是预后不好的表现[464]。小管周围的间质各异，从纤维结缔组织到伴有未分化性腺间质的不成熟间叶组织，如同发育中的性腺（图 13A.61）。出现不成熟的 Sertoli 细胞和间质是区分高分化与中低分化 Sertoli-Leydig 细胞瘤的主要特征[555]。低分化肿瘤的间质最丰富，构成肿瘤的主体（图 13A.62）[571]。间质细胞一般没有显著的非典型性，但易见核分裂象，平均 4～5 个/10HPF。多数肿瘤出现单个或小到中等大小的 Leydig 细胞簇。在细胞丰富的肿瘤结节周边 Leydig 细胞常常最为明显。Leydig 细胞为多角形，核圆形，位于中央，胞浆丰富，嗜酸性。已有证据提示 Leydig 细胞是反应性的，不是肿瘤性病变的组成部分[572]，但这种提法还没有得到证实。20%～25% 的中低分化 Sertoli-Leydig 细胞瘤有异源性成分。最常见的是肠型黏液性上皮（图 13A.63），但是类癌、神经母细胞、软骨和横纹肌母细胞也有描述[555,573,574]。Sertoli-Leydig 细胞瘤中常常出现分泌甲胎蛋白的具有嗜酸性胞浆的多角形细胞簇。尽管这些细胞被某些作者解释是 Leydig 细胞[562,566,575]，但目前多数作者将其视为局灶性异源性肝的分化[560,565,576-578]。

多数成熟和不成熟的 Sertoli 细胞细胞角蛋白免疫组化染色阳性[579,580]，但这些细胞上皮膜抗原染色通常阴性[520,579]。角蛋白染色特别有助于确定这些肿瘤中不成熟的 Sertoli 细胞巢和细胞索。Sertoli 细胞显示 CD99 膜染色[581]，而且据报道多数肿瘤出现 WT-1 染色，尽管可能取决于所用的抗体[520]。间质细胞和 Leydig 细胞 vimentin 阳性[483,484]。在 Sertoli-Leydig 细胞瘤中，Sertoli 细胞和 Leydig 细胞的 inhibin 和 calretinin 免疫组化染色几乎总是阳性[275,493,495,497,500,520,580]。腺癌 inhibin 或

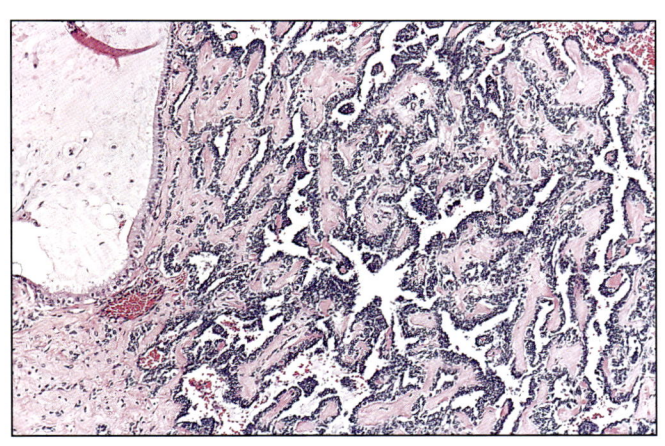

图 13A.60　中分化 Sertoli-Leydig 细胞瘤。分支状的网状小管伴有局灶性乳头状表现。

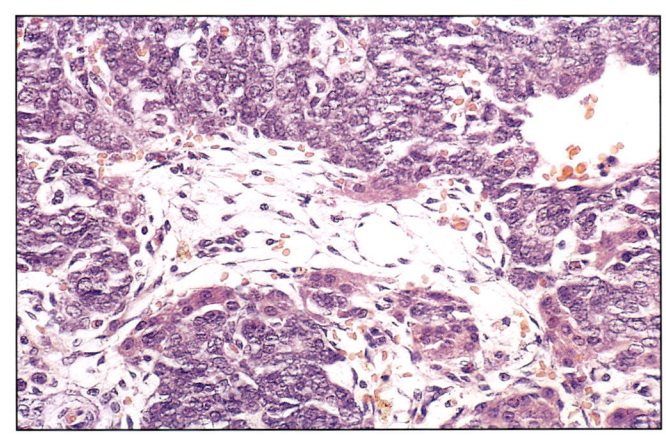

图 13A.62　低分化 Sertoli-Leydig 细胞瘤。纤维性间质中可见不成熟的间质细胞巢。少数具有嗜酸性胞浆的 Leydig 细胞呈小簇状生长。

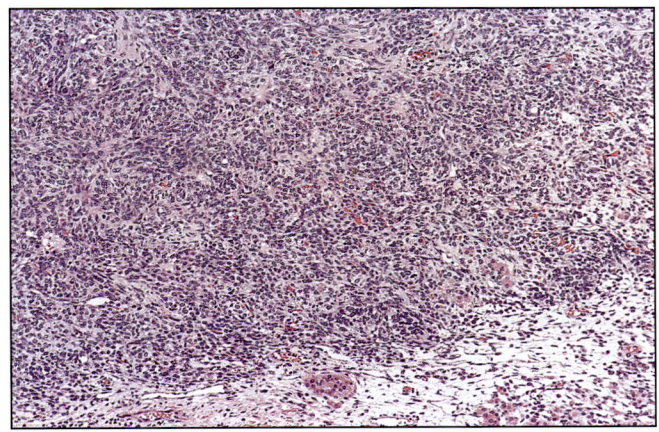

图 13A.61　中分化 Sertoli-Leydig 细胞瘤。淡染的 Sertoli 细胞和深染的不成熟间质细胞呈片块样结构，在其周围可见具有明显嗜酸性胞浆的 Leydig 细胞巢。

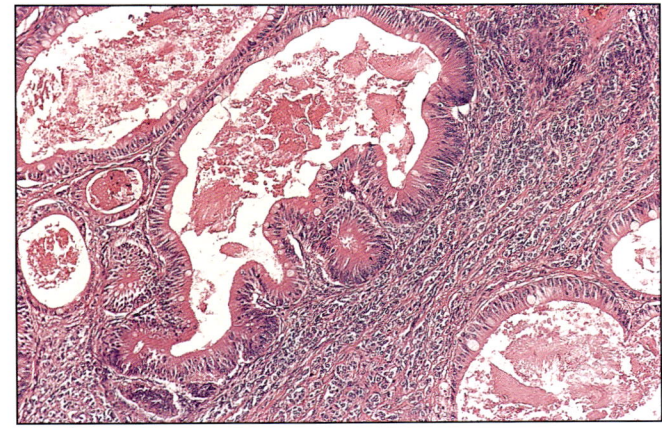

图 13A.63　伴有异源性肠上皮的中分化 Sertoli-Leydig 细胞瘤。大的腺体内衬包括杯状细胞在内的肠型细胞。在肠型腺体之间的间质可以见到 Sertoli-Leydig 细胞瘤的典型特征。

calretinin 染色偶尔阳性，因此，当用于 Sertoli-Leydig 细胞瘤的诊断时，inhibin 和 calretinin 总是应该作为包括细胞角蛋白和上皮膜抗原在内的抗体的一部分，而且可能还要包括诸如癌胚抗原（CEA）等着染腺癌的其他抗体。甲胎蛋白免疫染色显示分泌甲胎蛋白肿瘤中的肝样细胞胞浆染色阳性，此外，某些肿瘤血清甲胎蛋白水平并不升高，这种肿瘤应用抗肝细胞抗体进行免疫染色可显示肝样细胞胞浆染色阳性[562-566,575-578]。异源性肿瘤的胃肠上皮含有嗜银细胞，这些嗜银细胞嗜铬素、5-羟色胺和其他肽类染色阳性[582]，异源性类癌成分嗜铬素或突触素染色阳性[576]。Leydig 细胞、Sertoli 细胞和间质细胞 P-450 细胞色素（P-450 cytochromes）免疫反应阳性，说明所有这些细胞都可能是类固醇生成的部位[583]。

Sertoli 细胞瘤　Sertoli cell tumor

Sertoli 细胞瘤是最罕见的性索-间质肿瘤[584]。与 Sertoli-Leydig 细胞瘤的区别在于，它们不含有 Leydig 细胞或未成熟性腺间质。

临床特征　Sertoli 细胞瘤最常发生于生育期年龄的妇女，偶尔也发生于儿童和绝经后妇女。患者平均年龄大约 30 岁[584,585]。偶尔，Sertoli 细胞瘤发生于 Peutz-Jeghers 综合征的患者[584,586,587]，尽管正如下面讨论的，伴有环状小管的性索肿瘤是 Peutz-Jeghers 综合征患者比较特征性的表现。2/3 的 Sertoli 细胞瘤分泌类固醇激素。多数肿瘤分泌雌激素，少数分泌雄激素。伴有激素活性肿瘤的女孩表现早熟性假青春期和阴道出血。老年妇女有不规则流血、绝经后出血，或在少数情况下表现为男性化，取决于激素分泌的类型和量[584]。激素不活跃性肿瘤患者具有非特异性的症状，例如腹痛或腹胀，或者偶尔发现肿瘤。Sertoli 细胞瘤单侧发生，并且临床上多数表现为良性，可通过单侧输卵管-卵巢切除术治疗[585,588]。少数低分化或侵袭性 Sertoli 细胞瘤复发或转移，并引起患者死亡[584]。多数患者在诊断时肿瘤已播散到卵巢外，少数 Ia 期 Sertoli 细胞瘤已经转移。

病理学　Sertoli 细胞瘤是单侧性有包膜的肿瘤，平均直径 8cm；大多数在 4~12cm 之间。切面灰色、褐色、棕色或黄色，以实性为主，尽管某些肿瘤有小的囊肿。

显微镜下，肿瘤由 Sertoli 细胞组成，在成熟的纤维性或透明间质中生长。小管结构是其特征[584]。小管结构倾向于是单管性，由圆形或卵圆形具有中央腔的开放性腺体，或长的 2 或 3 层细胞厚度的闭合条索样小管组成。常常出现混合性的小管结构。某些肿瘤有条索状、小梁状或弥漫性肿瘤生长区域。

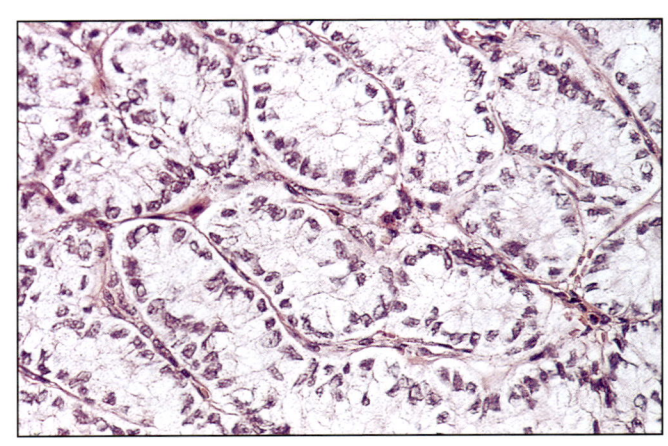

图 13A.64　Sertoli 细胞瘤。小管内衬柱状细胞，具有一致的位于基底的细胞核和丰富的透明胞浆。

Sertoli 细胞是立方的或柱状细胞，具有圆形到卵圆形的细胞核，有时含有小的核仁。奇异但不是变性的细胞核对于预后好像并无不利影响。胞浆从透明到嗜酸性不一（图 13A.64）。不常见的 Sertoli 细胞瘤亚型包括富于脂质型（lipid rich type），其细胞具有丰富的透明、泡沫状胞浆[584,585]；以及嗜酸细胞型（oxyphilic type），由具有丰富的嗜酸性颗粒状胞浆的细胞组成[586]。多数 Sertoli 细胞瘤为高分化，具有一致的温和的细胞核，几乎没有核分裂象。少于 10% 的 Sertoli 细胞瘤临床上表现为恶性。这些肿瘤具有发育不好的小管结构，Sertoli 细胞具有增大的非典型性细胞核，有 5 个或更多核分裂象 /10HPF[584,589,590]。在诊断时局限于卵巢的，以及几乎没有核非典型性和核分裂活性的 Sertoli 细胞瘤可以被视为良性肿瘤。

Sertoli 细胞瘤倾向于 vimentin 和 cytokeratin 免疫反应阳性[579]，但是上皮膜抗原阴性，而且 inhibin、calretinin 和 CD99 阳性[494,500,584]。少数肿瘤显示平滑肌肌动蛋白、S-100 蛋白或神经元特异性烯醇化酶局灶弱阳性，但缺乏嗜铬素染色[584]。

伴有环状小管的性索肿瘤（SCTAT）Sex cord tumor with annular tubules (SCTAT)

SCTAT 被认为是一种"未分类"的性索-间质肿瘤，这是因为它的组织学发生具有争议。然而，它的组织学表现和临床特征是有特色的[591]。

临床特征　SCTAT 发生在两种临床状况下。大约 1/3 发生于 Peutz-Jeghers 综合征的妇女[466]，是一种常染色体显性遗传性疾病，表现为 19 号染色体上的 *STK11* 肿瘤抑制基因突变[592-594]。受累的患者有黏膜皮肤黑色素沉着和错构瘤性肠息肉[595]。在 10%~20% 的 Peutz-Jeghers 综合征患者中，发现有可触及的不同类型的卵巢肿瘤[596]，但是如果在显微镜下检查卵巢，实际上所有的卵巢都含有 SCTAT[597]。在这种临床情况下，肿瘤通常很小，在显微镜下才能见到，多中心性，双侧发生，并有 *STK11* 突变[598]。SCTAT 几乎总是 Peutz-Jeghers 综合征妇女的偶然发现，因为它们太小以致不能触及，少数患者分泌足够量的类固醇激素而引起症状。在 Peutz-Jeghers 综合征患者见到的显微镜下 SCTAT，临床上是良性的，无症状的患者不需要做卵巢切除术[597]。临床上发现 Peutz-Jeghers 综合征患者有 SCTAT，通常可以通过单侧输卵管-卵巢切除术进行治疗，尽管已有少数双侧性或恶性 SCTAT 的病例报告[599]。少数 Peutz-Jeghers 综合征妇女发生高分化宫颈内膜腺癌，因此由妇科医师进行终生监护是恰当的[596,597,600-602]。发生于 Peutz-Jeghers 综合征儿童的一种非常罕见的卵巢性索-间质肿瘤，能够引起性早熟[603]。Sertoli 细胞瘤，包括不常见的嗜酸细胞型或含有脂质胞浆的亚型，在少数情况下也可发生于 Peutz-Jeghers 综合征的患者[584,586]。

大约 2/3 的 SCTAT 发生在没有 Peutz-Jeghers 综合征的患者（非综合征性 SCTAT，non-syndromic SCTAT）[585,597,604-606]。在非综合征性 SCTAT 中通常检测不到 *STK11* 突变[598]。非综合征性 SCTAT 发生的年龄范围广泛，从 6 岁到 76 岁不等，平均年龄 36 岁[597]。出现的症状取决于患者的年龄。月经前女孩经常有早熟的假青春期[597,605]。老年妇女可以有月经紊乱或绝经后出血。有证据显示这些肿瘤可以产生黄体酮和雌激素，因有某些患者的子宫内膜显示有黄体酮的影响，而另外一些患者可见腹膜蜕膜反应[585,607,608]。大约 50% 的患者可以触及单侧附件肿物。少数 SCTAT 妇女血清中抗 Müller 激素（Müller 抑制物质）和 inhibin 浓度增高。研究证明，这些物质是随访 SCTAT 患者有用的肿瘤标志物[609,610]。伴有局限性肿瘤的年轻妇女可以通过单侧输卵管-卵巢切除术进行治疗，而老年妇女和处于疾病晚期的妇女则需通过子宫切除术、双侧输卵管-卵巢切除术以及卵巢外肿瘤切除来治疗。大约 15% 的非综合征性 SCTAT 在临床上是恶性的[597,604]。某些患者复发出现较早[597]，但多数复发较晚，于最初治疗后 5 年或更多年以后发生[604,606,607,610]。肿瘤转移很难预测。某些患者联合化疗有效，至少短期内有效[610]，但在其他一些患者化疗无效[607]。

病理学 在 Peutz-Jeghers 综合征的患者，SCTAT 较小，大体检查通常不能发现。那些能被见到的 SCTAT 为实性褐色或黄色肿瘤，可能包含钙化。肿瘤倾向于多灶性和双侧性发生。非综合征性 SCTAT 通常为单侧性，大小不同，从显微镜下可以见到的肿瘤或直径小于 1cm 的小结节，到直径超过 20cm 的巨大肿瘤。肿瘤以实性为主，尽管某些肿瘤可见囊肿，切面呈鱼肉状，褐色或黄色。

显微镜下，可见圆形有时是融合性的肿瘤细胞巢，形成单一或复合的闭合环状小管，其核心为嗜酸性透明物质（图 13A.65）。肿瘤细胞在纤维性间质内生长，周围绕以基底膜样物质，这些基底膜样物质与核心的透明物质相连续。环状小管的核心和基底膜样物质 PAS 染色阳性。一般有"成对细胞"排列在小管内，并列细胞的胞核位于细胞相反方向的末端。肿瘤细胞为柱状，具有透明或泡沫状胞浆、圆形或卵圆形深染的细胞核和小的核仁。偶尔可见核沟。非典型性和核分裂象不常见。来自不伴有 Peutz-Jeghers 综合征患者的大的肿瘤可能含有长而闭合的小管、融合的肿瘤细胞巢、局灶性实性生长区域、囊肿或无定形透明物质的无细胞区域（图 13A.66）。偶见小面积的颗粒细胞或 Sertoli 细胞分化[597,605,606,611]。来自某些 SCTAT 的转移性肿瘤类似于颗粒细胞瘤[606]，而来自某些颗粒细胞瘤的转移性肿瘤类似于 SCTAT[612]，强调了这两种类型的性索-间质

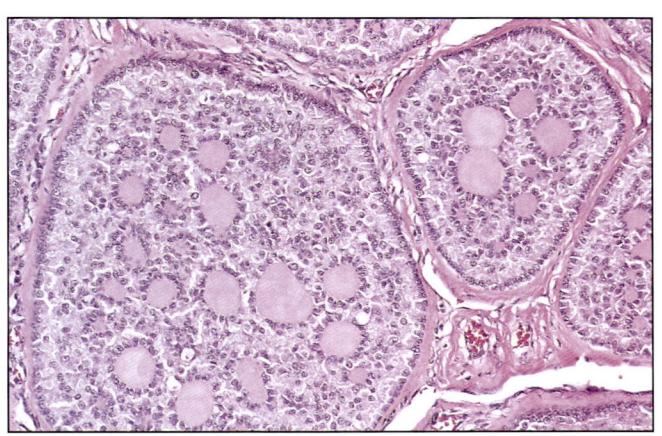

图 13A.65 伴有环状小管的性索肿瘤（SCTAT），来自 Peutz-Jeghers 综合征患者。肿瘤细胞巢被纤维性间质围绕。复杂的环状小管围绕着由基底膜样物质构成的透明核心。注意肿瘤细胞核完全反向的排列。

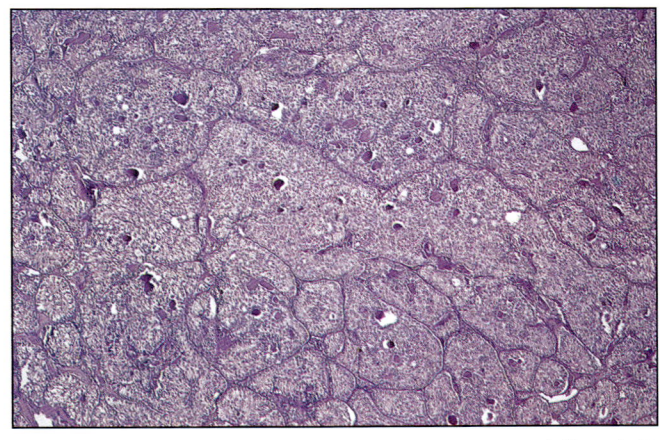

图 13A.66 伴有环状小管的性索肿瘤。大的肿瘤中的融合性肿瘤细胞巢，来自不伴有 Peutz-Jeghers 综合征的患者。

肿瘤之间的密切关系。一种独特的肿瘤含有子宫内膜样腺体分化的区域[608]。与侵袭性行为相关的特征包括间质浸润和核分裂象数目增多[585,604]。

SCTAT的免疫表型类似于Sertoli细胞瘤。Vimentin、inhibin和calretinin染色阳性，细胞角蛋白阳性而上皮膜抗原阴性[275,520,613]。很多学者研究过SCTAT的电子显微镜特征，希望从中获得一些有关SCTAT组织学发生的线索[514,585,606,614-616]。肿瘤细胞巢周围以及充满细胞巢中央腔隙的基底膜样物质，形成了光学显微镜下见到的透明核心。许多肿瘤细胞含有胞浆内微丝，微丝在某些细胞中形成核周聚集体。这些微丝被某些人解释为Charcot-Böttcher微丝，这导致他们得出结论，即SCTAT是Sertoli细胞瘤[514,585,611-616]。其他作者没有发现Charcot-Böttcher微丝，他们的结论是，肿瘤细胞的形态表示SCTAT是颗粒细胞瘤的一种亚型[606,614,615]。

Leydig细胞瘤　Leydig cell tumor

多数卵巢Leydig细胞瘤起源于卵巢门，推测来自于门细胞，导致偶尔将发生于卵巢门的Leydig细胞瘤（hilar Leydig cell tumors）称作"门细胞瘤"（hilus cell tumors）[617]。发生于卵巢门部位以外卵巢间质的Leydig细胞瘤少见。这种类型的肿瘤包括非门Leydig细胞瘤和间质Leydig细胞瘤[521,618,619]。

临床表现　Leydig细胞瘤一般发生于绝经后妇女。平均年龄58岁，几乎所有的患者都超过30岁[617]。常见的临床表现为多毛症或有男性化的征象，例如痤疮、脱发、声音变粗、男性体态或阴蒂肥大。男性化患者血清睾酮浓度升高，但尿17-酮类固醇一般在正常范围[617,620]。非男性化患者出现闭经或绝经后出血，取决于她们的年龄。某些Leydig细胞瘤是在由于其他一些疾病而手术时偶然发现的。子宫内膜可有增生甚或有腺癌[621]，很可能是继发于外周的睾酮向雌激素的转变。在做出诊断之前，症状常常持续多年。这是因为Leydig细胞瘤通常很小而难以定位。在某些病例，不能触及的肿瘤通过影像学研究可以发现，但在另外一些病例，则需要测量通过选择性卵巢静脉导管插入术而获得的血液中激素的浓度[622,623]。多数Leydig细胞瘤是单侧发生，但是少数双侧发生的肿瘤也有报道[624]。实际上，所有Leydig细胞瘤都是良性的，通过手术可以治愈[521,617-619]。肿瘤切除之后男性化征象可以消退。恶性Leydig细胞瘤非常少见，仅有几例报道[617]。

病理学　Leydig细胞瘤是单侧性小的实性肿瘤，呈棕色或棕黄色，位于卵巢门，或在少数情况下位于卵巢髓质或皮质。平均直径在3～5cm之间，但是小到0.7cm和大到15cm的肿瘤也有报道。

显微镜下，卵巢门Leydig细胞瘤界限清楚但无包膜。肿瘤细胞类似于睾丸Leydig细胞，在正常情况下，门细胞出现在卵巢门神经的周围[617]。门细胞为圆形或多角形，具有丰富的颗粒状嗜酸性胞浆（图13A.67）。许多细胞含有黄色或棕色脂色素。细胞核小而一致，从空泡状到深染不一，并可含有显著的核仁。Reinke结晶是Leydig细胞的特征，但是仅见于50%的卵巢门Leydig细胞瘤。Reinke结晶是胞浆内嗜酸性杆状小体，两端钝圆或变细（图13A.68）。胞浆内常常易于发现嗜酸性透明小球，被认为是Reinke结晶的前体。其他显著的特征包括肿瘤内血管周围成簇的细胞核以及血管壁特有的纤维素样改变[617]。

有两种类型的非卵巢门Leydig细胞瘤（non-hilar Leydig cell tumors）。单纯性非卵巢门Leydig细胞瘤是局限性的肿瘤，类似于卵巢门Leydig细胞瘤，除了部位不同以外；它们通常位于髓质中央[619,625]。间质Leydig细胞瘤（stromal Leydig cell tumors）是含有成簇、成巢或片块状Leydig细胞的纤维瘤或卵泡膜细胞瘤[521,618,626,627]。根据

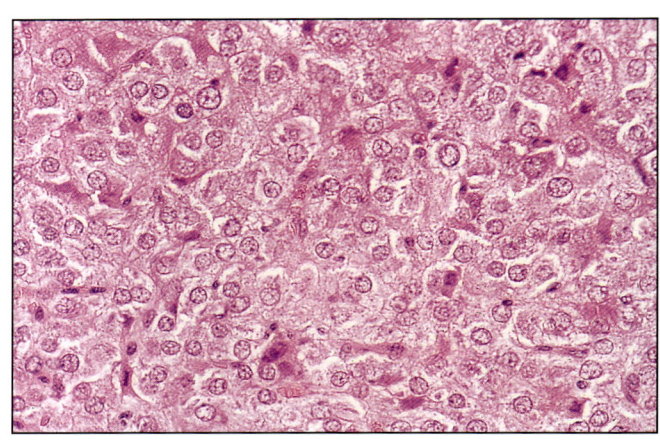

图13A.67　Leydig细胞瘤。肿瘤细胞具有丰富的嗜酸性胞浆和均匀一致的位于中心的圆形细胞核。

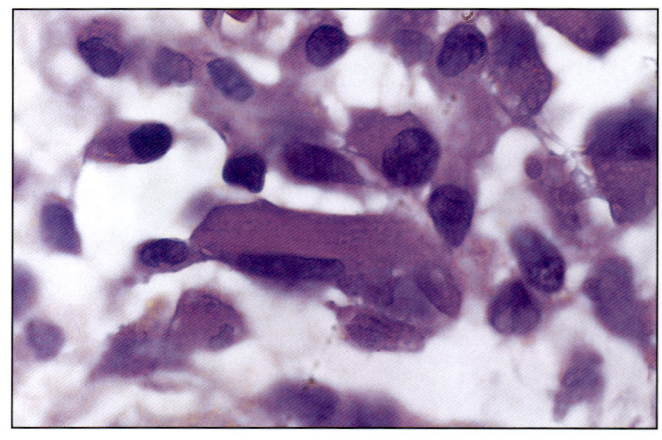

图13A.68　Leydig细胞瘤。嗜酸性杆状Reinke结晶出现在视野中央的细胞中。

定义，为了诊断非卵巢门 Leydig 细胞瘤，肿瘤细胞内必须发现 Reinke 结晶。因为仅有 50% 的卵巢门 Leydig 细胞瘤含有 Reinke 结晶，某些非卵巢门 Leydig 细胞瘤未被认识而被误诊为间质黄体瘤（stromal luteoma）[628]或黄素化卵泡膜细胞瘤[521]。

不管它们在卵巢中的起源部位如何，Leydig 细胞瘤显示 inhibin 和 calretinin 的强阳性染色[629]。

类固醇细胞瘤 Steroid cell tumors

这种类型的卵巢肿瘤包括有些异质的不能特异分类的间质肿瘤。这种肿瘤也叫"脂质细胞瘤"（lipid cell tumors）。类似于 Leydig 细胞但是缺乏 Reinke 结晶的细胞，以及类似于肾上腺皮质细胞的细胞，以不同的比例出现在多数肿瘤中[630,631]。

临床特征 类固醇细胞瘤发生的年龄范围广泛，从 3 岁到 80 岁不等。患者多为中年人，平均年龄是 45 岁，但类固醇细胞瘤偶尔也发生于儿童和年龄较高的患者[509,632,633]。多数类固醇细胞瘤分泌男性类固醇激素，在数量上足以引起多毛症和男性化。男性化患者血清睾酮浓度和尿 17-酮类固醇增高[630,631]。一种不常见的肿瘤分泌肾素和睾酮，而且伴有继发性红细胞增多症[634]。非男性化患者表现为腹胀或腹痛、月经不规律或绝经后出血。少数类固醇细胞瘤分泌皮质醇，并引起 Cushing 综合征[630,635,636]。

多数肿瘤在诊断时局限于卵巢内，双侧发生罕见（6%）[630]。诊断时有 10%～20% 的患者已发生盆腔、腹膜或远处转移[630,631]。IA 期肿瘤的年轻患者可通过输卵管-卵巢切除术治疗。老年患者和晚期肿瘤通过子宫切除术和双侧输卵管-卵巢切除术治疗。在肿瘤切除之后，多毛症和男性化的征象消退。相当比例的（25%～43%）类固醇细胞瘤在临床上是恶性的，其中包括多数引起 Cushing 综合征的病变[630,631,635]。复发一般在治疗后的头几年内发现，但是大约 20% 在 5 年之后发现[630]。

病理学 类固醇细胞瘤是实性肿瘤，直径从小于 1cm 到大于 20cm 不等，平均 7cm。切面褐色、黄色或桔黄色，大约 25% 的病例有出血和坏死区。已有少数卵巢旁类固醇细胞瘤的报告，可能起源于异位的卵巢组织[637-639]。

显微镜下，一般混合出现 Leydig 样细胞和肾上腺皮质样细胞，虽然可能以一种成分为主。Leydig 样细胞为圆形或多角形，具有丰富的有时是空泡状的嗜酸性胞浆（图 13A.69）。核圆，位于中央，典型者具有小的核仁。从未发现 Reinke 结晶。肾上腺皮质样细胞也是圆形或多角形，具有丰富的浅淡或透明的空泡状胞浆（图 13A.70）。核呈空泡状，可有小至中等大小的明

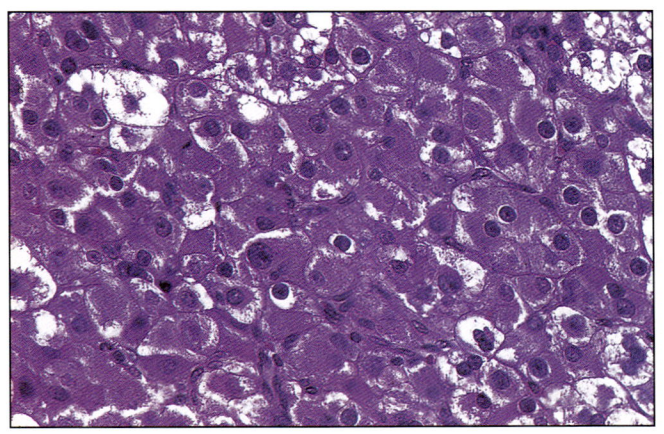

图 13A.69 类固醇细胞瘤。肿瘤细胞类似于 Leydig 细胞，具有丰富的嗜酸性胞浆，但缺乏 Reinke 结晶。

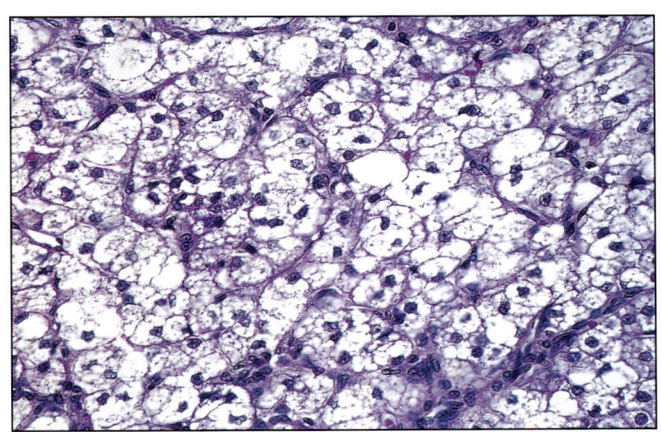

图 13A.70 类固醇细胞瘤。肾上腺样细胞，具有丰富的空泡状透明胞浆。

显的核仁。肾上腺型细胞脂肪染色阳性。多数病例核分裂象少见，核的非典型性缺乏或轻微。见于恶性类固醇细胞瘤的病理学特征包括肿瘤较大、出血或坏死、有 2 个或 2 个以上核分裂象/10HPF，以及中到重度核的非典型性[630,631]。

Vimentin、inhibin 和 calretinin 免疫组化染色通常阳性[492-494,613,640]。多数类固醇细胞瘤 melan-A 染色阳性，但相关的标志物 MART-1 染色通常缺乏[640,641]。30%～50% 的肿瘤细胞角蛋白染色阳性，通常为局灶性，有时是核周球状染色方式，大约 1/3 的病例平滑肌肌动蛋白染色阳性[642]。

其他性索-间质肿瘤 Other sex cord-stromal tumors

两性母细胞瘤（gynandroblastoma）是罕见的肿瘤，伴有 Sertoli 或 Sertoli-Leydig 细胞的实质性区域和颗粒细胞分化（每种成分≥10%）[643-648]。这种类型的肿瘤被某些学者放在未归类的性索-间质肿瘤中[649]。两性母细胞瘤患者一般出现男性化，虽然外周睾酮转化成雌激

素可能导致子宫内膜增生，从而引起异常阴道出血[648]。治疗方法是手术切除。报告的所有病例均呈良性临床经过，但是由于其特定的肿瘤成分，或许应该将其看作具有与颗粒细胞瘤或中分化Sertoli-Leydig细胞瘤同样的恶性潜能。两性母细胞瘤单侧发生，直径在1～18cm[643]。肿瘤可以为实性或部分囊性。实性区域呈白色、褐色或黄色。显微镜下，内衬Sertoli细胞的开放或闭合的小管和条索混合有巢状或片状的颗粒细胞（图13A.71）。可能出现微卵泡和颗粒细胞瘤的其他典型结构。颗粒细胞成分通常是成年型的，虽然少数病例为幼年型[650-652]。间质可能含有类似于卵泡膜细胞、黄素化细胞或Leydig细胞的梭形细胞。在已报道的两性母细胞瘤的病例中，既无明显的细胞非典型性也无常见的核分裂象。这些肿瘤表达inhibin和calretinin。Vimentin和雄激素受体主要在颗粒细胞成分中表达，而低分子量角蛋白和CD10多半在Sertoli细胞成分中表达[652]。

硬化性间质瘤（sclerosing stromal tumor）是不常见的良性肿瘤，主要发生于青少年和二十多岁的年轻女性[653-657]。常见的症状是月经紊乱或盆腔疼痛，虽然少数病例出现男性化[658,659]。硬化性间质瘤是与Meigs综合征有关的肿瘤类型之一[660]。硬化性间质瘤偶尔在妊娠期间发现[661,662]，这时可能引起男性化[663]。硬化性间质瘤是良性肿瘤，因为多数病例发现于年轻妇女，所以最好采取手术切除或单侧输卵管-卵巢切除术治疗。硬化性间质瘤直径从1.5cm到17cm不等。多数是实性的，或者以实性为主，伴有小的囊肿，但是偶尔也有以囊性为主的肿瘤[654,657]。实性区域质硬，分叶状，白色或黄色。显微镜下，硬化性间质瘤具有斑驳的表现，这是由于富于细胞的结节以及水肿区域或细胞稀少的纤维性间质并列出现。血管显著，常常呈"鹿角"或"血管外皮细胞瘤样"表现。肿瘤细胞包括梭形纤维母细胞、肌样细胞和具有空泡状嗜酸性胞浆的多角形卵泡膜样细胞（图13A.72）。免疫组化染色，vimentin、inhibin、calretinin和melan-A阳性[494,495,535,641,664]，多数肿瘤含有肌样细胞，其平滑肌肌动蛋白或desmin免疫染色阳性[535,657,665]。常常可能发现肿瘤细胞核雌激素或孕激素受体阳性；孕激素受体阳性通常是最突出的[657,666]。最近，在卵泡膜样细胞中已经发现血管内皮生长因子（VEGF），其受体定位于血管内皮细胞，提示VEGF在这种肿瘤特征性的血管结构和水肿中可能具有一定的作用[657]。

间质黄体瘤（stromal luteoma）是罕见的分泌雌激素的肿瘤，主要发生于绝经后妇女[628]。最常见的症状是异常子宫出血，子宫内膜活检经常显示有增生表现。少数情况下，间质黄体瘤有男性化表现。1/3的病例是手术或尸检时偶然发现。临床上表现为良性。间质黄体瘤是小的单侧发生的肿瘤；报告的所有病例直径都小于3cm。切面灰色、白色、黄色或棕色。肿瘤位于卵巢间质，由黄素化间质细胞组成。肿瘤细胞呈多角形，具有颗粒状嗜酸性胞浆和小圆形位于中央的细胞核。与Leydig细胞瘤的鉴别是基于间质黄体瘤位于非卵巢门部位和胞浆缺乏Reinke结晶。一般具有其他卵巢异常，包括常常是双侧性发生的间质卵泡膜细胞增生和门细胞增生。

不符合任何命名分类的肿瘤叫做未分类的性索-间质肿瘤（unclassified sex cord-stromal tumors）[8]。临床表现倾向于非特异性，伴有异常出血和腹部肿块，或腹部疼痛。从妊娠妇女切除的性索-间质肿瘤常常难以分类，其中某些肿瘤必须被归入"未分类"[447]。多数病例诊断时肿瘤局限于卵巢，预后较好。少数肿瘤相关性死亡已见报道，因此应该将这些肿瘤看作是具有低度恶性潜能的，沿着颗粒细胞分化或中分化Sertoli-Leydig细胞瘤[649,669]。未分类的性索-间质肿瘤由不同数量的梭形细胞、条索状或小梁状的性索细胞以及不明确的小管样结构混杂组成[649-667]。这些肿瘤不具有足够的特异性生长方式，无法归类为颗粒细胞瘤或Sertoli-Leydig细胞瘤，

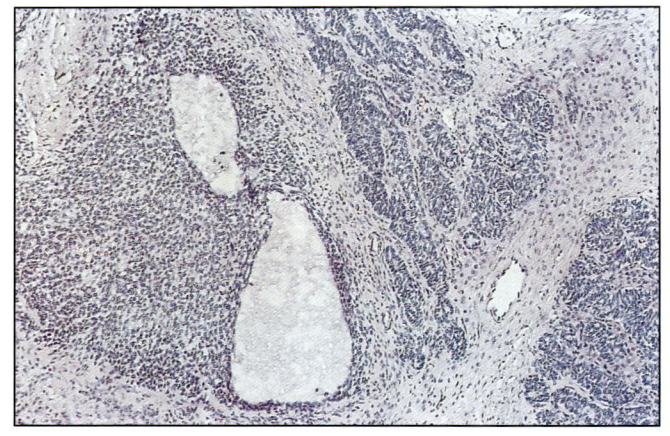

图13A.71 两性母细胞瘤。含有卵泡的颗粒细胞成分（左）以及Sertoli小管和Leydig细胞（右）紧密混合。

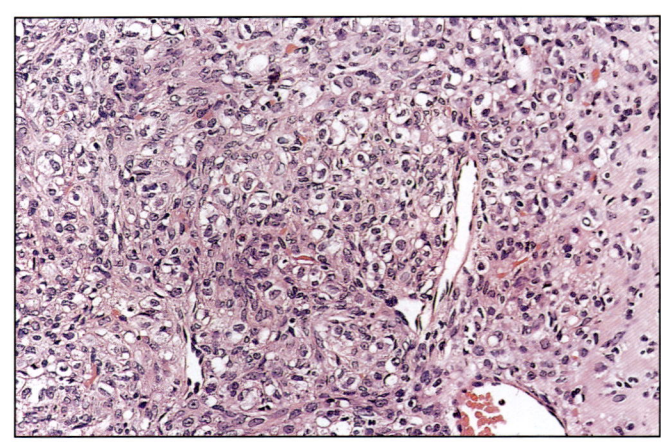

图13A.72 硬化性间质瘤。富于细胞的部位由肥胖的圆形细胞组成。

尽管正如上面提到的一样，某些学者将两性母细胞瘤归入这个范畴[649]。

非特异性间叶性肿瘤
Non-specific mesenchymal tumors

所有类型的间叶性肿瘤均可发生于卵巢。这些肿瘤的大体和显微镜下形态与发生在软组织或子宫的间叶性肿瘤相同，临床行为也是如此。平滑肌瘤是最常见的卵巢间叶性肿瘤[668-671]。脂肪平滑肌瘤是平滑肌瘤的一种亚型，表现为平滑肌与脂肪组织混合存在[672-673]。其他偶尔发生于卵巢的良性软组织肿瘤是血管瘤[674,675]和黏液瘤[676,677]。卵巢黏液瘤的细胞和血管比软组织黏液瘤丰富。某些学者认为黏液瘤是纤维瘤-卵泡膜细胞瘤组中的一个肿瘤[678]，但是主要的观点认为它是一个独立的疾病[676]。

卵巢原发性肉瘤罕见[679]。上面所讨论的纤维肉瘤和子宫内膜样间质肉瘤是最常见的卵巢肉瘤。平滑肌肉瘤可以发生于卵巢，可以通过用于评估子宫平滑肌肉瘤的类似的特征来诊断。卵巢平滑肌肉瘤显示中到重度的核非典型性，常见核分裂象和肿瘤细胞坏死。报告病例数最大的一项研究发现，具有弥漫性显著的核非典型性以及5个或5个以上核分裂象/10HPF的肿瘤，其行为可能像平滑肌肉瘤；多数但不是所有的肿瘤可有局灶性肿瘤细胞坏死[671]。其他类型的原发性卵巢肉瘤是横纹肌肉瘤[680]、软骨肉瘤[681]、骨肉瘤[682,683]、恶性神经鞘瘤[684]和血管肉瘤[685,686]。

恶性淋巴瘤　Malignant lymphoma

临床特征　在卵巢肿瘤中淋巴瘤的数量少于1%[687-689]。这种病例的临床表现是盆腔或腹部疼痛、腹胀、月经紊乱，或出现"B"型淋巴瘤的发热、夜汗或体重降低等症状。检查时，可触及单侧或双侧附件肿块。尽管临床上表现为卵巢肿瘤，但是淋巴瘤通常也累及盆腔或腹部淋巴结、肝或脾、或其他器官，说明卵巢受累是播散性疾病的一部分[689,690]。少数仅仅通过卵巢切除术治疗的患者从不发生卵巢外的淋巴瘤，提示这种罕见的淋巴瘤原发于卵巢[687,688,690-692]。Ann Arbor淋巴瘤分期能比FIGO分期提供更多的预后信息[693]。接受现代联合化疗患者的生存率大于50%，与分级和分期类似的淋巴瘤总的存活率相似[687,689,691,693]。

病理学　50%以上的病例双侧卵巢受累[689]，虽然卵巢原发性淋巴瘤倾向于单侧发生[692]。大小从显微镜下可见到直径大于20 cm，平均直径10～15cm。少数卵巢淋巴瘤是在显微镜下检查由于其他原因而切除的卵巢时偶然发现的[692]。切面鱼肉样，粉红色、褐色或灰白色。显微镜下，几乎均为非Hodgkin淋巴瘤[687,688,690,691,694]。Burkitt淋巴瘤和Burkitt样淋巴瘤最常见于儿童和年轻妇女，但也可发生于老年妇女。肿瘤细胞均匀一致，圆形，具有小到中等大小的核，染色质粗，伴有1～3个核仁。核分裂象常见。胞浆稀少呈嗜碱性。细胞成片生长，散在含有吞噬性组织细胞的间隙，形成了Burkitt淋巴瘤典型的"星空"(starry sky)现象，或以条索的形式出现[688]。它们倾向于环绕而不是取代卵泡和其他卵巢结构。大B细胞淋巴瘤是成人最常见的卵巢淋巴瘤。肿瘤细胞具有圆形、卵圆形或有裂的细胞核和少量到中等量的双染性胞浆（图13A.73）。核深染，染色质粗，或为具有显著核仁的空泡状核。核分裂象多见。细胞成片生长，或呈条索状局灶浸润间质。其他类型的非Hodgkin淋巴瘤偶尔累及卵巢，包括淋巴母细胞淋巴瘤、滤泡性淋巴瘤以及T细胞淋巴瘤。血管浸润和局灶间质硬化常见于所有类型的淋巴瘤。最有用的免疫组化标志物是标记B细胞的CD45（白细胞共同抗原，LCA）和CD20，以及标记T细胞的CD3。当最初的标志物染色结果模糊时，其他的B细胞和T细胞分化标志物也有帮助，例如CD79a、CD45RA、CD45RO和CD43，而且，对于不常见的卵巢淋巴瘤，必须应用各种另外的染色以确定其免疫表型。免疫组化研究一般显示为B细胞表型[688,693]。

白血病　Leukemia

白血病经常累及卵巢，但很少表现为卵巢肿瘤。粒细胞肉瘤（granulocytic sarcoma）是不成熟髓细胞的髓外肿块。它是单侧或双侧卵巢增大的罕见原

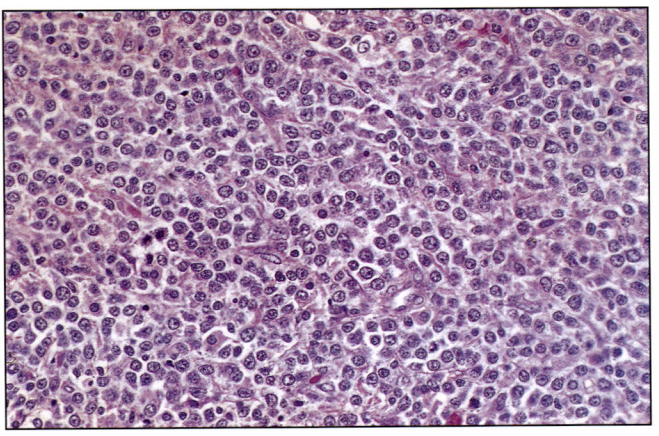

图13A.73　淋巴瘤。伴有空泡状核的成片的大淋巴细胞，核染色质粗，胞浆稀少，符合大细胞淋巴瘤。

因[695,696]。切面呈分叶状，质硬或呈鱼肉样，颜色范围从白色或褐色到绿色不定，虽然这是粒细胞肉瘤的特征，但是很少能够见到。显微镜下，粒细胞肉瘤由成片或成条索的不成熟的造血细胞组成，伴有中等大小的圆形细胞核，核染色质细，核仁不明显，胞浆稀少，双染性。髓细胞分化的证据一般不显著，容易漏掉，例如胞浆嗜酸性或混合有嗜酸性髓细胞。萘基氯乙酸酯酶组织化学染色通常阳性，虽然常常仅是局灶阳性。粒细胞肉瘤各种不同类型的免疫组化染色阳性，比组织化学染色容易解释。髓过氧化物酶和溶菌酶最敏感和最特异。B 和 T 淋巴细胞分化标志物免疫染色阴性，例如 CD20 和 CD3。在诊断粒细胞肉瘤时，白血病可能累及或不累及外周血和骨髓；如果诊断时没有出现白血病，白血病一般随后发生。

生殖细胞肿瘤　　Germ cell tumors

这一组肿瘤来自于生殖细胞（表 13A.9）。某些肿瘤由未分化细胞组成（无性细胞瘤、胚胎性癌），而另外一些肿瘤具有向胚胎性（畸胎瘤）或胚胎外（绒毛膜癌、卵黄囊瘤）分化的结构。良性囊性畸胎瘤常见，但是其他类型的生殖细胞肿瘤罕见，包括所有的恶性肿瘤。

表13A.9　卵巢生殖细胞肿瘤

生殖细胞肿瘤

无性细胞瘤
卵黄囊瘤（内胚窦瘤）
胚胎性癌
多胚瘤
绒毛膜癌
畸胎瘤
　　成熟性畸胎瘤
　　　实性
　　　囊性（良性囊性畸胎瘤；皮样囊肿）
　　未成熟性畸胎瘤
　　神经外胚层肿瘤
　　来源于成熟性畸胎瘤的恶性肿瘤
　　单胚层畸胎瘤
　　　卵巢甲状腺肿
　　　类癌
混合性生殖细胞瘤
性腺母细胞瘤
未分类生殖细胞肿瘤

无性细胞瘤　　Dysgerminoma

无性细胞瘤是卵巢最常见的恶性生殖细胞肿瘤[1,3,4,697]，但它仅占所有恶性卵巢肿瘤的 1%~2%。

临床特征　无性细胞瘤是一种好发于儿童和年轻女性的肿瘤[698,702]。平均年龄 22 岁，90% 的患者在 30 岁以下[703-705]。在妊娠期间发现的恶性卵巢肿瘤大约 20% 是无性细胞瘤[706,707]。典型的临床表现是腹胀、腹部肿块或腹痛。某些患者有月经异常或胃肠道或泌尿道症状。少数患者有高钙血症[708-711]。血清乳酸脱氢酶（LDH）经常升高，可以作为一个有用的肿瘤标志物[705,712-714]。血清甲胎蛋白或人绒毛膜促性腺激素水平增高往往提示存在其他生殖细胞成分，尽管少数单纯性无性细胞瘤患者血液中这些物质的量也有所增加[714-717]。在性腺发育不全患者，无性细胞瘤是最常见的恶性性腺肿瘤[704,718,719]。

诊断时，60%~80% 患者的无性细胞瘤局限于卵巢（I 期）[698,700,702,712]。通常单侧发生，但是 5%~15% 的病例双侧卵巢含有肿瘤（IB 期）[698-700,702,705]。在双侧发生的病例中，对侧卵巢肿瘤半数是在显微镜下发现的，因此某些肿瘤医师建议，如果要进行单侧输卵管-卵巢切除术，一个明显正常的对侧卵巢需要进行活检[698,699,720]。无性细胞瘤通过淋巴道转移至主动脉旁淋巴结，随后播散到纵隔淋巴结，而且可以通过腹膜播散到盆腔和腹腔[699,712,719]。

包膜完整的单侧无性细胞瘤（FIGO Ia 期）可以通过输卵管-卵巢切除术治疗，5 年生存率大于 90%[698,700,702,712,720,721]。单纯进行手术治疗的患者约 20%~35% 复发，所以提倡这些患者术后还要进一步治疗[700,722]。所幸的是，复发通常可以得到成功治疗，而常规的辅助治疗常常被拒绝，因其对于生育具有不良的影响。当无性细胞瘤来源于发育不全的性腺时，恰当的治疗是双侧性腺切除术。晚期疾病（>IA 期）的标准治疗是腹式子宫切除术、双侧输卵管-卵巢切除术、有限的减瘤术以及术后化疗或放疗[723]。如果肿瘤没有累及子宫和对侧卵巢，晚期病例也可以予以保留，因为保存这些患者的生育能力是非常重要的[712,724]。以铂为基础的化疗方案对无性细胞瘤非常有效，而且比放疗引起卵巢衰竭和不育的可能性小[725-729]。根据报告化疗的有效率达到 90%，而且长期存活率在 80% 以上，即使是在晚期或复发的病例。任何复发通常都是在初次治疗两年内出现[701,725,729-731]。

病理学　无性细胞瘤是大的实性肿瘤，直径通常大于 10cm，表面光滑。切面呈鱼肉状，同质性或结节状，灰色、褐色或白色。大的肿瘤常常出现出血和坏死。

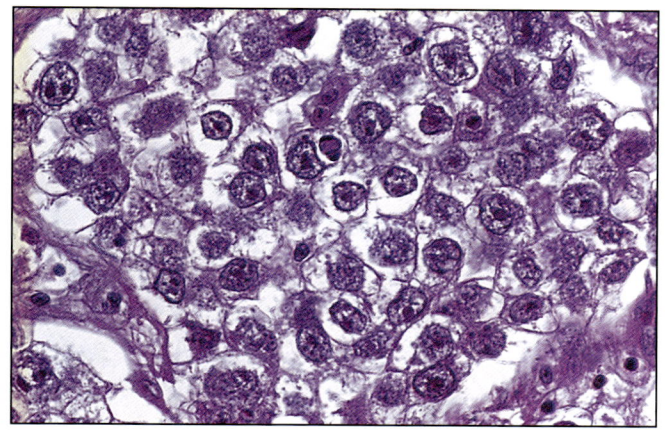

图13A.74 无性细胞瘤。细胞核呈空泡状，伴有显著的核仁、丰富的透明胞浆和清楚的细胞膜。

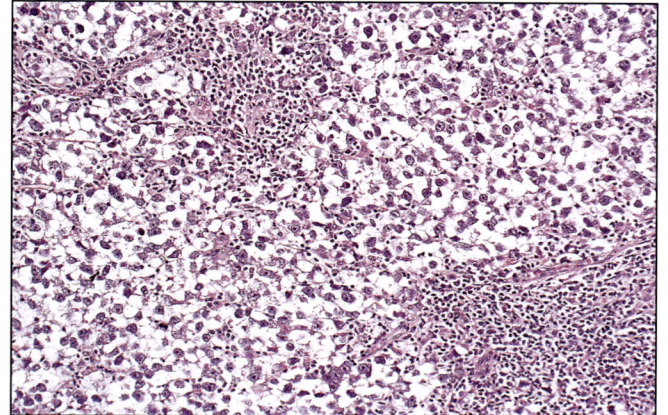

图13A.75 无性细胞瘤。具有丰富透明胞浆的肿瘤细胞小叶，被含有大量淋巴细胞的纤维性间隔分隔。

无性细胞瘤的显微镜下表现与睾丸精原细胞瘤相同。肿瘤细胞多角形，具有明显的细胞膜和丰富的颗粒状到透明的胞浆（图13A.74）。PAS染色常常可以证实胞浆中的糖原。核位于中央，圆形，空泡状，含有突出的核仁。核分裂象一般多见。细胞呈巢状、小叶状、小梁状生长，周围绕以纤维性间隔。细胞内黏着力偶尔丧失，伴有腺样间隙形成。纤维间隔内通常可见淋巴细胞，偶尔在肿瘤细胞中也能见到淋巴细胞（图13A.75）。某些肿瘤淋巴细胞数量较多，形成片块或结节，可能含有反应性的生发中心。经常可见上皮样细胞和多核Langhans巨细胞，某些肿瘤含有结节病样肉芽肿（sarcoid-like granuloma）。纤维性或肉芽肿性反应可能非常明显，以致掩盖了肿瘤细胞。某些无性细胞瘤可以出现坏死区域，特别是较大的肿瘤。非典型性程度比普通肿瘤明显而且核分裂率高（核分裂象多于30个/10HPF）的肿瘤称为"间变性无性细胞瘤"（anaplastic dysgerminoma）。这种病例的预后与典型的无性细胞瘤相似[700,716]。大约3%的无性细胞瘤含有合体滋养巨细胞，但是并不显示其他非无性细胞瘤的分化。这些肿瘤被称为伴有合体滋养巨细胞的无性细胞瘤（dysgerminoma with syncytiotrophoblastic giant cells），与缺乏合体滋养巨细胞的肿瘤具有同样的预后[716]。已有1例无性细胞瘤发生于发育不全的性腺的报告[732]。

无性细胞瘤与睾丸的精原细胞瘤有相似的免疫表型。最有特征性的发现是肿瘤细胞胎盘碱性磷酸酶（placental alkaline phosphatase，PLAP）、CD117和OCT4阳性染色[733,734]。PLAP和CD117是膜染色，通常较强而弥漫。OCT4是核转录因子的蛋白产物，因此核染色阳性；OCT4一般也呈弥漫性强染色。抗细胞角蛋白的单克隆抗体，特别是抗低分子量细胞角蛋白的抗体，在无性细胞瘤中可以阳性[735]，但染色通常为局灶性，可有点状或轮圈样外观。合体滋养巨细胞人绒毛膜促性腺激素染色阳性，这种细胞偶尔可在无性细胞瘤中见到[716,732]，而且偶尔单核肿瘤细胞也可阳性[735,736]。甲胎蛋白（AFP）染色几乎总是阴性。显微镜下可见无性细胞瘤转化为卵黄囊瘤的病灶，这样的病例已有几例报告，并且显示卵黄囊分化区域甲胎蛋白和细胞角蛋白染色阳性，而典型的无性细胞瘤区域阴性[717]。无性细胞瘤中浸润的淋巴细胞是T细胞，各种T细胞分化标志物免疫组化染色阳性[737]。

卵黄囊（内胚窦）瘤
Yolk sac (endodermal sinus) tumor

卵黄囊瘤是恶性生殖细胞肿瘤，肿瘤分化为卵黄囊结构[738-741]。这种肿瘤以往被称为内胚窦瘤。卵黄囊瘤是第二个最常见的卵巢恶性生殖细胞肿瘤，大约占卵巢恶性肿瘤的1%[697]。

临床特征 卵黄囊瘤主要发生于儿童和年轻女性，虽然少数病例报告本病发生于45岁以上的妇女[742-748]。平均年龄19岁。

最常见的症状是腹痛、腹部增大或腹部肿块[744,746]。大约10%的患者由于肿瘤破裂或扭转而引起急腹症。多数卵黄囊瘤患者血清甲胎蛋白（AFP）水平增高[742,749,750]，而且某些患者CA-125水平也增高[749]。

诊断时,大约50%的患者卵黄囊瘤局限于卵巢[742-744]。当肿瘤播散到卵巢外时，可播散到腹膜和网膜、腹主动脉旁淋巴结和肝。大约10%的病例肿瘤好像局限于盆腔(Ⅱ期)，其余40%发生广泛转移（Ⅲ期和Ⅳ期）。

推荐的卵黄囊瘤初始手术治疗是单侧输卵管-卵巢切除术伴有卵巢外肿瘤的局限性减瘤术。局灶性（Ⅰ期）肿瘤患者双侧卵巢受累罕见，因此对侧卵巢没有必要进行活检[744]。如果没有受累，晚期患者也无需切除对侧卵巢和子宫。尽管表面上看来手术充分，但在得到联合化疗之前，卵黄囊瘤患者的预后极差[744,751,752]。临床经过以迅速发生转移和高死亡率为特征，即使手术时肿瘤局限于卵巢的患者也是如此。研究证实，放疗对于治疗这些肿瘤无效[742,753]。1975年前一项大宗经过治疗的病例研究显示，患者的3年存活率仅为13%[744]。VAC[长春新碱(vincristine)、放线菌素D(actinomycin D, dactinomycin)和环磷酰胺(cyclophosphamide)]联合化疗完全改变了卵黄囊瘤患者的前景。当用VAC化疗治疗时，大约80%的Ⅰ期患者存活，大约50%的晚期患者存活[742,754,755]。含有铂的化疗方案对于Ⅰ期患者效果更好，而且晚期患者的生存率也有改善[731,756-762]。血清AFP水平可用于监控治疗反应和检测肿瘤复发[749,757]。卵黄囊瘤患者不需要进行二次剖腹探查[763]，即使在少数具有正常血清AFP水平的有肿瘤残留的患者中[764]。

病理学 卵黄囊瘤体积大，平均直径16cm[742,744]，切面褐色、白色或灰色，伴有小囊腔以及出血和坏死区。

卵黄囊瘤主要有5种生长方式，还有许多罕见的生长方式。多数肿瘤为混合性的生长方式。两种最常见和最具有特征性的形态是网状或微囊性结构以及内胚窦结构[744]。网状结构是由疏松的微囊性网状间隙组成的，内衬单层扁平或立方细胞（图13A.76）。这些细胞具有透明或双染性的胞浆以及非典型性深染的细胞核。内胚窦结构也叫花彩状或假乳头状结构，由内衬柱状细胞的相互吻合的腺体或乳头组成，胞浆透明或双染性，核呈梭形，深染。Schiller-Duval 小体是内胚窦结构的特征性表现，它是由被覆柱状肿瘤细胞的纤维血管乳头突入内衬立方细胞的腺体或囊性间隙组成的（图13A.77），见于大约2/3的病例。Schiller-Duval 小体是卵黄囊瘤的诊断特征。内胚窦结构常常合并成与之密切相关的腺泡状-腺体结构，其中相互吻合的小管和腺体被黏液样或梭形细胞间质围绕。腺体内衬立方形或柱状细胞，而且常为多层或形成小的乳头。实性结构的特征是成巢或成片的小至中等大小的未分化细胞，伴有中等量的双染性或透明的胞浆。多囊泡状卵黄结构的囊肿类似于卵黄囊小泡，内衬立方、柱状或黏液性上皮细胞（图13A.78）。囊肿由不成熟的富于细胞的间叶性间质围绕[765]。罕见的结构包括肝样结构，由片块状或小梁状的大细胞组成，核呈空泡状，位于中心，核仁突出，胞浆丰富，嗜酸性颗粒状[424,741,766,767]。这些细胞类似于在肝细胞癌中所见的细胞。虽然某些卵黄囊瘤出现大面积的肝样分化，但是这种结构经常是局灶性的显微镜下所见[768]。腺体结构罕见，但它是卵黄囊瘤的重要结构，其中具有子宫内膜样或肠型腺体区域。子宫内膜样亚型可能被误诊为子宫内膜样癌，腺体内衬单层柱状细胞，具有透明的核上或核下胞浆空泡（图13A.79）[769,770]。肠型结构可能类似于原发性或转移性黏液性肿瘤，它以原始的内胚层腺体聚集为

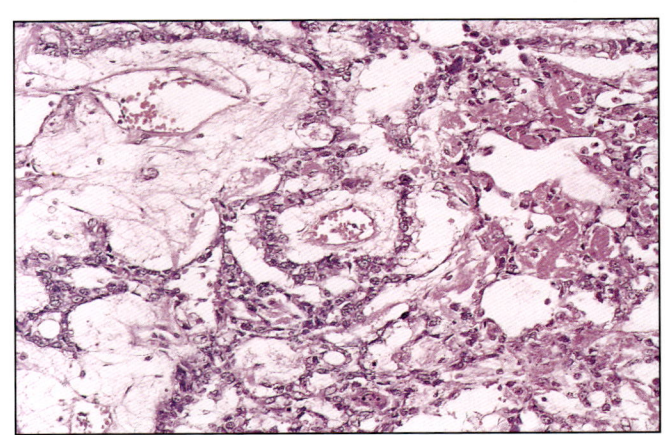

图13A.77 卵黄囊瘤。视野中心可见伴有Schiller-Duval小体的内胚窦结构。Schiller-Duval小体是长入囊性间隙的乳头状结构。乳头被覆肿瘤细胞，中央为毛细血管。

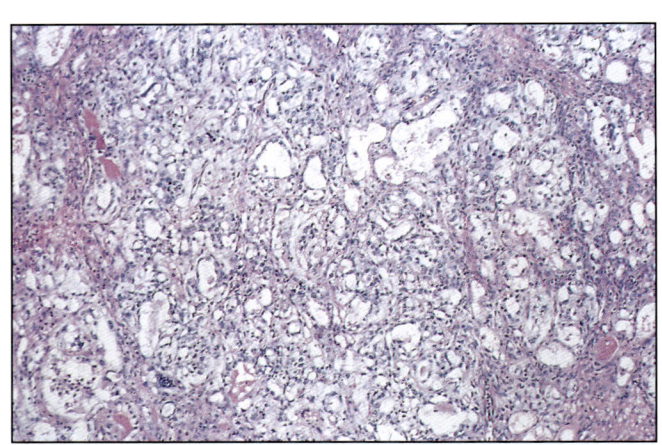

图13A.76 卵黄囊瘤。典型的微囊性或网状结构。

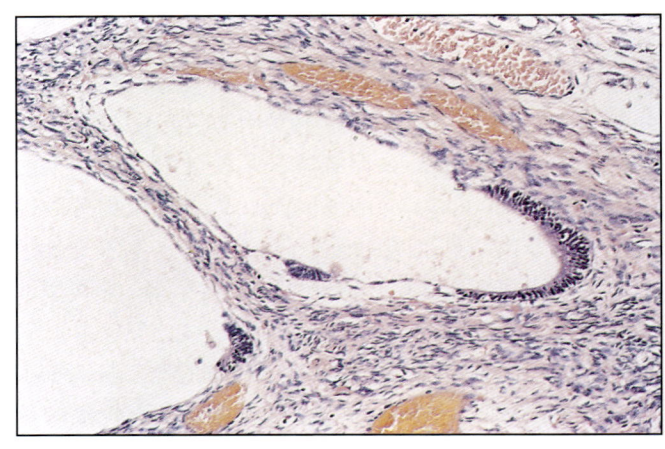

图13A.78 卵黄囊瘤。多囊泡状卵黄结构，其中囊肿部分内衬柱状肿瘤细胞，部分内衬扁平细胞，周围绕以不成熟的间质。

特征，腺体内衬矮柱状细胞，生长在疏松的或细胞丰富的间质中[771,772]。卵黄囊瘤还可能含有类似于胎儿肺的腺体。这些生殖细胞起源的卵黄囊瘤的腺体分化结构，必须与发生于老年妇女的罕见肿瘤相鉴别，这种肿瘤中的卵黄囊瘤来源于或伴有子宫内膜样或黏液性上皮性肿瘤[276,277,429,773]。

嗜酸性 PAS 阳性的抗淀粉酶的玻璃样小体是卵黄囊瘤的一个特征性表现，这种小体最常见于网状结构和内胚窦结构（图 13A.80）。网状和实性区域一般也含有大量的细胞外玻璃样 PAS 阳性物质，这些物质由层粘连蛋白和Ⅳ型胶原组成，其超微结构类似于基底膜[745,768]。某些作者将这些物质解释为腔壁的卵黄囊分化（parietal yolk sac differentiation）[768]。50% 的卵黄囊瘤可见内衬柱状和杯状细胞的小而温和的肠腺体，而且描述了两例罕见的肿瘤，其中卵黄囊瘤与黏液性类癌混合存在[774]。25% 的卵黄囊瘤有突出的含有梭形或星形细胞的黏液样间质，这些细胞的细胞角蛋白和 vimentin 染色均呈阳性反应[742,775]。这些间质细胞可以分化为诸如软骨、横纹肌和骨等间叶性成分，偶尔见于卵黄囊瘤。15%~20% 的病例，卵黄囊瘤内或其附近的间质细胞出现黄素化。极少数病例存在合体滋养巨细胞[745,746,776]。

卵黄囊瘤最重要的免疫组化表现是 AFP 呈阳性表达。75% 以上的卵黄囊瘤细胞胞浆、囊肿和腺体内的分泌物、某些玻璃样小体 AFP 阳性染色，但是这种表达通常微弱和呈局灶性[364]。卵黄囊瘤细胞 α_1- 抗胰蛋白酶[424,777]和胎盘碱性磷酸酶[778,779]免疫组化染色阳性，细胞外的玻璃样物质层粘连蛋白阳性[768]。卵黄囊瘤细胞角蛋白阳性而上皮膜抗原阴性[364]。细胞角蛋白 AE1/AE3 胞浆阳性，相反胚胎性癌呈特征性的膜染色。卵黄囊瘤细胞角蛋白 7 阴性；这个结果加上缺乏上皮膜抗原染色和 AFP 染色阳性，可将卵黄囊瘤与透明细胞癌区别开来[364]。卵黄囊瘤 OCT4 和 CD117 阴性，这与细胞角蛋白及 AFP 阳性染色一起，可将卵黄囊瘤的实性结构与无性细胞瘤鉴别开来。人绒毛膜促性腺激素免疫染色为阴性，除了那些罕见的含有合体滋养巨细胞的肿瘤以外[745,746]。卵黄囊瘤中或小或大的肝样分化区域抗肝细胞抗体染色阳性，然而这不是一个特异性的表现，因为肝样癌和转移性肝细胞癌抗肝细胞抗体也阳性[420]。

胚胎性癌 Embryonal carcinoma

胚胎性癌是一种少见的卵巢肿瘤，它在形态学上与睾丸的胚胎性癌相同。

临床特征 胚胎性癌几乎全部发生于儿童和年轻女性[745,746,780]，虽然有一些发生于老年女性的报道[781]。平均年龄大约为 15 岁。典型表现是盆腔或腹部疼痛或腹部可触及肿块。月经异常常见于青春期后患者。大部分患者妊娠试验阳性或血清 β-HCG 浓度升高，大约 50% 的月经初潮前期患者出现早熟性假青春期[780]。

在诊断时胚胎性癌局限于卵巢的患者，恰当的外科治疗方法为单侧输卵管-卵巢切除。胚胎性癌实际上从不双侧发生，因此没有必要进行对侧卵巢的活组织检查。晚期肿瘤（FIGO IA 期以上）通常进行腹式子宫全切术、双侧输卵管-卵巢切除术及限制性的减瘤术。胚胎性癌患者通常年轻，因此如果对侧卵巢及子宫没有受累，可以进行单侧输卵管-卵巢切除术及限制性的减瘤术。

在应用有效的联合化疗之前，胚胎性癌通常迅速致死，即使是 Ⅰ 期患者，存活率也只限于 50%[780]。目前，胚胎性癌完全被切除的患者术后应用以顺铂为基础的辅

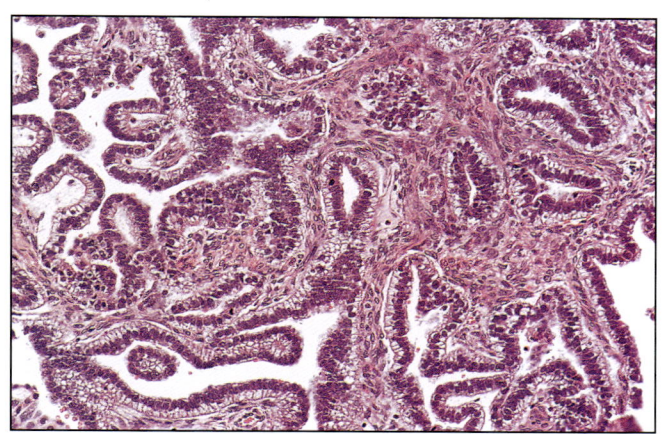

图13A.79　卵黄囊瘤。子宫内膜样亚型，腺体内衬具有明显核下空泡的柱状肿瘤细胞。

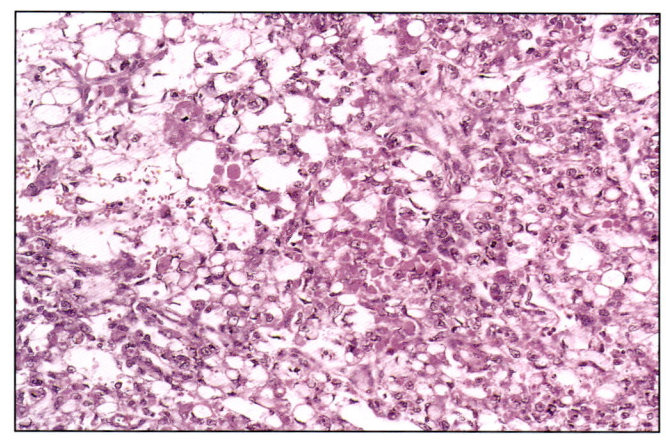

图13A.80　卵黄囊瘤。具有许多嗜酸性透明小体的网状结构。

助化疗，可以获得近乎完全的成功[758]。许多伴有残留或复发性肿瘤的患者可以应用联合化疗治愈[782]。

血清β-HCG和AFP分析可用于评估治疗效果。如果治疗之后两种标志物之一或两者同时升高，或在随访过程中标志物升高，代表患者出现复发或转移性肿瘤。

病理学 胚胎性癌是一种大的实性肿瘤，平均直径为15～17 cm。切面呈鱼肉样，褐色或灰色，伴有小囊、出血和坏死区域。

卵巢胚胎性癌的显微镜下结构与睾丸胚胎性癌相似。肿瘤细胞具有大的空泡状核，核染色质粗，有一或两个显著的核仁（图13A.81）。胞浆丰富，双染性或透明。肿瘤细胞呈巢状或片块状生长，偶尔可见散在的裂隙、腺体或乳头状结构。多数胚胎性癌含有局灶性合体滋养巨细胞。间质疏松水肿，或由富于细胞的增生性小的原始梭形细胞组成。

免疫染色细胞角蛋白和CD30阳性，细胞膜着色。胚胎性癌显示OCT4核的阳性染色，但是CD117和上皮膜抗原阴性。合体滋养巨细胞和偶尔出现的类似于中间滋养细胞的大的单核细胞，绒毛膜促性腺激素免疫反应阳性[745,746,780]。在70%的病例中，单核胚胎性癌细胞有弥漫性的胞浆AFP染色。

多胚瘤（polyembryoma）是一种少见的恶性生殖细胞肿瘤，它的特征介于胚胎性癌和相对比较分化的恶性生殖细胞肿瘤之间；它通常是作为混合性生殖细胞肿瘤的一种成分[783-786]。显微镜下，多胚瘤由许多胚胎样小体（embryoid body）组成，生长在原始的胚胎性间质内。胚胎样小体类似于14～20周的胚胎。它们含有由高柱状细胞组成的胚盘（embryonic disc），细胞核深染，有些类似于内衬胚胎性癌裂隙和腺体的细胞。胚盘的一侧是羊膜腔，而另外一侧是内衬甲胎蛋白阳性细胞的卵黄囊[787]。胚胎样小体通常扭曲或不完整，难以辨认。

绒毛膜癌 Choriocarcinoma

生殖细胞起源的单纯性卵巢原发性绒毛膜癌极其少见[697,788-790]。一篇有关恶性卵巢生殖细胞肿瘤的综述指出，绒毛膜癌少于1%[697]。绒毛膜癌最常见于作为混合性生殖细胞肿瘤的一种成分。

临床特征 卵巢绒毛膜癌发生于儿童和年轻妇女[791,792]。临床表现是腹痛和异常阴道出血。妊娠试验阳性，血清β-HCG升高[788,793,794]。经前期儿童可有早熟性假青春期[788]。手术时经常可见腹腔积血。

卵巢绒毛膜癌为单侧发生，可通过输卵管-卵巢切除术治疗。只有当对侧卵巢或子宫受累时，才需要进行腹式子宫切除及双侧输卵管-卵巢切除术。术后予以以顺铂为基础的联合化疗方案[758]。即使应用次佳化疗方案，也能取得令人满意的结果[788]。妊娠期绒毛膜癌的化疗和预后是不同的，所以鉴别妊娠期绒毛膜癌和生殖细胞来源的绒毛膜癌十分重要。如果患者处于经前期，绒毛膜癌一定是来源于生殖细胞。妊娠期卵巢绒毛膜癌，或从子宫或输卵管转移而来或原发于卵巢，与来源于生殖细胞的绒毛膜癌相似，易发生于生育期的年轻女性[789]。妊娠期绒毛膜癌与来源于生殖细胞的绒毛膜癌在形态学上没有区别，虽然出现妊娠黄体支持前一种诊断。临床病史可能有助于鉴别诊断。如果通过DNA分析或HLA分型能够发现父系成分，那么绒毛膜癌就来源于妊娠[791,795-797]。

病理学 绒毛膜癌是单侧性质软的紫红色肿瘤，切面可见出血和坏死。直径从4cm到25cm不等。

显微镜下，大多数肿瘤有出血和坏死。成活的细胞滋养细胞和合体滋养巨细胞在肿瘤周边呈丛状生长（图13A.82）。细胞滋养细胞有丰富的透明胞浆和清楚的细胞边界。它们的核不规则，呈空泡状，有些细胞含有巨大核仁。合体滋养巨细胞含有丰富的空泡状嗜碱性或双染性胞浆，内有多个深染的细胞核。所有的滋养细胞细胞角蛋白阳性，合体滋养巨细胞细胞角蛋白染色致密。β-HCG免疫组化染色合体滋养巨细胞胞浆阳性[794]。

畸胎瘤 Teratoma

良性囊性畸胎瘤（皮样囊肿）是最常见的卵巢肿瘤，占所有卵巢肿瘤的25%或25%以上[1,3,4]。其他类型畸胎瘤少见。多数畸胎瘤具有46XX核型，被认为是由单个单倍体生殖细胞通过单性生殖（parthenogenesis）发展而成[798-801]。

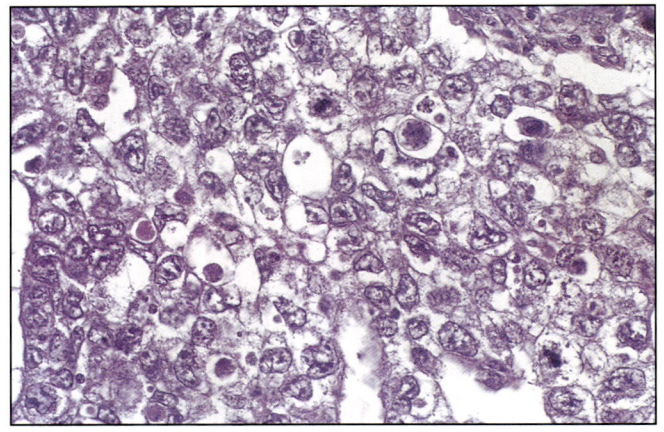

图13A.81 胚胎性癌。间变性恶性生殖细胞成片块状生长。肿瘤其他部位有腺体和合体滋养巨细胞。

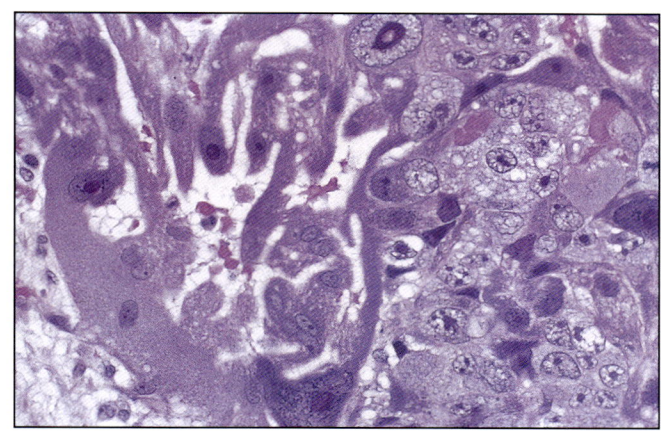

图13A.82 绒毛膜癌。细胞滋养细胞具有淡染的胞浆和伴有明显块状染色质的空泡状核。合体滋养细胞具有多个较小的细胞核,位于合胞体细胞的嗜碱性胞浆内。

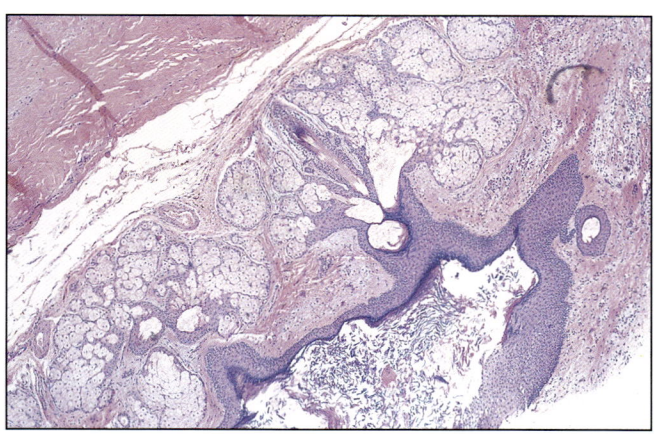

图13A.83 良性囊状畸胎瘤("皮样囊肿")。囊肿内衬皮肤和表皮附件。表皮为复层鳞状上皮,其下为毛干和皮脂腺。囊腔内有角质碎屑。

成熟性(良性)畸胎瘤 Mature (benign) teratoma

成熟性畸胎瘤是囊性,或在少数情况下是实性肿瘤,含有来自一个或一个以上胚层(即外胚层、中胚层和内胚层)的各种成熟组织。

临床特征 良性畸胎瘤发生于所有年龄的患者。多数见于20~50岁之间的妇女;只有大约20%发生于绝经后的妇女[802-805]。高峰发病年龄在20~29岁之间[1,806]。许多患者没有症状,肿瘤是在常规检查或在评估或治疗某些其他病变时发现的。当肿瘤大小达到很大时,患者会出现盆腔压迫或疼痛症状。最常见的严重并发症是扭转,见于3%~10%的病例,破裂大约见于1%的病例[806]。扭转可引起急腹症。自发性破裂的后遗症是急性腹膜炎,或在少数情况下发生慢性肉芽肿性腹膜炎。成熟性畸胎瘤为良性肿瘤,可以保守治疗。通过腹腔镜或剖腹进行囊肿切除术是充分的治疗[807-810],尤其是在儿童和年轻的妇女[806]。双侧良性畸胎瘤见于10%~15%的患者。由成熟神经胶质组织(0级)组成的腹膜种植发生在少数卵巢成熟性畸胎瘤的患者。这种腹膜种植对于生存率没有不利影响。

病理学 良性畸胎瘤几乎总是囊性肿瘤。它们的大小从几个厘米到重达几千克不等;平均直径为7~8 cm。在体温条件下囊内容物为液体,但在室温下变成固体,柔软或质硬。切面为单房性囊肿,少数为多房性,囊壁上有被称为皮样乳头(dermoid papilla)的实性突起。囊内含有毛发、凝块状物质,或为油性或为浆液性的液体。可能发现软骨、骨或牙齿。局灶性类似于脑的灰褐色软组织以及亮绿色或棕色的甲状腺组织也较常见。在囊性畸胎瘤中,致密的实性区域少见;出现这些区域提出了是否存在未成熟性畸胎瘤的问题,必须仔细取材用于组织学检查。完全实性的成熟性(良性)畸胎瘤罕见,只有通过显微镜检查才能与未成熟性畸胎瘤相区分[813]。

良性畸胎瘤是含有不同比例的外胚层、中胚层和内胚层结构的混合性肿物,这些结构以器官样的生长方式分布于肿瘤之中。在2/3的成熟性畸胎瘤中,至少可以见到来源于两个胚层的组织,而大约1/3的成熟性畸胎瘤出现所有三个胚层的组织[4,803]。外胚层衍生物最常见,例如皮肤、毛囊、皮脂腺和汗腺,当这些结构在组织学图像中占主导地位时,肿瘤通常被称为"皮样囊肿"(dermoid cyst)(图13A.83)。常常出现的其他外胚层成分包括脑(通常为神经胶质)、脉络膜丛、外周神经以及牙的结构。常见的内胚层组织有包括内分泌细胞在内的消化道黏膜[814]、呼吸道黏膜、肾组织和甲状腺组织。最常见的中胚层衍生物是脂肪组织、平滑肌或横纹肌、骨或软骨,以及围绕其他成分的疏松的结缔组织框架。出人意料的是,男性的组织偶尔也可出现在良性畸胎瘤中,例如前列腺[815-818]。在皮样乳头的切片中,最有可能找到外胚层和中胚层衍生的成分。在某些肿瘤中,单一成分十分显著,将其分类为单胚层畸胎瘤是恰当的(例如卵巢甲状腺肿,struma ovarii)。囊腔内衬扁平上皮或为周围绕以多核巨细胞的肉芽组织,在某些畸胎瘤中还有噬脂细胞(lipophages)。上皮破坏,囊内容物释放到周围组织,可能引起异物肉芽肿性反应。

未成熟性畸胎瘤 Immature teratoma

未成熟性畸胎瘤是最常见的卵巢恶性生殖细胞肿瘤之一,在大的癌症中心中,占这类肿瘤的20%~30%[754,819]。

临床特征 未成熟性畸胎瘤主要发生于儿童及年轻

女性。患者平均年龄大约为 20 岁，几乎没有年龄小于 7 岁或大于 40 岁的患者[820-826]。临床表现为非特异性。患者主诉为盆腔或腹部疼痛、腹部肿胀或可触及的腹部肿块。少数患者由于肿瘤扭转或破裂而引起急腹症[827]。单纯性未成熟性畸胎瘤患者可有血清甲胎蛋白水平升高，而且肿瘤标志物 CA-125 水平常常轻度升高[819,827-829]。多数患者（50%～80%）在诊断时肿瘤为局限性（Ⅰ期）。虽然晚期患者可以发生对侧卵巢转移，但双侧卵巢受累罕见[821,822,827,830]。未成熟性畸胎瘤播散主要是通过盆腔和腹腔腹膜以及网膜种植[831]。10%～15% 的病例对侧卵巢有良性囊性畸胎瘤[821,827,830]。

局限性肿瘤（ⅠA 期）患者可行单侧输卵管-卵巢切除术。少数患者通过囊肿切除术以及术后化疗获得成功[832]。较晚期的肿瘤可以进行单侧输卵管-卵巢切除术及卵巢外肿瘤切除术治疗[724,819]。如果不存在保存生育能力的问题，或对侧卵巢或子宫受累，治疗方法为子宫及双侧输卵管-卵巢切除术。ⅠA 期 1 级未成熟性畸胎瘤患者预后很好，可以单独通过手术治疗。ⅠA 期 3 级未成熟性畸胎瘤患者或晚期疾病患者需要术后化疗。ⅠA 期 2 级肿瘤患者的辅助化疗问题尚有争议；有些作者提倡化疗[758,827,828,833,834]，但是另外一些作者并不提倡[819,820,824]。儿童的预后似乎较好，而与肿瘤分级无关[835]。在转移灶缺乏未成熟组织或诸如卵黄囊瘤等其他恶性生殖细胞成分时，不管肿瘤分级如何，儿科肿瘤医师往往拒绝应用化疗[836]。对于手术后没有肿瘤残留的患者，含有顺铂的化疗方案非常有效，例如 BEP（顺铂、依托泊甙和博来霉素）方案，生存率可以达到 90%～100%[758,831]。肉眼可见肿瘤残留或复发性未成熟性畸胎瘤预后较差。

在有卵巢外肿瘤扩散的患者，转移灶的显微镜下表现具有重要预后意义。有些腹膜种植或淋巴结转移只含有成熟组织，对于预后不会产生不良影响[812,821,822,827,837-840]。这些 0 级种植通常是由部分或全部成熟的神经胶质组成（图 13A.84）。新近关于神经胶质种植的分子研究显示，它们在遗传学上不同于卵巢肿瘤，但是与其具有同样的遗传方式[841,842]。推测是肿瘤产生的物质导致腹膜或腹膜下组织化生为神经胶质。这种起源就为在种植中偶尔发现子宫内膜异位和神经胶质组织混合存在提供了一个似乎合理的解释[843,844]。没有完全切除的未成熟性畸胎瘤患者化疗后二次手术可能显示残留的未成熟性畸胎瘤、没有肿瘤残留、小的神经胶质种植或巨大成熟性畸胎瘤结节[763]。切除这些大的结节可以避免粘连或压迫邻近组织，并阻止"种植性畸胎瘤综合征"（growing teratoma syndrome）的发生[763,819,845,846]。在少数情况下，长期存在的未完全切除的低级别畸胎瘤种植可以发生恶性肿瘤[847]。

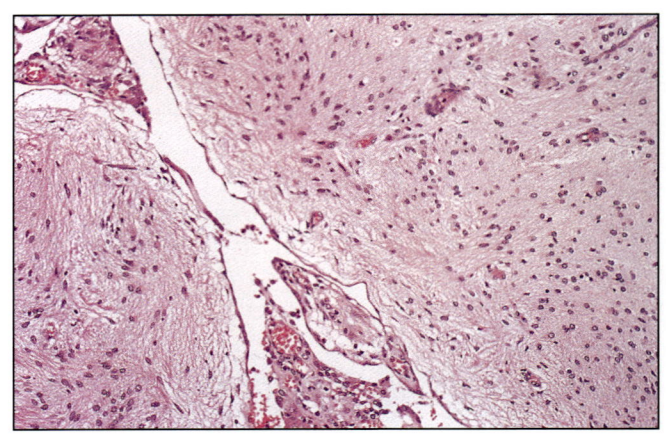

图 13A.84　网膜的神经胶质种植。在这个 0 级种植灶中，良性表现的神经胶质结节被腹膜覆盖。

病理学　未成熟性畸胎瘤是一种以实性为主的单侧性肿瘤，直径平均为 18cm。实性部分为灰色或棕色，可以质软或质硬，有砂砾感。切面一般可见散在的小囊。大约四分之一的病例可见一个或多个含有角质碎屑或毛发的大囊肿，类似于皮样囊肿[830]。

多数肿瘤可以见到由所有三个胚层衍生而来的组织，而且成熟和未成熟成分混合存在。这些组织通常杂乱分布，而且常常缺乏良性囊性畸胎瘤的器官样生长方式。外胚层和中胚层衍生物一般主要位于未成熟成分中。未成熟神经外胚层成分是最容易辨认和定量的未成熟组织[821,822]。其中包括成片的核分裂活跃的不成熟神经上皮细胞、内衬具有复层深染细胞核的柱状胚胎细胞的腺体和小管、含有无核原纤维区域的成巢和成片的神经母细胞以及 Homer Wright 菊形团、核分裂活跃的不成熟神经胶质，以及伴有黑色素沉着的原始视网膜（图 13A.85 和 13A.86）[848]。在未成熟性畸胎瘤的神经成分中，偶尔可见显著的良性血管增生[849]。不成熟的间叶

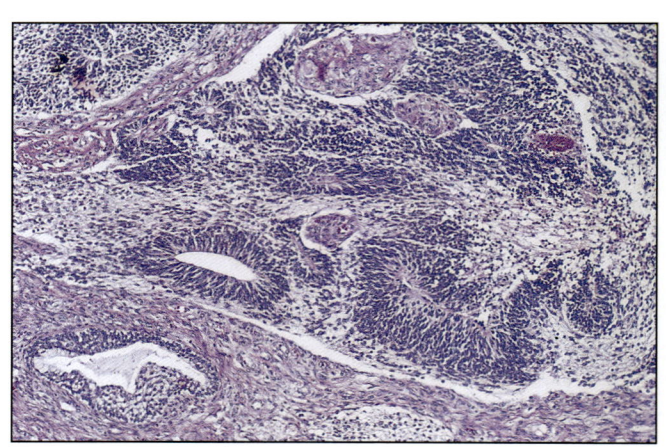

图 13A.85　未成熟性畸胎瘤。不成熟的神经组织（上）是最容易辨认和定量的不成熟成分。这张照片还可见到不成熟的内胚层成分（左下）。

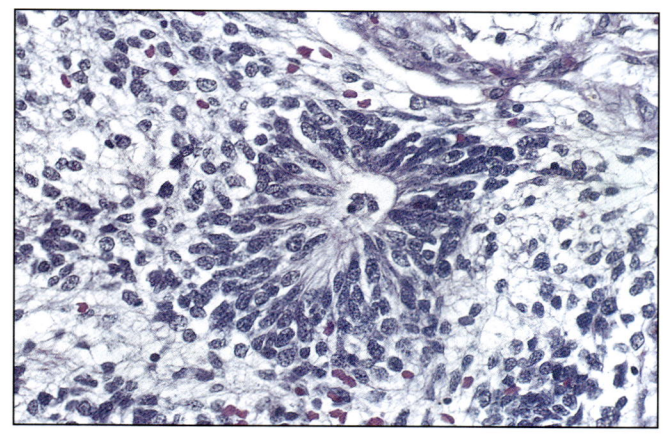

图13A.86 未成熟性畸胎瘤。不成熟性神经组织中小圆形神经母细胞围绕原始神经管。

表13A.10	未成熟性畸胎瘤的组织学分级	
级别	不成熟组织	神经上皮数量
0	缺乏	没有
1	+	罕见，不大于1 lpf/每张切片
2	++	常见，不大于3 lpf/每张切片
3	+++	显著，≥4 lpf/每张切片

lpf= 低倍视野（low power field）

性间质细胞丰富，由小的梭形细胞组成，细胞核深染（图.13A.87）。通常可见核分裂象。在未成熟性畸胎瘤中常常出现软骨，而且可能难以确定软骨是否为不成熟性。当有许多含有小的软骨细胞的陷窝，以及软骨样分化灶被不成熟的小圆形间质细胞包绕时，将这种软骨解释成不成熟的间叶成分是恰当的。一种少见的伴有横纹肌肉瘤性间叶成分的侵袭性未成熟性畸胎瘤已有报告[850]。不成熟性内胚层组织并不常见，而且很少见于缺乏不成熟性外胚层衍生物的病例。可能见到的不成熟性内胚层结构的类型包括内衬具有核下和核上空泡的柱状细胞的原始腺体、部分分化的分层的伴有杯状细胞的柱状肠上皮，以及岛屿状胎儿肝组织[766,851]。不成熟性肾（生后肾）结构，例如胚胎样肾小球，是未成熟性畸胎瘤罕见的成分[852]。显微镜下，未成熟性畸胎瘤中偶尔可见灶状卵黄囊瘤，只要仅有几个（≤3）小灶而且直径小于3 mm，好像并不影响预后[822,853]。儿科病理医师提出，胎儿型肝和具有核下空泡的分化性腺体类似于不成熟的内胚层或胎儿肺，是高分化类型的卵黄囊瘤[835]，而妇科病理医师趋向于将数量有限的这些成分视为畸胎瘤的组成部分。未成熟性畸胎瘤的分级方法将其定为4级，从完全由成熟组织组成的0级肿瘤，到含有丰富的不成熟组织的3级肿瘤（表13A.10）[822]。未成熟性畸胎瘤可以发生0级转移，但是原发性卵巢肿瘤必须根据定义分为1、2或3级。在两级分类系统中，提出1级肿瘤为低级别，而2级和3级肿瘤为高级别肿瘤，但是一般并不应用[853]。

少数生殖细胞肿瘤含有神经外胚层细胞，形成类似于各种中枢神经系统肿瘤的生长方式。这种类型的肿瘤也可发生在常常伴有畸胎瘤的睾丸。睾丸神经外胚层肿瘤的诊断仅限于神经外胚层成分直径至少有1 cm的肿瘤[854]。似乎有理由将这种大小标准应用于卵巢肿瘤，虽然在卵巢肿瘤，神经外胚层成分一般是多数或所有大的肿瘤的组成成分。有三种主要结构[855]。原始神经外胚层肿瘤（primitive neuroectodermal tumors）由成巢或成片的小细胞组成，这些小细胞核深染，核分裂活跃（图13A.88）[330,820,855,856]。某些细胞含有原纤维性胞浆，某些肿瘤含有伴有中心腔的菊形团、神经纤维网、神经母细胞性菊形团，或有局灶性神经胶质分化。这种

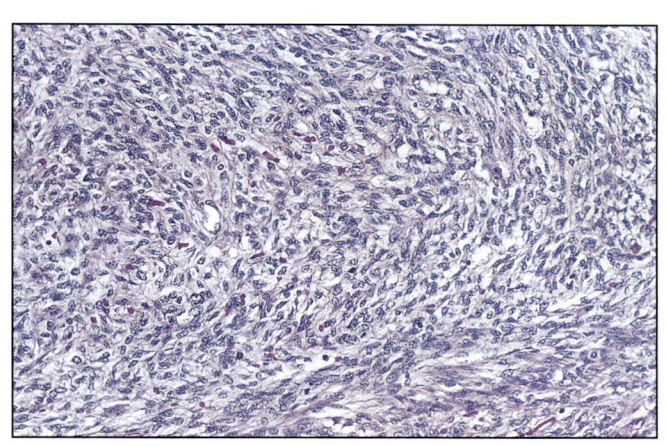

图13A.87 未成熟性畸胎瘤。不成熟性间叶组织。这种类型的不成熟组织可能难以辨认和定量。

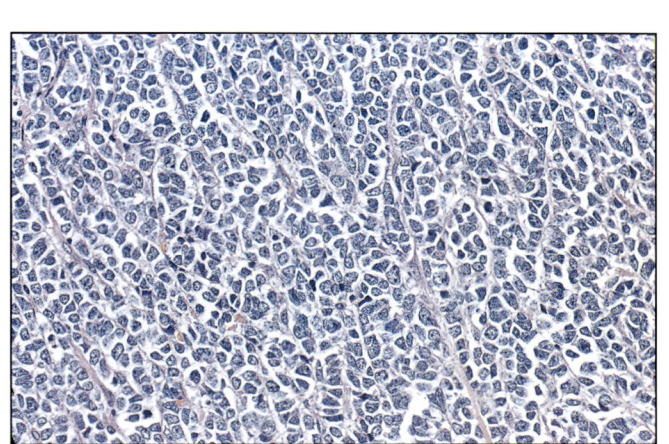

图13A.88 原始神经外胚层肿瘤。弥漫成片的小圆形细胞，细胞核深染，胞浆稀少。

类型的肿瘤类似于髓上皮瘤、室管膜母细胞瘤或神经母细胞瘤。第二种类型的神经外胚层肿瘤表现为广泛的神经胶质分化，类似于多形性胶质母细胞瘤（glioblastoma multiforme）[855]。第三种类型的神经外胚层肿瘤类似于室管膜瘤（ependymoma）[855,857-859]。伴有原纤维性胞浆的圆形或柱状细胞构成了血管周围的假菊形团结构以及伴有中央腔的真正的室管膜菊形团。在某些肿瘤中，室管膜细胞内衬腺体、囊肿或被覆在乳头周围，可能导致误诊为上皮性肿瘤。原始神经外胚层肿瘤和类似于多形性胶质母细胞瘤的肿瘤常常含有畸胎瘤成分，但室管膜细胞瘤通常没有畸胎瘤成分。如果神经外胚层肿瘤和恶性胶质瘤播散到卵巢以外，则预后不好，但是室管膜瘤即使出现转移似乎也是一个惰性的肿瘤。这些肿瘤一般被分类为单胚层畸胎瘤，尽管也可以将其视为未成熟性畸胎瘤的亚型。

在未成熟性畸胎瘤的诊断上，免疫组化检查的作用有限。神经胶质原纤维酸性蛋白（GFAP）染色可以标记神经胶质原纤维和胞体，可能有助于辨认神经胶质分化[813,860,861]。原始神经上皮细胞 GFAP 染色阴性，虽然有些肿瘤应用神经细丝和神经元特异性烯醇化酶（NSE）抗体染色阳性[860,861]。肠道和呼吸道上皮含有嗜银细胞，这些嗜银细胞与多种神经激素肽类抗体产生反应[861]。不成熟的内胚层结构 AFP 染色阳性，例如孤立的卵黄囊样小泡、未成熟性腺体和肠上皮以及肝[829,861,862]。免疫染色还可能有助于确定某些不成熟成分的存在。例如，原始神经上皮 CD99 和 bcl-2 染色阳性，未成熟的软骨 CD34 和 bcl-2 阳性表达[862]。

成熟性（良性囊性）畸胎瘤的继发性肿瘤 Secondary neoplasms in mature (benign cystic) teratoma

发生于良性囊性畸胎瘤的良性或恶性肿瘤罕见。恶性变仅发生于 1%～3% 的良性囊性畸胎瘤[805,863-866]。

临床特征 继发性恶性肿瘤一般发生于绝经后的妇女，但是可以见于任何年龄患者。主诉为非特异性，包括腹部或盆腔疼痛、腹胀或可以触及的腹部肿块。在 50%～75% 的患者，肿瘤局限于卵巢（Ⅰ期），这些患者预后较好[867]。晚期肿瘤患者预后不好[868]。多数病例化疗或放疗没有反应，在诊断后的一或两年之内死亡。

病理学 大体上，继发性肿瘤可以在囊壁内面形成结节状或乳头状肿物，或者可能有囊壁增厚或硬结。在某些情况下，只有通过显微镜下检查才能发现继发性肿瘤。继发性肿瘤通常为单侧性，但对侧卵巢可能含有

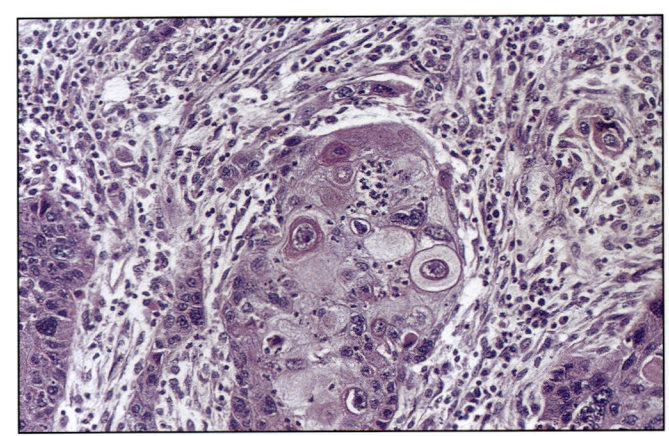

图13A.89 鳞状细胞癌。图示角化性鳞状细胞癌是良性囊性畸胎瘤的继发性肿瘤。

一个良性囊性畸胎瘤。痣[869]、皮质腺腺瘤和其他皮肤附件肿瘤、良性涎腺型肿瘤、脑脊膜瘤[870]、血管球瘤[871]以及血管瘤性血管增生[849,872]，是发生于良性囊性畸胎瘤的良性肿瘤[873]。已经报道的原位恶性肿瘤包括原位鳞状细胞癌和 Paget 病[418,874-876]。浸润性鳞状细胞癌大约占良性囊性畸胎瘤中继发性恶性肿瘤的 85%（图 13A.89）[418,865-868]。余下的是其他类型的皮肤癌，例如基底细胞癌或皮脂腺癌[877,878]、黑色素瘤[879-882]、腺癌[864,883-886]、各种类型的肉瘤[887,888]以及其他罕见类型的肿瘤。来自畸胎瘤的罕见的黏液性上皮性肿瘤可以引起腹膜假黏液瘤[889]。

卵巢甲状腺肿 Struma ovarii

卵巢甲状腺肿是一种畸胎瘤，其中以甲状腺组织为主要成分[890]。50% 以上的肿瘤由甲状腺组织组成才能诊断卵巢甲状腺肿。根据这个定义，卵巢甲状腺肿在良性卵巢畸胎瘤中占 1%～3%[4,803,891]。

临床特征 卵巢甲状腺肿主要发生于 40 岁以上的妇女。通常是一个偶然发现，或在伴有非特异性症状的患者中发现，例如腹部或盆腔疼痛或腹胀。少数患者有腹水或腹水和胸水（假 Meigs 综合征）[892-896]。偶尔有患者出现激素介导的症状，例如异常阴道出血[894]。不到 10% 的卵巢甲状腺肿患者出现甲状腺功能亢进症状，其中有些患者同时有甲状腺肿大[891,893,897]。多数卵巢甲状腺肿为良性肿瘤，囊肿切除术或单侧输卵管-卵巢切除术是恰当的治疗方法。根据组织学结构诊断为恶性卵巢甲状腺肿的肿瘤在临床上很少为恶性，不需要进行根治性的治疗[891,898-902]。少数恶性甲状腺肿局部转移到腹膜或网膜，或转移到诸如淋巴结、肝、骨或肺等远隔部位[890,903-906]。这种情况最好是通过子宫切除术和双侧输卵管-卵巢切除术、甲状腺切除术，以及给予放射性碘治疗[893,904,907]。

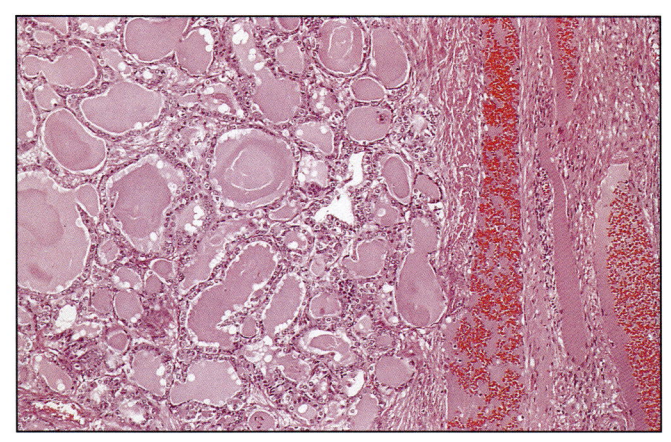

图13A.90 卵巢甲状腺肿。这种类型的单胚层畸胎瘤主要由成熟的甲状腺滤泡组成。

病理学 卵巢甲状腺肿是一个局限性的肿瘤,大小从直径只有 1 或 2cm 的小结节,到直径大于 10 cm 的大肿块。平均大小为 5～10 cm。切面,卵巢甲状腺肿为红色、绿色或褐色,伴有黏滑的肉样外观,常常出现小的囊腔,偶尔肿瘤主要或完全为囊性[908]。显微镜下,卵巢甲状腺肿由充满嗜酸性胶质的滤泡组成,内衬立方形或柱状细胞,细胞核圆形,均匀一致(图 13A.90)。可以出现退行性改变,例如纤维化、钙化和充满含铁血黄素的巨噬细胞聚集。卵巢甲状腺肿的囊性亚型几乎不含有滤泡,难以辨认[908]。可能出现诊断问题的其他生长方式包括:由透明细胞、嗜酸性细胞或印戒细胞组成的肿瘤;肿瘤细胞呈条索样排列;以及细胞丰富的肿瘤,其中肿瘤细胞表现为微滤泡性、小梁状或实性方式生长,类似于甲状腺的滤泡腺瘤[891,909]。卵巢甲状腺肿细胞丰富的亚型可以称为增生性卵巢甲状腺肿(proliferative struma ovarii)[891]。甲状腺球蛋白免疫染色胶质和滤泡细胞胞浆阳性,甲状腺转录因子 -1(thyroid transcription factor-1,TTF-1)肿瘤细胞核阳性[910]。这些表现可以确定疑难病例的诊断。如果仔细寻找,许多病例可以发现其他的畸胎瘤性成分。某些卵巢甲状腺肿病例的周围出现黄素化的卵巢间质细胞[909]。这些细胞可能是引起某些患者内分泌症状的激素来源,通过 inhibin 免疫染色可以识别。

任何类型的甲状腺癌都可以发生于卵巢甲状腺肿。最常见的是乳头状癌,与发生在甲状腺的乳头状癌具有同样的组织学表现[891]。乳头状癌呈浸润性生长,通常含有发育好的乳头,由具有大而密集且有核沟的核的细胞组成,伴有小的核仁[898,911]。某些细胞核透明,而另外一些细胞含有核内胞浆包涵体。细胞浆中等量或丰富而致密。滤泡内的胶质常常为实性,强嗜酸性表现。如同甲状腺一样,卵巢甲状腺肿也有滤泡状亚型乳头状癌的描述[912]。滤泡癌少见。它是一种细胞丰富的肿瘤,其中肿瘤细胞呈微滤泡性、小梁状或实性方式生长。滤泡癌与增生性卵巢甲状腺肿难以鉴别,但是核非典型性、常见核分裂象、特别是浸润性生长方式或血管浸润均支持滤泡癌的诊断[891]。类似于髓样癌的罕见的肿瘤也有描述。多数恶性卵巢甲状腺肿病例单独根据组织学背景被称为癌,但从不发生卵巢外播散。不过,临床上已经发生转移的恶性卵巢甲状腺肿病例也有充分的记载。

甲状腺肿病(strumosis)是一种模糊的病变,以良性卵巢甲状腺肿患者出现腹膜和网膜高分化甲状腺组织种植为特征[913,914]。有人认为是甲状腺肿破裂的结果。鉴别甲状腺肿病和来自高分化滤泡癌的转移性恶性甲状腺肿主要依靠临床(例如缺乏进行性种植),因为种植的组织学特征是相似的,并不总是能够明确地正确诊断卵巢原发。事实上,并不是所有作者都接受甲状腺肿病是一种确凿有据的疾病[894]。

类癌 Carcinoid tumor

类癌是不常见的卵巢肿瘤,被归类为单胚层畸胎瘤,因为许多病例伴有其他畸胎瘤的成分[915]。单纯性卵巢类癌多半是过度生长的畸胎瘤,类癌发生在畸胎瘤内,而其他可能的来源包括黏液性肿瘤的神经内分泌细胞或异源性 Sertoli-Leydig 细胞瘤的黏液成分[593,916,917]、卵巢内分泌细胞或新化生的非内分泌性卵巢细胞。

临床特征 多数患者是围绝经期或绝经后的妇女,具有非特异性症状,例如盆腔或腹部疼痛、腹部增大、月经不规律或异常阴道出血。1/4～1/3 的卵巢类癌患者有类癌综合征[918]。其中多数有大的岛屿状类癌;这种综合征很少发生于其他类型的类癌[919]。类癌综合征的典型症状包括面部潮红、腹泻、支气管痉挛、高血压和继发于类癌心脏病的水肿[920]。某些小梁状或甲状腺肿类癌患者发生严重的慢性便秘,是由肿瘤分泌的肠激素 YY 肽引起的[921-923]。少数甲状腺肿类癌患者有甲状腺功能亢进[924]。

在诊断时,类癌通常为单侧性并局限于卵巢内[919]。10%～15% 的患者对侧卵巢有良性囊性畸胎瘤。标准的治疗是子宫切除术及双侧输卵管 - 卵巢切除术,但是对于年轻患者,单侧输卵管 - 卵巢切除术已经足够。一旦肿瘤切除,症状通常迅速减轻,但是类癌心脏病患者可能有进行性心脏病,尽管类癌已被完全切除[918,925]。类癌预后通常较好。转移和肿瘤相关性死亡罕见,主要发生在诊断时伴有卵巢外播散的患者[916,918,919,926]。甲状腺肿类癌的甲状腺肿成分和类癌成分好像都有可能发生转移[927]。

胃肠道类癌常常转移到卵巢,原发部位一般是小肠或阑尾[928]。转移性类癌可能引起如同原发性卵巢类癌一样的症状，包括类癌综合征。类癌可能是转移性的线索包括双侧发生、多结节状以及出现腹膜转移。

病理学 类癌是单发性、质硬、褐色或黄色的实性肿瘤，从显微镜下可见到直径8～10cm，而且似乎常发生在良性囊性畸胎瘤或黏液性肿瘤的壁上。

所有的卵巢类癌完全或部分由圆形或立方形的神经内分泌细胞组成，细胞核均匀一致，染色质粗，伴有小的核仁（图13A.91）。胞浆中等量，从透明到嗜酸性不一。在苏木素-伊红染色的切片中胞浆一般呈颗粒状。亲银染色或嗜银染色胞浆颗粒通常阳性。发生在卵巢的类癌有4种组织学类型；某些肿瘤中可见这些类型混合存在[407]。岛屿型（insular type）是最常见的类型[919]。细胞成巢、成片或呈岛屿状方式，或内衬小的管状腺泡。显微镜下表现类似于中肠类癌。小梁状（trabecular）类癌由高柱状细胞组成，核位于中心，胞浆颗粒状嗜酸性[916,929]。肿瘤细胞呈条索状、带状或小梁状生长，其形态类似于前肠或后肠类癌。甲状腺肿类癌（strumal carcinoid）是混合性肿瘤，含有类癌和甲状腺肿（甲状腺）两种成分[924,930-932]。类癌成分通常呈小梁状结构，虽然某些病例可见局灶性岛屿状或黏液性结构[933]。甲状腺肿成分由甲状腺滤泡组成，滤泡充满胶质，内衬柱状滤泡细胞。大约50%的病例胶质中有草酸钙结晶。在两种成分混合存在的部位，类癌细胞在滤泡间或滤泡内生长，似乎破坏并取代滤泡细胞[932]。因此，某些滤泡内衬甲状腺细胞，某些内衬混合性的甲状腺和类癌细胞，而另外一些内衬类癌细胞[924,930,934]。少数甲状腺肿类癌病例出现淀粉样物[935]。最后，卵巢可以发生非常少见的原发性黏液性类癌（mucinous carcinoid）[926,936,937]。在黏液性类癌中，内衬柱状或立方细胞以及杯状细胞的圆形或管状腺体，浸润间质或漂浮在黏液池中。典型的黏液性类癌的亚型显示很大程度的腺体密集，伴有筛状或微囊状结构，以及核的非典型性程度增加。黏液性类癌可以与癌混合，这种混合类型的癌是最容易播散到卵巢外的一种黏液性类癌[937]。某些类癌的周围可以见到黄素化的间质细胞。卵巢类癌附近常常可以发现良性畸胎瘤性成分。发现畸胎瘤性成分是类癌原发于卵巢的重要证据。总是应该考虑卵巢类癌是转移而来的可能性。转移性类癌通常为多结节性、双侧发生，而且不伴有畸胎瘤[928,938]。通过适当的临床检查，常常能够发现卵巢外的原发性肿瘤。

确定类癌诊断最有用的免疫组化染色是嗜铬素和突触素。如同后肠类癌一样，小梁状和甲状腺肿类癌一般还有前列腺特异性酸性磷酸酶（prostate specific acid phosphatase，PSAP）染色，但是前列腺特异性抗原（prostate specific antigen，PSA）染色阴性[912,931,932]。通过免疫组化检查，可以发现类癌细胞中有各种肽类激素，包括5-羟色胺、胃泌素、胰多肽（PP）、血管活性肠多肽（VIP）、胰岛素、胰高血糖素、P物质、促肾上腺皮质激素（ACTH）和生长抑素[939,940]。伴有慢性便秘的小梁状和甲状腺肿类癌患者蛋白YY染色（protein YY）一般阳性[922,923,941]。少数类癌降钙素阳性，包括某些甲状腺肿类癌[929,935]。虽然与甲状腺型组织有关，但是甲状腺肿类癌似乎与（甲状腺型）髓样癌并无密切关系。这些肿瘤的组织学表现和临床行为均有较大区别。除了少数例外，几乎所有的甲状腺肿类癌病例均缺乏降钙素和淀粉样物，而且甲状腺肿类癌CEA免疫染色阴性，而髓样癌一般阳性[924]。甲状腺肿类癌的甲状腺成分，胶质和滤泡上皮细胞浆中甲状腺球蛋白染色阳性[930,932,942,943]，而且滤泡上皮细胞核甲状腺转录因子-1（TTF-1）阳性[912]。

恶性混合性生殖细胞肿瘤
Malignant mixed germ cell tumor

恶性混合性生殖细胞肿瘤含有混合性的各种单纯性生殖细胞肿瘤。它们占所有恶性生殖细胞肿瘤的5%～20%[762,944,945]。含有良性畸胎瘤性成分的恶性生殖细胞肿瘤不包括在这个范畴内。

临床特征 混合性生殖细胞肿瘤发生于儿童和年轻女性。平均年龄为16岁。通常的临床表现是腹痛或腹部肿胀，或可触及腹部肿块。有些患者有急腹症。大约1/3患有混合性生殖细胞肿瘤的经前期儿童具有早熟性假青春期，而月经初潮后儿童和成人则经常有闭经或异常阴道出血[944]。血清标志物研究结果取决于存在的生殖细胞成分。大约50%的患者妊娠试验阳性或血清β-HCG水平增高。50%的患者甲胎蛋白水平增高。在

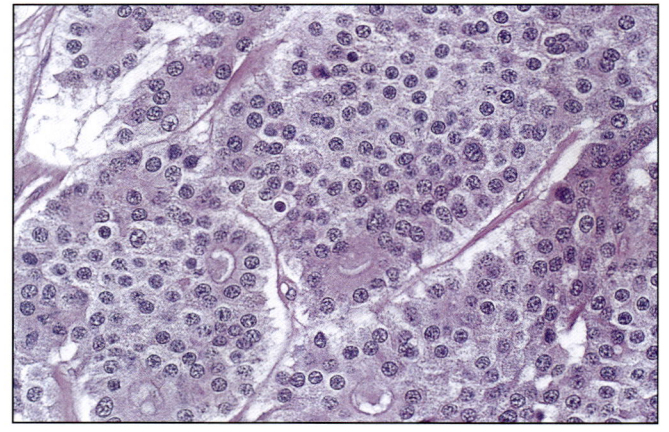

图13A.91 岛屿状类癌。肿瘤细胞形成小管或界限清楚的巢状结构。肿瘤细胞具有颗粒状嗜酸性或双染性胞浆，细胞核均匀一致，圆形，位于中央，伴有独特的染色质形态。

诊断时大约 2/3 患者的肿瘤处于 I 期[944,945]。

有包膜的单侧肿瘤（IA 期）通过输卵管 - 卵巢切除术治疗。较晚期的肿瘤采用腹式全子宫切除术和双侧输卵管 - 卵巢切除术，或者如果要保留生育能力，而且子宫和对侧卵巢没有受累，则进行单侧输卵管 - 卵巢切除术和限制性的减瘤术。仅仅通过手术治疗的 I 期肿瘤患者半数以上复发[944-946]。因此，除了仅仅含有无性细胞瘤的 IA 期和 I 级未成熟性畸胎瘤患者外，多数患者都需要化疗。多数 I 期患者应用辅助性化疗治疗可以治愈[758,945]。较晚期肿瘤患者的生存率大约为 50%[945,947]。早期报道显示预后似乎取决于肿瘤大小、存在的各种生殖细胞成分的类型和数量以及肿瘤分期[944,946]。现有的结果指出，对于应用现代联合化疗治疗的患者来说，分期是唯一有意义的决定预后的因素[762,945]。

病理学 混合性生殖细胞瘤倾向于体积较大，平均直径 15cm。肿瘤的大体表现取决于出现的肿瘤成分。无性细胞瘤呈鱼肉状，灰色、褐色或白色。卵黄囊瘤颜色不一，含有小的囊肿，经常有坏死区。未成熟性畸胎瘤呈白色或褐色，可能含有囊肿和质硬的骨或软骨灶。绒毛膜癌区域可见出血和坏死。混合性生殖细胞瘤一般为单侧性，但当出现无性细胞瘤时，可为双侧发生[945]。

80% 的混合性生殖细胞瘤有两种恶性成分（图 13A.92），15% 有三种，其余的有四种或四种以上的恶性成分。这些成分可以混合存在，也可以分开生长，但是病灶彼此相邻。无性细胞瘤是最常见的成分，其次是卵黄囊瘤和未成熟性畸胎瘤。胚胎性癌、绒毛膜癌和多胚瘤少见[783,944,945]。除了作为混合性生殖细胞瘤的一种成分外，绒毛膜癌和多胚瘤在卵巢罕见。

性腺母细胞瘤 Gonadoblastoma

性腺母细胞瘤是一种罕见的肿瘤，由生殖细胞和性索细胞混合而成，几乎全都发生在异常的性腺[948-953]。

临床特征 性腺母细胞瘤可以发生在任何年龄的患者，但是主要发生在年轻女性。诊断时的平均年龄是 18 岁；80% 的性腺母细胞瘤在 20 岁以前发现[948]，而且可以见于小儿[954]。少数肿瘤为偶然发现，或者是在腹部或盆腔 X 线检查时见到附件钙化时发现的。多数性腺母细胞瘤是在评估原发性或继发性闭经或异常生殖道形成时发现的。多数患者为女性表型，但也有出现男性表型的病例。女性表型患者具有正常或短的阴道，宫颈小。75% 的患者子宫小，35% 的患者输卵管小或不发育。多数患者轻度男性化[952]。最常见的核型是 46XY 和 45X/46XY。90% 以上的患者出现一个 Y 染色体或 Y 染色体片段。某些患者的 Y 染色体物质通过常规核型分析检测不到[948,955]，但是应用较为敏感的分子生物学技术可以发现[956]。对于具有镶嵌核型的患者进行性腺母细胞瘤的原位杂交研究发现，性腺母细胞瘤是由具有 Y 染色体的细胞衍化而来的。新近研究提示，接近着丝粒的 Y 染色体长臂有一个区域，称为 GBY 区域（GonadoBlastoma locus on the Y chromosome，Y 染色体上的性腺母细胞瘤位点），这个区域含有一个与性腺发育不全患者性腺母细胞瘤易感性相关的基因[955,957]。最可能的候选基因被认为是 Y 编码的睾丸特异性蛋白（TSPY）[958]。

性腺母细胞瘤是良性肿瘤，除非无性细胞瘤或某些其他类型的恶性生殖细胞瘤过度生长。治疗采取性腺切除术，因为性腺异常，没有正常生育功能。性腺母细胞瘤通常为双侧性，所以需要进行双侧性腺切除术，以防止男性化或恶性生殖细胞肿瘤发展[948,953]。具有 Y 染色体的性腺异常患者，发生性腺母细胞瘤或恶性生殖细胞肿瘤的危险性大约为 25%[959]。筛查 Y 染色体物质可能有助于确定处于性腺肿瘤危险的患者[960]。多数发生在性腺母细胞瘤的恶性肿瘤是无性细胞瘤[948,952,961]，而大约 10% 是卵黄囊瘤或胚胎性癌[948,952,961,962]。

病理学 性腺母细胞瘤来源于异常性腺，包括条索状性腺、不确定的性腺和发育不全的睾丸[952]。肿瘤一般较小，从显微镜下可见到直径 2～3cm。40% 以上是双侧性的。切面褐色或白色，经常含有砂质感的钙化区域。

显微镜下，生殖细胞巢和性索细胞巢由纤维性间质围绕（图 13A.93）。两种类型的生殖细胞在性腺母细胞瘤中均有描述[963,964]。某些性腺母细胞瘤是不成熟的，表现为核浆比例增高，染色质粗，某些细胞核核仁突出以及胞浆稀少，而另外一些比较成熟，细胞核较小而致密，胞浆丰富透明。性索细胞包围生殖细胞。颗粒细胞和 Sertoli 细胞具有重叠的特征，难以分类。这些细胞围

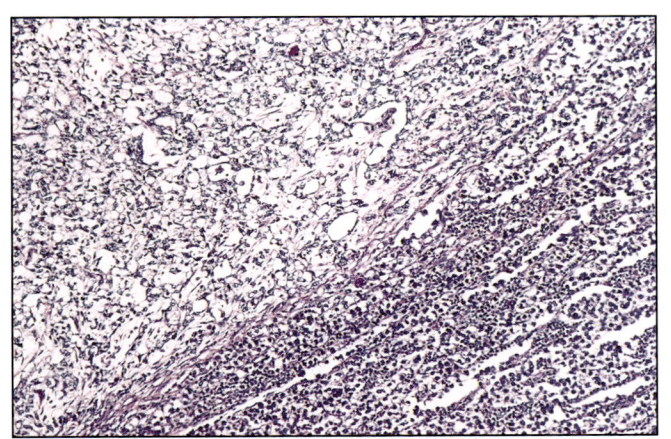

图13A.92 恶性混合性生殖细胞瘤。肿瘤含有两种恶性生殖细胞成分。视野左上为卵黄囊瘤，右下为无性细胞瘤。

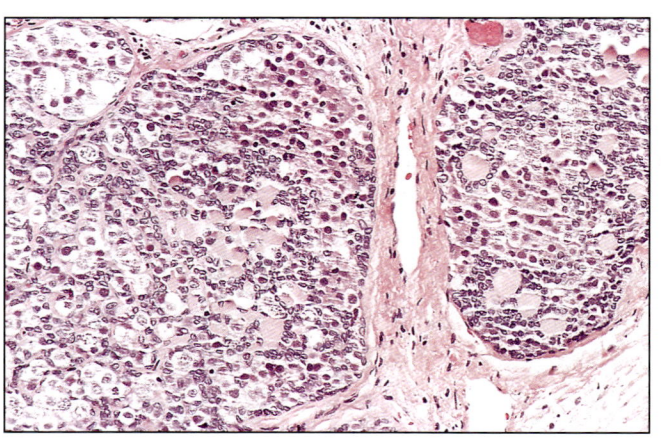

图13A.93 性腺母细胞瘤。肿瘤细胞巢由纤维性间质围绕，细胞巢含有透明的基底膜样型物质、大的生殖细胞，以及小而深染的性索-间质细胞。

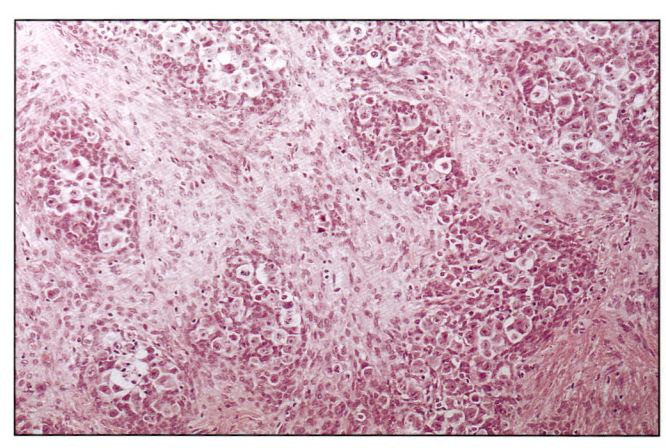

图13A.94 混合性生殖细胞-性索-间质肿瘤。这种类型的肿瘤发生于具有正常核型的患者，含有混合性的大的生殖细胞和较小的、深染的性索-间质细胞。注意缺乏性腺母细胞瘤可见的巢状生长方式和透明核心。

绕生殖细胞和透明的嗜酸性基底膜样物质圆柱体，或在性腺母细胞瘤细胞巢的周围呈栅栏状排列。青春期后患者，性腺母细胞瘤周围的间质常常含有黄素化或Leydig样细胞。间质可能含有不同大小的微小钙化。

性索成分免疫组化染色 inhibin、vimentin 和 cytokeratin 阳性。透明物质抗-Laminin 抗体阳性[965]。生殖细胞胎盘碱性磷酸酶、CD117（c-kit）、OCT-4 和 TSPY 有不同程度的阳性表达[963,964,966,967]。有人提出，那些共同表达 TSPY 和 OCT-4 的细胞是原位癌细胞，可以进展为浸润性生殖细胞肿瘤，通常是精原细胞瘤，其中 TSPY 表达可能丢失[964]。性腺母细胞瘤细胞巢之间间质中的黄素化细胞，inhibin 和 calretinin 染色强阳性。

少数其他类型的混合性生殖细胞-性索-间质肿瘤病例已有描述（图13A.94）[968]，包括伴有上皮成分的肿瘤[969]。这些肿瘤发生于基因型正常的女性，缺乏含有透明核心的散在的细胞巢可以将其与性腺母细胞瘤鉴别开来。一例性腺母细胞瘤伴有9cm的性索-间质肿瘤，类似于Sertoli细胞瘤，除了无性细胞瘤外[970]。显微镜下可见的性腺母细胞瘤样病变发生在缺乏基因异常的胎儿和婴儿的卵巢。它们常常见于滤泡囊肿壁上。它们与真正的性腺母细胞瘤的关系并不清楚[971,972]。

其他罕见的卵巢肿瘤
Other rare tumors of the ovary

小细胞癌（高钙血症型）
Small cell carcinoma (of hypercalcemic type)

小细胞癌是不能确定组织发生的具有侵袭性生物学行为的肿瘤，主要发生于年轻女性[330,973-976]。

临床特征 根据报告，小细胞癌的年龄范围从儿童到55岁[977]，但是主要发生于年轻女性，患者平均年龄24岁。少数病例好像是家族性的[979]。临床表现一般具有非特异性症状，例如腹胀、腹部或盆腔疼痛、恶心或呕吐，或者有可以触及的腹部肿块。大约2/3的患者具有高钙血症，但高钙血症通常没有症状[351]。血清甲状旁腺激素水平并不升高。大约50%的患者在诊断时疾病局限。小细胞癌通常单侧发生。双侧性肿瘤主要见于广泛转移的患者，对侧卵巢可能是转移播散的肿瘤[975]。小细胞癌具有侵袭性，即使诊断时肿瘤局限于卵巢，也有较高的死亡率[975,978]。有局限性肿瘤的妇女经子宫切除术和双侧输卵管-卵巢切除术治疗后，有较好的生存率，因此这是标准的手术治疗[975]。辅助性化疗或放疗的作用并不清楚，晚期或复发患者对放疗和化疗有局限性反应[980]。据报告少数患者具有良好的治疗反应[981,982]。在最大的一宗报告中，33%的Ia期肿瘤患者在最后随访期间存活且无疾病存在的证据，相比之下，Ic期患者的存活率为10%，而II、III、IV期患者的存活率仅为6.5%[975]。

病理学 小细胞癌是实性、结节状、灰色或褐色的肿瘤，大小为6～27cm不等，平均直径15cm。某些肿瘤的切面可见小的囊肿以及出血和坏死区。

显微镜下，典型的表现之一是均匀一致的小细胞呈弥散性片块状分布，偶见不规则的充满淡嗜酸性物质的滤泡样结构（图13A.95）[976]。某些肿瘤的肿瘤细胞呈巢状或条索状生长。肿瘤细胞圆形或梭形，胞浆稀少，核深染，圆形、卵圆形或梭形，染色质细颗粒状，核仁不明显或缺乏核仁（图13A.96）。核分裂象常见，一般超过20个/10HPF。流式细胞检查显示肿瘤细胞是DNA

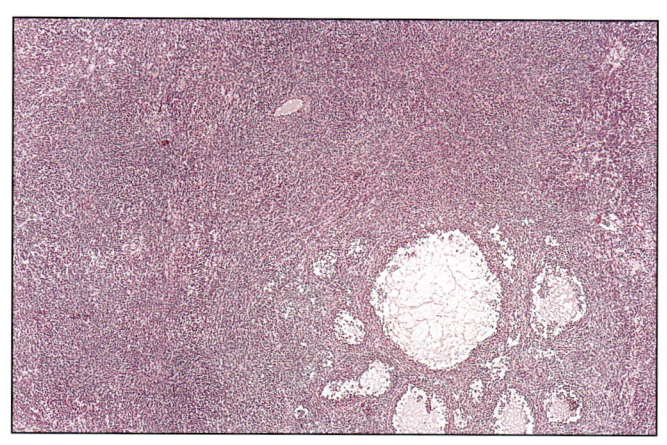

图13A.95 小细胞癌。弥散性生长形态伴有一些充满嗜酸性物质的滤泡。

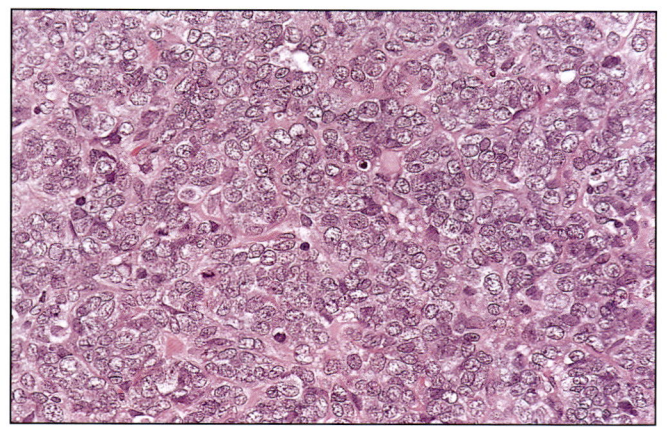

图13A.96 小细胞癌。肿瘤细胞胞浆稀少,细胞核单形性,小圆形或卵圆形,染色质细,核仁不明显。

二倍体[983]。大约50%的病例出现具有丰富的嗜酸性胞浆、空泡状核和显著核仁的较大的细胞。当这些大细胞占优势时,肿瘤被称为小细胞癌的"大细胞亚型"[351,984]。12%的小细胞癌中,可见内衬良性或恶性黏液上皮的腺体。

低分子量细胞角蛋白免疫染色显示斑块状阳性,多数肿瘤上皮膜抗原(EMA)免疫反应阳性[489,984-986]。多数小细胞癌显示p53蛋白阳性核染色,虽然这种染色可能是中等强度或仅为局灶阳性[978,985]。小细胞癌倾向于WT-1弥散性强阳性核染色,calretinin细胞核和细胞浆染色以及CD10细胞膜斑块状染色[985]。仅有少数肿瘤显示诸如CD56、嗜铬素和突触素等神经内分泌标志物阳性染色,而CD99、desmin、inhibin和TTF-1染色阴性[493,985,986]。尽管血清中缺乏甲状旁腺激素,但是根据报告少数肿瘤甲状旁腺激素和甲状旁腺激素相关蛋白免疫反应阳性[489,987,988]。Inhibin染色阴性,加上EMA和WT-1染色阳性有助于与幼年性颗粒细胞瘤鉴别,后者inhibin阳性,而EMA阴性。重要的是应该注意,小细胞癌和幼年性颗粒细胞瘤calretinin染色均可阳性。

小细胞癌具有上皮性肿瘤的超微结构特征[973,984,987,989-991]。成群的肿瘤细胞周围有不连续的基底膜围绕,而且相邻细胞之间有桥粒样连接。少数病例存在有腔的小管,内衬表面具有微绒毛的细胞。最具特征性的超微结构是显著扩张的粗面内质网的水池,其中充满无定形的中等电子密度的物质。一组研究的4例肿瘤中,3例见到具有致密轴心的神经分泌颗粒[987],但是其他研究没有这样的发现[973,984,989]。

小细胞癌曾被认为是一种类型的性索-间质肿瘤[989]、生殖细胞起源的神经内分泌肿瘤[987]、与卵黄囊瘤相关的生殖细胞肿瘤[984]以及上皮性肿瘤[992],但它的肿瘤谱系目前尚未确定。缺乏Inhibin免疫染色,加之某些病例EMA阳性,不同于性索-间质肿瘤inhibin阳性而EMA阴性的典型的免疫表型,提示小细胞癌不能归入这个范畴。

纤维组织增生性小圆细胞肿瘤
Desmoplastic small round cell tumor

纤维组织增生性小圆细胞肿瘤(DSRCT)(也见第15章)是一种恶性的腹腔内肿瘤,主要发生于年轻男性[993-995]。然而,这些肿瘤也有非常少数发生在女性,而且罕见的病例临床上表现为原发性卵巢肿瘤[996-1000]。诊断时,腹腔内总是有广泛的肿瘤生长,尽管进行积极治疗,但多数患者仍死于肿瘤。采用包括手术切除、化疗和放疗在内的多种治疗方式的患者,好像有最好的预后,3年生存率大约50%[1001,1002]。细胞来源尚不清楚,但肿瘤细胞显示t(11;22)(p13;q12)染色体易位,其中有Ewing肉瘤和Wilms瘤基因融合(EWS-WT1)[1003-1005]。

肿瘤实性,灰色、褐色或白色,伴有坏死区。显微镜下,肿瘤细胞小,细胞核均匀一致,圆形,深染,核仁不明显,胞浆稀少到中等量[330,1006]。肿瘤细胞呈片块状或巢状生长,被硬化的纤维性间质分开(图13A.97)。DSRCT具有特征性的多表型免疫反应[993,996,997]。肿瘤细胞细胞角蛋白和上皮膜抗原、神经元特异性烯醇化酶、desmin、WT-1、胎盘碱性磷酸酶染色阳性,CD99偶尔阳性[995,1007-1009]。其他神经内分泌和肌肉标志物通常阴性。

可能Wolff起源的女性附件肿瘤
Female adnexal tumor of probable Wolffian origin

这种独特的肿瘤通常发生于阔韧带或输卵管系膜(见628页)[1010],但是少数病例发生于卵巢[1011-1015]。最可能的起源是来自中肾管(Wolff)残余。肿瘤主要

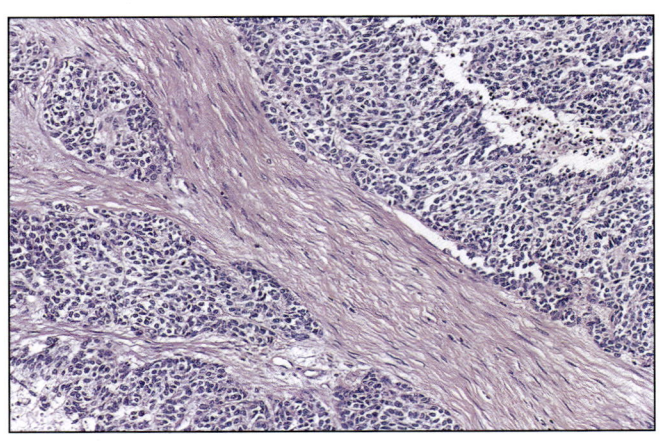

图13A.97　纤维组织增生性小圆细胞肿瘤。成巢或成片的小圆形肿瘤细胞被纤维组织增生性纤维性间质分隔。

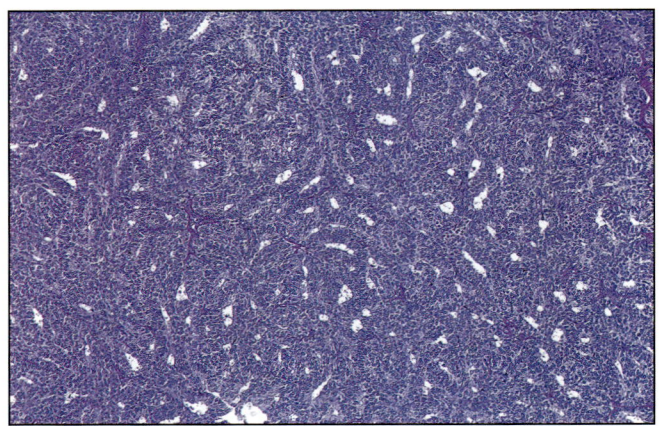

图13A.98　Wolff起源的女性附件肿瘤。均匀一致的温和的肿瘤细胞，呈混合性弥漫性和小管状生长方式。

发生于中年妇女。某些肿瘤是在无症状妇女中偶然发现的，但当肿瘤较大时，出现的症状是盆腔肿块。肿瘤实性，灰色、褐色或黄色。直径从 2cm 到 20cm，平均 11～12cm。显微镜下表现为均匀一致的、小到中等大小的上皮细胞呈弥散性、小梁状、小管状、微囊状或筛状生长（图 13A.98）。小管周围明显的基底膜具有特征性，而且有不等量的纤维性间质。肿瘤细胞 vimentin、cytokeratin、雄激素受体、inhibin 和 calretinin 免疫反应阳性，但是上皮膜抗原阴性[1015,1016]。核分裂象通常罕见，几乎没有细胞非典型性。这些肿瘤多数是良性的，但也有少数发生在卵巢或接近卵巢区域的恶性病例报告[1011]。后者显示核分裂活性或细胞非典型性增加、梭形细胞过度生长或淋巴管浸润。

腺瘤样瘤　Adenomatoid tumor

腺瘤样瘤最常见于输卵管和子宫肌层，但也有发生于卵巢门或邻近卵巢门的罕见病例报告[1017]。某些肿瘤为显微镜下所见，而另外一些为质硬的灰色或褐色结节。直径一般小于 2cm。显微镜下表现类似于其他部位的腺瘤样瘤（见第 14 章）。它们是间皮来源的良性肿瘤，肿瘤界限清楚但无包膜。腺瘤样瘤由内衬立方细胞的小管和囊肿组成，周围围绕不等量的纤维性或纤维肌性间质。Cytokeratin 和 calretinin 免疫染色阳性。

卵巢转移性肿瘤
Metastatic tumors in the ovary

卵巢转移性肿瘤比女性生殖道任何其他部位都常见[1018,1019]。卵巢转移性肿瘤占所有恶性卵巢肿瘤的 5%～10%[1020-1022]。可能的转移途径包括逆行性淋巴管播散、经腹膜播散和血行转移[1023]。根据受累卵巢的病理学以及临床和手术所见，多数卵巢转移可以用淋巴管和经腹膜播散来解释，特别是来自腹部原发部位的转移[1024]。乳腺、大肠、子宫内膜和胃的腺癌是最常见的原发部位，但是各种各样的恶性肿瘤偶尔也能引起卵巢转移[1025]。这些包括宫颈[1026,1027]、阑尾[1028]、胰腺[1029]、胆管和胆囊[1030]、肝[420,425,1031]、肾[360,404,1032-1034]、泌尿道[404,405]和肺[412,413]等部位的癌，以及黑色素瘤[880,1035]、恶性淋巴瘤和不同类型的软组织肉瘤及胃肠道肉瘤[1036-1039]。卵巢转移性子宫内膜腺癌与子宫内膜和卵巢同时发生的原发性子宫内膜样腺癌常常很难鉴别。这个问题在子宫内膜样腺癌（见 581 页）一节中讨论。

临床特征　具有临床意义的卵巢转移最常发生于有卵巢外癌症病史的妇女，通常是结肠或直肠癌[1040]，从原发性肿瘤手术到发现卵巢转移的平均时间大约是 2 年，但间隔长度不同，从几个月到 5 年以上[1041]。有些患者没有原发性卵巢外肿瘤的病史[1018,1042]。患者表现为盆腔肿瘤的症状，例如盆腔或腹部疼痛、胃肠或泌尿道功能紊乱、腹胀或异常子宫出血，而且经常被认为有原发性卵巢癌[1043-1045]。发现其中多数患者有局灶性晚期胃肠道原发癌，同时伴有卵巢转移，但是在少数情况下，原发部位在卵巢肿瘤切除数月或数年之后才被发现。当具有结直肠癌病史的妇女出现新的盆腔肿块时，最可能的诊断是转移性腺癌，但有相当比例的病例发现有良性或原发性恶性卵巢肿瘤（一项研究显示 26% 为良性，17% 为原发性卵巢癌）[1041]。2%～13% 的结直肠癌妇女发生卵巢转移[1046,1047]，导致某些作者提倡在切除原发性肿瘤时，进行预防性地卵巢切除[1048,1049]。然而，卵巢切除并没有改善生存率，其有效性目前还不清楚[1050-1053]。卵巢转移的妇女预后不好[1040,1054,1055]，但是手术切除似乎能够延长生存期并减轻症状。某些研究者发现，卵巢转移多半发生在绝经前妇女，但是这种发现并没有被其他学者证实[1042,1048,1056]。

卵巢最常见的转移性肿瘤是乳腺癌，但它很少具有临床意义。组织学上，在因为乳腺癌激素治疗而切除的卵巢中，发现多数转移性乳腺癌病灶小，有时仅在显微镜下才能见到[1018,1057]。有乳腺癌病史的妇女发现附件肿块，很可能是原发性卵巢肿瘤而不是转移癌[1058]。临床表现如同原发性卵巢肿瘤的转移性乳腺癌，在乳腺原发性肿瘤发现之前，常常出现诊断问题[1040,1059]。

病理学 卵巢转移性肿瘤的表现不同，取决于原发部位。50%～70%的转移性结直肠癌病例为双侧性。卵巢肿瘤平均直径为10～11cm，表面光滑，倾向于囊性或实性和囊性[1044,1060]。一项研究显示，假定所有的双侧性黏液性肿瘤或小于10cm的黏液性肿瘤为转移性肿瘤，而所有大于10cm的单侧性黏液性肿瘤为原发性肿瘤，那么90%的黏液性肿瘤可以被正确地分为原发性或转移性[211]。囊肿为单房性或多房性，其中充满黏液。转移性胃癌通常有Krukenberg瘤的表现，卵巢倾向于保持自身的形状，但会有对称性或非对称性增大。卵巢质硬，表面上有结节状的区域。切面灰色、褐色或白色，呈水肿性和蜂窝状，伴有小的黏液性囊肿。多数其他类型的转移性肿瘤表现为实性，并且在卵巢皮质和髓质内形成多发性结节，常常伴有浆膜种植。

镜下提示卵巢肿瘤可能是转移性病变的一般特征包括：双侧性、多结节性生长方式；卵巢表面种植；淋巴管内许多转移性癌栓，尤其是卵巢门和卵巢系膜；以及出现原发性卵巢肿瘤不常见的组织学形态，例如印戒细胞表现或呈单行排列的浸润方式[1061]。某些转移性肿瘤周围的间质发生黄素化[1044,1060]，但是它也发生在原发性肿瘤的周围，黄素化并不意味着肿瘤是转移性的。偶尔，黄素化细胞分泌足够量的雌激素或雄激素，从而引起临床症状[1062]。

转移性结直肠腺癌常常类似于卵巢原发性腺癌[1020,1044,1046,1060,1063]。典型的结直肠腺癌以吸收细胞为主，杯状细胞缺乏或不显著，类似子宫内膜样腺癌（图13A.99）。转移性结直肠腺癌形成大而复杂的腺体和囊肿，内含坏死碎屑。这些碎屑呈粗颗粒状，含有核碎片和炎症细胞，从而形成了一种独特的表现，经常被称之为"污秽性"坏死（"dirty" necrosis）（图13A.100）[1060]。虽然广泛坏死是转移性结直肠腺癌的特征，但它也可以见于卵巢原发性腺癌[1020,1064]。内衬腺体和囊肿的恶性细胞分层，或呈车轮状、花环状或筛状生长方式，伴有节段性上皮坏死灶（图13A.100）。

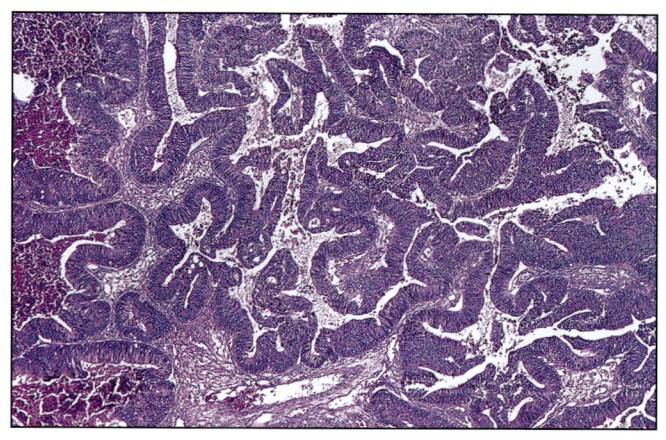

图13A.99 卵巢转移性结直肠腺癌。肿瘤性腺体内衬伴有致密胞浆的柱状细胞，杯状细胞不明显。组织学图像类似于卵巢子宫内膜样癌。

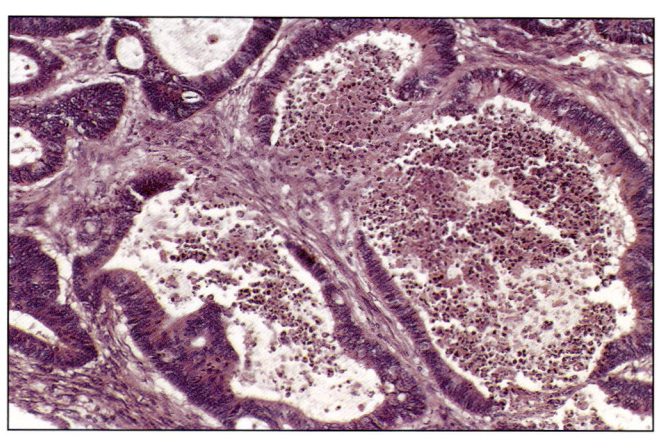

图13A.100 卵巢转移性结直肠腺癌。恶性腺体充满黏液以及细胞和细胞核的碎屑，即所谓的"污秽性"坏死。某些腺体显示节段性坏死。

核的非典型性程度高于相似结构分级的子宫内膜样腺癌。一般缺乏原发性子宫内膜样癌的典型表现，例如鳞状化生、局灶性腺纤维瘤生长方式和邻近的子宫内膜异位症。当杯状细胞较多并产生大量黏液时，转移性结直肠癌类似于卵巢原发性黏液性癌[211]。来自胰腺和胆道的转移性腺癌也可以表现为黏液性腺癌，因此应该加以鉴别诊断[1029,1063]。转移灶内偶尔出现类似于良性或交界性黏液性肿瘤的区域，这种现象并不可靠，也不一定代表是原发性卵巢黏液性癌。转移性黏液性腺癌显示一般转移性肿瘤的显微镜下特征，包括表面种植和至少局灶性的浸润性生长[1061]，但是可能仍有必要对比转移和原发的显微镜下表现，并且进行免疫组化研究，以便得出正确诊断。

几种免疫组化染色可能有助于卵巢原发性腺癌和转移性结直肠腺癌的鉴别诊断，但是没有一种染色是决定性的（表13A.11）[733,1023]。Cytokeratin亚型免疫染色

表13A.11	原发性和转移性卵巢腺癌的免疫表型						
肿 瘤	CK 7	CK 20	CDX-2	Villin	GCDFP-15	CA125	WT-1
原发性卵巢癌							
浆液性	+	−	−	−	−	+	+
子宫内膜样	+	−	−	−	−	+	−
黏液性	+	V	V	+	−	NV	−
转移性癌							
结直肠	−	+	+	+	−	−	−
阑尾	NV	+	+	V	−	−	−
胃	+	V	NV	na	−	−	−
乳腺	+	−	−	−	V	NV	−

CK7：细胞角蛋白7；CK20：细胞角蛋白20；GCDFP-15：大囊肿病液体蛋白15；na：资料不足；+：通常阳性；−：通常阴性；V：可为阳性或阴性，但常常阳性；NV：可为阳性或阴性，但常常阴性。

是最有用的染色。原发性卵巢腺癌CK7染色几乎总是强阳性，而结直肠腺癌CK7通常阴性[219,1064-1067]。子宫内膜样癌CK20免疫染色通常阴性[202,1064]。卵巢黏液性腺癌CK20可以阳性[202,1066]，但是染色一般较弱并呈局灶性[219]。相反，结直肠腺癌CK20呈弥漫强阳性表达。因此，CK7阳性/CK20阴性这种免疫表型强烈提示为原发性卵巢癌，而CK7阴性/CK20阳性的免疫表型则高度支持为转移性腺癌（见表13A.11）[1067-1069]。虽然结肠腺癌几乎总是CK7阴性，但是某些直肠腺癌和来自胃肠道较近端部分的腺癌CK7可能阳性，包括阑尾、小肠和胃[1065,1069,1070]。可能有助于鉴别原发性和转移性肿瘤的其他免疫组化染色包括CDX-2[216,218,220,221,1071,1072]，结直肠癌CDX-2染色核呈阳性，而子宫内膜样癌一般阴性，仅少数黏液性癌阳性；某些结直肠癌和子宫内膜样癌β-连环蛋白（β-catenin）染色核呈阳性，但原发性黏液性癌通常阴性[217,221]；子宫内膜样癌OC125（CA125）显示阳性膜染色，而原发性黏液性癌和转移性结直肠癌通常阴性[130,1073-1075]。某些转移性结直肠腺癌和原发性黏液性腺癌中α-甲酰基-CoA消旋酶（alpha-methylacyl-CoA racemase）（也叫P504S）染色显示颗粒状胞浆染色，而子宫内膜样癌倾向于阴性[2221]；癌胚抗原（CEA）阴性或弱阳性支持卵巢原发而不是转移性结直肠腺癌[397,1044,1064,1066,1076]。

来自阑尾的转移性肿瘤罕见，仅占卵巢转移性肿瘤的1%[1077]。转移到卵巢的阑尾肿瘤多数是印戒细胞腺癌，它发生于黏膜基底并浸润阑尾壁。肿瘤含有不同比例的印戒细胞、小管和杯状细胞[1028]。伴有内衬杯状细胞的明显小管成分的癌已被分类为杯状细胞或黏液性类癌，或在过去被称为混合性类癌-腺癌[1077,1078]。这种肿瘤的生物学行为具有侵袭性，而且并不总是显示类癌典型的染色方式[亲银阳性、嗜铬素和（或）突触素免疫反应阳性]。如果转移伴有卵巢间质增生，这种转移可以满足典型的或腺管状Krukenberg瘤的诊断标准（见下文）[1079,1080]。其他转移性阑尾腺癌是结直肠或黏液性肠型腺管状腺癌[1028,1077,1081]。这些转移性肿瘤CK20免疫染色通常阳性，但CK7也有大约50%的病例阳性[1028]。伴有阑尾和卵巢肿瘤的女性腹膜假黏液瘤的问题将在下面讨论。

转移性类癌在显微镜下与原发性卵巢类癌相同，但它们不伴有其他畸胎瘤性成分[928]。此外，转移性类癌通常双侧性和多灶性发生。最常见的原发部位是小肠。

转移性乳腺腺癌常常是偶尔发现，但在大约1/3的病例，因实性弥散性或结节性转移而使卵巢增大[1057,1059]。显微镜下，多数转移癌类似于浸润性导管癌或小叶癌，容易辨别出来是从乳腺转移而来的。可能难以与原发性肿瘤或来自其他器官的转移性肿瘤鉴别的不常见的显微镜下结构包括：单个细胞生长、弥漫性实性生长方式，以及筛状生长方式[1057]。转移性乳腺癌CK7通常阳性，CK20阴性，可能显示雌激素和孕激素受体核的阳性染色，这种免疫表型与许多原发性卵巢癌重叠。大囊肿病液体蛋白-15（GCDFP-15）免疫染色阳性支持转移性乳腺癌的诊断（表13A.11），但是根据个人的经验，卵巢转移性癌中这种抗体的免疫反应不如文献报道中的常见[1082]。来自印戒细胞型浸润性小叶癌的卵巢转移可以形成Krukenberg瘤[1083]。

Krukenberg瘤是转移性腺癌的一种形式，有时见于年轻女性，肿瘤中可见恶性的印戒细胞生长于细胞丰富的间质中[1084-1086a]。原发癌通常在胃[1086,1087]，但是乳腺[1083,1087]、结肠[1086,1087]、胆囊或其他部位的印戒细胞癌也可以引起这种类型的转移癌。Krukenberg瘤在美国和欧洲相对少见，但常见于胃癌高发地方的人群，例如日本和日本女性移民[1027,1087]。显微镜下，印戒细胞呈单个细胞、不同大小的细胞巢或条索状生长，或表现为广泛散在的小管（图13A.101）。恶性细胞含有胞浆黏液小体，深染的细胞核受压变扁并移向细胞膜。某些肿瘤出现伴有嗜酸性胞浆和偏心细胞核的小的多角形或立方形细胞。除了印戒细胞以外，少数Krukenberg瘤含有明显的管状腺体。这些肿瘤被称为小管状Krukenberg瘤[1088,1089]。卵巢门淋巴结常常含有聚合在一起或形成腺体的肿瘤细胞。Krukenberg瘤间质丰富，细胞多，局灶水肿，而且可能含有黏液池。恶性肿瘤细胞可被间质掩盖，但切片通过PAS或黏蛋白卡红中性黏蛋白染色，或cytokeratin或上皮膜抗原免疫组化染色容易辨认。肿瘤细胞CK7倾向于阳性，而CK20染色不定。反应性的间质细胞可能显示inhibin强阳性。少数Krukenberg瘤被称为"原发的Krukenberg瘤"，因为不能发现卵巢外有原发性肿瘤[1090,1091]。胃肠道原发癌，特别是胃的原发癌，即使经过仔细的检查依然不能发现肿瘤，因此最好将所有的Krukenberg瘤都看成是转移性肿瘤，直到被临床随访或尸检证实之后。不过，少数患者在Krukenberg瘤切除后长期生存，或在尸检时也不能发现原发部位，这就提出了存在原发性印戒细胞Krukenberg瘤的可能性[1085,1086]。

腹膜假黏液瘤　Pseudomyxoma peritonei

腹膜假黏液瘤（也见第15章）是不常见的病变，其中黏液性腹水引起进行性腹胀和胃肠功能失常[1092]。黏液黏稠，分为小腔，黄棕色或红色，含有纤维性机化灶，并与邻近器官粘连。女性腹膜假黏液瘤常常伴有类似于交界性黏液性肿瘤的卵巢肿瘤（图13A.102），或在少数情况下伴有黏液性囊腺瘤，有人提出腹膜假黏液瘤几乎是所有交界性黏液性肿瘤妇女的死亡原因[1093]。腹膜假黏液瘤也可以发生在胃肠道肿瘤患者中，特别是阑尾的肿瘤，少数病例伴有其他部位的肿瘤。

腹膜假黏液瘤有三种不同的显微镜下形态[191,1094,1095]。第一，黏液表浅，位于卵巢、腹膜或网膜表面，可能含有炎症细胞、巨噬细胞、纤维母细胞，并有向内生长的毛细血管。某些病例没有上皮，而另外一些有少量的低级别黏液性上皮。这些病变被命名为"无细胞性"（acellular）或"表面机化性"（superficial organizing）腹膜假黏液瘤，取决于是否出现上皮组织。第二，最常见的结构是黏液贯穿在整个受累的组织中。黏液由

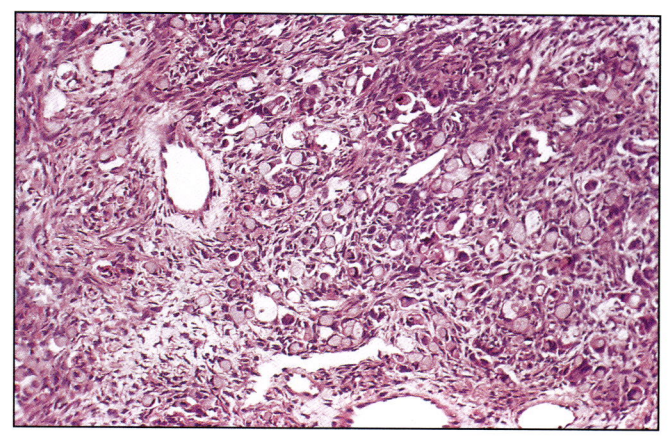

图13A.101　Krukenberg瘤。伴有胞浆黏液空泡的印戒细胞浸润增生的卵巢间质。

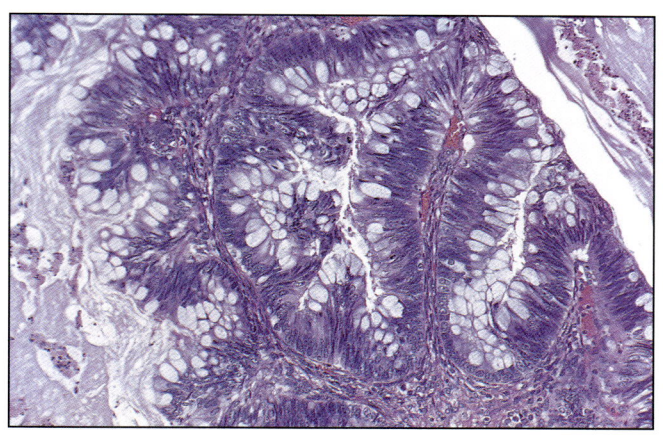

图13A.102　伴有腹膜假黏液瘤妇女的卵巢黏液性肿瘤。肿瘤类似于交界性黏液性肿瘤。患者具有双侧卵巢肿瘤、腹膜假黏液瘤和原发性横结肠腺癌。

束状纤维组织围绕，并有机化，伴有纤维母细胞和毛细血管向内生长。偶尔，黏液或邻近的纤维束中可见条带状的低级别黏液性上皮（图13A.103）[1096]。这种形态被某些作者称为播散性腹膜腺黏蛋白沉积症（disseminated peritoneal adenomucinosis，DPAM）[1095]，见于良性或交界性卵巢黏液性肿瘤的妇女。第三，黏液含有较多的上皮细胞，这些细胞显示高级别核的非典型性，或有明确的黏液性腺癌的特征，例如增生性恶性腺体，呈实性生长或有印戒细胞。这种结构可以称为转移性黏液性癌或腹膜黏液性癌病（peritoneal mucinous carcinomatosis）。预后与存在的腹膜黏液性病变的类型有关。伴有无细胞性或表面机化性黏液的患者预后最好[191,1094]。诊断"无细胞性黏液"需要仔细的研究，因为如果多做切片通常可以发现上皮细胞。所谓的播散性腹膜腺黏蛋白沉积症患者的预后介于中

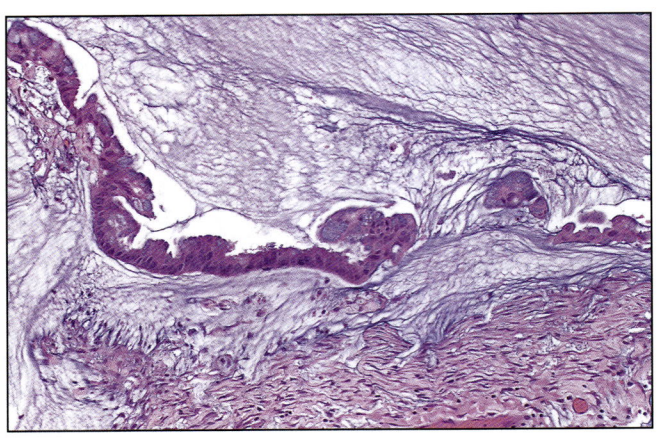

图13A.103　腹膜假黏液瘤。网膜中机化分割的黏液和温和的黏液性上皮。这种组织学结构被某些学者称为"播散性腹膜腺黏蛋白沉积症"。

间状态，比较容易复发，临床经过漫长，某些病例最终死于腹膜假黏液瘤的并发症[1094,1097-1099]。黏液中出现显著非典型性或恶性细胞的患者预后不良，通常在诊断之后几年内死于癌病[1095,1099,1100]。腹膜假黏液瘤的根治方式包括腹膜切除术和近年来出现的腹腔内化疗，看起来有一些治疗效果[1101-1104]。

发生在腹膜假黏液瘤患者的卵巢肿瘤的组织发生一直存在争论。最近的临床病理研究显示，几乎所有的腹膜假黏液瘤妇女均有阑尾肿瘤，或在少数几个病例有胃肠道其他部位的肿瘤。这些研究使得多数学者得出卵巢肿瘤是继发性肿瘤这一结论，原发部位通常是阑尾[1094,1105,1106]。支持这种理论的表现包括：卵巢和阑尾肿瘤通常是同时发生的；卵巢和阑尾肿瘤组织学表现相似；卵巢肿瘤通常为双侧性，这个发现更加符合是继发性肿瘤而不是原发性交界性黏液性肿瘤；当单侧发生时，卵巢肿瘤最常见于靠近阑尾的右侧；卵巢表面可出现种植，这种发现是转移的特征；大体和显微镜下表现并不完全是典型的原发性黏液性肿瘤；受累卵巢病变可能表浅；腹膜假黏液瘤几乎总是出现，常常含有上皮细胞，其表现与腹腔内黏液中的上皮细胞相同；某些卵巢肿瘤CK7免疫染色阴性[1107,1108]；卵巢和阑尾肿瘤显示免疫组化染色和分子标记物MUC2阳性表达，MUC2是肠肿瘤的标记物，而原发性卵巢黏液性肿瘤表达MUC5AC而不是MUC2[1109,1110]；某些病例卵巢和阑尾肿瘤的分子生物学表现相似[1111-1113]。并非所有病理医师和妇产医师都同意卵巢肿瘤是继发的；某些学者认为某些或所有的卵巢肿瘤都是原发性肿瘤，可能是引起腹膜假黏液瘤的黏液上皮的来源[1093,1114]。这些学者中有人发现，来自阑尾良性或增生性病变的卵巢转移这种概念很难接受[1093]。支持将卵巢和阑尾肿瘤解释为同时发生的原发性肿瘤的特征包括：卵巢肿瘤比阑尾肿瘤大；卵巢肿瘤常常含有良性表现的黏液性上皮，通常伴有与交界性黏液性肿瘤的移行；有相当比例的病例找不到阑尾破溃的部位；除了卵巢之外，没有其他脏器转移（尽管脾受累现在已有报道）[1115]；阑尾肿瘤有时发现于卵巢肿瘤之后；腹膜假黏液瘤偶尔发生在数年之前具有阑尾切除病史的患者，或发现在腹膜假黏液瘤手术时切除的阑尾组织学正常[1093]；孤立性腹膜假黏液瘤和卵巢肿瘤患者可以治愈，尽管未能切除阑尾[1093]；以及有些患者，卵巢和阑尾肿瘤在分子水平上存在差异[1111]。

目前总的看法是，腹膜假黏液瘤患者所发生的卵巢肿瘤是继发于胃肠道肿瘤，而且几乎所有的病例一般均位于阑尾[1096,1116,1117]。病理医师应该记住，腹膜假黏液瘤患者倾向于有阑尾的异常，即使大体检查以及卵巢出现肿瘤时没有发现异常。如果可能，应该切除阑尾并进行充分的组织学检查。阑尾肿瘤的类型以及腹膜黏液中肿瘤细胞的组织学形态是腹膜假黏液瘤的重要预后因素，应在病理学报告中加以描述。多数患者，阑尾肿瘤是低级别的黏液性肿瘤，有时伴有憩室[1118]，尽管少数患者表现为腺癌[1119,1120]。少数患者没有发现卵巢外原发性肿瘤。其中部分患者，腹膜假黏液瘤的解释可能是来自良性畸胎瘤肠型黏液性肿瘤的腹膜播散，从而引起腹膜假黏液瘤[889]。这样的肿瘤具有肠的免疫表型（CK7阴性，CK20阳性，CDX-2阳性），而不是卵巢黏液性肿瘤的免疫表型（CK7阳性，CK20和CDX-2染色不定）。在少数病例，腹膜假黏液瘤的衍化并不符合现今疾病的概念，在这样的病例中，腹膜假黏液瘤可来自卵巢黏液性肿瘤或某些其他器官隐匿性的原发性黏液性肿瘤。

卵巢良性瘤样病变
Benign tumor-like conditions of the ovary

高反应性黄素化(多发性双侧性卵泡膜黄体囊肿)
Hyperreactio luteinalis (multiple bilateral theca lutein cysts)

高反应性黄素化是一种妊娠相关性重度卵巢增大，是由许多大的卵泡膜黄体囊肿引起的，通常为双侧性。

临床特征　高反应性黄素化是卵巢增大的少见原因，发生在人绒毛膜促性腺激素（HCG）血清浓度增高的女性[1121,1122]。它见于大约 25% 的妊娠滋养细胞疾病女性患者[1123]，并偶尔发生在伴有胎儿水肿或多次妊娠的妇女[1124,1125]。本病很少发生在单胎妊娠的妇女[1126-1128]。它可以发生于任何一个妊娠三月期，通常没有症状而于超声检查时发现。合并囊内出血的患者可以有腹痛，而伴有卵巢扭转或破裂的患者会出现急腹症[1129]。女性男性化在妊娠滋养细胞疾病患者中罕见，但大约 25% 发生在其余的患者中。女性婴儿并不发生男性化。分娩后囊肿消退，因此应该尽量采取保守的治疗措施。

病理学 卵巢充血增大，有时非常显著，许多囊肿直径可达 3~4 cm。显微镜下，囊肿是卵泡膜黄体囊肿。囊肿内衬几层显示不同程度黄素化的颗粒细胞，被一圈黄素化的卵泡膜细胞所环绕（图 13A.104）。黄素化细胞较大，多角形，伴有丰富的嗜酸性胞浆，核圆形，位于中央。囊肿周围的间质水肿。

妊娠黄体瘤　Luteoma of pregnancy

妊娠黄体瘤是性腺间质细胞的结节性增生，出现于妊娠末三个月，并于分娩之后消退[1121,1123,1130,1131]。它的产生受人绒毛膜促性腺激素（HCG）的影响，但是与高反应性黄素化不同，通常没有 HCG 水平异常增高[1130]。

临床特征 黄体瘤主要发生于经产妇女，其中黑人占大多数，平均年龄 27~28 岁。黄体瘤常常不能触及，通常是在超声检查、剖宫产或输卵管结扎时无意中发现的[1130,1132,1133]。大约 1/3 的患者在妊娠末三个月出现男性化[1130]，这些男性化母亲所生的女婴中 50% 以上出现男性化[1121,1130,1134]。治疗上应尽量保守，因为未经治疗的黄体瘤会自发退化。在分娩之后 5 天内出现明显的退行性改变[1131]。最佳的处理是通过活检确定诊断，如果病理医师通过冰冻切片可以确诊，而且没有其他复杂的因素，例如破裂或扭转引起的坏死，则没有必要进行另外的手术。

病理学 妊娠黄体瘤表现为单侧（大约 2/3 的病例）或双侧卵巢的结节性增生。切面显示皮质或髓质有一个或多个质软的褐色、棕色或黄色结节。结节平均 6~10 cm，可能含有出血或坏死灶。常见大小不一的囊肿。

显微镜下，妊娠黄体瘤是由成片或成巢的黄素化细胞组成的。它们含有丰富的嗜酸性颗粒状胞浆和圆形的空泡状细胞核（图 13A.105）。没有核的非典型性，但是容易找到核分裂象（1~2 个 /10HPF）。没有发现 Reinke 结晶。在邻近的卵巢经常可以见到卵泡膜黄体囊肿，而且间质或囊肿壁或闭锁卵泡内可能出现黄素化细胞增生结节。

妊娠期显微镜下可见的颗粒细胞增生　Microscopic granulosa cell proliferations in pregnancy

在妊娠妇女的卵巢中，显微镜下偶尔发现灶状颗粒细胞增生，类似于小的颗粒细胞瘤[478,1135,1136]。增生的颗粒细胞排列成小梁状、岛屿状、弥散分布或呈微滤泡状结构。颗粒细胞增生也会发生在具有妊娠黄体瘤或高反应性黄素化的卵巢中。这种现象通常被认为是对于 HCG 的良性增生性反应，而不是小的颗粒细胞瘤，因为它们发生在妊娠期间，呈多灶性，局限于闭锁卵泡的中央，而且没有发生于妊娠妇女颗粒细胞瘤的形态学变化（如黄素化、水肿等）。没有复发的病例报道。

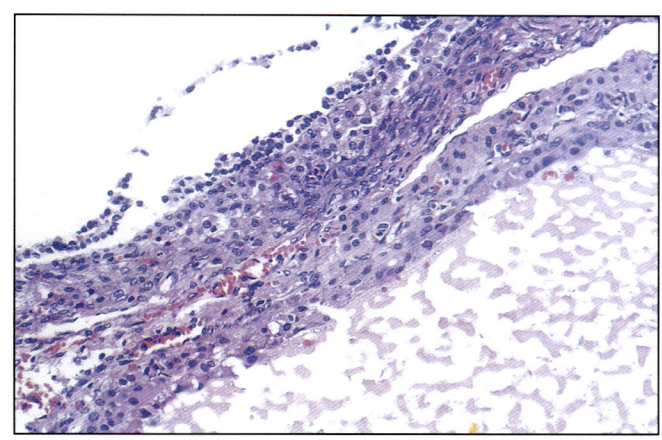

图 13A.104 高反应性黄素化。顶部囊肿内衬颗粒细胞，其下为黄素化卵泡膜细胞。底部囊肿内衬黄素化的颗粒细胞和卵泡膜细胞。

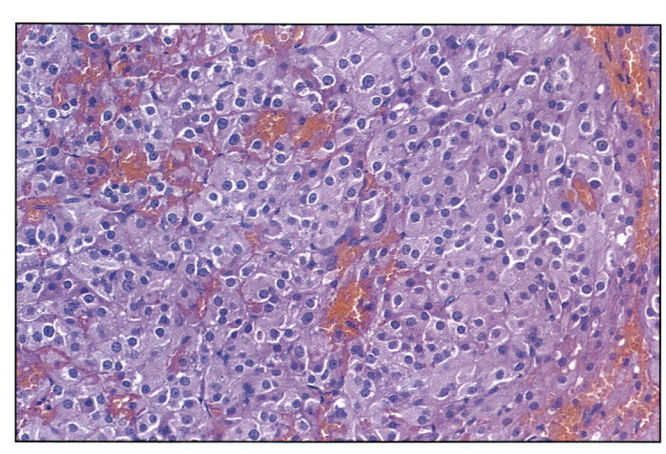

图 13A.105 妊娠黄体瘤。黄体瘤由圆形到多角形细胞组成，含有丰富的嗜酸性胞浆，核圆形，位于中心。

重度水肿和纤维瘤病
Massive edema and fibromatosis

卵巢重度水肿是年轻妇女单侧卵巢增大的一种罕见的原因，被认为是由于卵巢间断性扭转伴有蒂部淋巴管和静脉梗阻造成的[1137-1141]。少数卵巢重度水肿发生在老年妇女，是由转移癌引起卵巢门淋巴管梗阻引起的[1142,1143]。临床表现为急腹症和实性附件肿块。受累卵巢切面水肿，粉色到黄色，平均直径 11.5 cm[1140]。显微镜下，间质水肿是主要表现。某些病例出现黄素化细胞聚集。血管扩张充血，提示部分性或间断性扭转也许是水肿的原因。卵巢纤维瘤病可能与卵巢病变有关，这种病变表现为小的纤维母细胞增生，围绕和分隔正常卵巢结构，从而引起卵巢增大[1140]。胶原纤维数量不定，可见水肿。组织学图像类似于纤维瘤，但是纤维母细胞增生呈多灶性和弥散性而不是局灶性。

输卵管肿瘤
Tumors of the fallopian tube

相对于卵巢和子宫而言，输卵管原发性肿瘤少见。发生在卵巢的许多同样类型的肿瘤可以发生在输卵管（表 13A.12）。某些可能累及卵巢的肿瘤，例如腺瘤样瘤以及 Wolff 管起源的女性附件肿瘤（FATWO），较常见于输卵管及输卵管旁区域。最常见的输卵管肿瘤是各种类型的癌。鉴别输卵管原发性肿瘤与来自女性生殖道其他部位（特别是卵巢或生殖道外）的转移癌至关重要。

输卵管良性肿瘤
Benign tumors of the fallopian tube

腺瘤样瘤　Adenomatoid tumor

腺瘤样瘤来源于间皮，是最常见的输卵管良性肿瘤[1144-1146]。大部分是中年或老年妇女因为其他原因手术时偶然发现的，但大的肿瘤可能引起症状。腺瘤样瘤小，平均直径 1～2 cm。肿瘤为灰白色或黄色的界限清楚的结节，恰好位于浆膜面的下方。

显微镜下，肿瘤由内衬扁平细胞的腺样囊性或微囊性空隙，或被覆具有丰富嗜酸胞浆的立方细胞的条索或小管组成（图 13A.106）。某些肿瘤细胞具有显著的胞浆空泡，类似于印戒细胞。胞浆空泡和腺样间隙含有富于透明质酸的 Alcian 蓝阳性物质，是间皮肿瘤的特征。浸润性的显微镜下表现有时提出有无腺癌的问题。然而，腺瘤样瘤大体局限，细胞学形态温和，

表13A.12	最常见的输卵管肿瘤的分类
恶性上皮性肿瘤	
浆液性腺癌	
子宫内膜样腺癌	
移行细胞癌	
其他	
交界性上皮性肿瘤	
交界性浆液性肿瘤	
交界性子宫内膜样肿瘤	
其他	
原位癌	
良性上皮性肿瘤	
乳头状瘤（具体类型）	
囊腺瘤（具体类型）	
腺纤维瘤（具体类型）	
囊腺纤维瘤（具体类型）	
化生性乳头状息肉	
子宫内膜样息肉	
其他	
上皮性瘤样病变	
输卵管上皮增生	
结节性输卵管峡炎	
输卵管子宫内膜异位	
混合性上皮-间叶性肿瘤	
恶性混合性Müller管肿瘤（癌肉瘤）	
腺肉瘤	
软组织肿瘤	
平滑肌肉瘤	
平滑肌瘤	
其他	
间皮肿瘤	
腺瘤样瘤	
生殖细胞肿瘤	
成熟性畸胎瘤	
未成熟性畸胎瘤	
其他	
滋养细胞疾病	
绒毛膜癌	
胎盘部位滋养细胞肿瘤	
上皮样滋养细胞肿瘤	
水泡状胎块	
胎盘部位结节	
其他	
血液和淋巴组织肿瘤	
淋巴瘤	
白血病	
继发性肿瘤	

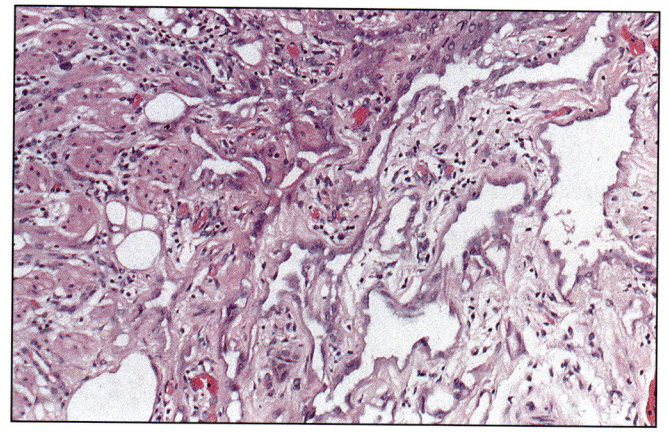

图103A.106 输卵管的腺瘤样瘤。小管（右）和微囊状间隙（左）内衬立方到扁平的具有温和细胞核的间皮细胞。

没有核分裂象。腺瘤样瘤偶尔梗死，可能难以诊断，除非有残余的存活区域或在梗死区内能够找到典型的组织形态证据[1147]。细胞角蛋白免疫染色常常能够突出显示腺瘤样瘤的典型结构，即使在大部分梗死的标本中。细胞角蛋白和间皮标志物 calretinin 以及细胞角蛋白 5/6 免疫组化染色阳性[1148]。腺瘤样瘤 WT-1 染色显示核呈阳性，类似于其他间皮肿瘤[1149]，腺癌标志物 Ber-EP4、CEA、B72.3 染色阴性，或至多是弱阳性或局灶阳性。免疫表型支持腺瘤样瘤是间皮来源，有助于与腺癌的鉴别诊断。

良性上皮性肿瘤 Benign epithelial tumors

浆液性或子宫内膜样囊腺瘤、腺纤维瘤和囊腺纤维瘤很少发生于输卵管[1151-1155]。少数交界性浆液性和子宫内膜样肿瘤已有报道[1151,1156]。良性和交界性黏液性肿瘤也有报道，但不能完全除外其中某些可能是转移性肿瘤[1157]。

平滑肌瘤和其他间叶性肿瘤 leiomyomas and other mesenchymal tumors

平滑肌瘤是输卵管最常见的间叶性肿瘤[1158,1159]。通常较小，为孤立性病变，常常是偶然发现的。其大体和组织学表现都与子宫平滑肌瘤相似。显微镜下，肿瘤由交织成束的梭形平滑肌细胞组成，具有温和的梭形细胞核和原纤维性嗜酸性胞浆。在子宫平滑肌瘤发生的变性改变同样可以见于输卵管平滑肌瘤，包括水肿改变、玻璃样变性和纤维化。

已经报道的在输卵管发生的其他良性软组织肿瘤包括脂肪瘤、血管平滑肌脂肪瘤[1160]、血管瘤[1161-1163]、血管肌纤维母细胞瘤[1164]、孤立性纤维瘤[1165]、神经鞘瘤[1166,1167]、神经节瘤[1168]和软骨瘤[1169,1170]。

畸胎瘤 Teratoma

输卵管畸胎瘤罕见，而且大部分都是良性囊性畸胎瘤[1171-1173]，少数实性成熟性[1174,1175]和未成熟性畸胎瘤[1176,1177]也有所报道。输卵管畸胎瘤患者年龄从21岁到60岁不等[1171]。多数输卵管畸胎瘤是有蒂的肿块，位于输卵管峡部或壶腹部的腔内，虽然壁内和浆膜的畸胎瘤也有报道。显微镜下，良性畸胎瘤含有成熟性的外胚层、中胚层和内胚层组织，而不成熟性成分出现在未成熟性畸胎瘤中。单胚层畸胎瘤也可发生于输卵管。一例完全由甲状腺组织组成的畸胎瘤被称为"输卵管甲状腺肿"（struma salpingis），而且伴有同侧卵巢甲状腺肿[1178]。在另外一个病例中，类癌发生于成熟性畸胎瘤[1179]。最后，未成熟性畸胎瘤可以作为输卵管混合性生殖细胞肿瘤的一部分[1180]。

输卵管恶性肿瘤 Malignant tumors of the fallopian tube

腺癌 Adenocarcinoma

原发性输卵管腺癌大约占所有女性生殖道恶性肿瘤的1%[1181]。在美国平均年发病率为每一百万妇女每年有3.6人患病。这个发病率很可能是低估的数字，因为那些已经扩展到卵巢的晚期肿瘤常常被诊断为卵巢癌。

临床表现 输卵管癌主要发生在中年以上的妇女。患者平均年龄55岁，虽然输卵管癌发生年龄广泛，从20岁到80岁以上不等[1182,1183]。常见的临床表现是异常阴道出血或排液、腹痛、腹部或盆腔肿块[1184]。少数患者表现为提示盆腔炎症性疾病的症状和体征[1185]。术前一般很少能够做出诊断，因为症状和体征不具有特异性，而且很难定位一个附件肿块是输卵管肿块。有人提出慢性输卵管炎是发病因素[1186]。大约15%的输卵管癌患者有 BRCA1 或 BRCA2 种系突变[1187-1189]。评估来自 BRCA1 或 BRCA2 种系突变或有乳腺癌及卵巢癌家族史妇女的预防性输卵管-卵巢切除标本发现，这些患者输卵管上皮异型增生/原位癌和隐匿性输卵管浸润性腺癌的发生率增加[166-168,1190-1192]。隐匿癌见于2.5%～17%的行预防性输卵管-卵巢切除术的患者[165,166,1193,1194]。输卵管上皮异常与卵巢异常相同，甚或更为常见[164,167]，某些在双侧卵巢切除术后被认为具有发生原发性腹膜浆液性癌的高危患者，事实上可能已经发生了隐匿性输卵管癌的腹膜播散[1193]。对于病理医师来说，将输卵管标本连续切片并将所有切片进行镜检是非常重要的[168]。小的输卵管癌的治疗是由一些标准参数决定的，例如肿瘤部位、分级和分期。

输卵管癌的治疗与卵巢癌相似。主要的治疗是手术切除肿瘤，通常采取腹式子宫切除和双侧输卵管-卵巢切除术。最佳的手术包括完整的手术分期，即网膜切除术、盆腔和主动脉旁淋巴结清扫以及腹膜活检。根据肿瘤分级、部位、浸润深度或破裂确定的处于复发高危险的早期肿瘤患者，通常要辅以化疗。晚期肿瘤患者进行肿瘤细胞减灭术，随后进行以铂为基础的化疗[1195-1198]。肿瘤分期（表13A.13）是最重要的预后参数。系列报告显示，Ⅰ期肿瘤患者的5年生存率为32%～80%，Ⅱ期为16%～58%，而Ⅲ-Ⅳ期0～29%[1184,1195,1199-1203]。监察、流行病学和最终结果方案（SEER）数据库患者的研究显示，生存率似乎较高，Ⅰ期肿瘤患者为95%，Ⅱ期75%，Ⅲ期69%，而Ⅳ期为45%[1204]。在Ⅰ期患者，预后不利的因素包括深层浸润到输卵管壁和破裂[1199]。输卵管伞端肿瘤比具有同样浸润深度的壶腹部和峡部肿瘤预后要差。治疗前血清CA125水平与肿瘤分期有关，而且可以用于监测治疗反应[1199,1205]。

病理学 大体上，输卵管肿胀，浆膜面光滑或有颗粒状出血，取决于浸润深度。外科医师或病理医师最初可能怀疑为输卵管积水、输卵管积血或输卵管积脓，而不是肿瘤。输卵管伞端是小肿瘤最常发生的部位，可能容易漏诊[1205a]。根据报告，双侧输卵管肿瘤的发生率在3%～30%之间，平均20%。切面显示为褐色到黄色的实性或乳头状肿瘤，部分或完全充满输卵管腔。大的肿瘤一般含有出血和坏死区域。

两种类型的输卵管上皮内非典型性已有描述：原位癌和增生。在原位癌，上皮细胞具有增大深染的具有恶性特征的细胞核（图13A.107）。某些细胞核含有核仁，而且可见核分裂象，有时为异常核分裂象。异

表13A.13	输卵管癌的FIGO分期。（Reprinted from International Journal of Gynecology and Obstetrics. Benedet JL, Pecorelli S. Staging Classifications and Clinical Practice guidelines of gynaecologic cancers. p 81, ©2000. With permission from International Federation of Gynecology and Obstetrics.）
0期	原位癌
Ⅰ期	肿瘤仅限于输卵管
ⅠA	肿瘤局限于一侧输卵管，没有穿透浆膜面，而且没有腹水
ⅠB	肿瘤局限于双侧输卵管，没有穿透浆膜面，而且没有腹水
ⅠC	肿瘤局限于一侧或双侧输卵管，蔓延至或穿透浆膜，或者在腹水或腹膜冲洗液中找到恶性细胞
Ⅱ期	肿瘤累及单侧或双侧输卵管，伴有盆腔扩散
ⅡA	扩散或转移至子宫或卵巢
ⅡB	扩散至其他盆腔脏器
ⅡC	盆腔扩散伴有腹水或腹腔冲洗液中找到恶性细胞
Ⅲ期	肿瘤累及单侧或双侧输卵管，伴有盆腔外腹膜种植
ⅢA	显微镜下可见盆腔外腹膜转移
ⅢB	大体可见盆腔外腹膜转移，直径≤2cm
ⅢC	腹膜转移，直径≥2cm
Ⅳ期	远处转移

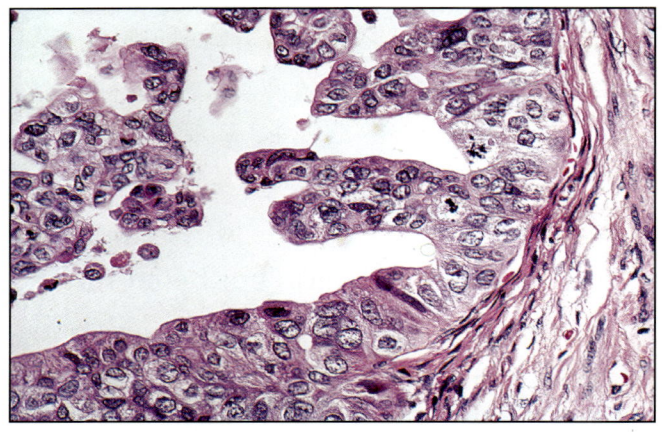

图13A.107 输卵管原位腺癌。输卵管内衬极性消失的复层非典型性柱状细胞。细胞核具有非典型性，核浆比例增高，可见核分裂象。

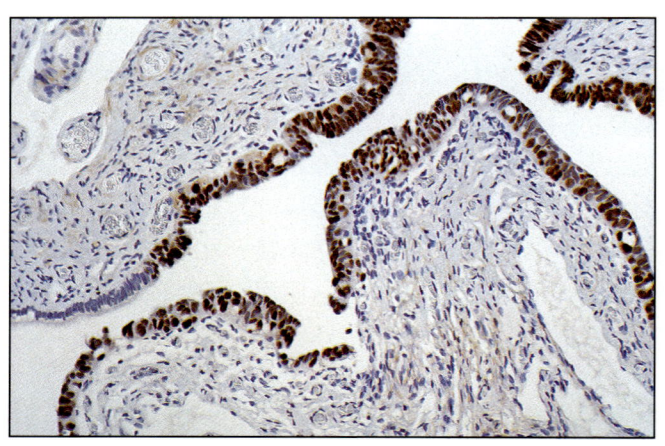

图13A.108 原位腺癌p53免疫染色。原位腺癌细胞核呈强阳性染色，但其余正常输卵管上皮（左下）阴性。

常细胞为矮柱状，具有嗜酸性或双染性胞浆，核浆比例一般增高。异常细胞通常分层，伴有极性消失，偶尔成簇生长。纤毛细胞减少或消失。原位癌部位 p53 蛋白染色通常呈强阳性反应（图 13A.108），有助于识别而且支持原位癌的诊断。原位癌仅仅被接受为输卵管腺癌的前体病变。这是一种在 BRCA 突变或有乳腺癌或卵巢癌家族史的妇女行预防性输卵管-卵巢切除术标本中可以发现的异常之一[166,1191]。广泛的非典型性不明显的输卵管上皮增生已有报道。大部分被命名为非典型性增生的异常以细胞密集、复层、极性消失，而且至少具有中度的核非典型性为特征。核非典型性的程度不如原位癌，而且核分裂象缺失或稀疏。增生的临床意义还不清楚。p53 染色通常阴性，而且不是原位癌或浸润性腺癌的前体病变[1191,1206]。

发生在卵巢的同样类型的癌也可以出现在输卵管。浆液性癌是最常见的输卵管癌。在预防性输卵管-卵巢切除术标本中发现的隐匿性浆液性癌一般较小（1～2 mm 或更小），可以发生在黏膜、伞端或浆膜。这些小癌通常只有在组织学检查时才能发现，为了发现这些小癌需要将输卵管连续切片并全部提交进行显微镜下检查[166]。子宫内膜样癌是第二个最常见的输卵管癌，随后是移行细胞癌和未分化癌。卵巢常见的某些类型的癌，例如透明细胞癌和黏液性癌，只是偶尔发生于输卵管。一项有关输卵管癌的大宗研究发现，50% 为浆液性癌，25% 为子宫内膜样癌，11% 为移行细胞癌，8% 为未分化癌，4% 为混合细胞型癌，2% 为透明细胞癌[1182]。其他研究显示浆液性癌的百分数较高[1183,1199,1207]。输卵管浆液性癌与卵巢浆液性癌的组织学表现相同（图 13A.109）。子宫内膜样癌倾向于向腔内生长，几乎没有输卵管壁浸润，因此预后可能相对较好。输卵管子宫内膜样癌表现出几种生长方式。最常见的生长方式是融合性或背靠背的腺体，内衬复层柱状细胞（图 13A.110）。某些病例出

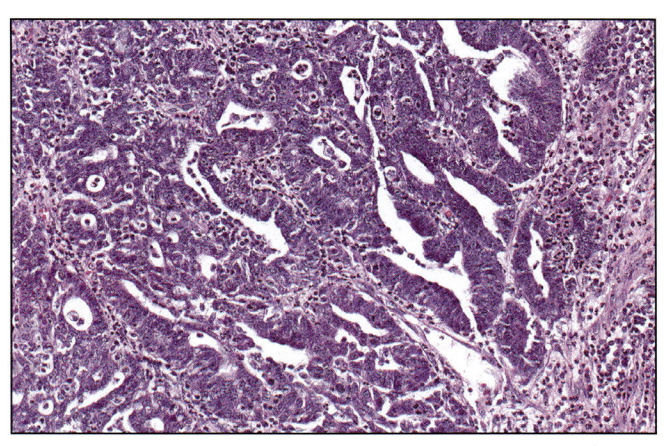

图13A.110 输卵管子宫内膜样癌。子宫内膜样癌主要呈腺样生长方式。肿瘤细胞呈柱状，伴有非典型性深染的细胞核。可见核分裂象。

现鳞状分化。第二种形态类似于可能来源于 Wolff 管的女性附件肿瘤（FATWO），见下[1208-1211]。它由成片的小的多角形或梭形细胞组成，伴有提示鳞状分化的局灶性旋涡状结构。成片的细胞中夹杂有小的腺体、囊肿或筛状间隙，其中含有 PAS 阳性的嗜酸性物质。这种类型的子宫内膜样癌与可能来源于 Wolff 管的女性附件肿瘤（FATWO）的不同之处在于，它含有可识别的灶状鳞状分化和较大程度的核非典型性和核分裂活性。少见类型的输卵管癌包括透明细胞癌[1212-1214]、鳞状细胞癌[1215]、黏液性癌[1216]、玻璃样细胞癌[1217]、肝样癌[1218]、神经内分泌癌[1219]和淋巴上皮样癌[1182]。

输卵管腺癌的免疫表型类似于组织学类型相同的卵巢癌。原发性输卵管癌一般 CK7 阳性，而 CK20 阴性。输卵管浆液性癌 WT-1 染色核呈弥漫强阳性[133]。

肿瘤分期是最重要的预后因素。病理医师应当注意肿瘤是否破裂，以及是否扩散到输卵管浆膜。在 I 期肿瘤中，肿瘤起源部位（伞端还是其他部位）和管壁浸润深度具有预后意义[1199,1220]。组织学分级与生存率几乎无关[1182,1199]。

腺肉瘤和癌肉瘤
Adenosarcoma and carcinosarcoma

腺肉瘤是一种双相性肿瘤，其中良性上皮腺体混合有恶性间叶成分，通常是非特异性梭形细胞肉瘤。原发性输卵管腺肉瘤已有少数病例报道[1221,1222]。

癌肉瘤又叫恶性混合性 Müller 瘤（MMMT），是一种双相性肿瘤，其中恶性上皮和间叶成分混合存在。上皮成分一般是浆液性或子宫内膜样癌。间叶成分是圆形或梭形细胞肉瘤，可能含有异源性成分，例如横纹肌肉瘤或软骨肉瘤。少数输卵管原发性癌肉瘤已有报道[1223-1231]。癌肉瘤附近的输卵管黏膜存在原位癌支持输卵管来源[1232]。癌肉瘤必须与伴有梭形细胞成分

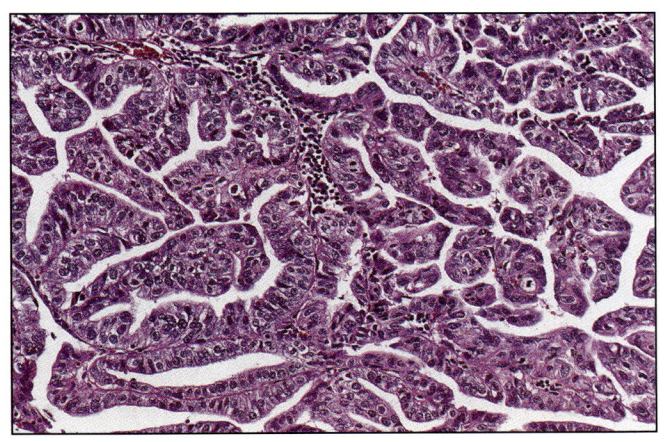

图13A.109 输卵管浆液性癌。癌的乳头状突起被覆矮柱状细胞，具有增大的非典型性细胞核。

的子宫内膜样癌相鉴别。输卵管癌肉瘤主要发生于绝经后妇女，并且临床上表现为侵袭性，但是早期肿瘤患者可以治愈[1223-1225,1233]。

恶性间叶性肿瘤
Malignant mesenchymal tumors

输卵管肉瘤罕见，但是也有几例报道，包括平滑肌肉瘤[1234,1235]、子宫内膜间质肉瘤[328]、胚胎性横纹肌肉瘤[1236]以及所谓的恶性纤维组织细胞瘤[1237]。作为系统性疾病，淋巴瘤也可以累及输卵管。淋巴瘤倾向于累及同侧卵巢和输卵管。输卵管原发性淋巴瘤非常罕见[1238-1240]。

妊娠滋养细胞疾病
Gestational trophoblastic disease

输卵管妊娠滋养细胞疾病少见，其临床表现与输卵管妊娠相似。部分性和完全性水泡状胎块均可以发生于输卵管[1241-1245]，如同绒毛膜癌一样[1241,1246-1248]。它们的组织学表现类似于子宫的相应肿瘤（见第13章第三部分）。输卵管水泡状胎块罕见，应用严格的诊断标准十分重要；一项研究证实，诊断为输卵管水泡状胎块的多数病例是早期胎盘形成或水肿性流产[1245]。胎盘部位滋养细胞肿瘤（PSTT）和上皮样滋养细胞肿瘤（ETT），是两种不常见的中间滋养细胞肿瘤，少数发生在输卵管和阔韧带附近[1249-1252]。输卵管异位妊娠后胎盘部位结节也有少数病例报告[1250,1253-1255]。这些良性结节是由纤维素、结缔组织和非增生性中间滋养细胞组成的。

转移性肿瘤　Metastatic tumors

输卵管转移性肿瘤比原发性肿瘤常见。多数病例来自卵巢或子宫内膜腺癌，沿着腹膜表面或通过输卵管腔播散。也可以通过输卵管的淋巴管或血管发生转移。来自生殖器外原发性肿瘤的输卵管转移并不常见。

阔韧带和圆韧带肿瘤
Tumors of the broad and round ligaments

发生在卵巢的许多肿瘤也可以见于阔韧带（表13A.14），还可以出现于卵巢附件组织、子宫内膜异位症或腹膜。所有类型的间叶性肿瘤偶尔也可发生于阔韧带。这些肿瘤与卵巢或软组织的相应肿瘤相同，这里不再进一步讨论。这里集中讨论的是比起卵巢或输卵管更常发生于阔韧带和圆韧带的肿瘤和瘤样病变。

表13A.14　阔韧带和圆韧带肿瘤

Müller管型上皮性肿瘤
浆液性腺癌
子宫内膜样腺癌
黏液性腺癌
透明细胞腺癌
交界性肿瘤（具体类型）
腺瘤和囊腺瘤（具体类型）
其他肿瘤
Wolff管来源的附件肿瘤（FATWO）
室管膜瘤
伴有von Hippel-Lindau病的乳头状囊腺瘤
子宫样肿块
腺肉瘤
肾上腺残余
其他
间叶性肿瘤
平滑肌肉瘤
平滑肌瘤
其他
继发性肿瘤

肾上腺皮质残余和肿瘤
Adrenal cortical rests and tumors

在阔韧带的常规切片中偶尔可以见到肾上腺皮质结节，但是充分研究表明这种现象相对常见，可见于20%以上的妇女[1256]。肾上腺皮质残余是黄色的小结节，最大径通常只有几个毫米。位于腹膜下方，可以是单侧性，也可以是双侧性。显微镜下，肾上腺残余组织完全由肾上腺皮质细胞组成。这些细胞呈多角形，具有丰富的透明空泡状胞浆和小的空泡状核（图13A.111）。增生性肾上腺残余组织可以见于肾上腺已被结核等疾病破坏或摘除的患者的阔韧带。据报告几例Nelson综合征患者（因Cushing综合征而切除双侧肾上腺后发生分泌ACTH的垂体肿瘤）有男性化的增生性肾上腺残余[1257,1258]。有报道少数卵巢外类固醇细胞瘤发生于阔韧带[637,1259,1260]。如同在卵巢一样，它们也是由肾上腺皮质细胞或Leydig样细胞组成的，或最常见的是由这两种细胞混合组成的。少数其他类型的性索-间质肿瘤见于阔韧带，包括卵泡膜细胞瘤和颗粒细胞瘤[1261-1263]。

Wolff管来源的女性附件肿瘤
Female adnexal tumor of Wolffian origin (FATWO)

FATWO发生于阔韧带，或在少数情况下发生于卵

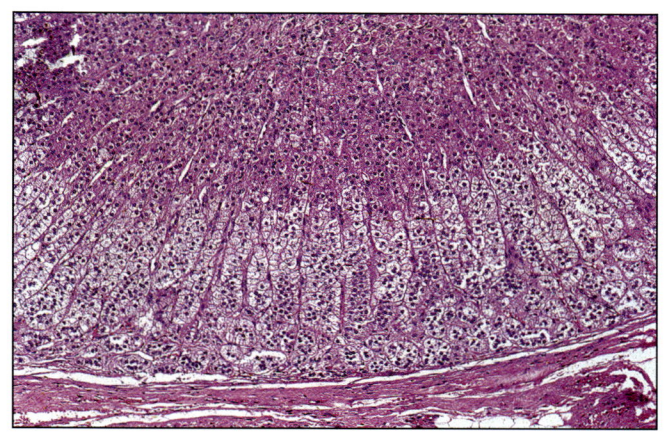

图13A.111 阔韧带的肾上腺残余。带状结构，周围的细胞具有泡沫状透明胞浆，而中央的细胞具有致密的嗜酸性胞浆。

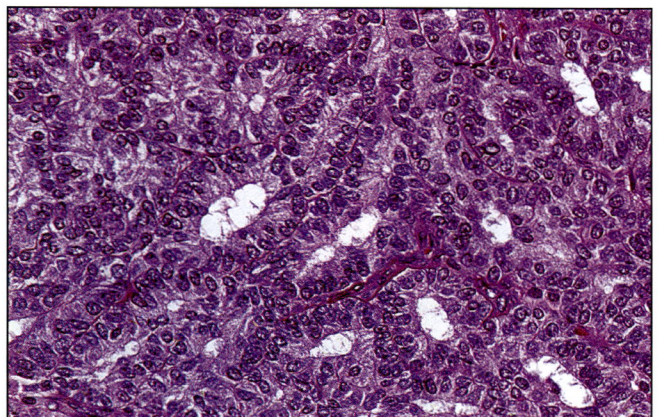

图13A.112 阔韧带的Wolff肿瘤。呈小管状和小梁状混合性结构。肿瘤细胞核均匀一致，深染，核位于基底，顶部胞浆为嗜双色性。未见核分裂象。

巢和盆腔其他部位[1010-1012]。一般认为它是来源于中肾的残余，常见于阔韧带。大部分患者是中年人，中位年龄大约50岁，但是年龄分布较广，从15岁到83岁均可发病[1264]。临床表现为非特异性，那些较小的肿瘤通常是无意中发现的。肿瘤为实性，切面白色或灰色，直径从2cm到20cm不等。显微镜下，多角形或梭形上皮细胞呈弥漫片块状生长，或表现为小梁状、小管状、网状、微囊状或筛状结构（图13A.112）。一般表现为不同结构的混合性生长，尽管可能以一种或另外一种结构为主。肿瘤细胞核一般深染，而且形态一致。显著的核非典型性和核分裂活性少见，如果出现提示有恶性的可能。FATWO通常是良性的，尽管大约15%的病例在临床上有恶性行为[1264-1266]。提示恶性的显微镜下表现包括核分裂活性增加、显著的核非典型性、梭形细胞过度生长以及淋巴管血管浸润；如果患者表现为或发生转移，那么无论组织学形态如何，肿瘤显然都是恶性的[1266-1270]。恶性FATWO一般进展缓慢，中位复发时间大约为4年。

肿瘤部位和独特的显微镜下表现通常允许病理医师做出FATWO的正确诊断。鉴别诊断包括类似于FATWO的输卵管子宫内膜样癌亚型，这在上面输卵管腺癌一节中已经做过讨论[1209,1211,1271]，以及性索-间质肿瘤，例如颗粒细胞瘤或Sertoli细胞瘤。FATWO的免疫表型在上皮性肿瘤和性索-间质肿瘤之间具有重叠，因此免疫组化研究并不一定总有帮助；FATWO的免疫表型类似于卵巢网[1015]。FATWO显示vimentin、cytokeratin、CK7、cytokeratin CAM5.2、CK19免疫染色阳性，但多数上皮膜抗原（EMA）阴性[1015,1016,1272]。Inhibin、calretinin和melan-A免疫染色通常阳性[613,1015,1273]。CD10免疫染色FATWO阳性，有助于与某些其他疾病的鉴别诊断[363]。

阔韧带上皮性囊肿和肿瘤
Epithelial cysts and tumors of the broad ligament

Müller管、中肾或间皮来源的良性囊肿偶尔发生在阔韧带。Müller管和中肾来源的囊肿最常见。Müller囊肿内衬纤毛或无纤毛的柱状细胞，而中肾囊肿内衬扁平上皮细胞[1274]。阔韧带原发性上皮性肿瘤少见，但无论良性[1275]、交界性[1276]还是恶性[1277]阔韧带上皮性肿瘤的组织学表现均与卵巢的同类肿瘤相同。多数良性和交界性上皮性肿瘤是浆液性肿瘤[1276,1278]，虽然已有Brenner瘤的病例报告[1279]，不同类型的腺癌在阔韧带已有报道，包括子宫内膜样腺癌、透明细胞腺癌、黏液性腺癌、浆液性腺癌和未分类癌[1277,1280-1282]。良性和交界性肿瘤患者预后较好[1276]，而阔韧带腺癌可能具有侵袭性，治疗上与卵巢或输卵管癌相似[1277]。

von Hippel-Lindau病是常染色体显性遗传综合征，与13号染色体短臂上的肿瘤抑制基因VHL突变有关[1283]。本病患者易患肿瘤，包括视网膜血管瘤、小脑血管母细胞瘤、嗜铬细胞瘤和肾细胞癌[1284]。某些男性von Hippel-Lindau病患者发生附睾透明细胞乳头状囊腺瘤，当肿瘤为双侧性时，与这种综合征的关系尤其密切[1285]。少数女性von Hippel-Lindau病患者阔韧带发生类似的乳头状肿瘤[1285-1289]。阔韧带肿瘤是多囊状的，乳头具有明显的纤维血管或透明间质轴心，向囊内生长。乳头被覆单层立方到柱状细胞，具有温和的圆形细胞核和中等量的透明或嗜酸性胞浆。偶尔，组织学结构可能类似于转移性肾透明细胞癌，应该认真对待von Hippel-Lindau病患者。免疫组化染色可以用于区分阔韧带良性乳头状肿瘤与转移性肾细胞癌，因为乳头状肿瘤CK7阳性，而CD10和肾细胞癌抗原阴性[1285]，而转移性肾细胞癌的染色结果正好相反。

阔韧带和圆韧带的间叶性肿瘤
Mesenchymal tumors of the broad ligament and round ligament

平滑肌瘤是阔韧带和圆韧带最常见的间叶性肿瘤[1290]。平滑肌瘤是质硬的白色或褐色圆形结节，切面呈旋涡状结构。显微镜下，阔韧带和圆韧带的平滑肌瘤与子宫平滑肌瘤相似。平滑肌瘤的亚型可以发生于阔韧带，例如脂肪平滑肌瘤[1291]。透明细胞上皮样平滑肌瘤和可能相关的肿瘤——血管周围上皮样细胞肿瘤 (perivascular epithelioid cell tumor，PEComa) 和血管肌肉脂肪瘤，在阔韧带和圆韧带已经有所报道[1292-1294]。原发性阔韧带平滑肌肿瘤必须与长入阔韧带的子宫平滑肌肿瘤相鉴别，包括平滑肌瘤、平滑肌瘤变型 [如分割性 (dissecting) 和分叶性 (cotyledonoid) 平滑肌瘤][1295,1296]以及静脉内平滑肌瘤[1297]。阔韧带很少发生平滑肌肉瘤[1298,1299]。"子宫样肿块"（uterus-like masses）在附件已有描述，看起来很像平滑肌瘤。然而，它们具有带状生长结构，中央为子宫内膜组织，周围为平滑肌[1300]。

从理论上讲，任何类型的软组织肿瘤均可发生在阔韧带。已经报道一些肿瘤是副神经节瘤[1301]——所谓的恶性纤维组织细胞瘤[1302]、伴有巨大菊形团的玻璃样梭形细胞肿瘤（hyalinizing spindle cell tumor with giant rosettes）[1303]和腺泡状软组织肉瘤[1304]。

室管膜瘤　Ependymoma

中枢神经系统以外的室管膜瘤罕见，但是已经有几例阔韧带[1305-1307]和卵巢[855,858,1308,1309]室管膜瘤的报道。阔韧带肿瘤直径从1cm到大于15cm不等，通常有囊性和实性两种区域。显微镜下，附件室管膜瘤类似于中枢神经系统室管膜瘤，并与卵巢室管膜瘤一样（见612页）。肿瘤细胞立方形到柱状，伴有嗜酸性胞浆和均匀一致的圆形或卵圆形细胞核。细胞成片生长，形成室管膜性菊形团和小管、血管周围假菊形团和线状乳头。乳头状结构往往导致误诊为上皮性肿瘤。然而，肿瘤细胞GFAP阳性[1305]。阔韧带室管膜瘤是惰性肿瘤，但具有转移播散能力。卵巢室管膜瘤可能来源于畸胎瘤，但阔韧带室管膜瘤的来源尚不清楚[1306]。

参考文献

1. Koonings P P, Campbell K, Mishell D R Jr et al. 1989 Relative frequency of primary ovarian neoplasms: a 10-year review. Obstet Gynecol 74: 921–926
2. Gee D C, Russell P 1981 The pathological assessment of ovarian neoplasms. IV: The sex cord-stromal tumours. Pathology 13: 235–255
3. Katsube Y, Berg J W, Silverberg S G 1982 Epidemiologic pathology of ovarian tumors: a histopathological review of primary ovarian neoplasms diagnosed in the Denver Standard Metropolitan Statistical Area, 1 July–31 December 1969 and 1 July–31 December 1979. Int J Gynecol Pathol 1: 3–16
4. Russell P, Painter D M 1982 The pathological assessment of ovarian neoplasms. V. The germ cell tumours. Pathology 14: 47–72
5. Russell P 1979 The pathological assessment of ovarian neoplasms. I. Introduction to the common "epithelial" tumours and analysis of benign "epithelial" tumours. Pathology 11: 5–26
6. Serov S F, Scully R E, Sobin L H 1973 Histological typing of ovarian tumours. World Health Organization, Geneva
7. Seidman J D, Russell P, Kurman R J 2002 Surface epithelial tumors of the ovary. In: Kurman RJ (ed) Blaustein's pathology of the female genital tract 5th edn. Springer-Verlag, New York, p 791–904
8. Tavassoli F A, Devilee P 2003. World Health Organization. Pathology and genetics of tumours of the breast and female genital organs. International Agency for Research on Cancer, Lyon
9. Prat J 2003 Serous tumors of the ovary (borderline tumors and carcinomas) with and without micropapillary features. Int J Gynecol Pathol 22: 25–28
10. Hart W R 2005 Borderline epithelial tumors of the ovary. Mod Pathol 18 Suppl 2: S33–S50
11. Lawrence W D 1995 The borderland between benign and malignant surface epithelial ovarian tumors. Current controversy over the nature and nomenclature of "borderline" ovarian tumors. Cancer 76: 2138–2142
12. Diamond M P, Baxter J W, Peerman C G Jr et al. 1988 Occurrence of ovarian malignancy in childhood and adolescence: a community-wide evaluation. Obstet Gynecol 71: 858–860
13. Schultz K A, Sencer S F, Messinger Y et al. 2005 Pediatric ovarian tumors: a review of 67 cases. Pediatr Blood Cancer 44: 167–173
14. Menczer J, Sadetzki S, Murad H et al. 1999 Childhood and adolescent ovarian malignant tumors in Israel. A nationwide study. Acta Obstet Gynecol Scand 78: 813–817
15. Hassan E, Creatsas G, Deligeorolgou E et al. 1999 Ovarian tumors during childhood and adolescence. A clinicopathological study. Eur J Gynaecol Oncol 20: 124–126
16. Morowitz M, Huff D, Von Allmen D 2003 Epithelial ovarian tumors in children: A retrospective analysis. J Pediatr Surg 38: 331–335
17. Kennedy A W, Hart W R 1996 Ovarian papillary serous tumors of low malignant potential (serous borderline tumors) – A long term follow-up study, including patients with microinvasion, lymph node metastasis, and transformation to invasive serous carcinoma. Cancer 78: 278–286
18. Sayedur R M, Al-Sibai M H, Rahman J et al. 2002 Ovarian carcinoma associated with pregnancy. A review of 9 cases. Acta Obstet Gynecol Scand 81: 260–264
19. Webb P M, Purdie D M, Grover S et al. 2004 Symptoms and diagnosis of borderline, early and advanced epithelial ovarian cancer. Gynecol Oncol 92: 232–239
20. McLemore M R, Aouizerat B 2005 Introducing the MUC16 gene: implications for prevention and early detection in epithelial ovarian cancer. Biol Res Nurs 6: 262–267
21. Verheijen R H, Von Mensdorff-Pouilly S, van Kamp G J 1999 CA 125: fundamental and clinical aspects. Semin Cancer Biol 9: 117–124
22. Yin B W T, Dnistrian A, Lloyd K O 2002 Ovarian cancer antigen CA125 is encoded by the MUC16 mucin gene. Int J Cancer 98: 737–740
23. Moss E L, Hollingworth J, Reynolds T M 2005 The role of CA125 in clinical practice. J Clin Pathol 58: 308–312
24. Kaern J, Tropé C G, Abeler V M 1993 A retrospective study of 370 borderline tumors of the ovary treated at the Norwegian Radium Hospital from 1970 to 1982: A review of clinicopathologic features and treatment modalities. Cancer 71: 1810–1820
25. Camatte S, Morice P, Atallah D et al. 2002 Lymph node disorders and prognostic value of nodal involvement in patients treated for a borderline ovarian tumor: An analysis of a series of 42 lymphadenectomies. J Am Coll Surg 195: 332–338
26. Malpica A, Deavers M T, Gershenson D et al. 2001 Serous tumors involving extra-abdominal/extra-pelvic sites after the diagnosis of an ovarian serous neoplasm of low malignant potential. Am J Surg Pathol 25: 988–996
27. Russell P, Merkur H. 1979 Proliferating ovarian "epithelial" tumours: a clinicopathological analysis of 144 cases. Aust NZ J Obstet Gynaecol 19: 45–51
28. Kurman R J, Trimble C L 1993 The behavior of serous tumors of low malignant potential: are they ever malignant? Int J Gynecol Pathol 12: 120–127
29. Siriaunkgul S, Robbins K M, McGowan L et al. 1995 Ovarian mucinous tumors of low malignant potential: a clinicopathologic study of 54 tumors of intestinal and mullerian type. Int J Gynecol Pathol 14: 198–208
30. Kehoe S, Powell J 1996 Long-term follow-up of women with borderline ovarian tumors. Int J Gynaecol Obstet 53: 139–143
31. Longacre T A, McKenney J K, Tazelaar H D et al. 2005 Ovarian serous tumors of low malignant potential (borderline tumors): outcome-based study of 276 patients with long-term (≥5-year) follow-up. Am J Surg Pathol 29: 707–723

32. Seidman J D, Kurman R J 2000 Ovarian serous borderline tumors: A critical review of the literature with emphasis on prognostic indicators. Hum Pathol 31: 539–557
33. Prat J, De Nictolis M 2002 Serous borderline tumors of the ovary: a long-term follow-up study of 137 cases, including 18 with a micropapillary pattern and 20 with microinvasion. Am J Surg Pathol 26: 1111–1128
34. Slomovitz B M, Caputo T A, Gretz H F III et al. 2002 A comparative analysis of 57 serous borderline tumors with and without a non-invasive micropapillary component. Am J Surg Pathol 26: 592–600
35. Zanetta G, Rota S, Chiari S et al. 2001 Behavior of borderline tumors with particular interest to persistence, recurrence, and progression to invasive carcinoma: A prospective study. J Clin Oncol 19: 658–664
36. Crispens M, Bodurka D, Deavers M et al. 2002 Response and survival in patients with progressive or recurrent serous ovarian tumors of low malignant potential. Obstet Gynecol 99: 3–10
37. Morris R T, Gershenson D M, Silva E G et al. 2000 Outcome and reproductive function after conservative surgery for borderline ovarian tumors. Obstet Gynecol 95: 541–547
38. Lim-Tan S K, Cajigas H E, Scully R E 1988 Ovarian cystectomy for serous borderline tumors: a follow-up study of 35 cases. Obstet Gynecol 72: 775–781
39. Rice L W, Berkowitz R S, Mark S D et al. 1990 Epithelial ovarian tumors of borderline malignancy. Gynecol Oncol 39: 195–198
40. Casey A C, Bell D A, Lage J M et al. 1993 Epithelial ovarian tumors of borderline malignancy: long-term follow-up. Gynecol Oncol 50: 316–322
41. Barnhill D, Kurman R, Brady M et al. 1995 Preliminary analysis of the behavior of stage I ovarian serous tumors of low malignant potential: A Gynecologic Oncology Group study. J Clin Oncol 13: 2752–2756
42. Ji H, Yliskoski M, Anttila M et al. 1996 Management of stage-I borderline ovarian tumors. Int J Gynaecol Obstet 54: 37–44
43. Deffieux X, Morice P, Camatte S et al. 2005 Results after laparoscopic management of serous borderline tumor of the ovary with peritoneal implants. Gynecol Oncol 97: 84–89
44. Maneo A, Vignali M, Chiari S et al. 2004 Are borderline tumors of the ovary safely treated by laparoscopy? Gynecol Oncol 94: 387–392
45. Camatte S, Morice P, Pautier P et al. 2002 Fertility results after conservative treatment of advanced stage serous borderline tumour of the ovary. BJOG 109: 376–380
46. Gilks C B, Alkushi A, Yue J J et al. 2003 Advanced-stage serous borderline tumors of the ovary: a clinicopathological study of 49 cases. Int J Gynecol Pathol 22: 29–36
47. Fauvet R, Boccara J, Dufournet C et al. 2004 Restaging surgery for women with borderline ovarian tumors: results of a French multicenter study. Cancer 100: 1145–1151
48. Winter W E III, Kucera P R, Rodgers W et al. 2002 Surgical staging in patients with ovarian tumors of low malignant potential. Obstet Gynecol 100: 671–676
49. Eichhorn J H, Bell D A, Young R H et al. 1999 Ovarian serous borderline tumors with micropapillary and cribriform patterns – A study of 40 cases and comparison with 44 cases without these patterns. Am J Surg Pathol 23: 397–409
50. Silva E G, Tornos C, Zhuang Z et al. 1998 Tumor recurrence in stage I ovarian serous neoplasms of low malignant potential. Int J Gynecol Pathol 17: 1–6
51. Parker R L, Clement P B, Chercover D J et al. 2004 Early recurrence of ovarian serous borderline tumor as high-grade carcinoma: a report of two cases. Int J Gynecol Pathol 23: 265–272
52. Lackman R D, Carey M S, Kirk M E et al. 2003 Surgery as sole treatment for serous borderline tumors of the ovary with non-invasive implants. Gynecol Oncol 90: 407–412
53. Trope C, Kaern J, Vergote I B et al. 1993 Are borderline tumors of the ovary overtreated both surgically and systemically? A review of four prospective randomized trials including 253 patients with borderline tumors. Gynecol Oncol 51: 236–243
54. Barakat R R, Benjamin I, Lewis J L Jr et al. 1995 Platinum-based chemotherapy for advanced-stage serous ovarian carcinoma of low malignant potential. Gynecol Oncol 59: 390–393
55. Link C J J, Reed E, Sarosy G et al. 1996 Borderline ovarian tumors. Am J Med 101: 217–225
56. Sherman M E, Mink P J, Curtis R et al. 2004 Survival among women with borderline ovarian tumors and ovarian carcinoma: a population-based analysis. Cancer 100: 1045–1052
57. Awada A, Klastersky J 2004 Ovarian cancer: state of the art and future directions. Eur J Gynaecol Oncol 25: 673–676
58. Cannistra S A 2004 Cancer of the ovary. N Engl J Med 351: 2519–2529
59. Averette H E, Donato D M 1990 Ovarian carcinoma. Advances in diagnosis, staging, and treatment. Cancer 65: 703–708
60. Baker T R, Piver M S, Hempling R E 1994 Long term survival by cytoreductive surgery to less than 1 cm, induction weekly cisplatin and monthly cisplatin, doxorubicin, and cyclophosphamide therapy in advanced ovarian adenocarcinoma. Cancer 74: 656–663
61. Le T, Krepart G V, Lotocki R J et al. 1997 Does debulking surgery improve survival in biologically aggressive ovarian carcinoma? Gynecol Oncol 67: 208–214
62. Bristow R E, Montz F J, Lagasse L D et al. 1999 Survival impact of surgical cytoreduction in stage IV epithelial ovarian cancer. Gynecol Oncol 72: 278–287
63. Leitao M M Jr, Boyd J, Hummer A et al. 2004 Clinicopathologic analysis of early-stage sporadic ovarian carcinoma. Am J Surg Pathol 28: 147–159
64. Schilder J M, Thompson A M, DePriest P D et al. 2002 Outcome of reproductive age women with stage IA or IC invasive epithelial ovarian cancer treated with fertility-sparing therapy. Gynecol Oncol 87: 1–7
65. Ayhan A, Celik H, Taskiran C et al. 2003 Oncologic and reproductive outcome after fertility-saving surgery in ovarian cancer. Eur J Gynaecol Oncol 24: 223–232
66. Pectasides D, Farmakis D, Koumarianou A 2005 The role of neoadjuvant chemotherapy in the treatment of advanced ovarian cancer. Oncology 68: 64–70
67. Johnston S R 2004 Ovarian cancer: review of the National Institute for Clinical Excellence (NICE) guidance recommendations. Cancer Invest 22: 730–742
68. Muggia F M 2004 Recent updates in the clinical use of platinum compounds for the treatment of gynecologic cancers. Semin Oncol 31(Suppl 14): 17–24
69. Bookman M A, Greer B E, Ozols R F 2003 Optimal therapy of advanced ovarian cancer: carboplatin and paclitaxel vs. cisplatin and paclitaxel (GOG 158) and an update on GOG0 182-ICON5. Int J Gynecol Cancer 13: 735–740
70. NIH Consensus Dev Panel Ovarian Cancer 1995 Ovarian cancer: Screening, treatment, and follow-up. JAMA 273: 491–497
71. Hoskins P J 1995 Treatment of advanced epithelial ovarian cancer: Past, present and future. Crit Rev Oncol Hematol 20: 41–59
72. Ozols R F 1995 Current status of chemotherapy for ovarian cancer. Semin Oncol 22 Suppl. 12: 61–66
73. McGuire W P, Hoskins W J, Brady M F et al. 1996 Cyclophosphamide and cisplatin compared with paclitaxel and cisplatin in patients with stage III and stage IV ovarian cancer. N Engl J Med 334: 1–6
74. Partridge E E, Phillips J L, Menck H R 1996 The National Cancer Data Base report on ovarian cancer treatment in United States hospitals. Cancer 78: 2236–2246
75. Ozols R F, Vermorken J B 1997 Chemotherapy of advanced ovarian cancer: Current status and future directions. Semin Oncol 24: S1–S9
76. Lambert H E, Gregory W M, Nelstrop A E et al. 2004 Long-term survival in 463 women treated with platinum analogs for advanced epithelial carcinoma of the ovary: life expectancy compared to women of an age-matched normal population. Int J Gynecol Cancer 14: 772–778
77. Fujiwara K, Sakuragi N, Suzuki S et al. 2003 First-line intraperitoneal carboplatin-based chemotherapy for 165 patients with epithelial ovarian carcinoma: results of long-term follow-up. Gynecol Oncol 90: 637–643
78. Rothenberg M L, Liu P Y, Braly P S et al. 2003 Combined intraperitoneal and intravenous chemotherapy for women with optimally debulked ovarian cancer: Results from an intergroup phase II trial. J Clin Oncol 21: 1313–1319
79. Soper J T, Berchuck A, Dodge R et al. 1992 Adjuvant therapy with intraperitoneal chromic phosphate (^{32}P) in women with early ovarian carcinoma after comprehensive surgical staging. Obstet Gynecol 79: 993–997
80. Mychalczak B R, Fuks Z 1992 The current role of radiotherapy in the management of ovarian cancer. Hematol Oncol Clin North Am 6: 895–913
81. Einhorn N. 1996 Ovarian cancer. Acta Oncol 35: 86–92
82. Randrianjafisamindrakotroka N S, Gasser B, Philippe E 1993 [The malignant potential of adenofibroma and cystadenofibroma of the ovary and mesovarium. 118 cases including 13 proliferative and 5 carcinomatous.] J Gynecol Obstet Biol Reprod (Paris) 22: 33–38
83. Cheng E J, Kurman R J, Wang M et al. 2004 Molecular genetic analysis of ovarian serous cystadenomas. Lab Invest 84: 778–784
84. Seidman J D, Mehrotra A 2005 Benign ovarian serous tumors: a re-evaluation and proposed reclassification of serous "cystadenomas" and "cystadenofibromas". Gynecol Oncol 96: 395–401
85. Silverberg S G, Bell D A, Kurman R J et al. 2004 Borderline ovarian tumors: key points and workshop summary. Hum Pathol 35: 910–917
86. Seidman J D, Soslow R A, Vang R et al. 2004 Borderline ovarian tumors: diverse contemporary viewpoints on terminology and diagnostic criteria with illustrative images. Hum Pathol 35: 918–933
87. De Nictolis M, Montironi R, Tommasoni S et al. 1992 Serous borderline tumors of the ovary: A clinicopathologic, immunohistochemical, and quantitative study of 44 cases. Cancer 70: 152–160
88. Tavassoli F A 1988 Serous tumor of low malignant potential with early stromal invasion (serous LMP with microinvasion). Mod Pathol 1: 407–414
89. Bell D A, Scully R E 1990 Ovarian serous borderline tumors with stromal microinvasion: a report of 21 cases. Hum Pathol 21: 397–403
90. Nayar R, Siriaunkgul S, Robbins K et al. 1996 Microinvasion in low malignant potential tumors of the ovary. Hum Pathol 27: 521–527
91. Hanselaar A G J M, Vooijs G P, Mayall B et al. 1993 Epithelial markers to detect occult microinvasion in serous ovarian tumors. Int J Gynecol Pathol 12: 20–27
92. Katzenstein A L, Mazur M T, Morgan T et al. 1978 Proliferative serous tumors of the ovary. Histologic features and prognosis. Am J Surg Pathol 2: 339–355
93. Mooney J, Silva E, Tornos C et al. 1997 Unusual features of serous neoplasms of low malignant potential during pregnancy. Gynecol Oncol 65: 30–35

94. Buttin B M, Herzog T J, Powell M A et al. 2002 Epithelial ovarian tumors of low malignant potential: the role of microinvasion. Obstet Gynecol 99: 11–17
95. Silva E G, Tornos C S, Malpica A et al. 1997 Ovarian serous neoplasms of low malignant potential associated with focal areas of serous carcinoma. Mod Pathol 10: 663–667
96. Segal G H, Hart W R 1992 Ovarian serous tumors of low malignant potential (serous borderline tumors): The relationship of exophytic surface tumor to peritoneal "implants". Am J Surg Pathol 16: 577–583
97. Diebold J, Seemueller F, Loehrs U. 2003 K-RAS mutations in ovarian and extraovarian lesions of serous tumors of borderline malignancy. Lab Invest 83: 251–258
98. Sieben N L G, Kolkman-Uljee S M, Flanagan A M et al. 2003 Molecular genetic evidence for monoclonal origin of bilateral ovarian serous borderline tumors. Am J Pathol 162: 1095–1101
99. Ortiz B H, Ailawadi M, Colitti C et al. 2001 Second primary or recurrence? Comparative patterns of p53 and K-ras mutations suggest that serous borderline ovarian tumors and subsequent serous carcinomas are unrelated tumors. Cancer Res 61: 7264–7267
100. Krishnamurti U, Sasatomi E, Swalsky P A et al. 2005 Microdissection-based mutational genotyping of serous borderline tumors of the ovary. Int J Gynecol Pathol 24: 56–61
101. Gu J, Roth L M, Younger C et al. 2001 Molecular evidence for the independent origin of extra-ovarian papillary serous tumors of low malignant potential. J Natl Cancer Inst 93: 1147–1152
102. Lu K H, Bell D A, Welch W R et al. 1998 Evidence for the multifocal origin of bilateral and advanced human serous borderline ovarian tumors. Cancer Res 58: 2328–2330
103. Bell D A, Weinstock M A, Scully R E 1988 Peritoneal implants of ovarian serous borderline tumors. Histologic features and prognosis. Cancer 62: 2212–2222
104. Deavers M T, Gershenson D M, Tortolero-Luna G et al. 2002 Micropapillary and cribriform patterns in ovarian serous tumors of low malignant potential: a study of 99 advanced stage cases. Am J Surg Pathol 26: 1129–1141
105. Lee K R, Castrillon D H, Nucci M R 2001 Pathologic findings in eight cases of ovarian serous borderline tumors, three with foci of serous carcinoma, that preceded death or morbidity from invasive carcinoma. Int J Gynecol Pathol 20: 329–334
106. Gershenson D M, Silva E G, Tortolero-Luna G et al. 1998 Serous borderline tumors of the ovary with non-invasive peritoneal implants. Cancer 83: 2157–2163
107. Seidman J D, Kurman R J 1996 Subclassification of serous borderline tumors of the ovary into benign and malignant types – A clinicopathologic study of 65 advanced stage cases. Am J Surg Pathol 20: 1331–1345
108. Gershenson D M, Silva E G, Levy L et al. 1998 Ovarian serous borderline tumors with invasive peritoneal implants. Cancer 82: 1096–1103
109. Bell K A, Sehdev A E S, Kurman R J 2001 Refined diagnostic criteria for implants associated with ovarian atypical proliferative serous tumors (borderline) and micropapillary serous carcinomas. Am J Surg Pathol 25: 419–432
110. Rota S M, Zanetta G, Ieda N et al. 1999 Clinical relevance of retroperitoneal involvement from epithelial ovarian tumors of borderline malignancy. Int J Gynecol Cancer 9: 477–480
111. Leake J F, Rader J S, Woodruff J D et al. 1991 Retroperitoneal lymphatic involvement with epithelial ovarian tumors of low malignant potential. Gynecol Oncol 42: 124–130
111a. McKenny J K, Balzer B L, Longacre T A 2006 Lymph node involvement in ovarian serous tumors of low malignant potential (borderline tumors): pathology, prognosis, and proposed classification. Am J Surg Pathol 30: 614–624
112. Clement P B, Young R H, Oliva E et al. 1996 Hyperplastic mesothelial cells within abdominal lymph nodes: mimic of metastatic ovarian carcinoma and serous borderline tumor – a report of two cases associated with ovarian neoplasms. Mod Pathol 9: 879–886
113. Ordonez N G 1998 Role of immunohistochemistry in distinguishing epithelial peritoneal mesotheliomas from peritoneal and ovarian serous carcinomas. Am J Surg Pathol 22: 1203–1214
114. Chamberlin M D, Eltabbakh G H, Mount S L et al. 2001 Metastatic serous borderline ovarian tumor in an internal mammary lymph node: a case report and review of the literature. Gynecol Oncol 82: 212–215
115. Reich O, Tamussino K, Haas J et al. 2000 Benign mullerian inclusions in pelvic and paraaortic lymph nodes. Gynecol Oncol 78: 242–244
116. Moore W F, Bentley R C, Berchuck A 2000 Some mullerian inclusion cysts in lymph nodes may sometimes be metastases from serous borderline tumors of the ovary. Am J Surg Pathol 24: 710–718
117. Prade M, Spatz A, Bentley R et al. 1995 Borderline and malignant serous tumor arising in pelvic lymph nodes: evidence of origin in benign glandular inclusions. Int J Gynecol Pathol 14: 87–91
118. Tan L K, Flynn S D, Carcangiu M L 1994 Ovarian serous borderline tumors with lymph node involvement: clinicopathologic and DNA content study of seven cases and review of the literature. Am J Surg Pathol 18: 904–912
119. Burks R T, Sherman M E, Kurman R J 1996 Micropapillary serous carcinoma of the ovary – a distinctive low-grade carcinoma related to serous borderline tumors. Am J Surg Pathol 20: 1319–1330
120. Smith Sehdev A E, Sehdev P S, Kurman R J 2003 Non-invasive and invasive micropapillary (low-grade) serous carcinoma of the ovary: a clinicopathologic analysis of 135 cases. Am J Surg Pathol 27: 725–736

121. Goldstein N S, Ceniza N 2000 Ovarian micropapillary serous borderline tumors – clinicopathologic features and outcome of seven surgically staged patients. Am J Clin Pathol 114: 380–386
122. Mills S E, Andersen W A, Fechner R E et al. 1988 Serous surface papillary carcinoma. A clinicopathologic study of 10 cases and comparison with stage III–IV ovarian serous carcinoma. Am J Surg Pathol 12: 827–834
123. White P F, Merino M J, Barwick K W 1985 Serous surface papillary carcinoma of the ovary: a clinical, pathologic, ultrastructural, and immunohistochemical study of 11 cases. Pathol Annu 20 Pt 1: 403–418
124. Rutledge M L, Silva E G, McLemore D et al. 1989 Serous surface carcinoma of the ovary and peritoneum. A flow cytometric study. Pathol Annu 24 Pt 2: 227–235
125. Gooneratne S, Sassone M, Blaustein A et al. 1982 Serous surface papillary carcinoma of the ovary: a clinicopathologic study of 16 cases. Int J Gynecol Pathol 1: 258–269
126. Mulhollan T J, Silva E G, Tornos C et al. 1994 Ovarian involvement by serous surface papillary carcinoma. Int J Gynecol Pathol 13: 120–126
127. Che M, Tornos C, Deavers M T et al. 2001 Ovarian mixed-epithelial carcinomas with a microcystic pattern and signet-ring cells. Int J Gynecol Pathol 20: 323–328
128. Bell D A, Scully R E 1994 Early de novo ovarian carcinoma: a study of fourteen cases. Cancer 73: 1859–1864
129. Cathro H P, Stoler M H 2002 Expression of cytokeratins 7 and 20 in ovarian neoplasia. Am J Clin Pathol 117: 944–951
130. Keen C E, Szakacs S, Okon E et al. 1999 CA125 and thyroglobulin staining in papillary carcinomas of thyroid and ovarian origin is not completely specific for site of origin. Histopathology 34: 113–117
131. Multhaupt H A, Renas-Elliott C P, Warhol M J 1999 Comparison of glycoprotein expression between ovarian and colon adenocarcinomas. Arch Pathol Lab Med 123: 909–916
132. Hwang H, Quenneville L, Yaziji H et al. 2004 Wilms tumor gene product: sensitive and contextually specific marker of serous carcinomas of ovarian surface epithelial origin. Appl Immunohistochem Mol Morphol 12: 122–126
133. Hashi A, Yuminamochi T, Murata S et al. 2003 Wilms tumor gene immunoreactivity in primary serous carcinomas of the fallopian tube, ovary, endometrium, and peritoneum. Int J Gynecol Pathol 22: 374–377
134. Goldstein N S, Bassi D, Uzieblo A 2001 WT1 is an integral component of an antibody panel to distinguish pancreaticobiliary and some ovarian epithelial neoplasms. Am J Clin Pathol 116: 246–252
135. Goldstein N S, Uzieblo A 2002 WT1 immunoreactivity in uterine papillary serous carcinomas is different from ovarian serous carcinomas. Am J Clin Pathol 117: 541–545
136. Shimizu M, Toki T, Takagi Y et al. 2000 Immunohistochemical detection of the Wilms' tumor gene (WT1) in epithelial ovarian tumors. Int J Gynecol Pathol 19: 158–163
137. Otis C N, Krebs P A, Quezado M M et al. 2000 Loss of heterozygosity in $P53$, BRCA1, and estrogen receptor genes and correlation to expression of p53 protein in ovarian epithelial tumors of different cell types and biological behavior. Hum Pathol 31: 233–238
138. Anttila M A, Ji H, Juhola M T, Saarikoski S V et al. 1999 The prognostic significance of p53 expression quantitated by computerized image analysis in epithelial ovarian cancer. Int J Gynecol Pathol 18: 42–51
139. Wen W H, Reles A, Runnebaum I B et al. 1999 p53 mutations and expression in ovarian cancers: correlation with overall survival. Int J Gynecol Pathol 18: 29–41
140. Eltabbakh G H, Belinson J L, Kennedy A W et al. 1997 p53 overexpression is not an independent prognostic factor for patients with primary ovarian epithelial cancer. Cancer 80: 892–898
141. Diebold J, Suchy B, Baretton GB et al. 1996 DNA ploidy and MYC DNA amplification in ovarian carcinomas – Correlation with p53 and bcl-2 expression, proliferative activity and prognosis. Virchow' Arch 429: 221–227
142. Klemi PJ, Pylkkänen L, Kiilholma P et al. 1995 P53 protein detected by immunohistochemistry as a prognostic factor in patients with epithelial ovarian carcinoma. Cancer 76: 1201–1208
143. Acs G, Pasha T, Zhang P J 2004 WT1 is differentially expressed in serous, endometrioid, clear cell, and mucinous carcinomas of the peritoneum, fallopian tube, ovary, and endometrium. Int J Gynecol Pathol 23: 110–118
144. Al Hussaini M, Stockman A, Foster H et al. 2004 WT-1 assists in distinguishing ovarian from uterine serous carcinoma and in distinguishing between serous and endometrioid ovarian carcinoma. Histopathology 44: 109–115
145. Singer G, Shih I, Truskinovsky A et al. 2003 Mutational analysis of K-ras segregates ovarian serous carcinomas into two types: invasive MPSC (low-grade tumor) and conventional serous carcinoma (high-grade tumor). Int J Gynecol Pathol 22: 37–41
146. Haas C J, Diebold J, Hirschmann A et al. 1999 In serous ovarian neoplasms the frequency of Ki-ras mutations correlates with their malignant potential. Virchow's Arch 434: 117–120
147. Bell D A 2005 Origins and molecular pathology of ovarian cancer. Mod Pathol 18 Suppl 2: S19–S32
148. Meinhold-Heerlein I, Bauerschlag D, Hilpert F et al. 2005 Molecular and prognostic distinction between serous ovarian carcinomas of varying grade and malignant potential. Oncogene 24: 1053–1065
149. Singer G, Stohr R, Cope L et al. 2005 Patterns of p53 mutations separate ovarian serous borderline tumors and low- and high-grade carcinomas and provide support for a new model of ovarian carcinogenesis: a mutational analysis with immunohistochemical correlation. Am J Surg Pathol 29: 218–224

150. Bristow R E, Gossett D R, Shook DR et al. 2002 Micropapillary serous ovarian carcinoma: surgical management and clinical outcome. Gynecol Oncol 86: 163–170
151. Sieben N L, Macropoulos P, Roemen G M et al. 2004 In ovarian neoplasms, BRAF, but not KRAS, mutations are restricted to low-grade serous tumours. J Pathol 202: 336–340
152. Moran C A, Suster S, Silva E G 2005 Low-grade serous carcinoma of the ovary metastatic to the anterior mediastinum simulating multilocular thymic cysts: a clinicopathologic and immunohistochemical study of 3 cases. Am J Surg Pathol 29: 496–499
153. Recine M A, Deavers M T, Middleton L P et al. 2004 Serous carcinoma of the ovary and peritoneum with metastases to the breast and axillary lymph nodes: a potential pitfall. Am J Surg Pathol 28: 1646–1651
154. Silverberg S G 2000 Histopathologic grading of ovarian carcinoma: a review and proposal. Int J Gynecol Pathol 19: 7–15
155. Shimizu Y, Kamoi S, Amada S et al. 1998 Toward the development of a universal grading system for ovarian epithelial carcinoma – Testing of a proposed system in a series of 461 patients with uniform treatment and follow-up. Cancer 82: 893–901
156. Shimizu Y, Kamoi S, Amada S et al. 1998 Toward the development of a universal grading system for ovarian epithelial carcinoma. I. Prognostic significance of histopathologic features – problems involved in the architectural grading system. Gynecol Oncol 70: 2–12
157. Piek J M, Torrenga B, Hermsen B et al. 2003 Histopathological characteristics of BRCA1- and BRCA2-associated intraperitoneal cancer: a clinic-based study. Fam Cancer 2: 7–8
158. Kauff N D, Satagopan J M, Robson M E et al. 2002 Risk-reducing salpingo-oophorectomy in women with a BRCA1 or BRCA2 mutation. N Engl J Med 346: 1609–1615
159. Rebbeck T R, Lynch H T, Neuhausen S L et al. 2002 Prophylactic oophorectomy in carriers of BRCA1 or BRCA2 mutations. N Engl J Med 346: 1616–1622
160. Rutter J L, Wacholder S, Chetrit A et al. 2003 Gynecologic surgeries and risk of ovarian cancer in women with BRCA1 and BRCA2 Ashkenazi founder mutations: an Israeli population-based case-control study. J Natl Cancer Inst 95: 1072–1078
161. Casey M J, Synder C, Bewtra C et al. 2005 Intra-abdominal carcinomatosis after prophylactic oophorectomy in women of hereditary breast ovarian cancer syndrome kindreds associated with BRCA1 and BRCA2 mutations. Gynecol Oncol 97: 457–467
162. Piver M S, Jishi M F, Tsukada Y et al. 1993 Primary peritoneal carcinoma after prophylactic oophorectomy in women with a family history of ovarian cancer: A report of the Gilda Radner Familial Ovarian Cancer Registry. Cancer 71: 2751–2755
163. Lu K H, Garber J E, Cramer D W et al. 2000 Occult ovarian tumors in women with BRCA1 or BRCA2 mutations undergoing prophylactic oophorectomy. J Clin Oncol 18: 2728–2732
164. Colgan T J, Murphy J, Cole D E C et al. 2001 Occult carcinoma in prophylactic oophorectomy specimens – Prevalence and association with BRCA germline mutation status. Am J Surg Pathol 25: 1283–1289
165. Powell C B, Kenley E, Chen L M et al. 2005 Risk-reducing salpingo-oophorectomy in BRCA mutation carriers: role of serial sectioning in the detection of occult malignancy. J Clin Oncol 23: 127–132
166. Leeper K, Garcia R, Swisher E et al. 2002 Pathologic findings in prophylactic oophorectomy specimens in high-risk women. Gynecol Oncol 87: 52–56
167. Agoff S N, Mendelin J E, Grieco V S et al. 2002 Unexpected gynecologic neoplasms in patients with proven or suspected BRCA-1 or -2 mutations: implications for gross examination, cytology, and clinical follow-up. Am J Surg Pathol 26: 171–178
168. Colgan T J 2003 Challenges in the early diagnosis and staging of fallopian-tube carcinomas associated with BRCA mutations. Int J Gynecol Pathol 22: 109–120
169. Lakhani S R, Manek S, Penault-Llorca F et al. 2004 Pathology of ovarian cancers in BRCA1 and BRCA2 carriers. Clin Cancer Res 10: 2473–2481
170. Shaw P A, McLaughlin J R, Zweemer R P et al. 2002 Histopathologic features of genetically determined ovarian cancer. Int J Gynecol Pathol 21: 407–411
171. Werness B A, Ramus S J, DiCioccio R A et al. 2004 Histopathology, FIGO stage, and BRCA mutation status of ovarian cancers from the Gilda Radner Familial Ovarian Cancer Registry. Int J Gynecol Pathol 23: 29–34
172. Ferenczy A, Talens A, Zoghby et al. 1977 Ultrastructural studies on the morphogenesis of psammoma bodies in ovarian serous neoplasia. Cancer 39: 2451–2459
173. Gilks C B, Bell D A, Scully R E 1990 Serous psammocarcinoma of the ovary and peritoneum. Int J Gynecol Pathol 9: 110–121
174. Powell J L, McDonald T J, White W C 1998 Serous psammocarcinoma of the ovary. South Med J 91: 477–480
175. Giordano G, Gnetti L, Milione M 2005 Serous psammocarcinoma of the ovary: a case report and review of literature. Gynecol Oncol 96: 259–262
176. Weir M M, Bell D A, Young R H 1998 Grade 1 peritoneal serous carcinomas – A report of 14 cases and comparison with 7 peritoneal serous psammocarcinomas and 19 peritoneal serous borderline tumors. Am J Surg Pathol 22: 849–862
177. Chao A, Chao A, Yen Y S et al. 2004 Abdominal compartment syndrome secondary to ovarian mucinous cystadenoma. Obstet Gynecol 104: 1180–1182
178. Tenti P, Aguzzi A, Riva C et al. 1992 Ovarian mucinous tumors frequently express markers of gastric, intestinal, and pancreatobiliary epithelial cells. Cancer 69: 2131–2142
179. Shiohara S, Shiozawa T, Shimizu M et al. 1997 Histochemical analysis of estrogen and progesterone receptors and gastric-type mucin in mucinous ovarian tumors with reference to their pathogenesis. Cancer 80: 908–916
180. Ball N J, Robertson D I, Duggan M A et al. 1990 Intestinal differentiation in ovarian mucinous tumours. Virchow's Arch [A] 417: 197–201
181. Klemi P J 1978 Pathology of mucinous ovarian cystadenomas. I. Argyrophil and argentaffin cells and epithelial mucosubstances. Acta Pathol Microbiol Scand [A] 86: 465–470
182. Ishikura H, Sasano H 1998 Histopathologic and immunohistochemical study of steroidogenic cells in the stroma of ovarian tumors. Int J Gynecol Pathol 17: 261–265
183. Bell D A 1991 Mucinous adenofibromas of the ovary. A report of 10 cases. Am J Surg Pathol 15: 227–232
184. Kao G F, Norris H J 1979 Unusual cystadenofibromas: endometrioid, mucinous, and clear cell type. Obstet Gynecol 54: 729–736
185. De Nictolis M, Montironi R, Tommasoni S et al. 1994 Benign, borderline, and well-differentiated malignant intestinal mucinous tumors of the ovary: a clinicopathologic, histochemical, immunohistochemical, and nuclear quantitative study of 57 cases. Int J Gynecol Pathol 13: 10–21
186. Guerrieri C, Högberg T, Wingren S et al. 1994 Mucinous borderline and malignant tumors of the ovary: A clinicopathologic and DNA ploidy study of 92 cases. Cancer 74: 2329–2340
187. Hart W R 2005 Mucinous tumors of the ovary: a review. Int J Gynecol Pathol 24: 4–25
188. Hart W R, Norris H J 1973 Borderline and malignant mucinous tumors of the ovary: Histologic criteria and clinical behavior. Cancer 31: 1031–1045
189. Ronnett B M, Kajdacsy-Balla A, Gilks C B et al. 2004 Mucinous borderline ovarian tumors: points of general agreement and persistent controversies regarding nomenclature, diagnostic criteria, and behavior. Hum Pathol 35: 949–960
190. Rodriguez I M, Prat J 2002 Mucinous tumors of the ovary: a clinicopathologic analysis of 75 borderline tumors (of intestinal type) and carcinomas. Am J Surg Pathol 26: 139–152
191. Lee K R, Scully R 2000 Mucinous tumors of the ovary: a clinicopathologic study of 196 borderline tumors (of intestinal type) and carcinomas, including an evaluation of 11 cases with "pseudomyxoma peritonei". Am J Surg Pathol 24: 1447–1464
192. Nomura K, Aizawa S, Hano H 2004 Ovarian mucinous borderline tumors of intestinal type without intraepithelial carcinoma: are they still tumors of low malignant potential? Pathol Int 54: 420–424
193. Nomura K, Aizawa S 2000 Non-invasive, microinvasive, and invasive mucinous carcinomas of the ovary – A clinicopathologic analysis of 40 cases. Cancer 89: 1541–1546
194. Khunamornpong S, Russell P, Dalrymple J C 1999 Proliferating (LMP) mucinous tumors of the ovaries with microinvasion: morphologic assessment of 13 cases. Int J Gynecol Pathol 18: 238–246
195. Ludwick C, Gilks C B, Miller D et al. 2005 Aggressive behavior of stage I ovarian mucinous tumors lacking extensive infiltrative invasion: a report of four cases and review of the literature. Int J Gynecol Pathol 24: 205–217
196. Michael H, Sutton G, Roth L M 1987 Ovarian carcinoma with extracellular mucin production: reassessment of "pseudomyxoma ovarii et peritonei". Int J Gynecol Pathol 6: 298–312
197. Rutgers J L, Scully R E 1988 Ovarian mullerian mucinous papillary cystadenomas of borderline malignancy. A clinicopathologic analysis. Cancer 61: 340–348
198. Nomura K, Aizawa S 1996 Clinicopathologic and mucin histochemical analyses of 90 cases of ovarian mucinous borderline tumors of intestinal and mullerian types. Pathol Int 46: 575–580
199. Rodriguez I M, Irving J A, Prat J 2004 Endocervical-like mucinous borderline tumors of the ovary: a clinicopathologic analysis of 31 cases. Am J Surg Pathol 28: 1311–1318
200. Shappell H W, Riopel M A, Smith Sehdev A E et al. 2002 Diagnostic criteria and behavior of ovarian seromucinous (endocervical-type mucinous and mixed cell-type) tumors: atypical proliferative (borderline) tumors, intraepithelial, microinvasive, and invasive carcinomas. Am J Surg Pathol 26: 1529–1541
201. Dube V, Roy M, Plante M et al. 2005 Mucinous ovarian tumors of Mullerian-type: an analysis of 17 cases including borderline tumors and intraepithelial, microinvasive, and invasive carcinomas. Int J Gynecol Pathol 24: 138–146
202. Miettinen M 1995 Keratin 20: immunohistochemical marker for gastrointestinal, urothelial, and Merkel cell carcinomas. Mod Pathol 8: 384–388
203. Rutgers J L, Bell D A 1992 Immunohistochemical characterization of ovarian borderline tumors of intestinal and mullerian types. Mod Pathol 5: 367–371
204. Abu-Jawdeh G M, Jacobs T W, Niloff J et al. 1996 Estrogen receptor expression is a common feature of ovarian borderline tumors. Gynecol Oncol 60: 301–307
205. Sasaki E, Sasano N, Kimura N et al. 1989 Demonstration of neuroendocrine cells in ovarian mucinous tumors. Int J Gynecol Pathol 8: 189–200
206. Aguirre P, Scully R E, Dayal et al. 1984 Mucinous tumors of the ovary with argyrophil cells: an immunohistochemical study. Am J Surg Pathol 8: 345–356

207. DeBoer W G, Ma J, Nayman J 1981 Intestine-associated antigens in ovarian tumours: an immunohistochemical study. Pathology 13: 547–555
208. Louwerens J K, Schaberg A, Bosman F T 1983 Neuroendocrine cells in cystic mucinous tumours of the ovary. Histopathology 7: 389–398
209. Sporrong B, Alumets J, Clase L et al. 1981 Neurohormonal peptide immunoreactive cells in mucinous cystadenomas and cystadenocarcinomas of the ovary. Virchow's Arch [A] 392: 271–280
210. Watkin W, Silva E G, Gershenson D M 1992 Mucinous carcinoma of the ovary: pathologic prognostic factors. Cancer 69: 208–212
211. Seidman J D, Kurman R J, Ronnett B M 2003 Primary and metastatic mucinous adenocarcinomas in the ovaries: incidence in routine practice with a new approach to improve intraoperative diagnosis. Am J Surg Pathol 27: 985–993
212. Lee K R, Nucci M R 2003 Ovarian mucinous and mixed epithelial carcinomas of mullerian (endocervical-like) type: a clinicopathologic analysis of four cases of an uncommon variant associated with endometriosis. Int J Gynecol Pathol 22: 42–51
213. Kikkawa F, Kawai M, Tamakoshi K et al. 1996 Mucinous carcinoma of the ovary – Clinicopathologic analysis. Oncology (Basel) 53: 303–307
214. Chen S, Leitao M M, Tornos C et al. 2005 Invasion patterns in stage I endometrioid and mucinous ovarian carcinomas: a clinicopathologic analysis emphasizing favorable outcomes in carcinomas without destructive stromal invasion and the occasional malignant course of carcinomas with limited destructive stromal invasion. Mod Pathol 18: 903–911
215. Hart W R 1977 Ovarian epithelial tumors of borderline malignancy (carcinomas of low malignant potential). Hum Pathol 8: 541–549
216. Raspollini M R, Amunni G, Villanucci A et al. 2004 Utility of CDX-2 in distinguishing between primary and secondary (intestinal) mucinous ovarian carcinoma: an immunohistochemical comparison of 43 cases. Appl Immunohistochem Mol Morphol 12: 127–131
217. Chou Y Y, Jeng Y M, Kao H L et al. Differentiation of ovarian mucinous carcinoma and metastatic colorectal adenocarcinoma by immunostaining with beta-catenin. Histopathology 43: 151–156
218. Groisman G M, Meir A, Sabo E 2004 The value of Cdx2 immunostaining in differentiating primary ovarian carcinomas from colonic carcinomas metastatic to the ovaries. Int J Gynecol Pathol 23: 52–57
219. Ji H, Isacson C, Seidman J D et al. 2002 Cytokeratins 7 and 20, Dpc4, and MUC5AC in the distinction of metastatic mucinous carcinomas in the ovary from primary ovarian mucinous tumors: Dpc4 assists in identifying metastatic pancreatic carcinomas. Int J Gynecol Pathol 21: 391–400
220. Tornillo L, Moch H, Diener P A et al. 2004 CDX-2 immunostaining in primary and secondary ovarian carcinomas. J Clin Pathol 57: 641–643
221. Logani S, Oliva E, Arnell P M et al. 2005 Use of novel immunohistochemical markers expressed in colonic adenocarcinoma to distinguish primary ovarian tumors from metastatic colorectal carcinoma. Mod Pathol 18: 19–25
222. Moskaluk C A, Zhang H, Powell S M et al. 2003 Cdx2 protein expression in normal and malignant human tissues: an immunohistochemical survey using tissue microarrays. Mod Pathol 16: 913–919
223. Prat J, Scully R E 1979 Ovarian mucinous tumors with sarcoma-like mural nodules. A report of seven cases. Cancer 44: 1332–1344
224. Baergen R N, Rutgers J L 1995 Classification of mural nodules in common epithelial tumors of the ovary. Adv Anat Pathol 2: 346–351
225. Bague S, Rodriguez I M, Prat J 2002 Sarcoma-like mural nodules in mucinous cystic tumors of the ovary revisited – A clinicopathologic analysis of 10 additional cases. Am J Surg Pathol 26: 1467–1476
226. Matias-Guiu X, Aranda I, Prat J 1991 Immunohistochemical study of sarcoma-like mural nodules in a mucinous cystadenocarcinoma of the ovary. Virchow's Arch A Pathol Anat Histopathol 419: 89–92
227. Hamada T, Sasaguri T, Tanimoto A et al. 1995 Ovarian mucinous cystadenocarcinoma with sarcoma-like mural nodules. J Surg Oncol 58: 201–207
228. Sondergaard G, Kaspersen P 1991 Ovarian and extraovarian mucinous tumors with solid mural nodules. Int J Gynecol Pathol 10: 145–155
229. Czernobilsky B, Dgani R, Roth L M 1983 Ovarian mucinous cystadenocarcinoma with mural nodule of carcinomatous derivation: a light and electron microscopic study. Cancer 51: 141–148
230. Prat J, Young R, Scully R 1982 Ovarian mucinous tumors with foci of anaplastic carcinoma. Cancer 50: 300–304
231. Nichols G E, Mills S E, Ulbright T M et al. 1991 Spindle cell mural nodules in cystic ovarian mucinous tumors: A clinicopathologic and immunohistochemical study of five cases. Am J Surg Pathol 15: 1055–1062
232. Baergen R N, Rutgers J L 1994 Mural nodules in common epithelial tumors of the ovary. Int J Gynecol Pathol 13: 62–71
233. Chang W C, Sheu B C, Lin M C et al. 2005 Carcinosarcoma-like mural nodule in intestinal-type mucinous ovarian of borderline malignancy: a case report. Int J Gynecol Cancer 15: 549–553
234. Prat J, Scully R E 1979 Sarcomas in ovarian mucinous tumors. A report of two cases. Cancer 44: 1327–1331
235. Bruijn J A, Smit V T, Que D G et al. 1987 Immunohistology of a sarcomatous mural nodule in an ovarian mucinous cystadenocarcinoma. Int J Gynecol Pathol 6: 287–293
236. Collins R J, Cheung A, Ngan H Y et al. 1991 Primary mixed neuroendocrine and mucinous carcinoma of the ovary. Arch Gynecol Obstet 248: 139–143
237. Eichhorn J H, Young R H, Scully R E 1992 Primary ovarian small cell carcinoma of pulmonary type: a clinicopathologic, immunohistologic, and flow cytometric analysis of 11 cases. Am J Surg Pathol 16: 926–938
238. Khurana K K, Tornos C, Silva E G 1994 Ovarian neuroendocrine carcinoma associated with a mucinous neoplasm. Arch Pathol Lab Med 118: 1032–1034
239. Jones K, Diaz J A, Donner L R 1996 Neuroendocrine carcinoma arising in an ovarian mucinous cystadenoma. Int J Gynecol Pathol 15: 167–170.
240. Eichhorn J H, Lawrence W D, Young R H et al. 1996 Ovarian neuroendocrine carcinomas of non-small-cell type associated with surface epithelial adenocarcinomas. A study of five cases and review of the literature. Int J Gynecol Pathol 15: 303–314
241. Ishikura H, Shibata M, Yoshiki T 1999 Endocrine cell micronests in an ovarian mucinous cystadenofibroma: a mimic of microinvasion. Int J Gynecol Pathol 18: 392–395
242. Snyder R R, Norris H J, Tavassoli F 1988 Endometrioid proliferative and low malignant potential tumors of the ovary. A clinicopathologic study of 46 cases. Am J Surg Pathol 12: 661–671
243. Bell K A, Kurman R J 2000 A clinicopathologic analysis of atypical proliferative (borderline) tumors and well-differentiated endometrioid adenocarcinomas of the ovary. Am J Surg Pathol 24: 1465–1479
244. Gaing A A, Kimble C C, Belmonte A H et al. 1988 Invasive ovarian endometrioid adenofibroma with omental implants and collision with endometrial adenocarcinoma. Obstet Gynecol 71: 440–444
245. Kline R C, Wharton J T, Atkinson E N et al. 1990 Endometrioid carcinoma of the ovary: retrospective review of 145 cases. Gynecol Oncol 39: 337–346
246. Aure J C, Hoeg K, Kolstad P 1971 Clinical and histologic studies of ovarian carcinoma. Long-term follow-up of 990 cases. Obstet Gynecol 37: 1–9
247. Makar A P, Baekelandt M, Trope C G et al. 1995 The prognostic significance of residual disease, FIGO substage, tumor histology, and grade in patients with FIGO stage III ovarian cancer. Gynecol Oncol 56: 175–180
248. McMeekin D S, Burger R A, Manetta A et al. 1995 Endometrioid adenocarcinoma of the ovary and its relationship to endometriosis. Gynecol Oncol 59: 81–86
249. Fukunaga M, Nomura K, Ishikawa E et al. 1997 Ovarian atypical endometriosis: its close association with malignant epithelial tumours. Histopathology 30: 249–255
250. DePriest P D, Banks E R, Powell D E et al. 1992 Endometrioid carcinoma of the ovary and endometriosis: the association in postmenopausal women. Gynecol Oncol 47: 71–75
251. Stern R C, Dash R, Bentley R C et al. 2001 Malignancy in endometriosis: frequency and comparison of ovarian and extraovarian types. Int J Gynecol Pathol 20: 133–139
252. Heaps J M, Nieberg R K, Berek J S 1990 Malignant neoplasms arising in endometriosis. Obstet Gynecol 75: 1023–1028
253. Modesitt S C, Tortoler-Luna G, Robinson J B et al. 2002 Ovarian and extraovarian endometriosis-associated cancer. Obstet Gynecol 100: 788–795
254. Erzen M, Rakar S, Klancar B et al. 2001 Endometriosis-associated ovarian carcinoma (eaoc): an entity distinct from other ovarian carcinomas as suggested by a nested case-control study. Gynecol Oncol 83: 100–108
255. Roth L M, Czernobilsky B, Langley F A 1981 Ovarian endometrioid adenofibromatous and cystadenofibromatous tumors: benign, proliferating, and malignant. Cancer 48: 1838–1845
256. Eichhorn J H, Scully R E 1996 Endometrioid ciliated-cell tumors of the ovary: a report of five cases. Int J Gynecol Pathol 15: 248–256
257. Kao G F, Norris H J 1978 Cystadenofibromas of the ovary with epithelial atypia. Am J Surg Pathol 2: 357–363
258. Bell D A, Scully R E 1985 Atypical and borderline endometrioid adenofibromas of the ovary: a report of 27 cases. Am J Surg Pathol 9: 205–214
259. Norris H J 1993 Proliferative endometrioid tumors and endometrioid tumors of low malignant potential of the ovary. Int J Gynecol Pathol 12: 134–141
260. Roth L M, Emerson R E, Ulbright T M 2003 Ovarian endometrioid tumors of low malignant potential: a clinicopathologic study of 30 cases with comparison to well-differentiated endometrioid adenocarcinoma. Am J Surg Pathol 27: 1253–1259
261. Brescia R J, Dubin N, Demopoulos R I 1989 Endometrioid and clear cell carcinoma of the ovary. Factors affecting survival. Int J Gynecol Pathol 8: 132–138
262. Russell P 1979 The pathological assessment of ovarian neoplasms. III. The malignant "epithelial" tumours. Pathology 11: 493–532
263. Zaino R J, Kurman R J, Diana K L et al. 1995 The utility of the revised International Federation of Gynecology and Obstetrics histologic grading of endometrial adenocarcinoma using a defined nuclear grading system: A Gynecologic Oncology Group study. Cancer 75: 81–86
264. Kim K R, Scully R E 1990 Peritoneal keratin granulomas with carcinomas of endometrium and ovary and atypical polypoid adenomyoma of endometrium. A clinicopathological analysis of 22 cases. Am J Surg Pathol 14: 925–932
265. Kurman R J, Craig J M 1972 Endometrioid and clear cell carcinoma of the ovary. Cancer 29: 1653–1664
266. Tornos C, Silva E G, Khorana S M et al. 1994 High-stage endometrioid carcinoma of the ovary: Prognostic significance of pure versus mixed histologic types. Am J Surg Pathol 18: 687–693

267. Young R H, Prat J, Scully R E 1982 Ovarian endometrioid carcinomas resembling sex cord-stromal tumors. A clinicopathologic analysis of 13 cases. Am J Surg Pathol 6: 513–522
268. Roth L M, Liban E, Czernobilsky B 1982 Ovarian endometrioid tumors mimicking Sertoli and Sertoli-Leydig cell tumors: Sertoliform variant of endometrioid carcinoma. Cancer 50: 1322–1331
269. Ordi J, Schammel D P, Rasekh L et al. 1999 Sertoliform endometrioid carcinomas of the ovary: a clinicopathologic and immunohistochemical study of 13 cases. Mod Pathol 12: 933–940
270. Pitman M B, Young R H, Clement P B et al. 1994 Endometrioid carcinoma of the ovary and endometrium, oxyphilic cell type: a report of nine cases. Int J Gynecol Pathol 13: 290–301
271. Tornos C, Silva E G, Ordonez N G 1995 Endometrioid carcinoma of the ovary with a prominent spindle-cell component, a source of diagnostic confusion – A report of 14 cases. Am J Surg Pathol 19:1343–1353
272. Dabbs D J, Sturtz K, Zaino R J 1996 The immunohistochemical discrimination of endometrioid adenocarcinomas. Hum Pathol 27: 172–177
273. Guerrieri C, Franlund B, Malmstrom H et al. 1998 Ovarian endometrioid carcinomas simulating sex cord-stromal tumors: a study using inhibin and cytokeratin 7. Int J Gynecol Pathol 17: 266–271
274. Matias-Guiu X, Pons C, Prat J 1998 Mullerian inhibiting substance, alpha-inhibin, and CD99 expression in sex cord-stromal tumors and endometrioid ovarian carcinomas resembling sex cord-stromal tumors. Hum Pathol 29: 840–845
275. Hildebrandt R H, Rouse R V, Longacre T A 1997 Value of inhibin in the identification of granulosa cell tumors of the ovary. Hum Pathol 28: 1387–1395
276. Nogales F F, Bergeron C, Carvia R E et al. 1996 Ovarian endometrioid tumors with yolk sac tumor component, an unusual form of ovarian neoplasm – Analysis of six cases. Am J Surg Pathol 20: 1056–1066
277. Lopez J M, Malpica A, Deavers M T et al. 2003 Ovarian yolk sac tumor associated with endometrioid carcinoma and mucinous cystadenoma of the ovary. Ann Diagn Pathol 7: 300–305
278. Sheu B C, Lin H H, Chen C K et al. 1995 Synchronous primary carcinomas of the endometrium and ovary. Int J Gynaecol Obstet 51: 141–146
279. Falkenberry S S, Steinhoff M M, Gordinier M et al. 1996 Synchronous endometrioid tumors of the ovary and endometrium – A clinicopathologic study of 22 cases. J Reprod Med 41: 713–718
280. Eifel P, Hendrickson M, Ross J et al. 1982 Simultaneous presentation of carcinoma involving the ovary and the uterine corpus. Cancer 50: 163–170
281. Pearl M L, Johnston C M, Frank T S et al. 1993 Synchronous dual primary ovarian and endometrial carcinomas. Int J Gynaecol Obstet 43: 305–312
282. Soliman P T, Slomovitz B M, Broaddus R et al. 2004 Synchronous primary cancers of the endometrium and ovary: a single institution review of 84 cases. Gynecol Oncol 94: 456–462
283. Zaino R, Whitney C, Brady M F et al. 2001 Simultaneously detected endometrial and ovarian carcinomas – a prospective clinicopathologic study of 74 cases: a gynecologic oncology group study. Gynecol Oncol 83: 355–362
284. Ulbright T M, Roth L M 1985 Metastatic and independent cancers of the endometrium and ovary: a clinicopathologic study of 34 cases. Hum Pathol 16: 28–34
285. Shenson D L, Gallion H H, Powell D E et al. 1995 Loss of heterozygosity and genomic instability in synchronous endometrioid tumors of the ovary and endometrium. Cancer 76: 650–657
286. Fujita M, Enomoto T, Wada et al. 1996 Application of clonal analysis – Differential diagnosis for synchronous primary ovarian and endometrial cancers and metastatic cancer. Am J Clin Pathol 105: 350–359
287. Emmert-Buck M R, Chuaqui R, Zhuang Z et al. 1997 Molecular analysis of synchronous uterine and ovarian endometrioid tumors. Int J Gynecol Pathol 16: 143–148
288. Ricci R, Komminoth P, Bannwart F et al. 2003 PTEN as a molecular marker to distinguish metastatic from primary synchronous endometrioid carcinomas of the ovary and uterus. Diagn Mol Pathol 12: 71–78
289. Fujii H, Matsumoto T, Yoshida M et al. 2002 Genetics of synchronous uterine and ovarian endometrioid carcinoma: Combined analyses of loss of heterozygosity, PTEN mutation, and microsatellite instability. Hum Pathol 33: 421–428
290. Irving J A, Catasus L, Gallardo A et al. 2005 Synchronous endometrioid carcinomas of the uterine corpus and ovary: alterations in the beta-catenin (CTNNB1) pathway are associated with independent primary tumors and favorable prognosis. Hum Pathol 36 605–619
291. Barakat R R, Rubin S C, Wong G et al. 1992 Mixed mesodermal tumor of the ovary: analysis of prognostic factors in 31 cases. Obstet Gynecol 80: 660–664
292. Boucher D, Tetu B 1994 Morphologic prognostic factors of malignant mixed mullerian tumors of the ovary: a clinicopathologic study of 15 cases. Int J Gynecol Pathol 13: 22–28
293. Brown E, Stewart M, Rye T et al. 2004 Carcinosarcoma of the ovary: 19 years of prospective data from a single center. Cancer 100: 2148–2153
294. Bicher A, Levenback C, Silva E G et al. 1995 Ovarian malignant mixed Müllerian tumors treated with platinum-based chemotherapy. Obstet Gynecol 85: 735–739
295. Chang J, Sharpe J C, A'Hern R P et al. 1995 Carcinosarcoma of the ovary: incidence, prognosis, treatment and survival of patients. Ann Oncol 6: 755–758
296. Harris M A, Delap L M, Sengupta P S et al. 2003 Carcinosarcoma of the ovary. Br J Cancer 88: 654–657
297. Pfeiffer P, Hardt-Madsen M, Rex S et al. 1991 Malignant mixed Müllerian tumors of the ovary: report of 13 cases. Acta Obstet Gynecol Scand 70: 79–84
298. Sreenan J J, Hart W R 1995 Carcinosarcomas of the female genital tract: a pathologic study of 29 metastatic tumors: Further evidence for the dominant role of the epithelial component and the conversion theory of histogenesis. Am J Surg Pathol 19: 666–674
299. DiSilvestro P A, Gajewski W H, Ludwig M E et al. 1995 Malignant mixed mesodermal tumors of the ovary. Obstet Gynecol 86: 780–782
300. Tate T J, Blessing J A, DeGeest K et al. 2004 Cisplatin as initial chemotherapy in ovarian carcinosarcomas: a Gynecologic Oncology Group study. Gynecol Oncol 93: 336–339
301. Barnholtz-Sloan J S, Morris R, Malone J M Jr et al. 2004 Survival of women diagnosed with malignant, mixed mullerian tumors of the ovary (OMMMT). Gynecol Oncol 93: 506–512
302. Duska L R, Garrett A, Eltabbakh G H et al. 2002 Paclitaxel and platinum chemotherapy for malignant mixed mullerian tumors of the ovary. Gynecol Oncol 85: 459–463
303. Sit A S, Price F V, Kelley J L et al. 2000 Chemotherapy for malignant mixed Müllerian tumors of the ovary. Gynecol Oncol 79: 196–200
304. Muntz H G, Jones M A, Goff B A et al. 1995 Malignant mixed Mullerian tumors of the ovary – Experience with surgical cytoreduction and combination chemotherapy. Cancer 76: 1209–1213
305. Le T, Krepart G V, Lotocki R J et al. 1997 Malignant mixed mesodermal ovarian tumor treatment and prognosis: a 20-year experience. Gynecol Oncol 65: 237–240
306. Ariyoshi K, Kawauchi S, Kaku T et al. 2000 Prognostic factors in ovarian carcinosarcoma: a clinicopathological and immunohistochemical analysis of 23 cases. Histopathology 37: 427–43.
307. Hellstrom A C, Tegerstedt G, Silfversward C et al. 1999 Malignant mixed mullerian tumors of the ovary: histopathologic and clinical review of 36 cases. Int J Gynecol Cancer 9: 312–316
308. Dehner L P, Norris H J, Taylor H B 1971 Carcinosarcomas and mixed mesodermal tumors of the ovary. Cancer 27: 207–216
309. Barwick K W, Livolsi V A 1980 Malignant mixed mesodermal tumors of the ovary: a clinicopathologic assessment of 12 cases. Am J Surg Pathol 4: 37–42
310. Terada K Y, Johnson T L, Hopkins M et al. 1989 Clinicopathologic features of ovarian mixed mesodermal tumors and carcinosarcomas. Gynecol Oncol 32: 228–232
311. Ehrmann R L, Weidner N, Welch W R et al. 1990 Malignant mixed mullerian tumor of the ovary with prominent neuroectodermal differentiation (teratoid carcinosarcoma). Int J Gynecol Pathol 9: 272–282
312. Barua R, Richmond D 1988 Trophoblastic differentiation in a malignant mixed mesodermal tumor of the ovary. Hum Pathol 19: 1235–1236
313. Rebischung C, Pautier P, Morice P et al. 2000 Alpha-fetoprotein production by a malignant mixed mullerian tumor of the ovary. Gynecol Oncol 77: 203–205
314. Deligdisch L, Plaxe S, Cohen C J 1988 Extrauterine pelvic malignant mixed mesodermal tumors. A study of 10 cases with immunohistochemistry. Int J Gynecol Pathol 7: 361–372
315. Plaxe S C, Dottino P R, Goodman H M et al. 1990 Clinical features of advanced ovarian mixed mesodermal tumors and treatment with doxorubicin- and cis-platinum-based chemotherapy. Gynecol Oncol 37: 244–249
316. Amant F, Vloeberghs V, Woestenborghs H et al. 2003 Transition of epithelial toward mesenchymal differentiation during ovarian carcinosarcoma tumorigenesis. Gynecol Oncol 90: 372–377
317. Sahin A, Benda J A 1988 An immunohistochemical study of primary ovarian sarcoma. An evaluation of nine tumors. Int J Gynecol Pathol 7: 268–279
318. Costa M J, Khan R, Judd R 1991 Carcinosarcoma (malignant mixed mullerian [mesodermal] tumor) of the uterus and ovary. Correlation of clinical, pathologic, and immunohistochemical features in 29 cases. Arch Pathol Lab Med 115: 583–590
319. Clarke T J 1990 Histogenesis of ovarian malignant mixed mesodermal tumours. J Clin Pathol 43: 287–290
320. Dellers E A, Valente P T, Edmonds P R et al. 1991 Extrauterine mixed mesodermal tumors: an immunohistochemical study. Arch Pathol Lab Med 115: 918–920
321. Mukai K, Varela-Duran J, Nochomovitz L E 1980 The rhabdomyoblast in mixed Müllerian tumors of the uterus and ovary. An immunohistochemical study of myoglobin in 25 cases. Am J Clin Pathol 74: 101–104
322. Eichhorn J H, Young R H, Clement P B 2002 Mesodermal (mullerian) adenosarcoma of the ovary: a clinicopathologic analysis of 40 cases and a review of the literature. Am J Surg Pathol 26: 1243–1258
323. Fukunaga M, Nomura K, Endo Y et al. 1997 Ovarian adenosarcoma. Histopathology 30: 283–287
324. Oliva E, Clement P B, Young R H 2000 Endometrial stromal tumors: an update on a group of tumors with a protean phenotype. Adv Anat Pathol 7: 257–281
325. Baiocchi G, Kavanagh J J, Wharton J T 1990 Endometrioid stromal sarcomas arising from ovarian and extraovarian endometriosis: report of two cases and review of the literature. Gynecol Oncol 36: 147–151

326. Silverberg S G, Nogales F F 1981 Endolymphatic stromal myosis of the ovary: a report of three cases and literature review. Gynecol Oncol 12: 129–138
327. Young R H, Prat J, Scully R E 1984 Endometrioid stromal sarcomas of the ovary. A clinicopathologic analysis of 23 cases. Cancer 53: 1143–1155
328. Chang K L, Crabtree G S, Lim-Tan S K et al. 1993 Primary extrauterine endometrial stromal neoplasms: a clinicopathologic study of 20 cases and a review of the literature. Int J Gynecol Pathol 12: 282–296
329. Geas F L, Tewari D S, Rutgers J K et al. 2004 Surgical cytoreduction and hormone therapy of an advanced endometrial stromal sarcoma of the ovary. Obstet Gynecol 103: 1051–1054
330. McCluggage W G 2004 Ovarian neoplasms composed of small round cells: a review. Adv Anat Pathol 11: 288–296
331. Fukunaga M, Ishihara A, Ushigome S 1998 Extrauterine low-grade endometrial stromal sarcoma: report of three cases. Pathol Int 48: 297–302
332. Scully R E, Barlow J F 1967 "Mesonephroma" of ovary: tumor of Mullerian nature related to endometrioid carcinoma. Cancer 20: 1405–1417
333. Roth L M, Langley F A, Fox H et al. 1984 Ovarian clear cell adenofibromatous tumors: benign, low malignant potential, and associated with invasive clear cell carcinoma. Cancer 53: 1156–1163
334. Bell D A, Scully R E 1985 Benign and borderline clear cell adenofibromas of the ovary. Cancer 56: 2922–2931
335. Montag A G, Jenison E L, Griffiths C et al. 1989 Ovarian clear cell carcinoma. A clinicopathologic analysis of 44 cases. Int J Gynecol Pathol 8: 85–96
336. Kennedy A W, Biscotti C V, Hart W R et al. 1989 Ovarian clear cell adenocarcinoma. Gynecol Oncol 32: 342–349
337. Aure J C, Hoeg K, Kolstad P 1971 Mesonephroid tumors of the ovary. Clinical and histopathologic studies. Obstet Gynecol 37: 860–867
338. Crozier M A, Copeland L J, Silva E G et al. 1989 Clear cell carcinoma of the ovary: a study of 59 cases. Gynecol Oncol 35: 199–203
339. Doshi N, Tobon H 1977 Primary clear cell carcinoma of the ovary. An analysis of 15 cases with review of the literature. Cancer 39: 2658–2664
340. Norris H J, Rabinowitz M 1971 Ovarian adenocarcinoma of mesonephric type. Cancer 28: 1074–1081
341. Rogers L W, Julian C G, Woodruff J D 1972 Mesonephroid carcinoma of the ovary: a study of 95 cases from the Emil Novak Ovarian Tumor Registry. Gynecol Oncol 1: 76–89
342. Shevchuk M M, Winkler-Monsanto B, Fenoglio C M et al. 1981 Clear cell carcinoma of the ovary: a clinicopathologic study with review of the literature. Cancer 47: 1344–1351
343. Klemi P J, Meurman L, Gronroos M et al. 1982 Clear cell (mesonephroid) tumors of the ovary with characteristics resembling endodermal sinus tumor. Int J Gynecol Pathol 1: 95–100
344. Kennedy A W, Biscotti C V, Hart W R et al. 1993 Histologic correlates of progression-free interval and survival in ovarian clear cell adenocarcinoma. Gynecol Oncol 50: 334–338
345. Recio F, Piver M S, Hempling R E et al. 1996 Lack of improved survival plus increase in thromboembolic complications in patients with clear cell carcinoma of the ovary treated with platinum versus nonplatinum-based chemotherapy. Cancer 78: 2157–2163
346. Goff B, Sainz de la Cuesta R, Muntz H et al. 1996 Clear cell carcinoma of the ovary: a distinct histologic type with poor prognosis and resistance to platinum-based chemotherapy in stage III disease. Gynecol Oncol 60: 412–417
347. Sugiyama T, Kamura T, Kigawa J et al. 2000 Clinical characteristics of clear cell carcinoma of the ovary – A distinct histologic type with poor prognosis and resistance to platinum-based chemotherapy. Cancer 88: 2584–2589
348. Omura G A, Brady M F, Homesley H D et al. 1991 Long-term follow-up and prognostic factor analysis in advanced ovarian carcinoma: the Gynecologic Oncology Group experience. J Clin Oncol 9: 1138–1150
349. Itamochi H, Kigawa J, Sugiyama T et al. 2002 Low proliferation activity may be associated with chemoresistance in clear cell carcinoma of the ovary. Obstet Gynecol 100: 281–287
350. Ho C M, Huang Y J, Chen T C et al. 2004 Pure-type clear cell carcinoma of the ovary as a distinct histological type and improved survival in patients treated with paclitaxel-platinum-based chemotherapy in pure-type advanced disease. Gynecol Oncol 94: 197–203
351. Clement P B, Young R H, Scully R E 1991 Clinical syndromes associated with tumors of the female genital tract. Semin Diagn Pathol 8: 204–233
352. Kitazawa R, Kitazawa S, Matui T et al. 1997 In situ detection of parathyroid hormone-related protein in ovarian clear cell carcinoma. Hum Pathol 28: 379–382
353. Al-Nafussi A I, Hughes D E, Williams A R 1993 Hyaline globules in ovarian tumours. Histopathology 23: 563–566
354. Kwon T J, Ro J Y, Tornos C et al. 1996 Reduplicated basal lamina in clear-cell carcinoma of the ovary: An immunohistochemical and electron microscopic study. Ultrastruct Pathol 20: 529–536
355. Mikami Y, Hata S, Melamed J et al. 1999 Basement membrane material in ovarian clear cell carcinoma: correlation with growth pattern and nuclear grade. Int J Gynecol Pathol 18: 52–57
356. Young R H, Scully R E 1987 Oxyphilic clear cell carcinoma of the ovary. A report of nine cases. Am J Surg Pathol 11: 661–667
357. Sato Y, Shimamoto T, Amada et al. 2003 Prognostic value of histologic grading of ovarian carcinomas. Int J Gynecol Pathol 22: 52–56
358. Ohkawa K, Amasaki H, Terashima Y et al. 1977 Clear cell carcinoma of the ovary: light and electron microscopic studies. Cancer 40: 3019–3029
359. Jenison E L, Montag A G, Griffiths C T et al. 1989 Clear cell adenocarcinoma of the ovary: a clinical analysis and comparison with serous carcinoma. Gynecol Oncol 32: 65–71
360. Cameron R I, Ashe P, O'Rourke D M et al. 2003 A panel of immunohistochemical stains assists in the distinction between ovarian and renal clear cell carcinoma. Int J Gynecol Pathol 22: 272–276
361. Nolan L P, Heatley M K 2001 The value of immunocytochemistry in distinguishing between clear cell carcinoma of the kidney and ovary. Int J Gynecol Pathol 20: 155–159
362. Vang R, Whitaker B P, Farhood A I et al. 2001 Immunohistochemical analysis of clear cell carcinoma of the gynecologic tract. Int J Gynecol Pathol 20: 252–259
363. Ordi J, Romagosa C, Tavassoli F A et al. 2003 CD10 expression in epithelial tissues and tumors of the gynecologic tract: a useful marker in the diagnosis of mesonephric, trophoblastic, and clear cell tumors. Am J Surg Pathol 27: 178–186
364. Ramalingam P, Malpica A, Silva E G et al. 2004 The use of Cytokeratin 7 and EMA in differentiating ovarian yolk sac tumors from endometrioid and clear cell carcinomas. Am J Surg Pathol 28: 1499–1505
365. Yoonessi M, Abell M R 1979 Brenner tumors of the ovary. Obstet Gynecol 54: 90–96
366. Balasa R W, Adcock L L, Prem K A et al. 1977 The Brenner tumor: a clinicopathologic review. Obstet Gynecol 50: 120–128
367. Fox H, Agrawal K, Langley F A 1972 The Brenner tumour of the ovary. A clinicopathological study of 54 cases. J Obstet Gynaecol Br Commonw 79: 661–665
368. Silverberg S G 1971 Brenner tumor of the ovary. A clinicopathologic study of 60 tumors in 54 women. Cancer 28: 588–596
369. Jorgensen E O, Dockerty M B, Wilson R B et al. 1970 Clinicopathologic study of 53 cases of Brenner's tumors of the ovary. Am J Obstet Gynecol 108: 122–127
370. Carpen E 1976 Brenner tumours of the ovary. A clinicopathological study. Acta Obstet Gynecol Scand 50 Suppl: 1–41
371. Ehrlich C E, Roth L M 1971 The Brenner tumor. A clinicopathologic study of 57 cases. Cancer 27: 332–342
372. Waxman M 1979 Pure and mixed Brenner tumors of the ovary: clinicopathologic and histogenetic observations. Cancer 43: 1830–1839
373. Yoshida M, Obayashi C, Tachibana M et al. 2004 Coexisting Brenner tumor and struma ovarii in the right ovary: case report and review of the literature. Pathol Int 54: 793–797
374. Burg J, Kommoss F, Bittinger F et al. 2002 Mature cystic teratoma of the ovary with struma and benign Brenner tumor: a case report with immunohistochemical characterization. Int J Gynecol Pathol 21: 74–77
375. Lamping J D, Blythe J G 1977 Bilateral Brenner tumors: a case report and review of the literature. Hum Pathol 8: 583–585
376. Trebeck C E, Friedlander M L, Russell P et al. 1987 Brenner tumours of the ovary: a study of the histology, immunohistochemistry and cellular DNA content in benign, borderline and malignant ovarian tumors. Pathology 19: 241–246
377. Roth L M, Dallenbach-Hellweg G, Czernobilsky B 1985 Ovarian Brenner tumors: I. Metaplastic, proliferating, and low malignant potential. Cancer 562: 582–591
378. Hallgrimsson J, Scully R E 1972 Borderline and malignant Brenner tumours of the ovary. A report of 15 cases. Acta Pathol Microbiol Scand [A] 80 Suppl. 233: 56–66
379. Roth L M, Sternberg W H 1971 Proliferating Brenner tumors. Cancer 27: 687–693
380. Woodruff J D, Dietrich D, Genadry R et al. 1981 Proliferative and malignant Brenner tumors. Review of 47 cases. Am J Obstet Gynecol 141: 118–125
381. Miles P A, Norris H J 1972 Proliferative and malignant Brenner tumors of the ovary. Cancer 30: 174–186
382. Roth L M, Gersell D J, Ulbright T M 1993 Ovarian Brenner tumors and transitional cell carcinoma: recent developments. Int J Gynecol Pathol 12: 128–133
383. Baker P M, Young R H 2003 Brenner tumor of the ovary with striking microcystic change. Int J Gynecol Pathol 22: 185–188
384. Austin R M, Norris H J 1987 Malignant Brenner tumor and transitional cell carcinoma of the ovary: a comparison. Int J Gynecol Pathol 6: 29–39
385. Roth L M, Czernobilsky B 1985 Ovarian Brenner tumors. II. Malignant. Cancer 56: 592–601
386. Silva E G, Robey-Cafferty S S, Smith T L et al. 1990 Ovarian carcinomas with transitional cell carcinoma pattern. Am J Clin Pathol 93: 457–465
387. Eichhorn J H, Young R H 2004 Transitional cell carcinoma of the ovary: a morphologic study of 100 cases with emphasis on differential diagnosis. Am J Surg Pathol 28: 453–463
388. Kommoss F, Kommoss S, Schmidt D et al. 2005 Survival benefit for patients with advanced-stage transitional cell carcinomas vs. other subtypes of ovarian carcinoma after chemotherapy with platinum and paclitaxel. Gynecol Oncol 97: 195–199
389. Hollingsworth H C, Steinberg S M, Silverberg S G et al. 1996 Advanced stage transitional cell carcinoma of the ovary. Hum Pathol 27: 1267–1272
390. Robey S S, Silva E G, Gershenson D M et al. 1989 Transitional cell carcinoma in high-grade high-stage ovarian carcinoma. An indicator of favorable response to chemotherapy. Cancer 63: 839–847

391. Gershenson D M, Silva E G, Mitchell M F et al. 1993 Transitional cell carcinoma of the ovary: a matched control study of advanced-stage patients treated with cisplatin-based chemotherapy. Am J Obstet Gynecol 168: 1178–1187
392. Costa M J, Hansen C, Dickerman A et al. 1998 Clinicopathologic significance of transitional cell carcinoma pattern in nonlocalized ovarian epithelial tumors (stages 2–4). Am J Clin Pathol 109: 173–180
393. Seldenrijk C A, Willig A P, Baak J P et al. 1986 Malignant Brenner tumor. A histologic, morphometrical, immunohistochemical, and ultrastructural study. Cancer 58: 754–760
394. Santini D, Gelli M C, Mazzoleni G et al. 1989 Brenner tumor of the ovary: a correlative histologic, histochemical, immunohistochemical, and ultrastructural investigation. Hum Pathol 20: 787–795
395. Prat J 2005 Ovarian carcinomas, including secondary tumors: diagnostically challenging areas. Mod Pathol 18 Suppl 2: S99–111
396. Soslow R A, Rouse R V, Hendrickson M R 1996 Transitional cell neoplasms of the ovary and urinary bladder: a comparative immunohistochemical analysis. Int J Gynecol Pathol 15: 257–265
397. Charpin C, Bhan A K, Zurawski V R J et al. 1982 Carcinoembryonic antigen (CEA) and carbohydrate determinant 19-9 (CA 19-9) localization in 121 primary and metastatic ovarian tumors: an immunohistochemical study with the use of monoclonal antibodies. Int J Gynecol Pathol 1: 231–245
398. Logani S, Oliva E, Amin M B et al. 2003 Immunoprofile of ovarian tumors with putative transitional cell (urothelial) differentiation using novel urothelial markers: histogenetic and diagnostic implications. Am J Surg Pathol 27: 1434–1441
399. Riedel I, Czernobilsky B, Lifschitz-Mercer B et al. 2001 Brenner tumors but not transitional cell carcinomas of the ovary show urothelial differentiation: immunohistochemical staining of urothelial markers, including cytokeratins and uroplakins. Virchow's Arch 438: 181–191
400. Ogawa K, Johansson S L, Cohen S M 1999 Immunohistochemical analysis of uroplakins, urothelial specific proteins, in ovarian Brenner tumors, normal tissues, and benign and neoplastic lesions of the female genital tract. Am J Pathol 155: 1047–1050
401. Ordonez N G 2000 Transitional cell carcinomas of the ovary and bladder are immunophenotypically different. Histopathology 36: 433–438
402. Croft P R, Lathrop S L, Feddersen R M et al. 2005 Estrogen receptor expression in papillary urothelial carcinoma of the bladder and ovarian transitional cell carcinoma. Arch Pathol Lab Med 129:94–199
403. Young R H, Scully R E 1988 Urothelial and ovarian carcinomas of identical cell types: problems in interpretation. A report of three cases and review of the literature. Int J Gynecol Pathol 7: 197–211
404. Oliva E, Musulen E, Prat J et al. 1995 Transitional cell carcinoma of the renal pelvis with symptomatic ovarian metastases. Int J Surg Pathol 2: 231–236
405. Groutz A, Gillon G, Shimonov M et al. 1996 Late, isolated, secondary ovarian transitional cell carcinoma: An unusual course of bladder malignancy. Br J Urol 78(5): 795–796
406. Silva E G, Tornos C, Bailey M A et al. 1991 Undifferentiated carcinoma of the ovary. Arch Pathol Lab Med 115: 377–381
407. Eichhorn J H, Young R H 2001 Neuroendocrine tumors of the genital tract. Am J Clin Pathol 115 Suppl: S94–112
408. Fukunaga M, Endo Y, Miyazawa Y et al. 1997 Small cell neuroendocrine carcinoma of the ovary. Virchow's Arch 430: 343–348
409. Chen K T 2000 Composite large-cell neuroendocrine carcinoma and surface epithelial-stromal neoplasm of the ovary. Int J Surg Pathol 8: 169–174
410. Ohira S, Itoh K, Shiozawa T et al. 2004 Ovarian non-small cell neuroendocrine carcinoma with paraneoplastic parathyroid hormone-related hypercalcemia. Int J Gynecol Pathol 23: 393–397
411. Eichhorn J H, Young R H, Scully R E 1993 Nonpulmonary small cell carcinomas of extragenital origin metastatic to the ovary. Cancer 71: 177–186
412. Young R H, Scully R E 1985 Ovarian metastases from cancer of the lung: problems in interpretation. A report of seven cases. Gynecol Oncol 21: 337–350
413. Irving J A, Young R H 2005 Lung carcinoma metastatic to the ovary: a clinicopathologic study of 32 cases emphasizing their morphologic spectrum and problems in differential diagnosis. Am J Surg Pathol 29: 997–1006
414. Agoff S N, Lamps L W, Philip A T et al. 2000 Thyroid transcription factor-1 is expressed in extrapulmonary small cell carcinomas but not in other extrapulmonary neuroendocrine tumors. Mod Pathol 13: 238–242
415. Kaufmann O, Dietel M 2000 Expression of thyroid transcription factor-1 in pulmonary and extrapulmonary small cell carcinomas and other neuroendocrine carcinomas of various primary sites. Histopathology 36: 415–420
416. Ordonez N G 2000 Value of thyroid transcription factor-1 immunostaining in distinguishing small cell lung carcinomas from other small cell carcinomas. Am J Surg Pathol 24: 1217–1223
417. Tetu B, Silva E G, Gershenson D M 1987 Squamous cell carcinoma of the ovary. Arch Pathol Lab Med 111: 864–866
418. Pins M R, Young R H, Daly W J et al. 1996 Primary squamous cell carcinoma of the ovary. Report of 37 cases. Am J Surg Pathol 20: 823–833
419. Ishikura H, Scully R E 1987 Hepatoid carcinoma of the ovary. A newly described tumor. Cancer 60: 2775–2784
420. Pitman M B, Triratanachat S, Young R H et al. 2004 Hepatocyte paraffin 1 antibody does not distinguish primary ovarian tumors with hepatoid differentiation from metastatic hepatocellular carcinoma. Int J Gynecol Pathol 23: 58–64
421. Tochigi N, Kishimoto T, Supriatna Y et al. 2003 Hepatoid carcinoma of the ovary: a report of three cases admixed with a common surface epithelial carcinoma. Int J Gynecol Pathol 22: 266–271
422. Senzaki H, Kiyozuka Y, Mizuoka H et al. 1999 An autopsy case of hepatoid carcinoma of the ovary with PIVKA-II production: immunohistochemical study and literature review. Pathol Int 49: 164–169
423. Tsung J S, Yang P S 2004 Hepatoid carcinoma of the ovary: characteristics of its immunoreactivity. A case report. Eur J Gynaecol Oncol 25: 745–748
424. Prat J, Bhan A K, Dickersin G R et al. 1982 Hepatoid yolk sac tumor of the ovary (endodermal sinus tumor with hepatoid differentiation): a light microscopic, ultrastructural and immunohistochemical study of seven cases. Cancer 50: 2355–2368
425. Young R H, Gersell D J, Clement P B et al. 1992 Hepatocellular carcinoma metastatic to the ovary: A report of three cases discovered during life with discussion of the differential diagnosis of hepatoid tumors of the ovary. Hum Pathol 23: 574–580
426. Civantos F, Rywlin A M 1972 Carcinomas with trophoblastic differentiation and secretion of chorionic gonadotrophins. Cancer 29: 789–798
427. Matias-Guiu X, Prat J 1990 Ovarian tumors with functioning stroma. An immunohistochemical study of 100 cases with human chorionic gonadotropin monoclonal and polyclonal antibodies. Cancer 65: 2001–2005
428. Oliva E, Andrada E, Pezzica E et al. 1993 Ovarian carcinomas with choriocarcinomatous differentiation. Cancer 72: 2441–2446
429. Rutgers J L, Young R H, Scully R E 1987 Ovarian yolk sac tumor arising from an endometrioid carcinoma. Hum Pathol 18: 1296–1299
430. Stage A H, Grafton W D 1977 Thecomas and granulosa-theca cell tumors of the ovary: an analysis of 51 tumors. Obstet Gynecol 50: 21–27
431. Anikwue C, Dawood M Y, Kramer E 1978 Granulosa and theca cell tumors. Obstet Gynecol 51: 214–220
432. Bjorkholm E, Silfversward C 1981 Prognostic factors in granulosa-cell tumors. Gynecol Oncol 11: 261–274
433. Stenwig J T, Hazekamp J T, Beecham J B 1979 Granulosa cell tumors of the ovary. A clinicopathological study of 118 cases with long-term follow-up. Gynecol Oncol 7: 136–152
434. Malmstrom H, Hogberg T, Risberg B et al. 1994 Granulosa cell tumors of the ovary: prognostic factors and outcome. Gynecol Oncol 52: 50–55
435. King L A, Okagaki T, Gallup D G et al. 1996 Mitotic count, nuclear atypia, and immunohistochemical determination of Ki-67, c-myc, p21-ras, c-erbB2, and p53 expression in granulosa cell tumors of the ovary: mitotic count and Ki-67 are indicators of poor prognosis. Gynecol Oncol 61: 227–232
436. Segal R, DePetrillo A D, Thomas G 1995 Clinical review of adult granulosa cell tumors of the ovary. Gynecol Oncol 56: 338–344
437. Bjorkholm E, Pettersson F 1980 Granulosa cell and theca cell tumors. The clinical picture and long term outcome for the Radiumhemmet series. Acta Obstet Gynecol Scand 59: 361–365
438. Fox H, Agrawal K, Langley F A 1975 A clinicopathologic study of 92 cases of granulosa cell tumor of the ovary with special reference to the factors influencing prognosis. Cancer 35: 231–241
439. Evans A T I, Gaffey T A, Malkasian G D Jr et al. 1980 Clinicopathologic review of 118 granulosa and 82 theca cell tumors. Obstet Gynecol 55: 231–238
440. Aboud E 1997 A review of granulosa cell tumours and thecomas of the ovary. Arch Gynecol Obstet 259: 161–165
441. Pautier P, Lhomme C, Culine S et al. 1997 Adult granulosa-cell tumor of the ovary: A retrospective study of 45 cases. Int J Gynecol Cancer 7: 58–65
442. Nakashima N, Young R H, Scully R E 1984 Androgenic granulosa cell tumors of the ovary. A clinicopathologic analysis of 17 cases and review of the literature. Arch Pathol Lab Med 108: 786–791
443. Norris H J, Taylor H B 1969 Virilization associated with cystic granulosa tumors. Obstet Gynecol 34: 629–635
444. Martinez L, Salmeron M, Carvia R E et al. 1997 Androgen producing luteinized granulosa cell tumor. Acta Obstet Gynecol Scand 76: 285–286
445. Castro C V, Malpica A, Hearne R H et al. 2000 Androgenic adult granulosa cell tumor in a 13-year-old prepubertal patient: a case report and review of the literature. Int J Gynecol Pathol 19: 266–271
446. Sayegh R A, DeLellis R, Alroy J et al. 1999 Masculinizing granulosa cell tumor of the ovary in a postmenopausal woman – A case report. J Reprod Med 44: 821–825
447. Young R H, Dudley A G, Scully R E 1984 Granulosa cell, Sertoli-Leydig cell, and unclassified sex cord-stromal tumors associated with pregnancy: a clinicopathological analysis of thirty-six cases. Gynecol Oncol 18: 181–205
448. Sehouli J, Drescher F S, Mustea A et al. 2004 Granulosa cell tumor of the ovary: 10 years follow-up data of 65 patients. Anticancer Res 24: 1223–1229
449. Miller B E, Barron B A, Wan J Y et al. 1997 Prognostic factors in adult granulosa cell tumor of the ovary. Cancer 79: 1951–1955
450. Lauszus F F, Petersen A C, Greisen J et al. 2001 Granulosa cell tumor of the ovary: a population-based study of 37 women with stage I disease. Gynecol Oncol 81: 456–460
451. Ali S Z 1998 Metastatic granulosa-cell tumor in the liver: cytopathologic findings and staining with inhibin. Diagn Cytopathol 19: 293–297
452. Duhig E E, Riha R L, Clarke B E 2002 Test and teach. An unusual tumour presenting in the lungs. Metastatic adult granulosa cell tumour of the ovary, microfollicular patterns. Pathology 34: 78–81

453. Hines J F, Khalifa M A, Moore J L et al. 1996 Recurrent granulosa cell tumor of the ovary 37 years after initial diagnosis: a case report and review of the literature. Gynecol Oncol 60: 484–488
454. Gershenson D M, Morris M, Burke T W et al. 1996 Treatment of poor-prognosis sex cord-stromal tumors of the ovary with the combination of bleomycin, etoposide, and cisplatin. Obstet Gynecol 87: 527–531
455. Chiara S, Merlini L, Campora E et al. 1993 Cisplatin-based chemotherapy in recurrent or high risk ovarian granulosa-cell tumor patients. Eur J Gynaecol Oncol 14: 314–317
456. Pecorelli S, Wagenaar H C, Vergote I B et al. 1999 Cisplatin (P), vinblastine (V) and bleomycin (B) combination chemotherapy in recurrent or advanced granulosa(-theca) cell tumours of the ovary. An EORTC gynaecological cancer cooperative group study. Eur J Cancer [A] 35: 1331–1337
457. Lane A H, Lee M M, Fuller AF Jr et al. 1999 Diagnostic utility of Mullerian inhibiting substance determination in patients with primary and recurrent granulosa cell tumors. Gynecol Oncol 73: 51–55
458. Rodgers K E, Marks J F, Ellefson D D et al. 1990 Follicle regulatory protein: a novel marker for granulosa cell cancer patients. Gynecol Oncol. 37: 381–387
459. Lappohn R E, Burger H G, Bonma J et al. 1989 Inhibin as a marker for granulosa cell tumors. N Engl J Med 321: 790–793
460. Jobling T, Mamers P, Healy D et al. 1994 A prospective study of inhibin in granulosa cell tumors of the ovary. Gynecol Oncol 55: 285–289
461. Boggess J F, Soules M R, Goff B A et al. 1997 Serum inhibin and disease status in women with ovarian granulosa cell tumors. Gynecol Oncol 64: 64–69
462. Healy D L, Burger H G, Mamers P et al. 1993 Elevated serum inhibin concentrations in postmenopausal women with ovarian tumors. N Engl J Med 329: 1539–1542
463. Burger H G, Robertson D M, Cahir N et al. 1996 Characterization of inhibin immunoreactivity in post-menopausal women with ovarian tumours. Clin Endocrinol (Oxf) 44: 413–418
464. Young R H, Scully R E 1983 Ovarian sex cord-stromal tumors with bizarre nuclei: A clinicopathologic analysis of 17 cases. Int J Gynecol Pathol 1: 325–335
465. Gaffey M J, Frierson H F J, Iezzoni J C et al. 1996 Ovarian granulosa cell tumors with bizarre nuclei: an immunohistochemical analysis. Mod Pathol 9: 308–315
466. Young R H 2005 Sex cord-stromal tumors of the ovary and testis: their similarities and differences with consideration of selected problems. Mod Pathol 18 Suppl 2: S81–S98
467. Young R H, Oliva E, Scully R E 1994 Luteinized adult granulosa cell tumors of the ovary: a report of four cases. Int J Gynecol Pathol 13: 302–310
468. Young R H, Scully R E 1983 Ovarian stromal tumors with minor sex cord elements: a report of seven cases. Int J Gynecol Pathol 2: 227–234
469. Price A, Russell P, Elliott et al. 1990 Composite mucinous and granulosa-cell tumor of ovary: case report of a unique neoplasm. Int J Gynecol Pathol 9: 372–378
470. Doussis-Anagnostopoulou I A, Remadi S, Czernobilsky B 1996 Mucinous elements in Sertoli-Leydig and granulosa cell tumours: A revaluation. Histopathology 28: 372–375
471. Chandran R, Rahman H, Gebbie D 1993 Composite mucinous and granulosa-theca-cell tumour of the ovary: an unusual neoplasm. Aust NZ J Obstet Gynaecol 33: 437–439
472. McKenna M, Kenny B, Dorman G et al. 2005 Combined adult granulosa cell tumor and mucinous cystadenoma of the ovary: granulosa cell tumor with heterologous mucinous elements. Int J Gynecol Pathol 24: 224–227
473. Nogales F F, Concha A, Plata C et al. 1993 Granulosa cell tumor of the ovary with diffuse true hepatic differentiation simulating stromal luteinization. Am J Surg Pathol 17: 85–90
474. Ahmed E, Young R H, Scully R E 1999 Adult granulosa cell tumor of the ovary with foci of hepatic cell differentiation: a report of four cases and comparison with two cases of granulosa cell tumor with Leydig cells. Am J Surg Pathol 23: 1089–1093
475. Fox H 2003 Pathologic prognostic factors in early stage adult-type granulosa cell tumors of the ovary. Int J Gynecol Cancer 13: 1–4
476. Schumer S T, Cannistra S A 2003 Granulosa cell tumor of the ovary. J Clin Oncol 21: 1180–1189
477. Fujimoto T, Sakuragi N, Okuyama K et al. 2001 Histopathological prognostic factors of adult granulosa cell tumors of the ovary. Acta Obstet Gynecol Scand 80: 1069–1074
478. Clement P B, Young R H, Scully R E 1988 Ovarian granulosa cell proliferations of pregnancy: a report of nine cases. Hum Pathol 19: 657–662
479. McCluggage W G, Young R H 2004 Non-neoplastic granulosa cells within ovarian vascular channels: a rare potential diagnostic pitfall. J Clin Pathol 57: 151–154
480. Otis C N, Powell J L, Barbuto D et al. 1992 Intermediate filamentous proteins in adult granulosa cell tumors: An immunohistochemical study of 25 cases. Am J Surg Pathol 16: 962–968
481. Park S H, Kim I 1994 Histogenetic consideration of ovarian sex cord-stromal tumors analyzed by expression pattern of cytokeratins, vimentin, and laminin. Correlation studies with human gonads. Pathol Res Pract 190: 449–456
482. Chada S, van der Kwast T H 1989 Immunohistochemistry of ovarian granulosa cell tumors. The value of tissue specific proteins and tumour markers. Virchow's Arch A Pathol Anat Histopathol 414: 439–445
483. Miettinen M, Wahlstrom T, Virtanen I et al. 1985 Cellular differentiation in ovarian sex-cord-stromal and germ-cell tumors studied with antibodies to intermediate-filament proteins. Am J Surg Pathol 9: 640–651
484. Benjamin E, Law S, Bobrow L G 1987 Intermediate filaments cytokeratin and vimentin in ovarian sex cord-stromal tumours with correlative studies in adult and fetal ovaries. J Pathol 152: 253–263
485. Costa M J, DeRose P B, Roth L M et al. 1994 Immunohistochemical phenotype of ovarian granulosa cell tumors: Absence of epithelial membrane antigen has diagnostic value. Hum Pathol 25: 60–66
486. Santini D, Ceccarelli C, Leone O et al. 1995 Smooth muscle differentiation in normal human ovaries, ovarian stromal hyperplasia and ovarian granulosa-stromal cells tumors. Mod Pathol 8: 25–30
487. Loo K T, Leung A K F, Chan J K C 1995 Immunohistochemical staining of ovarian granulosa cell tumours with MIC2 antibody. Histopathology 27: 388–390
488. Choi Y L, Kim H S, Ahn G 2000 Immunoexpression of inhibin alpha subunit, inhibin/activin betaA subunit and CD99 in ovarian tumors. Arch Pathol Lab Med 124: 563–569
489. Aguirre P, Thor A D, Scully R E 1989 Ovarian small cell carcinoma. Histogenetic considerations based on immunohistochemical and other findings. Am J Clin Pathol 92: 140–149
490. McCluggage W G 2001 Value of inhibin staining in gynecological pathology. Int J Gynecol Pathol 20: 79–85
491. Zheng W, Senturk B Z, Parkash V 2003 Inhibin immunohistochemical staining: a practical approach for the surgical pathologist in the diagnoses of ovarian sex cord-stromal tumors. Adv Anat Pathol 10: 27–38
492. Flemming P, Grothe W, Maschek H et al. 1996 The site of inhibin production in ovarian neoplasms. Histopathology 29: 465–468
493. Rishi M, Howard L N, Bratthauer G L et al. 1997 Use of monoclonal antibody against human inhibin as a marker for sex cord stromal tumors of the ovary. Am J Surg Pathol 21: 583–589
494. Stewart C J R, Jeffers M D, Kennedy A 1997 Diagnostic value of inhibin immunoreactivity in ovarian gonadal stromal tumours and their histological mimics. Histopathology 31: 67–74
495. Costa M J, Ames P F, Walls J et al. 1997 Inhibin immunohistochemistry applied to ovarian neoplasms: A novel, effective, diagnostic tool. Hum Pathol 28: 1247–1254
496. Yao D X, Soslow R A, Hedvat C V et al. 2003 Melan-A (A103) and inhibin expression in ovarian neoplasms. Appl Immunohistochem Mol Morphol 11: 244–249
497. Cathro H P, Stoler M H 2005 The utility of calretinin, inhibin, and WT1 immunohistochemical staining in the differential diagnosis of ovarian tumors. Hum Pathol 36: 195–201
498. Shah V I, Freites N O, Maxwell P et al. 2003 Inhibin is more specific than calretinin as an immunohistochemical marker for differentiating sarcomatoid granulosa cell tumour of the ovary from other spindle cell neoplasms. J Clin Pathol 56: 221–224
499. Gurusinghe C J, Healy D L, Jobling T et al. 1995 Inhibin and activin are demonstrable by immunohistochemistry in ovarian tumor tissue. Gynecol Oncol 57: 27–32
500. Movahedi-Lankarani S, Kurman R J 2002 Calretinin, a more sensitive but less specific marker than alpha-inhibin for ovarian sex cord-stromal neoplasms – An immunohistochemical study of 215 cases. Am J Surg Pathol 26: 1477–1483
501. McCluggage W G, Maxwell P 2001 Immunohistochemical staining for calretinin is useful in the diagnosis of ovarian sex cord-stromal tumours. Histopathology 38(5): 403–408
502. Young R H, Dickersin G R, Scully R E 1984 Juvenile granulosa cell tumor of the ovary. A clinicopathological analysis of 125 cases. Am J Surg Pathol 8: 575–596
503. Zaloudek C J, Norris H J 1982 Granulosa tumors of the ovary in children: a clinical and pathologic study of 32 cases. Am J Surg Pathol 6: 503–512
504. Lack E E, Perez-Atayde A R, Murthy A S K et al. 1981 Granulosa-theca cell tumors in premenarchal girls: A clinical and pathologic study of ten cases. Cancer 48: 1846–1854
505. Vassal G, Flamant F, Caillaud J M et al. 1988 Juvenile granulosa cell tumor of the ovary in children: A clinical study of 15 cases. J Clin Oncol 6: 990–995
506. Biscotti C V, Hart W R 1989 Juvenile granulosa cell tumors of the ovary. Arch Pathol Lab Med 113: 40–46
507. Bouffet E, Basset T, Chetail N et al. 1997 Juvenile granulosa cell tumor of the ovary in infants: A clinicopathologic study of three cases and review of the literature. J Pediatr Surg 32: 762–765
508. Calaminus G, Wessalowski R, Harms D et al. 1997 Juvenile granulosa cell tumors of the ovary in children and adolescents: results from 33 patients registered in a prospective cooperative study. Gynecol Oncol 65: 447–452
509. Schneider D T, Janig U, Calaminus G et al. 2003 Ovarian sex cord-stromal tumors – a clinicopathological study of 72 cases from the Kiel Pediatric Tumor Registry. Virchow's Arch 443: 549–560
510. Plantaz D, Flamant F, Vassal G et al. 1992 [Granulosa cell tumors of the ovary in children and adolescents. Multicenter retrospective study in 40 patients aged 7 months to 22 years.] Arch Fr Pediatr 49: 793–798
511. Velasco-Oses A, Alouso-Alvaro A, Blanco-Pozo A et al. 1988 Ollier's disease associated with ovarian juvenile granulosa cell tumor. Cancer 62: 222–225

512. Tamimi H K, Bolen J W 1984 Enchondromatosis (Ollier's disease) and ovarian juvenile granulosa cell tumor: A case report and review of the literature. Cancer 53: 1605–1608
513. Tanaka Y, Sasaki Y, Nishihira H et al. 1992 Ovarian juvenile granulosa cell tumor associated with Maffucci's syndrome. Am J Clin Pathol 97: 523–527
514. Nomura K, Furusato M, Nikaido T et al. 1991 Ovarian sex cord tumor with annular tubules. Report of a case. Acta Pathol Jpn 41: 701–706
515. Frausto S D, Geisler J P, Fletcher M S et al. 2004 Late recurrence of juvenile granulosa cell tumor of the ovary. Am J Obstet Gynecol 191: 366–367
516. Powell J L, Otis C N 1997 Management of advanced juvenile granulosa cell tumor of the ovary. Gynecol Oncol 64: 282–284
517. Schneider D T, Calaminus G, Wessalowski R et al. 2002 Therapy of advanced ovarian juvenile granulosa cell tumors. Klin Padiatr 214: 173–178
518. Silverman L A, Gitelman S E 1996 Immunoreactive inhibin, mullerian inhibitory substance, and activin as biochemical markers for juvenile granulosa cell tumors. J Pediatr 129: 918–921
519. Nishida M, Jimi S, Haji M et al. 1991 Juvenile granulosa cell tumor in association with a high serum inhibin level. Gynecol Oncol 40: 90–94
520. Deavers M T, Malpica A, Liu J et al. 2003 Ovarian sex cord-stromal tumors: an immunohistochemical study including a comparison of calretinin and inhibin. Mod Pathol 16: 584–590
521. Zhang J, Young R H, Arseneau J et al. 1982 Ovarian stromal tumors containing lutein or Leydig cells (luteinized thecomas and stromal Leydig tumors) – a clinicopathological analysis of 50 cases. Int J Gynecol Pathol 1: 270–285
522. Roth LM, Sternberg W H 1983 Partly luteinized theca cell tumor of the ovary. Cancer 51: 1697–1704
523. Norris H J, Taylor H B 1968 Prognosis of granulosa-theca tumors of the ovary. Cancer 21: 255–263
524. Waxman M, Vuletin J C, Ureuyo R et al. 1979 Ovarian low-grade stromal sarcoma with thecomatous features: a critical reappraisal of the so-called "malignant thecoma". Cancer 44: 2206–2217
525. Karck U, Kommoss F, Henne K et al. 1991 [Recurrent theca cell tumor.] Geburtshilfe Frauenheilkd 51: 577–579
526. Clement P B, Young R H, Hanna W et al. 1994 Sclerosing peritonitis associated with luteinized thecomas of the ovary: a clinicopathological analysis of six cases. Am J Surg Pathol 18: 1–13
527. Werness B A 1996 Luteinized thecoma with sclerosing peritonitis. Arch Pathol Lab Med 120: 303–306
528. Spiegel G W, Swiger F K 1996 Luteinized thecoma with sclerosing peritonitis presenting as an acute abdomen. Gynecol Oncol 61: 275–281
529. Iwasa Y, Minamiguchi S, Konishi I et al. 1996 Sclerosing peritonitis associated with luteinized thecoma of the ovary. Pathol Int 46: 510–514
530. Reginella R F, Sumkin J H 1996 Sclerosing peritonitis associated with luteinized thecoma. Am J Roentgenol 167: 512–513
531. Young R H, Clement P B, Scully R E 1988 Calcified thecomas in young women. A report of four cases. Int J Gynecol Pathol 7: 343–350
532. Klemi P J, Gronroos M 1979 An ultrastructural and clinical study of theca and granulosa cell tumors. Int J Gynaecol Obstet 17: 219–225
533. Amin H K, Okagaki T, Richart R M 1971 Classification of fibroma and thecoma of the ovary. An ultrastructural study. Cancer 27: 438–446
534. McCluggage W G, Sloan J M, Boyle D D et al. 1998 Malignant fibrothecomatous tumour of the ovary: diagnostic value of anti-inhibin immunostaining. J Clin Pathol 51: 868–871
535. Tiltman A J, Haffajee Z 1999 Sclerosing stromal tumors, thecomas, and fibromas of the ovary: an immunohistochemical profile. Int J Gynecol Pathol 18: 254–258
536. Fletcher J A, Gibas Z, Donovan K et al. 1991 Ovarian granulosa-stromal cell tumors are characterized by trisomy 12. Am J Pathol 138: 515–520
537. Pejovic T, Heim S, Mandahl N et al. 1990 Trisomy 12 is a consistent chromosomal aberration in benign ovarian tumors. Genes Chromosom Cancer 2: 48–52
538. Mrózek K, Nedoszytko B, Babinska M et al. 1990 Trisomy of chromosome 12 in a case of thecoma of the ovary. Gynecol Oncol 36: 413–416
539. Shashi V, Golden W L, von Kap-Herr C et al. 1994 Interphase fluorescence in situ hybridization for trisomy 12 on archival ovarian sex cord-stromal tumors. Gynecol Oncol 55: 349–354
540. Scurry J, Allen D, Dobson J 1996 Ovarian fibromatosis, ascites and omental fibrosis. Histopathology 28: 81–84
541. Frigerio L, Taccagni G L, Mariani A et al. 1997 Idiopathic sclerosing peritonitis associated with florid mesothelial hyperplasia, ovarian fibromatosis, and endometriosis: a new disorder of abdominal mass. Am J Obstet Gynecol 176: 721–722
542. Sivanesaratnam V, Dutta R, Jayalakshmi P 1990 Ovarian fibroma – clinical and histopathological characteristics. Int J Gynaecol Obstet 33: 243–247
543. Dockerty M B, Masson J C 1944 Ovarian fibromas: a clinical and pathologic study of 283 cases. Am J Obstet Gynecol 47: 741–752
544. Prat J, Scully R E 1981 Cellular fibromas and fibrosarcomas of the ovary. A comparative clinicopathologic analysis of seventeen cases. Cancer 47: 2663–2670
545. Gargano G, De Lena M, Zito F et al. 2003 Ovarian fibroma: our experience of 34 cases. Eur J Gynaecol Oncol 24: 429–432
546. Lurie S 2000 Meigs' syndrome: the history of the eponym. Eur J Obstet Gynecol Reprod Biol 92: 199–204
547. Kimonis V E, Goldstein A M, Pastakia B et al. 1997 Clinical manifestations in 105 persons with nevoid basal cell carcinoma syndrome. Am J Med Genet 69: 299–308
548. Tsuji T, Kawauchi S, Utsunomiya T et al. 1997 Fibrosarcoma versus cellular fibroma of the ovary – A comparative study of their proliferative activity and chromosome aberrations using MIB-1 immunostaining, DNA flow cytometry, and fluorescence in situ hybridization. Am J Surg Pathol 21: 52–59
549. Dal Cin P, Pauwels P, Van den Berghe H 1998 Fibrosarcoma versus cellular fibroma of the ovary. Am J Surg Pathol 22: 508–510
550. Lee H Y, Ahmed Q 2003 Fibrosarcoma of the ovary arising in a fibrothecomatous tumor with minor sex cord elements. A case report and review of the literature. Arch Pathol Lab Med 127: 81–4
551. Kruger S, Schmidt H, Kupker W et al. 2002 Fibrosarcoma associated with a benign cystic teratoma of the ovary. Gynecol Oncol 84: 150–154
552. Leung W Y, Schwartz P E, Ng H T et al. 1990 Trisomy 12 in benign fibroma and granulosa cell tumor of the ovary. Gynecol Oncol 38: 28–31
553. Ayhan A, Tuncer Z S, Hakverdi A U et al. 1996 Sertoli-Leydig cell tumor of the ovary: a clinicopathologic study of 10 cases. Eur J Gynaecol Oncol 17: 75–78
554. Young R H, Scully R E 1985 Ovarian Sertoli-Leydig cell tumors. A clinicopathologic analysis of 207 cases. Am J Surg Pathol 9: 543–569
555. Zaloudek C, Norris H J 1984 Sertoli-Leydig tumors of the ovary. A clinicopathologic study of 64 intermediate and poorly differentiated neoplasms. Am J Surg Pathol 8: 405–418
556. Roth L M, Anderson M C, Govan A D T et al. 1981 Sertoli-Leydig cell tumors: a clinicopathologic study of 34 cases. Cancer 48: 187–197
557. Talerman A 1987 Ovarian Sertoli-Leydig cell tumor (androblastoma) with retiform pattern. A clinicopathologic study. Cancer 60: 3056–3064
558. Roth L M, Slayton R E, Brady L W et al. 1985 Retiform differentiation in ovarian Sertoli-Leydig cell tumors: a clinicopathologic study of six cases from a Gynecologic Oncology Group study. Cancer 55: 1093–1098
559. Young R H, Scully R E 1983 Ovarian Sertoli-Leydig cell tumors with a retiform pattern – A problem in diagnosis: a report of 25 cases. Am J Surg Pathol 7: 755–771
560. Mooney E E, Nogales F F, Bergeron C et al. 2002 Retiform Sertoli-Leydig cell tumours: clinical, morphological and immunohistochemical findings. Histopathology 41: 110–117
561. Talerman A, Haije W G 1985 Ovarian Sertoli cell tumor with retiform and heterologous elements (letter). Am J Surg Pathol 9: 459–460
562. Tiltman A, Dehaeck K, Soeters R et al. 1986 Ovarian Sertoli-Leydig cell tumour with raised serum alpha fetoprotein. A case report. Virchow's Arch [A] 410: 107–112
563. Tetu B, Ordóñez N G, Silva E G 1986 Sertoli-Leydig cell tumor of the ovary with alpha-fetoprotein production. Arch Pathol Lab Med 110: 65–68
564. Mann W J, Chumas J, Rosenwaks Z et al. 1986 Elevated serum alpha-fetoprotein associated with Sertoli-Leydig cell tumor of the ovary. Obstet Gynecol 67: 141–144
565. Young R H, Perez-Atayde A R, Scully R E 1984 Ovarian Sertoli-Leydig cell tumor with retiform and heterologous components. Report of a case with hepatocytic differentiation and elevated serum alpha-fetoprotein. Am J Surg Pathol 8: 709–718
566. Gagnon S, Tétu B, Silva E G et al. 1989 Frequency of alpha-fetoprotein production by Sertoli-Leydig cell tumors of the ovary: an immunohistochemical study of eight cases. Mod Pathol 2: 63–67
567. Young R H, Scully R E 1984 Well-differentiated ovarian Sertoli-Leydig cell tumors: a clinicopathological analysis of 23 tumors. Int J Gynecol Pathol 3: 277–290
568. Gershenson D M, Copeland L J, Kavanagh J J et al. 1987 Treatment of metastatic stromal tumors of the ovary with cisplatin, doxorubicin, and cyclophosphamide. Obstet Gynecol 70: 765–769
569. Mooney E E, Vaidya K P, Tavassoli F A 2000 Ossifying well-differentiated Sertoli-Leydig cell tumor of the ovary. Ann Diagn Pathol 4: 34–38
570. Omeroglu A, Husain A N, Siziopikou K 2002 Pathologic quiz case – A papillary ovarian tumor in a 4-year-old girl – Pathologic diagnosis: Sertoli-Leydig cell tumor, retiform type. Arch Pathol Lab Med 126: 377–378
571. Ching B, Klink A, Wang L 2004 Pathologic quiz case: a 22-year-old woman with a large right adnexal mass. Poorly differentiated Sertoli-Leydig cell tumor of the right ovary with retiform differentiation and heterologous elements (mucinous components). Arch Pathol Lab Med 128: e93–e95
572. Mooney E E, Man Y G, Bratthauer G L et al. 1999 Evidence that Leydig cells in Sertoli-Leydig cell tumors have a reactive rather than a neoplastic profile. Cancer 86: 2312–2319
573. Young R H, Prat J, Scully R E 1982 Ovarian Sertoli-Leydig cell tumors with heterologous elements. I. Gastrointestinal epithelium and carcinoid: A clinicopathologic analysis of 36 cases. Cancer 50: 2448–2456
574. Prat J, Young R H, Scully R E 1982 Ovarian Sertoli-Leydig cell tumors with heterologous elements. II. Cartilage and skeletal muscle. A clinicopathologic analysis of twelve cases. Cancer 50: 2465–2475
575. Chumas J C, Rosenwaks Z, Mann W J et al. 1984 Sertoli-Leydig cell tumor of the ovary producing alpha-fetoprotein. Int J Gynecol Pathol 3: 213–219
576. Hammad A, Jasnosz K M, Olson P R 1995 Expression of alpha-fetoprotein by ovarian Sertoli-Leydig cell tumors – Case report and review of the literature. Arch Pathol Lab Med 119: 1075–1079
577. Chadha S, Honnebier W J, Schaberg A 1987 Raised serum alpha-fetoprotein in Sertoli-Leydig cell tumor (androblastoma) of ovary: report of two cases. Int J Gynecol Pathol 6: 82–88

578. Mooney E E, Nogales F F, Tavassoli F A 1999 Hepatocytic differentiation in retiform Sertoli-Leydig cell tumors: distinguishing a heterologous element from Leydig cells. Hum Pathol 30: 611–617
579. Costa M J, Morris R J, Wilson R et al. 1992 Utility of immunohistochemistry in distinguishing ovarian Sertoli-stromal cell tumors from carcinosarcomas. Hum Pathol 23: 787–797
580. Kato N, Fukase M, Ono I et al. 2001 Sertoli-stromal cell tumor of the ovary: Immunohistochemical, ultrastructural, and genetic studies. Hum Pathol 32: 796–802
581. Gordon M D, Corless C, Renshaw A A et al. 1998 CD99, keratin, and vimentin staining of sex cord-stromal tumors, normal ovary, and testis. Mod Pathol 11: 769–773
582. Aguirre P, Scully R E, DeLellis R A 1986 Ovarian heterologous Sertoli-Leydig cell tumors with gastrointestinal-type epithelium. An immunohistochemical analysis. Arch Pathol Lab Med 110: 528–533
583. Sasano H, Okamoto M, Mason J I et al. 1989 Immunohistochemical studies of steroidogenic enzymes (aromatase, 17α-hydroxylase and cholesterol side-chain cleavage cytochromes P-450) in sex cord-stromal tumors of the ovary. Hum Pathol 20: 452–457
584. Oliva E, Alvarez T, Young R H 2005 Sertoli cell tumors of the ovary: a clinicopathologic and immunohistochemical study of 54 cases. Am J Surg Pathol 29: 143–156
585. Tavassoli F A, Norris H J 1980 Sertoli tumors of the ovary. A clinicopathologic study of 28 cases with ultrastructural observations. Cancer 46: 2281–2297
586. Ferry J A, Young R H, Engel G et al. 1994 Oxyphilic Sertoli cell tumor of the ovary: a report of three cases, two in patients with the Peutz-Jeghers syndrome. Int J Gynecol Pathol 13: 259–266
587. Zung A, Shoham Z, Open M et al. 1998 Sertoli cell tumor causing precocious puberty in a girl with Peutz-Jeghers syndrome. Gynecol Oncol 70: 421–424
588. Young R H, Scully R E 1984 Ovarian Sertoli cell tumors. A report of 10 cases. Int J Gynecol Pathol 2: 349–363
589. Watson B, Siegel C L, Ylagan L R 2003 Metastatic ovarian Sertoli-cell tumor: FNA findings with immunohistochemistry. Diagn Cytopathol 29: 283–286
590. Phadke D M, Weisenberg E, Engel G et al. 1999 Malignant Sertoli cell tumor of the ovary metastatic to the lung mimicking neuroendocrine carcinoma: report of a case. Ann Diagn Pathol 3: 213–219
591. Scully R E 2000 The prolonged gestation, birth, and early life of the sex cord tumor with annular tubules and how it joined a syndrome. Int J Surg Pathol 8: 233–238
592. Papageorgiou T, Stratakis C A 2002 Ovarian tumors associated with multiple endocrine neoplasias and related syndromes (Carney complex, Peutz-Jeghers syndrome, von Hippel-Lindau disease, Cowden's disease). Int J Gynecol Cancer 12: 337–347
593. Hemminki A 1999 The molecular basis and clinical aspects of Peutz-Jeghers syndrome. Cell Mol Life Sci 55: 735–750
594. Jenne D E, Reimann H, Nezu J et al. 1998 Peutz-Jeghers syndrome is caused by mutations in a novel serine threonine kinase. Nat Genet 18: 38–43
595. Westerman A M, Wilson J H 1999 Peutz-Jeghers syndrome: risks of a hereditary condition. Scand J Gastroenterol Suppl 230: 64–70
596. Srivatsa P J, Keeney G L, Podratz K C 1994 Disseminated cervical adenoma malignum and bilateral ovarian sex cord tumors with annular tubules associated with Peutz-Jeghers syndrome. Gynecol Oncol 53: 256–264
597. Young R H, Welch W R, Dickersin G R et al. 1982 Ovarian sex cord tumor with annular tubules. Review of 74 cases including 27 with Peutz-Jeghers syndrome and four with adenoma malignum of the cervix. Cancer 50: 1384–1402
598. Connolly D C, Katabuchi H, Cliby W A et al. 2000 Somatic mutations in the STK11/LKB1 gene are uncommon in rare gynecological tumor types associated with Peutz-Jegher's syndrome. Am J Pathol 156: 339–345
599. Lele S M, Sawh R N, Zaharopoulos P et al. 2000 Malignant ovarian sex cord tumor with annular tubules in a patient with Peutz-Jeghers syndrome: a case report. Mod Pathol 13: 466–470
600. Chen K T 1986 Female genital tract tumors in Peutz-Jeghers syndrome. Hum Pathol 17: 858–861
601. Podczaski E, Kaminski P F, Pees R C et al. 1991 Peutz-Jeghers syndrome with ovarian sex cord tumor with annular tubules and cervical adenoma malignum. Gynecol Oncol 42: 74–78
602. Mangili G, Taccagni G, Garavaglia E et al. 2004 An unusual admixture of neoplastic and metaplastic lesions of the female genital tract in the Peutz-Jeghers syndrome. Gynecol Oncol 92: 337–342
603. Young R H, Dickersin G R, Scully R E 1983 A distinctive ovarian sex cord-stromal tumor causing sexual precocity in the Peutz-Jeghers syndrome. Am J Surg Pathol 7: 233–243
604. Gloor E 1979 Ovarian sex cord tumor with annular tubules. Clinicopathologic report of two benign and one malignant cases with long follow-ups. Virchow's Arch [A] 384: 185–193
605. Anderson M C, Govan A D T, Langley F A et al. 1980 Ovarian sex cord tumours with annular tubules. Histopathology 4: 137–145
606. Hart W R, Kumar N, Crissman J D 1980 Ovarian neoplasms resembling sex cord tumors with annular tubules. Cancer 45: 2352–2363
607. Shen K, Wu P-C, Lang J-H et al. 1993 Ovarian sex cord tumor with annular tubules: a report of six cases. Gynecol Oncol 48: 180–184
608. Czernobilsky B, Gaedcke G, Dallenbach-Hellweg G 1985 Endometrioid differentiation in ovarian sex cord tumor with annular tubules accompanied by gestagenic effect. Cancer 55: 738–744
609. Gustafson M L, Lee M M, Scully R E et al. 1992 Müllerian inhibiting substance as a marker for ovarian sex-cord tumor. N Engl J Med 326: 466–471
610. Puls L E, Hamous J, Morrow M S et al. 1994 Recurrent ovarian sex cord tumor with annular tubules: tumor marker and chemotherapy experience. Gynecol Oncol 54: 396–401
611. Ahn G H, Chi J G, Lee S K 1986 Ovarian sex cord tumor with annular tubules. Cancer 57: 1066–1073
612. Matamala M F, Nogales F F, Lardelli P et al. 1987 Metastatic granulosa cell tumor with pattern of sex cord tumor with annular tubules. Int J Gynecol Pathol 6: 185–193
613. Kommoss F, Oliva E, Bhan A K et al. 1998 Inhibin expression in ovarian tumors and tumor-like lesions: an immunohistochemical study. Mod Pathol 11: 656–664
614. Kalifat R, de Brux J 1987 Ovarian sex cord tumor with annular tubules: an ultrastructural study. Int J Gynecol Pathol 6: 380–388
615. Crissman J D, Hart W R 1981 Ovarian sex cord tumor with annular tubules. An ultrastructural study of three cases. Am J Clin Pathol 75: 11–17
616. Astengo-Osuna C 1984 Ovarian sex cord-stromal tumor with annular tubules: case report with ultrastructural findings. Cancer 54: 1070–1075
617. Paraskevas M, Scully R E 1989 Hilus cell tumor of the ovary. A clinicopathological analysis of 12 Reinke crystal-positive cases and nine crystal-negative cases. Int J Gynecol Pathol 8: 299–310
618. Sternberg W H, Roth L M 1973 Ovarian stromal tumors containing Leydig cells. I. Stromal-Leydig tumor and non-neoplastic transformation of ovarian stroma to Leydig cells. Cancer 32: 940–951
619. Roth L M, Sternberg W H 1973 Ovarian stromal tumors containing Leydig cells. II. Pure Leydig cell tumors, non-hilar type. Cancer 32: 952–960
620. Baiocchi G, Manci N, Angeletti G et al. 1997 Pure Leydig cell tumour (Hilus cell) of the ovary: a rare cause of virilization after menopause. Gynecol Obstet Invest 44: 141–144
621. Ichinohasama R, Teshima K, Kishi K et al. 1989 Leydig cell tumor of the ovary associated with endometrial carcinoma and containing 17 beta-hydroxysteroid dehydrogenase. Int J Gynecol Pathol 8: 64–71
622. Regnier C, Bennet A, Malet D et al. 2002 Intraoperative testosterone assay for virilizing ovarian tumor topographic assessment: report of a Leydig cell tumor of the ovary in a premenopausal woman with an adrenal incidentaloma. J Clin Endocrinol Metab 87: 3074–3077
623. Gorgojo J J, Almodovar F, Lopez E et al. 2003 Coincidental diagnosis of an occult hilar steroid cell tumor of the ovary and a cortisol-secreting adrenal adenoma in a 49-year-old woman with severe hyperandrogenism. Fertil Steril 80: 1504–1507
624. Duun S 1994 Bilateral virilizing hilus (Leydig) cell tumors of the ovary. Acta Obstet Gynecol Scand 73: 76–77
625. Oler A, Singh M, Ural S H 1999 Bilateral ovarian stromal hyperplasia concealing a nonhilar, pure stromal-Leydig cell tumor. A case report. J Reprod Med 44: 563–566
626. Paoletti M, Pridjian G, Okagaki T et al. 1987 A stromal Leydig cell tumor of the ovary occurring in a pregnant 15-year-old girl. Ultrastructural findings. Cancer 60: 2806–2810
627. Takeuchi S, Ishihara N, Ohbayashi C et al. 1999 Stromal Leydig cell tumor of the ovary. Case report and literature review. Int J Gynecol Pathol 18: 178–182
628. Hayes M C, Scully R E 1987 Stromal luteoma of the ovary: a clinicopathological analysis of 25 cases. Int J Gynecol Pathol 6: 313–321
629. Cao Q J, Jones J G, Li M 2001 Expression of calretinin in human ovary, testis, and ovarian sex cord-stromal tumors. Int J Gynecol Pathol 20: 346–352
630. Hayes M C, Scully R E 1987 Ovarian steroid cell tumors (not otherwise specified). A clinicopathological analysis of 63 cases. Am J Surg Pathol 11: 835–845
631. Taylor H B, Norris H J 1967 Lipid cell tumors of the ovary. Cancer 20: 1953–1962
632. Lin C J, Jorge A A L, Latronico A C et al. 2000 Origin of an ovarian steroid cell tumor causing isosexual pseudoprecocious puberty demonstrated by the expression of adrenal steroidogenic enzymes and adrenocorticotropin receptor. J Clin Endocrinol Metab 85: 1211–1214
633. Powell J L, Dulaney D P, Shiro B C 2000 Androgen-secreting steroid cell tumor of the ovary. South Med J 93: 1201–1204
634. Stephen M R, Lindop G B M 1998 A renin secreting ovarian steroid cell tumour associated with secondary polycythaemia. J Clin Pathol 51: 75–77
635. Young R H, Scully R E 1987 Ovarian steroid cell tumors associated with Cushing's syndrome: a report of three cases. Int J Gynecol Pathol 6: 40–48
636. Elhadd T A, Connolly V, Cruickshank D et al. 1996 An ovarian lipid cell tumour causing virilization and Cushing's syndrome. Clin Endocrinol (Oxf) 44: 723–725
637. Roth L M, Davis M M, Sutton G P 1996 Steroid cell tumor of the broad ligament arising in an accessory ovary. Arch Pathol Lab Med 120: 405–409
638. Dumic M, Simunic V, Ilic-Forko J et al. 2001 Extraovarian steroid cell tumor "not otherwise specified" as a rare cause of virilization in twelve-year-old girl. Horm Res 55: 254–257
639. Liu A X, Sun J, Shao W Q et al. 2005 Steroid cell tumors, not otherwise specified (NOS), in an accessory ovary: a case report and literature review. Gynecol Oncol 97: 260–262

640. Deavers M T, Malpica A, Ordonez N G et al. 2003 Ovarian steroid cell tumors: an immunohistochemical study including a comparison of calretinin with inhibin. Int J Gynecol Pathol 22: 162–167
641. Stewart C J, Nandini C L, Richmond J A 2000 Value of A103 (melan-A) immunostaining in the differential diagnosis of ovarian sex cord stromal tumours. J Clin Pathol 53: 206–211
642. Seidman J D, Abbondanzo S L, Bratthauer G L 1995 Lipid cell (steroid cell) tumor of the ovary: immunophenotype with analysis of potential pitfall due to endogenous biotin-like activity. Int J Gynecol Pathol 14: 331–338
643. Jaworski R C, Fryatt J J, Turner T B et al. 1986 Gynandroblastoma of the ovary. Pathology 18: 348–351
644. Anderson M C, Rees D A 1975 Gynandroblastoma of the ovary. Br J Obstet Gynaecol 82: 68–73
645. Chalvardjian A, Derzko C 1982 Gynandroblastoma: its ultrastructure. Cancer 31: 664–670
646. Guo L, Liu T 1995 Gynandroblastoma of the ovary: review of the literature and report of a case. Int J Surg Pathol 3: 137–140
647. Fukunaga M, Endo Y, Ushigome S 1997 Gynandroblastoma of the ovary: A case report with an immunohistochemical and ultrastructural study. Virchow's Arch 430: 77–82
648. Yamada Y, Ohmi K, Tsunematu R et al. 1991 Gynandroblastoma of the ovary having a typical morphological appearance: a case study. Jpn J Clin Oncol 21: 62–68
649. Seidman J D 1996 Unclassified ovarian gonadal stromal tumors – A clinicopathologic study of 32 cases. Am J Surg Pathol 20: 699–706
650. McCluggage W G, Sloan J M, Murnaghan M et al. 1996 Gynandroblastoma of ovary with juvenile granulosa cell component and heterologous intestinal type glands. Histopathology 29: 253–257
651. Broshears J R, Roth L M 1997 Gynandroblastoma with elements resembling juvenile granulosa cell tumor. Int J Gynecol Pathol 16: 387–391
652. Vang R, Herrmann M E, Tavassoli F A 2004 Comparative immunohistochemical analysis of granulosa and sertoli components in ovarian sex cord-stromal tumors with mixed differentiation: potential implications for derivation of sertoli differentiation in ovarian tumors. Int J Gynecol Pathol 23: 151–161
653. Chalvardjian A, Scully R E 1973 Sclerosing stromal tumors of the ovary. Cancer 31: 664–670
654. Tiltman A J 1985 Sclerosing stromal tumor of the ovary. Int J Gynecol Pathol 4: 362–369
655. Gee D C, Russell P 1979 Sclerosing stromal tumours of the ovary. Histopathology 3: 367–376
656. Lam R M, Geittmann P 1988 Sclerosing stromal tumor of the ovary. A light, electron microscopic and enzyme histochemical study. Int J Gynecol Pathol 7: 280–290
657. Kawauchi S, Tsuji T, Kaku T et al. 1998 Sclerosing stromal tumor of the ovary. A clinicopathologic, immunohistochemical, ultrastructural, and cytogenetic analysis with special reference to its vasculature. Am J Surg Pathol 22: 83–92
658. Cashell A W, Cohen M L 1991 Masculinizing sclerosing stromal tumor of the ovary during pregnancy. Gynecol Oncol 43: 281–285
659. Ismail S M, Walker S M 1990 Bilateral virilizing sclerosing stromal tumours of the ovary in a pregnant woman with Gorlin's syndrome: implications for pathogenesis of ovarian stromal neoplasms. Histopathology 17: 159–163
660. Bildirici K, Yalcin O T, Ozalp S S et al. 2004 Sclerosing stromal tumor of the ovary associated with Meigs' syndrome: a case report. Eur J Gynaecol Oncol 25: 528–529
661. Gurbuz A, Karateke A, Kabaca C et al. 2004 Sclerosing stromal cell tumor of the ovary in pregnancy: a case report. Eur J Gynaecol Oncol 25: 534–535
662. Calabrese M, Zandrino F, Giasotto V et al. 2004 Sclerosing stromal tumor of the ovary in pregnancy: clinical, ultrasonography, and magnetic resonance imaging findings. Acta Radiol 45: 189–192
663. Duska L R, Flynn C, Goodman A 1998 Masculinizing sclerosing stromal cell tumor in pregnancy: report of a case and review of the literature. Eur J Gynaecol Oncol 19: 441–443
664. Kostopoulou E, Moulla A, Giakoustidis D et al. 2004 Sclerosing stromal tumors of the ovary: a clinicopathologic, immunohistochemical and cytogenetic analysis of three cases. Eur J Gynaecol Oncol 25: 257–260
665. Saitoh A, Tsutsumi Y, Osamura R Y et al. 1989 Sclerosing stromal tumor of the ovary. Immunohistochemical and electron microscopic demonstration of smooth-muscle differentiation. Arch Pathol Lab Med 113: 372–376
666. Lifschitz-Mercer B, Open M, Kushnir I et al. 1995 Hyaline globules and progesterone receptors in an ovarian sclerosing stromal tumour. Histopathology 27: 195–197
667. Simpson J L, Michael H, Roth L M 1998 Unclassified sex cord-stromal tumors of the ovary – A report of eight cases. Arch Pathol Lab Med 122: 52–55
668. Matamala M F, Nogales F F, Aneiros J et al. 1988 Leiomyomas of the ovary. Int J Gynecol Pathol 7: 190–196
669. Prayson R A, Hart W R 1992 Primary smooth-muscle tumors of the ovary: A clinicopathologic study of four leiomyomas and two mitotically active leiomyomas. Arch Pathol Lab Med 116: 1068–1071
670. Doss B J, Wanek S M, Jacques S M et al. 1999 Ovarian leiomyomas: clinicopathologic features in fifteen cases. Int J Gynecol Pathol 18: 63–68
671. Lerwill M F, Sung R, Oliva E et al. 2004 Smooth muscle tumors of the ovary: a clinicopathologic study of 54 cases emphasizing prognostic criteria, histologic variants, and differential diagnosis. Am J Surg Pathol 28: 1436–1451
672. Mira J L 1991 Lipoleiomyoma of the ovary: report of a case and review of the English literature. Int J Gynecol Pathol 10: 198–202
673. Dodd G D, Lancaster K T, Moulton J S 1989 Ovarian lipoleiomyoma: a fat-containing mass in the female pelvis. Am J Roentgenol 153: 1007–1008
674. Alvarez M, Cerezo L 1986 Ovarian cavernous hemangioma. Arch Pathol Lab Med 110: 77–78
675. Gucer F, Ozyilmaz F, Balkanli-Kaplan P et al. 2004 Ovarian hemangioma presenting with hyperandrogenism and endometrial cancer: a case report. Gynecol Oncol 94: 821–824
676. Eichhorn J H, Scully R E 1991 Ovarian myxoma: clinicopathologic and immunocytologic analysis of five cases and review of the literature. Int J Gynecol Pathol 10: 156–169
677. Tetu B, Bonenfant J L 1991 Ovarian myxoma. A study of two cases with long-term follow-up. Am J Clin Pathol 95: 340–346
678. Costa M J, Morris R, DeRose P B et al. 1993 Histologic and immunohistochemical evidence for considering ovarian myxoma as a variant of the thecoma-fibroma group of ovarian stromal tumors. Arch Pathol Lab Med 117: 802–808
679. Shakfeh S M, Woodruff J D 1987 Primary ovarian sarcomas: report of 46 cases and review of the literature. Obstet Gynecol Surv 42: 331–349
680. Nielsen G P, Oliva E, Young R H 1998 Primary ovarian rhabdomyosarcoma: a report of 13 cases. Int J Gynecol Pathol 17: 113–119
681. Talerman A, Auerback W M, Van Meurs A J 1981 Primary chondrosarcoma of the ovary. Histopathology 5: 319–324
682. Hines J F, Compton D M, Stacy C C et al. 1990 Pure primary osteosarcoma of the ovary presenting as an extensively calcified adnexal mass: a case report and review of the literature. Gynecol Oncol 39: 259–263
683. Sakata H, Hirahara T, Ryu A et al. 1991 Primary osteosarcoma of the ovary. A case report. Acta Pathol Jpn 41: 311–317
684. Stone G C, Bell D A, Fuller A et al. 1986 Malignant schwannoma of the ovary. Report of a case. Cancer 58: 1575–1582
685. Nucci M R, Krausz T, Lifschitz-Mercer B et al. 1998 Angiosarcoma of the ovary – Clinicopathologic and immunohistochemical analysis of four cases with a broad morphologic spectrum. Am J Surg Pathol 22: 620–630
686. Nielsen G P, Young R H, Prat J et al. 1997 Primary angiosarcoma of the ovary: a report of seven cases and review of the literature. Int J Gynecol Pathol 16: 378–382
687. Osborne B M, Robboy S J 1983 Lymphomas or leukemia presenting as ovarian tumors: an analysis of 42 cases. Cancer 52: 1933–1943
688. Monterroso V, Jaffe E S, Merino M J et al. 1993 Malignant lymphomas of the ovary. A clinicopathologic analysis of 39 cases. Am J Surg Pathol 17: 154–170
689. Dimopoulos M A, Daliani D, Pugh W et al. 1997 Primary ovarian non-Hodgkin's lymphoma: outcome after treatment with combination chemotherapy. Gynecol Oncol 64: 446–450
690. Fox H, Langley F A, Govan A et al. 1988 Malignant lymphoma presenting as an ovarian tumour: a clinicopathological analysis of 34 cases. Br J Obstet Gynaecol 95: 386–390
691. Paladugu R R, Bearman R M, Rappaport H 1980 Malignant lymphoma with primary manifestation in the gonad: a clinicopathologic study of 38 patients. Cancer 45: 561–571
692. Vang R, Medeiros L J, Warnke R et al. 2001 Ovarian non-Hodgkin's lymphoma: a clinicopathologic study of eight primary cases. Mod Pathol 14: 1093–1099
693. Vang R, Medeiros L J, Fuller G N et al. 2001 Non-Hodgkin's lymphoma involving the gynecologic tract: a review of 88 cases. Adv Anat Pathol 8: 200–217
694. Chorlton I, Norris H J, King F M 1974 Malignant reticuloendothelial disease involving the ovary as a primary manifestation: a series of 19 lymphomas and 1 granulocytic sarcoma. Cancer 34: 397–407
695. Oliva E, Ferry J A, Young R H et al. 1997 Granulocytic sarcoma of the female genital tract: A clinicopathologic study of 11 cases. Am J Surg Pathol 21: 1156–116
696. Pressler H, Horny H P, Wolf A et al. 1992 Isolated granulocytic sarcoma of the ovary: histologic, electron microscopic, and immunohistochemical findings. Int J Gynecol Pathol 11: 68–74
697. Kurman R J, Norris H J 1977 Malignant germ cell tumors of the ovary. Hum Pathol 8: 551–564
698. Asadourian L A, Taylor H B 1969 Dysgerminoma. An analysis of 105 cases. Obstet Gynecol 33: 370–379
699. DePalo G, Pilotti S, Kenda R et al. 1982 Natural history of dysgerminoma. Am J Obstet Gynecol 143: 799–807
700. Bjorkholm E, Lundell M, Gyftodimos A et al. 1990 Dysgerminoma. The Radiumhemmet Series 1927–1984. Cancer 65: 38–44
701. Buskirk S J, Schray M F, Podratz K C et al. 1987 Ovarian dysgerminoma: A retrospective analysis of results of treatment, sites of treatment failure, and radiosensitivity. Mayo Clin Proc 62: 1149–1157
702. Gordon A, Lipton D, Woodruff J D 1981 Dysgerminoma: a review of 158 cases from the Emil Novak Ovarian Tumor Registry. Obstet Gynecol 58: 497–504
703. Susnerwala S S, Pande S C, Shrivastava S K et al. 1991 Dysgerminoma of the ovary: review of 27 cases. J Surg Oncol 46: 43–47

704. Talerman A, Huyzinga W T, Kuipers T 1973 Dysgerminoma: clinicopathologic study of 22 cases. Obstet Gynecol 41: 137–147
705. Casey A C, Bhodauria S, Shapter A et al. 1996 Dysgerminoma: the role of conservative surgery. Gynecol Oncol 63: 352–357
706. Karlen J R, Akbari A, Cook W A 1979 Dysgerminoma associated with pregnancy. Obstet Gynecol 53: 330–335
707. Buller R E, Darrow V, Manetta A et al. 1992 Conservative surgical management of dysgerminoma concomitant wiht pregnancy. Obstet Gynecol 79: 887–890
708. Fleischhacker D S, Young R H 1994 Dysgerminoma of the ovary associated with hypercalcemia. Gynecol Oncol 52: 87–90
709. Inoue H, Kikuchi Y, Hirata J et al. 1995 Dysgerminoma of the ovary with hypercalcemia associated with elevated parathyroid hormone-related protein. Jpn J Clin Oncol 25: 113–117
710. Okoye B O, Harmston C, Buick R G 2001 Dysgerminoma associated with hypercalcemia: A case report. J Pediatr Surg 36: E10
711. Evans K N, Taylor H, Zehnder D et al. 2004 Increased expression of 25-hydroxyvitamin D-1alpha-hydroxylase in dysgerminomas: a novel form of humoral hypercalcemia of malignancy. Am J Pathol 165: 807–813
712. Thomas G M, Dembo A J, Hacker N F et al. 1987 Current therapy for dysgerminoma of the ovary. Obstet Gynecol 70: 268–275
713. Schwartz P E, Morris J M 1988 Serum lactic dehydrogenase: a tumor marker for dysgerminoma. Obstet Gynecol 72: 511–515
714. Hamm W, Bolte A 1995 Treatment of pure dysgerminomas with preservation of fertility. Onkologie 18: 126–129
715. Kapp D S, Kohorn E I, Merino M J et al. 1985 Pure dysgerminoma of the ovary with elevated serum human chorionic gonadotropin: Diagnostic and therapeutic considerations. Gynecol Oncol 20: 234–244
716. Zaloudek C J, Tavassoli F A, Norris H J 1981 Dysgerminoma with syncytiotrophoblastic giant cells: a histologically and clinically distinctive subtype of dysgerminoma. Am J Surg Pathol 5: 361–367
717. Parkash V, Carcangiu M L 1995 Transformation of ovarian dysgerminoma to yolk sac tumor: evidence for a histogenetic continuum. Mod Pathol 8: 881–887
718. Burkons D M, Hart W R 1978 Ovarian germinomas (dysgerminomas). Obstet Gynecol 51: 221–224
719. Gallion H H, van Nagell J R Jr, Donaldson E S et al. 1988 Ovarian dysgerminoma: report of seven cases and review of the literature. Am J Obstet Gynecol 158: 591–595
720. LaPolla J P, Benda J, Vigliotti A P et al. 1987 Dysgerminoma of the ovary. Obstet Gynecol 69: 859–864
721. Ayhan A, Bildirici I, Gunalp S et al. 2000 Pure dysgerminoma of the ovary: a review of 45 well staged cases. Eur J Gynaecol Oncol 21: 98–101
722. Santoni R, Cionini L, D'Elia F et al. 1987 Dysgerminoma of the ovary: A report on 29 patients. Clin Radiol 38: 203–206
723. Zaghloul M S, Khattab T Y 1992 Dysgerminoma of the ovary: Good prognosis even in advanced stages. Int J Radiat Oncol Biol Phys 24: 161–165
724. Low J J H, Perrin L C, Crandon A J et al. 2000 Conservative surgery to preserve ovarian function in patients with malignant ovarian germ cell tumors – A review of 74 cases. Cancer 89: 391–398.
725. Williams S D, Blessing J A, Hatch K D et al. 1991 Chemotherapy of advanced dysgerminoma: trials of the Gynecologic Oncology Group. J Clin Oncol 9: 1950–1955
726. Mitchell M F, Gershenson D M, Soeters R P et al. 1991 The long-term effects of radiation therapy on patients with ovarian dysgerminoma. Cancer 67: 1084–1090
727. Culine S, Lhomme C, Kattan J et al. 1995 Cisplatin-based chemotherapy in dysgerminoma of the ovary: thirteen-year experience at the Institut Gustave Roussy. Gynecol Oncol 58: 344–348
728. Williams S D, Kauderer J, Burnett A F et al. 2004 Adjuvant therapy of completely resected dysgerminoma with carboplatin and etoposide: a trial of the Gynecologic Oncology Group. Gynecol Oncol 95: 496–499
729. Brewer M, Gershenson D M, Herzog C E et al. 1999 Outcome and reproductive function after chemotherapy for ovarian dysgerminoma. J Clin Oncol 17: 2670–2675
730. Freel J H, Cassir J F, Pierve V K et al. 1979 Dysgerminoma of the ovary. Cancer 43: 798–805
731. Segelov E, Campbell J, Ng M et al. 1994 Cisplatin-based chemotherapy for ovarian germ cell malignancies: The Australian experience. J Clin Oncol 12: 378–384
732. Morimura Y, Nishiyama H, Yanagida K et al. 1998 Dysgerminoma with syncytiotrophoblastic giant cells arising from 46,xx pure gonadal dysgenesis. Obstet Gynecol 92: 654–656
733. Baker P, Oliva E 2005 Immunohistochemistry as a tool in the differential diagnosis of ovarian tumors: an update. Int J Gynecol Pathol 24: 39–55
734. Cheng L, Thomas A, Roth L M et al. 2004 OCT4: A novel biomarker for dysgerminoma of the ovary. Am J Surg Pathol 28: 1341–1346
735. Lifschitz-Mercer B, Walt H, Kushnir I et al. 1995 Differentiation potential of ovarian dysgerminoma: an immunohistochemical study of 15 cases. Hum Pathol 26: 62–66
736. Mullin T J, Lankerani M R 1986 Ovarian dysgerminoma: immunocytochemical localization of human chorionic gonadotropin in the germinoma cell cytoplasm. Obstet Gynecol 68: 80S–83S
737. Dietl J, Horny H-P, Ruck P et al. 1993 Dysgerminoma of the ovary: An immunohistochemical study of tumor-infiltrating lymphoreticular cells and tumor cells. Cancer 71: 2562–2568
738. Gonzalez-Crussi F 1979 The human yolk sac and yolk sac (endodermal sinus) tumors. A review. Perspect Pediatr Pathol 5: 179–215
739. Teilum G 1959 Endodermal sinus tumors of the ovary and testis: comparative morphogenesis of the so-called mesonephroma ovarii (Schiller) and extraembryonic (yolk sac-allantoic) structures of the rat's placenta. Cancer 12: 1092–1105
740. Nogales F F 1993 Embryologic clues to human yolk sac tumors: a review. Int J Gynecol Pathol 12: 101–107
741. Sasaki H, Furusato M, Teshima S et al. 1994 Prognostic significance of histopathological subtypes in stage I pure yolk sac tumour of the ovary. Br J Cancer 69: 529–536
742. Gershenson D M, del Junco G, Herson J et al. 1983 Endodermal sinus tumor of the ovary: the M.D. Anderson experience. Obstet Gynecol 61: 194–202
743. Kawai M, Kano T, Furuhashi Y et al. 1991 Prognostic factors in yolk sac tumors of the ovary. A clinicopathologic analysis of 29 cases. Cancer 67: 184–192
744. Kurman R J, Norris H J 1976 Endodermal sinus tumor of the ovary. A clinical and pathologic analysis of 71 cases. Cancer 38: 2404–2419
745. Langley F A, Govan A D T, Anderson M C et al. 1981 Yolk sac and allied tumours of the ovary. Histopathology 5: 389–401
746. Morris H H, La Vecchia C, Draper G J 1985 Endodermal sinus tumor and embryonal carcinoma of the ovary in children. Gynecol Oncol 21: 7–17
747. Kinoshita K 1990 A 62 year old woman with endodermal sinus tumor of the ovary. Am J Obstet Gynecol 162: 760–761
748. Oh C, Kendler A, Hernandez E 2001 Ovarian endodermal sinus tumor in a postmenopausal woman. Gynecol Oncol 82: 392–394
749. Kawai M, Furuhashi Y, Kano T et al. 1990 Alpha-fetoprotein in malignant germ cell tumors of the ovary. Gynecol Oncol 39: 160–166
750. Pliskow S 1993 Endodermal sinus tumor of the ovary: review of 10 cases. South Med J 86: 187–189
751. Jimerson G K, Woodruff J D 1977 Ovarian extraembryonal teratoma. I. Endodermal sinus tumor. Am J Obstet Gynecol 127: 73–79
752. Huntington R W J, Bullock W K 1970 Yolk sac tumors of the ovary. Cancer 25: 1357–1367
753. Ungerleider R S, Donaldson S S, Warnke R A et al. 1978 Endodermal sinus tumor: the Stanford experience and the first reported case arising in the vulva. Cancer 41: 1627–1634
754. Gershenson D M, Copeland L J, Kavanagh J J et al. 1985 Treatment of malignant nondysgerminomatous germcell tumors of the ovary with vincristine, dactinomycin, and cyclophosphamide. Cancer 56: 2756–2761
755. Slayton R E, Hreschyshyn M M, Silverberg S G et al. 1978 Treatment of malignant ovarian germ cell tumors: response to vincristine, dactinomycin, and cyclophosphamide (preliminary report). Cancer 42: 390–398
756. Gershenson D M, Kavanagh J J, Copeland L J et al. 1986 Treatment of malignant nondysgerminomatous germ cell tumors of the ovary by vinblastine, bleomycin, and cisplatin. Cancer 57: 1731–1737
757. Sessa C, Bonazzi C, Landoni F et al. 1987 Cisplatin, vinblastine, and bleomycin combination chemotherapy in endodermal sinus tumor of the ovary. Obstet Gynecol 70: 220–224
758. Williams S, Blessing J A, Liao S-Y et al. 1994 Adjuvant therapy of ovarian germ cell tumors with cisplatin, etoposide, and bleomycin: A trial of the Gynecologic Oncology Group. J Clin Oncol 12: 701–706
759. Peccatori F, Bonazzi C, Chiari S et al. 1995 Surgical management of malignant ovarian germ-cell tumors: 10 years' experience of 129 patients. Obstet Gynecol 86: 367–372
760. Zalel Y, Piura B, Elchalal U et al. 1996 Diagnosis and management of malignant germ cell ovarian tumors in young females. Int J Gynaecol Obstet 55: 1–10
761. Nawa A, Obata N, Kikkawa F et al. 2001 Prognostic factors of patients with yolk sac tumors of the ovary. Am J Obstet Gynecol 184: 1182–1188
762. Tewari K, Cappuccini F, DiSaia P J et al. 2000 Malignant germ cell tumors of the ovary. Obstet Gynecol 95: 128–133
763. Williams S D, Blessing J A, DiSaia P J et al. 1994 Second-look laparotomy in ovarian germ cell tumors: the gynecologic oncology group experience. Gynecol Oncol 52: 287–291
764. Curtin J P, Rubin S C, Hoskins W J et al. 1989 Second-look laparotomy in endodermal sinus tumor: a report of two patients with normal levels of alpha-fetoprotein and residual tumor at reexploration. Obstet Gynecol 74: 683–685
765. Nogales F F, Matilla A, Nogales-Ortiz F et al. 1978 Yolk sac tumors with pure and mixed polyvesicular vitelline patterns. Hum Pathol 9: 553–566
766. Nakashima N, Fukatsu T, Nagasaka T et al. 1987 The frequency and histology of hepatic tissue in germ cell tumors. Am J Surg Pathol 11: 682–692
767. Devouassoux-Shisheboran M, Schammel D P, Tavassoli F A 1999 Ovarian hepatoid yolk sac tumours: morphological, immunohistochemical and ultrastructural features. Histopathology 34: 462–469
768. Ulbright T M, Roth L M, Brodhecker C A 1986 Yolk sac differentiation in germ cell tumors. A morphologic study of 50 cases with emphasis on hepatic, enteric, and parietal yolk sac features. Am J Surg Pathol 10: 151–164
769. Clement P B, Young R H, Scully R E 1987 Endometrioid-like variant of ovarian yolk sac tumor. A clinicopathological analysis of eight cases. Am J Surg Pathol 11: 767–778

770. Kommoss F, Schmidt M, Merz E et al. 1999 Ovarian endometrioid-like yolk sac tumor treated by surgery alone, with recurrence at 12 years. Gynecol Oncol 72: 421–424
771. Cohen M B, Mulchahey K M, Molnar J J 1986 Ovarian endodermal sinus tumor with intestinal differentiation. Cancer 57: 1580–1583
772. Kim C R, Hsiu J G, Given F T 1989 Intestinal variant of ovarian endodermal sinus tumor. Gynecol Oncol 33: 379–381
773. Mazur M T, Talbot W H Jr, Talerman A 1988 Endodermal sinus tumor and mucinous cystadenofibroma of the ovary. Occurrence in an 82-year old woman. Cancer 62: 2011–2015
774. Nogales F F, Buritica C, Regauer S et al. 2005 Mucinous carcinoid as an unusual manifestation of endodermal differentiation in ovarian yolk sac tumors. Am J Surg Pathol 29: 1247–1251
775. Michael H, Ulbright T M, Brodhecker C A 1989 The pluripotential nature of the mesenchyme-like component of yolk sac tumor. Arch Pathol Lab Med 113: 1115–1119
776. Harms D, Janig U 1986 Germ cell tumours of childhood. Report of 170 cases including 59 pure and partial yolk-sac tumours. Virchow's Arch [A] 409: 223–239
777. Beilby J O W, Horne C H W, Milne G D et al. 1979 Alpha-fetoprotein, alpha-1-antitrypsin and transferrin in gonadal yolk sac tumours. J Clin Pathol 32: 455–461
778. Manivel J C, Jessurun J, Wick M R et al. 1987 Placental alkaline phosphatase immunoreactivity in testicular germ cell neoplasms. Am J Surg Pathol 11: 21–29
779. Bailey D, Marks A, Stratis M et al. 1991 Immunohistochemical staining of germ cell tumors and intratubular malignant germ cells of the testis using antibody to placental alkaline phosphatase and a monoclonal anti-seminoma antibody. Mod Pathol 4: 167–171
780. Kurman R J, Norris H J 1976 Embryonal carcinoma of the ovary: a clinicopathologic entity distinct from endodermal sinus tumor resembling embryonal carcinoma of the adult testis. Cancer 38: 2420–2433
781. Kammerer-Doak D, Baurick K, Black W et al. 1996 Endodermal sinus tumor and embryonal carcinoma of the ovary in a 53-year-old woman. Gynecol Oncol 63: 133–137
782. Williams S D, Blessing J A, Moore D H et al. 1989 Cisplatin, vinblastine, and bleomycin in advanced and recurrent ovarian germ-cell tumors. A trial of the Gynecologic Oncology Group. Ann Intern Med 111: 22–27
783. King M E, Hubbell M J, Talerman A 1991 Mixed germ cell tumor of the ovary with a prominent polyembryoma component. Int J Gynecol Pathol 10: 88–95
784. Chapman D C, Grover R, Schwartz P E 1994 Conservative management of an ovarian polyembryoma. Obstet Gynecol 83 Suppl.: 879–882
785. Jondle D M, Shahin M S, Sorosky J et al. 2002 Ovarian mixed germ cell tumor with predominance of polyembryoma: a case report with literature review. Int J Gynecol Pathol 21: 78–81
786. Nishida T, Oda T, Sugiyama T et al. 1998 Ovarian mixed germ cell tumor comprising polyembryoma and choriocarcinoma. Eur J Obstet Gynecol Reprod Biol 78: 95–97
787. Takemori M, Nishimura R, Yamasaki M et al. 1998 Ovarian mixed germ cell tumor composed of polyembryoma and immature teratoma. Gynecol Oncol 69: 260–263
788. Axe S R, Klein V R, Woodruff J D 1985 Choriocarcinoma of the ovary. Obstet Gynecol 66: 111–114
789. Jacobs A J, Newland J R, Green R K 1982 Pure choriocarcinoma of the ovary. Obstet Gynecol Surv 37: 603–609
790. Corakci A, Ozeren S, Ozkan S et al. 2005 Pure nongestational choriocarcinoma of ovary. Arch Gynecol Obstet 271: 176–177
791. Tsujioka H, Hamada H, Miyakawa T et al. 2003 A pure nongestational choriocarcinoma of the ovary diagnosed with DNA polymorphism analysis. Gynecol Oncol 89: 540–542
792. Goswami D, Sharma K, Zutshi V et al. 2001 Nongestational pure ovarian choriocarcinoma with contralateral teratoma. Gynecol Oncol 80: 262–266
793. Wheeler C A, Davis S, Degefu S et al. 1990 Ovarian choriocarcinoma: a difficult diagnosis of an unusual tumor and a review of the hook effect. Obstet Gynecol 75: 547–549
794. Vance R P, Geisinger K R 1985 Pure nongestational choriocarcinoma of the ovary. Report of a case. Cancer 56: 2321–2325
795. Grover V, Grover R K, Usha R et al. 1990 Primary pure choriocarcinoma of the ovary. Gynecol Obstet Invest 30: 61–63
796. Fisher R A, Newlands E S, Jeffreys A J et al. 1992 Gestational and nongestational trophoblastic tumors distinguished by DNA analysis. Cancer 69: 839–845
797. Shigematsu T, Kamura T, Arima T et al. 2000 DNA polymorphism analysis of a pure non-gestational choriocarcinoma of the ovary: case report. Eur J Gynaecol Oncol 21: 153–154
798. Dahl N, Gustavson K H, Rune C et al. 1990 Benign ovarian teratomas. An analysis of their cellular origin. Cancer Genet Cytogenet 46: 115–123
799. Linder D, McCaw B K, Hecht F 1975 Parthenogenetic origin of benign ovarian teratomas. N Engl J Med 292: 63–66
800. Surti U, Hoffner L, Chakravarti A et al. 1990 Genetics and biology of human ovarian teratomas. I. Cytogenetic analysis and mechanism of origin. Am J Hum Genet 47: 635–643
801. Vortmeyer A O, Devouassoux-Shisheboran M, Li G et al. 1999 Microdissection-based analysis of mature ovarian teratoma. Am J Pathol 154: 987–991
802. Gordon A, Rosenshein N, Parmley T et al. 1980 Benign cystic teratomas in postmenopausal women. Am J Obstet Gynecol 138: 1120–1123
803. Caruso P A, Marsh M R, Minkowitz S et al. 1971 An intense clinicopathologic study of 305 teratomas of the ovary. Cancer 27: 343–348
804. Wei F, Jiang Z, Yan C 2001 Analysis of 20 mature ovarian cystic teratoma cases in postmenopausal women. Chin Med J (Engl)114: 137–138
805. Ayhan A, Bukulmez O, Genc C et al. 2000 Mature cystic teratomas of the ovary: case series from one institution over 34 years. Eur J Obstet Gynecol Reprod Biol 88: 153–157
806. Comerci J T Jr, Licciardi F, Bergh P A et al. 1994 Mature cystic teratoma: a clinicopathologic evaluation of 517 cases and review of the literature. Obstet Gynecol 84: 22–28
807. Lin P, Falcone T, Tulandi T 1995 Excision of ovarian dermoid cyst by laparoscopy and by laparotomy. Am J Obstet Gynecol 173: 769–771
808. Albini S M, Benadiva C A, Haverly K et al. 1994 Management of benign ovarian cystic teratomas: laparoscopy compared with laparotomy. J Am Assoc Gynecol Laparosc 1: 219–222
809. Mecke H, Savvas V 2001 Laparoscopic surgery of dermoid cysts – intraoperative spillage and complications. Eur J Obstet Gynecol Reprod Biol 96: 80–84
810. Templeman C L, Fallat M E, Lam A M et al. 2000 Managing mature cystic teratomas of the ovary. Obstet Gynecol Surv 55: 738–745
811. Fanning J, Bates T S I 1996 Mature solid teratoma associated with gliomatosis peritonei. Am J Obstet Gynecol 155: 661–662
812. Robboy S J, Scully R E 1970 Ovarian teratoma with glial implants on the peritoneum. An analysis of 12 cases. Hum Pathol 1: 643–653
813. Steeper T A, Mukai K 1984 Solid ovarian teratomas: an immunocytochemical study of thirteen cases with clinicopathologic correlation. Pathol Annu 19: 81–92
814. Bosman F T, Louwerens J W K 1981 APUD cells in teratomas. Am J Pathol 104: 174–180
815. Nogales F F, Vergara E, Medina M T 1995 Prostate in ovarian mature cystic teratoma. Histopathology 26: 373–375
816. Vadmal M, Hajdu S I 1996 Prostatic tissue in benign cystic ovarian teratomas. Hum Pathol 27: 428–429
817. McLachlin C M, Srigley J R 1992 Prostatic tissue in mature cystic teratomas of the ovary. Am J Surg Pathol 16: 780–784
818. Halabi M, Oliva E, Mazal P R et al. 2002 Prostatic tissue in mature cystic teratomas of the ovary: a report of four cases, including one with features of prostatic adenocarcinoma, and cytogenetic studies. Int J Gynecol Pathol 21: 261–267
819. Bonazzi C, Peccatori F, Colombo N et al. 1994 Pure ovarian immature teratoma, a unique and curable disease: 10 years' experience of 32 prospectively treated patients. Obstet Gynecol 84:98–604
820. Nielsen S N, Gaffey T A, Malkasian G D Jr 1986 Immature ovarian teratoma: a review of 14 cases. Mayo Clin Proc 61: 110–115
821. Nogales F F, Favera B E, Major F J et al. 1976 Immature teratoma of the ovary with a neural component ("solid" teratoma). A clinicopathologic study of 20 cases. Hum Pathol 7: 625–642
822. Norris H J, Zirkin H J, Benson W L 1976 Immature (malignant) teratoma of the ovary. A clinical and pathologic study of 58 cases. Cancer 37: 2359–2372
823. Harms D, Janig U 1985 Immature teratomas of childhood. Report of 21 cases. Pathol Res Pract 179: 388–400
824. Koulos J P, Hoffman J S, Steinhoff M M 1989 Immature teratoma of the ovary. Gynecol Oncol 34: 46–49
825. Sen D K, Sivanesaratnam V, Sivanathan R et al. 1988 Immature teratoma of the ovary. Gynecol Oncol 30: 321–328
826. Doss B J, Jacques S M, Qureshi F et al. 1999 Immature teratomas of the genital tract in older women. Gynecol Oncol 73: 433–438
827. Gershenson D M, del Junco G, Silva E G et al. 1986 Immature teratoma of the ovary. Obstet Gynecol 68: 624–629
828. Kawai M, Kano T, Furuhashi Y et al. 1991 Immature teratoma of the ovary. Gynecol Oncol 40: 133–137
829. Perrone T, Steeper T A, Dehner L P 1987 Alpha-fetoprotein localization in pure ovarian teratoma. An immunohistochemical study of 12 cases. Am J Clin Pathol 88: 713–717
830. Yanai-Inbar I, Scully R E 1987 Relation of ovarian dermoid cysts and immature teratomas: an analysis of 350 cases of immature teratoma and 10 cases of dermoid cyst with microscopic foci of immature tissue. Int J Gynecol Pathol 6: 203–212
831. Li H, Hong W, Zhang R et al. 2002 Retrospective analysis of 67 consecutive cases of pure ovarian immature teratoma. Chin Med J (Engl) 115: 1496–1500
832. Beiner M E, Gotlieb W H, Korach Y et al. 2004 Cystectomy for immature teratoma of the ovary. Gynecol Oncol 93(2): 381–384
833. Vergote I B, Abeler V M, Kjrstad K E et al. 1990 Management of malignant ovarian immature teratoma. Role of adriamycin. Cancer 66: 882–886
834. Micha J P, Kucera P R, Berman M L et al. 1985 Malignant ovarian germ cell tumors: a review of thirty-six cases. Am J Obstet Gynecol 152: 842–846
835. Heifetz S A, Cushing B, Giller R et al. 1998 Immature teratomas in children: Pathologic considerations – A report from the combined Pediatric Oncology Group Children's Cancer Group. Am J Surg Pathol 22: 1115–1124

836. Marina N M, Cushing B, Giller R et al. 1999 Complete surgical excision is effective treatment for children with immature teratomas with or without malignant elements: A Pediatric Oncology Group/Children's Cancer Group Intergroup Study. J Clin Oncol 17: 2137–2143
837. Perrone T, Steiner M, Dehner L P 1986 Nodal gliomatosis and alpha-fetoprotein production. Two unusual facets of grade I ovarian teratoma. Arch Pathol Lab Med 110: 975–977
838. Harms D, Janig U, Göbel U 1989 Gliomatosis peritonei in childhood and adolescence. Clinicopathological study of 13 cases including immunohistochemical findings. Pathol Res Pract 184: 422–430
839. Nielsen S N J, Scheithauer B W, Gaffey T A 1985 Gliomatosis peritonei. Cancer 56: 2499–2503
840. El Shafie M, Furay R W, Chablani L V 1984 Ovarian teratoma with peritoneal and lymph node metastases of mature glial tissue: a benign condition. J Surg Oncol 27: 18–22
841. Ferguson A, Katabuchi H, Ronnett B M et al. 2001 Glial implants in gliomatosis peritonei arise from normal tissue, not from the associated teratoma. Am J Pathol 159: 51–55
842. Kwan M Y, Kalle W, Lau G T et al. 2004 Is gliomatosis peritonei derived from the associated ovarian teratoma? Hum Pathol 35: 685–688
843. Calder C J, Light A M, Rollason T P 1994 Immature ovarian teratoma with mature peritoneal metastatic deposits showing glial, epithelial, and endometrioid differentiation: a case report and review of the literature. Int J Gynecol Pathol 13: 279–282
844. Muller A M, Sondgen D, Strunz R et al. 2002 Gliomatosis peritonei: a report of two cases and review of the literature. Eur J Obstet Gynecol Reprod Biol 100: 213–222
845. Kattan J, Droz J P, Culine S et al. 1993 The growing teratoma syndrome: a woman with nonseminomatous germ cell tumor of the ovary. Gynecol Oncol 49: 395–399
846. Amsalem H, Nadjari M, Prus D et al. 2004 Growing teratoma syndrome vs chemotherapeutic retroconversion: case report and review of the literature. Gynecol Oncol 92: 357–360
847. Dadmanesh F, Miller D M, Swenerton K D et al. 1997 Gliomatosis peritonei with malignant transformation. Mod Pathol 10: 597–601
848. Ulbright T M 2005 Germ cell tumors of the gonads: a selective review emphasizing problems in differential diagnosis, newly appreciated, and controversial issues. Mod Pathol 18 Suppl 2: S61–S79
849. Baker P M, Rosai J, Young R H 2002 Ovarian teratomas with florid benign vascular proliferation: a distinctive finding associated with the neural component of teratomas that may be confused with a vascular neoplasm. Int J Gynecol Pathol 21: 16–21
850. Yanai H, Matsuura H, Kawasaki M et al. 2002 Immature teratoma of the ovary with a minor rhabdomyosarcomatous component and fatal rhabdomyosarcomatous metastases: the first case in a child. Int J Gynecol Pathol 21: 82–85
851. Nogales F F, Avila I R, Concha A et al. 1993 Immature endodermal teratoma of the ovary: Embryologic correlations and immunohistochemistry. Hum Pathol 24: 364–370
852. Nogales F F, Ortega J I, Rivera F et al. 1980 Metanephrogenic tissue in immature ovarian teratoma. Am J Surg Pathol 4: 297–299
853. O'Connor D M, Norris H J 1994 The influence of grade on the outcome of stage I ovarian immature (malignant) teratomas and the reproducibility of grading. Int J Gynecol Pathol 13: 283–289
854. Michael H, Hull M T, Ulbright T M et al. 1997 Primitive neuroectodermal tumors arising in testicular germ cell neoplasms. Am J Surg Pathol 21: 896–904
855. Kleinman G M, Young R H, Scully R E 1993 Primary neuroectodermal tumors of the ovary: a report of 25 cases. Am J Surg Pathol 17: 764–778
856. Block M, Gilbert E, Davis C 1984 Metastatic neuroblastoma arising in an ovarian teratoma with long-term survival. Case report and review of the literature. Cancer 54: 590–595
857. Dekmezian R H, Sneige N, Ordóñez N G 1986 Ovarian and omental ependymomas in peritoneal washings: cytologic and immunocytochemical features. Diagn Cytopathol 2: 62–68
858. Guerrieri C, Jarlsfelt I 1993 Ependymoma of the ovary: A case report with immunohistochemical, ultrastructural, and DNA cytometric findings, as well as histogenetic considerations. Am J Surg Pathol 17: 623–632
859. Carr K A, Roberts J A, Frank T S 1992 Progesterone receptors in bilateral ovarian ependymoma presenting in pregnancy. Hum Pathol 23: 962–965
860. Vance R P, Geisinger K R, Randall M B et al. 1988 Immature neural elements in immature teratomas. An immunohistochemical and ultrastructural study. Am J Clin Pathol 90: 397–411
861. Calame J J, Schaberg A 1989 Solid teratomas and mixed Mullerian tumors of the ovary: a clinical, histological, and immunocytochemical comparative study. Gynecol Oncol 33: 212–221
862. Cho N H, Kim Y T, Lee J H et al. 2005 Diagnostic challenge of fetal ontogeny and its application on the ovarian teratomas. Int J Gynecol Pathol 24: 173–182
863. Genadry R, Parmley T, Woodruff J D 1979 Secondary malignancies in benign cystic teratomas. Gynecol Oncol 8: 246–251
864. Stamp G W H, McConnell E M 1983 Malignancy arising in cystic ovarian teratomas. A report of 24 cases. Br J Obstet Gynaecol 90: 671–675
865. Hirakawa T, Tsuneyoshi M, Enjoji M 1989 Squamous cell carcinoma arising in mature cystic teratoma of the ovary. Clinicopathologic and topographic analysis. Am J Surg Pathol 13: 397–405
866. Peterson W F 1957 Malignant degeneration of benign cystic teratomas of the ovary. A collective review of the literature. Obstet Gynecol Surv 12: 793–830
867. Tseng C J, Chou H H, Huang K G et al. 1996 Squamous cell carcinoma arising in mature cystic teratoma of the ovary. Gynecol Oncol 63: 364–370
868. Kikkawa F, Ishikawa H, Tamakoshi K et al. 1997 Squamous cell carcinoma arising from mature cystic teratoma of the ovary: a clinicopathologic analysis. Obstet Gynecol 89: 1017–1022
869. Kuroda N, Hirano K, Inui Y et al. 2001 Compound melanocytic nevus arising in a mature cystic teratoma of the ovary. Pathol Int 51: 902–904
870. Takeshima Y, Kaneko M, Furonaka O et al. 2004 Meningioma in mature cystic teratoma of the ovary. Pathol Int 54: 543–548
871. Silver S A, Tavassoli F A 2000 Glomus tumor arising in a mature teratoma of the ovary – Report of a case simulating a metastasis from cervical squamous carcinoma. Arch Pathol Lab Med 124: 1373–1375
872. Itoh H, Wada T, Michikata K et al. 2004 Ovarian teratoma showing a predominant hemangiomatous element with stromal luteinization: report of a case and review of the literature. Pathol Int 54: 279–283
873. Chumas J C, Scully R E 1991 Sebaceous tumors arising in ovarian dermoid cysts. Int J Gynecol Pathol 10: 356–363
874. Tobon H, Surti U, Naus G J et al. 1991 Squamous cell carcinoma in situ arising in an ovarian mature cystic teratoma. Report of one case with histopathologic, cytogenetic, and flow cytometric DNA content analysis. Arch Pathol Lab Med 115: 172–174
875. Shimizu S, Kobayashi H, Suchi T et al. 1991 Extramammary Paget's disease arising in mature cystic teratoma of the ovary. Am J Surg Pathol 15: 1002–1006
876. Monteagudo C, Torres J V, Llombart-Bosch A 1999 Extramammary Paget's disease arising in a mature cystic teratoma of the ovary. Histopathology 35: 582–584
877. Vartanian R K, McRae B, Hessler R B 2002 Sebaceous carcinoma arising in a mature cystic teratoma of the ovary. Int J Gynecol Pathol 21: 418–421
878. Ribeiro-Silva A, Chang D, Bisson F W et al. 2003 Clinicopathological and immunohistochemical features of a sebaceous carcinoma arising within a benign dermoid cyst of the ovary. Virchow's Arch 443: 574–578
879. Davis G L 1996 Malignant melanoma arising in mature ovarian cystic teratoma (dermoid cyst). Report of two cases and literature analysis. Int J Gynecol Pathol 15: 356–362
880. Gupta D, Deavers M T, Silva E G et al. 2004 Malignant melanoma involving the ovary: a clinicopathologic and immunohistochemical study of 23 cases. Am J Surg Pathol 28: 771–780
881. Vimla N, Kumar L, Thulkar S et al. 2001 Primary malignant melanoma in ovarian cystic teratoma. Gynecol Oncol 82: 380–383
882. Watanabe Y, Ueda H, Nakajima H et al. 2001 Amelanotic malignant melanoma arising in an ovarian cystic teratoma – A case report. Acta Cytol 45: 756–760
883. Fujiwara K, Ginzan S, Silverberg S G 1995 Mature cystic teratomas of the ovary with intestinal wall structures harboring intestinal-type epithelial neoplasms. Gynecol Oncol 56: 97–101
884. Cobellis L, Schurfeld K, Ignacchiti E et al. 2004 An ovarian mucinous adenocarcinoma arising from mature cystic teratoma associated with respiratory type tissue: a case report. Tumori 90: 521–524
885. Kushima M 2004 Adenocarcinoma arising from mature cystic teratoma of the ovary. Pathol Int 54: 139–143
886. Levine D A, Villella J A, Poynor E A et al. 2004 Gastrointestinal adenocarcinoma arising in a mature cystic teratoma of the ovary. Gynecol Oncol 94: 597–599
887. Climie A R, Heath L P 1968 Malignant degeneration of benign cystic teratomas of the ovary. Review of the literature and report of a chondrosarcoma and carcinoid tumor. Cancer 22: 824–832
888. Aygun B, Kimpo M, Lee T et al. 2003 An adolescent with ovarian osteosarcoma arising in a cystic teratoma. J Pediatr Hematol Oncol 25: 410–413
889. Ronnett B M, Seidman J D 2003 Mucinous tumors arising in ovarian mature cystic teratomas: relationship to the clinical syndrome of pseudomyxoma peritonei. Am J Surg Pathol 27: 650–657
890. Hasleton P S, Kelehan P, Whittaker J S et al. 1978 Benign and malignant struma ovarii. Arch Pathol Lab Med 102: 180–184
891. Devaney K, Snyder R, Norris H J et al. 1993 Proliferative and histologically malignant struma ovarii: a clinicopathologic study of 54 cases. Int J Gynecol Pathol 12: 333–343
892. Amr S S, Hassan A A 1994 Struma ovarii with pseudo-Meigs' syndrome: report of a case and review of the literature. Eur J Obstet Gynecol Reprod Biol 55: 205–208
893. Kempers R D, Dockerty M B, Hoffman D L et al. 1970 Struma ovarii – ascitic, hyperthyroid, and asymptomatic syndromes. Ann Intern Med 72: 883–893
894. Willemse P H, Oosterhuis J W, Aalders J G et al. 1987 Malignant struma ovarii treated by ovariectomy, thyroidectomy, and 131I administration. Cancer 60: 178–182
895. Huh J J, Montz F J, Bristow R E 2002 Struma ovarii associated with pseudo-Meigs' syndrome and elevated serum CA 125. Gynecol Oncol 86: 231–234
896. Loizzi V, Cormio G, Resta L et al. 2005 Pseudo-Meigs syndrome and elevated CA125 associated with struma ovarii. Gynecol Oncol 97: 282–284

897. Matsuda K, Maehama T, Kanazawa K 2001 Malignant struma ovarii with thyrotoxicosis. Gynecol Oncol 82: 575–577
898. Berghella V, Ngadiman S, Rosenberg H et al. 1997 Malignant struma ovarii – A case report and review of the literature. Gynecol Obstet Invest 43: 68–72
899. Makani S, Kim W, Gaba A R 2004 Struma ovarii with a focus of papillary thyroid cancer: a case report and review of the literature. Gynecol Oncol 94: 835–839
901. Nahn P A, Robinson E, Strassman M 2002 Conservative therapy for malignant struma ovarii – A case report. J Reprod Med 47: 943–945
902. Bolat F, Erkanli S, Kayaselcuk F et al. 2005 Malignant struma ovarii: a case report. Pathol Res Pract 201: 409–412
903. Pardo-Mindan F J, Vazquez J J 1983 Malignant struma ovarii. Light and electron microscopic study. Cancer 51: 337–343
904. McDougall I R, Krasne D, Hanbery J W et al. 1989 Metastatic malignant struma ovarii presenting as paraparesis from a spinal metastasis. J Nucl Med 30: 407–411
905. Ribeiro-Silva A, Bezerra A M, Serafini L N 2002 Malignant struma ovarii: an autopsy report of a clinically unsuspected tumor. Gynecol Oncol 87: 213–215
906. Dardik R B, Dardik M, Westra W et al. 1999 Malignant struma ovarii: two case reports and a review of the literature. Gynecol Oncol 73: 447–451
907. DeSimone C P, Lele S M, Modesitt S C 2003 Malignant struma ovarii: a case report and analysis of cases reported in the literature with focus on survival and I131 therapy. Gynecol Oncol 89: 543–548
908. Szyfelbein W M, Young R H, Scully R E 1994 Cystic struma ovarii: a frequently unrecognized tumor. A report of 20 cases. Am J Surg Pathol 18: 785–788
909. Szyfelbein W M, Young R H, Scully R E 1995 Struma ovarii simulating ovarian tumors of other types. A report of 30 cases. Am J Surg Pathol 19: 21–29
910. Hamazaki S, Okino T, Tsukayama C et al. 2002 Expression of thyroid transcription factor-1 in strumal carcinoid and struma ovarii: an immunohistochemical study. Pathol Int 52: 458–462
911. Rosenblum N G, Livolsi V A, Edmonds P R et al. 1989 Malignant struma ovarii. Gynecol Oncol 32: 224–227
912. Brunskill P J, Rollason T P, Nicholson H O 1990 Malignant follicular variant of papillary struma ovarii. Histopathology 17: 574–576
913. Balasch J, Pahisa J, Márquez M et al. 1993 Metastatic ovarian strumosis in an in-vitro fertilization patient. Hum Reprod 8: 2075–2079
914. Karseladze A I, Kulinitch S I 1994 Peritoneal strumosis. Pathol Res Pract 190: 1082–1085
915. Soga J, Osaka M, Yakuwa Y 2000 Carcinoids of the ovary: an analysis of 329 reported cases. J Exp Clin Cancer Res 19: 271–280
916. Robboy S J, Scully R E, Norris H J 1977 Primary trabecular carcinoid of the ovary. Obstet Gynecol 49: 202–207
917. Robboy S J 1984 Insular carcinoid of ovary associated with malignant mucinous tumors. Cancer 54: 2273–2276
918. Davis K P, Hartmann L K, Keeney G L et al. 1996 Primary ovarian carcinoid tumors. Gynecol Oncol 61: 259–265
919. Robboy S J, Norris H J, Scully R E 1975 Insular carcinoid primary in the ovary. A clinicopathologic analysis of 48 cases. Cancer 36: 404–418
920. Chaowalit N, Connolly H M, Schaff H V et al. 2004 Carcinoid heart disease associated with primary ovarian carcinoid tumor. Am J Cardiol 93: 1314–1315
921. Yaegashi N, Tsuiki A, Shimizu T et al. 1995 Ovarian carcinoid with severe constipation due to peptide YY production. Gynecol Oncol 56: 302–306
922. Motoyama T, Katayama Y, Watanabe H et al. 1992 Functioning ovarian carcinoids induce severe constipation. Cancer 70: 513–518
923. Shigeta H, Taga M, Kurogi K et al. 1999 Ovarian strumal carcinoid with severe constipation: immunohistochemical and mRNA analyses of peptide YY. Hum Pathol 30: 242–246
924. Robboy S J, Scully R E 1980 Strumal carcinoid of the ovary. An analysis of 50 cases of a distinctive tumor composed of thyroid tissue and carcinoid. Cancer 46: 2019–2034
925. Wilkowske M A, Hartmann L C, Mullany C J et al. 1994 Progressive carcinoid heart disease after resection of primary ovarian carcinoid. Cancer 73: 1889–1891
926. Alenghat E, Okagaki T, Talerman A 1986 Primary mucinous carcinoid tumor of the ovary. Cancer 58: 777–783
927. Armes J E, Ostor A G 1993 A case of malignant strumal carcinoid. Gynecol Oncol 51: 419–423
928. Robboy S J, Scully R E, Norris H J 1974 Carcinoid metastatic to the ovary. A clinicopathologic analysis of 35 cases. Cancer 33: 798–811
929. Talerman A, Evans M I 1982 Primary trabecular carcinoid tumor of the ovary. Cancer 50: 1403–1407
930. Snyder R R, Tavassoli F A 1986 Ovarian strumal carcinoid: immunohistochemical, ultrastructural, and clinicopathologic analysis. Int J Gynecol Pathol 5: 187–201
931. Sidhu J, Sánchez R L 1993 Prostatic acid phosphatase immunoreactivity in strumal carcinoids of the ovary: An immunohistochemical study. Cancer 72: 1673–1678
932. Stagno P A, Petras R E, Hart W R 1987 Strumal carcinoids of the ovary. An immunohistologic and ultrastructural study. Arch Pathol Lab Med 111: 440–446
933. Matias-Guiu X, Forteza J, Prat J 1995 Mixed strumal and mucinous carcinoid tumor of the ovary. Int J Gynecol Pathol 14: 179–183
934. Ulbright T M, Roth L M, Ehrlich C E 1982 Ovarian strumal carcinoid. An immunocytochemical and ultrastructural study of two cases. Am J Clin Pathol 77: 622–631
935. Dayal Y, Tashjian A J Jr, Wolfe H J 1979 Immunocytochemical localization of calcitonin-producing cells in a strumal carcinoid with amyloid stroma. Cancer 43: 1331–1338
936. Wolpert H R, Fuller A F, Bell D A 1989 Primary mucinous carcinoid tumor of the ovary. A case report. Int J Gynecol Pathol 8: 156–162
937. Baker P M, Oliva E, Young R H et al. 2001 Ovarian mucinous carcinoids including some with a carcinomatous component – A report of 17 cases. Am J Surg Pathol 25: 557–568
938. Serratoni F T, Robboy S J 1975 Ultrastructure of primary and metastatic ovarian carcinoids: analysis of 11 cases. Cancer 36: 157–160
939. Sporrong B, Falkmer S, Robboy S J et al. 1982 Neurohormonal peptides in ovarian carcinoids: an immunohistochemical study of 81 primary carcinoids and of intraovarian metastases from six mid-gut carcinoids. Cancer 49: 68–74
940. Braunschweig R, Hurlimann J, Gloor E et al. 1994 [Ovarian carcinoid tumors: immunohistochemical and ultrastructural study of 8 cases.] Ann Pathol 14: 155–162
941. Matsuda K, Maehama T, Kanazawa K 2002 Strumal carcinoid tumor of the ovary: a case exhibiting severe constipation associated with PYY. Gynecol Oncol 87: 143–145
942. Greco M A, Livolsi V A, Pertschuk L P et al. 1979 Strumal carcinoid of the ovary: an analysis of its components. Cancer; 43: 1380–1388.
943. Senterman M K, Cassidy P N, Fenoglio C M et al. 1984 Histology, ultrastructure, and immunohistochemistry of strumal carcinoid: a case report. Int J Gynecol Pathol 3: 232–240
944. Kurman R J, Norris H J 1976 Malignant mixed germ cell tumors of the ovary. A clinical and pathologic analysis of 30 cases. Obstet Gynecol 48: 579–589
945. Gershenson D M, del Junco G, Copeland L J et al. 1984 Mixed germ cell tumors of the ovary. Obstet Gynecol 64: 200–207
946. Jimerson G K, Woodruff J D 1977 Ovarian extraembryonal teratoma. II. Endodermal sinus tumor mixed with other germ cell tumors. Am J Obstet Gynecol 127: 302–305
947. De Palo G, Zambetti M, Pilotti S et al. 1992 Nondysgerminomatous tumors of the ovary treated with cisplatin, vinblastine, and bleomycin: long-term results. Gynecol Oncol 47: 239–246
948. Troche V, Hernandez E 1986 Neoplasia arising in dysgenetic gonads. Obstet Gynecol Surv 41: 74–79
949. Garvin A J, Pratt-Thomas H R, Spector M et al. 1976 Gonadoblastoma: histologic, ultrastructural, and histochemical observations in five cases. Am J Obstet Gynecol 125: 459–471
950. Govan A D, Woodcock A S, Gowing N F et al. 1977 A clinico-pathological study of gonadoblastoma. Br J Obstet Gynaecol 84: 222–228
951. Woodcock A S, Govan A D, Gowing N F et al. 1979 A report of the histological features in 12 cases of gonadoblastoma. Tumori 65: 181–189
952. Scully R E 1970 Gonadoblastoma: a review of 74 cases. Cancer 25: 1340–1356
953. Deligdisch L, Richards C J, Reyniak V J 1988 Pure gonadal dysgenesis and gonadal tumors: report of three cases and review of literature. Mt Sinai J Med 55: 313–317
954. Pena-Alonso R, Nieto K, Alvarez R et al. 2005 Distribution of Y-chromosome-bearing cells in gonadoblastoma and dysgenetic testis in 45,X/46,XY infants. Mod Pathol 18: 439–445
955. Tsuchiya K, Reijo R, Page D C et al. 1995 Gonadoblastoma: molecular definition of the susceptibility region on the Y chromosome. Am J Hum Genet 57: 1400–1407
956. Mancilla E E, Poggi H, Repetto G et al. 2003 Y chromosome sequences in Turner's syndrome: association with virilization and gonadoblastoma. J Pediatr Endocrinol Metab 16: 1157–1163
957. Salo P, Kaariainen H, Petrovic V et al. 1995 Molecular mapping of the putative gonadoblastoma locus on the Y chromosome. Genes Chromosomes Cancer 14: 210–214
958. Lau Y, Chou P, Iezzoni J et al. 2000 Expression of a candidate gene for the gonadoblastoma locus in gonadoblastoma and testicular seminoma. Cytogenet Cell Genet 91: 160–164
959. Schellhas H F 1974 Malignant potential of the dysgenetic gonad. Part I. Obstet Gynecol 44: 298–309
960. Horn L C, Limbach A, Hoepffner W et al. 2005 Histologic analysis of gonadal tissue in patients with Ullrich-Turner syndrome and derivative Y chromosomes. Pediatr Dev Pathol 8: 197–203
961. Hart W R, Burkons D M 1979 Germ cell neoplasms arising in gonadoblastomas. Cancer 43: 669–678
962. Talerman A 1974 Gonadoblastoma associated with embryonal carcinoma. Obstet Gynecol 43: 138–142
963. Jorgensen N, Müller J, Jaubert F et al. 1997 Heterogeneity of gonadoblastoma germ cells: Similarities with immature germ cells, spermatogonia and testicular carcinoma in situ cells. Histopathology 30: 177–186
964. Kersemaekers A M, Honecker F, Stoop H et al. 2005 Identification of germ cells at risk for neoplastic transformation in gonadoblastoma: an immunohistochemical study for OCT3/4 and TSPY. Hum Pathol 36: 512–52.
965. Roth L M, Eglen D E 1989 Gonadoblastoma. Immunohistochemical and ultrastructural observations. Int J Gynecol Pathol 8: 72–81

966. Rajpert-De M E, Hanstein R, Jorgensen N et al. 2004 Developmental expression of POU5F1 (OCT-3/4) in normal and dysgenetic human gonads. Hum Reprod 19: 1338–1344
967. Hildenbrand R, Schröder W, Brude E et al. 1999 Detection of *TSPY* protein in a unilateral microscopic gonadoblastoma of a Turner mosaic patient with a Y-derived marker chromosome. J Pathol 189: 623–626
968. Talerman A 1972 A distinctive gonadal neoplasm related to gonadoblastoma. Cancer 30: 1219–1224
969. Tavassoli F A 1983 A combined germ cell-gonadal stromal-epithelial tumor of the ovary. Am J Surg Pathol 7: 73–84
970. Nomura K, Matsui T, Aizawa S 1999 Gonadoblastoma with proliferation resembling Sertoli cell tumor. Int J Gynecol Pathol 18: 91–93
971. Kedzia H 1983 Gonadoblastoma: structures and background of development. Am J Obstet Gynecol 147: 81–85
972. Safneck J R, deSa D J 1986 Structures mimicking sex cord-stromal tumours and gonadoblastomas in the ovaries of normal infants and children. Histopathology 10: 909–920
973. Dickersin G R, Kline I W, Scully R E 1982 Small cell carcinoma of the ovary with hypercalcemia: a report of eleven cases. Cancer 49: 188–197
974. Scully R E 1993 Small cell carcinoma of hypercalcemic type. Int J Gynecol Pathol 12: 148–152
975. Young R H, Oliva E, Scully R E 1994 Small cell carcinoma of the ovary, hypercalcemic type: a clinicopathological analysis of 150 cases. Am J Surg Pathol 18: 1102–1116
976. Clement P B 2005 Selected miscellaneous ovarian lesions: small cell carcinomas, mesothelial lesions, mesenchymal and mixed neoplasms, and non-neoplastic lesions. Mod Pathol 18 Suppl 2: S113–S129
977. Schleef J, Wagner A, Kleta R et al. 1999 Small-cell carcinoma of the ovary of the hypercalcemic type in an 8-year-old girl. Pediatr Surg Int 15: 431–434
978. Seidman J D 1995 Small cell carcinoma of the ovary of the hypercalcemic type: p53 protein accumulation and clinicopathologic features. Gynecol Oncol 59: 283–287
979. Longy M, Toulouse C, Mage P et al. 1996 Familial cluster of ovarian small cell carcinoma: a new mendelian entity? J Med Genet 33: 333–335
980. Tewari K, Brewer C, Cappuccini F et al. 1997 Advanced-stage small cell carcinoma of the ovary in pregnancy: long-term survival after surgical debulking and multiagent chemotherapy. Gynecol Oncol 66: 531–534
981. Sholler G L, Luks F, Mangray S et al. 2005 Advanced small cell carcinoma of the ovary in a pediatric patient with long-term survival and review of the literature. J Pediatr Hematol Oncol 27: 169–172
982. Rana S, Warren B K, Yamada S D 2004 Stage IIIC small cell carcinoma of the ovary: survival with conservative surgery and chemotherapy. Obstet Gynecol 103: 1120–1123
983. Eichhorn J H, Bell D A, Young RH et al. 1992 DNA content and proliferative activity in ovarian small cell carcinomas of the hypercalcemic type: Implications for diagnosis, prognosis, and histogenesis. Am J Clin Pathol 98: 579–586
984. Ulbright T M, Roth L M, Stehman F B et al. 1987 Poorly differentiated (small cell) carcinoma of the ovary in young women: evidence supporting a germ cell origin. Hum Pathol 18: 175–184
985. McCluggage W G, Oliva E, Connolly L E et al. 2004 An immunohistochemical analysis of ovarian small cell carcinoma of hypercalcemic type. Int J Gynecol Pathol 23: 330–336
986. Riopel M A, Perlman E J, Seidman J D et al. 1998 Inhibin and epithelial membrane antigen immunohistochemistry assist in the diagnosis of sex cord-stromal tumors and provide clues to the histogenesis of hypercalcemic small cell carcinomas. Int J Gynecol Pathol 17: 46–53
987. Abeler V, Kjrstad K E, Nesland J M 1988 Small cell carcinoma of the ovary. A report of six cases. Int J Gynecol Pathol 7: 315–329
988. Matias-Guiu X, Prat J, Young R H et al. 1994 Human parathyroid hormone-related protein in ovarian small cell carcinoma: an immunohistochemical study. Cancer 73: 1878–1881
989. McMahon J T, Hart W R 1988 Ultrastructural analysis of small cell carcinomas of the ovary. Am J Clin Pathol 90: 523–529
990. Dickersin G R, Scully R E 1993 An update on the electron microscopy of small cell carcinoma of the ovary with hypercalcemia. Ultrastruct Pathol 17: 411–422
991. Dickersin G R, Scully R E 1998 Ovarian small cell tumors: an electron microscopic review. Ultrastruct Pathol 22: 199–226
992. Idei Y, Kitazawa S, Fujimori T et al. 1996 Ovarian small cell carcinoma with K-*ras* mutation: a case report with genetic analysis. Hum Pathol 27: 77–79
993. Gerald W L, Miller H K, Battifora H et al. 1991 Intra-abdominal desmoplastic small round-cell tumor. Report of 19 cases of a distinctive type of high-grade polyphenotypic malignancy affecting young individuals. Am J Surg Pathol 15: 499–513
994. Hassan I, Shyyan R, Donohue J H et al. 2005 Intraabdominal desmoplastic small round cell tumors. Cancer 104: 1264–1270
995. Lae M E, Roche P C, Jin L et al. 2002 Desmoplastic small round cell tumor – A clinicopathologic, immunohistochemical, and molecular study of 32 tumors. Am J Surg Pathol 26: 823–835
996. Young R H, Eichhorn J H, Dickersin G R et al. 1992 Ovarian involvement by the intra-abdominal desmoplastic small round cell tumor with divergent differentiation: a report of three cases. Hum Pathol 23: 454–464
997. Zaloudek C, Miller T R, Stern J L 1995 Desmoplastic small cell tumor of the ovary: a unique polyphenotypic tumor with an unfavorable prognosis. Int J Gynecol Pathol 14: 260–265
998. Elhajj M, Mazurka J, Daya D 2002 Desmoplastic small round cell tumor presenting in the ovaries: report of a case and review of the literature. Int J Gynecol Cancer 12: 760–763
999. Parker L P, Duong J L, Wharton J T et al. 2002 Desmoplastic small round cell tumor: report of a case presenting as a primary ovarian neoplasm. Eur J Gynaecol Oncol 23: 199–202
1000. Slomovitz B M, Girotra M, Aledo A et al. 2000 Desmoplastic small round cell tumor with primary ovarian involvement: case report and review. Gynecol Oncol 79: 124–128
1001. Lal D R, Su W T, Wolden S L et al. 2005 Results of multimodal treatment for desmoplastic small round cell tumors. J Pediatr Surg 40: 251–255
1002. Goodman K A, Wolden S L, La Quaglia M P et al. 2002 Whole abdominopelvic radiotherapy for desmoplastic small round-cell tumor. Int J Radiat Oncol Biol Phys 54: 170–176
1003. Ladanyi M, Gerald W 1994 Fusion of the EWS and WT1 genes in the desmoplastic small round cell tumor. Cancer Res 54: 2837–2840
1004. Gerald W L, Haber D A 2005 The EWS-WT1 gene fusion in desmoplastic small round cell tumor. Semin Cancer Biol 15: 197–205
1005. Sandberg A A, Bridge J A 2002 Updates on the cytogenetics and molecular genetics of bone and soft tissue tumors. Desmoplastic small round-cell tumors. Cancer Genet Cytogenet 138: 1–10
1006. Ordonez N G 1998 Desmoplastic small round cell tumor I: a histopathologic study of 39 cases with emphasis on unusual histological patterns. Am J Surg Pathol 22: 1303–1313
1007. Sebire N J, Gibson S, Rampling D et al. 2005 Immunohistochemical findings in embryonal small round cell tumors with molecular diagnostic confirmation. Appl Immunohistochem Mol Morphol 13: 1–5
1008. Zhang P J, Goldblum J R, Pawel B R et al. 2003 Immunophenotype of desmoplastic small round cell tumors as detected in cases with EWS-WT1 gene fusion product. Mod Pathol 16: 229–235
1009. Ordonez N G 1998 Desmoplastic small round cell tumor II: An ultrastructural and immunohistochemical study with emphasis on new immunohistochemical markers. Am J Surg Pathol 22: 1314–1327
1010. Kariminejad M H, Scully R E. 1973 Female adnexal tumor of probable Wolffian origin: a distinctive pathologic entity. Cancer 31: 671–677.
1011. Young R H, Scully R E 1983 Ovarian tumors of probable Wolffian origin: a report of 11 cases. Am J Surg Pathol 7: 125–136
1012. Tavassoli F A, Andrade R, Merino M 1990 Retiform wolffian adenoma. In: Fenoglio-Preiser CM, Wolffe M, Rilke F (eds) Progress in surgical pathology. Field and Wood Medical Publishers, Inc, New York, vol. XI, p 121–136
1013. Inoue H, Kikuchi Y, Hori T et al. 1995 An ovarian tumor of probable Wolffian origin with hormonal function. Gynecol Oncol 59: 304–308
1014. Delaloye J F, Ruzicka J, De Grandi P 1993 An ovarian tumor of probable Wolffian origin. Acta Obstet Gynecol Scand 72: 314–316
1015. Devouassoux-Shisheboran M, Silver S A, Tavassoli F A 1999 Wolffian adnexal tumor, so-called female adnexal tumor of probable Wolffian origin (FATWO): immunohistochemical evidence in support of a Wolffian origin. Hum Pathol 30: 856–863
1016. Rahilly M A, Williams A R W, Krausz T et al. 1995 Female adnexal tumour of probable Wolffian origin: a clinicopathological and immunohistochemical study of three cases. Histopathology 26: 69–74
1017. Young R H, Silva E G, Scully R E 1991 Ovarian and juxtaovarian adenomatoid tumors: a report of six cases. Int J Gynecol Pathol 10: 364–372
1018. Mazur M T, Hsueh S, Gersell D J 1984 Metastases to the female genital tract. Analysis of 325 cases. Cancer 53: 1978–1984
1019. Abu-Rustum N R, Barakat R R, Curtin J P 1997 Ovarian and uterine disease in women with colorectal cancer. Obstet Gynecol 89: 85–87
1020. Ulbright T M, Roth L M, Stehman F B 1984 Secondary ovarian neoplasia. A clinicopathologic study of 35 cases. Cancer 53: 1164–1174
1021. Young R H, Scully R E 1991 Metastatic tumors in the ovary: a problem-oriented approach and review of the recent literature. Semin Diagn Pathol 8: 250–276
1022. Powari M, Dey P, Gupta S K et al. 2003 Metastatic tumours of the ovary: a clinico-pathological study. Indian J Pathol Microbiol 46: 412–415
1023. McCluggage W G, Wilkinson N 2005 Metastatic neoplasms involving the ovary: a review with an emphasis on morphological and immunohistochemical features. Histopathology 47: 231–247
1024. Chang T C, Changchien C C, Tseng C W et al. 1997 Retrograde lymphatic spread: a likely route for metastatic ovarian cancers of gastrointestinal origin. Gynecol Oncol 66: 372–377
1025. Moore R G, Chung M, Granai C O et al. 2004 Incidence of metastasis to the ovaries from nongenital tract primary tumors. Gynecol Oncol 93: 87–91
1026. Elishaev E, Gilks C B, Miller D et al. 2005 Synchronous and metachronous endocervical and ovarian neoplasms: evidence supporting interpretation of the ovarian neoplasms as metastatic endocervical adenocarcinomas simulating primary ovarian surface epithelial neoplasms. Am J Surg Pathol 29: 281–294
1027. Yada-Hashimoto N, Yamamoto T, Kamiura S et al. 2003 Metastatic ovarian tumors: a review of 64 cases. Gynecol Oncol 89: 314–317
1028. Ronnett B M, Kurman R J, Shmookler B M et al. 1997 The morphologic spectrum of ovarian metastases of appendiceal adenocarcinomas –

A clinicopathologic and immunohistochemical analysis of tumors often misinterpreted as primary ovarian tumors or metastatic tumors from other gastrointestinal sites. Am J Surg Pathol 21: 1144–1155
1029. Young R H, Hart W R 1989 Metastases from carcinomas of the pancreas simulating primary mucinous tumors of the ovary. A report of seven cases. Am J Surg Pathol 13: 748–756
1030. Young R H, Scully R E 1990 Ovarian metastases from carcinoma of the gallbladder and extrahepatic bile ducts simulating primary tumors of the ovary. A report of six cases. Int J Gynecol Pathol 9: 60–72
1031. De Groot M E, Dukel L, Chadha-Ajwani S et al. 2000 Massive solitary metastasis of hepatocellular carcinoma in the ovary two years after liver transplantation. Eur J Obstet Gynecol Reprod Biol 90: 109–111
1032. Young R H, Hart W R 1992 Renal cell carcinoma metastatic to the ovary: a report of three cases emphasizing possible confusion with ovarian clear cell adenocarcinoma. Int J Gynecol Pathol 11: 96–104
1033. Hammock L, Ghorab Z, Gomez-Fernandez C R 2003 Metastatic renal cell carcinoma to the ovary: a case report and discussion of differential diagnoses. Arch Pathol Lab Med 127: e123–e126
1034. Insabato L, De Rosa G, Franco R et al. 2003 Ovarian metastasis from renal cell carcinoma: a report of three cases. Int J Surg Pathol 11: 309–312
1035. Young R H, Scully R E 1991 Malignant melanoma metastatic to the ovary: a clinicopathologic analysis of 20 cases. Am J Surg Pathol 15: 849–860
1036. Young R H, Scully R E 1990 Sarcomas metastatic to the ovary: a report of 21 cases. Int J Gynecol Pathol 9: 231–252
1037. Young R H, Scully R E 1989 Alveolar rhabdomyosarcoma metastatic to the ovary. A report of two cases and a discussion of the differential diagnosis of small cell malignant tumors of the ovary. Cancer 64: 899–904
1038. Eltabbakh G H, Belinson J L, Biscotti C V 1997 Osteosarcoma metastatic to the ovary: a case report and review of the literature. Int J Gynecol Pathol 16: 76–78
1039. Irving J A, Lerwill M F, Young R H 2005 Gastrointestinal stromal tumors metastatic to the ovary: a report of five cases. Am J Surg Pathol 29: 920–926
1040. Demopoulos R I, Touger L, Dubin N 1987 Secondary ovarian carcinoma: a clinical and pathological evaluation. Int J Gynecol Pathol 6: 166–175
1041. Abu-Rustum N, Barakat R R, Curtin J P 1997 Ovarian and uterine disease in women with colorectal cancer. Obstet Gynecol 89: 85–87
1042. Miller B E, Pittman B, Wan J Y et al. 1997 Colon cancer with metastasis to the ovary at time of initial diagnosis. Gynecol Oncol 66: 368–371
1043. Herrera-Ornelas L, Natarajan N, Tsukada Y et al. 1983 Adenocarcinoma of the colon masquerading as primary ovarian neoplasia. An analysis of ten cases. Dis Colon Rectum 26: 377–380
1044. Daya D, Nazerali L, Frank G L 1992 Metastatic ovarian carcinoma of large intestinal origin simulating primary ovarian carcinoma: a clinicopathologic study of 25 cases. Am J Clin Pathol 97: 751–758
1045. Petru E, Pickel H, Heydarfadai M et al. 1992 Nongenital cancers metastatic to the ovary. Gynecol Oncol 44: 83–86
1046. Birnkrant A, Sampson J, Sugarbaker P H 1986 Ovarian metastasis from colorectal cancer. Dis Colon Rectum 29: 767–771
1047. Blamey S L, McDermott F T, Pihl E et al. 1981 Resected ovarian recurrence from colorectal adenocarcinoma: a study of 13 cases. Dis Colon Rectum 24: 272–275
1048. MacKeigan J M, Ferguson J A 1979 Prophylactic oophorectomy and colorectal cancer in premenopausal patients. Dis Colon Rectum 22: 401–405
1049. Graffner H O, Alm P O, Oscarson J E 1983 Prophylactic oophorectomy in colorectal carcinoma. Am J Surg 146: 233–235
1050. Ballantyne G H, Reigel M M, Wolff B G et al. 1985 Oophorectomy and colon cancer. Impact on survival. Ann Surg 202: 209–214
1051. Sielezneff I, Salle E, Antoine K et al. 1997 Simultaneous bilateral oophorectomy does not improve prognosis of postmenopausal women undergoing colorectal resection for cancer. Dis Colon Rectum 40: 1299–1302
1052. Banerjee S, Kapur S, Moran B J 2005 The role of prophylactic oophorectomy in women undergoing surgery for colorectal cancer. Colorectal Dis 7: 214–217
1053. Tentes A, Markakidis S, Mirelis C et al. 2004 Oophorectomy during surgery for colorectal carcinoma. Tech Coloproctol 8 Suppl 1: s214–s216
1054. Blamey S, McDermott F, Pihl E et al. 1981 Ovarian involvement in adenocarcinoma of the colon and rectum. Surg Gynecol Obstet 153: 42–44
1055. Ayhan A, Guvenal T, Coskun F et al. 2003 Survival and prognostic factors in patients with synchronous ovarian and endometrial cancers and endometrial cancers metastatic to the ovaries. Eur J Gynaecol Oncol 24: 171–174
1056. Taylor A E, Nicolson V M C, Cunningham D 1995 Ovarian metastases from primary gastrointestinal malignancies: The Royal Marsden Hospital experience and implications for adjuvant treatment. Br J Cancer 71: 92–96
1057. Gagnon Y, Têtu B 1989 Ovarian metastases of breast carcinoma. A clinicopathologic study of 59 cases. Cancer 64: 892–898
1058. Simpkins F, Zahurak M, Armstrong D et al. 2005 Ovarian malignancy in breast cancer patients with an adnexal mass. Obstet Gynecol 105: 507–513
1059. Young R H, Carey R W, Robboy S J 1981 Breast carcinoma masquerading as primary ovarian neoplasm. Cancer 48: 210–212
1060. Lash R H, Hart W R 1987 Intestinal adenocarcinomas metastatic to the ovaries. A clinicopathologic evaluation of 22 cases. Am J Surg Pathol 11: 114–121
1061. Lee K R, Young R H 2003 The distinction between primary and metastatic mucinous carcinomas of the ovary: gross and histologic findings in 50 cases. Am J Surg Pathol 27: 281–292
1062. Scully R E, Richardson G S 1961 Luteinization of the stroma of metastatic cancer involving the ovary and its endocrine significance. Cancer 14: 827–840
1063. Hart W R 2005 Diagnostic challenge of secondary (metastatic) ovarian tumors simulating primary endometrioid and mucinous neoplasms. Pathol Int 55: 231–243
1064. DeCostanzo D C, Elias J M, Chumas J C 1997 Necrosis in 84 ovarian carcinomas: a morphologic study of primary versus metastatic colonic carcinoma with a selective immunohistochemical analysis of cytokeratin subtypes and carcinoembryonic antigen. Int J Gynecol Pathol 16: 245–249
1065. Ueda G, Sawada M, Ogawa H et al. 1993 Immunohistochemical study of cytokeratin 7 for the differential diagnosis of adenocarcinomas in the ovary. Gynecol Oncol 51: 219–223
1066. Berezowski K, Stastny J F, Kornstein M J 1996 Cytokeratins 7 and 20 and carcinoembryonic antigen in ovarian and colonic carcinoma. Mod Pathol 9: 426–429
1067. Loy T S, Calaluce R D, Keeney G L 1996 Cytokeratin immunostaining in differentiating primary ovarian carcinoma from metastatic colonic adenocarcinoma. Mod Pathol 9: 1040–1044
1068. Wauters C C A P, Smedts F, Gerrits L G M et al. 1995 Keratins 7 and 20 as diagnostic markers of carcinomas metastatic to the ovary. Hum Pathol 26: 852–855
1069. Wang N P, Zee S, Zarbo R J et al. 1995 Coordinate expression of cytokeratins 7 and 20 defines unique subsets of carcinomas. Appl Immunohistochem 3: 99–107
1070. Park S Y, Kim H S, Hong E K et al. 2002 Expression of cytokeratins 7 and 20 in primary carcinomas of the stomach and colorectum and their value in the differential diagnosis of metastatic carcinomas to the ovary. Hum Pathol 33: 1078–1085
1071. Werling R W, Yaziji H, Bacchi C E et al. 2003 CDX2, a highly sensitive and specific marker of adenocarcinomas of intestinal origin: an immunohistochemical survey of 476 primary and metastatic carcinomas. Am J Surg Pathol 27: 303–310
1072. Fraggetta F, Pelosi G, Cafici A et al. 2003 CDX2 immunoreactivity in primary and metastatic ovarian mucinous tumours. Virchow's Arch 443: 782–786
1073. Loy T S, Quesenberry J T, Sharp S C 1992 Distribution of CA 125 in adenocarcinomas: An immunohistochemical study of 481 cases. Am J Clin Pathol 98: 175–179
1074. Koelma I A, Nap M, Rodenburg C et al. 1987 The value of tumour marker CA 125 in surgical pathology. Histopathology 11: 287–294
1075. Leake J, Woolas R P, Daniel J et al. 1994 Immunocytochemical and serological expression of CA 125: A clinicopathological study of 40 malignant ovarian epithelial tumours. Histopathology 24: 57–64
1076. Fleuren G J, Nap M 1988 Carcinoembryonic antigen in primary and metastatic ovarian tumors. Gynecol Oncol 30: 407–415
1077. Merino M J, Edmonds P, LiVolsi V 1985 Appendiceal carcinoma metastatic to the ovaries and mimicking primary ovarian tumors. Int J Gynecol Pathol 4: 110–120
1078. Burke A P, Sobin L H, Federspiel B H et al. 1990 Goblet cell carcinoids and related tumors of the vermiform appendix. Am J Clin Pathol 94: 27–35
1079. Klein E A, Rosen M H 1996 Bilateral Krukenberg tumors due to appendiceal mucinous carcinoid. Int J Gynecol Pathol 15: 85–88
1080. Mandai M, Konishi I, Tsuruta Y et al. 2001 Krukenberg tumor from an occult appendiceal adenocarcinoid: a case report and review of the literature. Eur J Obstet Gynecol Reprod Biol 97: 90–95
1081. McBroom J W, Parker M F, Krivak T C et al. 2000 Primary appendiceal malignancy mimicking advanced stage ovarian carcinoma: a case series. Gynecol Oncol 78: 388–390
1082. Monteagudo C, Merino M J, LaPorte N et al. 1991 Value of gross cystic disease fluid protein-15 in distinguishing metastatic breast carcinomas among poorly differentiated neoplasms involving the ovary. Hum Pathol 22: 368–372
1083. Le Bouëdec G, De Latour M, Levrel O et al. 1997 Ovarian carcinoma mucocellular (Krukenberg's tumor): ten cases of breast cancer metastasis. Presse Med 26: 454–457
1084. Yakushiji M, Tazaki T, Nishimura H et al. 1987 Krukenberg tumors of the ovary: a clinicopathologic analysis of 112 cases. Nippon Sanka Fujinka Gakkai Zasshi 39: 479–485
1085. Wong P C, Ferenczy A, Fan L D et al. 1986 Krukenberg tumors of the ovary. Ultrastructural, histochemical and immunohistochemical studies of 15 cases. Cancer 57: 751–760
1086. Holtz F, Hart W R 1982 Krukenberg tumors of the ovary. A clinicopathologic analysis of 27 cases. Cancer 50: 2438–2447
1086a. Kiyokawa T, Young R H, Scully R E 2006 Krukenberg tumors of the ovary: a clinicopathologic analysis of 120 cases with emphasis on their variable pathologic manifestatations. Am J Surg Pathol 30: 277–299
1087. Hale R W 1968 Krukenberg tumor of the ovaries. A review of 81 records. Obstet Gynecol 32: 221–225
1088. Bullon A, Arseneau J, Prat J et al. 1981 Tubular Krukenberg tumor: a problem in histopathologic diagnosis. Am J Surg Pathol 5: 225–232
1089. Fung M F, Vadas G, Lotocki R et al. 1991 Tubular Krukenberg tumor in pregnancy with virilization. Gynecol Oncol 41: 81–84

1090. Joshi V V 1968 Primary Krukenberg tumor of ovary. Review of literature and case report. Cancer 22: 1199–1207
1091. Woodruff J D, Novak E R 1960 The Krukenberg tumor: Study of 48 cases from the Ovarian Tumor Registry. Obstet Gynecol 15: 351–360
1092. Galani E, Marx G M, Steer C B et al. 2003 Pseudomyxoma peritonei: the "controversial" disease. Int J Gynecol Cancer 13: 413–418
1093. Kahn M A, Demopoulos R I 1992 Mucinous ovarian tumors with pseudomyxoma peritonei: a clinicopathological study. Int J Gynecol Pathol 11: 15–23
1094. Prayson R A, Hart W R, Petras R E 1994 Pseudomyxoma peritonei: a clinicopathologic study of 19 cases with emphasis on site of origin and nature of associated ovarian tumors. Am J Surg Pathol 18: 591–603
1095. Ronnett B M, Zahn C M, Kurman R J et al. 1995 Disseminated peritoneal adenomucinosis and peritoneal mucinous carcinomatosis – A clinicopathologic analysis of 109 cases with emphasis on distinguishing pathologic features, site of origin, prognosis, and relationship to "Pseudomyxoma peritonei". Am J Surg Pathol 19: 1390–1408
1096. Young R H 2004 Pseudomyxoma peritonei and selected other aspects of the spread of appendiceal neoplasms. Semin Diagn Pathol 21: 134–150
1097. Gough D B, Donohue J H, Schutt A J et al. 1994 Pseudomyxoma peritonei: Long-term patient survival with an aggressive regional approach. Ann Surg 219: 112–119
1098. Miner T J, Shia J, Jaques D P et al. 2005 Long-term survival following treatment of pseudomyxoma peritonei: an analysis of surgical therapy. Ann Surg 241: 300–308
1099. Ronnett B M, Yan H, Kurman R J et al. 2001 Patients with pseudomyxoma peritonei associated with disseminated peritoneal adenomucinosis have a significantly more favorable prognosis than patients with peritoneal mucinous carcinomatosis. Cancer 92: 85–91
1100. Yan H, Pestieau S R, Shmookler B M et al. 2001 Histopathologic analysis in 46 patients with pseudomyxoma peritonei syndrome: failure versus success with a second-look operation. Mod Pathol 14: 164–171
1101. Bryant J, Clegg A J, Sidhu M K et al. 2005 Systematic review of the Sugarbaker procedure for pseudomyxoma peritonei. Br J Surg 92: 153–158
1102. Guner Z, Schmidt U, Dahlke M H et al. 2005 Cytoreductive surgery and intraperitoneal chemotherapy for pseudomyxoma peritonei. Int J Colorectal Dis 20: 155–160
1103. Deraco M, Baratti D, Inglese M G et al. 2004 Peritonectomy and intraperitoneal hyperthermic perfusion (IPHP): a strategy that has confirmed its efficacy in patients with pseudomyxoma peritonei. Ann Surg Oncol 11: 393–398
1104. Glehen O, Mohamed F, Gilly F N 2004 Peritoneal carcinomatosis from digestive tract cancer: new management by cytoreductive surgery and intraperitoneal chemohyperthermia. Lancet Oncol 5: 219–228
1105. Young R H, Gilks C B, Scully R E 1991 Mucinous tumors of the appendix associated with mucinous tumors of the ovary and pseudomyxoma peritonei. A clinicopathological analysis of 22 cases supporting an origin in the appendix. Am J Surg Pathol 15: 415–429
1106. Ronnett B M, Kurman R J, Zahn C M et al. 1995 Pseudomyxoma peritonei in women: a clinicopathologic analysis of 30 cases with emphasis on site of origin, prognosis, and relationship to ovarian mucinous tumors of low malignant potential. Hum Pathol 26: 509–524
1107. Guerrieri C, Franlund B, Boeryd B 1995 Expression of cytokeratin 7 in simultaneous mucinous tumors of the ovary and appendix. Mod Pathol 8: 573–576
1108. Ronnett B M, Shmookler B M, Diener-West M et al. 1997 Immunohistochemical evidence supporting the appendiceal origin of pseudomyxoma peritonei in women. Int J Gynecol Pathol 16: 1–9
1109. O'Connell J T, Hacker C M, Barsky S H 2002 MUC2 is a molecular marker for pseudomyxoma peritonei. Mod Pathol 15: 958–972
1110. O'Connell J T, Tomlinson J S, Roberts A A et al. 2002 Pseudomyxoma peritonei is a disease of MUC2-expressing goblet cells. Am J Pathol 161: 551–564
1111. Chuaqui R F, Zhuang Z P, Emmert-Buck M R et al. 1996 Genetic analysis of synchronous mucinous tumors of the ovary and appendix. Hum Pathol 27: 165–171
1112. Cuatrecasas M, Matias-Guiu X, Prat J 1996 Synchronous mucinous tumors of the appendix and the ovary associated with pseudomyxoma peritonei – A clinicopathologic study of six cases with comparative analysis of c-Ki-ras mutations. Am J Surg Pathol 20: 739–746
1113. Szych C, Staebler A, Connolly D C et al. 1999 Molecular genetic evidence supporting the clonality and appendiceal origin of Pseudomyxoma peritonei in women. Am J Pathol 154: 1849–1855
1114. Seidman J D, Elsayed A M, Sobin L H et al. 1993 Association of mucinous tumors of the ovary and appendix: A clinicopathologic study of 25 cases. Am J Surg Pathol 17: 22–34
1115. Du Plessis D G, Louw J A, Wranz B 1999 Mucinous epithelial cysts of the spleen associated with pseudomyxoma peritonei. Histopathology 35: 551–557
1116. Misdraji J, Young R H 2004 Primary epithelial neoplasms and other epithelial lesions of the appendix (excluding carcinoid tumors). Semin Diagn Pathol 21: 120–133
1117. Mukherjee A, Parvaiz A, Cecil T D et al. 2004 Pseudomyxoma peritonei usually originates from the appendix: a review of the evidence. Eur J Gynaecol Oncol 25: 411–414
1118. Lamps L W, Gray G F Jr, Dilday B R et al. 2000 The coexistence of low-grade mucinous neoplasms of the appendix and appendiceal diverticula: a possible role in the pathogenesis of pseudomyxoma peritonei. Mod Pathol 13: 495–501
1119. Misdraji J, Yantiss R K, Graeme-Cook F M et al. 2003 Appendiceal mucinous neoplasms: a clinicopathologic analysis of 107 cases. Am J Surg Pathol 27: 1089–1103
1120. Kabbani W, Houlihan P S, Luthra R et al. 2002 Mucinous and nonmucinous appendiceal adenocarcinomas: different clinicopathological features but similar genetic alterations. Mod Pathol 15: 599–605
1121. Clement P B 1993 Tumor-like lesions of the ovary associated with pregnancy. Int J Gynecol Pathol 12: 108–115
1122. Scully R E, Young R H, Clement P B 1998 Tumors of the ovary, maldeveloped gonads, fallopian tube, and broad ligament. Armed Forces Institute of Pathology, Washington, DC
1123. Clement P B, Young R H, Scully R E 1989 Nontrophoblastic pathology of the female genital tract and peritoneum associated with pregnancy. Semin Diagn Pathol 6: 372–406
1124. Hatjis C G 1985 Nonimmunologic fetal hydrops associated with hyperreactio luteinalis. Obstet Gynecol 65: 11S–3S
1125. Reubinoff B E, Mor-Yosef S, Shushan A et al. 1994 Hyperreactio luteinalis associated with non-immune hydrops fetalis – the role of pituitary hormones. Eur J Obstet Gynecol Reprod Biol 53: 144–146
1126. Schnorr J A Jr, Miller H, Davis J R et al. 1996 Hyperreactio luteinalis associated with pregnancy: a case report and review of the literature. Am J Perinatol 13: 95–97
1127. Bidus M A, Ries A, Magann E F et al. 2002 Markedly elevated beta-hCG levels in a normal singleton gestation with hyperreactio luteinalis. Obstet Gynecol 99: 958–961
1128. Csapo Z, Szabo I, Toth M et al. 1999 Hyperreactio luteinalis in a normal singleton pregnancy – A case report. J Reprod Med 44: 53–56
1129. Upadhyaya G, Goswami A, Babu S 2004 Bilateral theca lutein cysts: a rare cause of acute abdomen in pregnancy. Emerg Med Australas 16: 476–477
1130. Garcia-Bunuel R, Berek J S, Woodruff J D 1975 Luteomas of pregnancy. Obstet Gynecol 45: 407–414
1131. Norris H J, Taylor H B 1967 Nodular theca-lutein hyperplasia of pregnancy (so-called "pregnancy luteoma"). A clinical and pathologic study of 15 cases. Am J Clin Pathol 47: 557–566
1132. Sternberg W H, Barclay D L 1966 Luteoma of pregnancy. Am J Obstet Gynecol 95: 165–184
1133. Choi J R, Levine D, Finberg H 2000 Luteoma of pregnancy: sonographic findings in two cases. J Ultrasound Med 19: 877–881
1134. Hensleigh P A, Woodruff J D 1978 Differential maternal-fetal response to androgenizing luteoma or hyperreactio luteinalis. Obstet Gynecol Surv 33: 262–271
1135. Satyanarayana S, Bohre J K 2001 Ovarian granulosa cell "tumorlet" and mature follicles with ectopic decidua in pregnancy – a case report. Indian J Pathol Microbiol 44: 149–150
1136. Piana S, Nogales F F, Corrado S et al. 1999 Pregnancy luteoma with granulosa cell proliferation: an unusual hyperplastic lesion arising in pregnancy and mimicking an ovarian neoplasia. Pathol Res Pract 195: 859–863
1137. Chervenak F A, Castadot M, Wiederman J et al. 1980 Massive ovarian edema: a review of world's literature and report of two cases. Obstet Gynecol Surv 35: 677–684
1138. Kanbour A I, Salazar H, Tobon H 1979 Massive ovarian edema. A non-neoplastic pelvic mass of young women. Arch Pathol Lab Med 103: 42–45
1139. Roth L M, Deaton R L, Sternberg W H 1979 Massive ovarian edema. A clinicopathologic study of five cases including ultrastructural observations and review of the literature. Am J Surg Pathol 3: 11–21
1140. Young R H, Scully R E 1984 Fibromatosis and massive edema of the ovary, possibly related entities: a report of 14 cases of fibromatosis and 11 cases of massive edema. Int J Gynecol Pathol 3: 153–178
1141. Lara-Torre E, Geist R R, Rabinowitz R et al. 2005 Massive edema of the ovary: a case report and review of the pertinent literature. J Pediatr Adolesc Gynecol 18: 281–284
1142. Krasevic M, Haller H, Rupcic S et al. 2004 Massive edema of the ovary: a report of two cases due to lymphatic permeation by metastatic carcinoma from the uterine cervix. Gynecol Oncol 93: 564–567
1143. Bazot M, Detchev R, Cortez A et al. 2003 Massive ovarian edema revealing gastric carcinoma: a case report. Gynecol Oncol 91: 648–650
1144. Youngs L A, Taylor H B 1967 Adenomatoid tumors of the uterus and fallopian tube. Am J Clin Pathol 48: 537–545
1145. Stephenson T J, Mills P M 1986 Adenomatoid tumours: an immunohistochemical and ultrastructural appraisal of their histogenesis. J Pathol 148: 327–335
1146. Salazar H, Kanbour A, Burgess F 1972 Ultrastructure and observations on the histogenesis of mesotheliomas, "adenomatoid tumors", of the female genital tract. Cancer 29: 141–152
1147. Skinnider B F, Young R H 2004 Infarcted adenomatoid tumor: a report of five cases of a facet of a benign neoplasm that may cause diagnostic difficulty. Am J Surg Pathol 28: 77–83
1148. Nogales F F, Isaac M A, Hardisson D et al. 2002 Adenomatoid tumors of the uterus: an analysis of 60 cases. Int J Gynecol Pathol 21: 34–40
1149. Schwartz E J, Longacre T A 2004 Adenomatoid tumors of the female and male genital tracts express WT1. Int J Gynecol Pathol 23: 123–128
1150. Delahunt B, Eble J N, King D et al. 2000 Immunohistochemical evidence for mesothelial origin of paratesticular adenomatoid tumour. Histopathology 36: 109–115

1151. Alvarado-Cabrero I, Navani S S, Young R H et al. 1997 Tumors of the fimbriated end of the fallopian tube: a clinicopathologic analysis of 20 cases, including nine carcinomas. Int J Gynecol Pathol 16: 189–196
1152. De la Fuente A A 1982 Benign mixed Mullerian tumour–adenofibroma of the fallopian tube. Histopathology 6: 661–666
1153. Chen K T 1981 Bilateral papillary adenofibroma of the fallopian tube. Am J Clin Pathol 75: 229–231
1154. Kayaalp E, Heller D S, Majmudar B 2000 Serous tumor of low malignant potential of the fallopian tube. Int J Gynecol Pathol 19: 398–400
1155. Gurbuz Y, Ozkara S K 2003 Immunohistochemical profile of serous papillary cystadenofibroma of the fallopian tube: a clue of paramesonephritic origin. Appl Immunohistochem Mol Morphol 11: 153–155
1156. Zheng W X, Wolf S, Kramer E E et al. 1996 Borderline papillary serous tumor of the Fallopian tube. Am J Surg Pathol 20: 30–35
1157. Seidman J D 1994 Mucinous lesions of the Fallopian tube: A report of seven cases. Am J Surg Pathol 18: 1205–1212
1158. Honore L H, Dunnett I P 1976 Leiomyoma of the Fallopian tube. A case report and review of the literature. Arch Gynakol 221: 47–50
1159. Moore O A, Waxman M, Udoffia C 1979 Leiomyoma of the fallopian tube: a cause of tubal pregnancy. Am J Obstet Gynecol 134: 101–102
1160. Katz D A, Thom D, Bogard P et al. 1984 Angiomyolipoma of the fallopian tube. Am J Obstet Gynecol 148: 341–343
1161. Talerman A 1969 Haemangioma of the Fallopian tube. J Obstet Gynaecol Br Commonw 76: 559–560
1162. Ebrahimi T, Okagaki T 1973 Hemangioma of the Fallopian tube. Am J Obstet Gynecol 115: 864–865
1163. Joglekar V M 1979 Haemangioma of the fallopian tube. Case report. Br J Obstet Gynaecol 86: 823–825
1164. Kobayashi T, Suzuki K, Arai T et al. 1999 Angiomyofibroblastoma arising from the fallopian tube. Obstet Gynecol 94: 833–834
1165. Berzal-Cantalejo F, Montesinos-Carbonell M, Montesinos-Carbonell M L et al. 2005 Solitary fibrous tumor arising in the fallopian tube. Gynecol Oncol 96: 880–882
1166. Okagaki T, Richart R M 1970 Neurilemoma of the fallopian tube. Am J Obstet Gynecol 106: 929
1167. Duran B, Guvenal T, Yildiz E et al. 2004 An unusual cause of adnexal mass: fallopian tube schwannoma. Gynecol Oncol 92: 343–346
1168. Weber D L, Fazzini E 1970 Ganglioneuroma of the Fallopian tube. A heretofore unreported finding. Acta Neuropathol 16: 173–175
1169. Spanta R, Lawrence W D 1995 Soft tissue chondroma of the fallopian tube. Differential diagnosis and histogenetic considerations. Pathol Res Pract 191: 174–176
1170. Han J Y, Hwang H S, Kim Y B et al. 2002 Extraskeletal chondroma of the fallopian tube. J Korean Med Sci 17: 276–278
1171. Mazzarella P, Okagaki T, Richart R M 1972 Teratoma of the uterine tube. A case report and review of the literature. Obstet Gynecol 39: 381–388
1172. Hurd J K Jr 1978 Benign cystic teratoma of the fallopian tube. Obstet Gynecol 52: 362–364
1173. Kutteh W H, Albert T 1991 Mature cystic teratoma of the fallopian tube associated with an ectopic pregnancy. Obstet Gynecol 78: 984–986
1174. Yoshioka T, Tanaka T 2000 Mature solid teratoma of the fallopian tube: case report. Eur J Obstet Gynecol Reprod Biol 89: 205–206
1175. Alenghat E, Sassone A M, Talerman A 1982 Mature, solid teratoma of the fallopian tube. J Reprod Med 27: 484–486
1176. Baginski L, Yazigi R, Sandstad J 1989 Immature (malignant) teratoma of the fallopian tube. Am J Obstet Gynecol 160: 671–672
1177. Sweet R L, Selinger H E, McKay G 1975 Malignant teratoma of the uterine tube. Obstet Gynecol 45: 553–556
1178. Hoda S A, Huvos A G 1993 Struma salpingis associated with struma ovarii. Am J Surg Pathol 17: 1187–1189
1179. Astall E C, Brewster J A, Lonsdale R 2000 Malignant carcinoid tumour arising in a mature teratoma of the fallopian tube. Histopathology 36: 282–283
1180. Li S, Zimmerman R L, Livolsi V A 1999 Mixed malignant germ cell tumor of the fallopian tube. Int J Gynecol Pathol 18: 183–185
1181. Ajithkumar T V, Minimole A L, John M M et al. 2005 Primary fallopian tube carcinoma. Obstet Gynecol Surv 60: 247–252
1182. Alvarado-Cabrero I, Young R H, Vamvakas E C et al. 1999 Carcinoma of the fallopian tube: a clinicopathologic study of 105 cases with observations on staging and prognostic factors. Gynecol Oncol 72: 367–379
1183. Piura B, Rabinovich A 2000 Primary carcinoma of the fallopian tube: study of 11 cases. Eur J Obstet Gynecol Reprod Biol 91: 169–175
1184. Obermair A, Taylor K H, Janda M et al. 2001 Primary fallopian tube carcinoma: the Queensland experience. Int J Gynecol Cancer 11: 69–72
1185. Romagosa C, Torne A, Iglesias X et al. 2003 Carcinoma of the fallopian tube presenting as acute pelvic inflammatory disease. Gynecol Oncol 89: 181–184
1186. Demopoulos R I, Aronov R, Mesia A 2001 Clues to the pathogenesis of fallopian tube carcinoma: a morphological and immunohistochemical case control study. Int J Gynecol Pathol 20: 128–132
1187. Aziz S, Kuperstein G, Rosen B et al. 2001 A genetic epidemiological study of carcinoma of the fallopian tube. Gynecol Oncol 80: 341–345
1188. Zweemer R P, Van Diest P J, Verheijen R H et al. 2000 Molecular evidence linking primary cancer of the fallopian tube to BRCA1 germline mutations. Gynecol Oncol 76: 45–50
1189. Levine D A, Argenta P A, Yee C J et al. 2003 Fallopian tube and primary peritoneal carcinomas associated with BRCA mutations. J Clin Oncol 21: 4222–4227
1190. Paley P J, Swisher E M, Garcia R L et al. 2001 Occult cancer of the fallopian tube in BRCA-1 germline mutation carriers at prophylactic oophorectomy: a case for recommending hysterectomy at surgical prophylaxis. Gynecol Oncol 80: 176–180
1191. Carcangiu M L, Radice P, Manoukian S et al. 2004 Atypical epithelial proliferation in fallopian tubes in prophylactic salpingo-oophorectomy specimens from BRCA1 and BRCA2 germline mutation carriers. Int J Gynecol Pathol 23: 35–40
1192. Piek J M J, Van Diest P J, Zweemer R P et al. 2001 Dysplastic changes in prophylactically removed Fallopian tubes of women predisposed to developing ovarian cancer. J Pathol 195: 451–456
1193. Olivier R I, van B M, Lubsen M A et al. 2004 Clinical outcome of prophylactic oophorectomy in BRCA1/BRCA2 mutation carriers and events during follow-up. Br J Cancer 90: 1492–1497
1194. Scheuer L, Kauff N, Robson M et al. 2002 Outcome of preventive surgery and screening for breast and ovarian cancer in BRCA mutation carriers. J Clin Oncol 20: 1260–1268
1195. Gadducci A 2002 Current management of fallopian tube carcinoma. Curr Opin Obstet Gynecol 14: 27–32
1196. Takeshima N, Hasumi K 2000 Treatment of fallopian tube cancer. Review of the literature. Arch Gynecol Obstet 264: 13–19
1197. Cormio G, Maneo A, Gabriele A et al. 1996 Primary carcinoma of the fallopian tube. A retrospective analysis of 47 patients. Ann Oncol 7: 271–275
1198. Gemignani M L, Hensley M L, Cohen R et al. 2001 Paclitaxel-based chemotherapy in carcinoma of the fallopian tube. Gynecol Oncol 80: 16–20
1199. Baekelandt M, Nesbakken A J, Kristensen G B et al. 2000 Carcinoma of the fallopian tube – Clinicopathologic study of 151 patients treated at the Norwegian Radium Hospital. Cancer 89: 2076–2084
1200. Schneider C, Wight E, Perucchini D et al. 2000 Primary carcinoma of the fallopian tube. A report of 19 cases with literature review. Eur J Gynaecol Oncol 21: 578–582
1201. Rosen A C, Klein M, Hafner E et al. 1999 Management and prognosis of primary fallopian tube carcinoma. Austrian Cooperative Study Group for Fallopian Tube Carcinoma. Gynecol Obstet Invest 47: 45–51
1202. Peters W A III, Andersen W A, Hopkins M P 1989 Results of chemotherapy in advanced carcinoma of the fallopian tube. Cancer 63: 836–838
1203. Tulunay G, Arvas M, Demir B et al. 2004 Primary fallopian tube carcinoma: a retrospective multicenter study. Eur J Gynaecol Oncol 25: 611–614
1204. Kosary C, Trimble E L 2002 Treatment and survival for women with Fallopian tube carcinoma: a population-based study. Gynecol Oncol 86: 190–191
1205. Hefler L A, Rosen A G, Graf A H et al. 2000 The clinical value of serum concentrations of cancer antigen 125 in patients with primary fallopian tube carcinoma. A multicenter study. Cancer 89: 1555–1560
1205a. Medeiros F, Muto M G, Lee Y et al. 2006 The tubal fimbria is a preferred site for early adenocarcinoma in women with familial ovarian cancer syndrome. Am J Surg Pathol 30: 230–236
1206. Yanai-Inbar I, Silverberg S G 2000 Mucosal epithelial proliferation of the fallopian tube: prevalence, clinical associations, and optimal strategy for histopathologic assessment. Int J Gynecol Pathol 19: 139–144
1207. di Re E, Grosso G, Raspagliesi F et al. 1996 Fallopian tube cancer: incidence and role of lymphatic spread. Gynecol Oncol 62: 199–202
1208. Navani S S, Alvarado-Cabrero I, Young R H et al. 1996 Endometrioid carcinoma of the fallopian tube: a clinicopathologic analysis of 26 cases. Gynecol Oncol 63: 371–378
1209. Daya D, Young R H, Scully R E 1992 Endometrioid carcinoma of the fallopian tube resembling an adnexal tumor of probable Wolffian origin: a report of six cases. Int J Gynecol Pathol 11: 122–130
1210. Williamson J M S, Armour A 1993 Microcystic endometrioid carcinoma of the Fallopian tube simulating an adnexal tumour of probable Wolffian origin. Histopathology 23: 578–580
1211. Fukunaga M, Bisceglia M, Dimitri L 2004 Endometrioid carcinoma of the fallopian tube resembling a female adnexal tumor of probable wolffian origin. Adv Anat Pathol 11: 269–272
1212. Barakat R R, Rubin S C, Saigo P E et al. 1991 Cisplatin-based combination chemotherapy in carcinoma of the fallopian tube. Gynecol Oncol 42: 156–160
1213. Hartley A, Rollason T, Spooner D 2000 Clear cell carcinoma of the fimbria of the fallopian tube in a BRCA1 carrier undergoing prophylactic surgery. Clin Oncol (R Coll Radiol) 12: 58–59
1214. Voet R L, Lifshitz S 1982 Primary clear cell adenocarcinoma of the fallopian tube: light microscopic and ultrastructural findings. Int J Gynecol Pathol 1: 292–298
1215. Cheung A N, So K F, Ngan H Y et al. 1994 Primary squamous cell carcinoma of fallopian tube. Int J Gynecol Pathol 13: 92–95
1216. Jackson-York G L, Ramzy I 1992 Synchronous papillary mucinous adenocarcinoma of the endocervix and fallopian tubes. Int J Gynecol Pathol 11: 63–67
1217. Herbold D R, Axelrod J H, Bobowski S J et al. 1988 Glassy cell carcinoma of the fallopian tube. A case report. Int J Gynecol Pathol 7: 384–390

1218. Aoyama T, Mizuno T, Andoh K et al. 1996 alpha-Fetoprotein-producing (hepatoid) carcinoma of the fallopian tube. Gynecol Oncol 63: 261–266
1219. Dursun P, Salman M C, Taskiran C et al. 2004 Primary neuroendocrine carcinoma of the fallopian tube: a case report. Am J Obstet Gynecol 190: 568–571
1220. Peters W A III, Andersen W A, Hopkins M P et al. 1988 Prognostic features of carcinoma of the fallopian tube. Obstet Gynecol 71: 757–762
1221. Benda J A, Veronezi-Gurwell A, Wilcox M et al. 1994 An unusual extrauterine variant of adenosarcoma with multiple recurrences over 16 years. Gynecol Oncol 53: 131–137
1222. Gollard R, Kosty M, Bordin G et al. 1995 Two unusual presentations of mullerian adenosarcoma: case reports, literature review, and treatment considerations. Gynecol Oncol 59: 412–422
1223. Carlson J A Jr, Ackerman B L, Wheeler J E 1993 Malignant mixed Müllerian tumor of the fallopian tube. Cancer 71: 187–192
1224. Weber A M, Hewett W F, Gajewski W H et al. 1993 Malignant mixed mullerian tumors of the fallopian tube. Gynecol Oncol 50: 239–243
1225. Horn L C, Werschnik C, Bilek K et al. 1996 Diagnosis and clinical management in malignant Mullerian tumors of the fallopian tube. A report of four cases and review of recent literature. Arch Gynecol Obstet 258: 47–53
1226. Imachi M, Tsukamoto N, Shigematsu T et al. 1992 Malignant mixed Mullerian tumor of the fallopian tube: report of two cases and review of literature. Gynecol Oncol 47: 114–124
1227. Muntz H G, Rutgers J L, Tarraza H et al. 1989 Carcinosarcomas and mixed Mullerian tumors of the fallopian tube. Gynecol Oncol 34: 109–115
1228. Buchino J J, Buchino J J 1987 Malignant mixed mullerian tumor of the fallopian tube. Arch Pathol Lab Med 111: 386–387
1229. Lim B J, Kim J W, Yang W I et al. 2004 Malignant mixed mullerian tumor of fallopian tube with multiple distinct heterologous components. Int J Gynecol Cancer 14: 690–693
1230. Manes J L, Taylor H B 1976 Carcinosarcoma and mixed mullerian tumors of the fallopian tube: report of four cases. Cancer 38: 1687–1693
1231. van Dijk C M, Kooijman C D, van Lindert A C 1990 Malignant mixed mullerian tumour of the fallopian tube. Histopathology 16: 300–302
1232. Gagner J P, Mittal K 2005 Malignant mixed Mullerian tumor of the fimbriated end of the fallopian tube: origin as an intraepithelial carcinoma. Gynecol Oncol 97: 219–222
1233. Ebert A D, Perez-Canto A, Schaller G et al. 1998 Stage I primary malignant mixed mullerian tumor of the fallopian tube. Report of a case with five-year survival after minimal surgery without adjuvant treatment. J Reprod Med 43: 598–600
1234. Jacoby A F, Fuller A F J, Thor A D et al. 1993 Primary leiomyosarcoma of the fallopian tube. Gynecol Oncol 51: 404–407
1235. Ebert A, Goetze B, Herbst H et al. 1995 Primary leiomyosarcoma of the fallopian tube. Ann Oncol 6: 618–619
1236. Buchwalter C L, Jenison E L, Fromm M et al. 1997 Pure embryonal rhabdomyosarcoma of the fallopian tube. Gynecol Oncol 67: 95–101
1237. Halligan A W, McGuinness E P 1990 Malignant fibrous histiocytoma of the fallopian tube. Br J Obstet Gynaecol 97: 275–276
1238. Noack F, Lange N, Lehmann V et al. 2002 Primary extranodal marginal zone B-cell lymphoma of the fallopian tube. Gynecol Oncol 86: 384–386
1239. Gaffan J, Herbertson R, Davis P et al. 2004 Bilateral peripheral T-cell lymphoma of the fallopian tubes. Gynecol Oncol 95: 736–738
1240. Goodlad J R, MacPherson S, Jackson R et al. 2004 Extranodal follicular lymphoma: a clinicopathological and genetic analysis of 15 cases arising at non-cutaneous extranodal sites. Histopathology 44: 268–276
1241. Muto M G, Lage J M, Berkowitz R S et al. 1991 Gestational trophoblastic disease of the fallopian tube. J Reprod Med 36: 57–60
1242. Newcomer J R 1998 Ampullary tubal hydatidiform mole treated with linear salpingotomy. A case report. J Reprod Med 43: 913–915
1243. Terada S, Suzuki N, Uchide K et al. 1993 Partial hydatidiform mole in the fallopian tube. Gynecol Obstet Invest 35: 240–242
1244. Montgomery E A, Roberts E F, Conran R M et al. 1993 Triploid abortus presenting as an ectopic pregnancy. Arch Pathol Lab Med 117: 652–653
1245. Burton J L, Lidbury E A, Gillespie A M et al. 2001 Over-diagnosis of hydatidiform mole in early tubal ectopic pregnancy. Histopathology 38: 409–417
1246. Dekel A, Van Iddekinge B, Isaacson C et al. 1986 Primary choriocarcinoma of the fallopian tube. Report of a case with survival and postoperative delivery. Review of the literature. Obstet Gynecol Surv 41: 142–148
1247. Lee S M, Kang J H, Oh S Y et al. 2005 A successfully treated case of primary tubal choriocarcinoma coexistent with viable intrauterine pregnancy. Gynecol Oncol 97: 671–673
1248. Bakri Y N, Amri A, Mulla J 1992 Gestational choriocarcinoma in a tubal ectopic pregnancy. Acta Obstet Gynecol Scand 71: 67–68
1249. Su Y N, Cheng W F, Chen C A et al. 1999 Pregnancy with primary tubal placental site trophoblastic tumor – A case report and literature review. Gynecol Oncol 73: 322–325
1250. Baergen R N, Rutgers J, Young R H 2003 Extrauterine lesions of intermediate trophoblast. Int J Gynecol Pathol 22: 362–367
1251. Parker A, Lee V, Dalrymple C et al. 2003 Epithelioid trophoblastic tumour: report of a case in the fallopian tube. Pathology 35: 136–140
1252. Kuo K T, Chen M J, Lin M C 2004 Epithelioid trophoblastic tumor of the broad ligament: a case report and review of the literature. Am J Surg Pathol 28: 405–409
1253. Campello T R, Fittipaldi H, O'Valle F et al. 1998 Extrauterine (tubal) placental site nodule. Histopathology 32: 562–565
1254. Kouvidou C, Karayianni M, Liapi-Avgeri G et al. 2000 Old ectopic pregnancy remnants with morphological features of placental site nodule occurring in fallopian tube and broad ligament. Pathol Res Pract 196: 329–332
1255. Nayar R, Snell J, Silverberg S G et al. 1996 Placental site nodule occurring in a fallopian tube. Hum Pathol 27: 1243–1245
1256. Falls J L 1955 Accessory adrenal cortex in the broad ligament. Incidence and functional significance. Cancer 8: 142–150
1257. Wild R A, Albert R D, Zaino R J et al. 1988 Virilizing paraovarian tumors: a consequence of Nelson's syndrome? Obstet Gynecol 71: 1053–1056
1258. Verdonk C, Guerin C, Lufkin E et al. 1982 Activation of virilizing adrenal rest tissues by excessive ACTH production. An unusual presentation of Nelson's syndrome. Am J Med 73: 455–459
1259. van Ingen G, Schoemaker J, Baak J P 1991 A testosterone-producing tumour in the mesovarium. Pathol Res Pract 187: 362–370
1260. Sasano H, Sato S, Yajima A et al. 1997 Adrenal rest tumor of the broad ligament: case report with immunohistochemical study of steroidogenic enzymes. Pathol Int 47: 493–496
1261. Keitoku M, Konishi I, Nanbu K et al. 1997 Extraovarian sex cord-stromal tumor: case report and review of the literature. Int J Gynecol Pathol 16: 180–185
1262. Lin H H, Chen Y P, Lee T Y 1987 A hormone-producing thecoma of broad ligament. Acta Obstet Gynecol Scand 66: 725–727
1263. Shone N, Duggan M A, Ghatage P 2003 Granulosa cell tumour of the broad ligament. Pathology 35: 265–267
1264. Steed H, Oza A, Chapman W B et al. 2004 Female adnexal tumor of probable wolffian origin: a clinicopathological case report and a possible new treatment. Int J Gynecol Cancer 14: 546–550
1265. Atallah D, Rouzier R, Voutsadakis I et al. 2004 Malignant female adnexal tumor of probable wolffian origin relapsing after pregnancy. Gynecol Oncol 95: 402–404
1266. Ramirez P T, Wolf J K, Malpica A et al. 2002 Wolffian duct tumors: case reports and review of the literature. Gynecol Oncol 86: 225–230
1267. Prasad C J, Ray J A, Kessler S 1992 Female adnexal tumor of wolffian origin. Arch Pathol Lab Med 116: 189–191
1268. Brescia R J, Cardoso de Almeida P C, Fuller A F J et al. 1985 Female adnexal tumor of probable Wolffian origin with multiple recurrences over 16 years. Cancer 56: 1456–1461
1269. Daya D 1994 Malignant female adnexal tumor of probable wolffian origin with review of the literature. Arch Pathol Lab Med 118: 310–312
1270. Sheyn I, Mira J L, Bejarano P A et al. 2000 Metastatic female adnexal tumor of probable wolffian origin – A case report and review of the literature. Arch Pathol Lab Med 124: 431–434
1271. Karpuz V, Berger S D, Burkhardt K et al. 1999 A case of endometrioid carcinoma of the fallopian tube mimicking an adnexal tumor of probable Wolffian origin. APMIS 107: 550–554
1272. Tiltman A J, Allard U 2001 Female adnexal tumours of probable Wolffian origin: an immunohistochemical study comparing tumours, mesonephric remnants and paramesonephric derivatives. Histopathology 38: 237–242
1273. Stewart G J R, Nandini C L, Richmond J A 2000 Value of A103 (melan-A) immunostaining in the differential diagnosis of ovarian sex cord stromal tumours. J Clin Pathol 53: 206–211
1274. Genadry R, Parmley T, Woodruff J D 1977 The origin and clinical behavior of the parovarian tumor. Am J Obstet Gynecol 15 129: 873–880
1275. Honore L H, O'Hara K E 1980 Serous papillary neoplasms arising in paramesonephric parovarian cysts. A report of eight cases. Acta Obstet Gynecol Scand 59: 525–528
1276. Aslani M, Ahn G H, Scully R E 1988 Serous papillary cystadenoma of borderline malignancy of broad ligament. A report of 25 cases. Int J Gynecol Pathol 7: 131–138
1277. Aslani M, Scully R E 1989 Primary carcinoma of the broad ligament. Report of four cases and review of the literature. Cancer 64: 1540–1545
1278. d'Ablaing G III, Klatt E C, DiRocco G et al. 1983 Broad ligament serous tumor of low malignant potential. Int J Gynecol Pathol 2: 93–99
1279. Hampton H L, Huffman H T, Meeks G R 1992 Extraovarian Brenner tumor. Obstet Gynecol 79: 844–846
1280. Kobayashi Y, Yamazaki K, Shinohara M et al. 1996 Undifferentiated carcinoma of the broad ligament in a 28-year-old woman – a case report and results of immunohistochemical and electron-microscopic studies. Gynecol Oncol 63: 382–387
1281. Altaras M M, Jaffe R, Corduba M et al. 1990 Primary paraovarian cystadenocarcinoma: clinical and management aspects and literature review. Gynecol Oncol 38: 268–272
1282. Mrad K, Driss M, Abdelmoula S et al. 2005 Primary broad ligament cystadenocarcinoma with mucinous component: a case report with immunohistochemical study. Arch Pathol Lab Med 129: 244–246
1283. Lonser R R, Glenn G M, Walther M et al. 2003 von Hippel-Lindau disease. Lancet 361: 2059–2067
1284. Friedrich C A 1999 Von Hippel-Lindau syndrome – A pleomorphic condition. Cancer 86: 1658–1662
1285. Aydin H, Young R H, Ronnett B M et al. 2005 Clear cell papillary cystadenoma of the epididymis and mesosalpinx: immunohistochemical differentiation from metastatic clear cell renal cell carcinoma. Am J Surg Pathol 29: 520–523

1286. Gersell D J, King T C 1988 Papillary cystadenoma of the mesosalpinx in von Hippel-Lindau disease. Am J Surg Pathol 12: 145–149
1287. Korn W T, Schatzki S C, DiSciullo A J et al. 1990 Papillary cystadenoma of the broad ligament in von Hippel-Lindau disease. Am J Obstet Gynecol 163: 596–598
1288. Werness B A, Guccion J G 1997 Tumor of the broad ligament in von Hippel-Lindau disease of probable mullerian origin. Int J Gynecol Pathol 16: 282–285
1289. Gaffey M J, Mills S E, Boyd J C 1994 Aggressive papillary tumor of middle ear/temporal bone and adnexal papillary cystadenoma: manifestations of von Hippel-Lindau disease. Am J Surg Pathol 18: 1254–1260
1290. Breen J L, Neubecker R D 1962 Tumors of the round ligament. A review of the literature and a report of 25 cases. Obstet Gynecol 19: 771–780
1291. Sonobe H, Ohtsuki Y, Iwata J et al. 1995 Myolipoma of the round ligament: report of a case with a review of the English literature. Virchow's Arch 427: 455–458
1292. Fink D, Marsden D E, Edwards L et al. 2004 Malignant perivascular epithelioid cell tumor (PEComa) arising in the broad ligament. Int J Gynecol Cancer 14: 1036–1039
1293. Chopra R, Al Mulhim A R, Hashish H 2003 Parametrial angiomyolipoma with multicystic change. Gynecol Oncol 90: 220–223
1294. Bakotic B W, Cabello-Inchausti B, Willis I H et al. 1999 Clear-cell epithelioid leiomyoma of the round ligament. Mod Pathol 12: 912–918
1295. Roth L M, Reed R J, Sternberg W H 1996 Cotyledonoid dissecting leiomyoma of the uterus – The Sternberg tumor. Am J Surg Pathol 20: 1455–1461
1296. Roth L M, Reed R J 2000 Cotyledonoid leiomyoma of the uterus: report of a case. Int J Gynecol Pathol 19: 272–275
1297. Mulvany N J, Slavin J L, Ostor A G et al. 1994 Intravenous leiomyomatosis of the uterus: a clinicopathologic study of 22 cases. Int J Gynecol Pathol 13: 1–9
1298. Cheng W F, Lin H H, Chen C K et al. 1995 Leiomyosarcoma of the broad ligament: a case report and literature review. Gynecol Oncol 56: 85–89
1299. Shah A, Finn C, Light A 2003 Leiomyosarcoma of the broad ligament: a case report and literature review. Gynecol Oncol 90: 450–452
1300. Ahmed A A, Swan R W, Owen A et al. 1997 Uterus-like mass arising in the broad ligament: a metaplasia or mullerian duct anomaly? Int J Gynecol Pathol 16: 279–281
1301. Al Jafari M S, Panton H M, Gradwell E 1985 Phaeochromocytoma of the broad ligament. Case report. Br J Obstet Gynaecol 92: 649–651
1302. Dieste M C, Lynch G R, Gordon A et al. 1987 Malignant fibrous histiocytoma of the broad ligament: a case report and literature review. Gynecol Oncol 28: 225–229
1303. Fras A P, Frkovic-Grazio S 2001 Hyalinizing spindle cell tumor with giant rosettes of the broad ligament. Gynecol Oncol 83: 405–408
1304. Nielsen G P, Oliva E, Young R H et al. 1995 Alveolar soft-part sarcoma of the female genital tract: a report of nine cases and review of the literature. Int J Gynecol Pathol 14: 283–292
1305. Duggan M A, Hugh J, Nation J G et al. 1989 Ependymoma of the uterosacral ligament. Cancer 64: 2565–2571
1306. Bell D A, Woodruff J M, Scully R E 1984 Ependymoma of the broad ligament. A report of two cases. Am J Surg Pathol 8: 203–209
1307. Grody W W, Nieberg R K, Bhuta S 1985 Ependymoma-like tumor of the mesovarium. Arch Pathol Lab Med 109(3): 291–293
1308. Komuro Y, Mikami M, Sakaiya N et al. 2001 Tumor imprint cytology of ovarian ependymoma – A case report. Cancer 92: 3165–3169
1309. Kleinman G M, Young R H, Scully R E 1984 Ependymoma of the ovary: report of three cases. Hum Pathol 15: 632–638.

第二部分

子宫内膜
Endometrium

George L. Mutter 和 Tan A. Ince 著

戴 林 译　回允中 校

子宫内膜		子宫内膜腺癌	660
子宫内膜腺体肿瘤形成	652	子宫内膜癌的预后因素	660
子宫内膜癌前病变标准和命名的变化过程	653	子宫内膜样腺癌	661
EIN，子宫内膜样（Ⅰ型）子宫内膜腺癌的前体病变	654	乳头状浆液性和透明细胞癌	662
		显示混合性分化的肿瘤	663
子宫内膜上皮内肿瘤形成	655	子宫内膜间质肿瘤	667
乳头状浆液性腺癌的前体病变	660	非Müller肿瘤	669

子宫内膜腺体肿瘤形成
Endometrial glandular neoplasia

发病率和发病机制

子宫内膜癌有不同的组织学亚型（表13B.1），是女性生殖道最常见的浸润性癌，除了皮肤癌以外，占所有女性浸润性癌的7%。从前子宫内膜癌比宫颈癌少见得多，但是随着宫颈鳞状上皮内病变（SIL）的早期诊断和治疗以及较年轻年龄组子宫内膜癌患者的增加，使这两个肿瘤的发生比例翻转过来。在美国现在每年新增子宫内膜癌患者40 100人，而新的浸润性宫颈癌12 200人[1]。尽管子宫内膜癌的发病率高，但它通常发生在绝经后的妇女，并引起异常（绝经后）出血。因此一般可以早期发现并在病变的早期阶段进行治疗[2]。

子宫内膜癌在40岁以前的女性患者中是不常见的。它的发病高峰在55～65岁。这个肿瘤较常见于肥胖、糖尿病（60%以上的患者有葡萄糖耐量异常）、高血压和不孕患者。发生子宫内膜癌的妇女倾向于是未经产和具有无排卵功能性月经不规则的病史。少数情况下，子宫内膜癌和乳腺癌可以发生在同一个患者[3]。

根据肿瘤可能存在的不同发病机制，一般可以将子宫内膜癌分为Ⅰ型和Ⅱ型[4]。第一种亚型（Ⅰ型癌）研究得最充分，发生在长期雌激素刺激的背景上，而且常有以诊断性病变[子宫内膜上皮内肿瘤形成（EIN），或非典型子宫内膜增生]为特征的癌前阶段。Ⅰ型子宫内膜肿瘤形成的两种病变（癌前病变和癌）似乎与肥胖和无排卵周期有关，无排卵周期的子宫内膜受到非对抗性雌激素刺激的作用。提示与激素病理生理学有关的其他证据包括：

1. 患有卵巢分泌雌激素肿瘤的妇女发生子宫内膜癌的危险性较高。
2. 卵巢发育不全和较早就将卵巢切除的妇女，发生子宫内膜癌的非常罕见。
3. 没有孕激素对抗的雌激素替代疗法与妇女发病的危险性增加有关，长期给实验动物投予己烯雌酚（DES）可以引起子宫内膜息肉、子宫内膜增生和癌。
4. 绝经后妇女，由肾上腺和卵巢产生的雄激素前体在体内脂肪中能够合成较多的雌激素，这种所见可以部分解释为什么子宫内膜癌危险性的增加与年龄和肥胖有关。

表13B.1　子宫内膜癌分类和分级

子宫内膜样癌
（根据肿瘤组织的结构分为1～3级，肿瘤细胞核具有明显非典型性增加一级）
- 伴有分泌分化
- 伴有纤毛分化
- 伴有鳞状分化

浆液性腺癌（根据定义为3级）
透明细胞癌（根据定义为3级）
黏液性腺癌（属于子宫内膜样癌，分1～3级）
鳞状细胞癌
混合性癌
未分化癌
其他罕见类型，例如移行细胞癌

与前述危险因素有关的子宫内膜癌倾向于高分化，而且其组织学表现酷似正常子宫内膜腺体（子宫内膜样）。在子宫内膜样或I型癌中，分泌性、鳞状上皮、黏液性和嗜酸性输卵管分化也可能是肿瘤的一种成分。如同下面描述的一样，这一组肿瘤一般具有较好的预后。

然而必须注意，应该避免将雌激素与子宫内膜癌之间的流行病学相关性，看成是所有与非对抗性雌激素作用有关的子宫内膜病变都是低危癌前病变的证据。对于围绝经期妇女来说，反复出现无排卵性月经周期是正常的，而这个时期正好就在子宫内膜癌发病高峰50～70岁之前，此时I型癌的发病率增加。有多少这样的患者由于与无排卵周期有关的子宫内膜病变而切除了子宫还不清楚。

第二种亚型的子宫内膜癌至关重要，患者年龄较大，先前并不伴随雌激素过多或癌前的EIN病变。这一组肿瘤（II型癌）一般分化较差，包括类似于卵巢癌亚型（乳头状浆液性癌）的肿瘤。总的来说，这些肿瘤的预后比子宫内膜样癌要差，其好发因素还不清楚[4]。

分子生物学研究已经证实，子宫内膜腺癌的子宫内膜样亚型与浆液性亚型具有不同的发病机制。位于10q23部位的 *PTEN* 肿瘤抑制基因失活与子宫内膜样肿瘤有关，而新近研究提示，1p 丢失可能主要发生在浆液性肿瘤[5,6]。*p53* 功能丢失（免疫组化检查显示异常蛋白聚集）在浆液性亚型也比子宫内膜样病变常见[7]，而透明细胞癌居于两者之间[8]。微卫星不稳定性在子宫内膜样癌比浆液性癌常见[9]。

子宫内膜样子宫内膜癌发生的时相
Phases of endometrioid endometrial carcinogenesis

基于肿瘤进展过程中基因突变驱使的连续克隆选择制作的子宫内膜肿瘤发生的动态模型（图13B.1），与已经提出的其他几个肿瘤相似[10-13]。每次连续克隆选择都是通过与亲体成分的成功竞争发生的。

在哺乳动物，特殊细胞谱系的克隆性增生发生在限定的环境下。例如，建立B细胞克隆能够产生大量的特殊抗体。另外，多数驱体组织为多克隆性，除非在损伤的周围组织中的部分增生细胞具有明显的生长优势。因此，子宫内膜组织的克隆性增生可以被看做是创建具有生长优势的一个细胞或一群细胞的证据，这就是肿瘤性病变的特征。

应用来自这个模型的各种分子标记系统，现在已经能够确定可辨认最早期子宫内膜样子宫内膜癌（I型）的癌前病变。其中包括单个患者在癌前和癌发生之间 *PTEN* 和 *K-ras* 基因突变谱系的持续（正向延续）[17-19] 以及证实癌前病变的单克隆性生长[14-16]。组织形态检查证实的子宫内膜前病变的分子生物学特征，已经允许用

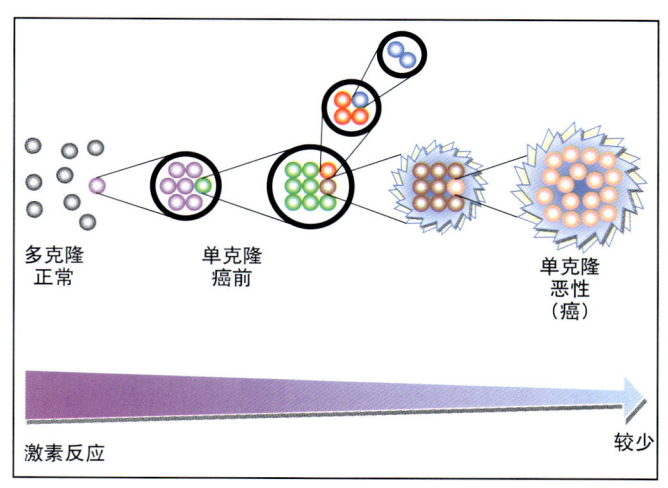

图13B.1　子宫内膜肿瘤发生过程的模型。癌前病变是单克隆性肿瘤，它开始于正常多克隆组织的突变，在非对抗性雌激素促有丝分裂的作用下，突变造成生长潜能轻度增加。通过突变和选择，癌前病变克隆得以发生和发展，最终达到不再需要激素支持而存在的阶段。足够的基因损伤积累造成这些癌前病变恶性转化，并浸润邻近的间质组织。

于描述癌前病变的组织病理学特征[20,21]。这些病变称作EIN，与以前应用的世界卫生组织（WHO）增生纲要相比，在生物学上是比较一致的具有高癌危险的子宫内膜。

子宫内膜癌前病变标准和命名的变化过程
Changing landscape of endometrial precancer criteria and terminology

长期以来，前瞻性研究支持子宫内膜样子宫内膜癌存在前驱病变这一假设，在出现其本身尚不足以诊断为癌的独特的组织病理学表现之后，随后发生癌的危险性增高。在子宫内膜增生的各种亚型中，患有子宫内膜非典型性增生的妇女发生癌的危险性最高。传统上，WHO根据细胞是否有非典型性和结构形态是单纯还是复杂，将子宫内膜增生分为4组[22-24]。在这4组中，患有非典型性腺瘤性增生的妇女，在子宫切除后发现25%同时存在有腺癌[24,25]，而且将来发生腺癌的危险性增加14倍[22]。这就形成了一种概念，诊断非典型性增生也就意味着病变达到了危险的阈值，有理由进行手术干预或激素治疗。相反，对于治疗这个诊断范畴内没有非典型性的增生却存在着明显的挑战，因为它具有较低但是仍然明显的发生癌的危险。

WHO子宫内膜增生亚型诊断的可重复性差，使得病理医师感到困扰，新近研究显示，诊断为子宫内膜非典型性增生的病例，经过第二个病理医师复检只有一半或少于一半得到证实[14,26-28]。最重要的也许是癌的结局

降低了这种方法的阴性预测价值，因为没有非典型性的子宫内膜增生患者癌的发生频率也高。总之，仅仅根据以前所采用的形态学方法很难将子宫内膜增生分为良性和癌前病变。因此，我们在这里提出了一种诊断子宫内膜癌前病变的替代方法，它结合了近十年来对这个病变相关认识的新的重要进展。

EIN，子宫内膜样（I型）子宫内膜腺癌的前体病变
EIN, a precursor to endometrioid (type I) endometrial adenocarcinoma

HE切片的计算机形态测量分析显示，这些癌前病变腺体的表面积均大于间质[15,20]。腺体结构特征在辨认癌前病变中具有重要作用，这一概念完全不同于WHO子宫内膜增生分类系统中长期强调的细胞核的改变。它推动了新的诊断模式的发展，其中癌前病变被命名为EIN，它是联合应用结构和细胞学标准进行诊断的，根本不同于过去用于增生分型的标准[15,16]。虽然发现这种结构特征是借助图像分析完成的，但是由此引出的诊断标准并不需要特殊的仪器。

为了清楚地了解早期阶段子宫内膜的致癌作用，对于EIN的分子生物学、临床和组织学特征要有充分的认识[29,30]。PTEN肿瘤抑制基因突变出现在常规光学显微镜下所见的任何明显的组织病理学变化之前[31]。有人认为（尚未特别提出），其他的基因变化引起形态学上已有改变的子宫内膜腺体出现局灶性亚克隆性膨胀性生长，表现为结构密集（腺体成分超过间质）和细胞学改变[20,32]。EIN病变的细胞学变化总是不同于周围背景正常子宫内膜的细胞学，早期阶段在低倍镜下观察容易发现，确定EIN病变的密集腺体和规则分布的不密集的正常子宫内膜腺体的细胞学不同。EIN病变基本的细胞学表现在不同患者之间有明显的差异，可能包括细胞浆分化（输卵管、黏液性、嗜酸性、乳头状）或细胞核大小、结构和形状的变化。结合形态测量和分子生物学分析显示，不是所有的EIN病变都具有显著的圆形细胞核和明显核仁等非典型性核的典型特征。相反，它的形状可能不同于背景，表现为细胞较长或大小不同。重要的表现是在结构形态发生了改变的腺体中细胞学具有一致的变化。

在临床上应用EIN标准预测癌的发生优于从前的WHO子宫内膜增生的标准[33]。477例长期随访患者子宫内膜详细形态测量评估显示，一旦细胞学改变和腺体密集符合EIN标准的病变最大径至少为1mm时，预期（至少一年后）患者发生子宫内膜癌的危险性增加45倍[34]。同时发生癌的危险性也高达大约27%[35]。没有EIN的阴性预测价值相对较高，达到99%[34]。这些对于非典型性子宫内膜增生发生癌的最大优势比为7～27倍，阴性预测价值98%[22,33,34]。病理医师将EIN纲要主观用于医院常规诊断的97例子宫内膜"增生"，显示EIN诊断具有非常好的可重复性，诊断者之间Kappa值为0.73～0.90，三位病理医师的诊断一致性为75%。所有8例（100%）存在EIN的病例最终诊断为癌，而这8例从前归在非典型性增生（n=5）和无非典型性（n=3）的子宫内膜增生范畴[36]。

EIN的诊断

命名法 nomenclature

表13B.2和13B.3显示EIN方案的诊断分类，其中每一类别均有不同的治疗策略[37]。在治疗策略方面可能存在局部差异，最重要的是要区分与之相关的诊断边界。例如在美国，将来打算生育的妇女如果患有癌前病变，经常考虑是应用伴有孕激素的激素治疗消除病变还是选择子宫切除。必须明确区分EIN和腺癌，因为后者常规处理是手术切除。在某些欧洲国家，子宫内膜癌前病变和癌在治疗上的这种差异关系不大，在那里对于这两种诊断的治疗标准都可以是子宫切除。根据这一治疗原则，欧洲人提议将高分化癌及其前驱病变合并为单一的诊断范畴，这在美国几乎没有得到支持[27]。

EIN的诊断方案是用来替代而不是补充过去的子宫内膜增生命名。应当记住的是，准确地应用这种或任何其他分类方法，取决于仔细地分析每一个样本的所有表现。与EIN表现相重叠的个别腺体结构或细胞学的变化，

表13B.2	子宫内膜上皮内肿瘤形成（EIN）：诊断方案			
EIN命名方法		分布	功能类型	治疗
非拮抗性雌激素引起的子宫内膜结构改变（增生紊乱、良性子宫内膜增生）		弥漫性	雌激素作用	激素治疗
EIN		局灶性到弥漫性	癌前病变	激素或外科
癌		局灶性到弥漫性	癌	根据外科分期

表13B.3 子宫内膜上皮内肿瘤形成（EIN）：诊断标准（必须全部符合）

EIN标准	评注
结构	腺体面积大于间质（VPS＜55%）
细胞学	结构密集灶与背景之间细胞学不同
大小＞1 mm	最大长径超过1 mm
除外相似病变	伴有重叠标准的良性病变：基底层子宫内膜、分泌、息肉、修复等
除外癌	如果有迷宫样腺体、实性区域或明显的筛状结构诊断为癌

VPS(volume percentage stroma)：间质体积百分数。

可能见于种种不相关的病变，鉴别这些子宫内膜病变和EIN在诊断上具有最大的挑战性。

子宫内膜上皮内肿瘤形成
Endometrial intraepithelial neoplasia

EIN方案中的一般诊断方法
General approach to diagnosis within the EIN schema

EIN是具有进展为子宫内膜腺癌高度危险性的癌前病变，必须与良性的激素影响、腺癌和各种各样的类似病变相鉴别，因为其组织病理学表现部分地与EIN重叠。后者尤其难于简单描述，因为准确辨认EIN的类似病变，需要了解各种各样应该做出特殊诊断的与之不相关的病变。良性子宫内膜息肉、孤立的子宫内膜基底层和子宫下段组织碎片，以及正切的分泌期子宫内膜都是容易错误诊断为"增生"或EIN的特殊例子。

伴有非子宫内膜样分化的子宫内膜，即所谓的化生，存在特殊的问题。主要诊断为化生而不伴有良性、癌前或癌的诊断是非常罕见的，因为子宫内膜腺体的非子宫内膜样分化一般被看作是良性、癌前和恶性病变的特征[38]。相反，病理医师应该应用清楚表明是良性（退化性、激素性）、癌前（EIN）或恶性（腺癌）病变的主要诊断术语，其次附加上非子宫内膜样分化的描述。例如，输卵管分化可以是伴有散在的输卵管变化的无排卵周期子宫内膜的一部分、EIN伴输卵管分化或腺癌伴输卵管状分化。诊断良性、癌前和恶性化生性病变的标准是分化状态特有的。应该仔细检查非子宫内膜样腺体的分布，继发于体内激素作用引起的变化倾向于随意散在分布于子宫内膜腔中，而由退变引起的改变在崩解或炎症部位最明显。伴有非子宫内膜样分化的癌前EIN病变，在病变早期就倾向于比较局限、地图状和膨胀性。

对于不好的标本，最好的诊断方法也无济于事。标本完整性、取样是否充分、局部关系（如位于息肉内或是子宫下段）以及患者的激素状态，常常影响对于子宫内膜活检和刮宫标本的解释。实际情况是，总有一些标本不能诊断，对于这些病例，病理医师应该清楚地指出出现问题的原因，指导临床对于不能完全做出诊断的病变，在适当的时候进行随访和重复进行子宫内膜取样。

非拮抗性雌激素导致结构变化的子宫内膜
Endometrium with architectural changes of unopposed estrogens

这些子宫内膜的特征是由异常延长的雌激素作用引起的整个子宫内膜腔的同质性区域效应，一般超出正常月经周期中滤泡期的12～14天。长期接触雌激素可能继发于排卵停止或应用外源性激素治疗。子宫内膜是由核分裂活跃的腺体组成的，其结构变化与接触雌激素的持续时间有关（图13B.2）。起初，结构变化可能轻微，由少数散在的囊肿组成["增生紊乱"(disordered hyperplasia)，图13B.2A]，但是随着接触雌激素持续时间的延长，囊肿变得比较明显，腺体分布较不规则，而且管状腺体可能出现分支[良性子宫内膜增生(benign endometrial hyperplasia)]。虽然不规则的腺体结构可能形成杂乱的彼此接近的腺丛，但是具有规律的不规则形态表现。这些随意分布的集中的腺体可能容易与EIN区分开来，因为其细胞学与不密集部位的腺体相似。输卵管改变表现为由伴有粉染胞浆的纤毛细胞组成的腺体，也可以随意分布于整个子宫内膜中，可以累及囊肿或非囊肿性腺体。在脆弱的小血管内形成的纤维素性血栓可以造成微小梗死，组织学上表现为散在的间质崩解，患者出现月经过多（图13B.2B）。间质塌陷产生退变腺体移位并列的人工假象，不要误诊为局灶性EIN病变。在无排卵周期期间或之后发生的子宫内膜崩解是常见的情况，可能被过诊断为EIN或非典型性子宫内膜增生。

子宫内膜上皮内肿瘤形成
Endometrial intraepithelial neoplasia

表13B.3列出了EIN的诊断标准，必须符合所有标准才能诊断。EIN是局灶性病变，在低倍镜下表现为密集排列的灶状腺体（图13B.3）。在具有许多组织碎片的

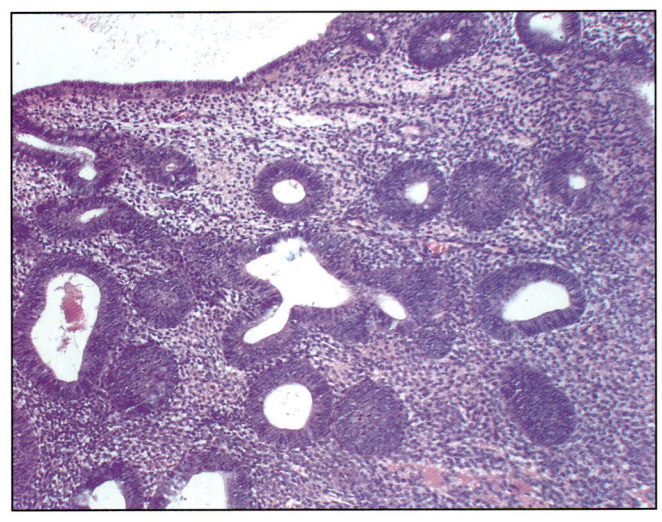

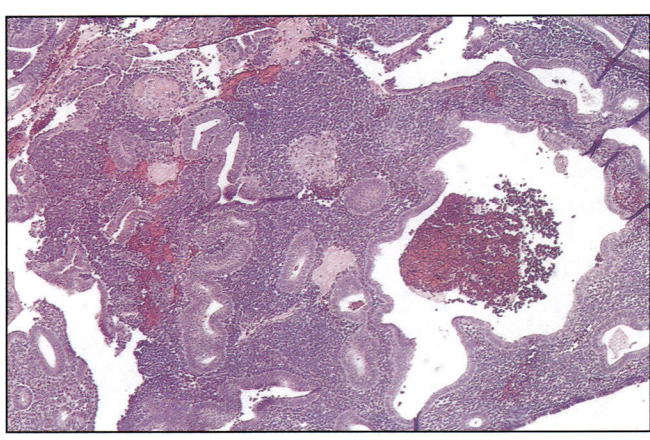

图13B.2 子宫内膜异常增生（无排卵子宫内膜）。在这些活检中容易见到接触雌激素的多种特征，包括输卵管化生和在增生背景下的散在的囊性扩张腺体。腺体密集区域的细胞学与其他部位的相似（A），当发生输卵管变化时，可以不规则地累及管状和囊状扩张的腺体。长期接触雌激素可以导致腺体与间质的比例增加，称作良性子宫内膜增生，伴有纤维素性血栓、微小梗死和间质崩解（B），引起月经过多。

标本中，首先全面检查整个标本，随后根据结构形态选择个别视野仔细观察，这是做出正确诊断的主要步骤。进一步的仔细的检查将会发现，密集腺体的细胞学与背景腺体不同。细胞学和结构的一致变化是 EIN 病变的关键成分，虽然评估这些改变的准确特征所应用的方法不同于从前应用的诊断增生的方法。

EIN 的密集结构可以简单地描述为腺体的表面积（包括上皮和腺腔）超过间质。应用精确定量的术语，可以将其描述为间质体积百分数（volume percentage stroma, VPS）> 55%，而应用某些技术，准确地辨认这种病变是可能的。腺体可能达到这种密度的非 EIN 病变包括分泌期子宫内膜、基底层子宫内膜和囊性改变的子宫内膜。

细胞学改变是 EIN 的基本特征，出现细胞学变化可以

表13B.4	子宫内膜癌的分期（FIGO）
分期	范围
I	癌局限于子宫体
Ia	肿瘤局限于子宫内膜
Ib	肿瘤浸润子宫肌层内半部分
Ic	肿瘤浸润子宫肌层外半部分
II	肿瘤累及子宫体和宫颈
IIa	肿瘤累及宫颈内膜腺体
IIb	肿瘤浸润宫颈间质
III	肿瘤扩散到子宫外，但没有超出真骨盆
IIIa	肿瘤穿透浆膜到附件，或伴有腹腔冲洗液阳性
IIIb	肿瘤累及阴道
IIIc	肿瘤累及骨盆或腹膜淋巴结
IV	癌已经扩散到真骨盆外，或明显累及膀胱或直肠黏膜
IVa	肿瘤累及膀胱和肠黏膜
IVb	肿瘤已经转移到远处，包括腹腔内或腹股沟淋巴结

Adapted from International Journal of Gynecology and Obstetrics. Benedet JL, Pecorelli S.Staging classifications and clinical practice guidelines of gynaecologic cancers, P60, ©2000. With permission from International Federation of Gynecology and Obstetrics.

确认密集区域不是正常腺体移位造成的人工假象。由此看来，主要是改变了陈旧的增生范例[33]。EIN 的细胞学改变见于那些伴有结构异常的腺体，可能包括细胞核和细胞浆的变化，有时甚至出现非子宫内膜样分化，形成黏液性、输卵管性或微乳头状的细胞学改变。EIN 病变的细胞形态变化是相对而言的，它是通过比较同一个标本中病变腺体与非病变腺体细胞之间的差异确定的（图 13B.4）。EIN 病变没有固定的共同的细胞学表现，而且那些具有非子宫内膜样分化、细胞核长或主要为细胞浆改变的病变，从经典的意义上来说并不具有"非典型性"（图 13B.5）。

EIN 病变扩大，最终可以占据整个子宫内膜腔，影响背景与病变细胞学的比较。这些病例通常有一些残留的腺体，数量或许很少，但仍适合作为比较的参考（图 13B.4）。当 EIN 占据了整个子宫内膜腔时，通常出现明显的细胞学异常，诊断并不困难。

细胞学上发生了变化的密集的腺体簇的大小至少必须达到 1mm。典型者要求几十个腺体（或更多）。过去的形态测量研究已经显示，这个临界大小确定的病变发生癌的危险性增加 45 倍[34]。包括 Pipelle 活检在内的大多数标本，组织碎片的大小完全超过了上述阈值，所以组织碎片并不妨碍应用最小在 1 mm 的大小标准。微小的宫腔镜活检是个例外。这种方式取得的标本经常伴有

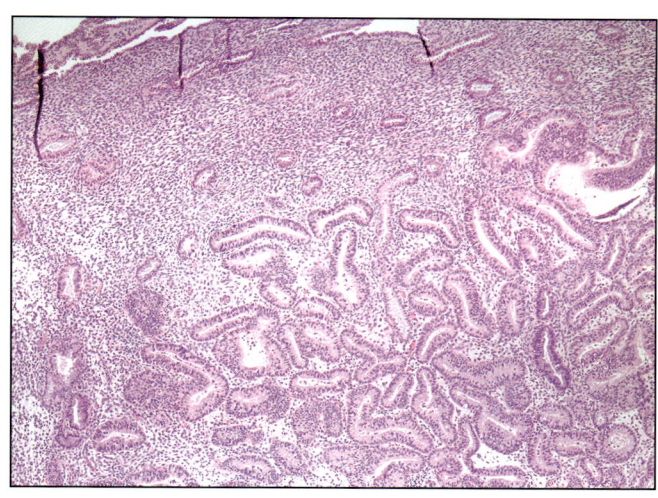
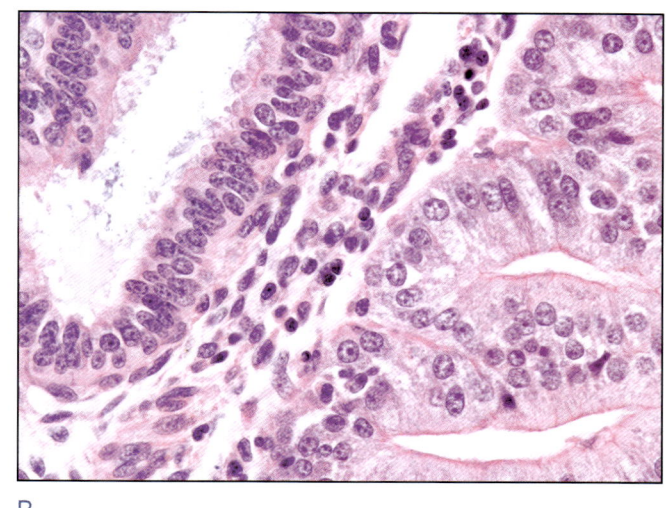

图13B.3 子宫内膜上皮内肿瘤形成（EIN）。局灶性EIN。低倍镜下显示局限性的成簇的密集腺体，其中腺体面积超过间质面积（A）。与这种结构变化一致的是细胞学改变。与背景腺体（B，左上）不同，病变腺体具有丰富的胞浆和圆形的细胞核（B，右下）。EIN病变由一群单个腺体组成，偶尔见腺体分支，但是没有真正的筛状或实性结构。

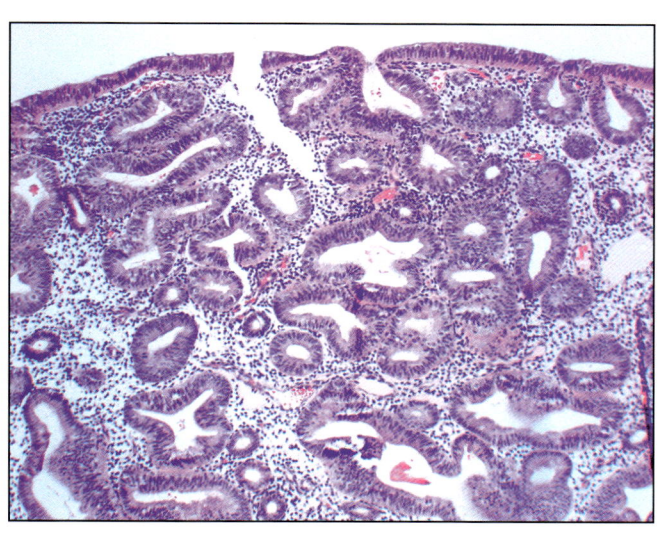
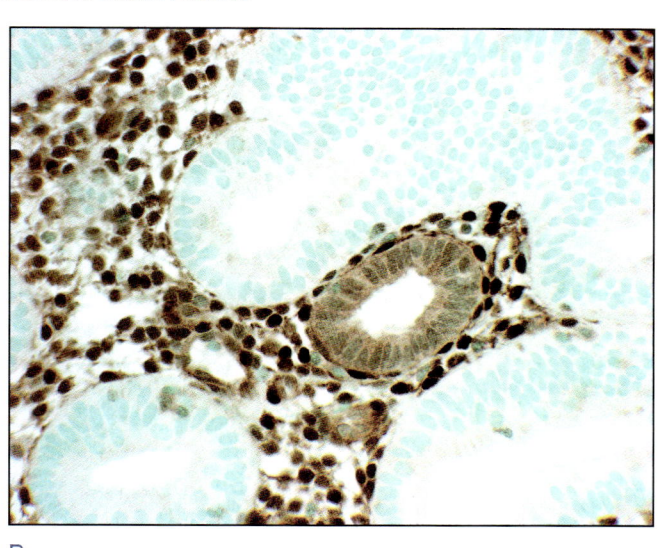

图13B.4 子宫内膜上皮内肿瘤形成（EIN）。（A）EIN病变累及整个子宫内膜。辨认这个遍布整个子宫内膜的癌前EIN病变的周界是困难的，但是它具有正常的直径较小的圆形的背景腺体。正常腺体PTEN蛋白（抗体6h2.1）呈明显的深棕色染色(B)，而遗传学发生改变的EIN病变缺乏PTEN染色。

人工挤压，不能对比检查病变与背景之间的交界部位，不适合用于评估是否存在子宫内膜癌前病变的可能性。大小不足1 mm的具有细胞学改变的成簇密集腺体（腺体面积＞间质面积）的诊断取决于组织碎片的状况。如果这样的病灶出现在一个较大的碎块中，可以简单地加以描述而不做出EIN的诊断。另一方面，如果是多数非常小的碎片，大小均小于1 mm，其中含有细胞学不同于其他碎片的密集腺体，则可能是破碎了的EIN的一部分。这种情况也可做出描述性的诊断，说明不能除外EIN，并建议重新取材进行评估。

虽然良性息肉必须与EIN鉴别，但不总是有排除性的特殊发现。大约15%的EIN病变发生在息肉的边缘。这些病例应该完全符合EIN所有的诊断标准，但要注意解释细胞学应以息肉本身作为背景，而不是与自身功能性子宫内膜进行比较。由多数内衬良性上皮的大体可见的扩张腺体组成的息肉，不要误诊为EIN。

除外子宫内膜腺癌
Excluding endometrial adenocarcinoma

通过出现实性肿瘤性上皮区域或迷宫样蔓延或变形的腺腔，以及代表正常腺体-间质相互关系破坏的间质受累可以识别癌（图13B.6）。低分化癌和浆液性癌可以通过其独特的细胞学表现进行诊断（见下文）。

癌应该与EIN鉴别，因为前者必须手术切除而不用

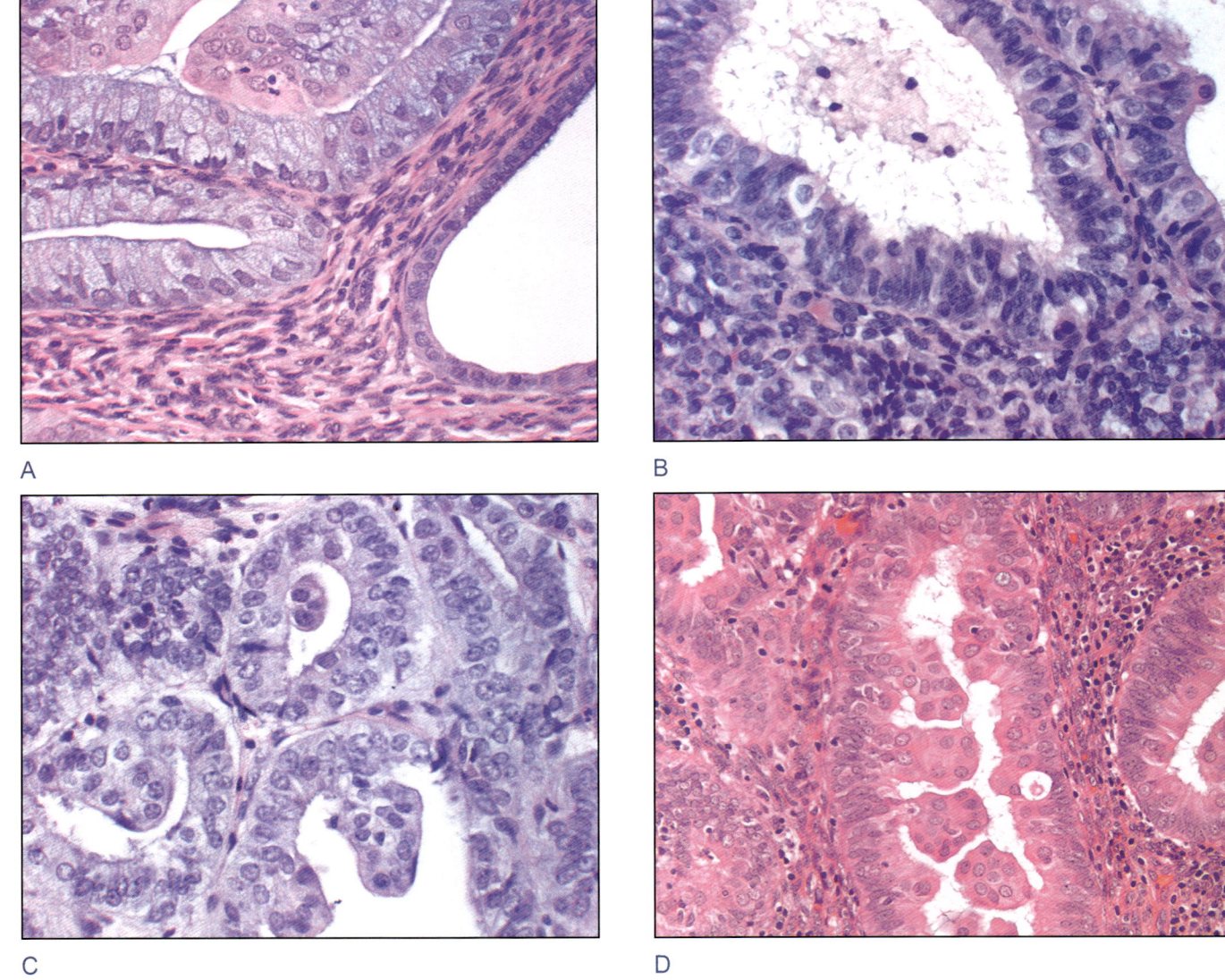

图 13B.5 子宫内膜上皮内肿瘤形成（EIN）的非子宫内膜样分化。这种改变了的分化可以是肿瘤性病变的一部分，包括胞浆和细胞核的变化。变性或激素作用可能类似于分化状态的改变。图中显示 4 例伴有非子宫内膜样分化的 EIN：（A）黏液性；（B）输卵管；（C）乳头状；（D）嗜酸细胞性。它们全都发生在伴有腺体高度密集的结构异常的部位，容易辨认异常的生长方式。注意这里缺少间质破坏，在某些情况下间质破坏可以引起继发性乳头状或嗜酸细胞性改变。在这些病例的诊断中应用"化生"一词可能引起误解。

激素治疗。如果肿瘤性上皮与间质分离或仅出现在非常小的组织碎片中，有时也许不可能解决这个鉴别诊断问题。在这些情况下，明确的诊断为"EIN 不能除外癌"将会提示临床医师对这个问题的警觉。最后，重要的是要强调子宫内膜癌的手术治疗可以根据病变的分布而加以改进。手术治疗完全位于息肉内的癌可能完全不同于已经扩散到子宫下段的高分化腺癌。

EIN的治疗

EIN 的治疗是直接去除病变。更喜欢选择子宫切除术；然而，希望保留生育能力的较为年轻的女性和手术风险大的患者可能不适合手术治疗。多数雌激素引起的子宫内膜改变和某些 EIN 病变孕激素治疗有效[39-42]。长期激素处理可以缓解伴有无排卵型子宫内膜病变妇女的症状，例如口服避孕药。通过规律活检监测子宫内膜（通常每 6 个月一次），可以早期发现伴有非拮抗性雌激素的患者自然发生的肿瘤性病变。EIN 患者的孕激素治疗是有争议的，必须考虑患者的情况和主治医师的临床判断。在撤退性出血之后总是应该进行随访活检，以避免孕激素对于细胞核形态学的混淆作用（图 13B.7）。证实对于孕激素治疗有抵抗的 EIN 患者，应该再次评估进行手术治疗的可能。

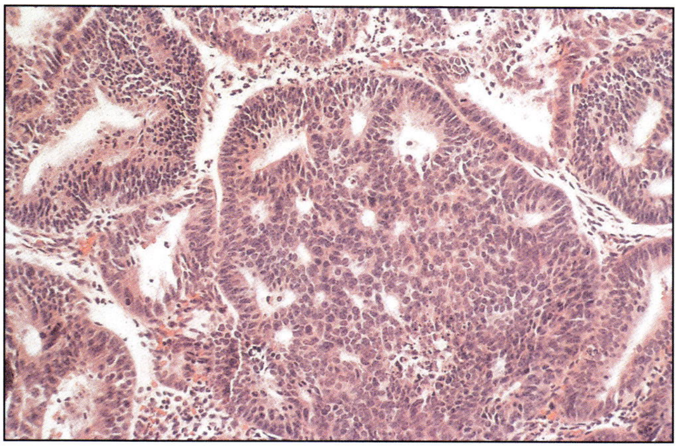

图13B.6 出现下列特征之一可将高分化腺癌与子宫内膜上皮内肿瘤形成鉴别开来：（A）筛状结构伴有正常腺体轮廓丧失；（B）不规则的迷宫样腺体；（C）绒毛腺管状结构；或（D）实性上皮或肌层浸润（没有显示）。

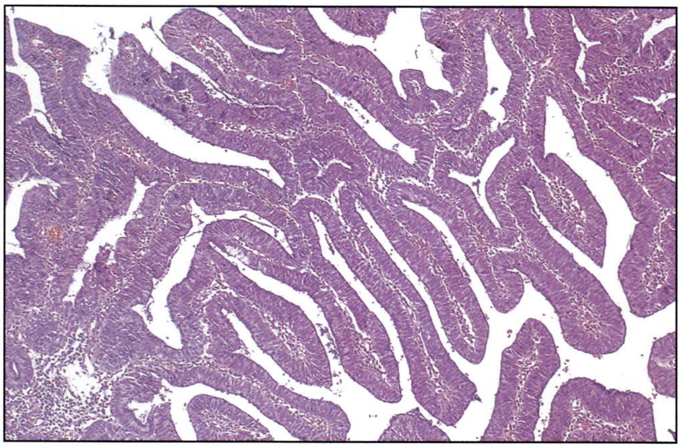

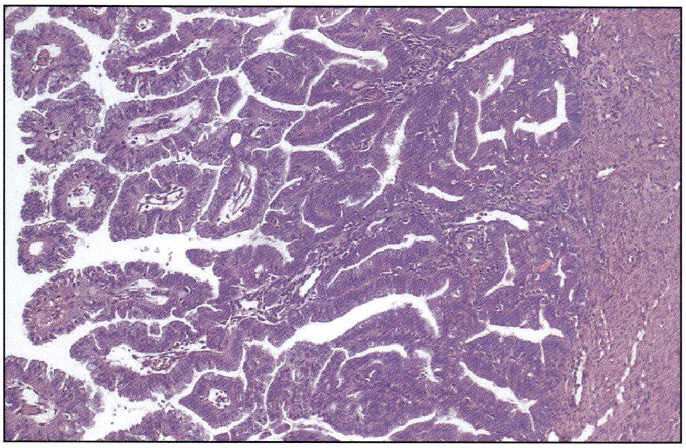

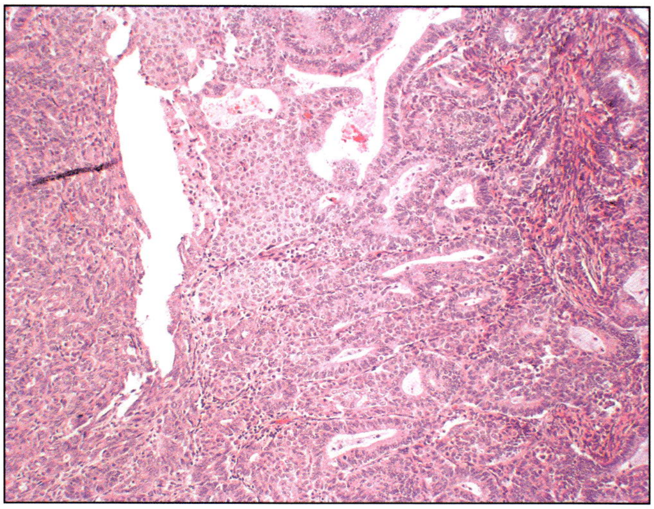

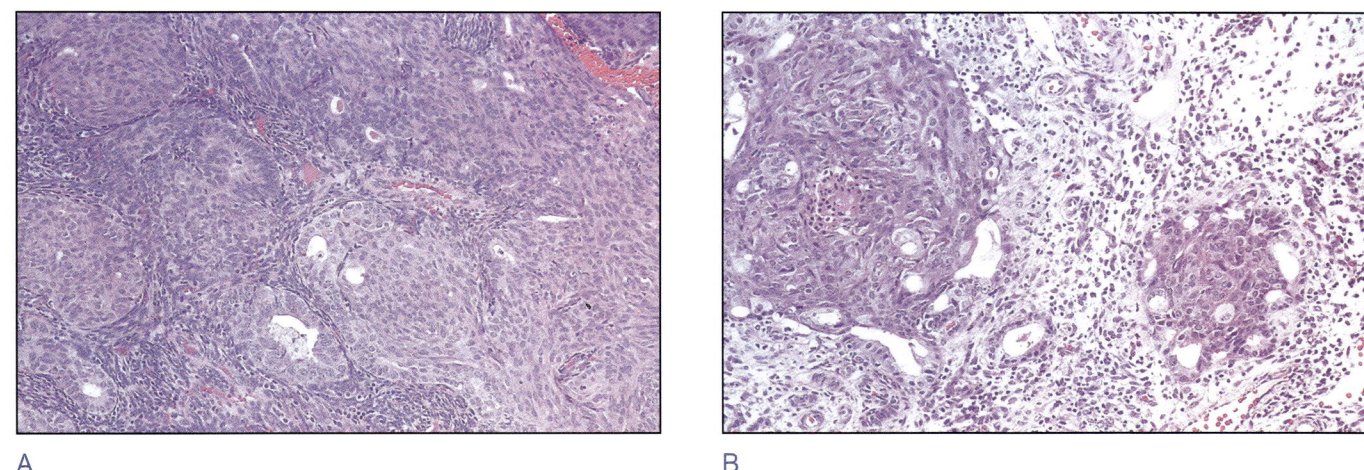

图13B.7 孕激素对于伴有桑葚化生的子宫内膜上皮内肿瘤形成（EIN）的作用。鳞状桑葚与子宫内膜腺体病变相互混合，甲地孕酮（Megace）治疗前（A）和治疗后6个月（B）进行比较，核的细胞学发生了引人注目的改变。桑葚化生常见于EIN。应用孕激素使得腺体细胞核变小，而且腺上皮变少。 对于仍然处于孕激素作用下的子宫内膜的解释要加以小心，因为细胞变得更加温和，而且由于间质膨胀造成结构改变。一种策略是主张在获得随访活检之前，应完成应用孕激素治疗后造成的撤退性出血。

乳头状浆液性腺癌的前体病变
Precursors to papillary serous adenocarcinoma

浆液性子宫内膜上皮内癌（serous endometrial intraepithelial carcinoma，"浆液性EIC"）是乳头状浆液性子宫内膜腺癌的原位病变，它常常与浸润性乳头状浆液性子宫内膜腺癌伴随发生，而不是先于其发生[7,43]。浆液性EIC不应该与相似的子宫内膜样型腺癌前驱病变的缩写词EIN混淆（见上文）。浆液性EIC具有非常高级别的核非典型性、脱落细胞或鞋钉样细胞形态学，以及表明细胞失活的p53异常染色（图13B.8）。浆液性EIC的行为如同腺癌，包括可以转移到腹膜部位，偶尔沿着表面生长。诊断浆液性EIC，尤其是当其作为一个孤立性病变发生时，应该仔细进行临床分期以除外这种可能性。

在非常罕见的情况下，p53突变发生于细胞形态介于正常和浆液性EIC之间的子宫内膜上皮细胞[44]。这些细胞可能具有p53异常和染色体17p和1p的缺失，它们持续存在于同一个患者的比较典型的浆液性EIC区域或乳头状浆液性腺癌中[45]。有人提示这种"子宫内膜腺体异型增生"可能是一个真正的癌前病变，但是它们的长期自然病史和发生癌的危险性还没有被充分证明。

子宫内膜腺癌
Endometrial adenocarcinoma

大体病理学　　Gross pathology

子宫内膜癌既可以表现为息肉样也可以弥漫性累及整个子宫内膜表面（图13B.9）。肿瘤播散一般是经过直接浸润肌层，最终扩散到邻近的子宫旁组织。肿瘤累及阔韧带可以形成临床上可触及的肿块。最后发生区域淋巴结转移；晚期肿瘤可能发生血行转移到肺、肝、骨和其他器官。在某些类型的肿瘤，特别是乳头状浆液性癌，相对表浅的子宫内膜受累就可以伴有广泛的腹膜病变，提示经由腹膜种植播散[46]。

子宫内膜癌的预后因素
Prognostic factors in endometrial carcinomas

几个作者已经提出了预示女性子宫内膜腺癌死亡率增加的标准。这些危险因素涉及几个方面，包括肿瘤的分期、分级、组织学亚型和其他一些特征。

子宫内膜癌的分期方法总结在表13B.4中。子宫内膜癌的分级是一个复杂而又有争议的问题[47]。简单地说，分级是根据肿瘤的生长方式、细胞核非典型性的程度和肿瘤的类型。

没有明显细胞核非典型性或其他浆液性癌特征的子宫内膜样型腺癌可以分成下列3级：

- G1：高分化腺癌，实性生长的腺体成分（除外鳞状细胞区域）少于5%
- G2：中分化腺癌，实性生长的腺体成分在5%～50%之间
- G3：低分化腺癌，实性生长的腺体成分大于50%

在这一组肿瘤中存在一些例外情况。出现显著的细胞核非典型性时，肿瘤的分级应该比单独根据结构的分级提高一级（例如G2而不是G1）。另外一个例外是肿

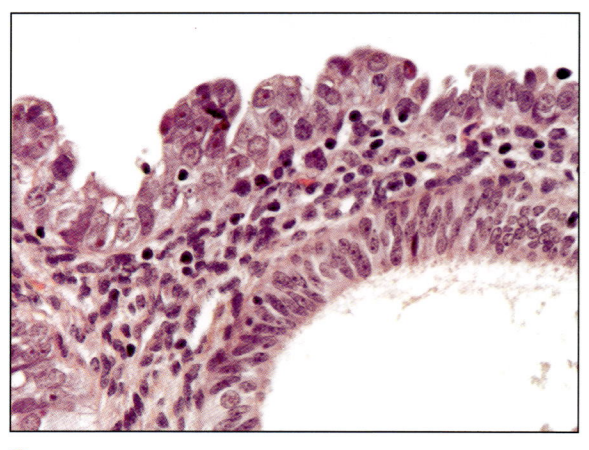

图13B.8　浆液性子宫内膜上皮内癌（EIC）。（A）p53突变（免疫组织化学染色）细胞累及浅表子宫内膜腺体和子宫腔的腔面。（B）乳头状浆液性癌的细胞学。这个病例是典型的非浸润性浆液性EIC，邻近区域伴有浸润性乳头状浆液性癌；然而，在少数情况下浆液性EIC可以是一个孤立的发现。

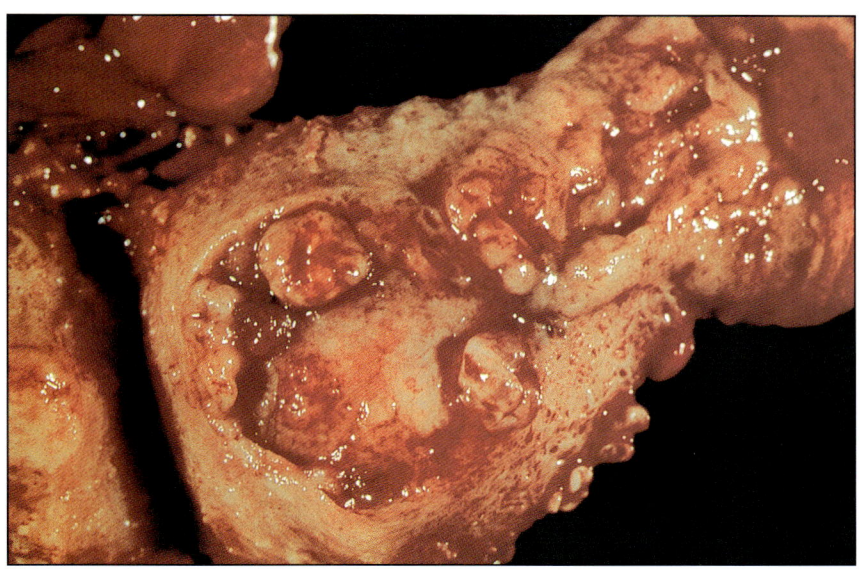

图13B.9 子宫内膜腺癌，表现为子宫表面弥漫性不规则的结节。

瘤明显的双向分化，其中两种独立而又各具特点的成分并列存在，两者均可以是高分化和低分化。在这种情况下，病理报告中两者的分级应该特别谨慎[2]。

其余的子宫内膜癌，特别是乳头状浆液性腺癌和透明细胞癌，肿瘤分级实际上并没有意义。诊断为这两种肿瘤就意味着是高危险的肿瘤，而且诊断乳头状浆液性腺癌要求注意治疗可能存在的腹膜病变[46]。

除了分级和细胞类型之外，其他的预后因素包括子宫肌层浸润的深度、血管浸润、腹膜冲洗液的状况和患者的年龄[48]。

子宫内膜样腺癌
Endometrioid adenocarcinoma

子宫内膜样腺癌可以被分成几个形态学亚型，其中每一种亚型均可能具有不同的分化程度。在评价这种类型肿瘤时要记住的三个重要参数是：(1)腺体形态和结构；(2)肿瘤细胞核非典型性的程度；(3)细胞分化的形态(或化生)。根据WHO的分级方法总结在第660页。

多数子宫内膜样癌的组织学特征是界限非常清楚的腺体，内衬细胞学上为恶性的复层柱状上皮细胞。典型者为高分化（I级）子宫内膜样腺癌，易于辨认腺体结构（图13B.10，左）；中分化（2级）癌显示形成完好的腺体混有恶性细胞实性片块；或低分化（3级）癌，以实性细胞片块为特征，几乎没有可以辨认的腺体，细胞核的非典型性比较明显，而且核分裂活跃（图13B.10，右）。其中5%～10%的病例有乳头状（绒毛腺管状）结构[49]。子宫内膜样腺癌的常规分级方法基本上是根据评估巨大腺体的生长结构。然而，子宫内膜癌的另外一种亚型表现为微小腺体的生长结构，它的表现不同于常见的伴有子宫内膜增生的分支状巨大腺体。这些微小腺体形态以小管状或筛状腺体排列为特征，分化可能不同，从非常高分化到中分化各异。当出现黏液化生时，前者可能与宫颈内膜上皮混淆[50-52]（图13B.11）。少数病例可能显示细胞条索位于玻璃样变的间质中，形成性索样表现[53]。伴有明显淋巴细胞浸润的低分化肿瘤可能提示与遗传性非息肉病结直肠癌相关的可能性[54]。

一般来说，子宫内膜样肿瘤表现为细胞核增大，复层排列，但是细胞核多形性的程度较轻。子宫内膜样癌的形态学亚型分类主要是根据肿瘤细胞分化的类型，可以是鳞状、黏液性、输卵管或分泌性上皮。

2%～20%的子宫内膜样腺癌可见鳞状分化。最常见的是组织学表现为良性的鳞状成分[所谓的"腺癌伴有鳞状上皮化生"，或比较传统的伴有高分化腺癌的"腺

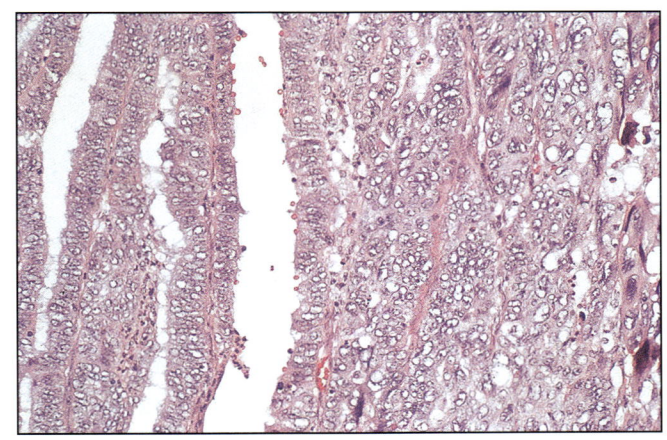

图13B.10 子宫内膜样腺癌，显示同一个肿瘤中高分化(左)和低分化(右)的成分。

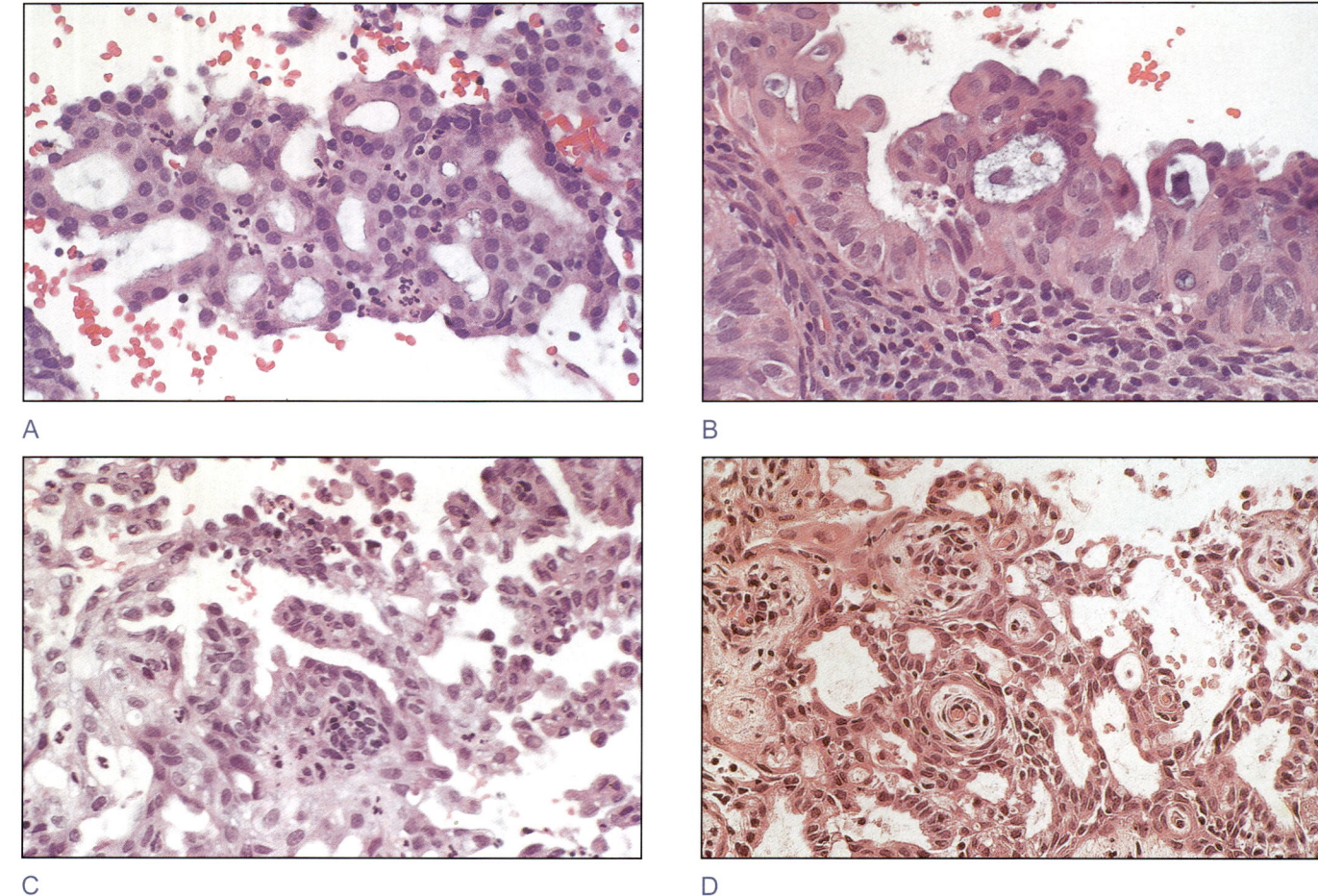

图13B.11 （A）子宫内膜癌的微小腺体亚型，呈现相互交错的小管状腺体，伴有轻度的细胞学非典型性。相比之下，（B）较大腺体单纯的黏液性化生，不伴有微小腺体结构，虽然可以出现微乳头状结构。（C）乳头状合体细胞"化生"呈现没有腺管状结构的表面生长结构。（D）宫颈内膜的微小腺体改变作为对照。

棘癌"（adenoacanthoma）]。较少见的是中或低分化子宫内膜样癌含有明显恶性表现的鳞状成分。这样的肿瘤过去称作"腺鳞癌"（adenosquamous carcinoma）。然而，过去有关鳞状分化的临床意义一直是争论的焦点，至于是否必须应用"腺鳞癌"这一术语的意见也不一致。最后决定，应以腺体分化的程度来确定肿瘤的分级，用"鳞状分化"一词取代"鳞状化生"（例如中分化腺癌，子宫内膜样型，伴有鳞状分化）[55]。还可以见到少数移行细胞癌伴有鳞状分化的病例[56]。

如同伴有鳞状分化的子宫内膜样癌一样，伴有黏液分化的肿瘤也可以表现出不同程度的非典型性。最微妙的表现是伴有轻度核非典型性的微小腺体肿瘤，它可能类似宫颈内膜肿瘤。与宫颈内膜不同的是肿瘤没有鳞状分化，而且细胞排列紧密，肿瘤细胞成筛状结构，伴有不同程度的黏液产物。比较容易区分的是生长方式，显示明显的非典型性、坏死和乳头状结构。一般来说，伴有轻度非典型性的病变倾向于是外生性，而且浸润轻微，而大约一半的病例伴有比较典型的子宫内膜样成分，它也可以是浸润性的[50-52]（图 13B.11A）。

输卵管性和分泌性子宫内膜癌是另外两种少见的形态。两者都伴有高分化上皮区域，通常预示具有良好的预后[57]。输卵管（纤毛）分化可以见于巨大腺体和微小腺体生长结构。对于子宫内膜复杂性生长结构一般均应持有怀疑态度，而不管上皮分化保留的程度。非常罕见的子宫内膜样腺癌病例可以显示Sertoli型特征[58]。

乳头状浆液性和透明细胞癌
Papillary serous and clear cell carcinomas

虽然作为低分化腺癌的分类一般要求失去腺体分化并出现实性结构，但是两种组织学形态的生物学行为如同低分化癌，不管其分化程度如何，它们是乳头状浆液性癌和透明细胞癌。尤其是浆液性癌，它是具有高度侵袭性的子宫癌，1982年提出要与子宫内膜样癌严格区别开来[59]。其他一些研究大都证实了这些最初的观察，而且浆液性肿瘤的类型得到了扩展，包括另外两个特殊的亚型：（1）混合性浆液性和子宫内膜样癌；（2）起源于子宫内膜息肉的浆液性癌。后者最具迷惑性，因为大部分肿瘤可能很小，却有明显的向子宫内膜和腹膜表面播散的倾向。

纯粹的浆液性癌十分少见，一项研究显示只占子宫内膜癌的1.1%[60]。作者们报告5年和10年生存率非常低，分别为27%和14%。Carcangiu和Chambers分析了三个参数：（1）肿瘤明显局限于息肉内；（2）肿瘤伴有子宫内膜样成分；（3）肿瘤与具有相似形态学的卵巢癌共存[61]。所有三组的预后都是差的，伴有子宫内膜样成分对于生存率并没有有利的影响。局限于息肉内的肿瘤与伴有肌层浸润的相似分期的肿瘤具有同样的侵袭性生物学行为，而伴有卵巢受累的癌的生物学行为如同高分期的癌，Silva和Jenkins以及Gallion等也有同样的观察结果[62,63]。Goff等得出同样的结论，特别提到肿瘤分级和肌层浸润范围与腹腔冲洗液阳性和肿瘤预后危险性的关系不大[46]。生存率与毛细淋巴管浸润呈负相关。部分患有小的子宫肿瘤的患者存活，Grice及其同事在随后的研究中发现，经过仔细分期之后的局限于子宫的肿瘤具有较好的预后[64]，Carcangiu等在Ia期病变的研究中也有同样的结论[65]。最近Hui等发现，任何局限于子宫内膜的这样的肿瘤（不管是否位于息肉内）一般都有非常好的预后[66]。

当病理医师面对一个浆液性癌时，重要的是对输卵管和卵巢充分取材进行组织学检查，同样要对腹膜进行随机取样，并注意有无毛细淋巴管浸润。

包括与子宫内膜样肿瘤混合存在的浆液性癌在内，所有的浆液性肿瘤都有一个共同的特征，即细胞核有明显的非典型性，并伴有巨核和突出的核仁（图13B.12）。某些肿瘤呈明显的乳头状结构，乳头通常伴有宽的基底和不规则的形状，并有大量单个肿瘤细胞从乳头上脱落下来。另外一些肿瘤表现为小管状或裂隙样的腺体，具有同样的细胞核的特征，或为规则的腺体，内衬一层或两层非典型性细胞，突出于腺腔中呈"鞋钉"样表现。共同的特征是肿瘤细胞呈微乳头状排列，以及没有间质支持的小而疏松黏合的肿瘤细胞簇。

子宫内膜透明细胞癌通过出现两个特征而与浆液性癌略有不同。其一，腺体或乳头被覆单层多角形细胞，细胞核一致，核仁明显（图13B.13）。其二，与浆液性癌不同，没有明显脱落的细胞出现。当肿瘤细胞排列成片块状时，细胞仍然保留清晰的界限，虽然如同浆液性癌一样可以有明显的细胞核非典型性。在透明细胞癌的小管状亚型，肿瘤腺体之间还可以出现嗜酸性PAS阳性的无细胞基质。透明细胞癌应该与偶尔出现透明胞浆的低分化子宫内膜样肿瘤鉴别。分泌空泡同样不要与透明细胞癌混淆，后者需要出现高级别的核和特征性的具有轻微复层的腺体生长方式[67]。

如同浆液性癌一样，透明细胞癌不易"分级"，而且这种分级对于临床治疗可能并不重要。子宫透明细胞癌一般比子宫内膜样癌的预后要差，但是没有累及腹膜表面的倾向。Abeler及其同事[68,69]报告5年和10年粗生存率分别是42%和39%。当出现毛细淋巴管浸润时，与伴有子宫深肌层浸润患者15%的5年生存率有关[68]。

显示混合性分化的肿瘤
Tumors showing mixed differentiation

癌肉瘤（包括恶性混合性Müller肿瘤）
Carcinosarcomas (includes malignant mixed müllerian tumors)

癌肉瘤由子宫内膜腺癌和恶性间叶（间质）成分共同组成。后者可以包括子宫内膜间质、平滑肌（平滑肌肉瘤）、骨骼肌（横纹肌肉瘤）、软骨（软骨肉瘤）甚至有骨样组织（骨肉瘤）。上皮和间叶成分的单克隆特性，提示它们起源于共同的干细胞，应用上皮细胞标志物染色间质细胞常常阳性支持这一概念。这些肿瘤作为"化生性癌"（metaplastic carcinomas）这一概念进一步得到免疫组化和临床上的支持；预后明显与浆液性或透明细胞的腺体组织学，以及诸如子宫肌层浸润、毛细淋巴管浸润和宫颈受累等其他参数有关。相反，间叶性成分的分化程度并不影响预后，而且转移通常是由上皮成分而不是间叶组织组成，提示肉瘤分化是侵袭的标志而不是肿瘤更具侵袭性的成分[70,71]。转移方式通常是经由淋巴管，与原发性肉瘤特征性的血源性播散相比，其行为比较类似于上皮性肿瘤。

大体上，癌肉瘤的外观比腺癌更似鱼肉状，可能巨大，呈息肉状，有时突入宫颈口（图13B.14）。组织学上，肿瘤通常由腺癌混合有间质（肉瘤性）成分组成；同时，肿瘤也可以由两种明显独立的上皮和间叶成分组成，类似于"碰撞瘤"（collision tumor）（图13B.15）。最常见的腺癌成分是子宫内膜样癌。传统上将癌肉瘤分为同源性或异源性恶性混合性Müller肿瘤，根据间叶成分表达的分化是子宫固有的（间质肉瘤或平滑肌肉瘤）还是子宫外的（横纹肌肉瘤、软骨肉瘤等）。这种区分是根据

显示混合性分化的肿瘤

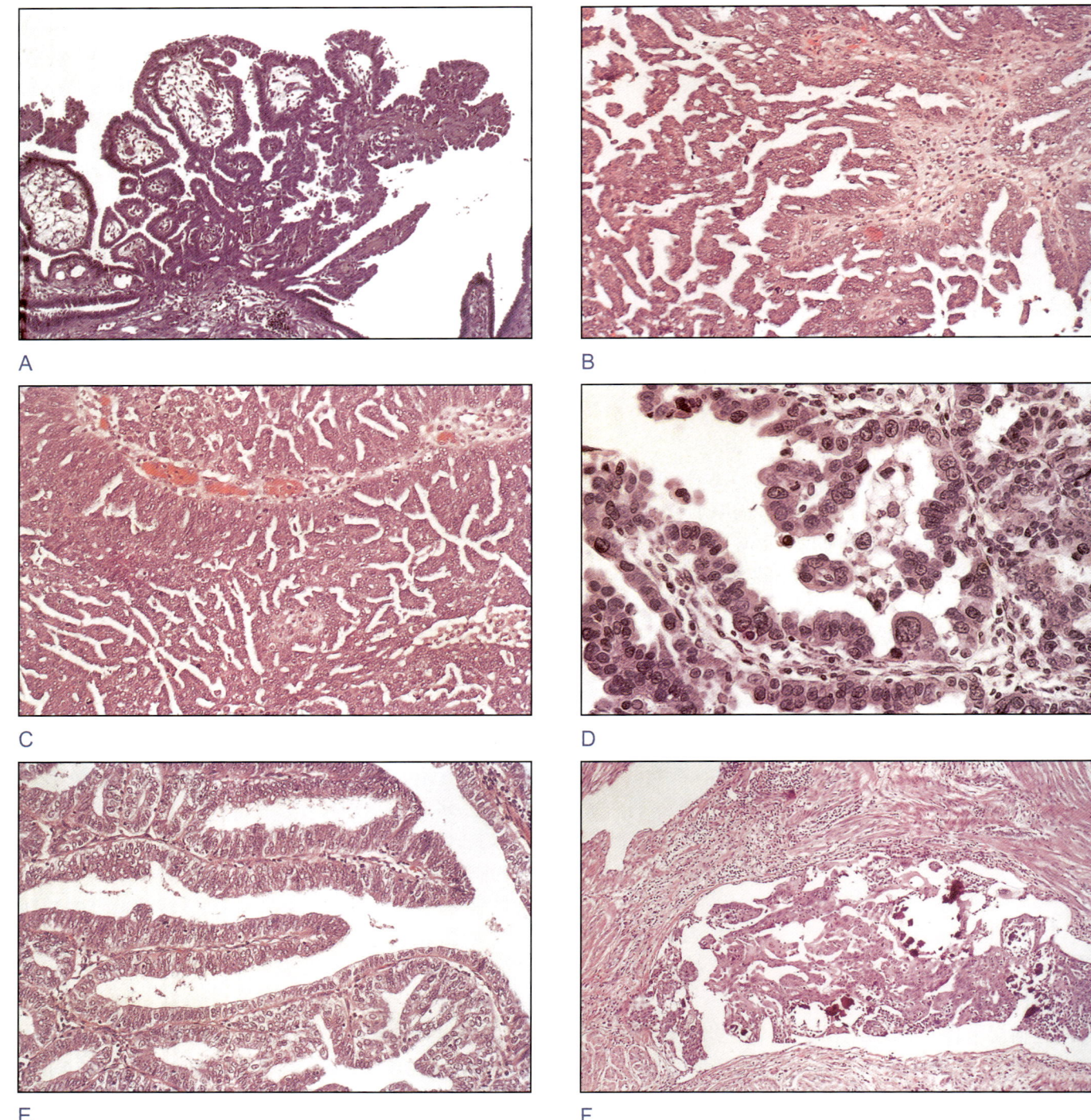

图13B.12 子宫内膜浆液性癌。这种病变组织学上可以表现为：（A）被覆肿瘤细胞的粗钝乳头；（B）犬牙交错的肿瘤性上皮排列成无序的微乳头；（C）不规则的小裂隙样腺体（D）内衬细胞伴有明显增大而深染的细胞核。微乳头状结构和巨核并存是浆液性癌的特征。偶尔，子宫内膜样癌（E）和浆液性癌（F）可以共同存在于同一个病例中。

有报告提示异源性肿瘤的预后更差。然而，普遍认为两者预后均差，现在将所有的肿瘤都称为"癌肉瘤"[70,71]。

癌肉瘤几乎全部发生于绝经后患者（最常见于60岁以上的妇女），其中某些患者从前有盆腔放射的病史。

这些肿瘤具有侵袭性，5年生存率是25%～30%，预后不良的主要因素是附件播散、淋巴结转移和癌的组织学类型[70,72]。对于晚期疾病，辅助治疗可能起到局部控制作用，但未得到证实。

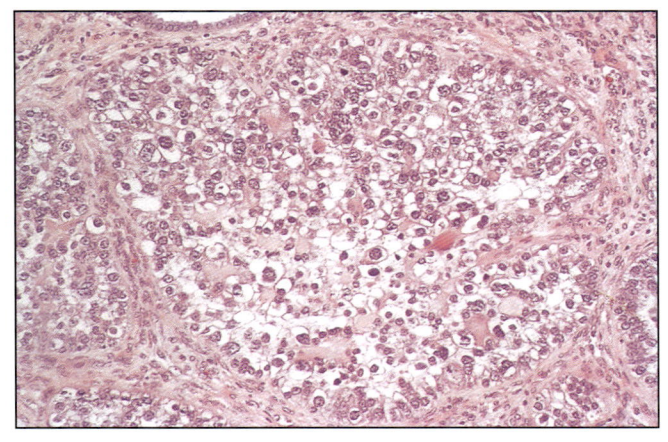

图13B.13 透明细胞癌，显示特征性的透明细胞，伴有清楚的细胞界限和灶状嗜酸性基质轴心。

腺肉瘤

如同癌肉瘤一样，Müller腺肉瘤由上皮和间质成分组成。然而，这些肿瘤与癌肉瘤不同，通常表现为良性上皮位于肉瘤性间质中。腺肉瘤的预后比癌肉瘤好得多，但是出于治疗的目的，将它与子宫内膜息肉、腺纤维瘤和腺肌瘤区分开来可能是重要的[73]。

如同癌肉瘤一样，腺肉瘤最常见于绝经后的妇女，虽然总的发病年龄分布宽广。典型者表现为巨大的肿瘤充满子宫内膜腔，少数情况下发生于宫颈内膜。鉴别腺

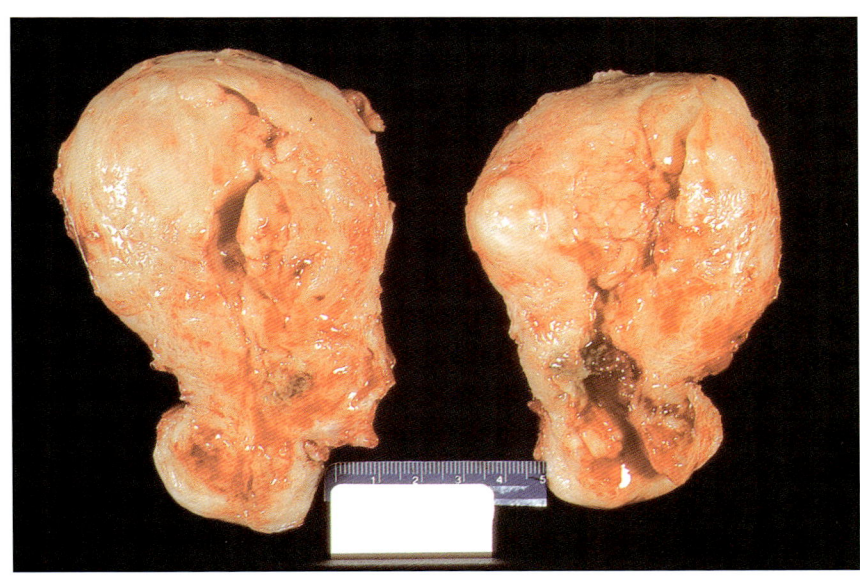

图13B.14 癌肉瘤。这个对切的子宫显示前壁和后壁表面被覆闪光的均质性肿瘤。

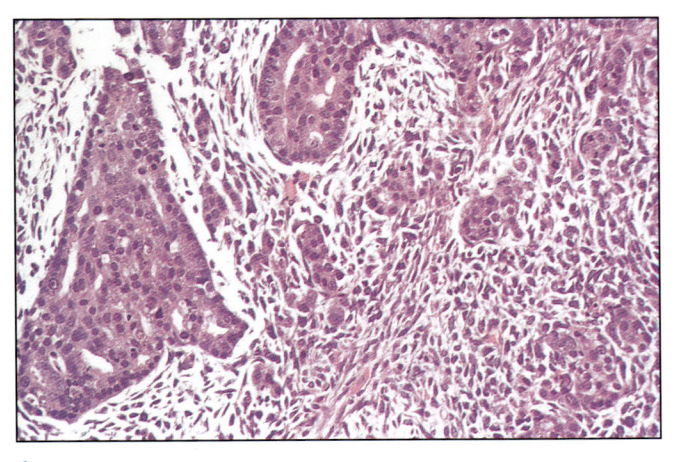

A

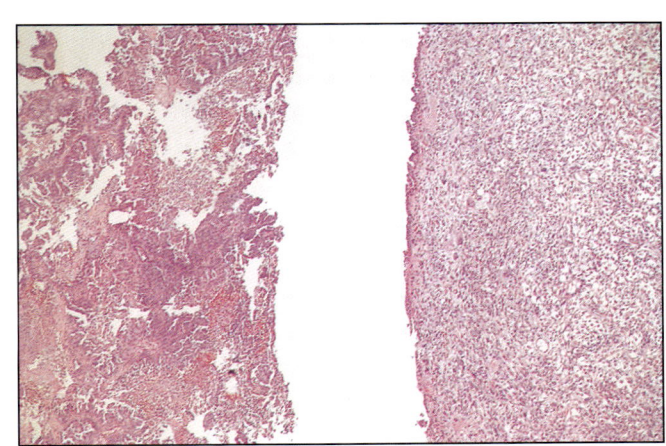

B

图13B.15 癌肉瘤的两种生长方式包括：（A）上皮和间质成分混合存在；（B）并列分开的上皮性（左）和间叶性（右）肿瘤。

显示混合性分化的肿瘤

肉瘤的重要组织学特征包括伴有裂隙样或叶状内折的不规则的腺体结构、间质上皮乳头和腺体内息肉样突起。上皮细胞可以不同，从假复层到纤毛细胞到鞋钉样细胞各异，类似于反应性的宫颈内膜上皮。偶尔，腺体出现非典型性。间质一般富于细胞，伴有腺体周围间质细胞套，这个特征可将这些肿瘤与子宫内膜息肉或腺肌瘤性息肉区别开来。间质成分可能显示广泛的分化，包括同源性分化和异源性分化（图13B.16），某些病例出现性索样成分[74]。

腺肉瘤一般具有良性生物学行为，但是的确存在局部复发的危险。Clement 和 Scully 报告的 100 例中有 23 例复发，其中 1/3 发生在 5 年后，而且绝大部分是局部复发，发生在阴道、盆腔或腹腔[73]。远处转移罕见，但是应该注意潜在的恶性行为，并将这些肿瘤与良性息肉鉴别开来。在与腺纤维瘤的鉴别诊断中，腺肉瘤间质细胞核分裂象通常为每 10 个高倍视野 1 个或 1 个以上；明显的间质细胞构成；以及间质细胞具有轻度以上的非典型性[74]。这个肿瘤的正确诊断显然是基于对于这些肿瘤的经验，其中某些肿瘤即使表现温和也可以复发，或者可能容易与子宫内膜息肉混淆。应用上述标准很少做出腺纤维瘤的诊断[73]。

与临床有关的一个重要决定是，是否切除患有腺肉瘤的年轻女性的卵巢。这一过程常常被认为是腺肉瘤病例治疗的标准程序，而且在伴有不常见的子宫内膜息肉的年轻女性诊断腺肉瘤应该十分小心。

其他间质-上皮性肿瘤包括腺肌瘤性息肉（adenomyomatous polyps）和非典型性息肉样腺肌瘤（atypical polypoid adenomyomas, APA）[75-78]。后者主要发生在绝经前患者，不要与腺肉瘤混淆，因为具有典型的肌瘤性间质。然而，APA 可能有伴有鳞状桑葚的异常腺上皮，偶尔有与 EIN 或腺癌不能区分的区域共存（图13B.17）。它与浸润癌共存的危险性低，但是处理这些肿瘤应该小心，并通过仔细随访或切除子宫以除外癌。

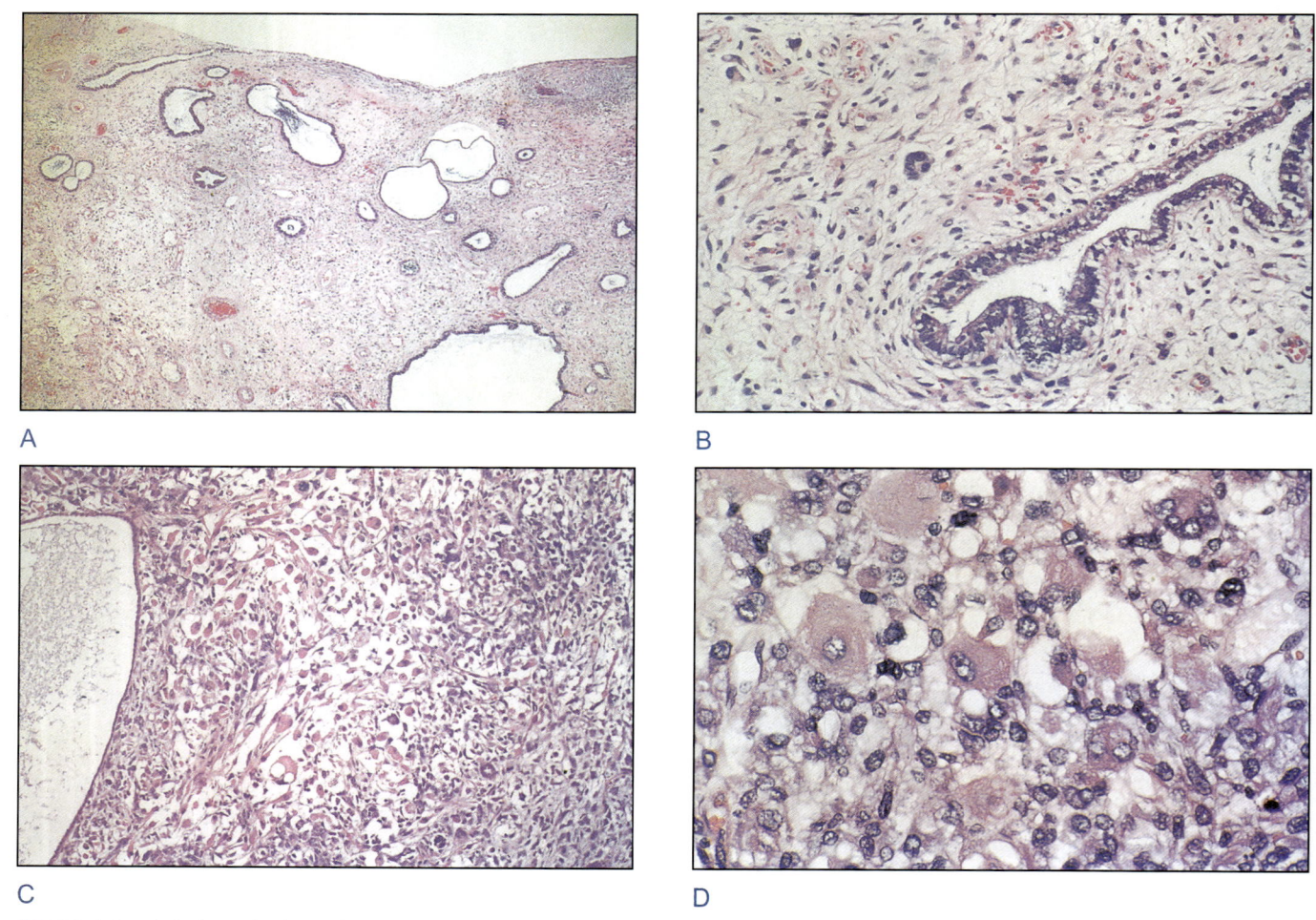

图13B.16 腺肉瘤。（A）低倍镜下观，不同大小的腺体与富于细胞的间质混合存在。（B）高倍镜下观，腺肉瘤显示良性表现的腺体与邻近的肉瘤性间质。（C 和 D）间质细胞分化可以包括伴有横纹肌母细胞的异源性分化。注意图（C）中良性表现的腺体。

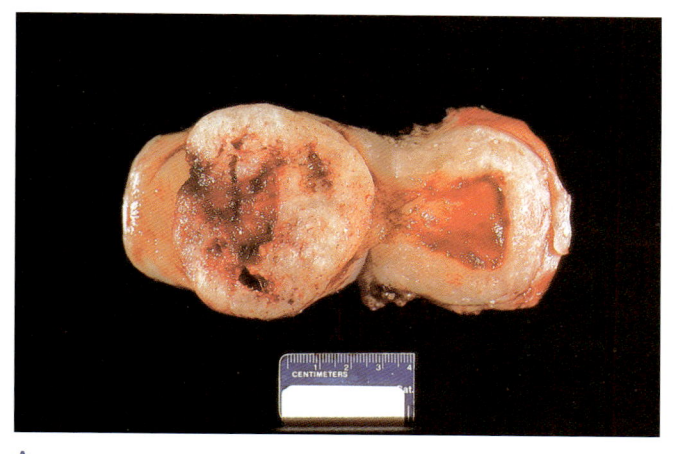
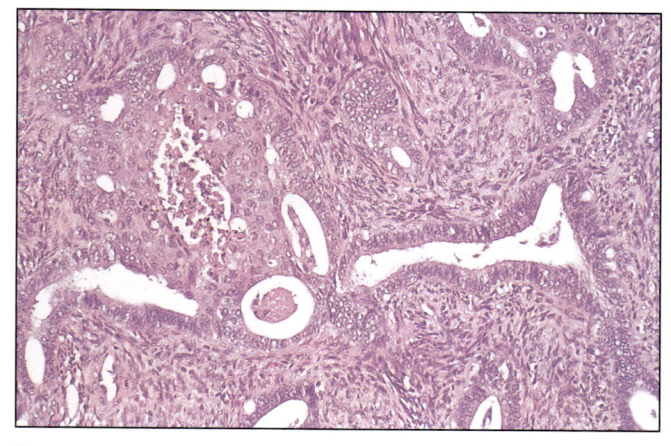

图13B.17 非典型性息肉样腺肌瘤。（A）这个肿瘤表现为子宫下段的一个独立性瘤块。（B）组织学检查，这些肿瘤是由肌瘤性间质和犬牙交错的子宫内膜样腺体混合组成的，而且常见鳞状桑葚。

子宫内膜间质肿瘤
Endometrial stromal tumors

子宫内膜间质偶尔可以发生肿瘤，这种肿瘤细胞可以类似于正常间质细胞，或与间质细胞略有差异。与大多数肿瘤类似，子宫内膜间质肿瘤可以是高分化或为低分化。间质肿瘤被分为三种类型：（1）良性子宫内膜间质结节；（2）低级别子宫内膜间质肉瘤[所谓的淋巴管内间质肌病 (endolymphatic stromal myosis)]；（3）未分化子宫内膜肉瘤。所有这些肿瘤都可以有高的核分裂率，过去认为应该特别注意这一特征，但是现在发现核分裂象对于鉴别这些肿瘤几乎没有价值[79]。

临床特征

与癌肉瘤相比，子宫内膜间质肿瘤一般发生在较年轻的患者，高峰发病年龄在30~50岁之间。子宫内膜间质结节是良性的；Tavassoli 和 Norris[80] 以及 Chang 等[81]报告这种肿瘤的5年生存率均为100%，这一点最近也被其他作者所证实[82]。低级别子宫内膜间质肉瘤的预后是值得警惕的，但是一般具有较好的预后。大约1/3的低级别子宫内膜间质肉瘤患者在10~15年内复发；大约15%的病例发生远处转移和死于转移性肿瘤[81]，但是也可以长期存活。子宫内膜未分化肉瘤死亡率高，预后差。

病理学特征

间质结节（stromal nodule）是一个界限清楚的肿瘤，起初检查时可能被误认为是平滑肌肿瘤；然而，典型的间质结节质地较软并呈黄色。大部分肿瘤小于10 cm。组织学检查肿瘤由子宫内膜间质细胞组成，肿瘤与周围子宫肌层之间有一个分离的界限分明的交界面，虽然两者之间可以出现轻微的局部交错（图13B.18A），但是其深度不应超过3 mm。间质细胞围绕着许多类似于螺旋小动脉的血管。间质结节不发生毛细淋巴管浸润。

低级别子宫内膜间质肉瘤（low-grade endometrial stromal sarcomas）大体可以表现为子宫肌壁内息肉样或弥漫浸润性肿物。组织学上，它们是由高分化子宫内膜间质细胞伴有丛状毛细血管网组成的。不同于子宫内膜间质结节，低级别子宫内膜间质肉瘤以"舌样"方式浸润子宫肌层肌束之间，而且可以累及淋巴管腔，因此过去称之为子宫内膜间质肌病 (endometrial stromal myosis)。重要的是要强调，根据细胞学或核分裂活性无法区分低级别子宫内膜间质肉瘤与子宫内膜间质结节，主要特征是看有无周围子宫肌层或脉管结构的浸润[81]（图13B.18B）。在分子遗传学水平，多数低级别子宫内膜间质肉瘤以染色体交互易位为特征，t (7;17)(p15;q21)[83]，它产生 JAZF1-JJAZ1 融合基因产物[84]。同样的基因畸变出现于间质结节。

在低级别子宫内膜间质肉瘤中，核分裂活性的预后意义不大。单一变量分析发现高手术分期和核分裂指数与肿瘤预后差有关，而在Ⅰ期肿瘤中核分裂指数不具有独立的预后价值。这是将子宫内膜间质肉瘤单独分为一组的原因。45%的Ⅰ期肿瘤表现为轻度细胞学非典型性和低核分裂指数，这些患者中45%出现一次或多次复发。这也就强调了根据分化程度、非典型性和核分裂活性评估间质肉瘤复发的危险性是困难的。许多低级别子宫内膜间质肉瘤可以显示其他类型的分化，包括平滑肌[85,86]和性索[87]分化。后者可以十分类似于卵巢颗粒细胞或其他性索间质肿瘤，具有小而一致的卵圆形细胞核和规则的排列方式。这样的肿瘤 inhibin 染色也可能阳性[88]，类似于与其对应的卵巢肿瘤。区分低级别子宫内膜间质肉瘤和平滑肌肿瘤有时可能是困难的，但是可以借助于免疫组织化学染色。虽然平滑肌肌动蛋白（SMA）和结

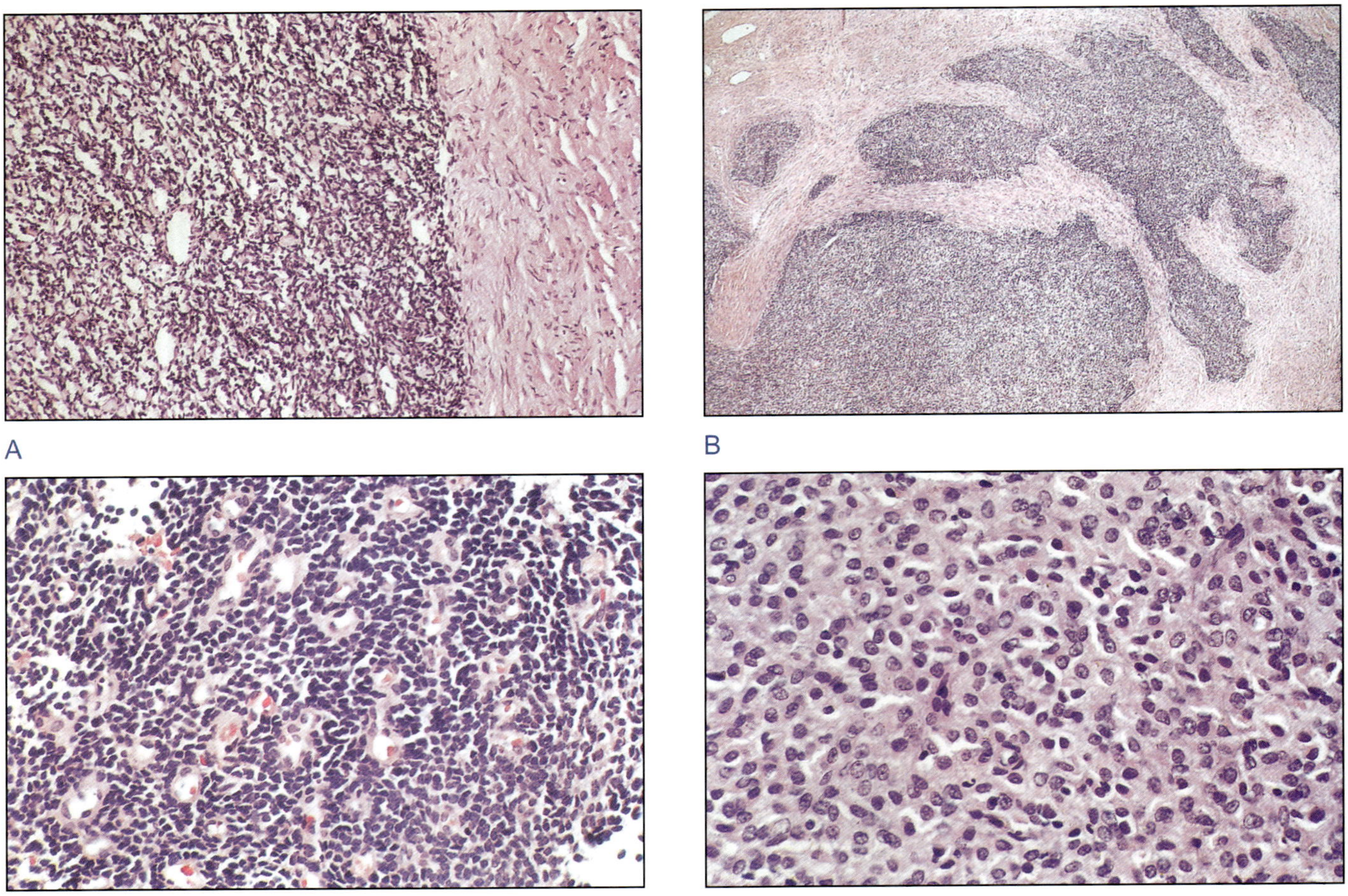

A

B

C

D

图13B.18 子宫内膜间质肿瘤。（A）诊断间质结节要求肿瘤与子宫肌层交界界限清楚，肿瘤和子宫肌层仅有轻微的交错。（B）低级别子宫内膜间质肉瘤表现为不规则的舌状肿瘤性间质浸润子宫肌层。在较高倍数下可见肿瘤细胞围绕血管的排列方式（C）或类似于性索间质肿瘤的条索样排列（D）。

蛋白（desmin）在两个肿瘤均可阳性，CD10 也一样，不过，间质肉瘤 SMA 和 desmin 通常只是局灶阳性，CD10 染色一般较强而且比较明确，另外 caldesmon 在绝大多数子宫平滑肌肿瘤中阳性而间质肉瘤阴性。

未分化子宫内膜肉瘤（undifferentiated endometrial sarcomas）（从前称高级别间质肉瘤）与子宫内膜间质几乎没有相似之处。这些肿瘤以高核分裂率、明显的细胞学非典型性、孕激素受体丧失和常见坏死为特征。Evans 根据严重的间变或多形性将这一组肿瘤与形态学上十分类似于子宫内膜间质的肿瘤（低级别子宫内膜间质肉瘤）分开[89]（图 13B.19）。这种肿瘤被恰当地描述为"未分化"，现在认为它与低级别子宫内膜间质肉瘤无关。因为未分化子宫内膜肉瘤发生在年龄较大的女性，其预后类似于癌肉瘤。Chang 等[81]建议将这一部分肿瘤与间质肉瘤分开，这一提议最近得到 WHO 的认可[79]。

总之，间质肿瘤的诊断是根据它们与子宫内膜间质相似的程度以及与邻近正常组织交界面的关系。良性间质结节与低级别子宫内膜间质肉瘤的区别是根据间质与子宫肌层之间是否有均匀一致的界限，因此，在刮宫标

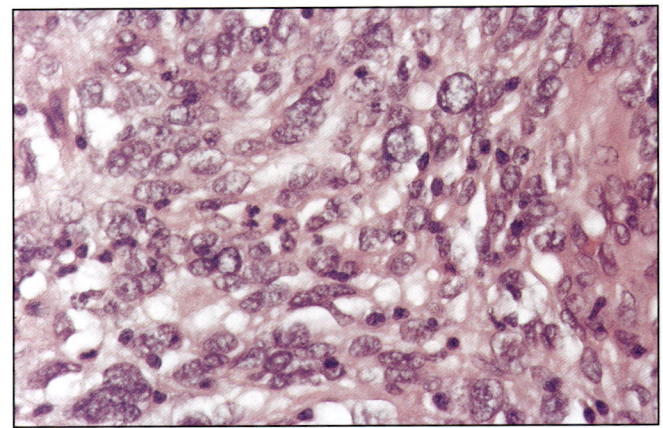

图13B.19 未分化间质肉瘤。这种间变性病变不同于普通的（低级别）子宫内膜间质肉瘤。

本中是不可能做出确切诊断的。低级别子宫内膜间质肉瘤浸润子宫肌层，并可以显示性索样、上皮样和腺体分化。其他有助于诊断的特征包括分支状的血管结构、泡沫细胞伴有坏死和"条索状"胶原。肿瘤医师应该知道低级别子宫内膜间质肉瘤复发率高，而且根据个例不能可靠预测肿瘤的预后。未分化子宫内膜肉瘤在组织学或

抗原表达上与子宫内膜间质少有相似之处，并且常有明显的坏死。

子宫内膜肿瘤形成与他莫西芬治疗
Endometrial neoplasia and tamoxifen therapy

近些年来发现，乳腺癌患者应用他莫西芬治疗与一系列的子宫内膜病变有关，包括良性息肉、黏液性癌、乳头状浆液性癌、腺肉瘤和平滑肌瘤[90-94]。可惜的是，多数研究是个例报告或是通过会诊获得的。此外，危险评估发现，从前患有乳腺肿瘤的妇女发生子宫内膜肿瘤的固有危险性较高，这可能造成混淆。现在推测，他莫西芬能使发生子宫内膜肿瘤的危险性增加。最常见的并发症是发生子宫内膜息肉。他莫西芬的弱雌激素作用可以造成患者易于患癌，但要确定这些妇女是否处于所有已报告肿瘤的高度危险之中，尚需进一步的长期研究。

非 Müller 肿瘤
Non-Müllerian neoplasms

列在这一节中的所有肿瘤并不一定都起源于子宫内膜，虽然偶尔全都可以发生在这个部位而不是子宫肌壁；然而，要确定它们在子宫的确切来源常常是不可能的。

血管肿瘤　　Vascular tumors

累及子宫内膜的良性血管瘤十分罕见[95]。所谓的子宫"血管外皮细胞瘤"可以发生于任何年龄，某些在子宫腔内形成息肉样肿块[96-99]。这些肿瘤的组织学表现与发生在其他部位的肿瘤一样（见第3章），虽然这种肿瘤的确切性质尚有争议。子宫血管外皮细胞瘤可能与子宫内膜间质肉瘤十分相似，可以通过肿瘤中出现不规则的窦样血管进行鉴别诊断，特别是那些显示分支状"鹿角"形态的血管（可以论证，但可能没有说服力）。

子宫血管肉瘤[100-102]是罕见的侵袭性肿瘤，组织学上与发生在皮肤和软组织的肿瘤没有不同（见第3章）。

神经外胚层肿瘤　　Neuroectodermal tumors

累及子宫内膜的良性神经鞘瘤非常罕见[103]。子宫可以发生原始神经外胚层肿瘤[104-106]和胶质瘤性肿瘤[107]，虽然它们的组织发生还不清楚。原始神经外胚层肿瘤（primitive neuroectodermal tumors）倾向于显示明显的神经母细胞或髓母细胞的结构，伴有局灶性神经胶质或神经元分化。子宫内膜单纯性胶质瘤性肿瘤仅有一例报告，类似于低级别原纤维性星形细胞瘤[107]。发生于子宫内膜的副神经节瘤也有少数报告[108,109]。

其他罕见肿瘤　　Miscellaneous rare tumors

所谓的"恶性纤维组织细胞瘤"[110,111]、巨细胞瘤[112,113]、恶性横纹肌样肿瘤[114-116]、腺泡状软组织肉瘤[117-119]、Brenner瘤[120]、成熟性囊性畸胎瘤[121]、未成熟畸胎瘤[122]、卵黄囊瘤[123]、Wilms瘤[124,125]和视网膜原基瘤（retinal anlage tumor）[126]偶尔均可发生于子宫。

淋巴瘤和白血病　　Lymphoma and leukemia

对于患有晚期淋巴瘤和白血病的妇女来说，淋巴瘤或白血病细胞浸润子宫内膜并不少见。然而，在罕见的情况下，淋巴瘤最初可以表现为子宫内膜病变，其中某些病变局限于子宫内膜，显然是原发于这个部位[127-129]。子宫内膜的淋巴瘤通常为非Hodgkin淋巴瘤，虽有一例子宫内膜Hodgkin淋巴瘤报告[130]。多数病例显示B细胞分化，分级可以不同[131,132]。颗粒细胞肉瘤也可以发生在子宫内膜[133]，还有骨髓瘤[134]；非常罕见的情况下慢性淋巴细胞性白血病也可以出现在这个部位[135]。

转移性肿瘤　　Metastatic tumors

生殖道外肿瘤发生子宫转移少见[136-138]。子宫转移性肿瘤的原发肿瘤按发病率递减顺序分别为乳腺癌、胃癌、结肠癌和胰腺癌；少见的转移性肿瘤来自肾、膀胱、胆囊或甲状腺，虽然恶性黑色素瘤也可以转移到子宫[139,140]。

参考文献

1. American Cancer Society 2004 American Cancer Society facts and figures. American Cancer Society, Atlanta, Georgia
2. Curry S, Kelly S 1990 Cancer of the female genital tract: overview. In: Osteen R (ed) Cancer manual. American Cancer Society, Boston, p. 253
3. Rose P G 1996 Endometrial carcinoma. N Engl J Med 335: 640–649
4. Deligdisch L, Holinka C 1987 Endometrial carcinoma: two diseases? Cancer Detect Prev 10: 237–246
5. Peiffer S, Herzog T J, Tribune D et al. 1995 Allelic loss of sequences from the long arm of chromosome 10 and replication errors in endometrial cancers. Cancer Res 55: 1922–1926
6. Arlt M F, Herzog T J, Mutch D G et al. 1996 Frequent deletion of chromosome 1p sequences in an aggressive histologic subtype of endometrial cancer. Hum Mol Genet 5: 1017–1021
7. Sherman M E, Bur M E, Kurman R J 1995 *P53* in endometrial cancer and its putative precursors: evidence for diverse pathways of tumorigenesis. Hum Pathol 26: 1268–1274
8. Lax S F, Pizer E S, Ronnett B M et al. 1998 Clear cell carcinoma of the endometrium is characterized by a distinctive profile of *p53, Ki-67,* estrogen and progesterone receptor expression. Hum Pathol 29: 551–558
9. Faquin W C, Fitzgerald J T, Lin M C et al. 2000 Sporadic microsatellite instability is specific to neoplastic and preneoplastic endometrial tissues. Am J Clin Pathol 113: 576–582
10. Shibata D, Navidi W, Salovaara R et al. 1996 Somatic microsatellite mutations as molecular tumor clocks. Nature Med 2: 676–681
11. Hopkin K 1996 Tumor evolution: survival of the fittest cells. J NIH Res 8: 37–41
12. Califano J, Van der Riet P, Westra W et al. 1996 Genetic progression model for head and neck cancer: implications for field cancerization. Cancer Res 56: 2488–2492

13. Rubin H 1985 Cancer as a dynamic developmental disorder. Cancer Res 45: 2935–2942
14. Zaino R J, Kauderer J, Trimble C L et al. 2006 Reproducibility of the diagnosis of atypical endometrial hyperplasia: a Gynecologic Oncology Group study. Cancer 106: 804–811
15. Mutter G L 2000 Endometrial precancer type collection. Available online at http:www.endometrium.org
16. Mutter G L 2000 Endometrial intraepithelial neoplasia (EIN): will it bring order to chaos? The Endometrial Collaborative Group. Gynecol Oncol 76: 287–290
17. Mutter G L, Boynton K A, Faquin W C et al. 1996 Allelotype mapping of unstable microsatellites establishes direct lineage continuity between endometrial precancers and cancer. Cancer Res 56: 4483–4486
18. Jovanovic A S, Boynton K A, Mutter G L 1996 Uteri of women with endometrial carcinoma contain a histopathologic spectrum of monoclonal putative precancers, some with microsatellite instability. Cancer Res 56: 1917–1921
19. Mutter G L, Chaponot M, Fletcher J 1995 A PCR assay for non-random X chromosome inactivation identifies monoclonal endometrial cancers and precancers. Am J Pathol 146: 501–508
20. Mutter G L, Baak J P A, Crum C et al. 2000 Endometrial precancer diagnosis by histopathology, clonal analysis and computerized morphometry. J Pathol 190: 462–469
21. Mutter G L 2000 Histopathology of genetically defined endometrial precancers. Int J Gynecol Pathol 19: 301–309.
22. Kurman R, Kaminski P, Norris H 1985 The behavior of endometrial hyperplasia: a long term study of "untreated" hyperplasia in 170 patients. Cancer 56: 403–412
23. Sherman A, Brown S 1979 The precursors of endometrial carcinoma. Am J Obstet Gynecol 135: 947–956
24. Tavassoli F, Kraus F 1978 Endometrial lesions in uteri resected for atypical endometrial hyperplasia. Am J Clin Pathol 70: 770–779
25. Colgan T J, Norris H J, Foster W et al. 1983 Predicting the outcome of endometrial hyperplasia by quantitative analysis of nuclear features using a linear discriminant function. Int J Gynecol Pathol 1: 347–352
26. Winkler B, Alvarez S, Richart R et al. 1984 Pitfalls in the diagnosis of endometrial neoplasia. Obstet Gynecol 64: 185–194
27. Bergeron C, Nogales F, Masseroli M et al. 1999 A multicentric European study testing the reproducibility of the WHO classification of endometrial hyperplasia with a proposal of a simplified working classification for biopsy and curettage specimens. Am J Surg Pathol 23: 1102–1108
28. Kendall B S, Ronnett B M, Isacson C et al. 1998 Reproducibility of the diagnosis of endometrial hyperplasia, atypical hyperplasia, and well-differentiated carcinoma. Am J Surg Pathol 22: 1012–1019
29. Mutter G L, Ince T A 2003 Molecular pathogenesis of endometrial cancer. In: Fuller A, Seiden M V, Young R (eds) Uterine cancer: American Cancer Society atlas of clinical oncology. B C Decker, Hamilton, Ontario, Canada, p.10–21
30. Mutter G L 2002 Diagnosis of premalignant endometrial disease. J Clin Pathol 55: 326–331
31. Mutter G L, Ince T A, Baak J P A et al. 2001 Molecular identification of latent precancers in histologically normal endometrium. Cancer Res 61: 4311–4314
32. Mutter G L 2001 Endometrial intraepithelial neoplasia: a new standard for precancer diagnosis. Cont Ob Gyn 46: 92–98
33. Baak J P A, Mutter G L 2005 Endometrial intraepithelial neoplasia (EIN) and the WHO 94 classification of endometrial hyperplasia. J Clin Pathol 58: 1–6
34. Baak J P A, Mutter G L, Robboy S et al. 2005 The molecular genetics and morphometry-based intraepithelial neoplasia classification system predicts disease progression in endometrial hyperplasia more accurately than the 1994 World Health Organization classification system. Cancer 103: 2304–2312
35. Dunton C, Baak J, Palazzo J et al. 1996 Use of computerized morphometric analyses of endometrial hyperplasias in the prediction of coexistent cancer. Am J Obstet Gynecol 174: 1518–1521
36. Hecht J L, Ince T A, Baak J P A et al. 2005 Prediction of endometrial carcinoma by subjective EIN diagnosis. Mod Pathol 18: 324–330
37. Silverberg S G, Mutter G L, Kurman R J et al. 2003 Tumors of the uterine corpus: epithelial tumors and related lesions. In: Tavassoli F A, Stratton M R (eds) WHO classification of tumors: pathology and genetics of tumors of the breast and female genital organs. IARC Press, Lyon, France, p 221–232
38. Nucci M, Crum C, Prasad N et al. 2000 Mucinous endometrial epithelial proliferations: a morphologic spectrum of changes with diverse clinical significance. Mod Pathol 12: 1137–1142
39. Amezcua C A, Lu J J, Felix J C et al. 2000 Apoptosis may be an early event of progestin therapy for endometrial hyperplasia. Gynecol Oncol 79: 169–176
40. Lindahl B, Alm P, Ferno M et al. 1990 Endometrial hyperplasia: a prospective randomized study of histopathology, tissue steroid receptors and plasma steroids after abrasion, with or without high dose gestagen treatment. Anticancer Res 10: 725–730
41. Randall T C, Kurman R J 1997 Progestin treatment of atypical hyperplasia and well-differentiated carcinoma of the endometrium in women under age 40. Obstet Gynecol 90: 434–440
42. Zheng W, Baker H E, Mutter G 2004 Involution of PTEN-null endometrial glands with progestin therapy. Gynecol Oncol 92: 1008–1013
43. Ambros R A, Sherman M E, Zahn C M et al. 1995 Endometrial intraepithelial carcinoma: a distinctive lesion specifically associated with tumors displaying serous differentiation. Hum Pathol 26: 1260–1267
44. Zheng W, Liang S X, Yu H et al. 2004 Endometrial glandular dysplasia: a newly defined precursor lesion of uterine papillary serous carcinoma. Part I: morphologic features. Int J Surg Pathol 12: 207–223
45. Liang S X, Chambers S K, Cheng L et al. 2004 Endometrial glandular dysplasia: a putative precursor lesion of uterine papillary serous carcinoma. Part II: molecular features. Int J Surg Pathol 12: 319–331
46. Goff B A, Kato D, Schmidt R A et al. 1994 Uterine papillary serous carcinoma: patterns of metastatic spread. Gynecol Oncol 54: 264–268
47. Zaino R J, Kurman R J, Diana K L et al. 1995 The utility of the revised International Federation of Gynecology and Obstetrics histologic grading of endometrial adenocarcinoma using a defined nuclear grading system, a Gynecologic Oncology Group study. Cancer 75: 81–86
48. Zaino R J, Kurman R J, Diana K L et al. 1996 Pathologic models to predict outcome for women with endometrial adenocarcinoma. The importance of the distinction between surgical stage and clinical stage. A Gynecologic Oncology Group study. Cancer 77: 1115–1121
49. Zaino R J, Kurman R J, Brunetto V L et al. 1998 Villoglandular adenocarcinoma of the endometrium: a clinicopathologic study of 61 cases. A Gynecologic Oncology Group study. Am J Surg Pathol 22: 1379–1385
50. Ross J C, Eifel P J, Cox R S et al. 1983 Primary mucinous adenocarcinoma of the endometrium. A clinicopathologic and histochemical study. Am J Surg Pathol 7: 715–729
51. Young R H, Scully R E 1992 Uterine carcinomas simulating microglandular hyperplasia: a report of six cases. Am J Surg Pathol 16: 1092–1097
52. Chumas J C, Nelson B, Mann W J et al. 1985 Microglandular hyperplasia of the uterine cervix. Obstet Gynecol 66: 406–409
53. Murray S K, Clement P B, Young R H 2005 Endometrioid carcinomas of the uterine corpus with sex cord-like formations, hyalinization, and other unusual morphologic features: a report of 31 cases of a neoplasm that may be confused with carcinosarcoma and other uterine neoplasms. Am J Surg Pathol 29: 157–166
54. van den Bos M, van den Hoven M, Jongejan E et al. 2004 More differences between HNPCC-related and sporadic carcinomas from the endometrium as compared to the colon. Am J Surg Pathol 28: 706–711
55. Zaino R J, Kurman R J 1988 Squamous differentiation in carcinoma of the endometrium: a critical appraisal of adenoacanthoma and adenosquamous carcinoma. Semin Diagn Pathol 5: 154–171
56. Lininger R A, Ashfaq R, Albores-Saavedra J et al. 1997 Transitional cell carcinoma of the endometrium and carcinoma with transitional cell differentiation. Cancer 79: 1933–1943
57. Hendrickson M R, Kempson R L 1983 Ciliated carcinoma – a variant of endometrial adenocarcinoma: a report of 10 cases. Int J Gynecol Pathol 2: 13–27
58. Eichhorn J H, Young R H, Clement P B 1996 Sertoliform endometrial adenocarcinoma: a study of four cases. Int J Gynecol Pathol 15: 119–126
59. Hendrickson M, Ross J, Eifel P et al. 1982 Uterine papillary serous carcinoma: a highly malignant form of endometrial adenocarcinoma. Am J Surg Pathol 6: 93–108
60. Abeler V M, Kjorstad K E 1990 Serous papillary carcinoma of the endometrium: a histopathological study of 22 cases. Gynecol Oncol 39: 266–271
61. Carcangiu M L, Chambers J T 1992 Uterine papillary serous carcinoma: a study on 108 cases with emphasis on the prognostic significance of associated endometrioid carcinoma, absence of invasion, and concomitant ovarian carcinoma. Gynecol Oncol 47: 298–305
62. Silva E G, Jenkins R 1990 Serous carcinoma in endometrial polyps. Mod Pathol 3: 120–128
63. Gallion H H, van Nagell J R Jr, Powell D F et al. 1989 Stage I serous papillary carcinoma of the endometrium. Cancer 63: 2224–2228
64. Grice J, Ek M, Greer B et al. 1998 Uterine papillary serous carcinoma: evaluation of long-term survival in surgically staged patients. Gynecol Oncol 69: 69–73
65. Carcangiu M L, Tan L K, Chambers J T 1997 Stage Ia uterine serous carcinoma. A study of 13 cases. Am J Surg Pathol 21: 1507–1514
66. Hui P, Kelly M, O'Malley DM et al. 2005. Minimal uterine serous carcinoma: a clinicopathological study of 40 cases. Mod Pathol 18: 75–82
67. Kurman R J, Scully R E 1976 Clear cell carcinoma of the endometrium. An analysis of 21 cases. Cancer 37: 872–882
68. Abeler V M, Kjrstad K E 1991 Clear cell carcinoma of the endometrium: a histopathologic and clinical study of 97 cases. Gynecol Oncol 40: 207–217
69. Abeler V M, Vergote I J, Kjorstad K E et al. 1996 Clear cell carcinoma of the endometrium. Cancer 78: 1740–1747
70. Silverberg S G, Major F J, Blessing J A et al. 1990 Carcinosarcoma (malignant mixed mesodermal tumor) of the uterus. A Gynecologic Oncology Group pathologic study of 203 cases. Int J Gynecol Pathol 9: 110
71. Bitterman P, Chun B, Kurman R J 1990 The significance of epithelial differentiation in mixed mesodermal tumors of the uterus. A clinicopathologic and immunohistochemical study. Am J Surg Pathol 14: 317–328
72. Major F J, Blessing J A, Silverberg S G et al. 1993 Prognostic factors in early-stage uterine sarcoma: a Gynecologic Oncology Group study. Cancer 71 (4 suppl.): 1702–1709
73. Clement P B, Scully R E 1990 Mullerian adenosarcoma of the uterus: a clinicopathologic analysis of 100 cases with a review of the literature. Hum Pathol 21: 363–381
74. Clement P B, Scully R E 1989 Mullerian adenosarcomas of the uterus with sex cord-like elements. A clinicopathologic analysis of eight cases. Am J Clin Pathol 91: 664–672

75. McCluggage W G, Haller U, Kurman R J et al. 2003 Tumors of the uterine corpus: mixed epithelial and mesenchymal lesions. In: Tavassoli F A, Devilee P (eds) WHO classification of tumors: pathology and genetics of tumors of the breast and female genital organs. IARC Press, Lyon, France, p 245–249
76. Mazur M T 1981 Atypical polypoid adenomyomas of the endometrium. Am J Surg Pathol 5: 473–482
77. Young R H, Treger T, Scully R E 1986 Atypical polypoid adenomyoma of the uterus: a report of 27 cases. Am J Clin Pathol 86: 139–145
78. Longacre T A, Chung M, Rouse R V et al. 1996 Atypical polypoid adenomyofibromas (atypical polypoid adenomyomas) of the uterus. A clinicopathologic study of 55 cases. Am J Surg Pathol 20: 1–20
79. Hendrickson M R, Tavassoli F A, Kempson R L et al. 2003 Tumors of the uterine corpus: mesenchymal tumors and related lesions. In: Tavassoli F A, Devilee P (eds) WHO classification of tumors: tumors of the breast and female genital organs. IARC Press, Lyon, France, p 233–244
80. Tavassoli F A, Norris H J 1981 Mesenchymal tumors of the uterus. VII. A clinicopathological study of 60 endometrial stromal nodules. Histopathology 5: 1–10
81. Chang K L, Crabtree G S, Lim-Tan S K et al. 1990 Primary uterine endometrial stromal neoplasms. A clinicopathologic study of 117 cases. Am J Surg Pathol 14: 415–438
82. Dionigi A, Oliva E, Clement P B et al. 2002 Endometrial stromal nodules and endometrial stromal tumors with limited infiltration: a clinicopathologic study of 50 cases. Am J Surg Pathol 26: 567–581
83. Micci F, Walter C U, Teixeira M R et al. 2003 Cytogenetic and molecular genetic analyses of endometrial stroma sarcoma: nonrandom involvement of chromosome arms 6p and 7p and confirmation of JAZF1/JJAZ1 gene fusion in t(7;17). Cancer Genet Cytogenet 144: 119–124
84. Koontz J I, Soreng A L, Nucci M et al. 2001 Frequent fusion of the JAZF1 and JJAZ1 genes in endometrial stromal tumors. Proc Natl Acad Sci USA 98: 6348–6353
85. Oliva E, Clement P B, Young R H et al. 1998 Mixed endometrial stromal and smooth muscle tumors of the uterus. A clinicopathologic study of 15 cases. Am J Clin Pathol 22: 997–1005
86. Yilmaz A, Rush D S, Soslow R A 2002 Endometrial stromal sarcomas with unusual histological features: a report of 24 primary and metastatic tumors emphasizing fibroblastic and smooth muscle differentiation. Am J Surg Pathol 26: 1142–1150
87. Clement P B, Scully R E 1976 Uterine tumors resembling ovarian sex-cord tumors. A clinicopathological analysis of 14 cases. Am J Clin Pathol 66: 512–525
88. Baker R J, Hildebrandt R H, Rouse R V et al. 1999 Inhibin and CD99 (MIC2) expression in uterine stromal neoplasms with sex-cord-like elements. Hum Pathol 30: 671–679
89. Evans H L 1982 Endometrial stromal sarcoma and poorly differentiated endometrial sarcoma. Cancer 50: 2170–2182
90. Cohen I, Rosen D J, Shapira J et al. 1994 Endometrial changes with tamoxifen: comparison between tamoxifen-treated and non-treated asymptomatic postmenopausal breast cancer patients. Gynecol Oncol 52: 185–190
91. Dallenbach-Hellweg G, Hahn U 1995 Mucinous and clear cell adenocarcinomas of the endometrium in patients receiving antiestrogens (tamoxifen) and gestagens. Int J Gynecol Pathol 14: 7–15
92. Silva E G, Tornos C S, Follen-Mitchell M 1994 Malignant neoplasms of the uterine corpus in patients treated for breast carcinoma: the effect of tamoxifen. Int J Gynecol Pathol 13: 248–258
93. Clement P B, Oliva E, Young R H 1996 Mullerian adenosarcoma of the uterine corpus associated with tamoxifen therapy: a report of six cases and a review of tamoxifen-associated endometrial lesions. Int J Gynecol Pathol 15: 222–229
94. Assikis V J, Jordan V C 1995 A realistic assessment of the association between tamoxifen and endometrial cancer. Endocr Rel Ca 2: 235–241
95. Shanberge J N 1994 Hemangioma of the uterus associated with heredity hemorrhagic telangiectasia. Obstet Gynecol 84: 708–710
96. Silverberg S G, Wilson M A, Board J A 1971 Hemangiopericytoma of the uterus: an ultrastructural study. Am J Obstet Gynecol 110: 397–404
97. Sooriyaarachchi G S, Ramirez G, Roley G L 1978 Hemangiopericytomas of the uterus: report of a case with a comprehensive review of the literature. J Surg Oncol 10: 399–408
98. Buscema J, Klein V, Rotmensch J et al. 1987 Uterine hemangiopericytoma. Obstet Gynecol 69: 104–108
99. Munoz A K, Berek J S, Fu Y S et al. 1990 Pelvic hemangiopericytomas: a report of five cases and literature review. Gynecol Oncol 36: 380–382
100. Ongkasuwan C, Taylor J E, Tang C W, Tang C Y et al. 1982 Angiosarcomas of the uterus and ovary. Cancer 49: 1469–1475
101. Witkin G B, Askin F B, Geratz J D et al. 1987 Angiosarcoma of the uterus: a light microscopic, immunohistochemical and ultrastructural study. Int J Gynecol Pathol 6: 176–184
102. Milne D S, Hinshaw K, Malcolm A J et al. 1990 Primary angiosarcoma of the uterus: a case report. Histopathology 16: 203–205
103. Gordon M D, Weilert M, Ireland K 1996 Plexiform neurofibromatosis involving the uterine cervix, endometrium, myometrium and ovary. Obstet Gynecol 88: 699–701
104. Hendrickson M R, Scheithauer B W 1986 Primitive neuroectodermal tumor of the endometrium: report of two cases, one with electron microscopic observations. Int J Gynecol Pathol 5: 249–259
105. Rose P G, O'Toole R V, Keyhani-Rofhaga S et al. 1987 Malignant peripheral primitive neuroectodermal tumor of the uterus. J Surg Oncol 35: 165–167
106. Daya D, Lukka H, Clement P B 1992 Primitive neuroectodermal tumors of the uterus: a report of four cases. Hum Pathol 23: 1120–1129
107. Young R H, Kleinman G W, Scully R E 1981 Glioma of the uterus: report of a case with comments on histogenesis. Am J Surg Pathol 5: 695–699
108. Young T W, Thrasher T V 1982 Non-chromaffin paraganglioma of the uterus: a case report. Arch Pathol Lab Med 106: 608–609
109. Tavassoli F A 1986 Melanotic paraganglioma of the uterus. Cancer 58: 942–948
110. Chou S T, Fortune D, Beischer N A et al. 1985 Primary malignant fibrous histiocytoma of the uterus – ultrasound and immunocytochemical studies of two cases. Pathology 17: 36–40
111. Fujii S, Kanzaki H, Konishi I et al. 1987 Malignant fibrous histiocytoma of the uterus. Gynecol Oncol 26: 319–330
112. Kindblom L G, Seidal T 1981 Malignant giant cell tumour of the uterus. Acta Pathol Microbiol Scand Sect A 89: 179–184
113. Kawai K, Senba M, Tagawa H et al. 1989 Osteoclast-like giant cell tumor of the endometrium. Zentralb Allg Pathol 135: 743–749
114. Cho K R, Rosenhein N B, Epstein J I 1989 Malignant rhabdoid tumor of the uterus. Int J Gynecol Pathol 8: 381–387
115. Fitko R, Brainer J, Schink J C et al. 1990 Endometrioid stromal sarcoma with rhabdoid differentiation. Int J Gynecol Pathol 9: 379–383
116. Niemann T 1997 Malignant rhabdoid tumor of the uterine corpus. Gynecol Oncol 64: 181–182
117. Gray D G, Glick A D, Kurtin P J et al. 1986 Alveolar soft part sarcoma of the uterus. Hum Pathol 17: 297–300
118. Nolan N P M, Gaffney E F 1990 Alveolar soft part sarcoma of the uterus. Histopathology 16: 97–99
119. Guillou L, Lamoureux E, Masse S et al. 1991 Alveolar soft-part sarcoma of the uterine corpus: histological, immunocytochemical and ultrastructural study of a case. Virchow's Arch [A] Pathol Anat Histopathol 418: 467–471
120. Arhleger R E, Bogian J J 1976 Brenner tumor of the uterus. Cancer 38: 1741–1743
121. Martin E, Scholes J, Richart R M et al. 1979 Benign cystic teratoma of the uterus. Am J Obstet Gynecol 135: 429–431
122. Ansah-Boateng Y, Wells M, Poole D R 1985 Coexistent immature teratoma of the uterus and endometrial adenocarcinoma complicated by gliomatosis peritoneii. Gynecol Oncol 21: 106–110
123. Joseph M G, Fellows F G, Hearn S A 1990 Primary endodermal sinus tumor of the endometrium: a clinicopathologic, immunocytochemical and ultrastructural study. Cancer 65: 297–302
124. Bittencourt A L, Britto J F, Fonseca L E 1981 Wilm's tumor of the uterus: the first report in the literature. Cancer 47: 2496–2499
125. Benatar B, Wright C, Freinkel A L et al. 1998 Primary extrarenal Wilms' tumor of the uterus presenting as a cervical polyp. Int J Gynecol Pathol 17: 277–280
126. Schultz D M 1957 A malignant melanotic neoplasm of the uterus, resembling the "retinal anlage" tumour. Am J Clin Pathol 28: 524–533
127. Fox H, More J R S 1965 Primary malignant lymphoma of the uterus. J Clin Pathol 18: 724–728
128. Harris N L, Scully R E 1984 Malignant lymphoma and granulocytic sarcoma of the uterus and vagina: a clinicopathologic analysis of 27 cases. Cancer 53: 2530–2545
129. Benjamin E, Isaacson P G 1996 Lymphoproliferative disease of the ovaries and female genital tract. In: Fox H, Wells M (eds) Haines and Taylor: obstetrical and gynaecological pathology, 4th edn. Churchill Livingstone, Edinburgh, p 1015–1041
130. Hung L H, Kurtz D M 1985 Hodgkin's disease of the endometrium. Arch Pathol Lab Med 109: 762–764
131. Van de Rijn M, Kamel O W, Chang P P et al. 1997 Primary low-grade endometrial B cell lymphoma. Am J Surg Pathol 21: 187–194
132. Vang R, Medeiros L J, Ha C S et al. 2000 Non-Hodgkin's lymphomas involving the uterus: a clinicopathologic analysis of 26 cases. Mod Pathol 13: 19–28
133. Garcia M G, Deavers M T, Knoblock R J et al. 2006 Myeloid sarcoma involving the gynecologic truct. A report of 11 cases and review of the literature. Am J Clin Pathol 125: 783–790
134. Smith N L, Baird D B, Strausbauch P M 1997 Endometrial involvement by multiple myeloma. Int J Gynecol Pathol 61: 173–175
135. Lucia S P, Mills H, Lowenhaupt E et al. 1952 Visceral involvement in primary neoplastic diseases of the reticuloendothelial system. Cancer 5: 1193–1200
136. Kaier W, Holm-Jensen S 1972 Metastases to the uterus. Acta Pathol Microbiol Scand 80: 835–840
137. Kumar N B, Hart W R 1982 Metastases to the uterine corpus from extragenital cancers: a clinicopathologic study of 63 cases. Cancer 50: 2163–2169
138. Kumar A, Schneider V 1983 Metastases to the uterus from extrapelvic primary tumors. Int J Gynecol Pathol 2: 134–140
139. Bauer R D, McCoy C P, Roberts D K et al. 1984 Malignant melanoma metastatic to the endometrium. Obstet Gynecol 63: 264–267
140. Luxman D, Jossiphov J, Cohen J R et al. 1997 Uterine metastasis from vulvar malignant melanoma. A case report. J Reprod Med 42: 244–246

第三部分

胎盘肿瘤和妊娠滋养细胞疾病
Tumors of the placenta and gestational trophoblastic disease

Christopher P. Crum、Yonghee Lee 和 David R. Genest 著

戴 林 译　回允中 校

胎盘肿瘤和妊娠滋养细胞疾病		滋养细胞起源	674
胎盘绒毛膜血管瘤	672	完全性和部分性水泡状胎块	675
其他罕见的良性胎盘肿瘤	672	侵袭性和转移性水泡状胎块	677
在胎盘内辨认胎儿恶性肿瘤	673	妊娠绒毛膜癌	677
来自母体的胎盘转移性肿瘤	673	胎盘内绒毛膜癌	679
妊娠滋养细胞疾病	674	胎盘部位滋养细胞肿瘤	679

引言　Introduction

发生在胎盘的肿瘤可以分为三种。第一种是胎盘实质的良性肿瘤，包括绒毛膜血管瘤；第二种是位于母体血管腔隙内（包括良性病变和转移性恶性肿瘤）或胎儿血管内（胎儿白血病或其他肿瘤）的母体或胎儿来源的肿瘤；第三种是滋养细胞肿瘤。

胎盘绒毛膜血管瘤
Placental chorangioma

绒毛膜血管瘤（血管瘤或所谓的胎盘血管黏液瘤）是良性肿瘤，大约见于1%的胎盘[1]。大多数绒毛膜血管瘤为孤立性质硬的实性结节，直径可达几个厘米，肿瘤位于接近胎儿面的胎盘表面实质内[1-3]。切面呈光滑的黏液样质地，为褐色、暗红色或呈花斑状表现（图13C.1）。

组织学上，肿瘤由多量薄壁胎儿型毛细血管或血窦组成，间质稀少，可以是纤维性、钙化或呈黏液样表现。绒毛膜血管瘤周围界限清楚（图13C.2）。

小而孤立的绒毛膜血管瘤通常没有临床意义，但多发性绒毛膜血管瘤可以伴有胎儿血管瘤。大的绒毛膜血管瘤（特别是直径大于5 cm）可以引起胎儿水肿、充血性心力衰竭和血小板减少症。

其他罕见的良性胎盘肿瘤
Other rare, benign placental tumors

与相对常见的胎盘绒毛膜血管瘤比较，已报告的其他良性胎盘肿瘤非常罕见；其中包括畸胎瘤[6-10]、肝腺瘤[11]以及肾上腺皮质腺瘤或残余[12-14]。所有这些肿瘤都是偶然的病理学所见，不伴有母体或胎儿异常。胎盘畸胎瘤通常为体积小的实性结节，附着于胎盘的胎儿面，

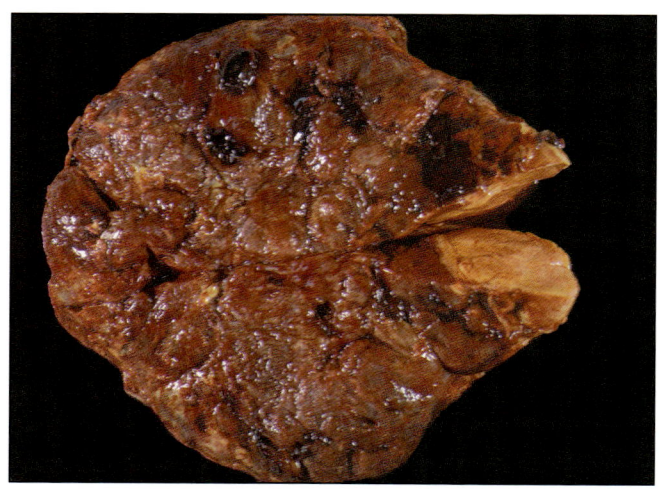

图13C.1　绒毛膜血管瘤的大体表现。

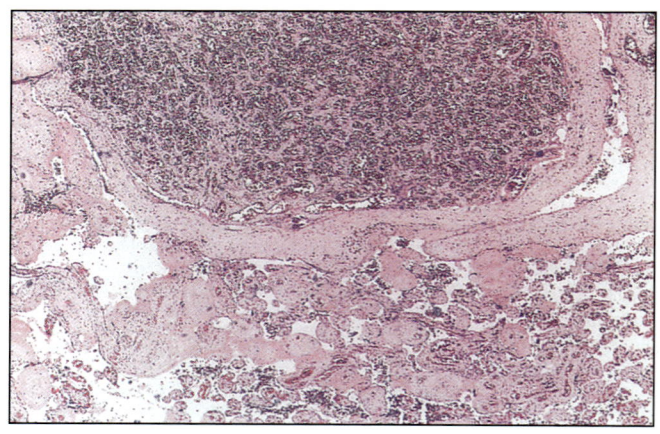

图13C.2　足月妊娠胎盘的良性绒毛膜血管瘤：类似于毛细血管瘤的胎儿毛细血管增生累及增大的干绒毛。

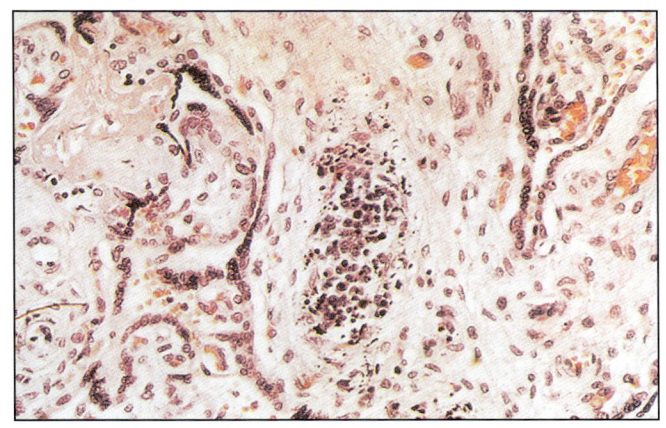

图13C.3 先天性肾上腺神经母细胞瘤广泛播散到足月胎盘的胎儿血管；本图可能类似于胎儿成红细胞增多症。

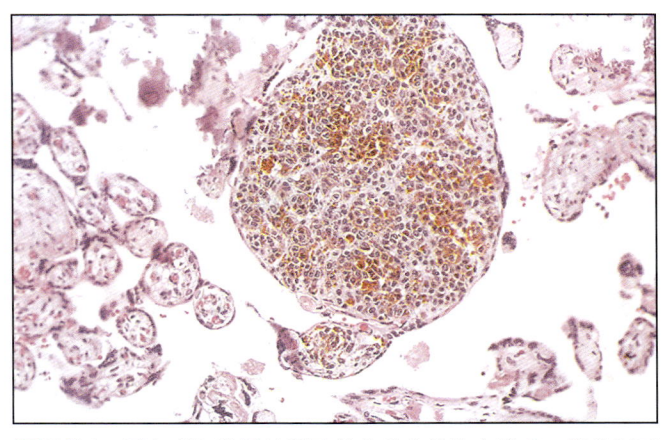

图13C.4 黑色素细胞局灶累及单个扩大的终末绒毛。婴儿躯干有一个巨大的先天性黑色素细胞痣，在4岁时病人情况良好。

由排列紊乱的来自所有三个胚层的成熟组织组成。大多数病例是以肠和皮肤组织分化为主。

恶性肿瘤细胞聚集。

胎儿的黑色素细胞病变很少累及胎盘，包括恶性黑色素瘤[19]和良性先天性黑色素细胞痣[20-22]。后者通常为位于绒毛间质内的体积小的孤立性色素痣细胞结节（图13C.4）；随访发现所有已报告的病例均为良性，符合神经外胚层细胞的异常迁移而不是转移。

在胎盘内辨认胎儿恶性肿瘤
Fetal malignancies identified in the placenta

先天性神经母细胞瘤是胎儿最常见的恶性肿瘤，偶尔转移到胎盘[15-18]。其特征为，大量小的肿瘤细胞播散到整个胎儿血管，非常类似于胎儿成红细胞增多症（erythroblastosis fetalis）（图13C.3）；胎盘水肿和绒毛水肿使之更加相似[15]。大部分病例肿瘤细胞局限于胎儿血管内，但绒毛间质浸润也有描述[16]。在胎盘可以辨认的另外一种恶性肿瘤是胎儿白血病，它与Down综合征有关。这个肿瘤表现为在绒毛干和终末绒毛的血管中出现胎儿髓母细胞，以及在绒毛实质中有

来自母体的胎盘转移性肿瘤
Maternal metastatic tumors in the placenta

母体恶性肿瘤转移到胎盘少见；已报告的少于100例[23-31]。最常见的转移到胎盘的4个肿瘤是：（1）黑色素瘤；（2）淋巴瘤/白血病；（3）乳腺癌；（4）肺癌[23-25,27,29-31]。胎盘的母体转移性肿瘤的特征是，局限于胎盘母体面绒毛之间的血管中，没有绒毛间质浸润

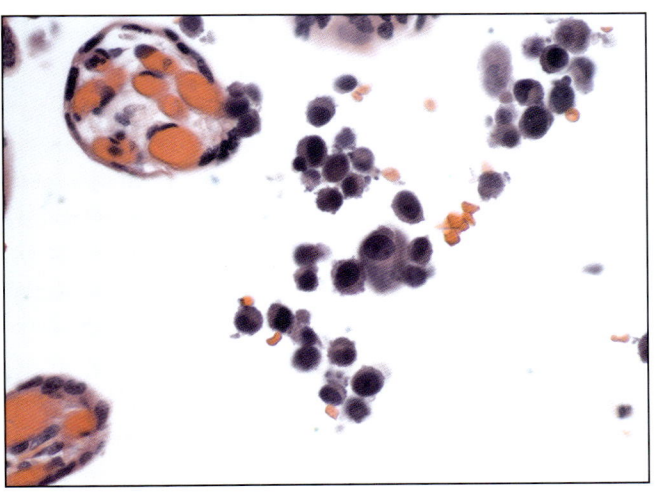

A

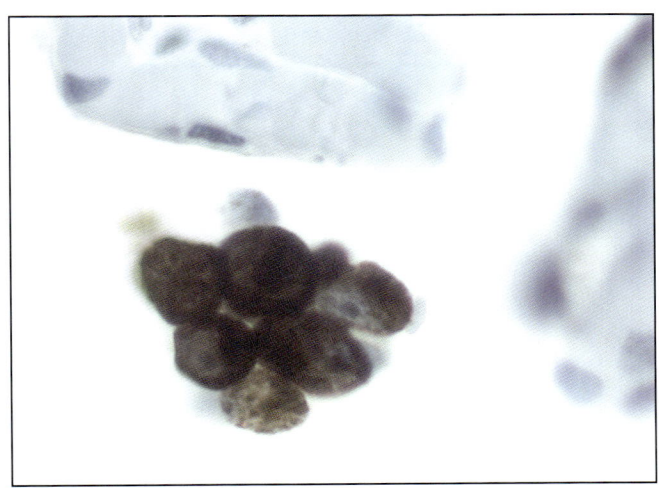

B

图13C.5 （A）绒毛间隙中散在来自母体黑色素瘤的恶性细胞。（B）肿瘤HMB-45强阳性。

（图 13C.5）。鉴别诊断包括胎盘内纤维蛋白中良性滋养细胞增生和胎盘内绒毛膜癌（见下）。

妊娠滋养细胞疾病 Gestational trophoblastic disease

引言 Introduction

世界卫生组织（WHO）的妊娠滋养细胞疾病分类将滋养细胞肿瘤分为以下几种类型，包括恶性肿瘤[妊娠绒毛膜癌和胎盘部位滋养细胞肿瘤（PSTT）]和瘤样病变、水泡状胎块（完全性、部分性、浸润性和转移性）、胎盘部位过度生长（过去称作合体细胞子宫内膜炎）以及胎盘部位结节或斑块[32,33]。不管怎样，肿瘤和瘤样病变的区分是根据定义。为了讨论的目的，将水泡状胎块看做是具有"前体"性质的肿瘤，即它们具有不同程度的进展为恶性肿瘤（绒毛膜癌）的危险性。

滋养细胞起源 Trophoblastic origins

妊娠期间滋养细胞的发展是从相对单一的胚外组织增生开始（绒毛前滋养细胞），随后进展为组织并区分为不同的分化途径。后一过程开始于胚胎发生并持续存在于整个妊娠期间。早期，滋养细胞密集于间质周围形成绒毛，在这个过程中形成绒毛细胞滋养细胞（villous cytotrophoblast），它表现为 p63 和增生性（MIB-1）免疫染色强阳性（图 13C.6）。这些阳性染色结果能将细胞滋养细胞与外围的绒毛外滋养细胞（extravillous trophoblast）（p63⁻、MIB-1⁻）区分开来。在胎盘细胞滋养细胞分化为绒毛合体滋养细胞（villous syncytiotrophoblast）（p63⁻、MIB-1⁻、inhibin⁺）和成熟的绒毛外滋养细胞，两者接近母体面的表面，位于绒毛之间。后者的发展经过一个由具有少量透明胞浆的绒毛外细胞（p63⁺/inhibin⁺）组成的中间阶段，随后细胞发育完全成熟，胞浆双染（p63⁻/inhibin⁺）。胎盘膜的透明细胞表型也很突出，由绒毛滋养细胞组成（图 13C.6）。最终，细胞滋养细胞被看做是增生的干细胞成分，沿着不同的分化途径变得成熟。完全性水泡状胎块和绒毛膜癌是以细胞滋养细胞增生为特征，部分性水泡状胎块仅为合体滋养细胞增生，而 PSTT 则是绒毛外基底滋养细胞（extravillous basal trophoblast）增生。部分 PSTT 含有上皮样滋养细胞（epithelioid trophoblast），p63 染色强阳性，推测是处于细胞滋养细胞和成熟绒毛外滋养细胞中间分化阶段的细胞的肿瘤性转化。一些作者提出这些肿瘤起源于膜滋养细胞（membranous trophoblastic cells）。然而，因为所有滋养细胞的形成都是一个连续分化的过程，所以可以认为这

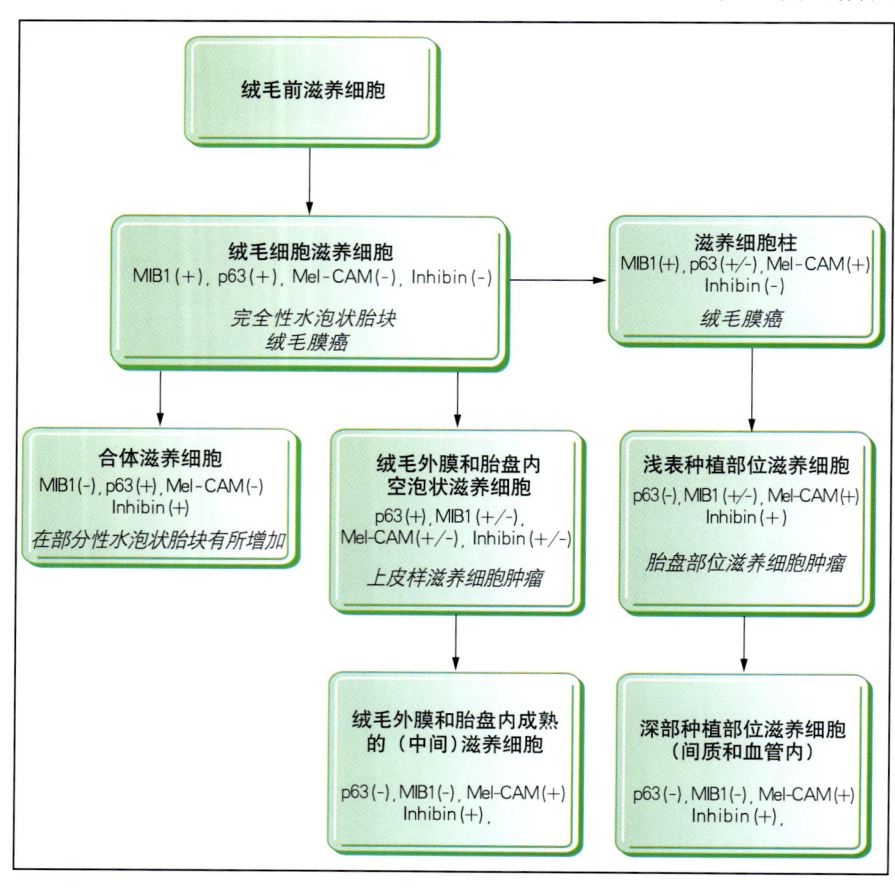

图13C.6 滋养细胞谱系及其肿瘤。

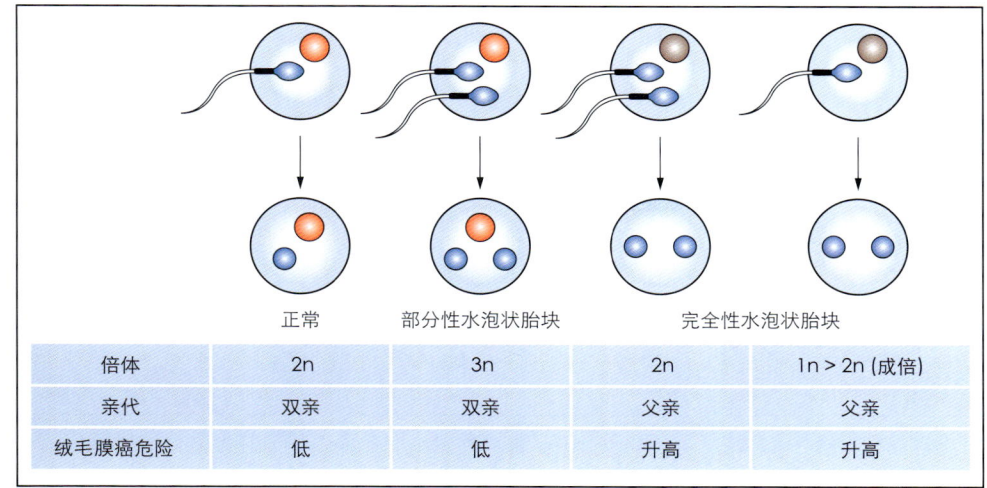

图13C.7 图示水泡状胎块的遗传学基础。

些肿瘤起源于胎盘内绒毛外滋养细胞。

完全性和部分性水泡状胎块
Complete and partial hydatidiform mole

水泡状胎块是具有绒毛水肿肿胀和滋养细胞增生的异常胎盘。所有水泡状胎块妊娠都是由异常受精引起的。完全性水泡状胎块是缺乏母体染色体的"空卵"（empty egg）受精，或是通过单个精子（90%的病例）复制其染色体成分变成46XX，或是通过两个精子（10%的病例）导致双精子46XX或46XY水泡状胎块[34-36]。相反，部分性水泡状胎块是三倍体，来自父体（雄异配性，diandric）基因组的另外两个复制，形成三倍体水泡状胎块（70%为69XXY；27%为69XXX；3%为69XYY）（图13C.7）[37-39]。雌异配性（digynic）（两个母体等位基因）三倍体妊娠是非水泡状胎块。除了这些细胞遗传学上的差别以外，完全性和部分性水泡状胎块在临床表现、生物学行为和病理学特征上也有不同[40-42]。

完全性水泡状胎块最常见于生育年龄两端的妇女和从前有过水泡状胎块的妇女。它的发病率在世界各地明显不同。发病率最高的地区是亚洲、拉丁美洲和中东（1:500妊娠者）。与之相比较，爱尔兰完全性水泡状胎块（1:2000妊娠者）和部分性水泡状胎块（1:700妊娠者）的发病率明显偏低[43]。

完全性水泡状胎块一般见于妊娠第一个三月期的晚期或第二个三月期的早期，伴有阴道出血、没有胎儿心跳、子宫不适当增大、βhCG水平显著升高和特征性的超声所见；水泡状胎块临床上容易诊断。近年来，随着超声检查的广泛使用，对完全性水泡状胎块典型表现的认识已经得到明显改进，使其能够较早诊断并终止异常妊娠。在1980年前，完全性水泡状胎块在平均妊娠16周被终止妊娠；现在，多数完全性水泡状胎块在8～12周即被终止妊娠，这些患者在临床上常常不被怀疑是水泡状胎块[44]。部分性水泡状胎块在临床上通常也不被怀疑，而是表现为过期流产，第一个三月期晚期出血，而且子宫小。

关于临床上的生物学行为，完全性水泡状胎块之后持续性妊娠滋养细胞肿瘤的发生率大约在20%～30%[45,46]，而部分性水泡状胎块后为1%～5%[41,47]。持续性滋养细胞肿瘤是一种临床诊断，这种诊断是根据βhCG促性腺激素未能自行降低做出的。持续性滋养细胞肿瘤的病理表现可以是子宫内残留的胎块绒毛、侵袭性水泡状胎块、转移性水泡状胎块、绒毛膜癌或PSTT。常常不能得到为准确病理学诊断所需的组织。完全性水泡状胎块后大约2%发生绒毛膜癌[46]，而部分性水泡状胎块极少发生绒毛膜癌，只有3例完整的病例报告[48]。

完全性水泡状胎块的大体标本通常表现为大量半透明葡萄样肿胀的绒毛（囊泡），直径可达2cm。没有妊

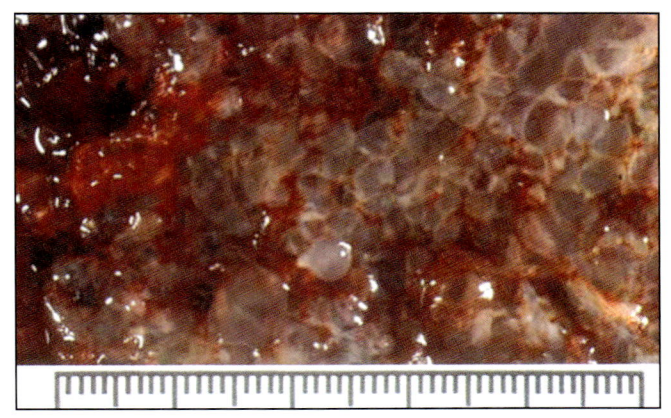

图13C.8 完全性水泡状胎块水肿绒毛的大体表现。

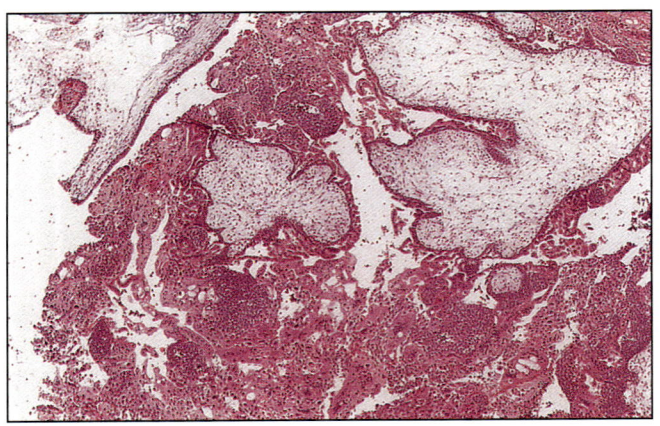

图13C.9 早期完全性水泡状胎块（妊娠8周排出物）伴有绒毛轻度水肿和小的空泡形成。但是两种滋养细胞出现明显增生和非典型增生。绒毛间质呈蓝色，富于细胞，伴有圆形球状突起。

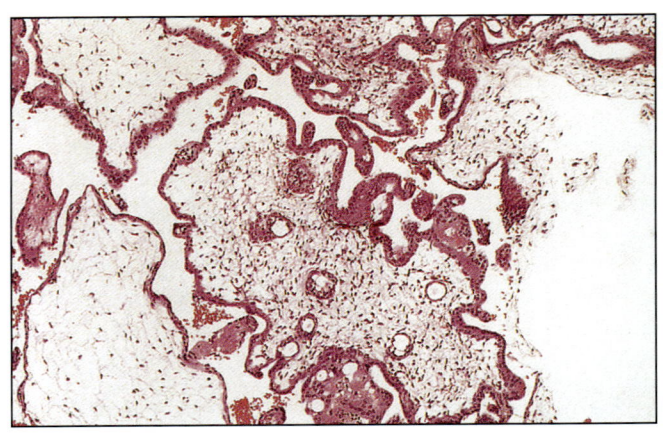

图13C.10 部分性水泡状胎块，伴有轻度滋养细胞增生。水肿绒毛边缘呈不规则"扇贝形"，并伴有许多滋养细胞内陷和"包涵体"形成。

娠囊、羊膜、脐索或胎儿组织（除了罕见的双胎病例）（图13C.8）。组织学上，绒毛弥漫性水肿，伴有大量充分发育的水池；间质中可见内衬原始内皮细胞的血管腔，但没有胎儿血细胞。细胞滋养细胞、绒毛外滋养细胞和合体滋养细胞总是出现增生和非典型性增生。常见细胞核分裂活跃，核明显增大和深染。增生的滋养细胞围绕绒毛杂乱排列（与正常早期胎盘中的"有极性"的滋养细胞增生不同）。种植部位滋养细胞也常显示明显的细胞非典型性，而且伴有大而奇异的深染细胞核；在绝大多数完全性水泡状胎块这种非典型性是明显的，但在部分性水泡状胎块不常见[49]。

上述病理学特征是>12周妊娠完全性水泡状胎块最特征性的表现。而较早期妊娠（<12周）的完全性水泡状胎块的表现通常比较轻微，使其病理诊断更具挑战性[44]。大体检查，早期完全性水泡状胎块的水池可以缺少或不明显。组织学上，虽然绒毛中的空泡可能不明显，但有显著的两种滋养细胞增生和非典型性增生（图13C.9）。提示早期完全性水泡状胎块病理学诊断的其他线索包括：种植部位滋养细胞明显非典型性，伴有微小星形间质细胞的异常原始绒毛间质，间质富于细胞和显著的核碎裂以及不常见的复杂球状突起的绒毛（"菜花样"绒毛）[44,50-52]。完全性水泡状胎块的组织学分级（根据滋养细胞非典型性和增生的程度）与临床生物学行为没有相关性[45,53]。

部分性水泡状胎块标本不如完全性水泡状胎块多。它由外观正常的不成熟胎盘组织组成，偶尔混合有水泡状胎块的水泡；此外，还经常可以见到羊膜、脐带和胚胎/胎儿组织。组织学上，部分性水泡状胎块由两种绒毛成分混合而成：(1) 小的纤维化的"正常"绒毛；(2) 大而不规则的水肿性绒毛，伴有多灶性轻到中度滋养细胞增生。某些增大的绒毛有中心水池，其他增大的绒毛有地图状、扇贝形的边缘，伴有不规则的滋养细胞内陷

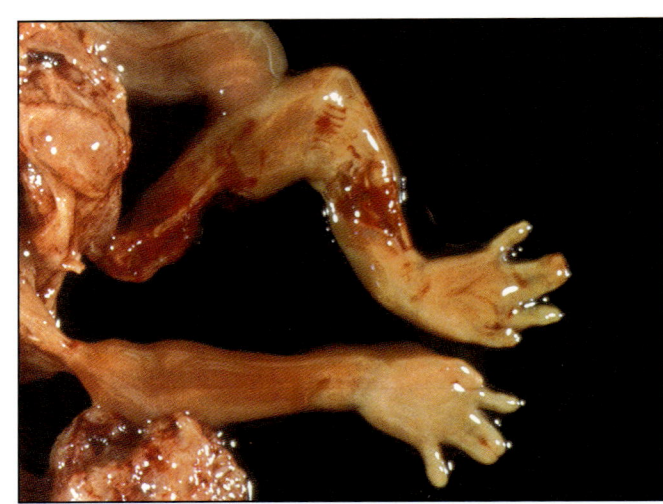

图13C.11 与部分性水泡状胎块和三倍体妊娠有关的并指（趾）畸形。

和包涵物形成（图13C.10）。部分性水泡状胎块滋养细胞的增生一般呈局灶状、轻度，并主要由合体滋养细胞组成，绒毛周围有许多杂乱排列的微小合体滋养细胞簇或"出芽"，或绒毛周围有大量合体滋养细胞聚集，具有明显胞浆陷窝，导致"花边状"或"蚕食样"表现。绒毛间质血管常常含有有核胎儿红细胞；另外，常见晚期胎儿发育的其他组织学证据，包括绒毛板、羊膜、脐带和胚胎/胎儿组织。当大体可见胎儿组织时，几乎总可发现胎儿畸形，特别是并指（趾）畸形（相邻的手指和脚趾融合）（图13C.11）[54,55]。

水泡状胎块的鉴别诊断包括：完全性还是部分性水泡状胎块；水肿性流产还是水泡状胎块；类似于水泡状胎块的特殊性胎儿综合征，包括18三体、Beckwith-Wiedemann综合征[56-58]和胎盘血管瘤性畸形[59]；以及部分性水泡状胎块还是水泡状胎块与双胎共存（图13C.12）[60-62]。

有关完全性和部分性水泡状胎块之间的鉴别诊断，

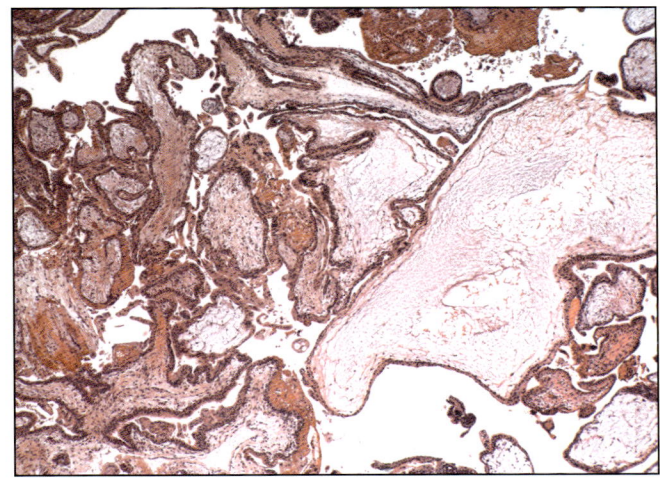

图13C.12 双胎性完全性水泡状胎块（右）和正常妊娠绒毛（左）。

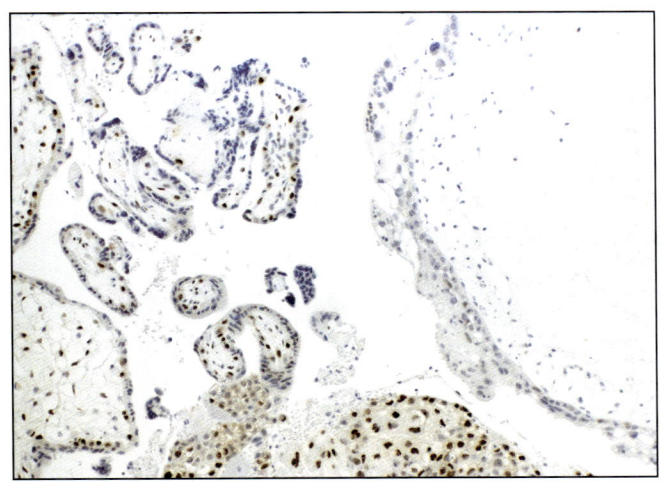

图13C.13 为图13C.12中的双胎性完全性水泡状胎块/正常妊娠绒毛的p57染色。完全性水泡状胎块绒毛组织中细胞滋养细胞和间质细胞 p57染色阴性（右），而正常绒毛p57染色阳性（左）。两者的绒毛外滋养细胞（底部）p57染色均为阳性，可作为阳性对照。

从前几项研究是应用 DNA 流式细胞技术，显示三倍体为部分性水泡状胎块[52,63-68]。然而，过去几年发表的一系列文章已经建立了免疫组织化学定位特异性基因的基因产物作为"金指标"，用以鉴别部分性与完全性水泡状胎块和完全性水泡状胎块与水肿性流产[69-73]。研究最多的是 p57KIP2，它表达的是来源于母体衍生的等位基因。因为这种后生的（epigenetic）调节机制，p57 在完全性水泡状胎块的细胞滋养细胞和绒毛间质细胞没有表达，不同于部分性水泡状胎块和水肿性流产（图13C.13）。有趣的是，所有妊娠的绒毛外滋养细胞均有p57 表达，可以将它作为一种有用的阳性对照。在个别例外情况下[74]，完全性水泡状胎块这个标志物阴性。由于不同观察者之间区分完全性水泡状胎块与部分性水泡状胎块或水肿性流产的可重复性存在差异，所以如果对水肿性妊娠的性质产生任何怀疑[75]，均应考虑做 p57KIP2 和其他相似标志物的免疫组织化学染色。

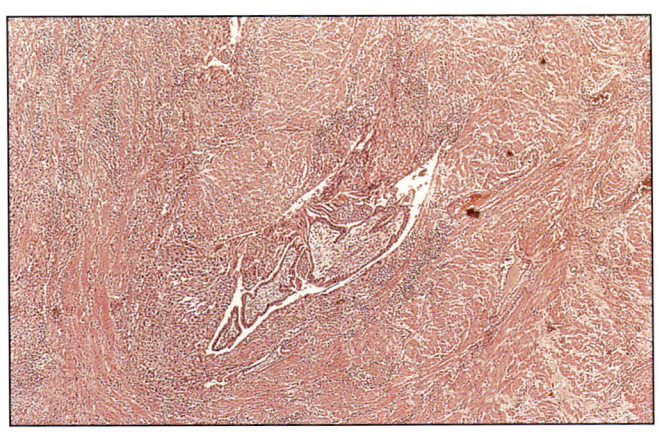

图13C.14 子宫切除标本中的侵袭性水泡状胎块；完全性水泡状胎块的绒毛出现在子宫肌壁深层的静脉管腔中。

侵袭性和转移性水泡状胎块
Invasive and metastatic mole

侵袭性水泡状胎块是指水泡状胎块（部分性或完全性）的绒毛组织出现在子宫肌层或子宫的血管中。在发生血管浸润之后，绒毛可以栓塞到远隔部位，包括阴道、肺和脑（转移性水泡状胎块）。当发展为持续性妊娠滋养细胞肿瘤时，如果宫腔内含有少量组织（经刮宫或超声检查确定），临床上可能需要怀疑侵袭性水泡状胎块的可能性。刮宫标本不能做出侵袭性水泡状胎块的病理学诊断，而要求外科手术标本才能诊断（即子宫切除、肺活检）；因为不经常使用外科手术方法治疗滋养细胞肿瘤，现在很少诊断浸润性和转移性水泡状胎块。

侵袭性水泡状胎块的大体表现是子宫肌壁内出血性结节，常没有可以辨认的绒毛。组织学上，在子宫肌壁或血管中可见伴有非典型性增生滋养细胞的水肿绒毛（图 13C.14）。侵袭性和转移性水泡状胎块采用化疗通常可以治愈，但是局部出血可能引起病人死亡，例如透壁性侵袭性水泡状胎块导致的腹腔内出血，或转移性水泡状胎块引起的肺出血。

妊娠绒毛膜癌
Gestational choriocarcinoma

妊娠绒毛膜癌可以发生于水泡状胎块妊娠（50%）、流产（25%）、异位妊娠（2.5%）或正常妊娠（22.5%）

之后[76]。绒毛膜癌通常发生在妊娠（水泡状胎块或其他）之后，其间隔为几个月；然而，发生在妊娠以后间隔很长（长达14年）的绒毛膜癌已有报告[77]。少数病例，可经胎盘病理学检查立即做出妊娠后胎盘内绒毛膜癌的诊断[78,79]。个别情况下，母亲的绒毛膜癌可以引起新生儿的转移[80,81]。

大多数妊娠后绒毛膜癌由于肿瘤累及子宫内膜而表现为异常子宫出血；一些症状也可以反映肿瘤转移，例如咯血和神经系统异常。在发生肿瘤转移的患者中，肺是最常受累的部位（90%），其次是脑和肝（50%）[82]。与先前不存在水泡状胎块的患者比较，水泡状胎块后的绒毛膜癌预后较好，可能与患水泡状胎块后密切监测使其可以早期诊断有关[83]。

绒毛膜癌大体表现为界限清楚的出血性结节（图13C.15）。组织学上，由于存活的肿瘤组织可能仅仅见于出血性结节的周边，因此可能需要广泛取材。肿瘤由合体滋养细胞、细胞滋养细胞和绒毛外滋养细胞混合组成，伴有明显的出血、坏死和血管浸润（图13C.16）。绒毛膜癌不引起间质反应或宿主的新生血管形成。恶性滋养细胞表现为明显的细胞非典型性和双向分化，伴有小巢状细胞滋养细胞（细胞界限清楚，胞浆透明）周围围绕多核合体滋养细胞（伴有紫色泡沫状胞浆）。合体滋养细胞 hCG 免疫组织化学染色强阳性，而人类胎盘催乳素（hPL）免疫反应弱阳性；成熟的绒毛外（中间性）滋养细胞免疫组织化学染色结果与之相反。所有类型的滋养细胞细胞角蛋白免疫组织化学染色结果强阳性。绒毛膜癌不进行组织学分级，因为它没有临床意义；然而，研究提示具有丰富的合体滋养细胞分化或明显慢性炎症的肿瘤预后较好[84]。某些肿瘤应用流式细胞技术研究显示为二倍体肿瘤，包括一些致死性病例[85]。

绒毛膜癌常经子宫内膜刮宫诊断，肿瘤表现为大量

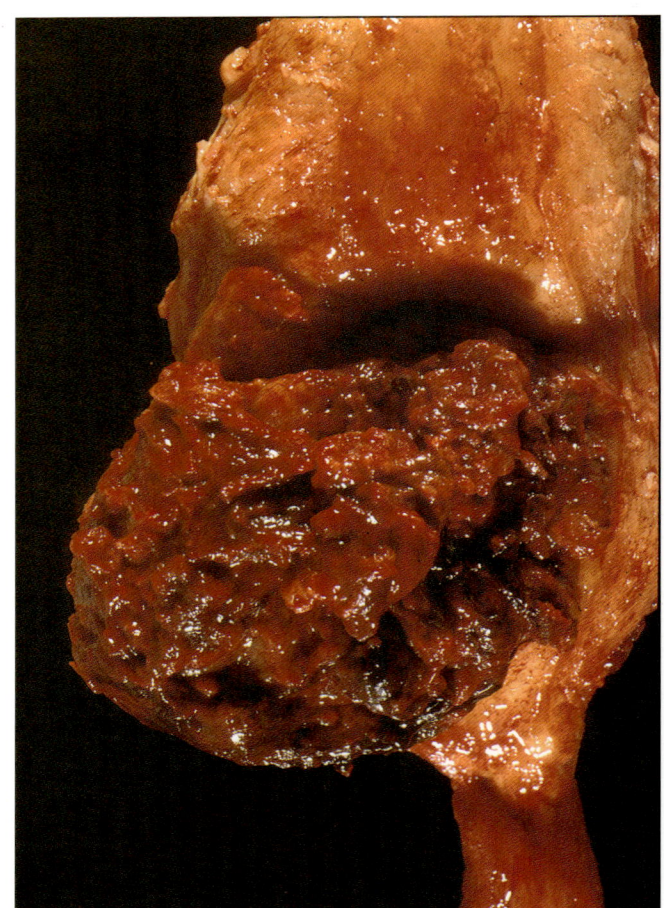

图13C.15 绒毛膜癌的大体表现，这里看到的是子宫内膜的出血性肿块。

出血和坏死，伴有大片双向型细胞，滋养细胞非典型性明显，核分裂活跃，没有绒毛组织（图13C.17）[86,87]。绒毛膜癌的鉴别诊断包括早期妊娠时的绒毛前滋养细胞、水泡状胎块后的持续性胎块组织、胎盘部位滋养细胞肿瘤（PSTT）和未分化癌。关于绒毛前滋养细胞，是少数缺乏明显细胞非典型性以及没有出血或坏死的

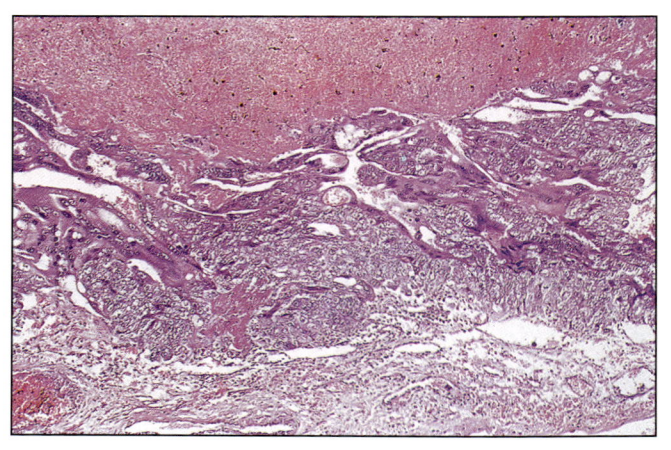

A

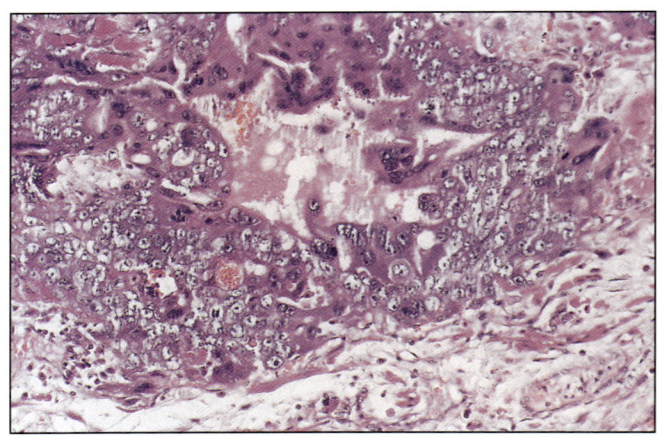

B

图13C.16 绒毛膜癌显示广泛出血（A），这是一个常见的现象。肿瘤呈现双向性，由细胞滋养细胞和多核合体滋养细胞组成（B），这种形态类似于正常种植的胚囊。绒毛膜癌显示这种程度的存活性是不常见的，因为大多数表现为广泛坏死。

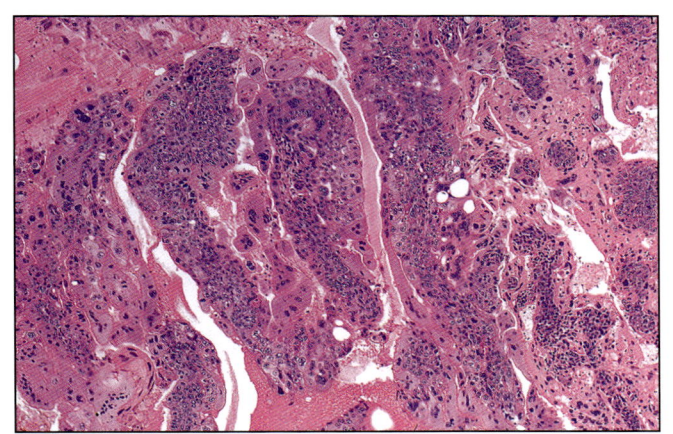

图13C.17　子宫内膜刮宫标本中的绒毛膜癌。

滋养细胞，它提示为早期妊娠。在水泡状胎块后的刮宫标本中，显微镜下可见散在的具有非典型性的滋养细胞灶；虽然这种表现提示绒毛膜癌，但也应该考虑来自侵袭性水泡状胎块的滋养细胞的可能性。PSTT基本上不含有合体滋养细胞，它是单形性中间滋养细胞肿瘤。hPL和hCG免疫组织化学染色可能更支持PSTT（如果以hPL染色阳性为主）。某些PSTT表现为hCG强阳性，但血清hCG水平低。

胎盘内绒毛膜癌
Intraplacental choriocarcinoma

多数妊娠绒毛膜癌发生在产后数周到数月。在罕见的情况下，绒毛膜癌与妊娠同时发生的病例已有报告[78,79,88-91]。胎盘内绒毛膜癌在婴儿出生前（因为转移）或在分娩时（在检查胎盘时偶然发现）诊断。足月胎盘中的绒毛膜癌在大体上通常表现为孤立性"梗死"结节，大小可达几个厘米；一例报告表现为多发性广泛播散的、5mm的白色小结节[90]。组织学上表现为位于母体面绒毛之间间隙的非典型性双向性的实性滋养细胞增生，并见多灶性粘附于绒毛间质（图13C.18）。细胞核深染，核分裂活跃，原始表现的细胞滋养细胞与合体滋养细胞混合，后者具有许多胞浆空隙。

胎盘内绒毛膜癌的鉴别诊断包括母体肿瘤转移到胎盘和良性胎盘内中间滋养细胞增生。后者表现为成簇的中间滋养细胞，细胞周围围绕纤维素样物质，胞浆嗜酸性，核深染，形状不规则，偶见核内包涵体，没有核分裂象。

胎盘部位滋养细胞肿瘤
Placental site trophoblastic tumor (PSTT)

PSTT是罕见的肿瘤，文献中大约有150例报告[92-107]。绒毛膜癌和PSTT之间在临床上具有几点区别：

1. 50%的绒毛膜癌发生在水泡状胎块之后，但水泡状胎块之后的PSTT很少有报告，大多数PSTT病例发生于正常妊娠之后。
2. 大多数绒毛膜癌发生在妊娠之后数周或数月，而PSTT发生的时间较短。
3. 绒毛膜癌是高度恶性的肿瘤，但对化疗和放射治疗非常敏感；相反，只有少数PSTT表现恶性生物学行为，它们对化疗和放疗不敏感。

大多数PSTT患者表现为不规则的阴道出血和低度阳性的βhCG。某些患者出现闭经、不孕或肾病综合征。

大体上，PSTT为棕红色实性结节，伴有不同程度的出血和坏死，典型者累及子宫内膜和肌层。组织学上，PSTT是中间滋养细胞或细胞滋养细胞的单向性增生，没有明显的合体滋养细胞。中间滋养细胞为中等大小到大的单核或多核细胞，细胞核有明显的非典型性（图

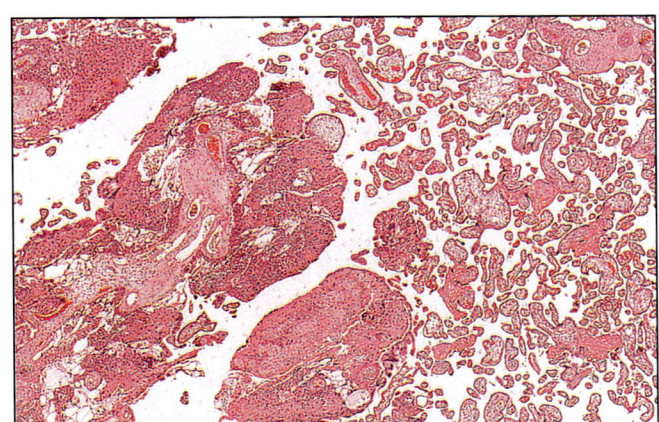

图13C.18　在足月胎盘中偶然发现的胎盘内绒毛膜癌；母体面绒毛之间的血管腔中可见高度非典型性增生的双向性滋养细胞，附着于绒毛间质。

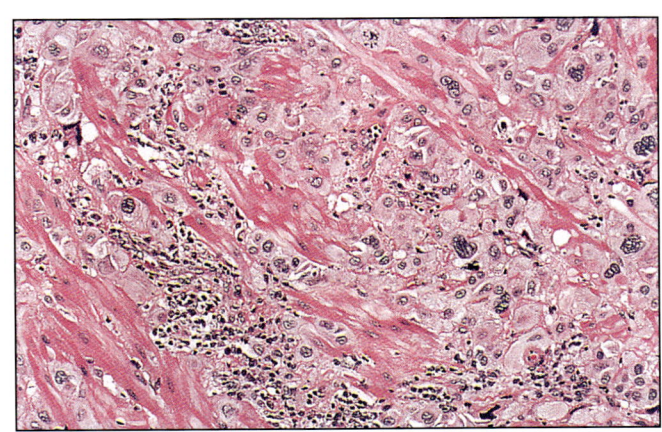

图13C.19　胎盘部位滋养细胞肿瘤。注意散在的非典型性和多核细胞。

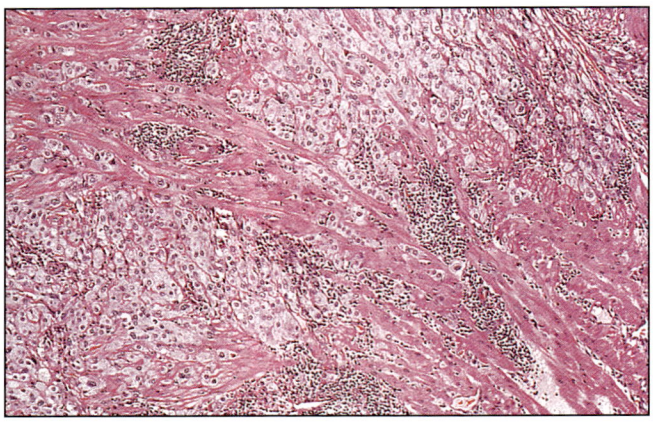

图13C.20 胎盘部位滋养细胞肿瘤。肿瘤性绒毛外细胞滋养细胞浸润子宫肌层；肿瘤细胞穿插在子宫肌层肌纤维之间，没有出血和坏死的证据。

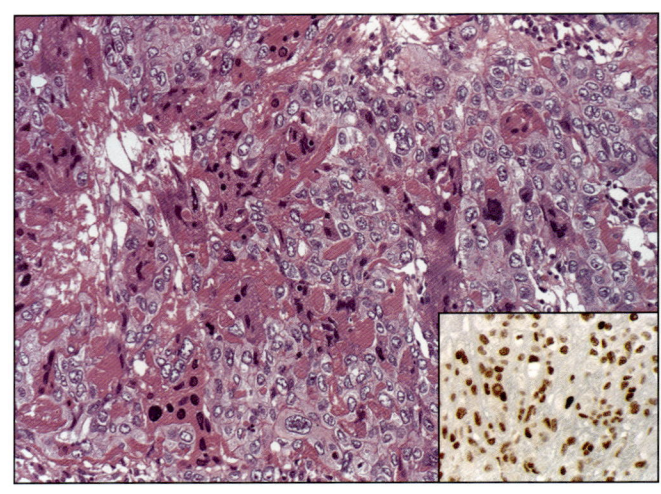

图13C.21 上皮样滋养细胞肿瘤和p63免疫组织化学染色（插图）。

13C.19），肿瘤细胞核仁明显，胞浆嗜酸到透明，散在核分裂象，而且偶见核内包涵体。肿瘤细胞特征性地浸润子宫肌壁全层（图 13C.20），伴有明显的血管性中心增生和血管内播散。高度活跃的核分裂（>4/10个高倍视野）表明预后差[103]。应用流式细胞学评估 PSTT 患者已有少数报告：8 例是二倍体（包括 3 例死亡病例），1 例是四倍体[85,101,107]。

上皮样滋养细胞肿瘤（epithelioid trophoblastic tumor, ETT）是近期描述的 PSTT 的一个亚型[108,109]。它的临床表现与 PSTT 十分相似。ETT 由单向增生的中间滋养细胞组成，它在几个方面不同于 PSTT（图 13C.21）：

1. 组成ETT的肿瘤性中间型滋养细胞较小，多形性不明显。
2. 除了单个细胞浸润之外，ETT以结节状方式生长，有时取代宫颈内膜表面上皮，十分相似于癌[109a]。
3. ETT 免疫组织化学染色hPL灶状阳性，但E-cadherin和表皮生长因子受体弥漫强阳性。此外，如同前面提到的一样，肿瘤细胞免疫表型类似于空泡状绒毛间滋养细胞和膜滋养细胞。

PSTT的鉴别诊断包括胎盘部位结节或斑块、种植部位超常反应、上皮样平滑肌肉瘤和低分化癌。广泛取材和CK、hCG以及hPL免疫组织化学染色有助于PSTT与非滋养细胞恶性肿瘤的鉴别诊断。胎盘部位结节或斑块[110,111]是一种界限清楚的病变，伴有丰富的玻璃样变的间质，其中散在有变性的中间滋养细胞浸润，这些细胞没有明显的细胞学非典型性，但是在少数情况下可能出现核分裂象[107]。胎盘部位结节发生在前次妊娠后数月到数年。相反，胎盘部位超常反应的发生在时间上与妊娠密切相关。这个诊断代表的是正常种植过程的一个非肿瘤性过度反应，通常与不成熟绒毛共存。

参考文献

1. Wallenburg H C S 1971 Choriangioma of the placenta: thirteen new cases and a review of the literature from 1939 to 1970 with special reference to the clinical complications. Obstet Gynecol Surv 26: 411–425
2. Fox H 1967 Vascular tumors of the placenta. Obstet Gynecol Surv 22: 697–711
3. Majlessi H F, Wagner K M, Brooks J J 1983 Atypical cellular choriangioma of the placenta. Int J Gynecol Pathol 1: 403–408
4. Arodi J, Auskender R, Atad J et al. 1985 Case report: giant choriangioma of the placenta. Acta Obstet Gynecol Scand 64: 91–92
5. Eldar-Geva T, Hochner-Celnikier D, Ariel I et al. 1988 Fetal high output cardiac failure and acute hydramnios caused by large placental choriangioma: case report. Br J Obstet Gynecol 95: 1200–1203
6. Smith L A, Pounder D J 1982 A teratoma-like lesion of the placenta: a case report. Pathology 14: 85–87
7. Sironi M, Declich P, Isimbaldi G et al. 1994 Placental teratoma with three-germ layer differentiation. Teratology 50: 165–167
8. Smith D, Majmudar B 1985 Teratoma of the umbilical cord. Hum Pathol 16: 190–193
9. Unger J L 1989 Placental teratoma. Am J Clin Pathol 92: 371–373
10. Block D, Cruikshank S, Kelly K et al. 1991 Placental teratoma. Int J Obstet Gynecol 34: 377–380
11. Chen K T K, Ma C K, Kassel S H 1986 Hepatocellular adenoma of the placenta. Am J Surg Pathol 10: 436–440
12. Cox J N, Chavier F 1980 Heterotopic adrenocortical tissue within a placenta. Placenta 1: 131–133
13. Labarrere C A, Caccamo D, Telenta M et al. 1984 A nodule of adrenocortical tissue within a human placenta: light microscopic and immunohistochemical findings. Placenta 5: 139–144
14. Qureshi F, Jacques S M 1995 Adrenocortical heterotopia in the placenta. Pediatr Pathol Lab Med 15: 51–56
15. Anders D, Kindermann G, Pfeifer U 1973 Metastasizing fetal neuroblastoma with involvement of the placenta simulating fetal erythroblastosis. J Pediatr 80: 50–53
16. Perkins D G, Kopp C M, Haust M D 1980 Placental infiltration in congenital neuroblastoma: a case study with ultrastructure. Histopathology 4: 383–389
17. Smith C R, Chan H S L, DeSa D J 1981 Placental involvement in congenital neuroblastoma. J Clin Pathol 34: 785–789
18. Strauss L, Driscoll S G 1964 Congenital neuroblastoma involving the placenta: reports of two cases. Pediatrics 34: 23–31
19. Schneidermann H, Yu-Yuan A, Campbell W A et al. 1987 Congenital melanoma with multiple prenatal metastases. Cancer 60: 1371–1377
20. Holaday W J, Castrow F F 1968 Placental metastasis from fetal giant pigmented nevus. Arch Dermatol 98: 486–488
21. Demian S D E, Donnelly W H, Frias J L et al. 1974 Placental lesions in congenital giant pigmented nevi. Am J Clin Pathol 61: 438–442

22. Jauniaux E, de Meeus M, Verellen G et al. 1993 Giant congenital melanocytic nevus with placental involvement: long-term follow-up of a case and review of the literature. Pediatr Pathol 13: 717–721
23. Potter J F, Schoeneman M 1970 Metastasis of maternal cancer to the placenta and fetus. Cancer 25: 380–388
24. Dildy G A, Moise K J, Carpenter R J et al. 1989 Maternal malignancy metastatic to the products of conception. Obstet Gynecol Surv 44: 535–540
25. Salamon M A, Sherer D M, Saller D N et al. 1994 Placental metastases in a patient with recurrent breast carcinoma. Am J Obstet Gynecol 171: 573–574
26. O'Day M P, Nielsen P, Al-Bozom I et al. 1994 Orbital rhabdomyosarcoma metastatic to the placenta. Am J Obstet Gynecol 171: 1382–1383
27. Pollack R N, Sklarin N T, Rao S et al. 1993 Metastatic placental lymphoma associated with maternal human immunodeficiency virus infection. Obstet Gynecol 81: 856–857
28. Pollack R N, Pollack M, Rochon L 1993 Pregnancy complicated by medulloblastoma with metastases to the placenta. Obstet Gynecol 81: 858–859
29. Tsujimura T, Matsumoto K, Aozasa K 1993 Placental involvement by maternal non-Hodgkin's lymphoma. Arch Pathol Lab Med 117: 325–327
30. Delrive C, Locquet E, Mallart A et al. 1989 Placental metastases from maternal bronchial oat cell carcinoma. Arch Pathol Lab Med 1123: 556–558
31. Read E J, Playzer P B 1981 Placental metastasis from maternal carcinoma of the lung. Obstet Gynecol 58: 387–391
32. Mazur M T, Kurman R J 1995 Gestational trophoblastic disease. In: Kurman R J (ed.) Blaustein's pathology of the female genital tract, 4th edn. Springer Verlag, New York, p 1049–1093
33. Silverberg S G, Kurman R J 1991 Gestational trophoblastic disease. In: Silverberg S G, Kurman R J (eds) Atlas of tumor pathology, 3rd series. Tumors of the uterine corpus and gestational trophoblastic disease. Armed Forces Institute of Pathology, Washington, DC, p 219–287
34. Azuma C, Saji F, Tokugawa Y et al. 1991 Application of gene amplification by polymerase chain reaction to genetic analysis of molar mitochondrial DNA: the genetic analysis of anuclear empty ovum as the cause of complete mole. Gynecol Oncol 40: 29–33
35. Kajii T, Ohama K 1977 Androgenetic origin of hydatidiform mole. Nature 268: 633–634
36. Ohama K, Kajii T, Okamoto E et al. 1981 Dispermic origin of XY hydatidiform moles. Nature 292: 551–552
37. Szulman A E, Surti U 1978 The syndromes of hydatidiform mole. II. Morphologic evolution of the complete and partial hydatidiform mole. Am J Obstet Gynecol 132: 20–27
38. Jacobs P A, Szulman A E, Funkhouser J et al. 1982 Human triploidy: relationship between parental origin of the additional haploid complement and development of partial hydatidiform mole. Ann Hum Genet 46: 223–231
39. Lawler S D, Fisher R A, Dent J 1991 A prospective genetic study of complete and partial hydatidiform moles. Am J Obstet Gynecol 164: 1270–1277
40. Szulman A E, Surti U 1978 The syndromes of hydatidiform mole. I. Cytogenetic and morphologic correlations. Am J Obstet Gynecol 131: 665–671
41. Berkowitz R S, Goldstein D P, Bernstein M R 1985 Natural history of partial molar pregnancy. Obstet Gynecol 66: 677–681
42. Vassilakos P, Riotton G, Kajii T 1977 Hydatidiform mole: two entities. Am J Obstet Gynecol 127: 167–170
43. Jeffers M D, O'Dwyer P, Curran B et al. 1993 Partial hydatidiform mole: a common but underdiagnosed condition. Int J Gynecol Pathol 12: 315–323
44. Mosher R, Goldstein D P, Berkowitz R et al. 1998 Complete hydatidiform mole: comparison of clinicopathologic features, current and past. J Reprod Med 43: 21–27
45. Genest D R, Laborde O, Berkowitz R S et al. 1991 A clinico-pathologic study of 153 cases of complete hydatidiform mole (1980–1990): histologic grade lacks prognostic significance. Obstet Gynecol 78: 402–409
46. Lurain J R, Brewer J I, Torok E E et al. 1983 Natural history of hydatidiform mole after primary evacuation. Am J Obstet Gynecol 145: 591–595
47. Rice L W, Berkowitz R S, Lage J M et al. 1990 Persistent gestational trophoblastic tumor after partial hydatidiform mole. Gynecol Oncol 36: 358–362
48. Bagshawe K D, Lawler S D, Paradinas F J et al. 1990 Gestational trophoblastic tumors following initial diagnosis of partial hydatidiform mole. Lancet 335: 1074–1076
49. Montes M, Roberts D, Berkowitz R S et al. 1996 Prevalence and significance of implantation site trophoblastic atypia in hydatidiform moles and spontaneous abortions. Am J Clin Pathol 105: 411–416
50. Keep D, Zaragoza M V, Hassold T et al. 1996 Very early complete hydatidiform mole. Hum Pathol 27: 708–713
51. Zaragoza M V, Keep D, Genest D R et al. 1997 Early complete hydatidiform moles contain inner cell mass derivatives. Am J Med Genet 70: 273–277
52. Paradinas F J, Browne P, Fisher R A et al. 1996 A clinical, histopathological and flow cytometric study of 149 complete moles, 146 partial moles and 107 non-molar abortions. Histopathology 28: 101–109
53. Elston C W, Bagshawe K D 1972 The value of histologic grading in the management of hydatidiform mole. J Obstet Gynaecol Br Commonw 79: 717–724
54. Doshi N, Surti U, Szulman A E 1983 Morphologic anomalies in triploid liveborn fetuses. Hum Pathol 14: 716–723
55. McFadden D E, Kalousek D K 1991 Two different phenotypes of fetuses with chromosomal triploidy: correlation with parental origin of the extra haploid set. Am J Med Genet 38: 535–538
56. Hillstrom M M, Brown D L, Wilkins-Haug L et al. 1995 Sonographic appearance of placental villous hydrops associated with Beckwith–Wiedemann syndrome. J Ultrasound Med 14: 61–64
57. McCowan L M E, Becroft D M O 1994 Beckwith–Wiedemann syndrome, placental abnormalities and gestational proteinuric hypertension. Obstet Gynecol 83: 813–817
58. Lage J M 1991 Placentomegaly with massive hydrops of placental stem villi, diploid DNA content, and fetal omphaloceles: possible association with Beckwith–Wiedemann syndrome. Hum Pathol 22: 591–597
59. Sander C M 1993 Angiomatous malformation of placental chorionic stem vessels and pseudo-partial molar placentas: report of five cases. Pediatr Pathol 13: 621–633
60. Choi-Hong S R, Genest D R, Crum C et al. 1995 Twin pregnancy with complete hydatidiform mole and coexisting fetus: utilization of fluorescent in situ hybridization to evaluate placental X- and Y-chromosomal content. Hum Pathol 26: 1175–1180
61. Steller M A, Genest D R, Bernstein M R et al. 1994 Natural history of twin pregnancy with complete hydatidiform mole and coexisting fetus. Obstet Gynecol 84: 35–42
62. Steller M A, Genest D R, Bernstein M R et al. 1994 Clinical features of multiple conception with partial or complete molar pregnancy and coexisting fetuses. J Reprod Med 39: 147–154
63. Koenig C, Demopoulos R I, Vamvakas E C et al. 1993 Flow cytometric DNA ploidy and quantitative histopathology in partial moles. Int J Gynecol Pathol 12: 235–240
64. Lage J M, Bagg A 1996 Hydatidiform moles: DNA flow cytometry, image analysis and selected topics in molecular biology. Histopathology 28: 379–382
65. Lage J M, Berkowitz R S, Rice L W et al. 1991 Flow cytometric analysis of DNA content in partial hydatidiform moles with persistent gestational trophoblastic tumor. Obstet Gynecol 77: 111–115
66. Lage J M, Driscoll S G, Yavner D L et al. 1988 Hydatidiform moles. Application of flow cytometry in diagnosis. Am J Clin Pathol 89: 596–600
67. Lage J M, Mark S D, Roberts D J et al. 1992 A flow cytometric study of 137 fresh hydropic placentas: correlation between types of hydatidiform moles and nuclear DNA ploidy. Obstet Gynecol 79: 403–410
68. Lage J M, Weinberg D S, Yavner D L et al. 1989 The biology of tetraploid hydatidiform moles: histopathology, cytogenetics, and flow cytometry. Hum Pathol 20: 419–425
69. Castrillon D H, Sun D, Weremowicz S et al. 2001 Discrimination of complete hydatidiform mole from its mimics by immunohistochemistry of the paternally imprinted gene product p57KIP2. Am J Surg Pathol 25: 1225–1230
70. Chilosi M, Piazzola E, Lestani M et al. 1998 Differential expression of p57kip2, a maternally imprinted cdk inhibitor, in normal human placenta and gestational trophoblastic disease. Lab Invest 78: 269–276
71. Genest D R, Dorfman D M, Castrillon D H 2002 Ploidy and imprinting in hydatidiform moles. Complementary use of flow cytometry and immunohistochemistry of the imprinted gene product p57KIP2 to assist molar classification. J Reprod Med 47: 342–346
72. Fisher R A, Hodges M D, Rees H C et al. 2002 The maternally transcribed gene p57 (KIP2) (CDNK1C) is abnormally expressed in both androgenetic and biparental complete hydatidiform moles. Hum Mol Genet 11: 3267–3272
73. Thaker H M, Berlin A, Tycko B et al. 2004 Immunohistochemistry for the imprinted gene product IPL/PHLDA2 for facilitating the differential diagnosis of complete hydatidiform mole. J Reprod Med 49: 630–636
74. Fisher R A, Nucci M R, Thaker H M et al. 2004 Complete hydatidiform mole retaining a chromosome 11 of maternal origin: molecular genetic analysis of a case. Mod Pathol 17: 1155–1160
75. Fukunaga M, Katabuchi H, Nagasaka T et al. 2005 Interobserver and intraobserver variability in the diagnosis of hydatidiform mole. Am J Surg Pathol 29: 942–947
76. Hertig A T, Mansell H 1956 Tumors of the female sex organs. Part I. Hydatidiform mole and choriocarcinoma. Atlas of tumor pathology, section 9, series I, fascicle 33. Armed Forces Institute of Pathology, Washington, DC
77. Lathrop J C, Watchel T J, Meissner G F 1978 Uterine choriocarcinoma fourteen years following bilateral tubal ligation. Obstet Gynecol 51: 477–478
78. Brewer J I, Mazur M T 1981 Gestational choriocarcinoma. Its origin in the placenta during seemingly normal pregnancy. Am J Surg Pathol 5: 267–277
79. Driscoll S G 1963 Choriocarcinoma. An "incidental finding" within a term placenta. Obstet Gynecol 21: 96–101
80. Aozasa K, Ito H, Kohro T et al. 1981 Choriocarcinoma in infant and mother. Acta Pathol Jpn 31: 317–322
81. Daamen C B, Bloem G W, Westerbeek A J 1961 Chorionepithelioma in mother and child. J Obstet Gynecol Br Commonw 68: 144–149
82. Mazur M T, Lurain J R, Brewer J I 1982 Fatal gestational choriocarcinoma. Cancer 50: 1833–1846
83. Soper J T, Evans A C, Conaway M R et al. 1994 Evaluation of prognostic factors and staging in gestational trophoblastic tumor. Obstet Gynecol 84: 969–973
84. Deligdish L, Driscoll S G, Goldstein D P 1978 Gestational trophoblastic neoplasms: morphologic correlates of therapeutic response. Am J Obstet Gynecol 130: 801–806
85. Elston C W, Bagshawe K D 1972 The diagnosis of trophoblastic tumors from uterine curettings. J Clin Pathol 25: 111–118

86. Fukunaga M, Ushigome S 1993 Malignant trophoblastic tumors: immunohistochemical and flow cytometric comparison of choriocarcinoma and placental site trophoblastic tumors. Hum Pathol 24: 1098–1106
87. Elston C W 1976 The histopathology of trophoblastic tumors. J Clin Pathol (suppl.) (R Coll Pathol) 29: 111–131
88. Mosher R, Genest D R 1996 Primary intraplacental choriocarcinoma: clinical and pathological features of seven cases (1967–1996) and discussion of the differential diagnosis. J Surg Pathol 2: 1–15
89. Fox H, Laurini R N 1988 Intraplacental choriocarcinoma: a report of two cases. J Clin Pathol 41: 1085–1088
90. Lage J M, Roberts D J 1993 Choriocarcinoma in a term placenta. Pathologic diagnosis of a tumor in an asymptomatic patient with metastatic disease. Int J Gynecol Pathol 12: 80–85
91. Olive D L, Lurain J R, Brewer J I 1984 Choriocarcinoma associated with term gestation. Am J Obstet Gynecol 148: 711–716
92. Kurman R J, Scully R E, Norris H J 1976 Trophoblastic pseudotumor of the uterus: an exaggerated form of "syncytial endometritis" simulating a malignant tumor. Cancer 38: 1214–1226
93. Duncan D A, Mazur M T 1989 Trophoblastic tumors: ultrastructural comparison of choriocarcinoma and placental-site trophoblastic tumor. Hum Pathol 20: 370–381
94. Eckstein R P, Paradinas F J, Bagshawe K D 1982 Placental site trophoblastic tumor (trophoblastic pseudotumor). Histopathology 16: 211–226
95. Eckstein R P, Russell P, Friedlander M L et al. 1985 Metastasizing placental site trophoblastic tumor: a case study. Hum Pathol 16: 632–636
96. Finkler N J, Berkowitz R S, Driscoll S G et al. 1988 Clinical experience with placental site trophoblastic tumors at the New England Trophoblastic Disease Center. Obstet Gynecol 71: 854–875
97. Gloor E, Dialdas J, Hurlimann J et al. 1983 Placental site trophoblastic tumor (trophoblastic pseudotumor) of the uterus with metastasis and fatal outcome. Clinical and autopsy outcome of a case. Am J Surg Pathol 7: 483–486
98. Gloor E, Hurlimann J 1981 Trophoblastic pseudotumor of the uterus: clinicopathologic report with immunohistochemical and ultrastructural studies. Am J Surg Pathol 5: 5–13
99. Heintz A P M, Schaberg A, Englesman E et al. 1985 Placental site trophoblastic tumor: diagnosis, treatment and biologic behavior. Int J Gynecol Pathol 4: 75–82
100. Hopkins M, Nunez C, Murphy J R et al. 1985 Malignant placental site trophoblastic tumor. Obstet Gynecol 66 (suppl.): 95S–100S
101. Kotylo P K, Michael H, Davis T E et al. 1992 Flow cytometric DNA analysis of placental-site trophoblastic tumors. Int J Gynecol Pathol 11: 245–255
102. Kurman R J, Young R H, Norris H J et al. 1984 Immunocytochemical localization of placental lactogen and chorionic gonadotropin in the normal placenta and trophoblastic tumors, with emphasis on intermediate trophoblast and the placental site trophoblastic tumor. Int J Gynecol Pathol 3: 101–121
103. Lathrop J C, Lauchlan S, Nayak R et al. 1988 Clinical characteristics of placental site trophoblastic tumor (PSTT). Gynecol Oncol 31: 32–42
104. Twiggs L B, Okagaki T, Phillips G L et al. 1981 Trophoblastic pseudotumor – evidence of malignant disease potential. Gynecol Oncol 12: 238–248
105. Young R H, Kurman R J, Scully R E 1988 Proliferations and tumors of intermediate trophoblast of the placental site. Semin Diagn Pathol 5: 223–237
106. Young R H, Scully R E, McCluskey R T 1985 A distinctive glomerular lesion complicating placental site trophoblastic tumor. Hum Pathol 16: 35–42
107. Fukunaga M, Ushigome S 1993 Metastasizing placental site trophoblastic tumor. An immunohistochemical and flow cytometric study of two cases. Am J Surg Pathol 17: 1003–1010
108. Shih I M, Kurman R J 1998 Epithelioid trophoblastic tumour. A neoplasm distinct from choriocarcinoma and placental site trophoblastic tumor simulating carcinoma. Am J Surg Pathol 22: 1393–1403
109. Shih I M, Kurman R J 2004 p63 expression is useful in the distinction of epithelioid trophoblastic and placental site trophoblastic tumors by profiling trophoblastic subpopulations. Am J Surg Pathol 28: 1177–1183
109a. Fadare O, Parkash V, Carcangiu M L, Hui P 2006 Epithelioid trophoblastic tumor: clinicopathological features with an emphasis on uterine cervical involvement. Mod Pathol 19: 75–82
110. Huettner P C, Gersell D J 1994 Placental site nodule: a clinicopathologic study of 38 cases. Int J Gynecol Pathol 13: 191–199
111. Young R H, Kurman R J, Scully R E 1990 Placental site nodules and plaques. A clinicopathologic analysis of 20 cases. Am J Surg Pathol 14: 1001–1009

第四部分

子宫肌层 Myometrium

Marisa R. Nucci 著

戴林 译　回允中 校

子宫肌层
- 引言　683
- 良性平滑肌肿瘤　683
- 恶性平滑肌肿瘤　688
- 不能确定恶性潜能的平滑肌肿瘤　692
- 伴有独特特征的平滑肌增生　692
- 罕见和独特的肿瘤　694

引言　Introduction

绝大多数子宫肌层肿瘤是由平滑肌细胞组成的。子宫平滑肌肿瘤在诊断上面临着挑战，而在学术上尚有困惑，主要是因为这个肿瘤包括了良性、恶性和不能确定生物学行为的具有各种组织病理学表现的肿瘤。这一节主要包括了良性平滑肌瘤和平滑肌肉瘤的组织学亚型，并讨论那些难于分类或生物学行为处于良性和明显恶性之间的平滑肌肿瘤。

良性平滑肌肿瘤　Benign smooth muscle neoplasms

临床特征

子宫平滑肌瘤（口语上称 fibroids，肌瘤）最常发生在育龄期妇女，是发生于子宫肌壁平滑肌的良性肿瘤。子宫平滑肌瘤十分常见，估计其发生率在经组织病理学仔细检查的子宫切除标本中为 77%（不管手术原因如何）[1]。子宫平滑肌瘤虽然常见，但能引起明显临床症状的仅占 25%[2]。伴随的临床症状与肿瘤大小和肿瘤在子宫壁所处的部位有关，其症状包括异常子宫出血、盆腔疼痛和压迫症状以及不孕。

肿瘤发生的危险因素包括种族和产次，黑人和未经产妇女更容易发生平滑肌瘤[2]。也有充分的证据支持平滑肌瘤是激素反应性和依赖性肿瘤：（1）这个肿瘤在青春期以前十分罕见；（2）妇女绝经后肿瘤有退化的倾向；（3）当体内激素水平发生变化时肿瘤可以迅速生长，比如妊娠、克罗米芬或孕激素治疗；（4）在月经周期的分泌期核分裂活性增加；以及（5）肿瘤细胞表达雌激素和孕激素受体。遗传倾向也是平滑肌瘤形成的一个因素，因为平滑肌瘤较常见于黑人女性，它的发生还可以作为 Reed 综合征的一部分，Reed 综合征是一种常染色体显性遗传性疾病，其特征是多发性皮肤和子宫平滑肌瘤，并且已经绘制出了 1 号染色体上延胡索酸水合酶的基因图[3-5]。

分子遗传学

平滑肌瘤是发生在子宫的具有独立克隆性的肿瘤[6]，40% 的肿瘤具有单一染色体畸变。其中最常见的是 7q 缺失、12q15 和 14q24 之间的易位、12 三体和 6p、10q22 或 13q 的重排[7]。可以发生各种不同的染色体畸变，提示肿瘤形成有多种不同的发病机制，t(12;14)(q15;q24) 涉及 12 号染色体上 HMGA2 基因（它编码一个转录调节蛋白），而 6p 重排已经显示影响相关基因 HMGA1，提示具有这两个不同畸变的肿瘤可以有共同的发病通路[8-11]。

病理学特征

典型的平滑肌瘤界限清楚，肿瘤呈白色，质地硬韧。在切开时由于肿瘤内压力释放而使切面明显膨出。平滑肌瘤有各种不同的组织学亚型。

平滑肌瘤，普通型　Leiomyoma, usual type

这些肿瘤显示典型的平滑肌分化的特征，是由成编织状排列的梭形细胞束组成的，胞浆嗜酸性，核呈良性表现，细长，两端钝圆（所谓的棚车形或雪茄形表现；图 13D.1）。核分裂活性可以不同，在月经周期的分泌期常常增加。但是每 10 个高倍视野通常小于 5 个。那些形态学良性但核分裂计数较高的平滑肌瘤将在核分裂活跃的平滑肌瘤项下讨论（见下）。

富于细胞性平滑肌瘤　Cellular leiomyoma

富于细胞性平滑肌瘤的诊断还没有精确的定义，而

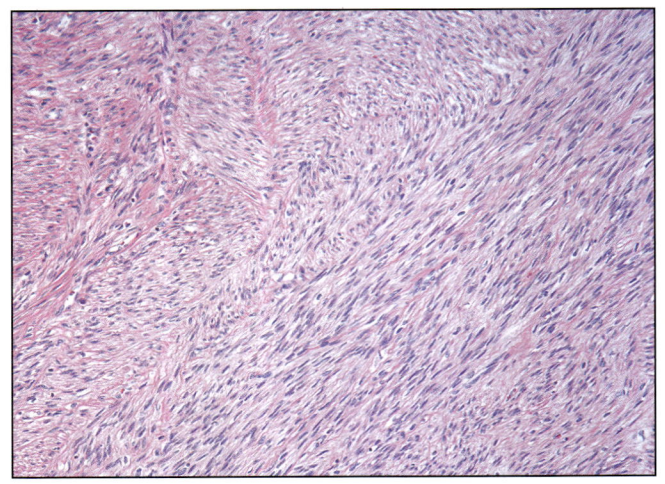

图13D.1 平滑肌瘤，普通型。良性梭形细胞编织状成束排列。

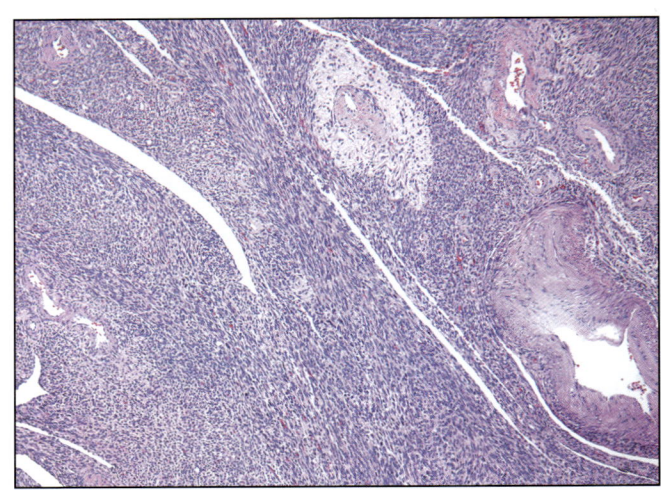

图13D.3 高度富于细胞性平滑肌瘤。束状结构、裂隙样腔隙以及大的厚壁血管是其特征。

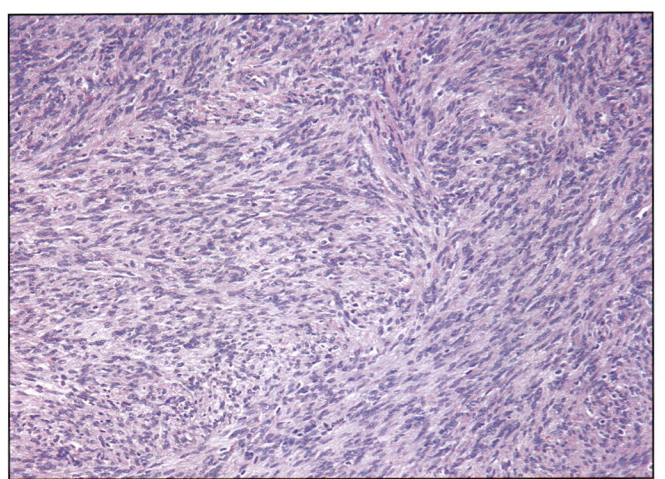

图13.D2 富于细胞性平滑肌瘤。与普通型平滑肌瘤不同，其肿瘤细胞比较丰富。

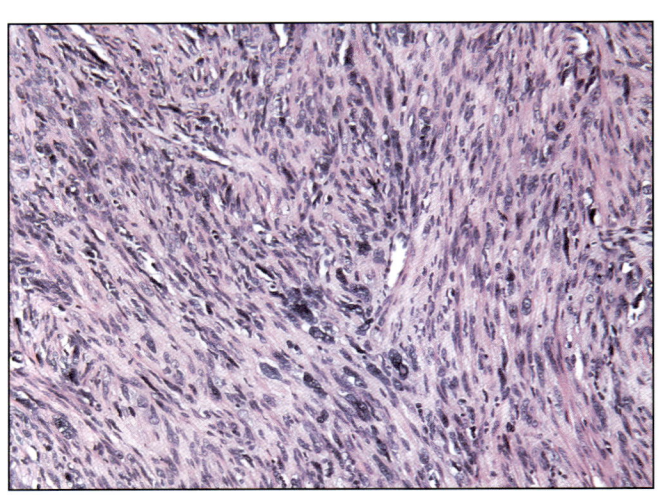

图13D.4 非典型性平滑肌瘤。增大的多形性细胞核弥漫性分布于整个肿瘤中。

且相当主观。按照世界卫生组织的定义，富于细胞性平滑肌瘤是指细胞比子宫肌层和普通型平滑肌瘤"明显"丰富的平滑肌瘤（图13D.2）。与普通型平滑肌瘤相似，富于细胞性平滑肌瘤界限清楚；然而，在大体检查时可能呈褐/棕或黄色，质地较软。富于细胞性平滑肌瘤具有均匀一致的良性细胞形态学特征，核分裂活性每10个高倍视野一般小于5个。核分裂数超出这个范围应该立即另外取材并仔细检查，看是否存在与恶性有关的其他组织学特征。

高度富于细胞性平滑肌瘤[12]
Highly cellular leiomyoma

这个亚型的定义是，一个平滑肌瘤细胞过于丰富，或细胞的丰富程度与子宫内膜间质肿瘤相当。这些肿瘤一般界限清楚，为褐/黄色的结节，质地一般比普通型平滑肌瘤软。组织学上，边缘常常不规则，加上肿瘤明显富于细胞以及形态上与子宫内膜肉瘤有重叠，可能类似于低级别子宫内膜间质肉瘤。然而，通过以下特征可以识别：(1)多数病例至少出现局灶性平滑肌肿瘤特征性的成束排列的区域；(2)大的厚壁血管；(3)裂隙样腔隙；(4)免疫组织化学染色desmin阳性/h-caldesmon阳性（图13D.3）。

核分裂活跃的平滑肌瘤[13-16]
Mitotically active leiomyoma

这种亚型的平滑肌瘤核分裂活跃，每10个高倍视野核分裂象大于5个，但在其他方面具有普通平滑肌瘤的典型特征，尤其是良性的细胞形态学特征、肿瘤界限清楚以及缺少（凝固性肿瘤细胞）坏死。这些肿瘤的年龄分布可能比较广泛，但不同于平滑肌肉瘤，一般见于生育年龄的妇女，中位年龄是40～50岁。核分裂活性增加可能是继发于激素的影响，因为这些肿瘤常见于妊娠期、月经周期的分泌期或使用激素治疗的妇女。大多数肿瘤每10个高倍视野核分裂象小于15个，超过这个核分裂数的组织学形态良性的肿瘤其生物学行为尚不清楚。

非典型性平滑肌瘤[15,17] Atypical leiomyoma

也叫合体细胞性、奇异性或多形性平滑肌瘤（但在最近的 WHO 分类中定义为非典型性平滑肌瘤）。这种亚型的特征是出现增大的、多形的、经常是多核的肿瘤细胞，这些细胞的分布可以是单灶性、多灶性或呈弥漫性（图 13D.4）。这些多形性细胞在低倍镜下总是可以辨认出来，细胞也可能具有丰富的嗜酸性胞浆、核内假包涵体和粗糙的染色质。大多数非典型性平滑肌瘤有与普通型平滑肌瘤相似的大体表现，但少数肿瘤颜色可能较黄，质地较软。其中多数肿瘤小于 5.5 cm，一般发生于育龄期妇女，中位年龄是 40 岁。肿瘤除了出现明显的核非典型性以外，限定的组织学表现是每 10 个高倍视野核分裂计数小于 7 个，尤其是肿瘤具有弥漫性非典型性时。这一标准是根据 Downes 和 Hart 的系列研究[17]，其中符合这些标准的肿瘤，随访结果（平均 11 年）显示为良性，在这一系列中大多数患者是通过子宫切除进行治疗的。重要的是应该注意，极少数长期随访的患者仅仅采用了肌瘤切除术；因此，对于这些肿瘤，特别是单单采取肌瘤切除术治疗的具有弥漫性非典型性的肿瘤，诊断时要加以小心。一个恰当的例子是，一例这样的肿瘤（每 10 个高倍视野核分裂象少于 2 个）仅仅采用肌瘤切除术治疗，术后 3 年肿瘤在子宫肌层手术部位复发（个人观察）。另外，在 Bell 等的系列研究中[15]，有一例患者的肿瘤具有弥漫性细胞核非典型性，每 10 个高倍视野核分裂象少于 2 个，在子宫切除后 24 个月腹腔内和盆腔内肿瘤复发。在他们的研究中原来肿瘤的大小不清楚，仅有 4 张 HE 切片被用以评估，在这种情况下，提出有平滑肌肉瘤取材不足的可能性，更为重要的是必须强调，对于所有伴有细胞核非典型性的肿瘤都要广泛取材。在充分足够取材（最少每个厘米取一块，包括与正常子宫肌层交界部位）之后，非典型性平滑肌瘤，特别是那些具有弥漫性细胞核非典型性的肿瘤可以通过缺少凝固性肿瘤细胞坏死和每 10 个高倍视野核分裂数少于 7 个与平滑肌肉瘤相鉴别；对于每 10 个高倍视野核分裂象 7~10 个的肿瘤，最好诊断为不能确定恶性潜能的肿瘤。在实际工作中，对于诊断为非典型性平滑肌瘤，但仅仅采用肌瘤切除手术的患者，要认真随访或考虑子宫切除。

继发于激素变化的平滑肌瘤[18-24] Leiomyoma with secondary hormonal changes

妊娠、口服避孕药或使用促性腺激素释放激素类似物治疗的患者平滑肌瘤，可能出现一些继发性退行性的组织学改变。也称为卒中性或出血性富于细胞性平滑肌瘤 (apoplectic or hemorrhagic cellular leiomyomata)，一般发生在

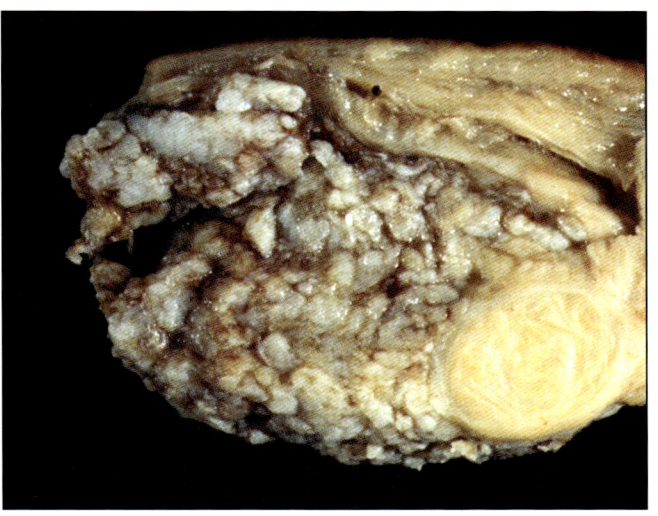

图 13D.5　水肿性平滑肌瘤。聚集的水肿液将平滑肌束分开，产生多结节的表现。

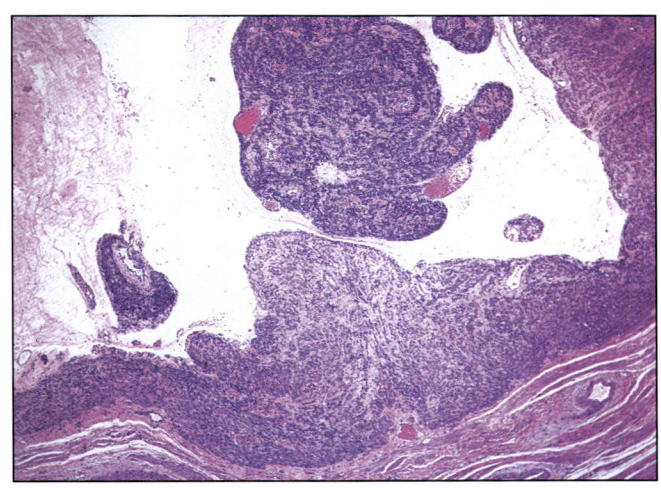

图 13D.6　水肿性平滑肌瘤。结节周围分布的水肿液具有特征性。

妊娠患者或口服避孕药的妇女，大体检查的特征为多发性出血灶，相当于组织学检查的新近出血和水肿的星形区域，周围围绕丰富的普通平滑肌细胞；核分裂象通常稀少。使用促性腺激素释放激素类似物治疗的患者，可能显示肿瘤中玻璃样变区域增加，细胞结构发生变化和肿瘤内血管的变化，包括宫腔狭窄和动脉硬化改变。

伴有水肿变性的平滑肌瘤[25] Leiomyoma with hydropic degeneration

水肿液聚集（水肿性改变）可以见于普通型平滑肌瘤中，呈局灶性或弥漫性分布。随着水肿性改变范围的扩大，平滑肌瘤的大体表现可以因为其切面有光泽而类似于黏液样平滑肌瘤，或由于肌束被水肿液分开形成突出物而类似于静脉内平滑肌瘤病（图 13D.5）。组织学上，细胞之间聚集的水肿液常常淡染，比黏液样变的嗜酸性强，而且通常导致水肿液分布于结节周围的特征性表现

（图 13D.6）。在一些病例中，由于水肿程度相当广泛以致掩盖了肿瘤的平滑肌本质（需要通过平滑肌标志物免疫组织化学染色加以证实）。水肿改变可以超出平滑肌瘤的边界，类似于黏液性肿瘤的浸润，然而，这些区域酸性黏蛋白染色通常阴性。肿瘤一般界限清楚，缺少平滑肌束突入内衬内皮的间隙（可能需要免疫组织化学染色证实），这有助于将伴有广泛水肿变性的平滑肌瘤与血管内平滑肌瘤病鉴别开来（见 692 页）。

丛状平滑肌瘤[26-28]　Plexiform leiomyoma

由于其在组织学检查时呈假上皮样表现，而认为它是上皮样平滑肌瘤的一个亚型。这个良性的平滑肌瘤也叫丛状小瘤（plexiform tumorlet），是子宫切除标本组织学检查时最常见的偶然发现。这些肿瘤可以单发或多发，典型病变小于 1 cm，组织学上以缎带样或成巢的多角形细胞为特征，胞浆稀少，核呈空泡状，被丰富的细胞外基质分开。细胞外基质的聚集引起细胞失去了典型的梭形细胞表现，而呈现上皮样细胞形态（图 13D.7）；核分裂象一般少见。免疫组织化学和超微结构分析显示，这些肿瘤具有平滑肌分化而不是上皮分化的特征。

上皮样平滑肌瘤[29-37]　Epithelioid leiomyoma

世界卫生组织（WHO）将上皮样平滑肌瘤定义为由具有上皮样表现的细胞组成的肿瘤。这些肿瘤在文献中也被描述为平滑肌母细胞瘤（leiomyoblastoma，提示肿瘤细胞具有一些不成熟的平滑肌细胞分化，类似于胎儿子宫平滑肌细胞）和透明细胞平滑肌瘤（clear cell leiomyoma，因为一些肿瘤细胞继发于线粒体或溶酶体的空泡化而具有透明胞浆）。上皮样平滑肌瘤患者的临床表现与普通型平滑肌瘤没有区别，最常见于育龄期妇女。大体检查，某些肿瘤的表现可以不同于普通型平滑

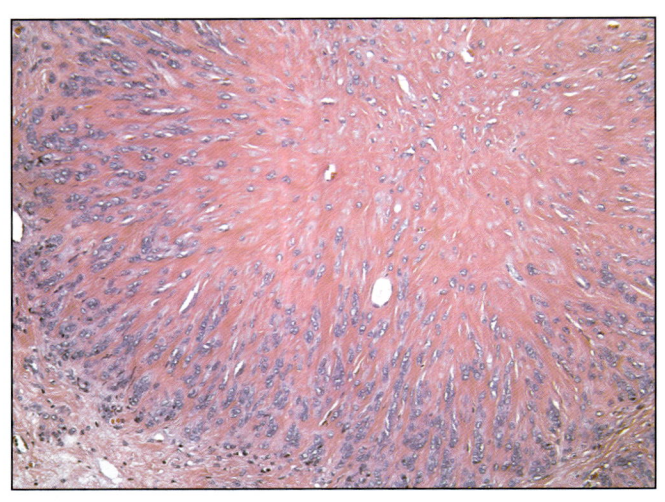

图13D.7　丛状平滑肌瘤。丰富的细胞外基质沉积将肿瘤细胞分开，呈现上皮样表现。

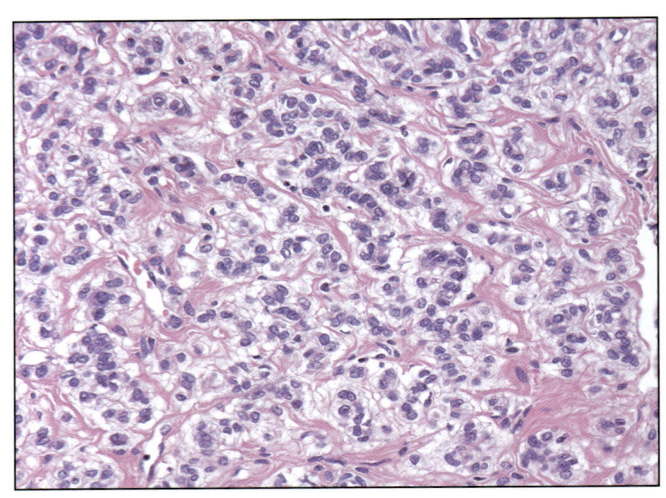

图13D.8　上皮样平滑肌瘤。具有嗜酸胞浆的圆形肿瘤细胞排列成缎带和条索状。

肌瘤，其质地较软和（或）呈褐色/黄色外观。显微镜下，这些肿瘤以圆形细胞增生为特征，细胞具有丰富的透明或嗜酸性胞浆，排列成片状，但有时也呈巢状和条索状（图 13D.8）。肿瘤细胞核可以位于中心，或位于周边而呈现印戒细胞形态。

由于具有上皮样分化的平滑肌肿瘤罕见，所以确定预测其生物学行为的可靠诊断标准受到限制。已经发表的文章数量非常有限，即使是在这些研究当中其分类和预后仍然是个问题。在已发表的文章中反映出对于这种肿瘤采取保守的态度，良性上皮样平滑肌瘤的诊断应该仅仅限于缺乏坏死、几乎没有核非典型性以及每 10 个高倍视野核分裂计数小于 3 个的肿瘤。其他与这一肿瘤良性生物学行为有关的特征包括肿瘤边界非常清楚和肿瘤大小小于 6cm。仅有少数几个上皮样平滑肌瘤进行了细胞遗传学分析，其中多数具有与普通型平滑肌瘤相似的异常表现，包括（7）（q21.1q31.2）缺失[33]，提示它们具有相似的发病机制。

黏液样平滑肌瘤[38]　Myxoid leiomyoma

这种非常罕见的平滑肌瘤亚型是以细胞外基质出现酸性黏液物质沉积为特征。大体检查一般显示肿瘤界限清楚，根据肿瘤中黏液样变化的程度肿瘤可以呈现灰色和凝胶状。组织学上，可见丰富的淡蓝色基质将平滑肌束纤维分开，阿辛蓝染色一般阳性（图 13D.9）。由于这种肿瘤罕见，区分良性黏液样平滑肌瘤和平滑肌肉瘤的诊断标准尚未确立。在实际工作中，根据有限的经验认为缺乏肿瘤细胞坏死、几乎没有核非典型性、缺乏肿瘤浸润以及每 10 个高倍视野核分裂象少于 2 个的肿瘤，为良性黏液样平滑肌瘤。

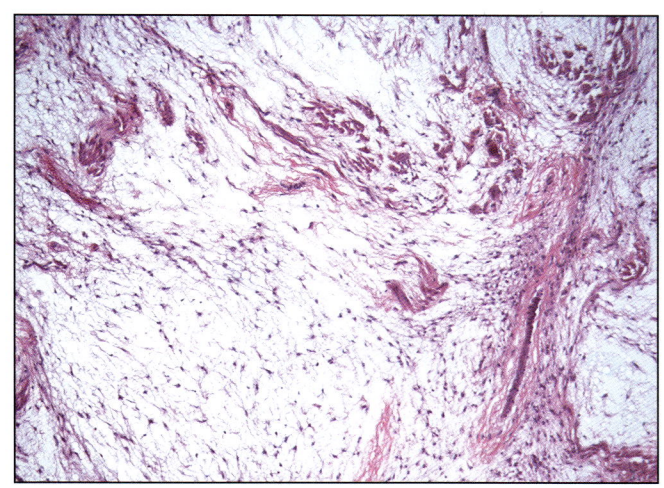

图13D.9　黏液样平滑肌瘤。平滑肌束纤维被丰富的淡蓝色黏液性基质分开。

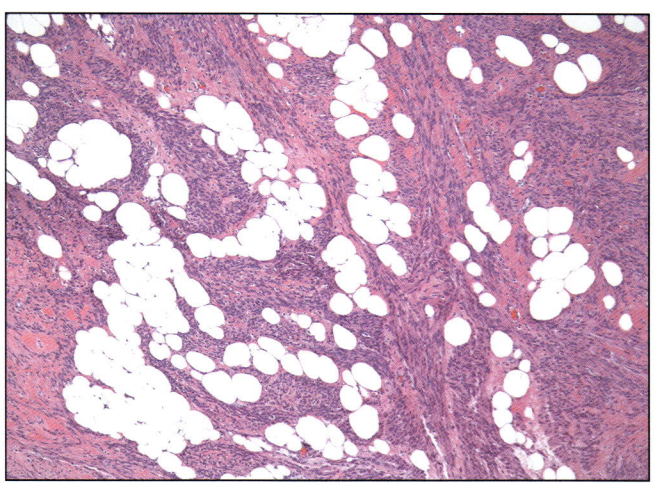

图13D.11　脂肪平滑肌瘤。典型表现的平滑肌瘤中混有脂肪细胞。

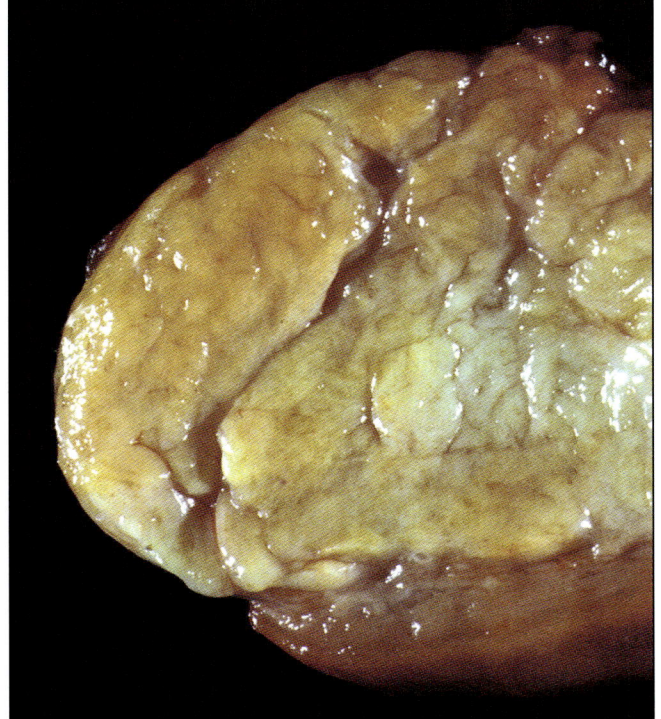

图13D.10　脂肪平滑肌瘤。出现明显的脂肪细胞成分，常常导致平滑肌瘤在大体上呈黄色表现。

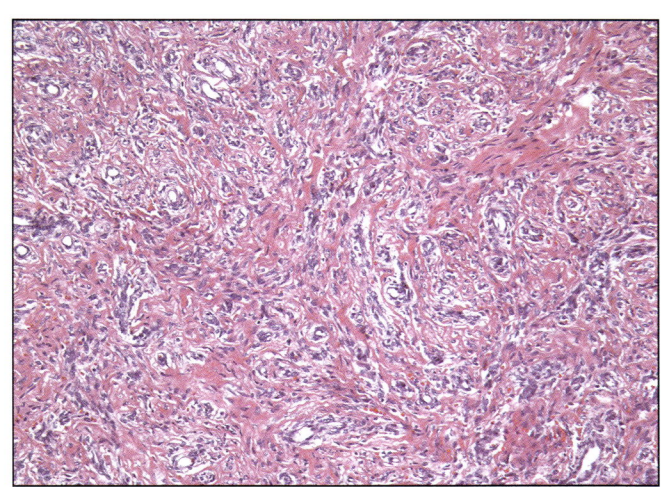

图13D.12　血管平滑肌瘤。血管数量增加是这个不常见平滑肌瘤亚型的特征。

脂肪平滑肌瘤[39-41]　Lipoleiomyoma

这个不常见的平滑肌瘤是以平滑肌细胞中混合出现数量不等的脂肪细胞为特征，当具有大量脂肪细胞时，大体检查时即可见肿瘤呈黄色（图13D.10和13D.11）。这种亚型的平滑肌瘤患者大多数是绝经后妇女，提出这种变化在本质上属于退行性变的可能；然而，有少数病例进行了细胞遗传学分析，显示位于基因 *HMGA2* 的12q15（40，41）的重排。涉及这个区域的基因 *HMGA2* 的异常表达也见于脂肪瘤（见第24章）。

血管平滑肌瘤[42]　Vascular leiomyoma

也叫血管肌瘤（angiomyoma）或 angioleiomyoma，这个不常见并且有些主观的良性平滑肌瘤亚型是以出现明显的血管成分为特征（图13D.12）。

平滑肌瘤伴有造血成分[43-49]
Leiomyoma with hematopoietic elements

偶尔，形态学上为普通型的平滑肌瘤可以出现多少不等、有时甚至是广泛的造血细胞浸润，包括淋巴细胞、肥大细胞、嗜酸性细胞和（或）组织细胞。大量淋巴细胞浸润，可能与促性腺激素释放激素促效药治疗有关，病变类似于淋巴瘤。但可以确定它是一个良性病变：（1）浸润的细胞局限于平滑肌瘤中；（2）浸润细胞的多克隆性本质。

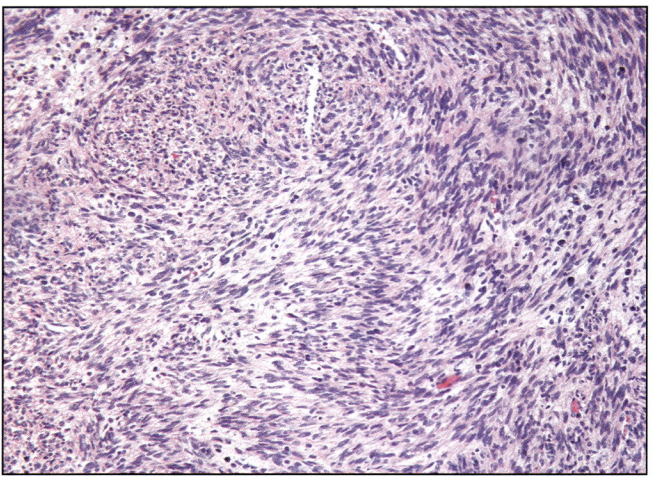

图13D.13 神经鞘瘤样平滑肌瘤。肿瘤细胞核呈栅栏状排列，可能类似于良性神经鞘肿瘤。

神经鞘瘤样平滑肌瘤[50,51]
Neurilemmoma(schwannoma)-like leiomyoma

平滑肌瘤的这一组织学亚型是以肿瘤细胞核呈栅栏状排列为特征，以致病变类似于良性神经鞘肿瘤（图13D.13）。虽然这种形态学上的类似可能非常离奇，但这些肿瘤并不显示神经鞘分化的超微结构特征。

腺肌瘤[52] Adenomyoma

虽然在此将其作为平滑肌瘤的一个亚型考虑，但是腺肌瘤是否为局限性腺肌症的一种变异还不清楚，而且其发病机制也尚未进行研究。与平滑肌瘤相似，这些病变一般发生在育龄期妇女，患者通常出现异常子宫出血。腺肌瘤最常表现为黏膜下病变（用于描述这个部位病变的替代术语包括腺肌瘤性息肉、息肉样腺肌瘤和带蒂的腺肌瘤），但它们可以位于子宫肌壁间或累及浆膜面。大体检查，典型病变与周围子宫肌层界限清楚，常常含有小的囊腔，而且可以有出血。

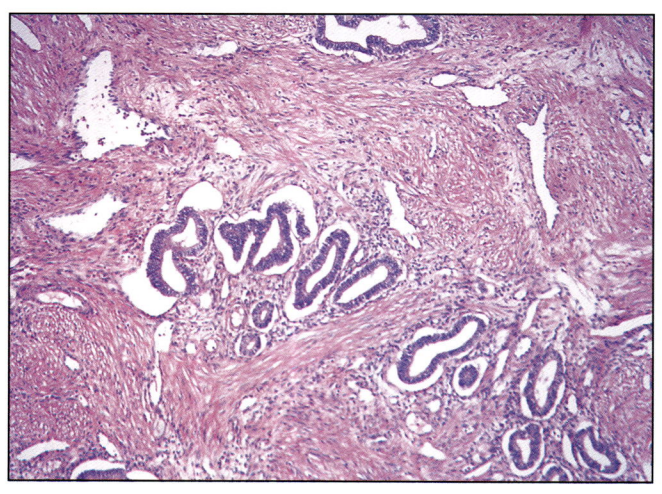

图13D.14 腺肌瘤。良性表现的子宫内膜腺体和间质位于肌瘤性间质中。

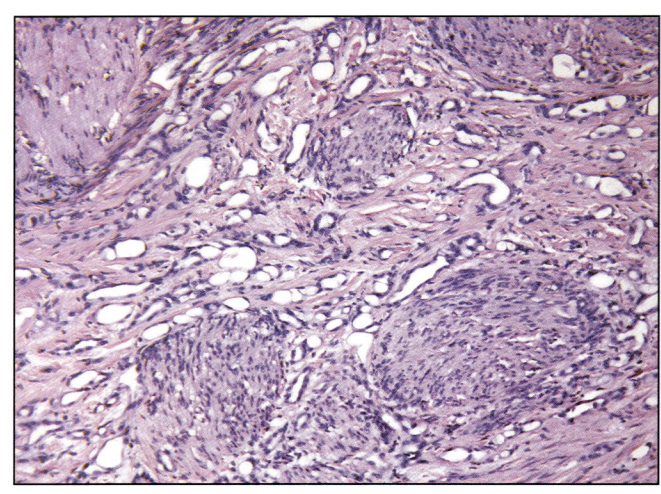

图13D.15 腺瘤样瘤。内衬良性立方至扁平上皮的假血管腔，周围围绕增生的平滑肌。

当病变位于黏膜下时，可以类似于子宫内膜息肉，但是质地通常较硬，切面呈肌瘤性表现。组织学上，这些病变由巢状或岛状分布的子宫内膜间质和形成完好或有时是囊状的良性子宫内膜样腺体组成，周围围绕增生的平滑肌，平滑肌成分一般占优势（图13D.14）。腺肌瘤与腺肌症的鉴别有时可能是人为的，一般来说，腺肌症倾向于是比较弥漫的病变，与子宫肌层界限不清。比较重要的是与非典型性息肉样腺肌瘤的鉴别（见第13章第二部分）。它与腺肌瘤类似，以肌瘤性间质为特征，但是非典型性息肉样腺肌瘤的不同之处在于具有比较复杂的腺体增生（在一些病例与高分化子宫内膜样腺癌无法区分），而且常常显示鳞状桑葚化生。

腺瘤样瘤[53-56] Adenomatoid tumor

这个肿瘤一般是在育龄期妇女子宫切除或肌瘤切除标本中偶然发现的。它本身不是平滑肌瘤的一个亚型，而是推测为起源于间皮的良性瘤性肿块，伴有明显的平滑肌成分，在大体和组织学检查时都可能类似于平滑肌瘤。腺瘤样瘤最常见于浆膜下区域，可以呈褐色、白色或黄色，与周围子宫肌层的界限一般不如平滑肌瘤清楚。大多数肿瘤小于5 cm；然而，偶尔肿瘤可以较大，而且多数这样的病例具有明显的囊性成分。组织学上，假血管腔隙内衬立方至扁平上皮细胞，细胞核呈良性表现，并被平滑肌束分开（图13D.15）。免疫表型支持这些肿瘤起源于间皮，上皮细胞成分表达calretinin、HMBE-1和WT-1[56]。

恶性平滑肌肿瘤
Malignant smooth muscle neoplasms

临床特征

子宫平滑肌肉瘤不常见，占所有子宫恶性肿瘤的2%

以下，年发病率估计为每100 000妇女中0.64例；然而，它却是最常见的子宫肉瘤，大约占子宫恶性间叶性肿瘤的25%[57,58]。因术前诊断良性平滑肌瘤而切除的子宫标本中，发现平滑肌肉瘤的也不常见，据估计为0.49%[59]。子宫平滑肌肉瘤的发生率似乎具有种族差异，黑人妇女发生肉瘤的危险性较大；其他潜在的危险因素包括口服避孕药和应用他莫昔芬（tamoxifen）[58,60]。诊断平滑肌肉瘤患者的中位年龄通常在40~60岁，最常见的症状是功能障碍性子宫出血和（或）下腹痛[57,59,61-64]。临床检查的典型表现是子宫增大，许多平滑肌肉瘤未被怀疑，而被推测为增大的平滑肌瘤。如果肿瘤不侵犯子宫内膜腔，术前刮宫标本不能提供信息。不过，对于绝经后患者，临床上发现较大而迅速生长的肿瘤时，应该怀疑有恶性的可能。

子宫平滑肌肉瘤是一种进展性的肿瘤，倾向于局部复发和（或）转移，最常见的转移部位是肝和肺。局部淋巴结转移并不常见，淋巴结转移一般仅仅见于晚期肿瘤患者，因此，通常仅在临床怀疑有淋巴结转移时才做淋巴结检查[65,66]。评估5年生存率差异较大。可能是因为在一些研究系列中病例数少，伴有早期病变的患者数量不同，以及平滑肌肉瘤的诊断标准发生变化；然而，多数研究评估5年生存率在45%~65%之间[57,60-62,64,67-69]。尽管肿瘤的生存率有所不同，但已经明确肿瘤分期与肿瘤预后明显相关[60-63,68-73]。标准的治疗方法是全子宫切除和双侧输卵管卵巢切除。病例对照研究已经提示，保留绝经前妇女的卵巢对于生存没有不良影响，尽管还有争议[63]。辅助治疗对于生存的影响也有争议[62-64,69,72]。

分子遗传学

与平滑肌瘤不同，平滑肌肉瘤的细胞遗传学特征是具有复杂的数量和结构异常，在同一个恶性肿瘤中，一个肿瘤细胞可以不同于另外一个肿瘤细胞，提示存在高度的基因组不稳定性[74-76]。其他的研究方法也支持这一观点，例如比较基因组杂交最常表现为10号和13号染色体长臂的杂合性缺失[77]。平滑肌肉瘤（典型的表现为基因表达下调）和平滑肌瘤转录特征不同，支持这些肿瘤具有不同的发病机制[78]。

病理学特征

典型的平滑肌肉瘤表现为孤立性的肿物或为子宫内主要的肿块，最常见于子宫肌壁间，但也可见于黏膜下或浆膜下，平均直径9 cm[62,63]。虽然某些肿瘤大体形态可能类似于平滑肌瘤，但大多数肉瘤具有明显不同的表现，边界不甚清楚，某些伴有明显的肌层浸润，质地较软，灰色到奶油色，并有多少不等的不规则分布的地图状出

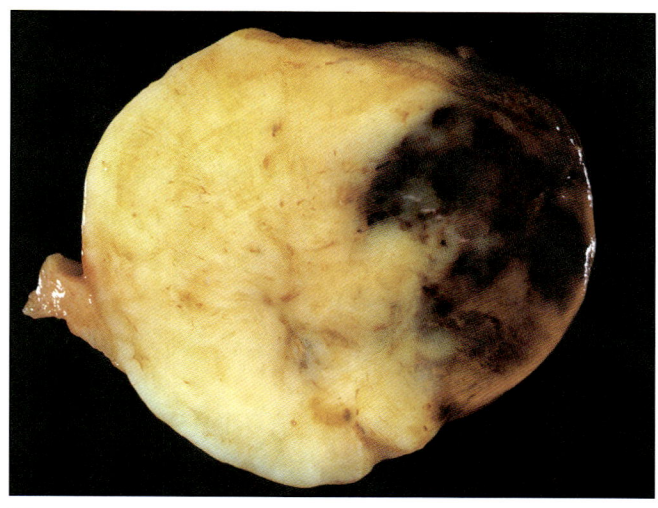

图13D.16　平滑肌肉瘤。肿瘤质地均匀，呈"鱼肉状"外观，伴有地图状出血和坏死是典型的大体表现。

血和坏死，后者在大体检查时常表现为黄色或绿色（图13D.16）。虽然这些不常见的大体特征都可能提出恶性的可能（并且应该立即扩大取材的范围），但平滑肌肉瘤的诊断完全是根据肿瘤的组织学表现。绝大多数平滑肌肉瘤为梭形细胞型；然而，也可出现上皮样和黏液样亚型，这些亚型具有不同的恶性诊断标准（表13D.1）。

梭形细胞平滑肌肉瘤
Spindle cell leiomyosarcoma

之所以称为平滑肌肉瘤的梭形细胞亚型，是因为其形态类似于良性平滑肌瘤，肿瘤由成束的具有不同程度嗜酸性胞浆的梭形细胞组成（图13D.17）。随着时间的延长，肿瘤细胞呈现非单一的组织学表现，例外的情况是肿瘤细胞坏死（可能难以辨认）对于恶性或许具有诊

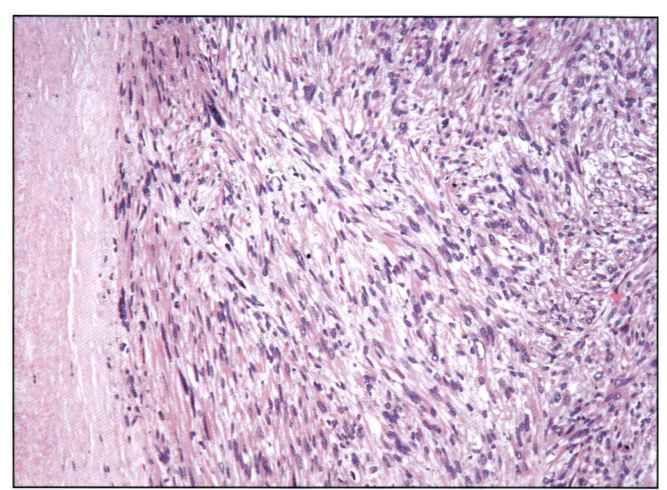

图13D.17　梭形细胞平滑肌肉瘤。伴有嗜酸性胞浆的梭形肿瘤细胞交错排列成束。注意核的非典型性和肿瘤细胞坏死（左）。

恶性平滑肌肿瘤

表13D.1　平滑肌肿瘤的诊断标准

梭形细胞平滑肌肿瘤伴有明显核的非典型性

弥漫性或多灶性中至重度核的非典型性 + 无肿瘤细胞坏死 + 核分裂象 ≥10/10个高倍视野 = **平滑肌肉瘤**

弥漫性、多灶性或局灶性中至重度核的非典型性 + 肿瘤细胞坏死 + 核分裂象 ≥1/10个高倍视野 = **平滑肌肉瘤**

弥漫性、多灶性或局灶性中至重度核的非典型性 + 无肿瘤细胞坏死 + 核分裂象 <7/10个高倍视野 = **非典型性平滑肌瘤**

弥漫性或多灶性中至重度核的非典型性 + 无肿瘤细胞坏死 + 核分裂象 >7但<10/10个高倍视野 = **不能确定恶性潜能的平滑肌肿瘤**

无明显核非典型性的梭形细胞平滑肌肿瘤

无或仅有轻度核的非典型性 + 肿瘤细胞坏死 + 核分裂象 ≥10/10个高倍视野 = **平滑肌肉瘤**

无或仅有轻度核的非典型性 + 肿瘤细胞坏死 + 核分裂象 <10/10个高倍视野 = **不能确定恶性潜能的平滑肌肿瘤**

无或仅有轻度核的非典型性 + 无肿瘤细胞坏死 + 核分裂象 >5但<15/10个高倍视野 = **核分裂活跃的平滑肌瘤**

无或仅有轻度核的非典型性 + 无肿瘤细胞坏死 + 核分裂象 >15/10个高倍视野 = **核分裂活跃的平滑肌瘤（不能确定生物学行为）**

黏液样平滑肌肿瘤

核分裂象 <2/10个高倍视野 + 无肿瘤细胞坏死 + 无至轻度核的非典型性 + 无子宫肌层浸润 = **黏液样平滑肌瘤**

核分裂象 >2/10个高倍视野或肿瘤细胞坏死或中至重度核的非典型性或浸润子宫肌层 = **黏液样平滑肌肉瘤**

上皮样平滑肌肿瘤

核分裂象 <3/10个高倍视野 + 无肿瘤细胞坏死 + 无至轻度核的非典型性 + 无血管浸润 + 肿瘤边界清楚 = **考虑上皮样平滑肌瘤**

核分裂象 >3/10个高倍视野或肿瘤细胞坏死或中至重度核的非典型性或血管浸润或肿瘤边界浸润 = **上皮样平滑肌肉瘤**

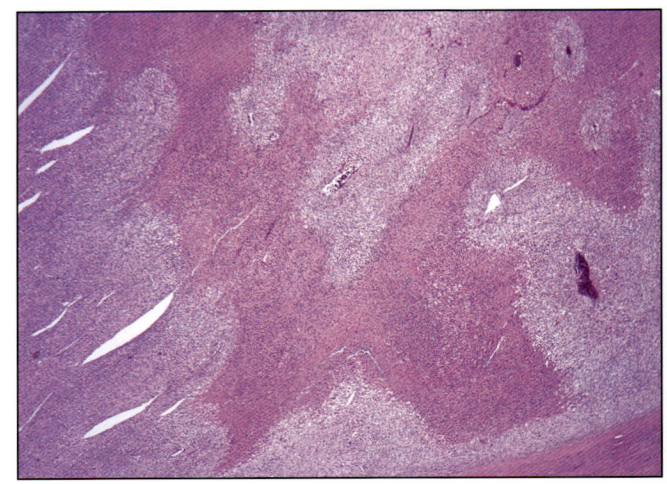

图13D.18　平滑肌肉瘤伴有肿瘤细胞坏死。注意肿瘤坏死边界不规则成角（"地图样"坏死）。

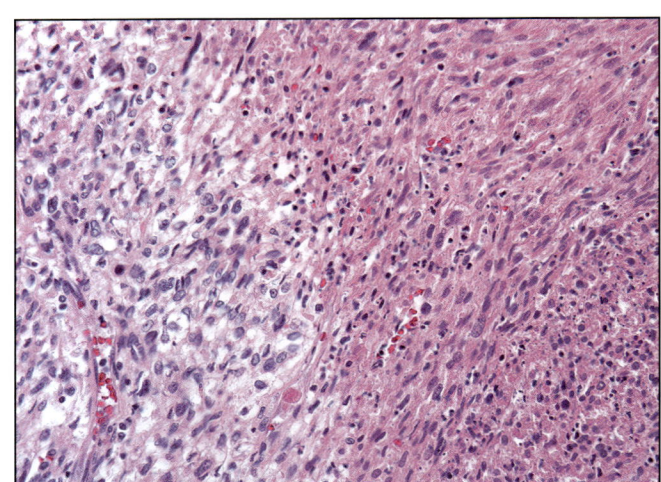

图13D.19　平滑肌肉瘤伴有肿瘤细胞坏死。其特征为存活细胞和坏死细胞分界清楚，而且伴有核碎片。

断意义。平滑肌肉瘤的诊断是根据 Bell 等的标志性研究资料做出的[15]，其中采用了联合的组织学特征进行评估。这些特征包括：（1）显著的核非典型的出现和范围（实际上，非典型性的定义是在低倍镜下就很显著，即应用 10 倍物镜）；（2）核分裂率；（3）是否有凝固性坏死。做出平滑肌肉瘤的诊断要求：（1）有弥漫性中度到重度细胞核非典型性和核分裂计数每 10 个高倍视野 10 个或大于 10 个；或（2）有弥漫性或多灶性中度到重度细胞核非典型性和肿瘤细胞坏死以及每 10 个高倍视野大于 1 个的任何程度的核分裂活性；或（3）无或仅有轻度细胞核非典型性和出现肿瘤细胞坏死以及核分裂计数每 10 个高倍视野大于 10 个。后一种情况非常少见，并且提出了十分重要的诊断问题，也就是是真正的肿瘤细胞坏死还是良性退行性改变的问题。凝固性肿瘤细胞坏死的特征是：（1）坏死边界不规则，成角状（"地图状"表现）；（2）存活细胞与坏死细胞界限清楚（相对于缺血引起的特征性的由肉芽组织或玻璃样变性构成的移行带）；（3）交界处出现细胞凋亡/核碎片；（4）坏死区域内见非典型性鬼影细胞（因为这些肿瘤细胞伴有非典型性）（图 13D.18 和 13D.19）。对于那些肿瘤细胞坏死模棱两可，而且没有或仅有轻度细胞非典型性的病例，应该考虑分类为不能确定恶性潜能的肿瘤（见下，不能确定恶性潜能的平滑肌肿瘤一节）。

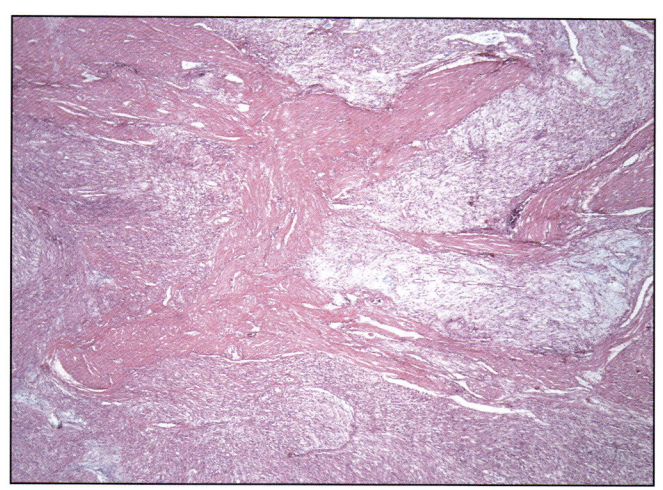

图13D.20 黏液样平滑肌肉瘤。丰富的细胞外基质沉积将肿瘤细胞分开。注意子宫肌层浸润。

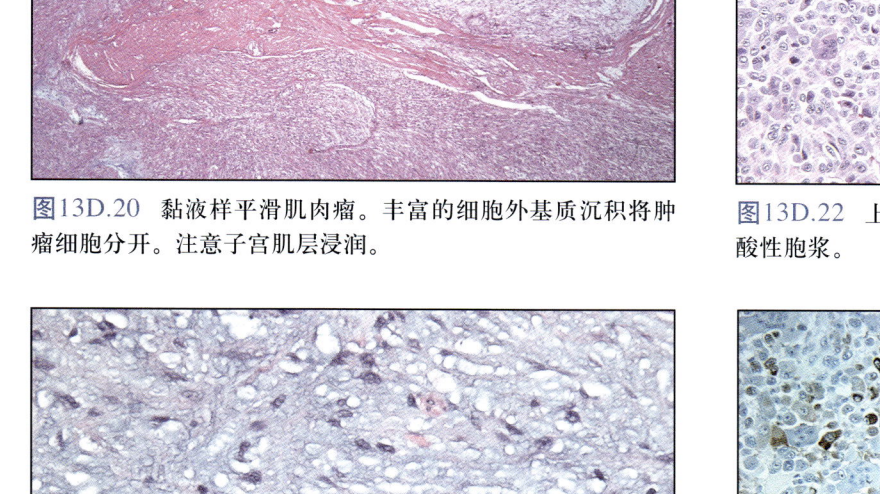

图13D.22 上皮样平滑肌肉瘤。圆形肿瘤细胞伴有丰富的嗜酸性胞浆。

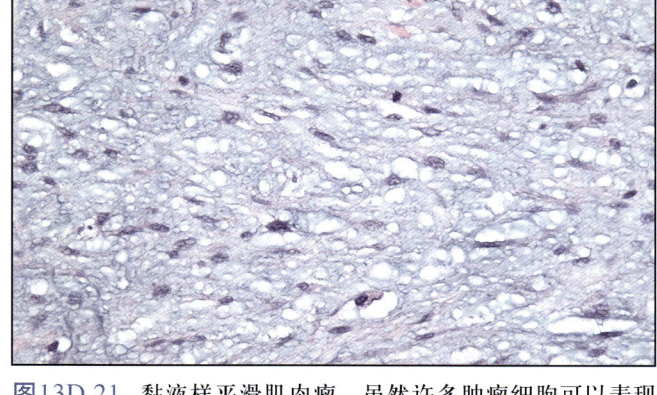

图13D.21 黏液样平滑肌肉瘤。虽然许多肿瘤细胞可以表现为良性，但大多数病例至少出现中度的核非典型性。

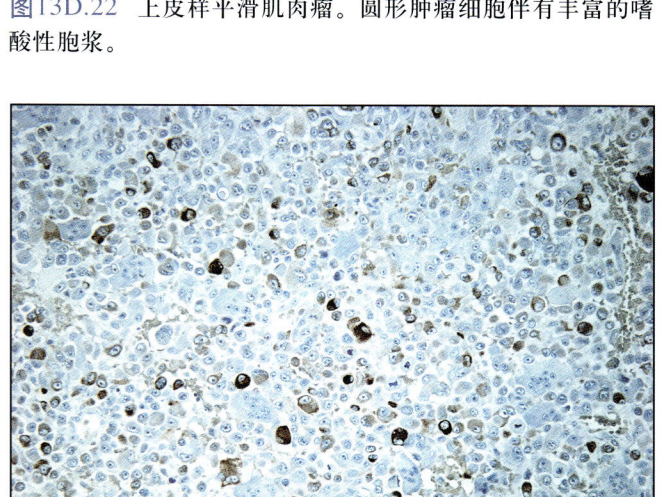

图13D.23 上皮样平滑肌肉瘤。肿瘤细胞desmin阳性。

黏液样平滑肌肉瘤[38,79-82]
Myxoid leiomyosarcoma

与梭形细胞平滑肌肉瘤相似，典型的黏液样平滑肌肉瘤也见于50～60岁的妇女，临床表现为异常出血、下腹痛和（或）盆腔肿块。所不同的是，黏液性平滑肌肉瘤大体呈胶样表现，切面有光泽，病变范围可能不同，取决于细胞外黏液物质的含量。组织学上，这些肿瘤以出现丰富的淡蓝色阿辛蓝染色阳性的细胞外黏液样物质为特征。肿瘤细胞可能为梭形或星形，细胞外黏液样基质的沉积可能使肿瘤的束状结构变得模糊（图13D.20）。虽然大部分肿瘤细胞呈良性的细胞形态学表现，但典型的至少表现局灶中度非典型性（图13D.21）。由于这个肿瘤罕见，鉴别黏液样平滑肌瘤与黏液样平滑肌肉瘤的诊断标准没有很好地建立。Atkins等提出，不管有无肿瘤细胞的非典型性或肿瘤细胞坏死，每10个高倍视野核分裂数大于2个可以用来区分良性和恶性黏液样肿瘤[38]。实际工作中，如果出现下列任何一条均应考虑黏液样平滑肌肉瘤的诊断：（1）中到重度细胞学非典型性；（2）凝固性肿瘤细胞坏死；（3）每10个高倍视野核分裂象大于2个；（4）肿瘤破坏性浸润周围子宫肌层。

上皮样平滑肌肉瘤[29,34,36,37]
Epithelioid leiomyosarcoma

上皮样平滑肌肉瘤的特征是以圆形肿瘤细胞为主，伴有丰富的嗜酸性或透明胞浆（图13D.22和13D.23）。与黏液样平滑肌肉瘤相似，由于这种肿瘤发病率低，所以用于可靠地预测上皮样平滑肌肿瘤生物学行为的诊断标准受到限制，文献中仅有有限数目的系列报告。在已发表的最大系列的上皮样平滑肌肉瘤中（80例，以摘要形式[37]），肿瘤恶性生物学行为与出现肿瘤细胞坏死、血管浸润、中到

不能确定恶性潜能的平滑肌肿瘤
Smooth muscle tumors of uncertain malignant potential

尽管大量的临床病理学研究强调了恶性子宫平滑肌肿瘤的诊断标准，但仍然有部分病变难于分类。例如上皮样和黏液样平滑肌肿瘤，因为它们罕见，所以难于确定有效的诊断标准用于预测其恶性生物学行为。那些接近但又不够诊断恶性的标准，或出现不明确的肿瘤细胞坏死，以及不能与良性病变明确区分开来的肿瘤，最好放在不能确定恶性潜能的类型中。另外，由 Bell 等[15]提出的那些提示肿瘤不能确定或具有低度恶性潜能的特征列于表 13D.1 中。实际上，仅有少数平滑肌肿瘤属于这一类型。

伴有独特特征的平滑肌增生
Smooth muscle proliferations with unusual features

伴有血管浸润的平滑肌瘤[83]
Leiomyoma with vascular invasion

伴血管浸润的平滑肌瘤是指普通的平滑肌瘤中出现不常见的显微镜下肿瘤血管内延伸。虽然这些肿瘤没有伴有长期随访的系列报告，但一般认为它们是良性肿瘤而没有复发的危险。这些病变与静脉内平滑肌瘤病不同，它们缺乏超出平滑肌瘤范围以外的血管浸润。

静脉内（血管内）平滑肌瘤病[83-85]
Intravenous (intravascular) leiomyomatosis

静脉内平滑肌瘤病是一种不常见的疾病，典型的见于晚期育龄期妇女，平均年龄在 40～50 岁。本病以血管内良性表现的平滑肌组织增生为特征。典型的临床表现是异常子宫出血、盆腔疼痛和（或）盆腔包块，临床检查通常表现为子宫增大。大体检查，子宫肌壁一般可见多发性肿物，而且在子宫旁血管内还能见到蠕虫样栓子（图 13D.24）。偶尔，肿瘤可以延伸到下腔静脉及其分支，包括累及心脏。子宫通常有普通型的平滑肌瘤；然而，某些病例表现为整个肿瘤位于血管腔中，在最初的大体检查中可能被忽视。组织学上，血管内肿瘤常呈分叶状或裂隙状，类似于典型的子宫平

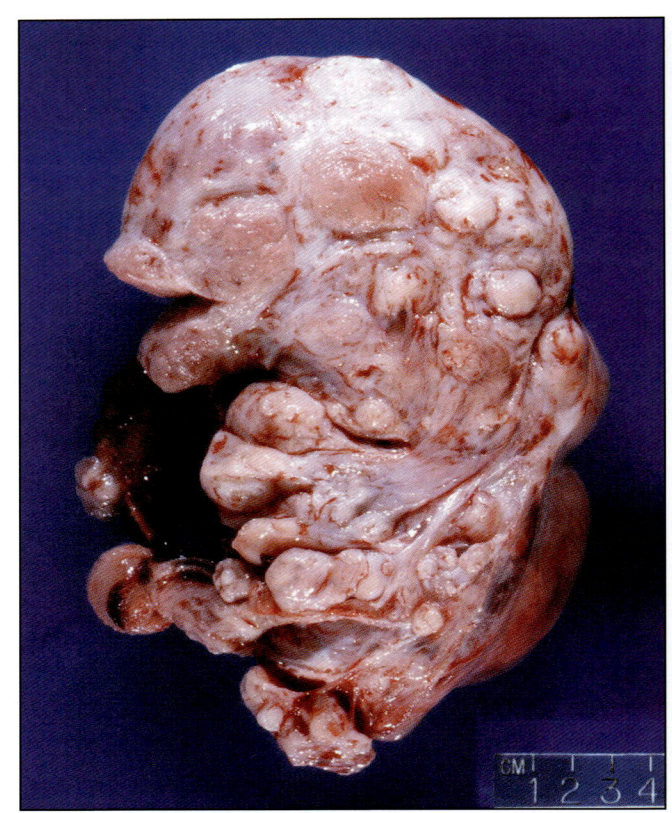

图13D.24 静脉内平滑肌瘤病。多发性肿瘤结节充满子宫肌壁内的血管腔。（Courtesy of Dr. Christopher Otis, Baystate Medical Center, Springfield, MA.）

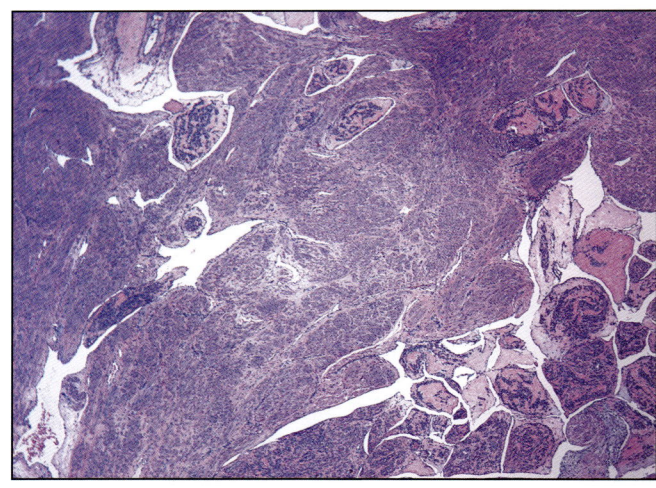

图13D.25 静脉内平滑肌瘤病。特征为多发性肿瘤结节位于呈现裂隙样外观的血管腔内。

滑肌瘤，许多病例还可能表现为广泛的水肿或玻璃样变（图 13D.25 和 13D.26）。可能出现其他的组织学变异，包括血管内肿瘤成分富于细胞，呈黏液样、上皮样或含有脂肪细胞成分（脂肪平滑肌瘤样）。虽然已经提出肿瘤来源于血管平滑肌，但是两例肿瘤的细胞遗传学分析显示，出现常见于子宫平滑肌瘤的派生染色体 der(14)t(12;14)(q15;q24)，支持为子宫起源[86]。尽管出现广泛的血管受累，但一般认为静脉内平滑肌瘤病预

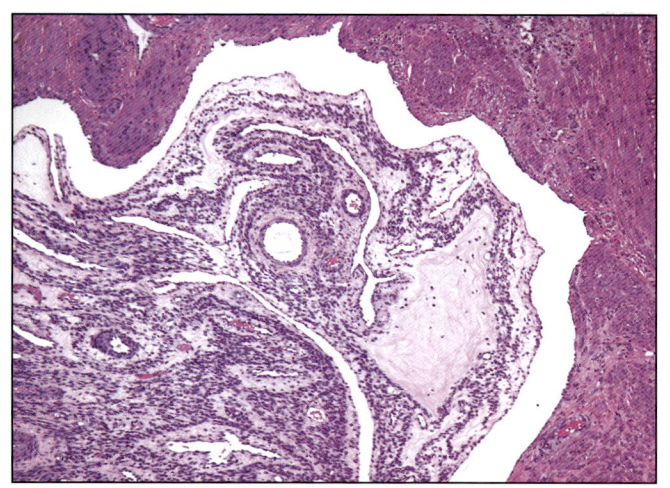

图13D.26 静脉内平滑肌瘤病。血管腔中的肿瘤结节伴有水肿改变。

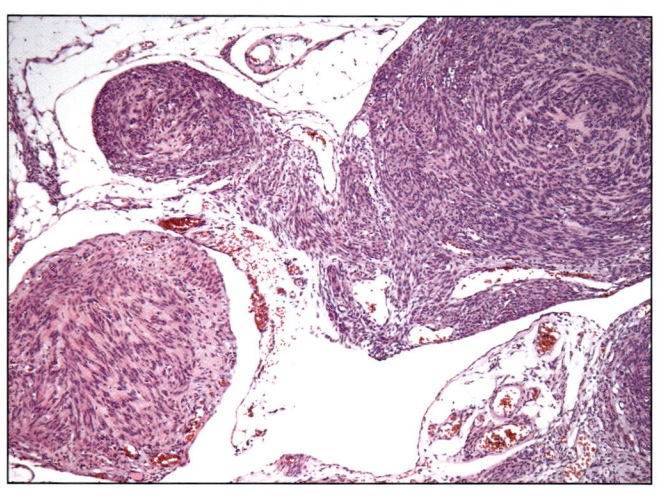

图13D.28 播散性腹膜平滑肌瘤病。组织学上,普通的平滑肌小瘤累及网膜。

后好,特别是在可以手术切除的病例。大部分病例呈良性的临床经过,盆腔复发或远处转移的危险性低,最常见的转移部位在肺。主要的鉴别诊断是将静脉内平滑肌瘤病与子宫内膜间质肉瘤区分开来,特别是富于细胞的亚型。后者血管内成分缺少裂隙状轮廓以及厚壁血管;对于诊断有困难的病例,缺乏肌肉标志物阳性,特别是h-caldesmon阴性,是子宫内膜间质肿瘤的特征。

播散性腹膜平滑肌瘤病[87-90]
Disseminated peritoneal leiomyomatosis

播散性腹膜平滑肌瘤病(英文又称leiomyomatosis peritonealis disseminata)是一种罕见的疾病,一般发生于育龄期的妇女,病变特征为大量伴有极少核分裂活性的组织学上良性的平滑肌瘤性小瘤分布于腹膜和网膜表面(图13D.27和13D.28)。小瘤的数量和大小变化很大,数量从几个到无数个瘤结节,大小从显微镜下可见到通常小于3 cm。病变广泛,临床上常常类似于播散性恶性肿瘤。常常同时伴有妊娠或外源性激素治疗,但并不是所有的病例。虽然这种相关因素提示了激素影响在肿瘤的发生中具有作用,但克隆性研究显示播散性腹膜平滑肌瘤病的瘤结节是克隆性的,具有相同的X染色体失活[90],提示它们全都来源于单一转化事件,而且全部都由同一个结节衍生而来(即为"转移性")。虽然这一发现是有趣的,但患者一般具有良性临床经过,一般提倡采取保守治疗并对患者进行长期随访。

子宫内弥漫性平滑肌瘤病[91-93]
Intrauterine diffuse leiomyomatosis

弥漫性平滑肌瘤病是罕见的良性疾病,由于出现大量大小不等、相互融合、界限常常不清的平滑肌瘤,因此子宫表现为特征性的弥漫性对称性增大。典型的患者年龄小于40岁,最常见的症状是异常子宫出血。大体检查显示子宫增大,可以超过1公斤,子宫肌壁几乎完全被大量的平滑肌瘤取代,肿瘤相互融合,肿瘤彼此之间不像普通型子宫平滑肌瘤界限那么清楚(图13D.29)。组织学上,平滑肌瘤结节多数为显微镜下所见,一般由良性的富于细胞的平滑肌组成。虽然某些肿瘤的界限可以清楚,但平滑肌瘤结节界限通常不清,而且常常彼此相互融合(图13D.30)。一例弥漫性平滑肌瘤病的克隆性分析显示,在8个独立的平滑肌瘤结节中有不同的、但是并非任意的X染色体失活,支持每个肿瘤结节起源于独立的转化事件这一假设[93]。这个发现类似于典型的子宫平滑肌瘤,提示弥漫性平滑肌瘤病的患者特别容易形成平滑肌瘤结节。

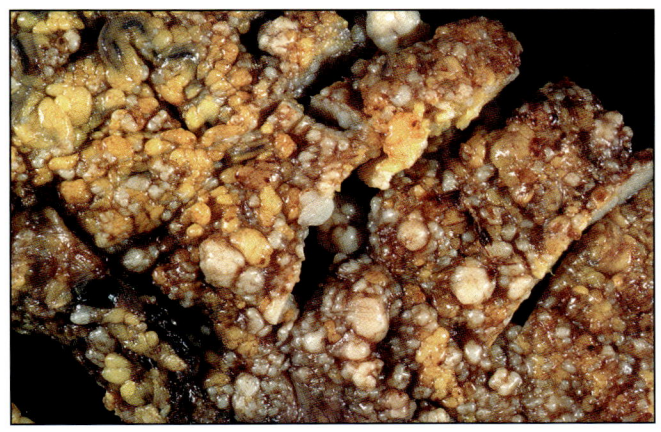

图13D.27 播散性腹膜平滑肌瘤病。大量的肿瘤结节分布于网膜上,类似于转移癌。

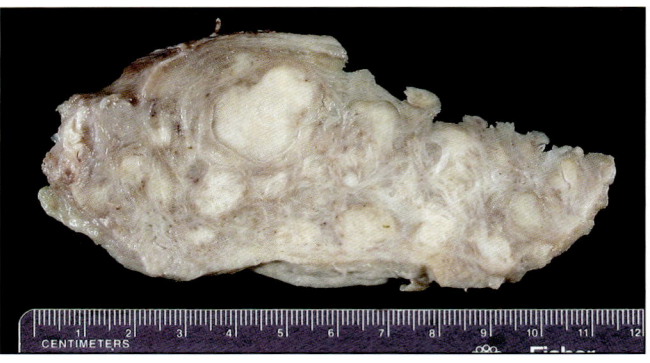

图13D.29　子宫内弥漫性平滑肌瘤病。界限不甚清楚的平滑肌瘤结节弥漫性累及子宫肌层。

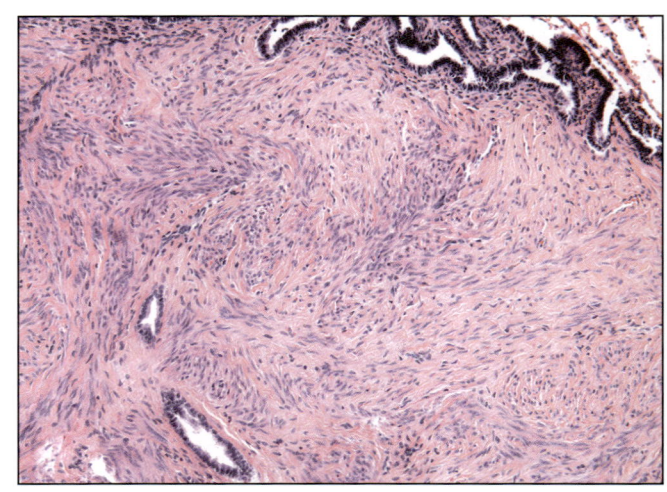

图13D.31　良性转移性平滑肌瘤。一个良性子宫平滑肌瘤患者的肺实质内见良性增生的平滑肌。

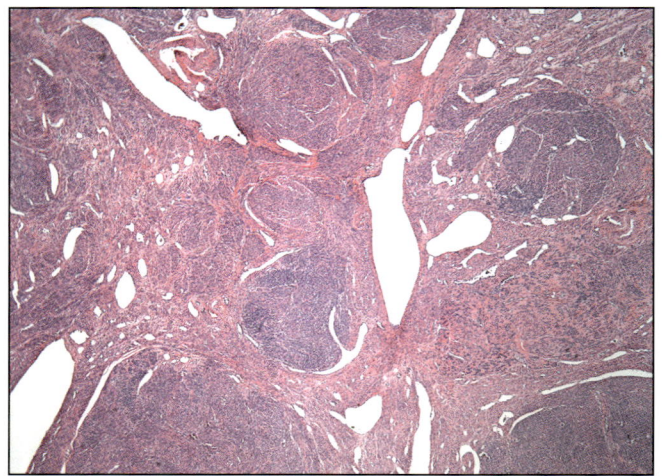

图13D.30　子宫内弥漫性平滑肌瘤病。大量且有些融合的平滑肌瘤弥漫性累及子宫肌层。

良性转移性平滑肌瘤[94-97]
Benign metastasizing leiomyoma

所谓的良性转移性平滑肌瘤是用于描述子宫平滑肌瘤患者的肺或淋巴结中出现类似于子宫平滑肌瘤的平滑肌增生，肿瘤细胞学呈良性，核分裂不活跃。这一命名的根据是这些肿瘤来源于组织学表现良性的子宫平滑肌肿瘤（平滑肌瘤）的播散，仅仅根据形态学标准不能确认肿瘤具有转移性潜能（平滑肌肉瘤）。然而，还不清楚这种病变是一种生物学上独特的临床病理学疾病，还是由组织学上相似但生物学上毫不相关的病变组成的疾病。本病患者通常有因子宫平滑肌瘤切除子宫/肌瘤切除的病史，或在诊断时同时有肿瘤存在。组织学上，"转移性"病灶由良性表现的增生性平滑肌细胞组成，没有核的多形性、坏死或明显核分裂活性的证据（图13D.31）。良性转移性平滑肌瘤的临床过程不一，有些病例临床表现呈惰性，而另一些表现为进展性（甚至可以致死）肺部累及。

罕见和独特的肿瘤
Rare and unusual neoplasms

横纹肌肉瘤[98-100]　Rhabdomyosarcoma

纯粹的子宫横纹肌肉瘤十分罕见，只有经广泛取材排除了癌肉瘤或腺肉瘤中肉瘤成分过度生长才能考虑诊断。子宫横纹肌肉瘤中最常见的是多形性横纹肌肉瘤；然而，梭形和腺泡亚型也有描述。在最大的一宗病例报告中，纯粹的多形性子宫横纹肌肉瘤患者临床表现为阴道出血、子宫增大或急腹症，诊断时的中位年龄为65岁[98]。肿瘤或表现为息肉样子宫内膜肿块或为子宫肌壁间肿块，组织学上，类似于软组织的多形性横纹肌肉瘤。肿瘤预后差，大多数患者2年内死于肿瘤。

子宫血管周围上皮样细胞肿瘤[101-104]
Uterine perivascular epithelioid cell tumor

血管周围上皮样细胞肿瘤（PEComas）是由具有丰富的透明到颗粒状胞浆的上皮样或多角形细胞组成的，具有围绕血管生长的倾向，肿瘤免疫组织化学染色显示HMB-45和desmin阳性。子宫血管周围上皮样细胞肿瘤是肿瘤家族中的一个成员，这个肿瘤家族包括上皮样血管平滑肌脂肪瘤、透明细胞"糖瘤"、圆韧带/镰状韧带的透明细胞肌黑色素细胞（myomelanocytic）肿瘤、盆腹腔血管周围上皮样细胞肉瘤以及淋巴管平滑肌瘤病，它们具有类似的组织形态学和免疫表型（也见第24章）。发生在子宫的这种病变已描述的有两种组织学形态。其中一种亚型肿瘤生长类似于低级别子宫内膜间质肉瘤，伴有子宫壁的指状浸润，其组成细胞具有丰富的嗜酸性、透明或颗粒状胞浆；这些肿瘤细胞 HMB-45 染色呈现弥漫阳性，而肌肉标志物仅呈局灶阳性[101]。另外一种亚型由上皮样细胞组成，肿瘤细胞较少透明胞浆，HMB-45 表达少见，肌肉标志物阳性表达比较广泛[101,102]。因此，子宫血管周围上皮样细胞肿瘤与上皮样平滑肌肿瘤的关系还不清楚，然而，它们可能是这一形态学谱系中的一部分。子宫血管周围上皮样细胞肿瘤最好考虑为不能确定恶性潜能的肿瘤，因为偶尔可以出现复发和晚期转移。由于报告的病例数目少，预测这一肿瘤生物学行为的明确而又有效的组织学标准还没有确立。

参考文献

1. Cramer S F, Patel A 1990 The frequency of uterine leiomyomas. Am J Clin Pathol 94: 435–438
2. Stewart E A 2001 Uterine fibroids. Lancet 357: 293–298
3. Alam N A, Bevan S, Churchman M et al. 2001 Localization of a gene (MCUL1) for multiple cutaneous leiomyomata and uterine fibroids to chromosome 1q42.3-q43. Am J Hum Genet 68: 1264–1269
4. Tomlinson I P, Alam N A, Rowan A J et al. 2002 Germline mutations in FH predispose to dominantly inherited uterine fibroids, skin leiomyomata and papillary renal cell cancer. Nat Genet 30: 406–410
5. Toro J R, Nickerson M L, Wei M H et al. 2003 Mutations in the fumarate hydratase gene cause hereditary leiomyomatosis and renal cell cancer in families in North America. Am J Hum Genet 73: 95–106
6. Mashal R D, Fejzo M L, Friedman A J et al. 1994 Analysis of androgen receptor DNA reveals the independent clonal origins of uterine leiomyomata and the secondary nature of cytogenetic aberrations in the development of leiomyomata. Genes Chromos Cancer 11: 1–6
7. Nilbert M, Heim S 1990 Uterine leiomyoma cytogenetics. Genes Chromos Cancer 2: 3–13
8. Schoenmakers E F, Wanschura S, Mols R et al. 1995 Recurrent rearrangements in the high mobility group protein gene, HMGI-C, in benign mesenchymal tumours. Nat Genet 10: 436–444
9. Gattas G J, Quade B J, Nowak R A et al. 1999 HMGIC expression in human adult and fetal tissues and in uterine leiomyomata. Genes Chromos Cancer 25: 316–322
10. Kazmierczak B, Dal Cin P, Wanschura S et al. 1998 HMGIY is the target of 6p21.3 rearrangements in various benign mesenchymal tumors. Genes Chromos Cancer 23: 279–285
11. Klotzbucher M, Wasserfall A, Fuhrmann U 1999 Misexpression of wild-type and truncated isoforms of the high-mobility group I proteins HMGI-C and HMGI(Y) in uterine leiomyomas. Am J Pathol 155: 1535–1542
12. Oliva E, Young R H, Clement P B et al. 1995 Cellular benign mesenchymal tumors of the uterus. A comparative morphologic and immunohistochemical analysis of 33 highly cellular leiomyomas and six endometrial stromal nodules, two frequently confused tumors. Am J Surg Pathol 19: 757–768
13. O'Connor D M, Norris H J 1990 Mitotically active leiomyomas of the uterus. Hum Pathol 21: 223–227
14. Prayson R A, Hart W R 1992 Mitotically active leiomyomas of the uterus. Am J Clin Pathol 97: 14–20
15. Bell S W, Kempson R L, Hendrickson M R 1994 Problematic uterine smooth muscle neoplasms. A clinicopathologic study of 213 cases. Am J Surg Pathol 18: 535–558
16. Dgani R, Piura B, Ben Baruch G et al. 1998 Clinical–pathological study of uterine leiomyomas with high mitotic activity. Acta Obstet Gynecol Scand 77: 74–77
17. Downes K A, Hart W R 1997 Bizarre leiomyomas of the uterus: a comprehensive pathologic study of 24 cases with long-term follow-up. Am J Surg Pathol 21: 1261–1270
18. Myles J L, Hart W R 1985 Apoplectic leiomyomas of the uterus. A clinicopathologic study of five distinctive hemorrhagic leiomyomas associated with oral contraceptive usage. Am J Surg Pathol 9: 798–805
19. Norris H J, Hilliard G D, Irey N S 1988 Hemorrhagic cellular leiomyomas ("apoplectic leiomyomas") of the uterus associated with pregnancy and oral contraceptives. Int J Gynecol Pathol 7: 212–224
20. Colgan T J, Pendergast S, LeBlanc M 1993 The histopathology of uterine leiomyomas following treatment with gonadotropin-releasing hormone analogues. Hum Pathol 24: 1073–1077
21. Rutgers J L, Spong C Y, Sinow R et al. 1995 Leuprolide acetate treatment and myoma arterial size. Obstet Gynecol 86: 386–388
22. Deligdisch L, Hirschmann S, Altchek A 1997 Pathologic changes in gonadotropin releasing hormone agonist analogue treated uterine leiomyomata. Fertil Steril 67: 837–841
23. Demopoulos R I, Jones K Y, Mittal K R et al. 1997 Histology of leiomyomata in patients treated with leuprolide acetate. Int J Gynecol Pathol 16: 131–137
24. Sreenan J J, Prayson R A, Biscotti C V et al. 1996 Histopathologic findings in 107 uterine leiomyomas treated with leuprolide acetate compared with 126 controls. Am J Surg Pathol 20: 427–432
25. Clement P B, Young R H, Scully R E 1992 Diffuse, perinodular, and other patterns of hydropic degeneration within and adjacent to uterine leiomyomas. Problems in differential diagnosis. Am J Surg Pathol 16: 26–32
26. Kaminski P F, Tavassoli F A 1984 Plexiform tumorlet: a clinical and pathologic study of 15 cases with ultrastructural observations. Int J Gynecol Pathol 3: 124–134
27. Seidman J D, Thomas R M 1993 Multiple plexiform tumorlets of the uterus. Arch Pathol Lab Med 117: 1255–1256
28. Nagel H, Brinck U, Luthje D et al. 1999 Plexiform leiomyoma of the uterus in a patient with breast carcinoma: case report and review of the literature. Pathology 31: 292–294
29. Kurman R J, Norris H J 1976 Mesenchymal tumors of the uterus. VI. Epithelioid smooth muscle tumors including leiomyoblastoma and clear-cell leiomyoma: a clinical and pathologic analysis of 26 cases. Cancer 37: 1853–1865
30. Mazur M T, Priest J B 1986 Clear cell leiomyoma (leiomyoblastoma) of the uterus: ultrastructural observations. Ultrastruct Pathol 10: 249–255
31. Hyde K E, Geisinger K R, Marshall R B et al. 1989 The clear-cell variant of uterine epithelioid leiomyoma. An immunohistologic and ultrastructural study. Arch Pathol Lab Med 113: 551–553
32. Kyriazis A P, Kyriazis A A 1992 Uterine leiomyoblastoma (epithelioid leiomyoma) neoplasm of low-grade malignancy. A histopathologic study. Arch Pathol Lab Med 116: 1189–1191
33. Karaiskos C, Pandis N, Bardi G et al. 1995 Cytogenetic findings in uterine epithelioid leiomyomas. Cancer Genet Cytogenet 80: 103–106
34. Prayson R A, Goldblum J R, Hart W R 1997 Epithelioid smooth-muscle tumors of the uterus: a clinicopathologic study of 18 patients. Am J Surg Pathol 21: 383–391
35. Watanabe K, Ogura G, Suzuki T 2003 Leiomyoblastoma of the uterus: an immunohistochemical and electron microscopic study of distinctive tumours with immature smooth muscle cell differentiation mimicking fetal uterine myocytes. Histopathology 42: 379–386
36. Atkins K, Bell S, Kempson R L et al. 2002 Epithelioid smooth muscle tumors of the uterus [abstract]. Mod Pathol 14: 132A
37. Oliva E, Nielsen G P, Clement P B et al. 1997 Epithelioid smooth muscle tumors of the uterus. A clinicopathologic analysis of 80 cases [abstract]. Lab Invest 76: 107A
38. Atkins K, Bell S, Kempson R L et al. 2002 Myxoid smooth muscle tumors of the uterus [abstract]. Mod Pathol 14: 132A
39. Shintaku M 1996 Lipoleiomyomatous tumors of the uterus: a heterogeneous group? Histopathological study of five cases. Pathol Int 46: 498–502
40. Hu J, Surti U, Tobon H 1992 Cytogenetic analysis of a uterine lipoleiomyoma. Cancer Genet Cytogenet 62: 200–202
41. Pedeutour F, Quade B J, Sornberger K et al. 2000 Dysregulation of HMGIC in a uterine lipoleiomyoma with a complex rearrangement including chromosomes 7, 12, and 14. Genes Chromos Cancer 27: 209–215
42. Hsieh C H, Lui C C, Huang S C et al. 2003 Multiple uterine angioleiomyomas in a woman presenting with severe menorrhagia. Gynecol Oncol 90: 348–352
43. Ferry J A, Harris N L, Scully R E 1989 Uterine leiomyomas with lymphoid infiltration simulating lymphoma. A report of seven cases. Int J Gynecol Pathol 8: 263–270
44. Bardsley V, Cooper P, Peat D S 1998 Massive lymphocytic infiltration of uterine leiomyomas associated with GnRH agonist treatment. Histopathology 33: 80–82
45. McClean G, McCluggage W G 2003 Unusual morphologic features of uterine leiomyomas treated with gonadotropin-releasing hormone agonists: massive lymphoid infiltration and vasculitis. Int J Surg Pathol 11: 339–344
46. Vang R, Medeiros L J, Samoszuk M et al. 2001 Uterine leiomyomas with eosinophils: a clinicopathologic study of 3 cases. Int J Gynecol Pathol 20: 239–243
47. Maluf H M, Gersell D J 1994 Uterine leiomyomas with high content of mast cells. Arch Pathol Lab Med 118: 712–714
48. Orii A, Mori A, Zhai Y L et al. 1998 Mast cells in smooth muscle tumors of the uterus. Int J Gynecol Pathol 17: 336–342
49. Adany R, Fodor F, Molnar P et al. 1990 Increased density of histiocytes in uterine leiomyomas. Int J Gynecol Pathol 9: 137–144
50. Gisser S D, Young I 1977 Neurilemoma-like uterine myomas: an ultrastructural reaffirmation of their non-Schwannian nature. Am J Obstet Gynecol 129: 389–392
51. Evans H L, Chawla S P, Simpson C et al. 1988 Smooth muscle neoplasms of the uterus other than ordinary leiomyoma. A study of 46 cases, with emphasis on diagnostic criteria and prognostic factors. Cancer 62: 2239–2247

52. Gilks C B, Clement P B, Hart W R et al. 2000 Uterine adenomyomas excluding atypical polypoid adenomyomas and adenomyomas of endocervical type: a clinicopathologic study of 30 cases of an underemphasized lesion that may cause diagnostic problems with brief consideration of adenomyomas of other female genital tract sites. Int J Gynecol Pathol 19: 195–205
53. Nogales F F, Isaac M A, Hardisson D et al. 2002 Adenomatoid tumors of the uterus: an analysis of 60 cases. Int J Gynecol Pathol 21: 34–40
54. Palacios J, Suarez M A, Ruiz V A et al. 1991 Cystic adenomatoid tumor of the uterus. Int J Gynecol Pathol 10: 296–301
55. De Rosa G, Boscaino A, Terracciano L M et al. 1992 Giant adenomatoid tumors of the uterus. Int J Gynecol Pathol 11: 156–160
56. Schwartz E J, Longacre T A 2004 Adenomatoid tumors of the female and male genital tracts express WT1. Int J Gynecol Pathol 23: 123–128
57. Friedrich M, Villena-Heinsen C, Mink D et al. 1998 Leiomyosarcomas of the female genital tract: a clinical and histopathological study. Eur J Gynaecol Oncol 19: 470–475
58. Harlow B L, Weiss N S, Lofton S 1986 The epidemiology of sarcomas of the uterus. J Natl Cancer Inst 76: 399–402
59. Leibsohn S, D'ablaing G, Mishell D R Jr et al. 1990 Leiomyosarcoma in a series of hysterectomies performed for presumed uterine leiomyomas. Am J Obstet Gynecol 162: 968–974
60. Brooks S E, Zhan M, Cote T et al. 2004 Surveillance, epidemiology, and end results analysis of 2677 cases of uterine sarcoma 1989–1999. Gynecol Oncol 93: 204–208
61. Mayerhofer K, Obermair A, Windbichler G et al. 1999 Leiomyosarcoma of the uterus: a clinicopathologic multicenter study of 71 cases. Gynecol Oncol 74: 196–201
62. Hsieh C H, Lin H, Huang C C et al. 2003 Leiomyosarcoma of the uterus: a clinicopathologic study of 21 cases. Acta Obstet Gynecol Scand 82: 74–81
63. Giuntoli R L, Metzinger D S, DiMarco C S et al. 2003 Retrospective review of 208 patients with leiomyosarcoma of the uterus: prognostic indicators, surgical management, and adjuvant therapy. Gynecol Oncol 89: 460–469
64. Dinh T A, Oliva E A, Fuller A F Jr et al. 2004 The treatment of uterine leiomyosarcoma. Results from a 10-year experience (1990–1999) at the Massachusetts General Hospital. Gynecol Oncol 92: 648–652
65. Leitao M M, Sonoda Y, Brennan M F et al. 2003 Incidence of lymph node and ovarian metastases in leiomyosarcoma of the uterus. Gynecol Oncol 91: 209–212
66. Goff B A, Rice L W, Fleischhacker D et al. 1993 Uterine leiomyosarcoma and endometrial stromal sarcoma: lymph node metastases and sites of recurrence. Gynecol Oncol 50: 105–109
67. Kahanpaa K V, Wahlstrom T, Grohn P et al. 1986 Sarcomas of the uterus: a clinicopathologic study of 119 patients. Obstet Gynecol 67: 417–424
68. Nordal R R, Thoresen S O 1997 Uterine sarcomas in Norway 1956–1992: incidence, survival and mortality. Eur J Cancer 33: 907–911
69. Chauveinc L, Deniaud E, Plancher C et al. 1999 Uterine sarcomas: the Curie Institut experience. Prognosis factors and adjuvant treatments. Gynecol Oncol 72: 232–237
70. Larson B, Silfversward C, Nilsson B et al. 1990 Prognostic factors in uterine leiomyosarcoma. A clinical and histopathological study of 143 cases. The Radiumhemmet series 1936–1981. Acta Oncol 29: 185–191
71. Gadducci A, Sartori E, Landoni F et al. 2002 The prognostic relevance of histological type in uterine sarcomas: a Cooperation Task Force (CTF) multivariate analysis of 249 cases. Eur J Gynaecol Oncol 23: 295–299
72. Bodner K, Bodner-Adler B, Kimberger O et al. 2003 Evaluating prognostic parameters in women with uterine leiomyosarcoma. A clinicopathologic study. J Reprod Med 48: 95–100
73. Pautier P, Genestie C, Rey A et al. 2000 Analysis of clinicopathologic prognostic factors for 157 uterine sarcomas and evaluation of a grading score validated for soft tissue sarcoma. Cancer 88: 1425–1431
74. Fletcher J A, Morton C C, Pavelka K et al. 1990 Chromosome aberrations in uterine smooth muscle tumors: potential diagnostic relevance of cytogenetic instability. Cancer Res 50: 4092–4097
75. Nilbert M, Mandahl N, Heim S et al. 1990 Complex karyotypic changes, including rearrangements of 12q13 and 14q24, in two leiomyosarcomas. Cancer Genet Cytogenet 48: 217–223
76. Sreekantaiah C, Davis J R, Sandberg A A 1993 Chromosomal abnormalities in leiomyosarcomas. Am J Pathol 142: 293–305
77. Quade B J, Pinto A P, Howard D R et al. 1999 Frequent loss of heterozygosity for chromosome 10 in uterine leiomyosarcoma in contrast to leiomyoma. Am J Pathol 154: 945–950
78. Quade B J, Wang T Y, Sornberger K et al. 2004 Molecular pathogenesis of uterine smooth muscle tumors from transcriptional profiling. Genes Chromos Cancer 40: 97–108
79. King M E, Dickersin G R, Scully R E 1982 Myxoid leiomyosarcoma of the uterus. A report of six cases. Am J Surg Pathol 6: 589–598
80. Kunzel K E, Mills N Z, Muderspach L I et al. 1993 Myxoid leiomyosarcoma of the uterus. Gynecol Oncol 48: 277–280
81. Chang E, Shim S I 1998 Myxoid leiomyosarcoma of the uterus: a case report and review of the literature. J Korean Med Sci 13: 559–562
82. Vigone A, Giana M, Surico D et al. 2005 Massive myxoid leiomyosarcoma of the uterus. Int J Gynecol Cancer 15: 564–567
83. Norris H J, Parmley T 1975 Mesenchymal tumors of the uterus. V. Intravenous leiomyomatosis. A clinical and pathologic study of 14 cases. Cancer 36: 2164–2178
84. Clement P B, Young R H, Scully R E 1988 Intravenous leiomyomatosis of the uterus. A clinicopathological analysis of 16 cases with unusual histologic features. Am J Surg Pathol 12: 932–945
85. Mulvany N J, Slavin J L, Ostor A G et al. 1994 Intravenous leiomyomatosis of the uterus: a clinicopathologic study of 22 cases. Int J Gynecol Pathol 13: 1–9
86. Dal Cin P, Quade B J, Neskey D M et al. 2003 Intravenous leiomyomatosis is characterized by a der(14)t(12;14)(q15;q24). Genes Chromos Cancer 36: 205–206
87. Tavassoli F A, Norris H J 1982 Peritoneal leiomyomatosis (leiomyomatosis peritonealis disseminata): a clinicopathologic study of 20 cases with ultrastructural observations. Int J Gynecol Pathol 1: 59–74
88. Valente P T 1984 Leiomyomatosis peritonealis disseminata. A report of two cases and review of the literature. Arch Pathol Lab Med 108: 669–672
89. Hardman W J III, Majmudar B 1996 Leiomyomatosis peritonealis disseminata: clinicopathologic analysis of five cases. South Med J 89: 291–294
90. Quade B J, McLachlin C M, Soto-Wright V et al. 1997 Disseminated peritoneal leiomyomatosis. Clonality analysis by X chromosome inactivation and cytogenetics of a clinically benign smooth muscle proliferation. Am J Pathol 150: 2153–2166
91. Clement P B, Young R H 1987 Diffuse leiomyomatosis of the uterus: a report of four cases. Int J Gynecol Pathol 6: 322–330
92. Mulvany N J, Ostor A G, Ross I 1995 Diffuse leiomyomatosis of the uterus. Histopathology 27: 175–179
93. Baschinsky D Y, Isa A, Niemann T H et al. 2000 Diffuse leiomyomatosis of the uterus: a case report with clonality analysis. Hum Pathol 31: 1429–1432
94. Abell M R, Littler E R 1975 Benign metastasizing uterine leiomyoma. Multiple lymph nodal metastases. Cancer 36: 2206–2213
95. Wolff M, Silva F, Kaye G 1979 Pulmonary metastases (with admixed epithelial elements) from smooth muscle neoplasms. Report of nine cases, including three males. Am J Surg Pathol 3: 325–342
96. Gal A A, Brooks J S, Pietra G G 1989 Leiomyomatous neoplasms of the lung: a clinical, histologic, and immunohistochemical study. Mod Pathol 2: 209–216
97. Esteban J M, Allen W M, Schaerf R H 1999 Benign metastasizing leiomyoma of the uterus: histologic and immunohistochemical characterization of primary and metastatic lesions. Arch Pathol Lab Med 123: 960–962
98. Ordi J, Stamatakos M D, Tavassoli F A 1997 Pure pleomorphic rhabdomyosarcomas of the uterus. Int J Gynecol Pathol 16: 369–377
99. Chiarle R, Godio L, Fusi D et al. 1997 Pure alveolar rhabdomyosarcoma of the corpus uteri: description of a case with increased serum level of CA-125. Gynecol Oncol 66: 320–323
100. McCluggage W G, Lioe T F, McClelland H R et al. 2002 Rhabdomyosarcoma of the uterus: report of two cases, including one of the spindle cell variant. Int J Gynecol Cancer 12: 128–132
101. Vang R, Kempson R L 2002 Perivascular epithelioid cell tumor ('PEComa') of the uterus: a subset of HMB-45-positive epithelioid mesenchymal neoplasms with an uncertain relationship to pure smooth muscle tumors. Am J Surg Pathol 26: 1–13
102. Silva E G, Deavers M T, Bodurka D C et al. 2004 Uterine epithelioid leiomyosarcomas with clear cells: reactivity with HMB-45 and the concept of PEComa. Am J Surg Pathol 28: 244–249
103. Greene L A, Mount S L, Schned A R et al. 2003 Recurrent perivascular epithelioid cell tumor of the uterus (PEComa): an immunohistochemical study and review of the literature. Gynecol Oncol 90: 677–681
104. Dimmler A, Seitz G, Hohenberger W et al. 2003 Late pulmonary metastasis in uterine PEComa. J Clin Pathol 56: 627–628

第五部分

宫颈　Cervix

Marisa R. Nucci, Kenneth R. Lee 和 Christopher P. Crum 著
回允中　韩桂萍　译

宫颈			
癌前疾病	697	神经内分泌癌	710
浸润性鳞状细胞癌	702	混合性上皮和间叶性肿瘤	711
浸润性腺癌	704	间叶性肿瘤	713
混合类型癌	709	黑色素细胞肿瘤	714
		其他罕见肿瘤	715

引言　Introduction

这一部分涵盖了发生于宫颈移行区或其附近的一系列宫颈肿瘤性病变。它被分为癌前上皮内肿瘤形成、上皮恶性肿瘤（包括鳞状上皮肿瘤、腺上皮肿瘤、混合类型癌和神经内分泌癌）、混合性上皮和间叶性肿瘤、间叶性肿瘤、黑色素细胞肿瘤和其他罕见的恶性肿瘤。

癌前疾病　Precancerous disease

鳞状上皮内肿瘤形成（鳞状上皮内病变；宫颈上皮内肿瘤形成）
Squamous intraepithelial neoplasia [Squamous intraepithelial lesions; Cervical intraepithelial neoplasia (CIN)]

引言

宫颈鳞状上皮内肿瘤形成指的是发生于移行区或其附近的，与人乳头状瘤病毒（HPV）有关的所有鳞状上皮改变，因此包括的术语有湿疣、CIN、异型增生（dysplasia）和鳞状上皮内病变。因为越来越明显地认识到，HPV 感染可以导致一系列鳞状上皮形态学改变，所以所有这些疾病均可以出现在鳞状上皮内病变的单一分类系统内。在这个分类系统中，低级别鳞状上皮内病变包括扁平和外生性、不成熟性和成熟性湿疣，以及在 CIN 分类方案中的 CIN1 病变。高级别鳞状上皮内病变相当于 CIN 2 和 CIN 3。

临床特征

鳞状上皮内肿瘤形成可以见于性活动开始后的任何年龄。现在已经明确，HPV 感染与宫颈肿瘤形成具有因果关系，包括浸润前和浸润性疾病。年轻人 HPV 感染普遍存在，在这个年龄组中，性活跃的妇女感染频率最高；感染通常是短暂的，没有任何相关的形态学改变，但是单一类型 HPV 的持续性感染却与宫颈肿瘤形成密切相关，不是同时发生就是随后发生[1-5]。已知生殖道 HPV 感染有许多类型，特别是宫颈，根据其与浸润性宫颈癌的关系分为低度危险和高度危险两组。HPV6 和 HPV11 是低度危险病毒的标准类型，因为它们与宫颈癌或高级别鳞状上皮癌前病变无关。相反，HPV16 被认为是高度危险性病毒，因为这种病毒与 50% 的浸润性鳞状细胞癌和高级别鳞状上皮癌前病变有关[6]。除了 HPV 感染之外，宫颈鳞状上皮内肿瘤形成的其他危险因素包括：（1）年龄（年轻、性活跃的妇女处于浸润前宫颈疾病最大的危险之中）；（2）免疫缺陷，例如人类免疫缺陷病毒（HIV）感染或治疗性免疫抑制；（3）吸烟[7-13]。

鳞状上皮内病变，低级别
Squamous intraepithelial lesion, low-grade

低级别鳞状上皮内病变可以分为 3 种形态学亚型：（1）尖锐湿疣（外生性湿疣）；（2）不成熟性湿疣（鳞状上皮乳头状瘤、乳头状不成熟性化生）；（3）扁平湿疣（CIN1）。**外生性湿疣**（exophytic condyloma）（图 13E.1）的特征是呈疣状生长，伴有粗钝的乳头、棘层增厚以及浅表挖空细胞非典型性（核深染，核大，双核形成，核的轮廓不规则）。这些外生性病变与 HPV6 和 HPV11 密切相关，在宫颈相对少见。**不成熟性湿疣**（immature condyloma）（图 13E.2）的特征是纤细的丝状乳头，被覆几乎不显示角化细胞成熟的鳞状上皮（酷似鳞状化生），但是显示轻度的细胞核密集和浅表挖空细胞轻度非典型性。这种不成熟性湿疣相对缺乏挖空细胞非典型性，很可能是反映了病毒细胞病变效应依赖于成

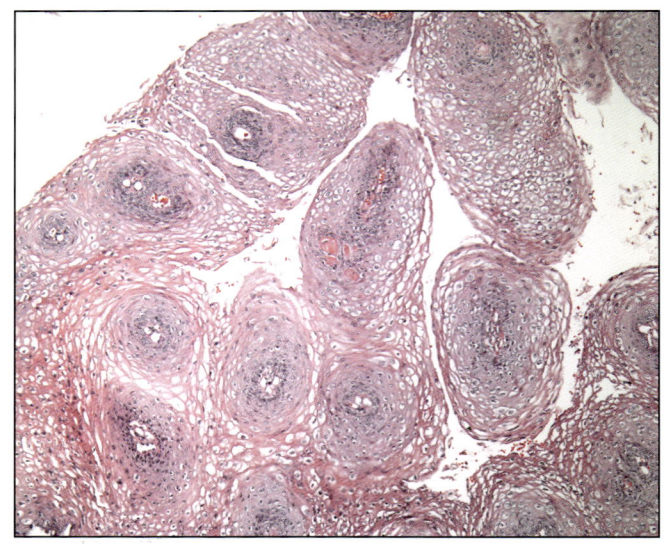

图13E.1　外生性湿疣。疣状生长方式伴有浅表挖空细胞非典型性。

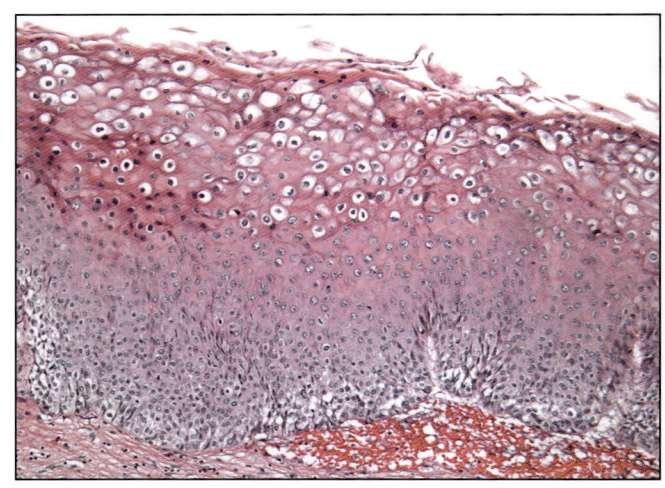

图13E.3　扁平湿疣。非典型性挖空细胞局限于上皮的上部。

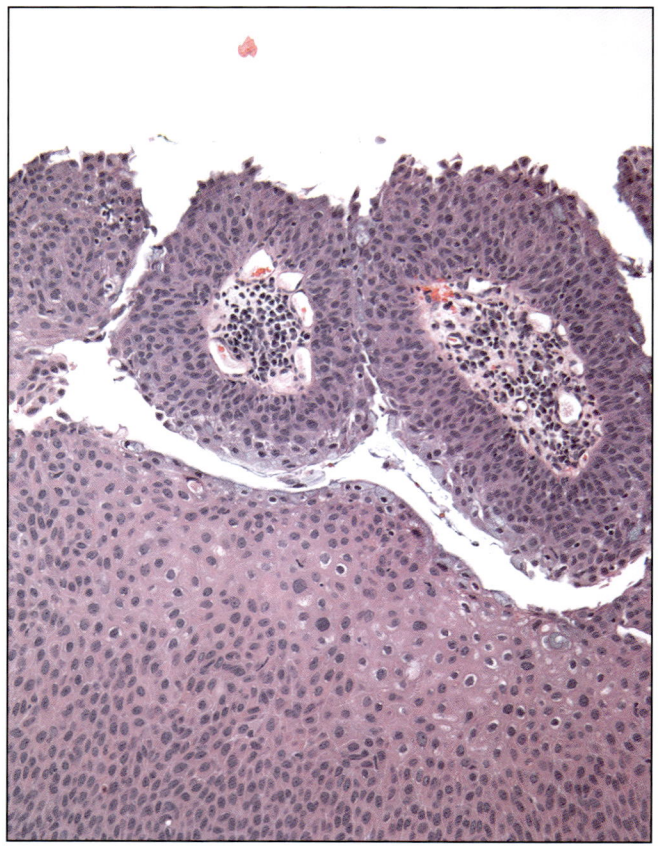

图13E.2　不成熟性湿疣。纤细的丝状乳头伴有浅表细胞轻度非典型性。

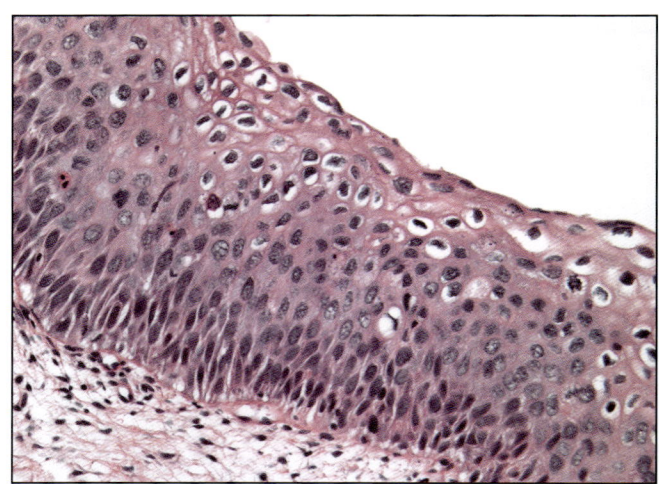

图13E.4　高级别鳞状上皮内病变（CIN 2）。注意表面挖空细胞改变。

熟，而这些病变的成熟是有限的。与外生性湿疣相似，不成熟性湿疣含有HPV6和11，支持将其包含在湿疣范畴内。乳头状不成熟性化生和鳞状上皮乳头状瘤的组织学表现与不成熟性湿疣相同，同样含有HPV6和11，因此，它们也包括在这个范畴内[14,15]。**扁平湿疣**（flat condyloma）的形态学特征类似于尖锐湿疣，但是缺乏外生性的生长方式（图13E.3）。非典型性挖空细胞的数量可能不同；然而，非典型性局限于上皮的上1/3，伴有基底细胞和副基底细胞核轻微的非典型性。这些病变通常与中度危险的HPV有关[6]。细胞增生标志物的表达，例如Ki-67，可能有助于将低级别鳞状上皮内病变与困难病例的反应性增生区分开来（主要的鉴别诊断），因为上层细胞阳性是HPV感染的上皮的特征，而正常黏膜这个标志物一般局限于下层[16-18]。

鳞状上皮内病变，高级别
Squamous intraepithelial lesion, high-grade

高级别鳞状上皮内病变的特征是上皮全层细胞核的非典型性，伴有不同程度的表面成熟。出现表面挖空细胞改变和上皮成熟的病变相当于CIN 2（图13E.4），而几乎没有成熟的那些病变相当于CIN 3（图13E.5）。这些病变与低级别鳞状上皮内病变的区别是：（1）上皮下

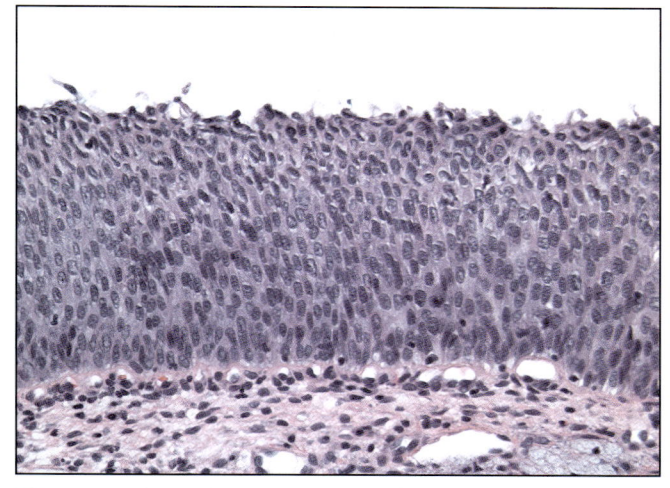

图13E.5 高级别鳞状上皮内病变（CIN 3）。全层细胞核非典型性，伴有轻微成熟。

层出现核的非典型性；（2）核分裂指数增加，上皮上半部分出现核分裂象；（3）细胞极性丧失；（4）异常核分裂象；以及在某些病例，（5）出现明显的非典型性奇异细胞。这些病变与高危险性 HPV 有关，特别是 HPV16。p16^{ink4} 是一种依赖细胞周期蛋白激酶抑制剂，似乎可以作为 HPV 感染的替代标志物，在中度和高度危险性 HPV 相关性病变有强烈表达。因为中度和高度危险性 HPV 与低级别和高级别鳞状上皮内病变均有关系，所以这个标志物不能将两者区分开来；然而，对于支持鳞状上皮内病变的诊断 p16^{ink4} 染色可能有用[19]。

腺上皮内肿瘤形成
Glandular intraepithelial neoplasia

引言

现在普遍认为，原位腺癌是多数浸润性宫颈腺癌的前体病变。这个结论的根据是：（1）原位癌和浸润癌的细胞形态学表现相似；（2）原位癌和早期浸润性腺癌的发生部位密切相关[20-22]；（3）伴随高危险性 HPV 类型的频率类似（主要是 HPV 16 和 18）[23]；（4）原位腺癌诊断时的平均年龄早于浸润性腺癌[22]；（5）从原位癌进展到浸润性腺癌的病例已有少数报告[24-27]。

临床特征

原位腺癌一般发生于生育年龄的年轻妇女，诊断时的平均年龄为 38 岁[22]。由于伴随的症状非常少见（如果存在，最常见的是异常阴道出血[28,29]），经由常规巴氏涂片检查通常可以辨认原位腺癌，要不然就是在组织取样时发现的，最常见的是处理鳞状上皮前体病变，或在随访的涂片中发现非典型性腺上皮细胞。与鳞状上皮前体病变不同，巴氏涂片检查对于检测原位腺癌和浸润性腺癌均不敏感，这或许与宫颈内膜取样不完全以及在细胞学涂片中鉴别良性和肿瘤性腺上皮困难有关[30-32]。因为患有原位腺癌的妇女多半年轻并且希望保留其生育能力，所以要是不切除子宫的话，最广泛推荐的治疗是宫颈锥形切除术。选择保守治疗的病人需要进行密切的临床随访，因为伴有清楚边缘的锥形活检并不能保证避免原位或浸润性癌的复发[33-42]。

病理学特征

原位腺癌几乎总是发生在鳞柱交界处（移行区），从部位上讲是一个连续的病变，但是在极少数情况下它可以发生在宫颈内膜的较上部分或为多灶性[43,44]。病变的范围可以不同，从局灶性到弥漫性累及宫颈一圈；偶尔可能延伸到子宫下段和子宫腔。30%～50% 的原位腺癌病例伴有鳞状上皮内病变[42,43,45]。组织学检查，宫颈腺体正常结构保留，内衬细胞密集，核大，深染，复层或假复层（图 13E.6）；在一个腺体内从正常到肿瘤的突然转化是其特征。核仁通常小而不明显，但是偶尔可以突出。出现核分裂象对于诊断是必需的，核分裂象通常位于腔面，具有"悬浮"的现象。基底部常见凋亡小体，见于多达 70% 的病例[46,47]。原位腺癌有时可能具有比较复杂的生长方式，伴有腔内乳头状内折或筛状结构（图 13E.7）；然而，总的良性腺体结构是保留的。

可能出现许多组织学亚型[33,43,48-50]，而且在一个病例中常常混合存在。虽然各种亚型的生物学行为或进展没有差异，但是了解原位腺癌的形态学差异对于诊断是重要的。

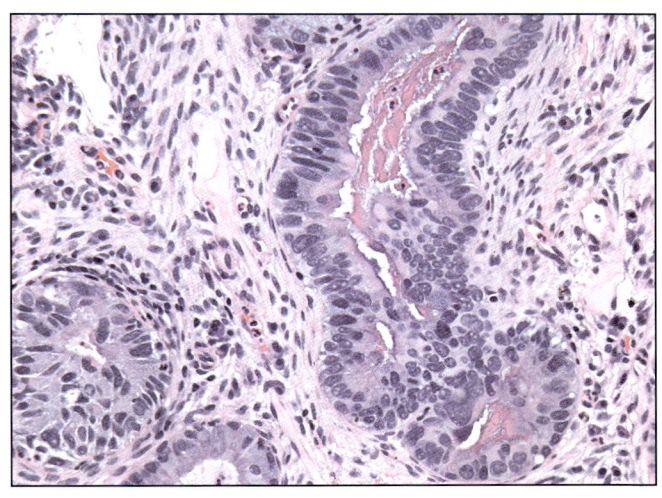

图13E.6 原位腺癌。核密集，增大，深染。

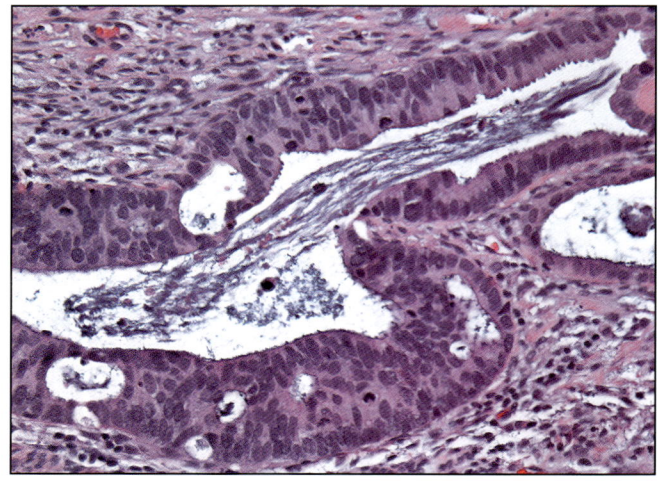

图13E.7 原位腺癌。注意复杂的筛状生长方式。

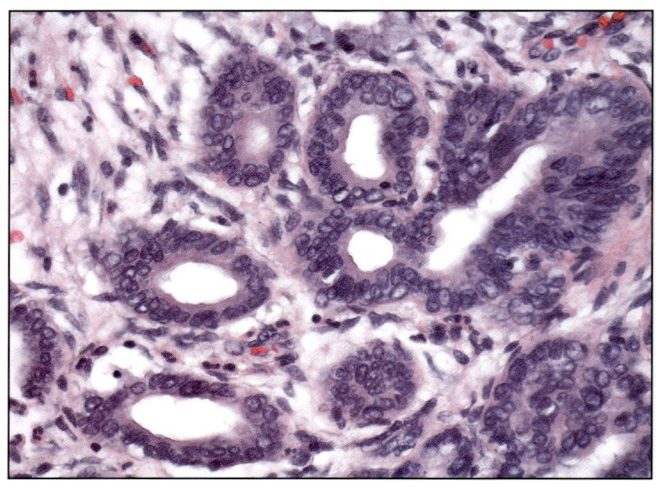

图13E.9 原位腺癌，子宫内膜样型。胞浆不丰富，类似于子宫内膜样腺体。

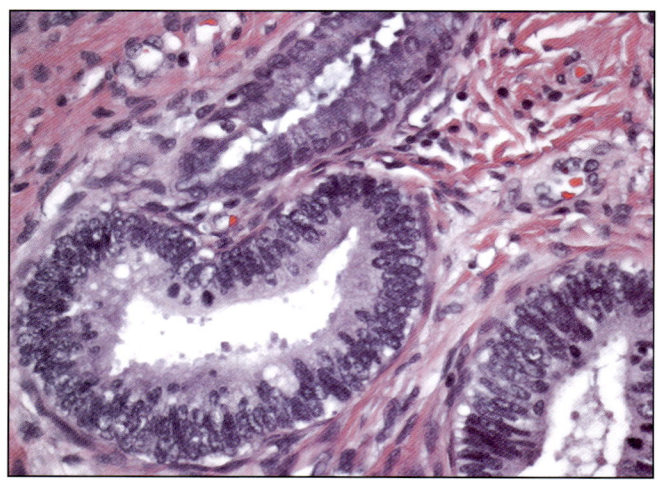

图13E.8 原位腺癌，宫颈内膜型。典型的黏液性胞浆酷似正常宫颈内膜分化的表现。

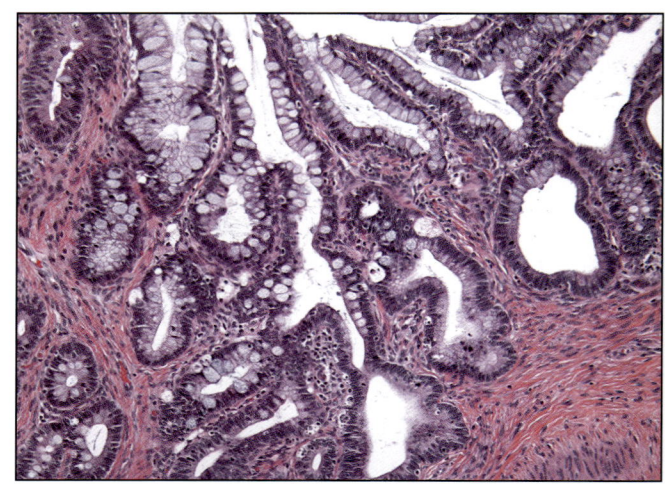

图13E.10 原位腺癌，肠型。注意肠型杯状细胞。

宫颈内膜型 (endocervical) 这种亚型最常见，其表现非常类似于具有柱状黏液性胞浆的宫颈内膜细胞（图13E.8）。

子宫内膜样型 (endometrioid) 这种亚型胞浆较少，细胞核较大，呈复层表现，类似于肿瘤性子宫内膜样腺体（图13E.9）。

肠型 (intestinal) 这种亚型常常没有显著的核密集和核深染，含有不同比例的肠型杯状细胞（图13E.10）。出现杯状细胞强烈提示病变可能为肿瘤，因为宫颈良性杯状细胞化生非常少见。

复层/鳞状黏液型 (stratified/squamomucinous) 复层肿瘤细胞呈现腺上皮和鳞状上皮两者的特征，是这种独特的原位腺癌亚型的特点。与高级别鳞状上皮内病变类似，肿瘤细胞为复层；然而，它们还含有黏液，表现为散在的胞浆空泡或特征性的"蜂窝状"结构（图13E.11）。

纤毛型 (ciliated) 这种罕见亚型的特征是纤毛细胞伴有显著的细胞非典型性和核分裂活性。它几乎总是伴有比较典型的宫颈内膜原位腺癌，这有助于其诊断并与良性输卵管化生鉴别。

原位腺癌与其最常见的良性类似病变的比较列在表13E.1中。

早期浸润性鳞状细胞癌
Early invasive squamous cell carcinoma

早期浸润性鳞状细胞癌（IA期）的定义是深度≤3mm，长度≤7mm，没有毛细淋巴管浸润，而且与较高分期的肿瘤病人不同，IA期浸润性鳞状细胞癌的病人可以保守治疗（仅仅切除）而不进行淋巴结清扫。早

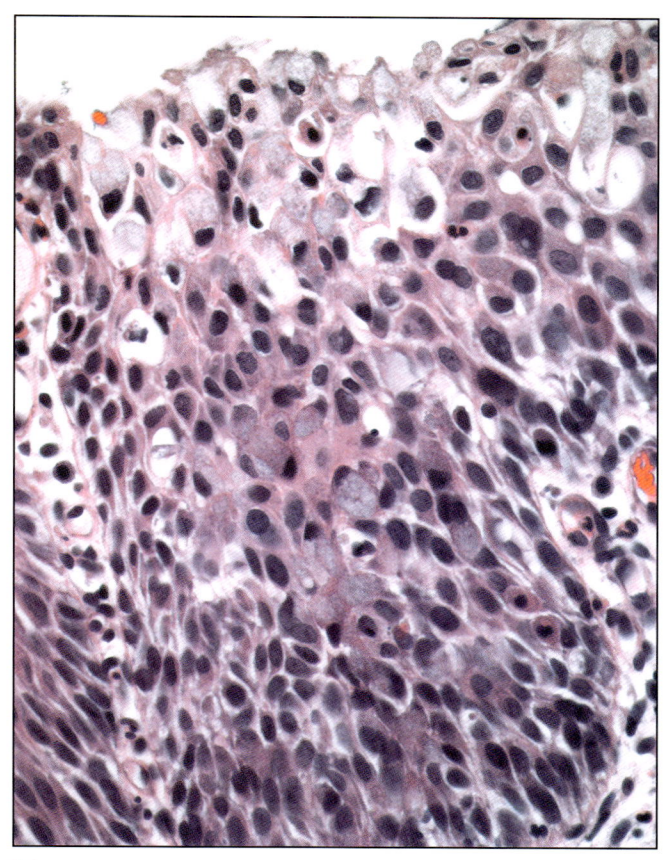

图13E.11 原位腺癌，鳞状黏液（复层）型。复层肿瘤细胞含有胞浆内黏液。

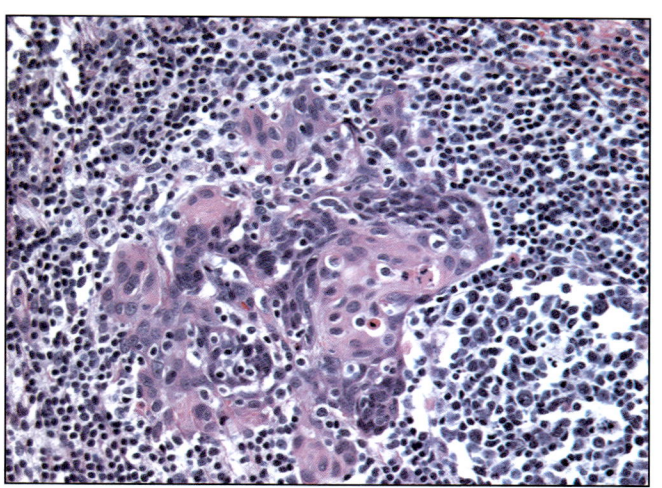

图13E.12 早期浸润性鳞状细胞癌。注意上皮间质交界模糊，极性丧失和显著的成熟。

期间质浸润是指肿瘤细胞破坏基底膜，而且有 < 3mm 的间质浸润，评估早期间质浸润是困难的。诊断早期浸润最常用的标准是：（1）邻近的间质有纤维组织增生性反应；（2）肿瘤性鳞状上皮有局灶性的显著的成熟；（3）上皮间质交界模糊；（4）在上皮间质交界部位核的极性丧失（图13E.12）。早期间质浸润最重要的类似病变包括：（1）正切的由高级别鳞状上皮内病变累及的宫颈内膜腺体；（2）从前活检的部位，可能伴有上皮移位和炎症反应；（3）继发于挤压或烧灼的人工变化；（4）对于高级别鳞状上皮内病变显著的炎症性反应造成上皮间质交界面不清；（5）错误解释宫颈胎盘种植部位。

表13E.1	原位腺癌（ACIS）与其类似病变的比较					
	ACIS	输卵管/输卵管子宫内膜样化生	子宫内膜异位症	Arias-Stella反应	放射影响	宫颈炎
部位	移行区；表面或深部腺体	通常在宫颈管上部；深度>浅表腺体	浅表或深部腺体	浅表>深部腺体；通常局灶	浅表或深部腺体	移行区
部分腺体受累	特征性	偶尔	少见	特征性	少见	少见
核复层	存在	不明显	存在	存在	缺乏	不明显
核深染	存在	不明显	存在	存在	存在	不明显
核增大	存在	不明显	不常见	存在	存在	存在
核仁	罕见	可能存在	可能存在	存在	存在	存在
核分裂活性	存在	不常见	存在	罕见	罕见	存在
凋亡	存在	罕见/缺乏	不常见	缺乏	缺乏	可能存在
纤毛	可能存在	存在	偶尔	缺乏	缺乏	缺乏
结构复杂	可能存在	缺乏	不常见	不常见	缺乏	缺乏
Mib-1增生指数	高	低	不定	低	低	不定

浸润性鳞状细胞癌
Invasive squamous cell carcinoma

在全世界范围内，宫颈癌是女性生殖道最常见的恶性肿瘤，而且是继乳腺癌后第二个最常见的女性恶性肿瘤（除了皮肤癌）[51]。在美国，宫颈癌少见得多，是位于子宫体和卵巢癌症之后第三个最常见的女性生殖道恶性肿瘤[52]。在全世界范围内，每年大约有 470 000 例宫颈癌，233 000 例死于本病，而在美国，每年大约有 13 000 例宫颈癌新病例，4800 例死亡[51,52]。总的来说，在过去几十年中，发达国家宫颈鳞状细胞癌的发病率在下降，部分原因好像是由于宫颈癌的普查[53]。从前认为宫颈癌是老年人的疾病，但是现在常见于 20～40 岁的病人。通过大量的实验、分子学和临床资料，现在已经明确宫颈浸润性鳞状细胞癌的发生与 HPV 感染具有因果关系。大约已从生殖道中分离出了 25 种不同类型的 HPV，其发生癌的危险性不同，HPV16 具有最大危险性。

宫颈浸润性鳞状细胞癌病人最常见的表现是异常阴道出血或异常巴氏涂片[54]。表现为异常巴氏涂片的病人（与有临床症状的病人相比，例如阴道出血或排液）可能有较好的预后，推测是发现较早的结果。早期浸润性肿瘤，在临床检查时可能仅仅表现为类似于高级别宫颈癌前病变的变化；较晚期的肿瘤可以是息肉状、蕈状，或引起宫颈弥漫性增大。浸润性鳞状细胞癌有许多组织学亚型。

角化型癌 (keratinizing) 这种类型的肿瘤具有突出的角化证据，表现为角化珠、角化透明颗粒、单个角化细胞以及伴有中心角化的鳞状细胞巢（图 13E.13）。这些肿瘤通常被归入高分化肿瘤，边缘浸润常呈推挤状。

大细胞非角化型癌 (large cell non-keratinizing) 组织学上这个肿瘤是由可以辨认的鳞状细胞组成的，细胞大，呈多角形，胞浆嗜酸性，可见细胞间桥，但是缺乏角化珠结构、角化透明颗粒或伴有中心角化的鳞状细胞巢（图 13E.14）。常常出现显著的细胞核多形性和伴有炎症的浸润性边缘，多数肿瘤通常被归入中分化肿瘤。

小细胞（低分化）非角化型癌 [small cell (poorly differentiated) non-keratinizing] 这种类型的肿瘤是由核浆比例高的肿瘤细胞构成的，组织学检查可见轻微的可以辨认的鳞状分化的证据（图 13E.15）。这些肿瘤一般被归入低分化肿瘤。在常规工作中不主张应用小细胞这一术语（代之以将其归入低分化非角化性鳞状细胞

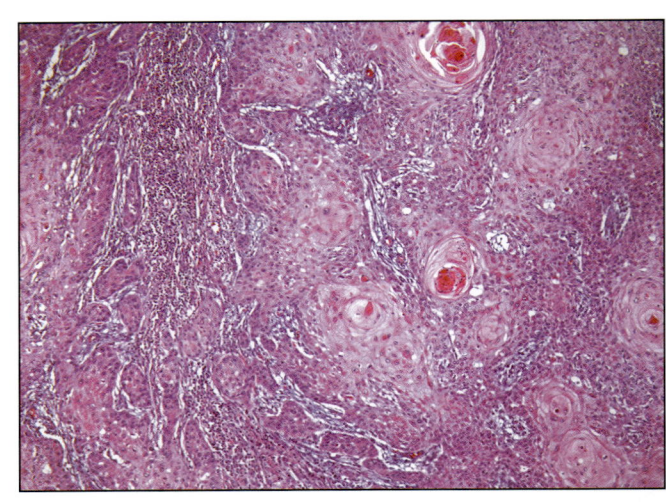

图13E.13 浸润性鳞状细胞癌，角化型。明显的角化珠和伴有中心角化的肿瘤细胞巢。

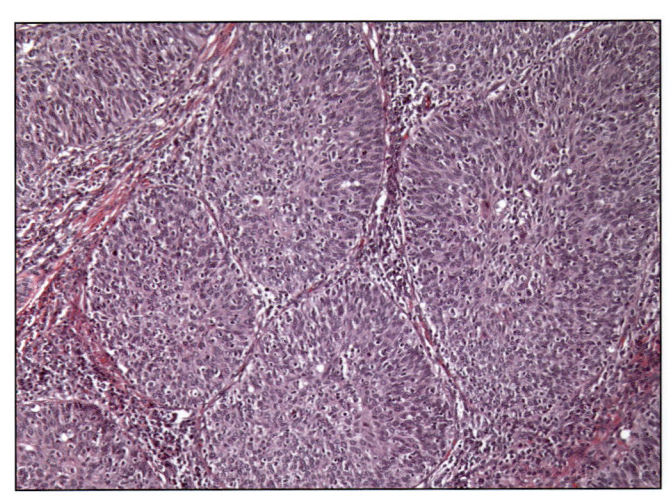

图13E.14 浸润性鳞状细胞癌，大细胞非角化型。缺乏显著的角化珠或中心角化的肿瘤细胞巢。

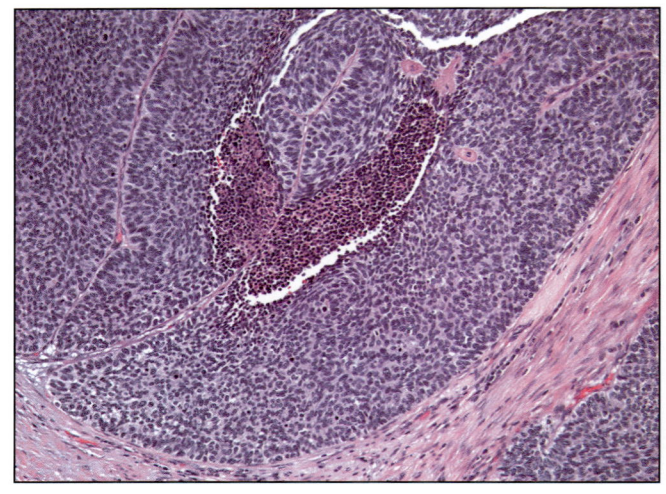

图13E.15 浸润性鳞状细胞癌，小细胞非角化型。轻微的可以辨认的鳞状分化。

癌），以防止与小细胞神经内分泌肿瘤混淆。

基底细胞样癌（basaloid） 某些浸润性鳞状细胞癌具有基底细胞样表现，肿瘤细胞巢有少量嗜酸性胞浆，周围的细胞核呈栅栏状排列，而且有不同程度的鳞状分化（图 13E.16）。这种类型的肿瘤应该诊断为浸润性鳞状细胞癌伴有基底细胞样特征，以免与腺样基底细胞癌混淆。

疣状癌（verrucous） 宫颈癌的这种亚型非常罕见，其特征为外生性，由被覆鳞状上皮的宽基底乳头组成，细胞几乎没有非典型性（图 13E.17）。这些肿瘤显示推挤性浸润边缘，上皮-间质交界均匀一致。必须严格应用诊断标准，诊断这些肿瘤应该小心（为了避免低诊断高分化鳞状细胞癌，高分化鳞状细胞癌与疣状癌不同，前者伴有局部淋巴结转移的危险）[55]。

湿疣性癌 [warty (condylomatous)]：这种亚型指的是具有 HPV 感染特征性表面上皮挖空细胞改变的外生性鳞状细胞癌。

乳头状癌（papillary） 宫颈乳头状癌的特征是乳头状生长方式，可以再分为三种组织学类型[56]：（1）乳头状未分化癌，被覆乳头的肿瘤细胞没有任何特殊类型分化的组织学证据；（2）乳头状移行细胞癌，与发生在泌尿道的病变具有类似的组织学表现；（3）乳头状鳞状移行细胞癌，它具有移行细胞和鳞状细胞两种特征（图 13E.18）。组织学区分后两种类型的临床重要性尚不清楚。

淋巴上皮样癌（lymphoepithelial-like） 这种亚型是由境界不清楚的非角化性肿瘤细胞聚集而成的，核大呈空泡状，核仁突出，胞浆嗜酸性，中等量，细胞边界不清楚，具有合体细胞的表现。肿瘤细胞的特征是混有许多淋巴细胞，形态类似于鼻咽部淋巴上皮样癌，这个术

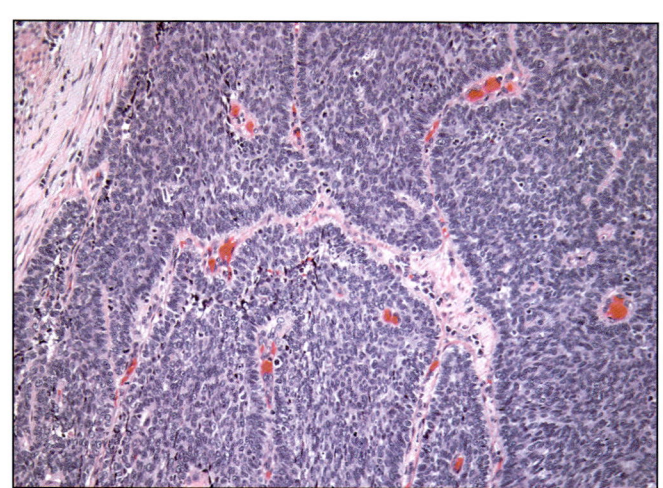

图13E.16 浸润性鳞状细胞癌，基底细胞样型。注意周围细胞核呈栅栏状排列。

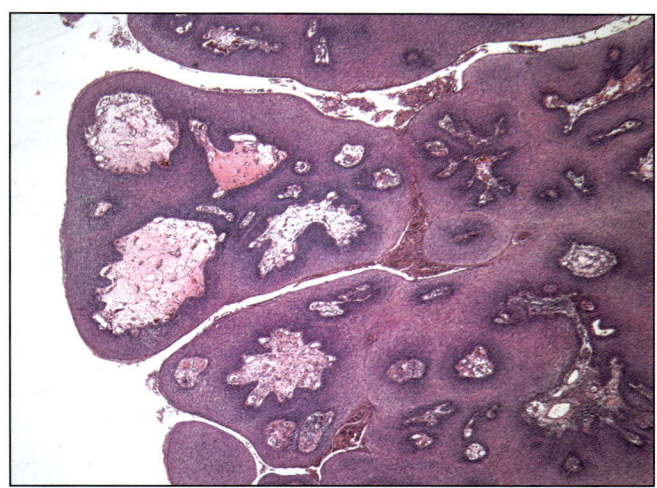

图13E.17 疣状癌。由宽基底乳头构成的外生性肿瘤，伴有轻度细胞学非典型性。

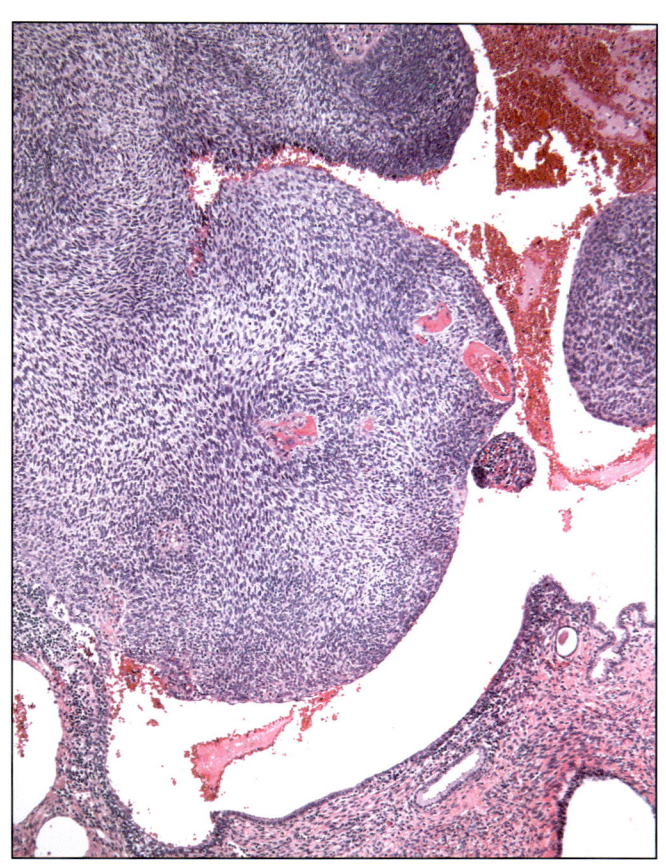

图13E.18 乳头状鳞状移行细胞癌。外生性乳头被覆兼有鳞状和移行细胞特征的肿瘤细胞。

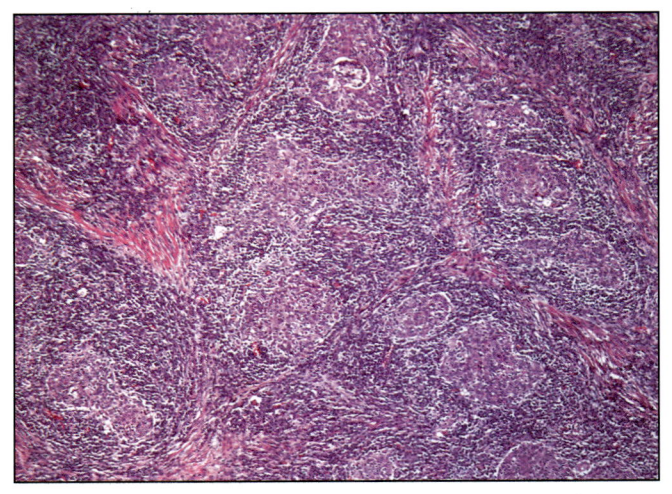

图13E.19 淋巴上皮样癌。边界不清楚的非角化性肿瘤细胞聚集，混有淋巴细胞并被许多淋巴细胞包绕。

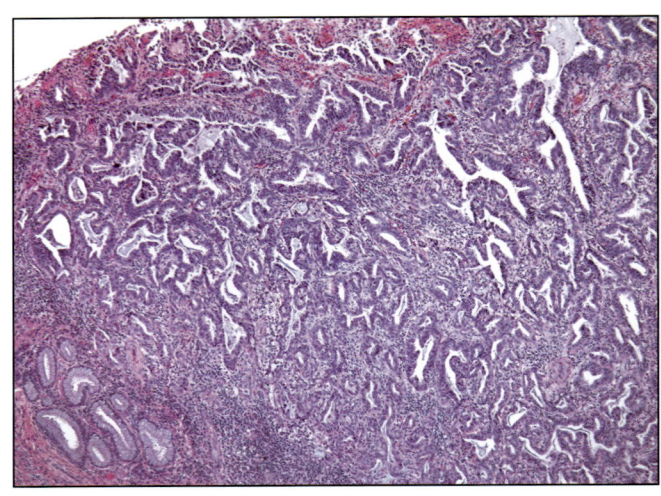

图13E.20 早期浸润性腺癌。注意纤维组织增生性间质中小而不规则形的腺体。

语是从鼻咽部淋巴上皮样癌借用而来的（图 13E.19）。

早期浸润性腺癌[20,21,22,33,57-68]
Early invasive adenocarcinoma

关于宫颈早期浸润性腺癌有许多组织病理学和生物学行为的描述。遗憾的是，对于微小浸润性腺癌的定义一般尚无公认而一致的看法；因此，这个术语不应该用于诊断报告，因为它的含义没有标准化。建议应用浅表浸润性腺癌这一术语，而且总是应该进行浸润深度的测量。评估早期浸润困难，因为原位腺癌可能有复杂的结构，而某些早期浸润性腺癌保持原位腺癌的结构表现。如果出现下面任何的组织学特征，就应该考虑浸润的可能性：（1）非典型性腺体比正常深；（2）小而形状不规则的腺体；（3）单个腺体；（4）炎症性或纤维组织增生性间质；（5）明显的腺体出芽；（6）腺体背靠背的融合性病灶；或（7）复杂的乳头状形态（图 13E.20）。预后与浸润深度密切相关，转移或复发的可能性随着浸润深度的增加而增加；然而，如果严格定义，早期浸润性病变淋巴结转移似乎非常少见[68,68a]。

浸润性腺癌　Invasive adenocarcinoma

浸润性宫颈腺癌的相对和绝对发病率均有明显增加，特别是在 35 岁以下的白人妇女[69,70]。现今，浸润性腺癌占所有浸润性宫颈癌的 20%～25%。与浸润性鳞状细胞癌发病率下降不同，浸润性腺癌的发病率有所增加，这可能是因为原位腺癌的发病率明显增加，而且巴氏涂片筛查对于辨认腺癌相对无效，这不同于鳞状上皮癌前病变。

普通的宫颈内膜（黏液性）腺癌和腺鳞癌与 HPV 感染密切相关[71]。在浸润性宫颈腺癌的组织病理学分类方面，有关宫颈内膜性腺癌和黏液性腺癌的区别尚有一些争论。有人坚持将宫颈内膜性腺癌归入黏液性腺癌（其中还包括微小偏离性腺癌、绒毛腺管状腺癌和肠型腺癌）的范畴，而另外一些人则认为，这种最常见的宫颈腺癌在 HE 切片上没有显著的黏液，因此应该被看成是一种单独的类型。这种争论主要是语义学上的争议，因为这种区别似乎并不具有任何临床意义。对于本章来说，将会分别讨论黏液性腺癌的每一种亚型。腺癌中出现第二种类型的腺癌，如果占据一个肿瘤的 10% 以上，则可诊断为混合性上皮性癌，并说明每一种成分的相对含量。

宫颈内膜腺癌（腺癌，普通宫颈内膜型）
Endocervical adenocarcinoma (adenocarcinoma, usual endocervical type)

临床特征

这种类型最常见，大约占宫颈腺癌的 80%[72]。最常见的症状是阴道出血，而且多数妇女临床上出现明显的宫颈肿块，通常为息肉样和外生性，但可以是硬结和溃疡[73]。偶尔，宫颈环周增大（所谓的桶状宫颈）。这些肿瘤绝大多数与高危险性 HPV 有关，特别是 HPV 16 和 18[74]。浸润性病变总的 5 年生存率为 50%～60%，年轻白人妇女的生存率似乎较好。

病理学特征

组织学检查，肿瘤细胞至少在某种程度上类似于宫颈内膜上皮，特别是原位肿瘤性宫颈内膜细胞，因此将这种类型的腺癌命名为宫颈内膜腺癌。肿瘤细胞胞浆含量不同，可以是黏液性、嗜酸性或两者联合存在（图13E.21）。核大深染，类似于原位腺癌，原位腺癌可能存在于浸润性腺癌的附近，常见许多凋亡小体和核分裂象。肿瘤可能有各种各样的生长方式。腺体大小可能各异，某些肿瘤具有显著的微囊成分。腺体可能密集排列，酷似微小腺体增生（图13E.22），或有较宽的间隙。肿瘤性腺体之间的间质常常（但不总是）显示纤维组织增生性或炎症性反应。

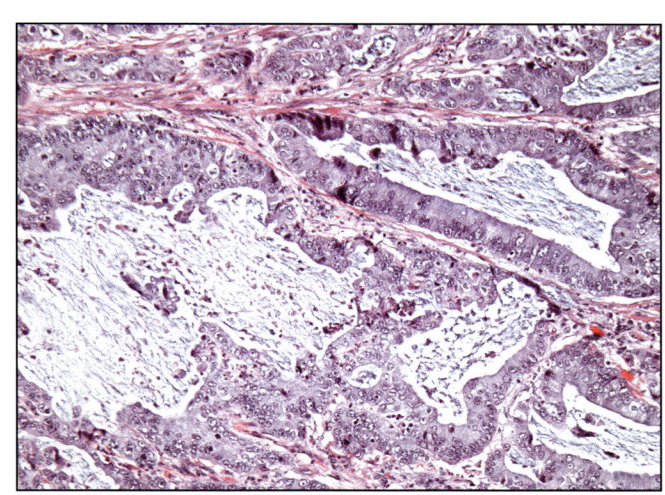

图13E.21 宫颈内膜腺癌。肿瘤细胞具有丰富的黏液性胞浆，类似于正常的宫颈内膜腺体。

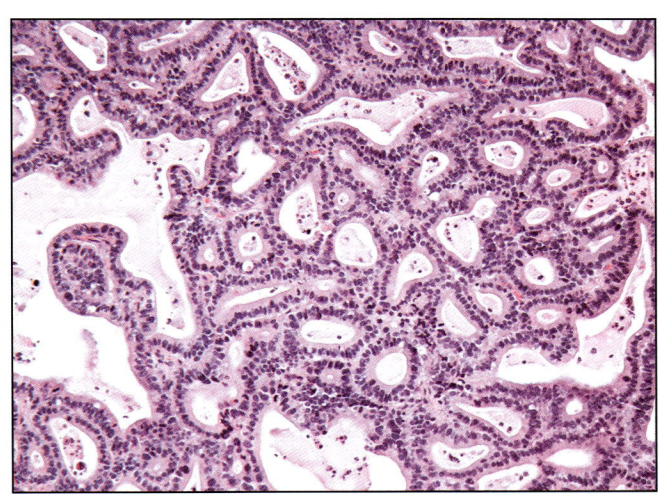

图13E.22 宫颈内膜腺癌。许多小腺体，类似于微小腺体增生。

微小偏离性腺癌（恶性腺瘤）[75-80]
Minimal-deviation adenocarcinoma (adenoma malignum)

临床特征

微小偏离性腺癌是一种罕见的、分化非常高的黏液性肿瘤，大约占宫颈腺癌的1%~2%。它发生在生育年龄的妇女（平均年龄42岁），如果有症状的话，最常见的是月经频多、阴道（常常是黏液样）排液或异常出血。大约10%~15%的恶性腺瘤病人伴有Peutz-Jeghers综合征。肿瘤抑制基因 *STK11*（丝氨酸苏氨酸激酶基因）突变是造成Peutz-Jeghers综合征的原因，在微小偏离性腺癌病例偶尔也可以见到这种改变[81,82]。临床检查通常发现宫颈异常，表现为增大和（或）变硬。恶性腺瘤病人倾向于出现高的分期，而且比普通宫颈内膜腺癌病人预后似乎要差，所有分期总的生存率是28%，1期肿瘤生存率是50%。恶性腺瘤可能伴有卵巢黏液癌，这在多数病例可能是转移性播散[83-85]。

病理学特征

微小偏离性腺癌的组织学特征是出现深部浸润的形状不规则的腺体，某些腺体可能有球状或指样突起，通常延伸到宫颈壁的外1/3（图13E.23）。虽然多数腺体内衬温和的黏液性上皮细胞，核小，位于基底，胞浆淡染呈柱状，但是许多细胞核大伴有核仁，不同于正常宫颈内膜腺体；通常出现恶性细胞学特征和炎症性、水肿性或纤维组织增生性间质反应，至少是局灶性。免疫组化检查，微小偏离性腺癌CEA可能阳性；然而，染色可能为局灶性，这就限制了它的应用。微小偏离性腺癌的腺体含有明显的中性黏液，类似于胃的黏液腺（而非肿

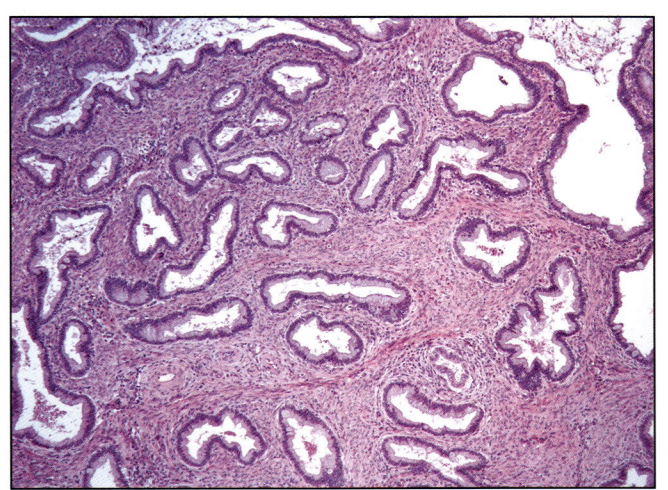

图13E.23 微小偏离性腺癌。腺体形状不规则，向宫颈壁深部延伸。

瘤性黏液性宫颈内膜上皮的特征是含有等量的中性和酸性黏液），这对于诊断可能是有用的[86,87]。这种类型的肿瘤仅有少数与 HPV 有关[74]。

微小偏离性腺癌的鉴别诊断包括种种非肿瘤性病变，其鉴别要点列在表 13E.2 中。这些病变要常见得多，在诊断微小偏离性腺癌之前，总是应该予以排除。

绒毛腺管状腺癌（高分化绒毛腺管状腺癌，高分化绒毛腺管状乳头状腺癌）[88-92]
Villoglandular adenocarcinoma (well-differentiated villoglandular adenocarcinoma; well-differentiated villoglandular papillary adenocarcinoma)

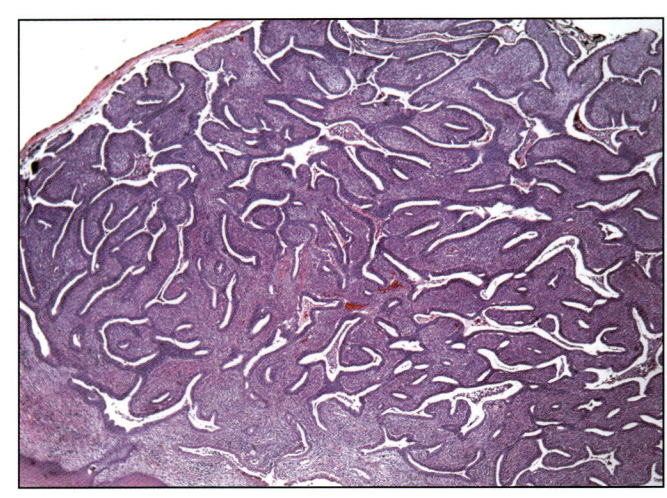

图 13E.24　绒毛腺管状腺癌。注意复杂的交错排列的腺体和富于细胞的纤维性间质。

这种亚型的腺癌不常见，一般发生于 30~40 岁的妇女，最常见的症状是阴道异常出血。临床上肿瘤通常明显，常常呈外生性息肉样或乳头状表现。这种肿瘤的组织学特点是表面出现由细的指样乳头组成的乳头状成分，伴有独特的纤维性梭形细胞间质。乳头下方常常混有由交错排列的分支状腺体组成的浸润性成分，与其下间质交界宽阔，呈推挤状（图 13E.24）。乳头被覆显示轻度至中度细胞核非典型性的复层柱状细胞，通常没有明显的黏液性胞浆。这种亚型与高危险性 HPV16 和 18 有关，而且常常伴有邻近的原位腺癌。因为某些较普通的乳头状腺癌具有乳头状绒毛腺管状成分，所以绒毛腺管状腺癌的诊断只能用于高分化，而且没有其他类型浸润性癌存在的病例。这常常只能在锥切活检或子宫切除标本中确定。虽然最初研究提示生物学行为良好，但是某些病例伴有局部淋巴结受累；因此，类似于普通的浸润性腺癌，考虑保守治疗应该注意诸如淋巴管/血管浸润和浸润深度等因素。

表 13E.2	微小偏离性腺癌及其常见类似病变的比较					
	微小偏离性腺癌	深部 Naboth 腺/囊肿	隧道状腺丛	腺肌瘤，宫颈内膜型	宫颈内膜异位症	分叶状宫颈内膜腺体增生
在宫颈的部位	通常延伸到外 1/2/透壁	可以出现在外 1/2	通常在内 1/3；少数累及外 1/2	位于宫颈壁的肿块	典型者仅仅累及外 1/2 和宫颈旁软组织	通常在内 1/2
宫颈异常表现	常见	不常见	不常见	常见	不常见	不常见
分叶状生长方式	罕见	不常见	特征性	常见	缺乏	特征性
叶样腺体	存在	缺乏	缺乏	存在	缺乏	存在
细胞学非典型性	存在，通常仅为局灶性	缺乏	不常见	不常见	不常见	不常见
核分裂活性	存在	不常见	不常见	不常见	不常见	不常见
纤维组织增生	存在，通常仅为局灶性	缺乏	缺乏	缺乏	缺乏	缺乏
肌瘤性间质	缺乏	缺乏	缺乏	存在	缺乏	缺乏

肠型腺癌[93-96] Enteric adenocarcinoma

普通型的宫颈内膜腺癌（以及某些腺鳞癌）可能出现灶状肠的分化，表现为杯状细胞、Paneth 细胞、嗜银细胞或印戒细胞。在非常罕见的情况下，可以这种形态为主。当出现这些形态时，应该排除转移性胃肠道腺癌。

子宫内膜样腺癌 Endometrioid adenocarcinoma

这个肿瘤非常类似于子宫内膜的子宫内膜样腺癌，细胞具有非黏液性胞浆，比宫颈内膜型腺癌细胞密集，层次较多（图13E.25）；偶尔出现鳞状化生，但是比子宫内膜原发性肿瘤少见得多。子宫内膜样腺癌与宫颈内膜型腺癌的区别有些主观；因此，这种亚型报告的频率不同[97,98]。与宫颈内膜亚型类似，子宫内膜样腺癌也伴有高危险性 HPV 和原位腺癌，支持具有共同的发病机制[22]。子宫内膜样腺癌的行为和预后似乎与普通的宫颈内膜型腺癌类似。主要的鉴别诊断是与子宫内膜原发性肿瘤区分，在活检/刮宫标本中的鉴别可能存在问题。支持宫颈内膜原发的特征包括：（1）出现宫颈肿块；（2）大部分肿瘤存在于宫颈内膜（与子宫内膜比较）样本；（3）存在宫颈原位腺癌；（4）病人小于 40 岁；（5）癌的 vimentin、雌激素受体（ER）和孕激素受体（PR）免疫染色阴性；以及（6）癌 HPV 阳性。支持子宫内膜原发的特征包括：（1）病人子宫增大，子宫内膜增厚，或月经异常；（2）肿瘤大部分出现在子宫内膜样本；（3）存在子宫内膜上皮内肿瘤形成；（4）肿瘤含有泡沫状间质细胞；（5）病人大于 50 岁；（6）肿瘤 vimentin、雌激素受体（ER）和孕激素受体（PR）免疫染色阳性；以及（7）肿瘤 HPV 阴性。

微小偏离性子宫内膜样腺癌[78,99,100] Minimal-deviation endometrioid adenocarcinoma

子宫内膜样宫颈腺癌的一种亚型，分化非常高，其生长方式和温和表现类似于微小偏离性宫颈内膜腺癌，除了内衬浸润性腺体的细胞是子宫内膜样而不同于黏液性细胞之外（图 13E.26）。这种亚型的子宫内膜样腺癌不同于子宫内膜异位症或输卵管子宫内膜样化生，它具有浸润性结构形态，并存在恶性细胞学特征和（或）纤维组织增生性间质，至少是局灶性。

透明细胞腺癌[101-105] Clear cell adenocarcinoma

宫颈透明细胞腺癌是一种罕见的恶性肿瘤，可以散在发生或与宫内接触己烯雌酚（diethylstilbestrol）有关。在任何一种情况下，似乎均有伴有两个高峰的双峰年龄分布，一个高峰年轻（平均 20～30 岁），一个高峰年老（平均 70～80 岁）[103]。病人通常表现为异常阴道出血或性交困难，临床上有一个明显的宫颈肿块。组织学检查，这些肿瘤类似于发生在女性生殖道其他部位透明细胞癌的表现，是由富于糖原的肿瘤细胞组成的，细胞核深染，形状不规则，排列成管囊状、实性，和（或）为乳头状生长方式。与其他组织学类型不同，透明细胞癌病人有时好像具有晚期局灶性或远处复发的较大倾向性。

鉴别诊断包括两个宫颈假肿瘤性病变：微小腺体增生和 Arias-Stella 反应。微小腺体增生不同于透明细胞癌的特征包括：（1）仅有局灶性的细胞核非典型性；（2）

图13E.25 子宫内膜样腺癌。肿瘤性腺体内衬细胞具有复层的细胞核，胞浆不显著，位于顶端，酷似子宫内膜原发性肿瘤。

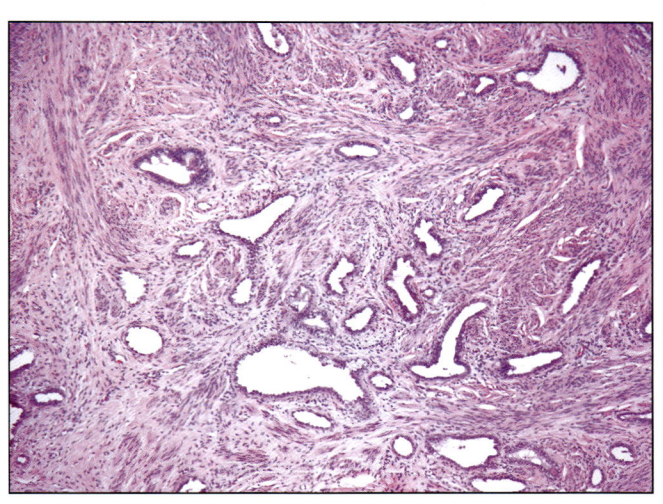

图13E.26 微小偏离性子宫内膜样腺癌。浸润深部的腺体缺乏位于顶端的黏液性胞浆，因此表现为子宫内膜样。

出现核下空泡和胞浆内黏液；(3) 缺乏糖原；(4) 缺乏浸润性生长方式；以及 (5) 出现储备细胞增生/鳞状化生。Arias-Stella 反应不同于透明细胞癌的特征包括：(1) 不伴有肿块性病变；(2) 通常为局灶性病变；以及 (3) 细胞核表现出一系列的细胞学非典型性。

乳头状浆液性腺癌[106]
Papillary serous adenocarcinoma

原发性宫颈乳头状浆液性腺癌非常少见。在最大的一组 17 例病人的研究中[106]，具有双峰年龄分布，病人或小于 45 岁，或大于 65 岁。最常见的症状是异常的阴道出血或排液，多数病人在临床上可见外生性或息肉样肿块。这些肿瘤在组织学上类似于发生在女性生殖道其他部位的普通的乳头状浆液性腺癌，具有复杂的分支状乳头，被覆细胞具有中到重度细胞学非典型性。常见细胞簇、微乳头和裂隙样结构；通常可见许多核分裂象。差不多半数的肿瘤伴有另外一种组织学亚型的腺癌，最常见的是绒毛腺管状腺癌，提示可能有共同的病因学。根据本人的经验，发生在较年轻妇女的乳头状浆液性腺癌 HPV 一般阳性，类似于绒毛腺管状腺癌。只有在排除了从子宫内膜或卵巢扩散而来的继发性肿瘤之后，才能诊断宫颈原发性乳头状浆液性腺癌，特别是在老年病人。宫颈 I 期乳头状浆液性腺癌病人的结果似乎与普通腺癌没有不同。

中肾腺癌[107-109]
Mesonephric adenocarcinoma

中肾腺癌是一种罕见的子宫恶性肿瘤，最常发生于宫颈。老的文献提到的中肾癌多数是透明细胞癌，最初认为透明细胞癌是中肾来源的。推测真正的中肾癌是来源于中肾残余——中肾管的残余成分，在男性中肾管发育成睾丸输出管、附睾、输精管、精囊和射精管；然而，在女性中肾管通常退化，但是小灶状中肾管可能持续存在于阔韧带、宫颈和阴道。中肾癌年龄分布广泛(34～73岁)，平均年龄为 50～60 岁。最常见的症状是异常阴道出血，而且多数病人有宫颈异常，最常见的是外生性息肉样肿块；然而，肿瘤还可能是结节状、溃疡性、或引起宫颈弥漫性增大 ["桶状宫颈"(barrel cervix)]。中肾癌的预后尚不确定，虽然提示它具有惰性的行为。早期以及晚期病人均可发生局灶性或腹腔内复发，但是复发可以发生于长时间内。

中肾癌通常累及宫颈壁的全层，具有浸润性的边缘，并向上延伸，有时侵及其上宫颈黏膜。常见中肾增生成分，但不总是出现。中肾癌具有种种组织学形态（图 13E.27 和 13E.28），最常见的是导管和小管，前者类似于子宫内膜样腺体肿瘤形成，后者由密集排列、不同大小、通常为小圆形的囊肿和(或)小管组成，其内常常含有明显嗜酸性的腔内物质（类似于中肾残余）。网状、实性、性索样和梭形形态也可以出现。梭形形态常常类似于子宫内膜间质肉瘤或非特异性梭形细胞肉瘤；因此，有人提出应用恶性混合性中肾肿瘤这一术语描述具有这种成分的肿瘤。因为这些梭形细胞灶上皮标志物通常阳性，所以它们很可能是梭形细胞癌。中肾癌 cytokeratin 7 和 EMA 阳性，calretinin 和 CD10 也可能阳性（表现

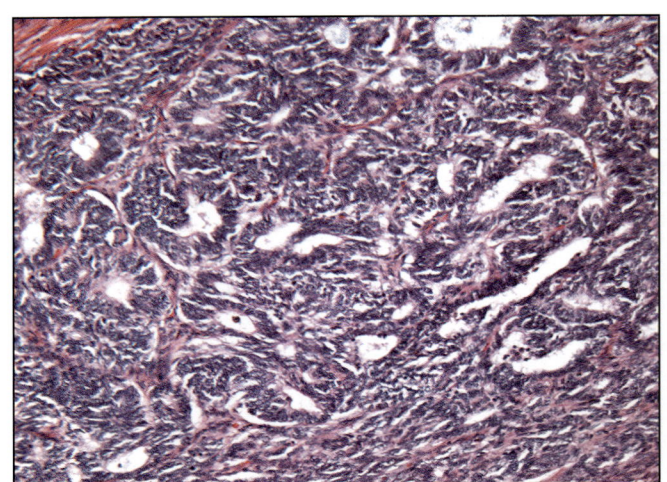

图13E.27 中肾腺癌伴有梭形间质。注意导管分化合并富于细胞的梭形间质。

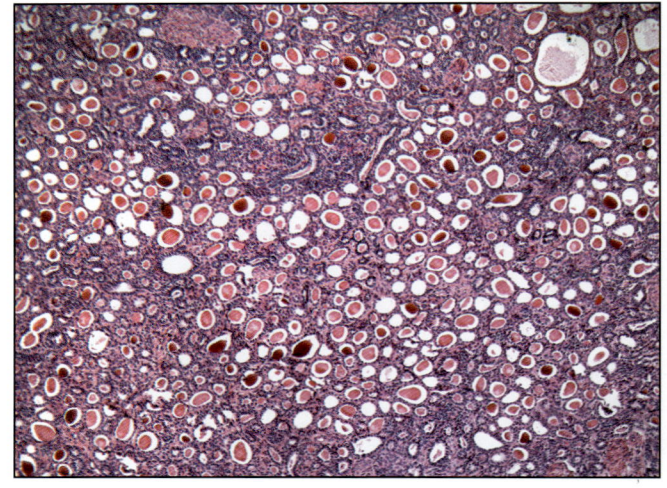

图13E.28 中肾腺癌，小管型。小管背靠背，没有提示浸润的交错排列的间质。

为顶端染色）。

中肾癌的鉴别诊断包括中肾增生（与小管亚型鉴别）和子宫内膜样癌（与导管亚型鉴别）。中肾癌不同于中肾增生的特征包括：（1）不规则的、紊乱的浸润；（2）腺体密集，背靠背；（3）核分裂活性；（4）核的非典型性；（5）淋巴管/血管/神经周围浸润；以及（6）存在其他组织学形态。导管亚型中肾癌与子宫内膜样癌的区别是腔内出现特征性的嗜酸性物质，而且前者伴有中肾增生。

混合类型癌　Mixed-type carcinomas

腺鳞癌　Adenosquamous carcinoma

如果严格地定义一个通过 HE 切片检查清楚显示可辨认的鳞状和腺体成分的肿瘤（图 13E.29），那么腺鳞癌大约占伴有腺体成分的宫颈癌的 1/3[97]。腺鳞癌这种术语不应该用于具有胞浆内黏液但是没有明显鳞状分化证据的低分化肿瘤。同样，伴有组织化学确定的胞浆内黏液的浸润性鳞状细胞癌也应该从这个类别中排除。与腺癌比较，腺鳞癌病人的预后尚不清楚；某些研究提示预后较差，尽管其他研究并非如此[97,110,111]。除了显示鳞状细胞癌和腺癌的典型形态学表现所显示的可清楚辨认的肿瘤性腺体和鳞状成分混合存在以外，已经公认腺鳞癌有两种组织学变型：玻璃状细胞癌和透明细胞腺鳞癌。

玻璃状细胞癌[112-116]　Glassy cell carcinoma

这种罕见的肿瘤被认为是腺鳞癌的一种变型，因为某些病例显微镜检查可能显示局灶性鳞状或腺体分化，而另外一些病例电镜检查证实有双相表现。这种肿瘤发生年龄可能广泛，但是与宫颈腺癌相比，一般说来好像发生于较年轻的年龄组。病人通常表现为阴道出血，临床检查时通常有一个大而显著的蕈状肿块。大细胞呈弥漫性片块状和巢状分布，具有丰富的嗜酸性到颗粒性胞浆，呈现毛玻璃状外观，核大，圆形到卵圆形，核仁突出，细胞界限清楚，这是玻璃状细胞癌的组织学特征（图 13E.30）。此外，有许多核分裂象和明显的炎症性间质浸润，常常由嗜酸细胞和浆细胞组成。因为某些典型的腺癌和大细胞非角化性鳞状细胞癌可以出现局灶性玻璃状细胞的特征，所以玻璃状细胞癌的诊断应该用于那些显示独特组织学特征的单纯性肿瘤。虽然认为这个肿瘤是腺鳞癌的一个变型，但是关于这个肿瘤是否可能是低分化癌的一种非特异的生长方式尚有争论，因为某些复发性腺癌和腺鳞癌放疗之后可能出现玻璃状细胞癌的形态学特征。总之，玻璃状细胞癌患者预后似乎较差，虽然由于这种类型的肿瘤罕见而生存资料有限。

透明细胞腺鳞癌[117]　Clear cell adenosquamous carcinoma

腺鳞癌这种罕见变型的组织学特征是，出现混合性腺体和鳞状成分，后者含有大量富于糖原的胞浆，呈现显著的透明细胞改变（图 13E.31）。这种肿瘤与 HPV18 密切相关，预后好像不良。

腺样基底细胞癌（腺样基底细胞上皮瘤）[118-128]　Adenoid basal carcinoma (adenoid basal epithelioma)

临床特征

腺样基底细胞癌是一种不常见的肿瘤，占宫颈癌的

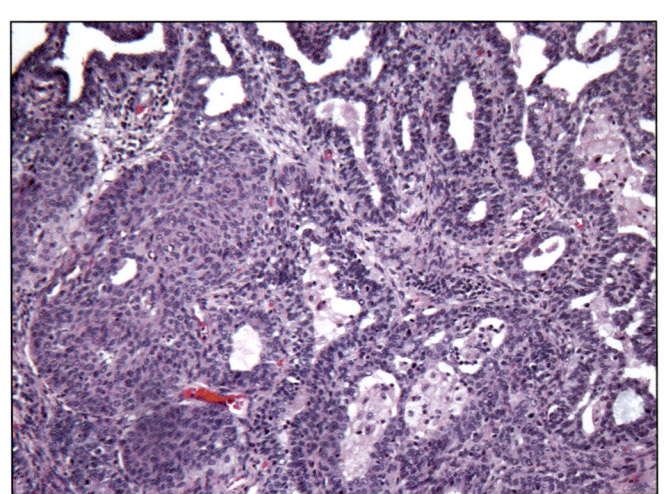

图 13E.29　腺鳞癌。出现明显的腺体和鳞状分化。

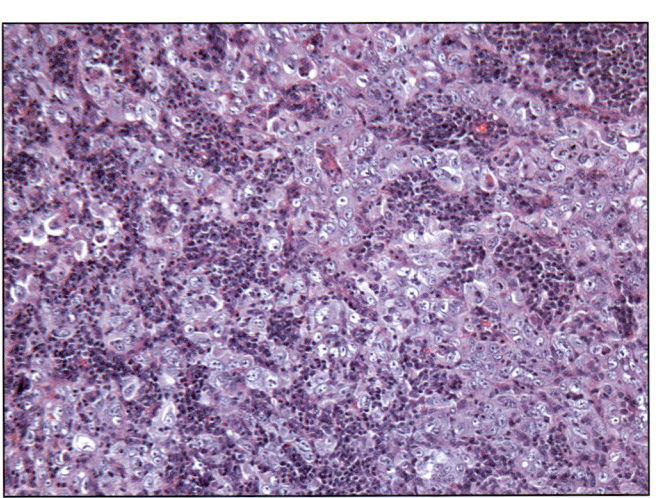

图 13E.30　玻璃状细胞癌。肿瘤细胞成巢聚集，胞浆丰富，嗜酸性，混有许多炎症细胞。

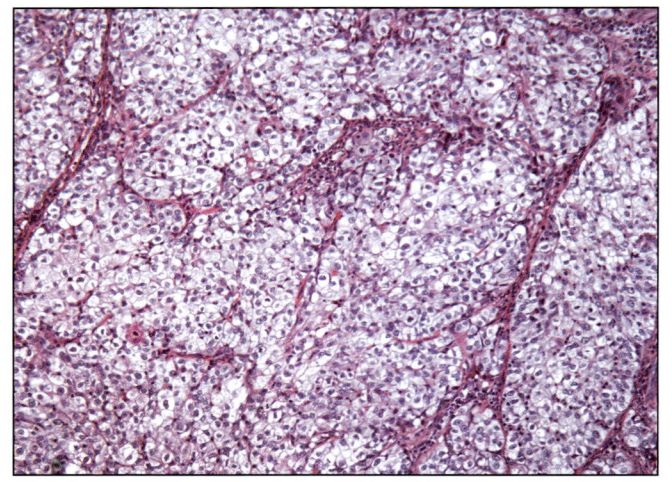

图13E.31 透明细胞腺鳞癌。注意丰富的透明胞浆。

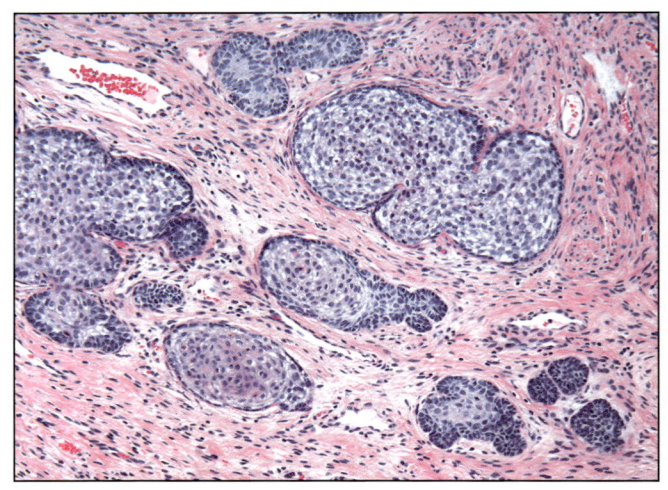

图13E.32 腺样基底细胞癌。注意周围的细胞核呈栅栏状排列，中心为非典型性鳞状分化。

不到5%。临床检查宫颈一般没有发现异常，通常是在锥切活检或子宫切除标本中偶然发现的，病人通常为绝经后的黑人妇女，伴有高级别鳞状上皮内病变。预后良好，具有典型的或单纯的组织病理学特征的肿瘤病人没有转移或复发。偶尔，腺样基底细胞癌可能伴有其他类型的肿瘤，特别是基底细胞样鳞状细胞癌、腺鳞癌、腺样囊性癌或癌肉瘤；这些复合性肿瘤的预后与较侵袭性的成分有关。因为预后非常良好，所以有人提出应用腺样基底细胞上皮瘤这一术语取代腺样基底细胞癌[121]；然而，这种形态并不总是能够预示其生物学行为。腺样基底细胞癌和腺样囊性癌的组织发生似乎有关[120]，因为两种肿瘤均发生于绝经后的妇女，具有偏离分化的能力，而且均伴有高危险性HPV感染。此外，极少数肿瘤可能具有腺样囊性癌和腺样基底细胞癌两者的特征，提示它们可能是这种形态学谱系中的一部分。

病理学特征

在大多数病例，被覆上皮有高级别鳞状上皮内病变（CIN），其下浸润性肿瘤可能出现三种形态分化：(1) 由具有不同程度非典型性的鳞状上皮构成的散在圆形细胞巢和细胞岛，周围的细胞核呈显著的栅栏状排列；(2) 基底细胞样细胞巢，胞浆稀少；(3) 基底细胞样细胞巢混有代表腺体分化的小的腺泡（图13E.32）。典型者不伴有间质反应。

腺样囊性癌 [120,124,125,128,129]
Adenoid cystic carcinoma

临床特征

腺样囊性癌是一种非常罕见的肿瘤（占宫颈癌的不到1%），一般发生于绝经后的妇女，通常为黑人，平均年龄70岁。病人通常表现为绝经后出血，临床检查宫颈可见脆而易碎的息肉样或溃疡性肿块。病人预后不好，因为腺样囊性癌常常伴有局部复发或转移性扩散。由于生物学行为不同，这种肿瘤应该与腺样基底细胞癌鉴别；然而，这两种肿瘤的组织发生似乎密切相关，因为两者均发生于绝经后妇女，并与高危险性HPV有关（通常是HPV 16）。此外，两种肿瘤均可出现具有另外一种肿瘤形态学特征的区域，而且极少数病例可能形成杂交性肿瘤。

病理学特征

组织学检查，宫颈腺样囊性癌与涎腺腺样囊性癌具有类似的表现，由密集排列的细胞构成细胞巢、细胞岛、细胞条索和小梁状结构，几无胞浆，细胞核深染。特征性的表现是，细胞巢具有筛状结构和栅栏状排列的细胞核，圆形间隙充满嗜酸性玻璃样或黏液性物质（图13E.33）。常见细胞多形性、多数核分裂象、坏死和纤维组织增生性间质反应。腺样囊性癌S-100蛋白染色常常阳性，而且肌肉特异性肌动蛋白（HHF35）也可能阳性，提示有肌上皮分化。

神经内分泌癌
Neuroendocrine carcinoma

归入宫颈神经内分泌癌范畴的肿瘤不常见，已被一个学术专题讨论会定义为类癌、非典型性类癌、小细胞癌和大细胞神经内分泌癌[130]。这些肿瘤没有明确的前体病变，但是可与较常见的宫颈鳞癌和腺癌的各

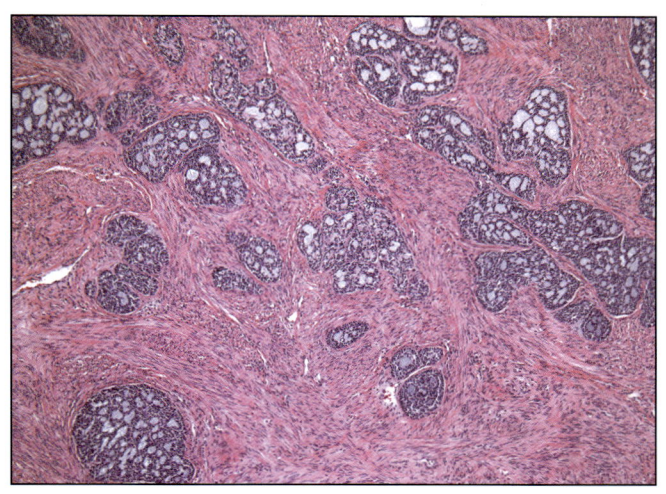

图13E.33 腺样囊性癌。注意筛状生长方式和中心圆形间隙，其内充满黏液性物质，类似于涎腺来源的肿瘤。

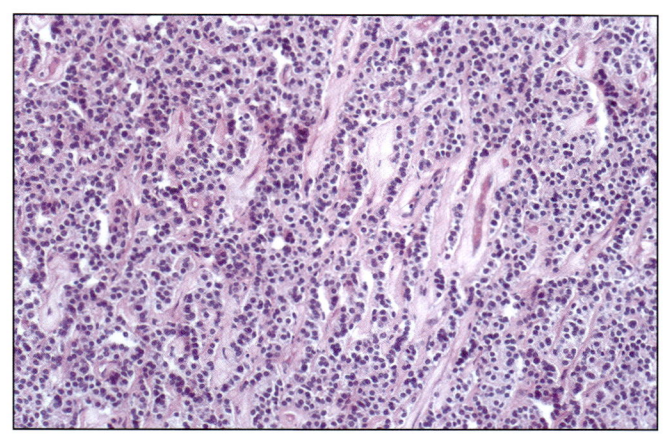

图13E.34 类癌。条索样生长方式。

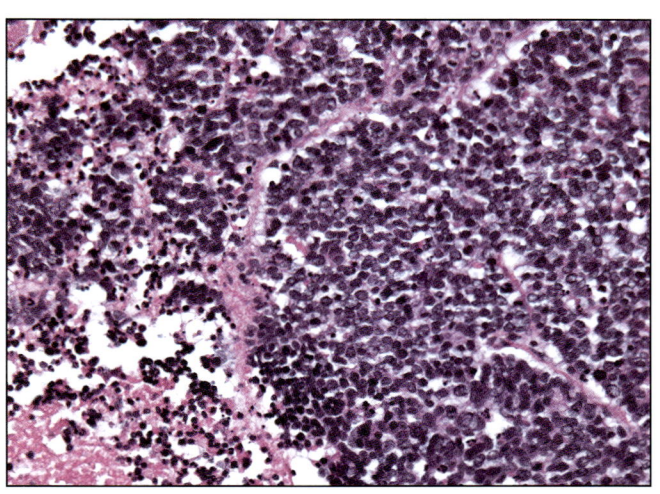

图13E.35 小细胞癌。致密的小细胞群，核深染，几无胞浆，可见许多核分裂象。注意图的左下部分有坏死。

种亚型共存，而且也与HPV18密切相关，提示有共同的起源[131]。仅仅是根据形态学的差异将其分为不同的亚型；然而，不同的形态结构可以共存，这些类型之间的诊断可重复性尚不清楚。因此，并不容易评估其生物学行为的不同，就临床而言，这些肿瘤的处理多数类似。此外，这些不同的形态学类型具有类似的分子生物学异常，最常见的是9p21杂合性丢失以及局灶性3p缺失，提示具有共同的发病机制[132]。总之，宫颈神经内分泌癌的结局是不良的，不管其形态学亚型如何[133-136]。

类癌　Carcinoid

宫颈类癌类似于其他部位的类癌，其组成细胞具有少量双染性到嗜酸性颗粒状胞浆，伴有小到中等大小的圆形到卵圆形细胞核，染色质呈细颗粒状。肿瘤细胞一般排列成小梁状、器官样、巢状、微腺泡状，或呈条索样生长方式（图13E.34）。缺乏坏死，每10个高倍视野核分裂数小于5个。

非典型性类癌　Atypical carcinoid

非典型性类癌具有与类癌同样的结构特征，区别在于具有坏死、细胞学非典型性，以及每10个高倍视野核分裂数在5～10个之间。

小细胞癌[131,137]　Small cell carcinoma

与肺的小细胞癌相似，典型的宫颈小细胞癌是由致密的小细胞群组成的，细胞核深染，几无胞浆，导致核浆比例增高（图13E.35）。肿瘤细胞排列成片块状、不规则聚集或没有黏着力的细胞巢，虽然偶尔可以出现玫瑰花结或不甚清楚的腺泡。细胞核变形具有特征性，常常出现坏死。这些病变一般具有侵袭性。

大细胞神经内分泌癌　Large cell neuroendocrine carcinoma

大细胞神经内分泌癌呈小梁状、巢状或岛屿状生长方式，构成细胞具有中等量到丰富的嗜酸性胞浆，核大，染色质空泡状，核仁明显（图13E.36）。其特征是出现多数核分裂象和坏死[138]。

混合性上皮和间叶性肿瘤　Mixed epithelial and mesenchymal tumors

Müller乳头状瘤[139,140]　Müllerian papilloma

Müller乳头状瘤是一种罕见的良性乳头状病变，较常发生于阴道（见725页），但是偶尔也可以发生于

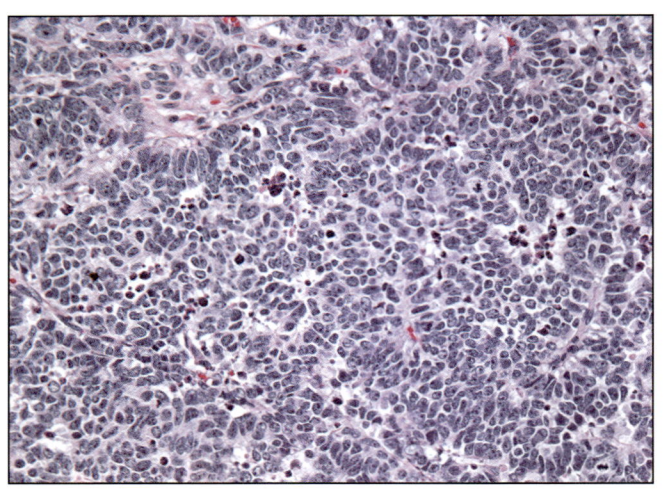

图13E.36　大细胞神经内分泌癌。肿瘤细胞核较大，染色质空泡状，核仁显著。

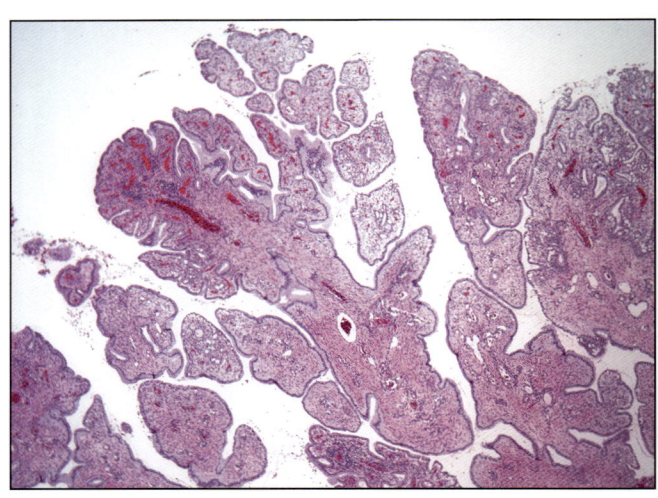

图13E.37　宫颈内膜息肉。外生性乳头伴有纤维性轴心。

宫颈。典型者发生于10岁以前的儿童，最常见的症状是阴道出血或排液。组织学家检查，病变由复杂的分支乳头组成，被覆没有纤毛的立方或柱状上皮，呈良性表现，没有核分裂活性。纤维间质轴心可能含有不同量的炎症细胞。这些病变通过局部切除治疗，偶尔可能复发。

宫颈内膜息肉　Endocervical polyp

宫颈内膜息肉一般是40～50岁妇女的偶尔发现；最常见的症状是引起阴道异常出血或排液[141,142]。宫颈内膜息肉虽然可以发生于沿着宫颈管的任何部位，但是最常见于宫颈口的附近。在绝经后的妇女，宫颈息肉与存在的子宫内膜息肉密切相关，而且建议考虑子宫内膜取样以便解释临床症状（并能排除共存的肿瘤）[143]。组织学检查，这些病变呈息肉样，伴有被覆良性表现的宫颈内膜上皮的间质轴心（图13E.37）。与腺上皮有关的间质的量可能不同，某些病例显示有明显的上皮，表现为微小腺体变化。最重要的鉴别诊断是排除腺肉瘤。宫颈腺肉瘤与宫颈内膜息肉的区别在于：(1) 腺体轮廓通常（但并不总是）有分叶样或叶状表现；(2) 腺体周围套袖；(3) 间质核分裂象每10个高倍视野大于2个；以及在某些病例(4) 出现非典型性间质细胞。肉瘤性过度生长和异源性间质分化也可以见于腺肉瘤。有些宫颈内膜息肉显示腺肉瘤的某些特征，但是不符合腺肉瘤的诊断标准（例如，伴有叶状结构的息肉，但是没有腺体周围套袖，间质核分裂不活跃）；在这些情况下，我们建议诊断为"宫颈内膜息肉伴有独特的组织学特征"，这是一种描述性的注释，提示临床随访并及时切除任何的复发性病变。

腺纤维瘤[144]　Adenofibroma

宫颈腺纤维瘤是一种混合性上皮和间叶肿瘤，其中上皮成分和纤维性间质成分均为良性。这些肿瘤非常罕见，至于其是否存在尚有某些争论，虽然在WHO宫颈肿瘤分类中已经得到承认。组织学检查，这些病变是由伴有纤维性轴心的乳头状叶丛组成的，乳头被覆良性立方和柱状上皮，上皮可能是黏液性、纤毛性或难以归类的上皮。与腺肉瘤的区别是腺纤维瘤缺乏腺体周围套袖、间质核分裂活性或间质非典型性。这些病变为良性，类似于良性宫颈息肉，但是有可能复发。治疗选择局部切除。

腺肌瘤，宫颈内膜型[145]　Adenomyoma, endocervical type

宫颈内膜型腺肌瘤是一种罕见的宫颈混合性上皮-间叶肿瘤，最常见的表现是无症状的肿块，受累妇女的平均年龄为40岁。肿瘤大小不定，可以大到23cm，多数病例小于8 cm。肿瘤一般发生于宫颈管，而且通常突入宫颈管，偶尔从宫颈口脱出；也可以发生壁内肿瘤。这种病变的特征是境界清楚的灰白色肿块，可能含有多发性黏液囊肿。组织学检查，腺肌瘤的腺体形状不规则，其中某些腺体可能显示乳头状内折和分叶样结构，周围绕以较小的圆形腺体，形成小叶状外观。腺体通常内衬良性高柱状宫颈内膜型黏液性上皮（偶尔出现局灶性输卵管分化和子宫内膜样腺体），核分裂象不常见。增生的良性平滑肌围绕腺体并将腺体分开，排列成交错的平滑肌束，类似于平滑肌瘤（图13E.38）。这些肿瘤为良性；在经子宫切除治疗的病人，可能存在

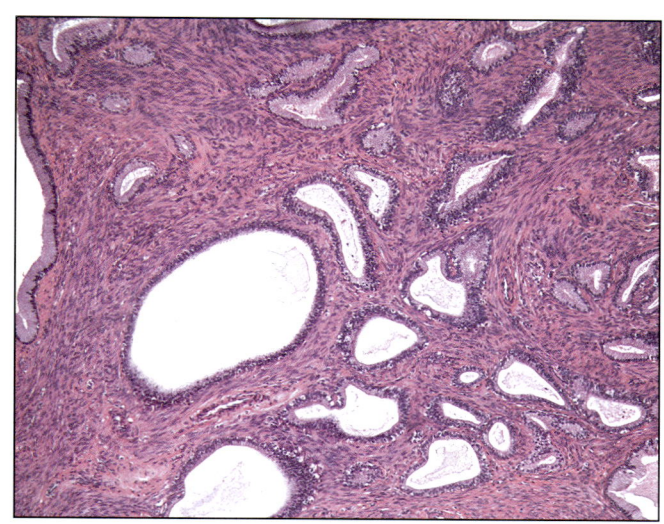

图13E.38 腺肌瘤,宫颈内膜型。腺体被肌瘤性间质分开。

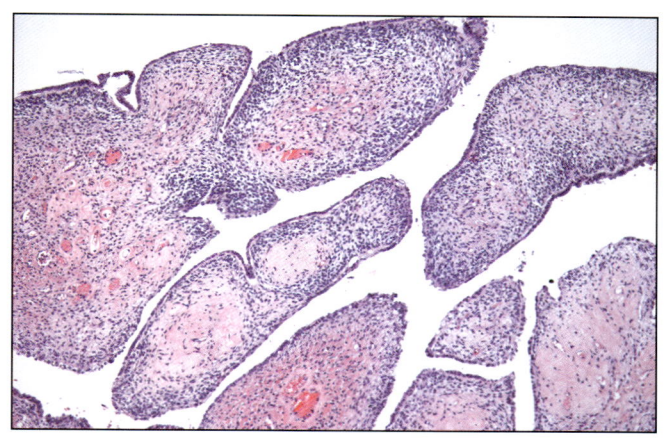

图13E.39 Müller腺肉瘤。息肉样分叶样生长方式伴有上皮下和腺体周围富于梭形细胞的间质。

残留的肿瘤,在仅仅通过局部切除治疗的病人,肿瘤可能再生长(不同于复发)。宫颈内膜型腺肌瘤与微小偏离性腺癌不同,其主要鉴别诊断要点在于:(1)境界清楚;(2)腺体排列成小叶状(微小偏离性腺癌小叶状结构少见);(3)存在平滑肌成分,缺乏纤维组织增生性间质;(4)均匀一致的良性细胞形态学特征。

子宫内膜型腺肌瘤和非典型性息肉样腺肌瘤偶尔可以累及宫颈,但是发生于子宫体的比较常见(见第13章第二部分)。

腺肉瘤(Müller腺肉瘤) Adenosarcoma (Müllerian adenosarcoma)

Müller腺肉瘤是一个双相性的肿瘤,由恶性间质成分混合良性上皮成分组成。这种肿瘤最常发生于子宫体(见第13章第二部分),但是,作为原发性肿瘤也可以发生于卵巢、盆腔和宫颈(以发生频率递减的顺序),在一项研究中,宫颈Müller腺肉瘤占病例的2%[146]。患有原发性宫颈肿瘤妇女的平均年龄为30~40岁(年龄范围为10~70岁),病人通常表现为复发性息肉或异常阴道出血[147,148]。肿瘤的特征是息肉样或乳头状,临床检查可见肿瘤从宫颈口突出。组织学检查,肿瘤呈息肉样,由复杂而不规则的分支腺体组成,伴有叶状或分叶样外观,内衬黏液性、纤毛性或子宫内膜样上皮(图13E.39)。腺体周围富于梭形细胞的间质套袖可能显示一系列的细胞核非典型性,这种表现具有特征性。每10个高倍视野至少应该有2个核分裂象,多数病例核分裂象超过4个。与子宫内膜腺肉瘤相似,这些肿瘤可能显示肉瘤性过度生长和异源性分化[149,150]。宫颈腺肉瘤病人的预后因素和结局尚不十分确定,因为发生在这个部位的腺肉瘤不常见;一项最大系列的12个病人的报告显示结局不良,1例于最初诊断之后1年死于本病,1例出现复发[147]。最近的研究显示与子宫内膜腺肉瘤相似,预后好像与出现深部浸润有关。

癌肉瘤(恶性Müller混合瘤)[151-155] Carcinosarcoma (malignant Müllerian mixed tumor)

癌肉瘤是由恶性上皮和间叶成分组成的,最常见于子宫体的肿瘤。宫颈原发性癌肉瘤罕见,一般发生在绝经后的妇女,通常为黑人,大多数病人年龄超过60岁。肿瘤一般呈息肉样或有蒂,最大系列报告显示肿瘤大小从1cm到10cm不等[151],但是已有大至17cm的个案报告。与子宫体癌肉瘤不同,宫颈癌肉瘤与HPV感染有关,特别是HPV16。这种伴随现象可能与宫颈原发性肿瘤存在(宫颈型)腺体或鳞状上皮有关,这不同于子宫原发性肿瘤。基底细胞样鳞状细胞癌、腺样囊性癌、腺样基底细胞癌和未分化癌(不同于子宫内膜样癌或乳头状浆液性癌)较常伴有宫颈原发性肿瘤(图13E.40)。间叶性成分倾向于同源性分化,伴有纤维肉瘤或子宫内膜间质肉瘤形态。与子宫内膜癌肉瘤相比,宫颈癌肉瘤好像多半局限于子宫,因此预后可能较好[151]。鉴别诊断包括伴有梭形细胞成分的中肾癌和Wilms瘤,这两种肿瘤均发生于较年轻的妇女。

间叶性肿瘤 Mesenchymal tumors

平滑肌瘤 Leiomyoma

宫颈平滑肌瘤少见,在因为有症状的子宫体肌瘤或其他原因而切除的子宫标本中仅占不到1%[156]。多数宫颈平滑肌瘤是偶然发现的,不是具有临床意义的病变。

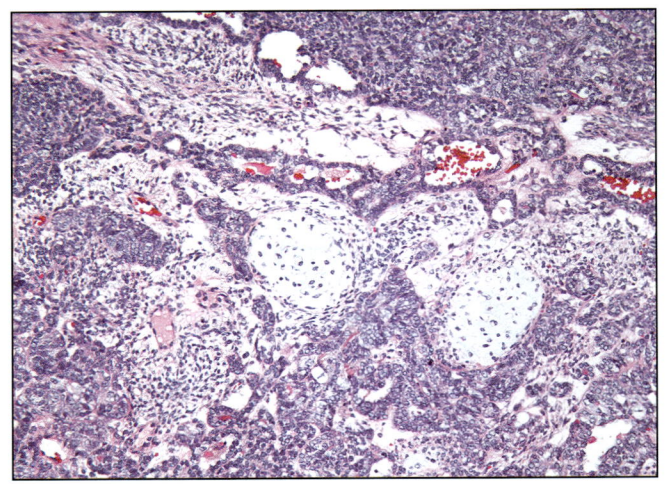

图13E.40　癌肉瘤。注意癌的成分是腺癌。

生殖道横纹肌瘤　Genital rhabdomyoma

生殖道横纹肌瘤是良性肿瘤，由成熟的横纹肌母细胞组成，偶尔可能累及宫颈，但是最常发生于阴道（见723页）。

胚胎性横纹肌肉瘤[157-160]　Embryonal rhabdomyosarcoma

胚胎性横纹肌肉瘤的葡萄状肉瘤（sarcoma botryoides）亚型较常累及阴道，但是在罕见的情况下也可能累及宫颈。宫颈葡萄状肉瘤的高发年龄一般在10～30岁，虽然个别病例发生于婴儿以及40～50岁的妇女。这种发病年龄不同于发生在阴道的肿瘤，阴道葡萄状肉瘤一般累及婴儿和幼儿。与阴道来源的肿瘤相似，宫颈葡萄状肉瘤也常常呈息肉样或具有"葡萄簇"的大体表现。最常见的症状包括阴道出血和感到阴道入口处有一个肿块。组织学检查，宫颈来源的肿瘤与发生于阴道的肿瘤具有同样的形态学表现（见724页）。然而值得注意的是，在某些病例可能出现软骨分化[158]。某些研究显示，与阴道原发性肿瘤相比，宫颈原发性肿瘤病人具有更加良好的结局[158]，这些病人可以采用保守的保留生育能力的治疗，即局部切除后接着进行化疗。

平滑肌肉瘤[161-164]　Leiomyosarcoma

宫颈原发性平滑肌肉瘤非常罕见。病人一般在围绝经期，平均年龄40～50岁，最常见的症状是异常阴道出血。恶性标准同用于子宫体平滑肌肿瘤的标准（见690页）。

子宫内膜间质肉瘤，低级别　Endometrioid stromal sarcoma, low-grade

在罕见的情况下，形态上类似于低级别子宫内膜间质肉瘤的肿瘤可以作为原发性肿瘤发生于宫颈，或为单纯性，或为复合性恶性混合性肿瘤或腺肉瘤[151,165]。主要的鉴别诊断是腺肌症，特别是单纯性肿瘤，腺肌症也可以表现为异常阴道出血。典型的宫颈腺肌症界限清楚，不出现间质肉瘤特征性的生长方式[166]。

腺泡状软组织肉瘤[167,168]　Alveolar soft part sarcoma

腺泡状软组织肉瘤较常发生于年轻成人的肢体，但在少数情况下可以发生于女性生殖道，包括阴道、宫颈和子宫体。病人年龄通常小于40岁，表现为异常阴道出血。宫颈原发性腺泡状软组织肉瘤与软组织腺泡状软组织肉瘤具有同样的特征性形态学表现和免疫表型（见第24章）。

恶性外周神经鞘肿瘤（恶性神经鞘瘤）[169]　Malignant peripheral nerve sheath tumor (malignant schwannoma)

宫颈恶性外周神经鞘肿瘤非常少见，最大系列病例报告仅有3个病人[169]。在这项研究中，病人年龄为25、65和73岁，其中两例表现为异常阴道出血。两例肿瘤呈息肉状，一例为溃疡性，大小为1.3、4.4和5.0cm。组织学检查，肿瘤由细胞丰富和细胞稀少的成束的梭形细胞带组成，类似于发生在软组织的恶性外周神经鞘肿瘤（见第27章）。所有肿瘤的核分裂均活跃，S-100蛋白阳性，肌肉标志物阴性。两例病人随访显示，一例在15个月时没有肿瘤证据，另外一例在子宫切除术后2年有多发性腹腔转移。

黑色素细胞肿瘤　Melanocytic tumors

蓝痣　Blue nevus

宫颈蓝痣类似于皮肤蓝痣，由增生的树突状黑色素细胞构成，常常有大量的色素，位于接近上皮界面的宫颈间质。最常见于宫颈管后部，通常是在中年妇女的子宫切除标本中偶然发现的。通过临床检查一般不能发现这些病变，但是可能有一种蓝黑色的大体表现。检查宫颈连续切片发现，多达29%的病例间质中可见灶状黑色素细胞，提示宫颈间质树突状黑色素细胞比最初评估的要常见。推测宫颈恶性黑色素瘤可能从这些细胞发生。

恶性黑色素瘤[170,171]　Malignant melanoma

宫颈原发性恶性黑色素瘤非常罕见，文献中大约有30例病例报告，其中某些病例记录不全。病人平均年龄 50～60 岁，通常表现为异常阴道出血。临床检查一般发现一个外生性脆而易碎的肿块，其外观可能有色素沉着，呈灰色、蓝色或黑色，或可能为无黑色素性。肿瘤的组织学表现与其他部位黑色素瘤类似，具有梭形和（或）上皮样表现；也可能发生酷似透明细胞癌的透明细胞变型。黑色素瘤标志物（S-100、HMB-45、Mart-1 和 Melan-A）阳性有助于黑色素瘤与类似肿瘤的鉴别。多数病人为 I 期或 II 期；然而，预后很差，多数病人在 2 年之内死于本病。

其他罕见肿瘤
Miscellaneous rare tumors

肾外 Wilms 瘤[172-177]
Extrarenal Wilms tumor

宫颈的肾外 Wilms 瘤罕见，文献中仅有 6 例发生于子宫的报告。病人年龄为 2、11、13、13、14 和 22 岁。2 例肿瘤来源于宫颈，其余的发生于子宫体。所有的病人均有息肉样肿块，大小从 2.2 到 17cm。组织学检查，这些肿瘤呈现特征性的 Wilms 瘤表现。1 例死于本病，1 例于切除之后 7 个月发生广泛腹腔内复发，3 例 2、5.6 和 9.6 年之后没有疾病的证据。

卵黄囊瘤（内胚窦瘤）[178]
Yolk sac tumor (endodermal sinus tumor)

在少数情况下，卵黄囊瘤可以累及下生殖道，较常见于阴道和宫颈。肿瘤一般呈息肉样，病人通常出现异常阴道出血。宫颈卵黄囊瘤的组织学表现类似于卵巢卵黄囊瘤（见 605 页）。

成熟囊性畸胎瘤　Mature cystic teratoma

发生于宫颈的成熟畸胎瘤已有少数病例报告，一般表现为一个息肉样肿块，组织学上由内胚层、中胚层和外胚层成分组成[179-181]。

造血肿瘤　Hematopoietic tumors

非 Hodgkin 淋巴瘤偶尔可以累及女性生殖道，作为原发性病变或有系统性扩散的证据。最常见的类型是弥漫性大 B 细胞淋巴瘤[182]。

粒细胞肉瘤（granulocytic sarcoma）[183-185]（急性髓细胞白血病累及软组织/器官）在少数情况下最初表现为一个宫颈原发性肿瘤，更为罕见的是这种表现可以在明显的白血病出现之前数周或数月发生。病人通常表现为异常出血（月经频多、性交后或绝经后出血），肿瘤易于造成其上黏膜变薄或有溃疡形成。累及女性生殖道的粒细胞肉瘤与其他部位髓外组织的粒细胞肉瘤具有同样的形态学特征和免疫表型（见第 21 章）。

参考文献

1. Rosenfeld W D, Rose E, Vermund S H et al. 1992 Follow-up evaluation of cervicovaginal human papillomavirus infection in adolescents. J Pediatr 121: 307–311
2. Melkert P W, Hopman E, van den Brule A J et al. 1993 Prevalence of HPV in cytomorphologically normal cervical smears, as determined by the polymerase chain reaction, is age-dependent. Int J Cancer 53: 919–923
3. Moscicki A B 1998 Genital infections with human papillomavirus (HPV). Pediatr Infect Dis J 17: 651–652
4. Moscicki A B, Shiboski S, Broering J et al. 1998 The natural history of human papillomavirus infection as measured by repeated DNA testing in adolescent and young women. J Pediatr 132: 277–284
5. Levert M, Clavel C, Graesslin O et al. 2000 [Human papillomavirus typing in routine cervical smears. Results from a series of 3778 patients.] Gynecol Obstet Fertil 28: 722–728
6. Lorincz A T, Reid R, Jenson A B et al. 1992 Human papillomavirus infection of the cervix: relative risk associations of 15 common anogenital types. Obstet Gynecol 79: 328–337
7. Koutsky L A, Holmes K K, Critchlow C W et al. 1992 A cohort study of the risk of cervical intraepithelial neoplasia grade 2 or 3 in relation to papillomavirus infection. N Engl J Med 327: 1272–1278
8. Brown M R, Noffsinger A, First M R et al. 2000 HPV subtype analysis in lower genital tract neoplasms of female renal transplant recipients. Gynecol Oncol 79: 220–224
9. Alloub M I, Barr B B, McLaren K M et al. 1989 Human papillomavirus infection and cervical intraepithelial neoplasia in women with renal allografts. BMJ 298: 153–156
10. Halpert R, Fruchter R G, Sedlis A et al. 1986 Human papillomavirus and lower genital neoplasia in renal transplant patients. Obstet Gynecol 68: 251–258
11. Wright T C Jr, Sun X W 1996 Anogenital papillomavirus infection and neoplasia in immunodeficient women. Obstet Gynecol Clin North Am 23: 861–893
12. Moscicki A B, Ellenberg J H, Vermund S H et al. 2000 Prevalence of and risks for cervical human papillomavirus infection and squamous intraepithelial lesions in adolescent girls: impact of infection with human immunodeficiency virus. Arch Pediatr Adolesc Med 154: 127–134
13. La Ruche G, You B, Mensah-Ado I et al. 1998 Human papillomavirus and human immunodeficiency virus infections: relation with cervical dysplasia-neoplasia in African women. Int J Cancer 76: 480–486
14. Trivijitsilp P, Mosher R, Sheets E E et al. 1998 Papillary immature metaplasia (immature condyloma) of the cervix: a clinicopathologic analysis and comparison with papillary squamous carcinoma. Hum Pathol 29: 641–648
15. Ward B E, Saleh A M, Williams J V et al. 1992 Papillary immature metaplasia of the cervix: a distinct subset of exophytic cervical condyloma associated with HPV-6/11 nucleic acids. Mod Pathol 5: 391–395
16. Resnick M, Lester S, Tate J E et al. 1996 Viral and histopathologic correlates of MN and MIB-1 expression in cervical intraepithelial neoplasia. Hum Pathol 27: 234–239
17. Mittal K 1999 Utility of proliferation-associated marker MIB-1 in evaluating lesions of the uterine cervix. Adv Anat Pathol 6: 177–185
18. Mittal K, Palazzo J 1998 Cervical condylomas show higher proliferation than do inflamed or metaplastic cervical squamous epithelium. Mod Pathol 11: 780–783
19. Keating J T, Cviko A, Riethdorf S et al. 2001 Ki-67, cyclin E, and p16INK4 are complimentary surrogate biomarkers for human papilloma virus-related cervical neoplasia. Am J Surg Pathol 25: 884–891
20. Kaku T, Kamura T, Sakai K et al. 1997 Early adenocarcinoma of the uterine cervix. Gynecol Oncol 65: 281–285
21. Ostor A, Rome R, Quinn M 1997 Microinvasive adenocarcinoma of the cervix: a clinicopathologic study of 77 women. Obstet Gynecol 89: 88–93
22. Lee K R, Flynn C E 2000 Early invasive adenocarcinoma of the cervix. Cancer 89: 1048–1055
23. Tase T, Okagaki T, Clark B A et al. 1989 Human papillomavirus DNA in adenocarcinoma in situ, microinvasive adenocarcinoma of the uterine cervix, and coexisting cervical squamous intraepithelial neoplasia. Int J Gynecol Pathol 8: 8–17
24. Boon M E, Baak J P, Kurver P J et al. 1981 Adenocarcinoma in situ of the cervix: an underdiagnosed lesion. Cancer 48: 768–773

25. Kashimura M, Shinohara M, Oikawa K et al. 1990 An adenocarcinoma in situ of the uterine cervix that developed into invasive adenocarcinoma after 5 years. Gynecol Oncol 36: 128–133
26. Boddington M M, Spriggs A I, Cowdell R H 1976 Adenocarcinoma of the uterine cervix: cytological evidence of a long preclinical evolution. Br J Obstet Gynaecol 83: 900–903
27. Hocking G R, Hayman J A, Ostor A G 1996 Adenocarcinoma in situ of the uterine cervix progressing to invasive adenocarcinoma. Aust NZ J Obstet Gynaecol 36: 218–220
28. Andersen E S, Arffmann E 1989 Adenocarcinoma in situ of the uterine cervix: a clinico-pathologic study of 36 cases. Gynecol Oncol 35: 1–7
29. Tobon H, Dave H 1988 Adenocarcinoma in situ of the cervix. Clinicopathologic observations of 11 cases. Int J Gynecol Pathol 7: 139–151
30. Krane J F, Granter S R, Trask C E et al. 2001 Papanicolaou smear sensitivity for the detection of adenocarcinoma of the cervix: a study of 49 cases. Cancer 93: 8–15
31. Schoolland M, Segal A, Allpress S et al. 2002 Adenocarcinoma in situ of the cervix. Cancer 96: 330–337
32. Lee K R, Minter L J, Granter S R 1997 Papanicolaou smear sensitivity for adenocarcinoma in situ of the cervix. A study of 34 cases. Am J Clin Pathol 107: 30–35
33. Ostor A G, Duncan A, Quinn M et al. 2000 Adenocarcinoma in situ of the uterine cervix: an experience with 100 cases. Gynecol Oncol 79: 207–210
34. Andersen E S, Nielsen K 2002 Adenocarcinoma in situ of the cervix: a prospective study of conization as definitive treatment. Gynecol Oncol 86: 365–369
35. Im D D, Duska L R, Rosenshein N B 1995 Adequacy of conization margins in adenocarcinoma in situ of the cervix as a predictor of residual disease. Gynecol Oncol 59: 179–182
36. Wolf J K, Levenback C, Malpica A et al. 1996 Adenocarcinoma in situ of the cervix: significance of cone biopsy margins. Obstet Gynecol 88: 82–86
37. Denehy T R, Gregori C A, Breen J L 1997 Endocervical curettage, cone margins, and residual adenocarcinoma in situ of the cervix. Obstet Gynecol 90: 1–6
38. Goldstein N S, Mani A 1998 The status and distance of cone biopsy margins as a predictor of excision adequacy for endocervical adenocarcinoma in situ. Am J Clin Pathol 109: 727–732
39. Azodi M, Chambers S K, Rutherford T J et al. 1999 Adenocarcinoma in situ of the cervix: management and outcome. Gynecol Oncol 73: 348–353
40. Poynor E A, Barakat R R, Hoskins W J 1995 Management and follow-up of patients with adenocarcinoma in situ of the uterine cervix. Gynecol Oncol 57: 158–164
41. Kennedy A W, Biscotti C V 2002 Further study of the management of cervical adenocarcinoma in situ. Gynecol Oncol 86: 361–364
42. Shin C H, Schorge J O, Lee K R et al. 2000 Conservative management of adenocarcinoma in situ of the cervix. Gynecol Oncol 79: 6–10
43. Jaworski R C, Pacey N F, Greenberg M L et al. 1988 The histologic diagnosis of adenocarcinoma in situ and related lesions of the cervix uteri. Adenocarcinoma in situ. Cancer 61: 1171–1181
44. Bertrand M, Lickrish G M, Colgan T J 1987 The anatomic distribution of cervical adenocarcinoma in situ: implications for treatment. Am J Obstet Gynecol 157: 21–25
45. Weisbrot I M, Stabinsky C, Davis A M 1972 Adenocarcinoma in situ of the uterine cervix. Cancer 29: 1179–1187
46. Biscotti C V, Hart W R 1998 Apoptotic bodies: a consistent morphologic feature of endocervical adenocarcinoma in situ. Am J Surg Pathol 22: 434–439
47. Moritani S, Ioffe O B, Sagae S et al. 2002 Mitotic activity and apoptosis in endocervical glandular lesions. Int J Gynecol Pathol 21: 125–133
48. Schlesinger C, Silverberg S G 1999 Endocervical adenocarcinoma in situ of tubal type and its relation to atypical tubal metaplasia. Int J Gynecol Pathol 18: 1–4
49. Willett G D, Kurman R J, Reid R et al. 1989 Correlation of the histologic appearance of intraepithelial neoplasia of the cervix with human papillomavirus types. Emphasis on low grade lesions including so-called flat condyloma. Int J Gynecol Pathol 8: 18–25
50. Park J J, Sun D, Quade B J et al. 2000 Stratified mucin-producing intraepithelial lesions of the cervix: adenosquamous or columnar cell neoplasia? Am J Surg Pathol 24: 1414–1419
51. Parkin D M, Bray F, Ferlay J et al. 2001 Estimating the world cancer burden: Globocan 2000. Int J Cancer 94: 153–156
52. Landis S H, Murray T, Bolden S et al. 1999 Cancer statistics, 1999. CA Cancer J Clin 49: 8–31
53. Vizcaino A P, Moreno V, Bosch F X et al. 2000 International trends in incidence of cervical cancer: II. Squamous-cell carcinoma. Int J Cancer 86: 429–435
54. Pretorius R, Semrad N, Watring W et al. 1991 Presentation of cervical cancer. Gynecol Oncol 42: 48–53
55. Wong W S, Ng C S, Lee C K 1990 Verrucous carcinoma of the cervix. Arch Gynecol Obstet 247: 47–51
56. Koenig C, Turnicky R P, Kankam C F et al. 1997 Papillary squamotransitional cell carcinoma of the cervix: a report of 32 cases. Am J Surg Pathol 21: 915–921
57. Qizilbash A H 1975 In-situ and microinvasive adenocarcinoma of the uterine cervix. A clinical, cytologic and histologic study of 14 cases. Am J Clin Pathol 64: 155–170
58. Christopherson W M, Nealon N, Gray L A Sr 1979 Noninvasive precursor lesions of adenocarcinoma and mixed adenosquamous carcinoma of the cervix uteri. Cancer 44: 975–983
59. Yeh I T, LiVolsi V A, Noumoff J S 1991 Endocervical carcinoma. Pathol Res Pract 187: 129–144
60. Noda K, Kimura K, Ikeda M et al. 1983 Studies on the histogenesis of cervical adenocarcinoma. Int J Gynecol Pathol 1: 336–346
61. Burghardt E 1984 Microinvasive carcinoma in gynaecological pathology. Clin Obstet Gynaecol 11: 239–257
62. Buscema J, Woodruff J D 1984 Significance of neoplastic atypicalities in endocervical epithelium. Gynecol Oncol 17: 356–362
63. Schorge J O, Lee K R, Flynn C E et al. 1999 Stage IA1 cervical adenocarcinoma: definition and treatment. Obstet Gynecol 93: 219–222
64. Webb J C, Key C R, Qualls C R et al. 2001 Population-based study of microinvasive adenocarcinoma of the uterine cervix. Obstet Gynecol 97: 701–706
65. Kaspar H G, Dinh T V, Doherty M G et al. 1993 Clinical implications of tumor volume measurement in stage I adenocarcinoma of the cervix. Obstet Gynecol 81: 296–300
66. Berek J S, Hacker N F, Fu Y S et al. 1985 Adenocarcinoma of the uterine cervix: histologic variables associated with lymph node metastasis and survival. Obstet Gynecol 65: 46–52
67. Teshima S, Shimosato Y, Kishi K et al. 1985 Early stage adenocarcinoma of the uterine cervix. Histopathologic analysis with consideration of histogenesis. Cancer 56: 167–172
68. Smith H O, Qualls C R, Romero A A et al. 2002 Is there a difference in survival for IA1 and IA2 adenocarcinoma of the uterine cervix? Gynecol Oncol 85: 229–241
68a. Ceballos K M, Shaw D, Daya D 2006 Microinvasive cervical adenocarcinoma (FIGO stage 1A tumors): results of surgical staging and outcome analysis. Am J Surg Pathol 30: 370–374
69. Peters R K, Chao A, Mack T M et al. 1986 Increased frequency of adenocarcinoma of the uterine cervix in young women in Los Angeles County. J Natl Cancer Inst 76: 423–428
70. Smith H O, Tiffany M F, Qualls C R et al. 2000 The rising incidence of adenocarcinoma relative to squamous cell carcinoma of the uterine cervix in the United States – a 24-year population-based study. Gynecol Oncol 78: 97–105
71. Pirog E C, Kleter B, Olgac S et al. 2000 Prevalence of human papilloma virus DNA in different histological subtypes of cervical adenocarcinoma. Am J Pathol 157: 1055–1062
72. Young R H, Clement P B 2002 Endocervical adenocarcinoma and its variants: their morphology and differential diagnosis. Histopathology 41: 185–207
73. Miller B E, Flax S D, Arheart K et al. 1993 The presentation of adenocarcinoma of the uterine cervix. Cancer 72: 1281–1285
74. An H J, Kim K R, Kim I S et al. 2005 Prevalence of human papillomavirus DNA in various histological subtypes of cervical adenocarcinoma: a population-based study. Mod Pathol 18: 528–534
75. McKelvey J L, Goodlin R R 1963 Adenoma malignum of the cervix. Cancer 16: 549–557
76. Silverberg S G, Hurt W G 1975 Minimal deviation adenocarcinoma ("adenoma malignum") of the cervix: a reappraisal. Am J Obstet Gynecol 121: 971–975
77. Kaku T, Enjoji M 1983 Extremely well-differentiated adenocarcinoma ("adenoma malignum") of the cervix. Int J Gynecol Pathol 2: 28–41
78. Kaminski P F, Norris H J 1983 Minimal deviation carcinoma (adenoma malignum) of the cervix. Int J Gynecol Pathol 2: 141–152
79. Gilks C B, Young R H, Aguirre P et al. 1989 Adenoma malignum (minimal deviation adenocarcinoma) of the uterine cervix. A clinicopathological and immunohistochemical analysis of 26 cases. Am J Surg Pathol 13: 717–729
80. Michael H, Grawe L, Kraus F T 1984 Minimal deviation endocervical adenocarcinoma: clinical and histologic features, immunohistochemical staining for carcinoembryonic antigen, and differentiation from confusing benign lesions. Int J Gynecol Pathol 3: 261–276
81. Lee J Y, Dong S M, Kim H S et al. 1998 A distinct region of chromosome 19p13.3 associated with the sporadic form of adenoma malignum of the uterine cervix. Cancer Res 58: 1140–1143
82. Kuragaki C, Enomoto T, Ueno Y et al. 2003 Mutations in the STK11 gene characterize minimal deviation adenocarcinoma of the uterine cervix. Lab Invest 83: 35–45
83. LiVolsi V A, Merino M J, Schwartz P E 1983 Coexistent endocervical adenocarcinoma and mucinous adenocarcinoma of ovary: a clinicopathologic study of four cases. Int J Gynecol Pathol 1: 391–402
84. Kaminski P F, Norris H J 1984 Coexistence of ovarian neoplasms and endocervical adenocarcinoma. Obstet Gynecol 64: 553–556
85. Young R H, Scully R E 1988 Mucinous ovarian tumors associated with mucinous adenocarcinomas of the cervix. A clinicopathological analysis of 16 cases. Int J Gynecol Pathol 7: 99–111
86. Hayashi I, Tsuda H, Shimoda T 2000 Reappraisal of orthodox histochemistry for the diagnosis of minimal deviation adenocarcinoma of the cervix. Am J Surg Pathol 24: 559–562
87. Utsugi K, Hirai Y, Takeshima N et al. 1999 Utility of the monoclonal antibody HIK1083 in the diagnosis of adenoma malignum of the uterine cervix. Gynecol Oncol 75: 345–348
88. Young R H, Scully R E 1989 Villoglandular papillary adenocarcinoma of the uterine cervix. A clinicopathologic analysis of 13 cases. Cancer 63: 1773–1779

89. Hopson L, Jones M A, Boyce C R et al. 1990 Papillary villoglandular carcinoma of the cervix. Gynecol Oncol 39: 221–224
90. Jones M W, Silverberg S G, Kurman R J 1993 Well-differentiated villoglandular adenocarcinoma of the uterine cervix: a clinicopathological study of 24 cases. Int J Gynecol Pathol 12: 1–7
91. Kaku T, Kamura T, Shigematsu T et al. 1997 Adenocarcinoma of the uterine cervix with predominantly villogladular papillary growth pattern. Gynecol Oncol 64: 147–152
92. Jones M W, Kounelis S, Papadaki H et al. 2000 Well-differentiated villoglandular adenocarcinoma of the uterine cervix: oncogene/tumor suppressor gene alterations and human papillomavirus genotyping. Int J Gynecol Pathol 19: 110–117
93. Mayorga M, Garcia-Valtuille A, Fernandez F et al. 1997 Adenocarcinoma of the uterine cervix with massive signet ring cell differentiation. Int J Surg Pathol 5: 95–100
94. Haswani P, Arseneau J, Ferenczy A 1998 Primary signet ring cell carcinoma of the uterine cervix: a clinicopathologic study of two cases with review of the literature. Int J Gynecol Cancer 8: 374–379
95. Fox H, Wells M, Harris M et al. 1988 Enteric tumours of the lower female genital tract: a report of three cases. Histopathology 12: 167–176
96. Lee K R, Trainer T D 1990 Adenocarcinoma of the uterine cervix of small intestinal type containing numerous Paneth cells. Arch Pathol Lab Med 114: 731–733
97. Schorge J O, Lee K R, Lee S J et al. 1999 Early cervical adenocarcinoma: selection criteria for radical surgery. Obstet Gynecol 94: 386–390
98. Zaino R J 2002 The fruits of our labors: distinguishing endometrial from endocervical adenocarcinoma. Int J Gynecol Pathol 21: 1–3
99. Young R H, Scully R E 1993 Minimal-deviation endometrioid adenocarcinoma of the uterine cervix. A report of five cases of a distinctive neoplasm that may be misinterpreted as benign. Am J Surg Pathol 17: 660–665
100. Rahilly M A, Williams A R, Al Nafussi A 1992 Minimal deviation endometrioid adenocarcinoma of cervix: a clinicopathological and immunohistochemical study of two cases. Histopathology 20: 351–354
101. Nordqvist S R, Fidler W J Jr, Woodruff J M et al. 1976 Clear cell adenocarcinoma of the cervix and vagina. A clinicopathologic study of 21 cases with and without a history of maternal ingestion of estrogens. Cancer 37: 858–871
102. Herbst A L, Cole P, Colton T et al. 1977 Age-incidence and risk of diethylstilbestrol-related clear cell adenocarcinoma of the vagina and cervix. Am J Obstet Gynecol 128: 43–50
103. Hanselaar A, van Loosbroek M, Schuurbiers O et al. 1997 Clear cell adenocarcinoma of the vagina and cervix. An update of the central Netherlands registry showing twin age incidence peaks. Cancer 79: 2229–2236
104. Reich O, Tamussino K, Lahousen M et al. 2000 Clear cell carcinoma of the uterine cervix: pathology and prognosis in surgically treated stage IB–IIB disease in women not exposed in utero to diethylstilbestrol. Gynecol Oncol 76: 331–335
105. Jones W B, Tan L K, Lewis J L Jr 1993 Late recurrence of clear cell adenocarcinoma of the vagina and cervix: a report of three cases. Gynecol Oncol 51: 266–271
106. Zhou C, Gilks C B, Hayes M et al. 1998 Papillary serous carcinoma of the uterine cervix: a clinicopathologic study of 17 cases. Am J Surg Pathol 22: 113–120
107. Ferry J A, Scully R E 1990 Mesonephric remnants, hyperplasia, and neoplasia in the uterine cervix. A study of 49 cases. Am J Surg Pathol 14: 1100–1111
108. Clement P B, Young R H, Keh P et al. 1995 Malignant mesonephric neoplasms of the uterine cervix. A report of eight cases, including four with a malignant spindle cell component. Am J Surg Pathol 19: 1158–1171
109. Silver S A, Devouassoux-Shisheboran M, Mezzetti T P et al. 2001 Mesonephric adenocarcinomas of the uterine cervix: a study of 11 cases with immunohistochemical findings. Am J Surg Pathol 25: 379–387
110. Look K Y, Brunetto V L, Clarke-Pearson D L et al. 1996 An analysis of cell type in patients with surgically staged stage IB carcinoma of the cervix: a Gynecologic Oncology Group study. Gynecol Oncol 63: 304–311
111. Alfsen G C, Kristensen G B, Skovlund E et al. 2001 Histologic subtype has minor importance for overall survival in patients with adenocarcinoma of the uterine cervix: a population-based study of prognostic factors in 505 patients with nonsquamous cell carcinomas of the cervix. Cancer 92: 2471–2483
112. Ulbright T M, Gersell D J 1983 Glassy cell carcinoma of the uterine cervix. A light and electron microscopic study of five cases. Cancer 51: 2255–2263
113. Littman P, Clement P B, Henriksen B et al. 1976 Glassy cell carcinoma of the cervix. Cancer 37: 2238–2246
114. Costa M J, Kenny M B, Hewan-Lowe K et al. 1991 Glassy cell features in adenosquamous carcinoma of the uterine cervix. Histologic, ultrastructural, immunohistochemical, and clinical findings. Am J Clin Pathol 96: 520–528
115. Pak H Y, Yokota S B, Paladugu R R et al. 1983 Glassy cell carcinoma of the cervix. Cytologic and clinicopathological analysis. Cancer 52: 307–312
116. Cherry C P, Glucksmann A 1956 Incidence, histology, and response to radiation of mixed carcinomas (adenoacanthomas) of the uterine cervix. Cancer 9: 971–979
117. Fujiwara H, Mitchell M F, Arseneau J et al. 1995 Clear cell adenosquamous carcinoma of the cervix. An aggressive tumor associated with human papillomavirus-18. Cancer 76: 1591–1600
118. Baggish M S, Woodruff J D 1966 Adenoid-basal carcinoma of the cervix. Obstet Gynecol 28: 213–218
119. Cviko A, Briem B, Granter S R et al. 2000 Adenoid basal carcinomas of the cervix: a unique morphological evolution with cell cycle correlates. Hum Pathol 31: 740–744
120. Grayson W, Taylor L F, Cooper K 1999 Adenoid cystic and adenoid basal carcinoma of the uterine cervix: comparative morphologic, mucin, and immunohistochemical profile of two rare neoplasms of putative 'reserve cell' origin. Am J Surg Pathol 23: 448–458
121. Brainard J A, Hart W R 1998 Adenoid basal epitheliomas of the uterine cervix: a reevaluation of distinctive cervical basaloid lesions currently classified as adenoid basal carcinoma and adenoid basal hyperplasia. Am J Surg Pathol 22: 965–975
122. Grayson W, Taylor L F, Cooper K 1997 Adenoid basal carcinoma of the uterine cervix: detection of integrated human papillomavirus in a rare tumor of putative "reserve cell" origin. Int J Gynecol Pathol 16: 307–312
123. Jones M W, Kounelis S, Papadaki H et al. 1997 The origin and molecular characterization of adenoid basal carcinoma of the uterine cervix. Int J Gynecol Pathol 16: 301–306
124. Ferry J A, Scully R E 1988 "Adenoid cystic" carcinoma and adenoid basal carcinoma of the uterine cervix. A study of 28 cases. Am J Surg Pathol 12: 134–144
125. van Dinh T, Woodruff J D 1985 Adenoid cystic and adenoid basal carcinomas of the cervix. Obstet Gynecol 65: 705–709
126. Daroca P J Jr, Dhurandhar H N 1980 Basaloid carcinoma of uterine cervix. Am J Surg Pathol 4: 235–239
127. Grayson W, Cooper K 2000 Adenoid basal epithelioma versus adenoid basal carcinoma. Am J Surg Pathol 24: 313–314
128. Grayson W, Cooper K 2002 A reappraisal of "basaloid carcinoma" of the cervix, and the differential diagnosis of basaloid cervical neoplasms. Adv Anat Pathol 9: 290–300
129. Albores-Saavedra J, Manivel C, Mora A et al. 1992 The solid variant of adenoid cystic carcinoma of the cervix. Int J Gynecol Pathol 11: 2–10
130. Albores-Saavedra J, Gersell D, Gilks C B et al. 1997 Terminology of endocrine tumors of the uterine cervix: results of a workshop sponsored by the College of American Pathologists and the National Cancer Institute. Arch Pathol Lab Med 121: 34–39
131. Stoler M H, Mills S E, Gersell D J et al. 1991 Small-cell neuroendocrine carcinoma of the cervix. A human papillomavirus type 18-associated cancer. Am J Surg Pathol 15: 28–32
132. Wistuba I I, Thomas B, Behrens C et al. 1999 Molecular abnormalities associated with endocrine tumors of the uterine cervix. Gynecol Oncol 72: 3–9
133. Delaloge S, Pautier P, Kerbrat P et al. 2000 Neuroendocrine small cell carcinoma of the uterine cervix: what disease? What treatment? Report of ten cases and a review of the literature. Clin Oncol (R Coll Radiol) 12: 357–362
134. Weed J C Jr, Graff A T, Shoup B et al. 2003 Small cell undifferentiated (neuroendocrine) carcinoma of the uterine cervix. J Am Coll Surg 197: 44–51
135. Boruta D M, Schorge J O, Duska L A et al. 2001 Multimodality therapy in early-stage neuroendocrine carcinoma of the uterine cervix. Gynecol Oncol 81: 82–87
136. Walker A N, Mills S E, Taylor P T 1988 Cervical neuroendocrine carcinoma: a clinical and light microscopic study of 14 cases. Int J Gynecol Pathol 7: 64–74
137. Connor M G, Richter H, Moran C A et al. 2002 Small cell carinoma of the cervix: a clinicopathologic and immunohistochemical study of 23 cases. Ann Diagn Pathol 6: 345–348
138. Gilks C B, Young R H, Gersell D J et al. 1997 Large cell neuroendocrine carcinoma of the uterine cervix: a clinicopathologic study of 12 cases. Am J Surg Pathol 21: 905–914
139. Schmedding A, Zense M, Fuchs J et al. 1997 Benign papilloma of the cervix in childhood: immunohistochemical findings and review of the literature. Eur J Pediatr 156: 320–322
140. Smith Y R, Quint E H, Hinton E L 1998 Recurrent benign Müllerian papilloma of the cervix. J Pediatr Adolesc Gynecol 11: 29–31
141. Caroti S, Siliotti F 1988 Cervical polyps: a colpo-cyto-histological study. Clin Exp Obstet Gynecol 15: 108–115
142. Golan A, Ber A, Wolman I et al. 1994 Cervical polyp: evaluation of current treatment. Gynecol Obstet Invest 37: 56–58
143. Vilodre L C, Bertat R, Petters R et al. 1997 Cervical polyp as risk factor for hysteroscopically diagnosed endometrial polyps. Gynecol Obstet Invest 44: 191–195
144. Zaloudek C J, Norris H J 1981 Adenofibroma and adenosarcoma of the uterus: a clinicopathologic study of 35 cases. Cancer 48: 354–366
145. Gilks C B, Young R H, Clement P B et al. 1996 Adenomyomas of the uterine cervix of endocervical type: a report of ten cases of a benign cervical tumor that may be confused with adenoma malignum. Mod Pathol 9: 220–224
146. Verschraegen C F, Vasuratna A, Edwards C et al. 1998 Clinicopathologic analysis of Müllerian adenosarcoma: the M.D. Anderson Cancer Center experience. Oncol Rep 5: 939–944
147. Jones M W, Lefkowitz M 1995 Adenosarcoma of the uterine cervix: a clinicopathological study of 12 cases. Int J Gynecol Pathol 14: 223–229
148. Kerner H, Lichtig C 1993 Müllerian adenosarcoma presenting as cervical polyps: a report of seven cases and review of the literature. Obstet Gynecol 81: 655–659

149. Ramos P, Ruiz A, Carabias E et al. 2002 Müllerian adenosarcoma of the cervix with heterologous elements: report of a case and review of the literature. Gynecol Oncol 84: 161–166
150. Park H M, Park M H, Kim Y J et al. 2004 Müllerian adenosarcoma with sarcomatous overgrowth of the cervix presenting as cervical polyp: a case report and review of the literature. Int J Gynecol Cancer 14: 1024–1029
151. Clement P B, Zubovits J T, Young R H et al. 1998 Malignant Müllerian mixed tumors of the uterine cervix: a report of nine cases of a neoplasm with morphology often different from its counterpart in the corpus. Int J Gynecol Pathol 17: 211–222
152. Grayson W, Taylor L F, Cooper K 2001 Carcinosarcoma of the uterine cervix: a report of eight cases with immunohistochemical analysis and evaluation of human papillomavirus status. Am J Surg Pathol 25: 338–347
153. Manhoff D T, Schiffman R, Haupt H M 1995 Adenoid cystic carcinoma of the uterine cervix with malignant stroma. An unusual variant of carcinosarcoma? Am J Surg Pathol 19: 229–233
154. Yannacou N, Gerolymatos A, Parissi-Mathiou P et al. 2000 Carcinosarcoma of the uterine cervix composed of an adenoid cystic carcinoma and an homologous stromal sarcoma. A case report. Eur J Gynaecol Oncol 21: 292–294
155. Takeshima Y, Amatya V J, Nakayori F et al. 2002 Co-existent carcinosarcoma and adenoid basal carcinoma of the uterine cervix and correlation with human papillomavirus infection. Int J Gynecol Pathol 21: 186–190
156. Tiltman A J 1998 Leiomyomas of the uterine cervix: a study of frequency. Int J Gynecol Pathol 17: 231–234
157. Brand E, Berek J S, Nieberg R K et al. 1987 Rhabdomyosarcoma of the uterine cervix. Sarcoma botryoides. Cancer 60: 1552–1560
158. Daya D A, Scully R E 1988 Sarcoma botryoides of the uterine cervix in young women: a clinicopathological study of 13 cases. Gynecol Oncol 29: 290–304
159. Bernal K L, Fahmy L, Remmenga S et al. 2004 Embryonal rhabdomyosarcoma (sarcoma botryoides) of the cervix presenting as a cervical polyp treated with fertility-sparing surgery and adjuvant chemotherapy. Gynecol Oncol 95: 243–246
160. Miyamoto T, Shiozawa T, Nakamura T et al. 2004 Sarcoma botryoides of the uterine cervix in a 46-year-old woman: case report and literature review. Int J Gynecol Pathol 23: 78–82
161. Kasamatsu T, Shiromizu K, Takahashi M et al. 1998 Leiomyosarcoma of the uterine cervix. Gynecol Oncol 69: 169–171
162. Grayson W, Fourie J, Tiltman A J 1998 Xanthomatous leiomyosarcoma of the uterine cervix. Int J Gynecol Pathol 17: 89–90
163. Gotoh T, Kikuchi Y, Takano M et al. 2001 Epithelioid leiomyosarcoma of the uterine cervix. Gynecol Oncol 82: 400–405
164. Irvin W, Presley A, Andersen W et al. 2003 Leiomyosarcoma of the cervix. Gynecol Oncol 91: 636–642
165. Boardman C H, Webb M J, Jefferies J A 2000 Low-grade endometrial stromal sarcoma of the ectocervix after therapy for breast cancer. Gynecol Oncol 79: 120–123
166. Clement P B, Young R H, Scully R E 1990 Stromal endometriosis of the uterine cervix. A variant of endometriosis that may simulate a sarcoma. Am J Surg Pathol 14: 449–455
167. Nielsen G P, Oliva E, Young R H et al. 1995 Alveolar soft-part sarcoma of the female genital tract: a report of nine cases and review of the literature. Int J Gynecol Pathol 14: 283–292
168. Sahin A A, Silva E G, Ordonez N G 1989 Alveolar soft part sarcoma of the uterine cervix. Mod Pathol 2: 676–680
169. Keel S B, Clement P B, Prat J et al. 1998 Malignant schwannoma of the uterine cervix: a study of three cases. Int J Gynecol Pathol 17: 223–230
170. Cantuaria G, Angioli R, Nahmias J et al. 1999 Primary malignant melanoma of the uterine cervix: case report and review of the literature. Gynecol Oncol 75: 170–174
171. Furuya M, Shimizu M, Nishihara H et al. 2001 Clear cell variant of malignant melanoma of the uterine cervix: a case report and review of the literature. Gynecol Oncol 80: 409–412
172. Bittencourt A L, Britto J F, Fonseca L E Jr 1981 Wilms' tumor of the uterus: the first report of the literature. Cancer 47: 2496–2499
173. Bell D A, Shimm D S, Gang D L 1985 Wilms' tumor of the endocervix. Arch Pathol Lab Med 109: 371–373
174. Comerci J T Jr, Denehy T, Gregori C A et al. 1993 Wilms' tumor of the uterus. A case report. J Reprod Med 38: 829–832
175. Benatar B, Wright C, Freinkel A L et al. 1998 Primary extrarenal Wilms' tumor of the uterus presenting as a cervical polyp. Int J Gynecol Pathol 17: 277–280
176. Babin E A, Davis J R, Hatch K D et al. 2000 Wilms' tumor of the cervix: a case report and review of the literature. Gynecol Oncol 76: 107–111
177. Massarelli G, Bosincu L, Costanzi G et al. 1999 Uterine Wilms' tumor. Int J Gynecol Pathol 18: 402–403
178. Copeland L J, Sneige N, Ordonez N G et al. 1985 Endodermal sinus tumor of the vagina and cervix. Cancer 55: 2558–2565
179. Iwanaga S, Ishii H, Nagano H et al. 1990 Mature cystic teratoma of the uterine cervix. Asia Oceania J Obstet Gynaecol 16: 363–366
180. Lim S C, Kim Y S, Lee Y H et al. 2003 Mature teratoma of the uterine cervix with lymphoid hyperplasia. Pathol Int 53: 327–331
181. Khoor A, Fleming M V, Purcell C A et al. 1995 Mature teratoma of the uterine cervix with pulmonary differentiation. Arch Pathol Lab Med 119: 848–850
182. Vang R, Medeiros L J, Ha C S et al. 2000 Non-Hodgkin's lymphomas involving the uterus: a clinicopathologic analysis of 26 cases. Mod Pathol 13: 19–28
183. Friedman H D, Adelson M D, Elder R C et al. 1992 Granulocytic sarcoma of the uterine cervix – literature review of granulocytic sarcoma of the female genital tract. Gynecol Oncol 46: 128–137
184. Kapadia S B, Krause J R, Kanbour A I et al. 1978 Granulocytic sarcoma of the uterus. Cancer 41: 687–691
185. Seo I S, Hull M T, Pak H Y 1977 Granulocytic sarcoma of the cervix as a primary manifestation: case without overt leukemic features for 26 months. Cancer 40: 3030–3037

第六部分

阴道 Vagina

Marisa R. Nucci 著
回允中 姜 影 译

阴道			
上皮性肿瘤	719	混合性上皮-间叶肿瘤形成	725
鳞状上皮肿瘤形成	719	黑色素细胞病变	726
腺上皮肿瘤形成	720	淋巴和造血肿瘤	727
罕见类型的上皮肿瘤形成	721	其他罕见的肿瘤	727
间叶性肿瘤形成和瘤样病变	722	转移性肿瘤	727

引言 Introduction

累及阴道的绝大多数癌前和恶性疾病是鳞状上皮亚型（阴道鳞状上皮内肿瘤形成和浸润性鳞状细胞癌）。腺上皮肿瘤形成、混合性上皮-间叶肿瘤、间叶肿瘤和黑色素细胞肿瘤也可能发生，但不常见。在这个部位列出的罕见肿瘤中，胚胎性横纹肌肉瘤是一个例外，它是儿童期最常见的阴道恶性肿瘤。

上皮性肿瘤 Epithelial tumors

鳞状上皮肿瘤形成
Squamous neoplasia

发生阴道鳞状上皮肿瘤形成的危险因素与宫颈类似，包括：(1) 首次性交的年龄；(2) 性伴侣的数目；(3) 伴随的免疫抑制状况；以及 (4) 吸烟[1]。阴道鳞状上皮肿瘤形成同样也与 HPV 感染密切相关[1,2]。与用于 HPV 相关性宫颈鳞状上皮病变的术语相比较，阴道上皮内病变 (vaginal intraepithelial lesion, VAIL) 这一术语分类包括湿疣（低级别 VAIL；VAIN 1）和阴道上皮内肿瘤形成 (vaginal intraepithelial neoplasia, VAIN)（高级别 VAIL；VAIN 2 和 3）的病变。

鳞状上皮内肿瘤形成（阴道上皮内病变；阴道上皮内肿瘤形成）
Squamous intraepithelial neoplasia (vaginal intraepithelial lesion; vaginal intraepithelial neoplasia)

临床特征

VAIN 比宫颈的 CIN 少见得多，这在很大程度上可能与宫颈移行区易感 HPV 有关；然而，可以累及这个部位的 HPV 类型比累及外阴的范围广泛，这与宫颈相似[2]。VAIN 病人最常见的表现是巴氏涂片异常，病人 40～60 岁，不伴有临床症状[3-5]。高级别病变倾向于发生在较大的年龄组，平均年龄比低级别病变大 15 岁[6,7]。临床/阴道镜检查通常显示多灶性病变，表现为白色上皮或白色上皮伴有斑点（点状），最常累及阴道的上 1/3[3,5,7,11]。累及宫颈和（或）外阴以及阴道的多中心性疾病常见[3,10]。有关 VAIN 自然病史的研究提示，进展为浸润性病变的危险性低（特别是对于低级别的病变），多数病变退化，只有少数持续存在[5,10,12]。进展危险最大的病人包括具有高级别、多灶性和（或）多中心病变的病人，以及那些免疫抑制的病人[1]。开始发生这种疾病的危险因素包括 HPV 感染、免疫抑制、接触己烯雌酚（虽然尚有争论）、放射治疗以及女性生殖道其他部位（宫颈、外阴）有鳞状上皮肿瘤形成[1,13,16]。这些病人的处理取决于病人的年龄和病变的形态学（低级别还是高级别）。患有低级别病变的年轻人可以单独通过观察进行保守治疗，因为这些病变多数通常自发性退化；对于治疗高级别和低级别病变的其他选择包括局部治疗、激光切除或手术切除。

病理学特征

阴道上皮内肿瘤形成 1（低级别阴道上皮内病变）
Vaginal intraepithelial neoplasia 1 (low-grade vaginal intraepithelial lesion)

低级别 VAIL 的组织学表现与宫颈相似，包括外生性和扁平湿疣 (VAIN 1)。外生性湿疣与 HPV6 和 11 密切相关，其组织学特征是疣状乳头状生长方式，伴有粗钝的乳头、棘层增厚和浅表挖空细胞非典型性，后者表现为核深染、核增大、双核形成以及核的轮廓不规则（图

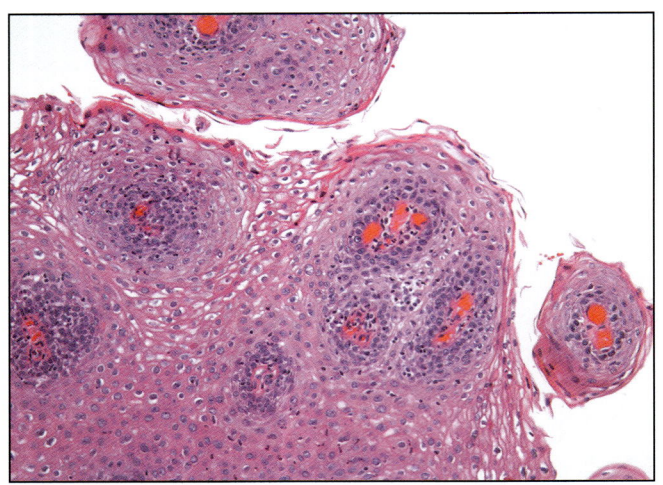

图13F.1 外生性湿疣。疣状乳头状生长和浅表挖空细胞非典型性。

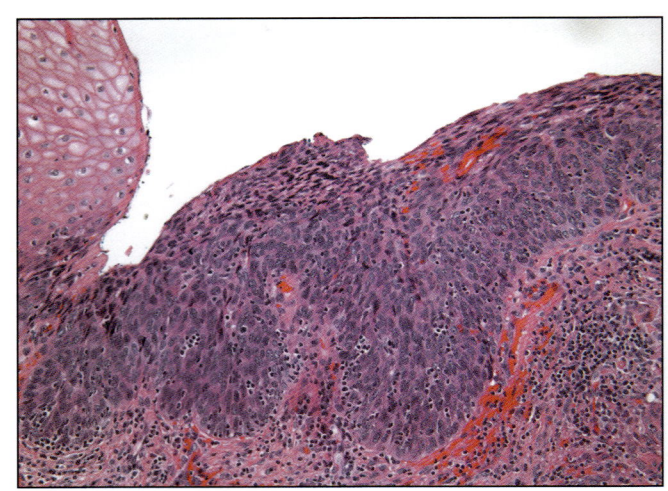

图13F.3 阴道上皮内肿瘤形成3。上皮全层核的非典型性，没有表面成熟。

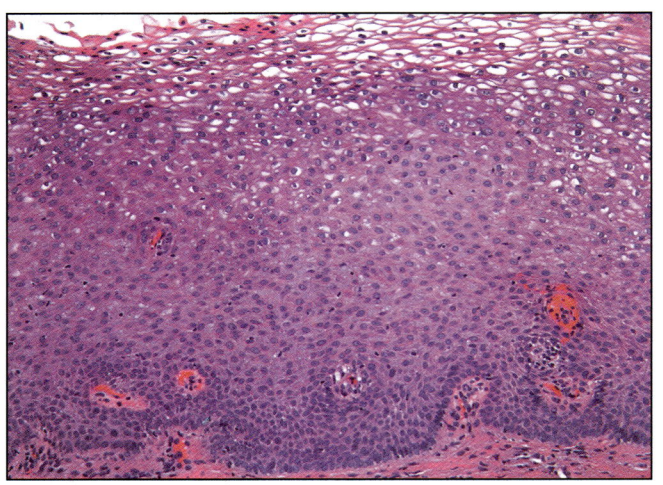

图13F.2 扁平湿疣。非典型性局限于上皮的上部。

13F.1）。扁平湿疣具有类似的形态学表现，但是缺乏乳头状结构（图13F.2）。

阴道上皮内肿瘤形成2-3（高级别阴道上皮内病变）Vaginal intraepithelial neoplasia 2-3 (high-grade vaginal intraepithelial lesion)

高级别VAIL的特征是上皮全层有细胞核的非典型性，伴有不同程度的表面成熟。显示表面挖空细胞改变和上皮成熟的病变相当于VAIN 2，而几乎没有成熟的病变相当于VAIN 3（图13F.3）。

鳞状细胞癌 Squamous cell carcinoma

与宫颈和外阴原发性病变不同，阴道浸润性鳞状细胞癌少见。它大约占所有女性生殖道肿瘤的2%，占2005年所有新诊断癌症病例的不到0.2%[17,18]。这些数字可能低估了原发性阴道鳞状细胞癌的实际发生率，因为按照惯例，阴道和宫颈均受累的肿瘤被认为是宫颈原发性肿瘤[17]。需要注意的是，先前5年之内有浸润性宫颈鳞状细胞癌的病人发生阴道浸润性鳞状细胞癌，被认为是宫颈原发性肿瘤的复发。发生阴道浸润性鳞状细胞癌的危险因素与原位鳞状上皮肿瘤形成类似，包括HPV感染、吸烟、免疫抑制以及女性生殖道其他部位的鳞状上皮肿瘤形成[1]。

阴道浸润性鳞状细胞癌发生的年龄范围可能广泛；然而，病人一般为绝经后妇女，诊断时的平均年龄为60～80岁[17,19,20]。出现的症状可能包括阴道出血、排液和（或）与肿块病变有关的症状。在晚期病例，邻近器官受累可能导致尿道梗阻。与原位鳞状上皮肿瘤形成相似，这些肿瘤最常见于阴道的上1/3，可能具有不同的临床表现，从扁平溃疡性病变，到外生性息肉样或蕈样肿块。组织学检查，其分化类型和范围类似于见于宫颈的病变（见702页）。治疗通常包括手术和放射治疗，生存与肿瘤分期有关，I期肿瘤（局限于阴道）的5年相对生存率为96%，II期（浸润阴道旁组织，但是未侵及盆壁）为73%，III期（延伸到盆壁）和IV期[浸润膀胱或直肠黏膜和（或）延伸到盆腔外]为36%（根据美国国家癌症中心资料）[17]。

腺上皮肿瘤形成 Glandular neoplasia

透明细胞腺癌[13,21-27] Clear cell adenocarcinoma

阴道透明细胞腺癌是一种罕见的恶性肿瘤，可以为散发性发生或与宫内接触己烯雌酚（DES）有关。根据来自荷兰登记中心的资料，它的发病好像有双峰年龄分布，一个年轻（平均20～30岁），一个年老（平均70～80岁），发生于接触或未接触己烯雌酚的病人。在宫内

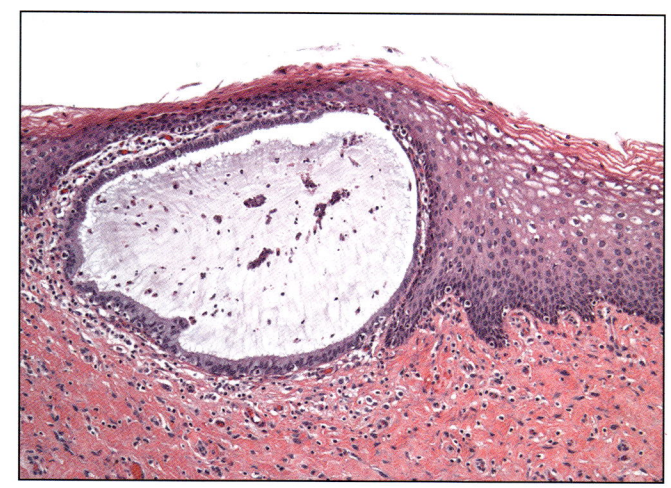

图13F.4 阴道腺病。鳞状上皮下黏液性腺体。

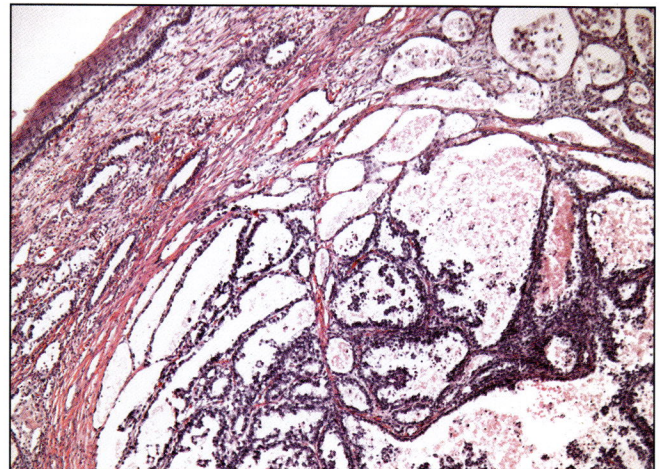

图13F.5 透明细胞癌。管囊性和乳头状生长方式。

接触己烯雌酚的病人，发生癌的危险性低（大约1000个妇女发生1例），危险增加与妊娠早期接触己烯雌酚和接触频率有关。考虑到接触己烯雌酚引起透明细胞癌的危险性低，提示其他一些因素与这些病人发生透明细胞癌有关，其他潜在的危险因素包括从前有流产和早产儿的病史。接触己烯雌酚还常常导致宫颈和阴道许多非恶性的改变，例如宫颈外翻和阴道腺病（图13F.4），阴道腺病常常伴有透明细胞癌或发生在阴道透明细胞癌的附近。

阴道透明细胞癌病人通常表现为异常阴道出血或性交疼痛，而且临床上具有明显的结节状或息肉样肿块；然而，在常规临床检测已知接触己烯雌酚的病人时，可以发现没有临床症状的较小的肿瘤。阴道和宫颈透明细胞癌病人总的预后非常好，5年和10年生存率分别为91%和85%。诊断时的分期是最好的预后指征，虽然较好的预后还与诊断时年龄大于19岁和主要呈管囊状组织学结构有关。

组织学检查，这些肿瘤的表现类似于发生于女性生殖道其他部位的透明细胞癌，由富于糖原的肿瘤细胞组成，核深染，形状不规则，排列成管囊状，实性和（或）呈乳头状生长方式（图13F.5）。鉴别诊断包括两个偶尔可能发生于阴道腺病的假肿瘤性病变：微小腺体增生和Arias-Stella反应。微小腺体增生不同于透明细胞癌的特征包括：（1）仅有局灶性核的非典型性；（2）存在核下空泡和胞浆内黏液；（3）缺乏糖原；（4）缺乏浸润性形态；以及（5）储备细胞增生/鳞状化生。Arias-Stella反应不同于透明细胞癌的特征包括：（1）没有相关的肿块性病变；（2）通常为局灶性；以及（3）细胞核呈现一系列的非典型性。

罕见类型的上皮肿瘤形成
Rare types of epithelial neoplasia

子宫内膜样、黏液性和肠型腺癌
Endometrioid, mucinous, and intestinal-type adenocarcinoma

累及阴道的转移性上生殖道或结直肠肿瘤很可能是这个部位腺癌的来源；然而，有少数原发性阴道腺癌的病例报告，原发性腺癌可能显示子宫内膜样、黏液性或肠型分化，或这些形态同时存在[28,35]。推测这些肿瘤来源于子宫内膜异位、宫颈内膜异位或肠型腺瘤（图13F.6），在某些病例，这些病变可能见于肿瘤成分附近或与之密切混合（图13F.7）。阴道出现子宫内膜异位或宫颈内膜异位并不奇怪；然而，出现肠型组织却令人迷惑，可能的病因包括肠化生、异位或泄殖腔源性残余。出现这些潜在的前体病变支持阴道原发；然而，在诊断原发性阴道腺癌之前，总是应该考虑除外来自其他部位的扩散。

其他罕见的上皮性恶性肿瘤
Other rare epithelial malignancies

各种各样癌的少数病例在阴道均有描述，其中包括腺鳞癌[36,37]、恶性混合性中肾瘤[38]以及小细胞神经内分泌癌[39]。在这些罕见的肿瘤中，最常见的是阴道原发性

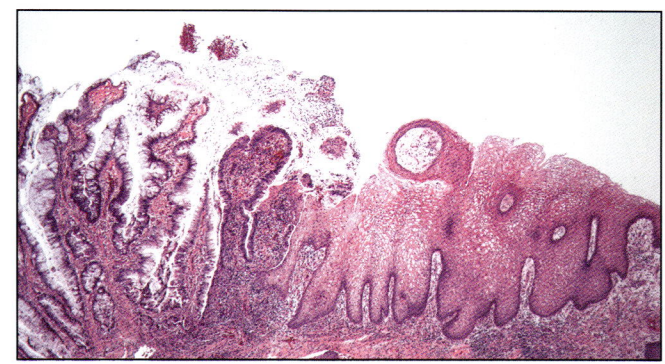

图13F.6 肠型腺瘤。这些病变在组织学上类似于发生在结肠的腺瘤。

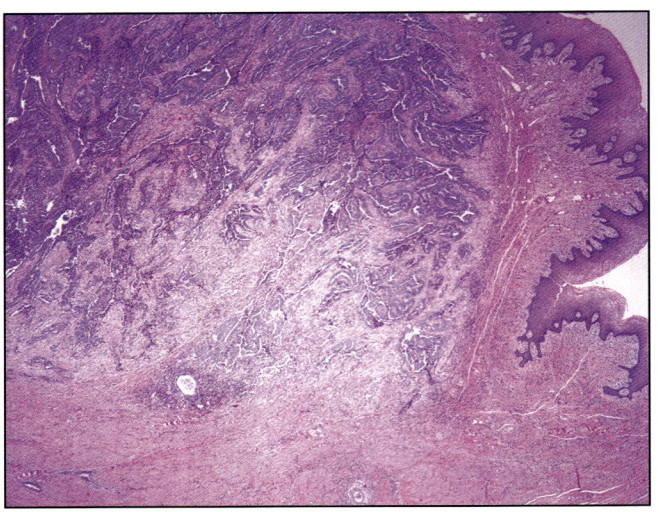

图13F.7　子宫内膜样腺癌。肿瘤的发生与其周围的子宫内膜异位有关。

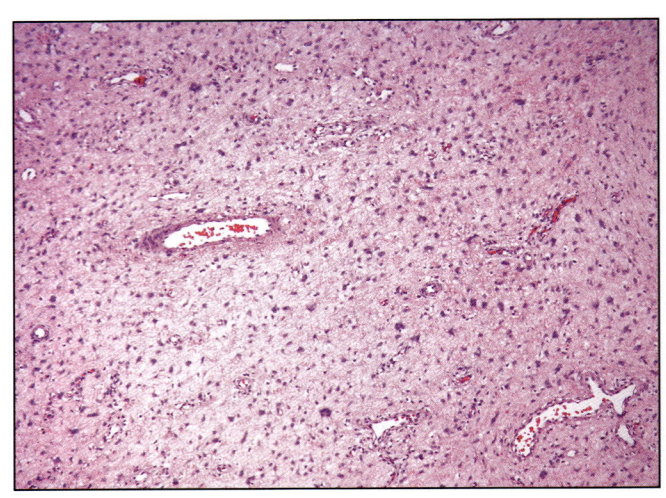

图13F.8　纤维上皮性间质息肉。假肉瘤性间质改变，伴有细胞成分增加和增大的非典型性间质细胞。

小细胞神经内分泌癌，它的平均发病年龄为50～60岁，通常小于5cm，组织学表现类似于肺小细胞癌[39]。由于这种肿瘤罕见，所以首先应该考虑来自肺转移的可能性。

间叶性肿瘤形成和瘤样病变
Mesenchymal neoplasia and tumor-like conditions

纤维上皮性间质息肉[40-51]
Fibroepithelial stromal polyp

纤维上皮性间质息肉可以发生于任何年龄，但是最常发生于生育年龄，青春期前罕见。这些病变最常发生于阴道，但是也可以累及外阴（见739页），偶尔累及宫颈。虽然通常为孤立性，但是可以为多发性息肉，这常常是与妊娠相关的一种特征。这些病变可以无蒂，或呈息肉样或丝状，大小可以不同，但是通常小于5cm。组织学检查，其特征为息肉样病变，被覆鳞状上皮，伴有纤维血管轴心。间质成分最为独特，形态各异，从细胞稀少到细胞丰富，这些细胞或为胞浆模糊的良性梭形细胞，或为具有显著增大而深染细胞核和丰富嗜酸性胞浆的细胞[51]（图13F.8）。后面这些假肉瘤性改变，最常发生于妊娠病人，促使某些作者应用假葡萄状肉瘤（pseudosarcoma botryoides）这一术语[41,44]。星形和多核细胞一般位于浅表部位，病变间质细胞和其上方上皮之间缺乏清楚的界限，这些也是特征性的组织学表现（图13F.9）。间质细胞desmin、vimentin、ER和PR染色通常阳性，actin阳性少见。在少数情况下，这些病变可能局部复发，特别是如果切除不完全或不断有激素刺激时（例如妊娠/激素替代疗法）。

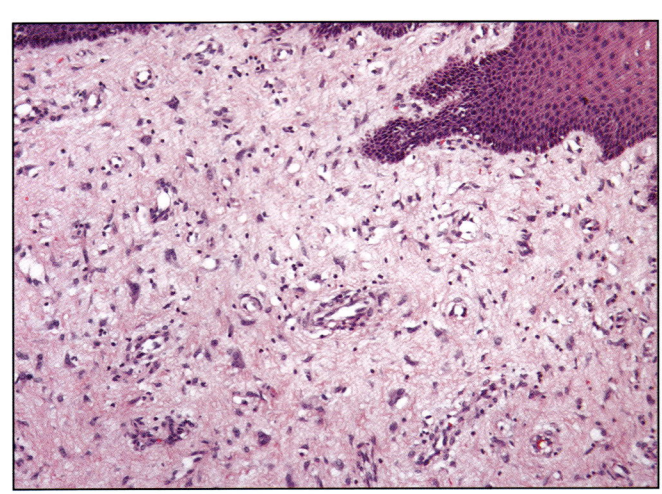

图13F.9　纤维上皮性间质息肉。星形和多核间质细胞具有特征性，位于上皮-间质交界的附近。

这些病变的发病机制尚不清楚，虽然它们很可能是一种反应性增生性病变，而不是肿瘤性病变，可能起源于女性生殖道远端独特的上皮下黏液样间质。激素受体的表达、发生于妊娠、妊娠期间可能为多发性而在妊娠之后可能自行退化，以及绝经后妇女与激素替代疗法有关，以上表现均支持其为反应性病变，在其发病机制中激素影响起着重要作用。

主要的鉴别诊断是侵袭性血管黏液瘤（对于那些细胞稀少和水肿的息肉）、肉瘤（对于那些显示假肉瘤性特征的病变）以及胚胎性横纹肌肉瘤（更多的是从历史而不是从实用的观点）。与纤维上皮性间质息肉相比，侵袭性血管黏液瘤位置较深，浸润明显，很少呈息肉状，而且具有比较显著的、间隔规则的血管成分。假肉瘤性间质息肉与肉瘤不同，缺乏明显的病变边缘，非典型性间质细胞延伸到间质-上皮交界，而且在接近间质-上皮交界处常常出现多核细胞，这是这种病变的特征。与葡萄状胚胎性横纹肌肉瘤不同，纤维上皮性间质息肉很少发生在青春期前，缺乏富于细胞的浅表新生层，缺乏横纹肌母细胞，而且缺乏骨骼肌特异性标志物的表达。

平滑肌瘤[52] Leiomyoma

阴道平滑肌瘤罕见，通常位于黏膜下，典型者为孤立性病变，较常累及阴道前壁，虽然可以发生于任何部位。它发生于生育年龄（类似于子宫平滑肌瘤），大小通常小于5cm。典型者小而没有症状，较大的肿瘤可以引起异常阴道出血、性交困难、疼痛或难产。组织学检查，阴道平滑肌瘤类似于子宫平滑肌瘤，界限清楚，没有浸润的证据，由交错排列的良性梭形细胞束组成，胞浆嗜酸性。确实没有浸润或显著细胞非典型性的证据，核分裂指数低（每10个高倍视野小于5个）的肿瘤被认为是良性平滑肌瘤（见下面平滑肌肉瘤一节中的恶性标准）。

生殖道横纹肌瘤[53-55] Genital rhabdomyoma

生殖道横纹肌瘤是一个显示明显骨骼肌分化的良性肿瘤，最常发生于阴道；然而，它也可以发生于外阴，偶尔发生于宫颈。这个肿瘤一般发生于中年妇女，通常呈息肉样，症状一般与肿块有关，包括性交困难和出血。组织学检查，其特征为黏膜下梭形或带状横纹肌母细胞成束增生，伴有丰富的嗜酸性胞浆，其中容易发现横纹（图13F.10和图13F.11）；核分裂象不常见，缺乏核的多形性。肿瘤细胞骨骼肌标志物阳性，尽管这对于诊断一般并不必要。生殖道横纹肌瘤与胚胎性横纹肌肉瘤不同，其主要鉴别诊断要点在于它缺乏核的非典型性/核深染，缺乏明显的核分裂活性，而且缺乏新生层，此外，生殖道横纹肌瘤发生于较大的年龄组。

手术后梭形细胞结节（假肉瘤性肌纤维母细胞增生）[56-58]
Postoperative spindle cell nodule (pseudosarcomatous myofibroblastic proliferation)

手术后梭形细胞结节最初在泌尿生殖道描述，特别是膀胱，但是偶尔可以发生于女性生殖道，包括阴道。虽然最初的描述是发生于应用手术器械之后（因此得名），但是这些病变可以发生于缺乏手术或任何其他外伤史的病人。它们一般形成息肉样肿块或结节，组织学检查以交错排列的肥胖梭形细胞束为特征，细胞核圆形到卵圆形，具有双极淡嗜酸性胞浆突起。这

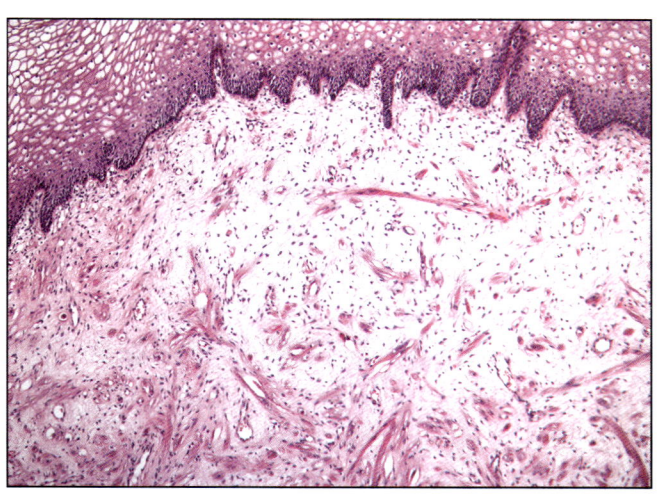

图13F.10　生殖道横纹肌瘤。黏膜下带状细胞增生，伴有丰富的嗜酸性胞浆。

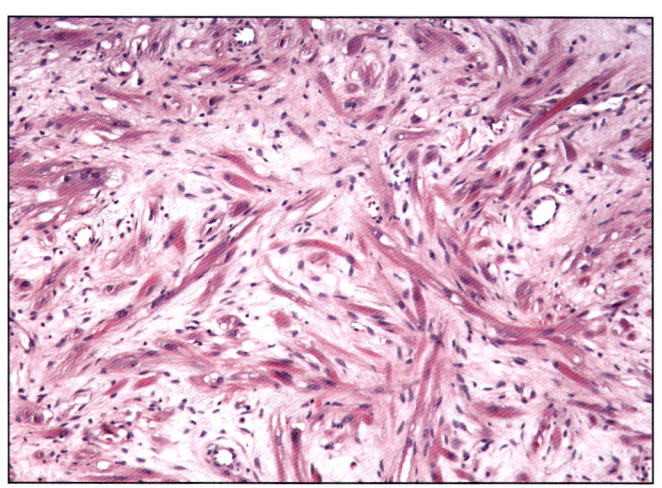

图13F.11　生殖道横纹肌瘤。肿瘤细胞排列成束状结构。

些肌纤维母细胞actin、desmin和（或）cytokeratin免疫染色可能阳性。可以出现散在的慢性炎症细胞、外渗的红细胞和含铁血黄素沉着。鉴别诊断主要是除外肉瘤，由于手术后梭形细胞结节常常出现许多核分裂象，而且其边界相对不很清楚，所以可能类似于肉瘤。缺乏明显的核非典型性和核深染，出现间质炎症，以及如果知道从前有手术史均有助于这个鉴别诊断。这些病变是良性病变，一般不复发，即使是在不完全切除之后。

血管肌纤维母细胞瘤　Angiomyofibroblastoma

血管肌纤维母细胞瘤是一种良性、非复发性间叶性肿瘤，可以发生于阴道，但是较常发生于生育年龄妇女的外阴（见740页）。

间叶性肿瘤形成和瘤样病变

深在性（侵袭性）血管黏液瘤
Deep (aggressive) angiomyxoma

深在性血管黏液瘤是一种非转移性、局部浸润性肿瘤，常常累及女性会阴和（或）盆腔软组织，平均年龄30～40岁（见742页）。

胚胎性横纹肌肉瘤[17, 59,60]
Embryonal rhabdomyosarcoma

横纹肌肉瘤（见第24章）是儿童期最常见的间叶恶性肿瘤，其中胚胎性横纹肌肉瘤是最常见的组织学亚型。当胚胎性横纹肌肉瘤累及黏膜部位时，例如累及阴道，它倾向于形成特征性的外生性葡萄样结构，获得了葡萄状肉瘤的命名；因此，在本质上，葡萄状肉瘤只不过是胚胎性横纹肌肉瘤肉眼检查时的一种独特亚型，具有特征性的临床表现，大概是由于肿物不受限制地向腔隙内生长。绝大多数患有阴道胚胎性横纹肌肉瘤的儿童小于5岁，大部分表现为阴道出血；在某些病人，第一个指征可能是肿瘤从阴道口脱出。在临床上，出现质软、脆而易碎、水肿性的息肉样突起，可能充满阴道。

组织学检查，胚胎性横纹肌肉瘤是圆形、梭形或带状细胞的息肉样增生，其中某些细胞具有鲜明的嗜酸性胞浆，位于鳞状上皮下的疏松黏液样基质内（图13F.12）。在HE切片上胞浆内可见明显的横纹。葡萄状肉瘤的一种特征性的、但并不一定出现的组织学特征是，相对未分化的肿瘤细胞聚集在黏膜表面下方[所谓的新生层（cambium layer）；图13F.13]。肿瘤细胞骨骼肌分化标志物一般阳性，包括MyoD1和肌细胞生成素（myogenin，myf 4），它们是直接抗骨骼肌特异性核

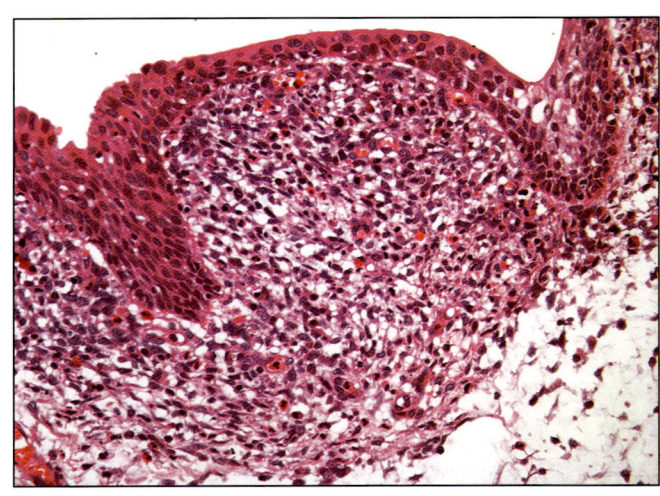

图13F.13 胚胎性横纹肌肉瘤。肿瘤细胞聚集在表面上皮下，形成所谓的新生层。

转录因子的抗体。发生于这个部位的胚胎性横纹肌肉瘤病人的预后良好，特别是葡萄状亚型，10年生存率大于90%。治疗通常采取手术和化疗，其中化疗可能引起肿瘤细胞显著的分化和成熟。鉴别诊断包括：（1）纤维上皮性间质息肉，与胚胎性横纹肌肉瘤不同，很少发生在青春期前，缺乏新生层，而且骨骼肌分化特异性标志物阴性；（2）生殖道横纹肌瘤，发生于成人，缺乏核的非典型性/核深染、明显的核分裂活性以及新生层；以及（3）Müller乳头状瘤（见下），可以是外生性和息肉样，但是缺乏上面描述的胚胎性横纹肌肉瘤特征性的组织学特征。

平滑肌肉瘤[17,52,61]   Leiomyosarcoma

虽然阴道平滑肌肉瘤罕见，文献中报告少于100例，但它是累及成人的最常见的阴道肉瘤。阴道平滑肌肉瘤发生的年龄范围广泛，从20～90岁不等，多数病人超过40岁。这些肿瘤最常累及阴道后壁或侧壁，一般表现为阴道出血/排液或与肿块有关的症状。因为这种肿瘤不常见，其恶性标准难以确定和证实。不过，大于3cm、有显著细胞学非典型性以及每10个高倍视野核分裂象超过5个的肿瘤，应该认为是恶性肿瘤；凝固性肿瘤细胞坏死和浸润性边缘也与恶性行为有关（图13F.14）。治疗主要是手术切除，预后与分期有关，总的生存率大约是43%。

其他罕见的肉瘤[62-64]   Other rare sarcomas

阴道偶尔可以见到原发性子宫内膜间质肉瘤，推测是由子宫内膜异位灶发生的。即使存在子宫内膜异位，也总是应该排除从子宫原发性肿瘤扩散而来的可能

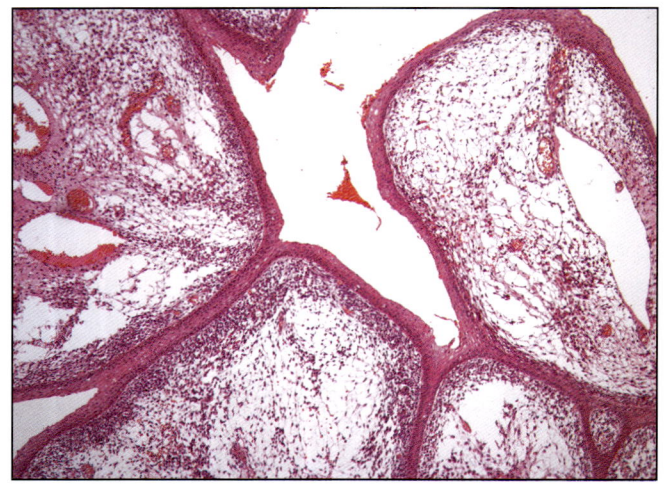

图13F.12 胚胎性横纹肌肉瘤。肿瘤的特征是呈息肉样，由圆形和梭形细胞组成，位于表面上皮下的疏松黏液样间质内。

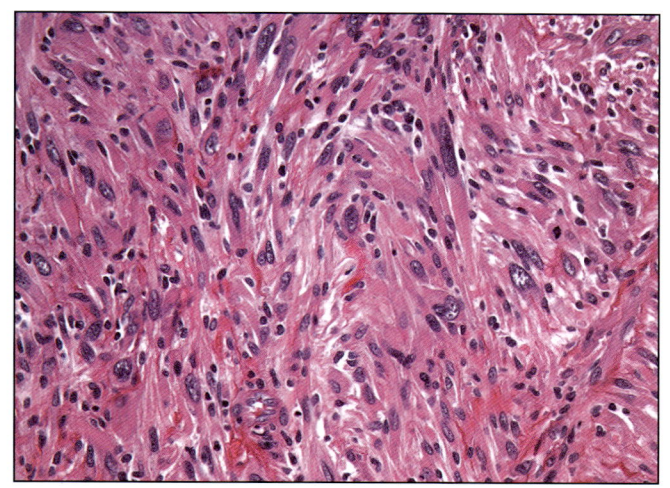

图13F.14 平滑肌肉瘤。弥漫性细胞学非典型性是诊断恶性的标准之一。

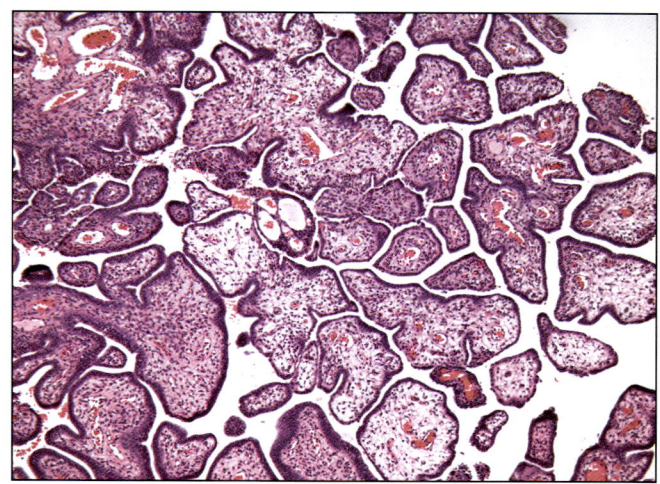

图13F.15 Müller乳头状瘤。复杂的分支乳头状突起具有特征性。

性。在少数情况下，Ewing 肉瘤、近端型上皮样肉瘤以及上皮样血管肉瘤可以原发于阴道；这些肿瘤与发生于其他部位的肿瘤具有同样的组织学表现和免疫表型（见第 24 章）。

混合性上皮-间叶肿瘤形成
Mixed epithelial-mesenchymal neoplasia

Müller乳头状瘤[65-71]　Müllerian papilloma

Müller 乳头状瘤是一种罕见的良性肿瘤，通常发生于 < 5 岁儿童的阴道和宫颈。从前文献中将其描述为中肾乳头状瘤，现在根据其形态学、免疫表型和超微结构特征认为来源于 Müller 管。这些主要以黏膜为基础的良性外生性乳头状肿瘤，最常表现为阴道出血，组织学表现为复杂的分支乳头状突起，被覆良性表现的矮柱状到立方上皮（图 13F.15 和 13F.16）。复发和个别恶性变的病例已有描述。

梭形细胞上皮瘤（良性混合瘤）[72-74]
Spindle cell epithelioma (benign mixed tumor)

梭形细胞上皮瘤是一种良性肿瘤，最常发生于阴道远端接近处女膜环的部位，表现为一个境界清楚、无痛性的黏膜下肿块，大小通常小于 5cm。诊断时的平均年龄为 30 ～ 40 岁，这些病变通常是在常规妇科检查时偶尔发现的，临床上多数被认为是囊肿或息肉。

组织学检查，这些肿瘤是界限清楚、没有包膜的肿块，接近上皮表面但并不与之连续，由增生的良性淡嗜酸性梭形细胞组成，细胞含量可以不同，伴有含有纤维母细

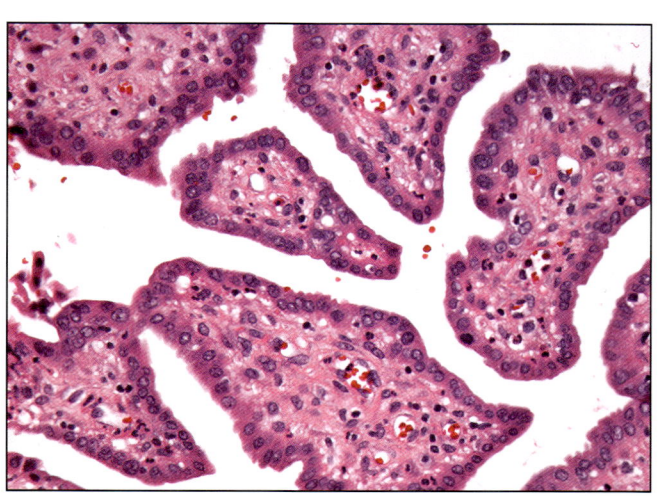

图13F.16 Müller乳头状瘤。乳头一般被覆立方到矮柱状上皮，伴有嗜酸性胞浆。

胞型细胞的较淡染的细胞稀少区，将细胞较为丰富的区域分隔成巢和互相连接的岛屿（图 13F.17）。通常出现小灶状的上皮分化，最常表现为鳞状上皮巢和交错排列的鳞状上皮条索，可能具有空泡状或糖原生成性外观（图 13F.18）。嗜酸性透明小球具有特征性，它是间质基质的凝聚（图 13F.19）。免疫组织化学检查，梭形细胞 keratin（图 13F.20）和平滑肌肌动蛋白（SMA）阳性，CD10 和激素受体可能阳性，但是 S-100 蛋白和 GFAP 阴性。虽然 keratin 和 SMA 共表达提示可能有肌上皮分化，并导致以前将这些病变命名为混合瘤（用于描述其他部位肌上皮性肿瘤的术语），根据免疫组化和超微结构特征，现在认为这些肿瘤并不显示真正的肌上皮分化，并且提出采用梭形细胞上皮瘤这一术语[72]。这些病变为良性，局部切除好像有效；首次切除之后 8 年复发的一个病例已

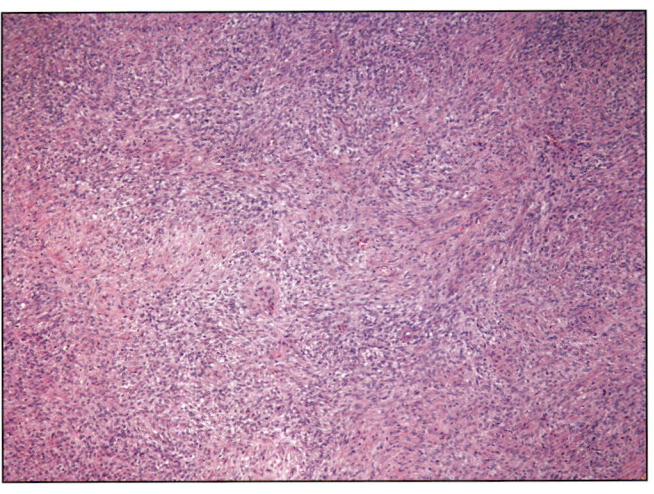

图13F.17 梭形细胞上皮瘤。不同细胞含量的梭形细胞增生，伴有淡染的细胞稀少区，将细胞比较丰富的区域分割成模糊的细胞巢。

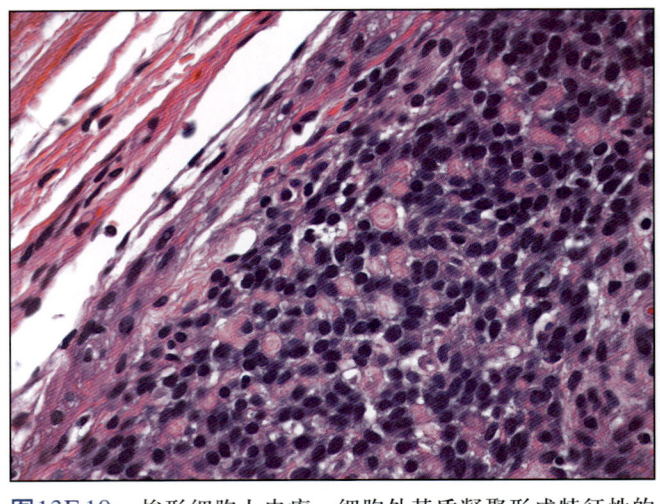

图13F.19 梭形细胞上皮瘤。细胞外基质凝聚形成特征性的嗜酸性透明小体。

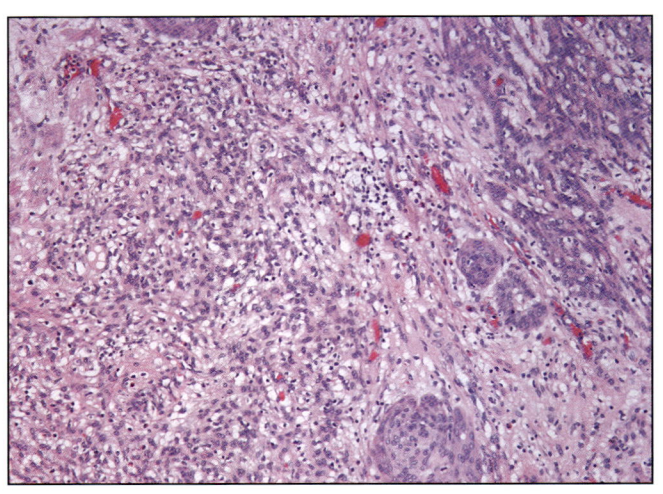

图13F.18 梭形细胞上皮瘤。上皮分化通常表现为鳞状上皮巢和交错排列的条索。

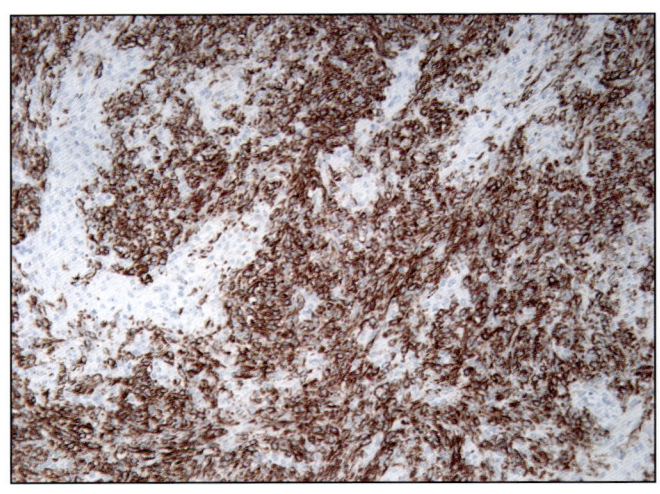

图13F.20 梭形细胞上皮瘤。富于梭形细胞的区域keratin弥漫阳性。

有报告[73]。鉴别诊断包括阴道恶性混合瘤，它含有恶性上皮和间质成分，梭形上皮细胞缺乏良性双相表现。

腺肉瘤[75-77]　Adenosarcoma

子宫外腺肉瘤最常累及卵巢或腹膜；然而，在阴道已有3例子宫外腺肉瘤的报告，发生在子宫内膜异位的基础上。病人年龄为42、45和56岁，全部有累及盆腔器官或软组织的广泛子宫内膜异位的病史，这使腺肉瘤的诊断提前了5年。肿瘤较大（6、10和16cm），最大的肿瘤表现为从阴道口脱出的肿块。组织学检查，类似于发生在子宫的腺肉瘤（见663页）。

癌肉瘤[78,79]　Carcinosarcoma

阴道原发性癌肉瘤（恶性混合性Müller瘤）罕见，在做出这个诊断之前，总是应该考虑是否从子宫原发性肿瘤扩散而来。与子宫癌肉瘤相似，阴道原发性癌肉瘤一般发生在病人绝经后，通常60～70岁，肿瘤显示类似的组织学表现（见661页）。虽然病例数目有限，总的预后似乎较差，多数病人诊断2年之内死于本病。

黑色素细胞病变　Melanocytic lesions

蓝痣[80,81]　Blue nevus

蓝痣很少累及阴道，表现为蓝黑色斑点或斑块，临床上可能类似于恶性黑色素瘤。组织学检查，这些病变类似于发生在其他部位的蓝痣，由黏膜下色素性树突状

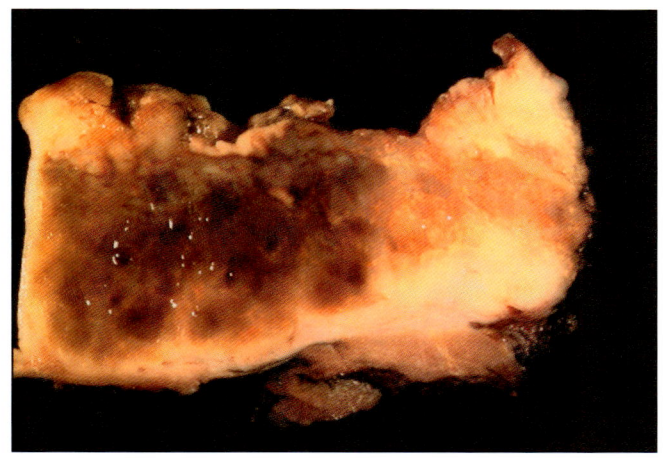

图13F.21　恶性黑色素瘤。色素性溃疡性肿块浸润阴道壁深部。

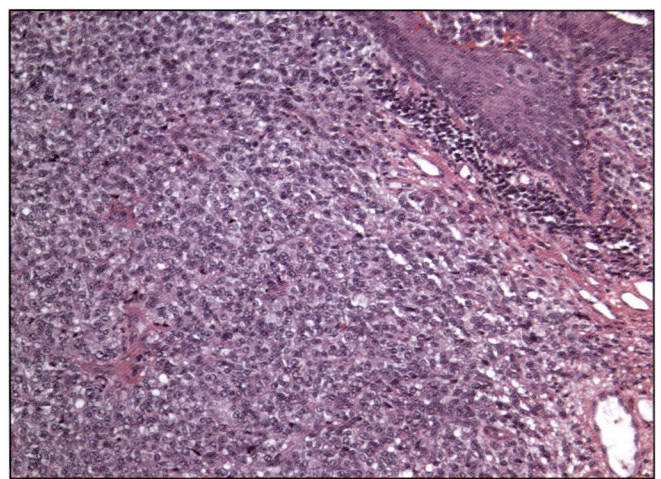

图13F.22　恶性黑色素瘤。伴有嗜酸性胞浆的上皮样肿瘤细胞片块具有特征性。

黑色素细胞组成（见第23章）。

恶性黑色素瘤[82-86] 　Malignant melanoma

阴道原发性恶性黑色素瘤非常少见，占发生于阴道部位恶性肿瘤的不到1%。这些肿瘤发生的年龄范围广泛，然而，多数病人为绝经后，平均年龄60～70岁。多数病人表现为阴道出血或出现与肿块相关的症状。临床检查一般显示息肉样或结节状肿块，可能为色素性或有溃疡形成，较常累及阴道的前壁或侧壁（图13F.21）。肿瘤与其他部位的黑色素瘤组织学表现类似，具有上皮样、梭形细胞或混合性形态学表现（图13F.22）。黑色素瘤标志物（S-100、HMB-45、Mart-1和Melan-A）阳性有助于这种肿瘤与潜在类似病变的鉴别，特别是无黑色素性或梭形细胞黑色素瘤与浸润性鳞状细胞癌或平滑肌肉瘤的鉴别。阴道黑色素瘤的预后均差，总的5年生存率小于20%；分期是最重要的预后因素。

淋巴和造血肿瘤　Lymphoid and hematopoietic tumors

淋巴瘤　Lymphoma

结外非Hodgkin淋巴瘤最常累及皮肤和胃肠道；然而，偶尔可以原发于阴道。在最大的系列研究中[87]，病人年龄从26岁到66岁不等（平均42岁），最常出现的症状是阴道出血，组织学检查，所有肿瘤均为弥漫性大B细胞淋巴瘤。在最后随访期间（1.8～18年）多数病人生存，没有疾病存在的证据。

白血病[88]　Leukemia

粒细胞肉瘤很少累及女性生殖道，女性生殖道的粒细胞肉瘤或为本病的第一个临床表现，或为急性粒细胞性白血病复发。卵巢是最常见的受累部位；然而，阴道，以及更少见的宫颈也可能受累。这些肿瘤与其他部位的粒细胞肉瘤具有类似的组织学表现（见第22章），氯乙酸酯酶（chloroacetate esterase）、溶菌酶、髓过氧化物酶（myeloperoxidase）、CD68和CD43一般阳性。主要的鉴别诊断是非Hodgkin淋巴瘤和低分化癌，通过免疫组化染色通常可以确立诊断。

其他罕见的肿瘤　Other rare tumors

内胚窦（卵黄囊）瘤[89,90]
Endodermal sinus (yolk sac) tumor

阴道内胚窦瘤的特征是发生于婴儿和5岁以下的小儿。病人通常表现为阴道出血，临床检查一般显示息肉样、脆而易碎的肿块，可能类似于葡萄状肉瘤。组织学检查，这些肿瘤与发生在较常见部位卵巢的肿瘤类似（见605页）。

转移性肿瘤　Metastatic tumors

阴道是来自生殖道和非生殖道原发性肿瘤转移的常见部位。在诊断原发性上皮恶性肿瘤之前，应该考虑来自宫颈、子宫和卵巢转移的可能性。根据女性生殖道转移频率和形式的大系列检查发现，来自非生殖道转移最常见的起源部位是结直肠[91]。

参考文献

1. Daling J R, Madeleine M M, Schwartz S M et al. 2002 A population-based study of squamous cell vaginal cancer: HPV and cofactors. Gynecol Oncol 84: 263–270
2. Sugase M, Matsukura T 1997 Distinct manifestations of human papillomaviruses in the vagina. Int J Cancer 72: 412–415
3. Lenehan P M, Meffe F, Lickrish G M 1986 Vaginal intraepithelial neoplasia: biologic aspects and management. Obstet Gynecol 68: 333–337
4. Mao C C, Chao K C, Lian Y C et al. 1990 Vaginal intraepithelial neoplasia: diagnosis and management. Zhonghua Yi Xue Za Zhi (Taipei) 46: 35–42
5. Aho M, Vesterinen E, Meyer B et al. 1991 Natural history of vaginal intraepithelial neoplasia. Cancer 68: 195–197
6. Audet-Lapointe P, Body G, Vauclair R et al. 1990 Vaginal intraepithelial neoplasia. Gynecol Oncol 36: 232–239
7. Diakomanolis E, Stefanidis K, Rodolakis A et al. 2002 Vaginal intraepithelial neoplasia: report of 102 cases. Eur J Gynaecol Oncol 23: 457–459
8. Petrilli E S, Townsend D E, Morrow C P et al. 1980 Vaginal intraepithelial neoplasia: biologic aspects and treatment with topical 5-fluorouracil and the carbon dioxide laser. Am J Obstet Gynecol 138: 321–328
9. Rome R M, England P G 2000 Management of vaginal intraepithelial neoplasia: a series of 132 cases with long-term follow-up. Int J Gynecol Cancer 10: 382–390
10. Dodge J A, Eltabbakh G H, Mount S L et al. 2001 Clinical features and risk of recurrence among patients with vaginal intraepithelial neoplasia. Gynecol Oncol 83: 363–369
11. Cardosi R J, Bomalaski J J, Hoffman M S 2001 Diagnosis and management of vulvar and vaginal intraepithelial neoplasia. Obstet Gynecol Clin North Am 28: 685–702
12. Sillman F H, Fruchter R G, Chen Y S et al. 1997 Vaginal intraepithelial neoplasia: risk factors for persistence, recurrence, and invasion and its management. Am J Obstet Gynecol 176: 93–99
13. Hatch E, Herbst A, Hoover R et al. 2000 Incidence of squamous neoplasia of the cervix and vagina in DES-exposed daughters. Ann Epidemiol 10: 467
14. Barzon L, Pizzighella S, Corti L et al. 2002 Vaginal dysplastic lesions in women with hysterectomy and receiving radiotherapy are linked to high-risk human papillomavirus. J Med Virol 67: 401–405
15. Fujimura M, Ostrow R S, Okagaki T 1991 Implication of human papillomavirus in postirradiation dysplasia. Cancer 68: 2181–2185
16. Robboy S J, Truslow G Y, Anton J et al. 1981 Role of hormones including diethylstilbestrol (DES) in the pathogenesis of cervical and vaginal intraepithelial neoplasia. Gynecol Oncol 12: S98–S110
17. Creasman W T, Phillips J L, Menck H R 1998 The National Cancer Data Base report on cancer of the vagina. Cancer 83: 1033–1040
18. Jemal A, Murray T, Ward E et al. 2005 Cancer statistics, 2005. CA Cancer J Clin 55: 10–30
19. Hellman K, Silfversward C, Nilsson B et al. 2004 Primary carcinoma of the vagina: factors influencing the age at diagnosis. The Radiumhemmet series 1956–96. Int J Gynecol Cancer 14: 491–501
20. Diakomanolis E, Rodolakis A, Stefanidis K et al. 2002 Primary invasive vaginal cancer. Report of 12 cases. Eur J Gynaecol Oncol 23: 573–574
21. Herbst A L, Ulfelder H, Poskanzer D C 1971 Adenocarcinoma of the vagina. Association of maternal stilbestrol therapy with tumor appearance in young women. N Engl J Med 284: 878–881
22. Herbst A L, Cole P, Colton T et al. 1977 Age-incidence and risk of diethylstilbestrol-related clear cell adenocarcinoma of the vagina and cervix. Am J Obstet Gynecol 128: 43–50
23. Herbst A L, Cole P, Norusis M J et al. 1979 Epidemiologic aspects and factors related to survival in 384 registry cases of clear cell adenocarcinoma of the vagina and cervix. Am J Obstet Gynecol 135: 876–886
24. Melnick S, Cole P, Anderson D et al. 1987 Rates and risks of diethylstilbestrol-related clear-cell adenocarcinoma of the vagina and cervix. An update. N Engl J Med 316: 514–516
25. Herbst A L 1981 The current status of the DES-exposed population. Obstet Gynecol Annu 10: 267–278
26. Herbst A L, Anderson D 1990 Clear cell adenocarcinoma of the vagina and cervix secondary to intrauterine exposure to diethylstilbestrol. Semin Surg Oncol 6: 343–346
27. Hanselaar A, van Loosbroek M, Schuurbiers O et al. 1997 Clear cell adenocarcinoma of the vagina and cervix. An update of the central Netherlands registry showing twin age incidence peaks. Cancer 79: 2229–2236
28. Kapp D S, Merino M, LiVolsi V 1982 Adenocarcinoma of the vagina arising in endometriosis: long-term survival following radiation therapy. Gynecol Oncol 14: 271–278
29. Haskel S, Chen S S, Spiegel G 1989 Vaginal endometrioid adenocarcinoma arising in vaginal endometriosis: a case report and literature review. Gynecol Oncol 34: 232–236
30. Mikami M, Nakamura M, Kurahashi T et al. 2003 A case of pT4 vaginal adenocarcinoma in which surgery prolonged disease-free interval. Arch Gynecol Obstet 268: 214–216
31. DeMars L R, Van Le L, Huang I et al. 1995 Primary non-clear-cell adenocarcinomas of the vagina in older DES-exposed women. Gynecol Oncol 58: 389–3192
32. Ebrahim S, Daponte A, Smith T H et al. 2001 Primary mucinous adenocarcinoma of the vagina. Gynecol Oncol 80: 89–92
33. Fox H, Wells M, Harris M et al. 1988 Enteric tumours of the lower female genital tract: a report of three cases. Histopathology 12: 167–176
34. Yaghsezian H, Palazzo J P, Finkel G C et al. 1992 Primary vaginal adenocarcinoma of the intestinal type associated with adenosis. Gynecol Oncol 45: 62–65
35. Mudhar H S, Smith J H, Tidy J 2001 Primary vaginal adenocarcinoma of intestinal type arising from an adenoma: case report and review of the literature. Int J Gynecol Pathol 20: 204–209
36. Rhatigan R M, Mojadidi Q 1973 Adenosquamous carcinomas of the vulva and vagina. Am J Clin Pathol 60: 208–217
37. Sulak P, Barnhill D, Heller P et al. 1988 Nonsquamous cancer of the vagina. Gynecol Oncol 29: 309–320
38. Bague S, Rodriguez I M, Prat J 2004 Malignant mesonephric tumors of the female genital tract: a clinicopathologic study of 9 cases. Am J Surg Pathol 28: 601–607
39. Bing Z, Levine L, Lucci J A et al. 2004 Primary small cell neuroendocrine carcinoma of the vagina: a clinicopathologic study. Arch Pathol Lab Med 128: 857–862
40. Norris H J, Taylor H B 1966 Polyps of the vagina. A benign lesion resembling sarcoma botryoides. Cancer 19: 227–232
41. Elliott G B, Reynolds H A, Fidler H K 1967 Pseudo-sarcoma botryoides of cervix and vagina in pregnancy. J Obstet Gynaecol Br Commonw 74: 728–733
42. Burt R L, Prichard R W, Kim B S 1976 Fibroepithelial polyp of the vagina. A report of five cases. Obstet Gynecol 47: 52S–54S
43. Chirayil S J, Tobon H 1981 Polyps of the vagina: a clinicopathologic study of 18 cases. Cancer 47: 2904–2907
44. O'Quinn A G, Edwards C L, Gallager H S 1982 Pseudosarcoma botryoides of the vagina in pregnancy. Gynecol Oncol 13: 237–241
45. Miettinen M, Wahlstrom T, Vesterinen E et al. 1983 Vaginal polyps with pseudosarcomatous features. A clinicopathologic study of seven cases. Cancer 51: 1148–1151
46. Maenpaa J, Soderstrom K O, Salmi T et al. 1988 Large atypical polyps of the vagina during pregnancy with concomitant human papilloma virus infection. Eur J Obstet Gynecol Reprod Biol 27: 65–69
47. Ostor A G, Fortune D W, Riley C B 1988 Fibroepithelial polyps with atypical stromal cells (pseudosarcoma botryoides) of vulva and vagina. A report of 13 cases. Int J Gynecol Pathol 7: 351–360
48. Hartmann C A, Sperling M, Stein H 1990 So-called fibroepithelial polyps of the vagina exhibiting an unusual but uniform antigen profile characterized by expression of desmin and steroid hormone receptors but no muscle-specific actin or macrophage markers. Am J Clin Pathol 93: 604–608
49. Mucitelli D R, Charles E Z, Kraus F T 1990 Vulvovaginal polyps. Histologic appearance, ultrastructure, immunocytochemical characteristics, and clinicopathologic correlations. Int J Gynecol Pathol 9: 20–40
50. Nucci M R, Fletcher C D 1998 Fibroepithelial stromal polyps of vulvovaginal tissue: From the banal to the bizarre. Pathol Case Rev 3: 151–157
51. Nucci M R, Young R H, Fletcher C D 2000 Cellular pseudosarcomatous fibroepithelial stromal polyps of the lower female genital tract: an underrecognized lesion often misdiagnosed as sarcoma. Am J Surg Pathol 24: 231–240
52. Tavassoli F A, Norris H J 1979 Smooth muscle tumors of the vagina. Obstet Gynecol 53: 689–693
53. Chabrel C M, Beilby J O 1980 Vaginal rhabdomyoma. Histopathology 4: 645–651
54. Hanski W, Hagel-Lewicka E, Daniszewski K 1991 Rhabdomyomas of female genital tract. Report on two cases. Zentralbl Pathol 137: 439–442
55. Iversen U M 1996 Two cases of benign vaginal rhabdomyoma. Case reports. APMIS 104: 575–578
56. Guillou L, Gloor E, De Grandi P et al. 1989 Post-operative pseudosarcoma of the vagina. A case report. Pathol Res Pract 185: 245–248
57. Proppe K H, Scully R E, Rosai J 1984 Postoperative spindle cell nodules of genitourinary tract resembling sarcomas. A report of eight cases. Am J Surg Pathol 8: 101–108
58. Young R H, Scully R E 1987 Pseudosarcomatous lesions of the urinary bladder, prostate gland, and urethra. A report of three cases and review of the literature. Arch Pathol Lab Med 111: 354–358
59. Leuschner I, Harms D, Mattke A et al. 2001 Rhabdomyosarcoma of the urinary bladder and vagina: a clinicopathologic study with emphasis on recurrent disease: a report from the Kiel pediatric tumor registry and the German CWS study. Am J Surg Pathol 25: 856–864
60. Andrassy R J, Hays D M, Raney R B et al. 1995 Conservative surgical management of vaginal and vulvar pediatric rhabdomyosarcoma: a report from the Intergroup Rhabdomyosarcoma Study III. J Pediatr Surg 30: 1034–1036
61. Ciaravino G, Kapp D S, Vela A M et al. 2000 Primary leiomyosarcoma of the vagina. A case report and literature review. Int J Gynecol Cancer 10: 340–347
62. Chang Y C, Wang T Y, Tzen C Y 2000 Endometrial stromal sarcoma of the vagina. Zhonghua Yi Xue Za Zhi (Taipei) 63: 714–719
63. Liao Y, Xin X, Lu X 2004 Primary Ewing's sarcoma – primitive neuroectodermal tumor of the vagina. Gynecol Oncol 92: 684–688
64. McAdam J A, Stewart F, Reid R 1998 Vaginal epithelioid angiosarcoma. J Clin Pathol 51: 928–930
65. Ulbright T M, Alexander R W, Kraus F T 1981 Intramural papilloma of the vagina: evidence of Mullerian histogenesis. Cancer 48: 2260–2266

66. Luttges J E, Lubke M 1994 Recurrent benign Mullerian papilloma of the vagina. Immunohistological findings and histogenesis. Arch Gynecol Obstet 255: 157–160
67. Cohen M, Pedemonte L, Drut R 2001 Pigmented mullerian papilloma of the vagina. Histopathology 39: 541–543
68. Dobbs S P, Shaw P A, Brown L J et al. 1998 Borderline malignant change in recurrent mullerian papilloma of the vagina. J Clin Pathol 51: 875–877
69. Abu J, Nunns D, Ireland D et al. 2003 Malignant progression through borderline changes in recurrent Mullerian papilloma of the vagina. Histopathology 42: 510–511
70. Arbo E, dos Reis R, Uchoa D et al. 2004 Vaginal Mullerian papilloma in a 2-year-old child. Gynecol Obstet Invest 58: 55–56
71. McCluggage W G, Nirmala V, Radhakumari K 1999 Intramural mullerian papilloma of the vagina. Int J Gynecol Pathol 18: 94–95
72. Branton P A, Tavassoli F A 1993 Spindle cell epithelioma, the so-called mixed tumor of the vagina. A clinicopathologic, immunohistochemical, and ultrastructural analysis of 28 cases. Am J Surg Pathol 17: 509–515
73. Wright R G, Buntine D W, Forbes K L 1991 Recurrent benign mixed tumor of the vagina. Gynecol Oncol 40: 84–86
74. Murdoch F, Sharma R, Al Nafussi A 2003 Benign mixed tumor of the vagina: case report with expanded immunohistochemical profile. Int J Gynecol Cancer 13: 543–547
75. Judson P L, Temple A M, Fowler W C Jr et al. 2000 Vaginal adenosarcoma arising from endometriosis. Gynecol Oncol 76: 123–125
76. Anderson J, Behbakht K, De Geest K et al. 2001 Adenosarcoma in a patient with vaginal endometriosis. Obstet Gynecol 98: 964–966
77. Liu L, Davidson S, Singh M 2003 Mullerian adenosarcoma of vagina arising in persistent endometriosis: report of a case and review of the literature. Gynecol Oncol 90: 486–490
78. Neesham D, Kerdemelidis P, Scurry J 1998 Primary malignant mixed Mullerian tumor of the vagina. Gynecol Oncol 70: 303–307
79. Shibata R, Umezawa A, Takehara K et al. 2003 Primary carcinosarcoma of the vagina. Pathol Int 53: 106–110
80. Tobon H, Murphy A I 1977 Benign blue nevus of the vagina. Cancer 40: 3174–3176
81. Heim K, Hopfl R, Muller-Holzner E et al. 2000 Multiple blue nevi of the vagina. A case report. J Reprod Med 45: 42–44
82. Chung A F, Casey M J, Flannery J T et al. 1980 Malignant melanoma of the vagina – report of 19 cases. Obstet Gynecol 55: 720–727
83. Weinstock M A 1994 Malignant melanoma of the vulva and vagina in the United States: patterns of incidence and population-based estimates of survival. Am J Obstet Gynecol 171: 1225–1230
84. DeMatos P, Tyler D, Seigler H F 1998 Mucosal melanoma of the female genitalia: a clinicopathologic study of forty-three cases at Duke University Medical Center. Surgery 124: 38–48
85. Gupta D, Malpica A, Deavers M T et al. 2002 Vaginal melanoma: a clinicopathologic and immunohistochemical study of 26 cases. Am J Surg Pathol 26: 1450–1457
86. Ragnarsson-Olding B, Johansson H, Rutqvist L E et al. 1993 Malignant melanoma of the vulva and vagina. Trends in incidence, age distribution, and long-term survival among 245 consecutive cases in Sweden 1960–1984. Cancer 71: 1893–1897
87. Vang R, Medeiros L J, Silva E G et al. 2000 Non-Hodgkin's lymphoma involving the vagina: a clinicopathologic analysis of 14 patients. Am J Surg Pathol 24: 719–725
88. Oliva E, Ferry J A, Young R H et al. 1997 Granulocytic sarcoma of the female genital tract: a clinicopathologic study of 11 cases. Am J Surg Pathol 21: 1156–1165
89. Young R H, Scully R E 1984 Endodermal sinus tumor of the vagina: a report of nine cases and review of the literature. Gynecol Oncol 18: 380–392
90. Copeland L J, Sneige N, Ordonez N G et al. 1985 Endodermal sinus tumor of the vagina and cervix. Cancer 55: 2558–2565
91. Mazur M T, Hsueh S, Gersell D J 1984 Metastases to the female genital tract. Analysis of 325 cases. Cancer 53: 1978–1984

第七部分

外阴 Vulva

Marisa R. Nucci 著

回允中　张艳梅　译

外阴

鳞状上皮肿瘤形成	730
良性肿瘤	730
癌前肿瘤形成	732
恶性鳞状上皮肿瘤	734
腺上皮肿瘤形成	735
良性肿瘤	735
恶性腺上皮肿瘤	736
黑色素细胞病变和肿瘤	738
间叶性肿瘤形成和瘤样病变	739
反应性病变	739
良性肿瘤	740
局部复发性间叶性肿瘤	742
恶性间叶性肿瘤	744
其他罕见的肿瘤	745

引言 Introduction

送来进行病理学检查的多数外阴标本是活检，部分切除或根治性切除的鳞状上皮肿瘤形成，这是本章第一节的主题。而腺上皮肿瘤形成、黑色素细胞肿瘤和间叶性肿瘤形成则少见得多，这些将在本章其余部分描述。

鳞状上皮肿瘤形成 Squamous neoplasia

发生在外阴的最常见的肿瘤前病变和肿瘤是鳞状上皮亚型。对于多数这些病变来说，主要病因是人乳头状瘤病毒（HPV）。与宫颈不同，只有某些 HPV 亚型（即 HPV 6、11 和 16）在外阴鳞状上皮肿瘤形成中占有优势。然而，不是所有类型的鳞状上皮肿瘤形成均与 HPV 感染有关，少数良性和恶性鳞状上皮病变尚有其他病因。

良性肿瘤 Benign neoplasms

前庭乳头状瘤（同义词：前庭乳头状瘤病、阴唇微乳头状瘤病、生理性乳头状瘤病）
Vestibular papilloma (synonyms: vestibular papillomatosis, micropapillomatosis labialis, physiologic papillomatosis)

临床特征

阴道前庭乳头是外阴检查时阴道入口周围的一种常见的正常发现；然而，在巴氏涂片异常的病人，这种表现可能促使活检以排除 HPV 相关病变的可能性，最常见的是尖锐湿疣。这些指样乳头状突起一般较小（通常小于 5mm），质软，常常围绕阴道开口排列，呈线样分布。如果出现症状的话，会表现为瘙痒或疼痛。其病因尚不清楚，似乎与 HPV 感染无关[1-3]。

病理学特征

鳞状上皮乳头状瘤一般是小的基底狭窄的指样乳头，被覆有光泽的黏膜。组织学检查，中心纤维轴心被覆复层鳞状上皮，典型者上皮糖原形成良好，没有棘层增厚或病毒细胞病变效应的证据（图 13G.1）。主要与尖锐湿疣进行鉴别诊断；然而，缺乏棘层增厚和细胞学非典型性可以排除这种可能性。

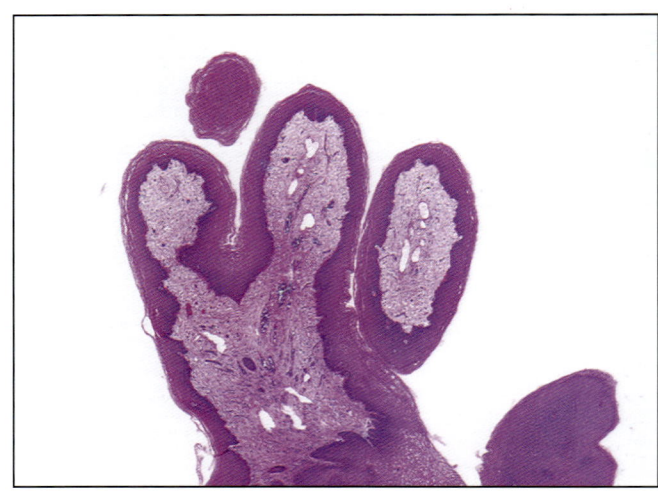

图13G.1　鳞状上皮乳头状瘤。复层鳞状上皮并不显示棘层增厚和病毒细胞病变效应。

脂溢性角化症　Seborrheic keratosis

临床特征

脂溢性角化症是一种良性表皮增生，较常发生在躯干和头颈部（见第23章），但是偶尔可以累及外阴皮肤。多数病变隆起，境界清楚，伴有蜡样外观；色素沉积并不少见。在生殖道脂溢性角化症已经发现HPV，特别是HPV6，HPV在这个部位的脂溢性角化症的发病机制中可能具有作用[4-6]。

病理学特征

这些病变的形态学类似于发生在生殖器外的脂溢性角化症（见第23章）。一般表现为鳞状上皮外生性增生，伴有棘层增厚、角化过度、疣状或网状生长方式。虽然一般不能发现病毒细胞病变效应，生殖道脂溢性角化症可以表现为角化过度症、乳头状瘤病和棘层增厚，这些是与尖锐湿疣共有的特征。考虑到这些生殖道病变常常与HPV有关，结合其形态学上的重叠，认为脂溢性角化症好像是尖锐湿疣的组织学亚型，或者至少是外阴HPV感染的另一种形态学表现，在治疗病人时应该考虑到这一点。

尖锐湿疣　Condyloma acuminatum

临床特征

尖锐湿疣作为一种与HPV感染（在外阴最常见的类型是HPV 6和11）相关的病变，一般发生在与性活动相伴的年龄，虽然偶尔可以发生在青春期前的儿童，提出性虐待的可能性[7]。这种病变可以为孤立性，但是较典型者为多发性，有时形成较大的融合性肿块。广泛性的外阴受累以及发病增加与免疫抑制有关[8]。尖锐湿疣是灰/粉/褐色乳头状或疣状增生，可能累及阴唇、会阴以及肛周皮肤或黏膜。如果有症状，可能出现局部刺激和瘙痒。治疗选择包括局部摘除疗法、切除或系统治疗[干扰素(interferon)]。复发并不少见，特别是在免疫抑制、糖尿病或妊娠的病人[9]；妊娠之后可能发生自发性消退。

病理学特征

尖锐湿疣的乳头状或疣状赘生物在肉眼检查时就很明显，组织学检查，乳头状结构被覆鳞状上皮并含有纤维血管轴心。棘层增厚、角化过度和角化不全常见；然而，与宫颈/阴道湿疣不同，挖空细胞非典型性可能轻微或仅为局灶性（图13G.2）。缺乏挖空细胞非典型性不能除外湿疣的可能性，因为显示棘层增厚和乳头状瘤病、但是缺乏明显病毒细胞病变组织学证据的病变与HPV6和11密切相关（表13G.1）[7]。在这些情况下，建议诊断鳞状上皮乳头状瘤，并且加上一个评注，说明这些病变常常与HPV有关；可能还要考虑基于分子学的HPV试验。缺乏挖空细胞非典型性的纤维上皮性息肉和扁平鳞状上皮增生与HPV感染无关。尖锐湿疣在组织学上不同于高级别外阴上皮内肿瘤形成（VIN 2-3），后者出

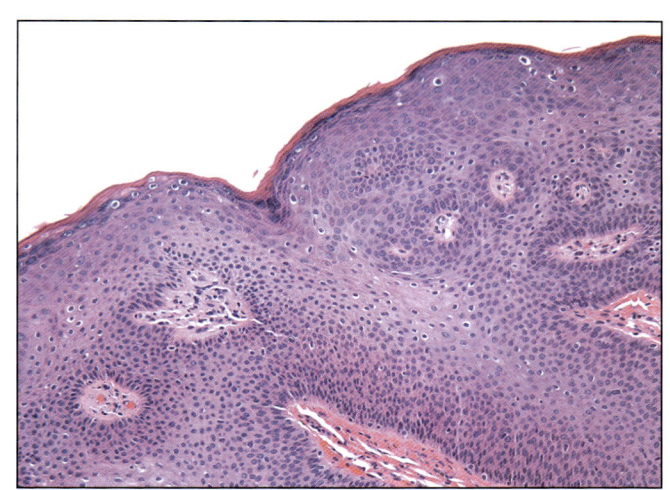

图13G.2　尖锐湿疣。挖空细胞非典型性可能轻微。

表13G.1　外阴鳞状上皮病变组织学特征比较

	乳头状瘤病	棘层增厚	挖空细胞形成	基底细胞非典型性
纤维上皮性间质息肉	+	–	–	–
鳞状上皮乳头状瘤	+	+	–	–
尖锐湿疣	+	+	+	–
Bowen样丘疹病（VIN 2-3）	+	+	±	+
分化性VIN	–	±	–	+

VIN：外阴上皮内肿瘤形成。

表13G.2	HPV相关性鳞状上皮内病变的鉴别诊断	
	尖锐湿疣	高级别VIN
临床表现	疣状乳头状	可变（扁平或乳头状）
核的特征	挖空细胞非典型性 核深染 外形不规则	挖空细胞非典型性 核深染 外形不规则
非典型性部位	中层到表面	基底到全层
伴随特征	棘层增厚 乳头状瘤病 角化不全	成熟异常 非典型性核分裂象
HPV类型	6，11	16

VIN：外阴上皮内肿瘤形成

现全层（或者接近全层）非典型性，以细胞核增大、核的轮廓不规则以及核深染为特征；VIN上皮全层出现核分裂活性以及异常核分裂象（表13G.2）。

癌前肿瘤形成　Premalignant neoplasia

外阴上皮内肿瘤形成
Vulvar intraepithelial neoplasia

VIN的诊断范畴涉及鳞状上皮的癌前改变；同义的其他术语（历史上较多应用）包括鳞状上皮异型增生、Bowen病和鳞状上皮原位癌。Bowen样丘疹病这一术语用于描述一种具有隆起的色素性病变的临床状况，通常发生在年轻妇女，常常自发性退化；这个术语不应该用于组织病理学诊断。对于外阴浸润性鳞状细胞癌的发生一般有两种公认而又非常独特的途径（与临床、形态学和病毒相关性参数有关）：（1）伴随典型性VIN的HPV相关性途径；（2）伴随分化（单纯）性VIN、硬化性苔藓和（或）外阴增生的非HPV相关性途径。

外阴上皮内肿瘤形成，典型性
Vulvar intraepithelial neoplasia, classic type

临床特征

在过去几十年中，典型性VIN的发生率有所增加，特别是在生育年龄的年轻妇女[10,11]。这可能与接触HPV的机会增加有关，特别是高危险性HPV 16、18和33，它们与这种类型的VIN密切相关。其他危险因素包括吸烟和人类免疫缺陷病毒（HIV）感染[12,13]。患有典型性VIN病人的主诉可能是外阴烧灼、瘙痒或疼痛。临床表现不同，具有一系列的变化，从扁平红斑性区域到深色素性或白色斑块、丘疹或疣状病变；这些表现还可以联合存在。外阴常常多灶性受累；大约30%的妇女还有宫颈和（或）阴道黏膜HPV相关性疾病[14,15]。治疗选择包括激光摘除和较常应用的广泛局部切除。因为VIN可能为亚临床的多灶性病变，所以复发并不少见。在HPV阳性的病人和大量吸烟者，切除不完全还有增加复发的危险性。边缘最好至少切除1cm；然而，为了维持性功能，不可能总是能够切除宽的组织或保证切缘阴性。临床上仅仅怀疑VIN的病例在组织病理学检查之后，发现多达20%的病例有浸润性鳞状细胞癌；多数病例为浅表浸润性癌[16,17]。

病理学特征

如同上面描述的一样，VIN的大体表现与其临床表现相同。组织学检查，VIN以全层或接近全层非典型性为特征。典型的表现包括核增大、核深染、凋亡和核分裂活性增加，伴有上皮上部出现核分裂象（包括异常核分裂象）（图13G.3）。可能存在不同程度的成熟和挖空细胞非典型性；角化过度和非典型性角化不全可能显著，与临床表现为白色有关。同样，上皮色素沉着以及间质和间质巨噬细胞内黑色素沉积可能明显，相当于临床显著的色素沉着部位。延伸到皮肤附件并不少见，不要误诊为浸润。

与宫颈前体病变相似，VIN也分为3级：1级、2级和3级。VIN 2和3相当于高级别前体病变，对于大多数病例来说区分两者是不恰当的，因为，在临床上它们的处理方式类似。一般来说，VIN 2相当于显示

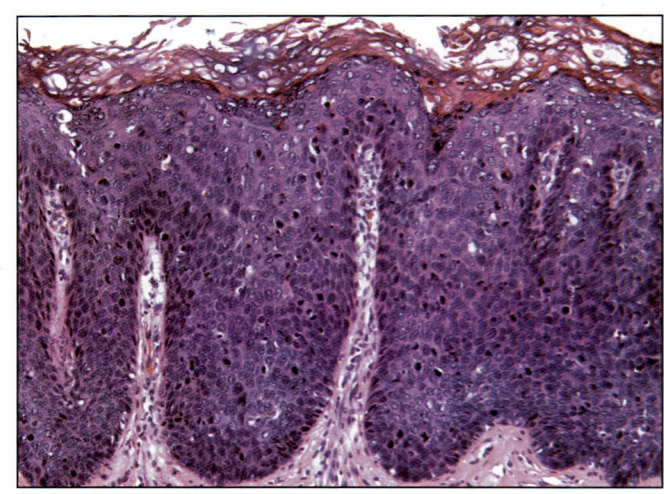

图13G.3　外阴上皮内肿瘤形成，典型性。上皮全层出现核增大、核深染、凋亡和核分裂活性。

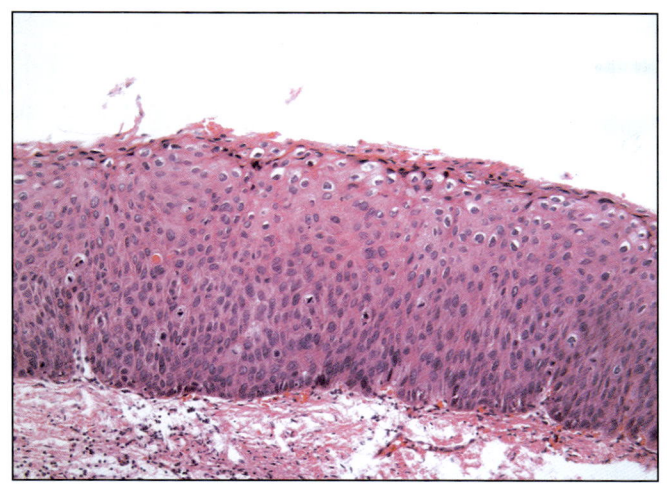

图13G.4 VIN 2。表面成熟伴有挖空细胞非典型性。

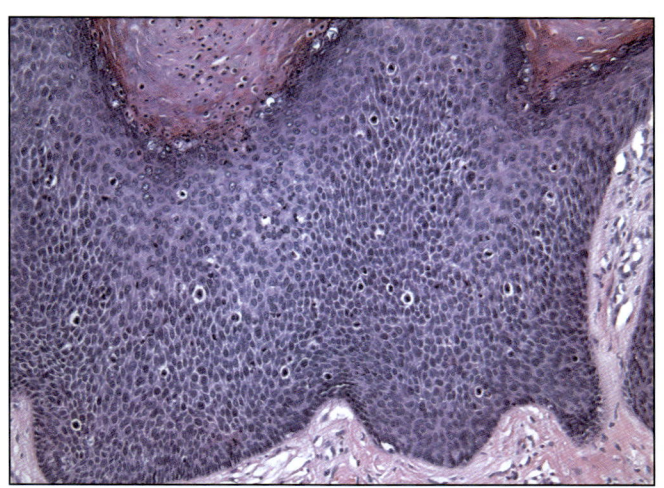

图13G.5 VIN 3。最低限度的表面成熟。

伴有表面角化和挖空细胞非典型性的成熟的病变（图13G.4）；VIN 3 显示最低限度的成熟（图13G.5）。与宫颈前体病变不同，VIN 1 并不相当于外生性或扁平湿疣，类似于低级别前体病变的组织学改变应该称为湿疣（尖锐）。根据定义，VIN 1 相当于局限于较下层的非典型性；然而，各种非肿瘤性炎症性疾病以及分化性 VIN（见下）也可能显示较下层的非典型性，而这些病变可能并不一定相当于低度危险/低级别病变。因此，不主张应用 VIN 1 这一术语。

VIN 的鉴别诊断包括色素性脂溢性角化症，特别是那些有炎症和显示轻度核增大的病例；不过，这些病变缺乏 VIN 特征性的核密集、核深染和非典型性。伴随反应性改变的多核细胞形成 [所谓的外阴多核细胞非典型性 (multinucleated atypia of the vulva)] 可能酷似 VIN；然而，受累的细胞核并不深染或增大，而且周围上皮表现正常[18]。

外阴上皮内肿瘤形成，分化（单纯）性
Vulvar intraepithelial neoplasia, differentiated (simplex) type

临床特征

与典型性 VIN 相比，分化（单纯）性 VIN 发生在年龄稍大的人群。此外，分化（单纯）性 VIN 不常见多灶性病变，而且伴随宫颈/阴道癌前病变的危险性低，推测是由于它缺乏与 HPV 的相关性。临床上，分化性 VIN 没有独特的表现；它常常伴有硬化性苔藓或其他外阴炎症性疾病，只有在组织学检查时才能评估。对于这种类型的 VIN 来说，最初是在临床上显著的浸润性鳞状细胞癌附近做出诊断的并不少见。因此，对于由于其他原因（主要是硬化性苔藓）活检而诊断为分化性 VIN 的病人，处理起来非常困难。一般来说，建议完全切除病变，临床密切随访，对于临床上明显的病变活检尺度要放宽，以便除外浸润。

病理学特征

与典型性 VIN 不同，分化性 VIN 的非典型性局限于上皮的下层，而且可能轻微（图 13G.6）。典型病变有棘层增厚、异常角化细胞成熟以及基底细胞核密集，伴有核深染和反常的突出的核仁（一般认为后者典型情况下出现在反应性病变中）。偶尔可能有明显的棘层松解。还可能出现硬化性苔藓相关性变化，即均质化的真皮胶原和这个硬化带下方的带样淋巴细胞浸润。

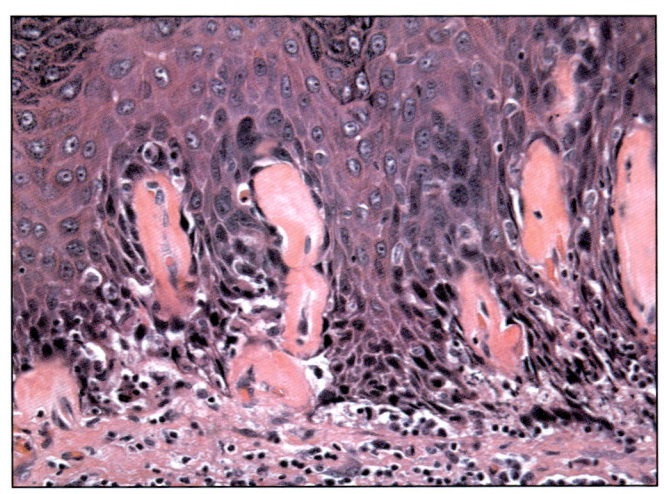

图13G.6 分化性VIN。核的非典型性局限于上皮的基底部分。

恶性鳞状上皮肿瘤
Malignant squamous neoplasms

鳞状细胞癌　Squamous cell carcinoma

浸润性鳞状细胞癌是外阴最常见的恶性肿瘤。发病率从 1:100 000 到 20:100 000 不等，发病率增加与年龄有关，高峰年龄在 70～80 岁[11,19]。新近研究发现，外阴鳞状细胞癌的发病机制有两个明显的途径：(1) 癌的发生与 HPV 感染和典型性 VIN 有关；(2) 癌发生于缺乏 HPV 感染的病人，或与分化性 VIN、硬化性苔藓（伴有或不伴有鳞状上皮增生）有关，或没有明显的癌前病变[19]。与由于非病毒性因素引起的外阴癌相比，典型性 VIN 和 HPV 感染相关性癌倾向于发生在相对较为年轻的年龄组；吸烟也是这个年龄组的危险因素[20]。

临床特征

浸润性鳞状细胞癌一般表现为一个孤立性的肿瘤，可以是外生性（结节状、疣状、蕈状）、内生性（溃疡伴有隆起质硬的边缘），或难以确定的黏膜增厚区。症状包括局部不适、疼痛、瘙痒和烧灼感，瘙痒和烧灼感可能与并发的感染有关，这两个症状并不少见。根据 FIGO 分类和结局的分期与疾病的分期有关；妇科肿瘤组的研究已经报告，I～IV 期疾病的 5 年生存率分别为 98%、85%、74% 和 31%[21]。治疗主要是外科手术。大于 FIGO IA 期（癌的直径小于 2 cm，伴有间质浸润小于 1mm）的病人通过切除（广泛局部、部分/全部外阴切除）治疗，并取腹股沟淋巴结。对于 FIGO IA 期的病人，广泛局部切除伴有 1 cm 的边缘已经足够；没有必要清扫淋巴结。下列情况考虑放射治疗：(1) 考虑有手术危险的病人；(2) 作为预后不好的肿瘤病人的辅助治疗；以及 (3) 不适合手术的复发或转移病人[22]；放射治疗对于预防局部淋巴结复发也可能起作用[23]。腹股沟淋巴结转移的危险因素包括：(1) 较高的肿瘤分级；(2) 临床上淋巴结可疑（例如固定、溃疡）；(3) 出现毛细淋巴管浸润；(4) 老年病人；以及 (5) 浸润较深；肿瘤大小和部位好像不是独立的危险因素[24]。与淋巴结状况有关的肿瘤复发危险因素包括淋巴结转移的数目和出现包膜外播散；HPV DNA 状况似乎没有预后意义[25]。

病理学特征

浸润性鳞状细胞癌有许多形态学亚型，包括角化性、非角化性、基底细胞样、湿疣样、梭形细胞和疣状癌。根据严格的定义疣状癌几乎没有转移的潜能，除此以外，将这些癌再从形态学上分为角化性、非角化性、基底细胞样和湿疣样并不具有临床意义。角化性癌具有显著的角化珠结构，而非角化性癌虽然可能存在伴有角化不良细胞的局灶性角化，但是没有角化珠形成（图 13G.7）。基底细胞样癌和湿疣样癌常常与 HPV 感染有关（特别是 HPV 16）；基底细胞样癌的组织学表现类似于 VIN，常常称为上皮内型浸润性鳞状细胞癌（intraepithelial type of invasive squamous cell carcinoma）（图 13G.8），而湿疣样亚型（warty variant）表面细胞具有挖空细胞非典型性。某些浸润性鳞状细胞癌，特别是在老年病人，可能有明显的梭形肿瘤细胞（图 13G.9）。这样一种表现常常提出肉瘤的可能性；然而，这个部位的梭形鳞状细胞癌常见得多，在诊断肉瘤之前首先应该予以除外（与黑色素瘤一道）。此外，棘层松解性病变可能类似于血管肉瘤。重要的是需要指出，某些梭形细胞鳞状细胞癌 keratin 染色可能仅仅局灶阳性，可能需要应用一系列的 keratins；邻

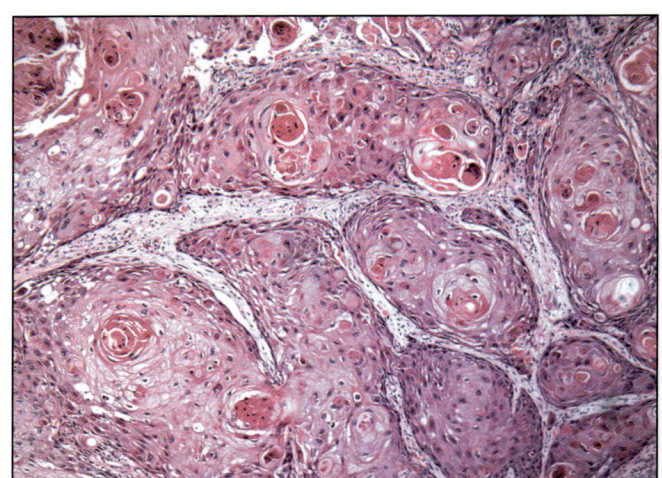

图13G.7　浸润性鳞状细胞癌，角化型。明显的角化珠结构和中心角化漩涡。

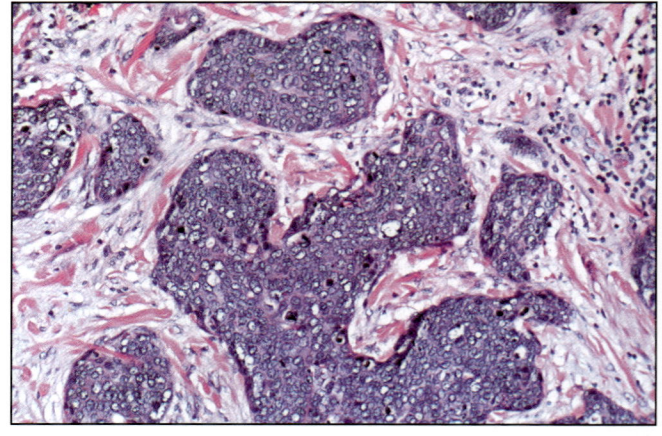

图13G.8　浸润性鳞状细胞癌，基底细胞样型。浸润的肿瘤细胞巢显示轻微的成熟。

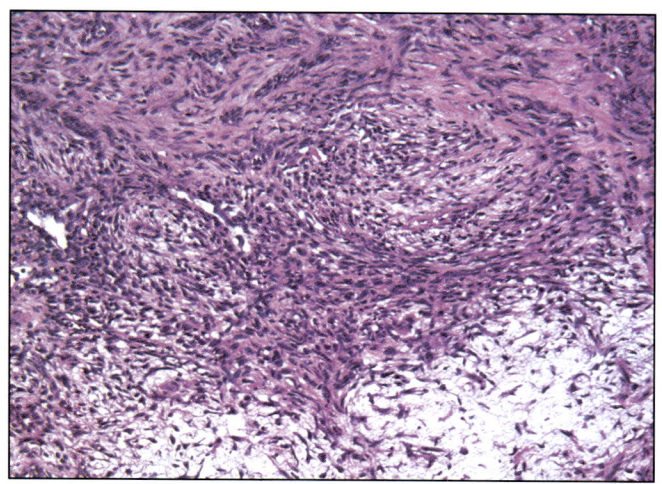

图13G.9 浸润性鳞状细胞癌，梭形细胞型。显著的梭形肿瘤细胞酷似肉瘤。注意图片上部出现肿瘤细胞巢，揭示了这个肿瘤的真正本质。

近的原位癌可能提示（而且支持）鳞状细胞癌的诊断。

疣状癌 Verrucous carcinoma

疣状癌是浸润性鳞状细胞癌的一种罕见的亚型，一般发生于老年妇女，通常在80～90岁。临床特征是预后特别好（几乎没有转移潜能），组织学特征是具有非常高分化的表现，伴有轻微的细胞学非典型性（图13G.10）和粗钝的浸润性边缘。疣状癌的发病机制尚不清楚，某些研究显示好像与HPV感染无关[26]。在某些病例，邻近的外阴黏膜可能显示不同程度的棘层增厚、疣状结构、颗粒细胞层消失、表层上皮细胞苍白以及角化不全；这些改变被称为外阴棘层增厚伴有分化改变（vulvar acanthosis with altered differentiation），可能是疣

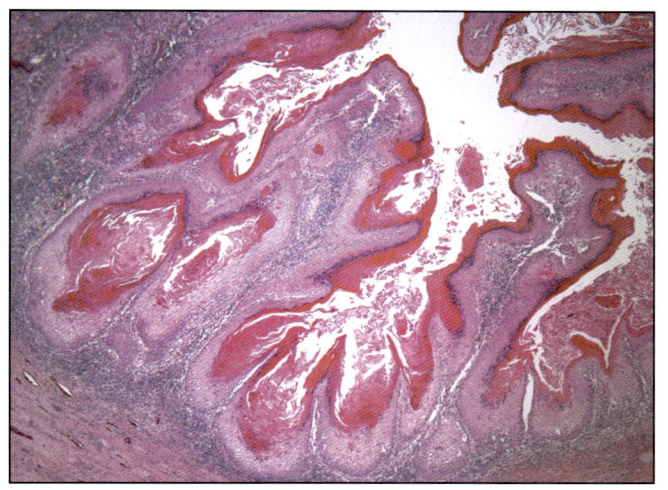

图13G.10 疣状癌。与间质的交界面粗钝以及几乎没有细胞学非典型性是其特征。

状癌的前体病变（或危险因素）[26]。

基底细胞癌 Basal cell carcinoma

外阴基底细胞癌[27-31]是一种少见的肿瘤，占外阴恶性肿瘤的2%～5%。它主要发生在绝经后的妇女，发病高峰年龄在70～80岁。最常见的症状包括瘙痒、疼痛和（或）刺激，可以持续不同的时间，从数月到数年。临床表现各异，可以是息肉样病变、结节或斑块，伴有或不伴有溃疡形成；还可能发生色素沉着过多或色素减退。肿瘤通常位于大阴唇，大小一般小于2 cm，虽然可以发生较大的肿瘤或多灶性的病变。组织学检查，外阴基底细胞癌与发生在长期暴露于阳光的皮肤的基底细胞癌表现类似。外阴基底细胞癌可为局灶侵袭性，但只偶尔发生转移；因此，广泛局部切除不进行淋巴结清扫是标准的治疗方法，除非临床上怀疑局部淋巴结受累。

腺上皮肿瘤形成 Glandular neoplasia

引言 Introduction

外阴腺上皮肿瘤形成可以从皮肤附件结构、特化的肛门生殖器乳腺型腺体、前庭大腺（Bartholin）和前庭小腺、尿道旁腺（Skene腺）发生，或者可能无法确定来源。

良性肿瘤 Benign neoplasms

前庭大腺腺瘤（腺肌瘤）Bartholin's gland adenoma (adenomyoma)

前庭大腺腺瘤是一种非常罕见的肿瘤[32]，直径平均2～3 cm，实性，临床检查常常被认为是囊肿。其特征为导管和腺泡不规则性增生，内衬分泌黏液的上皮，可以被肌瘤性间质分开。腺瘤和结节性增生的区别是后者保留了正常导管与腺泡的关系，虽然归入腺瘤的病变是否为真正的肿瘤尚有争论。在少数情况下，涎腺样癌的发生可能与腺瘤有关[32,33]。

乳头状汗腺腺瘤 Papillary hidradenoma

临床特征

乳头状汗腺腺瘤是一种良性附件（汗腺）肿瘤[34,35]，几乎毫无例外地发生于白人妇女的肛门生殖器部位。本病发生的年龄范围广泛，可以累及生育年龄妇女和绝经后妇女。乳头状汗腺腺瘤一般小于3 cm，为孤立性、位于大阴唇真皮的圆顶形结节；偶尔可以发生多发性结节（通常

小于3个)。如果有症状，可能包括疼痛或出血。偶尔，病人会注意到病变大小随着月经周期而变化。少数情况下，病人有外生性或溃疡性病变，临床上酷似恶性肿瘤。

病理学特征

乳头状汗腺腺瘤是境界清楚、位于真皮的实性或囊实性病变。组织学表现类似于乳腺导管内乳头状瘤（图13G.11）。肿瘤没有包膜，但是常常有一个假包膜，由周围一圈受压的间质组成。肿瘤含有复杂而不同的增生性成分，包括腺泡、小管、乳头和（或）囊肿。这些结构内衬两种细胞：外层基底细胞（类似于乳腺导管内乳头状瘤的肌上皮层）和内层分泌细胞，分泌细胞具有顶浆分泌腺分化的特征，胞浆嗜酸性颗粒状，伴有顶端突起，细胞核圆形，位于基底部。

前庭小腺腺瘤
Adenoma of minor vestibular glands

前庭小腺腺瘤[36,37]是一种罕见的良性肿瘤，最常见的是持续性性交困难和（或）疼痛（外阴前庭炎）病人接受小前庭附件切除治疗时偶然发现的。肿瘤通常小于2cm，由增生的腺体和导管组成，内衬立方到柱状细胞，顶端含有黏液性胞浆。

混合性肿瘤（多形性腺瘤、软骨样汗腺腺瘤）
Mixed tumor (pleomorphic adenoma, chondroid syringoma)

涎腺型混合瘤（多形性腺瘤）[38,39]被认为是起源于前庭大腺、前庭小腺或皮肤汗腺，很少发生于外阴。软组织肌上皮瘤归入混合瘤范畴，偶尔也可能累及腹股沟部位[40]。最常见的表现是境界清楚的皮下结节。组织学特征类似于涎腺混合性肿瘤。少数情况下，可以发生具有恶性细胞形态学特征的恶性混合瘤和肌上皮癌病例。几乎所有的混合瘤和肌上皮瘤均表达keratin，绝大多数还表达S-100、calponin和EMA。也可能表达GFAP、SMA、p63和desmin，但不太一致[40]。

其他良性皮肤附件肿瘤
Other benign skin appendage neoplasms

汗腺腺瘤（syringoma）是外分泌汗腺的良性肿瘤，好发于面部、颈部和躯干，但是也可能发生于外阴，外阴汗腺腺瘤一般表现为双侧多发性肤色丘疹[41-43]。它发生的年龄范围可能广泛，诊断时的平均年龄为20～30岁。如果出现症状，最常见的是瘙痒。组织学检查，外阴汗腺腺瘤的表现类似于发生在较普通部位的汗腺腺瘤（见第23章）。

其他皮肤附件肿瘤偶尔可以累及外阴，包括毛鞘（毛发）囊肿 [trichilemmal (pilar) cysts]、毛母细胞纤维瘤（trichoblastic fibroma）和毛上皮瘤（trichoepithelioma）[44-48]。

恶性腺上皮肿瘤
Malignant glandular neoplasms

外阴Paget病　Vulvar Paget's disease

临床特征

乳腺外Paget病[49-55]是一种罕见的肿瘤，可能仅仅累及表皮（伴有或不伴有真皮浸润），或是来自其下方恶性肿瘤的扩散。最常见的受累部位是外阴，但是即使是在这个部位，它也是一种罕见的肿瘤，不到所有外阴恶性肿瘤的1%～2%。与乳腺Paget病不同，外阴Paget病不常伴有其下方的恶性肿瘤，少数病例（通常少于10%～15%）与局部（最常见的是皮肤附件）癌有关[49-55]。这不同于肛周Paget病（表皮内肿瘤性病变主要累及肛周黏膜），肛周Paget病下面常常伴有直肠腺癌[56]。侵袭性Paget病（invasive Paget's disease）的肿瘤细胞越过基底膜侵入真皮，大约发生在15%～20%的病例[49-55]。浸润小于1 mm的病人预后类似于非侵袭性Paget病[49,50]，虽然个别病例伴有局部淋巴结转移[57,58]。浸润大于1 mm或其下方有癌的病人预后不好，而且具有较大的局部和远隔转移的危险[49-51,54]。总的复发率大约为30%，病变切除不完全者复发率最高[49-52,54,55]。

外阴Paget病一般发生在60～70岁，较常见于白人，最常表现为瘙痒[54]。临床检查一般显示表面呈红色，有不规则的抓痕，是一个界限清楚的病变，可能被误认为是一种湿疹性炎症性病变。外阴Paget病的特

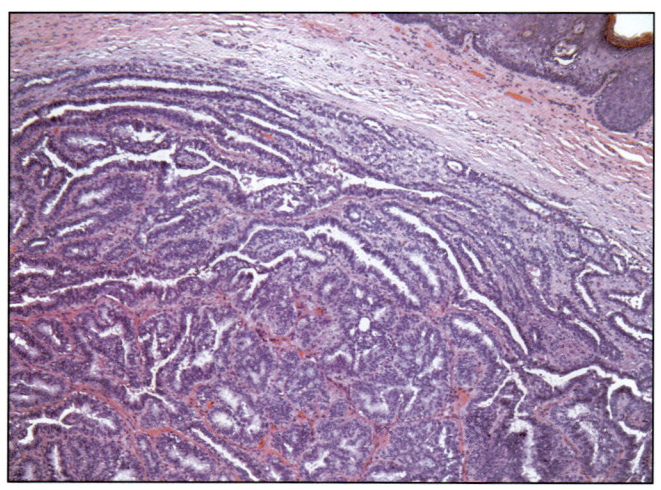

图13G.11　乳头状汗腺腺瘤。复杂增生的小管和腺泡类似于乳腺导管内乳头状瘤。

征是累及阴唇，两侧受累并不少见，而且可能延伸并累及肛周部位。本病可以进一步延伸，超出临床表现所提示的区域；因此，常常进行活检以便确定疾病范围，这有助于指导手术治疗。

病理学特征

外阴Paget病以表皮内大的表皮样细胞增生为特征，胞浆丰富，颗粒状或空泡状淡染，核圆形，核仁突出。表皮内细胞单个或成簇排列，多数细胞常常在副基底层，而某些细胞接近上层（图13G.12）。基底膜下方出现单个细胞或细胞簇表明有真皮浸润（侵袭性Paget病）。外阴Paget病与其他上皮内恶性肿瘤的免疫组化表现列在表13G.3中。肿瘤细胞胞浆内黏液、CK7、EMA、CEA和GCDFP一般阳性；罕见的病例也可能共同表达CK20[49,50]。CK7阴性、CK20阳性和GCDFP阴性的Paget病病例，强烈提示从隐匿的胃肠道（直肠）原发性肿瘤扩散而来的可能性[50,56]。主要应与原位恶性黑色素瘤进行鉴别诊断，通过黑色素瘤表达黑色素瘤标志物（S-100、HMB-45、MART-1）和缺乏keratins、CEA和GCDFP阳性表达可能容易鉴别。

前庭大腺癌 Bartholin's gland carcinoma

前庭大腺恶性肿瘤少见，占所有外阴恶性肿瘤的2%～7%[59-62]。多数病例发生于50～60岁的绝经后妇女，表现为一个无痛性的外阴肿块。如果具备下述条件，认为肿瘤是原发性前庭大腺肿瘤：（1）辨认出从良性前庭大腺转变为肿瘤性病变；（2）其他部位没有发现原发性肿瘤；以及（3）肿瘤组织学符合从前庭大腺来源。许多不同类型的癌可以起源于前庭大腺，最常见的是鳞状细胞癌、腺癌（黏液性、乳头状或胶样癌）以及腺样囊性癌；偶尔还可能发生腺鳞癌、移行细胞癌和小细胞癌[63-67]。

乳腺型腺癌 Mammary-type adenocarcinoma

乳腺型腺癌[68-77]是一个非常少见的恶性肿瘤，认为是来源于形态学上类似于乳腺的外阴良性腺体组织。最初认为是"异位"乳腺组织，但是这些腺体具有外分泌和顶浆分泌分化的特征，所以可能是肛门生殖器皮肤汗腺的一种乳腺样变型[78]。这些肿瘤一般发生于50～80岁的绝经后妇女，大小通常小于4cm。与原发性乳腺癌类似，在组织学检查时外阴乳腺型腺癌可以显示导管、小叶或顶浆分泌腺分化。可能存在伴随的原位癌；在罕见的情况下可能见到没有浸润的导管原位癌[79,80]。肿瘤ER、PR和GCDFP可能阳性。

尿道旁腺腺癌 Skene's gland adenocarcinoma

尿道旁腺位于尿道两侧的附近，由黏液腺组成，开口于内衬移行上皮的导管。根据其形态学和前列腺标志物的表达，这些腺体被认为是男性前列腺在女性的类似组织（或同源发生）。少数情况下可能发生来源于这些腺体的腺癌[81-83]。组织学检查，这些肿瘤享有与前列

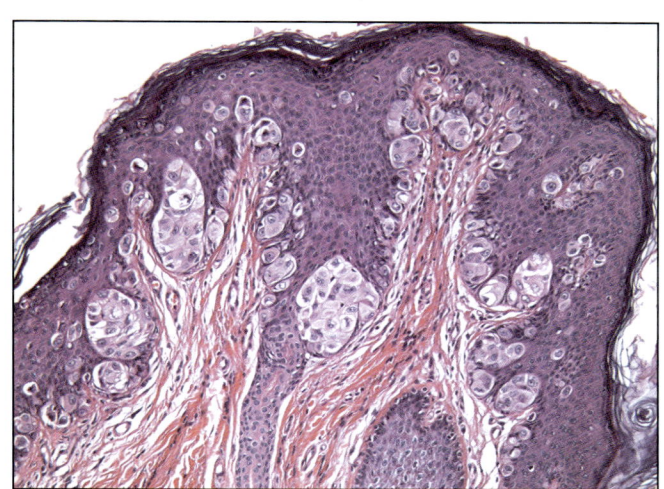

图13G.12 Paget病。表皮内细胞增生，伴有丰富的嗜酸性胞浆，核圆形，核仁突出。

表13G.3	不同类型外阴上皮内恶性肿瘤免疫组化所见比较								
	CK7	CAM5.2	CK20	EMA	CEA	GCDFP	S-100	HMB-45	Uroplakin
Paget病	+	+	-（+罕见）	+	+	+	-	-	-
原位黑色素瘤	-	-	-	-	-	-	+	+	-
Paget样鳞状细胞癌	+	-	-	+	-	-	-	-	-
Paget样直肠腺癌	-	+	+	+	+	-	-	-	-
Paget样移行细胞癌	±	+	±	+	+	-	-	-	+

EMA：上皮膜抗原（epithelial membrane antigen）；CEA：癌胚抗原（carcinoembryonic antigen）；GCDFP：大囊肿病液体蛋白（gross cystic disease fluid protein）。

腺癌共同的特征,高分化的肿瘤是由小腺体结构组成的,细胞核均匀一致,核仁突出,胞浆中等量,嗜酸性或颗粒状。与良性尿道旁腺相似,肿瘤细胞前列腺特异性抗原阳性。

其他罕见类型的腺癌 Other rare types of adenocarcinoma

绒毛腺管状(泄殖腔源性)腺癌 [villoglandular (cloacogenic) adenocarcinoma] 是一种非常罕见的肠型肿瘤,推测是来源于外阴的泄殖腔源性残余[84-88]。报告的病例非常之少,肿瘤通常发生于40岁以上的女性,大小<2cm,临床检查时呈现红色结节状或息肉样外观。组织学检查,肿瘤似乎与表皮直接连续,形态学类似于肠的腺癌。外阴腺管绒毛状腺瘤(tubulovillous adenoma of the vulva)也是非常少见,由此可以发生浸润性腺癌[87,89,90]。

子宫内膜异位症相关性腺癌(adenocarcinoma arising in association with endometriosis)在少数情况下可以发生于外阴;类似于其他部位的子宫内膜异位症的恶性转化,多数病例有子宫内膜异位症的形态学改变,但是也有发生透明细胞腺癌的报告[91-93]。

外阴可以遇到与Paget病无关的原发性汗腺癌(primary sweat gland carcinoma),但是非常罕见;其中包括外分泌汗腺腺癌(eccrine adenocarcinoma)、外分泌汗孔癌(eccrine porocarcinoma)、透明细胞汗腺腺癌(clear cell hidradenocarcinoma)和微囊性附件癌(microcystic adnexal carcinoma)[94-96]。

黑色素细胞病变和肿瘤 Melanocytic lesions and neoplasms

雀斑样痣 Lentigo

各种各样的术语已被用于描述生殖器部位的良性色素性斑,包括外阴黑变病(melanosis)和外阴雀斑样痣[生殖器雀斑样痣病(genital lentiginosis)]。前一个术语用于角化细胞基底色素沉着增加的外阴色素性病变,不伴有黑色素细胞增生。因为外阴色素斑与黑色素细胞增生无关的非常少见,所以常常应用外阴雀斑样痣这一术语,这样比较恰当。外阴雀斑样痣通常是一个孤立性、均匀一致的同质性色素斑,其大小<5mm;然而,有时在临床上生殖器雀斑样痣却令人担忧,呈花斑状表现,色素沉着不规则,比通常见到的要大[97]。外阴雀斑样痣的发生可能与LAMB综合征(黏膜皮肤雀斑样痣、心房黏液瘤和蓝痣)或多发性雀斑样痣(雀斑样痣和肥大性心肌病)有关[98,99]。外阴雀斑样痣好像不是原位黑色素

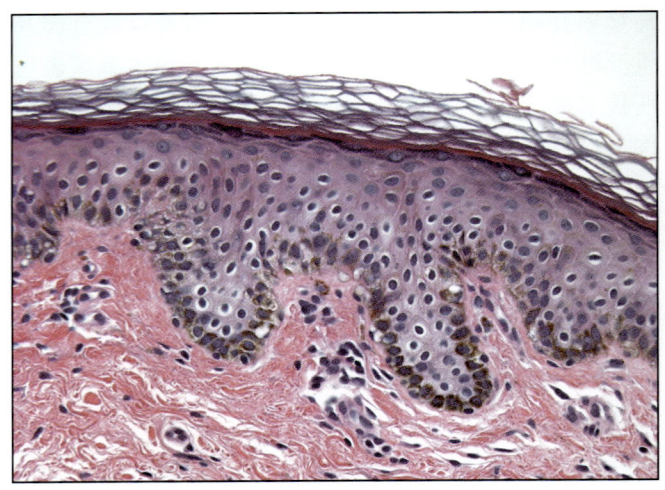

图13G.13 雀斑样痣。注意黑色素细胞增生和基底层色素沉着过度。

瘤或恶性黑色素瘤显著的前体病变。组织学检查,这些病变显示不同程度的棘层增厚、黑色素细胞增生以及基底层色素沉着过度(图13G.13);色素沉着失禁可能是突出的特征。不出现黑色素细胞非典型性。

生殖器型痣 Genital-type nevi

普通类型的黑色素细胞痣可以发生在外阴,包括获得性皮内痣、交界痣和复合痣、发育不良性痣以及蓝痣。外阴痣的这些亚型与见于生殖器外的痣相同,将在第23章进一步讨论。然而,生殖器痣的确具有独特的组织病理学特征[100,101]。这些痣也叫曲面痣(flexural nevi),因为它们可以发生在以冗余皮肤为特征的任何部位。生殖器型痣常常比普通型痣大,表现为比较不规则的色素沉着形态;然而,它们通常对称,而且境界清楚。组织学检查,表现为较大的交界痣细胞巢,伴有结构变异,包括痣细胞巢大小、形状和部位的差异以及痣细胞融合(图13G.14)。此外,常常伴有雀斑性黑色素细胞增生以及

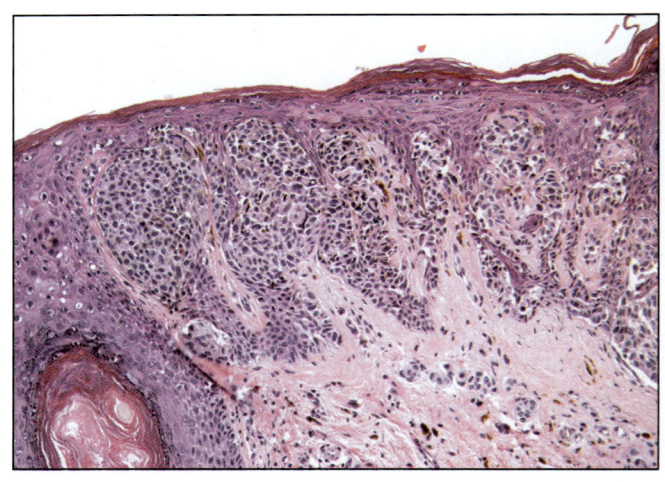

图13G.14 生殖器型痣。注意大的交界痣,痣细胞巢大小、形状和部位不同。

表皮内黑色素细胞巢。Paget 样扩散少见，如果出现应该高度关注有无黑色素瘤。虽然痣细胞常常出现细胞非典型性，通常只是见于少数细胞；出现弥漫性细胞学非典型性时也应该注意有无黑色素瘤。在提出具有黑色素瘤可能性特征的病例，应该考虑病人的年龄，因为外阴黑色素瘤一般是发生于老年女性的肿瘤。生殖器型痣与发育不良性痣具有某些重叠的组织学特征，但是后者倾向于呈现较为突出的雀斑样痣性生长方式，而且网嵴显著延长。此外，发育不良性痣比较常见间质纤维化和伴随慢性炎症浸润。

恶性黑色素瘤[102-117]　Malignant melanoma

恶性黑色素瘤不常累及外阴，但却是仅次于鳞状细胞癌的第二个最常见的外阴恶性肿瘤。生殖器外黑色素瘤病人的发病年龄高峰在 30~40 岁左右，与之不同的是外阴黑色素瘤一般发生在老年妇女，多数病人 50~80 岁。病人出现的症状通常与肿块有关；疼痛、出血或瘙痒也是常见的主诉。肿瘤累及外阴黏膜比皮肤常见，通常为明显的色素沉着；然而，无黑色素性肿瘤并不少见，在一项大的系列研究中占外阴黑色素瘤的 30%[107]。外阴黑色素瘤的发病机制了解较少；阳光照射、遗传因素以及产次好像不起作用。肿瘤厚度增加与预后不良有关；外阴黑色素瘤总的预后一般较差，因为与生殖器外黑色素瘤不同，多数外阴黑色素瘤病人处于疾病晚期。据报告 5 年生存率达 54%[105,108-110]；在一项 219 例大的系列研究中，5 年生存率为 47%[107]。组织学检查，外阴黑色素瘤的表现常常类似于肢端雀斑样痣黑色素瘤，其次为结节状黑色素瘤，浅表播散性黑色素瘤最不常见。在第 23 章中可以见到有关这些类型黑色素瘤组织病理学的详细描述。皮肤黑色素瘤已经做了显微镜下分期；然而，由于外阴黏膜没有真皮乳头和网嵴，所以不可能测定 Clark 分级。我们的惯例是报告仅仅用于黏膜黑色素瘤的 Breslow 厚度。Chung 描述的修订 Clark 分级也可以应用[114]。

间叶性肿瘤形成和瘤样病变
Mesenchymal neoplasia and tumor-like conditions

反应性病变　Reactive lesions

纤维上皮性间质息肉　Fibroepithelial stromal polyp

临床特征

纤维上皮性间质息肉[118-129] 是激素反应性病变，来源于女性生殖道远端上皮下的细胞。它们发生于生育年龄的妇女，一般发生在妊娠期间，但是也可能与激素替代疗法有关[119,124,125]。这些病变大小不同（但是一般小于 5cm），典型者呈息肉样或有蒂，通常为孤立性，虽然妊娠妇女可能发生多发性息肉[122,124]。妊娠之后，息肉常常退化，支持它们是良性反应性增生，是对激素环境改变的反应。这些病变有可能局部复发，特别是如果切除不完全，或继续有激素刺激时（例如妊娠），但是这相对少见[118,125,129]。

病理学特征

纤维上皮性间质息肉是息肉样病变，其特征为：(1) 纤维血管轴心；(2) 不同程度的富于细胞的间质；(3) 星形和多核间质细胞，最常出现在上皮-间质交界的附近或邻近明显的中心血管结构；以及 (4) 被覆鳞状上皮，可能显示不同程度的增生。这些病变没有明确的边缘，延伸至黏膜-黏膜下交界处，符合黏膜下组织增生性膨胀。发生在妊娠期间的息肉可见细胞构成增加，核有多形性，核分裂活跃，以致过去应用假葡萄状肉瘤这一术语。这些令人担忧的组织学所见不仅局限于妊娠相关性息肉，它们的出现可能提出恶性的可能[129]，然而，即使是在最活跃的病例，这些病变的形态学也与普通表现的息肉有所重叠，包括：(1) 病变缺乏可以辨认的边缘；(2) 非典型性间质细胞延伸到间质-上皮交界处；以及 (3) 这个部位普通息肉的间质-上皮交界附近常常出现多核细胞（图 13G.15）。与正常外阴间叶组织相似，这些病变的间质细胞 desmin、actin、vimentin、ER 和 PR 免疫染色可能阳性。虽然常常讨论，但是这些病变还是容易与葡萄状肉瘤鉴别；纤维上皮性间质息肉在青春期前罕见，并且缺乏上皮下细胞丰

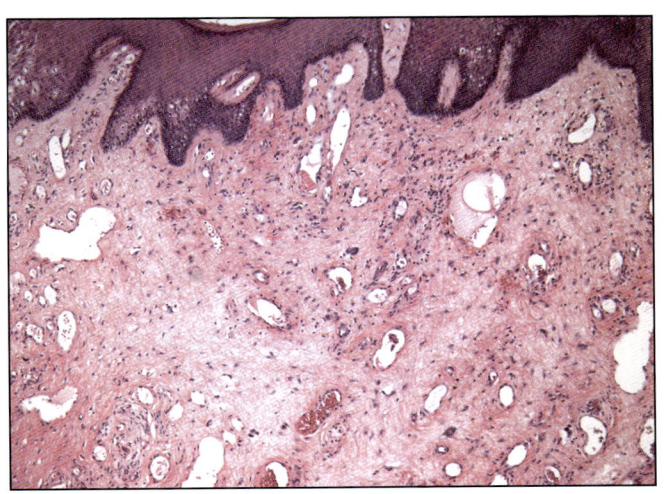

图 13G.15　纤维上皮性间质息肉。间质-上皮交界处出现特征性的星形和多核间质细胞。

富的新生层，缺乏横纹肌母细胞，以及缺乏骨骼肌标志物表达。

结节性筋膜炎　Nodular fasciitis

结节性筋膜炎是反应性肌纤维母细胞增生，比较典型的病变累及肢体；然而，它可以发生在诸多的部位，包括在个别情况下累及外阴[130-132]。知道这个不寻常的部位可以发生结节性筋膜炎，对于不要将其误认为恶性肿瘤至关重要。外阴结节性筋膜炎通常小于 3 cm，组织学检查与发生在其他部位的病例相同（见第 24 章），由境界相对清楚的疏松排列的梭形细胞增生组成，细胞具有两极胞浆突起，常常被比作组织培养的纤维母细胞。常见散在的炎症细胞和外渗的红细胞；核分裂活性常常显著。

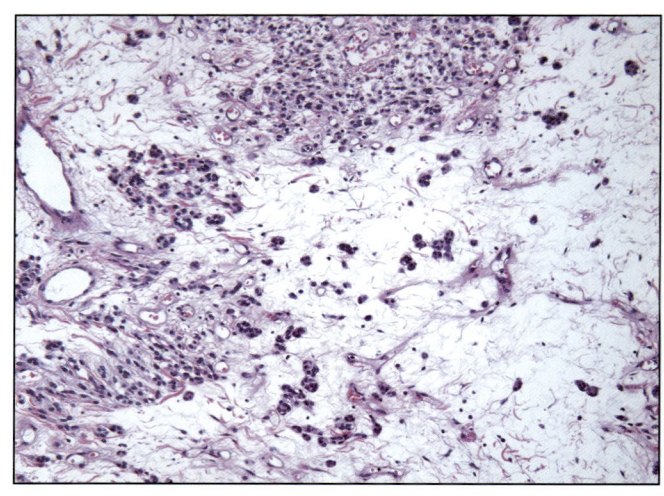

图13G.16　血管肌纤维母细胞瘤。注意许多毛细血管大小的血管和交替的细胞构成。

良性肿瘤　Benign neoplasms

血管肌纤维母细胞瘤　Angiomyofibroblastoma

临床特征

血管肌纤维母细胞瘤[133-138]是一种良性肿瘤，几乎完全发生在生育年龄妇女的外阴阴道部位；在少数情况下，类似的肿瘤也可以发生在绝经后的妇女以及男性的腹股沟/阴囊部位。肿瘤一般较小（小于 5 cm），境界清楚，临床检查可能被误诊为囊肿。这些肿瘤没有复发的潜能；因此，局部切除伴有清楚的边缘是适当的治疗。罕见的是，据说血管肌纤维母细胞瘤可以发生肉瘤性转变[139]。

病理学特征

血管肌纤维母细胞瘤是一种境界清楚的肿瘤，由许多纤细薄壁毛细血管大小的血管和肥胖的圆形到梭形细胞混合组成，肿瘤细胞一般围绕显著的血管结构成簇排列（图 13G.16）。间质细胞位于不同程度水肿到胶原性的基质中，伴有交替的细胞构成带，而且常常有一些上皮样表现（绝经后病人较常为梭形细胞，是个例外），具有中等量嗜酸性胞浆，核染色质细，核仁不明显。一般没有核分裂象。偶尔，病变内可见脂肪组织。间质细胞 desmin 染色一般阳性，actin 通常为阴性，但是可呈不同程度阳性反应。主要的鉴别诊断是侵袭性血管黏液瘤，两者必须区分开来，因为其生物学行为不同（见下文）；然而，它们在组织学表现上完全不同。侵袭性血管黏液瘤均一性地细胞稀少，具有浸润性的边缘，以及倾向于有较大的厚壁血管。表 13G.4 总结了常见外阴间叶性病变的临床和组织学区别。

富于细胞性血管纤维瘤　Cellular angiofibroma

临床特征

富于细胞性血管纤维瘤[140-142]是一种良性间叶性肿瘤，最常发生在外阴阴道部位。最初认为全部发生在女性，但是现在发现这些肿瘤还常常发生在男性的腹股沟阴囊部位，以及偶尔见于生殖器以外的部位。在女性，肿物平均 2.7 cm，发生年龄范围广泛（平均 53.5 岁），最常表现为一个境界清楚的无痛性皮下肿块[142]。如果完全切除，复发似乎非常罕见；一例复发性富于细胞性血管纤维瘤的个案报告很可能是残余肿瘤的继续生长[143]。局部保守切除伴有阴性边缘似乎是恰当的治疗。

病理学特征

富于细胞性血管纤维瘤一般质硬，具有橡皮样质地，外观呈灰/白色。组织学检查，多数病例边缘境界清楚；然而，一小部分病例边缘可能不清楚，并浸润周围正常组织。它是一个富于细胞的肿瘤，由下述成分构成：(1) 短而交错成束排列的良性梭形细胞，伴有短卵圆形到梭形的细胞核以及少量淡染的细胞浆，细胞界限清楚；(2) 许多小到中等大小的厚壁血管，常有玻璃样变性；以及 (3) 小束状胶原纤维（图 13G.17）。许多病例病变内还含有脂肪组织。核分裂象一般不常见，缺乏显著的核多形性，虽然偶尔出现变性核的非典型性。玻璃样变或水肿区域可能是造成细胞构成不同的原因。大约 60% 的病例间质成分 CD34 阳性；SMA 和 desmin 阳性少见，分别出现在大约 20% 和 8% 的病例[142]。

表13G.4 外阴间叶性病变鉴别诊断中常见的疾病

	侵袭性血管黏液瘤	血管肌纤维母细胞瘤	富于细胞性血管纤维瘤	纤维上皮性间质息肉	浅表血管黏液瘤
诊断时年龄	生育年龄	生育年龄	生育年龄	生育年龄	生育年龄
部位/形状	深在，非息肉状	皮下	皮下	通常息肉状，外生性	浅表，皮下或息肉状
大小	不定	通常<5 cm	通常<3 cm	不定	通常<3 cm
边缘	浸润性	境界清楚	境界通常清楚	与正常组织融合	局限性，清楚
细胞构成	细胞稀少	细胞过多与过少交替	富于细胞	不定	细胞过少
血管	中到大，厚壁	纤细，毛细血管大小，数量多	小到中，厚壁，常常玻璃样变	不定，通常大，厚壁，局限于轴心	纤细，薄壁，长
核分裂指数	罕见	通常少见	不定，可能活跃	不定	通常少见
生物学标志物	Desmin阳性	Desmin阳性	Desmin不定	Desmin阳性	Desmin阴性
临床经过	30%局部复发，可为破坏性	良性，无复发潜能	良性，复发非常罕见	良性，复发罕见（例如妊娠期间）	30%局部非破坏性复发

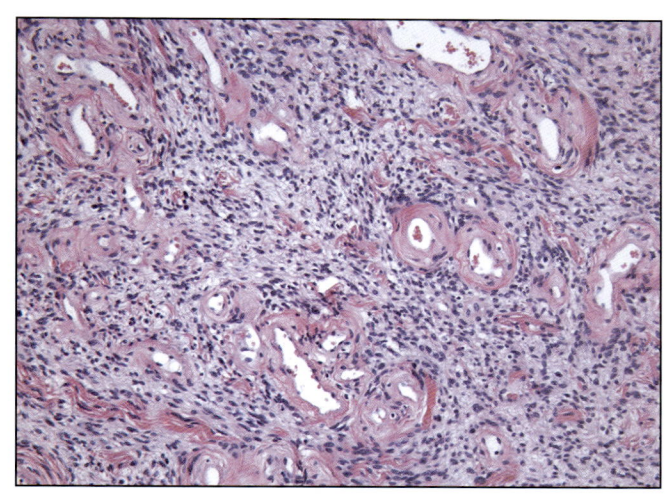

图13G.17 富于细胞性血管纤维瘤。短而交错排列的良性梭形细胞束、小束状胶原纤维和厚壁血管具有特征性。

皮肤纤维瘤（纤维组织细胞瘤）
Dermatofibroma (fibrous histiocytoma)

皮肤纤维瘤是真皮间质的良性肿瘤，最常发生于成人的肢体和躯干（见第23章），但是偶尔也可以累及外阴皮肤[144]。临床表现不同，多数病例表现为肤色或色素沉着性斑块、结节或丘疹。通过在病变一侧加压造成肿瘤小凹形成是特征性的临床征象。典型的组织学表现最常见于外阴，呈现境界相对清楚的梭形或组织细胞样细胞的席纹状增生，伴有陷入的玻璃样变真皮胶原，在偏振光显微镜下可见双折射。肿瘤上面的上皮出现增生并不少见。对于具有这种典型细胞形态学表现的肿瘤，通常不需要进一步治疗或考虑再次切除。

颗粒细胞瘤 Granular cell tumor

颗粒细胞瘤（见第27章）是一个少见的肿瘤，通常发生在头颈部；然而，这些肿瘤大约5%～15%发生在外阴，通常在大阴唇[145-147]。较常发生在黑人妇女，诊断时的平均年龄为50岁；偶尔可以发生在儿童[148,149]。典型的表现是缓慢生长的孤立性无症状的结节，常常是在常规检查时偶然发现的。如果有症状，最常见的是疼痛、肿物增大和瘙痒。少数情况下，如同其他部位一样，外阴可以发生多发性颗粒细胞瘤[150]。肿瘤复发罕见，即使是在不完全切除的情况下[145]；然而，通常选择的治疗方法是完全切除。恶性颗粒细胞瘤非常罕见，但在外阴已有报告[151]。

平滑肌瘤 Leiomyoma

虽然最初认为生殖器平滑肌肿瘤属于浅表平滑肌肿瘤的范畴，但是现在已经确定，女性生殖道远端的平滑肌肿瘤不同于皮肤（毛发）平滑肌肿瘤，而且不应该这样考虑或分类[152]。与子宫平滑肌肿瘤相比，外阴平滑肌瘤特别少见。它的发生年龄广泛，但是主要发生在30～50岁的妇女，一般表现为无痛性境界清楚的皮下肿块，通常小于3cm[152-154]。与子宫平滑肌瘤相似，肿

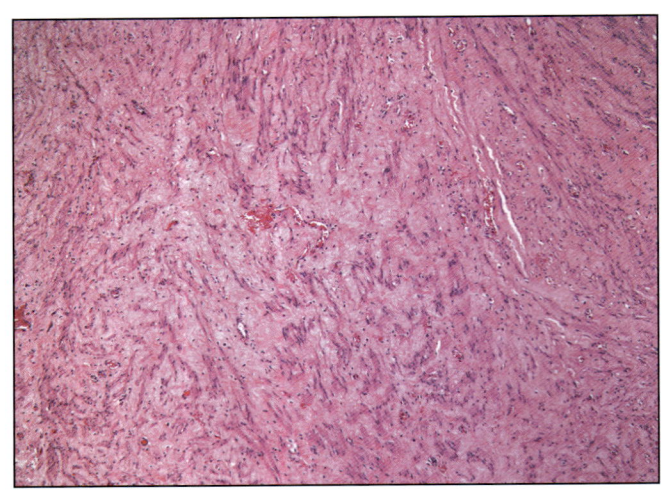

图13G.18 平滑肌瘤。注意突出的黏液玻璃样变，这是发生在女性生殖道远端的平滑肌肿瘤的特征。

瘤可以有梭形（通常）表现或（罕见）上皮样外观。外阴平滑肌瘤的梭形平滑肌细胞可以被不同量的黏液玻璃样物质分开，形成花边状或丛状外观（图13G.18）；偶尔可以出现明显的黏液池，以致掩盖了肿瘤的平滑肌本质[154]。虽然结合大小、界限、非典型性和核分裂计数已经提出了辨认这些平滑肌肿瘤具有恶性潜能的标准，但是现今确定的标准可能低诊了具有复发潜能的平滑肌肿瘤[152-154]。根据个人的经验，如果这个部位的平滑肌肿瘤具有任何核分裂活性、细胞核多形性或有显著的浸润性边缘，它就具有局部复发的潜能，常常发生在最初切除数十年之后[155]。

血管角质瘤 Angiokeratoma

累及外阴的血管角质瘤一般发生在50～60岁之前，表现为一个丘疹性、有时是湿疣性表现的病变，可以为孤立性或多发性，大小通常小于1 cm，颜色从红色到紫色不一[156]。多发性病变应该提出Fabry病的可能性，这是一种罕见的X-连锁染色体脂质障碍（溶酶体α-半乳糖苷酶缺乏）。病变通常没有症状；当出现症状时，可能包括出血、疼痛或瘙痒。组织学检查，血管角质瘤的特征是真皮乳头内出现紧密排列的充满血液的扩张血管。血管通常部分被表面上皮包绕，上皮可能表现为棘层增厚、角化过度，有时出现乳头状瘤病。

局限性淋巴管瘤 Lymphangioma circumscriptum

局限性淋巴管瘤是淋巴管的一种病变，或为先天性或为获得性（继发于淋巴管损伤），较常侵犯躯干、大腿和臀部皮肤和皮下组织（见第3章），但是也可以累及外阴[157]。许多充满透明液体的小囊泡具有特征性，症状可能包括肿胀、疼痛和继发于搔抓的感染。组织学检查可见许多扩张或囊性的淋巴管，其中某些淋巴管紧靠表面上皮附近，导致一种囊泡状的临床表现。

其他罕见的肿瘤 Other rare neoplasms

外阴平滑肌瘤病（leiomyomatosis of the vulva）是一种罕见的病变，其特征为界限不清的黏膜下多结节状平滑肌增生。外阴平滑肌瘤病病人同时或异时可能有食管病变（食管平滑肌瘤病）[158]。可能的发病机制包括激素反应性改变和家族性因素，包括伴随的Alport综合征[155,158]。

外阴脂肪母细胞瘤样肿瘤（lipoblastoma-like tumor of the vulva）是一种罕见的间叶性肿瘤，组织学检查类似于脂肪母细胞瘤病（见第24章），但是临床上不同，外阴脂肪母细胞瘤样肿瘤发生在年轻女性，而脂肪母细胞瘤病发生在年轻男孩（小于5岁）的躯干和肢端[159]。

生殖器横纹肌瘤（genital rhabdomyoma）是一种良性肿瘤，由成熟的横纹肌母细胞组成，较常发生于阴道（见723页）。

较常发生于生殖器外皮肤和皮下组织的各种其他良性间叶性肿瘤，偶尔也可能累及外阴，但是外阴不是特别好发的部位。它们的临床和组织学特征与发生在较常见部位的肿瘤相似。这些肿瘤包括脂肪瘤、神经纤维瘤、神经鞘瘤、毛细血管瘤和海绵状血管瘤。个别情况下，神经纤维瘤病累及女性生殖道，可能表现为阴蒂肥大[160,161]。

局部复发性间叶性肿瘤 Locally recurrent mesenchymal neoplasms

深在性（侵袭性）血管黏液瘤 Deep (aggressive) angiomyxoma

临床特征

深在性血管黏液瘤是一种局部浸润性非转移性的肿瘤，一般发生在女性的盆腔和会阴，平均年龄30～40岁，但是它也可能发生在男性的腹股沟阴囊部位[162-167]。类似于这个部位的其他软组织肿瘤，这个肿瘤可能被误诊为阴唇囊肿，最常见的是前庭大腺囊肿。肿瘤大小可能不同，但是常常相对较大（大于10 cm），而且可能有损毁的表现。深在性血管黏液瘤具有局部复发的倾向，大约发生在30%的病例，有时在最初切除之后许多年（常常是数十年）出现复发。少数情况下可能发生破坏性复发，但是至今遇到的一次以上的复发仍然非常少见。认为广泛局部切除伴有1 cm的边缘是恰当的治疗。

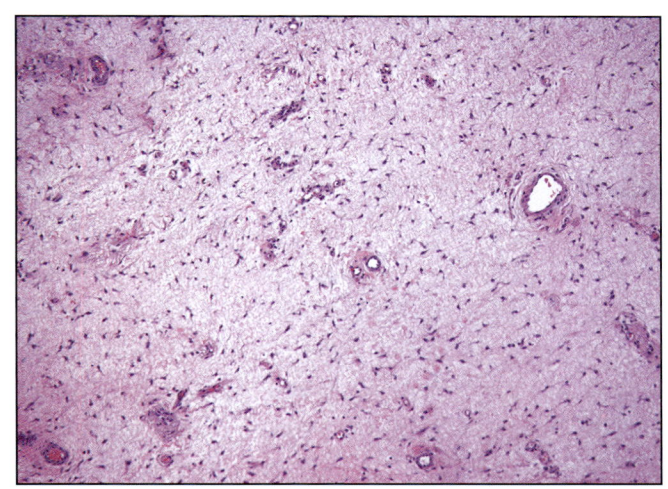

图13G.19 深在性（侵袭性）血管黏液瘤。良性梭形细胞位于黏液样基质中。注意大的厚壁血管。

病理学特征

侵袭性血管黏液瘤是一个特征性的质软的胶状肿瘤，肿瘤边界不清。组织学检查，它是一个细胞稀少的肿瘤，由梭形细胞组成，伴有纤细的胞浆突起，肿瘤细胞位于丰富的黏液样间质中，其中散在常常是厚壁和玻璃样变的中等到较大的血管（图13G.19）。疏松的胶原纤维和平滑肌细胞聚集 [所谓的肌样束 (myoid bundles)]，典型者或者排列成疏松的丛状，或者在血管附近排列成紧密的漩涡状结构。这种肿瘤具有不可靠的浸润性边缘，这是手术和病理检查确定边缘困难的原因；关于边缘状况的这种不确定性可能与复发倾向有关。侵袭性血管黏液瘤病变的间质细胞 desmin 和 actin 常常阳性，特别是肌样束。一例深在性血管黏液瘤的细胞遗传分析显示 t (8;12) 易位，而且反转录聚合酶链反应（RT-PCR）证实 HMGA2 异常表达，HMGA2 是一种 DNA 结构因子，在转录调节方面具有重要作用，它在其他伴有类似易位的肿瘤也有异常表达（例如子宫平滑肌瘤、脂肪瘤）[168]。虽然尚不清楚 HMGA2 如何表达才能导致肿瘤发生，但是有可能是靶基因转录的改变。

浅表性血管黏液瘤
Superficial angiomyxoma

临床特征

浅表性血管黏液瘤仅仅偶尔发生在生殖器部位，它较常见于头颈部和躯干（见第 24 章）；然而，因为它是一个黏液样的肿瘤，所以可能被误诊为侵袭性血管黏液瘤，有关侵袭性血管黏液瘤的讨论也包括在这一章中。这个肿瘤最常发生在 30～40 岁，典型者表现为缓慢生长的无痛性息肉样肿瘤，其大小通常小于 5 cm [169-171]。

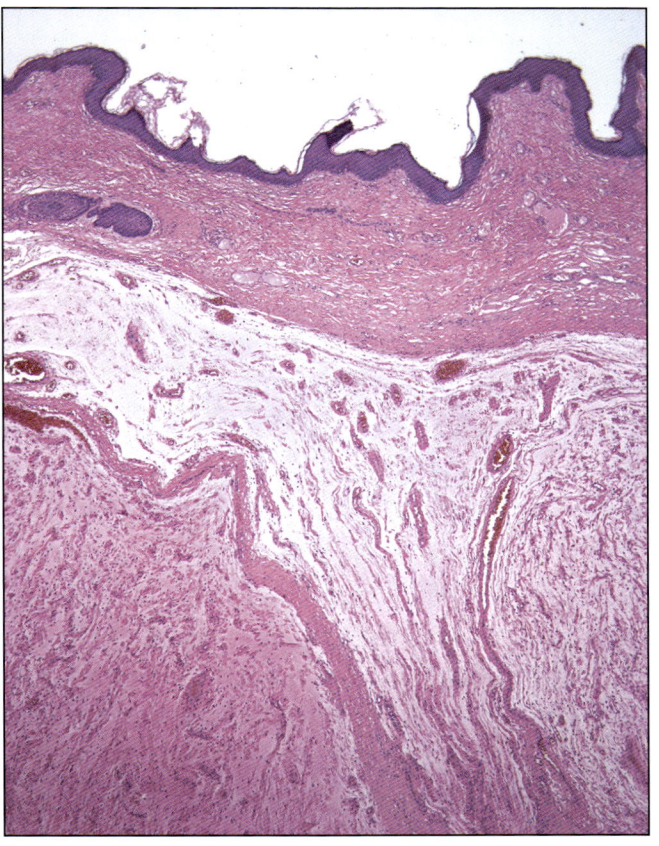

图13G.20 浅表性血管黏液瘤。良性梭形细胞多结节性黏液样增生。注意位于真皮表层。

虽然对于发生在生殖器部位的浅表性血管黏液瘤来说这种联系尚不清楚，但是其他部位出现多发性皮肤病变却与 Carney 综合征高度相关 [170]。

病理学特征

组织学检查，这个肿瘤是一个境界清楚（但是没有包膜）、多小叶的黏液样结节状增生，位于真皮和皮下组织浅层（图 13G.20）。黏液样结节是由梭形细胞和星形细胞、炎症细胞（特别是多形核白细胞），以及薄壁血管组成的。大约 1/3 的病例出现上皮成分，通常表现为内衬囊肿的鳞状上皮或基底细胞样上皮巢和条索，可能是来自皮肤附件。这些肿瘤大约 30% 的病例有局部非破坏性复发的潜能；应该进行完全切除，并伴有清楚的边缘。与侵袭性血管黏液瘤不同，浅表性血管黏液瘤一般累及真皮和皮下组织，缺乏显著的浸润性边缘或厚壁血管，而且其病变间质细胞 desmin 阴性。

隆凸性皮肤纤维肉瘤
Dermatofibrosarcoma protuberans

临床特征

隆凸性皮肤纤维肉瘤是一个纤维母细胞性肿瘤，只是偶尔发生在外阴[172-181]，较常位于躯干（见第 23 章）。它的临床表现可能不同，从肤色到不同程度色素沉着的斑块或结节，到外生性多结节性肿瘤。这个肿瘤具有高度局部复发的倾向，因此建议广泛局部切除。在典型的病例，转移非常罕见；然而，那些显示纤维肉瘤性改变的肿瘤具有转移高危险性（在一项研究中为 15%）[181]。

病理学特征

隆凸性皮肤纤维肉瘤是一个境界不清的梭形细胞单形性席纹状增生，一般浸润皮下脂肪组织。具有特征性花边状或蜂窝状结构。与上面正常表现或萎缩的表皮分离（Grenz 带），附件结构陷入，缺乏极性的胶原也是特征性的改变。少数这些肿瘤，包括外阴病例，显示出较高级别的纤维肉瘤性改变，最常见的特征是人字形的生长方式，伴有细胞构成和核分裂象增加[172,181]。隆凸性皮肤纤维肉瘤一般 CD34 弥漫阳性，XIIIa 因子阴性。

这些肿瘤一般具有 17 号染色体和 22 号染色体易位（常常表现为超多数量的环状染色体），导致 I 型胶原 α1（COL1A1）和血小板衍生生长因子β- 链（PDGFB）两个基因融合[182]。发生在外阴的隆凸性皮肤纤维肉瘤也可能含有 COL1A1- PDGFB 嵌合性融合转录物[173,174]。

隆凸性皮肤纤维肉瘤不同于皮肤纤维瘤，它倾向于浸润皮下组织，呈特征性的花边状结构，上面的上皮缺乏增生，当在偏振光显微镜下观察时缺乏双折光性胶原，倾向于环绕附件结构浸润，这在肿瘤实质内常常可以见到，而且典型者 CD34 弥漫阳性，XIIIa 因子阴性（虽然这两种肿瘤中这些标志物染色可能重叠）。

恶性间叶性肿瘤
Malignant mesenchymal neoplasms

平滑肌肉瘤　Leiomyosarcoma

平滑肌肉瘤是最常见的外阴肉瘤[183-185]。病人一般 30～50 岁，表现为一个肿块，通常大于 5 cm，虽然这些肿瘤大小可能不同。形态学上，这些肿瘤最常见的是普通的梭形细胞型，虽然黏液样变型也可能发生。因为外阴平滑肌肿瘤相对少见，而且长期随访的系列病例有限，所以难以可靠地确定这些肿瘤是否具有转移潜能。不过，仍然建议应用 Tavassoli 和 Norris 提出的标准[152-154]。具有 3 项或 3 项以上下述标准的肿瘤应该被分类为肉瘤：(1) 肿瘤大于 5 cm；(2) 浸润性边缘；(3) 每 10 个高倍视野核分裂象大于 5 个；以及 (4) 中到重度细胞学非典型性。虽然坏死没有列在标准之内，出现坏死应该强烈提出有肉瘤的可能。

横纹肌肉瘤　Rhabdomyosarcoma

在女性生殖道的远端，横纹肌肉瘤，特别是胚胎性横纹肌肉瘤的葡萄状肉瘤变型，较常发生在阴道（见 724 页）。然而，在少数情况下，横纹肌肉瘤的任何亚型也可能累及外阴[186-188]。类似于阴道横纹肌肉瘤，但是不如阴道横纹肌肉瘤常见，外阴胚胎性横纹肌肉瘤可以表现为息肉样、葡萄样肿块（葡萄状肉瘤），伴有相似的特征性临床和组织病理学表现。单纯性腺泡状横纹肌肉瘤也可能发生，其组织学特征为疏松粘着的细胞排列成巢状结构，但是也可以见到胚胎性、腺泡状、甚至多形性横纹肌肉瘤的混合性表现。出现腺泡状结构提示预后不良。

脂肪肉瘤　Liposarcoma

外阴脂肪肉瘤主要发生在中年妇女（平均年龄 52 岁），大小不同，最常见的组织学亚型是高分化脂肪肉瘤[189-193]。多数病例具有高分化脂肪肉瘤（非典型性脂肪瘤性肿瘤）的一般表现，脂肪细胞大小不同，脂肪细胞核非典型性，富于细胞的纤维间隔含有非典型性间质细胞。然而，某些病例可能具有不同的组织学表现，出现混合性良性梭形细胞、不同大小的脂肪细胞，以及许多具有两个空泡的脂肪母细胞（图 13G.21）。

近端型上皮样肉瘤
Proximal-type epithelioid sarcoma

近端型上皮样肉瘤[194] 是上皮样肉瘤的一种大细胞变型，较常发生于近端 / 中轴部位，特别是生殖器和会阴部位（见第 24 章）。外阴原发性近端型上皮样肉瘤病人的平均年龄为 30～40 岁，肿瘤通常小于 6cm，主要症状是出现肿块。在多数病例，这个肿瘤的组织学特征是显著增大的细胞呈多结节性或片块样增生，细胞具有丰富

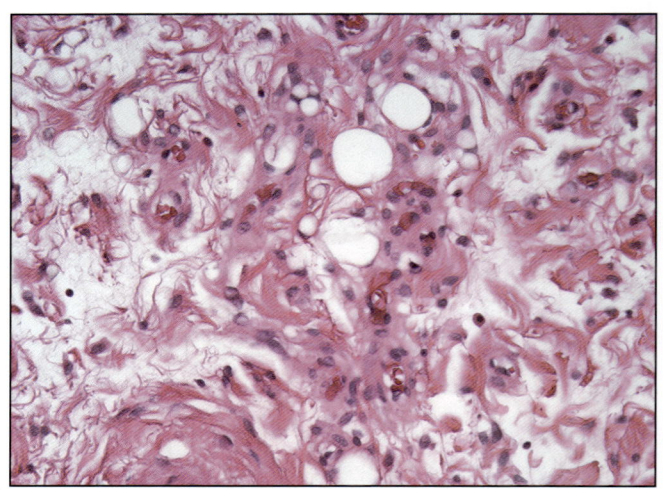

图13G. 21　脂肪肉瘤。不同寻常的变型，具有混合性良性梭形细胞、不同大小的脂肪细胞和两个空泡的脂肪母细胞。

的嗜酸性胞浆（呈现上皮样外观），核大呈空泡状，核仁突出；常常出现横纹肌样特征，伴有这种表现的细胞数量不定。这些肿瘤表达上皮标志物（keratin、EMA），常常表达CD34，而且还可能表达desmin或SMA。

其他罕见的肉瘤　Other rare sarcomas

腺泡状软组织肉瘤（alveolar soft part sarcoma）已有描述，发生在一个62岁的妇女，表现为右侧大阴唇有一个4cm的无症状的肿块[195]。组织学检查，这个肿瘤好像与发生在肢端的腺泡状软组织肉瘤一样，肢端是其较常见的部位，是由大的具有丰富颗粒性胞浆的多角形细胞组成的，排列成巢和腺泡状，被纤细的窦状血管分隔开。

骨外间叶性软骨肉瘤（extraskeletal mesenchymal chondrosarcoma）也有描述，发生在一个40岁的妇女，表现为左侧阴唇的肿块，肿块进行性增大，1年当中达到9cm[196]。组织学检查，肿瘤具有特征性的组织学表现，由低分化的梭形到圆形肉瘤细胞组成，伴有血管周细胞瘤样血管，而且突然融合到伴有软骨分化的区域。

滑膜肉瘤（synovial sarcoma）是肢端较常见的软组织肉瘤之一，偶尔也可能发生在外阴[197]。已有两例报告，发生在30岁和37岁的妇女，两个肿瘤均小于2cm，肿瘤具有双相结构。

血管肉瘤（angiosarcoma）偶尔可以累及外阴，具有发生在较常见部位的血管肉瘤的典型的生长方式和细胞形态学[184,185]。

Kaposi肉瘤（Kaposi's sarcoma）偶尔也可能累及外阴，在某些情况下可能是HIV感染和获得性免疫缺陷综合征（AIDS）的表现[198,199]。

其他罕见的肿瘤　Other rare neoplasms

非Hodgkin淋巴瘤（non-Hodgkin's lymphoma）偶尔累及外阴，或者作为这个部位的原发性肿瘤，或者为继发性受累，通常表现为一个外阴肿块，最常见的是弥漫性大B细胞淋巴瘤，在临床上具有侵袭性[200,201]。

内胚窦瘤（endodermal sinus tumor）最常发生在卵巢（单纯性或作为混合性生殖细胞肿瘤的一种成分）和阴道（见605页）。少数情况下，这种肿瘤可以发生在外阴[202]。这些肿瘤发生在婴儿，但是在20～30岁的年轻妇女也有描述。病人表现为在相对短的期间出现不同大小（可达7cm）的无痛性肿块。

Merkel细胞癌（Merkel cell carcinoma）本身是一种不常见的肿瘤，在非常罕见的情况下可以发生在外阴[203]。病人通常大于40岁，肿瘤大小<4cm。外阴Merkel细胞癌的细胞形态学和免疫表型一般类似于发生在其他较常见部位的肿瘤（见第23章）。预后不良。

皮脂腺癌（sebaceous carcinoma）一般发生在头颈部，特别是面部，但是可以发生在出现毛囊皮脂腺单位的任何部位，包括外阴，尽管罕见[204,205]。

外阴转移性肿瘤（metastatic tumors）[206]少见。大约50%由妇科原发性肿瘤播散而来，特别是宫颈。在其他诸多可能是原发性肿瘤的部位中，从胃肠道癌扩散而来好像最为常见。

参考文献

1. Pao C C, Hor J J, Fu Y L 1994 Genital human papillomavirus infections in young women with vulvar and vestibular papillomatosis. Eur J Clin Microbiol Infect Dis 13: 433–436
2. Gentile G, Formelli G, Pelusi G et al. 1997 Is vestibular micropapillomatosis associated with human papillomavirus infection? Eur J Gynaecol Oncol 18: 523–525
3. Moyal-Barracco M, Leibowitch M, Orth G 1990 Vestibular papillae of the vulva. Lack of evidence for human papillomavirus etiology. Arch Dermatol 126: 1594–1598
4. Zhu W Y, Leonardi C, Penneys N S 1992 Detection of human papillomavirus DNA in seborrheic keratosis by polymerase chain reaction. J Dermatol Sci 4: 166–171
5. Gushi A, Kanekura T, Kanzaki T et al. 2003 Detection and sequences of human papillomavirus DNA in nongenital seborrheic keratosis of immunopotent individuals. J Dermatol Sci 31: 143–149
6. Bai H, Cviko A, Granter S et al. 2003 Immunophenotypic and viral (human papillomavirus) correlates of vulvar seborrheic keratosis. Hum Pathol 34: 559–564
7. McLachlin C M, Kozakewich H, Craighill M et al. 1994 Histologic correlates of vulvar human papillomavirus infection in children and young adults. Am J Surg Pathol 18: 728–735
8. Chiasson M A, Ellerbrock T V, Bush T J et al. 1997 Increased prevalence of vulvovaginal condyloma and vulvar intraepithelial neoplasia in women infected with the human immunodeficiency virus. Obstet Gynecol 89: 690–694
9. Marshburn P B, Trofatter K F Jr 1988 Recurrent condyloma acuminatum in women over age 40: association with immunosuppression and malignant disease. Am J Obstet Gynecol 159: 429–433
10. Iversen T, Tretli S 1998 Intraepithelial and invasive squamous cell neoplasia of the vulva: trends in incidence, recurrence, and survival rate in Norway. Obstet Gynecol 91: 969–972
11. Sturgeon S R, Brinton L A, Devesa S S et al. 1992 In situ and invasive vulvar cancer incidence trends (1973 to 1987). Am J Obstet Gynecol 166: 1482–1485
12. Crum C P, McLachlin C M, Tate J E et al. 1997 Pathobiology of vulvar squamous neoplasia. Curr Opin Obstet Gynecol 9: 63–69
13. Spitzer M 1999 Lower genital tract intraepithelial neoplasia in HIV-infected women: guidelines for evaluation and management. Obstet Gynecol Surv 54: 131–137
14. Hording U, Daugaard S, Junge J et al. 1996 Human papillomaviruses and multifocal genital neoplasia. Int J Gynecol Pathol 15: 230–234
15. Sherman K J, Daling J R, Chu J et al. 1988 Multiple primary tumours in women with vulvar neoplasms: a case-control study. Br J Cancer 57: 423–427
16. Chafe W, Richards A, Morgan L et al. 1988 Unrecognized invasive carcinoma in vulvar intraepithelial neoplasia (VIN). Gynecol Oncol 31: 154–165
17. Husseinzadeh N, Recinto C 1999 Frequency of invasive cancer in surgically excised vulvar lesions with intraepithelial neoplasia (VIN 3). Gynecol Oncol 73: 119–120
18. McLachlin C M, Mutter G L, Crum C P 1994 Multinucleated atypia of the vulva. Report of a distinct entity not associated with human papillomavirus. Am J Surg Pathol 18: 1233–1239
19. Crum C P 1992 Carcinoma of the vulva: epidemiology and pathogenesis. Obstet Gynecol 79: 448–454
20. Haefner H K, Tate J E, McLachlin C M et al. 1995 Vulvar intraepithelial neoplasia: age, morphological phenotype, papillomavirus DNA, and coexisting invasive carcinoma. Hum Pathol 26: 147–154

21. Homesley H D, Bundy B N, Sedlis A et al. 1991 Assessment of current International Federation of Gynecology and Obstetrics staging of vulvar carcinoma relative to prognostic factors for survival (a Gynecologic Oncology Group study). Am J Obstet Gynecol 164: 997–1003
22. Blake P 2003 Radiotherapy and chemoradiotherapy for carcinoma of the vulva. Best Pract Res Clin Obstet Gynaecol 17: 649–661
23. Katz A, Eifel P J, Jhingran A et al. 2003 The role of radiation therapy in preventing regional recurrences of invasive squamous cell carcinoma of the vulva. Int J Radiat Oncol Biol Phys 57: 409–418
24. Homesley H D, Bundy B N, Sedlis A et al. 1993 Prognostic factors for groin node metastasis in squamous cell carcinoma of the vulva (a Gynecologic Oncology Group study). Gynecol Oncol 49: 279–283
25. Pinto A P, Schlecht N F, Pintos J et al. 2004 Prognostic significance of lymph node variables and human papillomavirus DNA in invasive vulvar carcinoma. Gynecol Oncol 92: 856–865
26. Nascimento A F, Granter S R, Cviko A et al. 2004 Vulvar acanthosis with altered differentiation: a precursor to verrucous carcinoma? Am J Surg Pathol 28: 638–643
27. Copas P R, Spann C O Jr, Majmudar B et al. 1996 Basal cell carcinoma of the vulva. A report of four cases. J Reprod Med 41: 283–286
28. Feakins R M, Lowe D G 1997 Basal cell carcinoma of the vulva: a clinicopathologic study of 45 cases. Int J Gynecol Pathol 16: 319–324
29. Benedet J L, Miller D M, Ehlen T G et al. 1997 Basal cell carcinoma of the vulva: clinical features and treatment results in 28 patients. Obstet Gynecol 90: 765–768
30. Gibson G E, Ahmed I 2001 Perianal and genital basal cell carcinoma: a clinicopathologic review of 51 cases. J Am Acad Dermatol 45: 68–71
31. Piura B, Rabinovich A, Dgani R 1999 Basal cell carcinoma of the vulva. J Surg Oncol 70: 172–176
32. Koenig C, Tavassoli F A 1998 Nodular hyperplasia, adenoma, and adenomyoma of Bartholin's gland. Int J Gynecol Pathol 17: 289–294
33. Padmanabhan V, Cooper K 2000 Concomitant adenoma and hybrid carcinoma of salivary gland type arising in Bartholin's gland. Int J Gynecol Pathol 19: 377–380
34. Woodworth H Jr, Dockerty M B, Wilson R B et al. 1971 Papillary hidradenoma of the vulva: a clinicopathologic study of 69 cases. Am J Obstet Gynecol 110: 501–508
35. Meeker J H, Neubecker R D, Helwig E B 1962 Hidradenoma papilliferum. Am J Clin Pathol 37: 182–195
36. Axe S, Parmley T, Woodruff J D et al. 1986 Adenomas in minor vestibular glands. Obstet Gynecol 68: 16–18
37. Punia R P, Bal A, Jain P et al. 2003 Minor vestibular gland adenoma: a case report. Aust NZ J Obstet Gynaecol 43: 322–323
38. Rorat E, Wallach R C 1984 Mixed tumors of the vulva: clinical outcome and pathology. Int J Gynecol Pathol 3: 323–328
39. Ordonez N G, Manning J T, Luna M A 1981 Mixed tumor of the vulva: a report of two cases probably arising in Bartholin's gland. Cancer 48: 181–186
40. Hornick J L, Fletcher C D M 2003 Myoepithelial tumors of soft tissue: a clinicopathologic and immunohistochemical study of 101 cases with evaluation of prognostic parameters. Am J Surg Pathol 27: 1183–1196
41. Huang Y H, Chuang Y H, Kuo T T et al. 2003 Vulvar syringoma: a clinicopathologic and immunohistologic study of 18 patients and results of treatment. J Am Acad Dermatol 48: 735–739
42. Isaacson D, Turner M L 1979 Localized vulvar syringomas. J Am Acad Dermatol 1: 352–356
43. Tay Y K, Tham S N, Teo R 1996 Localized vulvar syringomas – an unusual cause of pruritus vulvae. Dermatology 192: 62–63
44. Buchler D A, Sun F, Chuprevich T 1978 A pilar tumor of the vulva. Gynecol Oncol 6: 479–486
45. Avinoach I, Zirkin H J, Glezerman M 1989 Proliferating trichilemmal tumor of the vulva. Case report and review of the literature. Int J Gynecol Pathol 8: 163–168
46. Glusac E J, Hendrickson M S, Smoller B R 1994 Apocrine cystadenoma of the vulva. J Am Acad Dermatol 31: 498–489
47. Gilks C B, Clement P B, Wood W S 1989 Trichoblastic fibroma. A clinicopathologic study of three cases. Am J Dermatopathol 11: 397–402
48. Cho D, Woodruff J D 1988 Trichoepithelioma of the vulva. A report of two cases. J Reprod Med 33: 317–319
49. Crawford D, Nimmo M, Clement P B et al. 1999 Prognostic factors in Paget's disease of the vulva: a study of 21 cases. Int J Gynecol Pathol 18: 351–359
50. Goldblum J R, Hart W R 1997 Vulvar Paget's disease: a clinicopathologic and immunohistochemical study of 19 cases. Am J Surg Pathol 21: 1178–1187
51. Kodama S, Kaneko T, Saito M et al. 1995 A clinicopathologic study of 30 patients with Paget's disease of the vulva. Gynecol Oncol 56: 63–70
52. Fanning J, Lambert H C, Hale T M et al. 1999 Paget's disease of the vulva: prevalence of associated vulvar adenocarcinoma, invasive Paget's disease, and recurrence after surgical excision. Am J Obstet Gynecol 180: 24–27
53. Piura B, Rabinovich A, Dgani R 1999 Extramammary Paget's disease of the vulva: report of five cases and review of the literature. Eur J Gynaecol Oncol 20: 98–101
54. Parker L P, Parker J R, Bodurka-Bevers D et al. 2000 Paget's disease of the vulva: pathology, pattern of involvement, and prognosis. Gynecol Oncol 77: 183–189
55. Zollo J D, Zeitouni N C 2000 The Roswell Park Cancer Institute experience with extramammary Paget's disease. Br J Dermatol 142: 59–65
56. Goldblum J R, Hart W R 1998 Perianal Paget's disease: a histologic and immunohistochemical study of 11 cases with and without associated rectal adenocarcinoma. Am J Surg Pathol 22: 170–179
57. Fine B A, Fowler L J, Valente P T et al. 1995 Minimally invasive Paget's disease of the vulva with extensive lymph node metastases. Gynecol Oncol 57: 262–265
58. Feuer G A, Shevchuk M, Calanog A 1990 Vulvar Paget's disease: the need to exclude an invasive lesion. Gynecol Oncol 38: 81–89
59. Chamlian D L, Taylor H B 1972 Primary carcinoma of Bartholin's gland. A report of 24 patients. Obstet Gynecol 39: 489–494
60. Leuchter R S, Hacker N F, Voet R L et al. 1982 Primary carcinoma of the Bartholin gland: a report of 14 cases and review of the literature. Obstet Gynecol 60: 361–368
61. DePasquale S E, McGuinness T B, Mangan C E et al. 1996 Adenoid cystic carcinoma of Bartholin's gland: a review of the literature and report of a patient. Gynecol Oncol 61: 122–125
62. Cardosi R J, Speights A, Fiorica J V et al. 2001 Bartholin's gland carcinoma: a 15-year experience. Gynecol Oncol 82: 247–251
63. Rosenberg P, Simonsen E, Risberg B 1989 Adenoid cystic carcinoma of Bartholin's gland: a report of five new cases treated with surgery and radiotherapy. Gynecol Oncol 34: 145–147
64. Jones M A, Mann E W, Caldwell C L et al. 1990 Small cell neuroendocrine carcinoma of Bartholin's gland. Am J Clin Pathol 94: 439–442
65. Felix J C, Cote R J, Kramer E E et al. 1993 Carcinomas of Bartholin's gland. Histogenesis and the etiological role of human papillomavirus. Am J Pathol 142: 925–933
66. Milchgrub S, Wiley E L, Vuitch F et al. 1994 The tubular variant of adenoid cystic carcinoma of the Bartholin's gland. Am J Clin Pathol 101: 204–208
67. Obermair A, Koller S, Crandon A J et al. 2001 Primary Bartholin gland carcinoma: a report of seven cases. Aust NZ J Obstet Gynaecol 41: 78–81
68. Hendrix R C, Behrman S J 1956 Adenocarcinoma arising in a supernumerary mammary gland in the vulva. Obstet Gynecol 8: 238–241
69. Guerry R L, Pratt-Thomas H R 1976 Carcinoma of supernumerary breast of vulva with bilateral mammary cancer. Cancer 38: 2570–2574
70. Guercio E, Cesone P, Saracino A et al. 1984 [Adenocarcinoma occurring in an aberrant mammary gland located in the vulva.] Minerva Ginecol 36: 315–319
71. Cho D, Buscema J, Rosenshein N B et al. 1985 Primary breast cancer of the vulva. Obstet Gynecol 66: 79S–81S
72. Simon K E, Dutcher J P, Runowicz C D et al. 1988 Adenocarcinoma arising in vulvar breast tissue. Cancer 62: 2234–2238
73. Rose P G, Roman L D, Reale F R et al. 1990 Primary adenocarcinoma of the breast arising in the vulva. Obstet Gynecol 76: 537–539
74. Di Bonito L, Patriarca S, Falconieri G 1992 Aggressive "breast-like" adenocarcinoma of vulva. Pathol Res Pract 188: 211–214
75. Bailey C L, Sankey H Z, Donovan J T et al. 1993 Primary breast cancer of the vulva. Gynecol Oncol 50: 379–383
76. Levin M, Pakarakas R M, Chang H A et al. 1995 Primary breast carcinoma of the vulva: a case report and review of the literature. Gynecol Oncol 56: 448–451
77. Kennedy D A, Hermina M S, Xanos E T et al. 1997 Infiltrating ductal carcinoma of the vulva. Pathol Res Pract 193: 723–726
78. van der Putte S C, van Gorp L H 1994 Adenocarcinoma of the mammary-like glands of the vulva: a concept unifying sweat gland carcinoma of the vulva, carcinoma of supernumerary mammary glands and extramammary Paget's disease. J Cutan Pathol 21: 157–163
79. Pelosi G, Martignoni G, Bonetti F 1991 Intraductal carcinoma of mammary-type apocrine epithelium arising within a papillary hydradenoma of the vulva. Report of a case and review of the literature. Arch Pathol Lab Med 115: 1249–1254
80. Castro C Y, Deavers M 2001 Ductal carcinoma in-situ arising in mammary-like glands of the vulva. Int J Gynecol Pathol 20: 277–283
81. Pongtippan A, Malpica A, Levenback C et al. 2004 Skene's gland adenocarcinoma resembling prostatic adenocarcinoma. Int J Gynecol Pathol 23: 71–74
82. Dodson M K, Cliby W A, Keeney G L et al. 1994 Skene's gland adenocarcinoma with increased serum level of prostate-specific antigen. Gynecol Oncol 55: 304–307
83. Sloboda J, Zaviacic M, Jakubovsky J et al. 1998 Metastasizing adenocarcinoma of the female prostate (Skene's paraurethral glands). Histological and immunohistochemical prostate markers studies and first ultrastructural observation. Pathol Res Pract 194: 129–136
84. Kennedy J C, Majmudar B 1993 Primary adenocarcinoma of the vulva, possibly cloacogenic. A report of two cases. J Reprod Med 38: 113–116
85. Willen R, Bekassy Z, Carlen B et al. 1999 Cloacogenic adenocarcinoma of the vulva. Gynecol Oncol 74: 298–301
86. Zaidi S N, Conner M G 2001 Primary vulvar adenocarcinoma of cloacogenic origin. South Med J 94: 744–746
87. Rodriguez A, Isaac M A, Hidalgo E et al. 2001 Villoglandular adenocarcinoma of the vulva. Gynecol Oncol 83: 409–411
88. Dube V, Veilleux C, Plante M et al. 2004 Primary villoglandular adenocarcinoma of cloacogenic origin of the vulva. Hum Pathol 35: 377–379
89. Vitrey D, Frachon S, Balme B et al. 2003 Tubulovillous adenoma of the vulva. Obstet Gynecol 66: 1160–1163
90. Ghamande S A, Kasznica J, Griffiths C T et al. 1995 Mucinous adenocarcinomas of the vulva. Gynecol Oncol 57: 117–120

91. Mesko J D, Gates H, McDonald T W et al. 1988 Clear cell ("mesonephroid") adenocarcinoma of the vulva arising in endometriosis: a case report. Gynecol Oncol 29: 385–391
92. Hitti I F, Glasberg S S, Lubicz S 1990 Clear cell carcinoma arising in extraovarian endometriosis: report of three cases and review of the literature. Gynecol Oncol 39: 314–320
93. Bolis G B, Maccio T 2000 Clear cell adenocarcinoma of the vulva arising in endometriosis. A case report. Eur J Gynaecol Oncol 21: 416–417
94. Wick M R, Goellner J R, Wolfe J T III et al. 1985 Vulvar sweat gland carcinomas. Arch Pathol Lab Med 109: 43–47
95. Messing M J, Richardson M S, Smith M T et al. 1993 Metastatic clear-cell hidradenocarcinoma of the vulva. Gynecol Oncol 48: 264–268
96. Buhl A, Landow S, Lee Y C et al. 2001 Microcystic adnexal carcinoma of the vulva. Gynecol Oncol 82: 571–574
97. Barnhill R L, Albert L S, Shama S K et al. 1990 Genital lentiginosis: a clinical and histopathologic study. J Am Acad Dermatol 22: 453–460
98. Rhodes A R, Silverman R A, Harrist T J et al. 1984 Mucocutaneous lentigines, cardiomucocutaneous myxomas, and multiple blue nevi: the "LAMB" syndrome. J Am Acad Dermatol 10: 72–82
99. Voron D A, Hatfield H H, Kalkhoff R K 1976 Multiple lentigines syndrome. Case report and review of the literature. Am J Med 60: 447–456
100. Christensen W N, Friedman K J, Woodruff J D et al. 1987 Histologic characteristics of vulvar nevocellular nevi. J Cutan Pathol 14: 87–91
101. Rongioletti F, Ball R A, Marcus R et al. 2000 Histopathological features of flexural melanocytic nevi: a study of 40 cases. J Cutan Pathol 27: 215–217
102. Creasman W T, Phillips J L, Menck H R 1999 A survey of hospital management practices for vulvar melanoma. J Am Coll Surg 188: 670–675
103. Irvin W P Jr, Legallo R L, Stoler M H et al. 2001 Vulvar melanoma: a retrospective analysis and literature review. Gynecol Oncol 83: 457–465
104. Heller D S, Moomjy M, Koulos J et al. 1994 Vulvar and vaginal melanoma. A clinicopathologic study. J Reprod Med 39: 945–948
105. DeMatos P, Tyler D, Seigler H F 1998 Mucosal melanoma of the female genitalia: a clinicopathologic study of forty-three cases at Duke University Medical Center. Surgery 124: 38–48
106. Ragnarsson-Olding B K, Nilsson B R, Kanter-Lewensohn L R et al. 1999 Malignant melanoma of the vulva in a nationwide, 25-year study of 219 Swedish females: predictors of survival. Cancer 86: 1285–1293
107. Ragnarsson-Olding B K, Kanter-Lewensohn L R, Lagerlof B et al. 1999 Malignant melanoma of the vulva in a nationwide, 25-year study of 219 Swedish females: clinical observations and histopathologic features. Cancer 86: 1273–1284
108. Verschraegen C F, Benjapibal M, Supakarapongkul W et al. 2001 Vulvar melanoma at the M D Anderson Cancer Center: 25 years later. Int J Gynecol Cancer 11: 359–364
109. Raber G, Mempel V, Jackisch C et al. 1996 Malignant melanoma of the vulva. Report of 89 patients. Cancer 78: 2353–2358
110. Bradgate M G, Rollason T P, McConkey C C et al. 1990 Malignant melanoma of the vulva: a clinicopathological study of 50 women. Br J Obstet Gynaecol 97: 124–133
111. Khoo U S, Collins R J, Ngan H Y 1991 Malignant melanoma of the female genital tract. A report of nine cases in the Chinese of Hong Kong. Pathology 23: 312–317
112. Piura B, Rabinovich A, Dgani R 1999 Malignant melanoma of the vulva: report of six cases and review of the literature. Eur J Gynaecol Oncol 20: 182–186
113. Neven P, Shepherd J H, Masotina A et al. 1994 Malignant melanoma of the vulva and vagina: a report of 23 cases presenting in a 10-year period. Int J Gynecol Cancer 4: 379–383
114. Chung A F, Woodruff J M, Lewis J L Jr 1975 Malignant melanoma of the vulva: A report of 44 cases. Obstet Gynecol 45: 638–646
115. Trimble E L, Lewis J L Jr, Williams L L et al. 1992 Management of vulvar melanoma. Gynecol Oncol 45: 254–258
116. Johnson T L, Kumar N B, White C D et al. 1986 Prognostic features of vulvar melanoma: a clinicopathologic analysis. Int J Gynecol Pathol 5: 110–118
117. Wechter M E, Gruber S B, Haefner H K et al. 2004 Vulvar melanoma: a report of 20 cases and review of the literature. J Am Acad Dermatol 50: 554–562
118. Norris H J, Taylor H B 1966 Polyps of the vagina. A benign lesion resembling sarcoma botryoides. Cancer 19: 227–232
119. Elliott G B, Reynolds H A, Fidler H K 1967 Pseudo-sarcoma botryoides of cervix and vagina in pregnancy. J Obstet Gynaecol Br Commonw 74: 728–733
120. Burt R L, Prichard R W, Kim B S 1976 Fibroepithelial polyp of the vagina. A report of five cases. Obstet Gynecol 47: 52S–54S
121. Chirayil S J, Tobon H 1981 Polyps of the vagina: a clinicopathologic study of 18 cases. Cancer 47: 2904–2907
122. O'Quinn A G, Edwards C L, Gallager H S 1982 Pseudosarcoma botryoides of the vagina in pregnancy. Gynecol Oncol 13: 237–241
123. Miettinen M, Wahlstrom T, Vesterinen E et al. 1983 Vaginal polyps with pseudosarcomatous features. A clinicopathologic study of seven cases. Cancer 51: 1148–1151
124. Maenpaa J, Soderstrom K O, Salmi T et al. 1988 Large atypical polyps of the vagina during pregnancy with concomitant human papilloma virus infection. Eur J Obstet Gynecol Reprod Biol 27: 65–69
125. Ostor A G, Fortune D W, Riley C B 1988 Fibroepithelial polyps with atypical stromal cells (pseudosarcoma botryoides) of vulva and vagina. A report of 13 cases. Int J Gynecol Pathol 7: 351–360
126. Hartmann C A, Sperling M, Stein H 1990 So-called fibroepithelial polyps of the vagina exhibiting an unusual but uniform antigen profile characterized by expression of desmin and steroid hormone receptors but no muscle-specific actin or macrophage markers. Am J Clin Pathol 93: 604–608
127. Mucitelli D R, Charles E Z, Kraus F T 1990 Vulvovaginal polyps. Histologic appearance, ultrastructure, immunocytochemical characteristics, and clinicopathologic correlations. Int J Gynecol Pathol 9: 20–40
128. Nucci M R, Fletcher C D M 1998 Fibroepithelial stromal polyps of vulvovaginal tissue: from the banal to the bizarre. Pathol Case Rev 3: 151–157
129. Nucci M R, Young R H, Fletcher C D M 2000 Cellular pseudosarcomatous fibroepithelial stromal polyps of the lower female genital tract: an underrecognized lesion often misdiagnosed as sarcoma. Am J Surg Pathol 24: 231–240
130. LiVolsi V A, Brooks J J 1987 Nodular fasciitis of the vulva: a report of two cases. Obstet Gynecol 69: 513–516
131. Roberts W, Daly J W 1981 Pseudosarcomatous fasciitis of the vulva. Gynecol Oncol 11: 383–386
132. Gaffney E F, Majmudar B, Bryan J A 1982 Nodular fasciitis (pseudosarcomatous fasciitis) of the vulva. Int J Gynecol Pathol 1: 307–312
133. Fletcher C D M, Tsang W Y, Fisher C et al. 1992 Angiomyofibroblastoma of the vulva. A benign neoplasm distinct from aggressive angiomyxoma. Am J Surg Pathol 16: 373–382
134. Nielsen G P, Rosenberg A E, Young R H et al. 1996 Angiomyofibroblastoma of the vulva and vagina. Mod Pathol 9: 284–291
135. Ockner D M, Sayadi H, Swanson P E et al. 1997 Genital angiomyofibroblastoma. Comparison with aggressive angiomyxoma and other myxoid neoplasms of skin and soft tissue. Am J Clin Pathol 107: 36–44
136. Fukunaga M, Nomura K, Matsumoto K et al. 1997 Vulval angiomyofibroblastoma. Clinicopathologic analysis of six cases. Am J Clin Pathol 107: 45–51
137. Laskin W B, Fetsch J F, Tavassoli F A 1997 Angiomyofibroblastoma of the female genital tract: analysis of 17 cases including a lipomatous variant. Hum Pathol 28: 1046–1055
138. Hisaoka M, Kouho H, Aoki T et al. 1995 Angiomyofibroblastoma of the vulva: a clinicopathologic study of seven cases. Pathol Int 45: 487–492
139. Nielsen G P, Young R H, Dickersin G R et al. 1997 Angiomyofibroblastoma of the vulva with sarcomatous transformation ("angiomyofibrosarcoma"). Am J Surg Pathol 21: 1104–1108
140. Nucci M R, Granter S R, Fletcher C D M 1997 Cellular angiofibroma: a benign neoplasm distinct from angiomyofibroblastoma and spindle cell lipoma. Am J Surg Pathol 21: 636–644
141. Laskin W B, Fetsch J F, Mostofi F K 1998 Angiomyofibroblastomalike tumor of the male genital tract: analysis of 11 cases with comparison to female angiomyofibroblastoma and spindle cell lipoma. Am J Surg Pathol 22: 6–16
142. Iwasa Y, Fletcher C D M 2004 Cellular angiofibroma: clinicopathologic and immunohistochemical analysis of 51 cases. Am J Surg Pathol 28: 1426–1435
143. McCluggage W G, Perenyei M, Irwin S T 2002 Recurrent cellular angiofibroma of the vulva. J Clin Pathol 55: 477–479
144. Gonzalez S, Duarte I 1982 Benign fibrous histiocytoma of the skin. A morphological study of 290 cases. Pathol Res Pract 174: 379–391
145. Lack E E, Worsham G F, Callihan M D et al. 1980 Granular cell tumor: a clinicopathologic study of 110 patients. J Surg Oncol 13: 301–316
146. Horowitz I R, Copas P, Majmudar B 1995 Granular cell tumors of the vulva. Am J Obstet Gynecol 173: 1710–1713
147. Haley J C, Mirowski G W, Hood A F 1998 Benign vulvar tumors. Semin Cutan Med Surg 17: 196–204
148. Cohen Z, Kapuller V, Maor E et al. 1999 Granular cell tumor (myoblastoma) of the labia major: a rare benign tumor in childhood. J Pediatr Adolesc Gynecol 12: 155–156
149. Guenther L, Shum D 1993 Granular cell tumor of the vulva. Pediatr Dermatol 10: 153–155
150. Majmudar B, Castellano P Z, Wilson R W et al. 1990 Granular cell tumors of the vulva. J Reprod Med 35: 1008–1014
151. Robertson A J, McIntosh W, Lamont P et al. 1981 Malignant granular cell tumour (myoblastoma) of the vulva: report of a case and review of the literature. Histopathology 5: 69–79
152. Newman P L, Fletcher C D M 1991 Smooth muscle tumours of the external genitalia: clinicopathological analysis of a series. Histopathology 18: 523–529
153. Tavassoli F A, Norris H J 1979 Smooth muscle tumors of the vulva. Obstet Gynecol 53: 213–217
154. Nielsen G P, Rosenberg A E, Koerner F C et al. 1996 Smooth-muscle tumors of the vulva. A clinicopathological study of 25 cases and review of the literature. Am J Surg Pathol 20: 779–793
155. Nucci M R, Fletcher C D M 2000 Vulvovaginal soft tissue tumours: update and review. Histopathology 36: 97–108
156. Cohen P R, Young A W Jr, Tovell H M 1989 Angiokeratoma of the vulva: diagnosis and review of the literature. Obstet Gynecol Surv 44: 339–346
157. Vlastos A T, Malpica A, Follen M 2003 Lymphangioma circumscriptum of the vulva: a review of the literature. Obstet Gynecol 101: 946–954
158. Faber K, Jones M A, Spratt D et al. 1991 Vulvar leiomyomatosis in a patient with esophagogastric leiomyomatosis: review of the syndrome. Gynecol Oncol 41: 92–94

159. Lae M E, Pereira P F, Keeney G L et al. 2002 Lipoblastoma-like tumour of the vulva: report of three cases of a distinctive mesenchymal neoplasm of adipocytic differentiation. Histopathology 40: 505–509
160. Sutphen R, Galan-Gomez E, Kousseff B G 1995 Clitoromegaly in neurofibromatosis. Am J Med Genet 55: 325–330
161. Gersell D J, Fulling K H 1989 Localized neurofibromatosis of the female genitourinary tract. Am J Surg Pathol 13: 873–878
162. Steeper T A, Rosai J 1983 Aggressive angiomyxoma of the female pelvis and perineum. Report of nine cases of a distinctive type of gynecologic soft-tissue neoplasm. Am J Surg Pathol 7: 463–475
163. Begin L R, Clement P B, Kirk M E et al. 1985 Aggressive angiomyxoma of pelvic soft parts: a clinicopathologic study of nine cases. Hum Pathol 16: 621–628
164. Fetsch J F, Laskin W B, Lefkowitz M et al. 1996 Aggressive angiomyxoma: a clinicopathologic study of 29 female patients. Cancer 78: 79–90
165. Granter S R, Nucci M R, Fletcher C D M 1997 Aggressive angiomyxoma: reappraisal of its relationship to angiomyofibroblastoma in a series of 16 cases. Histopathology 30: 3–10
166. Tsang W Y, Chan J K, Lee K C et al. 1992 Aggressive angiomyxoma. A report of four cases occurring in men. Am J Surg Pathol 16: 1059–1065
167. Iezzoni J C, Fechner R E, Wong L S et al. 1995 Aggressive angiomyxoma in males. A report of four cases. Am J Clin Pathol 104: 391–396
168. Nucci M R, Weremowicz S, Neskey D M et al. 2001 Chromosomal translocation t(8;12) induces aberrant HMGIC expression in aggressive angiomyxoma of the vulva. Genes Chromos Cancer 32: 172–176
169. Allen P W, Dymock R B, MacCormac L B 1988 Superficial angiomyxomas with and without epithelial components. Report of 30 tumors in 28 patients. Am J Surg Pathol 12: 519–530
170. Fetsch J F, Laskin W B, Tavassoli F A 1997 Superficial angiomyxoma (cutaneous myxoma): a clinicopathologic study of 17 cases arising in the genital region. Int J Gynecol Pathol 16: 325–334
171. Calonje E, Guerin D, McCormick D et al. 1999 Superficial angiomyxoma: clinicopathologic analysis of a series of distinctive but poorly recognized cutaneous tumors with tendency for recurrence. Am J Surg Pathol 23: 910–917
172. Ghorbani R P, Malpica A, Ayala A G 1999 Dermatofibrosarcoma protuberans of the vulva: clinicopathologic and immunohistochemical analysis of four cases, one with fibrosarcomatous change, and review of the literature. Int J Gynecol Pathol 18: 366–373
173. Gokden N, Dehner L P, Zhu X et al. 2003 Dermatofibrosarcoma protuberans of the vulva and groin: detection of COL1A1-PDGFB fusion transcripts by RT-PCR. J Cutan Pathol 30: 190–195
174. Vanni R, Faa G, Dettori T et al. 2000 A case of dermatofibrosarcoma protuberans of the vulva with a COL1A1/PDGFB fusion identical to a case of giant cell fibroblastoma. Virchows Arch 437: 95–100
175. Moodley M, Moodley J 2000 Dermatofibrosarcoma protuberans of the vulva: a case report and review of the literature. Gynecol Oncol 78: 74–75
176. Soergel T M, Doering D L, O'Connor D 1998 Metastatic dermatofibrosarcoma protuberans of the vulva. Gynecol Oncol 71: 320–324
177. Davos I, Abell M R 1976 Soft tissue sarcomas of vulva. Gynecol Oncol 4: 70–86
178. Leake J F, Buscema J, Cho K R et al. 1991 Dermatofibrosarcoma protuberans of the vulva. Gynecol Oncol 41: 245–249
179. Barnhill D R, Boling R, Nobles W et al. 1988 Vulvar dermatofibrosarcoma protuberans. Gynecol Oncol 30: 149–152
180. Bock J E, Andreasson B, Thorn A et al. 1985 Dermatofibrosarcoma protuberans of the vulva. Gynecol Oncol 20: 129–135
181. Mentzel T, Beham A, Katenkamp D et al. 1998 Fibrosarcomatous ("high-grade") dermatofibrosarcoma protuberans: clinicopathologic and immunohistochemical study of a series of 41 cases with emphasis on prognostic significance. Am J Surg Pathol 22: 576–587
182. Naeem R, Lux M L, Huang S F et al. 1995 Ring chromosomes in dermatofibrosarcoma protuberans are composed of interspersed sequences from chromosomes 17 and 22. Am J Pathol 147: 1553–1558
183. DiSaia P J, Rutledge F, Smith J P 1971 Sarcoma of the vulva. Report of 12 patients. Obstet Gynecol 38: 180–184
184. Nirenberg A, Ostor A G, Slavin J et al. 1995 Primary vulvar sarcomas. Int J Gynecol Pathol 14: 55–62
185. Curtin J P, Saigo P, Slucher B et al. 1995 Soft-tissue sarcoma of the vagina and vulva: a clinicopathologic study. Obstet Gynecol 86: 269–272
186. Copeland L J, Gershenson D M, Saul P B et al. 1985 Sarcoma botryoides of the female genital tract. Obstet Gynecol 66: 262–266
187. Copeland L J, Sneige N, Stringer C A et al. 1985 Alveolar rhabdomyosarcoma of the female genitalia. Cancer 56: 849–855
188. Imachi M, Tsukamoto N, Kamura T et al. 1991 Alveolar rhabdomyosarcoma of the vulva. Report of two cases. Acta Cytol 35: 345–349
189. Nucci M R, Fletcher C D M 1998 Liposarcoma (atypical lipomatous tumors) of the vulva: a clinicopathologic study of six cases. Int J Gynecol Pathol 17: 17–23
190. Brooks J J, LiVolsi V A 1987 Liposarcoma presenting on the vulva. Am J Obstet Gynecol 156: 73–75
191. Gondos B, Casey M J 1982 Liposarcoma of the perineum. Gynecol Oncol 14: 133–140
192. Genton C Y, Maroni E S 1987 Vulval liposarcoma. Arch Gynecol 240: 63–66
193. Vecchione A, Palazzetti P 1967 [Anatomoclinical considerations on a case of liposarcoma with vulvar localization.] Riv Anat Patol Oncol 31: 177–193
194. Guillou L, Wadden C, Coindre J M et al. 1997 "Proximal-type" epithelioid sarcoma, a distinctive aggressive neoplasm showing rhabdoid features. Clinicopathologic, immunohistochemical, and ultrastructural study of a series. Am J Surg Pathol 21: 130–146
195. Shen J T, D'ablaing G, Morrow C P 1982 Alveolar soft part sarcoma of the vulva: report of first case and review of literature. Gynecol Oncol 13: 120–128
196. Lin J, Yip K M, Maffulli N et al. 1996 Extraskeletal mesenchymal chondrosarcoma of the labium majus. Gynecol Oncol 60: 492–493
197. Nielsen G P, Shaw P A, Rosenberg A E et al. 1996 Synovial sarcoma of the vulva: a report of two cases. Mod Pathol 9: 970–974
198. Hall D J, Burns J C, Goplerud D R 1979 Kaposi's sarcoma of the vulva: a case report and brief review. Obstet Gynecol 54: 478–483
199. Macasaet M A, Duerr A, Thelmo W et al. 1995 Kaposi sarcoma presenting as a vulvar mass. Obstet Gynecol 86: 695–697
200. Vang R, Medeiros L J, Malpica A et al. 2000 Non-Hodgkin's lymphoma involving the vulva. Int J Gynecol Pathol 19: 236–242
201. Vang R, Medeiros L J, Fuller G N et al. 2001 Non-Hodgkin's lymphoma involving the gynecologic tract: a review of 88 cases. Adv Anat Pathol 8: 200–217
202. Dudley A G, Young R H, Lawrence W D et al. 1983 Endodermal sinus tumor of the vulva in an infant. Obstet Gynecol 61: 76S–79S
203. Gil-Moreno A, Garcia-Jimenez A, Gonzalez-Bosquet J et al. 1997 Merkel cell carcinoma of the vulva. Gynecol Oncol 64: 526–532
204. Carlson J W, McGlennen R C, Gomez R et al. 1996 Sebaceous carcinoma of the vulva: a case report and review of the literature. Gynecol Oncol 60: 489–491
205. Rulon D B, Helwig E B 1974 Cutaneous sebaceous neoplasms. Cancer 33: 82–102
206. Neto A G, Deavers M T, Silvio E G et al. 2003 Metastatic tumors of the vulva. A clinicopathologic study of 66 cases. Am J Surg Pathol 27: 798–804

男性生殖道肿瘤
Tumors of the male genital tract

第一部分
前列腺和精囊 Prostate and seminal vesicles

Jae Y. Ro、Mahul B.Amin、Kyu-Rae Kim 和 Alberto G. Ayala 著

王功伟 译 高洪文 校

前列腺与精囊

前列腺 749	前列腺少见的良性上皮性病变 792
前列腺的癌前病变 750	前列腺间质病变 792
前列腺腺癌 755	恶性软组织肿瘤 798
其他类型的前列腺癌 774	累及前列腺的罕见的恶性肿瘤 800
与癌类似的病变 778	前列腺转移性实性肿瘤 801
与癌类似的其他病变 784	**精囊肿瘤和肿瘤性病变** 801
可能类似于前列腺腺癌的正常 788	精囊囊肿 801
组织解剖结构和非肿瘤性病变	其他良性肿瘤 801
萎缩 790	恶性肿瘤 802

前列腺 Prostate

前列腺癌和良性前列腺增生（benign prostatic hyperplasia，BPH）是前列腺的两个基本病变，这两种病变占所有前列腺疾病的90%以上。前列腺癌是美国男性中最常见的恶性肿瘤，是导致男性癌症死亡的第三个主要原因[1]，癌症的早期发现以及对癌前病变更好的认识为降低肿瘤的发病率和死亡率提供了可行的方法。90%以上的前列腺恶性上皮性肿瘤是普通的腺泡型癌，另外大约10%的前列腺癌与经典的组织学不同，被看作是特殊类型癌。

通常，前列腺病变的形态学诊断相对简单，尤其是区分良恶性病变。然而，在某些前列腺良性增生和正常的前列腺组织解剖结构表现为小腺体结构时，不论腺体伴有或不伴有细胞的非典型性，如果忽略了形态学上的细微差别，容易把这些小腺体误诊为恶性病变。绝大多数与癌相似的良性病变与前列腺癌发生年龄相同。这些病变没有特殊的临床表现，多数是在临床诊断为BPH患者的前列腺切除标本中遇到，或者是在前列腺穿刺活检组织中见到，这些腺体不同程度体现了激素的影响以及腺体的萎缩。与最新的世界卫生组织（WHO）分类[2]相同，前列腺肿瘤、瘤样病变以及前列腺增生的分类概括在表14A.1中。前列腺的良性病变可以分成上皮性和间质性病变。上皮性病变包括普通型BPH、基底细胞增生（basal cell hyperplasia，BCH）、透明细胞筛状增生（clear cell cribriform hyperplasia，CCCH）、萎缩和萎缩后增生（postatrophic hyperplasia，PAH）、硬化性腺病（sclerosing adenosis，SA）、中肾管残件增生、精阜黏膜腺体增生（verumontanum mucosal gland hyperplasia，VMGH）以及肾源性腺瘤（nephrogenic adenoma，NA）[3]。

前列腺最常见的间质性病变是前列腺间质增生；少见病变包括平滑肌瘤、非典型性间质增生以及与之紧密相关的非典型性平滑肌瘤（也称为奇异性或合胞体性平滑肌瘤）、叶状型非典型增生、手术后梭形细胞结节以及假肉瘤性纤维黏液样肿瘤。前列腺间质肉瘤以及其他类型肉瘤发生在成年人，相对少见；横纹肌肉瘤是儿童前列腺最常见的肿瘤。

表14A.1 世界卫生组织前列腺肿瘤的组织学分类[a]

上皮性肿瘤			血管瘤	9120/0
腺上皮性肿瘤			软骨瘤	9200/0
腺癌（腺泡型）		8140/3	平滑肌瘤	8890/0
萎缩性			颗粒细胞瘤	9580/0
假增生性			血管外皮细胞瘤	8150/1
泡沫细胞性			孤立性纤维性肿瘤	8815/0
胶样性		8480/3		
印戒细胞性		8490/3	**淋巴造血组织肿瘤**	
嗜酸细胞性		8290/3	淋巴瘤	
淋巴上皮瘤样性		8082/3	白血病	
具有梭形细胞分化的癌（癌肉瘤、肉瘤样癌）		8572/3		
			其他肿瘤	
前列腺上皮内肿瘤形成（PIN）			囊腺瘤	8440/0
前列腺上皮内肿瘤形成，III级（PIN III）		8148/2	肾母细胞瘤（Wilms瘤）	8960/3
			横纹肌样瘤	8963/3
导管腺癌		8500/3	生殖细胞肿瘤	
筛状		8201/3	卵黄囊瘤	9071/3
乳头状		8260/3	精原细胞瘤	9061/3
实性		8230/3	胚胎性癌和畸胎瘤	9081/3
			绒毛膜癌	9100/3
尿路上皮性肿瘤			透明细胞腺癌	8130/3
尿路上皮癌		8120/3	黑色素瘤	8720/3
鳞状细胞肿瘤			**转移性肿瘤**	
腺鳞状细胞癌		8560/3		
鳞状细胞癌		8070/3	**精囊肿瘤**	
基底细胞肿瘤			**上皮性肿瘤**	
基底细胞腺瘤		8147/0	腺癌	8140/3
基底细胞癌		8147/3	囊腺瘤	8440/0
神经内分泌肿瘤			**混合性上皮和间质肿瘤**	
腺癌伴有神经内分泌分化		8574/3	恶性	
类癌		8240/3	良性	
小细胞癌		8041/3		
副神经节瘤		8680/1	**间叶性肿瘤**	
神经母细胞瘤		9500/3	平滑肌肉瘤	8890/3
			血管肉瘤	9120/3
前列腺间质肿瘤			脂肪肉瘤	8850/3
恶性潜能未定的间质肿瘤		8935/1	恶性纤维组织细胞瘤	8830/3
间质肉瘤		8935/3	孤立性纤维性肿瘤	8815/0
			血管外皮细胞瘤	9150/1
间叶性肿瘤			平滑肌瘤	8890/0
平滑肌肉瘤		8890/3		
横纹肌肉瘤		8900/3	**其他肿瘤**	
软骨肉瘤		9220/3	绒毛膜癌	9100/3
血管肉瘤		9120/3	可能为Wolff来源的男性附属器肿瘤	
恶性纤维组织细胞瘤		8830/3		
恶性周围神经鞘肿瘤		9540/3	**转移性肿瘤**	

[a] 肿瘤疾病国际分类形态学编码（ICDO）和医学系统化专业术语（http://snomed.org）。生物学行为编码/0为良性肿瘤，/2为原位癌及III级上皮内肿瘤形成，/3为恶性肿瘤，/1为交界性或生物学行为不明确。

前列腺的癌前病变
Premalignant lesions of the prostate

虽然已经描述了两个公认的前列腺癌前病变：即前列腺上皮内肿瘤形成（prostatic intraepithelial neoplasia, PIN）（同义词：导管内异型增生、原发性非典型增生、大腺泡异型增生以及腺泡-导管异型增生）[4-9]和非典型性腺瘤性增生（atypical adenomatous hyperplasia, AAH）（同义词：腺病、小腺体增生），但是后者还没有被证实是癌前病变。首先，PIN 以细胞学非典型性为特征，结构得

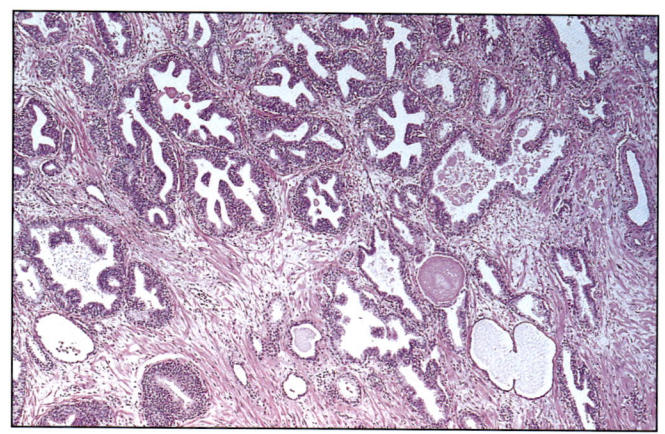

图14A.1 前列腺上皮内肿瘤形成（PIN）。PIN腺体结构复杂，以上皮增生和细胞核复层为特征。受累的腺体由增厚的细胞层组成，明显不同于正常或萎缩的腺体。

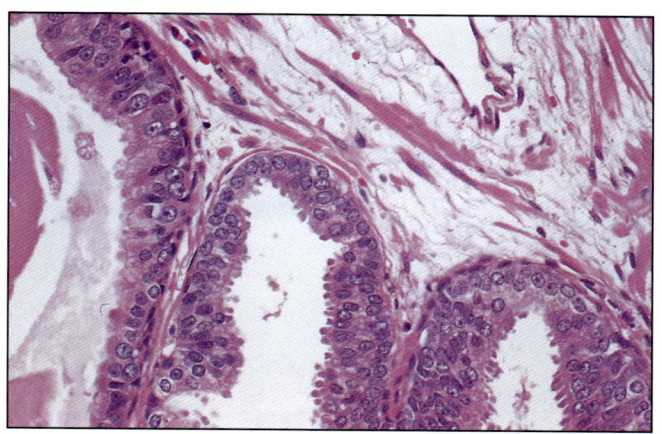

图14A.2 高倍镜下，前列腺上皮内肿瘤形成显示细胞数量增加，核大小不一，深染并有明显的核仁。

以保存；其次，PIN具有结构非典型性，其特征是新腺泡（neoacinar，即小腺体）增生，没有明显的细胞学非典型性。这将在下面前列腺癌的类似病变中讨论(见778页)。

前列腺上皮内肿瘤形成
Prostatic intraepithelial neoplasia

早在1965年[10]以及在随后的多年中[11,12] McNeal描述了这种癌前病变，但是直到20世纪80年代中期他的这一癌前病变的概念才被完全接受。在1986年，McNeal和Bostwick进一步提供了PIN是癌前病变性质的证据（当时命名为导管内异型增生），并介绍了分级系统[4]。1989年3月在美国马里兰州的Bethesda召开了前列腺癌前病变专题学术会议，会议采纳了前列腺上皮内肿瘤形成（PIN）为首选术语[13]。

PIN 的组织学特征

在低倍镜下PIN容易与正常的以及增生的腺上皮区别，因为受累的腺体或导管常常表现为明显的深染和细胞核复层（图14A.1）。高倍镜下，可见细胞核增大和深染（图14A.2）。根据细胞核变化的严重程度，PIN分为低级别PIN和高级别PIN[8,9]。

尽管马里兰Bethesda的全体会议[1,3]同意PIN仅有两个类型，即低级别PIN和高级别PIN，然而，为了更好地理解PIN，在这里按照McNeal和Bostwick建议的三级分级体系进行组织学描述[4]。低级别PIN（1级PIN）的特征是细胞数量轻度增加，细胞核大小不一、深染，见有小核仁。2级PIN表现为细胞核复层，有些细胞核增大伴有核仁，通常是局灶性的，尤其是核仁，并不是见于所有细胞中。许多时候很难区分低级别PIN（1级PIN）和2级PIN。相反，高级别PIN（3级PIN）上皮细胞可见恶性细胞学特征，与任何前列腺原位癌的所

表14A.2 前列腺上皮内肿瘤形成（PIN）的诊断标准

	低级别PIN（PIN1）	高级别PIN（PIN2和3）
结构	密集，复层，不规则间隙	变化多，伴有4种结构：簇状、微乳头状、筛状和扁平状
细胞核	轻度增大，大小差异明显（核大小不等）	明显增大，大小差异较小
染色质	正常	增加
核仁	很少见到明显的核仁	偶尔或常见大而明显的核仁

见相同。因此，高级别PIN的特征是细胞数量明显增加伴有细胞核复层及核深染。细胞核增大，在比较PIN上皮细胞和周围正常上皮细胞以及间质组织时容易证实这个特征；然而，有些病例因为固定或制片中人工假象的原因，或只是因为没有细胞核增大，而没有表现出这种特征。高级别PIN的标志是存在大核仁（2级PIN中很少，3级PIN中很多），直径大于1μm；在大核仁的周围常见有空晕。在PIN中核分裂象不常见，但可以见到（表14A.2）。

PIN 的分布

PIN主要见于前列腺的外周区（75%～80%），在移行区少见（10%～15%），在中央区极其少见（<5%），这种分布与前列腺癌的区域性分布相一致[4,5,14]。高级别PIN在穿刺活检组织中出现的频率为5%～16%，在经尿道前列腺切除（transurethral resection of the prostate，TURP）标本中为2.3%～4.2%[15-17]。

它可以累及部分腺泡腔或整个腺泡。起初，PIN的上皮增生表现为细胞数量增加排列成假复层，而随疾病进展，形成腔内乳头。PIN表现出多种结构形态：簇状、微乳头状、筛状或扁平状[8,18]。最常见的是乳头状和簇状结构，筛状结构少见；最少见的是扁平结构[8,18]。其他不常见的

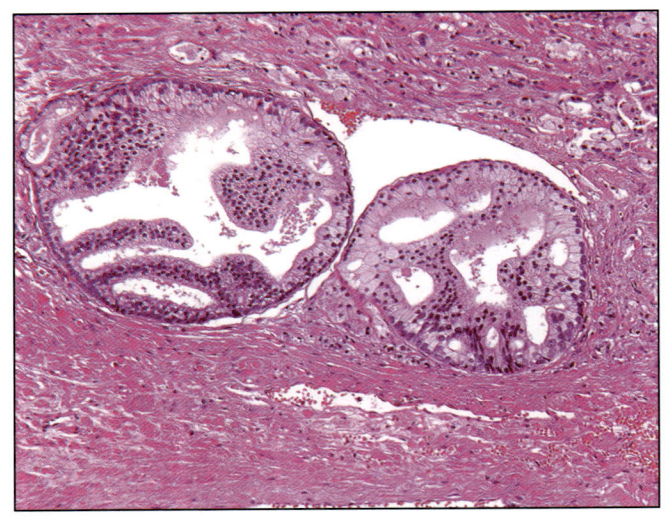

图14A.3 泡沫细胞高级别前列腺上皮内肿瘤形成（PIN）：PIN细胞有丰富的泡沫样胞浆，在腺体的上半部分较为明显。

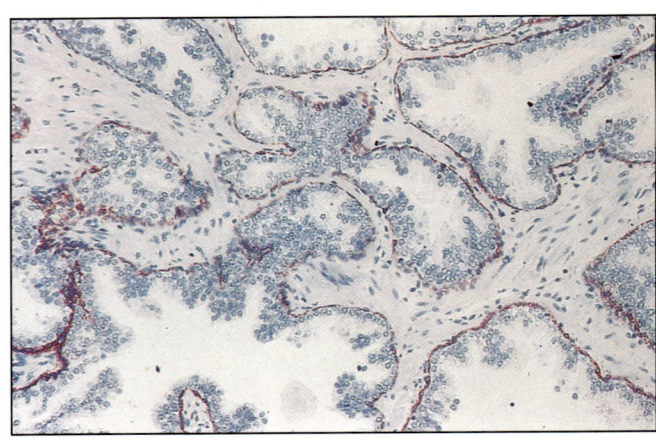

图14A.4 在低级别前列腺上皮内肿瘤形成中基底细胞层通常保留。34βE12免疫染色。

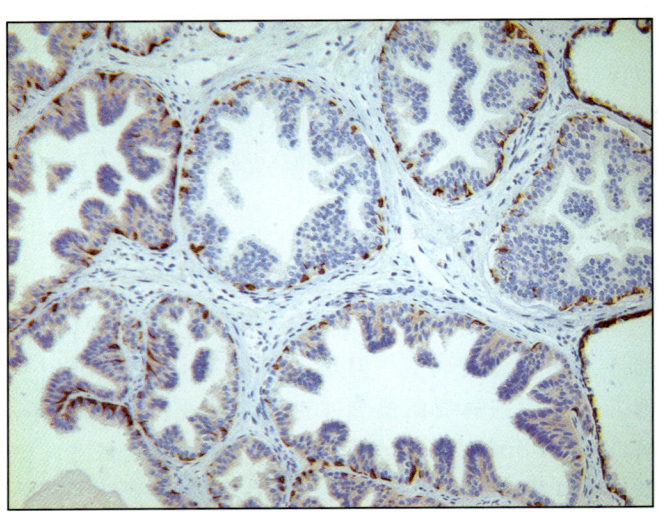

图14A.5 高级别前列腺上皮内肿瘤形成（PIN）的腺体通常显示基底细胞部分缺失。注意跳跃式的细胞核染色。与图14A.4 低级别PIN完整的基底细胞染色形成对比。

结构包括伴有黏液性细胞浆、印戒细胞改变、小细胞未分化特征[19]、泡沫细胞腺体型（图14A.3）以及内翻性（鞋钉样）PIN 特征[8, 20, 21]。除了泡沫细胞腺体型外，这些结构形态在高级别 PIN 中比低级别 PIN 中更为常见[18]。

PIN 的多中心性与癌前病变
Multifocality of PIN and precursor of malignancy

1969 年 McNeal[12] 提出了这种病变的多中心性；这个观察已经被其他学者所证实[4, 5, 22]。在一项从膀胱癌患者行膀胱前列腺切除手术获得的整个前列腺器官切片的研究中，Troncoso 等[14] 发现在 100 个前列腺中有 89 个发现有 PIN。绝大多数的 PIN 是多中心性的，伴有癌的前列腺比不伴有癌的前列腺有更多数量的 PIN 病灶。在 71% 伴有癌的前列腺中出现 10 个以上 PIN 病灶；而且多于 20 个 PIN 病灶的占有很大比例。

1986 年，McNeal 和 Bostwick[4] 研究了 100 例连续包埋的前列腺癌和 100 例尸检获得的良性前列腺，提供了有力的证据支持了高级别 PIN（当时称为导管内异型增生）是浸润性癌癌前病变的观点。他们报告了高级别病变（3 级）在有癌的前列腺（33%）中比无癌前列腺（4%）中更常见，并得出结论：在多数前列腺癌中 PIN 可能是前期病变[4]。这个发现被 Troncoso 等[14] 的研究所证实，他们发现在有癌的 61 个前列腺中 44 个（72.1%）出现高级别 PIN（3 级），在无癌的前列腺中仅 17.9% 发现有 PIN；因为高级别 PIN 与癌关系密切，所以它对癌有预测价值。有时可以看到直接从高级别 PIN 发生的癌[18,23,24]。

在低级别和高级别 PIN 中存在基底细胞层（图 14A.4 和 14A.5），但在高级别 PIN 中它可以局灶缺失（图 14A.5）。Bostwick 和 Brawer[5] 在 PIN 和癌的系列切片中使用对基底细胞特异的高分子量角蛋白（克隆 34βE12）染色，发现在 PIN 中基底细胞层存在，但在较高级别病变中有不同程度的缺失，尤其是在接近腺癌的腺泡中基底细胞缺失更加明显。这些发现使得这些作者推断前列腺癌发生早期浸润通常与高级别 PIN 有关，并且早期浸润是以基底细胞层的断裂为特征。McNeal 等把这些腺体命名为过渡性腺体[23]。在周围有非典型性小腺体的高级别 PIN 中，存在的问题是这些小腺体是来自周围高级别 PIN 的出芽或者是腺体横切，还是来自常与高级别 PIN 相连的浸润性癌。Kronz 等[25] 报告，在通过重复活检预测癌的情况下，周围伴有非典型性小腺体的 PIN 与单独的高级别 PIN 相比具有更大的危险性。尽管年龄和伴随的高级别 PIN 的主要结构可以帮助预测哪些伴有这种病变的男性在重复活检中会有癌，但是实际应用起来并不太可靠；因此，对所有周围伴有非典型性小腺体的 PIN 男性都应该反复活检。

免疫组织化学

在 PIN 的诊断中，基底细胞标志物是最常应用的标志物，如高分子量角蛋白（34βE12）、p63 以及细胞角蛋白 5/6。然而，已经进行了一整套免疫组织化学研究帮助分析高级别 PIN 和浸润性癌之间的关系。例如，超过 90% 的 PIN 和浸润性癌病例单克隆抗角蛋白抗体 KA4[26] 以及荆豆凝集素（UEA-I）染色阳性[26, 27]，而仅有 4% 的 BPH 对 KA4 有免疫反应，并且对 UEA-I 无反应；相比之下，在一个不同研究中发现凝集素结合体在局灶性异型增生中表达下降[28]。Vimentin 在绝大多数 BPH 和 15%PIN 的腺腔细胞中存在，但在浸润性腺癌中缺失[26]。其他研究，包括核仁组成区嗜银蛋白（AgNOR）以及静态 DNA 流式细胞术，表明高级别 PIN 和癌有相似的增生活性以及 DNA 含量，因此高级别 PIN 最有可能是癌前病变[29, 32]。另外还有很多研究支持 PIN 是癌症的前驱病变，其中免疫染色包括前列腺特异性抗原（prostate-specific antigen, PSA）、前列腺酸性磷酸酶（prostatic acid phosphatase, PrAP）、CD57、IV 型胶原、胶原酶、金属蛋白酶和基质溶素、上皮生长因子受体、增生细胞核抗原、Ki-67、MIB1 增生活性、p53 肿瘤抑制基因蛋白、c-myc 基因、bcl-2 癌蛋白等[22, 33-37]。在高级别 PIN 和癌中具有相似的细胞遗传学异常（涉及 7q、8q、10q、16q）和染色体数目的变化[38-41]。最近的一项研究[42]证实，在癌周围（距离小于 5mm）的孤立的高级别 PIN 腺体与远离癌（距离大于 5 mm）的腺体相比，前者 α-甲酰基辅酶 A 消旋酶（AMACR）/P504S 有更高的阳性率（56% vs. 14%；P＜0.0001）。邻近癌的高级别 PIN 的腺体也比那些远离癌的 PIN 腺体表现出更高的(P＜0.0004)AMACR/P504S 表达强度。这些资料表明，AMACR/P504S 强阳性的 PIN 比阴性或弱阳性的 PIN 与癌的关系更为密切，同时在这项研究中也提供了高级别 PIN 作为前列腺腺癌癌前病变的额外证据[42]。

鉴别诊断

良性/低级别病变最主要的鉴别诊断包括 1 级 PIN（低级别 PIN）与 2 级 PIN（认为是高级别 PIN）的鉴别，以及低级别 PIN 与前列腺中央区组织学形态的鉴别。高级别病变的鉴别诊断包括导管-子宫内膜样癌、筛状癌以及累及前列腺导管的移行细胞癌（transitional cell carcinoma, TCC）。在鉴别诊断中也包括其他病变，但它们更容易排除。下面简单讨论这些病变。

高级别 PIN 与低级别 PIN（High-grade PIN versus low-grade PIN） 低级别 PIN 与高级别 PIN 相鉴别的特征列在表 14A.2 中。然而，不幸的是，没有一个明确的组织学标准能够区分 1 级（低级别 PIN）和 2 级 PIN。两者相鉴别有主观性，一个病理医师可能只因为有核深染或存在一些核仁而错误地把一个病变简单地视为高级别 PIN。Sakar 等做了一项有趣的研究，他把 30 例含有不同程度结构非典型性腺体的前列腺穿刺活检切片，其中包括已诊断为高级别 PIN 的 22 个病例，交给 11 位泌尿病理医师诊断。在许多病例出现了不同的诊断后，作者得出结论："泌尿病理医师诊断 HGPIN（高级别 PIN）所使用的形态学标准一般来说较一致，但是对交界性病例应用的标准却有很大不同。这是导致文献中高级别 PIN 发生率不同的部分原因，这给患者带来明显不同的临床处理"[43]。

高级别 PIN 与中央区及移行细胞化生（High-grade PIN versus central zone and transitional metaplasia） 前列腺底部穿刺活检的组织中可以见到前列腺中央区的成分，其组织学特征容易与高级别 PIN 相混淆[44]。与前列腺外周区和移行区相比，中央区的特征是腺体之间存在较多的间质。前列腺中央区腺体常有细胞核复层，使导管表现异常，好像含有高级别 PIN。然而，其腺上皮细胞核单一、圆形，没有非典型性，偶尔可见到核仁，在中央区也可见类似于所谓罗马拱门和（或）形成筛状结构的小腺体结构。另外，腺体内可见乳头形成，含有中心性纤维血管轴心，上皮细胞没有非典型性。相反，高级别 PIN 的乳头没有中心性纤维血管轴心[44]。

移行细胞化生通常发生在邻近尿道的前列腺中央大导管，但是也可出现在前列腺外周区，这时可能与低级别 PIN 相混淆。存在卵圆形或轻度拉长的细胞核，常伴有核沟，是移行细胞化生的特征[45]。

高级别 PIN 与高级别肿瘤（High-grade PIN versus high-grade tumors） 在高级别的肿瘤中，前列腺导管的 TCC 以及伴有导管内筛状结构的病变是主要的鉴别诊断。

累及导管的 TCC 一般是高级别癌，可能显示中心粉刺型坏死，这个特征在高级别 PIN 中见不到。TCC 细胞表现为明显的细胞核间变，细胞大小形状不一，深染，核分裂活跃。这些细胞对 PSA、PrAP 和 AMACR/P504S 均无反应[46-48]。

含有导管内筛状结构的病变包括高级别 PIN、筛状癌、导管-子宫内膜样癌以及导管内原位癌。后三种病变的界限并不分明。筛状癌类似于导管-子宫内膜样癌，当其结构有重叠时很难区分。然而，一般来说导管-子宫内膜样癌细胞是立方形或高柱状，伴有明显的间变，而筛状癌细胞是单一圆形及高级别的。

导管-子宫内膜样癌类似于高级别 PIN，在穿刺活检标本中有时不能够鉴别二者。导管-子宫内膜样癌经常累及精阜周围的移行区，形态学上表现为复杂的背靠背腺体结构。有真正的乳头，常见坏死，细胞核明显间变，核分裂象常见[49,50]。如果见到粉刺样坏死可排除高级别 PIN。

高级别 PIN 常常扩展到导管，而导管的轮廓没有明显的变形。当筛状增生活跃，伴有明显地向受累导管/腺泡单位蔓延时，如果基底细胞消失则支持筛状癌或子宫内膜样癌而不是高级别 PIN。基底细胞的存在应该支持高级别 PIN 的诊断，但是应该慎重应用，因为导管-子宫内膜样癌或筛状癌可以逆行蔓延至导管/腺泡[49]。因此，基底细胞层的存在应该慎重解释。

原位癌这个术语已经应用于当导管/腺泡单位腺上皮被筛状癌取代的时候。McNeal 和 Yemoto[49] 认为前列腺癌累及导管是常见的现象，通常存在于肿瘤内，但在少数情况下可以远离它的浸润性区域，有鉴于此，他们使用了导管内癌这个术语，并且提出这种病变是前列腺癌发展的一部分而不是癌前病变。

应用上述导管内癌（定义为具有筛状、实性或粉刺结构的高级别 PIN）的标准，Wilcox 等[51] 研究了 252 名有导管内癌的 pT3N0 前列腺癌患者的整个切片，分析了导管内癌的存在与否与前列腺癌的 Gleason 评分、肿瘤总体积、手术边缘情况、精囊受累以及疾病进展的相关关系。结果发现，与没有导管内癌的前列腺癌患者相比，伴有导管内癌的前列腺癌患者 Gleason 评分较高和肿瘤总体积较大，而且更有可能出现精囊浸润和疾病进展。因此，所谓导管内原位癌的存在通常与浸润性前列腺癌有关，而很少出现诊断的问题。

Kronz 等也讨论了高级别 PIN 和累及导管的浸润性筛状癌的鉴别诊断[52]。他们报告了以下四个临床病理发现（两个临床和两个病理）有助于区分筛状高级别 PIN 和浸润性筛状癌：直肠指诊检查阳性（P=0.02）；经直肠前列腺超声检查阳性（P=0.02）；双侧非典型性筛状腺体（P=0.02）以及分离的筛状腺体（P=0.04）。包括筛状腺体数量、最大筛状腺体大小、坏死以及间质纤维化在内的其他发现在 PIN 和癌之间没有表现出差别。

高级别 PIN 和正常结构（High-grade PIN and normal structures） 正常结构，例如精囊和射精管可能类似于 PIN[53-55]。射精管/精囊上皮通常有散在的大而多形性的细胞核，常有核内包涵体和细胞浆内脂褐素沉着，尽管 PIN 上皮也可出现色素，但通常细腻且不明显[56]。在高级别 PIN 中细胞的多形性不常见。如果附近存在梗死或炎症（尤其是急性炎症）诊断高级别 PIN 应该谨慎，因为反应性病变诱导的细胞核非典型性可能类似于 PIN；在反应性前列腺上皮中通常并不出现 PIN 的各种结构特征。

高级别 PIN 的临床意义

一般认为，诊断为高级别 PIN 的患者大约 1/3（30%～35%）伴有浸润性前列腺癌，因此，在诊断高级别 PIN 后通常需要重复进行前列腺活检。遗憾的是，2/3 的患者在重复活检后没有发现浸润性癌，这其中的一些患者每年都在进行重复活检。泌尿科医师和病理医师逐渐意识到了这个问题。对于高级别 PIN 的认识观察者之间有良好的可重复性[57]，但是对于低级别 PIN 的认识却不是这样[58]。因此，有些低级别 PIN（1 级）病例可能被误诊为高级别 PIN。最近许多关于高级别 PIN 的文章已经提到其他一些相关的因素，或许有助于筛选有浸润性癌的高风险患者。

Kronz 等[25] 研究了在首次活检中仅有高级别 PIN 的 245 名男性（图 14A.6），他们至少有一次随访活检，32.2% 的男性重复活检证实有癌。唯一的独立性预测癌存在的组织学因子是伴有高级别 PIN 的活检点数。1 个或 2 个阳性活检点数，癌症存在的风险是 30.2%；3 个阳性活检点数，癌症存在的风险是 40%；超过 3 个阳性活检点数，癌症存在的风险是 75%。下面的因子不能预测癌的存在：活检组织中高级别 PIN 腺体的数量，活检组织中高级别 PIN 所占的最大百分比，明显的核仁，有明显核仁细胞的百分比，高级别 PIN 的类型（扁平、簇状、微乳头状、筛状），明显的多形性，直肠指诊，经直肠超声所见，前列腺癌家族史，高级别 PIN 诊断时血清 PSA 值以及血清 PSA 变化率。如果在前两次随访活检中没有发现癌，可能将来也不会发现。尽管在诊断高级别 PIN 时的临床发现对于预测谁可能会有前列腺癌没有帮助，但是组织学发现却有助于确认谁需要再次活检。

Bishara 等[59] 对 PIN 的组织学亚型分析显示，伴有簇状/扁平状 PIN（31.9%）比伴有微乳头状/筛状（22%）

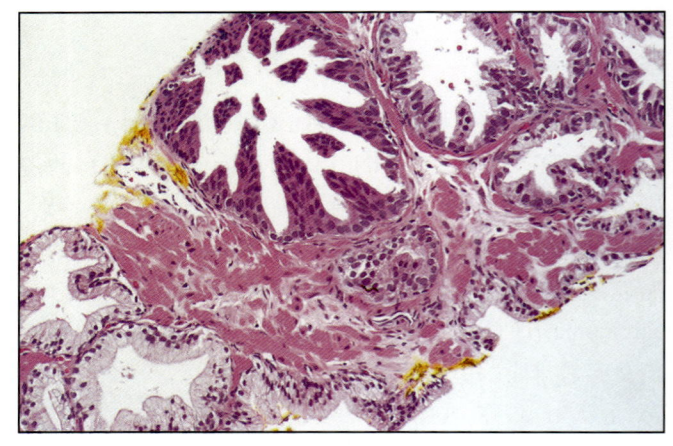

图 14A.6 穿刺活检中的前列腺上皮内肿瘤形成。前列腺上皮内肿瘤形成中增大的细胞核与邻近的良性腺体形成对比。

PIN 有更高的癌的风险，但是没有统计学差别。这一发现与另外一项提示微乳头和筛状高级别 PIN 伴有更高风险的研究有所不同[25]。Bishara 等[59] 也提出高级别 PIN 累及的活检组织点数是预测随访活检中有较高浸润性癌风险的因素。

高级别 PIN 的诊断会逐渐废弃吗？或许不会！然而，游戏规则可能随着扩大活检的引入而改变。这种方法称为"饱和"活检（"saturation" biopsies），与传统的前列腺六点活检不同，该方法针对 10 个或更多部位活检。用这样一种对前列腺的多点活检方法，发现前列腺癌的机会很高[60,61]。最近一项对 31 名经 12 点活检诊断为高级别 PIN 患者的研究，所有患者在重复活检前都随访 3 年，研究发现 8 名（28.8%）患者在重复活检中发现浸润性癌，11 名（35.5%）表现为高级别 PIN，12 名（38.7%）没有病变[62]。因此作者得出结论，高级别 PIN 是前列腺的癌前病变，并且推荐高级别 PIN 患者间隔一定时间后不管血清 PSA 水平是否变化都应重复活检[62]。其他作者认为在扩大活检中被诊断为高级别 PIN 的患者应该以临床为基础进行随访，如果临床提示有必要活检则应该进行重复活检[63,64]。对于通过 10 点或更多点活检诊断为高级别 PIN 的患者，最终决定是否进行重复活检应该由患者和泌尿科医师之间达成共识决定。

前列腺腺癌
Adenocarcinoma of the prostate

腺癌是迄今为止前列腺最常见的恶性肿瘤，是男性癌症相关死亡的主要原因之一。美国癌症协会估计 2006 年美国有 234 460 名男性诊断为前列腺癌，27 350 名男性死于该疾病[167]。前列腺癌是男性最常见的恶性肿瘤，占所有男性恶性肿瘤的 33%，占癌症死亡的 9%，是肺癌和直肠癌后第三个最主要的死亡原因[1]。在过去几年中前列腺癌的发病率和死亡率已经开始下降[65]。

前列腺癌发病率在不同种族之间差异很大，在美国、澳大利亚以及斯堪的纳维亚国家（可能是因为普查的原因）非常高。在美国，黑人人群的发病率最高，死亡率也很高。在欧洲的发病率不同，北欧和西欧国家的发病率高，而东欧和南欧国家的发病率较低。在亚洲人群中前列腺癌相对少见。除了因地域、种族和人种不同而造成的前列腺癌发病率不同之外，基因多态性因素也有可能导致不同的发病率[2]。虽然关于前列腺癌的原因和预防的一些重要问题还没有解决，但是随着对癌前上皮病变的充分认识以及临床先进技术的重大进展，例如经直肠前列腺超声检查和血清 PSA 水平检测[66,67]，明显提高了前列腺癌的早期发现。发现可导致发病和死亡的肿瘤仍然是主要问题：20% ~ 40% 的患者在诊断时已是高级别肿瘤。尽管前列腺癌发病率高，但是主要的临床矛盾是前列腺癌男性死亡时伴有该病，而不是死于肿瘤本身。

普通的前列腺腺癌占该器官上皮恶性肿瘤的 90% 以上。绝大多数病例表现为腺泡或腺泡/导管生长方式[2,68,69]。其余 10% 为特殊类型的前列腺癌，下面单独讨论。

癌可发生在前列腺任何区域，但在每个区域的相对分布是不同的：68% 的癌发生在外周区，24% 在移行区，8% 在中央区[70]。Mostofi 和 Price[71] 以及 Gleason[72] 很好地描述了前列腺癌不同的生长方式；其中包括腺泡状、融合性腺泡状、筛状、乳头状、小梁状以及实性。

绝大多数前列腺腺癌不难诊断；然而，还存在某些有问题的领域。首先是鉴别高分化腺癌与大量的良性或非典型性小腺体增生。其次是确认穿刺活检组织中微小癌灶的最低标准。最后，分化非常差的前列腺腺癌是组织形态学谱系的一个极端，可能难以与炎性浸润、转移癌以及累及前列腺的 TCC 鉴别。

高分化腺癌诊断标准包括在低倍镜下见到有分散的或局灶浸润的小腺体增生，仅有单层细胞被覆，完全缺乏基底层细胞，细胞核增大以及存在大的核仁[73-75]。小腺体增生通常表现为完整的腺泡结构，腺泡以背靠背方式排列（图 14A.7），边界清楚或有局灶浸润性边缘。核仁的大小至关重要，在癌中核仁的直径至少大于 1μm（图 14A.8）。我们通常不测量核仁大小，而是依赖于存在明显的核仁，有独特的樱桃红色。每个细胞核核仁的数量从 1 个到几个。当有多个核仁时，它们通常较小。被覆单层细胞（如基底细胞层缺如）对诊断前列腺高分化腺癌也是必需的[76]。腔内类晶体（图 14A.9）、蓝色黏液（图 A14.10）、肾小球样结构（图 14A.11）、黏液性纤维组织形成（胶原性微小结节）（图 14A.12）以及神经周围浸润（图 14A.13）的发现均有助于提示病理医

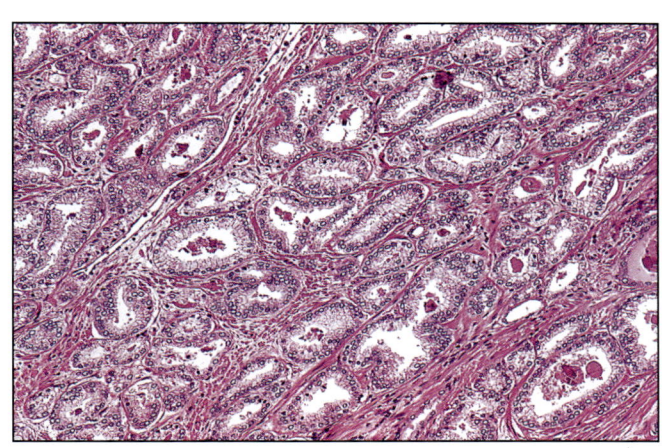

图14A.7　高分化腺癌。完整的小腺泡排列成背靠背结构。

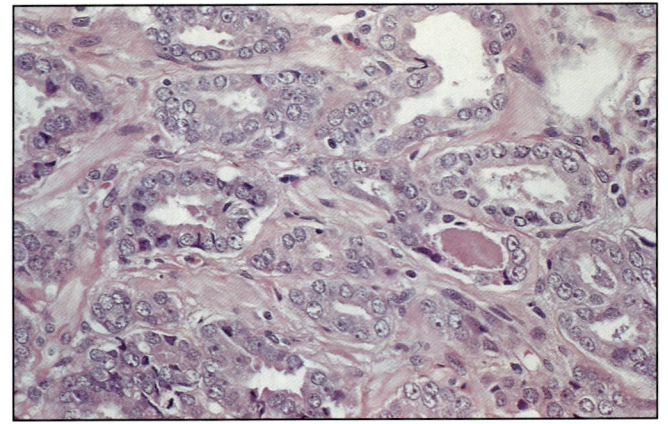

图14A.8　非典型性小腺体增生和前列腺腺癌的主要区别是后者存在明显的核仁以及缺乏基底细胞层。

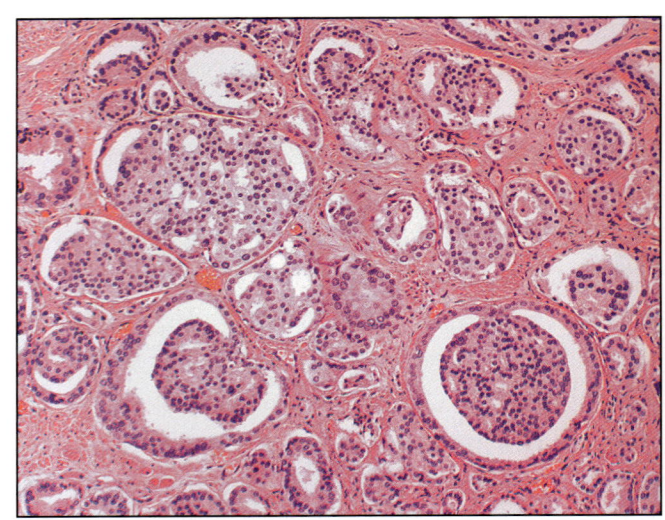

图14A.11　前列腺癌伴有肾小球样结构。肾小球样结构的特征是扩张的腺腔内恶性上皮呈筛状增生，仅附着于腺体的一侧。

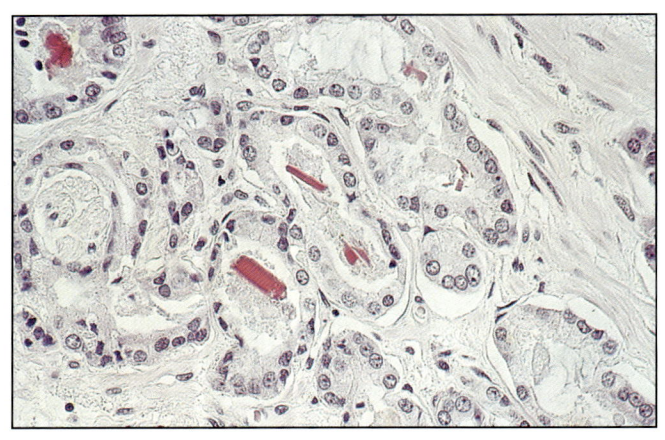

图14A.9　高分化腺癌腺腔内杆状类晶体。

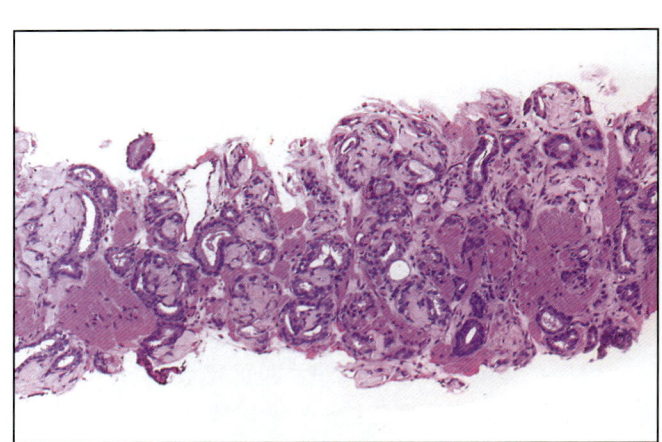

图14A.12　胶原性微小结节伴有前列腺腺癌。

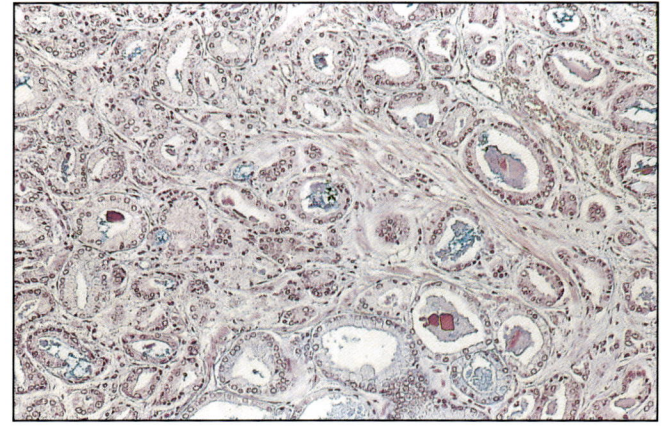

图14A.10　阿辛蓝染色显示腺腔内酸性黏液。腺腔内还有类晶体。

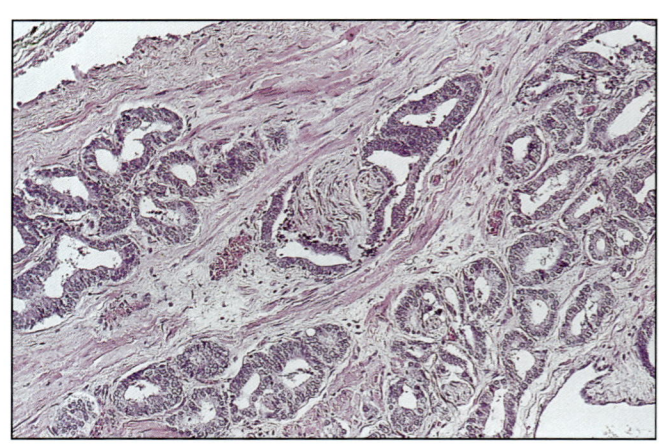

图14A.13　前列腺腺癌伴有神经周围浸润。腺体围绕整个神经，而且其细胞学特征符合癌的诊断标准。

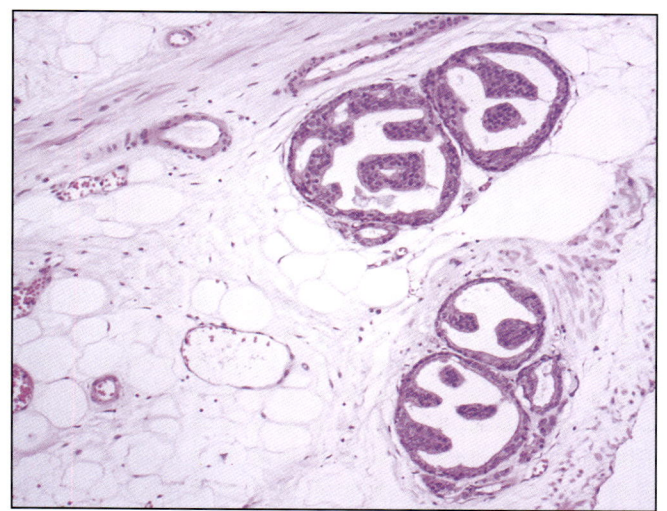

图14A.14 脂肪组织中存在恶性腺体提示癌向前列腺外蔓延。

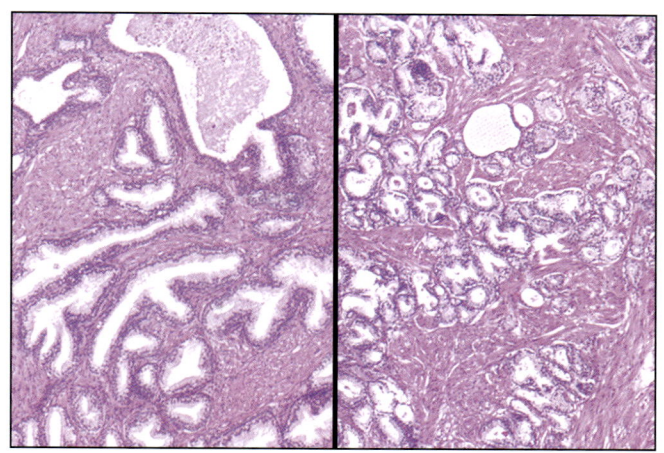

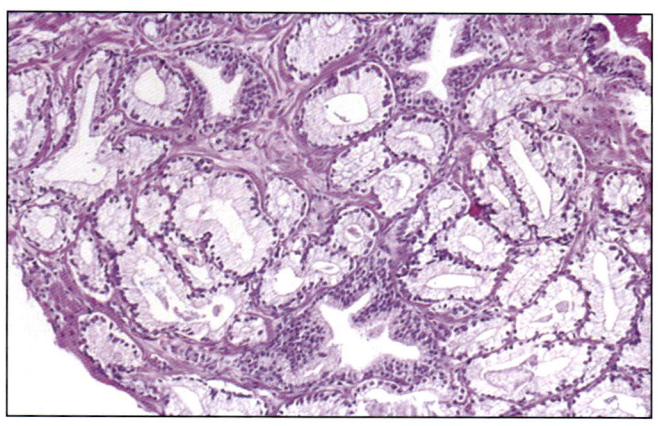

图14A.15 （A）图片左侧是正常前列腺，而右侧为可疑癌的腺体：腺体小（太小），并显示背靠背的排列（太密集）。（B）除了腺体小而密集之外，小腺体胞浆透明（太透明）。

师怀疑癌的诊断。腔内类晶体和蓝色黏液不具有病理诊断意义，但是它们通常与癌有关。然而，黏液性纤维组织形成、肾小球样结构、神经周围浸润以及脂肪组织内腺体（图14A.14）被认为具有诊断意义，可以确认前列腺癌的诊断[77]。对于在活检组织或TURP标本中筛查前列腺癌，"三太"原则（the rule of "three toos"）（即腺体太小、腺体太密集伴有背靠背排列，以及腺体太透明）非常有用（图14A.15）。要确定癌的诊断需具备三个诊断标准，即细胞核增大、明显的核仁以及缺乏基底细胞（图14A.16）。

类晶体 Crystalloids

在恶性腺泡腔内、癌周围的腺腔内（通常腺体结构表现为PIN或非典型性腺瘤性增生，在良性腺体中少见）以及前列腺硬化性腺病（SA）中可以发现类晶体[78-81]。它们一般是细长的，可以是菱形或针状，通常HE染色轻微嗜酸性（见图14A.9）。电镜下，它们是由电子致密物构成，缺乏真正结晶体的平行周期性，所以它们被称为类晶体[80,82]。在72.5%的癌中可以观察到它们，主要是在高分化性肿瘤腺泡或周围的良性腺泡内，它们也见于筛状癌内，在低分化癌中少见[80,81]。如果在穿刺活检组织中的良性腺体内见到类晶体的话，在随后的活检中发现癌的可能性低[83,84]。

黏液 Mucin

腔内黏液可发生在高分化和中分化前列腺腺癌中[75,85]。中性黏液可见于良性腺体，但是酸性黏液主要存在于前列腺腺癌中。癌中的黏液存在于腺腔内，黏蛋白卡红或阿辛蓝染色可以着色（图14A.10）；HE染色腔内黏液呈小束状及嗜碱性。肿瘤细胞浆通常不见黏液染色；这个参数在试图排除转移性腺癌时有帮助。然而，细胞浆内酸性黏液可见于增生性腺体。SA、PIN以及非典型性腺瘤性增生也有腔内酸性黏液，不能单独仅凭腔内黏液做出前列腺癌的诊断。因此，在日常诊断实践中酸性黏液组织化学染色意义不大，但是，在HE染色切片中发现蓝色黏液应该警示病理医师排除前列腺癌。

神经周围浸润、黏液性纤维组织形成（胶原性微小结节）或肾小球样结构
Perineural invasion, mucinous fibroplasia (collagenous micronodules), or glomerulation

除了脂肪组织内腺体外（图14A.14），根据报告神经周围浸润（图14A.13）、黏液性纤维组织形成/胶原性微小结节（在肿瘤性腺泡内或其周围的圆形密集玻璃样物质；图14A.12）以及肾小球样结构（筛状结构；图14A.11）均为恶性的特异性诊断特征，因为在良性前列

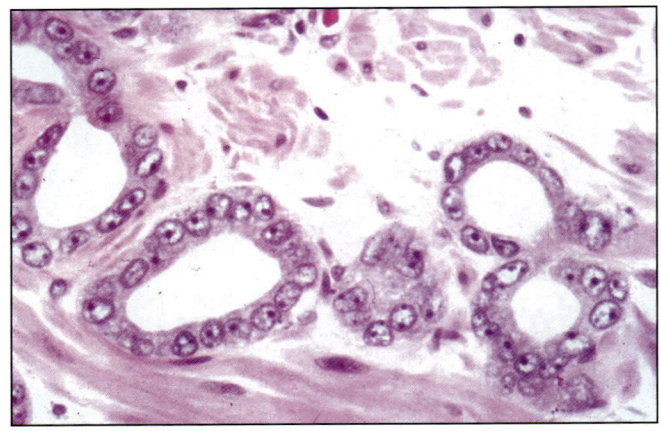

A

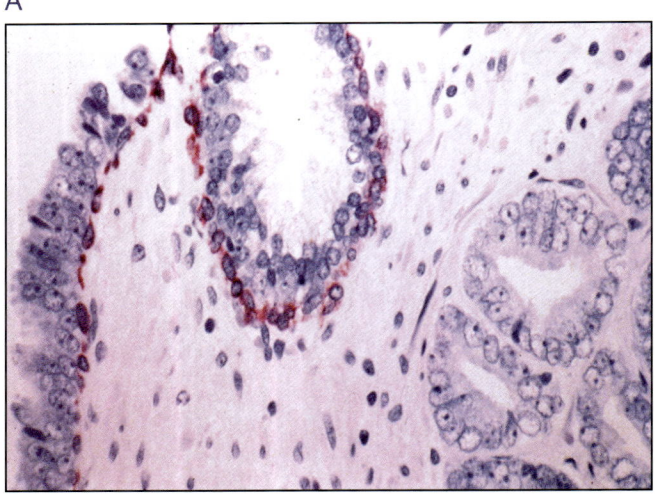

B

图14A.16　（A）为了证实前列腺癌的诊断，可疑腺体的细胞必须显示细胞核增大伴有明显的核仁，而且缺乏基底细胞。（B）本图显示癌的小腺体，没有基底细胞，而邻近的高级别前列腺上皮内肿瘤形成有明显的基底细胞。

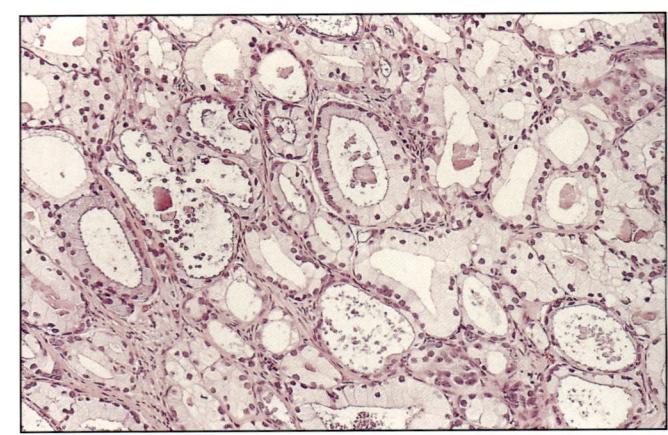

图14A.17　透明细胞（"移行区"）癌。小到中等大小背靠背的腺体内衬单层上皮细胞，细胞通常为高柱状，胞浆透明。

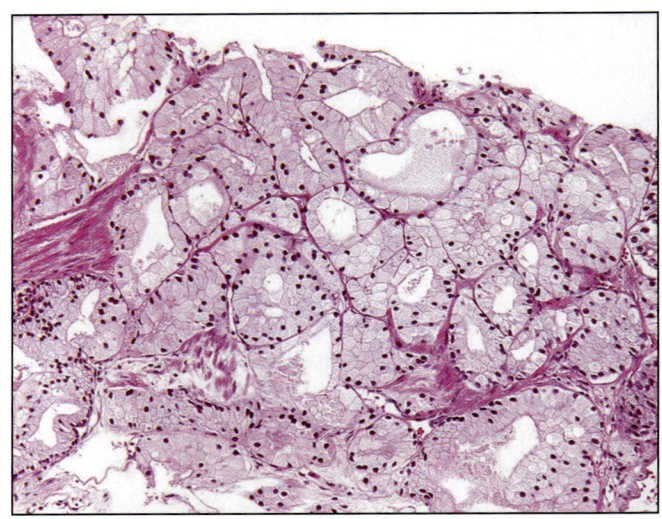

图14A.18　泡沫样腺体癌。肿瘤细胞高柱状，胞浆透明泡沫样，核深染位于基底部。

腺腺体中没有见过它们。淀粉样小体在良性腺泡中常见，但在腺癌中少见（发生率0.4%）。Christian等[86]认为腺癌中淀粉样小体少见（发生率0.4%），但见到淀粉样小体不能用于排除恶性肿瘤。

移行区癌　Transition-zone cancer

前列腺透明细胞（高柱状）癌是高分化腺癌一个有趣的形态学类型[70]。最近强调这种类型的癌类似于BPH，并且它已经被称为"假增生型"腺癌[87,88]。多数病例来源于移行区，但在穿刺活检标本中这种类型并不少见。它可能是经尿道切除标本中的一种类型。肿瘤由小到中等大小腺体构成，被覆单层上皮细胞。细胞形状通常是高柱状，但可以是立方的，其特征是有透明或双染性的细胞浆（图14A.17）。当腺体大小变化显著以及一些腺体出现囊性扩张时，导致病变结构与BPH相混

淆。一个类似的常见的高分化癌是所谓的泡沫样腺体癌（foamy gland carcinoma）[89]，通常由小腺体构成，有泡沫样细胞浆以及粉红色腔内分泌物（图14A.18）。泡沫样腺体癌是前列腺腺癌的独立的组织学类型，尽管它具有欺骗性的良性组织学表现[90]，但常有侵袭性行为。结构上类似于良性增生腺体的前列腺腺癌[假增生性前列腺腺癌（pseudohyperplastic prostatic adenocarcinoma）]是最近认识的病变（图14A.19）[88]。其良性表现的特征包括腺体有乳头状折叠、大腺体、有分支以及有淀粉样小体。在假增生性病灶内，有助于确立恶性诊断的特征是细胞核增大、粉红色无定形分泌物、偶尔或常见的核仁以及类晶体。其他与恶性相关的特征（核分裂象、淡蓝色黏液、周围高级别PIN以及神经周围浸润）可能并不常见。高分子量角蛋白、CK5/6和p63免疫组化染色显示假增生区域基底细胞缺乏，支持癌的诊断。认识假增

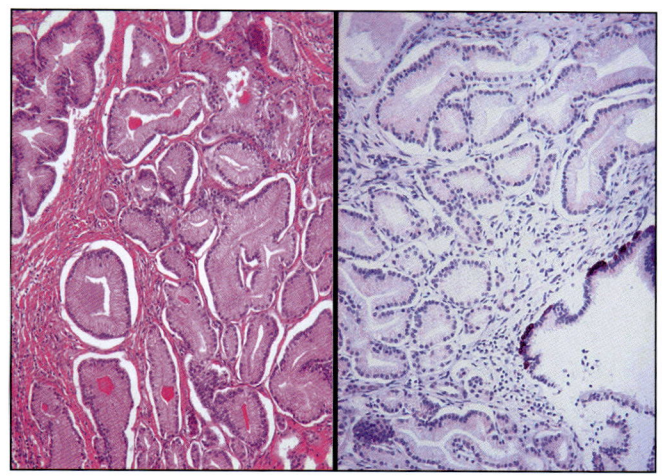

图14A.19 假增生性癌。分支状和乳头状的生长方式类似于良性增生性腺体（左）。右图高分子量角蛋白（34βE12）染色显示假增生性癌缺乏基底细胞，与邻近良性腺体存在基底细胞不同。

生性前列腺腺癌以及确立恶性诊断所必需的特征至关重要，目的是不要把这种癌误诊为良性病变[88]。

鉴别诊断

高分化腺癌一个重要的鉴别诊断是移行区小腺体增生，其中包括前列腺腺瘤性增生（腺病）、SA、BCH以及CCCH。这些良性小腺体增生的共同特点是存在基底细胞，而癌没有基底细胞，这可以通过使用高分子量角蛋白（34βE12）、CK5/6以及p63来证实。也有其他病变如NA、中肾和精阜增生以及正常解剖结构（如萎缩、射精管/精囊上皮和Cowper腺）与前列腺癌相似。这些病变在"癌类似病变"标题下讨论[3,73,91,92]。

最近研究比较多的是伴有萎缩结构的腺癌[腺癌的萎缩亚型（atrophic variant of adenocarcinoma）]，它可能被误诊为良性（图14A.20）[93-95]。尽管当存在萎缩样改变时必须考虑这种类型的癌，但是具有这种特殊类型萎缩结构的癌通常伴有典型的腺泡癌。对于疑难病例，在鉴别萎缩性前列腺癌和良性萎缩时，推荐使用包括AMACR、34βE12以及p63（在萎缩性癌中AMACR阳性染色，基底细胞标志物阴性）在内的免疫染色组合[96]。当前列腺癌为高级别恶性肿瘤时，膀胱TCC（累及前列腺）或前列腺导管和腺泡原发性TCC是其鉴别诊断[46,47,97,98]。高级别前列腺癌最常见的情况是有前列腺癌治疗史的患者，已经稳定几年，又出现了尿道梗阻。低分化前列腺癌通常细胞形态单一，并且常伴有少量腺泡结构；尽管细胞核大小不一，但变化不大，染色质均匀散在，多数细胞有明显核仁（图14A.21）。核分裂象少见。另一方面，TCC可能出现明显的细胞核多形性以及染色质不均匀分布，这包括许多深染细胞以及常见的核分裂象（图14A.22）。在与TCC鉴别诊断中免疫组化非常有价值[99,100]。PSA和PrAP染色是必做的项目，但重要的是要记住有激素治疗史的前列腺腺癌PSA可以阴性。而PrAP通常阳性，但是反应是局灶性的（图14A.23）。像这样的反应足以证实前列腺腺癌的诊断。血栓调节蛋白、Uroplakin以及尿路上皮标志物通常令人失望，可能是因为高级别TCC丢失了所有的抗原性[100]。

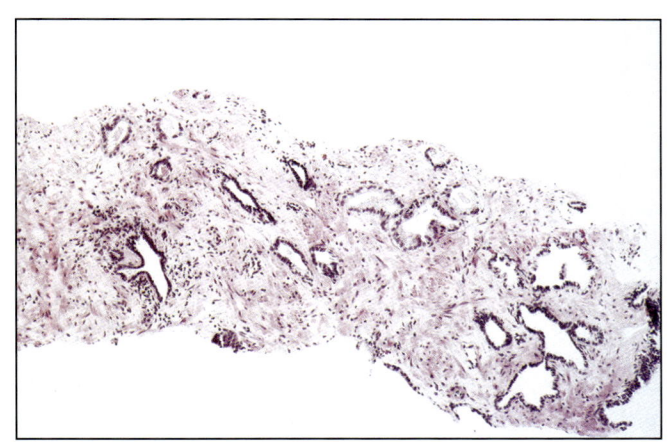

A

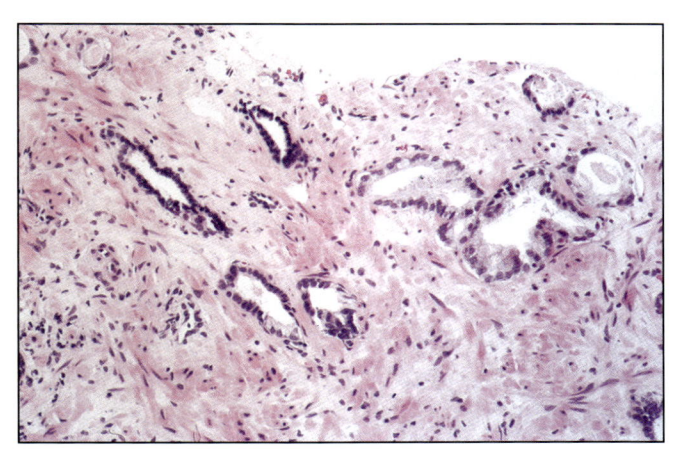

B

图14A.20 （A）伴有萎缩结构的腺癌。尽管许多腺体胞浆稀少，但在低倍镜下非小叶性及浸润性表现具有癌的特征。（B）高倍镜下某些腺体胞浆丰富，而另外一些腺体胞浆稀少（"萎缩"），但是具有浸润性结构。

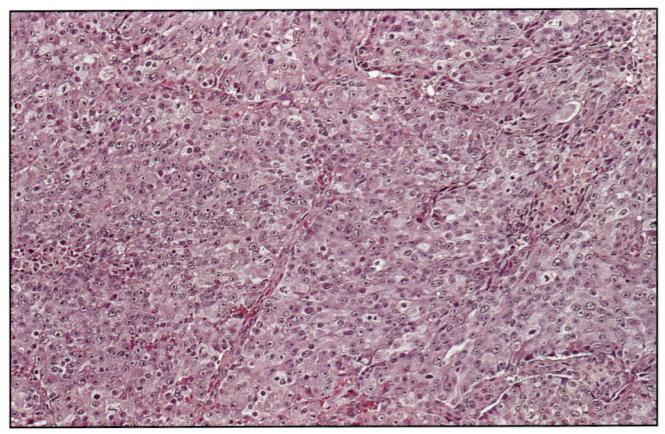

图14A.21 高级别实性前列腺腺癌。高级别前列腺腺癌可能与移行细胞癌混淆，但是前列腺腺癌肿瘤细胞通常呈单形性表现。

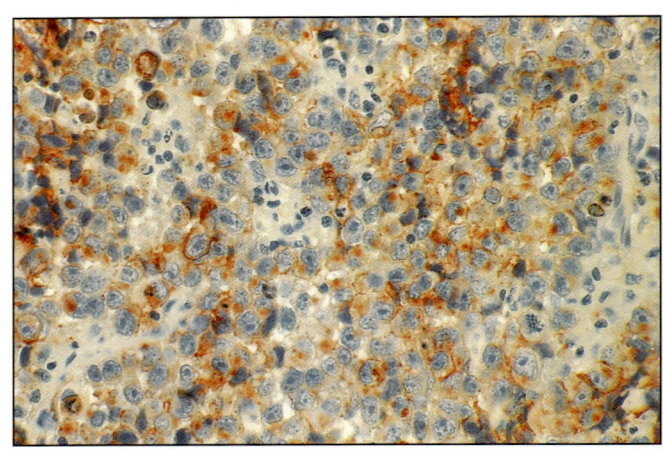

图14A.23 即使在实性高级别前列腺腺癌中，前列腺特异性抗原和前列腺酸性磷酸酶免疫染色通常也呈阳性，如同本图所示。

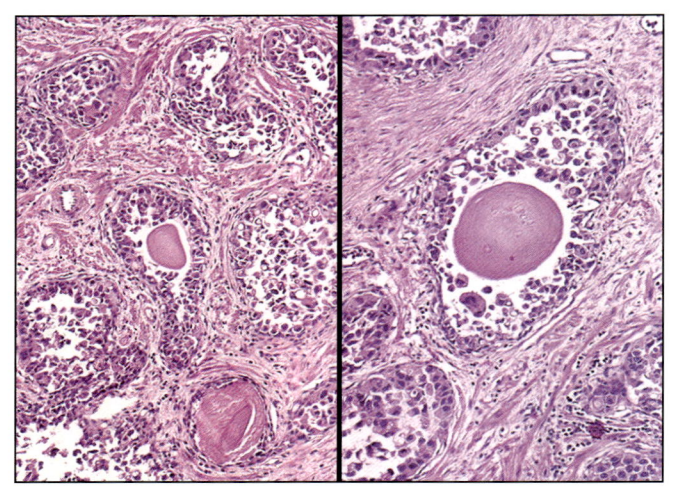

图14A.22 移行细胞癌累及前列腺导管。图中高级别恶性多形性细胞增生导致腺泡扩张。注意腺泡腔内存在淀粉样小体。肿瘤细胞比前列腺高级别腺癌多形性更加明显，核分裂活跃。

在20世纪90年代，外科病理医师的难点是在18G针穿刺活检中准确识别癌、鉴别与之相似的病变，以及确定诊断癌的非典型性腺体数量的最低标准。在书本上前列腺癌诊断标准的定义非常清楚，但是当在活检组织中仅有少量非典型性腺体时，使用这个标准常常有困难[101]。一个细致而系统的方法对诊断癌来说是必要的。这个过程涉及评价腺体的（1）结构特征；（2）细胞学特征；（3）在诊断中有帮助的线索。

结构上，在低倍镜和中倍镜下扫描时，发现小而散在成簇的密集排列的圆形、僵硬的腺体时，应该引起注意。癌的腺体大小可能不同，具有浸润性表现。它们必须是仅仅内衬分泌细胞。细胞学上，细胞是立方或柱状，

有嗜酸性、透明或不定形细胞浆以及圆形的细胞核，细胞核增大，并且明显大于周围良性腺体的核。一个重要的特征是存在明显的樱桃红色的核仁。其他诊断癌的线索包括腔内蓝染的黏液、类晶体、胶原性微小结节、肾小球样结构、核分裂象、神经周围或神经内浸润以及相关高级别PIN的存在[102-104]。如果存在明显的炎症、良性腺体出芽以及由挤压或切片厚造成的人工假象时，诊断应该谨慎。

免疫组织化学

在疑难病例中，免疫组化染色有很大帮助。可以做针对基底细胞层的高分子量角蛋白（克隆34βE12）、CK5/6或p63染色以及AMACR（P505S）染色。既然可疑病灶可能较小，并且深切会消失，有些医院为了可能进行的免疫染色提前把切片保存在涂有防脱胶的玻片上。在判定高分子量角蛋白、CK5/6或p63免疫染色时，一定要慎重，并且结合形态学，这就必须要求一个良好的内对照以及整个可疑病灶完全缺乏染色。34βE12和p63对基底细胞高度特异，前列腺癌区域内阴性。在良性基底细胞染色中p63比34βE12更敏感，尤其是TURP标本，在诊断富有挑战性的病例中稍微优于34βE12[105]。然而，基底细胞标志物混合应用鸡尾酒法（34βE12和p63）不仅增加了发现基底细胞的敏感性，而且也减小了染色的不稳定性，因此使基底细胞免疫染色更均匀[106]。当系统地进行这些步骤时，也许能够使人更有信心地诊断微小癌灶。

最近发现的前列腺癌肿瘤标志物、单克隆性（P504S）或多克隆性（AMACR-p）AMACR，结合HE组织学以及基底细胞标志物，在疑难的前列腺穿刺活检诊断中

应用得越来越多[107]。然而，还不知道根据常规 HE 组织学以及阴性基底细胞染色确定的恶性诊断中，仅应用 AMACR 阳性染色来支持这些恶性诊断的频率如何。最近，Zhou 等[108]对 307 例病理医师认为是非典型性病变而行会诊的前列腺穿刺活检组织，进行了 AMACR 的检测，检验其诊断效用。在综合评价 HE 染色切片、基底细胞标志物染色以及 AMACR 染色后，总计 215 例最终诊断为癌。在这 215 例中，176 例（81.9%）AMACR 染色阳性，39 例（18.1%）AMACR 染色阴性。当 AMACR 染色阴性时，没有一例最初诊断为癌、非典型性或良性的病变（根据常规组织学和阴性基底细胞标志物）因为 AMACR 染色结果而改变诊断。在专家会诊后确认为非典型性病变的 115 例中，76 例 AMACR 染色阳性；这 76 例中，34 例（44.7%）最终诊断为癌。在这 34 例中，11 例进行了根治性的前列腺切除术，所有的病例都发现癌。另外 3 个患者进行重复活检，2 个患者重复活检中有癌存在。专家会诊中把诊断从"非典型性"改为癌的病例，这些病例在 HE 切片和阴性基底细胞标志物基础上都高度怀疑癌。但是因为病灶小、缺乏细胞学非典型性或活检人工假象，不能确立明确的癌诊断。因此，当 AMACR 染色与仔细的组织学检查以及基底细胞标志物联合应用时，才有极大的诊断价值。然而，判定 AMACR 染色应该谨慎，因为大概 20% 根据 HE 染色结合阴性基底细胞标志物认为是癌的病例出现阴性 AMACR 染色。另外，良性前列腺病变，如 NA、非典型性腺瘤性增生、PIN 以及非前列腺肿瘤，AMACR 可以阳性[109,110]。

为了提高前列腺癌诊断的敏感性和特异性，已经联合应用了两种抗体的鸡尾酒法（p63/p504s）[111]。应用 p63/p504s 鸡尾酒法，89% 模棱两可的病变被清楚分类，而单应用 CK5/6 仅为 53%。两种抗体联合应用，一个（p504s）是阳性标志物，另一个（p63）是阴性标志物，用简单的免疫染色方法，便可以提高诊断绩效、敏感性和特异性，降低了假阴性风险；在非典型小腺体增生的病例中应用这种方法应该减少模棱两可病例的百分比以及再次活检的必要（图 14A.24）[48,111]。

Magi-Galluzzi 等[112]报道来自不同实验室的标本 AMACR 染色敏感性不同，可能与固定和处理不同有关。因此，重要的是每个实验室要充分利用这项技术，并且认识到有些穿刺活检的微小癌可能 AMACR 阴性。AMACR 对泡沫样腺体以及假增生性前列腺癌是一个很有用的诊断性标志物（图 14A.25），尽管这种阳性率比通常的小腺体腺癌低[113]。然而，当病理医师在 HE 染色切片以及基底细胞阴性染色基础上倾向这些特殊类型癌的诊断，而只因为似乎有良性外观还怀疑癌的诊断时，

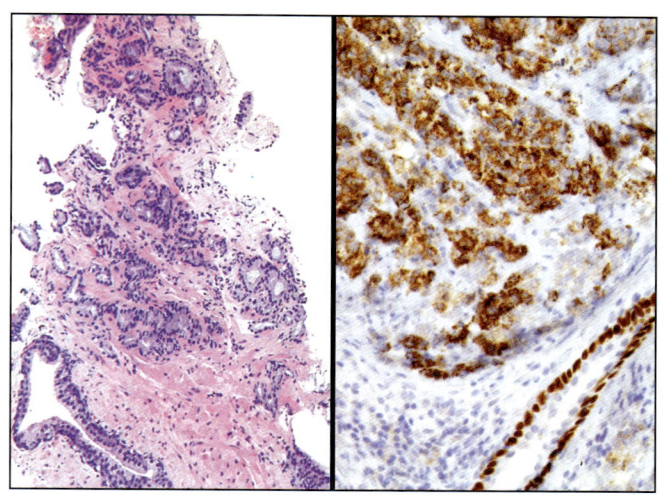

图 14A.24　α-甲酰基-辅酶A-消旋酶（AMACR）和 p63 联合（鸡尾酒法）染色。左图是微小腺泡癌的 HE 染色。右图是 AMACR/p63 鸡尾酒染色，p63 基底细胞核染色，而微小腺泡癌基底细胞阴性，AMACR 阳性。

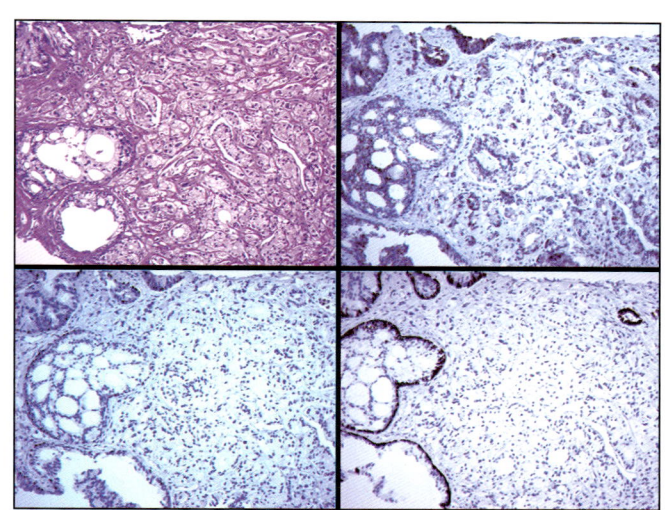

图 14.25　泡沫样腺体癌。HE（左上）显示泡沫样腺体癌，左侧伴有灶状高级别筛状前列腺上皮内肿瘤形成（PIN），右侧为浸润性癌，伴有具有泡沫样胞浆的高柱状细胞。癌及高级别 PIN 细胞浆 α-甲酰基-辅酶A-消旋酶（右上）染色阳性。高级别 PIN 的基底细胞 p63（左下）和高分子量角蛋白（右下）染色阳性。注意浸润性癌没有基底细胞染色。

AMACR 阳性染色可以提供另外的自信从而确立最后的恶性诊断。

另外判定 AMACR 染色时，需要谨慎，因为其他恶性肿瘤可以表达 AMACR。除淋巴瘤和黑色素瘤外，已经报道在结肠、卵巢、乳腺、膀胱、肺以及肾细胞癌中 AMACR 蛋白过表达。最高的过度表达见于结直肠癌和前列腺癌，分别在 92% 和 83% 病例中有阳性染色。

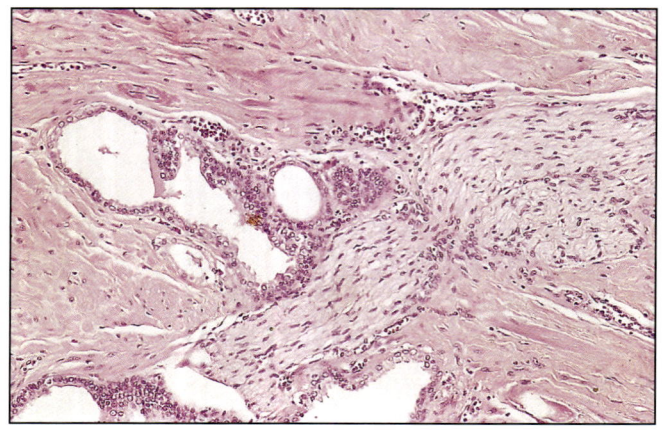

图14A.26 神经周围可见良性前列腺腺体。虽然良性腺体可以紧贴神经，但是从不完全围绕或侵犯神经。

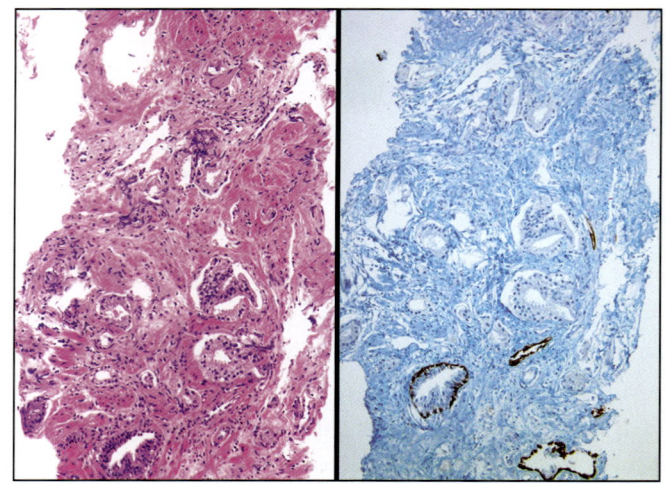

图14A.27 非典型性小腺泡增生。图示怀疑为癌的小腺体增生。结构上，左侧小腺体倾向于癌，但是细胞学表现不清楚。虽然小腺体缺乏基底细胞层（右侧，34βE12），但总的形态学特征不足以明确癌的诊断。因此，这种病变被怀疑为非典型性小腺体增生，而不诊断为恶性。

44%乳腺癌病例存在AMACR过度表达。64%高级别PIN和75%结肠腺瘤也过度表达AMACR[114]。

神经浸润 Nerve invasion

尽管可以看到良性前列腺腺体陷入神经周围，但是环周性神经周围浸润对前列腺癌有诊断价值（图14A.26）。前一种情况的腺体总是良性的，并且仅存在于神经一侧（图14A.26）。神经细胞粘附分子（Neural cell adhesion molecule，N-CAM）是一个众所周知的粘附分子免疫球蛋白超家族成员，参与前列腺癌的神经周围浸润和转移。Li等[115]研究N-CAM在前列腺癌中的表达。与没有神经周围浸润的神经相比，在73%（31/42）伴有神经周围浸润的神经中N-CAM上调（$P > 0.001$）。这些结果表明N-CAM可能参与前列腺癌的神经周围浸润。可以想象癌细胞通过有待建立的旁分泌环路向神经传递信号，增加N-CAM产生并提高粘附性。神经中N-CAM上调也帮助癌细胞向神经迁移，并促进神经周围扩散[115]。

疑为恶性的非典型性腺体（非典型性小腺泡增生）Atypical glands suspicious for malignancy (atypical small acinar proliferation, ASAP)

有一些腺体增生，达不到癌的最低诊断标准。如果不能做出癌的诊断，应该毫不犹豫地把这些腺体诊断为"疑为恶性的非典型性腺体（atypical glands suspicious for malignancy，AGSM）"或"非典型性小腺泡增生（atypical small acinar proliferation，ASAP）"。这个术语正越来越多应用于提示腺癌的一些小腺体增生，因为多种原因，例如缺乏核仁、缺乏细胞核增大、人工扭曲、腺体太少而不确切、组织用尽以及不能行基底细胞染色等，不能做出最终诊断（图14A.27）[116-119]。这个诊断不意味着一个独立疾病，而是仅指腺体的改变怀疑恶性。Chan和Epstein[117]研究144例AGSM（或ASAP）发现，48.9%在重复活检中发现浸润癌。作者也指出如果AGSM（或ASAP）倾向恶性而不支持良性，在重复活检中浸润性癌百分比提高到61%。同时他们推荐对这种诊断的患者应该重复活检，而不管其血清PSA水平的高低。其他作者也发现重复活检中相似或更高比例的浸润性癌[116,118,119]。既然在可疑区域发现浸润癌的机会大，建议可疑区域应该两点或多点活检，同时在前列腺其他部位多点活检[116,119]。

在前列腺穿刺活检标本中，单独依靠形态学区分良恶性前列腺腺体是有困难的，尤其是如果可疑病灶较小（ASAP）时。在诊断有困难的病例中，推荐基底细胞鸡尾酒法（34βE12和p63）与AMACR染色结合来提高诊断的准确性。然而，在小病变中，在一个切片上结合AMACR和基底细胞鸡尾酒染色应该优于单独应用每个标志物染色，因为多切片在小病变中丢失相关组织的机会大[120]。

分期系统 Staging systems

过去通常应用的Whitmore和Jewett分期系统（分类：A、B、C和D）基本上被使用更多参数的TNM系统所取代[121,122]（表14A.3和表14A.4）。A/T1期疾病是隐匿癌，见于临床上良性病变的前列腺切除标本中。A1/T1a期疾病由累及整个TURP标本小于5%的癌所组成；A2/T1b期疾病为累及切除组织多于5%的癌。对于TURP标本，我们建议报告微小癌灶的数量以及癌累及

表14A.3	北美（Whitmore-Jewett）前列腺癌分期系统
分期	所含标准的定义
A	没有可触及的肿瘤；在手术标本中偶然发现 A1癌累及3个碎片 A2癌累及超过3个碎片
B	可触及的肿瘤局限于前列腺 B1前列腺结节2 cm，局限于一叶 B2前列腺结节大于2 cm，但局限于一叶 B3前列腺结节累及两叶
C	蔓延到前列腺被膜外，但没有转移证据 C1肿瘤直径小于6 cm C2肿瘤直径6 cm
D	转移性疾病 D1盆腔淋巴结转移或尿道梗阻导致肾盂积水 D2骨或远处淋巴结或器官或软组织转移

标本的百分比。关于因良性疾病而行TURP中检查前列腺切除组织的数量问题，我们遵循Murphy等[123]的建议：任何送检标本包埋达到12克，可足以发现绝大多数的偶发癌，然后标本每增加10克另外包埋一盒。如果发现癌少于前列腺切除组织的5%，则应该对剩余的切除的前列腺进行组织学检查。

在临床T1期中，TNM系统包括第三个分类，即T1c，是指临床上不明显的癌症（直肠指诊阴性，超声检查阴性），只因PSA升高通过前列腺活检而发现。

可触及的癌或通过超声可见的癌若局限于前列腺划为B/T2期。既然针对B/T2期的根治性前列腺切除术是以治愈为目的，病理医师的作用是证实癌的诊断及肿瘤分级，提供病理分期，估计肿瘤体积，评价精囊及手术边缘，包括前列腺尖部和膀胱袖口。局限于器官内的肿瘤，即病理分期T2期肿瘤，根据侵犯的程度细分为T2a、T2b和T2c（分别是癌少于一个叶的1/2，多于一个叶的1/2但没有达到两个叶，以及侵犯两个叶）[124-126]。然而，是否真正存在T2b期肿瘤已经被质疑[127]。如果发现肿瘤超出前列腺的界限（如在精囊或前列腺周围结缔组织内），在病理上病变提高分期达到C/T3期。进一步的治疗取决于在根治性前列腺切除标本中的病理发现。

C/T3或T4期（表14A.3和表14A.4）病变是指癌症超出前列腺被膜侵犯精囊、膀胱、直肠或盆壁。在过去，有临床C/T3期病变的患者通常用盆腔局部放射治疗，5年生存率是60%～65%[128]。目前，临床医师决定最好的治疗是单独放射治疗或是与激素治疗相结合。如果患者出现尿路梗阻，手术通常限于TURP。有毒性的化学治疗通常用于激素治疗不敏感的病例。

D/N或M期是出现转移性病变时。这个分期在两个分期系统中也可以按照转移部位再细分期（表14A.3和表14A.4）。治疗主要包括用阻断剂的激素治疗、睾丸切除术，或两者相结合，从而阻断雄激素活性。在转移到骨的前列腺癌中，肿瘤的组织学以及PSA和嗜铬素A表达是不一样的。原发性肿瘤的Gleason分级不能预测转移的组织学结构。尽管大于70%的肿瘤细胞表达PSA，有些患者在不同的转移灶中PSA阳性细胞的比例变化较大。同样，转移灶中神经内分泌肿瘤细胞的比例变化大[129]。

在19 316例超过40岁男性的常规尸检中，有1589例（8.2%）前列腺癌[130]。这1589例前列腺癌患者35%存在转移，最常累及的部位是骨（90%）、肺（46%）、肝（25%）、胸膜（21%）以及肾上腺（13%）。基于这个尸检研究，作者们证实了几个重要的发现：首先，脊柱和肺转移存在相反的关系，前列腺癌脊柱转移不依赖于肺转移。其次，与最常见扩散到肺（6～8 cm）和肝（>8 cm）的前列腺肿瘤相比，最常见的脊柱转移发生在更小的前列腺肿瘤（4～6 cm），这表明在许多前列腺癌中脊柱转移早于肺和肝转移。第三，从腰椎水平到颈椎水平脊柱累及逐渐下降（从97%至38%），这与最初腰椎转移后继而沿椎静脉向上转移相一致。此项研究结果表明，骨、肺和肝是远处前列腺癌转移的最常见部位。除了通过肺的大静脉转移外，对于脊柱逆行性扩散的存在和临床意义有很大争议，它有可能发生在转移过程的早期[130]。至少一个标志物中有杂合性缺失，淋巴结阳性的前列腺癌比淋巴结阴性者常见，10q23.3可能是转移进展的一个标志物[130]。

分级系统 Grading systems

尽管文献中已经提出有许多前列腺癌的分级系统，而只有Gleason分级系统是普及的。因为M.D.Anderson癌症中心已经不再使用Gaeta和Mostofi分级系统[72, 131-134]，故本章不再讨论。

Gleason系统（Gleason system） Gleason系统[72]在美国和许多其他国家已被多数泌尿科医师和放射治疗医师所接受，这个系统是治疗决策的基础。Gleason设计这个系统是基于这样的事实，即前列腺癌具有不同的生长方式，从高分化到低分化，并且在前列腺癌中经常有多种生长方式同时存在。在Gleason系统中记录两种突出的结构（主要结构和次要结构）。这些结构的总和形成Gleason评分，范围从2到10[132-134]。然而最近一个

表14A.4 前列腺癌 2002 TNM分期

原发性肿瘤（T）
临床
- TX　原发肿瘤不能评价
- T0　没有原发肿瘤的证据
- T1　临床上肿瘤不明显，既不能触及，影像学也不能发现
  - T1a　在5%或更少的切除组织中组织学上偶然发现的肿瘤
  - T1b　在多于5%的切除组织中组织学上偶然发现的肿瘤
  - T1c　穿刺活检发现的肿瘤（如：因为PSA升高）
- T2　局限于前列腺的肿瘤*
  - T2a　肿瘤累及一个叶的1/2或更少
  - T2b　肿瘤累及超过一个叶的1/2，但没有达到2个叶
  - T2c　肿瘤累及2个叶
- T3　肿瘤突破前列腺被膜**
  - T3a　前列腺被膜外扩散（单侧或双侧）
  - T3b　肿瘤侵犯精囊
- T4　肿瘤固定或侵犯除精囊外的邻近结构：膀胱颈、肛门外括约肌、直肠、肛提肌和/或盆壁

*注释：一个或两个叶中穿刺活检发现的肿瘤，不能触及或通过影像学不能发现，分类为T1c。
**注释：浸润前列腺尖部或进入（但不是超过）前列腺被膜不能分类为T3而是T2。

病理（pT）
- pT2*　局限于器官内
  - pT2a　单侧，侵犯1/2个叶或更少
  - pT2b　单侧，侵犯多于1/2个叶，但没达到2个叶
  - pT2c　双侧病变
- pT3　前列腺外扩散
  - pT3a　前列腺外扩散**
  - pT3b　侵犯精囊
- pT4　侵犯膀胱、直肠

*注释：没有病理学T1分类。
**注释：阳性手术边缘应该用R1符号（残留微小病变）来说明。

局部淋巴结（N）
临床
- NX　区域淋巴结不能评价
- N0　无区域淋巴结转移
- N1　区域（多个）淋巴结转移

病理
- pNX　区域淋巴结不能评价
- pN0　无区域淋巴结转移
- pN1　区域（多个）淋巴结转移

远处转移（M）*
- MX　远处转移不能评价（不能通过任何方式评价）
- M0　无远处转移
- M1　远处转移
  - M1a　非区域性淋巴结转移
  - M1b　骨转移
  - M1c　其他部位转移，伴或不伴骨转移

*注释：当存在多于一个部位转移时，使用最高级别的分类。PM1c是最高级别的分类。

分期分组

期	T	N	M	G
I期	T1a	N0	M0	G1
II期	T1a	N0	M0	G2，3-4
	T1b	N0	M0	任何G
	T1c	N0	M0	任何G
	T1	N0	M0	任何G
	T2	N0	M0	任何G
III期	T3	N0	M0	任何G
IV期	T4	N0	M0	任何G
	任何T	N1	M0	任何G
	任何T	任何N	M1	任何G

Used with permission of the American Joint Committee (AJCC), Chicago, Illinois. The original source for this material is the AJCC Cancer Staging Manual, Sixth Edition (2002) published by Springer-Verlag New York, www.springeronline.com

---

重要的共识性会议推荐，穿刺活检中任何数量的高级别肿瘤成分均应作为Gleason评分的一部分，即使另外的次要结构范围较大[134a]。

Gleason 1型（Pattern 1）癌是单个、分离、圆形均一的腺体密集排列，伴有界限清楚的边缘。1型肿瘤的特征是：(1) 边界清楚的结节；(2) 腺体大小和形状相对一致；以及 (3) 腺体背靠背排列，其间伴有少量的间质（图14A.28）。与BPH和正常前列腺的分泌细胞不同，1型癌细胞均匀增大，侧面和腔面直而平坦。细胞核有时呈良性表现，但排列在基底，这不同于BPH或正常腺体核的不均匀分布。1型癌谷胱甘肽-S-转移酶免疫染色阴性，但BPH的分泌细胞呈弱阳性。有人提出这些细胞学所见可以用作诊断线索，尤其是在结构难以解释的小的穿刺活检标本[135]。

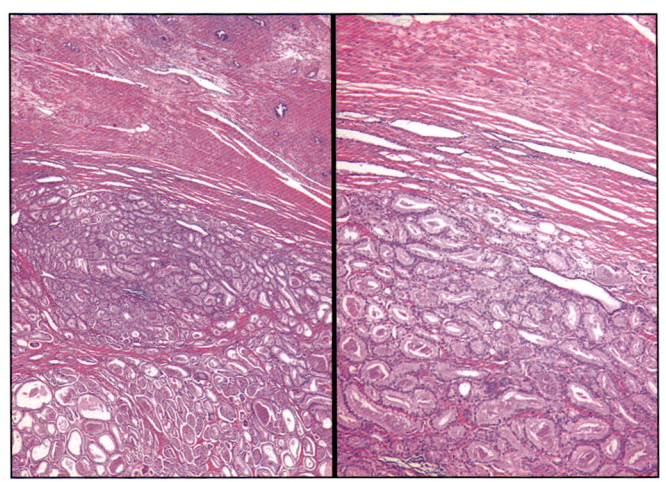

图14A.28 Gleason 1型癌。结节界限清楚，腺体大小形状相似，分布均匀，这是这种类型的特征。

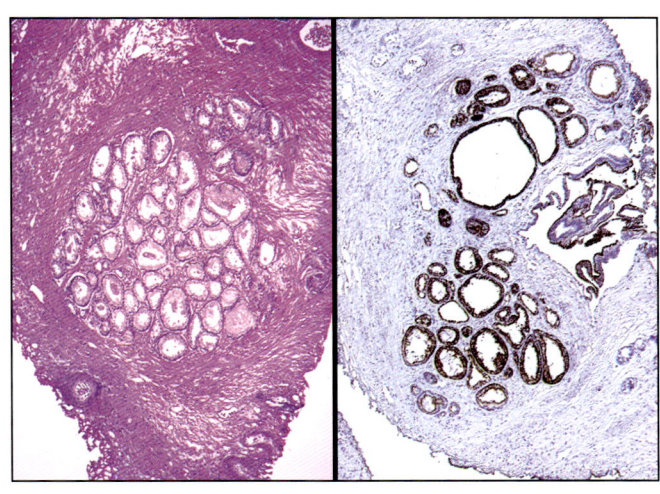

图14A.29 图示Gleason 2型癌。左侧的癌结节界限相对清楚，但有些腺体在结节外，单个腺体大小和形状有些差异。右图的小腺体α-甲酰基-辅酶A-消旋酶染色阳性，支持癌的诊断。

Gleason 2型（Pattern 2）癌类似于1型癌，但是：(1) 结节边缘不如1型癌清楚；(2) 腺体不如1型癌均匀一致；以及(3) 2型癌的间质比1型癌明显，但不如3型癌（小于一个腺体直径）（图14A.29）。Gleason 1型和2型癌在18号针（18-gauge）穿刺活检标本中罕见。众所周知，Gleason医师承认他的1型癌和2型癌可能是非典型性腺瘤性增生（腺病）。他在描述这个系统时，当时尚无可用的基底细胞染色标志物。最近会议达成共识，如果不经专家会诊普通病理医师在穿刺活检中不应做出Gleason 4分或4分以下的诊断[134a]。

Gleason 3型（Pattern 3）癌，腺体大小不等：出现小腺体和大腺体以及筛状或乳头状结构。边界不清。这是穿刺活检标本中最常见的类型，而且常常有伴有明显浸润性生长方式的灶状肿瘤性小腺体，或出现在良性腺体之间（提示浸润性生长）。

Gleason 3型癌有三个亚型。3A型（pattern 3A）以出现不规则的、成角、梨形或泪滴形的小到中等大小腺体为特征，这些腺体被胶原性间质分隔。3A型与2型的不同之处在于肿瘤性腺体在良性腺体之间浸润，而且间质比2型多（大于一个腺体直径），而且有较不规则的成角的腺体（图14A.30）。3B型（pattern 3B）由小而不规则的腺体构成，通常小于3A型的腺体，其中某些腺体呈条索状或变长，给人以腺腔消失的感觉。这种类型常常见到腺腔不明显的小细胞巢，但是可以勾画出

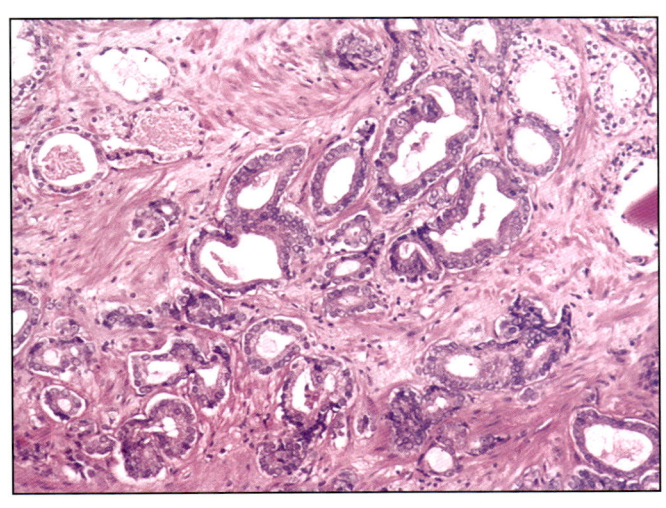

A

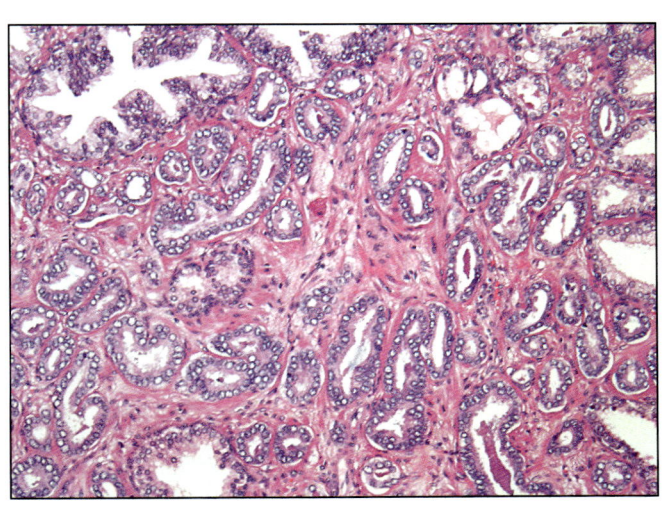

B

图14A.30 （A）Gleason 3A型癌，大腺体型。这种类型以小到中等大小的腺体为特征，腺体成角，变长，卵圆形，轮廓不规则，大小有些不同。它们往往在正常腺体之间浸润，并且有界限不清楚的浸润性边缘。（B）Gleason 3A型癌，大腺体型。这也是3A型的一种结构，由小而成角和不规则的腺体构成，其间有多少不等的胶原性结缔组织。注意左上角为高级别前列腺上皮内肿瘤形成。

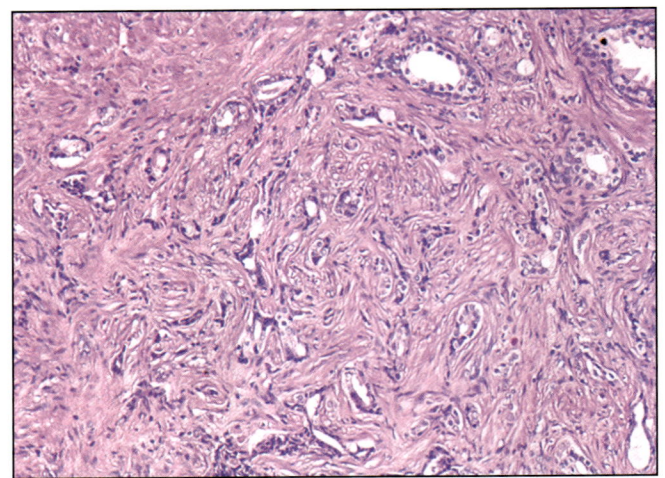

图14A.31　Gleason 3B型癌，小腺体型。这种类型的特征是存在丧失了腺腔的小腺体，给人以"融合"的假象。为了排除见于Gleason 4型癌的真正的融合，较深的切片通常能显示出腺腔。图中有些腺体见有腺腔，但是其他一些腺体形成条索，好像是塌陷的腺腔。这种类型一般很难与4型癌区分。

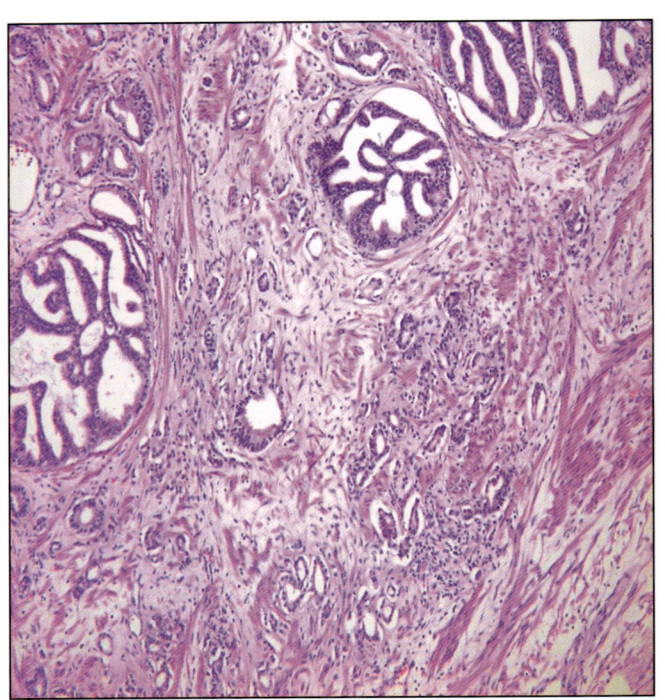

图14A.32　Gleason 3C型癌，筛状型。Gleason 3C型癌指的是伴有局灶乳头状/筛状结构的肿瘤。目前，这种亚型尚有争议，因为包括我们在内的某些病理医师不认为它是Gleason 3型癌，而应该考虑为Gleason 4型癌。本图确实显示了一些乳头状/筛状排列，但是这样的生长方式很可能是乳头状/筛状高级别PIN，在背景中有Gleason 3B型腺癌。

细胞巢的轮廓（图14A.31）。这种类型类似于Gleason 4型癌，但是没有真正的腺体融合或腺体链。3C型（pattern 3C）与3A型类似，但是具有局灶性筛状/乳头状结构（图14A.32）。推测这种类型包括伴有乳头状/筛状结构的高级别PIN病例。目前，多数病理医师认为Gleason 3C型癌仅有少量导管伴有筛状/乳头状结构，如果这种改变呈弥漫性，则很有可能是Gleason 4型癌。

Gleason 4型癌含有小而融合的腺体和浸润性条索；腺体增生可以形成大的乳头状或筛状结构，边界不清或融合性生长（4A型；图14A.33），肿瘤细胞胞浆可以透明（肾上腺样；4B型；图14A.34）。前列腺黏液性腺癌自动归为Gleason 4型癌。

Gleason 5型（pattern 5）癌多数肿瘤呈实性，仅有少量可识别的腺体。这种类型包括未分化小细胞癌以及任何出现坏死的癌，虽然最近有共识性会议提出小细胞癌不必进行Gleason分级[134a]。伴有粉刺样坏死的原型肿瘤是导管-子宫内膜样癌（5A；图14A.35）。然而，低分化前列腺癌可能呈实性方式生长，间质浸润表现为单个的细胞或界限不清的条索（5B；图14A.36）。

近些年来，这种分型已经显示出有预后意义：Gleason 7分或7分以上的肿瘤，即至少具有或为主要结构或为次要结构的Gleason 4型癌的肿瘤，比Gleason 6分或6分以下肿瘤的生物学行为要差[136]。某些研究者分析主要和次要结构在Gleason 7分的前列腺癌的预后上是否具有重要意义。一项研究[137]分析了823例Gleason 7分前列腺癌根治性切除标本的整体切片，Gleason 评分或为3+4分或为4+3分。总共643例患者

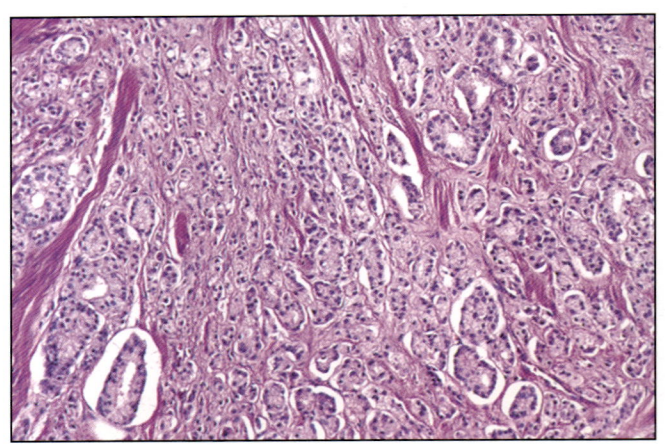

图14A.33　Gleason 4A型癌伴有腺体融合。本图显示大量不规则的和融合性的腺体，其中某些腺体相互融合在一起。

伴有Gleason 3+4分肿瘤，其余180例为Gleason 4+3分肿瘤患者。应用时序检验（log-rank test）进行统计学分析显示，在主要结构为Gleason 4分和主要结构为Gleason 3分患者之间无复发生存具有显著差异（$P < 0.0001$）。然而，应用术前PSA检查、肿瘤总体积、手术边缘情况、有无累及精囊、前列腺外蔓延以及淋巴结转移等多因素分析发现，主要Gleason结构没有独立的预后意义（$P=0.0557$）。Gleason 7分的前列腺癌是一

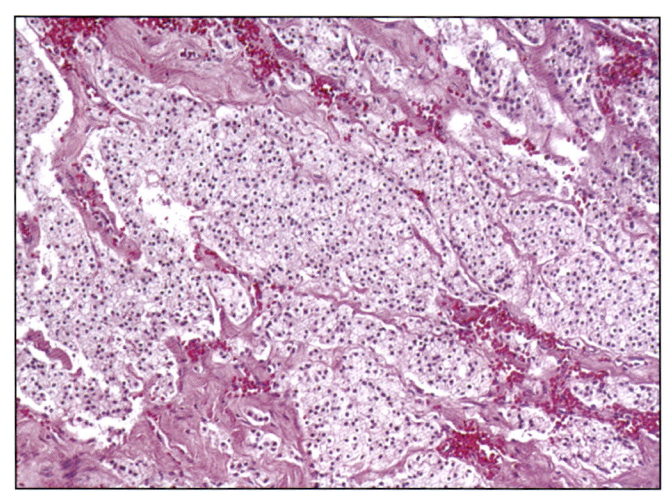

图14A.34 Gleason 4B型癌。本图显示丰富的单形性细胞增生,伴有明显的腺泡状结构,但在腺体之间没有结缔组织分隔。细胞显示透明和双染性的胞浆,表面上类似于透明细胞肾细胞癌(肾上腺样结构)。

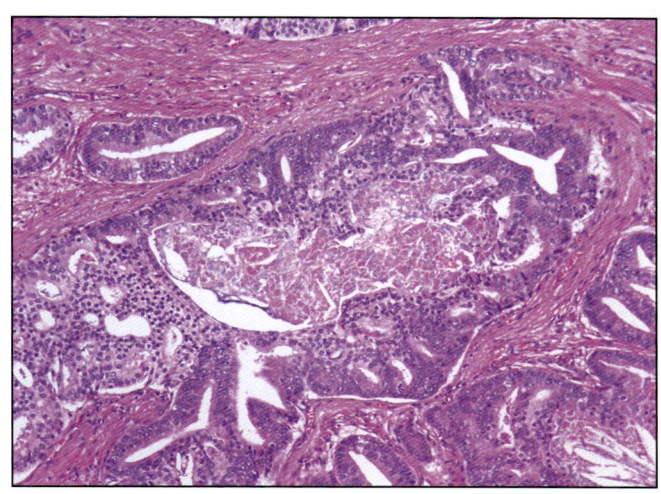

图14A.35 Gleason 5A型癌。本图显示轮廓不规则的膨胀的导管/腺泡,呈现筛状-乳头状结构,伴有中心粉刺样坏死。坏死总是代表Gleason 5型癌。

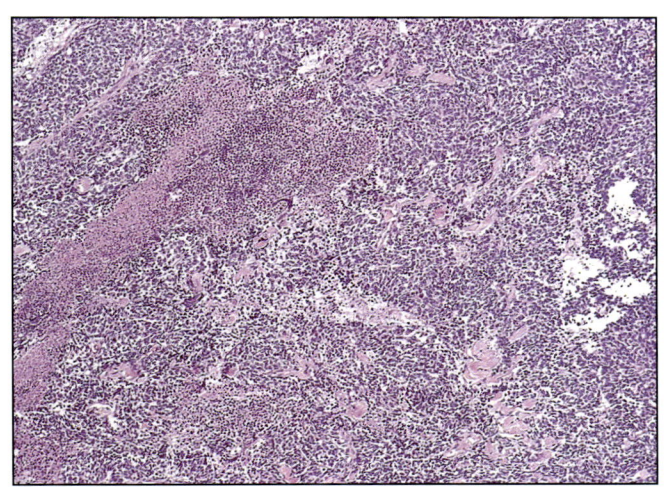

A

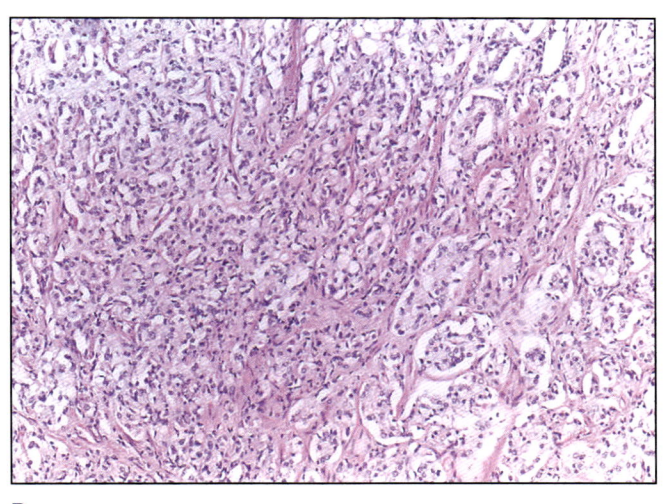

B

图14A.36 (A) Gleason 5B型癌,伴有实性小细胞增生和坏死区域。(B) Gleason 5B型癌。肿瘤呈实性生长伴有模糊的腺泡状结构。

组异质性的肿瘤。在这一组经耻骨后根治性前列腺切除术治疗的Gleason 7分肿瘤的男性中,显示Gleason主要结构与其他组织学和临床疾病进展预测因素具有显著相关性;然而,在多因素分析中它却不是疾病进展的独立预测因素(P=0.76)。

对于直径为0.6 mm的前列腺癌标本的组织芯片可能容易进行Gleason评分,前列腺癌组织芯片图像对于教授Gleason分级系统可能是一种好的方法,因为检查的是小的组织[138]。

在美国,Gleason系统已经成为临床报告的金标准,并与前列腺外蔓延、精囊浸润以及区域淋巴结转移有关[136, 139-141]。此外,前列腺癌DNA含量已与Gleason评分进行了对比研究[142]。Gleason评分达到5分的前列腺癌通常是二倍体肿瘤,而高级别癌(9~10分)通常是非整倍体肿瘤。中级别肿瘤(6~8分)既有二倍体又有非整倍体结构。

病理学报告以及与临床医师交流
Pathology report and communication with clinicians

在前列腺穿刺活检报告中最近的趋势是含有更多的信息以及新的诊断分类。Rubin等[143]设计了一项研究向外科泌尿肿瘤协会成员进行调查,以便确定什么样的信息对于泌尿科医师治疗前列腺癌患者是重要的。他们设计一个问卷来调查几个地区的前列腺穿刺活检报告,每个机构之间的报告各不相同。问卷发放给泌尿科医师,要求不记名回答后寄回;完整评价了42份问卷,占回问卷的76%(42/55)。参与这项调查的泌尿科医师经验丰富，平均有 22 年的临床实践（从 6 年到 35 年）。90% 以上的参与者在确定手术之前复习患者的活检；半数以上的回应者需要主要和次要 Gleason 评分。在针对不同部位有多个阳性点的活检的病例，80% 以上的回应者应用最高 Gleason 评分来决定他们的治疗方案，而不管受累标本总的百分比。回应者需要的其他病理学参数以递减的顺序排列为：癌累及穿刺标本的百分比（67%）、神经周围浸润存在与否（38%）、有癌的阳性活检点数（33%）以及累及标本的长度（29%）。仅有小部分回应者（24%）应用神经周围浸润情况来指导保留神经的手术。外科医师做的根治性前列腺切除术越多，他们越认为病理报告中神经周围浸润的信息在临床上越重要 [Mann-Whitney 检验，双尾检验（two-tailed），P=0.015]。98% 的泌尿科医师一致认为诊断报告中非典型性小腺泡增生（ASAP）这个术语足以提示临床重复活检。

在根治性前列腺切除组织中，癌症浸润神经周围独立预测病理分期的能力仍不清楚。应用单因素分析的多数研究发现，穿刺活检组织中神经周围浸润与检查整个根治性前列腺切除标本所发现的前列腺外蔓延有关。然而，当应用多因素分析时，仅有少数研究表明神经周围浸润具有明显的预测前列腺外扩散的能力 [144,145]。尽管存在争议，但仍推荐前列腺穿刺活检常规报告有无神经周围浸润。

Maru 等 [146] 报道神经周围浸润的直径是预后的独立预测因子（神经周围浸润 > 0.25 mm 而不是 < 0.25 mm），而且从前列腺切除标本中容易测量神经周围浸润的直径，这种测量能给前列腺癌患者提供重要的预后信息。他们的结论是，有关神经周围浸润意义的争论可能是由于以前研究神经周围浸润缺乏定量分析引起的。

淋巴血管浸润的存在与否同样重要。Herman 等 [147] 证实，在单因素分析中淋巴血管浸润是疾病进展的重要预测因素（P < 0.0001），与 Gleason 总分（P < 0.001）、前列腺外扩散（局灶性还是明确的；P=0.033）以及精囊受累（P < 0.001）明显相关。此外，在多因素分析中，淋巴血管浸润也是疾病进展重要的独立预测因素（P=0.0014）。

活检中微小癌的定义是小于 1 mm 或累及一个活检点 5% 的癌；这个定义意味着微小癌不包括含有两种 Gleason 结构和（或）多于一个活检穿刺点的癌。Rubin 等的研究 [148] 是为了确定微小腺癌病灶的 Gleason 评分是否具有预测价值。在微小癌病例中，治疗前 PSA 值是较高肿瘤分期唯一独立的预测因子，没有发现 Gleason 评分能够充分预测较高的肿瘤分期。这项研究结果证实，多数病例活检的 Gleason 评分可以预测前列腺切除标本的 Gleason 评分以及肿瘤分期。然而，对于活检组织微小癌的病例，其 Gleason 评分不能预测肿瘤的分期。为了把这种不确定性的信息准确地传递给临床医师，病理医师应该随微小癌灶 Gleason 评分的同时给出一个警示性注解。如果多个活检点含有不同 Gleason 评分的前列腺癌，应该给出每个点单独的 Gleason 评分，而不是整个的 Gleason 评分，尤其是在至少有一个活检点含有较高 Gleason 评分前列腺癌的病例中更应如此 [134a,149]。

病理医师通常把良性前列腺穿刺活检签发为"良性前列腺增生（BPH）"，此时活检并没有 BPH 特异性的组织学表现。虽然，在穿刺活检中偶尔可以发现提示是移行区的间质结节，但是穿刺活检很难做出腺体增生的诊断。因此，对良性前列腺活检不应该报告为 BPH，除非在活检组织中存在明确的间质结节 [150]。

治疗效果

前列腺癌放射治疗是导致前列腺反应性非典型性最常见的原因。据报道在大约 3/4 照射的前列腺中有非肿瘤性腺体细胞学非典型性，包括细胞核增大和深染，伴有明显的核仁（图 14A.37）[151]。然而，腺体结构保持相对正常，这是有助于排除前列腺癌的特征。放射治疗诱导的其他改变包括腺体与间质比例下降、萎缩、鳞状化生以及 BCH、伴有非典型性纤维母细胞的间质纤维化、异物巨细胞、动脉内膜增生以及血管壁内出现泡沫细胞。放射治疗类型影响组织学改变。应用组织内放射疗法（近距离放射疗法）/ 组织内和外照射联合放射疗法比单独应用外照射放射疗法引起的细胞学非典型性和间质纤维化更加明显。然而，治疗的类型与对血管的作用无关。应用组织内放射疗法（近距离放射疗法）/ 组织内和外照射联合放射疗法治疗的男性其上皮非典型性程度没有随时间而改变。而应用外照射治疗，在治疗超过 48 个月后进行活检的病例，其上皮非典型性比活检和治疗间隔时间较短的病例小。良性前列腺腺体的放射性非典型性可以在最初治疗后长时间持续存在，这是前列腺活检判断中的一个重要陷阱，因为明显的放射治疗反应可在组织内放射治疗（近距离放射疗法）后 72 个月的患者中见到 [152]。放射可以诱导肿瘤坏死和纤维化，但在许多情况下，治疗完成后仍有残留的活的肿瘤。当见到筛状结构、融合的腺体、实性片块和条索时，通常可以明确地做出前列腺癌的诊断。在穿刺活检组织中区别放射引起的非典型性小腺泡和微小腺泡癌可能是非常困难的。间质中腺泡分布不规则可以增加对癌的怀疑。缺乏基底细胞也有帮助，但有时基底细胞的存在与否因为腺泡皱缩和扭曲而很难判断。应用高分子量细胞角蛋白染色、CK5/6、p63 或基底细胞鸡尾酒（34βE12 和 p63）染色可能识别残留的基底细胞，这样能排除癌（图

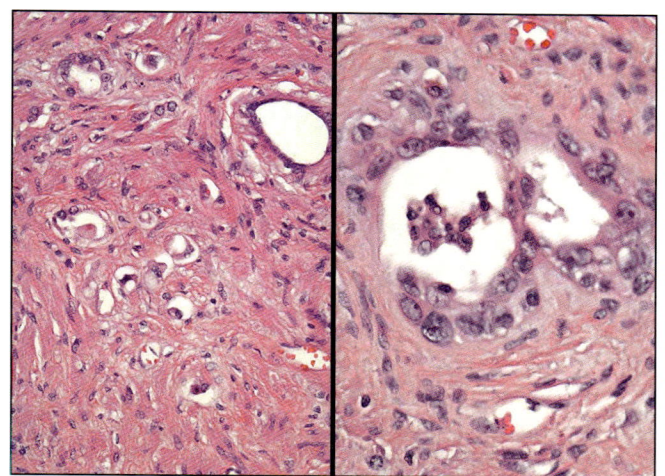

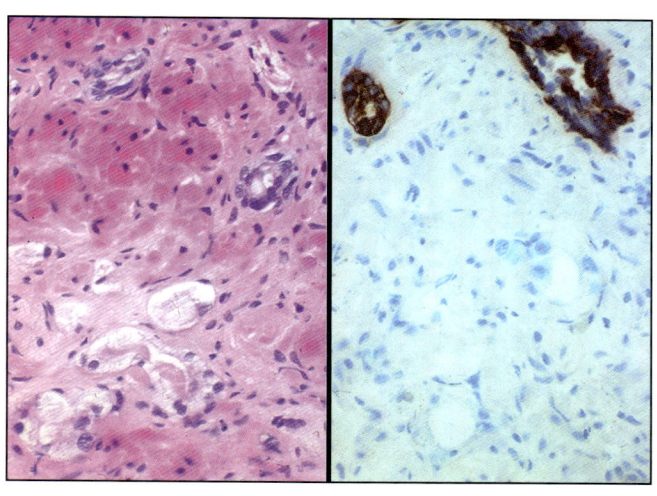

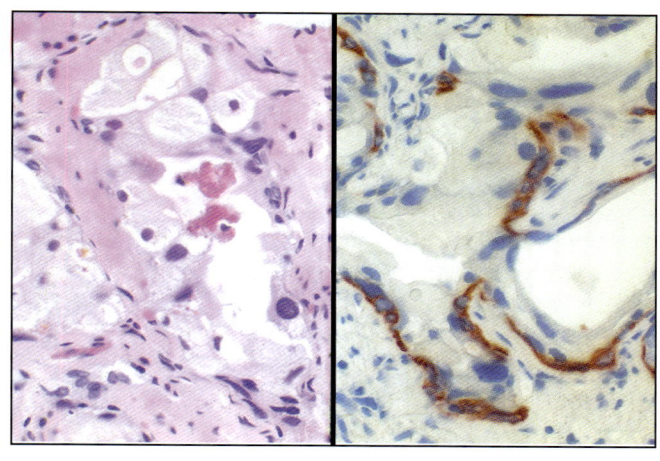

图14A.37 （A）放射治疗对于良性腺体的影响。左侧腺体扭曲并有单个细胞伴有细胞学非典型性。右侧见有非典型性腺体，伴有大而不规则的明显非典型性的细胞，提示为放射诱导的上皮非典型性。（B）良性腺体的放射治疗影响。左侧有一个腺体好像没有基底细胞，内衬细胞高度非典型性；这些细胞有异常的细胞核，细胞浆透明，类似于泡沫样腺体癌。然而，右图显示明显的基底细胞（34βE12染色），提示这是放射诱导的正常腺体改变。

14A.38）。放射引起的细胞非典型性可能类似于癌，尽管除了病史之外，非典型性的不规则分布可能是提示放射治疗反应的线索。放射可以诱导细胞的多形性，其程度常常超过癌。PSA免疫染色有助于识别间质中单个或空泡状的肿瘤细胞，这些细胞在常规光镜下可能类似于伴有空泡变的间质细胞。有人提出在放射治疗后12个月行前列腺穿刺活检价值不大，因为肿瘤细胞死亡表现滞后。据报道在三维外照射放射治疗后，前列腺的良性腺体和恶性腺体也有相似的放射性改变[153]。

50多年前就已认识到了诸如己烯雌酚等雌激素复合物引起的形态学改变。可能有鳞状化生，单个肿瘤细胞

图14A.38 放射治疗对于前列腺癌的影响。左侧显示2或3个内衬深染细胞核的腺体，以及几个扭曲的小腺体。图的右侧显示癌的区域缺乏基底细胞，不同于内衬基底细胞的良性腺体（上方），高分子量细胞角蛋白染色。

可以显示明显的胞浆、核固缩以及核仁消失。可以见到不规则"空的"间隙，这是皱缩肿瘤性腺体的残余，类似于去雄激素治疗引起的改变。最近研究分析了抗雄激素新辅助治疗的效果，包括应用诸如黄体激素释放激素促效剂、氟他胺以及醋酸环丙孕酮等药物完全阻断雄激素。最近报道，常常用于治疗增生和癌的5-α-还原酶抑制剂非那司提（finasteride）具有治疗作用[154]。与其他去雄激素方法相比，非那司提产生的形态学变化并不显著。在根治性前列腺切除标本中发现，新辅助治疗可使肿瘤体积减小，降低切缘阳性率，并有明显的降低分期的作用，但是后者可能具有欺骗性。

去雄激素治疗对于非肿瘤性组织和癌组织均有明显的影响。在非肿瘤区域，出现明显的腺体萎缩，伴有分泌细胞间隙皱缩，基底细胞明显（图14A.39）。灶状BCH常见，也可见到鳞状细胞和移行细胞化生。应用新辅助激素治疗比单独应用手术治疗的前列腺，其中高级别PIN出现的频率明显降低[155]。

癌性腺体表现为细胞浆量减少、细胞浆空泡、细胞核固缩、腺体直径减小以及黏液性破坏（图14A.40）。在许多病例中有明显的胶原性间质，掩盖了恶性腺体[155]。有时，肿瘤性腺泡完全消失留下间隙，有些间隙可能含有黏液物质，阿辛蓝染色更加明显。这种表现好像是卵巢假黏液瘤（图14A.41）。经常见到胶原性微小结节，这可能是外渗黏液的机化。可以见到呈血管外皮细胞瘤样外观的间质增生。细胞核改变包括核溶解、核固缩以及核碎裂。在治疗过的前列腺癌中，有时可见明显的Paneth细胞样改变，这与神经内分泌细胞数量增加有关。去雄激素治疗引起的相关的结构变化与术前活检相

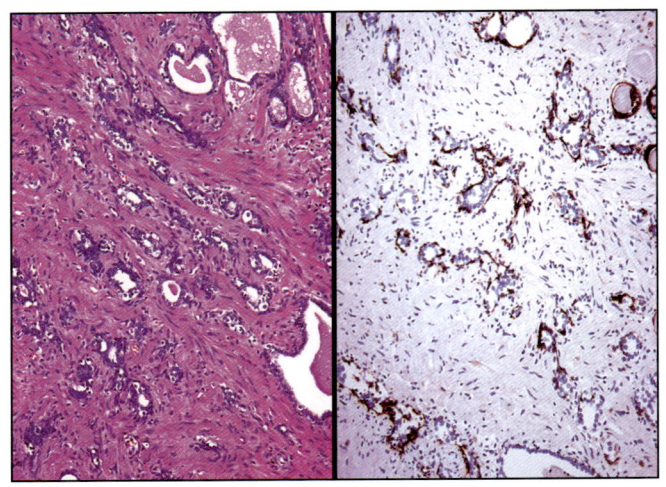

图14A.39 激素治疗引起的良性腺体萎缩和基底细胞增生。本图有明显的腺体萎缩，其特征是出现立方/扁平细胞（基底细胞），胞浆稀少，细胞核深染（左侧）。高分子量细胞角蛋白染色（34βE12）显示基底细胞的存在（右侧）。

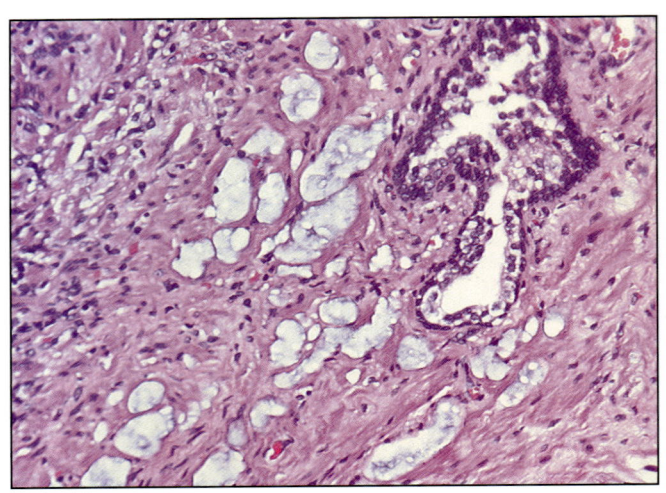

图14A.41 激素治疗的前列腺癌。在伴有明显基底细胞的大的良性腺体附近有扭曲而扩张的腺体结构，内衬扁平上皮，充满黏液性物质。间质中还有外渗的黏液池，与卵巢假黏液瘤十分相似。另外，间质中有弥漫性浸润的孤立性小簇状肿瘤细胞。

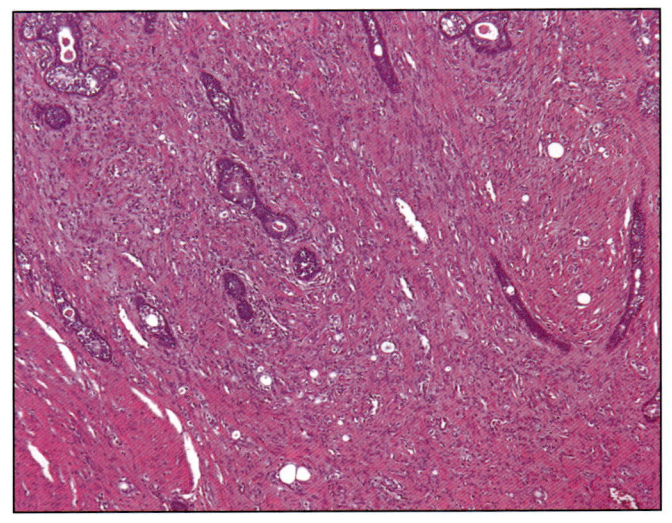

图14A.40 激素治疗的前列腺癌。注意在扭曲的深染肿瘤细胞条索背景中散在的良性腺体。癌性腺体表现为胞浆量减少、出现胞浆空泡、细胞核固缩以及腺体直径减小。

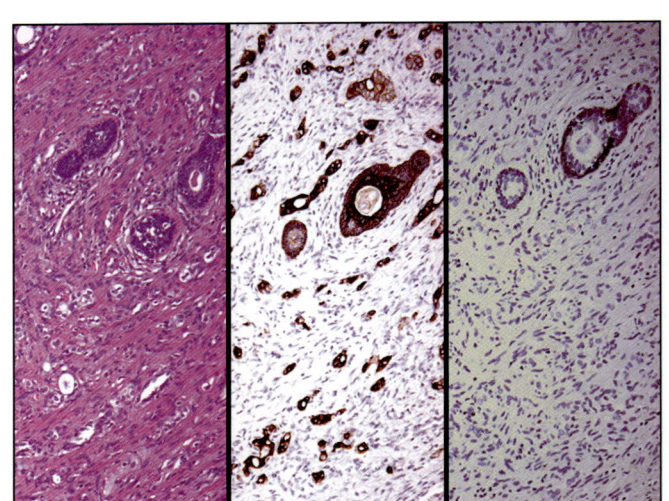

图14A.42 激素治疗的前列腺癌的免疫染色。最左侧为图14A.40的高倍放大，显示孤立性小簇状肿瘤细胞，中间图示其广谱CK阳性，而高分子量细胞角蛋白阴性（最右侧）。注意萎缩的正常腺体基底细胞阳性染色。

比导致明显更差的Gleason评分。这个改变可能是假的，主要与治疗过程中细胞浆减少和腺腔消失有关。应用DNA含量和增生细胞核抗原的某些研究显示，明显低分化区域的增生活性比含有类似结构而未经治疗的癌的增生活性低，表明这种"上调"是人为的。从实践的角度看，显示明显治疗效果的病例不应该分级。有些情况下，新辅助激素对于肿瘤结构的影响相对较小，这种情况可以进行分级，但要记住不要过度判定表面上类似于Gleason 5级的肿瘤。有些作者[155,156]提倡调整Gleason评分以补偿治疗的影响，但并不提倡应用这种方法，因为按照我们的观点，有些经过治疗的前列腺假4级和5级肿瘤不能可重复地与原本4级和5级的肿瘤区分开来。在有些病例中，治疗后前列腺组织中残留的癌很难评价，广谱CK和PSA免疫组化染色对于寻找癌细胞是必要的（图14A.42）。间质反应，包括组织细胞浸润，也可能类似于残留的癌细胞，有时需要应用巨噬细胞和前列腺上皮两种标志物来区分。

在许多医疗中心，治疗局部进展期肿瘤应用冷冻疗法。冷冻治疗后活检显示不同的组织学变化，取决于治疗后活检的时间。急性损伤表现为坏死、出血以及急性炎症。慢性改变包括纤维化、玻璃样变、钙化、含铁血黄素沉积、肉芽肿性炎、BCH 以及移行上皮和鳞状上皮化生[157,158]。有时存在残留的癌，通常保留其原来的形态学结构和分级。在冷冻治疗失败后补救性前列腺切除术的病理学分析中，被认为术中经直肠超声检查破坏了的区域可以见到存活的癌。

有一项关于前列腺癌患者应用单纯疱疹病毒胸苷激酶（HSV-tk）原位基因治疗，继之以更昔洛韦（ganciclovir）治疗的形态学研究[159]。前列腺切除标本显示以下形态学变化：（1）在癌灶中可见不同程度的坏死；（2）可见整个 Gleason 分级谱系的细胞改变；（3）正常前列腺很少发生坏死，但是含有密集的单核细胞浸润；（4）常见细胞核的细微结构消失。容积测量研究表明仅有部分肿瘤的形态受到影响，并证实受影响肿瘤的百分比与前列腺和肿瘤大小成反比关系。可见炎症反应，在正常的前列腺组织中以 CD20 阳性细胞为主，在肿瘤中以 CD8（细胞毒性 T 细胞）阳性细胞为主，在所有治疗过的前列腺区域以巨噬细胞为主[159]。

腺癌的变型　Variants of adenocarcinoma

前列腺腺癌的变型占所有病例的 5%～10%。识别这些亚型十分重要，因为其中许多亚型预后不良，而且其鉴别诊断常常不同于普通的微小腺泡癌。Gleason 分级常常可以用于这些亚型，这些亚型几乎总是 3 级或更高级别[160,161]。

黏液性腺癌　Mucinous adenocarcinoma

自从 1882 年 Boyd 首次报道第一例前列腺黏液性腺癌以来[162]，大约已经报告过 100 例原发性前列腺黏液性腺癌[50,163-165]。前列腺原发性黏液性腺癌的诊断标准是：（1）切除的肿瘤中至少 25% 必须是由细胞外黏液湖构成的；（2）非扩张性腺体含有黏液性物质不能看成是黏液性腺癌；（3）应该排除前列腺外部位肿瘤的扩散，或者肿瘤细胞 PSA 和 PrAP 免疫染色应该阳性。应用这些标准，Epstein 和 Lieberman[164] 以及 Ro 等[163] 报告黏液性腺癌的发生率大概占所有前列腺腺癌的 0.4%。

过去认为前列腺黏液性腺癌的侵袭性不如普通的前列腺腺癌[166-169]，不大可能转移到骨[167,168,170-172]，不伴有血清 PSA 水平升高[166,167,170,173]，并且是起源于前列腺的"女性"部分[166,169,171-173]。然而，最近研究发现其临床症状、转移方式、血清 PSA 水平以及对于激素治疗的反应与普通类型前列腺腺癌患者相似[163,164]。常见转移部位包括淋巴结、骨以及肺；有趣的是，一个病例表现为支气管内转移，最初与原发性支气管源性癌相混淆[174]。

组织学上，前列腺原发性黏液性腺癌伴有普通类型的前列腺腺癌（图 14A.43）；没有单纯性前列腺黏液性腺癌的病例报告。黏液性成分表现为细胞外黏液湖，常常含有肿瘤细胞形成的脑回状肿块，偶尔伴有腺泡或形成完好的腺体结构（图 14A.44）。不同标本之间以及同一肿瘤不同区域之间的非黏液性成分的形态有所不同。其形态主要是微小腺体，但也可以见到筛状、粉刺样、实性以及肾上腺样结构。一个显著的特征是漂浮在黏液湖中的肿瘤细胞具有非乳头状的生长方式，让人想起乳腺的胶样癌[163]。

在做出前列腺原发性黏液性腺癌的诊断之前，应该排除来自其他部位的转移或者从直肠、膀胱、前列腺尿道或 Cowper 腺黏液性腺癌的直接扩散[163-166,175,176]。前列腺原发性黏液性腺癌的几个特征有助于与非前列腺性黏液性腺癌的鉴别诊断。最具有特征性的改变是前列腺黏

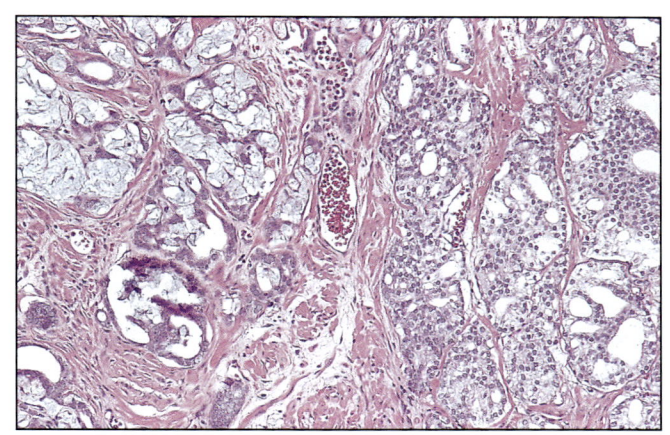

图14A.43　黏液性腺癌。左侧可见黏液性腺癌，右侧为普通类型的腺癌。在黏液性腺癌区域，肿瘤细胞漂浮在黏液湖中。

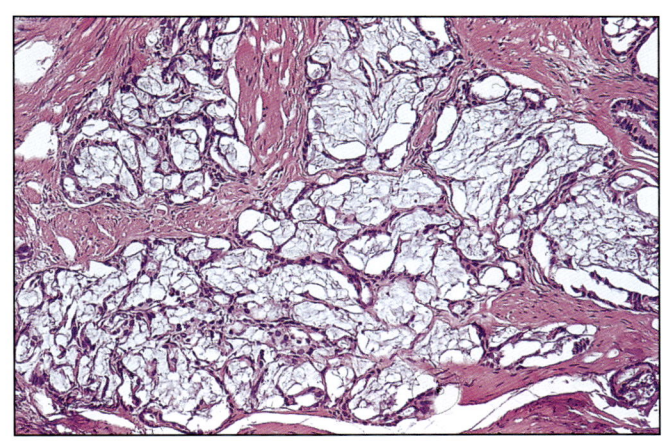

图14A.44　形成脑回状肿物的肿瘤细胞伴有丰富的细胞外黏液。

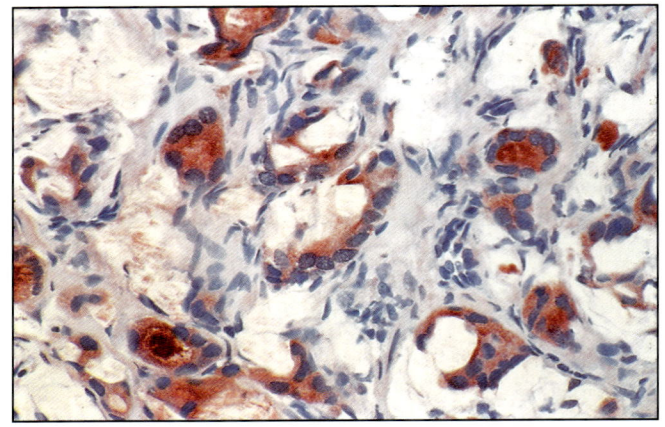

图14A.45 黏液性腺癌的肿瘤细胞前列腺特异性抗原和前列腺酸性磷酸酶免疫染色阳性。

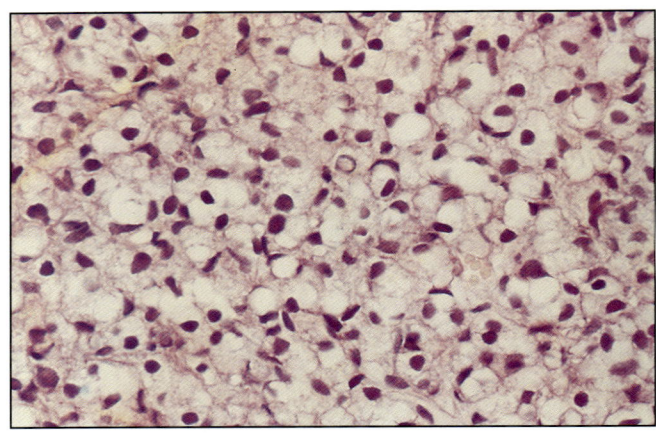

图14A.46 印戒细胞癌。这些肿瘤细胞的特征是胞浆透明，细胞核移位到周围。

液性腺癌几乎总是伴有"普通类型"的前列腺腺癌。此外，前列腺原发性黏液性腺癌与肠道或膀胱的黏液性腺癌不同，通常不含有柱状细胞或杯状细胞，或印戒细胞[163-165,175]，尽管有个别的报道[165,177]。

黏液性腺癌PSA和PrAP免疫染色阳性（图14A.45），但是癌胚抗原（CEA）染色阴性[163]。因为2/3以上的普通类型前列腺腺癌腔内含有黏液[75,85,178-180]，所以黏液局限在腺腔内的肿瘤不应该被分类为黏液性腺癌。

前列腺印戒细胞癌
Signet-ring cell carcinoma of prostate

前列腺原发性印戒细胞癌（signet-ring cell carcinoma，SRCC）极其罕见；文献中大约有24例报道[50,164,181-187]。所报道病例患者的年龄从50岁到80岁不等（平均67.5岁），症状和体征与普通前列腺癌没有不同。前列腺SRCC患者通常为晚期病变，患者或是pT3期或是pT4期，伴有或不伴有转移（C或D期）[181]。

SRCC表现为伴有印戒细胞形态学表现的未分化细胞的局灶性或弥漫性片块状生长，这样的肿瘤被认为是Gleason 5型癌。印戒细胞以细胞核偏位和胞浆透明为特征（图14A.46）。尽管有少数病例报道前列腺印戒细胞癌含有细胞浆内黏液，但是绝大多数病例却与之相反[181-183,185]。与诸如胃、结肠以及乳腺等其他部位SRCC的生长方式类似，肿瘤细胞弥漫性浸润前列腺间质（图14A.47）。所有前列腺SRCC均伴有其他类型的高级别前列腺癌，包括实性、粉刺样和筛状形式的癌[181]。文献中未见有单纯性SRCC的报道。与其他部位SRCC不同，前列腺SRCC通常不伴有黏液腺癌[75,163,164,175,177,181-183,185-187]。

印戒细胞前列腺标志物，包括PrAP和PSA阳

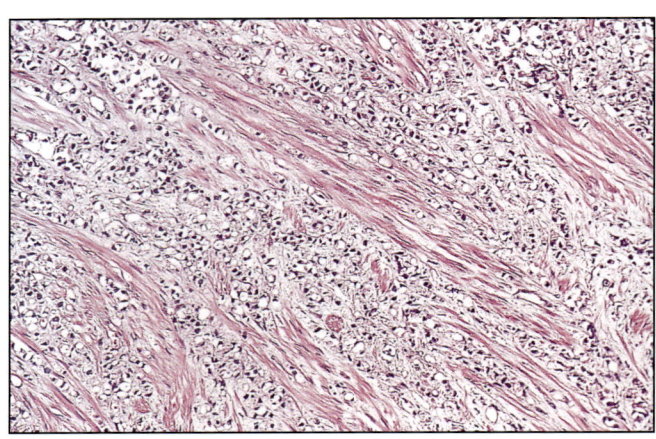

图14A.47 在印戒细胞癌中肿瘤细胞弥漫性浸润前列腺间质。

性[177,178]，但是CEA通常阴性。电镜检查，印戒细胞显示细胞浆内腔隙或胞浆空泡。一般不存在黏液或脂肪空泡[182]。

前列腺SRCC的鉴别诊断应该包括其他具有类似表现的肿瘤或伴有印戒细胞外观的细胞。慢性炎症区域出现的空泡状印戒表现的细胞是变形的淋巴细胞，可能类似于SRCC，因为它们在纤维平滑肌间质内浸润[188,189]。然而，缺乏PSA和PrAP免疫反应以及白细胞共同抗原阳性有助于排除癌[188]。在诊断前列腺原发性SRCC前，必须除外其他部位转移而来的肿瘤，包括由膀胱SRCC直接蔓延而来的肿瘤[181]。膀胱或其他器官的SRCC产生黏液，应用常规黏液染色可以证实。另外一个有助于确立原发性前列腺SRCC的发现是它伴有前列腺腺癌的其他组织学形态。激素治疗也可以导致印戒型肿瘤细胞的形成，但是常常伴有未受累及腺体的鳞状化生以及肿瘤细胞核的固缩，这提供了激素治疗的线索（图14A.48）[181,190]。

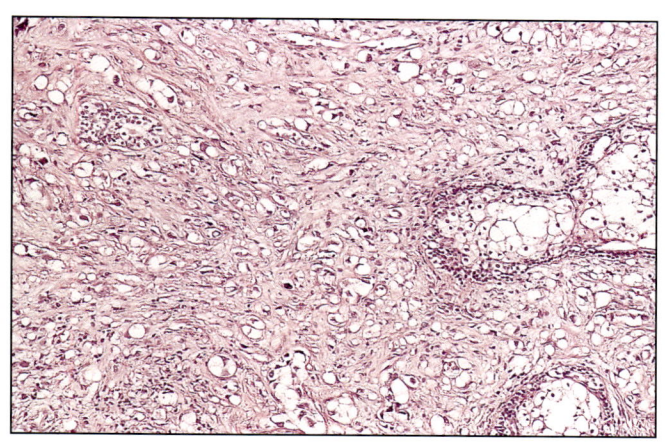

图14A.48 激素治疗可能引起肿瘤细胞胞浆透明，类似于印戒细胞癌。注意良性前列腺腺体鳞状化生。

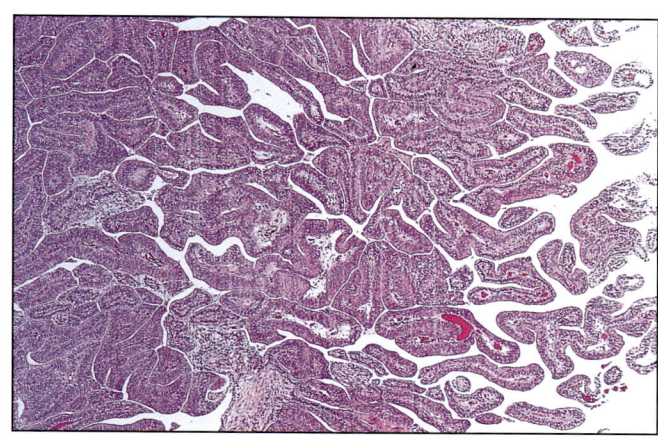

图14A.49 导管-子宫内膜样癌。A型结构显示明显的乳头状生长，伴有中央纤维血管轴心。

一般来说，前列腺 SRCC 患者的生存率低。多数患者在诊断之后 32～60 个月之间死于肿瘤，这些生存资料与高级别前列腺腺癌相似。其临床症状、转移方式以及血清 PrAP 和 PSA 水平也与普通的高级别前列腺腺癌患者相似[181,183,187]。

导管-子宫内膜样癌
Ductal-endometrioid carcinoma

前列腺子宫内膜样腺癌发生于前列腺精阜或其附近，1967 年由 Melicow 和 Pachter 首次描述[191]。他们认为其组织学形态和子宫腺癌相似，而且提出这种肿瘤来源于前列腺小囊，这种结构相当于女性子宫和阴道[191]。虽然有关这种病变的组织学发生还有某些争议，但是根据组织化学和超微结构发现，认为这种肿瘤是前列腺腺癌的导管亚型[50,192-195]。

导管-子宫内膜样癌有两种独特的组织学生长方式[192]。A 型结构显示明显的乳头状生长，以乳头状分叶为特征；肿瘤细胞被覆于中央的纤维血管轴心，从单层到复层高柱状上皮（图 14A.49）。细胞核位于基底，含有明显的大核仁以及丰富的嗜酸性胞浆（图 14A.50）。有些病例核分裂象常见（>10/10HPF），而少数病例可以有相当温和的细胞学特征。常见核下空泡和表现为腔内顶浆分泌的分泌活动。当肿瘤长入前列腺尿道或位于前列腺大导管中心时常常可以看到 A 型肿瘤。B 型的特征是导管内乳头状生长，伴有复杂的腺体、实性以及粉刺癌性结构（图 14A.51）。这种类型的肿瘤通常位于前列腺深部，在完整的或部分脱落的尿路上皮之下。肿瘤细胞与 A 型肿瘤相似。在大约半数的病例中这两种生长方式（A 型和 B 型）同时存在，两种成分往往相互混合。

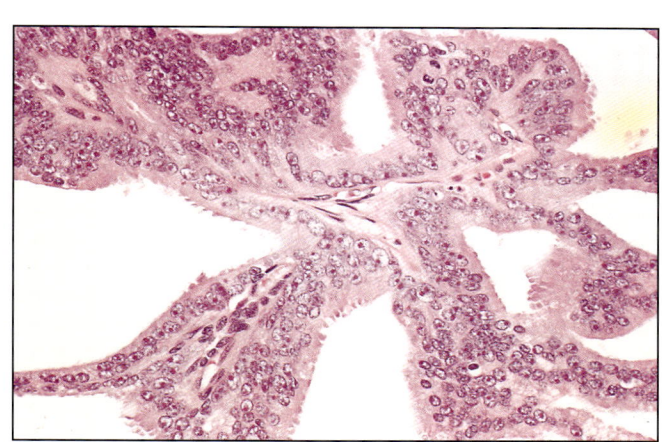

图14A.50 肿瘤细胞高柱状，伴有丰富的嗜酸性细胞浆。细胞核位于基底，伴有大而明显的核仁。

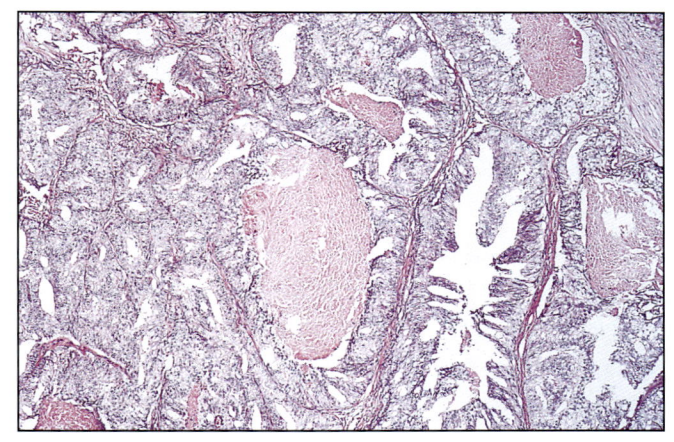

图14A.51 B 型导管-子宫内膜样癌的特征是导管内乳头状生长，伴有分支状腺体以及伴有粉刺样坏死的腺体。

微小腺泡癌常常伴有子宫内膜样癌，但通常是局灶性和低级别癌。前列腺导管癌是否为一个独立疾病一直存在争议[196]。根据我们的观点，当肿瘤完全或主要为这种组织学结构（超过80%）时，做出这种诊断是合适的。在穿刺活检标本中，导管癌的组织学所见可能并不代表前列腺内的肿瘤，因此，如果出现导管-子宫内膜样癌结构，可诊断为前列腺腺癌伴有导管-子宫内膜样组织学改变。所有导管-子宫内膜样癌PSA和PrAP免疫反应均呈阳性[192-195,197]。子宫内膜样癌CEA可以阳性，但为局灶弱阳性[192]。

已报道的发生这种肿瘤患者的年龄范围为50～86岁（平均65岁）。与普通前列腺腺癌相同，表现出的症状是尿道梗阻和血尿。血清PSA和PrAP水平常常正常，但可以升高。转移部位包括盆腔淋巴结、肺以及骨。然而，肿瘤在转移到骨之前更有可能转移到内脏。骨转移通常是成骨性的，但可以是溶骨与成骨混合性的。已经观察到一些客观存在的对激素治疗的反应（梗阻症状缓解，肿瘤体积减小，血清PSA和PrAP水平下降，骨疼痛减轻，新的骨转移的进展停止），这进一步支持了这种肿瘤是前列腺腺癌的特殊类型的观点[192,195]。

Melicow等[191,198]最初认为这种肿瘤通常是分期低的病变，侵袭性行为不如普通的前列腺腺癌。后来的报道还认为，可能是因为它位于尿道周围的中心部位以及易于出现早期症状，所以多数患者表现为前列腺局限性病变[199-202]。然而，最近几项大的研究已经证实这些肿瘤的分期比以前认为的要晚（T3/C或D）[192-195]。

在我们的研究中[192]5年生存率为30%，平均生存时间46.3个月，与文献中报道的生存率相似。Bostwick等[194]报道他们的10个患者平均生存37个月，粗略的5年生存率为15%；Dube等[203,204]报道5年生存率42.8%。Christensen等[205]报道了前列腺导管腺癌根治性手术治疗的结果。这项研究证实，前列腺导管腺癌的病理分期比临床上怀疑的分期要高，与相同分期的微小腺泡癌相比其根治性前列腺切除术后的复发率高。另外一项研究证实，穿刺活检所见前列腺导管腺癌提示是较晚期的癌，伴有短期内进展[206]。

鉴别诊断包括尿道乳头状腺瘤、前列腺型尿道息肉、PIN以及前列腺导管移行细胞癌（TCC）[46,47,97,98,192,207-212]。高级别PIN缺乏融合性生长、粉刺样坏死、核分裂活性以及伴随导管癌出现的某种程度的细胞核非典型性。累及前列腺导管及腺泡的TCC应该与实性前列腺导管腺癌（B型）相区别。前列腺导管-子宫内膜样腺癌PSA和PrAP阳性，这些染色解决了这个鉴别诊断问题[192-195]。某些导管-子宫内膜样癌有温和的细胞学表现，可能类似于尿道良性乳头状腺瘤。在这些病例中，临床-病理联系可以给病变的真正性质提供一些线索。前列腺型尿道息肉的细胞极其温和，腺体有两层细胞。

其他类型的前列腺癌
Other types of prostatic carcinoma

前列腺小细胞癌
Small cell carcinoma of the prostate

原发性前列腺小细胞癌少见。据报道它是一个高度侵袭性的肿瘤[213-218]，有些病例显示有神经内分泌分化[216-222]。多数患者年龄超过50岁（平均67岁），但少数患者年轻。症状和体征与普通前列腺腺癌患者相同，但是已经报道少数病例有副肿瘤综合征，包括Cushing综合征[214,221,222]、Eaton-Lambert综合征[220]、伴有抗利尿激素分泌紊乱的胰高血糖素血症性综合征、恶性高钙血症以及甲状腺毒症[50,216]。在有些患者中，前列腺腺癌早于小细胞癌发现，而在另外一些患者中小细胞癌表现为直接生成的肿瘤（de novo tumor）[213,214]。那些最初表现为普通微小腺泡性腺癌的小细胞癌患者生存7个月至9年（平均24个月）。在确认小细胞癌成分后，不管其有无腺癌病史，患者在1.5年内死亡（平均5个月）[213]。然而，最近应用的与肺小细胞癌相似的化学治疗方案有望延长患者的生命，尤其是对于那些仅有局部淋巴结扩散的患者[50,213,217,218,223]。

前列腺小细胞癌的组织学特征类似于肺和其他肺外部位的小细胞癌[213,217,219,222]。小细胞或为燕麦型或为中间型（图14A.52）。前列腺小细胞癌经常伴有普通的腺

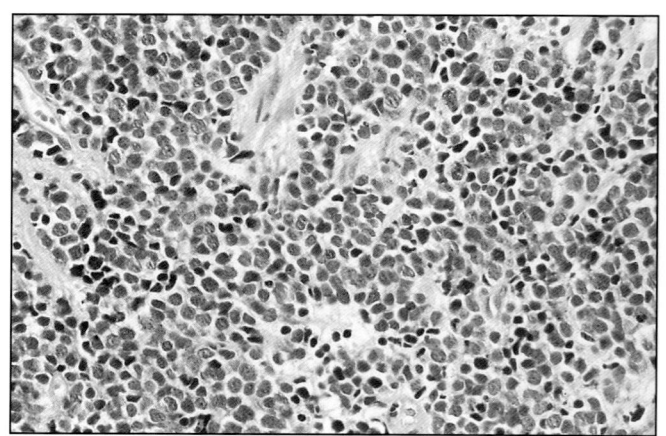

图14A.52 高倍放大的小细胞癌，肿瘤细胞表现为核深染以及明显的细胞核变形，这通常是小细胞癌的特征。

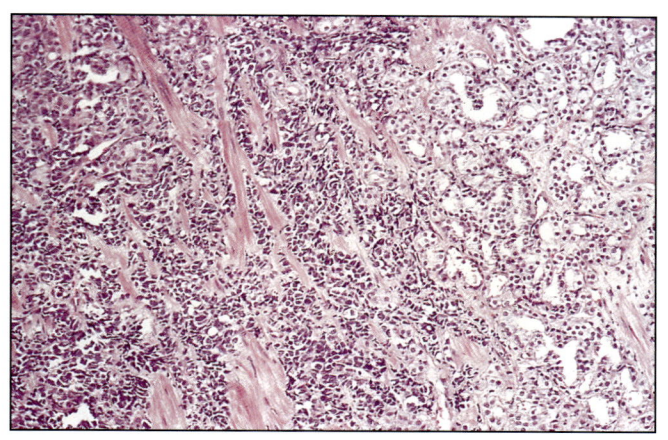

图14A.53 小细胞癌。左侧为小细胞癌，右侧为普通腺癌。

癌（多于50%病例）（图14A.53），在少数情况下可以伴有肉瘤样和鳞状细胞癌成分[213]。免疫组化和电镜研究证实前列腺小细胞癌的细胞是异源性的，与肺或肺外小细胞癌相同[214,216,219]。某些肿瘤细胞含有致密核心的神经内分泌颗粒，神经内分泌标志物免疫组化染色阳性（图14A.54），而另外一些肿瘤是低分化腺癌或可能是来源于基底（储备）细胞的癌[214,216,219,219a]。因为小细胞癌通常伴有其他类型前列腺癌，以及免疫组化和超微结构的异质性，所以我们相信前列腺小细胞癌来源于多潜能的前列腺上皮细胞；而且认为它不是来源于特化的神经内分泌细胞[214,216,219]。

PSA和PrAP水平均为播散性前列腺癌有用的临床

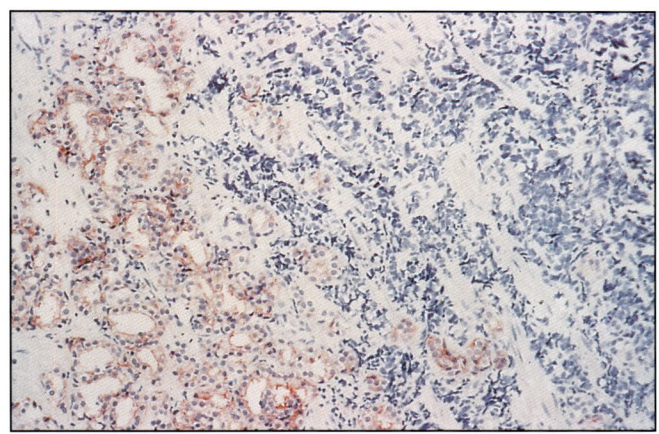

图14A.54 前列腺特异性抗原和前列腺酸性磷酸酶免疫染色腺癌成分阳性，而小细胞癌成分通常阴性。

标志物，但是前列腺小细胞癌常不伴有这些标志物的显著升高。前列腺小细胞癌往往早期转移到盆腔淋巴结、肺以及肝。不常见的转移部位，诸如网膜、声带、颞骨、腋窝淋巴结以及周围软组织也有报告[223]。

在前列腺原发性小细胞癌的鉴别诊断中必须考虑肺小细胞癌转移到前列腺。在尸检中发现前列腺转移性肿瘤占0.5%～2.2%，它们占前列腺所有恶性病变的1.2%[224,225]。仅有少数肺燕麦细胞癌转移到前列腺的病例报道[224-226]。因为前列腺小细胞癌和前列腺外小细胞癌形态学上没有差别，所以必须注意临床病理的相互关系[213]。虽然TTF-1不是肺小细胞癌的特异性标志物，但它可能有助于鉴别肺小细胞癌和肺外小细胞癌[227]。另一个有助于做出前列腺原发性小细胞癌诊断的表现是与前列腺腺癌密切相关；在许多病例中已经注意到这种关系[50,213]。累及前列腺的淋巴瘤少见，但是可能与前列腺小细胞癌相似。白细胞共同抗原和角蛋白免疫染色有助于鉴别诊断。前列腺胚胎性横纹肌肉瘤具有"圆形蓝染细胞的组织学"（round blue cell histology）特征，但是绝大多数病例发生在儿童人群。最近，在前列腺腺癌中描述了Paneth细胞样改变，可能是神经内分泌分化的一种形式[228,229]。

前列腺鳞状细胞癌和腺鳞癌
Squamous cell and adenosquamous carcinoma of prostate

前列腺鳞状细胞癌少见，占前列腺恶性肿瘤的0.2%[230-237]。文献中报道不足70例。它们或是单纯性鳞状细胞癌，或是与腺癌混合的鳞状细胞癌（腺鳞癌）。另外，已有TCC和肉瘤样癌伴有鳞状细胞癌和腺鳞癌的报道[237]。临床上，原发性鳞状细胞癌和腺鳞癌无法与前列腺腺癌区分。诊断单纯性鳞状细胞癌的标准是：（1）伴有无序生长、细胞间变和浸润的明显的恶性肿瘤；（2）伴有角化、角化珠以及细胞间桥证据的明确的鳞状特征；（3）缺乏任何腺体或腺泡成分；（4）没有其他部位的鳞状细胞癌，尤其是膀胱[238]。多数患者没有从前放射治疗或激素治疗的病史[237]，但是某些患者可以有先前的治疗史。单纯性鳞状细胞癌的组织学发生还不明确；推测前列腺尿道上皮、尿道周围导管的移行上皮、前列腺腺泡的基底（储备）细胞以及普通的腺泡细胞都可能是细胞的来源。然而，因为这种肿瘤罕见，很难接受任何单一的发病机制[230-235,237-241]。有一例发生于埃及血吸虫感染患者的前列腺鳞状细胞癌的报道[242]。

腺鳞癌（图14A.55）通常发生在普通前列腺腺癌放射治疗或激素治疗后几年之内，极少有例外[231-233,237,241,243]。Bennett和Edgerton[234]提出两个发生的假说：（1）激素

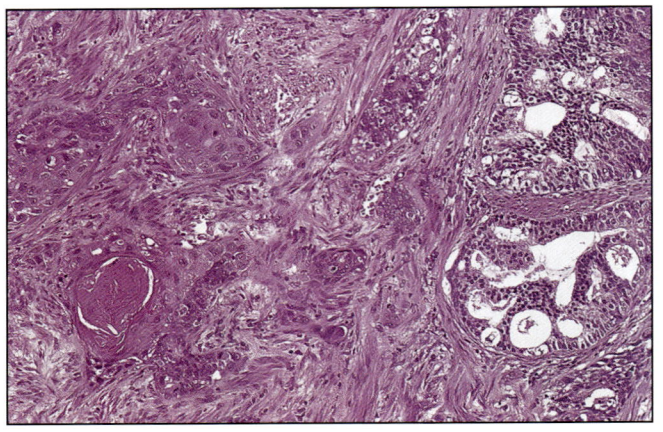

图14A.55 前列腺腺鳞癌。鳞状细胞癌（右侧）伴有腺癌（左侧）。

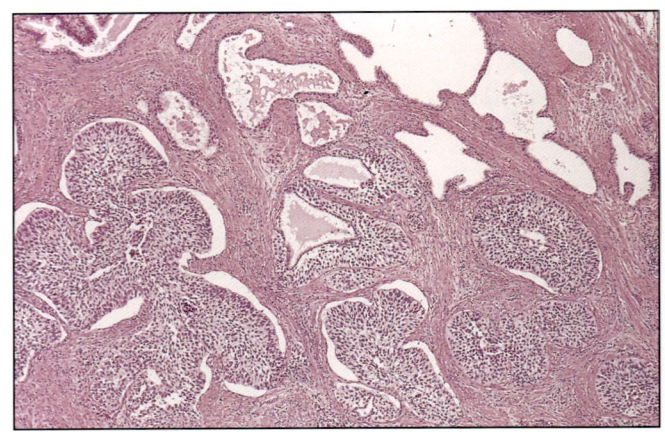

A

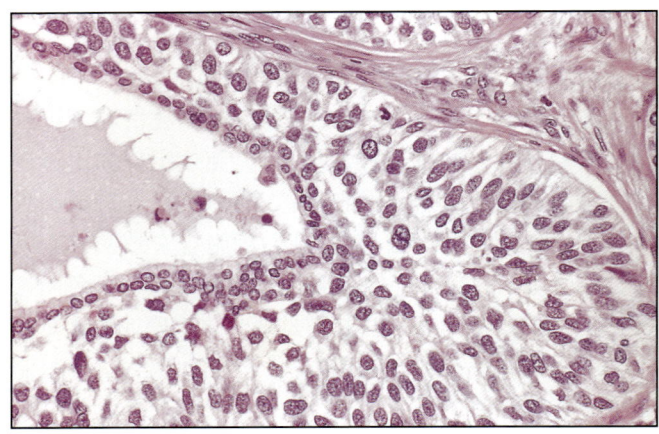

B

图14A.56 （A）移行细胞癌（TCC）累及前列腺导管和腺泡。TCC累及导管和腺泡腔面。没有间质浸润。（B）高倍镜下显示肿瘤细胞出现在基底层和前列腺上皮细胞之间。

和（或）放射治疗的影响改变了前列腺癌本身的性质转变为混合细胞型；或（2）在放射治疗或激素治疗的影响下，累及尿道周围导管的继发性腺癌、伴随的前列腺腺癌发生了鳞状细胞成分。

即使伴有转移，鳞状细胞癌患者血清PrAP和PSA水平通常也不升高[238,244,245]。骨转移通常是溶骨性的，而多数前列腺腺癌的骨转移是成骨性的[238,245]。前列腺鳞状细胞癌是有高度侵袭性的肿瘤[237]。在控制这种癌的过程中，许多治疗方法都没有很好的效果。雌激素治疗通常没有帮助[230-235,238-241]。在前列腺梗死和雌激素治疗的反应中，前列腺导管和腺泡的鳞状化生是一种常见的病变[233]。这种病变缺乏浸润和细胞间变，通常可与鳞状细胞癌鉴别。膀胱和尿道的TCC可以出现鳞状和腺体分化，可能类似于前列腺鳞状细胞癌和（或）腺鳞癌。另外，还应该除外肛管鳞状细胞癌的扩散或来自肺等远隔部位的转移。

前列腺移行细胞癌
Transitional cell carcinoma of prostate

根据不同的报道，前列腺TCC的发生率不一样，占所有前列腺癌的1%～5%[246]。尽管其所占比例低，但它是一个非常重要的病变，因为其生物学行为明显不同于普通的前列腺腺癌。TCC预后不良；TCC对于激素治疗没有反应[46,47,97,98,246]。虽然TCC可以原发于前列腺，但是大多数病例是膀胱TCC继发累及前列腺[50,246-249]。当膀胱TCC累及前列腺时，有两种累及方式：（1）通过前列腺尿道、前列腺导管及腺泡的黏膜Paget样扩散，伴有或不伴有间质浸润（图14A.56），和（2）通过膀胱壁直接浸润（图14A.57）[247,250-255]。

在前列腺原发性TCC中，最初累及的是尿道周围

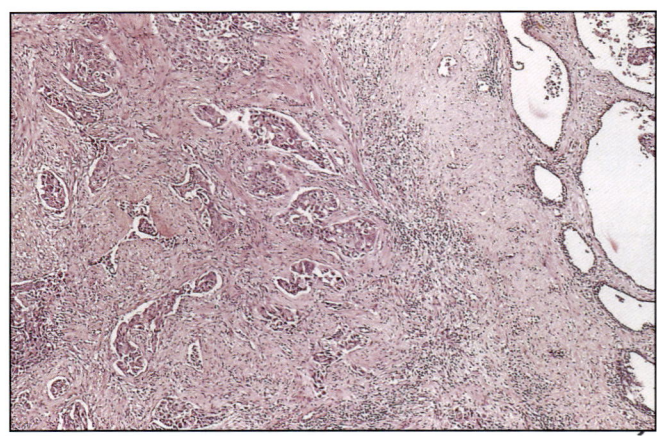

图14A.57 来自膀胱癌的移行细胞癌（TCC）直接蔓延。TCC累及前列腺间质。注意右侧是正常的前列腺腺体。

腺体和导管[46,47,256]。TCC可以沿导管和腺泡扩散，经常浸润纤维肌性间质。在继发性TCC中，位于膀胱颈部的深部浸润的膀胱癌直接侵犯前列腺。在有长期TCC病史的患者中，沿前列腺尿道和导管的Paget样扩散是

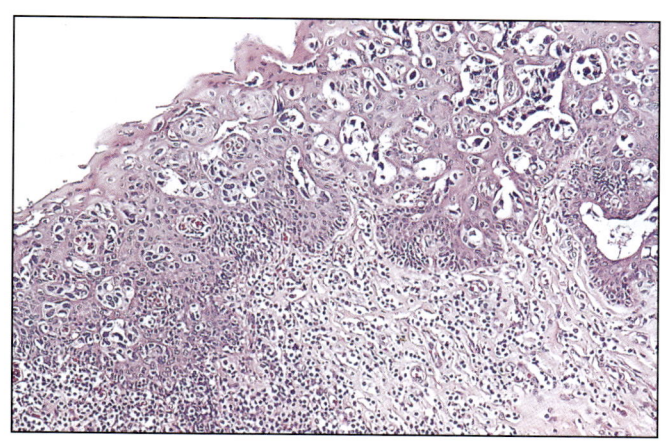

图14A.58 移行细胞癌在尿道口的鳞状上皮内蔓延。

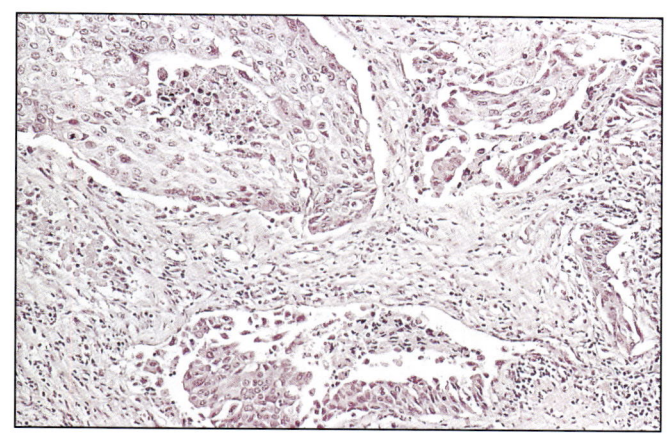

图14A.59 移行细胞癌通常表现为实性生长方式，常常伴有肿瘤坏死、核分裂象多以及细胞核的多形性。

前列腺受累的另外一种机制。正如原发性前列腺TCC一样，肿瘤开始以恶性Paget样细胞生长，发展成为局限于导管和腺泡的原位癌，最终可以浸润前列腺间质。TCC可以在上皮内扩散到射精管、精囊以及尿道口（图14A.58）[247,256,257]。在有长期膀胱癌病史的患者中TCC继发性累及前列腺的机制是，膀胱内疗法治疗膀胱内疾病是成功的，但是局部治疗对于移行细胞癌累及的前列腺尿道和尿道周围的导管以及腺泡没有影响，从而导致尿路上皮癌存在于前列腺内。

前列腺TCC通常表现为实性生长方式。另外，肿瘤周围的炎症、明显的细胞核多形性、含有高核分裂计数的实性细胞巢以及肿瘤坏死是诊断TCC的重要标准，上述表现都超过了前列腺腺癌（图14A.59）[47,246]。

在前列腺TCC中，间质浸润是一个非常重要的预后因素。在前列腺切除或膀胱前列腺切除术标本中，那些TCC局限于导管或腺泡的患者具有相对好的预后，但是伴有间质浸润的多数TCC患者会发生转移[248,251,253,254]。

因为前列腺TCC激素治疗无效，所以将前列腺TCC与普通前列腺腺癌和导管腺癌鉴别开来对于临床治疗十分重要。临床病史、仔细的显微镜检查以及免疫组化染色有助于鉴别TCC和普通前列腺腺癌及其导管亚型。TCC免疫染色PrAP和PSA阴性，而CEA、uroplakin以及血栓调节蛋白（thrombomodulin）常常阳性[99,246,258]。因为某些前列腺腺癌CK 7和CK 20阳性，以及某些尿路上皮癌CK 7和CK 20阴性，所以这些标志物在鉴别诊断中没有帮助[258]。

移行细胞化生容易与前列腺TCC鉴别，因为前列腺TCC细胞学上有间变，而移行细胞化生的细胞表现温和，伴有明显的核沟[45]。

肉瘤样癌　Sarcomatoid carcinoma

前列腺肉瘤样癌是一个双相性的肿瘤，含有癌和梭形或多形性肉瘤样成分（图14A.60），它是另外一种不常见的前列腺癌的变型。当普通的微小腺泡癌组织学结构少或者组织取样有限时，可能很难与真正的肉瘤区分。文献中曾经应用癌肉瘤、恶性混合性中胚层肿瘤、梭形细胞癌以及伴有假肉瘤样间质的癌来描述这种病变。严格地讲，传统上癌肉瘤的定义是伴有异源性肉瘤成分的双相性肿瘤。我们使用肉瘤样癌这个术语来描述所有表现为癌和肉瘤成分双相生长的肿瘤，而不管其是否存在异源性成分[259-263]。

文献中已有几例前列腺肉瘤样癌的病例报告，它们通常表现为梗阻症状，因此通常在经尿道前列腺切除术（TURP）标本中得到诊断[259,262-266]。这些肿瘤患者的年龄从58岁到85岁（平均71岁）。根据我们的经验，这些肿瘤总是伴有高级别前列腺腺癌，先于肉瘤成分或与之同时发生。多数患者在诊断时已有转移，50%有前列腺癌放射治疗或激素治疗的病史[266]。肉瘤样区域由梭形细胞构成，细胞核大，具有多形性，深染。这种形态属于高级别肉瘤（多数病例类似于所谓的恶性纤维组织细胞瘤）（图14A.61）。肉瘤样成分还可能类似于纤维肉瘤或平滑肌肉瘤。多达1/3的病例可见异源性肉瘤样成分（骨肉瘤、软骨肉瘤或横纹肌肉瘤）[259,264,265]。应用角蛋白、PrAP以及PSA抗体免疫染色可能有助于证明这些肿瘤的上皮性本质[99,259,264]。梭形细胞成分很少表达角蛋白，大概1/3的病例显示有局灶性PSA、PrAP或两

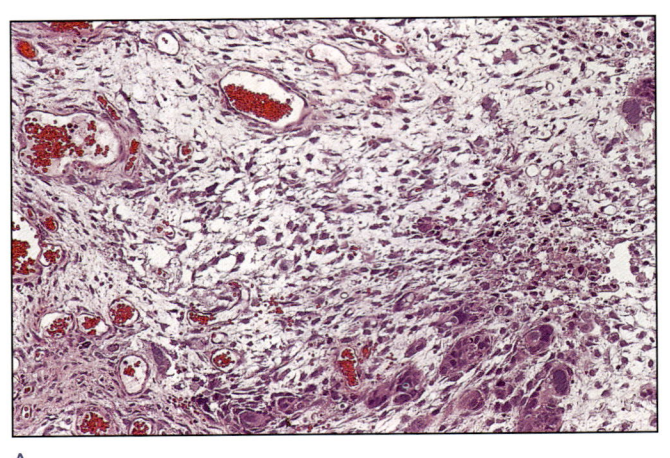
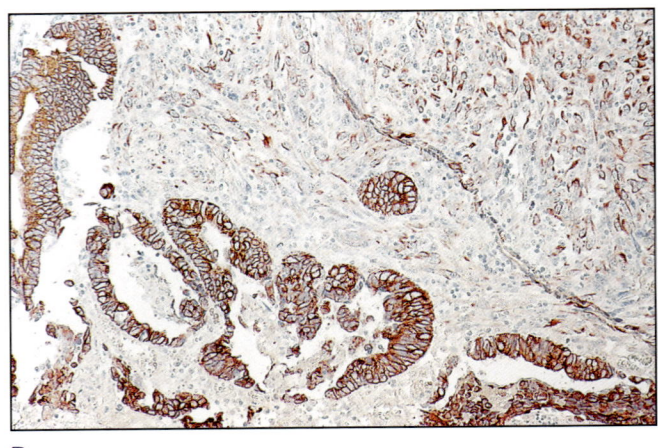

图14A.60 （A）肉瘤样癌。双相性肿瘤具有癌和梭形细胞肉瘤样成分；后者通常呈恶性纤维组织细胞瘤样结构，但常常具有一种不能分类的黏液样结构，如本例所见。（B）癌和肉瘤样成分角蛋白免疫染色均呈阳性反应。

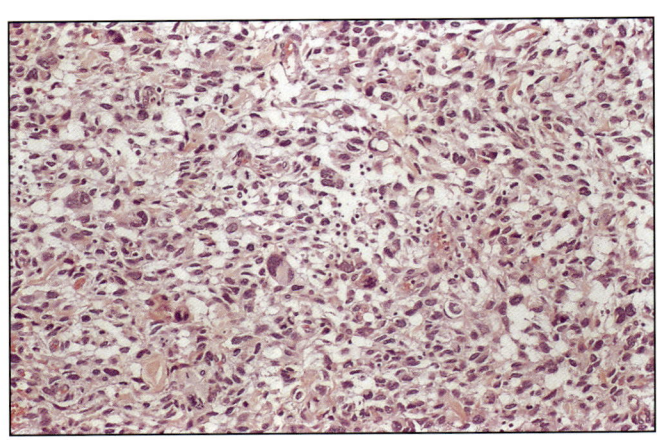

图14A.61 恶性纤维组织细胞瘤样结构是肉瘤样成分最常见的结构。

者的免疫反应[99,259,264]。

肉瘤样癌预后差。Shannon 等[259]报道的有随访资料的所有 9 例患者在诊断之后 3～48 个月（平均 12 个月）内死于本病。临床经过以侵袭性的局部复发为特征。Dundore 等[262]报道 5 年和 7 年癌特异性生存率分别为 41% 和 14%；86% 的患者死于本病（平均 9.5 个月）。

肉瘤样癌的鉴别诊断包括各种原发性前列腺肉瘤。与肉瘤样癌的区别在于其缺乏上皮成分（广泛取材之后），而且通常缺乏前列腺腺癌病史。在鉴别诊断中还应该考虑术后梭形细胞结节、叶状肿瘤以及假肉瘤性纤维黏液样肿瘤。在这些病变中，梭形细胞缺乏多形性或非典型性核分裂象。

其他类型的癌　Miscellaneous carcinomas

淋巴上皮瘤样癌[267]、嗜酸细胞癌[268]、巨细胞癌、肾型透明细胞癌[50,269]以及酷似女性生殖道肿瘤而不是典型前列腺腺癌的管囊状透明细胞腺癌[270]已有报道。

与癌类似的病变　Carcinoma mimics

多数类似于癌的腺泡增生来自移行区，因此最常见于因良性病变而行 TURP 或耻骨上/耻骨后前列腺切除术标本中，但在穿刺活检中这种改变也不少见。针对移行区的芯针活检（core biopsies）以及当前列腺太小或太大时针对周围区含有移行区的芯针活检，就导致了对移行区良性小腺泡增生的活检。因此，熟悉这些病变非常重要。

移行区腺泡增生：非典型性腺瘤性增生（腺病）Acinar proliferations of the transition zone: atypical adenomatous hyperplasia (adenosis)

前列腺非典型性腺瘤性增生（atypical adenomatous hyperplasia，AAH）或腺病很难与前列腺高分化腺癌鉴别。虽然 McNeal 认为这种病变可能是癌前增生，但是到目前为止多数研究没有提出令人信服的证据证明它是癌前病变[23,271-274]。1982 年 Brawn[92]提供了一项最好的具有临床随访资料的腺病患者的大样本研究。108 名非典型性腺瘤性增生（腺病）患者随访 5～15 年（平均 7.7 年），有 7 例发展成癌（6.5%）；在有类似随访时间的 2263 名增生患者中，有 84 名（3.7%）发展成癌。然而，许多专家认为 Brawn 图示的非典型性腺瘤性增生的病例可能是高分化癌。Lopez-Beltran 等[275]研究了非典型性腺瘤性增生、结节性增生以及高分化前列腺腺癌细胞核的三维体积。发现前列腺癌与非典型性腺瘤性增生或结节性增生之间存在明显差别，但是非典型性腺瘤性增生和良性增生之间的差别却不明显，这表明非典型性腺瘤性增生有可能是 BPH 组织学变型。然而，非典型性腺瘤性增生病变的基因变化各异[276,277]。非典型性腺瘤性增生是移行区病变，在穿刺活检中并不常见，因此除非有明显的 BPH 或需要特别针对这个区域取样，一般不进行活检。非典型性腺瘤性增生为多灶性；它在 TURP 标本中的发生率是 1.5%～19.6%，在根治性前列腺切除标本中达到 33%[278-280]。

非典型性腺瘤性增生是小至中等大小腺体的增生，似乎被覆单层上皮细胞，具有均匀一致的圆形细胞核，细腻而深染的染色质，既没有细胞核的非典型性，也没有明显的核仁（图 14A.62）[3,8,272]。基底细胞层通常不明显、变薄或是模糊，可能必须借助于高分子量细胞角蛋白（克隆性 34βE12）、p63 或 CK5/6 染色来证实基底细胞的存在，并证明这种病变是良性的（图 14A.63）。非典型性腺瘤性增生可有腔内类晶体、蓝色黏液以及局灶性浸润，使得与癌的鉴别更不可信。

非典型性腺瘤性增生的鉴别诊断包括高分化腺癌和所有其他有小腺体增生的病变。非典型性腺瘤性增生可以有局灶性 P504S 染色，但多数病例这个标志物阴性。相反，绝大多数前列腺癌呈弥漫性染色[109-111]。Yang 等[281]研究了 40 例非典型性腺瘤性增生病例的 P504S 表达，以便理解其作为前列腺腺癌癌前病变的意义。在所有 40 个非典型性腺瘤性增生病例中 34βE12 染色证实了碎片状基底细胞的存在。在多数（33/40，82.5%）非典型性腺瘤性增生没有发现 P504S 表达，4 例（10.0%）有局灶表达，仅有 3 例非典型性腺瘤性增生（7.5%）弥漫阳性。有趣的是，7 例 P504S 阳性的非典型性腺瘤性增生中 2 例发现周围有腺癌。相反，所有 BPH（20/20,100%）P504S 阴性，所有 20 例（100%）前列腺癌表现为 P504S 弥漫性阳性染色。这些发现表明非典型性腺瘤性增生是一种异质性病变。

基底细胞增生 Basal cell hyperplasia

前列腺基底细胞增生（BCH）是检查 TURP 标本中相对常见的病变[3,282,285]，但在穿刺活检中并不常见[286]。它通常见于 BPH 背景中，因此发生的年龄与 BPH 年龄组相同（范围 63～80 岁，平均 74 岁）；虽然多数病例同时出现 BPH 相关的组织学特征[283-287]，但是临床上也许表现为尿道梗阻。临床上其他的特征是与抗雄激素治疗有关[157]。

显微镜下其增生的程度不同：多数 BCH 病灶表现为单个或一小组腺泡的基底细胞增生，而小叶状或弥漫性 BCH 相当少见[3,282-284]。BCH 有与众不同的镜下表现。多数病例中认识这种疾病并不困难，但它可能酷似具有小腺泡结构的癌，尤其是不熟悉这种病变的组织学形态[3,73,282,283,288,289]和当出现明显的核仁时[3,290]。这种病变也被描述为前列腺"胎型化"（fetalization），因为在光镜下它类似于胎儿前列腺[291]。BCH 以巢状、管状以及条索状结节性生长为特征，充满了增生的小而深染的基底细胞。多数 BCH 细胞巢表现为周围的基底细胞呈垂直栅栏状排列。基底细胞细胞浆稀少，细胞核卵圆或短梭形，深染。通常没有核仁，或如果有的话也是不明显的小核仁（图 14A.64）。不存在核沟。核分裂象缺乏或极其少见，没有坏死。结节的边缘没有被膜，但在多数病例界限清楚[3,73,91,288,282-284,290]。BCH 通常与增生或正常的前列腺腺体混合。已经有伴有 SA[292] 和 CCCH 的报道[293]，SA 和 CCCH 是另外两种良性前列腺增生性病变。为了理解形态学，根据是否存在中心腔可以把 BCH 分为完全性和不完全性[91,284,288]。完全性 BCH 以实性基底

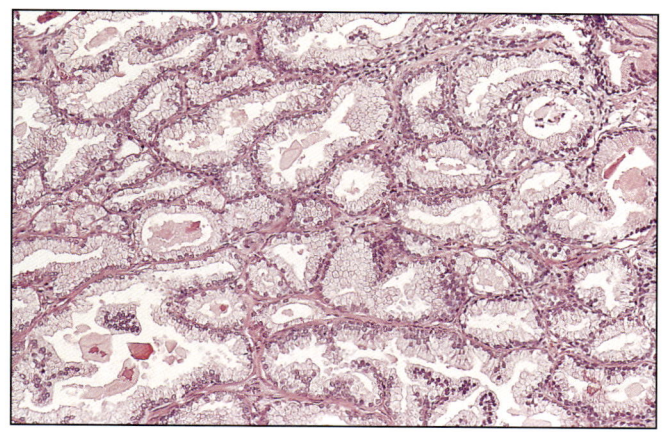

图 14A.62 非典型性腺瘤性增生（小腺体增生）。增生的小腺体背靠背排列。见不到明显的核仁。

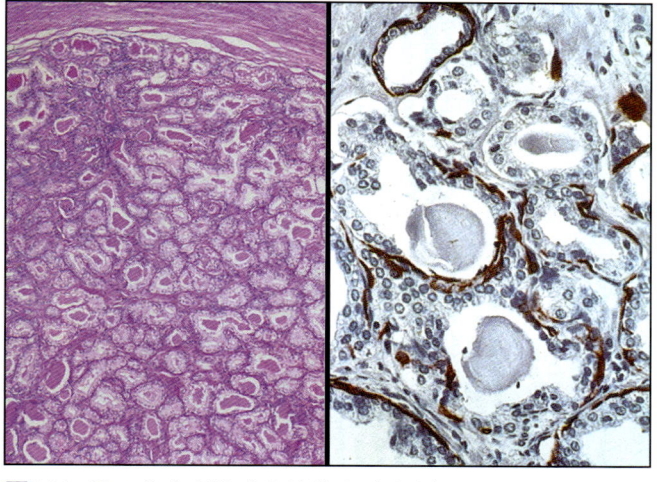

图 14A.63 非典型性腺瘤性增生（腺病）。界限清楚的结节（左侧）含有小腺体，腺体之间有少量间质，这种形态表面上类似于 Gleason 1 或 2 型前列腺癌，但腺病的腺体保留基底细胞层（34βE12 染色，右侧）。

与癌类似的病变

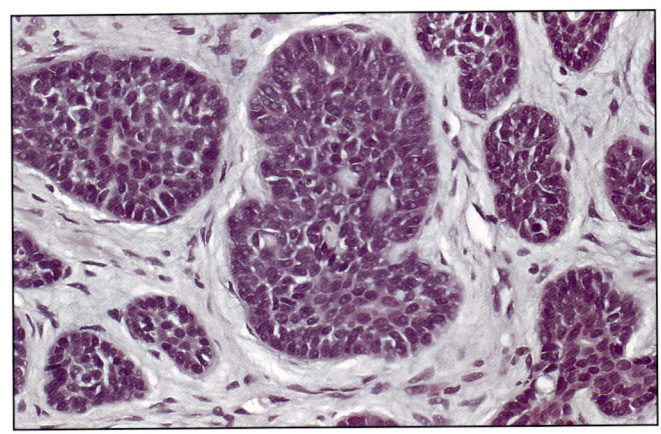

图14A.64 基底细胞增生。基底细胞实性增生，周围呈栅栏状排列，表面上类似于皮肤的基底细胞癌。

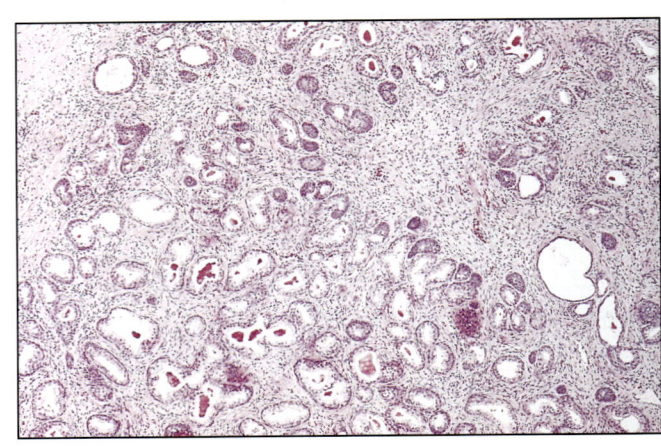

图14A.66 不完全性基底细胞增生（BCH）。本例显示多数基底细胞巢中存在腺腔，这是不完全性BCH的特征。

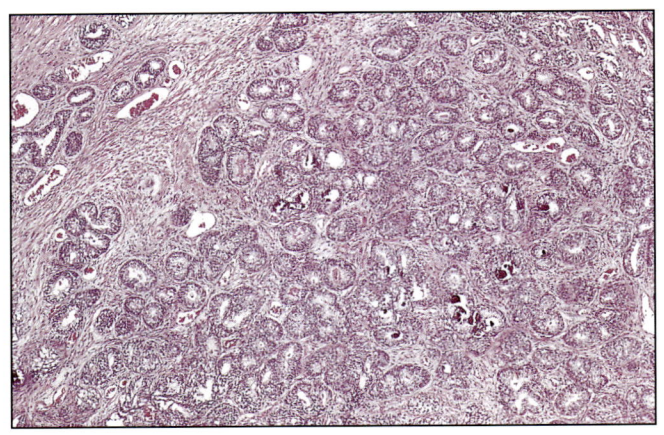

图14A.65 完全性基底细胞增生（BCH）。尽管有些细胞巢有腺腔，但多数是实性的。BCH中常见散在的钙化。

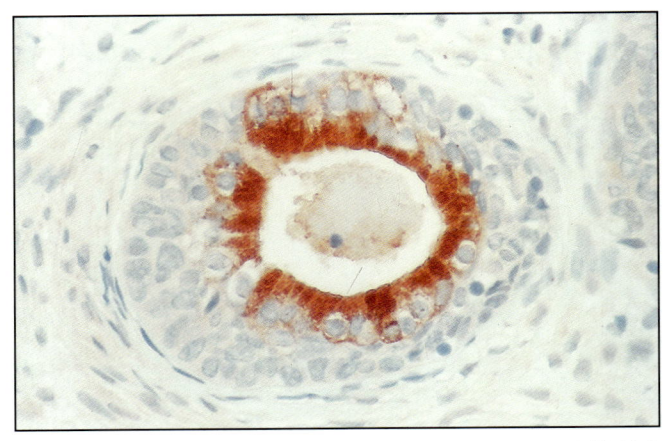

图14A.67 不完全性基底细胞增生显示腺腔分泌细胞前列腺特异性抗原（PSA）免疫反应。注意基底细胞缺乏PSA染色。

细胞巢为特征，没有腺腔分化（图14A.65），而不完全性BCH常常显示明显的伴有立方或柱状分泌细胞的中心腺体分化（图14A.66）；腺腔内可以含有中性和酸性黏液，PSA和阿辛蓝染色阳性[284]。腔内常见散在的微小钙化和淀粉样小体[91,283,284,288,294]。BCH的间质通常比周围正常的前列腺富于细胞，表现为纤维母细胞/肌纤维母细胞增生。BCH常见于梗死边缘，可能是对于缺血的反应[74,91,295]。

BCH中的基底细胞样细胞对高分子量细胞角蛋白（克隆性34βE12）、p63[105,296]以及CK5/6[296]有免疫反应，但PSA、PrAP以及AMACR[68,105,284,296,297]阴性。基底细胞样细胞和分泌细胞S-100蛋白、MSA或Vimentin免疫反应均呈阴性。在腺腔分化区域（不完全性BCH），腺腔分泌细胞PSA和PrAP阳性（图14A.67）[284]。不完全性BCH很有可能与癌混淆，因为其中某些病例显示小腺泡结构，伴有轻微的基底细胞增生。然而，不完全性BCH的腺泡由两种细胞构成，即内层的立方或柱状细胞以及外层的基底细胞样细胞，而根据定义前列腺癌则不含有基底细胞层[73,74,297]。低倍镜下BCH界限清楚的生长方式是这一鉴别诊断的最好线索，因为多数前列腺癌具有浸润性生长方式[91,283,284,288]。另外，癌显示细胞核增大并有明显的核仁[68,298-302]。BCH的基底细胞可以有核仁，但如上所述，它们一般是不明显的小核仁[283,284,303,304]。然而，非典型性BCH变型已有描述，它以细胞核增大、多形性、有核分裂象或明显的大核仁（平均直径1.96μm）为特征[305,306]。非典型性BCH这个命名没有临床意义或没有癌前病变的含义，这种改变部分可能与伴随的炎症有关[306]。

TCC累及前列腺容易与BCH鉴别，因为TCC显示明显的细胞学多形性，常见核分裂象并有坏死。另外，多数TCC患者有膀胱TCC的既往病史[246,307]。

其他良性病变，例如鳞状或移行细胞化生，也可能

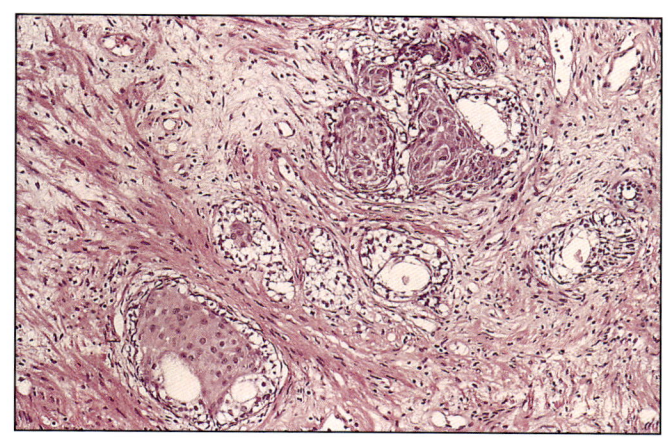

图14A.68 鳞状化生。鳞状化生细胞有丰富的嗜酸性细胞浆以及清楚的细胞边界。鳞状化生通常与雌激素治疗和梗死有关。

类似于BCH，但与BCH鉴别没有临床意义，而且在多数病例中因为具有特征性的组织学表现而容易鉴别。鳞状化生（图14A.68）通常见于梗死附近的区域或接受雌激素治疗的患者[230,233,239]。鳞状化生的细胞往往比基底细胞胞浆丰富，而且细胞界限清楚。移行细胞化生（图14A.69）在前列腺尿道周围的移行区相当常见，尽管它可以明显累及前列腺的周围区；回顾103例连续活检标本发现，34%的标本可见这种病变[45]。化生的移行细胞明显大于BCH的基底细胞，而且细胞浆更加丰富。在移行细胞化生中细胞核的染色质弥漫均匀地散在分布，而在BCH中更多呈团块状，化生的移行细胞细胞核有明显的核沟，在BCH的基底细胞却见不到核沟[304]。

Rioux-Leclercq和Epstein[294]描述了25例伴有少见特征的BCH，分成不同的四种类型：（1）BCH伴有细胞浆内小体（5例）；（2）BCH伴有钙化（8例），其中一个伴有胞浆内小体；（3）BCH伴有鳞状特征（3例）；以及（4）筛状BCH（9例），其中2例伴有胞浆内小体。总共5例含有明显的核仁和（或）细胞非典型性。在任何其他前列腺病变中没有描述过胞浆内玻璃样小体，好像对BCH具有诊断价值。BCH中所见到的钙化是沙粒体样钙化，不同于高级别前列腺癌坏死区域内偶尔见到的点状钙化。伴有鳞状特征的BCH不同于癌（腺鳞癌）的鳞状分化，也不同于伴随前列腺梗死或激素治疗出现的良性鳞状分化灶。筛状PIN和筛状癌腺体是伴有钻孔状腺腔的单一的腺体单位，而筛状BCH病灶内的许多腺体表现为单个BCH腺体的融合。疑难的病例应用34βE12、CK 5/6或p63染色可能有助于诊断。在筛状BCH中，高分子量细胞角蛋白、CK 5/6或p63染色显示某些腺体多层基底细胞染色以及一层连续的免疫反应。筛状PIN显示单层基底细胞有断续的免疫反应。认识BCH中不常见的形态学结构和细胞学特征有利于诊断以及与前列腺癌和高级别PIN的鉴别。

前列腺外周区可以发生BCH，存在于少数前列腺穿刺活检标本（10.2%）以及整个前列腺标本中（23%）[290]。BCH中存在明显核仁时，在诊断上可能要考虑肿瘤性增生。BCH细胞数量似乎随增生指数增加而增加，而同时凋亡指数下降。多数BCH病灶中存在炎症，提示未经治疗患者外周区的BCH可能是对于损伤的固定的反应[290]。

腺样基底细胞肿瘤
Adenoid basal cell tumor（ABT）

这是BCH的一种重要类型，其特征为增生的基底细胞形成较大的融合性结节，直径可达1 cm[284,308]。ABT细胞的细胞核通常比BCH大2~3倍，并且在大小和形状上有些变化。染色质均匀散在分布，细胞核偶尔含有小的核仁。ABT巢可出现腺腔分化区域，偶尔伴有筛状排列（图14A.70）。单个细胞巢常常被增厚的基底膜所围绕。ABT免疫组化发现与BCH类似，表明它们共同来源于前列腺的基底细胞。ABT被认为是局灶侵袭性病变，但有些病变在组织学上与腺样囊性/基底细胞样癌合并存在。

腺样囊性癌/基底细胞样癌
Adenoid cystic carcinoma(ACC)/basaloid carcinoma

这个肿瘤在前列腺中少见，有些研究者已经质疑它的存在，因为这些病变没有表现出浸润性生长或典型的神经周围浸润，而且它们常常含有典型的BCH。没有患者死于本病，并且认为已报道的病例可能是ABT[308]或

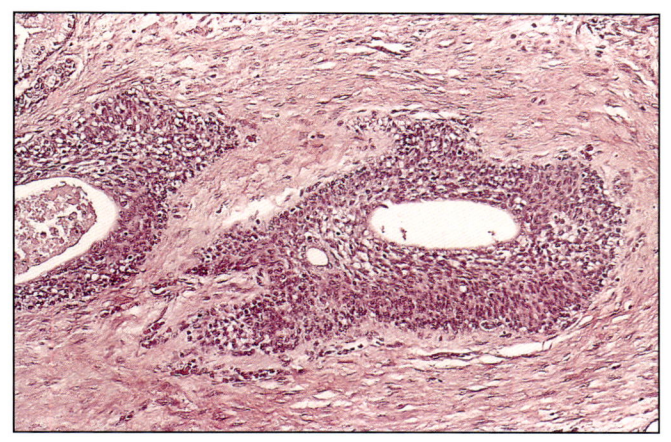

图14A.69 移行细胞化生。移行细胞化生通常见于前列腺尿道周围区。移行细胞化生的细胞比基底细胞增生的细胞大，细胞胞浆更多。

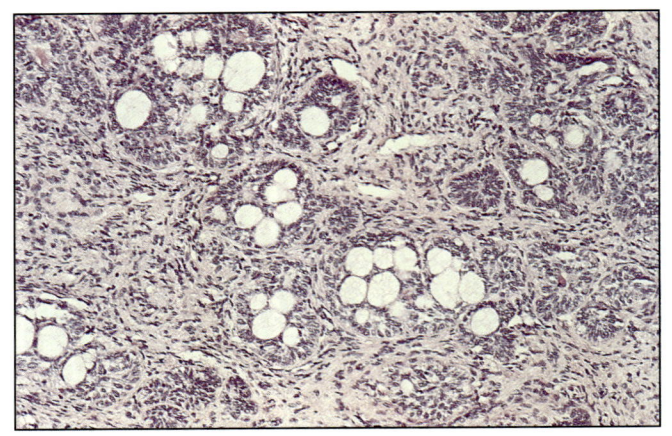

图14A.70 腺样基底细胞肿瘤。实性巢和伴有单个或多个腺腔的细胞巢存在于富于细胞的间质中。

腺样囊样肿瘤[309]。这种肿瘤被认为具有惰性生物学潜能。然而，最近一项19例患者的研究显示有前列腺外扩散（26%）、神经周围浸润（26%）（图14A.71）以及远处转移（21%）[310]。这些作者认为，前列腺ACC/基底细胞癌可能是一种具有侵袭性的肿瘤，需要切除治疗。

与典型的BCH或具有核仁的BCH相比，基底细胞样癌中bcl-2表达（P<0.0001）以及Ki-67指数（P=0.005）升高，而典型的BCH和具有核仁的BCH之间其表达没有显著差别。p53在区分良恶性前列腺基底细胞病变中没有鉴别意义。因此，bcl-2表达升高和较高的Ki-67指数可能有助于前列腺基底细胞增生性病变的诊断[311]。

因为基底细胞样肿瘤p63、CK 5/6以及34βE12常常阳性[284,310]，所以有人提出正常前列腺、BCH、ABT和ACC的基底细胞之间存在一种关系，代表从增生到良性然后进展到恶性肿瘤是一个连续的过程[284]。

McKenney等[312]最近报道一些前列腺基底细胞样细胞增生的病例，其形态学结构不是普通的BCH。前列腺绝大多数明显的基底细胞样细胞增生是两种类型中的一种。第一种类型，与结节性增生（腺样囊样增生）明显相关，尽管可见细胞非典型性和核分裂象，但是它们存在于一个有序的不明确的结节性（非浸润性）结构内。第二种类型（ACC和基底细胞样癌）表现为广泛而杂乱的浸润性生长方式。在行前列腺切除术后，ACC在生物学上是惰性的，但有低度远处转移的危险。

透明细胞筛状增生
Clear cell cribriform hyperplasia

前列腺CCCH是BPH的罕见形式[293,313]。1980年得到WHO认可[69]，1985年Gleason把它描述为前列腺显著的良性乳头状-筛状增生[74]。CCCH和BPH一样具有结节状的生长方式。其特征为累及BPH腺泡的复杂的透明细胞乳头状-筛状增生。在多数病例中，能见到从普通良性增生到CCCH的逐渐过渡[74,69,293]。正确认识它是一种良性病变对于避免它与恶性或癌前病变的混淆是非常重要的，尤其是对于伴有筛状-乳头状结构的病变。CCCH的临床特征基本上与BPH一样。患者年龄58～88岁（平均68岁）[290]。临床诊断几乎总是BPH，伴有尿道梗阻症状；在检查TURP或前列腺切除术标本时可以做出诊断[293,313]。

在组织学检查中，CCCH可以是局灶性或为广泛性，可以部分累及一个或几个前列腺碎片。低倍镜检查它呈结节性生长方式。由于外观温和的透明细胞增生而造成CCCH的腺泡单位扩张，呈乳头状-筛状排列（图14A.72）[293]。在扩张的腺泡周围有明显的由扁平细胞构成的基底细胞层，并与基底膜紧密接触。增生的细胞为圆形、立方形到高柱状，细胞浆多少不等，但通常丰富，

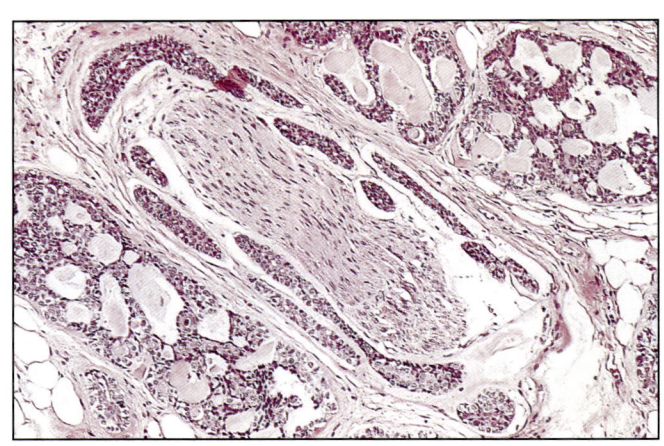

图14A.71 腺样囊性癌。可见腺样囊性癌的筛状结构伴有神经周围浸润。

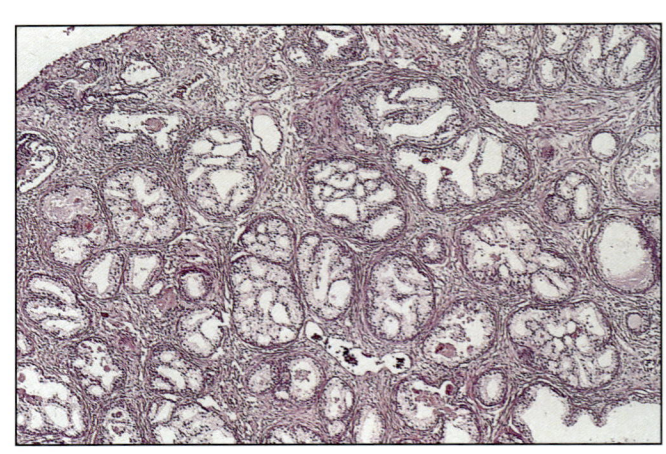

图14A.72 透明细胞筛状增生。这种病变的特征是伴有复杂的乳头状-筛状结构的扩张腺泡的结节性生长。

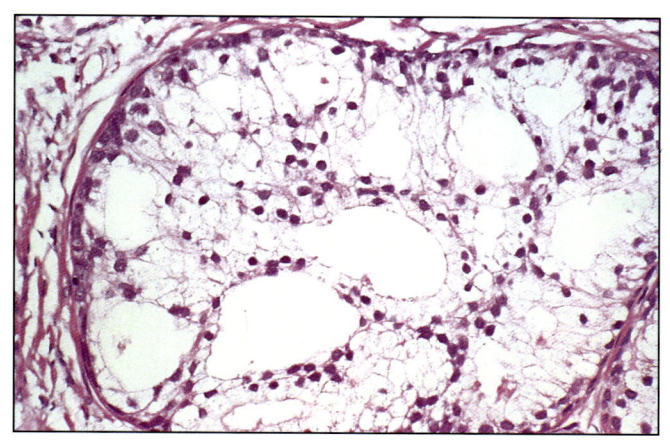

图14A.73 透明细胞筛状增生。腺泡周围存在基底细胞层。透明细胞形状从立方到高柱状，核仁缺乏或不明显。

最常见的是透明胞浆（图14A.73）。细胞核小，均匀一致，圆形到卵圆形，大小通常与周围增生腺泡中的上皮细胞核一致。周围细胞的细胞核略大于增生中心处细胞的细胞核，这表明向中心处的细胞成熟。核仁罕见，如果见到，也是不明显的小核仁。核分裂象缺乏。筛状腔隙内没有酸性黏液或类晶体。可以出现少量糖原，但细胞浆中通常见不到黏液。CCCH周围的间质不同于BPH或正常前列腺，没有纤维组织增生的迹象。CCCH可以伴有BCH；BCH可以存在于远离CCCH的区域，也可发生在CCCH相同的结节内。有些区域表现为两种成分的移行[293]。免疫过氧化物酶研究证实CCCH的透明细胞对PSA和PrAP显示出强阳性反应。高分子量细胞角蛋白（34βE12）、CK 5/6以及p63染色显示连续的基底细胞层（图14A.74）；虽然染色偶尔为局灶性，但是从不缺失或有问题存在[98,304,313]。

重要的是，不能把CCCH误认为是伴有乳头状-筛状结构的前列腺癌或癌前病变。CCCH鉴别诊断中的两个主要病变是筛状腺癌和高级别PIN[271,314]。前列腺腺癌的筛状变型虽然少见，但已得到公认[314]。当没有坏死时，Gleason在其分级系统中认为这种病变是Gleason 3型癌。当存在坏死时为Gleason 5型癌[72]。据报道以这种结构为主的癌，其肿瘤体积大且预后差，所以与CCCH的鉴别诊断有极其重要的意义。诊断CCCH的关键是结合其温和的细胞学特征和结构的均一性。除了均匀一致的透明细胞以及没有明显的细胞学非典型性或核仁以外，其膨胀性结节状生长方式、伴有界限清楚的边缘以及保留两种类型的细胞也是认识本病的主要特征[293]。虽然通过常规HE染色容易发现CCCH存在的基底细胞层，但是应用高分子量细胞角蛋白、CK 5/6或p63免疫染色可能更加易于识别，这些免疫染色在癌中均阴性。另一方面，筛状腺癌是以弥漫性的生长方式、细胞核增大、有明显的核仁以及偶尔出现坏死为特征。PIN可以表现为腔内分泌细胞乳头状突起，在高级别PIN病例中可有筛状结构。高级别PIN通常表现出一系列的形态结构，包括微乳头状、簇状、筛状以及扁平状，高倍镜下检查见细胞核增大，并有明显的核仁[4,5,271]。DNA流式细胞检查有时也可能有助于CCCH与筛状癌和高级别PIN的鉴别诊断，但是实际上没有必要。CCCH总是显示二倍体DNA含量，而筛状癌和高级别PIN可能显示非整倍体DNA含量[313]。

硬化性腺病 Sclerosing adenosis

前列腺硬化性腺病（SA）有许多不同的名称（腺瘤样瘤、纤维上皮性结节以及假腺瘤样瘤）[78,315-321]。Chen和Schiff[315]首次报道了这种病变，注意到其形态学类似于腺瘤样瘤，因此把这种病变命名为腺瘤样前列腺肿瘤。Hulman[316]也报道了相似的前列腺病变，应用组织化学和免疫组化的方法与典型腺瘤样瘤进行比较；他认为这种病变是前列腺源性，推荐使用假腺瘤样瘤这个词。Sesterhenn和Mostofi[317]提供25例SA的资料，他们以抽象的形式命名为前列腺纤维上皮性结节。根据组织学上与乳腺的SA相似，Young和Clement[318]使用了SA这个术语。SA是少见病变，以富于细胞的间质内含有大小不等的通常为小的增生的腺体为特征。SA在实践中和学术上都具有重要意义，因为它在组织学上明显类似于腺癌以及因为它的肌上皮细胞分化[78,79,309,318]（正常前列腺基底细胞无肌上皮特征，已经被Srigley[91]所证实）。Sakamoto等[319]回顾了263名前列腺癌患者的切片发现5例SA，其发生率为1.9%。

SA不是癌前病变。这种病变通常小，范围为

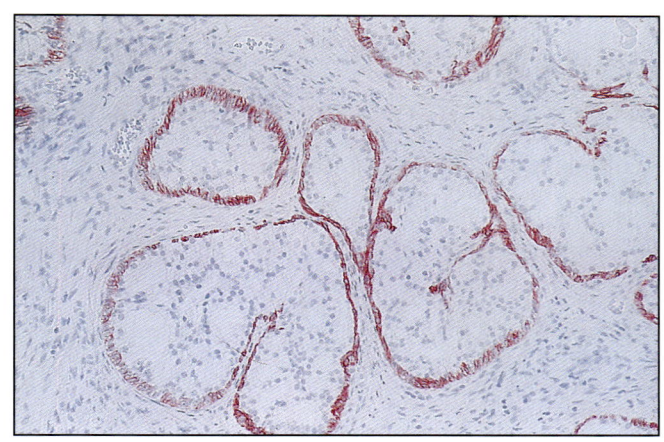

图14A.74 透明细胞筛状增生的基底细胞34βE12（K-903）染色阳性，而透明细胞阴性。

1.5～11.0 mm（平均 4.2 mm）。本病见于 TURP 或前列腺切除术标本（很少见于前列腺活检组织）[320]，与其他增生性良性病变一样位于移行区[78]。多数 SA 界限清楚，但没有被膜。某些病例病变的外周可见微小浸润。

显微镜下检查，SA 的特征为边界不清楚的结节，含有不规则的小腺泡以及细胞巢或细胞簇，位于富于细胞的间质中（图 14A.75）[78,315-318]。其中一些腺体轻微扩张，而另一些呈微小腺泡结构。评价被覆细胞的性质通常是困难的。多数基底细胞模糊不清或被挤压，但在多数病例中，有些腺体明确显示有基底细胞层的存在（图 14A.76）。腺腔细胞较大，细胞浆透明或嗜酸，细胞核位于基底部。位于基底部的细胞往往扁平或立方，细胞核平行于基底膜。浓厚的嗜酸性基底膜样物质围绕某些腺体。腺腔内可有阿辛蓝阳性酸性黏液以及类晶体[78]。间质是这种病变的组成部分，一般非常富于细胞，常常为黏液样[320,321]，由肥胖的纤维母细胞/肌纤维母细胞和平滑肌细胞组成。

免疫组化和超微结构分析显示，SA 腺体成分内的细胞广谱 CK、高分子量细胞角蛋白（克隆性 34βE12）、CK 5/6 以及 p63 阳性，提示为前列腺基底细胞来源。另外，在腺体成分和间质内可见明确的 MSA 和 S-100 蛋白阳性细胞团，提示肌上皮分化[319-321]。超微结构分析也证明在 SA 中有肌上皮分化，由此得出结论，SA 中的肌上皮细胞很可能是由前列腺基底细胞化生性改变过程所导致[78]。这些发现已被其他学者所证实[3,319,320]。

前列腺小腺泡腺癌是 SA 主要的鉴别诊断。与前列腺癌不同，SA 的特征是腺体和间质两种成分增生。SA 中小而密集排列的腺泡状结构伴有浸润性生长方式可能与肿瘤性腺体混淆，增生性间质可被误认为纤维组织增生性反应。在低倍镜下 SA 呈小叶性增生，腺体大小和形状常常不一，至少有些腺体有明确的双层细胞。基底细胞的存在可由高分子量细胞角蛋白（克隆性 34βE12）、CK 5/6 或 p63 染色所证实，这是排除腺癌诊断的关键特征[99,292,295]。然而，SA 基底细胞高分子量细胞角蛋白（克隆性 34βE12）、CK 5/6 或 p63 染色可以是局灶性的。与 SA 不同，小腺泡腺癌更常趋向于浸润周围的前列腺间质[73,74]。癌细胞的核仁通常明显。SA 的腺体和被挤压的小管可以被增厚的透明基底膜样物质所围绕，这在癌中见不到。SA 间质细胞丰富，由肥胖的梭形细胞构成，而浸润性腺癌通常不能引起间质反应或导致玻璃样变的细胞稀少的纤维组织增生性反应。腺腔内酸性黏液和类晶体在鉴别 SA 和癌的诊断中没有帮助，因为 SA 和癌都有这些特征[75,78-81]。

与癌类似的其他病变
Miscellaneous lesions that mimic carcinoma

中肾残件增生
Hyperplasia of mesonephric remnants

中肾残件增生少见，但是很重要，它是前列腺内的小腺体增生。一个误诊病例证实了这个诊断陷阱的严重性，这个病例误诊为癌，导致了根治性前列腺切除术，手术后没有发现癌的证据[322]。最近 Bostwick 等[323]指出不到 1% 的经尿道前列腺切除标本中存在中肾残件，在穿刺活检中更为少见。腺泡呈小叶状或浸润性，在结构上可以被误认为腺癌。这种细胞学上的良性发现可能导致低估诊断，并解释为良性前列腺腺泡，但是这没有明显的临床意义[323]。这种病变无症状，偶然发现，因此

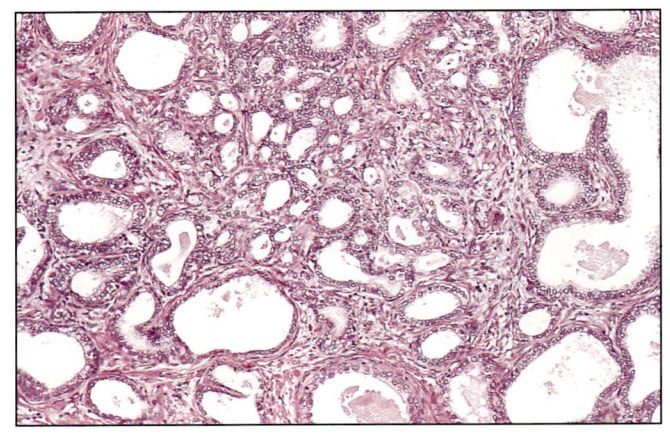

图 14A.75　硬化性腺病。小腺体增生伴有富于细胞的间质。

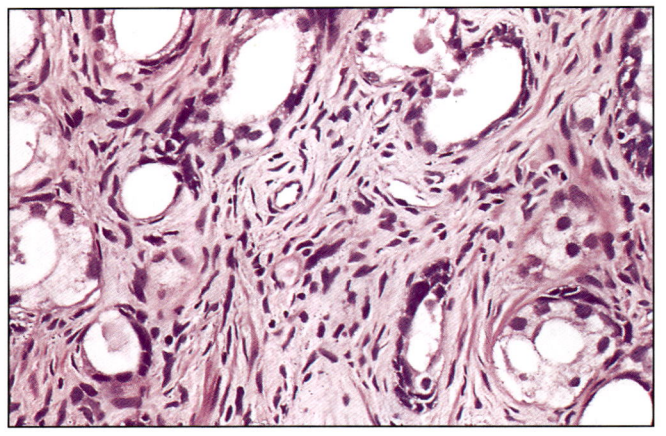

图 14A.76　硬化性腺病。至少有些小腺体有基底细胞。注意明显的富于细胞的间质。

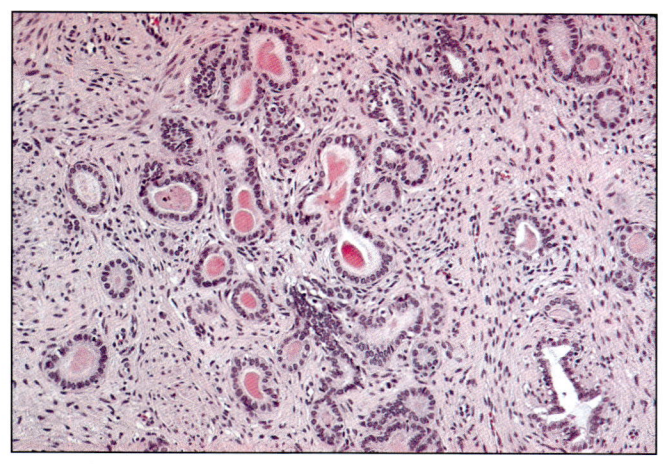

图14A.77 典型的中肾性增生。这种小腺体增生伴有内衬深染细胞核的小腺体和较大的腺体。腺腔内存在粉红色分泌物，间质是反应性的。

没有特征性的大体特征。显微镜下，其特征为内衬单层上皮的小管状结构呈小叶状增生或在平滑肌束和前列腺腺泡之间有浸润性腺体，没有纤维组织增生性间质反应[323]。小管大小不一，偶尔有囊肿形成及管内乳头状突起，扩张的腺体内有嗜酸性分泌物（图14A.77）[322-325]。细胞立方形，细胞浆稀少，因此好像是"萎缩"的细胞。病变细胞PSA和PrAP染色阴性，可以证实其为非前列腺谱系的细胞；病变细胞本身高分子量细胞角蛋白克隆性34βE12阳性[323]。细胞核温和没有明显的核仁。中肾残留可能伴有神经节和神经，类似于神经周围浸润，以致与癌混淆[322,324]。

Ayala等描述了以前不认识的中肾增生性病变[326]。这种病变由小管状结构组成，小管略大于正常导管，内衬深染的增生性长梭形上皮细胞；这些细胞PSA、PrAP、p63或高分子量细胞角蛋白阴性。这种病变的细胞核细长或梭形，密集深染以致看不清细胞核内的细节（图14A.78）。这种病变类似附睾，因此，在前列腺芯针活检中可能与高级别PIN相混淆。

精阜黏膜腺体增生
Verumontanum mucosal gland hyperplasia

精阜黏膜腺体增生（VMGH）是指精阜的小腺体增生，见于14%～29%的根治性前列腺切除标本中[327,328]。有资料显示可在穿刺活检组织中见到，有误诊为癌的可能性[329]。VMGH呈膨胀性生长，界限清楚，腺体腔小，排列呈背靠背方式。当在高倍镜下仔细观察细胞学的特征时，与癌的鉴别通常没有问题。腺体易见基底细胞层，并且含有淀粉样小体或橙棕色分泌物，细胞核不增大，无明显的核仁（图14A.79）。除癌之外，鉴别诊断包括NA、中肾残件增生以及非典型性腺瘤性增生。腺体PSA和PrAP阳性，基底细胞高分子量细胞角蛋白（克隆性34βE12）、CK 5/6或p63阳性。VMGH与正常精阜腺体的区别相对主观，需要认识这种病变的原因是可能将其误诊为癌[328]。一个研究报道VMGH的存在与非典型性腺瘤性增生有明显的相关性（$P < 0.001$，Fisher精确试验），并认为非典型性腺瘤

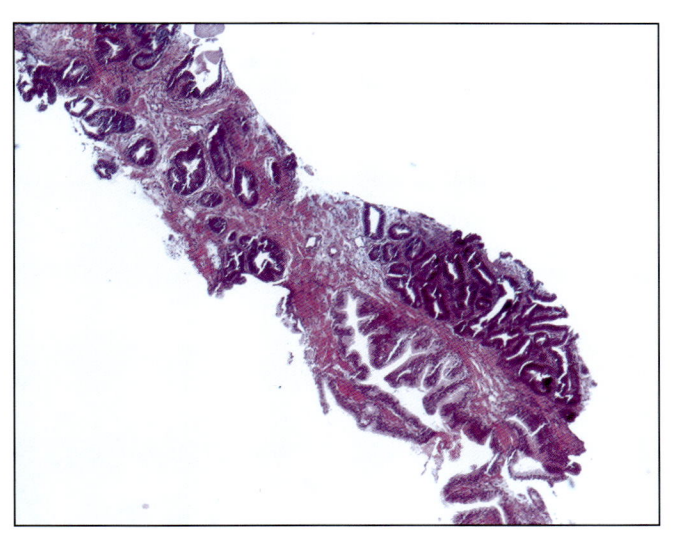

A

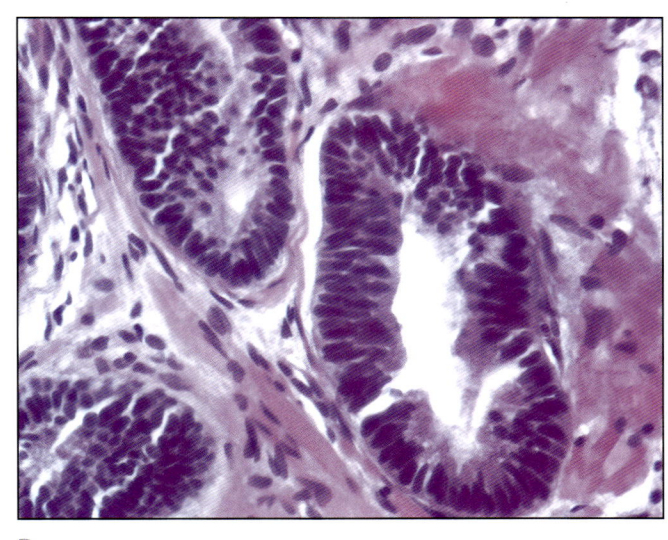

B

图14A.78 （A）中肾性增生，附睾型，类似于高级别前列腺上皮内肿瘤形成（PIN）。这种病变由略大于正常导管的管状结构构成，内衬增生的复层长梭形上皮细胞。（B）中肾性增生，附睾型，类似于高级别PIN。高倍镜下，腺体细胞核的特征是核深染，核的细节模糊，细胞与基底膜垂直。这种病变非常类似于横切的附睾，在前列腺芯针活检中可能与高级别PIN相混淆。

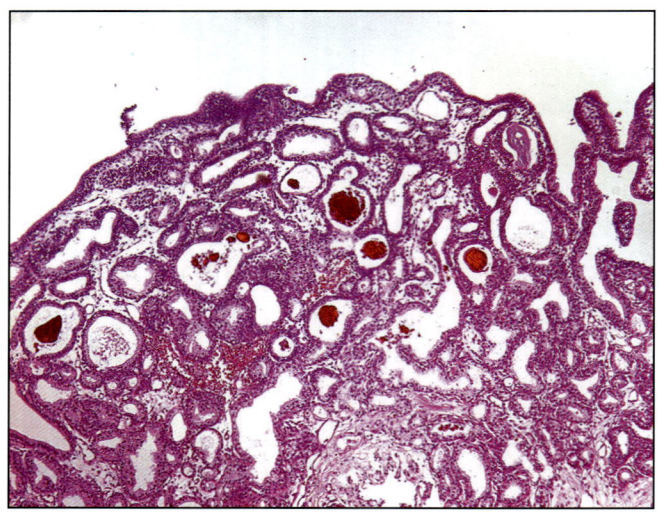

图14A.79 精阜黏膜腺体增生。这种病变是小到中等大小腺体的增生，基底细胞不明显。存在棕黄色腔内分泌物。

表现也是密集排列的小腺体增生[288,338,339]。

大体上，2/3 的 NA 是乳头状的；其余的是息肉样或无蒂[288]。显微镜下，NA 的特征是密集排列的小管状结构（内生性成分），伴有固有层水肿，而且好像在前列腺导管之间浸润，造成诊断上与癌的重叠。这些小管大小和形状差异很大，有时存在囊性扩张。这些小管通常较小，圆形到卵圆形，但可以弯曲，类似肾集合管或肾曲小管(图 14A.80)。可见乳头状突起，或者在表面（外生性成分）或者在扩张导管内[340]。小管、囊肿以及乳头主要被覆立方或柱状细胞。细胞浆通常缺乏，但偶尔可见中等到多量嗜酸或透明细胞浆。细胞核圆形，小或固缩，通常缺乏核仁，但有时核仁可以明显的。在某些区域，细胞核可以有"鞋钉"样外观（图 14A.81）。在罕见病例中，实性小管或被覆单层细胞的小管弥漫性增生，细胞核被细胞浆内腔隙挤压，类似于印戒细胞腺癌[288,333]。某些病例中细胞浆内可见糖原和黏液。尽管 NA 可见于

性增生和 VMGH 常常发生于其中一种病变存在时的前列腺中[328]。

肾源性腺瘤　Nephrogenic adenoma

肾源性腺瘤（NA）是从肾盂到尿道的被覆尿路上皮器官的良性病变（也见第 12 章）；本病在 1949 年由 Davis[330] 首先描述，他把这种病变命名为膀胱错构瘤，但是随后不久，Friedman 和 Kuhlenbeck[331] 根据它类似于发生中的肾小管以及可能具有肿瘤潜能，而把这种病变确定为现在的名字。虽然 NA 主要发生在膀胱，但是 10%～15% 病例累及尿道，在输尿管[332] 和肾盂[288,333] 少见。在尿道，NA 发生在球部和前列腺部，也可以发生在尿道憩室内[332-334]。在成人中男性占绝大多数，而在儿童中女性占多数，男女比例 1:3[288,333,335,336]。患者年龄范围 4～83 岁（平均 41 岁）。最常见的伴随状况包括手术史或创伤、感染、结石或肾移植病史[288,333]。这种病变通常单发，但可以多发[333]；病变通常小（0.5～2 cm），但是更大的甚至累及整个膀胱表面的病变已被报道[337]。大约 20% 的患者病变在膀胱镜检查时发现或偶然在显微镜下发现。其余患者的症状和体征为非特异性的，包括血尿、排尿困难、尿频、尿急以及耻骨上或胁腹部疼痛[333]。

NA 可见于 TURP 标本，因为在 TURP 操作过程中可能取到尿路上皮黏膜及上皮下组织。少见的是，它也可见于前列腺穿刺活检标本。当 NA 存在于前列腺尿道中，并且侵犯尿路上皮下组织而且似乎浸润前列腺固有实质时，可与前列腺腺癌混淆，因为 NA 常见的组织学

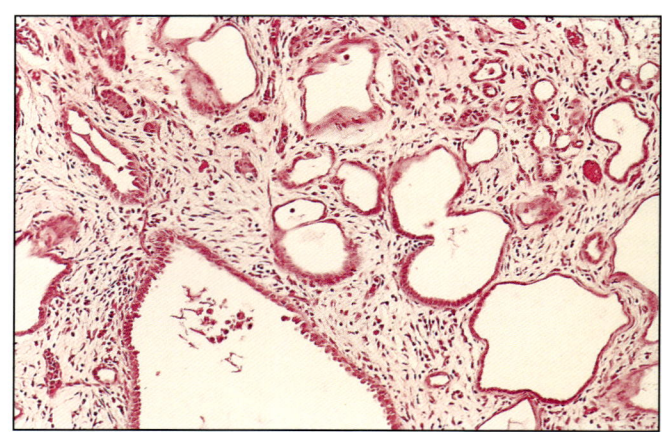

图14A.80 肾源性腺瘤。增生的小而扩张的腺体类似于肾小管。

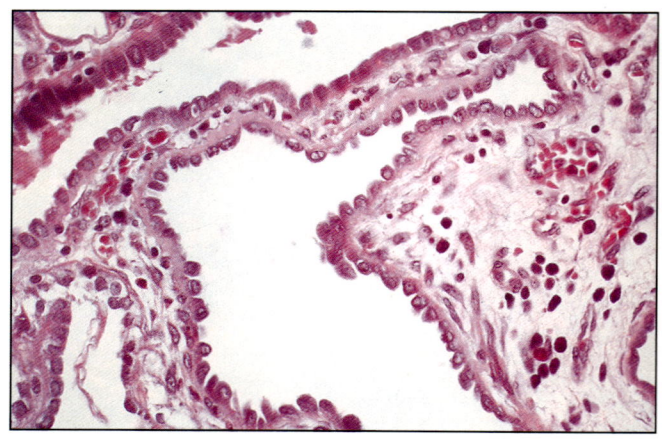

图14A.81 肾源性腺瘤。小管主要内衬伴有嗜酸性胞浆的立方细胞。某些细胞具有"鞋钉"样外观。

前列腺导管之间，但必须记住 NA 不是一个浸润性病变。前列腺尿道有黏膜下腺体，但前列腺导管的产物也排入尿道腔。因此 NA 可以与前列腺导管接触，产生 NA 浸润前列腺的假象。

超微结构和凝集素结合研究显示胚胎性肾小管和 NA 有某些相似性[341]；然而，其胚胎性来源还没有证实。目前多数研究者根据年龄范围广泛、部位分布、与创伤和炎症密切相关，以及有从尿路上皮向 NA 过渡的证据，支持化生性来源[333,338,342]。有些研究者提出 NA 是泌尿生殖道透明细胞癌的前体病变或对应的良性病变。尽管报道了几例与透明细胞腺癌同时存在的病例，但是没有证实两者有直接关系。NA 在保守治疗后可以复发，但是没有伴有明确恶性改变的病例。目前一致认为 NA 不是癌前病变[288,333,342-344]。

累及前列腺尿道的 NA 主要的鉴别诊断包括前列腺腺癌和尿道透明细胞癌[288,333,338,339,344]。NA 与透明细胞癌的鉴别通常不难，因为后者具有较弥漫的生长方式和较明显的细胞学非典型性；发生在男性尿道的透明细胞癌非常罕见，仅有 3 例报道（图 14A.82）[68,345]。当 NA 出现管状、条索或印戒样小管结构，有明显的核仁，下面的纤维平滑肌受累，有淡蓝色黏液性分泌物，局灶性 PSA 和 PrAP 阳性以及 34βE12 阴性（某些病例）时，NA 小而密集排列的小管可能与前列腺腺癌非常相似[346,347]。然而，用于诊断 NA 的特征包括：(1) 通常缺乏细胞核的非典型性或核仁；(2) 小管大小不一；(3) 典型的水肿或炎性间质；(4) 独特的中肾结构，例如乳头和"血管"；(5) 邻近尿路上皮；(6) 出现甲状腺样组织；(7) 小管周围鞘；(8) PrAP 和 PSA 阴性；(9) CK 7 阳性，在某些疑难的病例 34βE12 阳性[288,338,339,346,347]。细胞浆内黏液染色阳性提示 NA，因为前列腺腺癌的黏液往往位于腔内[75]。

最近确定的前列腺癌标志物 AMACR（P504S）在 NA 的细胞浆中呈强阳性反应，提示 NA 不仅在形态学上与前列腺癌相似，而且在免疫组化上也相似[346,348]。它编码 AMACR，这个蛋白参与脂肪酸支链的 β-氧化。在前列腺腺癌的鉴别诊断中 NA 是一个重要的诊断陷阱，而且仔细检查 HE 染色的切片仍然是正确诊断的关键，同时 PSA 染色阴性可支持这个诊断[348]。

前列腺型尿道息肉
Prostatic-type urethral polyp

含有前列腺组织的息肉样病变偶尔见于前列腺尿道，尤其是在精阜部位，少数情况下见于膜性尿道，尿道口以及膀胱三角区罕见（也见第 12 章）[207-212,349]。这些病变的患者通常年轻，发生于 20～30 岁或 30～40 岁，表现为与射精密切相关的血精或血尿[207-212,349]。这些病变被认为是年轻男性血尿的最常见原因。这些病变曾经被命名为前列腺尿道腺瘤性息肉[210]、前列腺尿道息肉[211]、前列腺尿道乳头状腺瘤[212,350]以及前列腺肉阜[349]。本病发病机制仍不明确，虽然有人提出是继发于发育异常的异位[209,212,349,351-354]、前列腺导管脱垂[349]、增生性病变[211,355]、黏膜过多[355]、化生[208]以及肿瘤形成[356]。

这些病变由乳头状或腺管状组织学结构组成（图 14A.83）。它们被覆柱状前列腺上皮或前列腺和移行上皮混合。在息肉间质内可见不同数量的腺体结构。在形态学上，它们与前列腺腺体相同，通常被覆两层细胞，由细胞核位于基底的高柱状上皮细胞和周围的扁平基底细胞层构成。偶尔，腔内可见淀粉样小体。没有见到细胞多形性、坏死、核分裂象增多或明显的核仁（图 14A.84）。PSA 和 PrAP 免疫组化染色强阳性，证实这些病变是前列腺来源[207-212,349,351-356]。所有这些病变的行为均为良性，并不被认为是癌前病变。主要的鉴别诊断包括前列腺导管-子宫内膜样癌。与前列腺息肉不同，导管-

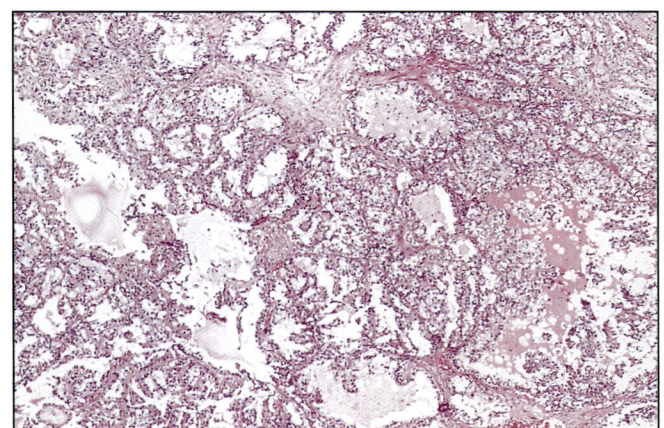

图 14A.82　透明细胞腺癌。这个低倍照片显示细胞丰富的肿瘤伴有小管和乳头状结构。

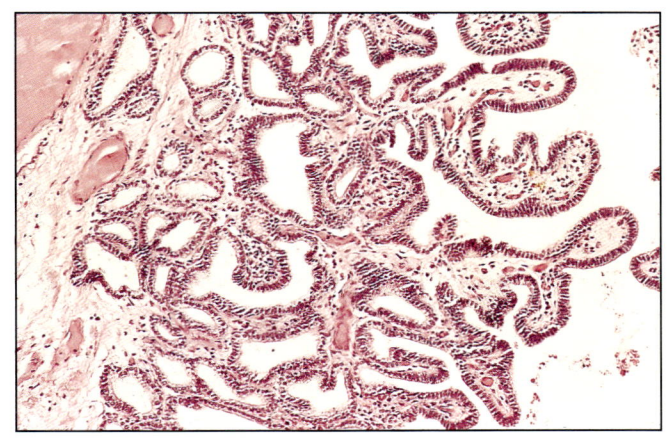

图 14A.83　前列腺息肉。这个息肉样病变是由乳头状和腺体结构组成的。

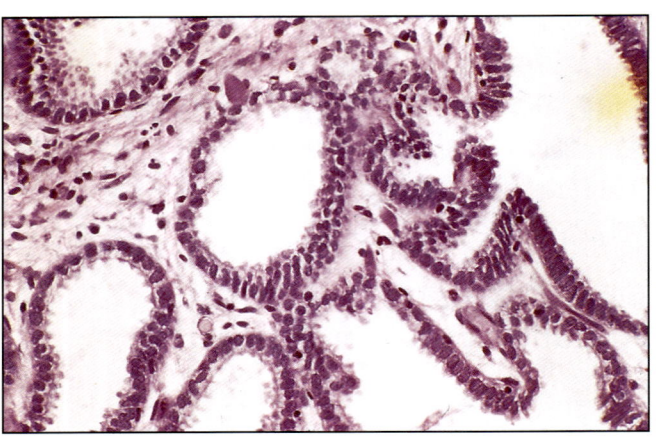

图14A.84 前列腺息肉。被覆细胞均匀一致，没有核的多形性、核分裂象增多或明显的核仁。

子宫内膜样癌通常表现为细胞核间变、明显的核仁、核分裂象以及肿瘤坏死[192]。

可能类似于前列腺腺癌的正常组织解剖结构和非肿瘤性病变
Normal histoanatomic structures and non-neoplastic lesions that may simulate adenocarcinoma of the prostate

射精管和精囊组织
Ejaculatory ducts and seminal vesicle tissue

在检查TURP或前列腺穿刺活检标本时偶尔可见来自精囊和射精管的组织碎片，在两项研究中报道其发生率是3%～23%[357,358]。精囊和射精管的组织学特征十分相似，在穿刺活检或TURP标本中有时很难区别。这两者都有管泡状腺体以及密集排列的小腺泡，内衬假复层高柱状分泌细胞以及一层小的基底细胞[53,54,357,358]。在活检中发现这些结构时，通常是来自中央区，常常是射精管而不是精囊。除非在超声引导下特异性定位精囊，否则精囊位置通常太深，通过随机活检或TURP不易取到。射精管和精囊上皮的特征是含有粗大颗粒状棕黄色脂褐素[53]。精囊和射精管上皮细胞常有大的非典型性细胞核；这些细胞核深染，因为染色质结构模糊，所以通常见不到细胞核的细节（图14A.85）。核仁和核分裂象很少出现[53,55,288]。Kuo和Gomez[53]在他们所检查的32例精囊中，24例（75%）显示有怪异的上皮细胞。因为这些结构常常为小腺体，呈背靠背排列，所以可与前列腺小腺泡癌混淆[53,55,73,282,288]。辨认精囊和射精管上皮的三个主要特征是：包括怪异细胞在内的明显的细胞核不规则性，核内包涵体和细胞浆内金黄色-棕色粗大折光性色素颗粒[53,54,73,282,288]。然而，必须记住的是极少数前列腺腺癌也含有脂褐素。这种色素往往比精囊的色素细腻，而且折光性小[56]。出现伴有明显核仁的规则的单形性细胞核以及缺乏基底细胞层支持癌的诊断。精囊分泌物相当常见，当呈液态时，由酸性黏多糖构成。分泌物浓缩好像伴有酸性丧失，可能导致致密的板片样分泌物和结晶形成。当诊断精囊上皮可能与前列腺癌混淆的前列腺穿刺活检时，了解精囊组织类晶体的形态学以及与前列腺类结晶的鉴别特征可能是重要的，因为小腺泡的形态学伴有细胞学非典型性和类晶体[359]。

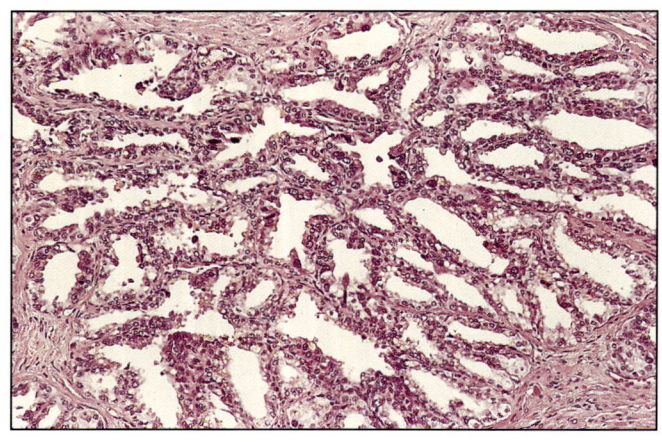
A

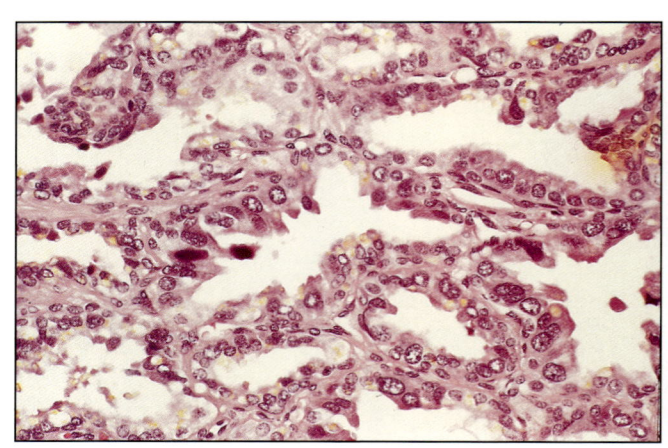
B

图14A.85 （A）精囊具有小腺泡结构。精囊的主要特征包括散在的多形性细胞核（怪异细胞）以及细胞浆内金黄色-棕色脂褐素颗粒。（B）高倍镜下显示怪异细胞和金黄色-棕色脂褐素颗粒。

精囊/射精管上皮PSA和PrAP阴性,但MUC6阳性,这种染色有助于精囊/射精管上皮与前列腺腺癌(MUC6阴性)的鉴别诊断[360]。

Cowper腺和副神经节组织
Cowper's glands and paraganglionic tissue

在TURP或穿刺活检标本中偶尔可以包含来自尿道球部Cowper腺体的组织[361,362]。Cowper腺是位于靠近前列腺尖端的尿生殖隔内的成对的结构,由呈背靠背排列的黏液性腺泡组成的小叶构成(图14A.86)。它们具有排泄导管,常被骨骼肌包绕。Cowper腺可与高分化前列腺腺癌相混淆;然而,Cowper腺表面上类似于小涎腺,温和的细胞核特征、缺乏明显的核仁、伴有骨骼肌、丰富的胞浆内黏液以及PSA和PrAP免疫反应阴性可以做出正确的诊断[91,73,282,361-363]。

前列腺黏液腺化生已被描述,并且可与Cowper腺相似(图14A.87)。然而,这种病变是随机分布于前列腺组织内;它可以局限于一个腺泡或累及成组的腺泡,但通常较小[364,365]。

存在于前列腺标本中的另外一种可能与癌混淆的正常结构是副神经节组织[91,282,366,367]。通常,副神经节组织存在于邻近外侧神经血管束的前列腺周围脂肪内,在少数情况下可见于前列腺外侧间质中。它由透明细胞团构成,伴有窦状血管结构、"细胞球(Zellballen)"外观、温和的卵圆形细胞核特征,通常有丰富的透明胞浆,并与神经纤维密切相关,上述特征可正确识别这种结构(图14A.88)。偶尔,存在伴有较大细胞核的较大的细胞。如果对它的真正本质存在任何的怀疑,前列腺(PSA和PrAP)和上皮(角蛋白和上皮膜抗原)标志物免疫染色阴性以及神经内分泌标志物[如神经元特异性烯醇化

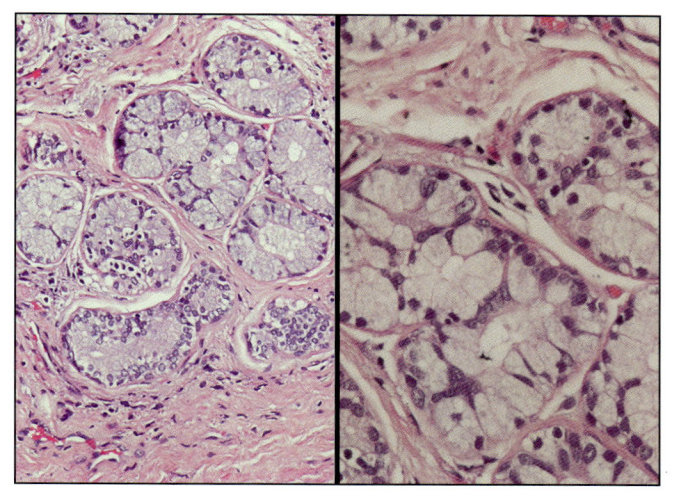

A

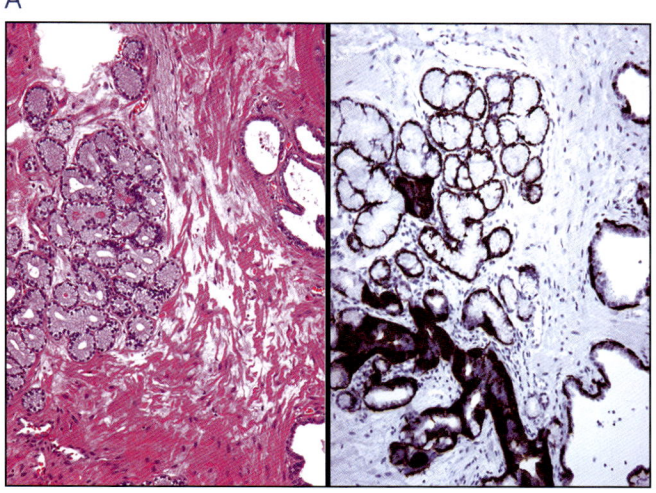

B

图14A.87 (A)黏液性化生。右图和左图显示圆形腺体,其特征是出现分泌黏液的细胞,伴有杯状空泡,表面上类似于Cowper腺。(B)黏液性化生。左图中的小腺体类似于Gleason 1或2型癌,但是右侧高分子量细胞角蛋白染色显示基底细胞层。

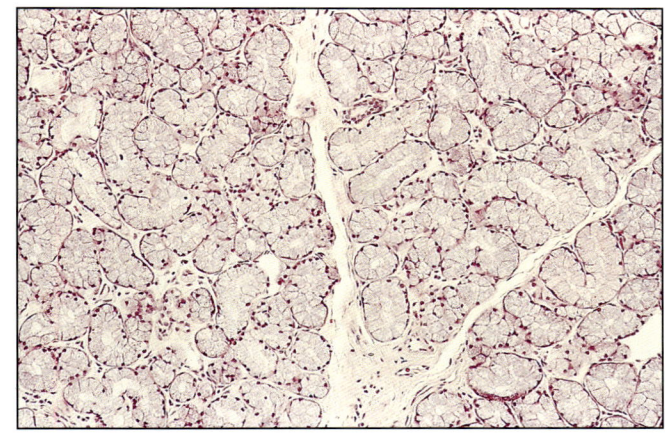

图14A.86 Cowper腺。分叶状的黏液性腺泡呈背靠背排列。细胞核形态温和,没有明显的核仁及丰富的黏液性胞浆,这是辨认Cowper腺的关键特征。

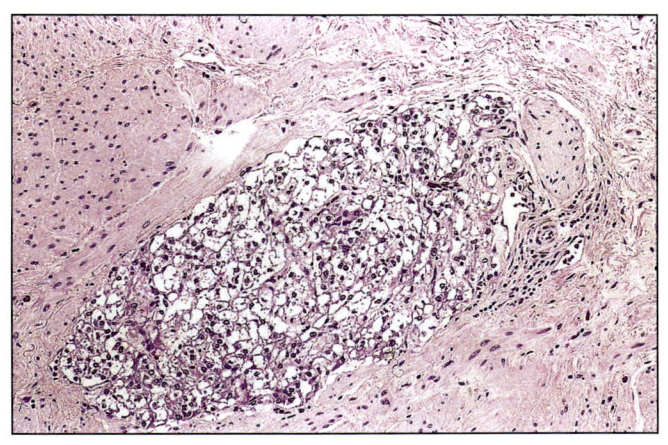

图14A.88 副神经节组织为胞浆透明的小细胞呈器官样排列,非常接近小神经和血管。

酶（NSE）、嗜铬素和突触素]染色阳性可以解决诊断问题[363]。已经报道了几例累及前列腺的副神经节瘤[368]。

萎缩　Atrophy

前列腺萎缩是老年男性相对常见的病变，但是也可见于20岁的成人[3,73,369-372]。萎缩可与增生共存，即使在同一个显微镜视野内[373]。它常常位于周围区，但在移行区和中央区也可出现[91,295]。在绝大多数病例中，萎缩的原因尚不清楚，推测是生理性和老年相关现象[370]。炎症[373]、营养缺乏、局部缺血[374]以及压迫被认为在萎缩的发病机制中起重要作用[11,372,375]。多数萎缩患者无症状，萎缩是在检查因为其他原因而行穿刺活检或TURP标本时偶然发现的。

显微镜下检查，萎缩可以是弥漫性或为局灶性。根据组织学表现，萎缩可以分为单纯性小叶萎缩、囊性萎缩或硬化性萎缩[373]。单纯性小叶萎缩是以密集排列的小腺泡聚集为特征，通常位于中央导管周围，保留正常小叶结构（图14A.89）。在囊性萎缩中，周围的腺泡变为囊性（图14A.90）。在硬化性萎缩中，小叶结构可以存在或不存在。萎缩性腺泡被硬化性间质成分不同程度地挤压和分离，导致腺体变长和扭曲，并被腺泡周围增生的纤维胶原组织所分隔（图14A.91）。这种类型的萎缩通常比单纯性小叶萎缩发生的年龄偏大[73,91,282,288,295]。前列腺间质弹力组织变性常常伴有萎缩[376]。

Gardner和Culberson[369]描述了另外一种类型的萎缩，表现为完全的发育不全。他们认为这不是真正的萎缩，而实际上是青春期后持续存在的腺体，它们保留了新生儿或青春期前未受刺激的前列腺形态。不管萎缩的形态如何，萎缩的腺体均内衬深染的矮立方到扁平细胞，伴有少量胞浆和温和的细胞核（图14A.92）。需要特别注意的是多数病例缺乏明显的核仁；当出现核仁时，它们总是小而不明显。通常存在基底细胞和分泌细胞双层细胞，但是，因为分泌细胞缺乏丰富的细胞浆，它们看

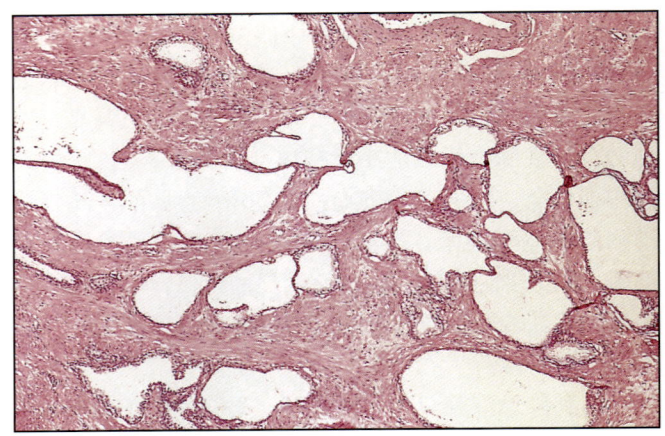

图14A.90　囊性萎缩。扩张的腺泡内衬扁平萎缩的细胞。

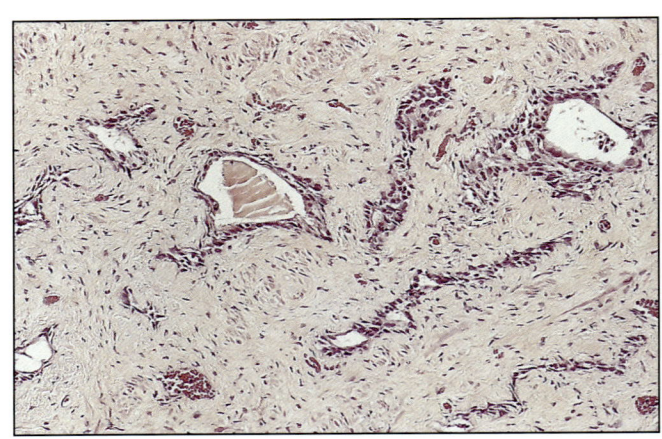

图14A.91　硬化性萎缩。内衬萎缩上皮细胞的不规则扭曲的裂隙样腺泡，位于宽带样的硬化性间质中。

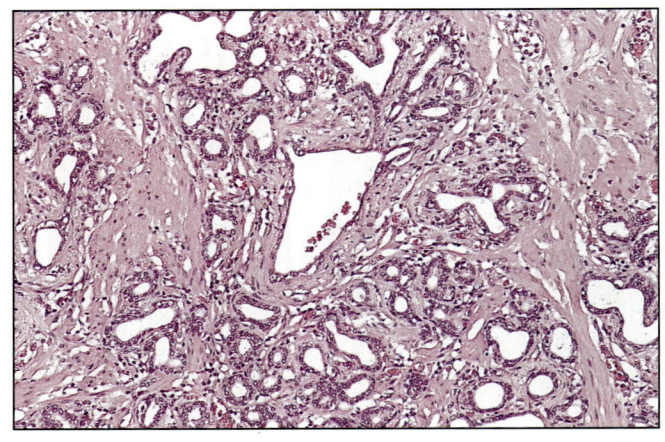

图14A.89　单纯性小叶萎缩。其特征是小腺体增生围绕中心扩张的导管，保存小叶结构。

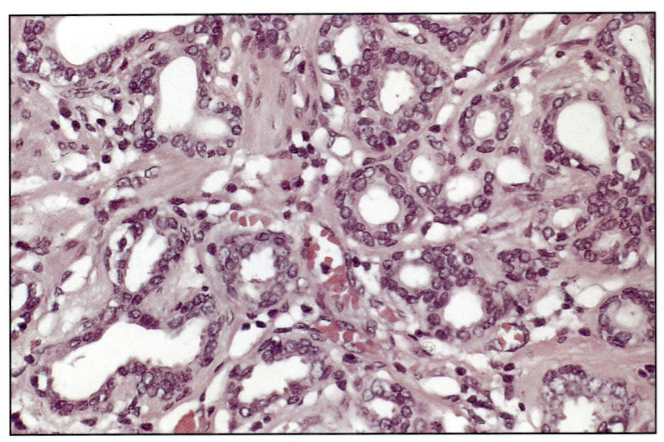

图14A.92　单纯性小叶萎缩的高倍放大。萎缩的腺体内衬均一的细胞，伴有深染的细胞核。核仁通常缺乏或不明显。

起来好像与基底细胞相似，这给辨认这两种类型的细胞造成了困难[73,91,282,288,295,371-373]。如果存在任何怀疑，应该做高分子量细胞角蛋白（克隆性34βE12）、CK 5/6或p63染色来证实基底细胞的存在，进而排除癌（图14A.93）[297,377,378]。萎缩有时伴有炎症和腺体周围纤维化，所以在周围的间质中经常见到散在的炎细胞[295,373]。在TURP或前列腺切除标本中见到萎缩时，做出诊断问题不大；而在穿刺活检中与腺癌鉴别或许会有困难。硬化性萎缩最常造成诊断困难，尤其是如果把间质反应当成肿瘤诱导的纤维组织增生时更是如此[91,288]。低倍镜下的结构特征、双层细胞以及温和的细胞学表明是一种良性病变。一种极具挑战性的情况是鉴别萎缩与伴有"萎缩"特征的癌。评价其浸润方式以及明智地应用免疫组化染色[高分子量细胞角蛋白（克隆性34βE12）、CK5/6、p63]对于诊断是有帮助的[93-95,379]。偶尔，萎缩的腺泡可以伴有继发性上皮增生性改变；这样的病变被某些研究者命名萎缩后增生（postatrophic hyperplasia，PAH）[371,372,380-382]。

萎缩后增生　Postatrophic hyperplasia

萎缩后增生（PAH）可发生在单纯性小叶萎缩或硬化性萎缩的背景中：小叶增生由单纯性小叶萎缩发展而来，而硬化后增生由硬化性萎缩发展而来。当小叶萎缩发生继发性增生性改变时，通常累及整个小叶，并且从萎缩的小腺体出芽形成密集排列的新腺泡。当在硬化性萎缩背景中发生继发性增生时，从萎缩的导管出芽形成小腺泡增生并穿透进入邻近致密的硬化性间质中。

在穿刺活检标本中，PAH与癌非常相似，见于2%～3%病例[380]。因为PAH存在萎缩和增生两种病变过程，所以如同普通的萎缩一样，腺体可以小而密集排列，胞浆稀少，或可能显示伴有增生腺泡的新的腺泡结构，可以见到透明的胞浆。诊断的线索是腺体大小和形状不同以及胞浆内容不等[380,381]。细胞学表现温和，没有明显的核仁，缺乏明显的浸润性生长或腺体融合，以及至少局部存在基底细胞层有助于避免误诊为癌。高分子量细胞角蛋白（克隆性34βE12）、CK 5/6或p63免疫染色有助于显示基底细胞，并证实良性病变的诊断[380]。

PAH和前列腺腺癌之间的关系存在争议。Anton等[382]根据系统的分区绘图研究坚持认为这两种病变没有关系。然而，Franks[371]和Liavag[372]提出硬化性萎缩后的PAH是小腺泡癌的前身，其根据是观察到两种病变同时发生在外周区，并且小腺泡增生（再生性）常见于萎缩的附近[371,372]（图14A.94）。相反McNeal报道，前列腺癌发生在上皮活跃的腺体，从来没有任何的萎缩[10,12,375,383,384]。最近的研究证实PAH中p53突变的频率与高级别PIN[385]相似，通过MIB-1标记显示的增生活性以及8号染色体的扩增明显高于BPH或单纯性萎缩，提示PAH和前列腺腺癌之间可能有关系[385-387]。然而，Anton等[382]没有证实PAH和前列腺癌之间有任何的关系。膀胱前列腺切除标本中PAH的发生率及其与偶发前列腺癌的关系与根治性前列腺切除标本没有明显的差异。PAH是相对常见的病变，最常见于前列腺尖端1/3的周围区。

前列腺内的骨骼肌和神经周围间隙的良性腺体　Skeletal muscle within prostate gland and benign glands in perineural space

传统的教科书上认为前列腺内不存在骨骼肌[288,388-391]；

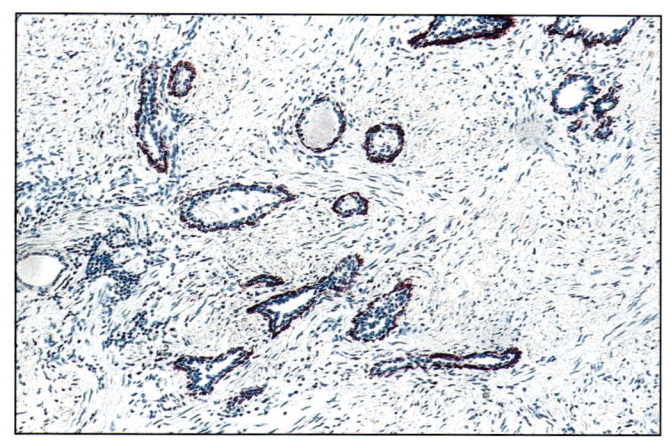

图14A.93　基底细胞特异性角蛋白34βE12（K903）免疫染色显示萎缩的腺体中保留基底细胞。

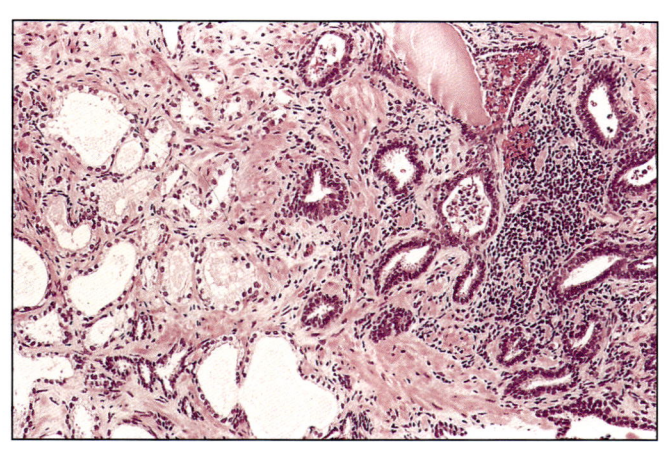

图14A.94　小腺体增生（左）伴有单纯性小叶萎缩（右）。内衬小腺体的细胞有丰富的透明胞浆，偶尔有核仁。

因此，在活检或TURP标本中发现前列腺内散在骨骼肌束，可能提出腺癌蔓延到前列腺外的可能性。然而，实际上在正常人类前列腺中来自盆底的骨骼肌可以进入前列腺。肌纤维在前部和侧部穿过尖端，向上延伸到前列腺的上面和基底，但在前列腺后面不存在肌纤维。因此，骨骼肌纤维常见于尖端、前部和侧部，向上可达前列腺基底部[288,295,388]。在这些部位骨骼肌纤维与前列腺正常腺体组织混合并不少见。因此，来自前部和前侧部的前列腺标本在前列腺腺体之间可以有散在的骨骼肌纤维。Manley[390]报道30.2%TURP标本中存在骨骼肌纤维。这个发现对不熟悉正常解剖学的医师会产生诊断困难，但是缺乏癌的细胞学标准以及腺体中存在基底细胞层，可以提供充足的良性证据并避免错误地诊断为癌（图14A.95）。了解存在骨骼肌纤维对于肿瘤正确分期也很重要。这样，出现癌累及横纹肌并不一定代表肿瘤有前列腺外蔓延[391]。

早些时候，几篇文章已经报道了神经周围可存在良性前列腺腺体（图14A.26），强调应用神经周围浸润作为前列腺腺癌诊断的单一标准存在潜在的危险[392-394]。McIntire和Franzini[392]报道的26例前列腺中6例神经周围间隙内有良性腺体。然而，在神经周围间隙内发现良性前列腺腺体时，腺体从不包绕神经或浸润神经。相反，前列腺癌常常包围整个神经，并且可以穿入神经（图14A.26）。非肿瘤性良性腺体不是真正浸润神经周围间隙，而只不过是与神经并列，给人以浸润的印象[288]。另外，神经周围间隙内的非肿瘤性腺体不具备癌的形态学标准。容易辨认良性腺体的双层细胞，这些细胞不含有明显的核仁。

前列腺少见的良性上皮性病变
Rare benign epithelial lesions of the prostate

囊腺瘤（巨大多房性囊腺瘤）
Cystadenoma (giant multilocular cystadenoma)

前列腺多房性囊腺瘤是前列腺唯一真正的良性上皮性肿瘤，报道的病例不足24例[395,396]。最常发生在20～80岁的患者（平均年龄64.5岁），伴有尿路梗阻的症状，伴有或不伴有可以触及的腹部肿物。肿瘤的最大径7.5～45 cm。影像学研究有助于确定病变浸润的范围。在报道的所有病例中，诊断都是在手术切除后做出的，但是肿物与前列腺的解剖关系却不一样。肿物界限清楚，部分与周围器官粘连。肿物大，有圆凸，多房性和囊性（图14A.96）。囊肿从几个毫米到大约4 cm不等，含有棕黄色或灰白色半固体到浓缩的物质。显微镜下肿瘤由腺体和囊肿构成，内衬立方到矮柱状上皮细胞，细胞核位于基底部（图14A.97）。可见化生性的鳞状和移行上皮。上皮细胞免疫组化染色PSA和PrAP阳性。治疗选择完全手术切除并保留正常盆腔结构[395,396]。

前列腺间质病变
Stromal lesions of the prostate

良性前列腺间质病变
Benign stromal lesions of the prostate

最常见的前列腺间质病变是良性间质增生，它通常

图14A.95 穿插在良性前列腺腺体中的横纹肌束。这种现象不应该解释为前列腺癌侵犯骨骼肌。

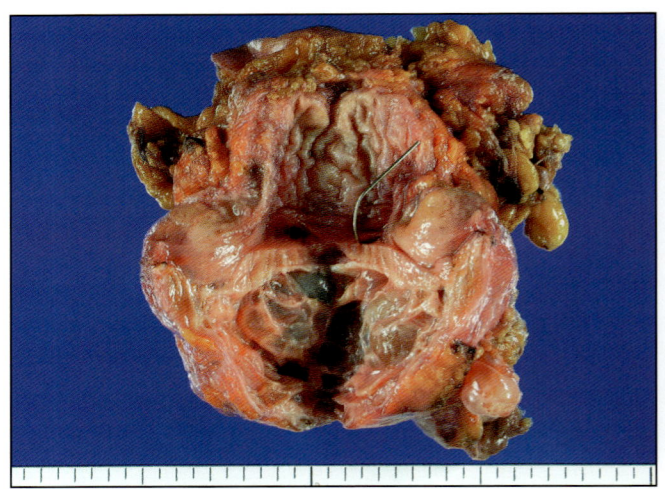

图14A.96 囊腺瘤。在这个根治性膀胱前列腺切除标本中，多房性囊性病变取代了整个前列腺。

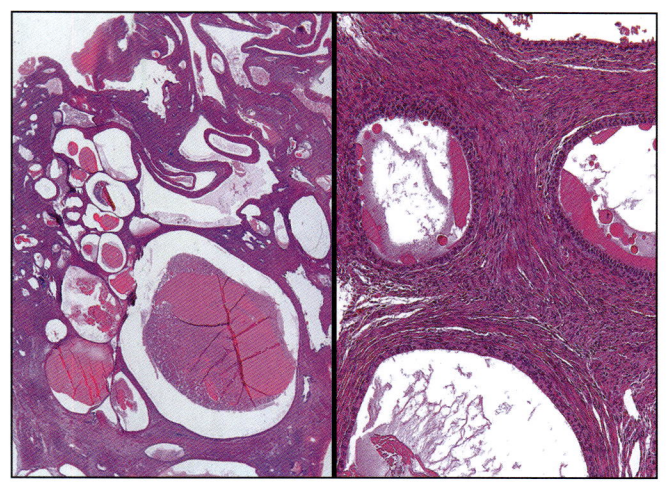

图14A.97 囊腺瘤。这个病变的特征是有许多大小不等的囊肿和细胞丰富的间质。高倍镜下，囊肿内衬扁平或立方上皮细胞，间质细胞非常丰富。

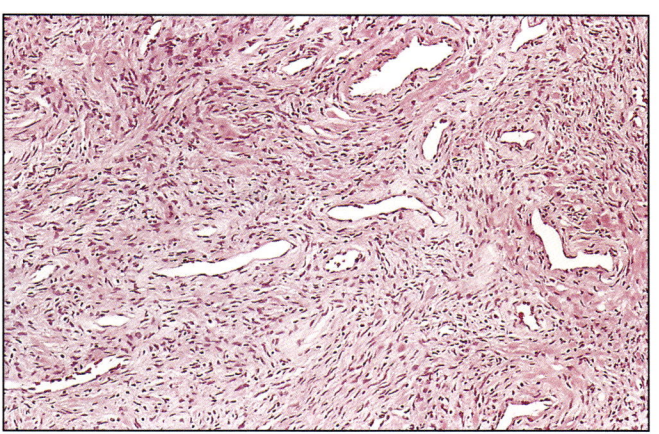

图14A.98 间质结节的特征是血管和梭形细胞增生。梭形细胞在血管周围排列成漩涡状结构。

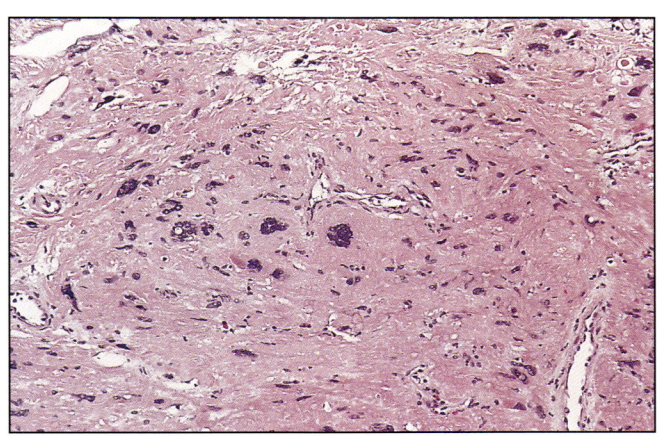

图14A.99 非典型性平滑肌瘤。在其他方面典型的平滑肌瘤背景中出现散在的非典型性梭形细胞。

伴有腺体增生区域，所以容易辨认，见于因临床上诊断BPH而行的TURP标本中。其他前列腺间质病变非常罕见，包括蓝痣、平滑肌瘤和叶状肿瘤。

前列腺的两种假肉瘤性病变——术后梭形细胞结节和假肉瘤性纤维黏液样肿瘤（炎性肌纤维母细胞肿瘤），已经逐渐得到公认。这些病变与肉瘤相似，因为它们富于细胞，有细胞多形性和（或）核分裂活性，可能错误地诊断为肉瘤。临床行为和治疗差别很大，意味着正确认识这些病变是非常重要的。

间质增生　Stromal hyperplasia

间质增生[间质结节（stromal nodule）]最常发生于BPH的情况下。它通常是在显微镜下发现，很少与恶性梭形细胞病变混淆，但是可与平滑肌瘤混淆[397-401]。间质增生是以温和的梭形细胞增生为特征，缺乏腺体成分。这种病变与周围前列腺组织的界限清楚，但没有包膜。梭形细胞排列成束状或漩涡状结构，类似于平滑肌瘤。这些病变常含有薄壁小血管，被梭形细胞成分围绕（图14A.98）。尽管间质可以见到黏液样变，而且可以很明显[402]，但是细胞核非典型性或核分裂象不是普通间质增生的特征。间质结节和平滑肌瘤的区分有些武断；平滑肌瘤被定义为直径超过1cm的病变，通常有被膜[403-405]。

非典型性间质增生 Atypical stromal hyperplasia

有几例罕见的平滑肌增生的报道，是以存在具有深染模糊细胞核的大的非典型性细胞为特征[406]。发生两种类型的增生：一种是非典型性细胞在正常前列腺腺体结构之间浸润，另一种是增生性改变形成单个结节。前一种类型称为非典型性间质增生，而第二种类型称为非典型性（奇异性或合体细胞性）平滑肌瘤[399,407-412]。无论这些病变是形成结节还是在正常腺体之间浸润，其特征都是"奇异"大细胞杂乱排列在间质平滑肌瘤性增生的背景中（图14A.99）。奇异细胞大小形状不一，具有深染的细胞核，常常表现为多核细胞；核分裂象少见或不存在，没有坏死。

已报道的患者年龄为49～69岁（平均53岁）。所有患者表现为由前列腺增大而导致的尿路梗阻症状，治疗采用TURP或耻骨上前列腺切除术。一个患者诊断为平滑肌肉瘤，并且接受了化学治疗[413]。随后进行TURP和耻骨上前列腺切除术，这名患者生存很好，随访36个月没有疾病复发。7例已报道的病例中6例随访14～96个月没有发现病变复发，1名患者手术后16个月死亡。尸检没有前列腺疾病的证据。尽管这些病变的临床行为好像是良性的，但是报道的病例数量非常少，因此研究者认为这些病变是恶性潜能未定的病

变 [399,409,411,412]。根据我们的经验（未发表资料），患者没有发展成恶性的迹象，尽管一个患者出现疾病复发，但是通过保守手术（TURP）成功治疗。

如果在穿刺活检中发现合体细胞性病变应该慎重做出诊断，因为退变表现的"合体细胞性"细胞可能代表手术切除时至少具有低度恶性潜能的间质肿瘤 [414]。主要的鉴别诊断包括间质肉瘤和肉瘤样癌。间质肉瘤除细胞多形性之外，通常表现为高度的核分裂活性以及肿瘤坏死 [415,416]。肉瘤样癌的肉瘤样成分一般为多形性，而且核分裂相当活跃。最重要的线索是证实伴随癌的成分 [259]。

平滑肌瘤　Leiomyoma

平滑肌瘤的定义是孤立的、边界清楚、有包膜的平滑肌增生性肿物，直径至少为 1 cm [403-405]。前列腺平滑肌瘤作为独立疾病没有被普遍接受：有些研究者认为报道的病例中，多数病例（如果不是全部的话）本质是增生性的间质结节 [343,397]。不到 70 例的单发性前列腺平滑肌瘤已被报道 [405,409,413,417,418]。多数病例发生在 48 岁以上的男性，但是少数患者低于 40 岁。发生在相对年轻患者的病例可能被认为是真正的肿瘤性病变，而不是增生性病变，但是还没有把这种病变定义为肿瘤性病变的组织学标准 [343]。这些肿瘤可以达到 12cm，切面质硬，漩涡状，白色。前列腺平滑肌瘤组织学上与发生在其他部位的平滑肌瘤相同，由嗜酸性梭形细胞组成，被数量不等的胶原所分隔。肿瘤细胞排列有序，交叉成束状。单个细胞有两端钝圆的细胞核，核染色质均匀分布。

因为报道的前列腺平滑肌肿瘤的病例很少，所以没有可靠的组织学标准来区分前列腺平滑肌瘤与平滑肌肉瘤。然而，浸润性生长、细胞丰富、细胞核非典型性、肿瘤坏死以及核分裂活性增加好像最为重要，如果至少出现两个或两个以上上述特征，则应做出肉瘤的诊断 [398,409]。

蓝痣、黑变病和前列腺上皮性色素
Blue nevus, melanosis and prostatic epithelial pigment

前列腺色素沉着性病变少见，包括蓝痣和黑变病 [419,420]。在前列腺中，"蓝痣"这个术语应用于当黑色素局限于间质中的黑色素细胞时（图 14A.100），而"黑变病"这个术语则应用于大体上可见有明显的病变和（或）显微镜下可见明显的黑色素，黑色素位于腺上皮和间质中的组织细胞内（图 14A.101）[419,421-423]。自从 1963 年 Nigogosyan 等 [424] 报道了第一例前列腺色素性病变以来，大约有 30 例前列腺蓝痣和（或）黑变病的病例报道。大约 2/3 的色素性病变是蓝痣，1/3 是黑变病。含有色素的前列腺病变的组织学发生尚不清楚 [419,425-431]。

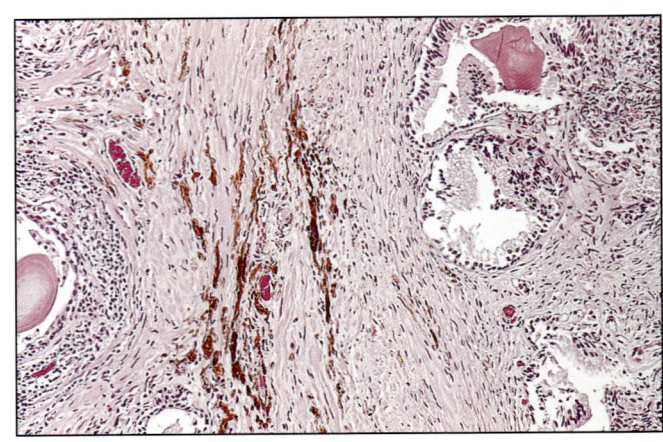

图14A.100　蓝痣。前列腺间质中存在含有色素的梭形细胞。

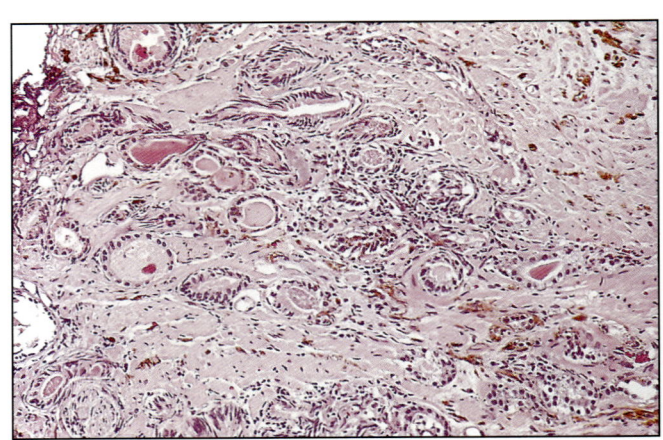

图14A.101　黑变病。间质梭形细胞和腺上皮细胞内均有棕黑色颗粒。

多数研究者认为黑色素是由间质中迁移的黑色素细胞产生的，然后迁移到腺上皮内 [419,427,431]。

文献记载蓝痣或黑变病患者的年龄从 20 岁到 80 岁（平均 68 岁），通常是偶然发现，最常见的临床表现是尿路梗阻；临床上通常诊断为 BPH。偶尔，在手术中怀疑为恶性黑色素瘤，是因为前列腺呈弥漫性的黑色改变。有些病变大体检查可见黑色或棕色 [419,424,427,429,431-434]。显微镜下，间质中可以见到散在的伴有长树突状突起的色素性梭形细胞，邻近前列腺腺泡。梭形细胞胞浆含有细颗粒状棕色或黑色色素。这种色素 Masson-Fontana 染色阳性，符合黑色素。超微结构分析，在白人男性的梭形细胞中含有不同阶段的黑色素小体，而在黑人男性的梭形细胞内仅含有成熟的 IV 型黑色素小体 [410]。虽然 Das Gupta 等 [435] 认为没有报道过令人满意的原发性前列腺恶性黑色素瘤的病例，但是 Berry 和 Reese [436] 描述的一例却可能是原发性前列腺恶性黑色素瘤。

最近对于色素比较关注，在仔细检查前列腺上皮时常常见到色素。这种色素具有脂褐素的特征，因为

Masson-Fontana、Ziehl-Nielsen 染色、Luxol 固蓝（Luxol fast blue）以及油红 O 染色阳性，见于 10%～100% 前列腺腺体中。如果检查整个前列腺或应用特殊染色检测，发现色素的几率更大。这种脂褐素存在于前列腺的所有部位、正常前列腺以及几种病理性情况，包括高级别 PIN 和癌[56,422]。这种色素通常细腻，金黄色，位于细胞核内或出现在整个细胞浆内；当色素明显时可以表现为黄棕色或蓝色。它比精囊的脂褐素细腻，折光性小。前列腺色素被认为是由于细胞内内源性副产品积累而形成的"消耗性"和"老年性色素"。了解前列腺内这些色素至关重要，尤其是在少量的活检标本中。伴有细胞核非典型性和色素的腺体不能被机械地解释为精囊/射精管上皮，应该考虑有 PIN 和癌的可能性。

纤维腺瘤样病变和叶状型肿瘤
Fibroadenoma-like lesion and phyllodes-type tumor

形态学上类似于乳腺纤维腺瘤的前列腺病变不常见到。Kafandaris 和 Polyzonis[437] 报道了 12 例前列腺病变，其特征是间质和腺体增生，没有细胞学非典型性，类似于管周型和管内型纤维腺瘤。Cox 和 Dawson[438] 报道了一种前列腺病变，其特征为没有非典型性的细胞丰富的纤维肌性间质围绕不规则形的增生的腺体，将其命名为囊腺瘤-平滑肌纤维瘤（巨大纤维腺瘤）。伴有间质细胞成分增多和细胞核非典型性的病变称为叶状型非典型性前列腺增生或前列腺叶状囊肉瘤，因为它们与乳腺叶状肿瘤相同[409,413,438-445]。这些肿瘤发生在 22 岁到 78 岁的成人（平均 52 岁），通常伴随前列腺增大而引起尿潴留、血尿以及排尿困难；多数患者临床上诊断为 BPH。这些病变最大径可以达到 5.8 cm[441,446,447]。

叶状型肿瘤在组织学上类似于乳腺的富于细胞性纤维腺瘤和叶状囊肉瘤。因为叶状结构可能不总存在，所以有些作者喜欢把这些肿瘤命名为前列腺混合性上皮-间质肿瘤[68]。存在上皮和间质细胞成分的双相生长方式，表现为不同程度的间质细胞构成和细胞学非典型性（图14A.102）。上皮细胞立方到柱状，有完整的基底细胞层；它们排列成腺体、裂隙样间隙或囊肿，由于间质增生，这些结构常常受压或变形。可以见到显著的上皮增生伴有叶样乳头状突起。间质细胞呈梭形，通常位于黏液样基质中，比腺体成分明显。偶尔可见缺乏腺体的单纯性间质增生。非典型性间质细胞主要存在于腺体周围。偶尔可见到异源性横纹肌母细胞分化[448]。

Bostwick 等[449] 研究了大量叶状肿瘤来阐述其组织学特征和临床预后的关系。他们把 23 例这样的肿瘤根据细胞丰富程度（1～3 级）、细胞非典型性（1～3 级）、

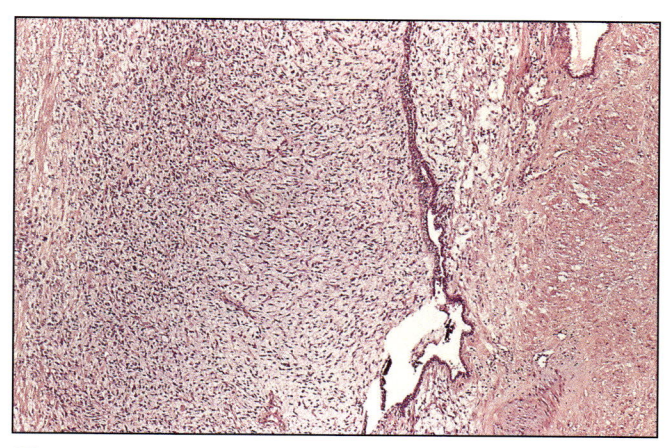

图14A.102 叶状肿瘤。这种病变的特征是伴有腺体和间质增生的双相性结构。

每 10 个高倍视野核分裂数量、间质/上皮比例（低或高）以及坏死（存在或缺乏）分为低级别（14 例）、中级别（7 例）和高级别（2 例）肿瘤。14 例低级别肿瘤中的 7 例（50%）复发，1 例病人出现了低级别肉瘤，这个患者在最初诊断后 5 次复发，14 年后出现转移。7 例中级别肿瘤中的 6 例可见复发，1 例出现低级别肉瘤，这个患者最初诊断后复发 3 次，11 年后出现腹壁转移。

除了 Bostwick 等报道的恶性叶状肿瘤病例之外，还有具有恶性组织学证据的叶状肿瘤的报道；这些病例的特征是间质过度生长、细胞核多形性、核分裂象多见[446,448,450-458] 以及在少数情况下出现横纹肌母细胞[448,454] 或平滑肌肉瘤性分化[459]。因为这些肿瘤生长迅速，初次治疗后复发，浸润邻近器官，或者转移到远隔器官，例如盆腔淋巴结、肺以及肝等[446,450,451,455]，以及至少已有 2 例患者死于本病[450,451]，所以它们表现为侵袭性的临床行为。

这种病变的发病机制尚不清楚。Attah 等[407,441] 根据肿瘤的部位（精阜）提出与雌激素有关；然而，还没有仔细检查激素失衡与前列腺叶状肿瘤发生之间的相互关系。

叶状型肿瘤与恶性叶状肿瘤和前列腺肉瘤不同，实际上它的间质细胞缺乏核分裂象，而且没有间质过度生长以及肿瘤坏死[442]。在鉴别诊断中还应该考虑前列腺肉瘤样癌，因为它具有双相性的本质。虽然肉瘤样癌的梭形间质成分可与叶状肿瘤相似，但肉瘤样癌的腺体成分是明确恶性的[259]。

报道的所有叶状型肿瘤病例均行手术治疗[438-445]；多数研究者提倡实行同治疗结节性增生一样的手术治疗。已经试用了化学治疗和放射治疗，可以获得部分缓解[454,455]。

术后梭形细胞结节
Postoperative spindle cell nodule

术后梭形细胞结节是一种组织学上类似于肉瘤的反应性纤维增生性病变。1984年Proppe等[460]首次描述了8例泌尿生殖道的术后梭形细胞病变。这些作者提出其中多数病变最初被诊断为肉瘤，或在鉴别诊断中主要考虑肉瘤的诊断，但是随访提示其为良性病变。这些病变是在因诸如BPH、前列腺腺癌或TCC等其他疾病而行膀胱镜检查后5周到3个月，发生在膀胱、前列腺以及前列腺尿道的[460-462]。

考虑到每年实施大量的下泌尿道检查，所以这种病变相对少见。患者年龄从29岁到79岁（平均60年）。多数无症状，但可以出现血尿和尿道梗阻症状。术后梭形细胞结节可以局部复发，需要再次切除，但是没有远处转移的病例报道。

术后梭形细胞结节病变通常较小，最大径从5mm到9mm，但可以较大（直径达到4cm）[460,462]。它由交错排列的肥胖梭形细胞束、散在的血管以及少量到中等数量的炎症细胞组成。梭形细胞核均匀一致，没有非典型性或多形性。在报道的病例中，核分裂象为1~25/10HPF（图14A.103）。见不到病理性核分裂象。可以见到核仁，但是小或者不明显。背景可有水肿或有局灶性玻璃样变，取决于手术操作和发现病变之间的时间间隔。一般来说，病变的边缘不清，经常表现为浸润性生长，取代胶原性间质并破坏周围的平滑肌[460-462]。免疫染色证实vimentin、SMA以及desmin阳性[461,462]。有趣的是，这些病变细胞角蛋白也可以阳性[461]。超微结构分析，这些梭形细胞表现为纤维母细胞/肌纤维母细胞分化[460-463]。许多良性和恶性肿瘤组织学上可以类似于术后梭形细胞结节。

最重要的鉴别诊断是前列腺肉瘤[460-462]。核分裂计数对于鉴别平滑肌肉瘤和术后梭形细胞结节没有帮助，因为后者核分裂象可以达到25个/10HPF[460-462]。此外，平滑肌肉瘤可以没有明显的细胞学非典型性。确认术后梭形细胞结节的关键特征是临床手术史或以前几个月内有器械检查史[460,462]。

可能与术后梭形细胞结节混淆的其他良性梭形细胞病变包括假肉瘤性纤维黏液样肿瘤[410,464-466]和间质结节[407,409]。与术后梭形细胞结节不同，这些病变是直接发生的，没有从前尿道器械检查的病史。这些病变是良性的，因此不应该导致治疗上的错误。

鉴别诊断还包括平滑肌肉瘤以外的恶性梭形细胞肿

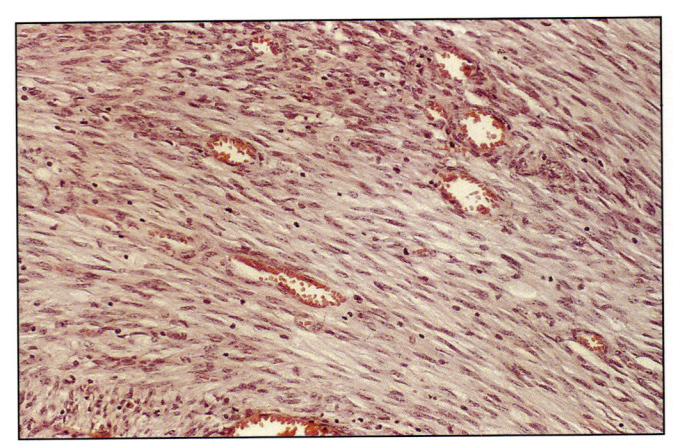

图14A.103 术后梭形细胞结节（PSCN）。核分裂象多见，但PSCN增生的细胞相对均匀一致，其细胞核缺乏恶性特征。

瘤：间质肉瘤、横纹肌肉瘤、神经纤维肉瘤和纤维肉瘤[414,461]。所谓的恶性纤维组织细胞瘤在前列腺也有描述[467]。这些肉瘤有足够的细胞学多形性，与术后梭形细胞结节鉴别一般不成问题。另外一个鉴别诊断是肉瘤样癌[259,264,468]。当这种肿瘤仅由肉瘤样成分组成时，可能要考虑与术后梭形细胞结节的鉴别诊断，例如穿刺活检或TURP取材有限的标本。然而，肉瘤样癌的梭形细胞成分一般有多形性，含有非典型性核分裂象，有些病例CK染色可能阳性，PSA和PrAP很少阳性[259,264,468]。临床医师和病理医师密切合作是正确诊断这种病变和避免不必要的根治性治疗的关键。当近期曾因其他疾病而行手术的患者被诊断为肉瘤时，临床医师应该提出术后梭形细胞结节的可能性。

假肉瘤性纤维黏液样肿瘤
Pseudosarcomatous fibromyxoid tumor

假肉瘤性梭形细胞增生类似于术后梭形细胞结节，可以发生在没有外科检查史的泌尿道内。这些病变被不同地命名为炎性假瘤、假性肉瘤以及炎性肌纤维母细胞瘤[410,464-466,469,470]。这种病变少见，诊断相当困难。它可以发生在沿泌尿道的任何部位，尤其是膀胱（见第12章）和前列腺。自从1980年Roth[470]首次描述了膀胱内的这种病变以来，文献中已经报道了膀胱和前列腺内大约50个病例[410,465,466,469-476]；在报道的病例中仅有6例累及前列腺部位[410,465,466,476]。

假肉瘤性纤维黏液样肿瘤确切的发病机制尚不清楚，但是具有包括肉芽组织型血管结构和明显炎细胞成分在内的组织学特征，并且报道病例所观察到的良性临床经过高度提示是反应性/假性肿瘤过程。它在组织学上类似于结节性筋膜炎[477]，并且Nochomovitz和

Orenstein[469]确实报道了这种病变是内脏类型的结节性筋膜炎。

组织学检查表现为黏液样病变，以非典型性纤维母细胞/肌纤维母细胞增生为特征，伴有明显的炎性成分和肉芽组织型血管结构（图14A.104）。它有界限不清的浸润性结构，可以延伸到周围结构。梭形细胞可以出现奇异性、包括带状或蝌蚪形细胞，伴有嗜酸性胞浆和明显的核仁（图14A.105）。可以存在核分裂活性，但不明显，异常核分裂象不是这种病变的特征[410,464-466,469-476]。最重要的鉴别诊断是各种黏液样病变（表14A.5）。其他恶性肿瘤，例如肉瘤样癌、恶性外周神经鞘肿瘤、纤维肉瘤、炎性纤维肉瘤[478]以及所谓的恶性纤维组织细胞瘤[467]在鉴别诊断中也应该考虑。然而，这些病变通常有足够的细胞学非典型性和核分裂活性，包括非典型性核分裂象，这些可以避免与良性病变混淆。

虽然假肉瘤性纤维黏液样肿瘤相当少见，但是它们的正确诊断对于避免不必要的根治性治疗意义重大。因为仅仅是最近才认识这种病变，仅有个案报道而且随访有限，所以对于治疗还没有统一的意见。没有患者发生转移或死于这种病变[410,464-466,469-476]。

根据经验，我们通常推荐保守治疗并密切随访。当病理医师在泌尿生殖道发现这种类型的病变时，必须将临床和病理联系起来。

其他良性间质病变
Other benign stromal lesions

在前列腺已经报道了少数几例嗜铬细胞瘤[479,480]、几例血管外皮细胞瘤[481]、孤立性纤维性肿瘤[482]、副神经节瘤[368]以及大概30例的软斑病[483]。我们认为有些血管外皮细胞瘤病例可能是间质肉瘤，其他病例可能是前列腺孤立性纤维性肿瘤[484]。它们的形态学特征与较常发生部位的相似。罕见的类似于透明细胞腺癌的前列腺黄色瘤病例已有报道[485]。

非特异性肉芽肿性前列腺炎通常伴有BPH，在临床上以及少数情况下在病理上可与前列腺癌相似。在TURP（图14A.106）或应用卡介苗（BCG）治疗表浅膀胱癌后（图14A.107）[486-488]，感染因子（组织胞浆菌病、隐球菌病、结核病）可能导致特异性肉芽肿性炎症。肉芽肿性前列腺炎的典型表现是伴有导管和腺泡破坏的肉芽肿形成以及慢性炎症反应；然而，伴有明显组织细胞和少量其他炎性成分的病变在组织学上可能与实性高级别前列腺癌相混淆[489-491]。仔细的组织学检查并借助于免疫组化染色（角蛋白、PSA和PrAP染色阴性，溶菌酶或KP-1阳性反应）可能有助于确立正确的诊断。

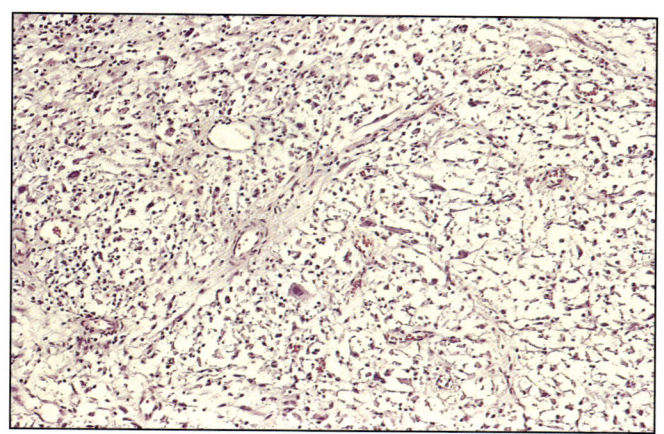

图14A.104 假肉瘤性纤维黏液样肿瘤。黏液样间质含有梭形细胞、裂隙样小血管以及炎性细胞，主要是淋巴细胞和浆细胞。

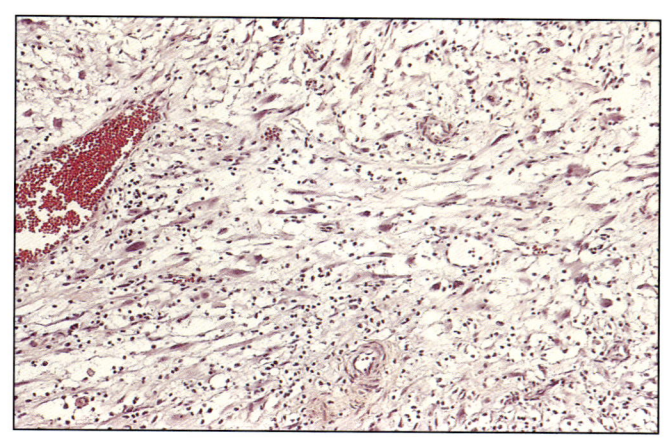

图14A.105 假肉瘤性纤维黏液样肿瘤。有一些奇异细胞，伴有一个或两个大的细胞核以及致密的嗜酸性胞浆。

表14A.5	假肉瘤性纤维黏液样肿瘤（PSFMT）和其他黏液样病变的鉴别特征			
特征	PSFMT	PSCN	ML	MR
细胞丰富程度	+/++	+++	+/++	+/++
生长方式	ND	束状	ND	新生层
多形性	+	−	±	+
核分裂象/10HPF	1~2	1~25	1~10	1~10
血管	裂隙样	ND	ND	ND
角蛋白	±	±	±	±
SMA	±	±	+	−
Desmin	±	±	+	+
Myogenin	−	−	−	+
EM	F/MF	F/MF	SM	STM
临床病程	I	I	R/M	R/M

PSCN：术后梭形细胞结节；ML：黏液样平滑肌肉瘤；MR：黏液样横纹肌肉瘤；ND：没有描述；SMA：平滑肌肌动蛋白；EM：电镜所见；F：纤维母细胞；MF：肌纤维母细胞；SM：平滑肌；STM：横纹肌；I：惰性；R/M：复发/恶性。

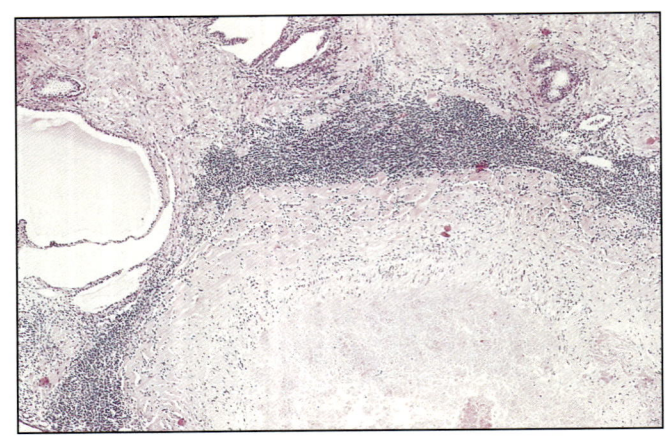

图14A.106 卵圆形、大而界限清楚的肉芽肿。密集的栅栏状排列的组织细胞带围绕着中心坏死。周围是密集的炎症细胞带，主要由淋巴细胞和浆细胞组成。

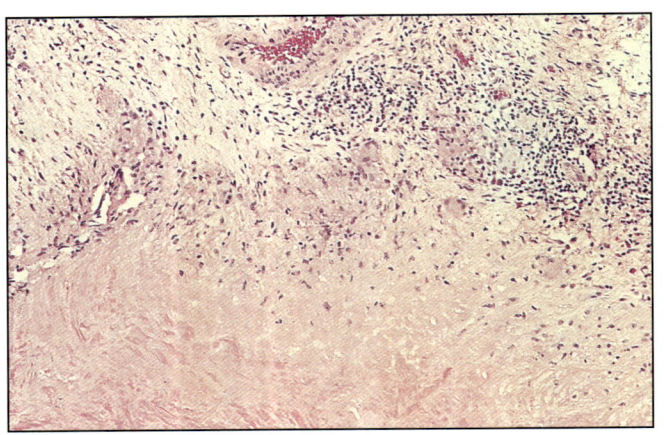

图14A.107 卡介苗（BCG）肉芽肿性炎症。中央无定形坏死区域被组织细胞和Langhans巨细胞所围绕。抗酸杆菌染色可以显示抗酸菌。

恶性软组织肿瘤
Malignant soft tissue tumors

前列腺肉瘤少见，在所有原发性前列腺肿瘤中占不到0.1%。多数前列腺肉瘤是特化的前列腺间质的肉瘤、平滑肌肉瘤或横纹肌肉瘤[414-416,492-502]。横纹肌肉瘤是最常见的前列腺肉瘤，常发生在婴儿、儿童以及青年人，而平滑肌肉瘤是第二个最常见的前列腺肉瘤，较常发生在较大的年龄组。实际上，前列腺肉瘤有两个年龄分布高峰：(1) 60 岁以上的患者；以及 (2) 婴儿、儿童和青年人。

横纹肌肉瘤　Rhabdomyosarcoma

横纹肌肉瘤（也见第 24 章）是最常见的前列腺肉瘤。虽然已有 18 例 50 岁以上患者的横纹肌肉瘤报道[494,503-509]，但是这种病变通常发生在 20 岁以下的人群。泌尿生殖系统，包括前列腺，占儿童横纹肌肉瘤的 21%，是继头颈部之后第二个好发部位[510]。

80% 以上的横纹肌肉瘤是胚胎性横纹肌肉瘤，包括葡萄状和梭形细胞亚型，其余的是腺泡状横纹肌肉瘤。腺泡状横纹肌肉瘤往往发生在稍大年龄组（中位年龄 22 岁）[499,511-514]。前列腺的多形性横纹肌肉瘤已有报道，但极其罕见[415,512]。

当肿瘤主要由圆形细胞构成时，可能必须应用诸如电镜和免疫组化等辅助检查来证实诊断。抗肌肉抗原的抗体最常用于横纹肌肉瘤的诊断，包括 MyoD1、肌细胞生成素（myogenin）、desmin 以及肌肉肌动蛋白（muscle actin）[99]。

最近，染色体分析已经应用于疑难病例的诊断，在腺泡状横纹肌肉瘤中应用 t(2;13) 或 t(1;13)，或在胚胎性横纹肌肉瘤中获得染色体 2、8 和 13[515]。

在成人群体中，单凭组织学结构去鉴别横纹肌肉瘤与前列腺小细胞癌[213,219]和淋巴瘤[516]可能是困难的。肿瘤的临床表现以及免疫组化和电镜分析通常可以确立正确诊断。在鉴别诊断中另外一个应该考虑的是假肉瘤性纤维黏液样肿瘤。与胚胎性横纹肌肉瘤一样，在黏液样背景中可以有带状或蝌蚪样细胞；然而，假肉瘤性纤维黏液样肿瘤没有新生层或细胞没有横纹，MyoD1、myogenin 染色阴性，而胚胎性横纹肌肉瘤的梭形细胞染色阳性[410,464,465]。

膀胱-前列腺横纹肌肉瘤发现相对早，因为它们产生与尿路有关的症状和体征，可以迅速得到医疗关注。横纹肌肉瘤可能较小，在诊断时明显局限于前列腺，但是可以迅速生长，侵犯邻近软组织和膀胱。相反，前列腺外的盆腔肿瘤在首次发现时通常较大并且有浸润[415,503-510,512-514]。因此，可以说膀胱-前列腺部位的横纹肌肉瘤比前列腺外腹膜后-盆腔软组织的肿瘤预后要好[512,517]。根据包括 54 例膀胱-前列腺横纹肌肉瘤的来自群间横纹肌肉瘤研究 IV（Intergroup Rhabdomyosarcoma Study IV）的结果，预后最好的相关因素是：在单因素分析中是诊断时年龄 1～9 岁；非浸润性肿瘤；肿瘤大小 < 5 cm；未累及淋巴结；I 或 II 期疾病；原发部位在眼眶或头颈部；以及胚胎性组织学特征（以上所有因素 P=0.001）。而多因素分析证实仅有年龄、临床上淋巴结的状况以及分期是独立的预后因素[517,518]。

横纹肌肉瘤的预后随联合治疗（多种药物化学治疗、手术和辅助放射治疗）的应用而有明显改善，至少在年轻患者，5 年无病生存率达 70%，总体生存率 75%[518]。因为联合治疗的出现，转移并不常见[511,512,517,518]。

平滑肌肉瘤　Leiomyosarcoma

平滑肌肉瘤是成人前列腺最常见的肉瘤[508,521]，而且在所有前列腺肉瘤中是继横纹肌肉瘤之后第二个最常见的肉瘤[415,493,508]。它占前列腺肉瘤的 25%。尽管多数患者为 40～50 岁至 70～80 岁（中位年龄 58 岁）[415,493,496,500,520]，但是平滑肌肉瘤累及患者的年龄范围广泛，包括小于 10 岁的患者[501]。

平滑肌肉瘤往往较大，可达到 21 cm（平均 9 cm），大体所见类似于相应的软组织肿瘤。它弥漫浸润前列腺和前列腺周围软组织。前列腺增大易被发现，临床诊断通常是 BPH 或前列腺炎[501,519-521]。

显微镜下，这个肿瘤组织学特征与软组织或内脏的平滑肌肉瘤一样（见第 24 章），由交错的梭形细胞束构成，细胞核末端钝圆，胞浆原纤维嗜酸性。总是存在不同程度的细胞核非典型性和核分裂象（图 14A.108）。肿瘤坏死和出血常见[415,511,522]。尽管平滑肌肉瘤的平滑肌本质通常靠常规光镜可以评价，但是通过免疫组化或电镜检查有助于进一步证实[492,519]。多数肿瘤是中级别到高级别的。在低度非典型性的肿瘤，尚未建立标准来区分平滑肌肉瘤和富于细胞性或合体细胞性平滑肌瘤。我们建议肿瘤至少具有下面两个不利的组织学参数才能做出平滑肌肉瘤的诊断：细胞丰富、多形性、细胞核的非典型性、坏死、浸润性生长以及核分裂活性。然而，有关评价前列腺平滑肌肿瘤生物学行为的可靠病理学特征的资料不足，因为这些肿瘤罕见，而且报道的病例随访不充分[492,501,522]。靠近前列腺的直肠胃肠道间质瘤病例要与前列腺平滑肌肉瘤鉴别也是困难的。在这种情况下，c-kit 和 CD34 免疫染色有助于它们的鉴别诊断。

已报道的平滑肌肉瘤患者的 5 年生存率是 50%～60%[416,521]；然而，随着对选择性患者进行的积极的联合治疗，包括根治性手术、术前和术后联合化学治疗以及放射治疗的应用，平滑肌肉瘤的预后是令人鼓舞的。Ahlering 等[522]报道，应用上述治疗方案平均随访 5 年的生存率为 90%。半数病例有局部复发和内脏转移[519,522]。

间质肉瘤（特异的前列腺间质肉瘤）　Stromal sarcoma (sarcoma of specialized prostatic stroma)

在成人前列腺软组织肉瘤相对少见的分类中，有一组肉瘤不同于平滑肌肉瘤，被认为是起源于特异的前列腺间质，这种看法是根据其孕激素和（或）雌激素受体阳性[414]。与前列腺叶状肿瘤一样，它们代表一个谱系。Gaudin 等[414]提出将不能确定恶性潜能的前列腺间质增生（prostatic stromal proliferation of uncertain malignant potential）这一名称用于没有明确肉瘤特征的病变，而前列腺间质肉瘤（prostatic stromal sarcoma）则用于伴有间质过度生长、核分裂象和坏死的肿瘤。局部复发导致患者死亡，也可发生转移，通常转移到肺。即使相对温和的不能确定恶性潜能的病变也可以复发，有时反复复发，并且可能需要根治性前列腺切除术。组织学上，肿瘤由原始的圆形、卵圆形或梭形细胞构成，偶尔伴有人字形结构，弥漫性浸润前列腺间质（图 14A.109）。这种肿瘤 CD34（干细胞标志物）和激素受体 [孕激素和（或）雌激素] 阳性，平滑肌标志物（SMA、HHF-35 和 desmin）染色不定（在明显的肉瘤中通常阴性）[414]。

其他肉瘤　Other sarcomas

Tannenbaum[493]曾经提到前列腺纤维肉瘤，但文献中没有详细描述这种病变。文献中已有 2 例前列腺骨肉瘤报道[523,524]。这两例均伴有前列腺腺癌：一例患者本

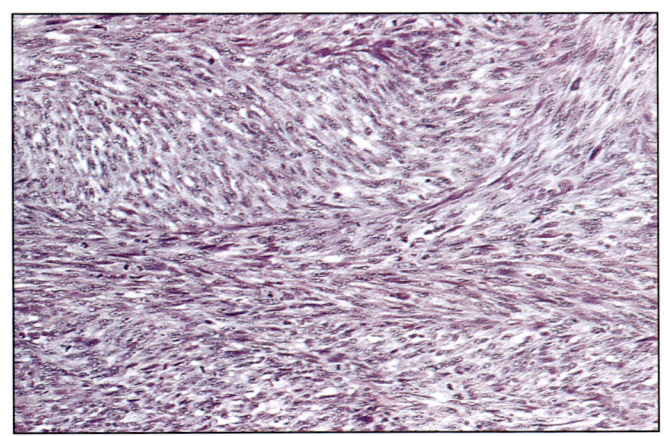

图 14A.108　平滑肌肉瘤梭形细胞交织成束。

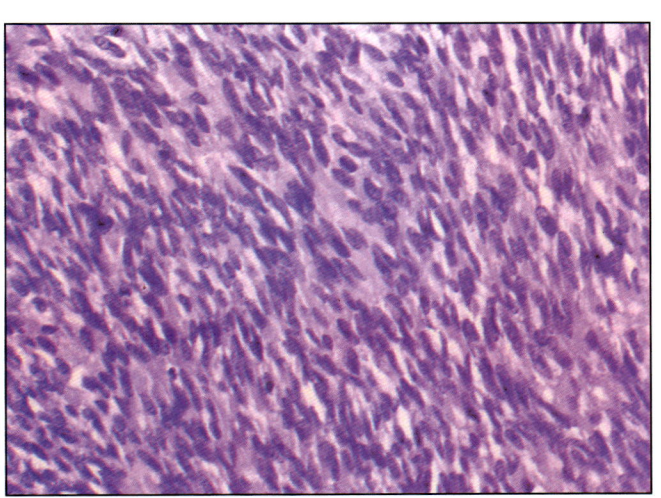

图 14A.109　间质肉瘤。这种病变的特征是密集排列的梭形细胞弥漫性增生，伴有模糊的胞浆和核分裂活性。

身发生骨肉瘤[523]，另一例在癌症放射治疗后发生骨肉瘤[524]。按照我们的定义这些病例可以归入肉瘤样癌而不是前列腺原发性骨肉瘤。我们在 12 例肉瘤样癌患者中遇到一例患者肉瘤样成分是骨肉瘤[259]。

已经报道了少数几例所谓的恶性纤维组织细胞瘤[467,525,526]。与软组织中类似的病变不同，这种肿瘤仅表现为中度的多形性，核分裂象少见。由于是个案报告加之随访时间太短，所以很难评价其恶性程度，但是预后似乎不良。

文献中已经描述了几例血管肉瘤，包括放射治疗后的血管肉瘤，并有充分的组织学描述[527,528]。患者年龄从 2 岁到 60 岁（平均 34.5 岁），一个患者肿瘤发生在前列腺腺癌放射治疗后 10 年。预后好像不好，因为其中 3 例在诊断后 6 个月内死亡[527]。肿瘤分化差；血管标志物免疫染色有助于鉴别血管肉瘤和低分化肉瘤[527,528]。Scully 等[529]报道了一例放射诱导的前列腺肉瘤。发生在前列腺的软骨肉瘤、恶性外周神经鞘肿瘤、神经母细胞瘤、原始周围神经外胚层肿瘤、恶性血管周围上皮样细胞肿瘤以及横纹肌样肿瘤均有报道[68,530,531]。

累及前列腺的罕见的恶性肿瘤
Rare malignant tumors involving the prostate

恶性淋巴瘤、白血病和浆细胞瘤
Malignant lymphoma, leukaemia, and plasmacytoma

前列腺恶性淋巴瘤罕见，不论是作为原发性肿瘤，还是继发于系统性受累的肿瘤。有 150 多例有完整资料的病例报道[516,532-535]。患者年龄从 14 岁到 86 岁（平均 61 岁）。淋巴瘤没有特异性的症状和体征。尿路梗阻症状、血尿或两者兼有是常见的症状。临床诊断几乎总是 BPH、前列腺炎或癌，即使是在以前诊断为淋巴瘤的患者也是如此[516,536-540]。

报道的病例包括见于其他部位的整个恶性淋巴瘤谱系；主要的类型是大细胞、混合细胞以及小裂细胞淋巴瘤[516]。仅有少数结节性、T 细胞、未分化 Burkitt 淋巴瘤以及非 Burkitt 淋巴瘤的病例报告[516,537]。Hodgkin 淋巴瘤、淋巴瘤样肉芽肿病以及亲血管性淋巴瘤在前列腺也有报道[415,541-543]。Bostwick 等[539]报道了最大系列（62 例）的累及前列腺的恶性淋巴瘤，35% 是原发性结外淋巴瘤，类型如下：B 细胞小淋巴细胞性（4 例），滤泡中心、滤泡性、I 级（小细胞）（1 例），滤泡中心细胞、滤泡性、II 级（大小细胞混合）（1 例），滤泡中心细胞、弥漫性、小细胞（2 例），弥漫性大 B 细胞淋巴瘤（12 例），高级别 B 细胞淋巴瘤、Burkitt 样（2 例）。48% 为以前证实的其他部位的淋巴瘤累及前列腺，包括：B 细胞慢性淋巴细胞白血病（8 例），滤泡中心、滤泡性、I 级（小细胞）（1 例），滤泡中心细胞、滤泡性、II 级（大小细胞混合）（1 例），滤泡中心细胞、弥漫性、小细胞（2 例），高级别 B 细胞淋巴瘤（11 例），外周 T 细胞淋巴瘤（2 例），高级别 B 细胞淋巴瘤、Burkitt 样（1 例），Burkitt 淋巴瘤（1 例），Hodgkin 淋巴瘤（2 例, 结节硬化型 1 例，混合细胞性 1 例）。17% 不能区分是原发性还是继发性淋巴瘤[539]。

由 King 和 Cox[534]制定的前列腺原发性淋巴瘤的标准是肿瘤局限于前列腺和邻近组织以及没有淋巴结受累。除了上述标准之外，Bostwick 和 Mann[516]还要求出现的主要症状应局限于前列腺，并且至少应有 1 个月的无病间隔期来完成分期程序。

不管患者年龄、肿瘤分期、组织学类型以及应用的治疗方案如何，累及前列腺的淋巴瘤预后不良[532-537]。Bostwick 等[539]报道的 62 例病例中 27 例患者死于恶性淋巴瘤，18 例患者诊断后生存 12～120 个月（8 例原发性和 10 例继发性），12 例死于其他或不明原因，5 例患者失访。累及前列腺的原发性和继发性淋巴瘤诊断之后平均生存时间没有统计学差异(9.8 个月和 12.7 个月)。

大约 20% 的白血病患者尸检发现有前列腺受累，但是由白血病直接导致前列腺临床症状者不足 1%[541,544,545]。慢性淋巴细胞性白血病是最常见的类型[541,544,545]。已经报道了 3 例前列腺粒细胞肉瘤病例[546-548]。

前列腺浆细胞瘤极其少见，浆细胞瘤累及前列腺是在系统性疾病诊断之后或尸检时得到证实的。有一个病例报道显示前列腺中度增大，无触痛，不规则，酷似原发性前列腺癌。镜下检查，成片肿瘤性浆细胞弥漫性浸润前列腺间质[549]。罕见的前列腺 Hodgkin 淋巴瘤和黏膜相关淋巴组织淋巴瘤已有报道[550]。

主要的鉴别诊断包括前列腺炎（尤其是小淋巴细胞性淋巴瘤[535]）和前列腺癌，尤其是小细胞癌和横纹肌肉瘤。临床病史和仔细的显微镜下评估加上包括免疫组化及电镜在内的辅助方法对于这些病变与淋巴瘤或白血病的鉴别诊断是必不可少的[99,219,497,516,551-553]。

生殖细胞肿瘤 Germ cell tumors

已经报道了几例累及前列腺的生殖细胞肿瘤。有些可能是原发性，但多数病变是来自腹膜后或膀胱后间隙的继发性受累。这些肿瘤发生在年轻或中年男性。前列腺原发性生殖细胞肿瘤的发病机制还不清楚，但可以解释为生殖细胞分离（sequestration）、未定型干细胞肿瘤性转化为生殖细胞、或者来自隐匿性睾丸原发性肿瘤的转移。在排除睾丸原发性肿瘤之后才能做出前列腺原发性生殖细胞肿瘤的诊断。精原细胞瘤和非精原细胞瘤性生殖细胞肿瘤，包括卵黄囊瘤、绒毛膜癌以及混合性生殖细胞肿瘤均有报道。已报道一例卵黄囊瘤混合小灶性的精原细胞瘤。精原细胞瘤患者的预后好，而非精原细胞瘤性生殖细胞肿瘤患者的预后不良[554]。

前列腺转移性实性肿瘤
Metastatic solid tumors to the prostate

当淋巴瘤、白血病以及从膀胱或直肠直接扩散而来的肿瘤被排除之后，转移性肿瘤不常累及前列腺。Johnson等[224]发现死于恶性肿瘤的男性患者中0.5%有前列腺转移。在相似的研究中，Zein等[225]和Bates[555]报道转移性前列腺癌发生率分别为2.2%和0.2%。结合这些报道[224,225]，继发性累及前列腺最常见的肿瘤是支气管癌，其次是黑色素瘤。其他常见的原发性部位包括胃肠道、胰腺和肾[556,557]。转移性睾丸生殖细胞肿瘤和来自甲状腺、阴茎及喉癌的转移也有报道[558]。

精囊肿瘤和肿瘤性病变
Tumors and tumorous conditions of seminal vesicles

精囊囊肿　Cysts of the seminal vesicle

精囊囊肿少见，有不到100例的报道。然而，这个数目没有反映真正的发生率。过去，临床上很少正确诊断这些病变，因为精囊影像检查困难。精囊囊肿通常伴有同侧肾发育不全[559-561]。有时认为感染后纤维化是其病因学因素[556]。获得性囊肿通常伴有射精管梗阻，因为泌尿道感染通常从前列腺尿道上行到精囊[559]。前列腺腺瘤性结节压迫射精管说明与BPH有关。囊肿通常单房，可能有出血。常为单侧性，但少数病例为双侧性[559-562]。有时精囊囊肿伴有睾丸缺失；少数伴有输精管异常。鉴别诊断包括脓肿、包虫囊肿、精囊或前列腺的实性和囊性肿瘤，以及射精管憩室[559,562,563]。

精囊囊肿最常见于20～30岁（范围18～59岁），多数无症状[559-563]。当囊肿有症状时，多数病例最初的表现是下泌尿道症状，例如灼痛、尿急和尿频。附睾炎、腹痛以及射精后会阴不适也不少见。报道的多数病例缺乏组织学描述。少数报道描述囊肿内衬一层均一的柱状到立方上皮，除了纤维性囊壁外没有间质成分[564-566]。

精囊淀粉样物质沉积
Amyloid deposition in seminal vesicle

精囊局限性淀粉样变被认为是老年性病变，在尸检或手术标本中偶有报道，其发生率大约为9%～16%[567]。文献中已经报道了输精管和射精管的淀粉样物质沉积。Jun等[568]最近报道了精囊淀粉样物质沉积，类似于癌的蔓延。大体上，精囊可能增厚，伴有腔隙变小或消失。显微镜下，淀粉样物质沉积往往呈结节状。由于上皮下细腻的原纤维性嗜酸性物质沉积，常常造成精囊变形（图14A.110）。见不到血管壁受累。刚果红染色阳性和苹果绿双折射证实嗜酸性物质的本质是淀粉样物质。

其他良性肿瘤　Other benign neoplasms

精囊平滑肌瘤极其少见；仅有少数报道病例[569]。它们好像是起源于精囊壁，并且表现为盆腔肿物。中肾错构瘤（mesonephric hamartoma）是另外一个少见的肿瘤，被认为是发生在输精管和精囊[570,571]。

其他良性肿瘤包括囊性肌瘤（cystomyoma）[572]、囊腺瘤[573-577]、神经鞘瘤、血管内皮细胞瘤和间叶瘤[577,578]。Mazur等[579]报道了一例不常见的伴有细胞学非典型性的精囊上皮-间质瘤。他们把这种病变命名为不能确定生物学潜能的囊性上皮-间质肿瘤。

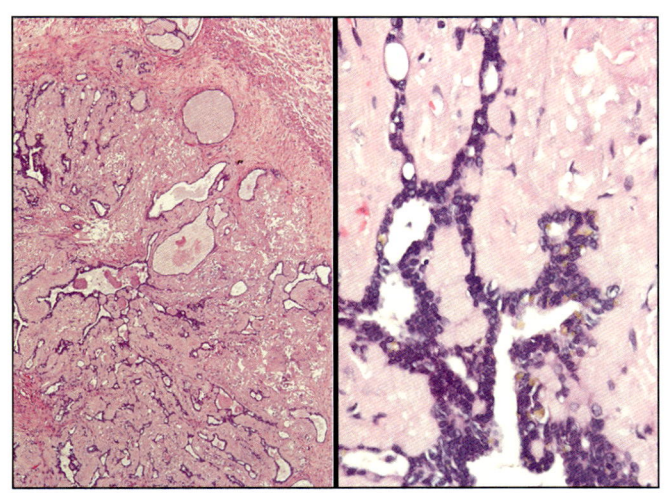

图14A.110　精囊淀粉样物质沉积。左图是精囊低倍镜图像。可能已经注意到淀粉样物质沉积，但右侧高倍镜图像中，淀粉样物质沉积更容易评价。典型的无定形/原纤维性嗜酸性物质取代固有层。精囊上皮内还可见到脂褐素。淀粉样物质没有累及血管壁。

恶性肿瘤　Malignant neoplasms

精囊腺癌　Adenocarcinoma of seminal vesicle

原发性精囊腺癌是少见的肿瘤：文献中大约报道50例[580-586]。患者年龄从19岁到88岁。多数患者发生在50岁之后。在手术前或死前很难确立原发性精囊癌的诊断，鉴别诊断包括前列腺癌、结肠癌或膀胱癌浸润精囊。为了做出原发性精囊癌的诊断，肿瘤应该位于精囊，PSA和PrAP阴性，而且应该没有其他原发性肿瘤[580-583]。

已经报道前列腺腺癌和正常前列腺结构MUC6（MUC6属于人类黏蛋白基因家族）阴性。相反，所有精囊和射精管MUC6抗体染色弥漫阳性。虽然没有应用MUC6研究精囊腺癌，但是这种标志物在与前列腺腺癌的鉴别诊断中可能具有价值[360]。

显微镜下所有肿瘤均为腺癌；它们通常显示乳头状生长或可能是低分化肿瘤，伴有实性、巢状以及条索样生长（图14A.111）。肿瘤细胞通常为高柱状或立方形。在正常精囊上皮附近通常可见原位癌。这种肿瘤黏蛋白、CA125和CEA染色阳性。

鉴别诊断包括由膀胱、前列腺或直肠蔓延而来的癌。膀胱TCC可以以两种不同的方式累及精囊，即黏膜扩散和肿瘤直接蔓延[247]（图14A.112）。当肿瘤累及黏膜面时，通常可见原位癌改变。因此，原位癌改变不一定是原发性癌真正的证据。前列腺腺癌也常常累及精囊（图14A.113）[587]。有时仅仅根据组织学形态不能将精囊原发性腺癌与由前列腺癌蔓延而来的癌区分开来。因此有

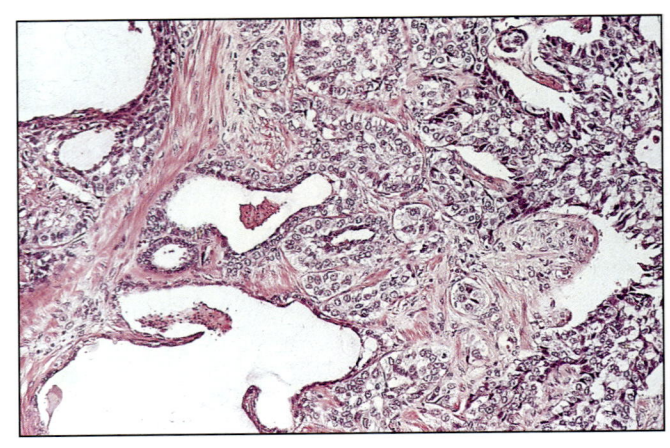

A

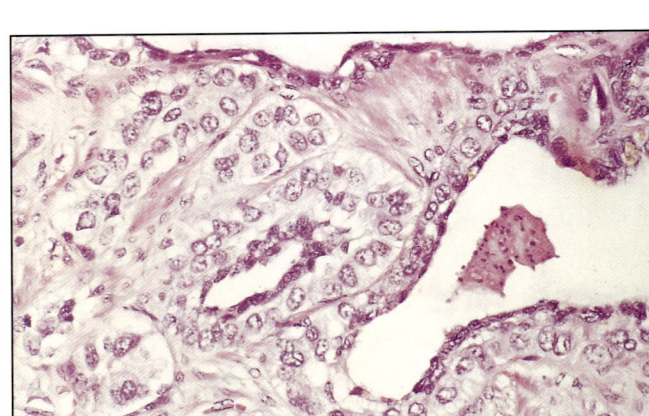

B

图14A.112　（A，B）膀胱移行细胞癌伴有精囊黏膜扩散。肿瘤细胞团以Paget样方式浸润于精囊上皮细胞和基底层之间。

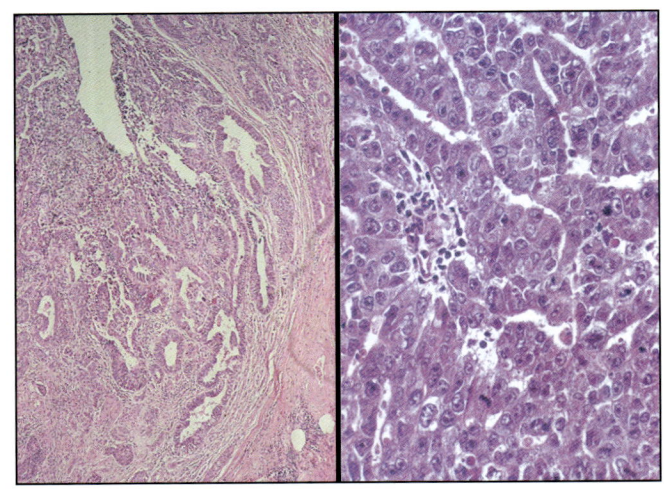

图14A.111　精囊腺癌。左图低倍镜下显示不规则排列的腺体结构。高倍镜下可见这种病变的恶性特征，表现为核的间变、明显的核仁以及多数核分裂象。

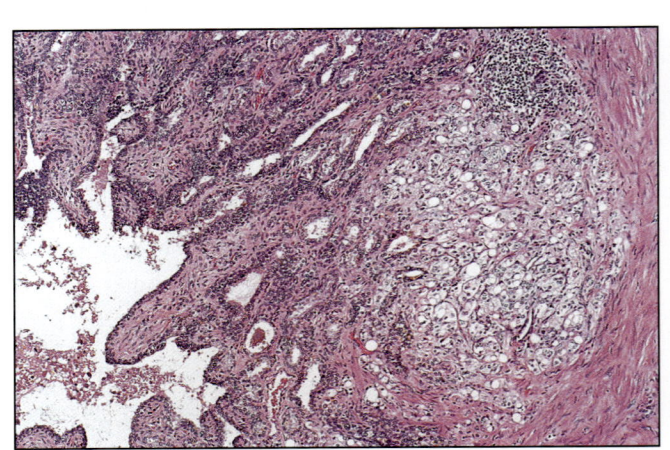

图14A.113　前列腺腺癌侵犯精囊。

必要进行前列腺标志物的免疫组化研究。

Ormsby 等最近的研究表明[586]，精囊腺癌具有独特的免疫表型，即 CK 7 阳性、CK 20 阴性、CA-125 阳性、PSA/PrAP 阴性，并且可以结合组织形态学来区分其他需要鉴别的肿瘤，包括前列腺腺癌（CA-125 阴性，PSA/PrAP 阳性）、膀胱 TCC（CK 20 阳性、CA-125 阴性）、直肠腺癌（CA-125 阴性、CK 7 阴性、CK 20 阳性）、膀胱腺癌（CA-125 阴性）以及发生在 Müller 管囊肿的腺癌（CA-125 阴性）。

精囊腺癌的预后差。根治性手术治疗已被尝试，但结果并不乐观。在应用放射治疗、睾丸切除或雌激素治疗的患者中，几乎没有长期生存者[580-583]。

其他恶性肿瘤　Other malignant neoplasms

已有一例发生于 29 岁男性的可能是 Wolff 管来源的男性附属器肿瘤的病例报告[588]。精囊肉瘤极其少见。文献中已经报道了"精囊"平滑肌肉瘤[589-591]、横纹肌肉瘤[592,593]、血管肉瘤[589,594-596]、纤维肉瘤、脂肪肉瘤以及叶状囊肉瘤[597]。这些肿瘤倾向于广泛侵犯邻近结构，常常掩盖了实际的来源部位。认识到这种困难，有些作者认为所有发生在膀胱和前列腺后面的肿瘤应该简单地归在一起，称为膀胱后肉瘤[589,594,595,598]。因为对于这些肿瘤缺乏经验，所以可推荐的治疗方法有限。已经应用手术切除，联合外部和植入放射治疗以及激素治疗。

参考文献

1. Jemal A, Siegel R, Ward E et al. 2006 Cancer statistics, 2006. CA Cancer J Clin 56: 106–130
2. Eble J N, Sauter G, Epstein J I et al. 2004 Pathology and genetics: Tumours of the urinary system and male genital organs. WHO classification of tumors. IARC Press, Lyon, p 160–215.
3. Srigley J R 2004 Benign mimickers of prostatic adenocarcinoma. Mod Pathol 17: 328–348
4. McNeal J E, Bostwick D G 1986 Intraductal dysplasia: a premalignant lesion of the prostate. Hum Pathol 17: 64–71
5. Bostwick D G, Brawer M K 1987 Prostatic intraepithelial neoplasia and early invasion in prostate cancer. Cancer 59: 788–794
6. Kastendieck H, Altenahr E, Husselmann H et al. 1976 Carcinoma and dysplastic lesions of the prostate. Z Krebsforsch 88: 33–54
7. Helpap B 1980 The biological significance of atypical hyperplasia of the prostate. Virchow's Arch [A] 387: 307–317
8. Amin M B, Ro J Y, Ayala A G 1993 Ideas in pathology. Putative precursor lesions of prostatic adenocarcinoma: fact or fiction? Mod Pathol 6: 476–483
9. Amin M B, Ro J Y, Ayala A G 1994 Prostatic intraepithelial neoplasia: relationship to adenocarcinoma of prostate. Pathol Annu 29: 1–30
10. McNeal J E 1965 Morphogenesis of prostate carcinoma. Cancer 18: 1659–1666
11. McNeal J E 1968 Regional morphology and pathology of the prostate. Am J Clin Pathol 49: 347–357
12. McNeal J E 1969 Origin and development of carcinoma in the prostate. Cancer 23: 24–34
13. Drago J R, Mostofi F K, Lee F 1989 Introductory remarks and workshop summary. Urology 34: 2–3
14. Troncoso P, Babaian R J, Ro J Y 1989 Prostatic intraepithelial neoplasia and invasive prostatic adenocarcinomas in cystoprostatectomy specimens. Urology 34: 52–56
15. Gaudin P B, Sesterhenn I A, Wojno K J et al. 1997 Incidence and clinical significance of high grade prostatic intraepithelial neoplasia in TURP specimens. Urology 49: 558–563
16. Pacelli A, Bostwick D G 1997 Clinical significance of high-grade prostatic intraepithelial neoplasia in transurethral resection specimens. Urology 50: 355–359
17. Bostwick D G, Qian J, Frankel K 1995 The incidence of high-grade prostatic intraepithelial neoplasia in needle biopsies. J Urol 154: 1791–1794
18. Bostwick D G, Amin M B, Dundore P 1993 Architectural patterns of high-grade prostatic intraepithelial neoplasia. Hum Pathol 24: 298–310
19. Reyes A O, Swanson P E, Carbone J M et al. 1997 Unusual histologic types of high-grade prostatic intraepithelial neoplasia. Am J Surg Pathol 21: 1215–1222
20. Argani P, Epstein J I 2001 Inverted (hobnail) high-grade prostatic intraepithelial neoplasia (PIN): report of 15 cases of a previously undescribed pattern of high-grade PIN. Am J Surg Pathol 25: 1534–1539
21. Berman D M, Yang J, Epstein J I 2000 Foamy gland high-grade prostatic intraepithelial neoplasia. Am J Surg Pathol 24: 140–144
22. Qian J, Jenkins R B, Bostwick D G 1997 Detection of chromosomal anomalies and c-myc gene amplification in the cribriform pattern of prostatic intraepithelial neoplasia and carcinoma by fluorescence in situ hybridization. Mod Pathol 10: 1113–1119
23. McNeal J E, Villers A, Redwine E A 1991 Microcarcinoma in the prostate: its association with duct-acinar dysplasia. Hum Pathol 22: 644–652
24. Bostwick D G 1995 High-grade prostatic intraepithelial neoplasia: the most likely precursor of prostate cancer. Cancer 75: 1823–1836
25. Kronz J D, Allan C H, Shaikh A A et al. 2001 Predicting cancer following a diagnosis of high-grade prostatic intraepithelial neoplasia on needle biopsy: data on men with more than one follow-up biopsy. Am J Surg Pathol 25: 1079–1085
26. Nagle R B, Brawer M K, Kittelson J 1991 Phenotypic relationships of prostatic intraepithelial neoplasia to invasive prostatic carcinoma. Am J Pathol 138: 119–128
27. Perlman E J, Epstein J I 1990 Blood group antigen expression in dysplasia and adenocarcinoma of the prostate. Am J Surg Pathol 14: 810–818
28. McNeal J E, Leav I, Alroy J 1988 Differential lectin staining of central and peripheral zones of the prostate and alterations in dysplasia. Am J Clin Pathol 89: 41–48
29. Deschenes J, Weidner N 1990 Nucleolar organizer regions (NOR) in hyperplastic and neoplastic prostate disease. Am J Surg Pathol 14: 1148–1155
30. Sesterhenn I A, Becker R L, Avallone F A 1991 Image analysis of nucleoli and nucleolar organizer regions in prostatic hyperplasia, intraepithelial neoplasia, and prostatic carcinoma. J Urogen Pathol 1: 61–74
31. Amin M B, Schultz D S, Zarbo R J 1994 Computerized static DNA ploidy analysis of prostatic intraepithelial neoplasia. Arch Pathol Lab Med 118: 260–264
32. Weinberg D S, Weidner N 1993 Concordance of DNA content between prostatic intraepithelial neoplasia and concomitant invasive carcinoma. Evidence that prostatic intraepithelial neoplasia is a precursor of invasive prostatic carcinoma. Arch Pathol Lab Med 117: 1132–1137
33. McNeal J E, Alroy J, Leav I et al. 1988 Immunohistochemical evidence for impaired cell differentiation in the premalignant phase of prostate carcinogenesis. Am J Clin Pathol 90: 23–32
34. Tamboli P, Amin M B, Xu H J et al. 1998 Immunohistochemical expression of retinoblastoma and p53 tumor suppressor genes in prostatic intraepithelial neoplasia: comparison with prostatic adenocarcinoma and benign prostate. Mod Pathol 11: 247–252
35. Tamboli P, Amin M B, Schultz D S et al. 1996 Comparative analysis of nuclear proliferative index (Ki-67) in benign prostate, prostatic intraepithelial neoplasia and prostatic carcinoma. Mod Pathol 9: 1015–1019
36. Zeng L, Rowland R G, Lele S M et al. 2004 Apoptosis incidence and protein expression of p53, TGF-beta receptor II, p27Kip1, and Smad4 in benign, premalignant, and malignant human prostate. Hum Pathol 35: 290–297
37. Zhang P J, Driscoll D L, Lee H K et al. 1999 Decreased immunoexpression of prostate inhibin peptide in prostatic carcinoma: a study with monoclonal antibody. Hum Pathol 30: 168–172
38. Emmert-Buck M R, Vocke C D, Pozzatti R O et al. 1995 Allelic loss of chromosome 8p12-21 in microdissected prostatic intraepithelial neoplasia. Cancer Res 55: 2959–2962
39. Macoska J A, Trybus T M, Benson P D et al. 1995 Evidence for three tumor suppressor gene loci on chromosome 8p in human prostate cancer. Cancer Res 55: 5390–5395
40. Qian J, Jenkins R B, Bostwick D G 1999 Genetic and chromosomal alterations in prostatic intraepithelial neoplasia and carcinoma detected by fluorescence in situ hybridization. Eur Urol 35: 479–483

41. Al-Maghrabi J, Vorobyova L, Toi A et al. 2002 Identification of numerical chromosomal changes detected by interphase fluorescence in situ hybridization in high-grade prostate intraepithelial neoplasia as a predictor of carcinoma. Arch Pathol Lab Med 126: 165–169
42. Wu C L, Yang X J, Tretiakova M et al. 2004 Analysis of alpha-methylacyl-CoA racemase (P504S) expression in high-grade prostatic intraepithelial neoplasia. Hum Pathol 35: 1008–1013
43. Sakar W A, Srigley J R, Dey J, et al. 2001 What features do urologic pathologists emphasize in diagnosing intraepithelial neoplasia (PIN)? A study of morphologic criteria and reproducibility. Mod Pathol 14: 122A (abstract)
44. Srodon M, Epstein J I 2002 Central zone histology of the prostate: a mimicker of high-grade prostatic intraepithelial neoplasia. Hum Pathol 33: 518–523
45. Yantiss R K, Young R H 1997 Transitional cell "metaplasia" in the prostate gland. A survey of its frequency and features based on 103 consecutive prostatic biopsy specimens. J Urol Pathol 7: 71–80
46. Greene L F, O'Dea M J, Dockerty M B 1976 Primary transitional cell carcinoma of the prostate. J Urol 116: 761–763
47. Rubenstein A B, Rubnitz M E 1969 Transitional cell carcinoma of the prostate. Cancer 24: 543–546
48. Molinie V, Fromont G, Sibony M et al. 2004 Diagnostic utility of a p63/alpha-methyl-CoA-racemase (p504s) cocktail in atypical foci in the prostate. Mod Pathol 17: 1180–1190
49. McNeal J E, Yemoto C E 1996 Spread of adenocarcinoma within prostatic ducts and acini. Morphologic and clinical correlations. Am J Surg Pathol 20: 802–814
50. Randolph T, Amin M B, Ro J Y 1997 Histologic variants of the prostatic adenocarcinoma and other carcinomas of the prostate. Mod Pathol 10: 612–629
51. Wilcox G, Soh S, Chakraborty S et al. 1998 Patterns of high-grade prostatic intraepithelial neoplasia associated with clinically aggressive prostate cancer. Hum Pathol 29: 1119–1123
52. Kronz J D, Shaikh A A, Epstein J I 2001 Atypical cribriform lesions on prostate biopsy. Am J Surg Pathol 25: 147–155
53. Kuo T, Gomez L G 1981 Monstrous epithelial cells in human epididymis and seminal vesicles: a pseudomalignant change. Am J Surg Pathol 5: 483–490
54. Arias-Stella J, Takano-Moron J 1958 Atypical epithelial changes in the seminal vesicles. Arch Pathol 66: 761–766
55. Coyne J D, Kealy W T, Annis P 1987 Seminal vesicle epithelium in prostatic needle biopsy specimens (letter). J Clin Pathol 40: 932
56. Amin M B, Bostwick D G 1996 Pigment in prostatic epithelium and adenocarcinoma: a potential source of diagnostic confusion with seminal vesicular epithelium. Mod Pathol 9: 791–795
57. Epstein J I, Grignon D J, Humphrey P A et al. 1995 Interobserver reproducibility in the diagnosis of prostatic intraepithelial neoplasia. Am J Surg Pathol 19: 873–886
58. Allam C K, Bostwick D G, Hayes J A et al. 1996 Interobserver variability in the diagnosis of high grade prostatic intraepithelial neoplasia and adenocarcinoma. Mod Pathol 9: 742–751
59. Bishara T, Ramnani D M, Epstein J I 2004 High-grade prostatic intraepithelial neoplasia on needle biopsy: risk of cancer on repeat biopsy related to number of involved cores and morphologic pattern. Am J Surg Pathol 28: 629–633
60. Eskew L A, Bare R L, McCullough D L 1997 Systematic 5 region prostate biopsy is superior to sextant method for diagnosing carcinoma of the prostate. J Urol 157: 199–202
61. Chen M E, Troncoso P, Johnston D A et al. 1997 Optimization of prostate biopsy strategy using computer based analysis. J Urol 158: 2168–2175
62. Lefkowitz G K, Taneja S S, Brown J et al. 2002 Followup interval prostate biopsy 3 years after diagnosis of high grade prostatic intraepithelial neoplasia is associated with high likelihood of prostate cancer, independent of change in prostate specific antigen levels. J Urol 168: 1415–1418
63. Babaian R J, Toi A, Kamoi K et al. 2000 A comparative analysis of sextant and an extended 11-core multisite directed biopsy strategy. J Urol 163: 152–157
64. San Francisco I F, Olumi A F, Kao J et al. 2003 Clinical management of prostatic intraepithelial neoplasia as diagnosed by extended needle biopsies. Br J Urol Int 91: 350–354
65. Hankey B F, Feuer E J, Clegg L X 1999 Cancer surveillance series: interpreting trends in prostate cancer – part I: evidence of the effects of screening in recent prostate cancer incidence, mortality, and survival rates. J Natl Cancer Inst 91: 1017–1024
66. Cooner W H, Mosley B R, Rutherford C L J 1988 Clinical application of transrectal ultrasonography and prostate specific antigen in the search for prostatic cancer. J Urol 139: 758–761
67. Lee F, Siders D B, Torp-Pedersen S T 1991 Prostate cancer: transrectal ultrasound and pathology comparison. A preliminary study of outer gland (peripheral and central zones) and inner gland (transition zone) cancer. Cancer 67: 1132–1142
68. Young R H, Srigley J R, Amin M B et al. 2000 Tumors of the prostate gland, seminal vesicles, male urethra, and penis. Atlas of tumor pathology, 3rd series. AFIP, Washington, DC
69. Mostofi F K, Sesterhenn I, Sobin L H (eds) 1980 Histological typing of prostate tumours. International histological classification of tumours. World Health Organization, Geneva, p 17–23
70. McNeal J E, Redwine E A, Freiha F S 1988 Zonal distribution of prostatic adenocarcinoma. Correlation with histologic pattern and direction of spread. Am J Surg Pathol 12: 897–906
71. Mostofi F K, Price E B J 1973 Tumors of the male genital system. Atlas of tumor pathology, 2nd series. Armed Forces Institute of Pathology, Washington, DC
72. Gleason D F 1977 Histologic grading and clinical staging of prostate carcinoma. In: Tannenbaum M (ed) Urologic pathology: the prostate. Lea & Febiger, Philadelphia, p 171–198
73. Kovi J 1985 Microscopic differential diagnosis of small acinar adenocarcinoma of prostate. Pathol Annu 20: 157–196
74. Gleason D F 1985 Atypical hyperplasia, benign hyperplasia and well differentiated adenocarcinoma of the prostate. Am J Surg Pathol 9 (suppl): 53–67
75. Ro J Y, Grignon D J, Troncoso P 1988 Mucin in prostatic adenocarcinoma. Semin Diagn Pathol 5: 273–283
76. Kramer C E, Epstein J I 1993 Nucleoli in low-grade prostate adenocarcinoma and adenosis. Hum Pathol 24: 618–623
77. Varma M, Lee M W, Tamboli P et al. 2002 Morphologic criteria for the diagnosis of prostatic adenocarcinoma in needle biopsy specimens. A study of 250 consecutive cases in a routine surgical pathology practice. Arch Pathol Lab Med 126: 554–561
78. Grignon D G, Ro J Y, Srigley J R 1992 Sclerosing adenosis of the prostate gland: a lesion showing myoepithelial differentiation. Am J Surg Pathol 16: 383–391
79. Holmes E J 1977 Crystalloids of prostatic carcinoma: relationship to Bence-Jones crystals. Cancer 39: 2073–2080
80. Ro J Y, Ayala A G, Ordonez N G et al. 1986 Intraluminal crystalloids in prostatic adenocarcinoma: immunohistochemical, electron microscopic and x-ray microanalytic studies. Cancer 57: 2397–2407
81. Ro J Y, Grignon D J, Troncoso P 1988 Intraluminal crystalloids in whole organ sections of prostate. Prostate 13: 233–239
82. Ohtsuki Y, Furihata M, Inoue K 1992 Immunohistochemical and ultrastructural studies of intraluminal crystalloids in human prostatic carcinomas. Virchow's Arch [A] 421: 421–425
83. Anton R C, Chakraborty S, Wheeler T M 1998 The significance of intraluminal prostatic crystalloids in benign needle biopsies. Am J Surg Pathol 22: 446–449
84. Henneberry J M, Kahane H, Humphrey P A et al. 1997 The significance of intraluminal crystalloids in benign prostatic glands on needle biopsy. Am J Surg Pathol 21: 725–728
85. Hukill P B, Vidone R A 1967 Histochemistry of mucus and other polysaccharides in tumors: carcinoma of the prostate. Lab Invest 16: 395–406
86. Christian J D, Lamm T C, Morrow J F et al. 2005 Corpora amylacea in adenocarcinoma of the prostate: incidence and histology within needle core biopsies. Mod Pathol 18: 36–39
87. Humphrey P A, Kaleem Z, Swanson P E et al. 1998 Pseudohyperplastic prostatic adenocarcinoma. Am J Surg Pathol 22: 1239–1246
88. Levi A W, Epstein J I 2000 Pseudohyperplastic prostatic adenocarcinoma on needle biopsy and simple prostatectomy. Am J Surg Pathol 24: 1039–1046
89. Nelson R S, Epstein J I 1996 Prostatic carcinoma with abundant xanthomatous cytoplasm. Foamy gland carcinoma. Am J Surg Pathol 20: 419–423
90. Tran T T, Sengupta E, Yang X J 2001 Prostatic foamy gland carcinoma with aggressive behavior: clinicopathologic, immunohistochemical, and ultrastructural analysis. Am J Surg Pathol 25: 618–623
91. Srigley J R 1988 Small-acinar patterns in the prostate gland with emphasis on atypical adenomatous hyperplasia and small-acinar carcinoma. Semin Diagn Pathol 5: 254–272
92. Brawn P N 1982 Adenosis of the prostate: a dysplastic lesion that can be confused with prostate adenocarcinoma. Cancer 49: 826–833
93. Egan A J, Lopez-Beltran A, Bostwick D G 1997 Prostatic adenocarcinoma with atrophic features: malignancy mimicking a benign process. Am J Surg Pathol 21: 931–935
94. Kaleem Z, Swanson P E, Vollmer R T et al. 1998 Prostatic adenocarcinoma with atrophic features: a study of 202 consecutive completely embedded radical prostatectomy specimens. Am J Clin Pathol 109: 695–703
95. Cina S J, Epstein J I 1997 Adenocarcinoma of the prostate with atrophic features. Am J Surg Pathol 21: 289–295
96. Farinola M A, Epstein J I 2004 Utility of immunohistochemistry for alpha-methylacyl-CoA racemase in distinguishing atrophic prostate cancer from benign atrophy. Hum Pathol 35: 1272–1278
97. Johnson D E, Hogan J M, Ayala A G 1972 Transitional cell carcinoma of the prostate. Cancer 29: 287–293
98. Rhamy R K, Buchanan R D, Spalding M J 1973 Intraductal carcinoma of the prostate gland. J Urol 109: 457–460
99. Ordonez N G, Ro J Y, Ayala A G 1990 Application of immunocytochemistry in the pathology of the prostate, In: Bostwick D G (ed) Pathology of the prostate. Churchill Livingstone, New York, p 137–160
100. Huang Q, Chu P G, Lau S K et al. 2004 Urothelial carcinoma of the urinary bladder with a component of acinar/tubular type differentiation simulating prostatic adenocarcinoma. Hum Pathol 35: 769–773
101. Epstein J I 2004 Diagnosis and reporting of limited adenocarcinoma of the prostate on needle biopsy. Mod Pathol 17: 307–315
102. Blaire B L, Kahane H, Epstein J I 1999 Perineural invasion, mucinous fibroplasia, and glomerulations. Diagnostic features of limited cancer on prostate needle biopsy. Am J Surg Pathol 23: 918–924

103. Bostwick D G, Wollan P, Adlakha K 1995 Collagenous micronodules in prostate cancer. A specific but infrequent finding. Arch Pathol Lab Med 119: 444–447
104. Pacelli A, Lopez-Beltran A, Egan A J et al. 1998 Prostatic adenocarcinoma with glomeruloid features. Hum Pathol 28: 543–546
105. Shah R B, Zhou M, LeBlanc M et al. 2002 Comparison of the basal cell-specific markers, 34betaE12 and p63, in the diagnosis of prostate cancer. Am J Surg Pathol 26: 1161–1168
106. Zhou M, Shah R, Shen R et al. 2003 Basal cell cocktail (34betaE12 + p63) improves the detection of prostate basal cells. Am J Surg Pathol 27: 365–371
107. Jiang Z, Wu C L, Woda B A et al. 2002 P504S/alpha-methylacyl-CoA racemase: a useful marker for diagnosis of small foci of prostatic carcinoma on needle biopsy. Am J Surg Pathol 26: 1169–1174
108. Zhou M, Aydin H, Kanane H et al. 2004 How often does alpha-methylacyl-CoA-racemase contribute to resolving an atypical diagnosis on prostate needle biopsy beyond that provided by basal cell markers? Am J Surg Pathol 28: 239–243
109. Beach R, Gown A M, De Peralta-Venturina M N et al. 2002 P504S immunohistochemical detection in 405 prostatic specimens including 376 18-gauge needle biopsies. Am J Surg Pathol 26: 1588–1596
110. Jiang Z, Fanger G R, Woda B A et al. 2003 Expression of alpha-methylacyl-CoA racemase (P504s) in various malignant neoplasms and normal tissues: a study of 761 cases. Hum Pathol 34: 792–796
111. Sanderson S O, Sebo T J, Murphy L M et al. 2004 An analysis of the p63/alpha-methylacyl coenzyme A racemase immunohistochemical cocktail stain in prostate needle biopsy specimens and tissue microarrays. Am J Clin Pathol 121: 220–225
112. Magi-Galluzzi C, Luo J, Isaacs W B et al. 2003 Alpha-methylacyl-CoA racemase: a variably sensitive immunohistochemical marker for the diagnosis of small prostate cancer foci on needle biopsy. Am J Surg Pathol 27: 1128–1133
113. Zhou M, Jiang Z, Epstein J I 2003 Expression and diagnostic utility of alpha-methylacyl-CoA-racemase (P504S) in foamy gland and pseudohyperplastic prostate cancer. Am J Surg Pathol 27: 772–778
114. Zhou M, Chinnaiyan A M, Kleer C G et al. 2002 Alpha-methylacyl-CoA racemase: a novel tumor marker over-expressed in several human cancers and their precursor lesions. Am J Surg Pathol 26: 926–931
115. Li R, Wheeler T, Dai H et al. 2003 Neural cell adhesion molecule is upregulated in nerves with prostate cancer invasion. Hum Pathol 34: 457–461
116. Allen E A, Kahane H, Epstein J I 1998 Repeat biopsy strategies for men with atypical diagnoses on initial prostate needle biopsy. Urology 52: 803–807
117. Chan T Y, Epstein J I 1999 Follow-up of atypical prostate needle biopsies. Urology 53: 351–355
118. Thorson P, Vollmer R T, Arcangeli C et al. 1998 Minimal carcinoma in prostate needle biopsy specimens: diagnostic features and radical prostatectomy follow-up. Mod Pathol 11: 543–551
119. Fadare O, Wang S, Mariappan M R 2004 Practice patterns of clinicians following isolated diagnoses of atypical small acinar proliferation on prostate biopsy specimens. Arch Pathol Lab Med 128: 557–560
120. Browne T J, Hirsch M S, Brodsky G et al. 2004 Prospective evaluation of AMACR (P504S) and basal cell markers in the assessment of routine prostate needle biopsy specimens. Hum Pathol 35: 1462–1468
121. Catalona W J 1984 Prostate cancer. Grune & Stratton, New York
122. Greene F L, Page D L, Fleming I D et al. 2002 AJCC cancer staging manual. Springer, New York, p 309–316
123. Murphy W M, Dean P J, Brasfield J A 1986 Incidental carcinoma of the prostate. How much sampling is adequate? Am J Surg Pathol: 170–174
124. Epstein J I 1991 The evaluation of radical prostatectomy specimens. Therapeutic and prognostic implications. Pathol Annu 26: 159–210
125. Mills S E, Bostwick D G, Murphy W M 1990 A symposium on the surgical pathology of the prostate. Pathol Annu 25: 109–158
126. Bastacky S I, Walsh P C, Epstein J I 1993 Relationship between perineural tumor invasion on needle biopsy and radical prostatectomy capsular penetration in clinical stage B adenocarcinoma of the prostate. Am J Surg Pathol 17: 336–341
127. Eichelberger L E, Cheng L 2004 Does pT2b prostate carcinoma exist? Critical appraisal of the 2002 TNM classification of prostatic carcinoma. Cancer 100: 2573–2576
128. Brawn P N, Ayala A G, von Eschenbach A C 1982 Histologic grading study of prostate adenocarcinoma: the development of a new system and comparison with other methods – a preliminary study. Cancer 49: 525–532
129. Roudier M P, True L D, Higano C S et al. 2003 Phenotypic heterogeneity of end-stage prostate carcinoma metastatic to bone. Hum Pathol 34: 646–653
130. Bubendorf L, Schopfer A, Wagner U et al. 2000 Metastatic patterns of prostate cancer: an autopsy study of 1589 patients. Hum Pathol 31: 578–583
131. Mostofi F K 1975 Grading of prostatic carcinoma. Cancer Chemother Rep 59: 111–117
132. Humphrey P A 2004 Gleason grading and prognostic factors in carcinoma of the prostate. Mod Pathol 17: 292–306
133. Gaeta J F, Asirwatham J E, Miller G et al. 1980 Histologic grading of primary prostatic cancer: a new approach to an old problem. J Urol 123: 689–693
134. Amin M B, Grignon D J, Humphrey P A et al. 2004 Gleason grading of prostate cancer. A contemporary approach. Lippincott, Williams and Wilkins, Philadelphia
134a. Epstein J I, Allsbrook W C Jr, Amin M B et al. 2005 The 2005 International Society of Urologic Pathology (ISUP) consensus conference on Gleason grading of prostatic carcinoma. Am J Surg Pathol 29: 1228–1242
135. McNeal J E, Cohen R J, Brooks J D 2004 Role of cytologic criteria in the histologic diagnosis of Gleason grade 1 prostatic adenocarcinoma. Hum Pathol 32: 441–446
136. Epstein J I, Pound C R, Partin A W et al. 1998 Progression following radical prostatectomy in men with Gleason score 7 tumor. J Urol 160: 97–101
137. Herman C M, Kattan M W, Ohori M et al. 2001 Primary Gleason pattern as a predictor of disease progression in Gleason score 7 prostate cancer: a multivariate analysis of 823 men treated with radical prostatectomy. Am J Surg Pathol 25: 657–660
138. De la Taille A, Viellefond A, Berger N et al. 2003 Evaluation of the interobserver reproducibility of Gleason grading of prostatic adenocarcinoma using tissue microarrays. Hum Pathol 34: 444–449
139. Bostwick D G 1994 Gleason grading of prostatic needle biopsies. Correlation with grade in 316 matched prostatectomies. Am J Surg Pathol 18: 796–803
140. Stamey T A, McNeal J E, Yemoto C M et al. 1999 Biological determinants of cancer progression in men with prostate cancer. JAMA 281: 1395–1400
141. Carlson G D, Calvanase C B, Kahane H et al. 1998 Accuracy of biopsy Gleason scores from a large uropathology laboratory: use of a diagnostic protocol to minimize observer variability. Urology 51: 525–529
142. Dejter S W, Cunningham R E, Noguchi P D 1989 Prognostic significance of DNA ploidy in carcinoma of prostate. Urology 33: 361–366
143. Rubin M A, Bismar T A, Curtis S et al. 2004 Prostate needle biopsy reporting: how are the surgical members of the Society of Urologic Oncology using pathology reports to guide treatment of prostate cancer patients? Am J Surg Pathol 28: 946–952
144. Bismar T A, Lewis J S J, Vollmer R T et al. 2003 Multiple measures of carcinoma extent versus perineural invasion in prostate needle biopsy tissue in prediction of pathologic stage in a screening population. Am J Surg Pathol 27: 432–440
145. Rubin M A, Bassily N, Sanda M et al. 2000 Relationship and significance of greatest percentage of tumor and perineural invasion on needle biopsy in prostatic adenocarcinoma. Am J Surg Pathol 24: 183–189
146. Maru N, Ohori M, Kattan M W et al. 2001 Prognostic significance of the diameter of perineural invasion in radical prostatectomy specimens. Hum Pathol 32: 828–833
147. Herman C M, Wilcox G E, Kattan M W et al. 2000 Lymphovascular invasion as a predictor of disease progression in prostate cancer. Am J Surg Pathol 24: 859–863
148. Rubin M A, Dunn R, Kambham N et al. 2000 Should a Gleason score be assigned to a minute focus of carcinoma on prostate biopsy? . Am J Surg Pathol 24: 1634–1640
149. Kunz G M J, Epstein J I 2003 Should each core with prostate cancer be assigned a separate Gleason score? Hum Pathol 34: 911–914
150. Viglione M P, Potter S, Partin A W et al. 2002 Should the diagnosis of benign prostatic hyperplasia be made on prostate needle biopsy? Hum Pathol 33: 796–800
151. Cheng L, Cheville J C, Bostwick D G 1999 Diagnosis of prostate cancer in needle biopsies after radiation therapy. Am J Surg Pathol 23: 1173–1183
152. Magi-Galluzzi C, Sanderson H, Epstein J I 2003 Atypia in nonneoplastic prostate glands after radiotherapy for prostate cancer: duration of atypia and relation to type of radiotherapy. Am J Surg Pathol 27: 206–212
153. Gaudin P B, Zelefsky M J, Leibel S A et al. 1999 Histopathologic effects of three-dimensional conformal external beam radiation therapy on benign and malignant prostate tissues. Am J Surg Pathol 23: 1021–1031
154. Bostwick D G, Qian J, Civantos F et al. 2004 Does finasteride alter the pathology of the prostate and cancer grading? Clin Prostate Cancer 2: 228–235
155. Bullock M J, Srigley J R, Klotz L H et al. 2002 Pathologic effects of neoadjuvant cyproterone acetate on nonneoplastic prostate, prostatic intraepithelial neoplasia, and adenocarcinoma: a detailed analysis of radical prostatectomy specimens from a randomized trial. Am J Surg Pathol 26: 1400–1413
156. Bentley G, Dey J, Sakr W A et al. 2000 Significance of the Gleason scoring system after neoadjuvant hormonal therapy. Mol Urol 4: 125–131
157. Shabaik A, Wilson S, Bidair M et al. 1995 Pathologic changes in prostate biopsies following cryoablation therapy of prostate cancer. J Urol Pathol 3: 183–193
158. Bahn D K, Lee F, Solomon M H et al. 1995 Prostate cancer: US-guided percutaneous cryoablation. Radiology 194: 551–556
159. Ayala A G, Wheeler T M, Shalev M et al. 2000 Cytopathic effect of in situ gene therapy in prostate cancer. Hum Pathol 31: 866–870
160. Grignon D J 2004 Unusual subtypes of prostate cancer. Mod Pathol 17: 316–327
161. Ro J Y, Grignon D J, Amin M B et al. 1997 Atlas of surgical pathology of the male reproductive tract. W B Saunders, Philadelphia
162. Boyd S 1882 A case of colloid scirrhus of the prostate. Trans Pathol Soc Lond 33: 200–203
163. Ro J Y, Grignon D J, Ayala A G 1990 Mucinous adenocarcinoma of the prostate: histochemical and immunohistochemical studies. Hum Pathol 21: 593–600
164. Epstein J I, Lieberman P H 1985 Mucinous adenocarcinoma of the prostate gland. Am J Surg Pathol 9: 299–308
165. Saito S, Iwaki H 1999 Mucin-producing carcinoma of the prostate: review of 88 cases. Urology 54: 141–144

166. Proia A D, McCarty K S, Woodard B H 1981 Prostatic mucinous adenocarcinoma: a Cowper gland carcinoma mimicker. Am J Surg Pathol 5: 701–706
167. Cricco R P, Kassis J 1979 Mucinous adenocarcinoma of prostate. Urology 14: 276–278
168. Alfthan O, Koivuniemi A 1970 Mucinous carcinoma of the prostate: case report. Scand J Urol Nephrol 4: 78–80
169. Sika J V, Buckley J J 1977 Mucus-forming adenocarcinoma of prostate. J Urol 118: 124–125
170. Elbadawi A, Craig W, Linke C A et al. 1979 Prostate mucinous carcinoma. Urology 13: 658–666
171. Patel R C, Dias R, Fernandes M et al. 1981 Adenocarcinoma of the prostate. Mucin secreting. NY State J Med 81: 936–937
172. Chica G, Johnson D E, Ayala A G 1977 Mucinous adenocarcinoma of the prostate. J Urol 118: 124–125
173. Lightbourn G A, Abrams M, Seymour L 1969 Primary mucoid adenocarcinoma of the prostate gland with bladder invasion. J Urol 101: 78–80
174. Lee D W, Ro J Y, Sahin A A 1990 Mucinous adenocarcinoma of the prostate with endobronchial metastasis. Am J Clin Pathol 94: 641–645
175. Odom D G, Donatucci C F, Deshon G E 1986 Mucinous adenocarcinoma of the prostate. Hum Pathol 17: 863–865
176. Manne R K, Haddad F S 1989 Mucinous adenocarcinoma of prostate. Urology 33: 247–249
177. Uchijima Y, Ito H, Takahashi M et al. 1990 Prostate mucinous adenocarcinoma with signet ring cells. Urology 36: 267–268
178. Franks L M, O'Shea J D, Thomson A E R 1964 Mucin in the prostate: a histochemical study in normal glands, latent, clinical, and colloid cancers. Cancer 17: 983–991
179. Pinder S E, McMahon R F T 1990 Mucins in prostatic carcinoma. Histopathology 16: 43–46
180. Nagakura K, Hayakawa M, Mukai K et al. 1986 Mucinous denocarcinoma of prostate: a case report and review of the literature. J Urol 135: 1025–1028
181. Ro J Y, El-Naggar A, Ayala A G 1988 Signet-ring-cell carcinoma of the prostate: electron-microscopic and immunohistochemical studies of eight cases. Am J Surg Pathol 12: 453–460
182. Hejka A G, England D M 1989 Signet ring cell carcinoma of prostate: immunohistochemical and ultrastructural study of a case. Urology 34: 155–158
183. Remmele W, Weber A, Harding P 1988 Primary signet ring cell carcinoma of the prostate. Hum Pathol 19: 478–480
184. Giltman L I 1981 Signet-ring adenocarcinoma of the prostate. J Urol 126: 134–135
185. Kums J J, van Helsdingen P J 1985 Signet-ring-cell carcinoma of the bladder and prostate. Urol Int 40: 116–119
186. Leong F J, Leong A S, Swift J 1996 Signet-ring cell carcinoma of the prostate. Pathol Res Pract 192: 1232–1238
187. Torbenson M, Dhir R, Nangia A et al. 1998 Prostatic carcinoma with signet ring cells: a clinicopathologic and immunohistochemical analysis of 12 cases, with review of the literature. Mod Pathol 11: 552–559
188. Alguacil-Garcia A 1986 Artifactual changes mimicking signet-ring-cell carcinoma of transurethral prostatectomy specimens. Am J Surg Pathol 10: 795–800
189. Schned A R 1987 Artifactual signet-ring cells (letter). Am J Surg Pathol 11: 736–737
190. Fergusson J D, Frank L M 1953 The response of prostatic carcinoma to estrogen treatment. Br J Surg 40: 422–428
191. Melicow M M, Pachter M R 1967 Endometrial carcinoma of prostate utricle (uterus masculinus). Cancer 20: 1715–1722
192. Ro J Y, Ayala A G, Wishnow K I 1988 Prostatic duct adenocarcinoma with endometrioid features: immunohistochemical and electron microscopic study. Semin Diagn Pathol 5: 301–311
193. Zaloudek C, Williams J W, Kempson R L 1976 "Endometrial" adenocarcinoma of the prostate: a distinctive tumor of prostatic duct origin. Cancer 37: 2255–2262
194. Bostwick D G, Kindrachuk R W, Rouse R V 1985 Prostatic adenocarcinoma with endometrioid features: clinical, pathologic, and ultrastructural findings. Am J Surg Pathol 9: 595–609
195. Epstein J I, Woodruff J M 1986 Adenocarcinoma of the prostate with endometrioid features: a light microscopic and immunohistochemical study of ten cases. Cancer 57: 111–119
196. Bock B J, Bostwick D G 1999 Does prostatic ductal adenocarcinoma exist? Am J Surg Pathol 23: 781–785
197. Lee S S 1994 Endometrioid adenocarcinoma of the prostate: a clinicopathologic and immunohistochemical study. J Surg Oncol 55: 235–238
198. Melicow M M, Tannenbaum M 1971 Endometrial carcinoma of uterus masculinus (prostatic utricle): report of 6 cases. J Urol 106: 892–902
199. Young B W, Lagios M D 1973 Endometrial (papillary) carcinoma of the prostatic utricle: response to orchiectomy. A case report. Cancer 32: 1293–1300
200. Sufrin G, Gaeta J, Staubitz W J 1986 Endometrial carcinoma of prostate. Urology 27: 18–29
201. Merchant R F, Graham A R, Bucher W C J 1976 Endometrial carcinoma of prostatic utricle with osseous metastases. Urology 8: 169–173
202. Rotterdam H Z, Melicow M M 1975 Double primary prostatic adenocarcinoma. Urology 6: 245–248
203. Dube V E, Farrow G M, Greene L F 1973 Prostatic adenocarcinoma of ductal origin. Cancer 32: 402–409
204. Dube V E, Joyce G T, Kennedy E 1972 Papillary primary duct adenocarcinoma of the prostate. J Urol 107: 825–826
205. Christensen W N, Steinberg C, Walsh P C et al. 1991 Prostatic duct adenocarcinoma: findings at radical prostatectomy. Cancer 67: 2118–2124
206. Brinker D A, Potter S R, Epstein J I 1999 Ductal adenocarcinoma of the prostate diagnosed on needle biopsy: correlation with clinical and radical prostatectomy findings and progression. Am J Surg Pathol 23: 1471–1479
207. Chan J K, Chow T C, Tsui M S 1987 Prostatic-type polyps of the lower urinary tract: three histogenetic types? Histopathology 11: 789–801
208. Remick D G, Kumar N B 1984 Benign polyps with prostatic-type epithelium of the urethra and the urinary bladder: a suggestion of histogenesis based on histologic and immunohistochemical studies. Am J Surg Pathol 8: 833–839
209. Butterick J D, Schnitzer B, Abell M R 1971 Ectopic prostatic tissue in urethra: a clinicopathological entity and a significant cause of hematuria. J Urol 105: 97–104
210. Stein A J, Prioleau P G, Catalona W J 1980 Adenomatous polyps of the prostatic urethra: a cause of hematospermia. J Urol 124: 298–299
211. Goldstein A M, Bragin S D, Terry R et al. 1981 Prostatic urethral polyps in adults: histopathologic variations and clinical manifestations. J Urol 126: 129–131
212. Baroudy A C, O'Connell J P 1984 Papillary adenoma of the prostatic urethra. J Urol 132: 120–122
213. Tetu B, Ro J Y, Ayala A G 1987 Small cell carcinoma of the prostate. Part 1: a clinicopathologic study of 20 cases. Cancer 59: 1803–1809
214. Schron D S, Gipson T, Mendelsohn G 1984 The histogenesis of small cell carcinoma of the prostate: an immunohistochemical study. Cancer 53: 2478–2480
215. Sarma D P, Weilbaecher T G 1989 Small-cell carcinoma of prostate. Urology 33: 332–335
216. Hagood P G, Johnson F E, Bedrossian C W 1991 Small cell carcinoma of the prostate. Cancer 67: 1046–1050
217. Amato R J, Logothetis C J, Hallinan R 1992 Chemotherapy for small cell carcinoma of prostatic origin. J Urol 147: 935–937
218. Oesterling J E, Hauzeur C G, Farrow G M 1992 Small cell anaplastic carcinoma of the prostate: a clinical, pathological and immunohistological study of 27 patients. J Urol 147: 804–807
219. Ro J Y, Tetu B, Ayala A G 1987 Small cell carcinoma of the prostate. II. Immunohistochemical and electron microscopic study of 18 cases. Cancer 59: 977–982
219a. Yao J L, Madeb R, Bourne P et al. 2006 Small cell carcinoma of the prostate: an immunohistochemical study. Am J Surg Pathol 30: 705–712
220. Tetu B, Ro J Y, Ayala A G 1989 Small cell carcinoma of prostate associated with myasthenic (Eaton–Lambert) syndrome. Urology 33: 148–152
221. Wenk R E, Bhagavan B S, Levy R 1977 Ectopic ACTH, prostatic oat cell carcinoma and marked hypernatremia. Cancer 40: 773–778
222. Ghali V S, Garcia R L 1984 Prostatic adenocarcinoma with carcinoidal features producing adrenocorticotropic syndrome: immunohistochemical study and review of the literature. Cancer 54: 1043–1048
223. Hindson D A, Knight L L, Ocker J M 1985 Small cell carcinoma of prostate: transient complete remission with chemotherapy. Urology 26: 182–184
224. Johnson D E, Chalbaud R, Ayala A G 1974 Secondary tumors of the prostate. J Urol 112: 507–508
225. Zein T A, Huben R, Lane W 1985 Secondary tumors of the prostate. J Urol 133: 615–616
226. Smedley H M, Brown C, Turner A 1983 Ectopic ACTH-producing lung cancer presenting with prostatic metastasis. Postgrad Med J 59: 371–372
227. Ordonez N G 2000 Value of thyroid transcription factor-1 immunostaining in distinguishing small cell lung carcinomas from other small cell carcinomas. Am J Surg Pathol 24: 1217–1223
228. Weaver M G, Abdul-Karim F W, Srigley J R 1992 Paneth cell-like change of the prostate gland. A histological, immunohistochemical, and electron microscopic study. Am J Surg Pathol 16: 62–68
229. Adlakha H, Bostwick D G 1994 Paneth cell-like change in prostatic adenocarcinoma represents neuroendocrine differentiation: report of 30 cases. Hum Pathol 25: 135–139
230. Accetta P A, Gardner W A 1982 Squamous metastases from prostatic adenocarcinoma. Lab Invest 46: 2A
231. Moyana T N 1987 Adenosquamous carcinoma of the prostate. Am J Surg Pathol 11: 403–407
232. Saito R, Davis B K, Ollapally E P 1984 Adenosquamous carcinoma of the prostate. Hum Pathol 15: 87–89
233. Lager D J, Goeken J A, Kemp J D 1988 Squamous metaplasia of the prostate: an immunohistochemical study. Am J Clin Pathol 90: 597–601
234. Bennett R S, Edgerton E O 1973 Mixed prostatic carcinoma. J Urol 110: 561–563
235. Gray G F, Marshall V F 1975 Squamous carcinoma of the prostate. J Urol 113: 736–738
236. Mai K T, Leahy C F 1996 Squamous cell carcinoma occurring as a circumscribed nodule in the transition zone of the prostate. J Urol Pathol 5: 85–92
237. Parwani A V, Kronz J D, Genega E M et al. 2004 Prostate carcinoma with squamous differentiation: an analysis of 33 cases. Am J Surg Pathol 28: 651–657
238. Mott L J 1979 Squamous cell carcinoma of the prostate: report of 2 cases and review of the literature. J Urol 121: 833–835
239. Sieracki J C 1955 Epidermoid carcinoma of the human prostate: report of three cases. Lab Invest 4: 232–240

240. Sarma D P, Weilbaecher T G, Moon T D 1991 Squamous cell carcinoma of prostate. Urology 37: 260–262
241. Wernert N, Goebbels R, Bonkhoff H 1990 Squamous cell carcinoma of the prostate. Histopathology 17: 339–344
242. Al Adnani M S 1985 Schistosomiasis, metaplasia and squamous cell carcinoma of the prostate: histogenesis of the squamous cells determined by localization of specific markers. Neoplasma 32: 613–622
243. Gattuso P, Carson H J, Candel A et al. 1995 Adenosquamous carcinoma of the prostate. Hum Pathol 26: 123–126
244. Corder M P, Cicmil G A 1976 Effective treatment of metastatic squamous cell carcinoma of the prostate with adriamycin. J Urol 115: 222
245. Thompson G J, Albers D D, Broders A C 1953 Unusual carcinomas involving the prostate gland. J Urol 69: 416–425
246. Goebbels R, Amberger L, Wernert N l 1985 Urothelial carcinoma of the prostate. Appl Pathol 3: 242–254
247. Ro J Y, Ayala A G, El-Naggar A 1987 Seminal vesicle involvement by in situ and invasive transitional cell carcinoma of the bladder. Am J Surg Pathol 11: 951–958
248. Wishnow K I, Ro J Y 1988 Importance of early treatment of transitional cell carcinoma of prostatic ducts. Urology 32: 11–12
249. Terris M K, Villers A, Freiha F S 1990 Transrectal ultrasound appearance of transitional cell carcinoma involving the prostate. J Urol 143: 952–956
250. Kirk D, Savage A, Makepeace M A et al. 1981 Transitional cell carcinoma involving the prostate – an unfavorable prognostic sign in the management of bladder cancer? Br J Urol 53: 610–612
251. Mahadevia P S, Koss L G, Tar I J 1986 Prostatic involvement in bladder cancer. Prostate mapping in 20 cystoprostatectomy specimens. Cancer 58: 2096–2102
252. Schellhammer P F, Bean M A, Whitmore W F J 1977 Prostatic involvement by transitional cell carcinoma: pathogenesis, patterns and prognosis. J Urol 118: 399–403
253. Amin M B, Murphy W M, Reuter V E 1997 Controversies in the pathology of transitional cell carcinoma of the urinary bladder, part II. In: Fechner F E, Rosen P P (eds) ASCP reviews in pathology, vol. 1. ASCP Press, Chicago, p 1–38
254. Cheville J C, Dundore P A, Bostwick D G 1998 Transitional cell carcinoma of the prostate. Clinical, pathological study of 50 cases. Cancer 82: 703–707
255. Wendelken J R, Schellhammer P F, Ladaga L E et al. 1979 Transitional cell carcinoma: cause of refractory cancer of the prostate. Urology 13: 557–560
256. Tomaszewki J E, Korat O C, LiVolsi V A 1986 Paget's disease of urethral meatus following transitional cell carcinoma of the bladder. J Urol 135: 368–370
257. Wood D P J, Montie J E, Pontes J E 1989 Transitional cell carcinoma of the prostate in cystoprostatectomy specimens removed for bladder cancer. J Urol 141: 346–349
258. Mhawech P, Uchida T, Pelte M F 2002 Immunohistochemical profile of high-grade urothelial bladder carcinoma and prostate adenocarcinoma. Hum Pathol 33: 1136–1140
259. Shannon R L, Ro J Y, Grignon D J 1992 Sarcomatoid carcinoma of the prostate: a clinicopathologic study of 12 patients. Cancer 69: 2676–2682
260. Ro J Y, Ayala A G, Sella A 1987 Sarcomatoid renal cell carcinoma: a clinicopathologic study of 42 cases. Cancer 59: 516–526
261. Ro J Y, Ayala A G, Wishnow K I 1988 Sarcomatoid bladder carcinoma: clinicopathologic and immunohistochemical study of 44 cases. Surg Pathol 2: 359–374
262. Dundore P A, Chevill J C, Nascimento A G et al. 1995 Carcinosarcoma of prostate. Report of 21 cases. Cancer 76: 1035–1042
263. Ohtsuki Y, Ro J Y, Ordonez N G 1996 Sarcomatoid carcinoma of the prostate with rhabdomyosarcomatous differentiation. J Urol Pathol 5: 157–163
264. Wick M R, Young R H, Malvesta R 1989 Prostatic carcinosarcomas. Clinical, histologic, and immunohistochemical data on two cases, with a review of the literature. Am J Clin Pathol 92: 131–139
265. Ogawa K, Kim Y C, Nakashima Y 1987 Expression of epithelial markers in sarcomatoid carcinoma: an immunohistochemical study. Histopathology 11: 511–522
266. Lauwers G Y, Schevchuk M, Armenakas N 1993 Carcinosarcoma of the prostate. Am J Surg Pathol 17: 342–349
267. Montironi R, Alexander E, Bostwick D G 1997 Prostate pathology case study seminar. Virchows Arch 430: 83–94
268. Ordonez N G, Ro J Y, Ayala A G 1992 Metastatic prostatic carcinoma presenting as an oncocytic tumor. Am J Surg Pathol 16: 1007–1012
269. Singh H, Flores-Sandoval N, Abrams J 2003 Renal-type clear cell carcinoma occurring in the prostate. Am J Surg Pathol 27: 407–410
270. Pan C C, Chiang H, Chang Y H et al. 2000 Tubulocystic clear cell adenocarcinoma arising within the prostate. Am J Surg Pathol 24: 1433–1436
271. Bostwick D G 1988 Premalignant lesions of the prostate. Semin Diagn Pathol 5: 240–253
272. Bostwick D G, Srigley J, Grignon D 1993 Atypical adenomatous hyperplasia of the prostate: morphologic criteria for its distinction from well-differentiated carcinoma. Hum Pathol 24: 819–832
273. Bostwick D G, Algaba F, Ayala A G 1994 Consensus statement on terminology: recommendation to use atypical adenomatous hyperplasia in place of adenosis of the prostate. Am J Surg Pathol 18: 1069–1071
274. Gaudin P B, Epstein J I 1994 Adenosis of the prostate: histologic features in transurethral resection specimens. Am J Surg Pathol 18: 863–870
275. Lopez-Beltran A, Artacho-Perula E, Luque-Barona R J et al. 2000 Nuclear volume estimates in prostatic atypical adenomatous hyperplasia. Anal Quant Cytol Histol 22: 438–444
276. Doll J A, Zhu X, Furman J et al. 1999 Genetic analysis of prostatic atypical adenomatous hyperplasia (adenosis). Am J Pathol 155: 967–971
277. Cheng L, Shan A, Cheville J C et al. 1998 Atypical adenomatous hyperplasia of the prostate: a premalignant lesion? Cancer Res 58: 389–391
278. Bostwick D G, Qian J 1995 Atypical adenomatous hyperplasia of the prostate. Relationship with carcinoma in 217 whole-mount radical prostatectomies. Am J Surg Pathol 19: 506–518
279. Mittal B V, Amin M B, Kinare S G 1989 Spectrum of histologic lesions in 185 consecutive prostatic specimens. J Postgrad Med 35: 157–161
280. Srigley J R, Toth P, Hartwick R W 1989 Atypical histologic patterns in cases of benign prostatic hyperplasia [abstract]. Lab Invest 60: 90A
281. Yang X J, Wu C L, Woda B A et al. 2002 Expression of alpha-methylacyl-CoA racemase (P504S) in atypical adenomatous hyperplasia of the prostate. Am J Surg Pathol 26: 921–925
282. Young R H 1988 Pseudoneoplastic lesions of the prostate gland. Pathol Annu 23: 105–128
283. Cleary K R, Choi H Y, Ayala A G 1983 Basal cell hyperplasia of the prostate. Am J Clin Pathol 80: 850–854
284. Grignon D J, Ro J Y, Ordonez N G et al. 1988 Basal cell hyperplasia, adenoid basal cell tumor, and adenoid cystic carcinoma of the prostate gland: an immunohistochemical study. Hum Pathol 19: 1425–1433
285. Sesterhenn I, Mostofi F K, Davis C J 1987 Basal cell hyperplasia and basal cell carcinoma. Lab Invest 56: 71A (abstract)
286. Hosler G A, Epstein J I 2005 Basal cell hyperplasia: an unusual diagnostic dilemma on prostate needle biopsies. Hum Pathol 36: 480–485
287. Van de Voorde W, Baldewijns M, Lauwerys J 1994 Florid basal cell hyperplasia of the prostate. Histopathology 24: 341–348
288. Sahin A A, Ro J Y, Troncoso P et al. 1990 Benign prostatic lesions with small acinar pattern mimicking adenocarcinoma. In: Damjanov I, Mills S E, Cohen A H et al. (eds) Progress in reproductive and urinary tract pathology. Field and Wood, Philadelphia, p 69–86
289. Yang X J, Tretiakova M S, Sengupta E et al. 2003 Florid basal cell hyperplasia of the prostate: a histological, ultrastructural, and immunohistochemical analysis. Hum Pathol 34: 462070
290. Thorson P, Swanson P E, Vollmer R T et al. 2003 Basal cell hyperplasia in the peripheral zone of the prostate. Mod Pathol 16: 598–606
291. Vales-Depena M A 1979 Prostate, Histology of the fetus and newborn. W B Saunders, Philadelphia, p 415–429
292. Ronnett B M, Epstein J I 1989 A case showing sclerosing adenosis and an unusual form of basal cell hyperplasia of the prostate. Am J Surg Pathol 13: 866–872
293. Ayala A G, Srigley J R, Ro J Y 1986 Clear cell cribriform hyperplasia of prostate: report of 10 cases. Am J Surg Pathol 10: 665–671
294. Rioux-Leclercq N C, Epstein J I 2002 Unusual morphologic patterns of basal cell hyperplasia of the prostate. Am J Surg Pathol 26: 237–243
295. McNeal J E 1988 Normal histology of the prostate. Am J Surg Pathol 12: 619–633
296. Molinie V, Herve J M, Lebret T 2004 Value of the antibody cocktail anti p63 + anti p504s for the diagnosis of prostatic cancer. Ann Pathol 24: 6–16
297. Hendrick L, Epstein J I 1989 Use of keratin 903 as an adjunct in the diagnosis of prostate carcinoma. Am J Surg Pathol 13: 389–396
298. Tannenbaum M, Becker S W 1977 Histopathology of the prostate gland. In: Tannenbaum M (ed) Urologic pathology: the prostate. Lea & Febiger, Philadelphia, p 303–397
299. Totten R S, Heinemann M W, Hudson P B et al. 1953 Microscopic differential diagnosis of latent carcinoma of prostate. Arch Pathol 55: 131–141
300. Harade M, Mostofi F K, Corle D K et al. 1977 Preliminary studies on histologic prognostic significance in cancer of the prostate. Cancer Treat Rep 61: 223–225
301. Myers R P, Neves R J, Farrow G M et al. 1982 Nucleolar grading of prostatic adenocarcinoma: light microscopic correlation with disease progression. Prostate 3: 423–432
302. Tannenbaum M, Tannenbaum S, DeSanctis P N et al. 1982 Prognostic significance of nucleolar surface area in prostate cancer. Urology 19: 546–551
303. Derme G B 1978 Basal cell proliferation in benign prostatic hyperplasia. Cancer 41: 1857–1862
304. Lin J I, Cohen E L, Villacin A B 1978 Basal cell adenoma of prostate. Urology 11: 409–410
305. Devaraj L T, Bostwick D G 1993 Atypical basal cell hyperplasia of the prostate: immunohistochemical profile and proposed classification of basal cell proliferations. Am J Surg Pathol 17: 645–659
306. Epstein J I, Armas O A 1992 Atypical basal cell hyperplasia of the prostate. Am J Surg Pathol 16: 1205–1214
307. Ayala A G, Ro J Y 1989 Premalignant lesions of the urothelium and transitional cell tumors. In: Young R H (ed) Pathology of the urinary bladder. Churchill Livingstone, New York, p 65–101
308. Reed R J 1984 Consultation case: prostate (prostatectomy) – adenoid basal cell tumor-multifocal basal cell hyperplasia. Am J Surg Pathol 8: 699–704
309. Young R H, Frierson H F, Mills S E 1988 Adenoid cystic-like tumor of the prostate gland. A report of two cases and review of the literature on "adenoid cystic carcinoma" of the prostate. Am J Clin Pathol 89: 49–56
310. Iczkowski K A, Ferguson K L, Grier D D et al. 2003 Adenoid cystic/basal cell carcinoma of the prostate: clinicopathologic findings in 19 cases. Am J Surg Pathol 27: 1523–1529

311. Yang X J, McEntee M, Epstein J I 1998 Distinction of basaloid carcinoma of the prostate from benign basal cell lesions by using immunohistochemistry for bcl-2 and Ki-67. Hum Pathol 29: 1447–1450
312. McKenney J K, Amin M B, Srigley J R 2004 Basal cell proliferations of the prostate other than usual basal cell hyperplasia: a clinicopathologic study of 23 cases, including four carcinomas, with a proposed classification. Am J Surg Pathol 28: 1289–1298
313. Frauenhoffer E E, Ro J Y, El-Naggar A K 1991 Clear cell cribriform hyperplasia of the prostate: immunohistochemical and DNA flow cytometric study. Am J Clin Pathol 95: 446–453
314. McNeal J E, Reese J H, Redwine E A 1986 Cribriform adenocarcinoma of the prostate. Cancer 58: 1714–1719
315. Chen K T, Schiff J J 1983 Adenomatoid prostatic tumor. Urology 21: 88–89
316. Hulman G 1989 "Pseudoadenomatoid" tumor of prostate. Histopathology 14: 317–319
317. Sesterhenn I A, Mostofi F K 1988 Fibroepithelial nodules of the prostate simulating carcinoma. Lab Invest 58: 83A
318. Young R H, Clement P B 1987 Sclerosing adenosis of the prostate. Arch Pathol Lab Med 111: 363–366
319. Sakamoto N, Tsuneyoshi M, Enjoji M 1991 Sclerosing adenosis of the prostate. Histopathologic and immunohistochemical analysis. Am J Surg Pathol 15: 660–667
320. Luque R J, Lopez-Beltran A, Perez-Seoane C et al. 2003 Sclerosing adenosis of the prostate. Histologic features in needle biopsy specimens. Arch Pathol Lab Med 127: e14–16
321. Jones E C, Clement P B, Young R H 1991 Sclerosing adenosis of the prostate gland. A clinicopathological and immunohistochemical study of 11 cases. Am J Surg Pathol 15: 1171–1180
322. Gikas P W, Del Buono E A, Epstein J I 1993 Florid hyperplasia of mesonephric remnants involving prostate and periprostatic tissue. Possible confusion with adenocarcinoma. Am J Surg Pathol 17: 454–460
323. Bostwick D G, Qian J, Ma J et al. 2003 Mesonephric remnants of the prostate: incidence and histologic spectrum. Mod Pathol 16: 630–635
324. Amin M B, Tamboli P, Varma M et al. 1995 Florid hyperplasia of mesonephric remnants: yet another differential diagnostic consideration under "small acinar proliferations of the prostate." Adv Anat Pathol 2: 108–113
325. Jimenez R E, Raval M F, Spanta R et al. 1998 Mesonephric remnants hyperplasia. Pitfall in the diagnosis of prostatic adenocarcinoma. J Urol Pathol 9: 83–92
326. Ayala A G, Tibbs R F, Tamboli P et al. 2004 High-grade prostatic intraepithelial neoplasia (PIN)-like lesion; a possible embryologic remnant mimicking carcinoma. Mod Pathol 17: 138A (abstract)
327. Gaudin P B, Wheeler T M, Epstein J I 1995 Verumontanum mucosal gland hyperplasia (VMGH) in prostatic needle biopsy specimens: a mimic of low-grade prostatic adenocarcinoma. Am J Clin Pathol 104: 620–626
328. Muezzinoglu B, Erdamar S, Chakraborty S et al. 2001 Verumontanum mucosal gland hyperplasia is associated with atypical adenomatous hyperplasia of the prostate. Arch Pathol Lab Med 125: 358–360
329. Gagucas R J, Brown R W, Wheeler T M 1995 Verumontanum mucosal gland hyperplasia. Am J Surg Pathol 19: 30–36
330. Davis T A 1949 Hamartoma of the urinary bladder. Northwest Med 48: 182–185
331. Friedman N B, Kuhlenbeck H 1950 Adenomatoid tumors of the bladder reproducing renal structures (nephrogenic adenomas). J Urol 64: 657–670
332. Peterson L J, Matsumoto L M 1978 Nephrogenic adenoma in urethral diverticulum. Urology 11: 193–195
333. Young R H, Scully R E 1986 Nephrogenic adenoma. A report of 15 cases, review of the literature, and comparison with clear cell adenocarcinoma of the urinary tract. Am J Surg Pathol 10: 268–275
334. Bhagavan B S, Tiamson E M, Wenk R E 1981 Nephrogenic adenoma of the urinary bladder and urethra. Hum Pathol 12: 907–916
335. Navarre R J J, Loening S A, Platz C 1982 Nephrogenic adenoma: a report of 9 cases and review of the literature. J Urol 127: 775–779
336. Rubin P, Murphy W M, Driver C 1985 Nephrogenic adenoma. Urology 25: 190–193
337. Newman J, Antonakopoulos G N 1985 Widespread mucous metaplasia of the urinary bladder with nephrogenic adenoma. Arch Pathol Lab Med 109: 560–563
338. McIntire T L, Soloway M S, Murphy W M 1987 Nephrogenic adenoma. Urology 29: 237–241
339. Malpica A, Ro J Y, Troncoso P 1994 Nephrogenic adenoma of prostatic urethra involving the prostate gland: a clinicopathological and immunohistochemical study of eight cases. Hum Pathol 25: 390–395
340. Oliva E, Young R H 1995 Nephrogenic adenoma of the urinary tract: a review of the microscopic appearance of 80 cases with emphasis on unusual features. Mod Pathol 8: 722–730
341. Devine P, Ucci A A, Krain H 1984 Nephrogenic adenoma and embryonic kidney tubules share PNA receptor sites. Am J Clin Pathol 81: 728–732
342. Murphy W M 1989 Diseases of the urinary bladder, urethra, ureters, and renal pelvis. In: Murphy W M (ed) Urological pathology. W B Saunders, Philadelphia, p 34–146
343. Peterson R O 1986 Urologic pathology. J B Lippincott, Philadelphia
344. Amin M B, Young R H 1997 Primary carcinomas of the urethra. Semin Diagn Pathol 14: 147–160
345. Drew P A, Murphy W M, Civantos F et al. 1996 The histogenesis of clear cell adenocarcinoma of the lower urinary tract. Case series and review of the literature. Hum Pathol 27: 248–252
346. Gupta A, Wang H L, Policarpio-Nicolas M L et al. 2004 Expression of alpha-methylacyl-coenzyme A racemase in nephrogenic adenoma. Am J Surg Pathol 28: 1224–1229
347. Allan C H, Epstein J I 2001 Nephrogenic adenoma of the prostatic urethra: a mimicker of prostate adenocarcinoma. Am J Surg Pathol 25: 802–808
348. Skinnider B F, Oliva E, Young R H et al. 2004 Expression of alpha-methylacyl-CoA racemase (P504S) in nephrogenic adenoma: a significant immunohistochemical pitfall compounding the differential diagnosis with prostatic adenocarcinoma. Am J Surg Pathol 28: 701–705
349. Hara S, Horie A 1977 Prostatic caruncle: a urethral papillary tumor derived from prolapse of the prostatic ducts. J Urol 117: 303–305
350. Mugler K C, Woods J E 2003 Pathologic quiz case: urethral mass in a 62-year-old man. Prostatic-type polyp of verumontanum. Arch Pathol Lab Med 127: e351–e352
351. Nesbit R M 1962 The genesis of benign polyps in the prostatic urethra. J Urol 87: 416–418
352. Walker A N, Mills S E, Fechner R E 1983 Epithelial polyps of the prostatic urethra. Am J Surg Pathol 7: 351–356
353. Craig J R, Hart W R 1975 Benign polyps with prostatic type epithelium of the urethra. Am J Clin Pathol 63: 343–347
354. Klein H Z, Rosenberg M L 1984 Ectopic prostatic tissue in bladder trigone: distinctive cause of hematuria. Urology 23: 81–82
355. Mostofi F K, Davis C J 1985 Male reproductive system and prostate. In: Kissane J M (ed) Anderson's pathology. C V Mosby, St. Louis, p 791–831
356. Eglen D E, Pontius E E 1984 Benign prostatic epithelial polyp of the urethra. J Urol 131: 120–122
357. Jensen K M, Sonneland P, Madsen P O 1983 Seminal vesicle tissue in "resectate" of transurethral resection of prostate. Urology 22: 20–23
358. Tsuang M T, Weiss M A, Evans A T 1981 Transurethral resection of the prostate with partial resection of the seminal vesicle. J Urol 126: 615–617
359. Shah R B, Lee M W, Giraldo A A et al. 2001 Histologic and histochemical characterization of seminal vesicle intraluminal secretions. Arch Pathol Lab Med 125: 141–145
360. Leroy X, Ballereau C, Villers A et al. 2003 MUC6 is a marker of seminal vesicle-ejaculatory duct epithelium and is useful for the differential diagnosis with prostate adenocarcinoma. Am J Surg Pathol 27: 519–521
361. Melcher M P 1986 Bulbourethral glands of Cowper. Arch Pathol Lab Med 110: 991 (letter)
362. Saboorian M H, Huffman H, Ashfaq R et al. 1997 Distinguishing Cowper's glands from neoplastic and pseudoneoplastic lesions of prostate. Immunohistochemical and ultrastructural studies. Am J Surg Pathol 21: 1069–1074
363. Cina S J, Silberman M A, Kahane H et al. 1997 Diagnosis of Cowper's glands on prostate needle biopsy. Am J Surg Pathol 21: 550–555
364. Shiraishi T, Kusano I, Watanabe M 1993 Mucous gland metaplasia of the prostate. Am J Surg Pathol 17: 618–622
365. Grignon D J, O'Malley F P 1993 Mucinous metaplasia in the prostate gland. Am J Surg Pathol 17: 287–290
366. Rode J, Bentley A, Parkinson C 1990 Paraganglial cells of urinary bladder and prostate: potential diagnostic problem. J Clin Pathol 43: 13–16
367. Ostrowski M L, Wheeler T M 1994 Paraganglia of the prostate: location, frequency, and differentiation from prostatic adenocarcinoma. Am J Surg Pathol 18: 412–420
368. Parwani A V, Cao D, Epstein J I 2004 Pathologic quiz case: a 35-year old man with hematuria. Paraganglioma involving the prostate. Arch Pathol Lab Med 128: e104–e106
369. Gardner W A J, Culberson D E 1987 Atrophy and proliferation in the young adult prostate. J Urol 137: 53–56
370. Moore R A 1936 The evolution and involution of the prostate gland. Am J Pathol 12: 599–624
371. Franks L M 1954 Atrophy and hyperplasia in the prostate proper. J Pathol Bacteriol 68: 617–621
372. Liavag I 1968 Atrophy and regeneration in the pathogenesis of prostate carcinoma. Acta Pathol Microbiol Scand 73: 338–350
373. Billis A, Magna L A 2003 Inflammatory atrophy of the prostate. Prevalence and significance. Arch Pathol Lab Med 127: 840–844
374. Meirelles L R, Billis A, Cotta A C et al. 2002 Prostatic atrophy: evidence for a possible role of local ischemia in its pathogenesis. Int Urol Nephrol 34: 345–350
375. McNeal J E 1983 The prostate gland: morphology and pathology. Monogr Urol 4: 3–33
376. Billis A, Magna L A 2000 Prostate elastosis: a microscopic feature useful for the diagnosis of postatrophic hyperplasia. Arch Pathol Lab Med 124: 1306–1309
377. O'Malley F P, Grignon D J, Shum D T 1990 Usefulness of immunoperoxidase staining with high molecular weight cytokeratin in the differential diagnosis of small acinar lesions of the prostate gland. Virchows Arch [A] 417: 191–196
378. Brawer M K, Nagle R B, Pitts W et al. 1989 Keratin immunoreactivity as an aid to the diagnosis of persistent adenocarcinoma in irradiated human prostates. Cancer 63: 454–460
379. Abrahams N A, Bostwick D G, Ormsby A H et al. 2003 Distinguishing atrophy and high-grade prostatic intraepithelial neoplasia from prostatic adenocarcinoma with and without previous adjuvant hormone therapy with the aid of cytokeratin 5/6. Am J Clin Pathol 120: 368–376
380. Amin M B, Tamboli P, Varma M et al. 1999 Postatrophic hyperplasia of the prostate gland: a detailed analysis of its morphology in needle biopsy specimens. Am J Surg Pathol 8: 925–931

381. Cheville J C, Bostwick D G 1995 Post-atrophic hyperplasia of the prostate. A histologic mimic of prostatic adenocarcinoma. Am J Surg Pathol 19: 1068–1076
382. Anton R C, Kattan M W, Chakraborty S et al. 1999 Postatrophic hyperplasia of the prostate: lack of association with prostate cancer. Am J Surg Pathol 23: 932–936
383. McNeal J E 1979 The origin and evolution of prostatic cancer. Cancer Detect Prev 2: 565–577
384. McNeal J E 1981 Normal and pathologic anatomy of prostate. Urology 17: 11–16
385. Tsujimoto Y, Takayama H, Nonomura N et al. 2002 Postatrophic hyperplasia of the prostate in Japan: histologic and immunohistochemical features and $p53$ gene mutation analysis. Prostate 52: 279–287
386. Ruska K M, Sauvageot J, Epstein J I 1998 Histology and cellular kinetics of prostatic atrophy. Am J Surg Pathol 22: 1073–1077
387. Shah R, Mucci N R, Amin A et al. 2001 Postatrophic hyperplasia of the prostate gland: neoplastic precursor or innocent bystander? Am J Pathol 158: 1767–1773
388. Ayala A G, Ro J Y, Babaian R 1989 The prostate capsule: does it exist? Am J Surg Pathol 13: 21–27
389. Graversen P H, England D M, Madsen P O 1988 Significance of striated muscle in curettings of the prostate. J Urol 139: 751–753
390. Manley C B 1966 The striated muscle of the prostate. J Urol 95: 234–240
391. Hasui Y, Shinkawa T, Osada Y 1989 Striated muscle in the biopsy specimen of the prostate. Prostate 14: 65–69
392. McIntire T L, Franzini D A 1986 The presence of benign prostatic glands in perineural spaces. J Urol 135: 507–509
393. Cramer S F 1981 Benign glandular inclusion in prostatic nerve. Am J Clin Pathol 75: 854–855
394. Carstens P H 1980 Perineural glands in normal and hyperplastic prostates. J Urol 123: 686–688
395. Choi Y H, Namkung S, Ryu B Y et al. 2000 Giant multilocular prostatic cystadenoma. J Urol 163: 246–247
396. Sung C O, Seo J, Song S Y 2004 Giant multilocular cystadenoma of the prostate. Kor J Pathol 38: 106–108
397. Franks L M 1954 Benign nodular hyperplasia of the prostate: a review. Ann R Coll Surg 14: 92–106
398. Regan J B, Barrett D M, Wold L E 1987 Giant leiomyoma of the prostate. Arch Pathol Lab Med 11: 381–382
399. Rosen Y, Ambiavagar P C, Vuletin J C 1980 Atypical leiomyoma of prostate. Urology 15: 183–185
400. Patch F S, Rhea L J 1935 Leiomyoma of the prostate gland. Br J Urol 7: 213–228
401. Michaels M M, Brown H E, Favino C J 1974 Leiomyoma of the prostate. Urology 3: 617–620
402. Begin L R 1993 Mucosubstance-rich myxoid stromal nodule of the prostate. Arch Pathol Lab Med 117: 318–320
403. Belis J A, Post G J, Rochman S C 1979 Genitourinary leiomyomas. Urology 13: 424–429
404. Kaufman J J, Berneike R R 1951 Leiomyoma of the prostate. J Urol 65: 297–310
405. Leonard A, Baert L, Van Praet F 1989 Solitary leiomyoma of the prostate. Br J Urol 60: 184–185
406. Wang X, Bostwick D G 1997 Prostatic stromal hyperplasia with atypia; a study of 11 cases. J Urol Pathol 6: 15–25
407. Attah E B, Powell M E 1977 Atypical stromal hyperplasia of the prostate gland. Am J Clin Pathol 67: 324–327
408. Leong S S, Vogt P J, Yu G S 1988 Atypical stromal smooth muscle hyperplasia of prostate. Urology 31: 163–167
409. Tetu B, Srigley J R, Bostwick D G 1990 Soft tissue tumors. In: Bostwick D G (ed) Pathology of the prostate. Churchill Livingstone, New York, p 117–135
410. Young R H, Scully R E 1987 Pseudosarcomatous lesions of the urinary bladder, prostate gland, and urethra; a report of three cases and review of the literature. Arch Pathol Lab Med 111: 354–358
411. Karolyi P, Endes P, Krasznai G 1988 Bizarre leiomyoma of the prostate. Virchow's Arch [A] 412: 383–386
412. Persaud V, Douglas L L 1982 Bizarre (atypical) leiomyoma of the prostate gland. West Ind Med J 31: 217–220
413. Tetu B, Ro J Y, Ayala A G 1988 Atypical spindle cell lesions of the prostate. Semin Diagn Pathol 5: 284–293
414. Gaudin P B, Rosai J, Epstein J I 1998 Sarcomas and related proliferative lesions of specialized prostatic stroma: a clinicopathologic study of 22 cases. Am J Surg Pathol 58: 43–50
415. Smith B H, Dehner L P 1972 Sarcoma of the prostate gland. Am J Clin Pathol 58: 43–50
416. Mottola A, Selli C, Carini M 1985 Leiomyosarcoma of the prostate. Eur Urol 11: 131–133
417. Muzafer M H 1987 Large leiomyoma of prostate. Br J Urol 5: 284–293
418. Vassilakis G B 1978 Pure leiomyoma of prostate. Urology 11: 93–94
419. Ro J Y, Grignon D J, Ayala A G 1988 Blue nevus and melanosis of the prostate: electron-microscopic and immunohistochemical studies. Am J Clin Pathol 90: 530–535
420. Lew S, Richter S, Jelin N 1991 A blue naevus of the prostate: a light microscopic study including an investigation of S-100 protein positive cells in the normal and in the diseased gland. Histopathology 18: 443–448
421. Langley J W, Weitzner S 1974 Blue nevus and melanosis of prostate. J Urol 112: 359–361
422. Brennick J B, O'Connell J X, Dickersin G R 1994 Lipofuscin pigmentation (so-called melanosis) of the prostate. Am J Surg Pathol 18: 446–454
423. Farid M K, Gahukamble L D 1995 Melanosis of the prostate in an elderly patient – a case report. Central Afr J Med 41: 101–102
424. Nigogosyan G, de la Pava S, Pickren J W 1963 Blue nevus of the prostate gland. Cancer 16: 1097–1099
425. Goldman R L 1968 Melanogenic epithelium in the prostate gland. Am J Clin Pathol 49: 75–78
426. Tannenbaum M 1974 Differential diagnosis in uropathology. III. Melanotic lesions of the prostate: blue nevus and prostatic epithelial melanosis. Urology 4: 617–621
427. Aguilar M, Gaffney E F, Finnerty D P 1982 Prostatic melanosis with involvement of benign and malignant epithelium. J Urol 128: 825–827
428. Block N L, Weber D, Schinella R 1972 Blue nevi and other melanotic lesions of the prostate: report of 3 cases and review of the literature. J Urol 107: 85–87
429. Gardner W A J, Spitz W U 1971 Melanosis of the prostate gland. Am J Clin Pathol 56: 762–764
430. Guillan R A, Zelman S 1970 The incidence and possible origin of melanin in the prostate. J Urol 104: 151–153
431. Rios C N, Wright J R 1976 Melanosis of the prostate gland: report of a case with neoplastic epithelium involvement. J Urol 115: 616–617
432. Jao W, Fretzin D F, Christ M L 1971 Blue nevus of the prostate gland. Arch Pathol Lab Med 91: 187–191
433. Kovi J, Jackson A G, Jackson M A 1977 Blue nevus of the prostate: ultrastructural study. Urology 9: 576–578
434. Martinez Marinez C J, Garcia Gonzalez R, Castaneda Casanova A L 1992 Blue nevus of the prostate: report of two new cases with immunohistochemical and electron-microscopic studies. Eur Urol 22: 339–342
435. Das Gupta T K, Brasfield R D, Paglia M A 1969 Primary melanomas in unusual sites. Surg Gynecol Obstet 128: 841–848
436. Berry N E, Reese L 1953 Malignant melanoma which had its first clinical manifestations in the prostate gland. J Urol 69: 286–290
437. Kafandaris P M, Polyzonis M B 1983 Fibroadenoma-like foci in human prostatic nodular hyperplasia. Prostate 4: 33–36
438. Cox R, Dawson M P 1960 A curious prostatic tumour: probably a true mixed tumour (cystadenoleiomyofibroma). Br J Urol 32: 306–311
439. Manivel C, Shenoy B V, Wick M R 1986 Cystosarcoma phyllodes of the prostate. Arch Pathol Lab Med 110: 534–538
440. Kirkland K L, Bale P M 1967 A cystic adenoma of the prostate. J Urol 97: 324–327
441. Attah E B, Nkposong E O 1976 Phyllodes type of atypical prostatic hyperplasia. J Urol 115: 762–764
442. Reese J H, Lombard C M, Krone K 1987 Phyllodes type of atypical prostatic hyperplasia: a report of 3 new cases. J Urol 138: 623–626
443. Ito H, Ito M, Mitsuhata N 1989 Phyllodes tumor of the prostate: a case report. Jpn J Clin Oncol 19: 299–304
444. Kendall A R, Stein B S, Shea F J 1986 Cystic pelvic mass: phyllodes-type variant of prostatic hyperplasia. J Urol 135: 550–553
445. Cummine H G, Johnson A S 1949 Report of a case of retrovesical polycystic tumour of probable prostatic origin. Aust NZ J Surg 19: 91–92
446. Lopez-Beltran A, Gaeta J F, Huben R et al. 1990 Malignant phyllodes tumor of prostate. Urology 35: 164–167
447. Kerley S W, Pierce P, Thomas J 1992 Giant cystosarcoma phyllodes of the prostate associated with adenocarcinoma. Arch Pathol Lab Med 116: 195–197
448. Yokota T, Yamashita Y, Okuzono Y 1984 Malignant cystosarcoma phyllodes of prostate. Acta Pathol Jpn 34: 663–668
449. Bostwick D G, Hossain D, Qian J et al. 2004 Phyllodes tumor of the prostate: long-term followup study of 23 cases. J Urol 172: 894–899
450. Agrawal V, Sharma D, Wadhwa N 2003 Case report: malignant phyllodes tumor of prostate. Int Urol Nephrol 35: 37–39
451. Watanabe M, Yamada Y, Kato H 2002 Malignant phyllodes tumor of the prostate: retrospective review of specimens obtained by sequential transurethral resection. Pathol Int 52: 777–783
452. Lam K C, Yeo W 2002 Chemotherapy induced complete remission in malignant phyllodes tumor of the prostate metastasizing to the lung. J Urol 168: 1104–1105
453. Probert J L, O'Rourke J S, Farrow R et al. 2000 Stromal sarcoma of the prostate. Eur J Surg Oncol 26: 100–101
454. De Raeve H, Jeuris W, Wyndaele J J et al. 2001 Cystosarcoma phyllodes of the prostate with rhabdomyoblastic differentiation. Pathol Res Pract 197: 657–662
455. Yamamoto S, Ito T, Miki M et al. 2000 Malignant phyllodes tumor of the prostate. Int J Urol 7: 378–381
456. De Siati M, Busolo A, Contin F et al. 1999 High grade phyllodes tumour of the prostate. Arch Ital Urol Androl 71: 225–227
457. Young J F, Jensen P E, Wiley C A 1992 Malignant phyllodes tumor of the prostate. A case report with immunohistochemical and ultrastructural studies. Arch Pathol Lab Med 116: 296–299
458. Gueft B, Walsh M A 1975 Malignant prostatic cystosarcoma phyllodes. NY State J Med 75: 2226–2228
459. Yum M, Miller J C, Agrawal B L 1991 Leiomyosarcoma arising in atypical fibromuscular hyperplasia (phyllodes tumor) of the prostate with distant metastasis. Cancer 68: 910–915
460. Proppe K H, Scully R E, Rosai J 1984 Postoperative spindle cell nodules of genitourinary tract resembling sarcomas. A report of 8 cases. Am J Surg Pathol 8: 101–108

461. Wick M R, Brown B A, Young R H 1988 Spindle-cell proliferations of the urinary tract: an immunohistochemical study. Am J Surg Pathol 12: 379–389
462. Huang W L, Ro J Y, Grignon D J 1990 Postoperative spindle cell nodule of the prostate and bladder. J Urol 143: 824–826
463. Young R H 1989 Non-neoplastic epithelial abnormalities and tumor-like lesions. In: Young R H (ed) Pathology of the urinary bladder. Churchill Livingstone, New York, p 44–49
464. Ro J Y, Ayala A G, Ordonez N G 1986 Pseudosarcomatous fibromyxoid tumor of the urinary bladder. Am J Clin Pathol 86: 583–590
465. Sahin A A, Ro J Y, El-Naggar A K et al. 1991 Pseudosarcomatous fibromyxoid tumor of the prostate; a case report with immunohistochemical, electron microscopic, and DNA flow cytometric analysis. Am J Clin Pathol 96: 253–258
466. Hafiz M A, Toker C, Sutula M 1984 An atypical fibromyxoid tumor of the prostate. Cancer 54: 2500–2504
467. Bain G O, Danyluk J M, Shnitka T K 1985 Malignant fibrous histiocytoma of prostate gland. Urology 26: 89–91
468. Ordonez N G, Ayala A G, von Eschenbach A C et al. 1982 Immunoperoxidase localization of prostatic acid phosphatase in prostatic carcinoma with sarcomatoid changes. Urology 19: 210–214
469. Nochomovitz L E, Orenstein J M 1985 Inflammatory pseudotumor of the urinary bladder – possible relationship to nodular fasciitis. Am J Surg Pathol 9: 366–373
470. Roth J A 1980 Reactive pseudosarcomatous response in urinary bladder. Urology 15: 635–637
471. Olsen S 1984 Tumors of the kidney and urinary tract. Color atlas and textbook. W B Saunders, Philadelphia, p 203–205
472. Hughes D F, Biggart J D, Hayes D 1991 Pseudosarcomatous lesions of the urinary bladder. Histopathology 18: 67–71
473. Coyne J D, Wilson G, Sandhu D 1991 Inflammatory pseudotumor of the urinary bladder. Histopathology 18: 261–264
474. Jones E C, Clement P B, Young R H 1993 Inflammatory pseudotumor of the urinary bladder: a clinicopathological, immunohistochemical, ultrastructural, and flow cytometric study of 13 cases. Am J Surg Pathol 17: 264–274
475. Ro J Y, El-Naggar A K, Amin M B 1993 Pseudosarcomatous fibromyxoid tumor of the urinary bladder and prostate: immunohistochemical, ultrastructural and DNA flow cytometric analysis of nine cases. Hum Pathol 24: 1203–1210
476. Jensen J B, Langkilde N C, Lundbeck F et al. 2003 Pseudosarcomatous fibromyxoid tumor of the prostate. Scand J Urol Nephrol 37: 85–87
477. Das S, Upton J D, Amar A D 1988 Nodular fasciitis of the bladder. J Urol 140: 1532–1533
478. Meis J M, Enzinger F M 1991 Inflammatory fibrosarcoma of the mesentery and retroperitoneum. A tumor closely simulating inflammatory pseudotumor. Am J Surg Pathol 15: 1146–1156
479. Voges G E, Wippermann F, Duber C et al. 1990 Pheochromocytoma in the pediatric age group: the prostate – an unusual location. J Urol 144: 1219–1221
480. Dennis P J, Lewandowski A E, Rohner T J J 1989 Pheochromocytoma of the prostate: an unusual location. J Urol 141: 130–132
481. Chen K T, Schiff J J 1987 Hemangiopericytoma of the prostate. J Surg Oncol 35: 42–43
482. Pins M R, Campbell S C, Laskin W B et al. 2001 Solitary fibrous tumor of the prostate a report of 2 cases and review of the literature. Arch Pathol Lab Med 125: 274–277
483. Sujka S K, Malin B T, Asirwatham J E 1989 Prostatic malakoplakia associated with prostatic adenocarcinoma and multiple prostatic abscesses. Urology 34: 159–161
484. Takeshima Y, Yoneda K, Sanda N et al. 1997 Solitary fibrous tumor of the prostate. Pathol Int 47: 713–717
485. Sebo T J, Bostwick D G, Farrow G M et al. 1994 Prostatic xanthoma. A mimic of prostatic adenocarcinoma. Hum Pathol 25: 386–389
486. Mies C, Balogh K, Stadecker M 1984 Palisading prostatic granulomas following surgery. Am J Surg Pathol 8: 217–221
487. Oates R D, Stilmant M M, Freedlund M C et al. 1988 Granulomatous prostatitis following bacillus Calmette–Guerin immunotherapy of bladder cancer. J Urol 140: 751–754
488. Dhundee J, Maciver A G 1991 An immunohistological study of granulomatous prostatitis. Histopathology 18: 435–441
489. Presti B, Weidner N 1991 Granulomatous prostatitis and poorly differentiated prostate carcinoma. Their distinction with the use of immunohistochemical methods. Am J Clin Pathol 95: 330–334
490. Helpap B 1994 Histological and immunohistochemical study of chronic prostatic inflammation with and without benign prostatic hyperplasia. J Urol Pathol 2: 49–64
491. Oppenheimer J R, Kahane H, Epstein J I 1997 Granulomatous prostatitis on needle biopsy. Arch Pathol Lab Med 121: 724–729
492. Carmel M, Masse S R, Lehoux J G 1983 Leiomyosarcoma of prostate. Urology 22: 190–193
493. Tannenbaum M 1975 Sarcomas of the prostate gland. Urology 5: 810–814
494. Narayana A S, Loening S, Weimar G W 1978 Sarcoma of the bladder and prostate. J Urol 119: 72–76
495. Rogers C P, Howards S L, Komp D M 1976 Urogenital rhabdomyosarcoma in childhood. J Urol 115: 738–739
496. Schmidt J D, Welch M J 1976 Sarcoma of the prostate. Cancer 37: 1908–1912
497. Tungekar M F, Al Adnani M S 1986 Sarcomas of the bladder and prostate: the role of immunohistochemistry and ultrastructure in diagnosis. Eur Urol 12: 180–183
498. Hays D M, Raney R B, Lawrence W J 1982 Bladder and prostatic tumors in the intergroup rhabdomyosarcoma study (IRS-1). Results of therapy. Cancer 50: 1472–1482
499. McDougal W S, Persky L 1980 Rhabdomyosarcoma of the bladder and prostate in children. J Urol 123: 882–885
500. Camuzzi F A, Block N L, Charyulu K 1981 Leiomyosarcoma of prostate gland. Urology 18: 295–297
501. Christoffersen J 1973 Leiomyosarcoma of the prostate. Acta Chir Scand 433: 75–84
502. Muller H-A, Wunsch P H 1981 Features of prostatic sarcomas in combined aspiration and punch biopsies. Acta Cytol 25: 480–484
503. Miettinen M 1988 Rhabdomyosarcoma in patients older than 40 years of age. Cancer 62: 2060–2065
504. King D G, Finney R P 1977 Embryonal rhabdomyosarcoma of the prostate. J Urol 117: 88–90
505. Waring P M, Newland R C 1992 Prostatic embryonal rhabdomyosarcoma in adults. A clinicopathologic review. Cancer 69: 755–762
506. Keenan D J, Graham W H 1985 Embryonal rhabdomyosarcoma of the prostatic urethral region in an adult. Br J Urol 57: 241
507. Nabi G, Dinda A K, Dogra P N 2002–2003 Primary embryonal rhabdomyosarcoma of prostate in adults: diagnosis and management. Int Urol Nephrol 34: 531–534
508. Sexton W J, Lance R E, Reyes A O et al. 2001 Adult prostate sarcoma: the M D Anderson Cancer Center Experience. J Urol 166: 521–525
509. Dalal D D, Tongaonkar H B, Krishnamurthy S et al. 2000 Embryonal rhabdomyosarcoma of prostate in an adult – a diagnostic dilemma. Ind J Cancer 37: 50–53
510. Newton W A J, Soule E H, Hamoudi A B 1988 Histopathology of childhood sarcomas, Intergroup Rhabdomyosarcoma studies I and II. Clinicopathologic correlation. J Clin Oncol 6: 67–75
511. Ghavimi F, Herr H, Jereb B 1984 Treatment of genitourinary rhabdomyosarcoma in children. J Urol 132: 313–319
512. Raney B J, Carey A, Snyder H M 1986 Primary site as a prognostic variable for children with pelvic soft tissue sarcomas. J Urol 136: 874–878
513. Fleischmann J, Perinetti E P, Catalona W J 1981 Embryonal rhabdomyosarcoma of the genitourinary organs. J Urol 126: 389–392
514. Kaplan W E, Firlit C F, Berger R M 1983 Genitourinary rhabdomyosarcoma. J Urol 130: 116–119
515. Gordon N, McManus A, Anderson J et al. 2001. Cytogenetic abnormalities in 42 rhabdomyosarcomas: a United Kingdom Cancer Cytogenetics Group study. Med Pediatr Oncol 36: 259–267
516. Bostwick D G, Mann R B 1985 Malignant lymphomas involving the prostate. A study of 13 cases. Cancer 56: 2932–2938
517. Raney R B, Anderson J R, Barr F G et al. 2001 Rhabdomyosarcoma and undifferentiated sarcoma in the first two decades of life: a selective review of intergroup rhabdomyosarcoma study group experience and rationale for Intergroup Rhabdomyosarcoma Study V. J Pediatr Hematol Oncol 23: 215–220
518. Donaldson S S, Meza J, Breneman J C et al. 2001 Results from the IRS-IV randomized trial of hyperfractionated radiotherapy in children with rhabdomyosarcoma – a report from the IRSG. Int J Radiat Oncol Biol Phys 51: 718–728
519. Aragona F, Serretta V, Marconi A 1985 Leiomyosarcoma of the prostate in adults. Ann Chir Gynaecol 74: 191–194
520. Cheville J C, Dundore P A, Nascimento A G 1995 Leiomyosarcoma of the prostate. Report of 23 cases. Cancer 76: 1422–1427
521. Fitzpatrick T J, Stump G 1960 Leiomyosarcoma of the prostate: case report and review of the literature. J Urol 83: 80–83
522. Ahlering T E, Weintraub P, Skinner D G 1988 Management of adult sarcomas of the bladder and prostate. J Urol 140: 1397–1399
522a. Herawi M, Epstein J I 2006 Specialized stromal tumors of the prostate: a clinicopathologic study of 50 cases. Am J Surg Pathol 30: 694–704
523. Meeter U L, Richards J N 1960 Osteogenic sarcoma of the prostate. J Urol 84: 654–657
524. Locke J R, Soloway M S, Evans J 1986 Osteogenic differentiation associated with x-ray therapy for adenocarcinoma of the prostate gland. Am J Clin Pathol 85: 375–378
525. Chin W, Fay R, Ortega P 1986 Malignant fibrous histiocytoma of prostate. Urology 27: 363–365
526. Oesterling J E, Epstein J I, Brendler C B 1990 Myxoid malignant fibrous histiocytoma of the bladder. Cancer 66: 1836–1842
527. Chandan V S, Wolsh L 2003 Postirradiation angiosarcoma of the prostate. Arch Pathol Lab Med 127: 876–878
528. Smith D M, Manivel C, Kapps D 1986 Angiosarcoma of the prostate: report of 2 cases and review of the literature. J Urol 135: 382–384
529. Scully J M, Uno J M, McIntyre M et al. 1990 Radiation-induced prostatic sarcoma: a case report. J Urol 144: 746–749
530. Colecchia M, Dagrada G, Poliani P L et al. 2003 Primary primitive peripheral neuroectodermal tumor of the prostate. Arch Pathol Lab Med 127: e190–e193
531. Pan C C, Yang A H, Chiang H 2003 Malignant perivascular epithelioid cell tumor involving the prostate. Arch Pathol Lab Med 127: E96–E98
532. Kerbl K, Pauer W 1988 Primary non-Hodgkin lymphoma of prostate. Urology 32: 347–349

533. Patel D R, Gomez G A, Henderson E S 1988 Primary prostatic involvement in non-Hodgkin lymphoma. Urology 32: 96–98
534. King L S, Cox T R 1951 Lymphosarcoma of the prostate. Am J Pathol 27: 801–823
535. Chu P G, Huang Q, Weiss L M 2005 Incidental and concurrent malignant lymphomas discovered at the time of prostatectomy and prostate biopsy. A study of 29 cases. Am J Surg Pathol 29: 693–699
536. Boe S, Nielsen H, Ryttov N 1981 Burkitt's lymphoma mimicking prostatitis. J Urol 125: 891–892
537. Cos L R, Rashid H A 1984 Primary non-Hodgkin lymphoma of prostate presenting as benign prostatic hyperplasia. Urology 23: 176–179
538. Doll D C, Weiss R B, Shah S 1978 Lymphoma of the prostate presenting as benign prostatic hypertrophy. South Med J 71: 1170–1171
539. Bostwick D G, Iczkowski K A, Amin M B et al. 1998 Malignant lymphoma involving the prostate: report of 62 cases. Cancer 83: 732–738
540. Ferry J A, Young R H 1997 Malignant lymphoma of the genitourinary tract. Curr Diagn Pathol 4: 145–169
541. Sridhar K N, Woodhouse C R J 1983 Prostatic infiltration in leukaemia and lymphoma. Eur Urol 19: 153–156
542. Banerjee S S, Harris M 1988 Angiotropic lymphoma presenting in the prostate. Histopathology 12: 667–670
543. Feinberg S M, Leslie K O, Colby T V 1987 Bladder outlet obstruction by so-called lymphomatoid granulomatosis (angiocentric lymphoma). J Urol 137: 989–990
544. Lewi H J E, White A, Cassidy M et al. 1984 Lymphocytic infiltration of the prostate. Br J Urol 56: 301–303
545. Cachia P G, McIntyre M A, Dewar A E et al. 1987 Prostatic infiltration in chronic lymphatic leukaemia. J Clin Pathol 40: 342–345
546. Garcia-Gonzalez R, Bellas-Mendez C, Llorente-Abarca C 1964 Leukemic infiltration of the prostate causing acute urinary retention. Eur Urol 10: 356–357
547. Chan Y F 1990 Granulocytic sarcoma (chloroma) of the kidney and prostate. Br J Urol 65: 655–656
548. Frame R, Head D, Lee R 1987 Granulocytic sarcoma of the prostate: two cases causing urinary obstruction. Cancer 59: 142–146
549. Hollenberg G M 1978 Extraosseous multiple myeloma simulating primary prostatic neoplasm. J Urol 119: 292–294
550. Jhavar S, Agarwal J P, Naresh K N et al. 2001 Primary extranodal mucosa associated lymphoid tissue (MALT) lymphoma of the prostate. Leuk Lymphoma 41: 445–449
551. Yao J C T, Wang W C C, Tseng H H et al. 1988 Primary rhabdomyosarcoma of the prostate: diagnosis by needle biopsy and immunocytochemistry. Acta Cytol 32: 509–512
552. Henkes D N, Stein N 1987 Fine-needle aspiration cytology of prostatic embryonal rhabdomyosarcoma: a case report. Diagn Cytol 3: 163–165
553. Kodet R, Kasthuri N, Marsden B et al. 1986 Gangliorhabdomyosarcoma: a histopathological and immunohistochemical study of three cases. Histopathology 10: 181–193
554. Han G, Miura A, Takayama T et al. 2003 Primary prostatic endodermal sinus tumor (yolk sac tumor) combined with a small focal seminoma. Am J Surg Pathol 27: 554–559
555. Bates A W, Baithun S I 2002 Secondary solid neoplasms of the prostate: clinicopathological series of 51 cases. Virchows Arch 440: 392–396
556. Green L K 1990 Metastatic neoplasms to the prostate: a review of 43 cases. Am J Clin Pathol 94: 509
557. Leung C S, Srigley J R, Robertson A R 1997 Metastatic renal cell carcinoma presenting as solitary bleeding prostatic metastasis. J Urol Pathol 7: 1–6
558. Motley R C, Utz D C, Farrow G M 1986 Testicular seminoma metastatic to the prostate. J Urol 135: 801–802
559. Gevenois P A, Van Sinoy M L, Sintzoff S A 1990 Cysts of the prostate and seminal vesicles: MR imaging findings in 11 cases. AJR 155: 1021–1024
560. Ejeckam G C, Govatsos S, Lewis A S 1984 Cyst of seminal vesicle associated with ipsilateral renal agenesis. Urology 24: 372–374
561. Haeney J A, Pfister R C, Maeres E M J 1987 Giant cysts of the seminal vesicles with renal agenesis. AJR 149: 139–140
562. Kenney P J, Leeson M D 1983 Congenital anomalies of the seminal vesicles: spectrum of computed tomographic findings. Radiology 149: 247–251
563. Shabsigh R, Lerner S, Fishman I J 1989 The role of transrectal ultrasonography in the diagnosis and management of prostatic and seminal vesicle cysts. J Urol 141: 1206–1209
564. Ornstein M H, Kershaw D R 1985 Cysts of the seminal vesicle are Mullerian in origin. J R Soc Med 78: 1050–1051
565. Stenos J, Pavlakis A, Rebelakos A 1985 Cysts of the seminal vesicle. A case report and review of the literature. Acta Urol Belg 53: 718–723
566. Van Lerberghe E, Beeckman P, Roelens J et al. 1987 Seminal vesicle cyst: report of a case. J Belg Radiol 70: 137–139
567. Coyne J D, Kealy W F 1993 Seminal vesicle amyloidosis. Histopathology 22: 173–176
568. Jun S Y, Kim K R, Cho K S et al. 2003 Localized amyloidosis of seminal vesicle and vas deferens: report of two cases. J Kor Med Sci 18: 447–451
569. Bahn D K, Brown R K J, Shei K Y 1990 Sonographic findings of leiomyoma of seminal vesicle. J Clin Ultrasound 18: 517–519
570. Kinas H, Kuhn M J 1987 Mesonephric hamartoma of the seminal vesicle: a rare cause of a retrovesical mass. NY State J Med 87: 48–49
571. Tamayo J L, Ruffolo E H 1967 Spermatic cord tumor. Mesonephric hamartoma of the vas deferens. Arch Surg 94: 430–431
572. Plaut A L, Standard S 1944 Cystomyoma of seminal vesicle. Ann Surg 119: 253–261
573. Lundhus E, Bundgaard N, Sorensen F B 1984 Cystadenoma of the seminal vesicle. Scand J Urol Nephrol 18: 341–342
574. Bullock K N 1988 Cystadenoma of the seminal vesicle. J R Soc Med 81: 294–295
575. Damjanov I, Apic R 1974 Cystadenoma of the seminal vesicles. J Urol 111: 808–809
576. Peker K R, Hellman B H J, McCammon K A et al. 1997 Cystadenoma of the seminal vesicle: a case report and review of the literature. J Urol Pathol 6: 213–221
577. Kan D V 1963 Benign tumors of the seminal vesicles. Urologia 28: 27–30
578. Islam M 1979 Benign mesenchymoma of seminal vesicles. Urology 13: 203–205
579. Mazur M T, Myers J L, Maddox W A 1987 Cystic epithelial-stromal tumor of the seminal vesicle. Am J Surg Pathol 11: 210–217
580. Kawahara M, Matsuhashi M, Tajima M 1988 Primary carcinoma of seminal vesicle. Diagnosis assisted by sonography. Urology 32: 269–272
581. Davis N S, Merguerian P A, Dimarco P L 1988 Primary adenocarcinoma of seminal vesicle presenting as bladder tumor. Urology 32: 466–468
582. Benson R C, Clark W R, Farrow G M 1984 Carcinoma of the seminal vesicle. J Urol 132: 483–485
583. Oguchi K, Takeuchi T, Kuriyama M 1988 Primary carcinoma of the seminal vesicle. Br J Urol 62: 383–384
584. Chinoy R F, Kulkarni J N 1993 Primary papillary adenocarcinoma of the seminal vesicle. Ind J Cancer 30: 82–84
585. Ohmori T, Okada K, Tabei R 1994 CA 125-producing adenocarcinoma of the seminal vesicle. Pathol Int 44: 333–337
586. Ormsby A H, Haskell R, Jones D et al. 2000 Primary seminal vesicle carcinoma: an immunohistochemical analysis of four cases. Mod Pathol 13: 46–51
587. Jun S Y, Kim K R, Ro J Y 2003 Mucosal spread of prostate adenocarcinoma to seminal vesicle. Pathol Case Rev 8: 78–81
588. Middleton L P, Merino M J, Popok S M et al. 1998 Male adnexal tumour of probable Wolffian origin occurring in a seminal vesicle. Histopathology 33: 269–274
589. Schned A R, Ledbetter J S, Selikowitz S M 1986 Primary leiomyosarcoma of the seminal vesicle. Cancer 57: 2202–2206
590. Muentener M, Hailemariam S, Dubs M et al. 2000 Primary leiomyosarcoma of the seminal vesicle. J Urol 164: 2027
591. Amirkhan R H, Molberg K H, Wiley E L et al. 1994 Primary leiomyosarcoma of the seminal vesicle. Urology 44: 132–135
592. Berger A P, Bartsch G, Horninger W 2002 Primary rhabdomyosarcoma of the seminal vesicle. J Urol 168: 643
593. Sanghvi D A, Purandare N C, Jambhekar N A et al. 2004 Primary rhabdomyosarcoma of the seminal vesicle. Br J Radiol 77: 159–160
594. Chiou R K, Limas C, Lance P H 1985 Hemangiosarcoma of the seminal vesicle: case report and literature review. J Urol 134: 371–373
595. Panageas E, Kuligowska E, Dunlop R 1990 Angiosarcoma of the seminal vesicle: early detection using transrectal ultrasound-guided biopsy. J Clin Ultrasound 18: 666–670
596. Lamont J S, Hesketh P J, de las Morenas A et al. 1991 Primary angiosarcoma of the seminal vesicle. J Urol 146: 165–167
597. Fain J S, Cosnow I, King B F et al. 1993 Cystosarcoma phyllodes of the seminal vesicle. Cancer 71: 2055–2061
598. Lazarus J A 1946 Primary malignant tumors of the seminal vesicles: report of a case of retrovesical sarcoma. J Urol 55: 190–205

第二部分

睾丸和睾丸周围组织
Testis and paratesticular tissues

Jae Y. Ro、Mahul B. Amin、Kyu-Rae Kim、Alberto G. Ayala 著

唐建武 译

睾丸和睾丸周围组织		混合性生殖细胞和性索肿瘤	830
生殖细胞肿瘤	812	性索-间质肿瘤	833
小管内生殖细胞肿瘤形成	812	属于肾上腺生殖器综合征的肿瘤	838
精原细胞瘤性肿瘤	816	淋巴网状组织肿瘤	839
非精原细胞瘤性生殖细胞肿瘤	822	转移性肿瘤	840
成熟性畸胎瘤	826	睾丸罕见的肿瘤和瘤样病变	841
未成熟性畸胎瘤	827	睾丸周围组织肿瘤和肿瘤性病变	844
绒毛膜癌	827	睾丸周围区域良性肿瘤	844
混合性生殖细胞肿瘤	829	睾丸周围区域恶性肿瘤	849

睾丸肿瘤约占所有男性恶性肿瘤的1%[1]。2006年美国癌症协会估计有8250名患者发生睾丸恶性肿瘤，其中370人死于本病[2]。生殖细胞来源的肿瘤占所有睾丸肿瘤的94%～96%，而性索-间质来源的肿瘤仅占4%～6%，其余各种组织来源的睾丸肿瘤罕见，约占所有睾丸肿瘤的1%。表14B.1列出了新近出版的WHO睾丸及睾丸周围肿瘤和瘤样病变的分类[3]。

病理医师对于睾丸肿瘤患者的治疗起着重要作用，通过正确的肿瘤分类、提供恰当的病理分期以及确定预后参数，可能有助于决定是监测还是进行进一步的治疗（表14B.2）。因此，评价一个睾丸肿瘤必须包括仔细的大体检查，以测量肿瘤大小、确定肿瘤是否蔓延至精索和被膜、注意大体表现出现的包括坏死和出血在内的差异、并且充分取样进行显微镜下检查（一般来说，按照肿瘤直径大小，每1 cm做一张切片，包括表现不同的区域）。显微镜下检查必须确认组织学类型［例如生殖细胞还是非生殖细胞肿瘤，精原细胞瘤还是非精原细胞瘤性肿瘤，或混合性生殖细胞肿瘤（MGCT），包括不同的成分及其所占的比例］，确定是否累及精索和白膜，并证实有无血管或淋巴管浸润。报告中可能还应该包括有无肿瘤坏死、核分裂象、纤维化、合体滋养层巨细胞、淋巴浆细胞浸润、肉芽肿性反应等其他特征以及睾丸的背景情况，包括小管内生殖细胞肿瘤形成（ITGCN）[4-8]。

生殖细胞肿瘤　Germ cell neoplasms

关于生殖细胞肿瘤组织发生的不同观点及其广泛的组织学表现反映在已经提出的不同的分类中（表14B.3）[3,9]。然而，为了治疗的目的，传统上将这些肿瘤分成两种主要类型：精原细胞瘤和非精原细胞瘤性生殖细胞肿瘤（NSGCT）[4-6]。

如果是非精原细胞瘤性肿瘤，必须进一步分类为单纯性或混合性肿瘤。对于混合性生殖细胞肿瘤来说，应该报告肿瘤中出现的所有成分以及每种成分大致所占的比例。为了治疗的目的，将含有精原细胞瘤性和非精原细胞瘤性两种成分的肿瘤看成是非精原细胞瘤性生殖细胞瘤（NSGCT）[4-6]。

小管内生殖细胞肿瘤形成
Intratubular germ cell neoplasia

普遍认为小管内生殖细胞肿瘤形成（ITGCN）是大多数浸润性生殖细胞肿瘤的前体。虽然Wilms[10]在1896年描述，浸润性癌附近的小管内存在非典型性细胞，但是Skakkebaek[11]在1972年首次报道了生精小管内的非典型性生殖细胞实际上就是浸润性睾丸生殖细胞肿瘤的前体。这种原位阶段的生殖细胞肿瘤发生于0.5%～1%的伴有严重精子减少的不育患者、2%～8%的隐睾症患

表14B.1　睾丸肿瘤的WHO组织学分类[a]

生殖细胞肿瘤
小管内生殖细胞肿瘤形成，未分类　　　　　　　9064/2
其他类型

一种组织学类型的肿瘤（单纯性）
精原细胞瘤　　　　　　　　　　　　　　　　　9061/3
　伴有合体滋养细胞的精原细胞瘤
精母细胞性精原细胞瘤　　　　　　　　　　　　9063/3
　伴有肉瘤的精母细胞性精原细胞瘤
胚胎性癌　　　　　　　　　　　　　　　　　　9070/3
卵黄囊瘤　　　　　　　　　　　　　　　　　　9071/3
滋养细胞肿瘤
　绒毛膜癌　　　　　　　　　　　　　　　　　9100/3
　绒毛膜癌以外的滋养细胞肿瘤
　　单相性绒毛膜癌
　　胎盘部位滋养细胞肿瘤　　　　　　　　　　9104/1
畸胎瘤　　　　　　　　　　　　　　　　　　　9080/3
　皮样囊肿　　　　　　　　　　　　　　　　　9084/0
　单胚层畸胎瘤
　伴有体细胞型恶性肿瘤的畸胎瘤　　　　　　　9084/3

一种以上组织学类型的肿瘤（混合性）
混合性胚胎性癌和畸胎瘤　　　　　　　　　　　9081/3
混合性畸胎瘤和精原细胞瘤　　　　　　　　　　9085/3
绒毛膜癌和畸胎瘤/胚胎性癌　　　　　　　　　 9101/3
其他

性索/性腺间质肿瘤

单纯性
Leydig细胞瘤　　　　　　　　　　　　　　　　8650/1
恶性Leydig细胞瘤　　　　　　　　　　　　　　8650/3
Sertoli细胞瘤　　　　　　　　　　　　　　　　8640/1
　富于脂质的Sertoli细胞瘤　　　　　　　　　　8641/0
　硬化性Sertoli细胞瘤
　大细胞钙化性Sertoli细胞瘤　　　　　　　　　8642/1
恶性Sertoli细胞瘤　　　　　　　　　　　　　　8640/3
颗粒细胞瘤　　　　　　　　　　　　　　　　　8620/1
　成人型颗粒细胞瘤　　　　　　　　　　　　　8620/1
　幼年型颗粒细胞瘤　　　　　　　　　　　　　8622/1
卵泡膜瘤/纤维瘤组
　卵泡膜瘤　　　　　　　　　　　　　　　　　8600/0
　纤维瘤　　　　　　　　　　　　　　　　　　8810/0

性索/性腺间质肿瘤：
　分化不完全　　　　　　　　　　　　　　　　8591/1
　性索/性腺间质肿瘤，混合性　　　　　　　　　8592/1
　恶性性索/性腺间质肿瘤　　　　　　　　　　　8590/3
含有生殖细胞和性索/性腺间质两种成分的肿瘤
　性腺母细胞瘤　　　　　　　　　　　　　　　9073/1
　生殖细胞-性索/性腺间质肿瘤，未分类

其他睾丸肿瘤
类癌　　　　　　　　　　　　　　　　　　　　8240/3
卵巢上皮性肿瘤
　交界性恶性浆液性肿瘤　　　　　　　　　　　8442/1
　浆液性癌　　　　　　　　　　　　　　　　　8441/3
　高分化子宫内膜样癌　　　　　　　　　　　　8380/3
　黏液性囊腺瘤　　　　　　　　　　　　　　　8470/0
　黏液性囊腺癌　　　　　　　　　　　　　　　8470/3
　Brenner瘤　　　　　　　　　　　　　　　　　9000/0
肾母细胞瘤　　　　　　　　　　　　　　　　　8960/3
副神经节瘤　　　　　　　　　　　　　　　　　8680/1

造血组织肿瘤

集合管和睾丸网肿瘤
腺瘤　　　　　　　　　　　　　　　　　　　　8140/0
癌　　　　　　　　　　　　　　　　　　　　　8140/3

睾丸周围组织肿瘤　　　　　　　　　　　　 9054/0
腺瘤样瘤　　　　　　　　　　　　　　　　　　9050/3
恶性间皮瘤
良性间皮瘤　　　　　　　　　　　　　　　　　9052/0
　高分化乳头状间皮瘤　　　　　　　　　　　　9055/0
　囊性间皮瘤　　　　　　　　　　　　　　　　8140/3
附睾腺癌　　　　　　　　　　　　　　　　　　8450/0
附睾乳头状囊腺瘤　　　　　　　　　　　　　　9363/0
黑色素性神经外胚层肿瘤　　　　　　　　　　　8806/3
纤维组织增生性小圆细胞肿瘤

精索和睾丸附件的间叶性肿瘤

睾丸继发性肿瘤

[a] 肿瘤学疾病国际分类的形态学编码（ICDO）和医学系统化专业术语（http://snomed.org）。生物学行为编码为：/0良性肿瘤，/2原位癌和Ⅲ级上皮内肿瘤形成，/3恶性肿瘤，以及/1交界性或生物学行为不确定的肿瘤。

者以及5%伴有睾丸恶性肿瘤病史的患者[12-23]。伴有睾丸未降和睾丸癌病史的患者，其对侧睾丸发生ITGCN的危险性为15%～20%[16,24]。性腺发育不全和睾丸女性化综合征的患者ITGCN的发病率也增高[25-27]。大约50%的ITGCN患者在5年内将会发展为浸润性癌，如果不切除睾丸，则有90%或90%以上的患者发展为浸润性癌[13,16,20]。大多数ITGCN患者发生精原细胞瘤，实际上原位精原细胞瘤和原位癌[或原位生殖母细胞瘤(gonocytoma in situ)]这两个名词可以和ITGCN交换使用。由于生精小管没有完全被非典型性细胞取代，而且随访研究表明，如果不切除睾丸甚至可以发生非精原细胞瘤性肿瘤，所以认为原位精原细胞瘤这个术语并不恰当。同时，也不提倡使用原位癌这个术语，因为生殖细胞不是上皮细胞，而且在所有的病例中均未确定其恶性潜能。不过，这种病变的表现和行为与其他部位的原位癌一样，显然是一种浸润前的病变[13,28]。

病理学特征

大体检查，除了可能含有ITGCN的疾病之外，ITGCN本身并不引起异常表现。显微镜下显示生精小管

表14B.2 睾丸生殖细胞肿瘤的TNM分类

原发性肿瘤（T）

在根治性睾丸切除术后常常要对原发性肿瘤的范围进行分类，因此还要进行病理学分期。

- *pTX　原发性肿瘤不能评估
- pT0　没有原发性肿瘤的证据（例如睾丸内组织学瘢痕）
- pTis　小管内生殖细胞肿瘤形成（原位癌）
- pT1　肿瘤局限于睾丸和附睾，没有血管/淋巴管浸润；肿瘤可以浸润白膜但没有浸润鞘膜
- pT2　肿瘤局限于睾丸和附睾，伴有血管/淋巴管浸润，或肿瘤穿透白膜，伴有鞘膜受累
- pT3　肿瘤侵犯精索，伴有或不伴有血管/淋巴管浸润
- pT4　肿瘤侵犯阴囊，伴有或不伴有血管/淋巴管浸润

注意：除了pTis和pT4外，原发性肿瘤的范围依据根治性睾丸切除术分类。在缺乏根治性睾丸切除术的情况下，TX可以用于其他分类。

局部淋巴结（N）

临床

- NX　局部淋巴结不能评估
- N0　无局部淋巴结转移
- N1　一个淋巴结转移，最大径≤2 cm；或多个淋巴结转移，最大径均＜2 cm
- N2　一个淋巴结转移，最大径＞2 cm但≤5 cm；或多个淋巴结转移，任何一个最大径均＞2 cm，但≤5 cm
- N3　一个淋巴结转移，最大径＞5 cm

病理学（pN）

- pNX　局部淋巴结不能评估
- pN0　无局部淋巴结转移
- pN1　一个淋巴结转移，最大径≤2 cm，以及≤5个淋巴结转移，最大径均＜2 cm
- pN2　一个淋巴结转移，最大径＞2 cm，但≤5 cm；或＞5个淋巴结转移，最大径均≤5 cm；或有肿瘤蔓延至淋巴结外的证据
- pN3　淋巴结转移，最大径＞5 cm

远处转移（M）

- MX　远处转移不能评估
- M0　无远处转移
- M1　远处转移
  - M1a　非局部淋巴结或肺转移
  - M1b　非局部淋巴结和肺以外部位的远处转移

血清肿瘤标志物（S）

- SX　得不到标志物研究资料或未进行标志物检测
- S0　标志物水平在正常范围内
- S1　LDH＜1.5×N*和
  hCG（mIu/ml）＜5000 和
  AFP（ng/ml）＜1000
- S2　LDH 1.5～10×N 或
  hCG（mIu/ml）5000～50 000 或
  AFP（ng/ml）1000～10 000
- S3　LDH＞10×N 或
  hCG（mIu/ml）＞50 000 或
  AFP（ng/ml）＞10 000

*N指血清LDH正常值上限

分期（Stage Grouping）

期	T	N	M	S
0期	pTis	N0	M0	S0
Ⅰ期	pT1-4	N0	M0	SX
ⅠA期	pT1	N0	M0	S0
ⅠB期	pT2	N0	M0	S0
	pT3	N0	M0	S0
	pT4	N0	M0	S0
ⅠS期	任何pT/Tx	N0	M0	S1-3
Ⅱ期	任何pT/Tx	N1-3	M0	SX
ⅡA期	任何pT/Tx	N1	M0	S0
	任何pT/Tx	N1	M0	S1
ⅡB期	任何pT/Tx	N2	M0	S0
	任何pT/Tx	N2	M0	S1
ⅡC期	任何pT/Tx	N3	M0	S0
	任何pT/Tx	N3	M0	S1
Ⅲ期	任何pT/Tx	任何N	M1	SX
ⅢA期	任何pT/Tx	任何N	M1a	S0
	任何pT/Tx	任何N	M1a	S1
ⅢB期	任何pT/Tx	N1-3	M0	S2
	任何pT/Tx	任何N	M1a	S2
ⅢC期	任何pT/Tx	N1-3	M0	S3
	任何pT/Tx	任何N	M1a	S3
	任何pT/Tx	任何N	M1b	任何S

Used with permission of the American Joint Committee on Cancer (AJCC), Chicago, Illinois. The original source for this material is the AJCC Cancer Staging Manual, Sixth Edition (2002) published by Springer-Verlag New York, www.springeronline.com

---

直径变小，而且管壁增厚。在早期阶段，有散在的伴有明显核仁和丰富透明胞浆的非典型性大细胞（大小为正常生殖细胞的两倍）（图14B.1A），这些细胞位于其他明显正常成熟的细胞之间。在晚期阶段，非典型性细胞（图14B.1B）常沿基底膜呈环状排列，而且随着病变进展异常细胞数量增加，最后占据整个生精小管。高倍镜下显示，大而明显的细胞呈Paget样表现；这些细胞核大、染色质粗、有大而明显的不规则形核仁。可见核分裂象，包括异常核分裂象，有丰富的透明胞浆，内含脂质和糖原。

表14B.3　睾丸生殖细胞肿瘤各种分类比较

AFIP（1999）	WHO（1977）	Dixon & Moore（1952）	Mostofi（1980）[4]	英国睾丸肿瘤专业组（Pugh 1976）
精原细胞瘤	精原细胞瘤	I 型精原细胞瘤	精原细胞瘤	精原细胞瘤
精母细胞性精原细胞瘤	精母细胞性精原细胞瘤	未列出	精母细胞性精原细胞瘤	精母细胞性精原细胞瘤
胚胎性癌	胚胎性癌	II 型胚胎性癌	成人型胚胎性癌	未分化型恶性畸胎瘤
卵黄囊瘤	卵黄囊瘤（内胚窦瘤）	未列出	婴儿胚胎性癌	儿童卵黄囊瘤（睾丸母细胞瘤）
多胚瘤	多胚瘤	未列出	多胚瘤	未列出
绒毛膜癌 胎盘部位滋养细胞肿瘤	单纯性绒毛膜癌	V 型绒毛膜癌	单纯性绒毛膜癌	恶性畸胎瘤，滋养细胞性
畸胎瘤： • 成熟性 • 未成熟性 • 单胚层	畸胎瘤： • 成熟性 • 未成熟性	III 型畸胎瘤 • 单纯性 ± 　精原细胞瘤	畸胎瘤： • 成熟性 • 未成熟性	分化性畸胎瘤
伴有第二种恶性成分的畸胎瘤（详细说明）	畸胎瘤伴有恶变	IV 型畸胎瘤，伴有EC和(或)C ± 精原细胞瘤	畸胎瘤伴有除了S、EC、C以外的恶性区	中间性恶性畸胎瘤
混合性生殖细胞肿瘤（指出成分）	胚胎性癌和畸胎瘤（畸胎癌） 绒毛膜癌和其他类型 其他组合	IV 型畸胎瘤伴有EC和(或)C ± S V 型绒毛膜癌伴有S和(或)EC 未列出	胚胎性癌和畸胎瘤（畸胎癌） 特殊肿瘤类型 特殊肿瘤类型	中间性恶性畸胎瘤 恶性畸胎瘤，滋养细胞性 复合性肿瘤

AFIP：美军病理学会；WHO：世界卫生组织；EC：胚胎性癌；C：绒毛膜癌；S：精原细胞瘤。

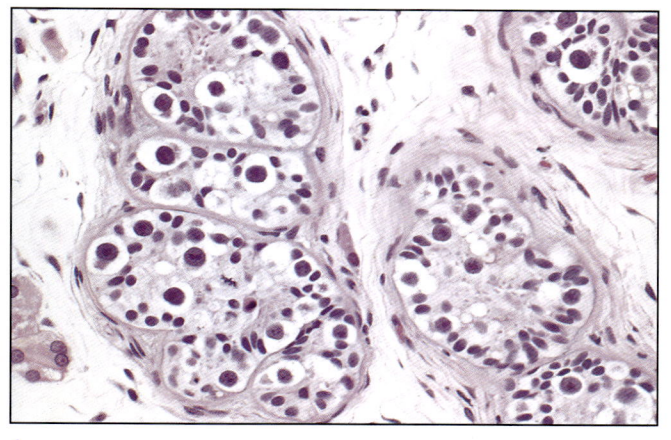

A

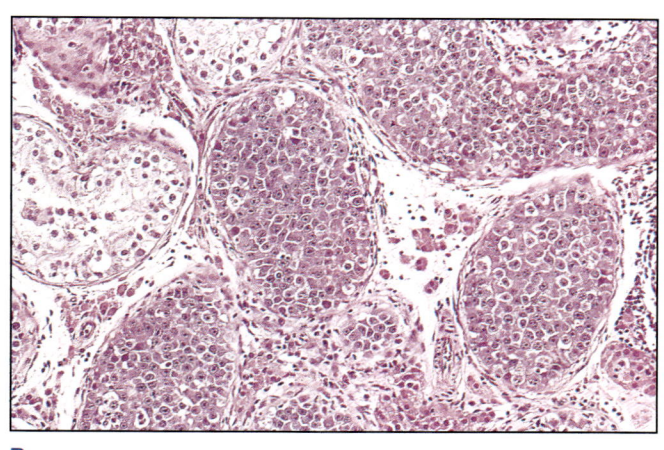

B

图14B.1　小管内生殖细胞肿瘤形成。（A）注意伴有丰富透明胞浆的非典型性大细胞，沿着生精小管的基底膜散在分布。（B）非典型性大细胞完全充满生精小管（原位精原细胞瘤）。

非典型性生殖细胞具有生成精子前体细胞或恶性精原细胞瘤细胞的超微结构特征。这些细胞的 DNA 成分呈非整倍体结构[14,29]。应用或不应用淀粉酶消化的 PAS 染色显示胞浆内含有丰富的糖原（图 14B.2）。

免疫组织化学　Immunohistochemistry

胎盘碱性磷酸酶（PLAP）是最有用的诊断性抗体，但是非典型性小管内生殖细胞其他标志物，包括 CD117（c-kit）、p53、神经元特异性烯醇化酶（NSE）、铁蛋白

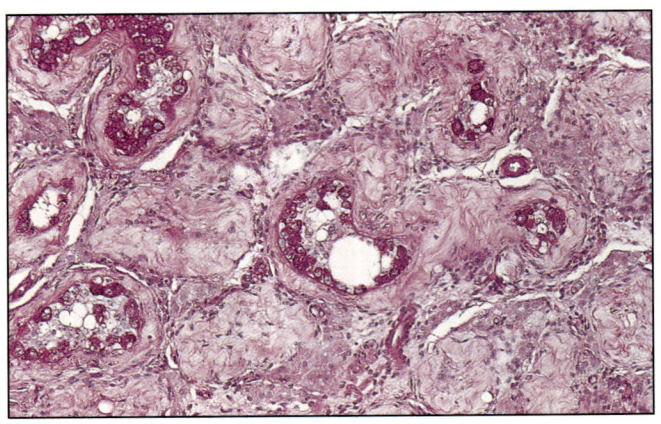

图14B.2 小管内非典型性生殖细胞含有丰富的糖原（PAS染色）。只有非典型性生殖细胞PAS染色阳性。

（ferritin）、单克隆抗体M2A（D2-40）以及43-9F也呈阳性反应[30-37]。新近OCT4的应用颇受欢迎，OCT4是在肿瘤性生殖细胞内发现的一种具有多向性潜能的转录因子[38]。

Giwercman等[37]报道ITGCN的细胞与43-9F抗体发生反应，而正常生殖细胞、Sertoli细胞、Leydig细胞和内皮细胞没有反应。

FHIT表达缺失（FHIT基因位于人染色体3p14.2）是ITGCN恒定的特征，提示在睾丸生殖细胞肿瘤发生的早期，FHIT表达缺失在成熟/分化缺损方面具有潜在作用。同样，精原细胞瘤缺乏FHIT表达也支持这个观点。然而，混合性生殖细胞肿瘤（MGCT）畸胎瘤成分中高分化腺体上皮有FHIT的再表达，提示在这一部分肿瘤中FHIT基因没有丢失，而是FHIT蛋白表达在生殖细胞肿瘤进展的整个过程中受到不同程度的调控[39]。细胞角蛋白（cytokeratin）、甲胎蛋白（AFP）和人绒毛膜促性腺激素（hCG）通常阴性。然而，小管内胚胎性癌与CD30、细胞角蛋白（AE1/AE3）、细胞角蛋白7局灶性以及p53发生免疫反应，但是细胞角蛋白20、p21和AFP阴性[40]。核型分析显示，ITGCN、精原细胞瘤和NSGCT常常出现等臂染色体(12p)这一标志染色体[41,42]。

RNA结合模体（RNA-binding motif, RBM）蛋白是一种新的标志物，正常男性生殖细胞持续表达，而恶性生殖细胞肿瘤或ITGCN不表达。因此，生殖细胞缺乏RBM表达是诊断睾丸侵袭前恶性病变的一种新的工具[43]。

在75%～99%的病例，浸润性生殖细胞肿瘤附近的小管内可见ITGCN；ITGCN与非精原细胞瘤性肿瘤（NSGCT）的关系比精原细胞瘤更加密切[32,44-46]。在大多数病例中，小管内肿瘤细胞缺乏进一步分化的证据，因此，只有在发生小管外蔓延后才能确定特殊的组织学亚型。是所有的浸润性生殖细胞肿瘤都要经过小管内病变阶段，还是有些肿瘤开始就是浸润性肿瘤，仍然不能确定，但是常常发现浸润性病变附近的小管内有异常生殖细胞，提示前者更有可能。

常见的小管内肿瘤包括小管内精原细胞瘤和小管内胚胎性癌[40]；其他类型包括小管内精母细胞性精原细胞瘤，还有罕见的小管内卵黄囊瘤或滋养细胞肿瘤[47]。尚无直接证据表明ITGCN是儿童卵黄囊瘤和畸胎瘤以及成人精母细胞瘤性精原细胞瘤的前体病变[48,49]。然而，新近有报告描述儿童和青少年发生ITGCN[50-53]。

治疗 Management

至于ITGCN是否应该治疗尚有争议。一些研究人员提倡给予低剂量的放疗；而其他一些人提倡监测，因为如果出现一个新的原发病灶，通过患者自查、体检或者是血浆标志物水平升高容易被发现。并且，如果发生肿瘤，目前的治疗手段非常有效。

精原细胞瘤性肿瘤 Seminomatous tumors

精原细胞瘤有两种类型：经典性精原细胞瘤和精母细胞性精原细胞瘤。

经典性精原细胞瘤 Classic seminoma

精原细胞瘤是最常见的睾丸肿瘤，占所有睾丸生殖细胞肿瘤的40%～50%[54-56]；85%～90%的精原细胞瘤为典型的或经典的精原细胞瘤，其余的由罕见的亚型组成，例如间变性精原细胞瘤和伴有合体滋养层巨细胞的精原细胞瘤[54,57,58]。双侧睾丸生殖细胞肿瘤（2%）患者中精原细胞瘤是最常见的生殖细胞肿瘤，并且常常发生在未下降的睾丸（5%～8%）[59-64]。

临床表现

精原细胞瘤最常发生于35～45岁的患者，50岁以上的男性相对少见，儿童罕见。这个年龄组比非精原细胞瘤性肿瘤晚10年。70%以上患者的临床表现包括睾丸增大，伴有或不伴有疼痛，10%的患者出现转移症状。有些精原细胞瘤患者无症状。男性乳腺发育、眼球突出和不孕症是很少出现的症状。血清PLAP和hCG升高分别见于40%和10%的患者；后者是男性乳腺发育的原因。在就诊时大约75%的精原细胞瘤患者局限于睾丸（5%～8%蔓延至精索和附睾）；相反，50%～70%的非精原细胞瘤性肿瘤在被诊断时已有转移[54]。

病理学特征

大体检查，肿瘤通常是境界清楚、均质状的质硬肿块，常常为灰白色，略呈分叶状，切面隆起（图

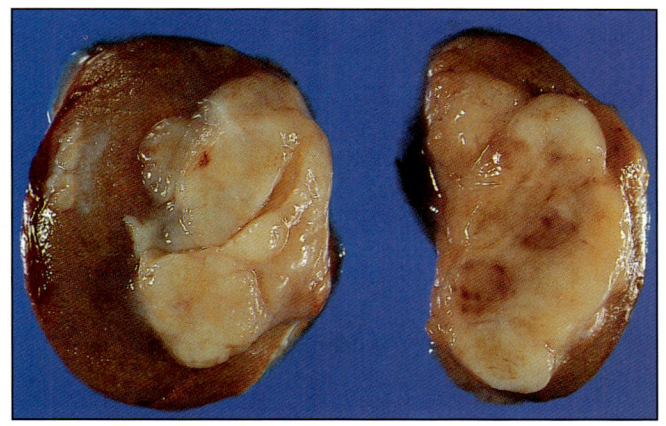

图14B.3 大体观,精原细胞瘤界限清楚,奶油色,均质,略呈分叶状。

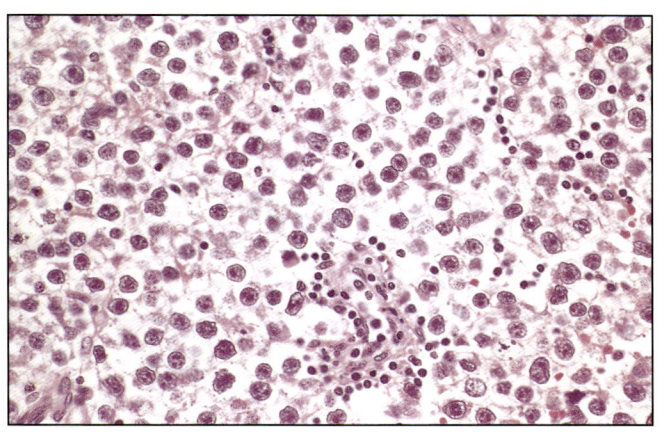

图14B.5 高倍镜下,精原细胞瘤细胞为均匀一致的大细胞,含有丰富的透明胞浆。肿瘤细胞胞膜清楚,分布均匀。

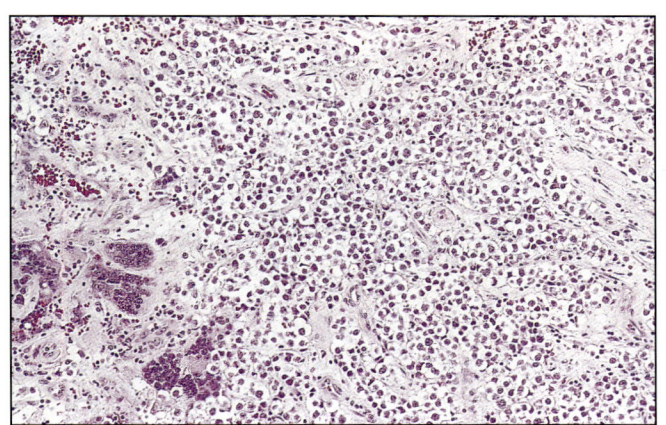

图14B.4 精原细胞瘤由单形性细胞群组成,被纤细的带状纤维血管间质分成小叶状。还可见到散在的合体滋养细胞。

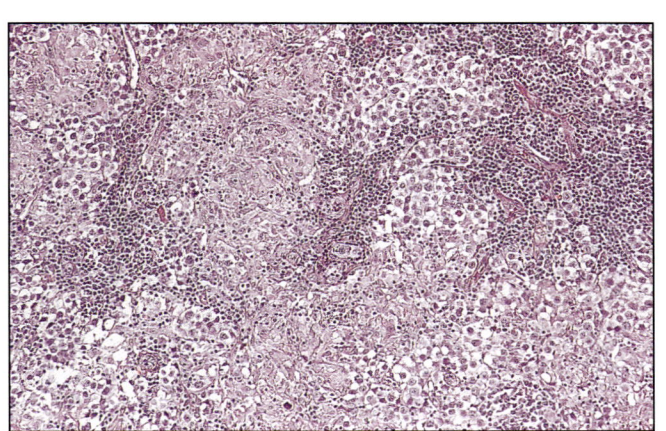

图14B.6 精原细胞瘤。这个精原细胞瘤内可见许多淋巴细胞和伴有上皮样组织细胞的界限不清的肉芽肿性反应。

14B.3)。出血和坏死并不常见,但可见于较大的肿瘤。肿瘤平均大小为5cm,少数病例超过10cm;在Ⅰ期精原细胞瘤中,61%的患者肿瘤大小为2~6cm[65]。

显微镜下检查显示大细胞弥漫性增生,排列成片块、巢状或条索状(图14B.4)。管状、网状、囊状、微囊状和筛状结构也曾有报道;管状精原细胞瘤(tubular seminoma)这个描述性术语曾用于假腺体变异[66-70]。具有这种变异的肿瘤总是存在经典性精原细胞瘤的区域。随着肿瘤的生长,精原细胞瘤常常破坏生精小管,但在肿块的周边肿瘤细胞之间可见陷入的生精小管。在极少数情况下,甚至可能有明显的小管间生长[71]。

肿瘤细胞分布均匀,相对较大但比较一致,具有明显的细胞膜(图14B.5)。细胞核大,圆形,位于中心,核膜清楚,染色质细条带状,伴有1或2个明显的核仁,胞浆丰富且常透明,但是可呈嗜酸性或嗜双色性。核分裂象常见。

精原细胞瘤常常(50%~60%病例)出现散在性或弥漫性肉芽肿性反应,伴有或不伴有多核巨细胞。转移性病灶可能以肉芽肿性炎症为主,造成诊断非常困难。在这种情况下,PLAP免疫组织化学染色非常有助于诊断。

10%~20%的病例出现散在的合体滋养层巨细胞[57,72]。可能出现在精原细胞瘤中的其他类型巨细胞包括桑葚细胞(mulberry cells)[73]和前面提到过的与肉芽肿相关的Langhans巨细胞。精原细胞瘤可以发生广泛的钙化和骨化[骨化性精原细胞瘤(ossifying seminoma)][74]。肿瘤被支持性间质分成小叶,间质内含有数量不等的淋巴细胞(图14B.6)。不同肿瘤之间以及同一肿瘤内的不同部分淋巴细胞浸润(以T淋巴细胞为主)的程度不同。间质的量也有不同,从稀少到丰富,而且表现不同,从纤细的纤维血管网到可能是玻璃样变的大的纤维束或间隔。某些肿瘤结缔组织的量可能十分丰富,以致难以辨认肿瘤细胞。多达1/3的精原细胞瘤可能显示远离肿瘤主体的小管间生长方式,这可能与睾丸网浸润有关[75a]。在少数情况下,精原细胞瘤瘤细胞不再出现,而是整个肿瘤被大量玻璃样变的纤维组织,偶尔被钙化组织所取代,这在某些情况下提示是耗尽的精原细胞瘤。出现ITGCN高度支持耗尽的精原细胞瘤的诊断。

累及睾丸网上皮的精原细胞瘤细胞的形态很难与ITGCN的形态区分。当出现睾丸网Paget样受累时，其腺管状结构可能与胚胎性癌混淆[76,77]。这种Paget样蔓延没有预后意义。

精原细胞瘤可以完全梗死，形成含有"鬼影"细胞的怀疑为肿瘤的肿块。当怀疑为精原细胞瘤的肿瘤出现结构改变时，特殊染色可能有助于诊断。Florentine等[78]报告，Masson三色染色可以明显改善核和细胞的结构，用以证实可疑的肿瘤。PLAP显示肿瘤细胞膜特异性的染色，并能确立精原细胞瘤的诊断。因此，Masson三色染色加上选择性的免疫染色有望为诊断某些坏死性肿瘤提供可靠的方法。

有争议的间变性亚型（anaplastic variant）占精原细胞瘤的5%～15%[58,72]。间变性精原细胞瘤和经典性精原细胞瘤在大体上没有区别。显微镜下，间变性精原细胞瘤的特征是核分裂活性增加（每一高倍视野有3个或3个以上的核分裂象）和核的多形性。Kademian等[72]报道8例间变性精原细胞瘤，认为这种亚型比经典性精原细胞瘤侵袭性强，即使是将两者按照分期对应比较时。Bobba等[79]报告有类似的结果，认为经典性和间变性精原细胞瘤具有不同的生存率和复发率。然而，其他学者持有不同意见，虽然间变性精原细胞瘤患者总的生存率比经典性患者低，但对同样的分期进行比较时，生存率并没有差别。在出现临床症状时，多数间变性精原细胞瘤已经发生转移，相反，经典性精原细胞瘤通常局限在睾丸内。这无疑是间变性精原细胞瘤患者总的生存率低的原因[58,80]。新近Tickoo等[81]在描述伴有非典型性的精原细胞瘤时发现，较大的肿瘤和伴有较多核分裂象的肿瘤具有较强的侵袭性行为。

组织化学和免疫组织化学
Histochemistry and immunohistochemistry

应用和不用淀粉酶消化的PAS染色显示肿瘤细胞内有糖原。这些细胞PLAP、D2-40和NSE免疫染色弥漫阳性（图14B.7）[82,83]。OCT4（POU5F1）是在胚胎干细胞和生殖细胞中有表达的转录因子，而且精原细胞瘤的瘤细胞核也呈阳性[84,85]。Vimentin可能阳性，但多数精原细胞瘤EMA、AFP和Ki-1（Ber-H2；CD30）阴性[86-88]。多数精原细胞瘤KIT（CD117）阳性，虽然ITGCN阴性[88a]。多达40%的肿瘤细胞细胞角蛋白可呈灶状阳性[88]。合体滋养层巨细胞细胞角蛋白和hCG阳性，这种所见不应错误地解释为代表癌的分化。最近一项研究表明，一种血管紧张素Ⅰ转换酶（CD143）的体细胞同工酶是向精原细胞瘤分化的肿瘤的合适的标志物，因为精母细胞性精原细胞瘤和NSGCT这个标志物阴性[36]。

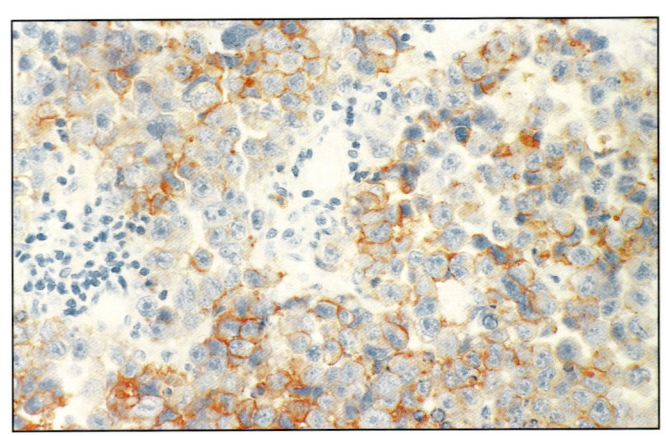

图14B.7 精原细胞瘤。胎盘碱性磷酸酶（PLAP）染色显示精原细胞瘤肿瘤细胞的细胞膜呈弥漫性免疫反应。

精原细胞瘤的hCG和AFP
hCG and AFP in seminoma

由于肿瘤内存在合体滋养层巨细胞，5%～60%的单纯性精原细胞瘤患者血清hCG水平轻度升高[89-93]，这些指标在睾丸切除术后恢复正常。hCG水平升高对于患者预后似乎并无不利影响。睾丸切除术后hCG水平持续升高提示有隐藏的绒毛膜癌病灶。

血清AFP水平升高实际上可以排除单纯性精原细胞瘤，尽管显微镜下评估可能仅仅显示精原细胞瘤成分而无任何其他非精原细胞瘤性生殖细胞成分；这些患者应按非精原细胞瘤方案进行治疗[94-96]。然而，血清AFP轻度升高（<16ng/ml）是可以接受的[96]。精原细胞瘤和非精原细胞瘤性肿瘤以及可能有局灶性非精原细胞瘤性成分的肿瘤在治疗上有所不同，因此在做出精原细胞瘤的诊断之前必须检查多个肿瘤切片。血清NSE水平是另外一种监测精原细胞瘤患者可能有用的标志物[97]。11例伴有转移性精原细胞瘤的患者发现8例血清NSE水平升高（73%），而54例没有转移证据的精原细胞瘤患者53例血清NSE水平正常。另外，化疗之后血清NSE水平恢复到正常。基于这些所见，Kuzmits等[97]认为测量NSE对于临床上监测转移性精原细胞瘤患者的化疗效果是有价值的。

细胞遗传学所见　Cytogenetic findings

精原细胞瘤最常见的细胞遗传学结构异常是出现等臂染色体12p。某些精原细胞瘤缺乏等臂染色体12p，但有其他染色体结构异常[98]。

在青少年和成人中，hiwi基因定位于12号染色体长臂的12q24.33条带，是一个显示与睾丸生殖细胞肿瘤、精原细胞瘤和非精原细胞瘤发生有关的基因组区。在正常人的睾丸中，hiwi基因特异地表达于生殖细胞，而且发现在精子发生过程中精母细胞和圆形的精子细胞有表达。在体细胞来源的睾丸肿瘤中 hiwi 基因没有表达，例如 Sertoli 细胞和 Leydig 细胞肿瘤（LCT）。Qiao 等[99]报道 19 例睾丸精原细胞瘤性肿瘤样本中发现 12 例有 hiwi 表达升高，而 10 例非精原细胞瘤性睾丸肿瘤中其表达并不升高，这些肿瘤和精原细胞瘤一样均来源于相同的前体细胞，只是丧失了其生殖细胞特征。最后，发现在 4 例精母细胞性精原细胞瘤性肿瘤中 hiwi 表达没有升高。

与正常睾丸相比，睾丸生殖细胞肿瘤生长激素变异型（GH-V）基因表达丢失，而且胎盘催乳素样（PLL）基因产物丢失（精原细胞瘤）或突变（NSGCT），对于这些肿瘤之间的相互关系和睾丸生殖细胞肿瘤的发生可能具有意义[100]。最近报道 16.6% 的精原细胞瘤中有 MAGE-1 抗原（黑色素瘤抗原编码基因家族的成员）表达。胚胎性癌、卵黄囊瘤或畸胎瘤均不含有 MAGE-1 蛋白。41.8% 的精原细胞瘤有 MAGE-3 抗原，而在胚胎性癌、卵黄囊瘤或畸胎瘤中没有发现这种蛋白。精原细胞瘤中出现 MAGE-1 和 MAGE-3 抗原与肿瘤大小、肿瘤分期、出现淋巴细胞浸润或患者的预后无关。人群中 MAGE 特异性人白细胞抗原（HLA）等位基因出现率低，肿瘤性生殖细胞 HLA Ⅰ 型抗原丢失，以及发现多数精原细胞瘤和所有的 NSGCT 缺乏 MAGE-1 和 MAGE-3 抗原肽，提示直接针对 MAGE-1 和 MAGE-3 抗原的免疫治疗可能不是治疗精原细胞瘤和 NSGCT 的最佳选择[101]。Zeeman 等[102]发现，在正常精子发生过程中、精原细胞瘤（经典性和精母细胞性）、原位癌（经典性精原细胞瘤和非精原细胞瘤的前体）、无性细胞瘤和性腺母细胞瘤均有 VASA mRNA（通过定量反转录 PCR）和蛋白（通过组织化学染色）表达。

鉴别诊断

鉴别诊断主要包括恶性淋巴瘤、胚胎性癌和内胚窦瘤。其他可能需要鉴别的疾病包括绒毛膜癌、肉芽肿性睾丸炎、Sertoli 细胞瘤和精母细胞性精原细胞瘤。大细胞性淋巴瘤相对容易排除，不管是原发性还是转移性。大细胞性淋巴瘤的特征是显示肿瘤细胞浸润生精小管之间的间质，缺乏小管内恶性生殖细胞增生，而且通常没有纤维化或肉芽肿性反应。淋巴瘤比精原细胞瘤更易累及白膜、附睾和精索。PLAP、CD20、CD3 和白细胞共同抗原（LCA）免疫染色有助于诊断。

胚胎性癌通常见于 20～30 岁的患者；它比精原细胞瘤细胞更加丰富，核的多形性明显，而且核分裂比较活跃。胚胎性癌也可出现乳头状和假腺体结构以及合体排列的细胞。与精原细胞瘤不同，胚胎性癌细胞角蛋白和 Ki-1（CD30）抗原阳性（表 14B.4）。单纯性内胚窦瘤通常见于儿童，而且多半排列成网状、黏液样及微囊状结构。肿瘤细胞之间有基底膜样物质沉积 [周缘卵黄囊分化（parietal yolk sac differentiation）] 是其特征。细胞角蛋白和 AFP 免疫染色有助于与精原细胞瘤的鉴别诊断。

精母细胞性精原细胞瘤发生于 50 岁以上的患者，通常由存在 3 种细胞类型的伴有明显多形性的圆形细胞组成，包括非常具有特征性的巨细胞。这种肿瘤通常没有纤维血管间隔、淋巴细胞浸润或肉芽肿性反应。伴有大量合体滋养层巨细胞的精原细胞瘤与绒毛膜癌的不同之处在于前者缺乏典型的双相性表现、发育不全的绒毛结构以及肿瘤出血和坏死。

精原细胞瘤内明显的肉芽肿性反应可能掩盖肿瘤细胞，而类似于肉芽肿性睾丸炎。病变周围出现 ITGCN、在高倍镜下仔细寻找肿瘤细胞以及 PLAP 免疫染色有助于解决诊断上的难题。

最后，精原细胞瘤的管状和假腺体结构（"管状精原细胞瘤"）和 Paget 样病变蔓延至睾丸网可能类似于 Sertoli 细胞瘤。前者总是伴有比较典型的经典性精原细胞瘤的区域。PLAP 免疫染色也有帮助，因为 Sertoli 细胞瘤 PLAP 染色阴性。

表 14B.4 恶性生殖细胞肿瘤的免疫组织化学所见

成分	病例数	PLAP	AFP	NSE	VIM	K	CEA	Leu-M1	EMA	hCG	Ki-1
Sem	(7)	6	−	7	−	−	−	−	−	−	−
EC	(33)	24	±	30	11	22	−	−	−	−	23
EST	(18)	±	15	3	−	18	−	−	−	−	1
IT	(23)	−	−	21	21	7	−	−	−	−	−
MT	(30)	±	−	24	14	30	22	22	21	18	−

Sem：精原细胞瘤；EC：胚胎性癌；EST：内胚窦瘤；IT：未成熟性畸胎瘤；MT：成熟性畸胎瘤；PLAP：胎盘碱性磷酸酶；AFP：甲胎蛋白；NSE：神经元特异性烯醇化酶；VIM：波形蛋白（vimentin）；K：细胞角蛋白；CEA：癌胚抗原；EMA：上皮膜抗原；hCG：人绒毛膜促性腺激素。

精原细胞瘤的治疗　Management of seminoma

经典性精原细胞瘤患者的治疗主要取决于疾病的分期[103,104]。Ⅰ期疾病（肿瘤局限于睾丸不伴有转移）采取根治性睾丸切除术后进行监测或放疗。睾丸切除术后推荐的治疗方案是低剂量放疗，99%的病例可以治愈。包括淋巴浆细胞浸润的密度、肉芽肿性反应的程度、肿瘤坏死、纤维化、浸润和间质细胞增生等病理学参数与生存率无关[105]。因此，当Ⅰ期经典性精原细胞瘤应用低剂量放疗时，这些肿瘤特征并不具有临床意义。血管-淋巴管浸润的确影响预后，它的出现就不能仅仅采取"单一监测"疗法[106]。

在监测方案中，研究发现原发性肿瘤的大小和睾丸网浸润是独立的预后因素[65,106,107]。小于3 cm、3～6 cm和大于6 cm的病变，在4年时其无复发的生存率分别为94%、82%和64%[65,107]。肿瘤大小＞6.0 cm与复发率高有关[107]。因此，对于监测方案这些因素是非常重要的。

Ⅱ期疾病的治疗一般根据病变的大小，是低容积（＜5 cm）或是高容积疾病（腹膜后＞6 cm）。前者接受放疗，而较大的病变接受化疗。Ⅲ期疾病应用化疗。

精原细胞瘤最重要的预后因素是诊断时的临床分期[103]。Ⅰ期、Ⅱ期和Ⅲ期的5年生存率分别为99%、89%和70%～85%[109,110]。

精母细胞性精原细胞瘤
Spermatocytic seminoma

精母细胞性精原细胞瘤是少见的肿瘤，占所有精原细胞瘤的3%～7%[109,110]。Masson于1946年最先将其描述为精原细胞瘤独立的组织学亚型[111]。他提出经典性精原细胞瘤起源于未分化的生殖细胞，而精母细胞性精原细胞瘤起源于正在形成精子的细胞，因此是一种比较分化的生殖细胞肿瘤[111]。

精母细胞和精原细胞高度表达的蛋白在精母细胞性精原细胞瘤也有表达，例如Chk2[112]、MAGE-A4[112]、NSE[112]、SSX[113]和NY-ESO-1[114]，但与从有丝分裂转化为减数分裂细胞周期可能有关的p19^{INK4d}没有表达[112]。基于这些结果，有人提出这种表达方式与精母细胞性精原细胞瘤来源于减数分裂前的生殖细胞、精原细胞或成人睾丸的初级精母细胞相符合，这些细胞丧失了胚胎特性，定向为精子生成系列细胞，但尚未通过减数分裂的关卡[112,114]。

临床特征

精母细胞性精原细胞瘤是一种睾丸独特的生殖细胞肿瘤，几乎总是为单纯性，虽然少数病例伴有肉瘤性去分化[115,116]。本病好发于50岁以上的男性（平均年龄55岁），表现为无痛性睾丸增大，但在少数情况下可以发生在较年轻的男性，年龄可以小到23岁[117-119]，这种肿瘤具有惰性的临床行为[109,110,116,120-122]。在已报道的150多例中只有1例真正的单纯性精母细胞性精原细胞瘤发生远处转移。相反，9例伴有肉瘤样去分化的精母细胞性精原细胞瘤中5例死于转移[110,115,116,122-124]。这种肿瘤与隐睾症或ITGCN无关。精母细胞性精原细胞瘤双侧发生（10%）比经典性精原细胞瘤（2%）常见。

病理学特征

肿瘤大小从3 cm至15 cm不等[110]。大体检查肿物呈灰黄色，质软，胶冻状，形成境界清楚的肿块，伴有囊性变和出血。与经典性精原细胞瘤相比，精母细胞性精原细胞瘤颜色更黄，质地更软，黏液样变更为明显[111]（图14B.8）。在伴有肉瘤性去分化的病例肿瘤可能表现为实性，并呈暗灰色。

低倍镜下，精母细胞性精原细胞瘤显示多形性细胞弥漫性增生，通常具有3种类型，伴有局灶性微囊和小管内以及间质性生长方式。缺乏明显的纤维血管间质，几乎没有淋巴细胞浸润和肉芽肿。细胞浆通常不含糖原。这个肿瘤不伴有其他生殖细胞成分。

高倍镜下，有3种类型细胞，每一种细胞具有独特的形态学（图14B.9）。大细胞（50～100 μm）最不常见，单核或多核。肿瘤细胞浆丰富，嗜酸性。肿瘤细胞核均匀一致，圆形，但是大小明显不同。细胞核含有"丝球状"染色质，类似于减数分裂前期的初级精母细胞。中等细胞（10～20 μm）核非常圆，伴有均匀散在分布的颗粒状染色质，或在少数情况下为丝球状染色质，胞浆嗜酸性。小细胞为淋巴细胞样细胞（6～8 μm），细胞核均匀一致，深染，胞浆量少。中等细胞和大细胞核所特有

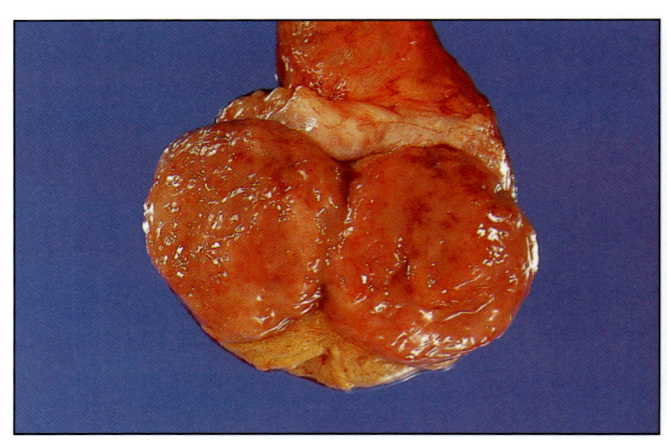

图14B.8　大体上，精母细胞性精原细胞瘤类似于经典性精原细胞瘤，但是较黄，胶冻状比较明显，质地较软。

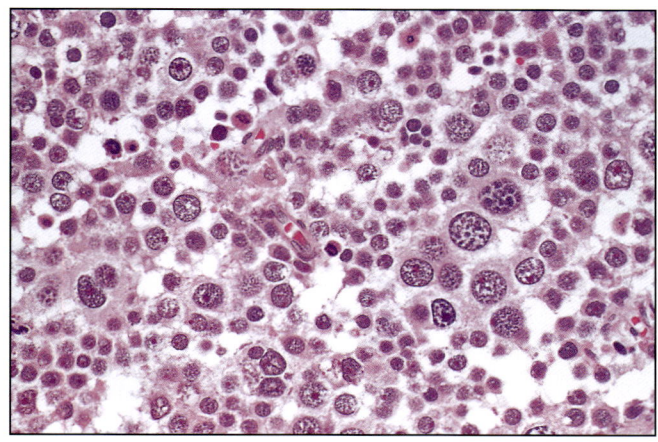

图14B.9 精母细胞性精原细胞瘤显示三种细胞类型：大细胞、中等大小细胞和小淋巴细胞样细胞。

的丝球状染色质可用于鉴别这个肿瘤和经典性精原细胞瘤。可有许多核分裂象。

虽然精母细胞性精原细胞瘤并不伴有其他生殖细胞成分，但是大约6%的病例伴有高级别的肉瘤，例如纤维肉瘤、横纹肌肉瘤或者未分化肉瘤[116,122,124]（图14B.10）。True等[122]提出这是精母细胞性精原细胞瘤发生间变性转化的表现，与其他器官肿瘤见到的状况相同。出现肉瘤性成分的精母细胞性精原细胞瘤通常转变为高度侵袭性的肿瘤[116,122,124]。报告的9例伴有肉瘤性转化的病例中5例死于转移，死亡发生在睾丸切除术后2年之内，而且只有肉瘤成分发生转移。据报道这种类型的精母细胞性精原细胞瘤化疗效果不好[116,122]。

"间变性"精母细胞性精原细胞瘤已有描述；其特征为明显占主导的单一形态的细胞，伴有显著的核仁，可能被误诊为胚胎性癌或精原细胞瘤[119]。诊断"间变性"精母细胞性精原细胞瘤没有明显的预后意义。

免疫组织化学

在其他类型生殖细胞肿瘤得到证实的各种肿瘤标志物，包括中间丝、OCT4和PLAP，在精母细胞性精原细胞瘤中均无表达[115,125,126]。有报道精母细胞性精原细胞瘤总是表达c-kit和VASA[102,126]。细胞角蛋白18（CK18）可呈点状阳性[115]。在生殖母细胞和精原细胞高表达的蛋白，例如Chk2、MAGE-A4和NSE，均可见于精母细胞性精原细胞瘤[112]。没有发现胚胎性生殖细胞表达而正常成人睾丸不表达的抗原，即TRA-1-60，而p53是个例外，它在80%的精母细胞性精原细胞瘤中阳性。在精母细胞性精原细胞瘤中没有发现原癌基因 $p19^{INK4d}$，$p19^{INK4d}$ 参与生殖细胞从有丝分裂转化为减数分裂。这种表达方式非常符合精母细胞性精原细胞瘤是来源于减数分裂前的生殖细胞，这种细胞已经丧失了胚胎特性，定向为精子生成系列，但还没有通过减数分裂的关卡，很可能是来源于成人睾丸细胞的精原细胞[112]。*NY-ESO-1* 基因是最近确认的癌/睾丸家族（cancer/testis family）的成员，其产物是一种高度致免疫性的肿瘤抗原。Satie等[114]报道，在59例睾丸肿瘤中Sertoli细胞、Leydig细胞、经典的精原细胞瘤或非精原细胞瘤性生殖细胞均不表达NY-ESO-1。相反，NY-ESO-1在原位癌（15例中7例阳性）和精母细胞性精原细胞瘤（16例中8例阳性）均有表达，前者是睾丸肿瘤的最早阶段，而后者被认为是起源于精原细胞或初级精母细胞。NY-ESO-1是一种可以用于追踪睾丸肿瘤发生早期进展的标志物，此时肿瘤出现与其来源细胞类似的表达方式，尽管肿瘤后来不再表达NY-ESO-1。

鉴别诊断

精母细胞性精原细胞瘤的鉴别诊断包括经典性精原细胞瘤、恶性淋巴瘤和实性胚胎性癌。经典性精原细胞瘤肿瘤细胞大，而且只有一种类型，伴有丰富的透明或嗜酸性胞浆；核呈空泡状，有1或2个明显的核仁。肿瘤细胞分布均匀，细胞边界清晰。纤维血管间隔将肿瘤细胞分成小叶状，表现为镶嵌结构。间质伴有淋巴浆细胞浸润和肉芽肿反应，并有未受累及的生精小管。

恶性淋巴瘤的特征是常常双侧发生。大细胞淋巴瘤由卵圆形到圆形淋巴细胞组成，伴有细胞和核的多形性。生长方式主要在间质，并破坏生精小管。LCA染色非常有用。

胚胎性癌通常见于20～30岁之间，这种肿瘤细胞核的多形性比精母细胞性精原细胞瘤明显，核分裂活跃，而且肿瘤细胞呈合体细胞性排列。它通常出现其他生长方式，包括乳头状、实性和假腺体成分。

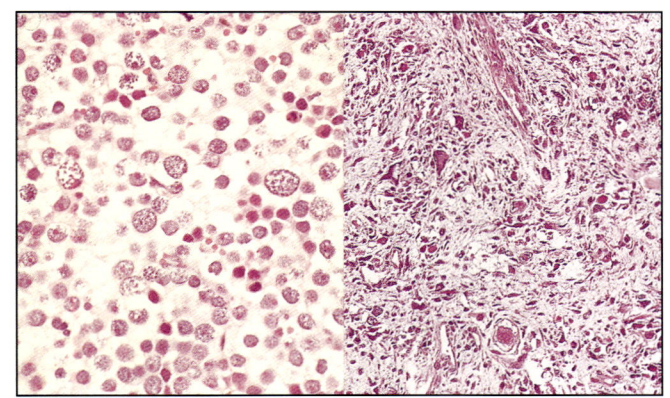

图14B.10 精母细胞性精原细胞瘤（左）伴有肉瘤样成分（右）。本图中的肉瘤样成分为横纹肌肉瘤。

治疗

治疗选择根治性睾丸切除术，腹膜后淋巴结切除没有作用。大部分患者接受下腹部小剂量放疗，但是进行术后放疗效果仍不明确，有待于未来的随机研究加以证实[117]。

非精原细胞瘤性生殖细胞肿瘤
Non-seminomatous germ cell tumors

命名为非精原细胞瘤性生殖细胞肿瘤（NSGCT）的肿瘤包括胚胎性癌、成熟性或未成熟性畸胎瘤、绒毛膜癌以及其他罕见的滋养细胞肿瘤、内胚窦瘤（卵黄囊瘤）、弥漫性胚胎瘤和多胚瘤；这些肿瘤可以单独出现或以不同的形式混合存在。为了治疗的目的，将含有精原细胞瘤性和非精原细胞瘤性两种成分的肿瘤，以及组织学检查为单纯性精原细胞瘤但血清 AFP 水平明显升高的肿瘤均看成是 NSGCT。曾有几例 AFP 轻度升高（＜18ng/ml）的单纯性精原细胞瘤病例报道[96]。

包括计算机断层摄影术（CT）、肿瘤标志物分析以及腹膜后淋巴结切除术在内的多学科诊断和分期程序已经证实，最初诊断时的疾病分期是重要的预后决定因素。新近的报告指出，在原发性肿瘤中有占整个肿瘤体积 80% 以上的胚胎性癌以及出现血管（图 14B.11）或淋巴管浸润是 I 期 NSGCT 的首要不利预后因素，在睾丸切除之后要选择适当的治疗[63,127-131]。肿瘤大小和其他组织学参数好像不具有预后意义，虽然其他研究人员发现肿瘤病理分期增加（肿瘤侵犯到白膜以外或进入附睾）、最初进行阴囊手术以及在不到 50% 的肿瘤出现畸胎瘤，均有不良的预后影响[130,131]。某些研究应用多元回归分析发现，只有胚胎性癌细胞成分和血管浸润是独立的变量；其他变量是相互联系的[132]。

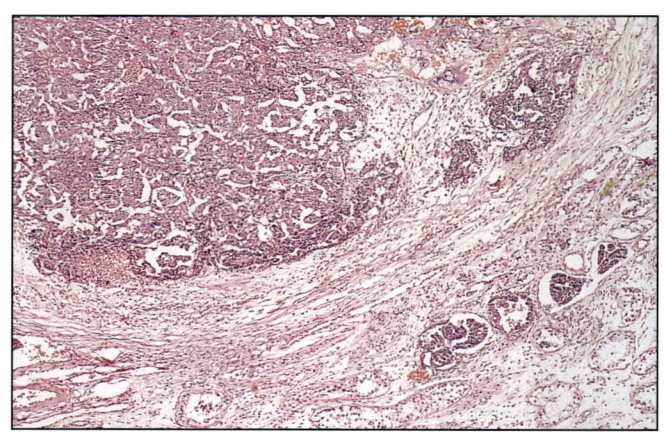

图14B.11　胚胎性癌伴有血管浸润。肿瘤细胞与血管的形状相吻合，代表真正的血管浸润。

胚胎性癌　Embryonal carcinoma

胚胎性癌是第二个最常见的单纯性睾丸生殖细胞肿瘤，占这些肿瘤的 15%～30%[133-135]。它最常发生于 25～35 岁之间的患者，平均年龄 32 岁。婴儿或儿童未见发生，40～50 岁以后非常罕见[130,136]。患者一般表现为无痛性睾丸增大，大部分为单侧发生；1/3 的患者表现为主动脉旁淋巴结、肺或肝转移[134]。这种肿瘤偶尔伴有男性乳腺发育，血清 AFP 和（或）hCG 水平可能升高[137,138]。

应用免疫组织化学检查重新评估 WHO 的材料，发现胚胎性癌有 20% 的发生率。"单纯性"胚胎性癌不允许出现根据 AFP 免疫反应确定的卵黄囊分化，根据这一标准，Mostofi 等[139]仅将 3.1% 的胚胎性癌病例归入"单纯性"范畴。目前的趋势是确定细胞或血清中有无 AFP 存在，因为不管肿瘤的细胞学表现如何，AFP 的出现都是卵黄囊分化的证据[140,141]；然而，发现 AFP 本身并不能改变诊断，除非通过光镜检查可以辨认出卵黄囊瘤特征性的组织学结构。

病理学特征

大体上，胚胎性癌可能是最小的生殖细胞肿瘤（就单纯性而言），大小平均 2.5 cm，但是也可以非常大；切面隆起，斑驳状，灰白色，颗粒状或光滑，境界不清，可见出血和坏死区域（图 14B.12）。在切除时，20% 的胚胎性癌侵犯邻近的附睾或白膜。

低倍镜下，胚胎性癌表现为腺泡状、管状、乳头状或实性结构，伴有合体性生长以及坏死、出血和纤维化区域（图 14B.13）。肿瘤内和肿瘤周围可见小管内胚胎性癌。受累的生精小管含有间变性肿瘤细胞，常常伴有中心坏死，伴有或不伴有钙化。

高倍镜下有明显的细胞多形性，核大而突出，不规则，略呈空泡状，胞浆丰富，细颗粒状，嗜酸性到嗜双色，细胞边界不清（图 14B.14）。瘤巨细胞和奇异性肿瘤细胞并不少见，如同深染的变性表现的破碎细胞（smudged cells）一样。核染色质粗糙，伴有清楚的核膜和明显的核仁，而且核分裂活跃，常常伴有非典型性核分裂象。间质淋巴细胞浸润和肉芽肿性反应少见。常常发生肿瘤周围血管淋巴管浸润，这是一种需要记录的重要特征。

免疫组织化学

免疫组织化学检查，广谱细胞角蛋白（CK cock-tail）、PLAP、Ki-1（CD30）和 OCT4 常常阳性（图 14B.15）。胚胎性癌肿瘤细胞核 OCT4 总是阳性[83,85]。肿瘤细胞 AFP 可能阳性。hCG 免疫染色仅见于合体滋

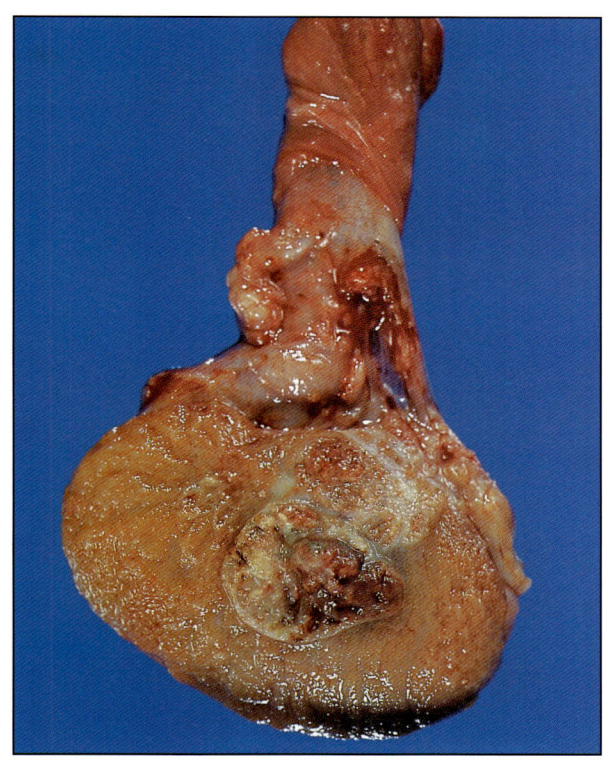

图14B.12 胚胎性癌。肿瘤境界不清，切面斑驳，呈灰白色颗粒状。注意肿瘤坏死和出血区。

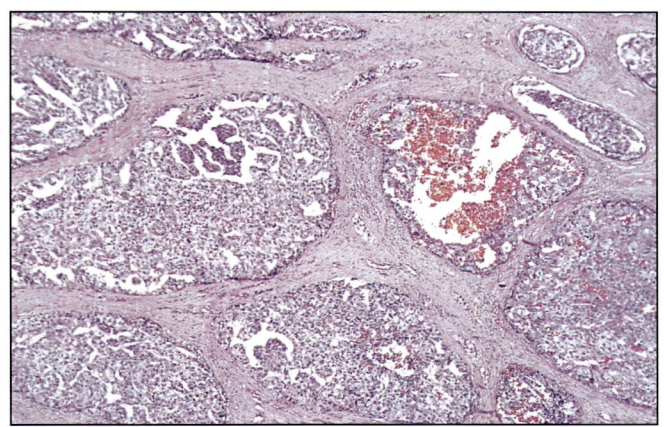

图14B.13 胚胎性癌伴有管状、乳头状和实性结构。

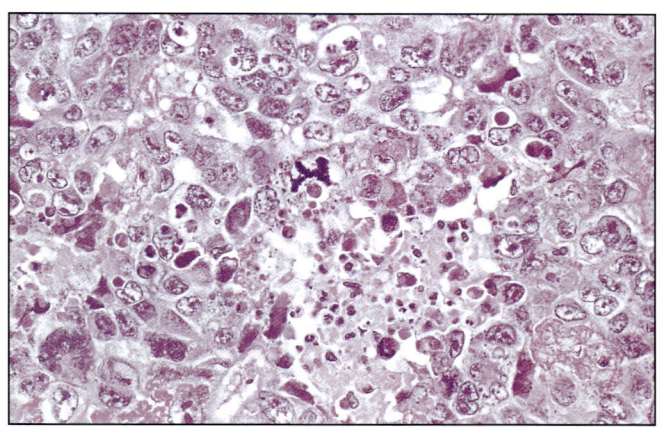

图14B.14 伴有实性结构的胚胎性癌。肿瘤细胞大，多形性，含有大的空泡状核和明显的核仁。细胞界限不清，常常有核的重叠，形成合体细胞结构。核分裂象常见，偶见非典型性核分裂象。

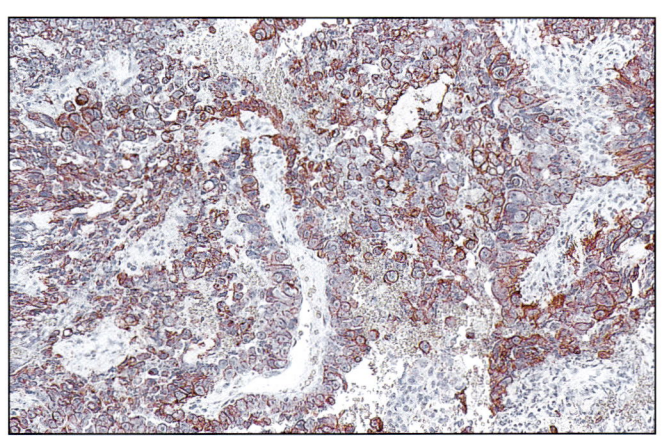

图14B.15 胚胎性癌Ki-1（CD30）免疫染色通常阳性。

养巨细胞，而不见于胚胎性癌的肿瘤细胞。CK 20、高分子量CK、CEA和Leu-M1通常阴性[86,88,90,125,142-148]。

Berney等[148]报道，CD30表达丧失常常发生于化疗之后的转移性胚胎性癌。这一发现的意义在于可应用CD30诊断转移性NSGCT，而且提示化疗可以改变胚胎性癌的免疫表型，尽管其特征性的组织学表现可以保留。

倍体分析显示平均指数为1.43×二倍体对照，小于精原细胞瘤的平均指数（1.66×二倍体对照）[149]。这些资料支持胚胎性癌起源于继发于肿瘤抑制基因缺失的精原细胞瘤。细胞遗传学分析证实，许多胚胎性癌病例出现等臂染色体12p[98,150]。

鉴别诊断

鉴别诊断包括精原细胞瘤、恶性淋巴瘤、内胚窦瘤和转移癌。虽然多数胚胎性癌易与精原细胞瘤区别，但在某些情况下，因为两者的组织学特征相似而非常难以鉴别。对于这样的病例应用CD30（Ki-1）免疫染色容易鉴别，因为这种标志物胚胎性癌常常阳性而精原细胞瘤阴性。广谱细胞角蛋白可能有所帮助，但是两者肿瘤均可阳性。精原细胞瘤倾向于显示单个细胞阳性，而且这种病变可以局灶阳性，但弥漫阳性可能罕见。出现Ki-1阳性细胞簇支持胚胎性癌的诊断。

大细胞淋巴瘤见于老年患者，常常双侧发生。较常累及附睾。淋巴瘤不存在见于胚胎性癌的乳头状、囊性、管状和腺泡状结构。CD20、CD3、CD5 和 LCA 可能显示肿瘤为淋巴细胞谱系，而 CK 阴性。免疫母细胞性淋巴瘤和 Ki-1 淋巴瘤问题最大；后者的诊断困难在于 Ki-1 淋巴瘤和胚胎性癌两者 Ki-1 均呈阳性而使诊断变得复杂。这时，PLAP 免疫染色有助于鉴别[86,151]。至于转移癌，几乎总有既往恶性肿瘤的临床病史，通常累及双侧睾丸，主要浸润睾丸间质。血管浸润在转移癌比较常见。转移性肿瘤可为多灶性或（和）双侧性。

卵黄囊瘤的细胞学和结构特征可能类似于胚胎性癌，但一般来说其多形性不明显，但有比较显著的结构多样性。卵黄囊瘤常常出现胞浆内和细胞外玻璃样小滴，细胞之间有基底膜样物质沉积（周缘卵黄囊分化）。卵黄囊瘤 AFP 免疫染色经常弥漫阳性，而 Ki-1（CD30）阴性。胚胎性癌含有较大和多形性比较明显的细胞核，伴有明显的核仁，核分裂比例高，经常为实性生长方式。

卵黄囊瘤（内胚窦瘤）
Yolk sac tumor （endodermal sinus tumor）

卵黄囊瘤是婴儿和小儿（出生至 5 岁）的肿瘤[152-160]，在这个年龄组，几乎总是发生单纯性卵黄囊瘤。卵黄囊瘤占全部儿童睾丸肿瘤的 75% ~ 80%，最常见于 1 岁和 2 岁的儿童（从新生儿到 8 岁）。在成人，单纯性卵黄囊瘤非常罕见，几乎总是混有其他肿瘤性生殖细胞成分[140,161,162]。患者表现为睾丸迅速增大和血清 AFP 升高。在儿科肿瘤中，卵黄囊瘤与隐睾症似乎没有令人信服的关联性。

病理学特征

大体检查，增大的睾丸内可见境界不清的分叶状灰白色或灰黄色的肿瘤，直径从 2 cm 到 6 cm 不等。它可能是局灶性囊性的肿瘤，或为质地不同的实性肿物，可以出现出血和坏死。切面通常有黏液性特征。

显微镜下，卵黄囊瘤的主要特点是同时出现多样组织学结构。网状-微囊性结构最常见，发生于 80% 的患者，由不规则的疏松间隙和相互吻合的细小条索以及内衬扁平或立方细胞的小管组成（图 14B.16）；微囊性结构的特征为显著的胞浆空泡（类似脂肪母细胞）和伴有乳头状细胞簇突向腔内的小囊腔（图 14B.17）。间质通常为黏液样（图 14B.18），而且网状/微囊状区域可以转化为梭形、实性结构或巨囊性区域。最具特征性的结构是形成 Schiller-Duval 小体（图 14B.19），其中心是纤

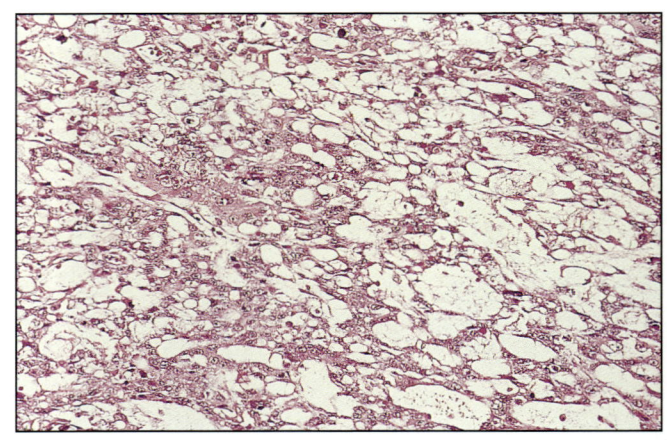

图 14B.16 伴有网状结构的内胚窦瘤，由不规则的相互吻合的腔隙组成，形成疏松的含有黏液样物质的囊腔。

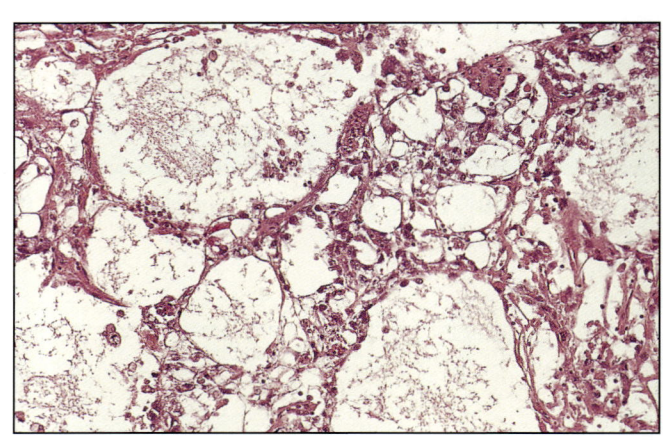

图 14B.17 伴有微囊和巨囊结构的内胚窦瘤。腔隙内衬扁平或立方细胞。

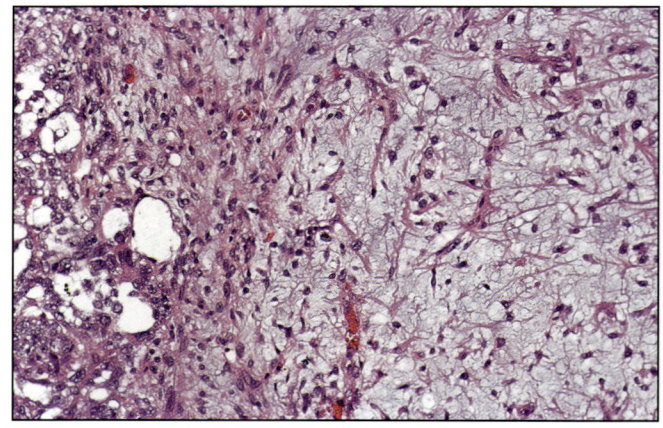

图 14B.18 内胚窦瘤的黏液样和梭形细胞结构。梭形肿瘤细胞被大量的黏液样间质分开。

维血管轴心，周围绕以恶性的立方形到柱状的上皮样细胞，这种结构可退变为内衬扁平细胞的囊性间隙。另外 10% 的肿瘤可见多囊性卵黄结构，含有伴有向心性缩窄

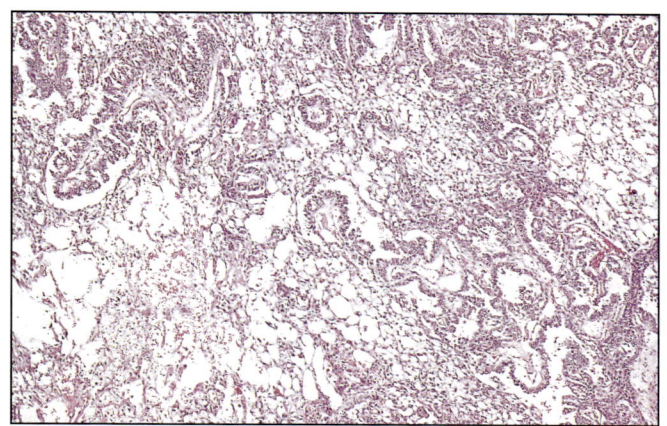

图14B.19 在网状背景下,内胚窦瘤可见横切和纵切的Schiller-Duval小体。

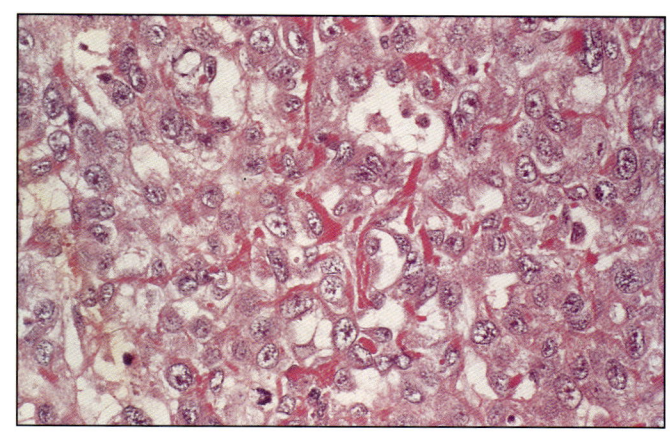

图14B.21 伴有实性生长方式的内胚窦瘤。还要注意大量的细胞外基底膜物质的出现(周缘卵黄囊分化)。

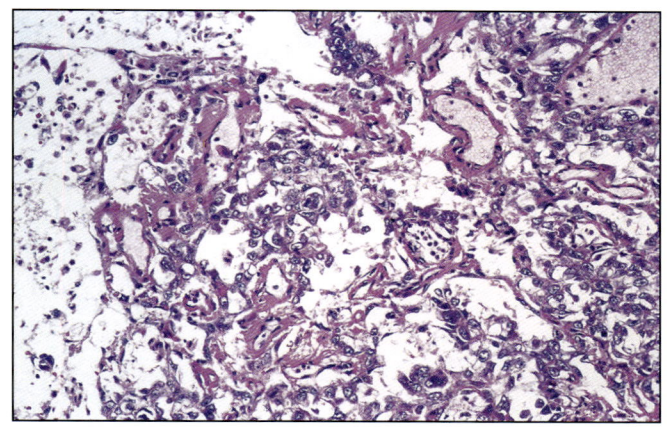

图14B.20 内胚窦瘤的周缘分化结构。注意肿瘤细胞周围生成大量嗜酸性基底膜样物质。

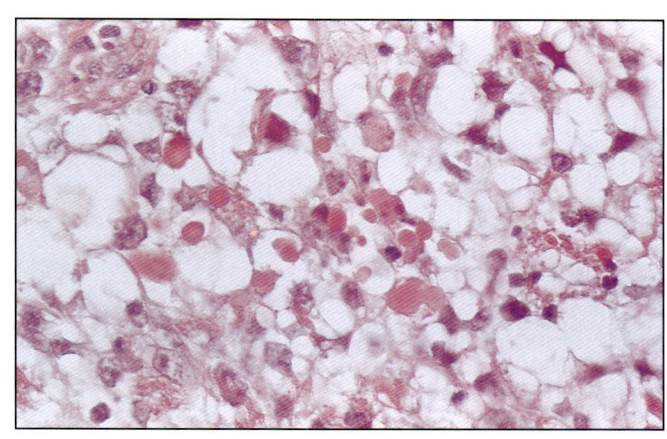

图14B.22 伴有细胞外嗜酸性玻璃样小体的内胚窦瘤。

的不规则的小管,类似于卵黄囊泡。周缘卵黄囊分化相当常见,特征为出现大量相当于基底膜物质的细胞外玻璃样物(图14B.20)[163]。其他变异包括实性(5%)(图14B.21)、乳头状(5%)、梭形细胞性、肠性(腺体-腺泡结构)以及肝细胞样结构[164-167]。内衬相互吻合小管的细胞通常为扁平或柱状细胞,可能被误认为是良性表现。细胞内或细胞外玻璃样小体是卵黄囊分化的特征,见于85%的病例(图14B.22)。这些小体PAS反应阳性,抗淀粉酶消化,而且含有AFP或α-抗胰蛋白酶。肿瘤细胞AFP、CK和PLAP阳性,Ki-1和hCG阴性[90,140,142,144,146,147,168-170]。周缘分化结构的基底膜物质AFP通常阴性。少数儿童病例与ITGCN有关;相反,几乎所有作为MGCT一种成分发生的伴有卵黄囊瘤的成人肿瘤均有ITGCN[171,172]。

小于2岁的患者预后最好[173]。在成人,伴有卵黄囊分化作为肿瘤一部分的NSGCT,其预后随着疾病分期不同而不同,但当应用目前的治疗模式时,卵黄囊分化的出现对预后似乎并无不利影响。因为成人单纯性卵黄囊瘤非常罕见,有关它的行为目前知之甚少。

多胚瘤 Polyembryoma

完全由胚胎样小体组成的单纯性多胚瘤是一种极其罕见的肿瘤,其中有胚胎性癌和卵黄囊瘤成分,有时还会有畸胎瘤成分,排列成类似于胚胎发生18天之前的体节前胚胎的结构。然而,比较常见的是伴有其他生殖细胞肿瘤成分,特别是卵黄囊瘤和畸胎瘤。血清AFP水平可明显升高。它表现为如同其他NSGCT一样的恶性行为,而且大多数专家将其视为非精原细胞瘤性(混合性)生殖细胞肿瘤[174-176]。肿瘤实性,质软,而且有些水肿;囊性区提示伴有畸胎瘤成分。低倍镜下可见大量胚胎样小体,周围被疏松的黏液瘤性间叶组织包绕。胚胎样小体由胚盘组成,一侧内衬立方细胞,背侧羊膜

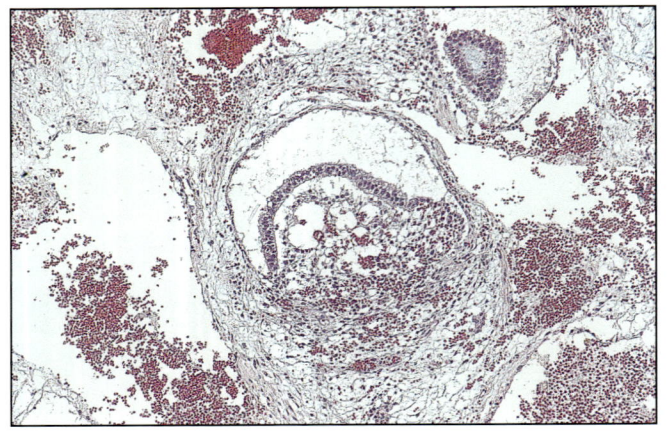

图14B.23 伴有一个胚胎样小体的多胚瘤。它由羊膜腔、胚盘、卵黄囊和黏液样胚外间叶组织组成。

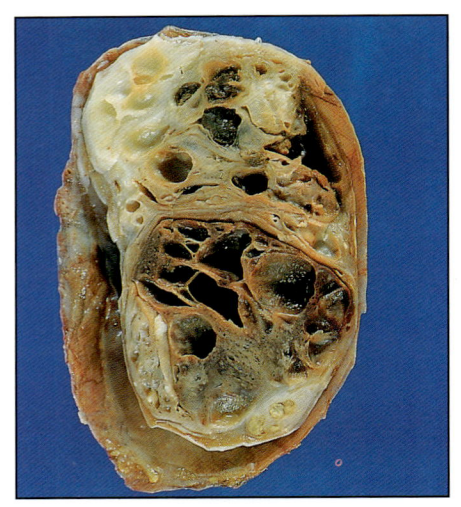

图14B.24 畸胎瘤伴有实性和多囊性区域

样腔内衬扁平上皮,而腹侧的卵黄囊样小泡由网状和黏液瘤性卵黄囊瘤组成(图14B.23)[174-176]。

胚胎样小体 AFP 和 CK 通常阳性,而 PLAP 可能阳性。周围间叶和黏液瘤性间质 vimentin 阳性。hCG 和 CEA 阴性。

成熟性畸胎瘤　Teratoma, mature

成熟性畸胎瘤是一种最常见的 MGCT。单纯性畸胎瘤罕见,仅占所有睾丸生殖细胞肿瘤的 2%～3%。它最常见于 1～20 岁。成熟性畸胎瘤是婴儿和儿童时期第二个最常见的肿瘤;诊断时的平均年龄为 20 个月[133,177-179]。患者表现为睾丸逐渐肿大,伴有或不伴有疼痛。青春期前患者的成熟性畸胎瘤几乎总是良性的,但在青春期后可呈侵袭性的临床经过,此时若这些患者发生转移,其中可能含有非畸胎瘤性恶性生殖细胞肿瘤成分。它见于大约 50% 的成人非精原细胞瘤性肿瘤[133,177,180-184]。

病理学特征

大体检查,肿瘤与周围未受累及的睾丸分界清楚,可能为实性或多囊性(图14B.24)。囊肿可能充满透明、角质的、胶冻状或黏液性物质,可见软骨、骨片、色素沉着组织和脑组织。

低倍镜下,可见外胚层、内胚层和中胚层组织混合存在,或杂乱排列或形成有序的结构(图14B.25)。外胚层成分通常包括表皮和神经组织,内胚层成分包括胃肠道和呼吸道黏膜以及其他部位黏液腺体,而中胚层包括骨、软骨和肌肉。可以出现其他成熟的体细胞成分。

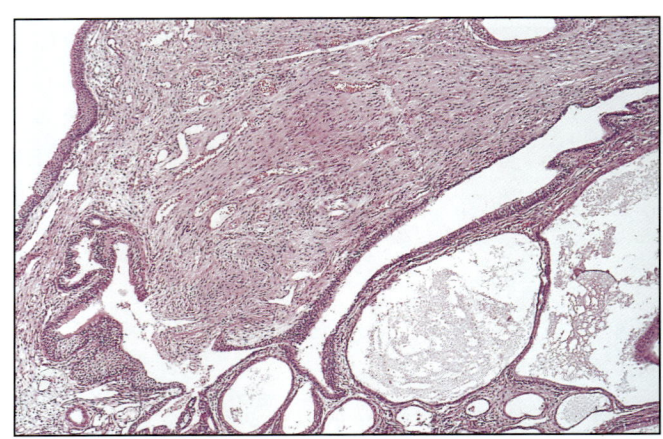

图14B.25 成熟性畸胎瘤伴有腺体和鳞状上皮以及平滑肌纤维。

最常见的成分是神经、软骨和各种类型的上皮[181]。虽然非常少见,但是可以出现色素沉着性视网膜型上皮、肾、肝、前列腺、脉络丛、胰腺组织和涎腺组织。大约 8% 的畸胎瘤可见含有 Langhans 型多核巨细胞的肉芽肿,这也可能是角质漏入间质引起的反应[185]。

罕见的睾丸皮样囊肿(dermoid cyst)应该归入成熟性畸胎瘤的一个亚型还是应该单独作为一种类型还有争论。形态学所见的范围也未完全明确,如同皮样囊肿与未分类型 ITGCN(IGCNU)的相互关系一样。Ulbright 和 Srigley[186] 报告,他们的 5 例睾丸皮样囊肿患者年龄为 17～42 岁,临床均表现为睾丸肿物。4 例病变由充满角质的囊肿组成,伴有囊壁增厚,而 1 例有岛状鳞状上皮细胞"阴影",伴有钙化和骨化(毛母质瘤样亚型)。2 例大体可见毛发。显微镜下检查,4 例有毛囊和皮脂腺,显示典型的向着表皮表面的皮肤型分化,虽然 2 例没有发现毛鞘。另外,纤维性囊壁含有平滑肌束(所有 5 例)以及外分泌汗腺或顶浆分泌腺(4 例)。某些病例还有内衬纤毛上皮的腺体（4个肿瘤，其中包括毛母质瘤样亚型）、肠黏膜（1个肿瘤）和骨（2个肿瘤）。没有细胞学非典型性或明显的核分裂活性，没有生精小管内有 IGCNU 的病例。所有患者均为临床 I 期，通过睾丸切除术治疗而无辅助治疗。随访从 1.5 年到 9.5 年不等，所有患者均健在。这项研究支持皮样囊肿可以有非皮肤性畸胎瘤成分，其重要的诊断标准为缺乏 IGCNU。它还支持皮样囊肿应从睾丸成熟性畸胎瘤中单独划分出来，因为后者在青春期后的患者具有恶性性质。这些观察支持青春期后患者的睾丸畸胎瘤至少有 2 种通路：比较常见的是通过 IGCNU，从浸润性恶性生殖细胞肿瘤分化而来；而少见的是通过皮样囊肿，直接从非恶性生殖细胞转化而来。因此，区别畸胎瘤和皮样囊肿非常重要，因为来自皮样囊肿的转移尚无报道[186]。

表皮样囊肿（epidermoid cyst）（见 843 页）不被认为是畸胎瘤，它在组织学上由至少部分内衬角化鳞状上皮的囊肿构成[187]。可能具有破裂的特征，伴有溃疡形成、异物肉芽肿反应和纤维化。未受累的睾丸组织应该广泛取材，因为出现 ITGCN 则不支持表皮样囊肿的诊断。

最近有 1 例睾丸黏液性囊腺瘤伴有肠分化的报道。作者认为这似乎是发表的第 1 例发生在睾丸内的良性黏液性囊腺瘤的报道。这个伴有肠分化的睾丸内肿瘤可能是良性单胚层性畸胎瘤[188]。

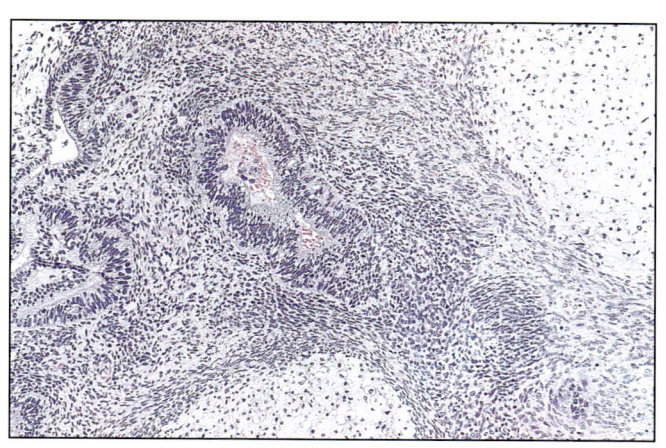

图14B.26 未成熟性畸胎瘤显示富于细胞的原始间充质、腺上皮和软骨组织。

睾丸畸胎瘤恶变少见。恶变的畸胎瘤一般含有在其他器官和组织遇到的恶性肿瘤，例如鳞状细胞癌、腺癌或肉瘤（例如横纹肌肉瘤、血管肉瘤）；伴有肉瘤性成分的患者预后通常不好[194,195]。

包含在睾丸畸胎瘤范畴内的肿瘤还包括单胚层和高度特化的肿瘤，例如类癌（见 841 页）和睾丸 PNET[193]。

未成熟性畸胎瘤　Teratoma,immature

未成熟性畸胎瘤是非精原细胞瘤性生殖细胞肿瘤（NSGCT）的一种常见成分。单纯性未成熟性畸胎瘤极其少见[189,190]。最常见的症状为无痛性睾丸肿大。肿瘤大小从 2 cm 至 4 cm 不等。它经常发生在出生到 7 岁之间的患者（平均 13 个月）[191]。畸胎瘤性成分未成熟并不是原发性肿瘤生物学行为不良的指征。睾丸畸胎瘤的侵袭性行为与患者年龄而不是与组织学类型直接相关。

畸胎瘤未成熟是指出现不能被辨认为正常成分的组织和类似于胚胎或胎儿组织的组织。因此，未成熟性畸胎瘤成分主要为富于细胞的梭形间叶性成分，但也可以见到未成熟的神经和上皮成分（图 14B.26）。梭形细胞常常出现核分裂象。其他类型的未成熟性成分包括类似于神经管的神经上皮和胚胎神经系统，以及类似于胚胎肾或肺的母细胞瘤性组织[192]。还可出现胚胎性横纹肌母细胞组织以及表现较成熟的骨骼肌[193]。类似于原始神经外胚层肿瘤（PNET）的微小病灶也可以见到[192]。肉瘤性成分（大于 1 个低倍视野）和 PNET 显著过度生长应予记录，虽然这些改变的预后意义还不完全清楚。

绒毛膜癌　Choriocarcinoma

单纯性绒毛膜癌极其罕见，占所有睾丸生殖细胞肿瘤的不到 1%[3,196]。比较常见的是作为 NSGCT 的一种成分，大约见于 8%～10% 的睾丸肿瘤。睾丸单纯性绒毛膜癌见于 10～30 岁的患者，是一种高度恶性的睾丸肿瘤。患者可能表现为诸如男性乳腺发育症（10%）等激素紊乱引起的症状、远处转移的症状以及血清 hCG 升高。患者也可表现为绒毛膜癌综合征，主要为由于广泛转移所致的内脏出血。睾丸通常小或大小正常，但可以增大和变硬，取决于出血的程度。肿瘤典型表现为广泛出血和坏死、周围可见存活的灰白色组织。偶尔，在出现广泛转移性肿瘤的病例，睾丸内出现充满含铁血黄素的瘢痕可能是唯一的特征。肿瘤通常由两种细胞成分构成——合体滋养细胞和细胞滋养细胞。排列成实性巢状或片块，偶尔呈绒毛样排列（图 14B.27）。合体滋养细胞是大的空泡状多核巨细胞，胞浆深嗜酸性。细胞滋养细胞是均匀一致的中等大小的多角形细胞，胞浆丰富透明，细胞界限清楚。除非与合体滋养细胞共存，细胞滋养细胞在组织学上难以归类，而且不能与精原细胞瘤或

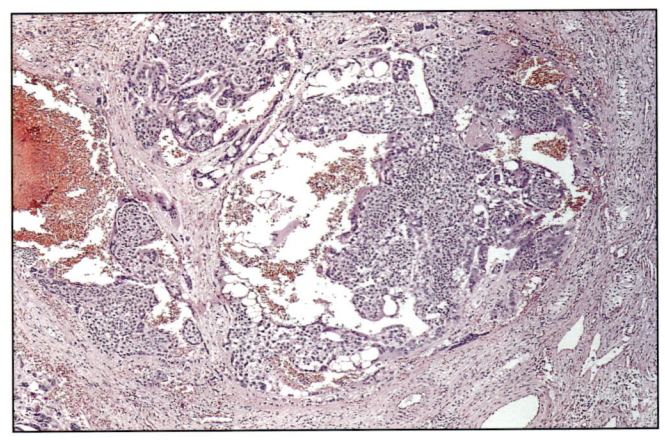

图 14B.27　绒毛膜癌。肿瘤的特征为绒毛样排列，外周为合体滋养细胞，而中心为细胞滋养细胞。常见出血和坏死。

胚胎性癌细胞可靠地鉴别开来。合体滋养细胞一般"覆盖"或包裹细胞滋养细胞，形成绒毛状结构。在非常少见的情况下，合体滋养细胞稀少，形成一种"单相性表现"。这些病例的多数细胞类似于中间性滋养细胞，具有大的单个核或双核，伴有丰富的胞浆[197,198]。

Ulbright 和 Loehrer[199] 描述了两种他们命名为绒毛膜癌样病变（choriocarcinoma-like lesions，CCLL）的有趣的病变，发生在 9 例伴有睾丸生殖细胞肿瘤的患者。其中一种亚型被认为是畸胎瘤性上皮不同寻常的增生，命名为畸胎瘤性 CCLL（5 例）。第二种亚型被认为是非双相性和囊性的绒毛膜癌，类似于 Mazur 等[200] 描述的非典型性绒毛膜癌。除了一例以外所有患者在切除 CCLL 之前均接受化疗。随访时间太短（平均 1.9 年）以至于不能确定其临床意义，但所有患者在手术切除之后都生存良好。胎盘部位滋养细胞肿瘤（PSTT）在女性生殖道是一种定义明确的疾病。在男性生殖道，曾有 2 例睾丸 PSTT 的报道[198,201]。虽然其发生非常罕见，但是睾丸 PSTT 还是被并入新近 WHO 男性生殖道肿瘤的分类中。第 1 例是 16 个月的男孩，其睾丸肿瘤含有单核中间性滋养细胞，人胎盘催乳素阳性，随访 8 年临床经过平稳（图 14B.28）[198]。第 2 例为成年男性患者，是在睾丸 NSGCT 晚期腹膜后复发而被发现的。肿瘤是因化疗之后 4 年血清 β-hCG 水平升高而被发现的。在回顾原发性睾丸肿物时，发现小灶状肿瘤性中间性滋养细胞。第二个病例提示类似于中间性滋养细胞的肿瘤细胞可以转移至区域性腹膜后淋巴结。

免疫组织化学

合体滋养细胞以及合体滋养细胞和细胞滋养细胞之间的过渡性细胞 hCG 阳性。人胎盘催乳素也呈阳性，但通常并不明显；细胞滋养细胞和合体滋养细胞两者细胞角蛋白（CK）均呈阳性。波形蛋白（vimentin）阴性，癌胚抗原（CEA）可能阳性[202]。合体滋养细胞和中间性滋养细胞抑制素（inhibin）阳性，而细胞滋养细胞阴性[203]。没有细胞滋养细胞的合体滋养细胞巨细胞团常常见于其他生殖细胞肿瘤，但它们并不是绒毛膜癌。单纯性绒毛膜癌预后不好，因其倾向于广泛播散。当绒毛膜癌作为 NSGCT 的一种成分时，命名为伴有绒毛膜癌成分的 NSGCT 比绒毛膜癌恰当。绒毛膜癌是生殖细胞肿瘤的一种成分，常常见于脑转移中。hCG 水平较高，较大量的绒毛膜癌和绒毛膜癌综合征均与预后不良有关；然而，绒毛膜癌成分的阈值尚未确定，低于这个阈值肿瘤就不会进展[204-206]。

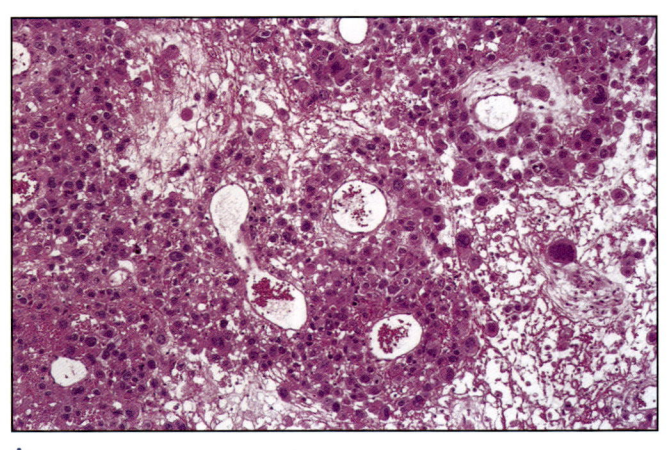

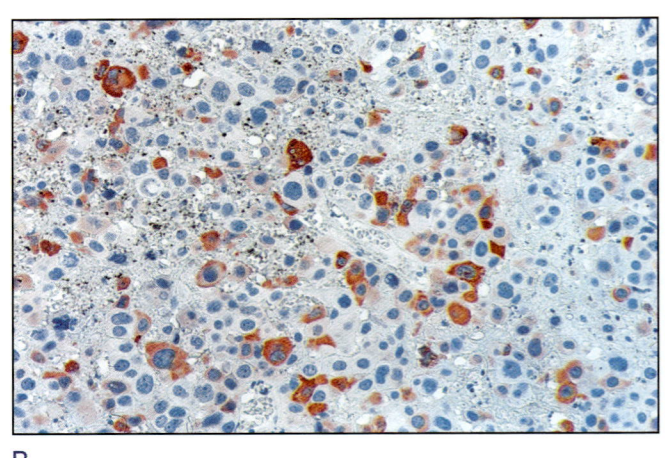

A　　　　　　　　　　　　　　　　　　　　B

图 14B.28　睾丸胎盘部位滋养细胞肿瘤。肿瘤细胞有丰富的深染嗜酸性胞浆和增大的细胞核，伴有裂隙和多核表现，类似于子宫胎盘部位滋养细胞肿瘤。（A）HE 染色；（B）人胎盘催乳素免疫染色。（Courtesy of Dr. Robert H. Young, Massachusetts General Hospital, Harvard Medical School.）

混合性生殖细胞肿瘤
Mixed germ cell tumors

混合性生殖细胞肿瘤（MGCT）是继精原细胞瘤之后第二个最常见的睾丸生殖细胞肿瘤，占所有原发性睾丸生殖细胞肿瘤的 40%～45%[3,4,207]。混合形式包括畸胎瘤和胚胎性癌（25%）、胚胎性癌和精原细胞瘤（15%）、畸胎瘤和胚胎性癌和精原细胞瘤（15%），以及在极少数情况下为精原细胞瘤和卵黄囊瘤。40% 的 MGCT 可见灶状卵黄囊瘤。畸胎癌（teratocarcinoma）这个名称用来表明临床上患有生殖细胞肿瘤的一组患者；并不表明它是 MGCT 的一种组织学亚型。遗憾的是，畸胎癌这个名称已被用于生殖细胞肿瘤的几种组合，包括胚胎性癌和畸胎瘤、卵黄囊瘤和畸胎瘤、胚胎性癌伴有卵黄囊瘤和畸胎瘤，以及胚胎性癌伴有精原细胞瘤和畸胎瘤。鉴于现今有关睾丸肿瘤组织病理学的知识以及当前处理和治疗的观念，畸胎癌这个名称已经没有什么价值。因此，我们建议使用不同的名称并标出不同生殖细胞肿瘤成分的相对比例。我们相信这种方法可以为预测预后和选择适当治疗提供必需的准确信息。MGCT 最常见于 20～40 岁的患者。睾丸增大是最常见的症状。

病理学特征

大体上，睾丸常常完全被肿瘤取代，一般呈现斑驳样外观，伴有囊性和实性区域以及出血和坏死区域（图 14B.29）。大体检查不能区分不同的成分，除了出现出血和坏死提示为胚胎性癌或绒毛膜癌，而出现巨囊、软骨或骨性区域提示为畸胎瘤性成分外。显微镜下，病变可以是囊性或为实性。低倍镜下通过其形态结构容易辨认出多种不同的生殖细胞成分。

胚胎性癌、未成熟性和成熟性畸胎瘤、卵黄囊瘤和绒毛膜癌在不同的肿瘤或同一肿瘤的不同区域出现的比例不同（图 14B.30）。在大多数病例中，这些成分杂乱地分布在整个肿瘤中。极少数情况下，卵黄囊瘤细胞弥漫地环绕在胚胎性癌周围，形成独特的"弥漫性胚胎瘤(diffuse embryoma)"结构（图 14B.31）[208,209]。

发生在睾丸 MGCT 的微囊型脑膜瘤已有 1 例报告，主要由成熟性和未成熟性畸胎瘤组成，伴有精原细胞瘤和胚胎性癌成分[210]。在睾丸畸胎瘤中辨认非生殖细胞肿瘤可能具有预后意义，取决于非生殖细胞成分的性质以及它是否播散到睾丸外。

免疫组织化学染色可以反映生殖细胞成分的分化。在卵黄囊瘤区域甲胎蛋白（AFP）通常阳性，胚胎性癌和精原细胞瘤细胞人绒毛膜促性腺激素（hCG）阴性，

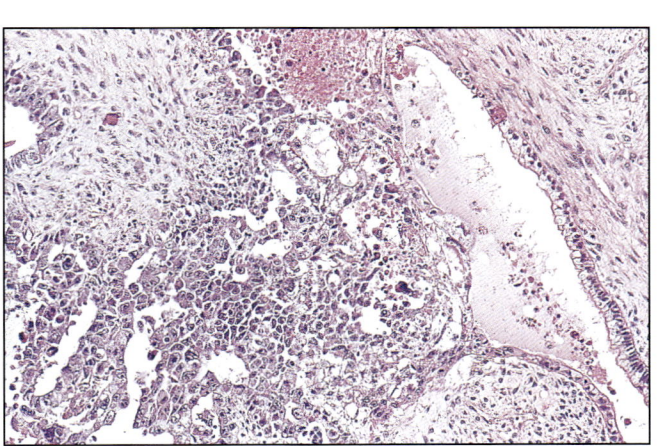

图 14B.30　混合性生殖细胞肿瘤。最常见的组合是胚胎性癌和畸胎瘤。

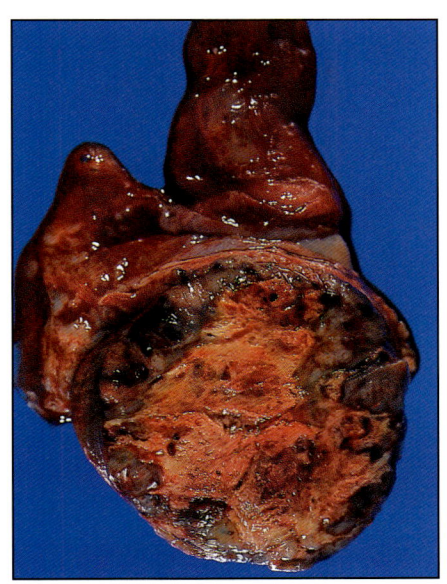

图 14B.29　混合性生殖细胞肿瘤。这个肿瘤是混合性胚胎性癌和畸胎瘤。坏死的中心部分为胚胎性癌，而周围黏液样区域为成熟性和未成熟性畸胎瘤。

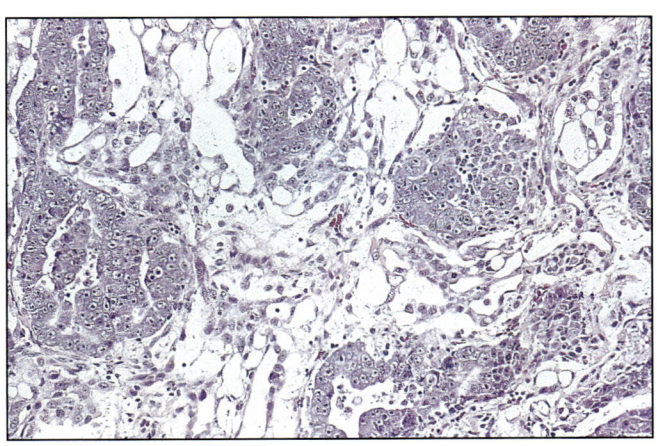

图 14B.31　混合性生殖细胞肿瘤。内胚窦瘤成分包绕在胚胎性癌周围，这种组合被称为弥漫性胚胎瘤。

而合体滋养巨细胞 hCG 阳性；所有生殖细胞肿瘤成分胎盘碱性磷酸酶（PLAP）通常阳性，虽然程度有所不同。胚胎性癌、畸胎瘤的上皮成分、卵黄囊瘤和绒毛膜癌细胞角蛋白（cytokeratin）阳性，但在精原细胞瘤通常阴性；胚胎性癌成分 Ki-1 阳性。癌胚抗原（CEA）和 Leu-M1 染色阴性（表 14 B.4）[211]。

Tezel 等[212] 报道，属于大 B-框环指蛋白家族的 RET 指蛋白（RET finger protein，RFP）在受检的 13 例单纯性精原细胞瘤中 12 例可见均一性和特异性地表达。它还见于 MGCT 中的精原细胞瘤成分，而单纯性非精原细胞瘤性生殖细胞肿瘤（NSGCT）RFP 表达阴性。男性生殖细胞和精原细胞瘤均有 RFP 表达加之高度侵袭性 NSGCT 缺乏 RFP 表达，提示 RFP 可能与生殖细胞增生的调节和（或）生殖细胞肿瘤的组织类型有关。最近 Jones 等[84] 报道，抗 OCT4 抗体免疫染色是辨认原发性睾丸胚胎性癌的一个有用的诊断工具，但是精母细胞性精原细胞瘤"通常"阴性。与 CD30 诊断胚胎性癌相比，OCT4 免疫染色具有类似的敏感性和较大的一致性。其他生殖细胞肿瘤成分（卵黄囊瘤、成熟性畸胎瘤、未成熟畸胎瘤和绒毛膜癌）OCT4 染色阴性。合体滋养细胞以及精母细胞性精原细胞瘤 OCT4 也完全阴性。睾丸非生殖细胞肿瘤 OCT4 免疫组化染色全部阴性[83,85]。

混合性生殖细胞和性索肿瘤
Mixed germ cell and sex cord tumors

性腺母细胞瘤 Gonadoblastoma

性腺母细胞瘤由 Scully 在 1953 年最初描述，患者是一名 8 岁的女孩[213]，它几乎总是见于发育不全的性腺或未下降的睾丸[214-218]，但在罕见的情况下可以发生在正常的性腺[219,220]。在受累的个体中，80% 为女性表型，20% 为男性表型。多数患者性染色质阴性，核型为 46XY 或为嵌合性 45XO/46XY[221]。患者性腺通常异常，并伴有隐睾症、尿道下裂和位于腹股沟或腹腔内的体内女性第二性器官。

性腺母细胞瘤通常是在对因其他原因切除的性腺进行组织学检查时偶然发现的[214]。1/3 的病例肿瘤呈双侧性，多数患者小于 20 岁。性腺母细胞瘤本身在临床上为良性肿瘤，但是许多人将其看作是"原位"生殖细胞肿瘤的一种形式[214-220]，因为 10%~50% 的病例伴有灶状恶性生殖细胞肿瘤，主要是精原细胞瘤，但有时为胚胎性癌、卵黄囊瘤、绒毛膜癌或畸胎瘤[214-220]。伴随的生殖细胞肿瘤的程度从原位癌到浸润癌[218]。

肿瘤呈灰白到棕黄色，大小不一，小到显微镜下可见的病灶（25%），大到直径数个厘米（可达 8 cm）。肿瘤可能质软呈鱼肉样，质硬，或类似于软骨，伴有钙化颗粒的斑点状，或几乎完全钙化。较大的肿瘤通常伴有其他恶性生殖细胞肿瘤成分。

低倍镜下显示肿瘤为由伴有空泡状透明胞浆的大圆形生殖细胞（类似于精原细胞瘤的细胞）组成的细胞巢，这些大细胞与性索衍化而来的较小的细胞密切混合，并常常被其包绕，周围为结缔组织间质（图 14B.32）。Sertoli 细胞和颗粒细胞排列在细胞巢的周围，而且包绕单个生殖细胞（滤泡）。这些细胞也可环绕含有无定形嗜酸性 PAS 阳性的玻璃样物质(Call-Exner 小体)的腔隙。细胞巢内可以出现许多 Call-Exner 小体和钙化。生殖细胞可见核分裂象，但性索-间质成分没有核分裂象。其他肿瘤性生殖细胞，通常是精原细胞瘤细胞的过度生长，可能引起性腺母细胞瘤病灶的变形和消失。在浸润性生殖细胞肿瘤中出现粗糙的钙化提示可能来源于性腺母细胞瘤。精原细胞瘤样细胞胎盘碱性磷酸酶（PLAP）阳性，而性索-间质细胞抑制素（inhibin）阳性[222,223]。性腺母细胞瘤患者的预后不同，似乎取决于其他生殖细胞成分的出现和范围[3,218]。单纯性性腺母细胞瘤患者的预后非常好。伴有精原细胞瘤的性腺母细胞瘤预后尚可，但伴有其他恶性生殖细胞成分的性腺母细胞瘤预后不好。性腺母细胞瘤的治疗选择性腺切除。是否进行进一步的放疗或化疗取决于其他恶性生殖细胞成分的出现和类型。当对侧性腺异常或未下降时，提倡切除双侧性腺，因为在性腺发育不全的性腺双侧性腺母细胞瘤的发病率高。

未分类的混合性生殖细胞和性索-间质肿瘤
Unclassified mixed germ cell and sex cord-stromal tumor

这种肿瘤发生在表型、解剖学和遗传学正常的成

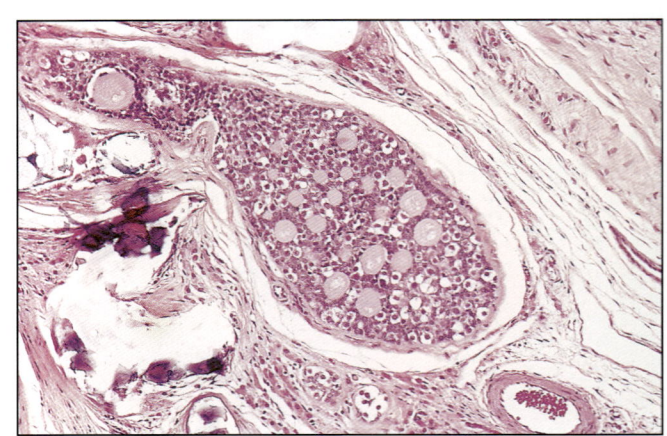

图 14B.32 性腺母细胞瘤。一个由伴有透明胞浆的大的生殖细胞和性索衍化而来的卵圆形细胞组成的细胞巢。也可出现玻璃样小体和散在的钙化。

年男性的下降的睾丸，年龄通常为 30～60 岁[217,224-228]。患者表现为渐进性无痛性的睾丸增大，不伴有内分泌异常。单纯性肿瘤局限于性腺，性腺外或对侧睾丸没有发现肿瘤[217]。小管内生殖细胞肿瘤形成（ITGCN）罕见。肿瘤不伴有转移性疾病，根治性切除受累的性腺之后患者预后良好。所有病例的对侧性腺都是正常的睾丸。

肿瘤通常较大，直径可达 12 cm，是境界清楚的实性质硬的结节，切面灰白色。睾丸常被肿瘤组织完全取代，没有出血或坏死。肿瘤周围的睾丸组织为正常组织但被挤压。

肿瘤由两种类型细胞构成——生殖细胞和性索衍生物（图 14B.33）。生殖细胞形成细胞团、细胞簇和小梁状结构，被纤维间隔包绕和分割。性索衍生物大多呈小梁状、实性、管状和条索样结构。在性索衍生物中，还可见到伴有许多 Call-Exner 小体的滤泡状结构或者缺乏任何特征性的结构。细胞丰富的程度不一，从细胞密集区域到玻璃样变的纤维组织。

高倍镜下，大的生殖细胞伴有透明胞浆和圆形淡染的细胞核，可见明显的核仁。性索衍化而来的肿瘤细胞界限不清，胞浆致密，核呈长梭形或短梭形，伴有散在颗粒状染色质，偶见核沟，中心常有单个不甚清楚的核仁。

生殖细胞 PLAP 通常阳性，但甲胎蛋白（AFP）、人绒毛膜促性腺激素（hCG）、Ki-1、癌胚抗原（CEA）和 Leu-M1 常呈阴性。生殖细胞来源的大细胞细胞角蛋白（cytokeratin）可能阴性，而性索-间质成分细胞角蛋白以及波形蛋白（vimentin）和抑制素（inhibin）可能阳性。由于非常罕见，诊断这种类型的肿瘤应当加以小心；一个常见的诊断陷阱是在性索-间质肿瘤的周围，偶尔在中心，出现陷入的非肿瘤性生殖细胞。一篇文章提示，开始被认为是具有未分类的混合性生殖细胞和性索-间质肿瘤特征的某些睾丸肿瘤，实际上是伴有陷入生殖细胞的性索-间质肿瘤[229]。

非精原细胞瘤性生殖细胞肿瘤的治疗 Management of NSGCT

在较大的医疗机构中，睾丸生殖细胞肿瘤的治疗存在某种程度的差异。下面是关于治疗策略的一个简要而粗略的讨论，其目的在于提供信息并着重强调一些具有临床意义的重要的病理学特征。

Ⅰ期非精原细胞瘤性生殖细胞肿瘤（Stage Ⅰ NSGCT）

Ⅰ期 NSGCT 睾丸切除术后传统的治疗策略包括腹膜后淋巴结切除术（retroperitoneal lymph node dissection, RPLND）、监测、高危患者的化疗以及腹膜后放疗。

治疗仍然选择 RPLND。因为传统的 RPLND 切除交感和副交感神经和神经节，术后会产生明显的后遗症和显著的不孕发生率。目前的 RPLND 损害较小，手术倾向于切除所有的淋巴结但保留交感和副交感神经节，即所谓的"保留神经"淋巴结切除术。

多数研究者普遍认为，以胚胎性癌为主（＞80%）和原发性肿瘤出现淋巴血管浸润是远处转移高度危险的组织学因素。M.D.Anderson 癌症中心认为血清 AFP＞80ng/ml 也是转移的高危因素[127]。根据是否存在这些因素将患者分为发生转移高危险组和低危险组。1981 年提出的监测疗法可以用于低危险组患者[6,127-132]。监测疗法昂贵，且需要患者充分配合。监测疗法包括经常检测血清标志物（LDH、hCG 和 AFP）的密切的临床跟踪、胸部 X 线检查和腹部 CT 扫描；此外，监测一般需要 2 年，因为监测失败 95% 发生在第 1 年，5% 发生在第 2 年。如果患者得到监测，其复发的机会大约为 27%。

Amato 等[230]评估了处于复发高危的 Ⅰ 期 NSGCT 患者在睾丸切除术后两个疗程的化疗是否可以避免再次化疗或手术。他们发现，睾丸切除术后两个疗程的辅助性化疗安全，而且患者的耐受性好，在不需要二次手术或延长化疗疗程的情况下，可明显降低临床 Ⅰ 期睾丸 NSGCT 高危组患者的复发率。因为仍然担心化疗在很长一段时间后可能引起另外一种肿瘤，所以这种治疗方案还需严密观察。Ⅰ 期 NSGCT 不需要腹膜后放疗。

Ⅱ期非精原细胞瘤性生殖细胞肿瘤（Stage Ⅱ NSGCT）

临床上 Ⅱ 期 NSGCT 患者是指放射影像学检查确定有腹膜后转移，或虽无淋巴结转移的放射学证据，但睾丸切除术后血清标志物水平升高。

对于 Ⅱ 期低体积疾病（最大直径＜5 cm）患者，标准的现今治疗选择包括：(1) RPLND 后定期随访观察或

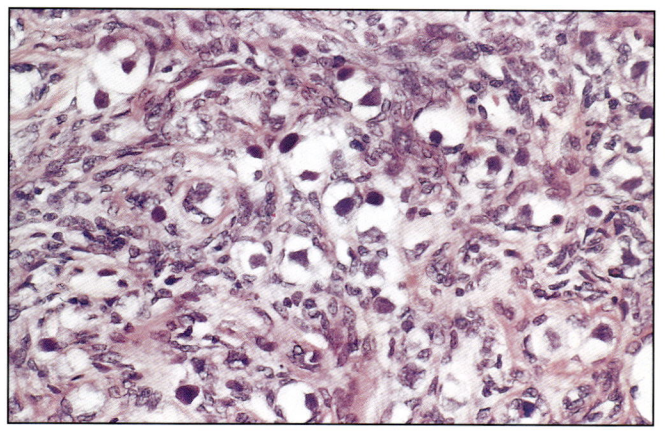

图 14B.33 未分类的混合性生殖细胞和性索-间质肿瘤。显示两种类型细胞：生殖细胞和性索衍生的细胞。生殖细胞具有大而圆形的细胞核和丰富的透明细胞浆。性索衍生的细胞为梭形细胞，胞浆稀少。核内可见纵行的核沟。

化疗[231]；(2) 对于伴有持续性肿块的患者化疗后可选择腹膜后淋巴结切除术[232]。

优先选择的治疗是 RPLND，尤其是如果原发性肿瘤有畸胎瘤成分者。理论基础是手术可以切除腹膜后淋巴结中所有的畸胎瘤成分。另一方面，化疗可以破坏高级别的畸胎瘤，但对低级别畸胎瘤性成分没有作用，这些成分将会继续生长（发展成畸胎瘤综合征）。与未行化疗的患者相比，化疗之后对于畸胎瘤成分进行 RPLND 更加困难。

对于接受过化疗的 II 期低体积疾病患者，进行放射学检查确定需要手术的腹膜后异常的次数与最初肿块的大小和原发性肿瘤的组织学类型（8%~26% 为胚胎性癌，36%~51% 为畸胎瘤）成比例。有趣的是，如果治疗前血清 AFP 水平正常，50% 接受过化疗的患者化疗后并不需要手术治疗。

转移性病灶的病理学所见可能不同于原发性肿瘤。不过，多达 15% 的病例转移灶内可见畸胎瘤，而原发性肿瘤却没有畸胎瘤[233-237]。

III 期非精原细胞瘤性生殖细胞肿瘤 (Stage III NSGCT)

晚期睾丸 NSGCT 的预后因素包括肿瘤的体积、转移部位和总数以及血清标志物（AFP、hCG 和 LDH）的水平[63,204,232,238-240]。

对于具有大块肿瘤的 II 期和 III 期 NSGCT 患者，治疗选择化疗；目前 60%~90% 处于这两期的患者通过化疗可以治愈[204,214,242]。治疗晚期 NSGCT 最常用的化疗方案是联合应用博来霉素、顺铂以及长春花碱或依托泊苷。应用这种方案进行治疗，导致 30% 的病例残余肿块需要手术切除。在这些病例中，15%~20% 可见残留的存活癌组织，36%~50% 为畸胎瘤以及 36%~40% 可见坏死或纤维化[242]。应用更加积极的化疗方案可使出现存活癌组织的频率进一步减少到 4%[243]；而且，多数伴有残余肿块的患者通过再次手术可以存活[232]。化疗之后的存活癌一般暗示预后堪忧；尽管手术后进行了化疗，但仍有 33%~75% 的受累患者死于本病[244,245]。

研究者普遍认为，如果 X 线检查未见异常，化疗后也未再进行 RPLND 的复发率会相对较低（4%~20%）[204,241,246]。Fossa 等[247] 对这种观点提出质疑，在他们研究的患者中尽管血清标志物正常并且 X 线无阳性发现，但仍有 30% 的患者镜下可见成熟性畸胎瘤（1 例有存活的癌）。

在化疗后大体仍能见到畸胎瘤的某些患者，意味着肿瘤复发。Indiana 大学的研究人员报告癌或畸胎瘤的复发率为 40%（各占 20%）[248]。他们的研究发现复发与原发性肿瘤的体积和出现伴有非生殖细胞成分的未成熟性畸胎瘤有关。提倡在化疗之后切除所有仍然可见的病变区域。来自 Royal Marsden 医院的一组报道显示，在畸胎瘤或纤维化未能完全切除的 12 例患者中，有 7 例复发[249]。Dexeus 等[250] 在 6 例没有完全切除畸胎瘤的病例中，也见到 3 例出现复发。

尽管成熟性畸胎瘤组织学表现为良性，但是流式细胞计数显示有非整倍体 DNA 成分，而且细胞遗传学分析有染色体结构畸变[251,252]。这些结果支持成熟性畸胎瘤具有恶变潜能；畸胎瘤未完全切除的患者常常复发更加强化了这种概念。在 Roth 等[241] 的一组病例中，所有晚期复发的患者（3~6 年后复发）从前均有畸胎瘤的证据。

手术最重要的作用是切除残留的成熟性畸胎瘤，这就表示 X 线检查仍有残留肿块患者的化疗可以停止。手术完全切除畸胎瘤仍然是最有效的治疗方法。此后，建议继续密切随访，特别是对未成熟性畸胎瘤伴有非生殖细胞成分、肿瘤体积大以及伴有可切除畸胎瘤的原发性纵隔肿瘤等高危险的患者。

化疗后的非生殖细胞恶性肿瘤
Non-germ cell malignancies following chemotherapy

在过去的几年中，研究者报道了生殖细胞肿瘤化疗后发生非生殖细胞恶性肿瘤[253-255]。他们将这些新的恶性肿瘤的发生归因于全能的生殖细胞部分分化为体细胞并伴有恶性转化，或先前存在的畸胎瘤性成分发生恶变。这些患者的预后取决于非生殖细胞恶性肿瘤的特性。Indiana 大学的 Ulbright 及其同事们遇到过几种类型的非生殖细胞恶性肿瘤，包括各种类型的肉瘤、来源于畸胎瘤的癌、肾母细胞瘤、PNET 和多形性胶质母细胞瘤[192,193,253,254,256,257]。发生横纹肌肉瘤的患者预后较差。与仅有畸胎瘤相比，其他类型的肉瘤、来源于畸胎瘤的癌和肾母细胞瘤对于预后似乎并无不良影响[253,254]。此时，化疗对于肉瘤成分的效果很难预测。然而，人们必须认识到的诊断困难是，没有一种术后评价方法能够可靠地排除化疗后存活癌的存在。化疗后的形态学改变包括坏死、纤维化、畸胎瘤和残留存活的生殖细胞肿瘤。持续性存在生殖细胞肿瘤，例如精原细胞瘤、胚胎性癌、卵黄囊瘤或绒毛膜癌，是需要进一步化疗的指征。然而，对于持续性存在的畸胎瘤、坏死和纤维化则并不认为是需要进一步治疗的指征。化疗后切除的标本含有坏死、纤维化或畸胎瘤的患者预后好。因此，正确辨认残留的恶性生殖细胞成分是重要的。尽管在生殖细胞肿瘤中绒毛膜癌转移的潜能最高，但它很少表现为 II 期疾病。

对于切除的转移性病灶的病理学评价
Pathologic evaluation of resected metastatic disease

化疗后完全切除的畸胎瘤性转移灶中有时上皮或间

叶成分表现出细胞学的非典型性，但这些改变并不影响随后的生物学行为。在畸胎瘤性转移灶中最重要的组织学参数是辨认畸胎瘤成分明显的恶变，而不是存在的高级别细胞学非典型性。辨认上皮成分恶变为癌相对容易。恶性间叶成分是根据单纯性间叶成分的量决定的；这样，应用4倍物镜观察超过一个视野的面积应该引起注意（图14B.34）。根据这些发现，Indiana大学研究组得出的结论是，在缺乏明显恶变的情况下，间叶性和上皮性成分出现细胞学非典型性并不足以改变伴有畸胎瘤性转移患者的常规的治疗方案[258]。

Chong等[259]回顾了16名晚期NSGCT患者的资料，这些病例先行化疗，后行延迟的睾丸切除术；在延迟性睾丸切除术时，13例完全缓解，3例部分缓解。13例患者中3例（23%）的睾丸中有存活的肿瘤。在3例部分缓解的患者中，1例睾丸内仍残存肿瘤组织，尽管做了进一步的治疗，但病情仍然进展。其他2例患者睾丸中未发现明显的肿瘤组织。这些资料提示原发部位和转移部位的生殖细胞肿瘤对治疗反应不同。

总的来说，由于病理学所见对于睾丸生殖细胞肿瘤患者的临床治疗很重要，所以病理报告应该包括以下信息：（1）大体特征，包括肿瘤大小、延伸到白膜外的范围、浸润到精索和精索边缘以及肿瘤坏死；（2）组织学分类：精原细胞瘤还是非精原细胞瘤（NSGCT）；（3）对于NSGCT，要描述肿瘤是单纯性还是混合性肿瘤，以及混合性肿瘤中各成分所占的比例；（4）描述是否存在血管或淋巴管浸润；（5）描述化疗后的切除标本中是否存在活的癌组织或含有非生殖细胞成分的畸胎瘤成分。恰当地解释化疗后持续存在的肿块对于决定这些患者进一步的治疗非常重要。显然，化疗后肿瘤生长方式改变并不少见，而且更多的经验和回顾这些标本将会进一步发现典型结构的改变[260]。

性索-间质肿瘤
Sex cord-stromal tumors

Leydig(间质)细胞瘤
Leydig (interstitial) cell tumor

Leydig细胞瘤（Leydig cell tumor，LCT）占所有睾丸肿瘤的1%～3%，可以发生于任何年龄，但最常见于10～20岁和50～60岁之间[3, 261-264]。大约20%病例见于青春期前年龄组。肿瘤常为单侧性，只有3%双侧发生[261]。成年人最常见的症状有睾丸肿大、性欲减低（20%）和男性乳腺发育（15%）。假性性早熟通常见于儿童。恶性临床行为发生在大约10%的病例，转移是判断恶性的唯一标准。在儿童，或在表现为内分泌异常的肿瘤均未见有恶性病例报告。

肿瘤为境界清楚的实性肿块，直径3～5 cm，质地均一柔软。颜色通常从黄色到红棕色，但少数可呈灰白色（图14B.35）。1/4的病例有灶状出血和（或）坏死，10%～15%病例可见肿瘤延伸到睾丸实质外。有少数睾丸外LCT的病例报道[263]。

弥漫性和结节状结构最常见；然而，也可见到小梁状、小管状和假滤泡性结构[261]。片块状或宽条索状肿瘤细胞被纤维性间质分隔，纤维性间质一般并不明显，但少数为玻璃样变、水肿性或黏液样间质。肿瘤有许多薄壁血管(图14B.36)。极少数病例可有微囊性生长方式，类似于卵黄囊瘤[264]。肿瘤细胞为大多角形细胞，核圆形，有丰富的嗜酸性或空泡状胞浆，后者反映了胞浆内有丰富的脂质（图14B.37）。极少数病例主要为伴有丰富嗜

图14B.34 未成熟性畸胎瘤伴有肉瘤样过度生长，来自因睾丸混合性生殖细胞肿瘤而接受治疗的患者。腹膜后病变显示弥漫性梭形细胞增生，与软组织的任何其他梭形细胞肉瘤不能区分。

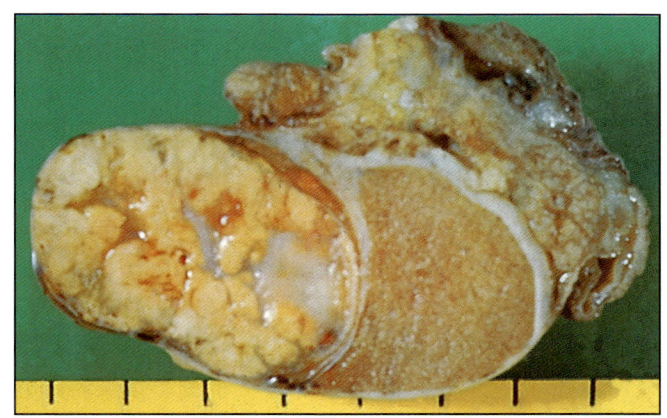

图14B.35 Leydig细胞瘤。肿瘤境界非常清楚、黄色，有灶状纤维性瘢痕。

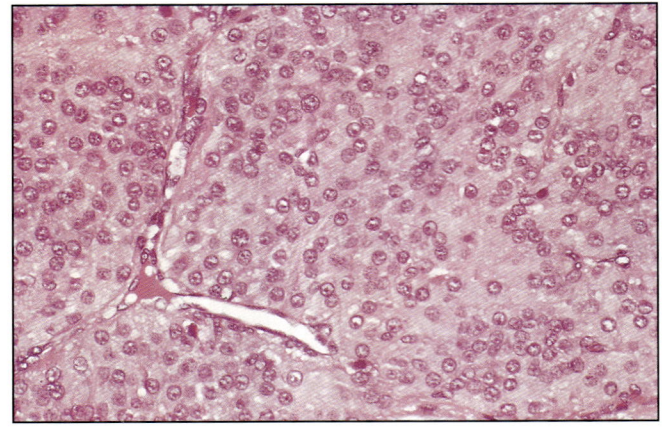

图14B.36　Leydig细胞瘤。肿瘤细胞弥漫分布，并由薄壁血管分隔。

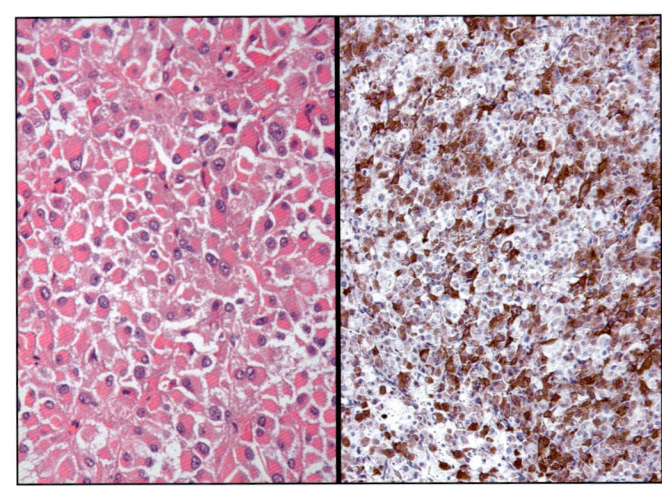

图14B.38　伴有横纹肌样细胞（左）的Leydig细胞瘤，肿瘤细胞inhibin染色阳性（右）。

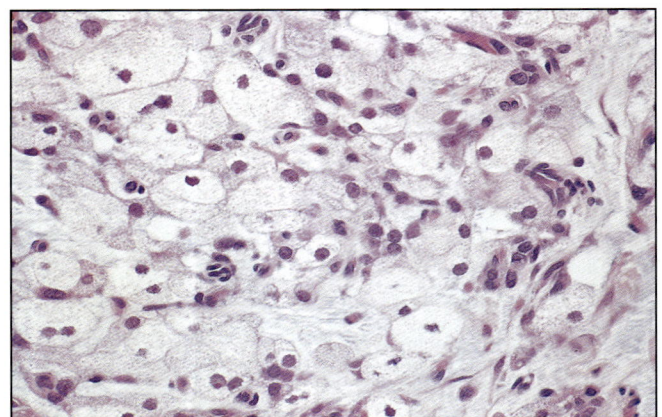

图14B.37　Leydig细胞瘤。肿瘤细胞呈大多角形。胞浆丰富，嗜酸性，由于富含脂质胞浆也可以透明。

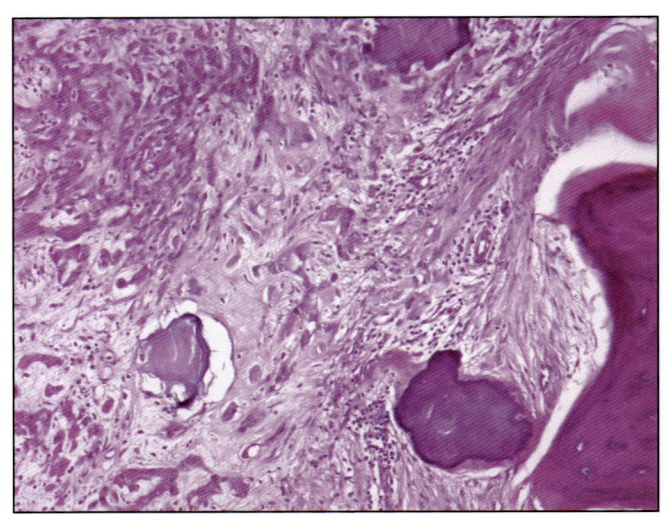

图14B.39　左侧可见Leydig细胞瘤，而右侧显示成熟的骨结构。

酸性胞浆的梭形细胞。核通常为圆形，伴有单个明显的核仁，可有核沟，类似于颗粒细胞的核。最近我们看到一例LCT伴有大量横纹肌样肿瘤细胞（图14B.38）。核分裂象极少或没有，但是极少数病例可以常见核分裂象[261]。一些病例核的多形性可能明显。25%～40%的病例可见具有诊断意义的Reinke结晶，10%～15%的病例可见脂褐素[261]。很少见到沙粒体和骨化[265, 266]。免疫组织化学染色可以检测出各种类固醇激素[267]。

最近Ulbright等[268]报道了19例伴有少见特征的睾丸LCT，包括脂肪分化、钙化伴有骨化（图14B.39）以及梭形肿瘤细胞。在LCT中认识这些少见的结构很重要，以防止把肿瘤性Leydig细胞混有脂肪组织错误地解释为睾丸外生长的证据（诊断恶性LCT的标准），而且可能有助于避免将LCT误诊为"肾上腺生殖器综合征的睾丸肿瘤"（其内可能含有脂肪），同时可以预防将伴有梭形细胞的LCT误诊为肉瘤或未分类的性索-间质肿瘤，以及将伴有钙化和骨化的LCT误诊为大细胞钙化性Sertoli细胞瘤（large cell calcifying Sertoli cell tumors, LCCSCT）。

这些胞瘤多数为良性，但可能有10%～20%病例为恶性[261,269,270]。遗憾的是，根据形态学检查没有单一的标准能够区分良性和恶性肿瘤。具有恶性结果的肿瘤往往较大，而且显示浸润性边缘、血管浸润、核的非典型性、坏死、高核分裂率以及缺乏脂褐素；单独一个特征不能诊断为恶性，伴有恶性结果的肿瘤通常表现出3种以上上述特征[261]。

Hekimgil等[271]报道，用于免疫组织化学分析的一组抗体，包括Ki-67、p53和bcl-2在鉴别恶性和交界性LCT方面可能具有诊断价值。肿瘤细胞抑制素(inhibin)、钙视网膜蛋白（calretinin）和波形蛋白（vimentin）阳性，但角蛋白（keratin）和S-100蛋白免疫组织化学染色阴性或局灶阳性[271-276]。LCT的鉴别诊断包括Leydig

细胞增生、大细胞钙化性Sertoli细胞瘤（LCCSCT）、肾上腺生殖器综合征的睾丸肿瘤（testicular tumor of the adrenogenital syndrome，TTAGS）、恶性黑色素瘤、淋巴瘤、浆细胞瘤、转移癌、肝样卵黄囊瘤以及软化斑。Leydig细胞增生的特点是大体检查缺乏散在的肿块，增生的细胞出现在萎缩睾丸的间质内。

TTAGS为双侧性、多灶性病变，发生在伴有肾上腺生殖器综合征的患者。镜下，肿瘤细胞类似于Leydig细胞，常常出现在间质中。丰富的脂褐素、在增生的肿瘤细胞之间出现生精小管以及临床病史有助于诊断。

LCCSCT常常为双侧性和多灶性，在肿瘤的周围可见小管内生长。肿瘤的特点是明显的钙化，通常遍布于整个肿瘤。LCCSCT的细胞与LCT的细胞非常相似，炎性成分以及小梁状、小簇状或实性小管状结构是有帮助的特征，连同钙化和小管内生长，也有助于区分LCCSCT和LCT。然而，LCT的间质也可出现明显的钙化，需要特别注意不要将其误诊为LCCSCT。

转移性恶性黑色素瘤通常为双侧性，伴有显著的间质浸润。肿瘤细胞多形性，伴有许多核分裂象，常常含有黄褐色黑色素。恶性黑色素瘤S-100蛋白和HMB45通常阳性。

恶性淋巴瘤常为双侧性；常常侵犯附睾和精索。肿瘤细胞浸润间质，也侵犯生精小管。淋巴瘤细胞LCA染色通常阳性。转移癌通常为双侧性或多灶性，常常伴有血管浸润和间质浸润。多数转移癌细胞角蛋白（cytokeratin）为强阳性。

因为胞浆明显嗜酸性，所以肝样卵黄囊瘤可能类似于LCT。肝样卵黄囊瘤总会表现出卵黄囊瘤的其他特征，可以非常容易地与LCT区分开来。软化斑含有组织细胞，并混有其他炎症细胞，而且伴有特征性的Michaelis-Gutmann小体。

Sertoli细胞瘤　Sertoli cell tumor

Sertoli细胞瘤占所有睾丸肿瘤的不到1%[3,277-280]。任何年龄都可发生，但30%的病例见于10岁之前。患者表现为阴囊肿块，通常为单侧性，但双侧发生的病例也有报道[3,278,279]。大约20%的患者出现男乳发育[3,278]，这种表现常与恶性Sertoli细胞瘤有关，而且这种肿瘤也可以见于隐睾未降[279]、Peutz-Jeghers综合征[281,282]和睾丸女性化综合征[283]的患者。大部分Sertoli细胞瘤为良性，但大约10%为恶性。恶性肿瘤最常转移至髂和主动脉旁淋巴结，很少转移至肺[284-286]。Sertoli细胞瘤有两种亚型——LCCSCT（见下）和硬化性Sertoli细胞瘤。没有硬化性Sertoli细胞瘤发生转移的报告。

病理学特征

大体检查显示一个小的（平均直径3.5 cm）境界清楚的肿瘤，通常为均质性，有时呈分叶状，肿瘤黄色到灰色或褐色到白色，极少呈囊性。出血、坏死和蔓延到睾丸外不常见[3,278,279]。除了LCCSCT外，双侧睾丸受累特别罕见。

普通性Sertoli细胞瘤由均匀一致的细胞组成，排列成小管状、实性巢、伴有或不伴有管腔的条索以及网状结构。纤细的纤维性间质包裹在肿瘤细胞巢的周围（图14B.40）。硬化性Sertoli细胞瘤（sclerosing Sertoli cell tumors）具有明显的间质硬化和玻璃样变，但在其他方面类似于普通性Sertoli细胞瘤的结构特征（图14B.41）[280]。硬化性肿瘤的小管偶有发育完好的基底膜。当以恶性梭形细胞成分为主时，称为肉瘤样Sertoli细胞瘤[287]。在高分化的肿瘤，小管内衬均匀一致的立方形或柱状细胞，伴有丰富的透明或嗜酸性胞浆。但在低分化的肿瘤，肿瘤细胞具有多形性特征[3,278-280]。肿瘤细胞核大呈空泡状，核仁明显，位于中心。少数病例具有比较明显的片块样

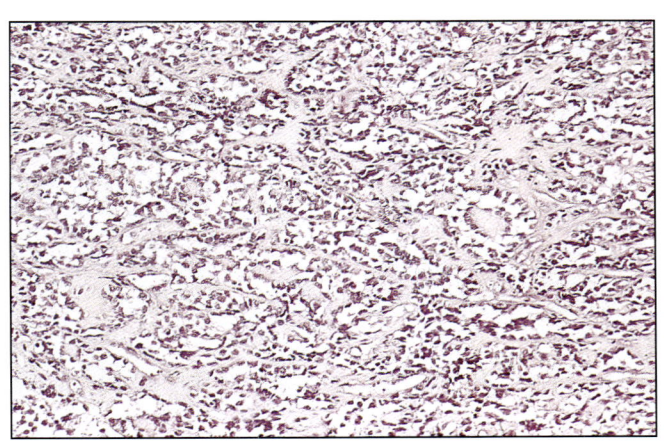

图14B.40　Sertoli细胞瘤。均匀一致的细胞在纤维性间质内排列成小管状。

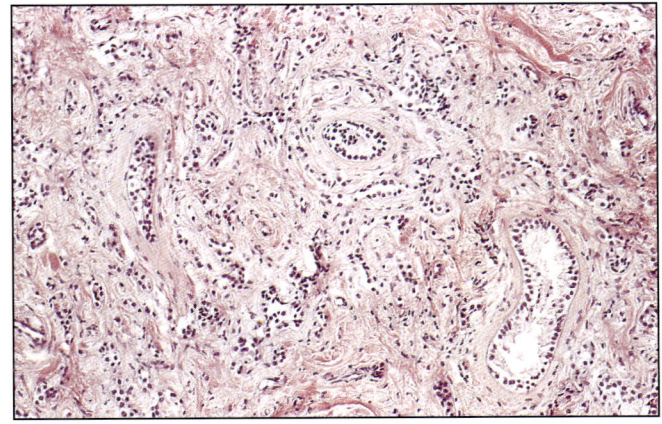

图14B.41　硬化性Sertoli细胞瘤。这种病变的典型表现是在致密的胶原化间质中肿瘤细胞形成散在的、小的、相互吻合的小管和条索。

结构，小管状结构不明显，可能类似于精原细胞瘤[288]。肿瘤较大（5 cm 或更大）、血管浸润、核分裂活性增加（每 10 个高倍视野超过 5 个核分裂象）、坏死、细胞多形性、实性结构以及梭形细胞分化是较常见于伴有恶性结局肿瘤的特征[289]。

免疫组织化学

高分化肿瘤 CK 常呈阳性；多数病例波形蛋白（vimentin）阳性[267,290]。抑制素（inhibin）和钙视网膜蛋白（calretinin）表达不稳定[272,274]。Sertoli 细胞以及颗粒细胞产生抗 Müller 激素（anti-Müllerian hormone, AMH）。因此，AMH 可以作为人颗粒细胞或 Sertoli 细胞来源的性腺肿瘤的特异性标志物，用免疫组织化学方法可与其他原发性或转移性肿瘤鉴别[291]。MIC-2 的标志物 CD99 与 sertoli 细胞瘤和颗粒细胞瘤有反应，可能有助于 Sertoli 细胞瘤和颗粒细胞瘤与癌的鉴别诊断[292]。

鉴别诊断

Sertoli 细胞瘤应与睾丸网的原发癌和睾丸转移癌相鉴别。转移癌通常会有混杂在一起的大小不等的腺体，伴有明显的核非典型性，而且常见核分裂象。在转移癌中常常出现黏蛋白，肿瘤细胞癌胚抗原（CEA）免疫染色常呈阳性。相反，Sertoli 细胞瘤显示大小相对均匀一致的腺体、实性小管状结构，以及混合性腺体、小梁状和肉瘤样生长方式。肿瘤细胞黏蛋白（mucin）和癌胚抗原（CEA）染色阴性。睾丸网癌主要位于睾丸网内。可见正常睾丸网的上皮向增生性上皮和肿瘤性上皮转化。通常见于隐睾症的灶状非肿瘤性细胞簇、Sertoli 细胞结节（Pick 腺瘤）以及腺瘤样瘤也可以类似于 Sertoli 细胞瘤。伴有大量透明细胞和"管状"结构的精原细胞瘤也可以类似于以实性为主的 Sertoli 细胞瘤；胎盘碱性磷酸酶（PLAP）和细胞角蛋白（cytokeratin）免疫染色有助于诊断。

大细胞性钙化性Sertoli细胞瘤
Large cell calcifying Sertoli cell tumor

大细胞性钙化性 Sertoli 细胞瘤（LCCSCT）是 Sertoli 细胞瘤的一个亚型，最常见于 10～20 岁的患者（年龄范围 2～51 岁，平均 21 岁）[293-295]。这种肿瘤的患者表现为睾丸肿块，常常为双侧性（40%）和多灶性（60%）[293]。这些肿瘤通常伴有男乳发育、性早熟、肢端肥大症、猝死和 Peutz-Jeghers 综合征[293]。多达 50% 的病例可能发现具有 Carney 综合征的特征，包括垂体腺瘤、心脏黏液瘤、肾上腺皮质结节性增生和皮肤色素沉着[293,296]。已经报告的大约 50 例 LCCSCT 中不到 10

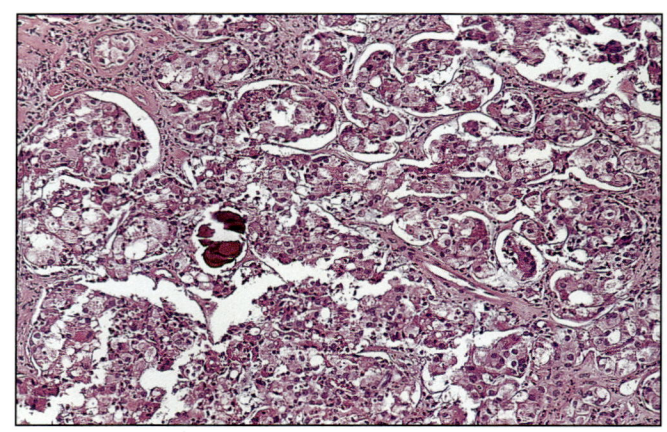

图14B.42　大细胞钙化性Sertoli细胞瘤。肿瘤细胞伴有丰富的嗜酸性胞浆，排列成巢状和簇状。还可见到层状钙化小体。

例具有恶性临床经过[296,297]。恶性肿瘤通常发生于非青春期患者和不伴有 Carney 或 Peutz-Jeghers 综合征的患者。这些病例常常为孤立性，体积较大，伴有坏死并蔓延到睾丸外[297]。

大体上，LCCSCT 直径通常 < 4 cm，质硬，黄褐色，境界清楚。显微镜下，伴有丰富嗜酸性胞浆的大的肿瘤细胞（15～35 μm）排列成弥漫性片块或细胞巢、小梁、条索、小管或成簇状，它们由纤维性间质分隔（图14B.42）[294]。通常有明显的钙化，并形成大的嗜碱性层状钙化小体[294]。伴有玻璃样变基底膜的灶性小管内肿瘤生长，见于 50% 的病例。小管内 Sertoli 细胞增生的双侧性和多中心性特征及其伴随的 LCCSCT 和 Peutz-Jeghers 综合征，提示它们是具有肿瘤生成潜能的增生性病变，或为某些睾丸 Sertoli 细胞瘤进展过程中的上皮内阶段。

肿瘤细胞常呈圆形，偶尔为立方形或柱状，少数情况下为梭形细胞。核圆形或卵圆形，伴有点彩状染色质和小的核仁。胞浆嗜酸性，呈毛玻璃样、细颗粒状或空泡状。核分裂象罕见。超微结构检查显示肿瘤细胞具有 Sertoli 细胞的特征[295,298,299,301,302]。

鉴别诊断包括 LCT 和 TTAGS[303]。LCT 通常为孤立性和单侧性病变，缺乏小管内生长和层状钙化小体。在 LCT 中可见 Reinke 结晶和脂褐素。近来一项研究显示，S-100-α 和 S-100-β 免疫阳性有可能作为 LCCSCT 的免疫组织化学标志物，尤其是当与 LCT 鉴别时；在常规组织病理学检查时 LCT 可能类似于 LCCSCT，但 LCT 只表达 S-100-α，而 S-100-β 染色阴性[304]。TTAGS 见于盐缺失性肾上腺皮质疾病的患者（见下）。实验室检查显示肾上腺生殖器综合征的典型所见。肿瘤含有大量脂褐素，但没有 Reinke 结晶。

颗粒细胞瘤　Granulosa Cell tumor

如同卵巢同类肿瘤一样，睾丸颗粒细胞瘤也有两种明

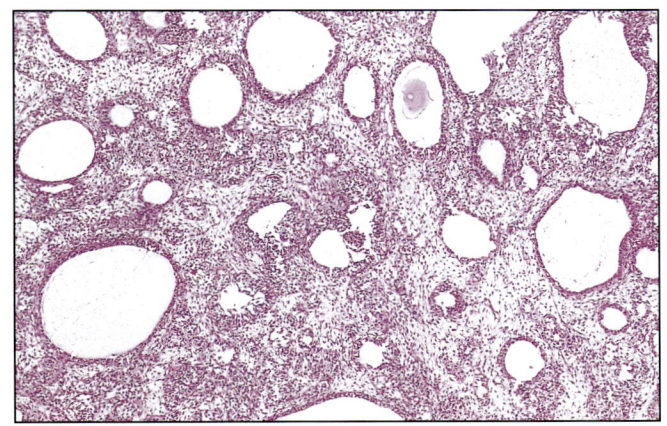

图14B.43 幼年性颗粒细胞瘤。多数肿瘤细胞弥漫排列，但也可形成含有嗜碱性黏液的滤泡结构，黏蛋白卡红染色阳性。

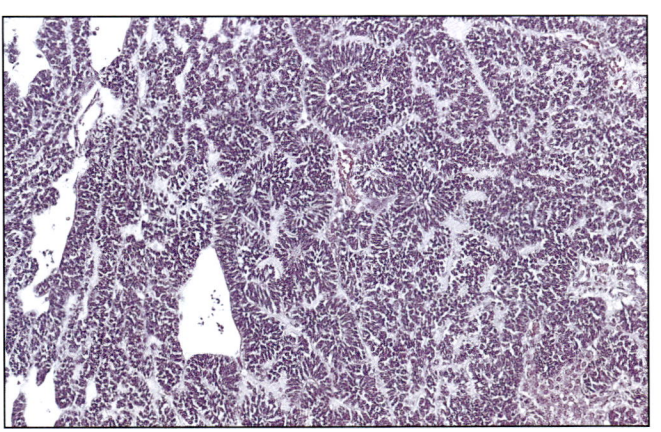

图14B.44 成年性颗粒细胞瘤。肿瘤排列成弥漫实性结构，并形成小的滤泡结构（Call-Exner小体）。

显不同的类型：幼年性和成年性。幼年性颗粒细胞瘤主要见于婴儿，是新生儿睾丸最常见的非生殖细胞肿瘤。它可能伴有睾丸未降或性腺发育不全。患者表现为阴囊肿块。从未见过幼年性肿瘤有恶性生物学行为的报告[305-310]。

4例成年性颗粒细胞瘤患者发生转移，具有恶性结局，通常转移至腹膜后淋巴结[311,312]。

幼年性颗粒细胞瘤直径通常6～8 cm，大多数呈囊性，或部分为实性，囊壁薄，囊内可见黏稠液体[305,313]。镜下，幼年性颗粒细胞瘤呈现滤泡状、实性或混合性结构，滤泡大小不等，可以很大（图14B.43）；常常有明显的玻璃样变性。滤泡内含有嗜碱性或嗜酸性液体，黏蛋白卡红和PAS染色阳性[305]。肿瘤由圆形到多角形细胞组成，核深染，通常有中等量到丰富的嗜酸性胞浆。核分裂活性可能显著。

成年性颗粒细胞瘤是最不常见的睾丸性索-间质肿瘤，文献报道的病例不足12例[3,278,311,312,314-317]。患者年龄从20岁到53岁。成年性颗粒细胞瘤可能伴有男性乳腺发育[314,315,317]。肿瘤为黄褐色、质硬、分叶状的肿块，大小可能从1cm到10 cm不等。显微镜下检查显示微滤泡性结构伴有Call-Exner小体或实性结构（图14B.44）。典型病例细胞核呈卵圆形到圆形，具有特征性的核沟。可以出现局灶性细胞学非典型性。

特殊染色和鉴别诊断

与幼年性颗粒细胞瘤不同，成年性颗粒细胞瘤黏蛋白卡红和PAS染色阴性。睾丸颗粒细胞瘤细胞角蛋白染色通常阴性或局灶阳性。波形蛋白（vimentin）、抑制素（inhibin）和钙视网膜蛋白（calretinin）通常阳性。成年性颗粒细胞瘤的鉴别诊断包括类癌、LCT和Sertoli细胞瘤。类癌具有卵圆形到圆形的细胞核，没有核沟，核染色质呈"椒盐状"（细颗粒状）。肿瘤有实性或岛屿状生长方式，伴有管状、小梁状和条索状结构。突触素（synaptophysin）、神经元特异性烯醇化酶（NSE）和嗜铬素（chromogranin）染色阳性，抑制素（inhibin）和钙视网膜蛋白（calretinin）染色阴性。

LCT和Sertoli细胞瘤与颗粒细胞瘤完全不同，鉴别诊断通常没有问题。幼年性颗粒细胞瘤的鉴别诊断包括卵黄囊瘤，后者没有明显的滤泡结构，缺乏明显的嗜碱性或嗜酸性分泌物，并且常常出现肿瘤的其他形态。其他可能需要鉴别诊断的有胚胎性横纹肌肉瘤和恶性淋巴瘤，然而前者并不发生在睾丸，而后者LCA阳性。

纤维瘤–卵泡膜细胞瘤组中的肿瘤
Tumors in the fibroma-thecoma group

纤维瘤-卵泡膜细胞瘤类的肿瘤非常罕见，与卵巢的同类肿瘤相似。平均年龄30岁，患者一般表现为睾丸肿块。随访结果平稳[3, 318-321]。

肿瘤大小从小于1 cm到大至7 cm不等。切面通常质硬，呈褐色到白色以至黄色。显微镜下特征类似于卵巢的相应肿瘤（见第13章第1部分）。富于细胞的肿瘤核分裂可能活跃，每10个高倍视野可见2个核分裂象。新近一项报告显示，纤维瘤的肿瘤细胞波形蛋白（vimentin）和平滑肌肌动蛋白（SMA）阳性，而细胞角蛋白、S-100蛋白、结蛋白（desmin）、CD99/MIC2（一种在Sertoli细胞和颗粒细胞有表达的蛋白）和CD34阴性[321]。

混合性或未分类的性腺间质肿瘤
Mixed or unclassified gonadal stromal tumor

某些睾丸性索-间质肿瘤具有两种或两种以上上面讨论的组织学亚型，因此被认为是混合性肿瘤。当这些肿瘤混有梭形细胞成分或主要由未分类的梭形细胞成分组成时，应用未分类性腺间质肿瘤这一术语。在这一讨论中，将混合性肿瘤和未分类性腺间质肿瘤放在一组，

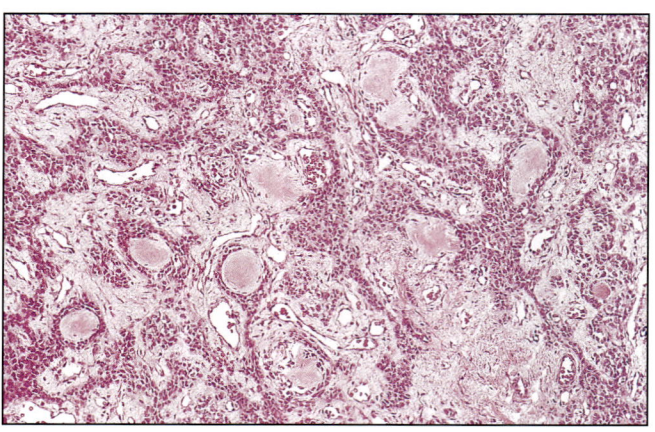

图 14B.45 未分类的性索-间质肿瘤。肿瘤细胞排列成小梁状和细胞巢,被纤维性间质分隔。

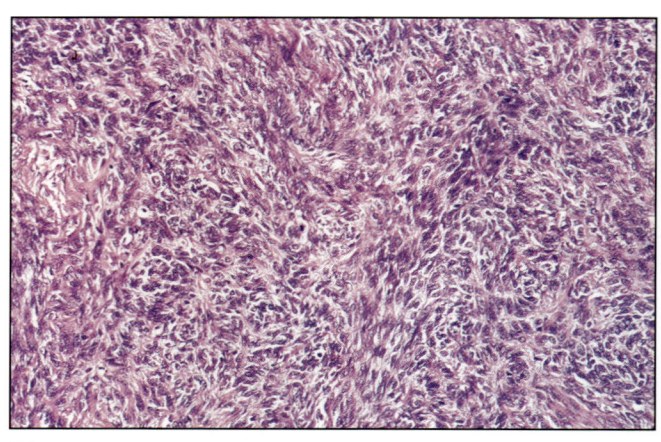

图 14B.46 未分类的性索-间质肿瘤。这个视野的肿瘤细胞呈梭形细胞外观,偶见核分裂象。

因为它们具有相似的临床病理学特征,而且在文献报告中也不可能准确地将混合性肿瘤与未分类的性腺间质肿瘤区分开。虽然这些肿瘤可以发生于任何年龄,但最常见于儿童(30% 的患者小于 1 岁)[3,278]。无痛性睾丸肿大是最常出现的症状,而且可能出现男性乳腺发育或其他激素相关性症状。发生在青春期前儿童(10 岁或小于 10 岁)的肿瘤行为多为良性,但在老年个体这些肿瘤有可能呈现恶性临床经过[278,322-324]。恶性肿瘤出现男性乳腺发育的频率高于良性肿瘤。

肿瘤的大体特征是不同大小、边界清楚的分叶状黄白色肿块,肿块可能取代整个睾丸。肿瘤内可见囊性区域,但出血和坏死并不常见。

低倍镜下可见各种形态结构,取决于组织学分化。最常见的是可见不同比例的上皮样和间质成分(图 14B.45)。在高分化肿瘤中,上皮样成分由发育良好的实性或中空小管或条索(Sertoli 细胞成分)组成;而在低分化肿瘤中,纤维性间质中有性索型细胞不规则的集聚或形成相互吻合的小梁。间质成分可以富于细胞,或为纤维组织。伴有少量胞浆的较小细胞的排列可能类似于 Call-Exner 小体(颗粒细胞成分)。

上皮样成分中的细胞通常具有嗜酸性、嗜双色性或空泡状胞浆,其内可能含有丰富的脂质。肿瘤一般具有圆形到卵圆形的空泡状细胞核,可能有明显的核仁,核分裂象罕见或缺如[278]。间质成分由梭形细胞构成,可能显示核沟和多形性,取决于分化的程度(图 14B.46)。间质成分可能常见核分裂象。免疫染色一般显示 S-100 蛋白和平滑肌肌动蛋白(SMA)阳性[318]。混合性 Ser-toli-LCT 在睾丸非常少见[325]。

影响预后的重要参数包括患者年龄、肿瘤大小、睾丸外浸润、坏死、多形性和核分裂活性。在成人,大约 25% 的肿瘤呈现恶性经过。良性性索-间质肿瘤可以通过腹股沟睾丸切除术治疗。如果临床和病理学特征支持有恶变可能,应该考虑进行仔细的分期检查,包括 CT 扫描和腹膜后淋巴管造影,密切随访和(或)腹膜后淋巴结切除术。恶性性索-间质肿瘤淋巴结转移率高,所以采用以上方法是正确的。

鉴别诊断包括指突状树突细胞肿瘤(interdigitating dendritic cell tumor),这是一种主要发生在淋巴结的非常罕见的肿瘤。Luk 等[326]报道过一例发生在睾丸的这样的肿瘤。显微镜下,它由漩涡状和成束的梭形细胞混有小淋巴细胞构成。然而,这样一种组织学表现可能类似于与各种其他肿瘤和瘤样病变,其中主要应与性索-间质肿瘤、间叶性肉瘤、梭形细胞癌、滤泡性树突细胞肿瘤和炎性假瘤进行鉴别诊断。病理医师应该了解这些病变,而且在遇到伴有明显小淋巴细胞背景的不常见的梭形细胞病变时,应该将其考虑在鉴别诊断中。然而,由于缺乏特异性的组织学表现,一般需要应用免疫组织化学和电镜检查明确诊断。这种肿瘤 S-100 蛋白和波形蛋白(vimentin)阳性,CD68 和 CD4 局灶阳性,但是抑制素(inhibin)、钙视网膜蛋白(calretinin)、melan-A 等性索间质肿瘤的标志物阴性。

属于肾上腺生殖器综合征的肿瘤
Tumor of adrenogenital syndrome

属于肾上腺生殖器综合征的睾丸肿瘤(testicular tumor of the adrenogenital syndrome,TTAGS)常常累及双侧睾丸,见于伴有盐丢失性肾上腺生殖器综合征的患者(21-羟化酶缺失)。肿块在儿童时期或年轻成人变得明显。边界清楚,暗褐色,分叶状,有纤维性间隔。病变可以为多灶性或单发,可以大到 10 cm;最常起源于

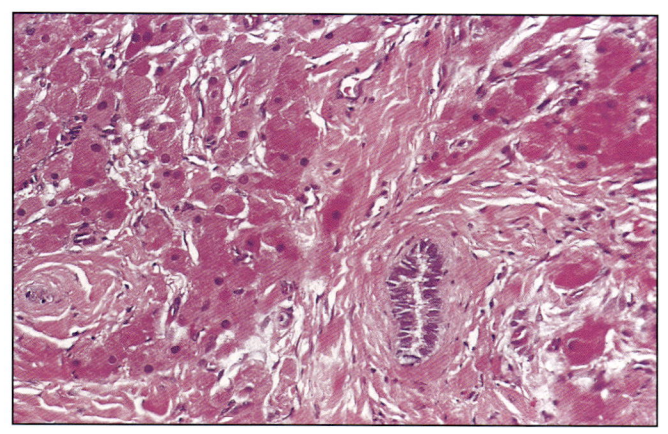

图14B.47 属于肾上腺生殖器综合征的肿瘤。伴有丰富的嗜酸性胞浆的大细胞弥漫性增生，被纤维血管间隔分开。

睾丸门的部位[327]。

低倍镜下，肿瘤内大细胞弥漫性增生，伴有被纤细的纤维血管间隔分开的宽条索状排列的肿瘤细胞（图14B.47）[327]。大细胞类似于Leydig细胞，胞浆丰富嗜酸，内含脂褐素，胞核位于中心，核仁明显[327-329]。

纤维化可能显著。肿瘤内可能存在生精小管。可见局灶性的核非典型性及核分裂象，缺乏Reinke结晶[327]。双侧性、多灶性、病变内存在生精小管以及对药物治疗有反应都表明这些肿瘤性病变可能不是真正的肿瘤，而是增生性病变。据报道，发生在肾上腺生殖器综合征患者的一个特殊的并被诊断为LCT的病例具有恶性行为；因此，必须慎重对待所有这些肿瘤都是良性的或"增生性"的观点[330]。这些肿瘤促肾上腺皮质激素（ACTH）抑制剂治疗有效，除非为了整形，否则无需切除睾丸。

鉴别诊断包括LCT和LCCST。多数病例单凭临床资料就足以将这种肿瘤与LCT和LCCST鉴别开来，虽然患者的睾丸病变可能出现在综合征其他症状出现之前。

淋巴网状组织肿瘤 Lymphoreticular neoplasms

淋巴瘤 Lymphoma

睾丸原发性恶性淋巴瘤罕见[331-333]。睾丸受累较常见于播散性疾病的晚期表现，在所有的淋巴瘤患者中，发生于大约20%的病例[331-336]。睾丸恶性淋巴瘤大约占所有睾丸肿瘤的5%[331,332]。它是60岁以上患者最常见的睾丸恶性肿瘤[337]，而且是第二个最常见的睾丸恶性肿瘤[331]。患者通常表现为无痛性睾丸肿大。弥漫性大B细胞淋巴瘤诊断时的平均年龄为66岁（范围19～91岁）[338]。90%的淋巴瘤是B细胞系淋巴瘤[332,335,339]。睾丸淋巴瘤倾向于伴有皮肤、中枢神经系统和Waldeyer环受累。双侧发生率从6%到38%不等（平均20%）[331-333,335,340]。

病理学特征

部分或整个睾丸实质被一个肿块或多发性融合性结节取代[331-333]。结节质硬或质软，鱼肉样和均质状，呈乳白色、褐色或淡粉色，与精原细胞瘤非常相似（图14B.48）[331,332]。坏死少见。多达50%的肿瘤扩散至精索或附睾[331-335]。肿瘤生长方式的特征是肿瘤细胞主要浸润间质，生精小管保持相对完整，虽然生精小管可以充满肿瘤细胞或消失（图14B.49）。多达2/3的病例可见血管浸润[332,333]。

高倍镜下，多数淋巴瘤可以进行亚型分类。一项最大系列研究表明，应用工作系统分类法发现大约80%

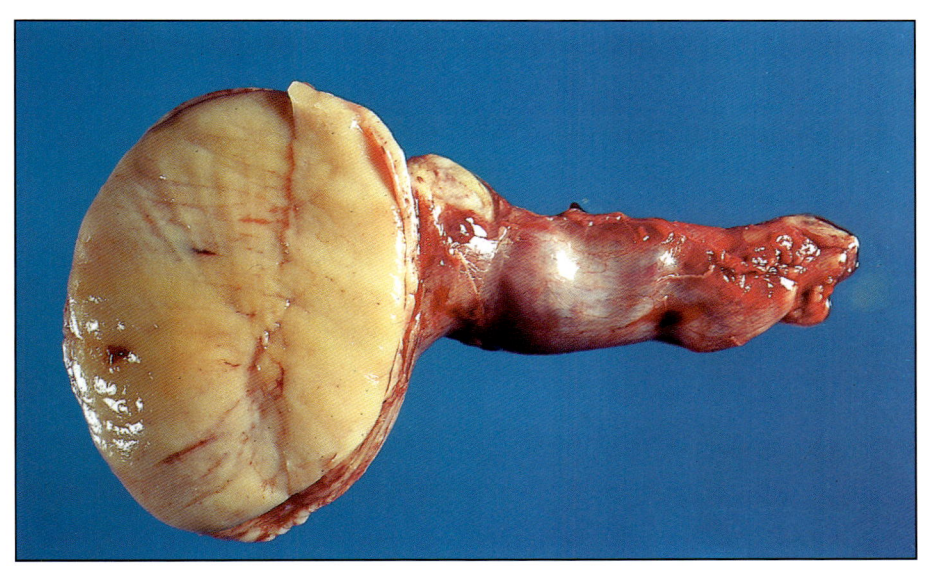

图14B.48 淋巴瘤。睾丸实质被质软的均质性棕褐色结节弥漫性取代，酷似精原细胞瘤。

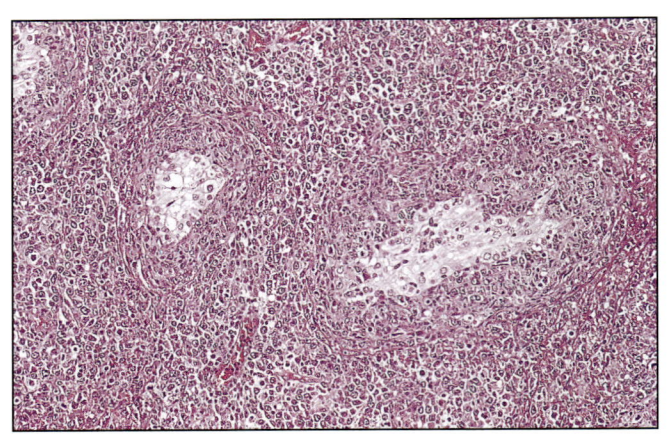

图14B.49 大细胞性淋巴瘤。肿瘤细胞主要浸润睾丸间质，但生精小管也可受累。

是弥漫性大细胞淋巴瘤，9% 是小无核裂细胞淋巴瘤；而用 Kiel 分类，62% 是中心母细胞性淋巴瘤，14% 是免疫母细胞性淋巴瘤，以及 9% 是 Burkitt 淋巴瘤[333]。也有间变性 Ki-1 淋巴瘤、T/ 自然杀伤细胞来源的淋巴瘤和 Hodgkin 病的病例报告[151,341-348]。在儿童和年轻人中，淋巴母细胞型 T 细胞淋巴瘤最常见[349]。如上所述，肿瘤细胞 cytokeratin 和 PLAP 染色阴性，而 LCA 通常阳性。

原发性儿童睾丸滤泡性淋巴瘤（primary pediatric follicular lymphoma of the testis，PPFLT）已有描述，但是病理学所见和临床特征提示它可能是滤泡性淋巴瘤的一个特殊亚型，同成人滤泡性淋巴瘤相比，其具有不同的发生机制和较好的预后[340,348]。分子生物学分析支持滤泡起源，显示单克隆免疫球蛋白重链基因重排和 BCL-6 突变，缺乏 BCL-2 主要断点和 BCL-2 小串区域重排，p53 突变和死亡相关蛋白激酶基因高度甲基化[340,348,350]。

生存率　Survival

在 2 年时总的生存率为 15%～30%[351]。一项大的系列研究发现，实际 5 年无病生存率是 35%，10 年总的生存率是 32%；平均总体生存时间是 4.4 年[337,352]。在 84 例患者中，42 例被分类为 Ⅰ 期，19 例为 Ⅱ 期，23 例为 Ⅲ-Ⅳ 期。整体平均存活 32 个月，Ⅰ 期 52 个月，Ⅱ 期 32 个月，Ⅲ-Ⅳ 期 12 个月（P < 0.0001）[337]。在所有的病例中，引起治疗失败的不良预后因素是血清白蛋白 ≤ 3.5g/dl（P=0.02）、年龄较大、疾病处于晚期以及缺乏含有蒽环类抗生素的化疗（每个 P ≤ 0.3）[340,352]。睾丸弥漫性大 B 细胞淋巴瘤的预后似乎比报告的其他部位弥漫性大 B 细胞淋巴瘤要差，即使是在 Ⅰ 期和有良好国际预后指数评分的病例[338]。在平均随访 7.6 年时，195 例患者（52%）复发。在诊断之后长达 10 年时发现 56 例（15%）患者有中枢神经系统复发。睾丸弥漫性大细胞淋巴瘤的特征是淋巴结外复发的危险性特别高，即使是诊断时伴有局灶性疾病的病例。以蒽环类抗生素为基础的化疗，中枢神经系统预防（因为复发最常见的部位是中枢神经系统）[338,353,354] 以及对侧睾丸照射似乎可以改善预后[338,353,354]。

白血病浸润　Leukemic infiltration

白血病广泛播散时可以累及睾丸。根据尸检报告，多达 65% 的急性白血病患者和 30% 的慢性白血病患者浸润睾丸[355-357]。现今，急性淋巴母细胞性白血病患者治疗之后活检最容易发现复发。伴有睾丸浸润的多数患者其他器官也有白血病浸润，支持睾丸浸润是白血病广泛播散的指征这种观点。白血病浸润总是双侧性的，但常常不对称，也可以累及附睾。

睾丸增大症状罕见；它仅见于 4.5% 的病例。在大体检查时，切面隆起，高出白膜。白血病浸润是一种比较常见的显微镜下所见[358]。当骨髓和脑膜疾病得到较长时间缓解时，睾丸受累的发生率增加[358-362]。睾丸浸润是全身复发的预兆，在患有淋巴母细胞性白血病的儿童尤其常见。

白血病细胞浸润间质，侵犯生精小管罕见。可能有血管壁浸润。浸润由原始淋巴细胞和未成熟的髓细胞组成，取决于白血病的类型[363]。

浆细胞瘤（多发性骨髓瘤）　Plasmacytoma (multiple myeloma)

睾丸部位的髓外浆细胞瘤罕见。它可以是多发性骨髓瘤的早期表现，或在患有多发性骨髓瘤的患者尸检时发现。没有骨髓受累证据的原发性睾丸浆细胞瘤只有几例报道[364-368]。睾丸增大可以单独出现[364,365]，或者伴有多发性骨髓瘤的系统性表现[369-374]。曾报道过一例获得性免疫缺陷综合征（AIDS）患者发生了睾丸原发性髓外浆细胞瘤[368]。它主要（75%）发生于 40～50 岁到 60～70 岁的患者，20%～30% 的病例为双侧性。

大体表现为粉褐色、分叶状、质硬、边界不清或散在的结节。肿瘤可为鱼肉样肿块，可达 8 cm，一般没有出血、坏死或囊肿形成。附件受累比淋巴瘤少见。

主要为未成熟性浆细胞在间质内呈浸润性生长，常常浸润生精小管、血管和白膜（图 14B.50）。肿瘤细胞均匀一致，由细胞学上未成熟的浆细胞构成。不伴有组织细胞、淋巴细胞或中性粒细胞。

转移性肿瘤　Metastatic neoplasms

睾丸转移性肿瘤相对罕见，在一家医院中只占睾丸

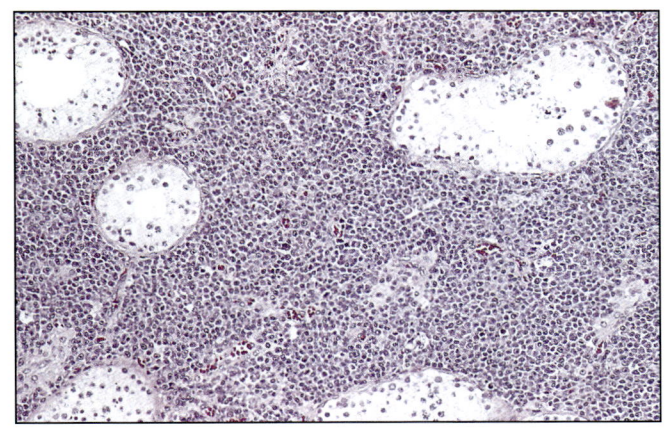

图14B.50　浆细胞瘤。未成熟性浆细胞浸润睾丸间质组织，将生精小管分开。

睾丸罕见的肿瘤和瘤样病变
Rare tumors and tumor-like conditions of the testis

类癌 Carcinoid tumor

大部分类癌发生于40～60岁之间的患者[384,385]。患者表现为疼痛性或无症状的睾丸增大，几乎均为单侧性发病。根据报告，不到15%的患者有类癌综合征的症状[386]。睾丸未下降一般与类癌的发生无关。但有一例报道[387]。睾丸类癌通常为原发性，但是确诊之前应该除外其他部位有原发性类癌。

类癌大多数为单纯性（大约75%），但有几例来源于睾丸畸胎瘤[385,387-390]。Berdjis和Mostofi[384]报告了12例原发性类癌，发生于7000例睾丸肿瘤中，其中2例来源于畸胎瘤。

病理学特征

肿瘤直径在3～5 cm之间，灰褐色到黄色，实性，呈分叶状，通常没有坏死和出血。当类癌伴有畸胎瘤时，出现畸胎瘤典型的大体特征。低倍镜下显示岛屿状、腺泡状或小梁状结构，均匀一致的肿瘤细胞排列成条索状、巢状或聚集成团，并被纤细或宽大的纤维性条带分隔（图14B.52）。高倍镜下肿瘤细胞显示均匀一致的圆形细胞核，含有细腻而散在的染色质（椒盐样结构）。胞浆呈嗜酸性细颗粒状。

除少数病例外，原发性睾丸类癌亲银反应阳性。Fontana-Masson和Grimelius染色通常阳性。肿瘤细胞细胞角蛋白（cytokeratin）、神经元特异性烯醇化酶

肿瘤的3.6%[375]。主要发生于50岁以上（平均55岁）的男性，表现为睾丸增大，伴有睾丸内结节或肿块[375-380]。双侧发生率为15%[375,376]。睾丸转移发生在2.5%的患有恶性肿瘤的男性，最常见的原发部位包括前列腺、肺、皮肤（恶性黑色素瘤）、结肠和肾（总共占这些肿瘤的80%）。罕见肿瘤包括神经母细胞瘤、Wilms瘤、视网膜母细胞瘤、间皮瘤和Merkel细胞瘤[375-377,381,382]。虽然大多数患者有其他部位原发性肿瘤的病史，但有罕见的病例（多达6%）最初可能表现为睾丸肿物[375-377]。

转移通常以单个或多个散在的结节发生。少数情况下可见整个睾丸实质弥漫性消失[375-377,383]。低倍镜下可见单个或多个结节，伴有坏死或出血区域。肿瘤细胞巢的周围有纤维组织增生性反应。高倍镜下转移性肿瘤细胞巢主要位于间质，生精小管相对很少受累（图14B.51）。常常可能有淋巴管和血管浸润[375,376]。转移肿瘤的组织学特征与原发性肿瘤相似[375]。

图14B.51　转移癌。肿瘤细胞巢主要位于间质，生精小管相对很少受累。

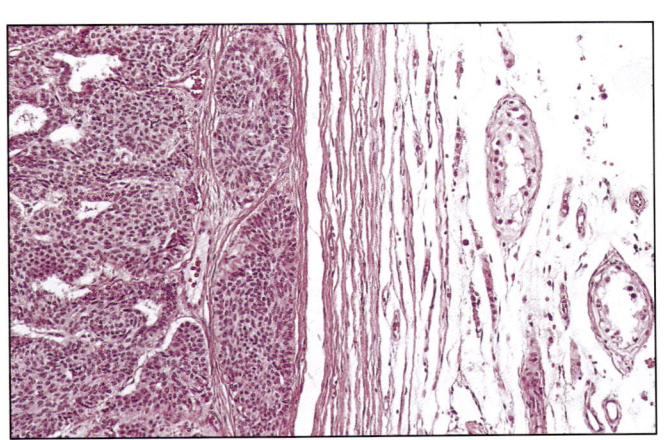

图14B.52　类癌。肿瘤显示岛屿状或小梁状结构，单形性细胞排列成条索状、巢状或细胞团。

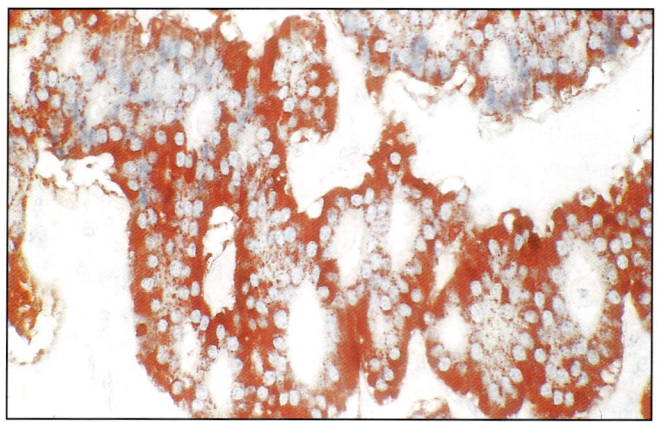

图14B.53 类癌。嗜铬素免疫染色肿瘤细胞呈强阳性。

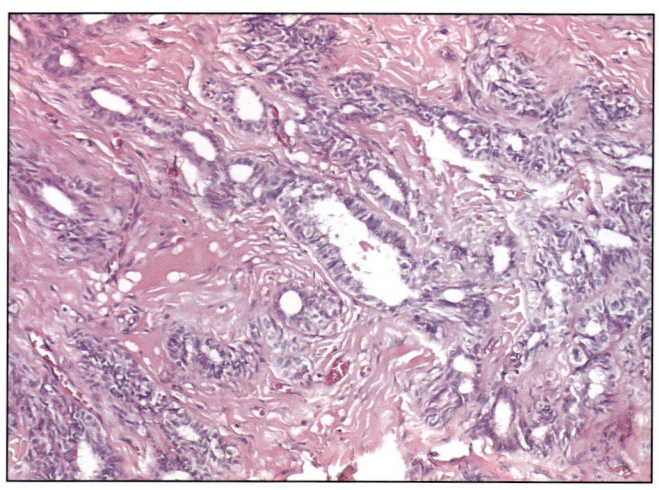

图14B.54 睾丸网显示腺瘤性增生。

(NSE)、突触素（synaptophysin）和嗜铬素（chromogranin）免疫染色阳性（图14B.53）。

单从组织学结构不能可靠地预测类癌的生物学行为，但是所有的睾丸类癌至少必须认为是低级别的恶性肿瘤。多数单纯性类癌具有良性临床经过[391]，但一项研究显示多达20%的病例有远处转移[385,386,392-394]，而且发生转移的肿瘤大于没有转移的肿瘤。

Reyes 等[391] 最近报道了另外 10 例睾丸原发类癌，并且依据 WHO 肺类癌分类标准将这些肿瘤分为低级别和中级别[395]。其中 9 例是低级别肿瘤，1 例是中级别肿瘤。所有低级别类癌患者生存良好，但是一例中级别肿瘤患者死于肿瘤。根据这一组病例的所见，他们提出应用神经内分泌癌代替睾丸类癌这一术语，神经内分泌癌能够较好地反映这些肿瘤的本质。推测原发性类癌或起源于单胚层畸胎瘤，或起源于性腺内的亲银或肠嗜铬细胞[390,396,397]。

Kato 等[386] 最近报道睾丸类癌并不显示 X 染色体明显的数目异常，而这种异常常见于睾丸生殖细胞肿瘤。因此，单纯性类癌的遗传性背景可能不同于一般的生殖细胞肿瘤。

睾丸网腺瘤性增生
Adenomatous hyperplasia of rete testis

由 Hartwick 等和其他人[398-402] 描述的睾丸网腺瘤性增生是一种不常见的病变。Hartwick 等报告来自两家医疗机构（M. D. Anderson Cancer Center, Houston,Texas 和 Sunnybrook Medical Center, Toronto, Canada）的 9 例腺瘤性增生[398]。其年龄范围从 30 岁到 74 岁（平均 59 岁，中位 66 岁）。虽然某些患者表现为大体可见的实性或囊性睾丸门肿物，但是大多数病例为显微镜下检查时偶然发现的。

显微镜下，增生由睾丸网上皮管状乳头状增生组成。内衬细胞为立方形到矮柱状，缺乏细胞核的多形性和核分裂象（图 14B.54）。睾丸网受累主要呈弥漫性，其周围的生精小管显示萎缩性改变。超微结构和免疫组织化学（角蛋白和上皮膜抗原阳性；波形蛋白、肌肉特异性肌动蛋白、结蛋白和 S-100 阴性）研究显示其特征类似于非增生性睾丸网上皮。睾丸网腺瘤性增生的患者没有局部复发或转移。作者报道可能的发病机制包括激素失衡或不明刺激的影响[398-401]。

Ulbright 和 Gersell[399] 报道 3 例生殖细胞肿瘤患者，描述伴随睾丸网增生出现嗜酸性透明小体。在较显著的病例，这种增生性病变形成实性或微囊性结构，酷似卵黄囊成分。然而，细胞具有温和的细胞学特征以及结构伴有睾丸网的构型是其反应性本质的关键。在同样的文章中，他们随后回顾了另外 48 例睾丸标本，发现 27 例生殖细胞瘤中 16 例的睾丸网或直细精管有透明小体形成，其他 5 例睾丸肿瘤（4 例间质肿瘤和 1 例浆细胞瘤）中 1 例有透明小体形成，而 16 例非肿瘤性病例均无透明小体形成。具有透明小体的许多病例也显示上皮增生。免疫染色支持这些增生性病变的非肿瘤性本质，而且表明这些透明小体是从内衬上皮细胞的睾丸网腔中吸收的没有分泌的各种蛋白。Ulbright 和 Gersell[399] 认为，这种假肿瘤性反应的形成是继发于肿瘤对睾丸网的浸润。

睾丸网和附睾的微小结石病
Microlithiasis of rete testis and epididymis

睾丸微小结石病是定义明确的临床和病理学疾病，通过睾丸超声检查容易诊断；然而，它与癌和不育的关系现在还有争论。近些年来人们力图弄清睾丸微小结石病的病变范围，但是，尚未发现有关附睾和睾丸网可能存在微小结石病的已发表的资料。

Nistal 等[401]在手术（8例附睾和6例睾丸）和尸检（12例）标本中已经观察到附睾和睾丸网的微小结石病。按着发病率递减的顺序，近端精子通路的微小结石依次见于睾丸网、附睾管和输精管。管腔内、上皮下和间质微小结石均定位于管道系统这些节段，上皮下微小结石最常见。在一例附睾间质微小结石的周围观察到类似于软斑病的肉芽肿性反应。微小结石的鉴别诊断包括淀粉样体（corpora amylacea）、Michaelis-Gutmann 小体、钙盐沉积、透明小体和寄生虫，例如巨大的肾蠕虫*肾膨结线虫*。在婴儿和年轻成人，附睾和睾丸网的微小结石病常常伴有近端导管系统改变。在年龄较大的成人，则与管道系统缺血和梗阻有关。

睾丸网腺癌 Adenocarcinoma of rete testis

睾丸网腺癌罕见，大约只有50例报道。肿瘤最常见于60岁以上的男性（年龄范围 20～90岁）[403-407]，25%的病例同时患有阴囊水肿[403,404]。疼痛性阴囊肿物是最常见的症状[403,404]，预后一般较差，大约有40%的无病生存率[404-406,408]。诊断睾丸网癌必须满足5项标准：（1）其他部位缺乏组织学相似的肿瘤；（2）肿瘤以睾丸门部为中心；（3）形态学与任何其他类型的睾丸或睾丸周围肿瘤不一致；（4）从未受累的睾丸网到肿瘤有移行；以及（5）以实性表现为主，伴有管状、乳头状和筛状生长方式[409]。

病理学特征

睾丸网腺癌通常呈实性，但偶尔也可呈囊性[403,404]。组织学形态包括管状、乳头状、筛状和实性结构（图14B.55）。间质可以明显，纤维组织广泛增生或透明变性。曾有1例报道含有梭形细胞肉瘤样成分[410]。肿瘤细胞为柱状到立方形，胞浆中等，嗜酸性或嗜双色性，细胞核复层，并有中度核的多形性。核分裂象常见。

应用淀粉酶处理的PAS染色、阿辛蓝（alcian blue）和黏蛋白卡红染色以及角蛋白（keratin）、癌胚抗原（CEA）和上皮膜抗原（EMA）免疫组织化学染色通常阳性。生殖细胞肿瘤标志物包括甲胎蛋白（AFP）、人绒毛膜促性腺激素（hCG）和胎盘碱性磷酸酶（PLAP）阴性。

睾丸网腺癌应与转移癌鉴别；然而，大多数病例单纯依赖组织学可能无法与之鉴别。恶性间皮瘤和浆液性癌是需要考虑的其他一些重要的鉴别诊断。

表皮样囊肿 Epidermoid cyst

表皮样囊肿占睾丸肿块的1%[187,411-413]。本病变为良性病变，见于任何年龄，但最常见于10～20岁到30～40岁的患者[411-413]。根据定义，肿瘤内应无其他生殖细胞成分。表皮样囊肿圆形到卵圆形，直径平均2 cm，但可大至10 cm[411,412]。病变为质软而境界清楚的囊性肿块，薄的纤维性囊壁内含有分层的干酪样物质（图14B.56）。

显微镜下检查睾丸内可见内衬稀疏鳞状细胞的囊肿，内含角化物和坏死物质（图14B.57）。与皮肤附件无关；然而，可见局灶性溃疡和异物巨细胞反应。

表皮样囊肿缺乏皮肤附件结构，可与皮样囊肿区分开来；与成熟性囊性畸胎瘤的不同在于缺乏其他成熟组织成分和ITGCN。最近研究表明，某些表皮样囊肿存在等位基因的丢失，与睾丸恶性生殖细胞瘤的某些位点相同。这些发现表明某些表皮样囊肿是肿瘤性的，尽管其杂合性缺失发生频率低也支持在遗传学上不同于恶性生殖细胞瘤[414]。

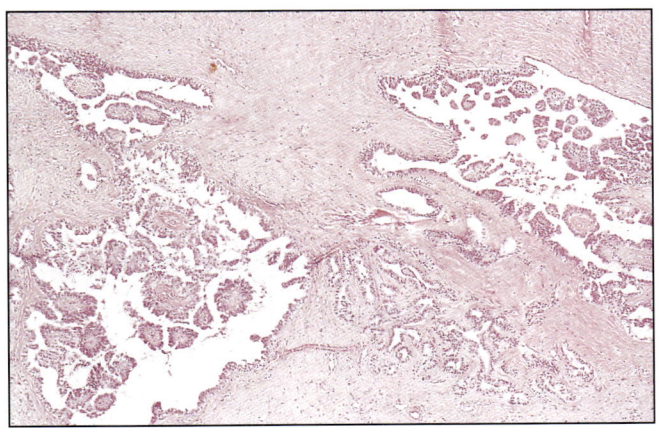

图14B.55 睾丸网腺癌。部分睾丸网被乳头状和小梁状肿瘤性增生上皮细胞占据。

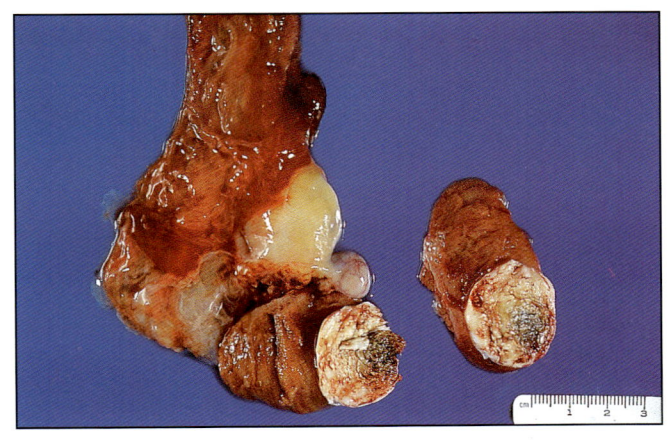

图14B.56 表皮样囊肿，肿瘤质软，境界清楚，囊性，内含分层的干酪样物质。

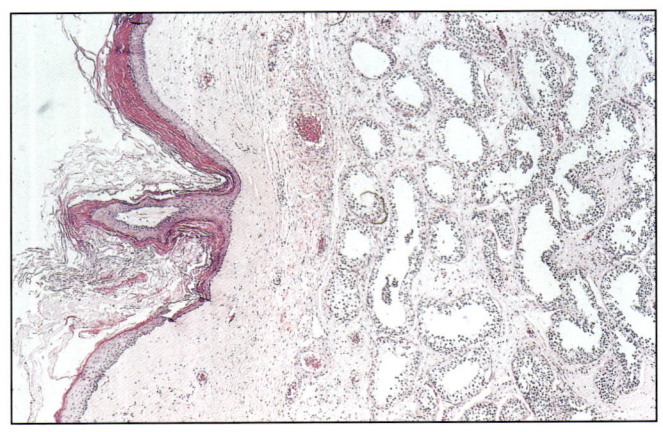

图14B.57 表皮样囊肿。内衬稀疏鳞状细胞的囊肿，内含角化物，无皮肤附件。

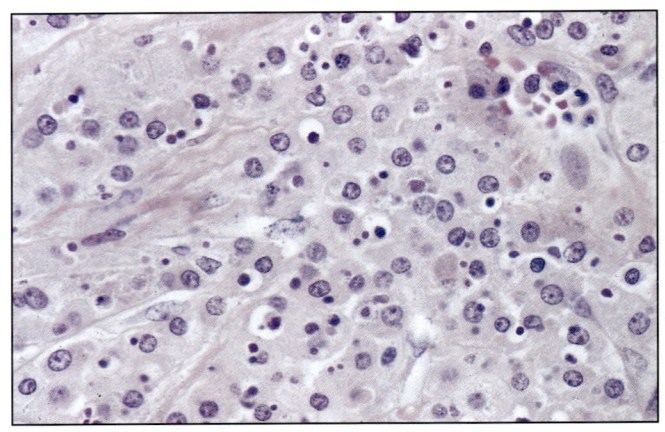

图14B.58 软斑病。其特征是伴有丰富的颗粒状嗜酸性胞浆的大的组织细胞弥漫性增生。有些细胞胞浆内含有嗜碱性包涵体，其周围有透明的空晕。

软斑病　Malakoplakia

软斑病可累及睾丸、附睾或二者同时受累。大约1/3的睾丸软斑病病例伴有附睾受累；12例附睾软斑病中6例同时有睾丸受累[415,416]。尽管软斑病可见于任何年龄，但在所有报道的病例中，75%的患者在40～69岁之间[415,416]。本病几乎总为单侧发生，而且较常累及右侧睾丸。患者常表现为疼痛性或无痛性睾丸增大，由于与周围组织发生纤维性粘连，所以固定于阴囊壁[415-417]。它可能引起睾丸梗死而没有扭转[418]。这些患者尿细菌培养可能阳性，最常见的是大肠杆菌[415]。大体检查睾丸实质被黄色、褐色或棕色的软到质硬的结节状肿块取代。纤维化可能明显，而且可见坏死区域[415-417]。

软斑病是一种破坏性炎症性病变，在睾丸实质中可有一个或多个脓肿[419]，白膜可见反应性炎症性改变。大的组织细胞取代生精小管和间质组织，这种组织细胞具有丰富的颗粒状嗜酸性胞浆（von Hansemann细胞），有些细胞胞浆中可能含有靶样嗜碱性包涵体（Michaelis-Gutmann小体）（图14B.58）[415-417]，病变背景中可见急性和慢性炎细胞浸润、肉芽组织以及纤维化。电镜检查显示这些包涵体是已经摄入了诸如大肠杆菌等细菌分解产物的吞噬溶酶体（phagolysosome）[415]。Michaelis-Gutmann小体von Kossa、PAS和铁染色均呈阳性反应[419,420]。鉴别诊断包括硬化性脂质肉芽肿、精子肉芽肿和肉芽肿性睾丸炎。硬化性脂质肉芽肿（sclerosing lipogranuloma）是由内源性或外源性油滴引起的异物炎症性反应构成的，缺乏Michaelis-Gutmann小体。精子肉芽肿（sperm granuloma）局限于附睾和精索，具有吞噬精子碎片的作用，缺乏Michaelis-Gutmann小体。非特异性肉芽肿性睾丸炎（non-specific granulomatous orchitis）累及生精小管，生精小管被由淋巴细胞、浆细胞和上皮样巨噬细胞等构成的炎症性浸润所取代。极少见到精子碎片。

睾丸周围组织肿瘤和肿瘤性病变 Tumors and tumorous conditions of paratesticular tissues

睾丸周围区域良性肿瘤 Benign tumors of paratesticular area

肾上腺残余　Adrenal rests

肾上腺残余被定义为出现在从腹腔到阴囊的睾丸下降路径上任何部位的异位的肾上腺皮质组织；可以发生于精索、睾丸网、附睾和白膜，偶尔见于3.8%的因睾丸未降或疝而接受手术的男性婴儿[421-423]。肾上腺残余由小的橙黄色结节（直径通常小于1 cm）构成，通常具有包膜。Czaplicki等[424]报道了一例发生于34岁男性的罕见的表现为精索肿块的精索肾上腺残余。切面可以出现正常肾上腺区域。

显微镜下检查，病变特征为有包膜的多角形细胞实性片块和巢状结构，多角形细胞具有丰富的胞浆和良性的细胞核特征（图14B.59），类似于正常肾上腺皮质组织，主要是束状带。少数情况下病变没有包膜。睾丸周围肾上腺残余的病变中未见有肾上腺髓质的报道。

脾-性腺融合　Splenic-gonadal fusion

脾-性腺融合是一种罕见的病变，通常累及左侧睾丸。文献报道病例不足100例[425-431]。脾-性腺融合的发生有两种形式：连续性和不连续性[432-433]。连续性脾-性腺融合，腹腔的脾和阴囊异位脾组织由一条索连接；条索可以是单纯性脾组织、纤维组织或两者都有。

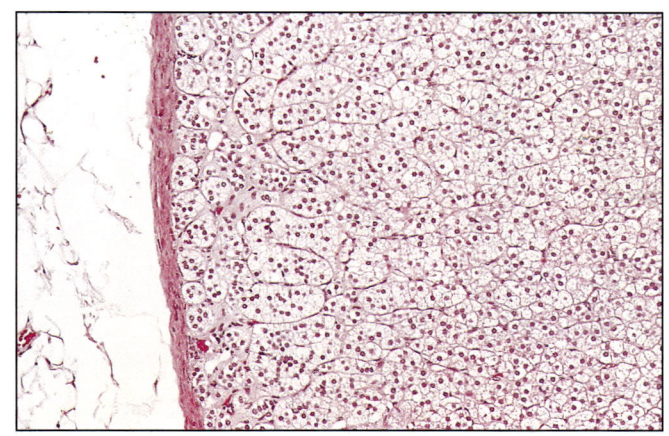
图14B.59 肾上腺残余。结节显示典型的正常肾上腺皮质组织的组织学特征。

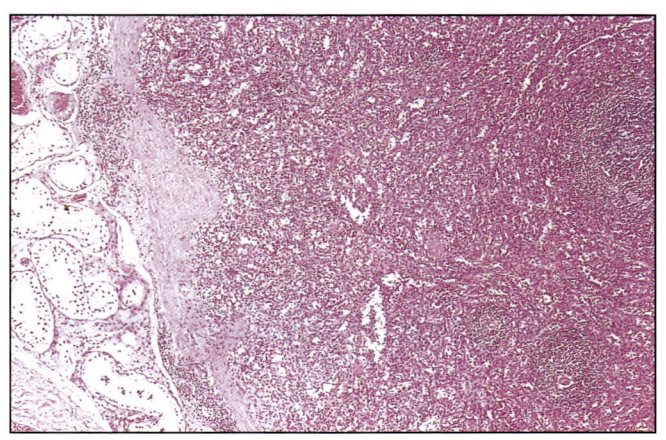
图14B.60 脾-性腺融合。睾丸组织通过白膜与脾组织连接。

不连续性脾-性腺融合，腹腔脾与阴囊副脾组织之间没有连接。脾-性腺融合被认为是发生在胎儿5～8周的发育异常，在此期间脾和性腺原基在局部解剖上非常接近。具有意义的是，脾-性腺融合经常伴有先天性异常，例如下颌过小和四肢不全畸形（严重的四肢缺陷）。

在已报道的病例中，患者年龄范围从婴儿至69岁不等，大部分为儿童或少年。脾-性腺融合主要见于白人人群。尽管它可以表现为阴囊或腹股沟肿块，或阴囊触痛，但通常为偶然发现。至今报道的病例大约25%伴有隐睾症。

脾-性腺融合的大体特征通常为散在的小肿物（但也可大至12 cm），几乎总是与睾丸上极或附睾头部融合。大体和显微镜下表现是正常脾组织通过纤维组织条带与睾丸组织分隔开来（图14B.60）；曾有纤维化、钙化、含铁血黄素沉着及脾小梁增厚的报道[429]。脾-性腺融合可以与成熟性畸胎瘤区分开来，因为脾-性腺融合缺乏其他类型的躯体组织。曾有几例脾-性腺融合的睾丸发生NSGCT的报道[431]。

精子肉芽肿　Sperm granuloma

精子肉芽肿几乎总是累及附睾或输精管。发生于18～74岁的患者；50%发生在20～30岁之间[434-436]。表现为疼痛性硬韧的结节[434-436]。15%～40%的患者曾有输精管切除术、外伤或附睾炎的病史；输精管切除术的患者1%～5%发生精子肉芽肿。与输精管切除术有关的精子肉芽肿90%位于输精管，其余的发生在附睾[435,437]。30%的精子肉芽肿与结节性输精管炎有关。精子肉芽肿偶尔被误认为睾丸肿瘤而实施睾丸切除术[438]。

典型的病变为质硬界限清楚的结节，大小2～3 mm，切面可见小而质软的黄色至奶白色灶。病变大小可以达到3 cm[434]。早期，以中性粒细胞浸润为主；病变逐渐被上皮样组织细胞取代，并伴有肉芽肿形成。晚期出现进行性纤维化和玻璃样变，伴有显著的脂色素沉着。输精管可见密集的炎症细胞浸润，伴有溃疡形成和坏死。炎性浸润由中性粒细胞、淋巴细胞、组织细胞和巨细胞组成。通常可见明显的组织细胞吞噬精子现象（图14B.61）。偶尔可见输精管上皮鳞状化生。多核巨细胞罕见[434-436]。抗酸染色可以显示精子的脂质成分，从而容易观察到精子碎片[439]。

硬化性脂质肉芽肿　Sclerosing lipogranuloma

这种独特的肉芽肿性反应最常发生在对于外源性脂质、石蜡或外伤的反应，少数是对腹腔镜疝修补术和曲张精索静脉切除术的反应[440]，主要见于40岁以下成人，通常位于睾丸周围，但偶尔也见于睾丸内。没有任何特殊病史的原发性硬化性脂质肉芽肿也有报告[441]。患者表现为可以触及的硬块，临床上疑为肿瘤。通常是由向

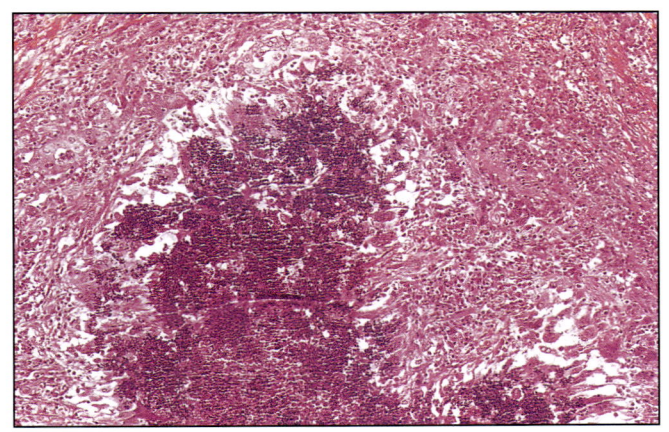
图14B.61 精子肉芽肿。伴有组织细胞、浆细胞、淋巴细胞和精子聚集的肉芽肿性炎症。

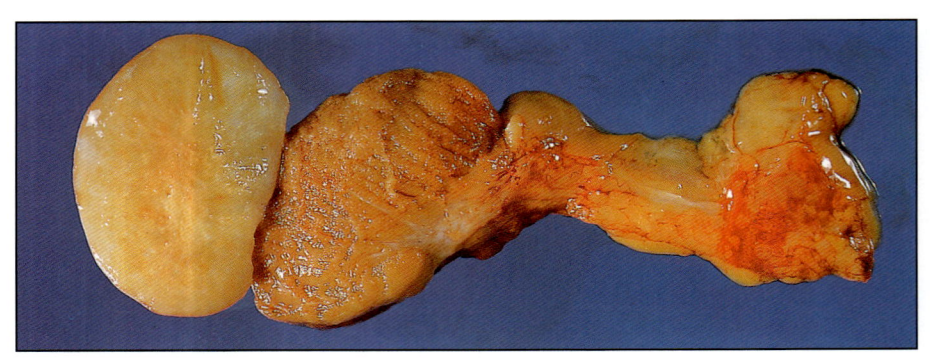

图14B.62 纤维性假瘤。附着于睾丸白膜上的一个卵圆形肿物，质硬，切面白色。

生殖器内注射外源性物质以增加其大小引起的；偶尔被归为由寒冷和外伤引起的病变[442-446]。这种病变也称为生殖器部位的石蜡瘤[443]。肿物境界不清、质硬且油腻。显微镜下可见大小不一的脂质空泡，周围可见异物巨细胞、慢性炎症、脂肪坏死和纤维化。

纤维性睾丸鞘膜炎（纤维性假瘤）
Fibrous periorchitis（fibrous pseudotumor）

纤维性睾丸鞘膜炎是弥漫性或局限性的反应性纤维瘤性增生，累及被膜、附睾和精索。在已报道的病例中，患者年龄从7岁至95岁不等；发病高峰为20～30岁[320,447-459]。

这种病变曾经用过的名称有纤维瘤、非特异性睾丸周围纤维化、结节性纤维性睾丸鞘膜炎、慢性增生性睾丸鞘膜炎、增生性精索炎、结节性纤维性假瘤、炎性假瘤、反应性睾丸鞘膜炎、假性纤维性睾丸鞘膜炎、睾丸周围纤维瘤病和纤维性间皮瘤[320,447,455]。文献一致认为这是一个反应性的非肿瘤性病变，临床上可能类似于睾丸或睾丸周围肿瘤[454,455,459]。有人限定将"假瘤"用于形成肿块的病变，而比较弥漫性的病变则应用"纤维性睾丸鞘膜炎"。

这种病变质硬，切面白色。弥漫性病变有鞘膜弥漫性增厚和条带状肌纤维母细胞增生包裹睾丸，称为纤维瘤性睾丸鞘膜炎（fibromatous periorchitis）。局灶性病变由单个或多个结节组成；结节直径从0.2cm至9.5cm不等（图14B.62）。病变呈现多种组织学表现；一些病例含有排列成漩涡状的梭形细胞和玻璃样变的胶原。可见局灶性钙化和骨化，代表是后期的病变。组织学检查可能比较富于细胞，伴有肉芽组织型纤维增生，可见显著的反应性间质细胞[456]，而且可能有炎症成分，包括淋巴细胞、浆细胞、组织细胞和散在的嗜酸性粒细胞（图14B.63）。

假瘤应与肉瘤鉴别。肉瘤一般细胞丰富，多形性明显，核分裂象增多，几乎没有炎细胞。

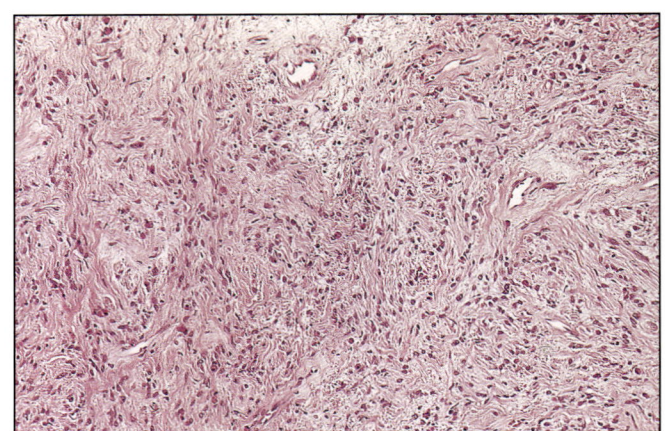

图14B.63 纤维性假瘤。病变特征为梭形细胞增生伴有炎细胞成分。

腺瘤样瘤 Adenomatoid tumor

腺瘤样瘤是睾丸周围组织最常见的良性肿瘤[460-470]。几乎总是单侧发生的不透光的孤立性肿物[461]。伴有或不伴有疼痛。可发生在任何年龄组，但最常见20～30岁到40～50岁之的患者。典型的部位为附睾，常见于下极，但也可见于睾丸白膜、精索、射精管、前列腺和肾上腺隐窝[460-470]。可见肿瘤局部延伸到睾丸实质[463]。临床行为均为良性。

病理学特征

肿瘤直径通常小于5 cm（大部分小于2 cm），典型者为单个、灰白色、境界清楚的质硬结节。少数可能形成斑块样病变。当肿瘤累及睾丸时，切面可能类似于精原细胞瘤。肿瘤由两种主要成分构成：上皮样细胞和纤维性间质。上皮样细胞排列成网状小管（圆形、卵圆形或裂隙状）、许多不规则的囊腔或小的条索或细胞簇[464,465]。纤维性间质有时可能玻璃样变，而且可能含有平滑肌。肿瘤边界可呈浸润性。当肿瘤出现广泛坏死时，可能引起诊断困难，推测是由于梗死造成的[466]。

小管内衬扁平至立方或矮柱状细胞，核圆形或卵圆

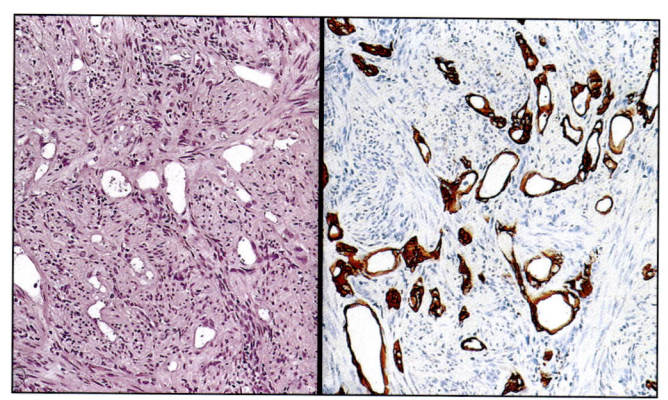

图14B.64 腺瘤样瘤。纤维性间质中出现不规则的裂隙样或腺腔结构（左）。内衬腔隙的细胞细胞角蛋白染色阳性（右）。

形，细胞浆丰富深染（图14B.64）。细胞浆可能含有大的胞浆内空泡，总的特征类似于印戒细胞。整个肿瘤或在其周围淋巴细胞聚集可能显著。最近有4例伴有广泛坏死的腺瘤样瘤（3例附睾肿瘤，1例睾丸内肿瘤）报道，推测是由于梗死引起的[466]。其中2例男性出现类似于附睾炎的急性阴囊疼痛，2例伴有可触及的肿块。显微镜下，肿瘤均以中心坏死为特征，至少可见局灶性淡染的干瘪的腺瘤样瘤，但是常常被不能归类的坏死组织遮掩。存活的腺瘤样瘤见于所有的病例，但是数量较少。坏死区域周围可见明显的胞核肥胖的（通常伴有明显的核仁，偶见核分裂象）纤维母细胞和肌纤维母细胞反应性病变。在2例附睾腺瘤样瘤中，邻近的睾丸网显示上皮增生，伴有透明小体形成。显微镜下表现常常提示有恶性肿瘤的可能，这是因为：（1）腺瘤样瘤与邻近组织的正常交界模糊；（2）反应性组织和腺瘤样瘤组织不规则地假性浸润脂肪；（3）由于梗死以及存活的肿瘤通常显示实性结构，因此缺乏典型的腺瘤样瘤；以及（4）伴随的反应性细胞呈非典型性。作者认为，如果不能正确解释腺瘤样瘤这种未被强调的特征，则有可能导致过度治疗。

电子显微镜观察显示腔面有许多微绒毛，细胞侧面有发育良好的桥粒[467]。经淀粉酶消化的PAS染色和黏蛋白卡红染色阴性。阿辛蓝（Alcian blue）染色可以阳性，但对透明质酸酶敏感。所有的肿瘤均表达细胞角蛋白AE1/AE3（图14B.64）、上皮细胞膜抗原（EMA）和波形蛋白（vimentin），某些肿瘤有细胞角蛋白34βE12弱表达[468]。癌胚抗原（CEA）、Leu-M1、Ⅷ因子和荆豆凝集素Ⅰ阴性[468-470]。血栓调节素（thrombomodulin）、HBME-1、CK5/6、OC125和calretinin阳性，提示病变具有间皮性质[468]。

鉴别诊断包括转移癌（包括印戒细胞癌）、睾丸网癌、恶性间皮瘤、硬化性脂质肉芽肿、睾丸周围卵黄囊瘤以及少见的睾丸组织细胞样血管瘤。转移癌一般都有先前癌的临床病史，最常见于40～50岁至60～70岁的患者，通常为双侧性。细胞通常明显为恶性。胞浆和管腔内抗透明质酸酶黏液染色可能阳性。睾丸网癌呈腺管乳头状结构，伴有细胞学上恶性的立方形或柱状细胞，CEA阳性，抗透明质酸酶黏液染色阳性。恶性间皮瘤则细胞数目较多，多形性明显，伴有较高的核分裂活性。硬化性脂质肉芽肿的胞浆空泡脂质染色阳性，而细胞角蛋白染色阴性。组织细胞样血管瘤血管免疫染色阳性，并且含有许多嗜酸性粒细胞[471]。

附睾乳头状囊腺瘤
Papillary cystadenoma of epididymis

附睾乳头状囊腺瘤是一种罕见的良性肿瘤[472,473]。它发生于16岁到81岁之间的男性，平均35岁。最常表现为阴囊肿物。大约2/3的病例发生在von Hippel-Lindau（VHL）综合征的患者，特别是双侧附睾受累的病例。总的来说，双侧受累大约为40%。肿瘤呈实性和囊性，发生于附睾的头部，最大径可达6 cm。

显微镜下，肿瘤由扩张的囊腔和小管组成，内衬具有单层或双层立方形到低柱状细胞的乳头。胞浆丰富而透明，内含糖原（图14B.65）。内衬细胞的表面可见纤毛。细胞核小，圆形至卵圆形，光滑，无核仁或核仁不明显。缺乏核分裂象。扩张的囊腔或管腔内常见嗜酸性胶样分泌物，原位杂交显示，VHL综合征附睾乳头状囊腺瘤的透明细胞有高水平的血管内皮生长因子（VEGF）mRNA。上述所见支持VEGF上调是由野生型VHL蛋白缺失引起的这种概念，推测VEGF水平升高可能是导致这些VHL相关性肿瘤囊肿形成和间质血管化的原因[474]。

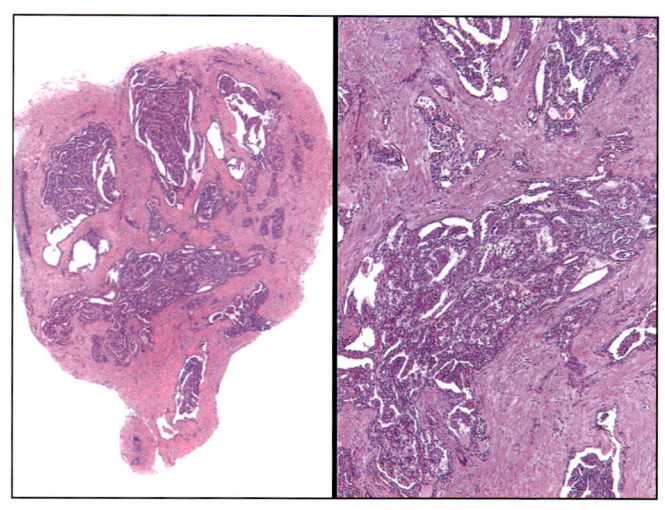

图14B.65 附睾囊腺瘤伴有乳头状生长（低倍）和透明细胞成分（高倍）。

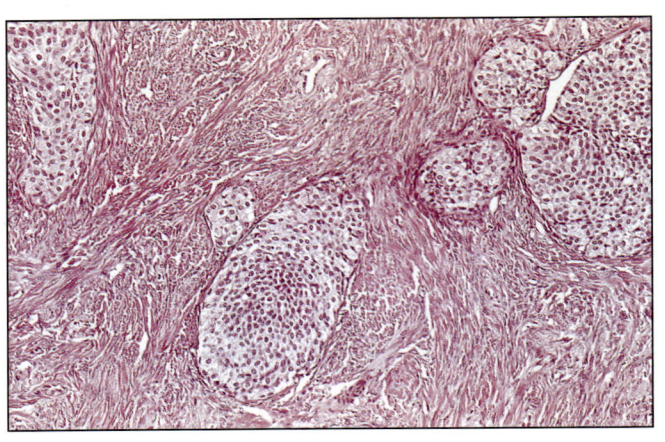

图14B.66 Brenner瘤。上皮细胞巢被胶原性间质分开。

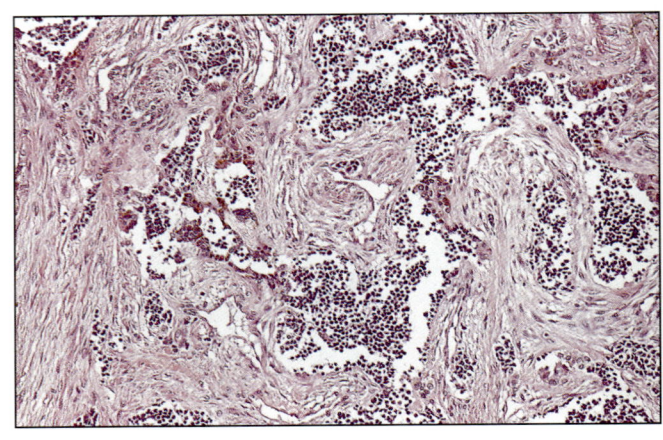

图16B.67 视网膜胚基瘤。肿瘤的特征是有两种类型细胞：小细胞和大的柱状到立方形的上皮样细胞。

鉴别诊断包括转移性肾细胞癌、Müller管来源的乳头状浆液性肿瘤、间皮瘤以及睾丸网或附睾腺癌。前列腺样上皮可见于附睾，可能与乳头状囊腺瘤混淆[472]。

Brenner瘤　Brenner tumor

这个部位的Brenner瘤非常罕见[475-478]，伴有腺瘤样瘤的Brenner瘤尤其罕见[479]。它可能来源于睾丸鞘膜的Walthard巢。在睾丸周围组织、白膜或睾丸鞘膜内可见小的（6 mm～2.7 cm）结节。

这些肿瘤的特征是境界清楚的细胞巢，主要为实性，偶尔为囊性，由多角形（移行细胞型）细胞组成，具有特征性的纵行核沟[475]。背景的胶原性间质将上皮细胞巢分开（图14B.66）。Brenner瘤是良性肿瘤，没有临床意义，但曾有1例罕见的睾丸和附睾恶性Brenner瘤的报道[480]。

睾丸或附睾的视网膜胚基瘤
Retinal anlage tumor of epididymis or testis

视网膜胚基瘤也叫黑色素性神经外胚层肿瘤（melanotic neuroectodermal tumor）、黑色素性突变瘤（melanotic progonoma）或黑色素性错构瘤（melanotic hamartoma）（也见第27章）。睾丸或附睾的视网膜胚基瘤报道不到10例[471-491]。大部分病例发生在10个月或更小的婴儿[481,482]。睾丸很少受累。最常见的症状为阴囊增大。这些肿瘤通常为良性，但据报告1例具有恶性行为，伴有腹股沟和腹膜后淋巴结转移。

肿瘤为色素沉着性境界清楚的圆形到卵圆形的实性结节，直径通常小于4cm。肿瘤紧靠睾丸，但很少侵犯睾丸实质。切面一般呈棕色、黑色或灰白色伴有深色色素沉着的区域；1例完全呈乳白色[492]。

低倍镜下，不规则形的细胞巢、条索以及裂隙样或肾小球样腔隙由两种类型的细胞组成或内衬两种类型的细胞，一种细胞为含有黑色素的色素性上皮样细胞，一种为神经母细胞瘤样小细胞（图14B.67）。典型病变可见明显的纤维性和玻璃样变的间质[481,482]。

高倍镜下可以区分两种类型的细胞[481,482,485]。一种类型是小的未分化性圆形到卵圆形深染的细胞，细胞核小而深染，胞浆稀少，类似于神经母细胞瘤细胞。可以出现核分裂活性，但是缺乏Homer Wright菊形团。另一种类型是大的柱状或立方形上皮样细胞，伴有丰富的嗜酸性胞浆，并且含有黑色素。细胞具有大的空泡状细胞核，伴有小的核仁。恶性视网膜胚基瘤可见血管浸润。小细胞和大细胞NSE、突触素（synaptophysin）和HMB-45染色均呈阳性。大细胞S-100染色可能阳性。大细胞细胞角蛋白阳性，小细胞细胞角蛋白和波形蛋白（vimentin）偶尔阳性[487]。

Müller型肿瘤　Tumors of Müllerian type

类似于卵巢常见上皮型肿瘤的睾丸和睾丸周围肿瘤十分少见[478,493-500]。患者年龄从11岁至68岁，平均年龄46岁。多数卵巢型上皮性肿瘤类似于交界恶性浆液性肿瘤，浸润性浆液性癌少见。睾丸周围交界性浆液性肿瘤在形态上和免疫表型上均与卵巢交界性浆液性肿瘤相同。迄今文献中尚无睾丸周围交界性浆液性肿瘤切除后复发或转移的报道[501]。

有关黏液性肿瘤的资料很少[478,495]。Ulbright和Young[499]最近报道9例黏液性肿瘤，其诊断标准和命名与卵巢相同。患者年龄为44～69岁（平均64岁）。表现为睾丸肿物（4例）或睾丸周围肿物（5例）。8例肿瘤呈囊性（平均大小3.5 cm），内含胶冻状物；1例（睾丸周围癌）表现为睾丸鞘膜增厚。2例被归类为黏液性囊腺瘤（均在睾丸周围），6例纯粹或主要为交界性肿瘤（4例睾丸；2例睾丸周围；1例为上皮内癌，1例为微小浸润性癌），1例为（睾丸周围）黏液性癌。囊腺瘤由子宫颈内膜样细胞组成，而肠样细胞是交界性肿瘤或癌的典型特征。常见囊肿破裂伴有黏液进入间质、炎症反应、营养不良性钙化伴有骨化。没有肿瘤伴有ITGCN或畸胎瘤性成分。一例癌的患者在出现腹膜播散之后不久死亡，尸检未能发现其他潜在的原发病灶。其余所有病例随访（1.8～12年）均无异常。睾丸和睾丸周围黏液性肿瘤类似于对应的卵巢肿瘤，具有相同的形态学表现，从良性到交界性到恶性，具有宫颈内膜样和肠样两种特征。临床特征对于除外转移特别重要，特别是在癌的病例，在一定程度上对于除外交界性肿瘤也很重要。

其他少见类型包括子宫内膜样腺癌[478]以及透明细胞腺癌[478,498]。每种类型的报道均少于10例[493]。

根据报告各种睾丸生殖细胞肿瘤伴有持续性Müller管综合征（其特征为正常男性出现持续性Müller管衍生）。然而，持续性Müller管结构恶变少有报道。有一例具有持续性Müller管结构的Müller管综合征患者发生透明细胞癌的报道[500]。这些肿瘤可能来源于发生Müller管肿瘤性化生的间皮、Müller管残存或畸胎瘤的黏液性上皮[494,499]。

组织学上，Müller型肿瘤类似于女性生殖道的Müller型肿瘤（见第13章）。因此，这些肿瘤通常并不存在诊断问题，但当其发生在不常见的部位或因其罕见，可以造成诊断错误。浸润性癌的诊断具有预后意义，因此必须辨认浸润，即使是局灶性浸润。

鉴别诊断包括睾丸网腺瘤、附睾腺癌、恶性间皮瘤以及转移癌。睾丸网癌位于睾丸门部，可见从正常上皮细胞转化为肿瘤细胞，而且具有裂隙样小管和实性区域以及乳头状结构。附睾腺癌极其少见[502]，具有管状或管状乳头状结构，常常伴有透明细胞特征。与间皮瘤不同，Müller型肿瘤没有双相性组织学结构或石棉接触史，并且具有较多的沙粒体。Müller（卵巢）型肿瘤CEA和CA125免疫染色阳性，而间皮瘤CK5/6、血栓调节素（thrombomodulin）和calretinin通常阳性。

良性软组织肿瘤　Benign soft tissue tumors

发生于其他部位的几乎所有类型的软组织肿瘤都可见于睾丸周围软组织[503]（见第3、24和27章）。这些软组织肿瘤包括平滑肌瘤、脂肪瘤、横纹肌瘤[504,505]、纤维瘤、血管瘤、神经鞘瘤和神经纤维瘤[455]。这个部位较特殊的软组织肿瘤包括组织细胞样血管瘤[471]、侵袭性血管黏液瘤[506,507]、血管肌纤维母细胞瘤和富于细胞性血管纤维瘤（也叫血管肌纤维母细胞瘤样肿瘤）[508,509,510]。也曾有过报道，睾丸周围或精索原有的平滑肌在血管或输精管之间或其周围呈非肿瘤性过度生长[511,512]。这种病变在临床上或病理学上均有可能与真性肿瘤混淆，特别是平滑肌瘤。病变由平滑肌束组成，生长在导管周围、血管周围和间质中，或呈混合性生长。所有病例均缺乏平滑肌瘤细胞互相黏着、交叉排列的生长方式，这种诊断特征有别于平滑肌瘤。这种病变的原因尚不清楚，虽然某些病例显微镜下可见附睾和输精管扩张，提示梗阻可能是其原因。切除并得到正确诊断的任何病例均为良性病变，没有临床意义。

睾丸周围区域恶性肿瘤
Malignant tumors of paratesticular region

附睾腺癌　Adenocarcinoma of epididymis

原发性附睾肿瘤罕见而且通常为良性，最常见的是腺瘤样瘤和平滑肌瘤，其次为乳头状囊腺瘤以及其他良性软组织肿瘤。

原发性附睾癌极其罕见，仅见散发的病例报道；某些已报告肿瘤的正确性值得怀疑，其中有些病例可能是其他类型的原发性或转移性癌。文献中报道的附睾腺癌不到12例[502]。患者年龄从27岁到82岁，平均60岁。所有病例均表现为阴囊肿物、疼痛或两者兼有，某些病例具有小的阴囊水囊肿。与附睾乳头状囊腺瘤不同，附睾腺癌没有VHL综合征的病史。大体上，所有的肿瘤均以附睾为中心。有些肿瘤侵犯附睾周围软组织、精索以及附近的睾丸。肿瘤最大径从2.0 cm至7.0 cm不等，可见出血和坏死灶。

病理学特征

显微镜下，大部分肿瘤为伴有单管性或比较复杂的管囊性或腺管乳头状结构的腺癌，内衬立方或柱状、以透明细胞为主的细胞，这些细胞浸润附睾平滑肌壁、附睾周围软组织，或浸润两者（图14B.68）。常见肿瘤坏死。伴有未分化片块样生长和鳞状细胞癌的病例也有报道[502,513]。与良性乳头状囊腺瘤不同，附睾癌细胞缺乏纤毛。免疫组织化学染色显示细胞角蛋白（AE1/3、Cam5.2）和EMA（仅是腔面）强阳性，但据报告CEA、Leu-M1、B72.3和Ber-EP4阴性。具有随访资料的大多数患者死于本病。

附睾腺癌的鉴别诊断包括附睾乳头状囊腺瘤、腺瘤

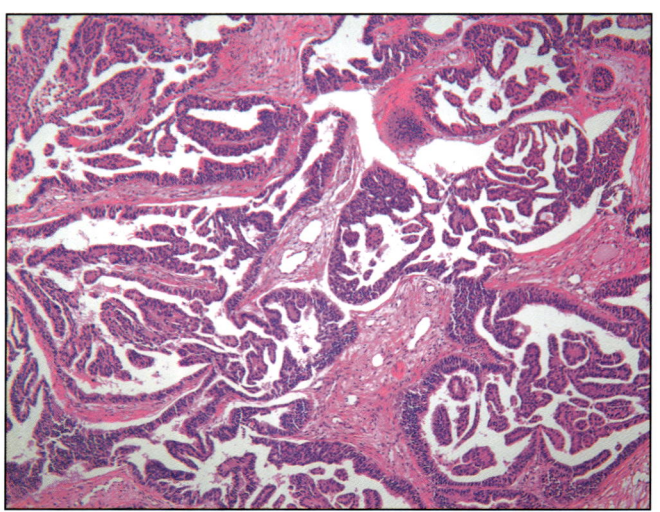

图14B.68 附睾腺癌。腺体不规则增生，伴有腺腔内乳头状内折和细胞非典型性。

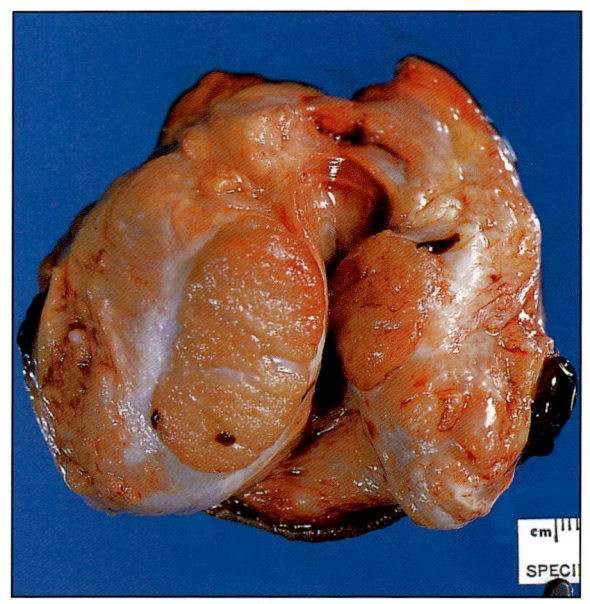

图14B.69 间皮瘤。睾丸鞘膜由于肿物而呈弥漫性增厚，肿物包裹睾丸鞘膜并浸润白膜和附睾。

样瘤、恶性间皮瘤、Müller型浆液性乳头状癌、睾丸网癌以及转移癌。附睾腺癌与转移癌的鉴别可能困难，而且可能主要依靠详细的临床检查。最后，为了避免不必要的过度诊断为癌，应该记住正常附睾常常显示伴有非典型性细胞的筛状结构。

睾丸鞘膜间皮瘤
Mesothelioma of tunica vaginalis

睾丸鞘膜恶性间皮瘤是一种侵袭性肿瘤，其特征为局部复发和远处转移。它与职业性接触石棉密切相关，40%的病例有石棉接触史[478,515]。肿瘤可能表现为长期的阴囊水囊肿，最常在穿刺抽液之后复发，但也可以形成质硬的肿块[515-523]。它发生于20～75岁之间，有20～40岁和50～80岁两个发病高峰年龄，虽然儿科年龄组的病例也有报道[478,520-522,524-527]。间皮瘤是一种实性或部分囊性的肿瘤，直径0.6～6.0 cm。肿瘤在睾丸鞘膜表面形成多发性凹凸不平的或乳头状结节，而且可能包裹整个鞘膜表面，伴有邻近精索、睾丸或附睾等软组织的浸润（图14B.69）[520-522,524-528]。

可以出现上皮性、肉瘤样或双相性（上皮性和肉瘤样）形态结构。上皮性间皮瘤较常见，占间皮瘤的75%，可以呈乳头状、腺管状（管泡状）或呈实性[515,528,529]。肉瘤样间皮瘤由界限不清的梭形细胞束组成。双相性间皮瘤显示上皮性和梭形细胞两种结构。上皮性间皮瘤的肿瘤细胞一般为立方形，伴有卵圆形空泡状的细胞核和中等量的嗜酸性胞浆。单纯性乳头状间皮瘤可见沙粒体。

还可见到高核分裂率、显著的核非典型性、突出的核仁和侵犯邻近结构[515,520,522]。在肉瘤样间皮瘤，梭形细胞排列成界限不清的束状或片块状。可见明显的细胞多形性和奇异细胞[523,528]。

高分化乳头状间皮瘤是上皮性间皮瘤一种少见的亚型，被认为具有低度恶性潜能。报告的大多数病例见于育龄女性的腹膜，但也可见于男性的睾丸鞘膜[530]。半数患者具有职业性石棉接触史。这些病变必须仔细地与伴有局灶外生性乳头生长方式的恶性间皮瘤鉴别。这种肿瘤没有间质浸润，或仅显示有限的间皮下层浸润[531]。

电子显微镜下显示有细长的微绒毛、糖原、张力原纤维、桥粒以及位于核周的线粒体[515,526]。肿瘤细胞黏液染色（PAS和黏蛋白卡红）以及CEA、Leu-M1、B72.3、MOC.31和Ⅷ因子免疫染色阴性。阿辛蓝（Alcian blue）染色阳性，但是透明质酸酶敏感。细胞角蛋白、CK5/6、EMA和calretinin阳性，尽管CK5/6染色不如胸膜间皮瘤稳定[531a]。间皮瘤总的预后不良。在随访超过2年的患者中，45%死于本病，17%带病生存，30%完全康复[528]。

小的乳头状间皮突起常常见于疝囊（见第15章）。这些病变要与间皮瘤区别。乳头状间皮突起通常为显微镜下所见的单个乳头。包括局灶性、伴有炎症性改变、轻度的细胞学非典型性以及缺乏坏死在内的组织学特征均支持其为反应性病变。间皮瘤还要与原发性或转移性腺癌区别。在转移性肿瘤，通常有从前癌症的临床病史，而且CEA、MOC.31和Leu-M1阳性。睾丸网癌也是重要的鉴别诊断。

横纹肌肉瘤　Rhabdomyosarcoma

横纹肌肉瘤是儿童最常见的肉瘤。它发生在7～36岁之间（平均年龄6.6岁）；60%发生在20岁以前[532-536]。大多数患者表现为阴囊肿物[533-536]；据报道成年患者还可出现腰痛、体重减轻、高钙血症和血小板减少症[537]。肿瘤常发生于精索和睾丸周围组织，但很少累及睾丸实质[538]。

肿瘤具有分叶状、光滑、灰白色有光泽的外观，通常造成睾丸移位而不取代睾丸（图14.B.70）[533,534]。最大径从1.5 cm到20 cm不等。最常见的（90%）组织学类型是胚胎性横纹肌肉瘤[533,535]。高倍镜下可见伴有或不伴有横纹的带状细胞以及奇异的"蝌蚪"细胞。肿瘤细胞为原始的肌母细胞型细胞，某些细胞具有强嗜酸性胞浆，位于黏液样间质中（图14B.71）。这个部位可见梭形细胞亚型的胚胎性横纹肌肉瘤，病变通常比较局限，而且预后明显好于典型的胚胎性横纹肌肉瘤[539,540]。睾丸周围横纹肌肉瘤大约6%为腺泡性横纹肌肉瘤。结蛋白（desmin）、肌肉特异性肌动蛋白（muscle-specific actin）、肌细胞生成素（myogenin）、myoD1和波形蛋白（vimentin）阳性。细胞角蛋白一般阴性。

预后主要取决于肿瘤的侵袭性、肿瘤大小、可否手术切除、淋巴结转移以及伴有局限性肿瘤的患者的年龄[541]。伴有局灶性疾病的患者预后很好，尽管对于低度危险患者化疗的强度和时间减少。一项系列报告显示总的5年生存率为85.5%，肿瘤局限的患者5年生存率为94.6%，而出现转移的患者为22.2%[541]。腹膜后淋巴结复发是治疗失败的主要原因。与儿童病例相比，成人患者肿瘤的行为更具侵袭性。胚胎性横纹肌肉瘤的5年生存率为80%，而梭形细胞亚型为95%[542]。然而，睾丸周围区域的腺泡状横纹肌肉瘤似乎并无不良的预后影响，其临床行为明显要好于其他部位同样类型的肿瘤[543]。Ⅲ期或Ⅳ期患者预后不良，尽管有少数长期存活的报道[544,545]。

其他软组织肉瘤　Other soft tissue sarcomas

平滑肌肉瘤是睾丸周围相对常见的肉瘤，特别是成人[455,546-551]。患者年龄从15岁至84岁不等（平均58岁）。平滑肌肉瘤起源于精索、附睾（精索与附睾的比例为5:1）、睾丸鞘膜、阴囊皮下组织和肉膜肌的软组织[549]。组织学特征类似于其他部位的平滑肌肉瘤，而且肿瘤可能呈现从高分化至低分化一系列的分化。与平滑肌瘤鉴别的标准尚不十分明确，尽管睾丸周围平滑肌肉瘤的诊断门槛要比其他部位更低。任何核分裂活性，特别是如果伴有细胞数目增加、坏死或浸润性生长方式，应被视为恶性征象。这个部位的多数平滑肌肉瘤在组织学上为低级别肿瘤，伴有高级别病变的肿瘤具有较强的侵袭性行为[549]。

文献报道睾丸周围脂肪肉瘤有100余例，年龄从16岁至90岁不等（平均56岁）[455,551-555]，但这一数字与其相对发生率相比显然是被低估了。肿瘤累及精索、睾丸被膜和附睾，大小从3 cm至30 cm（平均11.7 cm，中位数10 cm）[552]。Montgomery和Fisher[552]报道了30例睾丸周围脂肪肉瘤。19例为高分化，10例为去分化（5例伴有高级别、5例伴有低级别的去分化成分），1例为黏液样圆形细胞脂肪肉瘤。

大体检查为大块分叶状肿瘤，类似于脂肪瘤。组织学检查，大部分为高分化（脂肪瘤样或硬化型；也称非典型性脂肪瘤性肿瘤）或去分化肿瘤[552]。也可发生黏液样脂肪肉瘤、圆形细胞性（细胞性黏液样）脂肪肉瘤以及多形性脂肪肉瘤，但均少见。睾丸周围高分化脂肪肉瘤具有很长的临床经过，半数以上的病例复发，有时复发较晚，但总体预后良好。然而，去分化的脂肪肉瘤经常复发，而且可以发生转移，预后不良[552]。高分化

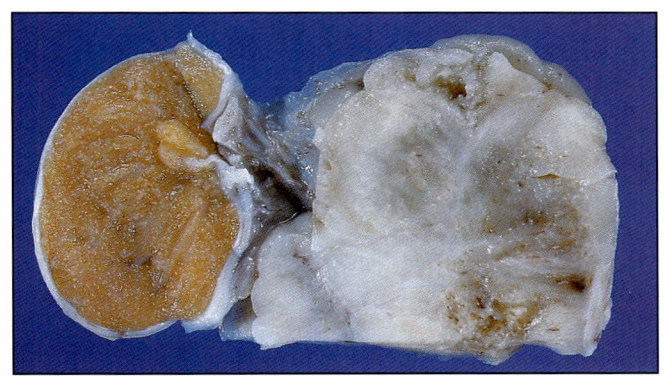

图14B.70　横纹肌肉瘤。肿瘤累及睾丸周围组织，呈分叶状，表面光滑，灰白色。

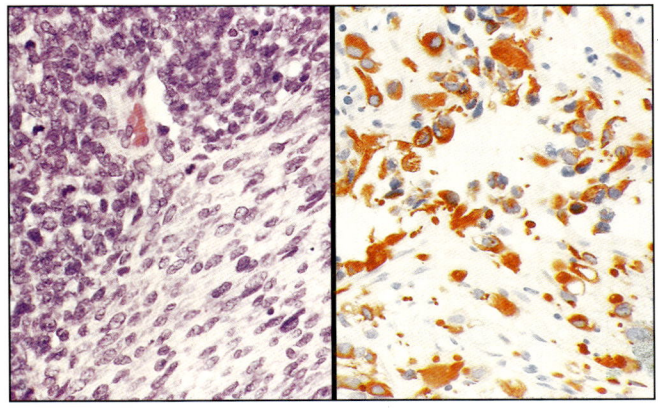

图14B.71　横纹肌肉瘤。胚胎性横纹肌肉瘤伴有富于细胞区域和黏液样区域（左），肿瘤细胞结蛋白（desmin）免疫染色强阳性（右）。

脂肪肉瘤主要的鉴别诊断有大的脂肪瘤和脂肪肉芽肿。

据报告发生在睾丸周围的其他软组织肉瘤包括纤维肉瘤、血管肉瘤、Kaposi 肉瘤[551]、所谓的恶性纤维组织细胞瘤[551]、恶性孤立性纤维性肿瘤[556]以及恶性横纹肌样肿瘤[557,558]。它们的大体和显微镜下特征与其较常见部位发生的相应肿瘤相似（见第 24 章）。

参考文献

1. Krain L S 1973 Testicular cancer in California from 1942 to 1969: the California Tumor Registry experience. Oncology 27: 45–51
2. Jemal A, Siegel R, Ward E et al. 2006 Cancer statistics, 2006. CA Cancer J Clin 56: 106–130
3. Eble J N, Sauter G, Epstein J I et al. 2004 Pathology and genetics: tumours of the urinary system and male genital organs. WHO classification of tumors. IARC, Lyon
4. Mostofi F K 1980 Pathology of germ cell tumors of testis. A progress report. Cancer 45: 1735–1754
5. Risdon R A 1973 Germ cell tumours of the testis. J Pathol Bacteriol 141: 355–361
6. Ro J Y, Dexeus F H, El-Naggar A 1991 Testicular germ cell tumors: clinically relevant pathologic findings. Pathol Annu 26: 59–87
7. Dry S M, Renshaw A A 1999 Extratesticular extension of germ cell tumors preferentially occurs at the hilum. Am J Clin Pathol 111: 534–538
8. Nazeer T, Ro J Y, Kee K H et al. 1996 Spermatic cord contamination in testicular cancer. Mod Pathol 9: 762–766
9. Damjanov I 1989 Tumors of the testis and epididymis, In: Murphy W M (ed) Urologic pathology. W B Saunders, Philadelphia, p 314–379
10. Wilms M 1896 Die teratoiden Geschwulste des Hoden mit Einschluss der sog: Cystoide und enchondrome. Beitr Pathol Anat Allg Pathol 19: 233–366
11. Skakkebaek N E 1972 Possible carcinoma-in-situ of the testis. Lancet 2: 516–517
12. Dorman S, Trainer T D, Lefke D 1979 Incipient germ cell tumor in a cryptorchid testis. Cancer 44: 1357–1362
13. Gondos B, Migliozzi J A 1987 Intratubular germ cell neoplasia. Semin Diagn Pathol 4: 292–303
14. Nistal M, Codesal J, Paniagua R 1989 Carcinoma in situ of the testis in infertile men: a histological, immunocytochemical, and cytophotometric study of DNA content. J Pathol Bacteriol 159: 205–210
15. Pryor J P, Cameron K M, Chilton C P 1983 Carcinoma in situ in testicular biopsies from men presenting with infertility. Br J Urol 55: 780–784
16. Skakkebaek N E, Berthelsen J G, Muller J 1982 Carcinoma-in-situ of the undescended testis. Urol Clin North Am 9: 377–385
17. Skakkebaek N E 1978 Carcinoma-in-situ of the testis: frequency and relationship to invasive germ cell tumours in infertile men. Histopathology 2: 157–170
18. Von der Maase H, Giwercman A, Muller J 1987 Management of carcinoma-in-situ of the testis. Int J Androl 10: 209–220
19. Von der Maase H, Rorth M, Walbom-Jorgensen S 1986 Carcinoma-in-situ of contralateral testis in patients with testicular germ cell cancer: study of 27 cases in 500 patients. Br Med J 293: 1398–1401
20. Von Eyben F E, Mikulowski P, Busch C 1981 Microinvasive germ cell tumors of the testis. J Urol 126: 842–844
21. Berthelsen J G, Skakkebaek N E, Mogensen P 1979 Incidence of carcinoma-in-situ of germ cells in contralateral testes of men with testicular tumors. Br Med J 2: 363–364
22. Skakkebaek N E, Berthelsen J G 1978 Carcinoma-in-situ of testis and orchiectomy. Lancet 2: 204–205
23. Berthelsen J G, Skakkebaek N E, von der Maase H 1982 Screening for carcinoma in-situ of the contralateral testis in patients with germinal testicular cancer. Br Med J 285: 1683–1686
24. Dieckmann K P, Loy V 1998 The value of the biopsy of the contralateral testis in patients with testicular germ cell cancer: the recent German experience. APMIS 106: 12–23
25. Muller J, Skakkebaek N E, Ritzen M 1985 Carcinoma in-situ of the testis in children with 45, X/46, XY gonadal dysgenesis. J Pediatr 106: 431–436
26. Nogales F F, Toro M, Ortega F 1981 Bilateral incipient germ cell tumours of the testis in the incomplete testicular feminization syndrome. Histopathology 5: 511–515
27. Muller J, Skakkebaek N E 1984 Testicular carcinoma in-situ in children with the androgen insensitivity (testicular feminization) syndrome. Br Med J 288: 1419–1420
28. Gondos B, Berthelsen J G, Skakkebaek N E 1983 Intratubular germ cell neoplasia (carcinoma in-situ): a preinvasive lesion of the testis. Ann Clin Lab Sci 13: 185–192
29. Giwercman A, Clausen O P F, Skakkebaek N E 1988 Carcinoma in-situ of the testis: aneuploid cells in semen. Br Med J 296: 1762–1764
30. Burke A P, Mostofi F K 1988 Placental alkaline phosphatase immunohistochemistry of intratubular malignant germ cells and associated testicular germ cell tumors. Hum Pathol 19: 663–670
31. Burke A P, Mostofi F K 1988 Intratubular malignant germ cells in testicular biopsies: clinical course and identification by staining for placental alkaline phosphatase. Mod Pathol 1: 475–479
32. Coffin C M, Ewing S, Dehner L P 1985 Frequency of intratubular germ cell neoplasia with invasive testicular germ cell tumors. Histologic and immunohistochemical features. Arch Pathol Lab Med 109: 555–559
33. Giwercman A, Marks A, Bailey D 1988 A monoclonal antibody as a marker for carcinoma in situ germ cells of the human adult testis. APMIS 96: 667–670
34. Jacobsen G K, Jacobsen M 1983 Ferritin (FER) in testicular germ cell tumours: an immunohistochemical study. Acta Pathol Microbiol Immunol Scand 91: 177–181
35. Bailey D, Marks A, Stratis M et al. 1991 Immunohistochemical staining of germ cell tumors and intratubular malignant germ cells of the testis using antibody to placental alkaline phosphatase and a monoclonal antiseminoma antibody. Mod Pathol 4: 167–171
36. Franke F E, Pauls K, Kerkman L et al. 2000 Somatic isoform of angiotensin I-converting enzyme in the pathology of testicular germ cell tumors. Hum Pathol 31: 1466–1476
37. Giwercman A, Lindenberg S, Kimber S J 1990 Monoclonal antibody 43-9F as a sensitive immunohistochemical marker of carcinoma in situ of human testis. Cancer 65: 1135–1142
38. Jones T D, Ulbright T M, Eble J N et al. 2004 OCT4: a sensitive and specific biomarker for intratubular germ cell neoplasia of the testis. Clin Cancer Res 10: 8544–8547
39. Eyzaguirre E, Gatalica Z 2002 Loss of Fhit expression in testicular germ cell tumors and intratubular germ cell neoplasia. Mod Pathol 15: 1068–1072
40. Rakheja D, Hoang M P, Sharma S et al. 2002 Intratubular embryonal carcinoma. Arch Pathol Lab Med 126: 487–490
41. van Echten J, van Gurp R J, Stoepker M et al. 1995 Cytogenetic evidence that carcinoma in situ is the precursor lesion for invasive testicular germ cell tumors. Cancer Genet Cytogenet 85: 133–137
42. Looijenga L H, Zafarana G, Grygalewicz B et al. 2003 Role of gain of 12p in germ cell tumour development. APMIS 111: 161–171
43. Lifschitz-Mercer B, Elliott D J, Leider-Trejo L et al. 2000 Absence of RBM expression as a marker of intratubular (in situ) germ cell neoplasia of the testis. Hum Pathol 31: 1116–1120
44. Jacobsen G K, Henriksen O B, Van der Maase H 1981 Carcinoma in situ of testicular tissue adjacent to malignant germ-cell tumors: a study of 105 cases. Cancer 47: 2660–2662
45. Reinberg Y, Manivel J C, Fraley E E 1989 Carcinoma in situ of the testis. J Urol 142: 243–247
46. Scully R E 1986 Testis. In: Hedson D E, Albores-Saavedra J (ed) The pathology of incipient neoplasia. W B Saunders, Philadelphia, p 329–343
47. Christensen T B, Daugaard G, Geertsen P F et al. 1998 Effect of chemotherapy on carcinoma in situ of the testis. Ann Oncol 9: 657–660
48. Manivel J C, Simonton S, Wold L E 1988 Absence of intratubular germ cell neoplasia in testicular yolk sac tumors in children: a histochemical and immunohistochemical study. Arch Pathol Lab Med 112: 641–645
49. Hartwick W, Ro J Y, Ordonez N 1990 Testicular germ cell tumors under age 5. Does intratubular germ cell neoplasia exist? Mod Pathol 3: 43A
50. Hu L M, Phillipson J, Barsky S H 1992 Intratubular germ cell neoplasia in infantile yolk sac tumor. Verification of tandem repeat sequence by in situ hybridization. Diagn Mol Pathol 1: 118–128
51. Ramani P, Yeung C K, Habeebu S S 1993 Testicular intratubular germ cell neoplasia in children and adolescents with intersex. Am J Surg Pathol 17: 1124–1133
52. Parkinson M C, Ramani P 1993 Intratubular germ cell neoplasia in an infantile testis. Histopathology 23: 99–100
53. Renedo D E, Trainer T D 1994 Intratubular germ cell neoplasia (ITGCN) with p53 and PCNA expression and adjacent mature teratoma in an infant testis. An immunohistochemical and morphologic study with a review of the literature. Am J Surg Pathol 18: 947–952
54. Jacobsen G K, Barlebo H, Oslen J 1984 Testicular germ cell tumors in Denmark 1976–1980: pathology of 1058 consecutive cases. Acta Radiol Oncol 23: 239–247
55. Ulbright T M, Roth L M 1987 Recent developments in the pathology of germ cell tumors. Semin Diagn Pathol 4: 304–319
56. Ulbright T M 1993 Germ cell neoplasms of the testis. Am J Surg Pathol 17: 1075–1091
57. Hedinger C, von Hochstetter A R, Egloff B 1979 Seminoma with syncytiotrophoblastic giant cells: a special form of seminoma. Virchow's Arch [A] 383: 59–67
58. Cockburn A G, Vugrin D, Batata M 1984 Poorly differentiated (anaplastic) seminoma of the testis. Cancer 53: 1991–1994
59. Giwercman A, Grindsted J, Hansen B 1987 Testicular cancer risk in boys with maldescended testis: a cohort study. J Urol 138: 1214–1216

60. Sokal M, Peckham M J, Hendry W F 1980 Bilateral germ cell tumours of the testis. Br J Urol 52: 158–162
61. Che M, Tamboli P, Ro J Y et al. 2002 Bilateral testicular germ cell tumors. Twenty-year experience at M D Anderson cancer Center. Cancer 95: 1228–1233
62. Fraley E E, Lange P H, Kennedy B J 1979 Germ-cell testicular cancer in adults. N Engl J Med 301: 1370–1377, 1420–1426
63. Javadpour N, Young J D J 1986 Prognostic factors in non-seminomatous testicular cancer. J Urol 135: 497–499
64. Scheiber K, Ackermann D, Studer U E 1987 Bilateral testicular germ cell tumors: a report of 20 cases. J Urol 138: 73–76
65. Jacobsen G K, von der Maase H, Specht L 1995 Histopathological features in stage I seminoma treated with orchiectomy only. J Urol Pathol 3: 85–94
66. Young R H, Finlayson N, Scully R E 1989 Tubular seminoma: report of a case. Arch Pathol Lab Med 113: 414–416
67. Damjanov I, Niejadlik D C, Rabuffo J V 1980 Cribriform and sclerosing seminoma devoid of lymphoid infiltrates. Arch Pathol Lab Med 104: 527–530
68. Zavala-Pompa A, Ro J Y, El-Naggar A K 1994 Tubular seminoma: an immunohistochemical and DNA flow-cytometric study of four cases. Am J Clin Pathol 102: 397–401
69. Takeshima Y, Sanda N, Yoneda K et al. 1999 Tubular seminoma of the testis. Pathol Int 49: 676–679
70. Ulbright T M, Young R H 2005 Seminoma with tubular, microcystic and related patterns. A study of 28 cases of unusual morphologic variants that often cause confusion with yolk sac tumor. Am J Surg Pathol 29: 500–505
71. Henley J D, Young R H, Wade C L et al. 2004 Seminomas with exclusive intertubular growth. A report of 12 clinically and grossly inconspicuous tumors. Am J Surg Pathol 28: 1163–1168
72. Kademian M, Bosch A, Caldwell W L 1977 Anaplastic seminoma. Cancer 40: 3082–3086
73. Thackray A C, Crane W A J 1976 Seminoma. In: Pugh R C P (ed) Pathology of the testis. Blackwell, Oxford, p 164–198
74. Kahn D G 1993 Ossifying seminoma of the testis. Arch Pathol Lab Med 117: 321–322
75. Bell D A, Flotte T J, Bhan A K 1987 Immunohistochemical characterization of seminoma and its inflammatory cell infiltrate. Hum Pathol 18: 511–520
75a. Browne T J, Richie J P, Gilligan T D, Rubin M A 2005 Intertubular growth in pure seminomas: associations with poor prognostic parameters. Hum Pathol 36: 640–645
76. Perry A, Wiley E L, Albores-Saavedra J 1994 Pagetoid spread of intratubular germ cell neoplasia into rete testis: a morphologic and immunohistochemical study of 100 orchiectomy specimens with invasive germ cell tumors. Hum Pathol 25: 235–239
77. Mai K T, Yazdi H M, Rippstein P 2001 Light and electron microscopy of the pagetoid spread of germ cell carcinoma in the rete testis: morphologic evidence suggestive of field effect as a mechanism of tumor spread. Appl Immunohistochem Mol Morphol 9: 335–339
78. Florentine B D, Roscher A A, Garrett J et al. 2002 Necrotic seminoma of the testis: establishing the diagnosis with Masson trichrome stain and immunostains. Arch Pathol Lab Med 126: 205–206
79. Bobba V S, Mittal B B, Hoover S V 1988 Classical and anaplastic seminoma: difference in survival. Radiology 167: 849–852
80. Johnson D E, Gomez J J, Ayala A G 1975 Anaplastic seminoma. J Urol 114: 80–82
81. Tickoo S K, Hutchinson B, Bacik J et al. 2002. Testicular seminoma: a clinicopathologic and immunohistochemical study of 105 cases with special reference to seminomas with atypical features. Int J Surg Pathol 10: 23–32
82. Manivel J C, Jessurun J, Wick M R 1987 Placental alkaline phosphatase immunoreactivity in testicular germ-cell neoplasms. Am J Surg Pathol 11: 21–29
83. Mostofi F K, Sesterhenn I A, Davis C J J 1987 Immunopathology of germ cell tumors of the testis. Semin Diagn Pathol 4: 320–341
84. Jones T D, Ulbright T M, Eble J N et al. 2004 OCT4 staining in testicular tumors: a sensitive and specific marker for seminoma and embryonal carcinoma. Am J Surg Pathol 28: 935–940
85. Looijenga L H, Stoop H, de Leeuw H P 2003 POU5F1 (OCT3/4) identifies cells with pluripotent potential in human germ cell tumors. Cancer Res 63: 2244–2250
86. Ferreiro J A 1994 Ber-H2 expression in testicular germ cell tumors. Hum Pathol 25: 522–524
87. Hittmair A, Rogatsch H, Hobisch A et al. 1996 CD30 expression in seminoma. Hum Pathol 27: 1166–1171
88. Cheville J C, Rao S, Iczkowski K A et al. 2000 Cytokeratin expression in seminoma of the human testis. Am J Clin Pathol 113: 583–588
88a. McIntyre A, Summersgill B, Grygalewicz B et al. 2005 Amplification and overexpression of the KIT gene is associated with progression in the seminoma subtype of testicular germ cell tumors of adolescents and adults. Cancer Res 65: 8085–8089
89. Butcher D N, Gregory W M, Gunter P A 1985 The biological significance of HCG-containing cells in seminoma. Br J Cancer 51: 473–478
90. Jacobsen G K 1983 Alpha-fetoprotein (AFP) and human chorionic gonadotropin (HCG) in testicular germ cell tumors. A comparison of histologic and serologic occurrence of tumor markers. Acta Pathol Microbiol Scand Sect A 91: 183–190
91. Paus E, Fossa S D, Risberg T 1987 The diagnostic value of human chorionic gonadotrophin in patients with testicular seminoma. Br J Urol 59: 572–577
92. Javadpour N 1980 Management of seminoma based on tumor markers. Urol Clin North Am 7: 773–781
93. Javadpour N 1984 Human chorionic gonadotropin in seminoma. J Urol 131: 407
94. Javadpour N 1980 Significance of elevated serum alphafetoprotein (AFP) in seminoma. Cancer 45: 2166–2168
95. Raghavan D, Vogelzang N J, Bosl G L 1982 Tumor classification and size in germ-cell testicular cancer. Influence on the occurrence of metastases. Cancer 50: 1591–1595
96. Nazeer T, Ro J Y, Amato B et al. 1998 Histologically pure seminoma with elevated alpha-fetoprotein (AFP): a clinicopathologic study of ten cases. Oncol Rep 5: 1425–1429
97. Kuzmits R, Schernthaner G, Krisch K 1987 Serum neuron-specific enolase: a marker for response to therapy in seminoma. Cancer 60: 1017–1021
98. Smolarek T A, Blough R I, Foster R S 1999 Cytogenetic analyses of 85 testicular germ cell tumors: comparison of postchemotherapy and untreated tumors. Cancer Genet Cytogenet 108: 57–69
99. Qiao D, Zeeman A M, Deng W et al. 2002 Molecular characterization of hiwi, a human member of the piwi gene family whose overexpression is correlated to seminomas. Oncogene 21: 3988–3999
100. Berger P, Untergasser G, Hermann M et al. 1999 The testis-specific expression pattern of the growth hormone/placental lactogen (GH/PL) gene cluster changes with malignancy. Hum Pathol 30: 1201–1206
101. Cheville J C, Roche P C 1999 MAGE-1 and MAGE-3 tumor rejection antigens in human germ cell tumors. Mod Pathol 12: 974–978
102. Zeeman A M, Stoop H, Boter M et al. 2002 VASA is a specific marker for both normal and malignant human germ cells. Lab Invest 82: 159–166
103. Babaian R J, Zagars G K 1988 Testicular seminoma: the MD Anderson experience. An analysis of pathological and patient characteristics and treatment recommendations. J Urol 139: 311–315
104. Zagars G K, Babaian R J 1987 The role of radiation in stage II testicular seminoma. Int J Radiat Oncol Biol Phys 13: 163–170
105. Johnson D E, Gomez J J, Ayala A G 1976 Histologic factors affecting prognosis of pure seminoma of the testis. South Med J 69: 1173–1174
106. Marks L B, Rutgers J L, Shipley W U 1990 Testicular seminoma: clinical and pathological features that may predict para-aortic lymph node metastases. J Urol 143: 524–527
107. Warde P, Specht L, Horwich A et al. 2002 Prognostic factors for relapse in stage I seminoma managed by surveillance: a pooled analysis. J Clin Oncol 20: 4448–4452
108. Warde P, Gospodarowicz M K, Banerjee D 1997 Prognostic factors for relapse in stage I testicular seminoma treated with surveillance. J Urol 157: 1705–1709
109. Farivari A, Mostofi F K 1984 Spermatocytic seminoma. J Urol 131: 226A
110. Talerman A 1980 Spermatocytic seminoma: clinicopathological study of 22 cases. Cancer 45: 2169–2176
111. Masson P 1946 Etude sur le seminome. Rev Can Biol 5: 361
112. Rajpert-De Meyts E, Jacobsen G K, Bartkova J et al. 2003 The immunohistochemical expression pattern of Chk2, p53, p19INK4d, MAGE-A4 and other selected antigens provides new evidence for the premeiotic origin of spermatocytic seminoma. Histopathology 42: 217–226
113. Stoop H, van Gurp R, de Krijger R et al. 2001 Reactivity of germ cell maturation stage-specific markers in spermatocytic seminoma: diagnostic and etiological implications. Lab Invest 81: 919–928
114. Satie A P, Rajpert-De Meyts E, Spagnoli G C et al. 2002 The cancer-testis gene, NY-ESO-1, is expressed in normal fetal and adult testes and in spermatocytic seminomas and testicular carcinoma in situ. Lab Invest 82: 775–780
115. Cummings O W, Ulbright T M, Eble J N et al. 1994 Spermatocytic seminoma: an immunohistochemical study. Hum Pathol 25: 54–59
116. Floyd C, Ayala A G, Logothetis C J 1988 Spermatocytic seminoma of testis with associated sarcoma of the testis. Cancer 61: 409–414
117. Chung P W, Bayley A J, Sweet J et al. 2004 Spermatocytic seminoma: a review. Eur Urol 45: 495–498
118. Burke A P, Mostofi F K 1993 Spermatocytic seminoma: a clinicopathologic study of 79 cases. J Urol Pathol 1: 21–32
119. Albores-Saavedra J, Huffman H, Alvarado-Cabrero I et al. 1996 Anaplastic variant of spermatocytic seminoma. Hum Pathol 27: 650–655
120. Rosai J, Siber I, Khodadoust K 1969 Spermatocytic seminoma: clinicopathologic study of six cases and review of the literature. Cancer 24: 92–102
121. Talerman A, Fu Y S, Okagaki T 1984 Spermatocytic seminoma: ultrastructural and microspectrophotometric observations. Lab Invest 51: 343–349
122. True L D, Otis C N, Delprado W 1988 Spermatocytic seminoma of testis with sarcomatous transformation. A report of five cases. Am J Surg Pathol 12: 75–82
123. Matoska J, Ondrus D, Hornak M 1988 Metastatic spermatocytic seminoma: a case report with light microscopic, ultrastructural and immunohistochemical findings. Cancer 62: 1197–1201
124. Matoska J, Talerman A 1990 Spermatocytic seminoma associated with rhabdomyosarcoma. Am J Clin Pathol 94: 89–95
125. Miettinen M, Virtanen I, Talerman A 1985 Intermediate filament proteins in human testis and testicular germ-cell tumors. Am J Pathol 120: 402–410
126. Decaussin M, Borda A, Bouvier R et al. 2004 Spermatocytic seminoma. A clinicopathological and immunohistochemical study of 7 cases. Ann Pathol 24: 161–166

127. Dunphy C H, Ayala A G, Swanson D A 1986 Clinical stage I non-seminomatous and mixed germ cell tumors of the testis: a clinicopathologic study of 93 patients on a surveillance protocol after orchiectomy alone. Cancer 62: 1202–1206
128. Dewar J M, Spagnolo D V, Jamrozik K D 1987 Predicting relapse in stage I non-seminomatous germ cell tumours of the testis. Lancet 1: 454
129. Koops H S, Sleijfer D T, Oosterhuis J W 1986 Wait-and-see policy in clinical stage I non-seminomatous germ cell tumors of the testis. Eur J Surg Oncol 12: 283–287
130. Rodriguez P N, Hafez G R, Messing E M 1986 Non-seminomatous germ cell tumor of the testicle: does extensive staging of the primary tumor predict the likelihood of metastatic disease? J Urol 136: 604–608
131. Fung C Y, Kalish L A, Brodsky G L 1988 Stage I non-seminomatous germ cell testicular tumour: prediction of metastatic potential by primary histopathology. J Clin Oncol 6: 1467–1473
132. Hoskin P, Dilly S, Easton D 1986 Prognostic factors in stage I non-seminomatous germ-cell testicular tumours managed by orchiectomy and surveillance: implicators for adjuvant chemotherapy. J Clin Oncol 4: 1031–1036
133. Nochomovitz L E, DeLa Torre F E, Rosai J 1977 Pathology of germ cell tumors of the testis. Urol Clin North Am 4: 359–378
134. Vugrin D, Chen A, Feigl P 1988 Embryonal carcinoma of the testis. Cancer 61: 2348–2352
135. Pierce G B J, Abell M R 1970 Embryonal carcinoma of the testis. Pathol Annu 5: 27–60
136. Tuttle J P J, Pratt-Thomas H R, Thomason W B 1977 Embryonal carcinoma of the testis in elderly men. J Urol 118: 1070–1072
137. Bosl G J, Lange P H, Nochomovitz L E 1981 Tumor markers in advanced non-seminomatous testicular cancer. Cancer 47: 572–576
138. Morinaga S, Ojima M, Sasano N 1983 Human chorionic gonadotropin and alpha-fetoprotein in testicular germ tumors: an immunohistochemical study in comparison with tissue concentrations. Cancer 52: 1281–1289
139. Mostofi F K, Sesterhenn I A, Davis C J J 1988 Developments in histopathology of testicular germ cell tumors. Semin Urol 6: 171–188
140. Talerman A, Haije W G, Baggerman L 1980 Serum alphafetoprotein (AFP) in patients with germ cell tumors of the gonads and extragonadal sites: correlation between endodermal sinus (yolk sac) tumor and raised serum AFP. Cancer 46: 380–385
141. Talerman A 1980 Endodermal sinus (yolk sac) tumor elements in testicular germ-cell tumors in adults: comparison of prospective and retrospective studies. Cancer 46: 1213–1217
142. Jacobsen G K, Jacobsen M, Clausen P P 1981 Distribution of tumor-associated antigens in the various histologic components of germ cell tumors of the testis. Am J Surg Pathol 5: 257–266
143. Battifora H, Sheibani K, Tubbs R R 1984 Antikeratin antibodies in tumor diagnosis. Distinction between seminoma and embryonal carcinoma. Cancer 54: 843–848
144. Jacobson G K 1986 Histogenetic considerations concerning germ cell tumours. Morphological and immunohistochemical comparative investigation of human embryo and testicular germ cell tumours. Virchow's Arch [A] 408: 509–525
145. Pallesen G, Hamilton-Dutoit S J 1988 Ki-1 (CD30) antigen is regularly expressed by tumor cells of embryonal carcinoma. Am J Pathol 133: 446–450
146. Shah V I, Amin M B, Linden M D et al. 1998 Utility of a selective immunohistochemical (IHC) panel in the detection of components of mixed germ cell tumors (GCT) of testis. Mod Pathol 11: 95A (abstract)
147. Shah V I, Amin M B, Linden M D et al. 1998 Immunohistologic profile of spindle cell elements in non-seminomatous germ cell tumors (NSGCT): histogenetic implications. Mod Pathol 11: 96A (abstract)
148. Berney D M, Shamash J, Pieroni K et al. 2001 Loss of CD30 expression in metastatic embryonal carcinoma: the effects of chemotherapy? Histopathology 39: 382–385
149. Oosterhuis J W, Castedo S M, de Jong B 1989 Ploidy of primary germ cell tumors of the testis. Pathogenetic and clinical relevance. Lab Invest 60: 14–21
150. Motzer R J, Rodriguez E, Reuter V E 1991 Genetic analysis as an aid in diagnosis for patients with midline carcinomas of uncertain histologies. J Natl Cancer Inst 83: 341–346
151. Ferry J A, Ulbright T M, Young R H 1997 Anaplastic large cell lymphoma presenting in the testis. J Urol Pathol 5: 139–147
152. Green D M 1983 The diagnosis and treatment of yolk sac tumors in infants and children. Cancer Treat Rev 10: 265–288
153. Harms D, Janig U 1986 Germ cell tumours of childhood: Report of 170 cases, including 59 pure and partial yolk-sac tumours. Virchows Arch [A] 409: 223–239
154. Griffin G C, Raney R B J, Snyder H M 1967 Yolk sac carcinoma of the testis in children. J Urol 137: 954–957
155. Gonzalez-Crussi F 1979 The human yolk sac and yolk sac (endodermal sinus) tumors: a review. Perspect Pediatr Pathol 5: 179–215
156. Kaplan G W, Cromie W C, Kelalis P P 1988 Prepubertal yolk sac testicular tumors: Report of the Testicular Tumor Registry. J Urol 140: 1109–1112
157. Kramer S A, Wold L E, Gilchrist G S 1984 Yolk sac carcinoma: an immunohistochemical and clinicopathologic review. J Urol 131: 315–318
158. Olsen M M, Raffensperger J G, Gonzalez-Crussi F 1982 Endodermal sinus tumor: a clinical and pathological correlation. J Pediatr Surg 17: 832–840
159. Pierce G B J, Bullock W K, Huntington R W J 1970 Yolk sac tumors of the testis. Cancer: 644–658
160. Wold L E, Kramer S A, Farrow G M 1984 Testicular yolk sac and embryonal carcinomas in pediatric patients: comparative immunohistochemical and clinicopathologic study. Am J Clin Pathol 81: 427–435
161. Logothetis C J, Samuels M L, Trinade A 1984 The prognostic significance of endodermal sinus tumor histology among patients treated for stage III non-seminomatous germ cell tumors of the testes. Cancer 53: 122–128
162. Talerman A 1975 The incidence of yolk sac tumor (endodermal sinus tumor) elements in germ cell tumors of the testis in adults. Cancer 36: 211–215
163. Ulbright T M, Roth L M, Broadhecker C A 1986 Yolk sac differentiation in germ cell tumors: a morphologic study of 50 cases with emphasis on hepatic, enteric, and parietal yolk sac features. Am J Surg Pathol 10: 151–164
164. Cohen M B, Friend D S, McInar J J 1987 Gonadal endodermal sinus (yolk sac) tumor with pure intestinal differentiation: a new histologic type. Pathol Res Pract 182: 609–616
165. Jacobsen G K, Jacobsen M 1983 Possible liver cell differentiation in testicular germ cell tumours. Histopathology 7: 537–548
166. Nakashima N, Fukatsu T, Nagasaka T 1987 The frequency and histology of hepatic tissues in germ cell tumors. Am J Surg Pathol 11: 682–692
167. Horie Y, Kato M 2000 Hepatoid variant of yolk sac tumor of the testis. Pathol Int 50: 754–758
168. Eglen D E, Ulbright T M 1987 The differential diagnosis of yolk sac tumor and seminoma: usefulness of cytokeratin, alpha-fetoprotein, and alpha-1-antitrypsin immunoperoxidase reactions. Am J Clin Pathol 88: 328–332
169. Noorgaard-Pedersen B, Albrechtsen R, Teilum G 1975 Serum alpha-fetoprotein as a marker for endodermal sinus tumour (yolk sac tumour) or a vitelline component of "teratocarcinoma." Acta Pathol Microbiol Scand [A] 83: 573–589
170. Tsuchida Y, Kaneko M, Yokomori K 1978 Alpha-fetoprotein, prealbumin, albumin, alpha-1-antitrypsin and transferrin as diagnostic and therapeutic markers for endodermal sinus tumors. J Pediatr Surg 13: 25–29
171. Koide O, Iwai S, Baba K et al. 1987 Identification of testicular atypical germ cells by an immunohistochemical technique for placental alkaline phosphatase. Cancer 59: 1325–1330
172. Ro J Y, Grignon- D J, Amin M B et al. 1997 Atlas of surgical pathology of the male reproductive tract. W B Saunders, Philadelphia
173. Grady R W, Ross J H, Kay R 1995 Patterns of metastatic spread in prepubertal yolk sac tumor of the testis. J Urol 153: 1259–1261
174. Gaillard J A 1972 Yolk sac tumour patterns and entoblastic structures in polyembryomas. Acta Pathol Microbiol Scand [A] 233: 18–25
175. Marin-Padilla M 1965 Origin, nature and significance of the "embryoids" of human teratomas. Virchow's Arch [A] 340: 105–121
176. Nakashima N, Murakami S, Fukatsu T 1988 Characteristics of "embryoid body" in human gonadal germ cell tumors. Hum Pathol 19: 1144–1154
177. Colodny A H, Hopkins T B 1977 Testicular tumors in infants and children. Urol Clin North Am 4: 347–358
178. Fraley E E, Ketcham A S 1968 Teratoma of testis in an infant. J Urol 100: 659–660
179. Hawkins E P 1990 Pathology of germ cell tumors in children. Crit Rev Oncol Hematol 10: 165–179
180. Leibovitch I, Foster R S, Ulbright T M et al. 1995 Adult primary pure teratoma of the testis. The Indiana experience. Cancer 75: 2244–2250
181. Pugh R C B, Smith J P 1964 Teratoma. Br J Urol 36: 28–44
182. Mahour G H, Wooley M M, Trivedi S N 1974 Teratomas in infancy and childhood: experience with 81 cases. Surgery 76: 309–318
183. Mosli H A, Carpenter B, Schillinger J F 1985 Teratoma of the testis in a pubertal child. J Urol 133: 105–106
184. Tapper D, Lack E E 1983 Teratomas in infancy and childhood: a 54 year experience at the Children's Hospital Medical Center. Ann Surg 198: 398–410
185. Tiltman A J 1974 Granulomatous reaction in testicular teratomas. S Afr Med J 48: 1231
186. Ulbright T M, Srigley J R 2001 Dermoid cyst of the testis: a study of five postpubertal cases, including a pilomatrixoma-like variant, with evidence supporting its separate classification from mature testicular teratoma. Am J Surg Pathol 25: 788–793
187. Dieckmann K P, Loy V 1994 Epidermoid cyst of the testis: a review of clinical and histogenetic considerations. Br J Urol 73: 436–441
188. Nokubi M, Kawai T, Mitsu S et al. 2002 Mucinous cystadenoma of the testis. Pathol Int 52: 648–652
189. Collins D H, Pugh R C P 1964 Classification and frequency of testicular tumours. Br J Urol 36: 1–11
190. Harms D, Janig U 1985 Immature teratomas of childhood. Report of 21 cases. Pathol Res Pract 179: 388–400
191. Kooijman C D 1988 Immature teratomas in children. Histopathology 12: 491–502
192. Michael H, Hull M T, Ulbright T M et al. 1997 Primitive neuroectodermal tumors arising in testicular germ cell neoplasms. Am J Surg Pathol 21: 896–904
193. Ulbright T M 1999 Testis risk and prognostic factors. The pathologist's perspective. Urol Clin North Am 26: 611–626
194. Comiter C V, Kibel A S, Richie J P et al. 1998 Prognostic features of teratomas with malignant transformation: a clinicopathologic study of 21 cases. J Urol 159: 359–363
195. Michael H 1998 Non-germ cell tumors arising in patients with testicular germ cell tumors. J Urol Pathol 9: 39–60

196. Cajal S R Y, Pinango L, Barat A 1987 Metastatic pure choriocarcinoma of the testis in an elderly man. J Urol 137: 516–519
197. Manivel J C, Niehans G, Wick M R et al. 1987 Intermediate trophoblast in germ cell neoplasms. Am J Surg Pathol 11: 693–701
198. Ulbright T M, Young R H, Scully R E 1997 Trophoblastic tumors of the testis other than classic choriocarcinoma: "monophasic" choriocarcinoma and placental site trophoblastic tumor: a report of two cases. Am J Surg Pathol 21: 282–288
199. Ulbright T M, Loehrer P J 1988 Choriocarcinoma-like lesions in patients with testicular germ cell tumors. Two histologic variants. Am J Surg Pathol 12: 531–541
200. Mazur M T, Lurain J R, Brewer J I 1982 Fatal gestational choriocarcinoma. Clinicopathologic study of patients treated at a trophoblastic disease center. Cancer 50: 1833–1846
201. Suurmeijer A J, Gietema J A, Hoekstra H J 2004 Placental site trophoblastic tumor in a late recurrence of a non-seminomatous germ cell tumor of the testis. Am J Surg Pathol 28: 830–833
202. Lind H M, Haghighi P 1986 Carcinoembryonic antigen staining in choriocarcinoma. Am J Clin Pathol 86: 538–540
203. Shih I M, Kurman R J 1999 Immunohistochemical localization of inhibin-alpha in the placental and gestational trophoblastic lesions. Int J Gynecol Pathol 18: 144–150
204. Logothetis C J, Samuels M L, Selig D E 1986 Cyclic chemotherapy with cyclophosphamide, doxorubicin, and cisplatin plus vinblastine and bleomycin in advanced germinal tumors: results with 100 patients. Am J Med 81: 219–228
205. Vaeth M, Schultz H P, von der Maase H 1984 Prognostic factors in testicular germ cell tumours: experiences with 1058 consecutive cases. Acta Radiol Oncol 23: 271–285
206. Stoter G, Sylvester R, Sleijfer D T 1988 A multivariate analysis of prognostic factors in disseminated non-seminomatous testicular cancer. Prog Clin Biol Res 269: 381–393
207. Pugh R C B, Thackray A C 1964 Combined tumour. Br J Urol 36: 45–51
208. De Almeida P C C, Scully R E 1983 Diffuse embryoma of the testis: a distinctive form of mixed germ cell tumor. Am J Surg Pathol 7: 633–642
209. de Peralta-Venturina M N, Ro J Y, Ordonez N G et al. 1994 Diffuse embryoma of the testis: an immunohistochemical study of two cases. Am J Clin Pathol 102: 402–405
210. Allen E A, Burger P C, Epstein J I 1999 Microcystic meningioma arising in a mixed germ cell tumor of the testis: a case report. Am J Surg Pathol 23: 1131–1135
211. Ro J Y, Han W, Ordonez N 1991 Non-seminomatous germ cell tumors of the testis: an immunohistochemical study of 46 cases. Lab Invest 64: 50A
212. Tezel G, Nagasaka T, Shimono Y et al. 2002 Differential expression of RET finger protein in testicular germ cell tumors. Pathol Int 52: 623–627
213. Scully R E 1953 Gonadoblastoma: a gonadal tumor related to the dysgerminoma (seminoma) and capable of sex-hormone production. Cancer 6: 455–463
214. Scully R E 1970 Gonadoblastoma: a review of 74 cases. Cancer 25: 1340–1356
215. Hughesdon P E, Kumarasamy T 1970 Mixed germ cell tumours (gonadoblastomas) in normal and dysgenetic gonads. Virchow's Arch [A] 349: 258–280
216. Ishida T, Tagatz G E, Okagaki T 1976 Gonadoblastoma: ultrastructural evidence for testicular origin. Cancer 37: 1770–1781
217. Talerman A 1980 The pathology of gonadal neoplasms composed of germ cells and sex cord stroma derivatives. Pathol Res Pract 170: 24–38
218. Hart W R, Burkons D M 1979 Germ cell neoplasms arising in gonadoblastomas. Cancer 43: 669–678
219. Chapman W H H, Plymyer M R, Dresner M L 1990 Gonadoblastoma in an anatomically normal man: a case report and literature review. J Urol 144: 1472–1474
220. Talerman A, Delemarre J F 1975 Gonadoblastoma associated with embryonal carcinoma in an anatomically normal man. J Urol 113: 355–359
221. Iezzoni J C, von Kap-Herr C, Golden W L et al. 1997 Gonadoblastomas in 45,X/46,XY mosaicism: analysis of Y-chromosome distribution by fluorescence in situ hybridization. Am J Clin Pathol 108: 197–201
222. Kommoss F, Oliva E, Bhan A et al. 1998 Inhibin expression in ovarian tumors and tumor-like lesions: an immunohistochemical study. Mod Pathol 11: 656–664
223. Jorgensen N, Muller J, Jaubert F et al. 1997 Heterogeneity of gonadoblastoma germ cells: similarities with immature germ cells, spermatogonia and testicular carcinoma in-situ cells. Histopathology 30: 177–186
224. Bolen J V 1981 Mixed germ cell–sex cord stromal tumor: a gonadal tumor distinct from gonadoblastoma. Am J Clin Pathol 75: 565–573
225. Matoska J, Talerman A 1989 Mixed germ cell–sex cord stromal tumor of the testis. Cancer 64: 2146–2153
226. Talerman A 1972 A distinctive gonadal neoplasm related to gonadoblastoma. Cancer 30: 1219–1224
227. Talerman A 1987 Tumors composed of germ cells and sex cord stromal derivatives. In: Talerman A, Roth L M (ed) Pathology of the testis and its adnexa. Churchill Livingstone, New York, p 59–62
228. Rames R A, Richardson M, Swiger F et al. 1995 Mixed germ cell–sex cord stromal tumor of the testis: the incidental finding of a rare testicular neoplasm. J Urol 54: 1479
229. Ulbright T M, Srigley J R, Reuter V E et al. 2000 Sex cord stromal tumors of the testis with entrapped germ cells: a lesion mimicking unclassified mixed germ cell sex cord stromal tumors. Am J Surg Pathol 24: 535–542
230. Amato R J, Ro J Y, Ayala A G et al. 2004 Risk-adapted treatment for patients with clinical stage I non-seminomatous germ cell tumor of the testis. Urology 63: 144–148
231. Johnson D E 1987 Improved survival results from early detection and diagnosis of testicular cancer. Oncology 32: 1
232. Logothetis C J, Swanson D A, Dexeus F 1987 Primary chemotherapy for clinical stage II non-seminomatous germ cell tumors of the testis: a follow-up of 50 patients. J Clin Oncol 5: 906–911
233. Pizzocaro G, Zanon-i F, Milani A 1984 Retroperitoneal lymphadenectomy and aggressive chemotherapy in non-bulky clinical stage II non-seminomatous germinal testis tumors. Cancer 53: 1363–1368
234. Pizzocaro G, Monfardini S 1984 No adjuvant chemotherapy in selected patients with pathologic stage II non-seminomatous germ cell tumors of the testis. J Urol 131: 677–680
235. Williams S D, Stablein D M, Einhorn L H 1987 Immediate adjuvant chemotherapy versus observation with treatment at relapse in pathological stage II testicular cancer. N Engl J Med 317: 1433–1438
236. Vugrin D, Whitemore W F, Cvitkovic E 1981 Adjuvant chemotherapy combination of vinblastine, actinomycin D, bleomycin, and chlorambucil following retroperitoneal lymph node dissection for stage II testis tumor. Cancer 47: 840–844
237. Moran C A, Travis W D, Carter D 1993 Metastatic mature teratoma in lung following testicular embryonal carcinoma and teratocarcinoma. Arch Pathol Lab Med 117: 641–644
238. Samuels M L, Johnson D E 1980 Adjuvant therapy of testis cancer: the role of vinblastine and bleomycin. J Urol 124: 369–371
239. Blacken R B, Johnson D E, Frazier O H 1983 The role of surgery following chemotherapy in stage III germ cell neoplasms. J Urol 129: 39–43
240. Peckham M J, Oliver R T D, Bagshawe K D 1985 Prognostic factors in advanced non-seminomatous germ-cell testicular tumours: results of a multicentre study. Report from the Medical Research Council Working Party on Testicular Tumours. Lancet 1: 8–11
241. Roth B J, Greist A, Kubilis P S 1988 Cisplatin-based combination chemotherapy for disseminated germ cell tumors: long-term follow-up. J Clin Oncol 6: 1239–1247
242. Williams S D, Birch R, Einhorn L H 1987 Treatment of disseminated germ-cell tumors with cisplatin, bleomycin, and either vinblastine or etoposide. N Engl J Med 316: 1435–1440
243. Lo R K, Friha F S, Torti F M 1989 Chemotherapy for advanced germ cell tumors of the testis: the Stanford experience. In: Johnson D E, Logothetis C J, von Eschenbach A C (eds) Systemic therapy for genitourinary cancers. Year Book, Chicago, p 338–341
244. Logothetis C J, Samuels M L 1984 Surgery in the management of stage III germinal cell tumors: observation in the MD Anderson Hospital experience, 1971–1979. Cancer Treat Rev 11: 27–37
245. Geller N L, Bosl G J, Chan E Y M 1989 Prognostic factors for relapse after complete response in patients with metastatic germ cell tumors. Cancer 63: 440–445
246. Peckham M J, Hendry W F 1985 Clinical stage II non-seminomatous germ cell testicular tumours: results of management by primary chemotherapy. Br J Urol 57: 763–768
247. Fossa S D, Ous S, Lien H H 1989 Post-chemotherapy lymph node histology in radiologically normal patients with metastatic non-seminomatous testicular cancer. J Urol 141: 557–559
248. Loehrer P J S, Hui S, Clark S 1986 Teratoma following cisplatin-based combination chemotherapy for non-seminomatous germ cell tumors: a clinicopathologic correlation. J Urol 135: 1183–1189
249. Tait D, Peckham M J, Hendry W F 1984 Post-chemotherapy surgery in advanced non-seminomatous germ-cell testicular tumours: the significance of histology with particular reference to differentiated (mature) teratoma. Br J Cancer 50: 601–609
250. Dexeus F M, Shirkhoda A, Logothetis C J 1989 Clinical and radiological correlation of retroperitoneal metastasis from non-seminomatous testicular cancer treated with chemotherapy. Eur J Cancer Clin Oncol 25: 35–43
251. Castedo S M M J, de Jong B, Oosterhuis J W 1989 Chromosomal changes in mature residual teratomas following polychemotherapy. Cancer Res 49: 672–676
252. Sella A, El-Naggar A, Ro J Y et al. 1991 Evidence of malignant features in histologically mature teratoma. J Urol 146: 1025–1028
253. Ulbright T M, Loehrer P J, Roth L M 1984 The development of non-germ-cell malignancies within germ cell tumors. A clinicopathologic study of 11 cases. Cancer 54: 1824–1833
254. Ulbright T M, Goheen M P, Roth L M 1986 The differentiation of carcinomas of teratomatous origin from embryonal carcinoma: a light and electron microscopic study. Cancer 57: 257–263
255. Ahlgren A D, Simrell C R, Triche T J 1984 Sarcoma arising in a residual testicular teratoma after cytoreductive chemotherapy. Cancer 54: 2015–2018
256. Michael H, Hull M T, Foster R S et al. 1998 Nephroblastoma-like tumors in patients with testicular germ cell tumors. Am J Surg Pathol 22: 1107–1114
257. Sahoo S, Ryan C W, Recant W M et al. 2003 Angiosarcoma masquerading as embryonal carcinoma in the metastasis from a mature testicular teratoma. Arch Pathol Lab Med 127: 360–363

258. Davey D D, Ulbright T M, Loehrer P J 1987 The significance of atypia within teratomatous metastases after chemotherapy for malignant germ cell tumors. Cancer 49: 533–539
259. Chong C, Logothetis C J, von Eschenbach A 1986 Orchiectomy in advanced germ cell cancer following intensive chemotherapy: a comparison of systemic to testicular response. J Urol 136: 1221–1223
260. Ro J Y, Amato R J, Ayala A G 1996 What does the pathology report really mean? Semin Urol Oncol 14: 2–7
261. Kim I, Young R H, Scully R E 1985 Leydig cell tumors of the testis. A clinicopathological analysis of 40 cases and review of the literature. Am J Surg Pathol 9: 177–192
262. Caldamone A A, Altebarmakian V, Frank I N 1979 Leydig cell tumor of testis. Urology 14: 39–43
263. Mauer R, Taylor C, Schmucki O 1980 Extratesticular gonadal stromal tumor of the pelvis. A case report with immunoperoxidase findings. Cancer 45: 985–990
264. Billings S D, Roth L M, Ulbright T M 1999 Microcystic Leydig cell tumors mimicking yolk sac tumor. A report of four cases. Am J Surg Pathol 23: 546–551
265. Minkowitz S, Soloway H, Soscia J 1965 Ossifying interstitial cell tumor of the testis. J Urol 94: 592–595
266. Balsitis M, Sokol M 1990 Ossifying malignant Leydig (interstitial) cell tumour of the testis. Histopathology 16: 597–601
267. Kurman R J, Andrade D, Goebelsmann U 1978 An immunohistological study of steroid localization in Sertoli–Leydig tumors of the ovary and testis. Cancer 42: 1772–1783
268. Ulbright T M, Srigley J R, Hatzianastassiou D K et al. 2002 Leydig cell tumors of the testis with unusual features: adipose differentiation, calcification with ossification, and spindle-shaped tumor cells. Am J Surg Pathol 26: 1424–1433
269. Cheville J C, Sebo T J, Lager D J et al. 1998 Leydig cell tumor of the testis: a clinicopathologic, DNA content and MIB-1 comparison of non-metastasizing and metastasizing tumors. Am J Surg Pathol 22: 1361–1367
270. Gulbahce H E, Lindeland A T, Engel W et al. 1999 Metastatic Leydig cell tumor with sarcomatoid differentiation. Arch Pathol Lab Med 123: 1104–1107
271. Hekimgil M, Altay B, Yakut B D et al. 2001 Leydig cell tumor of the testis: comparison of histopathological and immunohistochemical features of three azoospermic cases and one malignant case. Pathol Int 51: 792–796
272. Amin M B, Young R H, Scully R E 1998 Immunohistochemical profile of Sertoli and Leydig cell tumors of the testis [abstract]. Mod Pathol 11: 76A
273. Iczkowski K A, Bostwick D G, Cheville J C 1998 Inhibin is a sensitive and specific marker for testicular sex cord–stromal tumors. Mod Pathol 11: 774–779
274. McCluggage W G, Shanks J H, Whiteside C et al. 1998 Immunohistochemical study of testicular sex cord–stromal tumors, including staining with anti-inhibin antibody. Am J Surg Pathol 22: 615–619
275. Lugli A, Forster Y, Haas P et al. 2003 Calretinin expression in human normal and neoplastic tissues: a tissue microarray analysis on 5233 tissue samples. Hum Pathol 34: 994–1000
276. McCluggage W G, Maxwell P 2001 Immunohistochemical staining for calretinin is useful in the diagnosis of ovarian sex cord–stromal tumours. Histopathology 38: 403–408
277. Collins D H, Symington T 1964 Sertoli-cell tumor. Br J Urol 36: 52–61
278. Lawrence W D, Young R H, Scully R E 1986 Sex cord-stromal tumor. In: Talerman A, Roth L M (ed) Pathology of the testis and its adnexa. Churchill Livingstone, New York, p 67–92
279. Kaplan G W, Cromie W J, Kelalis P P 1986 Gonadal stromal tumors: a report of the prepubertal testicular tumor registry. J Urol 136: 300–302
280. Zukerberg L R, Young R H, Scully R E 1991 Sclerosing Sertoli cell tumor of the testis: a report of 10 cases. Am J Surg Pathol 15: 829–834
281. Dubois R S, Hoffman W H, Krishnan T H 1982 Feminizing sex cord tumor with annular tubules in a boy with Peutz–Jeghers syndrome. J Pediatr 101: 568–571
282. Wilson D M, Pitts W C, Hintz R L 1986 Testicular tumors with Peutz–Jeghers syndrome. Cancer 57: 2238–2240
283. Gabrilove J L, Freiberg E K, Leiter E 1980 Feminizing and non-feminizing Sertoli cell tumors. J Urol 124: 757–767
284. Talerman A 1971 Malignant Sertoli cell tumor of the testis. Cancer 28: 446–455
285. Rosvoll R V, Woodard J R 1968 Malignant Sertoli cell tumor of the testis. Cancer 22: 8–13
286. Godec C R 1985 Malignant Sertoli cell tumor of testicle. Urology 26: 185–188
287. Gilcrease M Z, Delgado R, Albores-Saavedra J 1998 Testicular Sertoli cell tumor with a heterologous sarcomatous component: immunohistochemical assessment of Sertoli cell differentiation. Arch Pathol Lab Med 122: 907–911
288. Henley J D, Young R H, Ulbright T M 2002 Malignant Sertoli cell tumors of the testis. A study of 13 examples of a neoplasm frequently misinterpreted as seminoma. Am J Surg Pathol 26: 541–550
289. Young R H, Koelliker D D, Scully R E 1998 Sertoli cell tumors of the testis, not otherwise specified. A clinicopathologic analysis of 60 cases. Am J Surg Pathol 22: 709–721
290. Nielsen K, Jacobsen G K 1988 Malignant Sertoli cell tumor of the testis: an immunohistochemical study and a review of the literature. APMIS 96: 755–760
291. Rey R, Sabourin J C, Venara M et al. 2000 Anti-Mullerian hormone is a specific marker of Sertoli- and granulosa-cell origin in gonadal tumors. Hum Pathol 31: 1202–1208
292. Gordon M D, Corless C, Renshaw A A et al. 1998 CD99, keratin, and vimentin staining of sex cord–stromal tumors, normal ovary, and testis. Mod Pathol 11: 769–773
293. Proppe K H, Scully R E 1980 Large-cell calcifying Sertoli cell tumor of the testis. Am J Clin Pathol 74: 607–619
294. Tetu B, Ro J Y, Ayala A G 1991 Large cell calcifying Sertoli cell tumor of the testis: a clinicopathologic, immunohistochemical and ultrastructural study of two cases. Am J Clin Pathol 96: 717–722
295. Chang B, Borer J G, Tan P E 1998 Large cell calcifying Sertoli cell tumor of the testis: case report and review of the literature. Urology 52: 520–522
296. De Raeve H, Schoonooghe P, Wibowo R et al. 2003 Malignant large cell calcifying Sertoli cell tumor of the testis. Pathol Res Pract 199: 113–117
297. Kratzer S S, Ulbright T M, Talerman A 1997 Large cell calcifying Sertoli cell tumor of the testis: contrasting features of six malignant and six benign tumors and a review of the literature. Am J Surg Pathol 21: 1271–1280
298. Waxman M, Damjanov I, Khapra A 1984 Large cell calcifying Sertoli cell tumor of testis: light microscopic and ultrastructural study. Cancer 54: 1574–1581
299. Proppe K H, Dickersin G R 1982 Large-cell calcifying Sertoli cell tumor of the testis: light microscopic and ultrastructural study. Hum Pathol 13: 1109–1114
300. Venara M, Rey R, Bergada I et al. 2001 Sertoli cell proliferations of the infantile testis: an intratubular form of Sertoli cell tumor? Am J Surg Pathol 125: 1237–1244
301. Horn T, Jao W, Keh P C 1983 Large-cell calcifying Sertoli cell tumor of the testis: a case report with ultrastructural study. Ultrastruct Pathol 4: 359–364
302. Perez-Atayde A R, Nunez A E, Carroll W L 1983 Large-cell calcifying Sertoli cell tumor of the testis: an ultrastructural, immunocytochemical, and biochemical study. Cancer 51: 2287–2292
303. Adesokan A, Adegboyega P A, Cowan D F et al. 1997 Testicular "tumor" of the adrenogenital syndrome: a case report of an unusual association with myelolipoma and seminoma in cryptorchidism. Cancer 80: 2117–2120
304. Tanaka Y, Carney J A, Ijiri R et al. 2002 Utility of immunostaining for S-100 protein subunits in gonadal sex cord–stromal tumors, with emphasis on the large-cell calcifying Sertoli cell tumor of the testis. Hum Pathol 33: 285–289
305. Lawrence W D, Young R H, Scully R E 1985 Juvenile granulosa cell tumor of the infantile testis: a report of 14 cases. Am J Surg Pathol 9: 87–94
306. Raju U, Fine G, Warrier R 1986 Congenital testicular juvenile granulosa cell tumor in a neonate with X/XY mosaicism. Am J Surg Pathol 10: 577–583
307. Crump W D 1983 Juvenile granulosa cell (sex-cord–stromal) tumor of fetal testis. J Urol 129: 1057–1058
308. Mostofi F K, Theiss E A, Ashley D J B 1959 Tumors of specialized gonadal stroma in human male subjects. Cancer 12: 944–957
309. Young R H, Lawrence W D, Scully R E 1985 Juvenile granulosa cell tumor: another neoplasm associated with abnormal chromosomes and ambiguous genitalia: a report of three cases. Am J Surg Pathol 9: 737–743
310. Harms D, Kock L R 1997 Testicular juvenile granulosa cell and Sertoli cell tumours: a clinicopathologic study of 29 cases from the Kiel Paediatric Tumor Registry. Virchows Arch 430: 301–309
311. Jimenez-Quintero L P, Ro J Y, Zavala-Pompa A 1993 Granulosa cell tumor of the adult testis: a clinicopathologic study of seven cases and a review of the literature. Hum Pathol 24: 1120–1125
312. Matoska J, Ondrus D, Talerman A 1992 Malignant granulosa cell tumor of the testis associated with gynecomastia and long survival. Cancer 69: 1769–1772
313. Groisman F M, Dische M R, Fine E M et al. 1993 Juvenile granulosa cell tumor of the testis: a comparative immunohistochemical study with normal infantile gonads. Pediatr Pathol 13: 389–400
314. Talerman A 1985 Pure granulosa cell tumour of the testis: report of a case and review of the literature. Appl Pathol 3: 117–122
315. Gaylis F D, August C, Yeldandi A 1989 Granulosa cell tumor of the adult testis: ultrastructural and ultrasonographic characteristics. J Urol 141: 126–127
316. Nistal M, Lazaro R, Garcia J et al. 1992 Testicular granulosa cell tumor of the adult type. Arch Pathol Lab Med 115: 284–287
317. Al-Bozom I A, El-Faqih S R, Hassan S H et al. 2000 Granulosa cell tumor of the adult type: a case report and review of the literature of a very rare testicular tumor. Arch Pathol Lab Med 124: 1525–1528
318. Renshaw A A, Gordon M, Corless C L 1997 Immunohistochemistry of unclassified sex cord-stromal tumors of the testis with a predominance of spindle cells. Mod Pathol 10: 693–700
319. Nistal M, Puras A, Perna C et al. 1996 Fusocellular gonadal stromal tumour of the testis with epithelial and myoid differentiation. Histopathology 29: 259–264
320. Jones M A, Young R H, Scully R E 1997 Benign fibromatous tumors of the testis and paratesticular region: a report of 9 cases with proposed classification of fibromatous tumors and tumor-like lesions. Am J Surg Pathol 21: 296–305
321. Deveci M S, Deveci G, Onguru O et al. 2002 Testicular (gonadal stromal) fibroma: case report and review of the literature. Pathol Int 52: 326–330
322. Gohji K, Higuchi A, Fujii A et al. 1994 Malignant gonadal stromal tumor. Urology 43: 244–247
323. Eble J N, Hull M T, Warfel K A et al. 1984 Malignant sex cord–stromal tumor of testis. J Urol 131: 546–550

324. Campbell C M, Middleton A W J 1981 Malignant gonadal stromal tumor: case report and review of the literature. J Urol 125: 257–259
325. Oosterhuis J W, Castedo S M, de Jong B 1989 A malignant mixed gonadal stromal tumor of the testis with heterologous components and i (12p) in one of its metastases. Cancer Genet Cytogenet 41: 105–114
326. Luk I S, Shek T W, Tang V W et al. 1999 Interdigitating dendritic cell tumor of the testis: a novel testicular spindle cell neoplasm. Am J Surg Pathol 23: 1141–1148
327. Rutgers J L, Young R H, Scully R E 1988 The testicular "tumor" of the adrenogenital syndrome: a report of six cases and review of the literature on testicular masses in patients with adrenocortical disorders. Am J Surg Pathol 12: 503–513
328. Fore W W, Bledsoe T, Weber D M et al. 1972 Cortisol production by testicular tumors in adrenogenital syndrome. Arch Intern Med 130: 59–63
329. Kirkland R T, Kirkland J L, Keenan B S et al. 1977 Bilateral testicular tumors in congenital adrenal hyperplasia. J Clin Endocrinol Metab 44: 369–378
330. Davis J M, Woodroof J, Sadasivan R et al. 1995 Case report: congenital adrenal hyperplasia and malignant Leydig cell tumor. Am J Med Sci 309: 63–65
331. Sussman E B, Hajdu S I, Lieberman P H 1977 Malignant lymphoma of the testis: a clinicopathologic study of 37 cases. J Urol 118: 1004–1007
332. Talerman A 1977 Primary malignant lymphoma of the testis. J Urol 118: 783–786
333. Ferry J A, Harris N L, Young R H 1994 Malignant lymphoma of the testis, epididymis, and spermatic cord. A clinicopathologic study of 69 cases with immunophenotypic analysis. Am J Surg Pathol 18: 376–390
334. Baldetorp L A, Brunkvall J, Cavallin-Stahl E 1984 Malignant lymphoma of the testis. Br J Urol 56: 525–530
335. Wilkins B S, Williamson J M, O'Brien C J 1989 Morphological and immunohistological study of testicular lymphomas. Histopathology 15: 147–156
336. Paladugu R R, Bearman R M, Rappaport H 1980 Malignant lymphoma with primary manifestation in the gonad. A clinicopathologic study of 38 patients. Cancer 45: 561–571
337. Lagrange J L, Ramaioli A, Theodore C H 2001 Non-Hodgkin's lymphoma of the testis: a retrospective study of 84 patients treated in the French anticancer centres. Ann Oncol 12: 1313–1319
338. Zucca E, Conconi A, Mughal T I 2003 Patterns of outcome and prognostic factors in primary large-cell lymphoma of the testis in a survey by the International Extranodal Lymphoma Study Group. J Clin Oncol 21: 20–27
339. Visco C, Medeiros L J, Mesina O M et al. 2001 Non-Hodgkin's lymphoma affecting the testis: is it curable with doxorubicin-based therapy? Clin Lymphoma 2: 40–46
340. Pileri S A, Sabattini E, Rosito P 2002 Primary follicular lymphoma of the testis in childhood: an entity with peculiar clinical and molecular characteristics. J Clin Pathol 55: 684–688
341. Akhtar M, Al-Dayel F, Siegrist K et al. 1996 Neutrophil-rich Ki-1 positive anaplastic large cell lymphoma presenting as a testicular mass. Mod Pathol 9: 812–815
342. Chan J K, Tsang W Y, Lau W H 1996 Aggressive T/natural killer cell lymphoma presenting as testicular tumor. Cancer 77: 1198–1205
343. Ng S B, Lai K W, Murugaya S et al. 2004 Nasal-type extranodal natural killer/T-cell lymphomas: a clinicopathologic and genotypic study of 42 cases in Singapore. Mod Pathol 17: 1097–1107
344. Ko Y H, Cho E Y, Kim J E et al. 2004 NK and NK-like T-cell lymphoma in extranasal sites: a comparative clinicopathological study according to site and EBV status. Histopathology 44: 480–489
345. Heller K N, Teruya-Feldstein J, La Quaglia M P et al. 2004 Primary follicular lymphoma of the testis: excellent outcome following surgical resection without adjuvant chemotherapy. Pediatr Hematol Oncol 26: 104–107
346. Kim Y B, Chang S K, Yang W I et al. 2003 Primary NK/T cell lymphoma of the testis. A case report and review of the literature. Acta Haematol 109: 95–100
347. van Droogenbroeck J, Altintas S, Pollefliet C et al. 2001 Intravascular large B-cell lymphoma or intravascular lymphomatosis: report of a case diagnosed by testicle biopsy. Ann Hematol 80: 316–318
348. Pakzad K, MacLennan G T, Elder J S et al. 2002 Follicular large cell lymphoma localized to the testis in children. J Urol 168: 225–258
349. Moller M B, d'Amore F, Christensen B E 1994 Testicular lymphoma: a population-based study of incidence, clinicopathological correlations and prognosis. The Danish Lymphoma Study Group. LYFO. Eur J Cancer 30A: 1760–1764
350. Lu D, Medeiros L J, Eskenazi A E et al. 2001 Primary follicular large cell lymphoma of the testis in a child. Arch Pathol Lab Med 125: 551–554
351. Doll D C, Weiss R B 1986 Malignant lymphoma of the testis. Am J Med 81: 515–524
352. Pectasides D, Economopoulos T, Kouvatseas G 2000 Anthracycline-based chemotherapy of primary non-Hodgkin's lymphoma of the testis. the Hellenic Cooperative oncology group experience. Oncology 58: 286–292
353. Seymour J F, Solomon B, Wolf M M et al. 2001 Primary large-cell non-Hodgkin's lymphoma of the testis: a retrospective analysis of patterns of failure and prognostic factors. Clin Lymphoma 2: 109–115
354. Lagrange J L, Ramaioli A, Theodore C H 2001 Radiation Therapy Group and the Genito-Urinary Group of the French Federation of Cancer Centres. Non-Hodgkin's lymphoma of the testis: a retrospective study of 84 patients treated in the French anticancer centres. Ann Oncol 12: 1313–1319
355. Givler R L 1969 Testicular involvement in leukemia and lymphoma. Cancer 23: 1290–1295
356. Reid H, Marsden H B 1980 Gonadal infiltration in children with leukemia and lymphoma. J Clin Pathol 33: 722–729
357. Miyoshi I, Saito T, Taguchi H et al. 2004 Granulocytic sarcoma of the testis. Br J Haematol 124: 695
358. Askin F B, Land V J, Sullivan M P 1981 Occult testicular leukemia: testicular biopsy at three years continuous complete remission of childhood leukemia. A Southwest Oncology Group Study. Cancer 47: 470–475
359. Eden O B, Hardisty R M, Innes E M 1978 Testicular disease in acute lymphoblastic leukemia in childhood. Report on behalf of the Medical Research Council's working party on leukemia in childhood. Br Med J 1: 334–338
360. Stoffel T J, Nesbit M E, Levitt S H 1975 Extramedullary involvement of the testes in childhood leukemia. Cancer 35: 1203–1211
361. Nesbit M E, Robinson L L, Ortega J A 1980 Testicular relapse in childhood acute lymphoblastic leukemia: association with pretreatment patient characteristics and treatment. Cancer 45: 2009–2016
362. Layfield L J, Hilborne L H, Ljung B M 1988 Use of fine needle aspiration cytology for the diagnosis of testicular relapse in patients with acute lymphoblastic leukemia. J Urol 139: 1020–1022
363. Ferry J A, Srigley J R, Young R H 1997 Granulocytic sarcoma of the testis. A report of two cases of a neoplasm prone to misinterpretation. Mod Pathol 10: 320–325
364. Terzian N, Blumenfrucht M J, Yook C R 1987 Plasmacytoma of the testis. J Urol 137: 745–746
365. Ferry J A, Ulbright T M, Young R H 1996 Anaplastic large cell lymphoma of the testis: a lesion that may be confused with embryonal carcinoma. J Urol Pathol 5: 139–147
366. Levin H S, Mostofi F K 1970 Symptomatic plasmacytoma of the testis. Cancer 25: 1193–1203
367. Suzuki K, Shioji Y, Morita T et al. 2001 Primary testicular plasmacytoma with hydrocele of the testis. Int J Urol 8: 139–140
368. Ramadan A, Naab T, Frederick W et al. 2000 Testicular plasmacytoma in a patient with the acquired immunodeficiency syndrome. Tumori 86: 480–482
369. Anghel G, Petti N, Remotti D et al. 2002 Testicular plasmacytoma: report of a case and review of the literature. Am J Hematol 71: 98–104
370. Cavanna L, Fornari F, Civardi G 1990 Extramedullary plasmacytoma of the testicle: sonographic appearance and ultrasonically guided biopsy. Blut 60: 328–330
371. Chica G, Johnson D E, Ayala A G 1978 Plasmacytoma of testis presenting as primary testicular tumor. Urology 11: 90–92
372. Weitzner S 1969 Metastatic plasma cell myeloma in testis. Report of a case and review of the literature. Rocky Mt Med J 66: 48–50
373. Soumerai S, Gleason E A 1980 Asynchronous plasmacytoma of the stomach and testis. Cancer 45: 396–400
374. Scully R E, Parham A R 1948 Testicular tumors. II. Interstitial cell and miscellaneous neoplasms. Arch Pathol 46: 229–242
375. Haupt H M, Mann R B, Trump D L 1984 Metastatic carcinoma involving the testis: clinical and pathologic distinction from primary testicular neoplasms. Cancer 54: 709–714
376. Tiltman A J 1979 Metastatic tumors in the testis. Histopathology 3: 31–37
377. Almagro U A 1988 Metastatic tumors involving testis. Urology 32: 357–360
378. Meares E M J, Ho T L 1973 Metastatic carcinomas involving the testis: a review. J Urol 109: 653–655
379. Young R H, van Patter H T, Scully R E 1987 Hepatocellular carcinoma metastatic to the testis. Am J Clin Pathol 87: 117–120
380. Ro J Y, Sahin A A, Ayala A G 1990 Lung carcinoma with metastasis to testicular seminoma. Cancer 66: 347–353
381. Salesi N, Fabi A, Di Cocco B et al. 2004 Testis metastasis as an initial manifestation of an occult gastrointestinal cancer. Anticancer Res 24: 1093–1096
382. Ro J Y, Ayala A G, Tetu B 1990 Merkel cell carcinoma metastatic to the testis. Am J Clin Pathol 94: 384–389
383. Dutt N, Bates A W, Baithun S I 2000 Secondary neoplasms of the male genital tract with different patterns of involvement in adults and children. Histopathology 37: 323–331
384. Berdjis C C, Mostofi F K 1977 Carcinoid tumors of the testis. J Urol 118: 777–782
385. Zavala-Pompa A, Ro J Y, El-Naggar A 1993 Primary carcinoid tumor of testis: immunohistochemical, ultrastructural, and DNA flow cytometric study of three cases with a review of the literature. Cancer 72: 1726–1732
386. Kato N, Motoyama T, Kameda N 2003 Primary carcinoid tumor of the testis: immunohistochemical, ultrastructural and FISH analysis with review of the literature. Pathol Int 53: 680–685
387. Finci R, Gunhan O, Celasun B 1987 Carcinoid tumor of undescended testis. J Urol 137: 301–302
388. Mason J C, Belville W D 1986 Primary carcinoid of the testis. Milit Med 151: 497–498
389. Ordonez N G, Ayala A G, Sneige N 1982 Immunohistochemical demonstration of multiple neurohormonal polypeptides in a case of pure testicular carcinoid. Am J Clin Pathol 78: 860–864
390. Wurster K, Brodner O, Rossner J A 1976 A carcinoid occurring in the testis. Virchow's Arch [A] 370: 185–192

391. Reyes A, Moran C A, Suster S et al. 2003 Neuroendocrine carcinomas (carcinoid tumor) of the testis. A clinicopathologic and immunohistochemical study of ten cases. Am J Clin Pathol 120: 182–187
392. Hosking D H, Bowman D M, McMorris S L 1981 Primary carcinoid tumor of the testis with metastases. J Urol 125: 255–256
393. Kaufman J J, Waisman J 1985 Primary carcinoid tumor of testis with metastasis. Urology 25: 534–536
394. Sullivan J L, Packer J T, Bryant M 1981 Primary malignant carcinoid of the testis. Arch Pathol Lab Med 105: 515–517
395. Travis W D, Colby T V, Corrin B 1999 Histological typing of lung and pleural tumours, 3rd edn. Berlin, Germany: Springer-Verlag
396. Bates R J, Perrone T L, Parkhurst E C 1981 Insular carcinoid arising in a mature teratoma of the testis. J Urol 126: 55–56
397. Talerman A, Gratama S, Miranda S 1978 Primary carcinoid tumor of the testis: case report, ultrastructure and review of the literature. Cancer 42: 2696–2706
398. Hartwick R W, Ro J Y, Srigley J R et al. 1991 Adenomatous hyperplasia of the rete testis: a clinicopathologic study of nine cases. Am J Surg Pathol 15: 350–357
399. Ulbright T M, Gersell D J 1991 Rete testis hyperplasia with hyaline globule formation. A lesion simulating yolk sac tumor. Am J Surg Pathol 15: 66–74
400. Nistal M, Garcia-Cabezas M A, Regadera J et al. 2004 Microlithiasis of the epididymis and the rete testis. Am J Surg Pathol 28: 514–522
401. Nistal M, Castillo M C, Regadera J et al. 2003 Adenomatous hyperplasia of the rete testis. A review and report of new cases. Histopathology 18: 741–752
402. Uguz A, Gonlusen G, Ergin M et al. 2002 Adenomatous hyperplasia of the rete testis: report of two cases. Int Urol Nephrol 34: 87–89
403. Haas G P, Ohorodnik J M, Farah R N 1987 Cystadenocarcinoma of the rete testis. J Urol 137: 1232–1233
404. Crisp-Lindgren N, Travers H, Wells M M 1988 Papillary adenocarcinoma of rete testis: autopsy findings, histochemistry, immunohistochemistry, ultrastructure, and clinical correlations. Am J Surg Pathol 12: 492–501
405. Sarma D P, Weilbaecher T G 1985 Adenocarcinoma of the rete testis. J Surg Oncol 30: 67–71
406. Nochomovitz L E, Orenstein J M 1984 Adenocarcinoma of the rete testis: case report, ultrastructural observations, and clinicopathologic correlates. Am J Surg Pathol 8: 625–634
407. Ballotta M R, Borghi L, Barucchello G 2000 Adenocarcinoma of the rete testis. Report of three cases. Adv Clin Pathol 4: 169–173
408. Gruber H, Ratschek M, Pummer K et al. 1997 Adenocarcinoma of the rete testis: report of a case with surgical history of adenomatous hyperplasia of the rete testis. J Urol 158: 1525–1526
409. Nochomovitz L E, Orenstein J M 1994 Adenocarcinoma of the rete testis: consolidation and analysis of 31 reported cases with a review of the literature. J Urol Pathol 2: 1–37
410. Visscher D W, Talerman A, Rivera L R 1989 Adenocarcinoma of the rete testis with a spindle cell component: a possible metaplastic carcinoma. Cancer 64: 770–775
411. Shah K H, Maxted W C, Chun B 1981 Epidermoid cysts of the testis: a report of three cases and analysis of 141 cases from the world literature. Cancer 47: 577–582
412. Price E B 1969 Epidermoid cysts of the testis: a clinical and pathologic analysis of 69 cases from the testicular tumor registry. J Urol 102: 708–713
413. Malek R S, Rosen J S, Farrow G M 1986 Epidermoid cyst of the testis: a critical analysis. Br J Urol 58: 55–59
414. Younger C, Ulbright T M, Zhang S et al. 2003 Molecular evidence supporting the neoplastic nature of some epidermoid cysts of the testis. Arch Pathol Lab Med 127: 858–860
415. McClure J 1980 Malakoplakia of the testis and its relationship to granulomatous orchitis. J Clin Pathol 33: 670–678
416. Diaz Gonzalez R, Levina O, Navas Palacias J J 1982 Testicular malakoplakia. J Urol 127: 325–328
417. Paquin F, Schick E, Parent C 1983 Malakoplakia of testis. Urology 21: 194–198
418. Grove J D, Harnden P, Clark P B 1993 Malakoplakia of epididymis associated with testicular infarction. Br J Urol 72: 656–657
419. Damjanov I, Katz S M 1981 Malakoplakia. Pathol Annu 16: 103–126
420. McClure J 1983 Malakoplakia. J Pathol Bacteriol 140: 275–330
421. Dahl E V, Bahn R C 1962 Aberrant adrenal cortical tissue near the testis in human infants. Am J Pathol 40: 587–598
422. Mares A J, Shkolnik A, Sacks M 1980 Aberrant (ectopic) adrenocortical issue along the spermatic cord. J Pediatr Surg 15: 289–292
423. Nelson A A 1939 Accessory adrenal cortical tissue. Arch Pathol 27: 955–965
424. Czaplicki M, Bablock L, Kuzaka B 1985 Heterotopic adrenal tissue. Int Urol Nephrol 17: 177–181
425. Andrews R W, Copeland D D, Fried F A 1985 Splenogonadal fusion. J Urol 133: 1052–1053
426. Ceccacci L, Tosi S 1981 Splenic–gonadal fusion: case report and review of the literature. J Urol 126: 558–559
427. Mendez R, Morrow J W 1969 Ectopic spleen simulating testicular tumor. J Urol 102: 598–601
428. Gouw A S, Elema J D, Bink-Boelkens M T et al. 1985 The spectrum of splenogonadal fusion: case report and review of 84 reported cases. Eur J Pediatr 144: 316–323
429. Pendse A K, Mathur P N, Sharma M M 1975 Splenic–gonadal fusion. Br J Surg 62: 624–628
430. Knorr P A, Borden T A 1994 Splenogonadal fusion. Urology 44: 136–138
431. Imperial S L, Sidhu J S 2002 Non-seminomatous germ cell tumor arising in splenogonadal fusion. Arch Pathol Lab Med 126: 1222–1225
432. Putschar W G, Manion W C 1956 Splenic–gonadal fusion. Am J Pathol 32: 15–34
433. McPherson F, Frias J L, Spicer D et al. 2003 Splenogonadal fusion–limb defect "syndrome" and associated malformations. Am J Med Genet 1: 518–522
434. Glassy F J, Mostofi F K 1956 Spermatic granulomas of the epididymis. Am J Clin Pathol 26: 1303–1313
435. Schmidt S S, Morris R R 1973 Spermatic granuloma: the complication of vasectomy. Fertil Steril 24: 941–947
436. Schmidt S S 1979 Spermatic granuloma: an often painful lesion. Fertil Steril 31: 178–181
437. Boorjian S, Lipkin M, Goldstein M 2004 The impact of obstructive interval and sperm granuloma on outcome of vasectomy reversal. J Urol 171: 304–306
438. Dunner P S, Lipsit E R, Nochomovitz L E 1982 Epididymal sperm granuloma simulating a testicular neoplasm. J Clin Ultrasound 10: 353–355
439. Berg J W 1954 An acid-fast lipid from spermatozoa. Arch Pathol 57: 115–120
440. Baladas H G, Ng B K 1997 Sclerosing lipogranuloma of the scrotum following a laparoscopic herniorraphy and varicocelectomy – a case report. Ann Acad Med Singapore 26: 238–240
441. Bussey L A, Norman R W, Gupta R 2002 Sclerosing lipogranuloma: an unusual scrotal mass. Can J Urol 9: 1464–1469
442. Oertel Y C, Johnson F B 1977 Sclerosing lipogranuloma of male genitalia: review of 23 cases. Arch Pathol Lab Med 101: 321–326
443. Brown A F, Joergensen E J 1974 Genital mammary paraffin oil granulomas in the male. Ann West Med Surg 1: 301–305
444. Smetana H F, Bernhard W 1950 Sclerosing lipogranuloma. Arch Pathol 50: 296–325
445. Marcil-Rojas R A, Colon J E, Figueroa J J 1956 Sclerosing lipogranulomas of the male genitalia: report of one case and review of the literature. J Urol 75: 334–338
446. Ricchiuti V S, Richman M B, Haas C A et al. 2002 Sclerosing lipogranuloma of the testis. Urology 60: 515
447. Benisch B, Peison B, Sobel H J 1981 Fibrous mesotheliomas (pseudofibroma) of the scrotal sac: a light and ultrastructural study. Cancer 47: 731–735
448. Gilchrist K W, Benson R C 1979 Multifocal fibrous pseudotumor of testicular tunics: possible clinical dilemma. Urology 14: 285–287
449. Nistal M, Paniagua R, Torres A 1986 Idiopathic periteticular fibrosis associated with retroperitoneal fibrosis. Eur Urol 12: 64–68
450. Sarlis I, Yakoymakis S, Rebelakos A G 1980 Fibrous pseudotumor of the scrotum. J Urol 124: 742–743
451. Strom G W 1977 Pseudotumor of testicular tunic. J Urol 118: 340
452. Turner W R J, Derrick F C, Sanders P I 1977 Benign lesions of the tunica albuginea. J Urol 117: 602–604
453. Young R H, Scully R E 1986 Miscellaneous neoplasms and non-neoplastic lesions. In: Talerman A, Roth L M (ed) Pathology of the testis. Churchill Livingstone, New York, p 93–130
454. Thompson J E, van der Walt J D 1986 Nodular fibrous proliferation (fibrous pseudotumor) of the tunica vaginalis testis. A light, electron microscopic and immunocytochemical study of a case and review of the literature. Histopathology 10: 741–748
455. Srigley J R, Hartwick R W 1990 Tumors and cysts of the paratesticular region. Pathol Annu 25: 51–108
456. Hollowood K, Fletcher C D M 1992 Pseudosarcomatous myofibroblastic proliferations of the spermatic cord ("proliferative funiculitis"). Histologic and immunohistochemical analysis of a distinctive entity. Am J Surg Pathol 16: 448–454
457. Fetsch J F, Montgomery E A, Meis J M 1993 Calcifying fibrous pseudotumor. Am J Surg Pathol 17: 502–508
458. Seethala R R, Tirkes A T, Weinstein S et al. 2003 Diffuse fibrous pseudotumor of the testicular tunics associated with an inflamed hydrocele. Arch Pathol Lab Med 127: 742–744
459. Oliva E, Young R H 2000 Paratesticular tumor-like lesions. Semin Diagn Pathol 17: 340–358
460. De Klerk D P, Nime F 1975 Adenomatoid tumors (mesothelioma) of testicular and paratesticular tissue. Urology 6: 635–641
461. Viprakasit D, Tannenbaum M, Smith A M 1974 Adenomatoid tumor of the male genital tract. Urology 4: 325–327
462. Williams S B, Han M, Jones R et al. 2004 Adenomatoid tumor of the testes. Urology 63: 779–781
463. Keily E A, Flanagan A, Williams G 1987 Intrascrotal adenomatoid tumors. Br J Urol 60: 255–257
464. Taxy J B, Battifora H, Oyasu R 1974 Adenomatoid tumors. A light microscopic, histochemical, and ultrastructural study. Cancer 34: 306–316
465. Yasuma T, Saito S 1980 Adenomatoid tumor of the male genital tract. A pathological study of eight cases and review of the literature. Acta Pathol Jpn 30: 883–909
466. Skinnider B F, Young R H 2004 Infarcted adenomatoid tumor: a report of five cases of a facet of a benign neoplasm that may cause diagnostic difficulty. Am J Surg Pathol 28: 77–83
467. Mackay B, Bennington J L, Skoglund R W 1971 The adenomatoid tumor. Fine structural evidence for a mesothelial differentiation. Cancer 27: 109–115

468. Delahunt B, Eble J N, King D G et al. 2000 Immunohistochemical evidence for mesothelial origin of paratesticular adenomatoid tumour. Histopathology 36: 109–115
469. Mucientes F, Govindarajan S, Burotto S 1985 Immunoperoxidase study on adenomatoid tumor of the epididymis using anti-mesothelial cell serum. Cancer 55: 363–365
470. Barwick K W, Madri J A 1982 An immunohistochemical study of adenomatoid tumor. Implications for histogenesis. Cancer 50: 931–938
471. Banks E R, Mills S E 1990 Histiocytoid (epithelioid) hemangioma of the testis. The so-called vascular variant of "adenomatoid tumor." Am J Surg Pathol 14: 584–589
472. Calder C J, Gregory J 1993 Papillary cystadenoma of the epididymis: a report of two cases with an immunohistochemical study. Histopathology 23: 89–91
473. Kragel P J, Pestaner J, Travis W D 1993 Papillary cystadenoma of the epididymis: a report of three cases with lectin histochemistry. Arch Pathol Lab Med 114: 672–675
474. Leung S Y, Chan A S, Wong M P et al. 1998 Expression of vascular endothelial growth factor in von Hippel–Lindau syndrome-associated papillary cystadenoma of the epididymis. Hum Pathol 29: 1322–1328
475. Goldman R L 1970 A Brenner tumor of the testis. Cancer 26: 853–856
476. Ross L 1968 Paratesticular Brenner-like tumor. Cancer 21: 722–726
477. Uzoaru I, Ray V H, Nadimpalli V 1995 Brenner tumor of the testis. Immunohistochemical comparison with its ovarian counterparts. J Urol Pathol 3: 249–253
478. Young R H, Scully R E 1986 Testicular and paratesticular tumors and tumor-like lesions of ovarian common epithelial and Mullerian types. Am J Clin Pathol 86: 146–152
479. Nogales F F J, Matilla A, Ortega I 1979 Mixed Brenner and adenomatoid tumor of the testis. An ultrastructural study and histogenetic considerations. Cancer 43: 539–543
480. Caccamo D, Socias M, Truchet C 1991 Malignant Brenner tumor of the testis and epididymis. Arch Pathol Lab Med 115: 524–527
481. Johnson R E, Scheithauer B W, Dahlin D C 1983 Melanocytic neuroectodermal tumor of infancy. A review of seven cases. Cancer 52: 661–666
482. Ricketts R R, Majmudar B 1985 Epididymal melanotic neuroectodermal tumor of infancy. Hum Pathol 16: 416–420
483. Frank R J, Koten J W 1967 Melanotic hamartoma ("retinal anlage tumor") of the epididymis. J Pathol Bacteriol 93: 549–554
484. Eaton W L, Ferguson J P 1956 Retinoblastic teratoma of the epididymis Case report. Cancer 9: 718–720
485. Cutler L S, Chaudhry A P, Topazian R 1981 Melanotic neuroectodermal tumor of infancy. An ultrastructural study, literature review and reevaluation. Cancer 48: 257–270
486. Zone R M 1970 Retinal anlage tumor of the epididymis. A case report. J Urol 103: 106–107
487. Pettinato G, Manivel J C, d'Amore E S 1991 Melanotic neuroectodermal tumor of infancy. A reevaluation of a histogenetic problem based on immunohistochemical, flow cytometric, and ultrastructural study of 10 cases. Am J Surg Pathol 15: 233–345
488. Henley J D, Ferry J, Ulbright T M 2000 Miscellaneous rare paratesticular tumors. Semin Diagn Pathol 17: 319–339
489. Toda T, Sadi A M, Kiyuna M et al. 1998 Pigmented neuroectodermal tumor of infancy in the epididymis. A case report. Acta Cytol 42: 775–780
490. Kobayashi T, Kunimi K, Imao T et al. 1996 Melanotic neuroectodermal tumor of infancy in the epididymis. Case report and literature review. Urol Int 57: 262–265
491. Calabrese F, Danieli D, Valente M 1995 Melanotic neuroectodermal tumor of the epididymis in infancy: case report and review of the literature. Urology 46: 415–418
492. Diamond D A, Breitfeld P P, Bur M et al. 1992 Melanotic neuroectodermal tumor of infancy; an important mimicker of paratesticular rhabdomyosarcoma. J Urol 147: 673–675
493. Jones M, Young R H, Srigley J R et al. 1995 Paratesticular serous papillary carcinoma. A report of six cases. Am J Surg Pathol 19: 1359–1366
494. Kernohan N M, Coutts A G, Best P V 1990 Cystadenocarcinoma of the appendix testis. Histopathology 17: 147–154
495. Remmele W, Kaiserling E, Zerban U 1992 Serous papillary cystic tumor of borderline malignancy with focal carcinoma arising in testis: case report with immunohistochemical and ultrastructural observations. Hum Pathol 23: 75–79
496. Axiotis C A 1988 Intratesticular serous papillary cystadenoma of low malignant potential: an ultrastructural and immunohistochemical study suggesting Mullerian differentiation. Am J Surg Pathol 12: 56–63
497. Blumberg H M, Hendrix L E 1991 Serous papillary adenocarcinoma of the tunica vaginalis of the testis with metastasis. Cancer 67: 1450–1453
498. Tulunay O, Gogus C, Baltaci S et al. 2004 Clear cell adenocarcinoma of the tunica vaginalis of the testis with an adjacent uterus-like tissue. Pathol Int 54: 641–647
499. Ulbright T M, Young R H 2003 Primary mucinous tumors of the testis and paratestis: a report of nine cases. Am J Surg Pathol 27: 1221–1228
500. Shinmura Y, Yokoi T, Tsutsui Y 2002 A case of clear cell adenocarcinoma of the mullerian duct in persistent mullerian duct syndrome: the first reported case. Am J Surg Pathol 126: 1231–1234
501. McClure R F, Keeney G L, Sebo T J et al. 2001 Serous borderline tumor of the paratestis: a report of seven cases. Am J Surg Pathol 25: 373–378
502. Jones M A, Young R H, Scully R E 1997 Adenocarcinoma of the epididymis. A report of four cases and review of the literature. Am J Surg Pathol 21: 1474–1480
503. Folpe A L, Weiss S W 2000 Paratesticular soft tissue neoplasms. Semin Diagn Pathol 17: 307–318
504. Tanda F, Rocca P C, Bosincu L et al. 1997 Rhabdomyoma of the tunica vaginalis of the testis: a histologic, immunohistochemical, and ultrastructural study. Mod Pathol 10: 608–611
505. Wehner M S, Humphreys J L, Sharkey F E 2000 Epididymal rhabdomyoma: report of a case, including histologic and immunohistochemical findings. Arch Pathol Lab Med 124: 1518–1519
506. Iezzoni J C, Fechner R E, Wong L S et al. 1995 Aggressive angiomyxoma in males. A report of four cases. Am J Clin Pathol 104: 391–396
507. Tsang W Y, Chan J K, Lee K C et al. 1992 Aggressive angiomyxoma. A report of four cases occurring in men. Am J Surg Pathol 16: 1059–1065
508. Laskin W B, Fetsch J F, Mostofi F K 1998 Angiomyofibroblastoma-like tumor of the male genital tract: analysis of 11 cases with comparison to female angiomyofibroblastoma and spindle cell lipoma. Am J Surg Pathol 22: 6–16
509. Ockner D M, Sayadi H, Swanson P E et al. 1997 Genital angiomyofibroblastoma. Comparison with aggressive angiomyxoma and other myxoid neoplasms of skin and soft tissue. Am J Clin Pathol 107: 36–44
510. Iwasa Y, Fletcher C D M 2004 Cellular angiofibroma: clinicopathologic and immunohistochemical analysis of 51 cases. Am J Surg Pathol 28: 1426–1435
511. Barton J H, Davis C J J, Sesterhenn I A et al. 1999 Smooth muscle hyperplasia of the testicular adnexa clinically mimicking neoplasia: clinicopathologic study of sixteen cases. Am J Surg Pathol 23: 903–909
512. Kikukawa T, Tanji N, Kurihara K et al. 2003 Smooth muscle hyperplasia of the epididymis: a case report. Pathology 35: 454–455
513. Rowlands R D, Nicholson G W 1909 A case of primary squamous-celled epithelioma of the epididymis. Lancet 1: 304–306
514. Shah V I, Ro J Y, Amin M B et al. 1998 Histologic variations in the epididymis: findings in 167 orchiectomy specimens. Am J Surg Pathol 22: 990–996
515. Grove A, Jensen M L, Donna A 1989 Mesotheliomas of the tunica vaginalis testis and hernial sacs. Virchows Arch [A] 415: 283–292
516. Antman K, Cohen S, Dimitrov N V 1984 Malignant mesothelioma of the tunica vaginalis testis. J Clin Oncol 2: 447–451
517. Carp N Z, Peterson R O, Kusiak J F 1990 Malignant mesothelioma of the tunica vaginalis testis. J Urol 144: 1475–1478
518. McDonald R E, Sago A L, Novicki D E 1983 Paratesticular mesotheliomas. J Urol 130: 360–361
519. Nistal M, Revestido R, Paniagua R 1992 Bilateral mucinous cystadenocarcinoma of the testis and epididymis. Arch Pathol Lab Med 116: 1160–1163
520. Chen K T, Arhelger R B, Flam M S 1982 Malignant mesothelioma of tunica vaginalis testis. Urology 20: 316–319
521. Eimoto T, Inoue I 1977 Malignant fibrous mesothelioma of the tunica vaginalis. A histologic and ultrastructural study. Cancer 39: 2059–2066
522. Fitzmaurice H, Hotiana M Z, Crucioli V 1987 Malignant mesothelioma of the tunica vaginalis testis. Br J Urol 60: 184
523. Abe K, Kato N, Miki K et al. 2002 Malignant mesothelioma of testicular tunica vaginalis. Int J Urol 9: 602–603
524. Khan M A, Puri P, Devaney D 1997 Mesothelioma of tunica vaginalis testis in a child. J Urol 158: 198–199
525. Fligiel Z, Kaneko M 1976 Malignant mesothelioma of the tunica vaginalis propria testis in a patient with asbestos exposure. A case report. Cancer 37: 1478–1484
526. Kamiya M, Eimoto T 1990 Malignant mesothelioma of the tunica vaginalis. Pathol Res Pract 186: 680–684
527. Linn R, Moskovitz B, Bolkier M 1988 Paratesticular papillary mesothelioma. Urol Int 43: 60–61
528. Jones M A, Young R H, Scully R E 1995 Malignant mesothelioma of the tunica vaginalis. A clinicopathological analysis of 11 cases with review of the literature. Am J Surg Pathol 19: 815–825
529. Sawada K, Inoue K, Ishihara T et al. 2004 Multicystic malignant mesothelioma of the tunica vaginalis with an unusually indolent clinical course. Hinyokika Kiyo 50: 511–513
530. Galateau-Salle F, Vignaud J M, Burke L et al. 2004 Well-differentiated papillary mesothelioma of the pleura: a series of 24 cases. Am J Surg Pathol 28: 534–540
531. Churg A 2003 Paratesticular mesothelial proliferations. Semin Diagn Pathol 20: 272–278
531a. Winstanley A M, Landon G, Berney D et al. 2006 The immunohistochemical profile of malignant mesotheliomas of the tunica vaginalis: a study of 20 cases. Am J Surg Pathol 30: 1–6
532. Arlen M, Grabstald H, Whitmore W F J 1969 Malignant tumors of the spermatic cord. Cancer 23: 525–532
533. Loughlin K R, Retik A B, Weinstein H J 1989 Genitourinary rhabdomyosarcoma in children. Cancer 63: 1600–1606
534. Cecchetto G, Grotto G, De Bernardi P 1988 Paratesticular rhabdomyosarcoma in childhood: experience of the Italian Cooperative Study. Tumori 74: 645–647
535. Fortune A, Bolton B R 1981 Rhabdomyosarcoma of the paratesticular tissues. J Urol 126: 563–564

536. Arean V M, Kreager J A 1965 Paratesticular rhabdomyosarcoma. Am J Clin Pathol 43: 418–427
537. Kattan J, Culine S, Terrier-Lacombe M J et al. 1993 Paratesticular rhabdomyosarcoma in adult patients: 16-year experience at Institut Gustave-Roussy. Ann Oncol 4: 871–875
538. Kumar P V, Khezri A A 1987 Pure testicular rhabdomyosarcoma. Br J Urol 59: 282
539. Leuschner I, Newton W A, Schmidt D 1993 Spindle cell variant of embryonal rhabdomyosarcoma in the paratesticular region: a report of the Intergroup Rhabdomyosarcoma Study. Am J Surg Pathol 17: 221–230
540. Cavazzana A O, Schmidt D, Ninfo V 1992 Spindle cell rhabdomyosarcoma. A prognostically favorable variant of rhabdomyosarcoma. Am J Surg Pathol 16: 229–235
541. Ferrari A, Bisogno G, Casanova M et al. 2002 Paratesticular rhabdomyosarcoma: report from the Italian and German Cooperative Group. J Clin Oncol 20: 449–455
542. Ferrari A, Casanova M, Massimino M et al. 1998 The management of paratesticular rhabdomyosarcoma: a single institutional experience with 44 consecutive children. J Urol 159: 1031–1034
543. Ferrari A, Bisogno G, Casanova M et al. 2004 Is alveolar histotype a prognostic factor in paratesticular rhabdomyosarcoma? The experience of Italian and German Soft Tissue Sarcoma Cooperative Group. Pediatr Blood Cancer 42: 134–138
544. Fleischmann J, Perinetti E P, Catalona W J 1981 Embryonal rhabdomyosarcoma of the genitourinary organs. J Urol 126: 389–392
545. Olive D, Flamat F, Zucker J M 1984 Paraaortic lymphadenectomy is not necessary in the treatment of localized paratesticular rhabdomyosarcoma. Cancer 54: 1283–1287
546. Kinjo M, Hokamura K, Tanaka K 1986 Leiomyosarcoma of the spermatic cord. A case report and review of the literature. Acta Pathol Jpn 36: 929–934
547. Soosay G N, Parkinson M C, Paradinas J et al. 1996 Paratesticular sarcomas revisited: a review of cases in the British Testicular Tumour Registry. Br J Urol 77: 143–146
548. Yashia P, Ausleaender L 1989 Primary leiomyosarcoma of the testis. J Urol 141: 955–956
549. Fisher C, Goldblum J R, Epstein J I et al. 2001 Leiomyosarcoma of the paratesticular region: a clinicopathologic study. Am J Surg Pathol 25: 1143–1149
550. Ptochos A, Iosifidis N, Papazafiriou G et al. 2003 Primary paratesticular epithelioid leiomyosarcoma. Urol Int 70: 321–323
551. Berkmen F, Celebioglu A S 1997 Adult genitourinary sarcomas: a report of seventeen cases and review of the literature. J Exp Clin Cancer Res 16: 45–48
552. Montgomery E, Fisher C 2003 Paratesticular liposarcoma: a clinicopathologic study. Am J Surg Pathol 27: 40–47
553. Ozkara H, Ozkan B, Alici B et al. 2004 Recurrent paratesticular myxoid liposarcoma in a young man. J Urol 171: 343
554. Kalyvas K D, Kotakidou R, Trantos A et al. 2004 Paratesticular well-differentiated, adipocytic type liposarcoma presenting as inguinal hernia. Urol Int 72: 264–268
555. Schwartz S L, Swierzewski S Jr, Sondak V K et al. 1995 Liposarcoma of the spermatic cord: report of 6 cases and review of the literature. J Urol 153: 154–157
556. Vallat-Decouvelaere W, Dry S M, Fletcher C D M 1998 Atypical and malignant solitary fibrous tumors in extrathoracic locations. Am J Surg Pathol 22: 1501–1511
557. Salamanca J, Rodriguez-Peralto J L, Azorin D et al. 2004 Paratesticular congenital malignant rhabdoid tumor diagnosed by fine-needle aspiration cytology. A case report. Diagn Cytopathol 30: 46–50
558. Kawanishi Y, Tamura M, Akiyama K 1989 Rhabdoid tumors of the spermatic cord. Br J Urol 63: 439–440

第三部分

阴茎和阴囊
Penis and scrotum

Jae Y. Ro、Mahul B. Amin、Kyu-Rae Kim、Alberto G. Ayala 著

李连宏 译

阴茎和阴囊		鳞状细胞癌的变异型	869
各种良性病变	861	腺鳞状细胞癌和其他罕见癌	872
肿瘤性病变	864	基底细胞癌	873
癌前病变	864	恶性黑色素瘤	873
良性肿瘤	866	肉瘤	873
恶性肿瘤	867	转移性肿瘤	873
鳞状细胞癌	867	**阴囊肿瘤和肿瘤性病变**	874

各种良性病变
Miscellaneous benign lesions

湿疣　Condyloma

湿疣是阴茎最常见的肿瘤性病变，由人类乳头状瘤病毒引起。湿疣通常见于年轻成人，在过去20年间，人类乳头状瘤病毒在年轻人中的感染率达到了流行的程度[1,2]。据报告在20～40岁的成人中湿疣的发病率大约为5%[3,4]。本病绝大多数是通过性传播的，男性的性伴侣如果患有HPV相关性宫颈病变，其阴茎湿疣的发病率高于平均水平[5]。当生殖道湿疣见于儿童时，应该怀疑性虐待的可能[6]。初次感染之后，常见自体感染。阴茎湿疣的潜伏期从数周到数月不等，甚至可达数年[7]。

这些病变最常见于阴茎头冠、舟状窝或阴茎开口处，也可见于阴囊皮肤或会阴（图14C.1）[7]。肉眼，湿疣为扁平或乳头状菜花样病变。镜下，主要是以成熟鳞状上皮增生为特征的鳞状上皮乳头状瘤。常常伴随的表现是角化过度、角化不全以及挖空细胞形成（图14C.2）[8]。普通的阴茎湿疣细胞学非典型性轻微，核分裂象局限于基底层。过去曾经认为，应用鬼臼树脂或激光治疗这些病变可能引起奇异的形态学变化，从而提出恶性的问题[9]。然而，现今有关HPV有不同类型、尤其是存在致癌性HPV的观点表明，非典型性改变很可能是由于病毒类型不同引起的，而与治疗无关。通过原位杂交或免疫组化方法可以检测HPV[10-13]。非异型增生性生殖器疣最常由HPV 6和HPV 11引起，而HPV

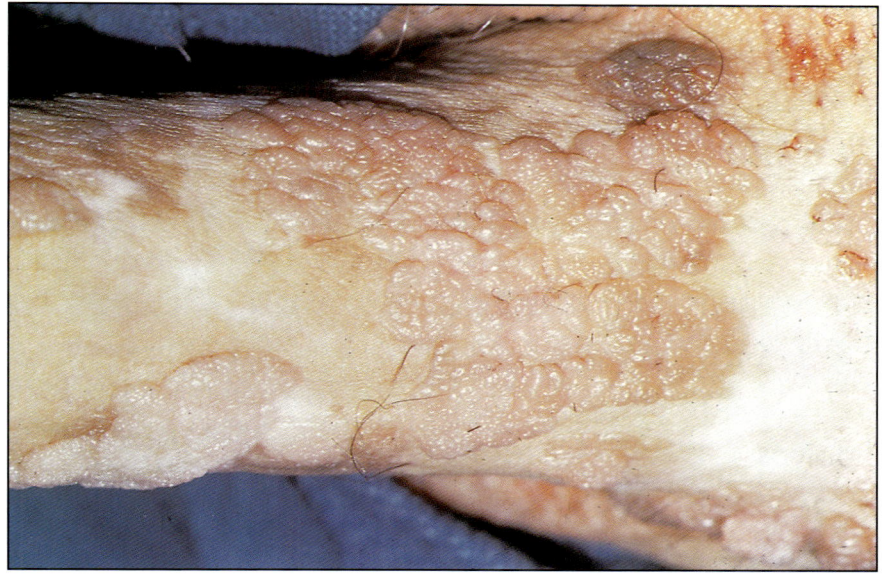

图14C.1　湿疣。阴茎体上可见多发性褐色-白色乳头状病变。

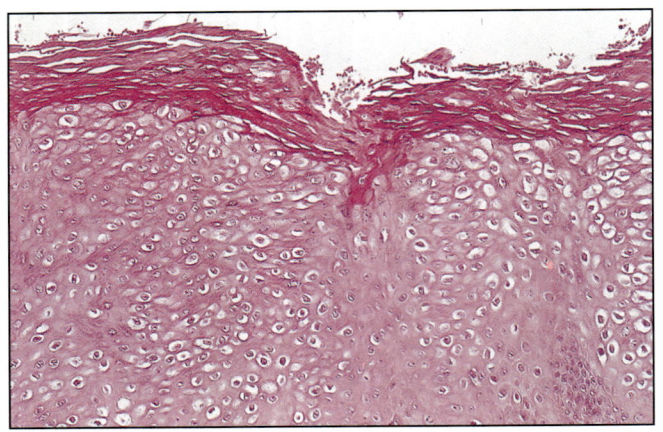

图14C.2 湿疣。高倍镜下显示挖空细胞形成和角化过度。注意缺乏显著的细胞学非典型性和核分裂象。

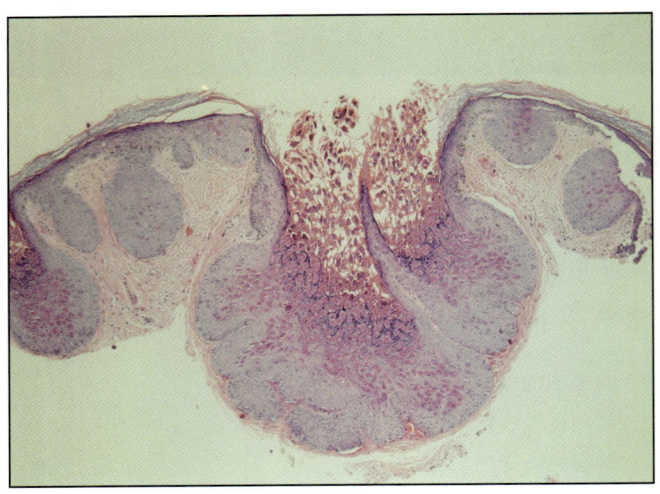

图14C.3 传染性软疣，可见许多球形软疣小体。

16和HPV 18常常与异型增生性湿疣有关[10-12]。虽然湿疣可以自行消退，但大约50%的受累病人病变持续存在。本病通常通过局部应用鬼臼树脂或激光进行治疗，绝大多数患者治疗有效[13]。

传染性软疣　Molluscum contagiosum

传染性软疣是一种相当常见的假瘤性病变，由传染性软疣病毒引起的，这种病毒是一种大的砖形DNA痘病毒。阴茎局限性淋巴管瘤（lymphangioma circumscriptum）罕见，仅见5例报道，临床上可能和传染性软疣相似[14]。

传染性软疣通常发生于儿童、青少年、年轻成人以及免疫损害的病人 [包括获得性免疫缺陷综合征（AIDS）病人]。在免疫损害病人中，病灶可达数百个，且不易消退。

组织学上，最具特征性的低倍镜下表现为棘层增厚的表皮杯状内陷进入真皮（图14C.3）[15]。病变并不累及基底层，但是表皮生发层细胞胞浆内出现包涵体，包涵体随着接近表面而进行性增大。这种包涵体被称为软疣小体（Henderson-Patterson小体），内含病毒颗粒。软疣小体开始为嗜酸性，当其逐渐增大并取代细胞核时变为嗜碱性且颗粒化。角质层最终破裂，并从中心破裂口释放出软疣小体。其下真皮通常缺乏显著的炎症，除非软疣小体和表皮成分破裂进入真皮。

绝大多数病变在6～12个月内自行消退，但仍需治疗以免自体接种和传染他人。治疗措施包括刮除术、应用鬼臼树脂、硝酸银或激光汽化疗法。

纤维上皮性息肉　Fibroepithelial polyps

阴茎纤维上皮性息肉十分少见，通常表现为一个息肉样或菜花样肿物，或为累及龟头或包皮的多个肿物[16,17]。息肉最大径从小于1cm到7.5cm不等，与长期应用避孕套导管（condom catheter）显著相关，在个别情况下，其发生可能与包茎有关。病人首次手术切除的年龄从4岁到58岁不等（中位年龄40岁），术前病程为6个月到10年。多数病变累及龟头腹侧，接近尿道口。

组织学检查，病变具有息肉样结构，被覆角化鳞状上皮。上皮下间质显著水肿，伴有原先存在的血管毛细血管扩张，而且在许多情况下，可见局灶性轻度小血管增生。间质细胞构成轻到中度增加，伴有单核和多核间叶细胞。常常可见轻度炎症浸润。免疫组织化学检查显示间质细胞免疫反应局限于肌肉特异性肌动蛋白（muscle-specific actin）、α-平滑肌肌动蛋白（α-SMA）和结蛋白（desmin），而S-100蛋白或CD34阴性。在所有的情况下，外科干预都应采用局部切除。虽然这些病变可能复发，但是复发病例仍可通过局部切除进行治疗[16]。

珍珠样乳头状瘤　Hirsutoid papillomas

珍珠样乳头状瘤，也叫做珍珠样阴茎丘疹（pearly penile papules），是一种常见的阴茎病变，没有临床意义，可见于大约20%～30%的正常男性[18]。珍珠样乳头状瘤很可能是交媾器官的胚胎性残留，这种交媾器官在其他哺乳动物中发育良好。特征性病变为黄白色丘疹（直径1～3 mm），通常位于阴茎冠，或偶尔见于阴茎系带处[19]。单个病变为圆顶状，类似于毛囊，通常排列成行。

组织学上，上皮增厚，伴有纤维血管轴心[血管纤维瘤（angiofibroma）][20]。因为珍珠样乳头状瘤与感染因子无关，而且没有恶变潜能，所以无需治疗。

阴茎囊肿　Penile cysts

在阴茎囊肿中表皮包涵囊肿（epidermal inclusion cyst）常见，通常见于阴茎体；囊肿直径通常从 1 mm 到 1 cm 不等，大的囊肿虽然少见，但有报道[21,.22]。阴茎黏液样囊肿（mucoid cyst）起源于异位尿道黏膜[23]。这些囊肿内含大量黏液样物质，内衬伴有黏液细胞的复层柱状上皮。一般位于包皮或龟头，多为单房性，大小从 2 mm 到 2 cm 不等。

中缝囊肿（median raphe cysts）是生殖道胚胎发育过程中的发育缺陷，可能是由生殖皱襞关闭不全引起的。组织学检查，囊肿内衬假复层柱状上皮。可能是单房性或为多房性[21,24,.25]。

Peyronie病　Peyronie's disease

Peyronie 病（也叫做阴茎海绵体硬结症、阴茎纤维硬化病和纤维性海绵体炎）表现为阴茎勃起疼痛伴有变形、弯曲和勃起紧绷感。虽然早在 1743 年就发现了本病，但其病因仍不清楚[26]。一些学者认为 Peyronie 病可能与纤维瘤病有关，因为大约 10% 的病人伴有其他形式的纤维瘤病，例如 Dupuytren 挛缩或掌跖纤维瘤病[26]。另外有人推测，本病是由继发于尿道炎的炎症/纤维性反应引起的。发生 Peyronie 病的其他致病因素包括反复的机械性损伤、高血压、糖尿病和免疫反应[27-30]。虽然较早的研究提示，特殊类型的人类白细胞抗原（human leukocyte antigen, HLA）可能与本病的发生有关，但是后来的研究并没有发现二者有关[30]。Bivens 等报道了 6 例伴有类癌综合征的 Peyronie 病病人，提示 5-羟色胺（serotonin）水平升高在本病的发生中可能具有作用[31]。在一项研究中，Guerneri 等[32]发现 14 例 Peyronie 病中 9 例存在染色体结构异常，最常见的是染色体 Y 丢失。

Peyronie 病累及中年或老年男性，在 40 岁以下的人群中很少发病，一般以在阴茎海绵体和白膜之间出现局限纤维组织为特征[26,33]。在勃起阴茎体的背侧常常可以触及质硬的斑块或结节。少数病例形成多发性斑块或可能是弥漫性病变。由于纤维组织没有弹性，导致阴茎在勃起时弯曲变性和疼痛[34]。组织学检查，纤维化是主要所见[26]。根据病变发展的时期不同，可见些许差异[35]。病变早期通常出现炎症细胞成分。晚期病变常常可见玻璃样变，伴有骨或软骨形成区域[26,36]。Peyronie 病的临床经过不同[37]。1/3 的病人病变可能自行消退。放射治疗、注射类固醇或手术切除可以缓解症状。

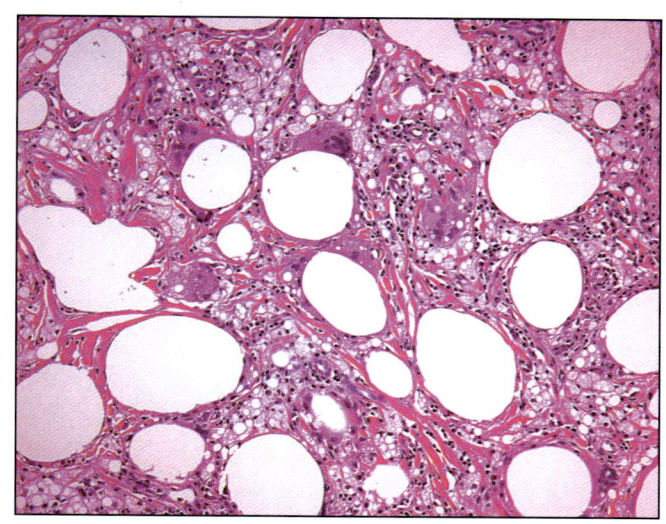

图14C.4　脂肪肉芽肿，可见大小不一的空隙和少数巨细胞。

脂肪肉芽肿（石蜡瘤）Lipogranulomas（paraffinomas）

脂肪肉芽肿几乎总是由于为了增大阴茎而注射异物造成的，例如石蜡、蜡、硅酮或油[38-42]。然而，偶有特发性病例报道[43]。临床上，病变表现为局部硬结，但表面没有变化。如果病人否认曾注射过异物，则诊断将很困难，可能需要活检。镜下检查显示典型的异物肉芽肿性炎症反应，伴有不同大小的埋在致密纤维组织中的脂质空泡（图 14C.4）。通过油红 O 染色可以证实存在脂质。本病应与腺瘤样瘤、脂肪肉瘤、转移癌和淋巴管瘤鉴别。在远东地区，可能将玻璃球植入阴茎以增加对于性伴侣的刺激，这种异物也可引起肉芽肿性反应并形成肿块（Tancho 小结）[44]。

干燥性闭塞性龟头炎（阴茎硬化性苔藓）Balanitis xerotica obliterans（penile lichen sclerosus）

干燥性闭塞性龟头炎是一种不明病因的慢性萎缩性黏膜皮肤病变，累及表皮及真皮结缔组织，最常受累的部位是男性和女性的生殖器和肛周皮肤。生殖器外病变可能伴有生殖器病变，尽管生殖器外病变可能单独存在。硬化性苔藓是龟头及包皮干燥性闭塞性龟头炎的同义词。本病与阴茎癌有关，推测至少是某些类型阴茎癌的癌前病变，尤其是非 HPV 变异型的鳞状细胞癌[45-50]。

干燥性闭塞性龟头炎常在老年男性包茎的包皮切除术中遇到。相反，在 117 例青春期的人群中，仅见 4%

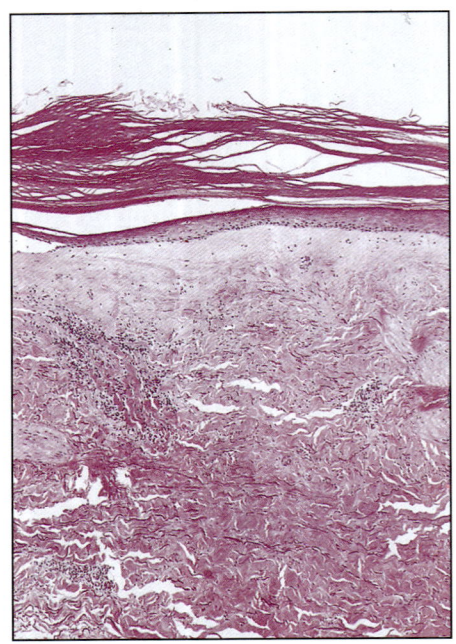

图14C.5 干燥性闭塞性龟头炎，可见表皮变薄、上皮脚变钝和消失以及角化过度。上皮下层胶原化。可见散在的淋巴细胞浸润。

患有本病[51]。特发性干燥性闭塞性龟头炎与包茎无关，而且具有典型的临床及病理学特点。这种典型类型病变的病因还不清楚，可能与自身免疫机制有关[51]。硬化性苔藓病人体内的器官特异性抗体（女性的甲状腺微粒体和壁细胞抗体，男性的平滑肌和壁细胞抗体）可能升高。与白斑病和局限性脱发等自身免疫性疾病有关，进一步证明了自身免疫发病机制在这些病变中可能起着重要作用这一假设。

临床上，病变的特征是累及包皮和龟头的白色丘疹或斑块，可能导致包茎、包皮开口狭窄、尿道口狭窄或裂隙形成。组织学检查显示病变特征类似于外阴硬化性苔藓，包括表皮萎缩、界面皮炎以及真皮水肿和纤维化（图14C.5）。

疣状黄瘤　Verruciform xanthoma

疣状黄瘤是一种疣状病变，病变特点为棘层增厚、角化过度、角化不全和钉突延长，伴有中性粒细胞浸润。上皮钉突之间的真皮有不同数量（常常显著）的黄瘤性细胞浸润（图14C.6）。本病常常为见于口腔的孤立性病变，生殖器（阴囊、阴茎和外阴部位）病变仅有少数报告。疣状黄瘤虽然在结构上与其他HPV感染相关性阴茎黏膜皮肤疣状病变相似，但是这个病变可能并不是HPV相关性阴茎病变。有报道显示黄瘤细胞CK、KP1、Mac387和XIIIa因子局灶弱阳性，而S-100蛋白和HPV免疫染

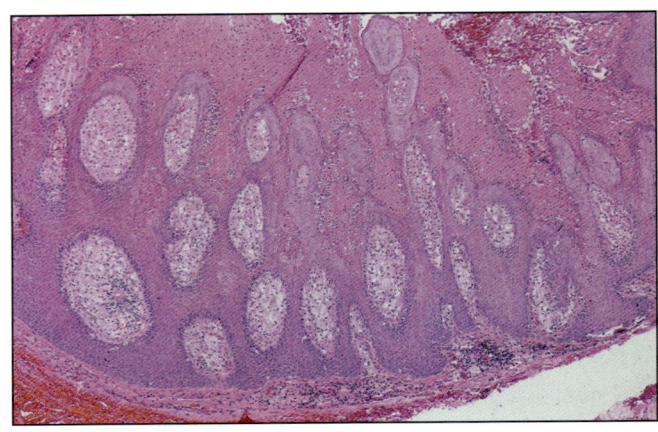

A

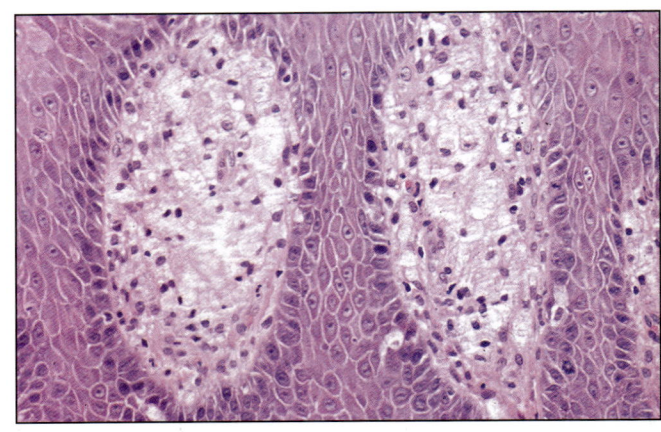

B

图14C.6 （A）疣状黄瘤。图示鳞状上皮增厚，真皮结缔组织可见乳头。（B）高倍镜下，乳头轴心可见许多黄瘤细胞。

色阴性。Mohsin等[52]推测，作为本病组织学标志的黄瘤细胞（泡沫细胞），可能来自皮肤的树突状细胞。

假上皮瘤性层状角化性龟头炎
Pseudoepitheliomatous keratotic and micaceous balanitis

这是一种罕见的龟头层状角化过度性病变[53]。本病最初由Lortat Jacob和Civatte报告[54]，描述为一种罕见的龟头隆起性脱屑性病变，以棘层增厚、角化过度和假上皮瘤性增生为特点。假上皮瘤性层状角化性龟头炎常可复发，可能为疣状癌的前驱病变。

肿瘤性病变　Neoplastic lesions

癌前病变　Premalignant lesions

阴茎癌前上皮内病变的命名是一个有争议的较大

问题。三个术语被用来描述组织学形态相似但临床表现和生物学行为不同的病变，分别为 Queyrat 增殖性红斑（erythroplasia of Queyrat, EQ）、Bowen 病（Bowen's disease, BD）和 Bowen 样丘疹病（Bowenoid papulosis, BP）[55-59]。有人建议可以用高级别阴茎上皮内病变（high-grade penile intraepithelial lesions）这样的术语来代替这三种疾病[56-58,60]。细胞学非典型性程度轻的病变（鳞状上皮增生或异型增生）可以有或没有临床表现，常常见于鳞状细胞癌的周围，证明它们具有癌前潜能[61]。

EQ 由 Queyrat 于 1911 年最先描述，是一种累及龟头和包皮的独特的病变[62]。据报告 EQ 患者年龄分布广泛，通常发生在 40~60 岁的病人。在 Graham 和 Helwig 报道的 100 例病人中，中位年龄为 51 岁[63]。包皮环切术可以预防 EQ 的发生，同样它也可以防止阴茎浸润性鳞状细胞癌的发生（详见浸润性鳞状细胞癌的病因讨论，867 页）。

临床上，Queyrat 增殖性红斑（EQ）表现为有光泽的红色隆起性柔软斑块，位于龟头或包皮[57,58,63,64]。本病有时可累及尿道口、包皮系带或阴茎颈部。半数以上的病人为孤立性病变；然而，也可能发生多发性病变[63]。组织学上，EQ 以鳞状上皮全层异型增生性改变为特征，伴有极性丧失、增生的大而深染的细胞、角化不良、多核细胞以及许多典型和非典型性核分裂象（图 14C.7）。上皮下间质可见带状慢性炎细胞浸润和血管增生。大约 10% 的 EQ 病人发展为浸润性鳞状细胞癌，2% 的 EQ 相关性癌发生远处转移[63]。

EQ 的病因基本上还不清楚。从前仅在极少数的典型病人中检测到 HPV 16 DNA。然而，最近 Wieland 等[65]报道在全部 8 名 EQ 患者中检测到了 HPV DNA，而在患炎性阴茎病变的对照组中没有检测到。尽管在这些病变中检测到了 HPV 8、16、39 和 51，但是在宫颈或外阴的癌前病变和癌中没有发现 HPV 8，在带有生殖器 HPV 类型的 Bowen 病也没有发现 HPV 8。这些资料提示，EQ 不同于其他生殖器肿瘤，存在 HPV 8 和致癌性生殖器 HPV 的共同感染。HPV 8 的存在与否可以帮助鉴别阴茎 EQ 和 BD。

许多不同的疾病可以引起阴茎病变，临床上可能类似于 EQ，包括 Zoon 龟头炎、其他炎症性病变，以及良性皮肤病的阴茎表现，例如药疹、银屑病和扁平苔癣[66]。

Bowen 病　Bowen's disease

Bowen 病（BD）这一术语用于表示一种组织学与 EQ（原位鳞状细胞癌）类似的病变，但这种病变累及阴茎体，或肉眼不像 EQ 那样发红[57,58,67,68]。BD 最常发生于 30~50 岁的病人，其发病年龄比 EQ 病人年轻 10 岁[68]。典型的病变出现有结痂的界限清楚的鳞屑性斑块。少数 BD 形成乳头状瘤性病变[69]。组织学上 BD 的特点实际上与 EQ 相同（图 14C.8）。虽然某些作者提出具有一些小的差别，但这些差别主要是由于解剖位置不同引起的[55]。BD 显示角化过度，但 EQ 没有角化过度；BD 常常累及毛囊皮脂腺单位，但这不是 EQ 的特征，因为 EQ 累及黏膜和皮肤上皮[70]。

EQ 和 BD 进展为侵袭性鳞状细胞癌的发生率相似（约 5%~10%）。将这两种病变区分开来的主要原因是二者具有不同的自然病史。研究表明，1/3 的 BD 病人发生皮肤或皮肤外恶性肿瘤[63]，但 EQ 患者并没有同样的发生全身恶性肿瘤的倾向[63,71-73]。然而，新近研究对于 BD 是否会发生内脏恶性肿瘤提出疑问。

Bowen 样丘疹病　Bowenoid papulosis

Bowen 样丘疹病（BP）这一术语是由 Wade 等[74]于 1978 年最先提出的，用来描述累及年轻男性阴茎体

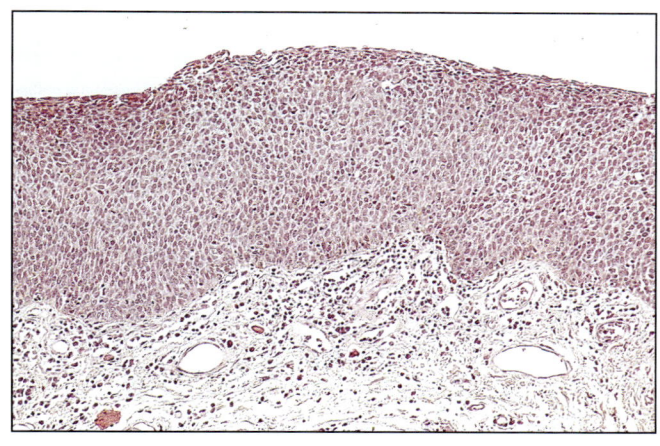

图 14C.7　Queyrat 增殖性红斑的镜下表现。异型增生的细胞累及上皮全层，核大深染，胞浆稀少。核分裂象多见。

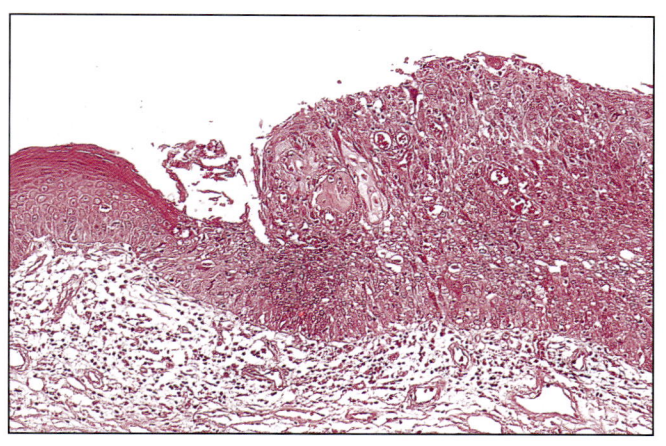

图 14C.8　鳞状细胞原位癌。Bowen 病和 Queyrat 增殖性红斑均显示上皮全层成熟障碍，伴有显著的细胞学非典型性。

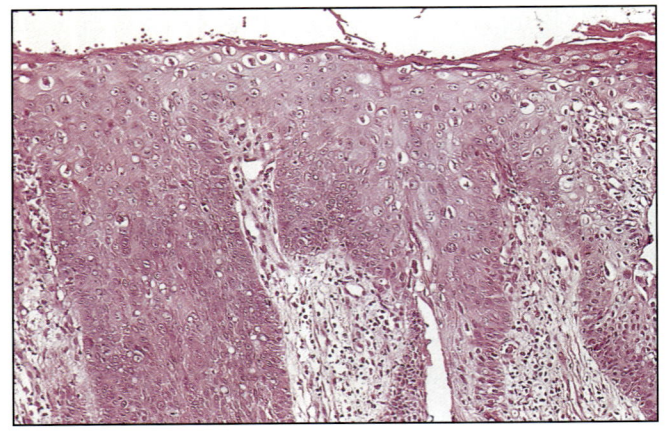

图14C.9 Bowen样丘疹病。组织学上，Bowen样丘疹病与原位癌（Bowen病和Queyrat增殖性红斑）基本相同。虽然有全层异型增生性变化，但也可见类似于湿疣的结构和细胞学变化。

或会阴的病变。这种病变组织学上与原位鳞状细胞癌相似；然而，它为多中心性，而且具有温和的临床过程[59,70,75]。在已报道的所有病例中，这种病变或对保守治疗（局部切除、局部或激光治疗）反应良好，或自行消退[70,76]。

BP通常发生在年轻成人，在Patterson等的一组51例男性BP病例中[70]，平均年龄为29.5岁，病变最常见于阴茎体；病灶通常为多中心性，以2～10 mm大小的丘疹为特征。有时丘疹可以融合形成斑块，类似于尖锐湿疣。

组织学上，BP的特点为不同程度的角化过度、角化不全、不规则的棘层肥厚和乳头状瘤病（图14C.9）[70]。虽然有时可见散在的非典型性角化细胞和核分裂象，甚至在表皮的顶层，但BP的角化细胞通常比BD或EQ的角化细胞成熟。Patterson等[70]指出，BP的非典型性角化细胞累及汗腺上部，而通常并不累及毛囊皮脂腺单位。但在BD这种情况恰好相反。

BP的病因还不清楚，但是推测病毒、免疫和化学刺激因子全都是其病因[70]。越来越多的证据表明BP与HPV有关。在某些BP病例中，发现了HPV DNA[77, 78-80]。另外，激素和免疫因素也可能具有重要病因作用[70]。

来自已报告病例的随访资料表明，BP的生物学行为与BD及EQ显著不同。某些病例病变可以自行消退。还没有发现任何一例进展为浸润性癌或发生全身恶性肿瘤[81]。新近的研究发现，BD和BP的形态测量评估结果显著不同。与BP相比，BD的细胞核较大，更接近卵圆形，边缘较不规则[82]。然而，BP与原位癌（BD/EQ）之间的组织学差异很小，不能单凭组织学表现做出正确的临床病理学诊断；相反，BP的诊断应该根据临床表现和大体所见以及组织学特征（表14C.1）。

良性肿瘤 Benign tumors

阴茎良性上皮性肿瘤罕见，曾有鳞状上皮乳头状瘤的报道。良性软组织肿瘤，例如平滑肌瘤、血管瘤（包括上皮样变异型）[83]、神经鞘瘤、神经纤维瘤、淋巴管瘤、血管球瘤、纤维组织细胞瘤和颗粒细胞瘤都曾有报道[83,84]。根据美军病理学会（AFIP）的经验，良性软组织肿瘤最常见于龟头，而恶性肿瘤则常见于阴茎体[83,84]。

血管角质瘤（angiokeratoma）是一种独特的良性血管病变，并不认为它是一种真正的肿瘤。这种病变的特点是累及阴囊，但也可累及阴茎。形态学上，这种病变显示表浅血管扩张，伴有被覆上皮疣状改变（图14C.10）。本病共有四种临床类型：（1）Fabry病相关性弥漫性体部血管角质瘤（angiokeratoma corporis diffusum），为发生于较大儿童的多发性血管角质瘤；（2）Mibelli血管角质瘤，是指累及双侧手指及脚趾背侧的血管角质瘤；（3）Fordyce血管角质瘤，特指发生在阴囊的血管角质瘤；以及（4）孤立性血管角质瘤。

新近描述的另外一种病变是肌内膜瘤(myointimoma)，

表14C.1	三种不同异型增生性病变的鉴别特征		
特征	Queyrat增殖性红斑	Bowen病	Bowen样丘疹病
部位	龟头、包皮	阴茎体	阴茎体
年龄	40～60岁	30～50岁	20～40岁
病变	红斑	鳞屑状斑块	斑块
角化过度	−	+	+
成熟	−	−	+
汗腺受累	−	−	+
毛囊皮脂腺受累	−	+	−
进展到癌	5%～10%	5%～10%	−
与内脏肿瘤的联系	−	10%	−
自行消退	−	−	+

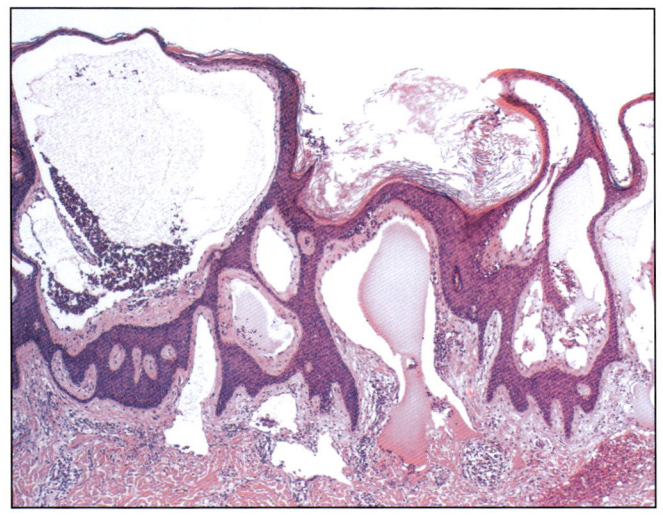

图14C.10 血管角质瘤以大而扩张的血管腔和疣状上皮改变为特征。

又叫肌内膜增生（myointimal proliferation），累及阴茎尿道海绵体[85]，病人年龄从2岁到61岁（中位年龄29岁），表现为一个肿块，其最大径从0.5 cm到1.9 cm不等。在手术治疗之前，病变可存在4天到6个月以上。显微镜下，尿道海绵体血管显示突出的纤维内膜增生，常常是闭塞性的，伴有丛状结构。这种增生是由星形的和梭形的细胞所组成，背景为丰富的纤维黏液样基质（图14C.11）。少数病变细胞具有成熟的黏液样特征，伴有中等量的嗜酸性胞浆，核的两端钝圆，可见核旁空泡，与黏液纤维瘤在形态学上具有相当程度的重叠。也可见到包括鬼影细胞在内的退行性变病灶。肌内膜病变免疫染色显示平滑肌肌动蛋白（SMA）、肌特异性肌动蛋白（HHF-35）和calponin弥漫阳性，但desmin为弱阳性。肌内膜细胞CD34、S100蛋白和角蛋白阴

性。VIIIrAg因子、CD31和CD34可以清楚显示内衬轻微闭塞血管的完整的内皮细胞、穿过增生部位的散在毛细血管和正常的未被累及的血管。随访资料表明本病为一种良性病变，没有转移的证据。需与肌纤维瘤、晚期血管内（结节性）筋膜炎、血管平滑肌瘤和丛状纤维组织细胞瘤进行鉴别诊断。

良性黑色素细胞病变也可发生在阴茎，例如黑色素细胞痣、黑变病和雀斑状黑变病。这些病变可能在阴茎黑色素瘤之前出现，也可与之同存。

恶性肿瘤 Malignant neoplasms

一般来说，阴茎恶性肿瘤的发生率很低（大约1/100 000），在西方国家占所有男性肿瘤的0.5%以下和所有生殖泌尿系统癌症的3%[86]。美国癌症学会估计，2006年1530名病人将会发生阴茎癌，其中280人将死于本病[87]。然而在某些国家，例如乌干达、巴西、牙买加、墨西哥和海地，阴茎癌很常见，占这些国家所有恶性肿瘤的10%～12%[86,88-90]。尽管有这些统计数据，阴茎癌的发病率在许多国家都在下降，部分原因在于个人卫生意识的提高[91]。阴茎最常见的恶性肿瘤是癌，迄今为止鳞状细胞癌是最常见的阴茎癌（表14C.2）[92]。

鳞状细胞癌 Squamous carcinoma

推测各种因素均与阴茎鳞状细胞癌发生的危险性增加有关，包括没有进行包皮环切、卫生差、包茎和病毒[86, 88-90, 93-96]。在婴儿期就做了包皮环切的人阴茎鳞状细胞癌的发病率极低。犹太人在出生时做包皮环切术，其阴茎鳞状细胞癌的发病率也极低[97]。晚至儿童期或青春期做包皮环切术好像可以起到一定但并不完全的预防作用[94-96]。穆斯林在儿童后期做包皮环切术，因此其阴茎鳞状细胞癌的发病率就要略高[97]。在印度，95%以上的阴茎癌发生在印度北部的印度人，因为这些人不做包皮环切，仅5%的病例为穆斯林[95]。虽然在出生时做包皮环切术可以很好地预防阴茎癌的发生，但是多数作者认为，在未做包皮环切术的男性，通过良好的卫生习惯也能获得同样低的阴茎癌的发生率。北欧国家阴茎癌的发生率很低，那里的男性并不常规做包皮环切术，但个人卫生习惯良好，支持这一观点[98]。

据报道几乎半数的阴茎癌患者与包茎共存[99]。实验表明包皮垢（脱落的上皮碎屑）在阴茎癌的发生中可能起重要作用[86]。包皮垢及其衍生物的潴留被认为对于阴

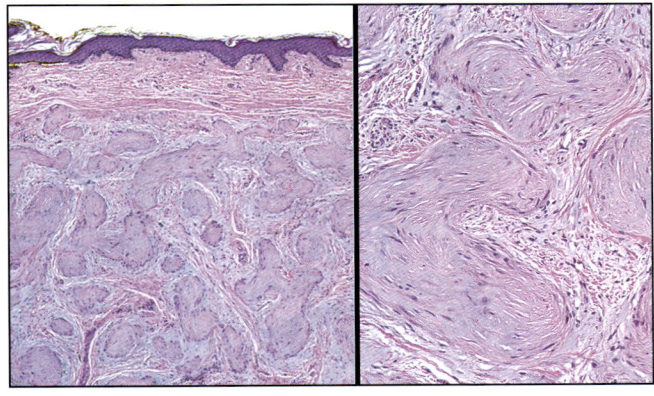

图14C.11 肌内膜瘤。这种血管病变以相互吻合的梭形细胞条索为特征，似乎起源于血管内膜。高倍镜下显示（右侧）伴有肌内膜增生的血管呈丛状分布。

表14C.2　世界卫生组织阴茎肿瘤组织学分类[a]

阴茎恶性上皮性肿瘤		癌前病变	
鳞状细胞癌	8070/3	上皮内瘤III级	8077/2
基底细胞样癌	8083/3	Bowen病	8081/2
湿疣性癌	8051/3	Queyrat增殖性红斑	8080/2
疣状癌	8051/3	Paget病	8542/3
乳头状癌，非特异性	8050/3		
肉瘤样癌	8074/3	黑色素细胞肿瘤	
混合性癌	8060/3	黑色素细胞痣	8720/0
腺鳞状细胞癌	8247/3	黑色素瘤	8720/3
Merkel细胞癌	8041/3		
神经内分泌型小细胞癌	8410/3	间叶性肿瘤	
皮脂腺癌	8310/3	造血系统肿瘤	
透明细胞癌	8090/3	继发性肿瘤	
基底细胞癌			

[a]肿瘤学疾病国际分类形态学编码（ICD-O）和医学系统化专业术语（http://snomed.org）。生物学行为编码：/0代表良性肿瘤，/2代表原位癌和上皮内瘤III级，/3代表恶性肿瘤。

茎上皮具有刺激作用。在未进行包皮环切和包茎的阴茎，这种影响可能更加严重[86]。

阴茎癌的发生与病毒也有关[100-105]。大约半数阴茎癌病例发现HPV 16和HPV 18[102-104]。某些研究提示，阴茎癌患者的妻子宫颈癌的发生率增高，支持性传播因子具有致癌作用这一理论[106,107]。然而，其他一些研究表明，阴茎癌患者的妻子生殖器癌的发生率并无显著升高[108]。HPV感染在阴茎癌的发生中可能起到一定作用，但是这种疾病可能具有多种病因；其他罕见的原因包括烟草、放射线、补骨脂素（psoralen）和紫外线A（PUVA）治疗，并且与疣状黄瘤有关[109-111]。

阴茎癌一般发生于老年男性[112-117]。诊断时病人年龄从20岁到90岁不等，但在40岁以下的男性中罕见[118]。病人通常表现为外生性或溃疡性肿物。也可出现阴茎疼痛、排液、排尿困难或淋巴结肿大等症状[86]。病变多数位于龟头和包皮[86]，也可位于包皮囊或冠状沟。发生在阴茎体和尿道口的癌罕见[114-119]。

多数阴茎癌起源于龟头黏膜的鳞状上皮，按发生的递减顺序还可累及包皮、冠状沟和阴茎体的皮肤[120]。生长方式可以为表面播散（水平生长的扁平肿瘤，伴有轻微表浅浸润）、纵向生长（纵向生长伴有深部穿透）[86]，或疣状生长（疣状/乳头状外生性生长，镜下与疣状癌、湿疣性癌或非特异性乳头状癌的组织学相关）[120,121]。还可见混合性生长或多中心生长方式（图14C.12）。表浅播散的肿瘤，如果手术边缘阴性，往往具有较好的预后，但纵向生长的肿瘤预后不良，常常

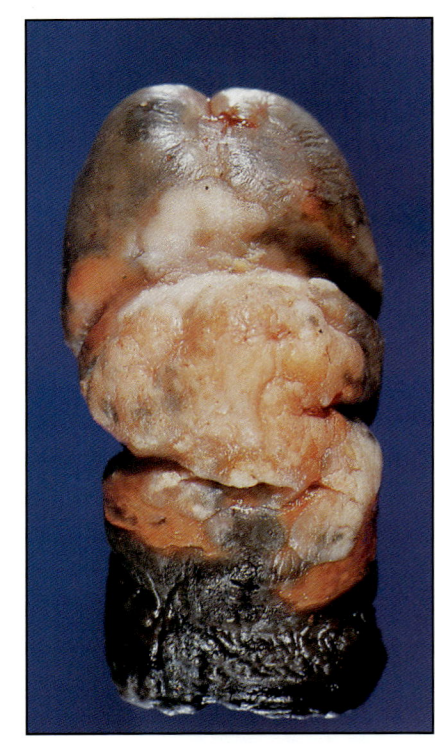

图14C.12　阴茎鳞状细胞癌。肿瘤形成大的广基息肉状肿块。

伴有淋巴结转移[122-125]。

组织学上，大多数阴茎鳞状细胞癌与其他器官的鳞状细胞癌相同，分为高、中、低分化（图14C.13和14C.14）。在鳞状细胞癌组织学亚型中（见下），疣状癌比湿疣性癌或非特异性乳头状癌预后好。基底细胞样癌和肉瘤样癌预后较差[121]。

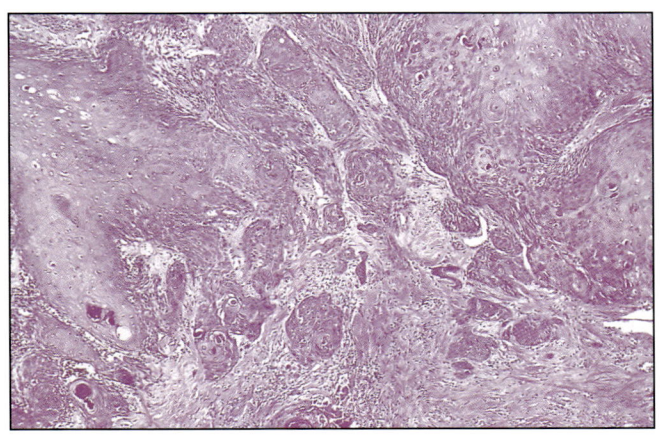

图14C.13　高分化浸润性鳞状细胞癌。虽然乳头状增生类似于疣状癌，但浸润的方式否定了这一诊断。

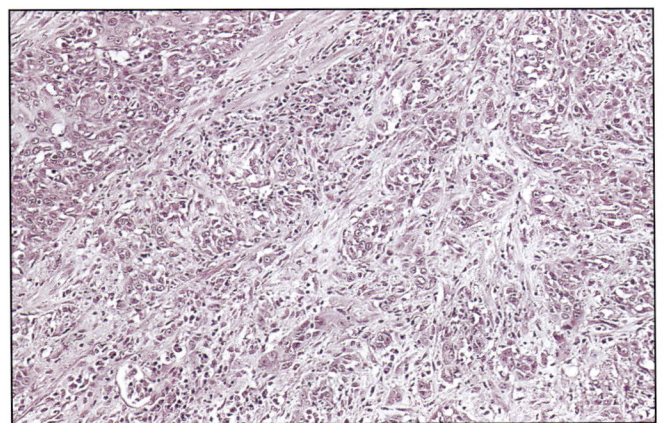

图14C.14　浸润性中分化鳞状细胞癌。

鳞状细胞癌的变异型
Variants of squamous cell carcinoma

疣状癌　Verrucous carcinoma

自从最初在口腔描述以来，疣状癌现已在很多器官中发现，包括喉、外阴、阴道、肛门和阴茎。疣状癌占阴茎恶性肿瘤的5%～16%[126]，它最常见于中年男性[126-131]。典型者为大的蕈伞状疣状病变，常有溃疡形成，并穿入正常组织。多数病变开始位于冠状沟，随后蔓延至龟头和包皮皮肤（图14C.15）。

镜下，疣状癌是一种高分化的鳞状细胞癌，伴有外生性和内生性的乳头状生长方式（图14C.16）。本病具有特征性的广基球根状浸润方式（图14C.17）。细胞学非典型性轻微，核分裂象十分少见，通常局限于肿瘤的深部。这些肿瘤倾向局部生长，不发生转移。如果疣状癌没有经过充分治疗，将会多次复发。主要的鉴别诊断包括尖锐湿疣（特别是巨大湿疣）、湿疣性癌和普通角化型鳞状细胞癌。当病变小时，区分疣状癌和尖锐湿疣仅仅具有学术上的意义，因为二者都为保守治疗。当病变大时，

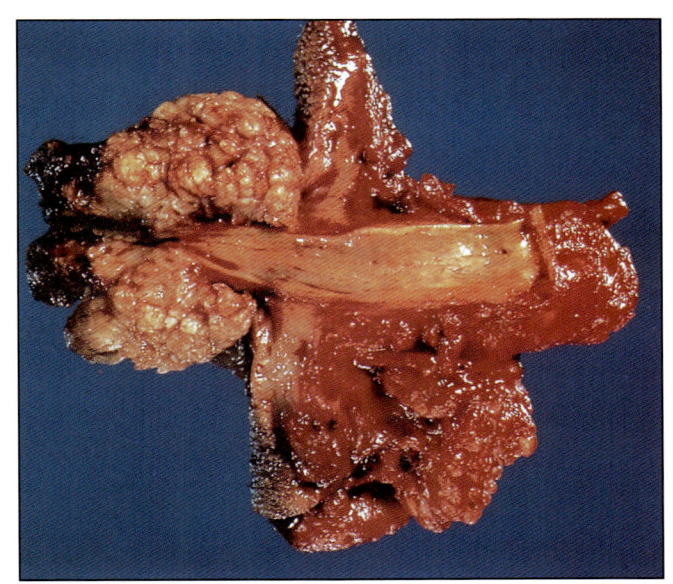

图14C.15　疣状癌，累及阴茎及尿道。

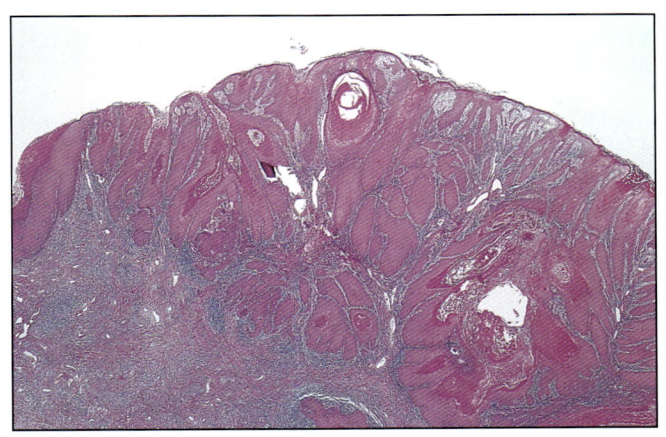

图14C.16　疣状癌。高分化鳞状细胞排列成蕨样乳头。肿瘤的特征是具有广基的浸润方式。

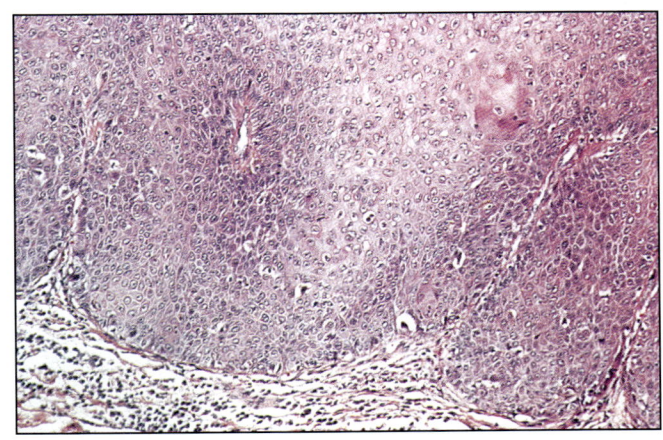

图14C.17　推挤式的浸润方式是鉴别疣状癌和高分化浸润性鳞状细胞癌的主要组织学标准。显示明显的推进式浸润边缘，伴有典型的局灶性浸润癌的混合性肿瘤并不少见。

应与 Buschke-Lowenstein 巨大湿疣鉴别。许多作者认为这些病变为同一种疾病[126,127]，但是组织学检查容易区分这两种病变，巨大湿疣可见 HPV 引起的改变，而疣状癌则少有或缺乏这些改变。无论是否决定区分二者，这两种病变的处理方法基本相似。然而，湿疣性癌和普通鳞状细胞癌必须与疣状癌相鉴别，因为它们的生物学行为不同，前者的处理常常需要前哨淋巴结活检或根治性腹股沟淋巴结清扫。疣状癌缺乏显著的细胞学非典型性、核分裂象和浸润生长方式，这些有助于将其与普通型鳞状细胞癌区分开来。湿疣性癌除了细胞学非典型性和破坏性浸润之外，还具有 HPV 相关性改变[121]。某些疣状癌病例可以检出 HPV DNA（6 型和 11 型），而且先前患有尖锐湿疣，提示病毒是疣状癌的病因[101,130]。

混合性癌　Mixed carcinomas

疣状/鳞状细胞癌（混合）
Verrucous/squamous carcinoma(hybrid)

大约 25% 的阴茎疣状癌病例在显微镜下可见局灶性细胞间变、核分裂活性增高和基底膜破裂[126,131]。这些肿瘤被称为混合性鳞状-疣状癌（hybrid squamous-verrucous carcinoma），类似的肿瘤在口腔也有描述。混合性鳞状-疣状癌与疣状癌在患者年龄、部位以及采取同样治疗措施之后的结局方面非常相似，尽管有关混合性鳞状-疣状癌的资料有限[126,131]。Masih 等[131] 应用 DNA 倍体和细胞周期分析发现，疣状癌和混合性鳞状-疣状癌均为二倍体，伴有类似的增生指数。

其他混合性癌包括湿疣性-基底细胞样癌、腺癌和基底细胞样癌 [腺基底细胞样癌 (adenobasaloid carcinoma)]，以及鳞状细胞癌和神经内分泌癌。

湿疣性癌
Warty（condylomatous）carcinoma

湿疣性癌是一种形态特殊的疣状肿瘤，其组织学特征与外阴同名肿瘤相似。这种肿瘤可以累及包括龟头、冠状窝和包皮在内的多个解剖部位，或仅累及阴茎的单一部位[121]。

大体特点为外生性菜花样肿物，灰白色，质硬。组织学检查，低倍镜下就有可能见到乳头状瘤病变，伴有棘层肥厚、角化过度和角质囊肿。伴有纤维血管轴心的长乳头显示 HPV 感染的细胞学特征以及浸润的结构特征。即使是在明显的浸润性癌灶中，也有明显的核非典型性，伴有挖空细胞和双核细胞形成（图 14C.18）[121]。进展性癌边缘可呈浸润、推挤或混合式生长[132]。大约 25%~45% 的湿疣性癌伴有 HPV DNA，远远高于普通的鳞状细胞癌[132]。

鉴别诊断包括其他疣状肿瘤，例如疣状癌、巨大湿疣和非特异性乳头状鳞状细胞癌。

与诸如典型的鳞状、乳头状、疣状或间变性癌等其他类型的阴茎癌相比，湿疣性癌与 HPV 联系更为密切；有人认为湿疣性癌是与巨大湿疣相对应的恶性病变[132]。湿疣性癌具有明显的局部淋巴结转移的危险，虽然不如典型的鳞状细胞癌的转移率高。因此，这种肿瘤应与疣状癌或其他类型的疣状癌区别[132,133]。

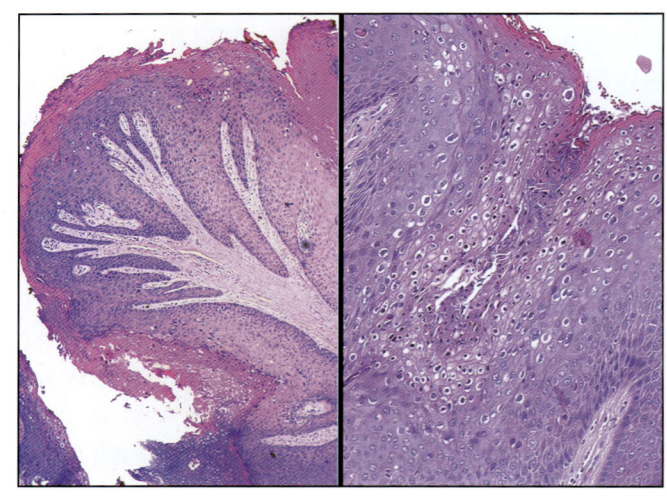

图14C.18　（A）湿疣性癌。低倍镜下显示乳头状生长方式。（B）左侧显示湿疣性癌伴有乳头状生长，右侧显示上皮细胞的非典型性挖空细胞改变。

非特异性乳头状癌 Papillary carcinoma, NOS

非特异性乳头状癌是一种外生性鳞状细胞癌，大体表现与湿疣性癌相似。这种肿瘤是由非典型性细胞组成的，没有HPV相关性特点，显示浸润性边缘。这种变型最常发生于40～60岁的病人。镜下，病变为高分化的角化过度性病变，伴有不规则的复杂乳头，有或没有纤维血管轴心。与疣状癌不同，乳头状癌呈浸润性生长，与间质的交界不规则。虽然这种肿瘤可以侵犯阴茎海绵体，但局部淋巴结转移非常罕见，因此预后很好。

基底细胞样癌 Basaloid carcinoma

这种肿瘤主要表现为垂直生长和深部浸润。组织学检查，肿瘤分化差，由基底细胞样细胞组成癌巢（图14C.19），伴有粉刺样坏死，可见较多核分裂象，角化很少见[134]。基底细胞样癌缺乏收缩人工假象或周边栅栏状排列以及高级别的细胞核，有助于与累及阴茎的罕见的基底细胞癌相鉴别。

假增生性非疣状鳞状细胞癌 Pseudohyperplastic non-verruciform squamous cell carcinoma

Cubilla等[135]报道了10例伴有假增生特点的阴茎高分化鳞状细胞癌，将其命名为假增生性非疣状鳞状细胞癌。在诊断时，本病的中位年龄是69岁。7例肿瘤为多中心性，主要累及包皮黏膜内面。大体上，肿瘤一般扁平或轻度隆起，呈白色颗粒状，大小约为2cm。镜下，显著的特点包括角化鳞状细胞巢，伴有轻度非典型性，周围由反应性纤维间质包绕（图14C.20）。在活检或切除标本的个别区域，与假上皮性瘤性增生的鉴别诊断非常困难，但当标本足够大时，就可以看到明确的浸润。周围的鳞状上皮一般显示与鳞状细胞癌有关的病变，从鳞状上皮增生到低级别鳞状上皮内病变，在少数病例可见高级别鳞状上皮内病变。在所有病例中都可见到明显的硬化性苔藓。本病可以通过包皮环切和部分阴茎切除术来治疗。除了1例于包皮环切术后2年龟头复发外，最初手术后随访没有异常所见。这些病例表明，存在少数伴有高度分化和假增生性特征的非疣状多中心性肿瘤，主要累及包皮[135]。

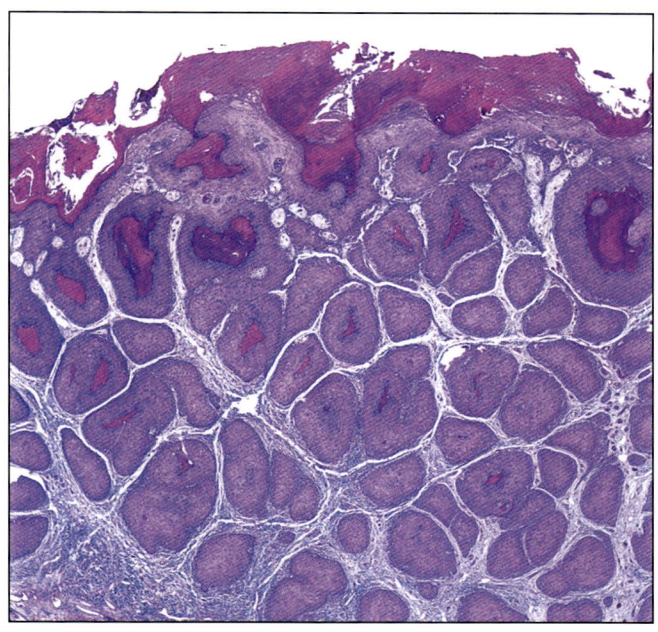

图14C.20 假增生性非疣状鳞状细胞癌。可见高分化癌向下增生，形成不同大小的癌巢，伴有轻度细胞非典型性，表面看来与假上皮瘤性增生相似。

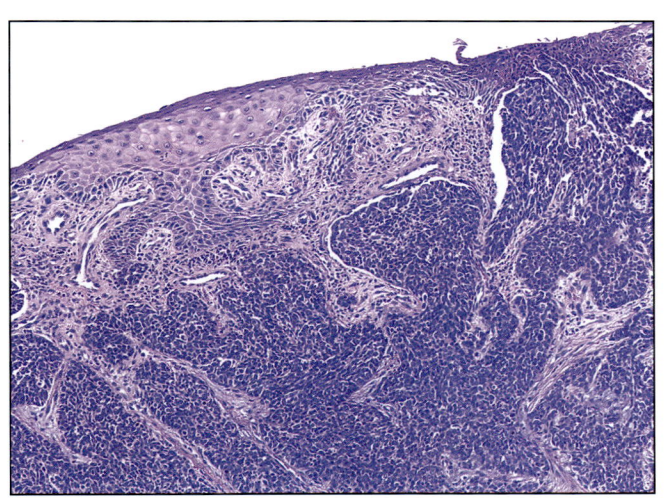

图14C.19 基底细胞样癌。肿瘤显示深染的基底细胞样细胞巢。（Courtesy of Dr G. Ayala, Baylor College of Medicine, Houston, TX）

肉瘤样癌（梭形细胞鳞状细胞癌） Sarcomatoid carcinoma (spindle cell squamous carcinoma)

虽然梭形细胞鳞状细胞癌常见于口腔、上呼吸道和食管，但在阴茎仅有几例报道[136-139]。在这些已报道的病例中，病变倾向于形成息肉样肿物。组织学上，肿瘤主要由梭形细胞构成，伴有局部鳞状细胞分化的区域（图14C.21）。梭形细胞成分常见明显的核多形性，核分裂

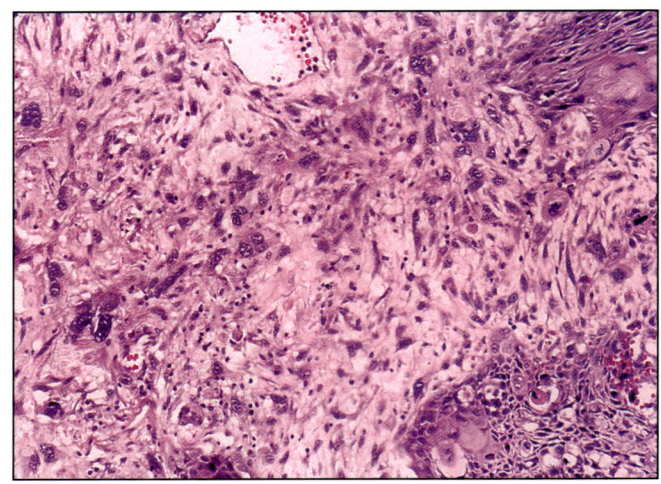

图14C.21 肉瘤样癌。这是一种双相性肿瘤，具有鳞状细胞癌和梭形肉瘤样成分。

象增加。也可见到棘层松解性假血管结构。

某些学者报道梭形细胞鳞状细胞癌呈局灶性生长，预后良好；然而，Velazquez 等[138]和 Lont 等[140]报道的病例具有高度侵袭的临床经过。因为报道的病例数量有限，本病的预后情况还不明了。虽然曾有报道疣状癌在经过放射治疗后发生了肉瘤样变，但其与放射治疗的关系还并不清楚[136]。

腺鳞状细胞癌和其他罕见癌
Adenosquamous carcinoma and other rare carcinomas

在龟头和冠状沟，曾报道过显示腺样和鳞状两种分化的肿瘤（腺鳞状细胞癌）[141]。这些肿瘤浸润往往很深[142,143]。罕见的阴茎腺癌和黏液表皮样癌也有报道[143,144]。其他少见的肿瘤包括小细胞癌[145]、Merkel细胞癌[146]、透明细胞癌[147]和皮脂腺癌[148]。

预后

有助于预测局部或全身转移的预后因素包括原发性肿瘤的大小、部位、形态学结构、组织学分级、肿瘤分期（表14C.3）、浸润深度和组织学类型[120,125,149-154]。Slaton 等[155]最近报道，阴茎肿瘤的病理学分期、血管浸润以及超过 50% 的肿瘤细胞分化差是腹股沟淋巴结转移的独立预测因素。因此，对于那些伴有 pT1 病变、没有血管浸润，而且分化差的肿瘤占 50% 或小于 50%的病人，好像没有理由进行预防性淋巴结切除术。

具有表浅播散生长方式的肿瘤主要问题在于获得阴性的手术切缘；手术切缘阴性预示预后良好。

表14C.3	阴茎癌的TNM分类[a]	
原发性肿瘤（T）		
TX	原发性肿瘤无法评估	
T0	未见原发性肿瘤	
Tis	原位癌	
Ta	非浸润性疣状癌	
T1	肿瘤侵及上皮下结缔组织	
T2	肿瘤侵及阴茎海绵体	
T3	肿瘤侵及尿道或前列腺	
T4	肿瘤侵及其他邻近器官	
局部淋巴结（N）		
NX	局部淋巴结无法评估	
N0	无局部淋巴结转移	
N1	单个表浅腹股沟淋巴结转移	
N2	多个或双侧表浅腹股沟淋巴结转移	
N3	腹股沟深部淋巴结或单侧或双侧盆腔淋巴结转移	
远处转移（M）		
MX	远处转移无法评估	
M0	无远处转移	
M1	远处转移	

附注：
后缀m代表存在多发性原发性肿瘤，记录在括弧内。例如 pTa (m) N0M0

分期分组			
0期	Tis	N0	M0
	Ta	N0	M0
Ⅰ期	T1	N0	M0
Ⅱ期	T1	N1	M0
	T2	N0	M0
	T2	N1	M0
Ⅲ期	T1	N2	M0
	T2	N2	M0
	T3	N0	M0
	T3	N1	M0
	T3	N2	M0
Ⅳ期	T4	任何 N	M0
	任何 T	N3	M0
	任何 T	任何 N	M1

Used with permission of the American Joint Committee on Cancer (AJCC), Chicago, Illinois. The original source for this material is the AJCC Cancer Staging Manual, Sixth Edition (2002) published by Springer-Verlag New York, www.springeronline.com

溃疡型肿瘤（垂直生长）具有很高的淋巴结转移率。阴茎癌首先局部扩散，破坏包皮和阴茎体。尿道受累通常继发于瘘管形成。Buck 筋膜富于弹力纤维，是抵御肿瘤侵袭的第一道屏障。然而，随着病变的进展，肿瘤可以穿过 Buck 筋膜和海绵体。远处转移最常通过淋巴

表14C.4	低危险和高危险阴茎癌
低危险组	高危险组
Tis	T2和T3肿瘤伴有3级肿瘤
疣状癌	肿瘤伴有血管浸润
T1伴有1级或2级肿瘤	基底细胞样癌
没有血管浸润的肿瘤	肉瘤样癌

管转移；腹股沟淋巴结一般最先受累。阴茎淋巴管在阴茎体和根部中线处形成丰富的吻合支；因此有时会发生交叉腹股沟淋巴结转移[156]。淋巴结是否转移以及转移的个数与预后相关[122-125]。然而，原发性肿瘤感染可能引起腹股沟淋巴结肿大而没有肿瘤转移，因此，肿瘤的正确分期常需做前哨淋巴结活检。血行播散很少见。少于2%的阴茎癌患者在诊断时就伴有远处内脏转移；然而，在未经治疗的病例，可能发生肝、肺、骨的转移。

疣状癌的预后比湿疣性癌和非特异性乳头状癌好，基底细胞样癌和肉瘤样癌的预后不良。表14C.4列出了高危险和低危险组。

基底细胞癌 Basal cell carcinoma

基底细胞癌（BCC）是身体其他部位皮肤最常见的恶性肿瘤（见第23章），但在阴茎和阴囊皮肤却非常少见[115,116]。本病可以累及龟头、包皮或阴茎体。一般会形成小的不规则形溃疡型肿物。镜下可见由小而一致的基底细胞样细胞组成的细胞巢，边缘呈栅栏状排列（图14C.22）。一般来说，基底细胞癌的临床病程具有惰性[157,158]。

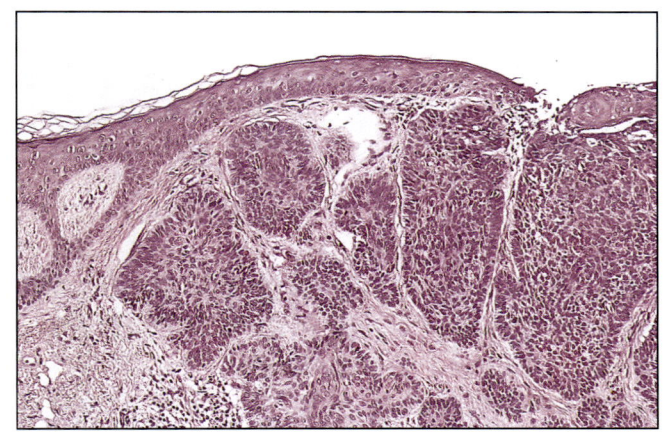

图14C.22　基底细胞癌。基底细胞癌的典型表现是由一致的基底细胞样细胞组成的界限分明的细胞巢。

恶性黑色素瘤 Malignant melanoma

阴茎原发性黑色素瘤罕见，文献报道不超过150例[159-167]。已报告的病例多数发生在40～60岁的病人[168]。大多数位于龟头，偶可发生于包皮和阴茎体。发生阴茎恶性黑色素瘤的危险因素是黑变病和先前存在的黑色素痣。阴茎黑色素瘤的组织学表现与发生在其他部位皮肤或黏膜的恶性黑色素瘤相同（见第23章）[68]。恶性黑色素瘤不同的组织类型，包括结节型、表浅扩散型和雀斑型均有报告[163-165,168,169]。

软组织恶性黑色素瘤[透明细胞肉瘤(clear cell sarcoma)]是一种少见肿瘤,常发生于四肢的腱鞘和腱膜。也有发生于阴茎的报道[170]。

阴茎恶性黑色素瘤的预后很差[68]。约有半数病人在发现本病时已发生了淋巴结转移[68]。预后不良的可能原因是本病表现特殊，或者说症状不特异，导致发现较晚以致延误了治疗。另外，解剖部位限制了手术切缘的大小，肿瘤富于血管、多个淋巴管引流通路都有利于肿瘤早期播散[166]。

肉瘤 Sarcoma

阴茎肉瘤是第二个最常见的阴茎肿瘤，但比癌要少见得多。血管肿瘤，尤其是上皮样血管内皮细胞瘤、血管肉瘤和Kaposi肉瘤是最常见的阴茎肉瘤[171,172]。肌源性（平滑肌肉瘤和横纹肌肉瘤）、神经源性、软骨样、骨样和纤维性肉瘤，以及所谓的恶性纤维组织细胞瘤和上皮样肉瘤都可发生[84,173-180]。这些病变的组织学特征与任何其他部位的同名肿瘤相似（见第24章）。

转移性肿瘤 Metastatic tumors

阴茎与盆腔脏器之间有丰富而复杂的血液循环通路，但阴茎转移性肿瘤十分少见。1985年Powell等[181]回顾文献发现仅有219例。1989年Perez-Mesa和Oxenhandler回顾文献又增加了6例新发病例[182]。在所有报道的病例中，最常见的原发部位为前列腺，其次为直肠乙状结肠、膀胱和肾[181-186]。不常见的原发部位包括肺、胰腺、鼻咽部和骨[181-185,187-189]。Tu等[190]最近的一篇报道称，在前列腺癌中，导管-子宫内膜样癌亚型最易发生阴茎转移。

最常见的转移部位为海绵体[183]。临床上，通常表现为多发性可以触及的疼痛性结节。这些结节可以累及皮肤发生溃疡，酷似梅毒性下疳。半数病人，可弥漫累及阴茎海绵体，引起阴茎异常勃起[183]。可以伴有血尿、排尿困难。在绝大多数病例中，阴茎转移一般发生于已知原发性肿瘤的晚期，所以不存在诊断困难。然而，在某些病例中，阴茎可能为癌转移的第一个部位[191,192]。

阴囊肿瘤和肿瘤性病变　Tumors and tumorous conditions of scrotum

非肿瘤性病变　Non-neoplastic lesions

表皮包涵囊肿　Epidermal inclusion cysts

表皮包涵囊肿（角化性囊肿）是发生在阴囊的常见病变。表现为单个或多个橡皮硬度的皮下或皮内结节。特点为内含灰白色乳酪样物质[68]。镜下，囊肿内衬角化鳞状上皮。

特发性阴囊钙质沉着症　Idiopathic scrotal calcinosis

特发性钙质沉着症是阴囊皮肤的一种少见的病变[193,194]。在两种情况下可以发生：先前存在的阴囊表皮囊肿或毛发囊肿钙化以及在缺乏囊肿的情况下真皮结缔组织钙化（特发性阴囊钙质沉着症）[195,196]。一种假设支持后者来源于外分泌汗腺导管粟粒疹，因为免疫组织化学发现外分泌汗腺的标志物癌胚抗原（CEA）阳性[196]。

病人一般为年轻人，但是也有老人和儿童。表现为多发性（可以多达50个）长期存在的质地硬韧的结节，大小不同，从几毫米到3 cm不等。被覆上皮一般完整，但可形成溃疡，释放出干酪样物。偶尔可表现为单个质硬结节。

组织学上，病变位于真皮，含有颗粒状和球状嗜苏木素的钙化物质。伴有或不伴有巨细胞性肉芽肿性炎症，并可见到囊肿壁（图14C.23）。特发性阴囊钙质沉着症也可能是"陈旧性"表皮囊肿的晚期表现，随着时间的推移，囊肿壁逐渐消失[197-199]。对于没有症状的病人，可能不需要治疗，但对于那些有感染、复发或广泛的病变则需要手术治疗。

硬化性脂肪肉芽肿　Sclerosing lipogranuloma

这种病变也可累及阴囊[39,40]。其临床表现及组织学所见均与阴茎或睾丸周围的硬化性脂肪肉芽肿相同（见845和863页）。

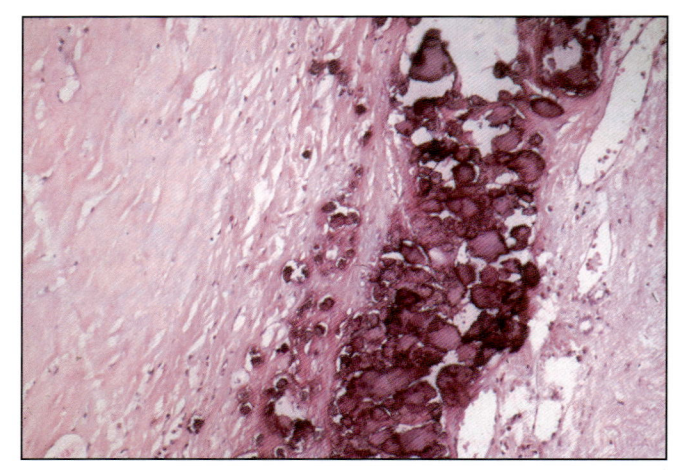

图14C.23　钙质沉着症，特征为在致密胶原间质中有广泛的磷酸钙沉积。

脂肪坏死　Fat necrosis

脂肪坏死最常见于儿童及青少年[200]。病人表现为阴囊壁的下部出现质硬结节。2/3的病人为双侧结节[200]。有人提示，当阴囊暴露在寒冷的环境中时，阴囊脂肪结晶化，造成脂肪坏死。

肿瘤性病变　Neoplastic lesions

阴囊的良性和恶性肿瘤均少见。绝大多数肿瘤性病变来源于皮肤和皮肤附件[201]。包括海绵状血管瘤和毛细血管瘤在内的血管瘤、淋巴管瘤、平滑肌瘤[202]和血管角质瘤为阴囊最常见的良性肿瘤[201]。鳞状细胞癌（见下）是阴囊最常见的恶性肿瘤。尖锐湿疣和疣状黄瘤是临床上表现为阴囊皮肤疣的两种病变；鳞状细胞癌偶尔可能酷似湿疣。疣状黄瘤最常见于口腔黏膜，其次为生殖器（阴囊和阴茎）皮肤。低倍镜下，这种病变与湿疣相似，可见棘层增厚、乳头状瘤病和角化不全，但本病在真皮乳头和变长的上皮脚顶端出现泡沫状巨噬细胞，有助于鉴别诊断（图14C.6）[52]。

具有血管平滑肌特点的错构瘤性病变（血管平滑肌瘤性增生）在阴囊有少数报道，偶尔会与恶性肿瘤相混淆。有关本病的描述很少，没有适当的特征化，所以有不同的诊断术语，包括错构瘤[203]、肌肉增生、平滑肌瘤和血管平滑肌瘤[204]。慢性阴囊淋巴水肿可能引起阴囊肉膜增生，形成平滑肌错构瘤的组织学表现。由于阴囊淋巴水肿造成的平滑肌增生是反应性病变而不是错构瘤性病变，所以在临床病理工作中应区别真正的错构瘤与反应性平滑肌增生[205]。阴囊非典型性纤维组织细胞瘤这种少见病例也曾有报道。这种病变在典型的纤维组织细胞瘤的背景下，可见大而深染外形不规则的细胞核、奇异的多核细胞 [怪异细胞 (monster cells)]，以及伴有大而突出细胞核的黄瘤性细胞，核分裂象罕见[206]。

鳞状细胞癌　Squamous carcinoma

鳞状细胞癌在阴囊的发病率远低于阴茎[207-211]。阴囊鳞状细胞癌的好发年龄为50~70岁[207,208]，在病变初期显示为孤立的小结节，常有溃疡形成。阴囊癌倾向于局部生长，向深部浸润。半数病人可发生腹股沟淋巴结转移。预后不良，预后与肿瘤分期有关。通用的分期系统为Lowe改良的Ray & Whitmore系统[207]。组织学上，多数肿瘤为中至高分化鳞状细胞癌。

阴囊癌是第一个公认的与职业暴露因素有关的肿瘤。在十八世纪，Percival Pott发现，接触煤烟和粉尘的人（例如扫烟囱的人和棉织厂工人）患阴囊癌的几率较高。后来发现3′,4′-苯并芘为致癌物质[212]。在过去的两个世纪，发现了很多与阴囊癌有关的工业和职业致癌物质。其他的危险因素包括HPV感染，以及补骨脂素和紫外线照射协同作用[109,213-215]。

某些学者提出，黑人阴囊恶性肿瘤少；然而，因为每个报道的系列中病例数少，是否存在种族差异性还有待于进一步研究[200]。

基底细胞癌　Basal cell carcinoma

发生于非阳光暴露部位的基底细胞癌，尤其是发生于肛周及生殖器部位的基底细胞癌十分少见。阴囊基底细胞癌的发病不到阴囊恶性肿瘤的5%[216]。在所有的非痣样基底细胞癌综合征（non-nevoid BCC syndrome）中，51例基底细胞癌（0.27%）发生在肛周和生殖器[217]。表现为无痛性溃疡结节[218,219]。组织学表现与皮肤和其他部位的基底细胞癌相同，包括Pinkus纤维上皮瘤在内的各种组织学亚型。在检测的标本中没有发现HPV。基底细胞癌预后相对较好。在30例有5年或更长随访时间的病例中，广泛切除之后7年只有一例复发。没有发现转移[217]。

Paget病　Paget's Disease

累及阴囊和阴茎皮肤的乳腺外Paget病很少见[220-226]。大部分病例与潜在的癌（或为皮肤附件或为内脏）有关。根据报告，膀胱、前列腺和尿道癌都可能伴有Paget病。阴茎和（或）阴囊Paget病常发生于50~70岁的人群。Paget病通常表现为鳞屑性湿疹样病变。镜下，其特征为上皮内非典型性细胞增生，这些细胞胞浆呈空泡状，伴有大的空泡状核（图14C.24）。这种非典型性细胞常在上皮脚顶端成簇出现。还常见到角化过度、角化不全

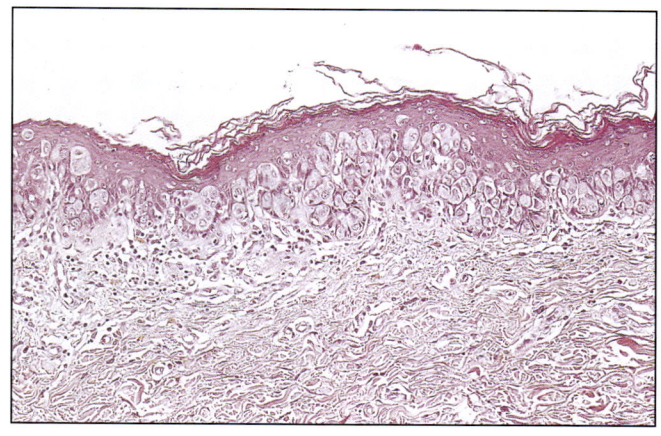

图14C.24　阴茎Paget病。黏膜内可见Paget细胞巢。细胞核大深染，胞浆淡染，偶尔呈空泡状。

和乳头状瘤病。上皮内肿瘤细胞的胞浆中含有中性和酸性黏多糖，可以PAS染色、黏蛋白卡红、阿辛蓝和醛品红染色加以证实。乳腺外Paget病的Paget细胞表达一致的黏蛋白（mucin）表型（MUC1$^+$MUC2$^-$MUC5AC$^+$），这与乳腺Paget病（MUC1$^+$MUC2$^-$MUC5AC$^-$）不同[227]。

Paget病的鉴别诊断包括鳞状细胞原位癌、Paget样Bowen病和恶性黑色素瘤。细胞浆内黏蛋白并非黑色素瘤和鳞状细胞原位癌的特点，所以黏蛋白染色有助于确定诊断。CEA免疫过氧化物酶染色也有帮助，因为Paget细胞CEA强阳性，而黑色素瘤细胞阴性[228]。在Paget样Bowen病，受累的表皮含有增生的肿瘤性上皮细胞，这些细胞呈Paget细胞样的巢状分布，但胞浆内缺乏黏蛋白。该病大囊肿病液体蛋白-15（GCDFP-15）、CEA、CAM5.2和c-erbB2阴性，细胞角蛋白（CK）20、S-100蛋白和Melan A也阴性[229]。虽然CK7被认为是Paget细胞的敏感标志物，但Paget样Bowen病的细胞也可显示阳性[229]。Williamson等[230]报道了两例Paget样Bowen病，一例为65岁男性，病变在大腿，另一例为25岁男性，病变部位为阴茎/阴囊部位。这两例病人都没有内脏器官恶性肿瘤的临床证据，两例病变的肿瘤细胞均显示CK7和CK19阳性，而CK18、CK20、CEA、GCDFP-15、c-erbB2、S-100和HMB-45阴性。总的来说，这些所见支持Paget样Bowen病的诊断。过去，其他人也证明CK7几乎总是Paget病的标志物。这两例Paget样Bowen病病变也表达CK7，在鉴别诊断中不要引起混淆[230]。

曾有乳腺外Paget病与邻近部位鳞状细胞原位癌并存的报道[231]。这种病人的结局取决于局部病变的范围以及伴随的恶性肿瘤的进展。

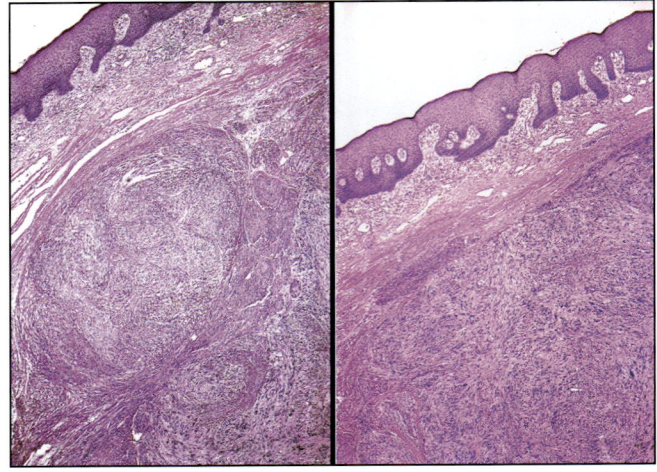

图14C.25　阴囊平滑肌肉瘤。皮肤下方可见梭形细胞增生，具有与常见部位的平滑肌肉瘤相同的特征。

肉瘤　Sarcoma

除了从精索蔓延而来的肉瘤以外，阴囊肉瘤十分罕见。最常见类型为平滑肌肉瘤（图14C.25），来源于阴囊肉膜；已报道的病例不超过30例[203, 232-234]。病人年龄35～89岁不等。曾有1例放射诱导的阴囊平滑肌肉瘤的报道[233]。只有5例病人有长期随访资料，其中4例最终发生远处转移[229]。阴囊平滑肌肉瘤与皮下平滑肌肉瘤的行为好像类似。淋巴管转移少见，但仍需要长期随访，因为晚期可能发生内脏转移或复发。在阴囊还曾报道过1例具有脂肪肉瘤和平滑肌肉瘤双重特点的病例[235]。曾报道过的发生在阴囊的肉瘤还包括脂肪肉瘤、所谓的恶性纤维组织细胞瘤、上皮样肉瘤及滑膜肉瘤[236-239]。其他恶性肿瘤非常罕见，包括恶性淋巴瘤和黑色素瘤。外伤后梭形细胞结节可能酷似肉瘤，这在阴囊已有报道[240]。为了避免误诊，需要仔细评估临床病理学资料。

参考文献

1. Rosenberg S K, Reid R 1987 Sexually transmitted papilloma viral infections in the male. I: Anatomic distribution and clinical features. Urology 29: 488–492
2. Chuang T Y 1987 Condyloma acuminata (genital warts). An epidemiologic view. J Am Acad Dermatol 16: 376–384
3. Chuang T Y, Perry H O, Kurland L T 1984 Condyloma acuminatum in Rochester, Minn, 1950–1978. I: Epidemiology and clinical features. Arch Dermatol 120: 469–475
4. Syrjanen K, Syrjanen S 1990 Epidemiology of human papilloma virus infections and genital neoplasia. Scand J Infect Dis Suppl 69: 7–17
5. Barrasso R, De Brux J, Croissant O 1987 High prevalence of papilloma virus-associated penile intraepithelial neoplasia in sexual partners of women with cervical intraepithelial neoplasia. N Engl J Med: 916–923
6. Schackner L, Hankin D E 1985 Assessing child abuse in childhood condyloma acuminatum. J Am Acad Dermatol 123: 157–160
7. Oriel J D 1971 Natural history of genital warts. Br J Vener Dis 47: 1–13
8. Margolis S 1984 Genital warts and molluscum contagiosum. Urol Clin North Am 11: 163–170
9. Goette D K 1976 Review of erythroplasia of Queyrat and its treatment. Urology 8: 311–315
10. Del Mistro A, Braunstein J D, Halwer M 1987 Identification of human papilloma virus types in male urethral condylomata acuminata by in situ hybridization. Hum Pathol 18: 936–940
11. O'Brien W M, Jenson A B, Lancaster W D 1989 Human papilloma virus typing of penile condyloma. J Urol 141: 863–865
12. Nuovo G J, Hochman H A, Eliezri H A 1990 Detection of human papilloma virus DNA in penile lesions histologically negative for condylomata. Analysis by in-situ hybridization and the polymerase chain reaction. Am J Surg Pathol 14: 829–836
13. Weaver M G, Abdul-Karim F M, Dale G 1989 Detection and localization of human papilloma virus in penile condylomas and squamous cell carcinomas using in-situ hybridization with biotinylated DNA viral probes. Mod Pathol 2: 94–100
14. Gupta S, Radotra B D, Javaheri S M et al. 2003 Lymphangioma circumscriptum of the penis mimicking venereal lesions. J Eur Acad Dermatol Venereol 17: 598–600
15. Epstein W L 1992 Molluscum contagiosum. Semin Dermatol 11: 184–189
16. Fetsch J F, Davis C J J, Hallman J R et al. 2004 Lymphedematous fibroepithelial polyps of the glans penis and prepuce: a clinicopathologic study of 7 cases demonstrating a strong association with chronic condom catheter use. Hum Pathol 35: 190–195
17. Yildirim I, Irkilata C, Sumer E et al. 2004 Fibroepithelial polyp originating from the glans penis in a child. Int J Urol 11: 187–188
18. Glicksman J M, Freeman R G 1966 Pearly penile papules. A statistical study of incidence. Arch Dermatol 93: 56–59
19. Johnson B L, Baxter D L 1964 Pearly penile papules. Arch Dermatol 90: 166–167
20. Tannenbaum M H, Becker S W 1965 Papillae of the corona of the glans penis. J Urol 93: 391–395
21. Elder D, Elenitsas R, Ragsdale B D 1997 Tumors of the epidermal appendages. In: Elder D, Elenitsas R, Jaworsky C et al. (ed) Lever's histopathology of the skin. Lippincott-Raven, Philadelphia. p 747–803
22. Rattan J, Rattan S, Gupta D K 1997 Epidermoid cyst of the penis with extension into the pelvis. J Urol 158: 593
23. Cole L A, Helwig E B 1976 Mucoid cysts of the penile skin. J Urol 115: 397–400
24. Golitz L E, Robin M 1981 Median raphe canals of the penis. Cutis 27: 170–172
25. Asarch R G, Golitz L E, Sausker W F 1979 Median raphe cysts of the penis. Arch Dermatol 115: 1084–1086
26. Enzinger F M, Weiss S W 2001 Fibromatoses. In: Enzinger F M, Weiss S W (ed) Soft tissue tumors. Mosby, St. Louis. p 309–346
27. Smith B H 1969 Subclinical Peyronie's disease. Am J Clin Pathol 52: 385–390
28. Nyberg L M, Bias W B, Hochberg M C 1982 Identification of an inherited form of Peyronie's disease with autosomal dominant inheritance and association with Dupuytren's contracture and histocompatibility B7 cross reacting antigens. J Urol 128: 48–51
29. Vande Berg J S, Devine C J, Horton C E 1981 Peyronie's disease: an electron microscopic study. J Urol 126: 333–336
30. Hinman F J 1980 Etiologic factors in Peyronie's disease. Urol Int 35: 407–413
31. Bivens C H, Marecek R L, Feldman J M 1973 Peyronie's disease – a presenting complaint of the carcinoid syndrome. N Engl J Med 289: 844–846
32. Guerneri S, Stioui S, Mantovani F et al. 1991 Multiple clonal chromosome abnormalities in Peyronie's disease. Cancer Genet Cytogenet 52: 181–185
33. Brock G, Hsu G L, Nunes L et al. 1997 The anatomy of the tunica albuginea in the normal penis and Peyronie's disease. J Urol 157: 276–281
34. McRoberts J W 1969 Peyronie's disease. Surg Gynecol Obstet 129: 1291–1294
35. Smith B H 1966 Peyronie's disease. Am J Clin Pathol 45: 670–678
36. Guileyardo J M, Sarma D P 1982 Human penile ossification. Urology 20: 428–429
37. Williams J L, Thomas G G 1970 The natural history of Peyronie's disease. J Urol 103: 75–76
38. Smetana H F, Bernhard W 1950 Sclerosing lipogranuloma. Arch Pathol 50: 296–325
39. Oertel Y C, Johnson F B 1977 Sclerosing lipogranuloma of male genitalia: review of 23 cases. Arch Pathol Lab Med 101: 321–326
40. Matsushima M, Tajima M, Maki A 1988 Primary lipogranuloma of the male genitalia. Urology 31: 75–77
41. Steward R C, Beason E S, Hayes C W 1979 Granulomas of the penis from self-injection with oils. Plast Reconstr Surg 64: 108–111
42. Lee T, Choi H R, Lee Y T et al. 1994 Paraffinoma of the penis. Yonsei Med J 35: 3440–3448
43. Matsuda T, Shichiri Y, Hida S 1988 Eosinophilic sclerosing lipogranuloma of the male genitalia not caused by exogenous lipids. J Urol 140: 1021–1024
44. Serour F 1993 Artificial nodules of the penis. Report of six cases among Russian immigrants in Israel. Sex Transm Dis 20: 192–193
45. Velazquez E F, Cubilla A L 2003 Lichen sclerosus in 68 patients with squamous cell carcinoma of the penis: frequent atypias and correlation with special carcinoma variants suggests a precancerous role. Am J Surg Pathol 27: 1448–1453

46. Powell J, Robson A, Cranston D 2001 High incidence of lichen sclerosus in patients with squamous cell carcinoma of the penis. Br J Dermatol 145: 85–89
47. Powell J, Robson A, Cranston D et al. 2003 High incidence of lichen sclerosus in patients with squamous cell carcinoma of the penis. Br J Dermatol 148: 1083–1084
48. Bouyssou-Gauthier M L, Boulinguez S, Dumas J P et al. 1999 Penile lichen sclerosus: follow-up study. Ann Dermatol Venereol 126
49. Nasca M R, Innocenzi D, Micali G 1999 Penile cancer among patients with genital lichen sclerosus. J Am Acad Dermatol 41: 911–914
50. Kumaran M S, Kanwar A J 2004 Squamous cell carcinoma in untreated lichen sclerosus: a rare complication. J Dermatol 31: 239–241
51. Campus G V, Alia F, Bosincu L 1992 Squamous cell carcinoma and lichen sclerosus et atrophicus of the prepuce. Plast Reconstr Surg 89: 692–694
52. Mohsin S K, Lee M W, Amin M B et al. 1998 Cutaneous verruciform xanthoma: a report of five cases investigating the etiology and nature of xanthomatous cells. Am J Surg Pathol 22: 479–487
53. Gray M R, Ansell I D 1990 Pseudo-epitheliomatous hyperkeratotic and micaceous balanitis: evidence for regarding it as pre-malignant. Br J Urol 66: 103–104
54. Lortat-Jacob E, Civatte J 1961 Balanite pseudoepitheliomateuse keratosique et micacée. Bull Soc Franc Dermatol Syph 68: 164–167
55. Rosai J 2004 Penis and scrotum. In: Rosai J (ed) Rosai and Ackerman's surgical pathology, 9th edn. Mosby, Edinburgh. p 1466–1482
56. Gerber G S 1994 Carcinoma in situ of the penis. J Urol 151: 829–833
57. Aynaud O, Lonesco M, Barrasso R 1994 Penile intraepithelial neoplasia. Specific clinical features correlate with histologic and virologic findings. Cancer 74: 1762–1767
58. Kaye V, Zhang G, Dehner L P et al. 1990 Carcinoma in situ of penis. Is distinction between erythroplasia of Queyrat and Bowen's disease relevant? Urology 36: 479–482
59. Su C K, Shipley W U 1997 Bowenoid papulosis: a benign lesion of the shaft of the penis misdiagnosed as squamous carcinoma. J Urol 157: 1361–1362
60. Cubilla A L, Meijer C J, Young R H 2000 Morphological features of epithelial abnormalities and precancerous lesions of the penis. Scand J Urol Nephrol Suppl 205: 215–219
61. Cubilla A L, Velazquez, E F, Young R H 2004 Epithelial lesions associated with invasive penile squamous cell carcinoma: a pathologic study of 288 cases. Int J Surg Pathol 12: 351–364
62. Queyrat L 1911 Erytroplasie du gland. Bull Soc Fr Dermatol Syphil 22: 378–382
63. Graham J H, Helwig E B 1973 Erythroplasia of Queyrat. A clinicopathologic and histochemical study. Cancer 32: 1396–1414
64. Anderson L, Johnson G, Brehmer-Anderson E 1967 Erythroplasia of Queyrat – carcinoma in situ. Scand J Urol Nephrol 1: 303–306
65. Wieland U, Jurk S, Weissenborn S 2000 Erythroplasia of Queyrat: coinfection with cutaneous carcinogenic human papillomavirus type 8 and genital papillomaviruses in a carcinoma in situ. J Invest Dermatol 115: 396–401
66. Davis-Daneshfar A, Trueb R M 2000 Bowen's disease of the glans penis. Cutis 65: 395–398
67. Hewan-Lowe L, Moreland A, Finnerty D P et al. 1990 Penis and scrotum, tumors and related disorders. In: Someren A (ed) Urologic pathology with clinical and radiological correlations. Macmillan, New York, p 640–659
68. Young R H, Srigley J R, Amin M B et al. 2000 Tumors of the prostate gland, seminal vesicles, male urethra, and penis. Atlas of tumor pathology, series 3, fascicle 28. AFIP, Washington, DC
69. Haneke E 1982 Skin diseases and tumors of the penis. Urol Int 37: 172–182
70. Patterson J W, Kao G F, Graham J H 1986 Bowenoid papulosis. A clinicopathologic study with ultrastructural observations. Cancer 57: 823–836
71. Graham J H, Helwig E B 1961 Bowen's disease and its relationship to systemic cancer. Arch Dermatol 83: 738–758
72. Chuang T Y, Tse J, Reizner G T 1990 Bowen's disease (squamous cell carcinoma in-situ) as a skin marker for internal malignancy. A case control study. Am J Prev Med 6: 238–243
73. Callen J P, Headington J T 1980 Bowen's and non-Bowen's squamous intraepithelial neoplasia of the skin: relationship to internal malignancy. Arch Dermatol 116: 422–426
74. Wade T R, Kopf A W, Ackerman A B 1978 Bowenoid papulosis of the penis. Cancer 42: 1890–1903
75. Taylor D R J, South D A 1981 Bowenoid papulosis: a review. Cutis 27: 92–98
76. Eisen R F, Bhawan J, Cahn T H 1983 Spontaneous regression of bowenoid papulosis of the penis. Cutis 32: 269–272
77. Endo M, Yamashita T, Jin H Y et al. 2003 Detection of human papillomavirus type 16 in bowenoid papulosis and nonbowenoid tissues. Int J Dermatol 42: 474–476
78. Reyes M, Moran C A, Suster S et al. 2003 Neuroendocrine carcinomas (carcinoid tumor) of the testis. A clinicopathologic and immunohistochemical study of ten cases. Am J Clin Pathol 120: 182–187
79. Zachow K R, Ostrow R S, Bender M 1982 Detection of human papilloma virus DNA in anogenital neoplasias. Nature 300: 771–773
80. Zelickson A S, Prawer S E 1980 Bowenoid papulosis of the penis, demonstration of intranuclear viral-like particles. Am J Dermatopathol 2: 305–308
81. Barnes R D, Sarembock L A, Abratt R P 1989 Carcinoma of the penis. J R Coll Surg Edinb 34: 44–46
82. Yu D S, Kim G, Song H J et al. 2004 Morphometric assessment of nuclei in Bowen's disease and bowenoid papulosis. Skin Res Technol 10: 67–70
83. Fetsch J F, Sesterhenn I A, Miettinen M et al. 2004 Epithelioid hemangioma of the penis: a clinicopathologic and immunohistochemical analysis of 19 cases, with special reference to exuberant examples often confused with epithelioid hemangioendothelioma and epithelioid angiosarcoma. Am J Surg Pathol 28: 523–533
84. Dehner L P, Smith B H 1970 Soft tissue tumors of the penis. A clinicopathologic study of 46 cases. Cancer 25: 1431–1447
85. Fetsch J F, Brinsko R W, Davis C J J et al. 2000 A distinctive myointimal proliferation ('myointimoma') involving the corpus spongiosum of the glans penis: a clinicopathologic and immunohistochemical analysis of 10 cases. Am J Surg Pathol 24: 1524–1530
86. Sufrin G, Huben R 1987 Benign and malignant lesions of the penis. In: Gillenwater J Y, Grayhack J T, Howards S S et al. (ed) Adult and pediatric urology. Year Book, Chicago, p 1448–1483
87. Jemal A, Siegel R, Ward E et al. 2006 Cancer statistics, 2006. CA Cancer J Clin 56: 106–130
88. Persky L, deKernion J 1986 Carcinoma of the penis. CA Cancer J Clin 36: 258–273
89. Dodge O G, Linsell C A 1963 Carcinoma of the penis in Uganda and Kenya Africans. Cancer 16: 1255–1263
90. Riveros M, Lebron R 1963 Geographic pathology of cancer of penis. Cancer 16: 798–811
91. Razdan S, Gomella L G 2005 Cancer of the genitourinary system. In: Devita V T, Hellman S, Rosenberg S A (ed) Cancer principles and practice of oncology. Lippincott, Williams and Wilkins, Philadelphia, p 1260–1267
92. Eble J N, Sauter G, Epstein J I et al. 2004 Pathology and genetics: tumours of the urinary system and male genital organs. WHO classification of tumors. IARC Press, Lyons, France
93. Brinton L A, Li J Y, Rong S D 1991 Risk factors for penile cancer: results from a case-control study in China. Int J Cancer 47: 504–509
94. Leiter E, Lefkovitis A M 1975 Circumcision and penile cancer. NY State J Med 75: 1520–1525
95. Dagher R, Selzer M L, Lapides J 1980 Carcinoma of the penis and the anti-circumcision crusade. J Urol 110: 79–80
96. Apt A 1965 Circumcision and penile cancer. Acta Med Scand 174: 493–504
97. Bissada N K, Morcos R R, El-Senoussi M 1986 Post-circumcision carcinoma of the penis. Clinical aspects. J Urol 135: 283–285
98. Jensen M S 1977 Cancer of the penis in Denmark 1942 to 1962 (511 cases). Dan Med Bull 24: 66–72
99. Reddy C R R M, Devendranath V, Pratap S 1984 Carcinoma of penis – role of phimosis. Urology 24: 85–88
100. Koutsky L A, Wolner-Hanssen P 1989 Genital papillomavirus infections: current knowledge and future prospects. Obstet Gynecol Clin North Am 16: 541–564
101. Loning T, Riviere A, Henke R P 1988 Penile/anal condylomas and squamous cell cancer. A HPV DNA hybridization study. Virchow's Arch [A] 413: 491–498
102. McCance D J, Kalache A, Ashdown K 1986 Human papillomavirus types 16 and 18 in carcinomas of penis from Brazil. Int J Cancer 37: 55–59
103. Cupp M R, Malek R S, Goellner J R 1995 The detection of human papillomavirus deoxyribonucleic acid in intraepithelial, in-situ, verrucous and invasive carcinoma of the penis. J Urol 154: 1024–1029
104. Masih A S, Stoler M H, Farrow G M 1993 Human papillomavirus in penile squamous cell lesions: a comparison of an isotopic RNA and two commercial nonisotopic DNA in situ hybridization methods. Arch Pathol Lab Med 117: 302–307
105. Gregoire L, Cubilla A L, Reuter V E et al. 1995 Preferential association of virus with high grade histologic variants of penile-invasive squamous cell carcinoma. J Natl Cancer Inst 87: 1705–1709
106. Graham S, Priore R, Graham M 1979 Genital cancer in wives of penile cancer patients. Cancer 44: 1870–1874
107. Iversen T, Tretli S, Johansen A et al. 1997 Squamous cell carcinoma of the penis and of the cervix, vulva and vagina in spouses: is there any relationship? An epidemiological study from Norway 1960–92. Br J Cancer 76: 658–660
108. Mainche A G, Pyrhonen S 1990 Risk of cervical cancer among wives of men with carcinoma of the penis. Acta Oncol 29: 569–571
109. Stern R S 1990 Genital tumors among men with psoriasis exposed to psoralens and ultraviolet A radiation (PUVA) and ultraviolet B radiation. The photochemotherapy follow up study. N Engl J Med 322: 1149–1151
110. Ravi R 1995 Radiation-induced carcinoma of the penis. Urol Int 54: 147–149
111. Takiwaki H, Yokota M, Ahsan K et al. 1996 Squamous cell carcinoma associated with verruciform xanthomas of the penis. Am J Dermatopathol 18: 551–554
112. Droller M J 1980 Carcinoma of penis: an overview. Urol Clin North Am 7: 783–784
113. Fraley E E, Zhang G, Sazama R 1985 Cancer of the penis. Prognosis and treatment plans. Cancer 55: 1618–1624
114. Jones W G, Hamers H, van den Bogaert W 1989 Penis cancer. A review by the joint radiotherapy committee of the European Organization for Research and Treatment of Cancer (EORTC) genitourinary and radiotherapy groups. J Surg Oncol 40: 227–231
115. Fossa S D, Hall K S, Johannessen N B 1987 Cancer of the penis. Eur Urol 13: 372–377

116. Narayana A S, Olney L E, Loening S A 1982 Carcinoma of the penis. Cancer 49: 2185–2191
117. Merrin C E 1980 Cancer of the penis. Cancer 45: 1973–1979
118. Derrick F C J, Lynch K M J, Kretkowski R C 1973 Epidermoid carcinoma of the penis: computer analysis of 87 cases. J Urol 110: 303–305
119. Hanash K A, Furlow W L, Utz D C et al. 1970 Carcinoma of the penis: a clinicopathologic study. J Urol 104: 291–297
120. Cubilla A L, Barreto J E, Caballero C et al. 1993 Pathologic features of epidermoid carcinomas of the penis. A prospective study of 66 cases. Am J Surg Pathol 17: 753–763
121. Cubilla A L, Velazques E F, Reuter V E et al. 2000 Warty (condylomatous) squamous cell carcinoma of the penis. A report of 11 cases and proposed classification of "verruciform" penile tumors. Am J Surg Pathol 24: 505–512
122. Johnson D E, Lo R K 1984 Management of regional lymph nodes in penile carcinoma. Five year results following therapeutic groin dissections. Urology 24: 308–311
123. Pow-Sang J E, Benavente V, Pow-Sang J M 1990 Bilateral inguinal lymph node dissection in the management of cancer of the penis. Semin Surg Oncol 6: 241–242
124. Ayyappan K, Anathakrishnan N, Sankaran V 1994 Can regional lymph node involvement be predicted in patients with carcinoma of the penis? Br J Urol 73: 549–553
125. Horenblas S, van Tinteren H 1994 Squamous cell carcinoma of the penis. IV. Prognostic factors of survival: analysis of tumor, nodes and metastasis classification system. J Urol 151: 1239–1243
126. Johnson D E, Lo R K, Srigley J 1985 Verrucous carcinoma of the penis. J Urol 133: 216–218
127. McKee P H, Lowe D, Haigh R J 1983 Penile verrucous carcinoma. Histopathology 7: 897–906
128. Kraus F T, Perez-Mesa C 1966 Verrucous carcinoma. Clinical and pathologic study of 105 cases involving oral cavity, larynx, and genitalia. Cancer 19: 26–38
129. Yeager J K, Findlay R F, McAleer I M 1990 Penile verrucous carcinoma. Arch Dermatol 126: 1208–1210
130. Blessing K, McLaren K, Lessells A 1986 Viral etiology for verrucous carcinoma. Histopathology 10: 1101–1102
131. Masih A S, Stoler M H, Farrow G M 1992 Penile verrucous carcinoma: a clinicopathologic, human papillomavirus typing and flow cytometric analysis. Mod Pathol 5: 48–55
132. Bezerra A L, Lopes A, Landman G et al. 2001 Clinicopathologic features and human papillomavirus DNA prevalence of warty and squamous cell carcinoma of the penis. Am J Surg Pathol 25: 673–678
133. Rubin M A, Kleter B, Zhou M et al. 2001 Detection and typing of human papillomavirus DNA in penile carcinoma: evidence for multiple independent pathways of penile carcinogenesis. Am J Pathol 159: 1211–1218
134. Cubilla A L, Reuter V, Ayala G et al. 1998 Basaloid squamous cell carcinoma of the penis: a distinctive human papilloma virus-related penile neoplasm. Am J Surg Pathol 22: 755–761
135. Cubilla A L, Velazquez E F, Young R H 2004 Pseudohyperplastic squamous cell carcinoma of the penis associated with lichen sclerosus. An extremely well-differentiated, nonverruciform neoplasm that preferentially affects the foreskin and is frequently misdiagnosed: a report of 10 cases of a distinctive clinicopathologic entity. Am J Surg Pathol 28: 895–900
136. Fukunaga M, Yokoi K, Miyazawa Y et al. 1994 Penile verrucous carcinoma with anaplastic transformation following radiotherapy. A case report with human papillomavirus typing and flow cytometric DNA studies. Am J Surg Pathol 18: 501–505
137. Morinaga S, Nakamura S, Moro K et al. 1995 Carcinosarcoma (carcinoma with sarcomatous metaplasia) of the penis. J Urol Pathol 3: 369–376
138. Velazquez E F, Melamed J, Barreto J E 2005 Sarcomatoid carcinoma of the penis. A clinicopathologic study of 15 cases. Am J Surg Pathol 29: 1152–1158
139. Wood E W, Gardner W A J, Brown F M 1972 Spindle cell squamous carcinoma of the penis. J Urol 107: 990–991
140. Lont A P, Gallee M P, Snijders P et al. 2004 Sarcomatoid squamous cell carcinoma of the penis: a clinical and pathological study of 5 cases. J Urol 172: 932–935
141. Lenowitz H, Graham A P 1946 Carcinoma of the penis. J Urol 56: 458–484
142. Cubilla A L, Ayala M T, Barreto J E et al. 1996 Surface adenosquamous carcinoma of the penis. A report of three cases. Am J Surg Pathol 20: 156–160
143. Masera A, Ovcak Z, Volavsek M et al. 1997 Adenosquamous carcinoma of the penis. J Urol 157: 2261
144. Layfield L J, Liu K 2000 Mucoepidermoid carcinoma arising in the glans penis. Arch Pathol Lab Med 124: 148–151
145. Galanis E, Frytak S, Lloyd R V 1997 Extrapulmonary small cell carcinoma. Cancer 79: 1729–1736
146. Tomic S, Warner T F, Messing E et al. 1995 Penile Merkel cell carcinoma. Urology 45: 1062–1065
147. Liegl B, Regauer S 2004 Penile clear cell carcinoma. A report of 5 cases of a distinct entity. Am J Surg Pathol 28: 1513–1517
148. Oppenheim A R 1981 Sebaceous carcinoma of the penis. Arch Dermatol 117: 306–307
149. Adeyoju A B, Thornhill J, Corr J et al. 1997 Prognostic factors in squamous cell carcinoma of the penis and implications for management. Br J Urol 80: 937–939
150. Heyns C F, van Vollenhoven P, Steenkamp J W et al. 1997 Cancer of the penis – a review of 50 patients. S Afr J Surg 35: 120–124
151. McDougal W S 1995 Carcinoma of the penis: improved survival by early regional lymphadenectomy based on the histologic grade and depth of invasion of the primary lesion. J Urol 154: 1364–1366
152. Ornellas A A, Seixas A L, Marota A et al. 1994 Surgical treatment of invasive squamous cell carcinoma of the penis: retrospective analysis of 350 cases. J Urol 151: 1244–1249
153. Soria J C, Fizazi K, Piron D 1997 Squamous cell carcinoma of the penis: multivariate analysis of prognostic factors and natural history in a monocentric study with a conservative policy. Ann Oncol 8: 1089–1098
154. Denkow T 1999 The treatment of penile carcinoma: experience in 64 cases. Int Urol Nephrol 31: 525–531
155. Slaton J W, Morgenstern N, Levy D A et al. 2001 Tumor stage, vascular invasion and the percentage of poorly differentiated cancer: independent prognosticators for inguinal lymph node metastasis in penile squamous cancer. J Urol 165: 1138–1142
156. Velazquez E F, Soskin A, Bock A 2004 Positive resection margins in partial penectomies: sites of involvement and proposal of local routes of spread of penile squamous cell carcinoma. Am J Surg Pathol 28: 384–389
157. Ladocsi L T, Siebert C F J, Rickert R R et al. 1998 Basal cell carcinoma of the penis. Cutis 61: 25–27
158. Kim E D, Kroft S, Dalton D P 1994 Basal cell carcinoma of the penis: case report and review of the literature. J Urol 152: 1557–1559
159. Stillwell T J, Zincke H, Gaffey T A 1988 Malignant melanoma of the penis. J Urol 140: 72–75
160. Oldbring J, Mikulowski P 1987 Malignant melanoma of the penis and male urethra. Report of nine cases and review of the literature. Cancer 59: 581–587
161. Begun F P, Grossman H B, Diokno A C 1984 Malignant melanoma of the penis and male urethra. J Urol 132: 123–125
162. Manivel J C, Fraley E E 1988 Malignant melanoma of the penis and male urethra: 4 case reports and literature review. J Urol 139: 813–816
163. Johnson D E, Ayala A G 1973 Primary melanoma of the penis. Urology 2: 174–177
164. Rashid A M, Williams R M, Horton L W 1993 Malignant melanoma of penis and male urethra. Is it a difficult tumor to diagnose? Urology 41: 470–471
165. de Bree E, Sanidas E, Tzardi M et al. 1997 Malignant melanoma of the penis. Eur J Surg Oncol 23: 277–279
166. Larsson K B, Shaw H M, Thompson J F et al. 1999 Primary mucosal and glans penis melanomas: the Sydney Melanoma Unit experience. Aust NZ J Surg 69: 121–126
167. Orlandini V, Kolb F, Spatz A et al. 2004 [Melanoma of the penis: 6 cases.] Ann Dermatol Venereol 131: 541–544
168. Konigsberg H A, Gray G F 1976 Benign melanosis and malignant melanoma of penis and male urethra. Urology 7: 323–326
169. aeger N, Wirtler H, Tschubel K 1982 Acral lentiginous melanoma of penis. Eur Urol 8: 182–184
170. Saw D, Tse C H, Chan J K C 1986 Clear cell sarcoma of the penis. Hum Pathol 17: 423–425
171. Waguespack R L, Fair K P, Svetec D A et al. 1996 Glomangioma of the penile and scrotal median raphe. J Urol 156: 179
172. Pacifico A, Piccolo D, Fargnoli M C et al. 2003 Kaposi's sarcoma of the glans penis in an immunocompetent patient. Eur J Dermatol 13: 582–583
173. Calonje E, Fletcher C D M, Wilson-Jones E et al. 1994 Retiform hemangioendothelioma. A distinctive form of low-grade angiosarcoma delineated in a series of 15 cases. Am J Surg Pathol 18: 115–125
174. Pow-Sang M R, Orihuela E 1994 Leiomyosarcoma of the penis. J Urol 151: 1643–1645
175. Ormsby A H, Liou L S, Oriba H A 2000 Epithelioid sarcoma of the penis: report of an unusual case and review of the literature. Ann Diagn Pathol 4: 88–94
176. Amin M B, Srigley J R, Ro J Y 1997 Leiomyosarcoma of the penis: a study of 7 cases. Mod Pathol 10: 68A (abstract)
177. Blasius S, Brinkschmidt C, Bier B 1995 Extraskeletal myxoid chondrosarcoma of the penis. J Urol Pathol 3: 73–80
178. Yantiss R K, Althausen A F, Young R H 1998 Malignant fibrous histiocytoma of the penis. Report of a case and review of the literature. J Urol Pathol 9: 171–180
179. Lowentrit B, Parsons J K, Argani P et al. 2004 Pediatric epithelioid sarcoma of the penis. J Urol 172: 296–297
180. Dominici A, Delle Rose A, Stomaci N et al. 2004 A rare case of leiomyosarcoma of the penis with a reappraisal of the literature. Int J Urol 11: 440–444
181. Powell B L, Craig J B, Muss H B 1985 Secondary malignancies of the penis and epididymis: a case report and review of the literature. J Clin Oncol 3: 110–116
182. Perez-Mesa C, Oxenhandler R 1989 Metastatic tumors of the penis. J Surg Oncol 42: 11–15
183. Haddad F S 1984 Penile metastases secondary to bladder cancer. Review of the literature. Urol Int 39: 125–142
184. Robey E L, Schellhammer P F 1984 Four cases of metastases of the penis and review of the literature. J Urol 132: 992–994
185. Khubchandani M 1986 Metachronous metastasis to the penis from carcinoma of the rectum. Report of a case. Dis Colon Rectum 29: 52–54
186. Philip A T, Amin M B, Cubilla A L et al. 1999 Secondary tumors of the penis: a study of 16 cases. Mod Pathol 12: 104A (abstract)

187. Hashimoto H, Saga Y, Watabe Y 1989 Case report: secondary penile carcinoma. Urol Int 44: 56–57
188. Ordonez N G, Ayala A G, Bracken R B 1982 Renal cell carcinoma metastatic to penis. Urology 19: 417–419
189. Perez L M, Shumway R A, Carson C C 1992 Penile metastasis secondary to supraglottic squamous cell carcinoma: review of the literature. J Urol 147: 157–160
190. Tu S M, Reyes A, Maa A 2002 Prostate carcinoma with testicular or penile metastases. Clinical, pathologic, and immunohistochemical features. Cancer 94: 2610–2617
191. Adjiman S, Flam T A, Zerbib M 1989 Delayed nonurothelial metastatic lesions to the penis. A report of two cases. Eur Urol 16: 391–392
192. Powell F C, Venencie P Y, Winkelmann R K 1984 Metastatic prostate carcinoma manifesting as penile nodules. Arch Dermatol 20: 1604–1606
193. Malcolm A 1982 Idiopathic calcinosis of the scrotum. Br J Urol 54: 190
194. Cecchi R, Giomi A 1999 Idiopathic calcinosis cutis of the penis. Dermatology 198: 174–175
195. Swinehart J M, Golitz L E 1982 Scrotal calcinosis. Dystrophic calcification of epidermoid cysts. Arch Dermatol 118: 985–988
196. Dare A J, Axelsen R A 1988 Scrotal calcinosis: origin from dystrophic calcification of eccrine duct milia. J Cutan Pathol 15: 142–149
197. Kaskas M, Dabrowski A, Sabbah M 1991 Idiopathic calcinosis of the scrotum. Apropos of a case. A review of the literature. J Urol (Paris) 97: 287–290
198. Song D H, Lee K H, Kang W H 1988 Idiopathic calcinosis of the scrotum: histopathologic observations of fifty-one nodules. J Am Acad Dermatol 97: 287–290
199. Akosa A B, Gilliland E A, Ali M H 1989 Idiopathic scrotal calcinosis: a possible aetiology reaffirmed. Br J Plast Surg 42: 324–327
200. Hollander J B, Begun F P, Lee R D 1985 Scrotal fat necrosis. J Urol 134: 150–153
201. Ulbright T M, Amin M B, Young R H 1999 Tumors of the testis, adnexa, spermatic cord, and scrotum, 3rd series. Atlas of tumor pathology. Armed Forces Institute of Pathology, Washington, D C
202. Newman P L, Fletcher C D M 1991 Smooth muscle tumours of the external genitalia: clinicopathological analysis of a series. Histopathology 18: 523–529
203. Quinn T R, Young R H 1997 Smooth muscle hamartoma of the tunica dartos of the scrotum: report of a case. J Cutan Pathol 24: 322–326
204. Nuciforo P G, Roncalli M 2003 Pathologic quiz case: a scrotal sac mass incidentally discovered during autopsy. Paratesticular hamartoma with angioleiomyomatous features (angioleiomyomatous hyperplasia). Arch Pathol Lab Med 127: 239–240
205. van Kooten E O, Hage J J, Meinhardt W et al. 2004 Acquired smooth-muscle hamartoma of the scrotum: a histological simulator? J Cutan Pathol 31: 388–392
206. Huan Y, Vapnek J, Unger P D 2003 Atypical fibrous histiocytoma of the scrotum. Ann Diagn Pathol 7: 370–373
207. Lowe F C 1983 Squamous cell carcinoma of the scrotum. J Urol 130: 423–427
208. McDonald M W 1982 Carcinoma of scrotum. Urology 19: 269–274
209. Ray B, Whitmore W F 1977 Experience with carcinoma of the scrotum. J Urol 117: 741–745
210. Gerber W L 1985 Scrotal malignancies: the University of Iowa experience and review of the literature. Urology 26: 337–342
211. Andrews P E, Farrow G M, Oesterling J E 1991 Squamous cell carcinoma of the scrotum: long-term follow-up of 14 patients. J Urol 146: 1299–1304
212. Waldron H A 1983 On the history of scrotal cancer. Ann R Coll Surg 65: 420–422
213. Oesterling J E, Lowe F C 1990 Squamous cell carcinoma of the scrotum. Am Urol Assoc Update Series 9: 178–183
214. Orihuela E, Tyring S K, Pow-Sang M 1995 Development of human papillomavirus type 16 associated squamous cell carcinoma of the scrotum in a patient with Darier's disease treated with systemic isotretinoin. J Urol 153: 1940–1943
215. de la Brassinne M, Richert B 1992 Genital squamous cell carcinoma after PUVA therapy. Dermatology 185: 316–318
216. Grossman H B, Sogani P C 1981 Basal cell carcinoma of scrotum. Urology 17: 241–242
217. Gibson G E, Ahmed I 2001 Perianal and genital basal cell carcinoma: a clinicopathologic review of 51 cases. J Am Acad Dermatol 45: 68–71
218. Greider H E, Vernon S D 1982 Basal cell carcinoma of the scrotum. A case report and literature review. J Urol 127: 145–146
219. Ho W S, King W W, Chan W Y 1995 Basal cell carcinoma of the scrotum. N Med J Ind 8: 195
220. Hoch W H 1984 Adenocarcinoma of the scrotum (extramammary Paget's disease). A case report and review of the literature. J Urol 132: 137–139
221. Mitsudo S, Nakanishi I, Koss L 1981 Paget's disease of the penis and adjacent skin. Its association with fatal sweat gland carcinoma. Arch Pathol Lab Med 105: 518–520
222. Helwig E B, Graham J H 1963 Anogenital extramammary Paget's disease. A clinicopathological study. Cancer 16: 387–403
223. Perez M A, Larossa D D, Tomaszewski J E 1989 Paget's disease primarily involving the scrotum. Cancer 63: 970–975
224. Takahashi Y, Komeda H, Horie M 1988 Paget's disease of the scrotum. Acta Urol Jpn 34: 1069–1072
225. Smith D J, Handy F C, Evans J W 1994 Paget's disease of the glans penis: an unusual urological malignancy. Eur Urol 25: 316–319
226. Koh K B, Nazarina A R 1995 Paget's disease of the scrotum: report of a case with underlying carcinoma of the prostate. Br J Dermatol 133: 306–307
227. Kuan S F, Montag A G, Hart J et al. 2001 Differential expression of mucin genes in mammary and extramammary Paget's disease. Am J Surg Pathol 25: 1469–1477
228. Ordonez N G, Awalt H, Mackay B 1987 Mammary and extramammary Paget's disease: an immunohistochemical and ultrastructural study. Cancer 59: 1173–1183
229. Raju R R, Goldblum J R, Hart W R 2003 Pagetoid squamous cell carcinoma in situ (pagetoid Bowen's disease) of the external genitalia. Int J Gynecol Pathol 22: 127–135
230. Williamson J D, Maria I, Colome M I et al. 2000 Pagetoid Bowen disease: a report of 2 cases that express cytokeratin 7. Arch Pathol Lab Med 124: 427–430
231. Quinn A M, Sienko A, Basrawala Z et al. 2004 Extramammary Paget disease of the scrotum with features of Bowen disease. Arch Pathol Lab Med 128: 84–86
232. Moon T D, Sarma D P 1989 Leiomyosarcoma of the scrotum. J Am Acad Dermatol 20: 290–292
233. Dalton D P, Rushovich A M, Victor T A et al. 1988 Leiomyosarcoma of the scrotum in a man who had received scrotal irradiation as a child. J Urol 139: 136–138
234. Desai S R, Angarkar N N 2003 Leiomyosarcoma of the scrotum. Ind J Pathol Microbiol 46: 212–213
235. Suster S, Wong T Y, Moran C A 1993 Sarcoma with combined features of liposarcoma and leiomyosarcoma. Study of two cases of an unusual soft-tissue tumor showing dual lineage differentiation. Am J Surg Pathol 17: 905–911
236. Watanabe K, Ogawa A, Komatsu H 1988 Malignant fibrous histiocytoma of the scrotal wall: a case report. J Urol 140: 151–152
237. Chan J A, McMenamin M E, Fletcher C D M 2003 Synovial sarcoma in older patients: clinicopathological analysis of 32 cases with emphasis on unusual histological fetures. Histopathology 43: 72–83
238. Bajaj P, Aiyer H, Sinha B K et al. 2001 Pitfalls in the diagnosis of epithelioid sarcoma presenting in an unusual site: a case report. Diagn Cytopathol 24: 36–38
239. Kochman A, Jablecki J, Rabczynski J 1999 Recurrent primary well-differentiated intrascrotal liposarcoma: case report and review of the literature. Tumori 85: 135–136
240. Papadimitrious J C, Drachenberg C B 1994 Posttraumatic spindle cell nodules. Immunohistochemical and ultrastructural study of two scrotal lesions. Arch Pathol Lab Med 118: 709–711

腹膜肿瘤
Tumors of the peritoneum

Philip B. Clement 著

郑红芳 译　回允中 校

瘤样病变	881	转移性肿瘤	891
间皮肿瘤	886	第二Müller系统肿瘤和瘤样病变	893
其他原发性肿瘤	889		

在这一章里，我们按照以下几个方面回顾一下腹膜病变：瘤样病变，间皮肿瘤，其他原发性肿瘤，转移性肿瘤，以及从所谓的第二Müller系统衍化而来的病变。腹膜后疾病，除了腹膜起源的以外，不在这里介绍。

瘤样病变　Tumor-like lesions

间皮增生　Mesothelial hyperplasia

间皮增生是一种对急性和慢性炎症以及慢性渗出的常见反应（图15.1～图15.4）[1-4]。增生性病变可以在手术中发现，呈孤立性或多发性，一般为小的结节或斑块，但是更常见的是在显微镜检查中的偶然发现。间皮增生常常发生在伴有慢性输卵管炎和子宫内膜异位症的妇女的附件[2]，并且在伴有卵巢肿瘤的患者常常在附件及其他区域（尤其是网膜）可见[3]。此外，在交界性上皮性肿瘤上面的卵巢表面或卵巢浅层间质内出现的间皮增生，可能被误认为是浸润性肿瘤（图15.5）[3]。间皮增生还可以出现在疝囊，在一些病例是由于损伤或嵌顿造成的（图15.2）[4]。

在显著间皮增生的病例中，可以出现实性、小梁状、管状、乳头状或管状乳头状等结构（图15.1～图

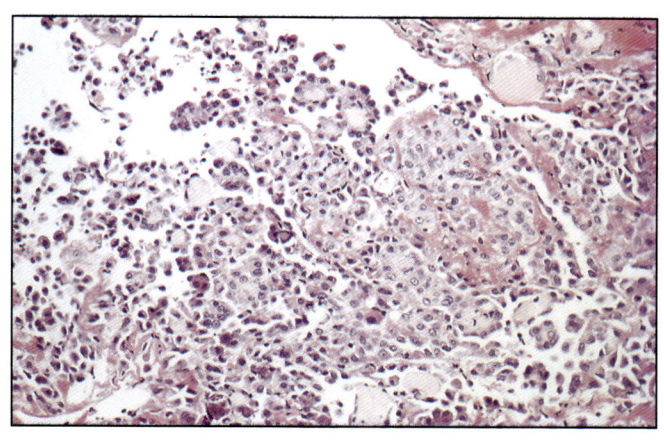

图15.2　累及疝囊的显著的乳头状间皮增生。

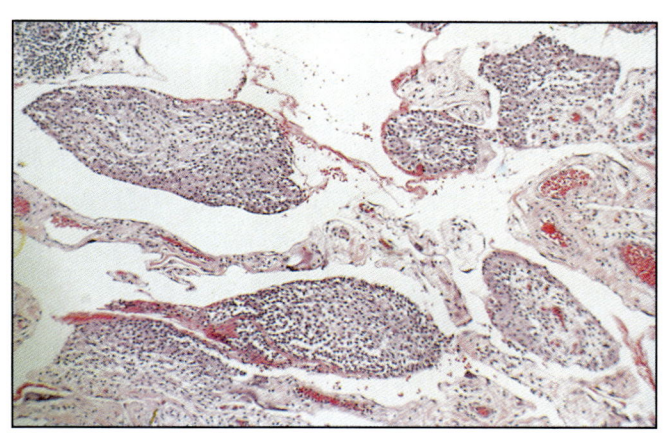

图15.1　累及网膜的结节状间皮增生。

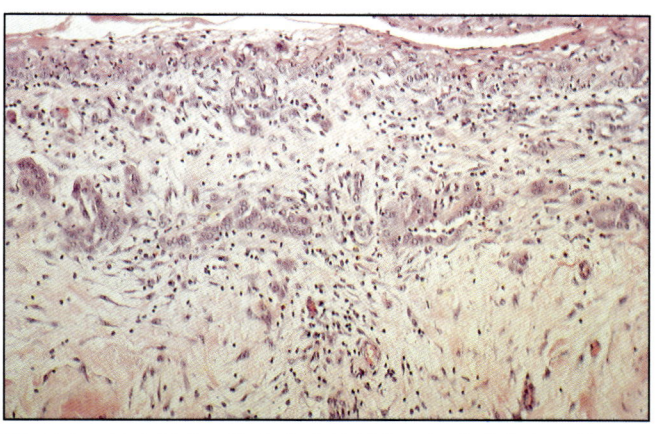

图15.3　间皮增生。注意炎症性纤维组织中线样排列的间皮细胞。

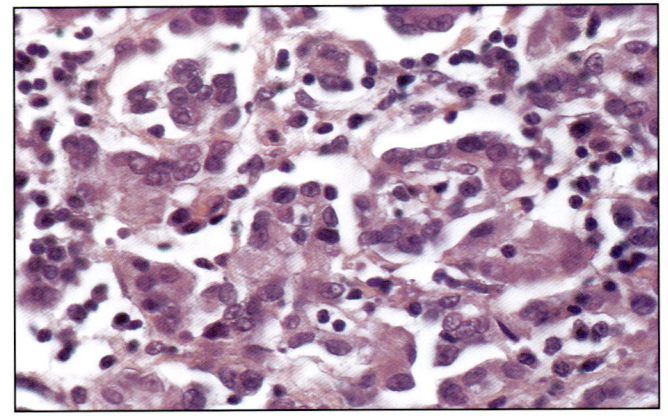

图15.4 卵巢周围乳头状间皮增生。注意轻微的核非典型性以及混合的炎症细胞。

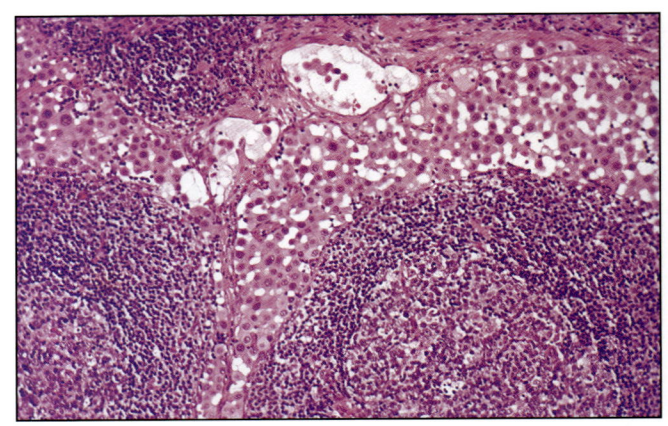

图15.6 盆腔淋巴结内增生性间皮细胞。间皮细胞充满被膜下淋巴管和淋巴窦。伴有腹膜间皮增生。

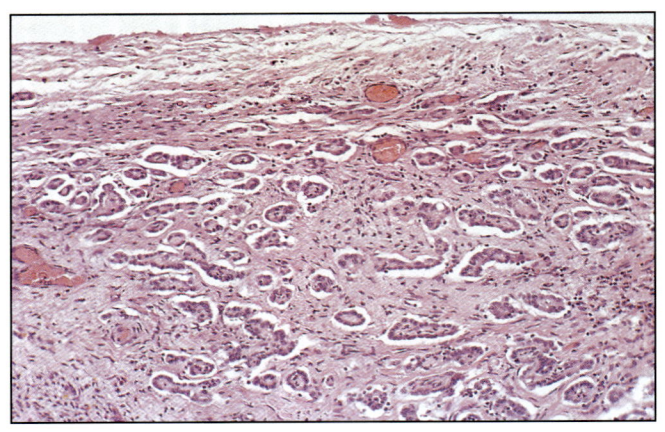

图15.5 卵巢间质内增生性间皮细胞巢（围绕细胞巢的空隙是人工假象）。增生性间皮细胞邻近黏液性交界性肿瘤，并且被误认为是浸润灶。

15.5），某些病例伴有间皮细胞向下延伸到浅表组织（图15.3和图15.5）。局灶细胞可以排列成线样，偶尔平行，呈薄层状分布，被纤维蛋白或纤维组织分隔，（图15.3）。间皮细胞可以含有充满酸性黏液（主要是透明质酸）的胞浆空泡，或者在少数情况下，其胞浆可以明显透明变。可以出现轻微到中度核非典型性、核分裂象，以及偶尔可出现多核细胞。可以见到沙粒体，在罕见的病例尚可见到类似于横纹肌母细胞的嗜酸性带状细胞[4]。在某些间皮增生的病例中，间皮细胞中可以混有不同数量的组织细胞（"结节性组织细胞/间皮细胞增生"），少数病例中组织细胞为主要成分[5,6]。区别这两种类型的细胞可能需要免疫组化检查，但未必具有临床重要性。

在罕见的情况下，增生的间皮细胞可能累及腹腔内淋巴结，这种情况伴有腹膜间皮增生，而且推测这样的病例是继发于腹膜间皮增生[7]。增生的间皮细胞可能主要累及被膜下淋巴管和结内的淋巴窦（图15.6），酷似窦组织细胞增生症、卵巢浆液性交界性肿瘤、转移癌或转移性间皮瘤累及淋巴结。在这样的病例，细胞角蛋白（cytokeratin）染色比常规染色切片更能显示间皮细胞广泛累及淋巴结。

间皮增生主要应与恶性间皮瘤进行鉴别诊断。出现大体可见的结节、坏死、显著增大的胞浆内空泡、重度核非典型性以及深部浸润倾向于间皮瘤而不是间皮增生[1]。然而，这些特征并不总是出现，或在间皮瘤中仅有局灶出现。虽然上皮膜抗原（EMA）和p53的免疫反应是恶性间皮瘤较为典型的特征，而结蛋白(desmin)的免疫反应是间皮增生较为典型的特征[8]，但是这些标记物在个别的病例可能不是完全可信的[1]。有时鉴别间皮增生性病变和间皮瘤可能是困难甚至是不可能的，尤其是在小的活检标本中。

除了间皮瘤，腹膜或淋巴结内间皮增生的鉴别诊断包括浆液性交界性肿瘤，或者表现为来自卵巢浆液性交界性肿瘤的播散，或者是原发性腹膜或淋巴结内浆液性交界性肿瘤（见第894页）。大体可见卵巢或腹膜肿瘤结节，可能具有纤毛的柱状细胞，出现细胞内或细胞外中性黏液以及大量沙粒体支持浆液性交界性肿瘤的诊断。对于"上皮性"抗原（见下文恶性间皮瘤一节）的免疫反应性在鉴别诊断中也是有用的。

腹膜包涵囊肿 Peritoneal inclusion cysts

腹膜包涵囊肿通常发生在育龄妇女[9-27]，同样的病变很少发生在男性或累及胸膜[16-18]。某些囊肿是在开腹手术中偶然发现的，呈单发性或多发性小而透明的薄壁单房性囊肿，附着或游离在腹腔内（图15.7）。它们偶尔累及圆韧带，可能类似于腹股沟疝。某些囊肿是在阑尾切除标本中浆膜的偶然发现。个别的病例位于腹膜后[25]。病理学检查发现，这些囊肿内衬一般光滑，含有黄色的水样或胶冻样内容物，有单层扁平良性表现的间皮细胞。某些病例可以见到成熟分层的鳞状上皮。大部分单房性间皮囊肿在本质上可能是反应性的，但某些累及结肠系膜、小肠系膜、腹膜后和脾包膜的病例，提示是来源于发育异常。

多房性囊肿肿块的直径可以达到20 cm（图15.8），内衬间皮细胞，被称作多房性腹膜包涵囊肿（multilocular peritoneal inclusion cysts，MPICs）、良性囊性间皮瘤、腹膜炎症性囊肿或术后腹膜囊肿[9-15,26]。MPICs常有临床表现，通常为下腹痛，可触及的肿块，或者两者都有。囊肿一般黏附在盆腔内脏，在临床上、手术中[13]或在病理检查时可能类似于囊性卵巢肿瘤；腹腔上部、脾[19]、肝[23]、腹膜后、腹股沟[24]和疝囊也可能受累。MPICs的间隔和囊壁可能含有相当多的纤维组织，其内容物可以类似于单房性囊肿的内容物，也可以是血清液或者完全为血性。

显微镜下检查显示，MPICs通常内衬单层扁平到立方上皮，少数情况下内衬鞋钉形细胞，间皮细胞一般具有良性细胞核的特征，但某些反应性非典型性改变并不少见(图15.9和图15.10)。间皮细胞可以增生进入囊腔，形成小的乳头或呈筛状结构，偶尔还可以发生鳞状上皮化生[14,15]。囊壁上可以出现典型的或非典型性间皮细胞增生，表现为单个的呈腺样或巢状分布（图15.11），或者可以出现类似于腺瘤样瘤的形态，导致可能提示为癌的浸润性结构[13-15]。在某些病例，间质内空泡状间皮细胞可能提出有无印戒细胞癌的可能性[15]。囊壁和分隔常

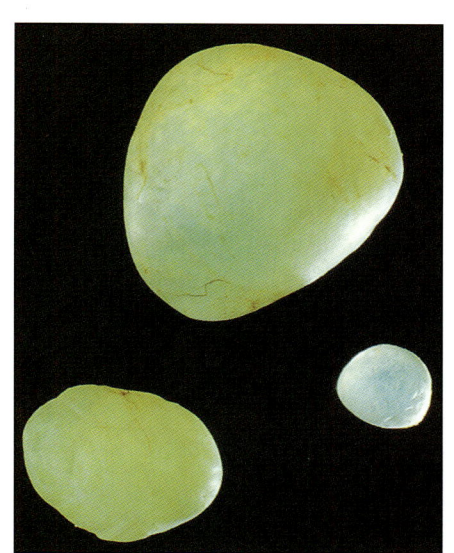

图15.7 单房性腹膜包涵囊肿。

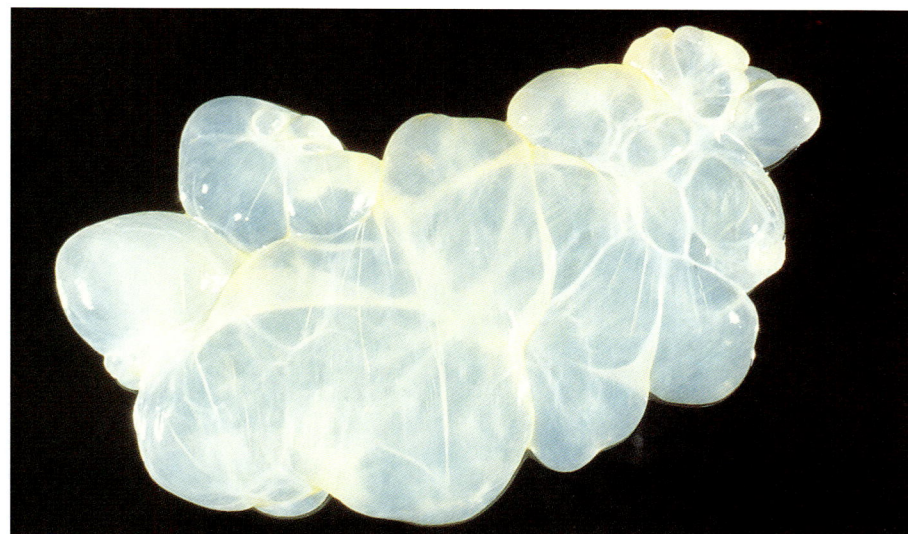

图15.8 多房性腹膜包涵囊肿。

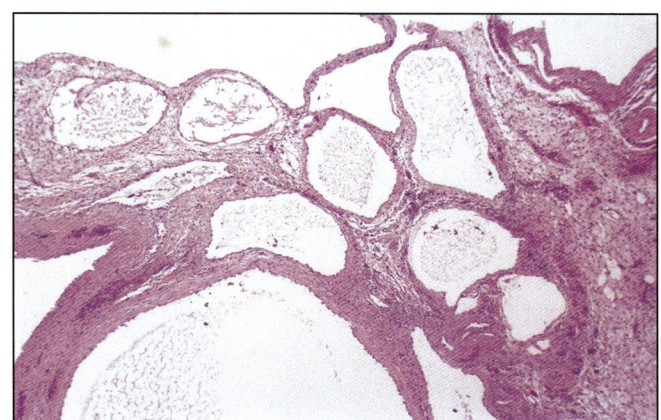

图15.9 多房性腹膜包涵囊肿。

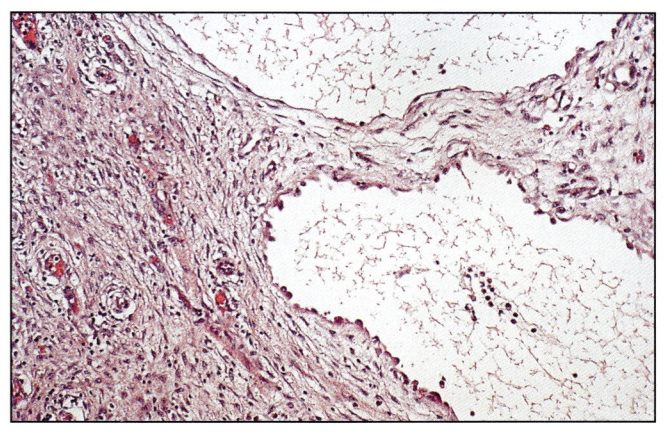

图15.10 多房性腹膜包涵囊肿。注意炎症性的间质以及偶见的内衬囊肿的鞋钉样间皮细胞。

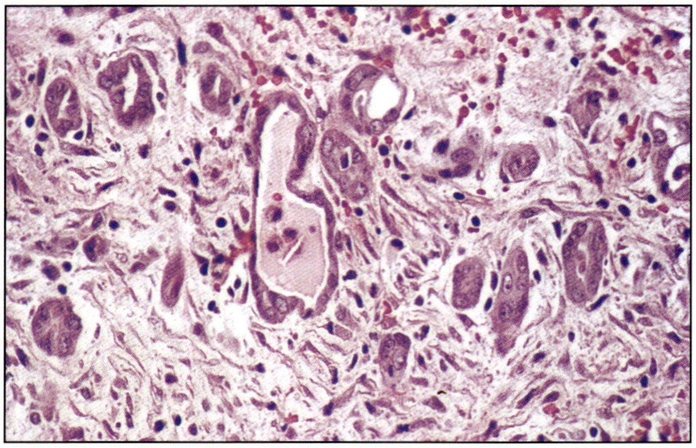

图15.11 多房性腹膜包涵囊肿，伴有囊壁间皮细胞。

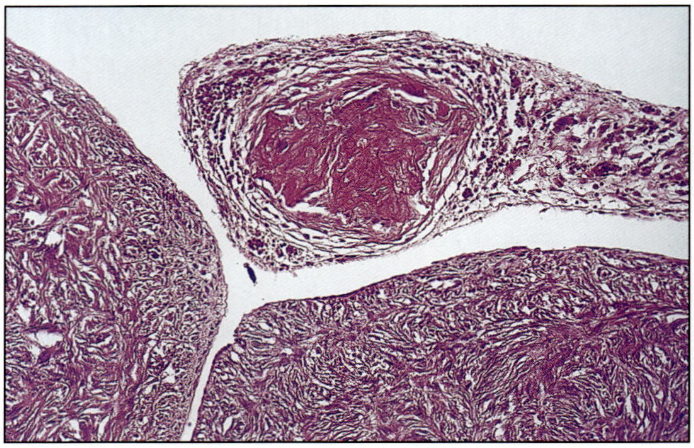

图15.12 卵巢表面角质肉芽肿。患者患有子宫内膜腺癌伴有广泛鳞状分化。

常由纤维血管结缔组织组成，伴有少量炎症细胞浸润，但在其他一些病例，可以见到严重的急性和慢性炎症（可能包括泡沫状组织细胞），纤维素，肉芽组织以及出血。

一项研究显示[15]，84%的患者具有一个或多个因素，例如腹部外科手术，盆腔炎症性疾病或子宫内膜异位症，指出炎症在MPICs发病机制中可能具有作用。有的病例可能难以区分是明显的黏连还是MPICs，这也符合炎症性的病因学。只有少数病例[18]与接触石棉有关。偶尔，MPICs对于雌激素和（或）孕激素受体具有免疫反应[26]，或在应用促性腺激素释放激素（GnRH）促效剂治疗之后变小[27]，提示某些病例激素因素可能具有一定作用。

对于我们认为是MPICs的病例进行随访显示，没有恶性行为的证据，但是多达50%的病变切除后数月到数年局部复发，某些病例多次复发[15]。然而，至少其中某些"复发"可能是由于新形成的术后黏连。因此对于这些病变，我们喜欢多房性腹膜包涵囊肿这一命名胜过良性囊性间皮瘤。

MPICs在大体和显微镜下检查都有可能与多房性囊性淋巴管瘤混淆[9]。不像MPICs，后者常常发生在儿童，一般是男孩，并且常常是位于盆腔外，大多数病例位于小肠系膜、网膜、结肠系膜或腹膜后。与MPICs不同，多房性囊性淋巴管瘤的内容物常常是乳糜样；显微镜下检查常常可以看到囊壁上有淋巴细胞聚集和平滑肌，内衬细胞染色示内皮标记物阳性而不是角蛋白。同样，脾内MPICs与脾的淋巴管瘤也有混淆[19]。在有问题的病例，区分内皮和间皮细胞的免疫组织化学染色具有诊断意义。MPICs的鉴别诊断还包括罕见的囊性腺瘤样瘤[28]。该肿瘤不同于MPICs，它常常发生在子宫，含有典型的腺瘤样瘤病灶，而且缺乏明显的炎症细胞浸润。

腹膜角质肉芽肿　Peritoneal keratin granulomas

在显微镜下，感染性和非感染性腹膜肉芽肿几乎总是很容易与肿瘤鉴别[29]。相反，继发于来源于女性生殖道肿瘤角蛋白种植的腹膜肉芽肿，可能与转移性肿瘤混淆[30]。肿瘤通常为子宫内膜（或者，不太常见的卵巢）伴有鳞状分化的子宫内膜样癌；此外，在少数情况下，宫颈鳞状细胞癌和子宫非典型性息肉样腺肌瘤也是角蛋白的来源[30]。肉芽肿由成层的角蛋白沉积构成，某些病例伴有坏死的鳞状细胞，被异物巨细胞和纤维组织包绕（图15.12）。

虽然随访资料显示，这些肉芽肿对于预后没有任何影响，但是这些病变的预后意义还没有被完全确定，因为某些病例随访时间较短，此外，某些患者术后还接受放疗、化疗，或联合放疗和化疗。如果能够看到角质肉芽肿，外科医师应该广泛取样，而病理医师应在显微镜下仔细检查，以便排除另外存在的任何存活癌细胞。鉴别诊断包括其他来源的角蛋白的反应性腹膜肉芽肿，包括羊水和卵巢皮样囊肿。在后一种情况中，囊肿破裂释放出皮脂样物质和角蛋白，典型者引起强烈的肉芽肿性，脂肪肉芽肿性以及纤维性腹膜炎症反应，在手术中可能类似于肿瘤[29]。

腹膜纤维化、硬化性腹膜炎和硬化性肠系膜炎　Peritoneal fibrosis, sclerosing peritonitis, and sclerosing mesenteritis

反应性腹膜纤维化（reactive peritoneal fibrosis）（包括纤维性黏连）是腹膜炎症和腹部手术的一种常见的后遗症，很少存在诊断问题。反应性腹膜纤维化性病变可能含有"多潜能浆膜下细胞"[31]，表现为肥胖的，常常为筋膜炎样的梭形细胞，对波形蛋白（vimentin）、SMA和CK具有免疫反应。

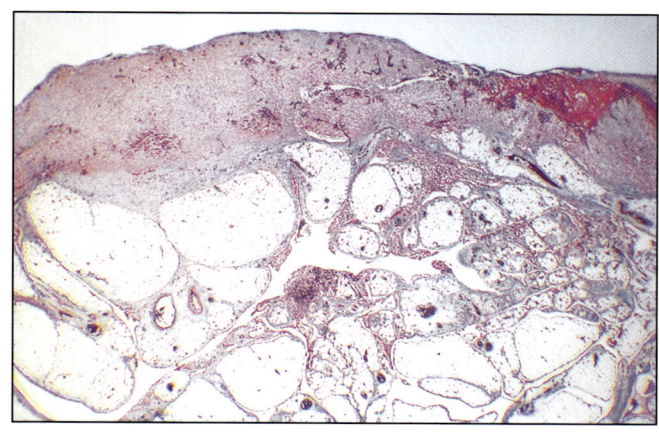

图15.13 硬化性腹膜炎，伴有卵巢黄素化卵泡膜细胞瘤。网膜表面和小叶间分隔纤维性增厚（Masson三色染色）。

硬化性腹膜炎（sclerosing peritonitis）是一种罕见的疾病，以腹膜纤维性增厚为特征，可以包裹小肠（"腹部茧"，abdominal cocoon），导致肠梗阻。虽然可以是特发的（这样的病例一般发生在青春期女孩），常见的相关病因包括普拉骆尔疗法（practolol therapy），长期动态腹膜透析，应用 LeVeen 腹腔静脉分流术，以及卵巢纤维卵泡膜性增生（典型者为黄素化的卵泡膜细胞瘤）（图 15.13）[32]。关于最后一个相关因素，手术中的表现可能类似于恶性卵巢肿瘤伴有腹膜播散，几个病例腹膜病变的显微镜下表现最初被误诊为转移性卵泡膜细胞瘤（图 15.13）。在这些病例中，硬化性腹膜炎的病因还不清楚。

硬化性肠系膜炎（sclerosing mesenteritis）（退缩性肠系膜炎，肠系膜脂膜炎，肠系膜脂质营养不良）是一种特发性疾病，以不同程度的脂肪坏死、慢性炎症以及纤维化为特征，通常累及小肠系膜。在最大的一项研究中[33]，患者年龄从 23 岁到 87 岁（平均 60 岁）；最常见的临床表现是腹痛或腹部包块。大体检查肠系膜最常见到的是孤立性肿块；多发性肿块或肠系膜弥漫性增厚不太常见。鉴别诊断包括多种良性病变和肉瘤[33]。与硬化性肠系膜炎不同，肠系膜纤维瘤病（腹腔内硬纤维瘤）浸润肠壁，具有束状结构，缺乏炎症和脂肪坏死。腹膜后纤维化在组织学上类似硬化性肠系膜炎，而且实际上可能是一种相关的疾病，但是这两种疾病常常可以通过它们不同的临床表现、部位以及手术中所见鉴别开来。不像硬化性肠系膜炎，炎性假瘤（浆细胞肉芽肿）的特征为密集的浆细胞浸润以及白细胞增多，红细胞沉降率升高和贫血。与硬化性肠系膜炎相比，累及肠系膜的肉瘤（特别是脂肪肉瘤）几乎总是有较多的细胞，间质或脂肪细胞核有非典型性以及核分裂活性。

在个别病例中，反应性纤维性腹膜病变可能难以与纤维组织增生性间皮瘤鉴别，尤其是在小的活检标本中。支持间皮瘤诊断的特征包括核的非典型性，坏死，胶原沉积呈器官样结构（束状，席纹状），以及浸润邻近组织[34]。

钙化性纤维性（假）瘤
Calcifying fibrous (pseudo) tumor

这是一种罕见的病变，典型者是一种偶然发现，累及成人小肠和胃的脏层腹膜[35-37]。罕见的病例呈现家族性[36]。在手术中，本病可能被误认为是转移癌，形成界限清楚的实性包块，直径常常小于 10 cm，切面呈沙砾感。组织学检查可见致密的玻璃样变的胶原，常常呈同心漩涡状排列，良性表现的纤维母细胞、淋巴细胞和浆细胞通常稀疏排列，偶见富于细胞的区域（可以聚集在血管周围），以及沙粒体。这些病变（推测为反应性）与有类似名称的似乎为肿瘤性的软组织肿块的关系还不清楚（见第 24 章），但有越来越多的证据提示，所有这些肿瘤可能有复发潜能[37]。

脾组织植入　Splenosis

脾组织植入，或者脾组织种植，常常在因外伤性脾破裂而进行的脾切除术数月到数年后的腹部手术中偶然发现[38,39]。几个到许多红蓝色腹膜结节，大小从勉强可见到直径 7 cm，散在分布于整个腹腔，某些病例位于盆腔（图 15.14）。手术中表现可能类似于腹膜子宫内膜异位症，良性或恶性血管肿瘤，或转移癌。

"黑变病"　"melanosis"

7 例腹膜褐色色素沉着（腹膜"黑变病"）病例伴有卵巢皮样囊肿；其中两例术前囊肿破裂[40]。剖腹手

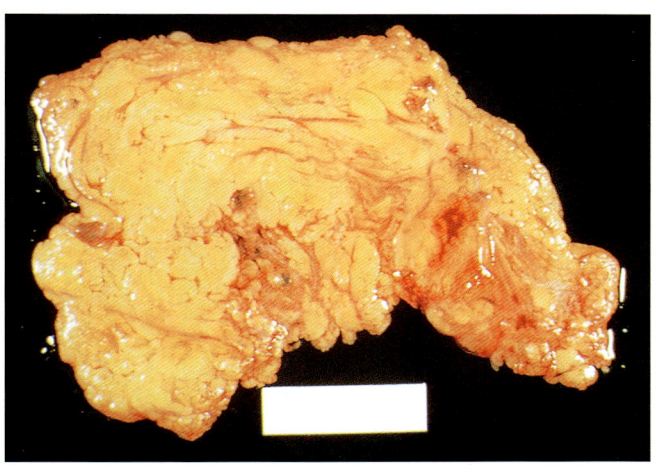

图15.14 网膜的脾组织植入。

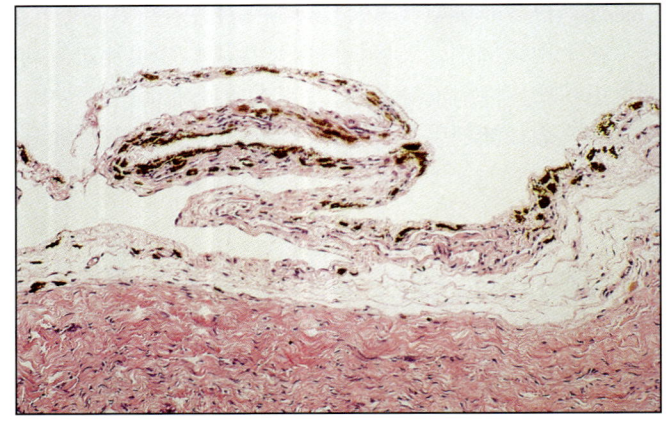

图15.15 腹膜黑变病。

术时发现，盆腔和网膜有局灶性或弥漫性褐色到黑色腹膜染色或色素沉着性瘤样结节。皮样囊肿中，某些子囊腔的内容物和内衬上皮有色素沉着。在显微镜下，卵巢和腹膜病变由纤维间质内充满色素的组织细胞组成（图15.15）。在报告的病例中，至少半数皮样囊肿中胃黏膜明显，有时伴有溃疡、坏死和出血。一项研究发现，色素既不是黑色素也不是含铁血黄素，而是含有高浓度的铁；提示皮样囊肿中的消化性溃疡与出血有关[40]。腹膜"黑变病"容易与转移性恶性黑色素瘤区别，因为色素性组织细胞具有温和的细胞核特征以及核分裂不活跃。

梗死性肠脂垂　　infarcted appendix epiploica

肠脂垂扭转和梗死，某些病例随后钙化，可能形成坚硬的瘤样肿块，黏附或游离于腹腔[41,42]。显微镜下检查发现，这些结构一般由分层的玻璃样变的纤维组织，围绕中心坏死和钙化的梗死脂肪组织组成（图15.16）。

软骨结节　　Cartilaginous nodules

腹膜软骨分化已有两例报告，均发生在绝经后妇女[43]。异位的腹膜病变为手术中偶然发现。一例为多发性结节，最大直径达到7 mm，而另外一例为直径2cm的单发性结节。两例结节均由成熟的透明软骨组成，周围绕以纤维组织。作者推测，结节可以是第二 Müller 系统的化生性病变，或为由间皮下组织衍化而来的软骨瘤。

间皮肿瘤　　Mesothelial neoplasms

孤立性纤维性肿瘤　　Solitary fibrous tumor

孤立性（或局限性）纤维性肿瘤较常累及胸膜（见第5章）或软组织（见第24章），在腹腔内罕见（图15.17）[44-46]。虽然这些肿瘤被称为"纤维性间皮瘤"，现在认为是来源于间皮下纤维母细胞。其临床和病理学特征类似于发生在胸膜和其他部位的同名肿瘤，包括对波形蛋白和CD34的强免疫反应以及CK阴性，这有助于与纤维组织增生性间皮瘤的鉴别[44-48]。偶尔，其他方面典型的肿瘤伴有细胞丰富的区域，显著的细胞核多形性或核分裂率高，被诊断为恶性肿瘤[47,48]。

腺瘤样瘤　　Adenomatoid tumor

这种间皮起源的良性肿瘤很少发生在生殖器外的腹膜，诸如网膜[49]或肠系膜[50]，而是较常见于男性和女性生殖道，将在第13章和第14章讨论。

高分化乳头状间皮瘤　　Well-differentiated papillary mesothelioma

腹膜高分化乳头状间皮瘤（well-differentiated papillary mesotheliomas, WDPMs）不太常见；大约已有50例的详细报告[51-56]，包括一个22个病例的系列报告[52]。大约75%的肿瘤发生在女性，通常在生育年龄，但是

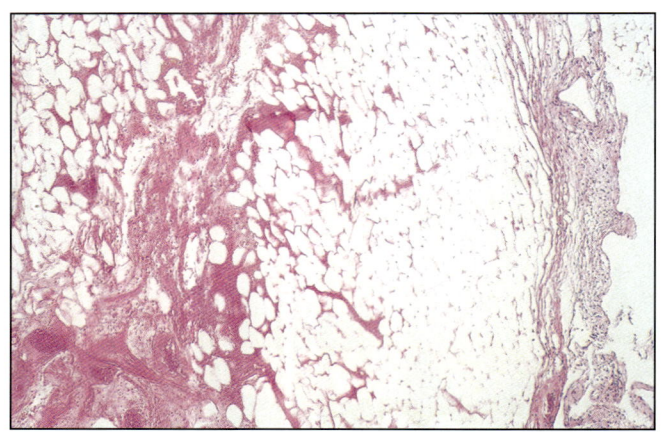

图15.16 梗死性肠脂垂。

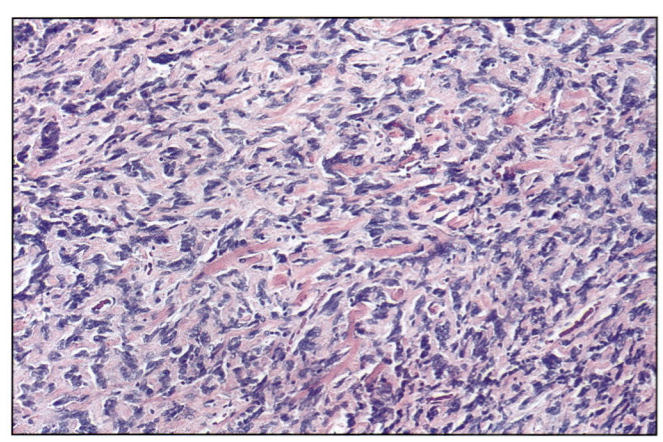

图15.17 腹膜孤立性纤维性肿瘤（"纤维性间皮瘤"）。

偶尔也可见于绝经后妇女[51,52]。WDPMs通常是剖腹手术的偶然发现，但是有的肿瘤伴有腹痛或腹水。然而，出现症状和（或）腹水更常见于恶性间皮瘤[54]。少数患者有石棉接触史[55]。

在剖腹手术和大体检查时，WDPMs可以为孤立性或多发性，表现为灰色到白色的质硬乳头状或结节状病变，直径常常小于2 cm。典型者累及网膜和盆腔腹膜[52,54]；几个肿瘤起源于胃、肠或肠系膜的腹膜[51]。

显微镜检查示，纤维性乳头被覆单层扁平到立方形间皮细胞（图15.18和图15.19），偶尔可能含有基底空泡；核呈良性特征，核分裂象稀少或缺乏。见到的不常见的其他形态包括管状乳头状（图15.18）、分枝索条状和实性片块状。某些肿瘤的间质广泛纤维化或偶尔呈黏液样；个别病例可见沙粒体。

多数孤立性WDPMs在临床上是良性的，虽然在少数情况下肿瘤可能持续长达数十年[52]。当出现多发性病变时，其临床经过还不十分确定。每个病变都应该取样进行显微镜检查，以排除恶性间皮瘤，因为Goldblum和Hart[54]发现，他们所有的伴有一个以上部位受累的腹膜间皮瘤，至少具有局灶性的恶性组织性特征。只有那些局限性和具有均一的良性组织学特征的病变，才能预示具有良性的临床经过。Butnor等报告了一系列WDPMs病例[55]，包括随访3年之后死于本病的具有多灶性WDPM的患者，但是尚不清楚肿瘤是否充分取样检查以排除恶性成分。

恶性间皮瘤　Malignant mesothelioma

临床特征

腹膜恶性间皮瘤（peritoneal malignant mesotheliomas，PMMs）比胸膜恶性间皮瘤少见得多（见第5章），仅占所有恶性间皮瘤的10%～20%[54,57-64]。PMMs在女性特别少见，在女性人群中，多数恶性乳头状腹膜肿瘤是卵巢外乳头状浆液性癌（见下文有关第二Müller系统肿瘤和瘤样病变一节）。

男女发病比例大约为2:1。患者常常为中年或老年人，但是个别PMM病例发生在年轻人或儿童[65-69]。患者常常出现非特异性症状，最常见的是腹部不适和腹胀，消化紊乱，以及体重下降。少数患者血清CA125水平升高[70]。多数病例出现腹水，腹水的细胞学检查偶尔具有诊断意义[61]。然而，诊断通常需要剖腹手术或者腹腔镜检查和活检。少数PMMs出现在疝囊或睾丸鞘膜积液囊壁内，表现为一个局限性腹膜后、肝、脐、肠、盆腔或卵巢肿瘤[61,64,71-74]，或表现为颈部或腹股沟淋巴结肿大[75]。某些病例出现炎症性包块，类似于阑尾炎或胆囊炎[76]。

文献中报告的多数PMMs男性病例具有石棉接触史，但在女性患者少有这样的病史[54,62-64]。在某些病例中，遗传因素、放射、慢性炎症、接触有机化学药品以及非石棉矿物纤维可能也起病因作用[77-79]。在大部分报告中，多数或全部患者为男性，诊断之后生存通常少于2年，虽然也有个别长期生存的病例[60,61,80,81]。相反，Kerrigan等在一项局限于女性的PMMs的研究中，发现40%的患者生存期为4年或更长，某些病例超过了10年。手术之后留有最小病变或者没有残留病变的比较年轻的患者显示其生存率有所改善[82]。

病理学特征

脏层和壁层腹膜弥漫增厚或者布满结节和斑块（图15.20），而且内脏常常被肿瘤包裹（并且可能被侵犯），虽然侵犯内脏以及淋巴结、肝、肺和胸膜转移比相当程度的癌的腹膜受累少见。然而，在尸检中可能见到明显

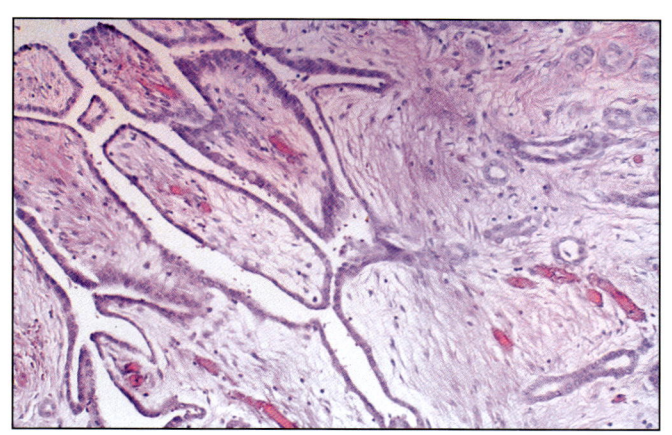

图15.18　高分化乳头状间皮瘤，伴有管状乳头状结构。

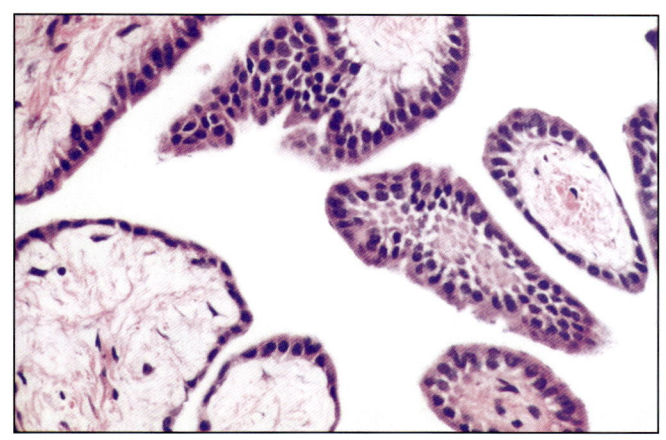

图15.19　高分化乳头状间皮瘤。

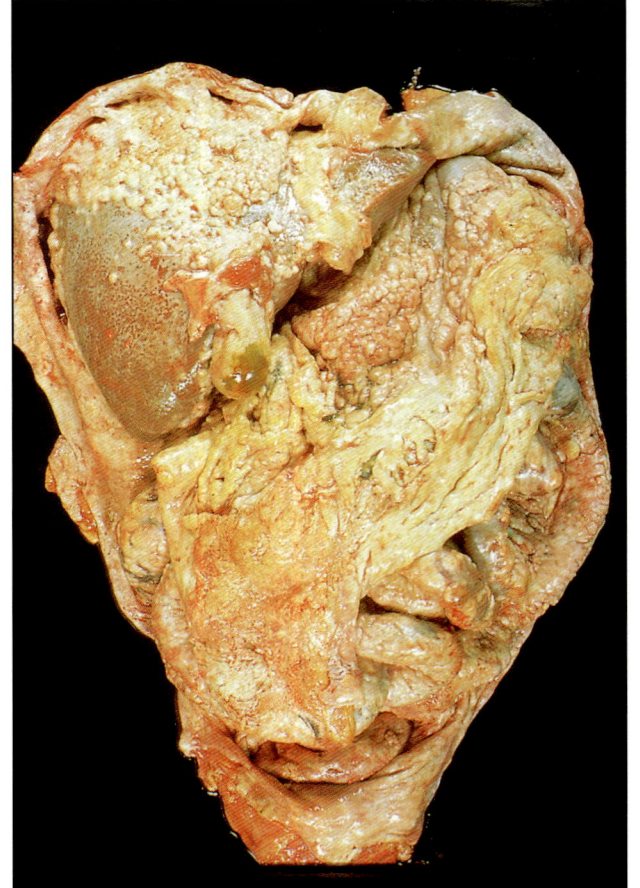

图15.20　腹膜弥漫性恶性间皮瘤。

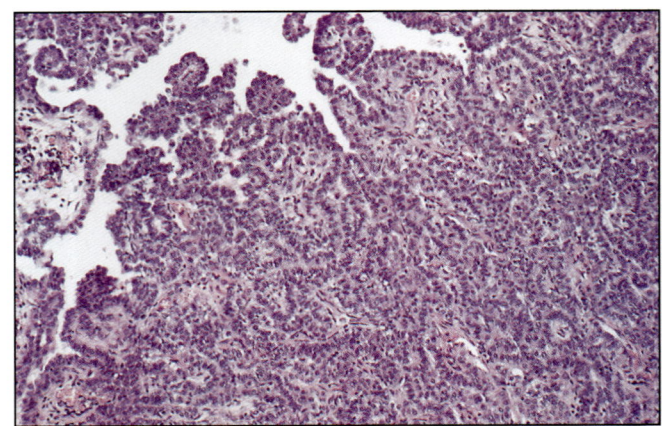

图15.21　弥漫性恶性间皮瘤。

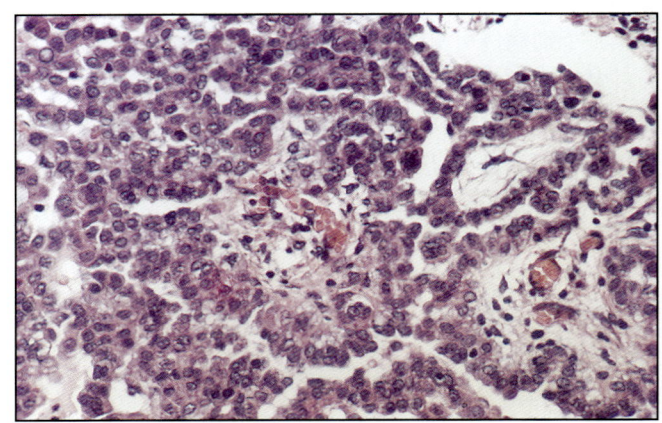

图15.22　弥漫性恶性间皮瘤。

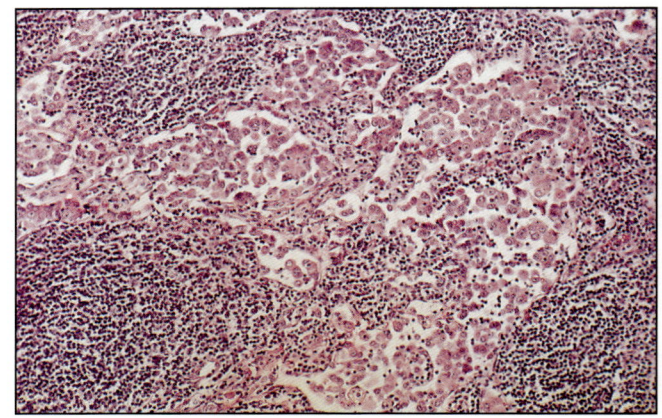

图15.23　腹部淋巴结的转移性恶性间皮瘤。

侵犯腹部器官和转移性病变。

显微镜下特征（图15.21～图15.23）一般类似于胸膜间皮瘤（见第5章），除了肉瘤样和双相性肿瘤特别少见以外。偶尔发生肉瘤样和双相性腹膜PMMs，并有一例双相性肿瘤报告，其中的肉瘤样成分含有横纹肌样细胞[74]。个别肿瘤具有明显的炎症反应，包括密集的淋巴细胞浸润[69]和许多泡沫状富含脂质的组织细胞[83]。可以出现沙粒体，但是在浆液性癌中更为常见，而且数量也常常更多。PMMs的免疫组织化学（见下文的鉴别诊断一节）和超微结构特征与胸膜的相应病变没有显著的差异。

少数PMMs以独特的片块样结构为特征，由具有丰富嗜酸性胞浆的多角形细胞组成（图15.24）[66-68]。这样的肿瘤被称为"蜕膜样间皮瘤"，强调它们类似于异位蜕膜（见下文第二Müller系统肿瘤和瘤样病变一节）。虽然最初认为较常见于年轻女性，但是女性只略占优势，而且年龄范围广泛[68]。这些肿瘤通常迅速致死。包括突出的嗜酸性核仁，核分裂活性，以及间皮瘤典型的免疫组织化学和超微结构所见（见下文）在内的种种特征支持间皮瘤的诊断。

鉴别诊断

伴有间皮增生的腹膜恶性间皮瘤（PMM）的鉴别诊断在别处讨论（见上文间皮增生一节）。与PMMs不同，高分化乳头状间皮瘤（WDPMs，上文已讨论）以均匀一致的良性组织学表现为特征，尽管PMMs可以是

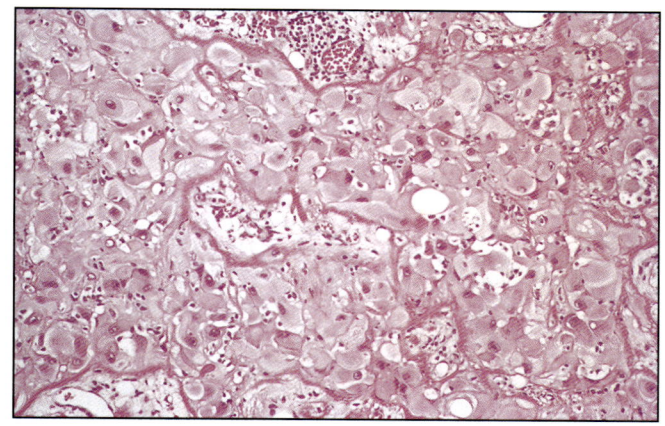

图15.24 "蜕膜样"恶性间皮瘤。

局灶高分化伴有类似 WDPM 的区域[54]。PMMs 还必须与浆膜恶性血管肿瘤(见第891页和第5章)以及弥漫累及腹膜的腺癌鉴别,包括转移性腺癌和女性腹膜原发性腺癌(见下面第二 Müller 系统肿瘤和瘤样病变一节)。伴有管状乳头状结构的肿瘤,以及病变细胞呈多角形伴有中等量的嗜酸性胞浆时,应该考虑到 PMM 的诊断。相反,出现柱状细胞支持腺癌的诊断。大部分腹膜原发性腺癌是浆液性乳头状癌,与发生于卵巢的浆液性乳头状癌不能区分,但与 PMMs 不同,其常常出现高级别甚至奇异核的特征以及许多沙粒体。类似的特征有助于将罕见的原发性腹膜恶性混合性中胚层肿瘤与罕见的双相性 PMMs 鉴别开来。

组织化学、免疫组织化学以及超微结构检查可能有助于 PMM 和腺癌的鉴别诊断[84-90]。与腺癌不同,PMMs(如同胸膜恶性间皮瘤)常以缺乏中性黏液和存在酸性黏液(主要为透明质酸)为特征,表现为阿利辛蓝(alcian blue)阳性,淀粉酶 PAS(D-PAS)阴性,胞浆小泡内有透明质酸酶敏感物质。然而,在少数情况下透明质酸可以滤入福尔马林中,导致假阴性的染色,或者出现细胞内或细胞外通过透明质酸酶预消化能够降低的 D-PAS 阳性物质。包括 PMMs 在内的大部分恶性间皮瘤,CK5/6 和钙结合蛋白(calretinin)阳性,而且缺乏种种"上皮性"抗原的反应性,其中最有用的是癌胚抗原(CEA)、B72.3、Leu-M1、Ber-EP4、S-100 以及胎盘碱性磷酸酶(PLAP)。在 PMMs 和浆液性腺癌的鉴别诊断中,Ber-EP4、B72.3、Leu-M1(CD15)、MOC-31 和 CA19-9 的免疫反应性支持浆液性癌,而血栓调节蛋白(thrombomodulin)、D2-40(或 podoplarin)以及钙结合蛋白的免疫反应性支持 PMM[89,90]。然而,没有一种单一的免疫组化染色在区分 PMM 和腺癌方面具有诊断性,而一系列的抗体染色结果应当结合 H.E. 和黏液染色进行诊断。

其他原发性肿瘤
Miscellaneous primary tumors

腹腔内纤维组织增生性小圆细胞肿瘤
Intra-abdominal desmoplastic small round cell tumor

临床特征

纤维组织增生性小圆细胞肿瘤(DSRCT)的组织发生不能确定[91-105]。它倾向于累及浆膜(包括罕见的累及胸膜的病例),提示可能是间皮来源的原始肿瘤[91],尽管有发生在非浆液性部位的例外情况,提示至少某些病例是非间皮起源。DSRCTs 的独特性是 22 号染色体上 Ewing 肉瘤(*EWS*)基因和 11 号染色体上 Wilms 肿瘤基因(*WT1*)融合,起因于 t(11;22)(p13;q12)染色体易位[94,96,101]。

DSRCT 更常见于男性患者(男女比例为 4:1),典型者发生在青春期和年轻成人(在最大的系列报告中中位年龄为 22 岁)。临床表现通常是腹胀、腹痛,以及可触及的腹部、盆腔或阴囊肿块,有时伴有腹水。有些患者血清神经元特异性烯醇化酶(NSE)水平升高[95]。剖腹手术可见不同大小的但常常是大的腹腔内肿块,伴有许多较小的腹膜"种植",可以累及腹腔的任何部位,或者偶尔累及腹膜后;少数肿瘤发生在胸膜[101]。在女性,肿瘤常常局限于盆腔,而且这样病例可能有明显的卵巢受累,可能类似于原发性卵巢肿瘤[92]。在男性,可能累及睾丸旁区域[99]。

DSRCTs 是高度侵袭性的肿瘤,在仅仅几年之内 90% 以上的患者死于肿瘤进展。典型者,最初对于减缩肿瘤体积的手术和化疗有部分反应,继而出现不能控制的肿瘤复发。即使在晚期阶段,多数肿瘤依然位于腹腔内;然而,偶尔有患者发生腹腔外转移,而且罕见的病例起初可能表现为淋巴结转移。

病理学特征

大体检查,肿瘤直径可达 40 cm。肿瘤表面光滑或有圆凸,切面质硬,灰白色,伴有灶状黏液变和坏死(图 15.25)。个别病例直接侵犯腹腔内或盆腔内脏器。显微镜下检查示,肿瘤细胞排列成大小和形状不同的界限清楚的基底样细胞巢和小梁,周围绕以富于细胞的纤维组织增生性间质(图 15.26 和图 15.27)。肿瘤细胞和间质成分的相对比例差异很大。某些细胞巢周围的栅栏状排列是一个常见的特征,中心坏死可以出现在某些较大的细胞巢中,伴有或不伴有钙化。个别病例可以出现菊形团样间隙[91,99]。肿瘤细胞均匀一致,胞浆稀少,细胞边

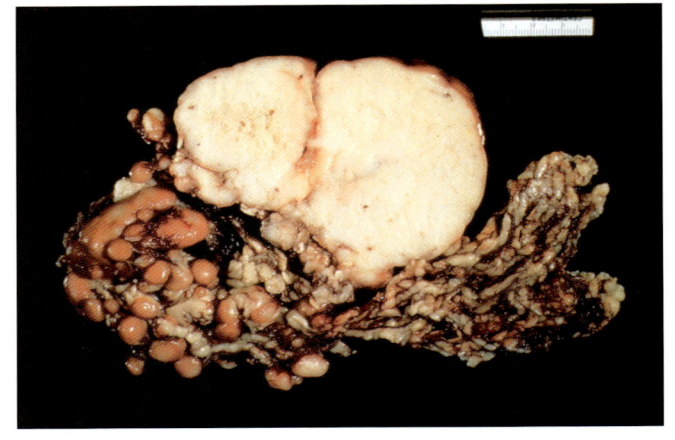

图15.25　腹腔内纤维组织增生性小圆细胞肿瘤。显示肿块切面呈白色鱼肉样，浸润网膜组织。还可见到许多小的卫星肿瘤结节。

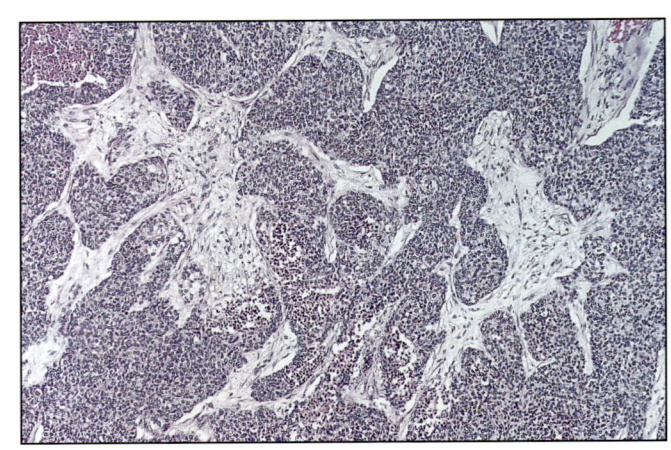

图15.26　腹腔内纤维组织增生性小圆细胞肿瘤。

图15.27　腹腔内纤维组织增生性小圆细胞肿瘤。

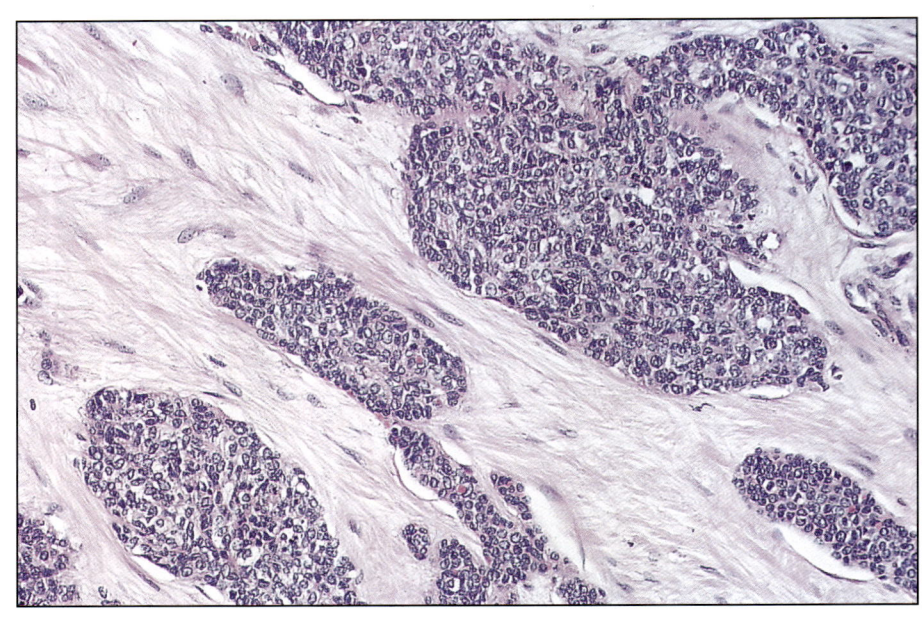

界不清，细胞核深染，小到中等大小，呈圆形或椭圆形，核仁通常不清楚。可见许多核分裂象和单个坏死细胞。在许多病例，某些肿瘤细胞以嗜酸性胞浆"包涵体"和偏心核为特征，导致横纹肌样表现（图15.28）。浸润脉管间隙常见，尤其是淋巴管。纤维组织增生性间质由位于胶原性基质内的纤维母细胞和肌纤维母细胞组成（没有细胞学非典型性）。不常见的特征[102]包括管状或腺体分化（有时伴有管腔内黏液），乳头，空泡状印戒样细胞，小灶状多形性肿瘤细胞，具有中等量胞浆的较大的细胞，以及仅有少量纤维组织增生性间质。

特殊技术表明，肿瘤为多向表型，包括对上皮（诸

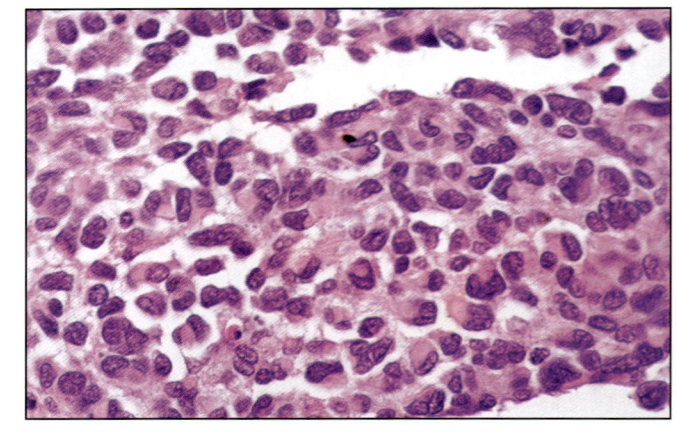

图15.28　腹腔内纤维组织增生性小圆细胞肿瘤。注意横纹肌样包涵体。

如 CAM5.2 的低分子量角蛋白，EMA），神经/神经内分泌（NSE，Leu-7）和肌肉（结蛋白，desmin）标记物以及波形蛋白的免疫反应性。典型者，结蛋白和波形蛋白阳性产物位于核旁并呈球形。新近一项研究显示[105]，差不多30%的病例出现局灶性肌红蛋白（myoglobin）免疫反应性（不能确定意义）。多数病例存在C末端部位 Wilms 肿瘤蛋白（WT1）核的免疫反应性[104,105]。对于 CD99 具有不同的反应。超微结构检查一般显示核旁胞浆内中等大小的细丝，不同类型的细胞连接，以及围绕肿瘤细胞巢的基底膜。少数病例还可以见到突入腔隙内的微绒毛样结构、有极向的细胞突起、微管、脂质小滴、糖原和致密轴心颗粒[91]。通过反转录酶多聚酶链反应检测到 *EWS/WT1* 基因融合具有诊断意义，而且当组织学特征不典型时尤其有用。

恶性血管肿瘤　Malignant vascular tumors

腹膜的恶性血管肿瘤近来已有描述，尤其是两例上皮样血管内皮瘤（epithelioid hemangioendotheliomas，EHE）和两例上皮样血管肉瘤（epithelioid angiosarcomas，EA），发生在 34～51 岁之间男性和女性患者[106,107]。这些肿瘤似乎不同于发生在肠系膜或腹膜后的血管肉瘤[108]，并且继发性累及腹膜。上文刚刚引用的研究中的四个肿瘤都是致命性的。肿瘤具有弥漫性片块状和巢状结构，伴有不同程度的血管分化，主要是以胞浆腔隙的形式存在。某些肿瘤最初得出腹膜恶性间皮瘤（PMM）印象的一些特征包括弥漫性分布，管状乳头状结构，形成双相结构的梭形细胞（包括反应性和肿瘤性细胞），波形蛋白和不同程度的角蛋白（cytokeratin）免疫反应性。通过肿瘤细胞至少对于两个内皮标记物的免疫性可以作出正确诊断，而对照组的 PMMs 则缺乏这种所见。

炎症性肌纤维母细胞瘤　Inflammatory myofibroblastic tumor

1986年，Day等最初报告了7例腹部"炎性假瘤"[109]，同义词还包括"浆细胞性肉芽肿"或"炎症性肌纤维母细胞瘤"[110]。随后发表的病例报告数量大得多[111,112]，并且提出这些病例最好被认为是炎症性纤维肉瘤[109]。在第24章中将更全面地论述这些肿瘤。腹部炎症性肌纤维母细胞瘤通常发生在20岁之前，患者表现为肿块，发热，生长障碍或体重下降，血红蛋白过少性贫血，血小板增多症，以及多克隆性γ球蛋白血症[109]。剖腹手术发现实性的肠系膜肿块，显微镜下检查发现其由肌纤维母细胞性梭形细胞、成熟的浆细胞以及小淋巴细胞组成（图15.29）。随访发现大部分患者术后经过良好，但是或许有 20%～25% 的患者出现局部复发，而

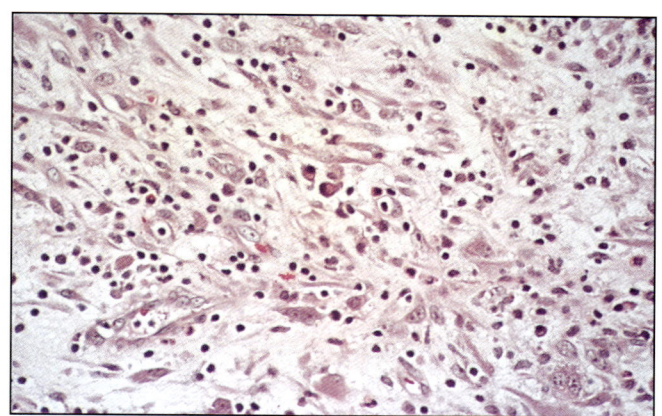

图15.29　腹腔内炎症性肌纤维母细胞瘤。

非常罕见的病例呈现真正恶性的行为[113]。

网膜-肠系膜黏液样错构瘤　Omental-mesenteric myxoid hamartoma

Gonzalez-Crussi 等[114] 将"网膜-肠系膜黏液样错构瘤"这个术语用于一种发生在婴儿的，以多发性网膜和肠系膜结节为特征的病变，结节由位于黏液样血管化间质内的肥胖间叶细胞组成。虽然某些病例最初考虑诊断为肉瘤，但是随访经过是良好的。随着时间的流逝，这些病变似乎应该属于炎症性肌纤维母细胞瘤这个范畴（见上文）。

转移性肿瘤　Metastatic tumors

腹膜的转移性受累通常是由于来自腹腔或盆腔内原发性肿瘤的种植，最常见的是来自女性生殖系统，尤其是卵巢（卵巢肿瘤累及腹膜在第13章讨论），但是偶尔也可以来自子宫内膜或输卵管。从这些部位转移到腹膜的浆液性癌的鉴别诊断包括原发性腹膜浆液性癌（PSCs；见下文第二 Müller 系统肿瘤和瘤样病变一节）。其他可以播散到腹膜的肿瘤是乳腺癌（乳腺癌转移可以出现在原发性肿瘤治疗之后数年）[115,116]，胃肠道（尤其是结肠和胃）癌和胰腺癌。某些病例的转移性肿瘤可能是印戒细胞癌，其中肿瘤细胞广泛分散于纤维性间质中（图15.30 和图15.31）。某些病例印戒细胞稀少，其细胞核具有相对温和的特征，可能导致良性表现的假象。

腹膜假黏液瘤　Pseudomyxoma peritonei

黏液性肿瘤累及腹膜可以伴有广泛的腹腔内黏液集聚（图15.32），即谓的"腹膜假黏液瘤"（PP）[117-123a]。文献中表明 PP 病变的显微镜下表现包括：腹腔内的游离黏液（黏液性腹水）；小的或大的黏液沉积物黏附到

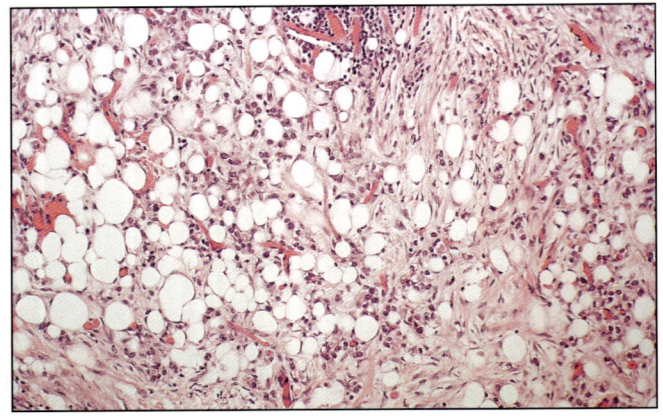

图15.30　网膜的转移性胃腺癌。肿瘤细胞具有相对一致的细胞核，在这个放大倍数下可能被误认为是炎症细胞。

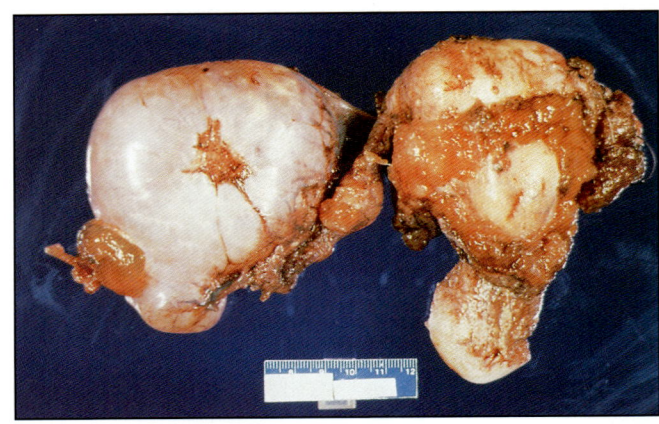

图15.32　腹膜假黏液瘤。黏液性物质累及卵巢黏液性肿瘤和子宫的浆膜。（Courtesy of Dr. W. Dwayne Lawrence.）

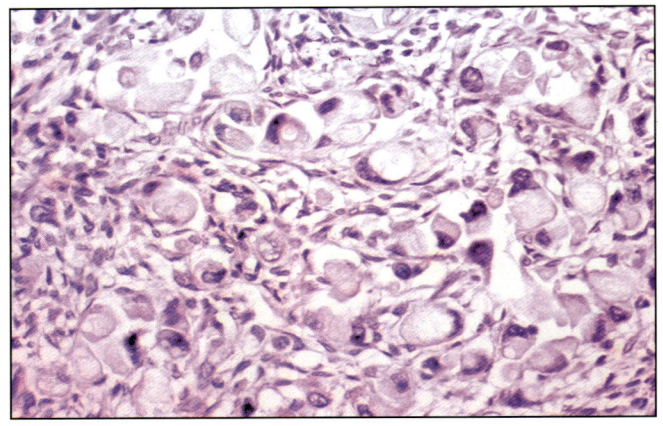

图15.31　网膜的转移性印戒细胞癌。

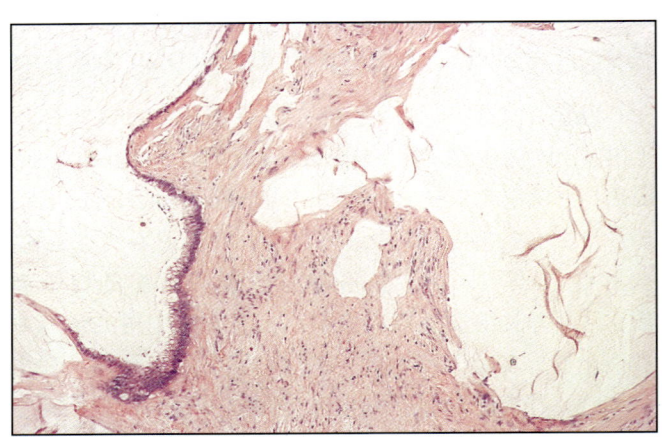

图15.33　腹膜假黏液瘤。

腹膜表面，含有炎症和间皮细胞，有时尚有机化的毛细血管和纤维母细胞，但是通常缺乏肿瘤性上皮细胞；以及黏液池，可能含有或不含有肿瘤细胞（图15.27和图15.28），周围绕以致密的胶原组织（分割性黏液）（图15.33）。如果在PP中出现肿瘤细胞，它们通常是高分化的肠型黏液性柱状细胞（图15.33）。至于腹腔内全部为黏液集聚，还是只有部分黏液集聚就能够诊断PP，现在还没有达成一致意见。

　　绝大多数PP病例的原发性肿瘤是阑尾低级别黏液性肿瘤，可能只有在显微镜下检查才能发现。因此，所有PP病例均应进行阑尾切除术，如果没有大体可见的病变，整个阑尾也应该送检进行组织学检查。在这种情况下，阑尾肿瘤和伴随的PP都显示一致的MUC2过表达[124]。不伴有阑尾肿瘤的PP病例，可能是由于来自胃肠道和胰胆管其他部位的黏液性肿瘤，卵巢黏液性肿瘤（尤其是那些发生于卵巢畸胎瘤的黏液性肿瘤）[125,126]，以及少数其他部位黏液性肿瘤的转移。在这样的病例中，一侧或典型者双侧卵巢可以被低级别黏液性囊性肿瘤所取代，认为这也是从阑尾肿瘤转移而来的。常常还可以出现无细胞的黏液分割整个卵巢间质（"卵巢假黏液瘤"）[117,118]。

　　腹膜假黏液瘤这个术语是临床和外科的名称，不应该出现在病理报告的病理学诊断中。报告应该包括：

- 评估肿瘤（阑尾，卵巢或其他）为良性，交界性或恶性，注明有无破裂。
- 分析腹膜病变为黏液性腹水（游离于腹腔内），机化的黏液性液体，或黏液分割伴有纤维化。
- 注明有无肿瘤性上皮细胞，以及它们是良性、交界性（非典型性）还是恶性。PP腹膜沉积物中无细胞，比沉积物中有分化较好的黏液性上皮的预后要好，而当腹膜沉积物由明显的癌细胞组成时，比那些由高分化黏液性上皮组成的肿瘤的预后要差的多，而且生存期也短[121,123,123a]。

第二 Müller 系统肿瘤和瘤样病变
Tumors and tumor-like lesions of the secondary müllerian system

这一节叙述的是共同起源于所谓的第二 Müller 系统的肿瘤和瘤样病变［除了子宫内膜异位症和发生于子宫内膜异位症的肿瘤（第 13 章）］，第二 Müller 系统即女性盆腔和下腹间皮及其邻近的间充质[127-129]。Müller 管起源于体腔上皮的内陷，这些组织的 Müller 潜能与它们和 Müller 管密切的胚胎起源相一致。第二 Müller 系统病变包括那些含有浆液性，子宫内膜样和黏液性上皮的病变，类似于正常或肿瘤性的输卵管、子宫内膜及宫颈内膜上皮。盆腔腹膜的化生潜能还包括可能向移行（尿路）和鳞状上皮分化。上皮性病变可能伴随下面间充质的增生，或可能引起多种由子宫内膜间质型细胞、蜕膜或平滑肌组成的真正的间质性病变。

腹膜浆液性病变 Peritoneal serous lesions

种种浆液性病变可以累及腹膜表面（而且某些病例累及腹膜后淋巴结），但是几乎不累及卵巢，这种形态提示为腹膜多灶起源。本节不认为阔韧带或腹膜后的局灶性单房性肿块是浆液性肿瘤。

输卵管内膜异位症 Endosalpingiosis

输卵管内膜异位症的定义是在腹膜或盆腔，或主动脉旁淋巴结出现内衬良性输卵管型上皮的腺体[130-140]。多数学者支持第二 Müller 系统起源，但是输卵管内膜异位症与输卵管损伤（慢性输卵管炎，输卵管积水，先前的输卵管妊娠，结节性输卵管峡炎，输卵管灌洗）有关，说明输卵管上皮种植是另外一种组织发生机制。输卵管内膜异位症是一种良性病变，具有良好的临床经过，但是常常伴有卵巢或腹膜的浆液性肿瘤，而这些肿瘤常常是交界性的[141,142]。

输卵管内膜异位症几乎全部发生在女性，一般发生在生育年龄，但个别患者发生在绝经后。这种年龄分布和输卵管内膜异位上皮中出现雌激素受体，提示这个病变是雌激素依赖性的。由于这种病变通常为显微镜下偶然发现，其报告的数目常常随着组织学取样范围的不同而不同。例如，Zinsser 和 Wheeler[130] 回顾性检查网膜，发现 12.5% 有输卵管内膜异位腺体，但是在前瞻性研究中比较全面地检查网膜时，这个数字增加了一倍。同样，在进行淋巴结切除术的患者中，淋巴结受累从 2% 到 41% 不等[134-137]。一项研究显示，因盆腔癌而进行淋巴结切除的患者中，每个淋巴结切 6 张切片，15.4% 的病例至少有一个淋巴结可以见到输卵管内膜异位腺

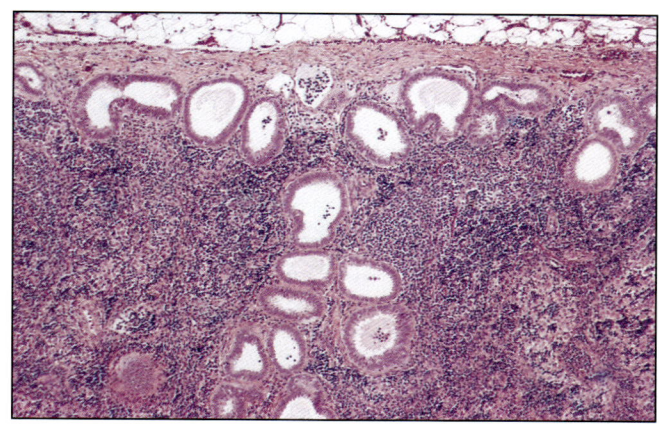

图 15.34　输卵管内膜异位症累及腹腔内淋巴结。注意包膜内有多数腺体。

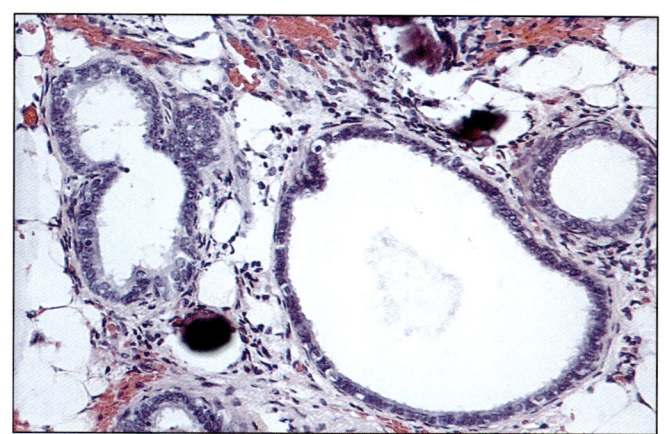

图 15.35　网膜输卵管内膜异位症。注意沙粒体。

体[137]。输卵管内膜异位症不常见的临床表现包括腹膜囊性肿块[143]；淋巴结肿大；子宫增大[143]；腹股沟肿块（代表输卵管内膜异位和可能由它发生的浆液性交界性肿瘤）[144]；放射学检查可见的盆腔钙化；以及子宫直肠陷凹液体，腹腔冲洗液[132]，或宫颈 Pap 涂片中出现沙粒体。

显微镜下见，输卵管内膜异位腺体一般位于间皮下间质内，或者位于淋巴结包膜或表浅皮质实质内（图 15.34 和图 15.35）。个别病例腺体位置较深，例如肠壁[140]、子宫[143] 或膀胱[145]，或淋巴结的髓质[134]。输卵管内膜异位腺体可以是囊性的，而且个别腔内含有间质乳头，腺体通常内衬单层纤毛柱状上皮细胞或者类似于输卵管内衬细胞的混合性细胞类型（纤毛细胞，没有纤毛的分泌细胞，钉细胞）（图 15.36）。细胞通常具有良性的细胞核的特征，并且缺乏核分裂活性。腔内或邻近的间质内常常出现沙粒体（图 15.35），偶尔沙粒体数量很大。输卵管内膜异位症可以混有其他良性 Müller 腺体（所谓的 Müller 病，müllerianosis）[145,146] 或含有化生的鳞状上皮[138]。

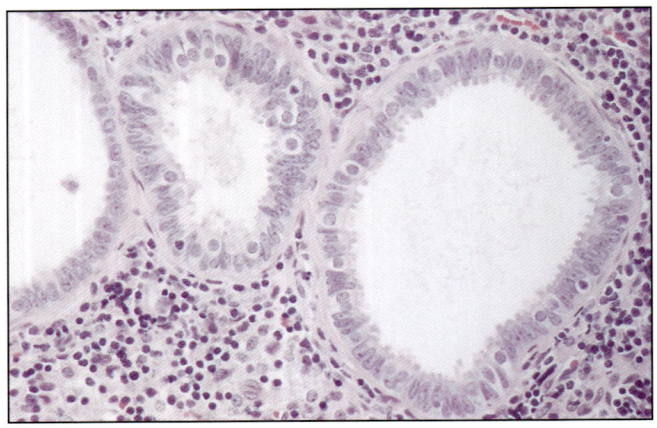

图15.36 淋巴结输卵管内膜异位症。注意多种类型细胞的混合，包括纤毛细胞。

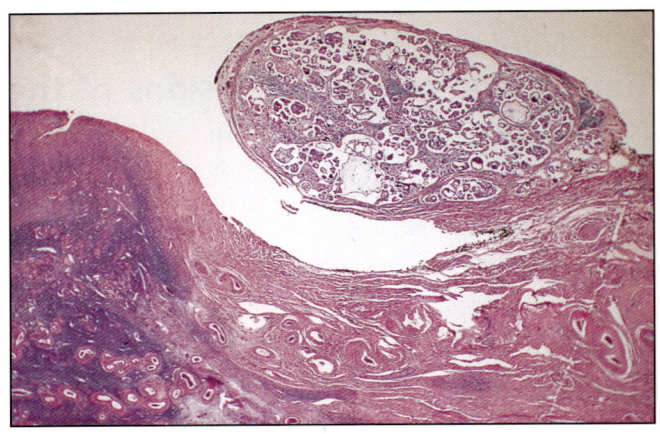

图15.38 腹膜浆液性交界性肿瘤。卵巢系膜上的肿瘤结节与卵巢（最左侧）相邻，卵巢没有异常。

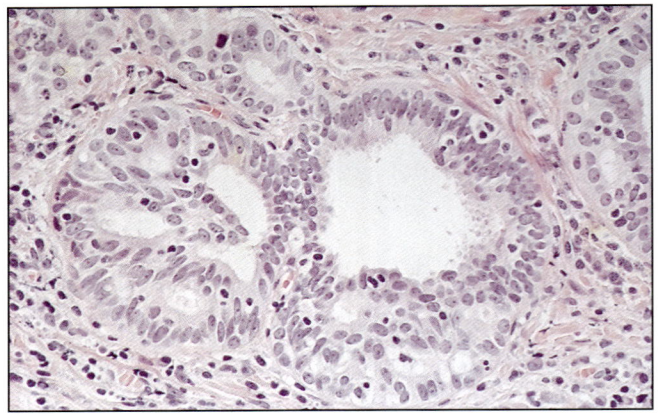

图15.37 淋巴结非典型性输卵管内膜异位症。注意细胞分层，腺腔内桥接。然而，细胞具有良性细胞核的特征。

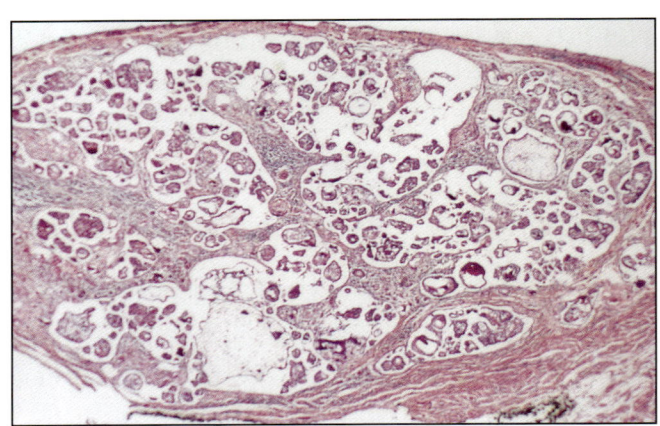

图15.39 腹膜浆液性交界性肿瘤。

非典型性输卵管内膜异位症这个术语已经被用于具有以下特征的输卵管内膜异位性病变，即内衬分层细胞，细胞出芽，筛状结构，以及有不同程度的细胞非典型性，而且发生在没有卵巢交界恶性浆液性肿瘤的情况下（图15.37）[141]。邻近淋巴结的非典型性输卵管内膜异位罕见，这样的病例很可能来源于淋巴结内浆液性肿瘤[147]。其他病例的淋巴结内输卵管内膜异位症可以伴有卵巢浆液性交界性肿瘤，提示在某些这样的病例中，前者是已经成熟了的转移性交界性浆液性肿瘤[142]。显微镜下检查时，非典型性输卵管内膜异位症应该与淋巴结内或腹膜浆液性交界性肿瘤鉴别（见下文），但是没有统一的可以接受的鉴别标准。当"由输卵管型上皮组成的病变出现乳头、丛生或分离的细胞簇时……即使它们是发生在输卵管内膜异位症的背景上"，Bell和Scully应用浆液性交界性肿瘤这个术语[141,148]。淋巴结包膜受累（而不是窦隙），非典型性腺体与典型的输卵管内膜异位症的腺体伴随出现，以及良性的细胞核的特征有助于输卵管内膜异位症和非典型性输卵管内膜异位症同转移性腺癌的鉴别。

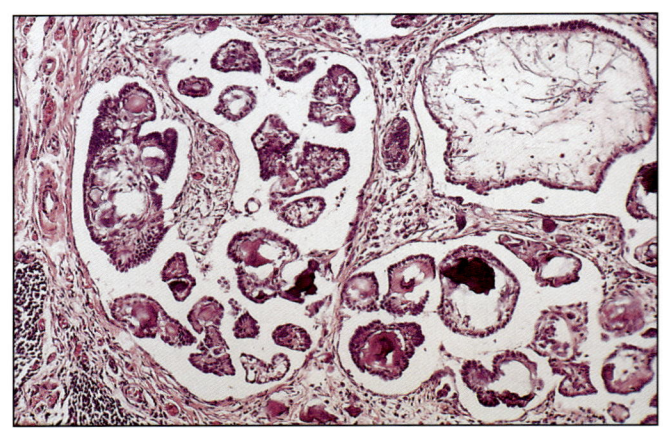

图15.40 腹膜浆液性交界性肿瘤。

腹膜交界恶性浆液性肿瘤
Peritoneal serous tumors of borderline malignancy（PSBT）

PSBTs的组织学表现与卵巢浆液性交界性肿瘤的非浸润性腹膜种植是相同的（图15.38～图5.40），只有当卵巢没有受累，相似的肿瘤仅仅轻微累及表面，或者伴有浆液性囊腺瘤时才能诊断 PSBTs[148,149]。多数病例可以看到输卵管内膜异位症。PSBTs 发生在年轻成年女性，表现为腹痛和不育；某些病例的腹膜病变是在剖腹手术中偶然发现的。典型的术中所见是腹膜表面黏连或呈颗粒性；肿块仅见于个别病例。多数病例仅仅累及盆腔腹膜，但是偶尔上腹部腹膜也可受累。

在 39 例具有随访资料的患者中[148,149]，4 例患者在切除持续性或复发性交界性肿瘤后生存良好，1 例发生腹膜浸润性低级别浆液性癌，1 例死于播散性浆液性肿瘤；其余患者随访中没有发现异常。这些资料表明，多数 PSBTs 具有良好的预后，类似于伴有非浸润性种植的可以进行比较的卵巢病变的患者，即使是为了保存生育能力而进行保守治疗的患者，预后也好。

高级别腹膜浆液性癌
High-grade peritoneal serous carcinomas

腹膜浆液性癌的临床表现与Ⅲ期卵巢癌患者相似[84,150-164]。某些腹膜浆液性癌发生在因为家族性卵巢癌先前预防性切除卵巢的妇女[150]，而有些发生在证明有 *BRCA-1* 突变的患者[161,165]。与散发性病例相比，*BRCA-1* 突变患者具有独特的较高的 *p53* 突变发生率[162]。在手术时发现腹膜癌病而卵巢大小和形状正常，提示弥漫性恶性间皮瘤或来自于隐匿性原发性肿瘤的癌病的诊断。至少在某些病例中，检查显示卵巢表面有不同程度的受累，这是腹膜浆液性癌腹膜多灶性受累的一部分（图 15.41）。这些肿瘤通常是高级别的，类似于典型的卵巢浆液性癌（图 15.42 和图 15.43），包括常常出现沙粒体。多数研究显示，当分期、分级和残留肿瘤体积都相当时，腹膜浆液性癌的行为类似于或者比Ⅲ期卵巢浆液性癌更差。

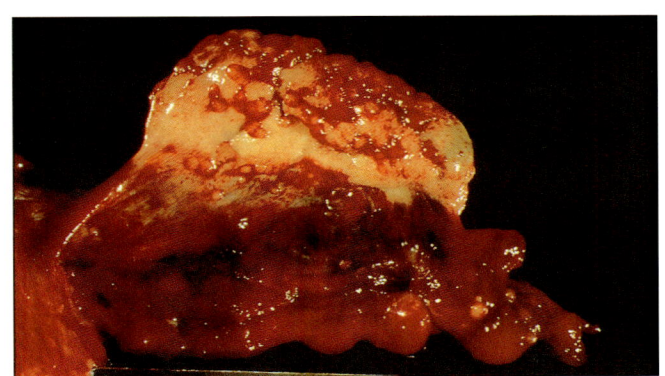

图15.41　累及卵巢和输卵管浆膜的腹膜浆液性癌。肿瘤广泛播散伴有显著的网膜疾病。注意卵巢和输卵管浆膜面小的赘生物。

低级别腹膜浆液性癌，包括沙粒体癌
Low-grade peritoneal serous carcinomas, including psammocarcinomas

这是一种罕见的腹膜浆液性癌，其特征是具有类似于浆液性交界性肿瘤的低级别的细胞核（见上文），与后者不同的是它能出现内脏和淋巴管浸润[166]。少

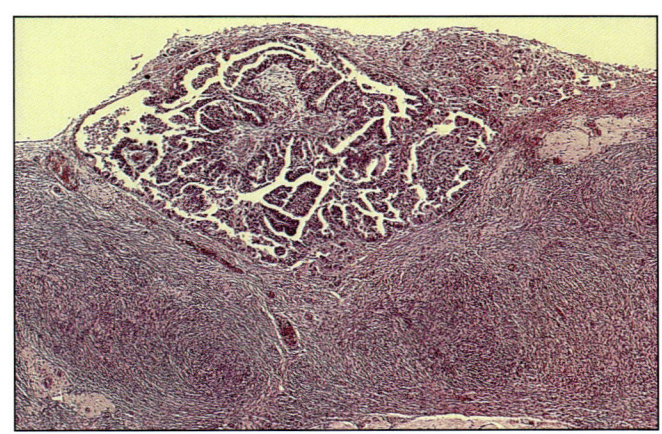

图15.42　累及卵巢的腹膜浆液性癌。肿瘤大部分位于卵巢外，卵巢受累局限在卵巢表面。

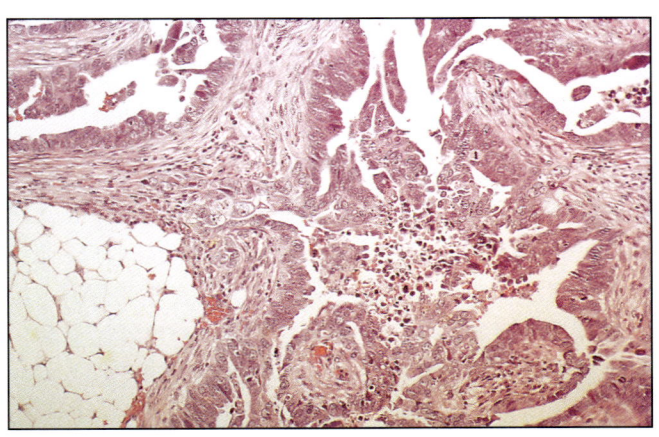

图15.43　累及网膜的浆液性表面乳头状癌。

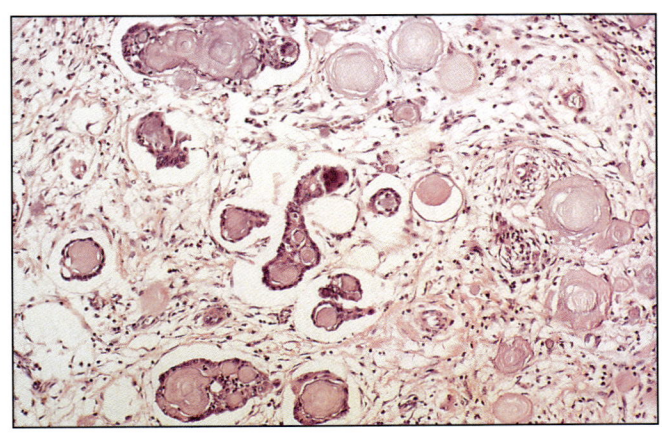

图15.44　腹膜沙粒体癌。

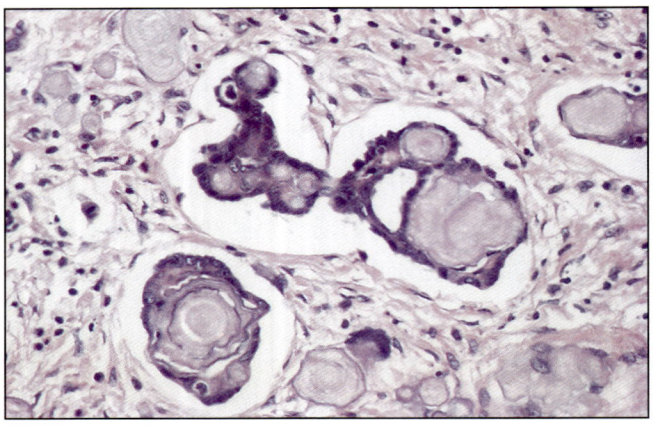

图15.45　腹膜沙粒体癌。

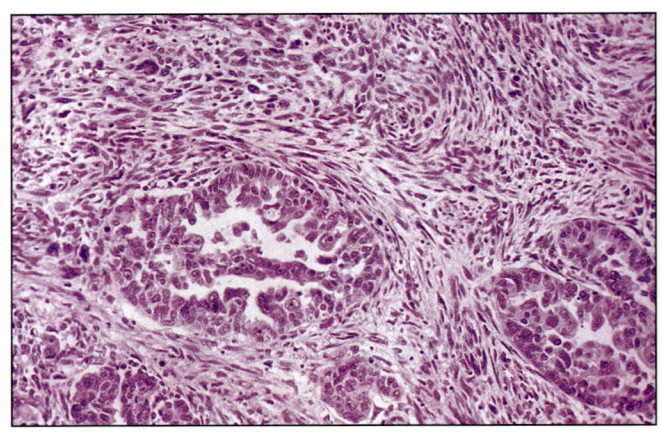

图15.47　腹膜恶性Müller混合瘤（癌肉瘤）。这个患者卵巢和子宫均无异常。

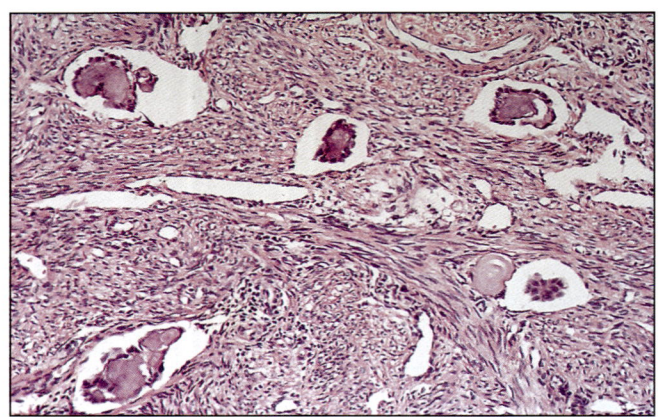

图15.46　腹膜沙粒体癌，累及子宫肌层淋巴管。

数低级别腹膜浆液性癌是腹膜沙粒体癌[166-168]，它以至少75%的乳头和细胞巢内出现沙粒体为特征（图15.44～图15.46）。如同浆液性交界性肿瘤一样，低级别腹膜浆液性癌常常是惰性肿瘤，具有良好的预后，虽然肿瘤偶尔复发、持续或致死。浆液性交界性肿瘤和低级别腹膜浆液性癌的显微镜下特征重叠，因此需要充分取样以作出正确诊断。

腹膜子宫内膜样肿瘤 Peritoneal endometrioid tumors

女性盆腔或腹膜后可以见到种种子宫内膜样肿瘤，但是没有类似的肿瘤累及卵巢或子宫的证据，也没有子宫内膜异位症的证据。虽然其中某些肿瘤可能发生在子宫内膜异位的病灶，而且之后掩盖了子宫内膜异位症的改变，但是其他肿瘤很可能是直接来源于间皮或间皮下间质。这些肿瘤包括子宫内膜样囊腺纤维瘤[169]和囊腺癌[170]，子宫内膜间质肉瘤（ESS）[171]，同源性和异源性恶性中胚层混合瘤（图15.47）[172-174]，以及中胚层腺肉瘤[175,176]。这些肿瘤在临床和病理学上都一般和发生在子宫体和卵巢的相应肿瘤相似。然而，原发性子宫外子宫内膜间质肿瘤的行为多半是高分期而不是低分期的子宫原发性子宫内膜间质肉瘤[171]。

腹膜黏液性病变 Peritoneal mucinous lesions

宫颈内膜型良性腺体累及腹膜（"宫颈内膜异位症"，endocervicosis）罕见，但有累及子宫后浆膜以及子宫直肠陷凹的病例报告[127]；类似的良性腺体还可以在盆腹腔淋巴结内见到[177]。有这样一个病例，某些淋巴结内的黏液性上皮呈乳头状，而且淋巴结内病变伴有子宫内膜黏液性化生和双侧卵巢黏液性交界性肿瘤[177]。宫颈内膜异位症还可以作为一种瘤样病变，发生在膀胱后壁或后部圆顶[178,179]，子宫宫颈外壁[180]，阴道顶部[181]和肠壁[182]。在这样的病例，腺体在平滑肌中的浸润形态，轻度的局灶性上皮非典型性，以及腺体周围有反应性间质，单独一项或联合存在均可能提示微小偏离型腺癌。出现混合性良性Müller型腺体（输卵管内膜异位性，子宫内膜样，所谓的"Müller病"（mülleria-nosis）[145,146]，子宫内膜间质[178]，或两者，可以帮助作出正确诊断。

类似于卵巢来源的黏液性肿瘤在卵巢外部位已有描述，通常位于肠系膜和腹膜后；还有发生于腹股沟区的个案报告[183-187]。这些肿瘤一般形成大的囊性肿块（图15.48），显微镜下检查类似于卵巢黏液性囊腺瘤、交界性肿瘤（图15.49）或囊腺癌。个别肿瘤含有间变性肿瘤的附壁结节[187]。虽然这些肿瘤的行为一般与卵巢的相应肿瘤没有区别（见第13章），一例其他方面典型的交界性肿瘤在切除之后4年发生转移[183]。

其他腹膜上皮性病变 Other peritoneal epithelial lesions

移行（尿路）上皮Walthard细胞巢常常出现在所有年龄妇女的盆腔腹膜，一般累及输卵管的浆膜面、输卵

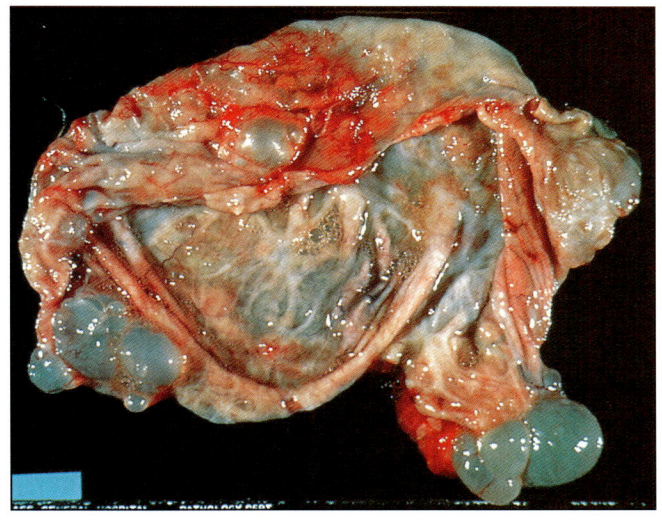

图15.48 卵巢外（腹膜后）黏液性囊腺瘤。这个患者卵巢没有异常。

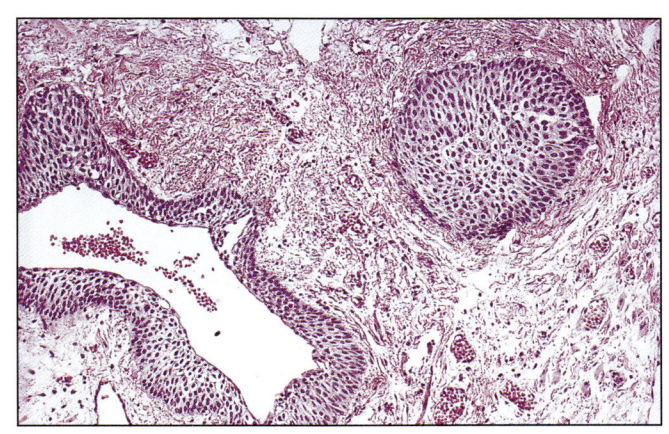

图15.50 囊性和实性Walthard细胞巢。

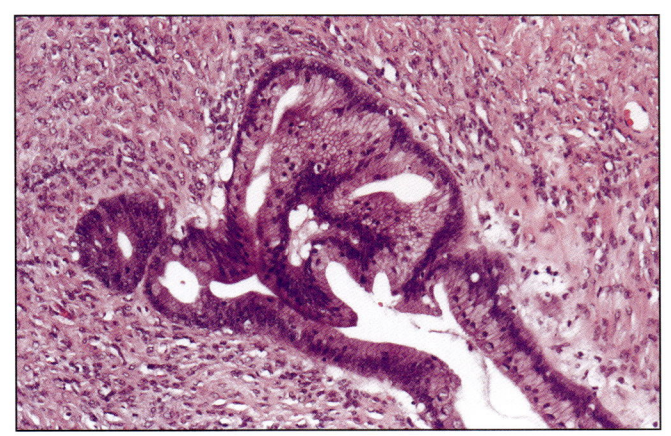

图15.49 卵巢外（腹膜后）具有交界恶性的黏液性肿瘤。

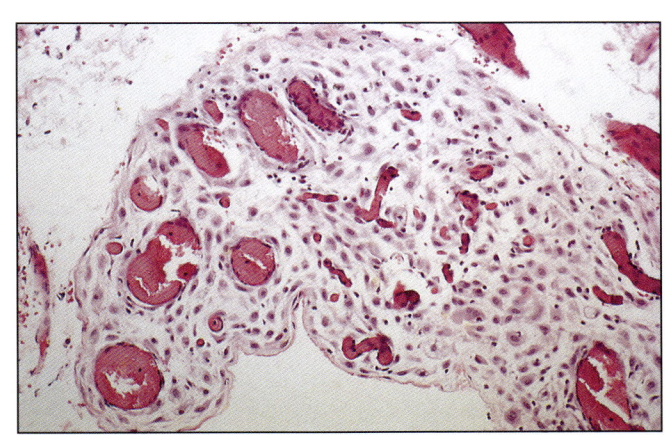

图15.51 卵巢周围黏连处的异位蜕膜。注意有许多小血管。

管系膜和卵巢系膜（图15.50）[188-190]。虽然Walthard细胞巢偶尔可以由具有鳞状表现的细胞组成，但是真正的腹膜鳞状化生非常罕见[191]。罕见的女性卵巢外Brenner瘤病例已有报告，通常发生在阔韧带，或者罕见的病例发生于子宫[192]。一般认为起源于盆腔腹膜，这种衍化类似于对于多数卵巢Brenner瘤所作的假设。

几乎所有发生在盆腔的Müller型生殖器外的透明细胞癌，均发生于子宫内膜异位灶内，在此不进行进一步的探讨。另外，遇到两例显然不伴有子宫内膜异位症的透明细胞癌，可能是腹膜起源。一例是乙状结肠系膜内的局限性肿块，而另外一例广泛累及腹膜。

异位蜕膜　Ectopic decidua

在妊娠妇女，异位蜕膜是盆腔腹膜和网膜间皮下间质内的一种常见的发现，少数异位蜕膜位于盆腹腔淋巴结的浅层皮质内[135,138,195-198]。异位蜕膜一般是显微镜下的偶然发现，但是当剖宫产或产后输卵管结扎时可见看到明显的腹膜病变，表现为散布于腹膜表面的多发性灰白色，伴有局状性出血的结节或斑块，类似于恶性肿瘤。几个病例在妊娠的第3个三月期，分娩时或产褥期伴有大量腹腔积血，偶尔导致死亡。一个腹膜蜕膜反应显著的病例伴有分娩受阻[199]。到了产后6周异位蜕膜通常消退。

显微镜下见，异位蜕膜细胞单个分布或排列成结节或斑块，一般类似于正常部位的蜕膜（图15.51～图15.53）。可以混有平滑肌细胞，可能是来源于间皮下肌纤维母细胞。蜕膜灶常常有丰富的血管（图15.51），而且可能含有散在的淋巴细胞。蜕膜细胞灶状出血性坏死和不同程度的核的多形性和核深染，在少数情况下可能提示恶性肿瘤，但是大部分细胞呈良性表现以及缺乏核分裂象，可以作出正确的诊断。然而应当注意，

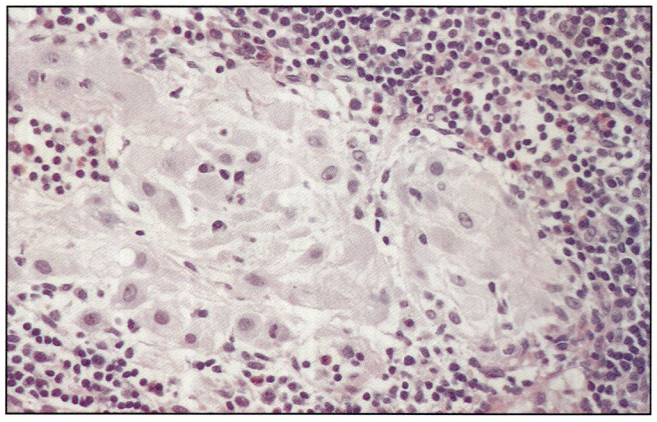

图15.52 盆腔淋巴结内的异位蜕膜。

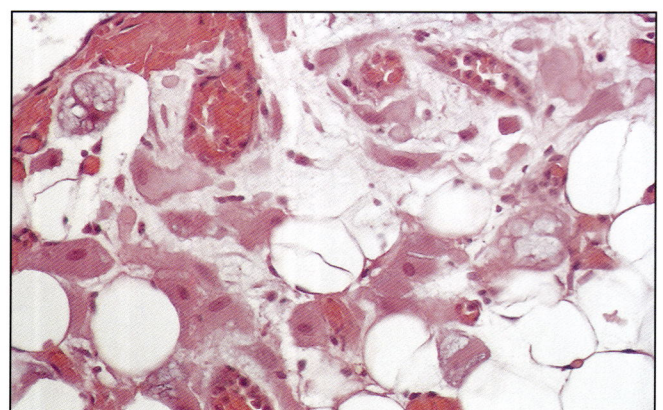

图15.53 网膜的异位蜕膜。某些细胞具有胞浆内空泡,含有嗜碱性黏液。

异位蜕膜和转移性鳞状细胞癌偶尔可以累及同一个淋巴结[197]。如同正常部位的蜕膜细胞一样,异位蜕膜细胞偶尔含有偏心的细胞核和伴有嗜碱性黏液的胞浆空泡(图15.53)。在这样的病例中,某些细胞可能类似于印戒细胞癌的细胞,但是与后者不同的是,特殊染色显示空泡中仅有酸性黏液。

腹膜平滑肌瘤病　Peritoneal leiomyomatosis

腹膜平滑肌瘤病(其同义词为腹膜播散性平滑肌瘤病,disseminated peritoneal leiomyomatosis,leiommyomatosis peritonealis disseminata)的特征是出现主要或完全由良性表现的平滑肌细胞组成的多发性腹膜结节[200-204]。大约已有60例病例报告,大部分发生在生育年龄的妇女(平均37岁),但是偶尔发生在绝经后的患者。报告的病例40%发生在黑人妇女。患者可以分为三组:(1)妊娠或产后妇女(43%);(2)口服避孕药的患者(27%);(3)不属于以上两组的妇女(30%);一例伴有颗粒细胞瘤。在妊娠妇女,本病通常是剖宫产或产后输卵管结扎时的偶然发现。非妊娠妇女以及某些

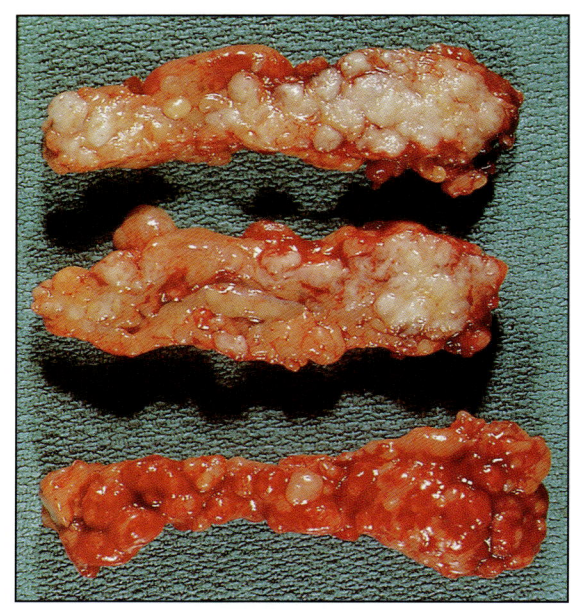

图15.54 累及网膜的腹膜平滑肌瘤病的切面。注意多发性结节。

有症状的妊娠妇女的症状常常与共存的子宫平滑肌瘤有关;其他一些病例由于触及盆腔结节,建议进行诊断性剖腹探查。数个到数不清的圆形实性质硬结节散在分布于盆壁腹膜和网膜,形成丛状结节或界限不清的片块状增厚,可能类似于转移性肿瘤(图15.54)。结节大小从显微镜下可见到直径10 cm不等,但是多数结节小于0.5 cm。类似的结节还可以累及子宫、卵巢、肠以及肠系膜的浆膜;上腹腹膜受累少见。还有一例报告盆腔淋巴结同时受累[201]。

显微镜下,结节通常具有典型平滑肌瘤的表现,或者少数为富于细胞性平滑肌瘤的表现(图15.55)。平滑肌细胞常常显示没有明显的细胞核的多形性和核分裂活性;然而,每10个高倍视野偶尔可能含有多达3个核分裂象[200]。在一例复发性病例的结节内可见性索样结

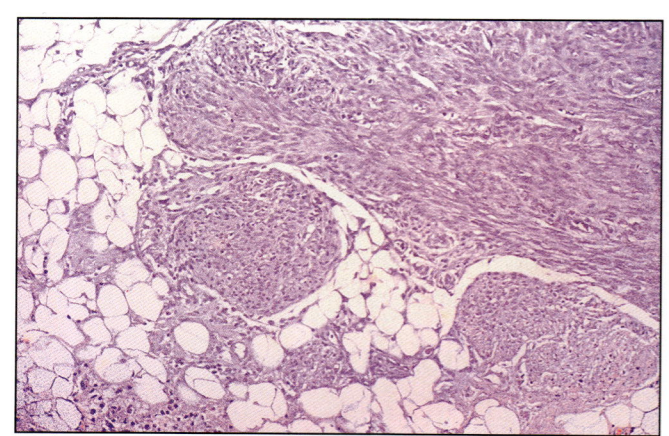

图15.55 累及网膜的腹膜平滑肌瘤病。

构[204]。在妊娠患者，蜕膜细胞和形态介于蜕膜和平滑肌之间的细胞可以混在平滑肌细胞之间（图 15.56）。在 10% 的病例中，可以见到与结节延续的子宫内膜异位症或输卵管内膜异位症病灶。超微结构研究证实存在平滑肌细胞，有时混有肌纤维母细胞、纤维母细胞，在妊娠患者还可以混有蜕膜细胞[200]。

除了下面提到的例外情况外，在随访检查中没有疾病进展的报告，尽管肿瘤切除不完全。几例妊娠患者当不再妊娠而进行二次检查时，结节已经完全或部分消退。冰冻切片确定诊断之后，需要进行保守治疗，虽然在以后妊娠时疾病可能复发。个别持续性腹膜平滑肌瘤病应用 GnRH 促效剂已经获得成功治疗[202,203]。

腹膜平滑肌瘤病发生平滑肌肉瘤转化已有 5 例报告[205]。每一例都是在典型的腹膜平滑肌瘤病诊断之后一年之内，腹腔内出现具有平滑肌肉瘤组织学表现的迅速生长的肿瘤（一例为转移性肿瘤）。其中 4 名妇女在开始有症状之后 2 年内死于本病。

腹膜平滑肌瘤病被认为是间皮下间充质细胞向平滑肌细胞化生性转化的一个结果。结节位于间皮下，而且偶尔与其他化生性病变（异位蜕膜，子宫内膜异位症，输卵管内膜异位症）并存，支持这种解释。70% 的病例

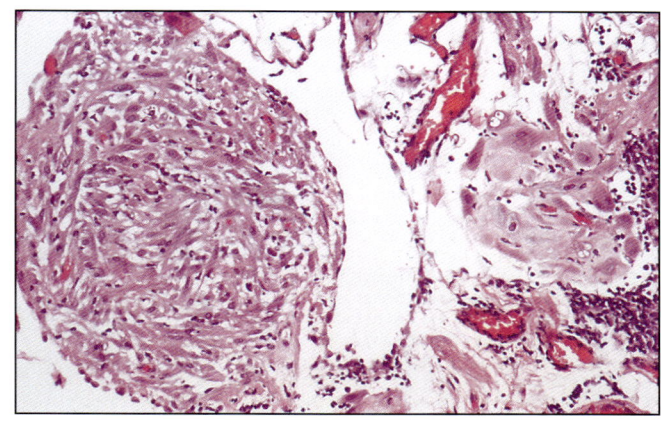

图15.56　腹膜平滑肌瘤病结节（左）邻近异位蜕膜灶(右)。

与妊娠或投予激素有关，提示本病具有激素背景；病变细胞内存在雌激素和孕激素受体[206]；在妊娠之后，卵巢切除术或应用 GnRH 促效剂治疗之后肿瘤变小[202,203]；单独给予雌激素或联合应用孕酮可以促使豚鼠产生类似的子宫和间皮下结节[207]。一项 4 例有关本病 X 染色体失活的研究分析显示[208]，在每个病例中检查的所有结节均为同一亲代 X 染色体非随机失活，符合单中心克隆性肿瘤，或在克隆性多中心病变中对 X 连锁等位基因的选择。

参考文献

1. Churg A, Colby T V, Cagle P et al. 2000 The separation of benign and malignant mesothelial proliferations. Am J Surg Pathol 24: 1183–1200
2. Kerner H, Gaton E, Czernobilsky B 1981 Unusual ovarian, tubal and pelvic mesothelial inclusions in patients with endometriosis. Histopathology 5: 277–282
3. Clement P B, Young R H 1993 Florid mesothelial hyperplasia associated with ovarian tumors: a potential source of error in tumor diagnosis and staging. Int J Gynecol Pathol 12: 51–58
4. Rosai J, Dehner L P 1975 Nodular mesothelial hyperplasia in hernia sacs. A benign reactive condition stimulating a neoplastic process. Cancer 35: 165–175
5. Ordonez N G, Ayala A G 1998 Lesions described as nodular mesothelial hyperplasia are primarily composed of histiocytes. Am J Surg Pathol 22: 285–292
6. Chikkamuniyappa S, Herrick J, Jagirdar J S 2004 Nodular histiocytic/mesothelial hyperplasia: a potential pitfall. Ann Diagn Pathol 8: 115–120
7. Clement P B, Young R H, Oliva E et al. 1996 Hyperplastic mesothelial cells within abdominal lymph nodes: a mimic of metastatic ovarian carcinoma and serous borderline tumor. A report of two cases associated with ovarian neoplasms. Mod Pathol 9: 879–886
8. Attanoos R L, Griffin A, Gibbs A R 2003 The use of immunohistochemistry in distinguishing reactive from neoplastic epithelium. A novel use for desmin and comparative evaluation with epithelial membrane antigen, p53, platelet-derived growth factor, P-glycoprotein, and bcl-2. Histopathology 43: 231–238
9. Carpenter H A, Lancaster J R, Lee R A 1982 Multilocular cysts of the peritoneum. Mayo Clin Proc 57: 634–638
10. Schneider V, Partridge J R, Gutierrez F et al. 1983 Benign cystic mesothelioma involving the female genital tract: report of four cases. Am J Obstet Gynecol 145: 355–359
11. Katsube Y, Mukai K, Silverberg S G 1982 Cystic mesothelioma of the peritoneum. A report of five cases and review of the literature. Cancer 50: 1615–1622
12. Moore J H Jr, Crum C P, Chandler J G et al. 1980 Benign cystic mesothelioma. Cancer 45: 2395–2399
13. McFadden D E, Clement P B 1986 Peritoneal inclusion cysts with mural mesothelial proliferation. A clinicopathological analysis of six cases. Am J Surg Pathol 10: 844–854
14. Weiss S W, Tavassoli F A 1988 Multicystic mesothelioma. An analysis of pathologic findings and biologic behavior in 37 cases. Am J Surg Pathol 12: 737–746
15. Ross M J, Welch W R, Scully R E 1989 Multilocular peritoneal inclusion cysts (so-called cystic mesotheliomas). Cancer 64: 1336–1346
16. Blumberg N A, Murray J F 1981 Multicystic peritoneal mesothelioma. S Afr Med J 59: 85–86
17. Sienkowski I, Russell A J, Dilly S A et al. 1986 Peritoneal cystic mesothelioma: an electron microscopic and immunohistochemical study of two male patients. J Clin Pathol 39: 440–445
18. Kjellevold K, Nesland J M, Holm R et al. 1986 Multicystic peritoneal mesothelioma. Pathol Res Pract 181: 767–771
19. Arber D A, Strickler J G, Weiss L M 1997 Splenic mesothelial cysts mimicking lymphangiomas. Am J Surg Pathol 21: 334–338
20. Harper G B Jr, Awbrey B J, Thomas C G Jr et al. 1986 Mesothelial cysts of the round ligament simulating inguinal hernia. Report of four cases and review of the literature. Am J Surg 151: 515–517
21. Demopoulos R I, Kahn M A, Feiner H D 1986 Epidemiology of cystic mesotheliomas. Int J Gynecol Pathol 5: 379–381
22. Gussman D, Thickman D, Wheeler J E 1986 Postoperative peritoneal cysts. Obstet Gynecol 68 53S–55S
23. Flemming P, Becker T, Klempnauer J et al. 2002 Benign cystic mesothelioma of the liver. Am J Surg Pathol 26: 1523–1527
24. Chen K T K 1998 Multicystic mesothelioma. Int J Surg Pathol 6: 43–48
25. Smith V C, Edwards R A, Jorgensen J L et al. 2000 Unilocular retroperitoneal cyst of mesothelial origin presenting as a renal mass. A report of 2 cases. Arch Pathol Lab Med 124: 766–769
26. Sawh R, Malpica A, Deavers M T et al. 2003 Benign cystic mesothelioma of the peritoneum: a clinicopathologic study of 17 cases and immunohistochemical analysis of estrogen and progesterone receptor status. Hum Pathol 34: 369–374
27. Letterie G S, Yon J L 1995 Use of a long-acting GnRH agonist for benign cystic mesothelioma. Obstet Gynecol 85: 901–903

28. Bisset D L, Morris J A, Fox H 1988 Giant cystic adenomatoid tumor (mesothelioma) of the uterus. Histopathology 12: 555–558
29. Clement P B 1995 Reactive tumor-like lesions of the peritoneum. Editorial. Am J Clin Pathol 103: 673–676
30. Kim K, Scully R E 1990 Peritoneal keratin granulomas with carcinomas of endometrium and ovary and atypical polypoid adenomyoma of endometrium. Am J Surg Pathol 14: 925–932
31. Bolen J W, Hammar S P, McNutt M A 1986 Reactive and neoplastic serosal tissue. A light microscopic, ultrastructural and immunohistochemical study. Am J Surg Pathol 10: 34–47
32. Clement P B, Young R H, Hanna W et al. 1994 Sclerosing peritonitis associated with luteinized thecomas of the ovary: a clinicopathological analysis of six cases. Am J Surg Pathol 18: 1–13
33. Emory T S, Monihan J M, Carr N J et al. 1997 Sclerosing mesenteritis, mesenteric panniculitis and mesenteric lipodystrophy: a single entity? Am J Surg Pathol 21: 392–398
34. McCaughey W T E, Al-Jabi M 1986 Differentiation of serosal hyperplasia and neoplasia in biopsies. Pathol Annu 21: 271–292
35. Kocova L, Michal M, Sulc M et al. 1997 Calcifying fibrous pseudotumor of visceral peritoneum. Histopathology 31: 182–184
36. Chen K T K 2003 Familial peritoneal multifocal calcifying fibrous tumor. Am J Clin Pathol 119: 811–815
37. Nascimento A F, Ruiz R, Hornick J L et al. 2002 Calcifying fibrous pseudotumor: clinicopathologic study of 15 cases and analysis of its relationship to inflammatory myofibroblastic tumor. Int J Surg Pathol 10: 189–196
38. Auerbach R D, Kohorn E I, Cornelius E A 1985 Splenosis: a complicating factor in total abdominal hysterectomy. Obstet Gynecol 65: 65S–68S
39. Matonis L M, Luciano A A 1995 A case of splenosis masquerading as endometriosis. Am J Obstet Gynecol 173: 971–973
40. Jaworski R C, Boadle R, Greg J et al. 2001 Peritoneal "melanosis" associated with a ruptured ovarian dermoid cyst: report of a case with electron-probe energy dispersive X-ray analysis. Int J Gynecol Pathol 20: 386–389
41. Elliott G B, Freigang B 1962 Aseptic necrosis, calcification and separation of appendices epiploicae. Ann Surg 155: 501–505
42. Vuong P N, Guyot H, Moulin G et al. 1990 Pseudotumoral organization of a twisted epiploic fringe or "hard-boiled egg" in the peritoneal cavity. Arch Pathol Lab Med 114: 531–533
43. Fadare O, Bifulco C, Carter D et al. 2002 Cartilaginous differentiation in peritoneal tissues: a report of two cases and a review of the literature. Mod Pathol 15: 777–780
44. Young R H, Clement P B, McCaughey W T E 1990 Solitary fibrous tumors ("fibrous mesotheliomas") of the peritoneum: a report of three cases. Arch Pathol Lab Med 114: 493–495
45. Flint A, Weiss S W 1995 CD-34 and keratin expression distinguishes solitary fibrous tumor (fibrous mesothelioma) of pleura from desmoplastic mesothelioma. Hum Pathol 26: 428–431
46. Fukunaga M, Naganuma H, Nikaido T et al. 1997 Extrapleural solitary fibrous tumor: a report of seven cases. Mod Pathol 10: 443–450
47. Hanau C A, Miettinen M 1995 Solitary fibrous tumor: histological and immunohistochemical spectrum of benign and malignant variants presenting at different sites. Hum Pathol 26: 440–449
48. Fukunaga M, Naganuma H, Ushigome S et al. 1996 Malignant solitary fibrous tumour of the peritoneum. Histopathology 28: 463–466
49. Hanrahan J B 1963 A combined papillary mesothelioma and adenomatoid tumor of the omentum. Report of a case. Cancer 16: 1497–1500
50. Craig J R, Hart W R 1979 Extragenital adenomatoid tumor. Evidence for the mesothelial theory of origin. Cancer 43: 1678–1679
51. Goepel J R 1981 Benign papillary mesothelioma of peritoneum: a histological, histochemical and ultrastructural study of six cases. Histopathology 5: 21–30
52. Daya D, McCaughey W T E 1990 Well-differentiated papillary mesothelioma of the peritoneum. a clinicopathologic study of 22 cases. Cancer 65: 292–296
53. Burrig K, Pfitzer P, Hart W 1990 Well-differentiated papillary mesothelioma of the peritoneum: a borderline mesothelioma. Virchow's Arch [Pathol Anat] 417: 443–447
54. Goldblum J, Hart W R 1995 Localized and diffuse mesotheliomas of the genital tract and peritoneum in women. A clinicopathologic study of nineteen true mesothelial neoplasms, other than adenomatoid tumors, multicystic mesotheliomas, and localized fibrous tumors. Am J Surg Pathol 19: 1124–1137
55. Butnor K J, Sporn T A, Hammar S P et al. 2001 Well-differentiated papillary mesothelioma. Am J Surg Pathol 25: 1304–1309
56. Diaz L K, Okronkwo A, Solans E P et al. 2002 Extensive myxoid change in well-differentiated papillary mesothelioma of the pelvic peritoneum. Ann Diagn Pathol 6: 164–167
57. Kannerstein M, Churg J 1977 Peritoneal mesothelioma. Hum Pathol 8: 83–94
58. Jones D E C, Silver D 1979 Peritoneal mesotheliomas. Surgery 86: 556–560
59. Plaus W J 1988 Peritoneal mesothelioma. Arch Surg 123: 763–766
60. Piccigallo E, Jeffers L J, Reddy R et al. 1988 Malignant peritoneal mesothelioma. A clinical and laparoscopic study of ten cases. Dig Dis Sci 33: 633–639
61. Asensio J A, Goldblatt P, Thomford N R 1990 Primary malignant peritoneal mesothelioma. A report of seven cases and a review of the literature. Arch Surg 125: 1477–1481
62. Kerrigan S A J, Turnnir R T, Clement P B et al. 2002 Diffuse malignant epithelial mesotheliomas of the peritoneum in women. A clinicopathologic study of 25 patients. Cancer 94: 378–385
63. Baker P M, Clement P B, Young R H 2005 Malignant peritoneal mesothelioma in women. A study of 75 cases with emphasis on their morphologic spectrum and differential diagnosis. Am J Clin Pathol 123: 724–737
64. Clement P B, Young R H, Scully R E 1996 Malignant mesotheliomas presenting as ovarian masses. A report of nine cases, including two primary ovarian mesotheliomas. Am J Surg Pathol 20: 1067–1080
65. Kane M J, Chahinian A P, Holland J F 1990 Malignant mesothelioma in young adults. Cancer 65: 1449–1455
66. Nascimento A G, Keeney G L, Fletcher C D M 1994 Deciduoid peritoneal mesothelioma. An unusual phenotype affecting young females. Am J Surg Pathol 18: 439–445
67. Shanks J H, Harris M, Banerjee S S et al. 2000 Mesotheliomas with deciduoid morphology. A morphologic spectrum and a variant not confined to young females. Am J Surg Pathol 24: 285–294
68. Shia J, Erlandson R A, Klimstra D S 2002 Deciduoid mesothelioma: a report of 5 cases and literature review. Ultrastruct Pathol 26: 355–363
69. Berry P J, Favara B E, Odom L F 1986 Malignant peritoneal mesothelioma in a child. Pediatr Pathol 5: 397–409
70. Almudevar Bercero E, Garcia-Rostan Y, Perez G M A et al. 1997 Prognostic value of high serum levels of CA-125 in malignant secretory peritoneal mesotheliomas affecting young women. A case report with differential diagnosis and review of the literature. Histopathology 31: 267–273
71. Chen K T K 1991 Malignant mesothelioma presenting as Sister Joseph's nodule. Am J Dermatopathol 13: 300–303
72. Mayall F G, Gibbs A R 1991 Malignant peritoneal mesothelioma giving rise to multiple intestinal polyps. Histopathology 18: 480–482
73. Fukayama M, Takizawa T, Koike M et al. 1987 Malignant peritoneal mesothelioma as a pelvic mass. Acta Pathol Jpn 37: 1149–1156
74. Matsukuma S, Aida S, Hata Y et al. 1996 Localized malignant peritoneal mesothelioma containing rhabdoid cells. Pathol Int 46: 389–391
75. Sussman J, Rosai J 1990 Lymph node metastasis as the initial manifestation of malignant mesothelioma. Report of six cases. Am J Surg Pathol 14: 818–828
76. Kerrigan S A J, Cagle P, Churg A 2003 Malignant mesothelioma of the peritoneum presenting as an inflammatory lesion. Am J Surg Pathol 27: 248–253
77. Gilks B, Hegedus C, Freeman H et al. 1988 Malignant peritoneal mesothelioma after remote abdominal radiation. Cancer 61: 2019–2021
78. Peterson J T Jr, Greenberg S D, Bufflier P A 1984 Non-asbestos-related malignant mesothelioma. A review. Cancer 54: 951–960
79. Huncharek M 1995 Genetic factors in the aetiology of malignant mesothelioma. Eur J Cancer 31A: 1741–1747
80. Brenner J, Sordillo P P, Magill G B 1981 Seventeen year survival in a patient with malignant peritoneal mesothelioma. Clin Oncol 7: 249–251
81. Norman P E, Whitaker D 1989 Nine-year survival in a case of untreated peritoneal mesothelioma. Med J Aust 150: 43–44
82. Feldman A L, Libutt S K, Pingpark J F et al. 2003 Analysis of factors associated with outcome in patients with malignant peritoneal mesothelioma undergoing surgical debulking and intraperitoneal chemotherapy. J Clin Oncol 21: 4560–4567
83. Kitazawa M, Kaneko H, Toshima M et al. 1984 Malignant peritoneal mesothelioma with massive foamy cells. Acta Pathol Jpn 34: 687–692
84. Bollinger D J, Wick M R, Dehner L P et al. 1989 Peritoneal malignant mesothelioma versus serous papillary adenocarcinoma. A histochemical and immunohistochemical comparison. Am J Surg Pathol 13: 659–670
85. Wick M R, Mills S E, Swanson P E 1990 Expression of "myelomonocytic" antigens in mesotheliomas and adenocarcinomas involving the serosal surfaces. Am J Clin Pathol 94: 18–26
86. McCaughey W T E, Colby T V, Battifora H et al. 1991 Diagnosis of diffuse malignant mesothelioma: experience of a US/Canadian mesothelioma panel. Mod Pathol 4: 342–353
87. Sheibani K, Esteban J M, Bailey A et al. 1992 Immunopathologic and molecular studies as an aid in the diagnosis of malignant mesothelioma. Hum Pathol 23: 107–116
88. Sheibani K, Stroup R M 1996 Immunopathology of malignant mesothelioma. Pathology 4: 191–212
89. Ordonez N G 2006 The diagnostic utility of immunohistochemistry and electron microscopy in distinguishing between peritoneal mesotheliomas and serous carcinomas: a comparative study. Mod Pathol 19: 34–48
90. Attanoos R L, Webb R, Dojcinov S D et al. 2002 Value of mesothelial and epithelial antibodies in distinguishing diffuse peritoneal mesothelioma in females from serous papillary carcinoma of the ovary and peritoneum. Histopathology 40: 237–244
91. Gerald W L, Miller H K, Battifora H et al. 1991 Intra-abdominal desmoplastic small round cell tumor. Am J Surg Pathol 15: 499–513
92. Young R H, Eichhorn J H, Dickersin G R et al. 1992 Ovarian involvement by the intra-abdominal desmoplastic small round cell tumor with divergent differentiation: a report of three cases. Hum Pathol 23: 454–464
93. Ordonez N G, El-Naggar A, Ro J Y et al. 1993 Intra-abdominal desmoplastic small cell tumor: a light microscopic, immunocytochemical, ultrastructural, and flow cytometric study. Hum Pathol 24: 850–865
94. Brodie S G, Stocker S J, Wardlaw J C et al. 1995 EWS and WT-1 gene fusion in desmoplastic small round cell tumor of the abdomen. Hum Pathol 26: 1370–1374

95. Schroder S, Padberg B 1993 Desmoplastic small-cell tumor of the peritoneum with divergent differentiation: immunocytochemical and biochemical findings (letter). Am J Clin Pathol 99: 353–354
96. Argatoff L H, O'Connell J X, Mathers J A et al. 1996 Detection of the EWS/WT1 gene fusion by reverse transcriptase-polymerase chain reaction in the diagnosis of intra-abdominal desmoplastic small round cell tumor. Am J Surg Pathol 20: 406–412
97. Dorsey B V, Benjamin L E, Rauscher F III et al. 1996 Intra-abdominal desmoplastic small round-cell tumor: expansion of the pathologic profile. Mod Pathol 9: 703–709
98. Amato R J, Ellerhorst J A, Ayala A G 1996 Intraabdominal desmoplastic small cell tumor. Report and discussion of five cases. Cancer 78: 845–851
99. Cummings O W, Ulbright T M, Young R H 1997 Desmoplastic small round cell tumors of the paratesticular region. A report of six cases. Am J Surg Pathol 21: 219–225
100. Charles A K, Moore I E, Berry P J 1998 Immunohistochemical detection of the Wilms' tumour gene WT1 in desmoplastic small round cell tumour. Histopathology 30: 312–314
101. Gerald W, Ladanyi M, de Alava E et al. 1998 Clinical, pathologic and molecular spectrum of tumors associated with t(11;22)(p13;q12): desmoplastic small round-cell tumor and its variants. J Clin Oncol 16: 3028–3036
102. Ordonez N G 1998 Desmoplastic small round cell tumor. I. A histopathologic study of 39 cases with emphasis on unusual histologic patterns. Am J Surg Pathol 22: 1303–1313
103. Lae M E, Roche P C, Jin L et al. 2002 Desmoplastic small round cell tumor. A clinicopathologic, immunohistochemical, and molecular study of 32 tumors. Am J Surg Pathol 26: 823–835
104. Ordonez N G 1998 Desmoplastic small round cell tumor. II. An ultrastructural and immunohistochemical study with emphasis on new immunohistochemical markers. Am J Surg Pathol 22: 1314–1327
105. Zhang P J, Goldblum J R, Pawel B R et al. 2003 Immunophenotype of desmoplastic small round cell tumors as detected in cases with EWS-WT1 gene fusion product. Mod Pathol 16: 229–235
106. Lin B T, Colby T, Gown A M et al. 1996 Malignant vascular tumors of the serous membranes mimicking mesothelioma. A report of 14 cases. Am J Surg Pathol 20: 1431–1439
107. Attanoos R L, Dallimore N S, Gibbs A R 1997 Primary epithelioid haemangioendothelioma of the peritoneum: an unusual mimic of diffuse malignant mesothelioma. Histopathology 30: 375–377
108. Meis-Kindblom J M, Kindblom L-G 1998 Angiosarcoma of soft tissue. A study of 80 cases. Am J Surg Pathol 22: 683–697
109. Day D L, Sane S, Dehner L P 1986 Inflammatory pseudotumor of the mesentery and small intestine. Pediatr Radiol 16: 210–215
110. Pettinato G, Manivel J C, De Rosa N et al. 1990 Inflammatory myofibroblastic tumor (plasma cell granuloma). Clinicopathologic study of 20 cases with immunohistochemical and ultrastructural observations. Am J Clin Pathol 94: 538–546
111. Meis J M, Enzinger F M 1991 Inflammatory fibrosarcoma of the mesentery and retroperitoneum. Am J Surg Pathol 15: 1146–1156
112. Coffin C M, Watterson J, Priest J R et al. 1995 Extrapulmonary inflammatory myofibroblastic tumor (inflammatory pseudotumor): a clinicopathologic and immunohistochemical study of 84 cases. Am J Surg Pathol 19: 859–872
113. Coffin C M, Humphrey P A, Dehner L P 1998 Extrapulmonary inflammatory myofibroblastic tumor: a clinical and pathological survey. Semin Diagn Pathol 15: 85–101
114. Gonzalez-Crussi F, deMello D E, Sotelo-Avila C 1983 Omental-mesenteric myxoid hamartomas. Am J Surg Pathol 7: 567–578
115. Merino M J, Livolsi V A 1981 Signet ring carcinoma of the female breast: a clinicopathologic analysis of 24 cases. Cancer 48: 1830–1837
116. Abu-Rustum N R, Aghajanian C A, Venkatraman E S et al. 1997 Metastatic breast carcinoma to the abdomen and pelvis. Gynecol Oncol 66: 41–44
117. Young R H, Gilks C B, Scully R E 1991 Mucinous tumors of the appendix associated with mucinous tumors of the ovary and pseudomyxoma peritonei. A clinicopathological analysis of 22 cases supporting an origin in the appendix. Am J Surg Pathol 15: 415–429
118. Michael H, Sutton G, Roth L M 1987 Ovarian carcinoma with extracellular mucin production: reassessment of "pseudomyxoma ovarii et peritonei." Int J Gynecol Pathol 6: 298–312
119. Seidman J D, Elsayed A M, Sobin L H et al. 1993 Association of mucinous tumors of the ovary and appendix. A clinicopathologic study of 25 cases. Am J Surg Pathol 17: 22–34
120. Costa M J 1994 Pseudomyxoma peritonei. Histologic predictors of patient survival. Arch Pathol Lab Med 118: 1215–1219
121. Prayson R A, Hart W R, Petras R E 1994 Pseudomyxoma peritonei. A clinicopathologic study of 19 cases with emphasis on site of origin and nature of associated ovarian tumors. Am J Surg Pathol 18: 591–603
122. Ronnett B M, Kurman R J, Zahn C M et al. 1995 Pseudomyxoma peritonei in women: a clinicopathologic analysis of 30 cases with emphasis on site of origin, prognosis, and relationship to ovarian mucinous tumors of low malignant potential. Hum Pathol 56: 509–524
123. Ronnett B M, Zahn C M, Kurman R J et al. 1995 Disseminated peritoneal adenomucinosis and peritoneal mucinous carcinomatosis. A clinicopathologic analysis of 109 cases with emphasis on distinguishing pathologic features, site of origin, prognosis, and relationship to "pseudomyxoma peritonei." Am J Surg Pathol 19: 1390–1408
123a. Bradley R F, Stewart J H 4th, Russell G B et al. 2006 Pseudomyxoma peritonei of appendiceal origin: a clinicopathologic analysis of 101 patients uniformly treated at a single institution, with literature review. Am J Surg Pathol 30: 551–559
124. O'Connell J T, Hacker C M, Barsky S H 2002 MUC2 is a molecular marker for pseudomyxoma peritonei. Mod Pathol 15: 958–972
125. Ronnett B M, Seidman J D 2003 Mucinous tumors arising in ovarian mature cystic teratomas. Relationship to the clinical syndrome of pseudomyxoma peritonei. Am J Surg Pathol 27: 650–657
126. McKenney J K, Soslow R A, Longacre T A 2004 Mucinous neoplasms arising in mature teratomas: a clinicopathologic study of ovarian and sacrococcygeal tumors. Mod Pathol 17: 206A (abstract)
127. Lauchlan S C 1972 The secondary mullerian system. Obstet Gynecol Surv 27: 133–146
128. Ober W B, Black M B 1955 Neoplasms of the subcoelomic mesenchyme. Arch Pathol Lab Med 59: 698–705
129. Clement P B 2002 Endometriosis, lesions of the secondary mullerian system, and pelvic mesothelial proliferations. In: Kurman R J (ed) Blaustein's pathology of the female genital tract, 5th edn. Springer Verlag, New York, p 729–789
130. Zinsser K R, Wheeler J E 1982 Endosalpingiosis in the omentum. A study of autopsy and surgical material. Am J Surg Pathol 6: 109–117
131. McCaughey W T E, Kirk M E, Lester W et al. 1984 Peritoneal epithelial lesions associated with proliferative serous tumours of the ovary. Histopathology 8: 195–208
132. Sidaway M K, Silverberg S G 1987 Endosalpingiosis in female peritoneal washings: a diagnostic pitfall. Int J Gynecol Pathol 6: 340–346
133. Copeland L J, Silva E G, Gershenson D M et al. 1988 The significance of mullerian inclusions found at second-look laparotomy in patients with epithelial ovarian neoplasms. Obstet Gynecol 71: 763–770
134. Kheir S M, Mann W J, Wilkerson J A 1981 Glandular inclusions in lymph nodes. The problem of extensive involvement and relationship to salpingitis. Am J Surg Pathol 5: 353–359
135. Yoonessi M, Satchindanand S K, Ortinez C G et al. 1982 Benign glandular elements and decidual reaction in retroperitoneal lymph nodes. J Surg Oncol 19: 81–86
136. Horn L-C, Bilek K 1995 Frequency and histogenesis of pelvic retroperitoneal lymph node inclusions of the female genital tract. Pathol Res Pract 191: 991–996
137. Maaben V, Hiller K 1994 Glandular inclusions in lymph nodes: pattern of distribution and metaplastic formation. Arch Gynecol Obstet 255: 1–8
138. Mills S E 1983 Decidua and squamous metaplasia in abdominopelvic lymph nodes. Int J Gynecol Pathol 2: 209–215
139. Reich O, Tamussino K, Haas J et al. 2000 Benign mullerian inclusions in pelvic and paraaortic lymph nodes. Gynecol Oncol 78: 242–244
140. McCluggage W G, Clements W D B 2001 Endosalpingiosis of the colon and appendix. Histopathology 39: 639–650
141. Bell D A, Scully R E 1989 Benign and borderline serous lesions of the peritoneum in women. Pathol Annu 24: 1–25
142. Moore W F, Bentley R C, Berchuk A et al. 2000 Some mullerian inclusion cysts in lymph nodes may sometimes be metastases from serous borderline tumors of the ovary. Int J Gynecol Pathol 24: 710–718
143. Clement P B, Young R H 1999 Tumor-like manifestations of florid cystic endosalpingiosis: a report of four cases including the first reported cases of mural endosalpingiosis of the uterus. Am J Surg Pathol 23: 166–175
144. Carrick K S, Mivenan J S, Albores-Saavedra J 2003 Serous tumor of low malignant potential arising in inguinal endosalpingiosis: report of a case. Int J Gynecol Pathol 22: 412–415
145. Young R H, Clement P B 1996 Mullerianosis of the urinary bladder. Mod Pathol 9: 731–737
146. Lim S, Kim J Y, Park K et al. 2003 Mullerianosis of the mesosalpinx: a case report. Int J Gynecol Pathol 22: 209–212
147. Prade M, Spatz A, Bentley R et al. 1995 Borderline and malignant serous tumor arising in pelvic lymph nodes: evidence of origin in benign glandular inclusions. Int J Gynecol Pathol 14: 87–91
148. Bell D A, Scully R E 1990 Serous borderline tumors of the peritoneum. Am J Surg Pathol 14: 230–239
149. Biscotti C V, Hart W R 1992 Peritoneal serous micropapillomatosis of low malignant potential (serous borderline tumors of the peritoneum). Am J Surg Pathol 16: 467–475
150. Tobacman J K, Tucker M A, Kase R et al. 1982 Intra-abdominal carcinomatosis after prophylactic oophorectomy in ovarian-cancer-prone families. Lancet 2: 795–797
151. White P F, Merino M J, Barwick K W 1985 Serous surface papillary carcinoma of the ovary: a clinical, pathologic, ultrastuctural, and immunohistochemical study of 11 cases. Pathol Annu 20: 403–418
152. Chen K T K, Flam M S 1986 Peritoneal papillary serous carcinoma with long-term survival. Cancer 58: 1371–1373
153. Lele S B, Piver M S, Matharu J et al. 1988 Peritoneal papillary carcinoma. Gynecol Oncol 31: 315–320
154. Mills S E, Andersen W A, Fechner R E et al. 1988 Serous surface papillary carcinoma. A clinicopathologic study of 10 cases and comparison with stage III–IV ovarian serous carcinoma. Am J Surg Pathol 12: 827–834
155. Dalrymple J C, Bannatyne P, Russell P et al. 1989 Extraovarian peritoneal serous papillary carcinoma. A clinicopathologic study of 31 cases. Cancer 64: 110–115

156. Raju U, Fine G, Greenawald K A et al. 1989 Primary papillary serous neoplasia of the peritoneum: a clinicopathologic and ultrastructural study of eight cases. Hum Pathol 20: 426–436
157. Wick M R, Mills S E, Dehner L P et al. 1989 Serous papillary carcinomas arising from the peritoneum and ovaries. A clinicopathologic and immunohistochemical comparison. Int J Gynecol Pathol 8: 179–188
158. Fromm G, Gershenson D M, Silva E G 1990 Papillary serous carcinoma of the peritoneum. Obstet Gynecol 75: 89–95
159. Ransom D T, Shreyaskumar R P, Keeney G L et al. 1990 Papillary serous carcinoma of the peritoneum. A review of 33 cases treated with platin-based chemotherapy. Cancer 66: 1091–1094
160. Truong L D, Maccato M L, Awalt H et al. Serous surface carcinoma of the peritoneum: a clinicopathologic study of 22 cases. Hum Pathol 1990; 21: 99–110
161. Bandera C A, Muto M G, Schorge J O et al. 1998 BRCA1 gene mutations in women with papillary serous carcinoma of the peritoneum. Obstet Gynecol 92: 596–600
162. Schorge J O, Muto M G, Lee S J et al. 2000 BRCAI-related papillary serous carcinoma of the peritoneum has a unique molecular pathogenesis. Cancer Res 60: 1361–1364
163. Halperin R, Zehavi S, Langer R et al. 2001 Primary peritoneal serous papillary carcinoma: a new epidemiologic trend? Int J Gynecol Cancer 11: 403–408
164. Halperin R, Zehavi S, Hadas E et al. 2001 Immunohistochemical comparison of primary peritoneal and primary ovarian serous papillary carcinoma. Int J Gynecol Pathol 20: 341–345
165. Barda G, Menczer J, Chetrit A et al. 2004 Comparison between primary peritoneal and epithelial ovarian carcinoma: a population-based study. Am J Obstet Gynecol 190: 1039–1045
166. Weir M M, Bell D A, Young R H 1998 Grade 1 peritoneal serous carcinomas: a report of 14 cases and comparison with 7 peritoneal serous psammocarcinomas and 19 peritoneal serous borderline tumors. Am J Surg Pathol 22: 849–862
167. McCaughey W T E, Schryer M J P, Lin X et al. 1986 Extraovarian pelvic serous tumor with marked calcification. Arch Pathol Lab Med 110: 78–80
168. Gilks C B, Bell D A, Scully R E 1990 Serous psammocarcinoma of the ovary and peritoneum. Int J Gynecol Pathol 9: 110–121
169. Hafiz M A, Toker C 1986 Multicentric ovarian and extraovarian cystadenofibroma. Obstet Gynecol 68: 94S–98S
170. Clark J E, Wood H, Jaffurs W J et al. 1979 Endometrioid-type cystadenocarcinoma arising in the mesosalpinx. Obstet Gynecol 54: 656–658
171. Chang K L, Crabtree G S, Lim-Tan S K et al. 1993 Primary extrauterine endometrial stromal neoplasms: a clinicopathologic study of 20 cases and a review of the literature. Int J Gynecol Pathol 12: 282–296
172. Mira J L, Fenoglio-Preiser C M, Husseinzadeh N 1995 Malignant mixed mullerian tumor of the extraovarian secondary mullerian system. Report of two cases and review of the English literature. Arch Pathol Lab Med 119: 1044–1049
173. Shen D, Khoo U, Xue W et al. 2001 Primary peritoneal malignant mixed mullerian tumors. A clinicopathologic, immunohistochemical, and genetic study. Cancer 91: 1052–1060
174. Sumathi V P, Murnaghan M, Dobbs S P et al. 2002 Extragenital mullerian carcinosarcoma arising from the peritoneum: report of two cases. Int J Gynecol Cancer 12: 764–767
175. Visvalingam S, Jaworski R, Blumenthal N et al. 2001 Primary peritoneal mesodermal adenosarcoma: report of a case and review of the literature. Gynecol Oncol 81: 500–505
176. Dincer A D, Timmins P, Fisher H et al. 2001 Primary peritoneal mullerian adenosarcoma with sarcomatous transformation. Int J Gynecol Pathol 21: 65–68
177. Baird D B, Reddick R L 1991 Extraovarian mucinous metaplasia in a patient with bilateral mucinous borderline ovarian tumors: a case report. Int J Gynecol Pathol 10: 96–103
178. Clement P B, Young R H 1992 Endocervicosis of the urinary bladder: a report of six cases of a benign mullerian lesion that may mimic adenocarcinoma. Am J Surg Pathol 16: 533–542
179. Nazeer T, Ro J Y, Tornos C et al. 1996 Endocervical-type glands in the urinary bladder: a clinocopathologic study of six cases. Hum Pathol 27: 816–820
180. Young R H, Clement P B 2000 Endocervicosis involving the uterine cervix: a report of four cases of a benign process that may be confused with deeply invasive endocervical adenocarcinoma. Int J Gynecol Pathol 19: 322–328
181. Martinka M, Allaire C, Clement P B 1999 Endocervicosis presenting as a painful vaginal mass: a case report. Int J Gynecol Pathol 18: 274–276
182. Chen K T K 2002 Endocervicosis of the small intestine. Int J Surg Pathol 10: 65–67
183. Banerjee R, Gough J 1988 Cystic mucinous tumours of the mesentery and retroperitoneum: report of three cases. Histopathology 12: 527–532
184. Pennell T C, Gusdon J P Jr 1989 Retroperitoneal mucinous cystadenoma. Am J Obstet Gynecol 160: 1229–1231
185. Pearl M L, Valea F, Chumas J et al. 1996 Primary retroperitoneal mucinous cystadenocarcinoma of low malignant potential: a case report and literature review. Gynecol Oncol 61: 150–152
186. Lee I, Ching K, Pang M et al. 1996 Two cases of primary retroperitoneal mucinous cystadenocarcinoma. Gynecol Oncol 63: 145–150
187. Mikami M, Tei C, Takehara K et al. 2003 Retroperitoneal primary mucinous adenocarcinoma with a mural nodule of anaplastic tumor: a case report and literature review. Int J Gynecol Pathol 22: 205–208
188. Bransilver B R, Ferenczy A, Richart R M 1974 Brenner tumors and Walthard cell nests. Arch Pathol Lab Med 98: 76–86
189. Roth L M 1974 The Brenner tumor and the Walthard cell nest. An electron microscopic study. Lab Invest 31: 15–23
190. Teoh T B 1953 The structure and development of Walthard nests. J Pathol 66: 433–439
191. Schatz J E, Colgan T J 1991 Squamous metaplasia of the peritoneum. Arch Pathol Lab Med 115: 397–398
192. Hampton H L, Huffman H T, Meeks G R 1992 Extraovarian Brenner tumor. Obstet Gynecol 79: 844–846
193. Evans H, Yates W A, Palmer W E et al. 1990 Clear cell carcinoma of the sigmoid mesocolon: a tumor of the secondary mullerian system. Am J Obstet Gynecol 162: 161–163
194. Lee K R, Verma U, Belinson J 1991 Primary clear cell carcinoma of the peritoneum. Gynecol Oncol 41: 259–262
195. Burnett R A, Millan D 1986 Decidual change in pelvic lymph nodes: a source of possible diagnostic error. Histopathology 10: 1089–1092
196. Zaytsev P, Taxy J B 1987 Pregnancy-associated ectopic decidua. Am J Surg Pathol 11: 526–530
197. Cobb C J 1988 Ectopic decidua and metastatic squamous carcinoma: presentation in a single pelvic lymph node. J Surg Oncol 38: 126–129
198. Buttner A, Bassler R, Theele C 1993 Pregnancy-associated ectopic decidua (deciduosis) of the greater omentum. An analysis of 60 biopsies with cases of fibrosing deciduosis and leiomyomatosis peritonealis disseminata. Pathol Res Pract 189: 352–359
199. Malpica A, Deavers M T, Shahab I 2002 Gross deciduosis peritonei obstructing labor: a case report and review of the literature. Int J Gynecol Pathol 21: 273–275
200. Tavassoli F A, Norris H J 1982 Peritoneal leiomyomatosis (leiomyomatosis peritonealis disseminata): a clinicopathologic study of 20 cases with ultrastructural observations. Int J Gynecol Pathol 1: 59–74
201. Hsu Y K, Rosenshein N B, Parmley T H et al. 1981 Leiomyomatosis in pelvic lymph nodes. Obstet Gynecol 57: 91S–93S
202. Clavero P A, Nogales F F, Ruiz-Avila I et al. 1992 Regression of peritoneal leiomyomatosis after treatment with gonadotropin releasing hormone analogue. Int J Gynecol Cancer 2: 52–54
203. Hales H A, Peterson C M, Jones K P et al. 1992 Leiomyomatosis peritonealis disseminata treated with a gonadotropin-releasing hormone agonist. Am J Obstet Gynecol 167: 515–516
204. Ma K F, Chow L T C 1992 Sex cord-like pattern leiomyomatosis peritonealis disseminata: a hitherto undescribed feature. Histopathology 21: 389–391
205. Raspagliesi F, Quattrone P, Grosso G et al. 1996 Malignant degeneration in leiomyomatosis peritonealis disseminata. Gynecol Oncol 61 272–274
206. Due W, Pickartz H 1989 Immunohistologic detection of estrogen and progesterone receptors in disseminated peritoneal leiomyomatosis. Int J Gynecol Pathol 8: 46–53
207. Lipschutz A, Vargas L Jr 1941 Structure and origin of uterine and extragenital fibroids induced experimentally in the guinea pig by prolonged administration of estrogen. Cancer Res 1: 236–243
208. Quade B J, McLachlin C M, Soto-Wright V et al. 1997 Disseminated peritoneal leiomyomatosis. Clonality analysis by X chromosome inactivation and cytogenetics of a clinically benign smooth muscle proliferation. Am J Pathol 150: 2153–2166

乳腺肿瘤
Tumors of the breast

16

Ian O. Ellis, Sarah E. Pinder, Andrew H.S. Lee 著
李香菊　薛卫成　阚秀 译

乳腺疾病分类	903	柱状细胞病变	917
纤维囊性变及相关疾病	903	增生性乳腺疾病/上皮增生	919
炎症性疾病	905	恶性肿瘤	924
纤维腺瘤、变异及相关病变	906	少见的上皮性肿瘤	951
硬化性病变	911	间质肿瘤	955
导管乳头状瘤及相关疾病	914	非固有肿瘤	960

乳腺疾病分类
Classification of breast disease

总的来说，乳腺疾病病理和临床分类应用的术语、定义和分类法 (systems) 现在较一致。WHO[1]、美国病理协会 (American Society of Pathology)[2]、病理学家皇家学院 (Royal College of Pathologists)[3-5] 和欧洲委员会 (European Commission)[6] 都提出了报告乳腺疾病的诊断标准。他们提出的这些标准实际上在良性疾病的分类上完全相同，病理学家们也应积极采纳[2-4,6]。皇家学院和欧洲委员会还提出了乳腺癌的分类标准及预后因素的评价[3-6]。

在这一章节，我们采用并认可了这些标准。乳腺良性肿瘤采用主要的已广为接受的分类，包括纤维囊性变、纤维腺瘤及变异、硬化性病变、乳头状瘤和增生性乳腺疾病；恶性上皮性肿瘤按类型分类，并对预后因素评估进行了相关描述。

纤维囊性变及相关疾病
Fibrocystic change and associated conditions

纤维囊性变　Fibrocystic change

病理学家喜欢使用纤维囊性变来描述囊肿形成、大汗腺化生、柱状细胞改变（盲管腺病）以及各种腺病等乳腺病变的组合。轻微病变被认为是正常形态的变异，归类为正常发展和退化的轻度异常或紊乱，这些病变包括纤维化、微囊形成、小叶退化和轻度硬化性腺病或柱状细胞病变[7]。应用包罗众多的分类 (umbrella category)，例如纤维囊性变，它包括不同病因或临床相关特征的多种乳腺病变，只有在缺乏主要的、独特的组织学病变时才使用。

随着乳腺癌风险与良性乳腺疾病相关性的回顾性研究发表，对纤维囊性变及其他良性病变（如乳头状瘤）中上皮增生的重要性也越来越了解。上皮增生的存在与否及其特征被看作纤维囊性变继续分类的必要形式[2,3]（见增生性乳腺疾病，第919页）。

临床特征

在有症状的乳腺临床病变中，纤维囊性变常表现为边界清楚程度不一和大小不一的包块。B超和影像学检查可见囊肿和微钙化。25岁之前少见，大多数病人35～50岁出现临床症状。绝经后病人罕见囊肿形成[8]。

大体表现

纤维囊性变的大体表现无特征性。一般说来，乳腺受累区域边界不清，含有质硬的纤维脂肪组织和大小不等的多发囊肿。

组织学表现

如前所述，纤维囊性变是由下述多种良性病变组合而来。

囊肿　Cyst

临床特征

囊肿被认为源于小叶"复旧"[9,10]，小叶腺泡内微囊肿形成和进展，通过扩张和融合成为大体可见的囊肿。

囊肿很常见，可占一般人群的19%[11]，7%可触摸到[8]。经常通过针吸处理。囊肿液可行细胞学检查，但除非囊肿液是血性或（液体吸出后）仍有肿物存在，否则这种方法被认为是没有价值的。因为囊肿内癌的发生率与囊肿相比是很低的。单个囊肿与乳腺癌之间没有相关性。

大体表现

囊肿可以单个或多个发生。一般不切除，除非反复发生的大囊肿或多个囊肿引起变形或不适，或者存在囊肿内病变。约77%的乳腺癌伴发囊肿[12]。它们大小不一，圆形，内容物可以是稀薄清亮的黄色液体或黏稠不透明的绿色或褐色物质。

组织学表现

囊肿主要分为两种，一种被覆单层立方上皮（图16.1）或扁平上皮；另一种囊肿更常见，被覆大汗腺化生上皮（图16.1）。这种上皮与正常的大汗腺上皮相似，细胞大，呈柱状，有丰富的颗粒状嗜酸性胞浆，核位于基底部。细胞浆以顶浆形式向管腔内突起。胞浆颗粒呈苏丹黑和抗淀粉酶的PAS阳性[10]。大汗腺上皮通常为单层，但不典型增生可导致乳头状结构形成。乳头状大汗腺改变与大汗腺化生的临床意义下文叙述。

囊肿液的生化研究有助于区分两种囊肿类型。高pH值和钠/钾比值低（与细胞内液相似）的囊肿更易复发，且常是大汗腺化生型；而低pH值和钠/钾比值高（与血浆相似）的囊肿不易复发，被覆立方形或扁平上皮[13,14]。

大汗腺化生　Apocrine metaplasia

大汗腺化生在乳腺常见，且与囊肿形成有关（见前）。普通型是由单层柱状细胞规则排列于正常的肌上皮层之上。大汗腺增生则增生旺盛，且呈乳头状，常形成纤细的纤维血管轴结构。罕见情况下，复杂型大汗腺增生形成片状或伴有多个不规则腔隙的复杂结构。

除常与囊肿相关外，大汗腺化生也可见于其他良性病变，包括硬化性腺病、乳头状瘤和纤维腺瘤。这种现象无特殊的临床意义。

尽管大汗腺化生中核和细胞学形态通常规则，但仍可检测到DNA四倍体[15]。可以解释为"大汗腺不典型性"，此时核增大、多形，核仁突出。目前大汗腺不典型性的临床意义尚不清楚。一些专家[16]认为这是一种单纯的良性状态，而其他专家则认为是大汗腺癌或髓样癌的前驱病变[8]。目前认为单纯的大汗腺改变继发乳腺癌的危险性轻度升高[2]。

鉴别诊断

一般来说，大汗腺化生易于辨认，可以和其他上皮增生性病变相区分。大汗腺不典型性和大汗腺化生可以伴发于硬化性腺病中，称为大汗腺腺病[17]。非典型大细胞若伴发于假浸润病变中（如硬化性腺病），可能被误诊为浸润癌。肌上皮成分的存在以及细胞的顶浆分泌特征可用于鉴别诊断。

柱状细胞改变（盲管腺病）
Columnar cell change (blunt duct adenosis)

柱状细胞改变（盲管腺病）得以在本章进行叙述的原因，是因为它是纤维囊性变的组成部分。与增生性改变相关的柱状细胞病变（columnar cell lesion）将在第917页描述。

临床特征

柱状细胞改变是乳腺很常见的良性改变。一些作者不认为这是一种正常现象[8]。它很少表现为明显的临床实体，常常是偶然发现或伴随纤维囊性变中的其他改变出现。尚未发现与乳腺癌有明确的相关性。

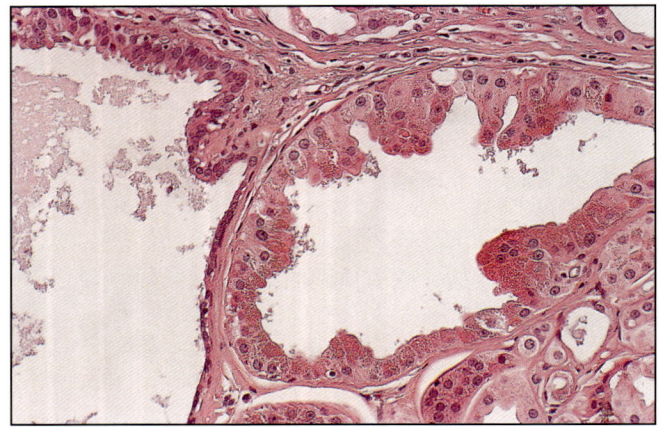

图16.1　囊肿。两个相邻的小囊肿。左侧被覆立方上皮，右侧被覆大汗腺上皮。

大体表现

柱状细胞改变通常是肉眼不可见的,少数情况下可表现为界限不清的微囊肿区。

组织学表现

单个的终末导管小叶单元(terminal duct lobular unit,TDLU)显示,正常管腔上皮被单层高柱状上皮细胞取代,其细胞核位于基底部,细胞浆有顶端突起。正常的圆形腺泡轮廓转变成较大的不规则分支状盲管结构(图16.2)。伴有轻度间质增生。肌上皮层和基底膜很容易见到。

鉴别诊断

柱状细胞改变不易误诊为其他乳腺病变。不同类型的上皮增生可发生于盲管腺病,尤其是男性乳腺发育上皮增生[18]。分泌期和泌乳期改变不易见到。

炎症性疾病 Inflammatory disorders

大多数乳腺炎症性疾病容易做出病理诊断,但硬化性淋巴细胞性乳腺炎在临床和病理上可能被误诊为恶性。

硬化性淋巴细胞性乳腺炎 Sclerosing lymphocytic lobulitis

硬化性淋巴细胞性乳腺炎也称为淋巴细胞性乳腺病(lymphocytic mastopathy),是近期才被确认的乳腺炎症性疾病[19,20],有证据支持其自身免疫发病机制。它与自身免疫性疾病,尤其是长期胰岛素依赖型糖尿病和甲状腺炎密切相关。炎症形态和乳腺上皮的HLA II型表达情况与自身免疫性疾病如Hashimoto甲状腺炎相似。

临床特征

硬化性淋巴细胞性乳腺炎常表现为与乳腺癌相似的肿物。肿物可多发或双侧发生。因此,认识了这种情况,可避免不必要的外科手术。此病可见于20~65岁妇女,但30多岁最常见。也可见于男性。

大体特征

典型病例表现为界限不清的质硬的灰白肿物,但有时外观像正常纤维乳腺组织。

组织学表现

特征性表现是在小叶和导管及血管周围形成圆形界清的淋巴细胞聚集灶(图16.3)。淋巴细胞通常以B细胞为主。生发中心可以出现。经常见到相关小叶萎缩。常有小叶间和小叶内纤维化形成。上皮样成纤维细胞可能会出现[21],非此病所特有。硬化性淋巴细胞性乳腺炎病人的连续活检常显示由密集的炎症进展为小叶萎缩、纤维化加剧、炎症减退的病程[20]。疾病晚期见到的改变(小叶萎缩、纤维化、轻度炎症)无特异性。病人无论有无糖尿病,其病理特征均相似。因此,一般的病理名称如硬化性淋巴细胞性乳腺炎或淋巴细胞性乳腺病比糖

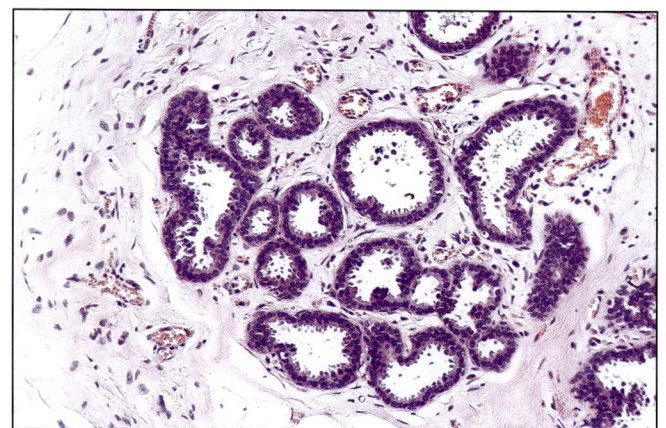

图16.2 柱状细胞改变。柱状细胞取代了正常腺泡衬覆细胞,终末导管小叶单元的正常形态变为一组不一致的扩张导管样结构。

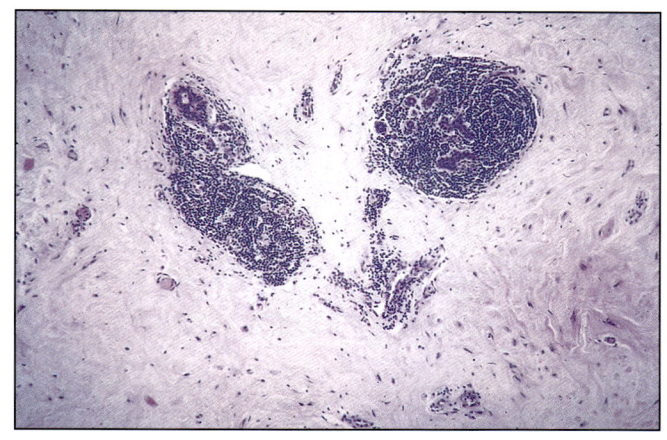

图16.3 硬化性淋巴细胞性乳腺炎显示特化性终末导管小叶间质中成熟小淋巴细胞浸润,形成圆形界清的浸润灶。

尿病性乳腺病更可取。

鉴别诊断

硬化性淋巴细胞性乳腺炎通常容易诊断。可能与淋巴瘤相混淆，但淋巴瘤通常具有不同的结构，由成片的细胞组成，细胞学常表现为中心母细胞型。淋巴瘤与硬化性淋巴细胞性乳腺炎的相关性在日本已有描述[22]，但近期欧洲[23]或美国[24]尚未见报道。像硬化性淋巴细胞性乳腺炎这样的炎症类型也可见于乳腺癌，尤其是浸润性小叶癌[25]，如果炎症过于显著可能会掩盖癌。

纤维腺瘤、变异及相关病变
Fibroadenoma, variants and related conditions

纤维腺瘤 Fibroadenoma

虽然在许多标准教科书中纤维腺瘤仍被看作是良性肿瘤[8,26-28]，但现在认为它们并非真正的肿瘤[29]，而是正常小叶增生的结果。这种观点是基于形态学[30]、形态测量学[31]和染色体[32]研究。在后者中，X-连锁的磷酸甘油激酶基因的限制性片段长度多态性（RFLP）可用于证明上皮细胞和间质细胞都是多克隆性。尽管大多数研究支持纤维腺瘤是由于血循环中雌激素相对于孕激素过多导致的激素反应性增生[33]，但病因尚不明确。在这里描述纤维腺瘤是因为它们形成可触及的乳腺肿物，临床上需要与癌鉴别。

临床特征

纤维腺瘤是最常见的乳腺良性肿瘤。可发生于青春期后的任何年龄，最常见于20～30岁。可单发或多发，可单侧或双侧发生。临床上表现为质硬或质韧的活动性界限清楚的无痛肿物。大多数直径1～2cm，但也常能达到4cm。随着乳腺癌筛查项目的发展，不可触及的纤维腺瘤通过乳腺影像学方法越来越多地能检测到。绝大多数在临床上呈良性行为，而且充分切除后不复发。因为纤维腺瘤常多发，新发病变很常见，甚至距原来活检部位很近。

对疑为纤维腺瘤的妇女，外科医生越来越倾向采用较为保守的方法处理，临床常用的三种检查方法为影像学、细针穿刺细胞学（fine needle aspiration cytology, FNAC）或粗针活检[34-36]。除非病人特别要求手术切除，如果所有指标都为良性，可以免除外科手术。

极少恶性变，目前仅有约120例纤维腺瘤相关的原位癌或浸润癌病例报道[37]。约50%的病例是小叶原位癌，不到40%为浸润癌，其余病例为导管原位癌。在许多病例中，肿瘤发生在相邻组织，很难判断与纤维腺瘤的关系是否仅仅出于巧合。流行病学研究表明，纤维腺瘤患者中继发浸润癌的相对危险性有轻微增加，约增加2倍[38,39]。"复杂"形态的纤维腺瘤（见下文）危险性增加到3倍，有乳腺癌家族史者危险性增加至4倍[38]。然而，单纯的纤维腺瘤绝对危险性为4%，仍然比较低。

大体表现

纤维腺瘤的大体表现具有特点（图16.4）。表现为界限清楚的球形或卵圆形结节，色泽灰白，与周围组织有明确的分界。切面通常略呈分叶状，呈光泽黏液样外观。多数病变手感较硬，但在老年妇女可能更加坚硬，甚至钙化。

组织学表现

主要表现为细胞稀疏的间质结缔组织围绕数量不等的导管共同增生（图16.5A,B和16.6）。间质核呈梭形，很少出现多形性，分裂象少见。间质成分变化显著，一些纤维腺瘤有明显的黏液样背景，而另一些病例则明显玻璃样变性。导管形态也常有变化，通常描述为两种典型类型：当导管被间质挤压成裂隙时称为管内型（图16.5B），而当间质围绕导管呈圆周状时称为管周型（图16.6）。事实上，两种类型可能在同一病变中见到，形

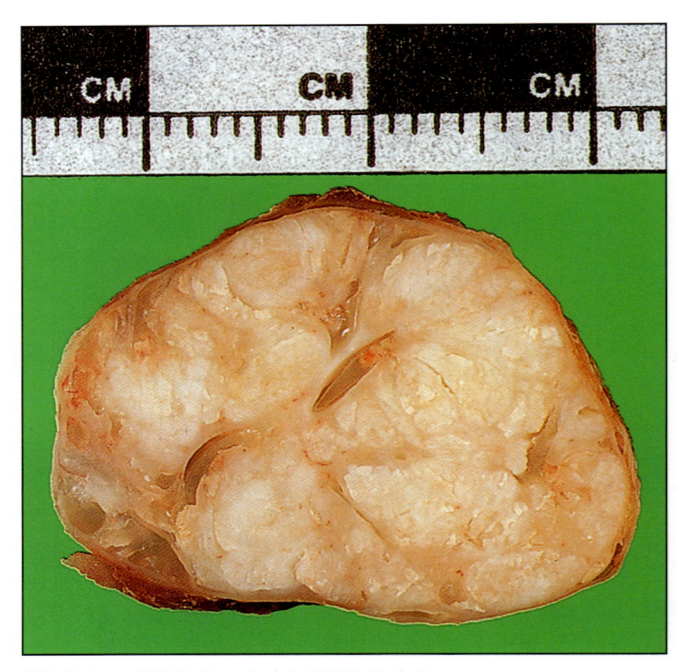

图16.4　纤维腺瘤。病变切面呈分叶状。

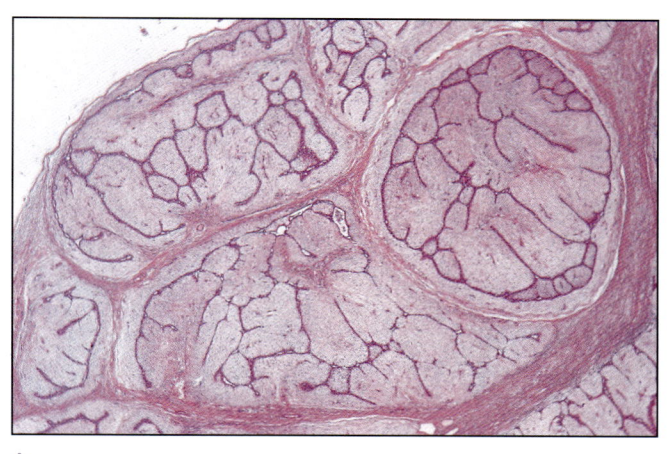 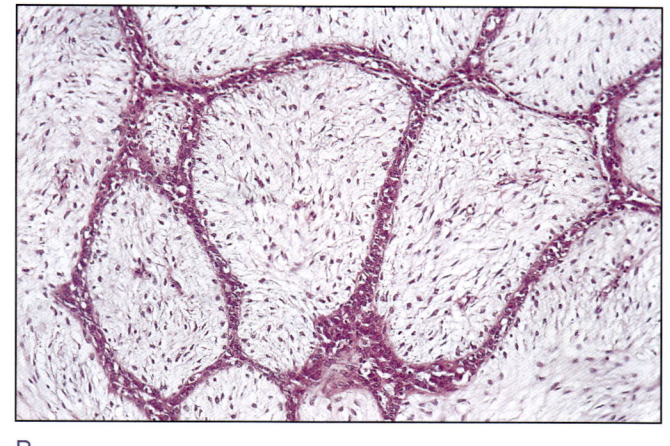

图16.5　纤维腺瘤。此病变表现为典型的管内型。有明显的结节状结构（A），（B）显示上皮裂隙和细胞丰富的小叶内间质特征性混合。

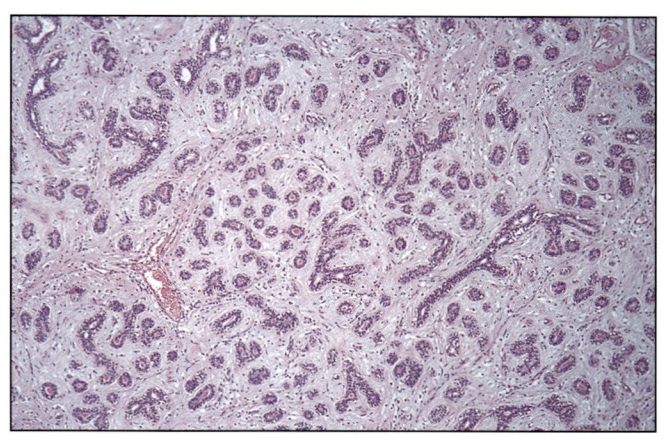

图16.6　管周型纤维腺瘤。

态的差异可能与切面有关。这些名称没有临床或预后意义，仅仅是描述性诊断。约20%的病例可分别或同时出现囊肿（直径超过3mm）、硬化性腺病、上皮钙化和乳头状大汗腺化生；这种病变被Page及其同事命名为复杂纤维腺瘤[38]。常见上皮增生，虽然侧切面（tangential sectioning）中可能出现令人担忧的增生形态，但不出现真正的不典型增生[27]。

年龄较大的患者，尤其是绝经后妇女，纤维腺瘤的间质细胞量减少，玻璃样变性明显。营养不良性钙化可随之发生，有些纤维腺瘤可以完全钙化。

鉴别诊断

鉴别诊断中最重要的病变是叶状肿瘤（见第909页）。尽管后者常见于年龄较大的人群，但在间质细胞丰富且上皮裂隙较多的大纤维腺瘤可能存在诊断困难。真正要区分纤维腺瘤和良性叶状肿瘤是不可能的，但间质核相对一致且缺乏分裂象更倾向于诊断纤维腺瘤。尽管我们不同意使用叶状纤维腺瘤这样的名称[40]，但有时给出这样一个有歧义的报告是难以避免的。对这样的病例完整切除可避免局部复发风险。

纤维腺瘤与乳腺错构瘤的鉴别在第909页讨论。

纤维瘤病（fibromatosis）[41]是引起乳腺肿物的少见病因，但导管周围纤维母细胞增生可能与纤维腺瘤类似。浸润性边缘、间质富于细胞和上皮成分相对稀少是支持纤维瘤病的诊断要点（见第959页）。

幼年性纤维腺瘤　Juvenile fibroadenoma

幼年性纤维腺瘤和巨大纤维腺瘤的名称滥用产生了许多困惑。事实上，后者不但用于描述大的纤维腺瘤，也被不恰当地用于良性叶状肿瘤。实际上，所有幼年性纤维腺瘤都很大，这个名称最好专门用于那些发生在青春期女孩且生长速度很快的纤维腺瘤。其表现为界限清楚的分叶状肿物（直径可达15～20厘米），牵拉皮肤并使乳头变形[42,43]。形态学上它与较为典型的纤维腺瘤完全相同。管周型和管内型生长方式都能见到，间质细胞丰富，很少玻璃样变性（图16.7），而且可能呈现假血管瘤样间质增生形态。上皮增生通常活跃[43]，Rosen已强调过可能遇到的各种增生形态[28,42]，不要误诊为导管不典型增生。幼年性纤维腺瘤完全良性，完整切除后不复发。

小管腺瘤　Tubular adenoma

虽然大多数专家现在已经接受单纯的乳腺腺瘤的存在[27,40,44]，但Rosen仍然认为小管腺瘤是纤维腺瘤的一种特殊类型[28]。确实有一些纤维腺瘤局灶呈管状结构，但我们依据Hertel及其同事制定的严格的形态学标准排

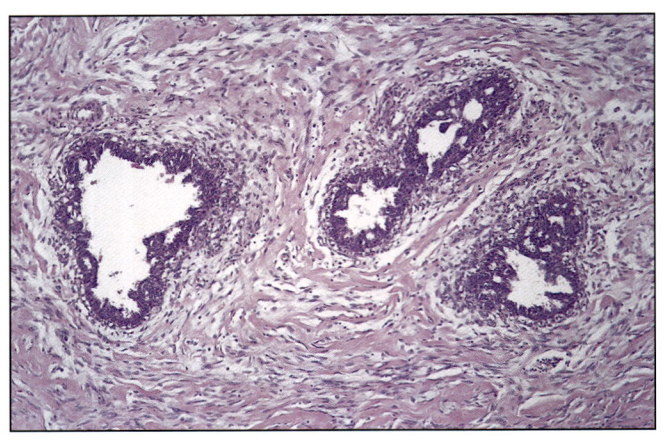

图16.7 幼年性纤维腺瘤。注意其间质细胞丰富，还可见轻度上皮增生。

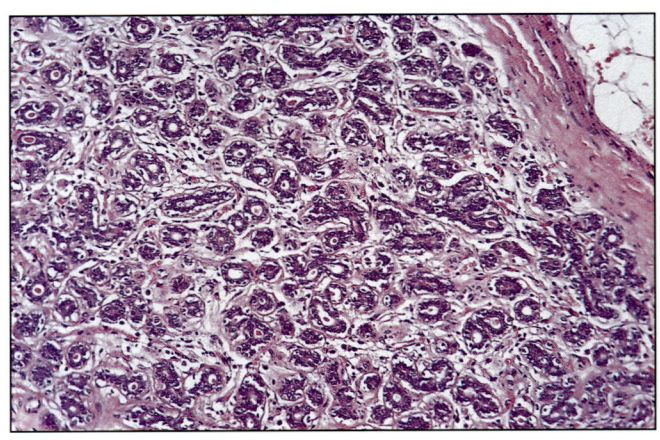

图16.8 小管腺瘤。许多小管状结构分布在纤细的细胞性间质中，小管主要由分泌性上皮细胞和较不明显的肌上皮细胞组成。

除了这些病变[45]。他们强调病变界限清楚，由排列紧密的小管组成，间质很少。所谓的妊娠腺瘤或泌乳腺瘤的特点还未确定。大多数病变有以下特点：生理性小叶增生形成单纯的结节，增生程度明显超过邻近乳腺组织，临床上可呈现明显的肿物[46]。少数情况下，它们因妊娠的激素刺激导致增生而形成真正的小管腺瘤[47]。

临床特征

小管腺瘤的临床表现与纤维腺瘤相似。

妊娠期可以出现多种良性非炎症性包块。在一项由28位患者组成的序贯性研究中（患者年龄16～48岁，平均23岁），可见3种病变类型[47]。纤维腺瘤样形态的腺瘤（16例）和小管腺瘤（2例）是最常见的病例，而通常表现为泌乳改变的"泌乳腺瘤"（10例）居于其次。病变出现在妊娠期或产后几个月，通常表现为无痛性肿物。

大体表现

小管腺瘤是直径介于1～4cm界限清楚的结节，大多数不超过2cm。切面呈细小结节状[48]。

组织学表现

病变区与邻近乳腺组织有明确的界限，但没有真正的包膜。由紧密排列的管状结构组成，与正常小叶的腺泡大小相近（图16.8）。小管被覆单层分泌细胞，也可出现稀少的扁平肌上皮细胞。没有细胞核不典型性，分裂象不常见。小管之间可见少量纤维结缔组织。

在"泌乳腺瘤"，可见大的扩张腺泡，呈现出泌乳组织典型的泡状结构。常见管腔内分泌物。

鉴别诊断

需要鉴别的病变仅有纤维腺瘤和小管癌。前者间质成分较突出，管状结构排列在小叶内。小管可见清楚的双层上皮。小管腺瘤一定不要误诊为小管癌。后者的小管围绕纤维化和弹性组织变性的核心呈特征性放射状排列。小管被覆单层上皮细胞，浸润周边间质和脂肪组织。

乳腺错构瘤　Mammary hamartoma

临床特征

乳腺错构瘤是相对少见的病变，主要发生在围绝经期人群[49-53]。表现为大的可触及的肿物，但令人吃惊的是它们常常不可触及，只有通过乳腺影像学检查才能发现。临床上可能与纤维腺瘤和叶状肿瘤相混淆。影像学表现为特征性的中心透明、界限清楚的大肿物。尽管可以引起乳腺明显变形，错构瘤完全良性，且充分切除后不会复发。

大体表现

病变大小差别很大，大小1～15cm，但大多数介于2～5cm。形成界限清楚的卵圆形肿物。质硬、肉样，见不到纤维腺瘤特征性的分叶状结构。

组织学表现

镜下，乳腺错构瘤尽管与邻近乳腺组织容易分离，但缺乏真正的包膜。由多种结缔组织间质与乳腺小叶组成（图16.9）。后者形态正常。偶见扩张的导管可以呈囊性。上皮增生不是其特征。常能见到岛状脂肪组织，通常出现在病变中心（图16.10）；腺脂肪瘤这个名称可以用于此类病变[28,50]。一些病例中间质出现假血管瘤样增生[52]。

鉴别诊断

对于可触及的包块，小的病变要与纤维腺瘤鉴别，大的则要与"幼年性"纤维腺瘤、假血管瘤样间质增生（PASH）和叶状肿瘤鉴别。镜下，大量间质伴有相对稀少的小叶可与纤维腺瘤鉴别，而富于细胞的间质围绕特征性的叶状上皮裂隙则提示叶状肿瘤。尽管假血管瘤样增生被描述为某些错构瘤的组成成分[52,53]，但通常只占一小部分，而不应与PASH病变形成的包块混淆[54]，后者以间质成分为主。乳腺影像学上，错构瘤可能会误诊为腺脂肪瘤。这种病变是由稀疏的乳腺小叶散布于成熟脂肪组织中形成界限清楚的结节，很少有其他间质[27,55]。

叶状肿瘤　Phyllodes tumor

这种不常见的乳腺肿瘤是由Müller[56]首先提出的，他用"叶状囊肉瘤"这个名词来描述大体检查呈叶状切面的乳腺大肿瘤（phyllos=leaf，希腊语）。因为多数病例都是良性的，这个名称易令人误解，就像巨大纤维腺瘤这个名词也令人误解一样，因为有一些巨大纤维腺瘤病例无疑是恶性的。基于这些原因，我们认可WHO（世界卫生组织）的分类[57]，其中指出应用较为广义的叶状肿瘤，根据组织学表现去评价"良性"或"恶性"[58]。

临床特征

叶状肿瘤通常发生于中老年妇女，40岁以下很少发生。形成分叶状质硬肿物，可能生长迅速，造成单侧乳房增大甚至引起皮肤溃疡，以前叶状肿瘤可以很大，但可能因为许多病人对乳腺关注程度提高，现在表现为直径≤2cm的肿物。

大体表现

叶状肿瘤为质硬的分叶状肿物，直径2～10cm不等（平均5cm）[58-60]。通常界限清楚，常有外凸性轮廓。切面呈特征性的漩涡状，与受压的叶芽相似，有肉眼可见的裂隙。较大的肿瘤常出现囊腔，出血和坏死灶也很常见。

组织学表现

镜下，叶状肿瘤包括两种主要成分：被覆上皮的裂隙和相关的富于细胞的间质（图16.11）。上皮成分通常包括肌上皮细胞和分泌性上皮细胞两层结构。局灶上皮增生常见，尽管有时可能呈旺炽型增生，但恶性变是极罕见的。小叶肿瘤形成和导管原位癌已有报道[8,61,62]，但相关的浸润癌极其罕见[63,64]。

间质成分的表现差别很大。大多数表现为良性。尽管间质细胞量明显多于纤维腺瘤，但这些梭形细胞不显示多形性，且核分裂象少见。偶然出现的怪异巨细胞（图16.12A）不能表明是恶性。在疾病形态的另一端，少数肿瘤会表现出明显的肉瘤样特征，表现为间质过度生长、细胞过度增加、核异型及核分裂象计数增加（图16.12B）。特殊情况下，横纹肌肉瘤、软骨肉瘤和骨肉

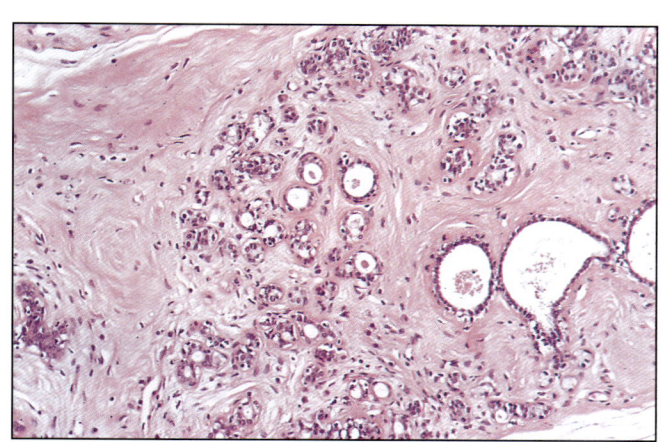

图16.9　乳腺错构瘤。不规则小叶结构及导管分布在玻璃样变性的结缔组织间质中。

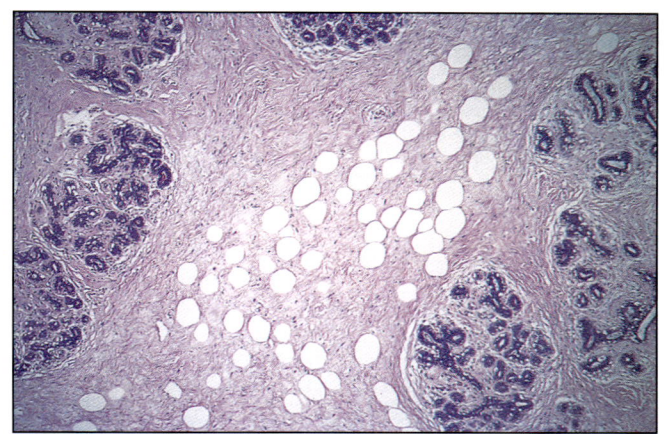

图16.10　错构瘤。切片取自大肿物的中心部分，呈现小叶结构、间质和脂肪组织的混合形态。

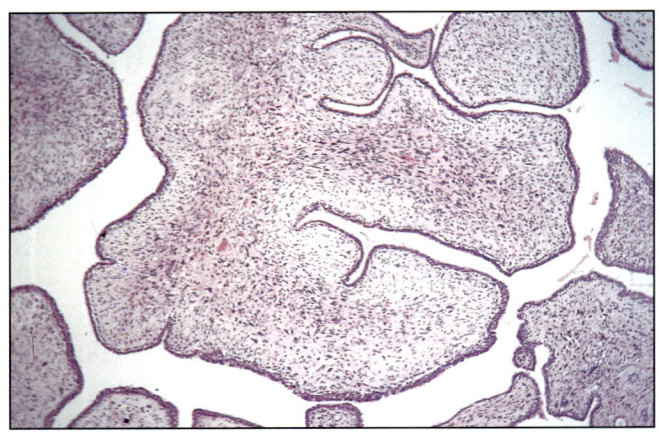

图16.11 叶状肿瘤。被覆上皮细胞的裂隙形成大的分叶状结构。有相关的富于细胞的间质。

瘤等特殊形态的出现是恶性变的明确指征。仍然存在一些中间状态的肿瘤，其形态对于病理和临床医师在判断局部复发和转移潜能方面造成困难。

Norris 和 Taylor[71] 首先提出浸润性边缘（与推挤性边缘相比）、细胞非典型性、分裂象增加和肿瘤较大者倾向恶性，其后一些研究也提出了预后问题[59,65-70]。这些研究的结果并不完全一致，原因包括病例数过少、数据不统一（多数来源于二级或三级会诊中心），有人分为良性和恶性两组，而有人则分为良性、交界性和恶性三组。然而，大多数研究肯定了由 Norris 和 Taylor[71] 提出并由 Pietruszka 和 Barnes[59] 改进的标准的重要性。其中一个研究是基于社区人群而不是会诊病例[58]，而且应用了 Pietruszka 和 Barnes[59] 及 Ward 和 Evans[67] 提出的半定量标准，把叶状肿瘤分为良性、交界性和恶性三组。良性组（22 例，68%）肿瘤为推挤性边缘，间质过度生长较轻微，细胞量及多形性相对较少，核分裂象计数不超过 10/10 个视野（视野区域 0.152mm）。恶性组（5 例，16%）有浸润性边缘，间质增生显著，细胞量丰富，多形性明显，核分裂象计数超过 10/10 个视野。另外 5 例呈中间特征，分类为交界组。我们发现上述这些因素在预测局部复发方面无意义，复发与局部切除的完整性密切相关。良性组复发者（4 例）全部发生在最初局部切除的病例，而后又做了彻底的局部再切除或乳腺切除术。在我们小病例组研究中，除 1 例局部切除后出现无法控制的胸壁复发外，最初行乳腺切除术的恶性组病人均未见复发或转移。

总之，上述组织病理学标准适用于把叶状肿瘤分为良性和恶性。良性肿瘤如果能完全切除，可实施局部保守手术。恶性肿瘤应施行乳腺切除术。叶状肿瘤很少转移，但毫无疑问也可发生。

鉴别诊断

鉴别诊断已在前面纤维腺瘤部分谈及（见第 907 页）。多数病例与纤维腺瘤的区别很明显，但在小的病变会遇到困难。分叶状表现和细胞性间质支持叶状肿瘤的诊断，但单凭大小不能作为鉴别点。另一个重要特点是一些叶状肿瘤表现出同一病变内的异质性，会出现像纤维腺瘤的良性区域。乳腺纤维瘤病、原发肉瘤和化生性癌，尽管非常罕见，也一定要与恶性叶状肿瘤相鉴别。多种成分混合存在，且出现其他病变中不可见的分叶裂隙是叶状肿瘤的特点。化生性癌可能需要免疫组化染色鉴别，其梭形细胞角蛋白抗体如 AE1/AE3、MNF116

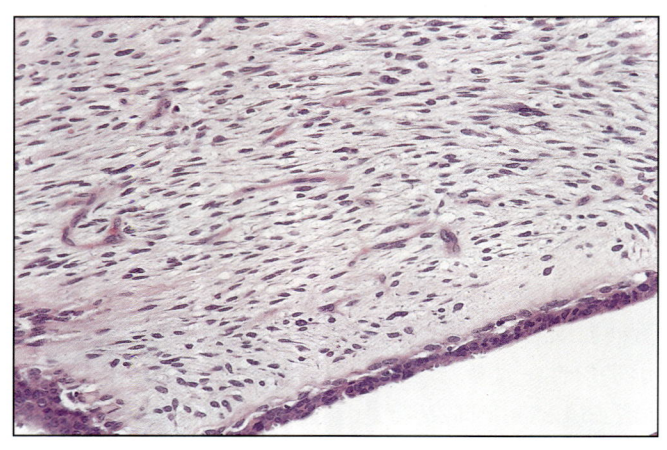

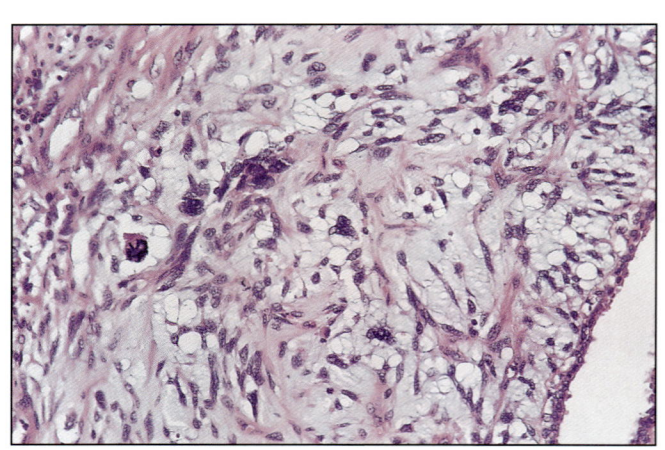

图16.12 叶状肿瘤。（A）此例良性病变中几乎见不到核多形性。（B）此例恶性病变的间质细胞可见到显著的核异型性及异常核分裂象。

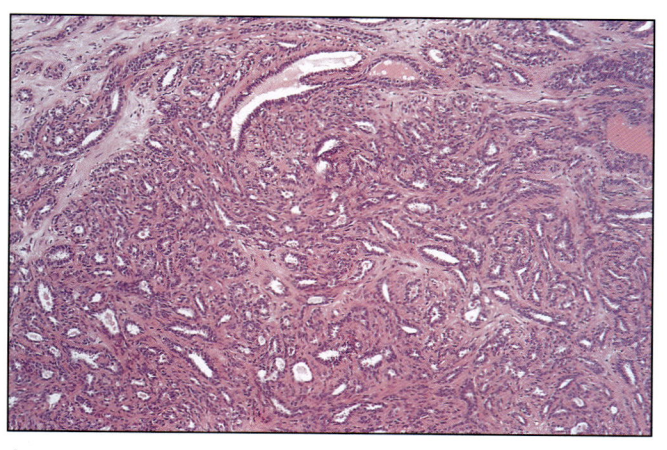
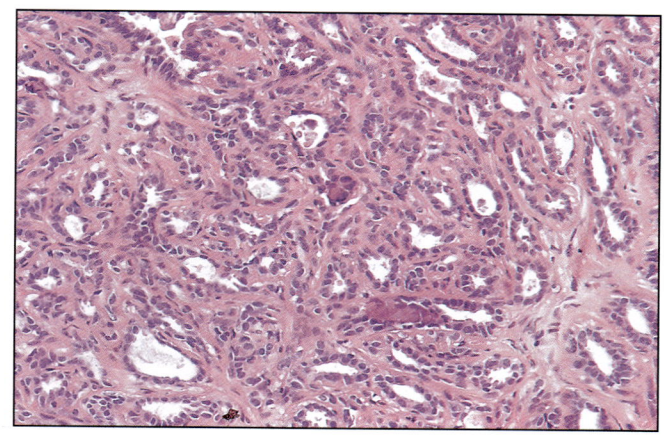

图16.13 硬化性腺病。（A）低倍视野显示腺上皮和小叶内间质呈结节状、杂乱无章的增生。（B）小管结构中可见微钙化灶。

和CAM 5.2免疫染色阳性。多数叶状肿瘤的间质成分表达CD34，但梭形细胞癌通常为CD34阴性[72]。

硬化性病变　Sclerosing lesions

这个广义的标题涵盖了由上皮增生和间质纤维化和硬化组成的病变，所形成的肿块在临床、乳腺影像学和组织学上可误诊为癌。具体病变包括硬化性腺病、微腺腺病、放射状瘢痕和复合硬化性病变。

硬化性腺病　Sclerosing adenosis

腺病和纤维腺病这类名词，笼统涵盖了腺体组织的病变，不具有特异性。由于病理学家过多地将其用于并无明显异常的乳腺组织，因此应该被摒弃。而硬化性腺病是指起源于终末导管小叶单位的相对特异的增生性病变。通常表现为纤维囊性变的组织学组成部分，但少数情况下也可表现为可触及的肿物[73]。后者被命名为腺病瘤（adenosis tumor）[74,75]。瘤在这里是用其最广义的概念，并不代表真正的肿瘤，而且已被普遍接受，尽管"结节性硬化性腺病"这个名称似乎更为合适。

临床特征

大多数临床上表现为可触及包块的患者是绝经前或围绝经期妇女，年龄范围20～70岁。肿物边界不清，但不会发生皮肤和深部筋膜固定。与乳腺癌相比，相关疼痛和触痛很常见。随着乳腺癌筛查项目的出现，由于微钙化的存在，硬化性腺病越来越多地通过乳腺影像学检查出来（见下文）。

大体表现

组织学上弥散的病变，大体没有明确的肿物。结节状或肿物型则形成界限不清的质硬肿块，大小0.5～3cm，平均1.5cm。没有特殊的颜色。

组织学表现

组织学上，小叶的正常轮廓被腺泡和小叶内间质细胞的不规则增生所破坏（图16.13），形成漩涡状外观。可以见到受压的小管结构，但腺泡腔通常消失。至少部分区域能见到双层结构，但上皮和肌上皮细胞可以分别增生。应用抗平滑肌肌动蛋白（SMA）（图16.14）或平滑肌肌球蛋白重链的免疫组化染色容易识别肌上皮成分。核小而规则，常无异型性，核分裂不常见。在小管腔内常可见细小的点状微钙化（图16.13B）。

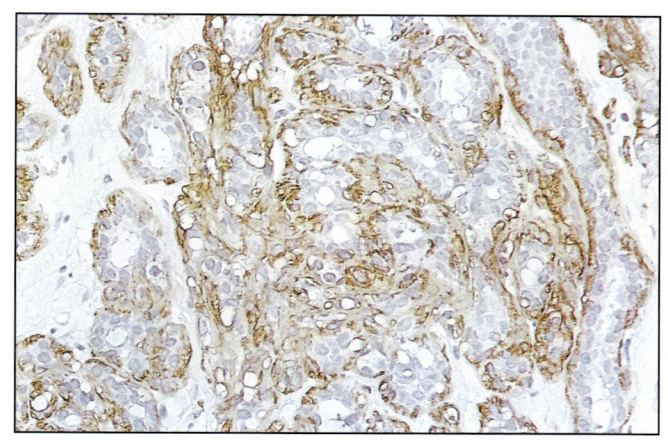

图16.14 硬化性腺病。通过抗平滑肌肌动蛋白的免疫组化染色可清晰地辨认肌上皮成分。

在弥漫型病变，可见到几个小而分散的小叶积聚，常与纤维囊性变的其他形态混合存在。在结节状病变中，扭曲变形的小叶可融合成"器官样"形态，形成境界清楚的肿物。

鉴别诊断

如果结节状病变形成足够大的可触及的肿物，临床上可能与癌难以区分。乳腺影像学上，与筛状导管原位癌的微钙化无法鉴别[76]。组织学上，主要的鉴别诊断是复合硬化性病变和浸润癌。中央弹力纤维变性伴有腺管内陷是复合硬化性病变的重要诊断特征，在硬化性腺病中也偶可见到[73]。与此相应，硬化性腺病病灶也常见于复合硬化性病变。这表明这两种病变代表增生性疾病的两极，如果你试图区分它们，势必会陷入一种语言上的争论。目前，决定哪种方式为主并用它作为诊断名词可能需要一定的经验。

与浸润性癌尤其是小管癌的鉴别更为重要。在少数硬化性腺病，病变可扩展到神经周间隙和血管[77-79]。大汗腺化生也可出现，伴有细胞学非典型性[80,81]，但如果没有确切的证据，这两个特征都不能作为诊断恶性的依据。与浸润性小管癌的主要鉴别点是小叶轮廓仍然存在，不规则增生的导管被覆双层上皮，缺乏孤立的空腔导管和纤维组织增生性间质。

尽管继发浸润癌的危险性很低[82]，但与结节状硬化性腺病相关的导管原位癌和小叶肿瘤形成已有报道[73,83]。导管原位癌的诊断应该不成问题，因为良性导管上皮增生在硬化性腺病中很罕见。小叶增生需引起更多重视，除非满足所有标准，否则不要做出小叶原位癌的诊断（见第923页）[60]。

微腺腺病　Microglandular adenosis

微腺腺病是一种少见的小管或腺泡结构的良性增生，可被误诊为浸润癌，尤其是小管癌[84-87]。

临床特征

微腺腺病常表现为可触及的包块，边界相对较清楚，直径可达几厘米。较小的病灶可能在因其他原因切除的乳腺组织中偶然发现。发病年龄变化较大，从20多岁到80多岁均能见到，但大多数病人在45～60岁发病。乳腺影像学特征不特异，但可能疑为恶性[87]。

多数专家把微腺腺病看作完全良性，没有发展为乳腺癌的危险[88]。但一些专家报道可以并存上皮增生性病变，包括非典型增生、原位癌和浸润癌[89,90]。另外一些人则认为没有确切的证据支持这种观点[86]。一些作者提出微腺腺病和腺泡细胞癌相关（见第954页），因为形态学和免疫表型有部分重叠，但这种观点还存在争议。

大体表现

受累乳腺组织切面边界不清，为普通的纤维脂肪组织。质地和外观的变化反映了其乳腺间质的特点。

组织学表现

微腺腺病定义为小圆形腺泡结构的增生，增生不以小叶为中心，而是无序排列，并可侵入纤维间质和脂肪组织。这些腺体通常由一致的单层立方上皮细胞形成，胞浆透明或嗜酸性，没有胞浆突起（图16.15），核分裂象缺如或非常罕见。最重要的是，基底的肌上皮细胞成分缺如[84]。见不到相关的间质反应，玻璃样变性偶会发生。网状纤维围绕腺体分布，腺体内有PAS阳性分泌物。伴有上皮增生的病例，腺体大小可有变化。腺体S-100蛋白阳性，但EMA、ER、PR和HER2/neu阴性。

鉴别诊断

微腺腺病最重要的鉴别诊断是单纯的小管型浸润癌，尤其是硬化变异型[91]。在这两种情况下在乳腺间质和脂肪组织中有异常排列的腺体。可用以下标准进行鉴

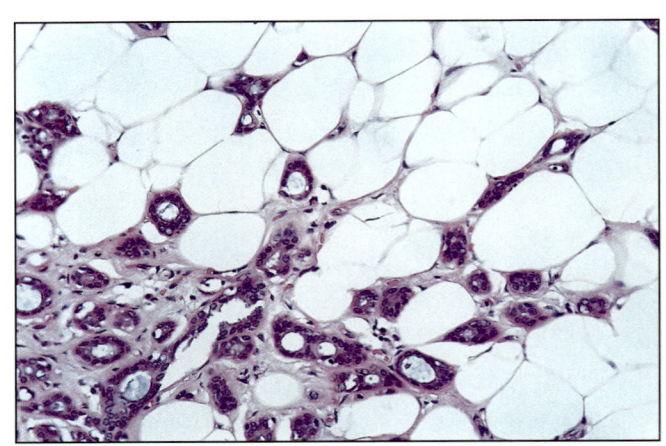

图16.15 微腺腺病。小圆形腺泡结构在纤维脂肪组织中不规则分布。

别；小管癌常有特征性的放射状形态，中央伴有弹力纤维变性和纤维化。它们引起一种特殊的异染性间质反应，而在微腺腺病中见不到。小管癌腺体大部分形状不规则，管腔变长，一些有分支。细胞学上，小管癌的细胞较大且胞浆丰富、嗜酸性，常形成特征性的顶端突起。小管癌罕见分泌现象。尽管多数研究强调微腺腺病以单层上皮细胞为特征[84,86,87]，一些作者报道在少数病例中存在肌上皮细胞（图 16.16）[92-94]。一些病例中使用抗平滑肌肌动蛋白（SMA）的免疫染色在鉴别微腺腺病和小管癌时具有辅助诊断意义。再者，小管癌常表达 EMA 和激素受体。

硬化性腺病可通过其有小叶中心性结构及存在较明显的肌上皮细胞层与微腺腺病区分。

由 Eusebi 和 Kiaer[95] 描述的罕见的腺肌上皮瘤可能具有与微腺腺病难以区分的成分，但典型形态具有肌上皮和上皮双重成分。其特征将在后面的章节详细介绍（见第 952 页）。

放射状瘢痕/复合硬化性病变
Radial scar / complex sclerosing lesion

这些具有弹力纤维中心的特殊的放射状病变有许多令人迷惑的名称，包括玫瑰花结样病变 (rosette-like lesions)[96]、硬化性乳头状增生[97]、良性硬化性导管增生[98]和浸润性上皮增生[10]。后者可能是最不合适的，而放射状瘢痕 (RS) 是由 Hamper 所提出的 "Strahlige Narben"[99] 翻译而来，得到广泛应用[60,100,101]。病变大小可有变化，较大的病例结构也更复杂，包括上皮过度增生。由于这个原因，Page 和 Anderson[60] 表示大小为 1～9mm 的病变命名为放射状瘢痕，而 ≥10mm 的病变应称为复合硬化性病变（CSL）。

临床特征

据报道 RS/CSL 发生于 15～80 岁的女性，多为绝经前和围绝经期妇女。最初认为此病变不常见，可能是因为不常表现为可触及的肿物。然而，对外科乳腺切除标本和活检乳腺组织的研究显示其为常见病变，多发且常为双侧[101-104]。在乳腺筛查项目中该病变越来越多地被检测出来，因为根据影像学区分它与微小浸润癌是不可能的[100,101,105]。因此，所有乳腺影像学检测出的放射状病变都应被切除。

大体表现

小的放射状瘢痕大体表现很不显著，3～4mm 以下的病变只有在组织学检查中才能发现。较大的放射状瘢痕及复合硬化性病变形成质硬的白色放射状结节，其中心致密，大小不一，为放射状纤细针状排列的纤维组织。中心弹力纤维变性可能表现为肉眼下的灰黄色斑点。

组织学表现

镜下表现取决于病变进展的阶段。小的早期放射状瘢痕是由细胞性结缔组织围绕放射状小导管组成的，弹力纤维变性轻微（图 16.17）。较大的病变中心出现致密

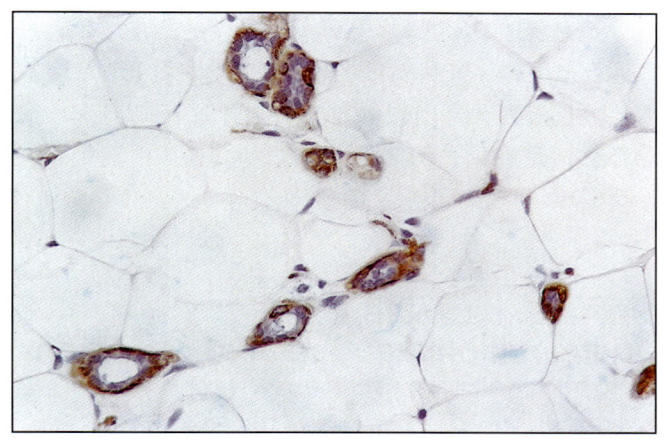

图16.16 此病例通过抗平滑肌肌动蛋白免疫组化染色显示了明确的肌上皮细胞层，表明这更像是硬化性腺病的一种形态，而不是微腺腺病。

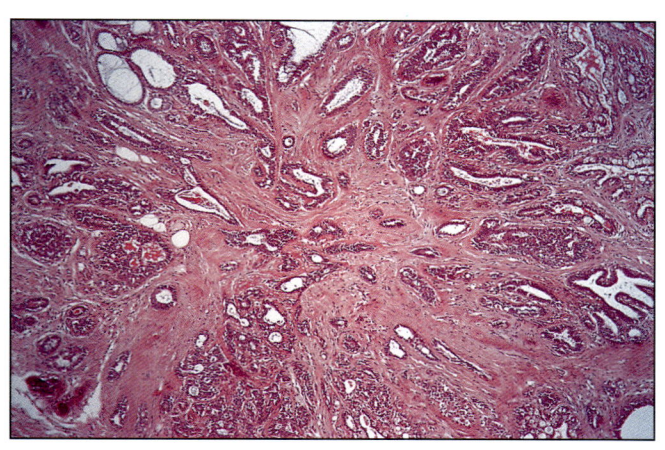

图16.17 放射状瘢痕显示中心瘢痕和放射状导管结构。

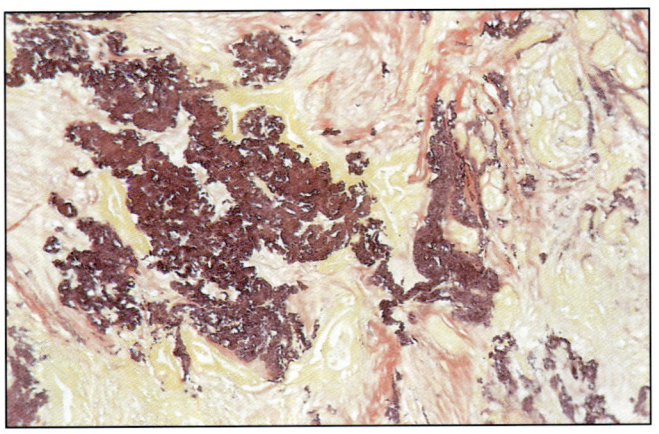

图16.18 复合硬化性病变，Van Gieson弹力纤维染色显示中心弹力纤维变性。

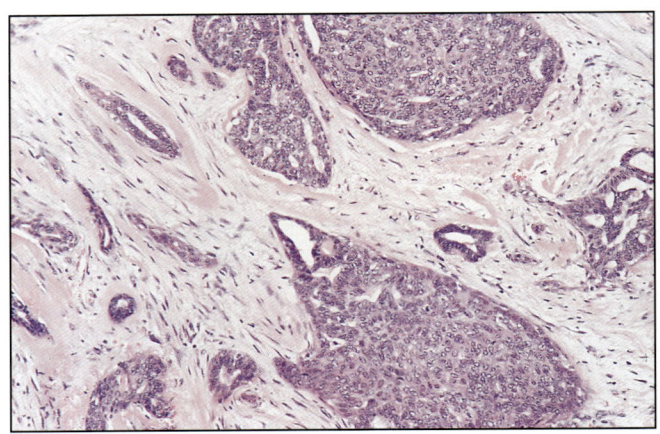

图16.20 普通型上皮增生与内陷的小导管可见于复合硬化性病变。

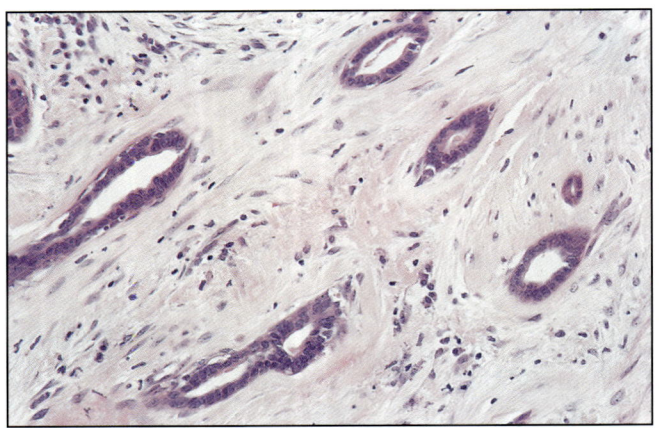

图16.19 此复合硬化性病变中，纤维和弹力纤维组织围绕内陷的导管，导管的双层上皮结构很明显。

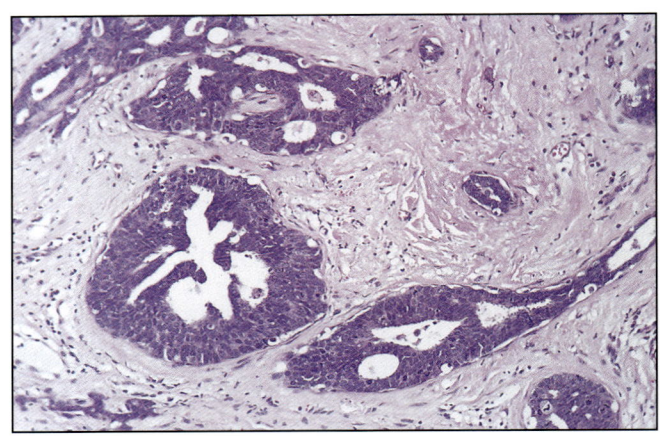

图16.21 放射状瘢痕中的非典型导管增生，附近可见弹力纤维变性和内陷的导管。

的硬化性纤维组织聚集，弹力纤维组织也更加显著（图16.18）。中心的导管被挤压，但正常的双层上皮结构仍然存在（图16.19）。导管结构在放射性结构中也会出现，常能见到囊性变（图16.17）。可以见到不同程度的上皮增生；通常是普通型增生（图16.20），但小心寻找导管和小叶非典型增生是很重要的（图16.21）。

除了病变较大外，复合硬化性病变正如其名称所示，显示多种组织形态。放射状瘢痕的所有基本组织特征都可存在，此外，还可出现硬化性腺病和乳头状瘤，伴有较明显的上皮增生。需要多个蜡块才能展示病变的完整结构。

鉴别诊断

组织学上，RS/CSL必须要与结节型硬化性腺病和小管癌鉴别。前者已在前文论述过（见第911页），这里主要强调与小管癌的鉴别。中心纤维-弹力纤维核心中出现内陷的导管导致了最大的鉴别难点。在RS/CSL中导管结构被覆双层上皮细胞，而小管癌的肿瘤性导管是单层结构（比较图16.19与图16.56）。平滑肌肌动蛋白免疫染色有助于确诊。RS/CSL中内陷的导管为扁平或拉长的，而小管癌中为圆形或卵圆形。相关的结缔组织间质特征也有辅助价值，RS/CSL中的间质致密，细胞较少，而小管癌是促纤维组织增生性间质。

如上所述，RS/CSL中有不同程度的上皮增生，从普通型增生到导管和小叶非典型增生均可见到。后者需要与原位癌区分，但很明显原位癌（图16.22）和浸润癌都会出现在相关的RS/CSL中[101,106]。如果满足恶性诊断标准，要记录下相应的名称。

导管乳头状瘤及相关疾病
Duct papilloma and related conditions

导管乳头状瘤 Duct papilloma

乳头状瘤被认为是导管增生性病变。主要发生在35～55岁妇女。多数病人表现为单个乳头导管溢液，

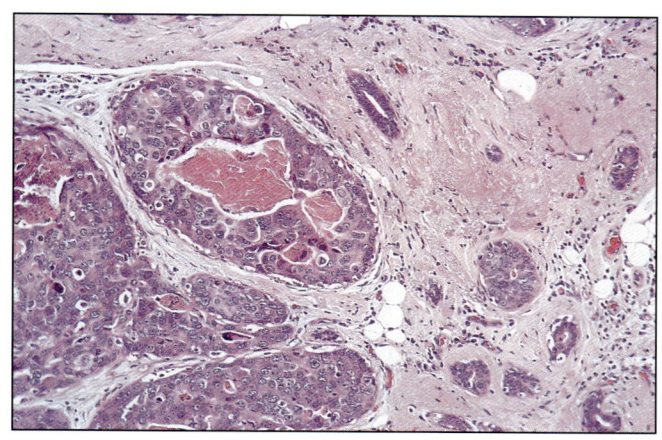

图16.22 复合硬化性病变。右侧为内陷导管周围弹力纤维组织增生；左侧为粉刺型导管原位癌（DCIS）。

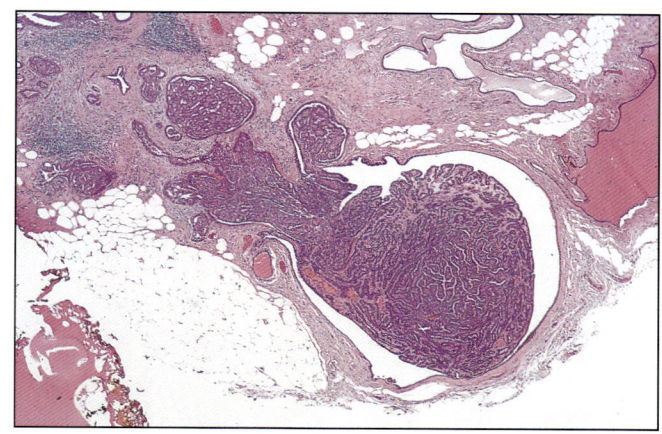

图16.23 导管乳头状瘤。一个大的导管乳头状瘤膨胀性生长并充满管腔。

常为血性，少数病例表现为可触及的包块，常邻近乳晕。导管乳头状瘤可分为两类，中央型（发生于主导管，通常单发）和外周型（发生于终末导管小叶单位，常多发）[8,107-109]。

现存的所有证据表明，发现一个孤立的中央型良性导管乳头状瘤并无继发癌的危险性，而多发乳头状瘤与并发导管原位癌相关，且继发癌的危险性增加[8,107-109]。

大体表现

大多数病例，导管乳头状瘤直径＜2～3mm，因此很难肉眼发现。通过附近的无定形坏死物（包括血凝块）能提示乳头状瘤在扩张导管中的位置，但是多数送检标本是纤维脂肪组织，其中无可识别的大体异常。需要多处取材来确定病变位置。较大的乳头状瘤直径可达1～2cm，可出现于囊内。

组织学表现

镜下，乳头状瘤具有分支状纤维血管轴心，通过蒂与导管壁相连（图16.23）。同一病变发出的多个分支可扩展到相邻的多个导管腔。偶尔为广基型。乳头被覆两种类型的上皮（图16.24），外层为立方或柱状分泌细胞层，内层为肌上皮层。有关两种类型细胞是否存在的疑问可以通过肌上皮标志物免疫染色解决，如抗平滑肌肌动蛋白、平滑肌肌球蛋白或p63。肌上皮层可能不完整，但在少数病例，它可能成为增生上皮的主要成分。单发的中央型导管乳头状瘤病例，邻近的导管通常没有明显病变，尽管可能扩张或充满血性坏死物。常见大汗腺化生，但通常非常局限。梗死和出血相对少见。

多发乳头状瘤通常作为局部或较弥漫的上皮增生性

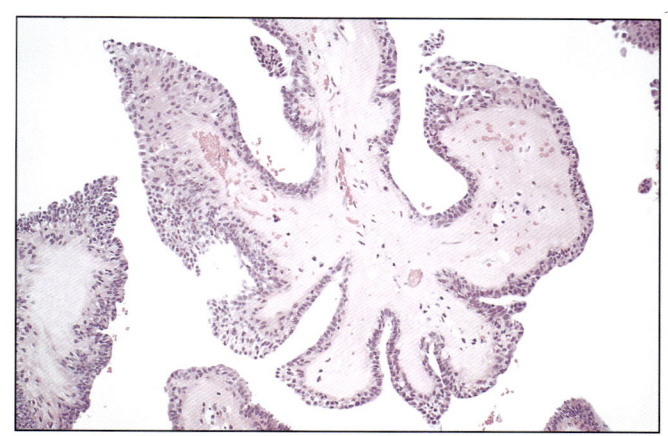

图16.24 导管乳头状瘤。乳头状分支具有纤维血管轴心，被覆肌上皮和上皮双层结构。

病变的一部分，发生于较小的外周导管，可伴有各种类型的上皮病变，包括普通型增生、导管非典型增生、小叶肿瘤形成和导管原位癌。

鉴别诊断

乳头状病变主要分为3类；形态学和肌上皮标志物（平滑肌肌动蛋白、p63和平滑肌肌球蛋白重链）以及基底角蛋白（CK5和CK14）的免疫组化染色可有助于区分类型。导管内乳头状瘤具有肌上皮层和普通型相关上皮增生，斑片状表达基底角蛋白。乳头状原位癌缺乏肌上皮层，且基底角蛋白常为阴性。第三种最少见的类型是良性乳头状瘤伴有导管原位癌或导管非典型增生，表现出肌上皮层依然存在，非典型区域基底角蛋白阴性。

硬化性乳头状瘤可能包括内陷的上皮结构，一定要小心地正确解释这些病变以避免过诊为恶性（见第929页）。应用免疫组化可有助于判断肌上皮层是否存留。平滑肌肌球蛋白重链和（或）p63是可供选择的标记，因其在肌上皮中表达，而在肌纤维细胞中不表达；平滑肌肌动蛋白在两种细胞类型中都表达，因此不能区分纤维化和肌上皮。

如果乳头状病变完全梗死，准确的分类常是不可能的。

乳头腺瘤 Adenoma of nipple

这个名称并非指某一特定的病变，过去将它用于描述乳头所有良性肿瘤。但是，主要病变包括上皮结构的过度增生，表现为乳头状和腺瘤样形态。由于组织学形态多变，关于合适的名称未能达成一致意见，一些人喜欢用乳头旺炽型乳头状瘤病（或乳晕下导管乳头状瘤病）[110-113]，而另一些人使用乳头腺瘤[60,114,115]或乳头状腺瘤[8,116]。

乳头腺瘤可发生于青春期后的任何年龄，但发病高峰是围绝经期。临床表现为乳头溢液或乳头下质硬小结节。后者可能发红甚或表皮结痂，与Paget病外观相似。

大体表现

病理学家常收到全部或部分乳头和乳晕标本，根据病变大小而定，很少超过1～1.5cm。结节界限不清，质硬，但没有特殊的明显表现。

组织学表现

镜下特征多变，但主要由弥散的乳头状导管上皮增生组成，常与腺瘤样区域混合存在（图16.25）。上皮为双层，伴有分泌上皮不同程度的增生，主要为普通型（图16.26）。病变中可见到正常的导管和小叶结构。细胞性间质同时增生，周围可见内陷导管的假浸润性形态。这种形态与核深染可导致误诊为恶性。

鉴别诊断

乳头腺瘤一定要与少见的乳头汗管瘤样腺瘤鉴别[85]。这一病变与乳头腺瘤的导管内乳头状增生相比，表现为小管结构在泌乳管间浸润（图16.27）。如上所示，乳头腺瘤的假浸润可导致诊断为恶性病变。整个病变中上皮结构规则且缺乏导管原位癌的特征性表现支持良性，存在双层上皮也支持良性。谨慎取材很重要，因为尽管发生相关癌的危险性较低，但已有一些相关报道[113,117]。

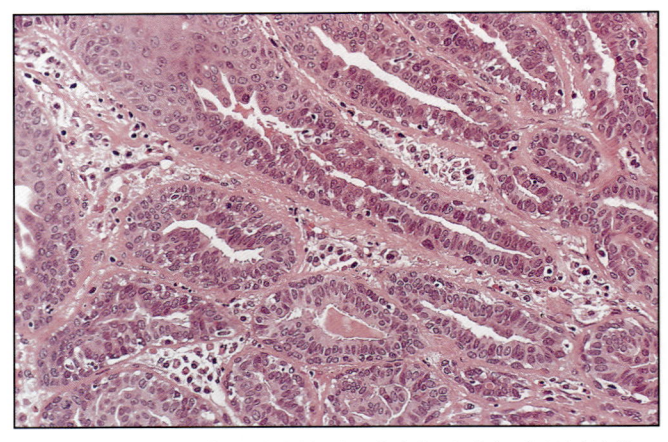

图16.26 乳头腺瘤。腺体被覆上皮和肌上皮细胞双层结构。常见上皮增生。

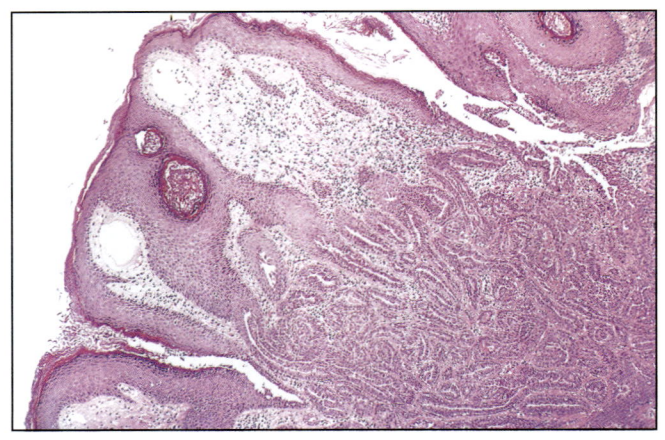

图16.25 乳头腺瘤。邻近表皮的乳头导管的腺性结构增生。

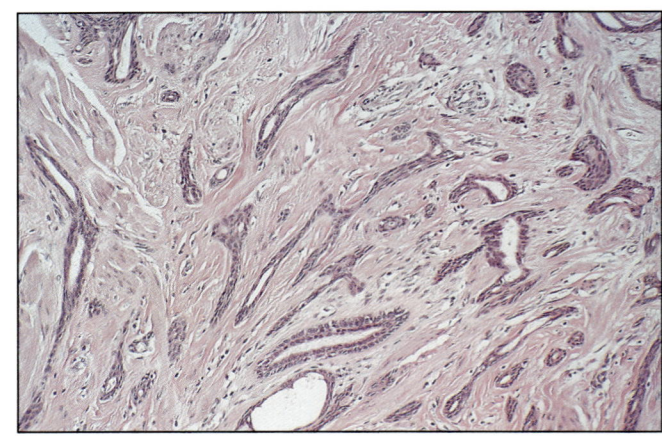

图16.27 乳头汗管瘤样腺瘤。明显的细胞性间质围绕浸润的细长或卵圆形腺体结构。

导管腺瘤　Ductal adenoma

这个名称是 Azzopardi 和 Salm 用来描述发生于乳腺大导管的具有硬化性腺瘤样或乳头状结构的实性良性病变[118]。随着越来越多的病例被描述，也越来越清楚其在形态学上与硬化性导管乳头状瘤、硬化性腺病和复合硬化性病变有很大重叠[60,119]，但病变发生在乳腺中心部位是多数病例的一个鉴别特征。多数病例被认为是导管乳头状瘤发生硬变所形成的[119]。

导管腺瘤不常见，可发生于青春期后的任何年龄，但多数发生于 45 岁以上妇女。尽管一些病变可能发生于外周，但多数表现为邻近乳头的可触及的实性肿块。

大体表现

大体上，多数导管腺瘤表现为界限清楚的灰褐或灰白结节，直径可达 3cm。在一些病例中，可见与导管腔或囊性结构明确相关。

组织学表现

根据肿物大小和纤维化的数量，镜下表现有所不同。可见单个或多个腺瘤样结节，由双层上皮结构组成：腔面的分泌性细胞和基底的肌上皮结构（图 16.28）。肌上皮细胞的免疫染色可识别这种结构[119,120]。一些病例中，上皮增生可形成乳头状形态。病变周围由致密纤维围绕，常含有断裂的弹力纤维组织，可能来源于原先的导管。

少部分导管腺瘤表现为中心放射状硬化。大汗腺改变常见于上皮成分中，这些上皮可以出现核异型性。

鉴别诊断

导管腺瘤是良性病变，需注意不要过诊为恶性，尤其是内陷导管具有明显上皮非典型性的病例。如上所述，此病变与硬化性腺病和复合硬化性病变的形态特征有许多重叠，在某些病例，要做出明确区分是不可能的[60]。

柱状细胞病变　Columnar cell lesions

临床特征

这种病变以前有多种名称，其命名尚需统一[121]。其他研究组以前所用的名称和术语包括盲管腺病、伴有明显顶浆突起和分泌的柱状改变（CAPSS）[122]、非典型囊性小叶[123]、伴有顶端突起的乳腺导管原位癌细胞在扩张小导管中的癌化[124]、高分泌性增生、乳腺导管上皮内平坦型肿瘤形成、单形性附壁导管原位癌、增生性开放性小叶、伴柱状改变的扩张小叶（ELUCA）。而我们对这组病变采用纯粹的描述性术语——柱状细胞病变。

柱状细胞病变的发生率明显增高，不仅是由于病理学家对此病变认识的提高，还因为乳腺影像学所见微钙化病变的粗针活检数量的增加。实际上，对柱状细胞病变最早的描述中，发现微钙化发生于几乎 3/4 的 CAPSS 病例[122]。

这些病变的临床意义还不清楚。尽管柱状细胞改变被认为是没有重要临床意义的良性病变，但是可以出现细胞非典型性（见下文）。尤其在粗针活检病例，这种情况需要关注，而在这些病例实施进一步的手术活检是明智的。这种病例与原位癌或浸润癌的相关性可达 25%~33%[125]。柱状细胞非典型性可能与导管内原位癌和浸润癌相关，后者常为小管癌[124]。病变的遗传相似性以及合并存在表明，在某些病例中柱状细胞非典型性可能是癌前病变[121,126]。

组织学表现

柱状细胞病变起源于终末导管小叶单元（TDLU），低倍镜下可见此病变的小叶中心性特点（图 16.29）。在高倍镜下，可见被覆这些 TDLU 的上皮细胞呈柱状，可轻度扩张和分泌，伴发钙化。柱状细胞厚度 1~2 层，垂直于基底膜排列，细胞特点较温和（图 16.30）。常可见顶端突起，表现为细胞腔面的"小泡"。细胞核一致，呈卵圆形。核分裂象罕见。

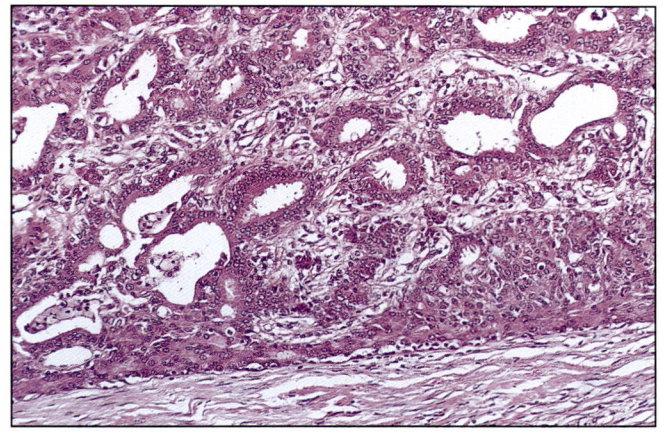

图 16.28　导管腺瘤。扩张的导管腔充满由被覆上皮的腺体结构、肌上皮细胞和间质组成的复杂结构。

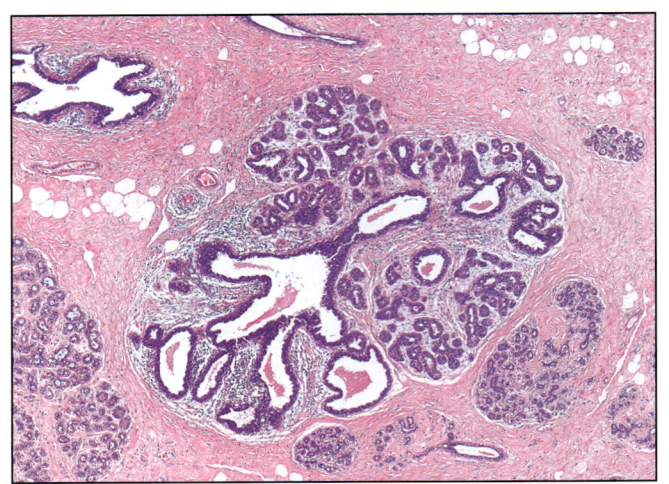

图16.29 柱状细胞改变导致终末导管扩张。

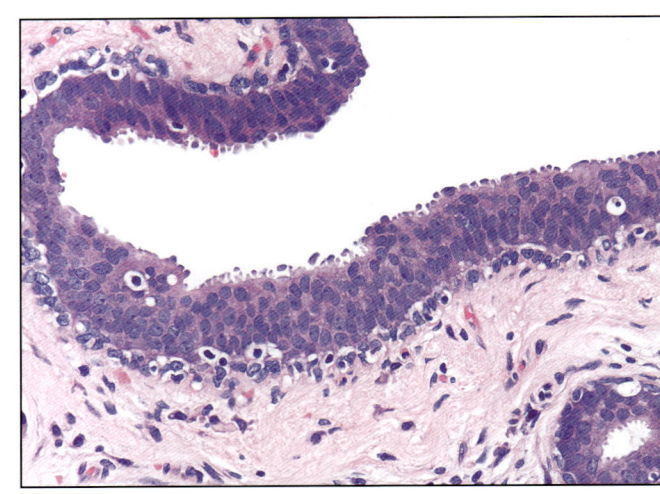

图16.31 伴有非典型性的柱状细胞增生，可归为平坦上皮非典型增生。细胞呈复层排列，表现出低度非典型性，具有圆形单一的细胞核。顶浆突起仍然存在。

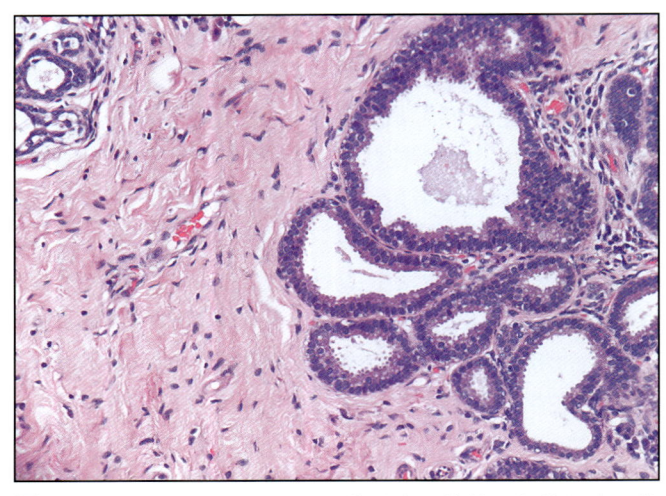

图16.30 柱状细胞改变。扩张的终末导管被覆柱状细胞，沿基底膜排列，有顶端胞浆突起和相对规则的卵圆性细胞核。

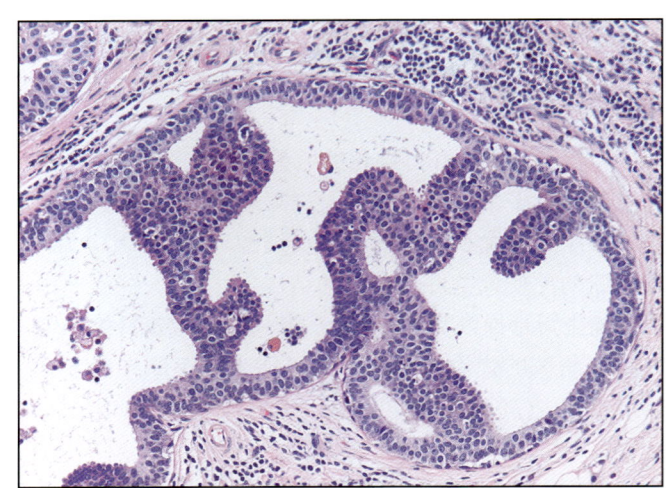

图16.32 平坦上皮非典型增生，局灶可见单一型细胞增生形成复杂的结构，应归入非典型导管增生。

柱状细胞增生由同样形态的细胞形成，超过2个正常细胞厚度，排列成簇状或形成突起。可见核拥挤和重叠，但细胞核特征与未增生型是相同的。顶端突起可能更明显，形成鞋钉样外观，管腔内有分泌现象，伴有较显著的沙粒体型微钙化。值得注意的是如果见到真正的微乳头、搭桥或筛状结构，应当诊断为非典型导管增生或导管癌，而不应诊断为柱状细胞增生。

柱状细胞改变和柱状细胞增生可显示细胞非典型性。这些病变也称为平坦上皮非典型性[127,128]。可以在柱状细胞改变或柱状细胞增生中发现。

在平坦上皮非典型性病例，低倍镜下TDLU常比一般的柱状细胞改变中所见颜色更深。细胞学特征不太令人担心的病例，小叶常呈轻至中度扩张。被覆于TDLU的细胞由一层或多层单一的立方细胞组成，类似于非典型导管增生/低级别导管内原位癌中的细胞。一些病例，柱状形态较明显，细胞仍然垂直于基底膜排列，但可以见到非典型细胞学特征，如染色质聚集、核仁明显或多形性（图16.31）。核分裂象非常罕见。

如果多形性明显或具有高度非典型性，就不应归为平坦上皮非典型增生，而应归为平坦型高级别导管原位癌（因为没有高度非典型导管增生这个名词）。同样，如果出现明显的结构非典型性，如实性搭桥或明确的微乳头结构，就应当考虑诊断为非典型导管增生/低级别导管癌（图16.32）。

鉴别诊断

柱状细胞病变起源于 TDLU，认识病变的局部解剖及柱状细胞形态可对大多数病例做出正确诊断。大汗腺化生可能与柱状细胞改变相似，而且也起源于 TDLU。在有疑问的病例可行雌激素受体评估；柱状细胞病变显著表达腺腔角蛋白（CK19）、雌激素受体和孕激素受体，而大汗腺化生细胞雌激素受体弱阳性或呈阴性。

增生性乳腺疾病/上皮增生
Proliferative breast disease / epithelial hyperplasia

临床特征

Page 和 Dupont 于 1985 年发表的回顾性研究中提出了上皮增生与癌有相关性的证据。这些作者研究了大量因良性乳腺疾病活检的妇女[129,130]。Page 此前还提出了上皮增生的预后分类[131]。美国病理界为此召开了一次会议。会议记录作为大家的统一意见发表[2,132]，概括指出良性疾病对继发乳腺癌有一定的临床危险性，而且对每一诊断类型的危险性给以适当的重视。

这些病变的危险性可概括如下[129,130,133-135]。约 70% 乳腺活检为良性的妇女，组织学并没有明显上皮增生。尽管可能出现其他病理形态，但与正常人群相比这组病人 15 年内继发乳腺癌的危险性并没有增加。25% 的良性活检表现为普通型上皮增生，其中 4% 在 15 年内发展为乳腺癌，危险性增加了 2 倍。非典型导管增生的妇女所占比例小，约占活检的 2%，其中 10% 在 15 年内继发乳腺癌，危险性增加了 5 倍。应该注意的是合并乳腺癌家族史的病人，非典型导管增生的危险性成倍增加。其危险程度与非典型小叶增生相似。继发肿瘤的危险性在同侧乳腺和对侧乳腺几率相等。

乳腺增生性疾病常与其他病变同时存在，例如纤维囊性变、乳头状瘤、硬化性病变。一般情况下它本身并无明显的临床特征。

大体表现

上皮增生通常是肉眼不可见的镜下异常。常与纤维囊性变或其他良性病变并发，受累乳腺在总体上显示出上述良性病变的特征。

组织学表现

普通型上皮增生（不伴有非典型性的增生性疾病）与非典型导管增生（伴有非典型性的增生性疾病）的组织学表现和鉴别诊断分别描述如下。

普通型上皮增生——不伴非典型性的增生性疾病
Usual-type epithelial hyperplasia — proliferative disease without atypia

组织学表现

超过管腔上皮和肌上皮细胞正常双层结构的任何细胞增生都称为上皮增生，但通常只有上皮层 ≥ 4 个细胞厚度（中度增生，见下文）才有临床意义。详细的组织学特征在下面鉴别诊断中描述（图 16.33 至 16.35）。进一步的分类要根据增生的程度和性质来决定。

导管上皮轻度增生（不会明显增加乳腺癌的危险性）用来指基底膜上方的增生细胞不超过 4 层。中度增生是指增生细胞超过 4 层，并可能形成管腔内搭桥（图 16.33）。在重度增生，导管腔扩张或被填满（图 16.34）。中度和重度普通型增生的区别相对主观。很明显，这是一组连续的病变。实际上，没有必要准确区分中度和重度增生这两个类型，因为一般合为一类来评价其危险性。

上皮增生可发生在终末导管、外周小导管或大导管，可以累及柱状细胞改变、乳头状瘤或其他良性病变区。病变部位以及与其他病变的相关性没有明确的额外临床意义。

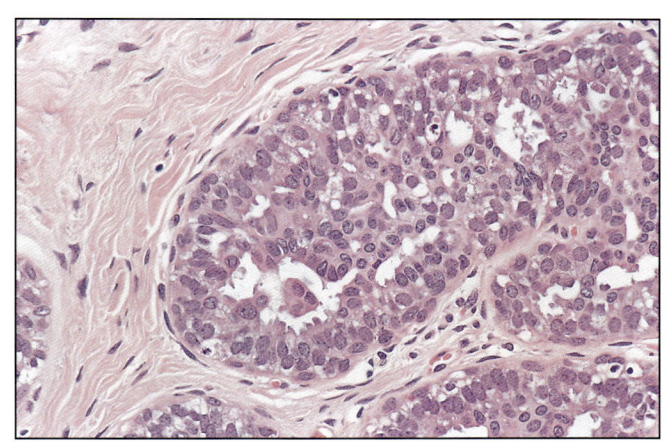

图16.33　普通型上皮增生。为轻度上皮增生。基底膜上的上皮细胞数目增加，肌上皮层存留。上皮细胞形成间桥横跨导管腔。残余腔隙形状、大小不规则，具有典型的裂隙样表现。

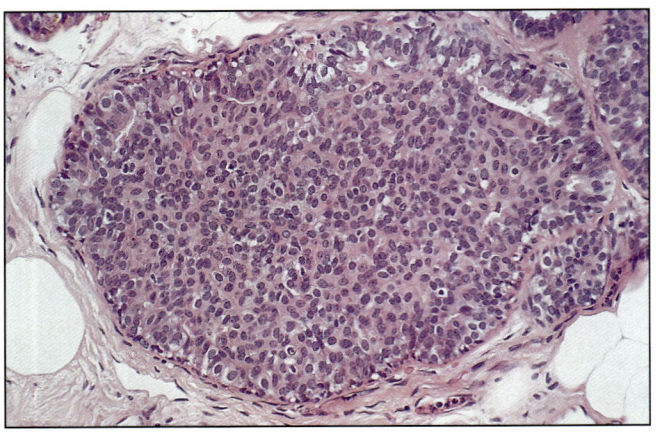

图16.34 普通型上皮增生。病变比图16.33中更活跃，导管腔基本消失。外周可见裂隙存留，可作为一个有用的诊断特征。细胞排列无极向，细胞界限不清。

鉴别诊断

普通型导管增生可根据低倍镜下结构和高倍镜下特征与非典型导管增生和原位癌区分。细胞种类混杂。上皮细胞占优势，但肌上皮细胞、基底细胞、中间上皮细胞和淋巴细胞也会出现（图16.35）。与ADH和DCIS中的管腔上皮细胞（CK8、18、19阳性）相比，基底/中间上皮细胞呈高分子量角蛋白（CK5/6、14）阳性[141,142]。上皮细胞通常较小，呈卵圆形，但大小和形态也有差别（图16.34和16.35）。作为一个增生病变，细胞排列杂乱、不规则（图16.34），呈漩涡状、片状，常形成微乳头、突起和搭桥，轮廓参差不齐。水流状特征可见于成片的细胞或细胞平行于乳头或搭桥排列时。新生或残留腺腔不规则，边界不清，常呈裂隙状（图16.35）。一个特别的诊断特征是裂隙状腔隙中保留了环形或部分环形结构（图16.35）。在特定的导管腔内，普通型上皮增生细胞排列不均匀，不同导管的密度也有变化。管腔内坏死、出血和周围间质改变可以出现，但很少见，且常局限于旺炽型病例。可发生微钙化，但对本病与非典型增生或导管原位癌的鉴别没有帮助。

非典型导管增生——伴有非典型性的增生性疾病
Atypical ductal hyperplasia—proliferative disease with atypia

组织学表现

Page概括的非典型导管增生（ADH）诊断标准被美国和皇家病理学院的共识会议[2,5,132]接受，作为界定具有乳腺癌危险性病变的公认标准。

病变是以筛状或微乳头状低级别/小细胞型导管原位癌为模型。具有DCIS的一些但并非全部特征的病变可归为ADH。要做出精确的诊断，需要观察低倍镜下（结构性）和高倍镜下（细胞学）特征（图16.36至16.38）。

Page采用的诊断DCIS和非典型导管增生的标准描述如下[135]：

1. 成群的形态一致的细胞。
2. 细胞间的腔隙均匀、光滑，或细胞均匀排列成微乳头。
3. 细胞核深染。

与导管原位癌的区分需要严格依据标准。Page及其同事[135,136]认为诊断低级别导管原位癌至少需要2个导管满足导管原位癌的全部特征。不满足这种特征者归

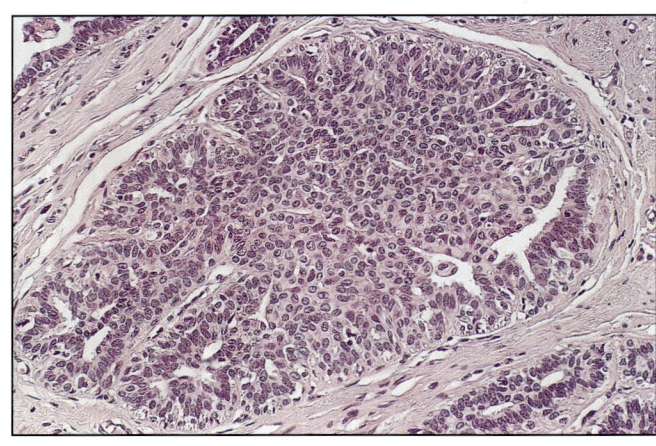

图16.35 普通型上皮增生。此病例显示了该病变所有的主要特征。虽然以上皮细胞增生为主，但也可见一些肌上皮细胞和淋巴细胞。

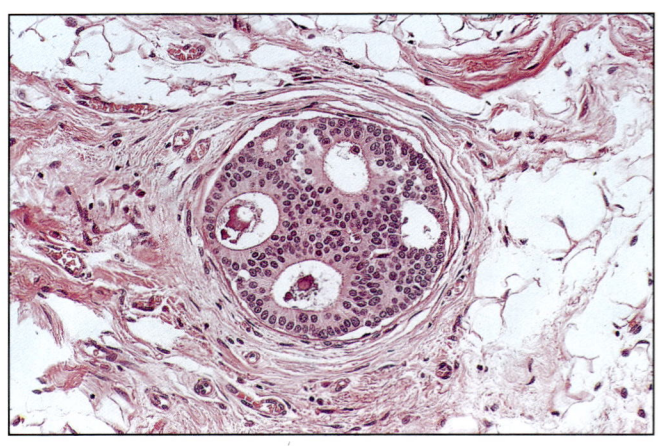

图16.36 非典型导管增生。形态单一的上皮细胞充满到导管腔，并形成特殊的穿凿状腺腔。外周肌上皮细胞缺失，围绕腺腔的细胞具有一些极性。

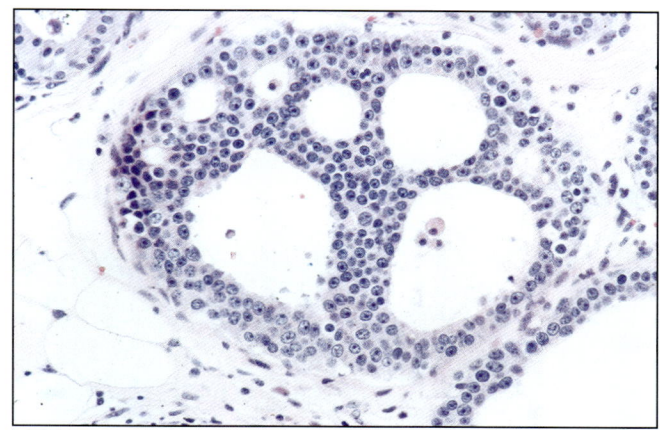

图16.37 非典型导管增生。扩张的导管内上皮细胞增生形成相对规则的圆孔。

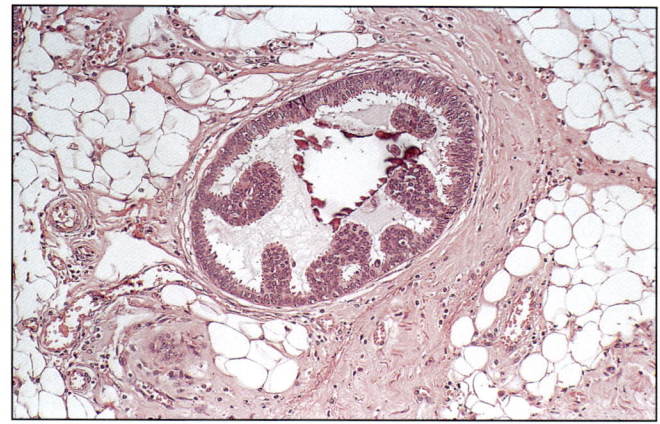

图16.38 非典型导管增生。形态一致的上皮细胞向腔内突起形成微乳头。

为非典型导管增生。该定义提供了一些区分这两种病变的客观依据。其他研究组也采用病变大小作为标准。Tavassoli及其同事[137]要求具有导管原位癌明确特征者，最大径至少扩展至2mm方可诊断导管原位癌，而较小的病变则归类为非典型导管增生。

我们认为要审慎采用这种诊断方法。我们的经验是这些病变（ADH）小（至少<5mm）而局限。非典型增生很轻微的病变，与乳腺癌危险性无关，在旺炽或中度上皮增生背景中可以被忽略。当增生病变较广泛（>1cm）并累及正常乳腺实质结构时，应当诊断为DCIS。

鉴别诊断

非典型导管增生是乳腺上皮增生性病变的交界区或灰区。采用规范化标准的某些研究，在一组专业病理医师中获得了满意的观察一致性[125]，但在另一些研究中，区分非典型增生和低级别原位癌的可重复性较差[138,139]。

区分非典型增生与普通型增生另一个有用的标准是非典型增生是由形态相对一致的克隆性、自主性细胞群形成[140]（图16.36），而普通型增生的细胞为多克隆性，大小和形态不一致（见图16.33至16.35）。除了形态规则外，非典型导管增生的结构排列也有序，而并非任意排列，均匀排列的细胞形成明显的筛孔或微乳头结构（见图16.36至16.38）。增生中见到的混杂细胞群消失，代之以单一的上皮细胞群（见图16.36至16.38）。

ADH（或低级别DCIS）的克隆性特点表现为增生上皮细胞中基底型角蛋白CK5/6和CK14的表达消失，而管腔角蛋白CK19一致阳性[141,142]。相反，普通型增生中可见管腔和基底型角蛋白混合表达。核分裂象、坏死、出血和钙化对于区分ADH、普通型增生、低级别DCIS通常没有意义。值得注意的是，基底和管腔型角蛋白免疫组化对于鉴别增生与高级别的克隆性病变（可能表达基底型上皮标志物）没有太大帮助，而低级别病变仅表达管腔型细胞角蛋白。

区分ADH与低级别DCIS可能很困难。与低级别DCIS一样，ADH通常呈雌激素受体一致强阳性，表达管腔型角蛋白，但HER2、p53和基底型角蛋白阴性。低级别DCIS与ADH的细胞遗传学特征也基本相似[140,141]。本质上讲，区分这两种病变要依据单个导管内增生的程度以及增生导管的数量。

我们认为要严格按照Page和其他专家的标准来进行界定。诊断DCIS需要满足上述全部诊断特征，而且病变必须累及至少两个导管腔。ADH缺乏其中某个或多个特征（见图16.36至16.38）。

如果在活检或粗针穿刺组织边缘诊断ADH，相邻组织可能有原位（或浸润）癌，因此应该施行再次切除[143]。据报道50%的类似病例在粗针活检后的切除标本中可见导管原位癌或浸润癌[143,144]。这种现象在检查较细的穿刺活检标本（如16G）时尤其明显；而用较粗的11G粗针活检时较少出现[145]。

一些专家发现了另一组非典型增生病变[88]，其缺乏特殊的结构形态，但可见到核浆比高、染色质深的多形性异常细胞。因为对这种病变还缺少长期随访研究，所以它与乳腺癌风险的相关性还没有明确的证据。其中一些病变，细胞呈大汗腺形态。能否归类为非典型增生尚未被一些专家接受[146]，尽管这种观点已有所流行[147,148]（也见于大汗腺DCIS，第927页）。目前我们将非典型导管增生的诊断局限于已证实有增加乳腺癌长期发病风险的病变，需要兼顾低级别导管原位癌的结构和细胞学特征。任何高级别细胞学非典型性都不应归入非典型导管增生中。

小叶肿瘤形成　Lobular neoplasia

临床特征

我们同意Haagensen[8,149]及其他人[146]的观点，认为这是一组发生于TDLU的特殊的上皮病变，形态范围从轻度非典型小叶增生（atypical lobular hyperplasia，ALH）到旺炽型小叶原位癌（lobular carcinoma in situ，LCIS）；有人也简单称为"小叶肿瘤形成"。将ALH和LCIS看作同一病变的人认为，这两种病变的细胞形态相同（图16.39至16.41），其区别主要在于TDLU受累的范围和程度。小叶肿瘤形成谱系内各病变的遗传学改变基本相似；与ALH相比，LCIS中未见到更大的遗传学和免疫组化异常。小叶原位癌这个术语某种程度上是个误称，目前并不将它看作是浸润癌必需的前驱病变。与LCIS相关的危险性评估认为这种病变更应该被看作是一种危险因素（或按危险因素来处理），而不是明确的癌。

两种形式的小叶肿瘤形成（ALH或LCIS）都是相对少见的病变，发生在约1%的活检标本。很少出现临床异常，切除组织的大体检查也很少发现异常。随着乳腺影像学筛查的应用，小叶肿瘤形成的发生率也随之升高，但小叶肿瘤形成常常是偶然发现，而不是乳腺影像学异常的特定原因[88]。但是，少数小叶肿瘤形成因为伴发的微钙化而被影像学发现。检出率很大程度上依赖于外科医师切除组织的大小和病理学家检查标本的仔细程度。切除的组织越多，检查的标本越大，检出率就越高。

ALH和LCIS继发癌的危险程度与ADH和DCIS相当，ALH的危险性增加4倍而LCIS增加10倍[130,133-135]。然而，LCIS的临床进展比DCIS更缓慢[151]。这些病变更常发现于围绝经期妇女，若年龄继续增长发病率将下降。与乳腺癌家族史也有协同作用；一级亲属（母亲、姐妹或女儿）有乳腺癌病史的ALH患者，其乳腺癌危险性将成倍增加，达到正常的9～10倍。ALH的Paget样扩散累及邻近导管（见下文）使乳腺癌危险性增加至7

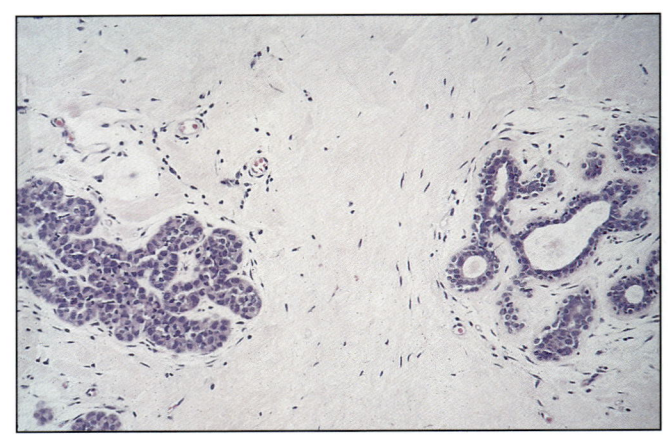

图16.39　小叶肿瘤形成。非典型小叶增生。两个相邻终末导管小叶单元(TDLU)。右侧的腺泡被覆正常双层细胞，左侧的细胞群与正常衬覆细胞相似，呈现轻度非典型小叶增生。

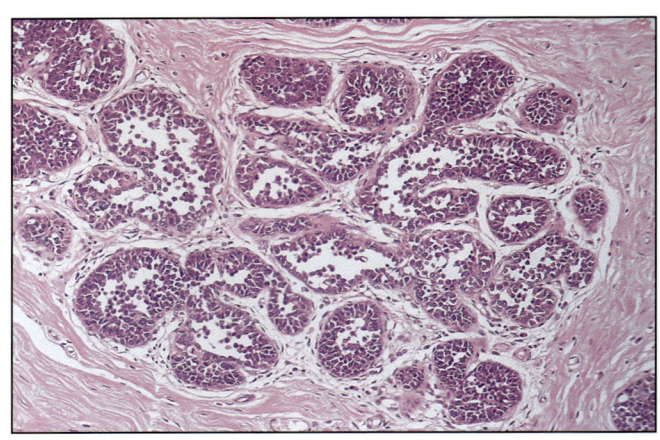

图16.40　小叶肿瘤形成。非典型小叶增生。终末导管小叶单元表现出一致的小细胞增生。一些腺泡被填满，但大多数仍有残留腔隙。

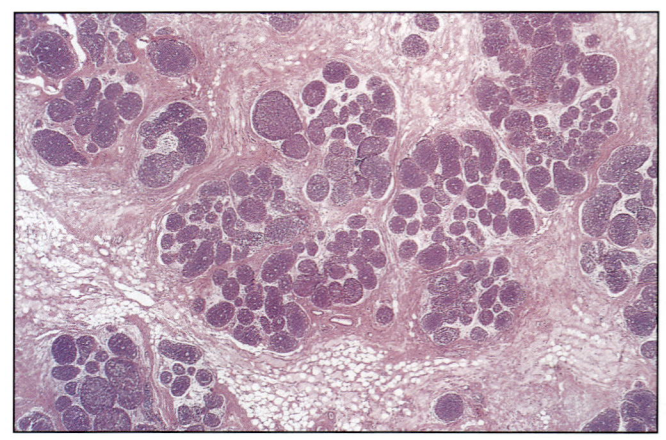

图16.41　小叶肿瘤形成。小叶原位癌(LCIS)。与正常腺泡细胞相似的小细胞完全充满腺腔，终末导管小叶单元明显扩张。

倍[134]。双侧乳腺都可发生癌，但近期分析显示同侧乳腺癌比对侧疾病的发生率高 3 倍[126]，专家称 ALH 的作用"在双侧乳腺界于局部癌前病变和一般危险性之间"[152]。在诊断 LCIS 后短时间内可发生肿瘤，但大多数在之后 15～20 年发生[149,153]。

小叶肿瘤形成实际上是个多灶性病变，许多病例在其他象限或对侧乳腺可以发现独立的病变（见综述[154]）。因此，约 1/3 的病人对侧乳腺出现病变，超过 50% 的病例在同侧乳腺发现其他多发病灶。

大体表现

除极少数旺炽型小叶原位癌形成明确的肿物病变外，ALH 和 LCIS 均不能通过肉眼发现。如上所述，小叶肿瘤形成常在因其他原因切除的组织中偶然发现。

组织学表现

小叶肿瘤形成的定义是 TDLU 腺泡内特征性细胞的一致性增生（图 16.39 至 16.41）。杂合性缺失研究显示小叶肿瘤形成是一种克隆性病变[155]。这种克隆性增生可以充满管腔并使 LCIS 的 TDLU 膨胀和扭曲。它可以在管腔上皮下以 Paget 样形式扩展，使邻近导管受累，或替代正常导管上皮层。

细胞有特征性外观，类似腺泡上皮细胞，细胞小，具有规则的圆形、浅染细胞核和一圈较窄的胞浆。核仁不明显或很小。细胞群的特点是小而一致，呈圆形。细胞松散而胞膜不明显。偶见细胞有胞浆内腔，这些是顶端微绒毛胞膜形成的充满黏液的小泡。通过上皮膜免疫反应或更传统的 AB-PAS 染色检测出来。

如上所述，小叶肿瘤形成可以典型的 Paget 样形态扩展至导管；单个或成群的肿瘤性小叶细胞在存留的管腔上皮层下扩展。更罕见情况下，受累更严重者，管腔上皮层可被取代，病变可充满导管腔，并造成与低级别实性导管原位癌鉴别困难（见下文）。

轻度小叶增生被看作轻度 ALH，尽管一些人把它分为"典型小叶增生"[88]。Page 发现此组病变继发癌的危险性没有明显增加，我们易于忽略轻度的小叶上皮增生[146]。大规模的 NSABP P1 临床试验证实，服用他莫昔芬作为预防性治疗的 LCIS 病人继发浸润癌的风险降低 56%，说明了组织学上诊断小叶肿瘤形成的重要性[156]。

一种多形性小叶原位肿瘤也见于报道[157]。此病变的结构形态与经典型相同，包括小叶中心性的低倍镜下表现。细胞疏松但是较大，多形性较明显，具有丰富的嗜酸性胞浆，细胞核较大，常有明显的核仁。分裂象较显著，免疫组化显示高增殖率和较高的 HER2 膜反应性，而小叶肿瘤形成典型的染色体改变（包括 16q 丢失、1q 获得）通常一致存在[158]。因为此型病变的形态更具侵袭性且免疫表型令人担忧，有人认为该类型与 DCIS 在临床上更相似，但对其行为尚不了解，需要进一步研究来明确此型小叶肿瘤形成的行为和处理方法。此外 LCIS 还有其他变异型，如透明细胞和印戒细胞型。大汗腺化生也可能与小叶原位癌并存[159]。

小叶肿瘤形成可能出现在良性病变中，如纤维腺瘤、放射状瘢痕和硬化性腺病。在上述某些情况下，采用 Page 制定的标准可能难以鉴别 ALH 和 LCIS，但可以根据受累程度进行主观判断。这些病变中 ALH 和 LCIS 的危险性与单独累及 TDLU 者相似[146]。

非典型小叶增生 (ALH) 与小叶原位癌 (LCIS) 的鉴别

ALH、ALH 伴导管受累以及 LCIS 的危险性很大程度上基于 Page 和 Dupont 的研究[133,150]。Page 报道采用以下标准诊断 LCIS 的符合率高[146]：

1. 小叶单位的所有细胞均为上述特征性的一致性细胞；
2. 必须充满（细胞之间没有散在的空隙）所有腺泡（TDLU）；
3. 小叶单位内至少有半数腺泡发生膨胀和扩张。

上述标准也适用于 ALH 的诊断，也就是当特征不能满足 LCIS 标准时。一些研究组认为"膨胀"的定义是腺泡宽度要 ≥ 8 个细胞。在 ALH，增生细胞可能与肌上皮细胞、白细胞及残留的腺泡上皮细胞混合存在。

鉴别诊断

LCIS 最常见的诊断困难是与导管原位癌累及小叶的鉴别，尤其当后者为低级别实性型时。所有类型的导管原位癌都可扩展侵犯 TDLU 的腺泡，以高级别病变更常见，不会引起诊断困难。诊断导管原位癌依靠 TDLU 导管中存在的特征性组织学表现。LCIS 和 ALH 常显示出小叶中心性，而当其扩散至邻近导管时通常呈 Paget 样形式。

小叶肿瘤形成通常粘附性差，伴 E-cadherin 弱表达或完全消失。这是一种钙依赖性细胞粘附分子，可由免疫组化检测出来。E-cadherin 已被认为是小叶肿瘤形成的特殊标记，实际上在一些交界性病变中 E-cadherin 免疫组化是非常有用的；E-cadherin 细胞膜着色减弱或消失可见于 95% 的小叶肿瘤形成病例。少数情况下，实性、规则的小细胞增生可以充满和破坏导管，并累及终末导管小叶单位（图 16.42）。在某些情况下，区分实性小细胞 DCIS 与 LCIS 几乎是不可能的。也有一些少见病变既有 DCIS 的特征同时又存在小叶中心性特征。当一些低级别实性上皮增生病例，需要鉴别 LCIS 与 DCIS 时，可见到交界形态的 E-cadherin 着色[160]。因此有一组交界性病变，常规 HE 染色和 E-cadherin 免疫染色呈混合形式，不能归入 LCIS 或 DCIS。我们认为把这两型病变（即中间型病变和具有两种病变特点的增生）报告为混合性 DCIS 和 LCIS 是明智的。这个办法可以提示临床医生患者可能具有与同侧乳腺癌相关的 DCIS 和与双侧乳腺癌相关的 LCIS。

如上所述，高级别导管原位癌侵犯小叶与小叶原位癌的鉴别没有太大困难[161]，因前者细胞学呈典型的恶性特征：高核浆比，细胞大，常见分裂象和坏死。当需要与多形性 LCIS 鉴别时，结构形态、病变主要累及导管以及 E-cadherin 胞膜阳性支持高级别 DCIS 诊断。

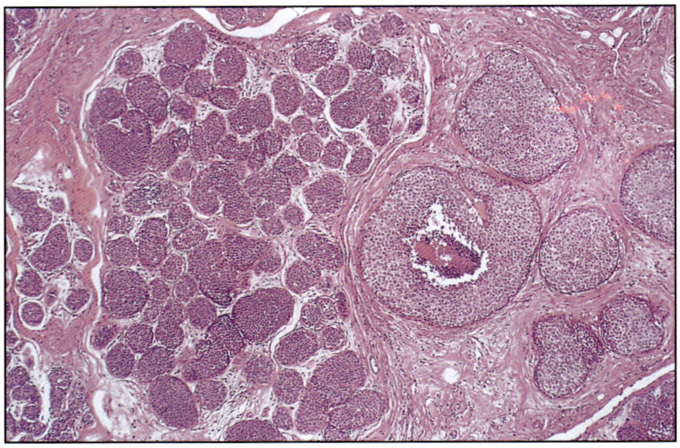

恶性肿瘤 Malignant tumors

癌 Carcinoma

乳腺癌是女性最常见的实性上皮恶性肿瘤，在一些国家乳腺癌与支气管癌发病率相当。可发生于任何年龄，但在 < 25 岁和 > 80 岁的女性罕见；发病高峰年龄在 45 ~ 60 岁。在大多数发达国家，尤其是英国和美国，发病率和死亡率都很高。发病率逐渐增加，尤其是在年轻组，而这并非完全由于"危险"人群的增加。女性乳腺癌比男性高出 200 倍以上。患病男性常常年龄较大[162]。

传统上将乳腺癌分为两个主要病理类型——原位癌和浸润癌。

原位癌 In situ carcinoma
导管原位癌 Ductal carcinoma in situ

临床特征

导管原位癌定义为乳腺实质结构内恶性上皮细胞增生，与浸润癌的区别在于显微镜下缺少基底膜外浸润。

传统上，根据 20 世纪 30 ~ 40 年代的研究结果，对 DCIS 施行乳腺切除术。引用最广的研究指出，如果只是实施活检术，3 年后进展为浸润癌的几率是 50%[163,164]。然而，值得注意的是那时只认识 DCIS 的大细胞/粉刺型。回顾最初诊断为良性且仅行活检术的病例[165,166]，结果显示复发率和进展为浸润癌的几率较低，约 20% ~ 30% 的病人在 15 ~ 20 年进展为浸润癌。近期研究发现，随着随访时间的延长进展为浸润癌的几率也增加，40% 的低级别 DCIS（以前大部分漏诊）之后 30 年发展为浸润癌[167]。

仅施行局部扩大切除（伴有或不伴有放射治疗）而不做乳腺切除术的 DCIS，其预后和最佳治疗方法仍不清楚，但相关的分级和生物学有差别。有关各型 DCIS 长期行为差别的进一步证据来自局灶 DCIS 的保守治疗试验，这些肿瘤常由乳腺影像学发现。对于接受保守外科治疗的 DCIS 病人，复发风险增加的因素包括年轻、边缘受累、病变级别高、坏死及生长方式等组织学特征[168-173]。原位癌通常在原活检部位或附近复

图 16.42 伴有实性导管受累的小叶肿瘤形成。旺炽型 LCIS 以实性非 Paget 样形式扩散至邻近导管。导管中的病变与小细胞实性 DCIS 不能鉴别，而且本例还可见到粉刺样中心坏死。

发，遗传学谱系与原肿瘤相似，表明是残留病变[174]。几个大规模研究显示乳腺放疗可以降低局部复发风险，但其中某些边缘情况难以定量[175,176]。继发性浸润癌也发生于同侧乳腺，邻近活检部位。这与三维重建研究[177]一起证实 DCIS 更像是一个局部性疾病[178]，不同于 LCIS[178]。

DCIS 的表现形式近年来有很大改变。传统上，DCIS 表现为一可触及的肿块或乳头溢液，常为血性。各种形式的 DCIS 都易形成微钙化，或者表现为管腔中央的粉刺型坏死，或者表现为筛状腺泡腔内分泌物浓缩，乳腺影像学分别表现为粗糙或细小的颗粒状密度影。随着乳腺影像学筛查的使用，通过微钙化检测 DCIS 已导致了病例数量的明显增加。在乳腺影像学检测广泛使用之前，DCIS 占乳腺癌的比例≤5%；而在乳腺影像学筛查中，其发生率增至 20%～25%[179-181]。

过去的临床实践中，粉刺型 DCIS 常表现为临床可触及的大包块，至少在某些病例[165,182]，而低级别/小细胞型 DCIS 呈局灶表现，从而导致误诊为良性乳腺疾病。这种有关生物学及累及范围的偏见，在实际筛查中没有什么帮助，因为高级别粉刺型 DCIS 可以早期出现粗糙钙化，常在检出时表现为局限的小病变。相反，低级别、非坏死型 DCIS 的钙化发生较晚，而且颗粒细小，不容易被乳腺影像学发现；50% 的病例其病变范围可能被低估[178]。低级别微乳头、筛状、非坏死型 DCIS 常表现为范围较广的病变，因此有可能不太适合保守治疗[178,183]。

在有症状的 DCIS 检查中，腋下淋巴结受累发生率约为 1%～2%，通常发生在病变广泛的病例，可能是漏取了浸润性小病灶。较小的 DCIS 通常由乳腺影像学筛查检出，这种病变能够全部取材进行组织学检查，根据现有资料和知识，尚未发现腋窝淋巴结受累的报道。因此，在前哨淋巴结活检技术广泛应用之前，局灶性 DCIS 不进行腋窝切除术[184]。然而，经粗针活检标本诊断的单纯性高级别 DCIS，若伴有广泛的放射学钙化（>40个点），约50%的病例存在浸润性病灶[185]，这些病例适合腋窝淋巴结切除或前哨淋巴结活检。

大体特征

表现为肿块的病变常显示边界不清的质硬的纤维组织，但通常见不到许多浸润癌中见到的边界清楚的实性肿物。伴有粉刺样坏死的 DCIS，尤其出现管腔扩张者，切面表现为肉眼可见的质软的奶酪样坏死物质。

乳腺影像学检出的病变通常肉眼不可见。需要使用标本影像学帮助选择适合组织学检查的部位，而且取材范围通常要比浸润癌更广泛[5]。

导管原位癌（DCIS）的分类

组织学上，DCIS 可分为不同的结构形态。辨认这些不同形态有助于 DCIS 的诊断，且 DCIS 的结构通常与疾病范围有关[183]。然而，在某个具体病变中常出现不止一种结构形态，使得分类难以重复。

有确凿的证据表明细胞学高级别的 DCIS 更易复发，且更易发展为浸润癌[169,170,172,183]。在 20 世纪 90 年代中期，对 DCIS 分类的重视逐渐增加；提出了几种分类系统。最重要的分类系统或者是根据分级，如英国[5]、美国、欧洲[6] 和 WHO[1] 推荐分类；或者是根据分级和结构/分化[186]；或者是对分级和坏死同时评估[169,170]。尚没有全球公认的最佳分类系统[187]，而且与可重复性有关的问题仍然存在[188]。

DCIS 分级的有效性通过生物学标记的研究得以进一步确认。高级别 DCIS 通常 HER2 和 P53 阳性，而雌激素受体、孕激素受体和 bcl-2 常为阴性，增殖率较高；而低级别 DCIS 的 HER2 和 P53 通常阴性，而雌激素受体、孕激素受体和 bcl-2 阳性，增殖率低[189-192]。与这些标志物在各级浸润癌中的表达结果相似。

不同级别的 DCIS 也存在遗传学差异[193]，表明它们进展为浸润癌的通路确实不一样。在浸润癌，原位成分和浸润成分的分级一致[194]。实际上，细胞核分级在 DCIS 与浸润性肿瘤之间或者在复发癌与转移癌之间倾向一致[195,196]。

大多数 DCIS 分级系统主要依据核分级，且采用三个级别；多数分级系统存在交叉。Van Nuys 系统结合核分级和坏死情况分类[169]。高级别是由核分级来确定。其余又分为伴有坏死的非高级别和不伴坏死的非高级别病变。欧洲病理学家工作组[186] 提出的分类办法兼顾核分级和细胞极性/分化。英国国家健康服务乳腺筛查组和 WHO[1] 推荐单独使用核分级[5]。我们采纳了这种方法，现介绍如下。

高核级导管原位癌
High nuclear grade DCIS

此病变由核浆比例高的多形性大细胞组成。染色质较粗糙，且常见大核仁。核分裂象多见，可出现异型核分裂。坏死常见。常表现为充满实性肿瘤细胞的导管中央坏死，以前称为粉刺型 DCIS（图 16.43）。坏死可能出现退行性钙化，乳腺影像学上钙化表现为分支状或线状形态。常可见导管周围纤维化和炎症细胞围绕血管聚集。除了伴有中心粉刺样坏死的实性 DCIS 外，高级别 DCIS 也可以出现筛状或微乳头状结构，偶尔也表现为不伴坏死的实性型（图 16.44）。

低核级导管原位癌
Low nuclear grade DCIS

此病变是由核较小的均匀分布的细胞组成。即使存在核仁，也不清楚。筛状（图 16.45）和微乳头状（图 16.46）结构比实性结构更常见。肿瘤细胞形成规则的穿凿性腔隙或球状突起，细胞围绕这些结构有序排列。核分裂象和坏死不常见。钙化的形成机制与高级别 DCIS 不同。钙化见于腺腔分泌物中，边界清楚且呈层状形态。

乳腺影像学上，呈典型的细颗粒状钙化聚集灶。

中等核级导管原位癌
Intermediate nuclear grade DCIS

中等核级 DCIS 的细胞核多形性低于高级别病变，但缺乏低级别 DCIS 的一致性。可以见到核仁，但通常不大。可以出现坏死，但不广泛。有一定的细胞极性。结构形态可呈实性、筛状或微乳头状。

导管原位癌的少见变异型
Rare variants of DCIS

有几种相对少见的变异型 DCIS，可单独出现或与较常见的亚型并存。

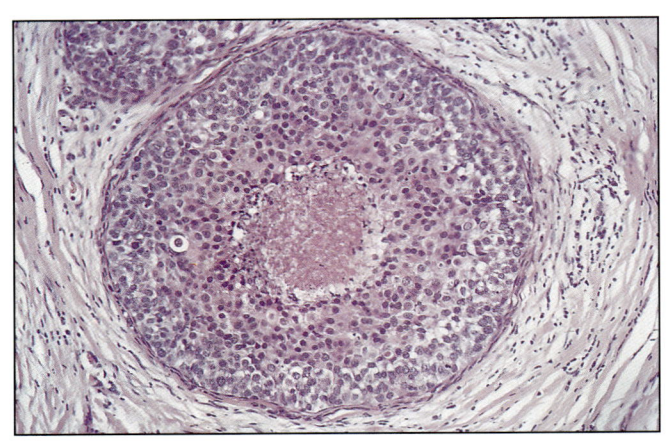

图 16.43 粉刺型 DCIS。肿瘤细胞表现出高级别恶性肿瘤的所有细胞学特征，包括核大、多形性和较多分裂象。这一亚型因导管腔中心的肿瘤细胞坏死而得名。

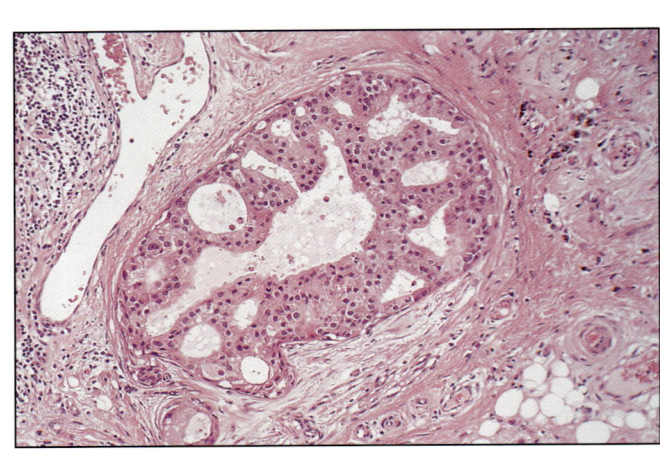

图 16.45 低级别筛状 DCIS。单一的细胞群形成明显的穿凿性腔隙。细胞界限清楚，分布均匀。

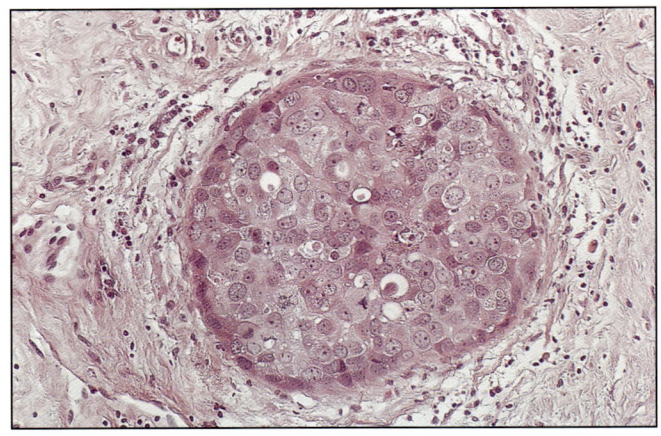

图 16.44 大细胞实性 DCIS。肿瘤细胞与粉刺型 DCIS 相同（图 16.43），但没有中心粉刺型坏死。

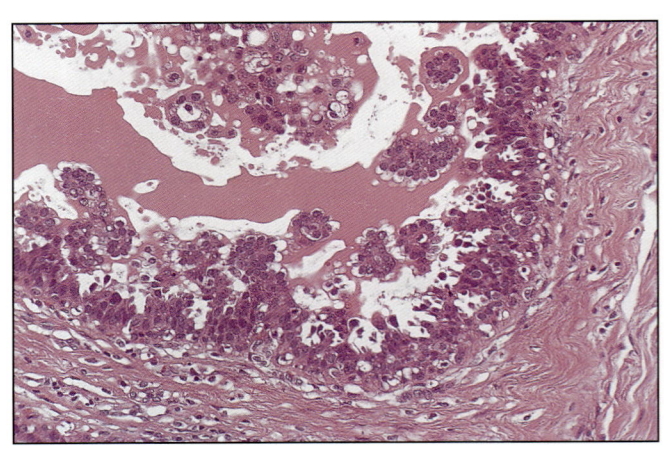

图 16.46 低级别微乳头状 DCIS。肿瘤细胞小而规则，排列成微乳头状。

小细胞实性导管原位癌
Small cell solid DCIS

这一病变中，导管腔充满了一致的细胞群，与低级别 DCIS 中见到的细胞相似，但缺乏有序的结构。如果这种病变累及终末导管小叶，可能与小叶原位癌无法区分（见第 922 页）。

大汗腺导管原位癌　　Apocrine DCIS

伴有明显核多形性和明显坏死的恶性大汗腺病变，容易诊断为高级别大汗腺 DCIS。对异型性不明显的大汗腺病变的分类要依据核形态和病变范围[147]；或者根据核形态、坏死、结构和病变范围[148,197]。实际上，诊断低级别大汗腺 DCIS 要谨慎；只有病变至少累及几个导管并有结构异常时我们才做此诊断，像在非大汗腺低级别 DCIS 中所见一样，常形成穿凿状、筛状腔隙，偶见微乳头状结构。病灶微小或细胞学异型性不明显的大汗腺增生，应小心诊断，可归类为大汗腺非典型增生。

神经内分泌导管原位癌
Neuroendocrine DCIS

这种伴有神经内分泌特征的 DCIS 变异型[198]通常见于 60 岁以上的妇女。因缺乏微钙化，这类病变常有临床症状，表现为肿块或乳头溢液。导管充满多角形小细胞或梭形细胞，至少局部可以经常见到纤维血管轴，常与 DCIS 实性区域混合存在。可见黏液。神经内分泌分化可由免疫组织化学证实，神经内分泌型 DCIS 常一致表达高水平的雌激素受体，有助于鉴别诊断，因为病变局部可能与普通型上皮增生相似。

印戒细胞导管原位癌　　Signet ring cell DCIS

伴有印戒细胞成分的混合型 DCIS 容易诊断；虽然据报道存在单一形态的印戒细胞型 DCIS，但非常罕见[199]，其临床意义尚不清楚。

囊性高分泌导管原位癌
Cystic hypersecretory DCIS

这一罕见类型的 DCIS[200,201]比较特殊，因其形成充满黏液物质的扩张性大囊腔。一些腔隙含有类似甲状腺类胶质的嗜酸性物质。被覆上皮可能大幅度萎缩，使得诊断性肿瘤细胞难以辨认。如果存在，这些细胞常排列成矮乳头状结构，与典型的微乳头型 DCIS 相似。细胞学显示胞浆丰富和分泌性改变。与囊性高分泌增生难以鉴别。

预后因素

传统上，DCIS 经乳腺切除治疗，治愈率为 98%~99%。现在对范围不超过 3~4cm 的 DCIS 采取较保守的外科手术，切除部分乳腺仍能保证美容效果。

最初的临床研究表明，保乳手术后的复发率比乳腺切除术高，因此，有关复发预测因素的研究引起了人们的兴趣。如上所述，高级别 DCIS 局部切除后更易复发[169,170,172]。一些研究表明较广泛的 DCIS 更易复发[170]。生长方式[173]和存在坏死[169,171]被认为有临床意义。

然而，复发最重要的预后因素是切除的完整性。切除的边缘越大，复发的危险越小[170]。DCIS 通常为单发，间隔 10mm 以上的跳跃性病变不常见[202]。这表明如果切缘带有足够的正常组织，大多数病例应该能够根除。

有关 DCIS 病灶周围理想的无瘤组织切除宽度还未达成一致。一些中心要求未受累组织的宽度为 20mm，另一些中心只要求 1~2mm。在 Nottingham，切缘距离 DCIS 为 10mm 者，在 58 个月的中位随访期后局部复发率为 6%[203]，其他专家也建议同样宽的边缘[204]。其他切缘较窄的病例，通过放疗可得到大致相同的局部复发率[175]。对边缘详细的评价需要较多的组织切片，而以上结果表明这是值得的。激素治疗在 DCIS 治疗中的作用还不清楚[205,206]。

鉴别诊断

小细胞 DCIS 和非典型导管增生的鉴别已在前面讨论过，DCIS 的诊断需要至少 2 个导管满足 DCIS 的所有形态特点（典型的筛状或微乳头状形态）。

DCIS 的扩展可以累及 TDLU，即所谓的"小叶癌化"[161]。这些细胞的细胞学特征与邻近导管中的细胞相似，区分高级别 DCIS 和小叶原位癌没有困难。

高级别 DCIS 常引起淋巴细胞反应和导管周围纤维化。相关特征可以解释 DCIS 形成肿块的原因，有时也能误导有经验的放射学家，误以为 DCIS 区域存在浸润癌。这种纤维化反应也会引起分类问题，导管周围结构变形与浸润性乳腺癌相似，尤其是存在小叶癌化时（图 16.47）。这也是不同的报道中微浸润癌和早期癌发生率不同的原因之一。

多数学者需要得到浸润的确切证据才诊断微浸润，即脂肪或间质中存在明确的 <1mm 的浸润灶。最好是在 DCIS 中通常存在的小叶中心性和器官样形态范围之外，伴有或不伴小叶癌化[146]。浸润灶超过 1mm 者应归为普

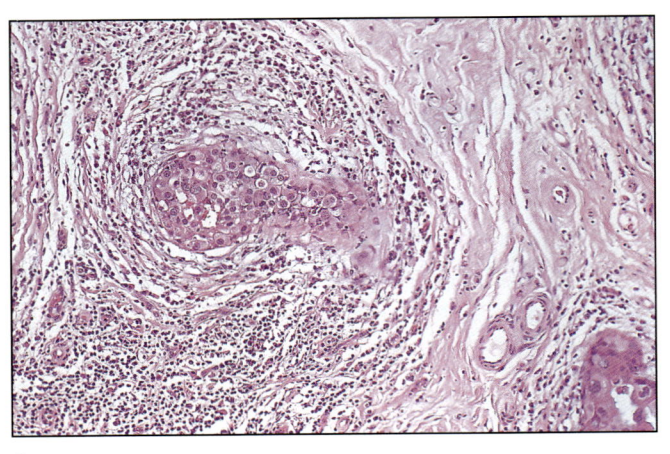
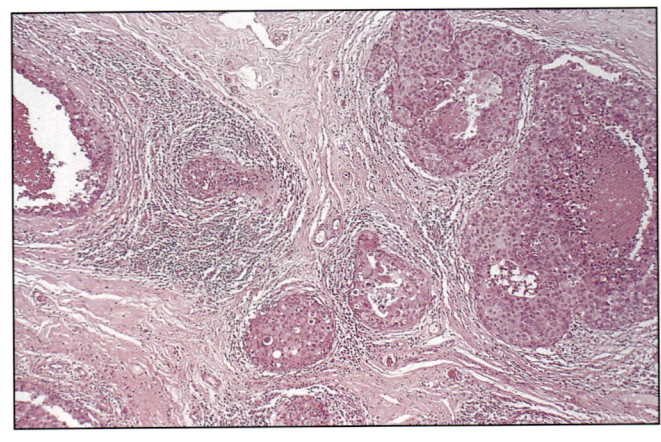

图16.47 大细胞粉刺型DCIS的假浸润。这是一种难以解释的现象。本例中高倍镜下的不规则肿瘤灶（A）可能代表浸润。而病灶周围由淋巴细胞和特化的小叶间质包绕（A，B）。小叶外间质未见肿瘤（B）。

通的浸润癌。

乳头Paget病
Paget's disease of the nipple

临床特征

乳头Paget病是高级别DCIS的一种表现，当累及乳晕下导管时，可沿着导管浸润表皮。这种观点的证据是，充分检查可以发现至少一个乳晕下导管具有高级别DCIS。早期报道中，35%~50%的患者伴发浸润癌[8]。Paget病发生于大约2%的乳腺癌患者，临床上表现为乳头红斑状或湿疹样皮疹[8]。这些临床特征可能与湿疹或其他慢性皮炎混淆。因此，任何有这种表现的乳头病变，尤其是不能迅速愈合时，应该怀疑Paget病并活检。

大体特征

乳头区皮肤表现为湿润的红斑状、湿疹样皮疹，可以出现结痂或角质化。

组织学特征

表皮包括单个或小团的多形性DCIS大细胞浸润，通常具有丰富而透明的胞浆，可伴有空泡形成（图16.48）。成群的细胞偶可形成腺泡结构。常伴随小的成

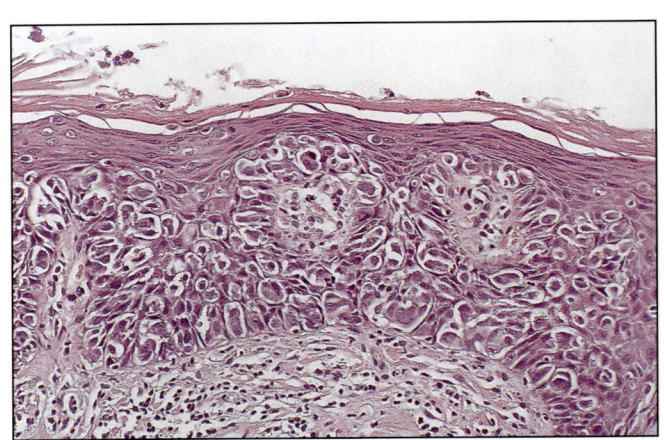

图16.48 乳头Paget病。多形性大细胞浸润乳头表皮，与粉刺型DCIS中的大细胞相同。

熟淋巴细胞浸润并累及表皮层；急性炎细胞也可出现。表皮可增生或表现为角化不良。

肿瘤细胞可表现为抗淀粉酶的PAS阳性染色，但免疫组织化学是更有价值的确诊手段[207]（见下文）。

鉴别诊断

在感染严重的乳头可能很难确定肿瘤细胞浸润。这些细胞也与黑色素细胞难以鉴别，尤其是胞浆空泡化或透明不明显时，它们还可能与其他慢性皮炎中见到的非典型角化细胞相似。在疑难病例中采用黏蛋白特殊染色并不可靠。而采用正常角化细胞不表达的低分子量角蛋白CK8、18、19（即CAM5.2）以及见于90%以上乳腺Paget病的HER2免疫组化染色，在疑难病例中意义重大[207]。

原位乳头状癌和囊内乳头状癌
Papillary carcinoma in situ and encysted papillary carcinoma

临床特征

原位乳头状癌的定义为发生在乳头状瘤基础上的原位恶性上皮病变。这些病变界限清楚；且形成"囊内"结构，周围有一界限清楚的胶原纤维带。病变通常发生于年龄较大的妇女，表现为包块或乳腺影像学上界限不清的肿块。如果 DCIS 没有超出纤维包膜且邻近乳腺组织没有 DCIS，保守治疗的预后非常好[208]。

大体特征

原位乳头状癌常为界限清楚的肿瘤性包块。常可见到含棕色或血性液体的囊性区域。大小不等，但常在 1～3cm 之间。

组织学特征

肿瘤呈界限非常清楚的圆形包块，周围常包绕厚薄不一的胶原性纤维囊。通过纤维血管轴心能发现乳头状结构背景。纤维血管轴心至少部分被覆正常的肌上皮和腔上皮双层结构或增生的上皮组织。在一些病例，纤维血管轴心周围是更加实性的增生上皮[209]。

典型原位乳头状癌的肿瘤细胞较高或呈柱状，垂直于乳头轴排列（图16.49）。排列紧密，有沿基底排列的卵圆形、浅染或深染细胞核。一些病例出现核极性消失和核多形性，这些细胞取代了正常的双层上皮，也就是说至少局部丢失了肌上皮层。

其他形式的 DCIS，尤其是微乳头状和筛状 DCIS，可以单独或混合出现。伴有典型筛状或实性 DCIS 的乳头状瘤也被归为原位乳头状癌。因此，由 Kraus 和 Neubecker[210] 提出的乳头状癌定义中包含微乳头状和筛状 DCIS。

在许多病例，尤其肿瘤较大的病例，会发生纤维血管轴广泛透明变性或纤维化。检查邻近乳腺组织和导管内有无扩散很重要，如果 DCIS 出现在邻近乳腺组织中，保守治疗后局部复发很常见。

鉴别诊断

相关的纤维组织成分，尤其是围绕乳腺组织的区域，可导致原位癌上皮结构内陷，表现为尖角状，与浸润癌相似。对于判定病变是否为浸润癌，我们会忽略这些包膜内病灶，只报告明确扩散至周围正常乳腺组织的浸润性病变。

浸润癌 Invasive carcinoma

临床特征

在没有乳腺影像学筛查时，绝大多数浸润癌是因为出现可触及的肿块被检测出来。发生于男性的病例总是很罕见。肿瘤1厘米到几厘米，质硬，边缘清楚或不清。被覆皮肤可出现凹陷，在进展性病例中，可见肿瘤固定于深筋膜。肿块可见于乳腺任何部位，但外上象限最常见。约 2% 的患者同时出现双侧浸润性癌[211]。乳头溢液是一种不常见的体征，乳腺疼痛也是

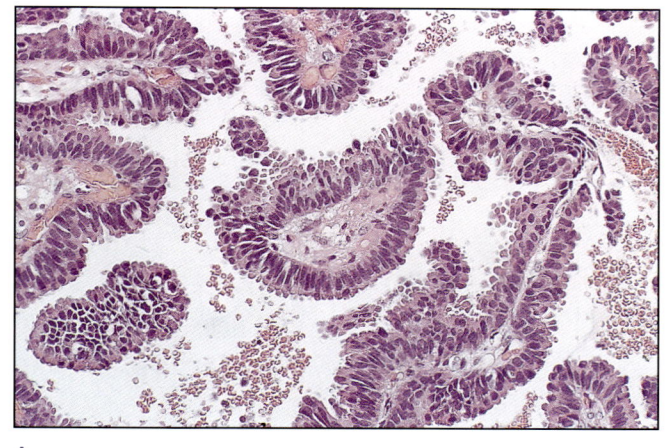

A

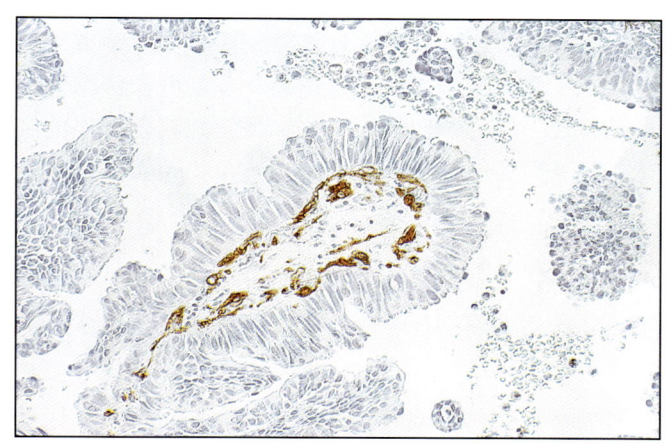

B

图16.49 原位乳头状癌。肿瘤细胞通常较高，柱状，垂直于基底膜排列（A）。平滑肌肌动蛋白免疫染色显示肌上皮细胞缺失（B）。

恶性肿瘤的罕见表现。乳腺影像学筛查的引入改变了乳腺癌的表现形式，目前许多病例是因不可触及的乳腺影像学异常而被检出。

尽管临床医生倾向于认为乳腺浸润癌是单一疾病，病理学家已分出越来越多的病理亚型[1,212-214]。组织学类型的重要性及其对预后的影响在下面讨论。每种主要类别也在随后描述。浸润癌的分级则在第942页单独讨论。

目前的分类方法是描述性的，相对有主观性，依赖于有经验的组织病理学家的评价。而且，肿瘤的组织学表现不能充分揭示潜在的复杂的基因改变和包含在其形成和进展中的生物学事件。因此，需要一种包括癌发生关键分子事件的新分类，从而为不同形态学表型和行为提供分子学解释。乳腺癌的细胞和分子异质性，以及包括细胞生长、分化、增生、浸润和转移调控的大量分子事件，都强调了统一研究多发性分子改变的重要性。近期的高通量基因研究已提供了挑战乳腺癌分子复杂性的机会，而且提供了根据基因表达模式进行生物学和临床分类的依据[215-219]。这些新的分子分类已分辨出许多基因，其中一些被作为乳腺癌亚型的代表基因。这些研究所用的肿瘤数量相对较少，需要扩大规模来证实，在进入临床使用前要与传统的分类系统进行比较。应用高通量组织芯片（TMA）筛查技术可以解决一些问题。这些研究已检查了乳腺癌相关蛋白（基因产物）的表达，从而辨认出与基因研究结果很相似的乳腺癌类型。值得注意的是要识别腺腔型与基底型分化，以及激素受体和HER-2表达。有基底上皮分化或HER-2表达的病例，其预后比腺腔分化和激素受体表达病例差[215,216]。近期提出了基底细胞型乳腺癌的概念，将在下文叙述。

除了识别乳腺癌新类型外，其他近期研究也对一些亚型的相关性提出挑战。乳腺髓样癌（medullary breast cancer）的诊断可重复性和预后相关性一直存在问题。一些研究认为，有髓样癌特征的肿瘤经常发生于*BRCA1*基因突变携带者[220]，值得放松髓样癌的定义，采用类髓样癌（medullary-like carcinoma）来区分这些肿瘤[5]。

非特殊型浸润癌（导管NST）
Invasive carcinoma of no special type (ductal NST)

这一组病例包含不符合其他任何类型诊断标准的乳腺癌，因此不能被看作是乳腺癌的一种具体类型。它是最常见的浸润癌"类型"，占所有浸润癌的47%～75%[212,213,221-223]。这也是男性最常见的类型[224]。以往使用过多种术语描述这些肿瘤，包括导管癌、非特指型癌（NOS）和非特殊型浸润癌（NST）。导管癌这一术语强调肿瘤来自导管而不是小叶上皮。尽管这种观点已不再严格固守，导管癌一词还在普遍使用，而且被WHO保留[1]。因此，现在我们选择的名称是非特殊型导管癌（ductal NST）。

大体表现

因为非特殊型导管癌是排除性诊断，没有特殊的形态学特征，可以见到多种表现。肿瘤大小差别很大，从0.5cm到≥10cm。大多数质硬，因此以前称为"硬"癌，切面有"砂砾"感。通常具有不规则的毛刺状轮廓，界限中等或不清。

组织学表现

组织学表现差异很大，部分取决于上皮和间质成分的相互关系，没有可用于分类的特征。癌细胞可以排列成合体片状、条索状或弥漫浸润（图16.50）。核可以出现高度多形性或者比较规则，腺体结构可以广泛或者缺失。多数病例可见灶状DCIS，一些专家提出伴有广泛原位成分者是一种亚型；这将在第946页讨论。偶尔，可见到鳞状化生区。约10%的病例显示神经内分泌分化的免疫组织化学证据，但没有临床或预

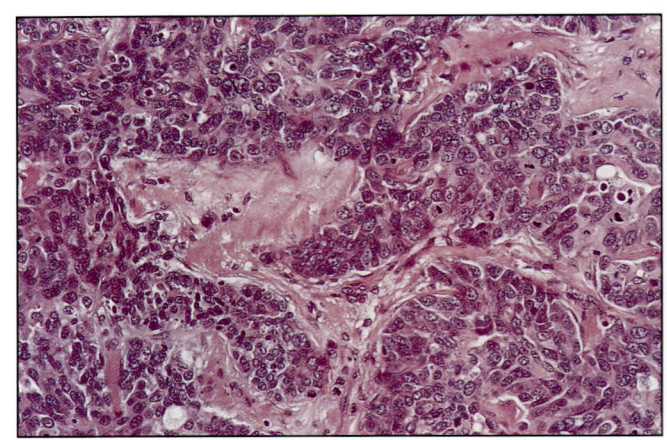

图16.50 非特殊型浸润癌。紧密排列的癌细胞呈片状和条索状侵入邻近的纤维组织。

后相关性[225]。要诊断非特殊型导管癌，要仔细检查几张有代表性的切片，必须有90%的区域由那种类型组成。如果非特殊型导管癌形态占肿瘤的50%～90%，而其余的是已知的特殊类型，那么就要归入下面介绍的混合类型之一[1,5]。有趣的是要注意雌激素受体阴性的非特殊型导管癌，通常表现为伴有明显淋巴间质和推挤性边缘的高级别病变[226]。

浸润性小叶癌
Infiltrating lobular carcinoma

经典型浸润性小叶癌由Foote和Stewart首先描述[227]。这种名称的使用是因为在形态特殊的弥漫单排浸润癌中，超过60%的病例伴有小叶原位癌[228]。尚未证实这些癌是否全部来源于小叶细胞。经典型的诊断标准已得到充分肯定[229,230]，一些变异型也被逐步确认[1]，被称为实性小叶癌[231]、腺泡型小叶癌[232]、小管小叶癌[233]和多形性小叶癌[234,235]。报道的浸润性小叶癌的发生率变化很大，从2%到15%不等[212,213,223,231]，这可能反映了诊断标准的应用有差别，而不是发生率真有不同。

浸润性小叶癌和小叶肿瘤形成（小叶原位癌和小叶非典型增生）都与E-cadherin蛋白表达的高频率缺失有关[83,236]。目前有关E-cadherin蛋白的缺失是否应该被视为小叶病变的特征表现仍有争议。有大量证据支持其作为辅助特征使用，有助于不明确病变的分类，但应该记住在其他形式的浸润癌中也可出现缺失[237]。

大体表现

通常有一种错误观念，由于肿瘤细胞浸润较弥散，会让人以为小叶癌也经常表现为边界不清的触摸不到的肿块。据我们的经验，大多数小叶癌形成与非特殊型导管癌相同的质硬包块，只有罕见病例表现为边界不清的硬化区。只有后者才会造成临床上通过触诊难以检出，或影像学检查不出异常。我们发现浸润性小叶癌和非特殊型导管癌的影像学特征无明显差异[238]。

组织学表现

有以下几种组织学亚型：

a **经典型** 经典型约占浸润性小叶癌的40%[213,230]。由小圆形或卵圆形细胞组成，胞浆少；细胞核通常偏位，形态一致，不常见分裂象。尽管在所有类型的乳腺癌均可见胞浆内腔，但在浸润性小叶癌更常见且更明显[239]。高碘酸-Schiff（PAS）/阿辛蓝组织化学染色或上皮膜抗原免疫染色中它们更易于观察[239]。肿瘤细胞弥漫浸润，在胶原纤维束之间形成特征性的单行排列（图16.51A）。如果残存正常的导管结构，这些单行的肿瘤细胞呈同心圆状浸润，形成"靶样"形态（图16.51B）。

b **腺泡型** 这种少见类型见于4%～5%的小叶癌[213,230]。细胞的组织学特征与经典型相同，但是由20个或更多的细胞积聚成圆形灶（图16.52）。

c **实性型** 约10%的小叶癌是这种类型[213,230]。肿瘤由典型的小叶细胞组成，但呈片状弥漫浸润，而不是呈单行条索，其间几乎没有间质（图16.53）。

d **管状小叶型** 这是另一少见变异型，占小叶癌的5%[213]。整体浸润方式类似经典型小叶癌，但在不同程

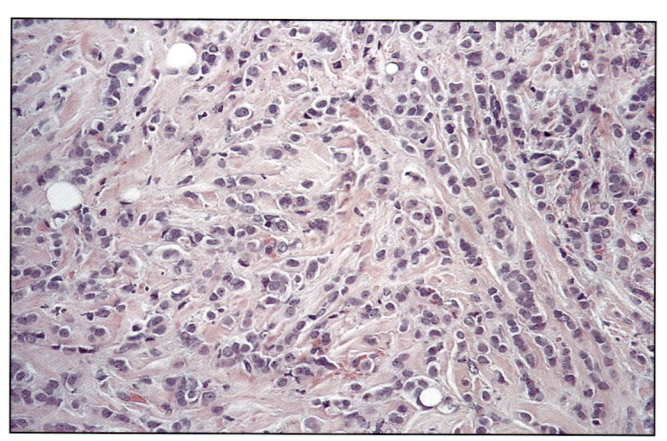

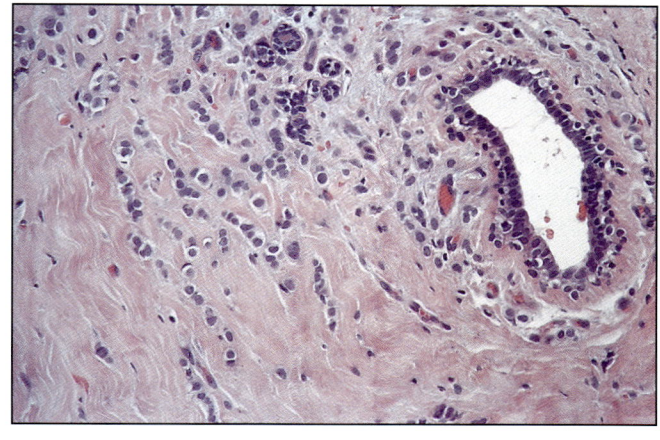

图16.51 浸润性小叶癌，经典型。肿瘤细胞单行排列浸润乳腺间质（A）。注意（B）中围绕一个正常导管结构的"靶样"形态。

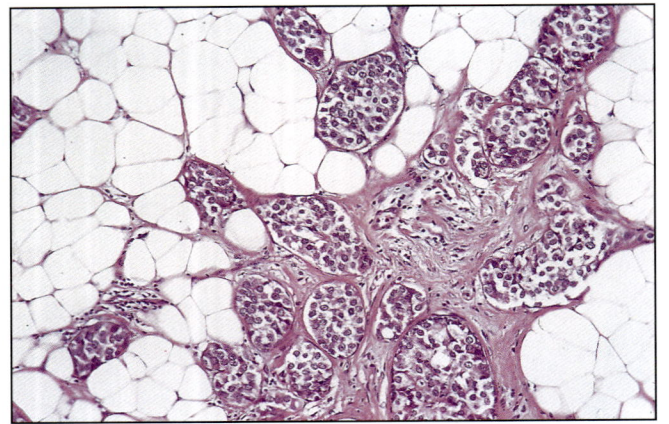

图16.52 腺泡型浸润性小叶癌。肿瘤由具有小叶癌形态特征的细胞组成圆形聚集灶。

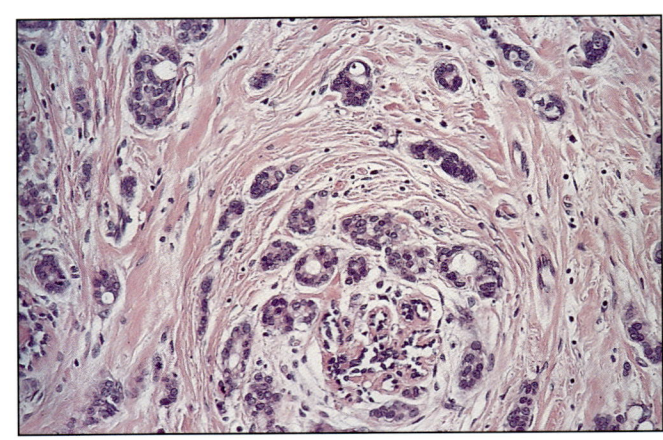

图16.54 小管小叶癌。可见单排的"靶样"浸润,但许多地方肿瘤细胞形成明确的微管状结构。

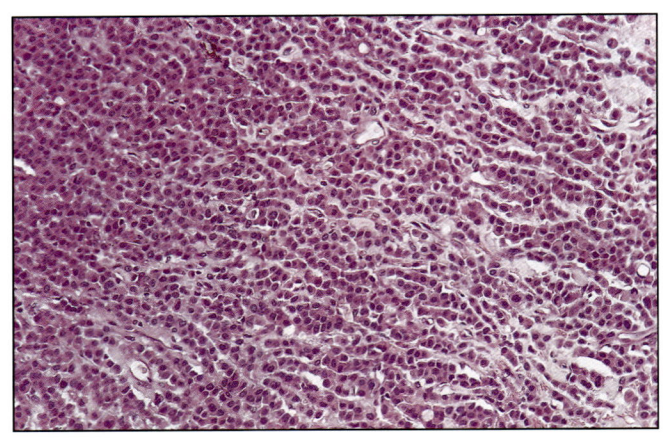

图16.53 实性型浸润性小叶癌。具有小叶癌细胞学特点的肿瘤细胞在结缔组织间质中成片浸润。

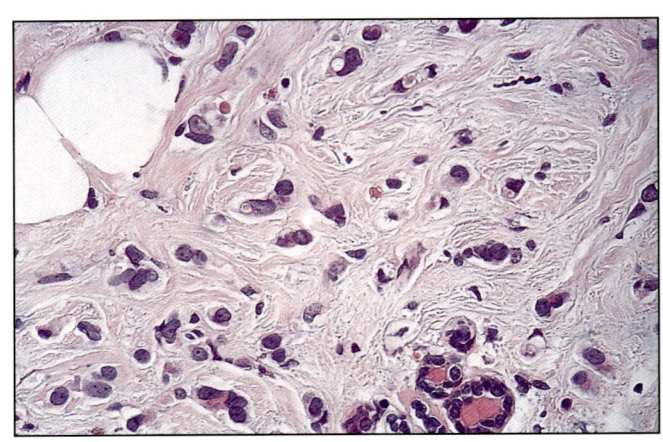

图16.55 多形性混合型小叶癌。这些肿瘤细胞可见明显的核异型,同时表现出典型的小叶形态。

度上,一些细胞条索形成明显的小管(图16.54),比小管癌中的小管小得多(比较图16.54与图16.56),也是由单层上皮细胞组成。常见原位癌,通常是筛状型或微乳头型。要诊断小管小叶癌,至少90%必须表现出相应的形态。

小管小叶癌的本质或来源,特别是这些肿瘤应该被看作小叶癌的变异型还是小管癌的变异型,仍然是一个问题,而且,某种程度上与所用诊断标准的差异有关。近期研究表明小管小叶癌常有 E-cadherin 表达,因其他类型的小叶癌没有这种情况,进一步对其包含在小叶癌亚型中提出异议[240]。尽管更常出现多灶性,它们确实与小管癌一样预后良好[241]。

e **多形性型** 多形性小叶癌的定义是具有经典性小叶癌的浸润方式但表现出细胞异型性,尤其是核多形性(图16.55)[230]的病例[1,157]。这一亚型的细胞比经典型大,胞浆更丰富,且常呈嗜酸性。需要强调的是这一型中可见大汗腺样分化[234,235,242]。尽管与其他小叶癌有相同的基因和免疫表型特征[158,243,244],此型更常出现不利的预后特征,如高核级和 *HER-2* 基因扩增[1,245]。

f **混合型** 如果以单一形态(如经典型)为主,病例就要归入某种具体亚型。其他归为混合型的病例约占浸润性小叶癌的40%[213]。

兼有小叶癌和非特殊型导管癌成分的肿瘤,只有小叶癌(或混合型小叶形态)超过90%才能归入这一类型。那些小叶成分占50%~90%的真正双向肿瘤被称为小叶-非特殊型导管混合癌(见下文)。

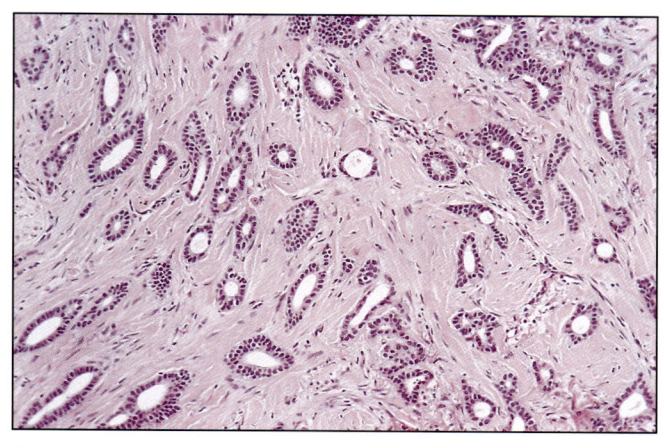 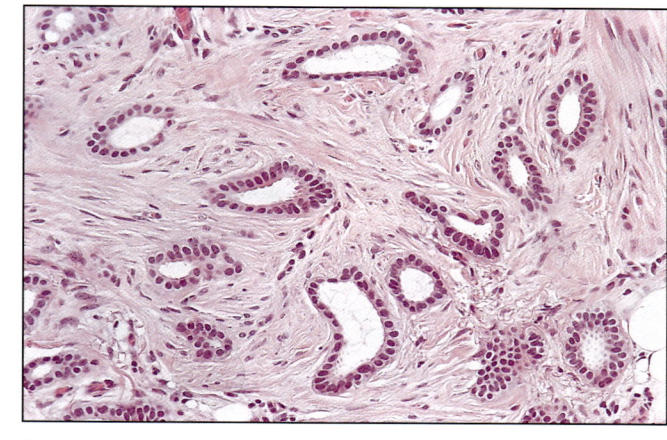

图16.56 小管癌。（A）低倍镜下表现为含有中心管腔的小管结构在硬化性间质中浸润。（B）同一病例高倍观，小管被覆单层上皮，核小而规则，异型性很小。

小管癌 Tubular carcinoma

在有症状的癌中，小管癌并不常见，发生率为1%～3%[212,213,221,222]，但在乳腺影像学筛查出的病例中发生率较高（9%～19%）[246-249]。当然，这是由于影像学能检出不可触及的小病变。普遍认为小管癌预后极好[213,250,251]。

大体表现

除肿瘤大小外，要鉴别小管癌和更常见的非特殊型导管癌或混合癌是不可能的。小管癌的直径通常为2mm～1.5cm，多数≤1cm，偶尔也可遇到≥2cm者。有两种主要的形态学亚型，"单纯"型（据报道其特点是放射状，由中心黄色弹力纤维增生和放射状分支组成）和"硬化"型（特点是较分散，结构不清）[91,252]。

组织学表现

单纯型小管癌的中心出现纤维化和弹力纤维增生，并有稀疏的小管状结构向外放射状排列，而周边小管状结构较丰富。硬化型小管癌的中心弹力纤维增生不明显，小管在结缔组织和脂肪中弥漫、无序分布。无论哪种类型，小管都具有卵圆形或圆形管腔，被覆单层上皮细胞（图16.56A）。细胞小而规则，核多形性不明显（图16.56B）。常见顶浆突起，但无特殊意义。分裂象少见。伴随的间质富于细胞，纤维组织增生；但在肿瘤周边小管可向邻近的脂肪组织浸润，不伴有相关的间质。常可见导管原位癌（通常是低级别，筛状型）。

一个肿瘤要确诊为小管癌，至少90%必须表现为明显的小管形态[91,103,212,213,252]。如果肿瘤包含的小管成分低于90%，就可归入混合性小管癌、导管癌、特殊型癌或未分类癌。唯一的例外是肿瘤由单纯的小管和单纯的筛状成分组成时，如果这种形态超过50%就可归为小管癌。

混合性小管癌 Tubular mixed carcinoma

如上所述，虽然普遍认为将90%作为小管癌的分界点，但一些作者提出如果肿瘤中出现≥75%的小管结构就应诊断为小管癌[101,253,254]。有人对小管占75%～90%的肿瘤采用混合性小管癌[91]或变异型小管癌[246,255]。这种定义排除了相当数量的肿瘤，包括小管成分所占比例少于75%者，将它们归入非特殊型导管癌中。由于这样做可能会丢失某些有用的预后信息，我们提出了一个相对宽泛的混合性小管癌定义[213]。这样可以识别14%有症状的癌，这些病例看来预后较好（见第942页）。就日常工作而言，我们将含有50%～90%特殊类型成分的癌诊断为混合性癌[5]。

大体表现

因为是小管癌和非特殊型导管癌的中间类型，其大体表现也与这些肿瘤相似。肿瘤大小约1.5～3cm，平均2cm。质硬，具有放射状外观，边界中等清楚或不清。

组织学表现

要诊断混合性小管癌，肿瘤必须具有放射状轮廓，由中心纤维化和包绕性小管结构以及周边非特殊导管癌的条索状或片状细胞组成的厚薄不一的浸润性边缘组成（图16.57）。通常中心有弹力纤维增生。从中心分化好

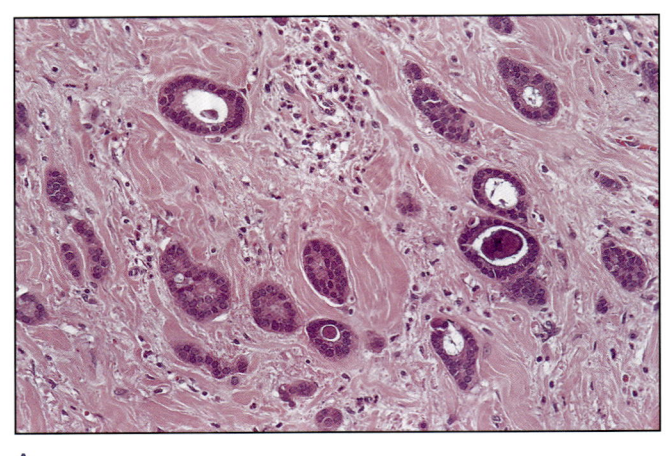
A

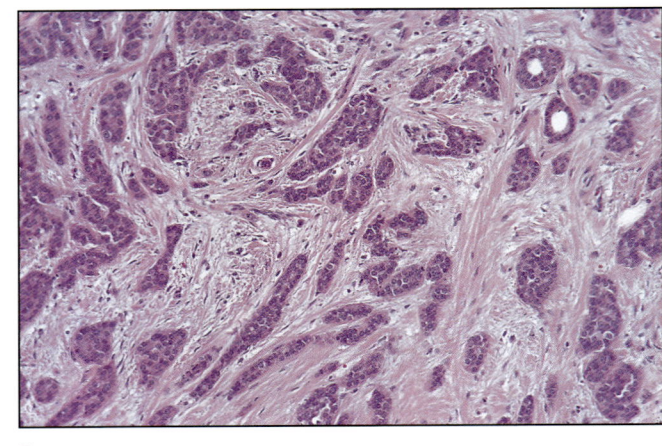
B

图16.57 混合性小管癌。(A) 中心区域表现为形态良好的小管结构。(B) 周边可见小管混入非特殊型导管癌实性条索中。

的小管癌向周边分化较差的非特殊导管癌渐进性发展，两种形态有过渡。通常要求小管成分至少达到50%，但是我们发现如果出现这种小管癌和非特殊型导管癌的特征性分布，尽管小管癌的数量很少，也可以归入混合性小管癌。

浸润性筛状癌 Invasive cribriform carcinoma

这些肿瘤被认为是与小管癌相近的特殊型乳腺癌[10,213,256,257]。因其形态学特殊而且预后极好，已经从非特殊型导管癌中分离出来。它们的有症状病例很少见，只占不到1%[213]，但在影像学筛查中较常遇到[246,248,249]。

大体表现

此型没有特殊的大体特征。肿瘤呈质硬的包块，常伴星芒状轮廓，大小在1～3cm之间。

组织学表现

浸润性筛状癌名称的使用，是因为构成浸润灶的规则小细胞与筛状型DCIS的细胞相似。核致密，多形性不明显，核分裂象少见。在浸润灶中，细胞排列成拱桥状，中间构成规整的、穿凿性空腔（图16.58）；常见上皮细胞"顶浆突起"。一些病例可见与小管癌相似的形态良好的小管结构，而另一些病例可见非特殊型导管癌的实性条索。一个肿瘤要诊断为筛状型，至少90%是这种形态。例外情况是如果病变的其余成分由单纯小管癌组成，那么筛状结构≥50%就可以诊断[212]。有人描述了浸润性筛状癌的一种罕见而特殊的变异型，其间质中含有破骨细胞样巨细胞[258-260]。免疫组织化学显示这种巨细胞为组织细胞源性，它们的出

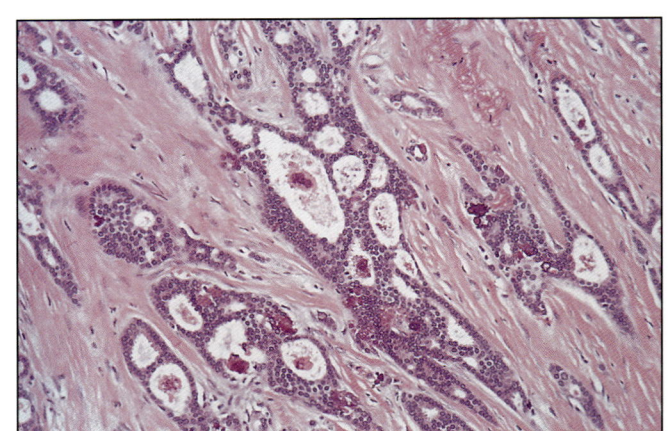

图16.58 浸润性筛状癌。肿瘤由具有筛状特征的浸润性小管结构组成。

现没有预后意义。

黏液癌 Mucinous carcinoma

这种类型也称为黏液样癌或胶样癌，正如名称所示，这些肿瘤的黏液成分肉眼就能看到。它们相对少见，占有症状病例的1%～4%[212,213,221-223]。乳腺筛查中的发生率并不增加[246]。

大体表现

黏液癌常形成边界十分清楚的瘤块，质软，切面呈有光泽的凝胶状。肿瘤直径1～4cm。

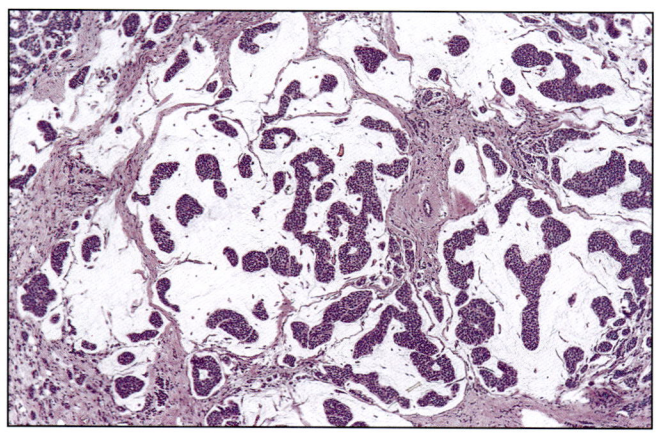
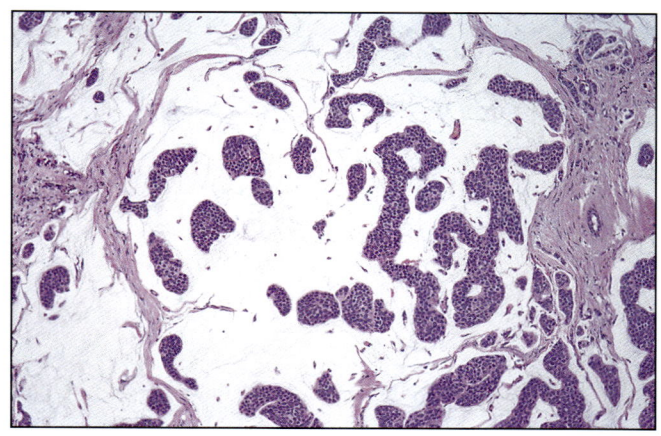

图16.59 黏液癌。（A）癌细胞团在大黏液湖中形成细胞岛。（B）细胞小，核规则、深染。

组织学表现

显微镜下，规则的上皮细胞（10～20个细胞）形成小岛或小团，漂浮在大量含MUC2和MUC6的细胞外黏液湖中（图16.59A）[261]。这些岛可以形成筛状或乳头状形态。细胞小，核深染，没有多形性，核分裂象少见（图16.59B）。在病变周边，肿瘤细胞岛可能被包埋在疏松的纤维间质中。坏死和血管浸润罕见。一些肿瘤由黏液癌和非特殊型导管癌混合组成，而过去对于这些病例如何分类一直没有统一意见。目前普遍认为黏液癌这个诊断应该用于单纯黏液癌形态≥90%的病例[212,213,262-264]。我们把非特殊型导管癌成分占10%～50%的病例归入混合型癌。

应用银染或神经内分泌标志物免疫组化可以检测黏液癌中的神经内分泌分化[10,265-267]，而且可能和预后较好有关[267]。

髓样癌　Medullary carcinoma

自从这种特殊型的浸润癌被描述以来，围绕其诊断标准和预后相关性的争论一直不断。髓样癌被作为独立类型提出是因为预后较好[268]，这种观点得到一些研究的支持[269-272]，但另一些研究则不支持[213,273-275]。一些可重复性研究表明，该肿瘤的发生率差异大（2%～10%不等），原因是诊断的可重复性差[269-272]以及诊断标准不一致[213,221-223]。有宽泛的类髓样癌特征而缺少绝对单形特征的肿瘤，可以发生在BRCA1基因突变携带者中[220]。一些研究组认为要放宽髓样癌的定义，使用"类髓样癌（medullary like carcinoma）"作为替代名称就是用来区分这些肿瘤[5]。近期资料表明这些肿瘤具有基底型角蛋白表型[279]，可能成为由基因表达和其他研究识别出的基底型乳腺癌的一部分[216,280]。

大体表现

大体上，典型的髓样癌边界清楚，质软、质地均一，大小为1～4cm。

组织学表现

普遍认为髓样癌诊断的形态学标准主要有3条（图16.60）：

1. 上皮细胞相互连接成片，形成合体网状结构。细胞大而多形，伴有一部分怪异核，分裂象计数高（即分化差）。这种形态至少占肿瘤的75%。

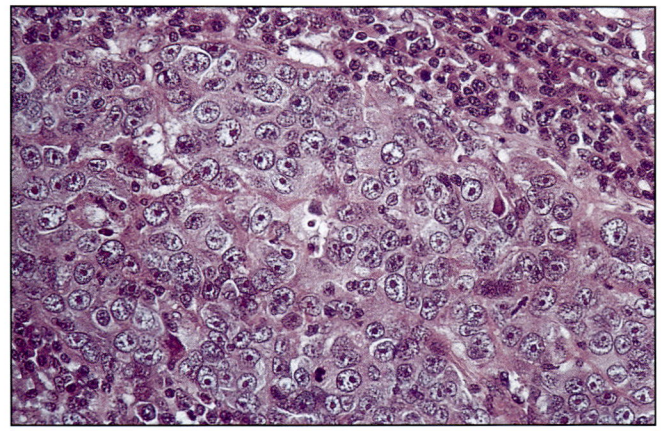

图16.60 髓样癌。高倍镜下显示肿瘤边界清楚，合体状生长，形态呈高级别，伴有密集的淋巴浆细胞浸润。

2. 相关间质有中-重度淋巴浆细胞浸润，但并非广泛存在于单个肿瘤细胞间。
3. 大体检查边界清楚，肿瘤边界呈推挤性而不是浸润性。

原位癌的存在并不影响髓样癌的诊断，但它只能是局部表现，肿瘤坏死也很少。

具有部分髓样癌特征的肿瘤被命名为非典型髓样癌[221,269]，尽管 Lidang Jensen 及其同事发现这样的分组对预后没有用处[272]。表现为淋巴浸润程度较轻，显微镜下浸润超出了主要界限或致密纤维化区。如果非特殊型导管癌占到 25% 而其余为经典型髓样癌，也可称为非典型髓样癌。最近，提出了类髓样癌这一术语[5]。具有类髓样癌特征的肿瘤已确认在 *BRCA1* 基因突变携带者中的发生率越来越高（见家族性乳腺癌章节，第 937 页）。

浸润性乳头状癌　Invasive papillary carcinoma

浸润性乳头状癌必须与原位乳头状癌鉴别清楚[242,281,282]。它是一种少见肿瘤，在有症状病例中所占比例 < 1%[213,222,255]，然而在年纪大的患者中可能更常见[281]。

大体表现

大体表现不恒定，多数乳头状癌分界清楚。质地较软或与非特殊型导管癌不易区分。肿瘤直径通常在 1~3cm 之间。

组织学表现

特征性表现是存在乳头状结构和相关的纤维血管轴心（图 16.61）。常可见黏液分泌，但我们把这些病例与黏液癌区分开来。细胞学特征差别很大，而且可能见到核多形性和核分裂象增加。大多数病例中，邻近导管可见到微乳头状或筛状原位导管癌。罕见"单纯的"浸润性乳头状癌，常与其他类型如非特殊型导管癌、黏液癌和浸润性筛状癌混合存在。

浸润性微乳头状癌
Invasive micropapillary carcinoma

根据上述定义，乳头状癌应该是一分叶状结构，中心有支持性纤维血管轴心。浸润性微乳头状癌被用来描述一种少见的、特殊的浸润性乳腺癌亚型，其中的上皮巢形成微乳头，但在透明腔隙内找不到纤维血管轴心（图 16.62）[283-285]。事实上这种肿瘤最先由 Peterse 正式描述，是具有意想不到的"翻转 (inside out)"生长模式的浸润癌[286]，用上皮膜抗原（EMA）免疫细胞化学染色可以更好地观察到（图 16.63）。所有观察者均注

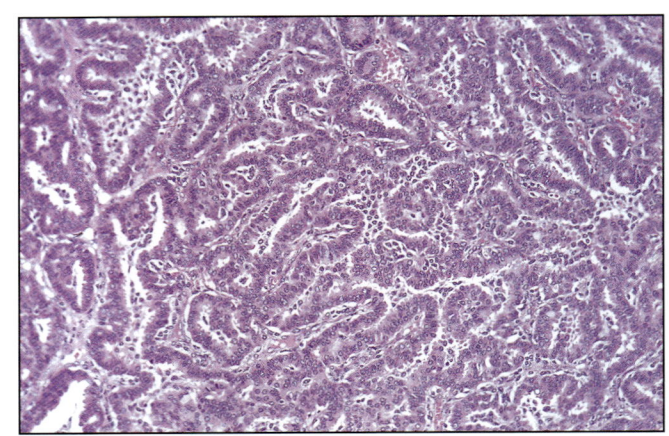

图 16.61　浸润性乳头状癌。尽管呈实性，肿瘤由中心伴有纤维血管轴心的乳头状结构组成。

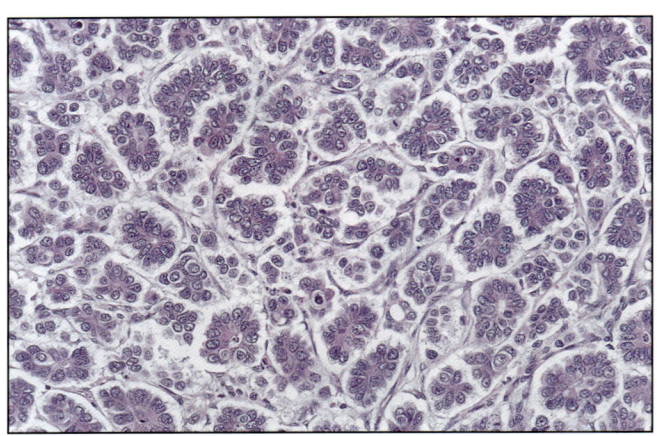

图 16.62　浸润性微乳头状癌。在透明空隙中可见"极向反转 (reverse polarity)"的上皮簇。

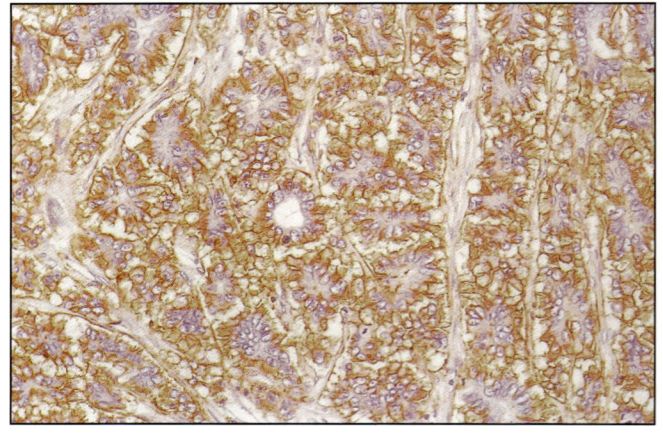

图 16.63　浸润性微乳头状癌的EMA免疫组化染色显示出极向反转（内外翻转）。

意到肿瘤周边血管浸润和淋巴结转移,一般预后很差[284,285]。至少部分与 *HER-2/neu* 的过表达率较高有关[287]。

混合型　Mixed types

除混合性小管癌被看作与小管癌密切相关的特殊肿瘤类型外,我们也注意到两种具有双向形态的混合型癌。

混合性导管 - 小叶癌有明确的非特殊型导管癌和浸润性小叶癌成分,前者占肿瘤的 10%～90%。这些肿瘤要与混合型浸润性小叶癌鉴别。

混合性导管 - 特殊型癌是由小管小叶癌、小管癌、浸润性筛状癌或黏液癌伴非特殊型导管癌混合形成的肿瘤,后者占肿瘤总体的 10% 以上。

家族性乳腺癌　Familial breast cancer

乳腺癌研究机构(the Breast Cancer Linkage Consortium group)详细研究了 *BRCA1*、*BRCA2* 基因胚系突变患者和非突变患者所发生乳腺癌的组织病理学和免疫组化特征[220,288-291]。发生于 *BRCA1* 突变患者的乳腺癌比散发癌组织学级别高,分裂象计数高,核多形性明显,管状结构较少。它们与同年龄组没有家族史的散发性乳腺癌相比更易出现类固醇受体和 HER2 阴性,发生 *p53* 基因突变。*BRCA2* 突变患者的乳腺癌因管状结构较少而分级也较高。就分裂象、多形性、类固醇受体表达或 *p53* 突变而言,它们与对照组没有显著差异。非 *BRCA1/2* 家族性乳腺癌的组织学与 *BRCA1* 和 *BRCA2* 乳腺癌不同,一般为低级别[220]。

对于原发性乳腺癌,进行组织学评估能否得出与家族性基因突变的联系?只评价形态学特征不足以给临床提供有用的准确信息。然而一项最近的研究[289]表明,形态学和免疫表型相结合可以提示 *BRCA1* 相关性癌。这组研究表明基底细胞标志物(包括 CK14、CK5/6、CK17、表皮生长因子和 osteonectin)在 *BRCA1* 肿瘤中更常见,而且在一项多变量分析中,CK14、CK5/6 和雌激素受体(ER)仍是 *BRCA1* 携带者重要的预后因素。相反,*BRCA2* 肿瘤中基底细胞标志物的表达与对照组相差不大。作者总结说综合年龄、家族史、基底细胞标志物和 ER 状态,可以很大程度上提高我们识别 *BRCA1* 突变患者的能力。

基底型乳腺癌　Basal type breast cancer

一般来说,乳腺癌大多起源于终末导管小叶单元的腺腔上皮细胞。近期的微阵列研究发现,少数有意义的乳腺癌具有基底细胞样基因表达谱[215,216,292]。早期一些研究表明一部分癌(2%～18%)有基底或肌上皮细胞表型,CK5 和 CK14 免疫组化染色阳性[293-295]。尽管基底型癌的定义尚不明确,有报道说某些特征与其有关。形态学上,它们通常为高级别[295],据报道某些病例包含大的中央无细胞区,由坏死、组织梗死、胶原和玻璃样物组成[296-298](图 16.64)。免疫组化除了表达一些肌上皮标志物外,常显示 ER、PR 和 HER-2 阴性[295,298],与 *BRCA1* 肿瘤免疫表型相似[3]。微阵列分析也表明散在的基底样癌与 *BRCA1* 突变的家族性乳腺癌相似[13,14,216,299]。近期的资料也提示,个别高级别 DCIS 具有基底细胞样表

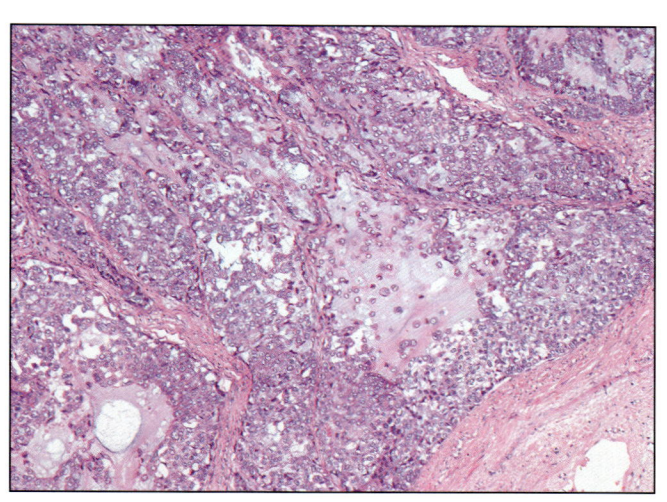

A

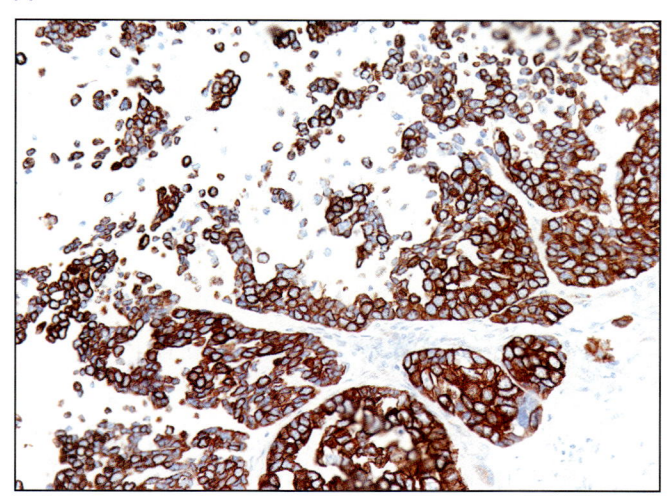

B

图 16.64　一例 3 级乳腺浸润癌表现出特征性的化生性基质(A)。这一肿瘤具有基底上皮表型,表达 CK5/6(B)。

型[299a]。

我们研究组[300]试图把基底型肿瘤按下列2组分型：
1. 具有基底表型的肿瘤（表达1或2个基底细胞标志物，如CK5/6和/或CK14）。
2. 具有肌上皮表型的肿瘤（表达SMA和/或p63）。

第1组进一步分为以下两个亚型：
A 基底细胞优势型（>50%的细胞阳性）
B 基底细胞特征型（10%～50%细胞阳性）

第1组肿瘤占病例的18.6%（1A和1B分别占10%和8.6%），第2组占13.7%。基底细胞（组1）表达与整体存活率下降以及无病生存中位时间下降相关，而且多变量分析表明基底细胞（而非肌上皮）表型具有独立的预后价值。

少见类型　　Rare type

这一部分简要叙述一组不常见的肿瘤类型，总体占浸润性癌的比例不足2%。值得注意的是单纯的大汗腺癌（像形态学描述的那样）非常罕见[301]，而大汗腺改变实际上可能是任何一种浸润癌的局部表现。更罕见的是乳腺的原发性小细胞癌[302]。

分泌性癌　　Secretory carcinoma

这些肿瘤在儿童首先描述[303]，但是也发生于任何年龄的成年人[304,305]。

大体上，它们界限清楚，直径通常≤2cm。组织学上，边界清楚，通常伴有外周纤维化。诊断性特征是存在细胞内和细胞外圆形空泡，整体上呈现透明细胞形态。空泡内分泌物经淀粉酶消化后PAS染色阳性，表明其为黏液性。遗传学上，它们明显不同于传统的导管癌[306]，尤其值得注意的是表达 *ETV6-NTRK3* 融合基因，这种改变也见于婴儿纤维肉瘤（见第24章）。在儿童，分泌性癌的预后极好，但有限的证据表明成人的预后并不那么乐观[307,308]。

鳞状细胞癌　　Squamous cell carcinoma

乳腺的单纯性鳞状细胞癌极罕见[308]，而且必须与非特殊型导管癌伴有局灶鳞状上皮化生和化生性癌（见下文）相鉴别。尽管一些实性肿瘤也见于报道[310]，大多数报道的乳腺鳞状细胞癌都含有囊性成分[309]。虽然可用于评价预后意义的病例较少，大多数属于高级别病变，具有凶险的临床过程[311]。

化生性癌　　Metaplastic carcinoma

化生性癌是指那些除了上皮成分外还表现出肉瘤样成分（如软骨、骨、黏液样间质和梭形细胞间质）的肿瘤。根据超微结构研究，大多数专家认为这些病例代表癌细胞的化生性改变[312,313]。这些肿瘤不常见，占浸润癌的0.3%[314]。大体上，它们常形成大而固定的结节状肿瘤，直径常达5cm。常常固定于皮肤或深筋膜。

显微镜下，可见两种主要的化生性癌亚型，而且据此分为：单相型"肉瘤样"癌或梭形细胞癌以及双相型"肉瘤样"癌（也称为"癌肉瘤"或"恶性混合性肿瘤"）[214,315-317]。单相型可以由单纯的梭形细胞或一些小的细胞粘附灶组成。双相型包括传统的癌区域，通常是非特殊型浸润癌或导管原位癌。

梭形细胞亚型可表现为片状多形细胞或类似纤维瘤病的温和梭形细胞等一系列形态（图16.65）[315,317-321]。间叶性成分通常没有清楚的分化方向；少数情况下可见血管肉瘤、平滑肌肉瘤、骨肉瘤、软骨肉瘤或横纹肌肉瘤成分。Wargotz和Norris描述了一种预后比其他化生性癌好的"基质形成"型[322]。分裂象多少不一，但通常在肿瘤细胞中很丰富。梭形细胞的上皮表型可通过一组标志物免疫染色检测出来，包括34βE12、CAM5.2、MNF116、CK7、CK19和CK20（图16.66）。重要的是用一组抗体进行检测，因为没有哪种角蛋白会出现于所有的梭形细胞癌中[72]。

由于化生性癌罕见，很难评价其预后，但多种证据

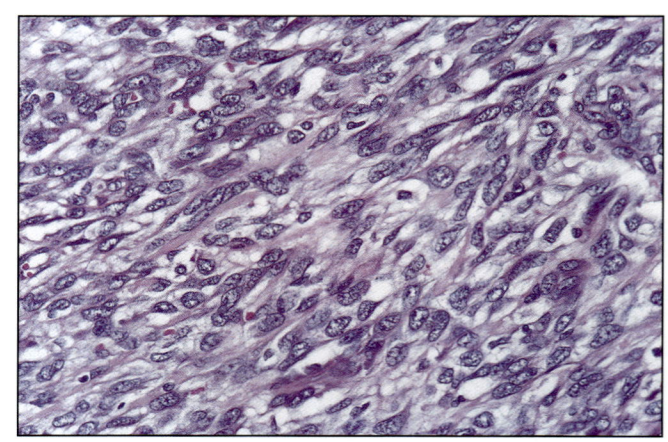

图16.65　化生性癌，由成片的梭形细胞组成，没有上皮分化形态。

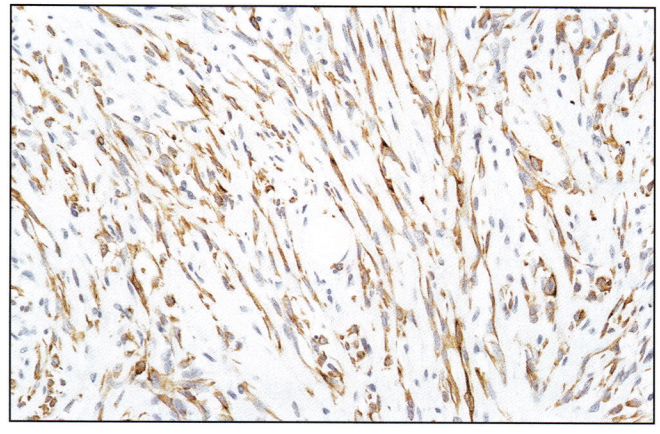

图16.66 化生性梭形细胞癌，肿瘤胞浆表达细胞角蛋白（MNF116）。

表明大多数化生性癌表现为复发早、生存差的高度恶性肿瘤[314-316,320,321]。化生性癌通常不表达雌、孕激素受体或HER-2，因此限制了可能的系统性治疗[314,321]。单相梭形细胞癌很少累及腋窝淋巴结。

低级别腺鳞癌
Low-grade adenosquamous carcinoma

低级别腺鳞癌是化生性癌的低级别变异型[308,323,324]。在这一罕见肿瘤中，某些汗管瘤样腺体成分显示鳞状分化，被富于细胞的纤维瘤病样梭形细胞间质包绕（图16.67）。在发表的文献中，低级别腺鳞癌大小为5～34mm，见于31～87岁妇女。据报道其发生与硬化性乳头状病变、放射状瘢痕和复合硬化性病变相关[323,325,326]。

低级别腺鳞癌由被覆上皮的小腺体和实性上皮条索组成，无序分布在浸润性梭形细胞间质中[324,326]。这3种成分的比例可以相差很大，有些可能以梭形细胞为主。实性巢中可以出现鳞状细胞、角化珠或鳞状上皮囊肿，表达高分子量细胞角蛋白。间质被描述为"纤维瘤病样"，细胞丰富，由形态良性的梭形细胞组成。间质成分可以出现胶原化、透明样变或细胞数量改变，罕见情况下可见骨软骨灶。与腺鳞癌相关的导管原位癌的发生率不恒定。与乳腺的涎腺样肿瘤相似，这些肿瘤的上皮成分缺乏雌激素受体表达。

上皮成分和一部分梭形细胞成分可以表达细胞角蛋白。在一些病例，梭形细胞对平滑肌肌动蛋白有反应。一般认为，此型化生性癌应该被看作是低级别癌，不完全切除者会局部复发，但转移的可能性较低。

乳腺癌的预后因素
Prognostic factors in breast cancer

对一些肿瘤来说，组织病理学在提供预后因素中的作用已建立了很多年（如在恶性黑色素瘤中测量肿瘤厚度，恶性淋巴瘤中组织学亚型的评估）。主要原因是治疗方法的多样性和病人的正确分流。然而，直到近期外科病理医师在乳腺疾病中的主要作用仍然是建立乳腺癌的基本诊断。除了检查局部淋巴结有无转移外，很少能提供其他预后信息。乳腺癌的治疗已经程序化，以手术治疗为主，很少再根据个体情况进行合适的治疗。然而，在最近二十年，乳腺癌的治疗发生了巨大变化，现在治疗方法的选择更加广泛。早期诊断，尤其是乳腺筛查检出的肿瘤预后较好，而且在治疗方案制定之前就评价每个患者的预后显得越来越重要。

大范围的预后因素研究已经展开，一些已被充分肯定，一些正在进展阶段，而其他的仍然只能作为研究手段。大致分为两组，传统因素和分子因素。传统因素可通过常规体检和肿瘤组织学检查进行评估。分子标志物的评估技术还没有广泛应用，但是其中一些（如激素受体）在治疗反应预测中越来越重要。本章中我们重点介绍传统因素，但我们也对治疗过程中有价值的那些分子标志物做一些简要介绍。

传统病理学因素

对常规乳腺癌标本进行仔细的组织病理学检查可以获得大量重要的预后信息。为了获得最精确的数据，要密切注意标本处理[5,327-329]。理想的情况是

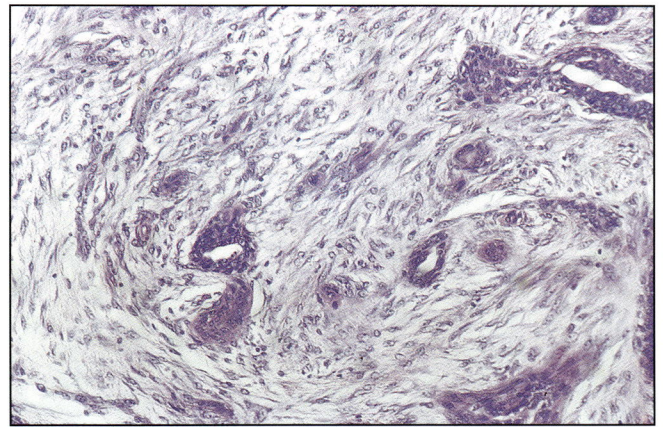

图16.67 低级别腺鳞癌，由一些显示鳞状分化的腺体结构组成，周围有良性形态的梭形细胞间质。

标本应该在新鲜时切开，以便肿瘤能够及时固定。固定好之后，要取足够的组织块进行常规石蜡包埋。然后切成标准的"薄"（4μm）切片，对于以下要描述的大多数参数，行 HE（苏木精 - 伊红）染色就可以了。

以下病理学因素（所有的这些评估都相对比较简单）都能或多或少地为临床提供有用的预后信息。

肿瘤大小

为了评估预后，肿瘤的大小应该只由病理学家来评价，因为临床测量不够精确。肿瘤三维直径的测量应当在新鲜状态下以毫米为单位进行。固定之后再进行核对，将最大直径作为肿瘤的大小。对于≤1cm的小肿瘤以及含大量原位癌成分的肿瘤，可能在组织切片上以微米为单位测量更为精确[330]。

作为时间依赖性因素，许多研究表明肿瘤大小与预后相关[331-334]，肿瘤小的患者比肿瘤大的生存率更高。而且，Nottingham/Tenovus 原发性乳腺癌研究（NTPBCS）已通过多变量分析证实肿瘤大小是一个重要的独立变量[335,336]，成为 Nottingham 预后指数（NPI）不可或缺的组成部分。

评价肿瘤大小在乳腺癌筛查中尤其重要。肿瘤直径≤10mm者，即所谓的轻微浸润癌（minimal invasive carcinoma, MIC）[337-339]，比≥15mm的肿瘤分期早（即淋巴结阴性）[121,246,333,338,340-343]。有趣的是，Nottingham Tenovus 研究对肿瘤大小类别分析指出，要获得长期的生存，较好的临界点实际上是 1.5cm。在英国国家乳腺癌筛查项目（National Breast Screening Program，NHSBSP）中，超过 50% 的浸润癌小于 15mm[344]。

淋巴结分期

在乳腺癌中淋巴结分期提供了很强的预后信息，目前一般认为淋巴结分期要依靠对切除淋巴结的组织学检查而不是依靠临床检查。

许多研究已表明，组织学上区域淋巴结受累的患者比没有淋巴结受累的患者预后差[331,335,345,346]。总体来说，淋巴结阴性患者的 10 年生存率为 75%，而淋巴结阳性患者下降到 25% ~ 30%。值得注意的是，淋巴结受累在男性患者更常见[162,224]。预后也与区域淋巴结受累的数目和水平有关。淋巴结受累的数目越多，预后越差[281,347]。在美国，NSABP 出于治疗目的将患者分为两组，1 ~ 3 个阳性淋巴结患者和≥4 个阳性淋巴结患者。这种方法被 UICC、AJCC、EU 和 UK 推荐使用[5,348]。同样，受累腋窝淋巴结水平"较高"或较远者，预后较差[8,349]，这对内乳淋巴结受累也同样适用[350]。我们和其他研究组已证实可以通过淋巴结摘除获得明显的预后信息，避免腋窝淋巴结清扫造成的致残性[335,336,351,352]。然而，关于腋窝淋巴结摘除和清扫的争论还在继续[353-357]。这里不再详述具体的争论，而是应该整理出现在所采用的治疗方法。淋巴结转移率的降低和前哨淋巴结活检的广泛实施（伴有或不伴其他淋巴结摘除）减少了腋窝清扫术的常规使用。乳腺内淋巴结摘除只适用于乳腺中心部位的肿瘤，对外侧的肿瘤不适用。低位腋清扫（在肋间臂丛神经之下）提供了准确预后所需的足够的淋巴结（通常 4 ~ 15 个），致残率低。淋巴结的分期如下：

1 期（N0）：没有淋巴结受累

2 期（N1）：1 ~ 3 个腋淋巴结或 1 个乳内淋巴结受累

3 期（N2，N3）：≥4 个腋淋巴结受累（N2=4 ~ 9 个受累淋巴结，N3=10 个以上淋巴结受累）

UICC、AJCC、UK 和 EU[5,348] 把单个淋巴结微转移性（转移灶大小 0.2 ~ 2mm）归为淋巴结阳性 2 期（N1）；而将孤立肿瘤细胞（转移灶<0.2mm）称为淋巴结阴性 1 期（N0）。尽管没有充分证据来支持这些建议，使用统一的淋巴结转移分类标准确实有实践意义。

这些建议也反应了大家最近对淋巴结转移大小的注意，尤其是所谓的隐性转移（传统 HE 染色漏诊的任何大小的转移）、微小转移（大小上限为 2mm）或孤立肿瘤细胞 [ITC(isolated tumor cell)，大小上限为 0.2mm]，就如 TNM 分类定义的一样。有一些证据表明大小不超过 2mm 的"微小转移"与淋巴结阴性的患者相比，并不对生存期造成负面影响[358-360]。有关孤立肿瘤细胞检测的数据，常常是通过连续切片和免疫组织化学染色发现，其结果并不一致。一些研究发现这些患者预后明显较差[361-364]，而另一些研究发现生存率没有差别[359,365,366]。Cserni 和 Dowlatshahi 已回顾了有关资料和临床期刊[367,368]。在 2002 年之前的文献中，微小转移的范围包括现在分类为 ITC 的病例。它们的预后相关性尚不肯定，还存在争论。Dowlatshahi[367] 认为只有通过大样本的随访资料研究才可以证实微小转移患者的预后较差。但是，一项最近的单中心回顾性研究（随访期限较长，且通过多变量分析）显示，伴有隐性转移的患者预后并不比没有淋巴结转移的患者差[360]，许多隐性转移病例已被称为组织学微小转移[367]。除了预后相关的问题，还有在小转移灶的分类中病理学家之间一致性的问题，表明需要更严格的标准[369]。

包绕腋窝淋巴结的脂肪组织中出现转移癌，即所谓结外扩散或包膜外转移（extracapsular metastasis，ECM）已成为公认的预后较差的因素[370,371]，而且一些放射肿瘤学家把它看作是术后腋窝放疗的指征。然而，一些研究已表明ECM不是一个独立因素，而是与受累淋巴结的数目紧密相关[372-374]。Donegan及其同事[374]已进一步得出结论，认为ECM本身不是腋窝清除术后放疗的指征。

前哨淋巴结活检 sentinel node biopsy

在黑色素瘤领域工作的Morton及其同事规定前哨淋巴结（第一站淋巴结）为原发病变直接回流通路上的第一个淋巴结[375]。目前前哨淋巴结（sentinel lymph node，SLN）作为乳腺癌淋巴结转移扩散的第一位置已被广泛接受[376]。这通过大量SLN和非SLN的详细组织病理学研究所证实[377-380]。当与传统方法比较时，SLN活检能使一部分病例的分期提高[381]。使用TNM分类系统，所见到的小转移通常为微小转移或ITC[348]，但也可能为较大的转移[382]。由于与淋巴结状态相关的大多数预后信息是通过单张常规的HE切片获得，因此以往所发现的转移通常较大（>2mm）。这种转移与预后较差明确相关。

检测SLN的病理方法差别很大；总体来说，方法越精确（如连续切片的数目和间距以及免疫细胞化学的使用）发现的转移灶越多（包括ITC、微小转移或较大的转移）[381-383]。

淋巴结病理学检查的实践指南 我们目前采用英国和欧洲的淋巴结检查标准[5]。乳腺癌患者切除的淋巴结（通常是腋窝，偶尔也可为乳内淋巴结）常规送病理学检查。这些标本可能为腋窝清扫标本、淋巴结摘除或前哨淋巴结活检。每个淋巴结都应该行组织学检查。采用的方法应该保证所有的淋巴结都能被评估，即每个淋巴结至少取一个组织块。这种最低标准允许多个淋巴结装入同一个蜡块进行检查。对前哨淋巴结和非引导的淋巴结标本（最好包括腋窝清扫标本），我们建议每个淋巴结都应该分别包埋进行组织学检查。通过HE染色组织切片光镜检查能够较大程度发现转移灶。任何大体上受累的淋巴结，取一块代表性的切片就足够了。大小超过5mm的淋巴结应该垂直于长轴每隔2～3mm切片。如果切割厚度不超过2mm，那么理论上说所有较大转移（>2mm）都可检出。因此组织块取材也提供一种替代性的间断切片。所有取材组织块均应该包埋并行组织学检查。较大的淋巴结可能需要多个包埋块。5mm以下的淋巴结可对半切开包埋，也可选择全部包埋，至少检查3个切面。

病理报告应当包括检查的淋巴结数目和有转移的淋巴结数目。特殊部位的淋巴结（腋尖淋巴结）可能由外科医师发现并单独记录，但也应该包括在总淋巴结数里面。

辅助技术 辅助技术包括多层面切片、应用免疫细胞化学和分子技术。这些检测能提高微转移的检出率，但意义尚不明确。除非有明确的证据支持并且有适当的方法来提高一致性，否则目前的资源还不允许常规推行这种详细的淋巴结检查技术。然而如果是出于兴趣或资源允许，可考虑以下方法。

微转移灶的检出率通过增加淋巴结的体积检查比例，以及增加淋巴结面积检查比例的方法得到提高。方法可包括连续切片或目前大多数研究所采用的间隔100μm进行切片，总共切取3个平面。Cserni[368]总结了这些研究并得出结论，大转移采用间隔1mm而微转移采用间隔200～250μm的间断切片（根据研究目的或资源），不需要再缩短切片的间隔距离。增加检查的平面数会提高检出率，但降低了实用性[368]。

免疫细胞化学检测是传统组织学的辅助技术，可通过直接标记肿瘤细胞群促使检出微转移灶。大多数研究使用广谱或低分子量细胞角蛋白，即AE1/AE3、MNF116、CAM5.2、CK19[367,384]。某些细胞角蛋白抗体能够和网状细胞、淋巴细胞发生交叉反应造成假阳性。应根据免疫反应并结合形态学进行评估。目前我们使用AE1/AE3抗体的免疫细胞化学染色来处理怀疑早期转移的病例。我们目前不采用免疫细胞化学常规筛查微转移。微转移（尤其是ITC）的临床和预后意义仍然不确定。

组织学类型

目前已经认识到某些特殊类型的浸润性乳腺癌预后良好。据报道小管癌[252,254,385,386]、黏液癌[262,387]、浸润性筛状癌[256]、髓样癌[269,388]、浸润性小叶癌[149]和小管小叶癌[233]的预后比非特殊型浸润性导管癌好。生存期与组织学类型的全面、长期的预后研究很少，但Dawson及其同事[389]发现乳腺切除后生存超过25年的患者与生存少于10年的患者相比，小管癌、黏液癌、髓样癌和浸润性小叶癌相对较多。这些发现已被爱丁堡的一项相似的研究所证实[263]，浸润性筛状癌也属于长期生存范畴。爱丁堡的研究组已表明，乳腺影像学筛查出的浸润癌病例中，"特殊型"所占比例也相对较多[246]，我们的研究也证实了这一点。

NTPBCS 报道也证实组织学类型能提供有力的预后信息[213]。在超过1500例的可手术的原发浸润癌患者中，至少随访10年后，发现特殊型（纯小管癌、浸润性筛状和黏液癌）的预后极好。研究也表明患有混合性小管癌以及混合性非特殊型-特殊型导管癌的患者预后较好，远好于非特殊型导管癌。在先前的研究中，这些混合型很少被发现，大多包括在一般的非特殊型导管癌中；由于它们至少占有症状肿瘤的15%，所以有价值的预后信息很容易丢失。

一般认为髓样癌的预后很好或较好[269,270, 272,387,390]，然而一些研究组并未证实比非特殊型导管癌生存期有优势[213,274,275]。然而，这些研究也发现髓样癌比对应的组织学3级的非特殊型导管癌预后好[213,274,275]。因此，我们认为髓样癌应被看作具有中等的预后，而不是很好的预后[213,391]。

虽然浸润性小叶癌的10年生存率为54%，仅属于中等预后，但它比非特殊型导管癌预后好[8,213]。然而，Dixon 及其同事[230]发现小叶癌不同组织亚型之间的生存率有明显差异，这在 NTPBCS 中也得到证实[392]。因此，经典型预后好（10年生存率为60%），混合型小叶癌中等预后（10年生存率为55%），而实性型预后差（10年生存率40%）。预后极好的小管小叶癌（10年生存率超过90%），尚不清楚到底归属小管癌还是小叶癌，目前认为是特殊的独立类型。

根据新近的 cDNA 芯片研究和应用基底细胞角蛋白的表型研究，已识别出了基底型乳腺癌，比其他类型预后差[300]。

乳腺浸润癌患者可以根据组织学类型进行粗略的预后分组：极好预后组由特殊型乳腺癌（小管癌、筛状癌、黏液癌）和小管小叶癌组成；较好预后组包括混合性小管癌、混合性非特殊型-特殊型导管癌和经典小叶癌；中等预后组包括混合性小叶癌、髓样癌和非典型髓样癌；差的预后组由非特殊型导管癌、混合性导管-小叶癌、实性小叶癌和3级基底型癌组成。

此外，乳腺癌的组织学类型增加了我们对乳腺癌生物学的理解。举例来说，浸润性小叶癌比非特殊型导管癌更常表达雌激素受体（ER）[393]，它们也有不同的转移模式，常出现后腹膜、浆膜表面等特殊部位转移[394,395]。目前的证据表明组织学类型与 BRCA1 和 BRCA2 基因表达之间有相关性。举例来说，2项重要的研究表明 BRCA1 比 BRCA2 相关病例更常出现髓样癌表现的高级别（3级）癌[290,291,396,397]（见上述家族性乳腺癌部分）。

组织学分级

肿瘤病理学的一个最基本特点是认识到肿瘤的形态学特征能够与其恶性程度相对应。有关乳腺癌组织学分化的分级研究首先由 Greenhough 完成[398]，除了方法的主观性和缺少临床资料外，他的结果显示了很好的预后相关性。从那时起已出现了多种不同的方法，但所有的方法都可追溯到 Greenhough 提出的方法。目前采用的主要方法分为两组，大多数沿袭最初的概念即参考多种细胞学因素[331,332,399-403]，另一些则专注于细胞核的特征[404-406]。尽管分类方法有差别，但许多研究表明分级与生存期显著相关，清楚地表明组织学分级是有力的预后因素；这些数据以前已有详细总结[330,403]。

尽管如此，采用世界卫生组织[1,409]提出的方法（即所谓的 Scarff-Bloom-Richardson 方法[399,400,407,408]），将组织学分级常规应用于诊断病理学中的推进速度缓慢。过去，主要是因为临床没有要求，此外方法的主观性和观察者的可重复性差也是不愿使用组织学分级的原因[410,411]，尽管有些研究认为不同观察者和同一观察者之间的可重复性并不太差[221,281,412,413]。

这些有争论的观点强调，组织学分级要在达成共识的情况下由受过训练的组织病理学家来进行。尽管组织学分级总会有一定的主观性，以往的研究可重复性差的一个主要原因是缺乏严格的定义和书面的形态学标准。因此，我们采用改良的 WHO 分级方法[399,400,409]，以产生更大的客观性[330,403]。目前这种方法已由 WHO 推荐使用[1]。

我们评估肿瘤的3个特征：作为腺体分化表现的腺管结构、核多形性和分裂象计数（表16.1，图16.68至16.70）。评分系统对每个因素均进行1~3分评估。根据以前的前瞻性研究，取75%和10%作为评估肿瘤区域腺体分化的分界点（图16.68）[414]。核多形性是以邻近乳腺组织中正常上皮细胞的形态为对照来评价的（图16.69）。核轮廓的不规则性以及核仁数目、大小都是有用的评分特征，但必须认识到这仍然是一项主观评估。最重要的变化与分裂活性有关。注意只能计数明确的核分裂象。核深染和碎裂的细胞要忽略掉，因为它们更可能代表凋亡而非增生。需要进行准确的定量评估而不是简单地以"每个高倍视野约2~3个分裂象"来表示[400]，因为不同显微镜的高倍视野面积可相差6倍[415]。然而，最精确的分裂指数计数法（计数分裂细胞所占的百分比）[416]费时费力，难以在日常工作中实施。根据分裂象计数的详细研究[417]，我们对固定视野采用标准化的分裂象计数（表16.2，图16.70）。使用这个系统，任何显微镜都能被校正，产生可重复和可对比的数据。

上述方法已得到 NTPBCS 的充分评价。根据 2000 例以上患者随访 3～18 年的生存结果分析，证实了组织学分级和预后的高度相关性；分级越高生存期越差[213,330]。其他研究中心也证实这种方法有很好的可重复性[418-420]，在英国 NHSBSP[5,327]、欧洲乳腺筛查病理组[6]、WHO[1] 和美国解剖和外科病理主任协会 (ADASP)[421] 已

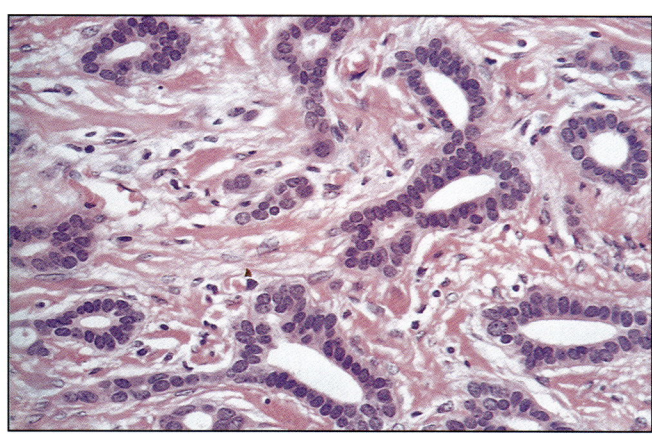

图16.68 组织学分级中腺管形成的评估。如同此处所示，只有出现明显中心腺腔的结构才能被计数。

表16.1	半定量法评估乳腺癌的组织学分级
腺管形成	
大部分肿瘤（>75%）	1分
中等程度（10%～75%）	2分
很少或无（<10%）	3分
核多形性	
细胞小而规则、一致	1分
大小和变异程度中等	2分
显著变异	3分
核分裂计数	
依据显微镜视野*	1～3分

*见表16.2

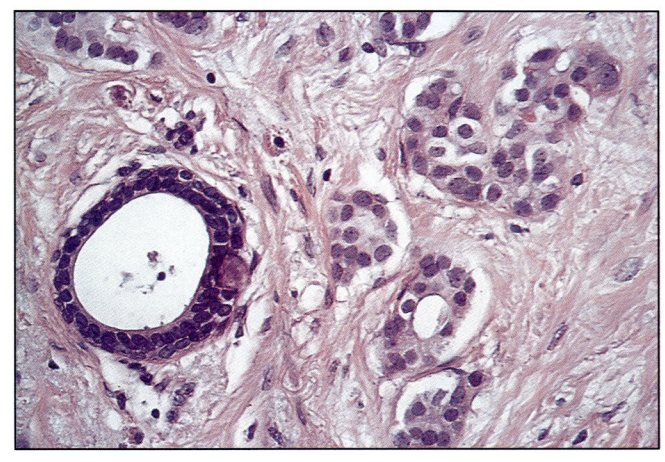

A

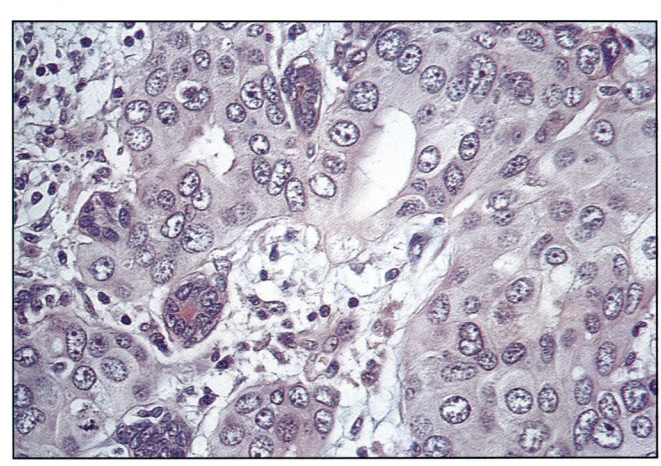

B

图16.69 组织学分级中通过与邻近正常上皮细胞的对比进行核多形性评估。（A）这个病例评为1分；核比正常上皮细胞略大，但大小和形状差别不大。（B）这个病例评为3分；细胞核比正常上皮细胞大得多，大小和形状有很大差别。

表16.2	根据显微镜视野评估核分裂象计数的得分		
视野直径 (单位：mm)	相应的核分裂象计数		
	1分	2分	3分
0.40	达到4	5~8	≥9
0.41	达到4	5~9	≥10
0.42	达到4	5~9	≥10
0.43	达到4	5~10	≥11
0.44	达到5	6~10	≥11
0.45	达到5	6~11	≥12
0.46	达到5	6~11	≥12
0.47	达到5	6~12	≥13
0.48	达到6	7~12	≥13
0.49	达到6	7~13	≥14
0.50	达到6	7~13	≥14
0.51	达到6	7~14	≥15
0.52	达到7	8~14	≥15
0.53	达到7	8~15	≥16
0.54	达到7	8~16	≥17
0.55	达到8	9~16	≥17
0.56	达到8	9~17	≥18
0.57	达到8	9~17	≥18
0.58	达到9	10~18	≥19
0.59	达到9	10~19	≥20
0.60	达到9	10~19	≥20
0.61	达到9	10~20	≥21
0.62	达到10	11~21	≥22
0.63	达到10	11~21	≥22
0.64	达到11	12~22	≥23
0.65	达到11	12~23	≥24
0.66	达到11	12~24	≥25
0.67	达到12	13~25	≥26
0.68	达到12	13~25	≥26
0.69	达到12	13~26	≥27
0.70	达到13	14~27	≥28

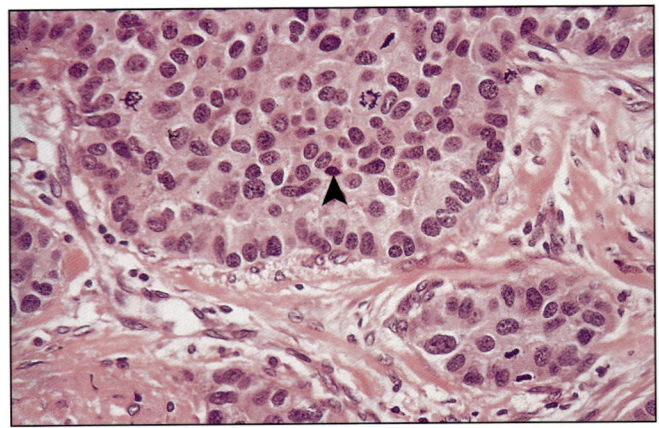

图16.70　组织学分级中核分裂象的定量评价。显示一些清楚明确的分裂象；深染的细胞核（箭头处）不应该计数。

将其作为最基本的病理数据。

在Nottingham，无论其形态学类型，我们对所有的乳腺浸润性癌均进行组织学分级，现在这种做法已被大家普遍接受[5,6,327,422]。一些病理学家批评这种做法，因为他们认为分级不适用于特殊型乳腺癌。我们认为分级实际上是评价组织学类型的一个组成部分；如小管癌总是组织学1级，而对小叶癌分级则产生了相应的生存曲线[330]。此外，对于一些特殊类型（如黏液癌和小管混合癌），分级比单纯的组织学分型更能提供准确的预后评价[391]。

脉管侵犯

有关乳腺癌脉管侵犯预后意义的看法仍不统一[423]。一些研究发现与临床结局无关[424,425]，而另一些则表明脉管侵犯的存在可预测患者的复发[353,426,427]和长期生存率[425,428-431]。这种差异体现在所报道的脉管侵犯的发生率差别很大，可能是因为真正的脉管与软组织间隙的鉴别存在问题。绝大多数的研究对象是特殊亚群（淋巴结阴性组），因此很难准确计算总发生率。报道的脉管侵犯的发生率为34%~54%。

尽管肌性血管偶可受侵，肿瘤栓子主要见于薄壁脉管；由于难以确定这些腔隙是淋巴管还是血管，就使用广义的脉管侵犯。为避免过诊断，必须小心避免把导管原位癌和出现收缩假象的浸润癌细胞索误诊为脉管浸润[432]。这些问题可以通过很好的组织固定和使用简单、严格的诊断标准而大大减少。确定脉管浸润应该是在肿瘤的邻近组织中进行，而不是在肿瘤

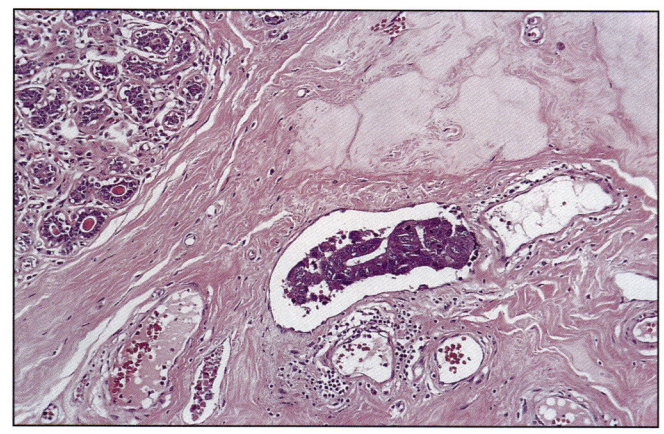

图16.71 乳腺癌中明确的脉管浸润。这一视野距离肿瘤主体结节几毫米，左侧显示一部分正常乳腺小叶，中心区域被覆扁平内皮细胞的血管内含有一个肿瘤栓子。

内。肿瘤栓子必须在被覆内皮细胞的腔隙中见到（图16.71）；这些腔隙通常位于结缔组织内，与乳腺小叶成分相隔离，而且常与小肌性血管距离很近。这些位置特征已由Örbo等评价过[432]。内皮标志物如CD31、CD34、层粘连蛋白、Ⅳ型胶原、Ⅷ因子相关抗原和荆豆凝集素Ⅰ的免疫染色，在鉴别脉管和导管结构没有帮助，但在除外收缩假象方面可能有用[433-437]。日常实践中，其应用局限于解决疑难病例。在一些研究中，评估脉管浸润的可重复性显示较满意[332,427]，而且是在存在疑问的病例[438]，3位观察者之间的完全符合率接近90%。

脉管浸润与局部淋巴结受累密切相关[430-432,439]，而且，可能由于这种相关性，使得它们能像淋巴结分期一样提供有力的预后信息[426]。在淋巴结阴性患者，脉管浸润的存在和早期复发有着明确的相关性[426,427,440,441]，而这些研究也表明较差的预后效果与隐性腋淋巴结受累无关。在NTPBCS研究中，我们不但肯定了脉管浸润在评估长期生存中的预后价值，而且在多变量分析中证实这种效果独立于淋巴结分期。最后，脉管浸润的存在是预示保乳治疗后局部复发[353,425,428-430]和乳腺切除后皮瓣复发的最重要因素之一[442]。

坏死

浸润性乳腺癌中出现局部坏死是相对常见的现象，偶尔表现为大体可见的界限清楚的灰暗区，常位于中心。显微镜下，像在任何组织中一样，坏死性肿瘤是以核碎裂、固缩和核溶解改变为特征，一般伴有中性粒细胞浸润。当肿瘤坏死存在足够长时间时，可以被纤维化替代。坏死几乎局限于非特殊组织学类型肿瘤（非特殊型导管癌），在那些高级别病变中最常见[359,443]，且与基底细胞表型相关[297]。很少有人研究出现坏死的浸润癌的实际比例。Carter等[444]给出的数据是40%，而Fisher等[359]的数据是60%。然而，后一组数据将原位癌的坏死也包括在内，所以是过高评估了。

一些研究已评估了肿瘤坏死作为潜在预后因素的作用。Carter等[444]显示有肿瘤坏死的患者10年生存率下降，Fisher等[332]发现坏死与早期的治疗失败有关。最近，Parham及其同事[445]在小范围形态学研究中发现广泛坏死与生存率低密切相关。遗憾的是这些研究都没有给出所用术语如广泛坏死的精确定义，因此限制了它们的价值。Parham及其同事根据肿瘤坏死和分裂象计数提出了乳腺癌的分级办法[446]。作者宣称与生存率有很好的相关性，但是仅提供了很少的数据，尤其是所采用的诊断标准，因此缺乏实用价值。

总之，有些证据指出肿瘤坏死是较差的预后指征，但是需要更详细的研究来产生可重复的坏死程度评判，并且与其他预后因素进行对照，尤其是组织学分级。

间质特征

在浸润性乳腺癌中，间质结缔组织的数量变化很大[445,447]。间质的预后意义还不肯定，发表的数据也不一致。因此，在主观或半定量研究中，间质纤维化与预后结果不一致，有的认为预后较好[448]，有的认为生存率较差[449]，有的则认为对短期和长期生存率没有显著影响[389]。最近，Parham及其同事[445]对少数患者进行了形态学测量，得出的结论是肿瘤/间质比高的病例比肿瘤/间质比低的病例预后好。肿瘤类型是一个混杂因素，因为广泛纤维化既可以出现在低级别肿瘤（如小管癌），又可以出现在高级别非特殊型导管癌。因此，间质纤维化可能不具有独立的预后意义。

乳腺癌间质中另一个可变成分是弹力组织。弹力纤维以两种基本形式分布：导管周和弥漫分布[450]。前者的弹力纤维围绕闭合的残留导管，呈同心圆状排列，而后者的纤维呈不同程度的聚集，特殊染色有助于发现（如Van Gieson弹力染色）。与间质纤维化病例一样，弹力纤维增生和预后的关系也不一致。一些研究显示存在弹力纤维增生的病例预后好[451,452]，但没有被其他研究证实[453,454]。Giri等[455]发现肿瘤中心弹力纤维增生有较大的临床意义，但结果是根据小样本研究得出，随访时间较短。弹力纤维增生与特殊类型肿瘤（如小管癌、混合型小管癌、浸润性筛状型）[213]有关，这些类型本身预后较好。这表明肿瘤中存在弹力纤维不是一个独立的预后因素。

广泛性原位癌　Extensive in situ component（EIC）

与浸润癌伴发的导管原位癌（DCIS）的量差别很大，评估其程度具有高度主观性。一些研究显示浸润癌中出现较多 DCIS 成分，其预后较好且淋巴结转移率较低[456,457]。然而，Millis 及其同事[458]发现大多数病例的原位癌和浸润癌分级一致（例如，低级别 DCIS 与低级别浸润癌相伴发），在评价 EIC 的独立预后作用中像是一个混淆因素。研究表明 EIC 在接受保守手术的浸润性癌患者的处理中可能有重要作用。1989 年欧洲癌症治疗研究组织共识会议上提出"乳腺保守治疗后复发的首要危险因素是肿瘤残留较多，而且主要来源于 EIC"[459]。这个观点是根据一些研究结果得出的[178,460-462]，但是后来波士顿研究组发表的文章对其正确性提出疑问[463]。他们发现切除的完整性是影响局部复发率的最有力因素，如果获得彻底切除，EIC 就不是预后因素。但是，EIC 确实能预示边缘受累的可能性，因而有一定参考价值。

乳腺癌的分子学预后因素(prognostic factor)和预测因素(predictive factor)

预后因素虽然不能作为治疗反应的特殊预言者，但可以为恶性肿瘤患者提供正确的治疗选择。那些肿瘤切除后预后很好的患者，可能不需要进行有害的辅助治疗，因辅助治疗本身就有明显的致病率。相反，那些预后差的患者可以得益于积极的辅助治疗。因为疾病的病程相差很远，发现浸润性乳腺癌的预后特征尤其重要[464]。一些"可治愈"的乳腺癌妇女，不会从辅助治疗中获得明显好处[465]，而另一些患者会迅速死于这种疾病。由于临床结局的差异和乳腺癌的普遍性，其预后因素在近期内得到了很广泛的研究。

乳腺癌中有关传统组织学预后因素的评估和作用已在前文论述。有关原发乳腺癌预后因素的许多最新研究是在检测新的变量。形态学、免疫组织化学或生物化学变量，至少在试验中表明与肿瘤的浸润、转移、分化或生长速度有关。因此，细胞粘附分子如整合素[466]和粘附素、蛋白酶、金属蛋白酶、生长因子及其受体[467]、激素受体[468]、肿瘤抑制基因如 $p53$[469]和包括 $c\text{-}erbB2$ 状态在内的癌基因[470]都已做过评估。其他研究也检测了肿瘤细胞 DNA 含量和乳腺癌增生指数。后者可以通过免疫组化检查，通过主观或图像分析显示 MIB1/Ki67 抗原的核阳性比例[471,472]，也可采用其他方法如胸苷和溴脱氧尿苷标记指数来评估。其中一些研究发现，在单变量分析中，这些分子学标志物与原发乳腺癌患者的预后有明显的相关性。然而，由于新的治疗方法针对特殊的细胞机制（例如生长控制或调节），需要相应的实验来识别肿瘤中这些通路的激活和放大。

乳腺癌中，雌激素受体（ER）是用于预测特殊治疗反应的最佳例证。由于它与组织学分级密切相关，在提示乳腺癌预后中不具有独立的意义。尽管如此，我们对所有浸润性乳腺癌常规进行 ER 评估，作为激素治疗反应的预测因素[473]。

雌激素受体　Estrogen receptor

类固醇激素能特异性地与细胞内受体密切结合。这些类固醇受体属于蛋白"超家族"，其功能是控制其他指定基因的转录[474]。类固醇受体如雌激素和孕激素受体定位于细胞核内。激素要弥散或转移至核内，与位于此处的类固醇受体二聚体形成复合体。一些由类固醇受体调节的基因在控制细胞生长中起作用，而目前大家认为这些作用与雌激素对乳腺癌行为和治疗的影响十分相关。

约 30% 的非选择性乳腺癌患者对激素治疗如卵巢切除术（或化学去势）或他莫昔芬治疗有反应。放射标记的雌二醇能与某些乳腺癌标本结合，这种效应与激素撤离反应有关[475]，导致了激素受体分析的发展，用于发现适合激素治疗的患者。通过单独对雌激素受体的分析（在组织细胞液标本中采用标准的放射配体结合分析），50%~60% 的雌激素受体阳性患者会出现治疗反应，而雌激素受体阴性的肿瘤患者仅观察到 <10% 的反应性[476]。历史上，激素受体 IHC 检测法出现之前，生化法检测雌激素受体的阳性阈值通常为 10fmol/mg 细胞液蛋白。我们发现如果肿瘤患者的受体水平高达数百 fmol/mg，治疗反应将超过 80%。反应的预测可通过联合雌激素与孕激素分析进一步得到提高[476]。ER、PR 均阳性的肿瘤患者有 78% 反应，ER 阳性 PR 阴性者有 34% 反应，ER 阴性 PR 阳性者有 45% 反应，ER 阴性 PR 阴性肿瘤有 10% 反应[476]。应该注意这些数据与配体结合分析系统有关，而且与 ER 和 PR 免疫组织化学分析所得结果可能不同。

分析方法

直到 20 世纪 80 年代后期，细胞液配体结合分析是标准的分析方法，但是有一些缺陷。尤其是它需要大量的组织匀浆，而且绝经前妇女高水平的内源性雌二醇也会影响受体的结合。20 世纪 80 年代，受体蛋白特异性单克隆抗体的出现[477]带动了酶免疫分析[478]和免疫细胞化学分析的发展[479,480]。最近，免疫细胞化学方法尽管还不容易计量，但是已经超越了配体结合和酶免疫生物化学分析，因为它们需要较少的组织，能够进行组织学评估，可减少取材失误[479,481-490]，而且可用于细针穿刺小标本[468,491]。所有这些形式的分析结果符合率很好[468,482,484,488,490,491]，但有些证据表明，免疫细胞化学结果与激素治疗反应的关系更密切[468,481,482]，可能是因为避免了取材失误和肿瘤细胞密度、类型的影响。

免疫细胞化学分析
Immunocytochemical assay

现代免疫细胞化学方法使用微波或压力锅进行抗原修复，高敏感性抗体和现代的 IHC 显色系统可成功地应用到常规制备的甲醛固定组织中[492-495]。

这些技术能将现代抗体成功应用于常规制备的组织标本中，使得雌激素受体状态的评估能作为乳腺癌组织学评估的一部分。在我们研究中心，这种方法[490]目前已为所有的原发性乳腺癌患者采用，使雌激素受体状态作为标准病理报告的一部分，而且这已成为英国皇家病理学院乳腺癌基本数据的一部分[5]。

用这些抗体评估 ER 状态，如果采用微波对组织进行预处理，与其他评估方式得出的结果相近，而且还有许多优点，尤其是可用于常规组织学标本[490]，方法简单、迅速。

雌激素受体是一种不耐热的不稳定核蛋白，为水溶性，肿瘤切除后半衰期很短。如果采用微波预消化，大多数组织固定液可用于保存受体反应性。然而，必须确保快速固定，肿瘤标本切除后应该立即切开以保证固定液能迅速穿透。此外，固定迅速的粗针活检样本可以作为外科切除组织的替代物。

对照 Controls

在激素受体分析中必需设立对照组织，因为会出现假阴性分级的危险。阳性对照组织不仅包括已知的强阳性组织块，还要有弱阳性组织块以确保敏感性；理想状态是受检组织块中有正常乳腺小叶和导管作为内对照，因为其中一部分应该表现阳性反应（见图 16.72）。采用内对照是为了防止固定不好导致的结果。

染色评估

雌激素和孕激素受体定位于乳腺上皮和癌细胞的细胞核（图 16.72）。目前对激素受体免疫细胞化学分析还没有国际认可的评分系统。肿瘤细胞阳性比例、反应强

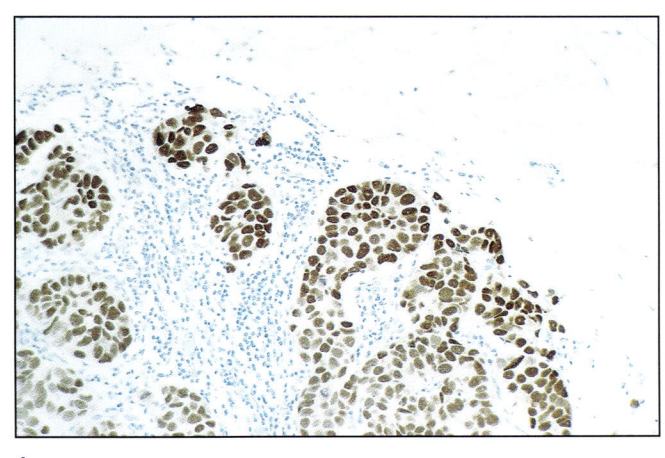

A

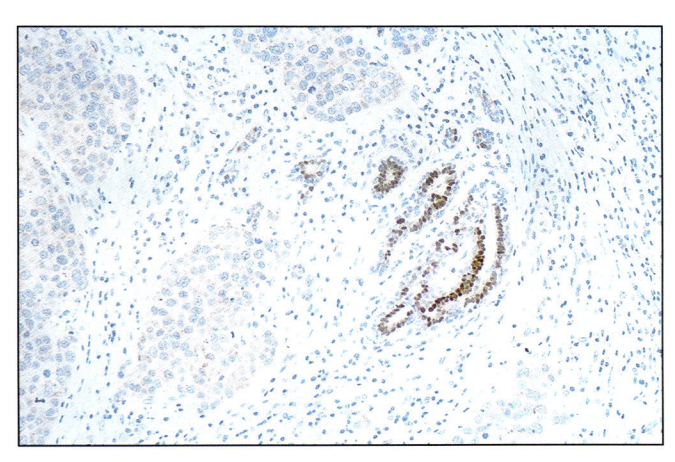

B

图16.72 雌激素受体免疫细胞化学反应，第一例显示核强阳性反应（A），而第二例没有核反应表明为阴性（B）。注意（B）中作为内对照的邻近正常乳腺上皮阳性。

度、二者联合评估（H-评分）[480]、简单分类[496]和"Quick评分"[497]系统都已提出过。目前的商业抗体可提供染色方法的帮助。欣慰的是实际上所有的评分方法都有预后作用[498]。

目前主要使用两种评分系统，H-评分和Quick评分系统，二者都兼顾反应细胞的强度和比例。H-评分依据肿瘤细胞阳性比例和反应强度乘积的总和；反应强度分为没有反应=0，弱反应=1，中等反应=2，强反应=3。如果100%肿瘤细胞都表现强阳性，那么就得出最高值300分。

许多实验室都采用相对简单的Quick评分系统。这是根据染色的比例和强度进行评估：

比例评分
0= 无着色
1= ＜1% 核着色
2= 1% ～ 10% 核着色
3= 11% ～ 33% 核着色
4= 34% ～ 66% 核着色
5= 67% ～ 100% 核着色

强度评分
0= 无着色
1= 弱着色
2= 中等着色
3= 强着色

总评分最大值为8。肿瘤评分≤2被认为ER阴性，几乎没有治疗反应。评价乳腺癌激素受体水平有以下几个原因：

1. 许多数据与转移癌的治疗相关，受体水平越高，对内分泌治疗反应的可能性越大；
2. 受体阴性的乳腺癌患者几乎没有激素治疗反应的可能；
3. 判定孕激素受体也有价值，即对于雌激素受体水平较低而孕激素受体水平较高的患者，内分泌治疗也有意义；
4. 染色水平很低（Quick评分=2）的乳腺癌患者，也可能从辅助内分泌治疗中获益[497]。这里强调需要有能检测很低水平蛋白表达的敏感性、可重复性技术。

临床应用

采用Quick评分或H-评分等半定量方法，能得到一个受反应强度影响的分值，这与通过生物化学方法评估出的受体量有关[490,487]。有经验的临床医生开始不仅关注基于常见临界点或阈值获得的标准结果，而且也关注敏感性和特异性等参数。评价在不同临界点的敏感性和特异性分析是可能的，因此不同的临床情况下要选择不同的阈值[490,487]。举例来说，当需要选择辅助激素治疗的敏感性时，低阈值可能比较合适；相反，年龄较大或患有进展性肿瘤的患者，选择一线激素治疗需要的是特异性，因此需要较高的阈值。

HER-2（C-erbB2 HER-2/neu）

研究证明HER-2/neu(c-erbB2)单克隆抗体trastuzumab（Herceptin）对HER-2蛋白过表达的肿瘤细胞有强效抑制作用。两项关键的大规模多中心试验报道，预先联合Herceptin化疗能使16%的c-erbB2过表达患者发生明确反应（8%完全缓解）[499]，当与其他化疗药物联合使用时反应率提高[500]。近期也在辅助性研究中发现了相似的明确结果[501]。适合这种靶向治疗的患者需要通过免疫细胞化学证实HER-2蛋白过表达（图16.73）或通过荧光原位杂交证实基因扩增。

HER-2免疫细胞化学分析　甲醛固定石蜡包埋的肿瘤组织样本可用于这种分析。最好使用缓冲甲醛溶液固定，Bouin固定液会影响荧光原位杂交。其他组织固定方法也可对抗原反应产生负面影响。

一些国家认为，提供检测服务的实验室应当每年都有一定数量的HER-2免疫组织化学检测；英国推荐每年最少250例[502]。有证据显示检测量较大的基准实验室(reference laboratory)，其检测结果的一致性较高[503,504]。这样一个检测数量能保证检测者的水平。检测数量较少（每年＜250例）的中心应当考虑采用基准实验室的服务。

免疫组织化学（IHC）和荧光原位杂交（FISH）是目前推荐使用的判定HER-2状态的方法[502]。其他HER-2检测技术[显色原位杂交(CISH)、聚合酶链反应、酶联免疫吸附分析、Southern印迹]也可使用，但没有被广泛采用。就免疫组织化学和FISH相关的HER-2检测而言，方法的全面标准化（包括评分监测、有效对照）都是必需的。参与外部质量评估与规范对保持结果的一致性也很重要[502,505]。

对于IHC为0/1+和3+的病例，IHC和FISH结果的一致性非常高，因此大多数病例不需要进行IHC和FISH双重检测[506,507]；而其余的研究显示较高的不一致性。这些资料表明，对于模糊的（2+）IHC结果需要进一步使用FISH检测来澄清HER-2状态。

对照　为了保证检测的准确性，对照的设置和监测是必需的。至少包括阳性对照、临界点对照和阴性对照。已知HER-2状态的多种细胞系样本可作为FISH和IHC

的有用对照[508]。如果可能，设立乳腺癌的组织对照更加合适，每批检查都应使用。通过评价作为内对照的正常乳腺上皮细胞可以监测抗原修复过度。如果在正常细胞出现膜反应，可能发生了抗原修复过度，应当考虑整批重新检测。

HER-2免疫组织化学分析评分 当进行IHC检测评分时，只有浸润性肿瘤的膜染色才被计数。如果使用商品化的试剂盒分析系统，应严格按照试剂盒分析步骤和评分方法。技术变更可导致假阳性和假阴性结果。推荐的评分方法是一种根据反应产物的强度和膜阳性细胞百分比的半定量系统，给出0~3+的分值范围（表16.3）。评分3+的样本看作明确的阳性，而评分0/1+的样本认为是阴性。交界性评分2+需要使用另一种分析系统，最好是FISH。

HER-2 FISH分析 对HER-2(ERBB2)的FISH检测应该符合以下标准[502]：

1. 方法的全面标准化。
2. 有效的对照设置，许多实验室将17号染色体对照包括在内，能够纠正17号染色体数目变化引起的HER-2信号变化（见于超过50%的病例）。
3. 有效的评分方法。

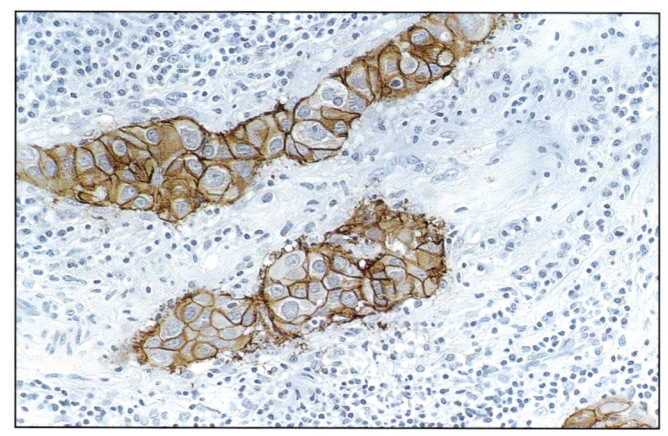

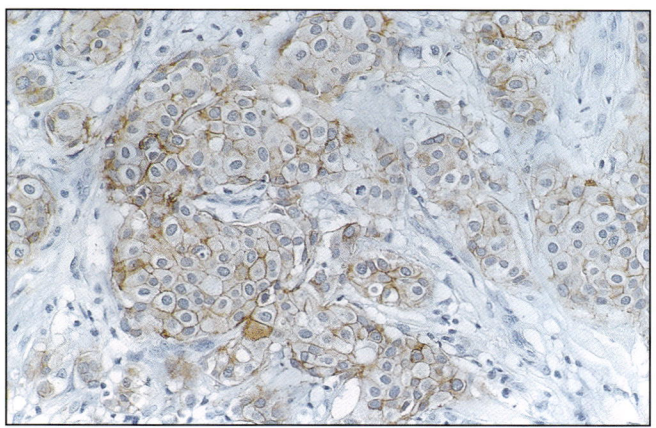

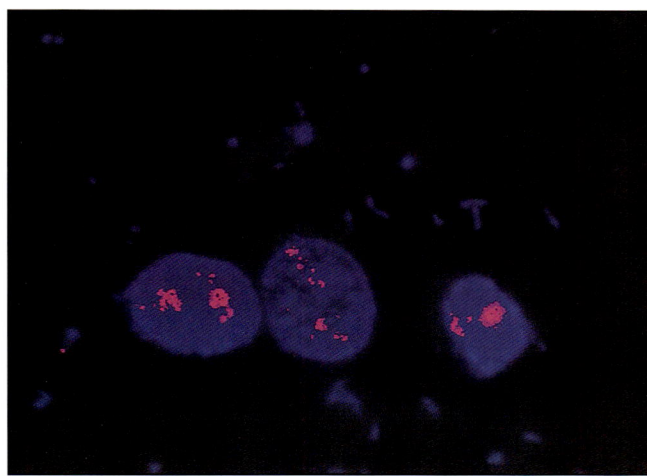

图16.73 两个肿瘤的HER-2 neu免疫细胞化学染色。（A）显示较强的完全的肿瘤细胞膜染色，这与基因扩增和Herceptin治疗反应有关。（B）表现为微弱的局灶的不完全膜反应，这与基因扩增无关，认为是阴性。（C）A例的FISH分析表明HER-2 ERBB2信号显著扩增。

表16.3	推荐的HER-2免疫组织化学评分方法	
报告评分	HER-2蛋白过表达评估	染色模式
0	阴性	无着色，或不到10%的肿瘤细胞膜着色
1+	阴性	超过10%的肿瘤细胞有微弱的/略能辨认的膜着色。仅部分细胞膜着色
2+	交界性	超过10%的肿瘤细胞可见微弱至中等的完全膜着色
3+	阳性	超过10%的肿瘤细胞可见强而完全的膜着色

组织消化应该标准化以保证核的形态，应严格遵守操作规程[509]。一些实验室发现杂交之前评估核结构并适当调整消化，对保存核的完整性很有帮助。这对疑难切片、细胞学样本、骨活检等尤其有用。杂交和冲洗步骤应该标准化。自动组织处理机和标准化商品化的组织消化试剂盒可提高一致性，应该考虑使用。推荐使用被认可的商品化探针或试剂盒。

HER-2 FISH 分析的评分 建议使用 HE 染色的连续切片来确定浸润性肿瘤的部位，检测后也用它定位要评分的肿瘤区域。应该小心避开导管原位癌区域，因为即使邻近的浸润癌细胞阴性它也可能显示扩增。如有经验，这些特征可在荧光显微镜下发现。然而，如果有任何不确定性，就要参考连续的 HE 切片。

HER-2 FISH 检测结果通常使用 HER-2 信号与 17 号染色体信号的比值来表示。比值 > 2 的肿瘤为阳性。对于不使用 17 号染色体探针的病例，HER-2 基因扩增的临界值还没有确定。计数 20～60 个细胞的 17 号染色体和 HER-2 信号，最好在 3 个不同的肿瘤视野中进行，从而计算 HER-2 与 17 号染色体的平均比值。大多数病例，当可见明显的扩增或比值低于 1.5 时，计数 20 个细胞就足够了。当肿瘤出现异质性(1%～2% 的病例)或比值接近 2.0（1.5～2.3）的肿瘤，要计数较多的细胞(达到 60 个)。每条 17 号染色体的 HER-2 复制数 > 2.0 的样本被认为是扩增。

预后因素的应用

病理学实验室在乳腺癌患者的诊断和预后判断中起主要作用。目前，最有价值的预后因素表现为能在常规固定、处理和染色的样本中进行评估的指标：组织学分级、淋巴结分期、肿瘤大小、脉管浸润和肿瘤类型。这些特征的准确评估需要高质量的 HE 切片。综合这些组织学特征能够预测每个患者的生存情况。预测特殊治疗反应的其他信息可以从免疫组化结果中获得；尤其是 ER 可以发现能够从激素治疗中获益的患者，与此相似，HER-2 阳性也是 HER-2 靶向治疗的一个必要条件。希望将来能发现对特殊治疗反应的其他标志物，使患者能根据各自的肿瘤及时开展最适合的治疗。

Nottingham 预后指数
Nottingham Prognostic Index

虽然某些单一预后因素可能非常有效，但目前逐渐认识到，以指数形式综合一系列预后变量的结果可能在判断预后方面有较高的准确性，而且可以区分适合不同治疗的各组患者。例如，长期预后很好的患者，其生存期与年龄匹配的对照妇女相似，不可能从辅助化疗中获益，只需要手术切除就能获得满意的结果。

Nottingham 预后指数得到最广泛的认可，其采用淋巴结分期、肿瘤大小和组织学分级这 3 个预后因素[335,336,510]。这是从一系列多变量分析中（包括时间依赖性和生物学变量）得出来的。指数公式很简单：

$$\text{Nottingham 预后指数（NPI）} = [\text{大小 (cm)} \times 0.2] + \text{淋巴结分期}（1\sim3）+ \text{分级}（1\sim3）$$

在临床实践中，可发现 3 个预后组：预后好组（评分 < 3.4）；中等预后组（评分为 3.4～5.4）；预后差组（评分 > 5.4）。三组的 15 年生存率分别为 80%、42% 和 13%。年龄相配的对照组妇女的 15 年生存率为 83%。NPI 的主要优势是得到 NTPBCS 的证实[510]。并且在 2 项大的多中心研究中进一步证实[511,512]。Danish 乳腺协作组研究[512]包括 9000 多个患者，值得注意的是组织学分级是在 32 个独立的病理科进行的，肯定了其作为预后因素的有效性。

对于这些预后因素的应用和整合已有正面的关键性评估[513]，NPI 被越来越多地应用于乳腺癌患者系统性治疗的分层，尤其是在英国[514]。因为是基于传统病理学因素，可以在大多数病理科施行。

最早的 NPI 相关研究来源于 1973～1987 年在 Nottingham 治疗的患者。在这段时间内辅助性治疗没有常规使用。1987 年，我们改变了 Nottingham 的治疗策略，要求对标本进行更仔细的病理检查，改良了手术程序，回顾了放疗原则，引入了真正适合的辅助激素治疗和辅助化疗。这些重要的治疗变革改善了所有预后组的生存期，包括那些目前不给予辅助性激素化疗的患者（表 16.4）。因此，我们认为生存率的提高是因为治疗策略的总体改善，而不是归因于任何单一因素（如辅助治疗的使用）。

治疗效果

化疗 Chemotherapy

对乳腺肿瘤多种药物化疗的效果少有描述。Kennedy 等描述了环磷酰胺、阿霉素、妊娠雌酮、甲氨蝶呤、5-氟尿嘧啶、他莫昔芬和甲酰四氢叶酸治疗前后的组织学特征[515]。在肿瘤附近的"正常"乳腺，常见类似于绝经后的退化改变，尤其是脂肪组织替代退化的小叶和间质。肿瘤细胞改变与临床反应有很强的相关性。反应不明显的患者很少出现治疗后改变。对化疗有反应的患者，最常见的是肿瘤细胞形态学和排列的改变。肿瘤细胞呈现良性组织细胞样表现，而且在间质中表现为

表16.4	NPI值与患者预后的关系		
预后组	NPI值	10年生存率（%）1973~1987年患者	10年生存率（%）1990~1996年患者
很好	≤2.4	94	95
好	≤3.4	83	91
中等1	≤4.4	70	80
中等2	≤5.4	51	70
差	≤6.4	19	45
很差	>6.4		33

单个散在细胞。其他特征还包括巨大核、多核、核深染、粗糙染色质聚集和核轮廓模糊。巨大核和多核并存良性上皮非典型性，但这些细胞有清楚的核膜，小核仁，核深染不明显。非典型性和正常细胞的混合出现、缺乏坏死、保留连续的肌上皮层等均有助于区分细胞学非典型性和残留癌。

激素治疗　　Hormone therapy

有关激素治疗组织学效果的报道也较少。上述研究结果也适用于激素治疗的研究[515]。在23%的病例中，作者见到肿瘤细胞呈泪滴样和空泡变，被认为是激素治疗（他莫昔芬）造成的，证据是月经周期中或接受高血压和抗精神病药物的正常乳腺也有类似的改变[516-518]。

放射治疗　　Radiotherapy

Schnitt等[519]描述了乳腺放射治疗后的表现。非肿瘤性乳腺显示与化疗后相似的改变，包括小叶硬化、萎缩和上皮非典型性，也会出现其他部位放疗后的相关改变，例如非典型性间质纤维母细胞和血管改变。TDLU中也可发现高度异型的细胞，如果并发明显的小叶纤维化，会呈现一种假浸润形态而酷似浸润癌。低倍镜下，小叶中心性轮廓对识别这些良性改变有用。尽管细胞核增大、深染，但核仁小，而且没有增生的证据。与残留导管内癌的鉴别也可能很困难。支持恶性诊断的特征是存在增生证据，如细胞重叠、极性消失、分裂象、受累导管和腺泡扩张、坏死等[60]。肿瘤细胞核有明显的核仁，染色质分布不规则。

少见的上皮性肿瘤　　Rare epithelial tumors

腺肌上皮瘤　　Adenomyoepithelioma

上皮和肌上皮细胞同时增生在乳头状瘤和硬化性腺病中很常见。近年来一些作者提出存在一种罕见的明确的实体肿瘤，称为腺肌上皮瘤[520-523]。肌上皮增生通常比其他病变（如乳头状瘤）更明显，但还没有统一的诊断标准，而且一些病例可能会被归入更常见类型，如导管腺瘤。

临床特征

实际上所有报道的腺肌上皮瘤病例都表现为可触及的肿物，偶尔伴有浆液性乳头溢液。年龄范围20~90岁。

腺肌上皮瘤通常为良性病变[524]，报道的复发率约10%[520,522]。恶性病变也很少发生转移扩散[525]。单纯的恶性肌上皮病变（肌上皮癌/恶性肌上皮瘤）也很少转移扩散[526-528]。

大体表现

腺肌上皮瘤通常呈结节状，界限清楚，切面灰白或棕褐色，大小可达7cm。

组织学表现

腺肌上皮瘤通常以实性而不是以腺体为主。有两种细胞类型。肌上皮细胞通常是主要成分。这些细胞多角形或梭形，细胞浆透明或嗜酸，形成腺体区的外层结构。免疫组织化学显示肌动蛋白和S-100阳性[524]。腺体成分由柱状或立方形细胞组成，细胞角蛋白和上皮膜抗原阳性。可出现坏死。

分类

Tavassoli[522]提出用肌上皮增生症（myoepitheliosis）这个术语来描述这样一种疾病，通常为多灶性，累及外周导管系统，以上皮下的圆形或梭形肌上皮细胞增生为特征。这些增生可以突向导管腔形成乳头状突起。肌上皮增生症与其他病变如乳头状瘤存在形态学交叉，使其意义受限。

Tavassoli及其同事[521]还描述了腺肌上皮瘤的梭形

细胞、小管状和分叶状亚型。在梭形细胞型中，肌上皮成分占优势，细胞呈梭形。与平滑肌瘤的鉴别在于发现衬覆上皮的腺腔。小管型实际上与小管腺瘤难以区分，因为它是由被覆双层肌上皮和上皮细胞的腺体结构聚集而成，境界清楚（图 16.74）。分叶型中，肌上皮细胞较肥胖，常有嗜酸性胞浆。它们成群排列，形成病变的结构特征。常伴有纤维化，同样呈分叶状形态。相似的纤维反应常包绕肿瘤。Tavassoli 认为小管型易于复发。

恶性腺肌上皮瘤有 2 种形式[525]。第一种是在典型的腺肌上皮瘤中可见明显的恶性区域。第二种是总体形态为腺肌上皮瘤，高倍镜下可见灶状细胞异型和分裂象增加。上述两型（包括转移灶）的恶性成分可以是上皮、肌上皮或两种的混合[521,522,525]。腺肌上皮瘤还与腺鳞癌相关[324]。

恶性肌上皮病变（肌上皮癌/恶性肌上皮瘤）[527,528]以梭形细胞肌上皮成分为主。这些异型细胞表现出多形性和较多分裂象。呈浸润性边缘。免疫组化显示肌动蛋白、细胞角蛋白阳性，有时 S-100 蛋白也呈阳性。相似的形态学和免疫表型可见于梭形细胞癌，使得鉴别诊断非常困难。

伴有大汗腺腺病的腺肌上皮瘤
Adenomyoepithelioma with apocrine adenosis

Eusebi 和 Kiaer 用腺肌上皮瘤这个术语来描述具有明显组织学特征的一组不同病变[95,523]。由 Eusebi 描述的两例发生于年龄较大的妇女，均表现为乳腺肿物。肿瘤切面质硬，一例境界清楚，另一例界限不清。肿瘤由两种不同类型的细胞巢组成（图 16.75）。多数细胞小而一致，伴有透明的细胞浆，有些区域细胞融合成片。在细胞巢中心出现第二种细胞，是具有大汗腺形态的柱状细胞，它们形成腺腔。透明细胞群表现肌动蛋白阳性反应，而且具有肌上皮细胞的超微结构。腺上皮细胞表达低分子量细胞角蛋白，产生丰富的耐淀粉酶消化的 PAS 阳性物质。腺上皮与肌上皮的比例在不同肿瘤之间以及同一肿瘤的不同区域差别很大。Eusebi 报道的病例缺少随访信息，但 Kiaer 等[95]描述的另一例表现为低度恶性，尽管经过了完整的局部切除还会多次复发。肿瘤表现为局部浸润，边界不清。

鉴别诊断

乳腺肌上皮肿瘤中描述的广泛的形态变化，会引起与其他良性肿瘤包括乳头状瘤、导管腺瘤、小管腺病、

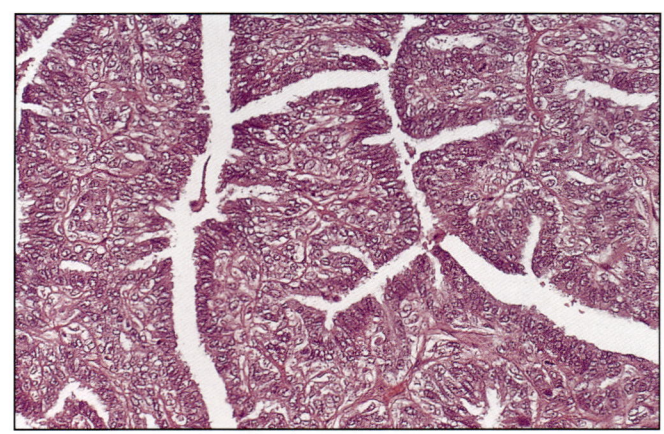

图16.74　腺肌上皮瘤。伴有显著肌上皮增生的导管内病变。

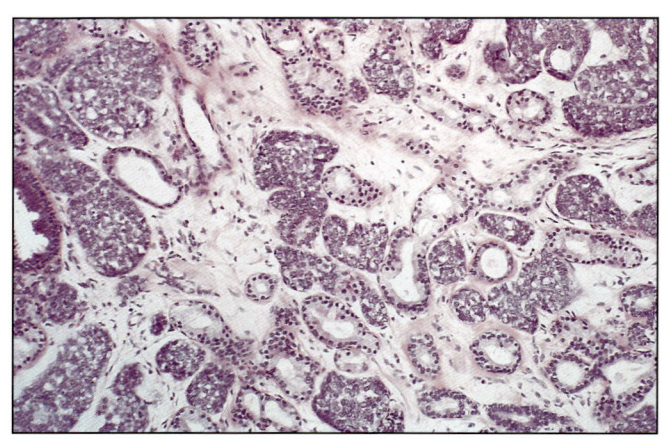

图16.75　伴有大汗腺腺病的腺肌上皮瘤。这是非常特殊的肿瘤，具有两种不同成分。腺体结构衬覆透明或大汗腺上皮细胞，而另一种小细胞（肌上皮）成群或成片排列。

硬化性腺病和复合硬化性病变的鉴别问题。某些病例的鉴别是主观的，取决于专家的经验和观点。我们的经验是对这些很好识别的、良性病变之外的病例，要采用严格的腺肌上皮瘤诊断标准。

当肿瘤细胞大而多形时，单纯的梭形细胞肌上皮肿瘤可能与梭形细胞癌相似；当肿瘤细胞小而规则时，则与平滑肌瘤或纤维瘤病相似。如上所述，与梭形细胞癌的鉴别很困难。纤维瘤病具有特征性的浸润形态，梭形细胞形态一致呈编织状。单纯梭形细胞肌上皮瘤的细胞通常比纤维瘤病见到的细胞大且不一致。

涎腺型肿瘤
Tumors of salivary gland type

乳腺可以发生多种类似涎腺腺体和支气管组织所发生的肿瘤。包括多形性腺瘤、腺样囊性癌和黏液表皮样癌。

多形性腺瘤（混合瘤）
Pleomorphic adenoma (mixed tumor)

临床特征

这些肿瘤表现为明确的可触及的肿物或影像学上的可疑包块[529]。患者年龄范围40～90岁，更常见于绝经后妇女。

尚不确定它们是真正的独特的肿瘤，还是伴有间质软骨化生的导管腺瘤或导管内乳头状瘤。

大体表现

病变单发或多发，直径大小在1～4cm之间。病变界限清楚，有时分叶状，切面白色或黄色，质韧。

组织学表现

根据定义，多形性腺瘤至少包括3种成分：上皮细胞、肌上皮细胞和软骨黏液样组织（图16.76）。上皮成分可形成腺泡状或导管状结构，可以呈岛状或条索状排列。细胞异型性轻微，没有明显的分裂活性。肌上皮成分邻近软骨黏液样组织区域，可以是肿瘤的主要成分。软骨黏液样间质组织可能包括已形成的透明软骨区域，可以出现局部钙化。50%病例可发现骨形成[530,531]。

病变一般境界清楚，可以出现一个胶原丰富的纤维性假包膜。有证据表明来源于伴残留腔隙的乳头状瘤。可以并存非特异性特征，包括上皮增生、硬化性腺病、囊性改变和大汗腺化生。

免疫细胞化学

上皮成分可用低分子量细胞角蛋白，肌上皮成分可用S-100或抗平滑肌肌动蛋白抗体来鉴别。

鉴别诊断

这些病变可以孤立发生，与复杂的导管内乳头状瘤或导管腺瘤不能区分。尝试鉴别这些病变并没有真正的益处。软骨形成可见于多种其他乳腺肿瘤中，如纤维腺瘤、错构瘤、导管内乳头状瘤和导管腺瘤；还可见于一些恶性肿瘤中，包括叶状肿瘤和化生性癌。诊断混合瘤要严格根据良性上皮组织、肌上皮增生和软骨黏液样间质的同时存在。

腺样囊性癌 Adenoid cystic carcinoma

临床特征

这是乳腺肿瘤的罕见类型，临床常表现为肿块性病变，最常见于绝经后患者[532]。肿瘤大小从＜2cm到＞10cm。有极好的长期预后[532]。少数情况下确实会发生转移扩散[533]。局部复发并不明显影响预后[534,535]。临床表现明确，偶尔可有疼痛[536]。

因为与浸润性筛状癌形态很相似，一些专家对乳腺中是否存在这种病变提出疑问[10]。然而，免疫细胞化学和超微结构证据支持乳腺内存在真正的腺样囊性癌[533,537]。

大体表现

肿瘤通常界限清楚，切面质硬、苍白，多数病例大小1～6cm，平均2.5cm[538]。

组织学表现

肿瘤类似浸润性筛状癌（图16.77A），但是可以出现实性区域。乳腺腺样囊性癌的特征与涎腺相应的肿瘤一样，由2种细胞类型组成。这两种细胞是：

1. 呈实性、筛状或小管样排列的小的基底样肌上皮细胞，包绕含基底膜样物质的假腺腔；
2. 围绕真腺腔排列的上皮细胞。

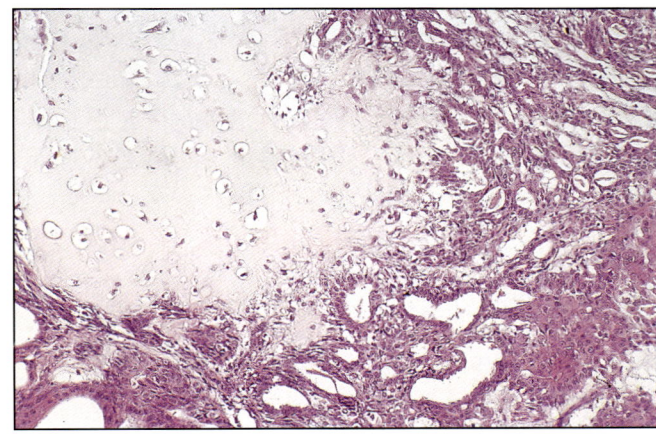

图16.76 多形性腺瘤（混合瘤）。表现为密切混合的腺体结构、肌上皮细胞和软骨黏液样间质。

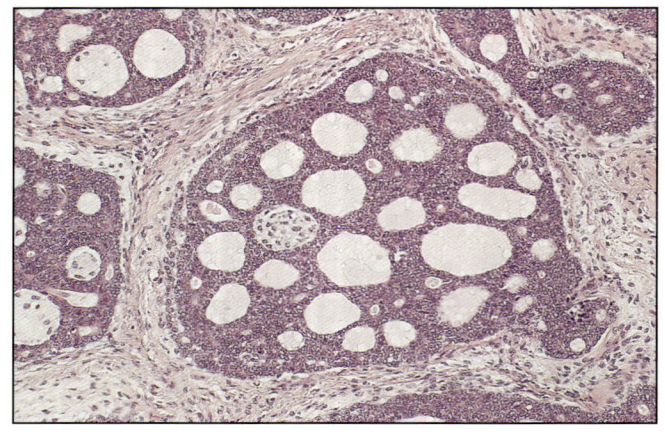

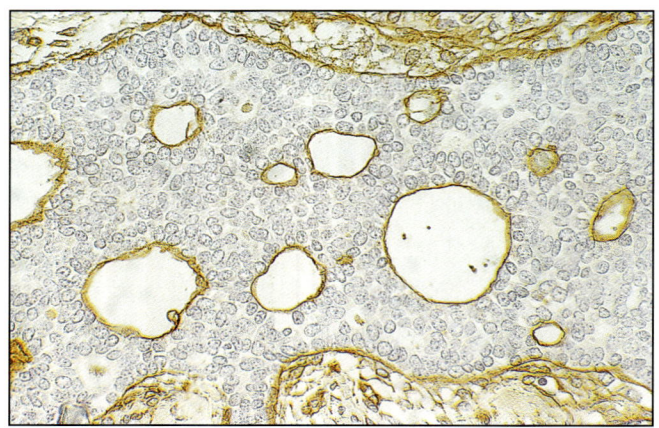

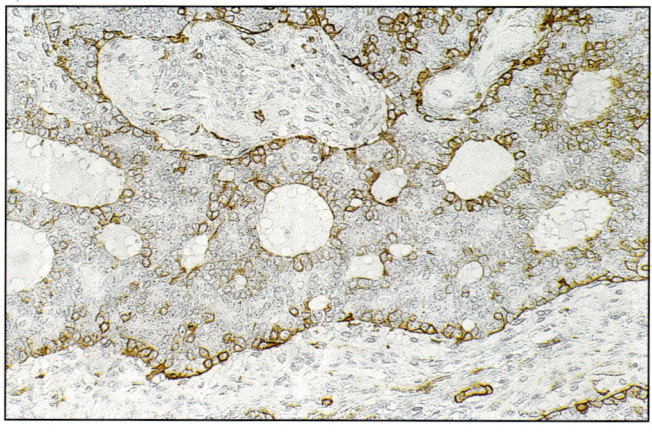

图16.77 腺样囊性癌。肿瘤细胞巢呈筛状结构。组织学可见诊断性的双相细胞群，应用免疫组化更容易发现。基底膜沉积物（层粘连蛋白）可围绕肿瘤细胞巢或位于腔内（B）。肌上皮细胞可应用肌动蛋白免疫染色（C）。

上皮细胞表达细胞角蛋白如 CAM5.2，而肌上皮细胞表达平滑肌肌动蛋白（图 16.77C）和 S-100 蛋白。此外，基底膜物质围绕在肿瘤巢周边或出现在假腺腔内，表达层粘连蛋白和Ⅳ型胶原（图 16.77B）。此型涎腺肿瘤通常不表达 ER、PR 和 HER2/neu。

超微结构

超微结构检查可肯定肿瘤的双相性，显示基底样腺腔和被覆上皮的真腺腔[533,538]。

鉴别诊断

主要的鉴别诊断是乳腺浸润性筛状癌。后者只有上皮细胞，通常有浸润性小管癌典型的小管成分混合存在，显示特征性的间质纤维反应。肿瘤细胞巢可以出现少量的基底膜，通常围绕在肿瘤巢周边。筛状癌通常是雌激素受体强阳性，而大多数腺样囊性癌雌激素受体阴性[539]。

腺泡细胞癌　Acinic cell carcinoma

临床特征

乳腺腺泡细胞癌（见第 7 章）是一种罕见肿瘤，只有 7 例报道[540-542]。累及 35～80 岁（平均 56 岁）的女性[541]，表现为 2～5cm 的可触及的结节。两例出现腋窝淋巴结转移。治疗方式不同，有的实施新辅助化疗加根治性乳腺切除，有的仅实施了肿物切除。有限的随访（最长为 5 年）表明 7 例均未死于肿瘤。

组织学表现

乳腺腺泡细胞癌与腮腺肿瘤相似，表现腺泡细胞（浆液性）分化，伴有酶原型（zymogen-type）细胞浆颗粒，还可出现淀粉酶、溶酶体和 α1-抗糜蛋白酶。

肿瘤并存实性（去分化）、微囊和微腺体区域（图 16.78A）。细胞学上，细胞具有丰富的、颗粒状、嗜碱或嗜酸性胞浆。颗粒粗糙、亮红色，与 Paneth 细胞相似（图 16.78B）。然而，也可出现透明的"肾上腺样"细胞浆。细胞核不规则，圆形或卵圆形，有单个核仁。分裂象计数差别大，可高达 15 个分裂象 /10 个高倍视野[541]。

免疫组织化学

大多数细胞表达抗淀粉酶、溶菌酶、糜蛋白酶、EMA 和 S-100 蛋白[541]。GCDFP-15（黏液顶浆标志物）也可局灶阳性。

组织学很难鉴别这两种细胞类型。黏蛋白染色很有用。假腺腔内容物阿辛蓝着色，而真腺腔则 PAS 阳性。

免疫组织化学

免疫组织化学在表现两种细胞类型方面特别有效。

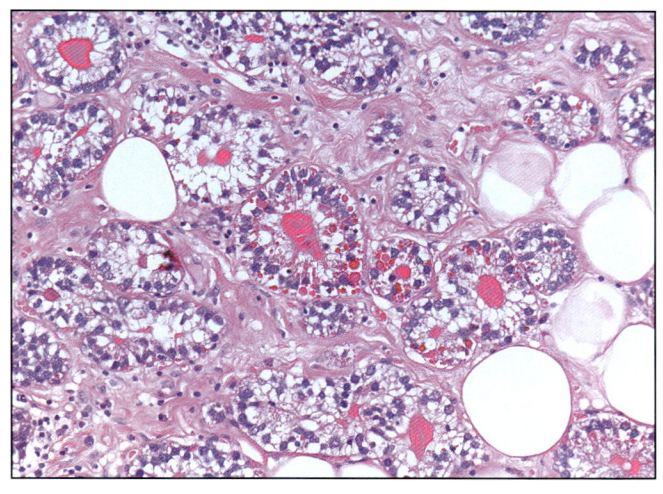

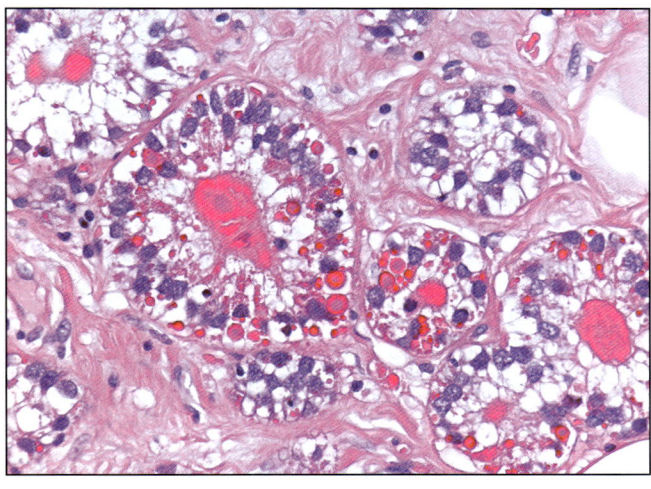

图16.78 一例乳腺腺泡细胞癌，表现为单层上皮细胞构成的腺体弥漫浸润间质。肿瘤没有间质反应。（A）肿瘤细胞具有透明的胞浆，许多含有明显的嗜酸性小球（B）。

乳腺多形性腺瘤和腺样囊性癌更具争议。乳腺黏液表皮样癌极罕见[543]。浸润性乳腺癌能发生局部鳞状分化或化生，尤其在年龄较大的妇女[10]。这两种特征的密切混合是对乳腺黏液表皮样癌的描述。这种肿瘤作为特殊类型的意义也存在疑问。低级别组织学特征与较好的长期预后相关[544,545]。更典型的是，高级别肿瘤中同时存在黏液和鳞状分化，对预后没有特殊的益处。某研究组[546]提出乳腺真正的黏液表皮样肿瘤可通过黏液分泌细胞、鳞状细胞、中间细胞和肌上皮细胞的混合出现来识别。其他研究者表明黏液分泌细胞为主是一个诊断特征[547]。不管怎样，这些病变与导管癌有相似的年龄分布。

大体表现

形态差异大，但是通常与传统的乳腺浸润性腺癌无法区分。

组织学表现

肿瘤呈浸润性，由不同比例的密切混合的肿瘤性鳞状、腺样和中间细胞成分组成。

免疫细胞化学

应用合适的低分子量和高分子量细胞角蛋白抗体可以鉴别鳞状和腺样成分。肌上皮成分可用抗平滑肌肌动蛋白和S-100蛋白抗体识别。角蛋白亚型特征与涎腺相应病变相似[543]。

鉴别诊断

有关这种肿瘤的争论依然存在，但是除了少见的低级别变异型外，没有特定的预后相关性。化生性癌常以未分化的肉瘤样梭形细胞为主，缺乏分化的鳞状成分。年龄较大的腺癌可表现非常多的鳞状化生，与单纯的鳞状细胞癌不能区分。

间质肿瘤　Stromal tumors

良性血管肿瘤　Benign vascular tumors

乳腺良性血管肿瘤罕见，约占乳腺血管病变的1/3。与血管肉瘤的鉴别可能存在问题，因为各级别的血管肉瘤至少局灶可以出现良性的组织学特征，尤其是在肿瘤周边。Rosen的研究组[548-551]已总结了有关乳腺血管肿瘤的经验，在一系列文章中描述了各种良性血管肿瘤。成为目前血管病变最全面的分类。

超微结构

所研究的3个病例，胞浆充满大小为0.08～0.9cm的酶原样颗粒[541]。

黏液表皮样癌
Mucoepidermoid carcinoma

临床特征

有关乳腺是否存在真正黏液表皮样癌的争论可能比

间质肿瘤

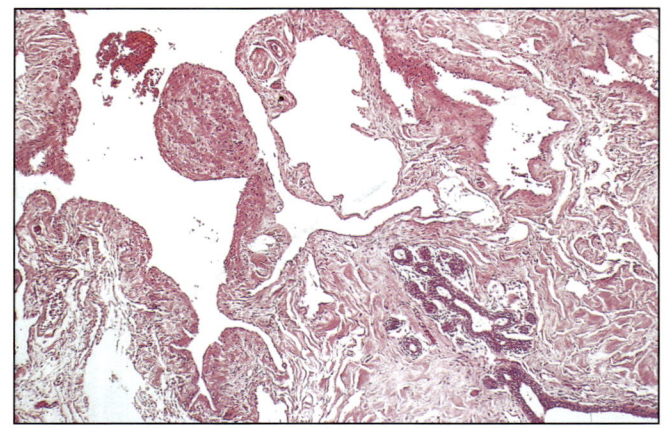

图16.79 静脉血管瘤。乳腺良性血管肿瘤由扩张的大血管组成，一些管壁含有平滑肌。

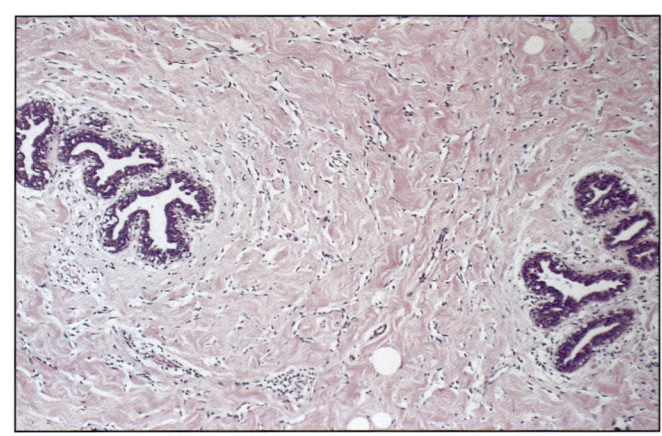

图16.80 乳腺间质的假血管瘤性增生。乳腺小叶外间质细胞丰富，高倍镜下显示类似血管腔的线样裂隙。

静脉血管瘤　Venous hemangioma

这是罕见的乳腺内间质肿瘤，大小1～5cm，由平滑肌围绕的大静脉组成（图16.79）[548]。

血管瘤或小叶周围血管瘤 Hemangioma or perilobular hemangioma

这是大小为2mm～2.5cm的小肿瘤，约半数是在显微镜下偶然发现。界限相对清楚，由梭形细胞套状围绕良性血管组成，附近常可见供血动脉[549]。许多病例局限于小叶周围纤维间质。有些可表现内皮细胞非典型性和吻合性血管腔，使其与1级血管肉瘤难以鉴别。通常小于2cm的乳腺血管肿瘤很少表现为恶性行为。

血管瘤病　Angiomatosis

这是一种非常罕见的（有时是先天的）较大的病变（中位直径9cm），由被覆扁平内皮细胞的非吻合性扩张血管或淋巴管组成，这种病变见于小叶间间质，不累及终末导管小叶单元[550]。

假血管瘤性间质增生 Pseudoangiomatous stromal hyperplasia

正如其名称表明的那样，这并非真正的血管病变。小叶间间质裂隙看上去似乎被覆一层良性的扁平上皮（图16.80）[54,552]。这被认为代表间质纤维母细胞改变，伴有局灶或弥漫的实质改变，如乳腺错构瘤[52]和男性乳腺发育[553]。如果不注意，病变可与血管肉瘤混淆。诊断线索是伴有其他病理改变，免疫组化表现为细胞波形蛋白和CD34阳性[52]，而其他内皮标志如von Willebrand因子、CD31为阴性。

皮下组织病变　Subcutaneous lesions

多种非实质的皮肤或皮下血管病变可误诊为乳腺血管肿瘤。病变包括血管瘤、动静脉畸形和错构瘤[551]。

血管肉瘤　Angiosarcoma

临床特征

乳腺血管肉瘤少见，但却是乳腺最常见的恶性间质肿瘤。常见表现为无痛性肿物，但在一些患者也表现为无肿物的弥漫性乳腺增大，临床表现为血管病变。双侧受累相对常见[554]。尽管血管肉瘤患者年龄跨度很大，但发病高峰在30多岁[554]。总体生存率很差，3年生存率仅为38%，5年生存率为33%[526,554]。组织学分级对于预后评估非常重要。1级（占病例的40%）和2级（占19%）预后好或中等，不同的研究结果不一致；一些研究报道预后很好[526]，而另一些则报道预后差[555]。3级肿瘤的5年生存率普遍认为很差，仅为15%[556]。转移扩散的部位很广泛，但肝、肺、皮肤和对侧乳腺更常见。

大体表现

大小为2cm至11cm之多。小于2cm的恶性肿瘤罕见，但大多数介于2～5cm。低级别肿瘤倾向具有相对均一的血管瘤样切面，而高级别肿瘤变化较大，外周为血管表现，中心实性区域伴有坏死和出血。

组织学表现

大多数乳腺血管肉瘤最重要的组织学特征是存在与血管瘤相似的低级别组织学表现，尤其是在周边部位。在活检或切除标本取材不充分时会导致低诊或误诊。

1级肿瘤由被覆1～2层内皮细胞的相互交通的血管组成，罕见或没有核分裂象（图16.81A）。可见局灶内皮细胞簇和血栓形成。常在脂肪细胞间穿插。没有乳头、实性未分化区、梭形细胞区和坏死。与良性血管瘤难以鉴别。辅助性鉴别特征如下：

1. 肿瘤大小：良性肿瘤一般<2cm，可能是显微镜下发现。血管肉瘤一般>2cm；
2. 良性病变中的血管是不连通的，常被覆扁平、非增生性内皮；
3. 约50%的良性血管瘤病例附近可见非肿瘤性肌性血管[549]；
4. 可见平滑肌围绕良性血管结构。

令人担忧的是，一种罕见的小叶周围血管瘤（大小<2mm）已有描述[549]，表现为一些内皮细胞核异型伴有一些吻合血管增生，而较大（3mm～2.5cm）的肿瘤伴有内皮核异型，但不出现吻合性血管。

2级血管肉瘤（图16.81B）具有混合性结构，显示内皮细胞突起伴有乳头形成和实性梭形细胞成分。乳头状结构中常见分裂象。形态以组织学1级为主，尤其是在肿瘤周边部。形态的多样性进一步强调需要对肿瘤充分取材。

3级肿瘤主要由实性、梭形细胞组成，常缺乏明显的血管腔。出血、坏死、细胞多形和分裂象明显。主要是与其他梭形细胞肿瘤鉴别。

应用免疫细胞化学辨认血管肉瘤已在第3章讨论。

放射后血管肉瘤
Post-radiation angiosarcoma

我们已充分认识到放射引起的肉瘤。保乳术加放射治疗越来越多地用于乳腺癌的治疗，其中大约0.1%会发生放射区的血管肉瘤[557]，皮肤最常见。放射暴露和发生血管肉瘤的时间间隔通常为2.5～10年，有时可能更短[558]。绝大多数病变发生于皮肤或皮下脂肪，少数发生于乳腺实质[558a]。放疗引起的血管肉瘤比原发肉瘤更常见，因为与乳腺癌治疗有关，多见于年龄较大的妇女。非典型血管病变也可发生于放疗后，必须与高分化血管肉瘤鉴别[558]。

淋巴管肉瘤（Stewart-Treves病变）
Lymphangiosarcoma(Stewart-Treves lesion)

这是根治性乳腺切除的少见并发症，通常是在术后10年发生于手术引起的淋巴水肿区，通常是在臂部（见第3章）。一些患者还进行了放疗，可能也是促进因素。肿瘤很具侵袭性，迅速扩散至整个淋巴水肿区并广泛播散全身[559,560]。5年生存率非常低。组织学上，肿瘤由乳头状或实性生长的未分化细胞或上皮样细胞组成。过

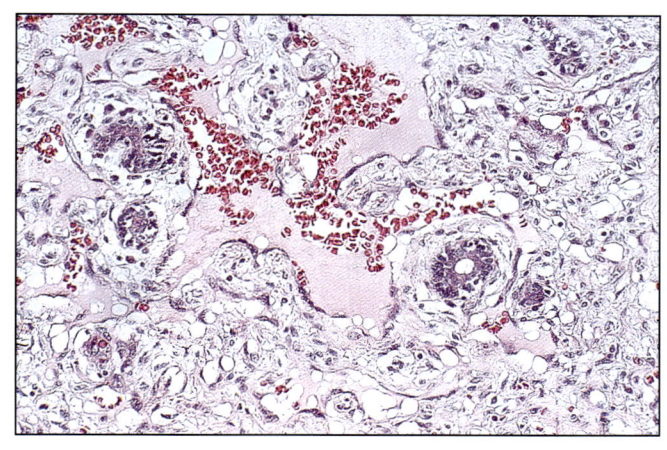

A

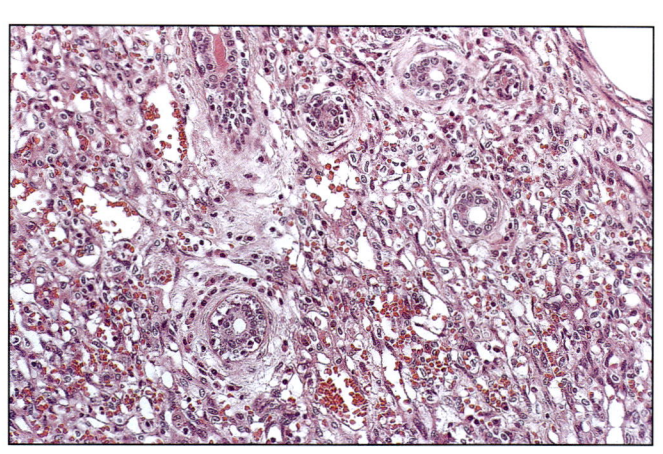

B

图16.81　血管肉瘤。乳腺血管肉瘤周边（A）和中心（B）的显微镜下表现。周边部肿瘤呈低级别表现，具有被覆内皮细胞的大血管。中心部肿瘤呈2级表现，伴有梭形细胞区。

去，这种形态被认为是代表乳腺癌细胞逆行性血管扩散，而不是真正的血管肉瘤。免疫组化和超微结构证实它们为脉管源性[561,562]，最好把它们看作级别很高的淋巴管肉瘤。

其他肉瘤　Other sarcomas

大多数类型的肉瘤均可以发生于乳腺。不具有乳腺特异性的肿瘤诊断标准，在本书各章分别介绍。需要记住的是乳腺是原发肉瘤的罕见部位（图16.82）。多数乳腺梭形细胞或未分化肉瘤病例，经认真取材和免疫组化研究，或者表现出叶状肿瘤特征性的上皮和间质双相结构，或者发现肿瘤性上皮分化而诊断为梭形细胞癌或化生性癌（见第938页）。发现肿瘤内或周围乳腺组织的导管原位癌对后者的诊断有帮助。

肌纤维母细胞瘤　Myofibroblastoma

临床特征

这种少见肿瘤[563]的发病年龄跨度很大。最初报道以男性为主[563]，之后的报道结果不一致[564]。临床上，肿瘤表现为病史较短的肿物，体检发现质硬，可活动。乳腺外相应的病变也有报道[565]。局部切除或乳腺切除后没有发现转移，被看作是良性病变。

大体特征

肿瘤大多发生在乳腺实质内。文献报道的平均大小为2.3cm，变化范围为1～4cm，也可见到孤立的更大的病例。肿瘤呈圆形，境界清楚，切面呈模糊的多结节状表现。

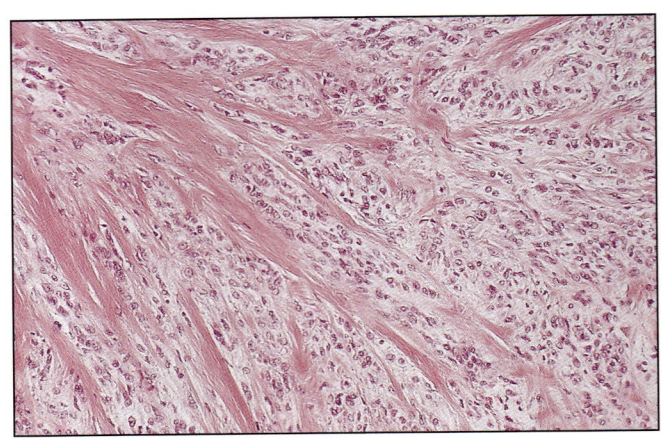

图16.82　间质肉瘤。伴有间叶表型（仅波形蛋白阳性）的浸润性单纯梭形细胞肿瘤。

组织学特征

肿瘤界限清楚，并有受压的乳腺组织形成的假包膜，通常没有内陷的乳腺实质结构。由胶原间质内排列成短束状的梭形细胞组成（图16.83）。像在梭形细胞脂肪瘤中一样，胶原束常常不完整。核卵圆形，轻度不规则，有小核仁，偶见核沟（图16.84）。细胞结构多样。可见平滑肌、软骨和脂肪[563,566]。分裂象不常见。梭形细胞表达结蛋白[567]、α-平滑肌肌动蛋白和CD34[568]，但是不表达细胞角蛋白和S-100。超微结构显示肿瘤细胞含有局灶密集的肌纤维束。

鉴别诊断

这种肿瘤与孤立性纤维瘤有一些形态学重叠，尽管后者结构更不典型（见第24章）。最近的研究[568]

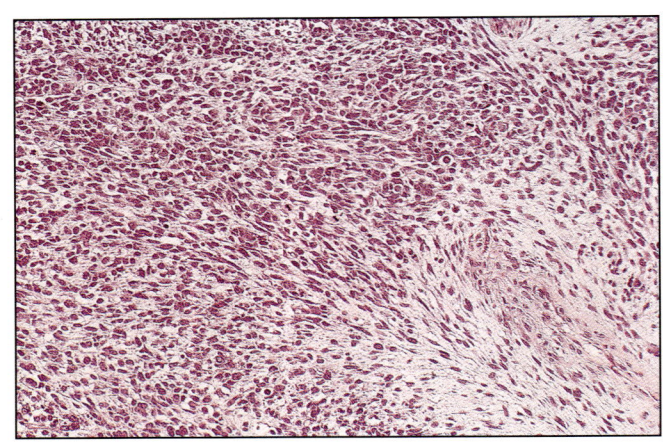

图16.83　肌纤维母细胞瘤。聚集成群的肥胖梭形细胞和透明变性的胶原条带是该肿瘤的两种特征性表现。

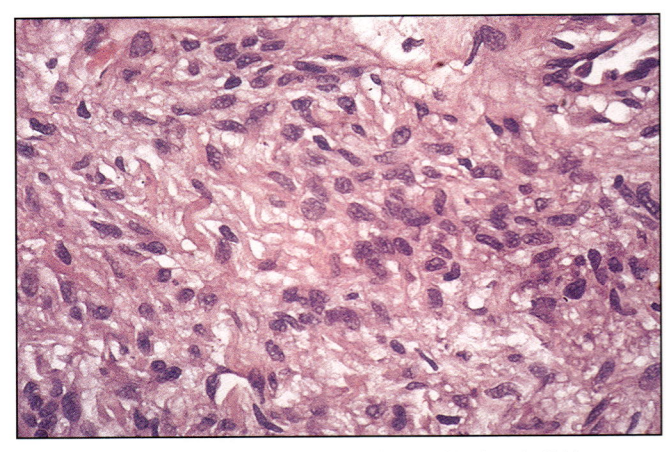

图16.84　肌纤维母细胞瘤。细胞小，呈梭形，有核沟。

显示孤立性纤维瘤的鉴别诊断特征为核仁不明显，胶原纤维束粗大，不表达结蛋白和 α-平滑肌肌动蛋白。而且，肌纤维母细胞瘤具有与梭形细胞脂肪瘤相同的核型。

纤维瘤病　Fibromatosis

临床特征

乳腺纤维瘤病是一种少见但已充分认识的疾病，实际上与其他部位的韧带样纤维瘤相同（见第 24 章）。文献中有较多的病例报道和一些系列报道[41,569-571]。几乎全部发生于女性。平均发病年龄为 25～45 岁，总体年龄分布为 15～80 岁。肿瘤通常表现为乳腺肿物，质硬，界限清楚或不清。可固定于深筋膜或表面皮肤。影像学上，病变与乳腺癌相同，表现为界限不清的致密肿物[572]。

切除不完全的乳腺纤维瘤病复发风险高。要仔细检查切缘，如果切缘仍有病变要立即扩大切除。与其他部位的纤维瘤病一样，其自然行为还不了解。侵袭性亚型已有报道，可以在乳腺内扩散并侵及胸壁和纵隔组织。然而，在一些诊断后复发但拒绝进一步治疗的患者中，病变处于静止状态。

大体表现

病变范围变化较大，从 < 1cm 到 > 10cm，平均 2～3cm。切面显示灰白色纤维组织形成的界限不清的质硬区。

组织学表现

纤维瘤病可有细胞和胶原丰富的透明变性区。诊断依靠发现温和的浸润性梭形细胞增生（图 16.85）。通常很少或没有分裂象。核多形性和异型可能给诊断带来疑问。细胞呈长束状、席纹状或编织状排列。肿瘤沿纤维间隔扩散，镜下病变可出现在肉眼病灶外很远的部位。细胞量最多的区域见于肿瘤周边部，而纤维化和透明变性位于中心。其他表现包括出现局灶淋巴细胞浸润，见于 50% 的病例[9,570]。被纤维瘤病包裹的导管和小叶等乳腺实质可表现出类似男性乳腺发育的微乳头状上皮增生特征。

鉴别诊断

80% 的乳腺纤维瘤病出现 β-catenin 核表达，这种表达在纤维腺瘤和叶状肿瘤中也有报道。梭形细胞癌需要用细胞角蛋白免疫组化来排除。纤维瘤病的免疫组化和超微结构特征细节在第 24 章叙述。

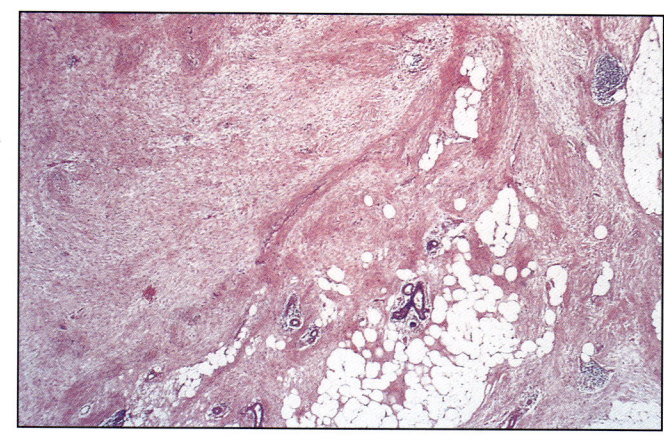

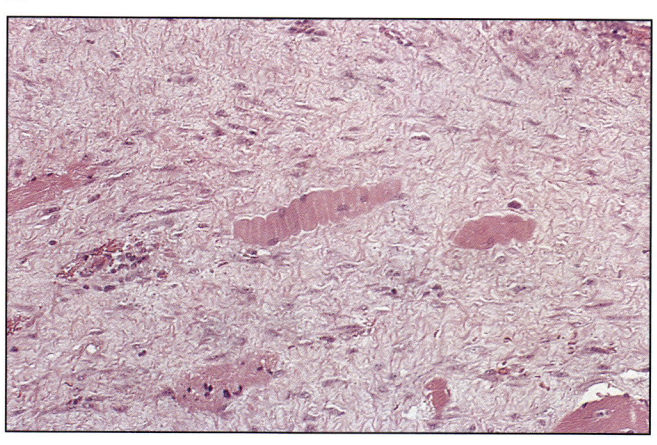

图 16.85　纤维瘤病。表现为界限不清的浸润性肿瘤，包绕原有的乳腺结构（A）。肿瘤由温和的梭形细胞组成（B）。

颗粒细胞瘤　Granular cell tumor

乳腺颗粒细胞瘤是一种罕见肿瘤，临床和影像学上类似恶性，但行为总是良性[573,574]。病理学实际上与其他部位的颗粒细胞瘤相同（见第 27 章）。大体上，边界不规则。组织学表现为多角形大细胞，伴有嗜酸性颗粒状胞浆。细胞核小而一致。有时间质显示广泛硬化，颗粒细胞不明显。偶尔，与脂肪坏死纤维化很难区分，尤其是在粗针活检。行为恶性的颗粒细胞瘤能够找到组织学线索[575]。免疫组化表达 S-100、CD68、抑制素、PGP9.5 和神经元特异性烯醇化酶 (NSE)[576]。细胞角蛋白阴性。

非固有肿瘤　Non-intrinsic tumors

恶性淋巴瘤　Malignant lymphoma

乳腺的原发恶性淋巴瘤可表现为肿物，临床上与癌不能区分。绝大多数具有B细胞表型，最常见的是弥漫大B细胞淋巴瘤、滤泡中心细胞淋巴瘤和黏膜相关淋巴组织淋巴瘤[23,24,577,578]。组织学上，淋巴细胞可呈线性"列兵"样排列，与经典型浸润性小叶癌相似（图16.86）。作为播散性疾病的一部分，淋巴瘤可继发性累及乳腺，大多数是低级别B细胞淋巴瘤。恶性淋巴瘤在第21章阐述。

转移性肿瘤　Metastatic tumors

其他部位的原发性肿瘤可以播散至乳腺，可发生于多种不同的癌[579]。当在乳腺中遇到一种少见肿瘤时，必须获得充足的临床病史，并查找其他部位是否存在肿瘤病史或播散性肿瘤。乳腺最常见的转移性肿瘤为淋巴瘤/白血病、黑色素瘤、肺癌（尤其是小细胞癌）、胃癌、前列腺癌和卵巢癌[580]。偶尔，肉瘤（尤其是腺泡状横

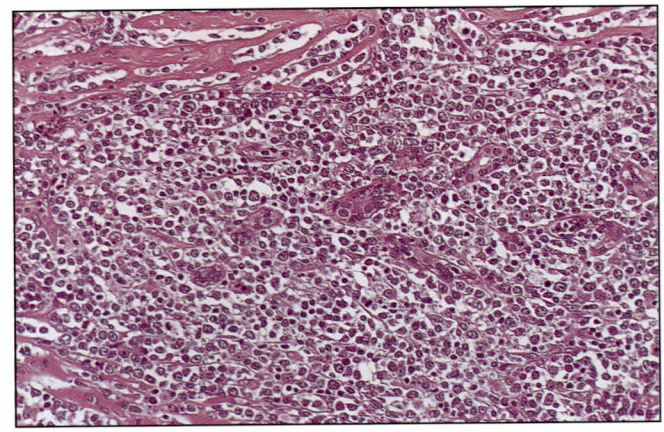

图16.86　恶性淋巴瘤。一群较大的转化淋巴细胞浸润终末导管小叶单元。注意原有的结构得到保留，与经典型浸润性小叶癌相似。

纹肌肉瘤）可转移至乳腺。如果采用保守治疗，原发性乳腺癌也可能转移至对侧或同侧乳腺。

鉴别原发和转移性癌一个有用的原则是如果并存原位癌，可支持原发性乳腺癌。

参考文献

1. Tavassoli F, Devilee, P 2003 Pathology and genetics of tumours of the breast and female genital organs. World Health Organisation classification of tumours. IARC Press, Lyon.
2. Hutter R V P 1986 Consensus meeting. Is fibrocystic disease of the breast precancerous? Arch Pathol Lab Med 110: 171–173
3. Royal College of Pathologists Working Group on Breast Screening 1990 Breast cancer screening guidelines for pathologists. NHSBSP Publications
4. Royal College of Pathologists Working Group on Breast Screening 1991 Pathology reporting in breast cancer screening. J Clin Pathol 44: 710–725
5. Pathologists, NBSPa.Rco 2005 Pathology reporting of breast disease 3rd edn. NHSBSP Publication No 58. NHS Cancer Screening Programmes, Sheffield
6. European Commission 1996 European guidelines for quality assurance in mammography screening 2nd edn. de Wolf CJM, Perry NM (eds) Office for Official Publications of the European Communities, Luxembourg
7. Hughes L E, Mansell R E, Webster D J T 1987 Aberrations of normal development and involution (ANDI): a new perspective on pathogenesis and nomenclature of benign breast disorders. Lancet ii: 1316–1319
8. Haagensen C D 1986 Diseases of the breast. WB Saunders, Philadelphia
9. Hayward J L, Parks A G 1958 Alterations in the microanatomy of the breast as a result of changes in the hormonal environment. In: Currie AR (ed) Endocrine aspects of breast cancer. Churchill Livingstone, Edinburgh, p. 133–134
10. Azzopardi J E 1979 Problems in breast pathology. WB Saunders, London
11. Frantz V K, Pickren J W, Melcher G W et al. 1951 Incidence of chronic cystic disease in so called normal breasts. Cancer 4: 762–783
12. Foote F W Jr, Stewart F W 1945 Comparative studies of cancerous versus non-cancerous breasts. Ann Surg 121: 574–585
13. Dixon J M, Scott W N, Miller W R 1985 Natural history of cystic disease: the importance of cyst type. Br J Surg 72: 190–192
14. Hughes L E, Mansel R E, Webster D J T 1989 Benign disorders and diseases of the breast. Baillière Tindall, London, 93–101
15. Izuo M, Okagaki T, Richart R M et al. 1971 DNA content in apocrine metaplasia of fibrocystic disease, complex and breast cancer. Cancer 27: 643–650
16. Page D L, Anderson T J, Johnson R L 1987 Sarcomas of the breast. In: Page DL, Anderson TJ (eds) Diagnostic histopathology of the breast. Churchill Livingstone, Edinburgh
17. Tesluk H, Amott T, Goodnight J E Jr 1986 Apocrine adenoma of the breast. Arch Pathol Lab Med 110: 351–352
18. Tham K T, Dupont W D, Page D L et al. 1989 Micropapillary hyperplasia with atypical features in female breasts, resembling gynecomastia. In Fenoglio-Preiser CM, Wolff M, Rilke F (eds) Progress in surgical pathology. Springer Verlag, Heidelberg
19. Schwartz I S, Strauchen J A 1990 Lymphocytic mastopathy. An autoimmune disease of the breast? Am J Clin Pathol 93: 725–730
20. Lammie G A, Bobrow L G, Staunton M D et al. 1991 Sclerosing lymphocytic lobulitis of the breast – evidence for an autoimmune pathogenesis. Histopathology 19: 13–20
21. Ashton M A, Lefkowitz M, Tavassoli F A 1994 Epithelioid stromal cells in lymphocytic mastitis – a source of confusion with invasive carcinoma. Mod Pathol 7: 49–54
22. Aozasa K, Ohsawa M, Saeki K et al. 1992 Malignant lymphoma of the breast. Immunologic type and association with lymphocytic mastopathy. Am J Clin Pathol 97: 699–704
23. Bobrow L G, Richards M A, Happerfield L C 1993 Breast lymphomas: a clinicopathological review. Hum Pathol 24: 274–278
24. Arber D A, Simpson J F, Weiss L M et al. 1994 Non-Hodgkin's lymphoma involving the breast. Am J Surg Pathol 18: 288–295
25. Lee A H, Happerfield L C, Millis R R et al. 1996 Inflammatory infiltrate in invasive lobular and ductal carcinoma of the breast. Br J Cancer 74: 796–801
26. Sloane J P 1987 Biopsy pathology of the breast. Chapman & Hall, London
27. Fechner R E 1987 Fibroadenoma and related conditions. In: Page DL, Anderson TJ (eds) Diagnostic histopathology of the breast. Churchill Livingstone, Edinburgh. p 72–85
28. Rosen P P (ed) 1996 Fibroepithelial neoplasms. In: Rosen's Breast pathology. Lipincott-Raven, Philadelphia, p 143–175
29. Dent D M 1989 Fibroadenoma. World J Surg 13: 706–710
30. Orcel L, Douvin D 1973 Contribution à l'étude histogénétique des fibro-adénomes mammaires. Ann Anat Pathol Paris 18: 255–276
31. Pesce C, Colacino R 1986 Morphometry of the breast fibroadenoma. Pathol Res Pract 181: 718–720
32. Noguchi S, Motomura K, Inaji H et al. 1993 Clonal analysis of fibroadenoma and phyllodes tumor of the breast by means of polymerase chain reaction. Cancer Res 53: 4071–4074
33. Martin P M, Kuttenn F, Serment H et al. 1979 Progesterone receptors in breast fibroadenomas. J Steroid Biochem 11: 1295–1298
34. Wilkinson S, Anderson T J, Rifkind E et al. 1989 Fibroadenoma of the breast: a follow-up of conservative management. Br J Surg 76: 390–391

35. Galea M H, Dixon A R, Pye G et al. 1993 Non-operative management of discrete breast lumps in women over 35 years of age (abstract). Breast 1: 164
36. Blamey R W 1998 Clinical aspects of benign breast lesions. In: Elston CW, Ellis IO (eds) Systemic pathology. The breast. Churchill Livingstone, London, p 231–238
37. Diaz N M, Palmer J O, McDivitt RW 1991 Carcinoma arising within fibroadenomas of the breast. Am J Clin Pathol 95: 614–622
38. Dupont W D, Page D L, Parl F F et al. 1994 Long term risk of breast cancer in women with fibroadenoma. New Engl J Med 331: 10–15
39. Levi F, Randimbison L, Te V C et al. 1994 Incidence of breast cancer in women with fibroadenoma. Int J Cancer 57: 681–683
40. Tavassoli F A (ed) 1992 Biphasic tumors. In: Pathology of the breast. Norwalk, Appleton and Lange, p. 425–481
41. Wargotz E S, Norris H J, Austin R M et al. 1987 Fibromatosis of the breast. A clinical and pathological study of 28 cases. Am J Surg Pathol 11: 38–45
42. Mies C, Rosen P P 1987 Juvenile fibroadenoma with atypical epithelial hyperplasia. Am J Surg Pathol 11: 184–190
43. Pike A M, Oberman H A 1985 Juvenile (cellular) adenofibromas. A clinicopathologic study. Am J Surg Pathol 9: 730–736
44. Elston C W, Ellis I O (eds) 1998 Fibroadenoma and related conditions. In Systemic pathology. The breast. Churchill Livingstone, London, p 147–186
45. Hertel B G, Zaloudek C, Kempson R L 1976 Breast adenomas. Cancer 37: 2891–2905
46. Slavin J L, Billson V R, Ostor A G 1993 Nodular breast lesions during pregnancy and lactation. Histopathology 22: 481–485
47. O'Hara M F, Page D L 1985 Adenomas of the breast and ectopic breast under lactational influences. Hum Pathol 16: 707–712
48. Moross T, Lang A P, Mahoney L 1983 Tubular adenoma of the breast. Arch Pathol 107: 84–86
49. Arrigoni M G, Dockerty M B, Judd E S 1971 The identification and treatment of mammary hamartoma. Surg Gynec Obstet 132: 259–262
50. Hessler C, Schnyder P, Ozzello L 1979 Hamartoma of the breast: diagnostic observation of 16 cases. Radiology 126: 95–98
51. Linell F, Ostberg G, Soderstrom J et al. 1979 Breast hamartomas. An important entity in mammary pathology. Virchow's Arch (A) Anat Pathol 383: 253–264
52. Fisher C J, Hanby A M, Robinson L et al. 1992 Mammary hamartoma – a review of 35 cases. Histopathology 20: 99–106
53. Daya D, Trus T, D'Souza T J et al. 1995 Hamartoma of the breast, an underrecognized breast lesion. A clinicopathologic and radiographic study of 25 cases. Am J Clin Pathol 103: 685–689
54. Powell C M, Cranor M L, Rosen P P 1995 Pseudoangiomatous stromal hyperplasia (PASH): a mammary stromal tumor with myofibroblastic differentiation. Am J Surg Pathol 19: 270–277
55. Spalding J E 1945 Adenolipoma and lipoma of the breast. Guys Hosp Rep 94: 80–84
56. Müller J 1838 Uber den feinern Bau und die Formen der krankhaften Geschwulste. Reimer, Berlin, p 54–60
57. World Health Organization 1981 International histological classification of tumours. Histologic types of breast tumours. World Health Organization, Geneva
58. Moffat C J, Pinder S E, Dixon A R et al. 1995 Phyllodes tumours of the breast: a clinicopathological review of 32 cases. Histopathology 27: 205–218
59. Pietruska M, Barnes L 1978 Cytosarcoma phyllodes. A clinico-pathologic analysis of 42 cases. Cancer 41: 1974–1983
60. Page D L, Anderson T J (eds) 1987 Radial scars and complex sclerosing lesions. In: Diagnostic pathology of the breast. Churchill Livingstone, Edinburgh, p 89–103
61. Grove A, Kirstensen L D 1986 Intraductal carcinoma within a phyllodes tumour of the breast – a case report. Tumori 72: 187–190
62. Knudsen P J T, Ostergaard J 1987 Cystosarcoma phylloides with lobular and ductal carcinoma in situ. Arch Pathol Lab Med 111: 873–875
63. Leong A S-Y, Meredith D J 1980 Tubular carcinoma developing within a recurring cystosarcoma phyllodes of the breast. Cancer 46: 1863–1867
64. Grimes M M 1992 Cystosarcoma phyllodes of the breast: histologic features, flow cytometry analysis and clinical correlations. Mod Pathol 5: 232–239
65. Hart W R, Bauer R C, Oberman H A 1978 Cystosarcoma phyllodes. A clinicopathologic study of twenty six hypercellular periductal stromal tumours of the breast. Am J Clin Pathol 70: 211–216
66. Hajdu S I, Espinosa M H, Robbins G F 1976 Recurrent cystosarcoma phylloides. A clinicopathologic study of 32 cases. Cancer 38: 1402–1406
67. Ward R M, Evans H L 1986 Cystosarcoma phylloides. A clinicopathologic study of 26 cases. Cancer 58: 2282–2289
68. Murad T M, Hines J R, Beal J et al. 1988 Histopathological and clinical correlations of cystosarcoma phyllodes. Arch Path Lab Med 112: 752–756
69. Cohn-Cedermark G, Rutqvist L E, Rosendahl I et al. 1991 Prognostic factors in cystosarcoma phyllodes. A clinicopathologic study of 77 patients. Cancer 68: 2017–2022
70. Tan P H, Jayabaskar T, Chuah K L et al. 2005 Phyllodes tumor of the breast: the role of pathologic parameters. Am J Clin Pathol 123: 529–540
71. Norris H J, Taylor H B 1967 Relationship of histologic features to behaviour of cystosarcoma phyllodes. Analysis of ninety four cases. Cancer 20: 2090–2099
72. Dunne B, Lee A H, Pinder S E et al. 2003 An immunohistochemical study of metaplastic spindle cell carcinoma, phyllodes tumor and fibromatosis of the breast. Hum Pathol 34(10): 1009–1015
73. Nielsen B B 1987 Adenosis tumour of the breast – a clinico-pathological investigation of 27 cases. Histopathology 11: 1259–1275
74. Haagensen C D, Lane N, Lattes R 1972 Neoplastic proliferation of the epithelium of the mammary lobules. Surg Clin N Am 52: 497–524
75. Linell F, Ljunberg O 1984 Atlas of breast pathology. Copenhagen, Munksgaard
76. Roebuck E J 1990 Clinical radiology of the breast. Heinemann Medical, Oxford
77. Taylor H B, Norris H J 1967 Epithelial invasion of nerves in benign diseases of the breast. Cancer 20: 2245–2249
78. Davies J D 1973 Neural invasion in benign mammary dysplasia. J Pathol 109: 225–231
79. Eusebi V, Azzopardi J G 1976 Vascular infiltration in benign breast disease. J Pathol 118: 9–16
80. Simpson J F, Page D L, Dupont W D 1990 Apocrine adenosis – a mimic of mammary carcinoma. Surg Pathol 3: 289–299
81. Carter D J, Rosen P P 1991 Atypical apocrine metaplasia in sclerosing lesions of the breast: a study of 51 patients. Mod Pathol 4: 1–5
82. Jensen R A, Page D L, Dupont W D et al. 1989 Invasive breast cancer risk in women with sclerosing adenosis. Cancer 64: 1977–1983
83. Rasbridge S A, Gillett C E, Sampson S A et al. 1993 Epithelial (E-) and placental (P-) cadherin cell adhesion molecule expression in breast carcinoma. J Pathol 169: 245–250
84. Clement P B, Azzopardi J G 1983 Microglandular adenosis of the breast – a lesion simulating tubular carcinoma. Histopathology 7: 169–180
85. Rosen P P 1983 Microglandular adenosis: a benign lesion simulating invasive mammary carcinoma. Am J Surg Pathol 7: 137–144
86. Tavassoli F A, Norris H J 1983 Microglandular adenosis of the breast. A clinicopathologic study of 11 cases with ultrastructural observations. Am J Surg Pathol 7: 731–737
87. Millis R R, Eusebi V 1995 Microglandular adenosis of the breast. Adv Anat Pathol 2: 10–18
88. Fechner R E, Mills S E 1990 Breast pathology. Benign proliferations, atypias and in situ carcinomas. ASCP Press, Chicago
89. Rosenblum M K, Purrazzella R, Rosen P P 1986 Is microglandular adenosis a precancerous disease? A study of carcinoma arising therein. Am J Surg Pathol 10: 237–245
90. James B A, Cranor M L, Rosen P P 1993 Carcinoma of the breast arising in microglandular adenosis. Am J Clin Pathol 100: 507–513
91. Parl F F, Richardson L D 1983 The histologic and biologic spectrum of tubular carcinoma of the breast. Hum Pathol 14: 694–698
92. Kay S 1985 Microglandular adenosis of the female mammary gland: Study of a case with ultrastructural observations. Hum Pathol 16: 637–640
93. Diaz N M, McDevitt R W, Wick M R 1991 Microglandular adenosis of the breast. An immunohistochemical comparison with tubular carcinoma. Arch Pathol Lab Med 115: 578–582
94. Elston C W, Ellis I O, Goulding H 1998 Sclerosing lesions. In Elston CW, Ellis IO (eds) Systemic pathology. The breast. Churchill Livingstone, London, p 501–513
95. Kiaer H, Nielson B, Paulsen S et al. 1984 Adenomyoepithelial adenosis and low grade malignant adenomyoepithelioma of the breast. Virchow's Arch A Pathol Ann 405: 55–67
96. Semb C 1928 Fibroadenomatosis cystic mammae. Acta Chirurg 10: 1–148
97. Fenoglio C, Lattes R 1974 Sclerosing papillary proliferations in the female breast. A benign lesion often mistaken for carcinoma. Cancer 33: 691–700
98. Tremblay G, Buell R H, Seemayer T A 1987 Elastosis in benign sclerosing ductal proliferations of the female breast. Am J Surg Pathol 1: 1155–1158
99. Hamperl H 1975 Strahlige Narben and Obliterierende mastopathie. Beitr pathol histol mamma. XI Virchow's Arch (A) 369: 55–68
100. Andersen J A, Carter D, Linell F 1986 A symposium on sclerosing duct lesions of the breast. Pathol Annu 1: 145–179
101. Linell F, Ljunberg O, Andersson I 1980 Breast carcinoma. Aspects of early stages, progression and related problems. Acta Path Microbiol Scand 272: 1–233
102. Welling S R, Alpers G E 1984 Subgross pathologic features and incidence of radial scars in the breast. Hum Pathol 15: 475–479
103. Nielsen M, Thomson J L, Primdahl S et al. 1987 Breast cancer and atypia among young and middle-aged women: a study of 110 medicolegal autopsies. Br J Cancer 56: 814–819
104. Nielsen M, Christensen L, Andersen J 1987 Radial scars in women with breast cancer. Cancer 59: 1019–1025
105. Ciatto S, Morrone D, Catarzi S et al. 1993 Radial scars of the breast: review of 38 consecutive mammographic diagnoses. Radiology 187(3): 757–760
106. Sloane J P, Mayers M M 1993 Carcinoma and atypical hyperplasia in radial scars and complex sclerosing lesions importance of lesion size and patient age. Histopathology 23: 225–231
107. Carter D 1977 Intraduct papillary tumors of the breast. A study of 78 cases. Cancer 59: 1689–1692
108. Ohuchi N, Abe R, Kasai M 1984 Possible cancerous change of intraductal papillomas of the breast. Cancer 54: 605–611
109. Papotti M, Gugliotta P, Ghiringhello B et al. 1984 Association of breast carcinoma and multiple intraductal papillomas: an histological and immunohistochemical investigation. Histopathology 8: 963–975
110. Jones D B 1955 Florid papillomatosis of the nipple ducts. Cancer 8: 315–319
111. Doctor V M, Sirsat M V 1971 Florid papillomatosis (adenoma) and other benign tumours of the nipple and areola. Br J Cancer 25: 1–9

112. Bhagavan B S, Patchefsy A, Koss L G 1973 Florid subareolar duct papillomatosis (nipple adenoma) and mammary carcinoma: report of three cases. Hum Pathol 4: 289–295
113. Rosen P P, Caicco J A 1986 Florid papillomatosis of the nipple. A study of 51 patients, including nine with mammary carcinoma. Am J Surg Pathol 10: 87–101
114. Handley R S, Thackray A C 1962 Adenoma of the nipple. Br J Cancer 16: 187–194
115. Ahmed A 1992 Diagnostic breast pathology. Churchill Livingstone, Edinburgh
116. Perzin K H, Lattes R 1972 Papillary adenoma of the nipple (florid papillomatosis, adenoma, adenomatosis). A clinico-pathologic study. Cancer 29: 996–1009
117. Gudjonsdottir A, Hagerstrand I, Ostberg G 1971 Adenoma of the nipple with carcinomatous development. Acta Pathol Microbiol Scand (A) 79: 676–680
118. Azzopardi J G, Salm R 1984 Ductal adenoma of the breast: a lesion which can mimic carcinoma. J Pathol 144: 15–23
119. Lammie G A, Millis R R 1989 Ductal adenoma of the breast – a review of fifteen cases. Hum Pathol 20: 903–908
120. Gusterson B A, Sloane J P, Middwood C et al. 1987 Ductal adenoma of the breast – a lesion exhibiting a myoepithelial/epithelial phenotype. Histopathology 11: 103–110
121. Schnitt S J, Vincent-Salomon A 2003 Columnar cell lesions of the breast. Adv Anat Pathol 10: 113–124
122. Fraser J L, Raza S, Chomy K et al. 1998 Columnar alteration with prominent apical snouts and secretions. A spectrum of changes frequently present in breast biopsies performed for microcalcifications. Am J Surg Pathol 22: 1521–1527
123. Oyama T, Maluf H, Koerner F 1999 Atypical cystic lobules: an early stage in the formation of low-grade ductal carcinoma in situ. Virchow's Arch 435: 413–421
124. Goldstein N S, O'Malley B A 1997 Cancerization of small ectatic ducts of the breast by ductal carcinoma in situ cells with apocrine snouts. A lesion associated with tubular carcinoma. Am J Clin Pathol 107: 561–566
125. Schnitt S J, Connolly J L, Tavassoli F A et al. 1992 Interobserver reproducibility in the diagnosis of ductal proliferative breast lesions using standardized criteria. Am J Surg Pathol 16: 1133–1143
126. Simpson P T, Gale T, Fulford L G et al. 2003 Pathology of atypical lobular hyperplasia and lobular carcinoma in situ. Breast Cancer Res 5: 258–262
127. Schnitt S J 2003 Flat epithelial atypia – classification, pathologic features and clinical significance. Breast Cancer Res 5: 263–268
128. Tavassoli F A, Hoefler H, Rosai J et al. 2003 Intraductal proliferative lesions. In: Tavassoli FA, Devilee P (eds) Pathology and genetics of tumours of the breast and female genital organs. IARC Press, Lyon
129. Dupont W D, Page D L 1989 Relative risk of breast cancer varies with time since diagnosis of atypical hyperplasia. Hum Pathol 20: 723–725
130. Page D L 1986 Cancer risk assessment in benign breast biopsies. Hum Pathol 17: 871–874
131. Page D L, Vander Zwaag R, Rogers L W et al. 1978 Relation between component parts of fibrocystic disease complex and breast cancer. J Natl Cancer Inst 61: 1055–1063
132. Hutter R V P 1985 Goodbye to "fibrocystic disease". New Eng J Med 312: 179–181
133. Dupont W D, Page D L 1985 Risk factors for breast cancer in women with proliferative breast disease. New Eng J Med 312: 146–151
134. Page D L, Dupont W E, Rogers L W 1986 Breast cancer risk of lobular-based hyperplasia after biopsy: "ductal" pattern lesions. Cancer Detec Prev 9: 441–448
135. Page D L, Dupont W D, Rogers L W et al. 1985 Atypical hyperplastic lesions of the female breast. A long-term follow-up study. Cancer 55: 2698–2708
136. Page D L, Rogers L W 1992 Combined histologic and cytologic criteria for the diagnosis of mammary atypical hyperplasia. Hum Pathol 23: 1095–1097
137. Tavassoli F A, Norris H J 1990 A comparison of the results of long term follow-up for atypical intraductal hyperplasia and intraductal hyperplasia of the breast. Cancer 65: 518–529
138. Rosai J 1991 Borderline epithelial lesions of the breast. Am J Surg Pathol 15: 209–221
139. Sloane J P, Amendoeira I, Apostolikas N et al. 1999 Consistency achieved by 23 European pathologists from 12 countries in diagnosing breast disease and reporting prognostic features of carcinomas. Virchow's Arch 434(1): 3–10
140. Lakhani S R, Collins N, Stratton M R et al. 1995 Atypical ductal hyperplasia of the breast: clonal proliferation with loss of heterozygosity on chromosomes 16q and 17p. J Clin Pathol 48: 611–615
141. Bocker W, Decker T, Ruhnke M et al. 1997 Ductal hyperplasia and ductal carcinoma in situ. Pathologie 18(1): 3–18
142. Bocker W, Moll R, Poremba C et al. 2002 Common adult stem cells in the human breast give rise to glandular and myoepithelial cell lineages: a new cell biological concept. Lab Invest 82: 737–746
143. Liberman L, Cohen M A, Dershaw D D et al. 1995 Atypical ductal hyperplasia diagnosed at stereotaxic core biopsy of breast lesions: an indication for surgical biopsy. Am J Roentgenol 164: 1111–1113
144. Dahlstrom J E, Jain S, Sutton T et al. 1996 Diagnostic accuracy of stereotactic core biopsy in a mammographic breast cancer screening programme. Histopathology 28: 421–427
145. Darling M L, Smith D N, Lester S C et al. 2000 Atypical ductal hyperplasia and ductal carcinoma in situ as revealed by large-core needle breast biopsy: results of surgical excision. Am J Roentgenol 175: 1341–1346.
146. Page D L, Anderson T J 1987 Diagnostic histopathology of the breast. Churchill Livingstone, Edinburgh
147. O'Malley F P, Page D L, Nelson E H, et al. 1994 Ductal carcinoma in situ of the breast with apocrine cytology: definition of a borderline category. Hum Pathol 25: 164–168
148. Tavassoli F A, Norris H J 1994 Intraductal apocrine carcinoma: a clinicopathologic study of 37 cases. Mod Pathol 7: 813–818
149. Haagensen C D, Lane N, Lattes R et al. 1978 Lobular neoplasia (so called lobular carcinoma in situ) of the breast. Cancer 42: 737–769
150. Page D L, Kidd T E Jr, Dupont W D et al. 1991 Lobular neoplasia of the breast: higher risk for subsequent invasive cancer predicted by more extensive disease. Hum Pathol 22: 1232–1239
151. Fisher E R, Land S R, Fisher B et al. 2004 Pathologic findings from the National Surgical Adjuvant Breast and Bowel Project. Twelve year observations concerning lobular carcinoma in situ. Cancer 100: 238–244
152. Page D L, Schuyler P A, Dupont W D et al. 2003 Atypical lobular hyperplasia as a unilateral predictor of breast cancer risk: a retrospective cohort study. Lancet 361: 125–129
153. Rosen P P, Kosloff C, Lieberman P H et al. 1978 Lobular carcinoma in situ of the breast: detailed analysis of 99 patients with average follow up of 24 years. Am J Surg Pathol 2: 225–251
154. Frykberg E R, Santiago F, Betshill W L Jr et al. 1987 Lobular carcinoma in situ of the breast. Surg Gynecol and Obstet 164: 285–301
155. Lakhani S R, Collins N, Sloane J P et al. 1995 Loss of heterozygosity in lobular carcinoma in-situ of the breast. J Clin Pathol Clin Mol Pathol 48(2): M74–M78
156. Fisher B, Costandino J P, Wickerham D L et al. 1998 Tamoxifen for prevention of breast cancer: report of the national Surgical Adjuvant Breast and Bowel Project P-1 Study. J Natl Cancer Inst 90: 1371–1388
157. Sneige N, Wang J, Baker B A et al. 2002 Clinical, histopathologic, and biologic features of pleomorphic lobular (ductal-lobular) carcinoma in situ of the breast: a report of 24 cases. Mod Pathol 15(10): 1044–1050
158. Reis-Filho J S, Simpson P T, Jones C et al. 2005 Pleomorphic lobular carcinoma of the breast: role of comprehensive molecular pathology in characterization of an entity. J Pathol 207: 1–13.
159. Eusebi V, Betts C, Haagensen D E Jr et al. 1984 Apocrine differentiation in lobular carcinoma of the breast. A morphologic, immunologic and ultrastructural study. Hum Pathol 15: 134–140
160. Jacobs T W, Pliss N, Kouria G et al. 2001 Carcinomas in situ of the breast with indeterminate features: role of E-cadherin staining in categorization. Am J Surg Pathol 25: 229–236
161. Kerner H, Lichtig C 1986 Lobular cancerization: incidence and differential diagnosis with lobular carcinoma in-situ of breast. Histopathology 10: 621–629
162. Donegan W L, Redlich P N, Lang P J et al. 1998 Carcinoma of the breast in males. A multi-institutional survey. Cancer 83: 498–509
163. Geschickter C F, Lewis D 1938 Comedo carcinomas of the breast. Arch Surg 33: 225–244
164. Geschickter C F 1943 Diseases of the breast. Lippincott, Philadelphia, p 502–507
165. Page D L, Dupont W D, Rogers L W et al. 1982 Intraductal carcinoma of the breast: follow up after biopsy alone. Cancer 49: 751–758
166. Rosen P P, Braun D W Jr, Kinne D W 1980 The clinical significance of preinvasive breast carcinoma. Cancer 46: 919–925
167. Page D L, Dupont W D, Rogers L W et al. 1995 Continued local recurrence of carcinoma 15–25 years after a diagnosis of low grade ductal carcinoma in situ of the breast treated by biopsy. Cancer 76: 1197–1200
168. Lagios M D 1990 Duct carcinoma in situ: pathology and treatment. Surg Clin North Am 70: 853–871
169. Silverstein M J, Poller D N, Waisman J R et al. 1995 Prognostic classification of breast ductal carcinoma-in-situ. Lancet 345: 1154–1157
170. Silverstein M J, Lagios M D, Craig P H et al. 1996 A prognostic index for ductal carcinoma in situ of the breast. Cancer 77: 2267–2274
171. Fisher E R, Costandino J, Fisher B et al. 1995 Pathologic findings from the National Surgical Adjuvant Breast Project (NSABP) Protocol B-17. Intraductal carcinoma (ductal carcinoma in situ). The National Surgical Adjuvant Breast and Bowel Project Collaborating Investigators. Cancer 75: 1310–1319
172. Lagios M D, Margolin F R, Westdahl P R et al. 1989 Mammographically detected duct carcinoma in situ. Frequency of local recurrence following tylectomy and prognostic effect of nuclear grade on local recurrence. Cancer 63: 618–624
173. Bijker N, Peterse J L, Duchateau L et al. 2001 Risk factors for recurrence and metastasis after breast-conserving therapy for ductal carcinoma-in-situ: analysis of European Organisation for Research and Treatment of Cancer Trial 10853. J Clin Oncol 19: 2263–2271
174. Waldman F M, DeVries R, Chew K L et al. 2000 Chromosomal alterations in ductal carcinomas in situ and their in situ recurrences. J Natl Cancer Inst 92: 313–320
175. Fisher B, Costandino J, Redmond C et al. 1993 Lumpectomy compared with lumpectomy and radiation therapy for the treatment of intraductal breast cancer. N Engl J Med 328: 1581–1586

176. Ottensen G L, Graversen H P, Blichert-Toft M et al. 2000 Carcinoma in situ of the female breast. 10 year follow-up results of a prospective nationwide study. Breast Cancer Res Treat 62: 197–210
177. Faverly D, Holland R, Burgers L 1992 Three dimensional imaging of mammary ductal carcinoma in situ. Virchow's Arch (A) Pathol Anat 421: 115–119
178. Holland R, Hendriks J H, Vebeek A L 1990 Extent, distribution, and mammographic/histological correlations of breast ductal carcinoma in situ. Lancet 335: 519–522
179. Smart C, Myers M, Gloecker L 1978 Implications from SEER data on breast cancer management. Cancer 41: 787–789
180. Anderssen I, Aspegren K, Janzon L et al. 1988 Mammographic screening and mortality from breast cancer: the Malmo mammographic screening trial. Br Med J 297: 943–948
181. Gibbs N M 1985 Comparative study of the histopathology of breast cancer in a screened and unscreened population investigated by mammography. Histopathology 9: 1307–1318
182. Bettshill W L Jr, Rosen P P, Leiberman P H et al. 1978 Intraductal carcinoma. Long term follow up after treatment by biopsy alone. J Am Med Assoc 239: 1863–1867
183. Bellamy C O, McDonald C, Salter D M et al. 1993 Noninvasive ductal carcinoma of the breast: the relevance of histologic categorization. Hum Pathol 24: 16–23
184. Van Dongen, J A, Holland R, Peterse J L et al. 1992 Ductal carcinoma in situ of the breast – 2nd Eortc Consensus Meeting. Eur J Cancer 28(2–3): 626–629
185. Bagnall M J, Evans A J, Wilson A R et al. 2001 Predicting invasion in mammographically detected microcalcification. Clin Rad 56: 828–832
186. Holland R, Peterse J L, Millis R R et al. 1994 Ductal carcinoma in situ: a proposal for a new classification. Semin Diagn Pathol 11(3): 167–180
187. Badve S, A'Hern R P, Ward A M et al. 1998 A long-term comparative study of the ability of five classifications of ductal carcinoma in situ of breast to predict local recurrence after surgical excision. Hum Pathol 29: 915–923
188. European Commission Working Group on Breast Screening Pathology 1998 Consistency achieved by 23 European pathologists in categorizing ductal carcinoma in situ of the breast using five classifications. Hum Pathol 29: 1056–1062
189. Bobrow L G, Happerfield L C, Gregory W M et al. 1994 The classification of ductal carcinoma in situ and its association with biological markers. Semin Diagn Pathol 11(3): 199–207
190. Poller D N, Roberts E C, Bell J A et al. 1993 p53 protein expression in mammary ductal carcinoma in situ: relationship to immunohistochemical expression of estrogen receptor and c-erbB-2 protein. Hum Pathol 24: 463–468
191. Allred D C, Clark G M, Molina R et al. 1992 Overexpression of HER-2/neu and its relationship with other prognostic factors change during the progression of in situ to invasive breast cancer. Hum Pathol 23: 974–979
192. Gupta S K, Douglas-Jones A G, Johnson R C et al. 1997 Classification of DCIS of the breast in relation to biological markers: p53, E-cadherin and MIB-1 expression. J Pathol 181(SS): A22
193. Buerger H, Otterbach F, Simon R et al. 1999 Comparative genomic hydridization of ductal carcinoma in situ of the breast – evicence of multiple genetic pathways. J Pathol 187: 396–402
194. Lampejo O T, Barnes D M, Smith P et al. 1994 Evaluation of infiltrating ductal carcinoma with a DCIS component: correlation of the histologic type of the in situ component with grade of the infiltrating component. Semin Diagn Pathol 11: 215–222
195. Millis R R, Barnes D M, Lampejo O T et al. 1998 Tumour grade does not change between primary and recurrent mammary carcinoma. Eur J Cancer 34: 548–553
196. Millis R R, Pinder S E, Ryder K et al. 2004 Grade of recurrent in situ and invasive carcinoma following treatment of pure ductal carcinoma in situ of the breast. Br J Cancer 90: 1538–1542
197. Leal C, Henrique R, Monteiro P et al. 2001 Apocrine ductal carcinoma in situ of the breast: histologic classification and expression of biologic markers. Hum Pathol 32: 487–493
198. Cross A S, Azzopardi J G, Krausz T et al. 1985 A morphological and immunocytochemical study of a distinctive variant of ductal carcinoma in-situ of the breast. Histopathology 9: 21–37
199. Fisher E R, Brown R 1985 Intraductal signet ring carcinoma: a hitherto undescribed form of intraductal carcinoma of the breast. Cancer 55: 2533–2537
200. Rosen P P, Scott M 1984 Cystic hypersecretory duct carcinoma of the breast. Am J Surg Pathol 8: 31–41
201. Guerry P, Erlandson R A, Rosen P P 1988 Cystic hypersecretory hyperplasia and cystic hypersecretory duct carcinoma of the breast. Pathology, therapy, and follow-up of 39 patients. Cancer 61: 1611–1620
202. Faverly D R, Burgers L, Bult P et al. 1994 Three dimensional imaging of mammary ductal carcinoma in situ: clinical implications. Semin Diagn Pathol 11: 193–198
203. Sibbering D M, Blamey R W 1997 Nottingham experience. In: Silverstein MJ (ed) Ductal carcinoma in situ of the breast. Williams and Wilkins, Baltimore, p 367–372
204. Silverstein M J, Lagios M D, Groshen S et al. 1999 The influence of margin width on local control of ductal carcinoma in situ of the breast. N Eng J Med 340: 1455–1461
205. Fisher B, Dignam J, Wolmark N 1999 Tamoxifen in the treatment of intraductal breast cancer: national Surgical Adjuvant Breast and Bowel Project B-24 randomised control trial. Lancet 353: 1993–2000
206. UK Coordinating Committee on Cancer Research Ductal Carcinoma in situ Working Party 2003 Radiotherapy and tamoxifen in women with completely excised ductal carcinoma in situ of the breast in the UK, Australia, and New Zealand: randomised controlled trial. Lancet 362: 95–102
207. Hitchcock A, Topham S, Bell J et al. 1992 Routine diagnosis of mammary Paget's disease. A modern approach. Am J Surg Pathol 16: 58–61
208. Carter D, Orr S L, Merino M J 1983 Intracystic papillary carcinoma of the breast. After mastectomy, radiotherapy or excisional biopsy alone. Cancer 52: 14–19
209. Maluf H M, Koerner F C 1995 Solid papillary carcinoma of the breast. Am J Surg Pathol 19: 1237–1244
210. Kraus F T, Neubecker R D 1962 The differential diagnosis of papillary tumours of the breast. Cancer 15: 444–455
211. Intra M, Rotmensz B, Viale G et al. 2004 Clinicopathologic characteristics of 143 patients with synchronous bilateral invasive breast carcinomas treated in a single institution. Cancer 101: 905–912
212. Page D L, Anderson T J, Sakamoto G 1987 Infiltrating carcinoma: major histological types. In: Page DL, Anderson TJ (eds) Diagnostic histopathology of the breast. WB Saunders, London, p 193–235
213. Ellis I O, Galea M, Broughton N et al. 1992 Pathological prognostic factors in breast cancer. II Histological type. Relationships with survival in a large study with long-term follow-up. Histopathology 20: 479–489
214. Pinder S E, Elston C W, Ellis I O 1998 Invasive carcinoma – usual histological types. In: Systemic pathology – the breast. Elston CW, Ellis IO (eds) Churchill Livingstone, London, p 283–338
215. Perou C M, Sorlie T, Eisen M B et al. 2000 Molecular portraits of human breast tumours. Nature 406: 747–752
216. Sorlie T, Tibshirani R, Parker J et al. 2003 Repeated observation of breast tumor subtypes in independent gene expression data sets. Proc Natl Acad Sci USA 100: 8418–8423
217. van't Veer L J, Dai H, van de Vijver M J et al. 2002 Gene expression profiling predicts clinical outcome of breast cancer. Nature 415: 530–536
218. van de Vijver M J, He Y D, van't Veer L J et al. 2002 A gene-expression signature as a predictor of survival in breast cancer. N Engl J Med 347: 1999–2009
219. Wang Y, Klijn J G, Zhang Y, et al. 2005 Gene-expression profiles to predict distant metastasis of lymph-node-negative primary breast cancer. Lancet 365: 671–679
220. Lakhani S R, Gusterson B A, Jacquemier J et al. 2000 The pathology of familial breast cancer: histological features of cancers in families not attributable to mutations in BRCA1 or BRCA2. Clin Cancer Res 6(3): 782–789
221. Fisher E R, Gregorio R M, Fisher B 1975 The pathology of invasive breast cancer. A syllabus derived from findings of the national surgical adjuvant breast cancer project (protocol no. 4). Cancer 36: 1–85
222. Rosen P P 1979 The pathological classification of human mammary carcinoma: past, present and future. Ann Clin Lab Sci 9: 144–156
223. Sakamoto G, Sugano H, Hartmann W H et al (eds) 1981 Comparative pathological study of breast carcinoma among American and Japanese women. Plenum, New York, p 211–231
224. Giordano S H, Cohen D S, Buzdar A. 2004 Breast carcinoma in men. A population-based study. Cancer 101: 51–57
225. Miremadi A, Pinder S E, Lees A H S et al. 2002 Neuroendocrine differentiation and prognosis in breast adenocarcinoma. Histopathology 40: 215–222
226. Putti T C, Abd El Rehim D, Pinder S E et al 2005 Estrogen receptor-negative breast carcinomas: a review of morphology and immunophenotypical analysis. Mod Pathol 46: 26–35
227. Foote F W Jr, Stewart F W 1946 A histologic classification of carcinoma in the breast. Surgery 19: 74–99
228. Foote F W Jr, Stewart F W 1941 Lobular carcinoma in situ. A rare form of mammary cancer. Am J Pathol 7: 491–496
229. Wheeler J E, Enterline H T 1976 Lobular carcinoma of the breast in situ and infiltrating. Pathol Annu 11: 161–188
230. Dixon J M, Anderson T J, Page D L et al. 1982 Infiltrating lobular carcinoma of the breast. Histopathology 6: 149–161
231. Fechner R E 1975 Histological variants of infiltrating lobular carcinoma of the breast. Hum Pathol 6: 373–378
232. Martinez V, Azzopardi J 1979 Invasive carcinoma of the breast: incidence and variants. Histopathology 3: 467–488
233. Fisher E R, Gregorio R M, Redmond C et al. 1977 Tubulolobular invasive breast cancer: a variant of lobular invasive cancer. Hum Pathol 8: 679–683
234. Eusebi V, Magalhaes F, Azzopardi J G 1992 Pleomorphic lobular carcinoma of the breast: an aggressive tumour showing apocrine differentiation. Hum Pathol 23: 655–662
235. Weidner N, Semple J P 1992 Pleomorphic variant of invasive lobular carcinoma of the breast. Hum Pathol 23: 1167–1171
236. Moll R, Mitze M, Frixen U H et al. 1993 Differential loss of E-cadherin expression in infiltrating ductal and lobular breast carcinomas. Am J Pathol 143(6): 1731–1742
237. Rakha E A, Abd El-Rehim D M, Pinder S E et al. 2005 E-cadherin expression in invasive non-lobular carcinoma of the breast and its prognostic significance. Histopathology 46: 685–693

238. Cornford E J, Wilson A R M, Athanassiou E 1995 Mammographic features of invasive lobular and invasive ductal carcinoma of the breast: a comparative analysis. Br J Radiol 68: 450–453
239. Quincey C, Raitt N, Bell J et al. 1991 Intracytoplasmic lumina – a useful diagnostic feature of adenocarcinomas. Histopathology 19: 83–87
240. Wheeler D T, Tai L H, Bratthauer G L et al. 2004 Tubulolobular carcinoma of the breast: an analysis of 27 cases of a tumor with a hybrid morphology and immunoprofile. Am J Surg Pathol 28: 1587–1593
241. Green I, McCormick B, Cranor M et al. 1997 A comparative study of pure tubular and tubulolobular carcinoma of the breast. Am J Surg Pathol 21(6): 653–657
242. Page D L, Anderson T J (eds) 1987 Uncommon types of invasive carcinoma. In: Diagnostic histopathology of the breast. Churchill Livingstone, Edinburgh
243. Wahed A, Connelly J, Reese T 2002 E-cadherin expression in pleomorphic lobular carcinoma: an aid to differentiation from ductal carcinoma. Ann Diagn Pathol 6(6): 349–351
244. Palacios J, Sarrio D, Garcia-Macias M C 2003 Frequent E-cadherin gene inactivation by loss of heterozygosity in pleomorphic lobular carcinoma of the breast. Mod Pathol 16(7): 674–678
245. Middleton L P, Palacios D M, Bryant B R et al. 2000 Pleomorphic lobular carcinoma: morphology, immunohistochemistry and molecular analysis. Am J Surg Pathol 24: 1650–1656
246. Anderson T J, Lamb J, Donnan P et al. 1991 Comparative pathology of breast cancer in a randomised trial of screening. Br J Cancer 64: 108–113
247. Patchefsky A S, Shaber G S, Schwartz G F et al. 1977 The pathology of breast cancer detected by mass population screening. Cancer 40: 1659–1670
248. Rajakariar R, Walker R A 1995 Pathological and biological features of mammographically detected invasive breast carcinomas. Br J Cancer 71: 150–154
249. Cowan W K, Kelly P, Sawan A et al. 1997 The pathological and biological nature of screen-detected breast carcinomas: a morphological and immunohistochemical study. J Pathol 182: 29–35
250. Diab S G, Clark G M, Osborne C K et al. 1999 Tumor characteristics and clinical outcome of tubular and mucinous breast carcinomas. J Clin Oncol 17(5): 1442–1448
251. Sullivan T, Raad R A, Goldberg S et al. 2005 Tubular carcinoma of the breast: a retrospective analysis and review of the literature. Breast Cancer Res Treat 93: 199–205
252. Carstens P H, Huvos A G, Foote F W Jr et al. 1972 Tubular carcinoma of the breast: a clinicopathological study of 35 cases. Am J Clin Pathol 58: 231–238
253. Peters, G N, Wolff M, Haagensen C D 1981 Tubular carcinoma of the breast – clinical pathologic correlations on 100 cases. Ann Surg 193: 138–149
254. McDivitt R W, Boyce W, Gersell G 1982 Tubular carcinoma of the breast. Am J Surg Pathol 6: 401–411
255. Dixon J M, Page D L, Anderson T J et al. 1985 Long term survivors after breast cancer. Br J Surg 72: 445–448
256. Page D L, Dixon J M, Anderson T J et al. 1983 Invasive cribriform carcinoma of the breast. Histopathology 7: 525–536
257. Venable J G, Schwartz A M, Silverberg S G 1990 Infiltrating cribriform carcinoma of the breast: a distinctive clinicopathologic entity. Hum Pathol 21: 333–338
258. Holland R, Van Haelst U J G M 1984 Mammary carcinoma with osteoclast-like giant cells. Cancer 53: 1963–1973
259. Saout L, Leduc M, Suy-Beng P T et al. 1985 Présentation d'un nouveau cas de carcinoma mammaire cribriforme associé à une réaction histiocytaire giganto-cellulaire. Arch Anat Cytol Pathol 33: 58–61
260. Tavassoli F A, Norris H J 1986 Breast carcinoma with osteoclast-like giant cells. Arch Pathol Lab Med 110: 636–639
261. Rakha E A, Boyce R W, Abd El-Rehim D et al. 2005 Expression of mucins (MUC1, MUC2, MUC3, MUC4, MUC5AC and MUC6) and their prognostic significance in human breast cancer. Mod Pathol 18: 1295–1304
262. Clayton F 1986 Pure mucinous carcinomas of the breast: morphologic features and prognostic correlates. Hum Pathol 17: 34–39
263. Rasmussen B B, Rose C, Christensen J B 1987 Prognostic factors in primary mucinous breast carcinoma. Am J Clin Pathol 87: 155–160
264. Komaki K, Sakamoto G, Sugano H et al. 1988 Mucinous carcinoma of the breast in Japan. A prognostic analysis based on morphologic features. Cancer 61: 989–996
265. Maluf H M, Koerner F C 1994 Carcinomas of the breast with endocrine differentiation: a review. Virchow's Arch 425(5): 449–457
266. Sapino A, Righi L, Cassoni P et al. 2000 Expression of the neuroendocrine phenotype in carcinomas of the breast. Semin Diagn Pathol 17(2): 127–137
267. Tse G M, Ma T K, Chu W C et al. 2004 Neuroendocrine differentiation in pure type mammary mucinous carcinoma is associated with favorable histologic and immunohistochemical parameters. Mod Pathol 17(5): 568–572
268. Moore O S, Foote F W Jr 1949 The relatively favourable prognosis of medullary carcinoma of the breast. Cancer 2: 635–642
269. Ridolfi R L, Rosen P P, Port A et al. 1977 Medullary carcinoma of the breast – a clinicopathological study with a ten year follow up. Cancer 40: 1365–1385
270. Rapin V, Contesso G, Mouriesse H et al. 1988 Medullary breast carcinoma. A re-evaluation of 95 cases of breast carcinoma with inflammatory stroma. Cancer 61: 2503–2510
271. Wargotz E S, Silverberg S G 1988 Medullary carcinoma of the breast. A clinicopathologic study with appraisal of current diagnostic criteria. Hum Pathol 19: 1340–1346
272. Jensen M L, Kiaer H, Andersen J et al. 1997 Prognostic comparison of three classifications for medullary carcinomas of the breast. Histopathology 30: 523–532
273. Cutler S J, Black M M, Friedall G H et al. 1966 Prognostic factors in cancer of the female breast. Cancer 19: 75–82
274. Pedersen L, Holck S, Schiodt T 1988 Medullary carcinoma of the breast. Cancer Treat Rev 15: 53–63
275. Fisher E R, Kenny J P, Sass R et al. 1990 Medullary cancer of the breast revisited. Breast Cancer Res Treat 16: 215–229
276. Pederson L, Zedeler K, Holck S et al. 1991 Medullary carcinoma of the breast, proposal for a new simplified histopathological definition. Br J Cancer 63: 591–595
277. Rigaud C, Theobald S, Noël P 1993 Medullary carcinoma of the breast. A multicenter study of its diagnostic consistency. Arch Path Lab Med 117: 1005–1008
278. Gaffey M J, Mills S E, Frierson H F 1995 Medullary carcinoma of the breast: interobserver variability in histopathologic diagnosis. Mod Pathol 8: 31–38
279. Jacquemier J, Padovani L, Rabayrol L et al. 2005 Typical medullary breast carcinomas have a basal/myoepithelial phenotype. J Pathol 207: 260–268
280. Jones C, Ford E, Gillett C et al. 2004 Molecular cytogenetic identification of subgroups of grade III invasive ductal breast carcinomas with different clinical outcomes. Clin Cancer Res 10: 5988–5997
281. Fisher E R, Palekar A S, Redmond C et al. 1980 Pathologic findings from the National Surgical Adjuvant Breast Project (protocol no. 4). VI. Invasive papillary carcinoma. Am J Clin Pathol 73: 313–322
282. Ellis I O, Elston C W, Pinder S E 1998 Papillary lesions. In: Elston CW, Ellis IO (eds) Systemic pathology. The breast. Churchill Livingstone, London, p 133–146
283. Siriaunkgul S, Tavassoli F A 1993 Invasive micropapillary carcinoma of the breast. Mod Pathol 6: 660–662
284. Luna More S, Gonzalez B, Acedo C et al. 1994 Invasive micropapillary carcinoma of the breast. A new special type of invasive mammary carcinoma. Pathol Res Pract 190: 668–674
285. Pettinato G, Manivel C J, Panico L et al. 2004 Invasive micropapillary carcinoma of the breast. Clinicopathologic study of 62 cases of a poorly recognized variant with highly aggressive behavior. Am J Clin Pathol 121: 857–866
286. Petersse J L 1993 Breast carcinomas with an unexpected inside out growth pattern. Rotation of polarisation associated with angio-invasion. Pathol Res Pract 189: 780
287. Varga Z, Zhao J, Ohlschlegel C et al. 2004 Preferential Her-2/neu overexpression and/or amplification in aggressive histological subtypes of invasive breast cancer. Histopathology 44: 332–338
288. Lakhani S R, Jacquemier J, Sloane J P et al. 1998 Multifactorial analysis of differences between sporadic breast cancers and cancers involving BRCA1 and BRCA2 mutations. J Natl Cancer Inst 90(15): 1138–1145
289. Lakhani S R, Reis-Filho J S, Fulford L et al. 2005 Prediction of BRCA1 status in patients with breast cancer using estrogen receptor and basal phenotype. Clin Cancer Res 11(14): 5175–5180
290. Lakhani S R 1999 The pathology of hereditary breast cancer. Dis Markers 15(1-3): 113–114
291. Lakhani S R, Van de Vijver M J, Jacquemier J et al. 2002 The pathology of familial breast cancer: predictive value of immunohistochemical markers estrogen receptor, progesterone receptor, HER-2, and p53 in patients with mutations in BRCA1 and BRCA2. J Clin Oncol 20(9): 2310–2318
292. Sorlie T, Perou C M, Tibshirani R et al. 2001 Gene expression patterns of breast carcinomas distinguish tumor subclasses with clinical implications. Proc Natl Acad Sci USA 98(19): 10869–10874
293. Dairkee S H, Ljung B M, Smith H et al. 1987 Immunolocalization of a human basal epithelium specific keratin in benign and malignant breast disease. Breast Cancer Res Treat 10(1): 11–20
294. Heatley M, Maxwell P, Whiteside C et al. 1995 Cytokeratin intermediate filament expression in benign and malignant breast disease. J Clin Pathol 48(1): 26–32
295. Jones C, Nonni A V, Fulford L et al. 2001 CGH analysis of ductal carcinoma of the breast with basaloid/myoepithelial cell differentiation. Br J Cancer 85(3): 422–427
296. Tsuda H, Takarabe T, Hasegawa T et al. 1999 Myoepithelial differentiation in high-grade invasive ductal carcinomas with large central acellular zones. Hum Pathol 30(10): 1134–1139
297. Tsuda H, Takarabe T, Hasegawa F et al. 2000 Large, central acellular zones indicating myoepithelial tumor differentiation in high-grade invasive ductal carcinomas as markers of predisposition to lung and brain metastases. Am J Surg Pathol 24(2): 197–202
298. Jimenez R E, Wallis T, Visscher D W 2001 Centrally necrotizing carcinomas of the breast: a distinct histologic subtype with aggressive clinical behavior. Am J Surg Pathol 25(3): 331–337
299. Hedenfalk I, Duggan D, Chen Y et al. 2001 Gene-expression profiles in hereditary breast cancer. N Engl J Med 344(8): 539–548

299a. Bryan B B, Schnitt S J, Collins L C 2006 Ductal carcinoma in situ with basal-like phenotype: a possible precursor to invasive basal-like breast cancer. Mod Pathol 19: 617–621
300. Rakha E A, Putti T C, Abd El-Rehim D M et al. 2006 Breast carcinomas with basal and myoepithelial differentiation: a review of morphology and immunophenotypical analysis. J Pathol 208: 495–506
301. Abati A D, Kimmel M, Rosen P P 1990 Apocrine mammary carcinoma. A clinicopathologic study of 72 cases. Am J Clin Pathol 94: 371–377
302. Shin S J, DeLellis R A, Ying L et al. 2000 Small cell carcinoma of the breast. A clinicopathologic and immunohistochemical study of nine patients. Am J Surg Pathol 24: 1231–1238
303. McDivitt R W, Stewart F W 1966 Breast carcinoma in children. J Am Med Assoc 195: 388–390
304. Oberman H A 1980 Secretory carcinoma of the breast in adults. Am J Surg Pathol 4: 465–470
305. Rosen P P, Cranor M L 1991 Secretory carcinoma of the breast. Arch Pathol Lab Med 115: 141–144
306. Diallo R, Schaefer K-L, Bankfalvi A et al. 2003 Secretory carcinoma of the breast: a distinct variant of invasive ductal carcinoma assessed by comparative genomic hybridization and immunohistochemistry. Hum Pathol 34: 1299–1305
307. Tavassoli F A, Norris H J 1980 Secretory carcinoma of the breast. Cancer 45: 2404–2413
308. Eusebi V, Foschini M P 1998 Rare carcinomas of the breast. In: Elston CW, Ellis IO (eds) Systemic pathology. The breast. Churchill Livingstone, London, p. 339–364
309. Hasleton P S, Misch K A, Vasudev K S et al. 1978 Squamous carcinoma of the breast. J Clin Pathol 31: 116–124
310. Eggers J W, McChesney T 1984 Squamous cell carcinoma of the breast: a clinicopathologic analysis of eight cases and review of the literature. Hum Pathol 15: 526–531
311. Hennessy B T, Krishnamurthy S, Giordano S et al. 2005 Squamous cell carcinoma of the breast. J Clin Oncol 23: 7827–7835
312. Kaufman M W, Marti J R, Gallager H S et al. 1984 Carcinoma of the breast with pseudosarcomatous metaplasia. Cancer 53: 1908–1917
313. Tavassoli F A 1992 Classification of metaplastic carcinomas of the breast. Pathol Ann 27: 89–119
314. Khan H N, Wyld L, Dunne B et al. 2003 Spindle cell carcinoma of the breast: a case series of a rare histological subtype. Eur J Surg Oncol 29(7): 600–603
315. Wargotz E S, Deos P H, Norris H J 1989 Metaplastic carcinomas. II. Spindle cell carcinoma. Hum Pathol 20: 732–740
316. Wargotz E S, Norris H J 1989 Metaplastic carcinomas. III. Carcinosarcoma. Cancer 64: 1490–1499
317. Foschini M P, Dina R E, Eusebi V 1993 Sarcomatoid neoplasms of the breast: proposed definitions for biphasic and monophasic sarcomatoid mammary carcinomas. Semin Diagn Pathol 10: 128–136
318. Gobbi H, Simpson J F, Borowsky A et al. 1999 Metaplastic breast tumors with a dominant fibromatosis-like phenotype have a high risk of local recurrence. Cancer 85(10): 2170–2182
319. Sneige N, Yaziji H, Mandavilli S R et al. 2001 Low-grade (fibromatosis-like) spindle cell carcinoma of the breast. Am J Surg Pathol 25(8): 1009–1016
320. Davis W G, Hennessy B, Babiera G et al. 2005 Metaplastic sarcomatoid carcinoma of the breast with absent or minimal overt invasive carcinomatous component. A misnomer. Am J Surg Pathol 29: 1456–1463
321. Carter M R, Hornick J L, Lester S et al. 2006 Spindle cell (sarcomatoid) carcinoma of the breast: a clinicopathologic and immunohistochemical analysis of 29 cases. Am J Surg Pathol 30: 300–309
322. Wargotz E S, Norris H J 1989 Metaplastic carcinomas of the breast. I. Matrix-producing carcinoma. Hum Pathol 20: 628–635
323. Rosen P P, Ernsberger D 1987 Low grade adenosquamous carcinoma. A variant of metaplastic mammary carcinoma. Am J Surg Pathol 11: 351–358
324. Van Hoeven K H, Drudis T, Cranor M L et al. 1993 Low-grade adenosquamous carcinoma of the breast. A clinicopathologic study of 32 cases with ultrastructural study. Am J Surg Pathol 17: 248–258
325. Denley H, Pinder S E, Tan P H et al. 2000 Metaplastic carcinoma of the breast arising within complex sclerosing lesion: a report of five cases. Histopathology 36(3): 203–209
326. Rosen P P 2001 Rosen's breast pathology. 2nd edn. Lippincott Williams and Wilkins, Philadelphia
327. National Coordinating Group for Breast Screening Pathology 1995 Pathology Reporting in Breast Cancer Screening. 2 edn. NHS BSP Publications No 3.
328. Davies J D, Bogomoletz W M 1987 Examination of breast specimens. ACP Broadsheet
329. Ellis I O, Elston C W, Evans A J et al. 1998 Diagnostic techniques and examination of pathological specimens. In: Elston CW, Ellis IO (eds) Systemic pathology. The breast. Churchill Livingstone, London, p, 21–46
330. Elston C W, Ellis I O, Goulding H et al. 1998 Role of pathology in the prognosis and management of breast cancer. In: Elston CW, Ellis IO (eds) Systemic pathology. The breast. Churchill Livingstone, London, p. 385–433
331. Elston C W, Gresham G A, Rao G S et al. 1982 The Cancer Research Campaign (Kings/Cambridge) Trial for Early Breast Cancer – pathological aspects. Br J Cancer 45: 655–669
332. Fisher E R, Sass R, Fisher B 1984 Pathologic findings from the National Surgical adjuvant Project for breast cancers (protocol No 4) X Discriminants for tenth year treatment failure. Cancer 53: 712–723
333. Carter C L, Allen C, Henson D E 1989 Relation of tumour size, lymph node status, and survival in 24 270 breast cancer cases. Cancer 63: 181–187
334. Neville A M, Bettelheim R, Gelber R D et al. 1992 Predicting treatment responsiveness and prognosis in node-negative breast cancer. J Clin Oncol 10: 696–705
335. Haybittle J L, Blamey R W, Elston C W et al. 1982 A prognostic index in primary breast cancer. Br J Cancer 45: 361–366
336. Todd J H, Dowle C, Williams M R et al. 1987 Confirmation of a prognostic index in primary breast cancer. Br J Cancer 56: 489–492
337. Gallager H S, Martin J E 1971 An orientation to the concept of minimal carcinoma. Cancer 28: 1505–1507
338. Beahrs O H, Shapiro S, Smart C et al. 1979 Summary report of the Working Group to review the National Cancer Institute – American Cancer Society Breast Cancer Demonstration Detection projects. J Nat Cancer Inst 62: 641–709
339. Hartman W H 1984 Minimal breast cancer: an update. Cancer 53: 681–684
340. Bedwani R, Vana J, Rosner D et al. 1981 Management and survival of female patients with "minimal" breast cancer: as observed in the long-term and short-term surveys of the American College of Surgeons. Cancer 47: 2769–2778
341. Rosen P P, Groshen S 1990 Factors influencing survival and prognosis in early breast carcinoma (TINOMO-TININO). Assessment of 644 patients with median follow up of 19 years. Surg Clin N Am 70: 937–962
342. Tabar L, Duffy S W, Krusemo V B 1987 Detection method tumour size and node metastases in breast cancers diagnosed during a trial of breast cancer screening. Eur J Cancer Clin Oncol 23: 959–962
343. Frisell J, Eklund G, Hellstrom L et al. 1987 Analysis of interval breast carcinomas in a randomised screening trial in Stockholm. Br Cancer Res Treat 9: 219–225
344. Royal College of Radiologists 1997 Quality Assurance Guidelines for Radiologists. Revised January 1997. NHSBSP Publications no 15
345. Fisher B, Slack N H, Katryk D 1975 Ten year follow up results of patients with carcinoma of the breast in a cooperative clinical trial evaluating surgical adjuvant chemotherapy. Surg Gynecol Obstet 140: 528–534
346. Ferguson D J, Meier P, Karrison T et al. 1982 Staging of breast cancer and survival rates: an assessment based on 50 years of experience with radical mastectomy. J Am Med Assoc 248: 1337–1341
347. Nemoto T, Vana J, Bedwani R N 1980 Management and survival of female breast cancer: results of a national survey by the American College of Surgeons. Cancer 45: 2917–2924
348. Sobin L H, Wittekind C 2002 TNM classification of malignant tumors 6th edn. Wiley, New York
349. Schottenfeld D, Nash A G, Robbins G F et al. 1976 Ten year results of the treatment of primary operable breast carcinoma. Cancer 38: 1001–1007
350. Handley R F 1972 Observations and thoughts on carcinoma of the breast. Proc R Soc Med 65: 437–444
351. Blamey R W, Davies C J, Elston C W et al. 1979 Prognostic factors in breast cancer: the formation of a prognostic index. Clin Oncol 5: 227
352. Du Toit R S, Locker A P, Ellis I O et al. 1990 Evaluation of the prognostic value of triple node biopsy. Br J Surg 77: 163–167
353. Locker A P, Ellis I O, Morgan D A et al. 1989 Factors influencing local recurrence after excision and radiotherapy for primary breast cancer. Br J Surg 76: 890–894
354. Steele R J C, Forrest A P M, Gibson T 1985 The efficacy of lower axillary sampling in obtaining lymph node status in breast cancer: a controlled randomized trial. Br J Surg 72: 368–369
355. Chetty U, Jack W, Dillon P et al. 1997 Axillary surgery in patients with breast cancer being treated by breast conservation: a randomised trial of node sampling and axillary clearance. Breast 6: 226
356. O'Dwyer P J 1992 Editorial. Axillary dissection in primary breast cancer; the benefits of node clearance warrant reappraisal. Br Med J 302: 360–361
357. Cabanes P A, Salmon R J, Vilcoq J R et al. 1992 Value of axillary dissection in addition to lumpectomy and radiotherapy in early breast cancer. Lancet 339: 1245–1248
358. Huvos A G, Hutter R V P, Berg J W 1970 Significance of axillary macrometastases and micrometastases in mammary cancer. Ann Surg 173: 44
359. Fisher E R, Palekar A, Rockette H et al. 1978 Pathologic findings from the National Surgical Adjuvant Breast Project (protocol no 4). V. Significance of axillary nodal micro and macro metastases. Cancer 42: 2032–2038
360. Millis R R, Springall R, Lee A H et al. 2002 Occult axillary lymph node metastases are of no prognostic significance in breast cancer. Br J Cancer 86(3): 396–401
361. Trojani M, de Mascarel I, Coindre J M et al. 1987 Micrometastases to axillary lymph nodes from invasive lobular caricnoma of breast: Detection by immunohistochemistry and prognostic significance. Br J Cancer 56: 838–839
362. Wells C A, Heryet A, Brochier J et al. 1984 The immunohistochemical detection of axillary micrometastases in breast cancer. Br J Cancer 50: 193–197
363. Springall R J, Ryina E R C, Millis R R 1990 Incidence and significance of micrometastases in axillary lymph nodes detected by immunohistochemical techniques. J Path 160: 174A
364. International Breast Cancer Study Group 1990 Prognostic importance of occult axillary lymph node micrometastases from breast cancers. Lancet 335: 1565–1568

365. Galea M, Athanassiou E, Bell J et al. 1991 Occult regional lymph node metastases from breast carcinoma: immunohistological detection with antibodies CAM 5.2 and NCRC-11. J Pathol 165: 221–227
366. McGuckin M A, Cummings M C, Walsh M D et al. 1996 Occult axillary node metastases in breast cancer: their detection and prognostic significance. Br J Cancer 73: 88–95
367. Dowlatshahi K, Fan M, Snider H C et al. 1997 Lymph node micrometastases from breast carcinoma: reviewing the dilemma. Cancer 80(7): 1188–1197
368. Cserni G 2004 A model for determining the optimum histology of sentinel lymph nodes in breast cancer. J Clin Pathol 57(5): 467–471
369. Cserni G, Bianchi S, Boecker W et al. 2005 Improving the reproducibility of diagnosing micrometastases and isolated tumor cells. Cancer 103(2): 358–367
370. Mambo N C, Gallager H S 1977 Carcinoma of the breast. The prognostic significance of extranodal extension of axillary disease. Cancer 39: 2280–2285
371. Cascinelli N, Greco M, Bufalino R et al. 1987 Prognosis of breast cancer with axillary node metastases after surgical treatment only. Eur J Cancer Clin Oncol 23: 795–799
372. Fisher E R, Gregorio R M, Redmond C et al. 1976 Pathologic findings from the National Surgical Adjuvant Breast Project (protocol no 4). III. The significance of extranodal extension of axillary metastases. Am J Clin Pathol 65: 439–444
373. Hartveit F 1984 Paranodal tumour in breast cancer: extranodal extension versus vascular spread. J Pathol 144: 253–256
374. Donegan W L, Stine S B, Samter T G 1993 Implications of extracapsular nodal metastases for treatment and prognosis of breast cancer. Cancer 72: 778–782
375. Morton D L, Wen D R, Wong J H et al. 1992 Technical details of intraoperative lymphatic mapping for early stage melanoma. Arch Surg 127(4): 392–399
376. Giuliano A E, Dale P S, Turner R R et al. 1995 Improved axillary staging of breast cancer with sentinel lymphadenectomy. Ann Surg 222(3): 394–399; discussion 399–401
377. Turner R R, Ollila D W, Krasne D L et al. 1997 Histopathologic validation of the sentinel lymph node hypothesis for breast carcinoma. Ann Surg 226(3): 271–276
378. Czerniecki B J, Scheff A M, Callans L S et al. 1999 Immunohistochemistry with pancytokeratins improves the sensitivity of sentinel lymph node biopsy in patients with breast carcinoma. Cancer 85(5): 1098–1103
379. Sabel M S, Zhang P, Barnwell J M et al. 2001 Accuracy of sentinel node biopsy in predicting nodal status in patients with breast carcinoma. J Surg Oncol 77(4): 243–246
380. Stitzenberg K B, Calvo B F, Iacocca M V et al. 2002 Cytokeratin immunohistochemical validation of the sentinel node hypothesis in patients with breast cancer. Am J Clin Pathol 117(5): 729–737
381. Cserni G, Amendoeira I, Apostolikas N et al. 2003 Pathological work-up of sentinel lymph nodes in breast cancer. Review of current data to be considered for the formulation of guidelines. Eur J Cancer 39(12): 1654–1667
382. Cserni G 2002 Complete sectioning of axillary sentinel nodes in patients with breast cancer. Analysis of two different step sectioning and immunohistochemistry protocols in 246 patients. J Clin Pathol 55(12): 926–931
383. Torrenga H, Rahusen F D, Meijer S et al. 2001 Sentinel node investigation in breast cancer: detailed analysis of the yield from step sectioning and immunohistochemistry. J Clin Pathol 54(7): 550–552
384. Dowlatshahi K, Fan M, Anderson J M et al. 2001 Occult metastases in sentinel nodes of 200 patients with operable breast cancer. Ann Surg Oncol 8(8): 675–681
385. Cooper H S, Patchefsky A S, Krall R A 1978 Tubular carcinoma of the breast. Cancer 42: 2334–2342
386. Carstens P H, Greenberg R A, Francis D et al. 1985 Tubular carcinoma of the breast. A long term follow up. Histopathology 9: 271–280
387. Lee B J, Hauser H, Pack G T 1934 Gelatinous carcinoma of the breast. Surg Gynecol Obstet 59: 841–850
388. Bloom H J C, Richardson W W, Fields J R 1970 Host resistance and survival carcinoma of the breast: a study of 104 cases of medullary carcinoma in a series of 1411 cases of breast cancer followed for 20 years. Br Med J 3: 181–188
389. Dawson P, Ferguson D J, Karrison T 1982 The pathologic findings of breast cancer in patients surviving 25 years after radical mastectomy. Cancer 50: 2131–2138
390. Richardson W W 1956 Medullary carcinoma of the breast. A distinctive tumour type with a relatively good prognosis following radical mastectomy. Br J Cancer 10: 415–423
391. Pereira H, Pinder S E, Sibbering D M 1995 Pathological prognostic factors in breast cancer. IV: Should you be a typer or a grader? A comparative study of two histological prognostic features in operable breast carcinoma. Histopathology 27: 219–226
392. Ellis I O 1991 Practical application of determinants of cell behaviour. Br Med Bull 42: 324–342
393. Domagala W, Markiewski M, Kubiak R et al. 1993 Immunohistochemical profile of invasive lobular carcinoma of the breast: predominantly vimentin and p53 protein negative, cathepsin D and oestrogen receptor positive. Virchow's Arch A Pathol Anat Histopathol 423: 497–502
394. Harris M, Khan M K 1984 Phyllodes tumour and stromal sarcoma of the breast: an ultrastructural comparison. Histopathology 8: 315–330
395. Lamovec J, Bracko M 1991 Metastatic pattern of infiltrating lobular carcinoma of the breast: an autopsy study. J Surg Oncol 48: 28–33
396. Breast Cancer Linkage Consortium 1997 Pathology of familial breast cancer: differences between breast cancer in carriers of BRCA1 or BRCA2 mutations and sporadic cases. Lancet 349: 1505–1510
397. Marcus J N, Watson P, Page D L et al. 1996 Hereditary breast cancer. Pathobiology, prognosis and BRCA1 and BRCA2 gene linkage. Cancer 77: 697–709
398. Greenough R B 1925 Varying degrees of malignancy in cancer of the breast. J Cancer Res 9: 452–463
399. Patey D H, Scarff R W 1928 The position of histology in the prognosis of carcinoma of the breast. Lancet i: 801–804
400. Bloom H J G, Richardson W W 1957 Histological grading and prognosis in breast cancer. Br J Cancer 11: 359–377
401. Elston C W 1987 Grading of invasive carcinoma of the breast. In: Page DL, Anderson T (eds) Diagnostic histopathology of the breast. Churchill Livingstone, Edinburgh, p 300–311
402. Contesso G, Mouriesse H, Friedman S et al. 1987 The importance of histologic grade in long-term prognosis of breast cancer: a study of 1010 patients, uniformly treated at the Institut Gustave-Roussy. J Clin Oncol 5: 1378–1386
403. Elston C W, Ellis I O 1991 Pathological prognostic factors in breast cancer. I. The value of histological grade in breast cancer: experience from a large study with long term follow up. Histopathology 19: 403–410
404. Black M M, Barclay T H C, Hankey B F 1975 Prognosis in breast cancer utilising histologic characteristics of the primary tumour. Cancer 36: 2048–2055
405. Hartveit F 1971 Prognostic typing in breast cancer. Br Med J 4: 253–257
406. Le Doussal V, Tubiana-Hulin M, Friedman S et al. 1989 Prognostic value of histologic grade nuclear components of Scarff Bloom Richardson (SBR). An improved score modification based on a multivariate analysis of 1262 invasive ductal breast carcinomas. Cancer 64: 1914–1921
407. Bloom H J G 1950 Prognosis in carcinoma of the breast. Br J Cancer 4: 259–288
408. Bloom H J G 1950 Further studies on prognosis of breast cancer. Br J Cancer 4: 347–367
409. Scarff R W, Torloni H 1968 Histological typing of breast tumours (International histological classification of tumours, no 2). World Health. Organization, Geneva
410. Stenkvist B, Westman-Naeser S, Vegelius J et al. 1979 Analysis of reproducibility of subjective grading systems for breast carcinoma. J Clin Pathol 32: 979–985
411. Gilchrist K W, Kalish L, Gould V E et al. 1985 Interobserver reproducibility of histopathological features in stage II breast cancer. An ECPG study. Breast Cancer Res Treat 5: 3–10
412. Hopton D S, Thorogood J, Clayden A D et al. 1989 Observer variation in histological grading of breast cancer. Eur J Surg Oncol 15: 21–23
413. Theissig F, Kunze K D, Haroske G et al. 1990 Histological grading of breast cancer – interobserver, reproducibility and prognostic significance. Pathol Res Pract 186: 732–736
414. Ellis I O, Broughton N, Elston C W et al 1987 The relationship of histological type to survival and oestrogen receptor status in primary operable breast carcinoma. J Pathol 152: 219A (abstract)
415. Ellis P, Whitehead R 1981 Mitosis counting – a need for reappraisal. Hum Pathol 12: 3–4
416. Quinn C M, Wright N A 1990 The clinical assessment of proliferation and growth in human tumours: evaluation of methods and applications as prognostic variables. J Pathol 160: 93–102
417. Mann R, Elston C W, Hunter S et al. 1985 Evaluation of mitotic activity as a component of histological grade and its contribution to prognosis in primary breast carcinoma. J Pathol 146: 271A
418. Dalton L W, Page D L, Dupont W D 1994 Histologic grading of breast carcinoma: a reproducibility study. Cancer 73: 2765–2770
419. Frierson H F Jr, Wolber R A, Berean K W et al. 1995 Interobserver reproducibility of the Nottingham modification of the Bloom and Richardson histological grading scheme for infiltrating ductal carcinoma. Am J Clin Pathol 103: 195–198
420. Robbins P, Pinder S, de Klerk N et al. 1995 Histological grading of breast carcinomas. A study of interobserver agreement. Hum Pathol 26: 873–879
421. Connolly J L, Fechner R E, Kempson R L et al. 1996 Recommendations for the reporting of breast carcinoma. Hum Pathol 27: 220–224
422. Page D L, Ellis I O, Elston C W 1995 Histologic grading of breast cancer. Let's do it. Am J Clin Pathol 103: 123–124
423. Lee A K, Delellis R A, Silverman M L et al. 1986 Lymphatic and blood vessel invasion in breast carcinoma: a useful prognostic indicator? Hum Pathol 17: 984–987
424. Sears H F, Janus C, Levy W et al. 1982 Breast cancer without axillary metastases. Are there subpopulations. Cancer 50: 1820–1827
425. Dawson P J, Karrison T, Ferguson D J 1986 Histological features associated with long-term survival in breast cancer. Hum Pathol 17: 1015–1021
426. Bettelheim R, Penman H G, Thornton-Jones H et al. 1984 Prognostic significance of peritumoral vascular invasion in breast cancer. Br J Cancer 50: 771–777
427. Roses D F, Bell D A, Flotte T J et al. 1982 Pathologic predictors of recurrence in stage I (T1N0M0) breast cancer. Am J Clin Path 78: 817–820

428. Nime F A, Rosen P P, Thaler H T et al. 1977 Prognostic significance of tumour emboli in intramammary lymphatics in patients with mammary carcinoma. Am J Surg Pathol 1: 25–30
429. Nealon T F Jr, Nkongho A, Grossi C E et al. 1981 Treatment of early cancer of the breast (T1N0M0 and T2N0M0) on the basis of histological characteristics. Surgery 89: 279–289
430. Rosen P P 1983 Tumour emboli in intramammary lymphatics in breast carcinoma: pathological criteria for diagnosis and clinical significance. Pathol Annu 18: 215–232
431. Pinder S E, Ellis I O, Galea M et al. 1994 Pathological prognostic factors in breast cancer. III. Vascular invasion: relationship with recurrence and survival in a large series with long-term follow-up. Histopathology 24: 41–47
432. Örbo A, Stalsberg H, Kunde D 1990 Topographic criteria in the diagnosis of tumor emboli in intramammary lymphatics. Cancer 66: 972–977
433. Bettelheim R, Mitchell D, Gusterson B A 1984 Immunocytochemistry in the identification of vascular invasion in breast carcinoma. J Clin Pathol 37: 364–366
434. Martin S A, Perez-Reyes N, Mendelsohn G 1987 Angioinvasion in breast carcinoma: an immuohistochemical study of factor VIII-related antigen. Cancer 59: 1918–1922
435. Lee A K C, DeLellis R A, Wolffe H J 1986 Intramammary lymphatic invasion in breast carcinomas. Evaluation using ABH isoantigens as endothelial markers. Am J Surg Pathol 10: 589–594
436. Ordonez N G, Brooks T, Thompson S et al. 1987 Use of *Ulex Europeus* agglutinin I in the identification of lymphatic and blood vessel invasion in previously stained microscopic slides. Am J Surg Pathol 11: 543–550
437. Saigo P E, Rosen P P 1987 The application of immunohistochemical stains to identify endothelial-lined channels in mammary carcinoma. Cancer 59: 51–54
438. Gilchrist K W, Gould V E, Hirschl S et al. 1982 Interobserver variation in the identification of breast carcinoma in intramammary lymphatics. Hum Pathol 13: 170–172
439. Cote R J, Rosen P P 1988 Monoclonal antibodies detect occult breast carcinoma metatases in the bone marrow of patients with early stage disease. Am J Surg Pathol 12: 333–340
440. Rosen P P, Saigo P E, Braun D W Jr et al. 1981 Predictors of recurrence in stage I (T1N0M0) breast carcinoma. Ann Surg 193: 15–25
441. Rosen P P, Saigo P E, Braun D W Jr et al. 1982 Occult axillary lymph node metastases from breast cancers with intramammary lymphatic tumour emboli. Am J Surg Path 6: 639–641
442. O'Rourke S, Galea M H, Morgan D et al. 1994 An audit of local recurrence after simple mastectomy. Br J Surg 81: 386–389
443. Page D L, Anderson T J, Connolly J et al. 1987 Miscellaneous features of carcinoma. In: Page DL, Anderson TJ (eds) Diagnostic histopathology of the breast. Churchill Livingstone, Edinburgh, p 51–61
444. Carter D, Pipkin R D, Shepard R H et al. 1978 Relationship of necrosis and tumour border to lymph node metastases and 10 year survival in carcinoma of the breast. Surg Pathol 2: 39–46
445. Parham D M, Robertson A J, Brown R A 1988 Morphometric analysis of breast carcinoma: association with survival. J Clin Pathol 45: 517–520
446. Parham D M, Hagen N, Brown R A 1992 Simplified method of grading primary carcinomas of the breast. J Clin Pathol 45: 517–520
447. Underwood J C 1972 A morphometric analysis of human breast carcinoma. Br J Cancer 26: 234–237
448. Sistrunk W E, MacCarty W C 1922 Life expectancy following radical amputation for carcinoma of the breast – a clinical and pathological study of 218 cases. Ann Surg 75: 61–69
449. Black R, Prescott R, Bers K et al. 1983 Tumour cellularity, oestrogen receptors and prognosis in breast cancer. Clin Oncol 9: 311–318
450. Parfrey N A, Doyle C T 1985 Elastosis in benign and malignant breast disease. Hum Pathol 16: 674–676
451. Shivas A A, Douglas J G 1972 The prognostic significance of elastosis in breast carcinoma. J Roy Coll Surg Edinb 17: 315–320
452. Masters J R, Millis R R, King R J et al. 1979 Elastosis and response to endocrine therapy in human breast cancer. Br J Cancer 39: 536–539
453. Robertson A J, Brown R A, Cree I A et al. 1981 Prognostic value of measurement of elastosis in breast carcinoma. J Clin Pathol 34: 738–743
454. Rasmussen B B, Pedersen B V, Thorpe S M et al. 1985 Elastosis in relation to prognosis in primary breast carcinoma. Cancer Res 45: 1428–1430
455. Giri D D, Lonsdale R N, Dangerfield V J et al. 1987 Clinicopathological significance of intratumoral variations in elastosis grades and the oestrogen receptor status of human breast cacinomas. J Pathol 151: 297–303
456. Silverberg S G, Chitale A R 1973 Assessment of the significance of the proportion of intraductal and infiltrating tumor growth in ductal carcinoma of the breast. Cancer 32: 830–837
457. Matsukuma A, Enjoji M, Toyoshima S 1991 Ductal carcinoma of the breast. An analysis of the proportion of intraductal and invasive components. Pathol Res Prac 187: 62–67
458. Millis R R, Thynne G S J 1975 In situ intraduct carcinoma of the breast: a long-term follow up study. Br J Surg 62: 957–962
459. Van Dongen J A, Fentiman I S, Harris J R et al. 1989 In situ breast cancer: the EORTC consensus meeting. Lancet ii: 25–27
460. Schnitt S J, Connolly J L, Harris J R et al. 1984 Pathologic predictors of early local recurrence in stage I and stage II breast cancer treated by primary radiation therapy. Cancer 53: 1049–1057
461. Fourquet A, Campana F, Zafrani B et al. 1989 Prognostic factors of breast recurrence in the conservation management of early breast cancer: a 25 year follow up. Int J Radiation Oncol Biol Phys 17: 719–725
462. Jacquemier J, Kurtz J M, Amalric R et al. 1990 An assessment of extensive intraductal component as a risk factor for local recurrence after breast-conserving therapy. Br J Cancer 61: 873–876
463. Gage I, Schnitt S J, Nixon A J et al. 1996 Pathologic margin involvement and the risk of recurrence in patients treated with breast-conserving therapy. Cancer 78: 1921–1928
464. Clark G M 1994 Do we really need prognostic factors for breast cancer? Br Cancer Res Treat 30: 117–126
465. Page D L 1991 Prognosis and breast cancer. Recognition of lethal and favorable prognostic types. Am J Surg Pathol 15: 334–349
466. Gui G P, Wells C A, Browne P D et al. 1995 Integrin expression in primary breast cancer and its relation to axillary nodal status. Surgery 117: 102–108
467. Harris A L 1994 What is the biological, prognostic, and therapeutic role of the EGF receptor in human breast cancer? Br Cancer Res Treat 29: 1–2
468. Robertson J F, Bates K, Pearson D et al. 1992 Comparison of two oestrogen receptor assays in the prediction of the clinical course of patients with advanced breast cancer. Br J Cancer 65: 727–730
469. Barbareschi M 1996 Prognostic value of the immunohistochemical expression of p53 in breast carcinomas. A review of the literature involving over 9000 patients. Appl Immunohistochem 4: 106–116
470. Lovekin C, Ellis I O, Locker A et al. 1991 C-erbB-2 oncoprotein in primary and advanced breast cancer. Br J Cancer 63: 439–443
471. Veronese S M, Gambacorta M, Gottardi O et al. 1993 Proliferation index as a prognostic marker in breast cancer. Cancer 71: 3926–3931
472. Pinder S, Wencyk P, Sibbering D M et al. 1995 Assessment of the new proliferation marker MIB1 in breast carcinoma using image analysis: Associations with other prognostic factors and survival. Br J Cancer 71: 146–149
473. Robertson J F, Ellis I O, Pearson D et al. 1994 Biological factors of prognostic significance in locally advanced breast cancer. Br Cancer Res Treat 29: 259–264
474. Parker M G 1991 Nuclear hormone receptors. Academic Press, London
475. Jensen E V, Jacobson H I 1962 Buyers guide to the mechanism of oestrogen action. Recent Prog Horm Res 18: 387
476. NIH consensus development conference on steroid receptors in breast cancer 1980 Cancer 46: 2759–2963
477. Greene G L, Nolan C, Engler J P et al. 1980 Monoclonal antibodies to human estrogen receptor. Proc Natl Acad Sci USA 77: 5115–5119
478. Jensen E V, Greene G L, De Sombre E R 1986 The estrogen-receptor immunoassay in the prognosis and treatment of breast cancer. Lab Manager 24: 25–42
479. King W J, Greene G L 1984 Monoclonal antibodies localise oestrogen receptor in nuclei of target cells. Nature 307: 745–747
480. McCarty K S Jr, Miller L S, Cox E B et al. 1985 Estrogen receptor analyses: correlation of biochemical and immunohistochemical methods using monoclonal antireceptor antibodies. Arch Pathol Lab Med 109: 716–721
481. Pertschuk L P, Eisenberg K B, Carter A C et al. 1985 Immunohistologic localization of estrogen receptors in breast cancer with monoclonal antibodies. Cancer 55: 1513–1518
482. Gaskell D J, Hawkins R A, Tesdale A L et al. 1992 The differing predictive values of oestrogen receptor assays for large breast cancers. Postgrad Med J 68: 900–903
483. McClelland R A, Berger U, Miller L S et al. 1986 Immunocytochemical assay for estrogen receptor in patients with breast cancer. Relationship to biochemical assay and to outcome of therapy. J Clin Oncol 4: 1171–1176
484. Seymour L, Meyer K, Esser K et al. 1990 Estimation of ER and PR by immunocytochemistry in breast cancer. Comparison with radioligand binding methods. Am J Clin Pathol 94: S35–40
485. Anderson J, Orntoft T, Skovgaard Poulson H 1986 Semiquantitive oestrogen receptor assay in formalin-fixed paraffin sections of human breast cancer tissue using monoclonal antibodies. Br J Cancer 53: 691–694
486. De Rosa C M, Ozzello L, Greene G L et al. 1987 Immunostaining of oestrogen receptor in paraffin sections of breast carcinoma using monoclonal antibody D753P: effects of fixation. Am J Surg Pathol 11: 943–950
487. Jackson D P, Payne J, Bell S et al. 1990 Extraction of DNA from exfoliative cytology specimens and its suitability for analysis and the polymerase chain reaction. Cytopathology 1: 87–96
488. Paterson D A, Reid C P, Anderson T J et al. 1990 Assessment of oestrogen receptor content of breast carcinoma by immunohistochemical techniques on fixed and frozen tissue and by chemical ligand binding assay. J Clin Pathol 43: 46–51
489. Snead D J, Bell J A, Dixon A R et al. 1993 Methodology of immunohistochemical detection of oestrogen receptor in human breast carcinoma in formalin fixed paraffin embedded tissue: a comparison with frozen section morphology. Histopathology 23: 233–238
490. Goulding H, Pinder S, Cannon P et al. 1995 A new method for the assessment of oestrogen receptor status on routine formalin-fixed tissue samples. Hum Pathol 26: 291–294
491. Hawkins R A, Sangster K, Tesdale A L et al. 1988 The cytochemical detection of oestrogen receptors in fine needle aspirates of breast cancer: correlation with biochemical assay and prediction of response to endocrine therapy. Br J Cancer 58: 77–80
492. Poulson H S, Jensen J, Hermansen C 1981 Human breast cancer: heterogeneity of estrogen binding sites. Cancer 43: 1791

493. Chiu K Y 1987 Use of microwave for rapid immunoperoxidase staining of paraffin sections. Med Lab Sci 44: 3–5
494. Shi S R, Key M E, Kalra K L 1991 Antigen retrieval in formalin-fixed, paraffin embedded tissues: an enhancement method for immunohistochemical staining based on microwave oven heating of tissue sections. J Histochem Cytochem 39: 741–748
495. Cuevas E C, Bateman A C, Wilkins B S et al. 1994 Microwave antigen retrieval in immunocytochemistry: a study of 80 antibodies. J Clin Pathol 47: 448–452
496. Barnes D M, Millis R R 1995 Oestrogen receptors: the history, the relevance and the methods of evaluation. In: Kirkham N, Lemoine NR (eds) Progress in pathology. Churchill Livingstone, Edinburgh, p 89–114
497. Harvey J M, Clark G M, Osborne C K et al. 1999 Estrogen receptor status by immunohistochemistry is superior to the ligand binding assay for predicting response to adjuvant endocrine therapy in breast cancer. J Clin Oncol 17: 1474–1481
498. Fisher E R, Anderson S, Dean S et al. 2005 Solving the dilemma of the immunohistochemical and other methods used for scoring estrogen receptor and progesterone receptor in patients with invasive breast carcinoma. Cancer 103: 164–173
499. Cobleigh M A, Vogel C L, Tripathy D et al. 1998 Efficacy and safety of Herceptin as a single agent in 222 women with HER2 overexpression who relapsed following chemotherapy for metastatic breast cancer. ASCO, Los Angeles
500. Slamon D, Leyland-Jones B, Shak S et al. 2001 Concurrent administration of anti-HER2 monochonal antibody and first-line chemotherapy for HER2-overexpressing metastatic breast cancer. A phase III multinational randomized controlled trial. N Engl J Med 344: 783–792
501. Piccart-Gebhardt M J, Proctor M, Leyland-Jones M et al. 2005 Trastuzumab after adjuvant chemotherapy in HER2-positive breast cancer. N Eng J Med 353: 1659–1672
502. Ellis I O, Bartlett J, Dowsett M et al. 2004 Best practice no 176: updated recommendations for HER2 testing in the UK. J Clin Pathol 57(3): 233–237
503. Paik S, Bryant J, Tan-Chiu E et al. 2002 Real-world performance of HER2 testing – National Surgical Adjuvant Breast and Bowel Project experience. J Natl Cancer Inst 94(11): 852–854
504. Roche P C, Suman V J, Jenkins R B et al. 2002 Concordance between local and central laboratory HER2 testing in the breast intergroup trial N9831. J Natl Cancer Inst 94(11): 855–857
505. Rhodes A, Jasani B, Anderson E et al. 2002 Evaluation of HER-2/neu immunohistochemical assay sensitivity and scoring on formalin-fixed and paraffin-processed cell lines and breast tumors: a comparative study involving results from laboratories in 21 countries. Am J Clin Pathol 118(3): 408–417
506. Dowsett M, Bartlett J, Ellis I O et al. 2003 Correlation between immunohistochemistry (HercepTest) and fluorescence in situ hybridization (FISH) for HER-2 in 426 breast carcinomas from 37 centres. J Pathol 199(4): 418–423
507. Lal P, Salazar P A, Hudis C A et al. 2004 HER-2 testing in breast cancer using immunohistochemical analysis and fluorescence in-situ hybridization. A single institution experience of 2279 cases and comparison of dual-color and single-color scoring. Am J Clin Pathol 121: 631–636
508. Rhodes A, Jasani B, Couturier J et al. 2002 A formalin-fixed, paraffin-processed cell line standard for quality control of immunohistochemical assay of HER-2/neu expression in breast cancer. Am J Clin Pathol 117(1): 81–89
509. Watters A D, Bartlett J M 2002 Fluorescence in situ hybridization in paraffin tissue sections: pretreatment protocol. Mol Biotechnol 24(3): 217–220
510. Galea M H, Blamey R W, Elston C E E et al. 1992 The Nottingham Prognostic Index in primary breast cancer. Br Cancer Res Treat 22: 207–219
511. Brown J M, Benson E A, Jones M 1993 Confirmation of a long-term prognostic index in breast cancer. Breast 2: 144–147
512. Balslev I, Axelsson C K, Zedeler K et al. 1994 The Nottingham Prognostic Index applied to 9149 patients from the studies of the Danish Breast Cancer Cooperative Group (DBCG). Br Cancer Res Treat 32: 281–290
513. Clark G M 1992 Integrating prognostic factors. Br Cancer Res Treat 22: 187–191
514. Miller W R, Ellis I O, Sainsbury J R et al. 1994 Prognostic factors. ABC of breast diseases. Br Med J 309: 1573–1576
515. Kennedy S, Merino M J, Swain S M et al. 1990 The effects of hormonal and chemotherapy on tumoral and non neoplastic breast tissue. Hum Pathol 21: 192–198
516. Longacre T A, Bartow S A 1986 A correlative study of human breast and endometrium in the menstrual cycle. Am J Surg Pathol 10: 382–393
517. Vogel P M, Georgiade N G, Fetter B F et al. 1981 The correlation of histologic changes in the human breast with the menstrual cycle. Am J Pathol 104: 23–34
518. Tavassoli F A, Tienyeh I 1987 Lactational and clear cell changes of the breast in non lactating, non pregnant women. Am J Clin Pathol 87: 23–29
519. Schnitt S J, Connolly J L, Harris J R et al. 1984 Radiation-induced changes in the breast. Hum Pathol 15: 545–550
520. Rosen P P 1987 Adenomyoepithelioma of the breast. Hum Pathol 18: 1232–1237
521. Loose J H, Patchefsky A S, Hollander I J et al. 1992 Adenomyoepithelioma of the breast. A spectrum of biologic behaviour. Am J Surg Pathol 16: 868–876
522. Tavassoli F A 1991 Myoepithelial lesions of the breast. Myoepitheliosis, adenomyoepithelioma, and myoepithelial carcinoma. Am J Surg Pathol 15: 554–568
523. Eusebi V, Casadei G P, Bussolati G et al. 1987 Adenomyoepithelioma of the breast with a distinctive type of apocrine adenosis. Histopathology 11: 305–315
524. McLaren B K, Smith J, Shuyler P A et al. 2005 Adenomyoepithelioma. Clinical, histologic and immunohistochemical evaluation of a series of related lesions. Am J Surg Pathol 29: 1294–1299
525. Rasbridge S A, Millis R R 1998 Adenomyoepithelioma of the breast with malignant features. Virchow's Arch 432: 123–130
526. Donnell R M, Rosen P P, Lieberman P H et al. 1981 Angiosarcoma and other vascular tumours of the breast. Pathologic analysis as a guide to prognosis. Am J Surg Path 5: 629–642
527. Schurch W, Seemayer T A 1985 Malignant myoepithelioma (myoepithelial carcinoma) of the breast – an ultrastructural and immunohistochemical study. Ultrastructural Pathol 8: 1–11
528. Thorner P S, Kahn H J, Baumal R et al. 1986 Malignant myoepithelioma of the breast – an immunohistochemical study by light and electron microscopy. Cancer 57: 745–750
529. Moran C A, Suster S, Carter D 1990 Benign mixed tumours (pleomorphic adenomas) of the breast. Am J Surg Pathol 40: 913–921
530. Smith B H, Taylor H B 1968 The occurrence of bone and cartilage in mammary tumours. Am J Clin Pathol 51: 610–618
531. Van der Walt J D, Rohlova B 1982 Pleomorphic adenoma of the human breast. A report of a benign tumour closely mimicking a carcinoma clinically. Clin Oncol 8: 361–365
532. Arpino G, Clark G M, Mohsin S et al. 2002 Adenoid cystic carcinoma of the breast. Molecular markers, treatment and clinical outcome. Cancer 94: 2119–2127
533. Wells C A, Nicoll S, Ferguson D J P 1986 Adenoid cystic carcinoma of the breast: a case with axillary lymph node metastasis. Histopathology 10: 415–424
534. Anthony P P, James P D 1975 Adenoid cystic carcinoma of the breast: prevalence, diagnostic criteria and histogenesis. J Clin Pathol 28: 647–655
535. Quizilbash A H, Patterson M C, Oliveria K F 1977 Adenoid cystic carcinoma of the breast. Arch Pathol Lab Med 101: 302–306
536. Jaworski R C, Kneale K L, Smith R C 1983 Adenoid cystic carcinoma of the breast. Postgrad Med J 59: 48–51
537. Bennett A K, Mills S E, Wick M R 2003 Salivary-type neoplasms of the breast and lung. Semin Diagn Pathol 20: 279–304
538. Ro J Y, Silva E G, Gallager H S 1987 Adenoid cystic carcinoma of the breast. Hum Pathol 18: 1276–1281
539. Kleer C G, Oberman H A 1998 Adenoid cystic carcinoma of the breast. Value of histologic grading and proliferative activity. Am J Surg Pathol 22: 569–575
540. Roncaroli F, Lamovec J, Zidar A et al. 1996 Acinic cell-like carcinoma of the breast. Virchow's Arch 429(1): 69–74
541. Damiani S, Pasquinelli G, Lamovec J et al. 2000 Acinic cell carcinoma of the breast: an immunohistochemical and ultrastructural study. Virchow's Arch 437: 74–81
542. Schmitt F C, Ribiero C A, Alvarenga S et al. 2000 Primary acinic cell-like carcinoma of the breast – a variant with good prognosis? Histopathology 36(3): 286–289
543. Di Tommaso L, Foschini M P, Ragazzini T et al. 2004 Mucoepidermoid carcinoma of the breast. Virchow's Arch 444: 13–19
544. Patchefsky A S, Frauenhoffer C M, Krall R A et al. 1979 Low grade mucoepidermoid carcinoma of the breast. Arch Pathol Lab Med 103: 196–198
545. Fisher E R, Palekar A S, Gregorio R M et al. 1983 Mucoepidermoid and squamous carcinoma of the breast with reference to squamous metaplasia and giant cell tumours. Am J Surg Pathol 7: 15–27
546. Hanna W, Kahn H J 1985 Ultrastructural and immunohistochemical characteristics of mucoepidermoid carcinoma of the breast. Hum Pathol 16: 941–946
547. Covi J, Duong J D, Leffall L D 1981 High grade mucoepidermoid carcinoma of the breast. Arch Pathol Lab Med 105: 612–614
548. Rosen P P, Jozefczyk M A, Boram L H 1985 Vascular tumours of the breast. IV. Venous haemangioma. Am J Surg Path 9: 659–665
549. Josefcyzk M A, Rosen P P 1985 Vascular tumours of the breast. II. Perilobular haemangiomas and haemangiomas. Am J Surg Path 9: 491–503
550. Rosen P P 1985 Vascular tumours of the breast. III. Angiomatosis. Am J Surg Pathol 9: 652–658
551. Rosen P P 1985 Vascular tumours of the breast. V. Non parenchymal haemangiomas of mammary subcutaneous tissues. Am J Surg Pathol 9: 723–729
552. Vuitch M F, Rosen P P, Erlandson R 1986 A pseudoangiomatous hyperplasia of mammary stroma. Hum Pathol 17: 185–191
553. Badve S, Sloane J P 1995 Pseudoangiomatous hyperplasia of the male breast. Histopathology 26: 463–466
554. Chen K T, Kirkegaard D D, Bocian J J 1980 Angiosarcoma of the breast. Cancer 46: 368–371
555. Merino M J, Carter D, Berman M 1983 Angiosarcoma of the breast. Am J Surg Pathol 7: 53–60
556. Rosen P P, Kimmel M, Ernsberger D 1988 Mammary angiosarcoma: the prognostic significance of tumour differentiation. Cancer 62: 2145–2152

557. Strobbe L J, Peterse H L, van Tinteren H et al. 1998 Angiosarcoma of the breast after conservation therapy for invasive cancer, the incidence and outcome. An unforeseen sequela. Br Cancer Res Treat 47: 101–109
558. Brenn T, Fletcher C D M 2005 Radiation-associated cutaneous atypical vascular lesions and angiosarcoma: clinicopathologic analysis of 42 cases. Am J Surg Pathol 29: 983–996
558a. Vorburger S A, Xing Y, Hunt K K et al. 2005 Angiosarcoma of the breast. Cancer 104: 2682–2688
559. Stewart R W, Treves N 1948 Lymphangiosarcoma in post mastectomy lymphoedema. A report of six cases in Elephantiasis Chirurgica. Cancer 1: 64–81
560. Martin M B, Kon N D, Kawamoto E H et al. 1984 Post mastectomy angiosarcoma. Am Surg 50(10): 541–545
561. Miettinen M, Lehto V P, Virtanen I 1983 Post mastectomy angiosarcoma (Stewart-Treves syndrome). Light microscopic, immunohistochemical and ultrastructural characteristics of two cases. Am J Surg Path 7: 329–339
562. McWilliam L J, Harris M 1985 Histogenesis of post mastectomy angiosarcoma – an ultrastructural study. Histopathology 9: 331–343
563. Wargotz E S, Weiss S W, Norris H J 1987 Myofibroblastoma of the breast. 16 cases of a distinctive benign mesenchymal tumour. Am J Surg Pathol 11: 493–502
564. McMenamin M E, DeSchryver K, Fletcher C D M 2000 Fibrous lesions of the breast: a review. Int J Surg Pathol 8: 99–108
565. McMenamin M E, Fletcher C D M. 2001 Mammary-type myofibroblastoma of soft tissue: a tumor closely related to spindle cell lipoma. Am J Surg Pathol 25: 1022–1029
566. Magro G, Michal M, Vasquez E, Bisceqlia M 2000 Lipomatous myofibroblastoma: a potential diagnostic pitfall in the spectrum of the spindle cell lesions of the breast. Virchows Arch 437: 540–544
567. Lee A H, Sworn M J, Theaker J M et al. 1993 Myofibroblastoma of the breast: an immunohistochemical study. Histopathology 22: 75–78
568. Salomao D R, Crotty T B, Nascimento A G 1997 Myofibroblastoma and solitary fibrous tumor of the breast: Histopathological and immunohistochemical comparative study. Lab Invest 76: 126
569. Gump F E, Sternschein M J, Wolff M 1981 Fibromatosis of the breast. Surg Gynaecol Obstet 15: 57–60
570. Rosen P P, Ernsberger D 1989 Mammary fibromatosis. A benign spindle cell tumour with significant risk for local recurrence. Cancer 63: 1363–1369
571. Devouassoux-Shisheboran M, Schammel M D, Man Y G et al. 2000 Fibromatosis of the breast: age-correlated morphofunctional features of 33 cases. Arch Pathol Lab Med 124: 276–280
572. Matherne T H, Green A Jr, Tucker J A et al. 2004 Fibromatosis: the breast cancer imitator. South Med J 97: 1100–1103
573. Adeniran A, Al-Ahmadie H, Mahoney M C et al. 2004 Granular cell tumor of the breast: a series of 17 cases and review of the literature. Breast J 10(6): 528–531
574. Gibbons D, Leitch M, Coscia J et al. 2000 Fine needle aspiration cytology and histological findings of granular cell tumor of the breast: review of 19 cases with clinical/radiologic correlation. Breast J 6: 27–30
575. Fanburg-Smith J C, Meis-Kindblom J M, Fante R et al. 1998 Malignant granular cell tumor of soft tissue: diagnostic criteria and clinicopathologic correlation. Am J Surg Pathol 22: 779–794
576. Le B H, Boyer P J, Lewis J E et al. 2004 Granular cell tumor: immunohistochemical assessment of inhibin-a, protein gene product 9.5, S-100 protein, CD68, and Ki-67 proliferative index with clinical correlation. Arch Pathol Lab Med 128: 771–775
577. Mattia A R, Ferry J A, Harris N L 1993 Breast lymphoma. A B-cell spectrum including the low grade B-cell lymphoma of mucosa associated lymphoid tissue. Am J Surg Pathol 17: 574–587
578. Domchek S M, Hecht J L, Fleming M D et al. 2002 Lymphomas of the breast. Primary and secondary involvement. Cancer 94: 6–13
579. Toombs B D, Kalisher L 1997 Metastatic disease in the breast; clinical, pathologic and radiographic features. Am J Roentgenol 129: 673–676
580. Georgiannos S N, Aleong J C, Goode A W 2001 Secondary neoplasms of the breast. A survey of the 20th century. Cancer 92: 2259–2266